Generic Name	Trade Name (Manufacturer)	Abbreviation
Hexalen	Altretamine (US Bioscience)	
Hydroxyurea	Hydrea (Squibb)	HU
Ifosfamide	Ifex (Bristol-Myers Squibb)	IFX
Idarubicin	Idamycin (Pharmacia Adria)	IDA
α-Interferon	Intron A (Schering) Roferon A (Roche)	α-IFN
Irinotecan	Camtosar (Pharmacia UpJohn)	CPT-11
Leuprolide acetate	Lupron (TAP)	LU
Levamisole HCl	Ergamisol (Janssen)	LEV
Megestrol acetate	Megace (Bristol-Myers Squibb)	MEG
Melphalan (L-phenylalanine mustard)	Alkeran (Glaxo Wellcome)	L-PAM
6-Mercaptopurine	Purinethol (Glaxo Wellcome)	6-MP
Methotrexate	Methotrexate (Lederle) Mexate (Bristol-Myers Squibb)	MTX
Mitomycin-C	Mutamycin (Bristol-Myers Squibb)	MITO
Mitotane	Lysodren (Bristol-Myers Squibb)	LYS
Mitoxantrone	Novantrone (Lederle)	NOV
Nitrogen mustard (mechlorethamine hydrochloride)	Mustargen (Merck & Co.)	HN_2
Octreotide	Sandostatin (Schering)	SAND
Paclitaxel	Taxol (Bristol-Myers Squibb)	TAX
Pegaspargase	Oncospar (Rhône-Poulenc Rorer)	PEG
Pentostatin (2'deoxycoformycin)	Nipent	PEN
Plicamycin	Mithracin (Miles)	MITH
Prednisone	Prednisone (Various)	PRED
Procarbazine	Matulane (Roche)	PCZ
Streptozotocin	Zanosar (UpJohn)	STN
Tamoxifen	Nolvadex (ICI Pharma)	TMX
Teniposide (VM-26)	Vumon (Bristol-Myers Squibb)	VM-26
6-Thioguanine	Tabloid-6 Thioguanine (Glaxo Wellcome)	6-TG
Thiotepa	Thiotepa (Lederle)	TT
Topetecan	Hycamtin (SmithKline Beecham)	TOPO
Trimetrexate	Neutrexin (US Bioscience)	TriMTX
Vinblastine	Velban (Lilly)	VLB
Vincristine	Oncovin (Lilly)	
Vinorelbine	Navelbine (Glaxo Wel	

THE
CHEMOTHERAPY
SOURCE BOOK

SECOND EDITION

THE
CHEMOTHERAPY
SOURCE BOOK

SECOND EDITION

Michael C. Perry, MD, FACP

Editor

Professor of Medicine
Nellie B. Smith Chair of Oncology
Director, Division of Hematology/Medical Oncology
University of Missouri/Ellis Fischel Cancer Center
Columbia, Missouri

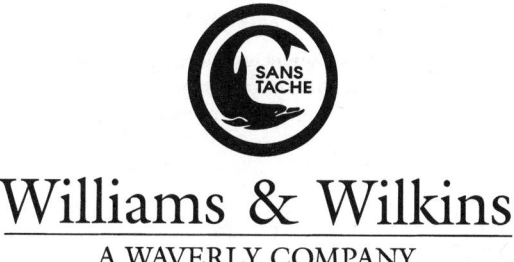

Williams & Wilkins
A WAVERLY COMPANY

BALTIMORE • PHILADELPHIA • LONDON • PARIS • BANGKOK
BUENOS AIRES • HONG KONG • MUNICH • SYDNEY • TOKYO • WROCLAW

Editor: Jonathan W. Pine, Jr.
Managing Editor: Molly Mullen
Production Coordinator: Barbara J. Felton
Copy Editor: Anne Schwartz
Designer: Wilma E. Rosenberger
Illustration Planner: Mario Fernandez
Cover Designer: Dan Pfisterer
Typesetter: University Graphics, Inc.
Printer/Binder: R. R. Donnelley & Sons
Digitized Illustrations: Publicity Engravers

Copyright © 1996 Williams & Wilkins

351 West Camden Street
Baltimore, Maryland 21201-2436 USA

Rose Tree Corporate Center
1400 North Providence Road
Building II, Suite 5025
Media, Pennsylvania 19063-2043 USA

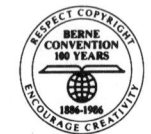

Accurate indications, adverse reactions and dosage schedules for drugs are provided in this book, but it is possible that they may change. The reader is urged to review the package information data of the manufacturers of the medications mentioned.

Printed in the United States of America

First Edition, 1992

Library of Congress Cataloging-in-Publication Data

The chemotherapy source book / Michael C. Perry, editor.—2nd ed.
   p. cm
   Includes bibliographical references and index.
   ISBN 0-683-06868-7
   1. Cancer—Chemotherapy.   2. Antineoplastic agents.   I. Perry, Michael C. (Michael Clinton), 1945–   .
   [DNLM: 1. Neoplasms—drug therapy.   2. Antineoplastic Agents—therapeutic use.   QZ 267 C5186 1996]
RC271.C5C446   1996
616.99'4061—dc20
DNLM/DLC
For Library of Congress   96-685
                                           CIP

The publishers have made every effort to trace the copyright holders for borrowed material. If they have inadvertently overlooked any, they will be pleased to make the necessary arrangements at the first opportunity.

To purchase additional copies of this book, call our Customer Service Department at **(800) 638-0672** or fax orders to **(800) 447-8438.** For other book services, including chapter reprints and large quantity sales, ask for the Special Sales department.

Canadian customers should call **(800) 268-4178,** or fax **(905) 470-6780.** For all other calls originating outside of the United States, please call **(410) 528-4223** or fax us at **(410) 528-8550.**

Visit Williams & Wilkins on the Internet: **http://www.wwilkins.com** or contact our Customer Service Department at **custserv @ wwilkins.com**. Williams & Wilkins customer service representatives are available from 8:30 am to 6:00 pm, EST, Monday through Friday, for telephone access.

96 97 98 99 00
1 2 3 4 5 6 7 8 9 10

9 780683 068689

Preface to Second Edition

One of life's more pleasant tasks is writing the preface to the second edition of a text. The obvious implication is that the first edition was at least a reasonable success, necessitating a second edition. Many of my colleagues have personally told me that they found the book useful, and I believe it has met many of my own expectations.

This edition features new chapters on differentiating agents and the chemotherapy of cancers of unknown origin and revisions of all other chapters from the first edition. A little less than one third, or twenty chapters, have new senior authors. Section Two, "Chemotherapeutic Agents," has been reorganized to reflect new knowledge of the mechanism of action of chemotherapeutic agents, and the chapter on investigational agents has been completely rewritten. Section Four, "Combination Chemotherapy Programs," has also been updated. Section Seven, "Hematologic Malignancies," has been subdivided into seven chapters, producing the opportunity to add new contributors and expand coverage.

I am thankful for the comments I have received regarding errors, omissions, and suggestions for additions or changes. Any new or remaining errors should be attributed to me. I am grateful to both the "old" contributors and the new, all of whom have made excellent contributions. The staff at Williams & Wilkins remains a pleasure to work with, and I am particularly indebted to my editor, Jonathan Pine; Molly Mullen, Managing Editor; and Barbara Felton, Production Coordinator; as well as the many other unseen individuals who make such a work possible. While giving out thank yous, I must also recognize Patty Moore, my administrative assistant, who has suffered through two versions of this book, as well as another text, and Sara Lowe, our student assistant. Perhaps my family will someday understand the inner drive that leads to entering into such projects.

MICHAEL C. PERRY
Columbia, Missouri

Preface to the First Edition

The idea for this book arose from my frustration at having to consult multiple sources for frequent, simple questions. I concluded that although there were many excellent texts for medical oncologists there was no one text to satisfy my needs. I developed the outline for the book over the next several months, bouncing ideas off of colleagues whenever they came into range.

In preparing this book I have been concerned with the practicing oncologist. I have imagined it as a well-worn text, growing dog-eared with use, rather than gathering dust on a shelf. With the possible exception of a reviewer, I doubt anyone will intentionally sit down to read it cover-to-cover. I anticipate that a reader may read a chapter here and there as his or her interest dictates or use it to look up a specific point. I have resisted the temptation to make a multi-authored book read as if it were written by a single individual, and I would prefer that each chapter be thought of as a scholarly essay by the contributor(s).

Section One deals in a practical way with the principles of chemotherapy, that is, the rationale, scientific basis, and various settings in which the drugs are currently used. The subsection on routes of administration explores the advantages and disadvantages of each route. As in other sections of the book, I have been fortunate to attract authors who are authorities in their areas.

Section Two, on chemotherapeutic drugs, discusses commercially available drugs by class, emphasizing their mechanisms of action, pharmacology, toxicity, etc. in nine chapters. There is also an extensive review on current investigational agents to aid the oncologist, nurse, pharmacologist, etc. who may need information regarding these agents. This information is not readily available in one source elsewhere.

Section Three includes 16 chapters by authorities on the management of chemotherapeutic drug toxicity by organ system and incorporates guidelines for dosage modifications in renal and hepatic failure. It also has chapters on gonadal toxicity and second malignancies, the most recently recognized toxicities of successful chemotherapy. The vexing problem of chemotherapy in pregnancy is also addressed.

The fourth section is a listing of combination chemotherapy programs and the appropriate references. It is one man's opinion (mine) of the most important historical and current regimens likely to be in use. I realize that this listing will not please everyone and that programs now in vogue may be replaced, hopefully by those offering higher complete response rates and improved survival.

The fifth section, drug administration, is aimed at the pharmacist or nurse preparing chemotherapy, and the nurse who administers the therapy and interacts with the pharmacist, patient, and physician.

In Section Six, selected authorities address the therapy of specific tumors based on current knowledge. I anticipate that this section will receive heavy and use and may elicit differing opinions.

I am grateful to my administrative assistants, Beth Van Hove and Patty Moore, for their assistance and patience, to my wife Nancy and daughters Rebecca and Katherine for allowing me to neglect them while I attempted to complete the text, to my contributors for their enthusiasm and expertise, and to my teachers whom I have tried to emulate. A special thanks also goes to the reference librarians, here and elsewhere, who helped with elusive references, sources, and searches. The editors and staff at Williams & Wilkins have been most helpful and supportive, especially Tim Satterfield, Jonathan Pine, Carol Eckhart, and Charles Zeller. Their advice and suggestions has made this a far better book than any effort of my own. I hope you enjoy our efforts.

MICHAEL C. PERRY, M.D.

Contributors

Joseph Aisner, M.D.
Professor of Medicine and Environmental &
  Community Medicine
Chief of Medical Oncology
Associate Director of Clinical Services
The Cancer Institute of New Jersey
New Brunswick, New Jersey

Karen H. Antman, M.D.
Professor of Medicine
Chief, Division of Medical Oncology
Columbia University
New York, New York

James O. Armitage, M.D.
Professor and Chairman
Department of Internal Medicine
University of Nebraska Medical Center
Omaha, Nebraska

Nancy L. Bartlett, M.D.
Assistant Professor, Department of Medical
  Oncology
Washington University
St. Louis, Missouri

Robert S. Benjamin, M.D.
Internist, Ashbel Smith Professor of Medicine
Chairman, Department of Melanoma/Sarcoma
  Medical Oncology
Chief, Sarcoma Section
Medical Director, Sarcoma Center
University of Texas M. D. Anderson Cancer
  Center
Houston, Texas

David Berd, M.D.
Professor of Medicine
Division of Neoplastic Diseases
Thomas Jefferson University
Philadelphia, Pennsylvania

Philip J. Bierman, M.D.
Associate Professor of Medicine
Department of Oncology/Hematology
University of Nebraska
Omaha, Nebraska

Jacob D. Bitran, M.D.
Director, Division Hematology/Oncology
Department of Medicine
Lutheran General Hospital
Park Ridge, Illinois
Professor of Clinical Medicine
University of Chicago School of Medicine
Chicago, Illinois

John D. Boice, Jr., Sc.D.
Chief, Radiation Epidemiology Branch
National Cancer Institute
Bethesda, Maryland

Ernest C. Borden, M.D.
Director, University of Maryland Cancer
  Center
University of Maryland
Baltimore, Maryland

Bruce E. Brockstein, M.D.
Fellow in Medicine
Section of Hematology/Oncology
University of Chicago Medical Center
Chicago, Illinois

Daniel R. Budman, M.D., F.A.C.P.
Associate Director, Don Monti Division of
  Oncology
North Shore University Hospital
Associate Professor of Clinical Medicine
Cornell University Medical College
Manhasset, New York

Linda J. Burns, M.D.
Assistant Professor of Medicine
Department of Medicine/Oncology
University of Minnesota
Minneapolis, Minnesota

Robert W. Carlson, M.D.
Associate Professor of Medicine
Division of Medical Oncology
Stanford University Medical Center
Stanford, California

Mario Castro, M.D.
Assistant Professor of Medicine
Department of Pulmonary & Critical Care
    Medicine
Washington University School of Medicine
St. Louis, Missouri

Majid Chahin, M.D.
Fellow, Division of Oncology
Emory University
Atlanta, Georgia

Bruce D. Cheson, M.D.
Head, Medicine Section
Clinical Investigations Branch
Cancer Therapy Evaluation Program
Division of Cancer Treatment
National Cancer Institute
Bethesda, Maryland

Gerald H. Clamon, M.D.
Professor of Internal Medicine
University of Iowa College of Medicine
Iowa City, Iowa

John T. Cole, M.D.
Staff Physician, Section of Hematology/
    Oncology
Department of Medicine
Ochsner Clinic
New Orleans, Louisiana

Barbara A. Conley, M.D.
Associate Professor, Department of Medicine
    and Oncology
The University of Maryland School of Medicine
Baltimore, Maryland

Jeffrey Crawford, M.D.
Associate Professor, Department of Medicine
Division of Hematology/Oncology
Duke University Medical Center
Durham, North Carolina

Alan S. Cross, M.D.
Professor, Department of Medicine
University of Maryland School of Medicine
Director of Infectious Diseases
University of Maryland Cancer Center
Baltimore, Maryland

Robert O. Dillman, M.D., F.A.C.P.
Medical Director, Hoag Cancer Center
Hoag Memorial Hospital Presbyterian
Newport Beach, California
Clinical Professor of Medicine
University of California, Irvine
Irvine, California

Donald C. Doll, M.D.
Chief, Hematology-Oncology
Harry S. Truman VAMC
Professor-University of Missouri
Columbia, Missouri

Ross C. Donehower, M.D.
Associate Professor of Oncology and Medicine
Division of Pharmacology and Experimental
    Therapeutics
The Johns Hopkins Oncology Center
Baltimore, Maryland

Victoria J. Dorr, M.D.
Assistant Professor of Medicine
Department of Internal Medicine-Hematology/
    Oncology
University of Missouri/Ellis Fischel Cancer
    Center
Columbia, Missouri

Mario A. Eisenberger, M.D.
Associate Professor, Department of Oncology
    and Urology
The Johns Hopkins University
Baltimore, Maryland

William D. Ensminger, M.D., Ph.D.
Professor of Internal Medicine and
    Pharmacology
University of Michigan Medical Center
Ann Arbor, Michigan

Marc S. Ernstoff, M.D.
Professor of Medicine
Section of Hematology/Oncology
Dartmouth-Hitchcock Medical Center
Lebanon, New Hampshire

Michael S. Ewer, M.D., M.P.H.
Internist, Associate Professor of Medicine
Special Assistant to the Vice President of
    Patient Care for Financial/Medical Concerns
Medical Specialties/Cardiology
University of Texas M.D. Anderson Cancer
    Center
Houston, Texas

Mehdi Farhangi, M.D.
Associate Professor of Medicine
Division of Hematology and Medical Oncology
University of Missouri-Columbia School of
    Medicine
Columbia, Missouri

Joseph A. Fontana, M.D. Ph.D
Professor of Medicine, Oncology and
    Biochemistry
University of Maryland at Baltimore
Chief of Hematology and Oncology
Veterans Administration Medical Center
Baltimore, Maryland

Arthur D. Forman, M.D.
Associate Professor, Department of Neuro-
    Oncology
University of Texas M.D. Anderson Cancer
    Center
Houston, Texas

Robert J. Fram, M.D.
Associate Director, Department of Oncology/
    Immunology
Knoll Pharmaceutical Company
Parsippany, New Jersey

Michael L. Friedland, M.D.
Dean
Professor of Medicine
Binghamton Clinical Campus
State University of New York Health Science
    Center at Syracuse
Binghamton, New York

Michael A. Friedman, M.D.
Deputy Commissioner for Operations
Food and Drug Administration
Rockville, Maryland
Formerly, CTEP, DCT
National Cancer Institute
Bethesda, Maryland

Marc B. Garnick, M.D.
Associate Professor of Medicine
Harvard Medical School
Boston, Massachusetts
Executive Vice President
Pharmaceutical Peptides, Inc.
Cambridge, Massachusetts

Dennis Gastineau, M.D.
Assistant Professor of Medicine
Mayo Medical School
Rochester, Minnesota

Teresa Gilewski, M.D.
Assistant Attending, Department of Medicine
Memorial Sloan Kettering Cancer Center
Assistant Professor, Department of Medicine
Cornell University
New York, New York

James H. Goldie, M.D.
Staff Physician, Department of Medical
    Oncology
B.C. Cancer Agency
Clinical Professor, Department of Medicine
University of British Columbia
Vancouver, British Columbia, CANADA

F. Anthony Greco, M.D.
Director, Sarah Cannon Cancer Center
Centennial Medical Center
Nashville, Tennessee

Louise B. Grochow, M.D.
Associate Professor, Oncology and Medicine
Acting Director, Division of Pharmacology and
    Experimental Therapeutics
Department of Oncology
The Johns Hopkins University School of
    Medicine
Baltimore, Maryland

John C. Gutheil, M.D.
Assistant Professor of Medicine and Oncology
University of Maryland Cancer Center
Baltimore, Maryland

John D. Hainsworth, M.D.
Associate Director, Sarah Cannon Cancer
    Center
Centennial Medical Center
Nashville, Tennessee

Nasrollah Hakami, M.D.
Professor of Child Health
Director, Pediatric Hematology/Oncology
Children's Hospital at University of Missouri
    Hospitals and Clinics
Columbia, Missouri

Bruce R. Harrison, M.S., R.Ph.
Clinical Pharmacy Specialist
Division of Hematology/Oncology/Bone
    Marrow Transplantation
St. Louis University School of Medicine and
    Veterans Affairs Medical Center
St. Louis, Missouri

Michael J. Hawkins, M.D.
Associate Professor of Medicine and
    Pharmacology
Division of Hematology and Oncology
Director, Experimental Therapeutics Program
Vincent T. Lombardi Cancer Research Center
Georgetown University Medical Center
Washington, D.C.

Meyer R. Heyman, M.D.
Associate Professor of Medicine and Oncology
University of Maryland Cancer Center
Department of Medicine
University of Maryland
Baltimore, Maryland

H. Clark Hoagland, M.D.
Professor of Medicine
Mayo Medical School
Chair, Division of Hematology
Mayo Clinic
Rochester, Minnesota

Antoinette F. Hood, M.D.
Professor of Pathology and Dermatology
Director of Dermatopathology
Department of Dermatology
Indiana University Medical Center
Indianapolis, Indiana

William J.M. Hrushesky, M.D.
Senior Attending Oncologist
Stratton Veterans Affairs Medical Center
Professor of Medicine and Immunobiology
Albany Medical College
Professor, Biomedical Sciences Department
School of Public Health
State University of New York (SUNY) at
   Albany
Albany, New York
Professor of Chemical Engineering
Rensselaer Polytechnic Institute
Troy, New York

Daniel C. Ihde, M.D.
Chief, Medical Oncology
Department of Internal Medicine
Washington University School of Medicine
St. Louis, Missouri

Mohammad Jahanzeb, M.D.
Assistant Professor, Department of Medicine
Division of Medical Oncology
Washington University School of Medicine
St. Louis, Missouri

**Mary H. Johnson, M.S., R.N., O.C.N.,
G.N.P.**
Advance Practice Nurse
University of Missouri/Ellis Fischel Cancer
   Center
Columbia, Missouri

Carl G. Kardinal, M.D., F.A.C.C.
Principal Investigator, Ochsner Community
   Clinical Oncology Program
Associate Head, Division of Hematology and
   Medical Oncology
Associate Director, Ochsner Cancer Institute
Ochsner Clinic and Alton Ochsner Medical
   Foundation
New Orleans, Louisiana

Christine M. Kearns, Pharm.D.
Assistant Professor of Pharmacy and Oncology
University of Maryland Cancer Center
University of Maryland School of Pharmacy
   and Medicine
Baltimore, Maryland

Ali Khojasteh, M.D., F.A.C.P.
President, Columbia Comprehensive Cancer
   Care Clinic
Clinical Associate Professor, Department of
   Medicine
University of Missouri School of Medicine
Columbia, Missouri

Paul King, M.D.
Assistant Professor of Internal Medicine
Division of Gastroenterology
University of Missouri
Columbia, Missouri

Catherine E. Klein, M.D.
Associate Professor of Medicine
Divisions of Hematology and Medical
   Oncology
University of Colorado Health Sciences Center
Denver Veterans Affairs Medical Center
Denver, Colorado

David Koh, M.D.
Pulmonary & Critical Care Fellow
Department of Pulmonary and Critical Care
   Medicine
Washington University School of Medicine
St. Louis, Missouri

William G. Kraybill, M.D.
Chief, Soft Tissue Sarcoma, Melanoma, and
   Bone Service
Roswell Park Cancer Institute
Associate Professor of Medicine
State University of New York at Buffalo
Buffalo, New York

Richard A. Larson, M.D.
Associate Professor, Department of Medicine
The University of Chicago
Chicago, Illinois

Victor A. Levin, M.D.
Professor of Medicine
Chairman, Department of Neuro-Oncology
Bernard W. Biedenharn Chair in Cancer
  Research
University of Texas M.D. Anderson Cancer
  Center
Houston, Texas

Stuart M. Lichtman, M.D., F.A.C.P.
Assistant Professor, Department of Medicine
North Shore University Hospital
Manhasset, New York

Dan L. Longo, M.D.
Scientific Director, National Institute on Aging
National Institutes of Health
Gerontology Research Center
Baltimore, Maryland

Mary Lorber, R.N., O.C.N., C.R.A.
Nurse Clinician
Department of Internal Medicine-Hematology/
  Oncology
University of Missouri/Ellis Fischel Cancer
  Center
Columbia, Missouri

Alan P. Lyss, M.D.
Director, Cancer Center and Clinical Research
Missouri Baptist Medical Center
Associate Professor of Clinical Medicine
Washington University School of Medicine
St. Louis, Missouri

David R. Macdonald, M.D.
Associate Professor of Medicine
Departments of Clinical Neurological Sciences
  and Oncology
University of Western Ontario
Victoria Hospital and London Regional
  Hospital
London, Ontario, Canada

Maurie Markman, M.D.
Director, Cleveland Clinic Cancer Center
Chairman, Department of Hematology/
  Medical Oncology
Cleveland Clinic Foundation
Professor of Medicine
Ohio State University School of Medicine
Cleveland, Ohio

Michael J. Mastrangelo, M.D.
Professor, Department of Medicine
Jefferson Medical College
Philadelphia, Pennsylvania

William F. Maule, M.D.
Section of Gastroenterology
Department of Medicine
Ochsner Clinic
Baton Rouge, Louisiana

Richard L. McKittrick, M.D.
Assistant Professor, Department of Internal
  Medicine
Division of Clinical Oncology
University of Kansas Medical Center
Kansas City, Kansas

Antonius A. Miller, M.D.
Associate Professor, Division of Hematology
  and Oncology
Department of Medicine
College of Medicine
The University of Tennessee, Memphis
Memphis, Tennessee

Debra Morris, R.N., M.N.
Oncology Nurse Practitioner
Division of Hematology/Oncology
University of Missouri/Ellis Fischel Cancer
  Center
Columbia, Missouri

Faith E. Nathan, M.D.
Clinical Assistant Professor of Medicine
Jefferson Medical College
Philadelphia, Pennsylvania

Larry Norton, M.D.
Chief, Breast Cancer Medicine Service
Department of Medicine
Memorial Sloan-Kettering Cancer Center
New York, New York

Howard Ozer, M.D.
Chairman and Director
Winship Cancer Center
Emory University
Atlanta, Georgia

Roy A. Patchell, M.D.
Associate Professor
Chief of Neuro-Oncology
Department of Surgery (Neurosurgery) &
  Neurology
University of Kentucky Chandler Medical
  Center
Lexington, Kentucky

Dilip V. Patel, M.D.
Attending Hematologist/Oncologist
Long Island Jewish Medical Center
New Hyde Park, New York
Assistant Professor of Medicine
Albert Einstein College of Medicine
Bronx, New York

William P. Patterson, M.D.
Division of Hematology
Harry S. Truman VAMC
Associate Professor, Department of Internal
   Medicine
University of Missouri
Columbia, Missouri

Michael C. Perry, M.D.
Professor of Medicine
Nellie B. Smith Chair of Oncology
Director, Division of Hematology/Medical
   Oncology
University of Missouri/Ellis Fischel Cancer
   Center
Columbia, Missouri

Douglas E. Peterson, D.M.D., Ph.D.
Professor and Head, Department of Oral
   Diagnosis
School of Dental Medicine
University of Connecticut Health Center
Farmington, Connecticut

Haralambos Raftopoulos, M.D.
Fellow, Division of Medical Oncology/
   Hematology
Columbia University
New York, New York

Kanti R. Rai, M.D.
Chief, Division of Hematology/Oncology
Division of Hematology Oncology
Long Island Jewish Medical Center
New Hyde Park, New York
Professor of Medicine
Albert Einstein College of Medicine
Bronx, New York

Mark J. Ratain, M.D.
Professor of Medicine
Chairman, Committee on Clinical
   Pharmacology
Department of Medicine
Section of Hematology/Oncology
University of Chicago
Chicago, Illinois

Garry P. Reams, M.D.
Associate Professor, Department of Internal
   Medicine
University of Missouri
Columbia, Missouri

Verna A. Rhodes, Ed.S., R.N., F.A.A.N.
Associate Professor of Nursing
Sinclair School of Nursing
University of Missouri
Columbia, Missouri

Charles E. Riggs, Jr., M.D.
Associate Professor, Division of Hematology/
   Oncology
Department of Internal Medicine
University of Iowa Hospitals and Clinics
Iowa City, Iowa

Eric K. Rowinsky, M.D.
Associate Professor of Oncology
Division of Pharmacology and Experimental
   Therapeutics
The Johns Hopkins Oncology Center
Baltimore, Maryland

Richard L. Schilsky, M.D.
Professor of Medicine and Clinical
   Pharmacology
Director, Cancer Research Center
University of Chicago
Chicago, Illinois

Mark M. Schubert, D.D.S., M.S.D.
Associate Professor, Department of Oral
   Medicine
University of Washington
Director, Department of Oral Medicine
Fred Hutchinson Cancer Research Center
Seattle, Washington

Nasir Shahab, M.D.
Fellow, Division of Hematology/Oncology
University of Missouri
Ellis Fischel Cancer Center
Columbia, Missouri

Matthew L. Sherman, M.D.
Clinical Assistant Professor of Medicine
Dana-Farber Cancer Institute
Harvard Medical School
Boston, Massachusetts
Director of Clinical Research
Genetics Institute
Cambridge, Massachusetts

Donna A. Shriner, PharmD
Research Pharmacist
Radiation Epidemiology Branch
National Cancer Institute
Bethesda, Maryland

Richard Simon, Ph.D.
Chief, Biometric Research Branch
National Cancer Institute
Bethesda, Maryland

Steven B. Standiford, M.D., F.A.C.S.
Assistant Professor of Clinical Surgery
University of Missouri/Ellis Fischel Cancer
    Center
Columbia, Missouri

Ronald L. Stephens, M.D.
Professor, Director of Clinical Oncology
Department of Internal Medicine
Division of Clinical Oncology
Kansas University Medical Center
Kansas City, Kansas

Donald K. Strickland, M.D.
Assistant Professor, Child Health
University of Missouri-Columbia
Columbia, Missouri

J. Tate Thigpen, M.D.
Professor, Department of Medicine
University of Mississippi Medical Center
Jackson, Mississippi

David A. Van Echo, M.D.
Associate Director of Clinical Research
Head, Hematology/Oncology
University of Maryland Cancer Center
University of Maryland Medical System
Baltimore, Maryland

Nicholas J. Vogelzang, M.D.
Professor of Medicine
Director, Genitourinary Oncology
Section of Hematology/Oncology
University of Chicago Medical Center
Chicago, Illinois

Everett E. Vokes, M.D.
Professor of Medicine and Radiation Oncology
Director for Clinical Affairs
Cancer Research Center
The University of Chicago Medical Center
Chicago, Illinois

Julie M. Vose, M.D.
Associate Professor, Department of Internal
    Medicine
University of Nebraska Medical Center
Omaha, Nebraska

Raymond P. Warrell, Jr., M.D.
Member, Memorial Sloan-Kettering Cancer
    Center
Professor of Medicine
Cornell University Medical College
New York, New York

Todd H. Wasserman, M.D.
Professor of Radiation Oncology
Washington University School of Medicine
Mallinckrodt Institute of Radiology
Radiation Oncology Center
St Louis, Missouri

James K. Weick, M.D., M.S.
Chairman, Department of Hematology,
    Medical Oncology
Cleveland Clinic Florida
Ft. Lauderdale, Florida

Raymond B. Weiss, M.D.
Chief of Medical Oncology
Walter Reed Army Medical Center
Washington, DC
Professor of Medicine
Uniformed Services University of the Health
    Services
Bethesda, Maryland

John D. Wilkes, M.D.
Assistant Professor of Medicine
Division of Hematology and Medical Oncology
University of Missouri-Columbia School of
    Medicine
Columbia, Missouri

Patricia A. Wood, M.D., Ph.D.
Assistant Professor of Medicine
Albany Medical College and Stratton
Veterans Affairs Medical Center
Albany, New York

Connie Henke Yarbro, R.N., B.S.N.
Clinical Associate Professor
Division of Hematology/Oncology
University of Missouri
Columbia, Missouri
and
Editor, Seminars in Oncology Nursing

John W. Yarbro, M.D., Ph.D.
Professor Emeritus
Division of Hematology/Oncology
University of Missouri
Columbia, Missouri

Clive S. Zent, M.D.
Clinical Fellow, Section of Hematology/
    Oncology
The University of Chicago Medical Center
Chicago, Illinois

Contents

Section Four/ **Combination Chemotherapy Programs**

Section Five/ **Drug Administration**

Section Six/ Current Therapy of Specific Solid Tumors

Section Seven/ Chemotherapy of Hematologic Malignancies

Section One: A

Principles of Chemotherapy:

Scientific Foundation of Chemotherapy

1

The Scientific Basis of Cancer Chemotherapy

John W. Yarbro

At the turn of the century, Paul Ehrlich observed that certain histologic stains were selectively concentrated in microorganisms and reasoned that such specificity might be used therapeutically if substances toxic to bacteria could be found. He coined the term *chemotherapy* during his search for a chemical that would cure syphilis. Thus began the search for "magic bullets" against disease, a search that met only limited success until the fortuitous discovery of penicillin launched an era of specific bacterial therapy. Unfortunately, to date, no anticancer agent has been found that even approaches the specificity of the agents used against bacteria.

The metabolism of the cancer cell has been thought to be so similar to that of the normal cell that we have been forced to utilize rather minute differences through which drugs might exert a differential effect. Traditionally. the most important such difference is the rapid rate of division of the cancer cell relative to most other body tissues. The pioneering work of Skipper demonstrated that even this small difference allowed chemotherapeutic cures in rapidly proliferating animal tumors such as the L1210 mouse leukemia.

In the past decade, many newly described differences between cancer cells and normal cells have been found on the basis of activation of growth pathways and inactivation of growth-control pathways by genetic alterations of oncogenes and cancer suppressor genes. These differences have provided multiple targets for effective therapy against the cancer cell. Unfortunately, to date only a few treatments have been based on this new cancer biology.

Two of the most important of these new biologic properties of the cancer cell, destined to play a major role in the future therapy of malignant disease, have recently received attention. Multicellular life forms could not exist if the cells of their bodies did not cooperate. Two key manifestations of this cooperation are cell senescence and programed cell death (apoptosis), both essential to the orderly course of multicellular life. Cancer cells, however, neither grow old nor do they die when the appropriate signals arrive. This is probably fundamental to malignant transformation.

Apoptosis is the cell suicide that normally follows genetic and other irreversible cell damage. Tumor cells become resistant to apoptosis and survive in spite of damage that renders normal cells nonviable. Loss of apoptosis not only accelerates the progression of the carcinogenic process by allowing mutant cells to persist but also renders cells resistant to chemotherapy, since the final common path of cell killing by toxic drugs is damage that initiates programed cell death mechanisms.

Cell senescence results when chromosomes can no longer replicate their DNA. Telomeres are multiple tandem repeats of guanine-rich sequences located at the ends of chromosomal DNA which grow shorter with each division until, eventually, the DNA polymerase machinery cannot initiate transcription of new DNA, and the cells become senescent (1). Telomerase is a ribonucleoprotein enzyme that elongates the telomeres by adding telomeric repeats. Normal somatic cells do not possess telomerase, whereas normal germ cells, cell lines immortalized by viral transformation, and most cancer cells are liberated from this biologic clock because they possess a telomerase (2) that uses an integral RNA template for reverse transcriptase synthesis of

3

the DNA telomeric motif (3). Both the resistance to apoptosis and the presence of telomerase promote tumor cell growth and offer tempting targets potentially exploitable in chemotherapy.

Beyond the presence of telomerase and resistance to apoptosis, human tumors have a number of major biologic impediments to chemotherapeutic cure, including Gompertzian growth, in which there are resting cells relatively resistant to chemotherapy; the use of alternate pathways when one source of metabolites is blocked; genetically acquired drug resistance; anatomic inaccessibility due to either sanctuary sites or inadequate circulation to the tumor; shedding of antigens or modulation of surface antigens to confound the host immune system; a variety of multidrug resistance devices; and no doubt many more, as yet undiscovered, strategies. This chapter discusses some of our attempts to circumvent tumor cell defense mechanisms, the major impediments to chemotherapeutic cure, and other features that form the scientific basis for cancer chemotherapy.

THE BIOCHEMICAL BULLET

Presently available drugs active against cancer cells are, with rare exceptions, the result of empiricism, luck, or trial and error. The discovery of nitrogen mustard during chemical warfare research is the well-reported first example, but even at that time, hydroxyurea had been on the shelf for over half a century with its activity undiscovered (4). In later years, agents discarded as excessively toxic were to prove a fertile source of anticancer drugs. The origin of the idea of the antifols is unclear or even disputed (5).

The first clearly successful "designer drug" for cancer was Heidelberger's 5-fluorouracil (5-FU) (6). Phenylalanine mustard, designed for melanoma because phenylalanine is the precursor of melanin, was ineffective in that tumor in spite of the indisputable biochemical logic of its construction. Over the years, numerous anticancer agents have been discovered, most by accident, a few by design, and a variety of metabolic inhibitors have been developed. Table 1.1 lists the presently available drugs classified by their mechanisms of action.

The largest family of anticancer drugs consists of agents that damage DNA directly by alkylation, platinum coordination cross-linking, double-strand cleavage by interrupting the action of topoisomerase II, single-strand cleavage by interrupting the action of topoisomerase I, blocking nucleic acid synthesis by intercalation into DNA, and other mechanisms. In cells with an intact response to genetic damage, cell proliferation is halted in G_2 until DNA repair takes place, or if damage is severe, the cell is induced to undergo apoptosis and cell death.

Two categories of spindle poisons are available: the vinca alkaloids, which depolymerize the spindle structure, and the taxanes, which render the spindle structure excessively stable. Both lead to a nonfunctional spindle and subsequent apoptosis.

The antimetabolites, for the most part, inhibit enzymes necessary for the DNA synthesis phase of the cell cycle and exert their maximum effect during this phase by inducing the formation of abnormal or fragmented DNA, which leads to arrested growth and apoptosis in cells retaining the capacity to so respond.

A variety of hormone agonists and antagonists are used to hamper the growth of tumors that have not yet lost their hormone response mechanisms.

This search for "magic bullets" during what has been called the pharmacologic era (7) failed to deliver agents with the specificity required to cure cancer. An early therapeutic triumph led perhaps to excessive enthusiasm. Hertz et al. demonstrated cure of choriocarcinoma using single-drug therapy facilitated by careful monitoring of the specific tumor marker chorionic gonadotropin (8). This seemed to offer an ideal model for curative therapy, but it could not be replicated for a quarter of a century, until the specificity of cisplatin against germ cell tumors provided a second model of a marker producing curable cancer.

Multiple combinations of various agents in different schedules have been used. Attempts have been made to schedule drugs at points in the cell cycle thought to be selectively sensitive. It was hoped that attention to mechanism and cell-cycle phase activity would allow greater cell kill. Attempts at scheduling drugs to synchronize cancer cells or otherwise take advantage of cell-cycle sensitivity have not yet proven very successful. A variety of techniques have been developed to determine cancer cell sensitivity in a manner analogous to that used in bacteria. Cells have been tested in monolayer culture, in explant culture, as xenographs in nude mice, and within microcapsules intraperitoneally in mice. The human tumor cloning assay in soft agar has been most thoroughly studied and provides clinically useful information, but it is cumbersome

Table 1.1. Chemotherapeutic Agents

Agents that damage the DNA template
  By alkylation
    nitrogen mustards: mechlorethamine, cyclophosphamide, melphalan, ifosfamide, chlorambucil
    nitrosoureas: carmustine (BCNU), lomustine (CCNU), semustine (mCCNU), streptozocin, chlorozotocin
    others: thiotepa, hexamethylmelamine, busulfan, dacarbazine, mitomycin C, procarbazine
  By platinum coordination cross-linking: cisplatin, carboplatin
  By double-strand cleavage via topoisomerase II:
    antibiotics: doxorubicin, daunorubicin, mitoxantrone, idarubicin, epirubicin, amsacrine
    podophyllotoxins: etoposide, teniposide
  By single-strand cleavage via topoisomerase I: camptothecins, topotecan, irinotecan
  By intercalation, blocking RNA synthesis: dactinomycin, mithramycin
  By uncertain mechanisms: bleomycin
Spindle poisons
  Vinca alkaloids: vincristine, vinblastine, vendesine, vinorelbine
  Taxanes: taxol, taxotere
Antimetabolites (enzyme inhibitors)
  Thymidylate synthase: 5-fluorouracil, 5-fluoro-2-deoxyuridine
  Dihydrofolate reductase: methotrexate, trimetrexate
  DNA polymerase: cytosine arabinoside (cytarabine), fludarabine, 2-chlorodeoxyadenosine (cladribine)
  Ribonucleotide reductase: hydroxyurea
  Phosphoribosylpyrophosphate amidotransferase: 6-mercaptopurine, 6-thioguanine
  Adenosine deaminase: deoxycoformycin (pentostatin)
Hormonal and antihormonal agents
  Agonists: estrogens, androgens, progestins, corticosteroids
  Antagonists: tamoxifen, aminoglutethimide, leuprolide, flutamide
Biological response modifiers
  Interferons, interleukins, BCG, levamisole
Miscellaneous
  Methyl-GAG, mitotane, asparaginase, prednimustine, estramustine, all *trans*-retinoic acid (ATRA)

---

and time consuming (9). A simpler dye exclusion assay has been developed that yields results in a few days (10). In spite of a great deal of research, it is fair to conclude that assays of tumor sensitivity have not played a significant role in cancer chemotherapy.

Our vast new knowledge of molecular biology may yet allow the design of agents to exploit unique features of malignancy. Drugs specific for telomerase might be highly tumor specific, since normal nongerm cells lack the enzyme. Antisense polynucleotides that bind to specific cell sequences have been suggested, and there is promise in chronic myeloid leukemia, in which the oncogene is well studied. Synthetic agents directed at membrane receptors whose structures we are just beginning to decode are also suggested, and the biologic molecules themselves offer promise. As it seemed 40 years ago, so too today it seems that there are more possibilities to investigate than investigators to frame the questions. To date, however, the biochemical "silver bullet" has eluded discovery.

This lack of success has led some to suggest that a new paradigm is needed (11). We have used the microbiologic model: the model that demands total cell kill of neoplastic cells, based on the assumption that the lesion inducing malignant change was irreversible. A number of observations have called this model into question: mucosa-associated lymphatic tissue lymphomas may be cured by antibiotic therapy of the *Helicobacter pylori* that is etiologic (12), persistence of the *bcr-abl* transcript in cells of chronic myelogenous leukemia after bone marrow transplant is not invariably associated with recurrent malignancy, graft-versus-host reaction may play a role in the cure of some leukemias, all *trans*-retinoic acid may induce differentiation of acute promyelocytic leukemia, levamisole may act through an immunologic mechanism. These observations and others suggest that host response may be more important than previously thought and that reversal of tumor cell phenotype may be possible. This offers a paradigm different from the total cell kill approach.

Others have suggested that the lack of chemotherapeutic success is due to the fact that neoplastic cells develop natural resistance to chemotherapeutic agents by a variety of mechanisms. The corollary of this is that we are unlikely to find agents specific for most cancers, and the most fruitful approach may be to turn our attention to the mechanisms by which tumor cells develop resistance to toxic agents.

TUMOR CELL RESISTANCE

Tumor cells become resistant to chemotherapeutic agents in a variety of ways, but resistance can be divided into two broad categories: kinetic resistance and genetic resistance. Kinetic resistance results from the fact that cells must be actively reproducing to be sensitive to most of the available antitumor agents. Resting cells are relatively resistant. Genetic resistance results from the natural selection of mutant clones that have acquired a mutation that renders them resistant to a particular chemotherapeutic agent, to groups of agents, or to some general mechanism used by most agents to induce cell death (e.g., apoptosis).

Kinetic Resistance

The first approach to overcoming tumor cell resistance was through a study of the kinetic differences between benign and malignant tissue. Cancer cells, at least *some* cancer cells, grow very rapidly and are susceptible to poisons directed at replicating cells. From the beginning, animal models offered promise.

SKIPPER'S LAWS

Several decades ago at the Southern Research Institute, Skipper and collaborators conducted a series of classic experiments using the L1210 mouse leukemia that established a set of laws concerning cancer chemotherapy (13). These laws still apply today, although our understanding of Gompertzian growth has made their application more complex. The L1210 tumor cells are in logarithmic (or exponential) growth; that is, all of the cells are in cycle and dividing, with no cells in a resting phase, and the cell number doubles at a tumor-specific rate. Skipper's laws apply only to the cells that are proliferating in this way.

The first of Skipper's laws is that the doubling time of proliferating cancer cells is a constant, forming a straight line on a semilog plot. Furth

had shown in 1937 that a single surviving cell will lead to treatment failure (14). Skipper showed that death results when the malignant cells reach a critical number or fraction of mouse body weight. Thus, survival is a function of the number of tumor cells injected into the mouse (or by analogy, the tumor body burden in man at the time of diagnosis).

The second law is that cell kill by drugs follows first-order kinetics; that is, the percentage of cells killed at a given drug dose in a given tumor is a constant, regardless of the body burden of tumor cells. Thus, a drug that kills 99% of tumor cells will kill this fraction regardless of the size of the tumor. By convention, one speaks of "log kill", the logarithm by which the original cell number must be reduced to equal the remaining cell number (e.g., 99% represents a 2-log kill). From these two simple laws, it is possible to understand mathematically how L1210 mouse leukemia is cured (or not cured). In the model system, it is even possible to calculate cure probabilities that can be confirmed experimentally. This work has had a continuing influence on the conceptual framework that dominates our approach to chemotherapy, as is illustrated by the current emphasis on high-dose chemotherapy with stem cell rescue.

GROWTH FRACTION

It may be that the simple Skipper model applies to an occasional human malignancy readily curable by chemotherapy in early-stage disease. Trophoblastic neoplasms, testicular germ cell tumors, and Burkitt's lymphoma come to mind. Many have even hoped that the micrometastases of some common tumors behave similarly. Unfortunately, few human cancers are composed of such highly responsive proliferating cells.

In solid tumors in animals and overwhelmingly in man, Skipper's laws apply only to the proliferating or stem cell compartment within the tumor—the fraction of cells within the total tumor that is actively growing. In 1960, Mendelsohn proposed the concept of the growth fraction (15). He suggested that perhaps tumors had cells equivalent to the stem cells present in normal tissues—a subpopulation of cells whose proliferation accounted for all of the growth of the tumor. Such a population, of course, would be the logical target for chemotherapy or radiation therapy. Destruction of the tumor stem cell population, it was argued, might eradicate the tumor as certainly as destruction of the marrow stem cell population terminated hematopoiesis. Using tritiated thymidine, it is possible to determine experimentally the fraction of cells in this proliferating population, but this is not clinically practical. Attempts to modify therapy on the basis of estimates of the growth fraction as determined by various techniques have not been successful.

GOMPERTZIAN GROWTH

The fact that the proliferating cell population is distinct from the nonproliferating population accounts in part for the therapeutic refractoriness of human tumors. Human tumors show a difference from the straight-line growth on a semilog plot seen by Skipper with L1210 mouse leukemia. Instead, human tumors follow a curve called Gompertzian, which describes a population increasing as a result of birth and decreasing as a result of death. Experimentally, tumor cell populations approximate this curve because in addition to proliferating cells, there are subpopulations that have ceased to proliferate, and cells that have died.

Tannock has shown that as cells accumulate into even a small mass, the diffusion process by which oxygen reaches the tumor cells is inadequate to supply cells in the center (16). Expanding solid tumors regularly outgrow their blood supply, the development of which lags behind the leading edge of invading tumor cells. This leads to anoxia, slowing of the cell cycle, exit of some cells into the G_0 nonproliferating phase, and cell death and necrosis. As the cell cycle slows and some cells exit the proliferating pool, Skipper's laws of cell kill no longer apply. The cells become temporarily resistant to chemotherapy. Drugs are available that act at different phases of the cell cycle, as noted above, but the resting or G_0 cell must be induced to enter the cell cycle before it becomes sensitive to chemotherapy or radiotherapy. Nonproliferating cells are less sensitive, in part perhaps because they have time to repair damaged DNA. A major rationale for fractionation of radiation therapy has always been that tumor shrinkage allows circulation to improve during therapy, thus causing resting cells to enter the proliferating radiation-sensitive pool.

The Gompertzian growth curve is sigmoid. Cell numbers accumulate slowly at first, because the number of dividing cells is small; then there is a rapid accumulation of cells, reaching a maximum growth rate at about one-third of maximum tumor volume. There follows a gradual slowing of the rate of growth, almost to a plateau, as the tumor approaches the volume necessary to kill the host. Tumor growth has been fit to a variety of model curves, and it is likely that no single equation describes all malignant growth. However, a sigmoid growth curve approximating Gompertzian growth is seen in many of the malignancies studied. Alternative models have been proposed that challenge Gompertzian growth, with temporarily dormant tumor cells, and computer modeling of these systems resembles actual survival data (17).

The dynamics of Gompertzian growth have been emphasized by Norton and Simon (18). Small tumors have the largest growth fraction, presumably because their supply of nutrients and oxygen is optimal. But since total cell number is small, even a large growth fraction yields only a small increase in tumor cell number. At the other extreme of the curve, total cell number is very large, but the growth fraction is at a minimum, probably because the number of anoxic and necrotic cells has reached a maximum. In the middle portion of the curve, growth reaches a maximum because, although neither the total cell number nor the fraction of proliferating cells is at a maximum, their *product* does reach a maximum (at about one-third of maximum tumor volume).

Since Skipper's laws apply only to the proliferating fraction, it is clear that our best opportunity (from a kinetic standpoint) to achieve total cell kill is in the early portion of the curve, when growth fraction is at a maximum. We see the maximum *measurable* tumor response at the midportion of the curve, where growth *rate* is greatest. This is the best place to estimate drug efficacy against a particular tumor. A comparable kill of proliferating cells at the upper portion of the curve will be unlikely to show a measurable response because the growth rate is so small.

Assuming they are not dormant, micrometastases are presumed to have a high growth fraction, so from kinetic considerations alone, our chance at total cell kill is highest, because fewer cells are in the nonproliferating phase of the cell cycle. Such reasoning as this led to the enthusiasm for adjuvant chemotherapy, and indeed, some success has been encountered in childhood malignancies and breast and colon cancer. These successes are, however, far less than was hoped for and less than theory had led us to believe possible. Why? Perhaps because we failed to give adequate importance to tumor progression and heterogeneity leading to the development of genetic resistance.

Genetic Resistance

Genetic resistance, unlike kinetic resistance, is a function of total body tumor burden, not simply the kinetics of a particular metastatic focus, because genetic resistance results from mutations that occur with cell doubling. Since micrometastases are clones from cells that have undergone many prior divisions within the primary tumor, genetic resistance becomes a dominant factor. Large tumors with many generations of tumor cells offer the best potential for the evolution of resistant clones of cells.

TUMOR PROGRESSION TO RESISTANCE

Tumor cell progression, like carcinogenesis itself, is dominated by the process of natural selection of mutations. The incidence of natural mutations, therefore, is of major interest. There are a few studies of genetic stability that allow estimation of the magnitude of the "normal" mutation rate (19–24). These studies are usually done in fibroblast cell cultures or with lymphocytes recently derived from human subjects. Usually either the X-linked hypoxanthine-guanine phosphoribosyl transferase locus or the autosomal sodium-potassium ATPase locus are studied by enumerating thioguanine-resistant or ouabain-resistant cells. Rates of mutation of an order of magnitude of 10^{-6} have been consistently found. If the few genes studied are typical, one might suggest a mutation rate of about one mutation per gene per 10^6 cells per generation, perhaps an order of magnitude higher in lymphocytes.

When malignant cells are compared with normal cells, the scanty data indicate about an order of magnitude increase in the mutation rate of malignant cells (20, 25, 26). Available data are consistent with an increased mutation rate in neoplastic cells to about one mutation per gene per 10^5 cells, or ten times normal. A similar rate is reported in Bloom's syndrome, a disease with an inherited increase in the mutation rate and an increase in the incidence of cancer (23). Chromosomal nondisjunction, mitotic recombination, or some other mechanism may result in loss of heterogeneity and loss of a normal cancer suppressor gene even more commonly, up to 10^{-4} per cell generation, based on data for the retinoblastoma gene (27). Legitimate methodologic issues have been raised (28), but it seems reasonable for present theoretic purposes to consider gene mutation rates of the order of 10^{-6} in normal cells and 10^{-5} in malignant cells. Hypermutation in human cancer is supported by the finding of a defective mismatch-repair gene in hereditary nonpolyposis colon cancer (HNPCC) families (29), associated with hypermutability (30). For reasons not yet fully elucidated, in HNPCC, the gene that is the target of this hypermutability is the receptor for TGF-β, a potent inhibitor of epithelial cell growth (31)

Foulds (32), Nowell (33), and Cairns (34) have emphasized the evolution of human tumors by natural selection of those mutations that predispose to malignant growth. Essential to such theories is the assumption that tumors have an inherently greater mutation rate than normal cells. Furthermore, with progression, there seems to be a continued increase in mutation rate (35). Our understanding of the increased mutation rate in cancer has been greatly augmented by the recent discovery of *p53*. This gene codes for a protein that delays cell division and stimulates DNA repair when damage to DNA is detected (36). When damage to DNA is severe, *p53* induces programed cell death. *p53* is inactivated in many tumor cells, and this undoubtedly allows very rapid mutation of neoplastic cells. Similarly, the discovery of germ line mutations of mismatch-repair genes leading to defective DNA repair in HNPCC patients (37) has added to our understanding of the increased mutation rate in malignancy. *bcl-2* is a gene that when induced will prevent the lymphocytes in nodular lymphoma from undergoing apoptosis. Clearly a pattern is emerging in which carcinogenesis, tumor progression, and resistance to chemotherapy (or radiotherapy) result from common mechanisms.

Natural resistance to chemotherapeutic agents occurs in mutant clones, in addition to other alterations in phenotypic behavior. Drug resistance produced by selection of mutant clones was first demonstrated in bacteria as long ago as 1943 in the classic work of Luria and Delbrück (38). It is virtually certain that drug resistance in human cancer cells evolves in this way.

There are multiple mechanisms for drug resistance, but the important point is that this resistance is different from the kinetic resistance encountered due to the cell cycle. Cell-cycle resistance is reversible when a cycling cell enters a sensitive phase or when a G_0 cell reenters the cell cycle. Genetic resistance is not usually considered reversible. Furthermore, since there is a ge-

Table 1.2. Mechanisms of Drug Resistance Developed during Cancer Progression and the Drugs Involved

1. *Decreased drug transport into cells:* methotrexate, melphalan, mechlorethamine, cytarabine
2. *Increased drug transport out of cells:* vinca alkaloids, antitumor antibiotics, etoposide (increased p-glycoprotein product of the *mdr* gene)
3. *Reduced activation of drug:* cytarabine (deoxycytidine kinase), 5-azacytidine (uridine-cytidine kinase), 5-fluorouracil (uridine kinase, orotic acid phosphoribosyl transferase, uridine phosphorylase), 6-mercaptopurine, 6-thioguanine (hypoxanthine-guanine phosphoribosyl transferase), methotrexate
4. *Increased inactivation of drug or active metabolite:* cytarabine (cytidine deaminase), all alkylating agents and agents acting through free radicals (glutathione, metallothioneins), 6-mercaptopurine, 6-thioguanine
5. *Increased DNA repair:* all alkylating agents, antitumor antibiotics, topoisomerase II–active drugs, cisplatin
6. *Use of alternate pathways as source of metabolites:* methotrexate and 5-fluorouracil (increased thymidine from salvage pathway), 6-mercaptopurine and 6-thioguanine (increased salvage pathway for purines)
7. *Gene amplification of enzyme target of drug action:* methotrexate (dihydrofolate reductase, 5-fluorouracil (thymidylate synthase), 2-deoxycoformycin (adenosine deaminase)
8. *Alteration of target to reduce drug binding:* vincristine (tubulin), methotrexate (dihydrofolate reductase), 5-fluorouracil (thymidylate synthase), hydroxyurea (ribonucleotide reductase), doxorubicin (topoisomerase II), daunomycin (topoisomerase II), etoposide (topoisomerase II)
9. *Loss of apoptosis:* loss of *p53* or *bcl-2* in a tumor cell can lead to resistance to all chemotherapeutic agents that act by inducing a cell to undergo programmed cell death

netic basis for the resistance, subsequent generations of cells remain resistant. As more is understood about impaired apoptosis as a mechanism of resistance, however, the possibility of reversal has been raised.

Because mutation is a random event, the number of drug-resistant clones increases as a direct function of the length of time a tumor has been present. The size of the tumor, or more precisely the number of resistant clones, is a direct function of the number of cell divisions that have occurred in the tumor. There is strong evidence that the size of the primary tumor in the best human model studied, breast cancer, is directly related to the incidence of metastasis and survival (39, 40). Resistance, then, is the major reason our therapy fails. There are numerous mechanisms of drug resistance as shown in Table 1.2 but each has natural selection of a growth-promoting mutation as a common origin.

THE GOLDIE-COLDMAN HYPOTHESIS

An important consequence of the development of drug resistance as tumors progress is that at the time of diagnosis most tumors possess resistant clones. Goldie and Coldman have estimated the role this might play in cancer therapy (41). If 1 g of tumor, 10^9 cells, is the minimum tumor size for detection, and 10^{-5} is a probable tumor mutation rate per gene, then such a tumor might contain 10^4 clones that might be resistant to a given drug. (This simple calculation does not

take into account a host of potential errors.) We would anticipate encountering drug resistance, therefore, even with small tumors. However, resistance to two drugs would be less likely, assuming the resistance involves independent mechanisms. Resistance by independent mechanisms should be seen in less than one cell in $10^5 \times 10^5$, or 10^{10}. This is only one doubly resistant clone per 10 g of tumor. Thus, a 3-g primary tumor with micrometastases might have no doubly resistant cells.

It follows that multidrug therapy should be substantially more effective than single-drug therapy. Combination chemotherapy has allowed cure of a number of cancers, especially childhood and hematologic malignancies. However, the common adult malignancies have eluded chemotherapeutic cure, probably in large part because of acquired multidrug resistance to antineoplastic drugs. Paradoxically, normal tissue *never* develops resistance to chemotherapy, emphasizing an important qualitative characteristic of the cancer cell, a characteristic that may depend on the presence of a functional *p53* gene product in normal cells.

MECHANISMS OF DRUG RESISTANCE

It is often true that a single mutation leads to resistance to a single drug. In some cases, there may be more than one mutation leading to resistance to a single agent such as 5-fluorouracil (42). Sometimes genetic resistance involves a mechanism that can produce resistance to more than one drug with a *single* mutation. For example, resistance to *all* alkylating agents may occur by overproduction of glutathione or metallothioneins, mechanisms for dealing with the free radicals produced by alkylating agents. Another common mechanism of drug resistance is the so-called pleotrophic drug resistance, or multiple drug resistance (MDR).

Ling et al. (43) noted that cancer cells may acquire resistance to multiple drugs by activation of a cellular excretion system, the p-glycoprotein membrane system. Bacteria have a membrane protein that functions to excrete toxins that enter the cell; this simple system has evolved in the mammalian cell to perform a complex excretory function dealing with a variety of hydrophobic natural products, including many of our chemotherapeutic agents (44). When activated, it protects the cancer cell from chemotherapy by excreting drugs that enter the cell. This gene, the *mdr* gene, codes for the membrane-bound p-glycoprotein that is the excretion channel. It may be activated by carcinogenesis (45). Some body tissues (e.g., colon and kidney) are rich in active p-glycoprotein, and tumors derived from such tissue are often initially resistant to drugs such as doxorubicin. Tumor progression leads to activation of the MDR phenotype in the absence of drug treatment because the *mdr* gene promoter is a target for the products of the *ras* oncogene and the *p53* cancer suppressor gene (46). This mechanism is thought to be important in the resistance of tumors to drug therapy. However, data suggest that clinical multidrug resistance may be seen in some tumors in the absence of the MDR phenotype (47).

Topoisomerase II represents another point at which mutations involving multiple drug resistance may occur. This enzyme is designed to allow long strands of DNA to pass through each other as they untangle. It is covalently bound by several drugs in such a way that it carries out the first step of its function, the cleavage of double-stranded DNA to allow another chain to pass through, but fails to rejoin the DNA. This leads to double-strand breaks. Strand cleavage is accomplished by splitting the phosphodiester bond and linking the 5′ of each cleaved strand to a tyrosine residue on topoisomerase II. Many anticancer drugs stabilize these DNA-enzyme complexes, blocking the second step, the rejoining of the cleaved DNA strands. Such complexes are reversible with removal of the drug (48). Doxorubicin, the podophyllotoxins, amsacrine,

5-iminodaunorubicin, and ellipticine are examples of topoisomerase II–active agents. Evidence that breaks are due to such a mechanism is the accumulation of protein-linked strand breaks. Such breaks do not arise by a free radical mechanism, although some topoisomerase-active drugs such as doxorubicin also produce free radicals. Free radical breaks are not reversible by removal of the drug.

There are derivatives of doxorubicin that do not intercalate but act the same way on topoisomerase II, so intercalation is not a prerequisite for this mechanism (49). A multidrug resistance phenotype may be acquired by a qualitative change in topoisomerase II (50). Resistance may also be associated with decreased amounts of topoisomerase II (51). Of note, cells made resistant to nitrogen mustard contain four times the preresistance amount of topoisomerase II, perhaps because this enzyme repairs monoadducts; such cells are hypersensitive to amsacrine, suggesting an interesting multidrug therapeutic strategy (52).

Topoisomerase II may explain why some slow-growing tumors are resistant to such agents as doxorubicin. Chronic lymphocytic leukemia has low levels of this enzyme (53). Perhaps many quiescent cells have low topoisomerase II levels.

APOPTOSIS

The term apoptosis was coined over two decades ago to describe a mechanism of cell death that differed markedly from necrosis in that the nucleus becomes pyknotic and the membrane remains intact. There is no release of cell contents to excite inflammation, and adjacent cells, not professional phagocytes, ingest the cell debris (54). The name of the phenomenon was derived from the Greek *apo*, meaning "apart," and *ptosis*, meaning "fallen." Drug-induced apoptosis was first observed when glucocorticoids were found to activate an endogenous endonuclease in thymocytes (55).

It now appears that the primary mechanism by which most chemotherapeutic agents induce cell kill is by causing cell damage, especially genetic damage, that results in the induction of apoptosis (56). Resistance to apoptosis, therefore, represents the most potent form of tumor cell resistance to chemotherapy. In this light, the inactivation of *p53* as a late step in tumor progression takes on great significance because *p53* plays a major role in the induction of apoptosis, although pathways to apoptosis independent of *p53* have been described (57). Since cells damaged by chemotherapeutic agents cannot be induced to undergo programed cell death in the absence of *p53*, they continue to replicate after severe genetic damage, and the increased mutation rate leads to accelerated tumor progression.

Another gene, *bcl-2*, was first described in nodular lymphoma and is one of a family of genes that control the apoptotic threshold. The protein that directly initiates apoptosis is Bax, and the protein product of *bcl-2*, Bcl-2, exerts its antiapoptotic action by forming heterodimers with Bax (58). Bcl-2 confers resistance to the chemotherapeutic agents commonly used in lymphoma (59).

When apoptosis is blocked, no drug or combination of drugs in any dose can be expected to eradicate all of the tumor cells. However, it has not yet been clearly established that all chemotherapeutic cell death, including that seen with very high dose therapy, depends on apoptosis.

COMBINATION CHEMOTHERAPY

Long before there was wide understanding of tumor progression, combination chemotherapy was discovered empirically and applied widely, and three principles for designing combinations were formulated almost by consensus. First, drugs known to be active as single agents should be selected, especially those that have produced some complete remissions. Second, drugs with different mechanisms of action should be combined. This should, in theory, allow multiple attacks on the biochemistry of the cancer cell, with additive, perhaps even synergistic, effect. Synergy is exceedingly difficult to document even in carefully controlled animal systems and essentially impossible to prove in man except under unusual circumstances. The third principle is that drugs with different dose-limiting toxicities should be combined so that each drug may be given at or near full therapeutic doses. Unfortunately, most chemotherapeutic agents have a significant overlap in toxic effects, with almost all having myelosuppression as the dose-limiting toxicity. Since most agents are myelosuppressive, dose reductions are common in combination regimens.

With our new understanding of the MDR type of resistance, we might add a fourth principle: Drugs with *different patterns* of resistance should be combined. The drugs excreted by the product of the mdr gene are a group of natural products, some of which have different mechanisms of action but a common mechanism of resistance. Obviously, we need more knowledge of the precise mechanisms of resistance. This is particularly true with apoptosis, since it is not yet clear whether some drugs, or some doses of drugs, kill cells without inducing programed cell death.

There are some biochemical principles that might apply. For example, we might exploit our knowledge of the influence of leucovorin on the binding of 5-fluorouracil to its target thymidine synthetase, or include considerations of sequential blockade of metabolic pathways such as combining hydroxyurea with cytarabine. Further, we might exploit clues such as the observation that in developing resistance to nitrogen mustard some malignant cells become increasingly sensitive to topoisomerase II inhibitors.

Such principles might lead to combinations of agents least likely to encounter cross-resistance, most likely to be additive or synergistic, and capable of being administered at the highest dose. Dose has always been a major consideration in chemotherapy because we have been exploiting such minor differences between the malignant and nonmalignant cell. In combinations, careful attention must be given to achieving maximum dose with minimum time intervals between doses.

DOSE INTENSITY

It is an article of faith among oncologists that most cancer chemotherapeutic agents show a steep dose-response curve. Even modest reductions in dose are felt to lead to substantial reductions in tumor cell kill. This has led to an emphasis on the intensity of treatment, expressed as average dose per week over the course of treatment. There are examples of correlations between dose intensity and response rate in advanced cancers, but of greater influence in practice has been the analysis by Hryniuk (60) of the relationship of survival to dose in adjuvant trials in breast cancer.

A variety of techniques have been developed to produce increased regional dose intensity. Intrathecal administration of methotrexate or cytarabine is one technique for dealing with privileged sanctuary sites by using an enhanced dose. Hepatic artery or portal vein infusion has been used to enhance dose to liver primary or secondary tumors (61). Limb perfusion has long been popular for melanoma. Intraperitoneal cisplatin for ovarian cancer, first described by Howell (62), has recently been reported to be superior to intravenous cisplatin in a randomized trial (63). Regional dose intensification has been associated with dramatic responses in numerous anecdotal reports. However, except for intrathecal therapy in acute lymphocytic leukemia and cisplatin in ovarian cancer, none of the regional methods has been reported in randomized trials to produce longer survival than conventional therapy.

It is generally accepted, though rigorous proof in man is sparse, that the most important parameter in dose level is the area under the curve in a plot of in vivo concentration versus time. Obviously the problem is complex, because there is a hierarchy of in vivo concentrations, starting with simple serum levels, then unbound or activated drug, activated-drug concentration within the target tumor cell, and so on. Unfortunately, there are few data from man to serve as a guide, and substantial data showing the poor correlation of animal models to man. Further, there may be unexpected complicating factors, as for example, the enhanced activation of cyclophosphamide induced by agents such as phenobarbital that stimulate the p450 system (64). Patterns of excretion, drug metabolism, protein binding, third-space sequestration, and other considerations come into play, but even with an agent such as methotrexate, where we have extensive experience with human dose levels that correlate with toxicity, there is still not good correlation between dose level and antitumor efficacy. Questions of dose intensity seem more likely to be resolved through careful clinical trials than by meticulous pharmacologic studies in animals.

Rescue as a Means of Increasing Dose Intensity

The focus on dose intensity derives from the wide assumption that present regimens are close to achieving total cancer cell kill. Data to support such an assumption are sparse, but there is no model except man likely to answer the question.

The classic rescue technique has been high-dose methotrexate followed by leucovorin. In theory, this allows massive doses of methotrexate to enter all cells; then normal cells, but not cancer cells, are rescued by the leucovorin. To date, it is clear that rescue allows very high doses of methotrexate to be well tolerated without myelotoxicity. Unfortunately, there are no published studies demonstrating that a randomized

population receiving high-dose methotrexate survives longer that a control population receiving conventional doses. Trimetrexate enters cells by diffusion, not by the active transport mechanism used for methotrexate and leucovorin. Thus, tumor cells that do not transport leucovorin into cells are not rescued.

The use of mesna in conjunction with high-dose ifosfamide is a form of rescue, since it prevents the acrolein metabolite of ifosfamide from damaging the bladder mucosa.

The ultimate in rescue techniques is, of course, stem cell rescue or bone marrow transplantation, which allows massive doses of myelotoxic drugs to be used. An allogeneic transplant may confuse the issue of dose intensity because graft-versus-tumor activity has been demonstrated. There is widespread use of high-dose therapy with stem cell rescue in the lymphomas (65), breast cancer (66), ovarian cancer (67), myeloma (68), and other tumors. Data to date are insufficient to allow a determination of the ultimate role of this technique, and the technique itself is under evolution as studies of tumor cell detection and purging in vitro continue.

It has long been assumed that high-dose therapy with stem cell rescue is indicated in first recurrence of aggressive non-Hodgkin's lymphoma, based on pilot studies showing up to 40% long-term survival in selected cases, compared with unselected historic controls, which do not show such survival. Patients who are sensitive to conventional doses are usually selected for high-dose therapy. High-dose therapy has also been used for patients who respond slowly to initial conventional therapy, based on the rationale that their tumors are relatively resistant. Two recent trials provide useful data. The first, reported in final form, demonstrates in a randomized trial that autologous bone marrow transplantation for patients who had only a partial remission after three cycles of CHOP (cyclophosphamide, doxorubicin, vincristine, prednisone) did not improve survival over that obtained with five additional courses of CHOP alone (69). A second study, reported in abstract form, supports the notion that treatment of first recurrent non-Hodgkin's lymphoma with high-dose therapy plus stem cell rescue improves survival (70). In view of the long interval between the claim that "second-" and "third-generation" chemotherapy regimens would improve survival and the disproof of this claim by randomized trials, it is encouraging to see randomized data begin to appear on the question of high-dose therapy with stem cell rescue.

The most important question that requires an answer is whether existing drugs *at any dose* can produce cures in the common neoplasms, given the fact that most of these cancers have lost the ability to undergo programed cell death as a result of mutations of the *p53* gene. If the answer is yes, then a line of research aimed at developing safe rescue using stem cells free of contaminating tumor cells might be productive.

MICROMETASTASES

It is generally assumed that micrometastases require the same high dose intensity for eradication as that required to produce regression in measurable tumors, because, although their cell number is small and they have a high growth fraction, the probability of encountering a drug-resistant clone is high. There are extensive data on various combinations of drugs used at high dose to eradicate micrometastases. It is fair to say that adjuvant therapy of micrometastases has not yet produced the kind of dramatic results our conventional theories have predicted. Are micrometastases dormant? Are they composed of cells sufficiently progressed to be unable to undergo apoptosis? Clearly metastatic tumor cells have undergone a series of mutations allowing them to grow independently of the basement membrane, to invade, to survive in the circulation, to grow in a new environment, and to stimulate the influx of new blood vessels. Changes in the gene *p53* usually occur late in this progression and render the cell unable to undergo programed cell death after damage by radiation or chemotherapy. Is this the reason adjuvant therapy so often fails? Or, is the resistance simply due to a lack of sufficiently active drugs?

NEOADJUVANT THERAPY

In approaching the question of why micrometastases are so seldom cured by intensive combination chemotherapy, many investigators are exploring the "neoadjuvant" approach, that is, chemotherapy before primary surgery. This gives, at best, a modest decrease of doubling times during which micrometastases might evolve genetic resistance. Might there be another advantage to neoadjuvant chemotherapy? Several animal models have shown a sudden growth spurt of metastases immediately after the primary tumor is removed (71). Can this offer a kinetic advantage? Human data are scanty,

with only a single unintentional observation by Nissen-Meyer providing long-term survival data (72). What causes the postoperative growth spurt? There is evidence in animals of communication between separate foci of cancer cells (73). This could be important to a kinetic explanation of the resistance of micrometastases to adjuvant chemotherapy.

It seems likely that the fundamental questions regarding neoadjuvant chemotherapy are sufficiently numerous and complex that several clinical trials will be required to produce the answers. Studies are presently in progress, but as yet there are no data indicating a significant survival advantage with the neoadjuvant approach.

POTENTIATORS OF CHEMOTHERAPY

It is possible to increase tumor cell kill by increasing the effects of a given dose of drug. A variety of drugs, while not themselves cytotoxic, potentiate the activity of cytotoxic agents in various ways. A potentiator may act by moving cells into a kinetic phase with greater susceptibility (androgens in prostate cancer), by accelerating mitosis so that there is insufficient time for G_2 repair of damaged DNA (aminophylline), by opposing acquired cellular resistance to cytotoxic attack (verapamil in MDR-pattern resistance), by altering cell membranes to increase drug influx (amphotericin B), by replacing molecular oxygen's role of facilitating free radical action (misonidazole), by promoting increased drug delivery to tumors (agents that improve red cell deformability), by facilitating entry into apoptosis in *p53* defective cells (no agent yet identified), and by as yet undiscovered mechanisms. This subject has recently been extensively reviewed (74). Potentiating agents are summarized in Table 1.3.

Of note, some anticancer drugs have a potentiating effect, so some of our present combinations may owe activity to this mechanism rather than to direct cytotoxicity. The observation that tamoxifen is an important ingredient in the combination regimen for melanoma, for example, may be due to either an additive cytotoxic effect or a potentiating effect (75). Further, some of our commonly used pharmaceuticals also have this action, which further confounds our interpretation of human trials. How many patient responses were related to concomitant therapy with, say, calcium channel blockers or aminophylline, or phenobarbital? To date, this is a relatively poorly investigated, but possibly useful,

Table 1.3. Potentiators of Cytotoxic Chemotherapy

Calcium channel blockers: (verapamil, diltiazem, flunarizine, amiodarone, nicardepine, nifedipine) There is
   evidence for a mechanism via p-glycoprotein with reversal of MDR-type resistance; however, other mechanisms
   are likely involved, since there is also potentiation of non-MDR drugs such as cisplatin, bleomycin, and 5-FU.
   Membrane alteration has been suggested. Tamoxifen, vincristine, vinblastine, reserpine, and quinidine have
   weak calcium channel blocking actions and also potentiate chemotherapeutic agents.

Calmodulin inhibitors: (phenothiazines including trifluopromazine, prochlorperazine, chlorpromazine, and
   thioridazine; nonphenothiazines including clomipramine, melittin, pimozide, lidocaine, propranolol,
   prenylamine, polysorbate, and others) There is evidence for a mechanism via reversal of MDR-type resistance,
   but as with calcium channel blockers, other factors are involved, since non-MDR-type drugs are also
   potentiated. Membrane alteration has been suggested.

Antifungal agents: (amphotericin B, ketoconazole, and others) This effect involves virtually all agents tested in
   vitro. The mechanism is probably via membrane alteration with increased cell uptake of cytotoxic agent.
   Cyclosporin A has weak antifungal activity and also potentiates chemotherapeutic agents.

Nitroimidazoles: (metronidazole, misonidazole, and related agents) Virtually all drugs and radiation tested in vitro
   have been potentiated. The mechanism is complex but probably involves potentiation of damage to anoxic cells
   as a common denominator. Depletion of glutathione may be involved.

Glutathione-depleting agents: (butathione sulfoximine, diethyl maleate, acetominophen, and others) Depletion of
   glutathione scavenging of free radicals necessary for action of many drugs and radiation is accomplished by
   binding to glutathione-S-transferase or by direct detoxification of the free radicals. Reduction of glutathione in
   normal tissues occurs but does not seem to significantly enhance toxicity.

Methylxanthines: (caffeine, theobromine, pentoxifylline, theophylline, aminophylline, and others) The mechanism
   is acceleration of damaged tumor cells through G_2, during which phase damaged cells usually delay entering
   mitosis so that repair of damaged DNA can take place; if damage is not repaired, cell death is more likely. Thus,
   these agents render the so-called "nonlethal" damage lethal by preventing repair. Some experiments show
   inconsistent results. The methylxanthine pentoxifylline may improve drug delivery by increasing red blood cell
   deformability.

Agents that improve drug delivery: (glycerol, mannitol, perfluorocarbons such as Fluosol-DA, angiotensin II, and
   others) The common denominator is increased blood flow with increased drug delivery and presumably better
   oxygenation.

Others: Perhexilene maleate may alter cell membranes of resistant cells to increase drug entry. Dipyridamole
   inhibits facilitated transport of purines and pyrimidines and increases sensitivity to methotrexate, 5-FU, cytosine
   arabinoside, and phosphonoacetyl-L-aspartate (PALA).

Agents that facilitate apoptosis in cells with defective p53: none identified as yet.

---

approach to chemotherapy, although since our
clinical protocols are already complex, it would
sorely tax the system to add data on all concurrent medications that might lead to insights relating to potentiation. Finally, interference is potentially just as important an area as potentiation
and far less studied.

To date we have only begun to investigate
methods of potentiating chemotherapy. In view
of the key role of apoptosis in the mechanism of
cell kill by chemotherapeutic agents, this would
seem to be the most fruitful area for study.

PRESENT STRATEGIES

The treatment strategies currently employed
in advanced disease involve combination regimens given at high dose intensities as early as
practical, utilizing a variety of techniques to increase the effective dose delivered. The goal is to
achieve a complete remission, following which,
further intensive chemotherapy is delivered, often for several cycles. Rarely is maintenance
therapy used except in acute lymphocytic leukemia. Adjuvant therapy regimens are increasingly patterned after regimens used for advanced disease. Terminology for these treatment
regimens is summarized in Table 1.4. This approach has proved modestly successful in that
we are able to cure several malignancies when
micrometastases are present or occasionally
even advanced disease as shown in Table 1.5.

Presently our emphasis is on intensive therapy. Inherent in this strategy is the assumption
that we are close enough to a total cell kill using
present drugs that if a small additional log kill
can be achieved we may obtain many more
cures. This strategy is based on the application
of the Skipper curve to the tumor stem cell population, the point being that as we approach total

Table 1.4. Terminology Used in Describing Chemotherapy

1. *Induction:* High-dose, usually combination, chemotherapy given with the intent of inducing complete remission when initiating a curative regimen. The term is usually applied to hematologic malignancies but is applicable to solid tumors.
2. *Consolidation:* Repetition of the induction regimen in a patient who has achieved a complete remission after induction, with the intent of increasing the cure rate or the remission duration.
3. *Intensification:* Chemotherapy after complete remission with higher doses of the same agents used for induction or with different agents at high doses, with the intent of increasing the cure rate or the remission duration.
4. *Maintenance:* Long-term, low-dose, single or combination chemotherapy in a patient who has achieved a complete remission, with the intent of delaying the regrowth of residual tumor cells.
5. *Adjuvant:* A short course of high-dose, usually combination, chemotherapy in a patient with no evidence of residual cancer after surgery or radiotherapy, given with the intent of destroying a small number of residual tumor cells.
6. *Neoadjuvant:* Adjuvant chemotherapy given in the preoperative or perioperative period.
7. *Primary chemotherapy:* Sometimes used as a synonym for neoadjuvant chemotherapy, but also applied to chemotherapy given in the absence of intended surgery or radiotherapy.
8. *Palliative:* Chemotherapy given to control symptoms or prolong life in a patient in whom cure is unlikely.
9. *Salvage:* A potentially curative, high-dose, usually combination, regimen given in a patient who has failed or recurred following a different curative regimen.

Table 1.5. Tumors in Which Chemotherapeutic Cure Is Possible

In an adjuvant setting
  Breast cancer
  Osteogenic sarcoma
  Soft tissue sarcoma
  Colorectal cancer
In advanced disease
  Choriocarcinoma
  Acute lymphocytic leukemia
  Hodgkin's disease
  Aggressive non-Hodgkin's lymphoma
  Germ cell cancer
  Acute myelogenous leukemia
  Wilms' tumor
  Embryonal rhabdomyosarcoma
  Ewing's tumor
  Neuroblastoma
  Small cell lung cancer
  Ovarian cancer

cell kill, the cure rate moves rapidly from very low to very high because it moves along a semilog curve.

A second theme in our present approach to therapy is that the biologic response modifiers will add several logs of cell kill to chemotherapy. The repeated failure of classic immunotherapy over the past 40 years notwithstanding, this view is widely held. The efficacy of interferon in several hematologic neoplasms has encouraged investigators to study its use more widely. At pres-

ent, the biologicals are in use primarily as single agents, but it is anticipated that combination with chemotherapeutic agents will quickly follow the discovery of a reliably active biologic agent.

Our strategies have allowed cure of a few pediatric and adult neoplasms, either as advanced disease or in the adjuvant mode, but unfortunately, most of the common cancers have escaped chemotherapeutic cure. It is likely that a major breakthrough will be required, perhaps even a paradigm shift, to substantially increase our cure rates in the common adult neoplasms. Absent this, we may incrementally improve our cure rates by study of present techniques.

FUTURE STRATEGIES

We are not yet exploiting our newly acquired knowledge of the new biology of cancer. We have only begun to evaluate high-intensity therapy requiring bone marrow transplantation, and until we have tested this approach on resistant tumors we will not know how close our present drugs are to total cell kill. All, or essentially all, of our chemotherapeutic agents have been selected for study because of their marked toxicity to rapidly growing cells, and we have yet to develop an effective screen to identify potential anticancer agents that do not fit this mold. Such a screen would qualify as a major breakthrough because it would imply the use of something other than proliferation rate to distinguish malignant from nonmalignant tissue. All *trans*-retinoic acid is a notable exception, and it is perhaps not surprising that this agent has recently been reported to increase the absolute cure rate in acute promyelocytic leukemia.

As retinoic acid illustrates, our rapidly expanding knowledge of oncogenes and their products offers a potential cornucopia of anticancer targets for exploitation. Membrane receptors, cytoplasmic signal mediators, and nuclear messenger receivers all provide grist for the mill of the synthetic chemist and molecular biologist. A primary challenge is to find a pharmacologic agent that mimics the action of the product of *p53* to allow damaged cells to undergo programed cell death after damage.

One area of intense interest is the antisense oligonucleotides (76). Because of the specificity of the Watson-Crick base pair structure, an oligonucleotide of 15 to 17 nucleotides would have a unique sequence relative to the entire human genome and be able to interfere in a highly specific manner with processes such as translation of mRNA. These agents show great promise for blocking specific gene expression (77). It is also possible to synthesize DNA-binding proteins that are site specific. One such peptide uses classical zinc-finger motifs to bind specifically to and repress a 9-base (three codon) target sequence spanning the fusion point of the *bcr-abl* fusion gene associated with chronic myelogenous leukemia, and this product suppresses the growth of murine cells in culture (78). Peptide nucleic acid chimeras (PNAs) are still another approach to specifically target cancer genes (79, 80).

The protein product Ras of the oncogene *ras* attaches to the cell membrane by a farnesyl group that is itself attached to Ras by the enzyme farnesyltransferase. Inhibitors of this enzyme inhibit the tumor growth–promoting action of Ras. Recently, new compounds have been synthesized that inhibit farnesyltransferase (81, 82).

New agents from natural sources continue to be developed. The enediynes are a new class of DNA-cleaving molecules with potent anticancer activity. Unlike the alkylating agents, which form intrastrand crosslinks, the enediynes are metabolized into active benzene diradicals that abstract hydrogen atoms from the sugar phosphate backbone, leading to cleavage of DNA (83).

If we can identify patterns of tumor cell progression that are predictable pathways of evolution, we might attempt anticipatory immunotherapy, that is, immunization of the patient against a surface marker we know the cancer cell

is likely to develop subsequently (p-glycoprotein for example).

We have only begun to investigate the numerous potentiators of chemotherapy, some of which may prove useful. Combinations of potentiators must be considered (84).

Autologous stem cell purification and transfusion is not beyond our present technology and would greatly facilitate study of autologous bone marrow transplantation because it would eliminate the question of contamination of the rescue stem cell population and allow a focus on the question of whether our present drugs are able to cure the common adult malignancies at myelotoxic doses.

Finally, there is no substitute for specificity. Our continued search for therapeutic agents may yet yield, by design or by chance, additional agents that bring to other neoplasms the specificity that methotrexate brought to trophoblastic neoplasms or that cisplatin brought to germ cell tumors. If agents that inhibit telomerase can be developed, we may achieve for the first time the level of specificity against tumor cells that penicillin exerts against organisms with cell walls. If agents that inhibit *ras* or *myc* or replace *p53* or *RB* can be developed, we might open the way to a new generation of anticancer drugs.

REFERENCES

1. Lundblad V, Szostak JW. A mutant with a defect in telomere elongation leads to senescence in yeast. Cell 1989;57:633–643.

2. Kim NW, Piatyszek MA, Prowse KR, et al. Specific association of human telomerase activity with immortal cells and cancer. Science 1994;266:2011–2015.

3. Cech TR. Chromosome end games. Science 1994; 266:387–388.

4. Yarbro JW. Inhibition of nucleic acid synthesis in mouse ascites tumor. Ph.D. thesis, University of Minnesota Graduate School, June 1965.

5. Wintrobe MW. Hematology, the blossoming of a science. Philadelphia: Lea & Febiger, 1985:512.

6. Heidelberger C. Fluorinated pyrimidines, a new class of tumor inhibitory compounds. Nature 1957; 179:663–666.

7. Carter SK. Some thoughts on resistance to cancer chemotherapy. Cancer Treat Rev 1984;11:(Suppl A)3–7.

8. Hertz R, Lewis J Jr, Lipsett M. Five years experience with chemotherapy of metastatic choriocarcinoma and related tropho-blastic tumors in women. Am J Obstet Gynecol 1961;82:631.

9. Hanauske AR, Hanauske U, Von Hoff D. The human tumor cloning assay in cancer research and therapy. Curr Probl Cancer 1985;9(12):1–66.

10. Weisenthal LM, Marsden JA, Dill PL, et al. A novel dye exclusion method for testing in vitro chemosensitivity in human tumors. Cancer Res 1983;43:749–757.

11. Schipper H, Goh CR, Wang TL. Shifting the cancer paradigm: must we kill to cure? J Clin Oncol 1995;13:801–807.

12. Wotherspoon AC, Doglioni C, Diss TC, et al. Regression of primary low-grade B-cell gastric lymphoma of mucosa associated lymphoid tissue type after eradication of *Helicobacter pylori*. Lancet 1993; 342:575–577.

13. Skipper HE. Historic milestones in cancer biology: a few that are important to cancer treatment (revisited). Semin Oncol 1979;6:506–514.

14. Furth J, Kahn MC. The transmission of leukemia of mice with a single cell. Am J Cancer 1937; 31:276–282.

15. Mendelsohn ML. The growth fraction: a new concept applied to tumors. Sci 1960;132:1496–1499.

16. Tannock IF. The relationship between cell proliferation and the vascular system in a transplanted mouse mammary tumor. Br J Cancer 1968;22:258–273.

17. Retsky MW, Swartzendruber DE, Bame PD, et al. Computer model challenges breast cancer treatment strategy. Cancer Invest 1994;12:559–567.

18. Norton L, Simon R. The Norton-Simon hypothesis revisited. Cancer Treat Rep 1986;70:163–169.

19. Dempsey JL, Seshadri RS, Morley AA. Increased mutation frequency following treatment with cancer chemotherapy. Cancer Res 1985;45:2873–2877.

20. Elmore E, Kakunaga T, Barrett JC. Comparison of spontaneous mutation rates of normal and chemically transformed human skin fibroblasts. Cancer Res 1983;43:1650–1655.

21. Albertini RJ, Castle KL, Borcherding WR. T-cell cloning to detect the mutant 6-thioguanine-resistant lymphocytes present in human peripheral blood. Proc Natl Acad Sci USA 1982;79:6617–6621.

22. Sanderson BJ, Morley AA. Mitogenic stimulation may induce an anti-mutagenic repair system in human lymphocytes. Mutagenesis 1986;1:131–133.

23. Warren ST, Schultz RA, Chang CC, et al. Elevated spontaneous mutation rate in Bloom syndrome fibroblasts. Proc Natl Acad Sci USA 1981; 78:3133–3137.

24. Harmon JM, Thompson EB. Isolation and characterization of dexamethasone-resistant mutants from human lymphoid cell line CEM-C7. Mol Cell Biol 1981; 1:512–521.

25. Seshadri R, Kutlaca RJ, Trainor K, et al. Mutation rate of normal and malignant human lymphocytes. Cancer Res 1987;15:407–409.

26. DeFazio A, Musgrove EA, Tattersall MH. Flow cytometric enumeration of drug-resistant tumor cells. Cancer Res 1988;48:6037–6043.

27. Weinberg RA. Tumor suppressor genes. Science 1991;254:1138–1146.

28. Kaden D, Gadi IK, Bardwell L, et al. Spontaneous mutation rates of tumorigenic and nontumorigenic Chinese hamster embryo fibroblast cell lines. Cancer Res 1989;9:3374–3379.

29. Bronner CE, Baker SM, Morrison PT, et al. Mutation in the DNA mismatch repair gene hMLH1 is associated with hereditary non-polyposis colon cancer. Nature 1994;368:258–261.

30. Parsons R, Li GM, Longley MJ, et al. Hypermutability and mismatch repair deficiency in RER tumor cells. Cell 1993;75:1227–1236.

31. Markowitz S, Wang J, Myeroff L, et al. Inactivation of the type II TGF-β receptor in colon cancer cells with microsatellite instability. Science 1995; 268:1336–1338.

32. Foulds L. The experimental study of tumor progression. A review. Cancer Res 1954;14:327–339.

33. Nowell PC. Chromosomal and molecular clues to tumor progression. Semin Oncol 1989;16:116–127.

34. Cairns J. Mutation selection and the natural history of cancer. Nature 1975;255:197–201.

35. Cifone MA, Fidler IJ. Increasing metastatic potential is associated with increasing genetic instability of clones isolated from murine neoplasms. Proc Natl Acad Sci USA 1981;78:6949–6952.

36. Smith ML, Chen IT, Zhan Q, et al. Interaction of the p53-regulated protein Gadd45 with proliferating cell nuclear antigen. Science 1994;266:1376–1380.

37. Fishel R, Lescoe MK, Rao MR, et al. The human mutator gene homolog MSH2 and its association with hereditary nonpolyposis colon cancer. Cell 1993; 75:1027–1038.

38. Luria SE, Delbrück M. Mutation of bacteria from virus sensitivity to virus resistance. Genetics 1943;28:491–511.

39. Koscielny S, Tubiana M, Le MG, et al. Breast cancer: relationship between the size of the primary tumour and the probability of metastatic dissemination, Br J Cancer 1984;49:709–715.

40. Fisher B, Slack NM, Bross IDJ. Cancer of the breast: size of neoplasm and prognosis. Cancer 1969; 24:1071–1080.

41. Goldie JH, Coldman AJ. A mathematical model for relating the drug sensitivity of tumors to their spontaneous mutation rate. Cancer Treat Rep 1979;63:1727–1733.

42. Mulkins MA, Heidelberger C. Biochemical characterization of fluoropyrimidine-resistant murine leukemia cell lines. Cancer Res 1982;42:965–973.

43. Ling V, Juranka PF, Endicott JA, et al. Multidrug resistance and p-glycoprotein expression. In: Woolley PW, Tew KD, eds. Mechanisms of drug resistance and neoplastic cells. New York: Academic Press, 1988.

44. Gerlach JH, Endicott JA, Juranka PF, et al. Homology between p-glycoprotein and a bacterial transport protein suggests a model for multidrug resistance. Nature 1986;324:485–488.

45. Fairchild CR, Ivy SP, Rushmore T, et al. Carcinogen induced mdr overexpression is associated with xenobiotic resistance in rat preneoplastic liver nodules and hepatocellular carcinomas. Proc Natl Acad Sci USA 1987;84:701:7705.

46. Chin KV, Ueda K, Pastan I, et al. Modulation of activity of the promoter of the human *MDR1* gene by Ras and p53. Science 1992;255:459–462.

47. Lai SL, Goldstein LJ, Gottesman MM, et al. MDR1 gene expression in lung cancer. J Natl Cancer Inst 1989;81:1144–1150.

48. Kohn KW, Pommier Y, Kerrigan D, et al. Topoisomerase II as a target of anticancer drug action in mammalian cells. NCI Monogr 1987;4:61–71.

49. Silber R, Liu LF, Israel M, et al. Metabolic activation of *N*-anthracyclines precedes their interaction with DNA topoisomerase II. NCI Monogr 1987;4:111–115.

50. Glisson BS, Sullivan DM, Gupta R, et al. Mediation of multi-drug resistance in a Chinese hamster ovary cell line by a mutant type of type II topoisomerase. NCI Monogr 1987;4:89–93.

51. Sullivan DM, Chow KC, Glisson BS et al. Role of proliferation in determining sensitivity to topoisomerase II active chemotherapy agents. NCI Monogr 1987;4:73–78.

52. Tan KB, Mattern MR, Boyce RA, et al. Elevated topoisomerase II activity and altered chromatin in nitrogen mustard resistant human cells. NCI Monogr 1987;4:95–98.

53. Potmesil M, Hsiang YH, Liu LF, et al. DNA topoisomerase II as a potential factor in drug resistance of human malignancies. NCI Monogr 1987;4:105–109.

54. Kerr JFR, Wyllie AH, Currie AR. A basic biological phenomenon with wide-ranging implications in tissue kinetics. Br J Cancer 1972;26:239–244.

55. Wyllie AH. Glucocorticoid induced thymocyte apoptosis is associated with endogenous endonuclease activation. Nature 1980;284:555–559.

56. Thompson CB. Apoptosis in the pathogenesis and treatment of disease. Science 1995;267:1456–1462.

57. Clarke AR, Pirdie CA, Harrison DJ, et al. Thymocyte apoptosis induced by p53-dependent and independent pathways. Nature 1993;362:849–852.

58. Yin XM, Oltvai ZN, Korsmeyer SJ. BH1 and BH2 domains of Bcl-2 are required for inhibition of apoptosis and heterodimerization with Bax. Nature 1994;369:321–323.

59. Miyashita T, Reed JC. Bcl-2 oncoprotein blocks chemotherapy induced apoptosis in a human leukemia cell line. Blood 1993;81:151–157.

60. Hryniuk WA, Figueredo A, Goodyear M. Applications of dose intensity to problems in chemotherapy of breast and colorectal cancer. Semin Oncol 1987; 14(Suppl 4):3–11.

61. Kemeny N, Schnwieder A. Regional treatment of hepatic metastases and hepatocellular carcinoma. Curr Probl Cancer 1989;13(4):197–284.

62. Howell SB. Intraperitoneal chemotherapy for ovarian carcinoma. J Clin Oncol 1988;6:1673–1675.

63. Alberts DS, Liu PY, Hannigan EV, et al. Phase III study of intraperitoneal cisplatin and intravenous cyclophosphamide versus intravenous cisplatin and intravenous cyclophosphamide in patients with optimal disease stage III ovarian cancer: a SWOG-GOG-ECOG intergroup study (INT 0051) (abstract 760). Proceedings of the annual meeting Am Soc Clin Oncol, 1995.

64. Alberts DS, Peng YM, Chen HS, et al. Effect of phenobarbital on plasma levels of cyclophosphamide and its metabolites in the mouse, Br J Cancer 1978; 38:316–324.

65. Cohen SC, Krigel RL. High dose therapy with stem cell infusion in lymphoma. Semin Oncol 1995; 22:218–229.

66. Crilley P, Goldstein LJ. Peripheral blood stem cell transplant in breast cancer. Semin Oncol 1995; 22:238–249.

67. Kotz KW, Schilder RJ. High dose chemotherapy and hematopoietic progenitor cell support for patients with epithelial ovarian cancer. Semin Oncol 1995;22:250–262.

68. Topolsky D, Biggs D. Transplantation in multiple myeloma. Semin Oncol 1995;22:230–237.

69. Verdonck LF, van Putten WL, Hagenbeek A, et al. Comparison of CHOP chemotherapy with autologous bone marrow transplantation for slowly responding patients with aggressive non-Hodgkin's lymphoma. N Engl J Med 1995;332:1045–1051.

70. Philip T, Guglielmi C, Chauvin F, et al. Autologous bone marrow transplantation versus conventional chemotherapy (DHAP) in relapsed non-Hodgkin's lymphoma: final analysis of the Parma randomized study (216 patients) (abstract 1220). Proceedings of the annual meeting, Am Soc Clin Oncol, 1995.

71. Gunduz N, Fisher B, Saffer EA. Effect of surgical removal on the growth and kinetics of residual tumor. Cancer Res 1979;39:3861–3865.

72. Nissen-Meyer R. One short chemotherapy course in primary breast cancer: 12 year follow-up in series 1 of the Scandinavian Adjuvant Chemotherapy Study Group. In: Jones SE, Salmon SE, eds. Adjuvant therapy of cancer II. New York: Grune & Stratton, 1979:207–213.

73. Heppner GH. Tumor cell societies. J Natl Cancer Inst 1989;81:648–649.

74. Stewart DJ, Evans WK. Non-chemotherapeutic agents that potentiate chemotherapy efficacy. Cancer Treat Rev 1989;16:1–40.

75. McClay EF, Mastrangelo MJ, Sprandio JD, et al. The importance of tamoxifen to a cisplatin-containing regimen in the treatment of metastatic melanoma. Cancer 1989;63:1292–1295.

76. Stein CA, Cheng YC. Antisense oligonucleotides as therapeutic agents: is the bullet really magical? Science 1993;261:1004–1012.

77. Wagner RW. Gene inhibition using antisense oligodeoxynucleotides. Nature 1994;372:333–335.

78. Choo Y, Sanchez-Gracia I, Klug A. In vivo repression by a site specific DNA-binding protein designed against an oncogene sequence. Nature 1994; 372:642–645.

79. Patel DJ. Marriage of convenience. Nature 1993; 365:490–492.

80. Egholm M, Buchardt O, Christensen L, et al. PNA hybridizes to complementary oligonucleotides obeying the Watson-Crick hydrogen bonding rules. Nature 1993;365:566–568.

81. Kohn NE, Mosser SD, deSolms SJ, et al. Selective inhibition of ras-dependent transformation by a farnesyltransferase inhibitor. Science 1993;260:1934–1937.

82. James GL, Goldstein JL, Brown MS, et al. Benzodiazepine peptidomimetics: potent inhibitors of Ras farnesylation in animal cells. Science 1993;260:1937–1942.

83. Nicolaou KC, Dai WM, Tsay SC, et al. Designed enediynes: a new class of DNA cleaving molecules with potent and selective anticancer activity. Science 1992;256:1172–1178.

84. Teicher BA, Herman TS, Holden SA, et al. Addition of misonidazole, etanidazole, or hyperthermia to treatment with Fluosol-DA/Carbinogen/Radiation. J Natl Cancer Inst 1989;81:929–934.

2

Antineoplastic Drug Development

Barbara A. Conley and David A. Van Echo

Although much progress has been made in the treatment of malignant disease with chemotherapy, there are still diseases for which no effective chemotherapy exists, and there are many initially responsive tumors that become resistant to previously effective therapy. In addition, as more is learned about the mechanisms of tumor resistance and factors influencing toxicity or response to chemotherapeutic agents in clinical use, there are additional reasons to learn to use these agents in the most rational and efficacious manner. Antineoplastic drug development is the process by which agents are discovered to have activity against neoplastic disease and are then evaluated for toxicity, activity, and efficacy. At some point, development also involves refinement in dosing strategies to compensate for patient factors such as age, altered hepatic or renal function, or interpatient variation in drug metabolism, excretion, or toxicity.

DRUG DISCOVERY

Discovery of agents that are active against malignant disease proceeds at a number of levels. The National Cancer Institute (NCI), the pharmaceutical industry, and individual researchers all contribute to this endeavor. Some drugs are designed and synthesized to have specific properties, such as inhibition of target enzymes. Others are similar in structure to known active drugs, but modification allows less toxicity or more activity. A great number of compounds are isolated from natural sources. In all, over 10,000 new potential anticancer drugs are screened for antitumor activity each year. Only a small fraction of these ever become useful clinically. Each drug whose development is spon-sored by the NCI must pass through a "decision network" prior to entering general clinical use. At each decision point (screening, animal toxicology, formulation, early clinical trials) data are presented to a committee, and the decision is made whether to continue with development of the particular drug or to "drop" it from future development.

SCREENING

To conserve financial, animal, and clinical resources, some sort of screening mechanism is necessary to allow only the most promising agents to be developed further. The selection of a screening model is important because an inadequate model could potentially lead to discarding a promising drug. From 1975 to 1985, the initial screen used by the NCI was a murine leukemia model (P388), and this model is still used as an initial screen by many pharmaceutical companies. Agents with significant activity in P388 leukemia are then tested against a panel of other human and animal tumors implanted into mice (1). Agents with broad activity in these initial screens then proceed to preclinical and clinical evaluation.

Recently, the NCI has instituted a new in vitro screen, which employs established human tumor cell lines (1). This effort was made possible by technical advances in cell culture, in the assay of cell viability, and in computer software that allows rapid screening of compounds against many tumor cell lines. This method also has the capability of comparing the activity of new agents with that of agents that have known activity. Agents that are active in the in vitro screen are then tested in vivo in animals implanted with human tumor cell lines. It is thus not necessary to test in vivo all the tumor types used in the in vitro screen; rather, only tumors found sensitive to the new drug in vitro will be used in the in vivo screen. This screen may be less sensitive for cytostatic drugs or differentiation inducers than for cytocidal drugs. Thus, even better initial screening methods are continually being sought (2).

New potential anticancer drugs are tested in animals bearing chemically induced, spontaneous, or implanted animal or human tumors. This type of investigation gives some idea of whether the doses necessary for antitumor activity can be tolerated by animals. Activity can be measured as a decrease in tumor growth or actual tumor size or as an increase in life span of tumor-bearing animals treated with the new agent, compared with the same measures performed in tumor-bearing animals who are not exposed to the new agent. The in vivo screens currently in use by the NCI differ from previous screens. Instead of a rigid protocol (i.e., single-dose or daily $\times$ 5 schedules) into which all new agents are fit, the newer studies modify protocols on the basis of preclinical studies to obtain the most data. New drugs are tested in athymic nude mice bearing fully established human tumors of interest. This is a more stringent measure of drug activity than measurement of growth inhibition or prolongation of life span measured when drug and tumor are injected simultaneously, for example.

ANIMAL TOXICOLOGY

Pharmacologic and toxicologic studies are performed in animals either simultaneously, with evaluation of in vivo efficacy, or after a drug shows promise in vitro and in vivo. Usually at least two species are tested. Monkeys, mice, rats, dogs, hamsters, or rabbits have been used in the past. Although fairly good correlations exist between doses that are toxic in animals and those that are toxic in humans, it is not yet possible to predict with great accuracy an initial human dose from data in only one species. Various toxic endpoints are described in these studies. Because lethality was considered to be the least variable of these endpoints, animal toxicology studies previously defined doses that were lethal in a certain percentage of the animals who received the same dose. Accordingly, the dose that was lethal to 10% of the animals given that dose was called the LD_{10}, and the dose lethal to 50% of the animals was called the LD_{50}, respectively.

Presently, the NCI uses a different study design to assess animal toxicity. A new drug is given in escalating doses to cohorts of mice. Instead of lethality, the endpoint currently sought is the dose that produces severe reversible toxicity (the maximum tolerable dose) for each schedule tested. These doses are then tested in dogs or rats to define interspecies variability for toxicity. If no toxicity is seen or it is different for the second species, then the maximum tolerable dose in the second species is defined. These studies are accompanied by pharmacokinetic measurements. This approach has resulted in a considerable savings in animal resources and in more useful dosing information prior to human clinical trials.

Pharmacokinetics are performed in animals to characterize the drug's absorption, bioavailability (if oral), clearance, half-life, metabolism, and excretion. These studies are generally done in more than one species as well, since there may be interspecies variation in absorption, excretion, metabolism, etc. If the animal toxicologic and pharmacokinetic studies are performed and analyzed prior to initiation of clinical trials in humans, they may be used to arrive at a logical schedule and initial dose for humans. At present, this initial dose is usually a fraction of either the lowest dose causing any toxicity in any species or a fraction (one-tenth or less) of the LD_{10} in the most sensitive species tested. Translating animal data to a dose appropriately close to the highest tolerable dose in humans involves upscaling doses from animal to humans and estimating toxicity from animal to humans. The area under the curve (AUC) of plasma drug concentration versus time at the maximum tolerable dose in animals is often similar to the AUC at the maximum tolerable dose in humans, but this is not always the case. The fundamental problem is to find an initial dose that will not cause prohibitive toxicity but yet will be close enough to the eventually recommended human dose so that as few patients as possible are treated at totally ineffective doses. This is an area of ongoing research, and the interested reader is referred to several articles dealing with this subject (3–12).

CLINICAL TRIALS

A drug that shows promising activity and acceptable toxicity in the preclinical screens and can be formulated for dosing in humans may then be chosen for clinical trial. The initial clinical evaluation of a drug proceeds in three steps, or phases. Phase I trials are concerned with the characterization of toxicity and with finding a tolerable dose for future trials. In addition, this phase may discover tumor types for which the drug has exceptional activity, as was the case for cisplatin and testicular cancer. Phase II trials evaluate the drug in specific tumor types for activity and some estimate of the magnitude of activity. Phase III trials compare the new treatment directly with standard therapy and evaluate efficacy. As with any experimental procedure, conduct of a clinical trial requires formulation of a hypothesis, design of methods to test the hypothesis, and evaluation of results.

Phase I Trials

Although therapeutic intent is present, phase I trials are designed to evaluate drug toxicity relative to dose. Although preclinical studies have shown a particular drug to be active in vitro against certain tumor types, this does not mean the drug will be active in patients. Thus, patients are chosen for phase I only if no other effective standard therapy is available for their tumor type, or, in other words, a new agent has as much chance of being active as any other treatment. Likewise, although animal toxicity studies may predict that the same toxicities will be seen in patients, this is not always the case. Eligibility requirements for phase I trials usually include the following: (a) a performance status such that patients are able to be out of bed and active at least half of the day (Eastern Cooperative Oncology Group ≤ 2 or Karnofsky performance status $\geq 60\%$) (13, 14); (b) normal hepatic, renal, and hematopoietic function; (c) no chemotherapy or radiation therapy for a specified time prior to receiving the new drug; (d) no uncontrolled concurrent medical illness; and (e) written informed consent. As stated above, the starting dose is defined as a fraction of the LD_{10} in the most sensitive animal species or by animal pharmacokinetic and toxicity studies.

Usually, dose escalation is planned in steps (modified Fibonacci scheme), such that the initial escalations represent a large percentage of the initial or previous dose, whereas subsequent escalations represent progressively smaller percentages of the previous dose. An example of a phase I dose escalation scheme is shown in Table 2.1. Usually three patients are treated at each dose level until significant toxicity is encountered. When a predefined proportion of the patients entered at a particular dose experience un-

Table 2.1 Example of Modified Fibonacci Search Scheme

Percentage Increase	Dose (mg/m²)	Anticipated No. of Patients
Starting dose	18	3
100	36	3
67	60	3
50	90	3
33.3	120	3
25	150	3
25	190	3
25	235	3

acceptable toxicity, that dose is defined as the maximum tolerable dose (MTD) *at that particular schedule*. Thus, an MTD is defined for each administration schedule of interest. Usually, additional patients are entered on the next lower dose in the escalation scheme, to evaluate toxicity further and arrive at a recommended dose for phase II trials. A dose approximately 10 to 25% less than the MTD is usually recommended for phase II trials. It should be emphasized that the MTD is currently defined in a small number of patients and thus does not give a good indication of inter- and intrapatient variability in pharmacokinetics or in response. Other escalation schemes have been proposed that may improve on the present study design, particularly the one proposed by Collins et al. (9), which would approach the MTD in humans as an area under the concentration-time curve (AUC) equivalent to the AUC obtained at the MTD for mice. For many drugs presently in use, this method would have eliminated some dose levels required by Fibonacci escalation, thus saving development time and reducing the number of patients treated at dose levels too low to have therapeutic value. Phase I drugs for cancer, unlike new drugs for other illnesses, are given to patients with cancer, as opposed to "normal" volunteers. This eliminates one source of variability, but other sources of interpatient (and intrapatient) variability exist. Sheiner et al. (15) have proposed an escalation scheme in which each patient can be given his or her own maximum tolerable dose, a method known as adaptive control.

Phase II Trials

After evaluation of phase I trials, which may include several schedules performed at different institutions, a decision is made whether to pursue phase II trials. This decision depends on the promise of the agent in preclinical trials and the toxicity encountered in phase I trials. The decision should not, however, be influenced by lack of antitumor activity in phase I trials. Many patients in phase I trials have extensive tumor burdens, and many have received previous therapy with one or several chemotherapeutic drugs and/or radiation therapy. Because of these factors, it is unusual for patients to respond to any regimen, and it is unusual for a new chemotherapeutic agent to show more than a 5 to 6% response rate in a phase I trial, even when it is found to be active subsequently.

The choice of tumor types against which the drug will be tested in phase II is empiric and may be guided by, but does not depend entirely on, which tumors have shown responses in previous preclinical and clinical trials. The goal of phase II trials is to discover tumor types for which the drug has some activity and to estimate the magnitude of that activity. Therefore, enough patients must be included in each trial so that one can confidently accept or reject the null hypothesis (i.e., that the drug has no activity). This requires a specification of a confidence level (90 to 95%) that the drug is not more effective than specified in producing responses. For example, if one wanted to know with 95% confidence that a drug is not more than 20% effective against a certain tumor type, one would need to enter 14 patients in the study without observing a single response (16). If a response was observed in the first 14 patients, then more patients would need to be entered to define the activity of the drug against that particular tumor. In a phase II trial, it is necessary to specify what degree of activity is of interest. For many epithelial tumors, such as colon carcinoma or non-small-cell lung cancer, an activity of 20% would be of interest. However, for tumors such as lymphomas or leukemias, where active single agents already exist, a drug may not be of interest unless it demonstrated an activity of 50% or greater. Statistical theory can provide an estimate of the minimum number of patients needed to demonstrate whether or not a drug can be expected to have the desired activity (17).

Once the number of patients needed has been specified, eligibility requirements need to be formulated. In contrast to patients entered on a phase I trial, phase II patients usually may not have received prior chemotherapy (except possibly adjuvant therapy). In addition, performance status requirements are usually more strict (ECOG performance status, 0 or 1; Karnofsky performance status ≥80%). At present, all patients are given the dose recommended from the phase I trials, although, as stated above, other study designs could also be considered.

Because the demonstration of activity is a major goal of the phase II trial, patients are required to have measurable disease. This usually means that the tumor(s) can be measured accurately in at least two dimensions. Patients whose disease is present in bone marrow, in bones, or in effusions or ascites alone do not have measurable disease as defined above and should not be included in phase II trials. Activity is defined precisely as complete response, partial response, or progression after a specified period of time. Complete response requires the disappearance of all evidence of disease and no new appearance of disease for a specified interval, usually 4 weeks. Partial response requires a reduction by at least 50% in the sum of the products of the two longest diameters of all lesions, maintained for at least one course of therapy, and no new appearance of disease. Minimal response or stable disease are categories sometimes reported but are inaccurate endpoints and generally should not be considered responses. Progression refers to the growth of disease while receiving chemotherapy. This is generally present if the sum of the products of the two longest diameters of all previously measured lesions increases by at least 25% or if new malignant lesions develop while the patient is on study.

In addition to clarifying the activity of an agent, one goal of phase II trials is to refine the toxicity data and dosing strategy arrived at in phase I trials and to evaluate cumulative toxicity.

Phase III Trials

Phase III studies are performed with agents that show significant activity in phase II trials. Here patients are usually randomized to receive a standard (control) treatment or the new treatment. Randomization tends to produce comparable study groups. Patients generally have not received previous treatment and should be stratified by any patient characteristics that are thought to influence response or survival, such as age, organ function, tumor characteristics, or extent of disease (16).

It is important that phase III trials have sufficient power to detect a difference between treatment groups if a difference exists. Therefore, the calculation of sample size is an essential part of the design of any phase III trial. Because the differences expected between treatment groups are usually fairly small, large numbers of patients are generally needed to demonstrate these differences. For this reason, phase III trials are probably best accomplished by large cooperative groups.

In addition to comparison of activity of two or more agents or combinations of agents, phase III trials increasingly are including quality-of-life analyses in their study designs. This is an important point, since efficacy may include an assessment of the cost (personal and financial) as well as the benefit of therapy.

PHARMACOKINETICS AND PHARMACODYNAMICS

Most phase I trials sponsored by the NCI and many studies sponsored by private concerns also define the pharmacokinetics of the drug under study. In other classes of drugs, phase I studies and pharmacokinetics are performed in normal volunteers. For antineoplastic drugs, phase I trials and pharmacokinetics are performed in patients with malignancy. Pharmacokinetic analysis defines the time course of the drug in the body. These studies characterize and model the absorption, distribution, and elimination and/or metabolism of the new agent. In addition, correlation of pharmacokinetic parameters with patient characteristics such as albumin, creatinine clearance, age, and hepatic function allows prediction of drug behavior in patients other than those of the original phase I group.

Pharmacodynamics refers to the action of the drug on the body and includes both toxic and therapeutic effects. In many classes of drugs, the relationship between some measure of drug exposure (peak plasma drug concentration, or area under the concentration $\times$ time curve) and the toxic or therapeutic effects of a drug are well defined. For example, it is known that there is a plasma concentration of theophylline below which most patients will not show any therapeutic response. It is also known that there is a plasma concentration of this drug above which a significant proportion of patients manifest toxicity due to the drug. Because a relatively fast and reliable assay is available for measuring theophylline in plasma and a therapeutic but non-toxic range of plasma concentrations can be specified, one can maintain each patient at his or her theoretically optimal dose of the theophylline. This strategy has not been consistently applied

to antineoplastic drugs, in part due to the lack, until recently, of plasma assays that are relatively simple and can be performed in a short period of time. In addition, previous phase I and II trials rarely looked for correlations between drug exposure (as opposed to dose) and toxic or therapeutic effects. However, few classes of drugs possess a narrower range between therapeutic and toxic doses than do antineoplastic drugs. Effects (toxic or therapeutic) of antineoplastic drugs often occur days to weeks after the drug has been given. This property and patient variability in pharmacokinetics (and even in pharmacodynamics) can make dosing a very inaccurate undertaking. Recently, phase I and II studies have documented relationships between drug exposure and toxicity. For example, severe and unacceptable toxicity of high-dose methotrexate has been related to the plasma concentration and time of exposure to this agent (18). Thrombocytopenia induced by the experimental differentiating agent HMBA was found to be related to the AUC (19). The grade of the most serious toxicity has also been related to the AUC for 5-fluorouracil given as a continuous infusion (20). The time above a threshold plasma concentration of paclitaxel has also been related to myelosuppression (21). Therapeutic effects have also been related to measures of drug exposure. For example, Evans et al. demonstrated a correlation between methotrexate AUC and response in children with acute lymphocytic leukemia (22).

Pharmacokinetic studies early in the clinical development of a drug have shown wide variability between patients but usually consistency in the same patient receiving multiple courses. Likewise, the response to the drug (toxic and therapeutic) has also been shown to have wide interpatient variability (23). Since dosing recommendations are heavily influenced by patients who are most sensitive to the drug, most patients may receive less drug than they can tolerate. If dose intensity is important, these patients may have less chance to respond than they would have if they could receive a larger dose.

Population pharmacokinetics defines patient pharmacokinetic parameters as means and variances (and covariances) in a population. Methods exist for modifying initial dosing by measuring plasma drug levels and adjusting each patient's dose to achieve a target (e.g., AUC or peak plasma concentration) defined in a similar population to achieve the desired result (increased efficacy and/or lower toxicity). To make dosage adjustment feasible in a large number of patients, methods need to be developed for reliably estimating drug exposure with only a few plasma samples, rather than the 20 to 30 usually obtained for each patient in a phase I trial. Such methods, called "optimal" or "limited" sampling strategies, are currently being evaluated (24–26).

CHEMOPREVENTION

Chemoprevention is the administration of an agent to prevent the onset of a malignancy. Candidate agents for chemoprevention are identified in several ways. Often, epidemiologic studies identify certain dietary components that may be preventive agents. Analysis of the diet can identify particular compounds that may have activity. Testing putative chemopreventive agents may take several forms. In vitro assays may test the ability of an agent to inhibit viral transformation or to affect certain cellular functions. Animal models have been developed in which cancer either develops spontaneously at an increased rate, or in which cancer can be induced by exposure to known carcinogens. Similar to the method used in development of antineoplastic agents, these preclinical studies can estimate appropriate exposures and toxicities prior to clinical trials. Clinical trials of cancer preventive agents differ substantially from clinical trials of antineoplastic agents, in that preventive agents must have little or no toxicity associated with them. These agents are given to people who are not ill at present and likely will have to be administered over a long period of time. In addition, some measure of efficacy other than development of frank malignancy is desirable, to decrease the time and expense involved in prevention trials. Therefore, these trials are often performed in patient populations with recognized premalignant lesions. Tissue biopsies or other putative markers indicating the state of the tissue relative to tissue that is frankly malignant are often followed. Chemoprevention is an active area of clinical research at present, and the interested reader is referred to several recently published reviews (27–29).

FUTURE DIRECTIONS

It is clear that new drugs will continue to be needed for cancer therapy. In addition, many exciting contributions have been, and probably will continue to be, made by biologic response modifiers. Targeted antibodies and gene therapy have also begun to be evaluated clinically.

Work continues to be done to find the most appropriate screening model for antitumor agents. New methods of translating animal dosing and toxicity data and better escalation schema are needed so that as few patients as possible receive doses that are far below those found to be effective, without creating undue toxicity. More recent trials are relating toxicity and efficacy to measures of drug exposure, and some are proposing individualized doses that are adjusted periodically to achieve a target (adaptive control).

Because technology is constantly expanding, we should not assume a drug is developed after it is in clinical use. Although the present development process is very time consuming, sometimes taking 10 years or more to complete, it is necessary to reevaluate constantly our clinical use of antineoplastic drugs in light of current knowledge. Thus 5-fluorouracil, "developed" over 30 years ago, needs to be reevaluated because today it is used in different regimens and with different biochemical response modifiers (methotrexate, leucovorin) as well as with cytotoxicity- and immune-modulating agents such as dipyridamole, interferons, and levamisole. Likewise, the anthracyclines, developed prior to current methods, are being evaluated with respect to rational dosing in patients with hepatic dysfunction, and with other agents that may decrease the cardiac toxicity associated with this class of agents. Oncology is a medical specialty closely tied to basic research. Future drug development will draw on many disciplines as our understanding of the cell biology of cancer increases. Exciting developments in many fields may be expected to contribute to the optimal medical management of the patient with malignancy.

References

1. Boyd MR. Status of the NCI preclinical antitumor drug discovery screen. PPO Updates 1989;3(10):1–12.

2. Scheithauer W, Clark GM, Moyer MP, et al. New screening system for selection of anticancer drugs for treatment of human colorectal cancer. Cancer Res 1986;46:2703–2708.

3. Freireich EJ, Gehan EA, Rall DP, et al. Quantitative comparison of toxicity of anticancer agents in mouse, rat, hamster, dog, monkey and man. Cancer Chemother Rep 1966;50:219–244.

4. Dedrick RL, Bischoff KB, Zaharko DS. Interspecies correlation of plasma concentration history of methotrexate. Cancer Chemother Rep 1970;54:95–101.

5. Boxenbaum H. Interspecies scaling, allometry, physiologic time, and the ground plan of pharmacokinetics. J Pharmacokinet Biopharm 1982;10:201–227.

6. Goldsmith MA, Slavik M, Carter SK. Quantitative prediction of drug toxicity in humans from toxicology in small and large animals. Cancer Res 1975; 35:1354–1364.

7. Guarino AM, Rosencweig M, Kline I, et al. Adequacies and inadequacies in assessing murine toxicity data with antineoplastic agents. Cancer Res 1979; 39:2204–2210.

8. Mordenti J. Man versus beast: pharmacokinetic scaling in mammals. J Pharm Sci 1986;75:1028–1040.

9. Collins JM, Zaharko DS, Dedrick RL, et al. Potential roles for preclinical pharmacology in phase I trials. Cancer Treat Rep 1986;70:73–80.

10. Scheithauer W, Clark GM, Salmon SE, Darda W, Shoemaker RH, Von Hoff DD. Model for estimation of clinically achievable plasma concentrations for investigational anticancer drugs in man. Cancer Treat Rep 1986;70(12):1379–1382.

11. Davis LE, Alberts DS, Plezia PM, Roe DJ, Griswold DP. Predictive model for plasma concentration-versus-time profiles of investigational anticancer drugs in patients. J Natl Cancer Inst 1988;80(11):815–819.

12. Graham MA, Kaye SB. New approaches in preclinical and clinical pharmacokinetics. Cancer Surv 1993;17:27–49.

13. Karnofsky DA, Burchenal JH. The clinical evaluation of chemotherapeutic agents in cancer. In: Macleod CM, ed. Evaluation of chemotherapeutic agents. New York: Columbia University Press, 1949:191–205.

14. Zubrod GC, Schneiderman M, Frei E III, et al. Appraisal of methods for the study of chemotherapy of cancer in man: comparative therapeutic trial of nitrogen mustard and triethylene thiophosphoramide. J Chronic Dis 1960;11:7–33.

15. Sheiner LB, Beal SL, Sambol NC. Study designs for dose-ranging. Clin Pharmacol Ther 46:63–77.

16. Wittes RE, Leventhal BG, eds. Research methods in clinical oncology. New York: Raven Press, 1988.

17. Snedecor GW, Cochran WG, eds. Statistical methods. 7th ed. Ames, IA: Iowa State University Press, 1980.

18. Favre R, Monjavel S, Alfonse M, et al. High dose methotrexate: a clinical and pharmacokinetic evaluation; treatment of advanced squamous cell carcinoma of the head and neck using a prospective mathematical model and pharmacokinetic surveillance. Cancer Chemother Pharmacol 1982;9:156–160.

19. Egorin MS, Sigman LM, Van Echo DA, Forrest A, Whitacre MY, Aisner J. Phase I clinical and pharmacokinetic study of hexamethylene bisacetamide (NSC 95580) administered as a five-day continuous infusion. Cancer Res 1987;49:617–623.

20. Trump D, Tutsch K, Willson J, Remick S, Egorin M. Pharmacodynamic and pharmacokinetic analysis of 5FU during 3 day continuous infusion (c.i.) with and without dipyridamole (Dp) (abstract). Proc Am Soc Clin Oncol 1989;8:66.

21. Giani L, Kearns CM, Giani A, et al. Nonlinear pharmacokinetics and metabolism of paclitaxel and its pharmacokinetic/pharmacodynamic relationships in humans. J Clin Oncol 1995;13:180–190.

22. Evans WE, Crom WR, Abromowitch M, et al. Clinical pharmacodynamics of high-dose methotrexate in acute lymphocytic leukemia: identification of a relationship between concentration and effect. N Engl J Med 1986;314:471–476.

23. Ratain MJ, Schilsky RL, Choi KE. Adaptive control of etoposide dosing: impact of interpatient pharmacodynamic variability. Clin Pharmacol Ther 1989; 45:226–233.

24. D'Argenio DZ. Optimal sampling time for pharmacokinetic experiments. J Pharmacokinet Biopharm 1981;9:739–755.

25. Ratain MJ, Vogelzang NJ. A limited sampling model for vinblastine pharmacokinetics. Cancer Treat Rep 1987;71:935–939.

26. Egorin MJ, Forrest A, Belani CP, Ratain MJ, Abrams JS, Van Echo DA. A limited sampling strategy for cyclophosphamide pharmacokinetics. Cancer Res 1989;49:3129–3133.

27. Sharma S, Stutzman JD, Kelloff GJ, Steele VE. Screening of potential chemopreventive agents using biochemical markers of carcinogenesis. Cancer Res 1994;54:5848–5855.

28. Boone CW, Steele VE, Kelloff GJ. Screening for chemopreventive (anticarcinogenic) compounds in rodents. Mutat Res 1992;267:251–255.

29. Kelloff GJ, Boone CW, Crowell JA, Steele VE, Lubet R, Sigman CC. Chemopreventive drug development: perspectives and progress (review with 226 refs). Cancer Epidemiol Biomarkers Prevention 1994; 3:85–98.

3
Principles of Pharmacology

Antonius A. Miller, Mark J. Ratain, and Richard L. Schilsky

The effective use of cancer chemotherapy benefits from a comprehensive understanding of the principles of pharmacology and tumor biology along with detailed knowledge of the natural history of the disease being treated and insight by the physician into the goals and expectations of the patient and family. In clinical practice, the selection of a particular chemotherapy program depends on many factors. These include clinical experience, an understanding of the pharmacology of the drugs to be used, the potential for drug interactions, the likelihood of drug-resistant cells in the tumor, the physiologic status of the patient, and the presence of sanctuary sites or other unusual characteristics of the tumor that may influence the dose, schedule, or route of administration of a particular drug. Of great importance is the recognition of those factors that may result in diminished antitumor activity (e.g., poor absorption of orally administered drugs) or excessive toxicity (e.g., abnormal renal function in a patient receiving methotrexate) in individual patients. This chapter reviews the principles of pharmacology as they apply to antineoplastic drugs and illustrates how an understanding of these principles can lead to an improvement in the therapeutic index of cancer chemotherapy.

GENERAL MECHANISMS OF DRUG ACTION

Membrane Transport

The initial requirement for drug action is adequate drug delivery to the target site (Fig. 3.1). This depends largely on blood flow in the tumor bed and the diffusion characteristics of the drug in tissue but may also be influenced by the extent of plasma protein binding and, for orally administered drugs, by absorption and first-pass metabolism in the liver. To produce cytotoxicity, most anticancer drugs require uptake into the cell. A notable exception is L-asparaginase, a bacterial enzyme that inhibits cell growth by depletion of circulating L-asparagine.

A number of mechanisms exist for the passage of drugs across the plasma membrane, including passive diffusion, facilitated diffusion, and active transport systems (1). Passive diffusion of drugs through the lipid bilayer structure of the plasma membrane is a function of the size and lipid solubility of the drug molecule. If the extracellular drug concentration is constant, then drug accumulation by the cell will continue until the rate of drug uptake from the extracellular space is equal to the rate of drug exit from the cell. At this point, a dynamic equilibrium is reached, and intracellular and extracellular drug levels are equal. As drug is cleared from the extracellular space, intracellular drug levels will decline if the drug is not bound or metabolized intracellularly. An important feature of the passive diffusion process is that it does not saturate (Fig. 3.2). That is, as the extracellular drug concentration increases, influx into the cell increases proportionally, and high intracellular drug levels can be achieved. Passive diffusion, however, is a highly inefficient and nonspecific process, although it may be particularly important when carrier-mediated processes are lost or nonfunctional, such as occurs in some cases of methotrexate resistance.

The passage of physiologically important hydrophilic compounds across the plasma membrane is usually mediated by a specific receptor or carrier in the plasma membrane that facilitates the translocation of the substance into or out of the cell. Carrier-mediated transport systems are distinguished from passive diffusion by having a high degree of specificity and by being saturable at high extracellular drug concentrations owing to the presence of a finite number of

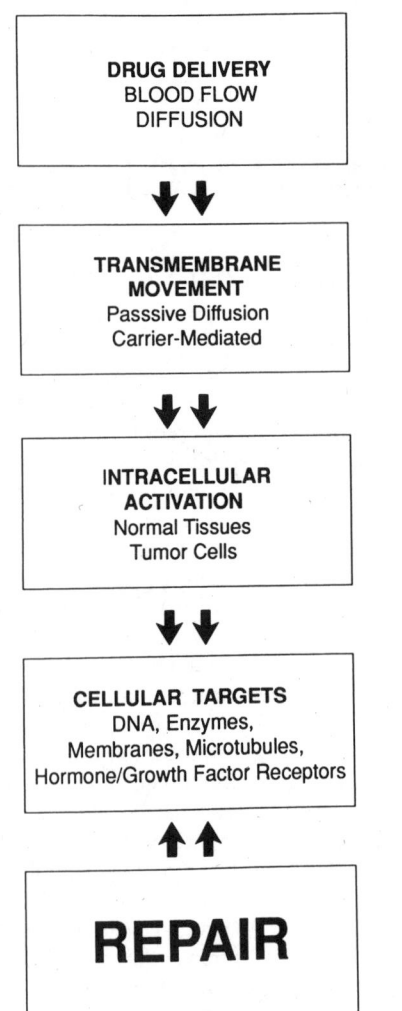

Figure 3.1.   Essential steps in drug action.

pling of carrier-mediated transport to an energy-generating reaction, usually hydrolysis of adenosine triphosphate (ATP).

Many antineoplastic drugs, particularly those that are structural analogues of natural compounds, gain entry into the cell by carrier-mediated mechanisms. Nucleosides such as cytosine arabinoside are transported by facilitated diffusion (2, 3), and methotrexate transport is an active energy-dependent carrier-mediated process (4). L-Phenylalanine mustard utilizes at least two amino acid transport systems, and its influx can be inhibited by the amino acid substrates specific for these transport carriers (5).

The importance of transmembrane movement of a drug to its pharmacologic effect depends on several factors, including the rate of drug delivery to the tissue, the affinity of the transport process, and the nature of the intracellular biochemical events required for drug action. Although membrane transport can be the rate-limiting event in drug action because it limits the rate at which the drug gains access to intracellular targets, this is not always the case. If drug delivery to a cell is slow relative to the rate of membrane transport, then the drug effect will be limited primarily by extracellular concentration, i.e., blood flow and diffusion of the drug. Similarly, if a drug requires intracellular activation—for example, phosphorylation—before it can exert a cytotoxic effect, then the rate-limiting step in drug action may be activation, rather than transport, if the rate of activation is slow relative to the rate of influx into the cell. Finally, it is important to remember that membrane transport is frequently bidirectional, with the final drug concentration in the cell representing the balance between drug influx and drug efflux. These processes may utilize different carrier systems and operate at different rates. While many efflux systems have not been carefully defined, one that appears to have great importance in cancer chemotherapy is the P-glycoprotein system that mediates multidrug resistance (6).

Intracellular Activation

Many anticancer drugs require activation intracellularly before they are able to exert a cytotoxic effect (Table 3.1). The activation process may occur by chemical or enzymatic reactions in either normal or tumor tissues. Cisplatin, for example, undergoes a chemical reaction with water molecules intracellularly, resulting in the generation of a positively charged aquated species

receptor molecules within the membrane. Once all carrier sites become occupied, further increases in extracellular drug concentration will not produce further increments in drug influx, unless a component of passive diffusion comes into play. The affinity of the carrier for the substrate can be estimated from the K_m, the drug concentration required to achieve one-half maximal transport. The lower the K_m, the higher the carrier affinity.

While all carrier-mediated systems enhance the rate of influx into the cell, not all carriers are able to translocate compounds against electrochemical forces and to ultimately develop gradients such that the intracellular concentration exceeds the extracellular drug level. To do so requires the expenditure of energy and the cou-

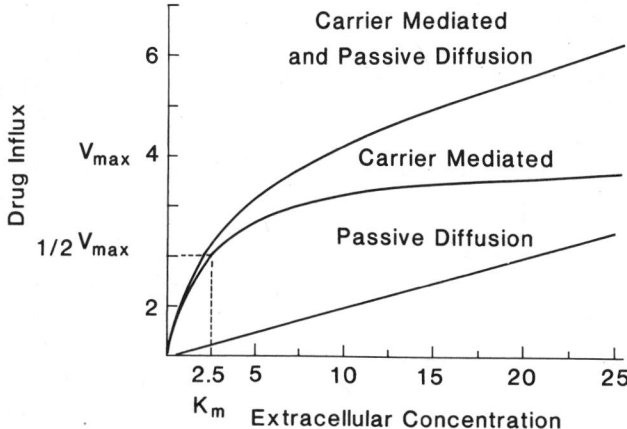

Figure 3.2.   Relationship between drug influx and extracellular concentration. The *lower line* illustrates the linear relationship for a passive diffusion process that does not saturate. For carrier-mediated processes, initial influx is rapid; K_m is equal to the extracellular concentration at which the influx rate is 1/2 maximal. Saturation occurs at high extracellular concentrations. For transport processes with a component of carrier-mediated influx and passive diffusion, the diffusion process dominates influx once saturation of the carrier occurs.

Table 3.1. Intracellular Activation of Anticancer Drugs

Drug	Activation Reaction	Site of Activation
Antimetabolites		
Methotrexate	Polyglutamation	Tumor cells
5-Fluorouracil	Phosphorylation	Tumor cells
Cytosine arabinoside	Phosphorylation	Tumor cells
6-Thioguanine	Phosphorylation	Tumor cells
6-Mercaptopurine	Phosphorylation	Tumor cells
Alkylating Agents		
Cisplatin	Aquation	Tumor cells
Cyclophosphamide	Enzymatic cleavage	Liver

that attacks nucleophilic sites on DNA (7). The activation of cyclophosphamide is mediated by hepatic microsomal enzymes with the release of active alkylating species into the systemic circulation (8).

Intracellular activation by tumor cells is a critical determinant of effect for virtually all antimetabolites. Cytosine arabinoside, 5-fluorouracil, and the purine antimetabolites (6-mercaptopurine and 6-thioguanine) all require phosphorylation to active nucleotide forms before they are able to exert a cytotoxic effect. Although methotrexate is an effective enzyme inhibitor in its native form, conversion of the drug to polyglutamate metabolites intracellularly significantly increases its potency and fa-

cilitates its binding to a number of enzymatic sites (9, 10).

The rate of formation of the activated drug species in the cell depends on a number of variables: the rate of transmembrane influx of the drug, the amount and affinity of the activating enzyme(s) in the cell, the amount and relative affinity of the naturally occurring enzyme substrates, and the rate of degradation of the activated drug by catabolic enzymes. For most antimetabolites, membrane transport is rapid relative to enzymatic activation and is therefore not rate limiting. Once inside the cell, antimetabolites must compete with the natural enzyme substrates for binding and activation, although pharmacologic concentrations of administered drugs (often in the range of 1 μM to 1 mM) frequently are far greater than the concentrations of their physiologic counterparts (1 nM to 1 μM), resulting in a competitive advantage for the drug. Finally, the activated drug is then a substrate for catabolic enzymes in the cell that tend to degrade the drug back to the parent compound or to an inactive metabolite. The concentration of active cytotoxic species in the cell is the result of all these processes. An excellent example is the pyrimidine nucleoside analogue, cytosine arabinoside (ara-C). Ara-C enters cells by a process of facilitated diffusion and is then metabolized in three successive phosphorylation reactions to the active triphosphate derivative, ara-CTP (Fig. 3.3). The first activating enzyme, deoxycytidine kinase, is found in lowest concen-

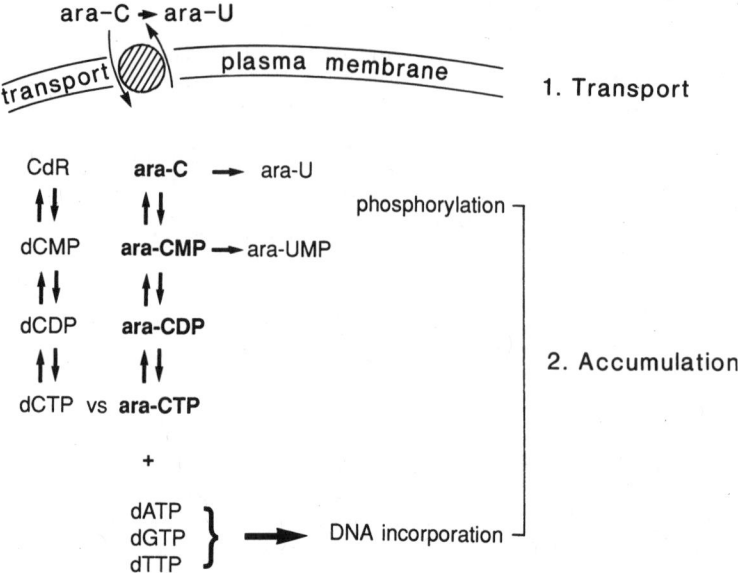

Figure 3.3.   Uptake and metabolism of cytosine arabinoside. Competition occurs between ara-C and the naturally occurring nucleotides at every enzymatic step. The rate-limiting step for drug activation is conversion of ara-C to ara-CMP by deoxycytidine kinase.

tration in cells and is believed to be the rate-limiting step in drug activation. Throughout the activation process, ara-C competes with endogenous substrates for enzyme binding. In the case of deoxycytidine kinase, the affinity for ara-C (K_m = 20 μM) is lower than that for the natural substrate, deoxycytidine (K_m = 7.8 μM) (11). However, the enzyme is strongly inhibited by dCTP but weakly inhibited by ara-CTP, allowing accumulation of ara-CTP to higher concentrations (12). Opposing the activation of ara-C are two deaminases, cytidine deaminase and dCMP deaminase, which convert ara-C and ara-CMP, respectively, to inactive uracil derivatives. The balance of these processes is crucial in determining the cytotoxicity of ara-C. Loss or diminished affinity of an activating enzyme may be responsible for drug resistance, as may enhanced activity of a catabolic enzyme.

Drug Interaction with Intracellular Targets

While anticancer drugs have traditionally been classified on the basis of their mechanism of action or their origins, they can also be grouped on the basis of the target of drug action. There are essentially five potential targets of drug action: nucleic acids, enzymes, membranes, microtubules, and hormone/growth factor re-

ceptors. When nucleic acids are the targets, it is generally DNA rather than RNA binding that is presumed to cause cell death. There are several mechanisms by which drugs can bind DNA, the best understood being alkylation of nucleophilic sites within the double helix. Most alkylating agents have two moieties capable of developing a charged carbon that binds covalently to negatively charged sites on DNA such as the O6 or N7 positions of guanine. Cross-linking of the two strands of DNA by the bifunctional alkylating agent prevents the use of that DNA as a template for further DNA synthesis (13, 14).

A second mechanism of drug binding to nucleic acids is intercalation, the insertion of a planar ring structure between two adjacent nucleotide bases of DNA. This mechanism is characteristic of many antitumor antibiotics. The antibiotic molecule is noncovalently, although firmly, bound to DNA and distorts the shape of the double helix, resulting in inhibition of RNA or DNA synthesis (15, 16). Recent data suggest that many classical intercalating agents such as doxorubicin may in fact be inhibitors of the enzyme topoisomerase II and may produce DNA strand breaks due to inhibition of the reannealing function of this enzyme (17, 18).

A third mechanism of nucleic acid damage is illustrated by the anticancer drug bleomycin. The amino-terminal tripeptide of the bleomycin molecule appears to intercalate between guanine-cytosine base pairs of DNA. The opposite end of the bleomycin peptide serves as a ferrous oxidase and is able to catalyze the reduction of molecular oxygen to superoxide or hydroxyl radicals that produce DNA breakage (19, 20).

Enzymes represent the second general category of targets for chemotherapeutic agents. Antimetabolites function as inhibitors of key enzymes in the purine or pyrimidine biosynthetic pathways or as inhibitors of DNA polymerase. Since most of these enzymes are active during DNA synthesis, antimetabolites tend to be cytotoxic only when present in sufficient concentration during the vulnerable S phase of the cell cycle. In general, the effectiveness of enzyme inhibitors also depends on the amount and affinity of the target enzyme and on the extent of competition by natural substrates for enzyme binding. In the case of methotrexate, for example, complete saturation of all dihydrofolate reductase binding sites is required before the enzyme is effectively inhibited. As methotrexate inhibits the function of this enzyme, dihydrofolate, the natural substrate, accumulates behind the metabolic block and is able to effectively compete with methotrexate for further enzyme binding (21). Thus, large amounts of methotrexate, well in excess of the enzyme-binding capacity, are required to effectively inhibit dihydrofolate reductase activity. If the enzyme is increased in amount, as in many resistant cells, it may not be possible to effectively deliver cytotoxic levels of methotrexate to the intracellular binding sites.

The microtubular spindle structure provides a third target for chemotherapeutic agents. The vinca alkaloids (vincristine, vinblastine, vinorelbine) exert their cytotoxic effects by binding to specific sites on tubulin, causing inhibition of assembly of tubulin into microtubules and ultimately leading to dissolution of the mitotic spindle structure (22). Although their principal function is the formation of the mitotic spindle during cell division, microtubules are also involved in many vital interphase functions, including the maintenance of shape, motility, signal transmission, and intracellular transport (23). The taxanes (paclitaxel, docetaxel), an important new class of anticancer agents, exert their cytotoxic effects by promoting polymerization of tubulin. Paclitaxel was the first in this group of novel plant alkaloids (24, 25). The microtubules formed in the presence of paclitaxel are extraordinarily stable and dysfunctional, thereby caus-

ing the death of the cell by disrupting the normal microtubule dynamics required for cell division and vital interphase processes. Paclitaxel has proven activity in ovarian and breast cancer and has recently shown promise in the treatment of other tumor types (26).

The search for specific inhibitors of tumor and growth factor receptors has been of great interest since the demonstration that antiestrogens can be effective in the treatment of breast cancers that contain the estrogen receptor. Recent studies have also demonstrated an important role for the antiandrogen, flutamide, in the treatment of prostate cancer (27). As more information becomes available concerning the growth regulatory properties of peptide oncogene products and their cellular receptors, these molecules are likely to become increasingly important as targets of novel chemotherapeutic agents (28).

Cellular Repair of Drug-Induced Injury

Cells that have been damaged by cytotoxic drugs frequently exhibit a variety of repair mechanisms. Indeed, the cytotoxic effects of a drug often represent the balance between injury and repair, and amplified repair mechanisms may account for cellular resistance to certain drugs. The cytotoxicity of alkylating agents reflects the balance between cross-link formation and removal by cellular repair processes. Many cells contain specific enzymes able to remove alkyl moieties from DNA, thereby repairing drug damage. A specific example is the protein O^6-alkyl-guanine transferase that repairs DNA injury produced by chloroethyl-nitrosoureas. Cells containing large amounts of this protein tend to be relatively resistant to these chemotherapeutic agents (29).

Cells also contain a variety of free radical–scavenging systems that protect them from the effects of ionizing radiation and drugs such as bleomycin and anthracyclines, which generate oxygen free radicals intracellularly. Catalase, superoxide dismutase, and glutathione peroxidase, key enzymes in the detoxification of reactive oxygen species, may be deficient in some tissues (e.g., cardiac muscle (30)), leading to excessive drug toxicity, or increased in others, leading to relative drug resistance. Recent studies suggest that expansion of intracellular reduced glutathione pools may be an important mechanism of alkylating-agent resistance in animal and human tumors (31, 32).

Finally, cells may be able to circumvent drug-induced injury by increased production of target enzymes. In experimental models, for example, exposure of cells to methotrexate or 5-fluorouracil can be shown to stimulate production of dihydrofolate reductase (33) or thymidylate synthase (34), respectively. New enzyme production occurs within minutes to hours of drug exposure and is presumed to represent enhanced translation of existing mRNA rather than transcription of additional message. Overexpression of DNA clearly does occur, however, and may be a fundamental mechanism of cellular resistance to antimetabolites and natural products due to increased constitutive production of target enzymes or P-glycoprotein (35).

As mentioned above, a prerequisite to drug effect at the target tissue is adequate drug delivery. Pharmacokinetics describes the concentration-time history of a drug in the body and can be used to answer fundamental questions concerning the optimal route and schedule of drug administration.

PRINCIPLES OF PHARMACOKINETICS

Definitions

Pharmacokinetics is the study of drug absorption, distribution, metabolism, and excretion. A fundamental concept in pharmacokinetics is drug clearance, i.e., elimination of drugs from the body, analogous to the concept of creatinine clearance. In clinical practice, clearance of a drug is rarely directly measured but is calculated as either

$$\text{Clearance} = \text{Dose}/\text{AUC} \qquad (\text{eq. } 3.1)$$
$$\text{or}$$
$$\text{Clearance} = \text{Infusion rate}/C_{ss} \qquad (\text{eq. } 3.2)$$

The AUC (or area under the concentration-time curve) represents the total drug exposure integrated over time and is an important parameter for both pharmacokinetic and pharmacodynamic analyses. As indicated in eq. 3.1, the clearance is simply the ratio of the dose to the AUC, so that the higher the AUC (for a given dose) the lower the clearance. If a drug is administered by continuous infusion *and* steady-state is achieved, the clearance can be estimated from a single measurement of plasma drug concentration as per eq. 3.2.

Clearance can be considered conceptually to be a function of both distribution and elimination. In the simplest pharmacokinetic model,

$$\text{Clearance} = VK \qquad (\text{eq. } 3.3)$$

where V is the volume of distribution, and K is the elimination constant. V is the volume of fluid in which the dose is initially diluted; thus the higher the V, the lower the initial concentration. K is the elimination constant, which is inversely proportional to the half-life, the period of time that must elapse to reach a 50% decrease in plasma concentration. When the half-life is short, K is high, and plasma concentrations decline rapidly. Thus, both a high V and a high K result in relatively low plasma concentrations and a high clearance.

Linear Pharmacokinetic Models

Although pharmacokinetic analysis can be conducted without specifying any mathematical model (noncompartmental methods), it is helpful to use such models as guides in therapeutic decision making. Drugs with linear pharmacokinetics have several important properties (Table 3.2). The key feature of a linear pharmacokinetic model is that

$$\frac{dC}{dt} = KC \qquad (\text{eq. } 3.4)$$

where C is the concentration, K is the elimination constant, t is the time, and dC/dt is the instantaneous rate of change in concentration. This indicates that the instantaneous rate of change in drug concentration depends only on the current concentration. The half-life will remain constant, no matter how high the concentration.

One implication of this principle is that the drug exposure (AUC) is not affected by changes in drug schedule. For example, the AUC after a 60 mg/m^2 bolus dose of doxorubicin equals the total AUC for three daily (or weekly) bolus doses of 20 mg/m^2, which equals the AUC for the same dose administered as a 96-hour infusion. A second implication is that the AUC is proportional to the dose. Thus, if one measures the AUC for a 60 mg/m^2 dose, one can estimate the AUC for

Table 3.2. Properties of Drugs with Linear Pharmacokinetics

Half-life is independent of concentration
Clearance is independent of dose
Clearance is independent of schedule

a 90 mg/m^2 dose in the same patient (50% higher).

The simplest linear pharmacokinetic model is

$$C(t) = \frac{\text{Dose}}{V} e^{-kt} \qquad \text{(eq. 3.5)}$$

shown graphically in Figure 3.4. This model assumes that the drug is administered as an instantaneous bolus and that complete distribution of the drug is also instantaneous.

These assumptions are often not valid. If the drug is administered as a slow bolus or infusion, the model must be corrected for the infusion duration. During the administration of the drug the concentration is increasing

$$C(t) = \left(\frac{\text{Total dose}}{\text{Infusion time}}\right)\left(\frac{1}{VK}\right) 1 - e^{-kt}$$

$$\text{(eq. 3.6)}$$

where $C(t)$ is the concentration at time t, and e is 2.718. After the infusion is terminated, the drug concentration decays at the same rate as if it had been administered as an instantaneous bolus. Thus, if T represents the infusion time, then the postinfusion drug concentrations can be represented as

$$C'(t) = C(T)e^{-k(t-T)} \qquad \text{(eq. 3.7)}$$

Often, the pharmacokinetic data are more complex than shown in Figure 3.4 and may be optimally fitted to a multicompartment model, usually two or three compartments (Fig. 3.5). It

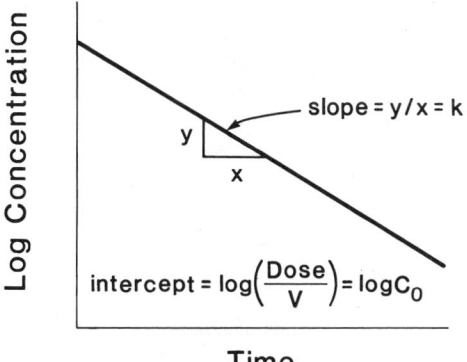

Figure 3.4. Concentration-time plot for 1-compartment linear pharmacokinetic model. C_0 represents the initial concentration, assuming instantaneous administration and distribution. The half-life is $\log_e(2)/k$.

must be emphasized that the compartments are theoretical and do not necessarily correlate with any anatomic space or physiologic process.

With the widespread availability of nonlinear regression programs, it has become quite easy to analyze pharmacokinetic data (36). Standard pharmacokinetic modeling programs are also available (37). The details of pharmacokinetic modeling are outside the scope of this chapter, however several caveats should be emphasized (38). The validity of pharmacokinetic modeling depends to a large extent on the quality of the data entered into the model. Thus, drug infusion must be precisely timed, plasma samples must be obtained on schedule, and analytical methods must be sensitive and specific. The data must be properly weighted to avoid bias due to the increased probability of analytical errors at drug concentrations near the detection limit. Results obtained using a specific model should be compared with those obtained by noncompartmental methods. Extrapolation of models outside the known time points must be done with great caution. Finally, there is a great risk of overparameterization in the use of multicompartmental models, and all parameter values should be checked for this problem.

Nonlinear Pharmacokinetic Models

Nonlinear pharmacokinetic models imply that some aspect of the pharmacokinetic behavior of the drug is saturable. The mathematics of nonlinear models are beyond the scope of this chapter (39, 40), but the principles are highly relevant to several anticancer agents. In contrast to drugs with linear pharmacokinetics, alteration of the schedule of drugs that display nonlinear kinetics may markedly affect the AUC and potentially alter clinical effects. Nonlinear pharmacokinetic behavior commonly occurs when there is saturation of a major metabolic pathway. This results in decreased clearance at higher doses, with a greater-than-proportional increase in the AUC. The AUC will also increase if the infusion duration is shortened, resulting from the slower clearance at the higher peak plasma concentrations. This is, for instance, relevant for 5-fluorouracil (41–43), probably owing to the saturability of its conversion to dihydrofluorouracil by the enzyme dihydropyrimidine dehydrogenase (44). Schaaf et al. (43) demonstrated that doubling of the 5-fluorouracil dose from approximately 7.5 mg/kg to 15 mg/kg (by i.v. bolus) resulted in a 135% increase in the mean AUC. Since 5-fluo-

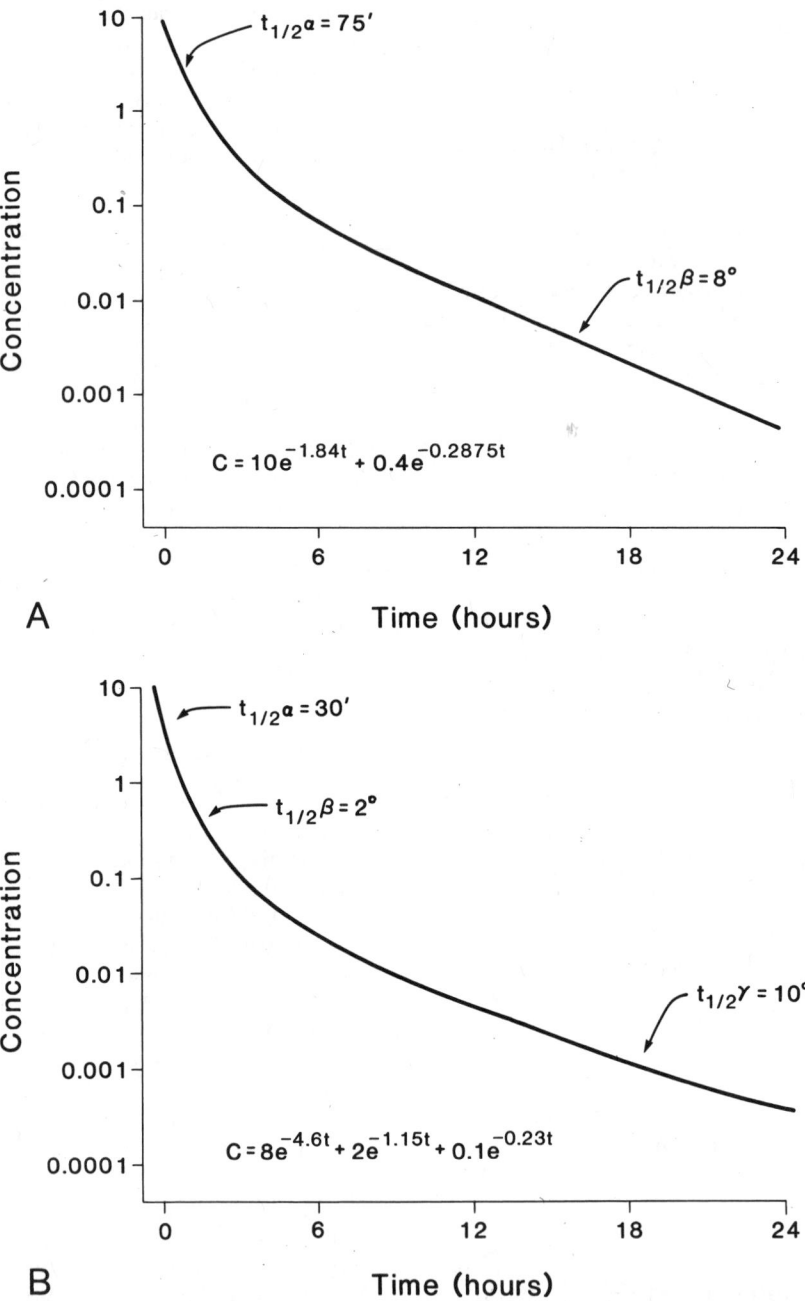

Figure 3.5.   Concentration-time plots for representative 2-compartment (A) **and 3-compartment** (B) **linear phar-macokinetic models.** The two curves are very similar, with $C_0 \approx 10$ for both models. Note that for each "compart-ment" there is one term, and the corresponding half-life equals $\log_e(2)/k_n$, where k_n is the nth term.

rouracil is used on a variety of schedules, its non-linear pharmacokinetic behavior is one factor in its highly schedule-dependent effects.

The opposite situation arises when a drug's absorption (or renal tubular reabsorption) is saturable. In this case, an increase in dose results in a less-than-proportional increase in the AUC. Examples of anticancer drugs with saturable kinetics include melphalan absorption from the gastrointestinal tract (45) and recombinant interleukin-2 absorption after subcutaneous administration (46). Cisplatin also appears to have nonlinear pharmacokinetics owing to saturability of its renal tubular reabsorption (47, 48). Forastiere et al. (48) demonstrated that free plasma platinum is increased by 42% when the drug is given as a 24-hour continuous infusion rather than as a short 20-minute infusion. Prolonged infusion was also associated with greater than a threefold increase in the free platinum half-life.

Interpatient Pharmacokinetic Variability

In describing a drug's pharmacokinetics, one must consider the extent of interpatient variability, often represented as the coefficient of variation (ratio of standard deviation to mean). Interpatient pharmacokinetic variability may be due to genetic differences in drug metabolism (49) or may result from acquired abnormalities. Cancer patients may have significant hepatic or renal dysfunction as well as other abnormalities that lead to alterations in pharmacokinetic parameters (Table 3.3).

Pharmacogenetics is the study of the influence of heredity on the fate of a drug in the body, drug response, and adverse drug reactions. Pharmacogenetic differences in drug metabolism may be relevant, for instance, for 5-fluorouracil. In humans, more than 85% of administered 5-fluorouracil is degraded through catabolism with dihydropyrimidine dehydrogenase controlling the initial, rate-limiting step. The clinical importance of this enzyme has recently been demonstrated with the identification of patients with severe toxicity due to dihydropyrimidine dehydrogenase deficiency (50, 51). Another example is the highly variable toxicity of amonafide, which is due to genetic differences in N-acetylation (52).

An understanding of interpatient pharmacokinetic variability is potentially of great importance for optimizing antineoplastic therapy. Variability in absorption is generally not consid-

Table 3.3. Potential Abnormalities in Cancer Patients Altering Pharmacokinetics of Anticancer Agents

Abnormalities of absorption
  Nausea/vomiting
  Prior surgery, radiotherapy, or chemotherapy
  Concurrent antiemetics affecting gut motility
  Patient compliance
Abnormalities of distribution
  Weight loss
  Obesity
  Decreased body fat (lipophilic drugs)
  Pleural effusions or ascites (methotrexate)
Abnormalities of elimination
  Hepatic dysfunction due to tumor replacement or
    prior (or concurrent) therapy
  Renal dysfunction due to malignant involvement or
    prior (or concurrent) therapy
Abnormalities in protein binding
  Hypoalbuminemia
  Concomitant medications

ered in the use of oral antineoplastic agents, even though oral therapy is commonly used for some diseases, such as chlorambucil for chronic lymphocytic leukemia or melphalan for multiple myeloma. The percentage of a drug absorbed is referred to as the bioavailability, the ratio of the AUC after oral administration to the AUC after intravenous administration of the same dose. Bioavailability of oral antineoplastics has not been well studied. The bioavailability of agents such as melphalan (53) and etoposide (54) is highly variable. It may also be accentuated by concomitant administration of other chemotherapeutic agents.

Variability in drug distribution may be attributed to changes in body size (55, 56) or to the ratio of fat to total mass. In the latter case, there may be altered distribution of lipophilic drugs, which includes most of the natural-product anticancer drugs and their analogues. The most commonly recognized abnormality of distribution is the delayed clearance of methotrexate, which results from accumulation of the drug in ascites or pleural effusions (57).

Many patients with advanced cancer have abnormalities of liver function tests or known mass lesions within the liver, often in association with significant malnutrition. Given that many antineoplastic agents are metabolized or excreted by the liver, recognizing altered elimination by the liver becomes important in the optimization of chemotherapy dosing. Unfortunately, altered hepatic elimination or metabolism is not easily predictable. Clearly, patients with severe hyperbilirubinemia owing to parenchymal replacement or obstruction are likely to have altered elimination. However, it is not often recognized that many patients with normal serum bilirubin levels may have a low drug clearance resulting in a high AUC and corresponding toxicity. A decrease in serum albumin (in patients with normal serum bilirubin concentrations) has been associated with a decrease in the hepatic elimination of antipyrine (58, 59)—a commonly used marker drug—as well as vinblastine (60) and trimetrexate (61). Thus, patients with a serum albumin less than 2.5 g/dL may be at increased risk of toxicity and are potentially candidates for dose reduction of agents requiring hepatic metabolism or excretion. At present, there are few firm guidelines useful for accurate dosing of antineoplastics in the setting of obvious hepatic disease (see Chapter 37).

In contrast, alterations in renal function generally correlate with renal clearance of drugs, since renal drug clearance tends to correlate with creatinine clearance. This has been well established for carboplatin (62, 63), where a firm relationship exists between renal function and carboplatin clearance, which can be used prospectively to modify the carboplatin dose and avoid excessive toxicity (62).

Abnormalities of protein binding are common but rarely affect clinical outcome. Many anticancer drugs, such as the vinca alkaloids (64) and etoposide (65), are highly protein bound. Changes in protein binding may affect drug clearance (66). Most importantly, protein binding must be considered in the interpretation of measured total plasma drug concentrations, since a decrease in protein binding will result in a relative increase in the pharmacologically active free drug (67).

Intrapatient Pharmacokinetic Variability

Although it is well established that interpatient pharmacokinetic variability may be significant, the importance of intrapatient variability (within a single patient) is less clear. Oncologists are commonly faced with the clinical situation of increasing myelosuppression after repetitive dosing. This is generally assumed to be due to the cumulative effects of chemotherapy, making the patient more sensitive to subsequent doses.

However, it is also possible that the patient's clearance of the drug(s) may have decreased, resulting in increased drug exposure.

Such a situation may arise when either hepatic or renal function changes. Renal function may change because of progressive disease (ureteral obstruction), complications of therapy (volume depletion), or as a direct toxic effect of therapy (cisplatin). Similarly, renal function may improve over time, reducing the actual drug exposure. Hepatic function may also change, producing changes in drug clearance. This may result in enhanced toxicity, as documented for vinblastine when given by prolonged continuous infusion (60). Thus, reviewing the outcome of prior doses helps to minimize the risk of an undesirable outcome due to intrapatient pharmacokinetic variability.

PRINCIPLES OF PHARMACODYNAMICS

Definitions

In a general sense, pharmacodynamics is the study of dose-response relationships. Thus, any laboratory or clinical study employing different doses of an agent is addressing a pharmacodynamic question. Examples include the exposure of tumor cells in vitro to varying doses of a new agent to evaluate its dose-response relationship and a phase I clinical trial to define the maximally tolerated dose and dose-limiting toxicities.

In the clinical setting, the results of treatment depend on both pharmacokinetics and pharmacodynamics. A patient may have excessive toxicity (at the usual dose) for one of two reasons. If the patient's pharmacokinetics are "abnormal," there may be decreased total body clearance, resulting in a higher-than-expected drug exposure. The second possibility is that the patient might simply be "sensitive" to an average drug exposure because of prior therapy, poor nutrition, or other less well defined reasons. It is important to distinguish between these two possibilities. In the first case, lowering the dose will result in an "average" drug exposure, whereas in the second case, lowering the dose will result in a lower-than-average drug exposure. The probability of tumor response in the patient with abnormal pharmacokinetics is higher than in the "sensitive" patient with unusual pharmacodynamics.

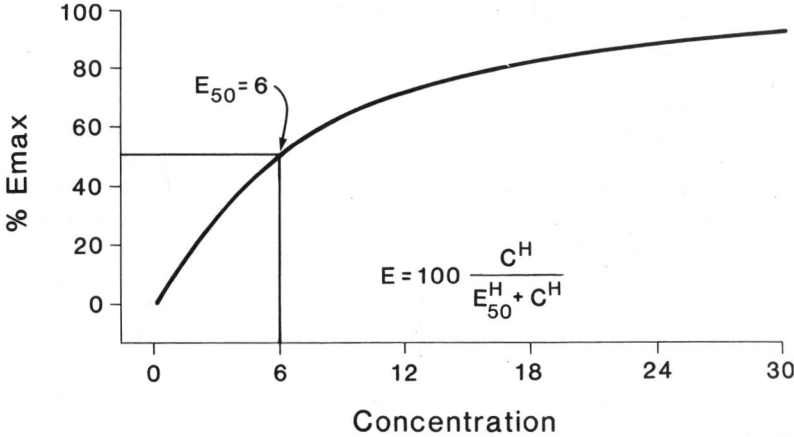

Figure 3.6.   Example of Emax model as proposed by Wagner (68). The maximum effect is 100%, and a concentration of 6 results in 50% effect. The exponent *H*, also known as the Hill constant, determines the shape of the curve and is usually between 1 and 2.

General Pharmacodynamic Principles

In the most general sense, any drug may be considered to have a maximal effect and a median dose (that required for 50% of the maximal effect). Wagner proposed a generalized sigmoidal model (Fig. 3.6), derived from the hypothesis that all drug effects require an initial interaction with a receptor (68).

Most studies addressing pharmacodynamic modeling of anticancer agents have separately addressed phase-specific agents (69–71). It may be adequate to use a simple log-linear model for non-phase-specific agents (70–72):

Survival fraction (*SF*)

$$= \frac{\text{Treated cells}}{\text{Control cells}} = e^{-KC} \quad \text{(eq. 3.8)}$$

This may be referred to as a steep dose-response curve, since the effect continues to increase as the concentration (*C*) increases. For any *K* (in eq. 3.8), an increase in *C* by 2.3/*K* will result in a 1-log increase in antitumor effect (Fig. 3.7*A*).

The issues for phase-specific agents, such as the antimetabolites, are much more complicated. By definition, some cells are out of "phase" and therefore not sensitive (or relatively insensitive) to the effects of the drug. This may not necessarily be overcome by increasing the dose, which

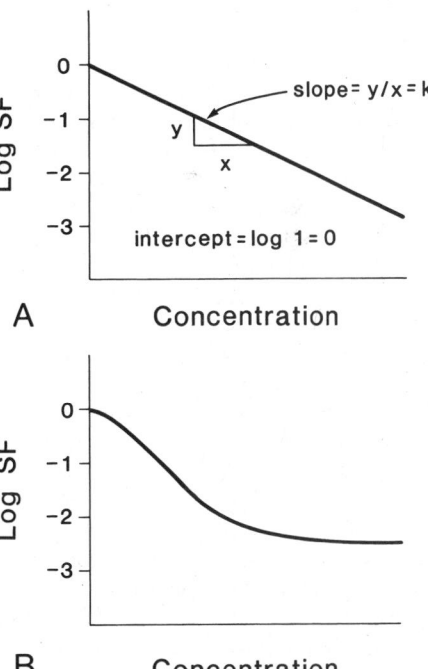

Figure 3.7.   Pharmacodynamic plots for drugs with nonsaturable (A) and saturable (B) effects. In the simplest pharmacodynamic model (**A**), there is a linear relationship between dose and log kill. In **B**, there is a maximal effect, resulting in a plateau in the dose-response curve.

results in a plateau in the dose-response curve (Fig. 3.7*B*), but could be overcome by increasing the duration of drug exposure.

The effects of antineoplastic agents depend on both the drug concentration and the duration of exposure to that concentration. For some agents, the effect is a function of the product of the concentration and the time, analogous to the area under the concentration-time curve, or AUC (71, 73). However, for antimetabolites and other phase-specific agents, the mathematical relationships are much more complex (70, 71, 74). Drug effect tends to be related to duration of exposure above a threshold concentration.

Pharmacodynamic Modeling of Cancer Chemotherapy

The introduction of pharmacodynamic modeling into clinical oncology has been a slow process. The relationship between toxicity subsequent to high-dose methotrexate and abnormalities in methotrexate clearance has led to the routine use of therapeutic drug monitoring of methotrexate to guide leucovorin dosing (75). However, studies of other drugs have not yet resulted in a change in clinical practice.

There is an expanding interest in trying to optimize cancer chemotherapy by individualizing dosing on the basis of measurements of plasma or tissue drug concentrations. One example is the titration of carboplatin dosing on the basis of the creatinine clearance, pretreatment platelet count, desired platelet nadir, and extent of prior chemotherapy (62). The potential usefulness of pharmacodynamics was demonstrated by studies correlating the clearance of methotrexate (76) and teniposide (77) with response or survival in children with acute lymphocytic leukemia. Other investigators have attempted to optimize the dosing of hexamethylene bisacetamide (78), 5-fluorouracil (79), and etoposide (67, 80–82). Pharmacodynamic studies have been hampered by the requirement to obtain numerous samples to accurately define the pharmacokinetics. Recent strategies have been developed with the aim of limiting the number of samples (83–86). Statistical approaches to pharmacodynamic modeling are also increasingly being refined (87).

The Future Role of Anticancer Pharmacodynamics

Should the clinical oncologist care about pharmacodynamics? Will therapeutic drug monitoring of antineoplastics be as useful as monitoring of theophylline or aminoglycoside dosing? How will these studies improve the therapeutic index? These are important issues that are currently being addressed.

Our true understanding of dosing of most anticancer drugs is primitive. Body surface area is generally the only value used to determine initial dosing (88). Prior toxicity may be used to adjust dosing for subsequent cycles, although doses are more often reduced than escalated, and the magnitude of dose changes is determined empirically and often arbitrarily.

For drugs with a relatively broad therapeutic index and/or minimal interpatient pharmacokinetic or pharmacodynamic variability, these strategies may not be necessary. As an example, therapeutic drug monitoring of α-interferon in hairy cell leukemia is unlikely to be useful (89). In contrast, adjuvant chemotherapy to treat breast cancer causes toxicity, but doses should not be reduced if the maximal benefit is to be achieved (90). Therapeutic drug monitoring of doxorubicin in this setting may potentially help to ensure adequate drug exposure and minimize the risk of toxicity.

In conclusion, medical oncologists are currently "empiric pharmacologists" using clinical experience as the care of an individual patient unfolds during the course of the disease. It is hoped that a better understanding of the clinical pharmacology of antineoplastic drugs (pharmacokinetics, pharmacogenetics, and pharmacodynamics) will provide a sound scientific basis for the improved care of patients with cancer.

REFERENCES

1. Goldman ID. Pharmacokinetics of antineoplastic agents at the cellular level. In: Chabner BA, ed. Pharmacologic principles of cancer treatment. Philadelphia: WB Saunders, 1982:15–44.
2. Wiley JS, Jones SP, Sawyer WD, Paterson ARP. Cytosine arabinoside influx and nucleoside transport sites in acute leukemia. J Clin Invest 1982;69:479–489.
3. Jarvis SM, Young JD. Nucleoside transport in rat erythrocytes: two components with differences in sensitivity to inhibition by nitrobenzylthioinosine and *p*-chloro-mercuriphenyl sulfonate. J Membr Biol 1986; 93:1–10.
4. Sirotnak FM. Correlates of folate analog transport, pharmacokinetics and selective antitumor action. Pharmacol Ther 1980;8:71–103.
5. Goldenberg GJ, Begleiter A. Membrane transport of alkylating agents. Pharmacol Ther 1980;8:237–274.
6. Beck WT. The cell biology of multiple drug resistance. Biochem Pharmacol 1987;36:2879–2887.

7. Lippard SJ. New chemistry of an old molecule: cis (Pt NH$_3$)$_2$ Cl$_2$). Science 1982;218:1075–1082.

8. Colvin M, Padgett CA, Fenselau C. A biologically active metabolite of cyclophosphamide. Cancer Res 1973;33:915–918.

9. Jolivet J, Schilsky RL, Bailey BD, Drake SC, Chabner BA. Synthesis, retention and biological activity of methotrexate polyglutamates in cultured human breast cancer cells. J Clin Invest 1982;70:351–360.

10. Allegra JC, Chabner BA, Drake JC. Enhanced inhibition of thymidylate synthase by methotrexate polyglutamates. J Biol Chem 1985;260:9720–9726.

11. Coleman CN, Stoller RG, Drake JC, Chabner BA. Deoxycytidine kinase: properties of the enzyme from human leukemic granulocytes. Blood 1975; 46:791–803.

12. Plagemann PGW, Marz R, Wohlhueter RM. Transport and metabolism of deoxycytidine and 1-β-D-arabinofuranosyl-cytosine into cultured Novikoff rat hepatoma cells, relationship to phosphorylation, and regulation of triphosphate synthesis. Cancer Res 1978; 38:978–989.

13. Kohn KW, Spears CL, Doty P. Inter-strand crosslinking of DNA by nitrogen mustard. J Mol Biol 1966;19:266–288.

14. Brookes P, Lawley PD. The reaction of mono- and bifunctional alkylating agents with nucleic acids. Biochem J 1961;80:496–503.

15. Pigram WJ, Fuller W, Hamilton LD. Stereochemistry of intercalation: interaction of daunomycin with DNA. Nature New Biol 1972;235:17–19.

16. Young RC, Ozols RF, Myers CE. The anthracycline antineoplastic drugs. N Engl J Med 1981; 305:139–153.

17. Tewey KM, Rowe TC, Yang L, Halligan BD, Liu LF. Adriamycin-induced DNA damage mediated by mammalian DNA topoisomerase II. Science 1984; 226:466–470.

18. Ross WE, Bradley MO. DNA double-stranded breaks in mammalian cells after exposure to intercalating agents. Biochim Biophys Acta 1981;654:129–134.

19. Takeshita M, Grollman AP, Ohtsubo E, et al. Interaction of bleomycin with DNA. Proc Natl Acad Sci USA 1978;75:5983–5987.

20. Giloni L, Takeshita M, Johnson F, et al. Bleomycin induced strand scission of DNA: mechanism of deoxyribose cleavage. J Biol Chem 1981;256:8608–8615.

21. White JC, Goldman ID. Mechanism of action of methotrexate. IV. Free intracellular methotrexate required to suppress dihydrofolate reduction to tetrahydrofolate by Ehrlich ascites tumor cells in vitro. Mol Pharmacol 1976;12:711–719.

22. Owellen RJ, Hartke CA, Dickerson RM, Hains FO. Inhibition of tubulin-microtubule polymerization by drugs of the vinca alkaloid class. Cancer Res 1976; 36:1499–1502.

23. Cass CE, Beck WT. Vinca alkaloid pharmacology and resistance. In: Kessel D, ed. Resistance to antineoplastic drugs. Boca Raton, FL: CRC Press, 1989:141–165.

24. Manfredi JJ, Horwitz SB. Taxol: an antimitotic agent with a new mechanism of action. Pharmacol Ther 1984;25:83.

25. Schiff PB, Horwitz SB. Taxol stabilizes microtubules in mouse fibroblast cells. Proc Natl Acad Sci USA 1980;77:1561.

26. Rowinsky EK, Donehower RC. Paclitaxel (Taxol). N Engl J Med 1995;332:1004–1014.

27. Crawford ED, Eisenberger MA, McLeod DG, et al. A controlled trial of leuprolide with and without flutamide in prostate carcinoma. N Engl J Med 1989; 321:419–424.

28. Goldenberg A, Masui H, Divgi C, Kamrath H, Pentlow K, Mendelsohn J. Imaging of human tumor xenografts with an indium-111-labeled anti-epidermal growth factor receptor monoclonal antibody. J Natl Cancer Inst 1989;81:1616–1625.

29. Dolan ME, Young GS, Pegg AE. Effect of O^6-alkylguanine pretreatment on the sensitivity of human colon tumor cells to the cytotoxic effects of chloroethylating agents. Cancer Res 1986;46:4500–4504.

30. Doroshow JH, Locker GY, Myers CE. Enzymatic defenses of the mouse heart against reactive oxygen: alterations produced by doxorubicin. J Clin Invest 1980;65:128–135.

31. Ahmad S, Okine L, Le B, Najarian P, Vistica DT. Elevation of glutathione in phenylalanine mustard-resistant murine L1210 leukemia cells. J Biol Chem 1987; 262:15048–15053.

32. Green JA, Vistica DT, Young RL, Hamilton TC, Rogan AM, Ozols RF. Potentiation of melphalan cytotoxicity in human ovarian cancer cell lines by glutathione depletion. Cancer Res 1984;44:5427–5431.

33. Domin BA, Grill SP, Bastow KF, et al. Effect of methotrexate on dihydrofolate reductase activity in methotrexate resistant human KB cells. Mol Pharmacol 1982;21:478–482.

34. Swain SM, Lippman ME, Egan EF, Drake JC, Steinberg SM, Allegra CJ. Fluorouracil and high dose leucovorin in previously treated patients with metastatic breast cancer. J Clin Oncol 1989;7:890–899.

35. Schimke RT. Gene amplification, drug resistance and cancer. Cancer Res 1984;44:1735–1742.

36. Garcia-Pena J, Azen SP. A user's experience with a standard non-linear regression program (BMDP 3R). Comput Programs Biomed 1979;10:185.

37. Metzler CM, Elfring GL, McEwen AJ. A user's manual for NONLIN and associated programs. Kalamazoo, MI: The Upjohn Co., 1974.

38. Metzler CM. Estimation of pharmacokinetics parameters: statistical conductions. Pharmacol Ther 1981;13:543–556.

39. Gibaldi M, Perrier D. Pharmacokinetics. 2nd ed. New York: Marcel Dekker, 1982:271–318.

40. Wagner JG, Szpunar GJ, Ferry JJ. A nonlinear physiologic pharmacokinetics model: i. Steady-state. J Pharmacokinet Biopharm 1985;13:73–92.

41. Collins J, Dedrick R, King F, Speyer J, Myers C. Nonlinear pharmacokinetics models for 5-fluorouracil in man: intravenous and intraperitoneal routes. Clin Pharmacol Ther 1980;28:235–246.

42. Wagner JG, Gyves JW, Stetson PL, et al. Steady-state nonlinear pharmacokinetics of 5-fluorouracil during hepatic arterial and intravenous infusions in cancer patients. Cancer Res 1986;46:1499–1506.

43. Schaaf LJ, Dobbs BR, Edwards IR, Perrier DG. Nonlinear pharmacokinetics characteristics of 5-fluorouracil (5-FU) in colorectal cancer patients. Eur J Clin Pharmacol 1987;32:411–418.

44. Mukherjee K, Heidelberger C. Studies on fluorinated pyrimidines, IX. The degradation of 5-fluorouracil-6-C^{14}. J Biol Chem 1960;235:433–437.

45. Choi KE, Ratain MJ, Williams SF, et al. Plasma

pharmacokinetics of high-dose oral melphalan in patients treated with trialkylator chemotherapy and autologous bone marrow reinfusion. Cancer Res 1989; 49:1318–1321.

46. Gustavson LE, Nadeau RW, Oldfield NF. Pharmacokinetics of teceleukin (recombinant human interleukin-2) after intravenous or subcutaneous administration to patients with cancer. J Biol Response Mod 1989;8:440–449.

47. Reece PA, Stafford I, Russell J, Grantley GP. Nonlinear renal clearance of ultrafilterable platinum in patients treated with cis-dichloradiammine platinum (II). Cancer Chemother Pharmacol 1985;15:295–299.

48. Forastiere AA, Belliveau JF, Boren MP, Vogel WC, Posner MR, O'Leary GP. Pharmacokinetics and toxicity evaluation of five-day continuous infusion versus intermittent bolus cis-diamminedichloropla tinum (II) in head and neck cancer patients. Cancer Res 1988; 48:3869–3874.

49. Vesell ES. Pharmacogenetic perspectives gained from twin and family studies. Pharmacol Ther 1989;41:535–552.

50. Diasio RB, Lu Z. Dihydropyrimidine dehydrogenase activity and fluorouracil chemotherapy. J Clin Oncol 1994;12:2239–2242.

51. Etienne MC, Lagrange JL, Dassonville O, et al. Population study of dihydropyrimidine dehydrogenase in cancer patients. J Clin Oncol 1994;12:2248–2253.

52. Ratain MJ, Rosner G, Allen SL, et al. Population pharmacodynamic study of amonafide: a Cancer and Leukemia Group B study. J Clin Oncol 1995;13:741–747.

53. Alberts DS, Chang SY, Chen H-SG, Evans TL, Moon TE. Oral melphalan kinetics. Clin Pharmacol Ther 1979;26:737–745.

54. Hande KR, Krozely MG, Greco FA, Hainsworth JD, Johnson DH. Bioavailability of low-dose oral etoposide. J Clin Oncol 1993;11:374–377.

55. Cheymol G. Drug pharmacokinetics in the obese. Fundam Clin Pharmacol 1988;2:239–256.

56. Rodvold KA, Rushing DA, Tewksbury DA. Doxorubicin clearance in the obese. J Clin Oncol 1988; 6:1321–1327.

57. Chabner BA, Stoller RG, Hande K, et al. Methotrexate disposition in human case studies in ovarian cancer and following high-dose infusion. Drug Metab Rev 1978;1:107–117.

58. Branch RA, Herbert CM, Read AE. Determinants of serum antipyrine half-lives in patients with liver disease. Gut 1973;14:569–573.

59. Sotaniemi EA, Pelkonen RO, Mokka RE, Huttunen R, Viljakainen E. Impairment of drug metabolism in patients with liver cancer. Eur J Clin Invest 1977;7:269–274.

60. Ratain MJ, Vogelzang NJ, Sinkule JA. Interpatient and intrapatient variability in vinblastine pharmacokinetics. Clin Pharmacol Ther 1987;41:61–67.

61. Fanucchi MP, Walsh TD, Fleisher M, et al. Phase I and clinical pharmacology study of trimetrexate administered weekly for three weeks. Cancer Res 1987;47:3303–3308.

62. Egorin MJ, Van Echo DA, Tipping SJ, et al. Pharmacokinetics and dosage reduction of cis-diammine (1,1-cyclobutane di-carboxylato)-platinum in patients with impaired renal function. Cancer Res 1984; 44:5432–5438.

63. Harland SJ, Newell DR, Siddik ZH, Chadwick R, Calvert AH, Harrap KR. Pharmacokinetics of cis-diammine-1,1-cyclobutane dicarboxylate platinum (II) in patients with normal and impaired renal function. Cancer Res 1984;44:1693–1697.

64. Donigian DW, Owellen RT. Interaction of vinblastine, vincristine and colchicine with serum proteins. Biochem Pharmacol 1973;22:2113.

65. Stewart CF, Pieper JA, Arbuck SG, Evans WE. Altered protein binding of etoposide in patients with cancer. Clin Pharmacol Ther 1989;45:49–55.

66. Smallwood RH, Mihaly GW, Smallwood RA, Morgan DJ. Effect of a protein binding change on unbound and total plasma concentrations for drugs of intermediate hepatic extraction. J Pharmacokinet Biopharm 1988;16:529–542.

67. Ratain MJ, Schilsky RL, Choi KE, et al. Adaptive control of etoposide administration: impact of interpatient pharmacodynamic variability. Clin Pharmacol Ther 1989;45:226–233.

68. Wagner JG. Kinetics of pharmacologic response: i. Proposed relationships between response and drug concentration in the intact animal and man. J Theoret Biol 1968;20:173–201.

69. Jusko WJ. A pharmacodynamic model for cell-cycle-specific chemotherapeutic agents. J Pharmacokinet Biopharm 1973;1:175–200.

70. Jusko WJ. Pharmacodynamics of chemotherapeutic effect: dose-time-response relationships for phase-nonspecific agents. J Pharm Sci 1987;60:892–895.

71. Ozawa S, Sugiyama Y, Mitsuhashi J, et al. Kinetic analysis of cell killing effect induced by cytosine arabinoside and cisplatin in relation to cell cycle phase specificity in human colon cancer and Chinese hamster cells. Cancer Res 49:3823–3838.

72. Skipper HE, Schabel FM, Mellett LB, et al. Implications of biochemical, cytokinetic, pharmacologic, and toxicologic relationships in the design of optimal therapeutic schedules. Cancer Chemother Rep 1970; 54:431–450.

73. Eichholtz-Wirth H. Dependence of the cytostatic effect of Adriamycin on drug concentration and exposure time in vitro. Br J Cancer 1980;41:886–891.

74. Eichholtz H, Trott KR. Effect of methotrexate concentration and exposure time on mammalian cell survival in vitro. Br J Cancer 1980;41:277–284.

75. Ackland SP, Schilsky RL. High-dose methotrexate: a critical reappraisal. J Clin Oncol 1987;5:2017–2031.

76. Evans WE, Crom WR, Stewart CF, et al. Clinical pharmacodynamics of high-dose methotrexate in acute lymphocytic leukemia. N Engl J Med 1986;314:471–477.

77. Rodman JH, Abromowitch M, Sinkule JA, Rivera GK, Evans WE. Clinical pharmacodynamics of continuous infusion teniposide: systemic exposure as a determinant of response in a phase I trial. J Clin Oncol 1987;5:1007–1014.

78. Conley BA, Forrest A, Egorin MJ, et al. Phase I trial using adaptive control dosing of hexamethylene bisacetamide (NSC 95580). Cancer Res 1989;49:3436–3440.

79. Milano G, Etienne MC, Renee N, et al. Relationship between fluorouracil systemic exposure and tumor response and patient survival. J Clin Oncol 1994; 12:1291–1295.

80. Karlsson MO, Port RE, Ratain MJ, Sheiner LB.

A population model for the leukopenic effect of etoposide. Clin Pharmacol Ther 1995;57:325–334.

81. Miller AA, Tolley EA, Niell HB, Griffin JP, Mauer AM. Pharmacodynamics of prolonged oral etoposide in patients with advanced non–small-cell lung cancer. J Clin Oncol 1993;11:1179–1188.

82. Miller AA, Tolley EA. Predictive performance of a pharmacodynamic model for oral etoposide. Cancer Res 1994;54:2080–2083.

83. Ratain MJ, Vogelzang NJ. A limited sampling model for vinblastine pharmacokinetics. Cancer Treat Rep 1987;71:935–939.

84. Ratain MJ, Staubus AE, Schilsky RL, Malspeis L. Limited sampling models for amonafide (NSC 308847) pharmacokinetics. Cancer Res 1988;48:4127–4130.

85. Egorin MJ, Forrest A, Belani CP, et al. A limited sampling strategy for cyclophosphamide pharmacokinetics. Cancer Res 1989;49:3129–3133.

86. Launay MC, Milano G, Iliadis A, Frenay M, Namer N. A limited sampling procedure for estimating Adriamycin pharmacokinetics in cancer patients. Br J Cancer 1989;60:89–92.

87. Mick R, Ratain MJ. Statistical approaches to pharmacodynamic modeling: motivations, methods, and misperceptions. Cancer Chemother Pharmacol 1993;33:1–9.

88. Reilly JJ, Workman P. Normalisation of anticancer drug dosage using body weight and surface area: is it worthwhile? Cancer Chemother Pharmacol 1993;32:411–418.

89. Golomb HM, Jacobs A, Fefer A, et al. Alpha-2 interferon therapy of hairy cell leukemia: a multicenter study of 64 patients. J Clin Oncol 1986;4:900–905.

90. Wood WC, Budman DR, Korzun AH, et al. Dose and dose intensity of adjuvant chemotherapy for stage II, node-positive breast carcinoma. N Engl J Med 1994;330:1253–1259.

4

The Norton-Simon Hypothesis

Larry Norton

WHY STUDY GROWTH CURVES?

Oncology is the study of the natural history and the means of perturbation of malignant growth. For this reason, concepts of growth, especially concepts of tumor growth, are fundamental to oncologic theory and practice. To the clinician, one particularly relevant group of questions concerns the relationship between a tumor's growth pattern and its response to anticancer pharmacotherapy. Such drug therapy is, after all, thought to work by disturbing mitosis. Does drug resistance emerge rapidly between the time the cancer is diagnosed and the time of initiation of chemotherapy? Can prognosis be improved by shrinking a tumor mass before surgical removal? What is the optimal scheduling of non-cross-resistant chemotherapies? What is the relationship between drug dose and the rate of tumor regression? These and similar issues are certainly important for practical applications but hold considerable theoretical interest as well.

The field of growth curve analysis approaches these issues by examining the rates of change of cell number over time in both the unperturbed and perturbed (e.g., therapeutic) environments. This field is closely allied with cellular cytokinetics—tritiated thymidine labeling and flow cytometry—because the kinetics of cellular proliferation underlie the kinetics of tumor growth. Both cellular proliferation and the pattern of tumor growth relate to such clinically relevant biologic characteristics as a cancer's tendencies to invade, to metastasize, and to respond to drug therapy. A fundamental concept is that cell proliferation generates tumor heterogeneity (1). Cell proliferation also generates tumor growth. Hence, the mathematical growth curves that summarize clinical course also relate to the rate of emergence of mutations toward metastatic potential and drug resistance. Understanding these growth curves, therefore, may provide important clues regarding better treatment, prognostication, and, ultimately, prevention.

THE SKIPPER-SCHABEL-WILCOX MODEL

The Skipper-Schabel-Wilcox growth curve model, also called the "log-kill" model, was the first to be considered seriously in modern oncology and is still most influential (2, 3). It was formulated from observations of leukemia L1210 in BDF1 or DBA mice. This tumor grows exponentially until it reaches a lethal tumor volume of 10^9 cells, equivalent to one cubic centimeter (4). The biologic fact is that 90% of the leukemia cells divide every 12 to 13 hours. This percentage does not change appreciably as the leukemia grows from a tiny number of cells to a number close to the lethal volume. As a result of this constancy in growth percentage (also called "growth fraction"), the doubling time is always constant. It takes about 11 hours for 100 cells to grow into 200 cells, a doubling of tumor size. Hence, it takes 11 hours for 10^7 cells to grow into 2×10^7 cells. This pattern applies to any constant fractional increase. That is, it takes 40 hours for 10^3 cells to grow into 10^4 cells, an increase of a factor of 10). So, increasing by a factor of 10 from 10^7 cells to 10^8 cells also takes 40 hours.

Exponential growth, with its constant doubling time and its constant "fractional increase" time, would have concrete clinical implications if this pattern of growth were clinically relevant (5). Doubling time can be measured in any tumor that doubles in size over a period of observation. (This does not mean that the doubling time so measured is constant, of course.) Doubling time has been measured in this way for many histologic types of cancer, and one of the key observations is that the results are heterogeneous both among cancers of the same type and between different types (5). However, there are some consistencies. The human cancers responding best to drug therapy, such as testicular cancer and choriocarcinoma, tend to have doubling times of less than 1 month. Less responsive cancers, such as squamous cell cancer of the head and neck, seem to double over about 2 months. The unresponsive cancers, like colon adenocarcinoma, have longer doubling times, 3 months or longer. This observation encouraged the notion that chemotherapy damages dividing cells, because shorter doubling time implies high growth fraction, perhaps coupled with low spontaneous death fraction.

Since the formulation of the log-kill model, little has happened to dispel the concept that mitotic rate and cell-kill rate are linked. However, it must be recognized that tumors with higher rates of cell loss will tend to have slower growth rates than tumors of similar proliferative rates but lower cell loss fractions. High cell production plus high cell loss means many mitoses per unit time. The probability of mutation correlates with the mitotic rate, so high growth fraction plus high death fraction should produce a higher rate of mutation toward drug resistance. (A mathematical formulation of this concept is discussed below under the heading "The Delbrück-Luria Concept.") Nevertheless, it is empirically observed that if a tumor grows exponentially and if it is homogeneous in drug sensitivity, the fraction of cells killed by a specific chemotherapy regimen is always the same regardless of the initial size of the malignant population. This is the essence of the log-kill model. One key assumption is exponential growth, but before we examine this assumption, let us further explore the implications of the log-kill model.

If a drug treatment reduces 10^6 cells to 10^5, the same therapy would reduce 10^4 cells to 10^3. Both 10^6 to 10^5 and 10^4 to 10^3 are examples of "one-log" kill, meaning a 90% decrease in cell number. For many drugs, the log-kill increases with increasing dose, so higher drug dosages are needed to eradicate larger inoculum sizes of transplanted tumors (6,7). Yet drug dose $3x$ may be thought of as drug dose $2x$ plus drug dose x. If another drug is given at dose y, and if the cell-kill from y equals the cell kill from x, then $2x$ plus y would be an equivalent therapy, in terms of log-kill, as $3x$. (The implications of drug resistance are considered below.) The superiority of $3x$ over x and of $2x$ plus y over x implies that if two or more drugs are used, the log-kills are multiplicative. If a given dose of drug A kills 90% of the cells (a one-log kill) and a given dose of drug B kills 90%, then drug A given with drug B should kill 90% of the 10% of cells left after B alone, resulting in a cell-kill of 99%, called a "two-log" kill. If C also kills 90%, then A plus B plus C should result in a three-log kill (99.9%), and so on. By this line of mathematical reasoning, based on the assumption of exponential growth, if enough drugs at adequate doses are applied against a tumor of sufficiently small size, fewer than one cell should be left, which means "cure." This global concept was of major value in the design of the early, indeed sometimes curative, treatments of childhood leukemia (8).

APPLICATION OF LOG-KILL TO MORE COMPLEX SITUATIONS

When log-kill concepts were first considered in the context of the postoperative adjuvant treatment of micrometastases, they generated much optimism (9, 10). Micrometastases are very small collections of cancer cells, and very small solid tumors in the laboratory contain a higher percentage of actively dividing cells than larger examples (11, 12). This is, of course, a violation of the assumptions of the log-kill model, because the growth fraction of micrometastases is not the same as that of larger tumors, but greater. Yet, if chemotherapy preferentially kills mitotic cells, the fraction of cells killed in these small tumors should be great. Therefore, if the assumptions of the log-kill model are wrong, the error should be in the direction of *underestimating* the impact of chemotherapy against micrometastases. Small-volume tumors should be more easily cured by combination chemotherapy than the model would have predicted.

The problem is that clinical experience has not confirmed these optimistic predictions. For example, let us examine the postoperative adjuvant chemotherapy of early-stage breast cancer. Such chemotherapy at conventional doses does reduce the probability of patients developing obvious distant metastases and does result in improved survival, but this effect is relatively modest (13). What are the reasons for this divergence between theory and data? Is it because the chemotherapy duration is too short? The log-kill model allows for this possibility. To illustrate this, let us assume that a given drug treatment causes a one-log kill with each application. Six cycles of that treatment should reduce tumors of 10^6 cells to just one cell. For this reason, six cycles should cure tumors of fewer than 10^6 cells. Tumors of more than 10^6 cells would merely need more cycles. Yet the hard fact is that adjuvant chemotherapy programs longer than 4 to 6 months do not improve results in the treatment of primary breast cancer (13). Hence, the failure of the log-kill model to predict the modest effect of adjuvant chemotherapy cannot be explained by insufficient duration of treatment.

Is there another explanation consistent with both the log-kill model and the data? Two major assumptions are exponential growth and homogeneous sensitivity to a given chemotherapy. The model does not work well if some cells in the tumor are biochemically refractory to the applied dose levels of the agents used. By "biochemically refractory" we do not have to mean resistance is also germane. Nevertheless, the assumption of the presence of absolutely resistant cells is a powerful concept. If such cells exist, once all sensitive cells are eliminated by a certain duration of treatment, more chemotherapy of the same type will not help. Skipper and colleagues dealt with this pitfall by invoking the concept that such resistance is acquired by random mutation during a cancer's growth history. In this case, the only way to guarantee the absence of resistant cells is to initiate therapy when the tumor is so small that recalcitrant mutants have not yet had time to emerge. Drug-resistant cells are indeed rarely found in small aliquots of Skipper's transplantable mouse leukemia. In human terms, this concept would mean that resistant cells would have to arise spontaneously between the time of the carcinogenic event and the appearance of larger, diagnosable tumors. The power of this idea is evident. To design universally effective drug therapies for cancer we need only answer two questions: When does drug resistance arise in the time-course of growth, and how can we diagnose cancer early enough to catch the disease before this happens (14, 18)?

THE DELBRÜCK-LURIA CONCEPT

To answer these two questions we consider quantitative models of the emergence of drug resistance. Drug resistance is a known fact in cancer therapeutics (15). The original theory of the rate of emergence of drug resistance was based on pioneering experiments in bacteriology in the 1940s by Luria and Delbrück. They discovered that different cultures of the same bacterial strain developed resistance to bacteriophage infection at different, random times prior to exposure to the viruses (16). They could measure the percentage of cells that had randomly acquired such

resistance by exposing each bacterial culture to the bacteriophage. The percentages varied from culture to culture, even though all cultures started off with the same number of the same bacteria. They reasoned that cultures that had experienced a mutation earlier in their growth histories had more time to develop a high percentage of resistant bacteria.

The mathematics of this phenomenon can be explained as follows: If a bacterium mutates toward property X with probability x at each mitosis, the probability of the cell not developing property X in one mitosis is $1 - x$. The probability of no mutations toward X occurring in y mitoses is $(1 - x)^y$. If each mitosis produces two viable cells (i.e., the assumption of no cell loss), it takes $N - 1$ mitoses for one cell to grow into N cells. Hence, the probability of not finding any bacteria with property X in N cells is exp $[(N - 1) * \ln(1 - x)]$, which is approximately exp $[-x(N - 1)]$, since, for small x, $\ln(1 - x)$ is approximately $-x$. In the case of cell loss, the probability will be smaller than exp$[-x(N - 1)]$.

Law found, within a decade of Delbrück and Luria's original observation in bacteria, that this same mathematical pattern applied to the emergence of methotrexate resistance in L1210 cells (17). Antimetabolite resistance was thus reasoned to be a trait acquired spontaneously at random times in the pretreatment growth of this cancer. Time has not diminished the enthusiasm of scientists for the quantitative concept of acquired mutations. Abnormalities in p53 or in other parts of the process regulating the entry of G^1 cells into S phase could disinhibit rereplication prior to M phase, so cells could produce aberrant levels of DNA (19–21). By this mechanism, aneuploidy as well as drug resistance should increase as a function of the number of passages through S phase. The presence of a significantly increased cell loss fraction would increase the probability of mutations per given cell number, since that cell number would then represent a significantly increased number of passages through S phase.

THE GOLDIE-COLDMAN MODEL

The genesis of combination chemotherapy— the foundation of modern medical oncology— was closely tied to the kinetic observations of Delbrück, Luria, Law, and others, at least in a qualitative sense (17). A therapist could be faced with a disease heterogeneous in drug sensitivity even at the time of first diagnosis if the tumor cells could acquire resistance to a drug prior to first exposure. In that case, the only hope for tumor eradication would rest with combinations of drugs. This hope was based on the improbability that any one cell could spontaneously become resistant to many different drugs with different biochemical sites of action (22). This statement was reexamined quantitatively in 1979 by Goldie and Coldman (23, 24), with later refinements to include multiple sublines with double or higher orders of drug resistance and the presence of cell loss (25). Their fundamental conclusion can be illustrated by reference to the expression $\exp[-x(N - 1)]$ derived above: At a tenable mutation rate $x = 10^{-6}$, the probability of no mutants in $N = 10^5$ cells is .905, but the probability of no mutants in 10^7 cells is .000045. Hence, a two-log growth can change a tumor from curable to incurable.

Although formulated to address the emergence of drug resistance, perhaps a better illustration of the power of this concept concerns the acquisition of metastatic ability, also a reflection of genetic lability (26). In primary breast cancer, the most reliable predictor of axillary metastases is tumor size. Only 17% of invasive ductal lesions under 1 cm in diameter are metastatic to the axilla, contrasted with 41% of lesions of 2 cm in diameter and 68% of tumors of 5 to 10 cm (27). The presence of axillary metastases, in turn, is the best predictor of eventual metastatic spread. For primary breast cancers that do not involve axillary lymph nodes, the probability of eventual distant metastases is also a function of tumor size. This probability increases sharply when the primary mass in the breast is found to be greater than 1 cm in diameter (28). The volume of 10^7 cancer cells is about 0.01 cc if the whole mass is cancer and about 1.0 cc if only 1% is cancer, 99% being benign host tissues like stromal cells, fibrosis, extracellular secretions, blood, and lymphatic vessels. A 1-cc spherical tumor, the critical size regarding prognostication in node-negative breast cancer, contains a volume of slightly over 0.5 cc. This is right in the middle of the range of 0.1 to 1.0 cc described above for 10^7 cells. Hence, clinical observations regarding the probability of metastases do fit the Goldie-Coldman model, although other explanations are possible, as described in the penultimate section of this chapter.

CLINICAL IMPLICATIONS OF THE GOLDIE-COLDMAN MODEL

The Goldie-Coldman model, focused on drug resistance, has generated testable predictions,

the foremost measure of the utility of a biomathematic formulation. The model predicts that a cancerous mass arising from a single drug-sensitive malignant cell has at most a 90% chance of being curable at 10^5 cells but almost no chance of being curable at 10^7 cells. Hence, even at the most liberal packing ratios of cancer cells to benign stroma, tumors larger than 1.0 cc should always be incurable with any single agent. The logical development of this idea is that the best strategy is to treat a cancer when it is as small as possible, before its cells can develop resistance. Once treatment is started, as many effective drugs as possible should be applied as soon as possible to prevent cells that are already resistant to one drug from mutating to resistance to others.

These recommendations are equivalent to the intuitive principles underlying combination chemotherapy, which were originally constructed to deal with drug resistance present at the time of first diagnosis (29). However, Goldie and Coldman went beyond this to suggest a novel treatment plan. They recognized that sometimes many drugs cannot be used simultaneously at good therapeutic levels because of overlapping toxicity or competitive interference. They reasoned that in this case, the drugs should be used in a strict alternating sequence. This hypothesis was based on several assumptions, concordant with the general mathematical term "symmetry." The first was that cells sensitive to a given therapy A (and resistant to therapy B) are as sensitive to therapy A as cells sensitive to therapy B (but resistant to therapy A) are sensitive to therapy B. The second was that the rate of mutation toward biochemical resistance is constant in both sublines, with cells sensitive to A mutating toward resistance to A, and cells sensitive to B mutating to resistance to B. The third assumption was that the growth pattern and growth rates of the two sublines were equivalent (30). With due respect, let us examine the assumptions, conclusions, and implications of this very important model.

However, before we turn to the specific aspects of the Goldie-Coldman model, we should reconsider the notion that all chemotherapeutic failure is rooted in *absolute* drug resistance. There is, indeed, much clinical experience to challenge this concept. When lymphomas and leukemias recur following chemotherapy-induced remission, they frequently respond to the same chemotherapy again! Patients with Hodgkin's disease who relapse 18 or more months after achieving complete remission from combination chemotherapy have an excellent chance of attaining complete remission again when the same chemotherapy is reapplied (31). Similarly, breast adenocarcinomas relapsing from postoperative adjuvant chemotherapy frequently respond to the same chemotherapy. For example, a Cancer and Leukemia Group B (CALGB) protocol treated patients with advanced breast cancer with cyclophosphamide, Adriamycin, and 5-fluorouracil (CAF) with or without tamoxifen (32). None of these patients had had prior chemotherapy for their advanced disease, but some had had prior adjuvant chemotherapy. Nevertheless, the odds of response, the duration of responses, and the overall probability of survival were unaffected by a patient's past history of adjuvant chemotherapy. A similar series of observations resulted from clinical trials at the National Cancer Institute in Milan. Patients who developed stage IV breast cancer after adjuvant cyclophosphamide, methotrexate, and 5-fluorouracil (CMF) responded as well to CMF for advanced disease as those who had been previously randomized to be treated with radical mastectomy alone (33). These findings mean that breast cancers that regrow after exposure to adjuvant CMF are not universally resistant to CMF (34), so all chemotherapeutic failure can not be due to permanent drug resistance. Although it is possible that some cancers escape cure because of a temporary absolute drug resistance that reverses over time, it is more likely that sensitive cells are somehow not completely eradicated by drugs to which they are still sensitive.

Before we consider the implications of this latter possibility, let us return to the specific conclusions of the Goldie-Coldman model. Are tumors larger than 1.0 cc always incurable with single drugs? The answer is no! Gestational choriocarcinoma and Burkitt's lymphoma, two rapidly growing cancers, have been cured with single drugs, even when therapy is initiated at tumor sizes much larger than 1.0 cc (35). Other counterexamples are childhood acute lymphoblastic leukemia, other pediatric cancers, adult lymphomas, and germ cell tumors, which are frequently cured with couplets and triplets of drugs. Hence, the presence of 10^7 cells does not always signify incurability. With respect to our previous discussion regarding metastatic potential, the presence of 10^7 cells does not always signify dissemination either.

In fact, the whole notion that cancers develop bad mutations rapidly as they grow is challenged by observations of the probability of metastatic disease. Standard practice until the late 19th century was not to operate on primary breast cancer, but to allow it to grow unperturbed, always to become metastatic (36). It has only recently been discovered that radical mastectomy in such cases, even without adjuvant treatment of any sort, interrupts the process; at 30 years of follow-up, more than 30% of patients are alive and free of disease (37, 38). The mortality rate, initially about 10% per year, drops gradually to about 2% per year by year 25 (39), and after 30 years is indistinguishable from that of the general population (40, 41). Hence, many, but not all, breast cancers have already developed metastases by the time of initial presentation, even though essentially all will develop metastases if left alone long enough. If local control is poor and the cancer cells in the breast are not completely removed or destroyed, will they mutate rapidly to produce metastatic clones? This question was asked by a protocol of the National Surgical Adjuvant Breast and Bowel Project (NSABP) in which some patients with primary disease were treated by lumpectomy without radiotherapy (42). The local relapse rate was significant, but survival was close to that of patients treated adequately de novo by lumpectomy plus immediate radiotherapy. Some metastases from residual cancer should be expected, even if the residual cells did not progress in their ability to release metastatic clones, so longer follow-up might eventually reveal a higher rate of distant metastases. However, the lack of a blatant difference so far indicates that tumor can remain in a breast, grow in the breast, and yet not develop metastatic cells at a very high rate as would be predicted by the Goldie-Coldman model.

What is the evidence that chemotherapy must be started as soon as possible after diagnosis to be effective? An early trial in the treatment of acute leukemia found that the response to an antimetabolite was the same if that drug was used first or sequentially after the use of a different antimetabolite (22). Hence, delay was not harmful, which contrasts with the prediction of the Goldie-Coldman model. A randomized trial by the International (Ludwig) Breast Cancer Study Group found a similar result. Node-positive breast cancer patients were given either 7 months of chemotherapy starting within 36 hours of surgery or 6 months of chemotherapy starting about 4 weeks after surgery (43). The results were the same, so the delay was not harmful here either. Stage B nonseminomatous testicular cancer patients were randomized after retroperitoneal lymph node dissection to either two cycles of cisplatin combination chemotherapy or to untreated observation (44). At a median follow-up of 4 years, 49% of patients randomized to observation relapsed, contrasted with only 6% of patients randomized to adjuvant chemotherapy. Yet the response of relapsing cases to subsequent chemotherapy was excellent, so there was no significant survival difference between the two approaches! Hence, most testicular carcinomas retained their chemosensitivity in spite of the delay in the initiation of treatment. In all of these examples, cells that are residual after surgery grow unimpeded without rapidly developing drug-resistant mutants.

Must all drugs in an adjuvant regimen be introduced early to have a biologic impact? A trial by the CALGB has concluded that this is not the case (45, 46). Patients with primary breast cancer and positive axillary lymph nodes were treated with 8 months of adjuvant CMF plus vincristine and prednisone (CMFVP) followed by either more CMFVP or 6 months of vinblastine, Adriamycin, thiotepa, and halotestin (VATH). Patients, especially those with four or more involved axillary nodes, receiving the crossover therapy experienced a significantly improved disease-free survival. Clearly, overwhelming resistance to VATH did not develop rapidly in the cells not eradicated by the CMFVP. The effect was not pronounced in patients with better prognoses. Similarly, a trial in Milan found no advantage to Adriamycin following CMF for patients with one to three involved nodes (47). This may be because of the impact of relative risk reduction: If the crossover works for all patients by reducing the rate of relapse by a certain percentage of that rate, those with lower rates of relapse without the crossover would experience a lower absolute benefit from the crossover than those at higher risk of relapse. Hence, the effect would exist in good-prognosis patients, but be more apparent in those with poorer prognoses (13).

The unique assertion of the Goldie-Coldman model concerns alternating chemotherapy sequences. In the clinic, however, this strategy has not demonstrated superiority. There has been little benefit in numerous attempts to use alternating chemotherapy sequences in the treatment of small cell lung cancer (48). In the treatment of diffuse aggressive non-Hodgkin's lymphoma, a National Cancer Institute trial found no advantage to a ProMACE-MOPP hybrid, which delivered eight drugs during each monthly cycle, over a full course of ProMACE (prednisone, methotrexate, Adriamycin, cyclophosphamide, etoposide) followed by MOPP (mechloreth-

amine, vincristine, procarbazine, prednisone) (49). In the treatment of advanced Hodgkin's disease, MOPP has been compared with MOPP alternating with Adriamycin, bleomycin, vinblastine, and decarbazine (ABVD), an effective first-line therapy and salvage regimen for patients refractory to MOPP (50, 51). MOPP-ABVD was found to be superior to MOPP in producing complete remission in chemotherapy-naive patients and in freedom from progression and survival (52, 53). An ABVD control arm was not studied. It is interesting, therefore, that the CALGB found that the complete remission rate and failure-free survival from MOPP-ABVD was better than that from MOPP alone but equivalent to ABVD alone (54). The superiority of MOPP-ABVD and ABVD over MOPP may have been due to differences in dose received. Only about 40% of MOPP patients received full doses of the cytotoxic agents by cycle three, compared with more than 70% on ABVD and on MOPP-ABVD. There was no advantage to the alternating scheme MOPP-ABVD over just ABVD alone. A similar result was found by the National Cancer Institute in its study of MOPP alternating with lomustine, Adriamycin, bleomycin, and streptozocin, which was equivalent to the use of MOPP alone (55). An Intergroup trial found that a hybrid of MOPP-ABVD was superior in complete remission duration, failure-free survival, and overall survival to MOPP followed by ABVD, but dose-received percentages were also an issue here (56). Patients treated with the hybrid regimen received higher doses because MOPP followed by ABVD required more dose modifications because of toxicity.

SEQUENTIAL CHEMOTHERAPY

As with the lymphomas, alternating strategies have not proven superior in the treatment of breast cancer. The VATH regimen is active against tumors relapsing from, or failing to respond to, CMF and thereby meets the criterion of non-cross-resistance (47). Yet in patients with advanced disease, the CALGB found no advantage to CMFVP alternating with VATH over CAF or VATH alone (58). In the adjuvant setting, a direct comparison of alternating and sequential chemotherapy was conducted in Milan. The sequential approach was previously described by reference to the use of VATH after CMFVP by the CALGB, also in the adjuvant setting. The National Cancer Institute in Milan had had a previous positive experience with sequential chemotherapy (59), but this was not a randomized trial testing the concept (60). To test the concept, Bonadonna and his colleagues randomized female patients with stage II breast cancer involving four or more axillary lymph nodes to one of two arms (61). Arm I prescribed four 3-week courses of doxorubicin (D) followed by eight 3-week courses of intravenous CMF (C), symbolized by DDDDCCCCCCCC. Arm II applied two courses of intravenous CMF alternating with one course of doxorubicin, repeated four times for a total of 12 courses. This may be symbolized by CCDCCDCCDCCD. The total amounts of doxorubicin and CMF in both arms were equal, as was the duration of therapy and the spacing of cycles. Remarkably, the patients who received arm I had a higher disease-free survival and a higher overall survival than those on arm II. At equivalent received doses, alternating courses of chemotherapy were found to be inferior to a crossover therapy plan (62).

The sequential chemotherapy strategy is also useful in the treatment of leukemia (63–66). In adult acute myelogenous leukemia, complete remission is obtained commonly with cytarabine plus anthracyclines. However, the median remission duration tends to be short. Given at low doses, postremission maintenance therapy is relatively ineffective, and this is not improved by a longer duration of treatment (32 months vs. 8 months of the same therapy). A more recent trial questioned the effectiveness of intensive rather than conventionally dosed postremission chemotherapy, basing its rationale on the steep dose-response curve for cytarabine. The trial studied 596 of 1088 patients who had achieved complete remission from standard induction chemotherapy and found that the highest-dose regimen was the best of three different dose schedules of cytarabine. In fact, the best results were comparable to those reported in patients with similar disease who were treated by allogeneic bone marrow transplantation during first remission. In support of this result, the Children's Cancer Study Group found that intensive induction followed sequentially by intensive consolidation and later intensification was superior to other strategies in the treatment of childhood acute lymphoblastic leukemia (67).

These observations in breast cancer and leukemia suggest that strategies other than repeated cycles of the same chemotherapy or strict alternation of conventionally dosed courses of chemotherapy may have significant clinical impact. They also illustrate that growth curve analysis is relevant to treatment design. Both the Skipper-Schabel-Wilcox and the Goldie-Coldman models illuminate aspects of aspects of cancer biology, including concepts of drug resistance. However, advances in the field of growth curve analysis may require a reevaluation of two assumptions intrinsic to these models: the concept of absolute drug resistance and the pattern of exponential growth.

IMPLICATIONS OF RELATIVE DRUG RESISTANCE

"Dose intensity," a term defined and popularized by the work of Hryniuk, is a method of classifying regimens using variables of dose level and time (77). It is, in essence, the total amount of drug received divided by the time over which it was administered. If regimen I gives x amount of drug over y days, and if regimen II gives $2x$ amount of drug over y days, then regimen II is clearly more dose intensive. Regimen III, giving x amount of drug over $y/2$ days, is as intensive as regimen II, by strict definition, but may be less effective in killing cancer cells if the total dose received is more important than the rate of drug delivery. Sometimes, once a certain minimal total dose is achieved, further increases in total dose are unimportant, as in the case of adjuvant breast cancer chemotherapy regimens longer than about 6 months (13, 68–70). It is important, in the discussion to follow, to distinguish dose intensity achieved by elevation of dose level (e.g., $2x$ over y days vs. x over y days) from that achieved by increased dose density (e.g., x over $y/2$ days vs. x over y days).

Extensive experimental evidence has established that much drug resistance is relative rather than absolute (71). In relative drug resistance, the probability of cell death depends upon the dose level employed (72, 73). In many animal experiments, log-kill is greater for the regimen with a higher dose intensity (72). In the clinic, even two-fold increases in dose level can have profoundly beneficial impact (74). This is not always seen with all drugs nor in all diseases (75). Yet in retrospective analyses, dose level seemed to be of major positive importance in adjuvant breast cancer chemotherapy (76, 77) and in the chemotherapy of advanced lymphoma (78). While the reliability of retrospective analyses is moot (79, 80), prospective trials are under way (81), and randomized trials in many diseases (childhood acute lymphoblastic leukemia (82), adult germ cell tumors (83), advanced breast cancer (84), and breast cancer in the adjuvant setting (85)) have found a rising dose-benefit curve.

While the shape of the dose-level versus cell-kill curve is not totally clear for any drug, some data suggest a strictly proportional relationship for some agents. A good example is a CALGB randomized trial in the adjuvant chemotherapy of breast cancer that treated node-positive patients by one of three plans of CAF (cyclophosphamide, doxorubicin, 5-fluorouracil) (85). Let z equal a certain total cumulative dose of CAF. Plan I gave $2z$ over 4 months, plan II gave $2z$ over 6 months, and plan III gave z over 4 months. Plan I was superior to plan III in reducing the rate of recurrence, but no difference has been reported between plans I and II. The total anticancer influence of CAF, therefore, seems to be strictly proportional to the total dose administered. For plan I, it was $2z$, the sum of $2z$ over the first 4 months plus zero for the 2 additional months. Plan II also gave $2z$ but spread out over 6 months. Plan III delivered z, which is half as much total anticancer influence, the sum of z over the first 4 months plus zero for the remaining 2 months. If CAF chemotherapy cures some patients, then plan I should eventually prove to be superior to plan II, because the log-kill accomplished at 4 months from $2z$ given over 4 months should be greater than the log-kill at 4 or 6 months from $2z$ given over 6 months, and that greater log-kill might be enough to cure some cancers.

The importance of this analysis rests in its suggestion that clinical treatment failure may be the consequence of insufficient dose density; $2z$ over 6 months, when it could have been given over 4 months, may not be the optimal way of using the drugs. By this hypothesis, a tumor may relapse because some of its cells (relatively, but not absolutely, insensitive to the agents applied) are not exposed to enough drug over a short enough time to be eradicated (18, 86). This may be analogous to the antibiotic chemotherapy of bacterial infections. Spreading an otherwise effective antibiotic regimen over too long a duration of treatment may not only allow bacteria to fail to be eradicated but also may give them the opportunity to develop drug resistance. The ability of increased dose density to improve clinical results depends highly on the shape or "steepness" of the dose-level versus cell-kill curve for each agent for each disease. It also depends on the shape of the tumor growth curve, which we have so far assumed to be exponential. However, as discussed below, growth curves that deviate significantly from exponentiality may be the rule, rather than the exception, in clinical cancer.

THE GOMPERTZIAN MODEL

Do all clinical cancers grow exponentially? Some lesions, particularly lung nodules, have been observed to follow exponential growth curves during periods of observation that are short in relationship to their total life histories (87–89). As previously noted, doubling times, a purely exponential concept, ranging from 1 week to 1 year, with a median of between 1 and 3 months, correlate with histologic type of cancer and some characteristics of clinical course. Yet measuring a doubling time does not prove that a tumor is growing exponentially, since that doubling time may not be constant over the whole range of sizes the tumor may assume over its life history.

It is now clear that many, if not all, human cancers do not grow exponentially (90–92). Examination of local recurrences of breast cancer has led some investigators to question the assumption that such cancers grow steadily (93). In these cases, the tumor size was measured at recurrence, and an extrapolation, following exponential kinetics, predicted the tumor size at a previous time when the patient had been examined. The absence of tumor noted at that previous time led these investigators to conclude that the regrowth had to have followed a period of dormancy. Another explanation concerns tumor geometry. If tumors always grow from a collection of cells outward like an expanding sphere, their reasoning would be correct. It would be similar to an army marching down a road, detectable from a great distance and appearing slowly. However, some cancers, especially skin metastases, first grow as reaching tendrils, later expanding to fill the space between the thin arms, like a tree filling out with leaves in the spring. This pattern is similar to an army hiding behind trees in a forest; each soldier need take only one step for the forest to seem suddenly saturated. In this case, estimation of population number at a previous time, based on measurements only at the time of diagnosis, would be unreliable.

A particular nonexponential growth pattern that has been found empirically to apply to many experimental and clinical cancers was first described by Benjamin Gompertz in 1825 (94). In Gompertzian growth, the doubling time increases steadily as the tumor grows larger, which means that the tumor grows progressively more slowly. This slowing may result more from decreased cell production than from increased cell loss as the tumor grows larger (12,

94). One important clinical characteristic of Gompertzian growth bears special mention. If a Gompertzian tumor is erroneously assumed to grow exponentially, the doubling time during the preclinical phase of growth will be assumed to be too long (95). Hence, the assumption of exponentiality had led to some unrealistically long estimates of the length of time from carcinogenesis to the appearance of clinical disease.

There is no commonly accepted theory that provides the biologic basis for Gompertzian growth. An old concept, now regarded as untenable, is that a solid tumor "outgrows" its supply of nutrients and, therefore, cannot sustain its otherwise natural tendency for exponential growth. Evidence against this is that large tumors, with relatively slow growth rates, often have adequate vascularity. Indeed, neovascularization is an important characteristic of malignancy (96). A newer, more molecular concept concerns the relationship between the cancer cell and its stromal environment (97, 98). Most biologic tissues, including cancers, are composed anatomically of fractals, or repeating elements. Examples are branching tree patterns, as in normal breasts and ductal adenocarcinomas of the breast, and multiple nodules, as in striated muscles and sarcomas. Fractals are self-similar over various scales of size, which means that a piece resembles the whole. A small branch of the ductal tree resembles a larger branch, which in turn resembles the whole tree. A characteristic of this type of structure is that the number of cells is proportional to the tissue volume raised to a power less than or equal to one. That power constant, called the *mass dimension*, is a function of the packing ratio, the percentage of the mass that is actually composed of cells. Low packing ratios (i.e., few cells per unit volume) translate to low power constants. It is apparent and may be profoundly meaningful biologically that loosely packed tumors, with relatively few cells per microscopic field, tend to be more benign, while cancers with densely packed cancer cells and little intervening stroma tend to be more malignant. This suggests a relationship between the fractal mass dimension, growth, and clinical aggressiveness.

Masses growing in a manner that preserves the power relationship between cell number and volume follow a Gompertzian curve (97, 98). The mass dimension, in fact, determines the shape of the Gompertzian curve, all else being equal. Values close to one give more aggressive growth, with little deviation from exponentiality. That is,

the doubling time stays close to constant. Mass dimensions much smaller than one produce Gompertzian curves with rapidly lengthening doubling times. Indeed, the doubling time can become so long that the mass can never double within the lifetime of the host. The mass hovers close to a plateau volume. A tumor with low mass dimension may plateau at a size so small that it is benign, as in ductal carcinoma in situ of the breast. (The other variable that determines the plateau size is the permissiveness of the stroma, how much the stroma will allow the tumor to grow or even support its growth. It is possible that a tumor can have a very high mass dimension and, therefore, a high packing ratio and still not grow very large because the allowance of the stroma is very low. This could account for densely packed benign tumors such as fibroadenomas.)

The mathematics of fractal growth presents an intriguing observation. Imagine that the mass dimension is not constant but changes, perhaps as a consequence of hormonal changes, multiple sequential mutations, or other genomic events. The interesting observation is that as a mass dimension increases slowly from very small toward one, the plateau size of the mass increases very slowly *until* the mass dimension crosses a threshold, at which time the plateau size suddenly becomes huge. This means that in a situation in which the mass dimension is slowly increasing, a precancerous mass can stay benign for a very long time but can suddenly become malignant with just a small additional increment in the power constant as it passes over a certain threshold. Hence, fractal geometry may provide some interesting clues regarding preneoplasia, malignant transformation, and Gompertzian growth kinetics. An important topic for study is the molecular basis of the mass dimension and the "allowance" characteristics of the cancer-stroma interaction. Indeed, there is now some evidence that mitotic disregulation (a putative determinant of mass dimension, i.e., cell packing) alone is not sufficient for neoplasia (99) but that a change in stromal allowance is also obligatory (100).

Gompertzian growth has many important biologic characteristics of direct relevance to the therapist. Some of these are illustrated below using a new model of human breast cancer (101). However, models more complex than simple exponential, or even simple Gompertzian, growth have been proposed. One in particular deserves note and consideration because it presents some interesting data and analysis.

THE SPEER-RETSKY MODEL

Speer, Retsky, and colleagues have presented a detailed study of several key data sets of relevance to the growth kineticist. The first is survival histories from 19th century breast cancer patients followed from diagnosis to death without surgery or any other effective treatment (36). The second is growth histories of mammographic shadows (102), and the third is data for disease-free survival following mastectomy (103). They fit a model in which tumors grow in randomly increasing steps of Gompertzian plateaus, so the overall growth pattern resembles an irregular Gompertzian curve (104). This work demonstrates that growth curves that deviate far from exponentiality can fit clinical data. However, it is questionable if the temporary plateaus that are predicted by the model are ever actually observed (105). Also, the Speer-Retsky model predicts a clinical plan of treatment that has proven ineffective in a clinical trial (106). Their suggestion was that postsurgical adjuvant chemotherapy should be applied intermittently over a prolonged duration so as to coincide with the anticipated growth spurts. While the failure of delayed "reinduction" with CMF after initial AC (doxorubicin plus cyclophosphamide) has been regarded as evidence against the Speer-Retsky model, a trial in high-dose chemotherapy of advanced breast cancer may be interpreted in a different light. In the latter study, patients with complete remissions induced by conventionally dosed chemotherapy were randomized to be treated immediately with high-dose chemotherapy or at the time of recurrence for complete remission. The patients who received the delayed chemotherapy "intensification" had a significantly improved overall survival (107). Many interpretations of these data are possible, so no firm conclusions regarding the validity or irrelevance of any model are appropriate at this time. Nevertheless, the notion that chemotherapy timed to coincide with tumor growth or regrowth is more effective than chemotherapy given during tumor growth quiescence may deserve further kinetic study.

The major criticism of the Speer-Retsky model was based on the philosophical concept of parsimony. The same clinical data used by Speer and Retsky can be fit more parsimoniously, and with greater accuracy, by a family of simple Gompertzian curves (101). Other curves, such as a family of exponential curves, could also be used to fit these data, but less successfully.

For example, exponential curves predict too short a time from relapse to death. The median curve from the family of simple Gompertzian curves would take just 3.5 months to increase by two logs from 10^2 to 10^4 but 5.5 months for 10^9 cells to grow just one log to 10^{10}. This is a realistic example of the increasing doubling time with increasing tumor volume that is characteristic of Gompertzian growth. Regardless of the validity of the Speer-Retsky model, since the overall growth curve predicted by their analysis may be smoothed to a Gompertzian curve, the clinical implications of Gompertzian growth are still germane.

THE NORTON-SIMON MODEL

Although Gompertzian growth, as a smooth function or as an approximation of an irregular growth pattern, is at least consistent with the growth of some human cancers, the problem of the pattern of regression of cancer in response to chemotherapy remains. A major reason why the Skipper-Schabel-Wilcox model is so meaningful is that it conceptualizes both tumor growth (exponential) and tumor regression (log-kill). We have seen that there are profound implications to the positive association between the rate of tumor regression and the dose intensity of chemotherapy. The rate of regression is also positively correlated with the growth rate just prior to treatment of the unperturbed tumor (32, 108, 109). If a tumor grew exponentially, its growth rate would always be proportional to tumor size. If an exponential tumor at size x is growing at rate y, the same tumor at size $2x$ would grow at rate $2y$. The rate of growth per tumor size (y/x) is the same in both cases. A rate of regression proportional to growth rate is, therefore, also proportional to tumor size; this results in a constant log-kill. For example, if an exponential tumor at size x shrinks at rate z to achieve a size $x/2$ in 1 week, this tumor or an identical tumor treated at size $2x$ with the same chemotherapy would shrink at rate $2z$ to achieve size x in 1 week, the same proportional change or log-kill.

The only important distinction between the Skipper-Schabel-Wilcox model and the Norton-Simon model is that in Gompertzian growth, unlike exponential growth, the growth rate of the unperturbed tumor is always changing. That is, if tumor at size x grows at rate y, the same tumor at size $2x$ would not grow at rate $2y$ but at a rate less than $2y$. Hence, the rate of regression relative to tumor size in response to an identical therapy would be proportional to y/x at size x and less than y/x at size $2x$. This means that the log-kill would be greater for very small cancers than for very large tumors.

The recognition of this phenomenon initially created much anticipation for the expected curative impact of chemotherapy against micrometastatic cancers. However, small cancers also regrow very quickly after perturbation. Gompertzian growth is, indeed, an efficient homeostatic system; at or close to plateau size, it is resistant to interference, but should it be reduced to small size, it can rebound quickly. As a consequence, Gompertzian tumors are difficult to eradicate, unless the impact of therapy is so great that regrowth is precluded.

For example, consider a tumor diagnosed at 10^{10} cells (about 100 cc at a packing ratio of 1:10, or 5 cm in diameter). Let 90% of the tumor be in the breast and axillary lymph nodes and the rest be scattered micrometastatically. If this primary tumor and the axillary contents are eradicated by surgery, with or without radiation therapy, there would still be 10^{9} metastatic cells in the body, invisible to our diagnostic tests. In the absence of adjuvant drug therapy, the tumor grows for 13.5 months, until it reaches about 10^{11} cells, large enough to be detected as metastases. Chemotherapy for advanced disease reduces the total cell number by two logarithms to about 10^{9}, but the same tumor eventually relapses, causing death at 10^{12} cells. If the same chemotherapy used in the advanced disease setting were given immediately after surgery, the relative rate of regression of the 10^{9}-cell tumor would be faster than that at 10^{11} cells. In fact, the same chemotherapy that caused a two-log kill of 10^{11} cells would be expected to cause instead a five-log kill of 10^{9} cells. These 10^{4} cells, however, can also regrow to relapse as stage IV disease at 10^{11} cells and to cause death at 10^{12} cells. The interesting observation is that while the time from surgery to stage IV is longer when the adjuvant chemotherapy is applied, the time from surgery to death would be identical in both circumstances. The greater fractional kill in the adjuvant setting is counterbalanced by a faster fractional regrowth. If some effective therapy is used when stage IV disease is diagnosed following the failure of adjuvant chemotherapy, the survival of the patient may be improved somewhat, so the patient who received adjuvant chemotherapy might live slightly longer than one who did not. But the adjuvant chemotherapy of breast cancer has less impact on overall survival than on dis-

ease-free survival. Gompertzian growth may explain why the survival of patients with stage IV breast cancer has improved just slightly in spite of more aggressive approaches to management in recent decades (110–112).

Would more aggressive (i.e., toxic) chemotherapy help? Imagine that such treatment reduces 10^{9} cells to 10^{2} cells instead of 10^{4}. By Gompertzian kinetics the growth from 10^{2} cells to 10^{4} cells is so rapid it would take just 3.5 months longer for the tumor to reach 10^{12}. For this reason, adjuvant drug therapies can differ greatly in log-kill but produce only marginal differences on survival results measured years later. The optimistic side of this analysis is that current adjuvant chemotherapies for breast cancer are probably bringing us much closer to total cellular eradication than we might otherwise be led to suspect from the modest clinical benefits observed.

By the Norton-Simon model, survival can be really improved only when tumor cell populations are precluded from regrowth, as by being eradicated. How can this be accomplished? Heterogeneity in drug sensitivity is a characteristic of neoplasia, so multiple drugs or multiple regimens are clearly needed in most settings. Gompertzian regression is often slow at macroscopic or large microscopic tumor sizes, so multiple cycles are rational. We have seen that the Goldie-Coldman concept of strictly alternating cycles has not yet proven useful clinically, but sequential chemotherapy has helped in some diseases. How can this be explained? In Gompertzian regression, slower-growing tumor cells tend to regress more slowly in response to a given therapy than faster-growing tumor cells of the same biochemical sensitivity (113). In a cancer heterogeneous in growth rate, therefore, the slower-growing clones are also the most kinetically resistant to chemotherapy. These slower-growing cells would likely be overgrown by faster-growing cells by the time of diagnosis, although they may increase in proportion in the selective environment of chemotherapy or, paradoxically, from a differentiating effect of subcurative chemotherapy (114).

How can we eradicate both the dominant, fast-growing, chemotherapy-responsive cells and the slower-growing, kinetically resistant cells? The Norton-Simon model suggests that the best way is to treat the faster-growing populations as efficiently as possible and then treat the numerically inferior, slower-growing populations as efficiently as possible (60). As shown by

Skipper and much clinical experience, the most efficient therapy is the most dose-intense therapy, giving as much drug as possible over as short a period as possible. Escalating dose level, however, may not be the optimal approach, especially if the dose-level/response relationship is not known. A more robust method of increasing dose intensity is to increase dose density, giving doses more closely together in time. This is accomplished by sequential therapy but not by strict alternation.

Sequential therapy has been successful in the laboratory. Alkylating agents seem particularly helpful as the crossover drugs; 10^8 L1210 cells may be cured by cytosine arabinoside plus 6-thioguanine for two or three courses, followed by one course of high doses of simultaneous cyclophosphamide and BCNU (115). BDF1 mice bearing the M5076 tumor experience a doubling of the complete remission rate and the median survival duration by the addition of one dose of L-phenylalanine mustard (L-PAM)—a drug that by itself is only weakly active—after four doses of methyl-CCNU (120). This latter effect is consistent with the hypothesis that the few cells left after methyl-CCNU induction are L-PAM sensitive, whereas in the untreated situation, most cells are methyl-CCNU sensitive but L-PAM resistant.

In the adjuvant breast cancer trial from Milan, the alternating plan, CCDCCDCCDCCD, gave eight cycles of CMF over 30 weeks and four cycles of doxorubicin over 33 weeks (62). The crossover plan, DDDDCCCCCCCC, gave eight cycles of CMF over 33 weeks and four cycles of doxorubicin over 9 weeks. The dose intensity of the CMF was almost the same; but for doxorubicin, it was significantly improved by the crossover. Using the doxorubicin earlier and more densely might also have minimized the expression of the multidrug-resistance gene, which tends to progress over time, independent of treatment (116, 117). Similarly, in the adjuvant chemotherapy of resected osteosarcoma, doxorubicin alone was superior to doxorubicin alternating with high-dose methotrexate; the dose density of the superior agent, doxorubicin, was impaired by the alternation (118). In other treatments previously described (ABVD following prolonged MOPP for advanced Hodgkin's disease (121) and doxorubicin following 6 months of CMF for primary breast cancer with low degrees of nodal involvement), the delayed use of doxorubicin might have compromised efficacy by this mechanism (47). A pilot study in breast cancer used Adria-

mycin following just 16 weeks of CMFVP in patients with node-positive primary disease, which might not have been long enough for multidrug resistance to be a problem (119). The results of trials in acute leukemia in adults (65) and children (67) are also consistent with the concept that sequential chemotherapy, by increasing dose density, improves clinical results. In these latter two examples, moreover, dose escalation was also accomplished, providing a double impact on dose intensity.

This double impact may be critical for further improvements in the efficacy of chemotherapy until agents or novel combinations of agents with higher cell-kill per dose are realized. As discussed above, the Goldie-Coldman model assumed symmetry: equal-sized tumor cell populations and equal rates of growth and mutation. Day extended the Goldie-Coldman model by performing computer simulations of mutation to drug resistance under asymmetrical conditions (121). His conclusion was similar to the Norton-Simon model in the expected superiority of a crossover plan (122). By his "worst drug rule," the therapy with a lower cell-kill per treatment (the worst drug) should be used either first or, if used second, for a longer duration. The Norton-Simon model finds that the induction therapy must be sufficiently cytoreductive for the residual tumor cell burden to be low. This might be why ABVD following dose-reduced MOPP was inferior to a hybrid MOPP/ABV delivered at fuller dosages (56). An efficient induction followed in sequence by one or more effective non-cross-resistant treatments would be ideal. Indeed, in the treatment of acute lymphocytic leukemia in children, a classic trial demonstrated that induction by vincristine plus prednisone facilitates the anticancer activity of methotrexate given in sequence (123). The Children's Cancer Study Group trial in childhood leukemia gave intensive induction, consolidation, and intensification, thereby illustrating the importance of initial cytoreduction (67).

At present, a large number of trials are seeking to improve clinical results by increasing dose density and dose escalation. Achieving dose density has been made easier by the use of granulocyte growth factors and other means of hematopoietic support (124, 125). In the adjuvant chemotherapy of breast cancer, the Southwest Oncology Group is coordinating an Intergroup study of doxorubicin followed by granulocyte colony-stimulating factor (G-CSF)-supported high-dose cyclophosphamide versus a more conventional, simultaneous doxorubicin plus cyclophosphamide combination (126). Investigators at Memorial Sloan-Kettering Cancer Center have piloted a regimen called ATC that gives dose-dense doxorubicin followed by dose-dense paclitaxel followed by dose-dense cyclophosphamide (126). The Intergroup plans to conduct a randomized comparison of this regimen with another form of dose intensification short-course high-dose combination chemotherapy with hematopoietic "stem cell" support in the treatment of women with stage II breast cancer and four to nine involved axillary lymph nodes. An ongoing adjuvant trial in Italy has randomized 718 early-stage breast cancer patients to a combination of cyclophosphamide, epirubicin, and 5-fluorouracil every 21 or every 14 days with G-CSF support (127). For diffuse large cell lymphoma, an experimental protocol has given induction doxorubicin, vincristine, plus prednisone followed in sequence by high-dose cyclophosphamide, then methotrexate plus vincristine, then etoposide, then L-PAM plus total body irradiation all with GM-CSF support. In a randomized comparison against a standard aggressive combination, this sequential plan has proven superior in complete remission rate, failure from relapse, failure from progression, and event-free survival (128).

BEYOND MITOTOXICITY

The Norton-Simon model does suggest that innovative dose-schedule schemes might be able to improve results in clinical anticancer chemotherapy. However, there is a dark side, and that is contained in the notion that failure to eradicate is tantamount to failure to cure or even to significantly alter long-term results in slow-growing cancers like breast cancer. However, a rapidly evolving modern view of anticancer therapy suggests that pharmacologic manipulations might be able to alter the biologic predeterminism of a cancer and thereby increase the odds that a cytoreduced tumor will never grow to become meaningful disease.

In fact, it is possible that the chemotherapy we currently use owes some of its beneficial impact to just such biologic modification. For example, we have seen that the rate of tumor regression is positively related to the rate of unperturbed growth. Tumors seem to regress most rapidly when they are growing most rapidly. In the past, we have used this observation to support the hypothesis that chemotherapy is a mitotic poison. In preparation for mitosis, cells

synthesize DNA and other macromolecules and are thereby at particular risk for cytotoxicity by drugs that interfere with such synthesis (129). The intuitive notion is that poisoning S phase renders cells incapable of progressing successfully through M phase. There is evidence to support this idea; hormones and growth factors increase both cell proliferation and cell kill from doxorubicin in MCF-7 cells in vitro (130). Estradiol enhances the cytotoxicity of melphalan in hormone-responsive cell lines (131). Hormone recruitment schemes have indeed resulted in high local response rates in locally advanced breast cancer in the clinic (132, 133). However, excluding data-driven subsets, hormone recruitment does not improve treatment results in stage III or in metastatic breast cancer (134–136). Hence, the assumed mitotoxicity of chemotherapy may merit further examination.

Contrary data, or at least data hinting at a deeper level of complexity, do exist. Tamoxifen causes a G^1-S arrest in sensitive cell lines and does antagonize the effects of melphalan and 5-fluorouracil, but this antagonism occurs at dose schedules that do not affect cell proliferation (131). Tamoxifen also augments chemotherapy in some cases; it actually enhances the cytotoxicity of doxorubicin and the alkylating agent 4-hydroxycyclophosphamide (131). When MCF-7 cells are exposed to low levels of doxorubicin, they do not show an immediate S-phase reduction but rather an accumulation of cells in late S, G^2, and M and a block of the G^1 to S transition starting 2 days after treatment (137). Clinically, only about 5% of the cells in an average breast cancer are in S phase. Hence, if chemotherapy were exclusively mitotoxic, the magnitude of the regressions seen in the clinic could not be explained (125). Nor could we explain the transient impact of chemotherapy on rapidly dividing bone marrow, alimentary mucosa, and hair follicles in contrast to its permanent impact on acute leukemias, malignant lymphomas, choriocarcinomas, and germ cell cancers. The magnitude of the thymidine labeling index of locally advanced breast cancer does not predict chemosensitivity (138), a topic under further study in node-negative patients (139).

While chemotherapy is assumed to be mitotoxic, hormonal therapies are known to modulate growth factor–stimulated transcription events upstream from the mitotic trigger (140). Yet the impact of adjuvant tamoxifen (141) and of adjuvant CMF (68) for breast cancer are qualitatively and qualitatively quite similar. Could chemotherapy and hormonal therapy share a similar mode of action, beyond mitotoxicity (142)? Breast cancer, for example, is modulated by endogenous growth factors secreted by a subset of tumor cells in an individual cancer (143) and by growth factors produced by the supporting stroma (144). For many cancers, malignant transformation alters gene expression for growth factors, their receptors, and intracellular signal transduction proteins (145). Leukemogenic drugs, such as alkylating agents, are known to cause cytogenetic abnormalities, frequently at loci coding for products related to growth factors (146).

Hematopoietic cells, deprived of essential growth factors, die by "apoptosis," an orderly process of programmed cell death (147, 148). Almost all chemotherapeutic drugs also cause apoptosis (149). The histologic analysis of breast cancers regressing after chemotherapy does not always reveal a high degree of necrosis, which is consistent with apoptosis (150). Consistent with an effect on host-tumor paracrine interactions is the observation that tumor resistance to alkylating agents could be operant in vivo but not in vitro (151).

Chemotherapy has, in fact, been observed to influence growth factor pathways in the laboratory. Doxorubicin upregulates epidermal growth factor receptors in HeLa and 3T3 cells (152). Activation of protein kinase C enhances the cytotoxicity of cisplatin without increasing drug uptake (153). In the treatment of human cancer xenografts, antibodies to the epidermal growth factor receptor, which can themselves inhibit growth (154), synergize with cisplatin (155). Such antibodies also synergize with doxorubicin in the treatment of A431 cells in athymic mice (156). Ongoing clinical trials are exploring the ability of antibodies to HER2 to synergize with doxorubicin plus cyclophosphamide and of antibodies to HER1 to synergize with paclitaxel.

If the pessimistic predictions of the Norton-Simon model prove valid and tumor regrowth precludes disease eradication in many cases, then the perturbation of growth factor pathways by agents designed for this purpose or by the biochemical modulation of existing chemotherapy effects may be a way of improving results in the clinic. Agents intended for this purpose are indeed coming to clinical trial: antibodies, kinase inhibitors, *ras* inhibitors, and other small molecules aimed at signal transduction and propagation. However, we already have on our side therapies that do cause tumor regression

and that do improve disease-free and overall survival and even, sometimes, cure. Their optimal use is still a priority in anticancer therapeutics. Hence, growth curve analysis has a place in modern oncology, to elucidate history, to explain data, to improve treatment with existing agents, and to predict a path toward the better treatments to come.

REFERENCES

1. Gilewski T, Norton L. Cytokinetics of neoplasia. In: Mendelsohn J, Howley P, Israel MA, Liotta LA, eds. The molecular basis of cancer. Philadelphia: WB Saunders, 1995:143–159.

2. Skipper HE, Schabel FM Jr, Wilcox WS. Experimental evaluation of potential anticancer agents XIII: on the criteria and kinetics associated with "curability" of experimental leukemia. Cancer Chemother Rep 1964;35:1–111.

3. Skipper HE. Laboratory models: the historical perspective. Cancer Treat Rep 1986;70:3–7.

4. Simpson-Herren L, Lloyd HH. Kinetic parameters and growth curves for experimental tumor systems. Cancer Chemother Rep 1970;54:143–174.

5. Frei E III. Models and the clinical dilemma. In: Fidler IJ, White RJ, eds. Design of models for testing therapeutic agents. New York: Van Nostrand Reinhold, 1982:248–259.

6. Goldin A, Venditti JM, Humphreys SR, Mantel N. Influence of the concentration of leukemic inoculum on the effectiveness of treatment. Science 1956;123:840.

7. Roosa R, Weaver CF, DeLamater ED. Importance of transplant size in chemotherapeutic assay with the use of the Gardner lymphosarcoma (abstract). Proc Am Assoc Cancer Res 1957;2:243.

8. Holland JF. Clinical studies of unmaintained remissions in acute lymphocytic leukemia. In: The proliferation and spread of neoplastic cells; 21st annual symposium on fundamental cancer research 1967, Univ. of Texas M. D. Anderson Hospital and Tumor Institute at Houston. Baltimore: Williams & Wilkins, 1968:453–462.

9. Schabel FM. Concepts for systemic treatment of micrometastases. Cancer 1975;35:15–24.

10. Shapiro DM, Fugmann RA. A role for chemotherapy as an adjunct to surgery. Cancer Res 1957; 17:1098–1101.

11. LaLa PK. Age-specific changes in the proliferation of Ehrlich ascites tumor cells grown as solid tumors. Cancer Res 1972;32:628–636.

12. Watson JV. The cell proliferation kinetics of the EMT6/M/AC mouse tumor at four volumes during unperturbed growth in vivo. Cell Tissue Kinet 1976; 9:147–156.

13. Early Breast Cancer Trialists' Collaborative Group. Treatment of early breast cancer: worldwide evidence in 1985–1990. A systematic overview of all available randomized trials in early breast cancer of adjuvant endocrine and cytotoxic therapy. New York: Oxford University Press, 1990.

14. DeVita VT. The relationship between tumor mass and resistance to treatment of cancer. Cancer 1983;51:1209–1220.

15. Givel JC, de Quay N, Albe X, Vassilakos P. Prognostic value of DNA ploidy of colorectal tumor cells. Helv Chir Acta 1989;55:679–683.

16. Luria SE, Delbrück M. Mutations of bacteria from virus sensitivity to virus resistance. Genetics 1943;28:491.

17. Law LW. Origin of resistance of leukaemic cells to folic acid antagonists. Nature 1952;169:628–629.

18. DeVita VT Jr. Dose-response is alive and well. J Clin Oncol 1986;4:1157–1159.

19. Hartwell LH, Weinert TA. Checkpoints: controls that ensure the order of cell cycle events. Science 1989;246:629–634.

20. Murray AW, Kirschner MW. Dominoes and clocks: the union of two views of the cell cycle. Science 1989;246:614–621.

21. Laskey RA, Fairman MP, Blow JJ. S phase of the cell cycle. Science 1989;246:609–614.

22. Frei E III, Freireich EJ, Gehan E, Pinkel D, Holland JF, et al. Studies of sequential and combination antimetabolite therapy in acute leukemia: 6-mercaptopurine and methotrexate. Blood 1961;18:431–454.

23. Goldie JH, Coldman AJ. A mathematic model for relating the drug sensitivity of tumors to their spontaneous mutation rate. Cancer Treat Rep 1979;63:1727–1733.

24. Goldie JH, Coldman AJ. Application of theoretical models to chemotherapy protocol design. Cancer Treat Rep 1986;70:127–131.

25. Goldie JH. Scientific basis for adjuvant and primary (neoadjuvant) chemotherapy. Semin Oncol 1987; 14:1–7.

26. Poste G, Fidler IJ. The pathogenesis of cancer metastases. Nature 1980;283:139–146.

27. National Cancer Institute (USA). Surveillance, Epidemiology and End Results (SEER) Program, 1974–1987.

28. Rosen PP, Groshen S. Factors influencing survival and prognosis in early breast carcinoma (T1N0M0-T1N1M0): assessment of 644 patients with median follow-up of 18 years. Surg Clin North Am 1990;70:937–962.

29. DeVita VT Jr, Young RC, Canellos GP. Combination vs. single agent chemotherapy: a review of the basis for selection of drug treatment of cancer. Cancer 1975;35:98–110.

30. Coldman AJ, Goldie JH. A mathematical model of drug resistance in neoplasms. In: Bruchovsky N, Goldie JH, eds. Drug and hormone resistance in neoplasia. Boca Raton, FL: CRC Press, 1982;1:55–78.

31. Dressler LG, Bartow SA. DNA flow cytometry in solid tumors: practical aspects and clinical applications. Semin Diagn Pathol 1989;6:55–82.

32. Kardinal CG, Perry MC, Korzun AH, Rice MA, Ginsberg S, Wood WC. Responses to chemotherapy or chemohormonal therapy in advanced breast cancer patients treated previously with adjuvant chemotherapy: a subset analysis of CALGB study 8081. Cancer 1988; 61:415–419.

33. Valagussa P, Tancini G, Bonadonna G. Salvage treatment of patients suffering relapse after adjuvant CMF chemotherapy. Cancer 1986;58:1411–1417.

34. Valagussa P, Brambilla C, Zambetti M, Bonadonna G. Salvage treatment after first relapse of breast cancer: a review. Third international conference on adjuvant therapy of primary breast cancer, St. Gallen, Switzerland, 1988:9.

35. Iversen OH, Iversen U, Ziegler JL, Bluming AZ. Cell kinetics in Burkitt's lymphoma. Eur J Cancer 1974; 10:155–163.

36. Bloom H, Richardson M, Harris B. Natural history of untreated breast cancer (1804–1933): comparison of treated and untreated cases according to histological grade of malignancy. Br Med J 1962;2:213–221.

37. Adair F, Berg J, Joubert L, Robbins GF. Long-term follow-up of breast cancer patients: the 30-year report. Cancer 1974;33:1145–1150.

38. Ferguson DJ, Meier P, Karrison T, Dawson PJ, Straus FH, Lowenstein FE. Staging of breast cancer and survival rates: an assessment based on 50 years experience with radical mastectomy. JAMA 1982;248:1337–1341.

39. Harris JR, Hellman S. Observations on survival curve analysis with particular reference to breast cancer. Cancer 1986;57:925–928.

40. Brinkley D, Haybittle JL. The curability of breast cancer. Lancet 1975;2:95–97.

41. Rutqvist LE, Wallgren A, Nilsson B. Is breast cancer a curable disease? A study of 14,731 women with breast cancer from the Cancer Registry of Norway. Cancer 1984;53:1793–1800.

42. Fisher B, Anderson S, Redmond CK, Wolmark N, Wickerham DL, Cronin WM. Reanalysis and results after 12 years of follow-up in a randomized clinical trial comparing total mastectomy with lumpectomy with or without irradiation in the treatment of breast cancer. N Engl J med 1995;333:1456–1461.

43. Ludwig Breast Cancer Study Group. Combination adjuvant chemotherapy for node-positive breast cancer. Inadequacy of a single perioperative cycle. N Engl J Med 1988;319:677–683.

44. Williams S, Stablein D, Einhorn L, Muggia F, Weiss R, et al. Immediate adjuvant chemotherapy versus observation with treatment at relapse in pathological stage II testicular cancer. N Engl J Med 1987; 317:1433–1438.

45. Korzun A, Norton L, Perloff M, Wood W, Carey R, et al. Clinical equivalence despite dosage differences of two schedules of cyclophosphamide, methotrexate, 5-fluorouracil, vincristine and prednisone (CMFVP) for adjuvant therapy of node-positive stage II breast cancer (abstract). Proc Am Soc Clin Oncol 1988;7:12.

46. Perloff M, Norton L, Korzun A, Wood W, Carey R, Weinberg V, Holland JF. Advantage of an adriamycin combination plus halotestin after initial CMFVP for adjuvant therapy of node-positive stage II breast cancer (abstract). Proc Am Soc Clin Oncol 1986;70:273.

47. Moliterni A, Bonadonna G, Valagussa P, Ferrari L, Zambetti M. Cyclophosphamide, methotrexate, fluorouracil with or without doxorubicin in the adjuvant treatment of resectable breast cancer with one to three positive axillary nodes. J Clin Oncol 1991;9:1124–1130.

48. Wampler GL, Heim WJ, Ellison NA, Ahlgren JD, Fryer JG, for the Mid-Atlantic Oncology Program. Comparison of cyclophosphamide, doxorubicin, vincristine with an alternating regimen of methotrexate, etoposide, cisplatin/cyclophosphamide, doxorubicin, vincristine in the treatment of extensive-disease small-cell lung cancer. J Clin Oncol 1991;9:1438–1445.

49. Longo DL, DeVita VT Jr, Duffey PL, Wesley MN, Ihde DC, et al. Superiority of ProMACE-CytaBOM over ProMACE-MOPP in the treatment of

advanced diffuse aggressive lymphoma: results of a prospective randomized trial. J Clin Oncol 1991;9:25–38.

50. Bonadonna G, Santoro A. ABVD chemotherapy in the treatment of Hodgkin's disease. Cancer Treat Rev 1982;9:21–35.

51. Santoro A, Bonfante V, Viviani S, Valagussa P, Bonadonna G. Salvage chemotherapy in relapsing Hodgkin's disease (abstract). Proc Am Soc Clin Oncol 1984;3:254.

52. Bonadonna G, Valagussa P, Santoro A. Alternating noncross-resistant combination chemotherapy or MOPP in stage IV Hodgkin's disease. Ann Intern Med 1986;104:739–746.

53. Valagussa P, Santoro A, Boracchi P, Viviani S, Bonadonna G. 9-year results of two randomized studies with MOPP and ABVD in Hodgkin's disease: multiple regression analysis (abstract). Proc Am Soc Clin Oncol 1989;8:976.

54. Canellos GP, Propert K, Cooper R, Nissen N, Andersen J, et al. MOPP vs. ABVD vs. MOPP alternating with ABVD in advanced Hodgkin's disease: a prospective randomized CALGB trial (abstract). Proc Am Soc Clin Oncol 1988;7:888.

55. Longo DL, Duffey PL, DeVita VT Jr, Wiernik PH, Hubbard SM, et al. Treatment of advanced-stage Hodgkin's disease: alternating noncrossresistant MOPP/CABS is not superior to MOPP. J Clin Oncol 1991;9:1409–1420.

56. Glick J, Tsiatis A, Schilsky R, Beck T, Oken M, Peterson B, Fisher R. A randomized phase III trial of MOPP/ABV hybrid vs. sequential MOPP-ABVD in advanced Hodgkin's disease: preliminary results of the Intergroup trial (abstract). Proc Am Soc Clin Oncol 1991;10:941.

58. Aisner J, Korsun A, Perloff M, Chiarieri D, Abrams J, et al. A randomized comparison of CAF, VATH, VATH alternating with CMFVP for advanced breast cancer, a CALGB study (abstract). Proc Am Soc Clin Oncol 1988;7:27.

59. Brambilla C, Rossi A, Valagussa P, Bonadonna G. Adjuvant chemotherapy in postmenopausal women: results of sequential noncross-resistant regimens. World J Surg 1985;9:728–737.

60. Norton L. Implications of kinetic heterogeneity in clinical oncology. Semin Oncol 1985;12:231–249.

61. Buzzoni R, Bonadonna G, Valagussa P, Zambetti M. Adjuvant chemotherapy with doxorubicin plus cyclophosphamide, methotrexate, fluorouracil in the treatment of resectable breast cancer with more than three positive axillary nodes. J Clin Oncol 1991; 9:2134–2140.

62. Bonadonna G, Zambetti M, Valgussa P. Sequential or alternating doxorubicin and CMF regimens in breast cancer with more than three positive nodes. Ten-year results. JAMA 1995;273:542–547.

63. Priesler H, Davis RB, Kirshner J, et al. Comparison of three remission induction regimens and two postinduction strategies for the treatment of acute nonlymphocytic leukemia: a Cancer and Leukemia Group B study. Blood 1987;69:1441–1449.

64. Cassileth PA, Lynch E, Hines JD, et al. Varying intensity of postremission therapy in acute myeloid leukemia. Blood 1992; 79:1924–1930.

65. Mayer RJ, Davis RB, Schiffer CA, et al. Intensive postremission chemotherapy in adults with acute myeloid leukemia. N Engl J Med 1994;331:896–903.

66. Bishop JF. Intensified therapy for acute myeloid leukemia (editorial). N Engl J Med 1994;331:941–942.

67. Tubergen D, Gilchrist G, Coccia P, Novak L, O'Brien R, et al. The role of intensified chemotherapy in intermediate risk acute lymphoblastic leukemia (ALL) of childhood (abstract). Proc Ann Mtg Am Soc Clin Oncol 1990;9:A835.

68. Bonadonna G, Valagussa P, Rossi A, Tancini G, Brambilla C, Zambetti M, Veronesi U. Ten-year experience with CMF-based adjuvant chemotherapy in resectable breast cancer. Breast Cancer Res Treat 1985; 5:95–115.

69. Henderson IC, Gelman RS, Harris JR, Canellos GP. Duration of therapy in adjuvant chemotherapy trials. NCI Monogr 1986;1:95–98.

70. Rivkin SE, Knight WA, McDivitt R, Cruz T, Foulkes M, et al. Adjuvant therapy for breast cancer with positive axillary nodes designed according to estrogen receptor status. J Steroid Biochem 1985;23:1151–1154.

71. Frei E, Teicher BA, Holden SA, Cathcart KN, Wang YY. Preclinical studies and clinical correlation of the effect of alkylating dose. Cancer Res 1988;48:6417–6423.

72. Bruce WR, Meeker BE, Valeriote FA. Comparison of the sensitivity of normal hematopoietic and transplanted lymphoma colony-forming cells to chemotherapeutic agents administered in vivo. J Natl Cancer Inst 1966;37:233–245.

73. Griswold DP Jr, Trader MW, Frei E III, Peters WP, Wolpert MK, Laster WR Jr. Response of drug-sensitive and -resistant L1210 leukemias to high-dose chemotherapy. Cancer Res 1987;47:2323–2327.

74. Franzini A, Broggi G, Giorgi C, Caiola L, Allegranza A. Predictive accuracy of cell kinetics data in glial tumors investigated by serial stereotactic biopsy. J Neurosurg Sci 1989;33:43–45.

75. Tattersall MHN, Parker LM, Pitman SW, Frei E III. Clinical pharmacology of high-dose methotrexate (NSC-740). Cancer Chemother Rep Part 3 1975;6:25–29.

76. Bonadonna G, Valagussa P. Dose-response effect of adjuvant chemotherapy in breast cancer. N Engl J Med 1981;304:10–15.

77. Hryniuk WM. The importance of dose intensity in the outcome of chemotherapy. In: DeVita VT Jr, Hellman S, Rosenberg SA, eds. Important advances in oncology 1988. Philadelphia: JB Lippincott, 1988:121–141.

78. DeVita VT, Hubbard SM, Longo DL. The chemotherapy of lymphomas: looking back, moving forward. The Richard and Hinda Rosenthal Foundation award lecture. Cancer Res 1987;47:5810–5824.

79. Henderson IC, Hayes DF, Gelman R. Dose-response in the treatment of breast cancer: a critical review. J Clin Oncol 1988;6:1501–1513.

80. Redmond C, Fisher B, Wieand HS. The methodological dilemma in retrospectively correlating the amount of chemotherapy received in adjuvant therapy protocols with disease-free survival. Cancer Treat Rep 1983;67:519–526.

81. Budman DR, Wood W, Korzun AH, Henderson IC, Cooper R, et al. CALGB 8541: a dose and dose intensity trial of cyclophosphamide, doxorubicin and 5-fluorouracil as adjuvant treatment of stage II, node positive female breast cancer (abstract). Proc Am Soc Clin Oncol 1991;10:129.

82. Pinkel D, Hernandez K, Borella L, Houlton C,

Aur R, Samoy G, Pratt C. Drug dosage and remission duration in childhood lymphocytic leukemia. Cancer 1971;27:247–256.

82a. Poste G, Fidler IJ. The pathogenesis of cancer metastases. Nature 1980;283:139–146.

83. Samson MK, Rivlin SE, Jones SE, Constanzi JJ, LoBuglio AF, et al. Dose-response and dose-survival advantage for high- vs. low-dose cisplatin combined with vinblastine and bleomycin in disseminated testicular cancer. Cancer 1984;53:1029–1035.

84. Tannock IF, Boyd NF, DeBoer G, Erlichman C, Fine S, et al. A randomized trial of two dose levels of cyclophosphamide, methotrexate, fluorouracil chemotherapy for patients with metastatic breast cancer. J Clin Oncol 1988;6:1377–1387.

85. Wood WC, Budman DR, Korzun AH, Cooper MR, Younger J, et al. Dose and dose intensity trial of adjuvant chemotherapy for stage II, node-positive breast carcinoma. New Engl J Med 1994;330:1253–1259.

86. Frei E III, Canellos GP. Dose: a critical factor in cancer chemotherapy. Am J Med 1980;69:585–594.

87. Collins VP, Loeffler K, Tivey H. Observations on growth rates of human tumors. Am J Roentgenol 1956;76:988–1000.

88. Steel GG. Growth kinetics of tumours—cell population kinetics in relation to the growth and treatment of cancer. Oxford: Clarendon Press, 1977:46–52.

89. Tubiana M. Tumor cell proliferation kinetics and tumor growth rate. Acta Oncol 1989;28:113–121.

90. Spratt JS, Greenberg RA, Heuser LS. Geometry, growth rates and duration of cancer and carcinoma in situ of the breast before detection by screening. Cancer Res 1986;46:970–974.

91. Demicheli R. Growth of testicular neoplasm lung metastases: tumor-specific relation between two Gompertzian parameters. Eur J Cancer 1980;16:1603–1608.

92. Sullivan PW, Salmon SE. Kinetics of tumor growth and regression in IgG multple myeloma. J Clin Invest 1972;51:1697–1708.

93. Demicheli R, Terenziani M, Valagussa P, Moliterni A, Zambetti M, Bonadonna G. Local recurrences following mastectomy: support for the concept of tumor dormancy. J Natl Cancer Inst 1994;86(1):45–48.

94. Laird AK. Dynamics of growth in tumors and normal organisms. NCI Monogr 1969;30:15–28.

95. Norton L. Mathematical interpretation of tumor growth kinetics. In: Greenspan EM, ed. Clinical interpretation and practice of cancer chemotherapy. New York: Raven, 1982:53–70.

96. Folkman J, Shing Y. Angiogenesis. J Biol Chem 1992;267:10931–10934.

97. Norton L. Introduction to clinical aspects of preneoplasia: a mathematical relationship between stromal paracrine autonomy and population size. In: Marks PA, Hans Türler H, Weil R, eds. Challenges of modern medicine, volume 1. Precancerous lesions: a multidisciplinary approach. Milan: Ares-Serono Symposia Publications, 1993:269–275.

98. Gilewski T, Norton L. Cytokinetics and breast cancer chemotherapy. In: Harris JR, Lippman ME, Morrow M, Hellman S, eds. Diseases of the breast. Philadelphia: Lippincott-Raven, 1995:751–768.

99. Norton L, Rosen PP, Rosen N. Refining the origins of breast cancer. Nature Med News Views 1995; 1:1250–1251.

100. Wakefield LM, Colletta AA, McCune BK, Sporn MB. Roles for transforming growth factors-beta in the genesis, prevention, treatment of breast cancer (review). Cancer Treat Res 1992;61:97–136.

101. Norton L. A Gompertzian model of human breast cancer growth. Cancer Res 1988;48:7067–7071.

102. Heuser L, Spratt J, Polk H. Growth rates of primary breast cancer. Cancer 1979;43:1888–1894.

103. Fisher B, Slack N, Katrych D, Wolmark N. Ten-year follow-up results in patients with carcinoma of the breast in a cooperative clinical trial evaluating surgical adjuvant chemotherapy. Surg Gynecol Obstet 1975;140:528–534.

104. Speer JF, Petrovsky VE, Retsky MW, Wardwell RH. A stochastic numerical model of breast cancer that simulates clinical data. Cancer Res 1984;44:4124–4130.

105. Norton L. Reply to letter to the editor. Cancer Res 1989;49:6444.

106. Fisher B, Brown AM, Dimitrov NV, Poisson R, Redmond C, et al. Two months of doxorubicin-cyclophosphamide with and without interval reinduction therapy compared with 6 months of cyclophosphamide, methotrexate, fluorouracil in positive-node breast cancer patients with tamoxifen-nonresponsive tumors: results from the National Surgical Adjuvant Breast and Bowel Project B-15. J Clin Oncol 1990; 8:1483–1496.

107. Peters WP, Jones RB, Vredenburgh J, Shpall EJ, Hussein A, et al. A large, prospective randomized trial of high-dose combination alkylating agents (CPB) with autologous cellular support (ABMS) as consolidation for patients with metastatic breast cancer achieving complete remission after intensive doxorubicin-based induction (AFM) (abstract 11). Br Cancer Res Treat 1995;37:35.

108. Norton L, Simon R. Growth curve of an experimental solid tumor following radiotherapy. J Natl Cancer Inst 1977;58:1735–1741.

109. Norton L, Simon R. Tumor size, sensitivity to therapy, and the design of treatment schedules. Cancer Treat Rep 1977;61:1307–1317.

110. Paterson AHG, Lees AW, Hanson J, Szafran O, Comish F. Impact of chemotherapy on survival in metastatic breast cancer (letter). Lancet 1980;2:312.

111. Powles TJ, Smith IE, Ford HT, Coombes RC, Jones JM, Gazet JC. Failure of chemotherapy to prolong survival in a group of patients with metastatic breast cancer. Lancet 1980;1:580–582.

112. Tormey D, Carbone P, Band P. Breast cancer survival in single and combination chemotherapy trials since 1968 (abstract). Proc Am Assoc Cancer Res 1977;18:64.

113. Norton L, Simon R. The Norton-Simon hypothesis revisited. Cancer Treat Rep 1986;70:163–169.

114. Ross DW, Capizzi RL. Differentiation vs. cytoreduction during remission induction in acute nonlymphoblastic leukemia treated with sequential high-dose ara-c and asparaginase. Cancer 1984;53:1651–1654.

115. Skipper HE. Analyses of multiarmed trials in which animals bearing different burdens of L1210 leukemia cells were treated with two, three, and four drug combinations delivered in different ways with varying dose intensities of each drug and varying average dose intensities. Southern Research Institute Booklet 7, 1986; 42:87.

116. Cordon-Cardo C, O'Brien JP. The multidrug

resistance phenotype in human cancer. In: DeVita VT Jr, Hellman S, Rosenberg SA, eds. Important advances in oncology 1991. New York: JB Lippincott, 1991:19–38.

117. Goldstein LJ, Galski H, Fojo A, Willingham M, Lai S-L, et al. Expression of multidrug resistance gene in human tumors. J Natl Cancer Inst 1989;81:116–124.

118. Cortes EP, Necheles TF, Holland JF, Carey RW, Blom J, et al. Adjuvant chemotherapy for primary osteosarcoma: a Cancer and Leukemia Group B experience. In: Salmon SE, Jones SE. Adjuvant chemotherapy of cancer III. New York: Grune & Stratton, 1981:201–210.

119. Bhardwaj S, Holland JF, Norton L. Intensive sequenced adjuvant chemotherapy for breast cancer (abstract). Proc Am Soc Clin Oncol 1991;10:75.

120. Griswold DP, Schabel FM Jr, Corbett TH, Dykes DJ. Concepts for controlling drug-resistant tumor cells. In: Fidler IJ, White RJ, eds. Design of models for testing cancer therapeutic agents. New York: Van Nostrand Reinhold, 1982:215–224.

121. Day RS. Treatment sequencing, asymmetry, uncertainty: protocol strategies for combination chemotherapy. Cancer Res 1986;46:3876–3885.

122. Norton L, Day R. Potential innovations in scheduling in cancer chemotherapy. In: DeVita VT Jr, Hellman S, Rosenberg SA, eds. Important advances in oncology 1991. New York: JB Lippincott, 1991:57–72.

123. Selawry OS, Hananian J, Wolman IJ, Abir E, Chevalier L, et al. New treatment schedule with improved survival in childhood leukemia. JAMA 1965; 194:187–193.

124. Frei E III, Antman K, Teicher B, Eder P, Schnipper L. Bone marrow autotransplantation for solid tumors—prospects. J Clin Oncol 1989;7:515–526.

125. Peters WP. High dose chemotherapy and autologous bone marrow support for breast cancer. In: DeVita VT Jr, Hellman S, Rosenberg SA. Important advances in oncology 1991. New York: JB Lippincott, 1991:135–150.

126. Hudis C, Lebwohl D, Crown J, Gilewski T, Surbone A, et al. Dose-intensive sequential crossover adjuvant chemotherapy for women with high risk node-positive primary breast cancer. In: Salmon SE, ed. Adjuvant therapy of cancer IV. Philadelphia: JB Lippincott, 1993:214–219.

127. Del Mastro L, Garrone O, Seroli MR, Canavese G, Catturich A, et al. A pilot study of accelerated cyclophosphamide, epirubicin, and 5-fluorouracil plus granulocyte colony stimulating factor as adjuvant therapy in early breast cancer. Eur J Cancer 1994;3A:606–610.

128. Gianni AM, Bregni M, Siena S, Brambilla C, Lombardi F, et al. Prospective randomized comparison of MACOP-B vs. rhGM-CSF-supported high-dose sequential myeloablative chemoradiotherapy in diffuse large cell lymphoma (abstract). Proc Am Soc Clin Oncol 1991;10:951.

129. Valeriote F, van Putten L. Proliferation-dependent cytotoxicity of anticancer agents: a review. Cancer Res 1975;35:2619–2630.

130. Hug V, Johnston D, Finders M, Hortobagyi G. Use of growth-stimulating hormones to improve the in vitro therapeutic index of doxorubicin for human breast cancer. Cancer Res 1986;46:147–152.

131. Osborne CK, Kitten L, Arteaga CL. Antago-nism of chemotherapy-induced cytotoxicity for human breast cancer cells by antiestrogens. J Clin Oncol 1989; 7:710–717.

132. Conte PF, Alama A, Bertelli G, Canavese G, Carnino F, et al. Chemotherapy with estrogenic recruitment and surgery in locally advanced breast cancer: clinical and cytokinetic results. Int J Cancer 1987; 40:490–494.

133. Swain SM, Sorace RA, Bagley CS, Danforth DN Jr, Bader J, et al. Neoadjuvant chemotherapy in the combined modality approach of locally advanced nonmetastatic breast cancer. Cancer Res 1987;47:3889–3894.

134. Conte PF, Pronzato P, Rubagotti A, Alama A, Amadori D, et al. Conventional vs. cytokinetic polychemotherapy with estrogenic recruitment in metastatic breast cancer: results of a randomized cooperative trial. J Clin Oncol 1987;5:339–347.

135. Lippman ME. Hormonal stimulation and chemotherapy for breast cancer (editorial). J Clin Oncol 1987;5:331–332.

136. Lippman ME, Cassidy J, Wesley M, Young RC. A randomized attempt to increase the efficacy of cytotoxic chemotherapy in metastatic breast cancer by hormonal synchronization. J Clin Oncol 1984;2:28–36.

137. Bontenbal M, Sieuwerts AM, Klijn JGM, Peters HA, Krijnen HLJM, Sonneveld P, Foekens JA. Effect of hormonal manipulation and doxorubicin administration on cell cycle kinetics of human breast cancer cells. Br J Cancer 1989;60:688–697.

138. Look AT, Robertson PK, Williams DL, Rivera G, Bowman WP, et al. Prognostic importance of blast cell DNA content in childhood acute lymphoblastic leukemia. Blood 1985;65:1079–1086.

139. Dressler LG. DNA flow cytometry measurements have significant prognostic impact in the node negative breast cancer patient: an intergroup study (INT 0076). Treatment of early stage breast cancer: program and abstracts. NIH concensus development conference, National Cancer Institute and the Office of Medical Applications of Research of the National Institutes of Health, June 18–21, 1990:99–101.

140. Lippman ME, Dickson RB. Growth control of normal and malignant breast epithelium. In: Ragaz J, Simpson-Herren J, Lippman ME, Fisher B, eds. Effects of therapy on biology and kinetics of the residual tumor, part A: pre-clinical aspects. New York: Wiley-Liss, 1990:147–178.

141. Wilson AJ, Baum M, Brinkley DM, Dossett JA, McPherson K, et al. Six-year results of a controlled trial of tamoxifen as single adjuvant agent in management of early breast cancer. World J Surg 1985;9:756–764.

142. Norton L. Biology of residual breast cancer after therapy: a kinetic interpretation. In: Ragaz J, Simpson-Herren J, Lippman ME, Fisher B, eds. Effects of therapy on biology and kinetics of the residual tumor, part A: Pre-clinical aspects. New York: Wiley-Liss, 1990:109–132.

143. Lippman ME, Dickson RB, Bates S, Knabbe C, Huff K, et al. Autocrine and paracrine growth regulation of human breast cancer. Breast Cancer Res Treat 1986;7:59–70.

144. Yee D, Rosen N, Favoni RE, Cullen KJ. The insulin-like growth factors, their receptors, and their binding proteins in human breast cancer. Cancer Treat Res 1991;53:93–106.

145. Weinberg RA, Bishop JM, Minna JD, Sharp PA. Gene regulation and oncogenes: AACR special conference in cancer research. Cancer Res 1989; 49:2188–2193.

146. Rowley JD, Golomb AM, Vardiman JW. Non-random chromosomal abnormalities in acute leukemia and dysmyelopoietic syndromes on patients with previously treated malignant disease. Blood 1981;58:759–767.

147. Koury MJ, Bondurant MC. Erythropoietin retards DNA breakdown and prevents programmed death in erythroid progenitor cells. Science 1990; 248:378–381.

148. Nishimura M, Sowa M, Chung YS, Yoshino H, Katoh Y, et al. An analysis of DNA histogram and the expression of carbohydrate antigens regarding the degree of malignancy in gastric cancer. Jpn J Gastroenterol 1989;86:843–850.

149. Barry MA, Behnke CA, Eastman A. Activation of programmed cell death (apoptosis) by cisplatin, other anticancer drugs, toxins and hyperthermia. Biochem Pharmacol 1990;40:2353–2362.

150. Kennedy S, Merino MJ, Swain SM, Lippman ME. The effects of hormonal and chemotherapy on tumoral and nonneoplastic breast tissue. Hum Pathol 1990;21:192–198.

151. Teicher BA, Herman TS, Holden SA, Wang Y, Pfeffer MR, Crawford JW, Frei E III. Tumor resistance to alkylating agents conferred by mechanisms operative only in vivo. Science 1990;247:1457–1461.

152. Zuckiet G, Tritton TR. Adriamycin causes upregulation of epidermal growth factor receptors in actively growing cells. Exp Cell Res 1983;148:155–161.

153. Isonishi S, Andrews PA, Howell SB. Increased sensitivity to cis-diamminedichloroplatinum (II) in human ovarian carcinoma cells in response to treatment with 12-O-tetradecanoylphorbol-13-acetate. J Biol Chem 1990;265:3623–3627.

154. Masui H, Kawamoto T, Sato JD, Wolf B, Sato G, Mendelsohn J. Growth inhibition of human tumor cells in athymic mice by antiepidermal growth factor receptor monoclonal antibodies. Cancer Res 1984; 44:1002–1007.

155. Mauer AM, Fisher V. Comparison of the proliferative capacity of leukemia cells in bone marrow and blood. Nature 1962;193:1085.

156. Aboud-Pirak E, Hurwitz E, Pirak ME, Fellot F, Schlessinger J, Sela M. Efficacy of antibody to epidermal growth factor receptor against KB carcinoma in vitro and in nude mice. J Natl Cancer Inst 1988; 80:1605–1611.

157. Norton L, Baselga J, Masui H, Hyman J, Kumar R, Mendelsohn J. Growth factor perturbation: a therapeutically exploitable mechanism for chemotherapy action (abstract). Proc Am Soc Clin Oncol 1991; 10:208.

5

Drug Resistance

James H. Goldie

At the present time, there are approximately 60 drugs generally available for the treatment of various types of malignancy. They are derived from a great variety of sources and act on a great many different biochemical processes within the cell. They have differing spectra of clinical activity and limiting toxicities. One thing that they all appear to have in common, however, is that cancer cells have the capacity to display resistance to every one of them. It seems apparent, therefore, that significant advances in the use of cancer chemotherapy will more likely depend on deeper understanding of drug resistance processes than upon simply adding to an already large inventory of drugs.

The first drugs that had a consistent therapeutic effect against some forms of metastatic malignancy were introduced into clinical practice shortly after the end of World War II (1). Even as the first, sometimes dramatic, clinical remissions were observed, it was noted that the patients' tumors almost invariably recurred and became unresponsive to repeat applications of the initial chemotherapy.

Antibiotics were coming into widespread clinical use at this time, and the similarities with acquired resistance in microbial populations immediately suggested themselves. The parallels with microbial drug resistance were reinforced by the studies of Law (2) in which he demonstrated that resistance to the folic acid antagonist methotrexate had the same biologic features that Luria and Delbrück had noted for bacterial resistance phenomena (3); that is, the drug-resistant phenotype appeared to arise randomly within the tumor cell population, consistent with a mutational origin. During the 1950s, a number of investigators were able to demonstrate biochemical changes in drug-resistant tumor cells in experimental systems, which were consistent with the cells having acquired a resistant phenotype (4, 5). For example, the resistant cells were shown to have impaired transport of the drug across the cell membrane or modification of the putative intracellular targets for the particular drug (6).

More recent studies have demonstrated a number of very broad mechanisms of drug resistance and, moreover, have demonstrated that some of the molecular events that lead to drug resistance are involved in the generation of the neoplastic state at a very fundamental level (7).

DEFINITIONS

The terms resistance and sensitivity are essentially relational statements and therefore, strictly speaking, should be defined in terms of some standard reference. In experimental, and particularly in in vitro, systems, this is relatively easy to establish, with the usual reference system being the parent cell line from which the resistant strain is developed. One can then pick an arbitrary concentration of drug and compare the amount of growth inhibition of the variant cell line with that of the parental line. Very simply, if growth is less inhibited in the variant cell line than in the parent, then we would define this as representing resistance. The resistance displayed by the variant cells is rarely absolute, and cells that are not inhibited by one concentration of a drug may well be inhibited by higher concentrations.

Cells that exhibit permanent drug resistance (i.e., show reduced growth inhibition essentially indefinitely) must be distinguished from cells that are temporarily less responsive to chemotherapeutic effect but may have their sensitivity restored under the right conditions and stimuli.

Distinction is also frequently made between so-called acquired drug resistance, which is the process whereby a tumor system progressively changes its degree of sensitivity to a particular drug, and intrinsic resistance, which implies that the cell line displays a high order of drug resistance from the beginning, without having initially undergone selection by the drug in question.

With in vivo tumors, either clinical or experimental, the definition of resistance is usually operational. That is, if a tumor fails to regress or progressively increases in size between treatment cycles of a drug given in the usual therapeutic dose, then the tumor can be considered "resistant." This need not mean that none of the tumor cells are being killed but simply that the number killed is lower than the net increase in cell number due to tumor growth, with the result that there is progressive increase in tumor burden over time. However, if the behavior of these treated tumors is compared with that of untreated controls, then some overall reduction in tumor doubling time may be noted, with some extension in average survival. Strictly speaking, any displacement of the untreated growth curve toward some degree of retardation implies less than absolute resistance. On a practical basis, though, small shifts in net growth rate of the tumor are unlikely to translate into clinically useful outcomes.

BIOLOGIC BASIS OF DRUG RESISTANCE

As mentioned above, there appear to be clear parallels between the development of resistance in tumor cell lines and the development of resistance to antibiotics by bacteria and other microbial species. Moreover, there are analogies to the phenomenon of intrinsic resistance in bacterial populations because different types of bacteria show variable degrees of inherent sensitivity to different antibiotics. For instance, *Mycobacterium tuberculosis* is poorly sensitive to penicillin and sulfanilamide but shows significant sensitivity to streptomycin and rifampicin (8). Even in the microbial systems, uniformly high sensitivity to all of the available antibiotics is not observed.

The origin of drug-resistant bacteria was the subject of considerable debate until the experimental studies of Luria and Delbrück in 1943 (3) demonstrated that acquired resistance in bacteria was compatible with a mutational origin for the resistant phenotypes (Fig. 5.1). The fluctuation test of Luria and Delbrück employed a statistical analysis of the distribution of resistant mutants in a bacterial population to distinguish between induction of, or selection for, resistant organisms. Application of this technique shows that agents such as antibiotics functioned in an essentially passive mode by eradicating the sensitive variants, leaving behind a resistant subpopulation. The work of Law referred to earlier (2) showed that essentially the same process was occurring in transplanted mouse lymphoma cells with respect to their capacity to develop resistance to methotrexate.

Recent studies have used fluctuation analysis to determine whether resistance to the commonly used agents etoposide and doxorubicin arises through mutational or inducible events. Jaffrezou et al. (9) found that in a line of human sarcoma cells, resistance to etoposide arose with a mutation rate ranging form 2.9×10^{-6} to 5.7×10^{-7}. The lowest concentration of etoposide was associated with the highest value for the mutation rate. The clones derived from the highest concentrations of drug used were unstable and reverted back to the sensitive mode. The other clones were stably resistant, and statistical analysis indicated that they had arisen by spontaneous mutation. In these cells, resistance was mediated by decreased expression of the target enzyme topoisomerase II.

Chen et al. (10), utilizing the same line of human sarcoma cells, found that doxorubicin resistance arose with a frequency of 1.8×10^{-6} per cell per generation. Analysis indicated that these clones had arisen from spontaneous mutation. The mechanism of resistance in these cell lines appeared to be overexpression of the *mdr*-1 gene (see below).

Other types of evidence are also strongly consistent with a genetic and mutational origin of the resistant phenotype (11, 12). These include studies in which a drug-sensitive and drug-resistant cell are fused together and the pattern of drug sensitivity in the resultant hybrid cell then examined. In these situations, the hybrid cells display patterns of drug resistance consistent with those predicted from Mendelian laws of genetic inheritance. Even more direct evidence can be obtained from DNA transfection studies in which DNA segments coding for specific genes can be transferred from a drug-resistant cell to a drug-sensitive one, conferring permanent and heritable drug resistance on the transfected cell (13).

It becomes relevant to ask why drug resistance appears to be so consistently associated

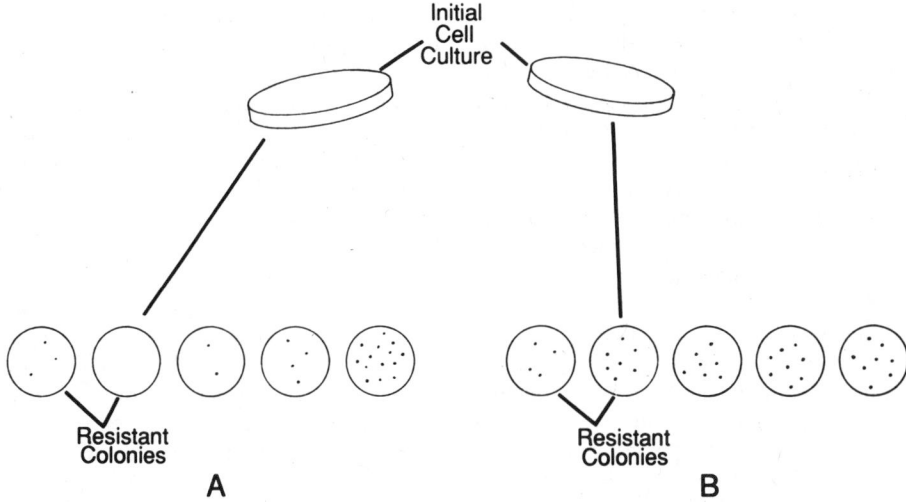

Figure 5.1.   The Luria-Delbrück fluctuation test to demonstrate the spontaneous nature of drug-resistant variant cells. In panel **A**, parallel subclonal populations of cells are grown up to a predetermined number. These are derived from a parent stock culture. The individual cultures are then exposed to a cytotoxic agent. A very substantial variation, or fluctuation, in numbers of resistant cells is noted per individual culture tube, with the variance among the tubes being significantly greater than the mean for the whole test population. When similar-size samples of cells are drawn directly from a stock culture, put in a parallel series of tubes, and then immediately treated with the cytotoxic agent, much less individual variation in resistant cell colonies is seen from one culture to the other. The difference in the two sets of experimental results is related to the random and spontaneous nature of mutational events. In any one individual subclonal culture displayed in panel **A**, there is a probability that a mutation may occur early in the growth of the clone, producing a large number of resistant colonies. Likewise, there is also a probability that no resistant colonies may have emerged in a specific individual clone. Since the cultures depicted in panel **B** are simply aliquots taken from a large representative population, little variation in the numbers of resistant cells from culture to culture is seen, and little would be expected. A positive result in a fluctuation test such as this is consistent with the spontaneous origin of the variant cells, as opposed to their direct induction by the toxic agent.

with the neoplastic state. As described above, many instances of specific drug resistance have been shown to be due to spontaneous mutations arising in the neoplastic cells. Why neoplastic cells should be so much more likely to express drug resistance mutations than are normal cells has been a puzzling question in cancer biology.

It has been postulated that cancer cells might be more "genetically unstable" than normal cells and thus more prone to evolve a great range of variant clones (14). Although chromosomal instability has been recognized in many types of cancer for some time (15), direct evidence of genetic instability has proven harder to establish. However, recent data point to a model of carcinogenesis that requires a "mutator phenotype" as an early event in the process toward transformation (16). These mutator phenotypes could arise through mutations of some of the genes that are involved in the fidelity of DNA replication. If this fidelity is impaired, then the cell will become highly vulnerable to a great variety of environmental mutagens, leading to an accumulation of mutations that may result in the malignant phenotype.

A commonly observed genetic lesion seen in malignancy (in some estimates, > 50% of all cases of human cancer) is inactivation of the *p53* gene, one of the so-called tumor suppressor genes (17). This inactivation can occur through mutation of the gene itself or through suppression of *p53* function by the inappropriate expression of certain types of oncogenes (*bcl-2*, *c-abl*, *ras*) (18). Hereditary disorders such as the Li-Fraumeni syndrome, which produce a variety of cancers at an early age, are associated with inheritance of a defective *p53* allele. The importance of *p53* in cancer development is related to the capacity of the normally functioning gene to cause G_1 arrest and promote DNA repair. If the degree of DNA damage is above a certain threshold, then *p53* appears to initiate a cellular self-destruction process usually called apoptosis, or programed cell death.

The process of apoptosis is also initiated during tissue modeling during normal growth and development and as the final event in terminal differentiation when a cell's useful life span is ended. The area of programed cell death is becoming extremely important in cancer biology and it has direct relevance to cancer chemotherapy.

Recent evidence suggests that chemotherapeutic agents commonly express their cell-killing effect by triggering apoptosis (7). Since apoptosis can be seen as one of the ways that cells prevent the accumulation of mutated and abnormal progeny, agents that produce genotoxic damage could be expected to be potent initiators of the process. It also implies that mutations affecting the apoptotic machinery could constitute another whole level where drug resistance changes might manifest themselves.

RESISTANCE DUE TO CELL KINETIC PHENOMENA

In addition to types of unambiguous genetic resistance, cells can exhibit reduced drug sensitivity by virtue of their position in the cellular division cycle. In the case of drugs that act primarily at one point in the cell cycle (e.g., during DNA synthesis), a cell may be quite invulnerable to the drug's effect if it does not pass through S phase during the period of drug exposure. Moreover, cells that are temporarily out of the division cycle in a so-called resting, or G_0, state may display significantly reduced drug sensitivity to a variety of agents (Fig. 5.2). In these examples of so-called "kinetic resistance," however, the phenomenon is generally only temporary. If the drug concentration is maintained long enough, then all of the cells in the tumor may pass through the vulnerable point in the cell cycle and become susceptible to the drug's effect. Likewise, cells that are in a resting state and are stimulated into division will become sensitive to drug effect.

That is, they will be sensitive if they are inherently sensitive to begin with. If a genetically drug-resistant cell switches from a resting to a proliferative phase, it will not become drug responsive. In the studies of Bruce et al. (19) described in Figure 5.2., it is important to note that the switch between a resting and proliferative state with associated changes in drug sensitivity is a phenomenon that was observed in the normal, as opposed to the malignant, cells in the test system. Under steady-state conditions, most of the hematopoietic stem cells in the mouse marrow were in a physiologic G_0 condition, with just

enough stem cells entering the division cycle to replenish the differentiated cells lost through normal attrition. Following perturbation by the chemotherapeutic agent, the surviving marrow stem cells all enter the generation cycle to replenish the marrow stem pool rapidly. Once this pool has regained its physiologic size, then further expansion of the normal stem cells is inhibited through a feedback process. The tumor cells in this system showed no such physiologic responses to external stimuli. Virtually all of the malignant stem cells appear to be in the generation cycle, so their drug sensitivity did not change because of kinetic alterations. One therefore has to exercise caution in extrapolating the behavior of resting normal cells to what may or may not occur in neoplastic systems.

There is certainly evidence that malignant cells can enter a nondividing state from which they can be recalled into division by appropriate stimuli (20). However, it is not clear from a mechanistic point of view if this is analogous to the physiologic G_0 state seen with the marrow stem cells. Indeed, if failure of so-called checkpoint arrest is one of the fundamental changes that occurs in malignancy, then the concept of the G_0 tumor cell needs to be questioned. Tumor cells may cease dividing under conditions in which nutrients and growth factors are limiting, but in vitro at least, this is a result of cells stopping at random points in the cell cycle (20).

A well-defined system for evaluating slowly dividing or nondividing tumor cells is the in vitro tumor microspheroid (22). This is a system in which tumor cells are grown as tiny cell aggregates ranging from a few hundred to over a million cells suspended in semisolid medium. As these tumor microspheroids get larger, they start to show some growth and kinetic properties that superficially resemble those seen with larger in vivo tumors. Different zones within the microspheroid show different growth rates; the outer layer of cells shows rapid proliferation, and the innermost layers show evidence of having ceased division.

If the spheroid is exposed to cytotoxic agents, resulting in removal of the outermost layer of cells, then the inner layers, now having access to an improved nutrient supply, enter into rapid division. In such test systems, most antitumor agents show preferential cytotoxicity for the rapidly dividing cells in the periphery of the tumor spheroid, but a few agents such as cisplatin, mitomycin C, and bleomycin still display significant cytotoxicity toward the nondividing cell

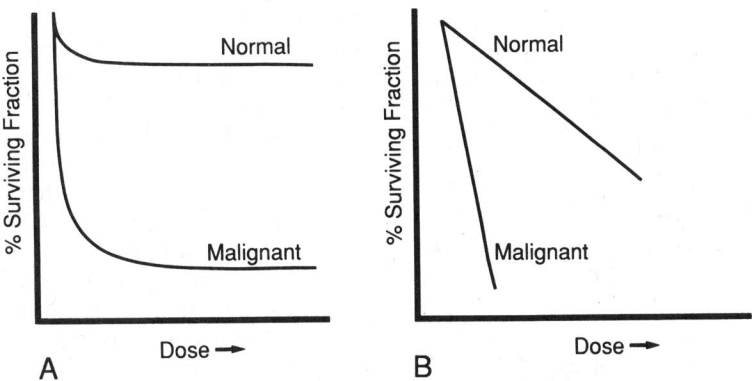

Figure 5.2.   The two principal types of dose-response curves for cytotoxic agents measured in vivo. The *left-hand panel* demonstrates so-called phase-specific or cell cycle stage–specific classes of agents. These include agents such as methotrexate, vincristine, and cytosine arabinoside. Such drugs exert their killing effects primarily during one phase of the cell cycle, so cells that do not pass through this particular vulnerable point are not killed during relatively short exposure. The normal cells of interest here are the colony-forming cells of the normal bone marrow. The fact that a significantly lower proportion of these cells are killed for any particular dose of drug (compared with rapidly proliferating lymphoma cells) indicates that a much lower proportion of the hemopoietic cells are in cell cycle during the period of exposure. The *right-hand panel* indicates a typical log-linear dose-response effect that is seen with alkylating agents and DNA intercalators. Increases in dose produce a linear increase in log kill of both normal and malignant cells, but again, there is a preferential killing effect on the malignant cells because a much higher percentage of these are in cell cycle at any given time. (Adapted from Bruce WR, Meaker BE, Valeriote FA. Comparison of the sensitivity of normal hematopoietic in transplanted lymphoma colony forming cells to chemotherapeutic agents administered in vivo. J Natl Cancer Inst 1966;37:233–245.)

elements (20). The exact contribution that nondividing or slowly dividing tumor cells make to clinical treatment failure is uncertain at this time, but since some antineoplastic agents are quite effective in eliminating such classes of cells, it would seem prudent to include them in developmental protocols.

Another phenomenon seen in multicell spheroids is the observation that when the spheroid is disaggregated to single-cell suspensions, the cells become sensitive to a variety of antineoplastic agents to which they were resistant as spheroids (23). These changes occur without major changes in kinetic parameters and would apparently point to some type of epigenetic mechanism being operative. It has been speculated that some diffusable substance can be transmitted from one cell to another while they are present as spheroids but not when the cells are more dispersed. (Whether such laboratory phenomena have clinical counterparts remains to be seen, and this is an area that needs further examination).

Tumor cells in vivo may display reduced drug sensitivity even though the individual cells themselves are constitutively sensitive. This has been reported in experimental systems utilizing mouse EMT-6 mammary carcinoma cells ren-

dered resistant to a number of cytotoxic agents in vivo (24). When the cells are removed from the animal and tested in suspension culture, they no longer display resistance. Purely in vivo resistance may also be seen if the tumor cells are present in locations in the body where it is difficult to achieve effective drug concentrations (e.g., central nervous system) or if there has been some alteration in the host's metabolism of the drug after it has been injected. With some drugs, enzyme systems may be induced in the liver and elsewhere that greatly enhance the rate of drug degradation, resulting in difficulty in achieving tumoricidal drug concentrations (23). These circumstances might be described as "pharmacologic resistance," and while undoubtedly constituting a serious clinical problem, it is of a different nature than acquired changes in the tumor cells themselves.

EXPERIMENTAL MODELS OF DRUG RESISTANCE

It is relatively easy to produce drug-resistant variant cell lines with established in vitro cell culture systems. A common method is to grow the cells in progressively increasing sublethal concentrations of a particular drug. When first

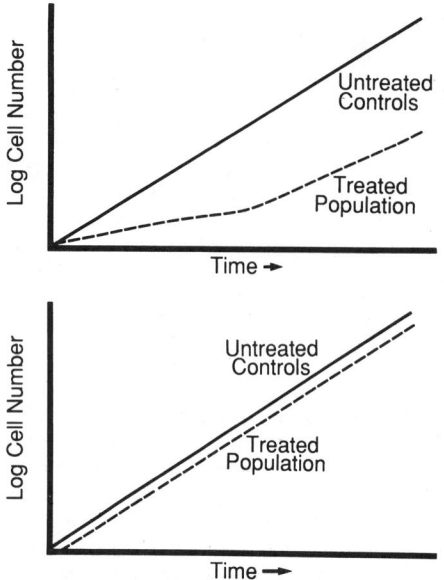

Figure 5.3.   Experimental method for producing drug-resistant cells in vitro. In the *upper diagram*, the growth rate of untreated control cells is measured over a standard period of time. A culture of cells identical to the control culture is then exposed to a predetermined concentration of a cytotoxic agent. Initially, the growth of the treated cells shows significant retardation, compared with the controls. After a variable period of time, cell numbers in the treated cultures increase, but the overall growth rate is slower than that of the untreated controls. In the *lower panel*, the treated cells have been repeatedly subcultured in the presence of the cytotoxic agent. After a variable period of time, the growth rate of the treated cells is equivalent to that of the untreated controls. At this point, the treated cells can be considered completely resistant to the particular concentration of agent, and they can be used for studies to determine any biochemical changes that have occurred within them, compared to the controls. If a more resistant phenotype is required, the concentration of drug in the treated cultures is increased, and the process is repeated.

exposed to the cytotoxic agent, the growth of the cell line is initially markedly inhibited, but over time, the cells appear to become adaptively resistant to the cytotoxic agent and begin growing at what is usually very close to their initial pretreatment doubling time. At this juncture, the concentration of the agent in the culture media can be increased, and the process then repeats itself. Depending upon the cell line, the particular anticancer agent that is being employed, and the degree of drug resistance that is desired, it generally takes from a few weeks to several

months to produce a cell line that will now grow unimpeded by concentrations of drug that would initially have been highly toxic (Fig. 5.3).

If the drug is now removed from the tissue culture environment, in most circumstances the cell line will maintain its resistance without continuous drug exposure, though it is not unusual to see a gradual reduction in drug resistance over time.

Such methods are very useful for obtaining stable cell culture lines that display high drug resistance to one or more antineoplastic agents. This, in turn, makes it easier to carry out biochemical characterization studies of the resistant cells. It can be legitimately argued that this process of producing drug-resistant cells differs appreciably from the usual methods of in vivo drug selection and also that the extremely high orders of drug resistance that can be developed with this approach may not be completely relevant to clinical situations.

If one uses an in vivo transplanted tumor as the experimental system, then the usual approach is to inoculate a known burden of tumor cells into a recipient host animal and then treat with a noncurative schedule of chemotherapeutic administration (24). Following an initial significant reduction in viable tumor cells in the treated animals, the tumor that grows back may display markedly reduced sensitivity to the initial chemotherapeutic drug.

When these resistant cells are harvested from the initial host animal and reinoculated into a second host, the cell lines continue to demonstrate diminished drug responsiveness (24). As with the in vitro systems, these resistant cells generally maintain their degree of resistance over many passages in recipient animals. Some decline in degree of resistance in the absence of periodic reselection may occur, however.

BIOCHEMICAL MECHANISMS INVOLVED IN DRUG RESISTANCE

If information is available about the action of a particular drug at the molecular level, then it becomes feasible to identify any intracellular changes that would tend to minimize the drug's cell-killing effects. The general principle is that for a drug to have some type of lethal action on a cell, it must first be transported across the cell membrane, may then require some form of intracellular activation, and then bind with some intracellular target. Whether the damage so produced is lethal to the cell will depend in part upon the capacity of the cell to repair or circumvent the biochemical lesion induced by the drug.

Drug-resistant states can arise from modification of any or all of the processes indicated. Highly drug resistant phenotypes may exhibit several changes toward minimizing drug cytotoxicity.

Impaired Transport of Drug across Cell Membrane

Although some agents appear to gain intracellular access through passive diffusion, many other classes of antineoplastic agents require some type of facilitated transport (25). If the drug has a chemical structure similar to that of a normal metabolite, it may use the same transport system that the normal substrate does. These processes generally involve the binding of the drug to a receptor protein on the cell membrane. Then, the protein-drug complex is translocated across the cell membrane, with release of drug into the intracellular milieu. If alterations occur in the structure of the protein receptor, or if there is a reduction in the amount of receptor on the cell membrane, then active transport of the drug is significantly impaired. This will result in a lower intracellular drug concentration, and there may not be enough drug inside the cell to cause cytotoxicity. Well-studied examples of this include methotrexate and nitrogen mustard (26, 27).

Another type of transport alteration that is now recognized as of increasing importance involves the increased activity of cellular mechanisms that result in extrusion of drug after it has been transported into the cell. This process also reduces the intracellular drug concentration to below cytocidal levels. This is seen in cell types displaying the so-called multidrug-resistant phenotype (28) and is discussed in greater detail below.

Reduced Intracellular Activation

A number of antineoplastic agents, primarily purine or pyrimidine analogues, must be converted into the appropriate nucleoside or nucleotide form to function as cytotoxic antimetabolites (29, 30). Since fully formed nucleotides are poorly transported across the cell membrane, it is not possible to bypass this step by administering the nucleotide of the drug systemically.

A common biochemical change that can occur within cells is loss of one or another of the enzymes responsible for converting the drug to its fully phosphorylated form (31). As these "enzyme deletions" are essentially nonlethal mutations from the cells' point of view, their occurrence can confer extremely high resistance to a particular antimetabolite. Examples of compounds affected by this mechanism include 6-mercaptopurine, 6-thioguanine, cytosine arabinoside, and 5-fluorouracil. Once this process has occurred, it cannot be circumvented by increasing the extracellular drug concentration. If the capacity to activate the drug intracellularly is lost, increasing the drug concentration will not compensate.

Altered or Increased Amounts of Intracellular Target

Many antineoplastic agents appear to exert their cytocidal effects by binding to a normal cell enzyme and rendering it nonfunctional. The drug may have a significantly higher affinity for the enzyme than the normal substrate does and bind tightly enough that it is not possible for the normal substrate to undergo metabolic conversion.

An excellent model system for this type of reaction involves the drug methotrexate, an extremely potent inhibitor of dihydrofolate reductase (32). By binding tightly to dihydrofolate reductase, methotrexate stops the generation of tetrahydrofolates within the cell. This, in turn, stops thymidine and purine biosynthesis, with consequent interruption of DNA synthesis. Cells that are resistant to methotrexate may show increased amounts of dihydrofolate reductase or, alternatively, may produce a variant dihydrofolate reductase that is no longer easily inhibited by the drug (33, 34). With these changes, effectively inhibiting all of the enzyme would require a much higher intracellular concentration of methotrexate, which may not be achievable.

Increased Intracellular Drug Detoxification

The glutathione-S-transferase system (GST) consists of a number of isozymes that are able to conjugate glutathione to a variety of different xenobiotic substances. Such conjugation may significantly reduce the cytotoxicity of the compound, and this appears to play a role in resistance to a number of alkylating agents (35).

Some investigators have found a correlation between increased GST expression and P-glycoprotein expression (see below), suggesting that the involved genes may be part of a system that is coordinately upregulated to protect cells from a variety of cytotoxic agents. Other investigators have been less convinced of this association.

Related to the GST system is the glutathione redox system, which involves a number of enzymes that can detoxify the harmful peroxide products that some antitumor agents (such as doxorubicin) produce. Although there is controversy over the precise role that the glutathione systems play in mediating drug resistance, it is probably reasonable to assume that they have some role in diminishing the cytotoxic effect of certain drugs and that they likely constitute a mechanism for generating broad degrees of drug resistance.

Increased Repair Capacity

Many of the antineoplastic agents exert their effect by directly damaging, in one way or another, the structural integrity of the cellular DNA (36, 37). Cells have evolved complex and highly effective mechanisms for repairing damaged DNA segments, and cell lines that show resistance to DNA-damaging agents such as alkylating agents and DNA intercalators display an enhanced capacity to repair the drug-induced damage (38). This may involve actually excising the segment of damaged DNA and replacing it with newly synthesized nucleotides that repair the areas of the drug-induced lesions (39).

Studies on cell lines that are alkylating-agent resistant have, in a number of circumstances, been able to document increased amounts or activity of some of the enzymes involved in DNA repair (40). An important determinant of alkylation resistance may be the cell's ability to specifically repair alkylation damage in the O_6 position of guanine residues in the DNA. Alkylation occurring at this site can be very efficiently removed by a specific methyl transferase (41). Cells that constitutively show a high methyl transferase repair capacity are designated as Mer$^+$. Cells with diminished activity of this enzyme are referred to as Mer$^-$, and they are particularly vulnerable to damage by nitrosourea-type alkylating agents. It has been suggested that measuring the methyl transferase activity in tumor cells might permit identification of individual patients who would be particularly susceptible to treatment by nitrosoureas.

Resistance to the agent cisplatin (cis-diamminedichloroplatinum (II)) has been shown in some instances to be due to enhanced activity of two of the DNA excision-repair enzymes (42). DNA-platinum adducts are removed by these enzymes with a greater efficiency than is seen in platinum-sensitive cells.

The Multidrug-Resistant Phenotype

In recent years, a very important mechanism of general biochemical drug resistance has been identified. A number of investigators in the early 1970s showed that in experimental systems, tumor cells that were rendered resistant to one type of antineoplastic agent (e.g., vinca alkaloids) would show a significant amount of collateral resistance to a number of other, apparently unrelated, types of antitumor drug (e.g., anthracyclines, epidiphylotoxins) (43, 44). This phenomenon was called pleiotropic resistance, and in 1976, Juliano and Ling (45) showed that pleiotropic resistance was mediated by a 170-kDa cell surface membrane glycoprotein. This protein, usually referred to as the P-glycoprotein (P-gp), is widely distributed in nature and functions as a cellular pump for extruding toxic molecules from inside the cell to the external environment.

The P-gp is present in a number of normal cells but in very low concentration. It appears that many tumor cells have the capacity to significantly increase the amount of P-gp present on their cell membranes, either by an increased rate of synthesis or by amplification of the genes coding for the P-gp.

Part of the P-gp molecule is located on the interior aspect of the cell membrane, and in this area, there is a binding site to which a number of different types of compounds can be bound through a process involving ATP (46). The compound is then translocated across the cell membrane, effectively removing it from the cell's interior.

The substances that can bind and be extruded by the P-gp pump mechanism tend to be large heterocyclic compounds that are derived from the natural environment, e.g., plant alkaloids and antibiotics. This suggests both the physiologic role of this drug-resistance marker and why it is capable of mediating resistance to a broad range of antineoplastic agents.

The P-gp associated with multidrug resistance is coded by the gene *mdr-1* and is one member of a large family of transport glycoproteins that have significant degrees of homology with each other (47). These proteins are known as ABC (ATP-binding cassette) proteins, and some of them mediate broad degrees of drug resistance. Related to P-gp is the recently described MRP (multidrug resistance protein) with a molecular weight of 190,000 (48). MRP is capable of effluxing a variety of antineoplastic agents and producing a multidrug-resistant phenotype.

The terminology used in describing the multidrug-resistant phenotypes is somewhat confusing. "Classical" MDR refers to the P-gp transporter described by Juliano and Ling, whereas "nonclassical" or "atypical" MDR can refer to an ever-expanding list of cellular phenotypes characterized by the capacity to display some type of pleiotropic resistance. In addition to MDR and MRP, multidrug resistance is also associated with mutations involving topoisomerase II, some of the general detoxifying enzyme systems (35) (glutathione-S-transferase), and many of the DNA repair systems (49). It might be helpful if the term multidrug resistance was confined to use in the "classical" case of MDR and the other broad categories of resistance were described as pleiotropic resistance, with the specific mediator substance named as well (e.g., pleiotropic resistance—topo II).

Since it was first identified in experimental systems, the P-gp has been found directly in clinical specimens. There does appear to be an approximate correlation between the amount and extent of expression of the P-gp and the resistance to natural product substances by the clinical tumor itself (50). Moreover, patients undergoing chemotherapeutic treatment may show, over time, the evolution of cell lines demonstrating enhanced P-gp concentration consistent with either selection or induction of the drug resistance marker (51).

The importance of P-gp expression in tumor cells is suggested by recent studies indicating that there may be an association between P-gp positivity and prognosis. In neuroblastoma and large cell lymphoma, patients who had a high proportion of P-gp-positive cells had a significantly poorer prognosis (52, 53). This is consistent with the hypothesis that P-gp is a clinical marker for drug resistance. However, the association is likely to be a complex with one with P-gp positivity coexisting with other markers of drug resistance. In addition, it is possible that P-gp expression may also be associated with other biologic changes (e.g., mutations in p53) that might be expected to confer a worse prognosis.

"GENERAL DRUG RESISTANCE"—A NEW CATEGORY OF RESISTANCE?

All of the drug resistance mechanisms mentioned in the previous section might be described as "upstream resistance," where there is interaction with the drug and the cell membrane, the drug's putative intracellular target, and finally intervention of cell repair processes. Any or all of these may be affected in drug-resistant states. However, there appears to be at least one further critical step in drug action that occurs downstream from the drug-target interaction—the process of apoptosis, mentioned above. There is considerable evidence accumulating that an important early event in apoptosis involves action of the *p53* product (17). This protein binds to specific areas on the DNA and is capable of initiating a number of complex sequences, including programed cell death or apoptosis. P-53 is not the only initiator of apoptosis, but it appears to be a very important one and, in particular, may be activated by relatively low levels of cell injury. Studies have shown that cells that are homozygous for wild type (normal) *p53* tend to be sensitive to a number of different types of antineoplastic agents plus radiation, whereas cells that are homozygous for mutated, or nonfunctional, *p53* are broadly resistant to many antineoplastic agents and radiation (7, 54). Heterozygotes appear to have intermediate-level resistance. Further, *p53*-associated drug resistance does not depend on other resistance mechanisms being present (55).

Certain oncogenes (such as *c-myc*) that produce positive growth signals may actually sensitize the cells to undergo apoptosis at very low levels of cell damage (18). If the apoptosis system is fully functional, such tumors may be exquisitely sensitive to both drugs and radiation. This appears to be the case with many germ cell tumors and some types of lymphoid malignancy. However, mutations affecting the *p53* system can induce resistance even in these very sensitive cell lines (7).

p53-based resistance carries with it a number of important implications for cancer chemotherapy, especially given the frequency with which *p53* mutations occur in human cancer. Apoptosis requires new protein synthesis for the cell death program to proceed, so presumably there are other steps that may be impaired even if *p53* and other initiators of apoptosis are functional. Alterations in any component of the apoptosis system might produce significant general drug and radiation resistance. Even if a drug successfully negotiates all of the upstream barriers to pharmacologic action, it can still fail because some part of the final common pathway of drug action is defective.

There are many unanswered questions about the general role of programed cell death systems as part of the cancer chemotherapy equation. There appear to be other mechanisms whereby apoptosis can be induced, and apoptosis may occur in the absence of functioning $p53$ by exposure to very high drug concentrations (7). Very little is known about these alternative pathways leading to programed cell death, including the critical threshold levels at which they can be initiated and if there are specific types of cell damage that are more prone to induce them. Likewise, it is not known whether combination chemotherapy treatments or combinations of drugs and radiation by interacting simultaneously with a number of intracellular targets may invoke different cell death programs than those seen with exposure to a single drug. As this whole area is now becoming an intensive field of investigation, answers to these questions may be forthcoming in the near future.

MATHEMATIC MODELING OF DRUG RESISTANCE

If the assumption is made that drug-resistant cancer cells arise as a consequence of spontaneous mutations, then it is possible to develop a mathematical theory that describes this process (56). The approach used is derived from the work of Luria and Delbrück and others, who studied the phenomenon of resistance development in bacteria. To adapt the theory to tumor cell populations, however, it is necessary to make a few more additional assumptions consistent with the more complex processes that appear to be involved in mammalian cells.

The basic Luria-Delbrück model predicted that there would be large variability in the numbers of resistant cells from one discrete sample to another. If a random mutation occurred early in the growth of a particular population, it would have time to produce large numbers of resistant progeny, resulting in a high fraction of resistant cells. In some cases, the mutation would, by chance, occur late, which would result in relatively few resistant cells appearing. There would also be the situation in which, by chance, no resistant cells would have appeared prior to the initiation of treatment. All of these different scenarios would be consistent with the same average mutation rate, and the marked variability in numbers of mutants from case to case simply reflects the randomness of the mutational process.

If we consider the circumstance in which no resistant cells appear until the time treatment has been started, these would represent the cases that would be potentially curable by appropriate chemotherapy. If we assume that we give sufficient courses of treatment to rapidly eradicate all of the sensitive cells in such cases, the probability of cure becomes (approximately) equal to the probability of no resistant cells being present. It is possible to develop a mathematical expression that precisely defines the probability of no resistant cells occurring, and if we set this as equal to the probability of cure, we can then examine which changes in which parameters will influence the overall probability of cure in a given hypothetical circumstance.

Very simply then, the probability (of cure) equals $e^{-\alpha(N-1)}$. In this equation, e is the base of natural logarithms, α is the mutation rate per cell generation, and N represents the total number of cells present in the tumor.

What this basically means is that the larger the tumor in cell numbers, or the higher the mutation rate, the lower the probability of cure. If this equation is plotted out for different values of α, the mutation rate, then we get a series of sigmoid curves, as in Figure 5.4. A relatively high mutation rate shifts the curve to the left, and a lower one will shift it to the right. The shape of the curve suggests that the probability of cure for a tumor will begin to decline fairly steeply at some point and will, within a relatively short period of time, become negligible.

Clearly, the probability of cure is strongly related to the absolute size of the tumor cell population at the time treatment is started. Smaller populations will be much more likely to be curable than will be larger ones.

The relationship predicts that for all clinically advanced tumors, cure by a single chemotherapeutic agent is probably nearly impossible. In contrast, therapy directed at minimal tumor burdens has a much greater likelihood of being successful.

This relationship would, on its own, strongly argue for the use of adjuvant chemotherapy in all circumstances in which it is feasible. Another inference regarding treatment strategy that can be readily deduced from the basic mathematical theory involves the superiority of combination

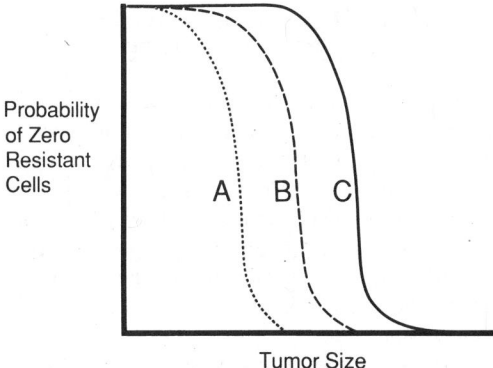

Figure 5.4.   Plot of the function P (zero resistant cells) $= e^{-\alpha(N-1)}$. This function represents the probability of finding no resistant cells in a particular colony (or tumor) of a known cell number. e equals base of natural logarithms; N, the size of the cell population in numbers; and α is the mutation rate per cell generation. This is the probability of finding zero resistant cells in the colony depicted in panel **A**, Figure 5.1. If the value for the mutation rate is fixed and different values for tumor size are used, this function will yield a sigmoid curve as illustrated in curve B above. Higher or lower values of the mutation rate will shift the curve to the left or the right (curves A and C). If the probability of zero resistant cells is considered equivalent to the probability of potential cure, then this function defines the relationship between tumor burden and curability. Low tumor burden and/or low mutation rates to resistance will be associated with a much greater probability of chemotherapy-induced cure.

chemotherapy over single-agent treatment, especially with respect to increasing cure rates.

If two non-cross-resistant agents are used simultaneously to treat a tumor, it is reasonable to assume that the probability of an individual tumor cell being resistant to both drugs simultaneously will be less than that of the cell being resistant to either one alone. This assumes that a mutation to resistance to one drug does not simultaneously cause resistance to the other (this would not be the case with the multidrug-resistant phenotype).

Under these circumstances, the effect of multiagent therapy can be considered equivalent in terms of the mathematical theory to having the mutation rate to resistance lowered. That is, for any particular tumor burden, the probability of cure will be greater if multiple agents are used rather than a single agent. Again, implicit in this assumption is the lack of cross-resistance between the two drugs and the assumption that each drug, on its own, has therapeutic activity against the sensitive cells of the tumor. That is,

if the particular tumor cell exhibited high intrinsic sensitivity to one of the drugs, therapeutic gain would not be expected by combining this drug with another to which the tumor cells were sensitive.

The basic mathematical theory can be made more complex to describe scenarios that more closely mimic the biology of actual tumors, including assumptions relating to the doubling time of the neoplasm, the proportion of clonogenic cells in the tumor, and the assumption of a number of different therapeutic agents of varying degrees of effectiveness (57, 58). However, even more complex versions of the model still yield the same general predictions regarding optimization of therapeutic strategy. These include the importance of commencing treatment as soon as feasible and when the tumor burden is least and exposing the tumor to as many therapeutically active agents as are available and practicable within as short a time frame as is tolerable. Deliberately withholding a potent agent to be used as second-line therapy after initial treatment failure can be easily perceived to be a very poor strategy, given the objective of attempting to eliminate the tumor as quickly as possible.

There is still ongoing debate about the utility of certain chemotherapy strategies such as the alternation of non-cross-resistant drugs in protocols rather than their sequential administration. A number of trials of alternating regimens have yielded either no increased benefit or, at best, only a small improvement in survival, much less than theoretic predictions (59).

There are probably a number of explanations for this finding, including the possibility (despite all the evidence) that mutations to resistance play no important part in clinical outcome. The drug combinations used in many studies have rarely been assessed for true equivalence of effect, a critical factor if alternation is to be effective. In addition, the whole issue of non-cross-resistance is clearly much more complex than was realized 15 years ago. Given the large number of mechanisms that exist to produce broad ranges of resistance, it is apparent that there is far less therapeutic diversity available than the 60 agents that we possess might imply. It would appear that the tumor cell sees a lot fewer drugs being aimed at it than the chemist does. This could account, in part, for some of the disappointing results seen in recent large-scale trials. A number of third-generation combination chemotherapy protocols were evaluated for the treatment of large cell lymphoma and were found to have no significant increased benefit as compared with the older, standard CHOP protocol (60). Essentially all of the multiagent protocols used produced similar results. Given the number of overlapping cross-resistance patterns that tumor cells express, in hindsight, the results might have been expected. From the perspective of drug resistance, the protocols were all very similar.

RELATIONSHIP BETWEEN DRUG AND RADIATION RESISTANCE

In the previous section, it was mentioned that defective *p53* function can simultaneously generate both drug and radiation resistance. This could help explain the frequent clinical instances in which tumors that are relatively radioresistant may be generally drug resistant as well (melanoma, glioblastoma, non-small-cell lung carcinoma, etc). Cancers that recur in radiation fields are often much more resistant to chemotherapy than if they had been treated with chemotherapy de novo.

Hill and coworkers have demonstrated that ionizing radiation can produce a number of drug-resistant phenotypes (61). The reverse sequence, in which chemotherapy produces radiation resistance, seems very rare (62). Given the biologic effect of radiation, the generation of drug-resistant phenotypes is likely a common consequence of treating tumor cell populations with radiation. It has been estimated that a clinical course of radiation (60 cGy) would generate up to 10^{15} DNA lesions in a 100-g tumor (63). This translates to an average of 10^7 DNA damaging events per cell. Given the fact that while tumor cells may have effective DNA repair processes, the fidelity of the repair tends to be deficient (15, 55), then the generation of a large number of mutations in the surviving radiated population is a predictable outcome.

This raises the question of the optimal sequence to be used when combining radiation and chemotherapy. On one hand, initial radiation may assist chemotherapy by (*a*) reducing overall tumor burden and (*b*) nonselectively killing a variety of drug-resistant cells already present. However, if the mutagenic effect of radiation results in the production of more drug-resistant cells than are killed, then this becomes a persuasive argument for using chemotherapy prior to radiation.

BIOCHEMICAL MODULATION OF DRUG RESISTANCE

As indicated in the previous section, one means of minimizing the likelihood of drug resistance is to adopt a chemotherapeutic strategy that uses the available agents in some type of maximally efficient manner. This approach basically involves using general biologic principles rather than discrete information about the biochemical composition of the resistant tumor cells themselves.

For some time, it has been the hope that as more was learned about specific mechanisms of resistance, it would be possible to directly develop treatment approaches that would specifically circumvent these mechanisms and thus restore sensitivity to the tumor cells. This would seem in theory to be the ideal approach, but in practice it has proved formidably difficult.

Various methods have been used in an attempt to augment drug transport or to inhibit cellular repair processes. With experimental in vitro systems, it has been possible in a number of instances to show that these approaches can indeed enhance drug responsiveness. Attempts to apply this at the clinical level have proven much more difficult, possibly in part because clinical drug resistance is likely multifactorial. Some of these resistance pathways may be poorly understood and not as yet identified; others may not be amenable (for one reason or another) to pharmacologic intervention.

An approach that does show some interesting potential utility involves cells that express the multidrug-resistant phenotype. Tsuro (64) has demonstrated that in vitro therapeutic concentrations of the calcium channel blocking agent verapamil are capable of inactivating the P-gp pump and preventing it from actively lowering intracellular drug concentration.

This demonstration has generated much interest in attempting to exploit this approach clinically. Until now, efforts have been hindered by the fact that the minimal effective concentrations of verapamil required are close to the toxic range for the drug. Also, it appears that there may be different species of P-gp, some of which are more effectively disabled by calcium channel blocking agents than are others.

A number of P-gp modulators have been evaluated, including analogues of verapamil and the immunosuppressive agent cyclosporine (64). These include calcium channel blockers, calmodulin antagonists such as chlorpromazine and trifluoperazine, antihormonal and hormonal agents such as tamoxifen and progesterone, and the naturally occurring agent cyclosporine and its synthetic analogues.

Some clinical activity has been noted, but complete restoration of sensitivity has not been seen, and the modulating agents themselves may have appreciable toxicity. Considering the multiple mechanisms of drug resistance that are probably operative in many tumor cells, it is unlikely that inactivating one mechanism of resistance will suffice to restore high levels of sensitivity. This would certainly be true for advanced tumors, but another possibility is to use the modulators early in the course of treatment to prevent certain mechanisms of resistance from evolving.

At an early investigative stage are experiments to evaluate the use of protein kinase inhibitors to reverse the multidrug-resistant state (65). A number of the proteins involved in mediating drug resistance, such as P-gp and topoisomerase II, are known to undergo posttranslational modification by being phosphorylated by protein kinases. Some of the processes associated with the function of certain oncogenes (e.g., *ras*) also require phosphorylation. In theory, interference with some of these steps by the appropriate inhibitor could modify multidrug resistance or even interrupt growth signals from the oncogenes themselves. Whether such compounds would display sufficient antitumor specificity is not known at this time.

The hypothesis that increased activity of the glutathione systems is responsible for multidrug resistance has lead to attempts to deplete intracellular glutathione by administration of agents such as butathionine sulfoximine (BSO), which inhibits the enzyme glutamyl cysteine synthetase. There is in vitro evidence that such techniques can increase drug sensitivity, but no compelling data are available, so far, to suggest that this can be exploited clinically.

Another biochemical modulation approach that may partly involve circumvention of resistance is the use of folinic acid concurrently with 5-fluorouracil. Although this technically might not be considered reversal of 5-FU resistance, the use of these two compounds in conjunction may overcome partial or moderate resistance to 5-FU to some extent. To exert some of its therapeutic effect, 5-FU must be converted into its nucleotide to bind to the enzyme thymidylate synthetase. The tightness of this binding is greatly enhanced if the intracellular concentration of reduced fo-

late is also increased. As at least some instances of 5-FU resistance may be associated with diminished affinity of the thymidylate synthetase for the 5-FU deoxyribonucleophosphate (DRP), then making large amounts of reduced folate available may partially overcome this phenomenon (66).

Presently, clinical evidence suggests that the combination of 5-FU plus folinic acid does result in significantly higher response rates than the use of 5-FU alone, suggesting that at least some instances of tumors that would have been considered "resistant" to 5-FU may have the sensitivity augmented by this biochemical maneuver (66).

CIRCUMVENTION OF RESISTANCE BY HIGH-DOSE CHEMOTHERAPY

A number of strategies have been found to play at least some role in overcoming drug resistance, including using combination chemotherapy, initiating treatment at the earliest time feasible (i.e., adjuvant chemotherapy) and, when available, using unique new compounds against drug-refractory tumors. Another approach is simply to greatly escalate the doses of the drugs used, a tactic that exploits the biologic fact that cells that are resistant to a particular dose level of drug may be sensitive to a higher level. The increased concentration of drug will overcome resistance by increasing net intracellular accumulation of drug and by saturating targets that may not be vulnerable to low concentrations of drug. The intriguing possibility has been suggested that the types of cellular injury induced by these high doses may mediate apoptosis even if *p53* and other critical genes are nonfunctional (7). If this can be confirmed, then it would be a strong additional rationale for the use of high-dose chemotherapy in association with bone marrow rescue techniques. Although there are many controversies to be resolved, high-dose chemotherapy plus marrow rescue undoubtedly can salvage some patients with otherwise incurable disease (67).

SUMMARY AND CONCLUSIONS

The problem of drug resistance in cancer chemotherapy can be approached from two rather different perspectives. The first defines the problem as being the consequence of a large number of interacting biologic phenomena. We might describe this as a "phenomenologic" or "epigenetic" model of drug resistance. Resistance is derived from a series of parallel events that occur during the development and spread of the cancer: changes in growth kinetics, alteration in tumor blood supply, pharmacokinetic effects, interaction between constituent cells of the tumor, direct induction of molecular changes in the cell in response to chemotherapeutic stress, and in addition, the development of mutations in some of the key genes that influence drug sensitivity.

The second viewpoint, which we can describe as the "genetic" model, would place genetic alterations (i.e., mutations) at the center of the process, with all the other mechanisms observed being epiphenomena derived from the fundamental genetic changes occurring within the tumor cells.

A pragmatic question to be asked is which model more readily leads to feasible therapeutic options. In this context, we should ask what lessons can be learned from the information that has been developed in the last few years about the nature of cancer itself.

Although there are still many unresolved questions, the author feels that a compelling and unifying model of carcinogenesis has emerged that places genetic mutation as the central driver of the neoplastic process. Early mutational events that reduce the accuracy of genetic information transmission will lead to a cascade of mutations, some of which will provide the mutant cells with a growth advantage. It appears that some of the mutations that release the cancer cell from proliferation constraints will simultaneously render the neoplasm less sensitive to many types of chemotherapy.

Paradoxically, it also seems that certain combinations of genetic events leading to cancer may in fact produce cells that display increased sensitivity to chemotherapy (compared with normal cells and many other types of tumor cells). For example, germ cell tumors of the testis usually have two normal alleles for *p53*, a circumstance that appears very rarely in other types of cancer, but which may well set the testicular cancer cell up for being hypersensitive to chemotherapy.

The genetic dysregulation displayed by the cancer cell will inevitably lead to a great deal of biologic and molecular heterogeneity. Application of chemotherapy at this point will quickly select for cells that show progressively more drug resistance. In fact, the surprising thing about cancer chemotherapy is not that it frequently fails, but that it is as effective as it is.

This chapter has distinguished between what we might call "upstream" drug action and sequelae of drug-target interaction such as apop-tosis. Virtually all of our present inventory of anticancer drugs might be described as upstream effectors, and we already have a large number of them. Differentiation inducers such as retinoids also appear to act remotely from the final differentiation or apoptosis pathways (69).

Unless nature has an unpleasant surprise for us, revealing another as yet unappreciated level of complexity in the cancer chemotherapy story, it appears that we are getting closer to being able to develop treatment strategies that will be based on the most fundamental processes operating within the cancer cell. The recent evidence linking chemotherapeutic effect to cell signal pathways that are responsible for initiating programed cell death points to new strategies for overcoming drug resistance. Preliminary studies in in vitro systems suggest that blocking expression of mutant *p53* with antisense oligonucleotides may trigger apoptosis in some tumor cell lines or, alternatively, sensitize cells to chemotherapeutic action (18). Translating these observations into clinically practical strategies is obviously a major challenge, but, at this point, there appears to be no reason in principle why such approaches might not work. Many things will need to be established, including whether such treatments will retain a useful therapeutic index with respect to effect on malignant cells versus normal ones. Theoretically, treatments directed at molecular abnormalities present only in cancer cells should be highly specific. Ascertaining whether this is the case is obviously going to be a matter of very high priority.

Drug-screening programs do not so far seem to have identified useful agents that act exclusively on the final steps in cell death. Agents of this type might be described as downstream effectors, and why some have not been found during random screening is puzzling. Unless such compounds have been missed in the screens, it may be that for some reason, natural selection has not favored such strategies in interspecies competition. Nature has been interested in producing efficient toxins against normal phenotypes rather than the category of mutants to which cancer cells belong. It is conceivable that the natural enviroment has few agents of this class and that new types of growth inhibitors will need to be synthesized. The next few years will see a determined search for such agents, and it seems not too optimistic to expect that some very useful drugs will emerge from this undertaking.

A final question to be considered is whether drugs that act by directly inhibiting the function of mutated oncogenes, antioncogenes, and promoter sequences will be subject to some of the same problems that have beset the conventional cytotoxic agents. That is, will the hetergeneity of loci of action produce resistance to these agents as well? The answer to this question must be a qualified "yes," as we know that the genes directly associated with cancer development exist in many mutant forms. Moreover, new classes of drugs will still need to be transported into the cell and escape detoxification. Nonetheless, it seems probable that a determined pharmacologic assault on these key targets, combined with standard treatment approaches, should start to yield treatment advances against broad spectrums of clinical malignancy.

REFERENCES

1. Rhoads CP. Nitrogen mustards in treatment of neoplastic disease. JAMA 1946;131:656–658.

2. Law LW. Origin of the resistance of leukemic cells to folic acid antagonists. Nature 1952;169:628–629.

3. Luria SE, Delbrück M. Mutations of bacteria from virus sensitivity to virus resistance. Genetics 1943;28:491–511.

4. Brockman RW. Mechanisms of resistance. In: Sartorelli AC, Jones DG, eds. Antineoplastic and immunosuppressive agents. Berlin: Springer-Verlag, 1974.

5. Hutchison DJ, Shmid FA. Cross resistance and collateral sensitivity. In: Mihich E, ed. Drug resistance and selectivity: biochemical and cellular basis. New York: Academic Press, 1973:73–126.

6. Hill BT. Biochemical and cell kinetic aspects of drug resistance. In: Bruchovsky N, Goldie JH, eds. Drug and hormone resistance in neoplasia. Boca Raton, FL: CRC Press, 1982:21–53.

7. Lowe SW, Ruley HE, Jacks T, Housman DE. p53 Dependant apoptosis modulates the cytotoxicity of anticancer agents. Cell 1993;74:957–967.

8. David HL. Probability distribution of drug resistant mutants in unselected populations of Mycobacterium tuberculosis. Appl Microbiol 1970;20:810–814.

9. Jaffrezou JP, Chen G, Duran GE, Kiihl JS, Sikic BI. Mutation rates and mechanisms of resistance to etoposide determined from fluctuation analysis. J Natl Cancer Inst 1994;86(15):1152–1158.

10. Chen G, Jaffrezou JP, Fleming WH, Duran GE, Sikic BI. Prevalence of multidrug resistance related to activation of the mdr1 gene in human sarcoma mutants derived by single-step doxorubicin selection. Cancer Res 1994;54:4980–4987.

11. Goldie JH, Coldman AJ. The genetic origin of drug resistance in neoplasms: implications for systemic therapy. Cancer Res 1984;44:3643–3653.

12. Ling V. Genetic basis of drug resistance mammalian cells. In: Bruchovsky N, Goldie JH, eds. Drug and hormone resistance in neoplasia, vol 1. Boca Raton, FL: CRC Press, 1982.

13. Bar-Eli M, Stang HD, Marcola KE, Cline NJ. Expression of a methotrexate resistant dihydrofolate reductase gene by transformed hematopoietic cells of mice. Somat Cell Genet 1983;9:55–67.

14. Nowell PC. The clonal evolution of tumor cell populations. Science 1978;194:23–28.

15. Cheng KC, Loeb LA. Genomic instability and tumor progression: mechanistic considerations. Adv Cancer Res 1993;60:121–156.

16. Loeb L. Mutator phenotype may be required for multistage carcinogenesis. Cancer Res 1991; 51:3075–3079.

17. Greenblatt MS, Bennett WP, Hollstein M, Harris CC. Mutations in the p53 tumor suppressor gene: clues to cancer etiology and molecular pathogenesis. Cancer Res 1994;54:4855–4878.

18. Martin SJ, Green DR. Apoptosis and cancer: the failure of controls on cell death and cell survival. Crit Rev Oncol Hematol 1995;18:137–153.

19. Bruce WR, Meaker BE, Valeriote FA. Comparison of the sensitivity of normal hematopoietic in transplanted lymphoma colony forming cells to chemotherapeutic agents administered in vivo. J Natl Cancer Inst 1966;37:233–245.

20. Durand RE. Chemosensitivity testing in V79 spheroids: role of drug delivery and cellular micro environment. J Natl Cancer Inst 1986;77:247–252.

21. Pardee AB. Growth dysregulation in cancer cells. Adv Cancer Res 1994;65:213–228.

22. Durand RE, Goldie JH. Interaction of etoposide and cisplatin in an in vitro tumor model. Cancer Treat Rep 1987;71:673–679.

23. Kobayushi H, Man S, Graham CH, et al. Acquired multicellular-mediated resistance to alkylating agents in cancer. Proc Natl Acad Sci USA 1993;90:3294–3298.

24. Teicher BA, Herman TS, Holden SA, et al. Tumor resistance to alkylating agents conferred by mechanisms operative only in vitro. Science 1990;247:1457–1461.

25. Goldman ID. Pharmacokinetics of antineoplastic agents at the cellular level. In: Chabner BA, ed. Pharmacologic principles of cancer treatment. Philadelphia: WB Saunders, 1982.

26. Goldman ID. The characteristics of the membrane transport of amethopterin and the naturally occurring folates. Ann NY Acad Sci 1971;186:400–422.

27. Goldenberg GJ, Begleiter B. Membrane transported alkylating agents. Pharmacol Ther 1980;8:237–274.

28. Gerlach JH, Kartner N, Bell DR, et al. Multi drug resistance. Cancer Surv 1986;5:25–46.

29. Evans RM, Laskin JD, Hakala MT. Assessment of growth limiting events caused by 5-fluorouracil in mouse cells and in human cells. Cancer Res 1980; 40:4113–4122.

30. Graham FL, Whitmore GF. Studies in mouse L-cells on the incorporation of 1b-D-arabinofuranosylcytosine into DNA and on the inhibition of DNA polymerase by 1b-D-arabinofuranosylcytosine-5' triphosphate. Cancer Res 1970;30:2636–2644.

31. Reichard P, Skold O, Klein G, et al. Studies on resistance against 5-fluorouracil. I. Enzymes of the uracil pathway during development of resistance. Cancer Res 1962;22:235–243.

32. Williams JW, Duggleby RG, Cutler R, et al. The inhibition of dihydrofolate reductase by folate analogues: structural requirements for slow and tight binding inhibitors. Biochem Pharmacol 1980;29:589–595.

33. Bertino JR, Donahue DR, Simmons B, et al. In-

duction of dihydrofolate reductase activity in leukocytes and erythrocytes in patients treated with methopterin. J Clin Invest 1963;42:466–475.

34. Flintooff WF, Asessani K. Methotrexate resistant Chinese hamster ovary cells contain a dihydrofolate reductase with an altered affinity for methotrexate. Biochemistry 1980;19:4321–4327.

35. Moscow JA, Dixon KH. Glutathione-related enzymes, glutathione and multi-drug resistance. In: Clynes M, ed. Multiple drug resistance in cancer. Norwell, MA: Kluver Academic, 1994:155–170.

36. Brookes P, Lawley PD. Evidence for the action of alkylating agents on deoxyribonucleic acid. Exp Cell Res 1963;(Suppl)9:521–524.

37. Kohn KW, Spears CL, Doty P. Intrastrand cross linking of DNA by nitrogen mustard. J Mol Biol 1966; 19:266–288.

38. Lawley PD, Brookes P. Cytotoxicity of alkylating agents towards sensitive and resistant strains of E. coli in relation to extent and mode of alkylation of cellular macromolecules and repair of alkylation lesions in deoxyribonucleic acid. Biochem J 1968; 109:433–447.

39. Roberts JJ, Brent TP, Crathorn AR. Evidence for the inactivation and repair of the mammalian DNA template after alkylation by mustard gas and half mustard gas. Eur J Cancer 1971;7:515–521.

40. Lindahl T. DNA repair enzymes. Annu Rev Biochem 1982;51:61–92.

41. Yarosh DB, Foote RS, Mitra S, Day RS. Repair of O (6)-methylguanine in DNA by demethylation is lacking in MER minus human tumor cell strains. Carcinogenesis 1983;4:199–205.

42. Taverna P, Hansson J, Scanlon KJ, Hill BT. Gene expression in x-irradiated human tumor cell lines expressing cisplatin resistance and altered DNA repair capacity. Carcinogenesis 1994;15:2053–2056.

43. Biedler JL, Riehm H. Cellular resistance to actinomycin D in Chinese hamster cells in vitro: cross resistance radioautographic and cytogenetic studies. Cancer Res 1970;30:1174–1179.

44. Ling V, Thompson LH. Reduced permeability in CHO cells as a mechanism of resistance to cultrasine. J Cell Physiol 1974;83:103–110.

45. Juliano RL, Ling V. A surface glycoprotein modulating drug permeability in Chinese hamster ovary cell mutants. Biochim Biophys Acta 1976; 455:152–159.

46. Bradley G, Juranka PF, Ling V. Mechanism of multidrug resistance. Biochim Biophys Acta 1988; 948:87–128.

47. Croop JM. P-glycoprotein structure and evolutionary homologous. In: Clynes M, ed. Multiple drug resistance in cancer. Norwell, MA: Kluwer Academic, 1994:1–32.

48. Cole SPC, Bhardway G, Gerbach JH, et al. Overexpression of a transporter gene in a multidrug resistant human lung cancer cell line. Science 1992; 258:1650–1654.

49. McClean S, Hill BT. An overview of membrane, cytosolic and nuclear proteins associated with the expression of multiple drugs in vitro. Biochim Biophys Acta 1992;1114:107–127.

50. Gerlach JH, Bell DR, Karakousis C, et al. P-glycoprotein in human sarcoma: evidence for multidrug resistance. J Clin Oncol 1987;5:1452–1460.

51. Ma DD, Davie RA, Harman DH, et al. Detection of a multidrug resistant phenotype in acute nonlymphoblastic leukemia. Lancet 1987;1:135–137.

52. Chan HS, Haddad G, Thorner PS, et al. P-glycoprotein expression as a predictor of outcome of therapy for neuroblastoma. N Engl J Med 1991;325:1608–1614.

53. Gascoyne RD, Tolcher A, Van Iderstine E, Connors JM. The prognostic sequence of p-glycoprotein expression in malignant lymphoma. Mod Pathol 1993; 6(1)A:5–18.

54. Xia F, Wang X, Wang YH, et al. Altered p53 status: correlation differences in sensitivity to radiation-induced mutations and apoptosis in two closely related human lymphoblast lives. Cancer Res 1995; 55:12–15.

55. Fisher TC, Milner AE, Gregory CD, et al. Bcl-2 modulation of apoptosis induced by anticancer drugs: resistance to thymidylate stress is independent of classical resistance pathways. Cancer Res 1993;53:3321–3326.

56. Goldie JH, Coldman AJ. A mathematic model for relating the drug sensitivity of tumors to their spontaneous mutation rate. Cancer Treat Rep 1979;63:1727–1733.

57. Coldman AJ, Goldie JH, Ng V. The effect of cellular differentiation on the development of permanent drug resistance. Math Biosci 1985;74:177–198.

58. Goldie JH, Coldman AJ. A model for tumor response to chemotherapy: an integration of the stem cell and somatic mutation hypothesis. Cancer Invest 1985; 3:553–564.

59. Goldie JH. Arguments supporting the concept of non-cross resistant combinations of chemotherapy. Cancer Invest 1994;12:324–328.

60. Fisher RJ, Gaynor ER, Dahlberg S, et al. Comparison of a standard regimen (CHOP) with 3 intensive chemotherapy regimens for advanced non-Hodgkin's lymphoma. N Engl J Med 1993;328:1002–1006.

61. Hill BT. Differing patterns of cross resistance from exposure to specific anti-tumor drugs or radiation in vitro. Cytotechnology 1993;12:265–288.

62. Powell SN, Abraham EH. The biology of radiation resistance: similarities, differences, and interactions with drug resistance. Cytotechnology 1993; 12:325–345.

63. Altman KI, Gerber GB, Okada S. Radiation biochemistry. Vol 1. London: Academic Press, 1970:52–56.

64. Tsuro T. Reversal of acquired resistance to vinca alkaloids and anthracycline antibiotics. Cancer Treat Rep 1983;67:889–894.

65. Grunicke H, Hofmann J, Utz I, Uberall F. Role of protein kinases in anti-tumor drug resistance. Ann Hematol 1994;69:s1–56.

66. Santi V. A biochemical rationale for the use of 5-fluorouracil in combination with leucovorin. Proceedings of symposium on the Current State of 5-Fluorouracil-Leucovorin Calcium Combinations. New York: Park Row, 1984:1–4.

67. Brandt SJ, Peters WP, Atwater SK, et al. Effect of recombinant human granulocyte-macrophage colony stimulating factor on hemopoietic reconstitution after high dose chemotherapy and autologous bone marrow transplantation. N Engl J Med 1988;318:869–876.

68. Lippman SM, Shin DM, Lee JJ, et al. P53 and retinoid chemoprevention of oral carcinogenesis. Cancer Res 1995;53:16–19.

6

Adjuvant Chemotherapy

Teresa Gilewski and Jacob D. Bitran

"All that we can do at the moment is speculate on the unknown but best we do this from a framework of the known—if the 'known' is truly known" (Anonymous). In 1971, Dr. H. Skipper applied this quote to his discussion of the cytokinetics of mammary tumor cells and its relevance toward the development of clinical therapeutic programs in the treatment of cancer (1). In the pursuit of new discoveries, it has often been characteristic of the medical community to build step by step upon factual information. This can be quite difficult to accomplish when treating human malignancies, since our understanding of tumor biology must, of necessity, often be obtained through the use of in vitro and in vivo animal models. The correlation of these models with the human counterpart has been subject to criticism. Can we assume the data and principles obtained from these studies can be applied to malignant tumors in humans? It is clear that while many therapeutic advances in man have arisen from knowledge acquired in experimental laboratory models, there are certainly many instances where the expected results did not occur. This latter situation has been especially noted in the exploration of adjuvant chemotherapy. Nevertheless, adjuvant therapy has proven to be beneficial in some human tumors and is based on several experimental concepts. A review of these concepts, in addition to factors that influence response to adjuvant chemotherapy, is presented, followed by an application of these ideas to human clinical trials.

DEFINITION AND HISTORY

Adjuvant chemotherapy involves the administration of chemotherapeutic agents, most often systematically, after removal of the primary tumor, at which point no evidence of residual disease exists. This treatment was founded on experimental data from the 1950s and 1960s that noted an inverse relationship between chemotherapeutic response and the number of tumor cells (2–4). The possibility of improved survival in patients with minimal disease after treatment with chemotherapy, coupled with the often poor responses documented in advanced disease, resulted in a considerable amount of enthusiasm for the utilization of adjuvant therapy. National clinical trials to address this issue were initiated in the mid-1950s and focused on cancers of gastrointestinal, lung, and breast origin (5, 6). Although, with the possible exception of breast cancer, the overall results were disappointing, it was suggested that the use of drugs ineffective for the specific tumors could account for these results. Therefore, studies from the following two decades employed a variety of supposedly effective chemotherapeutic agents in clinical as well as laboratory trials. Thus, a substantial amount of information concerning adjuvant therapy was produced, and although the outcome of these trials has been consistently positive in some diseases, such as Wilm's tumor, osteogenic sarcoma, colorectal cancer, and breast cancer, in many other solid tumors the results have not been as promising. The results of these clinical trials are reviewed later in this chapter.

Neoadjuvant chemotherapy also deserves mention at this point. This term, first used by Dr. E. Frei in 1982, refers to chemotherapy that is administered prior to local therapy in patients with localized disease for whom a completely effective treatment does not exist (7). It has been more recently defined as "primary chemotherapy," and the potential advantages and disadvantages of this therapy are described later (8, 9).

It is important to note that most laboratory and clinical studies have investigated the use of

79

adjuvant chemotherapy in a postoperative setting. However, the basic concepts of adjuvant therapy can also be applied to other forms of local treatment such as radiation therapy.

GENERAL CONCEPTS OF ADJUVANT CHEMOTHERAPY

Cell Kinetics

A general comprehension of cell kinetics and stem cell proliferation is fundamental to an understanding of adjuvant chemotherapy. The basic archetype of the cell cycle was documented in 1951 by Howard and Pelc using the technique of autoradiography (10). Since then, numerous investigators have contributed a substantial amount of information regarding cell kinetics and the cell cycle (11–14). The reproductive cycle of cells is controlled by external growth factors mediated through the activation of growth factor receptors and signal transduction to the nucleus. Cyclins are a family of proteins that regulate the normal cell cycles through cyclin-dependent kinases (13). Essentially, the cell cycle consists of several phases, including S, G_2, M, and G_1 (Fig. 6.1). DNA synthesis occurs during the S phase and is followed by the G_1 or postsynthetic phase; mitosis occurs during the M phase and is followed by the postmitotic or G_1 phase. The G_0 phase consists of nonproliferating or "resting" cells that under the appropriate conditions are capable of cell division. Most cell populations comprise both proliferating and nonproliferating cells. Some of the nonproliferating cells are capable of entering the active proliferating stage after stimulation (i.e., environmental changes), whereas other cells cannot undergo further cell division. The proportion of proliferating cells in relation to the total number of cells has been termed the growth fraction (14).

In the past, autoradiographic studies following the incorporation of tritiated thymidine (^{3}H-TdR) by cell nuclei synthesizing DNA allowed the determination of the labeling index (LI; ratio of labeled cells to total cells) and the percentage of labeled mitoses. However, autoradiography is time consuming, and other automated mechanisms such as flow cytometry have since been developed. At the present time, flow cytometry provides identical information. These values can then be applied to an estimation of the growth fraction and total cell cycle time or phase duration of a particular cell population (12). In an attempt to better delineate cell kinetics in human tumors, several studies have administered tritiated thymidine in vivo to patients with leukemia and solid tumors, either systematically, into neoplastic effusions, or into skin lesions (15–18). Unfortunately, many of the details of tumor cell kinetics remain unclear and under investigation.

Nonetheless, there is evidence to suggest that tumors grow because of differences in growth fractions between malignant and normal tissue, such that the rate of cell proliferation in malignant tissues is greater than the rate of cell death (18). Yet, even within the same tumor, a heterogeneous population of cells exists, which can exhibit varying cell cycle parameters (19). For example, Tannock, using a transplanted mouse mammary tumor, demonstrated that increasing tumor cell distance from the blood vessel could decrease the LI, perhaps by alteration of oxygen exposure (20). Other factors contributing to tumor heterogeneity include differences in drug sensitivity and stem cell characteristics.

Stem cells, those cells capable of unlimited proliferation, occur in normal tissue, and available data support the application of this concept to malignant tissues (20). In malignant disease the stem cells can potentially migrate to form metastases, in addition to promoting growth of the primary tumor. Since the development of in vitro soft agar colony-forming cell systems to maintain growth of human tumors, several studies have demonstrated that in human tumors, only a very small percentage (<1%) of cells may actually be clonogenic (stem cells) (22–23). How closely these systems approximate actual in vivo tumor growth is unknown, so caution must be used in interpreting the results.

Tumor Growth and Death

Knowledge of tumor growth and death patterns are essential to an understanding of adjuvant chemotherapy. Investigators from the Southern Research Institute and the National Cancer Institute have used a rapidly proliferating transplantable murine leukemia cell line

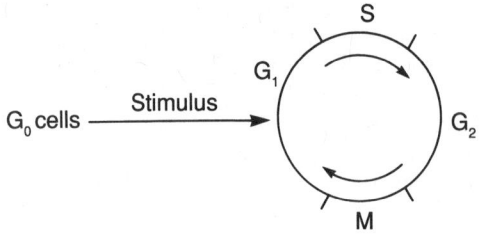

Figure 6.1.   Model of a cell cycle.

(L1210) to make the following observations with regard to tumor growth: (*a*) a single malignant cell can be lethal, (*b*) a relatively constant percentage of cells is destroyed after a specific dose of an effective drug, (*c*) a dose-response relationship can exist between an effective agent and its target cell population, and (*d*) treatment outcome is influenced by the number of malignant cells (3, 24). The growth fraction of this leukemia is nearly 100%, and it, therefore, provided a relatively predictable growth pattern, which followed exponential kinetics (25, 26). However, many animal tumors and human tumors do not follow such a pattern of growth and instead appear to proliferate by Gompertzian kinetics. As opposed to exponential kinetics, in which the growth factor is constant, the growth fraction in Gompertzian kinetics tends to reach its maximum when the tumor is approximately 37% of its greatest size. Thereafter, the growth fraction decreases exponentially and the tumor mass levels off (Fig. 6.2) (1, 9).

Early laboratory studies suggested several additional concepts regarding tumor development: (*a*) with progressive tumor expansion, growth fraction and sensitivity to antimetabolite agents decrease, and doubling time (time for the tumor to double in size) increases; (*b*) with a reduction in tumor mass, the growth fraction of the residual tumor cells subsequently increases; (*c*) rapidly growing tumors are more sensitive to chemotherapy; and (*d*) chemotherapy is often more effective on disseminated small foci of tumor cells than on "crowded" measurable solid tumors (11, 27). As Skipper succinctly stated: "The doubling time of tumors is often an ever changing value" (1). It is important to realize that the doubling time is not always an accurate reflection of the rate of cell proliferation (28). For example, it is possible that some tumors have a

high degree of cell loss, in addition to a high proliferation rate, so that the doubling time does not correlate with the extent of cell production. Therefore, a "slow-growing tumor" may not necessarily indicate a low "growth fraction" (22). This factor may partially explain the better than expected responsiveness of some tumors with long doubling times (28).

The concept of first-order kinetics in regard to cell kill is a critical principle in chemotherapy. As previously mentioned in the L1210 leukemia studies, this concept emphasizes that a constant percentage or fraction of a specific cell population, irrespective of size, will be destroyed with a constant dose of drug (29). Although this applies to tumors following exponential growth patterns, it may not pertain to many solid tumors that appear to have Gompertzian growth. To achieve a cure, all tumor cells actively dividing or capable of proliferation must be killed. However, the number of cells present, the cell kinetics, the chemotherapeutic agent administered, and the tumor growth rate can all play key roles in tumor response. For example, Shackney et al. have graphically demonstrated the difference in fractional cell kill that can occur between rapidly and slowly growing solid tumors (28) (Fig. 6.3). Treatment of rapidly growing tumors in early clinical stages may produce a complete response with a large fractional cell kill, whereas treatment of slowly growing tumors at a similar stage results in smaller cell kills and early recurrence. It may be necessary to treat the slowly growing tumors at a subclinical stage to achieve larger fractional cell kills and a possible complete response or cure.

Another concept that warrants reemphasis is the inverse relationship between growth fraction and tumor cell size. Laboratory studies have suggested an increase in growth fraction with tumor reduction. For example, Schabel detected minimal tumor cell kill in a transplantable plasmacytoma after treatment with cytosine arabinoside (ara-C) (29). However, if the hamsters received cyclophosphamide initially, resulting in a 3- to 4-log cell kill, followed by ara-C at the same dose and time, cure was achieved in more than 50% of the animals. It was suggested that the residual tumor cells were more sensitive to ara-C than previously because of a higher growth fraction. This observation can be applied to treatment of micrometastasis in adjuvant therapy, where the cells may be characterized by a higher growth fraction and greater sensitivity to drugs, particularly those that are cell-cycle specific. There-

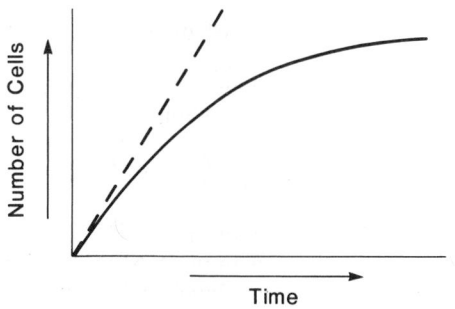

Figure 6.2. Patterns of tumor growth. Exponential kinetics, *dashed line*; Gompertzian kinetics, *solid line*.

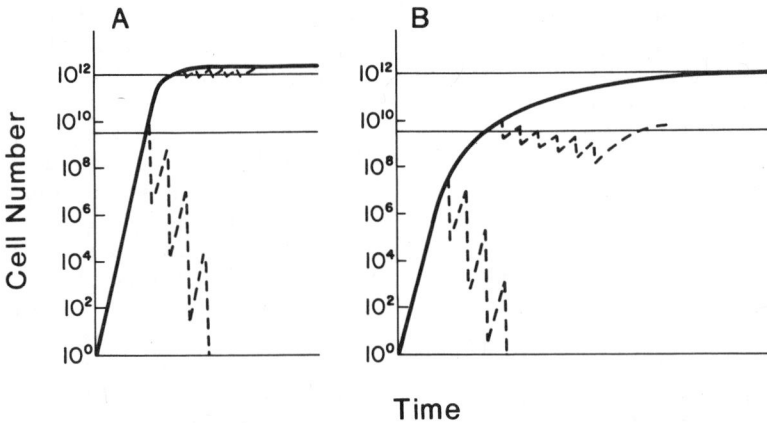

Figure 6.3.   Schematic representation of fractional cell kill in rapidly growing (A) and slowly growing (B) tumors. (From Schackney SE, McCormack GW, Cuchural GJ. Growth rate patterns of solid tumors and their relative responsiveness to therapy. Ann Intern Med 1978;89:107–121.).

fore, the patterns of tumor growth and destruction are critical to an understanding of adjuvant chemotherapy.

Drugs

Although the development and features of chemotherapeutic agents are detailed in other chapters, a brief overview is pertinent to this discussion of adjuvant therapy. Of the many factors involved in the ultimate effect of adjuvant chemotherapy, one of the most crucial elements is the choice of the anticancer drug. Several chemotherapeutic agents are relatively cell-cycle specific (e.g., antimetabolites and vinca alkaloids), implying that they are most active in certain phases of the proliferating cells (30). Other drugs may have a cytotoxic effect on both actively dividing and nonproliferating cells. Therefore, the antitumor response and toxicities induced by a drug may be greatly influenced not only by the intrinsic sensitivity of the cells to that agent but also by the cell cycle (23). The effectiveness of a drug for adjuvant therapy cannot always be based on the response that occurs in measurable advanced disease (31, 32). However, in general, drugs active in an adjuvant setting tend to be effective in advanced disease (33). Agents used adjuvantly must be active not only in controlling metastatic disease but in preventing local regrowth of tumor as well (34).

Although of interest, the use of in vitro assays for selection of chemotherapeutic agents for individual patients has not become prevalent owing to technical difficulties and expense (9, 35).

In addition, there is no evidence that the information from these assays, in comparison to currently available knowledge, significantly improves clinical management. Likewise, the screening of new drugs for use in clinical trials, employing animal models, human xenografts, and human tumor cell lines is a laborious process fraught with numerous difficulties (36, 37). Certainly, the lack of effective available agents can be a limiting factor to the potential benefit of adjuvant chemotherapy.

FACTORS INFLUENCING RESPONSE

Several significant factors in determining the effectiveness of adjuvant chemotherapy have been documented in animal laboratory experiments. These include tumor burden, dose and schedule of the administered chemotherapeutic agent, the use of combination chemotherapy, and the development of drug resistance.

Tumor Burden

As previously noted, a very important principle in adjuvant chemotherapy is the inverse relationship between number of tumor cells and chemotherapeutic response. In 1957, Shapiro and Fugmann reported the effect of intraperitoneal 6-mercaptopurine (6-MP) on a mammary adenocarcinoma in mice (2). The administration of 6-MP 24 hours after tumor transplantation resulted in an average of 57% "cures," whereas no cures were obtained if therapy was delayed until 15 days after tumor implantation. At 15 days neither surgery nor chemotherapy alone achieved a cure. However, 6-MP administration, after partial excision of a 15-day-old tumor to achieve the size of a tumor less than 8 days old, resulted in a 57% "cure" rate. This suggested that the age of the tumor was not a critical factor. To determine whether tumor mass or number of tumor cells was more significant, bilateral implants were evaluated (one was a 15-day-old larger mass and the other a smaller 5-day-old mass). Chemotherapy resulted in an average "cure" rate of 18% in the smaller tumor; however, if the larger tumor was excised on the day of the 6-MP administration, the "cure" rate for the smaller tumor markedly increased. This reinforced the idea that the number of tumor cells, regardless of "aggregate size," was the key factor in response, since the cure rate for the smaller tumor should have been similar in both situations if mass was the important element. These data and information from other early studies resulted in numerous trials over the next two decades to expand upon this concept (3, 4).

A variety of chemotherapeutic agents administered in a surgical adjuvant setting have been studied in other spontaneous and transplantable tumors such as Lewis lung carcinoma, colon carcinoma, B16 melanoma, and Ridgeway osteogenic sarcoma (1, 31, 34, 38–42). Adjuvant chemotherapy has achieved an increase in cure rates as well as an increased life span in numerous studies (1, 31, 34, 38, 40, 41). In addition, further studies suggest (a) an inverse relationship between cure rates and primary tumor mass at the time of surgery, (b) a direct relationship between primary tumor mass and incidence of metastatic disease, and (c) a direct relationship between primary tumor mass at the time of surgery and cure rates with surgical adjuvant chemotherapy (31, 34, 38, 40, 41).

Tumors of different histologic types do not uniformly metastasize, so that in some instances (e.g., B16 melanoma), large tumors may be curable with surgery alone or surgery plus chemotherapy, whereas a tumor of similar size in another model would be incurable with either therapeutic option (40). This may be due to the lack of metastatic disease or to the presence of a drug-sensitive low metastatic burden in the former model, despite the primary tumor size. Although many models support the concept of greater response with minimal disease (i.e., an adjuvant setting), an occasional model has demonstrated better chemotherapeutic response for a large primary tumor than for micrometastic

disease (32). Therefore, other factors besides tumor burden play a role in determination of ultimate chemotherapeutic effect.

Dose

The concept of dose or dose intensity (dose per unit of time) is critical in a discussion of chemotherapy, whether in the treatment of advanced disease or in an adjuvant setting. Several laboratory studies have demonstrated the importance of administration of maximum dose, as reduction in dose resulted in decreased therapeutic benefit (33, 38, 41–43). For example, in a mammary adenocarcinoma murine model, a 33% reduction in the doses of adjuvant cyclophosphamide and CCNU decreased the cure rate from greater than 80% to less than 50% and shortened the life span of the dying animals (31). Skipper found that in numerous animal models, dose was a significant factor in therapeutic outcome, and a reduction could produce a decrease in cure rate (44). In another experiment, using B16 melanoma cells, administration of methyl-CCNU 2 days after tumor implantation, when tumor was still unmeasurable, resulted in increased survival time and a delay in tumor appearance (40). Although no cures were achieved, better responses occurred at higher doses. Other experiments have documented numerous factors involved in dose-response curves, including the specific agents used, drug sensitivity of the tumor, and dose-schedule interactions (45). The drawback to higher doses is the development of toxicity that can potentially result in death. However, the dose-response curve is often steeper for tumors with a higher growth fraction, so the concept of dose intensity may be of considerable significance in treating micrometastases in an adjuvant setting, when cells may be more rapidly proliferating (39).

Combination versus Single-Agent Therapy

Combinations of chemotherapeutic agents have been administered in animal experiments, in both advanced and adjuvant settings, and the theory behind the use of combination chemotherapy is described elsewhere in this book. Therapeutic synergism with combinations of individually active drugs has been documented for many animal solid tumors in advanced disease (43). Adjuvant studies utilizing the Lewis lung carcinoma documented an increase in life span after postoperative administration of either bleomycin + methyl-CCNU or cisplatin + CCNU (34). The results were superior to those noted after surgery and single-agent therapy. However, if surgery was not performed, combination chemotherapy yielded effects similar to those obtained with single-agent chemotherapy. Several other studies have also demonstrated greater effectiveness with a particular adjuvant-combination chemotherapy regimen compared with single agents or other chemotherapy combinations (40, 46). However, the effectiveness of drug combinations may depend not only on the individual activity of each agent for the tumor but also on the proliferative rate of the tumor and scheduling of the drug administration (i.e., simultaneously or sequentially) (12, 43).

Schedule of Drug Administration

Chemotherapy can be administered either preoperatively, during surgery, or postoperatively. Obviously, drugs can also be used adjuvantly in a pre- or postradiation therapy setting, but most laboratory studies have involved surgery as the primary modality. Most laboratory trials have generally noted therapeutic effectiveness after administration of adjuvant chemotherapy within 1 to 5 days after surgery (1, 2, 31, 34). However, some studies have noted greater benefit with preoperative chemotherapy (34, 38). Survival may be affected by the timing of chemotherapy (i.e., preoperatively, same day as surgery, or postoperatively) in relation to the interval between tumor implantation and surgery (38). In addition, the duration of therapy and interval between doses of drugs may influence the effectiveness of adjuvant therapy (12, 47, 48). In many of these models, chemotherapy delays of several days could affect the outcome of therapy, since these tumors had relatively rapid doubling times, which could result in a prompt increase in tumor burden (41). Since timing of the initiation of adjuvant chemotherapy appears to influence therapeutic outcome, several studies have attempted to determine factors that may affect the development of postoperative metastases.

Evidence from animal models has documented an increase in the size of metastases after removal of the primary tumor, although both an increase and a decrease in the number of metastases have been noted (49, 50). Some data suggest that this postoperative growth may be due to release of tumor cells resulting from surgical manipulation of the tumor or progressive growth of already existing metastases, either from altera-

tions in the immune system or other effects of the surgery (49, 51–54). Simpson-Herren et al., utilizing Lewis lung carcinoma, demonstrated increases in the LI and growth rate, with minimal alteration in cell cycle parameters, of pulmonary metastases after a resection of the primary tumor (54). A decrease in life span occurred if the surgery was performed more than 6 days after initial tumor implantation, yet some cures and increased life spans occurred with earlier surgical excision. Interestingly, sham surgery (excision of normal tissue, thereby simulating tumor resection without actually disturbing the tumor) also resulted in a decrease in life span and increased the LI of both the primary tumor and the metastases. The life span of mice after establishment of artificial metastases (from intravenous injection of tumor cells) was increased after implantation of a subcutaneous tumor compared with that of mice receiving only the intravenous implant. This effect was related to the time of subcutaneous implantation relative to the intravenous infusion and suggested that the presence of a solid growing tumor inhibited the growth of the smaller metastatic foci. Therefore, these experiments indicated that a noncurative resection of the primary tumor could stimulate growth of residual disease.

Other studies have also evaluated the interaction between tumor foci. Using a mammary adenocarcinoma, Gunduz et al. simultaneously implanted two separate foci of tumor into several mice (55). With removal of one focus of tumor, the residual tumor was found to have a transient increase in the LI and growth fraction, with an increase in tumor size noted approximately 1 week later. The cell cycle parameters did not change significantly, indicating that the tumor growth was likely secondary to a shift of noncycling (G_0) cells to an activity dividing state. However, the tumor growth rate in mice initially injected with only one tumor focus did not differ from that of those implanted with two foci until the advanced stages of tumor growth. At that point, the single tumors developed at a more rapid rate. This experiment failed to document a significant interaction between growth patterns of two tumor foci until removal of one of the tumors.

A later study by the same group noted the influence of the time interval between primary tumor resection and chemotherapy on tumor growth and survival (56). In mice implanted with two different amounts of mammary carcinoma, resection of the larger focus resulted in a transient increase in LI (7-day duration) and an increase in growth of the residual tumor. Administration of cyclophosphamide on the day of surgery resulted in various effects on tumor growth depending on the dose. With 60 mg/kg, a transient rise (greater than in those treated with surgery alone) in labeling index followed by a depression occurred, and tumor growth was uninhibited. After doses of 120 or 240 mg/mg, a marked reduction in LI occurred in association with a suppression of tumor growth. Depression of LI was also noted with postoperative administration of cyclophosphamide, in association with a dose-related reduction of tumor growth. However, for the first 10 to 12 days after initiation of treatment, the greatest suppression of tumor growth and prolongation of survival occurred after preoperative administration of cyclophosphamide (5 or 7 days prior to surgery). During the first 4 weeks from start of therapy, postoperative chemotherapy was the least effective in improving survival, in comparison to preoperative or perioperative chemotherapy. However, even with postoperative chemotherapy, survival was greater than in untreated controls, although the benefit of chemotherapy decreased with progressive delays between its administration and removal of the primary tumor. For the lower dose of cyclophosphamide, the time interval between its administration and surgery was especially important. Of interest was the observation that suppression of metastatic tumor growth after administration of cyclophosphamide did not differ significantly between mice who underwent removal of the primary tumor and those who did not. This study suggests that tumor burden may not always be a critical factor in determining response to adjuvant therapy and that the timing of chemotherapeutic administration may be important. In addition to surgery, the possibility of an increase in metastases after radiation therapy has also been investigated (57). In summary, based on experimental models, the timing of adjuvant chemotherapy may significantly influence the therapeutic outcome.

Drug Resistance

Response to adjuvant chemotherapy can be influenced not only by the aforementioned factors but also by the presence of drug-resistant cells. Drug resistance can be temporary or permanent. Temporary resistance may arise in a situation where growth characteristics reduce cell sensitivity to a drug or physiologic limitations inhibit adequate exposure of the cancer cell to the drug (19). Early studies considered the growth and selection of drug-resistant tumor cells to be a significant factor in causing chemotherapeutic failure (58). The likelihood of an inadequate therapeutic outcome was felt to be greater with larger tumor burdens, where the existence of resistant cells was more probable because of their selection after repetitive cycles of drugs (39). This pattern was consistent with tumors that initially responded to therapy and subsequently developed drug resistance.

However, in 1943 Luria and Delbrück suggested that virus-resistant bacteria developed by spontaneous mutations independent of exposure to the virus (59). In 1979, Goldie and Coldman introduced a mathematical model to explain drug resistance based on this principle of spontaneous mutation (60). They proposed that resistant phenotypes are generated by random genetic alterations and that the presence of a resistant clone depends upon the mutation rate and growth curve of the tumor. The probability of resistant cells increases with tumor size, so that larger tumors have a greater potential for drug resistance. The ability to achieve cure is markedly reduced at a certain time in tumor growth when the cells increase by 1.77 logs (5.9 doublings). The point at which this critical period occurs depends on the mutation rate of the tumor. This model was later modified in 1983 to account for the variation in proliferative capacity of tumor cells and anticipated that slowly growing advanced tumors will have significant phenotypic heterogeneity with development of multiple levels of drug resistance (61). The size and the biologic age of the tumor (number of doublings to reach a certain size) have a significant impact on the extent of heterogeneity (62). However, even these very heterogeneous tumors are potentially curable at a certain time in their growth. This model would favor the early use of adjuvant therapy, as well as combination or alternating chemotherapy, in an attempt to circumvent drug resistance (63). For example, Skipper demonstrated in a murine sarcoma that alteration of cyclophosphamide and 6-mercaptopurine resulted in cures, whereas either agent alone produced resistance and treatment failure (64).

Another important concept is that of multidrug, or pleiotropic, drug resistance (MDR)—development of resistance to several unrelated drugs after exposure to a single agent. MDR has been associated with the presence of a surface glycoprotein (P-glycoprotein) and several other factors (9, 65, 66). Additional mechanisms for drug resistance include gene amplification and enzyme alteration. These are described in greater detail elsewhere (9, 67).

In summary, the presence of permanently resistant tumor stem cells at the time of treatment or their development during therapy is frequently the culprit of chemotherapeutic failure (40). One hopes that new strategies to circumvent drug resistance will result in improved therapeutic response (68). Finally, DeVita has noted that drug resistance in normal target tissue has not occurred in numerous studies (19). The explanation for this observation is unknown. It is clear that drug resistance is an important factor to consider in the use of adjuvant therapy.

ANIMAL MODELS

Most of the data in the prior sections was obtained from laboratory experiments utilizing murine tumor models. Much of this information has been applied toward the development of adjuvant therapy programs in humans. A criticism of this approach questions the validity of application of knowledge gained from animal studies to the human system. Griswold comments upon the importance of demonstrating that the "animal tumor system is not just another tumor but is indeed a model of some human cancer" (41). Such factors as tumor growth rates, patterns of metastatic growth, tumor sensitivity to certain drugs, and evaluation of response (i.e., endpoints) should ideally be similar when applying

information from one system to another (41). Many animal studies have utilized transplantable tumors, which may differ in many aspects from spontaneous malignancies in humans (33). In addition, the administration of surgical adjuvant chemotherapy in animal studies probably only approximates the biologic environment occurring in humans at that time. Nevertheless, despite all of these differences, basic generalizations regarding adjuvant therapy can be ascertained from these animal models and applied to the human system, with the realization that the unique characteristics of humans are yet to be identified. The development of new models may help to alleviate some of these difficulties (69).

HUMAN CLINICAL TRIALS

Cancers in humans often remain undetected until the tumor is palpable, at which point approximately 1 g or 10^9 malignant cells are present; to achieve this size, there have been approximately 30 doublings (19). Death often occurs when the tumor mass reaches 1 kilogram or 10^{12} cells (70) (Fig. 6.4). The development of metastases is a complex process and presumably a relatively inefficient one, since these cells must survive despite numerous prohibitive immunologic and environmental factors (71). Metastases tend to consist of heterogeneous population of cells, so that metastatic deposits may exhibit characteristics that differ not only from those of the primary tumor but from those of other metastatic foci as well. The purpose of adjuvant chemo-

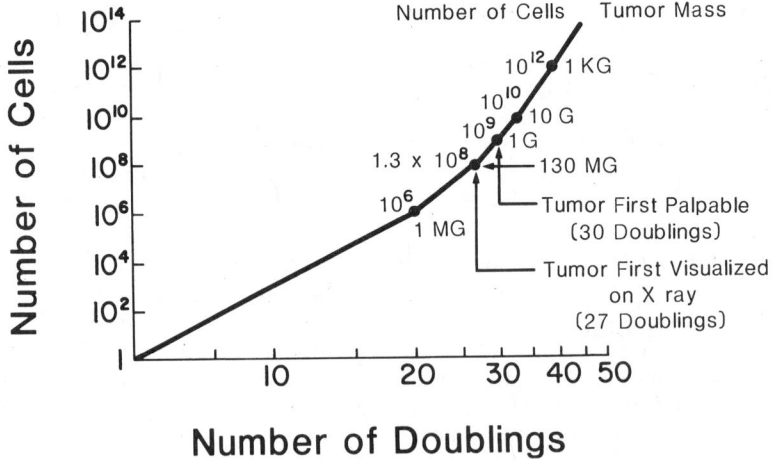

Figure 6.4. The life cycle of human cancers relating clinical events to the number of cells and population doublings. (From DeVita VT. The James Ewing lecture: relationship between tumor mass and resistance to chemotherapy. Cancer 1983;51:1209–1220.).

therapy is the destruction of a subclinical tumor stem cell population, whether microscopic local residual or micrometastatic disease. A 99.9 to 99.99% (3- to 4-log) decrease in human leukemic cells after single-agent chemotherapy has been estimated to result in complete remission (72). This figure has subsequently been used in other tumors as a guide to the amount of cell destruction necessary to achieve potential cure. Clinical trials using postoperative adjuvant chemotherapy were initiated in the 1950s, based on the premise that recurrences could develop as a result of surgical manipulation of the tumor (42). Several early studies evaluated the use of nitrogen mustard in lung cancer and thiotepa in gastric, colorectal, and breast carcinomas, administered the day of surgery and for several days postoperatively (6). With the exception of breast cancer, the results were generally discouraging. However, part of the explanation for these results was felt to be ineffective drugs. As new drugs were developed and found to be effective in advanced disease, they were subsequently tested in adjuvant settings. A review of several general concepts of adjuvant therapy as they specifically relate to human malignancies is presented below. These include the influence of dose, toxicities, timing of chemotherapy administration, drug resistance, and amount of tumor on therapeutic outcome. In addition, endpoints used in adjuvant trials and responses documented in various human malignancies are reviewed.

Dose

Adjuvant trials in the 1960s and 1970s did not emphasize dose intensity as a significant element in the quest for cure (73). Often doses were reduced in anticipation of decreasing toxicity, without much attention paid to the possibility of decreasing the chance for cure. Yet, as DeVita has mentioned, "dead patients don't complain of side effects" (73). It seems more apparent today that alterations in dose intensity and initial chemotherapy treatments may well be the most critical factor in causing therapeutic failure for drug-sensitive tumors (9). However, the practice of dose reduction in adjuvant chemotherapy is widespread in the oncologic community because of the desire to minimize toxicities in otherwise asymptomatic individuals, of whom a portion will be cured by local treatment alone (33).

Hryniuk and colleagues have developed a method of analyzing the influence of dose inten-

sity on therapeutic outcome (74). Dose intensity for single agents is defined as the amount of drug administered per unit time ($mg/m^2/week$), whereas a relative dose intensity is used for evaluation of multiagent chemotherapeutic programs. This latter calculation involves computing dose intensities for each individual drug in $mg/m^2/week$. These values are then used to obtain a decimal fraction for each drug, comparing the dose intensity in the standard regimen to that of the current regimen. An average relative dose intensity can then be obtained by averaging the individual components (75) (Table 6.1). Assumptions in this analysis of dose intensity included: (*a*) the schedule of drug administration does not significantly influence antitumor effect (although scheduling may effect toxicity); (*b*) various routes of administration are equivalent; (*c*) drugs administered simultaneously do not significantly interact with each other; and (*d*) individual drugs in a combination are equivalent in activity. It is important to distinguish between the projected dose and the dose actually received by the patient, as these may differ and can affect evaluation of a drug regimen through factors such as dose reduction of individual drugs and treatment delays. In multiagent trials, the impact of specific drugs on the overall drug combination can also be assessed by this analysis. Other factors that may influence the impact of dose intensity are the total amount of drug administered and the tumor burden (74, 75). Although a probable correlation between therapeutic outcome and dose intensity has been documented in advanced stages of lymphomas, breast cancer, colon cancer, and ovarian carcinoma, the impact of dose in adjuvant therapy trials is not as well defined (9, 75–78).

Information on a dose-response relationship for adjuvant therapy is lacking for most tumors, although this area has been evaluated to an extent in breast cancer. One of the earliest studies addressing this concept was a retrospective analysis reported by Bonadonna and Valagussa in 1981 (79). Patients received postoperative CMF (cyclophosphamide, methotrexate, 5-fluorouracil) for 6 to 12 months, with dose reductions for toxicities, patient refusal, age, and other reasons. Patients were subsequently categorized into one of the following groups depending on the percentage of projected dose actually administered: level I, >85%; level II, 65 to 84%; level III, <65%. Drug doses influenced the 5-year relapse-free survival (RFS) rate in both pre- and postmenopausal women, with greater responses noted for

Table 6.1. Sample Calculations: Dose Intensity, Relative Dose Intensity, and Average Relative Dose Intensity

	Dose Intensity	Relative Dose Intensity
Calculation of Dose Intensity		
Test Schedule		
Cyclophosphamide 80 mg/m^2/day (continuously)	560 mg/m^2/week	
Calculation of Relative Dose Intensity		
Standard		
Cyclophosphamide 80 mg/m^2/day (continuously)	560 mg/m^2/week	
		Test Schedule
Cyclophosphamide 100 mg/m^2/day	350 mg/m^2/week	350/560 = 0.62
(days 1–14, q 28 days)		
Calculation of Average Relative Dose Intensity		
Standard[a]		
Cyclophosphamide 2 mg/kg/day	560 mg/m^2/week	
Methotrexate 0.7 mg/kg/week	28 mg/m^2/week	
5-Fluorouracil 12 mg/kg/week	480 mg/m^2/week	
Test Regimen		
Cyclophosphamide 100 mg/m^2/day (days 1–14)	350 mg/m^2/week	350/560 = 0.62
Methotrexate 40 mg/m^2/days 1, 8	20 mg/m^2/week	20/28 = 0.71
5-Fluorouracil 600 mg/m^2/days 1, 8	300 mg/m^2/week	300/480 = 0.62
Repeat cycles every 28 days		*Average* 0.65

From Hryniuk WM. The importance of dose intensity in the outcomes of chemotherapy. In: DeVita VT, Hellman S, Rosenberg SA, eds. Important advances in oncology 1988. Philadelphia: JB Lippincott, 1988:121–142. With permission.
[a]Assume standard regimen to be CMF content of CMFVP regimen of Cooper and associates. To convert mg/kg to mg/m^2, multiply by 40.

level I patients. The number of involved lymph nodes within each group also had an impact upon RFS.

Another retrospective analysis by Hryniuk and others employed the previously described method of dose intensity to evaluate approximately 6000 stage II breast cancer patients with adjuvant CMF and melphalan coregimens (80, 81). The standard regimen used was the CMFVP combination developed by Cooper et al., although for this analysis it was assumed that vincristine (V) and prednisone (P) did not influence therapeutic outcome (80). Other assumptions included: (*a*) mg of cyclophosphamide = 40 × mg melphalan, (*b*) a dose intensity of 0 was allotted to drugs missing from the CMF combination, and (*c*) CMF and melphalan had equivalent antitumor effects for breast cancer. A relationship between projected dose intensity and 3-year RFS was noted for pre- and postmenopausal patients and all lymph node subsets. However, these data were later reanalyzed after restriction of trials to those realizing only CMF or CMFVP regimens, which resulted in the lack of a definite significant relationship between dose intensity and disease-free survival (45, 83).

A concise review of other retrospective analyses supporting or disproving a correlation between dose and disease-free or overall survival for adjuvant therapy in breast cancer has been compiled by Henderson et al. (45). Several randomized trials employing different doses of adjuvant chemotherapy for breast cancer have thus far not documented any dose-response relationship with disease-free or overall survival (84–86). High-dose chemotherapy followed by autologous bone marrow reinfusion, based on the assumption of steep dose-response curves for certain drugs, is also undergoing evaluation in both metastatic breast cancer and in an adjuvant setting for women at high risk for recurrence (more than 10 involved lymph nodes) (87–89). The administration of adjuvant high-dose chemotherapy is an intriguing concept, although the effectiveness relative to toxicity will require careful assessment.

The duration of adjuvant therapy in breast cancer has been addressed in studies from Italy. These studies documented no significant difference in therapeutic outcomes in 6 versus 12 months of therapy, although there was a trend in favor of the shorter course (90, 91). Administration of a higher percentage of projected dose was observed in the group receiving only 6 months of therapy. Other trials comparing various durations of therapy in breast cancer have not shown a consistent improvement in outcome with the longer durations (92).

A final comment regarding dose in clinical trials is the application of the Norton and Simon hypothesis to adjuvant therapy, which is presented in detail elsewhere in this book (93). This suggests that a "late intensification," or "spike," of chemotherapy (possibly a combination of drugs or an alternating schedule of chemotherapeutic agents) at the end of a planned course of treatment may eradicate microscopic tumor that would otherwise recur. This hypothesis has not been adequately tested in clinical trials thus far. In summary, at this time the impact of dose and duration of treatment on the outcome of adjuvant therapy has not been clearly defined.

Toxicities of Adjuvant Therapy

Toxicities due to adjuvant chemotherapy are an important issue, since, as previously mentioned, this may be a dose-limiting factor. The concept of cost-effectiveness—"Are the potential benefits worth the cost?" (i.e., monetary, morbidity/mortality)—is of significance in adjuvant therapy (94). Although most side effects from chemotherapy are transient and relatively well tolerated (e.g., alopecia, myelosuppression, gastrointestinal disturbances), long-term effects such as cardiac toxicity, as well as death, can occur as a result of adjuvant therapy. In addition, the possibility of increasing the risk of secondary malignancies does exist. Carcinogenic potential for numerous chemotherapeutic agents has been noted in animal models (95). In human studies, much information on the development of secondary malignancies has accumulated from studies in advanced breast cancer, Hodgkin's disease, non-Hodgkin's lymphoma, and ovarian cancer (96–98). However, evaluation of several adjuvant studies has yielded some data on the risk of secondary malignancies.

In breast cancer, Fisher et al. reported 27 cases of leukemia in 5299 patients (0.5%) treated with adjuvant L-phenylalanine mustard-containing regimens, with a cumulative risk of 1.29% ± 28% at 10 years for all patients; a cumulative risk of 0.27% at 10 years occurred in those treated with surgery alone (99). A statistically significant increased relative risk of acute myelogenous leukemia occurred following chemotherapy (24 ×

expected incidence). Several studies have also documented the development of leukemia after adjuvant therapy in breast cancer, utilizing drugs such as thiotepa, cyclophosphamide, chlorambucil, and nitrogen mustard, alone or in combination (99, 102). However, other analyses have failed to demonstrate an increased incidence of acute leukemia (103, 104). For example, at 10 years, Valagussa et al. did not observe any cases of acute leukemia in 666 patients treated with adjuvant CMF but did note development of 16 second solid tumors. The cumulative frequency of 4.2% ± 1.03, however, was similar to that observed after surgery alone (103). Adjuvant therapy of gastrointestinal cancers with methyl-CCNU resulted in a 4.0 ± 2.2% 6-year cumulative mean risk of developing acute leukemia or preleukemia (105).

In many diseases, longer follow-up is needed to evaluate the risk of secondary malignancies after adjuvant therapy. Numerous other factors may influence this risk, including total dose of drug administered, number of patients evaluated, types of drugs administered, preexistent risk of developing a malignancy, and other causes of death (106). Although it is also often difficult to evaluate quality-of-life issues, this is another important aspect of assessing cost-effectiveness, especially in an adjuvant setting. This type of analysis has been recently reported in postmenopausal women with breast cancer who received adjuvant therapy (107). In summary, the value of determining toxicities and means of circumventing these complications cannot be underestimated for adjuvant chemotherapy.

Timing of Therapy

Information from experimental models indicates that timing of drug administration may have an impact on the therapeutic outcome. In human trials, the best time to initiate adjuvant therapy is not clear. Most adjuvant regimens begin within 4 to 6 weeks of surgery; however, chemotherapy has also been used in a perioperative (immediately postoperative) or preoperative (primary/neoadjuvant) setting.

PERIOPERATIVE THERAPY

Wittes has observed several potential difficulties that probably inhibit the widespread use of this form of adjuvant therapy (31). First, the acute toxicities that often arise from chemotherapy may contribute to an increase in postoperative complications. Common side effects such as myelosuppression and nausea/vomiting may result in a greater frequency of infection and incidence of pain requiring sedation, respectively. This latter complication could potentially result in respiratory compromise. Second, inadequate wound healing may occur and may be influenced by the type of drug administered (108). Third, this may be a poor option for those diseases in which the choice of treatment depends upon classification of pathologic stage. Fourth, the feasibility of perioperative drug administration requires a coordinated effort between surgeon, medical oncologist, and ancillary services, which can often be difficult to achieve. Finally, the opportunity for extensive discussion of the disease and treatment options may be lost if a definite preoperative diagnosis cannot be established and therapy is immediately administered.

Despite these potential obstacles, several clinical perioperative trials have been conducted. One of the most supportive trials for the use of perioperative therapy is the Scandinavian trial in which breast cancer patients were randomized to no therapy or 6 days of cyclophosphamide beginning immediately postoperatively (109). An improvement in disease-free survival for the treated group remained after 20 years of follow-up. The British Cancer Research Campaign has noted similar results with a nearly identical regimen (110). Another Scandinavian study has compared a multidrug regimen in node-positive breast cancer patients given only perioperatively with treatment given for 1 year (109). After 1 year, a significant increase in relapse-free survival occurred in the group treated for 1 year, which persisted through follow-up of 8 years. The NSABP trial B01 randomized patients to no systemic therapy or to a perioperative course of thiotepa (111). At 5 years, there was a statistically significant increase in survival in the treatment group (primarily in the premenopausal node-positive patients), although at 10 years there was only a trend toward improved survival. Recent randomized trials from the Ludwig group and from Sertoli et al. have also explored the administration of (perioperative) chemotherapy in node-negative and -positive breast cancer patients. Early results indicate a benefit in some specific groups (112, 143). Other randomized trials in breast cancer are ongoing to determine the effects of timing of treatment initiation for adjuvant chemotherapy, and at this point, the optimal time has not been determined (92).

Evaluation of perioperative therapy in other common diseases such as non-small-cell lung cancer and colon cancer has not revealed signif-

icant improvement in therapeutic outcome, although ineffective drugs may have been used (113, 114). However, as Wittes notes, these trials indicate that using ineffective drugs perioperatively will not necessarily make them effective (33). In summary, there is some indication that perioperative therapy may be of clinical benefit, although well-designed trials with effective agents need to be performed before any final conclusions can be drawn.

PRIMARY (NEOADJUVANT) THERAPY

Primary chemotherapy, often used in childhood solid tumors, has recently become a more common approach in the treatment of adult solid tumors. The potential benefits of this therapy affect not only control of micrometastases but the primary tumor as well. Several experimental models using transplantable tumors have demonstrated an increase in cure rate with preoperative chemotherapeutic administration, as compared with postoperative administration, whereas other models have failed to produce this effect (115). Despite the previously discussed difficulties in applying information from laboratory studies to clinical trials, the concept of primary chemotherapy is an interesting one and worthy of further exploration.

Experimental factors possibly influencing the response to primary chemotherapy include those that may affect adjuvant therapy in general: growth rate of the tumor, presence of drug resistance, tumor burden, and type of drug used (116, 117). The diagram in Figure 6.5, based on the somatic mutation hypothesis of drug resistance by Goldie and Coldman (described above), demonstrates the relationship between probability of cure and tumor size (118). This concept can potentially be applied to the development of me-

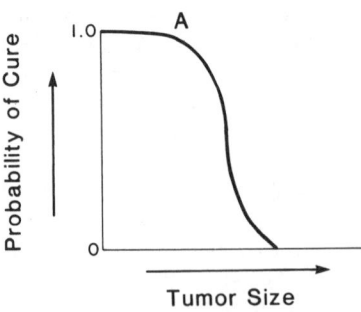

Figure 6.5.   Relationship between tumor size and probability of cure based on the somatic mutation hypothesis of drug resistance. (Modified from Goldie JH. Scientific basis for adjuvant and primary (neoadjuvant) chemotherapy. Semin Oncol 1987;14:1–7.).

tastases. For example, during primary tumor growth, it is postulated that metastases can either form gradually, independent of primary tumor size, or develop only after a critical tumor size is reached. If metastases develop by the latter mechanism, then they would be grouped around a certain point. If the micrometastatic tumor burden is primarily assembled on the curve at point *A* in Figure 6.5, then primary chemotherapy would be anticipated to significantly influence the cure rate. On the other hand, if micrometastases have been rather evenly distributed in their development and only a small portion exists along the steep section of the curve, a smaller impact of primary therapy on outcome would be expected. It is not clear which of these situations usually occurs, although some experimental data suggest that the generation of metastases occurs after the primary tumor attains a threshold size, at which point the development of metastatic variants occurs at a fast rate (119). Therefore, this process is similar to that for the occurrence of other spontaneous mutants, which would favor the use of primary chemotherapy (i.e., treatment as early as possible). However, there is some thought that metastases may be indolent with low growth fractions or be protected in fibrin "cocoons," which would make them less accessible to chemotherapy (120). In general, though, data from most laboratory models and some clinical trials advocate the early use of chemotherapy to contain micrometastatic disease.

Several advantages also exist for control of the primary neoplasm with primary chemotherapy (116, 120). First, local reduction of the tumor may facilitate the use of a more conservative approach for surgical procedures and/or radiotherapy. This can be especially important in head and neck tumors and sarcomas, where loss of functional use and cosmetic appearance can be devastating to the patient. Second, drug administration prior to local therapy avoids the potential for poor distribution of drug due to compromised vascularity from surgery or radiation therapy, in addition to the possibility of greater tumor heterogeneity from effects of radiation. Initial tumor reduction with chemotherapy may improve the vascularity of the tumor and its oxygen reserve and actually increase the subsequent response to radiation therapy. Third, some chemotherapeutic agents may also act as radiosensitizers through various mechanisms, and several trials are ongoing to evaluate the effects of alternating or simultaneous radiotherapy and chemotherapy (121, 123). Fourth, the tumor bi-

ology can be assessed by postchemotherapy surgery. This is a unique opportunity to determine the correlation between clinical measurements of tumor response and actual pathologic changes. Fifth, the response of the primary tumor to chemotherapy may indicate the response of micrometastases and influence further patient management. However, as with any therapy, there are also some potential adverse effects from primary chemotherapy. These include (*a*) selection of drug-resistant cells; (*b*) an increased toxicity with subsequent therapies; (*c*) an inability of chemotherapeutic agents to produce a significant reduction in the tumor, thereby possibly allowing further subclinical progression of disease; and (*d*) a loss of the advantage to attack micrometastases after surgery when they may exhibit more favorable cell kinetics. Despite these disadvantages, the use of primary chemotherapy certainly holds clinical promise for a variety of human solid tumors.

The response to primary chemotherapy may indicate a group of patients who will achieve prolonged disease-free survival. It is possible that with a greater number of well-designed clinical trials employing primary chemotherapy, correlations between initial response and ultimate outcome (i.e., survival), in combination with other prognostic factors, could alter the management of certain diseases (120). Trials utilizing primary chemotherapy, in combination with either surgery or radiation therapy, for solid tumors such as breast cancer, head and neck cancer, lung cancer, gastrointestinal cancers, genitourinary tract cancers, osteosarcomas, and pediatric malignancies have been conducted with some encouraging results (123–132). As DeVita notes, primary chemotherapy is becoming the "standard of treatment" in some groups of patients with diffuse large cell lymphomas, limited small cell lung cancers, pediatric cancers, and head and neck cancers (133). However, the concept of primary chemotherapy is generally applicable toward most tumors, and further investigation is needed to determine its ultimate role.

Avoiding Drug Resistance

Perhaps one of the most significant deterrents to achieving a cure after adjuvant chemotherapy is the presence of drug resistance. Early trials often administered only a single agent, and it was subsequently deduced that combinations of drugs could potentially improve the response. Using basic principles from the Goldie/Coldman hypothesis, one can conclude that exposure of the tumor cells to as many active agents as possible as early as possible may increase the cure rate. Although combination chemotherapy is presented elsewhere in this book, a few basic points are pertinent to this discussion of adjuvant therapy. In general, drugs used in combination should (a) be effective when used alone, (b) have few overlapping toxicities, (c) be administered at the optimal dose and schedule, and (d) be administered at constant intervals (9).

For most drug-sensitive malignancies, combination therapy tends to be more effective than single-agent therapy in producing cures, although this is not necessarily true for choriocarcinoma and Burkitt's lymphoma (134–136). Although most current adjuvant trials use combinations of chemotherapeutic agents, there is a paucity of randomized trials comparing single agents with combination chemotherapy. Ideally, one would want to use many effective agents simultaneously; however, because of toxicities, this is usually not possible. Therefore, a subsequent approach has been to alternate combinations of equally effective, non-cross-resistant drugs or to use half of the drugs from each combination to complete one cell cycle (i.e., days 1 and 8). This latter schedule has been termed a hybrid combination (9). Unfortunately, many of these alternating regimens have not been adequately assessed for true non-cross-resistance or equal efficacy with the standard therapy. Thus far, for most diseases, alternating regimens have not been more effective than conventional therapy, although randomized trials using these schedules need to be performed in an adjuvant setting to ultimately determine any benefit (33). Based on principles from the somatic mutation theory and our current understanding of resistance, emphasis should be placed on discovering new ways to administer active agents with minimal toxicity in the critical period when cure remains possible.

Amount of Disease

The tumor burden in humans cannot currently be accurately quantified, although clinical tests can provide information on the general extent of disease. Overall, subclinical metastases in the low TNM categories take longer to become clinically measurable than do those in tumors classified in the more advanced stages. Wittes has addressed the question of whether the low TNM stages may secure greater benefit from adjuvant therapy than the higher-staged resectable tumors (33). As noted earlier, the tumor burden in transplantable animal models has a significant impact on the chance for cure after adjuvant therapy, but in humans this association is not as evident. Does adjuvant chemotherapy have a greater impact on earlier stages of disease? This question has really not been adequately addressed to determine if there are certain subgroups where tumor burden is a significant factor in governing the effect of adjuvant therapy. In some tumors such as breast cancer, the use of adjuvant therapy has only recently been investigated in early-stage disease. Although both node-negative and node-positive patients benefit in terms of disease-free survival, it is not clear whether the benefit will be greater in the former group (137–139). Certainly, further evaluation of this area is of scientific interest.

Endpoints

Complete response rate is a significant element in determining the effectiveness of chemotherapy. However, in adjuvant chemotherapy administered after local treatment, there is no measurable disease, and relapse-free and overall survival become important endpoints. Survival statistics ultimately reflect the degree of cell kill achieved by adjuvant therapy, which may be complete eradication of micrometastases, reduction of the tumor burden but not complete eradication, or no effect on the micrometastatic lesions. Primary (neoadjuvant) chemotherapy, on the other hand, can measure complete response rates for the primary tumor, and one can postulate that a similar effect on micrometastases has occurred. With adjuvant therapy, the endpoints need to be followed over extended intervals, as recurrent disease may occur years after completion of therapy.

ADJUVANT THERAPY TRIALS

The results of adjuvant therapy in a variety of diseases are discussed in other chapters in this book, and the reader is referred to them for detailed information. However, a brief review of the effectiveness of adjuvant therapy in several diseases is in order, and where possible, review articles are referenced. International conferences are held every few years to review advances in the area of adjuvant therapy, and the results are published. Recent conference summaries have noted that although the effect of adjuvant therapy in many neoplasms has been disappointing, there have been some encouraging results (140, 141). However, it is imperative that these adjuvant trials continue, in the hope of identifying groups of patients who will benefit from therapy.

Breast Cancer

An extensive literature has been published and, in general, has indicated a benefit from postoperative adjuvant chemotherapy in stage I and II patients (138, 139, 142–148). It is important to stress that treatment of node-negative patients remains controversial for some subsets, and patients should be encouraged to enter clinical trials (149, 150). Two large overview analyses of postoperative therapy from pooled data have also been published (151, 152). The more recent study reported a definite reduction in mortality for women less than 50 years old, greater effectiveness with combination chemotherapy than with single-agent therapy, and no advantage of longer-duration therapy (152). Primary chemotherapy has also been used in locally advanced breast cancer as part of a multimodality approach (153). Current trials are focusing on primary chemotherapy for early-stage breast cancer (144, 145).

Lung Cancer

In general, results for non-small-cell lung cancer have been discouraging, although recent trials with cisplatin-based regimens and the use of primary (neoadjuvant) chemotherapy have provided some impetus for further evaluation (154–156). Some encouraging results have also been noted in limited small cell lung disease, using adjuvant chemotherapy with radiation therapy, surgery, or both (158–160).

Head and Neck Cancer

Chemotherapy in a postoperative or postradiation therapy setting has not been adequately evaluated, and therefore, its role is not clearly defined (161). However, the use of chemotherapy prior to surgery or radiation therapy or simultaneously with radiation therapy has resulted in significant response rates and encouraged further investigation of organ preservation (161–163). This is an exciting area, and patients should be encouraged to participate in investigational protocols when available.

Gastrointestinal Malignancies

Data exist to support the use of postoperative chemotherapy in rectal cancer (164, 165). Recent studies also indicate a benefit for adjuvant che-

motherapy in colon carcinoma, specifically with administration of 5-fluorouracil and levamisole in patients with stage C disease (166–168). There is a need for patients to be enrolled in clinical trials, as large numbers of patients are needed to determine the best adjuvant therapy. Chemotherapy and radiotherapy, occasionally followed by surgery, is indicated for anal cancer (166, 169).

Trials in pancreatic cancer are scarce, since this disease is often unresectable, although one trial has noted an improvement in survival with postoperative chemotherapy in completely resected tumors (166, 170). Most trials in gastric cancer have not demonstrated a consistent benefit with postoperative chemotherapy (166, 170). The recent emphasis in esophageal cancer has been on preoperative chemotherapy alone or with radiation therapy (129, 166). Further investigation is needed to determine the ultimate role of adjuvant chemotherapy in esophageal cancer and gastric cancer.

Sarcomas

Several studies have demonstrated an improvement in disease-free survival for adult extremity soft tissue sarcomas after adjuvant therapy, although in general, it has not been of benefit and should be viewed as investigational treatment (171–173). Response to primary chemotherapy in terms of tumor necrosis may be of prognostic significance (176, 177). Adjuvant therapy has been administered regionally as well as systematically.

Pediatric Solid Tumors

Childhood malignancies such as Wilms' tumor, Ewing's sarcoma, neuroblastoma, and rhabdomyosarcoma have shown improved results with the administration of systemic chemotherapy before or after local treatment (177).

Ovarian/Cervical Cancer

Most studies of adjuvant therapy in epithelial ovarian cancer have not shown significant clinical impact, although some subsets of patients may benefit (179). However, evidence exists to support the use of adjuvant therapy in ovarian germ cell tumors (180, 181), and some investigators feel it should be considered standard therapy (183). Trials in locally advanced cervical carcinoma indicate some benefit with adjuvant hydroxyurea, although numerous trials are ongoing to examine other potentially effective regimens (183).

Bladder Cancer

A paucity of randomized trials exists to adequately determine the role of pre- or postoperative systemic therapy in bladder cancer, although several studies have suggested a benefit in certain subgroups of patients (184–186). The use of chemotherapy with or without radiation to increase bladder preservation is also being evaluated (185).

Testicular Cancer

The need for adjuvant therapy in early-stage seminomatous testicular cancer is minimal and perhaps nonexistent, since most patients are cured with local therapy, and relapses can often be cured with chemotherapy at the time of recurrence (187). Adjuvant therapy may prevent relapse in nonseminomatous germ cell tumors, although equivalent cure rates can be obtained with optimal follow-up, using chemotherapy only at relapse (188, 189).

Melanoma

Adjuvant trials have not demonstrated a therapeutic benefit with chemotherapy for melanoma (190, 191). Preoperative treatment in stage II disease is also under investigation (192). Certainly, part of these poor results is due to a lack of effective chemotherapeutic agents.

Table 6.2. The Role of Adjuvant Chemotherapy in Human Solid Tumors

Definite benefit	Rectal cancer
Breast cancer	Anal cancer
Ovarian germ cell	Pediatric cancers (Wilms'
tumors	tumor, Ewing's sarcoma,
Osteosarcoma	neuroblastoma,
Colon cancer	rhabdomyosarcoma)
Possible benefit[a]	
Small cell lung cancer	
Head and neck cancer	
Non-small-cell lung	
cancer	
Soft tissue sarcomas	
Bladder cancer	
Esophageal cancer	
No definite benefit[a]	
Pancreatic cancer	Testicular cancer
Gastric cancer	Melanoma
Cervical cancer	

[a]It is important to note that the role of adjuvant chemotherapy in many of these tumors is undergoing active investigation, and patients should be entered on protocols.

In summary, as noted in Table 6.2, adjuvant chemotherapy has a definite role in the treatment of breast cancer, pediatric solid tumors (Wilms' tumor, Ewing's sarcoma, neuroblastoma), anal cancer, osteosarcoma, ovarian germ cell tumors, and more recently, in colon and rectal cancer. Groups of patients with other solid tumors appear to benefit from adjuvant therapy, although further evaluation is necessary before any final conclusions can be made.

CONCLUSION

The development of adjuvant chemotherapy regimens for malignant diseases is currently a very active and exciting area. The concept of adjuvant therapy is based on laboratory studies that documented an inverse relationship between the number of tumor cells present and chemotherapeutic response. Although most early trials investigated the postoperative administration of chemotherapy, recent enthusiasm in preoperative treatment has developed. The use of chemotherapy prior to local tumor management (surgery or radiation therapy) is termed neoadjuvant, or primary, chemotherapy. Characteristics of cell cycle kinetics, patterns of tumor growth, and the specific drugs administered are all important elements to consider when constructing effective adjuvant therapy programs. In laboratory models, several factors appear to influence the response to adjuvant chemotherapy. These include the amount of tumor present, the dose of drug administered, the use of combination of drugs as opposed to single agents, the timing of chemotherapy administration relative to primary tumor removal, and the development of drug-resistant tumor cells. Although the application of experimental laboratory data to treatment of human tumors has been criticized, valuable information has been acquired from these studies. This knowledge must be used with the realization that differences exist between the two systems, and therefore, caution must be exercised when generalizations are made.

Unfortunately, by the time a tumor is clinically apparent in humans, it has already undergone approximately 30 doublings and resulted in approximately one billion tumor cells. Despite this, some tumors are potentially curable with chemotherapy. It was hoped that with the use of adjuvant therapy, a large number of patients would be cured, since the amount of tumor present is smaller than in advanced disease. However, there are numerous factors that can potentially affect the response to adjuvant chemotherapy in humans. These include the dose of drug administered (total dose and dose intensity), the scheduling of drug administration relative to local primary therapy, and the presence of drug resistance (193). In addition, the development of toxicities from adjuvant therapy, both short-term and long-term, are critical factors in determining the cost-effectiveness of treatment. In particular, the risk of secondary malignancies and quality-of-life issues are key elements when administering treatment to patients, some of whom may be cured by local therapy alone. Nevertheless, the use of adjuvant chemotherapy remains an exciting area of investigation.

Although clinical trials have been disappointing in many tumors, a group of patients does appear to benefit from the use of adjuvant therapy. Current data support the use of adjuvant chemotherapy in breast cancer; colon, rectal, and anal cancer; osteosarcomas; some ovarian germ cell tumors; and pediatric malignancies such as Wilms' tumor, Ewing's sarcoma, rhabdomyosarcoma, and neuroblastoma. Other diseases that are undergoing active investigation with encouraging results include head and neck cancer, esophageal cancer, bladder cancer, non-small-cell and small cell lung cancer, and soft tissue sarcomas.

Unfortunately, the expected effects of adjuvant therapy have not been realized in many human tumors. However, with the development of new chemotherapeutic agents and biologic agents such as colony-stimulating factors, new regimens may provide additional information regarding dose intensity (194). A better understanding of the consequences of drug scheduling and tumor biology is also important. Despite many unanswered questions, adjuvant chemotherapy remains an intriguing concept and an exciting area worthy of further exploration.

REFERENCES

1. Skipper HE. Kinetics of mammary tumor cell growth and implications for therapy. Cancer 1971; 28:1479–1499.

2. Shapiro DM, Fugmann RA. A role of chemotherapy as an adjunct to surgery. Cancer Res 1957; 28:1098–1101.

3. Goldin A, Venditti JM, Humphreys SR, Mantel N. Influence of the concentration of leukemic inoculum on the effectiveness of treatment. Science 1956;123:840.

4. Martin DS, Fugmann RA. Clinical implications of the interrelationship of tumor size and chemotherapeutic response. Ann Surg 1960;151:97–100.

5. Shimkin MB, Moore GE. Adjuvant use of chemotherapy in the surgical treatment of cancer. JAMA 1958;1667:1710–1714.

6. Moore GE, Ross CA. Chemotherapy as an adjuvant to surgery. Annu Rev Med 1963;14:141–150.

7. Frei E. Clinical cancer research: an embattled species. Cancer 1982;50:1979–1992.

8. Muggia FM. Primary chemotherapy: concepts and issues. In: Wagner DJ, Blijhan GH, Smeets JBE, Wils JA, eds. Primary chemotherapy in cancer medicine. New York: Alan R Liss, 1985:377–383.

9. DeVita VT. Principles of chemotherapy. In: DeVita VT, Hellman S, Rosenberg SA, eds. Cancer: principles and practice of oncology. 3rd ed. Philadelphia: JB Lippincott, 1989:276–300.

10. Howard A, Pelc SR. Nuclear incorporation of P^{32} as demonstrated by autoradiographs. Exp Cell Res 1951;2:178–187.

11. Baserga R. Relationship of the cell cycle to tumor growth and control of cell division: a review. Cancer Res 1965;25:581–595.

12. Tannock I. Cell kinetics and chemotherapy: a critical review. Cancer Treat Rep 1978;62:1117–1133.

13. Hunter T, Pines J. Cyclins and Cancer. Cell 1991;66:1074.

14. Hunter T, Pines J. Cyclins and Cancer II: cyclin D and CDK. Cell 1994;79:573–584.

15. Mendelsohn ML. The growth fraction: a new concept applied to tumors. Science 1960;132:1496.

16. Clarkson B, Ota K, Ohkita T, O'Connor A. Kinetics of proliferation of cancer cells in neoplastic effusions in man. Cancer 1965;18:1189–1213.

17. Clarkson B, Fried J, Strife A, Sakai Y, Ota K, Ohkita T. Studies of cellular proliferation in human leukemia III. Behavior of leukemic cells in three adults with acute leukemia given continuous infusions of ^{3}H-thymidine for 8 or 10 days. Cancer 1970;25:1237–1260.

18. Young RC, DeVita VT. Cell cycle characteristics of human solid tumors in vivo. Cell Tissue Kinet 1970; 3:285–290.

19. DeVita VT. The James Ewing Lecture: relationship between tumor mass and resistance to chemotherapy. Cancer 1983;51:1209–1220.

20. Tannock IF. Experimental chemotherapy and concepts related to the cell cycle. Int J Radiat Biol 1986; 49:335–355.

21. Tannock IF. The relation between cell proliferation and the vascular system in a transplanted mouse mammary tumor. Br J Cancer 1968;22:258–273.

22. Hill BT. Implications of certain cell kinetic and biological parameters for preoperative chemotherapy. Recent Results Cancer Res 1986;103:41–53.

23. Salmon SE. Kinetics of minimal residual disease. Recent Results Cancer Res 1979;67:5–15.

24. Skipper HE, Schabel FM, Wilcox WS. Experimental evaluation of potential anticancer agents. XIII. On the criteria and kinetics associated with "curability" of experimental leukemia. Cancer Chemother Rep 1964;35:1–111.

25. Yankee RA, DeVita VT, Perry S. The cell cycle of leukemia L1210 cells in vivo. Cancer Res 1967; 27:2381–2385.

26. Skipper HE, Schabel FM, Mellett LB, et al. Implications of biochemical, cytokinetic, pharmacologic, and toxicologic relationships in the design of optimal

therapeutic schedules. Cancer Chemother Rep 1970; 54:431–450.

27. Schabel FM. The use of tumor growth kinetics in planning "curative" chemotherapy of advanced solid tumors. Cancer Res 1969;29:2384–2389.

28. Shackney SE, McCormack GW, Cuchural GJ. Growth rate patterns of solid tumors and their relation to responsiveness to therapy. Ann Intern Med 1978; 89:107–121.

29. Schabel FM. Concepts for systemic treatment of micrometastases. Cancer 1975;35:15–24.

30. Chabner BA, Myers CE. Clinical pharmacology of cancer chemotherapy. In: DeVita VT, Hellman S, Rosenberg SA, eds. Cancer: principles and practice of oncology. 3rd ed. Philadelphia: JB Lippincott, 1989;349–395.

31. Schabel FM. Surgical adjuvant chemotherapy of metastatic murine tumors. Cancer 1977;40:558–568.

32. van Putten LM, de Ruiter J, van de Velde CJ, Mulder JH, Gerritsen AF. Adjuvant chemotherapy: theoretical considerations and model studies. Recent Results Cancer Res 1979;67:119–125.

33. Wittes RE. Adjuvant chemotherapy–clinical trials and laboratory models. Cancer Treat Rep 1986; 70:87–103.

34. Merker PC, Wodinsky I, Cantor ML, Venditti JM. Effectiveness of clinically active antineoplastic drugs in a surgical-adjuvant chemotherapy treatment regimen using the Lewis lung (LL) carcinoma. Int J Cancer 1978;21:482–489.

35. Salmon SE, Hamburger AW, Soehnlen B, Durie BG, Alberts DS, Moon TE. Quantitation of differential sensitivity of human-tumor stem cells to anticancer drugs. N Engl J Med 1978;298:1321–1327.

36. Goldin A, Venditti JM. Progress report on the screening program at the division of cancer treatment, National Cancer Institute. Cancer Treat Rev 1980; 7:167–176.

37. Shoemaker RH. New approaches to antitumor drug screening: the human tumor colony-forming assay. Cancer Treat Rep 1986;70:9–12.

38. Karrer K, Humphreys SR, Goldin A. An experimental model for studying factors which influence metastasis of malignant tumors. Int J Cancer 1967; 2:213–223.

39. Skipper HE. Adjuvant chemotherapy. Cancer 1978;41:936–940.

40. Skipper HE. Experimental adjuvant chemotherapy: an overview. Recent Results Cancer Res 1986; 103:6–29.

41. Griswold DP. The potential for murine tumor models in surgical adjuvant chemotherapy. Cancer Chemother Rep 1975;5:187–204.

42. Burchenal JH. Adjuvant therapy–theory, practice, and potential. Cancer 1976;37:46–57.

43. Schabel FM, Griswold DP, Corbett TH, Laster WR, Mayo JG, Lloyd HH. Testing therapeutic hypotheses in mice and man: observations on the therapeutic activity against advanced solid tumors of mice treated with anticancer drugs that have demonstrated or potential clinical utility for treatment of advanced solid tumors of man. Methods Cancer Res 1979;17:3–51.

44. Skipper H. Data and analysis having to do with the influence of dose intensity and duration of treatment (single drugs and combinations) on lethal toxicity and the therapeutic response of experimental neoplasms. Birmingham: Southern Research Institute, booklets 13, 1986; 2–13, 1987, and 1, 1988.

45. Henderson IC, Hayes DF, Gelman R. Dose-response in the treatment of breast cancer: a critical review. J Clin Oncol 1988;6:1501–1515.

46. Fugmann RA, Martin DS, Hayworth PE, Stolfi RL. Enhanced cures of spontaneous murine mammary carcinomas with surgery and five-compound combination chemotherapy and their immunotherapeutic interrelationship. Cancer Res 1970;30:1931–1936.

47. Skipper HE, Schabel FM, Wilcox WS. Experimental evaluation of potential anticancer agents. XXI. Scheduling of arabinosylcytosine to take advantage of its S-phase specificity against leukemia cells. Cancer Chemother Rep 1967;51:125–165.

48. Neil GL, Homan ER. The effect of dose interval on the survival of L1210 leukemic mice treated with DNA synthesis inhibitors. Cancer Res 1973;33:895–901.

49. Schatten WE. An experimental study of postoperative tumor metastases. Cancer 1958;11:455–459.

50. Ketcham AS, Kinsey DL, Wexler H, Mantel N. The development of spontaneous metastases after the removal of a "primary tumor." Cancer 1961;14:875–882.

51. Riggins RS, Ketchman AS. Effect of incisional biopsy on the development of experimental tumor metastases. J Surg Res 1965;5:200–206.

52. Gershon RK, Carter RL, Kondo K. Immunologic defenses against metastases: impairment by excision of an allotransplanted lymphoma. Science 1968; 159:646–648.

53. Whitney RB, Levy JG, Smith AG. Influence of tumor size and surgical resection on cell-mediated immunity in mice. J Natl Cancer Inst 1974;53:111–116.

54. Simpson-Herren L, Sanford AH, Holmquist JP. Effects of surgery on the cell kinetics of residual tumor. Cancer Treat Rep 1976;60:1749–1760.

55. Gunduz N, Fisher B, Saffer EA. Effect of surgical removal on the growth and kinetics of residual tumor. Cancer Res 1979;39:3861–3865.

56. Fisher B, Gunduz N, Saffer EA. Influence of the interval between primary tumor removal and chemotherapy on kinetics and growth of metastases. Cancer Res 1983;43:1488–1492.

57. Baker D, Elkon D, Lim M, Constable W, Wanebo H. Does local x-radiation of a tumor increase the incidence of metastases? Cancer 1981;48:2394–2398.

58. Skipper HE, Schabel FM, Lloyd HH. Experimental therapeutics and kinetics: selection and overgrowth of specifically and permanently drug-resistant tumor cells. Semin Hematol 1978;15:207–219.

59. Luria SE, Delbrück M. Mutations of bacteria from virus sensitivity to virus resistance. Genetics 1943;28:491–511.

60. Goldie JH, Coldman AJ. A mathematic model for relating the drug sensitivity of tumors to their spontaneous mutation rate. Cancer Treat Rep 1979;63:1727–1733.

61. Goldie JH, Coldman AJ. Quantitative model for multiple levels of drug resistance in clinical tumors. Cancer Treat Rep 1983;67:923–931.

62. Goldie JH, Coldman AJ. Genetic origin of drug resistance in neoplasms: implications for systemic therapy. Cancer Res 1984;44:3643–3653.

63. Goldie JH, Coldman AJ, Gudauskas GA. Rationale for the use of alternating non-cross-resistant chemotherapy. Cancer Treat Rep 1982;66:439–449.

64. Skipper HE. Solid tumors in animals treated with surgery, chemotherapy, or surgery plus chemotherapy; variables which affect cure rates and the shapes and slopes of remission and survival curves (part II): Ridgeway osteogenic sarcoma. Birmingham: Southern Research Institute, booklet 14, 1982.

65. Biedler JL, Riehm H. Cellular resistance to actinomycin D in Chinese hamster cells in vitro: cross-resistance, radioautographic, and cytogenetic studies. Cancer Res 1970;30:1174–1184.

66. Deuchars KL, Ling V. P-glycoprotein and multidrug resistance in cancer chemotherapy. Semin Oncol 1989;16:156–165.

67. Frei E, Teicher B, Rosowsky A. Principles of adjuvant chemotherapy. In: Jones SE, Salmon SE, eds. Adjuvant therapy of cancer IV. Orlando: Grune & Stratton, 1984:61–69.

68. Salmon SE, Grogan TM, Miller TP, Dalton WS. Multidrug resistance: relevance to adjuvant therapy? In: Salman SE, ed. Adjuvant therapy of cancer VI. Philadelphia: WB Saunders, 1990:26–32.

69. Jasmin C, Judde JG, Georgoulias V, Smadja, Joffe F, Poupon MF. Models for adjuvant therapy. In: Jones SE, Salmon SE, eds. Adjuvant therapy of cancer IV. Orlando: Grune & Stratton, 1984:35–45.

70. Collins VP, Loeffler RK, Tivey H. Observations on growth rates of human tumors. Am J Roentgenol 1956;76:988–1000.

71. Fidler IJ, Hart IR. Biological diversity in metastatic neoplasms: origins and implications. Science 1982;217:998–1003.

72. Frei EA. Commentary: selected considerations regarding chemotherapy as adjuvant in cancer treatment. Cancer Chemother Rep 1966;50:1–8.

73. DeVita VT. Opening comments: only if you believe in magic. In: Jones SE, Salmon SE, eds. Adjuvant therapy of cancer IV. Orlando: Grune & Stratton, 1984:3–16.

74. Hryniuk WM. Average relative dose intensity and the impact on design of clinical trials. Semin Oncol 1987;14:65–74.

75. Hryniuk WM. The importance of dose intensity in the outcome of chemotherapy. In: DeVita VT, Hellman S, Rosenberg SA, eds. Important advances in oncology 1988. Philadelphia: JB Lippincott, 1988:121–142.

76. Carde P, MacKintosh FR, Rosenberg SA. A dose and time response analysis of the treatment of Hodgkin's disease with MOPP chemotherapy. J Clin Oncol 1983;1:146–153.

77. Levin L, Hryniuk WM. Dose intensity analysis of chemotherapy regimens in ovarian carcinoma. J Clin Oncol 1987;5:756–767.

78. Frei E, Canellos GP. Dose: a critical factor in cancer chemotherapy. Am J Med 1980;69:585–594.

79. Bonadonna G, Valagussa P. Dose-response effect of adjuvant chemotherapy in breast cancer. N Engl J Med 1981;304:10–15.

80. Hryniuk W, Levine MN. Analysis of dose intensity for adjuvant chemotherapy trials in stage II breast cancer. J Clin Oncol 1986;4:1162–1170.

81. Hryniuk WM, Bonadonna G, Valagussa P. The effect of dose intensity in adjuvant therapy of cancer V. Orlando: Grune & Stratton, 1987:13–23.

82. Cooper RG, Holland JF, Glidewell O. Adjuvant chemotherapy of breast cancer. Cancer 1979;44:793–798.

83. Gelman RS, Henderson IC. A reanalysis of dose intensity for adjuvant chemotherapy trials in stage II breast cancer. SAKK Bull 1987;1:10–12.

84. Abeloff MD, Mellits ED, Baumgardner R, Wilcox P, Watkins S. Prospective trial of standard vs low dose cytoxan, methotrexate, 5-FU (CMF) in adjuvant therapy of breast cancer—assessment of therapeutic efficacy and toxicity (abstract). Proc Am Assoc Cancer Res and Am Soc Clin Oncol 1981;22:440.

85. Ludwig Breast Cancer Study Group. A randomized trial of adjuvant combination chemotherapy with or without prednisone in premenopausal breast cancer patients with metastases in one to three axillary lymph nodes. Cancer Res 1985;45:4454–4459.

86. Korzun A, Norton L, Perloff M, et al. Clinical equivalence despite dosage differences of two schedules of cyclophosphamide, methotrexate, 5-fluorouracil, vincristine and prednisone (CMFVP) for adjuvant therapy of node-positive stage II breast cancer (abstract). Proc Am Soc Clin Oncol 1988;7:12.

87. Peters WP, Shpall EJ, Jones RB, et al. High-dose combination alkylating agents with bone marrow support as initial treatment for metastatic breast cancer. J Clin Oncol 1988;6:1368–1376.

88. Williams SF, Mick R, Desser R, Golick J, Beschorner J, Bitran JD. High dose consolidation therapy with autologous stem cell rescue in stage IV breast cancer. J Clin Oncol 1989;7:1824–1830.

89. Peters WP, Davis R, Shpall EJ, et al. Adjuvant chemotherapy involving high dose combination cyclophosphamide, cisplatin, carmustine (CPA, CDDP, BCNU) and autologous bone marrow support (ABMS) for stage II/III breast cancer involving ten or more lymph nodes. (CALGB 8782): a preliminary report (abstract). Proc Am Soc Clin Oncol 1990;9:22.

90. Tancini G, Bonadonna G, Valagussa P, Marchini S, Veronesi U. Adjuvant CMF in breast cancer: comparative 5-year results of 12 versus 6 cycles. J Clin Oncol 1983;1:2–10.

91. Bonadonna G, Valagussa P, Rossi A, et al. Ten-year experience with CMF-based adjuvant chemotherapy in resectable breast cancer. Breast Cancer Res Treat 1985;5:95–115.

92. Henderson IC. Adjuvant systemic therapy for early breast cancer. Curr Probl Cancer 1987;11:128–207.

93. Norton L, Simon R. New thoughts on the relationship of tumor growth characteristics to sensitivity to treatment. Methods Cancer Res 1979;17:53–90.

94. Gilewski T, Vogelzang NJ. Cost-effeciveness and reimbursement issues in renal cell carcinoma. Semin Oncol 1989;16(Suppl 1):20–26.

95. Weisburger EK. Bioassay program for carcinogenic hazards of cancer chemotherapeutic agents. Cancer 1977;40:1935–1949.

96. Kyle RA. Second malignancies associated with chemotherapeutic agents. Semin Oncol 1982;9:131–142.

97. Valagussa P, Santoro A, Fossati-Bellani F, Banfi A, Bonadonna G. Second acute leukemia and other malignancies following treatment for Hodgkin's disease. J Clin Oncol 1986;4:830–837.

98. Henne T, Schmahl D. Occurrence of second primary malignancies in man—a second look. Cancer Treat Rev 1985;12:77–94.

99. Fisher B, Rockette H, Fisher ER, Wickerham DL, Redmond C, Brown A. Leukemia in breast cancer patients following adjuvant chemotherapy or post-operative radiation: the NSABP experience. J Clin Oncol 1985;3:1640–1658.

100. Kapadia SB, Krause JR, Ellis LD, Pan SF, Wald N. Induced acute non-lymphocytic leukemia following long-term chemotherapy. Cancer 1980;45:1315–1321.

101. Rizzo SC, Ricevuti G, Gamba G, Grignani G. Multimodal treatment in operable breast cancer. Br Med J 1981:283–437.

102. Lerner HJ. Acute myelogenous leukemia in patients receiving chlorambucil as long-term adjuvant chemotherapy for stage II breast cancer. Cancer Treat Rep 1978;62:1135–1138.

103. Valagussa P, Tancini G, Bonadonna G. Second malignancies after CMF for resectable breast cancer. J Clin Oncol 1987;5:1138–1142.

104. Kardinal CG, Donegan WL. Second cancers after prolonged adjuvant thiotepa for operable carcinoma of the breast. Cancer 1980;45:2042–2046.

105. Boice JD, Greene MH, Killen JY, et al. Leukemia and preleukemia after adjuvant treatment of gastrointestinal cancer with semustine (methyl-CCNU). N Engl J Med 1983;309:1079–1084.

106. Henderson IC, Gelman R. Second malignancies from adjuvant chemotherapy? Too soon to tell. J Clin Oncol 1987;5:1135–1137.

107. Goldhirsch A, Gelber RD, Simes RJ, Glasziou P, Coates AS. For the Ludwig Breast Cancer Study Group. Costs and benefits of adjuvant therapy in breast cancer: a quality-adjusted survival analysis. J Clin Oncol 1989;7:36–44.

108. Ferguson MK. The effect of antineoplastic agents on wound healing. Surg Gynecol Obstet 1982; 154:421–429.

109. Nissen-Meyer R, Host H, Kjellgren K, Mansson B, Norin T. Neoadjuvant chemotherapy in breast cancer: as single perioperative treatment and with supplementary long-term chemotherapy. In: Salmon SE, ed. Adjuvant therapy of cancer V. Orlando: Grune & Stratton, 1987:253–261.

110. Riley D, Houghton J, Baum M. Cyclophosphamide and tamoxifen as adjuvant therapies in the management of early breast carcinoma. Br J Surg 1986; 73:1040.

111. Fisher B, Redmond CK, Wolmark N, and NSABP Investigators. Long term results from NSABP trials of adjuvant therapy for breast cancer. In: Salmon SE, ed. Adjuvant therapy of cancer V. Orlando: Grune & Stratton, 1987:283–295.

112. Sertoli MR, Pronzato P, Rubagotti A, et al. A randomized study of perioperative chemotherapy in primary breast cancer. In: Salmon SE, ed. Adjuvant therapy of cancer VI. Philadelphia: WB Saunders, 1990:196–203.

113. Slack NH. Bronchogenic carcinoma: nitrogen mustard as a surgical adjuvant and factors influencing survival. Cancer 1970;25:987–1002.

114. Dwight RW, Humphrey EW, Higgins GA, Keehn RJ. FUDR as an adjuvant to surgery in cancer of the large bowel. J Surg Oncol 1973;5:243–249.

115. van Putten LM. Experimental preoperative chemotherapy. Recent Results Cancer Res 1986;103:36–40.

116. Goldie JH, Coldman AJ. Theoretical considerations regarding the early use of adjuvant chemotherapy. Recent Results Cancer Res 1986;103:30–35.

117. Coldman AJ, Goldie JH. Factors affecting the development of permanent drug resistance and its impact upon neoadjuvant chemotherapy. Recent Results Cancer Res 1986;103:69–78.

118. Goldie JH. Scientific basis for adjuvant and primary (neoadjuvant) chemotherapy. Semin Oncol 1987;14:1–7.

119. Hill RP, Chambers AF, Ling V. Dynamic heterogeneity: rapid generation of metastatic variants in mouse B16 melanoma cells. Science 1984;224:998–1001.

120. Frei E, Miller D, Clark JR, Fallon BG, Ervin TJ. Clinical and scientific consideration in preoperative (neoadjuvant) chemotherapy. Recent Results Cancer Res 1986;103:1–5.

121. Coleman CN. Modification of radiotherapy by radiosensitizers and cancer chemotherapy agents. I. Radiosensitizers. Semin Oncol 1989;16:169–175.

122. Looney WB, Hopkins HA. Modification of radiotherapy by radiosensitizers and cancer chemotherapeutic agents. II. Cancer chemotherapeutic agents. Semin Oncol 1989;16:176–179.

123. Ervin TJ, Weichselbaum R, Miller D, Meshad M, Posner M, Fabian R. Treatment of advanced squamous cell carcinoma of the head and neck with cisplatin, bleomycin, and methotrexate (PBM). Cancer Treat Rep 1981;65:787–791.

124. Vokes EE, Moran WJ, Mick R, Weichselbaum RR, Panje WR. Neoadjuvant and adjuvant methotrexate, cisplatin, and fluorouracil in multimodal therapy of head and neck cancer. J Clin Oncol 1989;7:838–845.

125. Al-Sarraf M, Pajak TF, Jacobs J, et al. Combined modality therapy in patients with head and neck cancer: timing of chemotherapy. Radiation Therapy Oncology Group study. In: Salmon SE, ed. Adjuvant therapy of cancer VI. Philadelphia: WB Saunders, 1990:60–70.

126. Strauss G, Sherman D, Goustou M, et al. Neoadjuvant chemotherapy and radiotherapy followed by surgery in stage IIIA non-small cell carcinoma of the lung; a phase II study of the Cancer and Leukemia Group B. In: Salmon SE, ed. Adjuvant therapy of cancer VI. Philadelphia: WB Saunders, 1990:125–132.

127. Radosevich CA, Kies MS, Bannon DJ, Mira JG, Crowley JJ, Livingston RB. Long term follow-up after induction chemotherapy with or without chest radiation in limited small cell lung cancer. In: Salmon SE, ed. Adjuvant therapy of cancer V. Orlando: Grune & Stratton, 1987:179–188.

128. Jacquillat C, Weil M, Baillet F, et al. Neo-adjuvant chemotherapy in breast cancers: results in 381 patients. In: Salmon SE, ed. Adjuvant therapy of cancer VI. Philadelphia: WB Saunders, 1990:240–246.

129. Forastierre AA, Orringer MB, Perez-Tamayo C, Urba SG. Intensive pre-operative chemotherapy and radiation therapy for local-regional esophageal cancer. In: Salmon SE, ed. Adjuvant therapy of cancer VI. Philadelphia: WB Saunders, 1990:381–388.

130. Yagoda A. Neoadjuvant and adjuvant chemotherapy for urothelial tract tumors. In: Salmon SE, ed. Adjuvant therapy of cancer V. Orlando: Grune & Stratton, 1987:555–564.

131. Chawla SP, Benjamin RS, Jaffe N, et al. Preoperative intra-arterial cisplatin and limb-salvage surgery for patients with high-grade osteosarcoma of the extremities. In: Salmon SE, ed. Adjuvant therapy of cancer V. Orlando: Grune & Stratton, 1987:701–710.

132. Rosen G, Marcove RC, Caparros B, Nirenberg A, Kosloff C, Huvos AG. Primary osteogenic sarcoma: the rationale for preoperative chemotherapy and delayed surgery. Cancer 1979;43:2163–2177.

133. DeVita VT. On the value of response criteria in therapeutic research. Bull Cancer 1988;75:863–869.

134. Nathanson L, Hall TC, Schilling A, Miller S. Concurrent combination chemotherapy of human solid tumors: experience with a three-drug regimen and review of the literature. Cancer Res 1969;29:419–425.

135. DeVita VT, Schein PS. The use of drugs in combination for the treatment of cancer: rationale and results. N Engl J Med 1973;288:998–1006.

136. DeVita VT, Young RC, Canellos GP. Combination versus single agent chemotherapy: a review of the basis for selection of drug treatment of cancer. Cancer 1975;35:98–110.

137. Bonadonna G, Valagussa P. Adjuvant systemic therapy for resectable breast cancer. J Clin Oncol 1985;3:259–275.

138. Fisher B, Redmond C, Dimitrov NV, et al. A randomized clinical trial evaluating sequential methotrexate and fluorouracil in the treatment of patients with node-negative breast cancer who have estrogen-receptor-negative tumors. N Engl J Med 1989;320:473–478.

139. Fisher B, Constantino J, Redmond C, et al. A randomized clinical trial evaluating tamoxifen in the treatment of patients with node-negative breast cancer who have estrogen-receptor-positive tumors. N Engl J Med 1989;320:479–484.

140. Weiss GR, Coltman CA. Conference summary overview. In: Salmon SE, ed. Adjuvant therapy of cancer VI. Philadelphia: WB Saunders, 1990:623–629.

141. Einhorn LH. Conference summary. In: Salmon SE, ed. Adjuvant therapy of cancer V. Orlando: Grune & Stratton, 1987:795–801.

142. Mansour EG, Gray R, Shatila AH, et al. Efficacy of adjuvant chemotherapy in high-risk node-negative breast cancer. N Engl J Med 1989;320:485–490.

143. The Ludwig Breast Cancer Study Group. Prolonged disease-free survival after one course of perioperative adjuvant chemotherapy for node-negative breast cancer. N Engl J Med 1989;320:491–496.

144. Bonadonna G, Valagussa P, Moliterni A, et al. Milan adjuvant and neoadjuvant studies in stage I and II resectable breast cancer. In: Salmon SE, ed. Adjuvant therapy of cancer VI. Philadelphia: WB Saunders, 1990:169–173.

145. Fisher B, Wolmark N, Wickerham DL, Redmond CK, and other NSABP investigators. Current NSABP trials of adjuvant therapy for breast cancer. In: Salmon SE. Adjuvant therapy of cancer VI. Philadelphia: WB Saunders, 1990:275–285.

146. Wolmark N, Fisher B. Adjuvant chemotherapy in stage II breast cancer: a brief overview of the NSABP clinical trials. World J Surg 1985;9:699–706.

147. Bonadonna G, Valagussa P. The contribution of medicine to the primary treatment of breast cancer. Cancer Res 1988;48:2314–2324.

148. Glick JH. Meeting highlights: adjuvant therapy for breast cancer. JNCI 1988;80:471–475.

149. Glick JH. Adjuvant therapy for node-negative breast cancer: a proactive view. In: DeVita VT, Hellman S, Rosenberg SA, eds. Important advances in oncology 1990. Philadelphia: JB Lippincott, 1990:183–197.

150. Henderson IC. Adjuvant therapy for node-negative breast cancer: a cautious interpretation. In: DeVita VT, Hellman S, Rosenberg SA, eds. Important

advances in oncology 1990. Philadelphia: JB Lippincott, 1990:199–216.

151. Himmel HN, Liberati A, Gelber RD, Chalmers TC. Adjuvant chemotherapy for breast cancer—a pooled estimate based on published randomized control trials. JAMA 1986;256:1148–1159.

152. Early Breast Cancer Trialists' Collaborative Group. Effects of adjuvant tamoxifen and of cytotoxic therapy on mortality in early breast cancer. N Engl J Med 1988;319:1681–1692.

153. Hortobagyi GN, Ames FC, Buzdar AU, et al. Management of stage III primary breast cancer with primary chemotherapy, surgery, and radiation therapy. Cancer 1988;62:2507–2516.

154. Holmes EC. Adjuvant therapy of non-small cell lung cancer. In: Salmon SE. Adjuvant therapy of cancer VI. Philadelphia: WB Saunders, 1990:119–124.

155. Marangolo M, Fiorentini G. Adjuvant chemotherapy of non-small cell lung cancer: a review. Semin Oncol 1988;15(Suppl 7):13–17.

156. Gralla RJ. Preoperative and adjuvant chemotherapy in non-small cell lung cancer. Semin Oncol 1988;15(Suppl 7):8–12.

157. Ihde DC. Neoadjuvant chemotherapy for non-small cell lung cancer: current North American experience. Semin Oncol 1988;15(Suppl 7):3–7.

158. Seifter EJ, Ihde DC. Therapy of small cell lung cancer: a perspective on two decades of clinical research. Semin Oncol 1988;15:278–299.

159. Shepherd FA, Evans WK, Feld R, et al. Adjuvant chemotherapy following surgical resection for small-cell carcinoma of the lung. J Clin Oncol 1988; 6:832–838.

160. Minna JD, Pass H, Glatstein E, Ihde DC. Cancer of the lung—therapy of small cell carcinoma of the lung. In: DeVita VT, Hellman S, Rosenberg SA, eds. Cancer: principles and practice of oncology. 3rd ed. Philadelphia: JB Lippincott, 1989:666–687.

161. Jacobs C, Makuch R. Efficacy of adjuvant chemotherapy for patients with resectable head and neck cancer: a subset analysis of the head and neck contracts program. J Clin Oncol 1990;8:838–847.

162. Clerk JR, Fallon BG, Frei E. Induction chemotherapy as initial treatment for advanced head and neck cancer: a model for the multidisciplinary treatment of solid tumors. In: DeVita VT, Hellman S, Rosenberg SA. Important advances in oncology 1987. Philadelphia: JB Lippincott, 1987:175–195.

163. Al-Sarraf M. Head and neck cancer: chemotherapy concepts. Semin Oncol 1988;15:70–85.

164. O'Connell MJ, Gunderson LL, Fleming TR. Surgical adjuvant therapy of rectal cancer. Semin Oncol 1988;15:138–145.

165. Moertel CG, Foley J, Laurie J, et al. A new era of effective therapy for colorectal cancer. In: Salmon SE, ed. Adjuvant therapy of cancer VI. Philadelphia: WB Saunders, 1990:425–434.

166. Haller DG. Chemotherapy in gastrointestinal malignancies. Semin Oncol 1988;15(Suppl 4):50–64.

167. Moertel CG, Fleming TR, Macdonald JS, et al. Levamisole and fluorouracil for adjuvant therapy of resected colon carcinoma. N Engl J Med 1990;322:352–358.

168. Friedman MA, Hamilton JM. Progress in the adjuvant therapy of large bowel cancer. In: DeVita VT, Hellman S, Rosenberg SA, eds. Important advances in

oncology 1988. Philadelphia: JB Lippincott, 1988:273–296.

169. Powell BL, Craig JB. Review: adjuvant chemotherapy of solid tumors. Am J Med Sci 1987;294:33–41.

170. Douglass HO, Stablein DM. Ten year follow-up of first generation surgical adjuvant studies of the Gastrointestinal Tumor Study Group. In: Salmon SE, ed. Adjuvant therapy of cancer VI. Philadelphia: WB Saunders, 1990:405–415.

171. Antman K, Ryan L, Borden, et al. Pooled results from three randomized adjuvant studies of doxorubicin versus observation in soft tissue sarcoma: 10 year results and review of the literature. In: Salmon SE, ed. Adjuvant therapy of cancer VI. Philadelphia: WB Saunders, 1990:529–543.

172. Rosenberg SA. Adjuvant chemotherapy of adult patients with soft tissue sarcomas. Important Adv Oncol 1985:273–294.

173. Elias AD, Antman KH. Adjuvant chemotherapy for soft-tissue sarcoma: a critical appraisal. Semin Surg Oncol 1988;4:59–65.

174. Link MP. Adjuvant therapy in the treatment of osteosarcoma. In: DeVita VT, Hellman S, Rosenberg SA, eds. Important advances in oncology 1986. Philadelphia: JB Lippincott, 1986:193–207.

175. Rosen G. Neoadjuvant chemotherapy for osteogenic sarcoma: a model for the treatment of other highly malignant neoplasms. Recent Results Cancer Res 1986;103:148–157.

176. Prasad R, Baci G, Picci P. Neoadjuvant chemotherapy of high grade osteosarcoma and prognostic significance of percentage tumor necrosis and drug dose intensity. In: Salmon SE, ed. Adjuvant therapy of cancer VI. Philadelphia: WB Saunders, 1990:574–579.

177. Chawla SP, Rosen G, Eilber F, et al. Cisplatin and adriamycin as neoadjuvant and adjuvant chemotherapy in the management of soft tissue sarcomas. In: Salmon SE, ed. Adjuvant therapy of cancer VI. Philadelphia: WB Saunders, 1990:567–573.

178. Pizzo PA, Horowitz ME, Poplack DG, Hays DM, Dun LE. Solid tumors of childhood. In: DeVita VT, Hellman S, Rosenberg SA, eds. Cancer: principles and practice of oncology. 3rd ed. Philadelphia: JB Lippincott, 1989:1612–1670.

179. Alberts DS. Adjuvant therapy of epithelial ovarian cancer. In: Salmon SE, ed. Adjuvant therapy of cancer VI. Philadelphia: WB Saunders, 1990:491–500.

180. Slayton RE, Park RC, Silverberg SG, Shingleton H, Creasman WT, Blessing JA. Vincristine, dactinomycin, and cyclophosphamide in the treatment of malignant germ cell tumors of the ovary. Cancer 1985;56:243–248.

181. Smales E, Peckham MJ. Chemotherapy of germ cell ovarian tumors: first-line treatment with etoposide, bleomycin and cisplatin or carboplatin. Eur J Cancer Clin Oncol 1987;23:469–474.

182. Williams SD, Blessing JA, Slayton R, Berman BL, Homesley HD, Photopulos GJ. Ovarian germ cell tumors: adjuvant trials of the gynecologic oncology group. In: Salmon SE, ed. Adjuvant therapy of cancer VI. Philadelphia: WB Saunders, 1990:501–503.

183. Keys H, Bundy B, Stehman FB, DiSaia PJ, Larson J, Fowler WC. Adjuvants to radiation therapy in the treatment of locally advanced carcinoma of the cervix. The Gynecologic Oncology Group (GOG) experience. In: Salmon SE, ed. Adjuvant therapy of cancer VI. Philadelphia: WB Saunders, 1990:544–555.

184. Logothetis CJ, Johnson DE, Chong C, et al. Adjuvant cyclophosphamide, doxorubicin, and cisplatin chemotherapy for bladder cancer: an update. J Clin Oncol 1988;6:1590–1596.

185. Hall RR. Survival and neo-adjuvant chemotherapy in invasive bladder cancer. Prog Clin Biol Res 1988;269:569–575.

186. Daniels JR, Skinner DG, Russell CA, et al. The role of adjuvant chemotherapy following cystectomy for invasive bladder cancer: a prospective comparative trial. In: Salmon SE, ed. Adjuvant therapy of cancer VI. Philadelphia: WB Saunders, 1990:475–488.

187. Einhorn LH, Crawford ED, Shipley WU, Loehrer PJ, Williams SD. In: DeVita VT, Hellman S, Rosenberg SA, eds. Cancer: principles and practice of oncology. 3rd ed. Philadelphia: JB Lippincott, 1989:1071–1098.

188. Williams SD, Stablein DM, Einhorn LE, et al. Immediate adjuvant chemotherapy versus observation with treatment at relapse in pathological stage II testicular cancer. N Engl J Med 1987;317:1433–1438.

189. Einhorn LH. Adjuvant therapy of cancer VI. In: Salmon SE, ed. Adjuvant therapy of cancer VI. Philadelphia: WB Saunders, 1990:471–474.

190. Kaiser LR, Burk MW, Morton DL. Adjuvant therapy for malignant melanoma. Surg Clin North Am 1981;61:1249–1257.

191. Veronesi U, Adamus J, Aubert C, et al. A randomized trial of adjuvant chemotherapy and immunotherapy in cutaneous melanoma. N Engl J Med 1982;307:913–916.

192. Legha SS, Ring S, Balch CM, et al. Induction chemotherapy for the treatment of patients with stage II malignant melanoma. In: Salmon SE, ed. Adjuvant therapy of cancer VI. Philadelphia: WB Saunders, 1990:586–592.

193. Skipper HE. Dose intensity versus total dose of chemotherapy: an experimental basis. In: DeVita VT, Hellman S, Rosenberg SA. Important advances in oncology 1990. Philadelphia: JB Lippincott, 1990:43–64.

194. Gianni AM, Bregni M, Siena S, et al. Recombinant human granulocyte-macrophage colony-stimulating factor reduces hematologic toxicity and widens clinical applicability of high-dose cyclophosphamide treatment in breast cancer and non-Hodgkin's lymphoma. J Clin Oncol 1990;8:768–778.

7

Combination Chemotherapy

Michael L. Friedland

The modern era of chemotherapy, as noted in earlier sections of this text (1), was introduced during World War II as a result of the observations of Goodman, Wintrobe, and Dameshek on the treatment of Hodgkin's disease using mechlorethamine (2). In the following 10 to 15 years, many malignancies were also subjected to treatment with this and other drugs, with the disappointing observation that the regression of disease was only temporary. This period of chemotherapy was founded on presumptive biochemical mechanisms of action of the agents then available. Many of the available drugs were inactive when used singly and when used in combination, often produced significant additive toxicities. DeVita has described this era as the "period of total empiricism in cancer chemotherapy" (3). However, some encouraging results occurred, even though most patients treated had advanced solid tumors (4, 5).

Chemotherapy then entered the era of "enlightened empiricism" (1960–1975) (3). The studies of cancer chemotherapy and tumor cell growth by Skipper and his colleagues during this period added greatly to our understanding of tumor biology (6, 7). These elegant observations in the murine leukemia model offered an explanation for the observed failures to achieve cure. They confirmed that the growth of a single malignant cell could result in a lethal number of cells, that tumor growth was Gompertzian, that a given dose of a drug killed a given fraction of tumor cells ("fractional kill" hypothesis), and that there was an inverse relationship between tumor burden and curability.

These observations also provided a theoretical basis for the design of future combination chemotherapeutic approaches. Applying these principles, it was theoretically possible to induce complete remissions with combination chemotherapy. Unless chemotherapy was continued, however, recurrence and death would occur. The remarkable improvement in survival of patients with acute lymphocytic leukemia of childhood (8, 9) and Hodgkin's disease (10) evolved from the use of some of the concepts developed during this era.

Other approaches to the use of combinations of drugs in cancer treatment relied on efforts to "exploit biochemical differences between cancer and normal cells" (11). As noted, these differences may actually be a result of variation in tumor growth as well as biochemical differences. During the era of "enlightened empiricism," Sartorelli (12) reviewed the biochemical rationale for combination chemotherapy, developing the concept of "synergism," i.e., that these chemotherapeutic agents interfere with either differing metabolic pathways or act at different sites in the same pathway. This concept of synergism suggested that drugs might be used together to block the formation of essential cellular components, resulting in tumor cell death. In the development of the biochemical approach, several mechanistic concepts evolved (reviewed by Capizzi, Keiser, and Sartorelli (13)), including (a) sequential blockade, or the inhibition of two or more enzyme-mediated steps in the production of a necessary metabolite (14), e.g., the combination of hydroxyurea (an inhibitor of ribonucleotide reductase) and ara-C (an inhibitor of DNA polymerase); (b) concurrent blockade, or the inhibition of two or more parallel pathways in the synthesis of the necessary metabolite (15); and (c) complementary inhibition, or the interference with different but related biochemical processes. The use of the anthracycline daunorubicin (a DNA intercalator) and ara-C (a DNA polymerase inhibitor) in acute nonlymphocytic leukemia is an example of successful complementary inhibition (the interference with DNA repair and synthesis). Elucidation and design of treatment regimens based on these mechanisms did not result in the development of a great many successful combinations, although the use of thioguanine and ara-C in acute nonlymphocytic leukemia was a successful example of the application of these concepts (prior to the introduction of the anthracyclines).

Excellent reviews by Damon and Cadman dealing with the biochemical basis for combination chemotherapy provide an in-depth, lucid discussion of the development and utilization of these concepts of biochemical synergy (16, 17).

MODERN CONCEPTS

If the factors noted above (i.e., tumor cell growth characteristics, concepts of cell kill, the biochemical differences of cancer cells, and biochemically different drugs) were the only considerations necessary for the effective development of chemotherapy combinations, then more striking improvement in response and survival would have been observed than has been our current experience. An additional biologic phenomenon that must be considered in developing a rational approach to combination chemotherapy is tumor cell drug resistance (discussed in detail elsewhere in this text). Briefly, drug resistance in neoplasms has been observed for many years. Goldie and Coldman have attempted to explain the observations on the development of biochemical alterations in neoplastic cells that result in their diminished sensitivity to previously active chemotherapeutic agents (18). Goldie and Coldman also developed several concepts to further describe the problem of drug resistance (19). These relate closely to tumor cell growth and the hypotheses that early in growth there are few resistant cells and that over time (with increasing cell numbers), more resistant cells (mutants) are likely to develop.

These principles are based on the assumption that the "presence of resistant cells is assumed to be sufficient to cause treatment failure" (19). This has evolved into a practical approach that assumes that the more rapidly the sensitive cells are eliminated, the less likely it is that resistance will develop, resulting in a greater likelihood of attaining cure.

These observations led Goldie and Coldman to several additional inferences with regard to the development of effective combination chemotherapy: (a) a cell is less likely to be resistant to multiple drugs with independent modes of action; (b) heterogeneous populations of tumor cells require several drugs with independent modes of action (therefore not likely to be cross-resistant); and (c) the rate at which mutations (and therefore resistance) develop may be affected (retarded) by creating a more hostile environment for tumor cell growth through the use of higher drug concentrations. Multiple-drug regimens decrease the possibility that cells in the tumor will be resistant to all of them simultaneously, thus tending to reduce the number of cells capable of developing resistance.

A final generic comment relates to the principle of "nonoverlapping toxicity." Frei, in his 1972 presidential address to the American Association for Cancer Research (AACR), described this phenomenon as central to the development of effective combination chemotherapy of childhood acute lymphocytic leukemia (20). Agents "with qualitatively different toxicity and mechanisms of action could produce synergistic effects," while those with "similar dose limiting toxicity can be combined safely only by reducing the dose, resulting in a lessened effect." This concept of nonoverlapping toxicity and dose reduction has been incorporated into almost all existing treatment regimens. Only recently has the efficacy of this approach been questioned and (as explained in detail elsewhere in this text), full-dose therapy been proposed as an approach to combination chemotherapy (21). Further, the concept of total dose over time has been examined and suggested as a critical factor in attaining cure (22).

The era of "enlightened empiricism" saw some remarkable successes in the treatment of cancer. (The emergence of the oncologist's alphabet soup also occurred, with the introduction into our jargon of acronyms such as VAMP, POMP, and MOPP.) One could summarize this era as the period in which efforts to develop the scientific rationale for combination chemotherapy occurred. Several principles were derived, relating to the particular agents selected or to the biology of neoplasm. Generally, the agents used interacted with DNA to prevent DNA replication or RNA transcription or acted as inhibitors of nucleic acid synthesis. Agents selected for use in combinations had demonstrated activity when used as single agents, had different mechanisms of action, and had "minimally overlapping toxicities" (20). Also desirable was the selection of drugs that acted synergistically, so that their cytotoxic effects could be enhanced.

The objective of selecting agents with these properties was to increase the "fractional cell kill," that is, to increase the proportion of cells killed when the tumor burden is small enough to effect cure (this concept is also applied in combined modality therapy and adjuvant therapy, discussed elsewhere in this text). Other tumor cell kinetic information that has proven useful (and was derived in this era) included the use of agents administered at different time intervals to destroy tumor cells as they passed through the phases of the cell cycle (23, 24), the concept of schedule dependency. Agents may be used to "synchronize" cells so that a larger number are in a phase of the cell cycle where they are more sensitive to an additional drug or to "recruit" cells that are in the resting phase (usually when a large tumor burden is present), using a second agent to kill these cells as they are induced to proliferate.

Damon and Cadman (17) formulated a useful conceptual approach to the understanding and development of combination chemotherapy (Table 7.1). In the review cited they summarized, as well as proposed, new concepts of biochemical synergy useful in the further scientific development of combination chemotherapy. (One might use an oxymoronic term to describe this period, 1975 to date, as the era of "scientific empiricism.") Damon and Cadman's "planes of synergy" were based on observations of tumor biology and biochemical actions of drugs made over the last 30 years.

In their schema, the primary plane, or metabolic pathway inhibition, is postulated to be an intranuclear process that takes place via the inhibition of one component or metabolic product by the inhibition of two enzymes in sequence, the use of two noncompetitive inhibitors affecting one enzyme, or the inhibition of two pathways producing the same end product, obtaining higher levels of an inhibitor or promoting the conversion of a drug to its active form. The secondary plane, or macromolecule inhibition, involves the inhibition of DNA-directed RNA formation via the blocking of synthesis, repair, or processing of the macromolecule. The tertiary plane of synergy occurs at the level of cellular toxicity and involves concepts of tumor cell kinetics such as synchronization, recruitment, "resistance override," heterogeneous sensitivity override, and fractional cell kill. The importance of this latter concept cannot be overemphasized in understanding the principles of chemother-

Table 7.1. Conceptual Planes of Synergy[a]

Biochemical Plane	Title	Modulation	Components
1. (Primary)	Metabolic pathway inhibition	Yes	Cooperative blockade Sequential blockade Concurrent blockage Salvage pathway inhibition Intracellular drug level modulation Enhanced activation
2. (Secondary)	Macromolecule	Yes	Complementary (synthesis) inhibitor Complementary (repair) inhibition Complementary (processing) inhibition
3. (Tertiary)	Cellular (tumor) toxicity	No	Cell cycle synchronization Cell cycle recruitment Resistance override Heterogeneous sensitivity override Fractional cell kill
4. (Quaternary)	Host (selective) rescue	No	Selective toxicity Non-cross-host-toxic combination Selective rescues Dose intensity Sanctuary override (spatial cooperation)

From Damon LE, Cadmen EC. The metabolic basis for combination chemotherapy. Pharmacol Ther 1988;38:73–127.
[a]Synergy is a complex term. This table provides a conceptual framework from which questions of synergy can be addressed. Biochemical modulation is directly involved in only the first two planes, but is indirectly a component of all planes. Each plane contributes to the ultimate goal of therapeutic synergy (cure).

apy and synergy (cancer cell kill by drugs follows first-order kinetics, meaning that a given drug will eliminate a constant proportion of neoplastic cells). The implication of this level of synergy is that in order to "cure" a tumor, it is necessary to maximize doses or to start therapy when the tumor burden is small (19). The fourth plane of synergy is host rescue and cure; the features of this plane are selective toxicity, "non-cross-host toxic combinations" (permitting the use of full doses of all agents because of independent toxicities), selective rescue, dose intensity, and sanctuary override (17).

The application of these principles can be demonstrated by examining the clinical situations in which effective combination chemotherapy exists (Table 7.2). The information derived in the development of protocols used in the treatment of these malignancies includes many of those principles already discussed. All the neoplasms demonstrate responsiveness to a single agent that represents the cornerstone of the combinations, e.g., Adriamycin in the non-Hodgkin's lymphomas and cisplatin in testicular tumors. All use doses sufficient to induce toxicity. In childhood cancers, the combinations capitalize on the high tolerance that children exhibit to chemotherapy. Dose, schedule, and duration of therapy are considered critical in the case of pediatric hematologic neoplasms. All attempt to use the principles of nonoverlapping toxicities (more detailed examples of these principles are provided below); suffice it to say, the evidence is overwhelming that in many neoplasms, combination chemotherapy is more efficacious than single agents. Characteristics of the malignancies in Table 7.2 include high virulence, rapid growth, and drug sensitivity (and curability). The concept of the fourth plane of synergy, which includes sanctuary override and selective rescue, plays an important role in the design of several of these successful treatment regimens.

The implementation of this and the aforementioned concepts is illustrated in the protocols developed for treatment of the malignant lymphomas and some forms of acute leukemia. In the therapy of non-Hodgkin's lymphoma, third-generation regimens for the high-grade lymphomas have been developed. Laurence et al. (25), Klimo and Connors (26), and Skarin et al. (27) have developed and justified the multidrug, high-dose, and CNS prophylaxis approach quite cogently. These regimens employ the principles of non-cross-resistance, cycle specific activity, nonadditive toxicity, sanctuary override, host rescue, and drug resistance concepts. Preliminary data suggest that this approach will offer increased cure rates for these aggressive neoplasms. The treatment of pediatric acute lymphocytic leukemia has undergone several generations of treatment protocols (28, 29). These combination chemotherapeutic regimens have resulted in a median adverse-event-free survival of more than 5 years. In an effort to further enhance survival, a new intensive regimen has been developed (30). This regimen evolved because of the theoretical need for rapid, early, high fractional cell kill in poor-prognosis acute lymphocytic leukemia (ALL) patients. It also uses the principles of many drugs, short intervals between drugs, metabolic pathway inhibition, macromolecule inhibition, cellular toxicity, and host rescue. The projected 48-month event-free survival using this approach is 69 ± 5%.

A further example of these principles is the Vancouver seven-drug hybrid regimen for advanced Hodgkin's disease (31). The protocol is illustrated in Table 7.3. Klimo and Connors developed this regimen in an effort to apply the Goldie-Coldman principles of resistance (18). These principles, which included alternative modes of administration; briefer, more frequent dosage; non-cross-resistant agents; and cycle-active and marrow-sparing agents, have resulted

Table 7.2. Neoplasms in Which Combination Chemotherapy Has Proven Superior to Single Agents

Adult age group
  Head and neck cancer
  Small cell carcinoma of the lung
  Non-small-cell carcinoma of the lung
  Esophageal cancer
  Bladder cancer
  Testicular cancer
  Hodgkin's lymphoma
  Non-Hodgkin's lymphoma
  Acute lymphoblastic leukemia
  Ovarian cancer
  Breast cancer
  Acute nonlymphocytic leukemia
  Choriocarcinoma
Pediatric age group
  Wilms' tumor
  Neuroblastoma
  Burkitt's lymphomas
  Ewing's sarcoma
  Embryonal rhabdomyosarcoma
  Childhood germ cell tumors

Table 7.3. MOPP/ABV Hybrid

Drug	Dose	Route	Days Given
Nitrogen mustard	6 mg/m^2	i.v.	1
Vincristine	1.4 mg/m^2 (maximum 2 mg)	i.v.	1
Procarbazine	100 mg/m^2	p.o.	1–7
Prednisone	40 mg/m^2	p.o.	1–14
Adriamycin	35 mg/m^2	i.v.	8
Vinblastine	6 mg/m^2	i.v.	8
Bleomycin	10 mg/m^2	i.v.	8

in significant improvement in the observed remission rate in certain high-risk groups of patients.

Application of the synergistic biochemical approach has been less rewarding in the more "resistant" tumors, such as colorectal cancer, head and neck cancer, and advanced breast cancer. 5-Fluorouracil (5-FU) as a single agent has been the standard chemotherapeutic treatment for colorectal malignancy. By enhancing the ability of 5-FU to bind and then block thymidylate synthetase action, it was believed that its efficacy could be improved (32). The use of leucovorin (LV) prior to the administration of 5-FU does this effectively in animal models and has been incorporated into protocols that have yielded some promising responses (33). 5-FU is also an active agent in breast cancer. By combining 5-FU administration with LV, Doroshow et al. demonstrated a striking increase in efficacy in refractory metastatic breast cancer (34). Similarly, the combination of hydroxyurea and 5-FU has been used in poor-prognosis head and neck cancer. The principle involved in this approach is to increase the binding of 5-fluorodeoxyuridylate (5-FdUMP) to thymidylate synthetase by depleting cellular dUMP levels. Again, promising results have been obtained with this attempt at biochemical synergy (35). As we have learned more about mechanisms of resistance, more scientific approaches to combination chemotherapy have evolved. The approaches include dose intensification, alternative treatment schedules, newer combinations, physicochemical alterations (e.g., hyperthermia), cell membrane modifiers, and the use of a variety of chemotherapeutic agents with, or without, known antitumor activity (36, 37). The adaptation of these methods to clinical practice offers the potential for new and more active combination regimens. Elsewhere in this text, some of these new (and not so new) approaches are discussed in more detail.

Some of the problems encountered in developing new active combinations include identifying the mechanism of resistance involved and being able to reliably assay neoplastic tissue for appropriate markers. This was recently summarized by Yuen and Sikic, who review the problem of identifying the *mdr-1* gene marker and describe the treatment of patients with the modulators of MDR, cyclosporine and verapamil, as part of the chemotherapeutic combination (38). The authors indicated that while these lymphoma regimens show promise, toxicity of the modulators was a limiting factor.

One of the obvious problems in treatment with combination chemotherapy is the selection of resistant populations and the increase in the fraction of resistant cells over time. This elementary observation dictates that initial treatment must include agents that are directed at this problem. Regimens using cyclosporine and verapamil are excellent examples of this synergy and will probably shortly become first-line therapy in the treatment of some hematologic malignancies (Table 7.4) (38, 39). Other examples include the use of tamoxifen to modulate platinum therapy in the treatment of malignant melanoma

Table 7.4. Cyclosporine, Vincristine, Adriamycin and Dexamethasone in Refractory Myeloma

Drug	Dose	Route	Days Given
Vincristine	0.4 mg/day	i.v.	1–4
Adriamycin	9 mg/m/day	i.v.	1–4
Dexamethasone	40 mg	p.o.	1–4, 9–12, 17–20
Cyclosporine	7.5 mg/kg	i.v. (Cl)	1–4

Table 7.5. O^6-Benzylguanine (O^6BG) and BCNU Phase I Trial in Metastatic Solid Tumors[a]

Drug	Dose	Route	Time
O^6BG	10 mg/m	i.v.	T 0–1 (hours)
BCNU	13 mg/m	i.v.	T 21 days
PBM AT	NA	NA	T-24, 2, 6, 18, 24 hours and weekly
Tumor AT	NA	NA	T-24, 2, 18 hours

Modified from Gerson SL, Willson JKV. O^6-Alkylguanine-DNA alkyltransferase: a target for the modulations of drug resistance. Hematol Oncol Clin North Am 1995;9:431–450.
[a]This protocol involves assay of peripheral blood monocyte (PBM) and tumor alkyltransferase after the use of O^6BG to determine relationships between the two levels and to assess if PBM levels reflect tissue levels. Doses of O^6BG and BCNU will be escalated each cycle.

(40) and the recently proposed trial using O^6benzylguanine to deplete tumor alkyltransferase expression, a process that increases resistance to alkylating agents (41). This protocol is outlined in Table 7.5.

SUMMARY

In conclusion, combination chemotherapy has developed from an empiric to a reasonably scientific treatment modality in disseminated malignant disease. The concepts of combination chemotherapy have evolved from many years of painstaking laboratory and clinical efforts. Its principles involve

1. Biochemical synergy
2. Tumor cell kinetics
3. Fractional cell kill
4. Dose scheduling
5. Dose intensity and total dose
6. Nonoverlapping toxicity
7. Active agents
8. Tumor cell resistance
9. "Sanctuary override"
10. Non-cross-resistant agents
11. Host rescue
12. Identification of mechanisms of drug resistance

These principles have been used in the design of both primary and combined-modality chemotherapy combinations. Additionally, these principles form the basis for adjuvant and neoadjuvant approaches.

With our developing knowledge of molecular genetics and immunologic biology, we are likely to acquire new tools to study, identify, and develop appropriate therapeutic regimens. These methods suggest that we may be on the verge of leaving the era of "enlightened empiricism" and entering the realm of the true scientific basis for combination chemotherapy, far beyond the concepts of those "oncologists" in the "age of total empiricism."

REFERENCES

1. Yarbro J. Scientific basis of chemotherapy. In: Perry MC, ed. The chemotherapy sourcebook. Baltimore: Williams & Wilkins, 1991:2–14.
2. Goodman LS, Wintrobe MW, Dameshek W, et al. Nitrogen mustard therapy. JAMA 1946;132:126–132.
3. DeVita VT. Implications for surgical adjuvant treatment of cancer. Cancer 1983;51:1209–1220.
4. Li MC, Whitemore WF Jr, Goldby R, et al. Effects of combined drug therapy on metastatic cancer of the testis. JAMA 1960;174:1291–1299.

5. Li MC, Hertz R, Spencer DB. Effect of methotrexate therapy upon choriocarcinoma and chorioadenoma. Proc Soc Exp Biol Med 1956;93:361–366.
6. Skipper HE, Schobel FM Jr, Wilcox WS. Experimental evaluation of potential anticancer agents. XII. On the criteria and kinetics associated with "curability" of experimental leukemia. Cancer Chemother Rep 1964;35:1–111.
7. Skipper HE, Schobel FM Jr, Wilcox WS. Experimental evaluation of potential anticancer agents. XIV. Further study of certain basic concepts underlying chemotherapy of leukemia. Cancer Chemother Rep 1965; 45:5–28.
8. Freireich EJ, Karon M, Frei E III. Quadruple combined chemotherapy (VAMP) for acute lymphocytic leukemia in children (abstract). Proc Am Assoc Cancer Res 1964;5:20.
9. Pinke D, Hermoulex K, Borella L, et al. Drug dosage and remission duration in childhood lymphocytic leukemia. Cancer 1971;27:247–256.
10. DeVita VT Jr, Serpick AA, Carbone PP. Combination chemotherapy in the treatment of advanced Hodgkin's disease. Ann Intern Med 1970;73:881–895.
11. DeVita VT Jr, Young RC, Canellos GP. Combination versus single agent chemotherapy: a review of the basis for selection of drug treatment of cancer. Cancer 1975;35:98–110.
12. Sartorelli AC. Some approaches to the therapeutic exploitation of metabolic sites of vulnerability of neoplastic cells. Cancer Res 1969;29:2292–2299.
13. Capizzi RL, Keiser LW, Sartorelli AC. Combination chemotherapy: theory and practice. Semin Oncol 1977;4:227–253.
14. Potter VR. Sequential blocking of metabolic pathways in vivo. Proc Soc Exp Biol Med 1951;76:41–46.
15. Elion GB, Singer S, Hitchings GH. Antagonists of nucleic acid derivatives. VIII. Synergism in combinations of biochemically related antimetabolites. J Biol Chem 1954;208:477–488.
16. Damon LE, Cadman EC. Advances in rational combination chemotherapy. Cancer Invest 1986; 45:421–444.
17. Damon LE, Cadman EC. The metabolic basis for combination chemotherapy. Pharmacol Ther 1988; 38:73–127.
18. Goldie JH, Coldman AJ. A mathematical model for relating the drug sensitivity of tumors to their spontaneous mutation rate. Cancer Treat Rep 1979;63:1727–1733.
19. Goldie JE, Coldman AJ. The somatic mutation theory of drug resistance: the "Goldie-Coldman hypothesis revisited." PPO Updates, 1989, 5:1–12. In: DeVita VT Jr, Hellman S, Rosenberg SA, eds. Cancer: principles and practice of oncology. Philadelphia: JB Lippincott, 1989.
20. Frei E III. Combination cancer therapy: presidential address. Cancer Res 1972;32:2593–2607.
21. DeVita VT Jr. Dose response is alive and well. J Clin Oncol 1986;4:1157–1159.
22. Hryniuk WM. Is more better? J Clin Oncol 1986; 4:621–622.
23. Valeriote FA, Edelstein MB. The role of cell kinetics in cancer chemotherapy. Semin Oncol 1977; 4:217–226.
24. Valeriote FA, Lin HS. Synergistic interaction of anticancer agents: a cellular perspective. Cancer Chemother Rep 1975;59:895–900.

25. Laurence J, Coleman M, Allen SD, et al. Combination chemotherapy of advanced diffuse histiocytic lymphoma with the COP-BLAM regimen. Ann Intern Med 1982;97:190–195.

26. Klimo P, Connors JM. MACOP-B chemotherapy for the treatment of advanced diffuse large cell lymphoma. Ann Intern Med 1985;102:596–602.

27. Skarin AT, Canellos CP, Rosenthal DS, et al. Improved prognosis of diffuse histiocytic and undifferentiated lymphoma by the use of high dose methotrexate alternating with standard agents (M-BACOD). J Clin Oncol 1983;1:91–98.

28. Sallon SE, Weinstein JH, Nathan DG. The childhood leukemias. J Pediatr 1981;99:676–688.

29. Willoughby MLN. Childhood acute lymphoblastic leukemia: a review. J R Soc Med 1982;75:464–472.

30. Steinberg PG, Gaynor P, Miller DR. Improved disease-free survival of children with acute lymphoblastic leukemia at high risk for early relapse with the New York regimen—a new intensive therapy protocol: a report from the Children's Cancer Study Group. J Clin Oncol 1986;4:744–752.

31. Klimo P, Connors JM. MOPP/ABV hybrid program. Combination chemotherapy based on early introduction of seven effective drugs for advanced Hodgkin's disease. J Clin Oncol 1985;3:1174–1182.

32. Houghton J, Maroda S, Phillips J, et al. Biochemical determinates of responsiveness to 5-fluorouracil and its derivative in xenografts of human colorectal adenocarcinomas in mice. Cancer Res 1981;41:144–149.

33. Laufman LR, Krzeczowski KA, Roach R, Segal M. Leucovorin plus 5-fluorouracil: an effective treatment for metastatic colon cancer. J Clin Oncol 1987;5:1394–1400.

34. Doroshow JH, Leong L, Margolin K, et al. Refractory metastatic breast cancer: salvage therapy with fluorouracil and high dose continuous infusion leucovorin calcium. J Clin Oncol 1989;7:439–444.

35. Vokes EE, Panje WR, Schilsky RL, et al. Hydroxyurea, fluorouracil and concomitant radiotherapy in poor-prognosis head and neck cancer: a phase I-II study. J Clin Oncol 1989;7:761–768.

36. Marshall JL, Andrews PA. Preclinical and clinical experience with cisplatin resistance. Hematol Oncol Clin North Am 1995;9:415–429.

37. van Oosterom AT, Verweij JJ. New drugs for the treatment of sarcomas. Hematol Oncol Clin North Am 1995;9:909–925.

38. Yuen AR, Sikic BI. Multidrug resistance in lymphomas. J Clin Oncol 1994;12:2453–2459.

39. Sonneveld P, Schoester M, de Leeuw K. Clinical modulation of multidrug resistance in multiple myeloma: effect of cyclosporin on resistant tumor cells. J Clin Oncol 1994;12:1584–1591.

40. McClay EF, McClay MET, Albright KD, et al. Tamoxifen modulation of cisplatin resistance in patients with metastatic melanoma. Cancer 1993;72:1914–1918.

41. Gerson SL, Willson JKV. O^6-alkylguanine-dna alkyltransferase: a target for the modulations of drug resistance. Hematol Oncol Clin North Am 1995;9:431–450.

8

Combined Modality Therapy

Nancy L. Bartlett and Todd H. Wasserman

Unsatisfactory results with single modalities of therapy have led to the investigation of combined modality therapy (CMT) for many cancers. Classically, the concept of CMT referred to the concomitant use of irradiation (RT) and chemotherapy (CT). More recently, clinical investigators have used the term CMT to describe any combination of surgery, RT, or CT. While we agree with this broader definition, this chapter focuses specifically on the combination of RT and CT. We review the (*a*) clinical and theoretical rationale for CMT, including potential mechanisms of failure, (*b*) postulated mechanisms of specific RT-CT interactions, (*c*) sequencing strategies of CMT, (*d*) adverse RT-CT interactions, and (*e*) results of recent clinical trials designed to study the risks and benefits of using CMT to treat a variety of cancers.

CLINICAL RATIONALE FOR CMT

The initial goal of CMT was to increase overall survival by improving local control, decreasing distant metastases, or both. Over the last decade, the goals of combined CT-RT therapy have broadened to include organ and function preservation.

Improve Local Control

Local control of the primary tumor is required for cancer cure. Deaths due to locoregional failures constitute nearly all deaths from malignant gliomas, most deaths from head and neck and gynecologic cancers, and a significant minority of deaths from non-small-cell lung cancer and gastrointestinal and genitourinary cancers (1, 2). A significant increase in survival may result from better local and regional control. For example, in patients with locally recurrent cancers of the head and neck, uterus, cervix, bladder, and breast that are amenable to salvage surgery,

long-term disease control ranges from 10 to 80% (3). Uncontrolled studies in patients with medulloblastoma, prostate cancer, and bladder cancer also suggest that increased local control results in improved survival (2). If the addition of CT to RT can improve local control (either by independent cell kill or, ideally, by a beneficial interaction between RT and CT), then survival will be improved. Even in patients who succumb to distant disease, improved local control may result in significant palliation and improved quality of life.

Decrease Distant Failures

In addition to improving local control, administration of CT before (neoadjuvant), during, or after (adjuvant) surgery or RT may eliminate undetected micrometastases and decrease distant failure rates. Adjuvant CT is now the standard of care for all patients with node-positive breast and colon cancers, as large randomized trials have shown significantly improved survival rates with the addition of CT (4, 5). The use of either preoperative or postoperative CMT has improved overall survival rates and decreased both local and distant recurrences in patients with rectal cancer (6), while postoperative RT alone had no impact on overall survival despite decreased local failure rates (7).

In patients with systemic cancers such as non-Hodgkin's lymphoma, acute lymphoblastic leukemia, and small cell lung cancer, where CT is the mainstay of therapy, the addition of adjuvant RT to sanctuary sites such as the CNS and testes may decrease distant failure rates in these sites and consequently increase overall survival. Adding RT to sites of bulky disease may also decrease failure rates, as bulky sites may have the greatest likelihood of harboring resistant cells.

Organ and Function Preservation

The use of CMT to avoid debilitating surgery and preserve function is being applied to a growing number of cancers. Concurrent RT and infusional 5-fluorouracil (5-FU)-based CT cures 75 to 85% of patients with nonmetastatic anal carcinoma, with preservation of anal sphincter function in most patients (8, 9). Initial CT with cisplatin and 5-FU, followed by full-dose RT, will allow approximately half of patients with locally advanced laryngeal cancer to avoid laryngectomy, without an increase in local relapse or a decrease in survival (10). Extremity sarcomas (11), bladder cancer (12–15), esophageal cancer (16–19), and breast cancer (20, 21) are other malignancies in which preliminary studies suggest that overall survival and local control are not compromised when CMT is used in an attempt to avoid surgery.

THEORETICAL RATIONALE FOR CMT AND MECHANISMS OF FAILURE

Several recent reviews concisely summarize the theoretical rationale for CMT and why many of these exploitable mechanisms have not been realized clinically (22–25). Table 8.1 lists the commonly cited theoretical rationale for CMT, and Table 8.2 lists the potential mechanisms of failure of CMT. Both are discussed below in detail.

Table 8.1. Theoretical Rationale for Combined Modality Therapy

Prevention of emergence of resistant clones
Spatial cooperation
   CT treats disease outside RT field
   RT treats local disease and sanctuary sites
Direct biochemical and molecular interactions
   Modification of slope of dose-response curve
   Synchronization of cells by CT into a more RT-
     sensitive phase of the cell cycle
   Improved sensitization of hypoxic cells to RT by CT
   Improved killing of hypoxic cells by CT
   Inhibition of repair of potentially lethal and sublethal
     x-ray damage
Toxicity independence
Inhibition of tumor repopulation during fractionated RT
Tumor debulking by first modality leading to improved
   efficacy of second modality
   Improved chemotherapy delivery
   Improved oxygenation
   Smaller RT fields
Protection of normal tissues from RT damage

Table 8.2. Potential Mechanisms of Failure for Combined Modality Therapy

Inherent cross-resistance of CT and RT
Induction of common mechanisms of resistance during
   therapy
Enhanced normal tissue toxicity
   May lead to delay or dose reduction of potentially
     curative modality
   Acute and long-term complications may eliminate
     survival benefit of CMT
RT-induced vascular fibrosis resulting in decreased CT
   delivery

Prevent Emergence of Resistant Clones

The most fundamental principle behind CMT is that cells resistant to one modality may be sensitive to a different modality (22). The Goldie-Coldman hypothesis, which assumes that drug-resistant or radio-resistant populations arise spontaneously at a frequency that depends on the total number of clonogenic cells and the mutation frequency, suggests that early eradication of resistant cells by a second modality may prevent subsequent proliferation and improve tumor control (22, 26, 27). Because of inherent genetic instability, most tumors consist of many subclones with different levels of sensitivity to RT and CT (23, 28). If the mechanisms of resistance are independent, CMT may have an improved therapeutic index over either modality alone. For example, mechanisms of CT resistance such as changes in drug-activating enzymes, target enzymes, or drug-transport mechanisms are less likely to cause radiation resistance (23). Resistance mechanisms that lead to enhanced DNA repair and increased ability to scavenge free radicals are likely to cause cross-resistance of CT and RT. For example, the activated *ras* oncogene has been shown by Sklar to increase the intrinsic resistance of NIH 3T3 cells to both ionizing radiation and cisplatin (29, 30). These common resistance mechanisms may be one explanation for the disappointing results seen with CMT in the treatment of head and neck cancer. Wayne State University investigators retrospectively evaluated 57 patients with locally advanced head and neck cancer who had less than a complete response to cisplatin-based CT (31). Forty-one of 42 patients with a partial response to CT responded to RT, while only 1 of 18 patients with less than a partial response to initial CT responded to subsequent RT.

Spatial Cooperation

CMT may also result in improved outcome if one modality is able to treat disease at a site that is missed by another modality. This mechanism does not assume any interaction between CT and RT and was referred to by Steel and Peckham as spatial cooperation (32, 33). In preclinical experiments, both local RT and systemic cyclophosphamide are needed to control Lewis lung tumors implanted in the legs of C57 black mice (34). When used alone, RT will not prevent lung metastases, and cyclophosphamide will not control the primary tumor. This concept is the basis for administration of adjuvant CT following effective local therapy, for patients with a high likelihood of disease outside the radiation or surgical field. It is also the rationale for giving RT to limited areas of expected CT failure, such as the sanctuary sites of the testes and CNS in patients with hematologic malignancies. Since the two treatment modalities are expected to act entirely independently, scheduling strategies usually involve lengthening the time interval between RT and CT, in an attempt to give full doses of both.

Direct CT-RT Interactions

The most common reason for using CMT is to take advantage of the postulated direct biochemical and molecular interactions between CT and RT, which may result in an enhanced tumor response (25). Enhancement of tumor response implies that the administration of one agent (CT) increases the effect of another (RT), so that the combination produces better results than would be expected from the individual effects alone, that is $2 + 2 \geq 4$ (33). This term should be differentiated from sensitization, which is reserved for an effect of one agent that increases the effect of another, but which is inactive by itself (35). These interactions all involve CT enhancing RT effects, as opposed to RT having any effect on CT. The mechanisms of CT-RT interactions are not well understood, but potential mechanisms by which specific drugs may improve the effectiveness of RT are discussed in detail in the following section. These include increasing the slope of the radiation dose-response curve, synchronization of the cell cycle by CT into a more radiation sensitive phase such as G_2/M (e.g., paclitaxel), improved sensitization of hypoxic cells (e.g., cisplatin), direct toxicity to hypoxic cells (e.g., mitomycin), and inhibition of potentially lethal and sublethal x-ray damage repair by drugs such as cisplatin, actinomycin, and doxorubicin (36–38). Clinical application of these interactions requires a proportionally greater increase in antitumor efficacy than in normal tissue toxicity (23, 25). Most of these interactions probably result in additive cytotoxicity and not the hoped for supraadditive effect.

Toxicity Independence

Toxicity independence, a concept used to design combination CT regimens, is also potentially exploitable in combining CT and RT. By combining partially effective, noninteracting therapies with dissimilar toxicities, each can be given at or near full doses. While the same improvement in local control by CT can often be obtained by a relatively modest increase in radiation dose, this may not be the optimal strategy for decreasing acute and chronic toxicities. Assuming that a tumor mass weighs 100 g and contains 1% clonogenic cells, an RT dose of approximately 60 Gy in 30 fractions is needed for control if the tumor is radiosensitive. If CT alone resulted in a 90% response, the tumor-control dose would be reduced to 54 Gy. When CT results in a complete response (3-log kill), the radiation dose to achieve tumor control decreases to about 40 Gy (39). Even this modest decrease in RT dose may be desirable, as demonstrated in the treatment of pediatric Hodgkin's disease. Children and adolescents who received mediastinal irradiation doses greater than 30 Gy had a relative risk of acute myocardial infarction 45 times normal, while there was no increased risk in patients treated to lower total doses, although the patient cohort was much smaller (40). In adults, the relative risk of cardiac disease with mediastinal doses greater than 30 Gy was 3.5, while doses less than 30 Gy did not affect the risk (41). In tumors sensitive to both CT and radiation, combining lower cumulative doses of both RT and CT, in an effort to decrease long-term toxicities such as second malignancies, infertility, and cardiopulmonary damage without compromising cure rates may represent the optimal strategy.

Inhibit Tumor Repopulation during Fractionated RT

It has been postulated that repopulation between fractions may account for radioresistance in many tumors (42). As tumors shrink, improved blood flow and nutrition to the residual mass may result in a more rapid rate of proliferation, as evidenced by the increased radiation doses needed for tumor control when treatment duration is extended (23). Concurrent CT may slow the rate of repopulation if an active agent is available. However, as discussed previously, CMT would only lead to a therapeutic advantage if the rate of repopulation of tumor cells exceeds that of normal tissues in the RT field, such as the brain or lung. In rapidly proliferating tissues such as the gastrointestinal tract or skin, the increased toxicity to normal tissues may obviate any therapeutic gain. There is little clinical information on the influence of cytotoxic drugs on split-dose recovery of tumor cells after small fractionated doses, on drug-induced modification of clonogenic tumor cell repopulation when RT is given in a daily fractionation schedule, or on drug kinetics and the effects of reoxygenation.

Enhanced Efficacy of Second Modality Due to Decreased Tumor Bulk

Initial tumor shrinkage by CT may result in (a) smaller radiation fields with a sparing effect on normal tissues (e.g., the treatment of bulky mediastinal Hodgkin's disease) and (b) enhanced blood flow resulting in better oxygenation and less radioresistance. Several investigators have shown that up to 40% of clonogenic cells are hypoxic in experimental tumors and that they are two to three times more radioresistant than are oxygenated cells (43). As discussed below, the concept of neoadjuvant CT improving oxygenation and radiation sensitivity has been difficult to demonstrate clinically, perhaps because of induction of common mechanisms of resistance during initial CT. For example, while small-volume ovarian cancer is often controlled by initial RT, the same volume of disease after initial combination CT does not respond nearly as well (44, 45). In head and neck cancers, high complete response rates to neoadjuvant CT have not resulted in improved local control or survival.

In nonbulky tumors where radiation field size is not critical, shrinkage of tumors initially with RT could improve CT delivery and efficacy. Unfortunately, preclinical data show that exposure to RT may select for or induce drug resistance (46). Possible explanations for this detrimental effect include induction of the multidrug resistance gene by RT (47) or development of common mechanisms of resistance such as elevated levels of glutathione, which detoxify radiation-induced free radicals and repair damage of critical DNA sites (39, 48, 49). In addition, RT may induce vascular fibrosis and impair the blood supply, thereby decreasing delivery of drugs.

Protection from Radiation Effects to Normal Tissues.

In some experimental systems, CT increases the RT dose that is tolerated by normal tissue. For example, cyclophosphamide increased the survival of mice when given 1 to 3 days before whole-body RT (50), pretreatment with cytosine arabinoside protected the intestine against radiation damage (51), and pretreatment with vincristine induced transient reduction of bone marrow stem cell toxicity (52). Despite encouraging preclinical data, radiation protectors have not yet proven clinically useful.

EXPERIMENTAL BASIS OF CT-RT INTERACTIONS

Although a considerable amount of experimental data exploring the interactions between CT and RT exists, it is difficult to draw firm conclusions that can be reliably transferred to the clinic. This results from both the complexity of the questions asked and many methodologic limitations. Experimental systems have usually involved one or a limited number of fixed doses of CT and RT and cannot realistically test all possible combinations of sequence and schedule of CT and RT delivery. In most cases, the dose-response curves for each individual treatment are not known. An enhancement effect can only be deduced when dose-response curves for both modalities are known and these curves are either linear or can be made linear by mathematic transformation (e.g., changing exponential to linear by measuring log-cell kill) (32, 33). If the curves are not linear, isobolograms, or isoeffect plots, can be developed by using different assumptions about nonlinear additivity (33). These "envelopes of additivity" can be used to estimate RT-CT interactions (Fig. 8.1). Only points to the left of the envelope assure a supraadditive effect. While in vitro experiments use cellular and subcellular endpoints with linear dose-response curves, in vivo studies use gross tissue measurements, which usually have a steep shoulder effect in which no measurable tumor response or lethal events occur until a threshold

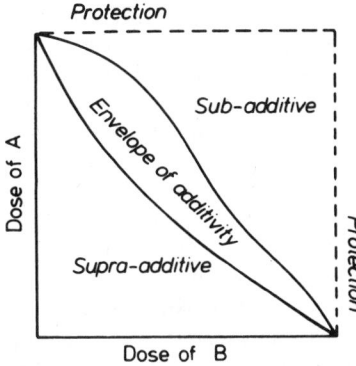

Figure 8.1. Isobologram approach when dose-response curves are not linear. Each point represents an identical survival or isoeffect under different assumptions of additivity. Only when experimental results occur to the left of the envelope can enhancement be definitely proven. (From Steele GG, Peckham MJ. Exploitable mechanisms in combined radiotherapy-chemotherapy: the concept of additivity. Int J Radiat Oncol Biol Phys 1979;5:85–91.)

dose is reached (53). Isobolograms have limited reliability when macroscopic endpoints are used.

Many of the in vitro tumor cell culture systems have been frequently passaged and must be considered as artificial tumor systems. Different sublines from the same parental tumor may behave differently. For example, conflicting results reported for the interaction of RT and doxorubicin on the L1210 cell line may be the result of differences between the sublines and unrelated to methodologic flaws (54). Cell lines may be heterogeneous in terms of cell cycle. Problems also exist with in vivo animal models. Some effects may depend on the strain of mice used. For example, BCNU causes significant skin toxicity when given before RT in some mouse strains but not others (55). Information gained by studying transplanted tumors may not be applicable to spontaneous tumors because of differences in blood supply, tumor-bed effects, pharmacokinetics, and other host factors.

Denekamp (56) and Dewey (57) have reviewed the advantages and disadvantages of different assay systems and endpoints. Monolayer systems are useful in obtaining cell kinetic information but are poor models for solid tumors. Spheroid cultures consisting of cells grown in suspension may be a better model. As the spheroids grow in size, they contain an outer zone of well-oxygenated and actively proliferating cells

and an inner zone of nutrient-deprived and hypoxic noncycling cells. Most assay systems have evolved from the study of RT alone. The addition of CT produces factors that are often difficult to control. RT can be delivered in seconds or minutes, which allows split-dose experiments, while CT has changing drug concentrations over several hours or days.

Steel (32) has reviewed the interaction between RT and several cytotoxic drugs against tumor cells. In certain systems, investigators have reported enhancement with almost every chemotherapeutic drug. However, the methodologic limitations previously cited and the lack of consistency from study to study make general statements difficult. Preclinical and clinical studies aimed at elucidating the mechanisms of CT-RT interactions for 5-FU, cisplatin, mitomycin C, hydroxyurea, paclitaxel, and camptothecin are discussed in detail below.

5-Fluorouracil–RT

5-FU interferes with DNA synthesis by inhibiting thymidylate synthetase and produces defective RNA by the incorporation of 5-fluorouridine triphosphate into RNA. In 1958, Heidelberger et al. noted greater regression of transplanted tumors treated with concomitant RT and 5-FU than of those treated with 5-FU alone (58). Vietti et al. (59) demonstrated that survival of a transplanted leukemia cell line in AKR/J mice treated with a single dose of RT and 5-FU depended on the time interval between the two modalities. Addition of 5-FU to RT had no significant effect when it was added more than 48 hours prior to irradiation. An enhanced effect was seen when 5-FU was given 20 to 48 hours prior to RT, but this effect significantly decreased when it was given less than 20 hours before RT. The greatest enhancement occurred when 5-FU was given 5 minutes to 8 hours after the dose of RT. These investigators speculated that the enhancement of cell kill when 5-FU was given after RT was due to inhibition of repair of sublethal damage. However, split-dose RT experiments have shown that 5-FU has no effect on repair of sublethal RT damage (60).

When 5-FU is present in concentrations sufficient to cause some cytotoxicity, it causes a significant change in the slope of the RT survival curve; this was interpreted as indicating enhanced cytotoxicity (54). Enhancement required continuous exposure for up to 48 hours.

As 5-FU appears equally toxic to aerobic and anaerobic cells, it may be useful against hypoxic cells that are relatively radioresistant (61). Thus, it appears that enhancement of RT by 5-FU is strongly dependent on both the 5-FU concentration and duration of exposure. As some degree of cytotoxicity appears to be necessary, CMT with 5-FU should be used with tumors that are at least partially sensitive to 5-FU, such as gastrointestinal and head and neck cancers.

Cisplatin-RT

Experimental and clinical data suggest that cisplatin enhances RT effects (62). Platinum complexes interact with DNA by both monofunctional and bifunctional cross-linking to bases (especially adjacent guanines in the helix) (63). Cisplatin given *prior* to RT has been shown to cause an increase in the slope of the RT dose-response curve (38, 64). Hypoxic conditions may enhance this interaction. Some studies have shown that cisplatin administered *after* RT may decrease the slope of the dose-response curve (36). Using in vivo transplanted tumors, the optimal strategy involves cisplatin given just prior to fractionated RT (65). Others have found that cisplatin may inhibit sublethal and potentially lethal RT damage repair (66, 67). Similar enhancing effects have been shown experimentally for the cisplatin analogue carboplatin (68). Since carboplatin can be given in higher platinum doses, clinical effects may be greater (68).

Importantly, most data suggest that increased damage to normal tissues by CMT employing cisplatin is a result of independent cell kill and not enhancement (36). Thus, the combined effect on bone marrow, skin, and lung does not appear to be substantially worse than with RT alone (38, 69). An exception appears to be a late effect of CMT on kidney function, which appears to be greater than expected by an additive effect alone (70, 71). Clinical trials designed to study the benefit of cisplatin-RT interactions in several tumors including head and neck, lung, esophageal, and bladder cancers are discussed below.

Mitomycin-RT Interactions

The alkylating agent mitomycin C is more toxic to hypoxic cells than to aerobic cells (72). This property makes it especially appealing for combining with RT, given that hypoxic cells are less responsive to radiation. Two preclinical studies showed supraadditive cell kill when mi-

tomycin C was administered 15 minutes or 24 hours prior to RT (73, 74). When the drug was given after RT, only an additive effect resulted (74). Because normal tissues do not contain hypoxic cells, the concomitant use of mitomycin C and RT should result in therapeutic gain without increasing normal tissue damage. Fu and Lam studied the effects of combined intraperitoneal mitomycin C and continuous low-dose-rate RT and observed no significant increase in early or late damage to mouse skin or soft tissues (75). A prospective randomized trial comparing RT alone to RT and mitomycin C in the treatment of head and neck cancer showed a significant increase in local regional control in the CMT arm, without any increase in normal tissue reactions (76).

Hydroxyurea-RT Interactions

Hydroxyurea (HU), another S-phase-specific agent, inhibits ribonucleotide reductase and impairs DNA synthesis. HU may have additive effects with RT by improving cell kill of S-phase cells, which are relatively radioresistant (25). Two preclinical studies suggest enhancement of RT effects by HU. Sinclair demonstrated that HU caused cell-cycle synchronization at the radiation-sensitive G_1/S interphase (77). Fram and Kufe showed that HU inhibited repair of radiation-induced single-strand breaks in vitro (78). Because HU has limited independent activity in solid tumors, few clinical trials have tested the HU-RT combination. Clinical studies are ongoing with 5-FU, HU, and RT in head and neck cancers.

Paclitaxel-RT Interactions

The microtubule inhibitor paclitaxel (Taxol) has significant activity in breast, ovarian, and lung cancer. Taxol acts by stabilizing microtubules and prevents mitosis by blocking cells in the G_2/M phase of the cell cycle. Several in vitro studies have investigated the ability of Taxol to enhance RT sensitivity by synchronizing cells in G_2/M, a more radiosensitive phase of the cell cycle. Taxol has enhanced RT sensitivity in a number of human tumor cell lines including astrocytoma, ovary, melanoma, and breast cancers (79–82). Steren et al. showed that treatment of three human ovarian cancer cell lines with Taxol 48 hours prior to RT had a greater sensitizing effect than treatment 24 hours prior to RT (81).

Clinical data testing Taxol-RT are not yet available.

Camptothecin-RT Interactions

Studies are under way to determine the activity of the camptothecin compounds (topotecan, CPT-11) for a variety of tumors including colon, ovarian, esophageal, and head and neck cancers. Camptothecins are topoisomerase I inhibitors that stabilize the topoisomerase I–DNA complex during S-phase, resulting in DNA damage and cytotoxicity. Preclinical data suggest that the camptothecins potentiate RT-induced cell killing. For example, in Chinese hamster ovary cells, topotecan reduced the D_{10} (radiation dose resulting in 10% survival) by approximately 50% (83). Enhancement of killing required exposing the cells to topotecan during the first 30 minutes after radiation therapy. In contrast, maximal enhancement of radiation-induced growth delay of implanted fibrosarcomas occurred when drug was given 2 to 4 hours prior to radiation (84). Proposed mechanisms of interaction between RT and the camptothecins include (*a*) inhibition of sublethal or potentially lethal damage repair following RT as shown in two human melanoma cell lines (85, 86) and (*b*) increasing the proportion of cells in S phase by slowing the rate of progression through S phase with radiation, thus increasing sensitivity to the camptothecins (87, 88). Hennequin showed supraadditivity of cell killing in both HeLa cells and V-79 fibroblasts following concomitant exposure to camptothecin and low-dose-rate irradiation (87). Clinical trials incorporating topotecan into a combined modality regimen are ongoing in advanced lung and head and neck cancers.

SEQUENCING STRATEGIES

Combined modality therapy can be given either concurrently or sequentially, with CT either before or after RT. Each of these approaches has potential advantages and disadvantages. Concomitant CT-RT exploits the direct biochemical and molecular interactions of the treatment modalities but often increases the toxicity to normal tissues. Normal tissue toxicity may result in treatment breaks or dose reductions that compromise the efficacy of the treatment. Sequential administration appears to lessen toxicity but prolongs treatment time and results in a delay of one modality of therapy. Studies using animal and human tumors have shown a faster dou-

bling rate after treatment with either CT or RT. In patients with cutaneous and pulmonary metastases, a 2.5- to 5-fold increase in doubling times has been demonstrated (89–91). Therefore, interruptions of therapy of only a few weeks may result in significant tumor repopulation. Neoadjuvant CT may induce common mechanisms of resistance, limiting the effectiveness of subsequent RT. Alternatively, neoadjuvant CT may increase oxygenation and RT efficacy by decreasing tumor volume. An additional concern with the use of neoadjuvant CT is that patients may refuse definitive RT because of side effects of initial CT (92).

Looney and Hopkins have suggested that rapid alternation of CT and RT may be a better strategy than either sequential or concurrent schedules (93–95). In this system, CT is given every 3 or 4 weeks (as usual), with RT starting approximately 7 days after CT and ending 7 days prior to the next CT treatment. This necessitates split-dose RT (93), which may be deleterious if the tumor is relatively chemoresistant. Alternating CT and RT may allow each modality to kill cells resistant to the other and prevent the emergence of doubly resistant populations, while minimizing the risk of normal tissue toxicity and maximizing doses of each modality.

Looney and Hopkins have presented data from a regrowth assay for the 392A hepatoma cell line injected into ACI rats (93–95). They showed that RT given as multiple fractions per day (MFD) was superior to the standard daily fractionation. When cyclophosphamide was given with daily fractionated doses, growth delay appeared additive; when cyclophosphamide was given with MFD, growth delay appeared greater than additive. The best cure rates were obtained when CT was alternated with MFD, with optimal separation at 6 or 7 days. This allowed the delivery of larger doses of RT over shorter intervals and allowed longer recovery times between treatment. As predicted by the Goldie-Coldman hypothesis, large doses of RT and CT given early in a treatment period proved to be optimal.

Tubiana and colleagues have tried this alternating approach in limited clinical studies (38, 39). In limited-stage small cell lung cancer, they showed a 79% complete response rate and a 3-year survival of 22% in 45 patients treated with CT (cyclophosphamide, doxorubicin, VP-16, and cisplatin) alternated with split-course radiotherapy to 55 Gy. CT was given over 6 days on a 30-

day schedule, with radiation interdigitated from days 13 through 25. These nonrandomized results appear to be superior to most standard therapies and were obtained with acceptable toxicity, but they need to be compared with standard therapy in randomized trials. Merlano et al. (96) and Taylor et al. (92) have published results of randomized trials in head and neck cancer showing better local control with the interdigitating approach than with sequential therapy. These results are discussed in detail below.

ADVERSE COMBINED MODALITY INTERACTIONS

Compared with either modality alone, CMT may cause increased damage to normal tissues. Possible interactions include enhancement of RT damage by CT; enhancement of CT damage by RT; additive effects of both modalities on the same tissue; effects on different tissues of the same organ, causing increased physiologic damage; or the production of injury usually not seen by either modality (97). Thus, careful analysis of normal tissue toxicity as well as tumor cell kill is necessary to fully assess the benefits of CMT. Enhancement of normal tissue toxicity usually appears to be most severe when the drug has a toxicity against that tissue in the absence of RT. Examples include the increased lung toxicity associated with cyclophosphamide and bleomycin and the increase in skin and mucosal damage seen with bleomycin when combined with RT. Enhancement usually appears greatest when RT and CT are given close together. Hematopoietic damage may be somewhat different, as peak enhancement appears when CT is given 1 to 3 days after RT administration (98).

In general, the toxicity to acutely proliferating tissues (early-reacting) such as bone marrow and intestine has been the main concern of medical oncologists. Conversely, toxicity to more slowly proliferating tissues (late-reacting) such as lung, liver, and the CNS are dose-limiting toxicities for RT. It is now clear that CT can cause overt or subclinical late effects that can seriously enhance RT-related toxicity. Similarly, mucositis and intestinal toxicity produced by CT are increased when CT is combined with RT. RT-induced toxicity is due to both parenchymal cell hypoplasia (causing both early and late toxicity) and fine vasculature and fibroconnective tissue damage (causing late toxicity). CT appears to affect both cycling and noncycling parenchymal cells, with

sparing of the microcirculation (99). Whether these interactions result in additive or enhanced toxicity depends on many factors, including the tissue involved, routes of administration of RT and CT, and timing (97).

Early-reacting tissues appear to respond to treatment in a manner determined by the number of surviving clonogenic target cells and are more amenable to in vitro analysis. For late-responding tissue, the problem is more complex, with effects on various cellular compartments (parenchyma, stroma, vascular) more difficult to quantitate. Unlike early-reacting tissues, there may be no simple relationship in late-reacting tissues between cell survival and a functional endpoint that can easily be quantitated or predicted (97).

One strategy to investigate the above effects is to compute CT-dependent dose-enhancement factors (DEFs) (defined as the RT dose required to produce a certain effect divided by the RT dose producing the same effect when combined with CT). As DEF calculations can be done for both normal tissues and tumors, therapeutic gain factors (TGFs) (defined as the DEF of the tumor divided by the DEF of normal tissue) can be generated. Theoretically, TGFs greater than one imply a greater effect on tumors than on normal tissue. As the endpoints used for toxicity to tumor and normal tissues can have varying sensitivities, and DEF calculations for the same tissue can differ depending on the assay, these calculations can only serve as rough guides for what can be expected clinically (98).

Experimental assay systems used to study the normal tissue toxicity of RT may be unreliable when CT is added. These assays use gross changes, physiologic changes, or survival curves to determine toxicity (100). Gross changes such as necrosis, paraplegia, or death tend to be reproducible and occur over narrow dose ranges. However, they rarely give insight into the pathophysiology of the interaction. Physiologic changes such as the respiratory rate are insensitive in tissues that have a large functional capacity such as the lung. Survival curve estimates of tissues such as bone marrow or intestine tend to be most useful, as they also allow the opportunity of estimating the capacity for accumulation of sublethal damage as well as repair. Unfortunately, techniques for obtaining cell survival data are not available for all tissues. Measured effects are not always due to interactions between CT and RT on the target tissue.

While lethality in certain experimental conditions correlates with specific RT-induced damage, the systemic effect of CT may hinder the ability to identify the etiology of the toxicity. For example, although doxorubicin appears to enhance RT-induced lung damage when measured by an increase in ventilatory rate, these results could be due to the effects of RT-doxorubicin-induced heart disease (101).

The large amount of experimental data on the effects of CMT on normal tissues has been reviewed recently by Steel (32). As in experiments studying CT-RT interactions against tumors, the lack of full dose-response curves in various assay systems makes conclusions difficult. One useful strategy has been the time-line approach, where fixed doses of CT and RT are used and only the timing interval between them varied. When therapeutic gain factors are calculated for drug administered simultaneously with RT, it becomes clear that it is unusual to have a better effect on tumor than on normal tissue (98). Often the interaction results in an overall detrimental effect.

Because of the inadequacies of experimental systems, careful documentation of clinical effects has produced the most useful information (97). Many of the most severe side effects, such as second malignancies in Hodgkin's disease and the leukoencephalopathy associated with combination CT and cranial RT in acute lymphocytic leukemia, were not predicted by experimental studies. Rubin et al. (102) reviewed the difficulties of toxicity-reporting systems. Radiotherapists and medical oncologists often have differing concerns. Clinical scoring cannot describe subclinical events and fundamental biologic interactions. The degree of clinically tolerable dysfunction varies between body organs. Confounding variables such as complications of surgery, the toxic effects of the tumor itself, and other comorbid conditions such as emphysema or diabetes mellitus hinder development of a uniform toxicity-scoring system. Despite these practical realities, careful, uniform scoring of toxicity including the grade, time frame, reversibility, and treatability is crucial to optimizing therapeutic outcome.

Doxorubicin-RT-Induced Heart Disease

The interaction between doxorubicin (Adriamycin) and RT is an example of one that produces late tissue damage. Doxorubicin's antitumor effect is felt to be due to intra-DNA intercalation or topoisomerase II–induced DNA cleavage. Its cardiac toxicity appears to be due to the generation of superoxide radicals by a doxorubicin-iron complex (103). The unique sensitivity of the heart to doxorubicin is due to decreased catalase and superoxide dismutase in the heart (104). The uncoupling of its cardiotoxic and antitumor effect is shown by treatment with the chelator ICRF-187, which protects against cardiotoxicity but does not lessen the antitumor effect (105). Studies in both animals (106) and humans (107) have shown that doxorubicin damages myocytes directly through myofibrillar degeneration and vacuolization, with sparing of the interstitial connective tissue and vasculature. Cardiac damage by RT is distinctly different, with diffuse interstitial fibrosis and a decrease in viable capillaries approximately 3 months after therapy. This leads to ischemia and secondary myocardial fibrosis (108, 109). Experiments in rabbits, using fractionated doses of doxorubicin and RT, suggest that the cardiotoxic effects are additive (106).

Billingham performed endomyocardial biopsies in 92 patients, 17 with previous mediastinal radiation (107). Patients with previous RT had worse endomyocardial biopsy scores for all levels of total doxorubicin dose, even when RT was given 5 to 10 years prior to CT. Fourteen of 17 patients with previous RT had swelling of capillary endothelial cells similar to that seen in acute radiation change. Retrospective nonrandomized studies by Gilladoga et al. (110) in children and Bristow et al. (111) in adults appear to substantiate the increased cardiotoxicity when doxorubicin and RT are given together. A review of 4000 patients who received doxorubicin, including 300 who received mediastinal RT, was unable to show a statistically significant increase in congestive heart failure in the combined group (112). Other clinical parameters such as dosing schedule, previous cardiac disease, and age may modify this risk (112).

CLINICAL TRIALS OF COMBINED MODALITY THERAPY

An exhaustive review of all clinical trials of CMT is beyond the scope of this chapter, and particular examples have already been discussed. However, a review of certain studies will illustrate both the promise and the difficulties in conducting trials of CMT. This section highlights recent randomized trials that support the use of CMT to improve overall survival because of im-

Table 8.3. Clinical Results of Combined Modality Therapy

CMT may improve local control[a] or survival[b]
    Rectal cancer[a,b]
    Limited stage small cell lung cancer[a,b(?)]
    Non-small-cell lung cancer[b]
    Hodgkin's disease[a]
    Limited-stage non-Hodgkin's lymphoma[a,b]
    Rhabdomyosarcoma[a,b]
    Anaplastic astrocytoma[a,b]
    Esophageal cancer[a,b]
CMT avoids debilitating surgery without compromising survival
    Anal cancer
    Bladder cancer
    Head and neck cancer
    Extremity sarcoma
    Breast cancer
Ineffective chemotherapy/no benefit from CMT
    Colon cancer
    Pancreatic cancer
    Gastric cancer
    Renal cancer
    Melanoma
    Uterine cancer

[a]May improve local control.
[b]May improve survival.

proved local control, decreased distant metastases, or both (Table 8.3). In addition, randomized trials and encouraging pilot data that support the use of CMT to avoid mutilating surgery and preserve function are discussed.

Improved Local Control and Decreased Distant Metastases

HEAD AND NECK CANCER

The role of CMT in the treatment of locally advanced head and neck cancers has come full circle and illustrates many of the theoretical points discussed earlier. Investigators initially tested the use of single-agent CT *concurrently* with RT in the postoperative setting, to take advantage of the synergy demonstrated in the laboratory between RT and many of the agents known to be active in head and neck cancer. Most of these studies resulted in better local control than with RT alone, including trials of bleomycin, methotrexate, cisplatin, mitomycin, and 5-FU (113, 114). In addition to improved local control, a survival advantage was reported in the cisplatin/RT (115) and 5-FU/RT (116) trials. These single-agent trials did not affect distant

failure rates, but they increased survival rates by improving local control alone.

To decrease distant failures, investigators next chose to administer combination CT instead of single agents. To avoid the excessive toxicity associated with concomitant administration of full-dose combination CT and RT, most trials administered full-dose CT either before or after definitive surgery and/or RT. Despite response rates as high as 90% with cisplatin and infusional 5-FU (117), most trials of neoadjuvant and adjuvant CT for locally advanced head and neck cancers have been disappointing (114, 118–120). Distant failure rates decreased but did not result in improved survivals, primarily because of higher local failure rates than were seen with concomitant therapy. The high incidence of noncompliance and severe concomitant comorbidity in this patient group may also eliminate any survival benefit derived from more intensive CT (114).

Recent efforts have turned again to concomitant CT and RT in an effort to improve locoregional control, which continues to be the major cause of treatment failure. Most investigators have chosen either split-course chemoradiotherapy or rapidly alternating chemoradiotherapy to limit mucosal and hematopoietic toxicity (114). For example, Taylor et al. showed that split-course concomitant cisplatin–5-FU and RT, administered every other week for seven courses, resulted in better local control than did neoadjuvant cisplatin–5-FU followed by RT (92). Survival rates were similar, but there were significantly fewer cancer deaths in the concomitant arm. Merlano et al. reported better survival rates with cisplatin–5-FU alternating with RT in three 2-week courses than with RT alone (96), as well as with three courses of vinblastine, bleomycin, and methotrexate alternating with three courses of RT compared with four cycles of neoadjuvant CT followed by definitive RT (121). The results of rapidly alternating therapy are encouraging, as it appears this approach may result in improved local and distant control without increasing toxic deaths, thereby improving overall survival. The use of CMT to avoid disfiguring surgery is discussed below in the section on organ preservation.

RECTAL CANCER

Several large randomized clinical trials for stage II and III rectal cancer completed during the last decade have led to significant improvements in the treatment of rectal cancer. In addition, these studies have confirmed in vitro data on RT-CT interactions in a clinical setting. The first randomized trials compared surgery alone with surgery plus postoperative RT. While some of these studies showed a decrease in local recurrence rates, none showed a survival advantage with the addition of RT (7, 122). In contrast, a large randomized trial comparing postoperative RT to postoperative RT and concomitant CT reported a significant decrease in both local recurrence rates and distant metastases, as well as an improvement in overall survival in the CMT arm (6). While additional cycles of adjuvant CT in the CMT arm may account for the decrease in distant metastases, CT alone has never been shown to decrease the incidence of local recurrence (7), suggesting a local synergistic effect of CT and RT. In 1990, a consensus conference of the NIH recommended that all patients with locally advanced rectal cancer receive postoperative CMT (123).

Current efforts are focused on refining the use of CMT in the treatment of rectal cancer by adjusting drug schedules and adding new drugs to enhance radiosensitization. A recently completed randomized trial showed a significant advantage to protracted venous infusion of 5-FU during the entire course of RT, compared with bolus 5-FU for 5 days during weeks 1 and 5 of RT (124). This study confirmed Byfield's in vitro data showing enhancement of 5-FU and RT cytotoxicity when tumor cells were continuously exposed to 5-FU for 24 to 48 hours after RT (60). An ongoing four-arm trial is studying the benefits of preoperative CMT versus preoperative RT alone, as well as the value of postoperative adjuvant CT (125). The concomitant CT in this trial is 5 days of bolus 5-FU plus low-dose leucovorin during weeks 1 and 5 of RT. The addition of leucovorin was based on both laboratory and clinical studies showing enhanced cytotoxicity of 5-FU by leucovorin (126) and laboratory studies showing enhanced radiosensitization with leucovorin (127, 128).

Current randomized trials in stage II and III rectal cancer are also trying to determine the value of preoperative versus postoperative CMT. Proponents of preoperative CMT cite improved tolerance, potential downstaging, increased resectability, a suggestion of improved local control, and the introduction of systemic therapy earlier in the course of treatment (129, 130). In addition, preoperative CMT may allow sphincter-sparing surgery in patients with early-stage rectal cancer. Proponents of postoperative

CMT cite the ability to adjust therapy on the basis of the pathologic stage and that tumor hypoxia associated with large rectal tumors would decrease the radiosensitivity (130). Large randomized trials in rectal cancer continue to move the field of CMT forward.

SMALL CELL LUNG CANCER (SCLC)

Because of frequent early dissemination, CT is the mainstay of therapy for patients with limited-stage SCLC. With CT alone, the complete response (CR) rate is approximately 50% (131, 132), but the 3-year survival is only 5 to 15% (133, 134). Up to 80% of patients treated with CT relapse in the chest, and some die of local disease without evidence of disseminated relapse (134). Two metaanalyses designed to determine the effect of chest RT on survival and local control in patients with limited-stage SCLC showed a 5% increase in the 2- and 3-year survival rates and a 25 to 30% increase in local control (135, 136). This modest improvement in survival with CMT, compared with CT alone, was not detected in most of the individual randomized trials because of small patient numbers. In both metaanalyses, CMT was significantly more toxic than CT alone, with increased hematologic, mucosal, skin, and pulmonary toxicity. Most of the trials used cyclophosphamide, doxorubicin, and (occasionally) methotrexate–drugs that are difficult to combine with RT because of overlapping toxicities and a high incidence of radiation recall. The introduction of the cisplatin-etoposide regimen in the last decade for SCLC has decreased the toxicity of CMT because these drugs do not have independent cardiac, pulmonary, or esophageal toxicity. Controversy continues regarding the optimal scheduling of RT and CT. Individual trials have shown advantages to both early (137) and late (138) introduction of RT. Introducing RT early may compromise subsequent CT dose intensity. Alternatively, early RT may effectively treat chemoresistant clones before they metastasize outside the local RT field (137). Because local recurrence rates still exceed 50% at 3 years, investigators continue to test new approaches, including hyperfractionated RT, new drugs, and high-dose therapy with peripheral blood progenitor cell or marrow rescue.

NON-SMALL-CELL LUNG CANCER (NSCLC)

Several randomized trials have compared RT alone with CMT for locally advanced NSCLC (139). Some trials have shown a modest survival benefit (5–10%) with CMT using cisplatin-based regimens, while others have shown no benefit. It may be that the negative trials were too small to detect a 5 to 10% difference in survival or that some trials used less-effective CT regimens. The Radiation Therapy Oncology Group (RTOG) and Eastern Cooperative Oncology Group (ECOG) recently reported a 1-year survival advantage for induction chemotherapy (cisplatin plus vinblastine) followed by RT, compared with standard RT alone or hyperfractionated RT alone (60% vs. 46% vs. 51%, respectively, $p = .03$) (140). This confirms a prior Cancer and Leukemia Group B study (141). The small survival advantage of CMT is likely due to a decrease in micrometastatic disease, since randomized trials have shown no difference in response rates between RT alone and CMT (140–142). Neither sequential nor concurrent CMT regimens have improved local control. A variety of new strategies are under investigation, including the use of newer agents such as Taxol, topotecan, navelbine, and gemcitabine; intensified RT protocols; and the possibility of resection after CMT.

ESOPHAGEAL CANCER

Less than 10% of patients with esophageal cancer survive for 5 years following surgery or RT. Because of these dismal results, the RTOG conducted a randomized trial comparing RT alone (64 Gy) versus CMT (four cycles of 5-FU–cisplatin plus 50 Gy given concurrently with the first two cycles of CT) (16). The 2-year survival rates were 10% for the RT arm and 38% for the CMT arm ($p < .01$). The patients who received CMT had fewer local ($p < .02$) and distant ($p < .01$) recurrences. There has been no randomized trial comparing surgery with chemoirradiation, but the results of the aforementioned trial compared with historic controls treated with surgery would suggest that CMT represents a reasonable alternative to esophagectomy (17). Forastiere et al. reported a 59% 2-year survival for 43 patients treated with CMT (concurrent 5-FU, cisplatin, vinblastine, and RT) followed by esophagectomy (18).

Organ and Function Preservation

ANAL CANCER

Since 1980, RT plus concurrent 5-FU and mitomycin has been the standard treatment for all stages of anal cancer. Overall and disease-free survival rates with CMT are at least as good as historic results with abdominoperineal resection, and CMT preserves anorectal function in 70 to 90% of patients (8). Several institutions have reported nonrandomized results showing better local control with CMT than with RT alone (8, 9). The advantage of CMT appears to be most marked for tumors larger than about 3 or 4 cm. The EORTC recently reported preliminary results of the first randomized trial comparing RT (60–65 Gy) alone with RT (60–65 Gy) plus 5-FU (750 mg/m^2/day on days 1–5 and 29–33) and mitomycin (15 mg/m^2 on day 1) for patients with locally advanced anal carcinoma. The CR rate was significantly better for patients treated with CMT (77 vs. 53%, $p < .01$), and consequently the need for colostomy was significantly lower with CMT (143a). The advantage of CMT in smaller tumors is less clear, as colostomy-free survivals with RT alone are generally at least 85%. However, these small tumors appear to be well controlled with a shorter course of radiation (30 Gy) when given in combination with 5-FU and mitomycin (144). This lower dose of RT may decrease the incidence of late damage to normal tissues in the field.

While pilot studies are under way to test other CT combinations (5-FU and cisplatin) in the treatment of anal cancer, 5-FU and mitomycin remain the standard of care. Due to the high incidence of hematologic toxicity with mitomycin, the RTOG and ECOG recently completed a randomized trial of 310 patients with anal cancer, comparing 5-FU (1000 mg/m^2/day for 4 days, weeks 1 and 4) alone with 5-FU and mitomycin (10 mg/m^2 on days 1 and 29). CT was administered concurrently with RT (45 Gy) in both arms. There was no difference in overall survival, however, there was a 50% decrease in locoregional failures (18 vs. 36%, $p < .01$) and colostomies (10 vs. 23%, $p < .01$) and an improved 4-year disease-free survival (75 vs. 51%, $p < .01$) in the mitomycin arm (145). Grade 4–5 toxicities were significantly higher in the mitomycin arm (26 vs. 7%), with 4 fatalities (3%) in the mitomycin arm.

It is still not clear whether the merits of CMT for anal cancer are simply additive or whether there is a clinically significant enhancing effect of 5-FU and mitomycin on RT. The inferior results of two small trials of sequential CT and RT support, but do not prove, a synergistic interaction. Administering 5-FU and mitomycin prior to RT resulted in CR rates of only 21 to 53% (146).

BLADDER CANCER

Cure rates for T$_{2-4}$ invasive bladder cancers range from 30 to 50% with radical cystectomy and 25 to 40% with radiation alone (12). In recent years, several centers have piloted combination chemoradiation protocols for these patients in an attempt to preserve the bladder without compromising survival. The RTOG reported a 3-year actuarial survival of 63% in a phase II study of concurrent RT and cisplatin (13). Forty percent of patients had bladder preservation without local failure. Kaufman et al. enrolled 53 patients with muscle-invading bladder cancers in a phase II study of transurethral resection and two courses of cisplatin-methotrexate-vinblastine followed by concurrent cisplatin and RT (40 Gy) (14). Incomplete responders underwent salvage cystectomy, and complete responders (53%) received an additional course of cisplatin and RT (25 Gy). Overall and disease-free survivals at 4 years were 53% and 45%, respectively, with 58% of patients having a well-functioning bladder free of invasive tumor. High complete response rates (74%) have also been reported for a 5-FU–cisplatin combination with concomitant bifractionated split-course radiation therapy (15). While these three pilot studies report results equivalent to those described for radical cystectomy, only a randomized trial will verify that CMT with bladder preservation is an acceptable alternative to radical cystectomy (14).

LARYNGEAL CANCER

While the results of CMT in advanced-stage head and neck cancer have not yielded improvements in disease-free or overall survival, organ preservation remains an important secondary endpoint (114, 118). Radical resections of advanced head and neck cancers often disfigure patients and may result in voice loss or alterations in swallowing. A prospective randomized trial comparing laryngectomy and postoperative RT with three cycles of induction CT (cisplatin and 5-FU) and RT showed no difference in 2-year survival (68%), but the larynx was preserved in 64% of patients in the CMT arm (10). Some investigators criticized the lack of a radiation alone arm, arguing that similar survivals and rates of larynx preservation can be obtained without the use of neoadjuvant CT (147). The current RTOG 91-11 trial for stage III or IV resectable cancer of the larynx compares three nonsurgical therapies to preserve the larynx, including RT alone, induction CT (cisplatin and 5-FU) followed by RT, and concurrent cisplatin and RT (148).

SARCOMA

Nearly 80% of patients with soft tissue or bone sarcomas of the extremity are candidates for limb-sparing surgeries, in part due to the introduction of multimodality therapy. The addition of adjuvant and neoadjuvant CT (doxorubicin, cisplatin, high-dose methotrexate) has increased the cure rate of osteosarcoma from less than 20% to nearly 60% (149). While this improvement in survival is largely due to a decrease in deaths from distant disease, the use of neoadjuvant CT has made limb salvage feasible for most patients (150). RT does not play a role in the initial therapy of osteosarcoma. For soft tissue sarcomas, conservative surgery and preoperative or postoperative RT produce local control rates equivalent to those achieved with amputation (151). However, more than half of patients with tumors greater than 5 cm will eventually succumb to distant disease. Adjuvant CT for soft tissue sarcoma remains investigational, with most randomized trials to date showing no survival advantage for patients treated with CT. CMT, with RT and (occasionally) conservative surgery sandwiched between courses of CT, is the treatment of choice for monostotic Ewing's sarcoma (152, 153). While good local control and limb preservation are a reality for most patients with extremity sarcomas, the challenge of distant disease remains.

BREAST CANCER

The combination of breast-conserving surgery and RT provides survivals equivalent to those of mastectomy for patients with early-stage breast cancer (154). In addition, adjuvant CT improves disease-free and overall survival rates for several groups of patients with stage I-III breast cancer (4). Consequently, many patients now receive combined RT and CT following conservative surgery. Harris and Recht recently reviewed the data on RT-CT sequencing in early-stage breast cancer (20). Conflicting data have made it difficult to determine if delaying RT or CT until after completion of the other modality affects survival or recurrence rates. One small randomized trial of postmastectomy patients compared (a) RT followed by CT, (b) CT (six cycles of CMF) followed by RT, or (c) a sandwich approach with three cycles of CT followed by RT, and then three additional cycles of CT (155). The best results were observed in patients treated with the sandwich approach. A retrospective study of node-positive patients treated with adjuvant CT and RT showed a 5-year local recurrence rate of 28% if RT was delayed more than 16 weeks after surgery, compared with only 5% if RT was given less than 16 weeks after surgery (20).

While simultaneous sequencing would avoid

the problem of delaying one modality, it may increase the early and late complications and decrease the cosmetic outcome. Some investigators have found an increased risk of acute skin reactions and radiation pneumonitis and a decrease in long-term cosmetic results when methotrexate was given concurrently with RT (20). Simultaneous RT and doxorubicin-containing CT may increase cardiac complications (156). One approach may be to omit the methotrexate and doxorubicin during RT. The question of RT-CT sequencing for the adjuvant treatment of breast cancer is the subject of ongoing randomized trials.

CONCLUSIONS

While combined modality therapy has improved survival and local control in some clinical situations, its most profound impact has probably been on function and organ preservation, a significant contribution to improving the quality of life of cancer patients. Much work remains in understanding the mechanisms of CT-RT interactions, both beneficial and detrimental, as well as the optimal sequencing and dosing. Experimental systems will not substitute for careful clinical observations concerning both the effect on tumor and the toxicity to normal tissues.

REFERENCES

1. Brady LW, Markoe AM, Micaily B, Fisher SA, Lamm FR. Innovative techniques in radiation oncology. Clinical research programs to improve local and regional control in cancer. Cancer 1990;65:610–624.

2. Suit HD, Westgate SJ. Impact of improved local control on survival. Int J Radiat Oncol Biol Phys 1986;12:453–458.

3. Suit HD. The scope of the problem of primary tumor control. Cancer 1988;61:2141–2147.

4. Bonadonna G, Valagussa P, Moliterni A, Zambetti M, Branbilla C. Adjuvant cyclophosphamide, methotrexate, and fluorouracil in node-positive breast cancer: the results of 20 years of follow-up. N Engl J Med 1995;332:901–906.

5. Moertel CG, Fleming TR, Macdonald JS, et al. Levamisole and fluorouracil for adjuvant therapy of resected colon carcinoma. N Engl J Med 1990;322:352–358.

6. Krook JE, Moertel CG, Gunderson LL, et al. Effective surgical adjuvant therapy for high-risk rectal carcinoma. N Engl J Med 1991;324:709–715.

7. Fisher B, Wolmark N, Rockette H, et al. Postoperative adjuvant chemotherapy or radiation therapy for rectal cancer: results from NSABP protocol R-01. J Natl Cancer Inst 1988;80:21–29.

8. Papillon J, Montbarbon JF. Epidermoid carci-noma of the anal canal: a series of 276 cases. Dis Colon Rectum 1987;30:324–333.

9. Cummings BJ, Keane TJ, O'Sullivan B, Wong CS, Catton CN. Epidermoid anal cancer: treatment by radiation alone or by radiation and 5-fluorouracil with and without mitomycin-C. Int J Radiat Oncol Biol Phys 1991;21:1115–1125.

10. The Department of Veterans Affairs Laryngeal Cancer Study Group. Induction chemotherapy plus radiation compared with surgery plus radiation in patients with advanced laryngeal cancer. N Engl J Med 1991;324:1685–1690.

11. Eilber FR, Eckhardt J, Morton DL. Advances in the treatment of sarcomas of the extremity. Current status of limb salvage. Cancer 1984;54:2695–2701.

12. Loehrer PJ Sr. Chemoradiotherapy in locally advanced bladder carcinoma. Semin Oncol 1992;19:92–95.

13. Tester W, Porter A, Asbell S, et al. Combined modality program with possible organ preservation for invasive bladder carcinoma: results of RTOG protocol 85-12. Int J Radiat Oncol Biol Phys 1993;25:783–790.

14. Kaufman DS, Shipley WU, Griffin PP, Heney NM, Althausen AF, Efird JT. Selective bladder preservation by combination treatment of invasive bladder cancer. N Engl J Med 1993;329:1377–1382.

15. Housset M, Maulard C, Chretien Y, et al. Combined radiation and chemotherapy for invasive transitional-cell carcinoma of the bladder: a prospective study. J Clin Oncol 1993;11:2150–2157.

16. Herskovic A, Martz K, al-Sarraf M, et al. Combined chemotherapy and radiotherapy compared with radiotherapy alone in patients with cancer of the esophagus. N Engl J Med 1992;326:1593–1598.

17. Coia LR. Esophageal preservation—the management of esophageal cancer with concurrent radiation and chemotherapy. Endoscopy 1993;25:664–669.

18. Forastiere AA, Orringer MB, Perez-Tamayo C, Urba SG, Zahurak M. Preoperative chemoradiation followed by transhiatal esophagectomy for cancer of the esophagus: final report. J Clin Oncol 1993;11:1118–1123.

19. Ilson DH, Kelsen DP. Combined modality therapy in the treatment of esophageal cancer. Semin Oncol 1994;21:493–507.

20. Harris JR, Recht A. How to combine adjuvant chemotherapy and radiation therapy. Recent Results Cancer Res 1993;127:129–136.

21. Chu FCH. Organ and functional preservation in the management of breast cancer. Cancer Invest 1995;13:75–85.

22. Vokes E. Interactions of chemotherapy and radiation. Semin Oncol 1993;20:70–79.

23. Tannock IF. Potential for therapeutic gain from combined-modality treatment. Front Radiat Ther Oncol 1992;26:1–15.

24. Fu KK. Interactions of chemotherapeutic agents and radiation. Front Radiat Ther Oncol 1992;26:16–30.

25. Schilsky RL. Biochemical pharmacology of chemotherapeutic drugs used as radiation enhancers. Semin Oncol 1992;19(4, Suppl 11):2–7.

26. Goldie JH, Coldman AJ. A mathematic model for relating the drug sensitivity of tumors to their spontaneous mutation rate. Cancer Treat Rep 1979;63:1727–1733.

27. Goldie JH, Coldman AJ, Gudauskas GA. Ra-

tionale for the use of alternating non-cross-resistant chemotherapy. Cancer Treat Rep 1982;66:439–449.

28. Tannock IF, Rotin D. Mechanisms of interaction between radiation and drugs with potential for improvements in therapy. NCI Monogr 1988;6:77–83.

29. Sklar MD. The *ras* oncogenes increase the intrinsic resistance of NIH 3T3 cells to ionizing radiation. Science 1988;239:645–647.

30. Sklar MD. Increased resistance to *cis*-diamminedichloroplatinum (II) in NIH 3T3 cells transformed by *ras* oncogenes. [Published erratum appears in Cancer Res 1988;48:3889] Cancer Res 1988;48:793–797.

31. Ensley JF, Jacobs JR, Weaver A, et al. Correlation between response to cisplatinum-combination chemotherapy and subsequent radiotherapy in previously untreated patients with advanced squamous cell cancers of the head and neck. Cancer 1984;54:811–814.

32. Steel GG. The search for therapeutic gain in the combination of radiotherapy and chemotherapy. Radiother Oncol 1988;11:31–53.

33. Steel GG, Peckham MJ. Exploitable mechanisms in combined radiotherapy-chemotherapy: the concept of additivity. Int J Radiat Oncol Biol Phys 1979; 5:85–91.

34. Steel GG, Hill RP, Peckham MJ. Combined radiotherapy-chemotherapy of Lewis lung carcinoma. Int J Radiat Oncol Biol Phys 1978;4:49–52.

35. Fu KK. Biological basis for the interaction of chemotherapeutic agents and radiation therapy. Cancer 1985;55:2123–2130.

36. Dewit L. Combined treatment of radiation and *cis*-diamminedichloroplatinum (II): a review of experimental and clinical data. Int J Radiat Oncol Biol Phys 1987;13:403–426.

37. Grau C, Overgaard J. Effect of cancer chemotherapy on the hypoxic fraction of a solid tumor measured using a local tumor control assay. Radiother Oncol 1988;13:301–309.

38. Double EB. Platinum-radiation interactions. NCI Monogr 1988;6:315–319.

39. Tubiana M. The 1987 Franz Buschke lecture: the role of radiotherapy in the treatment of chemosensitive tumors. Int J Radiat Oncol Biol Phys 1989;16:763–774.

40. Hancock SL, Donaldson SS, Hoppe RT. Cardiac disease following treatment of Hodgkin's disease in children and adolescents. J Clin Oncol 1993;11:1208–1215.

41. Hancock SL, Tucker MA, Hoppe RT. Factors affecting late mortality from heart disease after treatment of Hodgkin's disease. JAMA 1993;270:1949–1955.

42. Withers HR, Taylor JMG, Maciejewski B. The hazard of accelerated tumor clonogen repopulation during radiotherapy. Acta Oncol 1988;27:131–146.

43. Trott KR. The cellular interpretation of tumour radioresistance. Cancer Treat Rev 1984;11(Suppl A):81–83.

44. Dembo AJ. Radiotherapeutic management of ovarian cancer. Semin Oncol 1984;11:238–250.

45. Hoskins WJ, Lichter AS, Whittington R, Artman LE, Bibro MC, Park RC. Whole abdominal and pelvic irradiation in patients with minimal disease at second-look surgical reassessment for ovarian carcinoma. Gynecol Oncol 1985;20:271–280.

46. Hill BT. Interactions between antitumour agents and radiation and the expression of resistance. Cancer Treat Rev 1991;18:149–190.

47. Hill BT, Deuchars K, Hosking LK, Ling V, Whe-

lan RD. Overexpression of P-glycoprotein in mammalian tumor cell lines after fractionated x irradiation in vitro. J Natl Cancer Inst 1990;82:607–612.

48. Rice GC, Hoy C, Schimke RT. Transient hypoxia enhances the frequency of dihydrofolate reductase gene amplification in Chinese hamster ovary cells. Proc Natl Acad Sci USA 1986;83:5978–5982.

49. Ozols RF, Masuda H, Hamilton TC. Mechanisms of cross-resistance between radiation and antineoplastic drugs. NCI Monogr 1988;6:159–165.

50. Millar JL, Hudspith BN. Sparing effect of cyclophosphamide (NSC-26271) pretreatment on animals lethally treated with gamma-irradiation. Cancer Treat Rep 1976;60:409–414.

51. Phelps TA, Blackett NM. Protection of intestinal damage by pretreatment with cytarabine (cytosine arabinoside). Int J Radiat Oncol Biol Phys 1979;5:1617–1620.

52. Johnke RM, Kovacs CJ, Lovèn DP, Abernathy RS, Hooker JL. Altered radiosensitivity of hematopoietic stem cells by vincristine pretreatment: superoxide dismutase activity as a possible mechanism. NCI Monogr 1988;6:193–197.

53. Steel GG. Terminology in the description of drug-radiation interactions. Int J Radiat Oncol Biol Phys 1979;5:1145–1150.

54. Lelieveld P, Smink T, van Putten L. Experimental studies on the combination of radiation and chemotherapy. Int J Radiat Oncol Biol Phys 1978;4:37–41.

55. Lelieveld P, Brown JM, Goffinet DR, Schoeppel SL, Scoles M. The effect of BCNU on mouse skin and spinal cord in single drug and radiation exposures. Int J Radiat Oncol Biol Phys 1979;5:1565–1568.

56. Denekamp J. Experimental tumor systems: standardization of endpoints. Int J Radiat Oncol Biol Phys 1979;5:1175–1184.

57. Dewey WC. In vitro systems: standardization of endpoints. Int J Radiat Oncol Biol Phys 1979;5:1165–1174.

58. Heidelberger C, Griesbach L, Montag BJ, et al. Studies on fluorinated pyrimidines. II. Effects on transplanted tumors. Cancer Res 1958;18:305–317.

59. Vietti T, Eggerding F, Valeriote F. Combined effect of x radiation and 5-fluorouracil on survival of transplanted leukemic cells. J Natl Cancer Inst 1971; 47:865–870.

60. Byfield JE, Calabro-Jones P, Klisak T, Kulhanian F. Pharmacologic requirements for obtaining sensitization of human tumor cells in vitro to combined 5-fluorouracil or ftorafur and x-rays. Int J Radiat Oncol Biol Phys 1982;1923–1933.

61. Tannock IF. Toxicity of 5-fluorouracil for aerobic and hypoxic cells in two murine tumours. Cancer Chemother Pharmacol 1987;19:53–56.

62. Zak M, Drobnik J. Effects of *cis*-dichlorodiammine platinum (II) on the post-irradiation lethality in mice after irradiation with x-rays. Strahlentherapie 1971;142:112–115.

63. Double EB, Richmond RC. A review of platinum complex biochemistry suggests a rationale for combined platinum-radiotherapy. Int J Radiat Oncol Biol Phys 1979;5:1335–1339.

64. Richmond RC. Toxic variability and radiation sensitization by dichlorodiammine-platinum (II) complexes in *Salmonella typhimurium* cells. Radiat Res 1984; 99:596–608.

65. Kanazawa H, Rapacchietta D, Kallman RF.

Schedule-dependent therapeutic gain from the combination of fractionated irradiation and cis-diamminedichloroplatinum (II) in C3H/Km mouse model systems. Cancer Res 1988;48:3158–3164.

66. Carde P, Laval F. Effect of cis-dichlorodiammine platinum II and x rays on mammalian cell survival. Int J Radiat Oncol Biol Phys 1981;7:929–933.

67. Dritschilo A, Piro AJ, Kelman AD. The effect of cis-platinum on the repair of radiation damage in plateau phase Chinese hamster (V-79) cells. Int J Radiat Oncol Biol Phys 1979;5:1345–1349.

68. O'Hara JA, Double EB, Richmond RC. Enhancement of radiation-induced cell kill by platinum complexes (carboplatin and iproplatin) in V79 cells. Int J Radiat Oncol Biol Phys 1986;12:1419–1422.

69. Lelieveld P, Scoles MA, Brown JM, Kallman RF. The effect of treatment in fractionated schedules with the combination of x-irradiation and six cytotoxic drugs on the RIF-1 tumor and normal mouse skin. Int J Radiat Oncol Biol Phys 1985;11:111–121.

70. Stewart F, Bohlken S, Begg A, Bartelink H. Renal damage in mice after treatment with cisplatinum alone or in combination with x-irradiation. Int J Radiat Oncol Biol Phys 1986;12:927–933.

71. Stewart FA, Luts A, Oussoren Y, Begg AC, Dewit L, Bartelink H. Renal damage in mice after treatment with cisplatin and x-rays: comparison of fractionated and single-dose studies. NCI Monogr 1988;6:23–27.

72. Rockwell S. Use of hypoxia-directed drugs in the therapy of solid tumors. Semin Oncol 1992;19(4 Suppl 11):29–40.

73. Siemann DW, Keng PC. Responses of tumor cell subpopulations to single modality and combined modality therapies. NCI Monogr 1988;6:101–105.

74. Grau C, Overgaard J. Radiosensitizing and cytotoxic properties of mitomycin C in a C3H mouse mammary carcinoma in vivo. Int J Radiat Oncol Biol Phys 1991;20:265–269.

75. Fu KK, Lam, KN. Early and late effects of mitomycin C and continuous low-dose-rate irradiation on the mouse skin and soft tissues of the leg. Int J Radiat Oncol Biol Phys 1991;21:1523–1528.

76. Weissberg JB, Son YH, Papac RJ, et al. Randomized clinical trial of mitomycin C as an adjunct to radiotherapy in head and neck cancer. Int J Radiat Oncol Biol Phys 1989;17:3–9.

77. Sinclair WK. The combined effect of hydroxyurea and x-rays on Chinese hamster cells in vitro. Cancer Res 1968;28:198–206.

78. Fram RJ, Kufe DW. Inhibition of DNA excision repair and the repair of x-ray-induced DNA damage by cytosine arabinoside and hydroxyurea. Pharmacol Ther 1985;31:165–176.

79. Liebmann J, Cook JA, Fisher J, Teague D, Mitchell JB. In vitro studies of Taxol as a radiation sensitizer in human tumor cells. J Natl Cancer Inst 1994;86:441–446.

80. Geard CR, Jones JM, Schiff PB. Taxol and radiation. Monogr Natl Cancer Inst 1993;15:89–94.

81. Steren A, Sevin BU, Perras J, et al. Taxol sensitizes human ovarian cancer cells to radiation. Gynecol Oncol 1993;48:252–258.

82. Tishler RB, Geard CR, Hall EJ, Schiff PB. Taxol sensitizes human astrocytoma cells to radiation. Cancer Res 1992;52:3495–3497.

83. Mattern MR, Hofmann GA, McCabe FL, John-son RK. Synergistic cell killing by ionizing radiation and topoisomerase I inhibitor topotecan (SK&F 104864). Cancer Res 1991;51:5813–5816.

84. Kim JH, Kim SH, Kolozsvary A, Khil MS. Potentiation of radiation response in human carcinoma cells in vitro and murine fibrosarcoma in vivo by topotecan, an inhibitor of DNA topoisomerase I. Int J Radiat Oncol Biol Phys 1992;22:515–518.

85. Ng CE, Bussey AM, Raaphorst GP. Inhibition of potentially lethal and sublethal damage repair by camptothecin and etoposide in human melanoma cell lines. Int J Radiat Biol 1994;66:49–57.

86. Boothman DA, Wang M, Schea RA, Burrows HL, Strickfaden S, Owens JK. Posttreatment exposure to camptothecin enhances the lethal effects of x-rays on radioresistant human malignant melanoma cells. Int J Radiat Oncol Biol Phys 1992;24:939–948.

87. Hennequin C, Giocanti N, Balosso J, Favaudon V. Interaction of ionizing radiation with the topoisomerase I poison camptothecin in growing V-79 and HeLa cells. Cancer Res 1994;54:1720–1728.

88. Del Bino G, Bruno S, Yi PN, Darzynkiewicz Z. Apoptotic cell death triggered by camptothecin or teniposide: the cell cycle specificity and effects of ionizing radiation. Cell Proliferation 1992;25:537–548.

89. Tubiana M, Arriagada R, Cosset JM. Sequencing of drugs and radiation: the integrated alternating regimen. Cancer 1985;55(9 Suppl):2131–2139.

90. Van Peperzeel HA. Effects of single doses of radiation on lung metastases in man and experimental animals. Eur J Cancer 1972;8:665–675.

91. Malaise EP, Charbit A, Chavaudra N, Combes PF, Douchez J, Tubiana M. Change in volume of irradiated human metastases: investigation of repair of sublethal damage and tumour repopulation. Br J Cancer 1972;26:43–52.

92. Taylor SG, Murthy AK, Vannetzel JM, et al. Randomized comparison of neoadjuvant cisplatin and fluorouracil infusion followed by radiation versus concomitant treatment in advanced head and neck cancer. J Clin Oncol 1994;12:385–395.

93. Looney WB. Alternating chemotherapy and radiotherapy. NCI Monogr 1988;6:85–94.

94. Looney WB, Hopkins HA. Alternation of chemotherapy and radiotherapy in cancer management. III. Results in experimental solid tumor systems and their relationship to clinical studies. Cancer Treat Rep 1986;70:141–162.

95. Hopkins HA, Looney WB. Solid tumor models for the assessment of different treatment modalities: XXVI. Estimates of cell survival from tumor growth delay after alternating radiotherapy and chemotherapy. [Published erratum appears in Int J Radiat Biol Phys 1987;13(7):1123] Int J Radiat Oncol Biol Phys 1987;13(2):217–224.

96. Merlano M, Vitale V, Rosso R, et al. Treatment of advanced squamous cell carcinoma of the head and neck with alternating chemotherapy and radiotherapy. N Engl J Med 1992;327:1115–1121.

97. Howes AE. Models of normal tissue injury following combined modality therapy. NCI Monogr 1988; 6:5–8.

98. von der Maase H. Experimental studies on interactions of radiation and cancer chemotherapeutic drugs in normal tissues and a solid tumour. Radiother Oncol 1986;7:47–68.

99. Rubin P. The Franz Buschke lecture: late effects

of chemotherapy and radiation therapy: a new hypothesis. Int J Radiat Oncol Biol Phys 1984;10:5–34.

100. Field SB, Michalowski A. Endpoints for damage to normal tissues. Int J Radiat Oncol Biol Phys 1979; 5:1185–1196.

101. von der Maase H, Overgaard J, Vaeth M. Effect of cancer chemotherapeutic drugs on radiation-induced lung damage in mice. Radiother Oncol 1986; 5:245–257.

102. Rubin P, Constine LS, Van Ess JD. Scoring of late toxic effects—interaction of two modalities. NCI Monogr 1988;6:9–18.

103. Myers CE. Role of iron in anthracycline action. In: Hacker MP, Lazo JS, Tritton TR, eds. Organ directed toxicities of anticancer drugs. The Hague: Martinus Nijhoff, 1988:17–30.

104. Doroshow JH, Locker GY, Myers CE. Enzymatic defenses of the mouse heart against reactive oxygen metabolites: alterations produced by doxorubicin. J Clin Invest 1980;65:128–135.

105. Speyer JL, Green MD, Kramer E, et al. Protective effect of the bispiperazinedione ICRF-187 against doxorubicin-induced cardiac toxicity in women with advanced breast cancer. N Engl J Med 1988;319:745–752.

106. Eltringham JR, Fajardo LF, Stewart JR, Klauber MR. Investigation of cardiotoxicity in rabbits from Adriamycin and fractionated cardiac irradiation: preliminary results. Front Radiat Ther Oncol 1979; 13:21–35.

107. Billingham ME. Endomyocardial changes in anthracycline-treated patients with and without irradiation. Front Radiat Ther Oncol 1979;13:67–81.

108. Fajardo LF, Stewart JR. Experimental radiation-induced heart disease. I. Light microscopic studies. Am J Pathol 1970;59:299–316.

109. Fajardo LF, Stewart JR. Pathogenesis of radiation-induced myocardial fibrosis. Lab Invest 1973; 29:244–257.

110. Gilladoga AC, Manuel C, Tan CTC, Wollner N, Sternberg SS, Murphy ML. The cardiotoxicity of Adriamycin and daunomycin in children. Cancer 1976; 37(2 Suppl):1070–1078.

111. Bristow MR, Mason JW, Billingham ME, Daniels JR. Doxorubicin cardiomyopathy: evaluation by phonocardiography, endomyocardial biopsy, and cardiac catheterization. Ann Intern Med 1978;88: 168–175.

112. Von Hoff DD, Layard MW, Basa P, et al. Risk factors for doxorubicin-induced congestive heart failure. Ann Intern Med 1979;91:710–717.

113. Eisenberger M, Jacobs M. Simultaneous treatment with single-agent chemotherapy and radiation for locally advanced cancer of the head and neck. Semin Oncol 1992;19(4 Suppl 11):41–46.

114. Stupp R, Weichselbaum RR, Vokes EE. Combined modality therapy of head and neck cancer. Semin Oncol 1994;21:349–358.

115. Bachaud JM, David JM, Boussin G, Daly N. Combined postoperative radiotherapy and weekly cisplatin infusion for locally advanced squamous cell carcinoma of the head and neck: preliminary report of a randomized trial. Int Radiat Oncol Biol Phys 1991; 20:243–246.

116. Lo TC, Wiley AL Jr, Ansfield FJ, et al. Combined radiation therapy and 5-fluorouracil for advanced squamous cell carcinoma of the oral cavity and

oropharynx: a randomized study. Am J Roentgenol 1976;126:229–235.

117. Rooney M, Kish J, Jacobs J, et al. Improved complete response rate and survival in head and neck cancer after three-course induction therapy with 120-hour 5-FU infusion and cisplatin. Cancer 1985;55:1123–1128.

118. Dimery IW, Hong WK. Overview of combined modality therapies for head and neck cancer. J Natl Cancer Inst 1993;85:95–111.

119. Forastiere AA. Randomized trials of induction chemotherapy. A critical review. Hematol Oncol Clin North Am 1991;5:725–736.

120. Paccagnella A, Orlando A, Marchiori C, et al. Phase III trial of initial chemotherapy in stage III or IV head and neck cancers: a study by the Gruppo di Studio sui Tumori della Testa e del Collo. J Natl Cancer Inst 1994;86:265–272.

121. Merlano M, Corvo R, Margarino G, et al. Combination chemotherapy and radiation therapy in advanced inoperable squamous cell carcinoma of the head and neck. The final report of a randomized trial. Cancer 1991;67:915–921.

122. Balslev I, Pedersen M, Teglbjaerg PS, et al. Postoperative radiotherapy in Dukes' B and C carcinoma of the rectum and rectosigmoid. A randomized multicenter study. Cancer 1986;58:22–28.

123. NIH Consensus Conference. Adjuvant therapy for patients with colon and rectal cancer. JAMA 1990;264:1444–1450.

124. O'Connell MJ, Martenson JA, Wieand HS, et al. Improving adjuvant therapy for rectal cancer by combining protracted-infusion fluorouracil with radiation therapy after curative surgery. N Engl J Med 1994;331:502–507.

125. Bosset JF, Pelissier EP, Maniion G, et al. Plea for a preoperative adjuvant approach in the management of rectal cancer. Int J Radiat Oncol Biol Phys 1994; 29:205–208.

126. Petrelli N, Douglass HO Jr, Herrera L, et al. The modulation of fluorouracil with leucovorin in metastatic colorectal carcinoma: a prospective randomized phase III trial. Gastrointestinal Tumor Study Group. [Published erratum appears in J Clin Oncol 1990; 8(1):185] J Clin Oncol 1989;7:1419–1426.

127. Lawrence TS, Heimburger DK, Shewach DS. The effects of leucovorin and dipyridamole on fluoropyrimidine-induced radiosensitization. Int J Radiat Oncol Biol Phys 1991;20:377–381.

128. Kovacs CJ, Dainer PM, Evans MJ, Nyce J. Biochemical modulation of combined radiation and 5-fluorouracil treatment of murine tumors by d,1-leucovorin. Anticancer Res 1991;11:905–909.

129. Pahlman L, Glimelius B. Pre- or postoperative radiotherapy in rectal and rectosigmoid carcinoma. Report from a randomized multicenter trial. Ann Surg 1990;211:187–195.

130. Molls M, Fink U. Perioperative radiotherapy ± chemotherapy in rectal cancer. Ann Oncol 1994; 5(Suppl 3):105–113.

131. Feld R, Evans WK, DeBoer G, et al. Combined modality induction therapy without maintenance chemotherapy for small cell carcinoma of the lung. J Clin Oncol 1984;2:294–304.

132. Hong WK, Nicaise C, Lawson R, et al. Etoposide combined with cyclophosphamide plus vincristine compared with doxorubicin plus cyclophos-

phamide plus vincristine and with high-dose cyclophosphamide plus vincristine in the treatment of small-cell carcinoma of the lung: a randomized trial of the Bristol Lung Cancer Study Group. J Clin Oncol 1989;7:450–456.

133. Lichter AS, Bunn PA Jr, Ihde DC, et al. The role of radiation therapy in the treatment of small cell lung cancer. Cancer 1985;55(9 Suppl):2163–2175.

134. Osterlind K, Hansen HH, Hansen M, Dombernowsky P. Mortality and morbidity in long-term surviving patients treated with chemotherapy with or without irradiation for small-cell lung cancer. J Clin Oncol 1986;4:1044–1052.

135. Warde P, Payne D. Does thoracic irradiation improve survival and local control in limited-stage small-cell carcinoma of the lung? A meta-analysis. J Clin Oncol 1992;10:890–895.

136. Pignon J-P, Arriagada R, Ihde D, et al. A meta-analysis of thoracic radiotherapy for small-cell lung cancer. N Engl J Med 1992;327:1618–1624.

137. Murray N, Coy P, Pater JL, et al. Importance of timing for thoracic irradiation in the combined modality treatment of limited-stage small-cell lung cancer. The National Cancer Institute of Canada Clinical Trials Group. J Clin Oncol 1993;11:336–344.

138. Perry MC, Eaton WL, Propert KJ, et al. Chemotherapy with or without radiation therapy in limited small-cell carcinoma of the lung. N Engl J Med 1987;316:912–918.

139. Murren JR, Buzaid AC. Chemotherapy and radiation for the treatment of non-small-cell lung cancer. A critical review. Clin Chest Med 1993;14:161–171.

140. Sause WT, Scott C, Taylor S, et al. Radiation Therapy Oncology Group (RTOG) 88-08 and Eastern Cooperative Oncology Group (ECOG) 4588: preliminary results of a phase III trial in regionally advanced, unresectable non-small-cell lung cancer. J Natl Cancer Inst 1995;87:198–205.

141. Dillman RO, Seagren SL, Propert KJ, et al. A randomized trial of induction chemotherapy plus high-dose radiation versus radiation alone in stage III non-small-cell lung cancer. N Engl J Med 1990;323:940–945.

142. Le Chevalier T, Arriagada R, Quoix E, et al. Radiotherapy alone versus combined chemotherapy and radiotherapy in nonresectable non-small-cell lung cancer: first analysis of a randomized trial in 353 patients. J Natl Cancer Inst 1991;83:417–423.

143. Schaake-Koning C, van den Bogaert W, Dalesio O, et al. Effects of concomitant cisplatin and radiotherapy on inoperable non-small-cell lung cancer. N Engl J Med 1992;326:524–530.

143a. Roelofsen F, Bosset JF, Eschwége F, et al. Concomitant radiotherapy and chemotherapy superior to radiotherapy alone in the treatment of locally advanced anal cancer. Results of a phase III randomized trial of the EORTC radiotherapy and gastrointestinal cooperative groups (abstract). Proc Am Soc Clin Oncol 1995;14:454.

144. Nigro ND. The force of change in the management of squamous-cell cancer of the anal canal. Dis Colon Rectum 1991;34:482–486.

145. Flam MS, John M, Pajak T, et al. Radiation (RT) and 5-fluorouracil (5FU) vs. radiation, 5-FU, mitomycin-C (MMC) in the treatment of anal carcinoma: results of a phase III randomized RTOG/ECOG intergroup trial (abstract). Proc Am Soc Clin Oncol 1995; 14:443.

146. Cummings BJ. Anal canal carcinomas. Front Radiat Ther Oncol 1992;26:131–141.

147. Tannock IF, Cummings BJ. Neoadjuvant chemotherapy in head and neck cancer: no way to preserve a larynx. J Clin Oncol 1992;10:343–345.

148. Forastiere AA. Cisplatin and radiotherapy in the management of locally advanced head and neck cancer. Int J Radiat Oncol Biol Phys 1993;27:465–470.

149. Link MP, Goorin AM, Miser AW, et al. The effect of adjuvant chemotherapy on relapse-free survival in patients with osteosarcoma of the extremity. N Engl J Med 1986;314:1600–1606.

150. Gherlinzoni F, Picci P, Bacci G, Campanacci D. Limb sparing versus amputation in osteosarcoma. Correlation between local control, surgical margins and tumor necrosis: Istituto Rizzoli experience. Ann Oncol 1992;3:S23–S27.

151. Spiro IJ, Rosenberg AE, Springfield D, Suit H. Combined surgery and radiation therapy for limb preservation in soft tissue sarcoma of the extremity: the Massachusetts General Hospital experience. Cancer Invest 1995;13:86–95.

152. Gasparini M, Lombardi F, Ballerini E, et al. Long-term outcome of patients with monostotic Ewing's sarcoma treated with combined modality. Med Pediatr Oncol 1994;23:406–412.

153. Kinsella TJ, Miser JS, Waller B, et al. Long-term follow-up of Ewing's sarcoma of bone treated with combined modality therapy. Int J Radiat Oncol Biol Phys 1991;20:389–395.

154. Jacobson JA, Danforth DN, Cowan KH, et al. Ten-year results of a comparison of conservation with mastectomy in the treatment of stage I and II breast cancer. N Engl J Med 1995;332:907–911.

155. Lara Jimenez P, Garcia Puche J, Pedraza V. Adjuvant combined modality treatment in high risk breast cancer patients: ten year results (abstract). Proc 5th EORTC Breast Cancer Working Conference 1991; A293.

156. Buzzoni R, Bonadonna G, Valagussa P, Zambetti M. Adjuvant chemotherapy with doxorubicin plus cyclophosphamide, methotrexate, and fluorouracil in the treatment of resectable breast cancer with one to three positive axillary nodes. J Clin Oncol 1991; 9:2134–2140.

9

The Design and Interpretation of Clinical Trials

Richard Simon and Michael A. Friedman

The clinical trial is our most powerful tool for determining the value of an intervention—therapeutic, preventive, or diagnostic. Medicine contains many examples of expensive procedures of questionable value that have never been properly evaluated in clinical trials.

The history of medicine is filled with examples of ineffective and morbid treatments that persisted in practice on the basis of clinical impression and faulty theoretic arguments. It is often difficult to do a clinical trial; theoretic arguments for the value of a treatment often seem convincing, doctors like to offer newer alternatives to unsatisfactory treatments, and there are numerous psychologic, material, and bureaucratic disincentives to participation in clinical trials. Yet, it is clear that the practice of good medicine absolutely depends on the willingness of physicians to participate in properly designed and conducted clinical trials.

In this chapter we try to describe some of the most important components of good clinical trials. A therapeutic clinical trial is an experiment designed to determine the effectiveness of a treatment or the relative effectiveness of two treatments in a specified group of patients. A good clinical trial asks an important question and gets a reliable answer. As mentioned above, it is often difficult to ask an important question; each specialist may think his or her modality is the most effective and be unwilling to participate in a clinical trial comparing modalities. So we may get clinical trials comparing variations of each modality without ever asking fundamental questions. The treatment of patients will depend primarily on to whom they are referred. It is important to get a reliable answer because many new treatments are actually ineffective or harm-

ful. Although there are powerful incentives to use new therapies and to publish "positive" results, neither patient welfare nor the national pocketbook can afford a proliferation of useless treatments based on unreliable trends in immature data.

The essence of an experiment is planning. There is no question that valuable scientific information can be derived from observation of nonexperimental phenomena, but interpretation of nonexperimental data is often ambiguous and error prone. A clinical trial provides the opportunity to clearly attribute an effect to a treatment. The price of this clarity is careful planning. The scientific hypothesis must be specific: the patient population defined, the primary endpoint defined, the method of treatment administration defined, and the sample size and times of analysis defined. Some clinical trials are merely broad outlines for the management of a wide range of patients. Such protocols usually do not provide clear answers because, at the time of analysis, too many qualitative judgments have to be made about how to analyze the data. Treatment administration may be highly variable, and judgments are made about who to exclude and who to group with whom. The patient population may be quite varied, and so numerous subsets are analyzed. If no primary endpoint was initially identified, there are analyses with different endpoints, some of which have inadequate follow-up. These factors, combined with the lack of an adequate sample size and the practice of repeated analyses of accumulating data, result in the probability of finding at least one statistically significant false-positive conclusion of the order of 20 to 40% rather than the assumed 5%.

Planning good clinical trials is practically achievable, but it involves much more than just writing down how to treat a patient. The issues are the primary topic of this chapter. We hope that this information will be useful for evaluating the results of others' clinical trials as well as for planning our own. We have included nine guidelines for the reporting of clinical trial results. Generally, the evaluation of a treatment should be based on all good clinical trials that have addressed the question. It is a mistake to focus only on the positive and to assume that it was positive for some trivial reason, such as a slight variation in the way the treatment was administered. A section on metaanalysis and publication bias is included to emphasize these points.

INFORMED CONSENT

Fundamental to the conduct of clinical investigation is the practice of fully informed consent. A complete and comprehensible document not only is required by regulations of the U.S. Department of Health and Human Services but also is consistent with modern ethical clinical practice. By consenting to receive a certain therapy or to participate in a defined clinical trial, each individual (or designated representative) must be provided with adequate information concerning the nature of the treatment as well as alternative therapies that might be considered. This information should be presented in an understandable form, and there must be no coercion associated with participating in the treatment plan. Participation should be completely voluntary and relatively enlightened.

The eight elements crucial to the informed consent document and procedure include the following:

1. A full description of the therapy to be provided, with indications of which portions of the therapy are experimental (and are designed to address the research questions) and which procedures are standard. Information concerning the duration of participation, the schedule of therapy, and so forth are included.
2. The predictable risks and toxicities of the treatment.
3. The potential benefits not only for the individual patient but for others as well.
4. The alternative treatments that are reasonable options for the patient to consider. This does not include all conceivable treatment alternatives (including ineffective or highly speculative ones), but only treatment alternatives that are deemed reasonable for that patient to consider. Reasonable alternatives are those that according to the physician's best analysis, show solid evidence of benefit.
5. A pledge of confidentiality concerning the records of the patient's care, along with an indication of who will have access to this information; usually, the National Cancer Institute or other sponsors (such as private agencies or pharmaceutical industries) and the Food and Drug Administration.
6. Whether any compensation or treatment is available for those who suffer injury or toxicity of the treatment.
7. Specific health care professionals who can be contacted for more information about the treatment.
8. Indication that the therapy is to be accepted on a completely voluntary basis and that the patient may withdraw from therapy at any time without prejudicing his or her care in the future.

Not only must great care be taken in the construction and implementation of the informed consent document at the initiation of the study, but equal care must be given during the course of the research program to ensure that updated information is incorporated into the document. Should new clinical trial information become available that would materially affect the options available to a patient, such data should be incorporated into the document. In some sense, the formalized informed consent procedure for clinical investigation merely mimics the processes of education and assent that occur with any therapeutic compact between a physician and a patient.

PHASE I CLINICAL TRIALS

The purpose of a phase I clinical trial is to define, as carefully as possible, the toxicities associated with the presumed optimal therapeutic dose of a new agent. Because of the therapeutically speculative nature of such studies and the fact that clinical benefit cannot be predicted, generally it is those with disseminated and/or incurable disease who are recruited to phase I clinical trials. Reasonable performance status and physiologic organ function are often entry requirements, although exceptions are made for pharmacologic studies. Adequate qualitative toxicity information is the principal endpoint of a phase I trial. Increasingly, however, evidence of biologic effect associated with a particular dose is becoming an important study objective. The phase I testing of biologic agents, the so-called phase IB study, is an attempt to correlate particular doses of the agent with biologic parameters thought to be relevant (such as stimulation of a population of lymphocytes, generation of a cytotoxic antibody, and so forth). Performing a phase I study by merely looking at dose and cataloging types of toxicities is becoming less meaningful. More frequent is the evaluation of biochemical events associated with the administration of a new agent (such as intracellular concentrations of the drug, its metabolite(s), or its effect(s) on intracellular target enzymes or proteins) and the use of blood level monitoring. In such pharmacologic assessments, the serum concentration and the compartmentalization of the drug and its metabolites are assessed, and a threshold level associated with either activity or toxicity is documented. The pharmacokinetic- and pharmacodynamic-directed phase I studies provide considerable information and may indicate why a drug is ineffective or why it is toxic for populations of cancer patients.

Phase I studies are usually begun at a rather low initial dose based upon animal toxicology modeling, and the escalation of doses is based upon a predetermined sequence. Individual patients are usually not treated at different dose levels in a phase I study, since their data may not be fully assessable at both dose levels. However, it may be entirely appropriate for a patient who has had no meaningful associated toxicity at one dose level to subsequently receive a higher dose of that medication (if the intervening patients have been fully evaluated). This is not done to generate data for defining a maximum tolerated dose, but rather in a compassionate attempt to provide therapy to a patient with an otherwise desperate situation.

PHASE II CLINICAL TRIALS

There are two main types of phase II clinical trials. The first is the phase II trial of a new agent to determine whether it has any antitumor activity against a particular type of cancer. Such trials also provide rough estimates of the degree of activity. The main problems with many such trials are (*a*) the patients have received so much previous treatment that they cannot tolerate substantial doses of the new drug and (*b*) their tumors may have broad resistance mechanisms.

Placing such patients on a phase II trial generally does not provide them with much chance of benefit and does not represent a meaningful phase II evaluation of the activity of the drug. There has been a move to treat patients with much less prior therapy on phase II studies. The amount of prior therapy depends, of course, on the particular type of cancer (1).

The primary endpoint for most phase II studies of new agents is objective tumor shrinkage. For this reason, phase II studies are generally limited to patients with measurable disease. Even then, tumor measurements are variable, and it is important to have second-party review of response assessments. Variability in response assessment, definition of response, patient selection, treatment delivery, and small sample size result in a wide variation of reported response rates. Hence, the magnitude of a particular reported response rate should be interpreted cautiously. The most commonly used accrual plan for phase II studies was designed by Gehan (2) and aims to enroll 14 patients and terminates the trial if no responses are obtained. This is because the probability of getting no responses in 14 patients is less than 5% if the true-response probability is at least 20%. However, if even one response is obtained in the initial 14 patients, then a second stage of accrual should be performed to better estimate the response probability. Investigators usually accrue a total of 25 to 40 evaluable patients. The probability of getting at least one response in 14 patients is 51%, even when the true-response probability is as low as 5%. Hence, the second stage of accrual is essential.

An alternative approach to planning the accrual to a phase II trial has been the multistage approach described by Fleming (3). Fleming tests a null hypothesis that the true-response probability is less than some uninteresting level (p_0) against the alternative that the true-response probability is at least as great as a target level (p_1). A drug with response probability less than p_0 will be called inactive, and one with response probability greater than p_1 will be called highly active. If one specifies the number of stages desired, the target levels p_0 and p_1, and the error limits for accepting an inactive drug and rejecting a highly active drug, then designs of this type can be determined. Consider a design with $p_0 = .05$ and $p_1 = .20$, for which both error limits are to be <.10. These constraints can be met with a two-stage Fleming design having 15 patients in the first stage and 20 in the second stage. If no responses are observed among the first 15 patients, then the clinical trial is terminated, and the drug is rejected. If at least 3 responses are observed among the first 15 patients, then the trial is terminated with the conclusion that the drug is active. If 1 or 2 responses are observed in the first 15 patients, 20 more patients are accrued. After all 35 patients are evaluated, the drug is usually considered interesting if the response rate is at least 4/35 (11.4%) and rejected otherwise. Table 9.1 shows some other Fleming designs.

Fleming's design is attractive because it forces one to specify activity levels of interest and to attempt to define how decisions will be influenced by results. One must bear in mind, however, that acceptance of the drug for later study does not imply that it is highly active. For example, the drug is accepted in the above example if the observed response rate is 11.4%. Acceptance of the drug merely indicates that it is active, i.e., produces responses above a background rate of p_0. Rejection of the drug means that there is strong evidence that the drug is not highly active. The design provides a sample size large enough to ensure that if the drug is either inactive or highly active, then the appropriate decision will be reached. It is useful to employ confidence intervals for interpreting results after use of Fleming's design, (4). Such intervals make clear what is consistent with the results and avoid the potential misinterpretations that may result from accept-reject terminology. Simon's optimal two-stage designs (5) have also become popular because they minimize the expected number of patients exposed to inactive drugs but permit trials of active agents to continue accrual.

The second type of phase II trial is that of a combination of drugs that are known to be active against the tumor in question. Tannock and Warr have questioned whether such studies should even be called phase II trials because they differ in so many ways from the trials described above, which are merely clinical screens for activity (6). The objective of phase II trials of combinations is usually to determine whether the level of activity is substantially greater than that of the single agents or of other combinations. There is a role for such trials in selecting which phase III trials to conduct. The appropriate phase III trial to determine whether the combination is more "effective" than the single agents or another standard combination would generally use a direct measure of patient benefit as an endpoint, such as survival or quality of life. Unfortunately, high partial response rates in patient populations selected to tolerate intensive treatment are often reported without any explicit comparison group as the basis for concluding that the new treatment is highly "effective." Authors of such reports sometimes indicate that confirmation in a randomized clinical trial would be appropriate, but the sensational tone of their report makes it clear that they themselves would not participate in such a clinical trial. In this way, toxic and expensive treatments sometimes creep into standard practice without proper supporting evidence.

Phase II trials of combinations are inherently comparative and must be planned as such. Although they generally do not involve a randomized control group, a specific historic control group of patients should be used for interpreting the results. The comparability of the nonrandomized control group should be checked in detail and reported. The finite size of the historic control group should be taken into account in planning the study. Methods for planning studies in this way have been described (7, 8). For example, Table 9.2 shows the number of patients required in the experimental treatment group as a function of the size of a comparable historic control group and the response rate obtained for the historic controls. Phase II trials of combinations should generally be regarded as phase III

Table 9.1. Two-Stage Fleming Designs for Phase II Clinical Trials[a]

		First-Stage Sample Size	Maximum Sample Size	Reject Drug If Response Rate		Accept Drug If Response Rate		Probability of Early Termination[b]
p_0	p_1	N_1	N	$\leq r_1/N_1$	$\leq r/N$	$\geq a_1/N_1$	$\geq a/N$	
.05	.25	15	25	1/15	2/25	3/15	3/25	.83
.05	.20	15	35	0/15	3/25	3/15	4/35	.46
.10	.25	20	40	1/20	6/40	5/20	7/40	.74

[a]Type-I and type-II error probabilities approximately .10.
[b]Probability of early termination rejecting the drug after the first stage if the true response probability is .05.

Table 9.2. Required Sample Size for Detecting a 20 Percentage Point Improvement in Response Probability[a]

Observed Response Rate in Historic Controls	Number of Historic Controls				
	20	30	50	75	150
0.1	116	53	40	29	25
0.3	882	137	69	54	44
0.5	455	122	68	55	45

[a]One-sided type-I error of .05 and statistical power .80.

trials with specific historic controls. Phase II trials of combinations, as performed today, are probably our poorest category of clinical trials with regard to the manner in which they are designed, analyzed, and reported. False-positive reports from such trials are common and account in large part for the adoption into practice of ineffective regimens and the launching of phase III trials that demonstrate the ineffectiveness of the new treatment. Phase II trials of combinations can be important because they provide the opportunity to try innovative ideas in relatively small numbers of patients with short-term endpoints. More careful planning and reporting of such studies is necessary, however.

PHASE III CLINICAL TRIALS

The purpose of a phase III clinical trial is to determine whether a treatment is effective or is more effective than another treatment for a specified group of patients and to obtain an estimate of the degree of effectiveness or the difference in effectiveness of the two treatments. How do we determine whether a treatment is effective? This is inherently comparative. If the treatment cures the patient of a disease that never spontaneously remits, then the treatment is effective. If the treatment cures no one but causes partial shrinkages of tumors that do not spontaneously shrink, then the treatment is effective for shrinking tumors but may or may not be of benefit to the patient. If we want to know whether a noncurative treatment prolongs survival, then we need to compare survivals of a group of patients who receive the treatment to those of a group who do not receive it. In planning a phase III trial, we must define what group of patients to study, establish a comparison group that will provide an unbiased comparison, define the primary endpoint, and define the target sample size and a plan for interim monitoring that will provide a reliable

answer to the therapeutic questions posed. Some physicians do not understand that a protocol needs to be much more than just a prescription of how to treat patients. As stated in the introduction, such informal protocols are invitations to misleading conclusions.

Randomization

To determine whether a new treatment cures any patients with a disease that is uniformly and rapidly fatal, history provides a satisfactory control. In this situation, the patient population is completely homogeneous with regard to cure in the absence of the new therapy. Once we leave the setting of complete determinism of outcome, randomization is essential to ensure that the differences in outcome between the control group and the treatment group are attributable to treatment. Problems with historic controls have been enumerated and demonstrated many times (9). In the best of circumstances, historic controls are patients treated within the previous few years at the institution(s) performing the new study. The controls would have been treated on a protocol having exactly the same eligibility requirements, workup, supportive care, follow-up, and endpoint evaluation procedures as the current study. Referral patterns and accrual rates would be static, no patients in either group would be excluded from analysis because of ineligibility or nonevaluability, and an exhaustive demonstration of similarity in distribution of all suspected prognostic factors would be presented. These circumstances are actually rarely encountered. Pocock (10) has reported 19 unselected instances under circumstances approaching these, in which a collaborative group carried one treatment over for two successive studies. Even here, for 4 of the 19 pairs of trials, the differences in outcome were statistically significant at the $p <$ .02 level for the comparison of a treatment with itself.

It is sometimes said that randomization is unnecessary because matched historic controls can be selected. But one can confidently match only with regard to known prognostic factors, and these generally explain only a minor portion of the variability in prognosis among patients (11). Matching with regard to known factors gives no assurance that the distributions of unknown factors are similar between the treatment groups. It is also sometimes said that randomization is not effective in ensuring that the treatment groups are similar with regard to unknown prognostic factors unless the number of patients is large. This reflects a misunderstanding of randomization. Randomization does not ensure that the groups are medically equivalent, but it distributes the unknown biasing factors according to a known random distribution so that their effects can be rigorously allowed for in significance tests and confidence intervals. This is true regardless of the study size. A significance level represents the probability of obtaining such differences in outcome by random fluctuations.

Reports of nonrandomized phase II trials sometimes include a comparison of survivals between responders and nonresponders given the same treatment. The implication is that the treatment prolongs survival because the treatment causes responses and the patients with responses live longer. This is invalid reasoning for many reasons, and several journals have adopted editorial policies that prohibit such misleading analyses (12, 13). There is a time bias in this analysis because responders must live long enough for response to be observed. Also, responders may have more favorable prognostic factors than nonresponders have, leading to a difference in survival regardless of treatment. It is even possible that treatment may shorten the survival of nonresponders rather than lengthen that of responders. Improving partial response rates for patients with solid tumors may not result in improving survival. Demonstrating that a treatment prolongs survival requires comparing the survival of all patients receiving that treatment to the survival of an appropriate control group receiving some other treatment.

Whereas randomization has not been necessary for identifying some breakthroughs in diseases with uniformly fatal prognoses, it provides protection against misinterpretation of "dramatic" results in highly selected patients treated with regimens no better than the standard treatments and is essential for identifying moderate treatment improvements of great public health importance. Moderate treatment improvements can only be identified when moderate biases and moderate random variation are eliminated. The former is accomplished by using randomized treatment assignment, and the latter by using a large enough sample size.

Endpoint

The "endpoint" refers to the measure of patient benefit used in the clinical trial. The endpoint for a phase III trial should be either a direct assessment of patient benefit or a surrogate endpoint that has previously been shown to be highly correlated with a direct measure of patient benefit. For cancer trials, the main direct measures of patient benefit are survival and alleviation of symptoms of cancer. Easily administered functional assessment questionnaires are being developed and should be more widely utilized (14–16).

For some types of cancer, durable complete response or disease-free survival is an acceptable surrogate for survival as long as the treatments are not themselves lethal. In most cases, however, it has not been demonstrated that partial response is a good surrogate for survival. Partial response rates are often useful endpoints for phase II studies screening for antitumor activity, and it seems likely that in some cases partial response could be demonstrated to be a good surrogate for improvement in quality of life. But, to date, partial response has not been consistently demonstrated to be a satisfactory endpoint for phase III clinical trials.

One argument against the use of survival as an endpoint is that treatments subsequently administered after disease progression can influence survival. In many cases, however, such treatments have little effect on survival. If they do influence survival meaningfully and if one treatment group can be better "salvaged" than the other, then the lack of overall survival benefit is the important answer that should be obtained. When one wishes to determine whether an investigational drug has a beneficial influence on survival, however, the study should not be designed as a cross-over study. That is, if the usefulness of the drug in prolonging survival as a salvage treatment is not already established and if patients in the control arm get the drug on progression, then the potential usefulness of the drug may be masked.

Definition of endpoints is important for phase III trials. The required size and duration of the trial can vary substantially, based on the endpoint specified. The size of treatment effect that can be realistically expected may depend on the endpoint. Clear specification of the main endpoint enables the interpretation of final results to be clear-cut, without the ambiguities associated with interpreting multiple-endpoint analyses.

Eligibility Criteria

The purpose of a phase III clinical trial is to determine whether a treatment is beneficial for a well-defined group of patients. The eligibility criteria define the group of patients. The clearest analysis will be the comparison of outcomes for all patients randomized to one treatment to outcomes for all patients randomized to the other treatment. Analyses based on subsets of patients or analyses based on exclusions of some randomized patients are subject to much greater ambiguity of interpretation. Hence, eligibility criteria should be written with the intent of analyzing all eligible patients together as a whole. Patients who are very unlikely to tolerate one of the treatments should not be eligible.

Excluding patients from the analysis because of treatment deviations, early death, patient withdrawal, or other reasons may seriously bias the results. Excluded patients often have poorer outcomes than those not excluded. One can rationalize that patients not receiving treatment as specified in the protocol did worse because of that fact, but this is speculation. Canner (17) showed that patients with poor compliance to placebo pills in the Coronary Drug Project had much greater cardiovascular mortality than other placebo patients, and the difference could not be explained on the basis of known prognostic factors. Excluding patients (or "analyzing them separately," which is equivalent to excluding them) for reasons other than that they did not satisfy the eligibility criteria is a major defect in the analysis and reporting of phase III trials. If the conclusions of a study depend on exclusions, then these conclusions are suspect. Eligibility criteria for both patients and collaborators should be established in such a way that there will be few protocol deviations. Generally, the treatment plan should be viewed as a policy to be evaluated. When survival is the endpoint, the vital status of all patients can usually be traced, and there is little justification for exclusion of eligible patients. Censoring patients who go "off-study" or receive a nonprotocol treatment is a form of exclusion and should not be employed.

Some clinical trials go too far in defining very narrow eligibility criteria. Such rigid criteria restrict the entry of patients in two ways. First, the number of patients who satisfy all the criteria is limited. Second, the requirement of more detailed staging or workup than would normally be performed in general practice may reduce the willingness of physicians and patients to participate in the trial. The studies of Begg and Engstrom (18) indicated that eligibility criteria are the basis for excluding a large majority of patients from clinical trials and that "for many of the exclusion factors there exists little consensus on the precise nature of the exclusion or indeed whether the criterion should be used or not." The results of clinical trials with excessively restrictive eligibility criteria may not be applicable to the population at large. This is a serious concern. For most adult malignancies, only a small proportion of patients are entered on clinical trials. The results of clinical trials can, however, influence medical care nationwide or internationally. The discrepancy between broadly applied conclusions derived from a narrowly based study can have serious public health and financial implications.

Sample Size

Sample size and maturity of follow-up are major determinants of the reliability of a clinical trial. Most phase III clinical trials are planned to test a null hypothesis. That is, it is assumed that at a predetermined point in time, one will perform a statistical significance test of the null hypothesis of treatment equivalence with regard to the primary endpoint. If that significance level is less than some specified value (usually .05), then the null hypothesis will be rejected. The sample size is planned so that if the true difference in treatment efficacy is D instead of zero, then the probability (statistical power) for rejecting the null hypothesis will be some specified value (usually 80 to 90%).

To determine sample size, one must define the endpoint and the scale of measurement for expressing the difference (D). For example, D could be the difference in 5-year-survival probabilities or the logarithm of the ratio of medians. The technical aspects of scale of measurement are not of fundamental importance here. The main point is that the number of patients required depends critically on D. This can be seen in Table 9.3, in which the number of patients per treatment for detecting a difference in 5-year-survival probability is tabulated as a function of D and the expected 5-year-survival probability in the control group (19). In this table, a two-sided significance level of .05 is considered statistically significant, and a power of 90% is used. It is assumed that analysis occurs after all patients are followed for 5 years.

The parameter D does not represent the difference we hope exists; it represents the size of the difference that the study will be able to detect. For major phase III studies, it should generally represent the smallest difference that

Table 9.3. Required Sample Size for Comparing 5-Year Survival Proportions

Survival Proportion in Control Group	Difference in Survival Proportions[a]		
	0.10	0.15	0.20
0.05	198	106	69
0.10	281	143	89
0.20	410	197	117
0.30	496	231	133
0.40	533	244	141
0.50	533	242	133
0.60	496	216	117
0.70	410	172	89
0.80	281	106	—

[a]Number of patients per treatment to have power 0.90 for detecting difference in survival proportions. Type-I error α = .05 (two-sided).

would be clinically meaningful. Many studies are misreported as "negative" when, in fact, they are actually uninformative because they have a sample size sufficient only to detect unrealistically large differences. The inability to demonstrate a statistically significant difference does not imply that the treatments are equivalent. If D is chosen to be very large, then non-statistically-significant results will be consistent with both no difference and with major differences that are less than a "home run." For example, a complete response rate of 25/50 (50%) is not significantly different from one of 20/50 (40%) (p = .42), but an approximate 95% confidence interval for the true difference ranges from 13% favoring one treatment to 33% favoring the other treatment! The use of confidence intervals in reporting results would avoid much of the misinterpretation of "nonsignificant" results (4).

There have been few home runs in cancer therapeutics, and some of the major advances have come from stepwise improvements of moderate size. An absolute 15% increase in survival probability for a common type of cancer represents a major public health accomplishment that has rarely been achieved in oncology. Based on current concepts of the probability that a solid tumor has developed multiple resistance by the time of diagnosis, and based on the difficulty of substantially extending survival compared with temporarily shrinking a solid tumor, it is rarely plausible to expect a difference in survival probability of greater than 15% for adjuvant therapy studies. Small studies that report huge differences in survival probabilities are often statistical

flukes that will be nonconfirmable (see below). From Table 9.3 we see that to have 90% statistical power for detecting a 10 to 15% difference in survival probability generally requires a sample size in the range of 150 to 500 patients per treatment group for each set of patients that will be separately analyzed.

For diseases in which survival is short, it is not appropriate to speak in terms of differences in the proportion of patients who survive beyond a specified time. Unless the survival curves show a plateau, planning based on comparing the entire curves is a better approach. Table 9.4 shows the approximate total number of deaths necessary to provide 90% statistical power for detecting a specified ratio of median survivals for exponential distributions (20). For example, to detect a 50% increase in median survival, the combination of number of patients accrued and duration of follow-up must be such that a total of about 256 deaths are observed by the time of analysis. The 50% increase in median survival corresponds to at most a 15% absolute difference in proportion surviving beyond a specified time. Similarly, the 30% (1.3) and 75% (1.75) increases in medians correspond to maximum absolute differences in survival probabilities of about 10% and 20%, respectively. A 50% increase represents an increase of 1.5 years in median survival if the median in the control group is 3 years. To have 90% power for detecting an increase of this size, a study with about 256 total deaths would be required. With an accrual rate of 200 patients per year and a follow-up period of 3 years after the end of accrual, accrual for 2.4 years with entry of 480 patients is necessary (20).

Table 9.4. Required Sample Size for Comparing Survival Curves

Ratio of Median Survival	Number of Total Deaths to Observe
1.2	1268
1.3	612
1.4	372
1.5	256
1.6	190
1.7	150
1.8	122
1.9	102
2.0	88

[a]Total number of deaths in both groups to have power 0.90 for detecting ratio of median survivals. Type-I error α = .05 (two-sided).

In most studies comparing a new treatment with a standard treatment, it is implicit that the new treatment will be adopted only if it improves outcomes. There are an increasing number of studies, however, in which the new treatment is less debilitating and thus will be accepted as long as it does not have inferior efficacy. One can never demonstrate that two treatments are precisely equivalent with regard to outcome, but one can limit the size of the difference that might exist. Such studies need to be large because it is important to demonstrate that the loss in survival rate caused by the new therapy is very small at worst. Studies that reliably identify or exclude small differences must be very large. In reporting the results of such studies, it is important to calculate confidence limits for the survival differences that are consistent with the observed data, because significance tests can be very misleading. Confidence intervals are almost always more informative than significance tests, but the distinction is particularly important for studies of therapeutic equivalence because of the implications of a misinterpretation of nonsignificant differences. Although the use of confidence limits for reporting results is very important (21), sample sizes can be planned using conventional significance testing methods by requiring power at least 90% for the smallest difference of clinical significance. For 5-year survival, this difference should surely be no greater than 5 to 10%.

Interim Monitoring

Interim monitoring of accumulating data is important to ensure that the study remains safe and ethically appropriate. In some cases, early results will be sufficiently extreme so that the goals will have been accomplished with fewer patients than anticipated. Unfortunately, however, improper interpretation of interim results and publication of immature data are among the most frequent causes of misleading conclusions in the reporting of randomized clinical trials. This problem was well illustrated in a computer simulation by Fleming, Green, and Harrington (22), who assumed that patients were accrued to a two-armed randomized study at a constant rate of 40 patients per year over 3 years. The endpoint was survival, and the treatments were equivalent. If analyses were performed every 3 months, then the probability of obtaining a statistically significant ($p < .05$) result by chance alone at some point during the 4-year trial was

26%. This illustrates how misleading interim results can be.

To have reasonable assurance that an apparent interim treatment difference is not just a statistical anomaly due to repeated looks at accumulating data, a significance level much more stringent than $p < .05$ is required. A number of statistical approaches to interim monitoring of accumulating data have been developed. The simplest is recommended by Peto et al. (23). They proposed that the trial terminate if the two-sided significance level for the treatment comparison of the primary endpoint becomes less than .0025. If this did not occur, then the trial would end accrual at its preplanned target sample size. This approach was developed more fully by O'Brien and Fleming (24) and by Fleming, Green, and Harrington (25). It is a useful approach that requires large differences for early termination but does not substantially increase the maximum sample size. The decision to terminate a clinical trial is actually quite complex, and sequential statistical designs are oversimplifications of the true situation. Consequently, designs that are conservative early are desirable. Also, with survival data, early differences may not be representative of later effects. A more comprehensive discussion of statistical designs for interim monitoring is given by Pocock (26).

The cancer cooperative groups have adopted the use of data-monitoring committees to monitor interim results. With broadly based multidisciplinary representation, such committees can ensure that the patients are protected and that the interim data are carefully evaluated. The monitoring committee, generally, should have sole access to interim outcome results, to protect the participating physicians from the effects that superficial looks at those results could have on their ability to deal honestly with their patients. This also protects the study from early termination with inconclusive results based on unreliable judgments formed about relative treatment efficacy.

Green et al. (27). investigated the impact of data-monitoring committees by comparing results from two major cancer cooperative groups: one revealed interim outcome results only to the data-monitoring committee and the other made such results generally available to group members. Ten pairs of closely matched phase III trials of gastrointestinal, lung, and breast cancer were identified. Approximately one-half of the studies in the group without monitoring committees showed declining accrual rates over time, versus none in the group with monitoring committees. In the group without monitoring committees, two studies were terminated inappropriately, yielding equivocal results. Furthermore, the group without monitoring committees had two studies in which early positive results were published. Accrual then continued, and results from neither of the two were convincingly positive at the final analysis. Although all of these problems may not be due solely to the lack of monitoring committees, numerous cooperative group experiences show that such committees can contribute enormously to the protection of patients and the preservation of the integrity of prospective clinical trials.

Subset Analysis

The purpose of subset analysis is to determine which subtypes of patient benefit or fail to benefit from a new treatment. Although the motivation for subset analysis seems strong, such analyses are a frequent source of misleading claims in the medical literature. Unless the sample size of a clinical trial is made large enough for separate analysis of predefined subsets, the statistical power for finding real subset-specific treatment differences will be small. Unfortunately, the probability of finding a spurious subset-specific effect by chance alone is independent of the sample size and increases rapidly as the number of subsets examined increases. Consequently, most reported subset differences are spurious and are never confirmed by other studies.

To illustrate this point, Fleming and Watelet performed a computer simulation of 5000 clinical trials (28). Each trial had 400 patients, and the two treatments were equivalent. A modest subset analysis was performed for each trial. With age, sex, and performance status as the three covariates, six subset comparisons were performed: younger and older patients, males and females, and low- and high-performance-status groups. For each subset, the two equivalent treatments were compared. The results of the simulation demonstrated the unreliability of subset analyses. Even when the subset analyses were based on only three patient characteristics and were performed at only one time point, 20% of all trials yielded at least one false-positive ($p < .05$) subset comparison. When these subset analyses were performed at each interim analysis of a group sequential trial having up to four interim analyses, 39% of all trials had at least one false-positive significant subset result. Even if at-

tention were restricted to differences that were significant at the $p < .01$ level, nearly 15% of the group sequential trials had at least one false-positive subset comparison. Other simulated examples of spurious findings resulting from subset analyses are described by Lee et al. (29).

When major subset-specific treatment differences seem a priori likely, sample size should be established so that the subsets of interest can be analyzed separately with adequate statistical power. In other cases, subset analysis should be viewed as hypothesis generation to be tested in an independent trial before being believed. In either case, the strength of evidence favoring a subset-specific treatment effect should be evaluated by using appropriate statistical tools (30, 31). New Bayesian methods for subset analysis have recently been developed by Dixon and Simon (32).

IMPEDIMENTS TO CLINICAL TRIALS

One of the most substantial immediate obstacles to further progress in the therapy of malignant disease is the difficulty in recruiting adequate numbers of patients to clinical studies. Currently, in the United States, there are approximately 1 million new cancer patients diagnosed each year. Of that number, only a tiny fraction, between 25 to 35,000 patients per year, are enrolled on National Cancer Institute–sponsored clinical trials. In general, patients who have any common adult epithelial malignancies are rarely recruited to clinical studies (only 0.5% to 2.5% of such available patients). This is in sharp contrast to pediatric patients, among whom 40 to 70% of available children may be enrolled. The reasons for lethargic research participation are many but can be divided between those that affect the patient and those that affect the health care professional.

Patients may be reluctant to participate in a clinical investigation because they are disquieted at the concept of research. Also, a patient may only be able to receive the investigational therapy at a geographic site distant from familiar surroundings, family, and physicians, and this may be an impediment. Financial disincentive may exist because the patient's insurance may deny coverage for investigational therapies. More tests or evaluations may be required as part of a research program than otherwise would be standard or common practice. Patients may be uncomfortable with the concept that there is no single treatment that is known with assurance to be the best in that particular case.

From the physician's point of view, the disincentives to participation in clinical trials may include the following: genuine disagreement about the treatment options offered in a research program, discomfort with the concept of not being able to indicate to a particular patient a single therapy that is believed (by that physician) to be best, the financial disincentive in a referral practice where the physician cannot dictate what treatment will be provided to each individual patient, the extra time required for office staff to fill out paperwork associated with the clinical investigation, the extra time required by the physician to explain a clinical study, and the idea of performing research itself. Recognizing the extra burden associated with a clinical investigation and the extra cost in terms of time, energy, and dollars, participation in formal studies is fundamental to progress in clinical oncology. Not only does such participation help ensure high quality clinical care for the individual, but it also provides a vast societal benefit. The background for any such study is the belief that for each individual patient, optimal clinical care must be delivered. However, within that framework, considerable information can be gained for the whole population of patients with that disease. This is comforting to many patients, since it brings extra meaning to their own suffering and provides some linkage with a cohort of individuals who suffer from the same disease. From the physician's point of view, the value of participating in clinical trials is obvious.

INTERPRETING PUBLISHED REPORTS

The previous sections have presented key issues in the planning and conduct of a good clinical trial. Doctors who try to keep up with the medical literature are, however, faced with an even greater challenge—that of interpreting the results of the multiplicity of clinical trials published and determining whether and how those results should influence the treatment of their patients. This section discusses three facets of this issue. First, summary guidelines that physicians may use to evaluate a clinical trial report are reviewed.

Reporting Results of Clinical Trials

Effective reporting of results is an integral part of good research. Unfortunately, numerous surveys have indicated that the quality of reporting of clinical trial results is poor. Simon and Wittes developed a set of methodologic guidelines for reports of clinical trials, and these guidelines have been adopted by major cancer journals worldwide (12). The nine guidelines are listed below with brief comments.

1. Authors should briefly discuss the quality control methods used to ensure that the data are complete and accurate. A reliable procedure should be cited for ensuring that all patients entered on study are actually reported upon. If no such procedures are in place, their absence should be noted. Any procedures used to ensure that assessment of major endpoints is reliable should be mentioned (e.g., second-party review of responses) or their absence noted.

2. All patients registered on study should be accounted for. The report should specify for each treatment the number of patients who were not eligible, as well as who died or withdrew before treatment began. The distribution of follow-up times should be described for each treatment, and the number of patients lost to follow-up should be given.

3. The study should not have an inevaluability rate for major endpoints of greater than 15%. Not more than 15% of eligible patients should be lost to follow-up or considered inevaluable for response due to early death, protocol violation, missing information, etc. *Comment:* The 15% figure is obviously somewhat arbitrary, but inevaluability rates of 15% or more usually reflect inappropriate patient selection. For phase III studies, disqualifications are a source of potential bias; when the disqualification rate approaches the magnitude of the difference in outcomes being tested, the results are obviously not reliable.

4. In randomized studies, the report should include a comparison of survival and/or other major endpoints for all eligible patients as randomized, that is, with no exclusions other than those not meeting eligibility criteria.

5. The sample size should be sufficient to either establish or conclusively rule out the existence of effects of clinically meaningful magnitude. The adequacy of sample size should be demonstrated by either presenting confidence limits for true treatment differences or calculating statistical power for detecting differences.

6. Authors should state whether there was an initial target sample size, and if so, what it was. They should specify how frequently interim analyses were performed and how the decisions to stop accrual and report results were arrived at.

7. All claims of therapeutic efficacy should be based upon explicit comparisons with a specific control group, except in special circumstances in which each patient is his or her own control. If nonrandomized controls are used, the characteristics of the patients should be presented in detail and compared with those of the experimental group. Potential sources of bias should be adequately discussed. Comparison of survival between responders and nonresponders does not establish efficacy and should not generally be included. Reports of phase II trials that draw conclusions about antitumor activity but not therapeutic efficacy generally do not require a control group.

8. The patients studied should be adequately described. Applicability of conclusions to other patients should be carefully dealt with. Claims of subset-specific treatment differences must be carefully documented statistically as more than the random results of multiple-subset analyses. *Comment:* Care should be employed in extrapolating results to the general population of patients. Only a small fraction of patients enter clinical trials, and they are not a random sample. Proper statistical methodology is necessary to distinguish true subset-specific treatment differences from the random results of multiple-subset analyses. It is not generally recognized that, by chance alone, there is a 40% probability of finding at least 1 statistically significant false-positive treatment difference in the evaluation of 10 disjoint subsets.

9. The methods of statistical analysis should be described in sufficient detail so that a knowledgeable reader could reproduce the analysis if the data were available.

The Need for Confirmation of "Positive" Results

Independent confirmation is a widely accepted scientific principle, but its importance is sometimes overlooked when it comes to clinical trials. It is right to want to transfer effective treatments to the wide community of cancer patients as quickly as possible, but the reliability of a single unconfirmed study is often grossly overestimated.

Consider the expected results from 100 hypothetical clinical trials (33). Assume that in 90 cases, the two treatments are actually equivalent, and in 10, one is truly better than the other. Each trial outcome is categorized as to whether the observed treatment difference is statistically significant at the .05 level or not. The statistical power for detecting the true differences that exist is assumed to be 80%. Under these conditions, we expect that about 5% of the 90 trials of equivalent treatments will give statistically significant differences; this is about 5 trials. Of the 10 trials in which one treatment is more effective than the other, we expect to get a statistically significant difference in 8 of them. Hence, of the 13 trials that can be expected to give statistically significant results, 5 of 13 (38%) are false positives. The probability that a positive clinical trial result is a false positive is of the order of 38% if one accepts the premise that in most clinical trials, the experimental treatment is not more effective than the control or the degree of improvement is too small to be detected with the sample size used. This is often a reasonable premise, particularly as it applies to small, single-institution studies. This analysis and similar ones by Staquet et al. (34) and Zelen (35) demonstrate that positive findings require independent confirmation.

Publication Bias

Publication bias is the preference of medical journals for publishing "positive" clinical trial results rather than "negative" results. The bias does not result from an intent to deceive but from a desire to publish papers of greatest interest. Publication bias is not universal; major multicenter clinical trials, representing a great investment of effort and resources, are usually submitted for publication regardless of the results and accepted by some journal. Even for such studies, however, the results may determine which journal accepts the manuscript. The prestige and circulation of the journal in which an article is published can determine the influence that the article has on medical practice. Investigations by Begg and Berlin, however, indicated that publication bias is a major factor in the reporting of small studies (36). Hence, in reading the medical literature, particularly reports of small, single-institution studies, one must remember that negative trials of the same treatment may have been screened from publication or published in an obscure journal. This is disconcerting. Begg and Berlin conclude, "whereas many clinical studies are designed and conducted in a rigorous scientific manner, the manner of dissemination of the results via journal articles is primitive."

Combining Evidence from Several Clinical Trials

Often, more than a single clinical trial has evaluated the effectiveness of a specific treatment. Ultimate decision making about the value of the treatment should be based on evidence from all relevant clinical trials. In principle this seems obvious, but in practice it is often difficult to carry out. The available clinical trials often differ in details of treatment delivery, patient selection, study design, sample size, follow-up maturity, and in other aspects. Which trials are relevant? What variations of dose, schedule, patient selection, concurrent medication, etc. are important? Combining evidence from multiple clinical trials is also hampered by inadequacies of data reporting in publications.

Because of the above difficulties, there is a strong tendency to overinterpret the results of individual clinical trials and to attribute apparent differences in the outcomes of related trials to the differences in details of treatment delivery or patient selection. This is a dangerous practice that is almost certain to lead to erroneous conclusions when several related trials have been carried out.

Within the past several years, a more systematic and quantitative approach to combining evidence from several clinical trials has been employed, referred to as metaanalysis. Metaanalyses, like clinical trials, can be well or poorly performed. In a good metaanalysis, the results of all potentially relevant randomized clinical trials are assembled. Attention is limited to randomized trials because the bias from nonrandomized comparisons may swamp small-to-moderate therapeutic effects. Good metaanalyses, like good clinical trials, do not exclude any randomized patients. Attention should not be limited to published clinical trials because of the strong effect of publication bias—the effect that positive results have a greater chance of being published than negative results. The clinical trials should represent all initiated studies, all those initiated in a geographic region, or all those registered initially in a registry that is unbiased with regard to the results obtained (37).

There has been a great emphasis in published metaanalyses on calculating average treatment differences where the average is taken across randomized studies. This has been controversial because there is often disagreement over which studies are similar enough in design to combine in the average.

The National Cancer Institute held an international workshop on the methodology of metaanalysis (38) that discussed many of these issues. Accumulating the potentially relevant randomized studies by unbiased selection and obtaining the data in a manner that permits combination and exploration in several different ways represent valuable contributions. One can examine "all the evidence," free from the distortions of publication bias, patient exclusions, and variable endpoints. Confidence intervals can be calculated for the treatment differences found in each study to determine whether there are any real differences in outcome. Patient and study factors can be evaluated for their effect on outcome. Consistency of reported subset findings can be evaluated, and many other issues can be explored. This type of metaanalysis requires a great amount of effort and cooperation among the investigators who perform the clinical trials. However, it provides the medical community with an important perspective on treatment effectiveness.

REFERENCES

1. Wittes RE, Marsoni S, Simon R, et al. The phase II trial. Cancer Treat Rep 1985;69:1235–1239.
2. Gehan EA. The determination of the number of patients required in a preliminary and a follow-up trial of a new chemotherapeutic agent. J Chron Dis 1961; 13:346–353.
3. Fleming TR. One sample multiple testing procedure for phase II clinical trials. Biometrics 1982; 38:143–151.
4. Simon R. Confidence intervals for reporting clinical trial results. Ann Intern Med 1986;105:4429–4435.
5. Simon R. Optimal two-stage designs for phase II clinical trials. Controlled Clin Trials 1989;10:1–10.
6. Tannock I, Warr D. Nonrandomized clinical trials of cancer chemotherapy: phase II or III? J Natl Cancer Inst 1988;80:800–801.
7. Makuch RW, Simon RM. Sample size consideration for nonrandomized comparative studies. J Chron Dis 1980;33:175–181.
8. Dixon DO, Simon R. Sample size considerations for studies comparing survival curves using historical controls. J Clin Epidemiol 1988;41:1209–1214.
9. Simon RM. Design and conduct of clinical trials. In: DeVita VT Jr, Hellman S, Rosenberg SA, eds. Cancer: principles and practice of oncology. 3rd ed. Philadelphia: JB Lippincott, 1989:396–420.
10. Pocock SJ. Randomized clinical trials (letter). Br Med J 1977;1:1161.
11. Simon R. The importance of prognostic factors in cancer clinical trials. Cancer Treat Rep 1984;68:185–192.
12. Simon R, Wittes RE. Methodologic guidelines for reports of clinical trials. Cancer Treat Rep 1985; 69:1–3.
13. Anderson JR, Cain KC, Gelber RD, Gelman RS. Analysis and interpretation of the comparison of sur-

vival by treatment outcome variables in cancer clinical trials. Cancer Treat Rep 1985;10:1139–1146.

14. Wittes RE. Antineoplastic agents and FDA regulation: square pegs for round holes? Cancer Treat Rep 1987;71:795–806.

15. Ochs J, Mulhern R, Kun L. Quality-of-life assessment in cancer patients. Am J Clin Oncol 1988; 11:415–421.

16. Moinpour CM, Feigl P, Metch B, Haden KA, Meyskens FL, Crowley J. Quality of life endpoints in cancer clinical trials: review and recommendations. J Natl Cancer Inst 1989;81:485–495.

17. Canner PL. Influence of treatment adherence in the Coronary Drug Project (letter). N Engl J Med 1981; 304:612–613.

18. Begg CB, Engstrom PF. Eligibility and extrapolation in cancer clinical trials. J Clin Oncol 1987;5:962–968.

19. Simon R. The size of phase III cancer clinical trials. Cancer Treat Rep 1985;69:1087–1092.

20. Rubinstein LV, Gail MH, Santner TJ. Planning the duration of a comparative clinical trial with loss to follow-up and a period of continued observation. J Chron Dis 1981;36:469–474.

21. Makuch R, Simon R. Sample size requirements for evaluating a conservative therapy. Cancer Treat Rep 1978;62:1037–1040.

22. Fleming TR, Green SJ, Harrington DP. Considerations for monitoring and evaluating treatment effects in clinical trials. Controlled Clin Trials 1984;5:55–66.

23. Peto R, Pike MC, Armitage P, et al. Design and analysis of randomized clinical trials requiring prolonged observation of each patient. Br J Cancer 1976; 34:515–612, 1977;35:1–39.

24. O'Brien PC, Fleming TR. A multiple testing procedure for clinical trials. Biometrics 1979;35:549–556.

25. Fleming TR, Green SJ, Harrington DP. Designs for group sequential tests. Controlled Clin Trials 1984; 5:348–361.

26. Pocock SJ. Interim analyses for randomized clinical trials: the group sequential approach. Biometrics 1982;38:153–162.

27. Green SJ, Fleming TR, O'Fallon JR. Policies for study monitoring and interim reporting of results. J Clin Oncol 1987;5:1477–1484.

28. Fleming TR, Watelet L. Approaches to monitoring clinical trials. J Natl Cancer Inst 1989; 81:188–193.

29. Lee KL, McNeer JF, Starmer F, et al. Clinical judgment and statistics. Lessons from a simulated randomized trial in coronary artery disease. Circulation 1980;61:508–515.

30. Gail M, Simon R. Testing for qualitative interactions between treatment effects and patient subsets. Biometrics 1985;41:361–372.

31. Simon R. Patient subsets and variation in therapeutic efficacy. Br J Clin Pharmacol 1982b;14:473–482.

32. Dixon DO, Simon R. Bayesian subset analysis. Biometrics 1991;47:871–872.

33. Simon R. Randomized clinical trials and research strategy. Cancer Treat Rep 1982a;66:1083–1087.

34. Staquet MJ, Rozencweig M, Von Hoff DD, Muggia FM. The delta and epsilon errors in the assessment of cancer trials. Cancer Treat Rep 1979; 63:1917–1921.

35. Zelen M. Strategy and alternate randomized designs in cancer clinical trials. Cancer Treat Rep 1982; 66:1095–1100.

36. Begg CB, Berlin JA. Publication bias and dissemination of clinical research. J Natl Cancer Inst 1989; 81:107–115.

37. Simes RJ. Publication bias: the case for an international registry of clinical trials. J Clin Oncol 1986; 4:1529–1541.

38. Yusuf S, Simon R, Ellenberg SS, eds. Symposium on methodology for overviews of randomized clinical trials. Stat Med 1987;6:217–410.

10

Hematopoietic Growth Factors

Matthew L. Sherman and Marc B. Garnick

Hematopoietic growth factors, glycoproteins that regulate blood cell development, have become a potent and powerful tool for the medical oncologist (1–5) to alter outcomes following cancer chemotherapy administration and states associated with bone marrow dysfunction. In addition to their myelorestorative activities, hematopoietic growth factors have a wide spectrum of biologic activities on cells other than those regulating hematopoiesis. This chapter reviews the basic history, molecular biology, and preclinical and clinical applications of these very important classes of molecules.

General Introduction

Early pioneering investigators, including Till and McCulloch (6), Pluznik and Sachs (7), and Metcalf et al. (8) demonstrated the ability (either in vivo or in vitro) of progenitor hematopoietic cells to generate multilineage colonies. In animal systems in which lethally irradiated mice received syngeneic bone marrow, a group of cellular clusters and colonies developed in the spleens of the irradiated recipient mice. These "colonies" histologically resembled small islands of multilineage hematopoietic cells. The number of cells that were able to give rise to such colonies were expressed as colony-forming units (CFUs). In general, 1 per 10^5 nucleated cells injected yielded a "colony," usually appearing in the spleen. Subsequent in vitro work demonstrated that soluble factors were indeed able to stimulate individual bone marrow cells to yield colonies. For example, when bone marrow was plated in an agar-containing system, a colony (consisting of >50 cells) developing along predominantly granulocytic lines was named a colony-forming unit–granulocyte (CFU-G). Likewise, a CFU-M was a colony-forming units–monocyte/macrophage, and a CFU-MIX or CFU-GEMM consisted of a multilineage colony consisting of granulocyte, erythroid, macrophage, and megakaryocyte lineages. The lineage nomenclature of red cells included cells that gave rise to burst-forming units–erythroid (BFU-E) and colony-forming units–erythroid (CFU-E), both precursors of mature red blood cells.

Enormous investigative efforts have led to the characterization of these factors that give rise to colony formation. A group of colony-stimulating factors (CSFs), also known as hematopoietic growth factors, have emerged, which can modulate hematopoietic cells both in vitro and (recently) in vivo in both animal and human studies. Figure 10.1 represents a general schema of hematopoiesis, in which a primordial stem cell gives rise to early progenitors. Consequently, under the influence of various growth factors, cells of different stages of maturation and different lineages emerge as peripheral circulating blood cells. This chapter deals with the biologic activity of hematopoietic growth factors, ranging from the agents approved for clinical use (G-CSF, GM-CSF, and erythropoietin) to selected agents in investigational studies (IL-1, IL-3, IL-6, IL-11, PIXY321, and thrombopoietin). These now represent very important adjuncts to cancer chemotherapy and bone marrow transplantation.

G-CSF

Biology and Preclinical Pharmacology

G-CSF is a pleiotropic cytokine that has important regulatory effects on the proliferation, differentiation, and activation of hematopoietic precursors and cells of the neutrophilic lineage. The nonhuman primate model has been an excellent model for predicting human in vivo activity of hematopoietic growth factors (1–5, 9–16). The biologic activity, safety, and efficacy of hematopoietic growth factors in the nonhuman

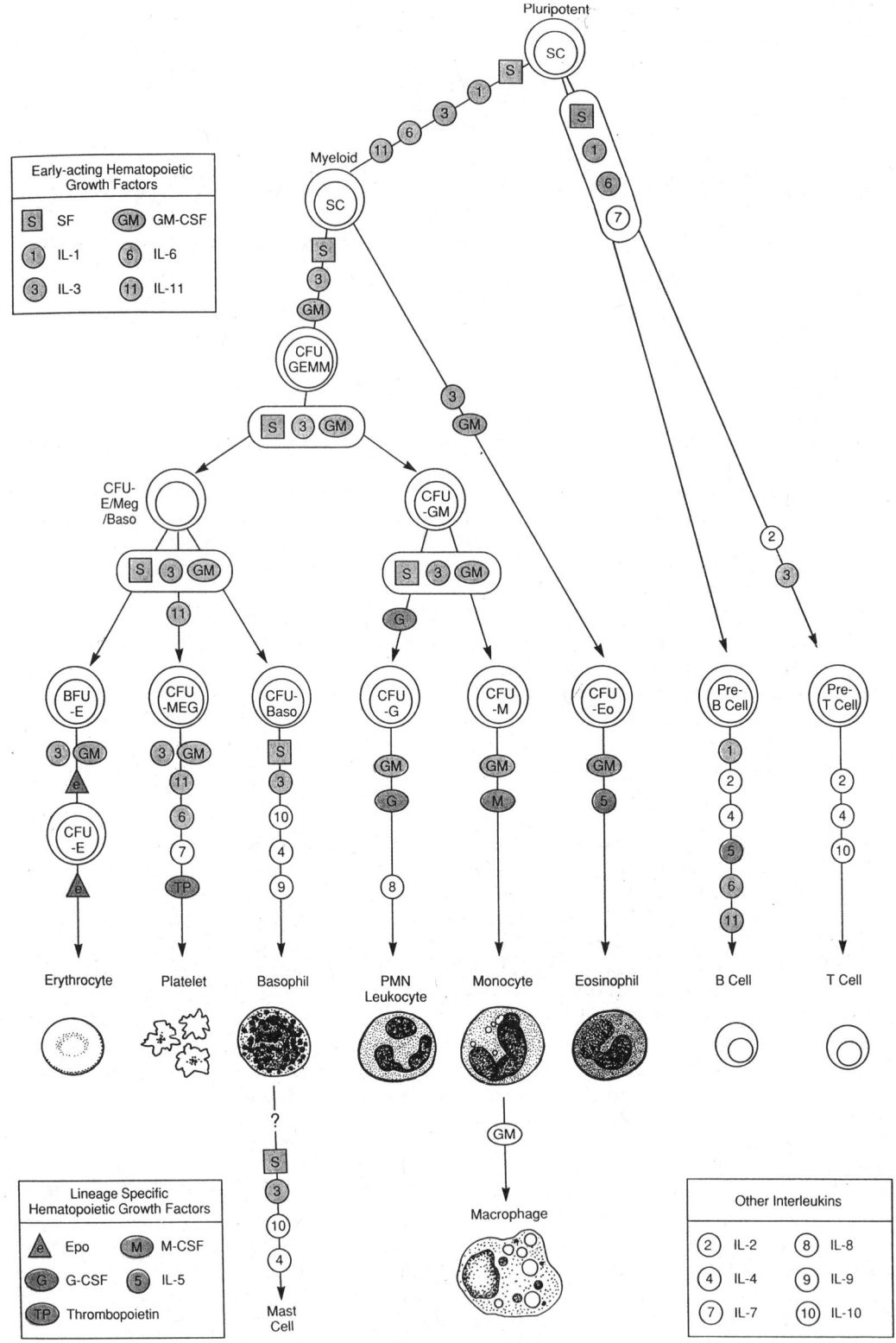

Figure 10.1. Major cytokine actions. The predominant actions of the different cytokines are indicated schematically. IL-3 and GM-CSF act broadly on most progenitor cells. IL-3, together with SF and IL-6, acts on more primitive cells than GM-CSF. The other cytokines are shown on the lineage pathways to which their actions are restricted. (From Sieff CA, Williams DA. Hematopoiesis. In: Handin RI, Lux SE, Stossel TP, eds. Blood: principles and practice of hematology. Philadelphia: JB Lippincott, 1995:194–195. With permission.)

primate, usually either cynomolgus or rhesus monkeys, have mirrored human responses. For example, the use of recombinant human (rh) G-CSF has been studied extensively in primates for its effects on normal hematopoiesis and in states associated with bone marrow dysfunction (8, 11, 14). There was a dose-dependent increase in the peripheral leukocyte count, usually occurring approximately 7 days following a 14- to 21-day intravenous or subcutaneous infusion. The preponderant cells in the periphery were neutrophils and monocytes, with little or no eosinophilia. Bone marrow evaluations from rhG-CSF-treated animals demonstrated hypercellularity with a proliferation of neutrophil precursors. Other sites of extramedullary hematopoiesis were occasionally noted.

Welte et al. (11, 14) have studied the effect of hematopoiesis in cyclophosphamide-treated primates. In these studies, the animals were treated either before and/or just shortly after receiving cyclophosphamide at a dose of 60 mg/kg/day for 2 consecutive days. The use of rhG-CSF shortened the time of leukocyte recovery in treated animals to approximately 1 week, compared with 4 weeks for control monkeys. Bone marrow evaluations of animals following rhG-CSF demonstrated multilineage responses, compared with control monkeys, in which persistent hypocellularity and aplasia were demonstrated. Other functional studies, such as nitroblue tetrazolium (NBT) reduction and chemotaxis, demonstrated marked enhancement in NBT reduction compared with that of control animals. The ability of cells to enhance phagocytosis of bacteria was also demonstrated with the use of rhG-CSF. Thus, the use of rhG-CSF decreased the time of recovery following relatively intensive doses of cyclophosphamide. Functional activity of neutrophils was maintained and enhanced during the administration of rhG-CSF. These authors suggested that rhG-CSF may be beneficial clinically in the myelodysplastic syndromes, congenital agranulocytosis, radiation-induced myelosuppression, and bone marrow transplantation.

Clinical Studies

rhG-CSF has been approved for use in a number of clinical indications, including ameliorating myelosuppression secondary to cancer chemotherapy. Bronchud et al. (17) studied 12 patients with advanced small cell carcinoma of the lung. Patients were treated with rhG-CSF at doses of 1 to 40 µg/kg/day for 5 days. Neutrophils rapidly increased to a maximum of approximately 100,000/mm^3 at a dose of 10 µg/kg/day. These patients were treated with rhG-CSF prior to the administration of combination chemotherapy, which included doxorubicin (Adriamycin), ifosfamide, mesna, and etoposide at relatively myelosuppressive doses. rhG-CSF was then administered for 14 days on alternate cycles of chemotherapy. The use of rhG-CSF in this population reduced the period of absolute neutropenia substantially, and neutrophil counts generally returned to normal within 2 weeks following initiation of therapy. In cycles in which patients were not treated with rhG-CSF, there were six episodes of documented infections, although no infectious episodes occurred during the rhG-CSF program. Functionally, neutrophil mobility and bactericidal ability were maintained during rhG-CSF therapy. Toxicity was minimal, and there were very few effects on other hematologic parameters aside from neutrophils. This study suggested a major role for the use of rhG-CSF in the amelioration of myelosuppression due to cancer chemotherapy.

Morstyn et al. (18) studied the use of rhG-CSF in individuals receiving melphalan. Patients were treated at rhG-CSF doses of 1 to 60 µg/kg/day intravenously both prior to and following chemotherapy. Prior to chemotherapy, there was a transient depression of circulating neutrophils, followed by a dose-dependent rise to levels up to 80,000 cells/mm^3. Following melphalan administration, the period of neutropenia was reduced when rhG-CSF was administered. In this study, melphalan was administered at a dose of 25 mg/m^2 by intravenous bolus injection. A day later, rhG-CSF was administered for 8 days following the melphalan administration. At high doses of rhG-CSF, early white blood cell progenitors appeared in the peripheral blood. The side-effect profile included the medullary expansion syndrome, resulting in bone pain, and some slight abnormalities of blood chemistries, including elevations of LDH, alkaline phosphatase, and uric acid levels. Pharmacokinetics revealed a half-life of approximately 8 minutes for the $t_{1/2}$-α; the $t_{1/2}$-β was approximately 110 minutes. This study suggested that rhG-CSF was well tolerated and could decrease the number of episodes of neutropenia following intensive chemotherapy and possibly allow dose intensification of chemotherapy.

Gabrilove et al. (19) studied individuals with

Table 10.1. Selected Studies Supporting the Approved Uses of rhG-CSF (Filgrastim)

Agent	Disease	Cytotoxic Regimen[a]	Reference
rhG-CSF	Small cell lung cancer	CAE	20
rhG-CSF	Small cell lung cancer	CAE	23
rhG-CSF	Non-Hodgkin's lymphoma	VAPEC-B	24
rhG-CSF	Severe chronic neutropenia	N/A	22

[a]Abbreviations: CAE: cisplatin, Adriamycin, etoposide; VAPEC-B: vincristine, doxorubicin, prednisolone, etoposide, cyclophosphamide, bleomycin; N/A: not applicable.

advanced forms of carcinoma of the urothelium, both prior to and following administration of M-VAC (methotrexate, vinblastine, doxorubicin (Adriamycin), and cisplatin) chemotherapy. In this study, 27 patients received up to 16 μg/kg of body weight of rhG-CSF before they received their first cycle of chemotherapy, during their cycle, or both. As in the previous studies, rhG-CSF resulted in a dose-dependent increase in the absolute neutrophil count and substantially reduced the number of patient days in which the absolute neutrophil count was below 1000/mm^3. In addition, fewer antibiotics were used to treat fever and neutropenia and the ability to give scheduled chemotherapy on time was greater in the rhG-CSF-treated cycles than in those cycles in which no rhG-CSF was administered. Further, the incidence of mucositis decreased in the rhG-CSF patients. These authors concluded that rhG-CSF had a major effect in ameliorating the hematologic and mucous membrane side effects of myelosuppressive chemotherapy.

Crawford (20) conducted a multicenter, randomized, double-blind, placebo-controlled study to examine the safety and efficacy of rhG-CSF in 210 patients, following cyclophosphamide, doxorubicin (Adriamycin), and etoposide chemotherapy for small cell lung cancer. rhG-CSF administration was associated with a significant reduction in the incidence, severity, and duration of neutropenia as well as the incidence and duration of infection, as demonstrated by the occurrence of fever. Furthermore, there were decreases in the number of days of hospitalization and intravenous antibiotic usage. Thus, the use of rhG-CSF has been exceptionally well tolerated and effective in ameliorating the side effects of myelosuppressive chemotherapy. These results were the basis for the approval of rhG-CSF for clinical use. In addition, data from human studies suggest that rhG-CSF is effective in ameliorating idiopathic cyclic neutropenia (21, 22). Selected randomized studies (23–25) supporting the approved uses of rhG-CSF are summarized in Table 10.1. Its role in other conditions, such as in combination with antibiotics to improve the outcome in community-acquired pneumonia, is currently being evaluated.

GM-CSF

Biology and Preclinical Pharmacology

GM-CSF stimulates the growth and differentiation of multiple lineages of hematopoietic cells. Specifically, GM-CSF stimulates cells committed to the neutrophil/macrophage lineage (CFU-GM) and cells of eosinophil colony-forming ability (CFU-Eo). In addition, GM-CSF in combination with erythropoietin stimulates multipotential progenitor cells that form granulocytic, erythroid, monocytic, and megakaryocytic colonies (CFU-GEMM) as well as erythroid colonies (BFU-E) (26–28). In addition to its effects on progenitor differentiation, GM-CSF also induces a number of functional changes in mature effector cells. GM-CSF can induce decreases in neutrophil migration (29) as well as increases in neutrophil phagocytosis and antitumor cytotoxicity for human target cells (30–32).

Several studies have evaluated effects on hematopoiesis following the parenteral administration of rhGM-CSF in nonhuman primates. In these studies (9), animals received continuous infusion rhGM-CSF over 7 to 10 days by the insertion of indwelling venous catheters. Doses of 1 to 2 × 10^7 units of rhGM-CSF/day, given as a continuous intravenous infusion over 7 days, resulted in dramatic increases (approximately seven times the preinfusion average) in the leukocyte count. Morphologic evaluation of bone marrows revealed marked hypercellularity. Typically, the increase in peripheral leukocyte count occurred in the first 1 to 3 days following initiation of the infusion and was maintained during rhGM-CSF administration. All formed elements, including neutrophils, band neutrophils, monocytes, lymphocytes, and eosinophils, were elevated. The most marked absolute rise was in the eosinophil count, but equally dramatic results were seen in the neutrophils and juvenile forms. In several additional studies, a reticulocytosis was occasionally observed. Platelet counts tended not to show any changes from baseline when rhGM-CSF was administered in a continuous intravenous infusion.

Several other preliminary experiments have also demonstrated that the duration of leukocytosis can be maintained for as long as 28 days with continuous infusion (9). Following rhGM-CSF cessation, there was a prompt decrease in the circulating white cell count, usually with return to baseline several days following discontinuation. A number of investigators have evaluated the use of rhGM-CSF in primate models exposed to high-dose chemotherapy, with or without total body irradiation (TBI), and supportive autologous bone marrow transplantation (12–14). Nienhuis et al. have performed efficacy studies with rhGM-CSF in autologous bone marrow transplantation in a primate model (12). In these studies, rhGM-CSF was either administered (a) for several days both before and after transplantation or (b) only following transplantation. The preparative bone marrow regimen included whole body radiation therapy, in which the animals received 1200 rads of absorbed TBI, given at a dose rate of 12 rad/min. Shortly thereafter, an autologous transplantation was effected by administering 2.0 to 5.0 × 10^8 cells/kg. Intensive supportive care was given to all animals. In the animals treated with rhGM-CSF, the neutrophil count reached 1000 cells/mm^3 by 8 to 9 days following the transplant, compared with an interval of 17 to 24 days for the controls. Four of the five animals tested showed an accelerated rate of platelet production. Following withdrawal of rhGM-CSF, the neutrophil count fell to values comparable to those observed in the untreated controls. Several additional animals who failed to engraft and who were part of an independent gene transfer experiment were treated with rhGM-CSF 5 to 7 weeks following transplantation. In both of the animals, there was a prompt and sustained elevation in bone marrow and peripheral myelopoiesis, with decreased requirements for both red cell and platelet transfusions.

In similar high-dose radiation studies, Monroy et al. (13) gave lethal doses of radiation therapy (800 Gy) to rhesus monkeys in a nonuniform radiation model in which a portion of the lower limbs are shielded. Following the administration of such lethal-dose radiation therapy, the bone marrow is unable to "regraft," and many animals die of bone marrow failure. However, the use of rhGM-CSF in the postradiation therapy period substantially increased granulocyte counts; to a lesser degree, platelet recovery was 4 to 7 days earlier than in the shielded animals to which no rhGM-CSF was given. Treatment

with rhGM-CSF leads to an early increase in bone marrow CFU-GM activity. In a small number of animals thus studied, overall survival has been improved in the rhGM-CSF-treated group.

Primate studies by Bonilla et al. (14) used subcutaneous rhGM-CSF following cyclophosphamide administration. In these studies, rhGM-CSF was administered either (a) prior to chemotherapy and daily throughout four cycles or (b) 72 hours after chemotherapy and then for 12-day intervals after each cycle. In the first treatment group, an absolute neutrophil count (ANC) nadir of 1.6 to 3.2 × 10^3/μL occurred on days 6 to 7, followed by a leukocytosis from 21,000 to 22,000/μL. This compared with a nadir of 0.2 to 1.1 × 10^3/μL for 18 days in control animals. The intermittently treated animals did not experience such profound protection effects. Thus, continuous infusion of rhGM-CSF had a major role in the amelioration of neutropenia.

Clinical Studies

rhGM-CSF IN AUTOLOGOUS BONE MARROW TRANSPLANTATION

rhGM-CSF has been evaluated under situations of cancer chemotherapy associated with autologous bone marrow transplantation. Brandt et al. (33) studied rhGM-CSF in individuals undergoing autologous bone marrow transplantation with high-dose combination chemotherapy consisting of carmustine (BCNU), cyclophosphamide, and cisplatin. Individuals with either breast cancer or melanoma were treated at doses ranging from 2 to 32 μg/kg of rhGM-CSF by continuous intravenous infusion for 14 days, beginning 3 hours after bone marrow infusion. The total leukocyte and granulocyte recoveries were accelerated over those of 24 concurrent historic controls (matched for age, diagnosis, and treatment regimen). Specifically, there was a dose-related increase in the white blood cell count, rising from 2575 ± 2304 at doses of 2 to 8 μg/kg. At doses of 16 μg/kg, the white blood cell count was 3120 ± 1744, compared with 863 ± 645 in the controls. There was no effect on platelet count. The main side effects of rhGM-CSF were weight gain, myalgias, and peripheral edema at the higher dose levels. At lower dose levels, which were very tolerable, there was accelerated myeloid recovery. There was an overall decrease in organ toxicity, as seen by serum creatinine and total bilirubin, compared with the historic controls. Likewise, the in-

Table 10.2. Selected Studies Supporting the Approved Uses of rhGM-CSF (Sargramostim)

Agent	Disease	Cytotoxic Regimen	Reference
rhG-CSF	Non-Hodgkin's lymphoma, Hodgkin's disease, acute lymphocytic leukemia	Total-body irradiation and cyclophosphamide-containing chemotherapies	35, 36

cidence of bacterial infections and overall mortality from the treatment was markedly reduced in the rhGM-CSF-treated patients. This study suggested that rhGM-CSF may decrease overall organ toxicity and hasten marrow engraftment in patients undergoing intensive chemotherapy or autologous bone marrow transplantation.

In another study (34), individuals with lymphoid malignancies who were undergoing autologous transplantation were treated with rhGM-CSF at doses ranging from 15 to 240 $\mu g/m^2/day$ for 14 days after transplant. Patients treated with rhGM-CSF had more rapid granulocyte and platelet recovery, fewer febrile days, and more rapid hospital discharges than did control patients not receiving rhGM-CSF. Hospitalization was reduced to 14 days in the treated group, compared with 6 to 7 weeks in controls.

On the basis of this and other studies (35–37), rhGM-CSF has been approved for use in myeloid reconstitution after autologous bone marrow transplantation. Treatment with rhGM-CSF has been associated with accelerating myeloid engraftment as well as decreasing the median duration of antibiotic administration, infectious episodes, and length of hospitalization (35–37). Other studies have demonstrated that rhGM-CSF can prolong the survival of patients who have undergone allogeneic or autologous bone marrow transplantation when engraftment is delayed (38–40). Table 10.2 lists recent studies that support the approved uses of rhGM-CSF. Prospective, comparative clinical studies of rhG-CSF and rhGM-CSF are necessary to determine both the relative efficacies and the toxicities of these two therapies.

RHGM-CSF WITH CANCER CHEMOTHERAPY

rhGM-CSF has been used to ameliorate chemotherapy-induced myelosuppression in indi-

viduals undergoing intensive chemotherapy with doxorubicin (Adriamycin), dacarbazine (DTIC), ifosfamide, and mesna (MAID). These patients were treated as part of an ongoing program for soft tissue sarcoma. Antman et al. (41) have been able to demonstrate physiologic activity of rhGM-CSF in individual patients prior to their receiving chemotherapy. In this study, patients were treated with rhGM-CSF to increase their white blood cell counts prior to the administration of chemotherapy. Shortly thereafter, rhGM-CSF was administered on the first cycle of MAID therapy. Following the second cycle, no rhGM-CSF was administered. Comparison of the rhGM-CSF cycle with the non-rhGM-CSF cycle showed a higher total white blood cell count, a higher neutrophil count, a shorter duration of neutrophils below 500/mm^3, and a higher platelet count in the rhGM-CSF cycle. Doses in this study started at 4 $\mu g/kg/day$, given as a continuous intravenous infusion, and continued through 64 $\mu g/kg/day$. Main toxicities were related to fluid retention and central venous thrombi (occurring at the highest dose). These side effects may have been related to the markedly elevated circulating leukocyte counts. rhGM-CSF was well tolerated at doses up to 32 $\mu g/kg/day$ and was able to ameliorate the leukopenia in patients undergoing intensive chemotherapy. Peripheral blood CFU-GM and BFU-E numbers were determined during each rhGM-CSF treatment. Most patients had increased levels of progenitor cells in response to rhGM-CSF.

MYELODYSPLASTIC SYNDROMES

rhGM-CSF derived from a yeast source has been evaluated in patients with myelodysplastic syndromes. In phase I study conducted by Vadhan-Raj et al. (42), rhGM-CSF was administered to eight patients with myelodysplastic syndromes. Many of these patients had abnormal karyotypes and had substantial previous therapy, including bone marrow transplantation, ara-C plus daunorubicin, and other alkylating agent therapy for their myelodysplastic syndromes. rhGM-CSF was given as a continuous intravenous infusion for 2 weeks, followed by a 2-week break. Cycles were repeated every 28 days. Doses of rhGM-CSF ranged from 300 to 500 $\mu g/m^2$ of body surface area. The main results in this study demonstrated marked increases in leukocyte count, as high as 5- to 70-fold over baseline. Granulocytes increased in all eight patients. The absolute number of monocytes, eosinophils, and lymphocytes also increased. Approximately 37% of patients also had a relatively substantial rise in platelet count and reticulocyte count, with reduced requirements for platelet transfusion and red cell transfusion. Bone marrow evaluation showed increased cellularity and a decreased number of blasts in the bone marrow of patients with refractory anemia with excess blasts (RAEB). As cycles were continued, doses required to maintain normal hematologic parameters lessened. Some patients were maintained off rhGM-CSF for a substantial time. The main side effect was bone pain, apparently related to medullary expansion syndrome from resultant leukocytosis. This study concluded that rhGM-CSF stimulated hematopoiesis markedly in vivo and produced a hematologic improvement in the short term follow-up of the study.

AIDS

Groopman et al. (43) first studied the clinical application of rhGM-CSF in 16 patients with AIDS and leukopenia. In this study, patients first received a single bolus intravenous dose. Forty-eight hours later, a 14-day continuous intravenous infusion of rhGM-CSF was initiated. This study indicated that rhGM-CSF could result in a dose-dependent increase in circulating leukocytes, with specific increases in circulating neutrophils, eosinophils, and monocytes. Individuals entering the study had a mean white count of 2225 ± 614 cells/μL; they ended with a range of 4575 ± 2397 cells/μL to a high of $48,700$ cells/μL in a patient receiving the highest dose. The side effects associated with administration of rhGM-CSF included low-grade fever, myalgias, phlebitis, and flushing. It was concluded that rhGM-CSF was well tolerated and biologically active in reestablishing normal white cell numbers in patients with AIDS. Bone marrow cellularity before and after treatment with rhGM-CSF demonstrated marked hypercellularity with a prominent increase in eosinophil counts. Hemoglobin, hematocrit, platelet count, and reticulocytes did not change during the course of administration. Additional studies have examined the use of subcutaneous rhGM-CSF in AIDS patients (44). Preliminary results indicate that all patients have more than tripled their predose white blood cell count to within 6 weeks of study entry. A dose response in leukocyte count was noted with increasing doses. Many lineages of white cells, including neutrophils, bands, eosinophils, and monocytes, were elevated. There has been no consistent change in viral activity in AIDS

patients receiving rhGM-CSF, suggesting that rhGM-CSF may lead to a decrease of the hematologic side effects associated with AZT administration.

INTERLEUKIN 1

IL-1α and IL-1β are structurally related proteins that recognize the same cell surface receptors. IL-1 exhibits a wide variety of biologic effects throughout the hematopoietic and immunologic systems (45–47). Clinical studies of rhIL-1 have shown accelerated hematopoiesis as monitored by neutrophil and platelet recovery after rhIL-1 alone and in combination with myelosuppressive chemotherapy (48–50). For example, Smith et al. (48) studied the effects of rhIL-1α administered intravenously to 28 patients with advanced malignancies at doses ranging from 0.01 to 1.0 μg/kg. rhIL-1α treatment was associated with increases in bone marrow cellularity and enhanced numbers of both myeloid cells and megakaryocytes (48). More recently, rhIL-1α was administered to 40 patients with non-Hodgkin's or Hodgkin's lymphoma after autologous transplantation. A trend to earlier neutrophil recovery and independence from RBC and platelet transfusion was associated with rhIL-1α therapy (51). However, the clinical toxicity of rhIL-1 is substantial, including fever, fatigue, chills, and dose-limiting hypotension. Taken together, these studies suggest that rhIL-1 will have limited value as a hematopoietic growth factor.

INTERLEUKIN 3

Biology and Preclinical Pharmacology

IL-3 is a pluripotent hematopoietin that acts at an earlier bone marrow progenitor level than either GM-CSF or G-CSF. The IL-3 gene is located very close to the GM-CSF gene on the long arm of chromosome 5. Its location here raises very interesting possibilities, in view of the association between leukemia, refractory anemia, and myelodysplastic syndrome that accompany chromosomal abnormalities involving the deletion of the long arm of chromosome 5.

Preclinical studies have shown that rhIL-3 functions as a multilineage hemopoietin in vivo by stimulating myelopoiesis, erythropoiesis, and thrombopoiesis in several murine and nonhuman primate models (16, 52–56). For example, previous studies have evaluated the use of rhIL-3 in nonhuman primates receiving multiple cycles of cyclophosphamide. rhIL-3 alone, when administered following cyclophosphamide, accelerated white blood cell and neutrophil recovery.

The hypothesis that various growth factors may act at different and overlapping stages of hematopoietic differentiation was based on in vitro data on stimulation of colony formation from murine, primate, and human bone marrow culture systems. Thus, factors such as rhIL-3, rhIL-6, or rhIL-1 may be necessary for early progenitor development or even possibly earlier to facilitate cells entering the cell cycle. Likewise, other factors, such as rhG-CSF or rhGM-CSF, may affect later stages of differentiation. Such terminology has led some investigators to consider the designation of factors as either class I (early acting) or class II (later acting) factors. Though this is an oversimplification, it does provide a framework for conceptualizing the sequential development, proliferation, maturation, and differentiation of bone marrow cells.

To test this hypothesis in vivo, investigations were set up in which growth factors were sequentially administered to primates. In such studies, the use of an early-acting growth factor, such as rhIL-3, was followed after a variable period of time by a later-acting factor, such as rhGM-CSF or rhGM-CSF administered both by continuous intravenous infusion and by subcutaneous administration.

In these studies, rhIL-3 has been administered for 7 to 21 days, followed by rhGM-CSF dosing. Specifically, a relatively lower dose of rhGM-CSF has been selected, which by itself would cause a moderate leukocytosis (e.g., a two- to threefold increase). A marked synergy was observed between the initial dose of rhIL-3 and rhGM-CSF, with which a relatively small dose (2 μg/kg intravenously for 8 to 14 days) results in a marked increase in white cells, including all lineages studied (16). A possible explanation for this phenomenon relates to the ability of rhIL-3 to expand the population of early progenitors that are sensitive to rhGM-CSF. Such studies are now being tested in states of marrow dysfunction. When similar experiments were done in which the order of drug administration was reversed (i.e., rhGM-CSF administered prior to rhIL-3), there was no additive or synergistic effect on myelopoiesis. Thus, there are a large number of possibilities for combination factor therapy, which are being evaluated preclinically and clinically.

Clinical Studies

Early phase I/II studies of rhIL-3 were conducted to investigate the effects of rhIL-3 in patients with normal hematopoiesis and advanced malignancies (57), bone marrow failure (57), aplastic anemia (58) or myelodysplastic syndrome (59, 60). Dose-dependent increases in neutrophils, eosinophils, and lymphocytes as well as platelet counts were observed in patients with normal hematopoietic function. Similarly, increases in circulating leukocytes and platelets were seen in patients with bone marrow failure secondary to chemotherapy, radiotherapy, or tumor infiltration. Side effects of rhIL-3 included fever, chills, headache, bone pain, and flushing.

Additional clinical testing of rhIL-3 has focused on its effects on chemotherapy-induced thrombocytopenia. D'Hondt et al. (61) performed a randomized double-blind, placebo-controlled trial of rhIL-3 alone, followed by combination chemotherapy with carboplatin, etoposide, and epirubicin, followed by a course of the same chemotherapy supported by rhIL-3 in 28 patients with small cell lung cancer. There were no significant differences between platelet nadirs or duration of nadirs of cycles 1 and 2; however, platelet counts after rhIL-3 rebounded higher (61).

Gianni et al. (62) examined the effects of rhIL-3 following cyclophosphamide chemotherapy in 12 patients with breast cancer. Again, there were no differences in platelet nadirs compared with historic controls. However, patients receiving rhIL-3 recovered platelets 3 days sooner, suggesting a modest effect of rhIL-3 on cyclophosphamide-induced thrombocytopenia. Biesma et al. (63) reported a decrease in chemotherapy treatment delays in patients with ovarian cancer who received cyclophosphamide, carboplatin, and rhIL-3 compared with patients not receiving rhIL-3. In contrast, Rusthoven et al. (64) showed no benefit of rhIL-3 in ovarian patients receiving carboplatin. Currently, phase III studies are under way to examine the effects of IL-3 on chemotherapy-induced thrombocytopenia.

INTERLEUKIN-6

IL-6 is a multifunctional cytokine that regulates the immune response, acute phase reaction, and hematopoiesis (65). Based on these various biologic activities, IL-6 has previously been named B-cell stimulatory factor-2, interferon-β2, hybridoma/plasmacytoma growth factor, and hepatocyte stimulatory factor. IL-6 stimulates murine and human granulocyte and granulocyte-macrophage colony formation and megakaryotic maturation in vitro (66–68). Early studies have shown that IL-6 acts synergistically with IL-3 to enhance the proliferation of murine multipotential progenitor cells (69). rhIL-6 also elevates platelet counts, bone marrow cellularity, and megakaryocyte size and ploidy in murine models and nonhuman primates (70, 71). Furthermore, rhIL-6 stimulates hematopoietic recovery after chemotherapy and radiation-induced myelosuppression (72, 73).

A phase I trial of rhIL-6 administered subcutaneously was performed in patients with advanced malignancies (74). Fever, chills, and fatigue were observed. Dose-dependent increases in platelet counts were seen in patients treated with 10 and 30 μg/kg rhIL-6. Similar results were seen in other phase I studies (75, 76). Demetri et al. (77) treated patients with sarcoma with doxorubicin (Adriamycin), ifosfamide, and DTIC and demonstrated a higher median platelet nadir in cycles with IL-6 and chemotherapy versus that with chemotherapy alone (77). A phase I/II trial of rhIL-6 and rhG-CSF was also performed in patients with non-small-cell lung cancer after chemotherapy with ifosfamide, carboplatin, etoposide, and mesna (78). Patients who received rhIL-6 had a more rapid platelet recovery, suggesting that rhIL-6 can decrease chemotherapy-associated thrombocytopenia. Additional clinical trials are ongoing to study the effects of rhIL-6 in accelerating hematopoiesis following myelosuppressive chemotherapy and bone marrow transplantation (79).

INTERLEUKIN-11

IL-11 is a bone marrow stroma–derived growth factor that stimulates hematopoiesis (80, 81). In combination with IL-3, IL-11 promotes megakaryocytopoiesis by stimulating the formation of colony-forming units–megakaryocyte (CFU-MKs) and burst-forming units–megakaryocyte (BFU-MKs). In addition, IL-11 promotes thrombopoiesis by increasing the size and ploidy of megakaryocytes (82). Other effects of IL-11 include stimulation of increases in DNA synthesis and immunoglobulin secretion by B cells (83), enhancement of CFU-E (84), production of acute-phase reactants (85), and inhibition of adipogenesis (86). The pharmacologic effects of IL-11 are summarized in Table 10.3.

Based on preclinical animal models in which

Table 10.3. Summary of Pharmacologic Effects of IL-11

- Increased platelet counts in all models examined
  Increased platelet progenitors (BFU-MK, CFU-MK)
  Shift to higher ploidy, when examined
- Increased leukocytes, primarily neutrophils, depending on model
  Increased myeloid progenitors in all models
- Data suggest potent effect on multilineage progenitor cell population in bone marrow
- Mild anemia in some models, although increased erythroid progenitors/precursors also seen in some models
- Increased acute-phase reactants noted in both in vitro and in vivo models

From Du XX, Williams DA. Interleukin-11: a multifunctional growth factor derived from the hematopoietic microenvironment. Blood 1994;83:2023–2030. With permission.

rhIL-11 significantly increases multilineage hematopoietic recovery after myelosuppressive therapy (87), Gordon et al. reported preliminary phase 1 results of IL-11 in women with advanced-stage breast cancer receiving high-dose cyclophosphamide and doxorubicin (88, 89). rhIL-11 was well tolerated and was associated with an increase in median platelet counts. rhIL-11 therapy was also associated with increases in the number and ploidy of megakaryocytes in the bone marrow (90). Recently, a phase II, randomized, double-blind, placebo-controlled study of rhIL-11 in patients with severe chemotherapy-induced thrombocytopenia demonstrated that significantly fewer rhIL-11-treated patients required platelet transfusions than did patients on placebo (J. Kaye, Genetics Institute, personal communication). The ultimate clinical benefit of rhIL-11 in the treatment and prevention of thrombocytopenia related to chemotherapy and bone marrow transplantation is undergoing further evaluation.

PIXY321

PIXY321 is a genetically engineered fusion protein consisting of the active domains of GM-CSF and IL-3 covalently linked by a synthetic amino acid linker sequence (91, 92). PIXY321 stimulates multipotential progenitor cells and colony-stimulating activity (90). Furthermore, PIXY321 enhances neutrophil and platelet recovery in sublethally radiated nonhuman primates (93). Vadhan-Raj et al. initiated a phase I/II study of PIXY321 in 24 patients with sarcoma who received chemotherapy with cyclophosphamide, doxorubicin, and dacarbazine (DTIC)

(CyADIC). Following chemotherapy, PIXY321 treatment was associated with a reduction in WBC nadir and duration of neutropenia. In addition, mean platelet nadirs were higher than those of historic controls (94). Other investigators have reported similar results in patients with breast, ovarian, or gastrointestinal cancer receiving chemotherapy and in patients with lymphoma following high-dose chemotherapy and autologous bone marrow transplantation (95–100). Phase III studies of PIXY321 in patients undergoing autologous bone marrow transplantation for lymphoma are ongoing.

THROMBOPOIETIN

In 1990, a retrovirus that induces an acute myeloproliferative syndrome in mice was described. The cellular homologue of the viral oncogene was named c-mpl (myeloproliferative leukemia) and found to encode for a hematopoietic growth factor receptor. Inhibition of the c-mpl receptor selectively reduced megakaryocyte proliferation. The recent isolation and cloning of the c-mpl ligand has led to the discovery of thrombopoietin (101–104). This purified protein stimulates the proliferation and polyploidization of megakaryocyte precursors, leading to increases in platelet counts when administered to normal mice. The clinical potential of this new growth factor to stimulate platelet recovery after chemotherapy or bone marrow transplantation remains to be shown.

ERYTHROPOIETIN

Erythropoietin (rhEpo) is an erythroid growth and differentiation factor that acts exclusively on committed erythroid progenitor and precursor cells. In vivo, erythropoietin produces an increase in erythropoiesis and new red blood cells. Patients with anemia and cancer have decreased serum levels of immunoreactive erythropoietin, compared with patients with iron-deficiency anemia (105). In addition, erythropoietin production is decreased after chemotherapy (105), suggesting a role for chemotherapy-associated nephrotoxicity.

Ludwig et al. (106) treated 13 patients with multiple myeloma and anemia with rhEpo. Eleven patients had a sustained increase in hemoglobin levels and improvement in the sense of well-being. The number of BFU-Es in both bone marrow and peripheral blood increased during rhEpo treatment (106). Oster et al. (107)

used rhEpo to treat 6 patients with non-Hodgkin's lymphoma or multiple myeloma with bone marrow involvement. Five patients had stimulation of erythropoiesis with significant increases in hemoglobin and hematocrit. Randomized, double-blind, placebo-controlled trials were conducted to evaluate rhEpo in cancer patients with anemia who received combination chemotherapy (108, 109). Statistically significant increases in hematocrits, improvement in energy level, and a trend toward reduction in RBC transfusions were associated with rhEpo treatment (108). rhEpo is also useful in the treatment of anemia in zidovudine (AZT)-treated patients infected with HIV (110).

SUMMARY

The use of hematopoietic growth factors in the practice of oncology has reduced the likelihood of complications related to bone marrow suppression following standard chemotherapy or high-dose cytotoxic therapy and bone marrow transplantation. In addition to their benefit for neutropenic fever and infection, other outcomes including chemotherapy dose intensity, quality of life, and cost benefit are under investigation. Recently, an expert panel convened by the American Society of Clinical Oncology published clinical practice guidelines on the use of hematopoietic growth factors (111). These recommendations as well as further research will provide additional information on the optimal use of hematopoietic growth factors in the adjuvant treatment of cancer.

REFERENCES

1. Clark SC, Kamen R. The human hematopoietic colony-stimulating factors. Science 1987;236:1229–1237.

2. Sieff CA. Hematopoietic growth factors. J Clin Invest 1987;79:1549–1557.

3. Golde DW, Gasson JC. Hormones that stimulate the growth of blood cells. Sci Am 1988;259:62–71.

4. Groopman JE, Molina J-M, Scadden DT. Hematopoietic growth factors. Biology and clinical applications. N Engl J Med 1989;321:1449–1459.

5. Laver J, Moore MAS. Clinical use of recombinant human hematopoietic growth factors. J Natl Cancer Inst 1989;81:1370–1382.

6. Till JE, McCulloch EA. A direct measurement of the radiation sensitivity of normal mouse bone marrow cells. Radiat Res 1961;14:213–222.

7. Pluznik DH, Sachs L. The cloning of normal "mast" cells in tissue culture. J Cell Comp Physiol 1965;66:319–324.

8. Metcalf D, Bradley TR, Robinson W. Analysis of

colonies developing in vitro from mouse bone marrow cells stimulated by kidney feeder layers or leukemic serum. J Cell Physiol 1967;69:93–108.

9. Donahue RE, Wang EA, Stone DK, et al. Stimulation of hematopoiesis in primates by continuous infusion of recombinant human GM-CSF. Nature 1986; 321:872–875.

10. Mayer P, Lam C, Obenaus H, Liehl E, Besemer J. Recombinant human GM-CSF induces leukocytosis and activates peripheral blood polymorphonuclear neutrophils in nonhuman primates. Blood 1987; 70:206–213.

11. Welte K, Bonilla MA, Gillio AP, et al. Recombinant human granulocyte colony-stimulating factor. Effects on hematopoiesis in normal and cyclophosphamide-treated primates. J Exp Med 1987;165:941–948.

12. Nienhuis AW, Donahue RE, Karlsson S, et al. Recombinant human granulocyte-macrophage colony stimulating factor (GM-CSF) shortens the period of neutropenia after autologous bone marrow transplantation in a primate model. J Clin Invest 1987;80:573–577.

13. Monroy RL, Skelly RR, Taylor P, Dubois A, Donahue RE, MacVittie TJ. Recovery from severe hematopoietic suppression using recombinant human granulocyte-macrophage colony-stimulating factor. Exp Hematol 1988;16:344–348.

14. Bonilla MA, Gillio AP, Potter GK, O'Reilly RJ, Souza LM, Welte K. Effects of recombinant human G-CSF and GM-CSF on cytopenias associated with repeated cycles of chemotherapy in primates (abstract). Blood 1987;70(Suppl 1):130a.

15. Donahue RE, Seehra J, Norton C, et al. Hematologic effects of recombinant human interleukin-3 (rhIL-3) and granulocyte/macrophage colony-stimulating factor (rhGM-CSF) in primates (abstract). Proc Am Soc Clin Oncol 1988;7:162.

16. Donahue RE, Seehra J, Metzger M, et al. Human IL-3 and GM-CSF act synergistically in stimulating hematopoiesis in primates. Science 1988;241:1820–1823.

17. Bronchud MH, Scarffe JH, Thatcher N, et al. Phase I/II study of recombinant human granulocyte colony-stimulating factor in patients receiving intensive chemotherapy for small cell lung cancer. Br J Cancer 1987;56:809–813.

18. Morstyn G, Souza LM, Keech J, et al. Effect of granulocyte colony stimulating factor on neutropenia induced by cytotoxic chemotherapy. Lancet 1988(Mar 26);667–672.

19. Gabrilove JL, Jakubowski A, Scher H, et al. Effect of granulocyte colony-stimulating factor on neutropenia and associated morbidity due to chemotherapy for transitional-cell carcinoma of the urothelium. N Engl J Med 1988;318:1414–1422.

20. Crawford J, Ozer H, Stoller R, et al. Reduction by granulocyte colony-stimulating factor of fever and neutropenia induced by chemotherapy in patients with small-cell lung cancer. N Engl J Med 1991; 325:164–170.

21. Bonilla MA, Gillio AP, Ruggeiro M, et al. Effects of recombinant human granulocyte colony-stimulating factor on neutropenia in patients with congenital agranulocytosis. N Engl J Med 1989;320:1574–1580.

22. Dale DC, Bonilla MA, Davis MW, et al. A randomized controlled phase III trial of recombinant human granulocyte colony-stimulating factor (filgrastim) for treatment of severe chronic neutropenia. Blood 1993;81:2496–2502.

23. Trillet-Lenoir V, Green J, Manegold C, et al. Recombinant granulocyte colony-stimulating factor reduces the infectious complications of cytotoxic chemotherapy. Eur J Cancer 1993;29A:319–324.

24. Pettengell R, Gurney H, Radford JA, et al. Granulocyte colony-stimulating factor to prevent dose-limiting neutropenia in non-Hodgkin's lymphoma: a randomized controlled trial. Blood 1992;80:1430–1436.

25. Stahel RA, Muller E, Pichert G, et al. Dose intensification with autologous marrow support in high-risk lymphoma: acceleration of hematopoietic recovery and reduction of days of hospitalization with granulocyte colony-stimulating factor (G-CSF) in randomized open-label trial (abstract). Proc Am Soc Clin Oncol 1992;11:331.

26. Metcalf D, Burgess A, Johnson G, et al. In vitro actions on hematopoietic cells of recombinant murine GM-CSF purified after production in *Escherichia coli*: comparison with purified native GM-CSF. J Cell Physiol 1986;128:421–431.

27. Sieff C, Emerson S, Donahue R, et al. Human recombinant granulocyte-macrophage colony-stimulating factor: a multilineage hemopoietin. Science 1985; 230:1171–1173.

28. Kaushansky K, O'Hara P, Berkner K, et al. Genomic cloning, characterization, and multilineage growth-promoting activity of human granulocyte-macrophage colony-stimulating factor. Proc Natl Acad Sci USA 1986;83:3101–3105.

29. Gasson J, Weisbart R, Kaufman S, et al. Purified human granulocyte-macrophage colony-stimulating factor: direct action on neutrophils. Science 1984; 226:1339–1342.

30. Metcalf D, Begley CG, Johnson GR, et al. Biologic properties in vitro of a recombinant human granulocyte-macrophage colony-stimulating factor. Blood 1986;67:37–45.

31. Fleischmann J, Golde D, Weisbart R, et al. Granulocyte-macrophage colony-stimulating factor enhances phagocytosis of bacteria by human neutrophils. Blood 1986;68:708–711.

32. Grabstein K, Urdal D, Tushinski R, et al. Induction of macrophage tumoricidal activity by granulocyte-macrophage colony-stimulating factor. Science 1986;232:506–508.

33. Brandt SJ, Peters WP, Atwater SK, et al. Effect of recombinant human granulocyte-macrophage colony-stimulating factor on hematopoietic reconstitution after high-dose chemotherapy and autologous bone marrow transplantation. N Engl J Med 1988;319:869–876.

34. Nemunaitis J, Singer JW, Buckner CD, et al. Use of recombinant human granulocyte-macrophage colony-stimulating factor in autologous bone marrow transplantation for lymphoid malignancies. Blood 1988;72:834–836.

35. Nemunaitis J, Rabinowe SN, Singer JW, et al. Recombinant granulocyte-macrophage colony-stimulating factor after autologous bone marrow transplantation for lymphoid cancer. N Engl J Med 1991; 324:1773–1778.

36. Rabinowe SN, Neuberg D, Bierman PJ. Long-term follow-up of a phase III study of recombinant hu-

man granulocyte-macrophage colony-stimulating factor after autologous bone marrow transplantation for lymphoid malignancies. Blood 1993;81:1903–1908.

37. Nemunaitis J, Singer JW, Buckner CD, et al. Long-term follow-up of patients who received recombinant human granulocyte-macrophage colony-stimulating factor after autologous bone marrow transplantation for lymphoid malignancy. Bone Marrow Transplant 1990;7:49–52.

38. Ester EH, Dixon D, Kantarjian H, et al. Treatment of poor-prognosis, newly diagnosed acute myeloid leukemia with Ara-C and recombinant human granulocyte-macrophage colony-stimulating factor. Blood 1990;75:1766–1769.

39. Buchner T, Hiddemann W, Koenigsmann M, et al. Recombinant human granulocyte-macrophage colony-stimulating factor after chemotherapy in patients with acute myeloid leukemia at higher age or after relapse. Blood 1991;78:1190–1197.

40. Blazar BR, Kersey JH, McGlave PB, et al. In vivo administration of recombinant human granulocyte-macrophage colony-stimulating factor in acute lymphoblastic leukemia patients receiving purged autografts. Blood 1989;73:849–857.

41. Antman KS, Griffin JD, Elias A, et al. Effect of recombinant human granulocyte-macrophage colony-stimulating factor on chemotherapy-induced myelosuppression. N Engl J Med 1988;319:593–598.

42. Vadhan-Raj S, Keating M, LeMaistre A, et al. Effects of recombinant human granulocyte-macrophage colony-stimulating factor in patients with myelodysplastic syndromes. N Engl J Med 1987;317:1545–1552.

43. Groopman JE, Mitsuyasu RT, DeLeo MJ, Oette DH, Golde DW. Effect of recombinant human granulocyte-macrophage colony-stimulating factor on myelopoiesis in the acquired immunodeficiency syndrome. N Engl J Med 1987;317:593–598.

44. Mitsuyasu RT, DeLeo M, Miles SA, et al. Effects of long term subcutaneous (SC) administration of recombinant granulocyte macrophage colony stimulating factor (GM-CSF) in patients with HIV-related leukopenia (abstract). Blood 1988;72(Suppl):356a.

45. Dinarello CA, Interleukin-1 and interleukin-1 antagonist. Blood 1991;77:1627–1652.

46. Dinarello CA, Wolff SM. The role of interleukin-1 in disease. N Engl J Med 1993;328:106–113.

47. Bagby GC Jr. Interleukin-1 and hematopoiesis. Blood Rev 1989;3:152–161.

48. Smith JW II, Urba WJ, Curti BD, et al. The toxic and hematological effects of interleukin-1 alpha administered in a phase I trial to patients with advanced malignancies. J Clin Oncol 1992;10:1141–1152.

49. Crown J, Jakubowski A, Kemeny N, et al. A phase I trial of recombinant human interleukin-1β alone and in combination with myelosuppressive doses of 5-fluorouracil in patients with gastrointestinal cancer. Blood 1991;78:1420–1427.

50. Smith JW II, Longo DL, Alvord WG, et al. The effects of treatment with interleukin-1α on platelet recovery after high-dose carboplatin, N Engl J Med 1993;328:756–761.

51. Weisdorf D, Katsanis, Verfaille C, et al. Interleukin-1α administered after autologous transplantation: a phase I/II clinical trial. Blood 1994;84:2044–2049.

52. Kindler V, Thorens B, de Kossodo S, et al. Stim-ulation of hematopoiesis in vivo by recombinant bacterial murine interleukin 3. Proc Natl Acad Sci USA 1986;83:1001–1005.

53. Metcalf D, Begley CG, Johnson GR, et al. Effects of purified bacterially synthesized murine multi-CSF (IL-3) on hematopoiesis in normal adult mice. Blood 1986;68:46–57.

54. Broxmeyer HE, Williams D, Hangoc G, et al. Synergistic myelopoietic actions in vivo after administration to mice of combinations of purified natural murine colony-stimulating factor 1, recombinant murine interleukin 3, and recombinant murine granulocyte/macrophage colony-stimulating factor. Proc Natl Acad Sci USA 1987;84:3871–3875.

55. Krumwieh D, Seiler FR. In vivo effects of recombinant colony stimulating factors on hematopoiesis in cynomolgus monkeys. Transplant Proc 1989; 21:2964–2967.

56. Mayer P, Valent P, Schmidt G, et al. The in vivo effect of recombinant human interleukin-3: demonstration of basophil differentiation factor, histamine-producing activity and priming of GM-CSF-responsive progenitors in nonhuman primates. Blood 1989; 74:613–621.

57. Ganser A, Lindemann A, Seipelt G, et al. Effect of recombinant human interleukin-3 in patients with normal hematopoiesis and in patients with bone marrow failure. Blood 1990;76:666–676.

58. Ganser A, Lindemann A, Seipelt G, et al. Effects of recombinant human interleukin-3 in aplastic anemia. Blood 1990;76:1287–1292.

59. Ganser A, Lindemann A, Seipelt G, et al. Effects of recombinant human interleukin-3 in patients with myelodysplastic syndromes. Blood 1990;76:455–462.

60. Kurzrock R, Talpaj M, Estrov Z, et al. Phase I study of recombinant human interleukin-3 in patients with bone marrow failure. J Clin Oncol 1991;9:1241–1250.

61. D'Hondt V, Weynants P, Humblet Y, et al. Dose-dependent IL-3 stimulation of thrombopoiesis and neutropoiesis in patients with small cell lung carcinoma before and following chemotherapy. A placebo controlled randomized phase Ib study. J Clin Oncol 1993;11:2063–2071.

62. Gianni AM, Siena S, Bregni M, et al. Recombinant human interleukin-3 hastens trilineage hematopoietic recovery following high-dose (7 mg/m²) cyclophosphamide cancer therapy. Ann Oncol 1993;4:759–766.

63. Biesma B, Willemse PHB, Mulden NH, et al. Effects of interleukin-3 after chemotherapy for advanced ovarian cancer. Blood 1992;80:1141–1148.

64. Rusthoven JJ, Eisenhauser E, Mazurka J, et al. Phase 1 clinical trial of recombinant human interleukin-3 combined with carboplatin in the treatment of patients with recurrent ovarian carcinoma. J Natl Cancer Inst 1993;85:823–825.

65. Kishimoto T. The biology of interleukin-6. Blood 1989;74:1–10.

66. Caraccido D, Clark SC, Rovera G. Human interleukin-6 supports granulocytic differentiation of hematopoietic cells and acts synergistically with GM-CSF. Blood 1989;73:666–670.

67. Gardner JD, Liechty KW, Christensen RD. Effects of interleukin-6 on fetal hematopoietic progenitors. Blood 1990;75:2150–2155.

68. Lotem J, Shabo Y, Sachs L. Regulation of mega-

karyocyte development by interleukin-6. Blood 1989; 74:1545–1551.

69. Ikebuchi K, Wong GG, Clark SC, et al. Interleukin-6 enhancement of interleukin-3-dependent proliferation of multipotential hematopoietic progenitors. Proc Natl Acad Sci USA 1987;84:9035–9039.

70. Asano S, Okano A, Ozawa K, et al. In vivo effects of recombinant human interleukin-6 in primates: stimulated production of platelets. Blood 1990; 75:1602–1605.

71. Ulich TR, del Castillo J, Guo K. In vivo hematologic effects of recombinant interleukin-6 on hematopoiesis and circulating numbers of RBCs and WBCs. Blood 1989;73:108–110.

72. Takatsuki F, Okano A, Suzuki C, et al. Interleukin-6 perfusion stimulator reconstitution of the immune and hematopoietic systems after 5-fluorouracil treatment. Cancer Res 1990;50:2885–2890.

73. Patchen ML, MacVittie TJ, Williams JL, et al. Administration of interleukin-6 stimulates multilineage hematopoiesis and accelerates recovery from radiation-induced hematopoietic depression. Blood 1991;77:472–480.

74. Weber J, Yang JC, Topalian SL, et al. Phase I trial of subcutaneous interleukin-6 in patients with advanced malignancies. J Clin Oncol 1993;11:499–506.

75. D'Hondt V, Humblet Y, Guillaume TH, et al. Thrombopoietic effects and toxicity of interleukin-6 in patients with ovarian cancer before and after chemotherapy: a multicentric placebo-controlled, randomized phase Ib study. Blood 1995;85:2347–2353.

76. Van Ganseren MM, Willemse PHB, Mulder NH, et al. Effects of recombinant human interleukin-6 in cancer patients: a phase I-II study. Blood 1994; 84:1434–1441.

77. Demetri GD, Bukowski RM, Samuels B, et al. Stimulation of thrombopoiesis by recombinant human interleukin-6 (IL-6) pre- and post-chemotherapy in previously untreated sarcoma patients with normal hematopoiesis (abstract). Blood 1993;82(Suppl 1):367a.

78. Ritch PS, Schiller J, Rivkin S, et al. Phase I elevation of recombinant human interleukin-6 (abstract). Blood 1993;82(Suppl 1):367a.

79. Willemse PHB, van Gamoren MM, Mulder NH, et al. Interleukin-6 as platelet stimulator in cancer patients (abstract). Proc Am Soc Clin Oncol 1994;13:448.

80. Paul SR, Bennett F, Calvetti JA, et al. Molecular cloning of a cDNA encoding interleukin 11, a stromal cell-derived lymphopoietic and hematopoietic cytokine. Proc Natl Acad Sci USA 1990;87:7512–7516.

81. Du XX, Williams DA. Interleukin-11. A multifunctional growth factor derived from the hematopoietic microenvironment. Blood 1994;83:2023–2030.

82. Yonemura Y, Kawakita M, Masuda T, et al. Synergistic effects of interleukin 3 and interleukin 11 on murine megakaryopoiesis in serum-free culture. Exp Hematol 1992;20:1011–1016.

83. Anderson KC, Morimoto C, Paul SR, et al. Interleukin-11 promotes accessory cell-dependent B-cell differentiation in humans. Blood 1992;80:2797–2804.

84. Quesniaux VFJ, Clark SC, Turner K, Fagg B. Interleukin-11 stimulates multiple phases of erythropoietin in vitro. Blood 1992;80:1218–1223.

85. Baumann H, Schendel P. Interleukin-11 regulates the hepatic expression of the same plasma protein genes as interleukin-6. J Biol Chem 1991;266:20424–20427.

86. Kawashima I, Ohsumi J, Mita-Honjo K, et al. Molecular cloning of cDNA encoding adipogenesis inhibiting factor and identity with interleukin-11. FEBS Lett 1991;283:199–202.

87. Leonard JP, Quinto CM, Kozitza MK, et al. Recombinant human interleukin-11 stimulates multilineage hematopoietic recovery in mice following a myelosuppressive regimen of sublethal irradiation and carboplatin. Blood 1994;83:1499–1506.

88. Gordon MS, Sledge GW, Battiato L, et al. The in vivo effects of subcutaneously (SC) administered recombinant human interleukin-11 (Neumega rhIL-11 growth factor; rhIL-11) in women with breast cancer (BC) (abstract). Blood 1993;82(Suppl 1):498a.

89. Gordon MS, Battiato L, Hoffman R, et al. Subcutaneously (SC) administered recombinant human interleukin-11 (Neumega rhIL-11 growth factor; rhIL-11) prevents thrombocytopenia following chemotherapy (CT) with cyclophosphamide (C) and doxorubicin (A) in women with breast cancer (abstract). Blood 1993; 82(Suppl 1):318a.

90. Orazi A, Cooper R, Tong J, et al. Recombinant human interleukin-11 (Neumega rhIL-11 growth factor; rhIL-11) has multiple profound effects on human hematopoiesis (abstract). Blood 1993;82(Suppl 1):369a.

91. Curtis BM, Williams DE, Broxmeyer HE, et al. Enhanced hematopoietic activity of a human granulocyte/macrophage colony-stimulating factor-interleukin 3 fusion protein. Proc Natl Acad Sci USA 1991; 88:5809–5813.

92. Williams DE, Park LS, Broxmeyer HE, et al. Hybrid cytokines as hematopoietic growth factors. Int J Cell Clon 1991;9:542–547.

93. Williams DE, Dunn JT, Park LS, et al. In vivo effects of a GM-CSF/IL-3 fusion protein (PIXY321) in sublethally irradiated monkeys. Biotechnol Ther 1993; 4:17–29.

94. Vadhan-Raj S, Papadopoulos NE, Burgess MA, et al. Effects of PIXY321, a granulocyte-macrophage colony-stimulating factor/interleukin-3 fusion protein, on chemotherapy-induced multilineage myelosuppression in patients with sarcoma. J Clin Oncol 1994; 12:715–724.

95. Collins D, Livingston RB, Ellis G, Caron D. Effect of PXY321 on hematologic recovery after high-dose cyclophosphamide (CTX), etoposide (VP-16) and cisplatin (CDDP)CEP) in women with breast carcinoma (abstract). Blood 1993;82(Suppl 1):366a.

96. Jakubowski A, Raptis G, Gilewski T, et al. Phase I/II trial of PIXY321 (PIXY) in patients (PTS) with metastatic breast cancer receiving doxorubicin and thiotepa (abstract). Blood 1992;80 (Suppl 1):88a.

97. Miller L, Smith J II, Urba W, et al. A phase I study of an IL-3/GM-CSF fusion protein (PIXY321) and high-dose carboplatin (CBDCA) in patients with advanced cancer (abstract). Proc Am Soc Clin Oncol 1993;12:138.

98. Runowicz CD, Mandeli J, Speyer J, et al. Phase I/II study of PIXY321 in combination with cyclophosphamide (CTX) and carboplatin (CP) in the treatment of patients (PTS) with ovarian cancer (OC) (abstract). Proc Am Soc Clin Oncol 1993;12:260.

99. Taylor C, Modiano M, Garrison L, et al. PIXY plus carboplatin (C) and Adriamycin (A) in patients with advanced gastrointestinal (GI) malignancy (abstract). Proc Am Soc Clin Oncol 1993;12:195.

100. Vose JM, Anderson J, Bierman PJ, et al. Initial

trial of PIXY321 (GM-CSF/IL-3 fusion protein) following high-dose chemotherapy and autologous bone marrow transplantation (ABMT) for lymphoid malignancy (abstract). Proc Am Soc Clin Oncol 1993;12:366.

101. de Sauvage FJ, Hass PE, Spencer SD, et al. Stimulation of megakaryocytopoiesis and thrombopoiesis by the cMpl ligand. Nature 1994;369:533–538.

102. Lok S, Kaushansky K, Holly RD, et al. Cloning and expression of murine thrombopoietin cDNA and stimulation of platelet production in vivo. Nature 1994; 369:565–568.

103. Kaushansky K, Lok S, Holly RD, et al. Promotion of megakaryocyte progenitor expansion and differentiation by the cMpl ligand thrombopoietin. Nature 1994;369:568–571.

104. Wendling F, Maraskovsky E, Debili N, et al. c-Mpl ligand is a humoral regulator of megakaryocytopoiesis. Nature 1994;369:571–574.

105. Miller CB, Jones RJ, Piantodosi S, et al. Decreased erythropoietin response in patients with the anemia of cancer. N Engl J Med 1990;322:1689–1692.

106. Ludwig H, Fritz E, Kotzmann H, et al. Erythropoietin treatment of anemia associated with multiple myeloma. N Engl J Med 1990;322:1693–1699.

107. Oster W, Herrmann F, Gamm H, et al. Erythropoietin for the treatment of anemia of malignancy associated with neoplastic bone marrow infiltration. J Clin Oncol 1990;8:956–962.

108. Case DC Jr, Bukowski RM, Carey RW, et al. Recombinant human erythropoietin therapy for anemic cancer patients on combination chemotherapy. J Natl Cancer Inst 1993;85:801–806.

109. Platanias LC, Miller CB, Mick R, et al. Treatment of chemotherapy-induced anemia with recombinant human erythropoietin in cancer patients. J Clin Oncol 1991;9:2021–2026.

110. Fischl M, Galpin JE, Levine JD, et al. Recombinant human erythropoietin for patients with AIDS treated with zidovudine. N Engl J Med 1990;322:1488–1493.

111. American Society of Clinical Oncology recommendations for the use of hematopoietic colony-stimulating factors. Evidence-based, clinical practice guidelines. J Clin Oncol 1994;12:2471–2508.

11

Biologic Response Modifiers: Principles of Immunotherapy

Majd Chahin and Howard Ozer

Cancer treatment has traditionally involved three modalities of therapy: surgery, radiotherapy, and chemotherapy. Over the past decade, a fourth modality of cancer treatment has emerged, biotherapy. While surgery and radiotherapy primarily deal with local treatment of cancer, chemotherapy and biotherapy generally deal with systemic control of metastatic disease. The field of biotherapy not only encompasses tumor immunology but also draws from the fields of molecular biology, recombinant genetics, and hybridoma technology. Biologic response modifiers (BRMs) refer to either natural biologic substances or methods by which the host-tumor interaction is altered, thus producing an antitumor effect. Their mechanisms of action are diverse but may include direct antitumor effects by interfering with cell growth and transformation or metastatic potential or by activating effector cells of the immune system, which then exhibit tumoricidal activity.

The earliest evidence suggesting the existence of an immune response to tumors occurred almost a century ago when Coley observed spontaneous regression of tumors in patients recovering from an acute infection and attempted to treat cancer patients with an extract called Coley's toxin (1). Spontaneous regression has occasionally, if rarely, been observed in a variety of malignancies, particularly melanoma and renal cell carcinoma (2, 3). This observation led to early attempts to immunize the tumor-bearing host by the administration of nonspecific immune adjuvants such as bacillus Calmette-Guerin (BCG), *Corynebacterium parvum*, or levamisole, or by the administration of tumor cells or their extracts used as vaccines. By and large, this form of active immunotherapy has been unsuc-

cessful in humans and hence has been abandoned (4).

However, as the understanding of tumor immunology progressed, new types of immunomodulators in the form of cytokines were discovered. Cytokines are soluble proteins secreted by cells of the immune system, either lymphocytes or monocytes, which then exert their growth regulatory action on other target cells. They may function as true hormones, for they circulate systemically, bind to specific receptors, and alter cellular activities (5). The two families of cytokines most extensively characterized and investigated are the interferons and the interleukins. Interferons, comprising three major species—α, β, and γ–were first discovered more than 30 years ago and initially characterized by their antiviral properties (6, 7). Much progress has been made in the understanding of how interferons exert their antiviral, antiproliferative, and immune modulator effects, and these are discussed below. The other group of cytokines is termed interleukins (meaning *between leukocytes*), and these comprise the means by which cells of the immune system communicate with each other. They were first identified by the function they exhibited in in vitro assays and were named accordingly—for example, macrophage-activating factor or T-cell growth factor (8).

Initial efforts to use cytokines in cancer therapy were hampered by cumbersome, difficult techniques of purification and characterization of these substances. Two important developments have occurred that have opened the doors for the investigation of biologic response modifiers. Recombinant DNA technology permitted the cloning and sequencing of specific genes of interest, which can then be inserted via plasmid transfection into a microorganism (usually *Escherichia coli* or yeast). The transformed microorganisms proliferate in vitro and then produce the desired gene product. This technique allows the large-scale production of extremely pure biologic substances that maintain their biologic activity. Hence, recombinant forms of cytokines can be mass produced for use in large clinical trials.

The other major technical advance in the field of immunotherapy was the discovery of hybridoma technology. Prior to this development, the use of antibody therapy was extremely limited because the only source of antibodies was from immunized animals and exhibited vast heterogeneity. The hybridoma technique, which fuses a reactive B lymphocyte to an immortal myeloma cell line, permits the production of highly purified and monospecific monoclonal antibodies (9). These monoclonal antibodies have proven to be powerful tools in the identification and characterization of tumor-associated antigens and, subsequently, in the diagnosis and treatment of tumors that express these antigens. In addition, monoclonal antibodies have aided tremendously in the characterization of various effector cells of the immune system and in the isolation of the biologic substances that they produce.

The development and application of interleukins have not only served to greatly increase our knowledge of the immune system but also opened novel avenues for cancer treatment, including the application of adoptive immunotherapy. Described and developed by Rosenberg and colleagues, this technique involves the generation ex vivo of lymphocytes called lymphokine-activated killer cells (LAKs) activated by interleukin-2 (IL-2) (10). Advances in this area have led to phase I/II clinical trials and show promise in treating certain types of cancer. Building on this technique of adoptive cellular immunotherapy, new directions are under way using IL-2 in conjunction with tumor-infiltrating lymphocytes, which appear to have even greater tumoricidal activity than LAK cells or IL-2 coupled to toxins.

Along with the identification and development of biologic response modifiers, new methodology has been required for the screening and evaluation of potential new agents. Preclinical screening of a biologic agent may require determination of its effects on normal immune effector-cell function rather than the cytotoxic effects on target tumor cells used in preclinical screening of cytotoxic agents. Both in vitro and in vivo models may be used in the initial screening, adding to time and cost in its development. After the initial evaluation of a BRM, it is then tested at various doses and schedules to determine the maximal enhancement of effector cell function without compromise to other immunologic responses. Phase I clinical trials with BRMs are designed to determine toxicities and side effects of the agent and the maximum tolerated dose (MTD). However, the MTD may not correlate with the most efficacious dose for biologic activity, or optimum biologic dose (OBD). For a BRM, dose escalation should be performed in cohorts of patients, because chronic administration of a BRM may produce tachyphylaxis or a cumulative toxicity, thus underestimating or overestimating the MTD of a single dose. Phase II trials to determine the efficacy of a BRM among various malignancies and phase III trials to compare a BRM to standard therapy, are conducted as with cytotoxic agents (11).

The field of biotherapy, though still in its infancy, has made vast progress in the past decade. Through techniques of genetic engineering, including recombinant DNA and hybridoma technology, highly purified biologics have been produced in large quantities and are now in clinical trials in a multitude of settings. A variety are now approved for general use or are in clinical trials, and many more are likely to be so over the next few years.

INTERFERONS

The interferons comprise a group of naturally occurring glycoproteins that have potent immunomodulating properties. They were first discovered in 1957 by Issacs and Lindenmann (6, 7). There are two categories of interferons: type I (IFN-α and IFN-β) and type II (IFN-γ) (12). These differ in their antigenic, biologic, and chemical properties, as well as their inducers and the cell source from which they are derived. Type I interferons are acid stable and could be produced by all human cells, although those used in clinical trials have been induced either in leukocytes or lymphoblastoid cell lines (α) or in fibroblasts or endothelial cells (β). Type II (IFN-γ) is produced only by T lymphocytes and natural killer (NK) cells. It is acid labile and its actions are mediated through separate receptors; IFN-α and IFN-β can compete for the same cell surface receptors. Genes for all types of IFNs have been sequenced and cloned (13). α-Interferons that are produced by recombinant DNA techniques are nonglycosylated and have a substitute amino acid at position 23 (arginine is IFN-α_{2a}, methionine is IFN-α_{2b}). Recombinant IFN-β is produced in *E. coli* using site-specific mutagenesis to replace serine for cysteine at the 17 position (14).

Mechanisms of Action

The specific mechanisms by which IFNs exert their antineoplastic effects remain unclear. IFN first binds to specific cell surface receptors. This complex is then internalized, where the receptors are reprocessed and returned to the cell surface. Intracellular IFN then acts by gene activation, resulting in decreased synthesis of some proteins while increasing synthesis of other proteins. IFN-α and IFN-β have a primary role in autocrine regulation of all growth and proliferation, but IFN-γ does not. Both IFN-α and IFN-β produce marked prolongation of each phase of the cell cycle, with a resultant increase in the percentage of cells arrested in the G_0 phase. They do not, however, greatly affect the rate of macromolecular synthesis. For example, IFN will decrease the rate of thymidine incorporation in a large number of cell types by affecting thymidine uptake and transport rather than by a direct effect on DNA synthesis (15). The resulting cytostatic and sometimes cytocidal effect produced by this prolongation of the cell cycle is felt to, in part, explain the antiviral and antiproliferative mechanism of IFNs.

Certain enzyme systems have been identified that implicate several biochemical pathways in the IFNs' mechanisms of action (16). For example, IFN induces 2',5'-oligoadenylate synthetase, an enzyme that catalyzes the synthesis of oligonucleotides that in turn activate an endoribonuclease that then catalyzes the cleavage of viral and cellular RNA. Rosenblum et al. showed that there is a correlation between the level of 2',5'-oligoadenylate synthetase in malignant lymphoid cells and in vivo sensitivity and resistance of CML cells to IFN-α (17). Indoleamine 2,3-deoxygenase, induced by IFN-α and IFN-β, degrades intracellular tryptophan, a precursor to certain physiologically important coenzymes.

IFN induces certain protein kinases and phosphodiesterases that degrade RNA or inhibit RNA transcription, leading to a halt in new protein synthesis (18). In addition, IFNs can modulate cell differentiation. They can reverse the malignant phenotype of tumor cells in vitro and have been shown to decrease their tumorogen-

icity in vivo. This effect is thought to be secondary to inhibition or downregulation of oncogene expression. IFNs are known to influence the expression of *c-myc*, *c-h ras*, and *c-abl* oncogenes (19). Similarly, IFN can influence the expression of endogenous or transfected *ras* oncogene expression; when murine 3T3 cells transformed by *HA-ras* oncogenes are exposed to IFN-α/β, a significant reduction in *ras* messenger RNA transcription and *ras* protein p21 production occurs, concomitant with a reversal of transformed phenotype and tumorogenicity (20).

Another primary IFN-induced effect on cell differentiation is thought to be modulation of the expression of major histocompatibility complex (MCH) antigens. These antigens play a primordial role in self-nonself recognition. Class I antigens, HLA-A, -B, and -C in humans, are normally expressed on the surface of most cells of the body and are involved in target recognition by cytotoxic/suppressor (CD8+) T cells. IFN-α and IFN-β primarily induce class I antigens.

Class II antigens, HLA-DP, -DQ, and -DR in humans, are found on certain cell types of the immune system, including macrophages, T cells, B cells, and Langerhans cells, and are important in all cell recognition and interaction of immune cells. Class II antigens are primarily induced by IFN-γ. Enhanced antigen expression in some tumor cells, by effect on (MHC) antigens, may play an important role in immune regulation of these tumors (21).

The effects of IFNs on cells of the immune system and their interactions are numerous and complex; virtually all immunologic cell types are affected by IFNs. Macrophages produce IFN-α and IFN-γ in response to virus double-stranded RNA and endotoxin and are themselves activated by IFNs, with resultant increase in both receptor-mediated and non-receptor-mediated phagocytosis and tumoricidal activity. IFN-mediated macrophage activation results in an increase in Fc receptors that bind antibody and present it to T helper cells, which in the presence of HLA class II antigens, then activate the T helper cell to cytotoxic activity. T cells also produce small quantities of IFN-α and IFN-β, as well as significant amounts of IFN-γ and are themselves induced by all three IFNs for increased cytotoxic activity.

T suppressor cells can either be up- or downregulated by IFNs. Likewise, natural killer (NK) cells are activated by IFNs and display increased cytotoxic activity against tumor cells. IFNs, as well, can work by augmenting the production and expression of other lymphokines, in particular interleukin-1 (IL-1), IL-2, and TNF.

Dosage and Toxicity

The initial clinical trials with IFN were designed to determine the MTD and toxicity profile. Human IFN-α was available in limited quantities, making it difficult to determine MTD, optimal dosing schedule, and optimal duration of treatment.

Patients enrolled in these studies generally had a diverse array of malignancies, including both hematologic and solid tumors, and were in the advanced stages of their disease, either because the tumor was refractory to conventional treatment or because of metastases at the time of presentation.

The MTD of IFN was reported in several studies to depend on the route of administration and schedule. The most pronounced acute dose-limiting toxicity is pyrexia with flulike symptoms (malaise, chills, and rigor). Intravenous administration results in peak serum levels at 30 minutes, with a half-life of approximately 1 hour, whereas intramuscular or subcutaneous administration yields peak serum levels at 6 and 8 hours with a half-life of about 6 to 8 hours. It was noted that either daily or thrice-weekly administration is better tolerated than intermittent administration at intervals greater than 3 days. This phenomenon appears to result from the development of tolerance or tachyphylaxis. For example, in a phase I trial, Laszlo et al. treated 17 patients with escalating doses of leukocyte IFN starting with an initial dose of 0.5 million units/m^2 IM thrice weekly and increasing the dose to a maximum of 15 million units/m^2 with the same schedule. They observed tachyphylaxis to fever and constitutional symptoms (22).

Using continuous intravenous infusion, Rohatiner et al. treated 37 patients with escalating doses of leukocyte IFN from 5 to 200 million units/m^2 per 24 hours for 5, 7, or 10 days (23). With doses below 58 million units/m^2 per 24 hours, constitutional symptoms tended to subside after 3 to 4 days. The MTD for continuous intravenous administration was 100 million units/m^2 per day given thrice weekly. A transient decrease in NK activity was observed after 12 to 24 hours, followed by an increase in NK activity after 1 week. However, after 3 to 4 weeks of administration, there was a decline in the NK activity to or below baseline level. At lower levels of 0.5 to 1 million units/m^2 per day either daily or thrice weekly, NK activity slowly rose after 7 days, with sustained activity after 4 to 5 weeks. No effect on monocyte activity or specific immunity was identified, and no correlation between NK activity and tumor response was observed.

With the advent of recombinant DNA technology, highly purified recombinant forms of IFN-α could be generated in large quantities. New clinical trials were initiated to assess maximum tolerated dosing schedules, routes of administration, and duration of treatments for various malignancies. These phase I trials with recombinant IFN-α demonstrated pharmacokinetic and toxicity profiles similar to those of natural human IFNs (24). With intravenous administration, peak serum levels in the range of 500 to 600 international units/mL occurred at 15 to 30 minutes, with a serum half-life of 2 hours. With intramuscular or subcutaneous administration, peak serum levels in the range of 100 to 200 international units per mL occurred at 4 to 6 hours, with a serum half-life of 6 to 8 hours. The most frequently identified MTD was 200 million units/m^2 intravenously in a single dose or 50 million units/m^2 per day for 5 days. For more continuous dosing, 15 million units/m^2 subcutaneously or intramuscularly, either daily or thrice weekly, was tolerated. The acute dose-limiting toxicity was pyrexia or flulike symptoms.

Sherwin et al. treated 81 patients with recombinant IFN by intramuscular administration thrice weekly for a total of 28 days with escalating doses in different patients ranging from 1 to 136 million units. They found excessive toxicities with body temperatures above 40°C and severe fatigue and anorexia at doses above 50 million units (25). At lower doses, tachyphylaxis to these constitutional symptoms occurred after 1 week of therapy. In one study, Miller et al. showed that indomethacin may be most useful to decrease the intensity of such reactions and that acetaminophen is of minimal efficacy, although commonly used (26, 27).

Other dose-related toxicities were myelosuppression with neutropenia, which is usually reversible, and thrombocytopenia. CNS toxicity and gastrointestinal toxicity, primarily with diarrhea and anorexia and some cardiovascular effects (tachycardia, hypertension) were reported as well. As with natural leukocyte IFN, the recombinant products were better tolerated when doses were escalated and titrated over time. Gutterman et al. escalated the doses after 72 to 96 hours, with an MTD ranging from 72 to 198 million units (28). Severe side effects were seen with doses exceeding 72 million units. As with the natural leukocyte products, common toxicities with recombinant IFN-α were dose-related and reversible. The abundance of recombinant material allowed prolonged continuous therapy to become a treatment option, leading to the observation that such long-term administration yielded no evidence of cumulative toxicities. Phase II trials of recombinant IFN have demonstrated equivalent clinical activity among various types of cancer, as had been observed with natural leukocyte IFN. Advances in the treatment of certain specific malignancies are summarized below.

Interferon in Chronic Myelogenous Leukemia

Chronic myelogenous leukemia (CML) is a hyperproliferative disorder of pluripotent hematopoietic stem cells that follows a triphasic clinical course, with a chronic phase lasting approximately 3.5 years, followed by an accelerated phase merging into a blast crisis. The Ph^1 chromosome is observed in 98% of CML patients. It results from a (9;22) (q^{34};q^{11})) translocation. The new fusion gene, called *bcr-abl*, produces an abnormal p210 tyrosine kinase that appears to be related to the pathogenesis of CML. In the past, busulfan and hydroxyurea were the most important drugs in the treatment of CML. However, these drugs only produced cytoreductions and did not alter the disease course. Bone marrow transplantation (BMT) was considered the only possible curative treatment. In recent years, IFN has been used for the treatment of CML for patients who are not candidates for BMT. Several clinical trials have been undertaken to study the effects of IFN-α on chronic-phase CML (29–31). The mechanism of action of IFN in CML is poorly understood. It was reported that the administration of IFN-α not only resulted in clinical response but also produced cytogenetic response with elimination of Ph^1 (29). The remission rate in one study was 77.9%, and complete disappearance of Ph^1 chromosome metaphases was confirmed in 18.8% of patients (32). This study suggested that disease-free survival improved with cytogenetic remission, and recent data suggest that this is true when that remission is achieved within the first year of treatment. Remissions were durable in patients with continued therapy and lasted more than 3 years. The effective doses of IFN-α used ranged from 3 to 9 million units intramuscularly or subcutaneously every day. Some reports indicated that higher doses produced additional elimination of chromosomal abnormalities (33).

More recently, clinical trials have been initiated following allogeneic BMT in an attempt to improve disease-free survival after BMT for CML. IFN has also been found to produce remission in patients with CML who had relapsed after allogeneic BMT (34).

HAIRY CELL LEUKEMIA

Hairy cell leukemia (HCL) is a relatively rare lymphoproliferative disorder with presenting signs of pancytopenia, a hypercellular marrow with the presence of hairy cells, and splenomegaly. Initial therapy has historically been splenectomy, with normalization of blood counts occurring in 40 to 60% of patients following surgery. In 1984, Quesada et al. treated seven patients with progressive HCL with human IFN-α at 3 million units intramuscularly per day and reported a 100% response, with three complete responses and four partial responses after 8 to 12 weeks of therapy (35). Responses were classified according to normalization of peripheral blood counts and of bone marrow morphology and cellularity. Therapy was continued either daily or thrice weekly for more than 6 months, with sustained duration of responses. This initial success sparked tremendous interest in the treatment of HCL as well as other leukemias and lymphomas with IFN.

Several single- and multiinstitutional phase II studies have been conducted using recombinant IFN-α_{2a} or IFN-α_{2b} in HCL and revealed similar efficacy between the two recombinant IFNs (36–40). Doses used in these studies ranged between 2 and 3 million units, subcutaneously or intramuscularly, daily to three times a week for a minimum duration of 6 months. Total response rates ranged from 80 to 90%, with most patients achieving a partial response. Time to response often took several months, with platelet counts normalizing after 1 to 2 months, granulocyte counts normalizing at 2 to 3 months, and normalization of hemoglobin at 3 to 6 months. Side effects and toxicity seen in these studies with low-to-moderate doses of IFN were acceptable and even absent in many patients.

The optimal duration of therapy, ranging from 6 to 18 months, has also been evaluated in these trials; at present, 12 months of therapy in responding patients is recommended (41). Following discontinuation of IFN therapy, the percentage of patients relapsing ranged from 13 to 45%, with a median duration until relapse of 7 to 24 months. Significant negative prognostic factors for relapsing patients include a high neutrophil alkaline phosphatase level while on study and an initial bone marrow HCL count above 30% (38). Prognostic factors found not to be related to early relapse include age, prior chemotherapy, bone marrow cellularity, hematologic parameters at the time of presentation, and duration of treatment. Although formal studies to assess the optimal dose-response relationship for IFN-α in HCL have not been conducted, a recent study to assess the efficacy of low-dose (0.2 million units/m² three times a week) IFN-α2b in an effort to minimize side effects revealed a poor response rate of 18%, with several patients progressing on this regimen, suggesting that the 2 million units/m² thrice-weekly dose is preferable (42).

Thus, it appears unequivocal that IFN-α is efficacious in the treatment of HCL and can be used as a second or alternate line of therapy following splenectomy or 2-deoxycoformicin. HCL patients who underwent splenectomy after achievement of complete response (CR) after IFN-α therapy were reported by Remgalis et al. (43). When results of several studies were combined, the partial response (PR) rate was 71%, and CR was about 9%, with minor response at 10% (44). The cost-benefit analysis of IFN therapy in HCL has also shown substantial clinical and cost advantages (45) over older supportive-care methods.

Interferon in Multiple Myeloma

In preclinical studies, both leukocyte and recombinant IFNs have demonstrated an antiproliferative effect on myeloma cell lines. When myeloma cells were incubated with IFN, their viability was generally suppressed (46), and the production of M-protein decreased in proportion to the amount of IFN added (47). In an early clinical trial, Mellstedt et al. achieved a high response rate in relapsing myeloma patients with human IFN (48). Since then, several large clinical trials with both human and recombinant IFN have been conducted, with response rates of 10 to 30% (49–56).

Though doses and regimens differed significantly, it appears that those patients who do respond do so at doses of 2 to 3 million units/m² per day thrice weekly. Relapsing patients respond better than do refractory patients (26 vs. 11%). If continued on maintenance therapy, about 50% of responding patients will continue to respond for more than 1 year. Maintenance therapy with IFN-α after remission following conventional induction chemotherapy was reported by Mandelli et al. with a dose of 3×10^6 U/m² thrice weekly, and remission and survival were prolonged, compared with no maintenance therapy (57).

In previously untreated patients, conventional chemotherapy with melphalan and prednisone is superior to IFN alone. However, preliminary studies comparing IFN in combination with cytotoxic chemotherapy (MP) with MP alone, reported a remission rate of 76% to 95% in the MP plus IFN group versus 48% to 68% with MP alone (58, 59). By analyzing subgroups of patients, it was noted that IFN-α and MP in combination were better in the subset of patients with IgA myeloma than MP alone, while no significant difference was found in IgG myeloma.

Lymphomas

Initial clinical trials with leukocyte and recombinant IFN-α in the treatment of non-Hodgkin's lymphoma have demonstrated considerable efficacy in selected histologic groups, including low-grade nodular lymphomas and cutaneous T-cell lymphomas (60–62). In contrast, high-grade diffuse lymphomas and advanced and refractory chronic lymphocytic leukemia do not respond appreciably to IFN-α (63–66). In low-grade non-Hodgkin's lymphoma trials, the doses of IFN employed ranged from 2 million units/m² thrice weekly up to 50 million units/m² thrice weekly, although significant dose reductions for toxicities were uniformly required at the higher doses. Total reported response rates ranged from 30 to 50%, with most being partial responses. The duration of treatment ranged from 4 to 36, months with a median duration of response of 8 months. Favorable prognostic factors for response to IFN included a follicular histology and no prior chemotherapy. Current trials are being conducted using IFN in combination with chemotherapy in a concomitant or maintenance fashion (67). In a National Cancer Institute (NCI) trial, patients with advanced-stage cutaneous T-cell lymphomas received IFN-α$_{2a}$ at high doses of 50 million units thrice daily and demonstrated a 45% response rate, with 10% complete and 35% partial responses and a median response duration of 5 months (68). Significant toxicities at these high doses required more than 50% dose reduction in all patients.

Renal Cell Carcinoma

Early clinical studies with human and recombinant IFN indicate small but definite response rates in metastatic renal cell carcinoma (29, 35, 48, 69–72). Several phase I/II clinical trials have been completed, with response rates ranging from 0 to 30% (73–76). However, these trials differ significantly in the dose, rate of administration, and schedule of IFN, as well as the total number of patients enrolled in the study. There appears to be a dose response, with the highest therapeutic index of 20% achieved with doses of at least 5 to 10 million units/day. Favorable prognostic factors for response include nephrectomy within 12 months preceding the start of therapy, discrete pulmonary metastases, and good performance status. Attempts to combine IFN with chemotherapeutic agents have so far produced marginal improvements at best (77). However, several trials combining IFN and IL-2 have shown potential benefit; this combination is tolerable and can be given in the outpatient setting (78).

Melanoma

Early empiric trials treating metastatic melanoma with leukocyte IFN-α were disappointing, possibly because of the low doses and the short duration of treatment. Phase I/II clinical trials using IFN-α_{2a} and IFN-α_{2b} permitted escalation of dose and longer duration of therapy and achieved response rates of 5 to 29%, with a median of 19% (73–76, 79–85). Some prognostic factors were found to correlate with responsiveness to IFN in these trials, suggesting that patients with visceral involvement were less likely to respond, whereas patients with only cutaneous or soft tissue disease with low tumor burdens demonstrated higher response rates. Overall, the best results were found with uninterrupted schedules at doses of 10–50 million units/m^2 daily or every other day. IFN has also been combined with a variety of other chemotherapeutic drugs in trials for the management of melanoma. So far, no clear superiority of any of the combination regimens has been noted in enhancing antitumor efficacy. Currently, several trials are attempting to define the role of IFN in the adjuvant management of melanoma (following resection of regional lymph node metastases). The results of these trials are not yet available.

Colorectal Cancer

Early studies on colon cancer cell lines demonstrated some added effect when IFN was combined with 5-FU, resulting in potentiation of the cytotoxic effects of 5-FU (86). Lindley et al. showed an increase in plasma levels of 5-FU when IFN was given during 5-FU infusion, suggesting that IFN may play a role in augmenting the cytotoxic capabilities of 5-FU (87). Phase II studies examined the role of this combination in the management of advanced colorectal carcinoma, and responses in the range of 26 to 63% were reported (88–90). In all these studies, an initial dose of 5-FU by infusion was followed by weekly 5-FU combined with 9 million units of IFN subcutaneously thrice weekly. The main drawback in each of these trials was the small number of patients included, and subsequent attempts to confirm these data in phase III studies proved unsuccessful.

Ovarian Cancer

Early studies suggested that intraperitoneal IFN in combination with cisplatin might be effective against minimal-residual-disease ovarian cancer following surgical resection (91), but further studies failed to confirm these results (92). Recent reports indicate that intraperitoneal combinations of IFN-α and cisplatin have more effect in the treatment of ascites due to recurrent/refractory ovarian cancer than either drug alone (93).

Other Neoplastic Diseases

IFN has been reported to be effective in various other malignancies. It has failed so far to elicit good response rates in most solid tumors, but IFN-α was recently reported to be effective in reducing the rate of local recurrence of superficial bladder cancer (94). A combination of IFN-α and mitomycin for superficial bladder cancer was reported to be more effective than either drug alone (95).

TUMOR NECROSIS FACTOR

TNF is a cytokine protein molecule consisting of 157 amino acids, with a molecular weight of approximately 17,000. It was first identified in mice primed with BCG and then challenged with endotoxin. When sera from these mice were introduced into mice bearing sarcomas, it resulted in hemorrhagic necrosis of the tumor, hence the name tumor necrosis factor. In a separate series of studies to elucidate the pathophysiology of cachexia, a protein factor that suppresses lipid metabolism was identified and subsequently named cachectin. Characterization of this protein revealed that cachectin was indeed identical to TNF. There are actually two species of TNF: TNF-α, which is produced by monocytes, and TNF-β (also called lymphotoxin), which is produced by stimulated lymphocytes. Both TNF-α and TNF-β have been cloned and sequenced and are now available in recombinant forms.

The mechanism of action of TNF is not clear. Many proposed mechanisms of action were described. These include activation of phospholipase A-Z, activation of lysosomes, activation of serine proteases, and generation of superoxides (96). Phase I trials have demonstrated toxicity profiles similar to those of other cytoxines/lymphokines, with the most common side effects being fever, fatigue, malaise, and hypotension (97, 98). Anaphylactic-like pulmonary toxicities were described, including ARDS and bronchospasm in one study when TNF infusion was used following treatment with IL-2 (99). Headache was the most common neurotoxicity. Other toxicities reported included declines in granulocytes, thrombocytes, and erythrocytes and coagulopathy (100). The MTD with intravenous administration is in the range of 200 mg/m^2 per day; dose-limiting toxicities are constitutional symptoms and hypotension. Intravenous administration appears to be more efficacious than subcutaneous or intramuscular administration. These phase I trials demonstrated responses in a variety of malignancies including colorectal carcinoma, breast carcinoma, renal carcinoma, and melanoma. In Kaposi's sarcoma, intralesional TNF administration at 25 μg/m^2 produced a significant response in terms of local tumor regression (101).

Other phase I trials have investigated concomitant administration of TNF with IFN-γ and have demonstrated major toxicity, with some partial responses seen in advanced solid tumors (102). Several phase II trials have been reported with TNF in various malignancies. One study of the National Cancer Institute of Canada Clinical Trials Group treated 26 patients with renal cell carcinoma with 150 mg/m^2 TNF intravenously for 5 consecutive days. Only one complete response was observed, in a patient with contralateral kidney and one lung metastasis, and one partial response of a primary kidney lesion, with complete regression of lung nodules and improved bone scans reported in others (103).

Other phase II trials failed to show responses to TNF in other solid tumors, including breast, colon, and sarcoma. Raeth et al. reported a phase II trial using rTNF in patients with ascites resulting from advanced ovarian cancer and non-ovarian tumors with intraperitoneal spread. Thirty-two patients were evaluated. Seventeen patients showed complete resolution of ascites with TNF 80 μg/m^2 weekly intraperitoneally. Fourteen others showed more than 50% decrease in ascites: all showed no reduction in primary tumor size (104). Other phase II studies using TNF in combination with other cytokines are in progress.

INTERLEUKIN-2

Like IFNs, the interleukins are lymphokines: proteins secreted by leukocytes that affect the growth and function of other leukocytes. IL-2 is secreted primarily by peripheral T helper lymphocytes as well as by tonsilar and splenic lymphocytes. A recombinant form of IL-2 has been cloned and differs from native IL-2 in two ways: it is not glycosylated and it differs in two amino acid positions. However, its biologic activity is essentially the same as that of the native molecule. IL-2 activity is mediated through a cell-surface receptor (the IL-2 receptor, IL-2R), which is expressed primarily on T cells but also found on B cells and macrophages. Though originally described as a T-cell growth factor, IL-2 has several biologic activities, including augmentation of cytolytic T-cell activity and induction of secretion of other lymphokines, including IFN-α, TNF, IL-1, IL-6, and growth factor for B cells and NK cells. In addition, IL-2 induces the proliferation and activation of certain cytolytic effector cells such as NK cells, cytotoxic T lymphocytes, and, in particular, LAK cells. The precursors of LAK cells found in the peripheral blood are phenotypically non-B, non-T lymphocytes. Following incubation with IL-2, these precursor cells develop the capacity to lyse tumor cells. These LAK cells represent a subpopulation of null cells and are phenotypically and functionally distinct from NK cells and cytolytic T lymphocytes.

Preclinical trials employing animal models used IL-2 in two ways: IL-2 infusion alone or IL-2 with LAK cell infusion. The so-called adoptive immunotherapy, in which ex vivo IL-2-expanded autologous LAK cells are reinfused to inhibit tumor growth, was first applied in clinical trials starting in 1981 using natural IL-2. In 1984, recombinant IL-2 was produced in large enough quantities to allow phase I trials to begin.

Initial studies at the NCI used recombinant IL-2 alone or IL-2 with autologous LAK cells (105). Though the infusion of LAK cells alone produced minimal toxicities, primarily fever and chills, the administration of IL-2 proved to have substantial cumulative toxicities, particularly when administered in high doses of up to 10,000 units/kg/hour (106, 107). Administration of high-dose IL-2 intravenously produced a capillary leak syndrome similar to that seen in septic shock, with significant hypotension, pulmonary edema, weight gain, and oliguria. Despite these substantial side effects, response rates on the order of 17–35% were shown to occur in patients with advanced malignancies (105,108–110). The highest response rates were seen in patients with renal cell carcinoma and melanoma, although responses were also seen in patients with colorectal, lung, and ovarian carcinomas, as well as Hodgkin's and non-Hodgkin's lymphomas. Additional phase I trials have sought to decrease the toxicity by altering the schedule and reducing the dose. Trials to evaluate constant intravenous infusion of escalating doses of IL-2 titrated to the individuals' tolerance have achieved similar response rates with significantly less toxicity (110, 111). A trial to evaluate weekly administration of lower doses of IL-2 demonstrated less toxicity but also less efficacy (112). A different avenue of adoptive immunotherapy currently under investigation uses tumor-infiltrating lymphocytes along with IL-2. Lymphoid cells isolated from solid tumors are composed of a variety of lymphocytes, the predominant phenotype being a cytotoxic/suppressor (CD8) T lymphocyte (113). When these lymphoid isolates are grown in culture in the presence of IL-2, an expansion of a subset of T lymphocytes emerges, which possesses tremendous cytotoxic activity against tumor or cells. Though investigations to characterize this IL-2–induced T lymphocyte have yielded somewhat different results, it appears that the predominant effector phenotype is a T cytotoxic/suppressor lymphocyte.

In 1986, Rosenberg et al. reported their results, using a murine sarcoma model, which demonstrated that tumor infiltrating lymphocytes (TILs) were 50 to 100 times more effective than LAK cells in mediating the regression of established cancer (114). The antitumor effect of TIL cells was enhanced by concomitant administration of IL-2 and by pretreatment with a single dose of cyclophosphamide. Based on this animal model, they conducted a phase II trial with 12 patients with metastatic cancer (melanoma, renal cell carcinoma, and colon cancer) (115). TIL

cultures, established from excisional biopsy or surgical specimen, were grown in conditional medium with IL-2 for a mean of 32 days. Patients were then stratified to receive pretreatment with cyclophosphamide (25 or 50 mg/kg) or no treatment, followed by TIL infusion (8×10^9 to 2.3×10^{11} cells per patient). Concomitant with the first TIL infusion, IL-2 was administered at doses of 10,000 to 100,000 µg/kg every 8 hours until dose-limiting toxicity was reached. TIL infusions were well tolerated, with most side effects related to the administration of IL-2. Partial responses were seen in a renal cell carcinoma and in a melanoma patient. Both responders had received cyclophosphamide and more than the median doses of TIL and IL-2. Duration of response was 3 months after treatment.

IL-2 has now been approved by the FDA for the treatment of metastatic renal cell carcinoma. This was based on studies done using bolus infusion of IL-2 at doses of 600,000 to 720,000 international units/kg on days 1 to 5 and 15 to 19, with about a 15% response rate and a CR rate of 4% (116, 117). Attempts to combine IL-2 and IFN-α have so far not shown increases in activity over IL-2 alone. In metastatic melanoma, the role of IL-2 is still unclear. Responses were of short duration, although long-term complete responders were reported (118).

The NCI group reported treating 20 patients with metastatic melanoma with a TIL protocol consisting of pretreatment with cyclophosphamide at 25 mg/kg followed 36 hours later by TIL infusion (range, 3×10^{10} to 75×10^{10}) over 1 to 2 days, along with IL-2 at 100,000 µg/kg every 8 hours until dose-limiting toxicity occurred (119). In six of these patients, an aliquot of indium-111–labeled TIL was infused and localized preferentially to tumor sites within 24 hours after injection (120). Of 15 patients never treated before with IL-2, 9 patients had objective regression of disease, including one complete response. In patients who had failed previous IL-2 treatment, 2 of 5 attained a partial response. Duration of response lasted from 2 to more than 13 months. Immunologic studies performed on the infused TIL suspensions demonstrated a predominance of CD3+ cells with variability of CD4+ and CD8+ cells among patients, along with varying patterns of cytotoxicity proliferation and lymphokine production. No pattern emerged to predict tumor regression in vivo.

Currently, attempts are underway to combine IL-2 with chemotherapy and/or other cytokines. Atzpodien et al. reported recently on 14 patients with progressive metastatic colorectal cancer treated using a combination of IL-2, IFN-α, and 5-FU. Only 4 patients achieved a PR; 8 had stable disease, with median response duration of 5.9 months. No toxic deaths were reported, and toxicity was moderate and included thrombocytopenia, leukopenia, nausea, malaise, and fever (121).

CYTOKINE GENE THERAPEUTICS

The recent advances in gene therapy and molecular biology have opened new doors for the use of cytokines in the treatment of malignancies. Gene therapy has been used as a way of delivering more localized antitumor effect of cytokines (e.g., GM-CSF) without the observed toxicities seen with systemic administration of these agents. The basic concept of this treatment modality is to modify tumor cells to produce immune-activating cytokines, which in turn would lead to immune responses mounted against the malignant cells, resulting in elimination of these cells and vaccination of the patient against recurrence of the tumor.

One approach was to transfer the cytokine genes retrovirally ex vivo into tumor cells grown in culture, then select the transduced cells and use them to inoculate cancer patients to produce immune responses. Early studies performed on murine animal models showed that localized enhanced secretion of cytokines may augment immune response by increasing the presentation of tumor-specific antigens. Retroviral transduction of the murine IFN-γ gene into nonimmunogenic, low class I–expressing murine sarcoma cell lines induced upregulation of MHC class I antigen expression and generated CD8+ TILs, which were therapeutic against parental tumor cells (122). Many other experimental studies based on this modality were reported, with tumor cells transduced with various cytokine genes including IL-2, IL-4, IL-7, TNF-α, IFN-γ, and GM-CSF (123). Another approach was to transduce TILs with cytokine genes, as a way of increasing the concentration of that cytokine in malignant tumors when the transduced TILs localized in the tumor deposits. Rosenberg et al. reported on the use of TILs tranduced with the TNF-α gene (124). A current clinical trial using this approach in melanoma patients is in progress.

MONOCLONAL ANTIBODIES

Antibodies are specific immunoglobulins produced by B lymphocytes or plasma cells in response to an antigenic stimulus (viral, bacterial, molecular, or cellular), and they participate in host immune reactions. By themselves, antibodies can be cytolytic by binding to an antigen on cell surfaces and triggering the classic complement cascade, thus producing cell membrane damage and, ultimately, cell death. They are also central to antibody-mediated or antibody-dependent cellular toxicity.

A variety of immunologic cells and effector cells possess Fc receptors, including macrophages, T lymphocytes, and large granular lymphocytes. In their monomeric form, these glycoproteins consist of two light and two heavy chains, which comprise different domains. The Fab domain serves as the antigen binding site; idiotypic diversity via gene recombination and somatic mutation in this domain accounts for the vast heterogeneity of immunoglobulins. The Fc domain serves as the binding site for complement or for lytic effector cells (macrophages, polymorphonuclear leukocytes). There are five classes of immunoglobulins (IgM, IgG, IgA, IgE, IgD), though IgM and IgG are by far the most abundant. They differ in their ability to fix complement and to bind to effector cells. IgM, a pentamer, is the first immunoglobulin produced following immunization, and while it binds complement most efficiently, it cannot bind to effector cells. Thus, IgM can participate in complement-mediated cytotoxicity but does not participate in antibody-dependent cellular cytotoxicity.

The predominant immunoglobulin found in the serum is IgG, which comprises four subclasses with somewhat different functions. The hierarchy of activity in regard to complement-mediated cytotoxicity is IgG3>IgG1>IgG4. For this reason, murine monoclonal antibodies developed for complement-mediated cytotoxicity are usually of the IgG3 subclass, while those developed for diagnostic reagents are of the IgG4 subclass. On the other hand, murine antibodies developed for antibody-dependent cell-mediated cytotoxicity are usually of the subclasses IgG2A and IgG3 because their Fc receptors bind effector cells well. Both complement-mediated and antibody-dependent cell-mediated cytotoxicity involves binding the effector cell to the Fc portion of the immunoglobulin; hence only intact monoclonal antibodies can be used for this approach.

In 1975, Kohler and Milstein described the hybridoma technique in which the fusion of B lymphocytes from mice immunized with sheep red blood cells were fused in vivo with an immortal, nonsecretory, murine myeloma cell line. This enabled the production of target-specific antibodies in milligram quantities, opening the door for new avenues for use of antibodies in cancer diagnosis and treatment (9). Some of the first monoclonal antibodies used in clinical trials were murine monoclonal antibodies raised against tumor-associated antigens because of the ease of obtaining large quantities of tumor cells as well as antigens previously identified and characterized with heterologous antibodies. Lymphoproliferative disorders, including leukemia and lymphomas, were among the first malignancies to be treated with monoclonal antibodies (125, 126). In these early studies, several major obstacles to therapy with monoclonal antibodies were identified (127–131): distribution and delivery of the antibody to the tumor site, hypersensitivity reactions, antigenic heterogeneity of tumor populations, and the development of human antimurine antibodies. In addition, antigenic modulations in which the tumor cell transiently loses the cell surface antigen following exposure to the antibody have been observed both in vitro and in vivo. This phenomenon may represent one of the mechanisms by which tumor cells can escape detection by antibody.

A review by Dillman regarding toxicities of intravenous murine monoclonal antibody brings up several observations (132). The most common toxicities observed with this intravenous murine antibody therapy were fever, rigors, chills, and diaphoresis occurring in approximately 20 to 25% of patients. Urticaria occurred in 15 to 20% of patients. However, anaphylaxis and serum sickness were rarely encountered. These allergic reactions occur almost exclusively in patients with hematologic malignancies with circulating target cells. Patients with solid tumors usually do not exhibit any severe allergic reactions. In addition, patients who develop an antimurine antibody do not have hypersensitivity reactions, presumably because of the blocking effect of host antibody. A clear correlation between toxicity and dose-infusion rate has been observed, with those patients receiving 0.5 to 1 mg/minute experiencing increased episodes of hypotension and bronchospasm.

An alternative use of monoclonal antibody therapy currently being explored involves the use of antiidiotype antibodies. In B-cell lymphoproliferative disorders, the tumor cells bear an idiotypic surface Ig antigen that can serve as a tumor-specific antigen to which a monoclonal

antibody can be developed. Repeated exposure to this murine monoclonal antibody (AB1) results in the production of a human antimouse antibody (AB2) that is directed against the idiotype region of the mouse immunoglobulin. This antiidiotype antibody (AB2) will in turn induce an anti-antiidiotype antibody (AB3), whose binding portion of the idiotype is the mirror image of the murine monoclonal antibody (AB1) and will bind to the tumor-specific antigen. The first reported clinical application of antiidiotype monoclonal antibody treatment was described by Miller et al. in 1982, in which a patient with a follicular B-cell lymphoma was treated with escalating doses from 1 to 150 mg of an idiotype-specific monoclonal antibody raised against his primary lymphoma idiotype; a dramatic and sustained complete remission was achieved (133).

Following this case report, additional clinical trials with antiidiotype monoclonal antibodies in treatment of B-cell malignancies yielded less dramatic responses of relatively short duration. A number of intriguing immunologic issues of therapy apply to the idiotype system. Obstacles to treatment include tumor-derived idiotypic protein in a patient's serum, which binds the antiidiotype monoclonal antibody; development of human antimurine antibodies; and spontaneous alteration of the idiotype by the lymphoma. Meeker et al. treated 11 patients with B-cell malignancies with escalating doses of antiidiotype monoclonal antibody infused intravenously every 2 to 3 days (134). At doses of 50 to 400 mg, the idiotype protein was eliminated from the serum, and antibody levels in the range of 300 μg/mL could be demonstrated, with a half-life of 2 to 4 days. Approximately 50% of patients developed a human antimurine antibody. Clinical responses were seen in 5 of 11 patients, with 4 partial and 1 minor response. All were of short duration, lasting only 1 to 6 months.

Further approaches using antiidiotypic monoclonal antibodies have incorporated antibody treatment in combination with other immunomodulators. Murine models using antibody with IL-2 have demonstrated synergistic effects on antibody-dependent cellular cytotoxicity and increased tumor responses, as well as survival (135). In an extension of the previous study from the Stanford group, Brown et al. reported 11 patients with B-cell lymphomas who were treated with antiidiotype monoclonal antibodies along with IFN-α at 12 million units thrice weekly (136). Following 12 courses of this combination, 2 complete responses and 7 partial responses were seen. The rationale behind this trial was based on the independent activities of antiidiotype antibodies and IFN-α in patients with B-cell lymphoma and their apparent synergy when combined in a murine lymphoma model. Such strategies may hold promise for future studies.

In addition to the use of native monoclonal antibodies in cancer therapy, another approach is the use of immunoconjugates in which monoclonal antibodies are used as carriers of cytotoxic substances such as radioisotopes, toxin, or chemotherapy agents. The idea of using radiolabeled antibodies for tumor localization dates back to the 1940s, when Pressman and Keighley demonstrated localization of radiolabeled antibodies in normal tissue and experimental tumors (127). Over the past several decades, numerous studies have used radiolabeled antibodies, and later monoclonal antibodies, in the detection and localization of various cancer types. Several trials have evaluated the use of radiolabeled antibodies in the treatment of cancer, so-called radioimmunotherapy. In an early phase I/II trial at Johns Hopkins, polyclonal ^{131}I-labeled antiferritin antibodies were used in the treatment of hepatoma. Induction therapy with external-beam radiation plus chemotherapy was followed by cyclic ^{131}I-labeled antibodies consisting of 30 mCi of ^{131}I on day 0 and 20 mCi on day 5, to yield a total 1200-rad tumor dose. Hematologic toxicity was acceptable with this regimen. There was a 50% response rate with four complete responses, one of longer than 3 years duration. The major toxicity seen in this study was myelosuppression (138). Other attempts concentrated on intralesional administration of radiolabeled monoclonal antibodies. Papanastassiou et al. treated patients with malignant gliomas by placing ^{131}I-labeled monoclonal antibodies in the postresection cavity. He noted marked reduction in the need for frequent aspiration prior to placement of the labeled antibodies (139). Epenetos et al. treated 24 patients with persistent ovarian carcinoma with intraperitoneally administered ^{131}I-labeled monoclonal antibody directed against the tumor-associated antigen (140). Nine of 16 patients with small volume of disease at the time of treatment responded, with four durable responses of more than 3 months duration. Doses above 140 mCi were most effective and treatment was well tolerated; the major side effects were mild abdominal pain, diarrhea, pyrexia, and moderate myelosuppression.

Intrathecal administration of ^{131}I monoclonal antibody for the treatment of leptomeningeal tumors has been reported by Lashford et al. (141). Doses ranging from 11 to 40 mCi of ^{131}I were administered with minimal acute toxicity, primarily aseptic meningitis. Good biodistribution in the CSF was demonstrated, and four of five patients achieved sustained clinical responses, with one partial response and three complete responses ranging from 7 months to 2 years duration. Radiolabeled monoclonal antibodies have been used in the treatment of hematologic malignancies as well. Press et al. reported on a phase I trial treating 19 patients with advanced non-Hodgkin's lymphoma with high doses of radiolabeled antibodies, followed by autologous stem cell rescue. Eighteen patients achieved a response, with 9 patients remaining in complete remission from 3 to 53 months (142). Currently, trials are attempting to establish the role of radiolabeled antibodies in the treatment of other hematologic malignancies including acute myelogenous leukemia (AML).

TOXIN-LINKED MONOCLONAL ANTIBODIES

Another approach to the use of immunoconjugates involves linking monoclonal antibodies to a highly lethal toxin, or so-called immunotoxins. A variety of protein toxins derived from plant or bacterial sources have been evaluated. Among the more popular are ricin, abrin, diphtheria toxin, gelonin, saporin, amanitin, and *Pseudomonas* exotoxin. These toxins are enzymes that require transport into the cytoplasm, where they act to inhibit protein synthesis (143). Hence, unlike most chemotherapy agents, they act on nondividing cells. The toxins are rendered lethal only when coupled to the antibody, which allows attachment to the cell surface and transport to the cytoplasm; this presumably confers specificity for cells targeted by the antibody. Amlot et al. reported five partial responses and one complete response (response duration, 30 to 78 days) using an anti-CD22 antibody conjugated to the deglycosylated ricin A chain in patients with relapsed Hodgkin's disease. Dose-limiting toxicity included vascular leak syndrome (weight gain, edema) and myalgias (144).

In another phase I trial, Spitler et al. treated 22 patients with malignant melanoma using a murine antimelanoma antibody–ricin A-chain immunotoxin (145). Doses ranged from 0.01 mg/kg/day for 5 days to 1 mg/kg/day for 4 days, with total doses ranging from 3.2 to 300 mg. The major dose-limiting toxicity again was capillary leak syndrome, fever, chills, and malaise. All appeared to be self-limiting after discontinuation of therapy. Following completion of therapy, almost all patients developed antimurine antibodies and anti–ricin A-chain antibodies. Of 22 patients treated, there was 1 CR that lasted longer than 26 months, and 4 mixed responses lasting from 2 to 17 months.

DRUG-LABELED MONOCLONAL ANTIBODIES

Obviously this approach has a major drawback—the development of drug resistance by tumor cells, the same problem facing use of systemic chemotherapy. This modality of treatment remains to be explored.

USE IN COMBINATION WITH CYTOKINES

Lane et al. treated 15 patients with refractory adenocarcinoma (5 breast, 5 lung, 5 colorectal) using murine monoclonal antibody L6 at 200 mg/m^2 intravenously daily on days 1 to 7, followed by a 1-week rest period. IL-2 was given subcutaneously for 4 consecutive days and was followed by 3 days of rest, for a total duration of 3 weeks. IL-2 was given at escalating doses of 2 $\times$ 10^6 μg/m^2, 3 $\times$ 10^6 μg/m^2 and 4.5 $\times$ 10^6 μg/m^2. The rationale for administration of L6 before Il-2 was to allow for tumor uptake before stimulating effector cells (macrophages, NK cells, and T cells). Side effects of L6 consisted of mild fever and chills along with rash and serum sickness in one patient. Dose-limiting toxicity was grade 4 fatigue and dyspnea. One patient with breast cancer had a transient mixed response, and one patient with a colorectal cancer had a partial response (146). Nevertheless, this study represents a new approach in the use of monoclonal antibodies with other BRMs.

USE OF MONOCLONAL ANTIBODIES IN BONE MARROW TRANSPLANTATION

Another intriguing approach to the application of monoclonal antibodies is in the area of BMT. Intensive therapy for certain hematologic malignancies as well as solid tumors is often limited by the toxicity to the patients' normal hematopoietic stem cells, whether the therapy is chemotherapy or radiotherapy. This dose-limiting toxicity can be circumvented by "rescuing" the patient with a BMT. Originally, high-dose chemotherapy followed by BMT was reserved for individuals who had an HLA-matched bone marrow donor (syngeneic or allogeneic donor). With the advent of monoclonal antibodies, techniques to eliminate malignant cells ex vivo have permitted autologous BMT in individuals with either minimal or occult bone marrow involvement. Several techniques have been employed involving monoclonal antibodies with complement in conjugation with toxins or chemotherapy or with physical separators such as magnetic particles.

Most experience in ex vivo purging of bone marrow has involved its use in hematologic malignancies, in particular B- and T-cell lymphomas and leukemia. Important issues involved in purging bone marrow of malignant cells include defining optimal conditions such as cell concentration, duration of treatment, and techniques for removal of neoplastic cells either by cell death or physically (147). In addition, the monoclonal antibody (or antibodies) used must be selective against tumor cells, thus sparing normal hematopoietic stem cells vital for proper engraftment. A variety of techniques have been developed that appear to meet these criteria. By far the most widely used technique for purging bone marrow involves complement-mediated cytotoxicity, using murine monoclonal antibody in the presence of rabbit complement. The ability to fix complement varies among the subclasses of IgG: IgG2 and IgG3 fix rabbit complement quite effectively. However, these monoclonal antibodies are technically more difficult to generate.

In 1983, Bast et al. reported on a clonogenic assay for elimination of a common acute lymphoblastic leukemia antigen (CALLA) positive leukemia cell line from human bone marrow by use of the J-5 murine monoclonal antibody plus complement (148). Under optimal conditions, more than 99% of ^{51}Cr-labeled leukemia lymphoblasts could be eliminated from a 100-fold excess of bone marrow cells, using three treatments for 30 minutes. Further developments in this clonogenic assay demonstrated that combinations of monoclonal antibodies proved more effective than single antibody, resulting in more than 4-log tumor cell lysis without significant loss of nonmalignant marrow stem cells (149). Other investigators have also demonstrated increased tumor kill by the use of multiple antibodies plus complement in the purging of marrow cells contaminated with CALLA plus leukemia cells or B-cell lymphoma cells.

At the University of Minnesota, investigators have used a combination of three monoclonal antibodies, BA-1, BA-2, and BA-3, which recognize surface antigens found on 70 to 80% of non-B/non-T acute lymphocytic leukemia (ALL) cells and 90% of B-cell lymphomas, and demonstrated more than 95% tumor lysis in the presence of a 100-fold excess of marrow cells with a single 60-minute treatment with the BA-1, -2, -3 cocktail (150). Thus, using a combination of monoclonal antibodies to purge marrow may help circumvent the phenotypic heterogeneity of lymphoma/leukemia cells, which may render them resistant to complement-mediated lysis (151). Other investigators have explored the application of bone marrow purging using malignant cells from solid tumors. Using the Fib-75 murine antibody, which binds complement and recognizes an antigen common to epithelial tumor cell lines, Buckman et al. developed a technique for eliminating more than 95% of tumor lysis in the presence of a 100-fold excess of marrow cells, without detriment to the marrow cells (152). Tumor lysis was inhibited by tumor clumps of more than 500 cells.

More sophisticated techniques have been developed using breast cancer or small cell lung cancer cell lines. Anderson et al. treated marrow contaminated with a clonogenic breast cancer cell line with a combination of immunoseparation with five different monoclonal antibodies linked to magnetospheres followed by chemoseparation with 4-hydroperoxycyclophosphamide (4-HC) (153). This resulted in elimination of up to 5 logs of tumor cells in the presence of a 10-fold excess of marrow cells but reduced the recovery of marrow colony-forming units (CFS-GM) by 50% or more. Similarly, Humblet et al. treated marrow contaminated with small cell lung cancer cell lines (SCLC) with two rat-anti-SCLC IgM antibodies (LCA1 and LC66) plus complement in the presence of a cyclophosphamide derivative and obtained 4- to 5-log reduction of malignant cells, but with significant toxicity to bone marrow stem cells (154).

Another technique for the elimination of malignant cells from bone marrow involves immunotoxin-mediated cytotoxicity. The toxin, most commonly ricin A chain, coupled to a monoclonal antibody, exerts its cytolytic action after internalization into the cell; hence, this technique takes considerably longer. In vitro studies have demonstrated results comparable to those with complement-mediated cytotoxicity. Using various monoclonal antibody–ricin A chain congregates, Bregni et al. treated Burkitt's lymphoma cell lines from 12 to 72 hours (155). Up to 4 logs of tumor cells in a 20-fold excess of marrow cells could be eliminated within 24 hours using 10^{-7} M immunotoxin, without significant compromise to normal bone marrow progenitor cells. Similar results were obtained by Strong et al. when T-cell ALL cell lines were treated with various monoclonal antibodies conjugated to intact ricin (156). Effective tumor cell kill of more than 4 logs was obtained with a combination of four immunotoxins. Their results suggest that these immunotoxins continued to act on target cells for 3 to 5 days.

Other techniques for immunoseparation or chemoseparation in bone marrow purging have been used. The use of magnetic immunobeads coupled to a monoclonal antibody has been shown to be effective in purging bone marrow of malignant cells (153, 157). Following incubation of the MoAb-magnetosphere with a bone marrow/tumor cell suspension the mixture is passed through a magnetic field. As with other techniques, multiple MoAb and multiple treatments improve the efficacy of tumor removal, as well as the ratio of tumor cells to beads. Finally, investigations combining monoclonal antibodies plus complement with chemotherapy (e.g. 4-hydroperoxycyclophosphamide or 2-deoxycorformycin) have shown additive effects in tumor cell elimination from bone marrow (153, 158, 159). Such new and innovative techniques developed in vitro are now being evaluated in clinical trials with autologous BMT.

The largest trials conducted to date are from the Dana Farber Institute in Boston. In 1982, Ritz et al. reported on the use of J-5 monoclonal antibody for ex vivo purging of marrow from pediatric CALLA-positive ALL patients in relapse (160). Following induction chemotherapy, bone marrow was harvested and treated at 2×10^7 cells/mL in three separate incubations with J-5 monoclonal antibodies plus complement, based on preclinical studies by Bast et al. (161). Of the four patients treated, all attained engraftment of normal myeloid cells, and two remained in unmaintained remission after 1 year. This trial was updated in 1987, at which time 31 patients with relapsed ALL had been treated in a similar fashion, though the protocol was modified to include a marrow treatment with two monoclonal antibodies (J5 and J2) (162). Disease-free survival at 5 years was 27%, although toxicity was high, with a mortality rate of 30%. In 1984, Nadler et al. reported eight patients with relapsing B-cell non-Hodgkin's lymphoma treated with intensive chemoradiotherapy followed by autologous bone marrow purged ex vivo with an anti–B cell monoclonal antibody plus complement. Following this therapy, six of eight patients were disease-free in unmaintained remission (163). Stable hematologic engraftment occurred by 8 weeks in all patients, and no significant acute toxic effects were seen. This trial was updated by Takvorian et al. in 1987, at which time, 49 patients with poor-prognosis non-Hodgkin's lymphoma had been treated in a similar fashion with autologous bone marrow purged ex vivo with a combination of monoclonal antibodies (J-5, J-2, anti-B5) or anti-B1 MoAb (164). Disease-free remission without maintenance therapy occurred in 34 patients at a median follow-up of more than 11 months (range, 2 to 22 months). Bone marrow involvement at the time of harvest did not appear to adversely affect disease-free survival.

At the University of Minnesota, investigators have used a combination of monoclonal antibodies plus complement in the treatment of ALL and non-Hodgkin's lymphoma (150, 159, 165). The three monoclonal antibodies BA-1, -2, and -3 have been discussed above. Ex vivo purging of bone marrow for autologous bone marrow transplantation (ABMT) following chemoradiotherapy in 13 patients with ALL resulted in effective engraftment in all patients and 50% disease-free remission at 6 months of follow-up (range, 2 to 16 months). Seventeen patients with non-Hodgkin's lymphoma treated in a similar fashion demonstrated effective engraftment after ex vivo purging and a 40% disease-free survival at 3 years in patients with disease in complete or partial remission at the time of BMT. Similar results in ALL patients have been confirmed by other investigators.

Alternate methods for ex vivo purging of bone marrow with immunotoxins prior to ABMT in ALL patients have demonstrated effective engraftment within the same time period as with nontreated bone marrow but a delay in recovery of cell-mediated immunologic response for up to 1 year. In one study, the actuarial relapse-free survival was 61% at 3 years (166). Recently, Ball et al. reported on their experience with ABMT for acute myeloid leukemia (167). On the basis of preclinical studies, they used a combination of two monoclonal antibodies (PM-81 and AML-2-23), which recognize antigens expressed on AML blast cells but not on pluripotent stem cells, plus complement to purge ex vivo bone marrow from remission patients. Of 30 patients treated with ablative chemoradiotherapy followed by ABMT, all patients experienced marrow engraftment, usually within 30 days. Median survival and relapse-free survival of first-complete-remission patients was 17 months post-ABMT and was 6 to 8 months for second- or third-remission patients. This method for ABMT in AML patients who are disease-free may prove to be of benefit, particularly in patients who have no suitable allogeneic donor.

Aside from their use in ABMT, ex vivo purging of bone marrow has been investigated for allogeneic bone marrow transplantation as a means of decreasing the incidence of graft-versus-host disease. The most widely investigated monoclonal antibodies for this purpose are in the Campath series. This series is composed of several types of rat antibodies (IgM and IgG2) that fix complement well and are effective in causing T-cell depletion. A few clinical trials have demonstrated a marked decrease in graft-versus-host disease to an incidence of approximately 14% (168, 169). However, significant problems remain in widespread application of these antibodies. One major problem is graft failure, which occurs in up to 15% of patients and remains a significant cause of death. A second problem that has been the source of considerable anxiety is the potential loss of the graft-versus-leukemia (GVL) effect, which may lead to an increased incidence of relapse following transplantation. To date, no randomized trials have been documented to assess the effectiveness of ex vivo purging in allogeneic bone marrow transplantation, and there are no data relating to the incidence of decreased GVL.

In summary, the use of monoclonal antibodies in ex vivo purging of bone marrow is exciting, but long-term clinical benefit is entirely unproven. It may be applicable in patients with minimal occult marrow involvement who are at high risk for relapse. Unfortunately, the absence of randomized phase III data continues to haunt any conclusions regarding efficacy. Several in vitro models have been developed combining monoclonal antibodies with complement, toxins, chemotherapy and/or physical separators, which demonstrate effective tumor reduction without deleterious effects to normal hematopoietic stem cells vital for proper engraftment. Though the initial clinical trials to date have been encouraging, randomized, double-blind studies are essential to confirm the necessity and efficacy of ex vivo bone marrow purging for ABMT.

REFERENCES

1. Coley WB. The treatment of malignant tumors by repeated inoculations of erysipelas, with a report of original cases. Am J Med Sci 1982;105:487–511.

2. Montie JE, Stewart BH, Straffon RA, et al. The role of adjunctive nephrectomy in patients with metastatic renal cell carcinoma. J Urol 1977;117:272–275.

3. Everson TC, Cole WH. Spontaneous regression of cancer. Philadelphia: WB Saunders, 1966.

4. Oldham RK, Smalley RV. Immunotherapy: the old and new. J Biol Response Mod 1983;2:1–37.

5. Rosenberg SA, Longo DL, Lotze MT. Principles and applications of biologic therapy. In: DeVita VT, Hellman S, Rosenberg SA, eds. Cancer: principles and practices of oncology. 3rd ed. Philadelphia: JB Lippincott 1989:301–347.

6. Issacs A, Lindenmann J. Virus interference. I. The interferon. Proc R Soc Lond (Biol) 1957;147:258–267.

7. Issacs A, Lindenmann J, Valentine RC. Virus interference. II. Some properties of interferon. Proc R Soc Lond (Biol) 1957;147:268–273.

8. Oldham RK. Biotherapy: general principles. In: Oldham RK, ed. Principles of cancer biotherapy. New York: Raven Press 1987:1–20.

9. Kohler G, Milstein C. Continuous cultures of fused cells secreting antibody of predefined specificity. Nature 1975;256:495–497.

10. Rosenberg SA. Adoptive immunotherapy of cancer using lymphokine activated killer cells and recombinant interleukin-2. In: DeVita VT, Hellman S, Rosenberg SA, eds. Important advances in oncology. Philadelphia: JB Lippincott 1986:55–91.

11. Hawkins MJ, Hoth DF, Wittes RE. Clinical development of biologic response modifiers: comparison with cytotoxic drugs. Semin Oncol 1986;13(2):144–152.

12. Clark JW, Longo DL. Interferons in cancer therapy. In: DeVita VT, Hellman S, Rosenberg SA, eds. Updates of cancer principles and practices of oncology. 2nd ed. Philadelphia: JB Lippincott 1987:1–16.

13. Pestka S. The human interferons—from protein purification and sequence to cloning and expression in bacteria: before, between and beyond. Arch Biochem Biophys 1983;221:1–37.

14. Mark DF, Lu SD, Creasy AA, Yamamoto R, Lin LS. Site specific mutogenesis of the human fibroblast interferon gene. Proc Natl Acad Sci USA 1984;81:5662–5666.

15. DeMaeyer EM, DeMaeyer-Guignard J. Interferons and other regulatory cytokines. New York: John Wiley & Sons, 1988:135–153.

16. Sen GC. Biochemical pathways in interferon action. Pharmacol Ther 1984;24:235–257.

17. Rosenblum MG, Maxwell BL, Talpaz M, et al. In vivo sensitivity and resistance of chronic myelogenous leukemia cells to α-interferon: correlation with receptor bending and induction of 2′,5′-oligoadenylate synthetase. Cancer Res 1986;46:4848–4852.

18. Samuel CE. Mechanism of interferon action: phosphorylation of protein synthesis initiation factor eIF-2 in interferon-treated cells by a ribosome-associated kinase possessing site specificity similar to hemin-regulated rabbit reticulocyte kinase. Proc Natl Acad Sci USA 1979;76:600–607.

19. Clemens M. Interferons and oncogenes. Nature 1985;313(14):531–532.

20. Contente S, Kenyon K, Rimoldi D, Friedman RM. Expression of gene rrg is associated with reversion of NIH 3T3 transformed by LTR-c-H-ras. Science 1990;249(4970):796–798.

21. Boyer CM, Dawson DV, Neal SE, Winchell LF, Leslie DS, et al. Differential induction by interferons of major histocompatibility complex-encoded and non-major histocompatibility complex encoded antigen in human breast cancer and ovarian carcinoma cell lines. Cancer Res 1989;49(11):2928–2934.

22. Laszlo J, Huang AT, Brenckman WD, et al. Phase I study of pharmacological and immunological effects of human lymphoblastoid interferon given to patients with cancer. Cancer Res 1983;43:4458–4466.

23. Rohatiner AZS, Balkwill FR, Griffin DB, Malpas JS, Lister TA. A phase I study of human lymphoblastoid interferon administered by continuous intravenous infusion. Cancer Chemother Pharmacol 1982;9:97–102.

24. Spiegel RJ. Intron A (interferon alfa-2b): clinical overview. Cancer Treat Rev 1985;12(Suppl B):5–6.

25. Sherwin SA, Knost JA, Fein S, et al. A multiple-dose phase I trial of recombinant leukocyte a interferon in cancer patients. JAMA 1982;248(19):2461–2466.

26. Miller RL, Steis RG, Clark JW, Smith JW 2d, Crum E, et al. Randomized trial of recombinant α-2b-IFN with or without indomethacin in patients with metastic malignant melanoma. Cancer Res 1989;49(7):1871–1876.

27. Witter FR, Woods AS, Griffin MD, Smith CR, et al. Effects of prednisone, aspirin and acetaminophen or an in vivo biologic response to IFN in humans. Clin Pharmacol Ther 1988;44(2):239–243.

28. Gutterman JU, Fine S, Quesada J, et al. Recombinant leukocyte a interferon: pharmacokinetics, single-dose tolerance and biologic effects in cancer patients. Ann Intern Med 1982;96(5):549–556.

29. Talpaz M, Kantarjian HM, McCredie KB, Keating MJ, Trujillo J, Gutterman J. Clinical investigation of human alpha interferon in chronic myelogenous leukemia. Blood 1987;69(5):1280–1288.

30. Talpaz M, Kantarjian HM, McCredie KB, Keating MJ, Trujillo J, Gutterman J. Hematologic remission and cytogenetic improvement induced by recombinant human interferon alpha a in chronic myelogenous leukemia. N Engl J Med 1986;314(17):1065–1069.

31. Ozer H. Biotherapy of chronic myelogenous leukemia with interferon. Semin Oncol 1988;15(5):14–20.

32. Talpaz M, Kantarjian HM, Kurzrock R, Trujillo JM, Gutterman J. Interferon-alpha produces sustained cytogenetic responses in chronic myelogenous leukemia. Ann Intern Med 1991;114:532–538.

33. Claxton D, Kantarjian H, Kurzrock R, Trujillo JM, Gutterman JU. Alpha-interferon dose-dependent suppression of secondary clones in patients with Philadelphia-positive chronic myelogenous leukemia. Acta Haematol 1990;83:149–151.

34. Higano CS, Raskind WI, Singer JW. The use of α interferon for the treatment of relapse of CML in chronic phase after allogeneic bone marrow transplantation. Blood 1992;80:1437–1442.

35. Quesada JR, Reuben J, Manning JT, Hersh EM, Gutterman JU. Alpha interferon for induction of re-

mission in hairy-cell leukemia. N Engl J Med 1984; 310(1):15–18.

36. Foon K, Maluish A, Abrams PG, et al. Recombinant leukocyte a interferon therapy for advanced hairy cell leukemia: therapeutic and immunologic results. Am J Med 1986;80:351–356.

37. Golomb HM, Fefer A, Golde DW, et al. Sequential evaluation of alpha-2b-interferon treatment in 128 patients with hairy cell leukemia. Semin Oncol 1987; 14(2 Suppl 2):13–17.

38. Ratain MJ, Golomb HM, Vardiman JW, et al. Relapse after interferon alfa-2b therapy for hairy-cell leukemia: analysis of prognostic variables. J Clin Oncol 1988;6(11):1714–1721.

39. Ratain MJ, Vardiman JW, Golomb HM. The role of interferon in the treatment of hairy cell leukemia. Semin Oncol 1986;13(3 Suppl 2):21–28.

40. Golomb H, Fefer A, Golde DW, et al. Report of a multi-institutional study of 193 patients with hairy cell leukemia treated with interferon-alfa 2b. Semin Oncol 1988;15(5 Suppl 5):7–9.

41. Golomb H, Ratain MJ, Fefer A, et al. Randomized study of the duration of treatment with interferon alfa-2b in patients with hairy cell leukemia. J Natl Cancer Inst 1988;80(5):np.

42. Moormeier JA, Ratain MJ, Westbrook CA, Vardiman JW, Daly KM, Golomb HM. Low-dose interferon alfa-2b in the treatment of hairy cell leukemia. J Natl Cancer Inst 1989;81:1172–1174.

43. Pangalis GA, Boussiotis VA, Kittas C, Panayiotidis PG, Loukopoulos D, Fessas P. Hairy cell leukemia: splenectomy after alpha 2b-interferon therapy (letter). Blood 1991;78:1385.

44. Saven A, Piro LD. Treatment of hairy cell leukemia. Blood 1992;79:1111–1120.

45. Ozer H, Golomb HM, Zimmerman H, Spiegal RJ. Cost-benefit analysis of interferon alfa-2b in treatment of hairy cell leukemia. J Natl Cancer Inst 1989; 81(8):594–602.

46. Grader D, von Stedingk KLV, von Steding KM, Wesserman J, Einhorn S. Influence of IFN on antibody production and viability of malignant cells from patients with multiple myeloma. Eur J Hematol 1991; 46:17–25.

47. Tanaka H, Tanabe O, Iwato K, Asaoku H, Ishikawa H, et al. Sensitive inhibitory effect of IFN-alfa on M protein secretion of human myeloma cells. Blood 1989;74(5):1718–1722.

48. Mellstedt H, Ahre A, Bjorkholm M, Holm G, Johansson B, Strander H. Interferon therapy in myelomatosis. Lancet 1979;3:245–247.

49. Wagstaff J, Scarffe JH, Crowther D. Interferon in the treatment of myeloma and the non-Hodgkin's lymphomas. Cancer Treat Rev 1985;12(Suppl B): 39–44.

50. Costanzi JJ, Cooper MR, Scarffe JH, et al. Phase II study of recombinant alpha-2 interferon in resistant multiple myeloma. J Clin Oncol 1985;3:654–659.

51. Costanzi JJ, Cooper MR, Scarffe JH, et al. Use in patients with resistant and relapsing multiple myeloma: a phase II study. In: Kisner DL, Smith JF, eds. Interferon alpha-2: preclinical and clinical evaluation. Boston: Martinus Nijhoff, 1985:75–85.

52. Cooper MR. Interferons in the management of multiple myeloma. Semin Oncol 1988;15(5):21–25.

53. Quesada JR, Alexanian R, Hawkins M, et al.

54. Ohno R, Kimura K, Amaki I, et al. Treatment of multiple myeloma with recombinant leukocyte A interferon. Cancer Treat Rep 1985;69:1433–1435.

55. Ohno R, Kimura K. Treatment of multiple myeloma with recombinant interferon alpha-2a. Cancer 1986;57:1685–1688.

56. Costanzi JJ, Pollard RB. The use of interferon in the treatment of multiple myeloma. Semin Oncol 1987; 14:24–28.

57. Mandelli F, Avvisati G, Amadori S, Boccadoro M, Gernone A, et al. Maintenance treatment with recombinant interferon alfa-2b in patients with multiple myeloma responding to conventional induction chemotherapy. N Engl J Med 1990;322(20):1430–1434.

58. Montuoro A, De Rosa L, De Blasio A, Pacilli L, Petti N, De Laurenzi A. Alpha-2a IFN/melphalan/prednisone versus melphalan/prednisone in previously untreated patients with multiple myeloma. Br J Haematol 1990;76(3):365–368.

59. Mellstedt H, Osterborg A, Bjoreman M, Benning G, Gahrton G, et al. Treatment of multiple myeloma with IFN-α: the Scandinavian experience. Br J Haematol 1991;79(Suppl 1):21–25.

60. Foon KA, Roth MS, Bunn PA. Alpha interferon treatment of low-grade B-cell non-Hodgkin's lymphomas, cutaneous T-cell lymphomas and chronic lymphocytic leukemia. Semin Oncol 1986;13(3 Suppl 2):35–42.

61. Foon KA, Sherwin SA, Abrams PG, et al. Treatment of advanced non-Hodgkin's lyphoma with recombinant leukocyte a interferon. N Engl J Med 1984; 311(18):1148–1152.

62. O'Connell MJ, Colgan JP, Oken MM, Ritts RE, Kay NE, Itri LM. Clinical trial of recombinant leukocyte a interferon as initial therapy for favorable histology non-Hodgkin's lymphomas and chronic lymphocytic leukemia: an Eastern Cooperative Oncology Group pilot study. J Clin Oncol 1986;4:128–136.

63. Kleiner P, Haber J, Hausner P. Alpha-2b interferon in the treatment of advanced chronic lymphocytic leukemia. Neoplasma 1989;36(2):215–220.

64. Pangalis GA, Griva E. Recombinant alfa-2b-interferon therapy in untreated stages A and B chronic lymphocytic leukemia: a preliminary report. Cancer 1988;61:869–872.

65. Foon KA, Bottino GC, Abrams PG, et al. Phase II trial of recombinant leukocyte a interferon in patients with advanced chronic lymphocytic leukemia. Am J Med 1985;78:216–220.

66. Canellos P. Interferon in the treatment of malignant lymphoma. Semin Oncol 1985;12(4):25–29.

67. Ozer H, Anderson JR, Peterson BA, et al. Combination trial of subcutaneous interferon alfa-2b and oral cyclophosphamide in favorable histology, non-Hodgkin's lymphoma. Invest New Drugs 1987; 5(Suppl):27–33.

68. Bunn PA, Foon KA, Ihde DC, et al. Recombinant leukocyte a interferon: an active agent in advanced cutaneous T-cell lymphomas. Ann Intern Med 1984;101:484–487.

69. Priestman TJ. Initial evaluation of human lymphoblastoid interferon in patients with advanced malignant disease. Lancet 1980;19:113–118.

70. Gutterman JU, Blumenschein GR, Alexanian R,

Treatment of multiple myeloma with recombinant alpha-interferon. Blood 1986;67:275–278.

et al. Leukocyte interferon-induced tumor regression in human metastatic breast cancer, multiple myeloma and malignant lymphoma. Ann Intern Med 1980; 93:399–406.

71. Merigan TC, Sikora K, Breeden JH, Levy R, Rosenberg SA. Preliminary observations on the effect of human leukocyte interferon in non-Hodgkin's lymphoma. N Engl J Med 1978;299(26):1449–1453.

72. Quesada JR, Swanson DA, Trindade A, Gutterman JU. Renal cell carcinoma: antitumor effects of leukocyte interferon. Cancer Res 1983;43:940–947.

73. Muss HB. The role of biological response modifiers in metastatic renal cell carcinoma. Semin Oncol 1988;15(5):30–34.

74. Neidhart JA, Gagen MM, Young D, et al. Interferon-a therapy of renal cancer. Cancer Res 1984; 44:4140–4143.

75. Umeda T, Nijima T. Phase II study of alpha interferon on renal cell carcinoma: summary of three collaborative trials. Cancer 1986;58:1231–1235.

76. deKernion JB, Sarna G, Figlin R, Linder A, Smith R. The treatment of renal cell carcinoma with human leukocyte alpha-interferon. J Urol 1983; 130:1063–1066.

77. Sertoli MR, Brunetti I, Ardizzoni A, Falcone A, et al. Recombinant α-2a IFN plus vinblastine in the treatment of metastatic renal cell carcinoma. Am J Clin Oncol 1989;12:43–45.

78. Hirsh M, Lipton A, Harvey H, Givant E, Hopper K, et al. Phase I study of IL-2 and IFN α-2a as outpatient therapy for patients with advanced malignancy. J Clin Oncol 1990;8(10):1657–1663.

79. Kirkwood JM, Ernstoff M. Potential applications of the interferons in oncology: lessons drawn from studies of human melanoma. Semin Oncol 1086; 13(3):48–56.

80. Sertoli MR, Bernengo MG, Ardizzoni A, et al. Phase II trial of recombinant alpha-2b interferon in the treatment of metastatic skin melanoma. Oncology 1989;46:96–98.

81. Legha SS, Papadopoulos NEJ, Plager C, et al. Clinical evaluation of recombinant interferon alfa-2a (Roferon-2) in metastatic melanoma using two different schedules. J Clin Oncol 1987;5(8):1240–1246.

82. Legha SS. Current therapy for malignant melanoma. Semin Oncol 1989;16(Suppl 1):34–44.

83. Creagan ET, Ahmann DL, Green SJ, et al. Phase II study of recombinant leukocyte a interferon (rIFN-aA) in disseminated malignant melanoma. Cancer 1984;54:2844–2849.

84. Creagan ET, Ahamnn DL, Frytak S, et al. Phase II trials of recombinant leukocyte A interferon in disseminated malignant melanoma: results in 96 patients. Cancer Treat Rep 1986;70:519–624.

85. Dorval T, Palangie T, Jouve M, et al. Clinical phase II trial of recombinant DNA interferon (interferon alfa 2b) in patients with metastatic melanoma. Cancer 1986;58:215–218.

86. Miyoshi T, Ogawa S, Kanamori T, et al. Interferon potentiates cytotoxic effects of 5-fluorouracil on cell proliferation of established human cell lines originating from neoplastic tissue. Cancer Lett 1983; 17:239–247.

87. Findley C, Bernard S, Gavigan M, et al. Interferon-alpha increases 5-fluorouracil plasma levels 64-fold within one hour Results of a phase I study (abstract). J Interferon Res 1990;10:16–31.

88. Wadler S, Schwartz EL, Goldman M, Lyver A, Rader M, et al. Fluorouracil and recombinant alfa-2a-interferon: an active regimen against advanced colorectal carcinoma. J Clin Oncol 1989;7(12):1769–1775.

89. Wadler S, Wiernik PH. Clinical update on the role of fluorouracil and recombinant interferon alfa-2a in the treatment of colorectal carcinoma. Semin Oncol 1990;17(Suppl 1):16–21.

90. Pazdur C, Ajani JA, Patt YZ, et al. Phase II study of fluorouracil and recombinant interferon alfa-2a in previously treated advanced colorectal carcinoma. J Clin Oncol 1990;8:2027–2031.

91. Berek JS, Hacker NF, Lichtenstein A, Jung T, Spina C, et al. Interperitoneal recombinant α-IFN for salvage immunotherapy in stage III epithelial ovarian cancer. Cancer Res 1985;45(9):4447–4453.

92. Markman M, Berek JS, Blessing JA, McGuire WP, Bell J, Homesley HD. Characteristics of patients with small-volume residual ovarian cancer unresponsive to cisplatin-based i.p. chemotherapy: lessons from a Gynecologic Oncology Group phase II trial of i.p. cisplatin and recombinant alpha interferon. Gynecol Oncol 1992;45(1):3–8.

93. Bezwoda WR, Golombick T, Dansey R, Keeping J. Treatment of malignant ascites due to recurrent/refractory ovarian cancer: the use of interferon-alpha or interferon-alpha plus chemotherapy in vivo and in vitro. Eur J Cancer 1991;27(11):1423–1429.

94. Sarosdy M. High-dose versus low-dose intervesical interferon-alpha 2b in the treatment of carcinoma in situ: a randomized, controlled study. Anticancer Drugs 1992;3(Suppl 1):13–17.

95. Engelmann U, Knopf HJ, Graff J. Interferon alpha 2b instillation prophylaxis in superficial bladder cancer—a prospective controlled three-armed trial. Anticancer Drugs 1992;3(Suppl 1):33–37.

96. Balkwill FR, Naylor MS, Malk S. Tumor necrosis factor as an anticancer agent. Eur J Cancer 1990; 26:641–644.

97. Jakubowski AA, Casper ES, Gabrilove JL, Templeton MA, Sherwin SA, Oettgen HF. Phase I trial of intramuscularly administered tumor necrosis factor in patients with advanced cancer. J Clin Oncol 1989; 7(3):293–303.

98. Feinberg B, Kurzrock R, Talpaz M, Blick M, Saks S, Gutterman JU. A phase I trial of intravenously-administered recombinant tumor necrosis factor-alpha in cancer patients. J Clin Oncol 1988;6(8):1328–1334.

99. Negrier MS, Pourreau CN, Palmer PA, Ranchere JY, et al. Phase I trial of recombinant interleukin-2 followed by recombinant tumor necrosis factor in patients with metastatic cancer. J Immunother 1992; 11(2):93–102.

100. Aulitzky WE, Tilg H, Vogel W, Aultzky W, Berger M, et al. Acute hematologic effects of interferon alpha, interferon gamma, tumor necrosis factor alpha and interleukin-2. Ann Hematol 1991;62(1):25–31.

101. Kahn J, Kaplan L, Ziegler J, et al. Phase II trial of intralesional recombinant tumor necrosis factor alpha (rTNF) for AIDS-associated Kaposi's sarcoma (KS) (abstract). Proc Am Soc Clin Oncol 8:4;1989.

102. Demetri GD, Spriggs DR, Sherman ML, Arthur KA, Imamura K, Kufe DW. A phase I trial of recombinant human tumor necrosis factor and

interferon-gamma: effects of combination cytokine administration in vivo. J Clin Oncol 1989;7(10):1545–1553.

103. Skillings J, Wierzbicki R, Eisenhauer E, Venner P, Letendre F, et al. A phase II study of recombinant tumor necrosis factor in renal cell carcinoma: a study of the National Cancer Institute of Canada Clinical Trials Group. J Immunother 1992;11(1):67–70.

104. Raeth U, Shmid H, et al. Phase II trial of recombinant human tumor necrosis factor in patients with malignant ascites from ovarian carcinoma and non-ovarian tumors with intraperitoneal spread (abstract). Proc Am Soc Clin Oncol 1991;10:187.

105. Rosenberg SA, Lotze MT, Muul LM, et al. A progress report on the treatment of 157 patients with advanced cancer using lymphokine-activated killer cells and interleukin-2 or high-dose interleukin-2 alone. N Engl J Med 1987;316:889–897.

106. Margolin KA, Rayner AA, Hawkins MJ, et al. Interleukin-2 and lymphokine-activated killer cell therapy of solid tumors: analysis of toxicity and management guidelines. J Clin Oncol 1989;7:486–498.

107. Thompson JA, Lee DJ, Cox WW, et al. Recombinant interleukin-2 toxicity, pharmacokinetics and immunomodulatory effects in a phase I trial. Cancer Res 1987;47:4202–4207.

108. Dutcher JP, Creekmore S, Weiss GR, et al. A phase II study of interleukin-2 and lymphokine-activated killer cells in patients with metastatic malignant melanoma. J Clin Oncol 1989;7:477–485.

109. Fisher RI, Coltman CA, Doroshow JH, et al. Metastatic renal cancer treated with interleukin-2 and lymphokine-activated killer cells: a phase II clinical trial. Ann Intern Med 1988;108:518–523.

110. Paciucci PA, Holland JF, Glidewell O, Odchimar R. Recombinant interleukin-2 by continuous infusion and adoptive transfer of recombinant interleukin-2 activated cells in patients with advanced cancer. J Clin Oncol 1989;7:869–878.

111. West WH, Tauer KW, Yannelli JR. Constant-infusion recombinant interleukin-2 in adoptive immunotherapy of advanced cancer. N Engl J Med 1987; 16:898–905.

112. Allison MA, Jones SE, McGuffey P. Phase II trial of outpatient interleukin-2 in malignant lymphoma, chronic lymphocytic leukemia and selected solid tumors. J Clin Oncol 1989;7:75–80.

113. Vose BM, Moore M. Human tumor-infiltrating lymphocytes: a marker of host response. Semin Hematol 1985;22(1):27–40.

114. Rosenberg SA, Speiss P, Lafreniere R. A new approach to the adoptive immunotherapy of cancer with tumor-infiltrating lymphocytes. Science 1986; 233:1318–1321.

115. Topalian SL, Solomon D, Avis FP, et al. Immunotherapy of patients with advanced cancer using tumor-infiltrating lymphocytes and recombinant interleukin-2: a pilot study. J Clin Oncol 1988;6(5):839–853.

116. Rosenberg SA, Lotze MT, Muul LM, Leitman S, Change AE, et al. A program report on the treatment of 157 patients with advanced cancer using lymphokine-activated killer cells and interleukin-2 or high dose interleukin-2 alone. N Engl J Med 1987; 316(15):889–897.

117. Abrams JS, Rayner AA, Wiernik PH, Parkinson DR, Eisenberger M, et al. High dose recombinant interleukin-2 alone. J Natl Cancer Inst 1990;82:1202–1206.

118. Parkinson DR, Abrams JS, Wiernik PH, Rayner AA, Margolin KA, et al. Interleukin-2 therapy in patients with metastatic malignant melanoma: a phase II study. J Clin Oncol 1990;8(10):1650–1656.

119. Rosenberg SA, Packard BS, Aebersold PM, et al. Use of tumor-infiltrating lymphocytes and interleukin-2 in the immunotherapy of patients with metastatic melanoma. N Engl J Med 1988;319(25):1676–1680.

120. Fisher B, Packard BS, Read EJ, et al. Tumor localization of adoptively transferred indium-[111] labeled tumor infiltrating lymphocytes in patients with metastatic melanoma. J Clin Oncol 1989;7(2):250–261.

121. Atzpodien J, Kirchner H, Hanninen EL, Menzel T, Deckert M, et al. Treatment of metastatic colorectal cancer using 5-FU in combination with recombinant subcutaneous human interleukin-2 and alpha-interferon. Oncology 1994;51(3):273–275.

122. Restifo MD, Spiese PJ, Karp SE, et al. A non-immunogenic sarcoma transduced with cDNA for interferon-γ elicits CD8+ T cells against the wild-type tumor: correlation with antigen presentation capability. J Exp Med 1992;175:1423–1431.

123. Tepper RI, Mule JJ. Experimental and clinical studies of cytokine gene modified tumor cells. Hum Gene Ther 1994;5:153–164.

124. Rosenberg SA. Gene therapy of patients with advanced cancer using tumor infiltrating lymphocytes transduced with the gene coding for tumor necrosis factor. Hum Gene Ther 1990;1:441–480.

125. Miller RA, Levy R. Response of cutaneous T cell lymphoma to therapy with hybridoma monoclonal antibody. Lancet 1981;1:226–230.

126. Foon KA, Schroff RW, Bunn PA, et al. Effects of monoclonal antibody therapy in patients with chronic lymphocytic leukemia. Blood 1984;64(5):1085–1093.

127. Larrick JW, Bourla JM. Prospects for the therapeutic use of human monoclonal antibodies. J Biol Response Mod 1986;5:379–393.

128. Schroff RW, Morgan AC, Woodhouse CS, et al. Monoclonal antibody therapy in malignant melanoma: factors effecting in vivo localization (abstract). J Biol Response Mod 1987;6:457–458.

129. Dillman RO, Beauregard JC, Halpern SE, Clutter M. Toxicities and side effects associated with intravenous infusion of murine monoclonal antibodies. J Biol Response Mod 1986;5:73–94.

130. Weinstein JN, Steller MA, Kennan AM, et al. Monoclonal antibodies in the lymphatics: selective delivery to lymph node metastases of a solid tumor. Science 1983;222:423–426.

131. Schroff RW, Foon KA, Beatty SM, Oldham RK, Morgan AC. Human anti-murine immunoglobulin responses in patients receiving monoclonal antibody therapy. Cancer Res 1985;45:879–885.

132. Dillman RO. Monoclonal antibodies for treating cancer. Ann Intern Med 1989;111:592–603.

133. Miller RA, Maloney DG, Warnke R, Levy R. Treatment of B-cell lymphoma with monclonal anti-idiotype antibody. N Engl J Med 1982;306(9):517–522.

134. Meeker TC, Lowder J, Maloney DG, et al. A clinical trial of anti-idiotype therapy for B-cell malignancy. Blood 1985;65(6):1349–1363.

135. Berinstein N, Levy R. Treatment of a murine

B cell lymphoma with monoclonal antibodies and IL-2. J Immunol 1987;139:971–976.

136. Brown SL, Miller RA, Horning SJ, et al. Treatment of B cell lymphomas with anti-idiotype antibodies alone and in combination with alpha interferon. Blood 1989;73(3):651–661.

137. Pressman D, Keighley G. The zone of activity of antibodies as determined by the use of radioactive tracers: the zone of activity of nephrotoxic anti-kidney serum. J Immunol 1948;59:141–146.

138. Order SE, Stillwagon GB, Klein JL, et al. Iodine 131 antiferritin, a new treatment modality in hepatoma: a Radiation Therapy Oncology Group study. J Clin Oncol 1985;3(12):1573–1582.

139. Papanastassiou V, Pizer BL, Coakham HB, Bullimore J, Zananiri T, Kemshead JT. Treatment of recurrent and cystic malignant gliomas by a single intracavitary injection of ^{131}I-monoclonal antibody: feasibility, pharmacokinetics and dosimetry. Br J Cancer 1993;67(1):144–151.

140. Epenetos AA, Munro AJ, Stewart S, et al. Antibody-guided irradiation of advanced ovarian cancer with intraperitoneally administered radiolabeled monoclonal antibodies. J Clin Oncol 1987;5:1890–1899.

141. Lashford LS, Davies AG, Richardson RB, et al. A pilot study of ^{131}I monoclonal antibodies in the therapy of leptomeningeal tumors. Cancer 1988;61:857–868.

142. Press OW, Early JF, Appelbaum FR, Martin PJ, Badger CC, et al. Radiolabeled-antibody therapy of B-cell lymphoma with autologous bone marrow support. N Engl J Med 1993;329(17):1219–1224.

143. Middlebrook JL, Dorland RB. Bacterial toxins: cellular mechanisms of action. Microbiol Rev 1984; 48(3):199–221.

144. Amlot PL, Stone MJ, Cunningham D, Fay J, Newman J, et al. A phase I study of anti-CD22-deglycosylated ricin A-chain immunotoxin in the treatment of B-cell lymphomas resistant to conventional therapy. Blood 1993;82(9):2624–2633.

145. Spitler LE, del Rio M, Khentigan A, et al. Therapy of patients with malignant melanoma using a monoclonal antimelanoma antibody-ricin A-chain immunotoxin. Cancer Res 1987;47:1717–1723.

146. Ziegler LD, Palazzolo P, Cunningham J, et al. Phase I trial of murine monoclonal antibody L6 in combination with subcutaneous interleukin-2 in patients with advanced carcinoma of the breast, colorectum and lung. J Clin Oncol 1992;10:1470–1478.

147. Krown SE, Real FX, Cunningham-Rundles S, et al. Preliminary observations on he effect of recombinant leukocyte A interferon in homosexual men with Kaposi's sarcoma. N Engl J Med 1983;308(18):1071–1076.

148. Bast RC, Ritz J, Lipton JM, et al. Elimination of leukemic cells from human bone marrow using monoclonal antibody and complement. Cancer Res 1983;43:1389–1394.

149. Bast RC, De Fabritiis P, Lipton J, et al. Elimination of malignant clonogenic cells from human bone marrow using multiple monoclonal antibodies and complement. Cancer Res 1985;45:499–503.

150. Hurd DD, LeBien TW, Lasky LC, et al. Autologous bone marrow transplantation in non-Hodgkin's lymphoma: monoclonal antibodies plus complement for ex vivo marrow transplant. Am J Med 1988;85:829–834.

151. Winter JN, Marder RJ, Mankad B, Epstein AL. Heterogeneity among the non-Hodgkin's lymphomas. Cancer 1988;61:1082–1090.

152. Buckman R, McIlhinney RAJ, Shepherd V, Patel S, Coombs RC, Neville AM. Elimination of carcinoma cells from human bone marrow. Lancet 1982; 25:1428–1430.

153. Anderson JC, Shpall EJ, Leslie DS, et al. Elimination of malignant clonogenic breast cancer cells from human bone marrow. Cancer Res 1989;49:4659–4664.

154. Humblet Y, Feyens A-M, Sekhavat M, Agaliotis D, Canon J-L, Syman ML. Immunological and pharmacological removal of small cell lung cancer cells from bone marrow autografts. Cancer Res 1989; 49:5058–5061.

155. Bregni M, De Fabritiis P, Raso V, et al. Elimination of clonogenic tumor cells from human bone marrow using a combination of monoclonal antibody: ricin A-chain conjugates. Cancer Res 1986;46:1208–1213.

156. Strong RC, Uckun F, Youle RJ, Kersey JH, Vallera DA. Use of multiple T cell-directed intact ricin immunotoxins for autologous bone marrow transplantation. Blood 1985;66(3):627–635.

157. Shimazaki C, Wisiniewski D, Scheinberg DA, et al. Elimination of myeloma cells for bone marrow by using monoclonal antibodies and magnetic immunobeads. Blood 1988;72(4):1248–1254.

158. De Fabritiis P, Bregni M, Lipton J, et al. Elimination of clonogenic Burkitt's lymphoma cells from human bone marrow using 4-hydroperoxycyclophosphamide in combination with monoclonal antibodies and complement. Blood 1985;65(5):1064–1070.

159. Schwartz CL, Minniti CP, Harwood P. Elimination of clonogenic malignant human T cells using monoclonal antibodies in combination with 2'-deoxycoformycin. J Clin Oncol 1987;5(12):1900–1911.

160. Ritz J, Sallan SE, Bast RC. Autologous bone-marrow transplantation in calla-positive acute lymphoblastic leukemia after in vitro treatment with J5 monoclonal antibody and complement. Lancet 1982; 10:60–63.

161. Bast RC, Ritz J, Lipton JM. Elimination of leukemic cells from human bone marrow using monoclonal antibody and complement. Cancer Res 1983; 43:1389–1394.

162. Niemeyer CM, Ritz J, Donahue K, Sallan SE. Monoclonal-antibody-purged autologous bone marrow transplantation for relapsed non-T-cell acute lymphoblastic leukemia in childhood. Haematol Blood Transfus 1987;31:67–74.

163. Nadler LM, Takvorian T, Botnick L. Anti-B1 monoclonal antibody and complement treatment in autologous bone-marrow transplantation for relapsed B-cell non-Hodgkin's lymphoma. Lancet 1984;25:427–430.

164. Takvorian T, Canellos GP, Ritz J. Prolonged disease-free survival after autologous bone marrow transplantation in patients with non-Hodgkin's lymphoma with a poor prognosis. N Engl J Med 1987; 316:1499–1505.

165. Ramsay N, LeBien T, Nesbit M. Autologous bone marrow transplantation (BMT) for acute lympho-

blastic leukemia (ALL) following marrow treatment with BA-1, BA-2, BA-3, and rabbit complement (C) (abstract). Blood 1983;62:228a.

166. Preijers FWMB, De Witte T, Wessels JMC. Autologous transplantation of bone marrow purged in vitro with anti-CD7-(WT1) ricin a immunotoxin in T-cell lymphoblastic leukemia and lymphoma. Blood 1989; 74(3):1152–1158.

167. Ball ED, Mills LE, Cornwell GG. Autologous bone marrow transplantation for acute myeloid leukemia using monoclonal antibody-purged bone marrow. Blood 1990;75(5):1199–1206.

168. Heit W, Bunjes D, Wiesneth M. Ex vivo T-cell depletion with the monoclonal antibody Campath-1 plus human complement effectively prevents acute graft-versus-host disease in allogeneic bone marrow transplantation. Br J Haematol 1986;64:479–486.

169. Tazzari PL, Barbieri L, Gobbi M. An immunotoxin containing a rat IgM monoclonal antibody (Campath 1) and saporin 6: effective on T lymphocytes and hemopoietic cells. Cancer Immunol Immunother 1988;26:231–236.

12

Circadian Timing of Cancer Chemotherapy

Patricia A. Wood and William J. M. Hrushesky

Temporal coordination of biologic processes with an approximately 24-hour cycle (circadian) is common throughout the animal and plant kingdoms. The fundamental importance of mechanisms to measure and anticipate time is demonstrated by the fact that many molecular strategies for keeping circadian time evolved in parallel among vastly different organisms. In all organisms studied, the capability to keep biologic time is an endogenous inherited characteristic. This temporal organization at the cellular, organ, and organismic levels results in predictable differences in the capacity of plants, animals, and human beings to respond to environmental demands and therapeutic interventions at different times throughout important biologic cycles. The emerging understanding of circadian biologic time structure is resulting in improved treatment of conditions as diverse as jet lag, worker performance and accidents in shift workers, depression, sleep disorders, peptic ulcer disease, cardiac ischemia, hypertension, peptic ulcer disease, and asthma. In the treatment of cancer, circadian timing of anticancer drugs, radiation therapy, and biologic agents can result in improved toxicity profiles, enhanced tumor control, and improved host survival.

Biologic Clocks Coordinate Circadian Time within the Organism

Teleologically, the organization of biologic function according to circadian time has provided an essential evolutionary advantage. Circadian time keeping helps the organism to use effectively energy forms that fluctuate with this daily cycle; to coordinate sleep/wake onset and integrity of sleep; to ensure biologic economy so that a cell or organ selectively expresses certain groups of genes at different critical times of day rather than all of its genes all the time; to coordinate photoperiodic behaviors (e.g., seasonal breeding, hibernation, migration); and perhaps to promote overall stability, since resonating systems are more resistant to disturbance. Circadian rhythms derive from both genetic determinants (oscillators that constitute the "clock(s)") located within the cell and the organism and from rhythmic external environmental inputs that affect and modify the endogenous oscillators. Common characteristics of all circadian clocks include a period length of about 24 hours under constant conditions (free from environmental input); the ability to be reset by environmental signals; the ability to maintain the same circadian period despite different ambient temperatures (temperature compensation); and an intracellular location (1). Studies of genetic clock mutants have identified mutational hot spots within a single or a few genes in several organisms ("clock genes") such as *frq* in *Neurospora*, *per* and *tim* in *Drosophila*, *tau* in hamsters, and *clock* in mice (2–6). The brief half-life, rapid response time, time lag between the appearance of the RNA and protein products of these genes, and an autoregulatory feedback loop appear to be able to generate and maintain these endogenous 24-hour rhythms (7). The product of these clock genes and their biochemical roles are not yet known; however, they appear not to work enzymatically but rather display stoichiometric behavior and effects.

In vertebrate animals the primary circadian clock is located mainly in the central nervous system (superchiasmatic nucleus (SCN) of the hypothalamus) and in the pineal gland. Circadian-dependent expression of appropriate clock genes has been localized in these oscillators. Circadian organismic time keeping has been depicted as the result of three separate but interacting components: the input pathways by which the environment can affect the central circadian clock(s) (e.g., retinal pathways to the central clock components); the central circadian clock (SCN and pineal), which comprises several oscillators; and the output pathways of the central clock(s) by which time keeping is imparted to cells and tissues outside the clock through effects on nonclock genes (e.g., clock-controlled genes).

Circadian Coordination of Physiology and Pathology

Predictable daily patterns (circadian rhythms plus regular daily exogenous influences) characterize the function of most organ systems (e.g., pulmonary, cardiovascular, renal, hematologic, immunologic, cognitive and motor function) at many levels. Physiologic functions such as temperature, organ blood flow, organ-coordinated rhythms in cell-cycle phase distribution, and drug metabolism each vary rhythmically throughout the day (8). At the cellular level, enzyme activities; protein phosphorylation; protein, hormone, and receptor concentrations; and gene expression vary predictably as a function of time of day. Many circadian variations in physiologic function are also preserved in common pathophysiologic states. The incidence and patterns of exacerbation of several diseases have a significant and predictable circadian time structure. For example, most cardiac ischemic events and actual myocardial infarctions occur between 8 AM and noon, coincident with the early morning rise in vascular resistance, sympathetic vascular tone, and platelet aggregability and nadir in plasma fibrinolytic activity (9–11).

Approaches to circadian-timed therapy have included the empiric study of several treatment times throughout a 24-hour span to evaluate differences in toxicity, efficacy, cost, and/or compliance. Other approaches have used circadian patterns of disease-specific activity to target therapy at the circadian time of highest risk for symptoms. In this approach, drug timing is used to optimize drug availability at the specific time when disease symptoms and complications are known to occur most frequently and reduce drug dosing at other times. Individuals who are active in the day and sleep in the night have been assumed to be fairly homogeneous with respect to the timing of their circadian-dependent physiology and pharmacology. When diseased patients have been studied as groups receiving different time-of-day therapies, reproducible time-of-day differences in drug toxicity, drug pharmacokinetics, and drug efficacy have been repeatedly observed. These results suggest that the assumption of some uniformity among patient circadian time structure is not totally inaccurate. Whether knowing the circadian time structure of each individual and using this to schedule drug therapy, rather than clock time, would further improve the outcome of circadian-based therapy is not yet clear.

BIOLOGIC BASIS FOR CIRCADIAN DEPENDENCE OF CANCER THERAPY

The rationale for applying circadian-timed therapy in cancer treatment is as follows. The balance between harm to the host and to the tumor, the toxic: therapeutic ratio, is not favorable for many cancer therapies. Therefore, approaches that might decrease toxicity while still maintaining the antitumor effect would be of great potential benefit. Response rates of established tumors to therapy are also not optimal; therefore, approaches to increase antitumor efficacy are also highly desirable. Many different approaches are being taken to address these problems. Circadian drug timing is one additional and unique approach to further enhancing the efficacy of cancer therapy.

Circadian Time Structure of the Host Relevant to Cancer

CIRCADIAN DRUG PHARMACOKINETICS

The pharmacokinetics of many drugs vary with the circadian time of their administration. This is a composite of endogenous circadian rhythms in addition to modulating factors such as posture, intake of solids and liquids, state of hydration, circulatory function, and physical activity. In terms of real-life therapy, both sets of daily rhythm inputs contribute meaningfully, and both are important for understanding, explaining, and most importantly for therapeutically utilizing circadian pharmacokinetics. These daily changes in the disposition of drugs can also be of clinical significance.

Absorption

Gastrointestinal motility, intraluminal pH, stomach blood flow, and digestive enzyme concentrations all affect drug absorption, and all vary as a function of the time of day (12–15). In addition, independent of meal timing or composition, there is evidence that a number of drugs, particularly the lipophilic ones, are absorbed more quickly in humans when administered in the early morning. This correlates with findings in rodents, where peak absorption of lipid soluble drugs occurs at the onset of activity. Outcome from childhood acute lymphoblastic leukemia (ALL) following oral maintenance chemotherapy with 6-mercaptopurine (6-MP) and

methotrexate is more favorable when these drugs are administered in the evening (16, 17). In this case, these differences may be partially attributable to improved absorption of the drugs at that time of day as well as to the interference of milk with the metabolism and absorption of the antipurine (18–20).

Distribution

In both rodents and humans, a circadian variation in free (non-protein-bound) plasma drug concentration has been reported for both acidic and basic drugs (21–23). This circadian variation will be most important for those drugs that are highly plasma protein bound with a small volume of distribution. A marked circadian variation in the degree of plasma protein binding of cisplatin has been reported, with a maximum in the afternoon (24) at a time associated with lower

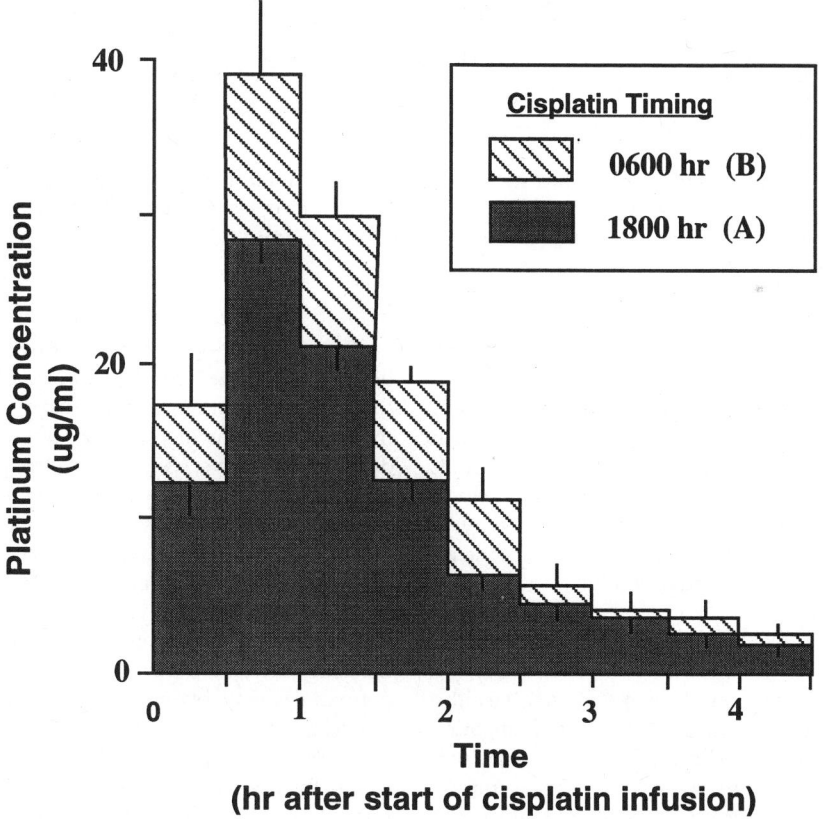

Figure 12.1. Kinetics of urine platinum concentration as a function of circadian time of cisplatin administration **(morning, 0600 hr, evening, 1800 hr).** Each *bar* represents the concentration of platinum ± SE in urine excreted in 30-min samples after evening (*shaded, A*) and morning (*hatched, B*) cisplatin administration in cancer patients (F, 7.4; $p < .01$). Greater renal tissue exposure to platinum is seen with morning cisplatin administration, which results in greater nephrotoxicity (see also Fig. 12.2).

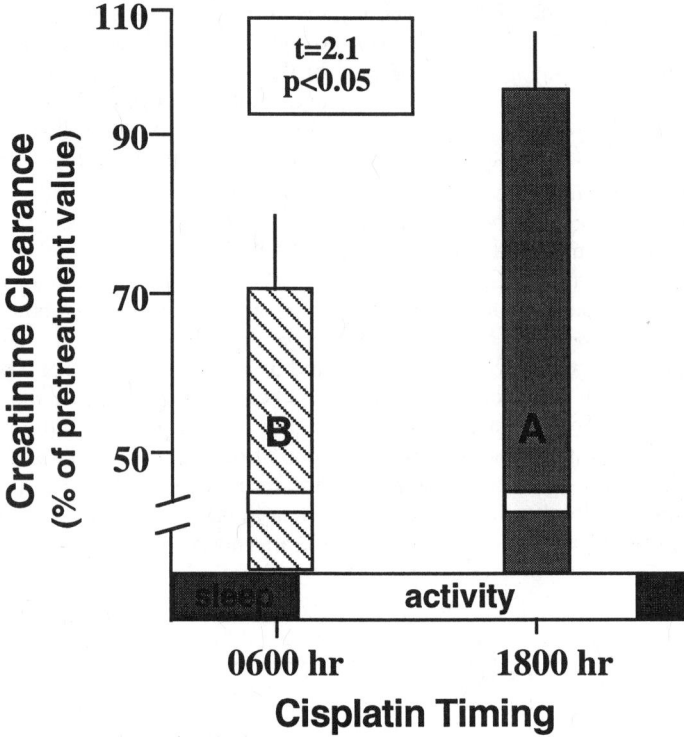

Figure 12.2.   Cisplatin-induced renal toxicity in cancer patients as a function of circadian time of cisplatin ad-ministration. Each bar is the mean ± SE of 24-hr creatinine clearance values (as % of pretreatment values) in patients receiving cisplatin in morning (*hatched, B*) and evening (*shaded, A*). Less nephrotoxicity results when cisplatin is administered in the evening.

nephrotoxicity. Hepatic portal transport efficacy varies in response to the concurrent consumption of nutrients and, in addition, has been shown to exhibit a clear circadian variation in fasting subjects (25). Under these conditions, maximum blood flow occurs in the early activity phase. For drugs that are largely extracted by the liver, such as antimetabolites, the rate of metabolism is largely dependent on the rate of hepatic blood flow.

Metabolism

Hepatic drug metabolism may involve either oxidation/reduction, hydrolysis, or conjugation, all of which have been documented to vary with circadian time (26). In rats, two peaks per 24-hour cycle in liver microsomal content of cytochrome P450 and NADPH–cytochrome C reductase have been described: midsleep and midactivity phase (27). Other rodent studies have shown circadian coordination in the activity of additional hepatic enzyme systems and levels of drug metabolites (28, 29).

The glutathione-mediated oxidation/reduction cycle may be circadian-time coordinated in that tissue glutathione levels vary throughout the day. The time of peak concentrations of reduced glutathione (GSH) concentration varies, however, depending upon the tissue studied; rodents have minimum liver GSH in early-activity and minimum heart GSH in late-activity span, while humans have minimum marrow GSH levels in the evening (30–32). The circadian pattern of GSH content in various tissues has also been inversely correlated with the circadian pattern of peroxidation by polyunsaturated fatty acids (33). Pretreatment of animals with adrenocorticotropic hormone (ACTH) to increase corticosteroid levels before administration of doxorubicin raises tissue GSH levels to the maximum daily concentration, making each time of administration equivalent to the optimal time of day for doxorubicin toxicity (34–36). These findings suggest the possibility that tissue GSH balance could be coordinated, in part, by the circadian pattern of adrenal corticosteroid.

Hydrolysis and conjugation reactions have also been shown to vary with circadian time. In rats, glucuronidation is higher during activity, and inversely, sulfation is twice as efficient in sleep (37). In a correlative clinical study using acetaminophen, which is eliminated by these pathways, plasma half-life was 15% longer when given at 6 AM than at 2 PM, with a similar pattern seen in the rat (38, 39).

Elimination

Large physiologic variations in renal function during a 24-hour period have been well described (40–42). Renal drug elimination is differentially affected by circadian differences in renal blood flow and glomerular filtration rate, pH, and renal tubular function. Both endogenous circadian rhythmic processes and exogenous circadian factors such as posture, intake, activity, and sleep contribute to daily differences in renal drug handling. Glomerular filtration is maximum during the activity cycle. The factors that account for these rhythms include circadian fluctuation in blood pressure, which covaries with atrial natriuretic peptide, which modifies renal function, vascular tone, the renal angiotensin system, and action of brain regulatory sites (43, 44). Urinary pH, which decreases during sleep, and urine concentration are similarly affected in the supine position, and both influence the concentration and rate of excretion of administered drugs (45, 46). Circadian-dependent variations in urinary excretion and concentration of cisplatin have been correlated with circadian-dependent drug-induced kidney damage (47). These studies demonstrated that in humans, the drug is more efficiently eliminated when administered in early activity (Fig. 12.1). This corresponds to the time of maximal nephrotoxicity, presumably because of the higher concentration of the drug in the kidney tubules (Fig. 12.2).

CIRCADIAN RHYTHMS IN HOST SUSCEPTIBILITY

Host Tissue Cytokinetic Rhythms

Reproducible temporal variation in the susceptibility to toxic insult of normal and tumor tissues follows from concepts of chronobiology. Most normal proliferating tissues examined in adult mammals appear to exhibit a marked and reproducible circadian variation in rate or numbers of cells in DNA synthesis and mitosis (48–51). For example, cell division of rodent hematopoietic marrow cells undergoes regular circadian variation (51–54). The number of rodent bone marrow stem cells and myeloid and erythroid colony-forming units (55–58) also has a predictable circadian variation. Smaaland confirmed a circadian variation in the DNA content (S phase) of normal human marrow by cytofluorometry, which had been previously reported using other methods (59, 60). Mitotic activity and number of colony-forming units in human marrow have also been shown to vary with circadian time (60–65). The percentage of marrow cells undergoing DNA synthesis was greatest during the first half of the activity phase and lowest during the first half of the night. Circadian organization in cell proliferation throughout the gastrointestinal mucosa has been documented in rodents (48, 66) and human beings (67). The highest gut DNA synthetic activity occurs around 7 AM in humans in both fed and fasted states, similar to the pattern in the bone marrow. This rough overlap of cytokinetic phasing between the two most important chemotherapy toxicity target tissues of human beings (marrow and gut) implies that S phase–specific cytotoxic agents that damage the gut and/or bone marrow might be expected to be less toxic if given during the nighttime.

Immune and Endocrine Rhythms

The immune and endocrine networks show coordination of functions with the time of day, which may also, in part, contribute to the circadian time dependence of some cancer therapies. Many studies in animals and humans have documented prominent circadian-dependent variations in peripheral blood T and B lymphocytes, T lymphocyte subpopulations, monocytes, and NK cells (52, 68). In vitro functional activities of these cells also vary as a function of circadian time, such as spontaneous NK cell activity, lymphocyte mitogenic response, and mixed lymphocyte response (52, 69–71). In vivo immune responsiveness varies with circadian time, including hypersensitivity reactions, acute graft rejection, and antibody responsiveness (72–75).

Circadian variations in serum corticosterone levels may be one mechanism by which circadian-dependent variations in the immune cells and cytokine networks could be coordinated; however, other mechanisms may also be operative. Endogenous serum ACTH and corticosteroid concentrations exhibit a prominent circadian rhythm with peak levels in early activity. Corticosteroids cause the redistribution of lymphocyte populations, modulate the functional activity of immune cells, inhibit the production and decrease the mRNA stability of cytokines such as tumor necrosis factor-α (TNF), interferon (IFN)-γ, interleukin-2 (IL-2), and IL-1 (76–79). Serum concentrations of IL-1 and IL-1 production by monocytes show maximal levels in midafternoon and minimal levels in the morning, the exact opposite pattern of circadian serum corticosteroid level (80, 81). IL-1 also acts to increase ACTH and therefore glucocorticoid levels in vivo, thereby creating an immunoregulatory, circadian-paced, feedback loop (82). Plasma levels of TNF, granulocyte-macrophage colony-stimulating factor, IL-2, IL-10, and erythropoietin also vary with circadian time (83–85). Plasma prolactin levels show circadian variations that could also modulate immune and hematologic functions in a circadian-dependent manner (86).

The administration of exogenous corticosteroids has a varying ability to perturb natural glucocorticoid rhythms, depending on the dose and the circadian schedule employed. Exogenous corticosterone also alters the ability of an animal to tolerate chemotherapy and could also theoretically alter its effect on the tumor. For example, administration of dexamethasone to animals prior to giving methotrexate suppressed their endogenous corticosterone levels, and all animals subsequently died earlier after methotrexate administration (87). Maximal toxicity of methotrexate was found to be in late activity at the time of lowest serum corticosterone levels, and elevating corticosterone levels decreased methotrexate toxicity. Exogenous corticosteroids administered prior to cyclophosphamide markedly decreased the antitumor effects in mice (88, 89). ACTH given before doxorubicin raised protective levels of GSH to the maximum circadian level in a variety of murine tissues, which subsequently protected these tissues from toxicity (36). Therefore, adjuvant use of steroids for amelioration of chemotherapy side effects may alter drug action in general and make the circadian pattern of drug effect less predictable.

CIRCADIAN TIME STRUCTURE OF TUMORS

Tumor Cytokinetic Rhythms

Circadian cytokinetic studies of human tumors are difficult because of the need for repeated biopsies. In two studies of patients with skin nodules from breast cancer, the mitotic index was determined over 24 hours (90, 91). A large interindividual variation was observed in the daily pattern of tumor mitotic indices, but a group circadian rhythm was, nonetheless, documented, with the maximum in the early afternoon near 3 PM and the minimum near 3 AM (92). A highly significant circadian rhythm in tumor cell DNA synthesis was found in both aneuploid and diploid ovarian tumor cells from peritoneal washings of ovarian cancer patients (93). The peak in ovarian tumor S phase (mid- to late morning) was found to be nearly 12 hours out of phase with the DNA synthesis in benign mesothelial cells (evening) in these patients. The circadian pattern of DNA synthesis in malignant lymph nodes of patients with non-Hodgkin's lymphoma is coordinated within the day, peaking during early sleep, being out of phase with normal bone marrow, which peaks in the first half or middle of each day (Fig. 12.3) (59, 94).

These data indicate that some cancer cells are to some extent in communication with the circadian cytokinetic pacemakers of the host and that cell-cycle phase-specific therapy might be likely to be more effective at certain specific times of the day. For example, in Figure 12.3, treatment at Rx1 with an S phase–active drug at noon would expose a much higher proportion of proliferating bone marrow cells to the agent and a corresponding relatively lower proportion of malignant lymphocytes. Treatment at Rx2 (midnight) would conversely expose a much higher relative proportion of proliferating malignant lymphoma cells than bone marrow cells to that S phase–active agent. In the former case, a great deal of bone marrow suppression with a corresponding lack of cytotoxicity to lymphoma might be expected. In the latter case, more tumor cell kill could be achieved with the same dose of S phase–active cytotoxic therapy, with relatively little bone marrow damage.

If tumor tissue susceptibility is coordinated during the day by host circadian rhythms, therapeutic gain can additionally be achieved by administering a drug at the time of day associated with maximal tumor susceptibility to that particular drug, resulting in greater tumor cell kill. This time-of-day difference in tumor cell kill can be further enhanced if the time of day of maximal tumor susceptibility is different from the time of day associated with maximum susceptibility for the most sensitive host tissue. If the susceptibility of tumor tissue to cytotoxic chemotherapy is not at all, or only weakly, coordinated during the day by the circadian rhythms of the host, therapeutic gain can be achieved by administering the cytotoxic drug at the time of day when the host tissues are least

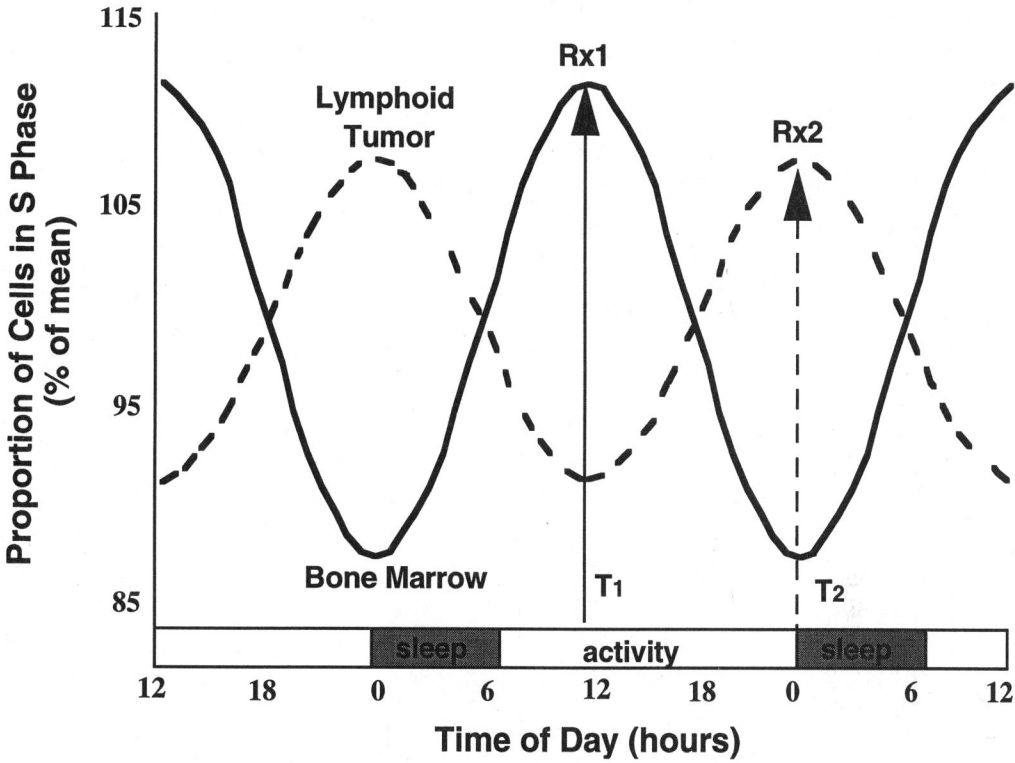

Figure 12.3. Circadian patterns of cytofluorometrically determined proportion of cells in DNA synthesis (S phase) in human nucleated bone marrow cells (*solid line*) (59) and malignant lymphocytes (*dashed line*) (94), obtained respectively from 16 normal subjects and 24 patients with malignant non-Hodgkin's lymphoma. Each subject had bone marrow sampled or a malignant lymph node aspirated every 3–4 hr for at least 24 hr. A highly statistically significant group circadian rhythm in the proliferate index of both tissues was found. This graph represents each series normalized to the circadian rhythm in cellular proliferation around their respective 24-hr means. While normal bone marrow DNA synthesis peaks each day around noon, DNA synthesis in lymphoma cells peaks near midnight.

damaged by that agent. This will allow escalation of dose intensity, with higher average doses delivered at correspondingly lower costs in terms of toxicity, possibly resulting in greater tumor cell kill.

Tumor Blood Flow Rhythms

The blood flow to subcutaneous tumors in rats has been shown to vary with circadian time, with twice the blood flow during the activity phase with no corresponding differences in tumor size or mean arterial blood pressure. This circadian rhythm in tumor blood flow was observed both early and late in the disease course. Angiotensin-induced hypertension elevated systemic arterial pressure equally but differentially increased tumor blood flow with greater increments during the activity phase (95). Since tumor blood flow is a major determinant of drug deliv-

ery to tumors (96) and oxygenation of tumors, this could contribute significantly to the circadian-dependent effects of chemotherapy and radiation therapy, respectively.

CIRCADIAN-TIMED THERAPY IN THE CANCER HOST

Most of the available data on chronopharmacology of cytotoxic agents have been obtained in rodents, but an increasing amount of data is now being amassed from organized human studies (Table 12.1). Each cytotoxic drug has an unique time-of-day efficacy pattern that depends on the compilation of several critical time-dependent factors discussed above. Drug analogues within the same class may or may not have similar circadian patterns, and combinations of drugs may or may not alter the optimal times of each drug. Therefore, empiric studies of drug

Table 12.1. Clinical Results Using Circadian-Timed Cancer Therapy

Drugs	n	Cancer	Schedule/Times Tested	Results	Author/Year
Fluoropyrimidine trials					
FUdR	54	Adv cancer	14 d flat v circ inf, peak 3–9 PM	Circ: less toxicity, > DI	(von Roemeling, Hrushesky 1989)
FUdR	63	Renal	14 d circ inf, peak 3–9 PM	OR: 24%	(Hrushesky et al. 1990)
FUdR	42	Renal	14 d circ inf, peak 3–9 PM	OR: 14%	(Damascelli et al. 1990)
FUdR	13	Renal	14 d circ inf, peak 3–9 PM	OR: 62%	(Huben et al. 1990)
FUdR	40	Renal	14 d circ inf, peak 3–9 PM	OR: 10%	(Dexeus et al. 1991)
FUdR	29	Renal	14 d flat v circ inf, peak 3–9 PM	Circ: > DI	(Wilkinson et al. 1993)
FUdR	28	Renal	14 d circ inf, peak 11 AM–11 PM	OR: 14%	(Conroy et al. 1993)
FUdR	20	Renal, GI	14 d circ inf, peak 3–9 PM	OR: 10%	(Natoli et al. 1994)
FUdR	26	Renal	14 d circ inf, peak 3–9 PM	OR: 8%	(Sampaio et al. 1994)
FUdR	104	Renal	14 d flat v circ inf, peak 2–8 PM	OR: 11%, Circ: less toxicity, > DI	(Bjarnason et al. 1995)
FUdR (ih)	48	GI (liver met)	14 d flat v circ inf, peak 3–9 PM	Same OR: 35%, circ: 70% > DI	(Wesen et al. 1992)
5FU (iv)/FUdR (ih)	38	GI (liver met)	5 d flat v circ inf; 5-FU peak 4 AM; FUDR peak 4 PM	OR: 43%; Circ: less neutropenia, alopecia	(Focan et al. 1994)
FUdR/LV	14	Adv cancer	5 d circ inf q 3 wk, peak 6 PM	Well tolerated	(Garufi et al. 1995)
5FU	35	GI	5 d circ inf, peak 4 AM	Higher DI (historical controls)	(Lévi et al. 1995)
5FU/LV	14	Adv cancer	14 d circ inf, peak 3–4 AM v 9–10 PM	Less toxicity, 9–10 PM	(Bjarnason et al. 1993)
5FU/LV	62	GI	14 d circ inf, peak 8 AM–4 PM v 4 PM-MN v MN-8 AM	OR: 29%	(Allegrini et al. 1995)
				Less toxicity, > DI, 4 PM-MN	(Falcone et al. 1995)
5FU/LV/Ox	93	GI	5 d circ inf q 3 wk; 5FU/LV, peak 4 AM; Oxaliplatin, peak 4 PM	OR: 58%	(Lévi et al. 1992b)
5FU/LV/Ox	37	GI (5FU resistant)	5 d circ inf q 3 wk; 5FU/LV, peak 4 AM; Oxaliplatin, peak 4 PM	OR: 43%	(Lévi et al. 1992a)
5FU/LV/Ox	48	GI (5FU resistant)	4 d circ inf q 2 wk; 5FU/LV, peak 4 AM; Oxaliplatin, peak 4 PM	OR: 38%	(Brienza et al. 1993)
5FU/LV/Ox	92	GI	5 d flat v circ inf q 3 wk; 5FU/LV, peak 4 AM; Oxaliplatin, peak 4 PM	OR: circ 53% v flat 32%; Toxicity: 2–8 fold lower, circ; DI(5FU/LV): 1.4 fold higher, circ; Improved survival (19 v 15 mo)	(Lévi et al. 1994)

Drugs	N	Cancer	Schedule	Results	Reference
5FU/LV/Mit	18	Breast	5 d circ inf q 3 wk 5FU/LV, peak 4 AM Mit, peak 4 PM	Well tolerated	(Deprés-Bummer et al. 1995)
5FU/LV/Carb	32	Lung	5 d circ inf q 3 wk 5FU/LV, peak 4 AM Carb, peak 4 PM	Well tolerated	(Focan et al. 1995)
Platinum trials					
Dox/Cisp	37	Ovary	A. Dox 6 AM, Cisp 6 PM v B. Dox 6 PM, Cisp 6 AM	Less toxicity, schedule A Survival A: 40% v. B: 11%	(Hrushesky 1985)
Dox/Cisp	23	Ovary, bladder	A. Dox 6 AM, Cisp 6 PM v B. Dox 6 PM, Cisp 6 AM	Less toxicity, schedule A	(Hrushesky et al. 1989)
Dox/Cisp	30	Endometrium	Dox 6 AM, Cisp 6 PM	OR: 60%	(Barrett et al. 1993)
THP-Dox/Cisp	31	Ovary	A. THP-Dox 6 AM, Cisp 4–8 PM B. THP-Dox 6 PM, Cisp 4–8 PM	A. OR: 73%, less toxicity B. OR: 57%, less DI	(Lévi et al. 1990)
Oxaliplatin	23	Adv cancer	5 d flat v circ inf, peak 4 PM	Circ: Less toxicity, 33% > DI	(Caussanel et al. 1990)
Carboplatin	7	Ovary	6 AM v 6 PM	Less thrombocytopenia, 6 PM	(Kerr et al. 1990)
VP16/Cisp	34	Adv cancer (previous Rx)	VP16, 7 AM or 7 PM	Less myelotoxicity, VP16 7 AM Cisplatin 6 PM	(Krakowski et al. 1988)
VP16/Cisp	124	Lung cancer	VP16, 6 AM v 6 PM Cisplatin, 6 PM	Less alopecia, VP16 at 6 AM Less nausea, ototoxicity VP16 6 PM Same marrow toxicity, DI	(Focan et al. 1990)
Methotrexate trials					
6-MP/MTX	118	ALL	Morning v evening	4-5 fold survival advantage, evening	(Rivard et al. 1985) (Rivard et al. 1993)
VB/CY/MTX	64	Adv cancer	A. 10 AM v B. 10 PM	OR: A > B (53 v 19%) Survival: A > B (8 v 4 mo)	(Focan 1979)
Biologic therapy					
Interferon-α	10	Renal, melanoma	21 d circ inf, peak 8 PM	Less toxicity, higher DI (historic controls)	(Deprés-Brummer et al. 1991)
Interferon-α	16	Adv cancer	7 d circ inf, peak 6 PM–3 AM	Less toxicity (historic controls)	(Iacobelli et al. 1995)
Melatonin	14	Breast cancer (tamoxifen failure)	melatonin, evening tamoxifen, midday	PR: 29%	(Lissoni et al. 1995)

aFUdR, fluorodeoxyuridine; 5-FU, 5-fluorouracil; LV, leucovorin; OX, oxaliplatin; Mit, mitoxantrone; Carb, carboplatin; Dox, doxorubicin; Cisp, cisplatin; THP-Dox, 4′ O-tetrahydropyranyldoxorubicin; VP16, etoposide; 6-MP, 6-mercaptopurine; MTX, methotrexate; VB, vinblastine, CY, cyclophosphamide; GI, colorectal cancer; met, metastases; Adv, advanced; ALL, acute lymphoblastic leukemia; v, versus; circ, circadian; inf, infusion; MN, midnight; DI, dose intensity; OR, overall response (complete plus partial responses).

timing around the clock are necessary to determine the optimal time for each drug, drug combination, and endpoint.

Cytotoxic Chemotherapy Drugs

FLUOROPYRIMIDINES
Biochemical Mechanisms

Multiple enzymes are involved in the anabolism of 5-fluorouracil (5-FU) and fluorodeoxyuridine (FUdR). The circadian pattern of activity of several of these enzymes has been carefully studied in rodents and human beings. Uridine phosphorylase, which converts administered 5-FU to FUdR, shows a circadian activity pattern in mouse liver, with a corresponding change in plasma uridine concentration, as does orotate phosphoribosyl-transferase (97, 98). On the other hand, thymidine phosphorylase, which under certain circumstances can also convert 5-FU to FUdR, has demonstrated little circadian variation in activity (98, 99). An important enzyme in fluorouracil activation is thymidine kinase, which anabolizes FUdR to FdUMP. FdUMP binds thymidylate synthase, thus blocking DNA synthesis through thymidine starvation. Thymidine kinase demonstrates a circadian variation in activity, with a similar pattern in rat spleen, marrow, intestine, and liver (100) that is in phase with the circadian variation in DNA synthesis in these tissues.

Circadian variation in dihydropyrimidine dehydrogenase (DPD) activity, the primary enzyme involved in fluoropyrimidine catabolism, was first demonstrated in human peripheral blood lymphocytes (101). Others subsequently demonstrated a circadian variation in DPD activity in rat and mouse liver (98, 99, 102). DPD activity in peripheral blood mononuclear cells has also been shown to vary with the time of day in cancer patients during a continuous steady-state infusion of 5-FU in a fashion similar to that in normal individuals (103). The circadian patterns of the rise and fall in enzyme activities of the anabolic and catabolic enzymes for fluoropyrimidines are exactly opposite to one another. Fluoropyrimidine effects may be extremely dependent upon their circadian timing because of (a) their very brief plasma half-life, (b) the dependence of antitumor effect and toxicity on anabolic clearance by DPD (104–106), (c) the marked circadian rhythm in their clearance, (d) the marked circadian variation in activities of the catabolic and anabolic enzymes for these drugs, and (e) the circadian variation in the fraction of cells in tissues in S phase, i.e., that are highly susceptible to fluoropyrimidine active metabolites.

Fluorodeoxyuridine (FUdR)

Preclinical trials in mice and rats and clinical chronotherapy trials in cancer patients have been fairly extensive (107–109). The toxicity of FUdR, given in mice as a bolus injection and in rats by circadian-shaped continuous infusion, has shown significant circadian-stage dependence in both its toxicology and antitumor efficacy (110–112). FUdR is most safely given and may be more effective against cancer during the later part of the daily activity cycle and the first half of the daily sleep span. Interestingly, the time of administration least likely to result in lethal toxicity is somewhat later with a continuous infusion schedule than when the bolus intravenous administration mode is employed.

A number of clinical studies have been performed using a 14-day intravenous infusion of FUdR by either flat infusion or by a quasi-sinusoidal circadian pattern (108). Up to severalfold better tolerance of the chemotherapy by the normal tissues was observed in the circadian arm of the studies, with FUdR peaking in the first half of the daily sleep cycle. Subsequent studies have confirmed the increased ability of patients to tolerate FUdR with the circadian schedule, with 50-100% more drug given with less toxicity (107, 113–116). An NCI-sponsored, multicenter trial in patients with renal cell cancer continues to accrue and randomize patients to a flat or circadian-shaped infusion of FUdR that confirms a significant difference in toxicity and dose intensity, favoring the circadian group (117, 118). Circadian-shaped administration of intraarterial hepatic FUdR has also improved and markedly (5-fold) diminished the frequency and severity of chemical cholangitis. These studies demonstrate that chronotherapy results in a safe 70% dose increase over flat schedules in one study, and more courses of treatment, at a higher dose intensity, with lower toxicity, in another study (109, 119).

5-Fluorouracil (5-FU)

A number of rodents studies have shown that the toxicity of 5-FU is markedly circadian-time dependent; however, there has not been consensus among studies as to the exact time of day that is the least toxic. Administration in the sleep span was found to be the safest in several studies

(120–122) while others found the safest time to be the sleep-wake interface (123). Other studies have found the least toxic time to be in midactivity (124, 125). Differences in endpoints, routes of drug administration, animal strain and species, drug dose, and schedule complicate the interpretation of these results. In aggregate, late activity to early sleep would appear to be the safest time for 5-FU. More studies are necessary to better resolve this. Only a few studies have looked at antitumor activity, with circadian-dependent efficacy found again, with the same limitations (122, 125). The exact relationship between circadian pattern of toxicity and efficacy is still not clear. Similar problems and questions of the exact best time of day for 5-FU are now being asked in clinical studies.

Infusional 5-FU.   One study in patients with colorectal cancer compared the toxicity of 5-FU using 5-day circadian-timed infusions with the majority of the dose given around 4 AM with historic studies in similar patients receiving 5-day flat infusions. Less toxicity and higher 5-FU dose intensity were achieved when most of the dose was given around 4 AM (126).

Infusional 5-FU and Leucovorin.   A 14-day infusion of escalating doses of 5-FU with leucovorin was performed with peak infusion of both agents at 4 AM. A cohort of patients, who developed more than grade II toxicity, had their peak infusion timing shifted from 4 AM to 10 PM. This trial found the maximum tolerated dose of the combination of 5-FU with leucovorin, administered in a circadian infusion pattern peaking at 4 AM, to be 250 mg/m^2/day for 5-FU and 20 mg/m^2/day for leucovorin. In the six patients who had their peak shifted from 4 AM to 10 PM, toxicity was subsequently reduced in all, at that same dose intensity, and further dose escalation was achieved in half of these patients (5-FU 300 mg/m^2/day and leucovorin 20 mg/m^2/day) (127). Another study, using 14-day infusion of 5-FU with leucovorin in colorectal patients, compared three times of day for peak delivery of equal doses, found lower toxicity and higher dose intensity when most of the drug was given between 4 PM and midnight, compared with peak delivery between 8 AM and 4 PM (second best), or midnight to 8 AM (worst for toxicity) (128, 129).

Infusional 5-FU, Leucovorin, and Oxaliplatin.   A series of studies with 5-FU with leucovorin combined with oxaliplatin (a cisplatin analogue) in a 5-day infusion with 5-FU/leucovorin

peaking at 4 AM and oxaliplatin peaking at 4 PM has been performed in patients with metastatic colorectal cancer. This regimen was well tolerated, with a 58% response in 93 patients and a 43% response in 37 previously treated patients (130). A randomized phase III multicenter trial compared this same 3 drug regimen of oxaliplatin, 5-FU, and leucovorin in previously untreated patients with metastatic colorectal cancer as either a 5-day continuous flat infusion or a 5-day circadian-timed infusion (peak 4 AM for 5-FU/leucovorin and 4 PM for oxaliplatin). Improved tolerability was reported with the circadian infusion, with a decreased incidence of stomatitis, hand-foot syndrome, neutropenia, and neuropathy. More importantly, increased response rates (49.5% vs. 30% $p = .007$) were also seen with the circadian infusion (131). These response rates in the circadian arm for metastatic colon cancer are better than most previously published rates for this disease. This is the largest study demonstrating that timing of cytotoxic drugs within the day determines their capacity to control metastatic cancer in human beings.

What Is the Best Timing for Fluoropyrimidines?   It is interesting to consider the possibility that concomitant use of a second agent such as leucovorin or platinum compounds that modulate the pharmacology of the first agent may cause a shift in the optimal chronobiologic timing of fluoropyrimidines. The addition of leucovorin to 5-FU may shift the optimum timing for the peak administration of 5-FU from the second half of the daily sleep span to the first half (132). The addition of cisplatin to 5-FU may also alter circadian patterns, which is supported by the finding of opposite circadian 5-FU pharmacokinetic profiles that have been reported with flat continuous infusions of 5-FU with or without platinum compounds. Two studies reported higher 5-FU plasma levels in early sleep during continuous 5-FU infusion when it was given concurrently with cisplatin (133, 134). Another study reported higher 5-FU plasma levels during early activity during 5-FU continuous infusion when it was given alone (103). The best time for peaking 5-FU and leucovorin infusion to minimize toxicity to the host may well be late in the daily activity span and first half of the sleep span. On the other hand, the best time for anticancer activity may not coincide with this time. Clearly this possibility is still open and critically important. It may well be that we need to pick a circadian pattern that is not minimally toxic to achieve maximal tumor control with fluoropy-rimidines. This very real possibility illustrates the need to plan multiarmed clinical studies to test several circadian times to evaluate toxicity and antitumor activity.

CYTOSINE ARABINOSIDE (Ara-C)

In mice who received an equal single dose of Ara-C at one of several different times of day, the lowest mortality was observed when the drug was given during the sleep span (135). Antitumor studies of Ara-C in leukemia-bearing mice have compared improvement in survival after equal doses of Ara-C every 3 hours for 24 hours, as opposed to the same total dose with Ara-C administration shaped at different times throughout the day (136). With the circadian, sinusoidally shaped Ara-C schedule, the long-term survival rate was 23%, compared with 11% for equal dosing throughout the day. In non-tumor-bearing mice, there was a clear advantage in lethal toxicity for animals given sinusoidal Ara-C in the rest span, with survival rates up to 80%, compared with 13% in the flat concentration schedule (137). Therefore, Ara-C is best administered to leukemic mice durng the midsleep span for optimal safety and antitumor efficacy. Analyses of the fraction of mouse bone marrow cells in DNA synthesis following circadian-timed Ara-C showed the greatest reduction when Ara-C was given in the second half of activity, near the time of lowest host tolerance (138). In studies combining Ara-C with other agents, including vincristine, cyclophospha-mide, cisplatin, and methylprednisolone, the optimal timing for Ara-C appears to remain relatively constant (139–141).

METHOTREXATE

A limited number of studies have been performed in a clinical setting. Intravenous metho-trexate has been studied in rats with peak toxicity in late activity/early rest phase (87). Methotrexate was found to have the longest half-life at the most toxic treatment time, which was at the time of lowest serum corticosterone. Interestingly, the toxicity could be blunted by the coadministration of corticosteroid (142). An enzymatic study showed that dihydrofolate reductase in the kidney was maximally inhibited by methotrexate in the early rest period, which correlates with the time of day of maximal toxicity (143). Clinical studies of several hundred children receiving oral methotrexate along with 6-MP as maintenance chemotherapy for ALL have

revealed that the drug may be better tolerated when given in the evening (16, 18, 19). More provocatively, the disease-free and overall survival of children receiving evening methotrexate along with 6-MP was found to be significantly better than that for children given their methotrexate in the morning. A small study in six lymphoma patients receiving methotrexate as a 30-minute infusion at either 6 AM or 6 PM found no differences in pharmacokinetics or clinical outcome (144).

PURINE ANALOGUES

In children with ALL in remission who were receiving maintenance chemotherapy with 6-MP daily and weekly methotrexate, together with monthly vincristine and prednisone, it was observed that of the 188 children in the study, 82 received their oral medications routinely in the morning and 36 received their medication each day in the evening, solely for reasons of convenience or compliance (16). Subsequent analysis determined that the relapse rate in those individuals who had survived free of disease for at least 78 weeks was likely to be 5 times greater in those given the chemotherapeutic agents in the morning than in those receiving the drugs in the evening (17). Conflicting results have been reported for pharmacokinetic studies in patients given oral 6-MP along with oral or intravenous methotrexate. In some of these studies, there have been no detectable drug concentration differences, regardless of the time of administration (145). In others, there appears to be a significantly larger area under the curve and a prolonged elimination half-life if 6-MP is administered in the evening rather than the morning hours (146, 147); this pharmacokinetic difference correlated with decrements in serum white blood cell counts (148, 149). Other data demonstrate interaction of milk enzymes (e.g., xanthine oxidase) with 6-MP (20). This may be relevant to 6-MP timing in ALL, since milk is an important constituent of many children's breakfast.

ANTHRACYCLINES

Chronopharmacodynamics Vary among Anthracyclines

Circadian studies with anthracyclines in animals demonstrate two- to threefold differences in lethal toxicity rates, depending on the time of day of their administration. The optimal circadian time varies, however, with both the route of drug administration and the particular drug analogue. Intraperitoneal administration of doxorubicin in rodents is the safest (e.g., mortality due to marrow and gut toxicity) when given during the second half of the sleep phase. The safest time for doxorubicin given intravenously, however, differs and is in mid to late activity (36, 150, 151). Circadian toxicology studies of other anthracycline analogues have demonstrated intraperitoneal mitoxantrone to be least toxic, with shortest drug half-life, when given in midactivity, while intraperitoneal epirubicin is least toxic when given in the midsleep span (152, 153).

Biochemical Mechanisms and Clinical Results

Drawing on results from several animal studies of the marked circadian-dependent toxicity and antitumor activity of doxorubicin and cisplatin, a sentinel study, reported in 1979, was designed in patients with metastatic bladder or ovarian cancer to receive doxorubicin and cisplatin, 12 hours apart, with cycles beginning at either 6 AM or 6 PM (154). A significant difference in nadir blood counts, time to nadir, and time to

blood count recovery was noted, with minimal myelotoxicity with morning doxorubicin and evening cisplatin (Fig. 12.4). In addition, nephrotoxicity was also markedly worse when cisplatin was administered at 6 AM, compared with 6 PM (Fig. 12.2).

In a similar study, patients with ovarian cancer were given doxorubicin and cisplatin at either 6 AM or 6 PM, respectively, with the second drug given 12 hours later (154, 155). In those patients who received doxorubicin at 6 AM and cisplatin at 6 PM, there were fewer dose reductions, episodes of infection, bleeding, treatment delays, and transfusion (Fig. 12.5). The average achievable dose intensity was also higher for the optimal schedule. This study confirmed the results of the earlier crossover study. The probability of 5-year survival was greater when doxorubicin was given 6 AM and cisplatin at 6 PM than when doxorubicin was given at 6 PM and cisplatin at 6 AM or when the same treatments were given at unspecified times (e.g., standard practice), similar to results obtained in tumor-bearing rats (Fig. 12.6) (154, 156).

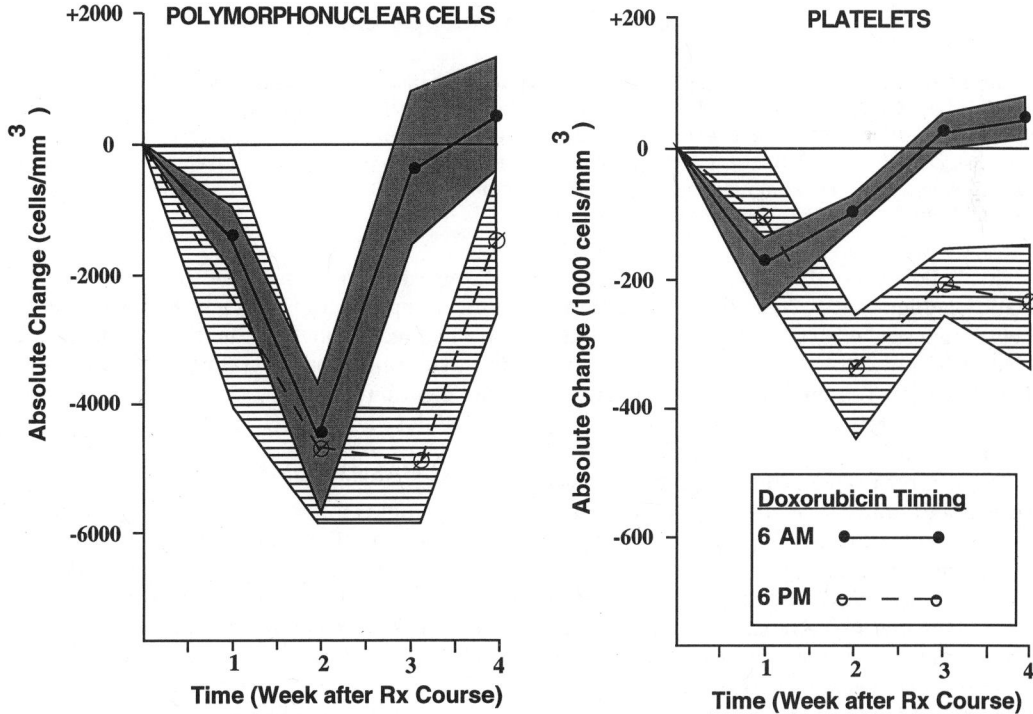

Figure 12.4.   Kinetics of peripheral blood count fall and recovery after doxorubicin-based chemotherapy (Rx) as a function of circadian time of doxorubicin administration. Data from a single patient showing change in neutrophil and platelet numbers from baseline after receiving morning doxorubicin (*closed circles,* 6 AM) and after receiving evening doxorubicin (*hatched,* 6 PM). *Shaded areas* represent two standard deviations.

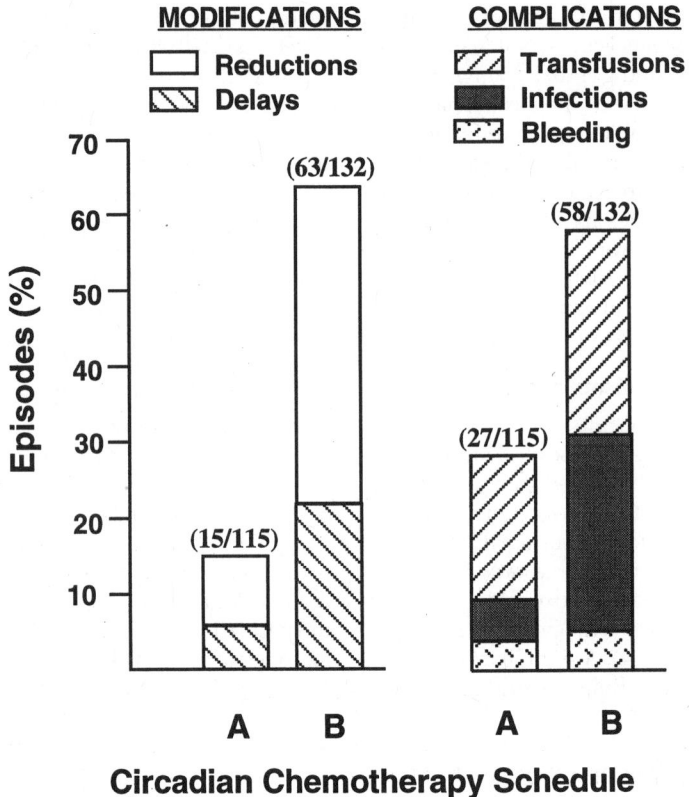

Figure 12.5.   The toxicities of two randomly assigned circadian treatment schedules (247 courses) in women with advanced ovarian cancer. Schedule A: doxorubicin 6 AM, cisplatin 6 PM; schedule B: cisplatin 6 AM, doxorubicin 6 PM. Dose reductions were three times more frequent when drugs were given on schedule B (31 vs. 9%, $\chi^2 = 17.4$, $p < .01$). Despite schedule B dose reductions and treatment delays, 44% of schedule B treatments were associated with bleeding, infection, or transfusion requirements, while only 23% of treatments given on schedule A were associated with these complications ($\chi^2 = 10.5$, $p < .01$).

In a follow-up study in 43 patients with metastatic bladder cancer, a similar randomization between these two schedules was performed, again with lower toxicity with the optimum timing (157). 4′-Tetrahydropyranyl doxorubicin (THP-doxorubicin) with cisplatin was studied in a similar manner, with two time-of-day schedules. Less renal and hematologic toxicity was seen in the optimal schedule, with response rates also felt to be improved (158). A single-armed chronobiologic study of doxorubicin and cisplatin in advanced endometrial cancer, performed by the Gynecologic Oncology Group, found overall response rates of 60%, three times the predicted response rate, with doxorubicin administered at 6 AM and cisplatin at 6 PM (159). Clearly, the anthracyclines appear to have a strong circadian stage dependency in terms of normal tissue toxicity and, perhaps as a result of maintained dose intensity, an improvement in

ultimate treatment outcome. In tumor-bearing animals, optimal timing at a fixed dose intensity also markedly enhanced the cure rates, indicating that optimal anthracycline circadian timing may contribute to better cancer control *independent* of dose intensity (160).

METAL-BASED COMPOUNDS

Platinum compounds each have very different toxicity profiles. Cisplatin, which is almost entirely excreted by the kidneys, is primarily a renal toxin and not primarily a marrow toxin. As a result of renal damange, cisplatin causes an isolated deficiency in red cells due to a progressive deficiency of erythropoietin (161). In contrast, carboplatin and oxaliplatin do not exhibit anywhere near the same degree of nephrotoxicity and act primarily as marrow toxins. Despite these differences, the circadian pattern of cisplatin and carboplatin drug-induced toxicity is

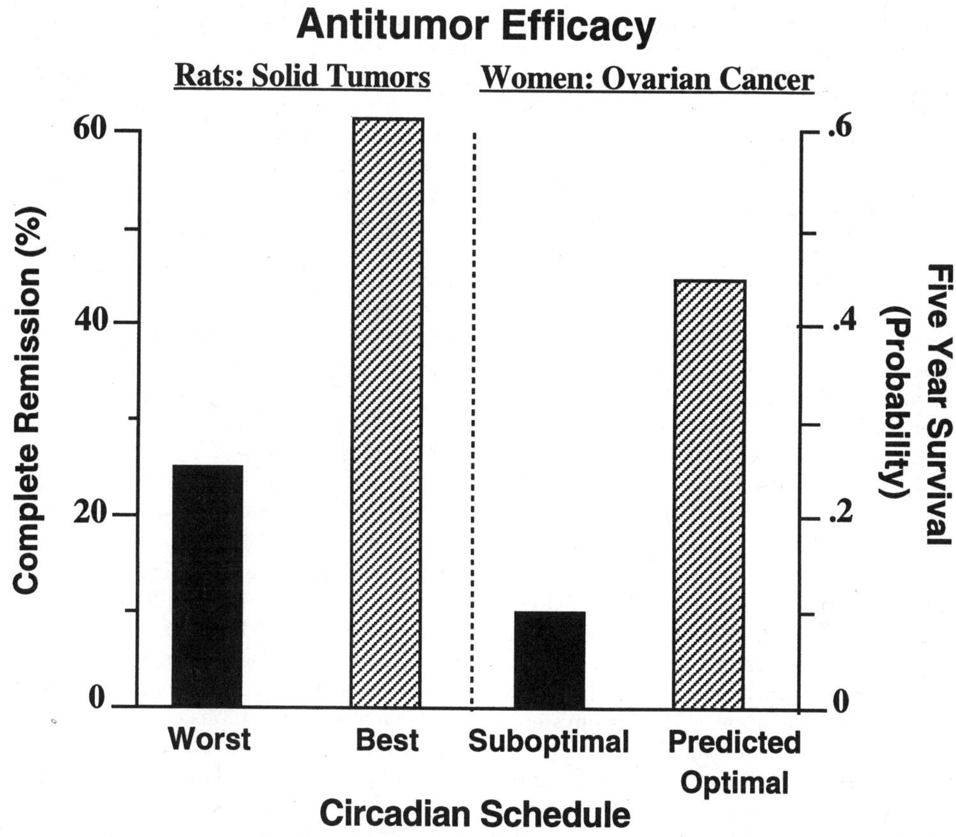

Figure 12.6.   The effect of circadian timing of doxorubicin/cisplatin circadian timing on antitumor efficacy and host toxicity. The ability of different circadian schedules of doxorubicin/cisplatin to control the growth of cancer in a transplanted rat tumor model and in women with advanced ovarian cancer is contrasted. In both studies, treatment timing was randomly assigned. In the rat system, if doxorubicin was given at usual daily awakening and cisplatin was given later in the daily activity span, 2.5 times as many complete tumor remissions were achieved compared with when cisplatin was given at usual awakening (Sothern et al. 1989). In women, the probability of 5-year survival was greater if the doxorubicin was given at 6 AM, just prior to usual daily awakening, and cisplatin was administered at 6 PM, than when doxorubicin was given at 6 PM followed by cisplatin at 6 AM (154, 155) (Modified from (247).

very similar (162–164). Because of the renal excretion of cisplatin and the fact that the plasma filtration rate is increased in the midactivity phase, one could hypothesize that the safest time to administer cisplatin would be during this span. This postulate was confirmed in a clinical study of urinary excretion kinetics that demonstrated that evening cisplatin administration is markedly less toxic than AM administration (165). Plasma protein binding of cisplatin is also circadian-stage dependent, with daily maximum around 4 PM (166). Studies of cisplatin given with anthracyclines have confirmed optimal dosing for reducing toxicity to be in the early evening hours (159, 160). This correlates well with animal studies, in which cisplatin was also better tolerated in mid to late activity (162, 165, 167) as were carboplatin and oxaliplatin (168). This chronopharmacology has been confirmed in humans; much greater thrombocytopenia was seen in patients when carboplatin was given at 6 AM than at 6 PM (169). Less toxicity and subsequently higher dose intensity were also demonstrated with a circadian infusion of carboplatin peaking at 4 PM, compared with a flat infusion (170).

ALKYLATING AGENTS

Although these agents have ultimately similar endpoints of action, they each require somewhat different metabolic steps for activation, and as a result, murine studies have demonstrated that the optimal timing of administration of these agents is quite different within this group. For example, cyclophosphamide given by the intraperitoneal route in a murine model is least toxic when given after daily arising (171–173). The optimal time for ifosfamide for the least toxicity is late in the activity phase (174). Mitomycin-C has been found to be least toxic, as measured by lethality, when administered to mice in mid- to late activity phase (175, 176). Histologically, this lethal toxicity may have been related to mitomycin-C-induced microangiopathic disease, which is a feared and often fatal clinical complication of this drug. Trough plasma concentrations of busulfan given in high dose to children for bone marrow transplantation show large circadian variation, with highest values in the early morning (177).

PLANT ALKALOIDS

Each of these drugs has a very different circadian optimum of delivery for least toxicity in mice. Vincristine has been found to be least toxic in early activity, vinblastine in midactivity, vinorelbine in late activity, and etoposide in late sleep (178–181). Vindesine, when administered by constant infusion over 48 hours in nine patients, exhibited a circadian variation in serum concentration, with maximum concentration at midday (182). In a study of patients given cisplatin at 6 PM and etoposide at either 6–7 AM or 6–7 PM, less alopecia occurred in the morning etoposide group, and less cisplatin toxicity (nausea, ototoxicity) occurred in the evening etoposide group in one study (183), while another study showed less marrow toxicity with morning etoposide (184).

Recombinant Protein Therapy in Cancer Patients

Circadian studies with recombinant proteins are beginning to provide support for the idea that the timing of cytokines within the day may affect both host toxicity and overall responses. For the antitumor cytokines TNF, IL-2, and IFN, substantial dose-related toxicities and limited antitumor response rates demand that these drugs be better understood and more optimally delivered. Clinical use of other less toxic cytokines is limited by their expense.

TUMOR NECROSIS FACTOR

Up to ninefold differences in the circadian-dependent lethal toxicity of human TNF in normal mice have been reported, with greatest toxicity when given just prior to daily awakening

(185). Consistent with the marked circadian dependence of TNF toxicity is the very similar circadian-dependent toxicity profile of endotoxin, whose toxicity is, in part, mediated by TNF (186–188). The antitumor activity of TNF appears also to vary with circadian timing, with greatest slowing of tumor growth and highest cures when given in late activity/early sleep (189). A circadian-dependent therapeutic window for maximal antitumor activity and yet lowered toxicity could be realized in this mouse tumor model by appropriate circadian timing of TNF in late activity.

INTERLEUKIN-2

The immune effects of IL-2 in mice are greater, as measured by increased spleen cell numbers and marrow natural killer cells, when IL-2 is administered in the activity phase (190). Toxicity of high-dose IL-2 in mice, as measured by survival, weight loss, and hypothermic effects, was the least when IL-2 was given during late activity (191). The antitumor response to IL-2 in mice with subcutaneous meth A sarcoma has been found to be biphasic, with inhibition of tumor growth when IL-2 was given in the late sleep phase and stimulation of tumor growth when given in midactivity phase (192). Rats with hepatomas transplanted into the liver, treated with hepatic arterial continuous infusion of IL-2, better tolerated the IL-2 and had higher tumor response rates with circadian-shaped IL-2 infusion weighted in late sleep, compared with those given IL-2 by a flat continuous infusion (193).

INTERFERON

The ability of IFN-α and -γ to augment NK cell activity in vitro shows a circadian susceptibility rhythm in mice and humans, with greatest activity in late activity/early sleep phase (194, 195). The ability of melatonin to stimulate IFN-γ production is greater in murine spleen cells obtained just after dark onset, which is the time of the endogenous rise in melatonin (196).

The circadian timing of IFN affects the degree of myelotoxicity in mice, with less white blood cell and marrow precursor suppression when IFN-α is administered in late sleep and when IFN-γ is administered in early activity (197, 198). Less suppression of blood lymphocyte numbers has been reported when IFN-α and -γ are given in early sleep (199). Reports of evening injections of IFN-α have claimed reduced toxicities in patients, compared with historic controls (200). Two clinical studies of circadian-timed IFN-α in advanced cancer have given large daily doses by continuous infusion over 21 days or 7 days with peak doses delivered in the evening (201, 202). Toxicities such as flulike symptoms, somnolence, and liver enzyme abnormalities were less severe than other previously reported continuous flat infusions of IFN, allowing a larger increment in dose intensity. The antitumor activity of IFN-α and -γ toward B16 melanoma in mice is greater in early sleep for IFN-α and greater in early activity phase for IFN-γ (203). Circadian timing in this model could produce maximal antitumor efficacy with less myelotoxicity for both of these interferons.

HEMATOPOIETIC GROWTH FACTORS

The response to erythropoietin (EPO), as measured by reticulocyte response, erythroid colony formation, and red cell mass expansion, varies with the circadian time of its subcutaneous administration in mice (57, 204, 205). Optimal circadian timing of EPO (late activity in mice) resulted in a twofold larger increment in red cell mass and required half the time to reach a target hematocrit.

INTERLEUKIN-1

IL-1 can modulate ACTH and glucocorticoid levels, each of which vary with circadian time, thereby creating a circadian-paced, immunoregulatory feedback loop (82). Serum levels of IL-1 (80) and IL-1 production by human blood monocytes (81) are substantially higher in the late activity phase of each day, the exact opposite to circadian glucocorticoid levels. The sleep-inducing effects and pyrogenic effects of intracerebral injections of IL-1-β in rats are reported to be greater at the time of sleep onset (206). IL-1 activity in the spinal fluid also varies with sleep-wake cycles in cats (207).

Radiation Therapy

Therapeutic results and patient tolerance to radiation are limited by the toxicity to normal tissues. The circadian timing of whole body radiation in mice has been shown to markedly affect overall toxicity, measured by lethality and the number of acutely surviving multipotent stem cells and nucleated marrow cells, with greater host tolerance when administered in sleep (208, 209). The efficacy of radiation therapy is highly dependent on the degree of tumor oxygenation and, therefore, tumor blood flow and hemoglobin concentration. Both tumor blood flow (95) and host hemoglobin concentrations vary with time of day and could therefore affect

radiation-induced antitumor responses. Clinical trials of circadian timing of radiation therapy have not been conducted.

Clinical Summary

Table 12.1 summarizes the current clinical data for circadian-timed therapy in cancer. Advantages for "optimal" circadian scheduling have been demonstrated for diminishing side effects and for increasing maximal safe dose intensity of drugs of diverse classes. Circadian scheduling advantage for three xenobiotics (doxorubicin, THP-doxorubicin, and etoposide) seems to favor early morning administration, perhaps because of a circadian synchrony of important oxidative defense mechanisms. Reactive nucleophilic platinum-based drugs (cisplatin and oxaliplatin) are more safely and effectively given in the evening, probably because of circadian variation in their protein binding, excretory pharmacokinetics, or other host cellular defense strategies. Antimetabolites (5-FU, FUdR, 6-MP, and methotrexate) are better tolerated and most effective when given in the evening hours or early in the daily sleep span, probably because these times of day are associated with the least DNA synthesis in bone marrow and gut. Circadian coordination of biochemical pathways relevant to both the anabolism and catabolism of these antimetabolites may also be, in part, responsible for the existence of prominent circadian rhythms in their toxicity and efficacy. Substantial advantages with circadian-timed chemotherapy have now been established in metastatic colon cancer, which double response frequency.

CURRENT LIMITATIONS IN CIRCADIAN-TIMED CANCER THERAPY

Chronobiology and Drug Development

The changes for successful anticancer drug development can be enhanced by taking chronopharmacology into account early in the drug development process. If the target of drug action is virtually present or absent at specific times of day, the results of in vivo screening studies will be divergent, depending upon when in the day they are performed. Preclinical studies are usually performed in the first half of the "working day," which corresponds to the first half of the mouse's sleep span (e.g., lights on during the sleep phase of these nocturnal animals). Phase I clinical trials are also carried out in the first half of the working day, the activity phase, exactly opposite to the circadian time studied in rodents, which might therefore be poorly predictive of drug toxicity. A poor therapeutic index could result from these preclinical and clinical circadian time discrepancies and cause an agent to be discarded as too toxic. The scenario would be different if preclinical studies demonstrated the optimum circadian time for therapy and subsequent phase I trials were performed at this time of day or at least several times of day. Since efficacy is also nonlinearly related to treatment timing, the circadian timing of drug administration in phase II and phase III studies is likewise relevant to maximizing drug efficacy.

Convenient and Predictable Delivery

To reliably and practically administer drugs at specific times within a 24-hour cycle, programable timed delivery mechanisms are needed to make this process more accurate, convenient, and less error prone. This has begun to be achieved with time-delayed pill formulations and computer-programable devices with clocks for timed parenteral deliveries. The issue is more complex when the drug or protein is delivered by a continuous infusion or in multiple and delayed timed pulses. In this case, not only is a programable delivery needed to administer the drug according to an optimal chronotherapeutic schedule, but the physical-chemical properties of the delivered agent and the surfaces of the device and tubing need to be understood. Not only can drugs adhere to the artificial surfaces and therefore be lost, but they may also be structurally altered by this interaction and loose biological activity. Recently the biologic activity of IL-2 was shown to be decreased by 90% during flow through a medical-grade silicone catheter, owing to conformational changes in the protein structure far beyond those losses attributable to adsorption (210). In the future, more sophisticated devices will be available, which may in addition respond via sensors to internal biologic rhythms (211–216). These may also include devices that deliver drugs through a transdermal route, using electric current or ultrasound waves to drive the agent through the skin or magnets to vary the release of drugs from implanted devices (217).

Relative Impact of Circadian Therapy

The benefits of circadian chemotherapy have been to reduce toxicity and hence improve quality of life, allow increased dose intensity, allow fewer days of hospitalization, and reduce treatment delays. The differences have ranged from 50% to eight- to tenfold in some studies. The survival advantage has been examined in several studies, but very few have been of adequate design or size to confirm these initial positive studies. Cost savings (less drug, less hospital admissions) have been implied from these results but have yet to be formally analyzed in these studies. How these and future circadian therapy results will compare with other strategies remains to be determined.

FUTURE DIRECTIONS

A better mechanistic understanding of circadian rhythms and drug action at the organ, cellular, and molecular level is needed to allow more rational design of circadian trials. Application of results from murine studies and the use of multiarm clinical designs with response surface analysis techniques will help to answer whether there is a best time for the treatment of particular cancers with specific drugs (218). Randomized clinical trials testing different times of day for therapies in cancer patients are necessary to actually determine what benefits can be derived (toxicity reduction, quality of life, response rates, survival) and the magnitude of such effects. In addition, to better understand circadian variations in the balance between a person and an established cancer, it will be invaluable to apply what we know and what we will learn about circadian biology toward preventing the development of a cancer.

Other biologic rhythms also appear relevant to the cancer problem. The ability to cure a transplanted mouse breast cancer by surgical resection has been shown to depend upon when in the fertility cycle the operation is performed (219). Twice as many mice are cured if the resection is performed at a time in the cycle near to follicle-stimulating hormone (FSH)/luteinizing hormone (LH) surges (proestrus). Cellular immune cancer defenses are much higher during this same phase (220). Ten retrospective studies of more than 2500 young women indicate that 10-year survival probability is enhanced by an average of 30% when the resection of the primary breast cancer is performed in the 7 to 10 days immediately following the FSH/LH surge (221–231). Several clinical studies, however, have failed to support these findings. These findings suggest that biologic rhythms other than the circadian cycle have profound influence over the host-cancer balance.

REFERENCES

1. Dunlap JC. Genetic analysis of circadian clocks. Annu Rev Physiol 1993;55:683–728.

2. Feldman JF, Hoyle M. Isolation of circadian clock mutants of *Neurospora crassa*. Genetics 1973; 75:605–613.

3. Konopka RJ, Benzer S. Clock mutants of *Drosophila melanogaster*. Proc Natl Acad Sci USA 1971; 68:2112–2116.

4. Ralph MR, Menaker M. A mutation of the circadian system in golden hamsters. Science 1988; 241:1225–1227.

5. Sehgal A, Price JL, Man B, Young MW. Loss of circadian behavioral rhythms and per RNA oscillations in the *Drosophila* mutant timeless. Science 1994; 263:1602–1606.

6. Vitaterna MH, King DP, Chang AM, et al. Mutagenesis and mapping of a mouse gene, *clock*, essential for circadian behavior. Science 1994;264:719–725.

7. Sassone-Corsi P. Rhythmic transcription and autoregulatory loops: winding up the biologic clock. Cell 1994;78:361–364.

8. Touitou Y, Haus E. Biologic rhythms in clinical and laboratory medicine. New York: Springer-Verlag, 1992.

9. Muller JE, Stone PH, Turi ZG, et al. Circadian variation in the frequency of onset of acute myocardial infarction. N Engl J Med 1985;313:1315–1322.

10. Tofler GH, Brezinski D, Schafer AI, et al. Concurrent morning increase in platelet aggregability and the risk of myocardial infarction and sudden death. N Engl J Med 1987;316:1514–1518.

11. Lemmer B. Cardiovascular chronobiology and chronopharmacology. In: Touito Y, Haus E, eds. Biologic rhythms in clinical and laboratory medicine. New York: Springer-Verlag, 1992;418–427.

12. Heading RCP, Tothill P, McGloughlin G, Sheaman DBC. Gastric emptying rate measurement in man. Gastroenterology 1976;71:45–50.

13. Lemmer B. Chronopharmacokinetics: In: Briemer D, Speiser P, eds. Topics in pharmaceutical sciences. New York: Elsevier, 1981:49–68.

14. Meyers JH. Motility of the stomach and duodenum. Physiology of the gastrointestinal tract. 2nd ed. New York: Raven Press, 1987:613–629.

15. Reinberg A, Smolensky MH. Circadian changes of drug disposition in man. Clin Pharmacokinet 1982; 7:401–402.

16. Rivard G, Infante-Rivard C, Hoyoux C, Champagne J. Maintenance chemotherapy for childhood acute lymphoblastic leukemia: better in the evening. Lancet 1985;ii:1264–1266.

17. Rivard GE, Infante-Rivard C, Dresse MF. Circadian time dependent response of childhood lymphoblastic leukemia to chemotherapy. A long term follow-up study of survival. Chronobiol Int 1993;10:201–204.

18. Riccardo R, Balis FM, Ferrara P, Lasorella A, Poplack DG, Mastrangelo R. Influence of food intake on bioavailability of oral 6-mercaptopurine in children with acute lymphoblastic leukemia. Pediatr Hematol Oncol 1986;3:319–324.

19. Pinkerton CR, Welshman SG, Glasgow JFT, Bridges JM. Can food influence the absorption of methotrexate in children with acute lymphoblastic leukemia? Lancet 1980;ii:944–945.

20. Rivard GE, Lin KT, Leclerc JM, David M. Milk could decrease the bioavailability of 6-mercaptopurine. Am J Pediatr Hematol Oncol 1989;11:402–206.

21. Bruguerolle B. Circadian phase dependent pharmacokinetics of disopyramide. Chronobiol Int 1984;1:267–271.

22. Bruguerolle B, Valli M, Jadot G, Bouyard L, Bouyard P. Circadian effect on carbamazepine kinetics in the rat. Eur J Drug Metab Pharmacokinet 1981; 6:189–194.

23. Bruguerolle B, Jadot G, Valli M, Bouyard L, Bouyard P. Etude chronocinetique de la lidocaine chex le rat. J Pharmacol (Paris) 1982;13:65–76.

24. Hecquet B, Bonneterre J. Cisplatin binding on plasma proteins. In: Reinberg A, Smolensky M, Labrecque G, eds. Annu Rev Chronopharmacol vol 1. New York: Pergamon Press, 1984;115–118.

25. Lemmer B, Nold G. Circadian changes in estimated hepatic blood flow in healthy subjects. Br J Pharmacol 1991;32:627–629.

26. Belanger MP, Labreque G. Temporal aspects of drug metabolism. In: Lemmer B, ed. Chronopharmacology: cellular and biochemical interactions. New York: Marcel Dekker, 1989:15–34.

27. Wielgus-Serafinska E, Plwka A, Ksminski M. Circadian variation of mitochondrial succinic dehydrogenase and microsomal cytochrome P-450 dependent monooxygenase activity in the liver of sexually immature and mature rats. J Physiol Pharmacol 1993; 44:55–63.

28. Radzialowski F, Bousquet W. Daily rhythmic variation in hepatic drug metabolism in rat and mouse. J Pharmacol Exp Ther 1968;163:229–238.

29. North C, Feuers RJ, Scheving LE, Pauli JE, Tsai TH, Casciano DA. Circadian organization of thirteen liver and six brain enzymes of the mouse. Am J Anat 1981;162:184–199.

30. Jaeger RJ, Conolly RB, Murphy SD. Diurnal variation of hepatic glutathione concentration and its correlation with 1,1-dichloroethylene inhalation toxicity in rats. Res Comm Chem Pathol Pharmacol 1973; 6:465–471.

31. Hrushesky WJM, Dell I, Eaton J, Halberg F. Circadian-stage-dependent effect of doxorubicin upon reduced glutathione in the murine heart (abstract). Proc Am Assoc Cancer Res 1982;23:12.

32. Smaaland R, Svardal AM, Lote K, Ueland PM, Laerum OD. Glutathione content in human bone marrow and circadian stage relation to DNA synthesis. J Natl Cancer Inst 1991;83:1092–1098.

33. Farooqui MYH, Ahmed AE. Circadian periodicity in tissue glutathione and its relationship with lipid peroxidation in rats. Life Sci 1984;34:2413–2418.

34. Haus E, Halberg F, Sothern RB, et al. Time-varying effects in mice and rats of several synthetic ACTH preparations. Chronobiologia 1980;7:211.

35. Lévi F, Hrushesky WJM, Holtzman J, Halberg G, Sanchez S, Kennedy BJ. ACTH 1-17 (A) raises cardiac-reduced glutathione (GSH) and protects mice from doxorubicin (D) lethal cardiotoxicity. Int J Chronobiol 1981;7:277.

36. Lévi F, Halberg F, Haus E, et al. Synthetic adrenocorticotropin for optimizing murine circadian

chronotolerance for adriamycin. Chronobiologia 1980; 7:227–244.

37. Belanger PM, Lalande M, Labrecque G, Dore FM. Diurnal variations in the transferases and hydrolases involved in glucuronide and sulfate conjugation of rat liver. Drug Metab Dispos 1985;13:386–389.

38. Shivley CA, Vesell ES. Temporal variations in acetaminophen and phenacetin half-life in man. Clin Pharmacol Ther 1975;18:413–424.

39. Belanger P, Lalande M, Dore F, Labreque G. Time-dependent variations in the organ extraction ratios of acetaminophen in rat. J Pharmacokinet Biopharm 1987;15:133–143.

40. Cambar J, Lemoigne F, Toussaint C. Diurnal variations evidence of glomerular filtration in the rat (author's transl) [French]. Experientia 1979;35:1607–1609.

41. Koopman MG, Krediet RT, Arisz L. Circadian rhythms and the kidney. Neth J Med 1985;28:416–423.

42. Waterhouse JM, Minors DS. Temporal aspects of renal drug elimination. In: Lemmer B, ed. Chronopharmacology: cellular and biochemical interactions. New York: Marcel Dekker, 1989:35–50.

43. Hermida RC, Ayeda DE, Fernandez JR, Major A. Time specified reference limits for ambulatory monitored blood pressure in clinical health. Biomed Instrum Technol 1993;27(3):235–243.

44. Portaluppi F, Vergnani L. Atrial natriuretic peptide and circadian blood pressure regulation: clues from a chronobiologic approach. Chronobiology 1993; 10(3):176–189.

45. Koopman MG, Kreiet RT, Zuyderhoudt FJM, deMoor EAM, Arisz L. A circadian rhythm of proteinuria in patients with a nephrotic syndrome. Clin Sci 1985;69:395–401.

46. Conroy RTWL, Mills JN. Human circadian rhythms. London: JA Churchill, 1970.

47. Lévi F. Chronopharmacologie de trois agents doués d'activité anticancéreuse chez le rat et/ou la souris (thesis). Paris: Université Paris VI, 1982.

48. Scheving LE, Tsai TS, Feuers RJ, Scheving LA. Cellular mechanisms involved in the action of anticancer drugs. In: Lemmer B, ed. Chronopharmacology: cellular and biochemical interactions. New York: Marcel Dekker, 1989:317–369.

49. Scheving LE. Circadian rhythms in cell proliferation: their importance when investigating the basic mechanism of normal versus abnormal growth. In: von Mayersbach H, Scheving LE, Pauli JE, eds. 11th International Congress of Anatomy, part C, Biological rhythms in structure and function. New York: Alan R Liss, 1981:39–79.

50. Durie BMG, Salmon SE, Russell DH. Polyamines as markers of response and disease activity in cancer chemotherapy. Cancer Res 1977;36:214–221.

51. Laerum OD, Sletvold O, Riise T. Circadian and circannual variation of the cell cycle distribution in the mouse bone marrow. Chronobiol Int 1988;5:19–35.

52. Haus E, Lakatua DJ, Swoyer J, Sackett LL. Chronobiology in hematology and immunology. Am J Anat 1983;168(4):467–517.

53. Laerum OD, Aardal NP. Chronobiological aspects of bone marrow and blood cells. In: von Mayersbach H, Scheving LE, Pauli JE, eds. 11th International Congress of Anatomy, part C, Biological rhythms in structure and function. New York: Alan R Liss, 1981:87–97.

54. Laerum OD, Smaaland R, Sletvold O. Rhythms in blood and bone marrow: potential therapeutic implications. In: Lemmer B, ed. Chronopharmacology: cellular and biochemical interactions. New York: Marcel Dekker, 1989:371–393.

55. Stoney PJ, Halberg F, Simpson HW. Circadian variation in colony-forming ability of presumably intact murine bone marrow cells. Chronobiologia 1975; 2:319–324.

56. Bartlett P, Haus E, Tuason T, Sacket-Lundeen L, Lakatua D. Circadian rhythm in number of erythroid and granulocytic colony forming units in culture (ECFU-C and GCFU-C) in bone marrow of BDF1 male mice. In: Haus E, Kabat HF, eds. Proc 15th International Conference on Chronobiology. Basel: S. Krager, 1984:160–164.

57. Wood P, Peace D, Hrushesky W. Endogenous erythropoiesis and erythropoietin responsiveness are circadian time dependent (abstract). Blood 1993;82:225.

58. Perpoint B, Le Bousse-Kerdiles C, Clay D, et al. In vitro chronopharmacology of recombinant mouse IL-3, mouse GM-CSF, and human G-CSF on murine myeloid progenitor cells. Exp Hematol 1995;23:362–368.

59. Smaaland R, Laerum OD, Lote K, Sletvold O, Sothern RB, Bjerknes R. DNA synthesis in human bone marrow is circadian stage dependent. Blood 1991; 77:2603–2611.

60. Mauer AM. Diurnal variation of proliferative activity in the human bone marrow. Blood 1965;26:1–7.

61. Killman SA, Cronkite EP, Fliedner TM, Bond VP. Mitotic indices of human bone marrow cells. I. Number and cytologic distribution of mitosis. Blood 1962;19:743–750.

62. Morley AA. A neutrophil cycle in healthy individuals. Lancet 1966;ii:1220–1222.

63. Ponassi A, Morra L, Bonanni F, et al. Normal range of blood colony forming cells (CFU-C) in humans. Blut 1979;39:257–263.

64. Ross DD, Pollak A, Akman SA, Bachur NR. Diurnal variation of circulating human myeloid progenitor cells. Exp Hematol 1980;8:954–960.

65. Smaaland R, Laerum O, Sothern R, Sletvold O, Bjerknes R, Lote K. Colony-forming unit-granulocyte-macrophage and DNA synthesis of human bone marrow are circadian stage dependent and show covariation. Blood 1992;79:2281–2287.

66. Scheving LE, Burns ER, Pauli JE, Tsai TH. Circadian variation in cell division of the mouse alimentary tract, bone marrow and corneal epithelium. Anat Rec 1978;191:479–486.

67. Buchi KN, Moore JG, Hrushesky WJM, Sothern RB, Rubin NH. Circadian rhythm of cellular proliferation in the human rectal mucosa. Gastroenterology 1991;101:410–415.

68. Lévi F, Canon C, Blum JP, Mechkouri M, Reinberg A, Mathe G. Circadian and/or circahemidian rhythms in nine lymphocyte-related variables from peripheral blood of healthy subjects. J Immunol 1985; 134:217–222.

69. Fernandes G, Halberg F, Yunis E, Good RA. Circadian rhythmic plaque-forming cell response of spleens from mice immunized by SRBC. J Immunol 1976;117:962–966.

70. Abo T, Kawate K, Itoh K, Kumagai K. Studies on the bioperiodicity of immune response. I. Circadian

rhythms of human T, B, and K cell traffic in the peripheral blood. J Immunol 1981;126:1360–1363.

71. Indiveri F, Perri I, Rogna S, et al. Circadian variations of autologous mixed lymphocyte reactions and endogenous cortisol. J Immunol Methods 1985;82:17–24.

72. Reinberg A, Zagulla-Mally Z, Ghata J, Halberg F. Circadian reactivity rhythms of human skins to house dust, penicillin and histamine. J Allergy 1989; 44:292–298.

73. Gervais P, Reinberg A, Gervais C, Smolensky M, DeFrance O. Twenty four hour rhythm in the bronchial hyperactivity to house dust in asthmatics. J Allergy Clin Immunol 1977;59:207–213.

74. Knapp MS, Pownall R, Cove-Smith JR. Circadian variation in cell-mediated immunity and the timing of human allograft rejection. In: Walker CA, Winget CM, Soliman KFA, eds. Chronopharmacology and chronotherapeutics. Tallahassee, FL: A&M University Foundation, 1981;329–338.

75. Fernandes G. Chronobiology of immune functions: cellular and humoral aspects. In: Touitou Y, Haus E, eds. Biologic Rhythms in Clinical and Laboratory Medicine. New York: Springer-Verlag, 1992: 493–503.

76. Beutler B, Krochin N, Milsark I, Luedke C, Cerami A. Control of cachectin (tumor necrosis factor) synthesis: mechanisms of endotoxin resistance. Science 1986;232:977–980.

77. Gessani S, McCandless S, Babglioni C. The glucocorticoid dexamethasone inhibits synthesis of interferon by decreasing the level of its mRNA. J Biol Chem 1988;263:7454–7457.

78. Arya SK, Wong-Staal F, Gallo RC. Dexamethasone-mediated inhibition of human T cell growth factor and gamma-interferon messenger RNA. J Immunol 1984;133:273–276.

79. Lee SW, Tsou AP, Chan H, et al. Glucocorticoids selectively inhibit the transcription of interleukin 1 beta gene and decrease the stability of interleukin 1 beta mRNA. Proc Natl Acad Sci USA 1988;85:1204–1208.

80. Bourin P, Lévi F, Mansour I, Doinel C, Joussemet M. Circadian rhythm of interleukin I (IL-1) in serum of healthy men. Annu Rev Chronopharmacol 1990;7:201–204.

81. Zabel P, Horst H, Kreiber C, Schlaak M. Circadian rhythm of interleukin-1 production of monocytes and the influence of endogenous glucocorticoids in man. Klin Wochenschr 1990;68:1217–1221.

82. Besedovsky H, Rey AD, Sorkin E, Dinarello CA. Immunoregulatory feedback between interleukin-1 and glucocorticoid hormones. Science 1986;223:652–654.

83. Young MRI, Matthews JP, Kanabrocki EL, Sothern RB, Roitman-Johnson B, Scheving LE. Circadian rhythmometry of serum interleukin-2, interleukin-10, tumor necrosis factor-α, and granulocyte-macrophage colony-stimulating factor in men. Chronobiol Int 1995;12:19–27.

84. Wide L, Bengtsson C, Birgegard G. Circadian rhythm of erythropoietin in human serum. Br J Haematol 1989;72:85–90.

85. Cotes PM, Brozovic B. Diurnal variation of serum immunoreactive erythropoietin in normal subject. Clin Endocrinol 1982;17:419–422.

86. Haus E, Lakatua DJ, Halberg F, et al. Chrono-

biological studies of plasma prolactin in women in Kyushu, Japan and Minnesota, USA. J Clin Endocrinol Metab 1980;51:632–640.

87. English J, Aherne GW, Marks V. The effect of timing of a single injection on the toxicity of methotrexate in the rat. Cancer Chemother Pharmacol 1982; 9:114–117.

88. Kodama M, Kodama T. Influence of corticosteroid hormones on the therapeutic efficacy of cyclophosphamide. Gann 1982;73:661–666.

89. Shepherd R, Harrap KR. Modulation of the toxicity and antitumor activity of alkylating drugs by steroids. Br. J Cancer 1982;45:413–420.

90. Voutilainen A. Über die 24-stunden-rhythmik der mitozfrequenz in malignen tumoren. Acta Path Micro Scan 1953;99(Suppl):1–104.

91. Tähti E. Studies of the effect of x-irradiation on 24 hour variations in the mitotic activity in human malignant tumours. Acta Path Microbiol Scand 1956; 117:1–61.

92. Garcia-Sainz M, Halberg F. Mitotic rhythms in human cancer reevaluated by electronic computer programs. Evidence for chronopathology. J Natl Cancer Inst 1966;37:279–292.

93. Klevecz RR, Shymko RM, Blumenfeld D, Braly PS. Circadian gating of S phase in human ovarian cancer. Cancer Res 1987;47:6267–6271.

94. Smaaland R, Lote K, Sothern RB, Laerum OD. DNA synthesis and ploidy in non-Hodgkin's lymphomas demonstrate variation depending on circadian stage of cell sampling. Cancer Res 1993;53:3129–3138.

95. Hori K, Suzuki M, Tanda S, Saito S, Shinozaki M, Zhang QH. Circadian dependent variation of tumor blood flow in rat subcutaneous tumors and its alteration by angiotensin II-induced hypertension. Cancer Res 1992;52:912–916.

96. Jain RK. Determinants of tumor blood flow: a review. Cancer Res 1988;48:115–126.

97. el Kouni MH, Naguib FNM, Park KS, Cha S, Darnowsk JW, Soong SJ. Circadian rhythm of hepatic uridine phosphorylase activity and plasma concentration of uridine in mice. Biochem Pharmacol 1990; 40:2479–2485.

98. Naguib HNM, Soong SJ, el Kouni MH. Circadian rhythm of orotate phosphoribosyltransferase, pyrimidine nucleoside phosphorylases and dihydroyracil dehydrogenase in mouse liver. Biochem Pharmacol 1993;45:667–673.

99. Daher GC, Harris BE, Zhang R, Willard EM, Soong SJ, Diasio RB. The role of dihydropyrimidine dehydrogenase (DPD) and thymidine phosphorylase (dThdPase) in the circadian variation of plasma drug levels of 5-fluorouracil (FUra) and 5-fluorodeoxyuridine (FdUrd) following infusion of FUra or FdUrd. Annu Rev Chronopharmacol 1990;7:227–230.

100. Zhang R, Lu Z, Diasio C, Liu T, Soong SJ, Diasio RB. Circadian rhythm of cytoplasmic thymidine kinase in rat bone marrow and intestinal mucosa: possible relevance to fluorodeoxyuridine (FdUrd) and 3'-azido-3'-deoxythymidine (AZT) chemotherapy (abstract). FASEB J 1993;7:689.

101. Tuchman M, Roemeling RV, Lanning R, Sothern RB, Hrushesky WJM. Sources of variability of dehydropyrimidine dehydrogenase (DPD) activity in human blood mononuclear cells. Annu Rev Chronopharmacol 1988;5:399–402.

102. Daher GC, Harris BE, Willard EM, Diasio RB.

Biochemical basis of circadian-dependent metabolism of fluoropyrimidines. In: Hrushesky WJM, Langer R, Theeuwes F, eds. Temporal control drug delivery. Ann NY Acad Sci 1991;618(Suppl):350–361.

103.　Harris BE, Song R, Soong SJ, Diasio RB. Relationship between dihydropyrimidine dehydrogenase activity and plasma 5-fluorouracil levels with evidence for circadian variation of enzyme activity and plasma drug levels in cancer patients receiving 5-fluorouracil by protracted continuous infusion. Cancer Res 1990; 50:197–201.

104.　Fleming RA, Milano G, Thyss A, et al. Correlation between dihydropyrimidine dehydrogenase activity in peripheral mononuclear cells and systemic clearance of fluorouracil in cancer patients. Cancer Res 1992;52:2899–2902.

105.　Zhang R, Lu Z, Liu T, Soong S, Diasio R. Relationship between circadian-dependent toxicity of 5-fluorodeoxyuridine and circadian rhythms of pyrimidine enzymes: possible relevance to fluoropyrimidine chemotherapy. Cancer Res 1993;53:2816–2822.

106.　Milano G, Eitenne MC, Renee N, et al. Relationship between fluorouracil systemic exposure and tumor response and patient survival. J Clin Oncol 1994; 12:1291–1295.

107.　Hrushesky WJM, von Roemeling R, Lanning RM, Rabatin JT. Circadian-shaped infusion of floxuridine for progressive metastatic renal cell carcinoma. J Clin Oncol 1990;8:1504–1513.

108.　von Roemeling R, Hrushesky WJM. Circadian patterning of continuous floxuridine infusion reduces toxicity and allows higher dose intensity in patients with widespread cancer. J Clin Oncol 1989;7:1710–1719.

109.　Wesen C, Hrushesky WJM, Roemeling RV, Lanning R, Rabatin J, Grage T. Circadian modification of intra-arterial 5-fluoro-2'-deoxyuridine infusion rate reduces its toxicity and permits higher dose intensity. J Infus Chemother 1992;2:69–75.

110.　von Roemeling R, Mormont MC, Walker K, Olshefski R. Cancer control depends upon the circadian shape of continuous FUDR infusion (abstract). Proc Annu Meet Am Assoc Cancer Res 1987;28:A1293.

111.　Von Roemeling R, Hrushesky WJM. Circadian pattern of continuous FUDR infusion reduces toxicity. In: Pauli JE, Scheving LE, eds. Advances in chronobiology, part B. New York: Alan R Liss, 1987:357–373.

112.　von Roemeling R, Hrushesky WJM. Determination of the therapeutic index of floxuridine by its circadian infusion pattern. J Natl Cancer Inst 1990; 82:386–393.

113.　Dexeus FH, Logothetis CJ, Sella A, Amato R, Kilbourn R, et al. Circadian infusion of floxuridine in patients with metastatic renal cell carcinoma. J Urol 1991;146;709–713.

114.　Huben RP, Dragone N, Perrapato SD. Continuous infusion FUDR chemotherapy in the treatment of metastatic renal cell carcinoma (abstract). Am Urol Assoc 1990:A413.

115.　Valvassori L, Bellegotti L, Marchiano A, et al. Continuous circadian-shaped infusion FUDR effectively reduces toxicity (abstract). Proc Am Soc Clin Oncol 1989;8:427.

116.　Wilkinson MJ, Frye JW, Small EJ, et al. A phase II study of constant-infusion floxuridine for the treatment of metastatic renal cell carcinoma. Cancer 1993;71:3601–3604.

117.　Hrushesky WJM, Bjarnson G, Harris G, Marsh R, Diasio R, et al. Circadian synchrony and stability: is time of day of cancer treatment meaningful? Proc Am Soc Clin Oncol 1993;12:460.

118.　Bjarnason GA, Hrushesky WJM, Diasio R, et al. Flat versus circadian modified 14 day infusion of FUDR for advanced renal cell cancer (RCC) (abstract). Proc Am Soc Clin Oncol 1994;13:223.

119.　Focan C, Krevitz F, Focan-Henrard D, et al. Treatment of hepatic metastases from colorectal cancer with continuous delivery of venous 5-fluorouracil (5FU) and arterial 5-fluorodeoxyuridine (FUDR). A randomized evaluation comparing combine flat versus chrono-modified infusion (abstract). Ann Oncol 1994; 5(Suppl 8):43.

120.　Burns RE, Beland SS. Effect of biological time on the determination of the LD50 of 5-fluorouracil in mice. Pharmacology 1984;28:296–300.

121.　Gonzalez RB, Sothern RB, Thatcher G, Nguyen N, Hrushesky WJM. Substantial difference in timing in murine circadian susceptibility to 5-fluorouracil and FUDR (abstract). Proc Amer Assoc Cancer Res 1989;30:2452a.

122.　Peters GJ, Van Dijk J, Nadal JC, Van Groeningen CJ, Lankelman J, Pinedo HM. Diurnal variation in the therapeutic efficacy of 5-fluorouracil against murine colon cancer. In Vivo 1987;1:112–118.

123.　Shakil A, Hirabayashi N, Toge T. Circadian variation of 5-fluorouracil and cis-platinum toxicity in mice. Hiroshima J Med Sci 1993;42:147–154.

124.　Gardner MLG, Plumb JA. Diurnal variation in the intestinal toxicity of 5-fluorouracil in the rat. Clin Sci 1981;61:717–722.

125.　Wood PA, Peace D, Torosoff M, Vyzula R, Hrushesky WJM. Can optimal circadian timing of 5-fluorouracil improve the therapeutic index (abstract)? Biol Rhythm Res 1995;26:460.

126.　Lévi F, Soussan A, Adam R, et al. A phase I–II trial of 5-day continuous intravenous infusion of 5-fluorouracil delivered at circadian rhythm modulated rate in patients with metastatic colorectal cancer. J Infus Chemother 1995;5:153–158.

127.　Bjarnason GA, Kerr IG, Doyle N, MacDonald M, Sone M. Phase I study of 5-fluorouracil and leucovorin by a 14-day circadian infusion in metastatic adenocarcinoma patients. Cancer Chemother Pharmacol 1993;33:221–228.

128.　Falcone A, Pfanner E, Lencioni M, et al. Chronoinfusion with 5-fluorouracil (5-FU) + L-folinic acid (L-FA): a randomized phase I study (abstract). Proc Am Soc Clin Oncol 1995;14:196.

129.　Allegrini G, Falcone A, Pfanner E, et al. Chronoinfusion with 5-fluorouracil plus L-folinic acid: a randomized phase I trial (abstract). Biol Rhythm Res 1995; 26:361.

130.　Lévi F, Misset JL, Brienza S, et al. A chronopharmacologic phase-II clinical trial with 5-fluorouracil, folinic acid, and oxaliplatin using an ambulatory multichannel programmable pump. Cancer 1992; 69(4):893–900.

131.　Lévi FA, Zidani R, Vannetzel JM, et al. Chronomodulated versus fixed-infusion-rate delivery of ambulatory chemotherapy with oxaliplatin, fluorouracil, and folinic acid (leucovorin) in patients with colorectal cancer metastases: a randomized multi-institutional trial. J Natl Cancer Inst 1994;86:1608–1617.

132.　Bjarnason GA, Kerr I, Doyle N, MacDonald M,

Sone M. Phase I study of 5-fluorouracil (5-FU) and leu-covorin (LV) by 14 days continuous infusion chrono-therapy in patients with metastatic adenocarcinoma (abstract). Eur J Cancer 1991;(Suppl 2):A528.

133. Petit E, Milano G, Levi F, Thyss A, Bailleul F, Schneider M. Circadian rhythm-varying plasma con-centration of 5-fluorouracil during a five day continu-ous infusion at a constant rate in cancer patients. Can-cer Res 1988;48:1676–1679.

134. Thiberville L, Compagnon P, Moore N, et al. Plasma 5-fluorouracil and a-fluorouracil-b-alanin ac-cumulation in lung cancer patients treated with con-tinuous infusion of cisplatin and 5-fluorouracil. Cancer Chemother Pharmacol 1994;35:64–70.

135. Cardoso SS, Scheving LE, Halberg F. Mortality of mice as influenced by the hour of the day of drug (ara-C) administration (abstract). Pharmacologist 1970; 12:302.

136. Haus E, Halberg F, Scheving L, et al. Increased tolerance of mice to arabinosylcytosine given on sched-ule adjusted to circadian system. Science 1972;177:80–82.

137. Scheving LE, Haus E, Kuhl JFW, Pauly FE, Halberg F, Cardoso SS. Different laboratories closely reproduce characteristics of circadian rhythm in tol-erance of mice for arabinofuranosylcytosine. Cancer Res. 1976;36:113–117.

138. Hromas RA, Hutchison JT, Markel DE, Scholes VE. Flow cytometric analysis of the effect of ara-C on the chronobiology of bone marrow DNA syn-thesis. Chronobiologia 1981;8:369–373.

139. Scheving LE, Burns R, Pauly JE, Halberg F, Haus E. Survival and care of leukemic mice after cir-cadian optimization of treatment with cyclophospha-mide and 1-β-D-arabinofuranosylcytosine. Cancer Res 1977;37:3648–3655.

140. Burns ER, Scheving LE. Circadian optimiza-tion of the treatment of L1210 leukemia with 1-β-D-arabinofuranasylcytosine, cyclophosphamide, vincris-tine and methylprednisolone. Chronobiologia 1980; 7:41–51.

141. Scheving LE, Burns ER, Halberg F, Pauly JE. Combined chronotherapy of L1210 leukemic mice using 1-β-D-arabinofuranosylcytosine, cyclophospha-mide, vincristine, methylprednisolone and cis-diam-minedichloroplatinum. Chronobiologia 1980;7:33–40.

142. English J, Aherne GW, Marks V. The effect of abolition of the endogenous corticosteroid rhythm on the circadian variation in methotrexate toxicity in the rat. Cancer Chemother Pharmacol 1987;19:287–290.

143. Malmary-Nebot MF, Labat C, Casanovas AM, Oustrin J. Aspect chronobiologique de l'action du méthotrexate sur la dihydrofolate réductase. Ann Pharm Fr 1985;43:337–343.

144. Robinson BA, Begg EJ, Colls BM, Jefferey GM, Sharman JR. Circadian pharmacokinetics of metho-trexate. Cancer Chemother Pharmacol 1989;24:397–399.

145. Balis FM, Jeffries SL, Lange B, et al. Chrono-pharmacokinetics of oral methotrexate and 6-mercap-topurine: is there diurnal variation in the disposition of antileukemic therapy. Am J Pediatr Hematol Oncol 1989;11(3):324–326.

146. Langevin AM, Koren G, Soldin S, Greenberg M. Pharmacokinetic case for giving 6-mercaptopurine maintenance doses at night. Lancet 1987;ii:505–506.

147. Koren G, Langevin AM, Olivieri N, Giesbrecht E, Zipursky A, Greenberg M. Diurnal variation in the pharmacokinetics and myelotoxicity of mercaptopu-rine in children with acute lymphocytic leukemia. Am J Dis Child 1990;144:1135–1137.

148. Lennard L, Lilleyman JS. Variable mercapto-purine metabolism and treatment outcome in child-hood lymphoblastic leukemia. J Clin Oncol 1989; 7(12)1816–1823.

149. Schmiegelow K, Pulczynska MK, Seip M. White cell count during maintenance chemotherapy for standard-risk childhood acute lymphoblastic leu-kemia: relation to relapse rate. Pediatr Hematol Oncol 1988;5:259–267.

150. Kuhl JFW, Grage F, Halberg F, Rosene G, Scheving LE, Haus E. Ellen-effect: tolerance of adria-mycin by mice and rats depends on circadian timing of injection. Int J Chronobiol 1973;1:335–336.

151. Sothern RB, Nelson WL, Halberg F. A circa-dian rhythm in susceptibility of mice to the anti-tumor drug adriamycin. 12th Conf Intern Soc Chronobiology. Milano: Il Ponte 1977:433–438.

152. Lévi F, Tampellini M, Metzger G, Bizi E, Le-maigre G, Hallek M. Circadian changes in mitoxan-trone toxicity in mice; relationship with plasma phar-macokinetics. Int J Cancer 1994;59:543–547.

153. Mormont MC, Roemeling RV, Sothern RB, et al. Circadian rhythm and seasonal dependence in the toxicological response of mice to epirubicin. Invest New Drugs 1988;6:273–283.

154. Hrushesky WJM, von Roemeling R, Sothern B. Circadian chronotherapy: from animal experiments to human cancer chemotherapy: In: Lemmer B, ed. Chronopharmacology: cellular and biochemical interactions. New York: Marcel Dekker, 1989:439–473.

155. Hrushesky WJM. Circadian timing of cancer chemotherapy. Science 1985;228(4695):73–75.

156. Sothern RB, Lévi F, Haus E, Halberg F, Hru-shesky WJM. Control of murine plasmacytoma with doxorubicin-cisplatin: dependence on circadian stage of treatment. J Natl Cancer Inst 1989;81(2):135–45.

157. Hrushesky WJM, Roemeling RV, Wood PA, Langevin TR, Lange P, Fraley E. High-dose intensity systemic therapy of metastatic bladder cancer. J Clin Oncol 1987;5(3):450–455.

158. Lévi F, Benavides M, Chevelle C, et al. Che-motherapy of advanced ovarian cancer with 4'-O-tetrahydropyranyl doxorubicin and cisplatin: a ran-domized phase II trial with an evaluation of circadian timing and dose-intensity. J Clin Oncol 1990;8(4):705–714.

159. Barrett R, Blessing J, Webster K, Twiggs L. Cir-cadian-timed combination doxorubicin-cisplatin che-motherapy for advanced endometrial carcinoma. Gy-necol Oncol 1990;36:285–297.

160. Sqalli A, Oustrin J, Houin G, Bugat R, Carton M. Clinical chronopharmacokinetics of doxorubicin. In: Reinberg A, Smolensky M, Labreque G, eds. Annu Rev Chronopharmacol. Oxford: Pergamon Press, 1988; 5:393–396.

161. Wood PA, Hrushesky WJM. Cisplatin-associ-ated anemia: an erythropoietin deficiency syndrome. J Clin Invest 1995;95:1650–1659.

162. Boughattas AN, Lévi F, Roulon A, et al. Sim-ilar circadian rhythm in murine host tolerance for two platinum analogs: carboplatin (cbdca) and oxaliplatin

(i-ohp) (abstract). Proc Am Assoc Cancer Res 1987; 28:451.

163. Boughattas N, Lévi F, Fournier C, et al. Circadian rhythm in toxicities and tissue uptake of 1,2-diammino-cyclohexane(*trans*-1)oxalatoplatinum(II) in mice. Cancer Res 1989;49:3362–3368.

164. Boughattas N, Lévi F, Hecquet B, et al. Circadian time dependence of murine tolerance for carboplatin. Toxicol Appl Pharmacol 1988;96:233–247.

165. Hrushesky WJM, Lévi F, Halberg F, Kennedy BJ. Circadian stage dependence of *cis*-diamminedichloroplatinum lethal toxicity in rats. Cancer Res 1982; 42:945–949.

166. Hecquet B, Maynadier J, Bonneterre J, Adenis L, Demaille A. Time dependency in plasmatic protein binding of cisplatin. Cancer Treat Rep 1985;69:79–83.

167. Halberg E, Halberg F, Venner KJ, et al. Twenty-four hour synchronized chronotolerance of *cis*-diamminedichloroplatinum (II) by rats on 8-h and 12-h photofraction gauged by acrophase and paraphase of rectal temperature. In: Reinberg A, Halberg F, eds. Chronopharmacology. New York: Pergamon Press, 1979:377.

168. Boughattas AN, Fournier C, Hecquet B, et al. Circadian time dependent tissue uptake of cisplatin and carboplatin following repeated administration: relationship with drug toxicities in mice. In: Reinberg A, Smolensky M, Labreque G, eds. Annual Review of Chronopharmacology. Oxford: Pergamon Press, 1990; 7:231–234.

169. Kerr DJ, Lewis C, O'Neil B, et al. The myelotoxicity of carboplatin is influenced by the time of its administration. Hematol Oncol 1990;8:59–63.

170. Caussanel JP, Lévi F, Brienza S, et al. Phase I trial of 5-day continuous venous infusion of oxaliplatin at circadian rhythm-modulated rate compared with constant rate. J Natl Cancer Inst 1990;82:1046–1050.

171. Haus E, Fernandes G, Kuhl JFW, Yunis EJ, Lee JP, Halberg F. Murine circadian susceptibility rhythm to cyclophosphamide. Chronobiologia 1974;1:270–277.

172. Hacker MP, Ershler WB, Newman RA, Fagan MA. Chronobiologic fluctuation of cyclophosphamide induced urinary bladder damage. Chronobiologia 1983;10:301–306.

173. Cardoso SS, Avery T, Venditti JM, Goldin A. Circadian dependence of host and tumor response to cyclophosphamide in mice. Eur J Cancer 1978;14:949–954.

174. Snyder NK, Smolensky M, Hsi BP. Circadian variation in the susceptibility of male Balb/c mice to ifosfamide. Chronobiologia 1981;8:33–44.

175. Klein F, Danober L, Roulon A, Lemaigre G, Mechouri M, Lévi F. Circadian rhythm in murine tolerance for the anticancer agent mitomycin C. In: Reinberg A, Smolensky M, Labrecque G, eds. Annual Review of Chronopharmacology. Oxford: Pergamon Press, 1988;5:367–370.

176. Sothern RB, Haus R, Langevin TR, et al. Profound circadian stage dependence of mitomycin-C toxicity. Oxford: Pergamon Press, 1988. In: Reinberg A, Smolensky M, Labrecque G, eds. Annual Review of Chronopharmacology 1988;5:389–392.

177. Vassal G, Challine D, Koscielny S, et al. Chronopharmacology of high-dose busulfan in children. Cancer Res 1993;53:1534–1537.

178. Halberg F, Gupta B, Haus E, et al. Steps toward a chronopolychemotherapy. Proc 14th International Congress of Therapeutics. Paris: L'Expansion Scientifique Francaise, 1977:151–196.

179. Lévi F, Mechkouri M, Roulon A, et al. Circadian rhythm in tolerance of mice for etoposide. Cancer Treat Rep 1985;69:1443–1445.

180. Mormont MC, Berestka J, Mushiya T, et al. Circadian dependence of vinblastine toxicity. In: Reinberg A, Smolensky M, Labrecque G, eds. Annual Review of Chronopharmacology. Oxford: Pergamon Press, 1986;3:187–190.

181. Tampellini M, Filipski E, Levi F. Circadian variation of vinorelbine toxicity in mice. Chronobiol Int 1995;12:195–198.

182. Focan C, Mazy JM, Zhou J, Rahmani R, Cano JP. Circadian variation of vindesine serum concentrations during continuous infusion. In: Reinberg A, Smolensky M, Labreque G, eds. Annual Review of Chronopharmacology, Oxford: Pergamon Press, 1988;5:411–414.

183. Focan C, Driesschaert P, Bastens B, et al. Circadian tolerance to etoposide and cisplatin as first line treatment for advanced lung carcinoma. In: Reinberg A, Smolensky M, Labreque G, eds. Annual Review of Chronopharmacology. Oxford: Pergamon Press, 1990; 7:219–222.

184. Krakowski I, Lévi F, Mechkouri M, et al. Dose intensity of etoposide (vp16)-cisplatin (cddp) depends upon dosing time (abstract). Proc Am Assoc Cancer Res 1988;29:776.

185. Hrushesky WJM, Langevin T, Kim YJ, Wood PA. Circadian dynamics of tumor necrosis factor-a (cachectin) lethality. J Exp Med 1994;180:1059–1065.

186. Halberg F, Johnson EA, Brown BW, Bittner JJ. Susceptibility rhythm to *E. coli* endotoxin and bioassay. Proc Soc Exp Biol Med 1960;103:142–144.

187. Elliot GT, Welty D, Kuo YD. The D-galactosamine loaded mouse and its enhanced sensitivity to lipopolysaccharide and monophosphoryl lipid A: a role for superoxide. J Immunol 1991;10:69–74.

188. Tracey KJ, Fong Y, Hesse DG, et al. Anti-cachectin-TNF monoclonal antibodies prevent septic shock during lethal bacteremia in baboons. Nature 1987; 330:662–664.

189. Hrushesky WJM, Langevin T, Nygaard S, Young J, Roemeling R. Circadian stipulation required for reduction of variability in TNF toxicity/efficacy. International Conference on Tumor Necrosis Factor and Related Cytokines. Heidelberg, Germany, 1987.

190. von Roemeling R, Salzer M, Connerty M, et al. Circadian stage dependent response to interleukin-2 in mouse spleen and bone marrow. Annu Rev Chronopharmacol 1990;7:173–176.

191. Lévi F, Bourin P, Pages N, et al. Dosing-time of IL-2 affects both lethal and central nervous system toxicity in mice. Proc Am Assoc Cancer Res 1992; 33:329.

192. Hrushesky WJM, Sánchez S, Wood PA, et al. Heterogeneity of interleukin-2 therapeutic activity (abstract). Proc Am Assoc Cancer Res 1992;33:300.

193. Kemeny M, Alava G, Oliver J. Improving responses in hepatoma with circadian patterned hepatic artery infusions of recombinant interleukin-2. J Immunother 1992;12:219–223.

194. Canon C, Lévi F. Immune system in relation to cancer. In: Touitou Y, Haus E, eds. Biologic rhythms in clinical and laboratory medicine. New York: Springer-Verlag, 1992:635–647.

195. Gatti G, Masera R, Cavallo R, et al. Circadian variation of interferon-induced enhancement of human natural killer (NK) cell activity. Cancer Detect Prevent 1988;12:431–438.

196. Biologic clocks. Cold Spring Harbor, New York: Long Island Biological Association, 1960. Cold Spring Harbor Symposia on Quantitative Biology; vol XXV.

197. Koren S, Fleischmann WR. Circadian variations in myelosuppressive activity of interferon-α in mice: identification of an optimal treatment time associated with reduced myelosuppressive activity. Exp Hematol 1993;21:552–559.

198. Koren S, Fleischmann WR. Optimal circadian timing reduces the myelosuppressive activity of rMuIFN-γ administered to mice. J Interferon Res 1993; 13:187–194.

199. Mann EA, Markovic SN, Murasko DM. Inhibition of lymphocyte recirculation by murine interferon: effects of various interferon preparations and timing of administration. J Interferon Res 1989;9:35–51.

200. Abrams PG, McClamrock E, Foon KA. Evening administration of alpha interferon. N Engl J Med 1985;312(7):443–444.

201. Després-Brummer P, Lévi F, Di Palma M, et al. A phase I trial of 21-day continuous venous infusion of α-interferon at circadian rhythm modulated rate in cancer patients. J Immunol 1991;10:440–447.

202. Iacobelli S, Garufi C, Itrelli L, et al. A phase I study of recombinant interferon-alpha administered as a seven-day continuous infusion at circadian-rhythm modulated rate in patients with cancer. Am J Clin Oncol 1995;18:27–31.

203. Koren S, Whorton EJ, Fleischmann WJ. Circadian dependence of interferon antitumor activity in mice. J Natl Cancer Inst 1993;85:1927–1932.

204. Wood PA, Hrushesky WJM. Chronopharmacodynamics of hematopoietic growth factors and antitumor cytokines. In: Hrushesky WJM, ed. Circadian cancer therapy. New York: CRC Press, 1994: 185–207.

205. Wood PA, Peace D, Troha T, Mann G, Hrushesky WJM. Efficacy of chronic erythropoietin is dependent upon the time of day of its administration (abstract). Exp Hematol 1994;22:707.

206. Opp M, Obal F, Krueger JM. Interleukin-1 alters rat sleep: temporal and dose-related effects. Am J Physiol 1991;260:R52–R58.

207. Lue FA, Bail M, Jephthat-Ochola J, Carayannoitis K, Gorczynski R, Moldofsky H. Sleep and cerebrospinal fluid interleukin-1-like activity in the cat. Int J Neurosci 1988;42:179–183.

208. Pizzarello DJ, Isaak D, Chua KE. Circadian rhythmicity in the sensitivity of two strains of mice to whole body radiation. Science 1964;145:286–291.

209. Ueno Y. Diurnal rhythmicity in the sensitivity of hematopoietic cells to whole-body irradiation of mice. Int J Radiat Biol 1968;14:307–312.

210. Tzannis ST, Pryzbycien TM, Hrushesky WJM, Wood P. The impact of formulated interleukin-2/delivery device surface interactions on bioefficacy. Materials Research Soc Symp Proc 1994;331:227–232.

211. Florence AT. Drug delivery systems of the future, vol 4. Greenford, Middlesex, United Kingdom: Duncan, Flockhard, 1988.

212. Theeuwes F, Yum SI, Haak R, Wong P. Systems for triggered, pulsed and programmed drug delivery. In: Hrushesky WJM, Langer R, Theeuwes F, eds. Temporal control of drug delivery. Ann NY Acad Aci, 1991;618:428–440.

213. Korsmeyer RW. Diffusion controlled systems: hydrogels. In: Tarchar PJ, ed. Polymers for controlled drug delivery. Boca Raton, FL: CRC Press, 1991:15–37.

214. Borodkin S. Ion-exchange resin delivery systems. In: Tarcha PJ, ed. Polymers for controlled drug delivery. Boca Raton, FL: CRC Press, 1991:215–230.

215. Pecosky DA, Robinson JR. Bioadhesive polymers and drug delivery. In: Tarcha PJ, ed. Polymers for controlled drug delivery. Boca Raton, F: CRC Press, 1991;99–125.

216. Mitragotri S, Blankschtein D, Langer R. Ultrasound-mediated transdermal protein delivery. Science 1995;269:850–853.

217. Ranney DF, Huffaker HH. Magnetic microspheres for the targeted controlled release of drugs and diagnostic agents. In: Juliano RL, ed. Biological approaches to the controlled delivery of drugs. Ann NY Acad Sci 1987;507:104–119.

218. Carter WH, Wampler GL. Review of the application of response surface methodology in the combination therapy of cancer. Cancer Treat Rep 1986; 70:133–140.

219. Ratajczak HV, Sothern RB, Hrushesky WJM. Estrous influence on surgical cure of a mouse breast cancer. J Exp Med 1988;168:88–96.

220. Hrushesky WJM, Gruber SA, Sothern RB, et al. Natural killer cell activity is age, estrous and circadian stage dependent and correlates inversely with metastatic potential. J Natl Cancer Inst 1988;80:1232–1237.

221. Hrushesky WJM, Bluming AZ, Gruber SA, Sothern RA. Menstrual influence on surgical cure of breast cancer. Lancet 1989;ii:949–952.

222. Fentiman I, Gregory WM, Richards MA. Effects of menstrual phase on surgical treatment of breast cancer (letter). Lancet 1994;344:402.

223. Senie R, Rosen P, Rhodes P, Lesser M. Timing of breast cancer excision during the menstrual cycle influences duration of disease-free survival. Ann Intern Med 1991;115:337–342.

224. Meyer K. Season and cycle: variation in presentation and response to therapy in premenopausal breast cancer (abstract). 7th Annu Clin Congress, October 21–24. Chicago, 1991.

225. Badwe RA, Gregory WM, Chaudary WM, et al. Timing of surgery during menstrual cycle and survival of premenopausal women with operable breast cancer. Lancet 1991;337:1261–1264.

226. Ville V, Lasry S, Spyratos F. Menstrual status and breast cancer surgery. Breast Cancer Res Treat 1990;16:119–121.

227. Ville V, Briere M, Lasry S, Spyratos F, Oglobine J, Brunet M. Timing of surgery in breast cancer. Lancet 1991;337:1604–1605.

228. Saad Z, Branwell JD, Girott M, et al. Timing of surgery in relation to the menstrual cycle in premenopausal women with operable breast cancer. Br J Surg 1994;31:217–220.

229. Spratt J, Zirnheld J, Yancey J. Breast cancer detection demonstration project data can determine whether the prognosis of breast cancer is affected by the time of surgery during the menstrual cycle. J Surg Oncol 1993;53:4–9.

230. Powles TJ, Jones AL, Ashley S, Tidy A. Men-

strual effect on surgical cure of breast cancer. Lancet 1989;ii:1343–1344.

231. Veronesi U, Luini A, Mariani L, et al. Effect of menstrual phase of surgical treatment of breast cancer. Lancet 1994;343:1545–1547.

232. Damascelli B, Marchiano A, Spreafico C, et al. Circadian continuous chemotherapy of renal cell carcinoma with an implantable, programmable infusion pump. Cancer 1990;66:237–241.

233. Dexeus FH, Logothetis CJ, Sella A, et al. Circadian infusion of floxuridine in patients with metastatic renal cell carcinoma. J Urology 1991;146:709–713.

234. Conroy T, Geoffrois L, Guillemin F, et al. Simplified chronomodulated continuous infusion of floxuridine in patients with metastatic renal cell carcinoma. Cancer 1993;72:2190–2197.

235. Natoli C, Irtelli L, Martino MT, et al. A phase II evaluation of 5-fluoro-2-deoxyuridine administered as a 14-day continuous venous infusion at circadian-rhythm modulated rate in gastrointestinal cancer and renal cell carcinoma. J Infus Chemother 1994;4:97–99.

236. Sampaio C, Olencki T, Murthy S, et al. Phase II trial of circadian infusion of the antimetabolite floxuridine in patients with metastatic renal cell carcinoma. J Infus Chemother 1994;4:100–103.

237. Bjarnason G, Hrushesky W, Marsh R, et al. Flat versus time-modified 14-day infusion of FUDR for advanced renal cell cancer: a phase-III study (abstract). Bio Rhythm Res 1995;26:369.

238. Garufi C, Lévi F, Giunta S, et al. Chronomodulated 5-day infusion of floxuridine and L-folinic acid in patients with advanced malignancies: a feasibility and tolerability study. J Infus Chemother 1995;5:134–137.

239. Lévi F, Brienza JL, Misset R, et al. Circumvention of clinical resistance of metastatic colorectal cancer to 5-fluorouracil (5-FU) with circadian rhythm modulated chemotherapy (abstract). Proc Am Soc Clin Oncol 1992;11:171.

240. Brienza S, Lévi F, Valori VM, et al. Intensified (every 2 weeks) chronotherapy with 5-fluorouracil (5-FU) folinic acid (FA) and oxaliplatin (L-OHP) in previously treated patients with metastatic colorectal cancer (abstract). Proc Am Soc Clin Onc 1993;12:197.

241. Deprés-Bummer P, Berthault-Cvitkovic F, Lévi F, et al. Circadian rhythm-modulated (CRM) chemotherapy of metastatic breast cancer with mitoxantrone, 5-fluorouracil, and folinic acid: preliminary results of a phase I trial. J Infus Chemother 1995;5:114–147.

242. Focan C, Denis B, Kreutz F, Focan-Henrard D, Lévi F. Ambulatory chronotherapy with 5-fluorouracil, floinic acid, and carboplatin for advanced non-small cell lung cancer: a phase II feasibility trial. J Infus Chemother 1995;5:148–152.

243. Barrett RJ, Blessing JA, Homesley HD, Twiggs L, Webster KD. Circadian-timed combination doxorubicin-cisplatin chemotherapy for advanced endometrial carcinoma. A phase II study of the Gynecologic Oncology Group. Am J Clin Oncol 1993;16:494–496.

244. Focan D. Sequential chemotherapy and circadian rhythm in human solid tumors. A randomized trial. Cancer Chemother Pharmacol 1979;3(3):197–202.

245. Lissoni P, Barni S, Meregalli S, et al. Modulation of cancer endocrine therapy by melatonin; a phase II study of tamoxifen plus melatonin in metastatic breast cancer patients progressing under tamoxifen alone. Br J Cancer 1995;71:854–856.

246. Wood P, Hrushesky W. Circadian rhythms and cancer chemotherapy. Crit Rev Eukaryotic Gene Expression 1996;6:103–146.

247. Hrushesky WJM, Bjarnason GA. Circadian cancer therapy. J Clin Oncol 1993;11:1403–1417.

Section One: B

Routes of Administration

13

Intraventricular Therapy

Arthur D. Forman and Victor A. Levin

Neoplasia in the meninges abuts the subarachnoid space and locally obliterates it and/or is bathed by the subarachnoid cerebrospinal fluid (CSF). Although not strictly meningeal neoplasia, leukemic cells and some metastatic foci can "seed" the choroid plexus or the ependymal surface of the ventricular system. In all cases, tumor cells lie in either direct contact or close approximation with the CSF.

DRUG DELIVERY

The delivery of many anticancer drugs from blood to brain (1, 2) and from blood to CSF is quite restricted. Table 13.1 shows the CSF:plasma ratios for some of the drugs studied in rhesus monkeys and humans. A CSF:plasma

Table 13.1. CSF:Plasma (or Serum) Drug Ratios following Intravenous Administration in Rhesus Monkeys or Humans

Drug	CSF:Plasma Ratio	Reference
TEPA	1.0	(84)
Thiotepa	1.0	(84)
Tiazofurin	0.28	(85)
6-Mercaptopurine	0.27	(26, 86)
Zidovudine (Azidothymidine)	0.24	(87)
5-Fluorouracil	0.155	(88)
Arabinosyl-5-azacytidine	0.15	(89)
Cytosine arabinoside	0.06–0.25	(26, 90)
Vincristine	0.05	(26)
Spiromustine	0.047	(91)
Dideoxycytidine	0.033	(92)
Cisplatin	0.029	(93)
Etoposide	0.018	(94)
Methotrexate	0.01–0.03	(95)
INF-α	0.01	(96)
Daunomycin	nd[a]	(26)
L-Asparaginase	nd	(26)

[a]nd, not detectable.

ratio below 0.05 signifies nonspecific leakage of drug. From Table 13.1 it can be seen that many drugs normally achieve CSF/plasma ratios below 0.05 in the settings of normal blood-brain and blood-CSF barriers. Obviously, once meningeal neoplasia has occurred, sites of blood-CSF leakage are present, drugs can more readily leak from blood into CSF, and higher ratios can thus be expected.

CSF PHYSIOLOGY

An understanding of CSF physiology will help in understanding intraventricular and intrathecal therapies. The greatest proportion of CSF is actively secreted by the choroid plexuses of the lateral and fourth ventricles. CSF is also produced, to a much lesser extent, from extrachoroidal sources that gain access to the CSF via the brain extracellular fluid (ECF). The CSF and ECF are in dynamic equilibrium, with the ependymal cells serving as a sieve rather than a barrier to exchange between the two. The ependymal cell cilia may have the further functions of reducing the impact of an "unstirred layer" at the interface of the CSF and cell surface and of expediting the mixing of metabolites, catabolites, and drugs between CSF and ECF.

The hydrostatically driven flow of CSF is from ventricles to basal cisterns to subarachnoid space and, ultimately, to the arachnoid granulations and into venous blood. This flow provides a strong diffusion gradient to lower ECF metabolites and catabolites being produced by brain parenchymal cells. This capacity to lower catabolites produced by cells has been referred to as the "sink effect" of the CSF. In addition to this CSF sink action, other functions that the CSF serves are (*a*) regulation of the brain extracellular environment, (*b*) movement of neuroendocrine hormones, and (*c*) buoyancy and protection of the brain from jarring associated with body movement and activity.

PHARMACOKINETICS

The CSF compartments and adjacent central nervous system (CNS) ECF constitute a regional cavity for the purposes of drug administration. This cavity is not closed, and drug administered into CSF can leave via (a) bulk absorption through the arachnoid granulations, (b) diffusion into ECF and surrounding cells, (c) diffusion into ECF and then across capillaries into the systemic circulation, and (d) biotransformation. Aside from biotransformation rates, which vary depending on the structure of the drug, the clearance of drugs from the CSF will be somewhat predictable, based on molecular size and partitioning into lipid (e.g., octanol/water partition coefficient) Figure 13.1 shows the observed relationship for K_{out} versus log $[(octanol/water)M_r^{-1/2}]$ as described by Levin and Landahl (3).

Just as the relationship between physical characteristics and K_{out} from the CSF is predictable, so is the distance that drug in the CSF can penetrate into adjacent brain parenchyma. The factors that determine the effective diffusing distance from the CSF-brain interface are (a) the tor-tuosity of the ECF, (b) the molecular size of the permeant drug, (c) the cell/ECF partitioning of the drug, and (d) the stability of the drug. Figure 13.2 shows the hypothetical relationship between drug half-life (a term that in this context includes biotransformation and the loss of drug from ECF to blood via permeation across capillaries), diffusion coefficient in cm^2/sec, and the distance into brain parenchyma that 10% of the CSF drug level will permeate. This bar graph was computed assuming diffusion from a planar surface.

A number of therapeutic points emerge for consideration. Drugs administered by intrathecal (spinal subarachnoid) administration will not reflux into the ventricular system unless a reversal of the normal hydrostatic gradient has occurred. Reversal of hydrostatic flow is observed in hydrocephalus. This is important, since it means that the intrathecal route is inferior when drug is required to reach the choroid plexuses or the ependymal surface. Other reasons to avoid the intrathecal route are the chance that drug will be injected subdurally and not enter the CSF and the risk of local damage to the spinal cord resulting from local high concentrations of drug at the injection site. Intraventricular drug administration with rapid but gentle barbotage four to six times will quickly dilute drug in a large ven-

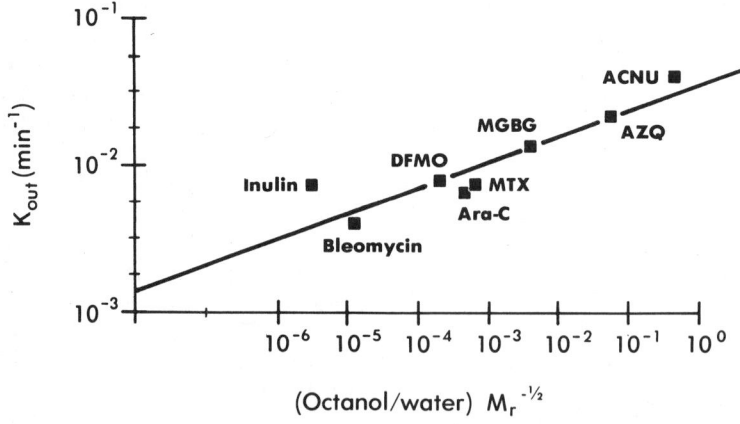

$$K_{out} = CL_{csf}/V_{csf}$$

$$\text{Log } K_{out} = -1.468 + 0.17 \text{ Log } [P(M_r)^{-1/2}]$$

Figure 13.1. These data were obtained from the literature (3, 9, 75, 114, 115, 116). $K_{out} = CL_{csf}/V_{csf}$ (3) and was plotted against the [log(octanol/water partition coefficient)$M_r^{-1/2}$]. The data were fit by a nonlinear least squares technique.

DIFFUSION FROM A PLANAR SURFACE

Distance for 10% of CSF Drug Level

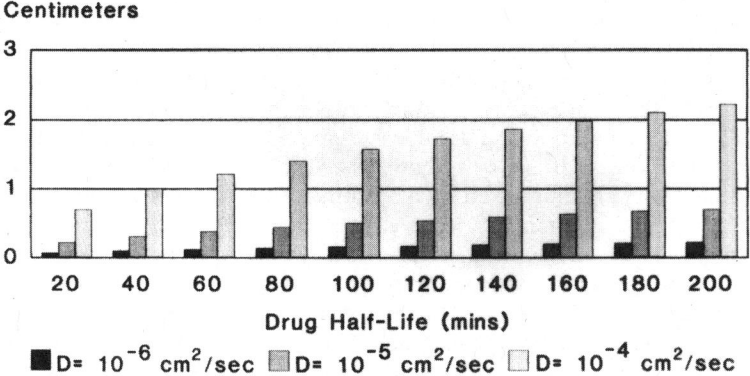

Figure 13.2. This bar graph shows the relationship between free water diffusion coefficient, D, drug half-life, and the distance into brain parenchyma attainable by 10% of the CSF drug level.

tricular fluid volume and will enhance egress from the ventricles to a half-time on the order of minutes (3).

DIFFUSION

Because drug diffusion into brain parenchyma is slow relative to its clearance from the CSF, the depth of effective drug concentration is small, and a therapeutic benefit for a nodular lesion on the surface or for a deeper parenchymal lesion is unlikely (Fig. 13.2). Further compromising drug delivery to a nodular tumor in the CSF pathway is the fact that when drug diffuses into a nodular lesion, as soon as it comes in contact with a tumor capillary, it crosses into the systemic circulation and reduces the potential tumor drug level. Pharmacokinetic calculations suggest that nodules greater than 5 mm in diameter are inadequately treated by regional therapies (4, 5). Thus, it is apparent that administration of drug into the CSF often fails because the drug does not make contact with tumor cells long enough to kill them. This is because (a) the tumor obliterates the subarachnoid space and drug cannot reach many of the cells; (b) the tumor is nodular and only the most superficial cells make contact with drug; and (c) the drug is too unstable or is small and nonionized and is cleared from the CSF before reaching distal sites in the CSF pathway. Sometimes these shortcomings can only be overcome by increasing the administered dose at the risk of CNS, toxicity or by

providing a carrier, such as a monoclonal antibody, to slow the drugs CSF clearance and to increase its targeting to tumor cells. To fully evaluate the potential of this last approach, further experimental study is required to ascertain optimal conditions for carrier-drug targeting.

REGIONAL DELIVERY

Regional delivery of chemotherapeutic agents to the CNS had its earliest use in the treatment of infectious meningitis. Antibiotics were percutaneously injected via a spinal needle through frontal burr holes into the frontal lobes and ventricles. In an effort to diminish the morbidity associated with this form of therapy, Ayub Ommaya developed an implantable closed delivery system while working at the National Institutes of Health (6). Using this system, the ease with which therapeutic agents could circumvent the blood-brain barrier opened new strategies for the treatment of CNS infections and malignancies. While great advances have been made in the 30 years since the introduction of the indwelling closed ventricular delivery system, major problems still face oncologic medicine in maximizing the benefit from these improvements.

Refinements, such as valves and shunt attachments, have permitted greater flexibility in the use of reservoirs. Lumbar reservoirs have been used more frequently for the delivery of analgesics than for chemotherapy. Although some studies have reported good results using lumbar reservoirs (7), their high rate of malfunction (8) and the better distribution of drug when delivered into a ventricle (9) have made the intraventricular route favored for chemotherapy for CNS malignancy.

Following percutaneous lumbar administration of methotrexate, the drug at times failed to reach the head and leaked into the epidural or subdural space; this complication was more likely with repeated lumbar administration (10). Even with successful lumbar administration, the intraventricular levels of methotrexate were highly variable, as indicated by a study measuring drug concentrations at both levels (4) (Fig. 13.3A). In that study, serum methotrexate levels were about 1×10^{-3} those achieved in the CSF (Fig. 13.3B).

Given the cell cycle–specific action of methotrexate, administering that drug by a pulse technique may limit its effectiveness while increasing the chances of neurotoxicity. One randomized study of children with leptomeningeal acute lymphocytic leukemia compared standard 12 mg/m², therapy twice weekly with "concentration × time" therapy (11). Using an Ommaya reservoir, 1 mg of methotrexate was administered every 12 hours for six doses, with the dosage adjusted to achieve a methotrexate level in lumbar spinal fluid prior to administration of the next dose of $5 \pm 2 \times 10^{-7}$ M. This course was repeated every 7 to 10 days until remission occurred and (as in standard pulse therapy) was repeated during the consolidation and maintenance periods. Less neurotoxicity was seen in patients who received the "concentration × time" therapy than in those who received the standard pulse therapy, with no difference in efficacy between the two approaches.

Numerous reports support the safety of intraventricular catheters; in one series of 387 patients, only 27 had complications (8), most of which were infections that were well controlled with antibiotics. Infected reservoirs can be successfully managed with antibiotic therapy without removal of the hardware (12), although in many cases, reservoir removal is required just as it is in other foreign-body infections. Skin bacteria are the most frequent cause of infection, but scrupulous attention to technique will lessen the incidence of this complication (12). An additional benefit of the reservoirs is the avoidance

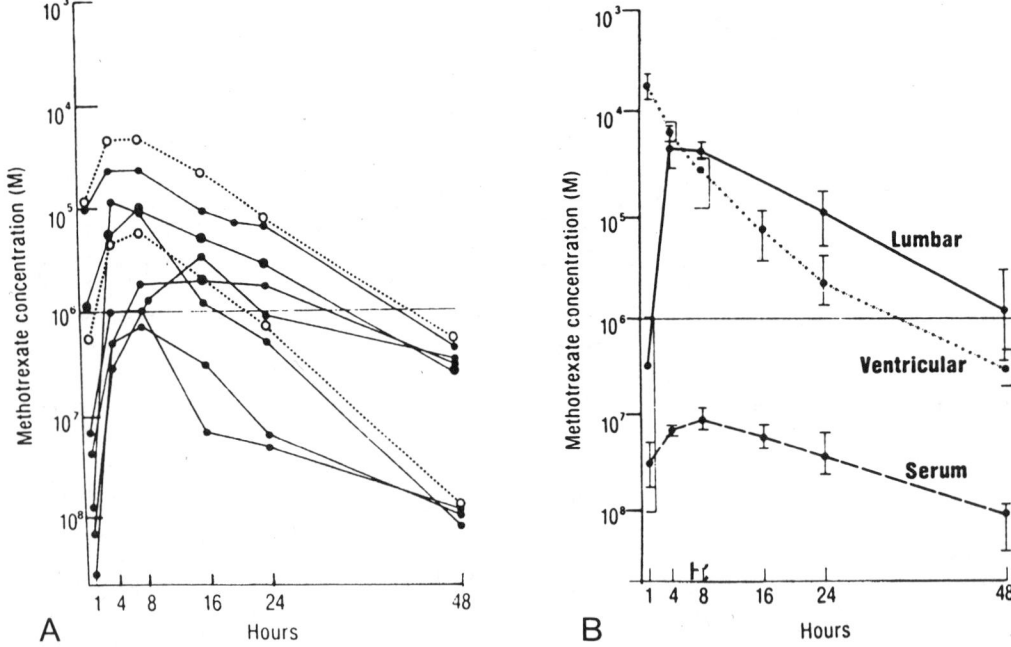

Figure 13.3.   A. Nine studies of intraventricular methotrexate concentration following lumbar administration. *Solid circles* represent a dose of 6.25 mg/m² and *open circles* a dose of 12.5 mg/m². **B.** Methotrexate distribution (mean ± range) in five studies following intraventricular administration of 6.25 mg/m². (Both from Shapiro W, Young D, Mehta B. Methotrexate distribution in cerebrospinal fluid after intravenous, ventricular and lumbar injection. N Engl J Med 1975;293:161–166. With permission.)

of repeated lumbar puncture, as that procedure poses an inconvenience to both patient and therapist.

Whether using lumbar puncture or an intraventricular reservoir, it is critical to establish the patency of the CSF pathways, as blockages are not uncommon in leptomeningeal malignancy. Local compromise of CSF flow may leave some areas untouched by the administered therapeutic agents and may increase local toxicity if CSF circulation is impaired. Radioisotopic scanning (e.g., with ^{111}In-albumin) can assure good flow, and focal radiation therapy can often ease areas of blockage once they have been identified.

Intraventricular therapy has been used to treat established leptomeningeal malignancy as well as for prophylaxis of tumors with a high incidence of CNS invasion, such as acute lymphocytic leukemia. The earliest widespread use of direct CNS therapy was for childhood acute lymphocytic leukemia (c-ALL). In the late 1960s, when advances in chemotherapy for c-ALL increased life expectancy in those patients from weeks to years, the prospects of long-term survival were diminished by an incidence of c-ALL relapse in the CNS as high as 75% (13). Often following this relapse, these patients would also develop a c-ALL relapse in bone marrow, which frequently proved fatal (14).

The blood-brain barrier prevents adequate levels of some systemically administered cytotoxic drugs from reaching the leukemic cells present in the CNS during induction, consolidation, and maintenance therapy. Leukemia can invade the CNS from the systemic circulation or it can develop de novo from hematopoietic rests in the choroid plexus and pia-arachnoid or from pluripotent microglia (15). Strategies to prophylactically treat the CNS have used irradiation and intraventricular therapy in varying combinations and have succeeded in decreasing the rate of relapse in the CNS to less than 10% of patients treated as well as in prolonging hematologic remission (16).

PROPHYLAXIS: CHILDHOOD ACUTE LYMPHOCYTIC LEUKEMIA

The first successful CNS prophylactic program, developed by the St. Jude's Cancer Research Hospital, consisted of 24 Gy of cranial irradiation in 14 to 15 fractions given over 17 to 18 days, with less irradiation given to children under 1 year of age. Intrathecal methotrexate at a dose of 12 mg/m^2 was given during radiation therapy every 3 to 4 days for a total of five doses. Evidence that during postnatal development body surface lagged behind CSF volume (Fig. 13.4) prompted the Children's Cancer Study Group (CCSG) to adopt a program using a fixed intraventricular dosage schedule of 6, 8, 10, and 12 mg of methotrexate for children of ages less than 1 year, 1 year, 2 years, and over 3 years, respectively. The intraventricular methotrexate

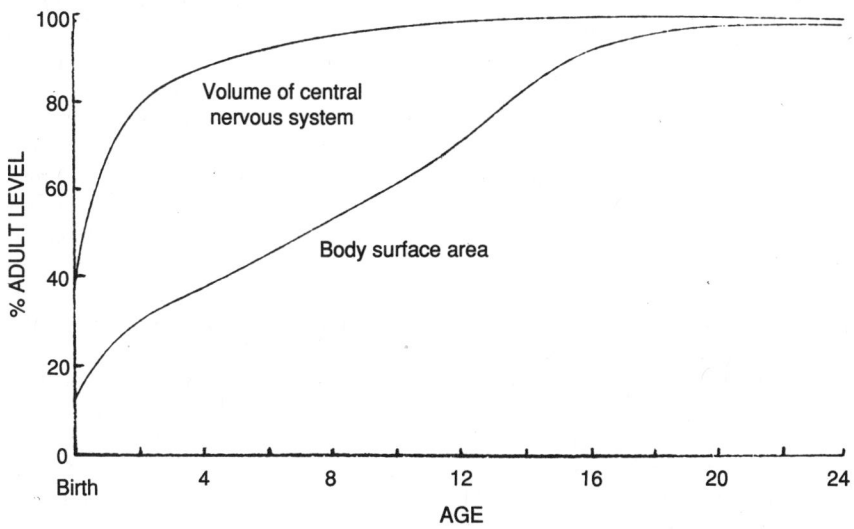

Figure 13.4. A comparison of body surface area and extracellular fluid volume of the CNS during childhood growth. (From Bleyer WA. Clinical pharmacology of intrathecal methotrexate: an improved regimen derived from age-related pharmacokinetics. Cancer Treat Rep 1977;61:1419–1425. With permission.)

was administered twice weekly during induction, then weekly, at which time 1800 rads of cranial irradiation was given. With this approach, the CNS relapse rate in average-risk patients fell to between 2 and 5%, and the relapse rate in high-risk patients to 6% (17) (Table 13.1).

Greater experience in treating c-ALL has allowed some risk factors for meningeal relapse to be identified (18, 19), perhaps eventually allowing therapy to be tailored to minimize the risk of toxicity without compromising prophylaxis. For example, patients who are young or black or those who have high white cell counts, lymphomatous characteristics, or thrombocytopenia are all at higher-than-average risk for leptomeningeal c-ALL relapse. Patients at low risk for leptomeningeal c-ALL recurrence should be treated prophylactically, but they can be treated with intraventricular methotrexate alone during both induction and maintenance therapy, thus avoiding cranial irradiation. Patients at intermediate risk have been treated with both cranial irradiation and chemotherapy regimens such as intraventricular methotrexate, cytosine arabinoside (ara-C), and hydrocortisone (20); intraventricular methotrexate and systemic intermediate-dose methotrexate (21); or high-dose intravenous methotrexate alone (22). Patients believed to be at high risk for meningeal c-ALL relapse have been treated with cranial irradiation combined with protracted intraventricular methotrexate or with intraventricular methotrexate and high-dose systemic methotrexate (23).

RADIOISOTOPES

Intraventricular radioactive gold (^{198}Au) (24) and radioactive chromium phosphate ($CrO_4^{32}P$) (25) without external radiation therapy have been used as prophylaxis in meningeal acute lymphocytic leukemia. ^{198}Au emits both γ and β energy, so scintigraphic evidence of its distribution can be obtained simply. The β rays, responsible for the bulk of the radioactivity delivered, on average penetrate tissues to only 3.6 mm, so the bulk of nervous system tissues are spared the effects of radiation. ^{32}P is a pure β emitter that has a half-life of 14.5 days and penetrates tissue to a maximum of 8 mm, with an average of 4 mm. In one series, $CrO_4^{32}P$ administered by lumbar puncture as maintenance therapy following induction of remission yielded a result that was not significantly different from that noted after intrathecal methotrexate prophylaxis (25). Cauda equina dysfunction was a complication of $CrO_4^{32}P$ therapy and was thought to be related to the intrathecal route of drug delivery. No studies have been published on the use of intraventricular therapy and radioactive $CrO_4^{32}P$ colloid.

PROPHYLAXIS: OTHER LEUKEMIAS

The well-established benefits of prophylactic intraventricular chemotherapy for c-ALL prompted interest in prophylaxis of other tumors in which CNS seeding commonly occurs. The decision to use prophylactic therapy must weigh the advantage to the patient against the risk of complications that include neurotoxicity and a decreased capacity for systemic chemotherapy, which may compromise definitive treatment. Though small amounts (about 0.001 of the CSF level for methotrexate) (26) of intraventricularly administered drugs enter the systemic circulation, these do not produce the marrow suppression associated with craniospinal irradiation and are thus less likely to compromise systemic chemotherapeutic efforts.

With longer survivals in patients with adult acute lymphocytic leukemia (a-ALL), the frequency of meningeal a-ALL has been increasing (27, 28), but its incidence, with rates ranging from 20 to 60%, appears more variable and probably less frequent than in c-ALL (29–33). Patients have been treated with intrathecal methotrexate and cranial irradiation (with a reduction in CNS relapse rate) (34), as well as with intraventricular methotrexate alone (15 mg every 4 weeks for six doses, with a renewal of therapy at bone marrow relapse) (35). With prophylaxis, a reduction in meningeal a-ALL relapse incidence similar to that achieved in c-ALL occurs but may not be associated with a survival advantage (34).

Prophylaxis for this condition remains controversial because few controlled studies have been performed and because differences in systemic protocols confound the studies that have been done. It may be better to give prophylaxis only to those patients at high risk for developing CNS disease. Patients who had an initially high white blood cell count, thrombocytopenia, a T-cell phenotype, B-cell leukemia, elevated lactic dehydrogenase levels, or a high proportion of leukemia cells in the S + G_2M compartment were at greater risk for development of CNS leukemia (36). An age less than 20 years and an L3 morphology may also place patients at increased risk for developing CNS a-ALL.

Compared with the number for a-ALL, even

fewer studies have carefully examined the incidence of meningeal involvement in acute non-lymphocytic leukemia (ANLL); however, given the poor prognosis with this condition, these patients' shorter survival likely gives them less time at risk to develop CNS disease than that for patients with ALL. One study demonstrated a CNS ANLL relapse rate of 11% but noted that only 2.6% had a relapse solely in the CNS (37), thus supporting the general concept that meningeal involvement portends a more aggressive phase of illness. Using prophylactic therapy for acute myelogenous leukemia, one group performed an uncontrolled study of cytosine arabinoside (100 mg) or methotrexate (15 mg) intraventricularly every 4 weeks for six doses. Only 2 of 28 patients developed CNS relapses, one of which occurred in a noncompliant patient (38).

Patients with myelomonocytic leukemia and 16 (p13q22) chromosomal inversion are at great risk of CNS involvement, especially malignant meningitis (39), despite their more generally favorable response to therapy. Prophylaxis has been demonstrated to be beneficial (40) for this subgroup of nonlymphocytic leukemia patients. Meningeal involvement may occur more frequently in other patients with acute monoblastic leukemia than in those with other ANLLs (41) as well, but the benefit of prophylactic intraventricular therapy has not yet been systematically examined with controlled studies. The role of prophylactic therapy in ANLL patients undergoing total body irradiation and bone marrow transplantation is uncertain at present (42); if the CNS is inadequately sterilized in preparation for bone marrow transplantation, the possibility of meningeal ANLL relapse will exist.

The relapse rates in the CNS in chronic lymphocytic and myelogenous leukemia are sufficiently low that prophylaxis would likely produce more toxicity than benefit (29).

PROPHYLAXIS: LYMPHOMA

African Burkitt's lymphoma is highly chemosensitive, with complete remissions achieved in over 80% of patients, but malignant meningitis occurs in about 40% of relapsing patients who receive no CNS prophylaxis (43). In a study using historic controls, patients received 15 mg of intrathecal methotrexate every 2 to 4 weeks; those treated prophylactically had a 13.7% CNS relapse rate compared with 25% in patients who received no prophylaxis. This difference was not significant, but when patients with the less-aggressive facial-only presentation were eliminated from the analysis, the difference in CNS relapse rate was significantly greater than 20%, and there was an almost 25% decrease in systemic relapse rate in patients prophylactically treated (44). Patients who have American Burkitt's lymphoma with minimal tumor at presentation or those who have had complete resection may have a lower incidence of CNS disease. Also, as with other lymphomas, there is a high correlation between bone marrow involvement and the development of malignant meningitis. Since American Burkitt's lymphoma patients with CNS relapse have a dismal prognosis, worse than that of patients with African Burkitt's lymphoma, prophylactic CNS therapy seems warranted (45).

Non-Hodgkin's lymphoma patients with lymphoblastic lymphoma (46) or diffuse histology and bone marrow involvement are at significant risk for CNS involvement (47); testicular involvement, epidural disease, malignant cells in the circulation (48), and extensive extra nodal disease also place these patients at high risk (49). These high-risk patients should receive prophylaxis if systemic remission is achieved. Intraventricular therapy has the advantage of not compromising systemic therapy, as does craniospinal irradiation, and may be less toxic than systemic high-dose methotrexate, which is used by some as CNS prophylaxis (49).

PROPHYLAXIS: OTHER TUMORS

Prophylaxis of other malignancies has been less well defined owing to the relative infrequency of CNS involvement in these tumors. Of the nonlymphomatous solid tumors responsive to therapy, small cell carcinoma of the lung has the greatest incidence of CNS involvement, with almost a quarter of these tumors associated with CNS disease. This figure increases to almost half of patients surviving more than 2 years. Prophylactic cranial irradiation decreases this incidence to less than 10% (50), but the impact of such irradiation on patient survival is unclear, and whether CNS chemotherapy will prove beneficial is, as yet, unanswered (51). Despite the belief that there is less neurotoxicity with prophylactic treatment programs that do not include irradiation, at least one study demonstrated no difference after 5 years between patients who had had prophylactic treatment that included irradiation and those who had received intraventricular and systemic therapy only (52). Establishing preventive therapies that maximize efficacy and minimize toxicity will require carefully designed prospective studies that take into consideration both the biologic behavior of the tumor and the unique pharmacokinetics of the CSF.

DIAGNOSIS OF ESTABLISHED LEPTOMENINGEAL CANCER

For treatment of leptomeningeal cancer to be successful, it is critical that diagnosis be made early, before there is bulk disease. Patients who are treated before developing significant deficits have a significantly greater chance of neurologic improvement than those with more advanced disease (53). The CNS has a vast surface area with many interstices in which asymptomatic tumor cells can lodge and remain undetected until their growth produces symptoms, by either local compression, hydrocephalus, or release of toxic substances. Though massive disease may be present without tumor cells being shed in the spinal fluid, and though tumor cells may not be found even with multiple samples, only rarely will protein and sugar levels and opening pressure all be normal in a patient suffering from meningeal carcinomatosis (54). Cytologic examination of CSF remains the single most important means of diagnosing leptomeningeal carcinomatosis, and the diagnostic accuracy with this technique is greatly improved if the sample is promptly (ideally within an hour) placed in preservative and if a large volume of fluid (about 10 mL) is sent for evaluation. In lymphoma (49), and perhaps other tumor types as well, there are small but significant false-positive and false-negative rates in cytologic diagnosis. Careful coordination between clinician and pathologist is needed to optimize diagnostic accuracy.

Because there is some correlation between a patient's overall burden of disease and the number of cells present in the fluid sample (15), earlier diagnosis will require improved diagnostic tools. Lactate dehydrogenase, β_2-microglobulin, β-glucuronidase, adenosine deaminase, and the CD9 and carinoembryonic antigens in CSF have all been examined as possible markers of leptomeningeal disease (55–58), but to date, all have shown disappointing abilities to make confident diagnoses. Comparison of serum and CSF levels may increase the sensitivity of these tests (59), but as these studies remain nonspecific, great care must be exercised in their interpretation, es-

pecially with regard to eliminating infection as a diagnostic possibility (60). A report (61) of 41 children found insulin-like growth factor binding protein-3 levels elevated in malignant meningitis from c-ALL, ependymoma, and medulloblastoma, yet elevated levels were also found in 15% of infectious meningitis cases. The levels also correlated with therapeutic effect, falling in patients whose tumors responded to treatment. In one study, the use of flow cytometry to detect DNA abnormalities in cells from patients with malignant meningitis added little diagnostically to routine cytology (62). In a study comparing the abilities of cytology and immunocytochemistry to diagnose meningeal carcinomatosis, immunocytochemistry was found to be a "minor help" in increasing the diagnostic yield of cytology (63). For lymphomatous meningitis, the use of electrostatically fixed poly-L-lysine-coated slides greatly improved immunocytologic diagnostic yield in one study of 26 patients with inconclusive routine cytology (64).

Three monoclonal antibodies that identify BCA-225 antigen, a cytoplasmic and surface glycoprotein found in breast cancer, have been used as a diagnostic assay in a small study (65). Four of five affected patients in that study had elevated BCA-225 levels, and data from a larger unreported series appear promising. Other monoclonal antibody panels have been used for the diagnosis of leptomeningeal malignant meningitis (66), but their effectiveness in diagnosing the commonly occurring tumors as yet remains unproven.

Magnetic resonance imaging (MRI) is not as accurate as myelography for diagnosing leptomeningeal carcinomatosis (67). Gadolinium enhancement greatly improves the sensitivity of MRI, though false-positive results are not uncommon. Clear-cut cases of leptomeningeal malignancy occur without MRI abnormality, and it is doubtful that MRI will ever confidently distinguish malignant from infectious chronic meningitides.

On rare occasions, the diagnosis of carcinomatous meningitis can be made without cytologic confirmation, but great care must be taken to eliminate infection as a diagnostic possibility. Causes of chronic meningitis that can mimic neoplastic spread include infection with a host of different agents as well as sarcoidosis and vasculitis (60). Careful microbacteriologic evaluation of CSF is critical in any suspected case of malignant meningitis. Meningeal biopsy should be considered for equivocal cases, particularly if imaging studies have demonstrated an accessible area of meningeal enhancement. In such cases, the diagnostic yield was 80% in one series (68).

THERAPY

The mainstay of therapy for established meningeal malignancy has been chemotherapy, usually methotrexate, delivered through an Ommaya reservoir coupled with focal radiotherapy to major sites of involvement (54). As in c-ALL, methotrexate may be given most effectively, and with less risk of leukoencephalopathy, when CSF is maintained at levels more constant than those achievable with pulse treatment (69). In one study of 19 patients with breast cancer, methotrexate was injected into an Ommaya reservoir whenever the CSF concentration fell below 10^3 nmol/L; more than half the patients had sustained neurologic relapse by 1 year, and all the patients had relapsed at 25 months (70). The median survival for these patients was 6 months, and despite the care taken to keep the CSF concentrations below 10^6 nmol/L, 3 of the 19 patients developed therapy-limiting encephalopathy, even though CNS irradiation was not used.

Using higher trough levels of methotrexate may improve control of the tumor cells, but this will likely be at the cost of greater encephalopathy (71). In another study, radiotherapy directed to sites of major clinical involvement and intraventricular methotrexate at a dose of 7 mg/m^2 plus citrovorum factor given twice weekly for five treatments achieved a median survival of 7.2 months in breast cancer patients, with 61% of these patients enjoying stabilization of their neurologic disease (54).

COMBINATION THERAPY

Combination intraventricular therapy for leptomeningeal disease has theoretic appeal, but few trials for solid tumors have been reported. In one study of 23 patients with a variety of solid tumors treated with a combination of methotrexate, ara-C, thiotepa, and hydrocortisone, results compared favorably with those of other reported series, but according to the authors, these patients may have suffered more neurotoxicity (53). Another randomized study comparing intraventricular methotrexate with the combination of methotrexate plus cytosine arabinoside failed to show an advantage for the combination

therapy (73). Hydrocortisone acetate given intrathecally has significant toxicity (74); as dexamethasone penetrates the CNS extremely well, there is little advantage in using direct steroid infusion into the CSF.

OTHER AGENTS

Ara-C, an antimetabolite, has activity in the rapidly proliferating lymphoreticular malignancies but, as should be anticipated, is less active in the more slowly growing solid tumors. In one study using ara-C at a dose of 12 to 20 mg intraventricularly either twice or three times weekly, the CSF was cleared of malignant cells in half the patients with leptomeningeal seeding from solid tumors (75). Another trial using intraventricular ara-C at a dose of 100 mg thrice weekly for leptomeningeal breast carcinomatosis failed to show any advantage over standard therapy (Dr. F. Holmes, personal communication, 1994). Both ara-C and methotrexate have been placed in liposomal formulation (76, 77) so that a continuous release of the drug can be obtained with achievement of therapeutically desired protracted low-level drug exposure and avoidance of peak levels that may contribute to toxicity. The liposomal ara-C preparation is presently under phase II multicenter evaluation for both solid and lymphoreticular malignant meningitis.

Thiotepa is an alkylating agent that can be given into the CSF, but in a clinical randomized trial (78) in patients with nonleukemic malignant meningitis, the drug showed no advantage over standard methotrexate therapy. It may be used in selective instances in which standard therapy failed.

New agents in early clinical trials offer theoretic promise, though none have yet demonstrated significant advantage over methotrexate therapy. Aziridinylbenzoquinone (AZQ), or diaziquone, is an alkylating agent that when given systemically causes severe myelosuppression (79), can be given safely into the CSF, and has activity against refractory acute lymphocytic leukemic meningitis (80, 81). As the drug is not cell-cycle specific, it has a theoretic advantage for treating more slowly growing solid-tumor malignant meningitis, though solid tumor trials with it have not yet been undertaken. Another alkylating agent, 4-hydroperoxycyclophosphamide, is presently undergoing phase 1 multicenter clinical evaluation (82).

Intrathecal melphalan has shown activity against rhabdomyosarcoma meningitis in an athymic nude rat model (83) and was well tolerated by the animals. The drug is presently undergoing phase 1 human clinical evaluation. Melphalan is a broad-spectrum nitrogen mustard derivative that has been designed to be carried by the L-amino acid transport system so that manipulation of CSF amino acid content may prove a means of improving its efficacy. Etoposide was well tolerated when given to two patients with nonleukemic meningitis and reportedly ameliorated their symptoms (84). Hormonal therapy can produce remission of carcinomatous meningitis (85) and should be considered as initial therapy for tumors that are hormonally responsive.

RADIOISOTOPES

Though radioisotopes instilled directly into the CSF have been used as prophylaxis against leptomeningeal leukemia (86) and lymphoma (87), the pharmacokinetics of presently used agents do not appear favorable to allow their use as therapy for leptomeningeal cancer from solid tumors (88). Because isotopes emit various types of energies with different depths of penetration, it is hoped that the different physical properties may be exploited to therapeutic advantage.

MONOCLONAL ANTIBODIES

Efforts to link radioisotopes or toxins to monoclonal antibodies that are immunoreactive to the patient's tumor and to instill this compound into the CSF offer hope for improved therapy of leptomeningeal carcinomatosis. In one study of monoclonal antibody–linked iodine-131, four to five patients with solid tumors responded to this therapy, with responses sustained for 7 months to 2 years (89). Unfortunately, monoclonal antibodies specific for common tumors are presently unavailable, and this study did not include patients with leptomeningeal metastasis from breast or lung cancer. Whether other isotopes or toxins would be more effective and what advantages the linkage to the antibody offers are presently unanswered questions. Theoretic models of monoclonal antibody–linked therapy suggest that the delivery of radioisotope may not be as specific as had been hoped, with significant hepatic and reticuloendothelial deposition being noted. In addition, these isotopes will likely have little penetration for tumor deposits greater than 5 mm in diameter (90, 91). Other problems include the patient forming antiantibodies (92) with the potential for serum sickness. Most importantly, therapy for the more commonly occurring tumors requires tumor-specific antibodies, which are as yet unavailable.

BIOLOGIC RESPONSE MODIFIERS

The purification and mass production of biologic response modifiers has offered new promise in the treatment of malignancy, but the clinical use of these agents is still in its infancy. Cytokines have protean actions in modulating inflammation and produce complex interactions with one another (93), such that an inflammatory cascade can result from the administration of a single agent. The direct effects of the biologic response modifiers on the nervous system (94, 95) may be as complex as their inflammatory effects (96); this is presently the subject of intensive investigations.

Of the therapeutic agents available, only α-interferon and interleukin-2 have been used to any extent against human leptomeningeal disease. Four patients with leptomeningeal tumor spread had intraventricular interferon therapy in a phase I study (97), with doses of 1 to 10 million units given three times weekly, up to a cumulative maximum dose of 113 million units administered to one patient. In all patients, the CSF was cleared of malignant cells for up to 10 weeks, but there was little improvement in neurologic symptoms. Therapy was discontinued because of progressive systemic disease or toxicity, either encephalopathy or progression of a preexisting leukoencephalopathy and myelopathy.

Interleukin-2 has been used in selective patients with leptomeningeal melanoma and renal cell carcinoma, with benefit in a few patients, but systemic disease progression has limited the duration of response. The meningitis and encephalopathy that the biologic response modifiers induce have been dose-limiting, and to date, responses have not been encouraging. Given the theoretic mechanisms of action of interleukin-2, meningeal inflammation may be unavoidable, and careful management of this iatrogenic meningitis will be mandatory if this form of therapy is to have benefit.

SUMMARY

Intraventricular therapy has been highly effective in treating established meningeal involvement in c-ALL, and prophylactic intraventricular therapy has been responsible for the prolonged survival achieved in patients with this condition. However, determining the least toxic form of effective therapy remains a challenge. The dismal results of treatment of leptomeningeal carcinomatosis can be attributed to multiple factors. First, adenocarcinomas and malignant melanoma predominate in most series (98, 99), and with the exception of breast cancer, these tumors are relatively insensitive to chemotherapy. As was seen in the experience with leukemia and lymphoma, CNS disease often heralds a more aggressive phase of malignancy (100), one in which systemic disease frequently becomes a pressing clinical problem. In most series reported in the literature, more than half the patients had advanced disease when their meningeal metastases were discovered. Also, these patients have commonly undergone prior therapies and are malnourished, thus limiting their ability to tolerate cytoreductive therapy. As with all therapeutic decisions in oncology, the clinician must consider the ability of the patient to tolerate the therapy as well as the biologic characteristics of the tumor. In addition, the protean sequelae of chronic meningitis pose enormous psychosocial stresses on both the patient and the family, thus requiring expert nursing care and counseling.

REFERENCES

1. Levin VA, Patlak CS, Landahl HD. Heuristic modeling of drug delivery to malignant brain tumors. J Pharmacokinet Biopharm 1980;8:257–296.

2. Levin VA. Relationship of octanol/water partition coefficient and molecular weight to rat brain capillary permeability. J Med Chem 1980;23:682–684.

3. Levin VA, Landahl HD. Pharmacokinetic approaches to drug distribution in the cerebrospinal fluid based on ventricular administration in beagle dogs. J Pharmacokinet Biopharm 1985;13:387–403.

4. Flessner MF, Fenstermacher JD, Dedrick RL, Blasberg RG. Peritoneal absorption of macromolecules studied by quantitative autoradiography. Am J Physiol 1985;248:H26–32.

5. Flessner MF, Fenstermacher JD, Dedrick RL, Blasberg RG. A distributed model of peritoneal-plasma transport: tissue concentration gradients. Am J Physiol 1985;248:F425–435.

6. Ommaya AK. Implantable devices for chronic access and drug delivery to the central nervous system. Cancer Drug Deliv 1984;1:169–179.

7. Dyck P. Lumbar reservoir for intrathecal chemotherapy. Cancer 1985;55:2771–2773.

8. Obbens E, Leavens M, Beal J, Lee Y. Ommaya reservoirs in 387 cancer patients: a 15 year experience. Neurology 1985;35:1274–1278.

9. Shapiro W, Young D, Mehta B. Methotrexate distribution in cerebrospinal fluid after intravenous, ventricular and lumbar injection. N Engl J Med 1975; 293:161–166.

10. Larson S, Schall G, Di Chiro G. The influence of previous lumbar puncture and pneumoencephalography on the incidence of unsuccessful radioisotope cisternography. J Nucl Med 1971;12:555–557.

11. Bleyer WA, Poplack DG, Simon RM. "Concentration × time" methotrexate via a subcutaneous reservoir: a less toxic regimen for intraventricular chemotherapy of central nervous system neoplasms. Blood 1978;51:835–842.

12. Dinndorf P, Bleyer W. Management of infectious complications of intraventricular reservoirs in cancer patients: low incidence and successful treatment without reservoir removal. Cancer Drug Deliv 1987;4:105–117.

13. Evans A, Gilbert E, Zandstra R. The increasing incidence of central nervous system leukemia in children. Cancer 1970;26:404–409.

14. Haghbin M, Zeulzer W. A long term study of cerebrospinal leukemia. J Pediatr 1965;67:23–30.

15. Bleyer W. Biology and pathogenesis of CNS leukemia. Am J Pediatr Hematol Oncol 1989;11:57–63.

16. Holland J, Glidewell O. Chemotherapy of acute lymphoblastic leukemia of childhood. 1972;30:1480–1487.

17. Bleyer W, Coccia P, Sather H, et al. and the Children's Cancer Study Group. Reduction in central nervous system leukemia with a pharmacokinetically derived intrathecal methotrexate dosage regimen. J Clin Oncol 1983;1:317–325.

18. Bleyer W, Poplack D. Prophylaxis and treatment of leukemia in the central nervous system and other sanctuaries. Semin Oncol 1985;12:131–148.

19. Poplack D. Acute lymphoblastic leukemia in childhood. Pediatr Clin North Am 1985;32:669–697.

20. Pinkel D. Patterns of failure in acute lymphocytic leukemia. Cancer Treat Symp 1983;2:259–266.

21. Freeman A, Weinberg V, Brecher M, et al. Comparison of intermediate dose methotrexate with cranial irradiation for the post-induction treatment of acute lymphocytic leukemia in children. N Engl J Med 1983; 308:477–484.

22. Poplack D, Reaman G, Bleyer W, et al. Central nervous system preventive therapy with high dose methotrexate in acute lymphoblastic leukemia: a preliminary report (abstract). Proc Am Soc Clin Oncol 1984;3:204.

23. Bleyer W. Central nervous system leukemia. Pediatr Clin North Am 1988;4:789–814.

24. Metz O, Stoll W, Plenert W. Meningiosis prophylaxis with intrathecal ^198Au-colloid and methotrexate in childhood acute lymphocytic leukemia. Cancer 1982;49:224–228.

25. Sackmann-Muriel F, Schere F, Barengols A, et al. Remission maintenance therapy for meningeal leukemia: intrathecal methotrexate and dexamethasone versus intrathecal craniospinal irradiation with a radiocolloid. Br J Haematol 1976;33:119–127.

26. Balis FM, Poplack DG. Central nervous system pharmacology of antileukemic drugs. Am J Pediatr Hematol Oncol 1989;11:74–86.

27. Stewart DJ, Keating MJ, McCreadie KB, et al. Natural history of central nervous system acute leukemia in adults. Cancer 1981;47:184–196.

28. Dawson DM, Rosenthal DS, Moloney WC. Neurologic complications of acute leukemia in adults: changing rate. Ann Intern Med 1973;79:541–544.

29. Weizsäcker M, Kölmel HW. Meningeal involvement in leukemias and malignant lymphomas of adults: incidence, course of disease and treatment for prevention. Acta Neurol Scand 1979;69:363–370.

30. Law IP, Blom J. Adult acute leukemia. Frequency of central nervous system involvement in long term survivors. Cancer 1977;40:1304–1306.

31. Gee TS, Haghbin M, Dowling MD, Cunningham I, Middleman M, Clarkson B. Acute lymphoblastic leukemia in adults and children: differences in response with similar therapeutic regimens. Cancer 1976; 37:1256–1264.

32. Baccarani M, Corbelli G, Amadori A, et al. Adolescent and adult lymphoblastic leukemia: prognostic features and outcome of therapy. A study of 293 patients. Blood 1982;60:677–684.

33. Clarkson B, Ellis S, Little C, et al. Acute lymphoblastic leukemia in adults. Semin Oncol 1985; 12:160–179.

34. Omura GA, Moffit S, Vogler WR, Salter MM. Combination chemotherapy of adult acute lymphoblastic leukemia with randomized central nervous system prophylaxis. Blood 1980;55:199–204.

35. Haaxma-Reiche H, Daenen S. Acute lymphoblastic leukemia in adults: results of intraventricular maintenance chemotherapy for central nervous system prophylaxis and treatment. Eur J Cancer Clin Oncol 1988;24:615–620.

36. Kantarjian HM, Walter RS, Smith TL, et al. Identification of risk groups for development of central nervous system leukemia in adults with acute lymphocytic leukemia. Blood 1988;72:1784–1789.

37. Strijckmans PA, Malarme M. Rationale and indications for the prophylactic treatment of leukemic meningitis. In: Hildebrand J, Gangji D, eds. Treatment of neoplastic lesions of the nervous system. Proceedings of an EORTC symposium, 1980. Oxford: Pergamon Press, 1980:1–8.

38. Haaxma-Reiche H, Daenen S, Witteveen R. Experiences with the Ommaya reservoir for prophylaxis and treatment of the central nervous system in adult acute myelocytic leukemia. Blut 1988;57:351–355.

39. Holmes R, Keating MJ, Cork A, et al. A unique pattern of central nervous system leukemia in acute myelomonocytic leukemia associated with inv(16) (p13q22). Blood 1985;65:1071–1078.

40. Larson RA, Williams SF, Le Beau MM, Bitter MA, Vardiman JW, Rowley JD. Acute myelomonocytic leukemia with abnormal eosinophils and inv(16) or t(16;16) has a favorable prognosis. Blood 1986;68:1242–1249.

41. Tobelem G, Jacquillat C, Chastang C, et al. Acute monoblastic leukemia. A clinical and biologic study of 74 cases. Blood 1980;55:71–76.

42. Seeldrayers P, Hildebrand J. Treatment of neoplastic meningitis. Eur J Cancer Clin Oncol 1984; 20:449–456.

43. Zeigler JL, Bluming AZ, Fass L, Morrow RH. Relapse patterns in Burkitt's lymphoma. Cancer Res 1972;321:1267–1272.

44. Nkrumah FK, Neequaye JE, Biggar R. Intrathecal chemoprophylaxis in the prevention of central nervous system relapse in Burkitt's lymphoma. Cancer 1985;56:239–242.

45. Sariban E, Edwards B, Janus C, Magrath I. Central nervous system involvement in American Burkitt's lymphoma. J Clin Oncol 1983;1:677–681.

46. Weinstein JH, Vance ZB, Jaffe N, Buell D, Cassady JR, Nathan DG. Improved prognosis for patients with mediastinal lymphoblastic lymphoma. Blood 1979;53:687–694.

47. Litam J, Cabanillas F, Smith T, Bodey G, Freireich E. Central nervous system relapse in malignant lymphomas: risk factors and implications for prophylaxis. Blood 1979;54:1249–1257.

48. Macintosh F, Colby T, Podolsky W, et al. Central nervous system involvement in non-Hodgkin's lymphoma: an analysis of 105 cases. Cancer 1982; 49:586–595.

49. Recht L, Straus DJ, Cirrincione C, Thaler HZ, Posner JB. Central nervous system metastases from non-Hodgkin's lymphoma: treatment and prophylaxis. Am J Med 1988;84:425–435.

50. Lucas CF, Robinson B, Hoskin PJ, Yarnold FR, Smith IE, Ford HT. Morbidity of cranial relapse in small cell lung cancer and the impact of radiation therapy. Cancer Treat Rep 1986;70:565–570.

51. Bleyer WA. Hobson's choice in the CNS radioprophylaxis of small cell lung cancer. Int J Radiat Oncol Biol Phys 1988;15:783–785.

52. Mulhern R, Wasserman A, Fairclough D, Ochs J. Memory function in disease-free survivors of childhood acute lymphocytic leukemia given CNS prophylaxis with or without 1,800 cGy cranial irradiation. J Clin Oncol 1988;6:315–320.

53. Stewart DJ, Maroun JA, Hugenholtz H, et al. Combined intraommaya methotrexate, cytosine arabinoside, hydrocortisone and thio-TEPA for meningeal involvement by malignancies. J Neurooncol 1987; 5:315–322.

54. Wasserstrom WR, Glass JP, Posner JB. Diagnosis and treatment of leptomeningeal metastases from solid tumors: experience with 90 patients. Cancer 1982;49:759–772.

55. Schold SC, Wasserstrom WR, Fleisher M, Schwartz MK, Posner JB. Cerebrospinal fluid biochemical markers of central nervous system metastases. Ann Neurol 1980;8:597–604.

56. van Zanten AP, Twijnstra A, Ongerboer de Visser BW, Hart AAM, Nooyen WJ. Tumour markers in the cerebrospinal fluid of patients with central nervous system metastases from extracranial malignancies. Clin Chim Acta 1988;175:157–166.

57. Pettersson T, Klockars M, Weber TH, Somer H. Diagnostic value of cerebrospinal fluid adenosine deaminase determination [see comments]. Scand J Infect Dis 1991;23:97–100.

58. Komada Y, Ochiai H, Shimizu K, Azuma E, Kamiya H, Sakurai M. Shedding of CD9 antigen into cerebrospinal fluid by acute lymphoblastic leukemia cells. Blood 1990;76:112–116.

59. Collins VP. Central nervous system tumors. Tumor Biol 1987;8:147–150.

60. Wilhelm C, Ellner JJ. Chronic meningitis. Neurol Clin 1986;4:115–140.

61. Muller HL, Oh Y, Gargosky SE, Lehrnbecher T, Hintz RL, Rosenfeld RG. Concentrations of insulin-like growth factor (IGF)-binding protein-3 (IGFBP-3), IGF, and IGFBP-3 protease activity in cerebrospinal fluid of children with leukemia, central nervous system tumor, or meningitis. J Clin Endocrinol Metab 1993;77:1113–1119.

62. Cibas ES, Malkin MG, Posner JB, Melamed MR. Detection of DNA abnormalities by flow cytometry in cells from cerebrospinal fluid. Am J Clin Pathol 1987; 88:570–577.

63. Boogerd W, Vroom TM, van Heerde P, Brutel de la Rivière G, Peterse JL, van der Sande JJ. CSF cytology versus immunocytochemistry in meningeal carcinomatosis. J Neurol Neurosurg Psychiatry 1988; 51:142–145.

64. Kranz BR, Thiel E, Thierfelder S. Immunocytochemical identification of meningeal leukemia and lymphoma: poly-L-lysine-coated slides permit multimarker analysis even with minute cerebrospinal fluid cell specimens. Blood 1989;73:1942–1950.

65. Fetell MR, Leon JA, Estabrook A, Yemul SS, Mesa-Tejada R. Diagnosis of meningeal carcinomatosis due to breast cancer by a specific antibody assay (abstract). American Neurological Association annual meeting, 1988.

66. Coakham HB, Brownell B, Harper EI, et al. Use of monoclonal antibody panel to identify malignant cells in cerebrospinal fluid. Lancet 1984;i:1095–1098.

67. Krol G, Sze G, Malkin M, Walker R. MR of cranial and spinal meningeal carcinomatosis: comparisonw ith CT and myelography. Am J Radiol 1988; 15:583–588.

68. Cheng TM, O'Neill BP, Scheithauer BW, Piepgras DG. Chronic meningitis: the role of meningeal or cortical biopsy. Neurosurgery 1994;34:590–595.

69. Bleyer WA, Poplack DG, Simon RM. "Concentration × time" methotrexate via a subcutaneous reservoir: a less toxic regimen for intraventricular chemotherapy of central nervous system neoplasms. Blood 1978;51:835–842.

70. Ongerboer de Visser BW, Somers R, Nooyen WH, van Heerde P, Hart AAM, McVie JG. Intraventricular methotrexate therapy of leptomeningeal metastasis from breast cancer. Neurology 1983;33:1565–1572.

71. Hryniuk WM, Bertino JR. Treatment of leukemia with large doses of methotrexate and folinic acid: clinical biochemical correlates. J Clin Invest 1969; 48:2140–2155.

72. Stewart DJ, Maroun JA, Hugenholtz H, et al. Combined intraommaya methotrexate, cytosine arabinoside, hydrocortisone and thio-TEPA for meningeal involvement by malignancies. J Neurooncol 1987; 5:315–322.

73. Hitchins RN, Bell DR, Woods RL, Levi JA. A prospective randomized trial of single agent versus combination chemotherapy in meningeal carcinomatosis. J Clin Oncol 1987;5:1655–1662.

74. Stratton I. Dangers of intrathecal hydrocortisone sodium succinate (letter). Med J Aust 1975;2:650.

75. Fulton DS, Levin VL, Gutin PH, et al. Intrathecal cytosine arabinoside for the treatment of meningeal metastases from malignant brain tumors and systemic tumors. Cancer Chemother Pharmacol 1982;8:285–291.

76. Kim S, Chatelut E, Kim JC, et al. Extended CSF cytarabine exposure following intrathecal administration of DTC 101. J Clin Oncol 1993;11:2186–2193.

77. Chatelut E, Kim T, Kim S. A slow-release methotrexate formulation for intrathecal chemotherapy. Cancer Chemother Pharmacol 1993;32:179–182.

78. Grossman SA, Finkelstein DM, Ruckdeschel JC, Trump DL, Moynihan T, Ettinger DS. Randomized prospective comparison of intraventricular methotrexate and thiotepa in patients with previously untreated

neoplastic meningitis. Eastern Cooperative Oncology Group. J Clin Oncol 1993;11:561–569.

79. Chamberlain MC, Prados MD, Silver P, Levin VA. A phase I/II study of 24 hour intravenous AZQ in recurrent primary brain tumors. J Neurooncol 1988; 6:319–323.

80. Zimm S, Holcenberg J, Balis F, Doherty K, Poplack DJ. Intrathecal diaziquone (AZQ): a new, clinically useful agent for the treatment of meningeal neoplasia (abstract). Proc Am Assoc Cancer Res 1988; 28:190.

81. Berg SL, Balis FM, Zimm S, et al. Phase I/II trial and pharmacokinetics of intrathecal diaziquone in refractory meningeal malignancies. J Clin Oncol 1992; 10:143–148.

82. Friedman HS, Ochs J, Finlay J, et al. Phase I trial of intrathecal 4-hydroperoxycyclophosphamide for neoplastic meningitis (abstract). Proc Annu Meet Am Assoc Cancer Res 1993;34:A1598.

83. Friedman HS, Archer GE, McLendon RE, et al. Intrathecal melphalan therapy of human neoplastic meningitis in athymic nude rats. Cancer Res 1994; 54:4710–4714.

84. van der Gaast A, Sonneveld P, Mans DR, Splinter TA. Intrathecal administration of etoposide in the treatment of malignant meningitis: feasibility and pharmacokinetic data. Cancer Chemother Pharmacol 1992;29:335–337.

85. Mencel PJ, DeAngelis LM, Motzer RJ. Hormonal ablation as effective therapy for carcinomatous meningitis from prostatic carcinoma. Cancer 1994; 73:1892–1894.

86. Reddeman H, Bartelt G, Blau H-J. Intrathekale radiogoldprohylaxe un liquorbefunde bei kindern mit akuter lymphoblastischer leukose. Folia Haematol 1986;113:466–473.

87. Rigon A, Sotti G, Zanesco L, et al. Profilassi meningea con radiocolloidi nell leucemia e nel linoofa non-Hodgkin dell'infanzia. Radiol Med 1985;71:517–520.

88. Doge H, Hliscs R. Intrathecal therapy with [198]Au-colloid for meningosis prophylaxis. Eur J Nucl Med 1984;9:125–128.

89. Lashford LS, Davies AG, Richardson RB, et al. A pilot study of ^{131}I monoclonal antibodies in the therapy of leptomeningeal tumors. Cancer 1988;61:857–868.

90. Wheldon TE, O'Donoghue JA, Hilditch TE, Barrett A. Strategies for systemic radiotherapy of micrometastases using antibody-targeted [131]I. Radiother Oncol 1988;11:133–142.

91. Bigler RE, Zanzonico PB, Cosma M, Sgouros G. Adjuvant radioimmunotherapy for micrometastases: a strategy for cancer cure. In: Srivastava SC, ed. Radiolabeled monoclonal antibodies for imaging and therapy. New York: Plenum, 1988:(75)409–429.

92. Hertler AA, Schlossman DM, Borowitz MJ, Poplack DG, Frankel AE. An immunotoxin for the treatment of T-acute lymphoblastic leukemic meningitis: studies in rhesus monkeys. Cancer Immunol Immunother 1989;28:59–66.

93. Kovacs EJ, Beckner SK, Longo DL, Varesio L, Young HA. Cytokine gene expression during the generation of human lymphokine-activated killer cells: early induction of interleukin 1 beta by interleukin 2. Cancer Res 1989;49:940–944.

94. Adams F, Quesada JR, Gutterman JU. Neuropsychiatric manifestations of human leukocyte inter-

feron therapy in patients with cancer. JAMA 1984; 252:938–941.

95. Smedley H, Katrak M, Sikora K, Wheeler T. Neurological effects of recombinant human interferon. Br Med J 1983;286:262–264.

96. Opp MR, Obal FR, Krueger JM. Effects of alpha-MSH on sleep, behavior, and brain temperature: interactions with IL 1. Am J Physiol 1988;255:R914–R922.

97. Obbens E, Feun LG, Leavens ME, Savaraj N, Stewart DJ, Gutterman JU. Phase 1 clinical trials of intralesional or intraventricular leukocyte interferon for intracranial malignancies. J Neurooncol 1985;3:61–67.

98. Henson RA, Urich H. Carcinomatous meningitis, In: Hanson RA, Urich H, eds. Cancer and the nervous system. Oxford: Blackwell Scientific Publications, 1982:100–119.

99. Wasserstrom WR, Glass JP, Posner JB. Diagnosis and treatment of leptomeningeal metastases from solid tumors: experience with 90 patients. Cancer 1982;49:759–772.

100. Freireich EJ. The clinical pharmacology of new agents related to the treatment of diffuse meningeal carcinomatosis. In: Whitehouse JMA, Kay HEM, eds. CNS complications of malignant disease. Baltimore: University Park Press, 1979:381–389.

101. Heideman RL, Cole DE, Balis F, et al. Phase I and pharmacokinetic evaluation of thiotepa in the cerebrospinal fluid and plasma of pediatric patients: evidence for dose-dependent plasma clearance of thiotepa. Cancer Res 1989;49:736–741.

102. Grygiel JJ, Balis FM, Collins JM, Lester CM, Poplack DG. Pharmacokinetics of tiazofurin in the plasma and cerebrospinal fluid of rhesus monkeys. Cancer Res 1985;45:2037–2039.

103. Zimm S, Ettinger LJ, Holcenberg JS, et al. Phase I and clinical pharmacological study of mercaptopurine administered as a prolonged intravenous infusion. Cancer Res 1985;45:1869–1873.

104. Balis FM, Pizzo PA, Murphy RF, et al. The pharmacokinetics of zidovudine administered by continuous infusion in children. Ann Intern Med 1989; 110:279–285.

105. Kerr IG, Zimm S, Collins JM, O'Neill D, Poplack DG. Effect of intravenous dose and schedule on cerebrospinal fluid pharmacokinetics of 5-fluorouracil in the monkey. Cancer Res 1984;44:4929–4932.

106. Heideman RL, Balis FM, McCully C, Poplack DG. Preclinical pharmacology of arabinosyl-5-azacytidine in nonhuman primates. Cancer Res 1988; 48:4294–4298.

107. Slevin ML, Piall EM, Aherne GW, Harvey VJ, Johnston A, Lister TA. Effect of dose and schedule on pharmacokinetics of high-dose cytosine arabinoside in plasma and cerebrospinal fluid. J Clin Oncol 1983; 1:546–551.

108. Heideman RL, Kelley JA, Packer RJ, et al. A pediatric phase I and pharmacokinetic study of spirohydantoin mustard. Cancer Res 1988;48:2292–2295.

109. Kelley JA, Litterst CL, Roth JS, et al. The disposition and metabolism of 2′,3′-dideoxycytidine, an in vitro inhibitor of human T-lymphotropic virus type III infectivity, in mice and monkeys. Drug Metab Dispos 1987;15:595–601.

110. DeGregorio MW, King OY, Holleran WM, et al. Ultrafiltrate and total platinum in plasma and cerebrospinal fluid in a patient with neuroblastoma. Cancer Treat Rep 1985;69:1441–1442.

111. Hande KR, Wedlund PJ, Noone RM, Wilkinson GR, Greco FA, Wolff SN. Pharmacokinetics of high-dose etoposide (VP-16-213) administered to cancer patients. Cancer Res 1984;44:379–382.

112. Thyss A, Milano G, Deville A, Manassero J, Renee N, Schneider M. Effect of dose and repeat intravenous 24 hr infusions of methotrexate on cerebrospinal fluid availability in children with hematological malignancies. Eur J Cancer Clin Oncol 1987;23:843–847.

113. Collins JM, Riccardi R, Trown P, O'Neill D, Poplack DG. Plasma and cerebrospinal fluid pharmacokinetics of recombinant interferon alpha A in monkeys: comparison of intravenous, intramuscular, and intraventricular delivery. Cancer Drug Deliv 1985; 2:247–253.

114. Zimm S, Collins JM, Curt GA, O'Neill D, Poplack DG. Cerebrospinal fluid pharmacokinetics of intraventricular and intravenous aziridinylbenzoquinone. Cancer Res 1984;44:1698–1701.

115. Levin VA, Byrd D, Campbell J, Davis RL, Borcich JK. CNS toxicity and CSF pharmacokinetics of intraventricular DFMO and MGBG in beagle dogs. Cancer Chemother Pharmacol 1984;13:200–205.

116. Levin VA, Byrd D, Sikic BI, et al. CNS toxicity and CSF pharmacokinetics of intraventricular bleomycin in beagle dogs. Cancer Res 1985;45:3810–3815.

117. Bleyer WA. Clinical pharmacology of intrathecal methotrexate: an improved dosage regimen derived from age-related pharmacokinetics. Cancer Treat Rep 1977;61:1419–1425.

14

Intraperitoneal Chemotherapy

Maurie Markman

The intraperitoneal administration of chemotherapeutic agents has evolved over the past 15 years from a pharmacologic concept to a procedure used by physicians in clinical practice. This chapter reviews the basic principles supporting the intraperitoneal delivery of antineoplastic agents, practical issues raised by the use of this technique, and results of single-agent and combination intraperitoneal chemotherapy trials in ovarian carcinoma, peritoneal mesothelioma, and gastrointestinal malignancies.

PRINCIPLES OF INTRAPERITONEAL CHEMOTHERAPY

The fundamental goal of the intraperitoneal administration of antineoplastic agents is to expose tumor present in the cavity to higher concentrations of drug for longer periods of time than can *safely* be accomplished following systemic drug delivery. Increased exposure is measured by demonstrating both higher peak levels and AUCs (area under the concentration versus time curve) in the *cavity* following intraperitoneal delivery, compared with those observed in the systemic circulation. Extensive preclinical evaluation has defined a number of characteristics considered important in optimizing any advantage associated with intraperitoneal drug delivery (Table 14.1) (1).

An important consideration in selecting drugs for intraperitoneal therapy of a previously treated tumor (e.g., small-volume residual ovarian carcinoma following systemically delivered cisplatin) is whether or not there is evidence of absolute, or only relative, resistance of the tumor to the agents in question. If the resistance that develops in tumors exposed to concentrations of drug achieved with systemic drug delivery can be overcome by exposing the tumor to the higher concentrations of the agent attainable following

intraperitoneal delivery, then there is a strong rationale for employing the *same* drug(s) administered by the intraperitoneal route following a major (but incomplete) response to the agent delivered intravenously.

This is the principal justification for the use of intraperitoneal cisplatin-based therapy in small-volume residual ovarian carcinoma following systemic treatment with this same agent. Under experimental conditions, it is difficult to induce more than a two- to fivefold resistance in ovarian carcinoma cell lines (2). With intraperitoneal delivery of this agent, concentrations achieved in the peritoneal cavity are 10 to 20 times higher than that observed following systemic drug administration (1, 3, 4). Thus, on the basis of these observations, responses of persistent or recurrent ovarian carcinoma to intraperitoneal cisplatin would be predicted to occur in patients who had previously demonstrated activity for the agent delivered systemically.

When antineoplastic agents are administered by the intravenous route, they reach the tumor by *capillary flow*. Any *advantage* for intraperitoneal treatment over that achieved with systemic drug delivery will be secondary to the direct *free surface diffusion* of the drug from the peritoneal surface into tumor. This is perhaps the major concern with the use of intraperitoneal therapy, because in general, the depth of penetration of chemotherapeutic agents into tumor tissue is extremely limited (1 to 3 mm). Thus, it is highly likely that if intraperitoneal treatment is to be shown to be superior to systemic drug administration, it will be in clinical situations in which only very small tumor nodules (<0.5 cm) or microscopic disease is present when intraperitoneal therapy is initiated.

Finally, there are several practical considerations involved in the potential use of intraperitoneal treatments. A number of investigators

Table 14.1. Desired Characteristics of Drugs Considered for Intraperitoneal Chemotherapy

1. No local toxicity to the peritoneum
2. Rapid metabolism to nontoxic metabolite during first passage through the liver, resulting in a major pharmacokinetic advantage for intraperitoneal administration, as drug uptake from the cavity is principally via the portal circulation
3. Slow exit from the peritoneal cavity
4. Rapid clearance from the systemic circulation
5. Clinical activity for the drug against the tumor
6. Experimental evidence of *concentration-dependent* cytotoxicity for the drug against the tumor
7. Experimental evidence of *concentration-dependent synergy* between the drugs against the tumor (for combination regimens)

have demonstrated both the safety and convenience of using surgically implanted, semipermanent, indwelling catheters through which the treatments are administered (5, 6). While percutaneous catheter placement with each treatment course may be used, there is legitimate concern that the bowel may be punctured during catheter insertion in patients without ascites and in individuals who have previously undergone one or more laparotomies with subsequent adhesion formation (7, 8).

In contrast to intravenous or intraarterial drug administration, where it can be assumed that blood flow will deliver the antineoplastic agent to the tumor following administration, use of large treatment volumes (≥ 2 L) is critical with intraperitoneal therapy, to optimize drug distribution (1). Unfortunately, even with the use of such volumes, there will always be portions of the peritoneal cavity which are not adequately bathed by the drug-containing fluid. Contrast CT scans and nuclear medicine scans may assist in identifying patients who cannot be treated by the intraperitoneal route because of mechanical difficulties encountered with intraperitoneal administration that prevent the high concentrations of drug present in the cavity from coming into direct contact with tumor. Such patients will need to be treated by alternative therapeutic strategies.

SINGLE AGENTS DELIVERED BY THE INTRAPERITONEAL ROUTE

A number of chemotherapeutic agents have been delivered by the intraperitoneal route in phase I trials designed to define the toxicity and pharmacokinetics associated with this route of

drug delivery. Table 14.2 outlines the pharmacokinetic advantage of intraperitoneal administration of selected agents (1). The results of trials involving several drugs of particular clinical interest are briefly summarized below.

Cisplatin and Carboplatin

As it is the single most important drug in the treatment of ovarian carcinoma, it is appropriate that considerable effort has been directed toward exploring the potential for cisplatin delivered by the intraperitoneal route. Several conclusions can be drawn from a review of a number of intraperitoneal cisplatin programs reported in the medical literature. First, following intraperitoneal delivery, the peritoneal cavity is exposed to concentrations of drug (peak and AUC levels) that are between 10 to 20 times higher than those in the systemic circulation (1, 3, 4). Second, there is little or no abdominal discomfort associated with intraperitoneal cisplatin delivery. This allows an escalation in intraperitoneal cisplatin dosage to *maximize* systemic delivery of the drug following intraperitoneal administration. Dose-limiting toxicity of intraperitoneal cisplatin will be the systemic side effects of the cytotoxic agent.

Third, the results of both single-agent and combination cisplatin-based intraperitoneal therapy, when delivered in the salvage setting to patients with ovarian cancer, have confirmed that patients can achieve surgically documented responses, including complete responses, through the use of this therapeutic strategy (9). A more critical examination of patients entered

Table 14.2. Pharmacokinetic Advantage Associated with Intraperitoneal Administration of Selected Chemotherapeutic Agents

Drug	Mean Peak Peritoneal Cavity/Plasma Concentration Ratio	Mean Peritoneal Cavity/Plasma AUC Ratio
Cisplatin	20	12
Carboplatin	18	—[a]
5-FU	298	376
Doxorubicin	474	—
Mitoxantrone	620	1408
Melphalan	93	65
Methotrexate	92	—
Cytarabine	664	474
Mitomycin C	71	—

[a]Not reported.

into these trials reveals two important factors that appear to define those individuals most likely to achieve benefit from the use of this approach (9).

Approximately 20 to 25% of ovarian cancer patients with microscopic disease only or those whose largest residual tumor nodules measure 0.5 cm or less in maximum diameter at the initiation of intraperitoneal therapy achieve a surgically documented complete response following second-line cisplatin-based therapy (9). However, as suggested by the preclinical data previously noted concerning the direct depth of penetration of cytotoxic agents into tissue (10–12), the complete response rate for patients with any nodule larger than 1 cm is less than 10% (9).

A second important factor influencing the chances for a favorable response is previous evidence of sensitivity to systemically administered platinum agents. Patients with small-volume disease when salvage therapy is initiated who have failed to respond to initial systemic platinum-based chemotherapy also experience a surgically documented response rate below 10% (9). In contrast, in individuals who have responded to front-line chemotherapy who also have small-volume disease at the initiation of salvage intraperitoneal cisplatin, the surgically documented complete response rate is approximately 30 to 35%.

Intraperitoneal cisplatin also appears to be of clinical utility in a subset of patients with peritoneal mesothelioma (13–15). While surgical assessment of responses in this disease setting is far more limited than that noted above in ovarian carcinoma, reduction in malignant ascites formation has been dramatic in many patients treated with intraperitoneal cisplatin. While responses may be of limited duration, some have persisted for longer than 2 to 3 years.

Investigators at the University of California, San Diego, have explored the use of intraperitoneal cisplatin along with the simultaneous intravenous administration of sodium thiosulfate, an agent demonstrated to protect against the nephrotoxic effects of cisplatin (3, 16). Using this approach, intraperitoneal cisplatin dosing has been escalated to 200 mg/m^2 with acceptable local and systemic toxicities. While clinical activity has been observed in both refractory ovarian carcinoma and peritoneal mesothelioma, it remains uncertain whether the responses observed are greater in number and of longer duration than those achieved with lower-dose intraperitoneal cisplatin without thiosulfate.

Carboplatin has been less extensively studied when administered by the intraperitoneal route than cisplatin. However, it has been shown that following intraperitoneal delivery, the drug has pharmacokinetic properties remarkably similar to those of cisplatin (1). Carboplatin is not locally toxic, and bone marrow suppression (principally thrombocytopenia) appears to be the dose-limiting side effect.

5-Fluorouracil (5-FU)

5-FU has been examined for intraperitoneal use in a number of trials, and as predicted on the basis of the known metabolic pathway of this agent, a major pharmacokinetic advantage for its administration by the intraperitoneal route has been demonstrated (17). The toxicity associated with intraperitoneal 5-FU delivery is both systemic and local (abdominal pain and adhesion formation). In general, local toxicity becomes the major side effect following several courses of treatment. A phase II trial of intraperitoneal 5-FU in ovarian carcinoma failed to show significant activity, but most patients treated in this program had previously received intravenous 5-FU (18). A phase III randomized trial comparing intraperitoneal 5-FU with intravenous 5-FU as adjuvant therapy in patients with colon carcinoma failed to reveal a survival advantage for intraperitoneal drug delivery (19). However, there was a statistically significant decrease in surgically defined peritoneal cavity recurrences in the group receiving intraperitoneal 5-FU. This would suggest that the high concentrations of drug achieved in the peritoneal cavity were effective in treating microscopic disease in that compartment, but the much lower drug delivery to the systemic circulation was ineffective therapy.

Doxorubicin and Mitoxantrone

Experimental observations have suggested that the activity of both doxorubicin and mitoxantrone against ovarian carcinoma might be substantially enhanced at the concentrations of the drugs achievable in the peritoneal cavity following intraperitoneal drug delivery (5, 20, 21). Unfortunately, despite a 2- to 3-log increased exposure of the peritoneal cavity to the two agents following intraperitoneal administration, dose-limiting toxicity is the development of significant abdominal pain and adhesion formation (1, 22).

Intraperitoneal mitoxantrone appears to cause less local toxicity than intraperitoneal doxorubicin (when dose levels corresponding to the relative concentrations used for systemic drug administration are compared). While the experience using intraperitoneal mitoxantrone in persistent ovarian carcinoma remains limited, surgically defined responses were observed in several phase I/II trials employing intraperitoneal mitoxantrone in this clinical setting (23–25). Of interest, responses to intraperitoneal mitoxantrone have been noted in patients previously treated with systemically delivered doxorubicin (24).

Melphalan

In several phase I trials, melphalan has been shown to be well tolerated when delivered by the intraperitoneal route (1, 26). Dose-limiting toxicity is bone marrow suppression. A moderate pharmacokinetic advantage for this route of drug delivery has been demonstrated. As melphalan does not require activation in the liver to become an active cytotoxic agent, it could be used in place of cyclophosphamide along with cisplatin in a combination intraperitoneal program in ovarian carcinoma (27).

INITIAL CHEMOTHERAPY OF OVARIAN CANCER

The first randomized trial examining a possible role for intraperitoneal therapy in the management of ovarian cancer has recently been reported (28). In this study, more than 600 patients with "small-volume" (largest residual tumor mass ≤2 cm) residual disease following staging/debulking surgery were randomized to receive six courses of intravenous cyclophosphamide (600 mg/m^2) plus either intravenous cisplatin *or* intraperitoneal cisplatin (both delivered at 100 mg/m^2). With a median follow-up for living patients of almost 4 years, survival was significantly longer for patients receiving the intraperitoneal treatment strategy ($p = .03$). In addition, there was less clinical hearing loss and neutropenia in the intraperitoneal treatment arm.

INTRAPERITONEAL CHEMOTHERAPY FOR GASTROINTESTINAL MALIGNANCIES

Several groups have begun to explore the potential for combination intraperitoneal therapy in patients with gastrointestinal malignancies. Combinations under evaluation include cisplatin–5-FU (29), 5-FU–leucovorin (30), and floxuridine (FUDR)-leucovorin (31). In general, combination regimens have been selected for testing by the intraperitoneal route on the basis of suggested efficacy following systemic drug administration. It is hoped that the higher concentrations of drugs present in the peritoneal cavity will result in higher response rates and improved survival for a subgroup of patients with a variety of gastrointestinal malignancies. Randomized trials will be required to address this important issue.

CONCLUSION

While intraperitoneal therapy can no longer be considered a highly experimental approach, especially in the management of ovarian carcinoma, a precise role for this technique in the standard treatment of any malignancy remains to be defined. Both theoretic considerations and increasing clinical experience strongly suggest that any advantage of this therapeutic strategy will be limited to those situations in which very small volume disease is present in the peritoneal cavity when treatment is initiated. Such clinical situations might include:

1. Treatment of patients with high-grade ovarian carcinoma who experience a surgically defined complete response, but where the risk of ultimate relapse approaches 50 to 60% (32, 33).
2. Treatment of patients with microscopic or very small volume residual ovarian carcinoma following systemically delivered therapy.
3. Initial treatment of patients with ovarian carcinoma who have only very small volume disease remaining following surgical debulking.
4. Treatment of patients with ovarian carcinoma following a *limited* exposure to systemically delivered drugs administered to further "debulk" the tumor.
5. Adjuvant therapy of patients with gastrointestinal malignancies where there is a great risk of relapse in the peritoneal cavity following primary curative surgical resection (e.g., gastric cancer).
6. Treatment of patients with gastrointestinal malignancies with small-volume intraperitoneal disease, either before or after surgical debulking.
7. Treatment of patients with peritoneal mesothelioma following a successful attempt at surgical debulking (to small-volume residual disease).

REFERENCES

1. Markman M. Intraperitoneal therapy for treatment of malignant disease principally confined to the peritoneal cavity. Crit Rev Oncol Hematol 1993;14:15–28.

2. Ozols RF, Corden BJ, Jacob J, Wesley MN, Ostchega Y, Young RC. High-dose cisplatin in hypertonic saline. Ann Intern Med 1984;100:19–24.

3. Howell SB, Pfeifle CL, Wung WE, et al. Intraperitoneal cisplatin with systemic thiosulfate protection. Ann Intern Med 1982;97:845–851.

4. Casper ES, Kelsen DP, Alcock NW, Lewis JL Jr. Ip cisplatin in patients with malignant ascites: pharmacokinetic evaluation and comparison with the iv route. Cancer Treat Rep 1983;67:235–238.

5. Piccart MJ, Speyer JL, Markman M, et al. Intraperitoneal chemotherapy: technical experience at five institutions. Semin Oncol 1985;12(3)(Suppl 4):90–96.

6. Pfeifle CE, Howell SE, Markman M, Lucas WE. Totally implantable system for peritoneal access. J Clin Oncol 1984;2:1277–1280.

7. Runowicz CE, Dottino PR, Shafir MK, Mark MA, Cohen CJ. Catheter complications associated with intraperitoneal chemotherapy. Gynecol Oncol 1986; 24:41–50.

8. Kaplan RA, Markman M, Lucas WE, Pfeifle CE, Howell SB. Infectious peritonitis in patients receiving intraperitoneal chemotherapy. Am J Med 1985;78:49–53.

9. Markman M, Reichman B, Hakes T, et al. Responses to second-line cisplatin-based intraperitoneal therapy in ovarian cancer: influence of a prior response to intravenous cisplatin. J Clin Oncol 1991;9:1801.

10. Ozols RF, Locker GY, Doroshow JH, et al. Pharmacokinetics of Adriamycin and tissue penetration in murine ovarian cancer. Cancer Res 1979;39:3209.

11. Nederman T, Carlsson J. Penetration and binding of vinblastine and 5-fluorouracil in cellular spheroids. Cancer Chemother Pharmacol 1984;13:131.

12. Los G, Mutsaers PHA, van der Vijgh WJF, et al. Direct diffusion of cis-diamminedichloroplatinum(II) in intraperitoneal rat tumors after intraperitoneal chemotherapy: a comparison with systemic chemotherapy. Cancer Res 1989;49:3380.

13. Markman M, Cleary S, Pfeifle C, et al. Cisplatin administered by the intracavitary route as treatment for malignant mesothelioma. Cancer 1986;58:18–21.

14. Markman M, Kelsen D. Intraperitoneal cisplatin and mitomycin as treatment of malignant peritoneal mesothelioma. Regional Cancer Treat 1989; 2(1):49–53.

15. Markman M, Kelsen D. Efficacy of cisplatin-based intraperitoneal chemotherapy as treatment of malignant peritoneal mesothelioma. J Cancer Res Clin Oncol 1992;118:547–550.

16. Howell SB, Zimm S, Markman M, et al. Long term survival of advanced refractory ovarian carcinoma patients with small-volume disease treated with intraperitoneal chemotherapy. J Clin Oncol 1987;5:689–695.

17. Speyer JL, Collins JM, Dedrick RL, et al. Phase 1 pharmacological studies of 5-fluorouracil administered intraperitoneally. Cancer Res 1980;40:567–572.

18. Ozols RF, Speyer JL, Jenkins J, Myers CE. Phase II trial of 5-FU administered Ip to patients with refractory ovarian cancer. Cancer Treat Rep 1984;68:1229–1232.

19. Sugarbaker PH, Gianola FJ, Speyer JC, Wesley R, Barofsky I, Myers CE. Prospective randomized trial of intravenous vs intraperitoneal 5-FU in patients with advanced primary colon or rectal cancer. Surgery 1985; 98:414–421.

20. Ozols RF, Grotzinger KR, Fisher RI, Myers CE, Young RC. Kinetic characterization and response to chemotherapy in a transplantable murine ovarian cancer. Cancer Res 1979;39:3202–3208.

21. Alberts DS, Young L, Mason N, Salmon SE. In vitro evaluation of anticancer drugs against ovarian cancer at concentrations achievable by intraperitoneal administration. Semin Oncol 1985;12(3)(Suppl 4):38–42.

22. Ozols RF, Young RC, Speyer JL, et al. Phase 1 and pharmacological studies of Adriamycin administered intraperitoneally to patients with ovarian cancer. Cancer Res 1982;42:4265–4269.

23. Alberts DS, Surwit EA, Peng YM, et al. Phase I clinical and pharmacokinetic study of mitoxantrone given to patients by intraperitoneal administration. Cancer Res 1988;48:5874–5877.

24. Markman M, George M, Hakes T, et al. Phase 2 trial of intraperitoneal mitoxantrone in the management of refractory ovarian carcinoma. J Clin Oncol 1990;8:146–150.

25. Markman M, Hakes T, Reichman B, et al. Phase 2 trial of weekly or biweekly intraperitoneal mitoxantrone in epithelial ovarian cancer. J Clin Oncol 1991; 9:978.

26. Howel SB, Pfeifle CE, Olshen RA. Intraperitoneal chemotherapy with melphalan. Ann Intern Med 1984;101:14–18.

27. Piccart MJ, Abrams J, Dodion PF, et al. Intraperitoneal chemotherapy with cisplatin and melphalan. J Natl Cancer Inst 1988;80:1118–1124.

28. Alberts DS, Liu PY, Hannigan EV, et al. Phase III study of intraperitoneal cisplatin/intravenous cyclophosphamide vs intravenous cisplatin/intravenous cyclophosphamide in patients with optimal disease stage III ovarian cancer: a SWOG-GOG-ECOG Intergroup Study (INT 0051) (abstract 760). Proc Am Soc Clin Oncol 1995;14:273.

29. Reichman B, Markman M, Hakes T, et al. Phase 1 trial of continuous intravenous infusion and intraperitoneal 5-fluorouracil and intraperitoneal cisplatin (abstract). Proc Am Soc Clin Oncol 1988;7:266.

30. Arbuck SG, Trave F, Douglass HO, Nava H, Zakrzewski S, Rustum YM. Phase 1 and pharmacologic studies of intraperitoneal leucovorin and 5-fluorouracil in patients with advanced cancer. J Clin Oncol 1986;4:1510–1517.

31. Smith JA, Markman M, Kelsen D, et al. Phase I study of intraperitoneal FUDR and leucovorin (abstract). Proc Am Soc Clin Oncol 1989;8:67.

32. Copeland LJ, Gershenson DM. Ovarian cancer recurrences in patients with no macroscopic tumor at second-look laparotomy. Obstet Gynecol 1986;68:873–874.

33. Rubin SC, Hoskins WJ, Saigo PE, et al. Prognostic factors for recurrence following negative second-look laparotomy in ovarian cancer patients treated with platinum-based chemotherapy. Gynecol Oncol 1991;42:137–141.

15

Continuous Intravenous Infusion Chemotherapy

Robert W. Carlson

The selection of an optimal dose and schedule of administration for cancer chemotherapeutic agents is particularly important as their therapeutic index is usually low. Multiple schedules for intravenous administration, including intermittent or frequent bolus infusions and continuous infusions, have been investigated in attempts to identify the optimal schedule of administration for many cancer chemotherapeutics.

Considerable interest and research into the value of continuous intravenous infusion chemotherapy has been generated by the availability of safe, reliable ambulatory chemotherapy infusion pumps (1–3). These studies have provided compelling clinical evidence that the toxicity of selected chemotherapeutic agents is decreased by the use of continuous infusion chemotherapy without loss of antitumor efficacy. In contrast, there is little clinical evidence documenting improvement in antitumor activity when chemotherapy is delivered by continuous intravenous infusion; in part this may be related to the paucity of prospective, randomized clinical trials comparing schedules of administration.

The use of continuous infusion therapy requires chronic venous access, a continuous infusion pump, and an appropriate drug reservoir and drug vehicle. Not all agents may be compatible for simultaneous mixture or infusion; potentially, therefore, multiple pump and multiple venous access channels may be required for combination therapy. All of these factors support the need for a sophisticated, committed health care team and patient/patient family for the successful application of the technology necessary to utilize continuous infusion chemotherapy.

The expense associated with continuous in-fusion therapy may be substantial, even in the ambulatory setting. Expenses not normally associated with bolus chemotherapy include the requirement for chronic venous access, a reliable pump apparatus, and replacement tubing or refill equipment.

In this chapter, the preclinical rationale for delivering selected chemotherapeutic agents by continuous infusion and representative clinical studies is reviewed. Unfortunately, few prospective, randomized clinical trials have been reported, so definitive conclusions regarding the role of continuous intravenous infusion cannot yet be made.

RATIONALE

Substantial preclinical rationale and evidence predicts that continuous infusion chemotherapy will provide superior antitumor activity compared with conventional single-bolus or intermittent bolus infusion chemotherapy. Most chemotherapeutic agents are either most effective against cycling cells or only effective then. Since only a fraction of a tumor cell population is actively cycling at any given time, prolonged infusion may expose a relatively larger proportion of the tumor cells to the cytotoxic agent as resting cells are recruited into the actively cycling pool. Further, the mechanism of action of many chemotherapeutic agents is restricted to a specific portion of the cell cycle. Thus, even actively cycling cells may be shielded from the cytotoxic agent if exposure occurs during a nonsensitive portion of the cell cycle.

In addition to cytokinetic factors that predict relative resistance to chemotherapeutic agents, the pharmacokinetics of most chemotherapeutic agents also predict limited cytotoxicity with intermittent bolus infusion. Most chemotherapeutic agents have short plasma half-lives. Bolus infusion thus provides effective drug exposure for short periods of time for most chemotherapeutic agents. With cell cycle phase–specific agents, bolus infusion results in a fraction of even the cycling proportion of cells being exposed to the agent during the sensitive portion of the cell cycle. Tumors with a small fraction of actively cycling cells or with a long cell-cycling time are predicted to be relatively resistant to intermittent bolus infusions of an agent with a short half-life; frequent bolus injections or continuous infusion chemotherapy would be predicted to have substantially greater antitumor efficacy.

The uptake of some cytotoxic agents may be a saturable process. Exposure of tumor cells for a prolonged time may thus increase the intracellular level of drug achieved in tumor cells. Rates of influx and efflux of cytotoxic agents may differ substantially between normal and malignant cells, and there may be substantial differences in the sensitivity of normal versus malignant cells to given levels of drug exposure. These factors predict that the potential enhancement of antitumor activity by continuous infusion may not be accompanied by commensurate enhancement of toxicity.

The antitumor efficacy of some chemotherapeutic agents appears to be related to delivered dose intensity. Because of diminished toxicity, some chemotherapeutic agents, such as 5-fluorouracil, may be given in more dose-intense schedules if delivered by continuous infusion. However, measured dose intensity between differing schedules of administration may not relate to antitumor activity.

In contrast, some theoretic or practical considerations predict that continuous infusion chemotherapy may be inferior to conventional bolus infusion. The measured plasma half-lives of chemotherapeutic agents assess the availability of drug for cellular uptake only. The most important component of drug half-life is the intracellular drug half-life. For most agents, the intracellular drug half-life is complex or unknown and likely varies significantly by patient and tumor type. How intracellular drug concentration is affected clinically by the schedule of administration for most agents is not known. In preclinical systems, exposure of cell cultures to low levels of many cytotoxic agents results in the development of acquired drug resistance, includ-

Table 15.1. Characteristics Predicting Superiority of Continuous Infusion Chemotherapy

Chemotherapeutic agent
  Phase specific
  Short half-life
  Reversible action
  Small volume of distribution
  Stable formulation
  Soluble in small volumes
  Time-dependent cellular uptake or tissue penetration
  Toxicity related to peak serum concentration
Patient
  Reliable central venous access
  Acceptable end organ function
Tumor
  Low growth fraction
  Slow drug uptake
  Rapid cellular excretion of drug

ing the multidrug resistance phenomenon. It is thus possible that the use of continuous infusion delivery may accelerate the emergence of resistant tumor cell subpopulations and diminish the effectiveness of some chemotherapeutic agents.

Characteristics of chemotherapeutic agents, patients, and tumors that predict favorable use of continuous infusion chemotherapy are provided in Table 15.1.

VENOUS ACCESS

The use of continuous intravenous infusion chemotherapy requires reliable, safe, long-term venous access. Many such venous access devices are currently available, including conventional peripheral intravenous catheters, subcutaneous tunneled silastic catheters (e.g., Hickman and Groshong catheters), and totally implantable subcutaneous access ports (e.g., Mediport, Portacath) (see Chapter 45). The subcutaneously tunneled and totally implantable access ports have the advantage of central venous delivery.

Central venous delivery is particularly important with continuous infusion of vesicants such as anthracyclines, vinca alkaloids, and mitomycin C. Despite the use of central venous catheters, occasional episodes of extravasation will nonetheless occur, because of the development of a fibrin sheath around the intravascular portion of the catheter with backtracking of the infusate, fracture or perforation of the subcutaneous portion of the catheter, or technical difficulties in accessing or maintaining access of subcutaneous infusion ports.

Some nonvesicant drugs, notably the fluoropyrimidines, cause a chemical phlebitis that may be severe when infusion is via low-flow, peripheral veins. Selected other agents, such as bleomycin and cytarabine, may be safely administered by continuous infusion via conventional peripheral catheter; indeed, these agents may be safely administered by continuous subcutaneous infusion.

The selection of a venous access device is based upon considerations of the chemotherapeutic agents to be infused, anticipated duration of infusion, willingness of patient and family to participate in catheter care, experience of the health care delivery team, and the rates of complications associated with each catheter type (see Chapter 45).

INFUSION PUMPS

Infusion pumps to deliver and control continuous infusions in the inpatient setting have existed for many years. Recently, infusion pumps for delivering and controlling ambulatory continuous intravenous infusion have become widely available. These infusion pumps include battery-driven syringe and peristaltic pumps, elastomeric balloon pumps, and implantable volatile liquid/vapor-powered pumps (Table 15.2)

(4). The ambulatory infusion pumps allow the delivery of continuous infusion chemotherapy on an outpatient basis with resulting cost savings and improved psychologic adjustment of the patient (5, 6).

The battery-powered pumps are the most versatile of the pumps and allow for wide ranges of reservoir size and infusion rate. The battery-powered pumps are, however, heavy and relatively complex to use. Flow-rate accuracy is usually excellent at flow rates of 5 mL/hr or greater but may be highly variable at rates of 1 mL/hr or less (7). The battery-powered pumps can be used for periods in excess of 48 hours without battery changes or recharging.

Alarm systems available on some pumps include low battery, high pressure, low volume, and system malfunction. Some of these pumps also generate significant background noise. Each individual pump may be utilized for many different patients, reducing the per patient cost of the pumps themselves. Nonreusable tubing for the peristaltic pumps or extension tubing for the syringe pumps is necessary for each patient.

Totally implantable pumps for intravenous infusion may have either fixed rates of infusion (e.g., Infusaid pump) or programable infusion rates (e.g., SynchroMed pump). These pumps are convenient and reliable, although they are each usable for only a single patient, are expensive, and require surgical implantation.

Table 15.2. Representative Ambulatory Infusion Pumps

Pump	Usable Reservoir Volume (mL)	Infusion rate (mL/hr)	Energy Source	Mechanism	Weight (g)
Bard Med Systems					
Ambulatory pump	1–250	0–20	Battery	Peristaltic	330
Provider 5500	External i.v. bag, any size	0.1–250	Battery	Peristaltic	400
Baxtor Healthcare					
Autosyringe					
AS20S	1–52	0.05–84.6	Battery	Syringe	680
AS2F	1–44	0.04–88.0	Battery	Syringe	550
Infusor	48	2 (fixed)	Elastomeric balloon	Elastomer balloon	35
Infusaid 400	47	0.04–0.25 (preset and fixed)	Volatile liquid/vapor	Totally implantable	275
Medtronic					
SynchroMed	18	0.025–0.9	Battery	Peristaltic, totally implantable	185

The elastomeric balloon pumps have a fixed and limited reservoir size and single, manufacturer-fixed infusion rate. These pumps are very simple to use, are light, produce no noise, and have a high degree of patient satisfaction. While each individual pump is relatively low-cost, each pump is disposed of following a single use; long-term use of these pumps for infusion therapy may therefore be relatively more expensive than other available devices.

Each of the available infusion pumps requires careful monitoring by a trained and experienced medical team. The selection of an infusion pump for an individual patient should include considerations of the agent to be infused, the anticipated duration of the infusional therapy, ability of the patient and family to participate in the monitoring of pump function, cost, and the expertise of the medical team.

CYTARABINE

The prototypic chemotherapeutic agent demonstrating strong schedule-dependent cytotoxicity is cytarabine. Numerous preclinical and clinical studies have demonstrated the schedule dependence of cytarabine's antitumor efficacy and toxicity. Cytarabine requires intracellular metabolic activation to arabinose-cytidine triphosphate (ara-CTP). ara-CTP exerts its cytotoxicity by fraudulent incorporation into DNA and by competitive inhibition of DNA polymerase and is highly S-phase specific. Cytarabine undergoes rapid in vivo deamination with a biphasic plasma disappearance curve with a $t_{1/2}$-α of 7 to 12 minutes and a $t_{1/2}$-β of 110 to 160 minutes (8). The S-phase specificity of cytarabine plus its rapid plasma disappearance predict schedule-dependent cytotoxicity.

Early experiments with L1210 leukemia in cell culture and in mice demonstrated that multiple frequent doses or continuous exposure to cytarabine had greater antitumor efficacy and toxicity than infrequent doses or short exposures and that schedule was more important than drug concentration (9–11). Recent evidence suggests that cytarabine uptake in human leukemia cells is a low-affinity, high-capacity process and that the duration and level of drug exposure may be limiting in intracellular drug accumulation (12). This suggests that prolonged exposure to high drug concentrations should optimize the antileukemic effects of cytarabine.

Doses of cytarabine 100 to 200 mg/m^2 every 12 hours by bolus injection or by continuous infusion for 5 to 7 days are widely used in the treatment of acute myelogenous leukemia. In attempts to overcome cytarabine resistance, higher doses have been used both in acute leukemia and in solid tumors (12). Recent evidence suggesting that low-dose cytarabine may induce differentiation has also led to the study of low-dose continuous infusion (13). Thus, both drug dose (concentration) and drug schedule (time of exposure) appear to be important considerations with cytarabine.

In a study that compared the toxicity of escalating doses of cytarabine given by continuous infusion or by single daily bolus injections for 5 days, continuous infusion produced greater myelosuppression than bolus injection at doses of 50 to 100 mg/m^2/day (14). Escalating from doses of 150 to 300 mg/m^2/day did not increase the myelosuppression with continuous infusion, and the myelosuppression was equivalent to that observed with daily bolus therapy at the same doses. Nonhematologic toxicity included anorexia with continuous infusion and mild nausea and vomiting with bolus injections.

Single bolus infusions of cytarabine with doses up to 4200 mg/m^2 produce no myelosuppression (15). Continuous infusions for 48 to 96 hours have similar and steep dose-response curves, with dose-limiting myelosuppression at 800 to 1000 mg/m^2. Shortening the infusion to 24 hours produces myelosuppression, beginning at doses of 600 mg/m^2 and increasing to doses of 1500 mg/m^2, above which no additional myelosuppression occurs.

With cytarabine administered as a 7-day continuous infusion, myelosuppression is not observed until a dose of 30 mg/m^2/day is reached (16). When the same total dose is administered as a 3.5-day continuous infusion, similar myelosuppression is observed; shorter infusion times were not associated with hematologic toxicity.

In a study of high-dose cytarabine 250 mg/m^2/hour (6 g/m^2/day) by continuous intravenous infusions of up to 24 hours, myelosuppression, usually thrombopenia, was found to be dose limiting (17). Nonmyelosuppressive toxicity consisted primarily of nausea and vomiting and was usually mild. Plasma levels of cytarabine (9 to 59 μM) of approximately 10- to 100-fold higher than that with standard-dose infusions were achieved. Others, using high-dose cytarabine by 36- to 72-hour continuous infusion, found the maximally tolerated dose to be 2 g/m^2/day (18, 19). Dose-limiting toxicities involved multiple organ systems including gastrointestinal tract, liver, kidney, and lung.

The plasma levels of cytarabine achieved with continuous subcutaneous infusion cytarabine have been studied in children and adults and are similar to those achieved by continuous intravenous infusion (20–22).

The preclinical schedule-dependent antitumor activity of cytarabine in the treatment of leukemia has led to a number of clinical studies. In an early study of 36 evaluable patients with acute leukemia treated with single-agent cytarabine 200 mg/m²/day, a 25% complete response and 11% partial response rate was observed. Myelosuppression, nausea, vomiting, and weight loss were observed in most patients (23).

The Southwest Oncology Group randomized 164 evaluable patients with acute leukemia to treatment with single-agent cytarabine 800 mg/m² by 48-hour continuous infusion or to 1000 mg/m² by 120-hour continuous infusion (24). The 120-hour continuous infusion regimen was superior in rate of complete response (38%), compared with 48-hour infusion (20%) ($p < .025$). The delivered dose intensities of the two regimens were remarkably similar, suggesting that the schedule of administration was more important than dose in the improvement in rate of complete response.

A study of 101 patients with previously untreated acute myelogenous leukemia compared cytarabine 200 mg/m²/day by continuous infusion for 7 days with cytarabine 500 mg/m² by 2-hour infusion every 12 hours for 6 days, both with daunorubicin 60 mg/m²/day for 3 days (25). No significant differences were observed in rates of complete response, number of induction courses to achieve remission duration, survival, or toxicity. However, the small number of patients in this study limits the power to detect potentially important differences between the treatment arms.

The Cancer and Leukemia Group B (CALGB) has studied cytarabine for 5 or 7 days by bolus versus continuous infusion in combination with daunorubicin in the treatment of acute myelogenous leukemia (Table 15.3) (26). Rates of complete response in both patients under 60 years of age and those 60 years of age and older were higher with the regimens including 7 days of cytarabine and were highest with the regimen using continuous infusion cytarabine.

Multivariate analysis of factors predicting complete response found the regimens using 7 days of cytarabine plus 3 days of daunorubicin to be superior to the regimens using 5 days of cytarabine plus 2 days of daunorubicin $p < .01$). Although the rates of complete response were higher with 7-day continuous infusion than with 7-day bolus injection cytarabine, the difference was not statistically significant.

Further study by the CALGB of 596 patients with acute myelogenous leukemia who had achieved complete remission following initial induction with daunorubicin and 7-day continuous infusion cytarabine assessed the importance of cytarabine dose and schedule in postremission therapy (27). Patients in complete remission were randomized to chemotherapy with single-agent cytarabine 100 mg/m²/day by 5-day continuous infusion, 400 mg/m²/day by 5-day continuous infusion, or 3 g/m² as a 3-hour infusion

Table 15.3. Cancer and Leukemia Group B Study of Dose and Schedule Effects of Cytarabine and Daunorubicin in the Treatment of Acute Myelogenous Leukemia

Induction Regimen	Age in Years	Complete Responses (%)
Cytarabine 100 mg/m² daily by continuous infusion × 7 days	<60	59
Daunorubicin 45 mg/m² daily × 3 days	≥60	45
Cytarabine 100 mg/m² every 12 hours × 7 days	<60	51
Daunorubicin 45 mg/m² daily × 3 days	≥60	38
Cytarabine 100 mg/m² daily by continuous infusion × 5 days	<60	45
Daunorubicin 45 mg/m² daily × 2 days	≥60	20
Cytarabine 100 mg/m² every 12 hours × 5 days	<60	39
Daunorubicin 45 mg/m² daily × 2 days	≥60	11

Data from Schiller J, Gajewski J, Nimer S, et al. A randomized study of intermediate versus conventional-dose cytarabine as intensive induction for acute myelogenous leukaemia. Br J Haematol 1992;81:170–177.

every 12 hours on days 1, 3, and 5. The disease-free survival rates were significantly different, with 4-year disease-free survival of 39% in the 3-g group, 25% in the 400-mg group, and 21% in the 100-mg group. The hazard ratios for relapse were not significantly different between the 400-mg and 3-g treatment groups. Survival rates were also different among the treatment groups, with 4-year survival of 46% in the 3-g group, 35% in the 400-mg group, and 34% in the 100-mg group. The higher dose regimens also had increased rates of toxicity. Hospitalization was required in 71% of the treatment courses in the 3-g group, 59% in the 400-mg group, and 16% of the 100-mg group. Serious central nervous system toxicity was observed in 12% of the patients in the 3-g group but in none of the other two treatment groups. This study suggests that increased doses of cytarabine postremission therapy result in improvement in disease-free and overall survival but with a substantial increase in toxicity. The variation of both dose and schedule in the three treatment arms does not allow direct conclusions about the relative value of dose versus schedule changes in cytarabine efficacy and toxicity.

High-dose cytarabine by rapid or continuous infusion, given alone or in combination with other agents, has been demonstrated to produce tolerable toxicity and response in patients refractory to conventional-dose cytarabine (12, 28–30). The high-dose regimens produce response rates of 35 to 70% in patients with refractory or relapsed acute myelogenous leukemia, including patients who have failed conventional-dose cytarabine (12, 29). In an early report of a study using cytarabine 3 g/m² over 2 hours followed by 1.5 g/m²/day by 4-day continuous infusion in combination with vincristine and prednisone, an 83% response rate was achieved in previously untreated patients with acute myelogenous leukemia (30). Moderate to severe diarrhea occurred in 35% of the patients. The 12% rate of toxic death was comparable to that of other aggressive regimens. Despite these encouraging rates of response, the role of high-dose cytarabine in the treatment of acute leukemia remains uncertain (31).

Low-dose continuous infusion cytarabine at doses of 5 to 20 mg/m²/day has been demonstrated to have activity in the treatment of primary and secondary acute nonlymphocytic leukemia and in the myelodysplastic syndromes (32). The rates of complete response, however, are relatively low. Toxicity is limited to the occurrence of myelosuppression but may be severe.

Thus, the substantial preclinical rationale predicting schedule-dependent antitumor activity of cytarabine has been confirmed in the clinic. Clinical experience demonstrates that the toxicity and antitumor activity of cytarabine is both dose and schedule dependent. The relative importance of schedule of administration versus the high-dose cytarabine regimens has not yet been established.

BLEOMYCIN

Bleomycin appears to exert its cytotoxicity by functioning as a mininuclease causing both single-strand and double-strand DNA breaks. Bleomycin appears to be cell cycle phase specific, exerting maximal cytotoxicity during the M and G_2 phases of the cell cycle (33) and blocking progression at the S-G_2 boundary (34). Bleomycin is used in the treatment of germ cell tumors, lymphomas, and squamous cell carcinomas. Plasma disappearance is rapid, with terminal half-lives of approximately 2 hours (8). Bleomycin produces chronic dose-related and dose-limiting pulmonary fibrosis.

In both the human tumor clonogenic assay and in human lymphoma and lung cancer cell lines, bleomycin produces dose-dependent reduction in colony formation with 1-hour exposure and further reduction in colony formation with continuous drug exposure (35–38). The dose-response curve in the study of Drewinko et al. was biphasic, suggesting a sensitive population of cells, probably reflecting the actively cycling fraction, and a more resistant population of cells (37). Prolonging the duration of exposure from 5 to 35 hours produced a 1000-fold reduction in colony formation.

The effects of alternation of the schedule of administration of bleomycin on antitumor activity in mice bearing Lewis lung carcinoma and on pulmonary toxicity in non-tumor-bearing mice have been studied (39). The mice were treated with three schedules delivering the same cumulative dose of bleomycin: (*a*) twice weekly injections, (*b*) 10 times weekly, or (*c*) continuous infusion. As assessed by antitumor activity, continuous infusion bleomycin was superior to both weekly schedules. Pulmonary fibrosis as detected by increase in pulmonary hydroxyproline content was observed with the two bolus schedules but was not detectable with bleomycin by continuous infusion. The absence of pulmonary toxicity with continuous infusion and the presence of pulmonary toxicity with therapy 10 times weekly suggests that a threshold level of bleomycin may be required before pulmonary toxicity is observed but that the threshold is probably quite low.

In another preclinical study, in mice bearing P388 lymphocytic leukemia, bleomycin by continuous intraperitoneal infusion was found to provide a fivefold reduction in leukemia colony-forming units, compared with intermittent bolus injection (40). Others have not found continuous infusion bleomycin to be superior to intermittent bolus in preclinical systems (41).

Pharmacokinetic studies of continuous infusion bleomycin in humans reveal that bleomycin plasma levels follow a two-compartment model with a $t_{1/2}$-α of 1.3 hours and a $t_{1/2}$-β of approximately 8.9 hours (42). Approximately 36 hours was required to achieve steady-state levels during infusion, suggesting that a loading dose of bleomycin at the initiation of infusion may be appropriate. In another study comparing plasma levels of bleomycin 15 mg given over 24 hours as a continuous intravenous versus subcutaneous infusion, steady-state plasma levels were achieved by approximately 8 hours and were similar by the two routes of administration (43).

A phase I study of continuous infusion bleomycin reported significant but acceptable toxicity and possible enhancement of antitumor activity (44). In this study, 119 patients were treated with 0.02 to 0.25 mg/kg/day of bleomycin by continuous intravenous infusion until dose-limiting toxicity was reached. Most patients were treated at 0.25 mg/kg/day dose of bleomycin continuously until limiting toxicity was reached. This represents a dose-intensive schedule of administration. The toxicity experience was similar to that in other series using bolus infusion bleomycin, except that alopecia was less common with continuous infusion. Dose-limiting mucocutaneous toxicity occurred after 7 to 11 days of infusion. Nearly all of the patients who had assessment of pulmonary function had a decrease in total lung capacity and in carbon monoxide diffusion lung capacity. Six patients experienced clinically overt pulmonary toxicity, which was fatal in five patients; comparison with the pulmonary toxicity in other series is difficult because of differing methods of monitoring and criteria for pulmonary toxicity. Thirty-two pa-

tients with ovarian carcinoma were treated in this study, and 10 (30%) achieved a partial or complete response with a 5.75-month median duration of response.

Prospective pulmonary function testing was performed in 13 patients treated with a bleomycin loading dose of 15 units/m^2 as an intravenous push followed by 15 units/m^2/day continuous intravenous infusion for 7 days (45). After a mean cumulative dose of 228 units of bleomycin, there was no change in pulmonary function as measured by mean vital capacity, forced expiratory volume in 1 second, total lung capacity, pulmonary diffusion capacity, PaO$_2$, or PaCO$_2$. While no patient received more than 289 units of bleomycin in this study, changes in total lung capacity and total pulmonary diffusion capacity are almost always seen in patients receiving intermittent bolus bleomycin at cumulative doses of 100 units or more.

The Southwest Oncology Group has reported a trial sequentially comparing three schedules of administration of bleomycin in combination with vincristine and mitomycin C in the treatment of advanced cervical cancer (46). Patients were treated with mitomycin C every 6 to 8 weeks, plus either twice-weekly bolus injections of bleomycin and vincristine for 12 weeks, or 2 weeks of twice-weekly injections of vincristine plus a weekly 4-day continuous infusion of bleomycin, or 24 weeks of weekly vincristine and bleomycin. The regimen using twice-weekly bleomycin had a response rate of 60%, that with continuous bleomycin, 39%, and that with weekly bleomycin, 25%. Median duration of response was short in all arms but favored the continuous infusion bleomycin regimen. The regimens incorporating twice-weekly or continuous infusion bleomycin were superior to that using weekly bleomycin in terms of survival ($p<.01$). The toxicity experience, especially leukopenia, of the patients treated with the infusion bleomycin regimen was felt to be less severe. While this trial provides suggestive evidence that frequent bolus or continuous infusion bleomycin is superior to intermittent bolus administration in the treatment of cervical cancer, the patient numbers are small, the study was not randomized, and the schedule of vincristine also differed among the three treatment groups.

A series has been reported of 111 patients with germ cell tumors treated with cisplatin, vinblastine, and doxorubicin in combination with either bleomycin 30 units/day by 3-day continuous infusion for three courses followed by bleomycin 15 units/day by 3-day continuous infusion for an additional three courses, or bleomycin 30 units/day by 3-day continuous infusion for only three courses (47). Formal pulmonary function testing was performed on most patients at baseline, prior to each cycle of chemotherapy, and during follow-up. A mean cumulative dose of 307 units of bleomycin was delivered. Bleomycin was terminated early in 15 patients because of a decrease in pulmonary diffusion capacity and in 1 patient because of dyspnea with a pulmonary infiltrate. Overall, a decrease of 25% or more of predicted diffusion capacity was detected in 32% of the patients. One patient experienced respiratory failure. The mean pulmonary diffusion capacity was 83% of baseline after six cycles of treatment. Of interest, the mean posttreatment diffusion capacity was 94% of baseline in 67 patients with determinations a mean of 20 months after treatment. While there was no control group, this suggests that pulmonary function, at least as measured by pulmonary diffusion capacity, may return to normal posttreatment in patients treated with continuous infusion bleomycin.

Substantial preclinical rationale and data predict schedule-dependent antitumor activity and pulmonary toxicity of bleomycin. Preclinical studies suggest that antitumor activity should be increased and pulmonary toxicity decreased with continuous infusion delivery. The available clinical studies do suggest diminished pulmonary toxicity with continuous infusion bleomycin, with little or no enhancement of antitumor activity. Appropriately designed randomized trials are needed in bleomycin-responsive tumors such as squamous cell cancer of the head and neck or germ cell tumors of the testis or ovary to further test the importance of schedule of administration.

DOXORUBICIN (ADRIAMYCIN)

The mechanism of action of the anthracycline antibiotics appears to be through intercalation between DNA base pairs and free radical formation, and they are more toxic to cycling, than to resting, cells. Of the two most widely used anthracycline antibiotics, doxorubicin has a broad spectrum of activity against lymphomas, carcinomas, and sarcomas, while daunorubicin is used primarily in the treatment of acute leukemia. Plasma disappearance of doxorubicin is triphasic with a mean $t_{1/2}$-α of 12 minutes,

$t_{1/2}$-β of 3.3 hours, and $t_{1/2}$-γ of 29.6 hours (8). Major acute toxicities associated with the anthracyclines are myelosuppression, nausea, vomiting, stomatitis, and alopecia. Cardiomyopathy is a major chronic toxicity of doxorubicin, is related to the total cumulative dose of doxorubicin, and occurs with significant frequency beginning at approximately 450 to 550 mg/m^2 of drug.

Studies performed on cell lines in culture reveal that doxorubicin cytotoxicity depends on both concentration and time of exposure (8, 48, 49). In mice implanted with either Lewis lung carcinoma or mammary carcinoma, divided-dose scheduling provided superior antitumor activity (50). In contrast, others have found no alteration in doxorubicin antitumor activity against L1210 leukemia, P388 leukemia, B-16 melanoma, or Lewis lung cancer by alteration in the schedule of administration (51). In non-tumor-bearing mice, rats, rabbits, and dogs, doxorubicin-associated cardiotoxicity is higher when treatment is given in high doses over a short period of time than when given in low doses over a long period of time (50, 52). Measurements of tissue doxorubicin levels in tumor-bearing mice reveal that peak levels and area under the concentration times time curves are not affected by the doxorubicin schedule of administration in tumor and spleen but are markedly reduced in the heart with divided-dose scheduling (50). This suggests that modifications in the schedule of administration of doxorubicin may result in enhanced antitumor activity with diminished cardiotoxicity.

Using conventional-dose-schedule doxorubicin at 60 to 75 mg/m^2 every 21 to 28 days, avoidance of doxorubicin-associated cardiomyopathy requires either empiric dose limitation at 450 to 550 mg/m^2 or careful monitoring of cardiac function and/or monitoring of morphologic changes by endomyocardial biopsy. Attempts to decrease the occurrence of doxorubicin-associated cardiomyopathy have included alterations in the schedule of administration, primarily through the use of weekly low-dose or continuous infusion doxorubicin. In nonrandomized studies, weekly low-dose doxorubicin appears to have antitumor activity equivalent to that of conventional high-dose intermittent doxorubicin (53–57). Weekly, low-dose doxorubicin also appears to be associated with a lower frequency of doxorubicin-associated congestive heart failure than standard-dose therapy every 3 weeks (53, 54, 56, 58). Doxorubicin-associated cardiac injury assessed by electron microscopy of endomyocardial biopsy specimens is also reduced by the use of the weekly low-dose schedule (59).

A randomized study in patients with non-small-cell lung cancer compared doxorubicin 20 mg/m² weekly versus doxorubicin 60 mg/m² every 3 weeks, both in combination with ftorafur, cyclophosphamide, and cisplatin (60). Rates of complete plus partial response were higher with weekly doxorubicin (31% vs. 19%, $p = .29$). Severe neutropenia and the occurrence of infectious complications were less frequent with the weekly schedule; this did not appear to be secondary to dose reductions in delivered chemotherapy. Cardiac toxicity, as measured by the endomyocardial biopsy score, appeared less severe with the weekly doxorubicin regimen.

Doxorubicin has been delivered by continuous infusion for periods ranging from 6 hours to 30 days. With increasing infusion times of 5 minutes to 96 hours, peak plasma levels of doxorubicin decrease while maintaining a constant area under the concentration times time curve (61–63). The use of continuous infusion doxorubicin requires the availability of central venous access because of the vesicant properties of doxorubicin.

Doxorubicin 50 mg/m² as a 6-hour continuous infusion has been given in combination with 5-fluorouracil and cyclophosphamide to 33 women with carcinoma of the breast (63). Antitumor activity appeared to be maintained with 6-hour infusion, but the mean resting radionuclide left ventricular ejection fraction declined with increasing cumulative doxorubicin dose, and use of a 6-hour doxorubicin infusion did not appear to protect against doxorubicin cardiac injury.

In a prospective randomized trial, doxorubicin 50 mg/m² every 3 weeks was administered as a 15- to 20-minute infusion versus a 6-hour infusion in patients with carcinoma of the breast

or ovary (64). Patients with breast cancer also received rapid-infusion cyclophosphamide and 5-fluorouracil, while patients with ovarian cancer also received rapid-infusion cisplatin and cyclophosphamide. No differences in response were observed between the two schedules of administration in either breast cancer or ovarian cancer. Cardiac toxicity was monitored by physical examination, resting radionuclide left ventricular ejection fraction, and electrocardiograms. Congestive heart failure developed in 14% of the patients treated with the rapid infusion and in none of the patients with 6-hour infusion. The decrease in mean left ventricular ejection fractions at both 300 mg/m² and 400 mg/m² was significantly greater with rapid-infusion doxorubicin (Table 15.4). Electrocardiographic changes were also less severe in the patients treated by 6-hour infusion. Thus, in this randomized study testing the duration of doxorubicin infusion, no difference in antitumor activity was demonstrated, but cardiac toxicity was significantly lower with 6-hour infusion doxorubicin.

In a study of continuous infusion doxorubicin for periods of 24 to 96 hours in patients with breast cancer or sarcomas, the antitumor activity and myelosuppression observed were similar to that expected with rapid-infusion doxorubicin (61). Nausea and vomiting appeared to be less frequent and less severe than with conventional rapid infusion. Compared with a nonrandomized control group, cardiac toxicity as assessed by endomyocardial biopsy was reduced by the use of continuous infusion therapy. More recently, sequential groups of patients with breast cancer were treated with doxorubicin by bolus, or 48-hour or 96-hour infusions in combination with 5-fluorouracil and cyclophosphamide (65). Rates of response and duration of response were equivalent with the three durations of doxorubicin infusion. Nausea and vomiting were less

Table 15.4. Cardiac Toxicity of Rapid versus Prolonged Infusion Doxorubicin

Doxorubicin Infusion Time (min)	No. of Patients	Mean Total Dose (mg/m²)	Mean % Change from Baseline in Left Ventricular Ejection Fraction		No. with Congestive Heart Failure
			After 300 mg/m² Doxorubicin	After 400 mg/m² Doxorubicin	
15–20	28	410	−17[d]	−21[b]	4
360	32	428	−4[a]	−6[b]	0

Data from Garnick MB, Weiss GR, Steele GD Jr, et al. Clinical evaluation of long-term, continuous-infusion doxorubicin. Cancer Treat Rep 1983;67:133–142.
[a]$p <.001$.
[b]$p <.001$.

with 48- or 96-hour infusions than with bolus infusion. The severity of mucositis was increased in the long-term infusion groups; in patients experiencing mucositis, shortening the duration of doxorubicin infusion without dose reduction reduced or prevented the recurrence of mucositis. An increase in the frequency of infectious complications was observed in the patients treated by 48- and 96-hour infusions and was felt to be secondary to the presence of long-term central venous catheters. The actuarial risk of clinical congestive heart failure was decreased at cumulative doxorubicin doses of approximately 400 mg/m² or more using 48- or 96-hour infusions.

Very long term continuous infusion doxorubicin has also been studied. In one study, patients with carcinomas or sarcomas were treated with doxorubicin 1 mg/m²/day by continuous infusion, escalating by 1 mg/m²/day every 3 weeks, until dose-limiting toxicity occurred (62). The longest duration of infusion was 22 weeks. The dose-limiting toxicities were found to be mucositis, leukopenia, thrombocytopenia, and conjunctivitis. A starting dose for further study of 4 mg/m²/day by continuous infusion was recommended. In a broad phase I–II study designed to identify the maximally tolerated doxorubicin dose for a minimum 30-day continuous infusion, patients were treated with escalating doses from 2 to 5 mg/m²/day of doxorubicin (66). Leukopenia and stomatitis were found to be dose limiting. The optimal dose was felt to be 3 mg/m²/day. Nausea, vomiting, diarrhea, and anorexia were not observed. The hand-foot syndrome, a syndrome of painful digital dysesthesia associated with an erythematous, desquamating dermatitis of the hands and feet, has been observed in patients treated with protracted continuous infusions of doxorubicin (67).

Thus, most clinical studies investigating the use of various schedules of administration of doxorubicin are nonrandomized. The prediction from preclinical systems that the antitumor activity of doxorubicin would be maintained or enhanced with a reduction in cardiac toxicity by the use of divided-dose scheduling has, in general, been confirmed. For the most part, the clinical studies demonstrate no alteration in antitumor activity of doxorubicin by divided-dose or continuous infusion schedules of administration. The results do consistently suggest, despite the nonrandomized nature of most studies, that the cardiac and gastrointestinal toxicity of doxoru-

bicin is decreased substantially by the use of low-dose, weekly or continuous infusion schedules of administration. While the data are limited, it appears that the longer the duration of continuous infusion, at least up to 96 hours, the greater the reduction in doxorubicin-related cardiac toxicity. The decrease in frequency of significant cardiac toxicity in practical terms is modest, however, as the early emergence of drug resistance continues to be a major problem.

5-FLUOROURACIL

5-Fluorouracil is a fluoropyrimidine antimetabolite that undergoes complex intracellular metabolic activation to fluorodeoxyuridine monophosphate (FdUMP), which inhibits thymidylate synthetase, and to fluorouridine triphosphate (FUTP), which is fraudulently incorporated into RNA. The cytotoxicity of 5-fluorouracil is relatively S-phase specific. The plasma disappearance of 5-fluorouracil is monoexponential, with a $t_{1/2}$ of 10 to 20 minutes (8). 5-Fluorouracil is used primarily in the treatment of carcinomas of the breast, gastrointestinal tract, and head and neck. Pharmacokinetic studies of 5-fluorouracil in plasma and bone marrow demonstrate 50- to 1000-fold lower levels of drug detected in the bone marrow of patients treated with continuous infusion compared with those after rapid bolus infusion, which may partially explain the toxicity differences observed with the varying schedules of administration (68). Studies of 5-fluorouracil pharmacokinetics have documented 10-fold variability in interpatient clearance, substantial circadian variation in plasma concentrations, and large variations in plasma concentrations depending on the infusion pump used for delivery (69–72).

Preclinical studies in the clonogenic assay document that time of exposure may be more important than concentration of drug in fluorouracil cytotoxicity (38). In mice bearing the L1210 leukemia, multiple doses of 5-fluorouracil produced superior durations of survival but did not increase the rate of cure (11).

Single-agent studies of dose schedule of administration demonstrate that 5-fluorouracil may be given safely in a wide variety of doses and schedules. The dose-limiting toxicities of bolus infusion 5-fluorouracil are myelosuppression, mucositis, and diarrhea; the dose-limiting toxicities of continuous infusion 5-fluorouracil are stomatitis and diarrhea. Studies of continuous infusion 5-fluorouracil consistently demonstrate that a higher total dose of 5-fluorouracil may be administered by continuous infusions of 8 hours or more than can be safely administered by bolus infusion. A randomized comparison of rapid infusion versus 2-hour infusion of 5-fluorouracil demonstrated similar toxicities for 15 mg/kg/day rapid infusion for 5 days and 25 mg/kg/day by 2-hour infusion for 5 days (73). In a dose-escalation study of 48-hour continuous infusion every 14 days, 30 mg/m^2/day was found to be the maximally tolerated dose (74). In studies of 5-fluorouracil given by 8- to 24-hour infusion for 5 days, doses of 22.5 to 30 mg/kg/day and 1 g/day are well tolerated; toxicity was limited primarily to stomatitis and diarrhea (75–81). Phase I studies of protracted continuous infusions of 5-fluorouracil have demonstrated that 300 to 350 mg/m^2/day of continuous infusion 5-fluorouracil may be given for more than 30 days (82, 83). Stomatitis and diarrhea were the major dose-limiting toxicities.

Recently, high-dose 24-to-48-hour continuous infusion 5-fluorouracil every 7 to 14 days has been evaluated (84–86). It appears that from 3000 to 3400 mg/m^2 of 5-fluorouracil by 24-to-48-hour continuous infusion may be administered with acceptable toxicity. With this dose schedule, the toxicity profile of 5-fluorouracil changes substantially, and central nervous system dysfunction (primarily ataxia) and leukopenia become dose limiting.

With protracted and high-dose continuous infusion 5-fluorouracil, the hand-foot syndrome or palmar-plantar erythrodysesthesia syndrome appears as a drug toxicity (87). The hand-foot syndrome begins with dysesthesias of the palms and soles that progress to pain and tenderness. There is associated symmetric swelling and erythema of the hands and feet. The syndrome resolves with cessation of drug infusion.

Cardiac toxicity also appears to be increased in patients treated with continuous infusion 5-fluorouracil. In a prospective study of 367 patients treated with chemotherapy that included 5-fluorouracil 600 to 1000 mg/m^2/day by 96- or 120-hour continuous infusion, cardiovascular events including including angina pectoris, hypotension, hypertension, arrhythmias, and sudden death occurred in 7.6% of the patients (88).

Nonrandomized studies of continuous infusion 5-fluorouracil in the treatment of colorectal cancer (79, 89–91), breast cancer (92, 93), and ovarian cancer (94) document significant antitumor activity and occasional responses in patients previously treated with bolus infusion 5-fluorouracil.

Few randomized studies testing the schedule of administration of 5-fluorouracil have been performed. Seifert et al. randomized patients with metastatic colorectal adenocarcinoma between 5-fluorouracil administered as a continuous 5-day infusion versus daily bolus injections for 5 days (81). Objective responses were observed in 44% of the patients treated by continuous infusion and 22% of the patients treated with bolus infusion. The median survival was 6 months in patients treated by continuous infusion and 2 months in those treated by bolus infusion. Although the continuous infusion schedule appeared superior, the authors state that some of the differences in this study were probably due to imbalances in patient characteristics at study entry.

The Mid-Atlantic Oncology Program has reported a randomized comparison of single-agent 5-fluorouracil by conventional bolus infusion versus protracted continuous infusion in the treatment of metastatic colorectal carcinoma (95). The response rate with continuous infusion was superior to that achieved with bolus infusion (30% vs. 6%; $p<.001$). Leukopenia less than 2000/μL was observed in 20% of the patients treated with bolus infusion and in 1% with continuous infusion, and the hand-foot syndrome developed in 23% of the patients treated with continuous infusion. Despite the increase in response rate with continuous infusion, survival did not differ between the two schedules.

The absence of significant myelosuppression observed with the use of continuous infusion 5-fluorouracil has resulted in the use of continuous infusion 5-fluorouracil in combination with other agents in the treatment of colorectal carcinoma (96–101), gastric carcinoma (100), pancreatic carcinoma (100), ovarian carcinoma (102), breast carcinoma (103), non-small-cell lung cancer (104), renal cell carcinoma (105), carcinoma of the prostate (106), and head and neck carcinoma (107–113). All of these studies have been either uncontrolled or nonrandomized comparisons of 5-fluorouracil schedule, and none provide rates of response and survival that are clearly superior to those achieved with bolus infusion 5-fluorouracil alone or in combination with the same agents. Recent studies using combination mitoxantrone, leucovorin, and continuous infusion 5-fluorouracil have proved encouraging rates of response in both previously treated and untreated patients (114–116). However, the importance of the schedule of administration of 5-fluorouracil in achieving the high rates of response in these studies is not known.

In summary, the therapeutic index of 5-fluorouracil is improved by the use of continuous infusion versus bolus infusion, primarily through a decrease in the severity of acute toxicity. In most studies, the antitumor activity of 5-fluorouracil does not appear to be increased. Two randomized studies in the treatment of metastatic colorectal carcinoma have been reported, and both demonstrate increased rates of response and either slight improvement or no difference in survival. Further randomized studies comparing continuous infusion versus bolus infusion 5-fluorouracil are necessary before the importance of schedule in antitumor activity will be defined.

VINCRISTINE AND VINBLASTINE

The vinca alkaloids vincristine and vinblastine are used in the treatment of lymphoma, leukemia, breast cancer, germ cell tumors, and selected pediatric tumors. They exert their primary antitumor activity by interfering with the microtubular mitotic spindle and are highly S-phase specific. Plasma pharmacokinetics are triphasic for both vincristine and vinblastine, with a $t_{1/2}$-α of less than 5 minutes, a $t_{1/2}$-β of 1 to 2.5 hours, and a $t_{1/2}$-γ of approximately 24 hours (8). When given by rapid infusion, the major toxicity of vincristine is peripheral neuropathy, while the dose-limiting toxicity of vinblastine is myelosuppression with occasional peripheral neuropathy. The vinca alkaloids are vesicants, and their delivery by continuous infusion is most safely accomplished with the use of secure central venous access.

In preclinical systems, the cytotoxic activity of vincristine and vinblastine depends on both drug concentration and time of exposure (35, 38, 117). As the spectrum of activity and toxicity differs between vincristine and vinblastine, the clinical experience with continuous infusion of these agents should be viewed separately.

In phase I studies of vincristine 0.5 to 1.0 mg/m^2/day by 5-day continuous infusion, dose-related neurotoxicity, leukopenia, and hyponatremia were observed. The toxicity was mild to moderate at 0.5 mg/m^2/day, unacceptable at 0.75 mg/m^2, and severe at 1.0 mg/m^2/day (118). Plasma pharmacokinetics of continuous infusion

vincristine 0.5 to 1.0 mg/m^2/day reveal similar steady-state concentrations and areas under the concentration times time curves, with superior area under the curve at all dose levels than with 2-mg bolus infusions (119, 120).

A study of vincristine, 0.5 mg rapid infusion followed by 0.25 mg/m^2/day by 5-day continuous infusion, was performed in 25 patients with various histologic types of refractory lymphomas. Twenty-four patients had previously received rapid infusion vincristine (121). A response rate of 36% was observed, although the median duration of response was only 2.1 months. Leukopenia and thrombocytopenia each were observed in only 12% of the patients. Neurotoxicity was common and included loss of deep tendon reflexes, paresthesias, constipation, myalgias, and decreased motor strength.

Continuous infusion vincristine 0.25 to 0.5 mg/m^2/day has been studied and found to be inactive in the treatment of refractory metastatic carcinoma of the breast (122–124) and refractory carcinoma of the cervix, ovary, and endometrium (125).

Continuous infusion vincristine has been incorporated in combination with other agents in the treatment of leukemia and myeloma. The combinations have demonstrated significant activity, although the importance of vincristine by continuous infusion in achieving the high rates of response is not known (126–130).

Early trials of vinblastine, 1 to 2 mg/m^2/day, by 5-day continuous infusion found myelosuppression to be dose limiting (131, 132). Disabling sensory-motor neuropathy was also observed in 3 of 10 patients in one study (132). Starting doses of 1.4 to 1.8 mg/m^2/day were associated with acceptable myelosuppression.

Protracted continuous infusions of vinblastine at doses of 0.5 to 0.9 mg/m^2/day were limited by leukopenia and peripheral neuropathy (133). In this study, there appeared to be no clear maximally tolerated dose, but plasma steady-state vinblastine levels were higher in patients experiencing leukopenia than in those without leukopenia. A dose of 0.7 mg/m^2/day by protracted continuous infusion was recommended for further study.

In an early phase II trial including 30 evaluable women with refractory metastatic breast cancer, vinblastine 1.4 to 2 mg/m^2/day by 5-day continuous infusion produced a 40% response rate, including a 50% response rate in patients with previous vinca alkaloid exposure (131). An update of this series with 106 evaluable patients reported an objective response rate of 37% (134). Leukopenia was the major toxicity, while non-hematologic toxicity including paresthesias, nausea and vomiting, and myalgias was observed in 11 to 14% of patients. In a retrospective analysis, the rates of response appeared to be dose-related; patients treated with more than 1.7 mg/m^2/day had a response rate of 49%; 1.7 mg/m^2/day, 32%; and less than 1.7 mg/m^2/day, 29%. In a study of vinblastine pharmacokinetics, from the same institution, the product of drug concentration times time of exposure was significantly greater in breast cancer patients who responded than in stable or progressing patients (135). The major source of this difference appeared to be differences in rates of drug clearance and not drug dose. Others have found 5-day continuous infusion vinblastine to be inactive in the treatment of breast cancer (136, 137).

Vinblastine by 5-day continuous infusion has been studied in a number of other tumor types and had minimal activity in renal cell carcinoma (138, 139), endometrial carcinoma (140), ovarian carcinoma (141), prostate carcinoma (142), cervical carcinoma (143), and lymphoma (144) and no activity in gastric carcinoma (145), sarcomas (146), ovarian carcinoma (147), or endometrial carcinoma (148). No clear advantage has been demonstrated from continuous infusion vinblastine in combination chemotherapy with interferon in the treatment of renal carcinoma (149) or either doxorubicin or cisplatin in the treatment of breast cancer (150, 151).

Continuous infusion therapy with either vincristine or vinblastine may be delivered with acceptable toxicity. There is no evidence that continuous infusion vincristine is superior to bolus vincristine in antitumor activity in the clinic. Continuous infusion vinblastine appears to have no or minimal activity in most tumor types. An exception is carcinoma of the breast, where high rates of response with continuous infusion vinblastine have been observed in some, but not all, studies.

CISPLATIN

Cisplatin is an inorganic heavy metal complex that exerts its cytotoxicity through the formation of intrastrand and interstrand DNA cross-links. Plasma pharmacokinetics are complex, with a prolonged decline of total platinum but a short plasma decline of the active, non-protein-bound, filterable platinum, with a $t_{1/2}$-α of 8 to 30 minutes and a $t_{1/2}$-β of 40 to 48 minutes (8). Nephrotoxicity, ototoxicity, nausea, and vomiting are the major toxicities of cisplatin administered under conventional rapid infusion dose schedules. Cisplatin has a broad spectrum of antitumor activity, including germ cell tumors, squamous carcinomas of the head and neck, lung cancer, ovarian cancer, bladder cancer, and a variety of other tumor types.

Cisplatin cytotoxicity is related to both drug concentration and time of exposure in cell culture (152, 153). In the clonogenic assay system, cisplatin inhibition of PC-7 colony-forming units is related to both drug concentration and time of exposure, but time of exposure appears relatively more important (38). In mice bearing L1210 leukemia, higher total doses of cisplatin were required with continuous infusion than with bolus infusion to achieve similar antitumor activity.

A comparison of plasma pharmacokinetics of the same daily dose of cisplatin delivered either as a 5-day continuous infusion or a daily bolus infusion for 5 days revealed that the area under the concentration times time curve of filterable platinum was 1.5 to 2.0 times higher with continuous infusion, while peak plasma levels of filterable platinum were eightfold lower with continuous infusion (154).

In early studies, cisplatin 60 to 125 mg/m^2 every 3 weeks was administered by 24-hour continuous infusion in patients with head and neck and ovarian cancers (155, 156). The nephrotoxicity observed in these studies was minimal, and nausea and vomiting may have been decreased. Although the studies were small, antitumor activity appeared to be similar to that of bolus infusion.

The Gynecologic Oncology Group subsequently randomized 331 evaluable patients with advanced or recurrent squamous cell carcinoma of the cervix to treatment with cisplatin 50 mg/m^2 every 3 weeks as a 24-hour continuous infusion or as a rapid, 1 mg/minute infusion (157). Rates of response, time to progression, and survival were not different with continuous versus rapid infusion. Patients treated by continuous infusion were significantly less likely to experience nausea and vomiting than those with rapid infusion (66% vs. 82%; $p = .002$). Nephrotoxicity was observed in 49% of the patients, but it was severe in only 2% and did not differ by treatment arm.

In early studies of cisplatin 20 mg/m^2/day for 5 days by continuous infusion, nephrotoxicity was observed in 21 to 33% of patients (158, 159). This high rate of nephrotoxicity may be related to what would now be considered inadequate rates of hydration. Subsequent studies of cisplatin 20 to 30 mg/m^2/day for 4 to 5 days, given with vigorous saline hydration, found significant nephrotoxicity in only 3 to 5% of the patients (160–162). One phase I study incorporating vigorous hydration found no nephrotoxicity at doses of 20 to 25 mg/m^2/day by 5-day continuous infusion, but 4 of 13 (31%) patients treated at 30 mg/m^2/day experienced nephrotoxicity (163). All of the studies of 5-day continuous infusion have documented decreased frequency and severity of nausea and vomiting. When delivered by continuous infusion, cisplatin doses higher than 30 mg/m^2/day for 5 days or infusions of 25 mg/m^2/day for longer than 5 days are associated with significant thrombopenia and neutropenia (160, 164). Peripheral neuropathy and ototoxicity occur with 4- or 5-day continuous infusion, although their frequency appears to be low (158, 160, 161, 163, 165).

In a phase I study designed to determine the optimal dose of cisplatin delivered over a minimum 30-day period, the dose-limiting toxicity was found to be nausea and vomiting at a daily dose of cisplatin 5 mg/m^2/day (166). Nephrotoxicity was observed in 3 of 14 (21%) patients.

Continuous infusion cisplatin, usually for 5 days, has been incorporated into a number of investigational combination chemotherapy regimens (167–174). In general, the toxicity experience in these studies has been substantial, and none of the continuous infusion cisplatin regimens has been compared with rapid infusion in a prospective, randomized clinical trial.

The use of continuous infusion cisplatin thus results in less nausea and vomiting than with bolus infusion and has a low frequency of significant nephrotoxicity when given with vigorous hydration. However, despite the relatively large number of phase I and phase II trials that document safety with vigorous hydration and selection of an appropriate dose schedule, there is no evidence to support the routine use of continuous infusion cisplatin for periods longer than 24 hours.

ETOPOSIDE

Etoposide (VP-16) is a semisynthetic derivative of podophyllotoxin that probably exerts its cytotoxicity by stabilizing the DNA–topoisomerase II complex and preventing the repair of single- and double-strand DNA breaks. Etoposide appears to be cell-cycle-phase specific, with maximal cell kill in the S and G$_2$ phases. The elimination half-life of conventional bolus infusion etoposide is approximately 7 hours, and the dose-limiting toxicity is myelosuppression. Etoposide is used in the treatment of germ cell tumors, lung cancer, and lymphoma.

Etoposide is poorly soluble in aqueous solutions, so that a final concentration for infusion of less than 0.4 mg/mL is required. Most investigators using continuous infusion have diluted the drug in normal saline because of concerns regarding compatibility with 5% dextrose. The relatively large volumes of normal saline required are of potential concern in patients with cardiovascular disease.

In preclinical systems, both etoposide dose and schedule of administration are important in determining cytotoxicity, with frequent, divided doses or continuous exposure producing superior cytotoxicity (38, 175, 176).

A phase I study of 5-day continuous infusion etoposide 20 to 80 mg/m^2/day found dose-limiting myelosuppression at 60 mg/m^2/day (177). Edema and congestive heart failure (as a consequence of the large volumes of normal saline required to deliver continuous infusion etoposide), stomatitis, and oral ulcerations were observed in some patients. Another phase I study found that etoposide 125 mg/m^2/day by 5-day continuous infusion had acceptable toxicity and that myelosuppression was dose limiting (178). Nonhematologic toxicities included nausea and vomiting, mucositis, diarrhea, myocardial infarction, and congestive heart failure.

Etoposide by 72-hour continuous infusion has been administered in escalating doses of 75 to 200 mg/m^2/day (179). Myelosuppression was dose limiting at 150 mg/m^2/day in patients with good performance status and 125 mg/m^2/day in those with poor performance status. Mucositis and cardiovascular events were not observed.

A phase I study of 14-day continuous infusion etoposide in patients with lung cancer found an MTD of 50 mg/m^2/day and a recommended phase II dose of 43 mg/m^2/day (180). Both leukopenia and stomatitis were dose limiting. Non-dose-limiting toxicity included alopecia and nausea.

Very long term continuous infusion etoposide has been administered for 21 or more days with a maximally tolerated dose of 25 mg/m^2/

day (181). Myelosuppression was dose limiting. Alopecia, nausea, fatigue, mucositis, and heart failure were also observed.

In phase I studies of continuous infusion etoposide and infusion or bolus cisplatin, the optimal dose schedule was found to be etoposide 75 mg/m^2/day and cisplatin 30 mg/m^2/day by 3-day continuous infusion (170), etoposide 30 mg/m^2/day and cisplatin 20 mg/m^2/day by 5-day continuous infusion (168), or etoposide 10 mg/m^2 bolus followed by 25 mg/m^2/day by 14-day continuous infusion with bolus cisplatin 30 mg/m^2/day on days 1 to 3 (182). Myelosuppression and renal failure were found to be dose limiting; no cardiovascular events were observed.

Three randomized studies of the schedule dependence of single-agent etoposide in the treatment of small cell lung cancer have been reported, and two document substantial schedule-dependent activity (Table 15.5) (183—

Table 15.5. Randomized Trials of the Schedule Dependence of Single-Agent Etoposide in Small Cell Lung Cancer

Series (Reference)	Etoposide Dose Schedule (mg/m^2)	Complete Response Rate (%)	Overall Response Rate (%)
Cavalli et al. (183)	250 i.v. weekly	5	20[a]
	500 divided over 3 days, p.o., weekly	12	65[a]
	850 divided over 5 days, p.o., every 3 weeks	11	42
Slevin et al. (184)	500 by 24-hour continuous infusion, every 3 weeks	0	10[b]
	500 divided over 5 days, by 2-hour infusion, every 3 weeks	5	89[b]
Clark et al. (185)	500 divided over 5 days, by 2-hour infusion, every 3 weeks	0	81
	500 divided over 8 days, by 75-minute infusion, every 3 weeks	9	87

[a]$p = .015$.
[b]$p = .001$.

185). The use of more frequent, divided-dose schedules appears to provide superior rates of response. The dose intensity of the two weekly regimens in the study of Cavalli et al. was equivalent, since the bioavailability of oral etoposide is approximately 50%. The overall response rate with the divided-dose weekly schedule was superior to that of the single weekly infusion ($p = .015$). In the study of Slevin et al., the same cumulative dose of etoposide was administered intravenously, making schedule the only difference between the regimens. Pharmacokinetic analysis of the two schedules of administration revealed similar half-times of elimination, areas under the concentration times time curves, and maximum drug concentrations. The superior rate of response with the divided-dose scheduling was accompanied by a significant survival advantage ($p = .01$). In the study of Clark et al., the same cumulative dose of etoposide was administered over 5 or 8 days by continuous infusion. Rates of response and survival did not differ between the study groups (185).

In contrast to the single-agent studies in small cell lung cancer, a randomized study in patients with extensive small cell lung cancer of combination chemotherapy incorporating single- versus divided-dose scheduling of etoposide failed to demonstrate differences in response, toxicity, or survival (186). In this study, patients were treated with combination chemotherapy with doxorubicin and cyclophosphamide plus etoposide for either 1 or 5 days to the same cumulative dose. It is possible that the failure to demonstrate differences was related to the concurrent use of other active agents in combination, so that the relative contribution of etoposide to the antitumor activity was reduced.

In a randomized phase II trial, patients with refractory metastatic breast carcinoma were randomized to treatment with 60 to 70 mg/m^2/day for 5 days of etoposide by either 1-hour rapid infusion or by continuous infusion (187). The rate of response was 13% to 1-hour infusion and was 14% to continuous infusion. Myelosuppression was similar in the two treatment groups. Reversible congestive heart failure occurred in 3% of the patients with 1-hour infusion and 16% with continuous infusion, presumably secondary to saline.

Forty-four evaluable patients with metastatic breast cancer who had failed one previous chemotherapy regimen were treated with 3-day continuous infusion etoposide in combination with 2-day continuous infusion cisplatin (188). A partial response rate of 25% was observed at the expense of considerable toxicity.

In summary, the cell-cycle-phase specificity and preclinical schedule-dependent cytotoxicity predict that etoposide will have strongly schedule-dependent cytotoxicity. Single-agent studies in small cell lung cancer demonstrate markedly schedule-dependent antitumor activity of etoposide. While etoposide can be safely administered by continuous intravenous infusion, there is no evidence that continuous infusion is superior to frequent rapid infusions in the treatment of any tumor, and the use of continuous infusion may be associated with a substantial risk of congestive heart failure.

METHOTREXATE

Methotrexate is a folate analogue that exerts cytotoxicity by inhibition of dihydrofolate reductase, resulting in the depletion of reduced intracellular folates necessary for thymidylate and purine biosynthesis. Methotrexate cytotoxicity is relatively S-phase specific. The spectrum of antitumor activity of methotrexate is broad, and it is used in the treatment of breast carcinoma, head and neck cancers, choriocarcinoma, lymphoma, bladder carcinoma, osteosarcomas, and other tumors. Drug clearance is primarily renal and therefore strongly depends upon renal function. With normal renal function, the plasma disappearance curve is triphasic, with a $t_{1/2}$-α of less than 1 hour, a $t_{1/2}$-β of 2 to 3 hours, and a $t_{1/2}$-γ of 8 to 12 hours (8). Methotrexate toxicities at usual doses include myelosuppression and mucositis, with renal insufficiency, hepatic dysfunction, and rash occasionally observed with high-dose methotrexate. Administration of the reduced folate leucovorin (leucovorin rescue), urinary alkalinization, and monitoring of methotrexate plasma levels are widely used to prevent or minimize the myelosuppression and mucositis observed with high-dose or infusional methotrexate (189, 190). The presence of third-space fluid or renal insufficiency greatly increases the frequency and severity of methotrexate toxicity, especially with the high-dose regimens.

Preclinical studies demonstrate that both drug concentration and time of exposure are important determinants in cytotoxicity to both normal and neoplastic cells but that time of exposure is relatively much more critical (38, 191, 192). A wide variety of dose schedules of methotrexate with or without leucovorin rescue have been used clinically. The intravenous dose schedules may be divided into those using low- to intermediate-dose methotrexate by rapid infusion without leucovorin rescue and those using intermediate- to high-dose methotrexate by up to 36-hour infusion with leucovorin rescue. The need for leucovorin rescue is determined by the plasma methotrexate level achieved, the duration of infusion, and the rate of decay of plasma levels (189). In general, methotrexate toxicity is more closely related to time of exposure than to level of exposure, as long as a certain threshold plasma concentration is exceeded. With high-dose or infusional methotrexate, leucovorin rescue must be initiated within 36 to 42 hours of the beginning of methotrexate exposure, to avoid or minimize drug-related toxicity (193).

Early experience with infusions of methotrexate documented antitumor activity in patients resistant to low-dose methotrexate but with substantial toxicity (194). These investigators used 18-hour continuous infusions of methotrexate of 48 mg/m^2/day for 1 to 3 days. The 18-hour continuous infusions were found to be toxic, especially when administered for 2 or 3 days, but with substantial antitumor activity in patients refractory to low-dose, intermittent methotrexate therapy. This suggested that alteration of the schedule of administration could overcome relative methotrexate resistance.

Pharmacokinetic studies comparing bolus infusion versus continuous infusion methotrexate demonstrate improved sustained methotrexate levels in plasma, tissue, and cerebrospinal fluid with the use of long-term infusion (195, 196). Comparison of the pharmacokinetics of intermediate-dose (0.5 g/m^2) and high-dose (2.5 g/m^2) methotrexate by 24-hour continuous infusion documents substantial interpatient variability in serum and cerebrospinal fluid levels (197). Cytotoxic cerebrospinal fluid methotrexate levels were not observed at the intermediate-dose level but were observed in 44% of the high-dose methotrexate cycles.

Phase I studies have demonstrated that 3 to 18 g of methotrexate as a 6-hour continuous infusion, 100 to 800 mg methotrexate as an 18-hour continuous infusion, or methotrexate 4.5 to 12.5 g/m^2 as a 24-hour continuous infusion, all with leucovorin rescue, are well tolerated (198, 199). Toxicity tends not to be related to dose but to methotrexate level at 48 and 72 hours and consists of myelosuppression, stomatitis, and elevated serum glutamic oxalacetic transaminase levels.

In a randomized phase I study comparing methotrexate at starting doses of 1 to 6.7 g/m^2 by either rapid infusion or 20-hour continuous infusion, both with leucovorin rescue, elevation in serum creatinine of more than 50% of baseline was observed in 58% of the adult patients, and 20% of the evaluable courses were associated with myelosuppression (200). The toxicity experience did not differ between the two schedules of administration. It is likely that the high rate of nephrotoxicity observed in this study was secondary to the lack of urinary alkalinization. Various dose schedules of methotrexate have been most systematically studied in the treatment of squamous cell carcinomas of the head and neck. An early study using methotrexate 2 mg/kg by 24-hour continuous infusion with leucovorin rescue demonstrated a 47% response rate in 19 patients with head and neck carcinoma (201). In a subsequent study, patients with recurrent or metastatic head and neck cancer were randomized between therapy with methotrexate given either weekly at a dose of 40 mg/m^2 intramuscularly or 1500 mg/m^2 by 24-hour continuous infusion with leucovorin rescue (202). The rate of response with the high-dose continuous infusion regimen was 32% versus 22% in the low-dose regimen (p = .52). The median time to progression favored the high-dose infusion regimen (11 weeks vs. 5 weeks; p = .04), but the toxicity of the infusion regimen was more severe (p = .01), and survival did not differ between the treatment arms. Another randomized study of three oral or bolus infusion dose schedules of methotrexate in the treatment of carcinoma of the head and neck, breast, and colon was performed by the Southeast Cancer Study Group (203). In this study, no meaningful differences in rates of response by dose schedule were observed in any of the disease sites.

The Eastern Cooperative Oncology Group has reported a trial of 237 evaluable patients with advanced recurrent stage III or IV squamous carcinomas of the head and neck that randomized patients between three treatment arms: (*a*) methotrexate 40 mg/m^2 bolus infusion every week; (*b*) methotrexate 250 mg/m^2 bolus infusion biweekly with leucovorin rescue; or (*c*) methotrexate 250 mg/m^2 bolus infusion with leucovorin rescue, cyclophosphamide 0.5 g/m^2, and cytarabine 300 mg/m^2, all biweekly (204). The weekly methotrexate regimen resulted in more frequent skin and mucosal toxicity, while the combination arm resulted in significantly more myelosuppression. The response rates for the weekly methotrexate arm, biweekly methotrexate with leucovorin rescue, and biweekly methotrexate with leucovorin rescue plus cyclophosphamide and cytarabine were 26%, 24%, and 18%, respectively. Methotrexate alone had a superior median duration of response of 105 days, compared with 42 or 49 days with the other treatment arms. Median survival also favored the weekly methotrexate regimen, but the differences between the three arms did not achieve statistical significance (p = .06).

Another trial of methotrexate in the treatment of advanced head and neck cancer randomized patients to three different dose levels of weekly methotrexate: 50 mg/m^2, 500 mg/m^2, or 5 g/m^2, all with leucovorin rescue (205). The high-dose regimen was found to produce more frequent myelosuppression, mucositis, nausea and vomiting, renal toxicity, and fatal toxicity than the other treatment arms. The response rate with the high-dose regimen was superior to the other treatment arms (50% vs. 21% vs. 31%), but the differences did not achieve statistical significance (chi-squared $p > .05$).

Early studies of intermediate-dose methotrexate in acute leukemia of childhood demonstrated that patients refractory to low-dose methotrexate could achieve remission with regimens using methotrexate 108 to 305 mg/m^2/day for 2 days as 4-hour continuous infusions (206). Subsequently, intermediate- and high-dose methotrexate has been incorporated into a number of combination regimens for the treatment of acute lymphocytic leukemia. In one such regimen, the pharmacokinetics of high-dose methotrexate as a component of the maintenance regimen in patients achieving a complete response were studied (207). The methotrexate was given as 1 g/m^2 by 24-hour continuous infusion with intravenous hydration, urinary alkalinization, and leucovorin rescue. Serum levels of methotrexate were found to vary widely within individual patients and among patients, even though the delivered dose of methotrexate was constant. Analysis of serum methotrexate levels revealed that patients with median steady-state serum concentrations of 16 μM or above had superior durations of hematologic and complete remission, compared with those with lower median steady-state concentrations. This suggested that monitoring of serum concentrations with escalation of methotrexate dose might produce improved outcome in patients with acute lymphocytic leukemia.

A phase I study designed to determine the maximally tolerated dose of methotrexate by a minimum 28 days of continuous infusion treated patients at doses of 0.75 to 2 mg/m²/day (208). The dose-limiting toxicity was thrombocytopenia or stomatitis in all patients who did not experience progressive disease. Mean steady-state serum methotrexate levels appeared related to the dose of methotrexate per day. The recommended dose of methotrexate for further study by 28-day continuous infusion was 0.75 mg/m²/day. This represents a dose intensity considerably lower than is tolerable with intermittent short-term infusion methotrexate, with or without leucovorin rescue, and confirms the importance of schedule in determining methotrexate toxicity. Subsequently, 14-day continuous infusion methotrexate has been incorporated into combination chemotherapy regimens with acceptable toxicity but has not yet been compared with bolus injection in either phase II or phase III trials (209, 210).

The relationship between dose and schedule for methotrexate thus appears complex in relation to both antitumor activity and toxicity. Despite a substantial number of clinical trials, comparisons of the various schedules of methotrexate administration are relatively few. For squamous cell carcinoma of the head and neck, there does not appear to be a strong schedule-response relationship in antitumor activity for intermediate to high doses of methotrexate. However, in acute lymphocytic leukemia, serum concentrations of methotrexate achieved are predictive for duration of remission maintenance. The toxicity of methotrexate is strongly schedule dependent, with increasing toxicity with increasing duration of exposure. However, the toxicity of high-dose methotrexate or methotrexate administered by continuous infusions of 36 hours or longer may be greatly reduced and often eliminated by the use of hydration, urinary alkalinization, and leucovorin rescue.

PACLITAXEL (TAXOL)

Paclitaxel produces an increased rate of microtubular formation and inhibition of microtubular depolymerization, resulting in the accumulation of disorganized microtubules, the failure to form a normal spindle apparatus, and blocking of cell cycling in the G_2 and M phases of the cell cycle. Paclitaxel has demonstrated substantial activity against carcinoma of the breast, ovary, and lung. Early studies of paclitaxel with short infusions and without premedication documented a high frequency of hypersensitivity reactions considered secondary to the cremophor vehicle. Other paclitaxel toxicities include neutropenia, thrombocytopenia, neuropathy, myalgias, diarrhea, mucositis, alopecia, and bradyarrhythmias.

Preclinical studies demonstrate both dose and schedule effects of paclitaxel cytotoxicity (211). Dosing every 3 hours is superior to single daily dosing against P388 leukemia, and prolonged exposure to frequent dosing is superior to less frequent dosing schedules. The dose-survival curve of paclitaxel reaches a plateau in some cell lines above which cells are more sensitive to increased time of exposure than to dose (212, 213).

Paclitaxel pharmacokinetics are complex, with a $t_{1/2}$-α of 0.2 hours, a $t_{1/2}$-β of 1.9 hours, and a $t_{1/2}$-γ of 20.7 hours (214). Linear pharmacokinetics are exhibited with infusions of 24 hours or longer, but nonlinear pharmacokinetics are exhibited with infusions of 6 hours or less at the higher doses.

Phase I trials have been completed in patients with solid tumors, using single-agent paclitaxel in a wide variety of schedules (Table 15.6) (215–227). Early studies with 1-hour infusions documented a high frequency of acute hypersensitivity reactions, most likely secondary to the cremophor vehicle (215–217). The frequency of hypersensitivity reactions led to the use of long-term infusions plus premedication with glucocorticoids, diphenhydramine, and H-2 blockers. These studies document that with premedication, hypersensitivity reactions are acceptable with infusions of 1 to 120 hours (Table 15.7) (228–230), and the dose-limiting toxicities are myelosuppression or neuropathy. Infusions of 24 hours or longer are associated with a low frequency of hypersensitivity reactions, with or without premedication.

Phase II studies have documented activity of paclitaxel in the treatment of epithelial ovarian carcinoma, breast cancer, and lung cancer. A multiinstitutional phase III study randomized 382 assessable patients with platinum-pretreated ovarian cancer to treatment in a 2 by 2 design with paclitaxel at a dose of either 135 mg/m² or 175 mg/m² as either a 3- or 24-hour infusion (231). Rates of response and the occurrence of

Table 15.6. Phase I Studies of Single-Agent Paclitaxel in Solid Tumors

Series	Recommended Phase II Dose	Dose-Limiting Toxicity	Premedication	Hypersensitivity Reactions (%)
1-hour infusion				
MD Anderson (215)	30 mg/m^2/day for 5 days	Myelosuppression	No	0
Johns Hopkins (216)	Not reached		No	28
University of Wisconsin (217)	Not reached		No	22
Sarah Cannon Cancer Center (218)	135 mg/m^2	Myelosuppression	Yes	11
	45 mg/m^2/day for 3 days		Yes	11
3-hour infusion				
Memorial Sloan-Kettering (219)	None	Hypersensitivity	No	18
University of Wisconsin (220)	210 mg/m^2 or 250 mg/m^2 + G-CSF	Myelosuppression, neuropathy	Yes	3
6-hour infusion				
Johns Hopkins (216)	170–212 mg/m^2	Myelosuppression	Yes	21
University of Wisconsin (217)	30 mg/m^2/day for 5 days	Myelosuppression	Yes	0
University of Texas, San Antonio (221)	225 mg/m^2	Myelosuppression	No	3
Albert Einstein (222)	250 mg/m^2	Myelosuppression, neuropathy	No/yes	75/3
24-hour infusion				
Mount Sinai (232)	135–170 mg/m^2	Myelosuppression	No	0
Albert Einstein (223)	250 mg/m^2	Neuropathy	Yes	4
National Cancer Institute (224)	250 mg/m^2 + G-CSF	Neuropathy	Yes	0
Pediatric Oncology Group (225)	350 mg/m^2	Neurotoxicity	Yes	6
96-hour infusion				
National Cancer Institute (226)	105–140 mg/m^2	Myelosuppression, mucositis	No	0
120-hour infusion				
Dana Farber (227)	30 mg/m^2/day	Myelosuppression	No/yes	0/0

Table 15.7. Phase II Studies of Single-Agent Paclitaxel in the Treatment of Breast Cancer

Series (Reference)	Dose (mg/m^2)	Infusion Duration	Patients With Prior Treatment (%)	Partial Response Rate (%)	Complete Response Rate (%)	Overall Response Rate (%)
MD Anderson (228)	250	24 hour	100	44	12	56
Memorial Sloan-Kettering (229)	250 + G-CSF	24 hour	62	50	12	62
	200 + G-CSF	24 hour	100	0	22	22
National Cancer Institute (230)	140	96 hour	100	48	0	48

severe hypersensitivity reactions were not affected by either dose or schedule of administration. Progression-free survival was superior in the high-dose group (median time to progression 19 vs. 14 weeks, $p = .06$; overall trend, adjusted $p = .02$) and in the 3-hour infusion group (overall trend, adjusted $p = .03$). Granulocytopenia was greater with 24-hour infusion (grade 4 granulocytopenia in 71% with 24-hour infusion, 18% with 3-hour infusion, $p<.0001$). Survival was not affected by dose or schedule. This suggests that paclitaxel by 3-hour infusion and at high dose may be superior to long-term infusions at lower doses in the treatment of ovarian cancer.

Considerable uncertainty exists regarding the optimal duration of infusion in patients with metastatic carcinoma of the breast. Nonrandomized clinical trials provide little evidence of schedule-related antitumor activity (Table 15.7), but randomized comparisons are required before definitive conclusions may be reached.

A number of phase II and phase III trials are now being conducted to define the activity and toxicity of a variety of dose schedules of paclitaxel as a single agent and in combination chemotherapy in the treatment of breast, lung, and ovarian cancers.

The available preclinical data suggest substantial schedule dependence of paclitaxel antitumor activity. Clinical studies document a lower frequency of hypersensitivity reactions with prolonged infusions when no premedication is administered. Moderate paclitaxel schedule dependence has been suggested in a randomized trial in epithelial ovarian cancer that favored 3-hour over 24-hour infusion. Further comparative studies are required before the true schedule dependence of paclitaxel is clearly defined.

SUMMARY

The mechanisms of action, pharmacokinetics, and available preclinical data predict that many cytotoxic agents will have schedule-dependent antitumor activity and toxicity. Particularly compelling is the schedule dependence of the cytotoxicity of cytarabine, where single large bolus injections have modest antitumor activity, while continuous exposure or multiple smaller bolus infusions have markedly enhanced antitumor activity. Similarly, in preclinical systems, it appears that the antitumor activity of bleomycin is improved and pulmonary toxicity decreased with continuous infusion therapy and that the use of frequent, low-dose doxorubicin decreases the severity of doxorubicin-associated cardiotoxicity.

The investigation of continuous intravenous schedules of administration in the clinic has been made possible by the availability of chronic venous access devices and of reliable ambulatory infusion pumps. The results of most trials demonstrate that the use of continuous infusion or frequent low-dose schedules of administration of most cytotoxic agents has not resulted in enhancement of antitumor activity. The most notable exception is the use of cytarabine in the treatment of acute leukemia, where continuous infusion or divided-dose scheduling appears to significantly enhance antitumor activity. Selected trials of continuous infusion bleomycin in cervical carcinoma, vinblastine in breast carcinoma, 5-fluorouracil in colon carcinoma, and methotrexate in acute lymphocytic leukemia have suggested increased antitumor activity, compared with conventional bolus infusion. Studies of continuous infusion doxorubicin, vincristine, cisplatin, and etoposide have not demonstrated enhancement of antitumor activity compared with that of conventional bolus infusion.

The use of continuous infusion or frequent divided-dose delivery has been demonstrated to decrease or alter the toxicity of a number of cytotoxic agents. The cardiotoxicity associated with the use of doxorubicin is decreased by schedules of administration, such as low-dose weekly or 48- or 96-hour continuous infusion, that reduce peak plasma levels. The myelosuppression associated with bolus infusions of 5-fluorouracil is reduced or eliminated, and the frequency and severity of mucositis and diarrhea are increased with the use of continuous infusions of 8 hours or more. There is suggestive evidence that nausea, vomiting, and renal toxicity are decreased when cisplatin is delivered by 24-hour continuous infusion and that the pulmonary toxicity of bleomycin is decreased with continuous infusion delivery. Hypersensitivity reactions to paclitaxel infusion may be minimized by the use of either premedication or prolongation of infusion to 24 or more hours.

In contrast, continuous infusions (compared with conventional single-bolus infusion) of cytarabine and methotrexate may have significantly enhanced toxicity, primarily myelosuppression and mucositis. The enhanced toxicity of 48-hour or longer continuous infusion methotrexate may be minimized or reduced by the use of hydration, urinary alkalinization, and leucovorin rescue.

Thus, the expectations based upon preclinical studies that alterations in the schedule of administration would enhance the antitumor activity and decrease the toxicity of many cytotoxic agents have been partially confirmed in the clinic. The known schedule dependence of many cytotoxic agents in preclinical systems and the results of selected early clinical trials confirm the need for further prospective clinical trials to better define the optimal schedule of administration for the available cytotoxic agents.

REFERENCES

1. Carlson RW, Sikic BI. Continuous infusion or bolus injection in cancer chemotherapy. Ann Intern Med 1983;99:823–833.

2. Vogelzang NJ. Continuous infusion chemotherapy: a critical review. J Clin Oncol 1984;2:1289–1304.

3. Lokich JJ, ed. Cancer chemotherapy by infusion. 2nd ed. Chicago: Precept Press, 1990.

4. Kwan JW. High-technology i.v. infusion devises. Am J Hosp Pharm 1989;46:320–335.

5. Plasse T, Ohnuma T, Bruckner H, Chamberlain K, Mass T, Holland JF. Portable infusion pumps in ambulatory cancer chemotherapy. Cancer 1982;50:27–31.

6. Magid DM, Vokes EE, Schilsky RL, et al. A randomized study of inpatient versus outpatient continuous intravenous infusion chemotherapy: psychological aspects. Sel Cancer Ther 1989;5:137–145.

7. Farrington EA, Stull JC, Leff RD. Flow rate variability from selected syringe and mobile infusion pumps. Drug Intell Clin Pharm 1988;22:687–690.

8. Balis FM, Holcenberg JS, Bleyer WA. Clinical pharmacokinetics of commonly used anticancer drugs. Clin Pharmacokinet 1983;8:202–232.

9. Kline I, Venditti JM, Tyrer DD, Goldin A. Chemotherapy of leukemia L1210 in mice with 1-βD-arabinofuranosylcytosine hydrochloride. I. Influence of treatment schedules. Cancer Res 1966;26:853–859.

10. Skipper HE, Schabel FM Jr, Wilcox WS. Experimental evaluation of potential anticancer agents. XXI. Scheduling of arabinosylcytosine to take advantage of its S-phase specificity against leukemia cells. Cancer Chemother Rep 1967;51:125–165.

11. Skipper HE, Schabel FM Jr, Mellett LB, et al. Implications of biochemical, cytokinetic, pharmacologic, and toxicologic relationships in the design of optimal therapeutic schedules. Cancer Chemother Rep 1970;54:431–450.

12. Capizzi RL, Yang J-L, Rathmell JP, et al. Dose-related pharmacologic effects of high-dose Ara-C and its self-potentiation. Semin Oncol 1985;2:65–75.

13. Kufe DW, Spriggs DR, Griffin JD. Pharmacologic studies of low-dose and high-dose continuous infusion cytosine arabinoside. Semin Oncol 1987;14:149–158.

14. Burke PJ, Serpick AA, Carbone PP, Tarr N. A clinical evaluation of dose and schedule of administration of cytosine arabinoside (NSC 63878). Cancer Res 1968;28:274–279.

15. Frei E III, Bickers JN, Hewlett JS, Lane M, Leary WV, Talley RW. Dose schedule and antitumor studies of arabinosyl cytosine (NSC 63878). Cancer Res 1969;29:1325–1332.

16. Ellison RR, Carey RW, Holland JF. Continuous infusions of arabinosyl cytosine in patients with neoplastic disease. Clin Pharmacol Ther 1967;8:800–809.

17. Spriggs DR, Robbins G, Takvorian T, Kufe DW. Continuous infusion of high-dose 1-βD-arabinofuranosylcytosine: a phase I and pharmacological study. Cancer Res 1985;45:3932–3936.

18. Donehower RC, Karp JE, Burke PJ. Pharmacology and toxicity of high-dose cytarabine by 72-hour continuous infusion. Cancer Treat Rep 1986;70:1059–1065.

19. Spriggs DR, Robbins G, Arthur K, Mayer RJ, Kufe D. Prolonged high dose ARA-C infusion in acute leukemia. Leukemia 1988;2:304–306.

20. Weinstein HJ, Griffin TW, Feeney J, Cohen HJ, Propper RD, Sallan SE. Pharmacokinetics of continuous intravenous and subcutaneous infusions of cytosine arabinoside. Blood 1982;59:1351–1353.

21. Slevin ML, Piall EM, Aherne GW, Johnston A, Lister TA. Subcutaneous infusion of cytosine arabinoside: a practical alternative to intravenous infusion. Cancer Chemother Pharmacol 1983;10:112–114.

22. Spriggs DR, Sokal JE, Griffin J, Kufe DW. Low dose ara-C administered by continuous subcutaneous infusion: a pharmacologic evaluation. Cancer Drug Delivery 1986;3:211–216.

23. Bodey GP, Freireich EJ, Monto RW, Hewlett JS. Cytosine arabinoside (NSC-63878) therapy for acute leukemia in adults. Cancer Chemother Rep 1969;53:59–66.

24. Southwest Oncology Group. Cytarabine for acute leukemia in adults: effect of schedule on therapeutic response. Arch Intern Med 1974;133:251–259.

25. Schiller J, Gajewski J, Nimer S, et al. A randomized study of intermediate versus conventional-dose cytarabine as intensive induction for acute myelogenous leukaemia. Br J Haematol 1992;81:170–177.

26. Rai KR, Holland JF, Glidewell OJ, et al. Treatment of acute myelocytic leukemia: a study by Cancer and Leukemia Group B. Blood 1981;58:1203–1212.

27. Mayer RJ, Davis RB, Schiffer CA, et al. Intensive postremission chemotherapy in adults with acute myeloid leukemia. N Engl J Med 1994;331:896–903.

28. Rudnick SA, Cadman EC, Capizzi RL, Skeel RT, Bertino JR, McIntosh S. High dose cytosine arabinoside (HDARAC) in refractory acute leukemia. Cancer 1979;44:1189–1193.

29. Early AP, Preisler HD, Slocum H, Rustum YM. A pilot study of high-dose 1-β-D-arabinofuranosyl cytosine for acute leukemia and refractory lymphoma: clinical response and pharmacology. Cancer Res 1982; 42:1587–1594.

30. Estey E, Keating MJ, Plunkett W, McCredie KB, Freireich EJ. Continuous infusion high-dose cytosine arabinoside without anthracyclines as induction and intensification therapy in adults under age 50 with newly diagnosed acute myelogenous leukemia. Semin Oncol 1987;14:58–63.

31. Peters WG, Colly LP, Willemze R. High-dose cytosine arabinoside: pharmacological and clinical aspects. Blut 1988;56:1–11.

32. Cheson BD, Jasperse DM, Simon R, Friedman MA. A critical appraisal of low-dose cytosine arabinoside in patients with acute non-lymphocytic leukemia and myelodysplastic syndromes. J Clin Oncol 1986;4:1857–1864.

33. Barranco SC, Humphrey RM. The effects of bleomycin on survival and cell progression in Chinese hamster cells in vitro. Cancer Res 1971;31:1218–1223.

34. Barranco SC, Luce JK, Romsdahl MM, Humphrey RM. Bleomycin as a possible synchronizing agent for human tumor cells in vivo. Cancer Res 1973; 33:882–887.

35. Wu P-C, Ozols RF, Hatanaka M, Boone CW. Anticancer drugs: effects on the cloning of Raji lymphoma cells in soft agar. J Natl Cancer Inst 1982; 68:115–121.

36. Ludwig R, Alberts DS, Miller TP, Salmon SE. Evaluation of anticancer drug schedule dependency using an in vitro human tumor clonogenic assay. Cancer Chemother Pharmacol 1984;12:135–141.

37. Drewinko B, Novak JK, Barranco SC. The response of human lymphoma cells in vitro to bleomycin and 1,3-bis (2-chloroethyl)-1-nitrosourea. Cancer Res 1972;32:1206–1208.

38. Matsushima Y, Kanzawa F, Hoshi A, et al. Time-schedule dependency of the inhibiting activity of various anticancer drugs in the clonogenic assay. Cancer Chemother Pharmacol 1985;14:104–107.

39. Sikic BI, Collins JM, Mimnaugh EG, Gram TE.

Improved therapeutic index of bleomycin when administered by continuous infusion in mice. Cancer Treat Rep 1978;2011–2017.

40. Peng Y-M, Alberts DS, Chen H-SG, Mason N, Moon TE. Antitumor activity and plasma kinetics of bleomycin by continuous and intermittent administration. Br J Cancer 1980;41:644–647.

41. Osieka R, Glatte P, Schmidt C-G. Continuous infusion versus intermittent bolus injection of bleomycin in a human embryonal testicular cancer xenograft. Cancer Treat Rep 1984;68:799–801.

42. Broughton A, Strong JE, Holoye PY, Bedrossian CWM. Clinical pharmacology of bleomycin following intravenous infusion as determined by radioimmunoassay. Cancer 1977;40:2772–2778.

43. Harvey VJ, Slevin ML, Aherne GW, Littleton P, Johnston A, Wrigley PFM. Subcutaneous infusion of bleomycin—a practical alternative to intravenous infusion. J Clin Oncol 1987;5:648–650.

44. Krakoff IH, Cvitkovic E, Currie V, Yeh S, LaMonte C. Clinical pharmacologic and therapeutic studies of bleomycin given by continuous infusion. Cancer 1977;40:2027–2037.

45. Cooper KR, Hong WK. Prospective study of the pulmonary toxicity of continuously infused bleomycin. Cancer Treat Rep 1981;65:419–425.

46. Baker LH, Opipari MI, Wilson H, Bottomley R, Coltman CA Jr. Mitomycin C, vincristine, and bleomycin therapy for advanced cervical cancer. Obstet Gynecol 1978;52:146–150.

47. Jensen JL, Goel R, Venner PM. The effect of corticosteroid administration on bleomycin lung toxicity. Cancer 1990;65:1291–1297.

48. Haskell CM, Sullivan A. Comparative survival in tissue culture of normal and neoplastic human cells exposed to Adriamycin. Cancer Res 1974;34:2991–2994.

49. Eichholtz-Wirth H. Dependence of the cytostatic effect of Adriamycin on drug concentration and exposure time in vitro. Br J Cancer 1980;41:886–891.

50. Pacciarini MA, Barbieri B, Colombo T, et al. Distribution and antitumor activity of Adriamycin given in a high-dose and a repeated low-dose schedule to mice. Cancer Treat Rep 1978;62:791–800.

51. Goldin A, Johnson RK. Experimental tumor activity of Adriamycin (NSC-123127). Cancer Chemother Rep 1975;6:137–145.

52. Solcia E, Ballerini L, Bellini O, et al. Cardiomyopathy of doxorubicin in experimental animals. Factors affecting the severity, distribution and evolution of myocardial lesions. Tumori 1981;67:461–472.

53. Weiss AJ, Metter GE, Fletcher WS, Wilson WL, Grage TB, Ramirez G. Studies on Adriamycin using a weekly regimen demonstrating its clinical effectiveness and lack of cardiac toxicity. Cancer Treat Rep 1976;60:813–822.

54. Weiss AJ, Manthel RW. Experience with the use of Adriamycin in combination with other anticancer agents using a weekly schedule, with particular reference to lack of cardiac toxicity. Cancer 1977;40:2046–2052.

55. Creech RH, Catalano RB, Shah MK. An effective low-dose Adriamycin regimen as secondary chemotherapy for metastatic breast cancer patients. Cancer 1980;46:433–437.

56. Chlebowski RT, Paroly WS, Pugh RP, et al. Adriamycin given as a weekly schedule without a loading course: clinically effective with reduced incidence of cardiotoxicity. Cancer Treat Rep 1980;64:47–51.

57. Torti FM, Aston D, Lum BL, et al. Weekly doxorubicin in endocrine-refractory carcinoma of the prostate. J Clin Oncol 1983;1:477–482.

58. Von Hoff DD, Layard MW, Basa P, et al. Risk factors for doxorubicin-induced congestive heart failure. Ann Intern Med 1979;91:710–717.

59. Torti FM, Bristow MR, Howes AE, et al. Reduced cardiotoxicity of doxorubicin delivered on a weekly schedule: assessment by endomyocardial biopsy. Ann Intern Med 1983;99:745–749.

60. Valdivieso M, Burgess MA, Ewer MS, et al. Increased therapeutic index of weekly doxorubicin in the therapy of non-small cell lung cancer: a prospective, randomized study. J Clin Oncol 1984;2:207–214.

61. Legha SS, Benjamin RS, MacKay B, et al. Reduction of doxorubicin cardiotoxicity by prolonged continuous intravenous infusion. Ann Intern Med 1982;96:133–139.

62. Garnick MB, Weiss GR, Steele GD Jr, et al. Clinical evaluation of long-term, continuous-infusion doxorubicin. Cancer Treat Rep 1983;67:133–142.

63. Speyer JL, Green MD, Dubin N, et al. Prospective evaluation of cardiotoxicity during a six-hour doxorubicin infusion regimen in women with adenocarcinoma of the breast. Am J Med 1985;78:555–563.

64. Shapira J, Gotfried M, Lishner M, Ravid M. Reduced cardiotoxicity of doxorubicin by a 6-hour infusion regimen: a prospective randomized evaluation. Cancer 1990;65:870–873.

65. Hortobagyi GN, Frye D, Buzdar AU, et al. Decreased cardiac toxicity of doxorubicin administered by continuous intravenous infusion in combination chemotherapy for metastatic breast carcinoma. Cancer 1989;63:37–45.

66. Lokich J, Bothe A, Zipoli T, et al. Constant infusion schedule for Adriamycin: a phase I–II clinical trial of a 30-day schedule by ambulatory pump delivery system. J Clin Oncol 1983;1:24–28.

67. Samuels BL, Vogelzang NJ, Ruane M, Simon MA. Continuous venous infusion of doxorubicin in advanced sarcomas. Cancer Treat Rep 1987;71:971–972.

68. Fraile RJ, Baker LH, Buroker TR, Horwitz J, Vaitkevicius VK. Pharmacokinetics of 5-fluorouracil administered orally, by rapid intravenous and by slow infusion. Cancer Res 1980;40:2223–2228.

69. Fleming RA, Milano GA, Etienne M-C, et al. No effect of dose, hepatic function, or nutritional status on 5-FU clearance following continuous (5-day), 5-FU infusion. Br J Cancer 1992;66:668–672.

70. Etienne MC, Milano G, Lagrange JL, et al. Marked fluctuations in drug plasma concentrations caused by use of portable pumps for fluorouracil continuous infusion. J Natl Cancer Inst 1993;12:1005–1007.

71. Metzger G, Massari C, Etienne M-C, et al. Spontaneous or imposed circadian changes in plasma concentrations of 5-fluorouracil coadministered with folinic acid and oxaliplatin: relationship with mucosal toxicity in patients with cancer. Clin Pharmacol Ther 1994;56:190–201.

72. Thiberville L, Compagnon P, Moore N, et al. Plasma 5-fluorouracil and α-fluoro-β-alanine accumulation in lung cancer patients treated with continuous infusion of cisplatin and 5-fluorouracil. Cancer Chemother Pharmacol 1994;35:64–70.

73. Moertel CG, Schutt AJ, Reitemeier RJ, Hahn

RG. A comparison of 5-fluorouracil administered by slow infusion and rapid injection. Cancer Res 1972; 32:2717–2719.

74. Hill GJ II, Grage TB, Wilson W, Ansfield FJ. 5-Fluorouracil intravenous infusion for 48 hours, repeated every two weeks. J Surg Oncol 1972;4:60–70.

75. Sullivan RD, Young CW, Miller E, Glatstein N, Clarkson B, Burchenal JH. The clinical effects of the continuous administration of fluorinated pyrimidines (5-fluorouracil and 5-fluoro-2'-deoxyuridine). Cancer Chemother Rep 1960;8:77–83.

76. Lemon HM. Reduction of 5-fluorouracil toxicity in man with retention of anticancer effects by prolonged intravenous administration in 5% dextrose. Cancer Chemother Rep 1960;8:97–101.

77. Reitemeier RJ, Moertel CG. Comparison of rapid and slow intravenous administration of 5-fluorouracil in treating patients with advanced carcinoma of the large intestine. Cancer Chemother Rep 1962; 25:87–89.

78. Staley CJ, Hart JT, Van Hagen F, Preston FW. Various methods of administering 5-fluorouracil. Cancer Chemother Rep 1962;20:107–112.

79. Hartman HA Jr, Kessinger A, Lemon HM, Foley JF. Five-day continuous infusion of 5-fluorouracil for advanced colorectal, gastric, and pancreatic adenocarcinoma. J Surg Oncol 1979;11:227–238.

80. Hum GJ, Bateman JR. 5-Day iv infusion with 5-fluorouracil (5-FU; NSC-19893) for gastroenteric carcinoma after failure on weekly 5-FU therapy. Cancer Chemother Rep 1975;59:1177–1179.

81. Seifert P, Baker LH, Reed ML, Vaitkevicius VK. Comparison of continuously infused 5-fluorouracil with bolus injection in treatment of patients with colorectal adenocarcinoma. Cancer 1975;36:123–128.

82. Lokich J, Bothe A, Fine N, Perri J. Phase I study of protracted venous infusion of 5-fluorouracil. Cancer 1981;48:2565–2568.

83. Spicer DV, Ardalan B, Daniels JR, Silberman H, Johnson K. Reevaluation of the maximum tolerated dose of continuous venous infusion of 5-fluorouracil with pharmacokinetics. Cancer Res 1988;48:459–461.

84. Spiers ASD, Kasimis BS, Janis MG. High-dose intravenous infusions of 5-fluorouracil for refractory solid tumors—the HI-FU regimen. Clin Oncol 1980; 6:63–69.

85. Ardalan B, Singh G, Silberman H. A randomized phase I and II study of short-term infusion of high-dose fluorouracil with or without N-(phosphonacetyl)-L-aspartic acid in patients with advanced pancreatic and colorectal cancers. J Clin Oncol 1988; 6:1053–1058.

86. Diaz-Rubio E, Aranda E, Martin M, Gonzalez-Mancha R, Gonzalez-Larriba J, Barneto I. Weekly high-dose infusion of 5-fluorouracil in advanced colorectal cancer. Eur J Cancer 1990;26:727–729.

87. Lokich JJ, Moore C. Chemotherapy-associated palmar-plantar erythrodysesthesia syndrome. Ann Intern Med 1984;101:798–800.

88. de Forni M, Malet-Martino MC, Jaillais P, et al. Cardiotoxicity of high-dose continuous infusion fluorouracil: a prospective clinical study. J Clin Oncol 1992; 10:1795–1801.

89. Hansen R, Quebbeman E, Ausman R, et al. Continuous systemic 5-fluorouracil infusion in advanced colorectal cancer: results in 91 patients. J Surg Oncol 1989;40:177–181.

90. Lokich JJ, Perri J, Bothe A, et al. Cancer chemotherapy via ambulatory infusion pump. Am J Clin Oncol 1983;6:355–363.

91. Rougier PD, Ammarguellat H, Ghosn M, et al. Phase II trial of 7-day continuous 5-fluorouracil infusion in the treatment of advanced colorectal carcinoma. Oncology 1992;49:35–39.

92. Huan S, Pazdur R, Singhakowinta A, Samal B, Vaitkevicius VK. Low-dose continuous infusion 5-fluorouracil: evaluation in advanced breast carcinoma. Cancer 1989;63:419–422.

93. Hansen R, Quebbeman E, Beatty P, et al. Continuous 5-fluorouracil infusion in refractory carcinoma of the breast. Breast Cancer Res Treat 1987;10:145–149.

94. Goodman HM, Dottino PR, Kredenster D, Mark M, Runowicz C, Cohen CJ. Continuous infusion fluoropyrimidines as salvage therapy for patients with advanced ovarian carcinoma. Gynecol Oncol 1988; 29:348–355.

95. Lokich JJ, Ahlgren JD, Gullo JJ, Philips JA, Fryer JG. A prospective randomized comparison of continuous infusion fluorouracil with a conventional bolus schedule in metastatic colorectal carcinoma: a Mid-Atlantic Oncology Program study. J Clin Oncol 1989; 7:425–432.

96. Greco FA, Richardson RL, Shulman SF, Oldham RK. Combination of constant-infusion 5-fluorouracil, methyl-CCNU, mitomycin C, and vincristine in advanced colorectal carcinoma. Cancer Treat Rep 1978; 62:1407–1408.

97. Kane RC, Cashdollar MR, Bernath AM. Treatment of advanced colorectal cancer with methyl-CCNU plus 5-day 5-fluorouracil infusion. Cancer Treat Rep 1978;62:1521–1525.

98. Bedikian AY, Staab R, Livingston R, Valdivieso M, Burgess MA, Bodey GP. Chemotherapy for colorectal cancer with 5-fluorouracil, cyclophosphamide, and CCNU: comparison of oral and continuous iv administration of 5-fluorouracil. Cancer Treat Rep 1978; 62:1603–1605.

99. Buroker T, Kim PN, Groope C, et al. 5-FU infusion with mitomycin-C versus 5-FU infusion with methyl-CCNU in the treatment of advanced colon cancer: a Southwest Oncology Group study. Cancer 1978; 42:1228–1233.

100. Buroker T, Kim PN, Groppe C, et al. 5-FU infusion with mitomycin-C vs. 5-FU infusion with methyl-CCNU in the treatment of advanced upper gastrointestinal cancer: a Southwest Oncology Group study. Cancer 1979;44:1215–1221.

101. Kemeny N, Israel K, Niedzwiecki D, et al. Randomized study of continuous infusion fluorouracil versus fluorouracil plus cisplatin in patients with metastatic colorectal cancer. J Clin Oncol 1990;8:313–318.

102. Izbicki RM, Baker LH, Samson MK, McDonald B, Vaitkevicius VK. 5-FU infusion and cyclophosphamide in the treatment of advanced ovarian cancer. Cancer Treat Rep 1977;61:1573–1575.

103. Abeloff MD, Beveridge RA, Donehower RC, et al. Sixteen-week dose-intense chemotherapy in the adjuvant treatment of breast cancer. J Natl Cancer Inst 1990;82:570–574.

104. Weiden PL, Einstein AB, Rudolph RH. Cisplatin bolus and 5-FU infusion chemotherapy for non-small cell lung cancer. Cancer Treat Rep 1985;69:1253–1255.

105. Kish JA, Wolf M, Crawford ED, et al. Evalu-

ation of low dose continuous infusion 5-fluorouracil in patients with advanced and recurrent renal cell carcinoma. Cancer 1994;74:916–919.

106. Kuzel TM, Tallman MS, Shevrin D, et al. A phase II study of continuous infusion 5-fluorouracil in advanced hormone refractory prostate cancer. An Illinois Cancer Center Study. Cancer 1993;72:1965–1968.

107. Coninx P, Nasca S, Lebrun D, et al. Sequential trial of initial chemotherapy for advanced cancer of the head and neck: DDP versus DDP + 5-fluorouracil. Cancer 1988;62:1888–1892.

108. Verweij J, de Long PC, de Mulder PHM, et al. Induction chemotherapy with cisplatin and continuous infusion 5-fluorouracil in locally far-advanced head and neck cancer. Am J Clin Oncol 1989;12:420–424.

109. Recondo G, Benhamed M, Cvitkovic E, Marandas P, Armand JP. 96-hour continuous infusion of cis-platinum, 5-fluorouracil and bleomycin in recurrent or metastatic head and neck squamous cell carcinoma, unexpected anemia. Eur J Cancer Clin Oncol 1989; 25:1529–1533.

110. Vokes EE, Schilsky RL, Choi KE, et al. A randomized study of inpatient versus outpatient continuous infusion chemotherapy for patients with locally advanced head and neck cancer. Cancer 1989;63:30–36.

111. Vokes EE, Panje WR, Mick R, et al. A randomized study comparing two regimens of neoadjuvant and adjuvant chemotherapy in multimodal therapy for locally advanced head and neck cancer. Cancer 1990; 66:206–213.

112. Dreyfuss AI, Clark JR, Wright JE, et al. Continuous infusion high-dose leucovorin with 5-fluorouracil and cisplatin for untreated stage IV carcinoma of the head and neck. Ann Intern Med 1990;112:167–172.

113. Fonseca E, Cruz JJ, Gomez A, et al. Neoadjuvant chemotherapy with cisplatin and 5-fluorouracil, both in continuous 96-hour infusion, in the treatment of locally advanced head and neck cancer. Am J Clin Oncol (CCT) 1994;17:6–9.

114. Jones SE, Mennel RG, Brooks B, et al. Phase II study of mitoxantrone, leucovorin, and infusional fluorouracil for treatment of metastatic breast cancer. J Clin Oncol 1991;9:1736–1739.

115. Hainsworth JD, Andrews MB, Johnson DH, Greco FA. Mitoxantrone, fluorouracil, and high-dose leucovorin: an effective, well-tolerated regimen for metastatic breast cancer. J Clin Oncol 1991;9:1731–1736.

116. Wils JA. Mitoxantrone, leucovorin and high-dose infusional 5-fluorouracil: an effective and well-tolerated regimen for the treatment of advanced breast cancer. Eur J Cancer 1993;29A:2106–2108.

117. Jackson DV Jr, Bender RA. Cytotoxic thresholds of vincristine in a murine and a human leukemia cell line in vivo. Cancer Res 1979;39:4346–4349.

118. Jackson DV Jr, Sethi VS, Spurr CL, et al. Intravenous vincristine infusion: phase I trial. Cancer 1981; 48:2559–2564.

119. Jackson DV Jr, Sethi VS, Spurr CL, et al. Pharmacokinetics of vincristine infusion. Cancer Treat Rep 1981;65:1043–1048.

120. Pinkerton CR, McDermott B, Philip T, et al. Continuous vincristine infusion as part of a high dose chemoradiotherapy regimen: drug kinetics and toxicity. Cancer Chemother Pharmacol 1988;22:271–274.

121. Jackson DV Jr, Paschold EH, Spurr CL, et al. Treatment of advanced non-Hodgkin's lymphoma with vincristine infusion. Cancer 1984;53:2601–2606.

122. Hopkins JO, Jackson DV Jr, White DR, et al. Vincristine by continuous infusion in refractory breast cancer: a phase II study. Am J Clin Oncol 1983;6:529–532.

123. Yau JC, Yap Y-Y, Buzdar AU, Hortobagyi GN, Bodey GP, Blumenschein GR. A comparative randomized trial of vinca alkaloids in patients with metastatic breast carcinoma. Cancer 1985;55:337–340.

124. Jackson DV, White DR, Spurr CL, et al. Moderate-dose vincristine infusion in refractory breast cancer. Am J Clin Oncol 1986;9:376–378.

125. Jackson DV Jr, Jobson VW, Homesley HD, et al. Vincristine infusion in refractory gynecologic malignancies. Gynecol Oncol 1986;25:212–216.

126. Barlogie B, Smith L, Alexanian R. Effective treatment of advanced multiple myeloma refractory to alkylating agents. N Engl J Med 1984;310:1353–1356.

127. Barlogie B, Alexanian R. Therapy of primary resistant and relapsed multiple myeloma. Onkologie 1986;9:210–214.

128. Walters RS, Kantarjian HM, Keating MJ, et al. Therapy of lymphoid and undifferentiated chronic myelogenous leukemia in blast crisis with continuous vincristine and Adriamycin infusions plus high-dose decadron. Cancer 1987;60:1708–1712.

129. Liso V, Specchia G, Pavone V, Capalbo S, Dione R. Continuous infusion chemotherapy with epirubicin and vincristine in relapsed and refractory acute leukemia. Acta Haematol 1990;83:116–119.

130. Stenzinger W, Blömker A, Hiddemann W, van de Loo J. Treatment of refractory multiple myeloma with the vincristine-Adriamycin-dexamethasone (VAD) regimen. Blut 1990;61:55–59.

131. Yap H-Y, Blumenschein GR, Keating MJ, Hortobagyi GN, Tashima CK, Loo TL. Vinblastine given as a continuous 5-day infusion in the treatment of refractory advanced breast cancer. Cancer Treat Rep 1980;64:279–283.

132. Young JA, Howell SB, Green MR. Pharmacokinetics and toxicity of 5-day continuous infusion of vinblastine. Cancer Chemother Pharmacol 1984;12:43–45.

133. Ratain MJ, Vogelzang NJ. Phase I and pharmacological study of vinblastine by prolonged continuous infusion. Cancer Res 1986;46:4827–4830.

134. Fraschini G, Yap H-Y, Hortobagyi GN, Buzdar A, Blumenschein G. Five-day continuous-infusion vinblastine in the treatment of breast cancer. Cancer 1985; 56:225–229.

135. Lu K, Yap H-Y, Loo TL. Clinical pharmacokinetics of vinblastine by continuous intravenous infusion. Cancer Res 1983;43:1405–1408.

136. Tannock I, Erlichman C, Perrault D, Quirt I, King M. Failure of 5-day vinblastine infusion in the treatment of patients with advanced refractory breast cancer. Cancer Treat Rep 1982;66:1783–1784.

137. Ingle JN, Ahmann DL, Gerstner JG, Green SJ, O'Connell MJ, Kvols LK. Evaluation of vinblastine administered by 5-day continuous infusion in women with advanced breast cancer. Cancer Treat Rep 1984; 68:803–804.

138. Kuebler JP, Hogan TF, Trump DL, Bryan GT. Phase II study of continuous 5-day vinblastine infusion

in renal adenocarcinoma. Cancer Treat Rep 1984; 68:925–926.

139. Crivellari D, Tumolo S, Frustaci S, et al. Phase II study of five-day continuous infusion of vinblastine in patients with metastatic renal-cell carcinoma. Am J Clin Oncol 1987;10:231–233.

140. Thigpen JT, Kronmal R, Vogel S, et al. A phase II trial of vinblastine in patients with advanced or recurrent endometrial carcinoma: a Southwest Oncology Group study. Am J Clin Oncol 1987;10:429–431.

141. Surwitt EA, Alberts DS, O'Toole RV, et al. Phase II trial of vinblastine in previously treated patients with ovarian cancer: a Southwest Oncology Group study. Gynecol Oncol 1987;27:214–219.

142. Dexeus F, Logothetis CJ, Samuels ML, Hossan E, von Eschenbach AC. Continuous infusion of vinblastine for advanced hormone-refractory prostate cancer. Cancer Treat Rep 1985;69:885–886.

143. Kavanagh JJ, Copeland LJ, Gershenson DM, Saul PB, Wharton JT, Rutledge FN. Continuous-infusion vinblastine in refractory carcinoma of the cervix: a phase II trial. Gynecol Oncol 1985;21:211–214.

144. Jackson DV Jr, Spurr CL, Caponera ME, et al. Vinblastine infusion in non-Hodgkin's lymphomas: lack of total cross-resistance with vincristine. Cancer Invest 1987;5:535–539.

145. Von Hoff DD, Goodman PJ, Presant CA, et al. A phase II trial of continuous infusion vinblastine in patients with gastric carcinoma: a Southwest Oncology Group study. Eur J Cancer 1990;26:405–407.

146. Yap B-S, Benjamin RS, Plager C, Burgess MA, Papadoupoulos N, Bodey GP. A randomized study of continuous infusion vindesine versus vinblastine in adults with refractory metastatic sarcomas. Am J Clin Oncol 1983;6:235–238.

147. Kavanagh JJ, Wharton JT, Rutledge FN. Continuous-infusion vinblastine for treatment of refractory epithelial carcinoma of the ovary: a phase II trial. Cancer Treat Rep 1984;68:1417–1418.

148. Kavanagh JJ, Saul PB, Wharton JT, Rutledge FN. A trial of continuous-infusion vinblastine in refractory endometrial adenocarcinoma. Gynecol Oncol 1987;26:236–239.

149. Trump DL, Ravdin PM, Boden EC, Magers CF, Whisnant JK. Interferon-α-n1 and continuous infusion vinblastine for treatment of advanced renal cell carcinoma. J Biol Response Mod 1990;9:108–111.

150. Tannir N, Yap H-Y, Hrotobagyi GH, Hug V, Buzdar AU, Blumenschein GR. Sequential continuous infusion with doxorubicin and vinblastine: an effective chemotherapy combination for patients with advanced breast cancer previously treated with cyclophosphamide, methotrexate, 5-FU, vincristine, and prednisone. Cancer Treat Rep 1984;68:1039–1041.

151. Fraschini G, Holmes FA, Buzdar AU, Hug V, Hortobagyi GN. Cisplatin in combination with continuous infusion vinblastine for refractory breast cancer. Am J Clin Oncol 1988;11:448–450.

152. Drewinko B, Brown BW, Gottlieb JA. The effect of cis-diamminedichloroplatinum (II) on cultured human lymphoma cells and its therapeutic implications. Cancer Res 1973;33:3091–3095.

153. Bergerat JP, Barlogie B, Drewinko B. Effects of cis-dichlorodiamminoplatinum (II) on human colon carcinoma cells in vitro. Cancer Res 1979;39:1334–1338.

154. Forastiere AA, Belliveau JF, Goren MP, Vogel WC, Posner MR, O'Leary GP Jr. Pharmacokinetic and toxicity evaluation of five-day continuous infusion versus intermittent bolus cis-diamminedichloroplatinum (II) in head and neck cancer patients. Cancer Res 1988; 48:3869–3874.

155. Jacobs C, Bertino JR, Goffinet DR, Fee WE, Goode RL. 24-hour infusion of cis-platinum in head and neck cancers. Cancer 1978;42:2135–2140.

156. Bozzino JM, Prasas V, Koriech OM. Avoidance of renal toxicity by 24-hour infusion of cisplatin. Cancer Treat Rep 1981;65:351–352.

157. Thigpen JT, Blessing JA, DiSaia PJ, Fowler WC Jr, Hatch KD. A randomized comparison of a rapid versus prolonged (24 hr) infusion of cisplatin in therapy of squamous cell carcinoma of the uterine cervix: a Gynecologic Oncology Group study. Gynecol Oncol 1989;32:198–202.

158. Salem P, Hall SW, Benjamin RS, Murphy WK, Wharton JT, Bodey GP. Clinical phase I-II study of cis-dichlorodiammineplatinum (II) given by continuous iv infusion. Cancer Treat Rep 1978;62:1553–1555.

159. Yap H-Y, Salem P, Hortobagyi GN, et al. Phase II study of cis-dichlorodiammineplatinum (II) in advanced breast cancer. Cancer Treat Rep 1978;62:405–408.

160. Lokich JJ. Phase I study of cis-diamminedichloroplatinum (II) administered as a constant 5-day infusion. Cancer Treat Rep 1980;64:905–908.

161. Salem P, Khalyl M, Jabboury K, Hashimi L. Cis-diamminedichloroplatinum (II) by 5-day continuous infusion: a new dose schedule with minimal toxicity. Cancer 1984;53:837–840.

162. Benahmed M, Renaux J, Spielman M, Rouesse J. Cis platine (CDDP) in continuous intravenous ambulatory infusion: a new method of administration. Cancer Drug Delivery 1986;3:183–188.

163. Posner MR, Skarin AT, Clark J, Ervin TJ. Phase I study of continuous-infusion cisplatin. Cancer Treat Rep 1986;70:847–850.

164. Posner MR, Ferrari L, Belliveau JF, et al. A phase I study of continuous-infusion cisplatin. Cancer Treat Rep 1987;59:15–18.

165. Sebille A, St-Guily JL, Angelard B, de Stabenrath A. Low prevalence of cisplatin-induced neuropathy after 4-day continuous infusion in head and neck cancer. Cancer 1990;65:2644–2647.

166. Lokich JJ, Zipoli TE. Phase-I study of protracted infusion of cisplatin. Cancer Drug Delivery 1984;1:247–250.

167. Posner MR, Belliveau JF, Weitberg AB, et al. Continuous-infusion cisplatin and bolus 5-fluorouracil in colorectal carcinoma. Cancer Treat Rep 1987;71:975–977.

168. Creagan ET, Richardson RL, Kovach JS. Pilot study of a continuous five-day intravenous infusion of etoposide concomitant with cisplatin in selected patients with advanced cancer. J Clin Oncol 1988;6:1197–1201.

169. Choksi AJ, Hong WK, Dimery IW, James P, Guillamondegui OM, Byers RM. Continuous cisplatin (24-hour) and 5-fluorouracil (120-hour) infusion in recurrent head and neck squamous cell carcinoma. Cancer 1988;61:909–912.

170. Lokich J, Anderson N, Bern M, Wallach S, Moore C, Williams D. Etoposide admixed with cisplatin: phase I clinical investigation of 72-hour infusion. Cancer 1989;63:818–821.

171. Kemeny N, Niedzwiecki D, Reichmaan B, et

al. Cisplatin and 5-fluorouracil infusion for metastatic colorectal carcinoma: differences in survival in two patient groups with similar response rates. Cancer 1989; 63:1065–1069.

172. LoRusso P, Pazdur R, Redman BG, Kinzie J, Vaitkevicius V. Low-dose continuous infusion 5-fluorouracil and cisplatin: phase II evaluation in advanced colorectal carcinoma. Am J Clin Oncol 1989;12:486–490.

173. Posner M, Slapak CA, Browne MJ, et al. A phase I–II trial of continuous-infusion cisplatin, continuous-infusion 5-fluorouracil, and VP-16 in colorectal carcinoma. Am J Clin Oncol 1990;13:455–458.

174. Saito K, Kiyoshi M, Keigo T, Kouhei Y, Miyazawa N. Phase II study of cisplatin as a 5-day continuous infusion with vindesine plus recombinant human granulocyte-colony-stimulating factor in the treatment of advanced non-small-cell lung cancer. Cancer Chemother Pharmacol 1992;31:81–84.

175. Dombernowsky P, Nissen NI. Schedule dependency of the antileukemic activity of the podophyllotoxin-derivative VP 16-213 (NCS-141540) in L1210 leukemia. Acta Pathol Microbiol Scand 1973; 81:715–724.

176. Wolff SN, Grosh WW, Prater K, Hande KR. In vitro pharmacodynamic evaluation of VP-16-213 and implications for chemotherapy. Cancer Chemother Pharmacol 1987;19:246–249.

177. Lokich J, Corkery J. Phase I study of VP-16-213 (etoposide) administered as a continuous 5-day infusion. Cancer Treat Rep 1981;65:887–889.

178. Aisner J, Van Echo DA, Whitacre M, Wiernik PH. A phase I trial of continuous infusion VP 16-213 (etoposide). Cancer Chemother Pharmacol 1982;7:157–160.

179. Bennett CL, Sinkule JA, Schilsky RL, Senekjian E, Choi KE. Phase I clinical and pharmacological study of 72-hour continuous infusion of etoposide in patients with advanced cancer. Cancer Res 1987;47:1952–1956.

180. Minami H, Shimokata K, Saka H, et al. Phase I clinical and pharmacokinetic study of a 14-day infusion of etoposide in patients with lung cancer. J Clin Oncol 1993;11:1602–1608.

181. Thompson DS, Hainsworth JD, Hande KR, Holzmer M, Greco FA. Prolonged administration of low dose infusional etoposide in patients with advanced malignancies. Cancer 1994;73:2824–2831.

182. Kunitoh H, Watanabe K. Phase I/II and pharmacologic study of long-term continuous infusion etoposide combined with cisplatin in patients with advanced non-small-cell lung cancer. J Clin Oncol 1994; 12:83–89.

183. Cavalli F, Sonntag RW, Jungi F, Senn HJ, Brunner KW. VP-16-213 monotherapy for remission induction of small cell lung cancer: a randomized trial using three dosage schedules. Cancer Treat Rep 1978; 62:473–475.

184. Slevin ML, Clark PI, Joel SP, et al. A randomized trial to evaluate the effect of schedule on the activity of etoposide in small-cell lung cancer. J Clin Oncol 1989;7:1333–1340.

185. Clark PI, Slevin ML, Joel SP, et al. A randomized trial of two etoposide schedules in small-cell lung cancer: influence of pharmacokinetics on efficacy and toxicity. J Clin Oncol 1994;12:1427–1435.

186. Mead GM, Thompson J, Sweetenham JW, Buchanan RB, Whitehouse JMA, Williams CJ. Extensive stage small cell carcinoma of the bronchus: a randomised study of etoposide given orally by one-day or five-day schedule together with intravenous Adriamycin and cyclophosphamide. Cancer Chemother Pharmacol 1987;19:172–174.

187. Schell FC, Yap HY, Hortobagyi GN, Issell B, Esparza L. Phase II study of VP16-213 (etoposide) in refractory metastatic breast carcinoma. Cancer Chemother Pharmacol 1982;7:223–225.

188. Krook JE, Loprinzi CL, Schaid DJ, et al. Evaluation of the continuous infusion of etoposide plus cisplatin in metastatic breast cancer: a collaborative North Central Cancer Treatment Group/Mayo Clinic phase II study. Cancer 1990;65:418–421.

189. Bleyer WA. Methotrexate: clinical pharmacology, current status and therapeutic guidelines. Cancer Treat Rev 1977;4:87–101.

190. Stoller RG, Hande KR, Jacobs SA, Rosenberg SA, Chabner BA. Use of plasma pharmacokinetics to predict and prevent methotrexate toxicity. N Engl J Med 1977;297:630–634.

191. Pinedo HM, Chabner BA. Role of drug concentration, duration of exposure, and endogenous metabolites in determining methotrexate cytotoxicity. Cancer Treat Rep 1977;61:709–715.

192. Eichholtz H, Trott K-R. Effect of methotrexate concentration and exposure time on mammalian cell survival in vitro. Br J Cancer 1980;41:277–284.

193. Levitt M, Mosher MB, DeConti RC, et al. Improved therapeutic index of methotrexate with "leucovorin rescue." Cancer Res 1973;33:1729–1734.

194. Djerassi I, Farber S, Abir E, Neikirk W. Continuous infusion of methotrexate in children with acute leukemia. Cancer 1967;20:233–242.

195. Liguori VR, Giglio JJ, Miller E, Sullivan RD. Effects of different dose schedules of amethopterin on serum and tissue concentrations and urinary excretion patterns. Clin Pharmacol Ther 1962;3:34–40.

196. Shapiro WR, Young DF, Mehta BM. Methotrexate: distribution in cerebrospinal fluid after intravenous, ventricular and lumbar injections. N Engl J Med 1975;293:161–166.

197. Thyss A, Milano G, Deville A, Manassero J, Renee N, Schneider M. Effect of dose and repeat intravenous 24 hr infusions of methotrexate on cerebrospinal fluid availability in children with hematological malignancies. Eur J Cancer Clin Oncol 1987;23:843–847.

198. Djerassi I, Rominger CJ, Kim JS, Turchi J, Suvansri U, Hughes D. Phase I study of high doses of methotrexate with citrovorum factor in patients with lung cancer. Cancer 1972;30:22–30.

199. Cohen HJ, Jaffe N. Pharmacokinetic and clinical studies of 1–4-h infusions of high-dose methotrexate. Cancer Chemother Pharmacol 1978;1:61–64.

200. Pitman SW, Parker LM, Tattersall MHN, Jaffe N, Frei E III. Clinical trial of high-dose methotrexate (NSC-740) with citrovorum factor (NSC-3590)—toxicologic and therapeutic observations. Cancer Chemother Rep 1975;6(Part 3):43–49.

201. Mitchell MS, Wawro NW, DeConti RC, Kaplan SR, Papac R, Bertino JR. Effectiveness of high-dose infusions of methotrexate followed by leucovorin in carcinoma of the head and neck. Cancer Res 1968; 28:1088–1094.

202. Taylor SG IV, McGuire WP, Hauck WW, Showel JL, Lad TE. A randomized comparison of high-dose infusion methotrexate versus standard-dose weekly therapy in head and neck squamous cancer. J Clin Oncol 1984;2:1006–1011.

203. Vogler WR, Jacobs J, Moffitt S, et al. Methotrexate therapy with or without citrovorum factor in carcinoma of the head and neck, breast, and colon. Cancer Clin Trials 1979;2:227–236.

204. DeConti RC, Schoenfeld D. A randomized prospective comparison of intermittent methotrexate, methotrexate with leucovorin, and a methotrexate combination in head and neck cancer. Cancer 1981; 48:1061–1072.

205. Woods RL, Fox RM, Tatersall MHN. Methotrexate treatment of advanced head and neck cancers: a dose response evaluation. Cancer Treat Rep 1981; 65(Suppl 1):155–159.

206. Djerassi I, Abir E, Royer GL Jr, Treat CL. Long-term remissions in childhood acute leukemia: use of infrequent infusions of methotrexate; supportive roles of platelet transfusions and citrovorum factor. Clin Pediatr 1966;5:502–509.

207. Evans WE, Crom WR, Abromowitch M, et al. Clinical pharmacodynamics of high-dose methotrexate in acute lymphocytic leukemia: identification of a relation between concentration and effect. N Engl J Med 1986;314:471–477.

208. Lokich JJ, Curt G. A phase I and pharmacology study of continuous-infusion low-dose methotrexate administration. Cancer 1985;56:2391–2394.

209. Lokich JJ, Phillips D, Green R, et al. 5-Fluorouracil and methotrexate administered simultaneously as a continuous infusion: a phase I study. Cancer 1985; 56:2395–2398.

210. Lokich J, Bern M, Anderson N, et al. Cyclophosphamide, methotrexate, and 5-fluorouracil in a three-drug admixture: a phase I trial of 14-day continuous ambulatory infusion. Cancer 1989;63:822–824.

211. Arbuck SG, Canetta R, Onetto N, Christian MC. Current dosage and schedule issues in the development of paclitaxel (Taxol). Semin Oncol 1993; 20(Suppl 3):31–39.

212. Lopes NM, Adams EG, Pitts TW, Bhuyan BK. Cell kill kinetics and cell cycle effects of taxol on human and hamster ovarian cell lines. Cancer Chemother Pharmacol 1993;32:235–242.

213. Rose WC, Crosswell AR, Casazza AM. Preclinical antitumor evaluation of taxol (abstract). Proc Am Assoc Cancer Res 1992;33:518.

214. Beijnen JH, Huizing MT, ten Bokkel Huinink WW, et al. Bioanalysis, pharmacokinetics and pharmacodynamics of the novel anticancer drug paclitaxel (Taxol). Semin Oncol 1994;21(Suppl 8):53–62.

215. Legha SS, Tenney DM, Irwin IR. Phase I study of taxol using a 5-day intermittent schedule. J Clin Oncol 1986;4:762–766.

216. Donehower RC, Rowinsky EK, Grochow LB, Longnecker SM, Ettinger DS. Phase I trial of taxol in patients with advanced cancer. Cancer Treat Rep 1987; 71:1171–1177.

217. Grem JL, Tutsch KD, Simon KJ, et al. Phase I study of taxol administered as a short iv infusion daily for 5 days. Cancer Treat Rep 1987;71:1179–1184.

218. Hainsworth JD, Greco FA. Paclitaxel administered by 1-hour infusion. Cancer 1994;74:1377–1382.

219. Kris MG, O'Connell JP, Gralla RJ, et al. Phase I trial of taxol given as a 3-hour infusion every 21 days. Cancer Treat Rep 1986;70:605–607.

220. Schiller JH, Storer B, Tutsch K, et al. Phase I trial of 3-hour infusion of paclitaxel with or without granulocyte colony-stimulating factor in patients with advanced cancer. J Clin Oncol 1994;12:241–248.

221. Brown T, Havlin K, Weiss G, et al. A phase I trial of taxol given by a 6-hour intravenous infusion. J Clin Oncol 1991;9:1261–1267.

222. Wiernik PH, Schwartz EL, Strauman JJ, Dutcher JP, Lipton RB, Paietta E. Phase I clinical and pharmacokinetic study of taxol. Cancer Res 1987; 47:2486–2493.

223. Wiernik PH, Schwartz EL, Einzig A, Strauman JJ, Lipton RB, Dutcher JP. Phase I trial of taxol given as a 24-hour infusion every 21 days: responses observed in metastatic melanoma. J Clin Oncol 1987; 5:1232–1239.

224. Sarosy G, Kohn E, Stone DA, et al. Phase I study of taxol and granulocyte colony-stimulating factor in patients with refractory ovarian cancer. J Clin Oncol 1992;10:1165–1170.

225. Hurwitz CA, Relling MV, Weitman SD, et al. Phase I trial of paclitaxel in children with refractory solid tumors: a Pediatric Oncology Group study. J Clin Oncol 1993;11:2324–2329.

226. Wilson WH, Berg S, Kang Y-K, et al. Phase I/II study of taxol 96-hour infusion in refractory lymphoma and breast cancer: pharmacodynamics and analysis of multi-drug resistance (mdr-1). Proc Am Soc Clin Oncol 1993;12:134.

227. Spriggs DR, Tondini C. Taxol administered as a 120 hour infusion. Invest New Drugs 1992;10:275–278.

228. Holmes FA, Valero V, Walters RS, et al. The M.D. Anderson Cancer Center experience with taxol in metastatic breast cancer. Monogr Natl Cancer Inst 1993;15:161–169.

229. Seidman AD, Norton L, Reichman BS, et al. Preliminary experience with paclitaxel (Taxol) plus recombinant human granulocyte colony-stimulating factor in the treatment of breast cancer. Semin Oncol 1993; 20(Suppl 3):40–45.

230. Wilson WH, Berg SL, Bryant G, et al. Paclitaxel in doxorubicin-refractory or mitoxantrone-refractory breast cancer: a phase I/II trial of 96-hour infusion. J Clin Oncol 1994;12:1621–1629.

231. Eisenhauer EA, ten Bokkel Huinink WW, Swenerton KD, et al. European-Canadian randomized trial of paclitaxel in relapsed ovarian cancer: high-dose versus low-dose and long versus short infusion. J Clin Oncol 1994;12:2654–2666.

232. Ohnuma T, Zimet AS, Coffey VA, Holland JF, Greenspan EM. Phase I study of taxol in a 24-hr infusion schedule (abstract). Proc Am Assoc Can Res 1985; 26:167.

16

Intraarterial Therapy

William D. Ensminger

The natural history of most solid tumors includes a period of confinement to a specific body region. Even with metastatic tumors, there may be one specific organ that is the primary (and sometimes sole) site of tumor growth and resultant morbidity and mortality. The limitation or concentration of metastases to a single or several organs has recently been highlighted as a clinically significant situation termed the "oligometastatic state" (1). Tumors generally induce a blood supply from the organ in which they grow; thus the arterial supply to such an organ provides direct access to the tumor. The objective of intraarterial therapy is to achieve increased tumor regression in the body region served by the artery infused relative to tumor regression possible with systemic intravenous therapies. Although decreased systemic toxicity is desirable, it is not the primary aim in most cases inasmuch as the dose is usually escalated to the maximum tolerated toxicity, whether regional or systemic. Decreased systemic toxicity is important, however, if one wants to add systemic therapy to intraarterial therapy without compromise of either. Factors influencing the achievement of the objective of intraarterial therapy are discussed below.

Surgical resection and radiotherapy share the same objective as intraarterial therapy. In most instances, these more conventional treatment modalities may compete for a segment of the patient population having regionally confined tumors. The constraints of these three regional treatment modalities are similar: inability to treat systemic disease in other organs, incomplete locoregional tumor eradication, and limiting regional tolerance. In patient populations where these are competing modalities, a comparative risk/benefit evaluation must take into consideration not only relative response rates, but also the degree to which the above constraints apply.

As described below, treatments combining intraarterial therapy with either surgical resection or radiotherapy have been applied to further regional tumor control.

REQUIREMENTS FOR SUCCESSFUL INTRAARTERIAL THERAPY

Anatomic Considerations

REGIONAL TUMOR CONFINEMENT

Several anatomic considerations bear on the appropriateness of intraarterial therapy. The first consideration is the necessity to have a regionally confined tumor. Thus, although the liver is frequently involved with metastatic lung cancer, breast cancer, and melanoma, these tumor types are almost uniformly systemic and involve other organs. Eradication of these tumors within the liver usually would have little benefit, as morbidity and mortality in other sites would quickly come to the fore. Although many patients with colorectal cancer metastatic to the liver seem to have metastases limited to the liver, effective control of the liver metastases allows time for other metastatic sites to develop and proliferate (2). Nonetheless, the fact that a minority of patients with three or less liver metastases from colorectal cancer can be cured with surgical resection suggests that the liver can sometimes be the only site of metastatic disease in this type of cancer (3). Such is not generally the case for lung cancer, breast cancer, and melanoma. Thus, regional tumor confinement is a major consideration in defining the potential benefit of intraarterial therapy.

TUMOR BLOOD SUPPLY

To obtain the benefits of intraarterial therapy, the tumor blood supply must be accessible and unique. It is obvious that agents must be given directly into the arterial supply feeding the tumor within an organ or body region. It is not sufficient, however, to assume that there is uniform distribution of an agent within the blood flowing through the artery into which the agent is injected or infused (4, 5). Streaming due to laminar flow can occur, leading to high concentrations of the therapeutic agent going into some tributaries of the artery being infused and negligible concentrations going into others. Tumors exposed to high concentrations of agent have the potential to respond, whereas others not being directly infused will not (6). Controversy exists as to the degree to which streaming within an artery in patients occurs and accounts for inhomogeneous tumor regression (5, 7).

A major problem in evaluating the confounding element of potential inhomogeneous flow of drug is the lack of agents that can be used to mimic the flow of the therapeutic agent. Flow rates of most intraarterial drug administrations are exceptionally low relative to those necessary in the use of radiographic contrast materials. Alternatively, the use of particulate tracer materials such as ^{99m}Tc-macroaggregated albumin (TcMAA), which can be administered slowly, may not faithfully reproduce flow patterns seen with soluble drugs. Thus, although TcMAA remains a useful agent with which to assess gross arterial flow distribution, its limitations include its particulate nature and a practical need to use flow rates greater than some drug infusion rates (which may be below 1 mL/day) (8, 9). When catheters are placed intraoperatively and the surface of the organ or area infused is directly observed, methylene blue or fluorescein can be used as a marker to document adequate flow throughout the organ or region (10).

In addition to ensuring flow to the tumor-bearing region, the tracer agents described above are important in preventing toxicity due to direct flow of the agent to other organs that may not be as tolerant as the target organ. A prime example of this role is in hepatic arterial chemotherapy where intraoperative methylene blue can be used to define the best catheter position and to facilitate the ligation of small vessels that branch off the hepatic artery and lead to the stomach and duodenum (10). Ligation of these small vessels can largely prevent gastric toxicity (10, 11). TcMAA can be used similarly with percutaneous angiographic catheter placement to define the best catheter position and provide guidance in the embolization/occlusion of vessels necessary to confine flow to the region desired (11, 12).

The distribution of tumor within the organ or region infused is an important consideration relative to the other two regional modalities, i.e., surgery and radiation. For example, whereas one to three hepatic tumor nodules in an accessible location might be excised readily, 25 small nodules throughout the liver would not be removable for cure but could be treated by intraarterial therapy. Similarly for external beam radiotherapy, where an isolated tumor or two might be effectively treated with refined dosimetry techniques, organ or regional tolerance might not allow enough dosage for radiotherapy alone to treat multiple, widely dispersed tumor nodules effectively (13). In this regard, comparison of the effectiveness of one regional modality with another must involve great care to make sure the disease processes being treated are similar. For example, patients having one to three resectable hepatic colorectal tumor metastases have a different intrinsic prognosis than those patients having 80% of their liver replaced by innumerable nodules of multifocal carcinoma (3).

DRUG DELIVERY MECHANISM

Arterial Access

RADIOLOGIC VERSUS SURGICAL CATHETER PLACEMENT

Intraarterial therapy requires a mechanism of access so that a therapeutic agent can be infused into the appropriate artery feeding the tumor confined to the specific body region (12). Short-term access (minutes to several weeks) is most conveniently achieved by using a plastic catheter percutaneously inserted into a major arm or leg artery with advancement and radiologic/fluoroscopic positioning of the tip into the appropriate regional artery to receive the therapeutic agent. The techniques involved in such catheter tip positioning and, initially, in defining the correct artery for infusion, fall within the domain of interventional angiography. For reasons outlined below, chronic arterial access (weeks to years) is usually achieved with surgically implanted silicone rubber catheters.

Three considerations are important in defining the ability to maintain arterial access. These are the stability of catheter tip position and the propensity for arterial thrombosis and infection. The mechanism of achieving access, radiologic versus surgical, and the associated catheter materials bear directly on these considerations.

As duration of access to the achieved increases, the three considerations above are increasingly influential in a corresponding shift from radiologic to surgical catheters. In the short run, radiologic catheters can be positioned precisely with minimal impact on the clinical state of the patient. The physiologic stress of surgical catheter placement is much greater. Radiologic catheter placement is generally considerably less costly than surgical catheter placement. Surgical catheters are usually connected to implanted access ports or pumps (see below), resulting in totally implanted systems that, once placed, are more acceptable to patients. Table 16.1 compares radiologic catheter placement with surgical catheter placement in terms of characteristics and advantages of each.

With percutaneously inserted, angiographically positioned catheters, there is rarely sufficient catheter tip stability to allow infusions beyond several weeks. One factor in catheter tip instability relates to catheter movement generated by motion of the insertion site. When the femoral artery is used, patients must refrain from walking, and such immobility carries the risk of deep venous thrombosis of leg veins. Insertion of angiographic catheters via the left brachial artery provides the safest route for protracted access in that patients remain mobile and right-handed patients can use their dominant arm. The left arm is preferable to the right because there is less risk of vertebral artery thrombosis or emboli, since the origin of the left vertebral artery is directly from the aorta.

Motion of the organ or body region being infused can lead to catheter tip displacement. For example, catheter tip motion occurs naturally with liver movement during diaphragmatic excursions with respiration. Movement of the he-patic artery so induced can lead to the tip migrating either distally or proximally in the artery. The position of the tip of surgically placed catheters relative to the artery being infused is generally defined at the time of operation, with the fixation site within several millimeters of the tip (11). For that reason, catheter tip migration is much less common, making surgical catheter placement the mechanism of choice for long-term intraarterial infusions. Even with surgically placed catheters, attention to the detailed arterial anatomy and the acquisition of sufficient surgical experience are prerequisites for a high success rate (14, 15).

THROMBOSIS

Thrombotic events influence arterial infusion in two ways. First, thrombosis of the vessel being infused removes the potential for further intraarterial therapy in most instances and may seriously compromise blood flow to the organ in question. For example, thrombosis of the internal carotid artery during a drug infusion of a brain tumor would be catastrophic. Second, clot formation on the catheter may lead to thrombotic emboli. Such emboli can cause strokes when they go to the brain (rare) and ischemia in the extremity bearing the insertion site (less rare) for percutaneously placed catheters. Thrombotic events bear a relationship to several factors, including intimal damage by the catheter tip, catheter material, area of the catheter exposed in the arterial stream, induction of turbulence by the catheter, duration of exposure to the catheter, and the thrombotic potential of the patient (which may be increased in some patients).

Intimal damage by the catheter tip occurs

Table 16.1. Comparative Characteristics of Radiologic versus Surgical Catheters

	Radiologic	Surgical
Catheter material	Polyethylene	Silicone rubber
Placement		
Trauma	Less	More
Cost	Less	More
Durability	Short (min-weeks)	Long (weeks-years)
Tip stability	Less	More
Arterial thrombosis	More likely	Less likely
Infections complications	More	Less
Pump used	Usually external	Usually implanted
Patient acceptance		
Convenience	Usually less	Usually more
Cosmetics	More noticeable	Less noticeable
Treatment location	In hospital	Outpatient

more frequently with radiologic catheters than with surgical catheters (11, 16). Polyethylene radiologic catheters are stiff, and the tip configuration and motion relative to the arterial wall is critical, with considerable potential for an angled tip to tear into the intima and lead to thrombosis. Radiologic catheters can cause arterial thrombosis at their percutaneous arterial insertion site, whereas surgically placed catheters cannot. Surgically placed silicone rubber catheters are much softer, and the tip is generally secured so that it does not abut into the arterial wall. In addition, lack of motion relative to the arterial wall (as is the case with surgically placed catheters) decreases the chance of intimal trauma. Essentially the entire length of the radiologic catheter (which may be 50 to 100 cm) is within the arterial system and rubbing on the arterial walls, whereas only 0.1 cm or so (the tip) of the surgical catheter is within the arterial flow. The potential for turbulence is variable and relates to catheter tip configuration relative to blood flow. It is difficult to evaluate turbulence in vivo. Turbulence that produces an increased chance of thrombosis and intimal damage would favorably influence drug mixing in the arterial flow (5). Comparative clinical data in controlled studies evaluating the intrinsic thrombogenic potential of polyethylene catheters versus silicone rubber catheters in intraarterial therapy are not available, although research continues on new catheter materials. The thrombotic potential of intraarterial therapy is certainly increased in some cancer patients, owing to a relative hypercoagulable state. Unfortunately, no easy test can evaluate the risk in a given patient.

One mechanism used to prevent arterial thrombosis is addition of low doses of heparin to the infusate. For radiologic catheters, constant infusion doses of 1000 to 5000 units of heparin per day can be used. With surgically placed catheters connected to subcutaneously placed infusion pumps, the standard dose rate is about 400 units per day, although 4000 units can be infused as well without induction of a bleeding diathesis. To further decrease the tendency for adverse thrombotic events during the use of radiologic catheters, for several years now we have administered a single enteric-coated aspirin per day to patients during their treatment and have had no adverse sequelae.

INFECTION

Considering the usual prolonged duration of use, intraarterial catheters have a low rate of infectious complications. Because radiologic catheters are percutaneously placed, there is a definite risk of infection, usually with *Staphylococcus aureus*, at the insertion site (16, 17). The risk of insertion site infection increases with the duration of radiologic catheter maintenance. Methods to prevent insertion site infection include strict aseptic technique in catheter placement and in dressing the site. We have had no insertion site infections in the last 300 patients treated with percutaneous catheters in whom oral antistaphylococcal agents (dicloxacillin, cephalexin, erythromycin) were administered prophylactically for the 7- to 14-day duration of catheter maintenance.

Surgically placed catheters are generally connected to subcutaneous devices (ports, pumps); these devices are intermittently or chronically accessed. Intermittent, short-term access, when conducted with sterile technique, is not associated with any appreciable infections risk. Infusion through a needle going into a subcutaneous port for 7 to 14 days carries a small risk of insertion site infection (18).

A second infectious risk is uniquely attributable to intraarterial therapy, namely, infection in the organ or region being infused. Tumor that is intrinsically necrotic or is made so by the treatment administered may be especially susceptible for bacterial growth. Thus, hepatic abscesses or even hepatic gas gangrene can be associated with hepatic arterial therapy (19). Cellulitis in head and neck cancer and in ulcerating tumors of the extremities may complicate regional therapy as well. Although intraarterial therapy may not be causal in a regional infection, the resultant bacteremia may seed the catheter, and catheter seeding may prevent effective antimicrobial treatment. With surgically implanted silicone rubber catheters, systemic antimicrobial therapy can often be successful without catheter removal. As a general principle, the threshold for institution of empiric broad-spectrum antibiotic coverage should be low in patients with indwelling intraarterial catheters, and treatment should take into consideration the potential infective etiologies operative in this setting.

Pumps

For cytokinetic and pharmacokinetic reasons (see below), many intraarterial therapy programs use protracted drug infusions requiring an infusion pump. There are two general types of infusion devices: external pumps and internal implanted pumps. All pumps applied to intra-arterial therapy must be able to work against arterial pressure dependably.

EXTERNAL PUMPS

There is a wide variety of commercially available external pumps, inasmuch as many of the devices used for intravenous infusions have sufficient pumping strength to work against arterial pressure (20, 21). For infusions in the hospital, larger pumps supported on wheeled i.v. stands are often used. These larger pumps generally have more built-in monitoring capabilities and can also infuse much larger fluid volumes. A number of smaller external pumps that are approximately wallet size can be used for intraarterial infusions, especially in outpatients. Outpatient intraarterial infusions with external pumps carry appreciable risks because of the likelihood of disruption of the continuity of the external tubing/catheter system, which is subject to arterial pressures. Such infusions should only be performed by experienced personnel in reliable, well-motivated patients who are cognizant of the risks of bleeding, infection, catheter migration (with radiologic catheters), extravasation (with infusion ports), and pump malfunction. The requirement for a team of support personnel to maintain intraarterial infusions and the intrinsic inconvenience and risks of the infusion systems restrict the widespread application of external devices to outpatient intraarterial therapy.

INTERNAL (IMPLANTED) PUMPS

The development of subcutaneously placed, totally implantable pumps attached to totally implanted, surgically placed silicone rubber catheters made it possible to more safely and reliably give chronic intraarterial infusions under defined conditions to many more patients (22, 23). The commercial availability of the Model 400 Infusaid pump in 1982 coupled with preliminary phase II data demonstrating response rates in the treatment of colorectal liver metastases of 70 to 80% provided the impetus for the implantation of some 20,000 pumps at over 1400 medical institutions worldwide (24). This totally implantable drug delivery system allowed patients to live relatively normal lives without the considerable inconvenience of external hardware. The safety and reliability of the implanted drug delivery system has proven to be more than adequate for the most hazardous of protracted intraarterial infusions, namely internal carotid

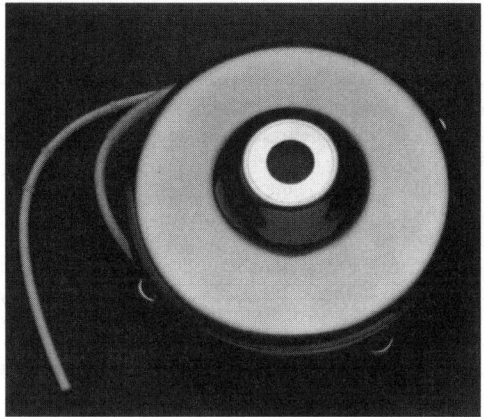

Figure 16.1.   Front view of second-generation implantable constant-rate infusion pump. (Photo courtesy of Therex Corporation.)

artery infusions for high-grade gliomas (25, 26). Individual patients have had implanted carotid arterial catheters and pumps for periods beyond 2 years. In addition, no embolic strokes have occurred in over 50 patients having such systems for chronic carotid arterial infusions.

There are two major categories of implantable pumps: those that deliver a constant flow rate and those that can be programed externally to deliver time-dependent flow rates. The Infusaid Model 400 pump, which has been commercially available for 13 years, represents the first generation of constant-flow devices. A second-generation constant-flow rate pump (Fig. 16.1), (Therex Corporation, Walpole, MA) is smaller and more streamlined in that the mechanism for direct catheter injection does not involve a protruding sideport as in the Model 400 Infusaid pump. Two programmable, variable-rate implanted pumps have been applied to intraarterial therapy, both for treatment of heptatic tumors. The Medtronic variable-rate pump is commercially available, with approval by the Food and Drug Administration based in part on data showing less toxicity with circadian-based hepatic arterial infusion of 5-fluoro-2'-deoxyuridine (FUDR) (27). The Infusaid Model 1000 programable pump uses a different pumping mechanism, but has similar capabilities to the Medtronic device.

Effective and Appropriate Drug

DOSE-RESPONSE EFFECT

As outlined in Table 16.2, there are a number of properties essential to the appropriateness of

Table 16.2. Properties of Drugs Suitable for Intraarterial Therapy

Tumor cytotoxicity proportionally to level of exposure, i.e., dose response (efficacy) in tumor
Ability to generate high regional, low systemic levels:
  High total body clearance
  High regional extraction
Absent or minimal regional toxicity
Systemic toxicity dose limiting

using a drug intraarterially in a given tumor type situated in a particular body region. One consideration is that tumor cytotoxicity be proportional to the level of exposure to the drug in question. Knowledge of the dose-response curve can allow assessment of the potential additional antitumor effect possible when intraarterial therapy can achieve definable increases in the level of regional drug exposure relative to those possible with conventional intravenous administration. Despite improved regional drug exposure, antitumor effect may not be significantly better for tumors that are too sensitive or too refractory (28). For tumors that are very sensitive to a given drug, intravenous administration may suffice to generate maximal antitumor effect (i.e., the dose-response curve is such that the response has already reached a plateau for concentrations achievable by the intravenous route). If a tumor is absolutely resistant to all concentrations of a given drug (a phenomenon seen in tumor cell culture systems), then the increased exposure generated through an arterial infusion of drug will be of no benefit. Unfortunately, few dose-response or response versus concentration data exist for most of the (heterogeneous) tumors in the clinical situation. Intraarterial chemotherapy trials with agents in which the drug exposure increase is defined relative to intravenous administration may contribute to such knowledge. Information from clinical trials comparing intravenous infusion of FUDR with hepatic arterial infusion of FUDR is colorectal liver metastases provided a major contribution in this regard (see below).

Consideration of the selectivity of dose-response effects must take into account the tolerance of the normal tissues within the distribution of the artery being infused. Although tolerance of a systemic tissue may ordinarily be dose limiting, regional infusions may raise the exposure of normal tissues in the region to such a level that they soon become dose limiting instead. For

example, hepatic arterial infusion of FUDR can lead to hepatobiliary toxicity, which is not seen with intravenous infusions (11, 29, 30). Intraarterial infusions of agents in head and neck cancer can generate mucositis, and arterial infusion of tumors of the extremities can lead to dermatitis in the distribution of the infused arteries (31, 32). The localized regional toxicities that develop from intraarterial infusion are indicative of higher local exposure being achieved with intraarterial treatment.

PHARMACOKINETICS AND INCREASED EXPOSURE

The exposure advantage of intraarterial administration must be evaluated with reference to concentrations that result from conventional intravenous administration. The total advantage of intraarterial administration is obtained on the first pass through the infused region. Any drug that leaves this region and reaches the systemic circulation will behave as if it had been given intravenously.

As developed by Collins (28), the combined advantage of increased local delivery and decreased systemic delivery achieved by intraarterial administration can be expressed as

$$\frac{[\text{Drug}]_{\text{Target region}}}{[\text{Drug}]_{\text{Systemic}}} = R_d = 1 + \frac{CL_{TB}}{Q(I - E)}$$

where CL_{TB} is the total body clearance of the drug, E the fraction of drug extracted during first pass through the region infused, and Q the blood flow through the artery infused. It can be seen that agents with a high total body clearance relative to the blood flow through the artery infused are essential for maximal regional effect.

Using the formula Table 16.3 gives an estimate of the exposure advantage for most agents that have been used for intraarterial infusion. Inasmuch as hepatic arterial infusion has been the most commonly utilized arterial route, estimated values taking into account the role of hepatic extraction are provided. Relative to the extraction across the liver, regional extraction for other sites is certainly small or nonexistent.

The regional advantage (in terms of the drug exposure increase possible) may diminish at higher dose rates for agents that display nonlinear pharmacokinetics with saturable elimination. For example, for fluorouracil (FU) given at a dose rate of 20 mg/kg/day as a constant infusion, the CL_{TB} is approximately 2 L/min and

Table 16.3. Estimated Intraarterial Exposure Advantage of Selected Anticancer Drugs

Drug	CL_{TB} (mL/min)	Estimated Exposure Advantage for $Q = 100$ mL/min	$E_{Hepatic}$	Estimated Exposure Advantage for HA Infusion ($Q = 250$ mL/min)	Ref.
FUDR	15,000	150	0.9	600	33
FU	4,000	40	0.8	80	34, 35
BUDR	3,500	35	0.8	70	36
BCNU	2,500	25		10	37
Adriamycin	900	9	0.3	6	38
Mitomycin	600	6	0.25	4	39
Cisplatin	400	4	0.25	3	40
Streptozocin	400	4	0.05	2	41

the hepatic extraction is 0.8 (34). At dose rates above 270 mg/kg/day, the CL_{TB} falls to less than 0.5 L/min and the hepatic extraction to 0.1. Hence, bolus or short, high-dose-rate hepatic arterial infusions of FU may have a markedly diminished regional selectivity that is only 5% of that possible at low dose rates. Recent studies with hepatic arterial infusions of the investigational radiosensitizer 5-bromo-2'-deoxyuridine, BUDR, indicate a fall in the regional exposure advantage by over 60% at high-dose rates (36).

Dose-response effects at the cellular level may lead to diminished regional selectivity at higher dose rates. Recent studies examining the tissue-dependent DNA incorporation profiles of the thymine analogue BUDR in a rabbit liver tumor model have demonstrated this phenomenon (42). Inasmuch as DNA incorporation of BUDR into tumor and bone marrow reaches a plateau at higher levels of exposure and the plateau is higher for bone marrow than for tumor, tumor incorporation at high-dose rates is less than that of marrow despite the achievement of higher tumor exposure (43, 44). The magnitude of this effect in clinical studies is yet to be determined. These results in an animal model system examining BUDR incorporation and the clinical pharmacokinetic studies cited above suggest that more is not always better, because of nonlinear pharmacokinetic and pharmacodynamic relationships.

Choice of Appropriate Agent

Thus, the choice of an appropriate agent for arterial administration must take into account all of the elements described above and outlined in Table 16.2. Because of the increased cost and risk of intraarterial therapies relative to more conventional intravenous or oral therapies, the agent used should have a rational basis insofar as that can be determined. Use of a drug to which the tumor is absolutely refractory or a drug that generates no increased regional exposure is to be avoided. On the other hand, when (*a*) there is a definite response to an agent, (*b*) the agent's pharmacokinetic properties generate increased regional exposure with intraarterial use, and (*c*) the agent generates dose-limiting toxicity in areas other than the tumor-bearing region to be infused, there is the chance that intraarterial administration will be of benefit.

AGENTS

Drugs

FUDR (floxuridine) is the only noninvestigational anticancer drug licensed for intraarterial use by the United States Food and Drug Administration (FDA). Although Table 16.3 is not inclusive, the drugs listed are likely to account for more than 95% of intraarterial drug use. In varying degrees, these drugs fulfill the criteria for being appropriate agents for intraarterial administration in tumor types that frequently are regionally confined where there is an accessible regional feeding artery (see below).

Therapeutic Microspheres

Therapeutic microspheres represent agents with a very high regional extraction. Intraarterially administered microspheres that have a larger diameter than the smallest-diameter afferent vessels (capillaries/sinusoids) will be entrapped and not pass through the region or organ. Entrapment of microspheres, when they are homogeneously mixed in the afferent artery, will occur within the infused tissue in a manner proportional to microcirculatory blood flow. To the degree that tumor nodules are hypervascular relative to surrounding tissue contained within the watershed of an artery, intraarterial microspheres represent a means for selective delivery of a therapeutic agent to such tumor nodules. For example, colorectal and other tumor nodules in the liver entrap on the average four times more tracer microspheres than does normal liver (45, 46).

Drugs and microspheres can be given together, a process termed chemoembolization. Chemoembolization using the hepatic artery has become a relatively standard procedure for the treatment of liver metastases from neuroendocrine neoplasms (47–49). Hepatic metastases from neuroendocrine tumors are generally quite hypervascular and display a tumor blush with angiographic contrast agents. Chemoembolization with coadministration of solutions of doxorubicin or cisplatin and small particles (Gelfoam, Ivalon) proceeds with sufficient administration of (50–350 micron) particles until loss of the tumor blush indicates cessation of blood flow to the tumor nodules. Recently, a similar approach using transcatheter chemoembolization has produced responses in hepatocellular carcinoma (50–52). Alternatively, drugs can be incorporated into the structure of the microsphere to then leach out locally once the microsphere becomes entrapped. Ethylcellulose microspheres (225 ± 55 micron in diameter) containing 80% by weight of biologically active mitomycin represent such a particle (53, 54). Preclinical studies in dogs demonstrated a slow drug release over hours, with a 60% reduction in systemic exposure to mitomycin when the drug-containing ethylcellulose microspheres were administered intraarterially (53). Clinical investigations initiated in Japan have generated minor responses in a small series of patients with regionally confined tumors (54). A second approach combining drugs and microspheres is exemplified by biodegradable starch microspheres (55). A concentrated suspension of drug and starch microspheres is injected together. Entrapment of microspheres leads to blockage of blood flow and entrapment as well as a high concentration of drug within the vascular bed so treated. Temporarily holding a concentrated drug solution in the arteriolar-capillary bed allows a high concentration gradient to be locally maintained for a controlled period of time. Microspheres employing this mechanism avoid the considerable formulation problems involved in incorporating the drug directly into the particle.

Carmustine (BCNU) and mitomycin have been examined in conjunction with 40-micron-diameter starch microspheres given via the hepatic artery (56, 57). By 30 minutes after hepatic arterial injection, the starch microspheres are completely lysed by serum amylase, and flow resumes through the hepatic vascular bed as ascertained by contrast angiography (56). Owing to their rapid tissue uptake/fixation and mechanism of action as alkylating agents where peak drug levels can be most relevant, carmustine and mitomycin were employed with starch microspheres. Due to increased drug delivery to the liver and hepatic tumor, systemic drug exposure was found to be reduced by 90% for carmustine and 70% for mitomycin. Although use of starch microspheres continues in Japan, interest in their application has waned in the United States. Although application of drugs with starch microspheres is investigational per FDA guidelines, the same operative principle has been applied by interventional angiographers using commercially available Ivalon and Gelfoam particles (see above).

Another type of therapeutic microsphere, yttrium-90 glass microspheres (Theragenics Corp., Atlanta, GA), is being applied clinically. Yttrium-90 microspheres give off a high energy electron with a short effective kill distance of 2 to 3 mm. Most of the radiation dose is given over a 7- to 10-day period, as the nuclide has a half-life of approximately 64 hours. Resin microspheres with yttrium-90 absorbed onto the surface were used in the 1970s to treat hepatic tumors, with some interesting responses and documentation in several treated patients (who died shortly after treatment) of three- to fourfold higher levels of yttrium-90 microspheres in tumor modules than in normal liver (58, 59). Due to leaching of yttrium-90 from these resin microspheres, several patients developed severe myelosuppression, leading to withdrawal of FDA permission for their further study. In 1985 another form of yttrium-90 microsphere became available, a 22-micron-diameter glass microsphere with the yttrium entrained with the glass originally as yttrium-89, then activated to yttrium-90 by neutron bombardment in a cyclotron. Preclinical studies of hepatic arterial yttrium-90 microspheres in dogs demonstrated that dogs could survive a 30,000 rad dose (based on liver weight) (60). Based on these animal studies, phase I clinical studies were initiated by us at the University of Michigan (61) and, subsequently, by others in Canada (62). The U.S. study demonstrated no dose-limiting toxicity through the 15,000 rad level, with no demonstrable hepatic or marrow toxicity. Despite patients not receiving a toxic dose, responses documented by CT scan were seen in patients who had failed hepatic arterial FUDR. The approach using intraarterial yttrium-90 microspheres has a number of advantages, including one-shot treatment requiring only 1 to 2 days of hospitalization and catheterization for only 1 to 2 hours, lack of cross-resistance of radiotherapy with intraarterial drugs, and potential for synergism with prior use of intraarterial BUDR as a radiosensitizer (63).

BODY REGIONS/ORGANS WHERE INTRAARTERIAL THERAPY IS APPLIED

Overview

Intraarterial therapy has a niche defined by competing alternative therapeutic approaches, by the limited tumor types that are confined to a single body region, by the blood supply to various regions of the body, and by normal tissue tolerance in the infused region. Surgery and radiotherapy are conventional approaches and curative in many regionally confined tumors. Some common tumor types such as breast cancer, lung cancer, and melanoma have such a propensity for widespread metastases as to preclude great success through tumor reduction in one location where many other sites are likely to be involved and to cause equivalent morbidity and mortality. When a tumor is fed by multiple arteries, it is usually impossible to treat the entire tumor mass intraarterially because of technical aspects of defining and controlling all the tumor blood supply. This is often the case with tumors within the peritoneal cavity. Intraarterial therapy is also not reasonable in lung cancer, as the pulmonary arterial flow is so great and the tumor blood supply can be partially from bronchial arteries as well. Normal tissue tolerance is a limiting factor for head and neck cancer and for tumors fed by the mesenteric arteries inasmuch as proliferating oral or gut mucosa is usually more sensitive than tumor cells to the agents employed. In the case of brain tumors, despite high normal tissue tolerance to most drugs, the thromboembolic potential from indwelling catheters heightens the risk of intraarterial treatments.

Liver

Hepatic arterial therapy for tumors metastatic to the liver and tumors primary in the liver accounts for most intraarterial therapies administered to cancer patients. Results and develop-

ments in hepatic arterial therapy are largely responsible for the continued interest in intraarterial therapy as a treatment modality. Many excellent reviews of hepatic arterial therapy have been written, usually with a focus on colorectal cancer (24, 64, 65). Discussion here cannot cover all of the details given in these reviews but will cover why hepatic arterial therapy has been important and define the current and probable future status of work in this area.

There are multiple reasons why hepatic arterial therapy is so widely practiced. Metastatic colorectal cancer in the liver is the primary cause of death of at least 12,000 patients per year. Some 2500 patients per year also die of primary hepatobiliary cancer localized only in the liver. Data from surgical resection of tumor nodules from the liver indicate that a small fraction of patients have cancer only in the liver and can be cured if such tumor is eradicated (3, 66). A wide variety of other solid tumors metastasize to the liver and may cause considerable morbidity and mortality (67). The liver is unique among large organs in having a dual body supply. Most of the nutrient supply to the normal liver is via the portal vein, and occlusion of the hepatic artery is fairly well tolerated (68–70). On the other hand, tumors within the liver receive some 95% of their blood supply from the hepatic artery. Chemotherapy given into the hepatic artery allows selective uptake into tumor, with sparing of uptake into normal liver (71). The relatively large size of the hepatic artery also makes its catheterization easier and safer than that for smaller arteries feeding other body regions.

The liver possesses two further unique properties: the ability to regenerate and the ability to catabolize and extract drugs. The ability to regenerate makes it possible for the liver to suffer considerable loss of normal cells and yet, subsequently, regenerate the cells and recover functional capabilities. As seen above (Table 16.3), the ability of the liver to extract drugs can account for as much as a 10-fold advantage (for FUDR, where hepatic extraction is 0.9 or 90%). This extraction ability is unique to the liver among organs that are reasonable to infuse therapeutically.

Hepatic arterial therapy can be divided into two eras, one before the implanted pump became available and one after it became available (1979 for investigational purposes, 1982 for widespread commercial application) (24). Angiographically positioned, percutaneously inserted catheters with external pumps were used from the early 1960s through the 1970s. The difficulty in placing and maintaining such angiographic systems limited the number of institutions involved; risks were very high for the inexperienced. Response rates (Table 16.4) in the hands of those with sufficient dedication were considerably higher than the 15 to 20% response rates seen with standard intravenous infusion of FU. The development of a totally implanted system utilizing the Infusaid Model 400 pump and surgical catheter placement did not employ a new drug and did not result in a higher rate of responses than were seen with angiographically placed catheters. Response rates for the initial phase II studies with the implanted drug delivery system generally ranged from 50 to 80% (24). Definition of the catheter implantation techniques combined with the high reliability of the implanted pump made it possible, however, for many more physicians to be involved in the treatment of patients with hepatic arterial chemotherapy.

The definition of a reliable drug delivery system, coupled with the results of early phase II studies, made it possible for the first time to perform randomized studies comparing intraarterial and intravenous therapy. Unfortunately, the speed with which these studies could be conducted was markedly inhibited by the widespread commercial availability of the Infusaid pump and by an increasingly competitive market for medical care delivery. Nonetheless, randomized studies confirm that hepatic arterial FUDR generates a higher rate of regression of colorectal liver metastases than does intravenous therapy with FUDR or FU (Table 16.5).

Despite these "positive" randomized studies, enthusiasm for the implanted drug delivery system waned somewhat with time for a number of reasons. The costs and risks of the implanted drug delivery system must be weighed against its benefits. In addition, the skill and dedication essential to correctly implant the drug delivery system and monitor for hepatic toxicity are higher and vary from the usual practice of many surgical and medical oncologists.

Although the studies cited in Table 16.5 were not designed to define a survival effect for treatment, two recently published studies demonstrate an improved survival in patients with colorectal liver metastases receiving hepatic arterial infusion of FUDR with a totally implanted system (81, 82). In the most recent study, patients treated with hepatic arterial FUDR had significantly prolonged overall survival and normal quality survival along with associated reductions in the size of metastases and in carcinoembryonic antigen levels, compared with patients randomized to conventional symptom palliation (82).

The ability to administer hepatic arterial FUDR chronically gave rise to regional toxicities. Gastric injury was seen when FUDR was infused inadvertently to the stomach through unligated branching arteries off the hepatic artery (10, 83, 84). More serious, however, was the biliary sclerosis seen as part of the hepatobiliary toxicity generated by hepatic arterial FUDR (25, 26). Although these regional toxicities can be managed, they play a role in any risk/benefit assessment.

Table 16.4. Hepatic Arterial Therapy with FUDR Using External Pumps for Colorectal Liver Metastases

Investigators (reference)	No. of Evaluable Patients	Response Rate (%)
Watkins et al. (72)	82	73
Cady et al. (73)	51	57
Buroker et al. (74)	21	35
Oberfield et al. (75)	48	75
Patt et al. (76)	12	83
Reed et al. (77)	77	76

Table 16.5. Randomized Studies of Hepatic Arterial versus Systemic Chemotherapy for Colorectal Liver Metastases

Group (reference)	No. Pts.	Response Rate (%)	
		Hep. Art.	Systemic
Memorial Sloan-Kettering (78)	100	50	20
Northern California Oncol. Group (79)	143	37	10
National Cancer Institute (80)	64	62	17
Hepatic Tumor Study Group (65)	43	58	38[a]
City of Hope (65)	41	56	0

[a]5-day infusional FU used.

Recently, the addition of leucovorin (LV) to FUDR has been shown to improve response rates, albeit with an increased risk of hepatobiliary toxicity (85, 86). The addition of dexamethasone to hepatic arterial FUDR/LV was shown to result in a response rate of 78% and a median survival of 24.8 months with 3% rate of biliary sclerosis in previously untreated patients with unresectable hepatic metastases from colorectal cancer (86).

Thus, at this juncture it is possible to say that implanted drug delivery systems administering hepatic arterial FUDR can generate a high response rate in colorectal liver metastases, but such therapy should only be applied to patients with no or minimal extrahepatic cancer and then only with careful monitoring to prevent severe toxicity.

One hopes that future investigations will address the current problems. New agents are needed, as FUDR is not enough. The aim must be complete eradication of the hepatic tumor. Inasmuch as hepatic arterial therapy can be viewed in many instances as a debulking approach, systemic therapies must be added to deal with extrahepatic micrometastases. In this regard, hepatic arterial FU may be better suited to give an additional systemic effect than the more highly hepatically extracted FUDR (87). It will take more effective hepatic arterial therapy, possibly combined with adjuvant systemic therapy, along with better patient selection to achieve a demonstrable survival advantage and to cure at least a minority of patients. In an attempt to increase the cure rate, a number of investigators are examining the use of adjuvant hepatic arterial chemotherapy after surgical resection of hepatic tumor in metastatic colorectal cancer and in primary liver cancer (88–90).

Brain/Gliomas

Whereas metastatic tumors to brain generally involve other organ sites, primary gliomas rarely metastasize outside the central nervous system. Despite the use of surgical resection plus high-dose radiotherapy with BCNU, median survival is less than 1 year, and high-grade gliomas are always fatal. Approximately 75% of glioblastomas fall within the distribution of the carotid arteries (91). As seen in Table 16.3, the most widely used chemotherapeutic agent in malignant gliomas, BCNU, should generate an increased exposure when given into the internal carotid artery where the flow is approximately 250 mL/

min. Toxicity and drug uptake studies in monkeys indicated a two- to threefold improved uptake of BCNU by the arterial versus the intravenous route (92). Based upon these considerations, a number of institutions initiated studies with intraarterial BCNU (91, 93–96). Responses were noted in patients failing prior radiotherapy. Toxicities reflected the increased regional exposures achieved and consisted of retinal damage with visual loss and leukocephalopathy (94, 96, 97).

Based upon the results of single-institution studies outlined above, in December 1983 the Brain Tumor Cooperative Group (BTCG) initiated a randomized trial of intraarterial versus intravenous BCNU combined with external beam radiotherapy in malignant gliomas. An analysis has been presented for 283 patients (98). Toxicities unique to the intraarterial arm (155 patients) were significant encephalopathy in 13 patients and ipsilateral visual loss in 25 patients. Actuarial survival curves showed slightly worse survival in the intraarterial arm. The interim analysis did not prove that the intraarterial arm had worse survival, but made it unlikely that a statistically significant benefit favoring intraarterial BCNU would ultimately occur (2% chance of this result even after 300 deaths). The result of this BTCG trial would seem to effectively end carotid arterial BCNU as an option with any advantages.

Cisplatin has pharmacokinetic properties that would lead to a two- to threefold exposure advantage intraarterially (Table 16.3). This has been confirmed by a recent positron emission tomographic analysis (99). Cisplatin has some activity against gliomas when administered intravenously and, for these reasons, has been given via the carotid artery as a treatment for primary as well as metastatic brain tumors (100–104). Variable results have been seen, with some studies more encouraging than others (105). Regional toxicity has also occurred, with encephalopathy, visual loss, and ototoxicity developing (101, 105). Evaluation of the efficacy of cisplatin will require a group study such as the one conducted by the BTCG for BCNU.

The totally implantable drug delivery system (Infusaid Model 400 pump and surgically inserted silicone rubber catheter) has made it possible to perform continuous infusions of the internal carotid artery. This system has been applied to administer 5-bromo-2'-deoxyuridine (BUDR) as a constant 8-week internal carotid arterial infusion to radiosensitize gliomas during concurrent external beam radiotherapy. Inasmuch as gliomas are cytokinetically much more active than normal brain tissue, this thymidine analogue should be incorporated selectively into newly synthesized tumor DNA.

The first 23 patients entered into the study of carotid arterial BUDR with concurrent radiotherapy at the University of Michigan had an estimated median survival time of 23 months with a median follow-up of 20 months (106, 107). No vascular complications or encephalopathies were noted. Dose-limiting toxicity was ipsilateral blepharitis, iritis, and conjunctivitis due to BUDR delivery via the ophthalmic artery to the territory normally supplied by the external carotid artery, which is ligated during drug delivery system implantation. Investigations on the use of topical thymidine to prevent this regional toxicity are under way, as are other studies to biomodulate BUDR incorporation through use of concurrently administered thymidylate synthase inhibitors, FU and FUDR.

Head and Neck Cancer

As noted in a recent review, the use of intraarterial chemotherapy for treatment of head and neck cancer remains controversial despite 30 years of experience. Initial studies involved intraarterial methotrexate, usually with leucovorin. Using a variety of criteria, the regression rates noted in these studies ranged from 27 to 76% (31). Consistent with a minimal regional advantage expected on a pharmacokinetic basis with methotrexate, the results are not much different than those reported for systemic methotrexate, although a randomized comparison has never been conducted.

The recognition that cisplatin had substantial activity in head and neck cancer, coupled with a projected exposure advantage to intraarterial use, led to its use in external carotid arterial infusions in head and neck cancer (108–111). Response rates in previously untreated patients have ranged as high as 70 to 80%. Ipsilateral hemialopecia develops and indicates increased selective regional drug exposure in the half of the scalp directly infused. Catheter-related toxicity can cause central nervous system complications such as motor weakness, hemiparesis, and embolic strokes. Despite the high response rates possible with intraarterial cisplatin, similarly high rates in the range of 80% are seen with intravenous cisplatin plus infusional FU.

The implantable drug delivery system described previously for hepatic arterial and inter-nal carotid arterial infusions has been applied as well to external carotid arterial infusions for head and neck cancer (31, 112). For bilateral disease, dual catheter pumps were used to infuse both external carotid arteries. The sideport of the implanted pump was accessed for short-term, direct catheter infusions of cisplatin, and the central pumping mechanism can slowly infuse FUDR. In 26 evaluable patients treated with an implanted system there were 2 complete responses, 10 partial responses, 6 minor responses, and 8 progressions. Nineteen patients had failed prior therapy. Stomatitis was dose limiting for FUDR dosage escalation. The investigators noted that the results did not differ from those reported for systemically administered cisplatin and continuous infusional FU and that identification of new agents with antitumor activity, a high CL_{TB}, and a lack of toxicity to proliferating oral mucosa would be needed to exploit this mode of drug delivery.

Other Sites and Tumors

Intraarterial infusions have less commonly been administered in a variety of other sites. Sarcomas of the extremities have been treated with intraarterial infusions of doxorubicin (Adriamycin) and/or cisplatin (32, 113, 114). Intraarterial cisplatin has been administered for melanoma of the extremities as well (115). Innovative clinicians have applied intraarterial chemotherapy infusions to primary breast cancer (116, 117), bladder cancer (118), gastric cancer (119), lung cancer (120), and other tumors (121). A new journal, *Regional Cancer Treatment* (Springer International), has come into being to document the results of such therapy in these and other sites and tumors. It is of some concern that the vast majority of studies tend to describe improvements in response rate that fall within the upper bounds of response rates for the same drug given intravenously. Randomized studies of intraarterial versus intravenous therapy with a given drug at the maximum tolerated dose for the route chosen have not been conducted to examine outcome and survival. Such studies are crucial and must take into consideration other modalities for local control, namely, surgery and radiotherapy.

FUTURE ROLE FOR INTRAARTERIAL THERAPY

It is likely that the future role for intraarterial therapy will be increasingly in combination with the other regional approaches of surgery and radiotherapy to generate improved local control with lessened normal tissue toxicity. Surgery may be used to debulk regional tumor, to be followed by intraarterial chemotherapy to the region and radiotherapy to sterilize the margins of larger bulky tumors. The combination of conformal radiotherapy to target specifically intrahepatic tumor and hepatic arterial infusion of a radiosensitizing agent with regional selectivity is currently under investigation (13, 122, 123). Regional therapy should be combined with systemic therapy if survival is to be improved when micrometastic disease is likely. Combination approaches have more stringent requirements than any single approach alone. Regional therapy should be temporally defined and of shorter duration, so that resistant tumor cells or tumor cells outside the region do not multiply and clonally expand. Patients can often tolerate a defined intense therapy better than a prolonged chronic program. Toxicity of intraarterial therapy will need to be confined to the region infused, with no overlap with, or compromise to, systemic chemotherapy. All of these considerations are more likely to generate improved results if those investigators focusing on regional therapy are willing to recognize that cancer is usually a systemic disease (when unresectable for cure) and if those focusing on systemic therapy recognize that proportional cell kill holds for all chemotherapeutic agents. Larger tumor masses may have resistant cells not seen in micrometastases—hence the role for and need for locoregional tumor eradication.

IMPACT OF REGIONAL CHEMOTHERAPY ON DEVELOPMENT AND APPLICATION OF DRUG DELIVERY SYSTEMS

A major contribution of regional chemotherapy has been its impact on drug delivery device technology. Application of the Infusaid pump to hepatic arterial chemotherapy led to its commercial approval in 1982. Some 20,000 of these pumps have been implanted at over 1400 different institutions worldwide. Thousands of physicians, nurses, and patients learned to use, maintain, and live with an implanted pump. From a technologic standpoint, this phenomenon is a remarkable achievement that is certain to have an impact on other diseases besides cancer. Recently, based on a chronobiologic approach to hepatic arterial chemotherapy, an im-

planted, externally programable pump has become commercially available (27). Such a device will certainly prove beneficial not only in the chronobiologic approach to cancer therapy but to endocrinology and, perhaps, cardiology as well.

Implantable ports developed as a natural extension of the sideport of the Model 400 Infusaid pump; the first implantation of infusion ports into patients took place at the University of Michigan in 1981 (124, 125). Vascular access ports have filled a need, and by current industry estimates, more than 150,000 ports, produced by many different manufacturers, are being implanted annually. Experience with surgical implantation and use of the much larger Infusaid pump played a key role in the acceptance of surgically implanted ports. In keeping with the role of interventional radiology (angiography) in intraarterial therapy, a new central venous access port that can be placed and located on the inner aspect of the upper arm has recently become available (Bard Access Systems, Salt Lake City, UT) and may prove useful with angiographically placed arterial catheters (126, 127). The expanding variety of ports has fostered the development of multiple reliable infusion pumps. Coupling these pumps with implanted ports has allowed many infusional therapies to be given on an outpatient basis, with great savings in cost and improvement in patient lifestyles.

SUMMARY

Intraarterial therapy has a long history and has been applied in both appropriate and inappropriate situations. The development of a totally implanted drug delivery system for hepatic arterial therapy fostered expansion of interest and enthusiasm for such therapy and allowed randomized studies to be conducted. These studies have shown a significant improvement in response rate, as would be expected from dose-response effects and the exposure advantage generated. Until recently, these randomized studies have not demonstrated a survival impact over systemic therapy, owing (in part) to study design, to most hepatic tumor regressions being partial, and to frequent development of extrahepatic disease. Device technology has blossomed, but new agents designed for, and effective with, that technology have not been forthcoming as yet. The development of directed gene therapy approaches using intraarterial transcatheter vector delivery directed to regionally defined tumors may present the opportunity to explore many new therapeutic possibilities (128). Future progress in cancer therapy is likely to depend upon the potential for intraarterial therapy to facilitate locoregional tumor control and its ability to be combined with other treatment modalities for regional and systemic tumor eradication.

REFERENCES

1. Hellman S, Weichselbaum RR. Oligometastases. J Clin Oncol 1995;13:8–10.
2. Niederhuber JE, Ensminger W, Gyves J, Thrall J, Walker S, Cozzi E. Regional chemotherapy of colorectal cancer metastatic to the liver. Cancer 1984;53:1336–1343.
3. Hughes KS, Simon R, Songhorabodi S, et al. Resection of the liver for colorectal carcinoma metastases: a multi-institutional study of indications for resection. Surgery 1986;103:278–288.
4. Blacklock JB, Wright DC, Dedrick RL, et al. Drug streaming during intraarterial chemotherapy. J Neurosurg 1986;64:284–291.
5. Dedrick RL. Arterial drug infusion: pharmacokinetic problems and pitfalls. J Natl Cancer Inst 1988;80:84–89.
6. Mavlight GM, Patt YZ, Haynie TP, Carrasco CH, Charnsangavej C, Wallace S. Differential tumor regression in patients with bilobar hepatic metastases and dual arterial supply: evidence supporting the advantage of intra-arterial over intravenous route of drug delivery. Sel Cancer Ther 1989;5:37–45.
7. Junck L, Koeppe RA, Greenberg HS. Mixing in the human carotid artery during carotid drug infusion study with PET. J Cereb Blood Flow Metab 1989;9:681–689.
8. Kaplan WD, D'Orsi CJ, Ensminger WD, Smith EH, Levin DC. Intra-arterial radionuclide infusion: a new technique to assess chemotherapy perfusion patterns. Cancer Treat Rep 1978;62:699–703.
9. Kaplan WD, Ensminger WD, Come SE, et al. Radionuclide angiography to predict patient response to hepatic artery chemotherapy. Cancer Treat Rep 1980;64:1217–1222.
10. Hohn DC, Stagg RJ, Price DC, Lewis BJ. Avoidance of gastroduodenal toxicity in patients receiving hepatic arterial 5-fluoro-2'-deoxyuridine. J Clin Oncol 1985;3:1257–1260.
11. Niederhuber JE, Ensminger WD. Surgical considerations of management of hepatic neoplasia. Semin Oncol 1983;10:135–147.
12. Stephens FO, Waugh RC, Prest G. Radiological versus surgical placement of cannulas for delivery of intra-arterial chemotherapy. Reg Cancer Treat 1988;1:37–43.
13. Lawrence TS, Ten Haken RK, Kessler ML, et al. The use of 3-D dose volume analysis to predict radiation hepatitis. Int J Radiat Oncol Biol Phys 1992;23:781–788.
14. Curley SA, Chase JL, Roh MS, Hohn DC. Technical considerations and complications associated with the placement of 180 implantable hepatic arterial infusion devices. Surgery 1993;114:928–935.
15. Campbell KA, Burns RC, Sitzmann JV, Lipsett PA, Grochow LB, Niederhuber JE. Regional chemotherapy devices: effect of experience and anatomy on complications. J Clin Oncol 1993;11:822–826.
16. Clouse ME, Ahmed R, Ryan RB, Oberfield RA, McCaffrey JA. Complications of long term transbrachial hepatic arterial infusion chemotherapy. Am J Roentgenol 1977;129:799–803.
17. Ansfield FJ, Ramirez G, Davis HL, et al. Further clinical studies with intrahepatic arterial infusion with 5-fluorouracil. Cancer 1975;36:2413–2417.
18. Brothers T, Von Moll LK, Niederhuber JE, Roberts JA, Walker-Andrews S, Ensminger WD. Experience with subcutaneous infusion ports in 300 patients. Surg Gynecol Obstet 1988;166:295–301.
19. D'Orsi CJ, Ensminger WD, Smith EH, Lew M. Gas-forming intrahepatic abcess: a possible complication of arterial infusion chemotherapy. Gastrointest Radiol 1979;4:157–160.
20. Lokich J, Ensminger WD. Ambulatory pump infusion devices for hepatic artery infusion. Semin Oncol 1983;10:183–190.
21. Tucker EM. Drug administration systems for infusion chemotherapy. In: Lokich JJ, ed. Cancer chemotherapy by infusion. Chicago: Precept Press, 1987:41–58.
22. Buchwald H, Grage TB, Vassilopoulos PP, Rohde TD, Varco RL, Backshear PJ. Intraarterial infusion chemotherapy for hepatic carcinoma using a totally implantable infusion pump. Cancer 1980;45:866–869.
23. Ensminger W, Niederhuber H, Dakhil S, Thrall J, Wheeler R. Totally implanted drug delivery system for hepatic arterial chemotherapy. Cancer Treat Rep 1981;65:393–400.
24. Ensminger W. Intraarterial chemotherapy for the treatment of hepatic metastases. In: DeVita VT, Hellman S, Rosenberg SA, eds. Cancer: principles and practice of oncology update series. Philadelphia: JB Lippincott, 1987;1:1–11.
25. Phillips TW, Chandler WF, Kindt GW, et al. A new implantable continuous and bolus intra-carotid drug delivery system for the treatment of malignant gliomas. Neurosurgery 1982;11:213–218.
26. Chandler WF, Greenberg HS, Ensminger WD, et al. Use of implantable pump system for intra-arterial, intraventricular and intratumoral treatment of malignant brain tumors. In: Penn RD, ed. Neurological applications of implanted drug pumps. Ann NY Acad Sci, 1988;531:206–212.
27. Hrushesky WJM. Automatic chronotherapy: an integral part of the future of medicine. In: Ensminger WD, Salem J-L, eds. Update in drug delivery systems. New York: Futura, 1989:13–33.
28. Collins JM. Pharmacologic rationale for regional drug delivery. J Clin Oncol 1984;2:498–504.
29. Kemeny MM, Battifora H, Blayney DW, et al. Sclerosing cholangitis after continuous hepatic artery infusion of FUDR. Ann Surg 1985;202:176–181.
30. Hohn D, Melnick J, Stagg R, et al. Biliary sclerosis in patients receiving hepatic arterial infusions of floxuridine. J Clin Oncol 1985;3:98–102.
31. Wheeler RH, Baker S. Head and neck cancer. In: Lokich JJ, ed. Cancer chemotherapy by infusion. Chicago: Precept Press, 1987:399–414.
32. Eilber FR, Mirra J, Eckardt J, Kern D. Intraar-

terial adrimycin, radiation therapy, and surgical excision for extremity skeletal and soft-tissue sarcomas. In: Howell SB, ed. Intra-arterial and intracavitary cancer chemotherapy. Boston: Martinus Nijhoff, 1984:141–152.

33. Ensminger W, Rosowsky A, Raso V, et al. A clinical pharmacological evaluation of hepatic arterial infusion of 5-fluoro-2'-deoxyuridine and 5-fluorouracil. Cancer Res 1978;38:3784–3792.

34. Ensminger W, Stetson P, Gyves J, et al. Dependence of hepatic arterial flurouracil pharmacokinetics on dose rate and duration of infusion (abstract). Proc Am Soc Clin Oncol 1983;2:98.

35. Wagner JG, Gyves JW, Stetson PL, et al. Steady-state nonlinear pharmacokinetics of 5-fluorouracil during hepatic arterial and intravenous infusions of 5-fluorouracil in cancer patients. Cancer Res 1986;46:1499–1506.

36. Ensminger WD, Andrews JC, Walker-Andrews S, Johnson N, Wollner I, Stetson P. Clinical pharmacology of hepatic arterial 5-bromo-2'deoxyuridine (BUDR). In: Ensminger WD, Salem J-L, eds. Update in drug delivery systems. New York: Futura, 1989:215–224.

37. Ensminger WD, Thompson M, Come S, Egan EM. Hepatic arterial BCNU (NSC-409962): a pilot clinical pharmacologic study in patients with liver tumors. Cancer Treat Rep 1978;62:1509–1512.

38. Garnick MBV, Ensminger WD, Israel M. A clinical pharmacological evaluation of hepatic arterial infusion of adriamycin. Cancer Res 1979;39:4105–4110.

39. Hu E, Howell SB. Pharmacokinetics of intraarterial mitomycin C in humans. Cancer Res 1983;43:4474–4477.

40. Campbell TN, Howell SB, Pfeifle CE, Wung WE, Bookstein J. Clinical pharmacokinetics of intraarterial cisplatin in humans. J Clin Oncol 1983;1:775–762.

41. Gyves JW, Stetson P, Ensminger WD, Meyer M, Walker S, Gilbertson S. Hepatic arterial streptozocin: a clinical pharmacologic study in patients with liver tumors. Cancer Drug Deliv 1983;1:63–68.

42. Stetson PL, Maybaum J, Wagner JG, et al. Tissue-specific pharmacodynamics of 5-bromo-2'-deoxyuridine incorporation into DNA in VX2 tumor-bearing rabbits. Cancer Res 1988;48:6900–6905.

43. Knol JA, Stetson PL, Wagner JG. 5-bromo-2'-deoxyuridine incorporation into DNA in hepatic VX2 tumor-bearing rabbits. J Surg Res 1989;47:112–116.

44. Ensminger WD. Hepatic arterial chemotherapy for primary and metastatic liver cancers. Cancer Chemother Pharmacol 1989;23(Suppl):S68–S73.

45. Ensminger WD, Gyves JW. Regional cancer chemotherapy. Cancer Treat Rep 1984;68:101–115.

46. Gyves J, Ensminger WD, Thrall J, Ziessman H, Niederhuber J, Keyes J, Walker S. Definition of hepatic tumor microcirculation by single-photon emission tomography (SPECT). J Nucl Med 1984;25:972–977.

47. Ruszniewski P, Rougier P, Roche A, et al. Hepatic arterial chemoembolization in patients with liver metastases of endocrine tumors. A prospective phase II study in 24 patients. Cancer 1993;71:2624–2630.

48. Mavligit GM, Pollack RE, Evans HL, Wallace S. Durable hepatic tumor regression after arterial chemoembolization-infusion in patients with islet cell carcinoma of the pancreas metastatic to the liver. Cancer 1993;72:375–380.

49. Perry LJ, Stuart K, Stokes KR, Clouse ME. Hepatic arterial chemoembolization for metastatic neuroendocrine tumors. Surgery 1994;116:1111–1117.

50. Kanematsu T, Matsumata T, Shirabe K, et al. A comparative study of hepatic resection and transcatheter arterial embolization for the treatment of primary hepatocelluar carcinoma. Cancer 1993;71:2181–2186.

51. Higuchi T, Kikuchi M, Okazaki M. Hepatocellular carcinoma after transcatheter hepatic arterial embolization. Cancer 1994;73:2259–2267.

52. Murakami S, Yoshimatsu S, Yamashita Y, Sagara K, Arakawa A, Takahashi M. Thranscatheter hepatic subsegmental arterial chemoembolization therapy using iodized oil for small hepatocellular carcinomas. Acta Radiol 1994;35:576–580.

53. Kato T, Nemoto R, Mori H, et al. Sustained-release properties of microencapsulated mitomycin C with ethylcellulose infused into the renal artery of the dog kidney. Cancer 1980;46:14–21.

54. Kato T, Nemoto R, Mori H, et al. Arterial chemoembolization with mitomycin C microcapsules in the treatment of primary or secondary carcinoma of the kidney, liver, bone and intrapelvic organs. Cancer 1981;48:674–680.

55. Lindell B, Aronsen KF, Nosslin B, et al. Studies in pharmacokinetics and tolerance of substance temporarily retained in the liver by microspheres embolization. Ann Surg 1978;187:95–99.

56. Dakhil S, Ensminger W, Cho K, et al. Improved regional selectivity of hepatic arterial BCNU with degradable microspheres. Cancer 1982;50:631–635.

57. Gyves J, Ensminger WD, Van Harken D, et al. Improved regional selectivity of hepatic arterial mitomycin by starch microspheres. Clin Pharmacol Ther 1983;34:259–265.

58. Grady E. Internal radiation therapy of hepatic cancer. Dis Colon Rectum 1979;22:371–375.

59. Grady ED, Auda SP, Cheek WV. Vasoconstrictors to improve localization of radioactive microspheres to treat liver cancer. In: Proceedings of the 1980 Medical Association of Georgia Scientific assembly (Georgia Chapter, American College of Surgeons), Atlanta, November 21, 1980.

60. Wollner IS, Knutsen C, Smith P, et al. Effects of hepatic arterial yttrium[90] glass microspheres in dogs. Cancer 1988;61:1336–1344.

61. Andrews JC, Walker SC, Ackermann RJ, Cotton LA, Ensminger WD, Shapiro B. Hepatic radioembolization with yttrium[90] containing glass microspheres: preliminary results and clinical follow-up. J Nucl Med 1994;35:1637–1644.

62. Herba MJ, Illescas FF, Thirlwell MP, et al. Hepatic malignancies: improved treatment with intraarterial Y[90]. Radiology 1988;169:311–314.

63. Wollner IS, Knutsen CA, Ullrich KA, et al. Effects of hepatic arterial yttrium[90] microsphere administration alone and combined with regional bromodeoxyuridine infusion in dogs. Cancer Res 1987;47:3285–3290.

64. Daly JM, Kemeny N. Therapy of colorectal hepatic metastases. In: DeVita VT, Hellman S, Rosenberg SA, eds. Important advances in oncology 1986. Philadelphia: JB Lippincott, 1986:251–268.

65. Niederhuber JE, Grochow LB. Status of infusion chemotherapy for the treatment of liver metastases. In: DeVita VT, Hellman S, Rosenberg SA, eds. Can-

cer: principles and practice of oncology update series. 2nd ed. Philadelphia: JB Lippincott, 1989;3:1–9.

66. Sugarbaker PH, Kemeny N. Treatment of metastatic cancer to liver. In: DeVita VT, Hellman S, Rosenberg SA, eds. Cancer: principles and practices of oncology. 3rd ed. Philadelphia: JB Lippincott, 1989:2275–2298.

67. Pickren JW, Tsukada Y, Lane WW. Liver metastasis: analysis of autopsy data. In: Weiss L, Gilbert HA, eds. Liver metastasis. Boston: GK Hall, 1982:2–18.

68. Healy JE. Vascular patterns in human metastatic liver tumors. Surg Gynecol Obstet 1965;120:1187–1193.

69. Ramming KP, Sparks FC, Eilber FR, et al. Hepatic artery ligation and 5-fluorouracil infusion for metastatic colon carcinoma and primary hepatoma. Am J Surg 1976;132:236–242.

70. Karakousis CP, Couglass HO Jr, Holyoke ED. Technique of infusion chemotherapy, ligation of the hepatic artery and dearterialization in malignant lesions of the liver. Surg Gynecol Obstet 1979;149:403–407.

71. Ridge JA, Sigurdson ER, Daly JM. Distribution of fluorodeoxyuridine uptake in the liver and colorectal hepatic metastases of human beings after arterial infusion. Surg Gynecol Obstet 1987;164:319–323.

72. Watkins E, Khazei AM, Nahra KS. Surgical basis for arterial infusion chemotherapy of disseminated carcinoma of the liver. Surg Gynecol Obstet 1970; 130:581–605.

73. Cady B, Oberfield RA. Regional infusion chemotherapy of hepatic metastases from carcinoma of the colon. Am J Surg 1974;127:220–227.

74. Buroker T, Samson M, Correa J, Fraile R, Vaitkevicius VK. Hepatic artery infusion of 5-FUDR after prior systemic 5-fluorouracil. Cancer Treat Rep 1976; 60:1277–1279.

75. Oberfield RA, McCaffrey JA, Polio J, Clouse ME, Hamilton T. Prolonged and continuous percutaneous intraarterial hepatic infusion chemotherapy in advanced metastatic liver adenocarcinoma from colorectal primary. Cancer 1979;44:414–423.

76. Patt YZ, Mavligit GM, Chuang VP, et al. Percutaneous hepatic arterial infusion (HA) of mitomycin C and floxuridine (FUDR): an effective treatment of metastatic colorectal carcinoma in the liver. Cancer 1980;46:261–265.

77. Reed ML, Vaitkevicius VK, Al-Sarraf M, et al. The practicality of chronic hepatic artery infusion therapy of primary and metastatic hepatic malignancies. Cancer 1981;47:402–409.

78. Kemeny N, Daly J, Reichman B, Geller N, Botet J, Oderman P. Intrahepatic or systemic infusion of fluorodeoxyuridine in patients with liver metastases from colorectal carcinoma. Ann Intern Med 1987;107:459–465.

79. Hohn D, Stagg R, Friedman M, et al. The NCOG randomized trial of intravenous (IV) versus hepatic arterial (IA) FUDR for colorectal cancer metastic to the liver (abstract). Proc Am Soc Clin Oncol 1987; 6:85.

80. Chang AE, Schneider PD, Sugarbaker PH, Simpson C, Culnane M, Steinberg SM. A prospective randomized trial of regional versus systemic continuous FUDR chemotherapy in the treatment of colorectal liver metastases. Ann Surg 1987;206:685–693.

81. Rougier P, Laplanche A, Huguier M, et al. Hepatic arterial infusion of floxuridine in patients with liver metastases from colorectal carcinoma: long-term results of a prospective randomized trial. J Clin Oncol 1992;10:1112–1118.

82. Allen-Mersh TG, Earlam S, Fordy C, Abrams K, Houghton J. Quality of life and survival with continuous hepatic-artery floxuridine infusion for colorectal liver metastases. Lancet 1994;344:1255–1260.

83. Chuang VP, Wallace S, Stroehlein J, Yap H-Y, Patt YZ. Hepatic artery infusion chemotherapy: gastroduodenal complications. Am J Roentgenol 1981; 137:347–350.

84. Crowley ML. Penetrating duodenal ulcer associated with an operatively implanted arterial chemotherapy infusion catheter. Gastroenterology 1982; 83:118–120.

85. Kemeny N, Seiter K, Conti JA, et al. Hepatic arterial floxuridine and leucovorin for unresectable liver metastases from colorectal carcinoma. Cancer 1994;73:1136–1142.

86. Kemeny N, Conti JA, Cohen A, et al. Phase II study of hepatic arterial floxuridine, leucovorin, and dexamethasone for unresectable liver metastases from colorectal carcinoma. J Clin Oncol 1994;12:2288–2295.

87. Klotz HP, Weder W, Largiader F. Local and systemic toxicity of intra-hepatic-arterial 5-FU and high-dose or low-dose leucovorin for liver metastases of colorectal cancer. Surg Oncol 1994;3:11–16.

88. Curley SA, Roh MS, Chase JL, Hohn DC. Adjuvant hepatic arterial infusion chemotherapy after curative resection of colorectal liver metastases. Am J Surg 1993;166:743–748.

89. Kemeny MM. Chemotherapy after hepatic resection of colorectal metastases. Cancer Treat Res 1994; 69:121–128.

90. Uchino J, Une Y, Misawa K, et al. Postoperative intraarterial chemotherapy prevents the recurrence of the hepatocellular carcinoma (HCC) after hepatectomy (abstract). Proc Am Soc Clin Oncol 1994;13:1367.

91. Hochberg FH, Heros DO. Regional infusion for brain tumors. In: Lokich JJ, ed. Cancer chemotherapy by infusion. Chicago: Precept Press, 1987;467–478.

92. Levin VA, Jabra PM, Freeman-Dove M. Pharmacokinetics of intracarotid artery C^{14}-BCNU in the squirrel monkey. J Neurosurg 1987;48:587–593.

93. Greenberg HS, Ensminger WD, Seeser JF, et al. Intraarterial BCNU chemotherapy for the treatment of malignant gliomas of the central nervous system: a preliminary report. Cancer Treat Rep 1981;65:803–810.

94. Greenberg HS, Ensminger WD, Chandler WF, et al. Intraarterial BCNU chemotherapy for treatment of malignant gliomas of the central nervous system. J Neurosurg 1984;61:423–429.

95. Kapp J, Vance R, Parker JL, Smith RR. Limitations of high dose intraarterial 1, 3-bis (2-chloroethyl)-1-nitrosourea (BCNU) chemotherapy for malignant gliomas. Neurosurgery 1982;10:715–719.

96. Safdari H, Mompeon B, Dubois JB, Gros C. Intraarterial 1,3-bis(2-chloroethyl)-1-nitrosourea chemotherapy for the treatment of malignant gliomas of the brain: a preliminary report. Surg Neurol 1985;24:490–497.

97. Madajewicz S, West CR, Park HC, et al. Phase II study—intra-arterial BCNU therapy for metastatic brain tumors. Cancer 1981;47:653–657.

98. Shapiro WR. Reevaluating the efficacy of intraarterial BCNU. J Neurosurg 1987;66:313–315.

99. Rottenberg DA, Dhawan V, Cooper SC, Strother SC, Alcock N, Ginos JZ. Assessment of the pharmacologic advantage of intra-arterial versus intravenous chemotherapy using Ni-cisplatin and positron emission tomography (PET) (abstract). Neurology 1987;37(Suppl 1):335.

100. Stewart DJ, Wallance S, Feun L, et al. A phase I study of intracarotid cis-diamminedichloroplatinum (II) in patients with recurrent malignant intracerebral tumors. Cancer Res 1982;42:2059–2062.

101. Feun LG, Wallace S, Stewart DJ, et al. Intracarotid infusion of cis-diamminedichloroplatinum in the treatment of recurrent malignant brain tumors. Cancer 1984;54:794–799.

102. Lehane DE, Bryan RN, Horowitz B, et al. Intraarterial cisplatinum chemotherapy for patients with primary and metastatic brain tumors. Cancer Drug Deliv 1983;1:69–77.

103. Madajewicz S, Meek A, Davis R, et al. Novel first line therapy for malignant astrocytomas (abstract). Proc Am Soc Clin Oncol 1994;13:503.

104. Dropcho EJ, Rosenfeld SS, Morawetz RB, et al. Preradiation intracarotid cisplatin treatment of newly diagnosed anaplastic gliomas. J Clin Oncol 1992; 10:452–458.

105. Newton HB, Page MA, Junck L, Greenberg HS. Intraarterial cisplatin for the treatment of malignant gliomas. J Neurooncol 1989;7:39–45.

106. Greenberg HS, Chandler WF, Diaz RF, et al. Intraarterial bromodeoxyuridine radiosensitization and radiation in treatment of malignant astrocytomas. J Neurosurg 1988;69:500–505.

107. Greenberg HS, Chandler WF, Ensminger WD, et al. Radiosensitization with carotid arterial infusion bromodeoxyuridine and external radiation for gliomas. In: Ensminger WD, Salem J-L, eds. Update in drug delivery systems. New York: Futura, 1989:233–246.

108. Lee Y-Y, Wallace S, Dimery I, Goepfert H. Intraarterial chemotherapy of head and neck tumors. Am J Neuroradiol 1986;7:343–348.

109. Frustaci S, Barzan L, Tumolo S, et al. Intraarterial continuous infusion of cis-diamminedichloroplatinum in untreated head and neck cancer patients. Cancer 1986;57:1118–1123.

110. Mortimer JE, Taylor ME, Schulman S, Cummings C, Weymuller E, Laramore G. Feasibility and efficacy of weekly intraarterial cisplatin in locally advanced (stage III and IV) head and neck cancer. J Clin Oncol 1988;6:969–975.

111. Simunek A, Krajina A, Hlava A. Selective intraarterial chemotherapy of tumors in the lingual artery territory by a new approach. Cardiovasc Intervent Radiol 1993;16:392–395.

112. Forastiere AA, Baker SR, Wheeler R, Medvec BR. Intraarterial cisplatin and FUDR in advanced malignancies confined to head and neck. J Clin Oncol 1987;5:1601–1606.

113. Jaffe N, Robertson R, Ayala A, et al. Comparison of intraarterial cis-diamminedichloroplatinum II with high-dose methotrexate and citrovorum factor rescue in the treatment of primary osteosarcoma. J Clin Oncol 1985;3:1101–1104.

114. Stephens FO, Tattersall MHN, Marsden W, Waugh RC, Green D, McCarthy SW. Regional chemotherapy with the use of cisplatin and doxorubicin as primary treatment for advanced sarcomas in shoulder, pelvis, and thigh. Cancer 1987;60:724–735.

115. Pitchard JD, Mavligit GM, Benjamin RS, et al. Regression of regionally confined melanoma with intra-arterial cis-dichlorodiammineplatinum (II). Cancer Treat Rep 1979;63:555–558.

116. Stephens FO. Advanced breast cancer: primary intra-arterial induction chemotherapy. Reg Cancer Treat 1989;2:5–8.

117. Carter RD, Faddis DM, Krementz ET, Salwen WA, Puyau FA, Muchmore JH. Treatment of locally advanced breast cancer with regional intraarterial chemotherapy. Reg Cancer Treat 1988;1:108–111.

118. Jacobs S, Menashe DS, Mewissen MW, Lipchik EO. Intraarterial cisplatin infusion in the management of transitional cell carcinoma of the bladder. Cancer 1989;64:388–391.

119. Stephens FO. Management of gastric cancer with regional chemotherapy preceding gastrectomy—5-year survival results. Reg Cancer Treat 1988;1:80–82.

120. Muller H, Walther H, Aigner KR. Regional chemotherapy of lung tumors and metastases. Reg Cancer Treat 1988;1:44–49.

121. Calvo DB, Patt YZ, Wallace S, et al. Phase I-II trial of percutaneous intraarterial cis-diamminedichloroplatinum (II) for regionally confined malignancy. Cancer 1980;45:1278–1283.

122. Robertson JM, Lawrence TS, Dworzanin LM, Andrews JC, Walker S, et al. The treatment of primary hepatobiliary cancers with conformal radiation therapy and regional chemotherapy. J Clin Oncol 1993; 11:1286–1293.

123. Ensminger WD, Walker SC, Stetson PL, et al. Clinical pharmacology of hepatic arterial infusion of 5-bromo-2'-deoxyuridine. Cancer Res 1994;54:2121–2124.

124. Neiderhuber JE, Ensminger WD, Gyves JW, Liepman M, Doan K, Cozzi E. Totally implanted venous and arterial access system to replace external catheters in cancer treatment. Surgery 1982;92:706–712.

125. Ensminger WD, Wollner IS. Implantable drug delivery devices (pumps, ports) in cancer therapy. Rational Drug Ther 1988;22:1–7.

126. Ensminger WD, Walker SC, Knol JA, Andrews JC. Initial clinical evaluation of a new implanted port accessed by catheter-over-needle systems. J Infus Chemother 1993;3:200–203.

127. Ensminger WD. Regional chemotherapy. Semin Oncol 1993;20:3–11.

128. Nabel GJ, Chang AE, Nable EG, et al. Immunotherapy for cancer by direct gene transfer into tumors. Hum Gene Ther 1994;5:57–77.

17

Perfusion Therapy

William G. Kraybill

Isolation perfusion administers chemotherapy to specific anatomic sites by isolating the arterial inflow and venous outflow. This permits the administration of very high doses of chemotherapy or other therapeutics to the perfused site and protects the remaining circulation and the patient from the toxicity that results from systemic chemotherapy. While different anatomic locations have been perfused, it has been used most commonly in the extremities, where isolation of the vasculature is simpler and less problematic. An additional benefit of this technique is that it provides the opportunity to add heat to the system. A number of tumors are heat sensitive, and by using a heat exchanger to increase the temperature of the perfusate, these tumors may be heated as well as perfused with high doses of chemotherapy. Therefore, isolation perfusion provides the clinician with the opportunity to subject an appropriately situated tumor to high doses of chemotherapy and hyperthermia. This chapter reviews the use of this modality in the management of patients with various tumors in various anatomic locations. Most studies have been in malignant melanomas of the extremity; however, there is a significant experience with the use of this technique with other tumors and in other anatomic locations.

The use of intraarterial chemotherapy was first reported by Klopp et al. in 1950, when they demonstrated the feasibility and efficacy of intermittently injected intraarterial nitrogen mustard through surgically placed catheters (1). In 1957, Ryan et al. successfully isolated the limbs, midgut, and liver of a dog and perfused them without serious ill effects, using low flow rates and pressures below the mean systemic arterial pressure (2). Further isolation was obtained by applying an external tourniquet. The area was sustained by the circulation of whole blood through an extracorporeal oxygenated system

utilizing a heart-lung apparatus. This technique permitted the addition of chemotherapeutic agents to the perfusion circuit at doses higher than could be tolerated systemically.

The first human perfusion was accomplished in 1957. The patient had satellitosis of the thigh from a melanoma of the foot, which had been excised the previous year. Isolation perfusion was performed with L-phenylalanine mustard (L-PAM) (3, 4). The patient experienced a complete response and remained disease free for 16 years, dying of "old age" at 92. Experience with this patient led to the first human trials of isolation perfusion in malignant melanoma, using the pump oxygenator.

The use of isolation perfusion to heat extremity tumors was reported by Cavaliere et al. in 1967 (5). Isolation perfusion was used to heat extremity tumors without the addition of chemotherapeutic agents. Melanomas were identified as particularly sensitive to heat. In 1969, Stehlin used hyperthermia effectively in combination with regional chemotherapy in patients perfused for malignant melanoma (6). With the addition of hyperthermia to regional perfusion and chemotherapy using an oxygenated system, the final major component of the perfusion chemotherapy technique was available.

SURGICAL CONSIDERATIONS

Isolation perfusion of the extremities is technically simpler than perfusion of other organs or regions such as the liver, lung, and pelvis. While there has been clinical experience with isolation perfusion of other organs, the largest and most successful experience has been in patients with malignancies involving the extremities. The goals of perfusion are to maintain physiologic conditions in the isolated extremity and to treat the malignancy with effective chemotherapy and/or other therapeutics and (usually) hyper-thermia. In the extremities, major vessels are accessible for clamping, and collateral circulation may be interrupted with ligation and the use of a tourniquet. The upper extremity is usually perfused through the axillary vessels, reached through a muscle-splitting, infraclavicular incision. A tourniquet is used routinely. The lower extremity may be perfused through the external iliac vessels, the femoral vessels, or the popliteal vessels. Again, collateral circulation may be ligated or temporarily occluded, and a tourniquet used. In both axillary perfusions and iliac perfusions, lymphadenectomy may be completed synchronously, though an increased number of postoperative complications may result.

After isolation of the vasculature, heparin is administered intravenously, vascular clamps are applied, and the tourniquet is tightened proximally to the ends of the catheters (4). Venous blood is collected by gravity, pumped through an oxygenator, warmed, and pumped back into the limb via the artery. The chemotherapeutic agent may be injected into the efferent arm of the extracorporeal system. Papaverine may also be introduced into the system to reduce perfusion resistance; epidural anesthesia may be used to achieve the same end. Monitoring systems are used to identify leakage from the isolation perfusion circuit into the systemic circulation and to monitor skin and muscle temperature (7). Radioactively labeled serum albumin has been used to monitor leak rate with a precordial scintillation probe.

Other anatomic areas have been treated with isolation perfusion. Wile and Smolin have reported the use of isolation perfusion for recurrent pelvic cancer (8). Pelvic isolation perfusion was achieved by occluding the aorta and vena cava above the bifurcations and using tourniquets around the thighs. While the study demonstrated relative isolation of the pelvic vasculature, this intervention has not been widely accepted, since most tumors requiring this type of management have developed systemic metastasis. Wanebo and colleagues used a balloon occlusion technique to perfuse the pelvis in patients with unresectable cancer (9); pelvic pain was relieved in six of eight symptomatic patients.

In their early experiments, Ryan and Creech developed methods for isolating the liver for the purpose of perfusion (2, 4). More recently, Schwemmle et al. have used isolation perfusion in patients with malignant disease involving the

liver (10). Most of the tumors in their series were metastatic colon cancers. The liver vasculature is isolated by an intrapericardial tourniquet of the inferior vena cava, cannulation of the portal vein, cannulation of the hepatic artery, and cannulation of the inferior vena cava below the renal veins, with a tourniquet at that level. Although 50 patients were reported in this series, enthusiasm for this procedure has been tempered by the high incidence of lung metastases (20%) and local recurrences (10%). The lung has also been perfused (11). Thus, it is technically possible to perfuse other organs besides the extremities. While these may be areas of valid investigation, most of the experience with this modality has been in perfusion of patients with malignancies of the extremities. Perfusion of organs other than the extremities should be viewed as experimental and should only be performed in centers where there is a special interest in developing and evaluating these specific therapeutic modalities.

ISOLATION PERFUSION IN THE MANAGEMENT OF EXTREMITY MELANOMAS

The most extensive experience with extremity perfusion has been in patients with malignant melanomas. Isolation perfusion has been used for all stages of malignant melanomas of the extremities, from primary localized tumors to locally advanced and recurrent tumors. Most clinical studies reporting results with isolation perfusion in melanomas have used the M. D. Anderson staging system (Table 17.1). Recent reports have used the American Joint Committee on Cancer (AJCC) staging system (12).

Table 17.1. M. D. Anderson Melanoma Staging

Stage	Description
IA	Intact primary melanoma
IB	Primary melanoma excised
IC	Multiple primary melanoma
II	Local recurrence within 3 cm of primary site
IIIA	Satellite or in-transit metastases excluding regional nodes
IIIB	Positive regional nodes
IIIAB	Satellite or in-transit metastases with positive regional nodes
IV	Distant metastases

From Cumberlin R, De Moss E, Lassus M, Friedman M. Isolation perfusion for malignant melanoma of the extremity: a review. J Clin Oncol 1985;3:1022–1031. With permission.

A number of technical factors affect the results and morbidity of isolation perfusion. Specifically, the use of heat, the perfusate chosen, the flow rates, the drug dosage, and the methods of determining drug dosage are critical factors in isolation perfusion. Leak rate is important for patients, especially for those being perfused with tumor necrosis factor (TNF). Prior to the report by Stehlin in 1969, most isolation perfusions using L-PAM were done without hyperthermia (6). Response rates with normothermic isolation perfusion using L-PAM were 30 to 62% (Table 17.2) (7). In the small number of patients who have undergone hyperthermic perfusion with L-PAM and have objective response rates reported, response rates of about 80% have been described (Table 17.2). Analysis of the relative merits of hyperthermic and normothermic perfusion is complicated by differing descriptions of what constitutes hyperthermia. Kroon, in his review of isolation perfusion for malignant melanoma with L-PAM, points out that a number of the so-called normothermic perfusions were actually done with tissue temperatures in the limb as low as 32 to 33°C (13). The situation is further complicated because many reports describe the temperature of the perfusate without reporting the tissue temperatures. Kroon's review correlates reports of complete and partial response rates with the reported temperatures of the tissue or, when this is not available, the temperatures of the priming fluid and the heat exchanger. This review clearly correlates complete response rates to tissue temperature in patients undergoing isolation perfusion with L-PAM. In

series with temperatures ranging from 41 to 42°C, response rates vary between 81 and 96% (Table 17.3). Viewed together, the reviews of Cumberlin et al. and Kroon demonstrate a definite advantage to the use of hyperthermia (defined as tissue temperatures of 40 to 42°C) in combination with L-PAM (Tables 17.2 and 17.3) (7, 13).

The perfusate used during isolation perfusion is important as a vehicle for the distribution of the chemotherapeutic agent and heat and in providing oxygenation and removal of metabolic waste products. In most centers, the extracorporeal circuit is primed with a mixture of whole blood and physiologic electrolyte solution to achieve an hematocrit of approximately 25%. The consensus has been that hemodilution is essential, since the viscosity of whole blood hampers rapid circulation in the extracorporeal system.

High flow rates in the isolated system are thought to produce a significant reduction in toxicity, but assessment and comparison of flow rates is also complicated by differences in the reporting methods used. Most authors report flow rates in milliliters per minute, while others use the perhaps more accurate milliliters per minute per liter of perfused tissue. Animal experiments, as well as some clinical studies, suggest that preperfusion tissue oxygen levels determined by transcutaneous PO_2 electrodes can only be maintained with abnormally high perfusion rates (600 to 1000 mL/min for the lower extremity) (13).

Drug dosages of L-PAM have varied between

Table 17.2. Objective Response Rates in Perfusion of Melanoma Patients

Author (Reference)	No. of Patients	Objective Response[a]	Comments
Normothermic perfusion with L-PAM			
Ryan (35)	83	30	Nodes and local recurrence
Steblin et al. (36)	11	55	Primary lesion
Bulman and Jamieson (37)	29	45	Local recurrence
Rosin and Westbury (38)	80	62	26% CR nodes and local recurrence
Total	203	47	
Hyperthermic perfusion with L-PAM			
Halstrom and Johnsson (39)	10	80	10% CR nodes and local recurrence
Steblin (6)	12	83	Advanced local disease
Total	22	82	

From Cumberlin R, De Moss E, Lassus M, Friedman M. Isolation perfusion for malignant melanoma of the extremity; a review. J Clin Oncol 1985;3:1022–1031. With permission.
[a]Complete remission (CR).

Table 17.3. Objective Response Rates[a] in Melanoma Patients after Isolation Perfusion with Melphalan

Author (Reference)	Total	No. of Patients CR	PR	Percentage CR + PR	Tissue Temperature
Hansson et al. (1977) (40)	14	3	3	43	?[b]
Bulman and Jamieson(1980) (39)	29	?	?	48	hypothermic (?)[c]
Couture (1982) (41)	13	?	?	46	?[d]
Kroon et al. (1987) (42)	18	7	8	83	37–38°C
Rochlin and Smart (1965) (43)	17	?	?	65	37–39°C
Jonsson et al. (1983) (44)	15	1	10	73	38–?°C[e]
Rosin and Westbury (1980) (38)	80	21	29	62	39–40°C
Lejeune et al. (1983) (45)	23	15	6	91	39–41°C
Vaglini et al. (1985) (46)	32	18	8	81	40–41°C
Storm and Morton (1985) (47)	26	21	0	81	40.5–42°C
Cavaliere et al. (1987) (48)	72	26	43	96	41–42°C

From Kroon BBR. Regional isolation perfusion in melanoma of the limbs: accomplishments, unsolved problems, future. Eur J Surg Oncol 1988;14:101–110. With permission.
[a]CR, complete remission; PR, partial remission.
[b]"Temperature in the heat exchanger between 40–42°C"; tissue temperatures not given.
[c]"Temperature of priming 37°C"; tissue temperatures not given.
[d]No temperature given.
[e]Maximum temperature not given.

0.45 and 1.5 mg/kg of body weight in the upper extremity and from 0.9 to 2.0 mg/kg in the lower extremity. Perfusion times have ranged from 45 to 120 minutes. While most L-PAM dosages have been described in mg/kg, some investigators have suggested that dosimetry should be based on the volume of the limb to be perfused (13–15). This value may easily be determined by immersion. On the basis of grading systems for toxic reactions of normal tissue, L-PAM doses of 10 mg/liter of perfused tissue have proved to be the maximum dose tolerated. The pharmacokinetics of isolation perfusion are further complicated because the dosimetric schedule must take into account the volume of the perfused region and the priming volume of the extracorporeal circuit. The other controversial dosimetric factor relates to whether or not drugs should be given once in a bolus dose or sequentially over the time of perfusion. Different centers vary these factors on the basis of their own experience. More pharmacologic studies to evaluate different methods of measuring dosage and evaluating dosing schedules are required.

Isolation Perfusion of Malignant Melanoma: Clinical Results

An accurate assessment of the clinical results of isolation perfusion in malignant melanoma of the extremities is difficult, as most available data are retrospective. Much of the data was collected

prior to the availability of the Breslow classification of malignant melanomas, and consequently, stratification according to those criteria is not available. Frequently, other risk factors such as sex, age, ulceration, and specific anatomic location have not been considered. In spite of these deficiencies, considerable retrospective data are available for review.

Isolation Perfusion of Malignant Melanoma: Therapeutic

It is useful to stratify patients undergoing perfusion into those who have locally advanced extremity melanomas and are undergoing perfusion primarily for palliation (M. D. Anderson stages II and IIIA melanomas) and patients undergoing prophylactic perfusion (M. D. Anderson stage I melanomas). Response rates to hyperthermic perfusion previously discussed (Tables 17.2 and 17.3) support the use of isolation perfusion for palliation of patients with locally advanced malignant melanoma who might otherwise require amputation. Cumberlin et al. have suggested that in combination with surgical excision, isolation perfusion in patients with stages II and IIIA melanomas may improve local control and survival (7). In a review by Kroon, the 2-year recurrence rate for patients with stage II disease was 20% (4 of 20) (13). In patients with stage IIIA lesions that were observed instead of excised following perfusion, a recurrence rate of

Table 17.4. Isolation Perfusion in Palliation

Author (Reference)	No. of Patients	Effective Palliation (%)	Duration
Normothermic perfusion			
Krementz and Ryan (49)	93	50	2+ months
Bulman and Jamieson (37)	29	49	7 months (mean)
Hyperthermic perfusion			
Rosin and Westbury (38)	80	63	23 months (mean)

From Cumberlin R, De Moss E, Lassus M, Friedman M. Isolation perfusion for malignant melanoma of the extremity: a review. J Clin Oncol 1985;3:1022–1031.

35% was noted. Five-year survival rates after perfusion for stages II and IIIA patients have ranged from 32 to 74%. For patients treated with surgery alone, 5-year survival rates have varied from 9 to 50%. While firm conclusions cannot be drawn from these retrospective data, most melanoma experts agree that local control (and probably survival) is improved in patients with stage II or IIIA recurrent melanomas.

The role of isolation perfusion in the management of patients with clinically positive lymph nodes (stages IIIAB and IIIB) seems less clear (13). These patients have an increased risk of hematogenous spread and, ultimately, systemic metastasis. Although some of these patients may benefit from isolation perfusion to palliate and prevent local recurrence in high-risk tumors of the extremity, there is little evidence that isolation perfusion improves survival.

Isolation perfusion is well documented as a method of providing palliation for patients with malignant melanoma (7). The morbidity of this treatment in skilled hands is low. Approximately 50 to 63% of patients perfused for palliation have satisfactory results, with decreased pain and avoidance of amputation (Table 17.4).

Isolation Perfusion of Malignant Melanoma: Prophylactic

A number of authors have recommended the use of isolation perfusion to decrease the risk of local recurrence and improve survival in patients with high-risk, stage I melanomas (7). While there appears to be some survival benefit for patients undergoing isolation perfusion, especially hyperthermic isolation perfusion with L-PAM, these recommendations are made al-

most exclusively on the basis of retrospective data. Final recommendations must await the results of randomized prospective trials.

There have been two randomized prospective trials using hyperthermic isolation perfusion in patients with malignant melanoma. In one, 107 patients with Clark's level III or greater malignant melanoma and a tumor thickness greater than 1.5 mm were randomized (16). Those in the control group were managed with wide local excision and regional lymph node dissection. The perfusion group was treated identically, except they received regional hyperthermic perfusion in addition (16). In this study, the recurrence rate in the control group was 27.8% in stage I patients, 31.6% in stage II patients, and 58.8% in stage III patients. In the perfusion group, recurrences were observed in 5.6% of stage I patients, 5.5% in stage II patients, and 12.5% in stage III patients. Differences in disease-free survival reached statistical significance: $p = .09$ in stage I, $p = .03$ in stage II, and $p = .003$ in stage III tumors. In a small second trial performed by the Swedish Melanoma Study Group, 69 patients with recurrent melanoma of the extremities were randomized to surgery or surgery with hyperthermic isolation perfusion (17). Tumor-free survival was better in the perfusion group ($p = .044$), though there was no improvement in survival ($p = .28$). While the Breslow level and lymph node status are provided in these trials, the extent of recurrent disease is not. Because the total number of patients is small in these series, most authors feel that final conclusions must await the results of more extensive randomized studies.

Isolation Perfusion of Malignant Melanoma: Complications

Severe complications secondary to isolation perfusion include amputations, compartment syndromes, nerve palsies, and contractures and have occurred in 2.7 to 7.1% of patients perfused (18–20). Complications resulting in death have occurred in up to 2.5% of patients undergoing isolation perfusion. While severe complications are relatively uncommon, mild-to-moderate morbidity is not. Erythema and occasional minimal blistering in the perfused limb occur frequently but usually resolve without significant disability. Edema, usually mild, occurs in up to 40% of patients undergoing isolation perfusion and may be exacerbated by concurrent lymphadenectomy. While edema can usually be con-

trolled with compression stockings and elevation, rare patients will develop massive edema
following isolation perfusion. The more frequently associated mild-to-moderate edema,
blistering, and erythema are usually tolerable.
Compared with the complications of other major
cancer interventions, the incidence and severity
of these complications are not inordinately
great, especially when the alternative may be
amputation.

ISOLATION PERFUSION: DRUGS AND THERAPEUTICS OTHER THAN L-PAM

Most experience with perfusion has been obtained with the use of L-phenylalanine mustard
(L-PAM), the first drug used by Creech in 1958
(4). It has been used extensively, even though
until recently its use in this country in its parenteral form has been limited by restrictions of
the Food and Drug Administration. Work done
in this country and in Europe has resulted in an
extensive database on the pharmacokinetics of
normothermic and hyperthermic isolation perfusion. The drug distribution, metabolism, tumor uptake, and leak rate and the effects of temperature have been extensively studied.

Recombinant Tumor Necrosis Factor-alpha (rTNF-α), Interferon-gamma (IFN-γ) and Melphalan

A potential major advance has been the use
of rTNF-α, IFN-γ, and melphalan in combination

to perfuse extremity melanomas and, to a lesser
degree, sarcomas (21, 22). Preclinical studies suggested that rTNF-α might be useful therapy in
malignancies, but the use of rTNF-α in humans
was inhibited by systemic toxicity (23–25). Liénard recognized the potential of perfusing this
highly effective but toxic drug (21, 22). Table 17.5
shows early responses in murine models, clinical
systemic trials, and early results using rTNF-α
with melphalan and IFN-γ in perfusion systems
(21, 23). Liénard and Lejeune initially reported
29 patients who underwent 31 isolation perfusions with 26 complete responses (90%) and 3
partial responses (10%) (21). This high response
rate appears to be secondary to a synergistic relation between TNF and melphalan.

Regional toxicity following perfusion with
TNF, IFN-γ, and melphalan occurs because of
the direct impact of these drugs on normal tissue
(23). Systemic toxicity can occur by a combination of effects: absence of complete isolation, persistence of some drug in the perfused extremity
after the perfusion, and the fact that the perfused
drugs may induce host mediators that may be
toxic. Virtually all patients have fevers and chills
approximately 5–6 hours after perfusion. Hypotension requiring dopamine occurs in 23 to
40% of patients perfused with TNF (21–23).
Other complications include adult respiratory
distress syndrome (ARDS), hyperbilirubinemia,
leukopenia, and thrombocytopenia (22). Thus,
while response rates are high, toxicity may be
significant. Perfusion with TNF appears to be a
major advance in the management of patients

Table 17.5. Dose, Route of Administration, and Clinical Responses with Various Types of Regional Therapy with TNF

Tumor Sites	TNF Doses	TNF MTD[a]	Manufacturer	No. CR[b]	PR[b]	MR (Ref)
		Direct Intralesional Injection				
Palpable skin or nodal	25–300 μg	>300 μg	Genentech	14	0	14	21 (50)
Palpable and visceral	43–522 μg/m²	391 μg/m²	Asahi	21	0[c]	19	19 (51)
Kaposi's sarcoma	5–100 μg/m²	25 μg/m²	Genentech	26[d] 19	35	35 (52)
Hepatic	100–350 μg/m²	>350 μg/m²	Knoll	15	0	0	0 (53)
		Intrahepatic Artery Infusion				
Hepatic	12.5–175 μg/m²/d × 5d	150 μg/m²/d	Genentech	14	0	14	21 (54)
		Isolated Limb Perfusion (ILP)				
Extremity	3 mg arm; 4 mg leg[e]	>4 mg	Boehringer	29	90	10	0 (21)

From Fraker DL, Alexander HR. Isolated limb perfusion with high-dose tumor necrosis factor for extremity melanoma and sarcoma.
In: DeVita VT, Hellman S, Rosenberg SA, eds. Important advances in Oncology 1994. Philadelphia: JB Lippincott, 1994:179–192.
[a]MTD, maximally tolerated dose.
[b]CR, complete response; PR, partial response; MR, minimal response.
[c]One patient with a partial response at site of injection of a hepatic tumor had a complete response at a distant bony metastasis.
[d]Responses reported for individual lesions treated.
[e]ILP performed with TNF plus melphalan and interferon-γ.

with locally advanced melanoma and possibly sarcoma. Clinical trials are ongoing in Europe and the United States seeking to confirm these early results.

There has also been significant experience with other drugs. Table 17.6 presents a review of response data in melanoma after isolation perfusion with drugs other than L-PAM (13). Because of the small number of patients in each study and the different perfusion conditions, it is difficult to compare response rates among different combinations of perfusion drugs. While significant responses have been noted with the use of dacarbazine (DTIC), cisplatin, and other combinations, none of the responses has represented a significant improvement over the use of L-PAM in hyperthermic isolation perfusion. When cisplatin is used at temperatures over 40°C, severe and sometimes permanent nerve damage may occur (18). The toxicity of DTIC is reported to be mild. While responses to DTIC have been reported, there are theoretical reasons to suggest that it might not be active in isolation perfusion because the active drug is formed by biotransformation and methylation in the liver (26). Edema and blistering have been reported with the use of nitrogen mustard (1, 20). Adriamycin and L-PAM have been used in the management of soft tissue sarcomas (11). The pharmacology of perfusion with these and other combinations has not been as carefully studied as L-PAM alone. Evaluation of new drugs and combinations for isolation perfusion is an area for potentially useful research.

ISOLATION PERFUSION: TUMORS OTHER THAN MALIGNANT MELANOMA

Most tumors managed with isolation perfusion have been malignant melanomas, but other tumors have also been treated with this modality, notably soft tissue sarcomas of the extremity. The most exciting results in tumors other than melanomas have been in patients perfused with TNF, IFN-γ, and melphalan for sarcomas. Recent results from Europe (27) report limb salvage in 91% (21/23) of patients whose tumors were deemed unresectable prior to perfusion. The level of perfusion is as distal as possible to allow perfusion of the entire tumor. Tumor softening begins almost immediately. If there are no pulmonary metastases, the tumor is resected 6–12 weeks after perfusion. Drugs used in the management of soft tissue sarcomas have been more varied than those used in malignant melanomas (28). Many authors have added actinomycin D to L-PAM when perfusing soft tissue sarcomas (29, 30). Nitrogen mustard has also been used in the management of these patients (29).

Radiation therapy combined with isolation

Table 17.6. Objective Response Rates in Melanoma Patients after Isolation Perfusion with Drugs Other Than Melphalan or with Drug Combinations

Author (Reference)	Drug (Combination)	No. of Patients[a]		
		Total	CR	PR
Cox (1975) (55)	Thiotepa Melphalan	28	10	?
Colomb (1976) (56)	Thiotepa Actinomycin D Melphalan	54	7	32
Aigner et al. (1983) (57)	Dacarbazine	4	1	0
Aigner et al. (1983) (58)	Cisplatin	12	2	4
Aigner et al. (1983) (58)	Cisplatin Actinomycin D	6	0	2
Aigner et al. (1984) (59)	Vindesine Dacarbazine Cisplatin	14	0	14
Shiu et al. (1986) (20)	Nitrogen mustard	19	6	6
Vaglini et al. (1987) (60)	Dacarbazine	24	3	7

From Kroon BBR. Regional isolation perfusion in melanoma of the limbs: accomplishments, unsolved problems, future. Eur J Surg Oncol 1988;14:101–110. With permission.
[a]CR, complete remission; PR, partial remission.

perfusion and local excision in patients with soft tissue sarcoma has resulted in 5-year survival rates of 65 to 75% (31). Results of isolation perfusion, radiation therapy, and excision of soft tissue sarcomas have been comparable to results reported for soft tissue sarcomas managed by radiation therapy and excision and those managed with intraarterial Adriamycin infusion, radiation therapy, and excision (32, 33). Most of the perfusion series were not stratified according to tumor grade, making comparisons of series difficult. Isolation perfusion with radiation therapy and excision is an alternative in the management of patients with soft tissue sarcomas of the extremities; however, it would appear to have no advantage over other multimodality methods of managing these extremity tumors. There has been a recent report of an intractable and progressive cutaneous non-Hodgkin's lymphoma of the lower extremity that was treated with sequential regional isolation perfusion with L-PAM (34). The therapy was temporarily effective in this patient. While most tumors managed with isolation perfusion have been malignant melanomas, this modality may be useful in selected patients with other tumors.

SUMMARY

Isolation perfusion with melphalan and hyperthermia appears to provide palliation for patients with locally advanced and recurrent malignant melanoma (stages II and IIIA). The recent development of perfusion using TNF, IFN-γ, and melphalan in the management of locally advanced sarcomas and melanomas is exciting, but the precise role of this modification of perfusion in the management of advanced neoplasms of the extremities and other perfusable organ sites awaits further study.

REFERENCES

1. Klopp CT, Alford TC, Bateman J, Berry GN, Winship T. Fractionated intra-arterial cancer chemotherapy. Ann Surg 1950;132:811–832.

2. Ryan RF, Krementz ET, Creech O, Winblad JW, Chamblee W, Check W. Selected perfusion of isolated viscera with chemotherapeutic agents using extracorporeal circuit. Surg Forum 1957;8:158.

3. Creech OJ Jr, Krementz ET. Cancer chemotherapy by perfusion. In: Haddow A, Weinhouse S, eds. Advances in cancer research. New York: Academic Press, 1961:111.

4. Creech OJ Jr, Krementz ET, Ryan RF, Winblad JN. Chemotherapy of cancer: regional perfusion utilizing an extracorporeal circuit. Ann Surg 1958;148:616–632.

5. Cavaliere R, Di Filippo F, Santori FS, et al. Role of hyperthermic perfusion in the treatment of limb osteogenic sarcoma. Oncology 1967;44:1–5.

6. Stehlin JS Jr Hyperthermic perfusion with chemotherapy for carcinoma of the extremity. Surg Gynecol Obstet 1969;129:305–308.

7. Cumberlin R, De Moss E, Lassus M, Friedman M. Isolation perfusion for malignant melanoma of the extremity: a review. J Clin Oncol 1985;3:1022–1031.

8. Wile A, Smolin M. Hyperthermic pelvic isolation perfusion in the treatment of refractory pelvic cancer. Arch Surg 1987;122:1321–1325.

9. Tuck B, Belliveau JF, Darnowski JW, Weinberg MC, Leenen L, Wanebo HS. Isolated pelvic perfusion for unresectable cancer using a balloon occlusion technique. Arch Surg 1993;128:533–539.

10. Schwemmle K, Link KH, Rieck B. Rationale and indications for perfusion in liver tumors: current data. World J Surg 1987;11:534–540.

11. Krementz ET. Regional perfusion: current sophistication, what next? Cancer 1986;57:416–432.

12. Beahrs OH, Henson DE, Hutter RVP, Kennedy BJ, eds. American Joint Committee on Cancer manual for staging of cancer. 4th ed. Philadelphia: JB Lippincott, 1992.

13. Kroon BBR. Regional isolation perfusion in melanoma of the limbs: accomplishments, unsolved problems, future. Eur J Surg Oncol 1988;14:101–110.

14. Koops HS, Oldhoff J, Oosterhuis JW, Beekhuis H. Isolated regional perfusion in malignant melanoma of the extremities. World J Surg 1987;11:527–533.

15. Wieberdink J, Benckhuijsen C, Braat RP, van Slooten EA, Olthuis GAA. Dosimetry in isolation perfusion of the limbs by assessment of perfused tissue volume and grading of toxic reactions. Eur J Cancer Clin Oncol 1982;18:905–910.

16. Ghussen F, Nagel K, Groth W, Muller JM, Stutzer H. A prospective randomized study of regional extremity perfusion in patients with malignant melanoma. Ann Surg 1984;200:764–768.

17. Hafstrom L, Rudenstow CM, Blomquist E, Ingrar C. Regional hyperthermic perfusion with melphalan after surgery for recurrent malignant melanoma of the extremities. J Clin Oncol 1991;9:2091–2094.

18. Janoff KA, Moseson D, Nohlgren J, Davenport C, Richards C, Fletcher WS. The treatment of stage I melanoma of the extremities with regional hyperthermic isolation perfusion. Ann Surg 1982;196:316–323.

19. Stehlin JS Jr, Giovanella BC, de Ipolyi PD, Anderson RF. Eleven years' experience with hyperthermic perfusion for melanoma of the extremities. World J Surg 1979;3:305–307.

20. Shiu MH, Knapper WH, Fortner JG, et al. Regional isolated limb perfusion of melanoma in-transit metastases using mechlorethamine (nitrogen mustard). J Clin Oncol 1986;4:1819–1826.

21. Liénard D, Lejeune FJ, Ewalenko P. In-transit metastases of malignant melanoma treated by high-dose rTNF-α in combination with interferon-γ and melphalan in isolation perfusion. World J Surg 1992;16:234–240.

22. Liénard D, Ewalenko P, Delmotte JJ, Renard N, Lejeune FJ. High-dose recombinant tumor necrosis factor alpha in combination with interferon gamma and melphalan in isolation perfusion of the limbs for melanoma and sarcoma. J Clin Oncol 1992;10:52–60.

23. Fraker DL, Alexander HR. Isolated limb perfusion with high-dose tumor necrosis factor for extremity melanoma and sarcoma. In: DeVita VT, Hellman S, Rosenberg SA, eds. Important advances in oncology 1994. Philadelphia: JB Lippincott, 1994:179–192.

24. Asher A, Mulé JJ, Reichert CM, Shiloni E, Rosenberg SA. Studies on the anti-tumor efficacy of systemically administered recombinant tumor necrosis factor against several murine tumors in vivo. J Immunol 1987;138:963–974.

25. Havell EA, Fiers W, North RJ. The antitumor function of tumor necrosis factor (TNF). I. Therapeutic action of TMF against an established murine sarcoma is indirect, immunologically dependent, and limited by severe toxicity. J Exp Med 1988;167:1067–1085.

26. Ariyan S, Mitchel MS, Kirkwood JM. Regional isolated perfusion of high risk melanoma of the extremities with imidazole carboxamide. Surg Gynecol Obstet 1984;158:238–242.

27. Schraffordt Koops H, Liénard D, Eggermont AM, Hoekstra HJ, van Geel BN, Lejeune FJ. Isolated limb perfusion with high-dose TNF-α, gamma-IFN, and melphalan in patients with irresectable soft tissue sarcomas: a highly effective limb salvage procedure (abstract). Soc Surg Oncol 1993;46:1.

28. Di Filippo F, Calabrò AM, Cavallari A, et al. The role of hyperthermic perfusion as a first step in the treatment of soft tissue sarcoma of the extremities. World J Surg 1988;12:332–339.

29. Krementz ET, Carter RD, Sutherland CM, Hutton I. Chemotherapy of sarcomas of the limbs by regional perfusion. Ann Surg 1977;185:555–563.

30. Stehlin JS Jr, de Ipolyi PD, Giovanella BC, Gatierrez AE, Anderson RF. Soft tissue sarcomas of the extremity: multidisciplinary therapy employing hyperthermic perfusion. Am J Surg 1975;130:643–646.

31. Lehti PM, Moseley HS, Janoff K, Stevens K, Fletcher WS. Improved survival for soft tissue sarcoma of the extremities by regional hyperthermic perfusion, local excision and radiation therapy. Surg Gynecol Obstet 1986;162:149–152.

32. Wood WC, Suit HD, Mankin HJ, Cohen AM, Proppe K. Radiation and conservative surgery in the treatment of soft tissue sarcoma. Am J Surg 1984;147:537–541.

33. Denton JW, Dunham WK, Salter M, Urist MM, Balch CM. Preoperative regional chemotherapy and rapid-fraction irradiation for sarcomas of the soft tissue and bone. Surg Gynecol Obstet 1984;158:545–551.

34. Jansen RFM, van Geel BN, van der Zee J, Hagenbeek A, Levendag PC. Intractable cutaneous non-Hodgkin's lymphoma of the lower limb: complete remission after sequential regional isolated hyperthermic perfusion and perfusion with 1-phenylalanine mustard (melphalan, l-PAM). Cancer 1989;64:392–395.

35. Ryan RF. Chemotherapy perfusion techniques and problems. Surg Clin North Am 1962;42:389–402.

36. Stehlin JS Jr, Clark RL, Vickers WE, Monges A. Perfusion for malignant melanoma of the extremities. Am J Surg 1963;105:607–614.

37. Bulman AS, Jamieson CW. Isolated limb perfusion with melphalan in the treatment of malignant melanoma. Br J Surg 1980;67:660–662.

38. Rosin RD, Westbury G. Isolated limb perfusion for malignant melanoma. Practitioner 1980;224:1031–1036.

39. Hafström L, Jönsson PE. Hyperthermic perfusion of recurrent malignant melanoma of the extremities. Acta Chir Scand 1980;146:313–318.

40. Hansson JA, Simert G, Vang J. The effect of regional perfusion treatment on recurrent melanoma of the extremities. Acta Chir Scand 1977;143:33–39.

41. Couture J. Melanoma: the management of local recurrence and in-transit metastasis. Can J Surg 1982;25:698–700.

42. Kroon BBR, van Geel AN, Benckhuijsen C, Wieberdink J. Normothermic isolation perfusion with melphalan for advanced melanoma of the limbs. Anticancer Res 1987;7:441–442.

43. Rochlin DB, Smart CR. Treatment of malignant melanoma by regional perfusion. Cancer 1965;18:1544–1550.

44. Jönsson PE, Hafström L, Hugander A. Results of regional hyperthermic perfusion for primary and recurrent melanomas of the extremities. Recent Results Cancer Res 1983;86:277–282.

45. Lejeune FJ, Deloof T, Ewalenko P, et al. Objective regression of unexcised melanoma in-transit metastases after hyperthermic isolation perfusion of the limbs with melphalan. Recent Results Cancer Res 1983;86:268–276.

46. Vaglini M, Andreola S, Attili, et al. Hyperthermic antiblastic perfusion in the treatment of cancer of the extremities. Tumori 1985;71:355–359.

47. Storm FK, Morton DL. Value of therapeutic hyperthermic limb perfusion in advanced recurrent melanoma of the lower extremity. Am J Surg 1985;150:32–35.

48. Cavaliere R, Calabrò AM, Di Filippo F, Carlini S, Giannarelli D. Prognostic parameters in limb recurrent melanoma treated with hyperthermic antiblastic perfusion (abstract). ICRCT Ulm 1987;G7:163.

49. Krementz ET, Ryan RF. Chemotherapy of melanoma of the extremities by perfusion: fourteen years of clinical experience. Ann Surg 1972;175:900–917.

50. Bartsch HH, Pfizenmaier K, Schroeder M, Nagel GA. Intralesional application of recombinant human tumor necrosis factor-alpha induces local tumor regression in patients with advanced malignancies. Eur J Cancer Clin Oncol 1989;25:287–291.

51. Pfreundschuh MG, Steinmetz HT, Tuschen R, Schenk V, Diehl V, Schaadt M. Phase I study of intratumoral application of recombinant human tumor necrosis factor. Eur J Cancer Clin Oncol 1989;25:379–388.

52. Kahn JO, Kaplan LD, Volberding PA, et al. Intralesional recombinant tumor necrosis factor-α for AIDS-associated Kaposi's sarcoma: a randomized, double-blind trial. J Acquir Immune Defic Syndr 1989;2:217–223.

53. Ijzermans JNM, van der Schelling GP, Scheringa M, Splinter RAW, Marquet RL, Jeekel J. Local treatment of liver metastases with recombinant tumour necrosis factor (rTNF): a phase one study. Neth J Surg 1991;43:121–125.

54. Mavligit GM, Zukiwski AA, Charnsargavej C. Regional biologic therapy: hepatic arterial infusion of recombinant human tumor necrosis factor in patients with liver metastases. Cancer 1992;69:557–561.

55. Cox KR. Survival after regional perfusion for limb melanoma. Aust NZ J Surg 1975;45:32–36.

56. Colomb FM. Perfusion of melanoma: 133 isolated perfusions in 114 patients. Panminerva Med 1976;17:8–10.

57. Aigner K, Hild P, Breithaupt H, et al. Isolated extremity perfusion with DTIC: an experimental and clinical study. Anticancer Res 1983;3:87–93.

58. Aigner K, Hild P, Henneking K, Paul E, Hundeiker M. Regional perfusion with *cis*-platinum and dacarbazine. Recent Results Cancer Res 1983;86:239–245.

59. Aigner K, Jungbluth A, Link KH et al. Die iso-lierte hypertherme Extremitäten Perfusion mit Vindesin, Dacarbazin und Cisplatin bei der Behandlung maligner Melanoma. Onkologie 1984;7:348–353.

60. Vaglini M, Belli F, Marolda R, Prada A, Santinami M, Cascinelli N. Hyperthermic antiblastic perfusion with DTIC in stage IIIA-IIIAB melanoma of the extremities. Eur J Surg Oncol 1987;13:127–129.

18

Bone Marrow Transplantation

Julie M. Vose and James O. Armitage

Many effective cancer chemotherapeutic agents are destructive to the normal bone marrow cells. Therefore, bone marrow toxicity is often a limiting factor in administration of adequate chemotherapy doses for curative intent. Hematopoietic stem cell transplantation allows the administration of "supralethal" chemo/radiotherapy to increase the percentage of malignant cells destroyed while rescuing the patient from hematopoietic toxicity with the transplant. Additionally, the healthy new cells transplanted may allow the replacement of an intact immune system to provide an antitumor effect or, in the case of bone marrow transplants for congenital diseases, to provide cells that are no longer deficient in certain vital components.

The first report of a procedure similar to a transplant was in 1939, when a patient received 18 mL of intravenous marrow from his brother as a treatment for aplastic anemia (1). The beginning of modern bone marrow transplantation can be traced to work showing that rodents could be protected against lethal hematopoietic injury by the intravenous infusion of bone marrow (2). The subsequent identification of the HLA system and the development of adequate storage techniques for hematopoietic cells laid the groundwork for clinical trials.

High-dose chemotherapy with bone marrow or peripheral blood progenitor (stem cells) transplant is now increasingly used for the treatment of many hematologic, immunologic, and neoplastic diseases (3–6). There are several sources of hematopoietic stem cells that can be used for the transplant. These include allogeneic bone marrow cells from an HLA-identical sibling donor, from a partially matched family donor, or from an unrelated donor from the national marrow donor program; syngeneic bone marrow from an identical twin donor; or autologous cells derived from either the bone marrow or the peripheral blood progenitor compartment. The chemo/radiotherapy regimen and the source of the hematopoietic stem cells used for reconstitution are chosen on the basis of the disease type and other patient characteristics.

The use of this treatment has been growing over the past several years. The most recent figures from the International Bone Marrow Transplant Registry demonstrate that approximately 12,000 autologous transplants were performed and reported to the registry in 1994, and approximately 8,000 allogeneic transplants were performed and reported to the registry in 1994 (Fig. 18.1) (7).

This chapter outlines the various diseases treated with high-dose therapy and transplantation, the therapy and supportive care used during the transplant, and the complications that may occur during the various types of transplantation.

ALLOGENEIC AND SYNGENEIC TRANSPLANTATION

Allogeneic bone marrow transplantation involves the transfer of stem cells from a donor to another person. A syngeneic transplant is the special case of a donor and a recipient who are genetically identical—an identical twin. Allogeneic transplants are considered for patients up to age 45–55 years, and occasionally, older patients are treated. The results tend to be poorer in older patients because of the increasing incidence of graft-versus-host disease with age. However, the decision in any individual patient must take into account all factors, including the patient's physiologic age, not just the chronologic age. The chances of having an HLA-match from a sibling would be one in four for each sibling. However, due to the relatively small size of families in the United States, only about

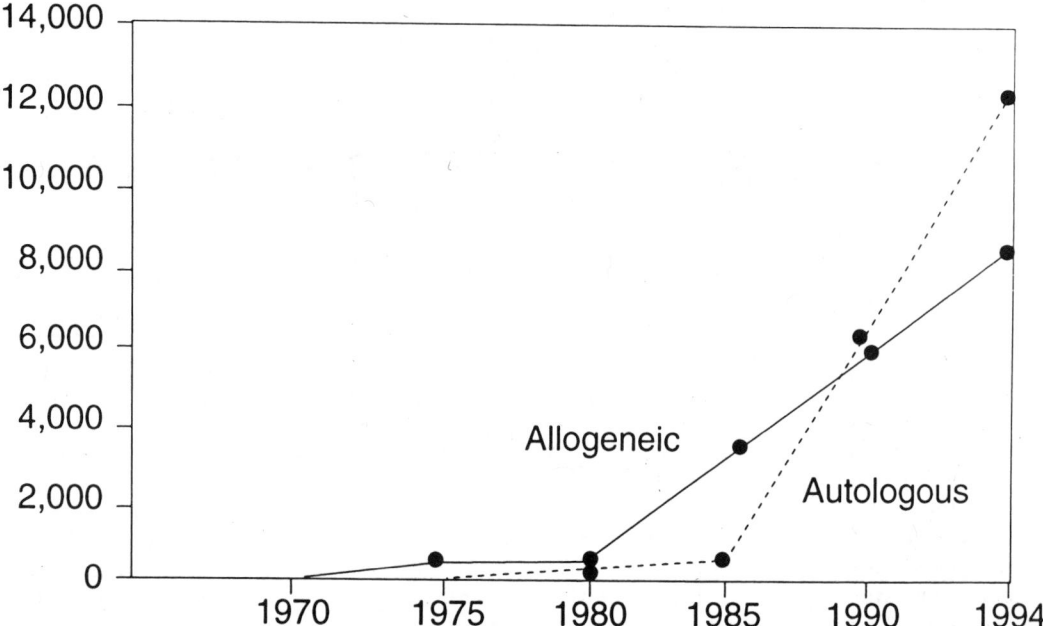

Figure 18.1.   Increasing use of blood and marrow transplantation. (Information reprinted with permission of the International Bone Marrow Transplant Registry—IBMTR).

30% of patients will have an HLA-matched sibling.

For patients who lack an HLA-identical sibling donor, there are two possible solutions: to identify an unrelated but closely HLA-matched person through the National Marrow Donor Program or to use a partially matched related donor. There are many possible HLA phenotypes, which makes the identification of a matched unrelated donor difficult and time consuming. For Caucasians of similar Northern European ethnic descent, it has been estimated that a registry of 200,000 potential donors would provide a 40–50% chance of finding an HLA-matched donor (8, 9). The National Marrow Donor Program has been developed to facilitate the search for unrelated donors in the United States (10).

An alternative approach is to identify a related person who shares some, but not all, of the patient's HLA antigens (11). Successful allogeneic transplantation can be performed with marrow from such donors, although the risks of graft rejection and graft-versus-host disease may be increased.

Once a suitable donor has been identified, the patient is prepared for the allogeneic or syngeneic transplant with high doses of chemotherapy alone or combined radio/chemotherapy. The purpose of this treatment is to destroy any remaining malignant cells, to provide sufficient immunosuppression to allow engraftment of the new cells, and to clear the marrow space for engraftment of the new cells. Only certain chemotherapeutic agents can be dose-escalated in this fashion. The agents chosen must have toxicities (other than hematologic ones) that are dose limiting at levels well above the hematologic effects that allow adequate escalation. For example, high doses of some anthracyclines are difficult to use in transplantation because of the cardiac toxicity that is apparent at relatively low doses. Most regimens consist of total body irradiation (TBI) combined with alkylating agents, etoposide, and/or cytarabine. Some non-TBI-containing regimens have also been developed using multiple alkylating agents.

AUTOLOGOUS BONE MARROW TRANSPLANTATION

Autologous bone marrow transplantation involves the use of the patient's own hematopoietic cells to reestablish hematopoietic cell function after the administration of high-dose chemo/radiotherapy. These reinfused hematopoietic cells can come from the patient's bone marrow, peripheral blood, or a combination of the two. This approach has several advantages and a number of disadvantages, compared with allogeneic transplantation. Since a major limitation to the use of allogeneic bone marrow transplantation is that only a minority of patients will have an HLA-matched sibling donor, the use of autologous hematopoietic cells greatly increases the number of patients eligible for transplantation. Autologous transplantation can also safely be used in an older patient population because of the increased safety profile and the lack of risk of graft-versus-host disease, which is always a concern as the age of the patient rises. The relative increases in autologous transplantation and allogeneic transplantation are shown in Figure 18.1.

However, a primary concern in using autologous hematopoietic cells is the risk of contamination of the graft with viable tumor cells. Most studies demonstrate that populations undergoing autologous transplant have higher relapse rates than those with allogeneic transplants. However, with the increased risk and complications of allogeneic transplantation, the outcome is often similar in the long-term follow-up (12). Numerous methods, including in vitro treatment with chemotherapeutic agents, monoclonal antibodies and complement, or "positive selection," have been attempted to decrease the tumor contamination and therefore decrease the possibility of relapse (13–17).

Retrospective analyses have suggested that patients receiving autologous grafts that were negative by molecular testing for residual disease may have better outcomes than patients with grafts that were positive by these techniques do (14). However, most relapses occur at sites of previous disease, raising the question of

whether resistance to treatment and overall increased tumor burden resulted in the relapse or the reinfusion of tumor cells caused the relapse. There have been initial trials demonstrating with gene-marking experiments that in at least some of the patients undergoing autologous transplantation for leukemia and neuroblastoma, marked reinfused cells did contribute to the relapse in some of the patients (18). Because of this controversy, studies evaluating the need for purging are ongoing, and no randomized trial has been published to date. Allogeneic and autologous transplantation are compared in Table 18.1.

INDICATIONS FOR TRANSPLANTATION

The indications for transplantation are not always clear-cut in each patient's clinical situation. However, there are a number of diseases that are generally accepted as indications for transplantation. The relative use of allogeneic and autologous transplantation for various diseases is outlined in Figure 18.2 according to information supplied to the American Bone Marrow Transplant Registry for the calendar year 1994 (7).

Malignant Conditions

NON-HODGKIN'S LYMPHOMA

A number of publications have evaluated allogeneic, syngeneic, and autologous transplantation for the treatment of intermediate and high-grade non-Hodgkin's lymphoma (NHL) (19–22). The patients with relapsed disease appear to benefit most from this therapy if they are transplanted when they still have chemotherapy-sensitive disease (19, 23). In addition, patients who have high-risk characteristics and are transplanted as part of their planned therapy early in the course of their disease in first partial or complete response appear to have an better outcome than similar patients treated with conventional therapy do (20, 21, 24). This concept must be tested in controlled randomized trials to analyze the impact of early transplantation.

The use of high-dose chemo/radiotherapy and transplantation in indolent NHL has only been evaluated in recent years. Studies using autologous transplantation for the treatment of relapsed indolent NHL have demonstrated a failure-free survival of 40–60% at a median follow-up of 3 years (22, 25, 26). Because late relapses are more likely to occur with these histo-

Table 18.1. Comparison of Autologous and Allogeneic Transplantation

Feature	Allogeneic	Autologous
Age limits	45–55 years	60–70 years
Availability	¼–⅓ of pts	Limited only by ability to collect adequate cells
Cause of failure	Complications of BMT GVHD[a] Disease relapse	Disease relapse Complications of BMT

[a]GVHD, graft-versus-host disease.

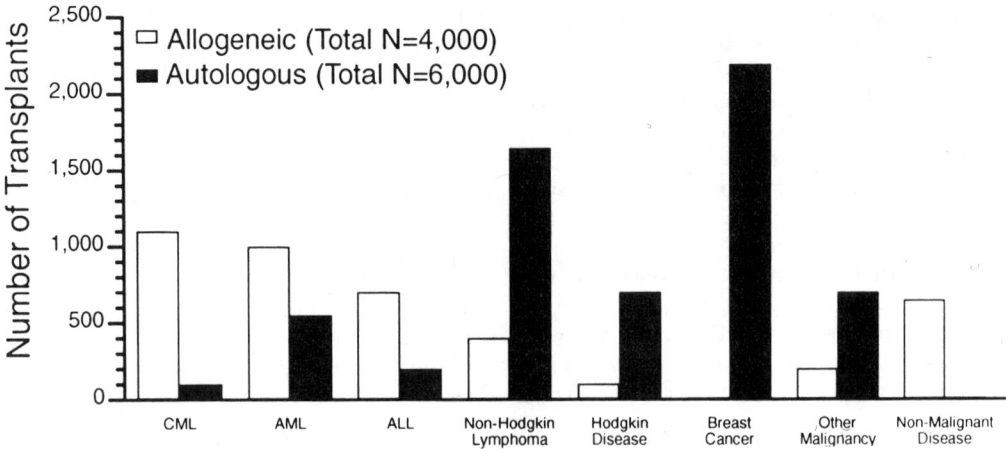

Figure 18.2.   Indications for blood and marrow transplants in North America, 1994. (Information reprinted with permission of the American Bone Marrow Transplant Registry—ABMTR).

logic types of lymphoma, much longer follow-up will be necessary to assess the long-term results of this treatment. The use of autologous transplantation in a cohort of patients in first complete remission was also recently tested at the Dana Farber Cancer Institute and at Stanford University. The long-term results of transplants in this patient population will be evaluated to assess the effect on changing the natural history of the illness (27). In addition, some centers are now evaluating allogeneic transplants in indolent lymphoma patients because of the possibility of decreased relapse rates.

HODGKIN'S DISEASE

High-dose therapy followed by autologous hematopoietic stem cell transplantation has now been widely accepted for patients with relapsed Hodgkin's disease. The use of allogeneic transplantation for patients with relapsed Hodgkin's disease has not been used as extensively because of the increased morbidity and mortality with this type of transplant (28). In patients who have received multiple chemotherapy regimens prior to coming to transplant, the outcome is poorer than that in less heavily pretreated patients (29). Although no large prospectively randomized trials are available, one study in Europe that randomized patients to receive BEAM (carmustine, etoposide, cytarabine, and melphalan) either as lower doses (mini-BEAM) or as a high-dose regimen with autologous transplant, did demonstrate a better outcome in the 20 patients randomized to the high-dose arm than that in those randomized to the mini-BEAM arm (30). An initial pilot trial of transplantation as part of the initial therapy for high-risk Hodgkin's patients demonstrated better results than those in historic controls (31).

MULTIPLE MYELOMA

Both autologous and allogeneic transplantation have been successfully performed in patients with multiple myeloma. A large series of allogeneic transplants in multiple myeloma patients demonstrated a 31% complete remission rate, with 43% of patients alive with a median follow-up of 24 months (32). Autologous transplantation for this disease can result in long-term disease-free survival in a percentage of patients and is more successful in patients who are less heavily pretreated and have a smaller tumor burden, similar to transplants in lymphoma patients (33–34).

ACUTE MYELOGENOUS LEUKEMIA (AML)/MYELODYSPLASTIC SYNDROME (MDS)

Because patients with good- or average-risk AML have the potential for cure with conventional induction and intensification therapy, most centers would use transplantation only for relapsed AML in adults or as part of the initial therapy for patients with known poor prognosis characteristics such as certain high-risk chromosomal abnormalities. The use of autologous versus allogeneic transplantation is controversial; most studies demonstrate a decreased relapse rate with allogeneic transplant but not as much difference in long-term outcome, because of increased morbidity and mortality with an allogeneic source of hematopoietic cells (35, 36).

Myelodysplastic syndromes are best treated with an allogeneic transplant from an HLA-identical sibling donor in young, otherwise healthy, patients (37). Unfortunately, most patients with MDS are elderly, which precludes this successful therapy in many patients.

ACUTE LYMPHOBLASTIC LEUKEMIA

The results of induction and consolidation therapy for ALL in children are excellent except in a few clinical circumstances such as ALL associated with the Philadelphia chromosome (38). Therefore, the use of transplantation for ALL in children is usually reserved for this high-risk group of patients or patients who relapse after their initial therapy. In adults, the indications for transplantation are similar, although a higher percentage of adults will fail after their initial therapy.

CHRONIC MYELOGENOUS LEUKEMIA (CML)

Allogeneic transplantation from an HLA-matched sibling donor for early-chronic-phase CML can produce long-term disease-free survival in 50–75% of patients (39–41). The results appear to be better when the patients are transplanted within the first year of diagnosis (39, 42), have received hydroxyurea rather than busulfan (42), and have not received extensive interferon (43). The use of alternative donors has also demonstrated promise in the treatment of CML.

BREAST CANCER

In the last several years, breast cancer has replaced NHL as the most common indication for an autologous transplant. However, its use for the treatment of this malignancy remains controversial. The use of high-dose chemotherapy for the treatment of metastatic breast cancer can result in a higher complete response rate than the use of conventional treatment (44, 45). However, the reported disease-free survival in chemotherapy sensitive stage IV breast cancer is 10–25% in most series (44–46). Current ongoing randomized trials may help to answer the question of the role of transplantation in the treatment of metastatic disease. The use of transplantation as adjuvant therapy in high-risk 10+ node-positive disease also appears promising (47). This treatment is also currently being compared with conventional therapy in randomized trials.

SOLID TUMORS

In addition to breast cancer, high-dose chemotherapy and transplant has had success in the treatment of some chemotherapy-sensitive solid tumors such as testicular cancer (48, 49), sarcoma (50), ovarian carcinoma (50), small cell lung cancer (50), and childhood tumors such as neuroblastoma or Wilm's tumor (51, 52). Other solid tumors that are chemotherapy refractory, such as melanoma or many gastrointestinal malignancies, are poor potential targets for this therapy.

Nonmalignant Conditions

IMMUNODEFICIENCY DISORDERS

Several inherited immunodeficiency disorders in children have now been successfully treated with high-dose chemotherapy and allogeneic transplantation. Disorders such as Wiskott-Aldrich syndrome or severe combined immunodeficiency syndrome (SCID) have been successfully treated with HLA-matched sibling transplants or transplants from alternative donors (53, 54).

GENETIC DISORDERS

Other genetic disorders such as osteopetrosis (55), Gaucher's disease (56), or Hurler's syndrome (57) can also be successfully treated with an allogeneic transplant. Other indications for allogeneic transplant are inherited hemoglobinopathies or other blood disorders such as sickle cell anemia, thalassemia, or acquired disorders such as paroxysmal nocturnal hemoglobinuria (58–60). The transplant must be performed prior to the onset of secondary organ failure or excess damage from the disorder.

APLASTIC ANEMIA

Allogeneic transplant can also lead to long-term disease-free survival in over half of the patients with aplastic anemia (61). Compared with standard immunosuppressive therapy, allogeneic transplant is more likely to produce a complete reversal of hematologic abnormalities. However, depending on the severity of aplastic anemia, the age of the patient, and the availability of a donor, a trial of other therapies may be appropriate before consideration of a transplant.

COMPLICATIONS

In addition to the acute toxicities associated with prolonged cytopenias, other organ toxicities can be associated with transplantation. The late toxicities must always be kept in mind when choosing therapies for patients.

CARDIAC TOXICITY

Most transplant centers screen potential patients for underlying cardiac abnormalities that would place them at potential increased risk during the procedure. Despite this screening, however, a small number of patients experience cardiotoxicity, either acutely during the transplant or at a later time, manifested as a cardiac arrhythmia, congestive heart failure, or cardiac ischemia due to the large volumes of fluids administered during the procedure or from the added physiologic stress. Complications associated with a pericardial effusion can be seen in some patients during or after transplant and are more common in patients with disease near that area and those receiving radiation therapy in that field. An idiosyncratic cardiomyopathy associated with the administration of high doses of cyclophosphamide can be demonstrated in a small number of patients. In addition, viral cardiomyopathies can also be seen in a small number of patients.

PULMONARY TOXICITIES

Pulmonary toxicities are common both during and after transplantation. In autologous transplant patients, complications include infections from bacterial, fungal, or viral sources during the transplant process. In addition, patients receiving certain chemotherapy agents such as BCNU (carmustine) have an increased incidence of chemotherapy-induced lung tissue damage posttransplant. This can usually be successfully treated with the prompt initiation of steroid therapy (62). In addition to these complications, patients undergoing allogeneic transplant are at increased risk for pneumonitis caused by cytomegalovirus, fungal infections due to the patient's increased immunosuppression, and adult respiratory distress syndrome or interstitial pneumonia of unknown etiology. Graft-versus-host disease can also manifest itself as bronchiolitis obliterans in the lung (63).

LIVER TOXICITY

The most frequent liver complication associated with transplantation is venoocclusive disease of the liver. Symptoms associated with this complication include jaundice, tender hepatomegaly, ascites, and weight gain. Progressive hepatic failure and multiorgan system failure can develop in the most severe cases. Predisposing factors appear to be previous hepatic injury, the use of certain agents in the conditioning regimen for transplant, and perhaps the use of alternative donors (64).

RENAL TOXICITY

Acute renal failure requiring dialysis during the transplant occurs infrequently. However, patients with underlying renal dysfunction are clearly at risk for this complication. The judicious use of nephrotoxic agents can decrease the incidence of this complication. The need for dialysis is typically a short-term complication, since the patient's underlying problem (e.g., a septic event) either improves with time or becomes life threatening, with fatal consequences.

GRAFT-VERSUS-HOST DISEASE

In the allogeneic transplant setting, complications associated with both acute and chronic GVHD are also of concern. Acute GVHD is manifested by symptoms in several organs systems including the skin, gastrointestinal tract, and liver. This complication occurs within the first 100 days following transplantation. The skin manifestations range from a maculopapular rash up to generalized erythroderma or desquamation. The severity of liver GVHD is scored on the basis of the bilirubin, and the gastrointestinal severity on the quantity of diarrhea per day.

Patients receiving transplants from alternative donors are at a much increased risk for this complication, and GVHD incidence and severity rise with the age of the patient. Other risk factors for the development of GVHD include a female donor (particularly a multiparous donor) and a male recipient and CMV seropositivity of the donor or patient. Patients receive prophylaxis for GVHD prevention most commonly with cyclosporine, with or without methotrexate and corticosteroids (65–67). Treatment for acute GVHD includes high-dose corticosteroids, antithymocyte globulin, and various monoclonal antibodies (68–70).

Chronic GVHD occurs after day 100 from the transplant and has some similar features. It is most likely to develop in older patients who also had acute GVHD (71). Symptoms associated with chronic GVHD include sicca syndrome, chronic sinusitis, rashes or skin thickening, diarrhea and a wasting syndrome, or liver function abnormalities (72). Patients are also at greatly increased risk for infectious complications, due to either the GVHD itself or the treatment administered. Adverse prognostic factors include thrombocytopenia, a progressive clinical presentation, and an elevated bilirubin (73). Treatment for the chronic form of the disease includes corticosteroids, cyclosporine, thalidomide, ultraviolet light treatments, or other immunosuppressive agents (74, 75).

GRAFT REJECTION

Graft rejection occurs when immunologically competent cells of host origin destroy the transplanted cells of donor origin. This complication occurs more commonly in patients receiving transplants from alternative donors, in T-cell-depleted transplants, and in patients with aplastic anemia receiving a non-TBI-containing regimen (76). Graft rejection is less likely in nontransfused aplastic anemia patients. This complication is uncommon with the use of HLA-matched sibling donors.

INFERTILITY

Many of the preparative regimens used for transplant are associated with a high incidence of permanent sterility. The use of TBI is almost always associated with sterility. However, successful pregnancies have occurred after the use of non-TBI-containing regimens (77). This is particularly true in patients who have been less heavily retreated prior to the transplant and are under the age of approximately 25 years at the time of transplant.

SECONDARY MALIGNANCIES

As there are more long-term survivors from transplantation, complications that develop years later are beginning to be recognized. One complication of the chemotherapy and/or radiotherapy used to treat malignancy is the development of a secondary malignancy. There have now been several reports of the development of secondary AML or MDS following transplantation (78, 79). Some studies have suggested that the use of TBI may increase the risk of these complications (79). It is unclear what role the transplant itself played in the development of the AML/MDS, since all patients received chemotherapy and/or radiotherapy prior to the transplant and, in some cases, following the transplant. Secondary solid tumors are also being recognized more frequently following transplantation, and the rates will most likely increase with further follow-up of surviving patients.

THE FUTURE OF TRANSPLANTATION

We have had tremendous success over the past two decades in the use of transplantation and the application of this treatment to more patient populations. Areas currently under development that may improve transplantation further include newer broader hematopoietic cytokines, ex vivo expansion of progenitors, genetic marking and modulation of cells, improved supportive care for transplant patients, and broadened use of alternative donors. The recognition of the best patient populations for treatment with transplantation as well as newer agents to assist in their treatment will be essential in the refinement of this therapy.

REFERENCES

1. Osgood EE, Riddle MC, Mathews TJ. Aplastic anemia treated with daily transfusions and intravenous marrow; case report. Ann Intern Med 1939; 13:357–367.
2. Lorenz E, Uphoff D, Reid TR, et al. Modification of irradiation injury in mice and guinea pigs by bone marrow injections. J Natl Cancer Inst 1951;12:197–201.
3. Thomas ED, Storb R, Clift A, et al. Bone marrow transplantation. N Engl J Med 1973;292:832–843.
4. Cheson BD, Lacern L, Leyland-Jones B, et al. Autologous bone marrow transplantation: current grafting and future directions. Ann Intern Med 1989;110:51–56.
5. Champlin RE, Gale RP. Bone marrow transplantation for acute leukemia: recent advances and comparison with alternative therapies. Semin Hematol 1987;24:55–67.
6. Ringden O, Groth CG, Erikson A, et al. Long-term follow-up of the first successful bone marrow transplantation in Gaucher's disease. Transplantation 1988;46:66–70.
7. IBMTR Newsletter. 1995;2:1–12.
8. Gahrton G. Bone marrow transplantation with unrelated volunteer donors. Eur J Cancer 1991; 27:1537–1539.
9. Beatty PG, Dahlberg S, Mickelson EM, et al. Probability of finding HLA-matched unrelated marrow donors. Transplantation 1988;45:714–718.
10. McCullough J, Hansen J, Perkins H, et al. The National Marrow Donor Program: how it works, accomplishments to date. Oncology 1989;3:63–68.
11. Beatty PG, Clift RA, Mickelson EM, et al. Marrow transplantation from related donors other than HLA-identical siblings. N Engl J Med 1985;313:765–771.
12. Chopra R, Goldstone AH, Pearce R, et al. Autologous versus allogeneic bone marrow transplantation for non-Hodgkin's lymphoma: a case-controlled analysis of the European Bone Marrow Transplant Group Registry data. J Clin Oncol 1992;10:1690–1695.
13. Gorin NC, Aegerter P, Auvert B, et al. Autologous bone marrow transplantation for acute myelocytic leukemia in first remission: a European survey of the role of marrow purging. Blood 1990;75:1606–1614.
14. Gribben JG, Freedman AS, Neuberg D, et al. Immunologic purging of marrow assessed by PCR before autologous bone marrow transplantation for B-cell lymphoma. N Engl J Med 1991;325:1525–1533.
15. Atzpodien J, Gulati SC, Strife A, et al. Photoradiation models for the clinical ex vivo treatment of autologous bone marrow grafts. Blood 1987;70:484–489.

16. Chang J, Coutinho L, Morgenstern G, et al. Reconstitution of haemopoietic system with autologous marrow taken during relapse of acute myeloblastic leukaemia and grown in long-term culture. Lancet 1986;1:294–295.

17. Shpall EJ, Stemmer SM, Johnston CR, et al. Purging of autologous bone marrow transplantation: the protection and selection of the hematopoietic progenitor cell. J Hematother 1992;73:835–840.

18. Brenner MK, Rill DR, Moen RC, et al. Gene-marking to trace origin of relapse after autologous bone-marrow transplantation. Lancet 1993;341:85–86.

19. Vose JM, Anderson JR, Kessinger A, et al. High-dose chemotherapy and autologous hematopoietic stem-cell transplantation for aggressive non-Hodgkin's lymphoma. J Clin Oncol 1993;11:1846–1851.

20. Gulati SC, Shank B, Black P, et al. Autologous bone marrow transplantation for patients with poor-prognosis lymphoma. J Clin Oncol 1988;6:1303–1313.

21. Nademanee A, Schmidt GM, O'Donnell MR, et al. High-dose chemoradiotherapy followed by autologous bone marrow transplantation as consolidation therapy during first complete remission in adult patients with poor-risk aggressive lymphoma: a pilot study. Blood 1992;80:1130–1140.

22. Freedman AS, Ritz J, Neuberg D, et al. Autologous bone marrow transplantation in 69 patients with a history of low-grade B-cell non-Hodgkin's lymphoma. Blood 1991;77:2524–2529.

23. Philip T, Armitage JO, Spitzer G, et al. High-dose therapy and autologous bone marrow transplantation after failure of conventional chemotherapy in adults with intermediate-grade or high-grade non-Hodgkin's lymphoma. N Engl J Med 1987;316:1493–1498.

24. Santini G, Coser P, Chisesi T, et al. Autologous bone marrow transplantation for advanced stage adult lymphoblastic lymphoma in first complete remission: a pilot study of the Non-Hodgkin's Lymphoma Cooperative Study Group (NHLCSG). Bone Marrow Transplant 1989;4:399–404.

25. Bierman P, Vose JM, Armitage JO. High-dose therapy followed by autologous hematopoietic rescue for follicular low-grade non-Hodgkin's lymphoma (NHL) (abstract). Proc Am Soc Clin Oncol 1992; 11:317a.

26. Rohatiner AZS, Johnson PWM, Price CGA, et al. Myeloablative therapy with autologous bone marrow transplantation as consolidation therapy for recurrent follicular lymphoma. J Clin Oncol 1994; 12:1177–1184.

27. Freedman A, Nadler L. Bone marrow transplantation in low-grade non-Hodgkin's lymphoma. Issues Hematol Oncol Immunol 1992;2(3):33–38.

28. Phillips G, Reece DE, Barnett MJ, et al. Allogeneic marrow transplantation for refractory Hodgkin's disease. J Clin Oncol 1989;7:1039–1045.

29. Bierman PJ, Bagin RG, Jagannath S, et al. High-dose chemotherapy followed by autologous hematopoietic rescue in Hodgkin's disease: long term follow-up in 128 patients. Ann Oncol 1993;4:767–773.

30. Linch DC, Winfield D, Goldstone AH, et al. Dose intensification with autologous bone-marrow transplantation in relapsed and resistant Hodgkin's disease: results of a BNLI randomized trial. Lancet 1993;341:1051–1054.

31. Carella AM, Carlier P, Congiu A, et al. Autologous bone marrow transplantation as adjuvant treatment for high-risk Hodgkin's disease in first complete remission after MOPP/ABVD protocol. Bone Marrow Transplant 1991;8:99–103.

32. Vesole DH, Jagannath S, Tricot G, et al. Allogeneic bone marrow transplantation (AlloBMT) in refractory multiple myeloma (MM) (abstract). Blood 1994;84:2128a.

33. Fermand JP, Ravaud PH, Chevret S, et al. High dose therapy and autologous blood stem cell transplantation (ABSCT) in multiple myeloma: preliminary results of a randomized clinical trial in 167 patients (abstract). Blood 1994;84:2125a.

34. Vesole DH, Jagannath S, Tricot G, et al. 400 Autotransplants (AT) for multiple myeloma (MM) (abstract). Blood 1994;84:2126a.

35. Zittoun R, Mandelli F, Willemze R, et al. Autologous or allogeneic bone marrow transplantation compared with intensive chemotherapy in acute myelogenous leukemia. N Engl J Med 1995;332:217–223.

36. Carella AM, Frassoni R, Van Lint MT, et al. Autologous and allogeneic BMT in acute myeloid leukemia in first complete remission: an update of the Genoa experience with 159 patients. Ann Hematol 1992; 64:128–131.

37. Anderson JE, Appelbaum FR, Fisher LD, et al. Allogeneic bone marrow transplantation for 93 patients with myelodysplastic syndrome. Blood 1993; 82:677–681.

38. Barrett AJ, Horowitz MM, Ash RC, et al. Bone marrow transplantation for Philadelphia chromosome-positive acute lymphoblastic leukemia. Blood 1992; 79:3067–3070.

39. Fefer A, Cheever MA, Thomas ED, et al. Disappearance of Ph[1]-positive cells in four patients with chronic granulocytic leukemia after chemotherapy, irradiation and marrow transplantation from an identical twin. N Engl J Med 1979;300:333–337.

40. Thomas ED, Clift RA, Fefer A, et al. Marrow transplantation for the treatment of chronic myelogenous leukemia. Ann Intern Med 1986;104:155–163.

41. Goldman JM, Apperley JF, Jones L, et al. Bone marrow transplantation for patients with chronic myeloid leukemia. N Engl J Med 1986;314:202–207.

42. Goldman JM, McGlave P, Szydlo P, et al. Impact of disease duration and prior treatment on outcome of bone marrow transplants for chronic myelogenous leukemia (CML) (abstract). Blood 1992;80(Suppl 1):170a.

43. Beelen DW, Graeven U, Elmaagacli AH, et al. Prolonged administration of interferon-alpha in patients with chronic-phase Philadelphia chromosome-positive chronic myelogenous leukemia before allogeneic bone marrow transplantation may adversely affect transplant outcome. Blood 1995;85:2981–2990.

44. Peters WP, Shpall EJ, Jones RB, et al. High-dose combination alkylating agents with bone marrow support as initial treatment for metastatic breast cancer. J Clin Oncol 1988;6:1368–1376.

45. Antman K, Ayash L, Elias A, et al. A phase II study of high-dose cyclophosphamide, thiotepa, and carboplatin with autologous marrow support in women with measurable advanced breast cancer responding to standard dose therapy. J Clin Oncol 1992; 10:102–110.

46. Williams SF, Gilewski T, Mick R, et al. High-dose consolidation therapy with autologous stem-cell rescue in stage IV breast cancer; follow-up report. J Clin Oncol 1992;10:1743–1747.

47. Peters W, Ross M, Vredenburgh J, et al. High-dose chemotherapy and autologous bone marrow sup-

port as consolidation after standard-dose adjuvant therapy for high-risk primary breast cancer. J Clin Oncol 1993;11:1132–1143.

48. Broun ER, Nichols CR, Kneebone P, et al. Long-term outcome of patients with relapsed and refractory germ cell tumors treated with high-dose chemotherapy and autologous bone marrow rescue. Ann Intern Med 1992;227:124–128.

49. Nichols CR, Andersen J, Lazarus HM, et al. High-dose carboplatin and etoposide with autologous bone marrow transplantation in refractory germ cell cancer: an Eastern Cooperative Oncology Group protocol. J Clin Oncol 1992;10:558–563.

50. Cheson BD. Autologous bone marrow transplantation for miscellaneous tumors. In: Armitage JO, Antman KH, eds. High-dose cancer therapy: pharmacology, hematopoietins, stem cells. Baltimore: Williams & Wilkins, 1992:763–771.

51. Philip T, Zucker JM, Bernard JL, et al. Improved survival at 2 and 5 years in the LMCE1 unselected group of 72 children with stage IV neuroblastoma older than 1 year of age at diagnosis: is cure possible in a small subgroup? J Clin Oncol 1991;9:1037–1044.

52. Pole JG, Casper J, Elfenbein G, et al. High-dose chemoradiotherapy supported by marrow infusions for advanced neuroblastoma: a Pediatric Oncology Group study. J Clin Oncol 1991;9:152–158.

53. Bortin MM, Rimm AA. Severe combined immunodeficiency disease: characterization of the disease and results of transplantation. JAMA 1977;238:591–600.

54. Parkman R, Rappeport J, Geha R, et al. Complete correction of the Wiskott-Aldrich syndrome by allogeneic bone marrow transplantation. N Engl J Med 1978;298:921–927.

55. Coccia PF, Krivit W, Cervenka J, et al. Successful bone-marrow transplantation for infantile malignant osteopetrosis. N Engl J Med 1980;302:701–708.

56. Rappeport JM, Ginns EI. Bone-marrow transplantation in severe Gaucher's disease. N Engl J Med 1984;311:84–88.

57. Field RE, Buchanan JA, Copplemans MG, et al. Bone-marrow transplantation in Hurler's syndrome. Effect on skeletal development. J Bone Joint Surg Br 1994;76:975–981.

58. Szer J, Deeg HJ, Witherspoon RP, et al. Long-term survival after marrow transplantation for paroxysmal nocturnal hemoglobinuria with aplastic anemia. Ann Intern Med 1984;101:193–195.

59. Thomas ED, Buckner CD, Sanders JE, et al. Marrow transplantation for thalassemia. Lancet 1982;2:227–229.

60. Vermylen C, Fernandez Robles E, Ninane J, et al. Bone marrow transplantation in five children with sickle cell anaemia. Lancet 1988;1:1427–1428.

61. Gluckman E, Horowitz MM, Champlin RE, et al. Bone marrow transplantation for severe aplastic anemia: influence of conditioning and graft-versus-host disease prophylaxis regimens on outcome. Blood 1992;79:269–275.

62. Chao NJ, Duncan SR, Long GD, et al. Corticosteroid therapy for diffuse alveolar hemorrhage in autologous bone marrow transplant recipients. Ann Intern Med 1991;114:145–146.

63. Deeg HJ, Storb R. Graft-versus-host disease: pathophysiological and clinical aspects. Annu Rev Med 1984;35:11–24.

64. Shulman HM, Hinterberger W. Hepatic veno-occlusive disease—liver toxicity syndrome after bone marrow transplantation. Bone Marrow Transplant 1992;10:197–214.

65. Storb R, Deeg HJ, Whitehead J, et al. Methotrexate and cyclosporine compared with cyclosporine alone for prophylaxis of acute graft versus host disease after marrow transplantation for leukemia. N Engl J Med 1986;314:729–735.

66. Ramsay NKC, Kersey JH, Robinson LL, et al. A randomized study of the prevention of acute graft-versus-host disease. N Engl J Med 1982;306:392–397.

67. Storb R, Deeg HJ, Pepe M, et al. Methotrexate and cyclosporine versus cyclosporine alone for prophylaxis of graft-versus-host disease in patients given HLA-identical marrow grafts for leukemia: long-term follow-up of a controlled trial. Blood 1989;73:1729–1734.

68. Martin PJ, Schoch G, Fisher L, et al. A retrospective analysis of therapy for acute graft-versus-host disease: initial treatment. Blood 1990;76:1464–1472.

69. Kennedy MS, Deeg HJ, Storb R, et al. Treatment of acute graft-versus-host disease after allogeneic marrow transplantation: randomized study comparing corticosteroids and cyclosporine. Am J Med 1985;78:978–983.

70. Herve P, Wijdenes J, Bergerat JP, et al. Treatment of corticosteroid resistant acute graft-versus-host disease by in vivo administration of anti-interleukin-2 receptor monoclonal antibody (B-B10). Blood 1990;75:1017–1023.

71. Atkinson K, Horowitz MM, Gale RP, et al. Risk factors for chronic graft-versus-host disease after HLA-identical sibling bone marrow transplantation. Blood 1990;75:2459–2464.

72. Shulman HM, Sullivan KM, Weiden PL, et al. Chronic graft-versus-host syndrome in man: a long-term clinicopathologic study of 20 Seattle patients. Am J Med 1980;69:204–217.

73. Sullivan KM, Witherspoon RP, Storb R, et al. Prednisone and azathioprine compared with prednisone and placebo for treatment of chronic graft-versus-host disease: prognostic influence of prolonged thrombocytopenia after allogeneic marrow transplantation. Blood 1988;72:546–554.

74. Sullivan KM, Witherspoon RP, Storb R, et al. Alternating-day cyclosporine and prednisone for treatment of high-risk chronic graft-versus-host disease. Blood 1988;72:555–561.

75. Vogelsang GB, Farmer ER, Hess AD, et al. Thalidomide for the treatment of chronic graft-versus-host disease. N Engl J Med 1992;326:1055–1058.

76. Champlin RE, Horowitz MM, van Bekkum DW, et al. Graft failure following bone marrow transplantation for severe aplastic anemia: risk factors and treatment results. Blood 1989;73:606–613.

77. Bociek G, Bierman P, Stewart D, et al. Pregnancy after autologous bone marrow transplantation (ABMT) (abstract). Proc ASCO 1994;13:1296a.

78. Stone RM, Neuberg D, Soiffer R, et al. Myelodysplastic syndrome as a late complication following autologous bone marrow transplantation for non-Hodgkin's lymphoma. J Clin Oncol 1994;12:2535–2542.

79. Darrington DL, Vose JM, Anderson JR, et al. Incidence and characterization of secondary myelodysplastic syndrome and acute myelogenous leukemia following high-dose chemoradiotherapy and autologous stem-cell transplantation for lymphoid malignancies. J Clin Oncol 1994;12:2527–2534.

Section Two

Chemotherapeutic Drugs

19

Covalent DNA-Binding Drugs

Louise B. Grochow

Chemotherapy drugs are included in the alkylating-agent drug class if they contain reactive alkyl groups capable of forming covalent bonds with DNA. These compounds all form chemically reactive intermediates and interact to form strong bonds with many cellular constituents. Drugs that contain two alkylating groups (bifunctional alkylating agents) are more cytotoxic than monofunctional compounds that can only produce single-strand DNA breaks. Using current sensitive techniques to detect cross-links in cells exposed to pharmacologic concentrations of alkylating compounds, the formation of cross-links between DNA strands is well correlated with cytotoxicity (1, 2). Some drugs included in this class, procarbazine and dacarbazine, do not produce cross-links, although the single-strand breaks produced at apurinic sites may result in chromosome breaks (3). The cytotoxicity for neoplastic cells relative to that for normal cells is not yet fully elucidated, but relative S-phase activity is partly explanatory. Cells that do not replicate immediately following exposure to alkylating agents may repair the cross-links that have been formed (4). Although a single unrepaired cross-link can sterilize a cell, unrepaired DNA strand breaks can result in activation of poly(ADP-ribose) polymerase and consumption of NAD^+, limiting ATP generation and causing energy-limited cell death (5).

Alkylating agents are an example of turning swords into plowshares: oncologists initiated trials of sulfur mustard after use of this toxic gas produced bone marrow aplasia. After activity was demonstrated in patients with lymphoma, subsequent investigations yielded not only the nitrogen mustards, with improvements in therapeutic index, but a series of congeners and prodrugs with chemical and pharmacologic properties that offer specific alterations in drug disposition, cellular uptake, reactivity, and re-

sistance, with resultant differences in efficacy and toxicity.

Nitrogen mustard was the first alkylating agent developed to treat malignancies (6). The class of alkylating agents based on nitrogen mustard reacts via a bis-chloroethyl group, which produces a three-membered ring—the highly reactive aziridine ion intermediate. This intermediate attacks electrophilic atoms such as the N^7 position of guanine (the site of alkylation for the bis-chloroethyl moieties, such as the active metabolite of cyclophosphamide) or the O^6 po-. sition of cytosine (the site of alkylation for the nitrosoureas (7)). Single adducts formed can be repaired by a series of repair enzymes: glycosylase cleaves the altered base from the deoxyribose, apurinic endonuclease excises the apurinic site, and DNA polymerase fills in the defect, based on the complementary strand (3). Unrepaired adducts at the O^6 guanine position result in base-pair substitution; these lesions can be repaired by O^6-alkylguanine DNA alkyl transferase.

Most alkylating agents are not charged and are not susceptible to exclusion by the multidrug resistance phenotype. Other mechanisms of resistance, such as the presence of aldehyde dehydrogenase (which catabolizes the active metabolite of cyclophosphamide), may be critical in protecting normal tissues from toxicity. Glutathione and glutathione-S-transferase together protect several classes of tissues from cytotoxicity from alkylating agents (and other sources of electrophiles) by providing alternative attractive nucleophilic targets (8). The rate of reaction of the aziridinium ion of melphalan with intracellular water is $\frac{1}{5}$ to $\frac{1}{10}$ that for glutathione alone, but the reaction with glutathione in the presence of glutathione-S-transferase is much more avid (9). Use of buthionine sulfoxime (BSO) to deplete glutathione is being explored as a mode of overcoming resistance mediated by glutathione. In parallel to attempts to inhibit multidrug resistance, this strategy may also increase normal tissue toxicity (10, 11).

Alkylating agents all share dose-related myelosuppression as a common toxicity. The steep dose-response curves demonstrated in vitro and the absence of a plateau in cytotoxic effect (such as that demonstrated by antimetabolites) makes these agents particularly suitable for dose-intense preparative regimens used in bone marrow transplantation (BMT). Thus, cyclophosphamide, melphalan, carmustine, and thiotepa are myeloablative drugs common to many BMT induction regimens.

NITROGEN MUSTARDS

The structures for the alkylating agents containing bischloroethyl alkylating groups are shown in Fig. 19.1.

Mechlorethamine
Nomenclature

Generic name: mechlorethamine, nitrogen mustard, HN_2

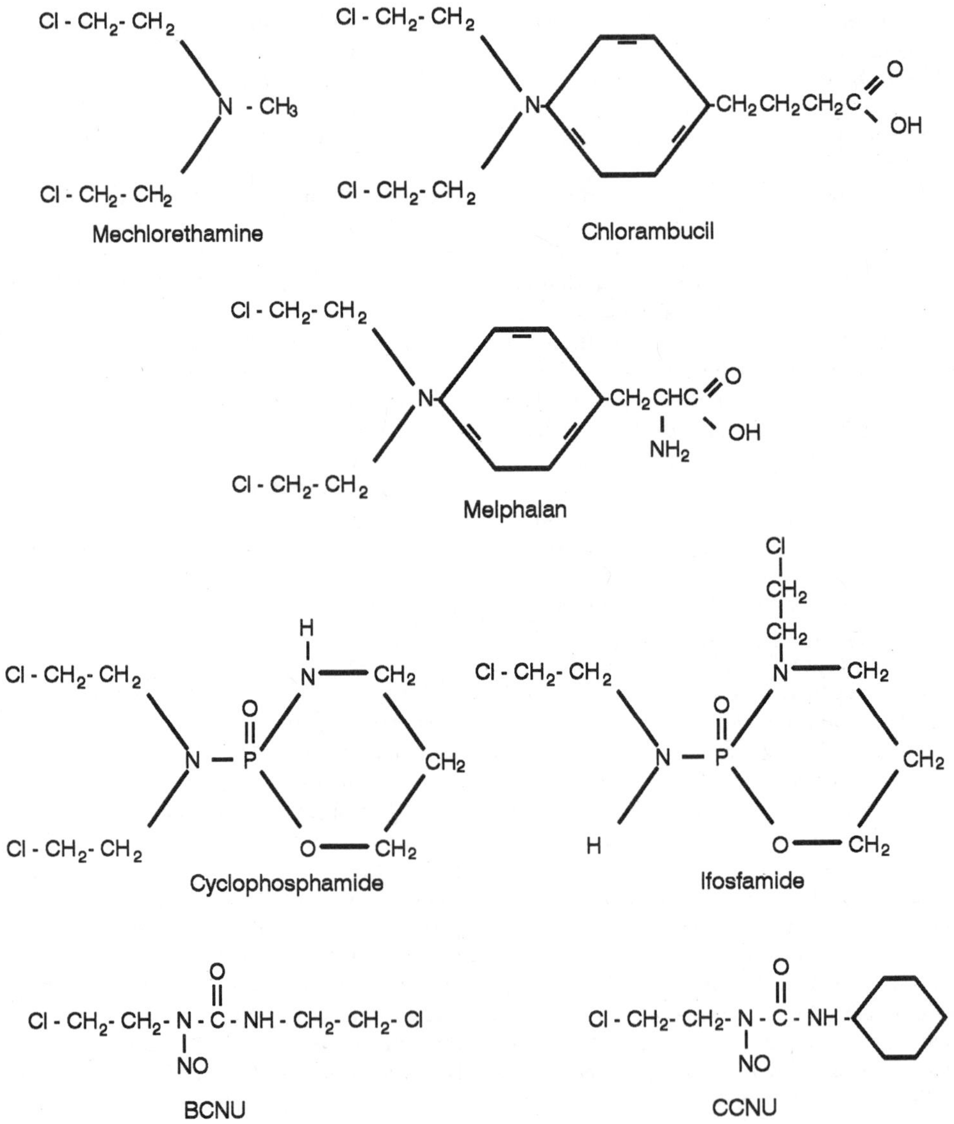

Figure 19.1.   Structures of bischloroethyl-based compounds.

Chemical name: 2-chloro-*N*-(2-chloro-ethyl)-*N*-methylethamine hydrochloride

Availability: Dry powder (10 mg) is available triturated with sodium chloride to 100 mg.

Preparation: Powder is dissolved with 10 mL of sterile water for injection or sodium chloride for injection. It must be administered promptly after dissolution, since it is unstable in aqueous solution.

Form: Mechlorethamine is a white, crystalline, hygroscopic powder. It is extremely water soluble. The molecular weight is 192.5

Administration: This highly reactive compound is given via a rapidly running i.v. as a slow push (1–3 min). Extreme care must be taken with handling to avoid skin, eye, or aerosol contact, as well as avoiding extravasation of this highly reactive compound. Prompt irrigation with water followed as soon as possible by sodium thiosulfate is recommended for any skin contact. Sodium thiosulfate is also used at ⅙ M for any drug infiltrations/extravasations.

Metabolism/Pharmacokinetics: Mechlorethamine is actively transported intracellularly by the choline transporter (12). Because the chloroethyl groups are so highly reactive, total body clearance for mechlorethamine is very rapid, with a half-life so short it has not been characterized.

Toxicity: Myelosuppression is dose limiting for mechlorethamine and may become more severe with ongoing treatment (13). Rapid decreases in lymphocyte count occur within 24 hours of administration. Nausea and vomiting occur within minutes of administration. Even when administered with a freely running i.v., patients may develop thrombosis and/or thrombophlebitis at the injection site (14). Secondary malignancies and infertility are late toxicities seen after treatment of Hodgkin's disease with MOPP (nitrogen mustard, vincristine (Oncovin), procarbazine, and prednisone) therapy: mechlorethamine and procarbazine are both presumed to contribute significantly to these delayed toxicities (15–18). Infertility with histologic evidence of depletion of germ cells was reported after treatment with mechlorethamine as early as 1948 (19). Alopecia is less prominent with mechlorethamine than with cyclophosphamide. Allergic reactions, nonallergic maculopapular rashes, and erythema multiforme have been rarely reported after treatment with mechlorethamine.

Indications: Nitrogen mustard has been used as part of MOPP combination therapy for Hodgkin's disease, but its difficulty of administration and late sequelae have led to other regimens being more widely used.

Chlorambucil
Nomenclature
Commercial name: Leukeran

Chemical name: 4-[bis (2-chloroethyl)-amino]benzene butanoic acid

Availability: Sugar-coated 2-mg tablets with excipients including lactose and corn and wheat starch.

Preparation: Oral tablets must be stored in light-resistant containers.

Form: Chlorambucil is an off-white slightly granular powder, and is only slightly water soluble. Its molecular weight is 304.23.

Administration: Orally

Metabolism: Chlorambucil undergoes rapid hepatic metabolism to the active alkylating compound bischloroethylphenylacetic acid (phenylacetic acid mustard) (20, 21).

Pharmacokinetics: Chlorambucil is consistently highly bioavailable, with peak concentrations reached within 1 hour. Its absorption is delayed and diminished by food (22). Although less reactive than melphalan, chlorambucil itself has a half-life of only 1.5 hours, and the active alkylating moiety, phenylacetic acid mustard, has a half life of 2.5 hours (20, 23–27). Clearance of chlorambucil and phenylacetic acid mustard occurs almost entirely by metabolism, principally in the liver. The inactive metabolites are extensively cleared by renal mechanisms. Chlorambucil is 99% protein bound (28).

Toxicity: Myelotoxicity is dose limiting for chlorambucil, and cumulative doses may result in sustained pancytopenia. After a single high dose, typical neutropenia is seen between days 8 and 15, with recovery by day 28; thrombocytopenia develops later, and the platelet count normalizes later. When given in divided doses, nausea and vomiting are unusual. Reversible neurologic toxicities, including twitching, agitation, confusion, and seizures have been reported in patients receiving chlorambucil (29). Maculopapular rashes as well as more severe progressive rashes have also been reported (30). Pulmonary damage has been reported in patients receiving multiple courses of chlorambucil (31). Premenopausal women may become amenorrheic or enter menopause after receiving chlorambucil (18, 32). Decreases in the motile sperm count may progress to infertility with cumulative doses greater than 400 mg (17, 33). Secondary leukemia has been reported in patients receiving chlorambucil for nonmalignant as well as malignant diseases (34).

Indications: Chlorambucil is generally used for the treatment of chronic lymphocytic leukemia, Waldenstrom's macroglobulinemia, and as second- or third-line therapy for patients with malignant lymphomas. It is also active in choriocarcinoma and ovarian neoplasms and has been used with prednisone for children with minimal change nephrotic syndrome.

Melphalan
Nomenclature
   Generic: melphalan, (L)-phenylalanine mustard, L-PAM, *l*-sarcolysin
   Commercial: Alkeran
   Chemical: 4-[bis (2-chloroethyl)amino]-L-phenylalanine

Availability: 2-mg tablets and 50-mg parenteral vials are available.

Preparation: Melphalan hydrochloride for injection is provided as a sterile lyophilized powder containing povidone. The manufacturer provides sterile diluent of water, sodium citrate, propylene glycol, and ethanol; the vial must be quickly shaken after dilution to ensure dissolution.

Form: Melphalan is an off-white to buff powder. It is insoluble in water. Its molecular weight is 305.2

Administration: Melphalan is given parenterally or orally. The parenteral formulation should be used as soon as possible after preparation, since hydrolysis rapidly occurs. The initial dilution is only stable for 90 minutes at room temperature; further dilution in 0.9% saline to prepare a solution with a maximal concentration of 0.45 mg/mL is made prior to administration. This diluted solution is only stable for 1 hour. Precipitates may form if the solution is refrigerated. Melphalan is usually given as a short infusion over 15–20 minutes.

Metabolism: Melphalan is one of several alkylating agents synthesized for reasons that are unrelated to its eventual utility: it was originally synthesized to exploit the uptake of phenylalanine in melanoma (35). Melphalan enters cells through active transport mechanisms, as it is an amino acid analogue. Spontaneous hydrolysis to monohydroxy- and dihydroxymelphalan occurs rapidly; these derivatives are much less potent than the parent compound. Melphalan is converted in the presence of intracellular glutathione and glutathione-S-transferase to 4-(glutathionyl)phenylalanine (36).

Pharmacokinetics: The mean values reported for the clearance of melphalan range from 320 to 730 mL/min (37, 38). The mean elimination half-life has been reported between 53 to 83 minutes; it is shorter in children and in patients receiving hyperhydration (39–43). After high doses (40–150 mg/m^2), the mean $t_{1/2\beta}$ was 3 hours in one study (44), but 6–12 hours in other studies (42, 43). The apparent bioavailability of melphalan is incomplete and variable, ranging from 25 to 89% (37, 45, 46). Absorption of melphalan can be inhibited by the presence of food or leucine (48, 49). At high doses used in preparative regimens for BMT, even greater variability in the extent of absorption is found (49, 50). Plasma protein binding is moderate (60–90%) and includes binding to both albumin and α_1-acid glycoprotein (39, 40, 51). Renal clearance has been shown to account for the disposition of 5 to 34% of the parent compound (39). However, in patients with renal insufficiency, myelosupression was more severe, and dose reductions are recommended for such patients (52). There is substantial interindividual variation in melphalan clearance, and good correlation between melphalan AUC (area under the curve) and myelosuppression, leading some authors to recommend pharmacokinetically guided dosing (53).

Toxicity: The dose-limiting toxicity for melphalan at conventional doses is neutropenia: the nadir WBC usually occurs between day 14 and day 21, with recovery by days 28 to 35. Unlike the oxazophosphorines, cyclophosphamide and ifosfamide, melphalan is associated with mucositis and enterocolitis when used at high doses as a single agent (54) or when combined with other alkylating agents (57, 58). Hepatic venoocclusive disease, hyponatremia due to the syndrome of inappropriate antidiuretic hormone (SIADH), and mental status changes have also been reported. Interstitial pneumonitis and subsequent fibrosis have been reported in patients receiving melphalan and prednisone for myeloma (57). The incidence of secondary leukemia is reported to be higher in patients treated with melphalan than in patients treated with cyclophosphamide (58, 59). Chromosomal aberration and an increased incidence of secondary solid malignancies have also been reported (60). Hypersensitivity reactions, including urticarial rashes, pruritus, and anaphylaxis, have occurred in a small number of patients receiving repeated doses of melphalan.

Indications: Melphalan has been used in the treatment of multiple myeloma, ovarian carcinoma, and breast cancer.

Cyclophosphamide
Nomenclature

Commercial names: Cytoxan, Neosar

Chemical name: 2-[bis (2-chloroethyl) amino] tetrahydro-2H-1,3,2-oxazaphosphorine 2-oxide monohydrate

Availability: For oral use, 25- and 50-mg tablets. For i.v. use, 100-mg, 200-mg, 500-mg, 1000-mg, and 2000-mg vials. Both dry anhydrous powder containing 45 mg of sodium chloride per 100 mg of drug and the lyophilized form containing 75 mg of mannitol per 100 mg of drug are available.

Preparation: The i.v. preparation can be dissolved in sterile water for injection or bacteriostatic water for injection (paraben preserved only) to provide a concentration of 20 mg/mL. The drug can then be further diluted in D5W, NS, or D5 Ringer's solution. For moderate-to-high doses, NS is recommended to minimize hyponatremia associated with SIADH (see below). Once diluted, the i.v. preparation is stable for 24 hours at room temperature or up to 6 days if refrigerated. There is no antimicrobial preservative.

Form: Cyclophosphamide is a white crystalline powder with a molecular weight of 279.1. It is soluble in water, saline, or ethanol.

Administration: Prior to the initial administration of any alkylating agent, a baseline white blood count should be assessed. Patients receiving conventional parenteral or oral doses of cyclophosphamide should be euvolemic and able to maintain an adequate urinary output of 1500 mL/day to minimize the risk of acute and chronic damage to the urothelium. Parenteral cyclophosphamide is normally infused over 15 to 60 minutes; rapid administration (<5–10 minutes) may cause acute lightheadedness, tearing, nausea, and perioral numbness. Since cyclophosphamide is a prodrug, no special precautions to minimize the risk of extravasation are needed for i.v. administration. When used in high doses, hydration with normal saline is provided concurrently for 24 hours after a dose to minimize bladder toxicity and hyponatremia.

Metabolism: The addition of a heterocyclic moiety to the bischloroethyl side chains of nitrogen mustard dramatically altered the reactivity, disposition, and effects of this class of agents, producing a drug with a 10-fold improved therapeutic index in murine models compared with nitrogen mustard. Cyclophosphamide is an inactive prodrug. Although originally designed to be specifically activated in tumors, it is actually metabolized by specific cytochrome P450s in the liver by microsomal oxidation to produce 4-hydroxycyclophosphamide (61). In vitro evidence for metabolism by prostaglandin H synthase and lipoxygenases to produce acrolein has also been presented, but the extent of metabolism by these pathways may be clinically insignificant (62, 63). Both 4-hydroxycyclophosphamide (4-HC) and its tautomer, aldophosphamide, are nonpolar, circulate freely, and enter cells by diffusion; at physiologic pH, the equilibrium between these forms favors 4-HC (64). 4-HC is further metabolized to the nontoxic 4-ketocyclophosphamide. Aldophosphamide decomposes to phosphoramide mustard and acrolein, the principal active and toxic products, respectively. Phosphoramide mustard (PM) and possibly nor-nitrogen mustard are the alkylating moieties that produce cross-links. PM is very polar, limiting cellular uptake; the 4-HC/aldophosphamide metabolites serve as delivery compounds for PM.

In addition to decomposition to PM, aldophosphamide is also efficiently catabolized to carboxyphosphamide by aldehyde dehydrogenase. Aldehyde dehydrogenase is present in high concentration in hepatocytes, intestinal mucosa, hematopoietic stem cells, and megakaryocytes (65). This enzyme, therefore, protects these normal tissues from cyclophosphamide toxicity.

Pharmacokinetics

Assay: The parent compound, cyclophosphamide, is most frequently assayed by gas chromatography with nitrogen-phosphorus detection after derivatization to form a stable, volatile compound (66, 67). A variety of techniques have been applied to the measurement of the intermediate and final alkylating moieties, including (a) a colorimetric assay measuring total alkylating activity by reaction with 4-(4-nitrobenzyl)-pyridine (68), (b) assays that derivatize the alkylating moieties with fluorescent side chains (69–71), and (c) gas chromatography with mass-spectral detection (72, 73).

Absorption: Cyclophosphamide is well absorbed orally in conventional divided doses such as those used for adjuvant therapy of breast carcinoma. The bioavailability after administration of 100- to 200-mg doses ranges from 74 to 97% (74–76). With larger doses, absorption has been found to be more variable (66).

Disposition and Elimination: Plasma concentrations of cyclophosphamide increase roughly linearly with parenteral dose, ranging from 4 nmol/L after a dose of 1 mg/kg to 500 nmol/L after 60 mg/kg (66, 77, 78). However, at the high doses used in BMT (2400 mg/m^2 or 60 mg/kg), many patients will exhibit Michaelis-Menten kinetics (78). The clearance rate for conventional doses of cyclophosphamide ranges from 35–200 mL/min, with a mean total body clearance rate of 80 mL/min (67, 78, 79). The renal clearance of cyclophosphamide is approximately 15 mL/min; a mean of 20% of administered cyclophosphamide is excreted as unmetabolized parent compound, but the amount of cyclophosphamide eliminated unchanged in the urine can be variable (78, 80). The terminal elimination half-life of cyclophosphamide ranges from 108 to 960 minutes, with a mean of 7 hours in adults (74, 81). In children, shorter half-lives are reported (70, 82). Cyclophosphamide appears to temporarily induce its own clearance, with more rapid clearances reported on subsequent days of multiday regimens (78, 83).

Measurements of the kinetics of specific metabolites have been limited by the non-specificity of the assays available. After high doses of cyclophosphamide (40–60 mg/kg) the overall alkylating activity has been reported as 10 to 80 μmol/L (70, 72, 73, 75). Concentrations of alkylating metabolites peak within 1 to 3 hours after drug administration, and the apparent terminal elimination half-life may be somewhat longer than for cyclophosphamide itself, with most reporting a mean half-life of approximately 8 hours, although the half-life for the initial tautomer pair of 4-HC/aldophosphamide is 1 to 5 hours.

Prior treatment with phenobarbital may induce the activity of the specific CYP450 isoenzymes identified as metabolizing cyclophosphamide (CYP 2B family and CYP2C9 (61)) and enhance the metabolism of cyclophosphamide, resulting in a shorter half-life for the parent compound (78, 84, 85). Concurrent administration of cimetidine may reduce the clearance of active metabolites (86).

Full doses of cyclophosphamide can be administered to patients in either renal or hepatic failure. Although there is an alteration in the elimination rate constant, there is no evidence that this results in more profound myelosuppression. Renal clearance contributes only modestly to the elimination of cyclophosphamide, and hepatic injury may result in decreased, rather than increased, exposure to active metabolites (87, 88). Patients who are obese (>20% over ideal body weight) may have a decreased clearance of cyclophosphamide (89, 90).

If further studies confirm a possible relationship between rapid metabolism of cyclophosphamide to its active metabolites and cardiac toxicity and duration of survival, therapeutic monitoring of cyclophosphamide or its metabolites in the setting of high-dose administration may become routine clinical practice (91).

Toxicity: In the absence of BMT or growth factors, myelosuppression is the principal dose-limiting toxicity for cyclophosphamide. Thrombocytopenia is less significant than granulocytopenia and lymphopenia until very high doses are used. WBC nadir generally occurs between days 9 and 15, with recovery by day 21. If used as a single agent, WBC recovery occurs even at very high doses, confirming the stem-cell-sparing importance of aldehyde dehydrogenase. Cyclophosphamide is also a very potent immunosuppressive drug, depleting B lymphocytes and suppressing T-lymphocyte function (92). Nausea and vomiting are generally delayed for 4 to 8 hours after the administration of cyclophosphamide and are generally well controlled with single agents such as dexamethasone or lorazepam. Altered mental status and seizures due to hyponatremia can occur in patients receiving moderate-to-high doses of cyclophosphamide and receiving free water (e.g., less than 0.9% saline), because of an antidiuretic effect similar to SIADH (93–95). Although no changes in ADH have been measured, urine output drops within 6 to 8 hours after administration. Furosemide promotes clearance of free water and can be used to correct hyponatremia if it occurs despite restriction of free water administration (96). Gonadal failure is observed acutely in men receiving cyclophosphamide, and aspermia or oligospermia may persist for years (17). Early menopause has been reported in women receiving cyclophosphamide combined with other drugs as adjuvant therapy for breast cancer, associated with both older age and more extended drug treatment (18). Cardiac toxicity is reported in a small percentage of patients receiving 60 to 75 mg/m^2 and may be associated with the nonlinear clearance observed in patients receiving these doses; higher doses, even when given by continuous infusion over 4 days, have resulted in permanent or lethal cardiotoxicity (91, 97). Pulmonary toxicity is infrequently reported (98, 99). Hemorrhagic cystitis occurs most commonly with repeated oral doses (when adequate urine output may not be maintained in outpatients) or at very high doses. The risk of hemorrhagic cystitis may be reduced by maintaining adequate bladder irrigation by parenteral hydration, via an indwelling catheter, or by the use of the thiol precursor mesna. Mesna is administered parenterally. In vivo, mesna is partially oxidized to the inert disulfide (sodium 2-mercaptoethanesulfonate disulfide, dimesna), is not taken up by cells, and is rapidly excreted to produce high concentrations of active mesna in the urine, reacting avidly with both alkylating metabolites such as phosphoramide mustard and nor-nitrogen mustard as well as with acrolein.

Indications: Cyclophosphamide is widely used in combinations with curative intent for the treatment of aggressive lymphomas, limited-stage small cell lung cancer, Ewing's sarcoma, neuroblastoma, acute lymphocytic leukemia, postoperative breast carcinoma, and esthesioneuroblastoma (100). At very high doses, it is the most common drug used in combination with other agents or radiation therapy in preparative regimens for BMT as curative therapy for acute myelocytic leukemia, lymphomas, and breast carcinoma. For palliation, it is used in combination for indolent lymphomas, breast carcinoma, neuroblastoma, retinoblastoma, endometrial carcinoma, multiple myeloma, chronic leukemias, and mycosis fungoides. Cyclophosphamide is also widely used as an immunosuppressant in nonmalignant diseases.

Ifosfamide
Nomenclature
  Generic name: Ifosfamide
  Commercial name: Ifex
  Chemical name: 3-(2-chloroethyl)-2-[(2-chloroethyl)amino]-tetrahydro-2H-1,3,2-oxazophosphorine 2-oxide
Availability: Single-dose vials containing either 1000 mg or 3000 mg of sterile ifosfamide are provided in combination packages with 200-, 400-, or 1000-mg ampules of mesna.
Preparation: Vials are prepared by adding either sterile water for injection or bacteriostatic water for injection (benzyl alcohol or paraben preserved) to provide a final solution of 50 mg/mL; 20 mL of diluent is added to the 1000-mg vials or 60 mL to the 3000-mg vials. Further dilution with 5% dextrose, 0.9% NaCl, lactated Ringer's, or sterile water, or admixtures of such solutions (e.g., 5% dextrose in 0.45% NaCl) is used to produce final concentrations of 0.6 to 20 mg/mL. Diluted solutions are physically and chemically stable for at least 1 week at 30°C or 6 weeks at 5°C; however, if the initial reconstitution is not with bacteriostatic water for injection, the dilution should be refrigerated and used within 6 hours.
Form: Ifosfamide is a white crystalline powder that is soluble in water, with a molecular weight of 261.1.
Administration: Prior to the initial administration of any alkylating agent, a baseline white blood count should be assessed. Patients receiving ifosfamide should be euvolemic and should receive at least 2 L per 24 hours of supplemental hydration. To minimize the risk of acute and chronic damage to the urothelium, ifosfamide is always given in conjunction with mesna (see discussion under cyclophosphamide toxicity above). A mesna dose of 10 to 20% of the ifosfamide dose is given as a loading dose, followed by a 24-hour infusion at the same total dose as the ifosfamide. Alternatively, mesna (10–20% of the ifosfamide dose) can be given with the ifosfamide (and can be admixed in the administration bottle), followed by additional doses (equal to 10–20% of the ifosfamide dose) 4 and 8 hours later. Parenteral ifosfamide is normally infused over 30 to 60 minutes. Since ifosfamide is an inactive prodrug, no special precautions to minimize the risk of extravasation are needed for intravenous administration. Ifosfamide is not administered orally because of high rates of production of the neurotoxic metabolite chloroacetaldehyde,

which produces encephalopathy and (reversible) coma (101–103). Ifosfamide is more effective when given as fractionated doses rather than single doses (104–106).

Metabolism: The metabolic pathways for ifosfamide parallel those used by cyclophosphamide, but as much as 50% of ifosfamide may undergo oxidation of the chloroethyl side chains, producing the dechloroethylated metabolites 2- and 3-dechloroethylifosfamide and releasing chloroacetaldehyde (101, 107). In addition, the aziridine groups of ifosfamide are less reactive, and the rate of formation of aziridine is slower. This results in an apparent 3- to 4-fold difference in potency for ifosfamide, compared with cyclophosphamide.

Ifosfamide has a chiral center and is administered as a mixture of the R- and S- enantiomers. S-ifosfamide has a 15 to 50% more rapid clearance than R-ifosfamide (108). Like cyclophosphamide, ifosfamide appears to induce its own metabolism (109).

Pharmacokinetics: Analytic methodology for ifosfamide parallels that for cyclophosphamide, with nitrogen phosphorus flame ionization detection by gas chromatography widely used for measurement of the parent compound. The mean total body clearance of ifosfamide at doses of 1500 to 3000 mg/m² has been reported from 69 to 84 mL/min/m² (recently reviewed in 110, 111), with higher rates being reported in children (109, 113). The elimination half-life is longer than that of cyclophosphamide, with the reported mean ranging from 5.5 to 7.7 hours. The alkylating activity reported after administration of 3.8 g of ifosfamide is similar to that reported after 1.1 g of cyclophosphamide (113). Renal clearance accounts for 14 to 50% of an administered dose (114).

Plasma ifosfamide and cisplatin concentrations have been monitored in patients receiving the preparative regimen of ifosfamide, carboplatin, and etoposide. Elevated plasma concentrations of ifosfamide (>153 µM at 16 to 22 hours into the continuous infusion of 4 g/m²/day × 4 days) were correlated with the subsequent development of renal insufficiency (115).

Toxicity: Nephrotoxicity rather than neutropenia is the dose-limiting toxicity of ifosfamide if used without mesna (see discussion under cyclophosphamide toxicity above). Alopecia, nausea, and vomiting occur with ifosfamide treatment at the same frequency seen after cyclophosphamide; emesis can usually be controlled with standard regimens. As with cyclophosphamide, when ifosfamide is used at very high doses, acute cardiotoxicity is reported (116). However, ifosfamide exhibits some toxicities not seen with cyclophosphamide. Encephalopathy has been dose limiting for ifosfamide at high doses (117, 118). Methylene blue has been used as an electron receptor to reduce encephalopathy (118a). Renal toxicity has also been significant, even when mesna is used in conjunction with ifosfamide (119–121). Fanconi's syndrome with severe wasting of potassium, magnesium, phosphorus, and bicarbonate has also been reported with high-dose ifosfamide (122). When used in BMT doses, the dose-limiting toxicities for ifosfamide (in combination with carboplatin and etoposide) are altered mental status progressing to coma and acute renal failure (123).

Indications: Ifosfamide has been approved for use in combination as salvage therapy for patients with germ cell neoplasia who have progressed after conventional cisplatin/bleomycin/etoposide therapy. Ifosfamide also has activity in many of the diseases treated with cyclophosphamide: sarcomas, refractory lymphomas, non-small-cell lung carcinoma, ovarian cancer, and head and neck carcinoma. The difference in toxicity and responses between the two compounds has recently been discussed (124).

Aziridines

Aziridines are analogues of the very reactive aziridinium moiety produced by the chloroethyl moiety of the nitrogen mustard compounds after loss of the chlorine atom and formation of the positively charged cyclic ion. They are much less reactive than the aziridinium intermediates. The structure of thiotepa is shown in Figure 19.2.

Thiotepa

Nomenclature

> *Generic name:* Thiotepa, TESPA, TSPA; TEPA is the major metabolite
> *Commercial name:* Thiotepa
> *Chemical name:* 1,1',1''-phosphinothioylidynetris-aziridine

Availability: Thiotepa powder for parenteral injection is available in 15-mg vials admixed with sodium chloride and sodium bicarbonate for reconstitution with sterile water.

Preparation: After initial dilution with sterile water to 10 mg/mL, further dilution in all conventional parenteral solutions produces stable

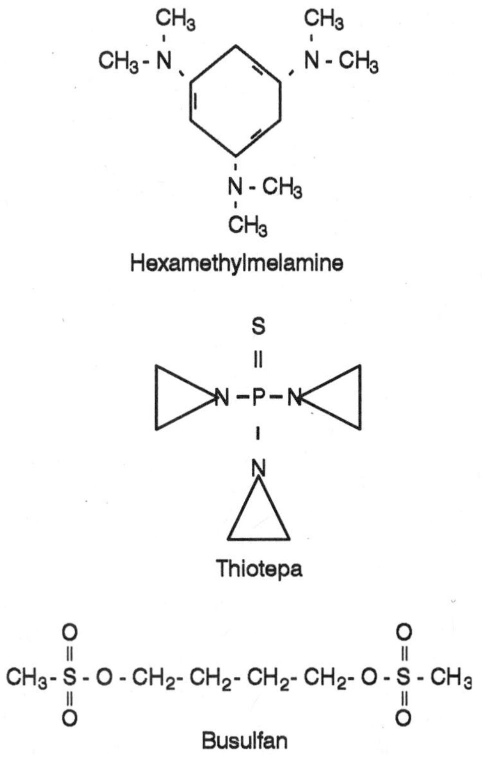

Hexamethylmelamine

Thiotepa

Busulfan

Figure 19.2.   Structures of hexamethylmelamine, thiotepa, and busulfan.

solutions. However, there is no preservative present, so despite chemical stability for at least 5 days at 2 to 8°C, solutions should be used promptly.

Form: Thiotepa is a fine, white crystalline flake, freely soluble in water. Its molecular weight is 189.23.

Administration: For conventional parenteral doses, thiotepa may be administered rapidly intravenously. For local administration, thiotepa may be admixed with 2% procaine or 0.1% epinephrine. Thiotepa has been given intravesically in small volumes. It is also administered via ventricular catheters for carcinomatous meningitis.

Metabolism: Thiotepa is extensively metabolized to TEPA (125, 126).

Pharmacokinetics: The mean elimination half-life for thiotepa is 2 to 3 hours, and the mean total body clearance has been reported between 316 to 340 mL/min (127). Some patients have higher peak plasma concentrations and larger exposures, measured as the AUC, of the metabolite, TEPA, than of thiotepa itself. At the high doses used in BMT, the ratio of the

AUC of the metabolite, TEPA, to the AUC of thiotepa is 0.15, rather than the ratio of 0.33 reported in patients receiving conventional doses of thiotepa, although these authors also reported 10-fold interpatient variability (128–130). Neither thiotepa nor TEPA is measurable in a human urine sample; although alkylating activity is measurable in the urine 48 hours after high-dose therapy, it has declined by 90 to 95% by 72 hours. Thiotepa is rapidly cleared from the CSF after intrathecal administration (131). Thiotepa protein binding is minimal (132).

Toxicity: The dose-limiting toxicity of thiotepa is myelosuppression. Patients who receive intravesical and intrathecal drug may have substantial systemic exposure to active drug and develop neutropenia, which may be delayed in onset. Nausea and vomiting can usually be controlled with conventional antiemetic regimens. Thiotepa produces alopecia, mucositis, stomatitis, and severe erythematous rash with subsequent hyperpigmentation at high doses. Headache and a tight sensation in the throat occur if it is administered rapidly. Altered mental status may occur at very high doses.

Indications: Thiotepa is an active alkylating agent used as second- or third-line treatment for patients with breast or ovarian carcinoma or lymphomas and as part of preparative BMT regimens. It has been used for local administration in multiple sites: in the spinal fluid for carcinomatous meningitis from breast or lung carcinoma, in the bladder for the treatment of superficial bladder carcinomas, and in the pleural and peritoneal spaces.

Altretamine (Fig. 19.2)
Nomenclature
Generic name: Altretamine, (hexamethylmelamine, HMM, HXM, NSC-13875)
Commercial name: Hexalen
Chemical name: N,N,N',N',N'',N''-hexamethyl-1,3,5-triazene-2,4,6-triamine
Availability: 50- and 100-mg oral capsules
Form: Altretamine is a white crystalline powder. Its molecular weight is 210.28. It is insoluble in water.
Administration: Oral; the parenteral formulation remains investigational.
Metabolism: Hexamethylmelamine undergoes hydroxylation of the methyl group via hepatic and intestinal cytochrome P450, followed by microsomal N-demethylation (133). The N-hy-

droxy metabolite, *N*-hydroxymethyl-penta-methyl-melamine (HMPMM) has been postulated as the active cytotoxic intermediate (134–136).

Pharmacokinetics: Peak concentrations after oral administration occur at 0.5 to 3 hours, but first-pass metabolism is highly variable, with 100-fold variations in peak blood concentrations (137). The elimination half-life ranges from 5 to 13 hours (137, 138). Although HMM crosses into the CSF poorly, in one patient, the demethylated metabolites were found in the CSF at concentrations proportional to plasma concentrations (139). HMM is 94% protein bound in mice (140).

Toxicity: Neurologic toxicity is dose limiting (141). Peripheral neuropathy, mood disorders, ataxia and vertigo, depression, agitation, and hallucinations have been reported. Nausea and vomiting, anorexia, and diarrhea may become progressively severe after several weeks of therapy, which limits the feasibility of prolonged courses of treatment. Myelosuppression is mild to moderate, and thrombocytopenia is less frequent. Rashes have been reported as hypersensitivity reactions

Indications: Altretamine is used as second-line therapy for ovarian carcinoma. It also has shown antineoplastic activity in breast cancer, lymphomas, and small cell carcinoma of the lung.

Mitomycin
Nomenclature
Generic name: Mitomycin, mitomycin-C
Commercial name: Mutamycin

Availability: Mitomycin is available in 5-, 20-, and 40-mg vials with mannitol (10, 40, and 80 mg, respectively).

Preparation: Mitomycin is reconstituted by adding sterile water to prepare a solution of 0.5 mg/mL. Dissolution may be delayed despite shaking. Mitomycin is less stable in D5W than in saline and is most stable (up to 24 hours) in sodium lactate.

Form: Mitomycin is a blue-violet crystalline powder; it is water soluble. It has a molecular weight of 334.32.

Administration: Mitomycin is one of the most potent vesicants administered to patients, possibly causing more extensive local toxicity than nitrogen mustard. A freshly placed, freely running i.v. should be used for administration, with frequent checks for blood return or local swelling. Extravasation can cause severe cellulitis leading to tissue sloughing that may require extensive skin grafting.

Metabolism: Mitomycin is activated in aqueous solution and in all tissues; enzymatic reduction via cytochrome P450, DT-diaphorase, and other hepatic reductases also occurs. Toxic hydroxyl and superoxide radicals are generated in an aerobic environment (142–144), but alkylation is more likely to occur in a reducing environment (145).

Pharmacokinetics: The mean elimination half-life for mitomycin is 54 minutes (146, 147). The total body clearance is high, 200 to 800 mL/min/m^2. Only 10% of the administered dose is recovered unchanged in the urine (147).

Toxicity: Myelosuppression is dose limiting and may be severe and prolonged after a single dose of 15 to 20 mg. Delayed neutropenia and thrombocytopenia may occur as long as 8 weeks after treatment, suggesting potent toxicity at an early precursor or stem cell. As many as 25% of patients do not have recovery of myeloid function. Nausea occurs with 1 to 2 hours of dosing; although emesis subsides after a few hours, nausea may persist for several days. Dexamethasome is commonly used as premedication for nausea. As noted above, mitomycin is a severe vesicant (148). Patients have even reported cellulitis with ulceration in locations distant from the administration site, such as venipuncture sites in the opposite arm that were still fresh (and presumably oozing subcutaneously) at the time of mitomycin administration. Mucositis and alopecia are common. Renal toxicity is seen in 2 to 5% of patients who have received less than 50 mg/m^2. The hemolytic uremic syndrome, which may be lethal, has occurred in patients receiving repeated doses of mitomycin (149). Infrequent reports of cough and pulmonary infiltrates indicate the potential for serious pulmonary toxicity; oxygen toxicity progressing to adult respiratory distress syndrome (ARDS) has been reported after mitomycin treatment.

Indications: Even compared with other alkylating agents, mitomycin has a low therapeutic index. It is not currently used in first-line therapy of any malignancy, although it has a critical role in combined-modality treatment of anal carcinoma in combination with radiation and 5-FU. It also has activity in gastric carcinoma, breast carcinoma, and head and neck carcinoma. It has not been shown to increase response rates over 5-FU alone in pancreatic or colon carcinoma.

ALKANE SULFONATES

Busulfan (Fig. 19.2)
Nomenclature
Generic name: Busulfan, busulphan
Commercial name: Myleran
Chemical name: 1,4-butanediol dimethanesulfonate
Availability: 2-mg tablets
Form: Busulfan is a white crystalline powder. It is only slightly soluble in water or ethanol. The molecular weight of busulfan is 246.31.
Administration: Orally. Busulfan has been crushed and mixed in a slurry for pediatric use. Although food may delay absorption, it does not appear to change the overall AUC after an oral dose.
Metabolism: Busulfan, like the nitrogen mustards, alkylates preferentially the N^7 position of guanine, but at a much slower rate (150). Busulfan is nearly entirely eliminated by metabolism, but the major metabolic products of busulfan (there have been at least a dozen identified) are inactive. The major metabolites result after reaction with glutathione: 3-hydroxysulfolane and 3-hydroxytetrahydrothiophene-1,1-dioxide (151, 152). Intermediate sulfonium ion metabolites (glutathione or *N*-acetyl-L-cysteine sulfonium ions) could cause toxic monoalkylations, although their contribution to drug activity or toxicity has not been demonstrated (153).
Pharmacokinetics: Busulfan is well absorbed orally, although variability in absorption, with bioavailability ranging from 47 to 120%, has been reported (154). The clearance rate (Cl/F) for busulfan is 175 mL/min in adults (155, 156); it is 2 to 4 times higher in infants, 450 to 700 mL/min, even when adjusted for body surface area (157–159). The elimination half-life is about 2.5 hours, but there is wide interpatient variability (155, 156, 160). Busulfan metabolism may vary with circadian rhythm, resulting in higher clearance rates and lower concentrations in the evening in some patients; this is more prominent in younger patients than in adults (156, 161, 162). Busulfan is lipophilic and crosses into CSF; concentrations at steady state in patients receiving BMT doses are 0.95 to 1.3 times plasma concentrations (163, 164). Reversible protein binding is negligible for busulfan (163, 164).

In the high doses used in BMT, a correlation has been shown between increased busulfan exposure and the occurrence of lethal hepatotoxicity in adults; many centers provide therapeutic monitoring and dose adjustment for busulfan in this setting (155, 162). In infants, therapeutic monitoring identified relative underdosing when providing doses on a per kg rather than a per m² regimen (165, 166). The rationale for therapeutic monitoring in this setting has recently been reviewed (167).
Toxicity: Busulfan is a potent hematopoietic stem cell toxin; after repeated conventional doses, some patients develop very prolonged pancytopenia, as well as an unusual wasting syndrome, bronchopulmonary dysplasia, and interstitial fibrosis. In high doses, hyperpigmentation, seizures, and hepatic venoocclusive disease (VOD) complicate its use. Prophylactic anticonvulsant therapy is routinely used with BMT preparative regimens (168, 169). Most centers monitor busulfan exposure and modify doses to minimize the risk of VOD (see under pharmacokinetics).
Indications: Although busulfan was widely used for chronic myelogenous leukemia, it is no longer used as a first-line drug for this disease. It is widely used as myeloablative therapy in combination for BMT, particularly in pediatric populations in which the growth-inhibitory effects of total body irradiation are unacceptable (170, 171).

Nitrosoureas
Lipid-soluble derivatives of bischloroethyl nitrosoureas are a second class of bischloroethyl compounds with antitumor activity. They include the derivatives of *N*-methyl-*N*-nitrosourea, carmustine and lomustine, and the naturally occurring methyl nitrosourea streptozocin (165). Although both BCNU and CCNU form DNA cross-links by chloroethylation of a nucleophilic DNA site, streptozocin does not form cross-links; it can, however, methylate DNA. Their structures are shown in Fig. 19.1.

Carmustine
Nomenclature
Generic name: Carmustine, BCNU, NSC-409962
Commercial name: BiCNU
Chemical name: 1,3-bis (2-chloroethyl)-1-nitrosourea
Availability: 100-mg vials are supplied with dehydrated alcohol diluent to be added.
Preparation: Carmustine is initially dissolved in 3 mL of absolute alcohol, and then admixed with 27 mL of sterile water; this produces 3.3

mg/mL BCNU in 10% ethanol, with a pH of 5.6 to 6.0. The initial solution may be clear to slightly yellow. It must be protected from light.

Form: Carmustine is a white lyophilized powder, It is only slightly soluble in water, is freely soluble in ethanol, and is highly lipid soluble. If exposed to temperatures higher than 30.5°, the powder may decompose to an oily liquid. The drug should only be used if it appears as dry flakes or a dry congealed mass. The molecular weight is 214.06.

Administration: Carmustine is highly reactive and can cause burning and hyperpigmentation of exposed skin. The 10% ethanol solution may be further diluted in saline or D5W and infused over 1 to 2 hours. For extended infusions, drug stability has been established after dilution for only 4 to 8 hours. Solutions must be prepared in glass containers.

Metabolism: In aqueous solution at physiologic pH, BCNU decomposes rapidly to form an isocyanate and a chloroethyldiazonium hydroxide ion, which preferentially alkylates the O^6 group of guanine (7, 173). Active hydroxylated metabolites represent the major circulating form for the nitrosoureas (174). Microsomal denitrosation, which can be induced by pretreatment with phenobarbital, may contribute to the clearance of BCNU and cause decreased activity (175, 176).

Pharmacokinetics: The clearance rate for BCNU is very high: it has been reported between 3000 mL/min and 5400 mL/min (177–179). The degradation half-life for BCNU in plasma is only 15 to 21 minutes, and even after high-dose BCNU, the elimination half-life is only 22 minutes (177, 179). BCNU is found in CSF at concentrations that are 30 to 97% of plasma concentrations (180). A correlation has been found between the AUC of high-dose BCNU and pulmonary toxicity (181).

Toxicity: Delayed hematologic toxicity is dose limiting for carmustine. Nadir platelet counts generally occur 4 weeks after administration, and nadir neutrophil counts occur 4 to 6 weeks after treatment (182). Cumulative myelosuppression may limit the number of treatment cycles that are tolerated. Nausea and vomiting are dose related, beginning shortly after treatment and lasting for 6 hours to 2 days. Pulmonary infiltrates and fibrosis occur after cumulative doses and may be rapidly progressive; although most patients had received cumulative doses in excess of 1500 mg/m², total doses as low as 600 mg/m² have been associated with pulmo-

nary toxicity (183–185). Reversible alterations in liver injury tests are seen in a small percentage of patients. Renal toxicity has been reported in patients receiving extended therapy with BCNU. Secondary acute leukemia occurs in 5 to 10% of patients previously treated with BCNU (186, 187).

Indications: Carmustine is widely used in the treatment of glioblastoma multiforme. It is included in combination therapy for both Hodgkin's and non-Hodgkin's lymphomas. It is also used in myeloma, lymphoma, melanoma, and mycosis fungoides.

Lomustine

Nomenclature

Generic name: Lomustine, CCNU

Commercial name: CeeNU

Chemical name: 1-(2-chloroethyl)-3-cyclohexyl-1-nitrosourea

Availability: Lomustine is available in 10-, 40-, and 100-mg capsules, to provide individualized dosing.

Preparation: Capsules

Form: Lomustine is a yellow powder that is insoluble in water (<0.05 mg/mL), soluble in alcohol (70 mg/mL), and very lipid soluble. Its molecular weight is 233.71.

Administration: Oral

Metabolism: In phosphate-buffered saline, the chemical half-life of CCNU is much longer than that of BCNU, about 2 hours. Microsomal metabolism has also been documented for CCNU (188–190).

Pharmacokinetics: Although radiolabeled drug studies indicate rapid absorption, parent drug is undetectable in plasma after oral dosing (191). CCNU is relatively unionized at physiologic pH and is highly lipid soluble. CNS levels are presumed to parallel plasma levels; CSF concentrations of drug and metabolite are more than 50% of concurrent plasma concentrations.

Toxicity: Delayed hematologic toxicity is dose limiting for lomustine, as it is for carmustine. Thrombocytopenia nadirs may occur before the delayed neutrophil nadir. Refractory pancytopenia may develop after cumulative doses. Nausea and vomiting occur in more than 50% of patients receiving lomustine. Delayed renal and pulmonary toxicity that may progress to fibrosis have occurred.

Indications: Lomustine is used in the treatment of malignant astrocytoma, glioblastoma multiforme, and lymphomas.

Streptozocin

This methylnitrosourea derivative was isolated from *Streptomyces* broth. It is minimally marrow toxic (192).

Nomenclature

Generic name: Streptozocin, streptozotocin, 1-methyl nitrosourea glucosamine, NSC-85998

Commercial name: Zanosar

Chemical name: 2-deoxy-2-[(methylnitrosoamino)carbonyl]amino-α-D-glucopyranose

Availability: 1000-mg vials admixed with 220 mg citric acid anhydrous.

Preparation: Solutions are stable for at least 48 hours at room temperature after reconstitution, but contain no antibacterial preservative.

Form: Streptozocin is a ivory crystalline powder. It is soluble in water and alcohol. The commercially available preparation is pale yellow lyophilized powder after admixture with anhydrous citric acid and sodium hydroxide to adjust pH. The molecular weight is 265.2.

Administration: Streptozocin is a severe vesicant. It is normally given by slow observed infusion over 15 to 60 minutes.

Metabolism: The drug is extensively metabolized in liver and kidneys.

Pharmacokinetics: Streptozocin is poorly bioavailable in preclinical models and has not been evaluated orally in man. The mean clearance of streptozocin is 480 mL/min. The elimination half-life is 35 to 85 minutes (193, 194). Less than 10% of the dose is excreted unchanged in the urine (193, 195).

Toxicity: Nephrotoxicity is dose limiting for streptozocin. (Not all alkylating agents have neutropenia as their dose-limiting toxicity; see cisplatin below.) The nephrotoxicity is cumulative and may be irreversible (192, 196, 197). Hypophosphatemia and mild proteinuria may herald nephrotoxicity; this may progress to severe azotemia, proximal renal tubular acidosis, and anuria. Severe nausea and vomiting won this drug the epithet "vomitocin." Emesis occurs within 1 to 4 hours of treatment. It may persist for 24 to 48 hours and be difficult to control, even with the full armament of dopamine and serotonin antagonists (197). Continuous infusion may reduce the severity of emesis but has been reported to cause confusion and lethargy (198). Myelosuppression does occur, but is usually mild to moderate (192, 199).

Indications: Streptozocin is used in the treatment of islet cell carcinoma and carcinoid tumors.

PLATINUM COMPOUNDS

The platinum antitumor compounds were discovered by taking advantage of a serendipitous opportunity. Rosenberg and colleagues, studying bacterial growth in the presence of electrical current, noticed growth inhibition in the water bath, where electrolysis with the platinum electrode had produced a previously undescribed complex with ammonia and chloride (200). Like the alkylating agents described above, platinum coordination complexes form strong covalent bonds by displacement of nucleophilic atoms such as the N^7 guanine to form interstrand cross-links that correlate with cytotoxicity (201, 202). The specific DNA-platinum adducts that have been identified are between adjacent guanine DNA bases, cross-strand cross-links to the adjacent complementary guanine, or between adjacent guanine and adenine DNA bases (203). DNA replication can be inhibited by as few as two platinum adducts in the DNA (204).

Cisplatin, the most active of the original group of compounds, is based on a platinum with an oxidation state of +2, with four ligands (Fig. 19.3). Compounds with a +4 oxidation

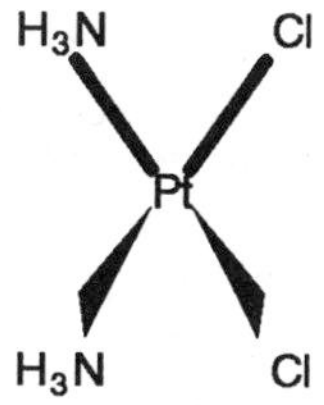

Cisplatin

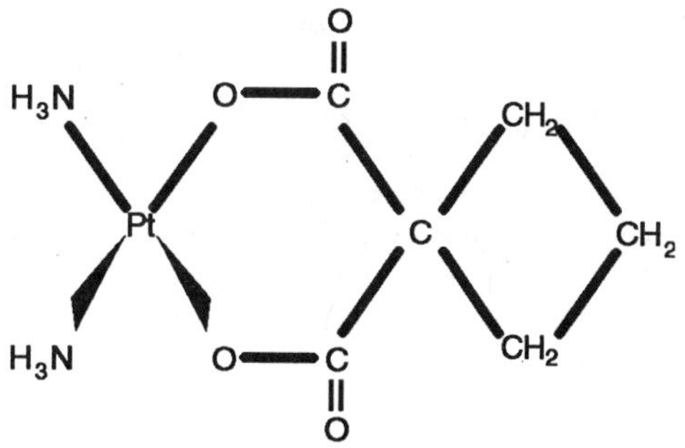

Carboplatin

Figure 19.3.   Structures of platinum compounds.

state have 6 ligands and are less reactive, but are likely to be reduced in vivo to +2 complexes (205). Less readily displaced ligands like the carboxyl ester groups in carboplatin also result in compounds that are less chemically reactive than cisplatin. *Cis*-dichloro (cisplatin) or *cis*-carboxylester (carboplatin) compounds form stereospecific cross-links; the *trans* analogues are inactive. The initial displacement of the chloride ligand by water to form the aquo ligand is thought to take place intracellularly where the chloride content is much lower; thus, the high-chloride extracellular fluid stabilizes cisplatin in its less reactive form for effective transport to cells, where the aquo ligand is formed.

Cisplatin

Nomenclature

Generic name: cisplatin (CDDP, NSC-119875)
Commercial name: Platinol
Chemical name: cis-diamminedichloroplatinum II

Availability: 10- and 50-mg vials for intravenous use, with mannitol, sodium chloride, and HCl.

Preparation: Cisplatin is diluted to 1 mg/mL with 10 or 50 mL of sterile water for injection. After dilution in 0.9% saline, cisplatin is less than 90% potent after 6 hours. (206). Aluminum needles/intravenous sets should not be used because of precipitate formation.

Form: Cisplatin is a white, lyophilized powder with a molecular weight of 300.1. It is moderately soluble in water (1 mg/mL).

Administration: Cisplatin is generally administered with forced diuresis, particularly with excess chloride, to minimize nephrotoxicity. Prehydration with normal saline, dilution in normal saline, and infusion over 1 to 24 hours with additional saline provided intravenously minimizes renal toxicity and emesis. Although mannitol has been widely used to support sustained diuresis, administration in hypertonic saline may be preferable because of the provision of additional chloride (207). Furosemide should only be used for patients who become clinically overhydrated.

Metabolism: In plasma, the high chloride concentration minimizes the aquation hydrolysis of cisplatin to the much more reactive aquo species. Intracellularly, cisplatin reacts with water to form the mono- and di-aquo platinum complexes, which react with nucleophilic sites. The energetically favorable DNA alkylation sites for cisplatin are the N^7s of guanine and adenine (208).

Pharmacokinetics: Assay: Cisplatin has been measured as the original drug as well as by measurement of ultrafiltrable platinum by flameless atomic absorption spectroscopy (209); cisplatin itself represents 60 to 80% of measured ultrafiltrable platinum, and the disposition of the two measurements are parallel (210).

The total body clearance of parent cisplatin is 400 to 500 mL/min; renal clearance represents 50 to 60 mL/min/m^2. The elimination half-life for cisplatin is greater than 24 hours (210, 211). Approximately 15% of administered cisplatin is excreted unchanged in the urine, but up to 90% of the administered platinum dose is recovered in the urine (212).

Toxicity: Nephrotoxicity is dose limiting for cisplatin administration (213, 214). Cisplatin nephrotoxicity is manifested early by wasting of potassium and magnesium, acute reductions in glomerular filtration rate, and urinary enzyme secretion (215). It is cumulative, and administration of other nephrotoxic agents such as aminoglycosides, even between courses, can potentiate its toxicity (216, 217). Focal acute tubular necrosis, dilated convoluted tubules, thickened tubular basement membranes, casts, and epithelial atypia are seen on kidney biopsy (218, 219). Investigators have postulated that alkylation with the sulfhydryl groups of critical enzymes may be responsible for some toxic effects (220). Cisplatin has been shown to suppress Na$^+$K$^+$-ATPase activity in renal tissue as well as Ca^{2+} channel function (221, 222). Peripheral neuropathy develops with repeated administration of cisplatin (223, 224). It may progress from paresthesias and a stocking-glove hypesthesia to weakness, if treatment is continued. Severe local neuropathy has been reported after regional administration of cisplatin (225–227). Nausea and vomiting made treatment with cisplatin very difficult prior to the advent of high-dose metoclopramide regimens and the development of serotonin antagonists such as ondansetron and granisetron (228, 229). Irreversible ototoxicity increases with increasing cisplatin cumulative dose (230–232). Organ culture has demonstrated the sensitivity of cochlear hair cells to cisplatin (233). Raynaud's syndrome occurs as a delayed complication of cisplatin treatment (234). Hypersensitivity reactions including urticaria, angioneurotic edema, and anaphylaxis have been reported. These may be managed with antihistamines and corticosteroids; for more severe reactions, epinephrine has been used with success. Pretreatment for allergic reactions has made retreatment feasible (235). Although azoospermia is universal within 3 to 6 weeks of cisplatin treatment, ⅓ of patients treated for germ cell malignancy successfully father children (236). Acute ischemic events have been reported in patients receiving cisplatin (237).

Indications: Cisplatin in used in curative regimens for germ cell malignancies, limited small cell carcinoma of the lung, osteogenic sarcoma, and carcinoma of the anus. It is also used in combinations for small cell carcinoma, non-small-cell lung cancer, bladder cancer, cervical cancer, ovarian cancer, glioblastoma, neuroblastoma, head and neck cancer, and esophageal, gastric, and endometrial cancers.

Carboplatin
Nomenclature
Generic name: Carboplatin (CBDCA, JM-8, NSC-241240)
Commercial name: Paraplatin
*Chemical name: cis-*diammine (1,1-cyclobutane dicarboxylato-(2-)OO') platinum II

Availability: Sterile lyophilized powder in vials containing 50, 150, or 450 mg of carboplatin with an equal weight of mannitol.

Preparation: Carboplatin is reconstituted by dilution to 10 mg/mL with sterile water or 5% dextrose in water. It can be further diluted to 0.5 mg/mL with 5% dextrose. Dilution in saline may result in conversion of some drug to cisplatin. Needles or intravenous sets with aluminum should not be used because of the formation of precipitates. Solutions may be maintained for up to 8 hours without refrigeration.

Form: Carboplatin is a crystalline powder with a molecular weight of 371.25. It is water soluble.

Administration: Carboplatin is usually infused over 15 to 60 minutes.

Metabolism: Like cisplatin, carboplatin undergoes aquation with elimination of the chlorine and cross-links DNA; it is 100 times less reactive than cisplatin (238).

Pharmacokinetics: Total body clearance of carboplatin is 73 mL/min in patients with normal renal function. Carboplatin elimination is slower than that of cisplatin, with a terminal half-life between 2 and 6 hours (239, 240). Carboplatin is extensively cleared (67%) by the kidneys; dose adjustment is required for renal insufficiency. There is a good correlation between the AUC of carboplatin and dose-limiting thrombocytopenia; a formula is available to select the dose of carboplatin desired to produce a given degree of thrombocytopenia on the basis of creatinine clearance, body surface area, and pretreatment platelet count (241, 242).

In the setting of BMT preparative regimens including carboplatin, the measurement of increased concentrations of ultrafiltrable platinum in the plasma at 16 to 22 hours into an infusion of 400 mg/m^2/day for 4 days (>14 μM) predicted the development of subsequent renal injury (115).

Toxicity: Unlike cisplatin, thrombocytopenia is dose limiting for carboplatin. Both thrombocytopenia and neutropenia are maximum between days 21 and 25, somewhat later than for the nitrogen mustard–based alkylating agents, but earlier than for nitrosoureas. Patients with extensive prior myelotoxic therapy may require up to 6 weeks for recovery of hematologic parameters. Emesis is much less severe and easier to ameliorate with carboplatin than with cisplatin. Rash, alopecia, and hepatotoxicity are unusual complications of carboplatin, reported more frequently in studies using escalating doses of carboplatin.

Indications: Carboplatin activity has been confirmed for many of the diseases that are treated with cisplatin: advanced ovarian carcinoma, small cell lung carcinoma, testicular cancer, medulloblastoma, and head and neck and genitourinary cancers.

METHYLATING AGENTS (FIG. 19.4)

Dacarbazine
Nomenclature
Generic name: Dacarbazine, DTIC, DIC, NSC-45388
Commercial name: DTIC-Dome
Chemical name:
5-(3,3-dimethyl-1-triazenyl)-1H-imidazole-4-carboxamide

Availability: 100-mg and 200-mg vials prepared with anhydrous citric acid and mannitol.

Preparation: Sterile water (9.9 or 19.7 mL) is added to the 100- or 200-mg vials, respec-

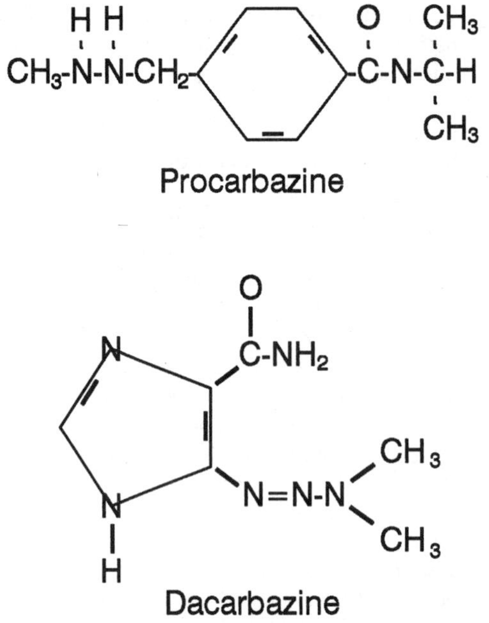

Procarbazine

Dacarbazine

Figure 19.4. Structures of methylating agents.

tively, to produce 10 mg/mL solutions. These solutions are stable up to 8 hours at room temperature, protected from heat and light.

Form: Dacarbazine is a colorless to ivory crystalline solid. Pink coloration indicates decomposition. It has a molecular weight of 182.18.

Administration: Dacarbazine may be administered as a rapid intravenous injection into a freely flowing freshly initiated i.v. or may be further diluted in 250 mL of D5W or normal saline and infused over 15 to 30 minutes.

Metabolism: Dacarbazine is metabolized by microsomal enzymes in the liver to MTIC (5-(3-monomethyl-1-triazenyl)-1H-imidazole-4-carboxamide (243, 244). MTIC spontaneously decomposes to AIC, a purine precursor, and a reactive methyl diazonium cation. MTIC is an inhibitor of nucleoside incorporation; the ultimate mode of action of dacarbazine may be multifactorial (245, 246).

Pharmacokinetics: The elimination half-life for the parent compound is only 41 to 110 minutes (247–249). Dacarbazine has a high total body clearance: the reported mean clearance is 1080 mL/min (247). Renal excretion of unchanged dacarbazine and AIC account for 1/3 to 1/2 of administered drug. The renal clearance rate has been estimated between 350 to 700 mL/min (247, 250). DTIC is minimally protein bound (20%) (251).

Toxicity: Dose-limiting toxicity for dacarbazine alone is myelosuppression. It is also a potent cause of emesis, but nausea can be frequently controlled with aggressive antiemetic regimens. Some clinicians gradually increase the dose over a course of treatment to minimize vomiting. A flulike syndrome with fever, malaise, and myalgias occasionally occurs (252). Hepatic vein thrombosis has been reported. Dacarbazine causes pain on infusion, and extravasation may produce severe vesicant effects. Patients must be cautioned to minimize sun exposure because of photosensitivity reactions seen in patients receiving moderate-to-high doses of dacarbazine (252).

Indications: Dacarbazine is used in combination for the treatment of metastatic melanoma and in the ABVD (doxorubicin (Adriamycin), bleomycin, vinblastine, and dacarbazine) regimen for Hodgkin's lymphoma. It is also included in the MAID (mesna, doxorubicin, ifosfamide, and dacarbazine) regimen for sarcoma.

Procarbazine

Nomenclature

Generic name: Procarbazine, NSC-77213

Commercial name: Matulane

Chemical name: N-isopropyl-α-(2-methylhydrazino)-p-toluamide monohydrochloride

Availability: Preparation: The oral hydrochloride salt is unstable in aqueous solution and is light sensitive.

Form: Procarbazine is a pale yellow crystalline powder; it is water soluble, but rapidly hydrolyzes. The molecular weight is 257.76.

Administration: Oral

Metabolism: Procarbazine is a congener of the MAO inhibitor 1-methyl-2-benzyl hydrazine (253). It is metabolized to azoprocarbazine and subsequently to methylazoxyprocarbazine and benzylazoxyprocarbazine by cytochrome P450 in the liver, but human leukemia cells can form cytotoxic species from the parent compound (254–256). Aldehyde dehydrogenase and xanthine oxidase are also catalysts for further activation of the azoxy metabolites (257). Methylation at the O^6 and N^7 positions of guanine has been demonstrated (258).

Pharmacokinetics: Procarbazine is promptly absorbed after oral administration, with a peak concentration about 1 hour after a dose; the methylazoxy isomer concentration peaks at 90 minutes (259). The half-life of the parent compound is only minutes (260). The half-life of the major metabolite is approximately 1 hour (261). This hydrazine derivative easily crosses the blood-brain barrier and produces CNS toxicity (262).

Toxicity: Dose-limiting toxicity after oral dosing is myelosuppression. Procarbazine can produce hemolysis in G6PD-deficient patients (263). Mild nausea and vomiting develop shortly after administration, making this oral formulation difficult to use consistently, but this often diminishes with ongoing treatment. Stepwise dose increments over the first few days of drug administration may minimize GI intolerance. Paresthesias and peripheral neuropathies, myalgias, arthralgias, and altered mental status also occur, including psychotic reactions, which may be related to its MAO inhibitory activity. Allergic reactions, including fulminant hyperpyrexia, have been reported. Interstitial pneumonitis has been reported. Procarbazine produces a disulfiram-like reaction if ethanol is ingested by patients. Acute hypertensive reactions may occur with coadministration of tricyclic antidepressants, sympathomimetic drugs, or tyramine-rich foods, as with any MAO inhibitor. Azoospermia and infertility after treatment with MOPP are presumed to be partly due to procarbazine. Patients who survive 10 years after the treatment of Hodgkin's lymphoma with MOPP have a 5 to 10% incidence of secondary leukemia (264), perhaps due to the combination of nitrogen mustard and procarbazine. Intravenously, neurotoxicity is dose limiting (265).

Indications: Procarbazine was included in the original curative therapy for Hodgkin's lymphoma, MOPP. It also has activity in non-Hodgkin's lymphoma, small cell carcinoma of the lung, glioblastoma, and melanoma.

REFERENCES

1. Ross WE, Ewig RA, Kohn KW. Differences between melphalan and nitrogen mustard in the formation and removal of DNA cross-links. Cancer Res 1978; 38:1502–1506.

2. Erickson CC, Bradley MO, Ducore JM, et al. DNA cross-linking and cytotoxicity in normal and transformed human cells treated with antitumor nitrosourea. Proc Natl Acad Sci USA 1980;77:467–471.

3. Bohr VA, Phillips DH, Hanawalt PC. Heterogeneous DNA damage and repair in the mammalian genome. Cancer Res 1987;47:6426–6436.

4. Tannock IF. Cell kinetics and chemotherapy: a critical review. Cancer Treat Rep 1978;62:1117–1133.

5. Berger NA, Sikorski GW, Petzold SH, Kurohara KK. Association of poly(adenosine diphosphoribose) synthesis with DNA damage and repair in normal human lymphocytes. J Clin Invest 1979;63:1164–1171.

6. Goodman LS, Wintrobe MM, Dameshek W, et al. Nitrogen mustard therapy: use of methylbis(B-chloroethyl)aminohydrochloride for Hodgkin's disease, lymphosarcoma, leukemia and certain allied and miscellaneous disorders. JAMA 1946;132:126–132.

7. Brent TP, Houghton PJ, Houghton JA. 06-Alkylguanine-DNA alkyltransferase activity correlates with the therapeutic response of human rhabdomyosarcoma xenografts to 1-(2-chlorethyl)-3-(trans-4-methylcyclohexyl)-1-nitrosourea. Proc Natl Acad Sci USA 1985;82:2985–2989.

8. Crook TR, Souhami RL, Whyman GD, McLean AEM. Glutathione depletion as a determinant of sensitivity of human leukemia cells to cyclophosphamide. Cancer Res 1986;46:5035–5038.

9. Bolton MG, Hilton J, Robertson KD, et al. Kinetic analysis of the reaction of melphalan with water, phosphate and glutathione. Drug Metab Dispos 1993; 21:986–996.

10. Ozols RF, Louie KG, Plowman J, et al. Enhanced melphalan cytotoxicity in human ovarian cancer in vitro and in tumor-bearing nude mice by buthionine sulfoximine depletion of glutathione. Biochem Pharmacol 1987;36:147–152.

11. Friedman HS, Colvin OM, Aisaka K, et al. Glutathione protects cardiac and skeletal muscle from cyclophosphamide-induced toxicity. Cancer Res 1990; 50:2455–2462.

12. Goldenberg GJ, Vanstone CL, Bihler I. Transport of nitrogen mustard on the transport carrier for choline in L5178Y lymphoblasts. Science 1971; 172:1148–1149.

13. DeVita VT, Serpick AA, Carbone PP. Combination chemotherapy in the treatment of advanced Hodgkin's disease. Ann Intern Med 1970;73:881–895.

14. Schneider SM, Distelhorst CW. Chemotherapy induced emergencies. Semin Oncol 1989;16:572–578.

15. Pedersen-Bjergaard J, Larsen SO. Incidence of acute non-lymphocytic leukemia, preleukemia, and acute myeloproliferative syndrome up to 10 years after treatment of Hodgkin's disease. N Engl J Med 1982; 307:965–970.

16. Pedersen-Bjergaard J, Larsen SO, Strack J, et al. Risk of therapy related leukemia and preleukemia after Hodgkin's disease. Lancet 1987;2:83–88.

17. Schilsky R. Male fertility following cancer chemotherapy. J Clin Oncol 1989;7:295–297.

18. Damewood MD, Grochow LB. Prospects for fertility after chemotherapy or radiation for neoplastic disease. Fertil Steril 1986;45:443–459.

19. Spitz S. The histological effects of nitrogen mustards on human tumors and tissues. Cancer 1948; 1:383–398.

20. Alberts DS, Chang SY, Chen HSG, et al. Pharmacokinetics and metabolism of chlorambucil in man: a preliminary report. Cancer Treat Rev 1979;6:9–17.

21. Dulik DM, Colvin OM, Fenselau C. Characterization of glutathione conjugates of chlorambucil by fast atom bombardment and thermospray liquid chromatography/mass spectrometry. Biomed Environ Mass Spectrom 1990;19:248–252.

22. Adair CG, Bridges JM, Desai ZR. Can food affect the bioavailability of chlorambucil in patients with hematologic malignancies? Cancer Chemother Pharmacol 1989;17:99–102.

23. Alberts DS, Chang SY, Chen HSG, et al. Comparative pharmacokinetics of chlorambucil and melphalan in man. Recent Results Cancer Res 1980;74:124–127.

24. Newell DR, Calvert AH, Harrap KR. Studies on the pharmacokinetics of chlorambucil and prednimustine in man. Br J Clin Pharmacol 1983;15:253–258.

25. Greig NH, Daly EM, Sweeney DJ, Rapaport SI. Pharmacokinetics of chlorambucil tertiary butyl ester, a lipophilic chlorambucil derivative that achieves and maintains high concentrations in the brain. Cancer Chemother Pharmacol 1990;25:320–325.

26. Bastholt L, Johansson CJ, Pfeiffer P. A pharmacokinetic study of prednimustine as compared with prednisone and chlorambucil in cancer patients. Cancer Chemother Pharmacol 1991;28:205–210.

27. Hartvig P, Simonsson B, Oberg G, Wallin J, Ehrsson H. Inter and intra-individual differences in oral chlorambucil pharmacokinetics. Eur J Clin Pharmacol 1998;35:551–554.

28. Ehrsson H, Lonroth U, Wallin I, Ehrnebo H, Nilsson SO. Degradation of chlorambucil in aqueous solution: influence of human albumin binding. J Pharm Pharmacol 1981;33:313–315.

29. Ciobanu N, Runowicz C, Gucalp R, et al. Reversible central nervous system toxicity associated with high dose chlorambucil in autologous bone marrow transplantation for ovarian carcinoma. Cancer Treat Rep 1987;71:1324–1325.

30. Pietrantonio F, Moriconi L, Torino F, Romano A, Gargovich A. Unusual reaction to chlorambucil; a case report. Cancer Lett 1990;54:109–111.

31. Cole SR, Myers TJ, Klatsky AU. Pulmonary disease with chlorambucil therapy. Cancer 1978;41:455–459.

32. Morganfield MC, Goldberg V, Parisier H, et al. Ovarian lesions due to cytostatic agents during the treatment of Hodgkin's disease. Surg Gynecol Obstet 1972;134:826–828.

33. Gradishar WJ, Schilsky RL. Effects of cancer treatment on the reproductive system. CRC Crit Res Oncol Hematol 1988;8:153–171.

34. Palmer RG, Denman AM. Malignancies induced by chlorambucil. Cancer Treat Rev 1984;11:121–129.

35. Bergel F, Stock JA. Cytoactive amino acid and peptide derivatives: part I: substituted phenylalanines. J Chem Soc 1954:76:2409–2411.

36. Dulik DL, Fenselau C. Conversion of melphalan to 4-(glutathionyl)phenylalanine: a novel mechanism for conjugation by glutathione-S-transferases. Drug Metab Dispos 1987;15:195–199.

37. Woodhouse KW, Hamilton P, Lennard A, Rawlins MD. The pharmacokinetics of melphalan in patients with multiple myeloma: an intravenous/oral study using a conventional dose regimen. Eur J Clin Pharmacol 1983;24:283–285.

38. Zucchetti M, D'Incalci M, Willems Y, Cavalli F, Sessa C. Lack of effect of cisplatin on i.v. L-PAM plasma pharmacokinetics in ovarian cancer patients. Cancer Chemother Pharmacol 1988;22:87–88.

39. Reece PA, Hill HS, Green RM, et al. Renal clearance and protein binding of melphalan in patients with cancer. Cancer Chemother Pharmacol 1988;22:348–352.

40. Gera S, Musch E, Osterheld HKO, Loos U. Relevance of the hydrolysis and protein binding of melphalan to the treatment of multiple myeloma. Cancer Chemother Pharmacol 1989;23:76–80.

41. Loos U, Musch E, Engel M, et al. The pharmacokinetics of melphalan during intermittant therapy of multiple myeloma. Eur J Clin Pharm 1988;35:187–193.

42. Gouyette A, Hartmann O, Pico JL. Pharmacokinetics of high-dose melphalan in children and adults. Cancer Chemother Pharmacol 1986;16:184–189.

43. Ardiet C, Tranchand B, Biron P, et al. Pharmacokinetics of high-dose intravenous melphalan in children and adults with forced diuresis: report in 26 cases. Cancer Chemother Pharmacol 1986;16:300–305.

44. Ninane J, Baurain R, deSelys A, Trout A, Cornu G. High dose melphalan in children with advanced malignant disease: a pharmacokinetic study. Cancer Chemother Pharmacol 1985;15:263–267.

45. Alberts DS, Chang SY, Chen H-SG, et al. Kinetics of intravenous melphalan. Clin Pharmacol Ther 1979;26:73–80.

46. Pallante SL, Fenselau C, Mennel RG, et al. Quantitation by gas chromatography-chemical ionization mass spectrometry of phenylalanine mustard in the plasma of patients. Cancer Res 1980;40:2268–2272.

47. Reece PA, Kotasek D, Morris RG, Dale BM, Sage RE. The effect of food on oral melphalan absorption. Cancer Chemother Pharmacol 1986;16:194–197.

48. Reece PA, Dale BM, Morris RG, et al. Effect of L-leucine on oral melphalan kinetics in patients. Cancer Chemother Pharmacol 1987;20:256–258.

49. Boros L, Peng YM, Alberts DS, et al. Pharmacokinetics of very high-dose oral melphalan in cancer patients. Am J Clin Oncol 1990;13:19–22.

50. Choi KE, Ratain MJ, Williams SF, et al. Plasma pharmacokinetics of high-dose oral melphalan in patients treated with trialkylator chemotherapy and autologous bone marrow reinfusion. Cancer Res 1989;49:1318–1321.

51. Gera S, Musch E, Osterheld HKO, Loos U. Relevance of the hydrolysis and protein binding of melphalan to the treatment of multiple myeloma. Cancer Chemother Pharmacol 1989;23:76–80.

52. Cornwell GO, Pajak TF, McIntyre OR, et al. Influence of renal failure on myelosuppressive effects of melphalan: cancer and Leukemia Group B experience. Cancer Treat Rep 1982;66:475–481.

53. Ploin YD, Tranchand B, Guastella JP, et al. Pharmacokinetically guided dosing for intravenous melphalan: a pilot study in patients with advanced ovarian carcinoma. Eur J Cancer 1992;28:1311–1315.

54. Vincent MD, Powles TJ, Coombes RC, McElwain TJ. Late intensification with high-dose melphalan and autologous bone marrow support in breast cancer patients responding to conventional chemotherapy. Cancer Chemother Pharmacol 1988;21:255–260.

55. Antman K, Eder JP, Elias A, et al. High-dose thiotepa alone and in combination regimens with bone marrow support. Semin Oncol 1990;17(Suppl 3):33–38.

56. Thatcher D, Lind M, Morgenstern G, et al. High-dose, double alkylating agent chemotherapy with DTIC, melphalan, or ifosfamide and marrow rescue for metastatic malignant melanoma. Cancer 1989;63:1296–1302.

57. Codling BW, Chakera TM. Pulmonary fibrosis following therapy with melphalan for multiple myeloma. J Clin Pathol 1972;25:668–673.

58. Einhorn N. Acute leukemia after chemotherapy (melphalan). Cancer 1978;41:444–447.

59. Greene MH, Harris EL, Gershenson DM, etl. Melphalan may be a more potent leukemogen than

cyclophosphamide. Ann Intern Med 1986;105:360–367.

60. Einhorn N, Eklund G, Lambert B. Solid tumors and chromosome aberrations as late side effects of melphalan therapy in ovarian carcinoma. Acta Oncol 1988; 27:215–219.

61. Chang TKH, Weber GF, Crespi CL, Waxman DJ. Differential activation of cyclophosphamide and ifosphamide by cytochromes P450 2B and 3A in human liver microsomes. Cancer Res 1993;53:5629–5637.

62. Kanekal S, Kehrer JP. Evidence for peroxidase-mediated metabolism of cyclophosphamide. Drug Metab Dispos 1993;21:37–41.

63. Kanekal S, Kehrer JP. Metabolism of cyclophosphamide by lipoxygenases. Drug Metab Dispos 1994;22:74–78.

64. Zon G, Ludeman SM, Brandt JM, et al. NMR spectroscopic studies of intermediary metabolites of cyclophosphamide. J Med Chem 1984;27:466–485.

65. Russo JE, Hilton J, Colvin OM. The role of aldehyde dehydrogenase isoenzymes in cellular resistance to the alkylating agent cyclophosphamide. Prog Clin Biol Res 1989;290:65–79.

66. Juma FD, Rogers HJ, Trounce JR. Pharmacokinetics of cyclophosphamide and alkylating activity in man after intravenous and oral administration. Br J Clin Pharmacol 1979;8:209–217.

67. Juma FD, Rogers HJ, Trounce JR. The pharmacokinetics of cyclophosphamide, phosphoramide mustard and nor-nitrogen mustard studied by gas chromatography in patients receiving cyclophosphamide therapy. Br J Clin Pharmacol 1980;10:327–335.

68. Epstein R, Rosenthal RW, Ess RJ. Use of gamma-(4-nitrobenzyl)pyridine and analytical reagents for ethyleneamines and alkylating agents. Anal Chem 1955;27:1435–1439.

69. Wagner T, Heydrich D, Jork T, Voelcker G, Hohorst HJ. Comparative study of human pharmacokinetics of activated ifosfamide and cyclophosphamide by a modified fluorometric test. J Cancer Res Clin Oncol 1981;100:95–104.

70. Sladek NE, Doeden D, Powers JF, Krivit W. Plasma concentrations of 4-hydroxycyclophosphamide and phosphoramide mustard in patients repeatedly given high doses of cyclophosphamide in preparation for bone marrow transplantation. Cancer Treat Rep 1984;68:1247–1254.

71. Phillips PC, Than TT, Cork LC, et al. Intrathecal 4-hydroxycyclophosphamide: neurotoxicity, pharmacokinetics and antitumor activity in a rabbit model of VX2 leptomeningeal carcinomatosis. Cancer Res 1992; 52:6168–6174.

72. Jardine I, Fenselau C, Appler M, Kan M-N, Brundrett RB, Colvin M. Quantitation by gas chromatography-chemical ionization mass spectrometry of cyclophosphamide, phosphamide mustard, and nornitrogen mustard in the plasma and urine of patients receiving cyclophosphamide therapy. Cancer Res 1978; 38:408–415.

73. Anderson LW, Ludeman SM, Colvin OM, Grochow LB, Strong JM. Quantitation of 4-hydroxycyclophosphamide/aldophosphamide in whole blood. J Chromatog Biomed Appl 1995;667:247–257.

74. D'Incalci M, Bolis G, Facchinetti T, et al. Decreased half-life of cyclophosphamide in patients under continual treatment. Eur J Cancer 1979;19:7–10.

75. Struck RF, Alberts DS, Horne K, Phillips JG, Peng YM, Roe DJ. Plasma pharmacokinetics of cyclophosphamide and its cytotoxic metabolites after intravenous versus oral administration in a randomized, crossover trial. Cancer Res 1987;47:2723–2726.

76. Wagner T, Fenneberg K. Pharmacokinetics and bioavailability of cyclophosphamide from oral formulations. Arzneimittelforschung 1984;3:313–316.

77. Egorin MJ, Forrest A, Belani CP, Ratain MJ, Abrams JS, Van Echo DA. A limited sampling strategy for cyclophosphamide pharmacokinetics. Cancer Res 1989;49:3129–3133.

78. Chen TL, Passos-Coelho JL, Noe DA, et al. Nonlinear pharmacokinetics of cyclophosphamide in patients with metastatic breast cancer receiving high-dose chemotherapy followed by autologous bone marrow transplantation. Cancer Res 1995;55:810–817.

79. Bramwell V, Calvert RT, Edwards G, Scarffe H, Crowther D. The disposition of cyclophosphamide in a group of myeloma patients. Cancer Chemother Pharmacol 1979;3:253–259.

80. Grochow LB, Colvin M. Clinical pharmacokinetics of cyclophosphamide. Clin Pharmacokinet 1980; 4:380–394.

81. Ottolenghi L, Morasca L, Marsoni S, et al. Plasma levels of cyclophosphamide in patients under polychemotherapeutic regimens. Biomedicine 1980; 32:123–127.

82. Tasso MJ, Boddy AA, Price L, Wyllie RA, Pearson A, Idle JR. Pharmacokinetics and metabolism of cyclophosphamide in pediatric patients. Cancer Chemother Pharmacol 1992;30:207–211.

83. Erlichman C, Soldin SJ, Hardy RW, et al. Disposition of cyclophosphamide on two consecutive cycles of treatment in patients with ovarian carcinoma. Arzneimittelforschung 1988;38:839–842.

84. Alberts DS, van Daalen Wetters T. The effects of phenobarbital on cyclophosphamide antitumor activity. Cancer Res 1976;36:2785–2789.

85. Waxman DJ, Azaroff L. Phenobarbital induction of cytochrome P450 gene expression. Biochem J 1992;281:577–592.

86. Anthony LB, Long QC, Struck RF, Handke KR. The effect of cimetidine on cyclophosphamide metabolism in rabbits. Cancer Chemother Pharmacol 1990; 27:125–130.

87. Humphrey RL, Kvols LK. The influence of renal insufficiency on cyclophosphamide-induced hematopoietic depression and recovery (abstract). Proc Am Assoc Cancer Res 1974;5:84.

88. Juma FD, Koech DK, Kasili EG, Ogada T. Pharmacokinetics of cyclophosphamide in Kenyan African children with lymphoma. Br J Clin Pharmacol 1984; 18:106–107.

89. Powis G, Reece P, Ahmann DL, Ingle JN. Effects of body weight on the pharmacokinetics of cyclophosphamide. Eur J Clin Pharmacol 1987;20:219–222.

90. Baker SD, Grochow LB, Donehower RC. Should anticancer drug doses be adjusted in the obese patient? J Natl Cancer Inst 1995;87:333–335.

91. Ayash LJ, Wright JE, Tretyakov O, et al. Cyclophosphamide pharmacokinetics: correlation with cardiotoxicity and tumor response. J Clin Oncol 1992; 10:995–1000.

92. Makinodan T, Santos GW, Quinn RP. Immunosuppressive drugs. Pharmacol Rev 1970;22:189–247.

93. DeFronzo RA, Braine HG, Colvin M, Davis PJ. Water intoxication in man after cyclophosphamide therapy; time course and relationship to drug activation. Ann Intern Med 1973;78:861–869.

94. Bode U, Seif SM, Levine AA. Studies on the antidiuretic effect of cyclophosphamide: vasopressin release and sodium excretion. Med Pediatr Oncol 1980; 8:295–302.

95. Bressler RB, Huston DP. Water intoxication following moderate-dose intravenous cyclophosphamide. Arch Intern Med 1985;145:548–549.

96. Green TP, Mirkin BL. Prevention of cyclophosphamide-induced antidiuresis by furosemide infusion. Clin Pharmacol Ther 1981;29:634–642.

97. Braverman AC, Antin JH, Plappert MT, Cook EF, Lee RT. Cyclophosphamide cardiotoxicity in bone marrow transplantation: a prospective evaluation of new dosing regimens. J Clin Oncol 1991;9:1215–1223.

98. Patel AR, Shah PC, Rhee HL, Sassoon H, Roo KP. Cyclophosphamide therapy and interstitial pulmonary fibrosis. Cancer 1976;38:1542–1549.

99. Patel JM. Metabolism and pulmonary toxicity of cyclophosphamide. Pharmacol Ther 1990;47:137–146.

100. Eden BV, Debo RF, Larner JM, et al. Esthesioneuroblastoma. Long-term outcome and patterns of failure—the University of Virginia experience. Cancer 1994;73:2556–2562.

101. Goren MP, Wright RK, Pratt CB, Pell FE. Dechloroethylation of ifosfamide and neurotoxicity. Lancet 1986;2:1219–1220.

102. Lewis LC, Meanwell CA. Ifosfamide pharmacokinetics and neurotoxicity. Lancet 1990;I:175–176.

103. Watkin SW, Husband DJ, Green JA, Wareniums HM. Ifosfamide encephalopathy: a reappraisal. Eur J Cancer Clin Oncol 1989;25:1303–1310.

104. Klein OH, Wickramanyake PD, Christian E, Corper C. Therapeutic effects of single push or fractionated injections or continuous infusions of oxazaphosphorines (cyclophosphamide, ifosfamide, Asta Z 7557). Cancer 1984;54(Suppl 6):1193–1203.

105. Morgan LR, Harrison EF, Hawke JE, et al. Toxicity of single vs fractionated-dose ifosfamide in non small cell lung cancer: a multicenter study. Semin Oncol 1982;9(Suppl 1):66–70.

106. Brade WP, Herdrich K, Varini M. Ifosfamide—pharmacology, safety and therapeutic potential. Cancer Treat Rev 1985;12:1–47.

107. Colvin M. The comparative pharmacology of cyclophosphamide and ifosfamide. Semin Oncol 1982; 9:2–7.

108. Prasad VK, Corlett SA, Abaasi K, et al. Ifosfamide enantiomers: pharmacokinetics in children. Cancer Chemother Pharmacol 1994;34:447–449.

109. Kurowski V, Wagner T. Comparative pharmacokinetics of ifosfamide, 4-hydroxyifosfamide, chloroacetaldehyde, and 2- and 3-dechloroethylifosfamide in patients on fractionated intravenous ifosfamide therapy. Cancer Chemother Pharmacol 1993;33:36–42.

110. Wagner T. Ifosfamide clinical pharmacokinetics. Clin Pharmacokinet 1994;26:439–456.

111. Kaijser GP, Beijnen JH, Bult A, Underberg WJM. Ifosfamide metabolism and pharmacokinetics (review). Anticancer Res 1994;14:517–532.

112. Boddy AV, Yule SM, Wyllie R, et al. Pharmacokinetics and metabolism of ifosfamide administered as a continuous infusion in children. Cancer Res 1993; 53:3758–3764.

113. Creaven PJ, Allen LM, Alford DA, Cohen MH. Clinical pharmacology of ifosfamide. Clin Pharmacol Ther 1974;16:77–86.

114. Gilard V, Malet-Martino MC, de Forni M, et al. Determination of the urinary excretion of ifosfamide and its phosphorated metabolites by phosphorus-31 nuclear magnetic resonance spectroscopy. Cancer Chemother Pharmacol 1993;31:387–394.

115. Wright JE, Elias A, Tretyakov O, et al. High-dose ifosfamide, carboplatin and etoposide pharmacokinetics: correlation of plasma drug levels with renal toxicity. Cancer Chemother Pharmacol 1995;36:345–351.

116. Quezado ZMN, Wilson WH, Cunnion RE, et al. High dose ifosfamide is associated with severe, reversible cardiac dysfunction. Ann Intern Med 1993; 118:31–36.

117. Klein HO, Wickramanayake PD, Coerper C, et al. High dose ifosfamide and mesna as continuous infusion over five days—a phase I/II trial. Cancer Treat Rev 1983;10(Suppl A):167–173.

118. Meanwell CA, Blake AF, Kelly KA, Honigsberger L, Blackledge G. Prediction of ifosfamide/ mesna associated encephalopathy. Eur J Cancer Clin Oncol 1986;22:815–819.

118a. Kupfer A, Aeschlimann C, Wermuth B, Cerny T. Prophylaxis and reversal of ifosfamide encephalopathy with methylene-blue. Lancet 1994; 343:763–764.

119. Elias AD, Eder JP, Shea T, et al. High dose ifosfamide with mesna uroprotection: a phase I study. J Clin Oncol 1990;8:170–178.

120. Skinner R, Sharkey IM, Pearson ADJ, et al. Ifosfamide, mesna and nephrotoxicity in children. J Clin Oncol 1993;11:173–190.

121. Arndt C, Morganstern B, Wilson D, Liedtke R, Miser J. Renal function in children and adolescents following 72 g/m2 of ifosfamide. Cancer Chemother Pharmacol 1994;34:431–433.

122. Beckwith C, Flaharty KK, Cheung AK, Beatty PG. Fanconi's syndrome due to ifosfamide. Bone Marrow Transplant 1993;11:71–73.

123. Fields KK, Elfenbein GJ, Lazarus HM, et al. Maximum-tolerated doses of ifosfamide, carboplatin and etoposide given over 6 days followed by autologous stem-cell rescue: toxicity profile. J Clin Oncol 1995;13:323–332.

124. Kamen B, Frenkel E, Colvin OM. Ifosfamide: should the honeymoon be over? J Clin Oncol 1995; 19:307–309.

125. Hagen B, Dale O, Neverdal G, Azri S, Nilsen OG. Metabolism and alkylating activity of thio-TEPA in rat liver slice incubation. Cancer Chemother Pharmacol 1991;28:441–447.

126. Ng SF, Waxman DJ. N,N',N''-triethylenethiophosphoramide (thio-TEPA) oxygenation by constitutive hepatic P450 enzymes and modulation of drug metabolism and clearance in vivo by P450-inducing agents. Cancer Res 1991;51:2340–2345.

127. Cohen BE, Egorin MJ, Kohlhepp EA, Aisner J, Gutierrez PL. Human plasma pharmacokinetics and urinary excretion of thiotepa and its metabolites. Cancer Treat Rep 1986;70:859–864.

128. Ackland SP, Choi KE, Ratain MJ, et al. Human plasma pharmacokinetics of thiotepa following administration of high-dose thiotepa and cyclophosphamide. J Clin Oncol 1988;6:1192–1196.

129. Egorin MJ, Cohen BE, Herzig RH, Ratain MJ, Peters WP. Human plasma pharmacokinetics and urinary excretion of thiotepa and its metabolites in pa-

tients receiving high-dose thiotepa therapy. Advances in Cancer Chemotherapy (symposium), Projects in Medicine, 1987:3–8.

130. O'Dwyer PJ, LaCreta FP, Schilder R, et al. Phase I trial of thiotepa in combination with recombinant human granulocyte-macrophage colony-stimulating factor. J Clin Oncol 1992;10:1352–1358.

131. Heideman RL, Cole DE, Balis F, et al. Phase I and pharmacokinetic evaluation of thiotepa in the cerebrospinal fluid and plasma of pediatric patients: evidence for dose-dependent plasma clearance of thiotepa. Cancer Res 1989;49:736–741.

132. Hagen B, Nilsen OG. The binding of thio-TEPA in human serum and to isolated serum protein fractions. Cancer Chemother Pharmacol 1987;20:319–323.

133. Borm PJA, Mingels MJ, Frankhuijzen-Sierevogel AC, et al. Cellular and subcellular studies of the biotransformation of hexamethylmelamine in rats and isolated hepatocytes and intestinal epithelial cells. Cancer Res 1984;44:2820–2826.

134. Gescher A, D'Incalci M, Fanelli R, Farina P. N-hydroxymethylpenta-methylmelamine, a major in vitro metabolite of hexamethylmelamine. Life Sci 1980; 26:147–154.

135. Miller KJ, McGovern RM, Ames MM. Effect of a hepatic activation system on the antiproliferative activity of hexamethylmelamine against human tumor cell lines. Cancer Chemother Pharmacol 1985;15:49–53.

136. Ross D, Langdon SP, Gescher A, Stevens MFG. Studies of the mode of action of antitumor triazenes and triazines. V. The correlation of the in vitro cytotoxicity and in vivo antitumor activity of hexamethylmelamine analogues with their metabolism. Biochem Pharmacol 1984;33:1131–1136.

137. D'Incalci M, Bolis G, Mangioni C, Morasca L, Garattini S. Variable oral absorption of hexamethylmelamine in man. Cancer Treat Rep 1978;62:2117–2119.

138. D'Incalci M, Farina P, Sessa C, Mangioni C, Garattini S. Hexamethylmelamine distribution in patients with ovarian and other pelvic cancers. Cancer Treat Rep 1982;66:231–235.

139. D'Incalci M, Sessa C, Beggiolin G, Mangioni C. Cerebrospinal fluid levels of hexamethylmelamine and N-demethylated metabolites. Cancer Treat Rep 1981;65:350–351.

140. Broggini M, Colombo T, D'Incalci M, et al. Pharmacokinetics of hexamethylmelamine and pentamethylmelamine in mice. Cancer Treat Rep 1981; 65:669–672.

141. Foster BJ, Harding BJ, Leyland-Jones B, Hoth D. Hexamethylmelamine. A critical review of an active drug. Cancer Treat Rev 1986;13:197–217.

142. Bachur NR, Gordon SL, Gee MV. A general mechanism for microsomal activation of quinone anticancer agents to free radicals. Cancer Res 1978; 38:1745–1750.

143. Adams GE, Stratford IJ. Bioreductive drugs for cancer therapy: the search for tumor specificity. Int J Radiat Oncol Biol Phys 1994;29:231–238.

144. Ross D, Siegel D, Beall H, Prakash AS, Mulcahy RT, Gibson NW. DT-diaphorase in activation and detoxification of quinones. Bioreductive activation of mitomycin C. Cancer Metastasis Rev 1993;12:83–101.

145. Tomasz M, Chawla AK, Lipman R. Mechanism of monofunctional and bifunctional alkylation of

DNA by mitomycin C. Biochemistry 1988;27:3182–3187.

146. Verweij J, den Hartigh J, Stuurman M, et al. Relationship between clinical parameters and pharmacokinetics of mitomycin C. J Cancer Res Clin Oncol 1984;113:91–94.

147. Dorr RT. New findings in the pharmacokinetics, metabolic and drug-resistance aspects of mitomycin C. Semin Oncol 1988;15:32–41.

148. Argenta LC, Manders EK. Mitomycin C extravasation injuries. Cancer 1983;51:1080–1082.

149. Verweij J, van der Burg MEL, Pinedo HM. Mitomycin C induced hemolytic uremic syndrome: six case reports and review of the literature on renal, pulmonary and cardiac side effects of the drug. Radiother Oncol 1987;8:33–41.

150. Tong WP, Ludlum DB. Crosslinking of DNA by busulfan formation of diguanyl derivatives. Biochim Biophys Acta 1980;608:174–180.

151. Bishop JB, Wassom JS. Toxicological review of busulfan (Myleran). Mutat Res 1986;168:15–45.

152. Hassan M, Ehrsson H. Urinary metabolites of busulfan in the rat. Drug Metab Dispos 1987;15:399–402.

153. Hassan M, Ehrrson H. Metabolism of ^{14}C-busulfan in isolated perfused rat liver. Eur J Drug Metab Pharmacokinet 1987;12:71–76.

154. Hassan M, Ljungman P, Bolme P, et al. Busulfan bioavailability. Blood 1994;84:2144–2150.

155. Grochow LB, Jones RJ, Brundrett RB, et al. Pharmacokinetics of busulfan: correlation with venoocclusive disease in patients undergoing bone marrow transplantation. Cancer Chemother Pharmacol 1989; 25:55–61.

156. Hassan M, Oberg G, Bekassy AN, et al. Pharmacokinetics of high-dose busulphan in relation to age and chronopharmacology. Cancer Chemother Pharmacol 1991;28:130–134.

157. Vassal G, Gouyette A, Hartmann O, Pico JL, Lemerle J. Pharmacokinetics of high-dose busulfan in children. Cancer Chemother Pharmacol 1989;24:386–390.

158. Grochow LB, Krivit W, Whitley CB, Blazar B. Busulfan disposition in children. Blood 1990;75:1723–1727.

159. Regazzi MB, Locatelli F, Buggia I, et al. Disposition of high dose busulfan in pediatric patients undergoing bone marrow transplantation. Clin Pharmacol Ther 1993;54:45–52.

160. Shaw PJ, Scharping CE, Brian RJ, Earl JW. Busulfan pharmacokinetics using a single daily high-dose regimen in children with acute leukemia. Blood 1994; 84:2357–2362.

161. Vassal G, Challine D, Koscielny S, et al. Chronopharmacology of high-dose busulfan in children. Cancer Res 1993;53:1534–1537.

162. Grochow LB. Busulfan disposition: the role of therapeutic drug monitoring in bone marrow transplantation induction regimens. Semin Oncol 1993; 20(Suppl 4):18–25.

163. Ehrsson H, Hassan M. Binding of busulfan to plasma proteins and blood cells. J Pharm Pharmacol 1984;36:694–696.

164. Hassan M, Oberg G, Ehrsson H, et al. Pharmacokinetic and metabolic studies of high dose busulphan in adults. Eur J Clin Pharmacol 1989;36:525–530.

165. Yeager AM, Wagner JE Jr, Graham ML, Jones

RJ, Santos GW, Grochow LB. Optimization of busulfan dosage in children undergoing bone marrow transplantation: a pharmacokinetic study of dose escalation. Blood 1992;80:2425–2428.

166. Vassal G, Deroussent A, Challine D, et al. Is 600 mg/m² the appropriate dosage of busulfan in children undergoing bone marrow transplantation? Blood 1992;79:2475–2479.

167. Vassal G. Pharmacologically-guided dose adjustment of busulfan in high-dose chemotherapy regimens—rationale and pitfalls. Anticancer Res 1994; 14:2363–2370.

168. Vassal G, Deroussent A, Hartmann O, et al. Dose-dependent neurotoxicity of high dose busulfan in children; a clinical and pharmacologic study. Cancer Res 1990;50:6203–6207.

169. Grigg AP, Shepherd JD, Phillips GL. Busulfan and phenytoin. Ann Intern Med 1989;11:1049–1050.

170. Urban C, Schwingshandl J, Slavic I, et al. Endocrine function after bone marrow transplantation without the use of preparative total body irradiation. Bone Marrow Transplant 1988;3:291–296.

171. Wingard JR, Plotnick LP, Freemer CS. Growth in children after bone marrow transplantation; busulfan plus cyclophosphamide versus cyclophosphamide plus total body irradiation. Blood 1992;79:1068–1073.

172. Skinner WA, Gram HF, Greene MO, et al. Potential anticancer agents. XXXI. The relationship of chemical structure to antileukemic activity with analogues. J Med Pharm Chem 1960;2:299–333.

173. Colvin M, Brundrett RB, Cowens W, Jardine I, Ludlum DB. A chemical basis for the antitumor activity of chloroethylnitrosoureas. Biochem Pharmacol 1976;25:695–699.

174. Wheeler GP, Johnston TP, Bowdon BJ, et al. Comparison of the properties of metabolites of CCNU. Biochem Pharmacol 1977;26:2331–2336.

175. Hill DL, Kirk MC, Struck RF. Microsomal metabolism of nitrosoureas. Cancer Res 1975;35:296–301.

176. Levin VA, Stearns J, Byrd A, Finn A, Weinkam RJ. The effect of phenobarbital on the antitumor activity of 1,3-bis (2-chloroethyl)-1-nitrosourea (BCNU), 1-(2-chlorethyl)-3-cyclohexyl-1-nitrosourea (CCNU) and 1-(2-chloroethyl)-3-(2,6-dioxo)-1-piperidyl-1-nitrosourea (PCNU), and on the plasma pharmacokinetics and biotransformation of BCNU. J Pharmacol Exp Ther 1979;208:1–6.

177. Mbidde EK, Selby PJ, Perren TJ, et al. High dose BCNU chemotherapy with autologous bone marrow transplantation and full dose radiotherapy for grade IV astrocytoma. Br J Cancer 1988;58:779–782.

178. Levin VA, Hoffman W, Weinkam RJ. Pharmacokinetics of BCNU in man: a preliminary study of 20 patients. Cancer Treat Rep 1978;62:1305–1312.

179. Henner WD, Peters WP, Eder JP, Antman K, Snipper L, Frei E III. Pharmacokinetics and immediate effects of high-dose carmustine in man. Cancer Treat Rep 1986;70:877–880.

180. DeVita VT, Denham C, Davidson JD, Oliverio VT. The physiologic disposition of the carcinostatic 1,3 bis (2-chloroethyl)-1-nitrosourea (BCNU) in man and animals. Clin Pharmacol Ther 1967;8:566–577.

181. Jones RB, Matthes S, Kemme D, Dufton C, Kernan S. Cyclophosphamide, cisplatin, and carmustine: pharmacokinetics of carmustine following multiple alkylating-agent interactions. Cancer Chemother Pharmacol 1994;35:59–62.

182. DeVita VT, Carbone PP, Owens AH Jr, et al. Clinical trials with 1,3-bis (2-chloroethyl)-1-nitrosourea, NSC-409962. Cancer Res 1965;25:1876–1881.

183. Crittenden D, Tranum BL, Haut A. Pulmonary fibrosis after prolonged therapy with 1,3-bis (chloroethyl)-1-nitrosourea. Chest 1977;72:372–373.

184. Litam JP, Dail DH, Spitzer G, et al. Early pulmonary toxicity after administration of high-dose BCNU. Cancer Treat Rep 1981;65:39–44.

185. O'Driscol BR, Hasleton PS, Taylor PM, et al. Active lung fibrosis up to 17 years after chemotherapy with carmustine (BCNU) in childhood. N Engl J Med 1990;232:378–382

186. Cohen RJ, Wiernik PH, Walker MD. Acute nonlymphocytic leukemia associated with nitrosourea chemotherapy: report of two cases. Cancer Treat Rep 1976;60:1257–1261.

187. Michels SD, McKenna RW, Arthur DC, Brunning RD. Therapy related acute myeloid leukemia and myelodysplastic syndrome: a clinical and morphologic study of 65 cases. Blood 1985;65:1364–1372.

188. Schein PS. Nitrosourea antitumor agents. In: Umeza H, ed. Advances in cancer chemotherapy. Baltimore: University Park Press, 1968:95–106.

189. May HE, Boose R, Reed DJ. Hydroxylation of the carcinostatic 1-(2-chloroethyl)-3-cyclohexyl-1-nitrosourea (CCNU) by rat liver microsomes. Biochem Biophys Res Commun 1974;57:426–433.

190. Reed DJ, May HE. Alkylation and carbamoylation intermediates from the carcinostatic 1-(2-chloroethyl)-3-cyclohexyl-1-nitrosourea (CCNU). Life Sci 1975;16:1263–1270.

191. Lee FYF, Workman P, Roberts JJ, Bleehen NM. Clinical pharmacokinetics of oral CCNU (lomustine). Cancer Chemother Pharmacol 1985;14:125–131.

192. Schein PS, O'Connell MJ, Blom J, et al. Clinical antitumor activity and toxicity of streptozotocin (NSC-85998). Cancer 1974;34:993–1000.

193. Adolphe AB, Glasofer ED, Troetel WM, et al. Preliminary pharmacokinetics of streptozotocin, an antineoplastic antibiotic. J Clin Pharmacol 1977;379–388.

194. Bhuyan BK, Kuentzel SL, Gray LG, et al. Tissue distribution of streptozotocin (NSC-85998). Cancer Chemother Rep 1974;58:157–165.

195. Goel R, McClay EF, Kirmani S, et al. Pharmacokinetic study of intraperitoneal streptozotocin. Clin Invest Med 1992;15:420–426.

196. Broder LE, Carter SK. Pancreatic islet cell carcinoma II. Results of therapy with streptozotocin in 52 patients. Ann Intern Med 1973;79:108–118.

197. Hritik DE, Goldsmith GH. Uric acid nephropathy and acute renal failure secondary to streptozocin nephrotoxicity. Am J Med 1988;84:153–156.

198. Kahn CR, Levy AG, Gardner JD, Miller JV, Gorden P, et al. Pancreatic cholera: beneficial effects of treatment with streptozotocin. N Engl J Med 1975; 292:941–945.

199. Seibert K, Golub C, Smiledge P, et al. Continuous streptozotocin infusion; a phase I study. Cancer Treat Rep 1979;63:2035–2037.

200. Rosenberg B, Van Camp L, Krigas T. Inhibition of cell division in *Escherichia coli* by electrolysis products from a platinum electrode. Nature 1965; 205:698–699.

201. Zwelling LA, Anderson T, Kohn KW. DNA-protein and DNA interstrand cross-linking by *cis*- and *trans*-platinum (II) diamminedichloride in L1210

mouse leukemia cells and its relation to cytotoxicity. Cancer Res 1979;39:365–369.

202. Eastman A. Re-evaluation of interaction of *cis*-dichloro(ethylenediamine)platinum (II) with DNA. Biochemistry 1986;25:3912–3915.

203. Poirier MC, Egorin MJ, Fichtinger-Schepman AM, Yuspa SH, Reed E. DNA adducts of cisplatin and carboplatin in tissues of cancer patients. In: Bartsch H, Hemminke K, O'Neill IK, eds. DNA damaging agents in humans: applications in cancer epidemiology and prevention (IARC Scientific Publication no. 89). 1988:313–320.

204. Heiger-Bernays WJ, Essigmann JM, Lippard SJ. Effect of the antitumor drug *cis*-diamminedichloroplatinum (II) and related platinum complexes on eukaryotic DNA replication. Biochemistry 1990;29:8461–8466.

205. Blatter EE, Vollano JE, Krishnan BS, Dabrowiak JC. Interaction of the antitumor agents *cis, cis, trans*-Pt(NH3)C12(OH)2 and *cis, cis, trans*-Pt IV{(CH3)2CHNH2}2Cl2(OH)2 and their reduction products with PM2 DNA. Biochemistry 1984;23:4817–4820.

206. Cheung Y, Cradock JC, Vishnuvajjala BR, Flora K. Stability of cisplatin, iproplatin, carboplatin and tetraplatin in commonly used intravenous solutions. Am J Hosp Pharm 1987;44:124–130.

207. Ozols RF, Corden BF, Jacob J, et al. High-dose cisplatin in hypertonic saline. Ann Intern Med 1984;100:19–24.

208. Pinto AL, Lippard SJ. Binding of the antitumor drug *cis*-diamminedichloroplatinum (II) (cisplatin) to DNA. Biochim Biophys Acta 1985;780:167–168.

209. Goel R, Andrews PA, Pfeifle CE, Abramson IS, Kirmani S, Howell SB. Comparison of the pharmacokinetics of ultrafilterable cisplatin species detectable by derivatization with diethyldithiocarbamate or atomic absorption spectroscopy. Eur J Cancer 1990;26:21–27.

210. Himmelstein KJ, Patton TF, Belt RJ, Taylor S, Repta AJ, Sternson LA. Clinical kinetics on intact cisplatin and some related species. Clin Pharmacol Ther 1981;29:658–664.

211. Belt RJ, Himmelstein KJ, Patton TF, Bannister SJ, Sternson LA, Repta AJ. Pharmacokinetics of nonprotein-bound platinum species following administration of *cis*-dichlorodiammineplatinum (II). Cancer Treat Rep 1979;63:1515–1521.

212. Weiner MW, Jacobs C. Mechanism of cisplatin nephrotoxicity. Fed Proc 1983;42:2974–2978.

213. Gottlieb JA, Drewinko B. Review of the current clinical status of platinum coordination complexes in cancer chemotherapy. Cancer Chemother Rep 1975;59:621–628.

214. Safirstein R, Winston J, Goldstein M, Moel D, Dickman S, Guttenplan J. Cisplatin nephrotoxicity. Am J Kidney Dis 1986;8:356–367.

215. Schilsky RL, Anderson T. Hypomagnesemia and renal magnesium wasting in patients receiving cisplatin. Ann Intern Med 1979;90:929–931.

216. Tanaka H, Ishikawa E, Tashima S, Shimizu E. Histopathological study of human cisplatin nephropathy. Toxicol Pathol 1986;14:247–257.

217. Fjeldborg P, Sorenson J, Helkjaer PE. The long-term effect of cisplatin on renal function. Cancer 1986;58:2214–2217.

218. Gonzales-Vitale JC, Hayes DM, Cvitkovic E, Sternberg SS. The renal pathology in clinical trials of *cis*-platinum(ll) diamminedichloride. Cancer 1977;39:1362–1371.

219. Madias NE, Harrington JT. Platinum nephrotoxicity. Am J Med 1978;65:307–314.

220. Dedon PC, Borch RF. Characterization of the reactions of platinum antitumor agents with biologic and nonbiologic sulfur-containing nucleophiles. Biochem Pharmacol 1987;36:1955–1964.

221. Uozumi J, Litterst CL. The effect of cisplatin on renal ATPase activity in vivo and in vitro. Cancer Chemother Pharmacol 1985;15:93–96.

222. Vasssilev PM, Kanazirska MP, Charmamella IJ, Dimitrov NV, Tien HT. Changes in calcium channel activity in membranes from *cis*-diamminedichloroplatinum (II)-resistant and -sensitive L1210 cells. Cancer Res 1987;47:519–522.

223. Von Hoff DD, Schilsky R, Reichert CM, et al. Toxic effects of *cis*-dichlorodiammineplatinum(ll) in man. Cancer Treat Rep 1979;63:1527–1531.

224. Grunberg SM, Sonka S, Stevenson LL, Muggia FM. Progressive paresthesias after cessation of therapy with very high-dose cisplatin. Cancer Chemother Pharmacol 1989;25:62–64.

225. Pomes A, Frustaci S, Cattaino G, et al. Local neurotoxicity of cisplatin after intra-arterial chemotherapy. Acta Neurol Scand 1986;73:302–303.

226. Frustaci S, Barzan L, Comoretto R, Tumolo S, LoRe G, Monfardini S. Local neurotoxicity after intra-arterial cisplatin in head and neck cancer. Cancer Treat Rep 1987;71:257–259.

227. Busse O, Aigner K, Wilimzig H. Peripheral nerve damage following isolated extremity perfusion with *cis*-platinum. Recent Results Cancer Res 1983;86:264–267.

228. Kovach JS, Moertel CG, Schutt AJ, Reitemeier RG, Hahn RG. Phase II study of *cis*-diamminedichloroplatinum (NSC-119875) in advanced carcinoma of the large bowel. Cancer Chemother Rep 1973;57:357–359.

229. Gralla RJ, Itri LM, Pisko SE, et al. Antiemetic efficacy of high-dose metoclopramide: randomized trials with placebo and prochlorperazine in patients with chemotherapy-induced nausea and vomiting. N Engl J Med 1981;305:905–909.

230. Vermorken JB, Kapteijn TS, Hart AA, Pinedo HM. Ototoxicity of *cis*-diamminedichloroplatinum(ll): influence of dose, schedule and mode of administration. Eur J Cancer Clin Oncol 1983;19:53–58.

231. Skinner R, Pearson AD, Amineddine HA, Mathias DB, Craft AW. Ototoxicity of cisplatinum in children and adolescents. Br J Cancer 1990;61:927–931.

232. Kretschmar CS, Warren MP, Lavally BL, Dyer S, Tarbell NJ. Ototoxicity of preradiation cisplatin for children with central nervous system tumors. J Clin Oncol 1990;8:1191–1198.

233. Anniko M, Sobin A. Cisplatin: evaluation of its ototoxic potential. Am J Otolaryngol 1986;7:276–282.

234. Fossa SD, Aass N, Ous S, Waehre H. Long-term morbidity and quality of life in testicular cancer patients. Scand J Urol Nephrol 1991;138(Supp):241–246.

235. Loehrer PJ, Einhorn LH. Drugs five years later: cisplatin. Ann Intern Med 1984;100:704–719.

236. Roth BJ, Einhorn LH, Greist A. Long-term

complications of cisplatin based chemotherapy for testis cancer. Semin Oncol 1988;15:345–350.

237. Doll DC, List AF, Greco FA, et al. Acute vascular ischemic events after cisplatin-based combination chemotherapy for germ-cell tumors of the testis. Ann Intern Med 1986;105:48–51.

238. Knox RJ, Friedlos F, Lydall DA, Roberts JJ. Mechanism of cytotoxicity of anticancer platinum drugs: evidence that cisdiamminedichloroplatinum(II) and cis-diammine-(1,1-cyclobutanedicarboxylato) platinum(II) differ only in the kinetics of their interaction with DNA. Cancer Res 1986;46:1972–1979.

239. Curt GA, Grygiel JJ, Corden BJ, et al. A phase I and pharmacokinetic study of diaminocyclobutane-dicarboxylatoplatinum (NSC-241240). Cancer Res 1983;43:4470–4473.

240. Reece PA, Bishop JF, Oliver IN, Stafford I, Hillcoat BL, Morstyn G. Pharmacokinetics of unchanged carboplatin (CBDCA) in patients with small cell lung carcinoma. Cancer Chemother Pharmacol 1987; 19:326–330.

241. Egorin MJ, Van Echo DA, Olman EA, et al. Prospective validation of a pharmacologically based dosing scheme for the cisdiamminedichloroplatinum (II) analogue diamminecyclobutane dicarboxylatoplatinum. Cancer Res 1985;45:6502–6506.

242. Vanwarmerdan LJ, Rodenhuis S, van Tellinghen O, Mats RA. Validation of a limited sampling model for carboplatin in a high dose chemotherapy combination. Cancer Chemother Pharm 1994;35:179–181.

243. Skibba JL, Ramirex G, Beal DD, Bryan GT. Metabolism of 4(5)-(3,3-dimethyl-1-triazeno)-imidazole-5(4)-carboxamide to 4(5)amino-imidazole-5(4)-carboxamide in man. Biochem Pharmacol 1970;19:2043–2051.

244. Vaughan K, Tang Y, Llanos G, et al. Studies of the mode of action of antitumor triazenes and triazines. 6. 1-aryl-3-(hydroxymethyl)-3-methyltriazine synthesis, chemistry and antitumor properties. J Med Chem 1984;27:357–363.

245. Hayward IP, Parson PG. Epigenetic effects of the methylating agent 5-(3,3-dimethyl-1-triazeno)-imidazole-4-carboxamide in human melanoma cells. Aust J Exp Biol Med Sci 1984;62:597–606.

246. Lee SM, Margison GP, Thatcher N, O'Connor PJ, Cooper DP. Formation and loss of O6-methyldeoxyguanosine in human leucocyte DNA following sequential DTIC and fotemustine chemotherapy. Br J Cancer 1994;69:853–857.

247. Breithaupt H, Dammann A, Aigner K. Pharmacokinetics of dacarbazine (DTIC) and its metabolite 5-aminoimidazole-4-carboxamide (AIC) following different dose schedules. Cancer Chemother Pharmacol 1982;9:103–109.

248. Loo TL, Householder GE, Gerulath AH, Saunders PH, Farquhar D. Mechanism of action and pharmacology studies with DTIC (NSC-45388). Cancer Treat Rep 1976;60:149–152.

249. Farina P, Benfenati BR, Reginato R, et al. Metabolism of the anticancer agent 1-(4-acetylphenyl-3,3-dimethyltriazene. Biomed Mass Spectrom 1983;10:485–488.

250. Fiore D, Jackson AJ, Didolkar MS, Dandu VR. Simultaneous determination of dacarbazine, its photolytic degradation product, 2-azahypoxanthine and the metabolite 5-aminoimidazole-4-carboxamide in plasma and urine by high-pressure liquid chromatography. Antimicrob Agents Chemother 1985;27:977–979.

251. Loo TL, Luce JK, Jardine JH, Frei E. Pharmacologic studies of the antitumor agent 5-(3,3-dimethyltriazeno)imidazole-4-carboxamide. Cancer Res 1968 28:2448–2452.

252. Buesa JM, Gracia M, Valle M, et al. Phase I trial of intermittent high-dose dacarbazine. Cancer Treat Rep 1984;68:499–504.

253. Bollag W. The tumor-inhibitory effects of the methylhydrazine derivative Ro 4–6467/1 (NSC-77213). Cancer Chemother Rep 1963;33:1–4.

254. Moloney SJ, Wiebkin P, Cummings SW, Prough RA. Metabolic activation of the terminal N-methyl group of N-isopropyl-alpha-(2-methylhydrazino)-p-toluamide hydrochloride (procarbazine). Carcinogenesis 1985;6:397–401.

255. Prough RA, Tweedie DJ. Procarbazine. In: Powis G, Prough RA, eds. Metabolism and action of anticancer drugs. London: Taylor and Francis, 1987:29.

256. Swaffar DS, Pomerantz SC, Harker WG, Yost GS. Non-enzymatic activation of procarbazine to active cytotoxic species. Oncol Res 1992;4:49–52.

257. Tweedie DJ, Fernandez D, Spearman ME, et al. Metabolism of azoxy derivatives of procarbazine by aldehyde dehydrogenase and xanthine oxidase. Drug Metab Dispos 1991;19:793–803.

258. Souliatis VL, Kaila S, Boussiotis VA, Pangulis GA, Kyrtopoulos SA. Accumulation of O^6 methylguanine in human blood leukocyte DNA during exposure to procarbazine and its relationships with dose and repair. Cancer Res 1990;50:2759–2764.

259. Shiba DA, Weinkam RJ. Quantitative analysis of procarbazine, procarbazine metabolites and chemical degradation products with application to pharmacokinetic studies. J Chromatogr 1982;229:397–407.

260. Raaflaub J, Schwartz DE. Uben den metabolismus eines cytostatisch wirksamen methylhydrazinderivates (Natulan). Experientia 1965;21:44–45.

261. Shiba DA, Weinkam RJ. The in vivo cytotoxic activity of procarbazine and procarbazine metabolites against L1210 ascites leukemia cells in CDF1 mice and the effects of pretreatment with procarbazine, phenobarbital, diphenylhydantoin and methylprednisolone upon in vivo procarbazine activity. Cancer Chemother Pharmacol 1983;11:124–129.

262. Oliverio VT, Denham C, Devita VT, Kelly MG. Some pharmacologic properties of a new antitumor agent N-isopropyl-α-(2-methylhydrazino)-p-toluamide hydrochloride (NSC-77213). Cancer Chemother Rep 1964;42:1–7.

263. Sponzo RW, Arseneau J, Canellos GP. Procarbazine induced oxidative haemolysis: relationship to in vivo red cell survival. Br J Haematol 1974;27:587–595.

264. Tucker MA, Coleman CN, Cox RS, Varghese A, Rosenberg SA. Risk of second cancers after treatment for Hodgkin's disease. N Engl J Med 1988;318:76–81.

265. Chabner BA, Sponzo R, Hubbard S, Canellos GP, Young RC, et al. High dose intermittent intravenous infusion of procarbazine (NSC-77213). Cancer Chemother Rep 1973;57:361–363.

20

Antimetabolites

John Gutheil and Christine Kearns

Antimetabolites are similar in structure to naturally occurring compounds required for the normal function of a cell (Fig. 20.1). This structural similarity allows many of the antimetabolites to serve as substrates for important cellular enzymes (Figs. 20.2 and 20.3). Many antimetabolites may only inhibit cell division after first being converted to a more toxic compound by a series of enzymatic steps. Each enzyme involved in this stepwise process is a potential site for the activity of an antimetabolite. Likewise, each enzyme in this process is also a potential site for the development of cellular resistance to an antimetabolite.

All antimetabolites covered in this chapter ultimately inhibit the replication or repair of DNA. This inhibition is brought about by either (*a*) the direct inhibition of the enzymes needed for DNA replication or repair or (*b*) the incorporation of an antimetabolite (or a compound derived from the antimetabolite) directly into DNA. The ability of an antimetabolite to inhibit DNA synthesis makes it most effective in the S phase of cell growth, and thus, an antimetabolite is generally more effective when given by prolonged infusions. Tumors with a high percentage of cells in S phase would be expected to be most sensitive to the effects of an antimetabolite, and likewise, normal cells with high growth fractions (the gastrointestinal (GI) tract and bone marrow) are also sensitive to antimetabolites. As a result, GI tract and bone marrow toxicity is common with this group of drugs. Antimetabolites are, as a rule, not mutagenic, and many have been used during pregnancy without apparent ill effect on the fetus (methotrexate is a notable exception).

Folate Antagonists
Methotrexate (MTX)
Nomenclature
Generic name: Methotrexate, NSC-740

Commercial names: Mexate, Folex, Rheumatrex
Availability
Tablets: Methotrexate sodium tablets contain 2.5 mg of methotrexate in bottles of 100.

Solutions: Methotrexate sodium for injection, preservative protected, is available at 25 mg/mL in 2-mL (50 mg) and 10-mL (250 mg) vials. Vials also contain 0.9% w/v benzyl alcohol as a preservative. Methotrexate LPF (sodium for injection, preservative free, is available as 25 mg/mL in 2-mL (50 mg), 4-mL (100 mg), 8-mL (200 mg) and 10-mL (250 mg) vials.

Powder: Methotrexate sodium for injection, freeze dried, preservative free, is available in 20-mg, 50-mg, and 1-g vials.

Storage: Both tablets and vials of methotrexate should be stored protected from light at room temperature. Both tablets and vials are stable for 2 years from the date of manufacture.
Preparation
Solutions: Methotrexate sodium for injection, preservative protected, may be further diluted with any compatible fluid such as sterile water, dextrose 5% water or 0.9% saline. Methotrexate LPF sodium for injection, preservative free, may be further diluted just prior to use with any compatible fluid such as sterile water, dextrose 5% water, or 0.9% saline.

Powder: Methotrexate sodium for injection, freeze dried, preservative free, can be reconstituted with any sterile, preservative-free fluid, such as sterile water, dextrose 5% water, or 0.9% saline. The 20-mg and 50-mg vials should be reconstituted to a concentration no greater than 25 mg/mL. The 1-g vial may be reconstituted to a concentration of 50 mg/mL. For intrathecal

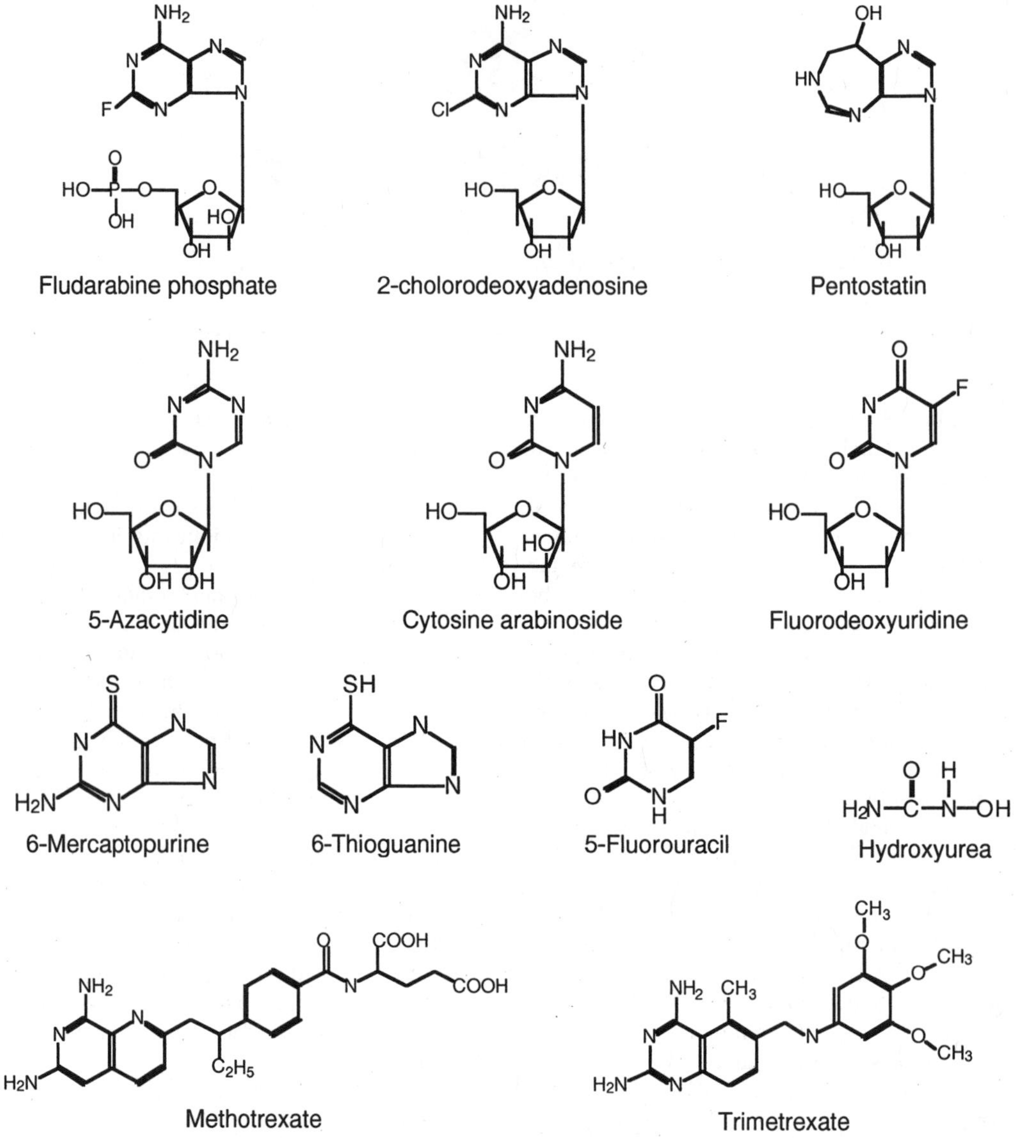

Figure 20.1.   Chemical structures of the antimetabolites.

administration, reconstitute to a concentration of 1 mg/mL in preservative-free fluid such as Elliott's B solution.

Pharmacology

Cellular: At conventional concentrations, methotrexate enters cells by facilitated transport via the folate transporter (1). At higher concentrations, methotrexate will enter cells via passive diffusion. Once within the cell, methotrexate undergoes the sequential addition of glutamyl residues via the same enzymes responsible for the polyglutamylation of folate. Methotrexate polyglutamates are both more highly charged and larger than methotrexate and are therefore less likely to diffuse out of the cell. In addition, methotrexate polyglutamates exhibit higher affinity than methotrexate for the binding sites of dihydrofolate reductase and thymidylate synthase (2).

The principal action of methotrexate (or methotrexate polyglutamate) appears to be binding tightly but reversibly to dihydrofolate reductase (3). However, methotrexate

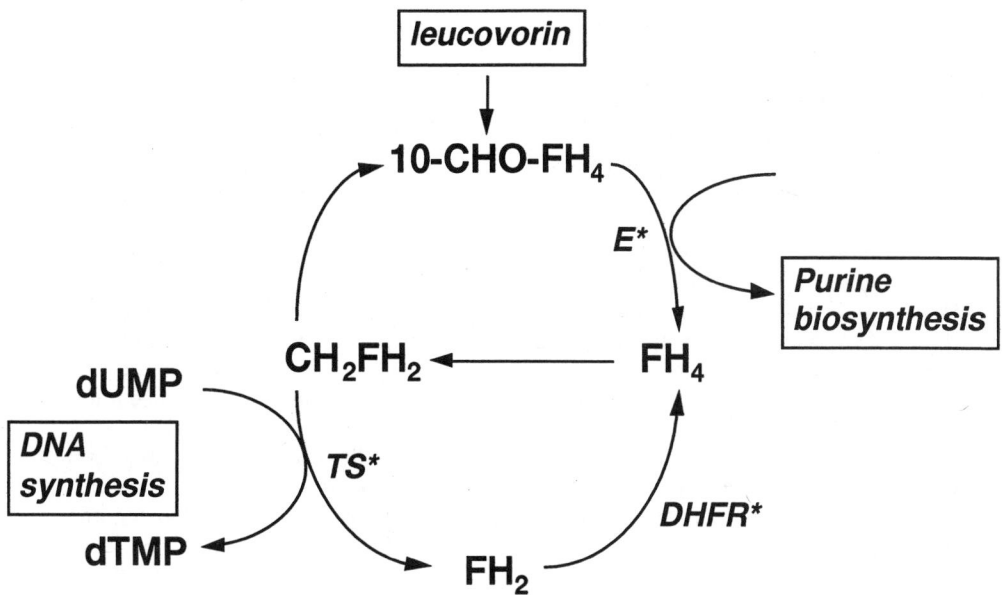

Figure 20.2.   Sites of action of methotrexate and methotrexate polyglutamates. Enzymes inhibited by MTX or MTX polyglutamates are indicated with an asterisk. Abbreviations: *E**, GAR and AICAR transformylases; *TS**, thymidylate synthetase; *DHFR**, dihydrofolate reducatase; *FH$_2$*, dihydrofolate; *F$_4$*, tetrahydrofolate; *dUMP*, deoxyuridylate; *dTMP*, thymidylate; *CH$_2$FH$_2$*, methylene tetrahydrofolate; *10-CHO-F$_4$*, 10-formyl tetrahydrofolate.

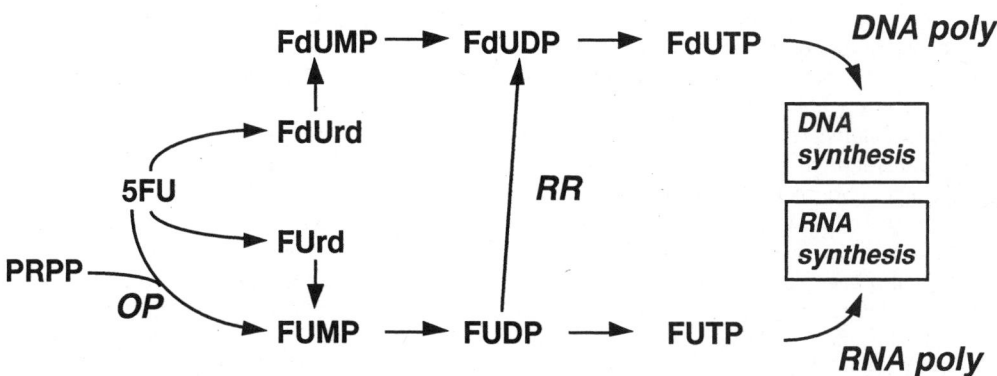

Figure 20.3.   Intracellular pathways for 5FU. Abbreviations: *RNA poly*, RNA polymerase; *DNA poly*, DNA polymerase; *RR*, ribonucleotide reductase; *OP*, orotate phosphoribosyltransferase.

polyglutamate also affects other cellular enzymes that collectively inhibit the cell's ability to use folate in one-carbon transfers (thymidylate synthase, AICAR transformylase, and GAR transformylase) (4). Methotrexate levels within a cell must be much higher than cellular folate levels for effective inhibition of cell growth. This has been attributed to the reversible nature of binding of methotrexate and dihydrofolate reductase. As methotrexate inhibits the ability of

dihydrofolate reductase to convert dihydrofolate to tetrahydrofolate, dihydrofolate levels within the cell increase. Increased levels of dihydrofolate compete with cellular methotrexate for binding to available dihydrofolate reductase. Cellular levels of dihydrofolate reductase also increase following exposure of a cell to methotrexate, thus making more dihydrofolate reductase available for binding to cellular dihydrofolate (5).

Decreases in cellular concentrations of

tetrahydrofolate lead to a decrease in the cellular concentrations of thymidine. The lack of cellular thymidine impairs the cell's ability to synthesize DNA. Synthesis of certain amino acids (i.e., those requiring the addition of single carbons during their synthesis) is also inhibited.

Certain compounds diminish the effect of methotrexate. The compound most commonly used in this respect is leucovorin. In cells made deficient in reduced folates as a result of exposure to methotrexate, leucovorin serves as an alternate supply of reduced folates. While dihydrofolate reductase remains inhibited from the presence of methotrexate, cells treated with leucovorin can again generate thymidine and will continue to synthesize DNA. If leucovorin is removed while cells remain exposed to therapeutic concentrations of methotrexate, cellular synthesis of DNA is once again inhibited (6, 7).

Resistance to methotrexate has been demonstrated from several mechanisms in vitro: (a) decreased transport of methotrexate into the cell (8), (b) decreased polyglutamylation of methotrexate within the cell allowing loss of methotrexate from the cell (9), (c) an increased level of dihydrofolate reductase within the cell (usually based on amplification of the gene) (10, 11), and (d) an alteration in the affinity of dihydrofolate reductase for methotrexate (12, 13). Resistance based on gene amplification (14, 15) and on decreased polyglutamation (16, 17) has also been demonstrated in humans.

Methotrexate has been shown to modulate the effect of 5-fluorouracil (5-FU) on cells via inhibition of purine biosynthesis. As with most antimetabolites, methotrexate is cell cycle–specific for the S phase.

Clinical: Oral absorption of methotrexate is rapid but unpredictable. Oral absorption is generally less than 50% and tends to decrease with increasing doses and in the presence of food (18). Plasma levels following oral administration peak at about 1 hour. Oral administration (generally doses less than 25 mg/m^2) is largely limited to low-dose regimens used in the treatment of non-neoplastic diseases (psoriasis and rheumatoid arthritis).

Methotrexate distributes widely in body tissues and is approximately 50% bound to plasma proteins (19). Elimination of methotrexate from plasma has been reported to be both age and dose dependent, with an α half-life of 0.75 to 2 hours and a β half-life of 3.5 to 10 hours. Some authors have also reported a γ half-life of approximately 27 hours (20, 21). Patients with pleural or peritoneal effusions may trap methotrexate within these third spaces and then slowly release methotrexate back into the circulation over time (22). Such prolonged low levels of methotrexate may lead to severe toxicity, and for this reason, it is recommended that large effusions be drained prior to treatment with methotrexate (22).

Methotrexate enters the cerebrospinal fluid poorly at conventional doses, with cerebrospinal fluid levels ranging from 3% to 10% of concomitant plasma levels. Cytotoxic levels of methotrexate can be achieved in the cerebrospinal fluid following either direct instillation of methotrexate into the cerebrospinal fluid or with the use of high-dose methotrexate therapy (>500 mg/m^2). Following administration directly into the intrathecal space, methotrexate will slowly leak back into the systemic circulation, with a half-life of 8 to 10 hours (23). With both high-dose therapy and administration of intrathecal methotrexate, patients are often treated with systemic leucovorin to protect against systemic toxicity. Leucovorin is commonly administered until the serum methotrexate level drops below 0.05 × 10^{-6} M (24).

Most methotrexate (50 to 80%) is eliminated unchanged in the urine in the first 12 hours (20). Methotrexate clearance approximates creatinine clearance. Methotrexate should therefore be used with caution in patients with renal impairment and should probably be avoided in patients with a creatinine clearance below 50 mL/min (25). Major metabolites of methotrexate include 7-OH methotrexate and DAMPA (4-amino-4-deoxy-N10-methylpteroic acid), which are both much less active than methotrexate. These metabolites may both be more prominent at later time points (>24 hours) during methotrexate elimination. Biliary excretion is generally a minor component of methotrexate excretion. However, in the face of renal failure, the addition of activated charcoal or cholestyramine may significantly increase the clearance of methotrexate from plasma (26, 27).

Indications

Therapy with methotrexate can be curative when used to treat choriocarcinoma (28) and hydatidiform mole (29). Methotrexate has also been used for intrathecal therapy in acute lymphocytic leukemia (ALL) (30). Methotrexate has been used in a large number of combination regimens including those for the treatment of breast cancer (31), head and neck cancer (32), lymphoma (33), osteosarcoma (34), and lung cancer (35). Methotrexate has been used in the treatment of both rheumatoid arthritis (36) and severe psoriasis (37). Additional conventional indications include ALL (38), bladder cancer (39), CNS lymphomas (40), ovarian carcinoma (41), colon carcinoma (42), and rhabdomyosarcoma (43).

Administration

General: Methotrexate may be administered either via oral, intravenous, intraarterial, or intrathecal routes. Both high-dose intravenous administration and intrathecal administration require special precautions and procedures.

Intrathecal Administration: Intrathecal administration generally requires the use of an Ommaya reservoir, which allows administration directly into the lateral ventricles. Methotrexate intended for intrathecal administration must be diluted in preservative-free fluid or the patient's own cerebrospinal fluid. A quantity of cerebrospinal fluid equal to the amount to be administered is removed prior to administration, and the drug is injected over 5 to 10 minutes. Patients are instructed to remain supine for 30 minutes following drug administration (44). Intrathecal methotrexate has been safely administered in combination with both cytarabine (ara-C) and dexamethasone (so-called triple intrathecal therapy).

High-Dose Methotrexate with Leucovorin Rescue: High-dose treatment with methotrexate should only be performed under the supervision of an experienced physician. The level of nursing care must also be adequate to ensure that the patient's urinary output and pH will be monitored rigorously and that treatment with leucovorin will be initiated at the specific time ordered. Patients considered for treatment with high-

dose methotrexate should be determined to have adequate marrow, liver, and renal function prior to therapy. Urinary output is maintained at more than 100 mL/hour and urinary pH is maintained above 7.0 until the serum methotrexate level is demonstrated to be below 0.05 μM (5 $\times$ 10^{-8} M). High doses of leucovorin are started 6 to 42 hours following treatment with high-dose methotrexate and are maintained until the serum methotrexate level has decreased below 0.05 μM. High-dose methotrexate given in the absence of an alkaline pH and adequate urine output results in a high incidence of renal failure from crystallization of both methotrexate and leucovorin in the renal tubules. High-dose methotrexate given in the absence of leucovorin would result in a high incidence of systemic toxicity (mucositis, diarrhea, and marrow failure) related to the direct toxicity of methotrexate on rapidly dividing cells (GI tract and bone marrow).

Dosage

Single Agent: Owing to erratic absorption, oral dosing is largely limited to the low-dose chronic treatment of psoriasis and rheumatoid arthritis. Weekly intravenous administration is used in the maintenance therapy of ALL (20 to 30 mg/m^2 twice a week), and single-agent high-dose therapy has been used in the treatment of CNS lymphomas (3.5 g/m^2 every 2 weeks) (40).

Combination Regimens: Methotrexate is used in a variety of combination regimens, making generalization about any particular dose and schedule difficult. In combination with certain agents (i.e., 5-FU, asparaginase, 6-mercaptopurine (6-MP), and ara-C), the schedule of administration may be important. Standard-dose methotrexate regimens generally use doses of 20 to 40 mg/m^2 every 1 to 2 weeks and 200 to 500 mg/m^2 every 2 to 4 weeks. Substantially higher doses have been used in various high-dose regimens. Doses in excess of 80 mg/week generally require leucovorin rescue to reduce systemic toxicity.

Intrathecal: Intrathecal doses range from 10 to 15 mg/m^2 in 4 to 15 mL of preservative-free solution. For adults, a maximum dose of 15 mg is recommended. When administered via Ommaya reservoir, smaller volumes (3 mL) are generally used. Methotrexate has been combined with both ara-C and dexamethasone for intrathecal administration.

High Dose: Methotrexate has been used at doses up to 15 gm/m^2 in conjunction with leucovorin rescue as part of high-dose methotrexate regimens.

Toxicity: The predominant toxicity with methotrexate is neutropenia, but anemia and thrombocytopenia can also be seen. Nadirs usually occur 10 days following drug administration, with recovery by day 14 to 21. Myelotoxicity is increased in the presence of clinical folate deficiency or impaired renal function. With high-dose treatment, leucovorin given within 42 hours of methotrexate will prevent or diminish myelotoxicity.

Mucositis is common and is seen 3 to 5 days following treatment with methotrexate. Diarrhea can be severe, and when associated with neutropenia, may place patients at a high risk for sepsis and death. Nausea and vomiting are usually mild, and most patients do not require antiemetics.

Renal toxicity with high-dose regimens is thought to be due to precipitation of methotrexate and its metabolite 7-OH methotrexate in the kidney. This can be diminished with both alkalinization of the urine (urine pH >7.0) and vigorous hydration (>100 mL/hr of urine output). Hemodialysis and peritoneal dialysis have proven ineffective in removing methotrexate from the circulation.

Methotrexate has been associated with both portal fibrosis and frank cirrhosis. These are generally seen with continuous low-dose administration. Brief elevation of transaminases is common after high-dose therapy but is not associated with subsequent liver failure.

Common side effects from intrathecal therapy include headache, fever, meningismus, vomiting, and cerebrospinal fluid pleocytosis. More serious side effect of intrathecal methotrexate include paralysis, cranial nerve palsies, seizures, and coma. Children treated prophylactically with intrathecal methotrexate have demonstrated demyelinating encephalopathy. This is usually seen in children who have also received CNS irradiation. Irradiation followed by methotrexate may lead to an increased incidence of leukoencephalopathy. Interestingly, this is seen less frequently if methotrexate precedes the use of CNS irradiation.

Both pulmonary infiltrates and fibrosis have been reported. An erythematous rash is seen in 5 to 10% of patients. This usually lasts for several days and resolves without incident.

Overdose

Intravenous Administration: Very high serum levels of methotrexate can generally be managed by the addition of leucovorin within 42 hours. However, serum levels in excess of 10^{-5} M are difficult to manage, even with leucovorin. Serious toxicity has been seen with methotrexate given in the presence of renal insufficiency, especially if the creatinine clearance is less than 50 mL/min. In the presence of renal insufficiency, biliary excretion may play a more prominent role in the total body clearance of methotrexate. Biliary clearance may be increased by the use of either cholestyramine or activated charcoal.

Intrathecal Administration: Inadvertent overdose of methotrexate given via the intrathecal route has resulted in death. This should probably be treated with removal of methotrexate from the intrathecal space and high doses of leucovorin (45). Carboxypeptidase-G2 has been reported to increase methotrexate clearance from the intrathecal space in preclinical studies and may prove useful in the future treatment of intrathecal methotrexate overdoses (46).

Trimetrexate (TMTX)

Nomenclature

Generic names: NSC-249008, NSC-352122

Commercial name: Trimetrexate

Availability: Trimetrexate is available for injection in 6-mL vials containing 25 mg of trimetrexate (Warner-Lambert).

Storage: Intact vials are stable for at least 24 months at room temperature. Following reconstitution, trimetrexate solutions are stable for 48 hours at either room temperature or under refrigeration.

Preparation: Trimetrexate in 25-mg vials should be reconstituted with sterile water for injection to a concentration of 12.5 mg/mL. Further dilution to a concentration of 0.1 mg/mL can be performed with dextrose 5% water. Trimetrexate is not compatible with saline-containing solutions.

Pharmacology

Cellular: Trimetrexate is similar to methotrexate in its ability to inhibit dihydrofolate reductase (Fig. 20.1). This leads to inhibition of several of the enzymes involved in one-carbon transfer reactions and ultimately to inhibition of DNA synthesis. Trimetrexate differs most notably from methotrexate in its mechanism of uptake into cells. Trimetrexate does not interact with the folate transporter used by both methotrexate and leucovorin. Instead, cellular uptake of trimetrexate appears to be based on passive diffusion across the cell membrane (47, 48). Trimetrexate also differs from methotrexate in that it is not polyglutamylated inside the cell (48). As expected, cells demonstrating resistance to methotrexate based on either an altered folate transporter or an inability to polyglutamylate methotrexate remain sensitive to trimetrexate. However, trimetrexate remains subject to resistance based on increased levels of dihydrofolate reductase. Unlike methotrexate, trimetrexate is affected by expression of the classical multi-drug-resistance phenotype (49).

Clinical: Oral trimetrexate has a mean bioavailability of 44% (19 to 67%) (50) and a terminal half-life of 6 to 18 hours (51). Distribution into the cerebrospinal fluid is generally poor, with only 1 to 2% of trimetrexate entering the cerebrospinal fluid (52, 53). Trimetrexate is significantly protein bound in human serum (>98%) (54). At least two metabolites of trimetrexate have been identified. Both appear to be *O*-demethylated glucuronide conjugates at the 4-position of the phenoxymethyl ring, and both appear to be active in vivo (55). Trimetrexate is cleared predominately by the liver, with only 9 to 22% recovered in the urine (53).

Indications: Trimetrexate has moderate activity against malignant mesothelioma (56), colorectal carcinomas (57), and bladder cancers (58). Minor responses or no responses have been demonstrated for non-small-cell lung cancers (59), esophageal cancers (60), cervical carcinoma (61), renal cell carcinomas (62), prostate cancers (63), malignant melanoma (64), adult gliomas (65), and refractory *Pneumocystis* pneumonia (66).

Administration: Trimetrexate has been administered by weekly bolus, daily × 5 days, daily × 9 days, and continuous infusional schedules. In general, the maximal tolerated dose is decreased by the use of infusional or repetitive daily schedules (52, 53, 67–70).

Dosage: Maximally tolerated doses depend on the route and schedule of administration. Shorter infusions are better tolerated, with a maximal tolerated dose of methotrexate of 220 mg/m^2 when given every 21 days (67). Alternatively, when given as a continuous infusion for 5 days, the maximal tolerated dose is 8 mg/m^2/day (69).

Toxicity: The dose-limiting toxicity of trimetrexate is myelosuppression. Recovery from myelosuppression is generally rapid and occurs by day 14. Toxicity is predominately leukocytopenia, with a less pronounced effect on platelets and red cells (71). Thrombocytopenia can become dose limiting with more frequent administration (54).

Mucositis can be severe; nausea, vomiting, anorexia, and diarrhea are infrequent. Dermatologic manifestations include maculopapular rashes with pruritis, hyperpigmentation, and mild alopecia. Hepatic toxicity includes transient elevations of hepatic enzymes. Renal toxicity has been limited to a transient elevation of serum creatinine. The presence of either low serum albumin levels or treatment with frequent, short infusions appears to be correlated with a higher incidence of significant toxicity (72, 73).

Pyrimidine Antagonists
5-Fluorouracil (5-FU)
Nomenclature

Generic names: 5-Fluoro-2,4 (1*H*,3*H*)-pyrimidinedione, NSC-19893

Commercial names: Adrucil (Adria), Fluoroplex (Allergan), Efudex (Roche), Fluorouracil injection (Roche)

Availability: Fluoroplex cream or topical solution contains 1% 5-FU in 30-g or 30-mL tubes. Efudex solution contains 2 or 5% 5-FU (w/w). Efudex cream contains 5% 5-FU (w/w). Fluorouracil injection in 10-mL vials contains 500 mg of 5-FU.

Storage: Vials should be protected from light and stored at room temperature. A slight discoloration may occur with storage but usually does not denote decomposition.

Preparation: All vials should be inspected for a visible precipitate prior to use. Gentle heating in a 140° water bath with shaking can sometimes clear a precipitate. 5-FU is compatible with either dextrose 5% water or 0.9% saline, and infusional solutions can be used for 24 hours after preparation. 5-FU should not be coadministered with either diazepam, doxorubicin, daunorubicin, idarubicin, cisplatin, or cytarabine. However, 5-FU and leucovorin are compatible for 14 days at room temperature. 5-FU is compatible with vincristine and methotrexate.

Pharmacology

Cellular: 5-FU acts as a false pyrimidine base. It differs from the naturally occurring base uracil by the addition of a fluoride at position 5. There is evidence for the entry of fluorouracil into cells via a carrier-mediated process. Intracellularly, 5-FU is converted to FUMP (fluorouridine monophosphate), FUTP (fluorouridine triphosphate), and FdUMP (fluorodeoxyuridine monophosphate). The cytotoxicity of fluorouracil is reported to be related to (a) inhibition of thymidylate synthetase by FdUTP, (b) incorporation of FUTP into cellular RNA, and (c) incorporation of FdUTP into cellular DNA (74–77). The relative contribution of each of these mechanisms to cellular cytotoxicity is not clear. As with other antimetabolites, 5-FU is most active in the S phase of cell growth. Resistance to 5-FU has been demonstrated to be based on either decreased activation of 5-FU to its active nucleotides (FUTP and FdUTP), increased clearance of FUMP through increased nucleotide phosphatase activity, or changes in cellular thymidylate synthetase resulting in reduced affinity of thymidylate synthetase for FdUMP (78).

Clinical: 5-FU demonstrates minimal systemic absorption following topical administration. Oral absorption is poor (25 to 30%), and 5-FU is therefore commonly administered intravenously (79). Approximately 10% of 5-FU is bound to plasma proteins. Most administered 5-FU is rapidly catabolized in the plasma and is therefore unavailable for inhibition of cellular growth. 5-FU is degraded to CO_2, urea, and α-fluoro-β-alanine (inactive), which are then excreted in the urine. Because most 5-FU is catabolized, minor changes in its catabolism can have profound effects on its cytotoxicity. 5-FU penetrates the blood-brain barrier well and distributes to all parts of the body by simple diffusion (80). Seven to 20% of the administered dose of 5-FU is excreted unchanged in the urine over 6 hours, and approximately 22 to 45% is metabo-

lized in the liver. The mean plasma half-life following intravenous administration is 16 minutes (range, 8 to 20 minutes) and generally follows first-order kinetics. Administered by intraarterial infusion, 5-FU has a first-pass clearance in the liver of 20 to 50% (81).

Modulation of Fluorouracil Therapy: The cytotoxicity of 5-FU may be modulated by a number of agents, including leucovorin, methotrexate, interferon, PALA, and cisplatin (DDP) (82). While the combination of 5-FU with various modulators has demonstrated increased toxicity, it is more difficult to demonstrate a survival advantage for patients treated in this fashion. With all schedules of 5-FU, it appears necessary to administer 5-FU at near toxic doses to achieve any clinical benefit. It is not clear that combination regimens purported to modulate 5-FU are necessarily more efficacious than an equitoxic (i.e., higher) dose of 5-FU given as a single agent (82). The modulation of 5-FU by leucovorin is secondary to the ability of leucovorin to increase cellular levels of reduced folates and thereby increase the stability of a ternary complex formed from the association of FdUMP, thymidylate synthetase, and reduced folate (83). Increased stability of the ternary complex results in prolonged inhibition of thymidylate synthetase and greater cytotoxicity. The modulation of 5-FU by methotrexate is sequence dependent and is based on the ability of methotrexate to increase the concentration of phosphoribosyl pyrophosphate (PRPP) prior to the administration of 5-FU. PRPP is a cofactor in the conversion of 5-FU to FUMP (84).

Indications: 5-FU has been used in a wide variety of tumors and regimens including colorectal carcinoma (85), breast cancer (86), gastric cancer (87), pancreatic cancer (88), bladder carcinoma (89), cervical carcinoma (90), head and neck tumors (91), and vulvar cancer (92). 5-FU has also been used as a radiation sensitizer (93) and for the treatment of liver metastases via direct intraarterial administration (94). Dermatologic indications for 5-FU include the treatment of multiple actinic keratoses, multiple solar keratoses, and superficial basal cell carcinomas (95).

Administration

Dermatologic: 5-FU is applied twice daily to lesions, with a usual duration of therapy of 2 to 4 weeks for keratoses and 3 to 6 weeks for basal cell carcinoma (with 5% cream).

Intravenous Push: Intravenous-push solutions do not require further dilution from that found in the commercial vial. The rate of administration is not critical and is only limited by the size of the vein used.

Intravenous Infusion: 5-FU may be administered as an infusion in either dextrose 5% water or 0.9% saline in an admixture calculated to be administered over no more than 24 hours.

Intraarterial Injection: Intrahepatic infusions of 5-FU have been delivered by schedules ranging from daily × 4 to continuous infusional schedules for 21 days (94).

Dosage: 5-FU has been given by a large number of schedules and as part of numerous regimens. When given as a bolus dose, doses range from 300 to 450 mg/m^2/day intravenously for 5 days every 28 days or 600 to 750 mg/m^2 intravenously weekly or every other week. Infusional 5-FU has also been used extensively with schedules ranging from 1 g/m^2/day for 4 to 5 days to 300 mg/m^2/day intravenously indefinitely (96). Intraarterial infusional schedules of 5-FU have used dosages ranging from 20 to 30 mg/kg/day × 4 followed by 15 mg/kg/day × 17 days (94).

Toxicity: Patients with a familial deficiency of dihydropyrimidine dehydrogenase should not receive 5-FU, as they are at risk for the development of severe toxicity (97). Hematologic effects are less pronounced with administration by continuous infusion than with bolus administration. Leukopenia (granulocytopenia) and thrombocytopenia are commonly seen, with lowest counts on days 9 to 14. Recovery is usually seen by the 30th day. GI toxicity (anorexia, nausea, and vomiting) is generally more severe with continuous-infusion schedules. When seen, stomatitis is an early sign of impending severe toxicity and indicates a need to delay further treatment. Stomatitis is rarely seen prior to the first week of therapy. Diarrhea can be life threatening when high doses of 5-FU are administered with leucovorin. Hepatitis has been seen with direct hepatic infusions.

Alopecia is mild, and hyperpigmentation of the nail beds and skin is common. A reversible maculopapular rash is common and is generally noted on the extremities but occasionally on the trunk. Increased sensitivity to sunlight is common, and exposure to sunlight may precip-

itate other dermatologic side effects such as hyperpigmentation. Hyperpigmentation over the vein used for the intravenous administration of 5-FU is common. Hand-foot syndrome (palmar-plantar erythrodysesthesia syndrome) is associated with the continuous infusion of 5-FU and has been reported to improve following treatment with pyridoxine.

Headache, minor visual disturbances, and cerebellar ataxia have been reported and can persist beyond the end of therapy. The toxic metabolite responsible for neurotoxicity may be fluorocitrate (98).

Asymptomatic ST wave changes on ECG suggestive of cardiac ischemia are common (68% of patients). The incidence is increased in patients with a prior history of ischemia. Both symptomatic myocardial ischemia and angina have been reported (99).

Anaphylaxis has been reported with 5-FU (100), as has lachrymal duct stenosis.

Overdose: Overdosage with 5-FU results in severe GI toxicity that is manifest as nausea, vomiting, severe diarrhea, GI ulceration and bleeding, and prolonged bone marrow depression.

Use in Pregnancy: 5-FU may cause fetal harm when administered to a pregnant woman. 5-FU has been shown to be teratogenic in laboratory animals.

Fluorodeoxyuridine (5-FUDR)
Nomenclature
　　5-Fluoro-2'-deoxyuridine, NSC-27640
　　NDC 4-1935–08
　　Floxuridine
　　FUDR (Roche)

Availability: FUDR is cmmercially available in vials containing 500 mg of lyophilized powder.

Storage: Unreconstituted FUDR is stored at room temperature and is stable for up to 36 months from the date of manufacture. Reconstituted FUDR at a concentration of 100 mg/mL in sterile water is stable for 2 weeks at room temperature (101). Solutions of 0.5 mg/mL in dextrose 5% water are stable for 7 days at room temperature (102).

Preparation: FUDR powder (500-mg vial) is reconstituted by the addition of 5 mL of sterile water. The final solution is 100 mg/mL and may be stored for up to 2 weeks under refrigeration. For use in infusion pumps, a solution containing FUDR (2.5 to 12 mg/mL) and heparin (200 units/mL) in bacteriostatic 0.9% saline is stable for 14 days. A solution containing FUDR (1 to 4 mg/mL) and leucovorin (0.03 to 0.96 mg/mL) is stable for 48 hours at room temperature. FUDR is compatible with dexamethasone, which is sometimes added to intrahepatic artery therapy.

Pharmacology

Cellular: FUDR may be considered a preactivated form of 5-FU in that it differs from 5-FU only by the addition of the deoxyribose sugar moiety. Like 5-FU, FUDR will bind to and inhibit thymidylate synthetase. FUDR is S-phase specific and is primarily toxic to DNA synthesis. FUDR can also inhibit RNA synthesis through incorporation of FUDR into RNA. Resistance to FUDR appears to include reduced metabolism to FdUMP, increased levels of thymidylate synthetase, and decreased binding to thymidylate synthetase (78, 103). The activity of FUDR can be modulated by leucovorin. This effect is thought to be based on the ability of leucovorin to increase the concentration of reduced folates in the cell and thereby increase the stability of the "ternary complex" of thymidylate synthetase, FdUMP, and reduced folate (104).

Clinical: FUDR is poorly absorbed from the GI tract and is administered primarily by intravenous infusion. About 29% of a dose is excreted in the urine as inactive metabolite (80). FUDR is more extensively metabolized to inactive metabolites by the liver during the first pass (90%) than is 5-FU and is therefore preferred over 5-FU for direct hepatic intraarterial administration. Greater extraction of FUDR during its pass through the liver results in lower systemic drug levels and fewer systemic side effects. Higher response rates are seen for direct intrahepatic infusion (intraarterial) of FUDR (50%) than for intravenous administration (20%). Some patients who fail to respond to intravenous FUDR respond to intrahepatic FUDR (25%) (105). The elimination half-life of FUDR is 20 to 40 minutes (80). FUDR is metabolized in the liver to its active metabolite FUDR-MP. FUDR can be catabolized directly to 5-FU. The relative distribution of FUDR between these two pathways may depend on the rate of infusion, with catabolism to 5-FU predominating when large bolus infusions are administered (81).

Indications: Intraarterial therapy of GI adenocarcinomas with metastasis to the liver (106).

Administration

Intraarterial Hepatic: Intrahepatic infusion of FUDR is carried out by continuous infusion for 7 to 14 days through a surgically placed hepatic arterial catheter (105). An H2 antagonist is administered during intraarterial administration of FUDR to decrease the incidence of peptic ulcer disease. Heparin (10,000 U/50 mL solution) is typically admixed with FUDR to prevent clotting in the catheter during infusion.

Intravenous: FUDR is administered intravenously in 100 to 500 mL of 0.9% saline or dextrose 5% water over at least 15 minutes (96).

Circadian Administration: The toxicity of FUDR appears to be decreased through the use of circadian administration; however, the response rate does not appear different from that with conventional administration (107).

Dosage

Intrahepatic Infusion: Doses are 0.1 to 0.6 mg/kg/day by intrahepatic infusion for 1 to 6 weeks. The length of infusion is generally dictated by the development of toxicity in a given patient (105).

Intravenous: Intravenous doses of FUDR from 0.5 to 1 mg/kg/day for 1 to 2 weeks by continuous administration have been used. Daily bolus schedules have used up to 30 mg/kg/day of FUDR for 5 days. FUDR has been used with cisplatin (7.5 mg/m²/day) at a dose of 0.075 mg/kg/day for 14 days (101). FUDR has also been used with 5-FU (350 mg/m²/day) at a dose of 0.1 mg/kg/day for 14 days (108).

Toxicity: Leukopenia and thrombocytopenia are dose related and more common with bolus administration. Nausea, vomiting, and anorexia are uncommon. Diarrhea is more common with infusional regimens. When severe diarrhea is seen, therapy should be discontinued (105). Mucositis is more common with infusional regimens, occurring in 10% of patients. Gastritis, enteritis, and abdominal cramps are more common with intrahepatic administration. Gastric ulcers have been reported in 17% of patients receiving intrahepatic infusion (105). It has been reported that careful surgical technique during the placement of the intrahepatic catheter may decrease the incidence of GI complications (109).

Alopecia is usually mild. Dermatitis and pigmentation changes are rare.

Increased bilirubin, increased transaminase levels, increased alkaline phosphatase, cholecystitis, and cirrhosis are dose limiting with intrahepatic administration. Hepatic toxicity is rare with intravenous administration. The addition of dexamethasone to intrahepatic injections may decrease the incidence of hepatic toxicity (105, 110).

Ataxia, blurred vision, fatigue, headache, depression, vertigo, nystagmus, seizures, and hemiplegia have been reported but are rare. When seen, neurologic toxicity is generally reversible and short-lived.

Fever, dysuria, hiccups, increased lacrimation, lethargy, malaise, and weakness are rare.

Azacytidine

Nomenclature

Generic names: 5-Azacytidine, NSC-102816, 5-AC ladakamycin

Commercial name: Mylosar

Availability: Azacytidine is available as 100-mg vials of lyophilized powder.

Storage: Unused vials, stored in the refrigerator, are stable for 4 years from the date of manufacture. Vials stored at room temperature are stable for 2 years. Following reconstitution, the drug becomes very unstable and must be further diluted within 30 minutes. Subsequent stability depends on both the concentration of azacytidine and the fluid composition (111). With dilution to 2 mg/mL, a solution will lose 10% of its activity in either 2.4 hours (0.9% saline) or 3 hours (dextrose 5% water) (112). With dilution to 0.2 mg/mL, a solution will lose 10% of its activity in either 1.9 hours (0.9% saline) or 0.8 hours (dextrose 5% water) (112).

Preparation: The 100-mg vial is reconstituted with 19.9 mL sterile water, resulting in a 5 mg/mL solution. Further dilution is then carried out with the appropriate fluid. All doses should be prepared immediately prior to use and discarded after 8 hours.

Pharmacology

Cellular: 5-Azacytidine acts as a false pyrimidine and thereby inhibits DNA and RNA synthesis and function. 5-azacytidine is activated to 5-azacytidine triphosphate by uridine-cytidine kinase and is deaminated by the liver to 5-azauridine (113). 5-Azacytidine triphosphate competes with cyti-

dine triphosphate for incorporation into both RNA and DNA (113). 5-Azacytidine triphosphate incorporated into DNA has been shown to inhibit DNA methylation and may thereby alter gene expression (114, 115). Resistance to 5-azacytidine may result from the decreased activity of uridine-cytidine kinase, which initially activates 5-azacytidine to 5-azacytidine triphosphate. While 5-azacytidine has activity in all phases of the cell cycle, it is most active during S phase.

Clinical: Subcutaneously administered 5-azacytidine results in plasma levels similar to those with intravenous administration at 2 hours. The elimination half-life is reported to be between 3.4 and 6.2 hours (116). About 90% of the drug is recovered in the urine by 24 hours. Twenty percent of administered 5-azacytidine is excreted as unchanged drug (116).

Indications: Azacytidine has been used in the treatment of both myelodysplastic syndrome (117) and acute nonlymphocytic leukemia (117, 118).

Administration: *Subcutaneous:* Solutions ranging from 50 to 100 mg/mL of 5-azacytidine have been used for subcutaneous administration. 5-Azacytidine is relatively nonirritating when used subcutaneously (119).

Continuous Infusion: Owing to its poor stability in solution, 5-azacytidine solutions must be prepared every 2 to 3 hours to facilitate long infusional schedules.

Dosage: In the treatment of myelodysplastic syndromes, 5-azacytidine has been used at 16.5 mg/m^2/day for 14 days (120). For the treatment of acute nonlymphocytic leukemia, reported schedules include the use of 5-azacytidine at 150 to 300 mg/m^2/day for 5 days, repeated every 3 weeks, and 150 to 200 mg/m^2 twice weekly for 2 to 8 weeks.

Toxicity: Leukopenia is common and is related to the dose and duration of therapy. The onset of leukopenia may be delayed, with a nadir in excess of 25 days. Thrombocytopenia is less common (121). Nausea and vomiting can be severe with bolus schedules and are much less common with infusional schedules (116). Diarrhea is seen in 50% of patients. Alopecia has been reported. Patients may experience a transient erythematous rash (122). Azotemia is common but usually transient. Renal tubular acidosis and proteinuria are rare. Hepatic toxicity has included elevations of transaminases, bilirubin, and alkaline phosphatase (121). Altered consciousness and coma have been reported (121). Hypotension may be seen following an intravenous bolus. Hypophosphatemia has been seen and can be associated with muscle weakness and myalgia (123). Restlessness, insomnia, fatigue, rhabdomyolysis (rare), conjunctivitis, and fever have been reported (124).

Purine Antagonists

6-Mercaptopurine (6-MP)

Nomenclature

Generic names: 6-Mercaptopurine, 1,7-Dihydro-6*H*-purine-6-thione, Mercaptopurine 6-MP

Commercial name: Purinethol

Availability: 6-MP is available as 50-mg tablets for oral administration. The lyophilized sodium salt of 6-MP for injection, in 500-mg vials, is available as an investigational agent.

Storage: 6-MP tablets should be kept at room temperature and protected from light.

Pharmacology

Cellular: 6-MP is an antimetabolite. It is thought to act as a false purine base. Structurally, 6-MP is similar to the naturally occurring purine guanine, differing by substitution of a sulfhydryl for the hydroxyl group on the 6-position of the purine ring. Intracellularly, 6-MP is phosphorylated to its active nucleotide derivatives by the enzyme hypoxanthine-guanine phosphoribosyl transferase (HGPRT). In its active forms, 6-MP is thought to exert its cytotoxic action by incorporation into DNA as a false nucleotide (125, 126) and through inhibition of de novo purine synthesis (127). 6-MP can be metabolized to 6-thioguanine nucleotides. Derivatives of 6-MP are further metabolized through oxidation by xanthine oxidase or, alternatively, through methylation by thiopurine methyl transferase (TPMT). Perturbations of these metabolic pathways can have significant clinical ramifications. The absence of HGPRT is thought to be one mechanism by which resistance to 6-MP is attained (128); however, increased activity of membrane-bound alkaline phosphatase may be of more importance clinically (129, 130).

Clinical: The bioavailability of oral 6-MP is poor. After oral dosing of 6-MP at 75 mg/

m², mean bioavailability was 16%, ranging from 5 to 37% (131). Simultaneous administration with food further decreases bioavailability (132, 133). The plasma half-life of 6-MP is approximately 1.5 hours (131). The major route of elimination of 6-MP is hepatic metabolism, and a hepatic first-pass effect is thought to contribute substantially to the poor oral bioavailability of the drug (131). Inhibition of the enzyme xanthine oxidase by allopurinol places patients at increased risk for significant 6-MP-associated toxicities (134, 135). Renal elimination is a minor route of elimination that may become significant with high-dose intravenous administration of 6-MP (134). Maintenance of remission in ALL in children has been associated with erythrocyte thioguanine nucleotide concentrations, with higher concentrations associated with more favorable outcomes (136). Low total plasma exposure of 6-MP has also been associated with an increased risk of relapse in children with ALL (137). High TPMT activity has also been correlated with an increased risk of relapse in pediatric ALL (138). Conversely, the constitutional absence of TPMT (a genetically polymorphic enzyme), an event that occurs in approximately 1 of every 300 persons, leads to excessive accumulation of 6-MP derivatives and is associated with extreme hematologic intolerance to 6-MP therapy. The dose of 6-MP in these patients must be significantly reduced (139, 140).

In light of the generally poor and variable oral bioavailability of 6-MP, coupled with the involvement of known highly variable enzymes in the metabolism of the drug, therapeutic drug monitoring and individualized dosing of 6-MP is suggested.

Indications: 6-MP has been used in combination-therapy regimens for remission induction and maintenance of remission of acute lymphoblastic leukemia in children. 6-MP has also been used in the treatment of chronic myelogenous leukemia.

Administration: 6-MP tablets are for oral administration. Sodium mercaptopurine for injection has been administered both intravenously and intrathecally (141–143).

Dosage: The usual oral 6-MP dose is 75 to 100 mg/m²/day. In the intravenous form, 6-MP has been administered at 50 mg/m²/hr by 48-hour continuous intravenous infusion (142). Intrathecally, 6-MP has been safely administered at a dose of 10 mg (143).

Drug Interactions: Allopurinol, an inhibitor of xanthine oxidase, interferes with the metabolism of oral 6-MP. The dose of 6-MP must be reduced by 50 to 75% when coadministered with allopurinol (144). In vitro data have suggested potential synergism, both schedule and sequence dependent, between 6-MP and methotrexate, and 6-MP and ara-C (145, 146).

Toxicity: The major toxicity of 6-MP is myelosuppression, primarily leukopenia and thrombocytopenia. Anorexia, nausea, and vomiting can occur and appear to be more common in adults (147). Hepatic dysfunction (mainly, reversible cholestatic jaundice) has been associated with 6-MP therapy (148). High-dose 6-MP therapy has been associated with acute hepatic necrosis (149).

6-Thioguanine (6-TG)

Nomenclature

Generic name: 6-Thioguanine, 2-Amino-1,7-dihydro-6H-purine-6-thiol, Thioguanine, 6-TG

Commercial name: Thioguanine Tabloid (Burroughs Wellcome)

Availability: 6-Thioguanine is available as 40-mg tablets for oral administration. The lyophilized sodium salt of 6-thioguanine for injection, in 75-mg vials, is available as an investigational agent.

Storage: 6-Thioguanine tablets should be stored at room temperature and protected from light.

Pharmacology

Cellular: 6-Thioguanine, like 6-MP, is a structural analogue of the naturally occurring purine guanine and is a purine antimetabolite. 6-Thioguanine is converted intracellularly to active 6-thioguanine nucleotides by the enzyme hypoxanthine-guanine phosphoribosyl transferase (HGPRT). The phosphorylated derivatives of 6-thioguanine are incorporated into DNA, inhibiting normal DNA replication (150). 6-Thioguanine also interferes with synthesis of RNA and can inhibit de novo purine synthesis (126, 151). A second mechanism of 6-thioguanine cytotoxicity, independent of activation by HGPRT, has been proposed based on observations of 6-thioguanine-induced growth arrest in cells deficient in

HGPRT (152–154). These studies provide evidence that cross-resistance between 6-MP and 6-thioguanine may not be complete. 6-Thioguanine is metabolized primarily by methylation via thiopurine methyl transferase. Unlike 6-MP, 6-thioguanine is not a substrate for xanthine oxidase.

Clinical: Oral absorption of 6-thioguanine is incomplete and highly variable (155, 156). As with 6-MP, food is thought to further decrease oral bioavailability (132). Peak plasma concentrations occur within 2 to 10 hours following an oral dose (156, 157). Estimates of the plasma half-life of 6-thioguanine range from 0.5 to 6 hours (158, 159). Renal elimination of 6-thioguanine and its metabolites accounts for 60 to 85% of bioavailable drug (155, 160). Unlike with 6-MP, oxidation of 6-thioguanine by xanthine oxidase is not a major metabolic pathway; thus, allopurinol does not affect 6-thioguanine metabolism.

Indications: 6-Thioguanine has demonstrated activity in induction and remission combination-therapy regimens for acute nonlymphocytic leukemia (161, 162). Activity has also been noted in chronic myelogenous leukemia (163). Recently, incorporation of 6-thioguanine in place of 6-MP into maintenance regimens for childhood ALL has been suggested on the basis of the more reliable accumulation of active intracellular metabolites (164). 6-Thioguanine has demonstrated little activity against a variety of solid tumors.

Administration: 6-Thioguanine tablets are for oral administration. Sodium thioguanine for injection has been administered both intravenously and intraperitoneally.

Dosage: The usual oral 6-thioguanine dose is 2 to 2.5 mg/kg/day, or approximately 75 mg/m²/day. Dose reduction may be necessary in patients with hepatic or renal dysfunction and can be titrated to hematologic tolerance. 6-Thioguanine does not require dose adjustment when administered with allopurinol. Intravenously, doses of up to 1000 mg/m² of 6-thioguanine have been administered (165). Intraperitoneal 6-thioguanine has been tolerated at doses up to 744 mg/m² (166).

Toxicity: The major toxicity of 6-thioguanine is myelosuppression, primarily leukopenia. GI toxicities are infrequent but can manifest as nausea, vomiting, and anorexia. Hepatotoxicity, although uncommon, can be severe. Fatal venoocclusive disease associated with 6-thioguanine therapy has been reported (167). Renal toxicity, in the form of elevated serum creatinine and crystalluria, has been described in patents receiving high-dose 6-thioguanine therapy (159).

Chlorodeoxyadenosine (2-CDA)

Nomenclature

Generic names: 2-Cladribine, 2-Chloro-6-amino-9-(2'-deoxy-β-D-erythropentofuranosyl)purine, 2-Chlorodeoxyadenosine, 2-Chloro-2'-deoxyadenosine, 2-Chloro-2'deoxy-β-D-adenosine
Commercial name: Leustatin

Availability: Cladribine is available in single-use vials containing 10 mg (1 mg/mL) of drug in sterile saline solution.

Storage: Cladribine solution should be stored under refrigeration and protected from light.

Preparation: Cladribine solution must be diluted for administration. Dilution in 0.9% sodium chloride for injection, USP, is recommended. Dilution in 5% dextrose results in increased degradation of the drug and is not advised.

Pharmacology

Cellular: Cladribine is a synthetic analogue of the naturally occurring purine deoxyadenosine. It differs by the substitution of a chlorine on the 2'-position of the adenosine ring. This substitution renders the compound resistant to deamination by adenosine deaminase (ADA) (168). Cladribine is readily taken up by cells, where it is phosphorylated by deoxycytidine kinase to predominantly the mono- and triphosphate forms (169). As with congenital adenosine deaminase deficiency, the accumulation of deoxynucleotide triphosphates mediates cellular toxicity (170). The mechanism of cladribine-induced cytotoxicity is thought to be multifactorial and includes inhibition of DNA synthesis and repair (171); inhibition of ribonucleotide reductase, resulting in disturbances of intracellular deoxynucleotide triphosphate pools (171, 172); incorporation into DNA (173); induction of DNA strand breaks (172, 174); and interference with the formation of nicotinamide adenine nucleotide (NAD) (174). Cellular sensitivity to cladribine is associated with a relatively high ratio of deoxycytidine kinase to deoxynucleotidase activity, which is characteristic of lymphocytes (173, 175). Cells sensitive to the effects of cladribine include resting and proliferating lymphocytes (173, 174), monocytes (176), and myeloid leukemia cells (169).

Clinical: Cladribine has a linear biphasic pharmacokinetic profile. Studies in both children and adults have demonstrated a relatively short α half-life of 3 to 35 minutes, followed by a more prolonged β half-life of 6 to 20 hours (177, 178). Cladribine is approximately 25% protein bound. The oral bioavailability of cladribine is approximately 50% of the administered dose (179) and is not affected by either food or omeprazole (180). Cladribine appears to be 100% bioavailable after subcutaneous administration (179). Cladribine enters the cerebral spinal fluid, with cerebrospinal fluid concentrations reaching 12 to 38% of the concurrent plasma concentrations during continuous intravenous infusions (177, 181). Renal elimination of cladribine accounts for approximately 50% of the dose (177).

Indications: Cladribine is active against a variety of lymphoid and some myeloid malignancies. Cladribine is indicated in the treatment of hairy-cell leukemia, in which complete response rates of greater than 80% after a single course of therapy have been reported (182–185). Cladribine is active in patients with hairy-cell leukemia who have failed treatment with pentostatin (182, 186, 187). Cladribine has also demonstrated promising activity in the treatment of both childhood and adult acute myelogenous leukemia (181, 188, 189). Patients with Waldenstrom's macroglobulinemia have been shown to respond well to cladribine therapy, with response rates approaching 80% (190–192), although activity in fludarabine-resistant disease is not as great (193). Cladribine has been shown to have activity against a variety of low-grade lymphoproliferative disorders and lymphomas (194–199), although, again, activity in fludarabine-resistant diseases is diminished (193, 200). Although clinical responses to cladribine therapy have been demonstrated for chronic myelogenous leukemia, they are not accompanied by cytogenetic response and are generally of short duration (201).

Administration: Cladribine is generally administered by continuous intravenous infusion for 5 to 7 days. Investigation is continuing into the feasibility of intermittent short infusions, subcutaneous infusions, and oral preparations of cladribine.

Dosage: Cladribine is usually dosed at 0.09 to 0.1 mg/kg/day by 7-day continuous infusion. In pediatric patients, a dose of 8.9 mg/m²/day for 5 days has been used.

Toxicity: The major toxicity of cladribine is myelosuppression, primarily neutropenia and lymphopenia. Thrombocytopenia and anemia may develop, particularly after repeated courses of therapy. Fever and infection are not uncommon in patients receiving cladribine (194, 200, 202). Neutropenia generally resolves within 3 weeks of therapy, but prolonged and cumulative lymphopenia, particularly suppression of CD4+ lymphocytes, has been observed (185, 190, 201, 203). Serious opportunistic infections associated with cladribine-induced immunosuppression have been reported (190, 195, 201).

Cladribine-associated toxicity to other organs, including the GI tract, liver, and kidneys, is uncommon. However, severe neurotoxicities, in the forms of transient blindness and sensory-motor peripheral neuropathy, have been reported (189, 202).

Pentostatin (dCF)
Nomenclature

Generic names: 2'-Deoxycofomycin, (R)-3-(2-Deoxy-β-D-erythropentofuranosyl)-3,6,7,8-tetrahydroamid-azo[4,5][d][1,3]diazepin-8-ol, Covidarabine

Commercial name: Nipent

Availability: The lyophilized powder of pentostatin is available in 10-mg vials.

Storage: Storage of the unreconstituted vials of pentostatin under refrigeration is recommended.

Preparation: The lyophilized powder of pentostatin, in 10-mg vials, is to be reconstituted with 5 mL sodium chloride for injection, USP. This solution is stable at room temperature for 72 hours. Further dilutions for patient administration, in either 0.9% sodium chloride solution or lactated Ringer's, are stable for 48 hours at room temperature. When diluted in 5% dextrose solution, pentostatin is stable for only 24 hours at room temperature. Under refrigeration, both the 0.9% sodium chloride solution and the 5% dextrose solution are stable for 4 days.

Pharmacology

Cellular: Pentostatin is a tightly binding, irreversible inhibitor of the enzyme adenosine deaminase (ADA) (204). Intracellularly, ADA deaminates adenosine and deoxyadenosine and thus controls the amount of adenosine or deoxyadenosine available for phosphorylation. By inhibiting ADA, pentostatin allows accumulation of deoxyadenosine triphosphate (205). Cells most susceptible to the effects of ADA inhibition are those with a relatively high activity ratio of deoxynucleoside kinases (phosphorylating enzymes) to 5'-nucleotidase (a dephosphorylating enzyme), such as is seen in T lymphocytes (168, 206). The exact mechanism by which cytotoxicity occurs is not well established and may well be a combination of the biochemical effects of the drug. Suspected mechanisms of cytotoxicity include accumulation of deoxyadenosine triphosphate leading to inhibition of the enzyme ribonucleotide reductase, incorporation of triphosphate derivatives of deoxycoformycin into DNA (207), and interference with NAD formation (174). Congenital adenosine deaminase deficiency, characterized by severe T-lymphocyte deficiency and impaired B-lymphocyte function (208), is associated with increased intracellular concentrations of deoxyadenosine triphosphate (209).

Clinical: Pentostatin displays a biphasic pharmacokinetic profile after intravenous administration. The short α half-life of approximately 10 minutes is followed by a more prolonged β half-life of approximately 5 to 6 hours (210). Renal elimination is the major route of clearance, with up to 50 to 90% of a dose excreted in the urine (210). Pentostatin protein binding is minimal. Dose reduction is necessary in patients with renal dysfunction, with attention to the fact that pentostatin itself is a nephrotoxic agent.

Indications: Pentostatin is active mainly in lymphoid malignancies, including hairy-cell leukemia (211–214), chronic lymphocytic leukemia (215, 216), T- and B- cell prolymphocytic leukemia (217, 218), and Sezary syndrome

(217). Pentostatin has demonstrated activity in patients with hairy-cell leukemia who have failed therapy with α-interferon and or splenectomy (213, 219).

Administration: Pentostatin is usually administered by short intravenous infusion, although it has been given by both bolus infusion and prolonged continuous intravenous infusions. Adequate hydration is suggested.

Dosage: The usual dose of pentostatin is 4 to 5 mg/m²/week for 3 weeks or 4 mg/m² every other week. Because pentostatin is primarily excreted by the kidneys, dosage reduction in patients with renal dysfunction is necessary.

Drug Interactions: Pentostatin may potentially increase the toxicity of the antimetabolites cytarabine and fludarabine. Significant cardiotoxicity has been reported with pentostatin in combination with high-dose cyclophosphamide (220).

Toxicity: The major toxicity of pentostatin at usual doses is myelosuppression, primarily neutropenia, lymphocytopenia, and thrombocytopenia. Recovery from pentostatin-induced lymphopenia may be prolonged and incomplete (221). Severe infections associated with pentostatin-induced lymphopenia can occur (222).

Pentostatin is nephrotoxic, and at high doses of pentostatin, acute renal failure is dose limiting. Preexisting renal dysfunction may predispose patients to pentostatin-induced renal failure, and therapy must be carefully evaluated in these patients. The renal toxic effects of pentostatin are cumulative.

Other major toxicities include dose-dependent lethargy and fatigue, nausea and vomiting, and dry skin. Keratoconjunctivitis has been described and responds to glucocorticoid eye drops (223). High-dose pentostatin therapy has been associated with hepatic enzyme elevations, pulmonary edema, and seizures.

Sugar-Modified Analogues
Cytarabine (Ara-C)
Nomenclature

Generic names: Cytosine arabinoside, NSC-63878, arabinosyl

Commercial names: Tarabine, Cytarabine, Cytosar-U (Upjohn)

Availability: Cytosine arabinoside is commercially available in 100-, 500-, 1000-, and 2000-mg vials.

Storage: Intact vials of ara-C are stored at room temperature or under refrigeration. Vials are stable at room temperature for at least 2 years from the date of manufacture. With reconstitution, ara-C appears stable for 8 days at room temperature and for 15 days if refrigerated; however, use of prepared solutions within 48 hours has been recommended. Ara-C at 20 to 80 mg/mL is stable for 28 days in infusion pumps.

Preparation: The 100-mg vial of ara-C is reconstituted with 5 mL of bacteriostatic water for a final concentration of 20 mg/mL, the 500-mg vial with 10 mL of bacteriostatic water for a final concentration of 50 mg/mL, the 1-g vial with 10 mL of bacteriostatic water for a final concentration of 100 mg/mL, and the 2-g vial with 20 mL of bacteriostatic water for a final concentration of 100 mg/mL. For subcutaneous use, reconstitute ara-C powder with sterile water or saline to a final concentration of 50 to 100 mg/mL. For intrathecal use, use either lactated Ringer's solution or 0.9% saline without preservative. For infusional therapy, solutions can be further diluted in any convenient volume of either dextrose 5% water or 0.9% saline.

Pharmacology

Cellular: Ara-C differs from the natural pyrimidine cytidine by the substitution of arabinose for the sugar moiety ribose. Entry of cyarabine into cells is mediated by a transport system used in the cellular uptake of nucleosides (224). Ara-C is sequentially phosphorylated to Ara-CTP by the action of deoxycytidine kinases (225). Ara-C decreases cellular levels of deoxycytidine by competition for the enzymes involved in the activation of cytidine. The formation of Ara-CTP and the lower cellular levels of deoxycytidine act in concert to inhibit DNA synthesis. DNA polymerase α is further inhibited following the incorporation of ara-CTP into DNA (225). The amount of ara-CTP incorporated into DNA has been correlated with cytotoxicity (226). Like other antimetabolites, ara-C is S-phase specific. Resistance to ara-C has been reported to be mediated by either impaired cellular uptake, decreased activation to ara-CTP, increased deactivation through deaminase activity, or increased intracellular dCTP pools. The relation of each of these mechanisms to resistance seen in human leukemia is not clear (227).

Clinical: Ara-C is poorly absorbed orally (20%) owing to its rapid deamination in the

GI tract (228). It is also rapidly deaminated in the blood stream, liver, and peripheral tissues, owing to the wide distribution of the enzyme cytidine deaminase. Cytidine deaminase converts ara-C to uracil arabinoside (ara-U), which is inactive. The half-life of ara-C has been reported to range from 2 to 11 hours (229). Ara-C appears to demonstrate biphasic elimination with an α half-life of 15 minutes thought to represent initial elimination by the liver. The β half-life is reported to range from 2 to 3 hours (230). Plasma levels of at least 0.01 to 0.15 μg/mL are needed for cytotoxic effects (230). These levels appear to be achievable with infusional regimens using doses of 100 to 200 mg/m^2. Cerebrospinal fluid levels are about 40% of plasma levels. High levels of ara-C in the cerebrospinal fluid and the long half-life of ara-C in the cerebrospinal fluid (2 to 11 hours) may result from the absence of cytidine deaminase in the cerebrospinal fluid (229). Rapid deamination in the blood stream and S-phase specificity make the use of a continuous infusional schedule the preferred method of administration.

Drug Interactions: Ara-C may decrease the cellular uptake of methotrexate. Methotrexate may decrease the intracellular activation of ara-C (231). Granulocyte-macrophage colony-stimulating factor (GM-CSF) may increase the incorporation of ara-C into human AML cells in vitro (232). Hydroxyurea may increase the effectiveness of ara-C through a decrease in intracellular deoxycytidine triphosphate levels (233).

Indications: Ara-C has been used in the treatment of acute nonlymphocytic leukemia (234), ALL (235), chronic lymphocytic leukemia (236), and meningeal leukemia (237). Ara-C has also been used in the treatment of non-Hodgkin's lymphoma (238), myelodysplastic syndrome (239), the 5q- syndrome (240), and meningeal carcinomatosis (241).

Administration: Ara-C has been given as an intravenous push, an intravenous infusion, a constant infusion, subcutaneously, intrathecally, and intraperitoneally. High-dose ara-C is usually given in 250 to 500 mL of dextrose 5% water or 0.9% saline over 1 to 3 hours.

Dosage: Constant infusional schedules of ara-C have used from 60 to 200 mg/m^2 of ara-C as a constant infusion for 5 to 10 days. Bolus schedules have used from 100 mg/m^2 intravenously or subcutaneously twice a day for 5 days every 28 days, 3 g/m^2 intravenously for 1 to 3 hours every 12 hours for 3 to 6 days, or 10 mg/m^2 subcutaneously every 12 hours for 15 to 21 days. Intrathecal administration of ara-C has used from 10 to 30 mg/m^2 intrathecally up to 3 times per week. When given intrathecally, ara-C has been combined with methotrexate and/or hydrocortisone.

Toxicity: Leukopenia and thrombocytopenia are common, with nadirs occurring in 5 to 7 days and recovery in 2 to 3 weeks. Nausea/vomiting, anorexia, diarrhea, metallic taste in the mouth, dysphasia, stomatitis, GI ulceration, pancreatitis, peritonitis, and cholestasis have all been reported. Transient skin erythema, alopecia, and hidradenitis are generally mild and self-limiting (242). Conjunctivitis and keratitis can be severe and are reduced with the use of prophylactic steroid eye drops (243). Mild elevations of transaminases and bilirubin and intrahepatic cholestasis have been reported. Neurologic side effects are more common with high-dose regimens and generally involve cerebellar dysfunction. With high-dose regimens, approximately 10% of patients experience severe cerebellar toxicity, which usually begins on the 5th day of treatment and lasts about 1 week. Cerebellar toxicity related to ara-C is not always reversible, and patients with severe toxicity are less likely to reverse completely. The risk factors for cerebellar toxicity include age above 40, creatinine level above 1.2 mg/100 mL, and hepatic dysfunction (244). Less common neurotoxicities include an expressive aphasia, neuropathies, parkinsonism, dizziness, and somnolence. Intrathecal administration may induce nausea/vomiting, fever, headache, meningeal signs, paresthesia, paraplegia, seizures, blindness, and encephalopathy. CNS toxicity may be related to accumulation of ara-CTP in the CNS. Rapid onset of pulmonary edema and cardiomegaly have been seen with high-dose regimens. Cardiomegaly, pericarditis, and thrombophlebitis have also been reported. Urinary retention can be seen. A flulike syndrome consisting of fever, arthralgia, myalgia, malaise, bone pain, and rhabdomyolysis has been reported.

Fludarabine (FAMP)
Nomenclature
Generic names: Fludarabine phosphate (NSC-312887), 2-Fluoroadenine arabinoside-5-phosphate, 2-Fluoro-ara-AM
Commercial name: Fludara (Berlex)

Availability: Fludarabine is commercially available as a lyophilized powder in 50-mg vials.

Storage: Unreconstituted vials should be stored in the refrigerator. The drug is reconstituted at a concentration of 1 mg/mL in dextrose 5% water or 0.9% saline. Fludarabine is stable for at least 16 days at room temperature. Reconstituted to a concentration of 0.04 mg/mL in dextrose 5% water or 0.9% saline, fludarabine is stable for at least 48 hours either at room temperature or refrigerated.

Preparation: The 50-mg vial is reconstituted with 2 mL of sterile water to a final concentration of 25 mg/mL. Further dilution is carried out with either 0.9% saline or dextrose 5% water to a final concentration of 0.04 to 1 mg/mL. Vials contain no preservative and should be used within 8 hours of preparation.

Pharmacology

   Cellular: The mechanism of action of fludarabine is similar to that of other nucleotide analogues such as ara-C (245). Fludarabine is rapidly dephosphorylated in serum to 2-fluoro-ara-A. 2-Fluoro-ara-A enters cells through a carrier-mediated transport process, where it is phosphorylated to the triphosphate (2-fluoro-ara-ATP) by deoxycytidine kinase and other kinases (246). The reduction in cellular DNA synthesis is proportional to the cellular concentration of 2-fluoro-ara-ATP (247). DNA synthesis is inhibited through the inhibition of both ribonucleotide reductase and DNA polymerase by 2-fluoro-ara-ATP.

   Clinical: Fludarabine is extensively bound to body tissues and is eliminated primarily by the kidneys (60%), with 24% of the total dose eliminated as 2-fluoro-ara-A. The α half-life of 2-fluoro-ara-AMP is less than 30 minutes (248). The half-lives reported for 2-fluoro-ara-A in plasma are an α of 40 minutes and a β of 10 hours (248). The half-life of intracellular 2-fluoro-ara-ATP is 15 hours. Fludarabine demonstrates a β half-life of 9 to 10 hours (248). The degree of fludarabine-associated neutropenia has been correlated with total exposure as expressed by plasma AUC (248).

Indications: Fludarabine has been used for the treatment of relapsed or refractory B-cell chronic lymphocytic lymphoma (249), low-grade non-Hodgkin's lymphoma (250), newly diagnosed chronic lymphocytic leukemia (251), mycosis fungoides (250), and Waldenstrom's macroglobulinemia (251).

Administration: Fludarabine is usually administered by intravenous infusion (in 50 to 100 mL dextrose 5% water or 0.9% saline) over 30 minutes or longer. Fludarabine may be given by continuous infusion following a loading dose (249).

Dosage: A 30% dosage reduction is recommended for patients with renal impairment (creatinine clearance < 70 mL/min, serum creatinine > 1.5). Fludarabine as a single agent is given as a 5-day treatment at 25 mg/m²/day every 4 weeks. When combined with chlorambucil (15 mg/m² day 1), fludarabine is given as 20 mg/m²/day for 5 days (252). A 5-day infusional schedule appears superior to once-a-week administration (251).

Toxicity: The degrees of leukopenia (primarily lymphocytes), granulocytopenia, and thrombocytopenia seen are dose related. Marrow toxicity may be cumulative, and hematologic toxicity is dose limiting. Patients with prior chemotherapy should therefore be treated cautiously with fludarabine. Fludarabine will decrease T-cell subsets and increase a patient's risk for opportunistic infections (253). Both nausea and vomiting are rare with prophylactic antiemetics. Anorexia, stomatitis, diarrhea, constipation, and abdominal cramps have been reported. Alopecia, rashes, and dermatitis are rare. Increases in SGOT (mild, transient) and cholestasis are also rare. Neurologic toxicity including somnolence, seizures, fatigue, and peripheral neuropathy is rare, while delayed demyelinating CNS toxicity is sometimes seen with higher doses. Dyspnea has been reported, as have hypotension and chest pain. Metabolic acidosis and lactic acidemia with rapid tumor lysis, muscle weakness, and fever have rarely been reported.

Ribonucleotide Reductase Inhibitors
Hydroxyurea
Nomenclature

   Generic names: Hydroxyurea (NSC-32065), Hydroxycarbamide

   Commercial names: Hydrea (Immunex), Litalir (Chemische Fabrik von Heyden)

Availability: Hydroxyurea is commercially available as 500-mg tablets from Immunex (Seattle, Washington).

Storage and Preparation: Tablets require no preparation and should be stored in a desiccated environment at room temperature until use.

Pharmacology

Cellular: Hydroxyurea diffuses passively into cells, where it is a potent inhibitor of ribonucleotide reductase, resulting in a fall in cellular levels of deoxyribonucleotides and an immediate inhibition of DNA synthesis. RNA and protein synthesis remain largely unaffected. Hydroxyurea may also damage DNA directly and may inhibit DNA repair. The cellular effects of hydroxyurea are reversible in vitro following removal of drug or by the addition of deoxynucleotides. Hydroxyurea is lethal to cells in S phase and is therefore cell-cycle specific. Increasing toxicity is seen with prolonged exposure. Hydroxyurea may hold cells at the G_1/S junction. This activity may be related to ornithine decarboxylase induction, which blocks polyamine synthesis (254).

Clinical: Oral administration of hydroxyurea results in peak plasma levels in 1 to 2 hours and peak cerebrospinal fluid levels in 3 hours. The serum half-life of hydroxyurea is approximately 5.5 hours. Approximately half of an oral dose of hydroxyurea is recovered unchanged in the urine over 12 hours, and half is metabolized in the liver to urea. Minimal amounts of hydroxyurea remain in the body 24 hours after administration. Intravenous administration of hydroxyurea has been investigated, and high plasma levels can be achieved (>2 mM) by either a 24-hour or a 48-hour infusion (255). Pharmacodynamic analysis has demonstrated a correlation between steady-state plasma levels and the degree of marrow suppression (256). Clinical investigations of hydroxyurea have been aided by the availability of sensitive assays for hydroxyurea in plasma (257).

Indications: Hydroxyurea has been used for a wide variety of tumors and indications, including melanoma, resistant CML (258), ovarian carcinoma, acute leukemia (259), prostate cancers, head and neck tumors (260), primary brain tumors, transitional cell carcinoma of the urinary bladder, renal cell carcinomas, leukocytosis and/or thrombocytosis (258), essential thrombocytemia, polycythemia vera, and hypereosinophilia (261). Hydroxyurea has also been used as a radiation sensitizer in the treatment of primary brain tumors (262), cervical cancer (263), and head and neck cancers (264). More recently, hydroxyurea has been used to induce increased fetal hemoglobin synthesis in sickle cell disease and β-thalassemia (265).

Administration: Hydroxyurea is administered orally. Capsules may be given either as a single daily dose or in divided daily doses, as dictated by patient tolerance. Capsules may also be opened and administered in juice or food to increase patient tolerance.

Drug Interaction: Hydroxyurea has been shown to increase the cytotoxicity of 5-FU when given after administration of 5-FU, perhaps resulting from the ability of hydroxyurea to lower deoxyuridine monophosphate pools (266). Hydroxyurea can theoretically influence the activity of a variety of anticancer agents, owing to its ubiquitous effect on cellular deoxyribonucleotide pools and its ability to inhibit repair of DNA damage caused by both anticancer drugs and irradiation (267).

Dosage: The usual starting dose for the control of hyperleukocytosis is 20 to 50 mg/kg given daily until the WBC is below 50,000/mm^3. Following a decrease in the white count, the dose of hydroxyurea is adjusted downward to maintain an acceptable WBC or to avoid unwanted side effects. Changes in the WBC may not be reflected immediately with changes in the daily dose of hydroxyurea and may require 3 to 4 days to be fully apparent. For continuous daily administration, a dose range of 20 to 30 mg/kg has been recommended. High-dose regimens using continuous intravenous infusional schedules have been reported, using dosages of up to 1 g/hr and achieving blood levels above 1 mM. The maximal tolerated dose of oral hydroxyurea has been reported to be 800 mg/m^2 every 4 hours and 3 mg/m^2/min for the 72-hour continuous intravenous infusion.

Side Effects and Toxicity: Hydroxyurea will cause a dose-related leukopenia with a median onset of 10 days (range, 6 to 16 days posttreatment). Anemia and thrombocytopenia are less common and generally occur following the onset of leukopenia. Increases in the mean red cell volume (MCV) may be dramatic and are unrelated to a deficiency of either folate or vitamin B_{12}. Acute leukemia has been reported to develop following the use of hydroxyurea for polycythemia vera and essential thrombocythemia (268) but is less common than with the alkylating agents. Nausea, diarrhea, constipation, and stomatitis may develop with long-term administration. The incidence of stomatitis may be increased with high-dose administration (269). Pulmonary infiltrates and cavitary lung lesions have developed following therapy with hydroxyurea (270). Acute aveolitis was reported in a patient treated for myeloproliferative syndrome (271). Hydroxyurea has been reported to cause lower leg ulcers (272) and skin and nail hyperpigmentation (273).

Use in Pregnancy: Hydroxyurea has been used successfully to treat pregnant patients with both primary thrombocythemia (274) and CML (275), without apparent damage to the child.

REFERENCES

1. Sirotnak FM, Goutas LJ, Mines LS. Extent of the requirement for folate transport by L1210 cells for growth and leukemogenesis in vivo. Cancer Res 1985; 45:4732–4734.

2. Chabner BA, Allegra CJ, Curt GA, et al. Polyglutamation of methotrexate. Is methotrexate a prodrug? J Clin Invest 1985;76:907–912.

3. Osborne MJ, Freeman M, Huennekens FM. Inhibition of dihydrofolate reductase by aminopterin and amethopterin. Proc Soc Exp Biol Med 1958;97:429–431.

4. Chabner BA, Collins JM, eds. Cancer chemotherapy: principles and practice. Philadelphia: JB Lippincott, 1990:110–153.

5. Sirotnak FM, Donsbach RC. The intracellular concentration dependence of antifolate inhibition of DNA synthesis in L1210 leukemia cells. Cancer Res 1974;34:3332–3340.

6. Matherly LH, Barlowe CK, Goldman ID. Antifolate polyglutamylation and competitive drug displacement at dihydrofolate reductase as important elements in leucovorin rescue in L1210 cells. Cancer Res 1986;46:588–593.

7. Matherly LH, Barlowe CK, Phillips VM, et al. The effects of 4-amino-antifolates on 5-formyltetrahydrofolate metabolism in L1210 cells. A biochemical basis for the selectivity of leucovorin rescue. J Biol Chem 1987;262:710–717.

8. Sirotnak FM, Moccio DM, Kelleher LE, et al. Relative frequency and kinetic properties of transport defective phenotypes among methotrexate-resistant L1210 clonal cell lines derived in vivo. Cancer Res 1981; 41:4447–4452.

9. Cowan KH, Jolivet J. A methotrexate resistant human breast cancer cell line with multiple defects, including diminished formation of methotrexate polyglutamates. J Biol Chem 1984;259:10793–10800.

10. Alt FW, Kellems RE, Bertino JR, et al. Selective multiplication of dihydrofolate reductase genes in methotrexate resistant variants of cultured murine cells. J Biol Chem 1978;253:1357–1370.

11. Melera PW, Lewis JA, Biedler JL, et al. Antifolate-resistant Chinese hamster cells. J Biol Chem 1980; 255:7024–7028.

12. Goldie JH, Krystal G, Hartley D, et al. A methotrexate insensitive variant of folate reductase present in two lines of methotrexate resistant L5178Y cells. Eur J Cancer 1980;16:1539–1546.

13. Flintoff WF, Essani K. Methotrexate-resistant Chinese hamster ovary cells contain a dihydrofolate reductase with an altered affinity for methotrexate. Biochemistry 1980;19:4321–4327.

14. Trent JM, Buick RN, Olson S, et al. Cytologic evidence for gene amplification in methotrexate resistant cells obtained from a patient with ovarian adenocarcinoma. J Clin Oncol 1984;2:8–15.

15. Carman MD, Schornagel JH, Rivest RS, et al. Resistance to methotrexate due to gene amplification in a patient with acute leukemia. J Clin Oncol 1984; 2:16–20.

16. Li WW, Lin JT, Tong WP, et al. Mechanisms of natural resistance to antifolates in human soft tissue sarcomas. Cancer Res 1992;52:1434–1438.

17. Lin JT, Tong WP, Trippett TM, et al. Basis for natural resistance to methotrexate in human acute nonlymphocytic leukemia. Leukemia Res 1991;15:1191–1196.

18. Chungi VS, Bourne DW, Dittert LW. Drug absorption VIII: kinetics of GI absorption of methotrexate. J Pharm Sci 1978;67:560–561.

19. Steele WH, Lawrence JR, Stuart JF, et al. The protein binding of methotrexate by the serum of normal subjects. Eur J Clin Pharmacol 1979;15:363–366.

20. Stoller RG, Jacobs SA, Drake JC, et al. Pharmacokinetics of high-dose methotrexate (NSC-740). Cancer Chemother Rep 1975;6:19–24.

21. Huffman DH, Wan SH, Azarnoff DL, et al. Pharmacokinetics of methotrexate. Clin Pharmacol Ther 1973;14:572–579.

22. Wan SH, Huffman DH, Azarnoff DL, et al. Effect of route of administration and effusions on methotrexate pharmacokinetics. Cancer Res 1974;34:3487–3491.

23. Bode U, Magrath IT, Bleyer WA, et al. Active transport of methotrexate from cerebrospinal fluid in humans. Cancer Res 1980;40:2184–2187.

24. Bertino JR. "Rescue" techniques in cancer chemotherapy: use of leucovorin and other rescue agents after methotrexate treatment. Semin Oncol 1977;4:203–216.

25. Dorr RT, Von Hoff DD, eds. Cancer chemotherapy handbook. 2nd ed. Norwalk: Appleton & Lange, 1994:692–705.

26. Breithaupt H, Kuenzlen E. Pharmacokinetics of methotrexate and 7-hydroxymethotrexate following infusions of high-dose methotrexate. Cancer Treat Rep 1982;66:1733–1741.

27. Erttmann R, Landbeck G. Effect of oral cholestyramine on the elimination of high-dose methotrexate. J Cancer Res Clin Oncol 1985;110:48–50.

28. Li MC, Hertz R, Spencer DB. Effect of methotrexate therapy upon choriocarcinoma and chorioadenoma. Proc Soc Exp Biol Med 1956;93:361–366.

29. Smith EB, Weed JC Jr, Tyrey L, et al. Treatment of nonmetastatic gestational trophoblastic disease: results of methotrexate alone versus methotrexate–folinic acid. Am J Obstet Gynecol 1982;144:88–92.

30. Aur RJ, Simone J, Hustu HO, et al. Central nervous system therapy and combination chemotherapy of childhood lymphocytic leukemia. Blood 1971; 37:272–281.

31. Fisher B, Redmond C, Dimitrov NV, et al. A randomized clinical trial evaluating sequential methotrexate and fluorouracil in the treatment of patients with node-negative breast cancer who have estrogen-receptor-negative tumors. N Engl J Med 1989;320:473–478.

32. Browman GP, Levine MN, Goodyear MD, et al. Methotrexate/fluorouracil scheduling influences nor-

mal tissue toxicity but not antitumor effects in patients with squamous cell head and neck cancer: results from a randomized trial. J Clin Oncol 1988;6:963–968.

33. Rizzoli V, Mangoni L, Caramatti C, et al. High-dose methotrexate-leucovorin rescue therapy: selected application in non-Hodgkin's lymphoma. Tumori 1985;71:155–158.

34. Link MP, Goorin AM, Miser AW, et al. The effect of adjuvant chemotherapy on relapse-free survival in patients with osteosarcoma of the extremity. N Engl J Med 1986;314:1600–1606.

35. Broder LE, Sridhar KS, Selawry OS, et al. A randomized clinical trial in bronchogenic small-cell carcinoma evaluating alternating maintenance therapy of vincristine, Adriamycin, procarbazine, and etoposide (VAPE) with cyclophosphamide, CCNU, and methotrexate (CCM) versus CCM maintenance alone in complete responders following VAPE induction and late intensification. Am J Clin Oncol (CCT) 1994;17:527–537.

36. Bannwarth B, Labat L, Moride Y, et al. Methotrexate in rheumatoid arthritis. An update. Drugs 1994; 47:25–50.

37. Lewis HM. Therapeutic progress. II: Treatment of psoriasis. J Clin Pharm Ther 1994;19:223–232.

38. Esterhay RJ Jr, Wiernik PH, Grove WR, et al. Moderate dose methotrexate, vincristine, asparaginase, and dexamethasone for treatment of adult acute lymphocytic leukemia. Blood 1982;59:334–345.

39. Sternberg CN, Yagoda A, Scher HI, et al. M-VAC (methotrexate, vinblastine, doxorubicin and cisplatin) for advanced transitional cell carcinoma of the urothelium. J Urol 1988;139:461–469.

40. Glass J, Gruber ML, Cher L, et al. Preirradiation methotrexate chemotherapy of primary central nervous system lymphoma: long-term outcome. J Neurosurg 1994;81:188–195.

41. Obasaju CK, Cowan RA, Wilkinson PM. Recurrent cervical cancer treated with cisplatin and methotrexate. Clin Oncol (R Coll Radiol) 1993;5:203–206.

42. Meta-analysis of randomized trials testing the biochemical modulation of fluorouracil by methotrexate in metastatic colorectal cancer. Advanced Colorectal Cancer Meta-Analysis Project. J Clin Oncol 1994; 12:960–969.

43. Bode U. Methotrexate as relapse therapy for rhabdomyosarcoma. Am J Pediatr Hematol Oncol 1986;8:70–72.

44. Blaney SM, Poplack DG, Godwin K, et al. Effect of body position on ventricular CSF methotrexate concentration following intralumbar administration. J Clin Oncol 1995;13:177–179.

45. Jakobson AM, Kreuger A, Mortimer O, et al. Cerebrospinal fluid exchange after intrathecal methotrexate overdose. A report of two cases. Acta Paediatr 1992;81:359–361.

46. Adamson PC, Balis FM, McCully CL, et al. Rescue of experimental intrathecal methotrexate overdose with carboxypeptidase-G2. J Clin Oncol 1991;9:670–674.

47. Jackson RC, Fry DW, Boritzki TJ, et al. Biochemical pharmacology of the lipophilic antifolate, trimetrexate. Adv Enzyme Regul 1984;22:187–206.

48. Marshall JL, DeLap RJ. Clinical pharmacokinetics and pharmacology of trimetrexate. Clin Pharmacokinet 1994;26:190–200.

49. Li XK, Kobayashi H, Holland JF, et al. Expression of dihydrofolate reductase and multidrug resistance genes in trimetrexate-resistant human leukemia cell lines. Leuk Res 1993;17:483–490.

50. Rogers P, Allegra CJ, Murphy RF, et al. Bioavailability of oral trimetrexate in patients with acquired immunodeficiency syndrome. Antimicrob Agents Chemother 1988;32:324–326.

51. Dorr RT, Von Hoff DD, eds. Cancer chemotherapy handbook. 2nd ed. Norwalk: Appleton & Lange, 1994:933–939.

52. Balis FM, Patel R, Luks E, et al. Pediatric phase I trial and pharmacokinetic study of trimetrexate. Cancer Res 1987;47:4973–4976.

53. Allegra CJ, Jenkins J, Weiss RB, et al. A phase I and pharmacokinetic study of trimetrexate using a 24-hour continuous-injection schedule. Invest New Drugs 1990;8:159–166.

54. Fanucchi MP, Walsh TD, Fleisher M, et al. Phase I and clinical pharmacology study of trimetrexate administered weekly for three weeks. Cancer Res 1987;47:3303–3308.

55. Bertino JR, Lin JT, Cashmore AR, et al. Clinical pharmacology and metabolism of trimetrexate. Semin Oncol 1988;15(2 Suppl 2):8–9.

56. Vogelzang NJ, Weissman LB, Herndon JE, et al. Trimetrexate in malignant mesothelioma: a Cancer and Leukemia Group B Phase II study. J Clin Oncol 1994; 12:1436–1442.

57. Conti JA, Kemeny N, Seiter K, et al. Trial of sequential trimetrexate, fluorouracil, and high-dose leucovorin in previously treated patients with gastrointestinal carcinoma. J Clin Oncol 1994;12:695–700.

58. Witte RS, Elson P, Khandakar J, et al. An Eastern Cooperative Oncology Group phase II trial of trimetrexate in the treatment of advanced urothelial carcinoma. Cancer 1994;73:688–691.

59. Gesme DH Jr, Jett JR, Schreffler DD, et al. A randomized phase II trial of amonafide or trimetrexate in patients with advanced non-small cell lung cancer. A trial of the North Central Cancer Treatment Group. Cancer 1993;71:2723–2726.

60. Falkson G, Ryan LM, Haller DG. Phase II trial for the evaluation of trimetrexate in patients with inoperable squamous carcinoma of the esophagus. Am J Clin Oncol (CCT) 1992;15:433–435.

61. Weiss GR, Liu PY, O'Sullivan J, et al. A randomized phase II trial of trimetrexate or didemnin B for the treatment of metastatic or recurrent squamous carcinoma of the uterine cervix: a Southwest Oncology Group trial. Gynecol Oncol 1992;45:303–306.

62. Witte RS, Elson P, Bryan GT, et al. Trimetrexate in advanced renal cell carcinoma. An ECOG phase II trial. Invest New Drugs 1992;10:51–54.

63. Scher HI, Curley T, Geller N, et al. Trimetrexate in prostatic cancer: preliminary observations on the use of prostate-specific antigen and acid phosphatase as a marker in measurable hormone-refractory disease. J Clin Oncol 1990;8:1830–1838.

64. Iscoe NA, Eisenhauer EA, Bodurtha AJ. Phase II study of trimetrexate in malignant melanoma: a National Cancer Institute of Canada Clinical Trials Group study. Invest New Drugs 1990;8:121–123.

65. Cairncross JG, Eisenhauer EA, Macdonald DR, et al. Phase II study of trimetrexate in recurrent anaplastic glioma. National Cancer Institute of Canada Clinical Trials Group Study. Can J Neurol Sci 1990; 17:21–23.

66. Sattler FR, Frame P, Davis R, et al. Trimetrexate

with leucovorin versus trimethoprim-sulfamethoxazole for moderate to severe episodes of *Pneumocystis carinii* pneumonia in patients with AIDS: a prospective, controlled multicenter investigation of the AIDS Clinical Trials Group protocol 029/031. J Infect Dis 1994; 170:165–172.

67. Grochow LB, Noe DA, Ettinger DS, et al. A phase I trial of trimetrexate glucuronate (NSC 352122) given every 3 weeks: clinical pharmacology and pharmacodynamics. Cancer Chemother Pharmacol 1989; 24:314–320.

68. Grochow LB, Noe DA, Dole GB, et al. Phase I trial of trimetrexate glucuronate on a five-day bolus schedule: clinical pharmacology and pharmacodynamics. J Natl Cancer Inst 1989;81:124–130.

69. Stewart JA, McCormack JJ, Tong W, et al. Phase I clinical and pharmacokinetic study of trimetrexate using a daily ×5 schedule. Cancer Res 1988;48:5029–5035.

70. Bishop JF, Raghavan D, Olver IN, et al. A phase I study of trimetrexate (NSC 352122) administered by 5-day continuous intravenous infusion. Cancer Chemother Pharmacol 1989;24:246–250.

71. Lin JT, Cashmore AR, Baker M, et al. Phase I studies with trimetrexate: clinical pharmacology, analytical methodology, and pharmacokinetics. Cancer Res 1987;47:609–616.

72. Eisenhauer EA, Zee BC, Pater JL, et al. Trimetrexate: predictors of severe or life-threatening toxic effects. J Natl Cancer Inst 1988;80:1318–1322.

73. Grem JL, Ellenberg SS, King SA, et al. Correlates of severe or life-threatening toxic effects from trimetrexate. J Natl Cancer Inst 1988;80:1313–1318.

74. Klubes P, Connelly K, Cerna I, et al. Effects of 5-fluorouracil on 5-fluorodeoxyuridine 5'-monophosphate and 2-deoxyuridine 5'monophosphate pools, and DNA synthesis in solid mouse L1210 and rat Walker 256 tumors. Cancer Res 1978;38:2325–2331.

75. Laskin JD, Evans MR, Slocum HK, et al. Basis for natural variation in sensitivity to 5-fluorouracil in mouse and human cells in culture. Cancer Res 1979; 39:383–390.

76. Evans RM, Laskin JD, Hakala MT. Assessment of growth limiting events caused by 5-fluorouracil in mouse cells and human cells in culture. Cancer Res 1979;39:383–390.

77. Spiegelman S, Sawyer R, Nayak R, et al. Improving the antitumor activity of 5-fluorouracil by increasing its incorporation into DNA via metabolic modulation. Proc Natl Acad Sci USA 1980;77:4966–4970.

78. Bapat AR, Zarow C, Danenberg PV. Human leukemic cells resistant to 5-fluoro-2'-deoxyuridine contain a thymidylate synthetase with lower affinity for nucleotides. J Biol Chem 1983;258:4130–4136.

79. Christophidis N, Vajda FJE, Lucas I, et al. Fluorouracil therapy in patients with carcinoma of the large bowel: a pharmacokinetic comparison of various rates and routes of administration. Clin Pharmacokinet 1978;3:330–336.

80. Clarkson B, O'Connor A, Winston L. The physiologic disposition of 5-fluorouracil and 5-fluoro-2'-deoxyuridine in man. Clin Pharmacol Ther 1964;5:581–610.

81. Ensminger WD, Rosowsky A, Raso V, et al. A clinical-pharmacological evaluation of hepatic arterial infusions of 5-fluoro-2'-deoxyuridine and 5-fluorouracil. Cancer Res 1978;38:3784–3792.

82. Sotos GA, Grogan L, Allegra CJ. Preclinical and clinical aspects of biomodulation of 5-fluorouracil. Cancer Treat Rev 1994;20:11–49.

83. Mini E, Trave F, Rustum YM, et al. Enhancement of the antitumor effects of 5-fluorouracil by folinic acid. Pharmacol Ther 1990;47:1–19.

84. Kemeny NE, Ahmed T, Michaelson RA, et al. Activity of sequential low dose methotrexate and 5-fluorouracil in advanced colorectal carcinoma: attempt at correlation with tissue and blood levels of phosphoribosylpyrophosphate. J Clin Oncol 1984;2:311–315.

85. Forman WB. The role of chemotherapy and adjuvant therapy in the management of colorectal cancer. Cancer 1994;74(7 Suppl):2151–2153.

86. Cameron DA, Gabra H, Leonard RC. Continuous 5-fluorouracil in the treatment of breast cancer. Br J Cancer 1994;70:120–124.

87. Krook JE, O'Connell MJ, Wieand HS, et al. A prospective, randomized evaluation of intensive-course 5-fluorouracil plus doxorubicin as surgical adjuvant chemotherapy for resected gastric cancer. Cancer 1991;67:2454–2458.

88. Tepper JE. Combined radiotherapy and chemotherapy in the treatment of gastrointestinal malignancies. Semin Oncol 1992;19(4 Suppl 11):96–101.

89. Logothetis CJ, Hossan E, Recondo G, et al. 5-Fluorouracil and interferon-alpha in chemotherapy refractory bladder carcinoma: an effective regimen. Anticancer Res 1994;14:1265–1269.

90. Rose PG. Locally advanced cervical carcinoma: the role of chemoradiation. Semin Oncol 1994;21:47–53.

91. Browman GP, Cripps C, Hodson DI, et al. Placebo-controlled randomized trial of infusional fluorouracil during standard radiotherapy in locally advanced head and neck cancer. J Clin Oncol 1994; 12:2648–2653.

92. Koh WJ, Wallace HJ, Greer BE, et al. Combined radiotherapy and chemotherapy in the management of local-regionally advanced vulvar cancer. Int J Radiat Oncol Biol Phys 1993;26:809–816.

93. Schilsky RL. Biochemical pharmacology of chemotherapeutic drugs used as: radiation enhancers. Semin Oncol 1992;19(4 Suppl 11):2–7.

94. de Takats PG, Kerr DJ, Poole CJ, et al. Hepatic arterial chemotherapy for metastatic colorectal carcinoma. Br J Cancer 1994;69:372–378.

95. Jansen GT. Topical chemotherapy. Clin Dermatol 1992;10:305–307.

96. Leichman CG. Prolonged infusion of fluorinated pyrimidines in gastrointestinal malignancies: a review of recent clinical trials. Cancer Invest 1994; 12:166–175.

97. Harris BE, Carpenter JT, Diasio RB. Severe 5-fluorouracil toxicity secondary to dihydropyrimidine dehydrogenase deficiency. A potentially more common pharmacogenetic syndrome. Cancer 1991;68:499–501.

98. Tuxen MK, Hansen SW. Neurotoxicity secondary to antineoplastic drugs. Cancer Treat Rev 1994; 20:191–214.

99. Anand AJ. Fluorouracil cardiotoxicity. Ann Pharmacother 1994;28:374–378.

100. Weiss RB. Hypersensitivity reactions. Semin Oncol 1992;19:458–477.

101. Lokich J, Anderson N, Bern M, et al. Combined floxuridine and cisplatin in a fourteen day infusion. Phase I study. Cancer 1988;62:2309–2312.

102. Keller JH, Ensminger WD. Stability of cancer chemotherapeutic agents in a totally implanted drug delivery system. Am J Hosp Pharm 1982;39:1321–1323.

103. Zhang ZG, Harstrick A, Rustum YM. Mechanisms of resistance to fluoropyrimidines. Semin Oncol 1992;19(2 Suppl 3):4–9.

104. Yin MB, Zakrzewski SF, Hakala MT. Relationship of cellular folate cofactor pools to the activity of 5-fluorouracil. Mol Pharmacol 1983;23:190–197.

105. Kemeny N, Daly J, Reichman B, et al. Intrahepatic or systemic infusion of fluorodeoxyuridine in patients with liver metastases from colorectal carcinoma. A randomized trial. Ann Intern Med 1987; 107:459–465.

106. Oberfield RA, McCaffrey JA, Polio J, et al. Prolonged and continuous percutaneous intra-arterial hepatic infusion chemotherapy in advanced metastatic liver adenocarcinoma from colorectal primary. Cancer 1979;44:414–423.

107. von Roemeling R, Rabatin JT, Fraley EE, et al. Progressive metastatic renal cell carcinoma controlled by continuous 5-fluoro-2-deoxyuridine infusion. J Urol 1988;139:259–262.

108. Anderson N, Lokich J, Bern M, et al. Combined 5-fluorouracil and floxuridine administered as a 14-day infusion. A phase I study. Cancer 1989;63:825–827.

109. Hohn DC, Stagg RJ, Price DC, et al. Avoidance of gastroduodenal toxicity in patients receiving hepatic arterial 5-fluoro-2'-deoxyuridine. J Clin Oncol 1985; 3:1257–1260.

110. Rougier P, Laplanche A, Huguier M, et al. Hepatic arterial infusion of floxuridine in patients with liver metastases from colorectal carcinoma: long-term results of a prospective randomized trial [see comments]. J Clin Oncol 1992;10:1112–1118.

111. Notari RE, DeYoung JL. Kinetics and mechanisms of degradation of the antileukemic agent 5-azacytidine in aqueous solutions. J Pharm Sci 1975; 64:1148–1157.

112. Cheung YW, Vishnuvajjala BR, Morris NL, et al. Stability of azacitidine in infusion fluids. Am J Hosp Pharm 1984;41:1156–1159.

113. Glover AB, Leyland-Jones B. Biochemistry of azacitidine: a review. Cancer Treat Rep 1987;71:959–964.

114. Friedman S. The inhibition of DNA(cytosine-5)methylases by 5-azacytidine. The effect of azacytosine-containing DNA. Mol Pharmacol 1981;19:314–320.

115. Taylor SM. 5-Aza-2'-deoxycytidine: cell differentiation and DNA methylation. Leukemia 1993;7 (Suppl 1):3–8.

116. Israili ZH, Vogler WR, Mingioli ES, et al. The disposition and pharmacokinetics in humans of 5-azacytidine administered intravenously as a bolus or by continuous infusion. Cancer Res 1976;36:1453–1461.

117. Pinto A, Zagonel V. 5-Aza-2'-deoxycytidine (decitabine) and 5-azacytidine in the treatment of acute myeloid leukemias and myelodysplastic syndromes: past, present and future trends. Leukemia 1993; 7(Suppl 1):51–60.

118. Glover AB, Leyland-Jones BR, Chun HG, et al.

Azacitidine: 10 years later. Cancer Treat Rep 1987; 71:737–746.

119. Bellet RE, Mastrangelo MJ, Engstrom PF, et al. Clinical trial with subcutaneously administered 5-azacytidine (NSC-102816). Cancer Chemother Rep 1974; 58:217–222.

120. Chitambar CR, Libnoch JA, Matthaeus WG, et al. Evaluation of continuous infusion low-dose 5-azacytidine in the treatment of myelodysplastic syndromes. Am J Hematol 1991;37:100–104.

121. Von Hoff DD, Slavik M, Muggia FM. 5-Azacytidine. A new anticancer drug with effectiveness in acute myelogenous leukemia. Ann Intern Med 1976; 85:237–245.

122. Goldsmith SM, Sherertz EF, Powell BL, et al. Cutaneous reactions to azacitidine (letter). Arch Dermatol 1991;127:1847–1848.

123. Ho M, Bear RA, Garvey MB. Symptomatic hypophosphatemia secondary to 5-azacytidine therapy of acute nonlymphocytic leukemia (letter). Cancer Treat Rep 1976;60:1400–1402.

124. Koeffler HP, Haskell CM. Rhabdomyolysis as a complication of 5-azacytidine. Cancer Treat Rep 1978;62:573–574.

125. Elion GB. Biochemistry and pharmacology of purine analogs. Fed Proc 1967;26:898–904.

126. Nelson JA, Carpenter JW, Rose LM, et al. Mechanisms of action of 6-thioguanine, 6-mercaptopurine and 8-azaguanine. Cancer Res 1975;35:2872–2878.

127. Skipper HE. On the mechanism of action of 6-mercaptopurine. Ann NY Acad Sci 1954;60:315–321.

128. Higuchi T, Nakamura T, Wakisaka G. Metabolism of 6-mercaptopurine in human leukemic cells. Cancer Res 1976;36:3779–3783.

129. Wolpert MK, Damle SP, Brown JE, et al. The role of phosphohydrolases in the mechanism of resistance of neoplastic cells to 6-thiopurines. Cancer Res 1971;31:1620–1626.

130. Scholar EM, Calabresi P. Increased activity of alkaline phosphatase in leukemic cells from patients resistant to thiopurines. Biochem Pharmacol 1979; 28:445–446.

131. Zimm S, Collins JM, Riccardi R, et al. Variable bioavailability of oral mercaptopurine. Is maintenance chemotherapy in acute lymphoblastic leukemia being optimally delivered? N Engl J Med 1983;308:1005–1009.

132. Burton NK, Barnett MJ, Aherne GW, et al. The effect of food on the oral administration of 6-mercaptopurine. Cancer Chemother Pharmacol 1986; 18:90–91.

133. Riccardi R, Balis FM, Ferrara P, et al. Influence of food intake on bioavailability of oral 6-mercaptopurine in children with acute lymphoblastic leukemia. Pediatr Hematol Oncol 1986;3:319–324.

134. Coffey JJ, White CA, Lesk AB, et al. Effect of allopurinol on the pharmacokinetics of 6 mercaptopurine in cancer patients. Cancer Res 1972;32:1283–1289.

135. Berns A, Rubenfeld S, Rymzo WT. Hazard of continuing allopurinol and thiopurine. N Engl J Med 1972;286:730–731.

136. Lilleyman JS, Lennard L. Mercaptopurine metabolism and risk of relapse in childhood lymphoblastic leukaemia. Lancet 1994;343:1188–1190.

137. Koren G, Ferrazini G, Sulh H, et al. Systemic

exposure to mercaptopurine as a prognostic factor in acute lymphocytic leukemia in children [see comments]. N Engl J Med 1990;323:17–21.

138. Klemetsdal B, Wist E, Aarbakke J. Gender difference in red blood cell thiopurine methyltransferase activity. Scand J Clin Lab Invest 1993;53:747–749.

139. Lennard L, Gibson BE, Nicole T, et al. Congenital thiopurine methyltransferase deficiency and 6-mercaptopurine toxicity during treatment for acute lymphoblastic leukaemia. Arch Dis Child 1993;69:577–579.

140. Evans WE, Horner M, Chu YQ, et al. Altered mercaptopurine metabolism, toxic effects, and dosage requirement in a thiopurine methyltransferase-deficient child with acute lymphocytic leukemia. J Pediatr 1991;119:985–989.

141. Pinkel D. Intravenous mercaptopurine: life begins at 40. J Clin Oncol 1993;11:1826–1831.

142. Adamson PC, Zimm S, Ragab AH, et al. A phase II trial of continuous-infusion 6-mercaptopurine for childhood leukemia. Cancer Chemother Pharmacol 1992;30:155–157.

143. Adamson PC, Balis FM, Arndt CA, et al. Intrathecal 6-mercaptopurine: preclinical pharmacology, phase I/II trial, and pharmacokinetic study. Cancer Res 1991;51:6079–6083.

144. Coffey JJ, White CA, Lesk AB, et al. Effect of allopurinol on the pharmacokinetics of 6-mercaptopurine (NSC 755) in cancer patients. Cancer Res 1972;32:1283–1289.

145. Bokkerink JP, De Abreu RA, Stet EH, et al. Cell-kinetics and biochemical pharmacology of methotrexate and 6-mercaptopurine in human malignant T-lymphoblasts. Klin Padiatr 1992;204:293–298.

146. Kano Y, Akutsu M, Kasahara T, et al. Schedule-dependent synergism and antagonism between methotrexate and 6-mercaptopurine in a human acute lymphoblastic cell line. Eur J Cancer 1991;27:1141–1145.

147. Burchenal JH, Ellison RR. Pyrimidine and purine antagonists. Clin Pharmacol Ther 1961;2:523–541.

148. Esterhay RJ Jr, Aisner J, Levi JA, et al. High-dose 6-mercaptopurine in advanced refractory cancer. Cancer Treat Rep 1978;62:1229–1231.

149. Einhorn M, Davidsohn I. Hepatotoxicity of 6-mercaptopurine. JAMA 1964;188:802–806.

150. Ling YH, Chan JY, Beattie KL, et al. Consequences of 6-thioguanine incorporation into DNA on polymerase, ligase, and endonuclease reactions. Mol Pharmacol 1992;42:802–807.

151. Grindey GB. Clinical pharmacology of the 6-thiopurines. Cancer Treat Rev 1979;6:19–25.

152. Morgan CJ, Chawdry RN, Smith AR, et al. 6-Thioguanine-induced growth arrest in 6-mercaptopurine-resistant human leukemia cells. Cancer Res 1994;54:5387–5393.

153. Ishiguro K, Schwartz EL, Sartorelli AC. Characterization of the metabolic forms of 6-thioguanine responsible for cytotoxicity and induction of differentiation of HL-60 acute promyelocytic leukemia cells. J Cell Physiol 1984;121:383–390.

154. Gusella JF, Housman D. Induction of erythroid differentiation in vitro by purines and purine analogues. Cell 1976;8:263–269.

155. LePage GA, Whitecar JP Jr. Pharmacology of 6-thioguanine in man. Cancer Res 1971;31:1627–1631.

156. Brox LW, Birkett L, Belch A. Clinical pharmacology of oral thioguanine in acute myelogenous leukemia. Cancer Chemother Pharmacol 1981;6:35–38.

157. Denes A, Presant C. 6-Thioguanine (TG). A phase I study of intermittant oral (p.o.) and intravenous (i.v.) therapy in solid tumors (ST) (abstract). Proc Am Assoc Cancer Res 1979;20:107.

158. Key NS, Kelly PM, Emerson PM, et al. Oesophageal varices associated with busulphan-thioguanine combination therapy for chronic myeloid leukaemia. Lancet 1987;2:1050–1052.

159. Konits PH, Egorin MJ, Van Echo DA, et al. Phase II evaluation and plasma pharmacokinetics of high-dose intravenous 6-thioguanine in patients with colorectal carcinoma. Cancer Chemother Pharmacol 1982;8:199–203.

160. Lu K, Benvenuto JA, Bodey GP, et al. Pharmacokinetics and metabolism of beta-2'-deoxythioguanosine and 6-thioguanine in man. Cancer Chemother Pharmacol 1982;8:119–123.

161. Gale RP. Advances in the treatment of acute myelogenous leukemia. N Engl J Med 1979;300:1189–1199.

162. Armitage JO, Burns CP. Maintenance of remission in adult acute nonmyeloblastic leukemia using intermittent courses of cytosine arabinoside (NSC-752). Cancer Treat Rep 1976;60:585–589.

163. Spiers AS, Galton DA, Kaur J, et al. Thioguanine as primary treatment for chronic granulocytic leukaemia. Lancet 1975;1:829–832.

164. Lennard L, Davies HA, Lilleyman JS. Is 6-thioguanine more appropriate than 6-mercaptopurine for children with acute lymphoblastic leukaemia? Br J Cancer 1993;68:186–190.

165. Edelstein MB, Crowley JJ, Valeriote FA, et al. A-phase II study of intravenous 6-thioguanine (NSC-752) in multiple myeloma. A Southwest Oncology Group study. Invest New Drugs 1990;8(Suppl 1):s83–86.

166. Zimm S, Cleary SM, Horton CN, et al. Phase I/pharmacokinetic study of thioguanine administered as a 48-hour continuous intraperitoneal infusion. J Clin Oncol 1988;6:696–700.

167. Griner PF, Elbadawi A, Packman CH. Veno-occlusive disease of the liver after chemotherapy of acute leukemia. Report of two cases. Ann Intern Med 1976;85:578–582.

168. Carson DA, Wasson DB, Kaye J, et al. Deoxycytidine kinase-mediated toxicity of deoxyadenosine analogs toward malignant human lymphoblasts in vitro and murine L1210 leukemia in vivo. Proc Natl Acad Sci USA 1980;77:6865–6869.

169. Avery TL, Rehg JE, Lumm WC, et al. Biochemical pharmacology of 2-chlorodeoxyadenosine in malignant human hematopoietic cell lines and therapeutic effects of 2-bromodeoxyadenosine in drug combinations in mice. Cancer Res 1989;49:4972–4978.

170. Mitchell BS, Mejisa E, Daddona PE, et al. Purinogenic immunodeficiency diseases: selective toxicity of deoxyribonucleosides for T cells. Proc Natl Acad Sci USA 1978;75:5011–5014.

171. Griffig J, Koob R, Blakley RL. Mechanisms of inhibition of DNA synthesis by 2-chlorodeoxyadenosine in human lymphoblastic cells. Cancer Res 1989;49(24 Pt 1):6923–6928.

172. Hirota Y, Yoshioka A, Tanaka S, et al. Imbalance of deoxyribonucleoside triphosphates, DNA double-strand breaks, and cell death caused by 2-chloro-

deoxyadenosine in mouse FM3A cells. Cancer Res 1989;49:915–919.

173. Carson DA, Wasson DB, Taetle R, et al. Specific toxicity of 2-chlorodeoxyadenosine toward resting and proliferating human lymphocytes. Blood 1983; 62:737–743.

174. Seto S, Carrera CJ, Kubota M, et al. Mechanism of deoxyadenosine and 2-chlorodeoxyadenosine toxicity to nondividing human lymphocytes. J Clin Invest 1985;75:377–383.

175. Kawasaki H, Carrera CJ, Piro LD, et al. Relationship of deoxycytidine kinase and cytoplasmic 5′-nucleotidase to the chemotherapeutic efficacy of 2-chlorodeoxyadenosine. Blood 1993;81:597–601.

176. Carrera CJ, Terai C, Lotz M, et al. Potent toxicity of 2-chlorodeoxyadenosine toward human monocytes in vitro and in vivo. A novel approach to immunosuppressive therapy. J Clin Invest 1990;86:1480–1488.

177. Kearns CM, Blakley RL, Santana VM, et al. Pharmacokinetics of cladribine (2-chlorodeoxyadenosine) in children with acute leukemia. Cancer Res 1994; 54:1235–1239.

178. Liliemark J, Juliusson G. On the pharmacokinetics of 2-chloro-2′-deoxyadenosine in humans. Cancer Res 1991;51:5570–5572.

179. Liliemark J, Albertioni F, Hassan M, et al. On the bioavailability of oral and subcutaneous 2-chloro-2′-deoxyadenosine in humans: alternative routes of administration [see comments]. J Clin Oncol 1992; 10:1514–1518.

180. Albertioni F, Juliusson G, Liliemark J. On the bioavailability of 2-chloro-2′-deoxyadenosine (CdA). The influence of food and omeprazole. Eur J Clin Pharmacol 1993;44:579–582.

181. Santana VM, Hurwitz CA, Blakley RL, et al. Complete hematologic remissions induced by 2-chlorodeoxyadenosine in children with newly diagnosed acute myeloid leukemia. Blood 1994;84:1237–1242.

182. Saven A, Piro LD. 2-Chlorodeoxyadenosine in the treatment of hairy cell leukemia and chronic lymphocytic leukemia. Leuk Lymph 1993;11(Suppl 2):109–114.

183. Lauria F, Benfenati D, Raspadori D, et al. High complete remission rate in hairy cell leukemia treated with 2-chlorodeoxyadenosine. Leuk Lymph 1993; 11:399–404.

184. Tallman MS, Hakimian D, Variakojis D, et al. A single cycle of 2-chlorodeoxyadenosine results in complete remission in the majority of patients with hairy cell leukemia. Blood 1992;80:2203–2209.

185. Estey EH, Kurzrock R, Kantarjian HM, et al. Treatment of hairy cell leukemia with 2-chlorodeoxyadenosine (2-CdA). Blood 1992;79:882–887.

186. Jehn U, Gawaz M, Grunewald R, et al. Successful treatment of patients with hairy cell leukemia (HCL) using a single cycle of 2-chloro-2′-deoxyadenosine (CdA). Anticancer Res 1993;13:1809–1814.

187. Saven A, Piro LD. Complete remissions in hairy cell leukemia with 2-chlorodeoxyadenosine after failure with 2′-deoxycoformycin [see comments]. Ann Intern Med 1993;119:278–283.

188. Santana VM, Mirro J Jr, Kearns C, et al. 2-Chlorodeoxyadenosine produces a high rate of complete hematologic remission in relapsed acute myeloid leukemia. J Clin Oncol 1992;10:364–370.

189. Vahdat L, Wong ET, Wile MJ, et al. Therapeutic and neurotoxic effects of 2-chlorodeoxyadenosine in adults with acute myeloid leukemia. Blood 1994; 84:3429–3434.

190. Dimopoulos MA, Kantarjian H, Weber D, et al. Primary therapy of Waldenstrom's macroglobulinemia with 2-chlorodeoxyadenosine. J Clin Oncol 1994; 12:2694–2698.

191. Dimopoulos MA, O'Brien S, Kantarjian H, et al. Treatment of Waldenstrom's macroglobulinemia with nucleoside analogues. Leuk Lymph 1993; 11(Suppl 2):105–108.

192. Dimopoulos MA, Kantarjian H, Estey E, et al. Treatment of Waldenstrom macroglobulinemia with 2-chlorodeoxyadenosine. Ann Intern Med 1993;118:195–198.

193. Dimopoulos MA, Weber DM, Kantarjian H, et al. 2-Chlorodeoxyadenosine therapy of patients with Waldenstrom macroglobulinemia previously treated with fludarabine. Ann Oncol 1994;5:288–289.

194. O'Brien S, Kurzrock R, Duvic M, et al. 2-Chlorodeoxyadenosine therapy in patients with T-cell lymphoproliferative disorders. Blood 1994;84:733–738.

195. Betticher DC, Fey MF, von Rohr A, et al. High incidence of infections after 2-chlorodeoxyadenosine (2-CDA) therapy in patients with malignant lymphomas and chronic and acute leukaemias. Ann Oncol 1994;5:57–64.

196. Hoffman M, Tallman MS, Hakimian D, et al. 2-Chlorodeoxyadenosine is an active salvage therapy in advanced indolent non-Hodgkin's lymphoma. J Clin Oncol 1994;12:788–792.

197. Juliusson G, Liliemark J. High complete remission rate from 2-chloro-2′-deoxyadenosine in previously treated patients with B-cell chronic lymphocytic leukemia: response predicted by rapid decrease of blood lymphocyte count. J Clin Oncol 1993;11:679–689.

198. Saven A, Carrera CJ, Carson DA, et al. 2-Chlorodeoxyadenosine: an active agent in the treatment of cutaneous T-cell lymphoma. Blood 1992;80:587–592.

199. Kay AC, Saven A, Carrera CJ, et al. 2-Chlorodeoxyadenosine treatment of low-grade lymphomas [see comments]. J Clin Oncol 1992;10:371–377.

200. O'Brien S, Kantarjian H, Estey E, et al. Lack of effect of 2-chlorodeoxyadenosine therapy in patients with chronic lymphocytic leukemia refractory to fludarabine therapy [see comments]. N Engl J Med 1994; 330:319–322.

201. Saven A, Piro LD, Lemon RH, et al. Complete hematologic remissions in chronic-phase, Philadelphia-chromosome-positive, chronic myelogenous leukemia after 2-chlorodeoxyadenosine. Cancer 1994; 73:2953–2963.

202. Kobayashi K, Vogelzang NJ, O'Brien SM, et al. A phase I study of intermittent infusion cladribine in patients with solid tumors. Cancer 1994;74:168–173.

203. Seymour JF, Kurzrock R, Freireich EJ, et al. 2-chlorodeoxyadenosine induces durable remissions and prolonged suppression of CD4+ lymphocyte counts in patients with hairy cell leukemia. Blood 1994;83:2906–2911.

204. Agarwal RP. Inhibitors of adenosine deaminase. Pharmacol Ther 1982;17:399–429.

205. Mitchell BS, Edwards NL, Koller CA. Deoxyribonucleoside triphosphate accumulation by leukemic cells. Blood 1983;62:419–424.

206. Wortmann RL, Mitchell BS, Edwards NL, et

al. Biochemical basis for differential deoxyadenosine toxicity to T and B lymphoblasts: role for 5′-nucleotidase. Proc Natl Acad Sci USA 1979;76:2434–2437.

207. Siaw MF, Coleman MS. In vitro metabolism of deoxycoformycin in human T lymphoblastoid cells. Phosphorylation of deoxycoformycin and incorporation into cellular DNA. J Biol Chem 1984;259:9426–9433.

208. Giblett ER, Anderson JE, Cohen F, et al. Adenosine-deaminase deficiency in two patients with severely impaired cellular immunity. Lancet 1972₁:1067–1069.

209. Cohen A, Hirschhorn R, Horowitz SD, et al. Deoxyadenosine triphosphate as a potentially toxic metabolite in adenosine deaminase deficiency. Proc Natl Acad Sci USA 1978;75:472–476.

210. Major PP, Agarwal RP, Kufe DW. Clinical pharmacology of deoxycoformycin. Blood 1981;58:91–96.

211. Spiers AS, Moore D, Cassileth PA, et al. Remissions in hairy-cell leukemia with pentostatin (2′-deoxycoformycin). N Engl J Med 1987;316:825–830.

212. Annino L, Ferrari A, Giona F, et al. Deoxycoformycin induces long-lasting remissions in hairy cell leukemia: clinical and biological results of two different regimens. Leuk Lymph 1994;14(Suppl 1):115–119.

213. Catovsky D, Matutes E, Talavera JG, et al. Long term results with 2′deoxycoformycin in hairy cell leukemia. Leuk Lymph 1994;14(Suppl 1):109–113.

214. Kraut EH, Grever MR, Bouroncle BA. Long-term follow-up of patients with hairy cell leukemia after treatment with 2′-deoxycoformycin. Blood 1994; 84:4061–4063.

215. Grever MR, Leiby JM, Kraut EH, et al. Low-dose deoxycoformycin in lymphoid malignancy. J Clin Oncol 1985;3:1196–1201.

216. Keating MJ, O'Brien S, Kantarjian H, et al. Nucleoside analogs in treatment of chronic lymphocytic leukemia. Leuk Lymph 1993;10(Suppl):139–145.

217. Mercieca J, Matutes E, Dearden C, et al. The role of pentostatin in the treatment of T-cell malignancies: analysis of response rate in 145 patients according to disease subtype. J Clin Oncol 1994;12:2588–2593.

218. Dohner H, Ho AD, Thaler J, et al. Pentostatin in prolymphocytic leukemia: phase II trial of the European Organization for Research and Treatment of Cancer Leukemia Cooperative Study Group. J Natl Cancer Inst 1993;85:658–662.

219. Golomb HM, Dodge R, Mick R, et al. Pentostatin treatment for hairy cell leukemia patients who failed initial therapy with recombinant alpha-interferon: a report of CALGB study 8515. Leukemia 1994; 8:2037–2040.

220. Gryn J, Gordon R, Bapat A, et al. Pentostatin increases the acute toxicity of high dose cyclophosphamide. Bone Marrow Transplant 1993;12:217–220.

221. Steis RG, Urba WJ, Kopp WC, et al. Kinetics of recovery of CD4+ T cells in peripheral blood of deoxycoformycin-treated patients. J Natl Cancer Inst 1991;83:1678–1679.

222. O'Dwyer PJ, Spiers AS, Marsoni S. Association of severe and fatal infections and treatment with pentostatin. Cancer Treat Rep 1986;70:1117–1120.

223. O'Dwyer PJ, Wagner B, Leyland-Jones B, et al. 2′-Deoxycoformycin (pentostatin) for lymphoid malignancies. Rational development of an active new drug. Ann Intern Med 1988;108:733–743.

224. Wiley JS, Jones SP, Sawyer WH, et al. Cytosine arabinoside influx and nucleoside transport sites in acute leukemia. J Clin Invest 1982;69:479–488.

225. Momparler RL. Kinetic and template studies with 1-β-D-arabinofuranosylcytosine 5′-triphosphate and mammalian deoxyribonucleic acid polymerase. Mol Pharmacol 1972;8:362–370.

226. Major PP, Egan EM, Beardsley GP, et al. Lethality of human myeloblasts correlates with the incorporation of arabinofuranosylcytosine into DNA. Proc Natl Acad Sci USA 1981;78:3235–3239.

227. Flasshove M, Strumberg D, Ayscue L, et al. Structural analysis of the deoxycytidine kinase gene in patients with acute myeloid leukemia and resistance to cytosine arabinoside. Leukemia 1994;8: 780–785.

228. Finklestein JZ, Scher J, Karon M. Pharmacologic studies of tritiated cytosine arabinoside (NSC-63878) in children. Cancer Chemother Rep 1970;54:35–39.

229. Chabner BA, Myers CE, Oliverio VT. Clinical pharmacology of anticancer drugs. Semin Oncol 1977; 4:165–191.

230. Ho DH, Frei E. Clinical pharmacology of 1-beta-*d*-arabinofuranosyl cytosine. Clin Pharmacol Ther 1971;12:944–954.

231. Tattersall MH, Harrap KR. Combination chemotherapy: the antagonism of methotrexate and cytosine arabinoside. Eur J Cancer 1973;9:229–232.

232. Karp JE, Burke PJ, Donehower RC. Effects of rhGM-CSF on intracellular ara-C pharmacology in vitro in acute myelocytic leukemia: comparability with drug-induced humoral stimulatory activity. Leukemia 1990;4:553–556.

233. Kobayashi K, Schilsky RL. Update on biochemical modulation of chemotherapeutic agents. Oncology 1993;7:99–106:109;110–114,117.

234. Mayer RJ, Davis RB, Schiffer CA, et al. Intensive postremission chemotherapy in adults with acute myeloid leukemia. Cancer and Leukemia Group B [see comments]. N Engl J Med 1994;331:896–903.

235. Suki S, Kantarjian H, Gandhi V, et al. Fludarabine and cytosine arabinoside in the treatment of refractory or relapsed acute lymphocytic leukemia. Cancer 1993;72:2155–2160.

236. Robertson LE, Hall R, Keating MJ, et al. High-dose cytosine arabinoside in chronic lymphocytic leukemia: a clinical and pharmacologic analysis. Leuk Lymph 1993;10:43–48.

237. Morra E, Lazzarino M, Brusamolino E, et al. The role of systemic high-dose cytarabine in the treatment of central nervous system leukemia. Clinical results in 46 patients. Cancer 1993;72:439–445.

238. Palmieri G, Morabito A, Rea A, et al. Cytosine arabinoside (ara-C) plus alpha-interferon (alpha IFN) determine prolonged complete remissions in patients with aggressive non-Hodgkin's lymphoma partially responsive to first-line doxorubicin-containing regimens. Br J Haematol 1994;88:421–423.

239. Aul C, Gattermann N. The role of low-dose chemotherapy in myelodysplastic syndromes. Leuk Res 1992;16:207–215.

240. Juneja HS, Jodhani M, Gardner FH, et al. Low-dose ARA-C consistently induces hematologic responses in the clinical 5q- syndrome. Am J Hematol 1994;46:338–342.

241. Nakagawa H, Murasawa A, Kubo S, et al. Di-

agnosis and treatment of patients with meningeal carcinomatosis. J Neurooncol 1992;13:81–89.

242. Bernstein EF, Spielvogel RL, Topolsky DL. Recurrent neutrophilic eccrine hidradenitis. Br J Dermatol 1992;127:529–533.

243. Friedland S, Loya N, Shapiro A. Handling punctate keratitis resulting from systemic cytarabine. Ann Ophthalmol 1993;25:290–291.

244. Baker WJ, Royer GL Jr, Weiss RB. Cytarabine and neurologic toxicity [see comments]. J Clin Oncol 1991;9:679–693.

245. Plunkett W, Gandhi V. Evolution of the arabinosides and the pharmacology of fludarabine. Drugs 1994;47(Suppl 6):30–38.

246. Brockman RW, Cheng YC, Schabel FM Jr, et al. Metabolism and chemotherapeutic activity of 9-beta-D-arabinofuranosyl-2-fluoroadenine against murine leukemia L1210 and evidence for its phosphorylation by deoxycytidine kinase. Cancer Res 1980; 40:3610–3615.

247. Danhauser L, Plunkett W, Keating M, et al. 9-beta-D-arabinofuranosyl-2-fluoroadenine 5'-monophosphate pharmacokinetics in plasma and tumor cells of patients with relapsed leukemia and lymphoma. Cancer Chemother Pharmacol 1986;18:145–152.

248. Hersh MR, Kuhn JG, Phillips JL, et al. Pharmacokinetic study of fludarabine phosphate (NSC 312887). Cancer Chemother Pharmacol 1986;17:277–280.

249. Puccio CA, Mittelman A, Lichtman SM, et al. A loading dose/continuous infusion schedule of fludarabine phosphate in chronic lymphocytic leukemia. J Clin Oncol 1991;9:1562–1569.

250. Redman JR, Cabanillas F, Velasquez WS, et al. Phase II trial of fludarabine phosphate in lymphoma: an effective new agent in low-grade lymphoma. J Clin Oncol 1992;10:790–794.

251. Keating MJ, O'Brien S, Robertson LE, et al. New initiatives with fludarabine monophosphate in hematologic malignancies. Semin Oncol 1993;20(5 Suppl 7):13–20.

252. Elias L, Stock-Novack D, Head DR, et al. A phase I trial of combination fludarabine monophosphate and chlorambucil in chronic lymphocytic leukemia: a Southwest Oncology Group study. Leukemia 1993;7:361–365.

253. Wijermans PW, Gerrits WB, Haak HL. Severe immunodeficiency in patients treated with fludarabine monophosphate. Eur J Haematol 1993;50:292–296.

254. Yarbro JW. Mechanism of action of hydroxyurea. Semin Oncol 1992;19(3 Suppl 9):1–10.

255. Blumenreich, Kellihan MJ, Joseph UG, et al. Long-term intravenous hydroxyurea infusions in patients with: advanced cancer. A phase I trial. Cancer 1993;71:2828–2832.

256. Smith DC, Vaughan WP, Gwilt PR, et al. A phase I trial of high-dose continuous-infusion hydroxyurea. Cancer Chemother Pharmacol 1993;33:139–143.

257. Havard J, Grygiel J, Sampson D. Determination by high-performance liquid chromatography of: hydroxyurea in human plasma. J Chromatogr 1992; 584:270–274.

258. Hehlmann R, Heimpel H, Hasford J, et al.

Randomized comparison of busulfan and hydroxyurea in chronic myelogenous leukemia: prolongation of survival by hydroxyurea: the German CML Study Group. Blood 1993;82:398–407.

259. Slapak CA, Desforges JF, Fogaren T, et al. Treatment of acute myeloid leukemia in the elderly with low-dose cytarabine, hydroxyurea, and calcitriol. Am J Hematol 1992;41:178–183.

260. Haraf DJ, Vokes EE, Weichselbaum RR, et al. Concomitant chemoradiotherapy with cisplatin, 5-fluorouracil and hydroxyurea in poor-prognosis head and neck cancer. Laryngoscope 1992;102:630–636.

261. Donehower RC. An overview of the clinical experience with hydroxyurea. Semin Oncol 1992;19(3 Suppl 9):11–19.

262. Levin VA. The place of hydroxyurea in the treatment of primary brain tumors. Semin Oncol 1992; 19(3 Suppl 9):34–39.

263. Stehman FB, Bondy BN, Thomas G, et al. Hydroxyurea versus misonidazole with radiation in cervical carcinoma: long-term follow-up of a Gynecologic Oncology Group trial. J Clin Oncol 1993;11:1523–1528.

264. Vokes EE, Haraf DJ, Panje WR, Schilsky RL, Weichselbaum RR. Hydroxyurea with concomitant radiotherapy for locally advanced head and neck cancer. Semin Oncol 1992;19(3 Suppl 9):53–58.

265. Hajjar FM, Pearson HA. Pharmacologic treatment of thalassemia intermedia with hydroxyurea. J Pediatr 1994;125:490–492.

266. Muggia FM, Moran RG. Treatment of colon cancer based on biochemical modulation of fluoropyrimidines by hydroxyurea. Semin Oncol 1992;19(3 Suppl 9):90–93.

267. Schilsky RL, Ratain MJ, Vokes EE, et al. Laboratory and clinical studies of biochemical modulation by hydroxyurea. Semin Oncol 1992;19(3 Suppl 9):84–89.

268. Weinfeld A, Swolin B, Westin J. Acute leukaemia after hydroxyurea therapy in polycythaemia vera and allied disorders: prospective study of efficacy and leukaemogenicity with therapeutic implications. Eur J Haematol 1994;52:134–139.

269. Brincker H, Christensen BE. Acute mucocutaneous toxicity following high-dose hydroxyurea. Cancer Chemother Pharmacol 1993;32:496–497.

270. Kavuru MS, Gadsden T, Lichtin A, et al. Hydroxyurea-induced acute interstitial lung disease. South Med J 1994;87:767–769.

271. Hennemann B, Bross KJ, Reichle A, et al. Acute alveolitis induced by hydroxyurea in a patient with myeloproliferative syndrome. Ann Hematol 1993; 67:133–134.

272. Nguyen TV, Margolis DJ. Hydroxyurea and lower leg ulcers. Cutis 1993;52:217–219.

273. Gropper CA, Don PC, Sadjadi MM. Nail and skin hyperpigmentation associated with hydroxyurea: therapy for polycythemia vera. Int J Dermatol 1993; 32:731–733.

274. Cinkotai KI, Wood P, Donnai P, et al. Pregnancy after treatment with hydroxyurea in a patient with primary thrombocythaemia and a history of recurrent abortion. J Clin Pathol 1994;47:769–770.

275. Jackson N, Shukri A, Ali K. Hydroxyurea treatment for chronic myeloid leukaemia during pregnancy. Br J Haematol 1993;85:203–204.

21

Antitumor Antibiotics and Related Compounds

Charles E. Riggs, Jr.

ANTITUMOR ANTIBIOTICS

Classical antitumor antibiotics all share the feature of being natural products of microbial metabolism. Most were initially isolated from fermentation broths of various *Streptomyces* species, based on observed cytotoxic activities present in crude extracts of microbial cultures. Efforts to improve the antiproliferative actions and to reduce the large-animal toxicities of the original antibiotics have employed chemical modifications of the naturally derived molecules, genetic manipulations of parent organisms to produce analogues, and directed syntheses of rationally engineered analogues. These have yielded a vast array of candidate compounds. Despite this, the venerable natural antibiotics (Table 21.1) remain the mainstays of clinical anticancer therapies, and their pharmacology and clinical roles are further explored in this chapter.

There is considerable structural diversity among the naturally occurring antitumor antibiotics, and yet there are remarkable similarities in mechanisms of action, effects on cellular intermediary metabolism, and spectra of toxicities (1, 2). A general scheme for understanding the intracellular actions and common features of these compounds is offered, followed by individual descriptions of each agent and its relevant analogues.

STRUCTURES

The variety of fungal organisms that are the sources of antitumor antibiotics gives rise to a broad array of chemical structures. The singular purpose of these chemicals is to afford the organisms a selective advantage in hostile environments, by interfering with the growth or proliferation of competing life forms (3). This property has brought these agents to attention as anticancer therapies, wherein the desire is to inhibit selectively the growth of the autonomously proliferating cancerous tissues, which differ, in many instances, only slightly from the normal host.

A wide spectrum of chemical entities has evolved to accomplish the task of arresting cell growth, including the polypeptides of bleomycin and of the side chains of dactinomycin (4) and the brightly colored chromophores of most of the antibiotics (Table 21.2). A common characteristic of these structures is the capacity to bind metal cations or to transport electrons, features that are associated with an ability to generate active oxidant species (5–7). Particular note can be made of the quinone group, which is vital for electron transport (8) and found in doxorubicin, daunorubicin, and mitomycin C (Table 21.2). However, these ring structures are also capable of other chemical interactions, including intercalation into or binding to DNA and RNA, membrane binding, receptor (and other protein) binding, enzyme inhibition (especially, DNA topoisomerase II), and alkylation (4).

The variety of chemical structures available in the naturally occurring antibiotics has also facilitated the development of analogues. Some analogues involve the deletion or substitution of part of the parent molecule to produce a drug with enhanced antitumor activity or less toxicity than the parent compound (8). Active derivatives of doxorubicin, daunorubicin, and mitomycin C have been synthesized by bonding acetyl, benzyl, phenyl, or lipid molecules onto the intact parent compound. The chemical (lipid solubility), pharmacologic (membrane, protein

Table 21.1. Sources of Antitumor Antibiotics

Generic Name	Other and Trade Names (Manufacturer)	Microbial Source (S. = Streptomyces)	Color of Aqueous Solution
Doxorubicin	Adriamycin (Adria)	S. peucetius, var. caesius	Red to orange
Daunorubicin	Cerubidine (Wyeth-Ayerst)	S. peucetius	Red to orange
Dactinomycin	Actinomycin D; Cosmegen (Merck)	S. parvulus	Yellow
Bleomycin	Blenoxane (Bristol)	S. verticillus	Clear to yellow
Mitomycin C	Mutamycin (Bristol)	S. caespitosus	Purple
Plicamycin	Mithramycin Mithracin (Miles)	S. plicatus	Yellow
Idarubicin	Idamycin (Adria)	Semisynthetic	Yellow
Mitoxantrone	Novantrone (Lederle)	Synthetic	Dark blue

Table 21.2. Structural Features of Antitumor Antibiotics

Structure	Action	Comment
Polycyclic chromophore	Intercalates into DNA	Gives antitumor antibiotics their characteristic colors May contain other groups
Quinone ring	Participates in electron transport reactions; the quinone is reduced in accepting an electron and can transfer the electron to other entities	Quinone functions as an electron acceptor from NADH or NADPH; requires enzymes and flavoproteins for activity
Polypeptide chains	Stabilize intercalated drug in the DNA helix	The chains of dactinomycin mainly stabilize; that of bleomycin intercalates into DNA via bithiazole rings
Aziridinyl ring	Opens under reducing conditions to yield active alkylating species	Appears to function best attached to a quinone or unsaturated ring
Microbial sugars	Serve to stabilize drug chromophores in DNA helix	May be charged at intracellular pH Hydrolytic or reductive cleavage of sugars results in antibiotic aglycone

binding), and, consequently, cytotoxic properties of some of the resulting analogues are sufficiently interesting that they have been tested in animal models of human cancer and in clinical trials. Of special note is the ability of some analogues to circumvent tumor-cell resistance to the parent compound, as a result of physical changes or pharmacologic differences conferred by the altered structure.

MECHANISMS OF ACTION

The wealth of structural diversity of the antibiotics makes it difficult to characterize a common mechanism of antineoplastic or antiproliferative action. For instance, doxorubicin has been reported to have at least seven different means of producing cellular dysfunction or death (8); which of these is the single most important in inducing clinical response in a particular case is usually not discernible. The following discussion attempts to indicate the most relevant biochemical actions for this class of drugs (Table 21.3).

The focal point for the cytotoxicities of antitumor antibiotics is DNA. By virtue of structure, antibiotics can intercalate in between base pairs of DNA (doxorubicin, daunorubicin, idarubicin, dactinomycin, bleomycin), bind to DNA (mitomycin C, plicamycin), and generate toxic oxygen free radicals, which cause single- or double-stranded DNA breaks (doxorubicin, daunorubi-

Table 21.3. Mechanisms of Action of Antitumor Antibiotics

Drug	Identified Mechanisms Producing Cytotoxicity
Doxorubicin	Intercalation into DNA and RNA
Daunorubicin	Inhibition of DNA, RNA polymerases
Idarubicin	Generation of oxygen free radicals
Mitoxantrone	Single- and double-strand DNA breaks
	Peroxidation of cell membrane and mitochondrial lipids
	Cell surface cytotoxic action
	Inhibition of glutathione synthesis
Dactinomycin	Intercalation into DNA (G-C base pairs)
	Inhibition of DNA-directed RNA synthesis (ribosoma RNA)
Bleomycin	Generation of oxygen free radicals
	Intercalation into DNA (bithiazoles)
	Single- and double-strand DNA breaks
Mitomycin C	Generation of oxygen free radicals
	Alkylation of DNA (guanine bases)
	Crosslinking of DNA strands
	Single-strand DNA breaks
Plicamycin	Binding to DNA (G-C base pairs); requires divalent cation (magnesium)
	Inhibition of RNA synthesis
	Single-strand DNA breaks
	Inhibition of adenosine deaminase

cin, idarubicin, bleomycin, mitomycin C). From this primary DNA damage come some of the numerous observed cytotoxic actions of these agents, such as inhibition of DNA-directed RNA synthesis, protein synthesis, and glutathione synthesis, defective mitoses, and high rates of mutation (4).

Structural features of the antibiotics confer specific characteristics to the DNA binding. Dactinomycin and plicamycin preferentially intercalate into guanine-cytosine base pairs of DNA (G-C specificity), so those domains of DNA enriched in G-C sequences will be most affected by these drugs (9). One mechanism of action of mitomycin C is alkylation of DNA (similar to that with nonclassic alkylators), and this reaction is specific for guanine bases (10). Bleomycin, a large polypeptide molecule, can intercalate only with its two sulfur-containing bithiazole rings (11). This probably requires an uncoiled length of DNA for proper positioning of the molecule.

The properties of plicamycin's structure are such that divalent cations, usually magnesium, are essential for binding to DNA (12).

Generation of oxygen free radicals has the potential for damaging a variety of necessary macromolecules—proteins, lipids, DNA, RNA—in target cells, and several antitumor antibiotics can transport free electrons to molecular oxygen (8). This property is a probable reason why fungal and other organisms developed the capacity to synthesize antibiotics, as a defense mechanism against invading bacteria and viruses. Electrons for these reactions are derived from intracellular reduced pyridine nucleotides (NADH, NADPH, and other minor sources) and are shuttled via the electron-transport chain enzymes and flavoproteins (13). The antibiotics probably function as intermediate electron acceptors and facilitate the transfer of free electrons directly to oxygen. The resultant activated oxygen species—superoxide anion, hydrogen peroxide, and hydroxyl radical—are extremely toxic to macromolecules, producing single- and double-stranded breaks in DNA (and possibly RNA), alterations of protein structure with consequent loss of function, and peroxidation of membrane and other cellular lipids (6).

The abilities of these compounds to intercalate into DNA give the advantage of bringing the toxic principles (free radicals) in proximity to one target of the radicals. Bachur et al. have shown that doxorubicin and daunorubicin can produce free radicals when incubated with nuclei from intact tumor cells (14), and similar actions probably occur with bleomycin and mitomycin C (15). A reasonable explanation for the similarities among the observed cytotoxic effects, spectra of anticancer activities, and clinical toxicities of these antitumor antibiotics is their dependence on particular base sequences and conformations of DNA for binding and on the presence of necessary enzyme systems for activation (8).

Lipids have become an important focus for research into the mechanisms of action of several of the antibiotics. Outer membranes of cells and of mitochondria, as well as those membranes comprising endoplasmic reticulum and Golgi apparatus, appear to be targets for antibiotic actions (16), and studies on the effects of these drugs on other cellular lipids are beginning. The microscopic events that can be observed in cells after exposure to antitumor antibiotics—cell swelling, mitochondrial swelling and deformation, and fragmentation of organelles—are the morphologic consequence of lipid peroxidation by free radicals (6). Lipids may also be employed to encapsulate anthracycline antibiotics (doxorubicin, daunorubicin, idarubicin) and other anticancer drugs, resulting in therapeutic agents different from the unencapsulated parent drug in both efficacy and toxicity (17). Experimental examples of both approaches in preclinical and clinical settings indicate that they are feasible, but whether more selective antitumor effects or better antitumor efficacy can regularly be achieved remains unknown.

Direct effects of anthracycline antibiotics and other agents on various cellular enzymes are increasingly recognized as important means of killing tumor cells or modulating cellular activities (18, 19). The most common specific targets for these antibiotics are DNA-modifying enzymes, such as topoisomerases and helicases.

These various mechanisms of action provide a rationale for understanding the modes by which tumor cells acquire resistance to antitumor antibiotics. Cells that repair DNA rapidly and efficiently will more readily resist and recover from antibiotic-induced damage (6). Experimental evidence exists for synergy between some of the antibiotics (19) and other agents that paralyze DNA repair (caffeine, etoposide) via interactions with DNA topoisomerase II. Cells that can express the glutathione-S-transferase genes seem to resist the toxicities of doxorubicin, mitomycin C, and daunorubicin (20). This resistance is based on the radical-detoxifying properties of reduced sulfhydryls, such as those of glutathione, cysteine, and others. Interactions among doxorubicin, cellular peroxisomes, and peroxide-generating enzymes can be responsible for cell death, by increasing the quantities of toxic hydrogen peroxide produced in target tumor cells (21).

Since drug action depends on the drug concentration at the site of action, tumor cells that can transport drug out of the cell will suffer less damage from binding and activation of the agent. A transmembrane protein, P-glycoprotein (gp-170), appears to function as an extrusion pump for a variety of xenobiotic compounds, including numerous anticancer drugs (22). Expression of the gene for this protein, the *mdr* gene, by tumor cells has been shown to correlate with resistance to these drugs (23). Since many chemotherapy-resistant tumors, such as colon carcinoma, sarcomas, and renal carcinoma, express the *mdr* gene before ever being exposed to antitumor antibiotics, it would seem logical to try to block the pump, to increase intracellular drug

concentrations (24). Studies of inhibitors of the gp-170 protein, which include such diverse agents as tricyclic antidepressants and calcium-channel blockers, are in progress (25–27).

COMMON TOXICITIES

Antitumor antibiotics interfere with growth and function of cycling cells, so that normal cells that are actively dividing, metabolically active, or deficient in certain intracellular defenses may be subject to toxicities (28). The clinical manifestations of toxicity common to two or more of the antibiotics are reflections of how ubiquitous the sensitive intracellular processes are. In this section, clinical toxicities that are shared by several of the antibiotics are discussed. Side effects peculiar to particular antibiotics are mentioned in the relevant sections.

The earliest cells of the bone marrow and tissues of the aerodigestive mucosa normally are rapidly dividing, with average cell-cycling times of 3 to 4 days. That compartment of cells—basal epithelial cells in the pharynx, esophagus, stomach, and intestine, and the normoblasts, myelocytes, and megakaryoblasts in the bone marrow—will be impaired or killed by drugs interfering with cell proliferation. Since it requires about 6 to 10 days for maturation of the cells in these tissues, the peripheral effects (oral or gastrointestinal ulcers, blood count suppression) will appear about 7 to 14 days after the chemotherapy insult, with recovery in 3 to 6 days. The acute and chronic effects of the antibiotics on the bone marrow and mucosa are frequently the dose-limiting toxicities of this class of agents (2).

Other acute effects (Table 21.4) include alopecia, nausea, vomiting, diarrhea, anorexia, and fever. Alopecia results from interference with protein synthesis in basal hair cells, so that weakened hair shafts are produced. Slight force suffices to break the shaft off at the scalp, giving the appearance of hair loss. The other effects indicated are consequences of the chemical and pharmacologic properties of the antibiotics on central nervous system and local receptors in the gut (29). As such, they are exquisitely dependent on the concentration of drug at the effector site, and modifications of dose and schedule of some antibiotics have been advocated as a means of avoiding undesirable toxicities. Thus, protracted infusions of doxorubicin, daunorubicin, or dactinomycin have been shown to be better tolerated than large single doses (30–32). Scalp cool-

Table 21.4. Common Toxicities of Antitumor Antibiotics

General Type of Toxicity	Antibiotics Producing This Toxicity[a]
Bone marrow suppression	DAUNO; DOX; DACT; IDA; MITO; NOVA; PLICA
Nausea, vomiting, anorexia	DAUNO; DOX; DACT; IDA; MITO; NOVA; PLICA
Stomatitis, alopecia	DAUNO; DOX; DACT; IDA; MITO; NOVA; BLEO
Extravasation necrosis	DAUNO; DOX; DACT; IDA; MITO; PLICA
Pulmonary	BLEO; MITO
Renal	MITO; PLICA
Hepatic	PLICA; DACT
Skin	BLEO; DACT; DAUNO; DOX; IDA
Microangiopathic hemolytic anemia	MITO; PLICA
Cardiac	DAUNO; DOX; IDA; MITO; NOVA
Fever	BLEO; DACT; PLICA

[a]Key: BLEO, bleomycin; DACT, dactinomycin; DAUNO, daunorubicin; DOX, doxorubicin; IDA, idarubicin; MITO, mitomycin C; NOVA, mitoxantrone; PLICA, plicamycin.

ing has been cited as a means of limiting hair loss by decreasing blood flow (and resultant drug delivery) to the hair cells, but the associated concern must be whether any tumor cells in the region also avoid exposure to effective concentrations of drug (33).

Extravasation injury, with inflammation, ulceration, and necrosis (34), remains a potential problem for several of the antibiotics (Table 21.4). The etiology of the injury is probably multifactorial, depending on the quantity of drug extravasated, the physical-chemical properties of the drug, the capacity of the tissue infiltrated to metabolize or to activate the drug, and the rate of clearance of the active irritants from the site of extravasation (35). Mitomycin C, plicamycin, dactinomycin, and anthracycline antibiotics are rapidly accumulated by cells, accounting for their severe local reactions (36). The first two of these are direct chemical toxins, while the enzyme systems needed to activate the latter three compounds are present in most tissues (8). The anthracyclines are the most fearsome vesicants, and this may relate to the documented persistence of these agents in subcutaneous tissues and local inflammatory cells at the extravasation site (37). This is believed to involve the release of active drug molecules from dying cells, reuptake by inflammatory (and other) cells in the vicinity, and death of these cells with rerelease of the drug molecules. A vicious cycle is perpetuated, as evidenced by the enlarging ulcers that characterize anthracycline extravasations and the documentation of measurable drug levels in biopsied ulcer tissues even weeks after the event.

Prevention of extravasation injury requires scrupulous attention to intravenous technique, employing central venous access whenever possible, prompt recognition of potential extravasation, and prompt institution of therapy. Use of subcutaneous ports and tunneled central venous catheters has lessened the likelihood of extravasation, but cracks in catheters or ports and leakage of high-concentration drug from the percutaneous access needle to a subcutaneous port must be continuously sought by close monitoring. Withdrawing whatever fluid will return from the subcutaneous site of a suspected extravasation is the best initial management, as this limits the quantity of drug available to produce injury. Cooling the area reduces metabolic activity and limits local diffusion of drug to surrounding tissues (38). Injection of thiosulfate, as is recommended as an antidote for alkylating agent extravasations, is not advised, since thiosulfate may activate the antibiotics (39). Injection of corticosteroids is advocated by some, but clinical trials of this have yielded inconsistent results. Painting the skin over the extravasated site with 50% DMSO (available commercially as a bladder irrigant) has been shown in experimental and clinical situations to offer the best protection against subsequent development of an ulcer (40). The DMSO should never be injected into the subcutaneous tissues, as experimental data have shown that this form of treatment produces more ulcers (41).

While no completely reliable predictors of whether an extravasation will result in an ulcer have been identified, the presence of pain in the site for more than 3 to 4 days is associated with higher rates of ulceration (34). For those patients in whom pain persists, prompt surgical evaluation for possible full-thickness resection and skin grafting of the defect should be considered (42). With attention to the timing of the procedures, the extravasated site can be surgically excised and grafted before any substantial myelosuppression occurs, so the patient will not face the hazard of an open ulcer or wound during a neutropenic episode.

Another cutaneous toxicity common to several antibiotics is the radiation recall phenomenon. As originally described, this reaction consisted of pain, erythema, and blistering or ulceration occurring geographically in a previous field of irradiation, within 3 to 7 days after injection of an antitumor antibiotic (43). The recovery from this insult was similar to that following severe radiation injury to skin. The drugs most commonly associated with this reaction are doxorubicin, daunorubicin, dactinomycin, and bleomycin. The best available therapy continues to be the same as that for severe radiation dermatitis—avoidance of infection, topical corticosteroids, and dressings as appropriate. Whether radiation therapy given concurrently with, or some time after, injection of an antitumor antibiotic can produce a similar "recall" phenomenon has not been well studied. Clinical trials of chemotherapy with or without simultaneous irradiation have not demonstrated rates of skin reactions higher than those expected with irradiation alone.

Chronic toxicities of chemotherapy with antitumor antibiotics include effects on lungs, kidney, liver, and heart. The essential early features of the chronic toxicities are edema, infiltration of the organs by inflammatory cells, and drop-out of normal cells. That these are identified as chronic toxicities indicates some sort of threshold dose or exposure of the normal tissues to the offending agents, but it must be constantly remembered that some patients can develop one of the "chronic" toxicities after even a single dose of drug. These toxicities are elaborated on further in the relevant sections on each drug.

CLINICAL ANTICANCER ACTIONS

Antitumor antibiotics are active against leukemias, lymphomas, sarcomas, carcinomas of most organs, and germ cell tumors. Doxorubicin is, without question, the single most active antibiotic in cancer therapy, both in terms of the number of different neoplasms that respond to it and in the number for which it can be curative (44). The disease in which each of the antibiotics is active are listed in the relevant sections.

Curative-intent therapy typically involves administration of the antitumor antibiotic as part of a multiagent chemotherapy regimen or of a multimodality program. In combination with other agents, doxorubicin can cure acute lymphocytic and nonlymphocytic leukemias, large cell lymphomas, limited small cell lung carcinoma, germ cell tumors of the ovary or testis, and certain childhood sarcomas (44). Doxorubicin is also active as part of adjuvant chemotherapy programs for sarcomas, breast cancer, and bladder carcinoma. Daunorubicin continues to be recognized as a necessary component of those chemotherapy regimens that are curative for adult and pediatric acute nonlymphocytic leukemia (45). In conjunction with 5-fluorouracil and radiation therapy, mitomycin C can be curative in treating squamous cell carcinoma of the anus, obviating the need for surgery in some cases (46). Bleomycin is a regular component of many curative-intent lymphoma protocols (47), often with doxorubicin. Dactinomycin remains a component of primary and adjuvant treatment protocols for acute lymphocytic leukemia and childhood sarcomas, especially Wilm's tumor (48). Until recognition of the remarkable activity of cisplatin in testicular cancer and other germ cell tumors, dactinomycin helped to effect cure in some patients with these diseases. Early data from therapy of patients with esophageal carcinoma suggest that use of mitomycin and bleomycin, in combination with cisplatin, vinca alkaloids, and radiation therapy, may be able to effect cure in a small percentage (46).

The palliative-intent roles of antitumor antibiotics are numerous and include single-agent, combination, and regional chemotherapies. These are mentioned in sections for each agent. In general, while major antineoplastic responses can be seen with such regimens, no clear-cut improvement in survival can be demonstrated. Therapy of chronic lymphocytic leukemia, small cell lymphomas, multiple myeloma and other dysproteinemias, metastatic or recurrent sarcomas, mesothelioma, recurrent germ cell tumors, carcinoid and islet-cell tumors, and advanced or metastatic carcinomas of bladder, breast, colon, esophagus, head and neck, liver, pancreas, prostate, stomach, thyroid, and uterus may result in clinically meaningful shrinkage of tumor and amelioration of symptoms. In selecting such a therapeutic approach, the potential toxicities of the agent(s) chosen should be carefully weighed against realistic clinical outcomes.

Regional chemotherapy—intrapleural, intrapericardial, intraperitoneal, intravesical, and intraarterial—has a major palliative role in relieving specific local symptoms, and may be part of curative-intent programs for ovarian (49) and superficial bladder carcinomas (46) and for isolated sarcomas (50). The pharmacokinetics of most of the antibiotics are such that regional therapy results in high local tissue concentrations of drug, with the advantages therefrom as mentioned in the preceding section. Thus, doxorubicin in ovarian and bladder carcinomas (44), doxorubicin or mitomycin C for superficial bladder cancer (46), or doxorubicin preoperatively in extremity sarcomas (50) have contributed to long-term freedom from disease or cure in appropriately selected patients. The roles of bleomycin in treating malignant effusions of the pleural, pericardial, and peritoneal spaces (51) and of mitomycin C intraperitoneally (46) are established as effective palliative maneuvers. Newer means for using these agents, alone and in combined-therapy or multimodality schemes, in approaching hepatic lesions, cerebral disease, and isolated lesions in other organs, remain the object of clinical-pharmacologic trials.

INDIVIDUAL ANTITUMOR ANTIBIOTICS

Doxorubicin (Adriamycin)

Although doxorubicin is the most recently discovered antitumor antibiotic in standard clinical use, its spectrum of activity and manageable toxicities give it the distinction of being the most commonly prescribed agent of this class in oncologic practice. Originally isolated from a variant of the fungus that produces daunorubicin (44), doxorubicin has been found as a component of fermentation broths of several microorganisms, and total chemical synthesis of the molecule is being attempted. Doxorubicin is composed of a brightly fluorescing, tetracyclic chromophore, adriamycinone, which gives the drug its characteristic red color, linked via a glycosidic bond to the aminosugar, daunosamine (Figure 21.1). The chemical reactivity of this structure has made doxorubicin an object of study by organic chemists, biochemists, and pharmacologists, in addition to its considerable role in cancer treatment.

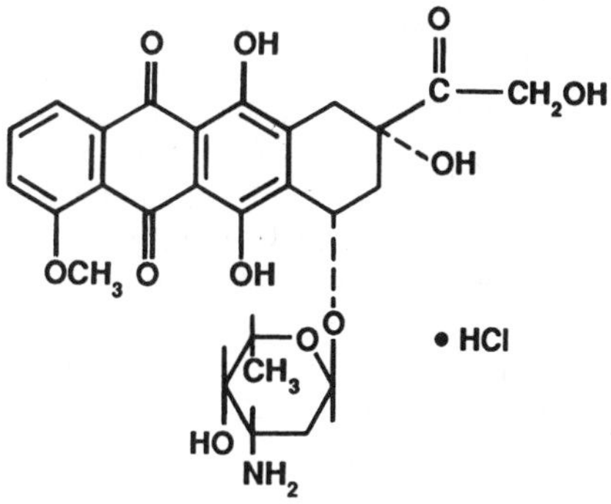

Doxorubicin

Figure 21.1.   Structure of doxorubicin. Note the quinone-semiquinone system (Table 21.2) in the central two rings of the chromophore, and the aminosugar, which is positively charged at intracellular pH. This positive charge may serve to stabilize the intercalated doxorubicin molecule, by electrostatic bonding to the phosphate groups of the DNA chain.

Doxorubicin can undergo three distinct chemical reactions in normal and cancer cells. Two of these involve interactions of the molecule with the cell's electron transport chain (52, 53), and the third is carbonyl reduction of the chromophore side chain (54, 55). This third reaction produces the alcohol metabolite of doxorubicin, doxorubicinol or adriamycinol, which has potent antiproliferative and antineoplastic actions, comparable to those of doxorubicin. The metabolism is catalyzed by a ubiquitous intracellular enzyme, daunorubicin reductase, and is dependent on the reduced cofactor, NADPH. Because adriamycinol is more polar than the parent drug molecule, it is less likely to traverse the cell membrane back to the extracellular space (56). This has given rise to the notion of "metabolic retention," by which the metabolism of doxorubicin makes it more likely to stay inside cells, increasing its cytotoxic effects.

The other two reactions begin with the transfer of a single electron to the quinone portion of the doxorubicin ring system (Table 21.2; Fig. 21.1), generating a free radical. In the presence of sufficient oxygen, doxorubicin can shuttle this electron to molecular oxygen, giving rise to superoxide anion radicals (57–59). These toxic intracellular radicals can be further converted to hydrogen peroxide and hydroxyl radicals, which can directly damage DNA, RNA, lipids, and proteins (16, 17, 21, 60, 61). In this process of shuttling electrons, the doxorubicin ring system is restored to its original state and can be available for additional redox cycling reactions. When oxygen concentrations are insufficient to allow the doxorubicin radical to transfer its unpaired electron, a molecule rearrangement can occur, producing a doxorubicin free radical that is hypothesized to be capable of directly damaging tissues (62, 63). The quinone system of adriamycinol can undergo the same redox cycling reactions, which probably contributes to its cytotoxic properties (64).

As suggested by the types of molecules doxorubicin radicals can damage, toxicity to nuclei, mitochondria, cytoplasmic structures, and cell membranes has been described as consequences of exposure of cells to doxorubicin (19, 63, 65–68). In 1972, Pigram demonstrated x-ray crystallographic evidence of doxorubicin intercalated in among DNA base pairs, with the aminosugar projecting into the minor groove of DNA (56). This could cause conformational changes in DNA structure, affecting the activities of DNA polymerase, DNA-directed RNA polymerase, and topoisomerases. Also, since nuclei have been shown to be able to metabolize doxorubicin to form free radicals (14), intercalation of doxorubicin into DNA may allow the site-specific formation of radicals toxic to DNA. Considerable argument remains as to which of these several possible doxorubicin reactions and interactions is primarily responsible for the remarkable cytotoxic activities of the drug, and much experimental work continues in this area.

Doxorubicin has a very broad spectrum of clinical anticancer activity and is one of the most frequently prescribed antineoplastic agents in therapy of human cancer. Definite activity (Table 21.5) has been reported in treating leukemias (acute lymphocytic, acute nonlymphocytic, and chronic lymphocytic), Hodgkin's disease, all subtypes of non-Hodgkin's lymphomas, multiple myeloma, osseous and nonosseous sarcomas, mesotheliomas, germ cell tumors of the ovary or testis, and carcinomas of the head and neck, thyroid, lung (both small cell and non-small-cell), breast, stomach, pancreas, liver, ovary, bladder, prostate, and uterus (44, 69). A variety of pediatric tumors are sensitive to it. However, antitumor activity appears to be lacking against malignant melanoma, primary malignant gliomas and astrocytomas, and carcinomas of the colon, small intestine, and esophagus. Curative potential exists for doxorubicin when it is included as part of multiagent and multimodality regimens against large cell non-Hodgkin's lymphomas, acute lymphocytic leukemia, testicular cancer, and a small percentage of small cell lung carcinomas and as part of adjuvant programs against breast cancers and sarcomas. Although doxorubicin-cytarabine combinations are active and potentially curative in therapy of acute nonlymphocytic leukemias, toxicities of doxorubicin, especially bowel mucositis with perforation, can be excessive (70). Most practitioners use daunorubicin in this setting, which offers the same complete remission rates with much less mucosal toxicity.

Clinical resistance of various cancers to doxorubicin has been the object of considerable laboratory (20–26) and clinical (26, 27) attention. Tsuruo et al. first reported collateral resistance to doxorubicin in mouse leukemia cells with induced resistance to vincristine (24). Numerous investigations have demonstrated the presence and genetics of a membrane glycoprotein, P-glycoprotein (gp-170), which functions as a drug-transport carrier to mediate efflux of doxorubicin from normal and tumor cells (22). A specific multidrug resistance gene, mdr, has been isolated, and its presence and specific activity in induced cells can be monitored. Its gene product, P-glycoprotein, appears to be inhibited by a variety of xenobiotic agents, including verapamil (and other calcium-channel blockers), tricyclic antidepressants, cyclosporine, and tamoxifen (22, 23, 27), and monoclonal antibodies directed at P-glycoprotein can also affect its inhibition (23). Despite promising basic research, clinical results in blocking P-glycoprotein activity and restoring sensitivity of resistant tumor cells to doxorubicin have been disappointing (23, 26, 27), and no practical, reliable clinical intervention can be presently recommended. Analogues of doxorubicin may be able to circumvent the multidrug transporter (20, 25), a notion which will be the object of clinical trials. Other patterns of resistance to doxorubicin involve alterations in (a) binding affinity to DNA topoisomerase II (19, 20), with decreased binding of doxorubicin to the enzyme complex; (b) cellular glutathione activity (20, 21), with amplification of glutathione-generating capacities in resistant cells; and (c) abilities of resistant cells to detoxify activated oxygen species (21), primarily hydrogen peroxide and hydroxyl radical.

For systemic therapy, doxorubicin must be administered intravenously. It is a chemical vesicant if extravasated. There are numerous dosage and schedule recommendations (69). Schedules most commonly encountered include intermit-

Table 21.5. Clinical and Pharmacologic Data for Doxorubicin

Molecular weight: 543.54
Plasma half-life: 16–24 hours (prolonged with hepatic dysfunction)
Total body clearance: 15–30 L/hr/m^2 (40–50% hepatic; 5–10% renal)

Diseases treated

Curative intent:	Acute lymphocytic leukemia
	Acute nonlymphocytic leukemia
	Non-Hodgkin's lymphomas (large cell)
	Hodgkin's disease
	Breast carcinoma (adjuvant only)
	Small cell lung carcinoma (limited stage)
	Osteogenic sarcoma (adjuvant only)
	Soft tissue sarcoma (adjuvant only)
	Germ cell tumors of testis, ovary
Palliative intent:	Relapsed leukemias—acute lymphocytic and nonlymphocytic types
	Chronic lymphocytic leukemia
	Multiple myeloma
	Non-Hodgkin's lymphomas (small-cell types)
	Metastatic/recurrent osteogenic and soft tissue sarcomas
	Malignant mesothelioma
	Carcinoid, islet-cell tumors
	Carcinomas of bladder, breast, head and neck, liver, lung, ovary (advanced), pancreas, prostate, stomach, thyroid, testis (recurrent), uterus

Toxicities

Acute	Bone marrow suppression
	Mucositis, stomatitis
	Alopecia
	Nausea, vomiting, anorexia
	Flushing of face, torso
	Vein itching
Chronic	Congestive cardiomyopathy
	Vein streaking
Special concerns	Radiation-recall dermatitis
	Extravasation necrosis of skin, subcutaneous tissue
	Reduce dose 50–75% in face of impaired liver function

tent intravenous injections given every 3 to 4 weeks (45 to 90 mg/m^2 per dose), divided doses given daily for 2 to 3 days during each course of therapy (25 to 40 mg/m^2 per dose), weekly single doses (15 to 30 mg/m^2 per dose), and continuous intravenous infusions lasting 72 to 144 hours (9 to 20 mg/m^2 per day). Of these, the intermittent bolus intravenous injections or 96-hour continuous infusions are usually employed, with selection of the schedule based on patient convenience, disease responsiveness, concomitant medications, and limiting toxicities (30).

Two routes of administration that have enjoyed more exposure in recent reports are intravesical and intraarterial doxorubicin. For superficial bladder cancer, intravesical doxorubicin

has induced long-term remissions in adjuvant treatment of primary and recurrent disease, with manageable toxicities (69). The doses have ranged from 50 to 90 mg every 3 weeks, for 4 to 8 cycles of therapy. Side effects have included dysuria, hematuria, bladder spasms, and frank cytitis, but discontinuation of therapy for these has been reported to be uncommon. Intraarterial doxorubicin has been employed in preoperative and radiotherapy-adjuvant settings for bone and soft tissue sarcomas (50, 69) and in therapy of advanced hepatic neoplasms (69). In the latter instance, the pharmacologic advantage for hepatic doxorubicin was calculated to be low, and the expense and morbidity of this mode of delivery were not offset by any definite improvement in response rates or durations. With sarcomas, adjuvant intraarterial doxorubicin has been an integral part of multimodality combined therapies, and cures of these aggressive neoplasms has been linked to this form of delivery. The initial response of an infused extremity sarcoma, as assessed by the degree of doxorubicin-induced necrosis, has been shown to correlate with the duration of disease-free and overall survivals and be directly linked to cure rates (69)

About 40 to 50% of doxorubicin and its active metabolites are excreted primarily in bile, and 5 to 10% in urine (71, 72). Most of the drug excreted during the first 24 to 48 hours after injection appears as doxorubicin or doxorubicinol, while after 48 hours, the principal species are sulfates and glucuronides of the doxorubicin aglycone. Individuals who have renal insufficiency may be treated at full dosages of doxorubicin, as compensatory increase in biliary elimination can prevent accumulation of active drug (73). However, in patients with impaired liver function, the dosage of doxorubicin must be decreased to prevent severe or fatal drug toxicities. Although the guidelines for dosage reduction vary, the following maximum dosages, based on levels of serum bilirubin and transaminases, can be recommended (74):

Bilirubin (mg/dL)	Transaminases (ALT or AST)	Maximum doxorubicin dosage (mg/m^2)
<2.0	>2–3 × normal	45–50
2.0–3.0	Any	30–40
>3.0	Any	15–20

Dosage escalations in patients with hepatic dysfunction should be considered in the event of improvement in measured liver function parameters or if there is no excessive mucositis or myelosuppression at the reduced dosage (75, 76).

Three general types of toxicities are recognized for doxorubicin—acute, chronic, and local (Table 21.5). The potential for the acute toxicities of nausea, vomiting, blood count suppression, and mucositis or stomatitis is the same as that for most antibiotics, as noted above, and these are typically dose limiting. Alopecia occurs in more than half of the patients receiving standard intermittent doses (44). The particular dose received per injection appears to play some role in whether alopecia complicates doxorubicin therapy, with lower, more frequent doses less likely to cause alopecia (33). There was a flurry of reports that scalp cooling could prevent alopecia

from doxorubicin (and other agents), but the protection afforded by scalp hypothermia seemed to be more a function of the dose per injection, the schedule of doxorubicin, and concomitant therapy than of the local remedy (33). There remains the additional concern that if the hair follicle survives a doxorubicin insult, then any focus of metastatic cancer in the scalp may be able to do likewise.

Facial flushing may occur and rarely be quite severe. The postulated mechanism is doxorubicin-induced histamine release (77), which has been shown to occur in animal models. Peripheral vein injections can be complicated by acute pain or itching locally. Controlling the rate of injection appears to be the best remedy for this, although some have advocated premedicating susceptible patients with antihistamines.

Congestive cardiomyopathy is a chronic toxicity of doxorubicin that has achieved much attention (78, 79) and generates much appropriate worry when patients have received large cumulative dosages. Acutely, doxorubicin (and daunorubicin) may produce atrial and ventricular dysrhythmias (80), which are ordinarily of little clinical significance in the absence of underlying heart disease. The clinical and pathologic pictures of chronic doxorubicin cardiomyopathy are those of cardiac dilation, biventricular heart failure refractory to usual management techniques, and primary myocyte damage and loss (82–85). Initial work in this area demonstrated an incidence of clinical cardiomyopathy of 10% at a cumulative doxorubicin dosage of 550 mg/m^2, with a sharp increase in the incidence curve at progressively higher dosages (78). Further experience has revealed that (a) the probability of clinical congestive heart failure is never zero with any dose of doxorubicin, with some patients developing this complication after a single dose (84); (b) there are definite risk factors to the earlier appearance of cardiotoxicity, including advanced age, history of uncontrolled hypertension or previous underlying congestive heart disease, mediastinal irradiation, and concomitant use of certain medications (78, 79); (c) altered schedules of doxorubicin delivery, including weekly and prolonged continuous infusion regimens, are less likely to produce congestive cardiomyopathy at any given dosage (30, 85–87), which is hypothesized to be due to the lower peak doxorubicin blood concentrations associated with such schedules (88); (d) there are no reliable predictive clinical tests for screening populations who might be at risk for cardiac damage with any particular dose of doxorubicin (89–92); and (e) there are no reliable antidotes to prevent or to reverse the cardiac injury (93–95). Recently, the U.S. Food and Drug Administration approved the use of Zinecard (dexrazoxane; ICRF-187) to prevent doxorubicin cardiac damage (96), based on results obtained from a sarcoma trial. In this study, dexrazoxane was coadministered with bolus-injection doxorubicin in study patients; compared with control patients, reductions in cardiac ejection fraction were lower in the study patients. However, the overall incidence of congestive heart failure was low in the entire study, and the significance of moderating any declines in cardiac ejection fractions on overall cardiac function and survival could be questioned. The recommendations that most clinicians follow are to limit the cumulative dosage of doxorubicin to 550 mg/m^2 with intermittent schedules or to 800 mg/m^2 with weekly or continuous infusion schedules (78, 79, 87); to perform the best-available screening—radionuclide ventriculography or endomyocardial biopsy—in those at high risk or whose therapy dictates exceeding the recommended cumulative dosage limits (81, 89); and to weigh carefully the need for each dose of doxorubicin in patients deemed at high risk for development of heart failure. Dexrazoxane is an attractive option to consider in those who might be felt to be at higher risk of cardiac decompensation initially, but it should be recognized that clinical trials in that specific population have not been reported.

The best hopes for new antidotes and approaches to these vexing problems likely reside in continuation of ongoing investigations into the basic mechanisms of the interactions of doxorubicin with cellular components. For instance, mitochondria are targets of anthracycline cardiotoxic effects (97), and the damage induced may be able to be blocked by free-radical scavengers or other compounds. Iron loading appears to play a role in experimental doxorubicin cardiotoxicity (98), and strategies for evaluating this in humans, or use of chelating therapies, may decrease the potential for damage.

Two local toxicities of doxorubicin with potentially devastating consequences are extravasation skin injury (necrosis) and the radiation recall reaction (30, 34, 36, 43, 99–102). These should ever be in mind when any doxorubicin dose is administered, with appropriate precautions taken to minimize the possibility of their occurrence. The potential for doxorubicin extravasa-

tions has increased, with increasing use of weekly divided-dose therapy given by peripheral vein and of continuous infusions given via subcutaneous ports and external pumps. Tunneled catheters should be employed whenever possible for long-term infusions or frequent-injection schedules. Patency of subcutaneous ports should be reassured by their adequacy for blood drawing, and if any question exists about patency, radiotracer or dye must be injected to seek out leaks.

The radiation recall phenomenon was noted early in the clinical testing of doxorubicin, as many of the patients studied had had prior irradiation for neoplastic disease (43). The observed reactions were painful, erythematous, and warm dermatitides located exactly in the previous field of irradiation, geographically reproducing radiation dermatitis. Infrequently, these reactions can go on to vesiculation, severe desquamation, and ulceration. The reactions typically occur 4 to 7 days after doxorubicin injection. Local therapy with topical corticosteroids and cooling have given the best relief of recall reactions (43). Resolution can take weeks, during which the patient suffers burning torment in the affected area. Occasionally, only redness and mild warmth characterize a recall reaction. Whether a "doxorubicin-recall" reaction occurs in patients receiving irradiation concurrently with or following doxorubicin chemotherapy remains a subject of debate. What few data exist suggest increased mucosal toxicities with doxorubicin-irradiation combinations but no greater skin reactions than those expected from irradiation alone (103).

Daunorubicin

The anthracycline antitumor antibiotic daunorubicin was discovered prior to doxorubicin and entered clinical trials in the early 1960s (104, 105). As the prototype anthracycline, daunorubicin was studied extensively, and most of the biochemical interactions, metabolic pathways, and toxicities described for doxorubicin had actually been worked out with daunorubicin (53, 55, 56). The remarkable clinical activity of daunorubicin against acute leukemias was recognized early (104–107), and it quickly became the standard by which new antileukemia therapies were judged.

The biochemistry and cellular pharmacology of daunorubicin are essentially the same as those for doxorubicin, with these slight differences.

The structural difference between the two drugs Fig. 21.2), which is the absence of one hydroxyl group, makes daunorubicin less polar and more lipid soluble than doxorubicin (64). Thus, it more readily enters cells and is available to intracellular enzymes, leading initially to higher levels of daunorubicin and its alcohol metabolite, daunorubicinol, inside cells exposed to ordinary pharmacologic concentrations of daunorubicin. Daunorubicinol is more polar than its parent, having about the same polarity as doxorubicin itself, and tends to accumulate in cells after their exposure to daunorubicin. This feature of daunorubicin, termed "metabolic retention" by Bachur (56), has an important clinical consequence. Daunorubicinol participates in many of the same biochemical reactions as do daunorubicin and doxorubicin, including interaction with DNA and generation of toxic oxygen free radicals (52). Cells that can metabolize the parent drugs to alcohol metabolites, including many tumor cells, will tend to concentrate the metabolites, giving rise to a ready source of intracellular oxidant stress. Since many tumor cells are deficient in antioxidant defenses, such as superoxide dismutase and the glutathione systems (108), metabolic retention of anthracyclines amplifies the potential for irreversible damage to important intracellular macromolecules, with resultant cell death.

The only practical clinical role for daunorubicin at present is as a component of remission-induction regimens for acute nonlymphocytic (daunorubicin-cytarabine) and acute lymphocytic (daunorubicin-vincristine-prednisone) leukemias (30, 75, 104, 107, 109). Although the usual circumstances find the drug used in the initial therapy of leukemias, many patients will still respond with remissions to daunorubicin after second, third, or fourth relapses (106, 109). In some patients, as occurs with doxorubicin, the necessity for stopping further daunorubicin therapy is cardiac toxicity, rather than resistance of the leukemia to anthracyclines (109). Daunorubicin also has antitumor activity against a variety of solid tumors (Table 21.6), perhaps more so with pediatric than adult solid tumors (30). The reason that doxorubicin is most commonly employed in solid tumors nowadays probably relates to the poor understanding of dose-schedule-toxicity relationships for daunorubicin during its initial clinical evaluations 20 to 25 years ago. Excessive mucositis and myelosuppression were routinely encountered as antileukemic dosages of daunorubicin were applied in therapy of solid tumors, and it became know on some hospital wards as "the red death." In more modern clinical trials, with better appreciation of its side effects and better supportive care procedures available, daunorubicin has been found to produce clinical responses in Hodgkin's disease, non-Hodgkin's lymphomas, malignant melanoma, sarcomas, and carcinomas of lung, breast, and the gastrointestinal tract (110).

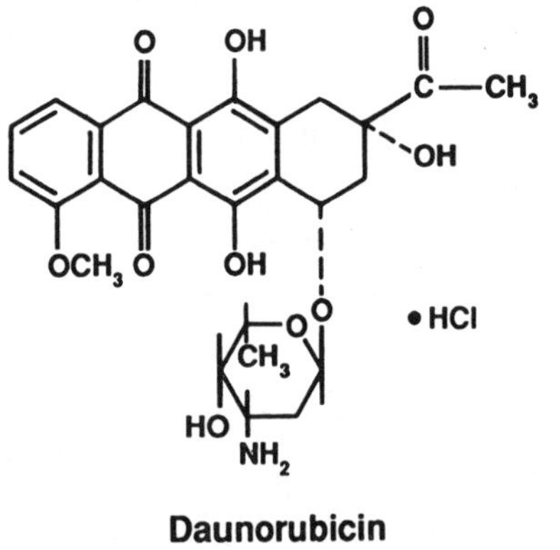

The dosages and toxicities of daunorubicin are nearly identical to those for doxorubicin, with these exceptions. For acute nonlymphocytic leukemias, dosages of 45 to 60 mg/m^2/day for 3 days are recommended (109), which are about 50% higher than those for doxorubicin. Randomized trials comparing daunorubicin with doxorubicin have shown a lesser incidence of mucositis, with a lower incidence of colonic damage and perforation with daunorubicin (70). It should remain the preferred anthracycline for this disease, pending reports on the antileukemia activities and toxicities of anthracycline analogues from trials in progress. The renal clearance for daunorubicin is about twice that for doxorubicin, with equivalent hepatic clearance, which has led to the suggestion that no dosage reductions are necessary for daunorubicin in the face of hepatic functional impairment (104–107, 109). Although no dosage modifications for daunorubicin are recommended in leukemia therapy, the situation in therapy of solid tumors and lymphomas must be clarified by further study.

Daunorubicin

Figure 21.2.   Structure of daunorubicin. Note the quinone-semiquinone system (Table 21.2) in the central two rings of the chromophore, and the aminosugar, which is positively charged at intracellular pH. This positive charge may serve to stabilize the intercalated daunorubicin molecule, by electrostatic bonding to the phosphate groups of the DNA chain.

Table 21.6. Clinical and Pharmacologic Data for Daunorubicin

Molecular weight: 527.5
Plasma half-life: 20 hours (may be prolonged with hepatic dysfunction)
Total body clearance: 34–67 L/hr/m^2 (40% hepatic; 10% renal)

	Diseases treated
Curative intent:	Acute lymphocytic leukemia
	Acute nonlymphocytic leukemia
Palliative intent:	Relapsed leukemias—acute lymphocytic and nonlymphocytic types
	Secondary acute leukemias (myelodysplastic, etc.)
	Carcinomas—experimental setting

	Toxicities
Acute:	Bone marrow suppression
	Mucositis, stomatitis
	Alopecia
	Nausea, vomiting, anorexia
	Flushing of face, torso
	Vein itching
Chronic:	Congestive cardiomyopathy
	Vein streaking
Special concerns:	Radiation-recall dermatitis
	Extravasation necrosis of skin, subcutaneous tissue
	Dose reduction probably not necessary in face of impaired liver function

---

Altered schedules and formulations of daunorubicin have been proposed and studied. As a weekly intravenous injection, dosages up to 50 mg/m^2/week were tolerated in one phase I trial (111). Whether this approach to daunorubicin therapy will give impetus to its use against neoplasia other than leukemia remains to be seen. In leukemia, continuous infusion daunorubicin has been tried, in efforts to maintain or to augment good antileukemic activity while decreasing the cardiac and, possibly, other toxicities (112). No enhancement of remission rates or lessening of acute toxicities was seen, and it is doubtful that further study of this schedule of administration is needed.

Liposomal daunorubicin, identical to a doxorubicin product, has been reported in phase I and other feasibility studies (17, 113, 114). In such formulations, the active anthracycline is encapsulated into one of several types of lipid-containing spheroids (either in the lipid membrane itself or in the aqueous contents of the spheroid) and infused intravenously (115). The major advantages appear to be a lessening of the potential for long-term or chronic toxicities, such as cardiac failure (17), with preservation of potent antitumor activity (113). Extravasation necrosis

may also be averted by the use of such formulations (116). Despite promising early results and the likelihood of approval of liposomal doxorubicin for human use in the near future, human studies of liposomal anthracycline therapy continue to be needed.

Dactinomycin (Actinomycin D)

The first clinically useful antitumor antibiotics were originally derived from *Actinomyces* species. Dactinomycin, which is presently obtained as a product of fermentation by *Streptomyces parvulus* (but produced by other *Streptomyces* species, as well) is the representative of the group that remains of clinical interest.

Unique structural features of actinomycins Fig. 21.3) have endeared these compounds to pharmacologists and cell biologists. The drug's yellow color is due to the tricyclic phenoxazone chromophore, which is linked to two short, identical cyclic polypeptides. The chromophore permits intercalation between base pairs in DNA, with a preference for guanine (4), while the polypeptide rings lie in the minor groove of DNA. This binding to DNA results in inhibition of RNA (117) and protein (118) syntheses, which

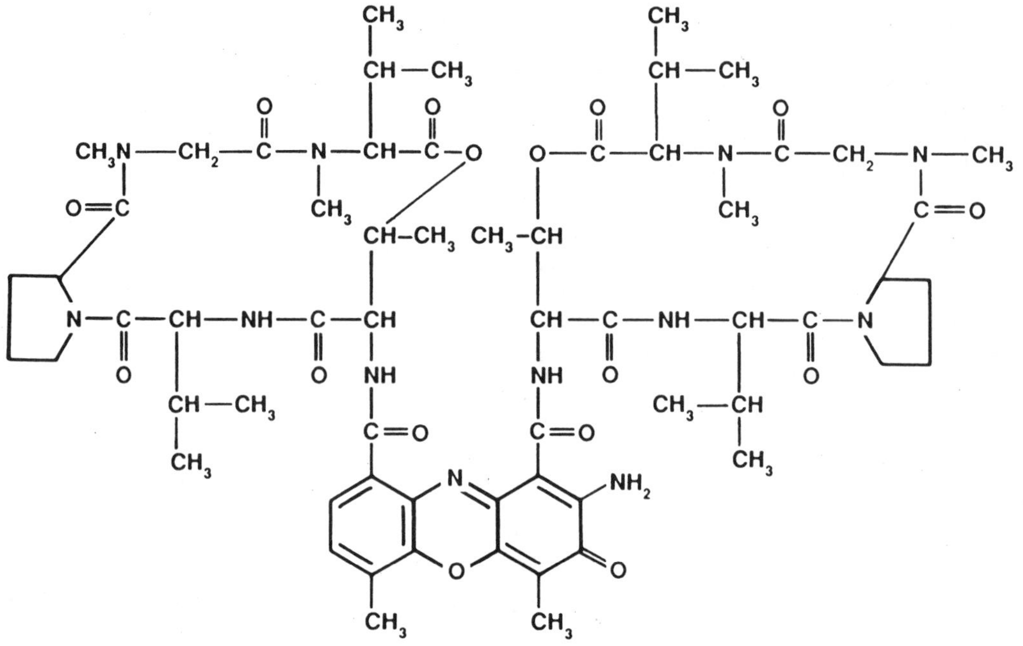

Dactinomycin

Figure 21.3.   Structure of dactinomycin. The three-ring chromophore is attached to two identical short peptide chains, which may serve to stabilize the molecule in its intercalation into or interactions with DNA and RNA.

activity has been used in the study of regulation of cell growth and of effects of other drugs on cellular function. Also, it has been show that dactinomycin can be activated to the free radical state (14) and, as such, may participate in the oxy-radical reactions described above.

Much is known about the uptake and intracellular disposition of dactinomycin. Sensitivity depends on the intracellular concentration of dactinomycin (119), while resistance to the drug appears to relate to reduced accumulation by tumor cells. Resistance can be reversed by treatments that alter membrane structure or permeability (120–122), and these observations may have applications in clinical situations. Two methods that are effective in reversing dactinomycin resistance in vitro are treating cells with the polyene antibiotic amphotericin B and encapsulating dactinomycin in lipid vesicles (liposomes). The amphotericin method (121) is presumed to depend on increased permeability of cell membranes after exposure to amphotericin B, with increased penetration of dactinomycin occurring by passive (temperature-dependent) diffusion. Dactinomycin-loaded liposomes can be phagocytosed by tumor cells, permitting in-

tracellular release of the encapsulated drug (114, 122). Both of these techniques should be able to be translated easily into clinical experience. The availability of antibiotics (doxorubicin, mitomycin C) and other antineoplastics with more manageable toxicities for use in the relevant neoplasms has removed much of the impetus for further definitive clinical trials aimed at reversing dactinomycin resistance.

Little is known about the human pharmacology of dactinomycin (Table 21.7), and most available information is based on studies with radioactive drug (123, 124). As with the other antibiotics, entry into nucleated (blood and tissue) cells is rapid, although a very long terminal elimination half-life has been suggested. This observation has led to the current clinical recommendations of giving dactinomycin by intermittent intravenous injection, rather than by daily divided-dose injections (48, 69). The dosage ranges are 0.4 to 0.6 mg/m^2/day (10 to 15 mg/kg/day) for 5 days, repeated every 4 to 6 weeks, or 1.25 to 2.0 mg/m^2 (50 mg/kg) every 3 to 4 weeks, with the latter schedule offering convenience at no higher toxicity. The usual route of administration is intravenous, but isolated limb perfu-

Table 21.7. Clinical and Pharmacologic Data for Dactinomycin

Molecular weight: 1255.5
Plasma half-life: 36–48 hours (prolonged with hepatic dysfunction)
Total body clearance: Unknown; human data suggest 15% hepatic, 20–30% renal

<table>
<tr><td colspan="2" align="center">Diseases treated</td></tr>
<tr><td>Curative intent:</td><td>Pediatric solid tumors
  Wilms' tumor
  Ewing's sarcoma
  Embryonal rhabdomyosarcoma
Gestational trophoblastic neoplasia
Osteogenic sarcoma (adjuvant only)
Soft tissue sarcoma (adjuvant only)
Germ cell tumors of testis, ovary</td></tr>
<tr><td>Palliative intent:</td><td>Relapsed leukemias—acute lymphocytic
Metastatic/recurrent osteogenic and soft tissue sarcomas
Regional perfusions of metastatic disease
Kaposi's sarcoma
Carcinomas of bladder, breast, ovary (advanced), testis (recurrent)
Paget's disease of bone</td></tr>
<tr><td colspan="2" align="center">Toxicities</td></tr>
<tr><td>Acute:</td><td>Bone marrow suppression (severe)
Mucositis, stomatitis
Alopecia (may include eyebrows)
Nausea, vomiting, anorexia
Flushing of face, torso
Vein itching, pain
Erythema, induration of skin</td></tr>
<tr><td>Chronic:</td><td>Aplastic anemia
Vein streaking
Hepatic function abnormalities</td></tr>
<tr><td>Special concerns:</td><td>Radiation-recall dermatitis, enteritis, stomatitis
Extravasation necrosis of skin, subcutaneous tissue
Perfused limbs may develop edema, ulceration
Reduce dose for concomitant radiation therapy</td></tr>
</table>

---

sions by intraarterial injections have been reported (125). A continuous intravenous infusion schedule has also been reported (31) and has allowed a substantial increase in delivered dose per treatment cycle.

The present clinical indications for dactinomycin include childhood tumors and refractory germ cell tumors (gestational trophoblastic neoplasms and testicular cancer; Table 21.7). The childhood tumors for which good activity has been described include Wilms' tumor, Ewing's sarcoma, and embryonal rhabdomyosarcoma (48, 125). Prior to recognition of the efficacy of doxorubicin in sarcomas, dactinomycin was an integral component of the VAC chemotherapy regimen, which was one of the first to demonstrate curative potential in sarcoma therapy (125). Dactinomycin was also an important

member of the early curative-intent VAB regimens for advanced testicular cancers and of the consolidation and maintenance chemotherapy programs in acute lymphocytic leukemia (125). In all cases mentioned, dactinomycin is employed as part of a multidrug combination regimen, which may also include radiation therapy, especially for the childhood tumors.

In the palliative setting, numerous single-agent and combination programs that include dactinomycin are known. Activity occurs against relapsed leukemias, recurrent lymphomas, sarcomas and germ cell tumors, nonepidemic Kaposi's sarcoma, and carcinomas of breast, bladder, and ovary (125). The extremity metastases from a variety of primary tumors can be treated by isolated limb perfusion with dactinomycin, with or without concomitant hyperthermia or irradiation of the limb lesions. The lesions and hypercalcemia of Paget's disease of bone respond to dactinomycin, and malignant hypercalcemia can improve (69). However, for this latter problem, effective less-toxic therapies are available, and dactinomycin should not be considered.

The toxicities of dactinomycin are quite severe, occasionally unpredictable, and always a prime source of worry when the drug is used. Severe bone marrow suppression occurs, primarily of leukocytes (125). Rarely, bone marrow suppression is severe enough to be in the range of aplastic anemia. Nausea, vomiting, alopecia, and mucositis are regular, as for most of the antibiotics, but their severity seems to be exaggerated with dactinomycin. Hepatic function can be compromised by long-term dactinomycin therapy (126). Edema and ulceration of perfused limbs is known (125). All of these side effects are enhanced by concurrent radiation therapy, including the possibility of fatal pulmonary fibrosis (127).

The skin and subcutaneous toxicities of dactinomycin can be particularly noxious (125). The radiation-recall phenomenon was first described in patients who received dactinomycin (43, 127) and developed the characteristic burning, erythema, and ulceration of the syndrome as long as 2 years after irradiation. Similar tissue toxicities are observed in the lungs and gastrointestinal mucosae, if they were in the radiation port. Dactinomycin also produces extravasation injury to skin and subcutaneous tissues (34, 36), and care must be given to ensuring patent, freely flowing intravenous access when the drug is administered by peripheral vein.

Bleomycin

Bleomycins are a family of related polypeptide antibiotics derived from *Streptomyces verticillus*, the members of which differ structurally primarily in the chemical side groups and functions attached to the parent peptide. They were described in 1966 by Umezawa (69), and the original microbial fermentation product was shown to be a mixture of at least 10 compounds. Modern purification techniques have permitted the isolation of enriched bleomycin A-2 (Fig. 21.4) for use as the clinical product (69), and

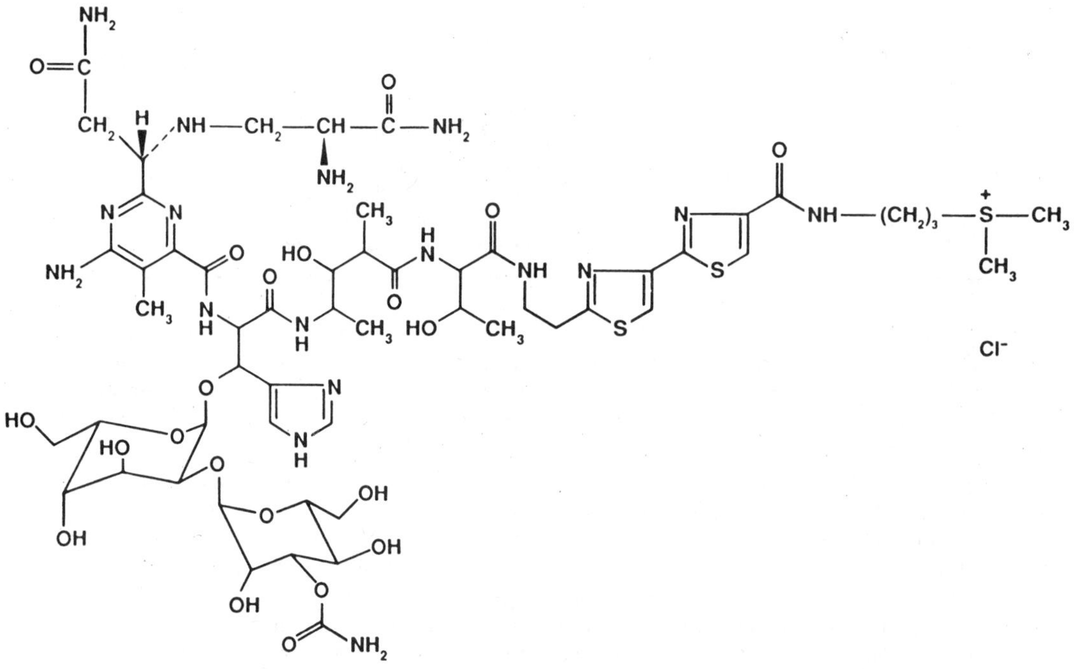

Bleomycin A$_2$

Figure 21.4.   Structure of bleomycin A$_2$. The amino acids of bleomycin contain amide groups (-NH-), which orient themselves to bind a metal ion. Once iron or copper is bound, bleomycin can participate in electron transport reactions, generating oxygen free radicals. The enzyme bleomycin hydrolase cleaves particular amide groups important for metal binding, and the metal-free peptide has no antiproliferative activity.

comments on bleomycin actions are based on results reported with this more purified material.

Experiments with DNA preparations and with intact cells (11) have shown that bleomycin produces strand scission of DNA, primarily single-strand breaks. Such breaks depend on the pH in the cell and are rapidly repaired by cells grown in bleomycin-free medium. Fragmentation of DNA by bleomycin may be enhanced by simultaneously irradiating the target cells (11). Other observed effects include inhibition of DNA-directed RNA polymerase in some systems (only when template DNA is preincubated with bleomycin), activation of DNases, and inhibition of thymidine incorporation into DNA (11). Mitochondrial damage can also be documented in cells exposed to bleomycin, with the characteristic histopathologic picture of swelling, hypertrophy, and alteration in number of mitochondria (128). Recent studies have demonstrated that bleomycin can damage mitochondrial DNA (128), with consequent impact on the respiratory chain enzymes and RNA for which it codes. In understanding the cytotoxic actions of this drug, it must be remembered that the particular toxic effect observed may depend on the experimental system employed. This suggests that bleomycin, like other antibiotics, has multiple means of exerting a deleterious impact on cell growth.

One feature essential to bleomycin's actions is the absolute requirement for a metal ion cofactor, without which DNA strand scission cannot occur. Copper or iron gives the most active fragmentation reactions when added to metal-stripped bleomycin, but nickel, manganese, cobalt, and others can alone restore at least some activity (129). In the presence of copper or iron, aerobic bleomycin solutions containing proper electron donors generate activated oxygen species, including superoxide anion, which can go on to damage DNA (130). These observations, along with knowledge of the synergy between bleomycin and irradiation (11), point to generation of reactive oxidants as the common mechanism for the cytotoxic effects of bleomycin. In this regard, bleomycin can be thought of as an enzyme similar to the iron-dependent cytochrome reductases, which, in site-specific manner near DNA, serves to reduce oxygen to toxic superoxides, the ultimate mediators of chemical damage to vital structures.

Inactivation of bleomycin by tissue homogenates occurs as a result of a particular detoxifying enzyme system. This enzyme activity, referred to as bleomycin hydrolase (69), catalyzes the removal of specific amide groups from the intact peptide. The important amides so cleaved are those necessary for the stereoselective binding of the metal cofactor (129), and the resulting inability of the bleomycin peptide to bind a metal ion is responsible for the loss of cytotoxic activity. Bleomycin hydrolase is found in every tissue, although its activities are lowest in skin and lung tissues (69). This may have implications for clinical bleomycin toxicities.

Bleomycin has cell cycle–specific cytocidal effects, and there is debate about whether it is phase specific (11). Although the most pronounced inhibition of cell growth is realized when bleomycin exposure occurs during S-phase, the drug can damage prophase chromosomes and induce a G_2-phase maturation arrest (11). As with many peptide pharmacologic agents, the serum half-life of bleomycin is relatively short after intravenous injection (131). This has advanced the notion of employing bleomycin as a prolonged infusion (69), to increase the likelihood that target tumor cells will pass through a sensitive phase of the cell cycle when therapeutic concentrations of the drug are present.

Phase II clinical trials of bleomycin revealed a single-agent antitumor spectrum that included squamous cell carcinomas, testicular carcinomas, Hodgkin's disease, and non-Hodgkin's lymphomas (69). The lack of appreciable bone marrow toxicity and its synergy with irradiation led quickly to inclusion of bleomycin in combination-therapy programs, and its present clinical utility portends a continued role in polychemotherapy and radiotherapy regimens (69).

Bleomycin is active against human cancer after intravenous, intramuscular, subcutaneous, or intracavitary (pleural, peritoneal, pericardial, bladder) administration (Table 21.8). The intravenous route is mostly commonly encountered, because the side effects are not increased compared with other routes, and other drugs requiring intravenous injection are usually simultaneously administered. The equivalence of intravenous and subcutaneous infusions of bleomycin in terms of pharmacokinetics and toxicities has been suggested (132), and subcutaneous infusion may be regarded as a practical alternative to intravenous infusion.

Schedules and dosages for bleomycin vary widely among regimens for different disease sites (69). Many programs employ single intravenous doses at 10 units/m², given as a weekly

Table 21.8. Clinical and Pharmacologic Data for Bleomycin

Molecular weight: 1414
Plasma half-life: 2–4 hours (may be prolonged with renal dysfunction); 3 hr (intrapleural); 5 hr (intraperitoneal)
Total body clearance: 3 L/hr/m² (50–70% renal)

Diseases treated

Curative intent:	Non-Hodgkin's lymphomas (large cell)
	Hodgkin's disease
	Germ cell tumors of testis, ovary
Palliative intent:	Intracavitary (pleura, pericardium, peritoneum)
	Non-Hodgkin's lymphomas (small cell types)
	Recurrent testicular carcinoma
	Mycosis fungoides
	Squamous cell carcinomas of head and neck, penis, skin, uterine cervix

Toxicities

Acute:	Anaphylaxis; anaphylactoid reactions
	Fever, chills, myalgias
	Mucositis, stomatitis
	Erythema, induration, scaling of skin
	Nausea, vomiting, anorexia
	Hypotension
	Urticaria; flushing of face, torso
	Vein itching; phlebitis
	Raynaud's phenomenon
Chronic:	Pulmonary fibrosis
	Cutaneous hypesthesia or hyperesthesia
	Hyperpigmentation
	Cutaneous hyperkeratosis
Special concerns:	Follow pulmonary diffusing capacity
	Radiation may potentiate pulmonary damage
	Reduce dose 50–75% in face of impaired renal function (creatinine clearance < 25 mL/min)

injection. References to doses of 30 units, irrespective of body size, are often encountered. In squamous cell carcinomas, the efficacy of bleomycin appears to be enhanced by using a continuous intravenous infusion of 72 to 96 hours' duration. The total dosage of 20 units/m² has been commonly cited for such infusions. Some confusion may exist in terminology for bleomycin dosing. Because the clinical product is a mixture of peptides differing slightly in structure, drug activity was originally expressed in units. Designation of milligram-activities occurred with the availability of more purified products. However, the currently preferred means for describing bleomycin doses is in units of bleomycin, and all standard references to bleomycin should use this format. Finally, it is important to remember that patients who receive bleomycin therapy for squamous cell cancers are frequently those with significant underlying lung disease, by virtue of long smoking histories, and they should be screened frequently for lung disease, as noted below. It has been recommended that bleomycin doses be reduced by 50 to 75 % in patients with creatinine clearance less than 25 mL/min (133), because of observations of increased incidence in pulmonary and other toxicities in such individuals.

The most common use for bleomycin is as a component of multiagent chemotherapy schemes in lymphomas. Three Hodgkin's disease combinations (ABVD, MOPP/ABV, SCAB) and numerous non-Hodgkin's lymphoma combinations (CHOP-Bleo, BACOP, M-BACOD, MACOP-B, ProMACE-Cyta BOM, and others) are routinely employed as first- and second-line therapies and most have demonstrated curative potential (69). In these, bleomycin is typically administered by direct intravenous injection at dosages of 10 to 15 units/m² every 2 to 3 weeks.

Occasionally, subcutaneous injection has been used to simplify the overall program, although this is less often done in current practice.

Bleomycin was a necessary component of the first widely acknowledge, curative-intent chemotherapy regimen for testicular carcinoma, cisplatin-vinblastine-bleomycin ("PVB"). This three-drug program, administered for a tolerably brief four monthly cycles, produced lasting complete remissions in 85 to 90% of those with lower volumes of metastatic testicular cancer and 50% of those with bulky, advanced disease (134). The effectiveness of short courses of therapy also made adjuvant therapy feasible for those with resected disease at high risk of recurrence. Careful studies demonstrated that exclusion of bleomycin from the combination or reducing its dosage lowered the cure rates in advanced disease. More recent studies have examined a PVB variant in which etoposide (VP16-213) is substituted for vinblastine ("PEB"). Direct comparisons of PVB with PEB have revealed equivalent anticancer efficacies, but lesser incidence and severity of neuromuscular toxicities with PEB (134). The PEB program is now regarded as the standard chemotherapy regimen for advanced testicular carcinomas. In PEB, the bleomycin is most commonly the source of irreversible toxicity, primarily pulmonary nodules and/or fibrosis. Current trials in testicular cancer are looking at cisplatin and etoposide, without or with added bleomycin. Preliminary results do not show any adverse impact on remission rate or extent, in contrast to the clear-cut advantage of adding bleomycin at full dosage to the cisplatin-vinblastine combination.

Regional chemotherapy with bleomycin has been established as a preferred means of approaching malignant effusions (135). Bleomycin sclerotherapy avoids the side effects of other medications (e.g., tetracyclines, alkylators) and the morbidity of repeated or prolonged intubations of the pleura, pericardium, or peritoneum. Several studies suggest that only a small drainage catheter need be placed, with removal of as much fluid as is feasible (136). Bleomycin, usually 60 units in 30 to 60 mL of preservative-free diluent, is then directly injected through the same tubing into the space. The catheter can be withdrawn, eliminating the need for prolonged drainage, as, for instance, with ordinary chest tubes. Toxicities can include local pain, fever, and allergic reactions (rash, bronchospasm), but many patients tolerate the procedure with minimal side effects. Response rates, defined as freedom from recurrent effusion for 3 to 6 months (135, 136), are high (50 to 75%). The most extensive experience is with malignant pleural effusion, but success rates with pericardial effusions and malignant ascites appear to be similar. Dose-response relations have been studied in pleural effusion, with 60 units giving results equivalent to those for 90 to 120 units, and better results than 30 units (136). Most reports have tended to use 60 units or more in the peritoneum, but 20 to 30 units for pericardial effusions. Cost considerations may have an impact on the decision to use bleomycin for malignant effusions, as this agent remains very expensive. A recent report suggests the equivalence of bleomycin and talc in relieving malignant effusions (137), with a much lower cost for the latter agent.

The toxicities of bleomycin are sufficiently unique and manageable that it can be included in combination chemotherapy regimens containing very myelosuppressive agents (2). Almost every patient will experience fever within the first 4 to 12 hours after bleomycin injection, which is usually brief and not clinically troublesome. Chills, myalgias, nausea, vomiting, and anorexia may accompany fever, but are less frequent. Urticaria, facial flushing, venous and cutaneous itching, and the Raynaud phenomenon may occur, and susceptible persons should be premedicated with antihistamines (69). Hypotension is seen with rapid intravenous infusions of higher bleomycin doses, although it may also be noted several hours after any dose or during continuous infusions. Three potentially serious bleomycin toxicities merit special consideration.

Anaphylactoid reactions and, rarely, anaphylaxis, were reported early on with bleomycin injections and were noted to present almost exclusively in lymphoma patients receiving their first doses of bleomycin (2). The recommendation was made to give one or two test doses of bleomycin, 0.5 to 1 unit intravenously on the 1 or 2 days prior to the first full dose, since some lymphoma patients manifested anaphylactoid reactions as long as 24 hours after the test dose. This recommendation was subsequently extended to include all patients receiving their first dose of bleomycin, although whether patients with cancers other than lymphoma are at high risk has never been adequately addressed. Bleomycin anaphylaxis is rare at present (69). Whether this is because susceptible patients are excluded from bleomycin therapy by a reaction to the test dose or the fact that bleomycin preparations are much more purified now than 2 decades ago (thus eliminating those antigenic materials responsible for anaphylaxis) is unclear. Patients who are to receive bleomycin for the first time should be test-dosed with 0.5 to 1 unit, prior to the first full dose. When possible, this should be done a full 24 hours before the full dose, but many practitioners give the test dose an hour or two before the full dose, carefully observing the patient for signs of reactions.

Chronic skin reactions following bleomycin therapy are common and can be troublesome. Activity of the enzyme bleomycin hydrolase is considerably less in skin (69) than in, for instance, bone marrow. It is believed that even low concentrations of bleomycin in skin can continue to form toxic radicals and produce DNA damage (11), if the drug is not inactivated by the enzyme. The types of toxicities observed include hyperpigmentation, especially at creases and folds in the areas of trauma, hyperkeratosis and thickening of skin, erythema, scaling, and, rarely, ulceration. Hypesthesia, hyperesthesia, and paresthesias have been reported, which may or may not resolve at discontinuation of therapy (137). Attempts to screen for susceptible individuals by measuring bleomycin hydrolase activities in skin have been unsuccessful because of the wide range of normal variation in the population (11). Topical corticosteroids remain the central focus of treatment strategies for affected patients, along with discontinuation of bleomycin therapy.

The most feared and potentially lethal toxicity of bleomycin is pulmonary fibrosis. Much is known about the problem (138). The pathology is interstitial fibrosis, similar to the pattern of idiopathic diffuse interstitial pneumonitis. The chest roentgenogram can show nodules and cavitary lesions, as well as the more familiar pattern of interstitial infiltrates and streaking. The incidence of fibrosis increases with increasing cumulative dose, with an inflection point in the incidence curve at 300 units total dose (69). Fibrosis appears earlier in those with impaired renal function who receive standard clinical doses of bleomycin (133, 139). Onset of a clinical picture of pulmonary fibrosis can occur during active bleomycin therapy or after cessation of bleomycin, and progression of pulmonary compromise may continue for months after discontinuation of the drug (140). Therapy of the disorder, in addition to stopping the drug, has encompassed local and systemic corticosteroids, bronchodila-

tors, and antioxidants (e.g., vitamin E). Responses to these have been inconsistent enough that no single recommendation can be made (138). In a number of cases, the respiratory disease picture improves, and clinical signs and symptoms may completely resolve. Most clinicians attempt to avoid the problem by ceasing bleomycin therapy at the first sign of toxicity or at 300 units total dose and employing corticosteroids for clinically apparent fibrosis.

There is presently no reliable predictive test for bleomycin pulmonary fibrosis. Physical examinations that seek fine inspiratory rales or pleural friction rubs are insensitive, and, by the time such signs are audible, the damage has been done. Blood gas analysis and pulmonary mechanics also identify only those persons with extant fibrosis, and, as noted, progression of the damage may occur despite intervention at that point. The carbon monoxide diffusing capacity (DL_{co}) has received great attention for its sensitivity, but it is an imperfect test (141). Studies that have examined DL_{co} have noted a low (15 to 20%) specificity in those persons who actually go on to have clinically significant bleomycin lung and, also, that most patients whose bleomycin is stopped because of a decline in DL_{co} never develop any evidence of fibrosis (69, 141). These studies suggest that many patients have bleomycin therapy discontinued inappropriately early and that clinical evidence for bleomycin lung may, in fact, be the best, early sign of toxicity. The safest course is to monitor both DL_{co} and the clinical presentation, stopping bleomycin in those in whom actual toxicity is suspected.

Mitomycin C

The mitomycins, a family of related antibiotics from *Streptomyces caespitosus*, are chemically similar to the porfiromycins. Both classes are of interest to cell biologists for their abilities to suppress bacterial replication and lymphocyte immune functions, for which they have been extensively utilized in the laboratory setting (4). Mitomycin C is the clinically approved entity.

The structural features (Fig. 21.5) of mitomycin C are of interest. Like the anthracyclines doxorubicin and daunorubicin, mitomycins possess a quinone ring (Table 21.2), which can be reduced by one-electron transfer to form free radicals (8, 142). Such activation by the electron-transport machinery of the cell appears to be required for drug activity. Quinone reduction is followed by opening of the three-membered

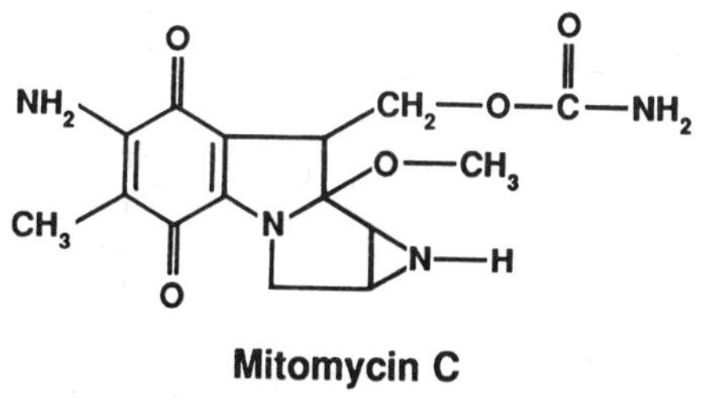

Mitomycin C

Figure 21.5.   Structure of mitomycin C. The molecule contains both quinone and aziridine functions (Table 21.2). The quinone ring may be reduced to generate free radicals of mitomycin, which can reduce oxygen to superoxide. The triangular aziridinyl group can open to generate an alkylating side chain.

aziridine ring (Table 21.2), which then functions as an alkylator (5, 8). The primary biochemical mechanism of action then appears to be alkylation of DNA, producing cross-linking and adduct formation. As with other antibiotics, guanine bases are the preferred sites of attachment (4, 10). It has been speculated that mitomycin may also participate in direct electron transfers to suitable acceptor molecules, such as molecular oxygen to give superoxide, but the impact of these reactions on cytotoxicity remains under investigation (5, 15).

Studies of mitomycin pharmacology were originally hampered by lack of a suitable assay, but recent development of high-performance liquid chromatographic methods has resulted in several good clinical reports (143–146). Disappearance from plasma is rapid, with metabolism, tumor cell uptake, and renal excretion accounting for this disposition. Pharmacokinetics do not appear to be dose dependent, with similar plasma half-lives for higher doses and lower doses.

Mitomycin is administered via the intravenous, intracavitary, and intraarterial routes. The usual dosage is 10 to 20 mg/m^2 every 4 to 8 weeks by intravenous or intraarterial injection (46, 69) or 20 mg total dose by the intravesical and intraperitoneal routes (51). Intravenous injections must be given with care through freely flowing access, as the drug is a vesicant (147). Intrapleural mitomycin seems to cause considerable local pain and is not recommended. However, intraperitoneal mitonmycin is well tolerated, causing neither significant local peritoneal irritation nor abdominal skin and subcutaneous problems (51).

The only circumstances in which mitomycin is considered to be curative are combination therapy for squamous cell carcinoma of the anus and intravesical therapy for superficial transitional cell carcinoma of the bladder (Table 21.9). Anal carcinomas are locally aggressive tumors, requiring morbid surgery for cure. A combination of mitomycin C by intravenous injection, 5-fluorouracil by continuous intravenous infusion, and radiation therapy to 50 to 65 Gy can produce magnificent shrinkage of local tumor, to the point of complete disappearance, in 60 to 80% of patients, with substantial numbers of cures (46, 148). Such excellent responses may obviate the need for disfiguring abdominoperineal resections that were required for cure previously.

Superficial bladder carcinomas can be prophylactically or therapeutically approached with mitomycin (149). As prophylaxis, mitomycin instilled monthly for two to six courses prevents recurrences in 30 to 40% of patients long-term. Shrinkage of superficial bladder tumors is also documented, but local recurrence tends to be common (150). However, in those patients for whom further local surgery is not an option and bladder preservation is important, intravesical therapy with mitomycin is well tolerated and beneficial.

In locally advanced, unresectable head and neck squamous cell carcinomas, the combination of mitomycin C by intravenous injection, 5-fluorouracil by infusion, and 50-Gy x-irradiation produce a 95% complete plus partial remission rate (151). This result is analogous to those with cisplatin-based regimens. In the cited study, patients having complete responses to the chemotherapy did not suffer recurrence of disease. No serious toxicities were encountered, and this approach to advanced head and neck cancer warrants further clinical study.

There are numerous palliative-intent situations for which mitomycin should be considered. As a single agent, it produces remissions in pleural mesothelioma (152) and in recurrent colorectal, breast, and bladder carcinomas (46). In advanced malignant pleural mesothelioma, mitomycin C alone gave a 20% partial remission rate, and cisplatin-mitomycin combination produce 25% responders, even in doxorubicin-refractory patients (152). Response rates of 40% are reported in recurrent breast cancer (46, 153), although a recent study (154) has questioned the value of mitomycin C as second- or third-line salvage therapy in this disease. Mitomycin is an integral component of combination regiments (FAM, SMF, FOMi, MVP, and others) for recurrent or metastatic carcinomas of the stomach,

Table 21.9. Clinical and Pharmacologic Data for Mitomycin C

Molecular weight: 334
Plasma half-life: 1–2 hours (may be prolonged with hepatic dysfunction)
Total body clearance: Probably about 30 L/hr; 9–20% renal excretion

Diseases treated

Curative intent:	Anal squamous cell carcinoma (with irradiation and 5-fluorouracil infusion)
	Superficial bladder carcinoma (intravesical)
Palliative intent:	Carcinomas of esophagus, pancreas, stomach
	Recurrent colon carcinoma
	Recurrent breast carcinoma
	Metastatic/recurrent osteogenic and soft tissue sarcomas
	Malignant mesothelioma
	Carcinomas of bladder, head and neck, liver, lung, uterine cervix
	Intracavitary—pleural, peritoneal, vesical—for recurrent, metastatic carcinoma, sarcoma

Toxicities

Acute:	Bone marrow suppression
	Severe thrombocytopenia
	Mucositis, stomatitis
	Paresthesias
	Nausea, vomiting, anorexia (prolonged)
	Extravasation injury and necrosis
	Vein pain, itching; phlebitis
	Skin induration, erythema, or ulceration
	Bronchospasm (with vinca alkaloids)
	Pulmonary infiltrates, cough, pneumonia
Chronic:	Microangiopathic hemolytic anemia
	Hemolytic uremic syndrome
	Pulmonary fibrosis, hemoptysis, dyspnea
	Cumulative bone marrow suppression
	Vein streaking or sclerosis, phlebitis
Special concerns:	May produce cardiac toxicities or potentiate doxorubicin cardiomyopathy
	Radiation-recall dermatitis possible
	Extravasation necrosis of skin, subcutaneous tissue
	Reduce doses 25–75% in face of significant prior leukocyte or platelet suppression

pancreas, esophagus, and lung (46, 155). Response rates of 15 to 45% are usual, and substantial relief of troubling symptoms may be the benefit. Recurrent sarcomas and gynecologic tumors may respond to combinations. Intraperitoneal mitomycin has been reported to be effective for peritoneal carcinomatosis, mesothelioma, and ovarian carcinoma (51, 156).

The toxicities of mitomycin are substantial, unpredictable, and always considered to be life threatening. The common toxicities are noted in the section above. Delayed myelosuppression, especially leukopenia and thrombocytopenia, frequently complicate mitomycin schedules (46), so that an 8-week interval between doses is frequently necessary after the second or third 4-week injection. Bone marrow suppression is cumulative, and marked, long-lasting thrombocytopenia and extreme sensitivity of blood counts to subsequent chemotherapy regimens are reported (157). Dosages of mitomycin should be reduced by 25 to 75% in the face of prior significant myelosuppression. Delayed nausea and vomiting, similar to those reported for cisplatin, occur, and prolonged anorexia is common (46). Mitomycin is a vesicant, and extravasation injury and necrosis may result (35, 147). Venous irritation, phlebitis, and phlebosclerosis are common. The dermatologic, cardiopulmonary, and hemostatic system toxicities of mitomycin are discussed in greater detail below.

Erythema, induration, and even ulceration of the skin have been reported to occur at a distance from the injection site and should be treated as with extravasation. Mitomycin has been responsible for the radiation-recall phenomenon (46), and the pattern of the reaction is similar to that seen with the anthracyclines and dactinomycin. Paresthesias may occur, which are felt to represent local damage to nerve endings in the dermis (46).

The pulmonary reactions produced by mitomycin can be fearsome and fatal. A peculiar syndrome of acute bronchospasm, occurring 4 to 12 hours after combined intravenous therapy with mitomycin and a vinca alkaloid, was noted in breast and lung cancer patients (158). Although pretreatment of susceptible individuals with bronchodilators helped to lessen the frequency and severity of this reaction, the possibility of fatal outcome still remained. Pulmonary fibrosis complicates mitomycin therapy, with a threshold dosage of about 50 to 60 mg/m^2. This amounts to three cycles of therapy at usual dosages, so careful attention must be paid to any pulmonary symptoms mentioned by patients receiving mitomycin. This reaction can be progressive and fatal, despite cessation of mitomycin (159, 160).

It has been suggested that congestive cardiomyopathy occurs with greater frequency and at lower cumulative drug dosages in patients receiving doxorubicin and mitomycin C in combination (161). Although synergistic cardiotoxicity with the combination has not been proven, scrupulous attention to pretreatment cardiac evaluation and prospective monitoring of cardiac function during therapy seem prudent practices in this setting.

Early in the experience with mitomycin in this country, a devastating syndrome with fever, thrombocytopenia, renal failure, anemia, and consumptive coagulopathy was noted. Features of the syndrome mimicked hemolytic uremic syndrome, and a high case-fatality rate ensued (46). This syndrome is now recognized as a form of microangiopathic hemolytic anemia with consumption, or thrombotic microangiopathy. Essential findings are intravascular hemolysis, activation of the fibrinolytic system, consumption of clotting factors, and the attendant clinical findings of renal failure with hypertension and other microvascular injuries (162, 163). While the precise pathophysiology remains uncertain, endothelial injury from mitomycin is suspected to be the initial insult, with other consequences cascading from that (164). There appears to be a threshold dosage of 50 to 60 mg/m^2, similar to that for the pulmonary lesions, although the syndromes are felt to be distinct entities (165). Attempts to control thrombotic microangiopathy from mitomycin have included corticosteroids, exchange transfusions, and the usual therapeutic maneuvers for disseminated intravascular coagulopathy (166). Hypertension seems to respond well to angiotensin-converting enzyme inhibitor therapy (e.g., captopril) in low doses (167), despite the potential concern of using such agents in states of compromised renal plasma flow. There remains a high fatality rate for this disastrous condition, although more recent use of intensive, combined prednisone-captopril-heparin therapy, with dialysis and vigorous blood component support, has produced survivors (166, 167).

Because of the activity of intravenous mitomycin C against hepatic metastases of colorectal carcinoma (46) and of the favorable pharmacokinetics of the drug (8), hepatic arterial mitomycin chemotherapy has been studied. Mitomycin C was admixed with starch microspheres and infused into the hepatic artery, in an effort to occlude the blood flow in tumor metastases and to maintain high local drug concentrations (168, 169). A partial response rate of 25% was observed, and the systemic toxicities were described as minimal. More recently, mitomycin C in an ethylcellulose microencapsulation matrix was infused intraarterially into livers of patients with cirrhosis and hepatoma (170). Responses, defined as reductions in tumor volume or in serum α-fetoprotein, occurred in 43% of patients, and systemic toxicities were minor. These newer therapeutic strategies may enjoy expanded roles in the future, in patients with locally advanced disease. They may be especially useful as components of combined-modality schemes. However, local reactions to mitomycin can occur, such as toxic epidermal necrolysis (171), when it is infused arterially into previously irradiated tissues.

Plicamycin (Mithramycin)

Although plicamycin was originally studied as a therapy for advanced testicular, bladder, and prostate cancers (172, 173), in which diseases investigators had originally noted good responses, its present role is almost exclusively confined to therapy of malignant hypercalcemia (174). Newer data (175) and the development of analogues of plicamycin have renewed interest in the antineoplastic properties of this family of drugs.

Plicamycin belongs to the chromomycin family and contains a central tricyclic aglycone (Fig. 21.6), to which are bonded several microbial sugars. The aglycone chromophore gives plicamycin solutions their characteristic yellow color, and the sugars confer water solubility. In vitro, plicamycin has antibacterial and anti-DNA-viral activities, and the major biochemical effect is inhibition of DNA-directed RNA synthesis (69). Binding to DNA occurs only in the presence of a divalent cation, such as magnesium (12), and appears to have preference for guanine-containing regions of DNA. Plicamycin does compete with dactinomycin for DNA binding, although the precise nature of its binding—intercalation versus other associations—is not clear. At high concentrations, single-strand DNA breaks and inhibition of DNA and protein syntheses are measurable (5). Which of these several effects are responsible for plicamycin's actions on cellular function are uncertain, since cell growth inhibition occurs at much lower drug concentrations than those necessary for the measured biochemical effects (5). Of potential interest for therapy

of certain lymphoid neoplams is the observation that plicamycin can inhibit the lymphoid marker enzyme, adenosine deaminase (176).

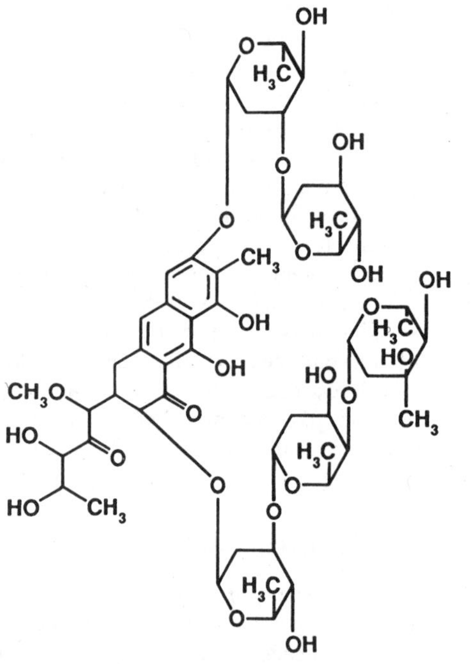

Human pharmacologic studies of plicamycin have been hampered by lack of a suitable assay method. Based on disappearance of radioactive plicamycin after injection in one patient, a relatively long elimination half-life of 12 to 24 hours has been suggested (69), and the major route of elimination appears to be renal (Table 21.10). The metabolic fate of the drug is unknown. As analogue development increases, suitable assays will need to be applied to plicamycin and analogues, for thorough understanding of pharmacokinetics and metabolism of the drugs.

The dosage recommendations for plicamycin vary with the indication. The two listed indications for the drug are therapy of refractory testicular cancer and of malignant hypercalcemia and hypercalciuria (69). Use of plicamycin in testicular cancer has waned since the advent of cisplatin-based regimens (134). Dosages from past trials were 25 to 30 mg/kg/day for 8 to 10 days, to be abbreviated if toxicities occurred. For the hypercalcemia and hypercalciuria of malignancy, lower dosages and briefer schedules have proven effective. The manufacturer recommends 25 mg/kg per day for 3 to 4 days, but a good hypocalcemic response can occur with 1.0 mg/m^2, every other day for 2 to 3 doses. Cautious delivery of additional every-other-day doses may be needed until the desired hypocalcemic effect or toxicity is reached (174). Caution in giving more than the recommended 2 to 3 doses must always be urged, with the benefits of relieving hypercalcemia carefully weighed against the considerable potential for severe toxicities.

Plicamycin has vesicant properties, and great care must be taken to avoid extravasation during intravenous injections (177). The potential for extravasation injury appears to depend on the concentration of the infused drug solution, so that low-volume, high-concentration injections are more hazardous than dilute preparations. A good recommendation is dilution of the desired drug dose in 100 to 250 mL of solution and administration over several hours by intravenous infusion.

The systemic toxicities of plicamycin are numerous, severe, and often unpredictable. Common toxicities of nausea, vomiting, mucositis, and bone marrow suppression are similar to those of dactinomycin and mitomycin. Platelet count depressions may be quite dramatic (178) and out of proportion to the declines in eryth-

Mithramycin

Figure 21.6.   Structure of plicamycin (mithramycin). It is uncertain if the three-ring chromophore participates in the cytotoxic or antihypercalcemic actions of the molecule. Note the unusual sugars bonded to the ring structure.

Table 21.10. Clinical and Pharmacologic Data for Plicamycin (Mithramycin)

Molecular weight: 1085.2
Plasma half-life: Unknown; probably 12–24 hours, based on disappearance of radioactivity in one patient
Total body clearance: Unknown; probably 50% renal

Diseases treated

Curative intent:	None
Palliative intent:	Germ cell tumors of testis, ovary
	Malignant hypercalcemia
	Paget's disease of bone
	Glioblastoma multiforme

Toxicities

Acute:	"Acute hemorrhagic syndrome"
	Severe thrombocytopenia
	Acute fibrinolysis, DIC
	Hypocalcemia
	Stomatitis
	Severe nausea, vomiting, anorexia
	Flushing of face, torso
	Renal—proteinuria, increased BUN, creatinine
	Hepatic—elevated transaminases, bilirubin
	Fever, vasculitic rash
Chronic:	Depressed hepatic synthetic activity with decreased albumin, clotting factors
	Vein streaking, phlebitis
Special concerns:	Rebound hypercalcemia after hypocalcemia
	Extravasation necrosis of skin, subcutaneous tissue (avoid by diluting in 150–500 mL infusate)
	Do not administer with renal, hepatic dysfunction

---

rocyte or leukocyte counts. Fever, rash, flushing, and local venous irritation or phlebitis are encountered.

The most worrisome side effect of plicamycin was originally termed "acute hemorrhagic syndrome." This was the precipitous presentation of diffuse hemorrhage, consumption of clotting factors, activation of the fibrinolytic system, hepatic and renal function abnormalities, and high death rate (28, 179). Dose and schedule dependence were recognized, with increased frequency of the syndrome for treatments above 30 mg/kg/day or given for longer than 10 days. It is imperative that patients receiving plicamycin be screened for adequacy of kidney and liver function, hemostatic abnormalities (prothrombin time, activated partial thromboplastin time, and thrombin time), and blood counts. The syndrome should be approached vigorously, with heparinization, blood component support, and, probably, corticosteroids (69). Associated infection should be sought.

Plicamycin may produce defects in platelet function and depression of hepatic synthesis of clotting factors, in the absence of the acute hem-

orrhagic syndrome (28, 180). The screening studies mentioned above should be repeated in the face of clinically apparent abnormalities or if more than three doses of plicamycin have to be administered for hypercalcemia. Plicamycin can affect the ability of the liver to synthesize clotting factors and to process bilirubin and can elevate serum hepatocellular enzymes, in the absence of the consumptive picture of the acute hemorrhagic syndrome (28, 180). These changes are usually reversible upon cessation of plicamycin therapy.

Other potentially serious complications are renal dysfunction and hypocalcemia (181). Elevated creatinine and blood urea nitrogen, proteinuria, and low serum phosphate, potassium, and calcium can occur, and are more frequent with daily dosing schedules. Acutely, hypocalcemia can complicate plicamycin therapy in the absence of other signs of renal injury, and the paradox of needing intravenous calcium replacement after plicamycin therapy of hypercalcemia is not rare (174).

The inhibitory effects of plicamycin on bone resorption and subsequent control of hypercalcemia have led to its use in treating Paget's disease of bone (182). Much lower doses, 10 mg/kg as single injections, seem effective. With the advent of calcitonin and bis-phosphonates, plicamycin should be considered an alternative only for refractory cases or in acute, dire situations.

IDARUBICIN

Recognition of the remarkable clinical antitumor activities of doxorubicin and daunorubicin and their favorable toxicity profiles, relative to existing antibiotics, prompted the search for additional agents with like actions. The two most fruitful of these searches have been the development of structural analogues of naturally occurring antibiotics and the identification of synthetic compounds whose chemical structures contain relevant prosthetic groups, such as the quinone rings or the aziridinyl ring. Two agents so identified have recently been approved for marketing: the daunorubicin analogue idarubicin (Idamycin) and the polar quinone-semiquinone compound mitoxantrone (Novantrone). The drugs are described below, as they indicate the potential benefits of present strategies for new-agent discovery and development.

Modifications of both the tetracyclic ring and the aminosugar of doxirubicin and daunorubicin by chemical additions, deletions, or substitutions have yielded a huge array of agents varying in their pharmacokinetics, spectra of anticancer activities, and clinical toxicities. The 4-demethoxy derivatives, in which the methoxy group on the "D" ring is chemically removed (Fig. 21.7), have attracted attention because of their abilities to be absorbed orally, their lessened potential for cardiac toxicities, and their longer half-lives, compared with the parent drugs (183, 184). Idarubicin, the signal member of this family of derivatives (Fig. 21.7), demonstrates well each of these advantages.

Idarubicin was described in 1976 by Arcamone, who had been instrumental in the basic and clinical development of doxorubicin. The activity of the demethoxyanthracyclines after oral administration was quickly discerned (184). Studies utilizing animal models confirmed that antitumor activity similar to that of doxorubicin occurred in the absence of the myocardial lesions typical for daunorubicin and doxorubicin. A host of derivatives were synthesized, and the best activity-toxicity relationships were seen with 4-demethoxydoxorubicin and idarubicin.

The stereochemistry of the chemically synthe-

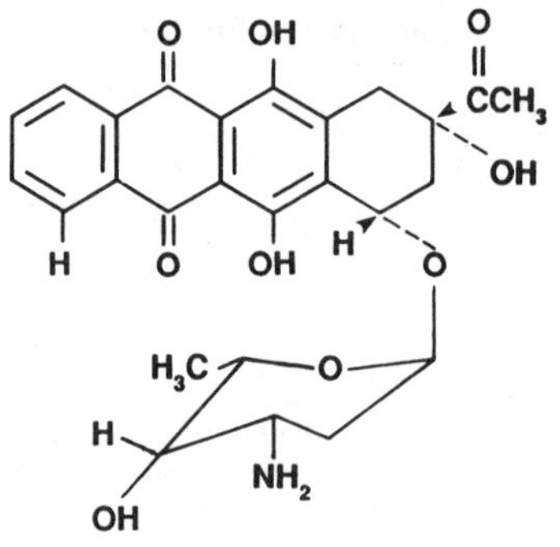

4-Demethoxydaunorubicin (Idarubicin)

Figure 21.7. Structure of idarubicin. This molecule differs from daunorubicin only in the substitution of a proton (-H) for the methoxy (-OCH₃) group of the "D" ring (*left side* of the pictured structure.) This minor alteration produces improvement in acid stability, permitting oral therapy, and changes the color of the molecule from red to yellow.

sized drugs is important in their metabolic and antitumor profiles (185), although the implications of this for therapy of human cancer is uncertain. The metabolic reactions that idarubicin can undergo appear to be the same as those for daunorubicin, namely, reduction of the side-chain carbonyl function to give the alcohol, idarubicinol, and reductive cleavage of the aminosugar to give the aglycone, 4-demethoxydaunomycinone. As with daunorubicin, the alcohol metabolite, idarubicinol, retains antitumor activity (64). This metabolite is also more polar than idarubicin and would be expected to be retained to greater degree intracellularly than the parent (metabolic retention, 56). The alteration of the ring structure in idarubicin confers a yellow color to aqueous solutions (Table 21.1), instead of the characteristic red of doxorubicin and daunorubicin.

Idarubicin induces time- and concentration-dependent increases in DNA breaks in tumor cells exposed to typical pharmacologic concentrations of the drug (186, 187). Cells resistant to doxorubicin may retain sensitivity to idarubicin (187), and the antiproliferative effects are not diminished by free-radical scavengers. These experiments lend additional credence to the notion that the primary mode of antineoplastic action of anthracyclines is by inhibition of DNA-processing reactions (5, 7, 8, 13, 14, 16, 17, 56), despite the evidence for additional modes of cell killing after exposures to these drugs (8, 18).

The pharmacokinetics of idarubicin in animal and human differ quantitatively from those for daunorubicin. After administration of equal doses of each drug to animals (188), higher amounts of idarubicin and metabolites are found in tissues, but after equitoxic doses, less idarubicin is found. These results suggest that idarubicin has higher tissue-binding capability and more potency than daunorubicin. After oral or intravenous administration of the same doses of idarubicin, lower levels of parent drug are found in serum and most tissues, but tumor content of drug is the same for each route (189). These results have implications for protection of the heart from anthracycline cardiotoxicity, as lower heart-to-tumor ratios for oral idarubicin indicate possible improvement in the therapeutic index.

Metabolism to idarubicinol is the primary fate of oral or intravenously administered idarubicin, with the liver quantitatively most important (190). Idarubicin is a less avid substrate for the aldoketo reductase enzyme mediating this reaction (55), but idarubicinol levels exceed idarubicin soon after drug administration. Aglycone metabolites, produced by microsomal reduction (52, 53), have been described (189, 190), but have not been adequately quantified. This class of metabolites is of concern, because algycones have

been indicted as possible mediators of anthracycline cardiac toxicities (58, 65, 67, 74, 98). In this regard, the observation that idarubicin can be converted to aglycones in the acidic milieu of the stomach (191) is germane to oral therapy. The practical impact of this finding on use of the oral route for idarubicin awaits clinical observations of the actual incidence of congestive cardiomyopathy in patients treated with oral idarubicin long-term.

The human pharmacokinetics of idarubicin after intravenous or oral administration have been extensively detailed (192–198) and are quite similar to those for daunorubicin (104, 105, 111, 116). The parent drug has a terminal elimination half-life of 10 to 30 hours after intravenous injection of single doses (Table 21.11) or 30 to 40 hours after oral doses. Combination chemotherapy (e.g., with cytarabine) does not appear to affect the half-life. The volume of distribution is quite large, 20 to 400 L/kg body weight, indicating substantial tissue uptake and binding. Total body clearance, 30 to 60 L/hr/m^2, is faster than that for daunorubicin, and the renal excretion is only 5% of dose, compared with 15 to 20% for daunorubicin. These data imply more rapid or extensive metabolism of idarubicin, and study of the metabolite, idarubicinol, confirm this. Ida-

Table 21.11. Clinical and Pharmacologic Data for Idarubicin

Molecular weight: 497.5
Plasma half-life: 10–30 hours after i.v. or oral dose (may be prolonged with hepatic dysfunction)
Total body clearance: 30–60 L/hr/m^2 (5% renal)

Diseases treated	
Curative intent:	Acute nonlymphocytic leukemia
Palliative intent:	Relapsed leukemias—acute lymphocytic and nonlymphocytic types
	Secondary acute leukemias (myelodysplastic, etc.)
	Breast carcinoma (no prior doxorubicin)
	Other carcinomas—experimental setting

Toxicities	
Acute:	Bone marrow suppression
	Mucositis, stomatitis
	Alopecia
	Nausea, vomiting, anorexia
	Flushing of face, torso
	Vein itching
Chronic:	Congestive cardiomyopathy (probably less than for daunorubicin)
	Vein streaking
Special concerns:	Radiation-recall dermatitis
	Extravasation necrosis of skin, subcutaneous tissue
	Dose reduction probably not necessary in face of impaired liver function

rubicinol is rapidly formed, and its levels in blood exceed those of idarubicin quickly after drug dosing. This metabolite persists for a long time and may be responsible for much of the antineoplastic effect of an idarubicin dose (192–194). After oral idarubicin doses, hepatic first-pass metabolism results predominantly in the appearance of idarubicinol in blood, with idarubicin concentrations being much lower and its presence short-lived (194). There may be prolongation of the half-life of idarubicin in the face of hepatic dysfunction, as occurs with doxorubicin, but the clinical importance of this phenomenon is uncertain.

Pharmacodynamic effects of idarubicin have been studied in acute leukemia (196, 197) and breast cancer (198). The leukemic cell content of idarubicin and idarubicinol were 400 and 200 times, respectively, the concentrations of these two species in plasma. In vitro sensitivity testing demonstrated the potency of idarubicin, with median inhibitory concentrations of 0.16 to 32 nM; these were about one-tenth of the corresponding inhibitory concentrations for daunorubicin. In breast cancer, lower plasma exposure to idarubicin, expressed as the area under plasma concentration-time plots, was encountered in patients with rapid progression of tumor than in responders. The same parameter correlated with depression in leukocyte counts, so that responding patients had higher drug exposures and lower leukocyte counts. While this is not a surprising finding in medical therapy of cancer, it does open the possibility of directing the intensity of therapy by pharmacokinetic monitoring, with a dosage-concentration-exposure relationship as a target for effective therapy.

Phase I and II studies of idarubicin have defined recommended dosages for both intravenous and oral therapy (199–206). In acute leukemia, daily intravenous dosages of 8 to 12 mg/m^2/day for 3 days have received widest attention. The same dosage has been given in conjunction with cytarabine in most studies. Oral doses are given at 45 to 60 mg/m^2 every 2 to 4 weeks on a single-day regimen, due to the very long persistence of the active metabolite, idarubicinol, in plasma. Daily-times-three oral regimens at 20 to 25 mg/m^2/day have been described for pediatric and adult leukemia patients (203, 205), and 4- to 5-day intravenous programs have been employed (202, 204), but there are no particular advantages in terms of response or toxicities with these modified schedules.

The approved clinical indication for idarubicin is in remission-induction therapy of acute nonlymphocytic leukemia (Table 21.11), but there are good data supporting its application to therapy of relapsed or refractory leukemias (201, 202, 204, 205), acute lymphocytic leukemia (203), and the myelodysplastic syndromes (206). Complete response rates of 40 to 80% are encountered in untreated leukemias, which is identical to results with daunorubicin, and survivals match those for patients responding to daunorubicin. In refractory/relapsed leukemias, response rates are 20 to 40%, again similar to the experience with daunorubicin. Adding cytarabine, as a daily injection, a continuous infusion, or on a high-dose schedule, to idarubicin has the same effect on response and survival as occurs with daunorubicin. In myelodysplastic syndrome, complete response rates of 50%, with partial responses of 50% have been reported. Again, this mimics the experience with daunorubicin, although the ability to give an oral therapy with a high therapeutic index to this group of typically elderly patients has quite an appeal.

Therapy of solid tumors with idarubicin must be regarded as palliative only. The best experience has been reported with breast cancer. In one study of oral idarubicin versus intravenous doxorubicin (207), the response rate for idarubicin was one-half that for doxorubicin (21 vs. 46%), and median survival was one-third shorter (14 vs. 20 months). In this study, the idarubicin was given orally and did not produce any cardiac toxicity or significant toxicities, in contrast to the notable alopecia, gastrointestinal damage, and cardiac damage that were seen with doxorubicin. Another study (208) of oral idarubicin found a 36% response rate in 50 patients, with one-quarter of these being complete remitters. Moderate toxicities, including alopecia and gastrointestinal signs, ensued. In seven patients receiving more than eight cycles of therapy, slight declines in cardiac ejection fraction occurred, in contrast to the other report. When the same oral dose, 45 mg/m^2/cycle, was divided into daily injections for 3 days, no objective tumor shrinkage was demonstrated in 22 patients (209). In all three trials, prior anthracycline chemotherapy was an exclusion for participation, so the discordant response rates and toxicity profiles are difficult to reconcile.

In lymphoma (210) and AIDS-related Kaposi's sarcoma (211), idarubicin failed to produce responders. However, all patients had progressed on prior chemotherapies, including doxorubicin, so the response rates in anthracycline-naive patients remains unknown. In non-small-cell lung cancer (212, 213), there were no responders to idarubicin among 38 participants, none of whom had had prior anthracyclines. For gastrointestinal cancers, response rates of 3 to 7% have been noted for colorectal (214), pancreatic (215), and esophagogastric (216) tumor patients. Genitourinary cancers are, likewise, poorly responsive to this agent, with no objective tumor regression in renal cell cancer (217) or ovarian carcinoma (218), and a very modest 10% partial remission rate in endometrial carcinoma (219), a disorder usually felt to be doxorubicin-sensitive (44). Finally, malignant melanoma is completely unresponsive to idarubicin (220).

The future of idarubicin depends on whether it can be applied to cancer therapies in novel ways—altered routes, schedules, or formulations—that distinguish it from daunorubicin. The oral route permits easy ambulatory therapy, and the interesting pharmacokinetics, with persistence of the cytotoxic metabolite, idarubicinol, for days after an oral dose, suggest possibilities for novel biochemical modulation schemes. The chemical reactivity of the carbonyl side chain of idarubicin, as with daunorubicin, permits linking of the drug to carrier molecules of interest. In one preclinical trial (221), the action of idarubicin linked to a monoclonal antibody was limited to the specific cells targeted by the antibody, while free idarubicin was cytotoxic to both targeted cells and other tumor cells not recognized by antibody. These kinds of modifications to drug activity may improve the selectivity of treatment sufficiently to stimulate studies in some of the unresponsive tumors noted above.

MITOXANTRONE

Directed searches for antitumor agents with certain chemical characteristics have yielded such medications as the benzoquinones (diaziquone [AZQ]), isobenzquinolines (amonafide), platinoids (carboplatin), nonclassic antifols (trimetrexate), and anthracenediones (mitoxantrone). That serendipity continues to play a substantial role in drug discovery and development is illustrated by the mitoxantrone story. Originally synthesized as stable dyes, the deeply colored anthracenediones languished until American Cyanamid researchers recognized that these compounds possessed the planar heterocyclic ring structure and basic side groups critical for effective intercalation into DNA (Fig. 21.8) and the quinone prosthetic group that could confer

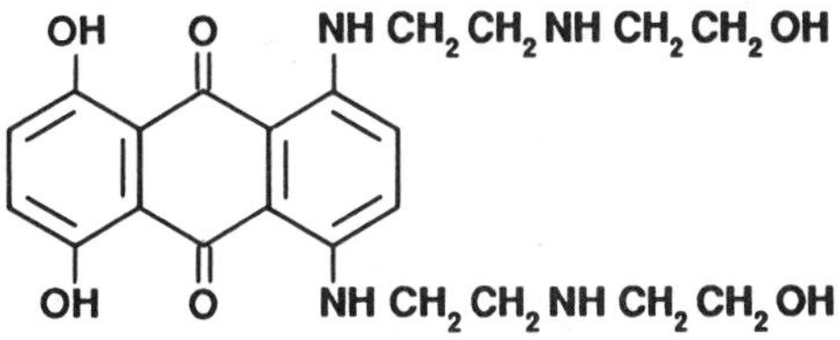

Mitoxantrone

Figure 21.8.   Structure of mitoxantrone. The tricyclic anthraquinone ring is planar, so it can intercalate into DNA. The positively charged, nitrogen-containing side chains project out from the molecule and serve to stabilize the ring in between DNA base pairs by interacting with the negatively charged phosphate backbone of DNA.

chemical reactivity (222). Three agents of this class—mitoxantrone, ametantrone, and bisantrene—have come to preclinical evaluation and clinical trial (223). Mitoxantrone was recently approved for therapy of acute leukemia and is the member of this class available for anticancer therapies now (Table 21.12).

Anthracenediones interact with DNA (224, 225), but the precise nature of the interactions and of the lesions produced is debated. Conflicting results indicate a high degree of (224), or very little (225), intercalation into DNA for mitoxantrone. There appears to be no base-specificity for intercalation (224). Alkaline elution assays of DNA integrity indicate both single- and double-stranded DNA breaks (225), most of which are protein associated. The frequency of DNA breaks in human leukemia cells exposed to combined mitoxantrone and cytarabine increased in a manner and to a degree suggesting true synergy between the drugs (226). The quinone-semiquinone structure of mitoxantrone initially led to the logical conclusion that generation of free radicals, with resultant intracellular oxidant stress, would be important in its mechanism of action. Subsequently, however, it has become clear that the capacity for free-radical production by mitoxantrone is limited (223, 227). Indeed, mitoxantrone inhibited the rate of lipid peroxidation in one model (227) and decreased the extent of doxorubicin-stimulated lipid peroxidation when both agents were included in the reaction mixture. The chemical rationale for this quenching effect and inability to activate mitoxantrone to the free-radical state may reside in the nitrogen-containing, basic side chains of mitoxantrone. Electrons transferred to the quinone-semiquinone nucleus can be redistributed into the

Table 21.12. Clinical and Pharmacologic Data for Mitoxantrone

Molecular weight: 444
Plasma half-life: 23–47 hours (prolonged with hepatic dysfunction)
Total body clearance: 13–34 L/hr/m^2 (40–50% hepatic; 5–10% renal)

	Diseases treated
Curative intent:	Acute lymphocytic leukemia
	Acute nonlymphocytic leukemia
	Non-Hodgkin's lymphomas (large cell)
Palliative intent:	Relapsed leukemias—acute lymphocytic and nonlymphocytic types
	Chronic myelocytic leukemia
	Multiple myeloma
	Non-Hodgkin's lymphomas
	Metastatic/recurrent osteogenic and soft tissue sarcomas
	Carcinomas of bladder, breast, head and neck, liver, lung, ovary (advanced), pancreas

	Toxicities
Acute:	Bone marrow suppression
	Mucositis, stomatitis
	Alopecia (less than for doxorubicin)
	Nausea, vomiting, anorexia
	Vein itching
Chronic:	Congestive cardiomyopathy (probably less risk than for doxorubicin)
	Bluish discoloration of veins, sclerae, nails
Special concerns:	Radiation-recall dermatitis
	Extravasation necrosis of skin, subcutaneous tissue (probably less than for doxorubicin)
	Reduce dose 50–75% in face of impaired liver function

electron-rich side chains via the process of intramolecular charge transfer and thus are not available to be transferred to molecular oxygen in the first critical steps of superoxide generation.

Mitoxantrone is not phase specific, having cytotoxic effects against cells in S-phase and inhibiting the G_2-M progression, but requires cycling cells for best action (223). The growth of a variety of animal and human cell lines is inhibited by mitoxantrone, including leukemias, adenocarcinomas, and sarcomas (223, 228, 229). In many cases, the therapeutic index or median inhibitory concentrations were much improved for mitoxantrone, compared with doxorubicin or other antitumor antibiotics (229). Overall, the spectrum of antitumor activity and the inhibitory concentrations of mitoxantrone required for activity compared well with those known for doxorubicin, suggesting the equivalence of the two agents in antineoplastic therapies.

Some of the numerous cell biologic effects are worth mentioning. In addition to interference with electron-transfer reactions, mitoxantrone inhibits hepatic microsomal cytochrome P-450

drug metabolism (230). The clinical impact of this as regards drug interactions in patients receiving mitoxantrone will be realized in postmarketing surveillance reports of unexpected or unusual toxicities. Platelet aggregation reactions are effectively inhibited by mitoxantrone, with potency comparable to that of aspirin (231). Although clinical bleeding is not likely to be enhanced by this interaction, the potential for tumor metastasis might be lessened in the face of local reductions in adhesiveness caused by inhibition of platelet aggregation. In like fashion, the effector arms of autoimmune functions appear to be paralyzed by mitoxantrone (232), with suppression of deleterious immunologic reactions.

Structural and other similarities between mitoxantrone and doxorubicin have fueled and directed investigations into mechanisms of resistance of tumor cells to mitoxantrone (25, 27, 223, 233, 234). Although cross-resistance to doxorubicin can be induced in tumor cells selected for resistance to mitoxantrone, such cells do not uniformly express the P-glycoprotein marker (233,

234) that is characteristic of doxorubicin resistance (25, 27). Also, uptake of mitoxantrone is much less affected than that of doxorubicin, suggesting there are alternative means by which the resistance is effected. Two groups (233, 234) have independently reported cytogenetic abnormalities in the mitoxantrone-resistance cells, with the chromosomal changes being found in different loci. It appears that there are novel gene expressions or amplification in mitoxantrone-resistant cells, which further distinguish this class of agents from the anthracyclines.

Study of the pharmacokinetics of mitoxantrone in humans has been hampered by the lack of assay techniques sensitive enough to detect drug concentrations encountered at typical clinical dosages. Simple absorbance methods can detect concentrations only as low as 1 ng/mL, which is the plasma level for mitoxantrone realized by 12 to 24 hours after single intravenous doses. Two methods with improved sensitivity have been reported, which should prompt reexamination of the human pharmacokinetics of mitoxantrone. Electrochemical detection of mitoxantrone (235) allowed measurement of concentrations as low as 0.1 ng/mL and permitted facile, on-line monitoring of parent drug. Whether metabolites could be as readily examined was not addressed. A radioimmunoassay (236) was developed by American Cyanamid investigators and gave a detection limit of 50 pg/mL (0.05 ng/mL). The major metabolite, a dicarboxylic acid of the side chains of mitoxantrone, was not detectable. Applications of these methods to clinical-pharmacologic trials may provide valuable insights into toxicities and potential drug interactions.

Because of the assay sensitivity problems mentioned above, the initial descriptions of human pharmacokinetics of mitoxantrone used observations from patients who received radioactive drug (237–239). The contribution of mitoxantrone and its metabolites to total plasma radioactivity of each sample was ascertained by high-performance liquid chromatographic separation of the components. The plasma disappearance half-life for mitoxantrone from these studies was about 40 hours, and recovery of unchanged drug in the urine was 6.5% of dose. Hepatic dysfunction or third-space fluid collections (ascites, etc.) prolonged the apparent half-life to 53 to 173 hours, suggesting the need for dosage reductions in patients so afflicted. Distribution of radioactivity occurred preferentially into cellular elements of blood and into tissues contributing to a high total-body clearance.

In one trial employing only absorbance detection of chromatographically analyzed serum samples, a very long terminal half-life of 217 hours was noted (240). Urinary studies demonstrated recovery of 6% of the administered dose, and urinary clearance amounted to only 6% of total-body clearance. Several metabolites were encountered in plasma and urine, and further analysis indicated the identity of two of these as the mono- and dicarboxylic acids of mitoxantrone. These metabolites are presumed to result from oxidation of the terminal hydroxyl groups present on the basic side chains of the parent molecule (241)

Distribution of mitoxantrone-derived radioactivity into tissue has revealed extensive tissue binding (239) and apparent correlation between the uptake of drug in the bone marrow and the level of myelosuppression. Long persistence of extractable mitoxantrone in tissues has been documented (239, 242), although the significance of this in light of mitoxantrone toxicities is speculative.

Phase I trials of mitoxantrone performed in cancer patients indicated the dosage of 10 to 12 mg/m^2 as single injection very 3 to 4 weeks was tolerated by patients with solid tumors (243). This can be compared with that for doxorubicin, 60 mg/m^2 every 3 weeks. Leukemia patients (244) could receive up to 5 days of treatment at that dosage level, as leukopenia was the dose-limiting toxicity in both trials. Prior to the demonstration of prolonged tissue persistence of mitoxantrone, a 24-hour continuous infusion schedule was examined, in the belief that such would increase the presence of the drug in tissues (245). The same maximally tolerated dosage, 12 mg/m^2/3 to 4 weeks was identified, so there appears to be no immediate advantage to this schedule. More recently, a protracted schedule of administration, continuous intravenous infusion for 21 days, was reported (246). The maximally tolerated dosage on this schedule was 1.1 mg/m^2/day, with leukopenia again dictating the limiting dosage. Since cycles were administered every 6 weeks in this study, the dosage rate of about 12 mg/m^2/3 weeks, identical to that for bolus injection, was achieved. In contrast, however, the total exposure to mitoxantrone, measured as area under plasma or leukocyte concentration-time curves, was twice as great for the prolonged infusion as for bolus injection. The application of these pharmacokinetic differences to therapy of human cancer would seem a fruitful clinical-pharmacologic enterprise.

Good clinical anticancer activity for mitoxantrone has been noted against acute leukemias (247–250), breast cancer (251–254), and lymphomas (255). Both as a single agent and in combination with cytarabine, mitoxantrone has induced responses in acute lymphocytic and nonlymphocytic leukemias. Response rates in relapsed leukemias are intimately tied to the chemoresponsiveness of the initial disease (247). The combination of mitoxantrone plus etoposide (VP16-213) has proven especially active in relapsed myeloid leukemias and may be of interest in the setting of acute leukemia complicating myelodysplastic syndromes (250).

In breast cancer, mitoxantrone as a single agent is comparable to doxorubicin, with responses occurring in 35 to 45% of anthracycline-naive patients (251). A large multicenter trial compared doxorubicin with mitoxantrone as second-line, single-agent therapy for advanced breast cancer (252). Participants were randomly allocated to receive doxorubicin, 75 mg/m^2, or mitoxantrone, 14 mg/m^2, repeated every 3 weeks. Response rates were 29% for doxorubicin and 20% for mitoxantrone, with about 10% of each responding group enjoying complete remission. However, the overall survivals were equivalent among the two groups, reflecting the limited numbers of responders. Toxicities were much less with mitoxantrone. In combination chemotherapy for metastatic breast cancer, similar results were obtained (253, 254). The response rates for cyclophosphamide and 5-fluorouracil, plus either doxorubicin (CAF) or mitoxantrone (CNF) were 37% and 29% respectively. No survival differences were encountered between the groups, and toxicities were somewhat less in the CNF group (253). A recently reported experience in lymphoma indicated more than 35% responders to mitoxantrone for Hodgkin's disease and non-Hodgkin's lymphomas, in patients relapsing from primary chemotherapy regimens, most having contained doxorubicin. As a single agent or a component of combination regimens, mitoxantrone has antilymphoma activity mimicking that of doxorubicin (223)

Mitoxantrone has demonstrated activity in ascites due to ovarian carcinoma (238, 239) and is active in metastatic disease recurring after cisplatin-based chemotherapies (256). Response has been noted in the occasional lung cancer patient (243), but most solid tumors other than those mentioned are relatively resistant to mitoxantrone (223). In most cases, antitumor activity less than that for doxorubicin has been recorded.

Because of the dose-limiting toxicity of myelosuppression and probably lesser degree of cardiac toxicity than for doxorubicin (see below), mitoxantrone has been included as a component of several high-dose chemotherapy regimens, delivered in the context of autologous bone marrow replacement. In combination with high-dose etoposide and thiotepa for relapsed breast cancer, mitoxantrone at 30 mg/m^2 contributed to the observed 61% response rate, of which 23% were complete remitters (257). The primary nonhematologic toxicity was mucosal, with high-grade mutositis in nearly 70%. Median duration of progression-free survival was 4 to 5 months. In conjunction with high-dose cyclophosphamide or high-dose melphalan (the latter substituted due to unacceptable urothelial toxicity with cyclophosphamide), mitoxantrone was studied in dose escalation with autologous marrow reconstitution (258). The maximally tolerated dosage of mitoxantrone with melphalan was 75 mg/m^2, delivered over 3 days. The limiting toxicity in this setting was, again, mucositis. Although patients with a variety of refractory solid tumors comprised the study group, 40% complete and 40% partial response rates were realized. Very high dose mitoxantrone can be delivered with manageable toxicities and should be the object of further study.

The toxicity spectrum for mitoxantrone is qualitatively similar to that of doxorubicin, but certain quantitative differences make mitoxantrone appealing as an alternative to its venerable cousin. The primary and dose-limiting side effects are leukopenia and thrombocytopenia, which has enhanced its role in therapy of acute leukemias. Anemia may also be seen, but is a later event. As with most agents in this class, nausea, vomiting, and anorexia occur and are usually less severe and as controllable as those complicating doxorubicin therapy. Delayed nausea seems less a problem than that with mitomycin or cisplatin. Stomatitis or other mucositis is uncommon at standard doses, but is more regularly observed with antileukemic dosages. All of these toxicities are more severe and more frequent in the face of pretherapy abnormalities of hepatic function (223). No data-based dosage reduction schemes have been elaborated, although 50 to 75% dose reductions have been described for patients with significant liver function impairment (253), apparently employing the same nomogram as reported for doxorubicin (74).

Mitoxantrone induces hepatic function abnormalities (223, 243, 247, 259, 260), typically of transaminases, and occasionally of alkaline phosphatase and bilirubin. These are usually of brief duration and entirely reversible. Although the significance of the observed changes in liver function is debated, more mucositis was detected in subsequent courses of therapy in individuals who had measurable hepatic toxicity with the first cycle of mitoxantrone (247, 259). Alopecia of lesser severity than that from anthracyclines is the rule with mitoxantrone. The curious circumstance of selective alopecia, with loss primarily of white hair, accompanied mitoxantrone therapy of chronic myelogenous leukemia (261). The more youthful appearance of the patients that resulted was regarded as a useful collateral benefit of therapy. The many other reported minor side effects of chemotherapy, such as rhinorrhea, headache, cough, constipation, and rash, occur with about the same frequency after mitoxantrone therapy as with anthracyclines.

The chemical effects of mitoxantrone give rise to other phenomena for which the clinician should be alert and about which the patient should be forewarned. The drug causes phlebitis in about 10% of veins injected and may impart a bluish discoloration to the vein (243). The bluenoses may be permanent. Although extravasation injury is a theoretic possibility with mitoxantrone, there appears to be a lesser incidence of this potential catastrophe than with the antibiotics. The small amount (5 to 7%) of mitoxantrone escaping unchanged into the urinary system imparts a green color to the urine for a day or two after therapy. Intraperitoneal therapy with mitoxantrone can be attended by serosal irritation and abdominal pain from the chemical vesicant properties of the agent (223, 238, 239).

The structural similarities between mitoxantrone and the anthracyclines aroused reasonable concern that mitoxantrone therapy might be associated with congestive cardiomyopathy. Animal studies (262, 263) suggested that mitoxantrone induces acute cardiac lesions that morphologically resemble those of doxorubicin. However, in contrast to the typically inexorable progression of doxorubicin-induced heart abnormalities, those pathologic lesions occurring after mitoxantrone therapy were frequently reversible. Mitoxantrone administered in the face of underlying doxorubicin heart damage (263) could worsen the pathologic lesions, but to a lesser degree than occurred with additional doxorubicin. There remained some evidence for reversibility, even with preexisting cardiac lesions.

Human trials of mitoxantrone have been carefully scrutinized for appearance of cardiac toxicity (243–256), with expectedly conflicting findings. In many cases, it has been difficult to separate the effects of prior doxorubicin, daunorubicin, mitomycin C, or mediastinal irradiation from mitoxantrone-induced cardiac changes. There now exist sufficient clinical observations and prospective monitoring to permit an assessment of the potential for mitoxantrone to cause cardiac damage (264–266). Cumulative dose-dependent declines in cardiac ejection fraction occur, in parallel with increases in systolic time interval measurements (264). These changes may improve with time, after cessation of mitoxantrone. The cumulative risk for cardiac toxicity was further estimated by evaluating patients receiving low, moderate, or high dosages of mitoxantrone per cycle (265) and adding in a factor reflecting prior doxorubicin therapy. Prior doxorubicin did increase the chances of developing mitoxantrone-related cardiotoxicity (congestive heart failure or decreased ejection fraction). Those on "high" dosage regiments were more likely to develop cardiotoxicity than those receiving "low" dosages. Examining only those patients with no prior doxorubicin, the incidence curve for cardiotoxicity rises gradually to a cumulative dosage of about 200 mg/m^2, then sharply increases. The level of 10% incidence of cardiotoxicity, which occurs at about 550 mg/m^2 for doxorubicin, is found with about 150 mg/m^2 for mitoxantrone. Given the equimyelotoxic comparative dosage ratio of 5:1 for doxorubicin to mitoxantrone, the equivalent dosage of doxorubicin causing 10% incidence of cardiomyopathy, as represented by the mitoxantrone curve, would be 750 mg/m^2. These data suggest that mitoxantrone has less potential for producing cardiotoxicity than does doxorubicin, but the reduction in risk is only moderate, at best. Great care and caution must be exercised in administering mitoxantrone to those with traditional risk factors for doxorubicin cardiac toxicity, and adhering to the same guidelines recommended for doxorubicin, as mentioned earlier in this chapter, would be prudent. The concern about long-term cardiac effects must be borne in mind, as cardiotoxicity has been reported to occur with respectable frequency in children (266). Delayed cardiotoxicity, as has been noted after doxorubicin (95), may yet be clinically recognized for mitoxantrone.

Regional chemotherapy with mitoxantrone was examined in early trials with the drug (238, 239) and has been expanded in two areas. In intraperitoneal therapy of ovarian carcinoma, dosages as high as 38 mg/m² could be administered with leukopenia as the major hematologic toxicity (49, 267). However, dosages in excess of 20 to 23 mg/m² induced a severe chemical peritonitis, usually necessitating narcotic analgesia for control. Although good effectiveness in controlling small residual disease masses was noted, with 33% surgically documented complete responders (49), the severe local toxicities would seem to militate against standard use of this therapeutic maneuver. Less toxic and equally effective intraperitoneal treatment with platinoid compounds is available.

Hepatic arterial mitoxantrone has been employed in hepatocellular carcinoma (268), analogous to the experience with doxorubicin. Approximately 25% of individuals had partial regressions of measurable tumor masses. However, marked leukopenia ensued and remained the dose-limiting toxicity. Of interest, some failing to respond to, or progressing on, mitoxantrone achieved a good response to salvage therapy with doxorubicin, which would indicate lack of complete cross-resistance between the agents.

The future for mitoxantrone as a reliable therapeutic agent will rest on identifying those regimens in which its lesser toxicities make it an attractive alternative to doxorubicin. In particular, the lessened cardiac toxicities may propel its use in the high-dose autologous transplantation setting for solid tumors, in which its substantial myelosuppression is not a liability. The intriguing notion of combined doxorubicin-mitoxantrone regimens should be further explored (223).

SUMMARY

Antitumor antibiotics are a diverse collection of drugs that share certain common structural features, mechanisms of action, toxicities, and anticancer activities. By appreciating the cellular pharmacologic and biochemical bases of their effects, a general understanding of the currently employed agents and their analogues can be achieved. This will allow better integration of these versatile drugs into present treatment programs and rational incorporation of future members of this class of agents into effective antineoplastic regimens. The striking differences among the antibiotics permit tailoring of investigational and treatment applications to maximize therapeutic responses, while minimizing the often substantial toxicities of individuals. Development of structural analogues of the existing agents and the identification of synthetic compounds whose mechanisms of action are similar to those of existing antibiotics will add valuable tools to cancer therapies that employ this class of drugs. Additional areas of research endeavor will include biochemical modulation, integrating treatment programs with biologic response modifiers, and new modifications of schedule and routes of administration.

REFERENCES

1. Robert J, Gianni L. Pharmacokinetics and metabolism of anthracyclines. Cancer Surv 1993;17:219–252.
2. Chabner BA, Myers CE, Coleman CN, Johns DG. The clinical pharmacology of antineoplastic agents. N Engl J Med 1975;292:1107–1113, 1159–1168.
3. Matney TS, Nguyen TV, Conner TH, et al. Genotoxic classification of anticancer drugs. Teratogenesis Carcinog Mutagen 1985;5:319–328.
4. Povirk, LF, Austin MJ. Genotoxicity of bleomycin. Mutat Res 1991;257:127–43.
5. Gutteridge, JMC, Quinlan GJ. Free radical damage to deoxyribose by anthracycline, aureolic acid, and aminoquinone antitumour antibiotics. Biochem Pharmacol 1985;34:4099–4103.
6. Southorn, PA, Powis, G. Free radicals in medicine. I. Chemical nature and biologic reactions. Mayo Clin Proc 1988;63:381–389.
7. Southorn, PA, Powis, G. Free radicals in medicine. II. Involvement in human disease. Mayo Clin Proc 1988;63:390–408.
8. Powis, G. Metabolism and reactions of quinoid anticancer agents. Pharmacol Ther 1987;35:57–162.
9. Sobell, HM, Jain, SC, Sakere, TD, et al. Stereochemistry of actinomycin-DNA binding. Nature (New Biol) 1971;231:200–205.
10. Dorr, RT, Bowden GT, Alberts DS, Liddil JD. Interactions of mitomycin C with mammalian DNA detected by alkaline elution. Cancer Res 1985;45:3510–3516.
11. Lazo, JS, Sebti SM. Bleomycin. Cancer Chemother Biol Resp Mod 1994;15:44–50.
12. Anyanwutaku, IO, Petroski RJ, Rosazza JP. Oxidative coupling of mithramycin and hydroquinone catalyzed by copper oxidases and benzoquinone. Implications for the mechanism of action of aureolic acid antibiotics. Bioorgan Med Chem 1994;2:543–551.
13. Fisher, J, Ramakrishnan K, Becvar JE. Direct enzyme-catalyzed reduction of anthracyclines by reduced nicotinamide adenine dinucleotide. Biochemistry 1983;22:1347–1355.
14. Bachur NR, Gee MV, Friedman RD. Nuclear catalyzed antibiotic free radical formation. Cancer Res 1982;42:1078–1081.

15. Pritsos, CA, Sartorelli, AC. Generation of reactive oxygen radicals through bioactivation of mitomycin antibiotics. Cancer Res 1986;46:3528–3532.

16. Mimnaugh EG, Trush MA, Bhatnagar, M, Gram TE. Enhancement of reactive oxygen-dependent mitochondrial membrane lipid peroxidation by the anticancer drug adriamycin. Biochem Pharmacol 1985; 34:847–856.

17. Gabizon AA. Liposomal anthracyclines. Hematol Oncol Clin North Am 1994;8:431–450.

18. Lown JW. Anthracycline and anthraquinone anticancer agents: current status and recent developments. Pharmacol Ther 1993;60:185–214.

19. Cummings J, Smyth JF. DNA topoisomerase I and II as targets for rational design of new anticancer drugs. Ann Oncol 1993;4:533–543.

20. van der Zee, AG, Hollema HH, de Bruijn HW, Willemse PH, Boonstra H, et al. Cell biological markers of drug resistance in ovarian carcinoma. Gynecol Oncol 1995;58:165–178.

21. Vamecq, J, Vallee L, Fontaine M, Nuyts JP, Lambert D, Poupaert J. Preliminary studies about novel strategies to reverse chemoresistance to Adriamycin regarding glutathione metabolism, peroxisomal and extraperoxisomal hydroperoxide and valproic acid metabolic pathways. Biol Cell 1993;77:17–26.

22. Nielsen D, Skovsgaard T. P-glycoprotein as multidrug transporter: a critical review of current multidrug resistant cell lines. Biochim Biophys Acta 1992; 1139:169–183.

23. Kruh GD, Goldstein LJ. doxorubicin and multidrug resistance. Curr Opin Oncol 1993;5:1029–1034.

24. Tsuruo T, Iida H, Tsukagoshi SY. Increased accumulation of vincristine and adriamycin in drug-resistant P388 tumor cells following incubation with calcium antagonists and calmodulin inhibitors. Cancer Res 1982;42:4730–4733.

25. Priebe W, Perez-Soler R. Design and tumor targeting of anthracyclines able to overcome mutidrug resistance: a double-advantage approach. Pharmacol Ther 1993;60:215–234.

26. Lum BL, Fisher GA, Brophy NA, Yahanda AM, Adler KM, et al. Clinical trials of modulation of multidrug resistance. Pharmacokinetic and pharmacodynamic considerations. Cancer 1993;72:3502–3514.

27. Ozols, RF, Cunnion RE, Klecker RW, et al. Verapamil and adriamycin in the treatment of drug-resistant ovarian cancer patients. J Clin Oncol 1987; 5:641–647.

28. Friedman MA, Carter SB. Serious toxicities associated with chemotherapy. Semin Oncol 1978;5:193–202.

29. Powis G. Anticancer drug pharmacodynamics. Cancer Chemother Pharmacol 1985;14:177–183.

30. DelaFlor-Weiss E, Uziely B, Muggia FM. Protracted drug infusions in cancer treatment: an appraisal of 5-fluorouracil, doxorubicin, and platinums. Ann Oncol 1993;4:723–733.

31. Blumenreich MS, Woodcock TM, Richman SP, et al. A phase I trial of dactinomycin intravenous infusion in patients with advanced malignancies. Cancer 1985;56:256–258.

32. Anderson N, Lokich JJ. Cancer chemotherapy and infusional scheduling. Oncology 1994;8:99–111.

33. Presser SE. Prevention of doxorubicin-induced hair loss. N Engl J Med 1980;302:921.

34. Rudolph R, Larson DL. Etiology and treatment

of chemotherapeutic agent extravasation injuries: a review. J Clin Oncol 1987;5:1116–1126.

35. Soble MJ, Dorr RT, Plezia P, Breckenridge S. Dose-dependent skin ulcers in mice treated with DNA binding antitumor antibiotics. Cancer Chemother Pharmacol 1987;20:33–36.

36. VanSloten Harwood K, Aisner J. Treatment of chemotherapy extravasation: current status. Cancer Treat Rep 1984;68:939–945.

37. Dahlstrom KK, Chenoufi H, Daugaard S. Fluorescence microscopic demonstration and demarcation of doxorubicin extravasation. Cancer 1990; 65:1722–1726.

38. Dorr RT, Alberts DS, Stone A. Cold protection and heat enhancement of doxorubicin skin toxicity in the mouse. Cancer Treat Rep 1985;69:431–437.

39. Powis G, Appel PL. Relationship of the single-electron reduction potential of quinones to their reduction by flavoproteins. Biochem Pharmacol 1980; 29:2567–2572.

40. Lawrence HJ, Walsh D, Zapotowski KA, et al. Topical dimethylsulfoxide may prevent tissue damage from anthracycline extravasation. Cancer Chemother Pharmacol 1989;23:316–318.

41. Dorr RT, Alberts DS. Failure of DMSO and vitamin E to prevent doxorubicin skin ulceration in the mouse. Cancer Treat Rep 1983;67:499–501.

42. Loth TS. Minimal surgical debridement for the treatment of chemotherapeutic agent-induced skin extravasations. Cancer Treat Rep 1986;70:401–404.

43. Donaldson SS, Glick JM, Wilbur JR. Adriamycin activating a recall phenomenon after radiation therapy. Ann Inter Med 1974;81:407–408.

44. Weiss RB. The anthracyclines: will we ever find a better doxorubicin? Semin Oncol 1992;19:670–686.

45. Berman E. Chemotherapy in acute myelogenous leukemia: high dose, higher expectations? J Clin Oncol 1995;13:1–4.

46. Doll DC, Weiss RB, Issell BF. Mitomycin: ten years after approval for marketing. J Clin Oncol 1985:3:276–286.

47. Bayer RA, Gaynor ER, Fisher RI. Bleomycin in non-Hodgkin's lymphoma. Semin Oncol 1992; 19(Suppl 5):46–53.

48. Mehta MP, Bastin KT, Wiersma SR. Treatment of Wilms' tumor. Current recommendations. Drugs 1991;42:766–780.

49. Markman M, George M, Hakes T, et al. Phase II trial of intraperitoneal mitoxantrone in the management of rafractory ovarian cancer. J Clin Oncol 1990; 8:146–150.

50. Blaney SM, Smith MA, Grem JL. Doxorubicin: role in the treatment of osteosarcoma. Cancer Treat Res 1993;62:55–73.

51. Schafers SJ, Dresler CM. Update on talc, bleomycin, and the tetracyclines in the treatment of malignant pleural effusions. Pharmacotherapy 1995; 15(2):228–235.

52. Bachur NR, Gordon SL, Gee MV. Anthracycline antibiotic augmentation of microsomal electron transport and free radical formation. Mol Pharmacol 1977; 13:901–910.

53. Bachur NR, Gee M. Microsomal reductive glycosidase. J Pharmacol Exp Ther 1976;197:681–686.

54. Huffman DH, Bachur NR. Daunorubicin metabolism by human hematological components. Cancer Res 1972;32:600–605.

55. Ahmed NK, Felsted RL, Bachur NR. Comparison and characterization of mammalian xenobiotic ketone reductases. J Pharmacol Exp Ther 1979;209:12–19.

56. Bachur NR. Adriamycin-daunorubicin cellular pharmacodynamics. Biochem Pharmacol 1974;23 (Suppl 2):207–216.

57. Cummings J, Anderson L, Willmott N, Smyth JF. The molecular pharmacology of doxorubicin in vivo. Eur J Cancer 1991;27:532–535.

58. Doroshow JH. Anthracycline antibiotic-stimulated superoxide, hydrogen peroxide, and hydroxyl radical production by NADH dehydrogenase. Cancer Res 1983;43:4543–4551.

59. Reif DW. Ferritin as a source of iron for oxidative damage. Free Rad Biol Med 1992;12:417–427.

60. Kanter PM, Schwartz HS. Adriamycin-induced DNA damage in human leukemia cells. Leuk Res 1979; 3:277–283.

61. Myers CE, McGuire WP, Liss RH, et al. Adrimycin: the role of lipid peroxidation in cardiac toxicity and tumor response. Science 1977;197:165–167.

62. Tannock I. Response of aerobic and hypoxic cells in a solid tumor to Adriamycin and cyclophosphamide and interaction of the drugs with radiation. Cancer Res 1982;42:4921–4926.

63. Potmesil M, Kirschenbaum S, Israel M, et al. Relationship of Adriamycin concentrations to the DNA lesions induced in hypoxic and euoxic L1210 cells. Cancer Res 1983;43:3528–3533.

64. Bachur NR, Steele M, Meriwether WD, Hildebrand RC. Cellular pharmacodynamics of several anthracycline antibiotics. J Med Chem 1976;19:651–654.

65. Keizer HG, Pinedo HM, Schuurhuis GJ, Joenje H. Doxorubicin (Adriamycin): a critical review of free radical-dependent mechanisms of cytotoxicity. Pharmacol Ther 1990;47:219–231.

66. Anderson RD, Berger NA. International Commission for Protection Against Environmental Mutagens and Carcinogens. Mutagenicity and carcinogenicity of topoisomerase-interactive agents. Mutat Res 1994;309:109–142.

67. Doroshow JH, Davies KJA. Redox cycling of anthracyclines by cardiac mitochondria. J Biol Chem 1986;261:3068–3074.

68. Goormaghtigh E, Ruysschaert JM. Anthracycline glycoside-membrane interactions. Biomed Biophys Acta 1984;779:271–288.

69. Riggs Jr. CE, Bennett JP. Clinical pharmacology of individual antineoplastic agents. In: Moossa AR, Schimpff SC, Robson MC, eds. Comprehensive textbook of oncology. 2nd ed. Baltimore: Williams & Wilkins, 1991:537–564.

70. Yates J, Glidewell O, Wiernik P, et al. Cytosine arabinoside with daunorubicin or adriamycin for therapy of acute myelocytic leukemia A CALGB study. Blood 1982;60:454–462.

71. Riggs CE, Benjamin RS, Serpick AA, Bachur NR. Biliary disposition of adriamycin. Clin Pharmacol Ther 1977;22:234–241.

72. Benjamin RS, Riggs CE, Bachur NR. Pharmacokinetics and metabolism of adriamycin in man. Clin Pharmacol Ther 1973;14:592–600.

73. Benjamin RS, Riggs CE, Bachur NR. Plasma pharmacokinetics of adriamycin and its metabolites in patients with normal hepatic and renal function. Cancer Res 1977;37:1416–1420.

74. Benjamin RS, Wiernik PH, Bachur NR. Adriamycin chemotherapy—efficacy, safety, and pharmacologic basis for an intermittent single high-dosage schedule. Cancer 1974;33:19–27.

75. Brenner DE, Wiernik PH, Wesley M, Bachur NR. Acute doxorubicin toxicity. Relationship to pretreatment liver function, response, and pharmacokinetics in patients with acute nonlymphocytic leukemia. Cancer 1984;53:1042–1048.

76. Sulkes A, Collins JM. Reappraisal of some dosage adjustment guidelines. Cancer Treat Rep 1987; 71:229–233.

77. Innis JD, Hurwitz A. Mechanism of hematocrit increase induced by the combined administration of morphine and adriamycin: role of histamine release. Toxicol Appl Pharmacol 1987;90:454–464.

78. Von Hoff DD, Layard MW, Basa P, et al. Risk factors for doxorubicin-induced congestive heart failure. Ann Intern Med 1979;91:710–717.

79. Dunn J. Doxorubicin-induced cardiomyopathy. J Pediatr Oncol Nurs 1994;11:152–160.

80. Steinberg JS, Cohen AJ, Wasserman AG, et al. Acute arrhythmogenicity of doxorubicin administration. Cancer 1987;60:1213–1218.

81. Billingham ME, Bristow MR. Evaluation of anthracycline cardiotoxicity: predictive ability and functional correlation of endomyocardial biopsy. Cancer Treat Symp 1984;3:71–76.

82. Pegelow CH, Popper RW, de Wit SA, et al. Endomyocardial biopsy to monitor anthracycline therapy in children. J Clin Oncol 1984;2:443–446.

83. Buzdar AU, Marcus C, Smith TL, Blumenschein GR. Early and delayed clinical cardiotoxicity of doxorubicin. Cancer 1985;55:2761–2765.

84. Bristow MR, Thompson PD, Martin RP, et al. Early anthracycline cardiotoxicity. Am J Med 1978; 65:823–832.

85. Speyer JL, Green MD, Dubin N, et al. Prospective evaluation of cardiotoxicity during a six-hour doxorubicin infusion regimen in women with adenocarcinoma of the breast. Am J Med 1985;78:555–563.

86. Weiss, AJ. Studies on cardiotoxicity and antitumor effect of doxorubicin administered weekly. Cancer Treat Symp 1984;3:91–94.

87. Anders RJ, Shanes JG, Zeller FP. Lower incidence of doxorubicin-induced cardiomyopathy by once-a-week low-dose administration. Am Heart J 1986;111:755–759.

88. Legha SS, Benjamin RS, Mackay B, et al. Reduction of doxorubicin cardiotoxicity by prolonged continuous intravenous infusion. Ann Inter Med 1982; 96:133–139.

89. Schwartz RG, McKenzie WB, Alexander J, et al. Congestive heart failure and left ventricular dysfunction complicating doxorubicin therapy: seven-year experience using serial radionuclide angiocardiography. Am J Med 1987;82:1109–1118.

90. Alexander J, Dainiak N, Berger HJ, et al. Serial assessment of doxorubicin cardiotoxicity with quantitative radionuclide angiocardiography. N Engl J Med 1979;300:278–283.

91. Borow KM, Henderson IC, Neuman A, et al. Assessment of left ventricular contractility in patients receiving doxorubicin. Ann Intern Med 1983;99:750–756.

92. Freter CE, Lee TC, Billingham ME, et al. Doxo-

rubicin cardiac toxicity manifesting seven years after treatment. Am J Med 1986;80:483–485.

93. Banks AR, Jones T, Koch TH, et al. Prevention of adriamycin toxicity. Cancer Chemother Pharmacol 1983:11:91–93.

94. Saini J, Rich MW, Lyss AP. Reversibility of severe left ventricular dysfunction due to doxorubicin cardiotoxicity. Ann Intern Med 1987;106:814–816.

95. Olson RD, Mushlin PS, Brenner DE, et al. Doxorubicin cardiotoxicity may be caused by its metabolite, doxorubicinol. Proc Natl Acad Sci USA 1988;85:3585–3589.

96. Curran CF, Narang PK, Reynolds RD. Toxicity profile of dexrazoxane (Zinecard, ICRF-187, ADR-529, NSC-169780), a modulator of doxorubicin cardiotoxicity. Cancer Treat Rev 1991;18:241–252.

97. Sokolove PM. Interactions of Adriamycin algycones with mitochondria may mediate Adriamycin cardiotoxicity. Int J Biochem 1994;26:1341–1350.

98. Hershko C, Link G, Tzahor M, Pinson A. The role of iron and iron chelators in anthracycline cardiotoxicity. Leuk Lymphoma 1993;11:207–214.

99. Rudolph R, Stein RS, Pattillo RA. Skin ulcers due to adriamycin. Cancer 1976;38:1087–1094.

100. Svingen BA, Powis G, Appel PL, Scott M. Protection by a-tocopherol and dimethylsulfoxide (DMSO) against adriamycin induced skin ulcers in the rat. Res Comm Chem Pathol Pharmacol 1981;32:189–192.

101. Forssen EA, Tokes ZA. Attenuation of dermal toxicity of doxorubicin by liposome encapsulation. Cancer Treat Rep 1983;67:481–484.

102. Gabel C, Eifel PJ, Tornos C, Burke TW. Radiation recall reaction to idarubicin resulting in vaginal necrosis. Gynecol Oncol 1995;57:266–269.

103. Perez CA, Einhorn L, Oldham RK, et al. Randomized trial of radiotherapy to the thorax in limited small-cell carcinoma of the lung treated with multiagent chemotherapy and elective brain irradiation: a preliminary report. J Clin Oncol 1984;2:1200–1208.

104. Greene W, Huffman D, Wiernik PH, et al. High-dose daunorubicin therapy for acute nonlymphocytic leukemia: correlation of response and toxicity with pharmacokinetics and intracellular daunorubicin reductase activity. Cancer 1972;30:1419–1427.

105. Huffman DH, Benjamin RS, Bachur NR. Daunorubicin metabolism in acute nonlymphocytic leukemia. Clin Pharmacol Ther 1972;13:895–905.

106. Weil M, Glidewell OJ, Jacquillat C, et al. Daunorubicin in the therapy of acute granulocytic leukemia. Cancer Res 1973;33:921–928.

107. Yates JW, Wallace HJ Jr, Ellison RR, Holland JF. Cytosine arabinoside (NSC-63878) and daunorubicin (NSC-83142) therapy in acute nonlymphocytic leukemia. Cancer Chemother Rep 1973;57:485–488.

108. Oberley LW, Schreiber AE, Rogers KL, et al. Antitumor therapies based on inhibition of antioxidant enzymes. In: Greenwald RA, Cohen G, eds. Oxy radicals and their scavenger systems. Vol 2: Cellular and medical aspects. Amsterdam: Elsevier, 1983:242–254.

109. Foon KA, Gale RP. Therapy of acute myelogenous leukemia. Blood Rev 1992;6:15–25.

110. Von Hoff DD. Use of daunorubicin in patients with solid tumors. Semin Oncol 1984;11(Suppl 3):23–27.

111. Woodcock TM, Allegra JC, Richman SP, et al.

Pharmacology and phase I clinical studies of daunorubicin in patients with advanced malignancies. Semin Oncol 1984;11(Suppl 3):28–32.

112. Lewis JP, Meyers FJ, Tanaka L. Daunomycin administered by continuous intravenous infusion is effective in the treatment of acute nonlymphocytic leukemia. Br J Hematol 1985;61:261–265.

113. Kim S. Liposomes as carriers of cancer chemotherapy. Current status and future prospects. Drugs 1993;46:618–638.

114. Lasic DD, Papahadjopoulos D. Liposomes revisited. Science 1995;267:1275–1276.

115. Amselem S, Cohen R. Barenholz Y. In vitro tests to predict in vivo performance of lipsomal dosage forms. Chem Phys Lipids 1993;64:219–237.

116. Gray A, Morgan J. Liposomes in haematology. Blood Rev 1991;5:258–272.

117. Bowen D, Goldman ID. The relationship among transport, intracellular binding, and inhibition of RNA synthesis by actinomycin D in Ehrlich ascites tumor cells in vitro. Cancer Res 1975;35:3054–3060.

118. Cooper HL, Braverman R. The mechanism by which actinomycin D inhibits protein synthesis in animal cells. Nature 1977;269:527–529.

119. Kessel D, Bosmann HB. On the characteristics of actinomycin D resistance in L5178Y cells. Cancer Res 1970;30:2695–2701.

120. Riehm H, Biedler JL. Potentiation of drug effect by Tween 80 in Chinese hamster cells resistant to actinomycin D and daunomycin. Cancer Res 1972; 32:1195–1200.

121. Medoff J, Medoff G, Goldstein MN, et al. Amphotericin B-induced sensitivity to actinomycin D in drug-resistant HeLa cells. Cancer Res 1975;35:2548–2552.

122. Papahadjopoulos D, Poste G, Vail WJ, et al. Use of lipid vesicles as carriers to introduce actinomycin D into resistant tumor cells. Cancer Res 1976; 36:2988–2994.

123. Tattersall MH, Sodergren JE, Dengupta SK, et al. Pharmacokinetics of actinomycin D in patients with malignant melanoma. Clin Pharmacol Ther 1975; 17:701–708.

124. Benjamin RS, Hall SW, Burgess MA. A pharmacokinetically based phase I-II study of single dose actinomycin D (NSC-3053). Cancer Treat Rep 1976; 60:289–291.

125. Frei E. The clinical use of actinomycin. Cancer Chemother Rep 1974;58:49–54.

126. Raine J, Bowman A, Wallendszus K, Pritchard J. Hepatopathy-thrombocytopenia syndrome—a complication of dactinomycin therapy for Wilms' tumor: a report from the United Kingdom Children's Cancer Study Group. J Clin Oncol 1991;9:268–273.

127. Cohen IJ, Loven D, Schoenfeld T, et al. Dactinomycin potentiation of radiation pneumonitis: a forgotten interaction. Pediatr Hematol Oncol 1991;8:187–192.

128. Lim LO, Neims AH. Mitochondrial DNA damage by bleomycin. Biochem Pharmacol 1987; 36:2769–2774.

129. Byrnes RW, Petering DH. Inhibition of bleomycin-induced cellular DNA strand scission by 1, 10-phenanthroline. Biochem Pharmacol 1991;41:1241–1248.

130. Takeshita M, Grollman AP, Ohtsubo E, et al.

Interaction of bleomycin with DNA. Proc Natl Acad Sci USA 1978;75:5983–5987.

131. Dorr RT. Bleomycin pharmacology: mechanism of action and resistance, and clinical pharmacokinetics. Semin Oncol 1992;19(Suppl 5):3–8.

132. Harvey VJ, Slevin ML, Aherne GW, et al. Subcutaneous infusion of bleomycin—a practical alternative to intravenous infusion. J Clin Oncol 1987;5:648–650.

133. Powis G. Effect of human renal and hepatic disease on the pharmacokinetics of anticancer drugs. Cancer Treat Rev 1982;9:85–124.

134. Williams SD, Birch R, Einhorn LH, et al. Treatment of disseminated germ-cell tumors with cisplatin, bleomycin, and either vinblastine or etoposide. N Engl J Med 1987;316:1435–1440.

135. Moffett MJ, Ruckdeschel JC. Bleomycin and tetracycline in malignant pleural effusions: a review. Semin Oncol 1992;19(Suppl 5):59–63.

136. Ostrowski MJ, Halsall GM. Intracavitary bleomycin in the management of malignant effusions: a multicenter study. Cancer Treat Rep 1982;66:1903–1907.

137. Schafers SJ, Dresler CM. Update on talc, bleomycin, and the tetracyclines in the treatment of malignant pleural effusions. Pharmacotherapy. 1995;15(2):228–235.

138. Hay J, Shahzeidi S, Laurent G. Mechanisms of bleomycin-induced lung damage. Arch Toxicol 1991;65:81–94.

139. McLeod BF, Lawrence HJ, Smith DW, et al. Fatal bleomycin toxicity from a low cumulative dose in a patient with renal insufficiency. Cancer 1987;60:2617–2620.

140. Ingrassia TS 3d, Ryu JH, Trastek VF, Rosenow EC 3d. Oxygen-exacerbated bleomycin pulmonary toxicity. Mayo Clinic Proc 1991;66:173–178.

141. McKeage MJ, Evans BD, Atkinson C, et al. Carbon monoxide diffusing capacity is a poor predictor of clinically significant bleomycin lung. J Clin Oncol 1990;8:779–783.

142. Bachur NR, Gordon SL, Gee MV. A general mechanism for microsomal activation of quinone anticancer agents to free radicals. Cancer Res 1978;38:1745–1750.

143. Van Hazel GA, Kovach JS. Pharmacokinetics of mitomycin C in rabbit and human. Cancer Chemother Pharmacol 1982;8:189–192.

144. Buice RG, Niell HB, Sidhu P, Gurley BJ. Pharmacokinetics of mitomycin C in non-oat cell carcinoma of the lung. Cancer Chemother Pharmacol 1984;13:1–4.

145. Schilcher RB, Young JD, Ratanatharathorn V, et al. Clinical pharmacokinetics of high-dose mitomycin C. Cancer Chemother Pharmacol 1984;13:186–190.

146. Hu E, Howell SB. Pharmacokinetics of intra-arterial mitomycin C in humans. Cancer Res 1983;43:4474–4477.

147. Dorr RT, Soble MJ, Liddil JD, Keller JH. Mitomycin skin toxicity studies in mice: reduced ulceration and altered pharmacokinetics with topical dimethyl sulfoxide. J Clin Oncol 1986;4:1399–1404.

148. Nigro ND, Seydel HG, Considine B, et al. Combined preoperative radiation and chemotherapy for squamous cell carcinoma of the anal canal. Cancer 1983;51:1826–1829.

149. Zincke H, Benson RC Jr, Hilton JF, Taylor WF. Intravesical thiotepa and mitomycin C treatment immediately after transurethral resection and later for superficial (stages Ta and Tis) bladder cancer: a prospective randomized, stratified study with crossover design. J Urol 1985;134:1110–1114.

150. Soloway MS. Treatment of superficial bladder cancer with intravesical mitomycin C: analysis of immediate and long-term response in 70 patients. J Urol 1985;134:1107–1109.

151. Dobrowsky D, Dobrowsky E, Strassl H, et al. Response to preoperative concomitant radio-chemotherapy with mitomycin C and 5-fluorouracil in advanced head and neck cancer. Eur J Cancer Clin Oncol 1989;25:845–849.

152. Bajorin D, Kelsen D, Mintzer DM. Phase II trial of mitomycin in malignant mesothelioma. Cancer Treat Rep 1987;71:857–858.

153. Konits PH, Aisner J, Van Echo DA, et al. Mitomycin C and vinblastine chemotherapy for advanced breast cancer. Cancer 1981;48:1295–1298.

154. Dees A, Verweij J, Van Putten WLJ, Stoter G. Mitomycin C is an inactive third-line treatment of hormone and chemotherapy refractory breast cancer. Eur J Cancer Clin Oncol 1987;23:1343–1347.

155. MacDonald JS, Woolley PV III, Smythe T, et al. 5-Fluorouracil, adriamycin, and mitomycin C (FAM): combination chemotherapy in the treatment of advanced gastric cancer. Cancer 1979;44:42–47.

156. Hagiwara A, Takahashi T, Lee R, et al. Selective delivery of high levels of mitomycin C to peritoneal carcinomatosis using a new dosage form. Anticancer Res 1986;6:1161–1164.

157. Rockwell S, Nierenburg M, Irvin CG. Effects of the mode of administration of mitomycin on tumor and marrow response and on the therapeutic ratio. Cancer Treat Rep 1987;71:927–934.

158. Luedke D, McLaughlin TT, Daughaday C, et al. Mitomycin C and vindesine associated pulmonary toxicity with variable clinical expression. Cancer 1985;55:542–545.

159. Verweij J, Van Zanten T, Souren T, et al. Prospective study on the dose relationship of mitomycin C-induced interstitial pneumonitis. Cancer 1987;60:756–761.

160. Chang AY, Kuebler JP, Pandya KJ, et al. Pulmonary toxicity induced by mitomycin C is highly responsive to glucocorticoids. Cancer 1986;57:2285–2290.

161. Buzdar AU, Legha SS, Tashima CK, et al. Adriamycin and mitomycin C: possible synergistic cardiotoxicity. Cancer Treat Rep 1978;62:1005–1008.

162. Cantrell JE Jr, Phillips TM, Schein PS. Carcinoma-associated hemolytic-uremic syndrome: a complication of mitomycin C chemotherapy. J Clin Oncol 1985;3:723–734.

163. Price TM, Murgo AJ, Keveney JJ, et al. Renal failure and hemolytic anemia associated with mitomycin C. Cancer 1985;55:51–56.

164. Sheldon R, Slaughter D. A syndrome of microangiopathic hemolytic anemia, renal impairment, and pulmonary edema in chemotherapy-treated patients with adenocarcinoma. Cancer 1986;58:1428–1436.

165. Valavaara R, Nordman E. Renal complications of mitomycin C therapy with special reference to the total dose. Cancer 1985;55:47–50.

166. Perry DJ. Reversible microangiopathic hemolytic anemia after mitomycin C. Cancer Chemother Pharmacol 1983;10:223.

167. Verweij J, Boven E, van der Meulen J, Pinedo HM. Recovery of mitomycin C-induced hemolytic uremic syndrome. Cancer 1984;54:2878–2881.

168. Ensminger WD, Gyves JW, Stetson P, Walker-Andrews S. Phase I study of hepatic arterial degradable starch microspheres and mitomycin. Cancer Res 1985;45:4464–4467.

169. Wollner IS, Walker-Andrews SC, Smith JE, Ensminger WD. Phase II study of hepatic arterial degradable starch microspheres and mitomycin. Cancer Drug Deliv 1986;3:279–284.

170. Audisio RA, Doci R, Mazaferro V, et al. Hepatic arterial embolization with microencapsulated mitomycin C for unresectable hepatocellular carcinoma in cirrhosis. Cancer 1990;66:228–236.

171. Rockwell S. Toxicity of intraarterial mitomycin C to previously irradiated tissues. Radiother Oncol 1986;6:75–76.

172. Kennedy BJ. Mithramycin therapy in testicular cancer. J Urol 1972;107:429–432.

173. Brown JH, Kennedy BJ. Mithramycin in the treatment of disseminated testicular neoplasms. N Engl J Med 1965;272:111–118.

174. Kiang DT, Loken MK, Kennedy BJ. Mechanism of the hypocalcemic effect of mithramycin. J Clin Endocr Metab 1979;48:341–344.

175. Hescock H Jr, Parker M, Wang TY, Ballinger R, Balducci L. Metastatic carcinoma of unknown primary: complete response to second-line treatment with plicamycin. Am J Med Sci 1989;298:34–37.

176. Evans JT, Tritsch GL, Mittelman A. Mithramycin inhibition of adenosine deaminase (ADA) activity (abstract). Proc Am Assoc Cancer Res Am Soc Clin Oncol 1979;20:85.

177. Purpura D, Ahern MJ, Shaverman N. Toxic epidermal necrolysis after mithramycin (letter). N Engl J Med 1978;299:1412.

178. Ahr DJ, Scialla SJ, Kimball DB Jr. Acquired platelet dysfunction following mithramycin therapy. Cancer 1978;41:448–454.

179. Monto RW, Talley RW, Caldwell MJ, et al. Observations on the mechanism of hemorrhagic toxicity in mithramycin (NSC-24559) therapy. Cancer Res 1969; 29:697–704.

180. Kennedy BJ. Metabolic and toxic effects of mithramycin during tumor therapy. Am J Med 1970; 49:494–503.

181. Weiss RB, Poster DS. The renal toxicity of cancer chemotherapeutic agents. Cancer Treat Rev 1982; 9:37–56.

182. Ryan WG, Schwartz TB, Fordham EW. Mithramycin and long remission of Paget's disease of bone. Ann Intern Med 1980;92:129–130.

183. Penco S, Casazza AM, Franchi G, et al. Synthesis, antitumor activity, and cardiac toxicity of new 4-demethoxyanthracyclines. Cancer Treat Rep 1983; 67:665–673.

184. DiMarco A, Casazza AM, Pratesi G, et al. Antitumor activity of 4-demethoxydaunorubicin administered orally. Cancer Treat Rep 1977;61:893–894.

185. Broadhurst MJ, Hassall CH, Thomas GJ. The total synthesis of 13(R)- and 13(S)-dihydro-4-demethoxydaunorubicin. Revision of stereochemistry of the microbial and mammalian reduction product of 4-demethoxydaunorubicin. Tetrahedron Lett 1984;25:6059–6062.

186. Capranico G, DeIsabella P, Penco S, et al. Role of DNA breakage in cytotoxicity of doxorubicin, 9-deoxydoxorubicin, and 4-demethyl-6-deoxydoxorubicin in murine leukemia P388 cells. Cancer Res 1989; 49:2022–2027.

187. Woods KE, Ellis AL, Randolph JK, Gewirtz DA. Enhanced sensitivity of the rat hepatoma cell to the daunorubicin analogue 4-demethoxydaunorubicin associated with the induction of DNA damage. Cancer Res 1989;49:4846–4851.

188. Formelli F, Casazza AM, DiMarco A, et al. Fluorescence assay of tissue distribution of 4-demethoxydaunorubicin and 4-demethoxydoxorubicin in mice bearing solid tumors. Cancer Chemother Pharmacol 1979;3:261–269.

189. Broggini M, Italia C, Colombo T, et al. Activity and distribution of iv and oral 4-demethoxydaunorubicin in murine experimental tumors. Cancer Treat Rep 1984;68:739–747.

190. Broggini M, Sommacampagna B, Paolini A, et al. Comparative metabolsim of daunorubicin and 4-demethoxydaunorubicin in mice and rabbits. Cancer Treat Rep 1986;70:697–702.

191. Cummings J, Milroy R. In vitro formation of a toxic aglycone metabolite of 4-demethoxydaunorubicin in conditions that parallel the stomach. Anticancer Res 1986;6:1177–1180.

192. Daghestani AN, Arlin ZA, Leyland-Jones B, et al. Phase I and II clinical and pharmacological study of 4-demethoxydaunorubicin (idarubicin) in adult patients with acute leukemia. Cancer Res 1985;45:1408–1412.

193. Tan CTC, Hancock C, Steinherz P, et al. Phase I and clinical pharmacological study of 4-demethoxydaunorubicin (idarubicin) in children with advanced cancer. Cancer Res 1987;47:2990–2995.

194. Berman E, Wittes RE, Leyland-Jones B, et al. Phase I and clinical pharmacology studies of intravenous and oral administration of 4-demethoxydaunorubicin in patients with advanced cancer. Cancer Res 1983;43:6096–6101.

195. Speth PAJ, van de Loo FAJ, Linssen PCM, et al. Plasma and human leukemic cell pharmacokinetics of oral and intravenous 4-demethoxydaunomycin. Clin Pharmacol Ther 1986;40:643–649.

196. Lu K, Savaraj N, Kavanagh J, et al. Clinical pharmacology of 4-demethoxydaunorubicin (DMDR). Cancer Chemother Pharmacol 1986;17:143–148.

197. Pui C-H, de Graff SSN, Dow LW, et al. Phase I clinical trial of orally administered 4-demethoxydaunorubicin (idarubicin) with pharmacokinetic and in vitro drug sensitivity testing in children with refractory leukemia. Cancer Res 1988;48:5348–5352.

198. Elbaek K, Ebbehoj E, Jakobsen A, et al. Pharmacokinetics of oral idarubicin in breast cancer patients with reference to antitumor activity and side effects. Clin Pharmacol Ther 1989;45:627–634.

199. Bonfante V, Verrari L, Villani F, Bonadonna G. Phase I study of 4-demethoxydaunorubicin. Invest New Drugs 1983;1:161–168.

200. Kaplan S, Sessa C, Willems Y, et al. Phase I trial of 4-demethoxydaunorubicin (idarubicin) with single oral doses. Invest New Drugs 1984;2:281–286.

201. Carella AM, Santini G, Martinengo M, et al. 4-Demethoxydaunorubicin (idarubicin) in refractory or relapsed acute leukemias. Cancer 1985;55:1452–1454.

202. Harousseau JL, Reiffers J, Hurteloup P, et al. Treatment of relapsed acute myeloid leukemia with idarubicin and intermediate-dose cytarabine. J Clin Oncol 1989;7:45–49.

203. Madon E, Grazia G, De Bernardi B, et al. Phase II study of idarubicin administered iv to pediatric patients with acute lymphoblastic leukemia. Cancer Treat Rep 1987;71:855–856.

204. Berman E, Raymond V, Daghestani A, et al. 4-Demethoxydaunorubicin (idarubicin) in combination with 1-B-D-arabinofuranosylcytosine in the treatment of relapsed or refractory acute leukemia. Cancer Res 1989;49:477–481.

205. Lowenthal RM, Chesterman CN, Griffiths JD, et al. Oral idarubicin as single-agent treatment of acute nonlymphocytic leukemia in poor-risk patients. Cancer Treat Rep 1987;71:1279–1281.

206. Johnson E, Parapia LA. Successful oral chemotherapy with idarubicin in refractory anemia with excess blasts. Eur J Haematol 1987;39:278–281.

207. Lopez M, Contegiacomo A, Vici P, et al. A prospective randomized trial of doxorubicin versus idarubicin in the treatment of advanced breast cancer. Cancer 1989;64:2431–2436.

208. Bastholt L, Dalmark M. Phase II study of idarubicin given orally in the treatment of anthracycline-naive advanced breast cancer patients. Cancer Treat Rep 1987;71:451–454.

209. Casper ES, Raymond V, Hakes TB, et al. Phase II evaluation of orally administered idarubicin in patients with advanced breast cancer. Cancer Treat Rep 1987;71:1289–1290.

210. Coonley CJ, Warrell RP Jr, Straus DJ, Young CW. Clinical evaluation of 4-demethoxydaunorubicin in patients with advanced malignant lymphoma. Cancer Treat Rep 1983;67:949–950.

211. Chachoua A, Green M, Laubenstein L, et al. Phase II study of oral idarubicin in patients with AIDS-associated Kaposi's sarcoma. Cancer Treat Rep 1987; 71:775–776.

212. Joss RA, Obrecht J-P, Alberto P, et al. Phase II trial of 4-demethoxydaunorubicin in patients with non-small cell lung cancer. Cancer Treat Rep 1984; 68:563–564.

213. Hochster HS, Green MD, Blum RH, et al. Oral 4-demethoxydaunorubicin (idarubicin) in bronchogenic lung cancer; phase II trial. Invest New Drugs 1986;4:275–278.

214. Harper HD, Kemeny NE, Ahmed T, et al. Phase II trial of 4-demethoxydaunorubicin in advanced colorectal carcinoma. Cancer Treat Rep 1984; 68:689–690.

215. Mittelman A, Magill GB, Raymond V, et al. Phase II trial of idarubicin in patients with pancreatic cancer. Cancer Treat Rep 1987;71:657–658.

216. Einzig A, Kelsen D, Cheng E, et al. Phase II study of 4-demethoxydaunorubicin in patients with adenocarcinoma of the upper gastrointestinal tract. Cancer Treat Rep 1984;68:1415–1416.

217. Scher HI, Yagoda A, Ahmed T, et al. Phase-II trial of 4-demethoxydaunorubicin (DMDR) for advanced hypernephroma. Cancer Chemother Pharmacol 1985;14:79–80.

218. Hakes TB, Daghestani AN, Dougherty JB, et al. Phase II study of 4-demethoxydaunorubicin in advanced ovarian carcinoma. Cancer Treat Rep 1985; 69:559–560.

219. Hakes TB, Raymond V. Phase II study of idarubicin in advanced endometrial carcinoma. Cancer Treat Rep 1987;71:535–536.

220. Stanton G, Casper ES, Friedman B. Phase II trial of 4-demethoxydaunorubicin in patients with advanced malignant melanoma. Cancer Treat Rep 1985; 69:915–916.

221. Pietersz GA, Smyth MJ, McKenzie AFC. Immunochemotherapy of a murine thymoma with the use of idarubicin monoclonal antibody conjugates. Cancer Res 1988;48:926–931.

222. White RJ, Durr FE. Development of mitoxantrone. Invest New Drugs 1985;3:85–93.

223. Faulds D, Balfour JA, Chrisp P, Langtry HD. Mitoxantrone. A review of its pharmacodynamic and pharmacokinetic properties, and therapeutic potential in the chemotherapy of cancer. Drugs 1991;41:400–449.

224. Kapuscinski J, Darzynkiewicz Z. Interactions of antitumor agents ametantrone and mitoxantrone (Novantrone) with double-stranded DNA. Biochem Pharmacol 1985;34:4203–4213.

225. Bowden GT, Roberts R, Alberts DS, et al. Comparative molecular pharmacology in leukemic L1210 cells of the anthracene anticancer drugs mitoxantrone and bisantrene. Cancer Res 1985;45:4915–4920.

226. Heinemann V, Murray D, Walters R, et al. Mitoxantrone-induced DNA damage in leukemia cells is enhanced by treatment with high-dose arabinosylcytosine. Cancer Chemother Pharmacol 1988;22:205–210.

227. Novak RF, Kharasch ED. Mitoxantrone: propensity for free radical formation and lipid peroxidation—implications for cardiotoxicity. Invest New Drugs 1985;3:95–99/

228. Wallace RE, Murdock KC, Angier RB, Durr FE. Activity of a novel anthracenedione,1,4-dihydroxy-5, 8-bis{{{2-[(2-hydroxyethyl)amino]ethyl}-amino}}-9, 10-anthracenedione dihydrochloride, against experimental tumors in mice. Cancer Res 1979;39:1570–1574.

229. Fujimoto S, Ogawa M. Antitumor activity of mitoxantrone against murine experimental tumors: comparative analysis against various antitumor antibiotics. Cancer Chemother Pharmacol 1982;8:157–162.

230. Kharasch ED, Wendel NK, Novak RF. Anthracenedione antineoplastic agent effects on drug metabolism in vitro and in vivo: relationship between structure and mechanism of inhibition. Fundam Appl Toxicol 1987;9:18–25.

231. Frank P, Novak RF. Effects of mitoxantrone and bisantrene on platelet aggregation and prostaglandin/thromboxane biosynthesis in vitro. Anticancer Res 1986;6:941–948.

232. Lublin FD, Lavasa M, Viti C, Knobler RL. Suppression of acute and relapsing experimental allergic encephalomyelitis with mitoxantrone. Clin Immunol Immunopathol 1987;45:122–128.

233. Dalton WS, Cress AE, Alberts DS, Trent JM. Cytogenetic and phenotypic analysis of a human colon carcinoma cell line resistant to mitoxantrone. Cancer Res 1988;48:1882–1888.

234. Harker WG, Slade DL, Dalton WS, et al. Multidrug resistance in mitoxantrone-selected HL-60 leukemia cells in the absence of P-glycoprotein overexpression. Cancer Res 1989;49:4542–4549.

235. Choi KE, Sinkule JA, Han DS, et al. High-performance liquid chromatographic assay for mitoxantrone in plasma using electrochemical detection. J Chromatogr 1987;420:81–88.

236. Nicolau G, Szucs-Myers V, McWilliams W, et al. Radioimmunoassay for mitoxantrone, a new antitumor agent. Invest New Drugs 1985;3:51–56.

237. Savaraj N, Lu K, Manuel V, Loo TL. Pharmacology of mitoxantrone in cancer patients. Cancer Chemother Pharmacol 1982;8:113–117.

238. Alberts DS, Peng YM, Bowden GT, et al. Pharmacology of mitoxantrone: mode of action and pharmacokinetics. Invest New Drugs 1985;3:101–107.

239. Alberts DS, Peng YM, Leigh S, et al. Disposition of mitoxantrone in cancer patients. Cancer Res 1985;45:1879–1884.

240. Ehninger G, Proksch B, Heinzel G, Woodward DL. Clinical pharmacology of mitoxantrone. Cancer Treat Rep 1986;70:1373–1378.

241. Chiccarelli FS, Morrison JA, Cosulich DB, et al. Identification of human urinary mitoxantrone metabolites. Cancer Res 1986;46:4858–4861.

242. Roboz J, Paciucci PA, Silides D, et al. Detection and quantification of mitoxantrone in human organs: a case report. Cancer Chemother Pharmacol 1984; 13:67–68.

243. Von Hoff DD, Pollard E, Kuhn J, et al. Phase I clinical investigation of 1, 4-dihydroxy-5,8-bis{{{2-[(2-hydroxyethyl)amino]ethyl}amino}}-9, 10-anthracenedione dihydrochloride (NSC 301739), a new anthracenedione. Cancer Res 1980;40:1516–1518.

244. Larson RA, Daly KM, Choi KE, et al. A clinical and pharmacokinetic study of mitoxantrone in acute nonlymphocytic leukemia. J Clin Oncol 1987;5:391–397.

245. Anderson KC, Garnick MB, Meshad MW, et al. Phase I trial of mitoxantrone by 24-hour continuous infusion. Cancer Treat Rep 1983;67:435–438.

246. Greidanus J, de Vries EGE, Mulder NH, et al. A phase I pharmacokinetic study of 21-day continuous infusion mitoxantrone. J Clin Oncol 1989;7:790–797.

247. Arlin ZA, Silver R, Cassileth P, et al. Phase I-II trial of mitoxantrone in acute leukemia. Cancer Treat Rep 1985;69:61–64.

248. Kaminer LS, Choi KE, Daley KM, Larson RA. Continous infusion mitoxantrone in relapsed acute nonlymphocytic leukemia. Cancer 1990;65:2619–2623.

249. Mittelman A, Rieber E, Friedland ML, Arlin ZA. Induction of remission in acute promyelocytic leukemia with mitoxantrone. Cancer Chemother Pharmacol 1985;14:81–82.

250. Ho AD, Lipp T, Ehninger G, et al. Combination of mitoxantrone and etoposide in refractory acute myelogenous leukemia: an active and well-tolerated regimen. J Clin Oncol 1988;6:213–217.

251. Stuart-Harris RC, Bozek T, Pavlidis NA, Smith IE. Mitoxantrone: an active new agent in the treatment of advanced breast cancer. Cancer Chemother Pharmacol 1984;12:1–4.

252. Henderson IC, Allegra JC, Woodcock T, et al. Randomized clinical trial comparing mitoxantrone with doxorubicin in previously treated patients with metastatic breast cancer. J Clin Oncol 1989;7:560–571.

253. Bennett JM, Muss HB, Doroshow JH, et al. A randomized multicenter trial comparing mitoxantrone, cyclophosphamide, and fluorouracil with doxorubicin, cyclophosphamide, and fluorouracil in the therapy of metastatic breast carcinoma. J Clin Oncol 1988;6:1611–1620.

254. Leonard RCF, Cornbleet MA, Kaye SB, et al. Mitoxantrone versus doxorubicin in combination chemotherapy for advanced carcinoma of the breast. J Clin Oncol 1987;5:1056–1063.

255. Silver RT, Case DC Jr, Wheeler RH, et al. Multicenter clinical trial of mitoxantrone in non-Hodgkin's lymphoma and Hodgkin's disease. J Clin Oncol 1991; 9:754–761.

256. Lawton F, Blackledge G, Mould J, et al. Phase II study of mitoxantrone in epithelial ovarian cancer. Cancer Treat Rep 1987;71:627–629.

257. Wallerstein R, Spitzer G, Dunphy F, et al. A phase II study of mitoxantrone, etoposide, and thiotepa with autologous marrow support for patients with relapsed breast cancer. J Clin Oncol 1990;8:1782–1788.

258. Mulder POM, Sleijfer DT, Willemse PHB, et al. High-dose cyclophosphamide or melphalan with escalating doses of mitoxantrone and autologous bone marrow transplantation for refractory solid tumors. Cancer Res 1989;49:4654–4658.

259. Paciucci PA, Sklarin NT. Mitoxantrone and hepatic toxicity (letter). Ann Intern Med 1986;105:805–806.

260. Shenkenberg TD. Mitoxantrone and hepatic toxicity (letter). Ann Intern Med 1986;105:806.

261. Arlin ZA, Friedland ML, Atamer MA. Selective alopecia with mitoxantrone (letter). N Engl J Med 1984;310:1464.

262. Tumminello FM, Leto G, Gebbia N, et al. Acute myocardial effects of mitoxantrone in the rabbit. Cancer Treat Rep 1987;71:529–531.

263. Tham P, Dougherty W, Iatropoulos MJ, et al. The effect of mitoxantrone treatment in beagle dogs previously treated with minimally cardiotoxic doses of doxorubicin. Am J Pathol 1987;128:121–130.

264. Unverferth DV, Unverferth BJ, Balcerzak SP, et al. Cardiac evaluation of mitoxantrone. Cancer Treat Rep 1983;67:343–350.

265. Mather FJ, Simon RM, Clark GM, Von Hoff DD. Cardiotoxicity in patients treated with mitoxantrone: Southwest Oncology Group phase II studies. Cancer Treat Rep 1987;71:609–613.

266. Ungerleider RS, Pratt CB, Vietti TJ, et al. Phase I trial of mitoxantrone in children. Cancer Treat Rep 1985;69:403–407.

267. Alberts DS, Surwit EA, Peng Y-M, et al. Phase I clinical and pharmacokinetic study of mitoxantrone given to patients by intraperitoneal administration. Cancer Res 1988;48:5874–5877.

268. Shepherd FA, Evans WK, Blackstein ME, et al. Hepatic arterial infusion of mitoxantrone in the treatment of primary hepatocellular carcinoma. J Clin Oncol 1987;5:635–640.

22

Microtubule-Targeting Drugs

Eric K. Rowinsky and Ross C. Donehower

Although the microtubule has been recognized as an important subcellular target of anticancer therapeutics, only two antimicrotubule agents, the vinca alkaloids vincristine and vinblastine, were widely utilized until the last decade. The recent identification of other classes of antimicrotubule agents that possess novel mechanisms of cytotoxic action and unique spectra of antitumor activity, such as the taxanes, semisynthetic vinca alkaloids like vinorelbine, and estramustine has resulted in a resurgence of interest in therapeutics directed at the microtubule. Most antimicrotubule agents are alkaloids, which are defined as structurally complex, plant-derived organic bases that possess pharmacologic activity. This chapter focuses on the two classes of alkaloids that have been widely incorporated into standard oncologic therapeutics—the vinca alkaloids and the taxanes. Estramustine, an agent rationally synthesized as an alkylating agent that affects microtubules, is also discussed.

Microtubules

Microtubules are composed of molecules of tubulin, each of which is a heterodimer consisting of two tightly linked subunits called α- and β-tubulin. Tubulin molecules assemble into microtubules by forming linear "protofilaments," with the β-tubulin subunit of one tubulin molecule in contact with the α-tubulin subunit of the next (1–3). Microtubules consist of 13 protofilaments aligned side by side around a seemingly hollow core. All protofilaments are aligned in parallel with the same polarity, that is, one end at which assembly is rapid (termed the "plus end") and one end in which assembly is slow or where net disassembly occurs (termed the "minus end"). Following polymerization, both α- and β-tubulin may undergo posttranslational modifications, which may account for the dis-

tinct functional differences of microtubules in various tissues (4, 5). Modified regions of polymerized tubulin also provide sites for the binding of microtubule-associated proteins (MAPs), which stabilize microtubules against disassembly, facilitate the initial nucleation step of tubulin polymerization, and mediate interactions with other cellular constituents (6, 7). The assembly and disassembly processes are in a dynamic equilibrium, the direction of which is influenced by both cellular and chemical mediators. In the intact cell, microtubules grow from a specific nucleating site or microtubule-organizing center, which is usually the centrosome. During rapid polymerization, the high concentration of free tubulin results in net assembly until a plateau phase is reached, at which time the rates of tubulin polymerization and depolymerization are balanced.

Each tubulin molecule is associated with two molecules of guanosine triphosphate (GTP); one is tightly bound to the α-tubulin subunit and the second, on the β-tubulin subunit, is readily exchangeable with free guanosine diphosphate (GDP) (8). GTP subunits are found only at the growing ends of microtubules, and the rate of growth depends on the availability of GTP. Microtubule growth at the plus end occurs spontaneously and results in the hydrolysis of GTP to GDP, which lowers the critical concentration required for polymerization and produces tighter binding of free tubulin (9, 10). In contrast, the minus end is bound tightly to the microtubule-organizing center, which prevents both assembly and disassembly at that end. The plus ends switch spontaneously from a slowing growing to a rapidly shrinking state, a process known as dynamic instability (11, 12). In mitosis, the rate of dynamic instability is accelerated, so that chromosomes can readily capture growing microtubules, thereby forming mitotic spindles;

MAPs suppress dynamic instability during many nonproliferative processes such as differentiation.

Vinca Alkaloids

The vinca alkaloids are naturally occurring or semisynthetic nitrogenous bases that are derived from the pink periwinkle plant, *Catharanthus roseus* G. Don (formerly *Vinca rosea* Linn). These compounds have a large dimeric asymmetric structure composed of a dihydroindole nucleus (vindoline), which is the major alkaloid in the periwinkle, linked by a carbon-carbon bond to an indole nucleus (catharanthine), which is found in much lower quantities. A single modification in the catharanthine ring, a methyl or formyl substitution (Fig. 22.1), is the only structural difference between vincristine (VCR) and vinblastine (VBL); however, the prototypic vinca alkaloids, VCR and VBL differ dramatically in their antitumor spectra and clinical toxicities. A third compound, vindesine (VDS; deacetyl VBL carboxamide), is a semisynthetic derivative and human metabolite of VBL that differs in two substituents attached to the vindoline nucleus and possesses somewhat unique toxicologic and pharmacologic properties. Although VDS is approved in Europe for the treatment of lung cancer, it has not been felt to have a unique role in cancer therapeutics in the United States and is therefore available only for investigational purposes. The semisynthetic VBL derivative vinorelbine (5'-norhydroVBL; VRL), which is structurally modified on the catharanthine nucleus and may not be completely cross-resistant with VCR and VBL, has also been approved in many countries for the treatment of non-small-cell lung cancer and is now approved in this country.

Mechanism of Action

Although the vinca alkaloids are capable of a wide range of biochemical and biologic activities that may or may not be related to their antimicrotubule effects, these agents mediate cytotoxicity principally by disrupting microtubules, particularly microtubules comprising the mitotic spindle apparatus, thereby facilitating metaphase arrest in dividing cells. Since microtubules are also involved in many nonmitotic functions, including chemotaxis, membrane and cellular scaffolding, intracellular transport, secretory processes, and transmission of receptor signals, it is not surprising that the vinca alkaloids also affect both nonmalignant and neoplastic cells in the G_1 and S phases of the cell cycle, in addition to mitosis (13–16).

The vinca alkaloids bind to sites on tubulin that appear to be distinct from the binding sites of the taxanes, GTP, colchicine, and many other synthetic compounds (17). At least two different sites, high-affinity and low-affinity sites, have been identified. The binding of the vinca alkaloids to high-affinity sites, which are found in low density at the ends of microtubules, results in the substoichiometric disruption of the microtubule assembly process (17–20). In fact, the binding of only one molecule of drug per micro-

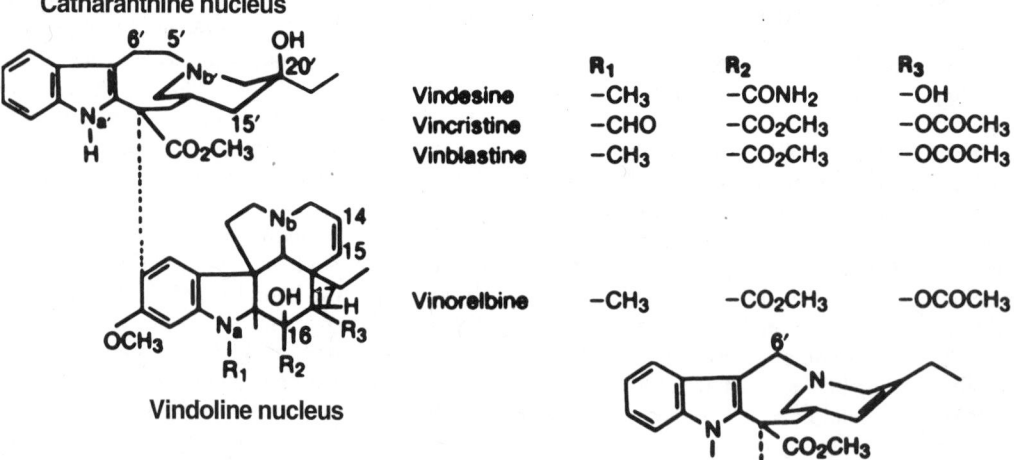

Figure 22.1.   Structural modifications of the vindoline nucleus and catharanthine nucleus in various *Vinca* alkaloids.

tubule may decrease the rate of microtubule assembly by as much as 50%. In essence, low concentrations of the vinca alkaloids, via binding to these high-affinity sites and modifying the dynamic equilibrium at the ends of microtubules, produce a "kinetic cap" at the plus end which accelerates the net disassembly of the microtubule at the minus end. The binding of the vinca alkaloids to low-affinity sites, which are situated along the wall of the microtubule, may induce the splaying of microtubules via a self-propagated mechanism into spiral aggregates or spiral protofilaments, leading to the formation of paracrystalline structures and the disintegration of microtubules (20). The cytototoxic effects of the vinca alkaloids are most clearly related to the induction of metaphase arrest by altering the dynamics of tubulin addition and loss at the ends of the mitotic spindle, which occurs at the lowest effective drug concentrations, with little or no microtubule depolymerization nor disorganization (21).

Mechanisms of Resistance

At least two different mechanisms that account for the rapid development of resistance to the vinca alkaloids in vitro have been elucidated; however, the clinical relevance of these mechanisms is not known. The best characterized mechanism is the phenomenon of pleiotropic, or multidrug, resistance (MDR), which results in decreased drug accumulation and retention and confers varying degrees of cross-resistance to other structurally bulky natural products, including the taxanes, anthracyclines, epipodophyllotoxins, actinomycin D, and colchicine (22). MDR is due to overexpression of the *mdr1* gene, which codes for a membrane P-glycoprotein (Pgp or P170) that functions as an energy-dependent plasma-membrane transport efflux pump. Pgp serves as a receptor for the vinca alkaloids, and drug resistance is proportional to the amount of Pgp (22–26).

Pgp is constitutively overexpressed by various normal tissues, including renal tubular epithelium, colonic mucosa, adrenal medulla, and other epithelial tissues (27). The protein has also been detected in several human cancers, particularly those derived from tissues in which the protein is constitutively overexpressed, such as kidney and large bowel carcinomas, posttreatment lymphomas, leukemias, and multiple myeloma. The specific Pgp associated with resistance to the vinca alkaloids differs slightly in amino acid sequence from Pgps from cells selected for resistance to other agents (28–30). These proteins also undergo posttranslational modifications, resulting in further structural diversity, which may explain the greater resistance to the specific agent used for selection and the variable degrees of resistance to other agents. Another important feature of MDR is that it is functionally reversible following treatment with various agents that have distinct structural and pharmacologic differences, such as the calcium channel blockers, calmodulin inhibitors, detergents, antibiotics, progestational and antiestrogenic agents, antihypertensives, antiarrhythmics, antimalarials, and immunosuppressives (22). These agents appear to bind directly to Pgp, thereby disrupting the pump's capacity to expel the vinca alkaloids and increasing intracellular drug concentrations.

The second mechanism of acquired drug resistance results from alterations in α- and β-tubulin proteins, possibly due to gene mutations or posttranslational modifications (31–34). These alterations result in either decreased drug binding or increased resistance to microtubule disassembly. Interestingly, these structural and functional alterations confer collateral sensitivity to the taxanes, which inhibit microtubule assembly.

Determinants of Sensitivity

There are undoubtedly other inherent, nonacquired factors that play a role in conferring differential cellular sensitivity and resistance to the vinca alkaloids. Several of these factors may explain the wide variability in tissue binding of the vinca alkaloids and, possibly, the substantial differences in their pharmacologic and toxicologic effects. Although the vinca alkaloids may demonstrate similar binding affinities and potencies against preparations of tubulin derived from any given tissue, these agents have different biologic activities in vivo, possibly because of their differential effects on various tubulin isoforms; differences in cofactors such as MAPs that influence interactions with tubulin; and differences in tissue permeation and cellular retention, which have been related to differences in cellular GTP content (35–46). There are also marked differences in cellular retention among the vinca alkaloids; VBL is accumulated to a much greater extent than either VCR or VDS. In addition, the degree of cellular accumulation of these compounds is directly related to drug lipophilicity, although a number of the aforementioned factors also undoubtedly play a role. Differences in pharmacologic characteristics may also account for differential sensitivity (see section on VCR pharmacology).

Vincristine (VCR)
Nomenclature and Structure

Generic name: vincristine sulfate

Commercial names: Oncovin, Vincasar, Vincrisul, Pericristine, Kyocristine

Chemical name: 22-oxovincaleukoblastine sulfate

Molecular weight: 923.0

Chemical formula: $C_{46}H_{56}N_4O_{10}H_2SO_4$

Availability: VCR for injection is available in 1-mL, 2-mL, and 5-mL vials for intravenous administration only. Each milliliter contains 1 mg of vincristine sulfate, the preservatives methylparaben and propylparaben or benzyl alcohol, citric acid and/or sodium citrate for pH adjustment, water, and occasionally mannitol.

Storage: VCR is sensitive to light and should be stored at 2 to 8°C; however, it is stable at room temperature for at least 1 month.

Administration: VCR is most commonly administered as a 1 mg/mL bolus injection through a freely running intravenous infusion. For administration of VCR as a longer infusion, drug concentrations of up to 16.7 mg/L in 5% dextrose have been maintained for 24 hours in glass and PVC containers with no loss of drug. When VCR solutions (1 mg/50 mL) in 5% dextrose or 0.9% sodium chloride are filtered at 3 mL/min through a 0.22 μm cellulose ester membrane filter (Ivex-2), 6.5% and 12% of drug, respectively, is bound and lost from solution.

Since VCR and the other vinca alkaloids are vesicants and may cause severe soft tissue injury, they should be administered only by trained oncology personnel. Every precaution should be made to ensure satisfactory placement of the indwelling venous catheter prior to drug administration, since extravasation of VCR into the dermal tissues may cause necrosis, cellulitis, and tissue sloughing. If extravasation occurs or is suspected, the infusion should be discontinued, and aspiration of any residual drug remaining in the tissues should be attempted. The application of local heat and injection of hyaluronidase 150 mg subcutaneously in a circumferential manner around the needle site are thought to minimize discomfort and the possibility of cellulitis (47). Inadvertent intrathecal administration is invariably fatal. Hepatic function should be evaluated prior to the administration of VCR (see sections on pharmacology and dosage).

Dosage: VCR is routinely administered to children (<10 kg) as an intravenous bolus injection at a dose of 2 mg/m² weekly; a dose of 0.05 mg/kg weekly is often used for smaller children. The standard weekly dose for adults is 1.4 mg/m² intravenously. A restriction of the absolute dose to 2 mg/m² (often referred to as "capping") has been largely adopted on the basis of early reports of severe neurotoxicity with higher doses. However, it has been suggested that "capping" be reconsidered in view of lack of supportive evidence (48). For most patients, the cumulative dose of VCR appears to be more critical than the magnitude of any single dose with respect to the development of severe neurotoxicity. In addition, significant interpatient variability exists, which may be due to large interindividual differences in drug exposure, and some patients are able to tolerate much higher VCR doses with little or no toxicity. VCR dose adjustments should be based on toxicity, particularly peripheral and autonomic neurotoxicity. However, VCR doses should not be reduced for the presence of mild neurotoxicity, especially if the drug is being used as part of a potentially curative treatment. VCR may have to be held for manifestations of a more serious neuropathy, such as painful paresthesias, peripheral motor weakness, cranial nerve palsies, or ileus, until resolution occurs. In clearly palliative settings, more liberal attitudes about modifying the therapeutic plan, such as dose reductions, lengthening of the intervals between doses, or selecting alternative drugs in the presence of moderate toxicity, may be justified in the event of moderate neurotoxicity.

Based on in vitro data suggesting that the duration of VCR treatment is an important variable in producing cytotoxicity, prolonged infusion schedules have been evaluated (49–51). Doses of 0.25 to 0.50 mg/m²/day as a continuous intravenous infusion for 5 days following a 0.5 mg/m² intravenous bolus dose have generally been well tolerated. Highly active combination chemotherapy regimens used in the primary and salvage treatments of patients with lymphoma (e.g., EPOCH [etoposide, prednisone, VCR, cyclophosphamide, and doxorubicin]) and multiple myeloma (VAD [VCR, doxorubicin, and dexamethasone]) have incorporated prolonged infusions of VCR (52,

53). In children, the administration of VCR as a 5-day infusion increases the dose that can be safely administered without major toxicity to twice that permitted with bolus schedules.

Since VCR is a potent vesicant, it should never be administered intramuscularly, subcutaneously, or intraperitoneally. Direct intrathecal injections of VCR or other vinca alkaloids (which have occurred as inadvertent clinical mishaps) induce a severe myeloencephalopathy, characterized by ascending motor and sensory neuropathies, encephalopathy, and rapid death. Administration of VCR 0.4 mg/day as a 5-day infusion into the hepatic artery has also been associated with profound toxicity, consisting of disorientation and diarrhea.

The major role of the liver in the disposition and metabolism of VCR dictates the need to consider dose modifications in patients with hepatic dysfunction (54); however, rigorous dosing guidelines have never been formally established. Standard guidelines stipulate a 50% reduction in dose for serum bilirubin concentrations between 1.5 and 3.0 mg/dL and a 75% reduction for a serum bilirubin concentrations above 3.0 mg/dL. Dose modifications for renal dysfunction are not indicated (55).

Pharmacology: Information regarding the pharmacologic behavior of the vinca alkaloids is limited for several reasons. Initially, the absence of sensitive and specific analytical assays capable of measuring the extraordinarily low drug concentrations in body fluids that result from the administration of milligram quantities of these agents precluded such analyses. To some extent, sensitive radioimmunoassay (RIA) and enzyme-linked immunosorbent assay (ELISA) methods that are capable of detecting picomolar drug concentrations have overcome this problem. However, early methods using polyclonal antisera were generally incapable of distinguishing between the parent compounds, metabolites, and degradation products, a task that is becoming feasible with high-performance liquid chromatography (HPLC), because of advances in HPLC extraction, separation, and detection methods.

Following standard doses of VCR as a bolus intravenous injection, peak plasma concentrations approach 0.4 μM (56). Plasma disposition is triphasic, with $T_{1/2\alpha}$ values below 5 minutes, due to rapid tissue binding, and $T_{1/2\beta}$ and $T_{1/2\gamma}$ values ranging from 50 to 155 minutes and 23 to 85 hours, respectively (49, 56–59). Similar pharmacokinetic parameters are noted in chil-

dren. Volumes of distribution (V_d) are high ($V_{d\gamma}$, 8.42 ± 3.17 L/kg), indicating extensive tissue binding (56, 57). Approximately 48% of VCR is bound to serum proteins. VCR also undergoes extensive binding to formed blood elements (especially platelets and red blood cells), which led in the past to the use of VCR-loaded platelets for treating disorders of platelet consumption such as idiopathic thrombocytopenia purpura. Poor drug penetration across the blood-brain barrier has been documented in most studies (60–64). In humans, VCR concentrations in cerebrospinal fluid are 20- to 30-fold lower than concurrent plasma concentrations and usually do not exceed 1.1 nM (64).

VCR is metabolized primarily by the liver and excreted in the stool and, to a lesser extent, in the urine. Seventy-two hours after the administration of radiolabeled VCR, approximately 12% of the radiolabel is excreted in urine (50% of which consists of metabolites), and approximately 70% is excreted in feces (40% of which consists of metabolites) (56). Metabolites appear rapidly in the bile, with only 46.5% present as unmetabolized VCR at 2 hours postinfusion. As many as 6 to 11 metabolites have been detected in both humans and animals; however, the structures of only two derivatives, 4-deacetylVCR and N-deformylVCR, have been identified (65, 66).

Differences in the biologic and toxicologic effects of the vinca alkaloids have been related to pharmacologic differences. In comparative studies of VCR, VBL, and VDS, VCR had the longest terminal $T_{1/2}$ and the lowest clearance rate; VBL had the shortest terminal $T_{1/2}$ and the highest clearance rate; and VDS had intermediate values (57, 58). It has been proposed that VCR's longer terminal $T_{1/2}$ and lower clearance rate account for its greater propensity to induce neurotoxicity. In addition to possible physiochemical determinants of sensitivity, cytotoxicity is directly related to the extracellular concentration of the vinca alkaloids when the duration of treatment is kept constant. However, the duration of drug exposure above a critical threshold concentration may be the most important determinant of cytotoxicity for the vinca alkaloids (49, 50, 67).

Indications: VCR has a broad antitumor spectrum and is an important component of combination chemotherapy regimens that commonly produce high remission rates in childhood and adult acute lymphocytic leukemias, Hodgkin's and non-Hodgkin's lymphomas, Wilms' tumor, Ewing's sarcoma, neuro-blastoma, and rhabdomyosarcoma (59). VCR is also commonly used in combination with other antineoplastic agents in multiple myeloma, chronic lymphocytic leukemia, lymphoblastic crisis of chronic myelogenous leukemia, sarcomas, and small cell lung carcinomas.

VCR has also been anecdotally reported to be useful in treating several nonmalignant hematologic disorders such as refractory autoimmune thrombocytopenia, hemolytic uremic syndrome, and thrombotic thrombocytopenia purpura (59, 68, 69).

Toxicities

Neurologic: Peripheral neurotoxicity is the principal toxicity of VCR (70–73). It is typically cumulative, and its severity is related to both total dose and duration of therapy. Initially, only symmetrical sensory impairment and paresthesias may be encountered, but neuritic pain, loss of deep tendon reflexes, ataxia, and motor dysfunction manifested by foot drop, wrist drop, paresis, and paralysis may develop with prolonged treatment. These signs may persist for months after treatment is discontinued. Severe motor dysfunction is usually irreversible or minimally reversible. Patients may also complain of bone, back, and limb pain. In adults, VCR-induced peripheral neuropathic effects may begin after cumulative doses of 5 to 6 mg and may be substantial after cumulative doses of 15 to 20 mg. Children may be less susceptible than adults; however, the elderly are particularly prone. Conventional doses of VCR have been associated with severe neurotoxicity in patients with antecedent neurologic disorders such as hereditary motor and sensory neuropathy type I, Charcot-Marie-Tooth disease, and childhood poliomyelitis (74, 75).

Despite the principal pathologic findings of primary axonal degeneration, peripheral nerve conduction velocities are generally normal except in patients with severe motor dysfunction. A VCR-induced acute necrotizing myopathy has also been reported (76).

Electroneurophysiologic studies typically reveal diminished amplitude of sensory and motor nerve action potentials and normal or slightly prolonged distal sensory and motor latencies (71–73, 77). Unmyelinated fibers may be the most sensitive to VCR, which may account for the early loss of deep tendon reflexes.

Cranial nerves may also be disrupted by VCR, resulting in hoarseness, diplopia, nerve deafness, jaw pain, pharyngeal pain, parotid gland pain, and facial palsies (71–73, 78). Although the uptake of the vinca alkaloids into the brain is low, VCR may rarely cause various central nervous system effects, including confusion, depression, agitation, insomnia, hypertension, hallucinations, seizures, coma, and the syndrome of inappropriate secretion of antidiuretic hormone (SIADH; see section on toxicity, endocrine). Visual disturbances, such as transient cortical blindness, retinal changes, and optic atrophy associated with blindness have also been observed (78, 80). Drug-induced neurologic syndromes characterized by ataxia and athetosis have also been associated with VCR.

Acute, severe effects of VCR on the autonomic nervous system are uncommon but may arise as a consequence of high-dose therapy (>2 mg/m^2) or in patients with altered hepatic function (81–83). Autonomic neurotoxic effects may include paralytic ileus, urinary retention, orthostatic hypotension, hypotension, and hypertension.

The potential for additive or synergistic effects of other neurotoxic chemotherapy agents (e.g., cisplatin) on vinca alkaloid–induced neurotoxicity have not been rigorously evaluated. The only known remedy for neurotoxicity associated with VCR is drug discontinuation or reduction of the dose and/or treatment interval. However, there have been attempts to ameliorate or prevent neurotoxicity with various agents such as thiamine, vitamin B$_{12}$, pyridoxine, and folinic acid, with no convincing successes (84–86). Folinic acid has been shown to protect mice against an otherwise lethal dose of VCR and has been used successfully in several cases of VCR overdosage in man; however, prospective studies have never been performed. Suggested doses for folinic acid for the treatment of overdosage are 15 mg every 3 hours for 24 hours and then every 6 hours for at least 48 hours. In a double-blinded, placebo-controlled randomized trial, coadministration of glutamic acid with VCR has been demonstrated to decrease VCR-induced neurotoxic effects such as loss of the Achilles tendon reflex and parasthesias (87). Glutamic acid also decreases the myelotoxicity of VBL. Although the mechanisms by which glutamic acid may inhibit the development of these toxic effects are unknown, possible mechanisms include interactions between the vinca alkaloids and glutamic acid at the microtubule level, since glutamic acid has been demonstrated to stabilize and polymerize tubulin, and competition for carrier-mediated transport or intracellular uptake at the level of the cell membrane.

Gastrointestinal: Constipation, abdominal cramps, weight loss, nausea, vomiting, oral ulcerations, diarrhea, paralytic ileus, intestinal necrosis and/or perforation, and anorexia may occur following the administration of VCR (88). Constipation due to autonomic nervous system dysfunction may be associated with impaction of stool in the upper colon; therefore, the rectum may be empty on digital examination, and an abdominal radiograph may be useful in diagnosing this entity. This condition may be responsive to high enemas and laxatives. A routine prophylactic regimen against constipation is therefore recommended for all patients receiving VCR. Paralytic ileus may also occur, particularly in pediatric patients. The ileus, which mimics a "surgical abdomen," will usually resolve with conservative therapy and temporary discontinuation of treatment.

Patients who receive high doses of VCR or have hepatic dysfunction may be especially prone to develop severe gastrointestinal complications due to autonomic neurotoxicity. Although success with drugs used prophylactically to minimize toxicity, including lactulose, caerulein, metoclopramide, and the cholecystokinin analogue sincalide, has been reported anecdotally, these agents may also alter the pharmacokinetic behavior of the vinca alkaloids by affecting biliary excretion and/or enterohepatic recirculation, which may ultimately result in increased drug clearance (89–93).

Genitourinary: VCR may cause bladder atony that can result in polyuria, dysuria, incontinence, and acute urinary retention because of drug-induced effects on the autonomic nervous system (82). Other drugs that are known to cause urinary retention,

particularly in the elderly, should, if possible, be discontinued for the first few days following VCR.

Cardiovascular: Hypertension and hypotension have been observed (see section on toxicity, neurologic). There have also been reports of acute myocardial infarctions following therapy with VCR (94).

Endocrine: VCR has been implicated as a cause of SIADH secretion by directly affecting either the hypothalamus, neurohypophyseal tract, or posterior pituitary gland and may cause symptomatic hyponatremia with seizures, particularly in patients receiving intensive hydration as part of their treatment (95). This drug-induced entity is accompanied by an actual increase in the serum ADH concentrations and usually remits within 2 to 3 days after onset. With fluid restriction, the hyponatremia improves as does SIADH due to other causes.

Hematologic: Severe myelosuppression is rare but may be a major feature of inadvertent VCR overdosage (96). However, mild to modest anemia, leukopenia, and thrombocytopenia may occur with conventional doses. VCR may induce an increase in circulating platelets as the result of endoreduplication of megakaryocytes (97).

Dermatologic: VCR-induced alopecia and rashes occur in approximately 20% of patients. VCR is considerably irritating to dermal tissues, and extreme care should be taken to prevent extravasation (see section on administration). Corticosteroids have also been reported to be useful in treating drug extravasation (98).

Miscellaneous: Fever without any other obvious etiology has occurred after treatment with VCR (99).

Vinblastine (VBL)
Nomenclature and Structure
Generic name: vinblastine sulfate
Commercial name: Velban, Velbe
Chemical name: vincaleukoblastine sulfate
Molecular weight: 909.1
Chemical formula: $C_{46}H_{58}N_4O_9H_2SO_4$
Availability: VBL is supplied in 10-mg and 25-mg vials at a concentration of 1 mg/mL with the preservatives phenol or benzyl alcohol and a 0.9% sodium chloride diluent. It is also available as 10 mg of lyophilized powder, which is

reconstituted with 10 mL of 0.9% sodium chloride (phenol or benzyl alcohol preservatives) to yield a concentration of 1 mg/mL at a pH of 3.5 to 5.

Storage: VBL, in its dry state or in solution, should be protected from light and stored at 2 to 8°C. At room temperature, intact vials are stable for at least 1 month. Once reconstituted and refrigerated, VBL may retain its potency for 30 days.

Administration: VBL is most commonly administered as a bolus injection through a freely running intravenous infusion. The solution for administration is usually prepared by adding 10 mL of 0.9% sodium chloride for injection to the 10-mg vial, which results in a solution with a VBL concentration of 1 mg/mL and a pH of 3.5 to 5. If protected from light, solutions prepared with preserved sodium chloride may be stored in the refrigerator for up to 30 days without significant loss of potency. The use of other solutions is generally not recommended. Alternatively, the drug may diluted in a larger volume of fluid (100 mL) and infused over longer periods (30 minutes).

VBL is occasionally infused over even longer periods, but as much as 10% of VBL at concentrations of up to 170 mg/L in 5% dextrose (glass and plastic containers) may be lost over 24 hours at room temperature (100). Solutions that contain 10 mg of VBL in 50 mL of 5% dextrose or 0.9% sodium chloride show no significant reduction in potency due to binding to 0.22-μm cellulose ester membrane filters (Ivex-2) when infused at 3 mL/min. However, 24% of drug is lost over 24 hours in solutions with drug concentrations of 1 mg/mL in 0.9% sodium chloride contained in an implantable pump (Infusaid 400); 48% is lost at 12 days, compared with a 0% and 20% loss of drug at 24 hours and 12 days, respectively, in glass containers. These data suggest that interactions between VBL and some component of the infusion device may occur (101).

Every precaution should be taken to ensure satisfactory placement of the indwelling venous catheter prior to the administration of VBL, since extravasation of drug into dermal tissues may cause necrosis, cellulitis, and sloughing. The catheter should be flushed before VBL is administered, to ensure patency. In addition, the site should be flushed again after the dose to ensure that all of the drug is delivered into the vein. If extravasation occurs or is suspected, the infusion should be discontin-

ued, and one should attempt to aspirate any residual drug remaining in the tissues. Application of local heat and injection of hyaluronidase 150 mg subcutaneously in a circumferential manner around the needle site are thought to minimize discomfort and the possibility of cellulitis (47). Like the other vinca alkaloids, VBL is a potent vesicant and should not be given intramuscularly, subcutaneously, or intraperitoneally. It is anticipated that intrathecal VBL would be fatal, as is the case with VCR. An oral preparation of VBL has been studied, but due to erratic absorption, oral administration is impractical.

Dosage: Since large variations in the degree of myelosuppression occur with VBL, the drug should not be given more frequently than once every 7 days. The most commonly used schedule utilizes a bolus injection at a dose of 6 mg/m² weekly in combination chemotherapy regimens. Approved recommendations for initial weekly dosing are 2.5 and 3.7 mg/m² for children and adults, respectively, followed by gradual dose escalation in increments of approximately 1.8 and 1.25 mg/m² each week. Dose escalations and modifications should be governed by hematologic tolerance. It is also recommended that doses of 18.5 mg/m² in adults and 12.5 mg/m² in children not be exceeded, although these doses are substantially higher than the doses that most patients can tolerate, even with less frequent schedules of administration. In VBL-containing chemotherapy combinations used to treat Hodgkin's disease, such as ABVD or the MOPP-ABV "hybrid," the individual VBL doses are 6 mg/m².

VBL has also been administered on prolonged infusion schedules to take advantage of the dependence of cytotoxicity on the duration of vinca alkaloid exposure (49, 50). Five-day continuous infusions of VBL have been utilized at doses ranging from 1.5 to 2 mg/m²/day, which achieve plasma concentrations of approximately 2 nM (102–104). However, there is little clinical evidence to support the notion that prolonged infusion schedules are more effective than bolus schedules.

As with VCR, dose modifications should be made for significant liver dysfunction. Although specific recommendations have not been rigorously formulated, standard guidelines stipulate a 50% dose reduction for serum bilirubin concentrations between 1.5 and 3.0 mg/dL, and a 75% reduction for serum bilirubin concentrations above 3.0 mg/dL. Dose reductions for renal dysfunction are not indicated (55).

Pharmacology: The pharmacologic behavior of VBL is similar to that described for VCR and principally reflects the extensive binding of VBL to plasma proteins and tissues. Although plasma protein binding has been reported to range from 43 to 99.7%, it most likely approaches the high end of this range (105–107). VBL is also extensively bound to formed peripheral blood elements, with 50% of radiolabeled drug bound to platelets and red and white blood cells within 20 minutes (107–109). Binding of VBL to platelets is extensive and probably the result of the high concentrations of tubulin in platelets.

As with the other vinca alkaloids, VBL's disposition in plasma is optimally fit by a triphasic pharmacokinetic model (105, 106). Distribution is rapid, with an initial half-life ($T_{1/2\alpha}$) of less than 5 minutes, due to extensive binding to tissues. VBL also appears to be more avidly sequestered in tissues than is VCR, in that 73% of the label is retained in the body 6 days after administration of radiolabeled drug (106). Values for β and terminal half-lives range from 53 to 99 minutes and 20 to 24 hours, respectively (57–59, 107, 110). Following an intravenous bolus injection of VBL at standard doses, peak plasma concentrations are approximately 0.4 μM (57–59, 110). Extended terminal half-lives and high steady-state drug levels have been reported following continuous intravenous infusions of VBL: 1.1 nM at 1 mg/m^2/day ($T_{1/2}$, 28 days); 3.3 nM at 1.7 mg/m^2/day ($T_{1/2}$, 3 days), and 6.6 nM at 2 mg/m^2/day (terminal $T_{1/2}$, 6 days) (111).

Disposition of VBL occurs primarily through hepatic metabolism and biliary excretion, which suggests that toxicity may be increased in patients with concurrent hepatic insufficiency and/or biliary obstruction (59, 107). Less than 15% of an administered dose is excreted in the urine, but fecal excretion of the parent compound is also low, which indicates that hepatic metabolism is significant. In dogs, 30 to 36% of radioactivity was found in the bile, and 12 to 17% in the urine over a 9-day period following administration of drug (59). In vitro studies suggest that the cytochrome P450 isoform CYP3A is involved substantially with VBL metabolism. DesacetylVBL (VDS), which may be as active as the parent compound, is the principal hepatic metabolite of VBL (59, 107, 110).

Indications: VBL has been an integral component of curative treatment regimens for testicular carcinomas and Hodgkin's and non-Hodgkin's lymphomas. A regimen termed PVB, consisting of cisplatin, VBL, and bleomycin, has until recently been the standard treatment for advanced carcinomas of the testes (112). VBL has been largely replaced by etoposide in this combination because of its more favorable toxicity profile (113). For Hodgkin's lymphoma, VBL is often used in combination with doxorubicin, bleomycin, and dacarbazine (ABVD). This regimen is either administered alone or alternated with MOPP (nitrogen mustard, VCR, procarbazine, and prednisone), which is "non-cross-resistant" to ABVD (114, 115). A MOPP/ABV "hybrid" regimen that includes both VCR and VBL has also been studied (116). Antineoplastic activity is also observed with VBL as a single agent or in combination with other antineoplastic drugs in carcinomas of the breast, bladder, and lung, Kaposi's sarcoma, choriocarcinoma, terminal phase of chronic myelogenous leukemia, mycosis fungoides, Letterer-Siwe disease (histiocytosis X), and choriocarcinomas that are resistant to other chemotherapy agents (117–124). Infusions of VBL or VBL-loaded platelets have been effective in some cases of refractory autoimmune thrombocytopenias, because of its avidity to platelets (125, 126).

Toxicities

Hematologic: Myelosuppression (in particular, neutropenia) is the principal toxicity of VBL. Thrombocytopenia and anemia are less common. Blood count nadirs occur within 4 to 10 days, with recovery in 7 to 21 days.

Gastrointestinal: Mucositis, pharyngitis, and stomatitis occur more frequently with VBL than with VCR, especially in patients receiving VBL on protracted schedules. VBL may also occasionally produce nausea and vomiting, anorexia, pain, diarrhea, and hemorrhagic enterocolitis. Other gastrointestinal effects, which may be related to direct drug effects on the autonomic nervous system, include constipation, ileus, and abdominal pain. These effects are more common with high single doses (e.g., >20 mg) or when VBL is used in combination with other neurotoxic agents such as cisplatin in chemotherapy regimens for patients with germ cell malignancies.

Neurologic: Neurologic effects are much

less common and severe than with VCR; however, the neurotoxic effects of vinca alkaloids are qualitatively similar, with sensory dysfunction and loss of deep tendon reflexes predominating (see section on VCR neurologic toxicities). Psychomotor depression, headaches, parotid gland pain, jaw pain, weakness, bone pain, adynamic ileus, urinary retention, orthostatic hypotension, ataxia, neuromyopathy, vocal cord paralysis, and convulsions may also occur. These effects are usually more pronounced in patients receiving VBL on protracted schedules.

Cardiovascular: Hypertension is the most common cardiovascular toxicity of VBL. Myocardial infarctions and cerebrovascular accidents suspected of being drug-related have occurred in patients undergoing chemotherapy with VBL given either alone or in combination with other antineoplastic agents, particularly cisplatin and bleomycin (94, 127). Raynaud's phenomenon has been reported to be a lingering toxic effect of this combination chemotherapy regimen (128). In one long-term follow-up study of patients who had received VBL, cisplatin, and bleomycin for germ cell cancer, symptomatic Raynaud's phenomenon had developed in 44%; however, an even higher percentage of patients had abnormal vasoconstrictive responses to cold stimuli (129). This does not appear to occur as frequently when etoposide is substituted for VBL. Improvement in symptoms has been reported with calcium channel–blocking agents such as nifedipine, but this therapy has not been evaluated prospectively in a randomized study (129).

Pulmonary: Acute pulmonary edema has occurred rarely after treatment with VBL (130). Other pulmonary effects, including acute bronchospasm, acute respiratory distress, interstitial pulmonary infiltrates, and dyspnea, have been noted, particularly in patients who have received or are receiving mitomycin (131).

Dermatologic: Mild and reversible alopecia is common. VBL induces photosensitivity reactions and may cause severe irritation to local tissues, including the cornea, following extravasation or contact. Like VCR, VBL is a vesicant, and the procedures used to administer drug and manage extravasation are similar to those described for VCR (47). Similar antidotes have also been recommended for VBL extravasation, including corticosteroids, diethylstilbestrol, and hyaluronidase, as well as a conservative approach (132).

Endocrine: A syndrome of inappropriate antidiuretic hormone (SIADH) secretion may occur that is similar to that described for VCR (133).

Miscellaneous: Pain in tumor-containing tissues may occur.

Vinorelbine (VRL)
Nomenclature and Structure
Generic names: vinorelbine ditartrate
Commercial names: Navelbine
Chemical name: 3',4'-didehydro-4'-deoxy-8'-norvincaleukoblastine [R-(R,R)-2,3-dihydroxybutanedioate (1:2)(salt)]
Molecular weight: 1079.12
Chemical formula: $C_{45}H_{54}N_5O_8:2C_4H_6O_6$

Availability: VRL for injection is a clear colorless to pale yellow solution in sterile water for injection, containing 10 mg of VRL per mL. It is available for injection in single-use, clear glass 1-mL (10 mg) or 5-mL (50 mg) vials. No preservatives or other additives are present.

Storage: The vials should be refrigerated at 2 to 8°C (36 to 46°F) and protected from light in the carton. Unopened vials are stable at temperatures up to 25°C (77°F) for up to 72 hours. Reconstituted VRL may be used for up to 24 hours under normal room light when stored in polypropylene syringes or polyvinyl chloride bags at 5 to 30°C (41 to 86°F).

Administration: The manufacturer recommends that the calculated dose of VRL be diluted to concentrations between 1.5 and 3.5 mg/mL in a syringe with either 5% dextrose or 0.9% sodium chloride or to concentrations between 0.5 and 2.0 mg/mL in an intravenous bag with either 5% Dextrose Injection, USP, 0.45% or 0.9% Sodium Chloride Injection, USP, 5% Dextrose and 0.45% Sodium Chloride Injection, USP, Ringer's Injection, USP, or Lactated Ringer's Injection, USP.

VRL is usually administered as a slow injection through a side-arm port into a running intravenous infusion or as a short intravenous infusion over 20 minutes. Shorter infusions over 6 to 10 minutes, which appear to be associated with a lower rate of inflammatory venous reactions, have also been recommended by the manufacturer. Oral administration has also been evaluated and appears to be well tolerated; however, an acceptable oral formulation is not yet available.

Dosage: VRL is most commonly administered intravenously at a dose of 30 mg/m^2 on a weekly or biweekly schedule. It is recommended that VRL should not be administered if the neutrophil count is below 1000/μL. Oral doses of 80 to 100 mg/m^2 given weekly are generally well tolerated (134). Other dosing schedules that have been evaluated include chronic oral administration of low doses and intermittent high-dose and prolonged intravenous infusions. As with other vinca alkaloids, the clearance of VRL is impaired in patients with hepatic dysfunction, and dose reductions should be considered in this setting (135). Approved recommendations include a 50% dose reduction for patients with serum bilirubin concentrations between 2 and 3 mg/dL and a 75% dose reduction for patients with serum bilirubin concentrations above 3.0 mg/dL. Dose reductions are not recommended for patients with renal insufficiency.

Indications: VRL is approved in the United States as either a single agent or in combination with cisplatin for the first-line treatment of patients with unresectable, advanced non-small-cell lung cancer. It has also demonstrated prominent antitumor activity in both minimally and heavily pretreated patients with metastatic breast carcinoma and activity in patients with advanced Hodgkin's and non-Hodgkin's lymphomas and ovarian carcinoma.

Pharmacology: VRL disposition in plasma has been described by both biexponential and triexponential pharmacokinetic models (134–141). As with the other vinca alkaloids, a rapid decay of VRL concentrations occurs in the first hour posttreatment, followed by slower elimination phases (T$_{1/2\gamma}$, 18 to 49 hours). Consequently, the plasma clearance rate is high, approaching hepatic blood flow. The V$_d$ at steady-state is large (20 to 75.6 L/kg).

VRL is extensively bound to platelets, lymphocytes, and plasma proteins, including α$_1$-acid glycoprotein, albumin, and lipoprotein (142). The magnitude of protein binding ranges from 80 to 91%, and the unbound fraction averages 0.14. Because of substantial binding to platelets, the percentage of drug bound in blood is approximately 98%. VRL is widely distributed, and high levels are found in all tissues

(tissue:plasma ratios of 20:80) except brain. Tissue distribution, except for fatty tissues, is greater than with other vinca alkaloids. VRL concentrations achieved in human lung are approximately 300-fold greater than plasma levels, and 3.4- and 13.8-fold higher than lung tissue concentrations achieved with VDS and VCR, respectively (143).

As with the other vinca alkaloids, the principal organ involved with drug disposition is the liver, with excretion into the feces (33 to 80%); urinary excretion represents only 16 to 30% of total drug disposition (138, 139). After treatment with radiolabeled drug, approximately 95% of the radioactivity excreted in the urine is in the form of unmetabolized VRL. Fecal excretion occurs slowly (>3 to 4 weeks in monkeys and humans), while complete urinary excretion occurs rapidly (>50% within 24 hours) (141). The recovery of VRL is incomplete (approximately 80% of total dose), even after prolonged collections, indicating substantial tissue binding and/or metabolism (138, 139). The liver plays a major role in drug metabolism. In vitro studies using liver extracts suggest that VRL is metabolized to both deacetylNVB and N-oxide (139, 141). Although VRL N-oxide does not appear to be an active cytotoxic agent, deacetyl-VRL may be as active as VRL (144). However, this may be of limited clinical significance, since metabolites have not been detected in blood and only small quantities have been found in urine.

VRL is active when given orally. Although 100% of total radioactivity is absorbed in animals after the ingestion of ^{3}H-VRL, the bioavailability of VRL formulated in powder-filled and liquid-filled gelatin capsules is 43% and 27%, respectively, in humans (134, 145). In patients with advanced cancers, peak plasma levels are achieved within 1 to 2 hours after an oral dose, and erratic pharmacokinetic behavior is not noted, indicating that oral administration may be feasible.

Toxicities

VRL shares many of the principal toxicities of VCR and VBL, particularly hematologic toxicity and neurotoxicity.

Hematologic: The dose-limiting toxicity of VRL on all schedules is neutropenia (146). Neutrophil count nadirs occur at 7 to 10 days posttreatment, and recovery is usually complete in 7 to 14 days. Myelosuppression is not cumulative and is readily reversible soon after the treatment is discontinued. Mild-to-moderate anemia is common, and clinically significant thrombocytopenia is rare. Thrombocytosis that is not associated with a coagulopathy may also occur.

Neurologic: VRL has been shown to have a lower affinity for axonal microtubules than for mitotic spindle microtubules, compared with both VCR or VBL, which seems to be confirmed by clinical results to date (146–148). A mild-to-moderate peripheral neuropathy, principally characterized by sensory symptoms, occurs in 7 to 31%, and gastrointestinal autonomic effects such as constipation are noted in as many as 30% of patients, with severe toxicity (e.g., paralytic ileus) in 2 to 3% (58, 148). As with the other vinca alkaloids, the incidence of neurotoxicity is related to the duration of treatment. In a study in patients with non-small-cell lung cancer randomized to treatment with either VRL alone, VRL and cisplatin, or VDS and cisplatin, the rate of severe neurotoxicity was lower in both the single-agent VRL and VRL-cisplatin arms than in the VDS/cisplatin arm (149). Furthermore, the addition of cisplatin did not significantly increase the incidence of severe toxicity above that observed with VRL alone. Reversible muscle weakness is occasionally noted after 3 to 6 months of treatment. Tumor pain and jaw pain have also been noted.

Gastrointestinal: The most common gastrointestinal toxicity of VRL is constipation. Although as many as 38% of patients experience nausea and vomiting, the incidence of severe toxicity is low (2 to 8%). Stomatitis and diarrhea of modest severity may occur in less than 20% of patients. Gastrointestinal effects are more common with oral administration.

Local Toxicity: Like other vinca alkaloids, VRL is a vesicant. Injection site reactions, including erythema, pain, and venous discoloration, occur in approximately 33% of patients (59, 148); however, severe local toxicity is uncommon (< 2%). The risk of phlebitis may increase if veins are not adequately flushed after treatment.

Miscellaneous: Six percent of patients have experienced chest pain with or without electrocardiographic changes suggestive of ischemia (148). However, many of the patients who experience chest pain have a history of either cardiovascular disease or thoracic neoplasms, and it has not been possible to determine whether the chest pain is due to drug-related phenomena, cancer, or exacerbation of underlying atherosclerotic cardiovascular disease. Pulmonary effects, characterized by dyspnea, have also been reported in approximately 5% of patients. Acute bronchospasm, which resembles an allergic reaction, typifies the most common pulmonary reaction. The second type is a subacute reversible reaction that is often associated with cough, dyspnea, and occasionally interstitial infiltrates. Corticosteroids have been felt to be beneficial in severe cases, and several patients have been retreated without sequelae. There is no evidence that VRL causes chronic pulmonary toxicity. Asymptomatic and transient abnormalities in liver function tests, particularly alkaline phosphatase, have been noted. Alopecia occurs in approximately 10% of patients.

Vindesine (VDS)

Nomenclature and Structure

Generic names: vindesine sulfate
Commercial names: Eldisine, Enisone. Although available in Europe and other areas, VDS is approved only for investigational use in the United States.
Chemical name: 3-carbamoyl-4-*O*-deacetyl-3-de(methoxycarbonyl)vincaleukoblastine; desacetyl vinblastine amide sulfate
Molecular weight: 851.9
Chemical formula: $C_{43}H_{55}N_5O_8H_2SO_4$

Availability: VDS for injection is supplied for investigational use in vials containing 5 mg of VDS as a lyophilized powder and 25 mg of mannitol, along with 5 mL of sterile diluent for reconstitution. The diluent contains 0.9% sodium chloride and benzyl alcohol for reconstitution to a drug concentration of 1 mg/mL and a pH of approximately 4.2 to 4.5.

Storage: VDS should be stored between 2 and 8°C (36 to 46°F). Reconstituted solutions retain their potency for 30 days when stored in this fashion.

Administration: VDS is commonly administered as a bolus injection through a freely running intravenous infusion. Precipitation will occur in solutions with pHs above 6. Therefore, dilution in multielectrolyte infusion solutions is not recommended. VDS has also been administered as a prolonged infusion. For prolonged intravenous infusions, the reconstituted solution can be further diluted with 5% dextrose or 0.9% sodium chloride, which results in solutions in which the drug is stable for at least 24 hours at room temperature (22 to 25°C) under normal lighting conditions. It is anticipated that intrathecal use of VDS would be fatal, as is the case with VCR.

Every precaution should be taken to ensure satisfactory placement of the indwelling venous catheter prior to the administration of VDS because extravasation into dermal tissues may cause necrosis, cellulitis, and sloughing. A 10-mL normal saline flush is recommended before and after drug administration to ensure the patency of the vein and flush any remaining drug from the tubing. Administration of 50 to 100 mL of fluid before and after the VDS infusion is recommended to minimize any delayed inflammation that may occur without apparent infiltration. If extravasation occurs or is suspected, the infusion should be discontinued, and one should attempt to aspirate any residual drug that may remain in tissues. Local heat application and injection of hyalouronidase 150 mg subcutaneously, circumferentially around the needle site, may minimize the discomfort resulting from extravasation of vinca alkaloids (47, 133).

Dosage: VDS is most commonly administered intravenously, as either a bolus injection or a brief infusion at a dose of 2 to 4 mg/m² every 7 to 14 days. It has also been administered in fractionated doses given as either an intermittent or continuous infusions over 1 to 5 days. Intermittent or continuous infusion schedules usually employ VDS doses of 1 to 2 mg/m²/day for 1 to 2 days or 1.2 mg/m²/day for 5 days every 3 to 4 weeks. As with the other vinca alkaloids, the relative therapeutic benefits of the various dosing schedules of VDS have not been rigorously evaluated.

Both hematopoietic and liver functions should be evaluated before treatment. Although firm dose modifications have not been established for VDS in patients with hepatic or renal dysfunctions, dose reductions should be considered in the presence of moderate-to-severe hepatic dysfunction, because of pharmacologic similarities with other vinca alkaloids and evidence suggesting that the liver has a significant role in its disposition and metabolism (See section on VCR dosage). Dose reductions for renal dysfunction are not indicated.

Pharmacology: The pharmacologic behavior of VDS is similar to that of the other vinca alkaloids. Following intravenous administration, plasma disposition is characterized by a triexponential model (57–59, 150). The drug is rapidly distributed to body tissues, as reflected in its brief α half-life of less than 5 minutes (3.2 minutes); β and terminal $T_{1/2}$s range from 55 to 99 minutes and 20 to 24 hours, respectively. VDS's relatively low clearance indicates that drug accumulation may occur with short-interval repetitive dosing schedules. VDS's very large V_d (58 L for the second phase and 600 L for the terminal phase), low renal clearance, and prolonged serum $T_{1/2}$s indicate that extensive tissue binding and delayed drug elimination may occur. Following intravenous bolus administration, peak plasma VDS concentrations range from 0.1 to 1.0 μM, approximately 16-fold higher than levels achieved with prolonged infusions (151–156). However, prolonged infusion schedules are associated with longer periods of drug exposure exceeding drug concentrations that induce cytotoxicity in vitro.

The liver is the principal organ responsible for the metabolism and excretion of VDS (151, 157, 158). Renal excretion accounts for only 1 to 13% of drug disposition (152, 154, 159). This disposition pattern indicates that dose reductions of VDS should be considered for patients with hepatic dysfunction (see section on dosage).

Indications: VDS is available only for investigational use in the United States. In some reports, response rates in non-small-cell lung cancer with combinations of VDS and cisplatin or mitomycin appear to be superior to those achieved with standard combinations or with either agent alone (160, 161). In addition, antineoplastic activity has been seen in acute lymphocytic leukemia, blast crisis of chronic myeloid leukemia, malignant melanoma, pediatric solid tumors, and metastatic renal, breast, esophageal, and colorectal carcinomas (162, 163); however, a unique role for VDS in oncology remains to be defined.

Toxicities: VDS exhibits varying degrees of the toxicities that occur with VCR and VBL. Major dose-limiting toxicities are hematologic and neurologic. These effects are increased in patients with preexisting hepatic dysfunction (164).

Hematologic: Neutropenia is the most common toxicity of VDS, with the nadir from single doses occurring in 7 days, with recovery in 14 days, and the nadir from 5-day continuous infusions in approximately 11 to 13 days, with recovery in 16 to 18 days. Thrombocytopenia is less severe than neutropenia, with platelet count depressions and recovery occurring in a time span that is similar to that of leukocytes. Ineffective erythropoiesis and thrombocytosis have also been reported.

Neurologic: Neurotoxic effects, including peripheral and autonomic nervous system manifestations, are similar to those described for VCR (see VCR, section on neurologic toxicities). Neurotoxicity is generally observed after 3 to 4 courses at conventional doses, but it is dose-limiting in only a small proportion of patients.

Gastrointestinal: Stomatitis and mucositis have occurred rarely. Nausea and vomiting have been observed. Gastrointestinal toxicity due to autonomic dysfunction (e.g., constipation, paralytic ileus) has also been described.

Dermatologic: Alopecia is relatively common. Rashes are noted in a small proportion of patients. As with the other vinca alkaloids, VDS is a potent vesicant, and care must be taken to avoid extravasation into the subcutaneous tissues during administration (see section on administration) (47, 132).

Miscellaneous: Fever, lethargy, cellulitis, and phlebitis have been infrequently associated with VDS. Acute ischemic events and myocardial infarctions have been described in the peritreatment period.

Drug Interactions: L-Asparaginase may modulate the clinical pharmacologic characteristics of VCR by decreasing its hepatic clearance, thereby increasing toxicity. To minimize this effect, VCR should be given 12 to 24 hours before L-asparaginase. VCR may also reduce the bioavailability of digoxin. Seizures associated with reduced plasma phenytoin concentrations by 50% have also been observed during treatment with the vinca alkaloids. Reduced phenytoin levels have been noted within 24 hours after dosing with both VCR and VBL, and low levels may persist for as long as 10 days (165, 166). The concurrent use of erythromycin and the vinca alkaloids, especially VBL, has also been associated with unusually severe toxicity, possibly due to the inhibitory effects of erythromycin on the cytochrome P450–mediated metabolism of the vinca alkaloids (167). On the other hand, VDS has been demonstrated to increase the plasma clearance of methotrexate (MTX) (168). In another study, VDS was also shown to decrease the hydroxylation of MTX (169). However, VDS did not affect cerebrospinal fluid levels of MTX (170).

Both VCR and VBL inhibit the efflux of MTX from leukemia cells in vitro, resulting in the intracellular accumulation of MTX (171, 172). However, the minimal concentrations of the vinca alkaloids required to achieve this effect in vitro (0.1 μM) are realized only momentarily during clinical treatment. In addition, the schedule that is most likely to achieve this effect, VCR followed by MTX, has not demonstrated therapeutic synergism in the L1210 murine leukemia model (173). Therapeutic synergism is noted with the sequence of MTX followed by VCR, but this interaction is not likely to be due the enhancement of MTX uptake. Thus, there seems to be very little justification for routine use of VCR pretreatment in high-dose MTX protocols. The vinca alkaloids and other antimicrotubule agents (e.g., taxanes) have also been demonstrated to inhibit the influx of the epipodyllotoxins into cells, resulting in less cytotoxicity in vitro (174); however, the clinical implications of this effect have not been evaluated. The rationale for the combination of the vinca alkaloids, particular VBL, with bleomycin in urologic malignancies was based on the possibility that therapeutic synergism may result from the synchronization of tumor cells by the vinca alkaloids in the G_2 and M cell-cycle phases (175), thereby facilitating the cytotoxic effects of bleomycin, which are G_2 phase–specific.

TAXANES

Although the taxanes affect microtubules, they are substantially different from the vinca alkaloids with respect to principal mechanisms of action, pharmacology, clinical indications, and toxicology.

The prototypic taxane, paclitaxel, was discovered as part of a National Cancer Institute program in which extracts of thousands of plants were screened for anticancer activity (176). It was initially isolated and supplied from the bark of the Pacific yew *Taxus brevifolia*. However, paclitaxel is also derived from alternate sources, including nonbark biomass, ornamental *Taxus* species, fungi, and especially semisynthetic processes. Currently commercial supplies of Taxol (Bristol-Myers Squibb) are manufactured using an approved partial synthetic process in which paclitaxel is made from a readily available precursor, 10-deacetylbaccatin III, derived from the needles of more abundant yew species such as the European yew *Taxus baccata*. Docetaxel, which is also derived semisynthetically from 10-deacetylbaccatin III, is slightly more water soluble than paclitaxel and is a more potent antimicrotubule agent in vitro; however, the clinical ramifications of this difference in potency is not known at this time (177). Docetaxel has recently been approved for treatment of anthracycline-refractory breast cancer in the United States, but it is approved for broader indications in breast and non-small-cell lung cancer in other countries.

The structures of paclitaxel and docetaxel are shown in Figure 22.2. Both are complex alkaloid esters consisting of a taxane system linked to a four-member oxetan ring at positions C-4 and C-5. The taxane rings of both paclitaxel and docetaxel, but not 10-deacetylbaccatin III, are linked to an ester at the C-13 position. Structure-function studies suggest that the moieties at the C-2' and C-3' positions on the C-13 side chain are crucial for the antimicrotubule properties of the taxanes (178). Neither the acetyl group at C-10 nor the phenyl group at C-5' on the C-13 side chain are required for in vitro activity, and the structures of paclitaxel and docetaxel differ in linkages at these positions.

Mechanism of Action: The binding site for paclitaxel on microtubules is different from the binding sites for exchangeable GTP, colchicine, podophyllotoxin, and vinblastine. Paclitaxel binds to the N-terminal 31 amino acids of the β-tubulin subunit in tubulin oligomers or polymers, rather than tubulin dimers (179, 180). Unlike colchicine and the vinca alkaloids, which prevent microtubule assembly, submicromolar concentrations of the taxanes

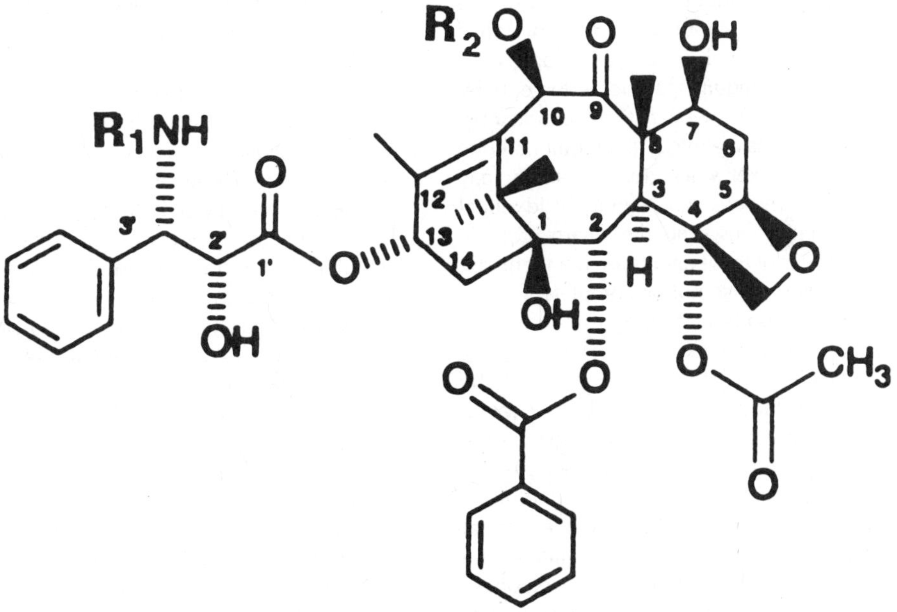

Taxotere : R_1 = -COOC(CH$_3$)$_3$; R_2 = H
Taxol : R_1 = -COC$_6$H$_5$; R_2 = -COCH$_3$

Figure 22.2.   Structures of the taxanes.

decrease the lag time, shift the dynamic equilibrium between tubulin dimers and microtubules toward polymerization, and stabilize microtubules against depolymerization (181–185). This excessive stability inhibits the dynamic reorganization of the microtubule network. The taxanes induce polymerization of tubulin in the presence or absence of factors that are usually essential for this function, such as exogenous GTP or MAPs. Docetaxel, which most likely shares the same tubulin binding site as paclitaxel, has a 1.9-fold higher effective affinity for the site (186, 187). The assembly of GDP- or GTP-tubulin induced by docetaxel also proceeds with a critical protein concentration that is 2.1-fold lower than that of paclitaxel.

At identical drug concentrations, the initial slope of the assembly reaction and the amount of polymer formed is greater for docetaxel. The cytotoxic effects of docetaxel are also several-fold greater than paclitaxel in vitro and in tumor xenografts (186, 188). The taxanes induce microtubule bundling in cells and in cell-free tubulin preparations (179, 182, 186, 187, 189). The agents also induce the formation of numerous abnormal mitotic asters, which, unlike mitotic asters formed under physiologic conditions, do not require centrioles for enucleation (188, 189). However, these characteristics may not translate into a greater therapeutic index for docetaxel, since greater potency may also result in more severe toxicity at identical drug concentrations, and the pharmacologic characteristics of these agents are not identical. The taxanes may also not be completely cross-resistant, but reports relating to cross-resistance are anecdotal at this juncture.

The taxanes inhibit proliferation of cells by inducing a sustained mitotic block at the metaphase/anaphase boundary at much lower concentrations than those required to increase microtubule polymer mass and microtubule bundle formation (191–192). These effects at low drug concentrations are associated with the formation of an incomplete metaphase plate of chromosomes and an arrangement of spindle microtubules resembling the abnormal organization that is induced by the vinca alkaloids (192). Aberrant mitotic spindle morphology and the mitotic block resulting from the stabilization of microtubule dynamics may be due to the inhibitory effects of the taxanes on intrinsic microtubule processes such as dynamic instability and "treadmilling" (i.e., the balanced net addition of tubulin at one end of the microtubule and the net loss of tubulin at the other end).

Following the disruption of microtubules and other cellular processes by the taxanes, the precise means by which cell death occurs are not clear. Morphologic features and a DNA fragmentation pattern that is characteristic of programed cell death, or apoptosis, in paclitaxel-treated human myeloid leukemia cells treated with paclitaxel indicate that the taxanes, like many other chemotherapeutic agents, may trigger apoptosis (193).

Both paclitaxel and docetaxel have been shown to enhance the cytotoxic effects of ionizing radiation in vitro at clinically achievable concentrations (<50 nM), which may be due to the inhibition of cell cycle progression in the G_2 and M phases, the most radiosensitive period of the cell cycle (194–196).

Mechanisms of Resistance: As with the vinca alkaloids, two mechanisms of acquired taxane resistance have been described in cells made resistant by prolonged treatment at low drug concentrations; however, both mechanisms have not been shown to develop in human tumors treated with the taxanes. Several mutant cell lines have structurally altered α- and β-tubulins and an impaired ability to polymerize tubulin dimers into microtubules (See section on vinca alkaloids, mechanisms of resistance) (33, 34, 197, 198). These cells lack normal microtubules in their interpolar mitotic spindles and have an inherently slow rate of microtubule assembly when grown in the absence of drug. The continuous presence of the taxanes is required for microtubule assembly to proceed. These mutants are also collaterally sensitive to the vinca alkaloids.

The second mechanism of acquired taxane resistance fits the general pattern of MDR (22–30, 199, 200, 203). Several different Pgps are overexpressed in taxane-resistant cells that exhibit MDR. Some Pgps from paclitaxel-resistant murine cells are similar, but not identical, to those found in vinblastine- and colchicine-resistant cells derived from the same parental line. These cells are cross-resistant with many other natural products, and resistance to both paclitaxel and docetaxel conferred by *mdr* can be reversed by many classes of drugs including the calcium channel blockers, tamoxifen, cyclosporin A, antiarrhythmic agents, and even the principal component of the vehicle used to formulate paclitaxel, Cremophor EL (polyoxyethylated castor oil) (199–203). In fact, plasma concentrations of Cremophor EL achieved with 3-hour infusions of paclitaxel 135 to 175 mg/m^2 in most patients are capable of reversing MDR in vitro (203). The early results of studies evaluating the role of MDR in conferring resistance to the taxanes in the clinic also suggest a lack of complete cross-resistance between the taxanes and anthracyclines (204).

Although the precise mechanisms for inherent taxane resistance are not known, cytotoxicity has been related to the propensity of human leukemia cells to form irreversible microtubule bundles in vitro and indirectly related to DNA polyploidy (189). Microtubule bundles and DNA polyploidy may prove to be useful correlates of lethal drug effects in the clinic (205).

Resistance to the taxanes may also be related to pharmacologic determinants. Perhaps the most important determinant of sensitivity to the taxanes in terms of cytotoxicity in vitro, toxicity, and perhaps clinical antitumor activity is the duration of drug exposure above a biologically relevant drug concentration or "threshold." For paclitaxel, the severity of neutropenia has been shown to be related to the duration of pharmacologic exposure above biologically relevant plasma concentrations ranging from 0.05 to 0.10 μM (206–208). In uncontrolled single-arm trials of paclitaxel in previously treated patients with breast cancer, the use of prolonged (96 hour) infusion schedules has resulted in impressive response rates and activity (209). In addition, impressive activity has been noted in patients with metastatic breast cancer treated with prolonged 96-hour infusions after disease progression shortly after treatment with paclitaxel on shorter schedules (210).

Paclitaxel

Nomenclature and Structure

Generic name: paclitaxel

Commercial names: Taxol, Anzatax

Chemical name: 5β,20-epoxy-1,2α,4,7β, 10β,13α-hexahydroxytax-11-en-9-one 4, 10-diacetate 2-benzoate 13-ester with (2R, 3S)-N-benzoyl-3-phenylisoserine

Molecular weight: 853.9

Availability: Paclitaxel for injection is available as a concentrated sterile solution in a 5-mL ampule. Each milliliter contains 6 mg of paclitaxel (30 mg/ampule) in polyoxyethylated castor oil (Cremophor EL) 50% and dehydrated alcohol, USP 50%. The contents of the ampule must be diluted before use.

Storage: Unopened vials should be refrigerated at 2 to 8°C (36 to 46°F). It is recommended that the vials be protected from light. Freezing does not adversely affect the agent. Upon refrigeration, components in the original vial may precipitate but will redissolve upon reaching room temperature, with little or no agitation. If the solution remains cloudy or if an insoluble precipitate is noted, the vial should be discarded.

Administration: Paclitaxel must be diluted in either 0.9% Sodium Chloride Injection, USP, 5% Dextrose Injection, USP, or 5% Dextrose and 0.9% Sodium Chloride Injection, USP, or 5% Dextrose in Ringers Injection, USP, to a final concentration of 0.3 to 1.2 mg/mL. The solutions are physically and chemically stable for up to 27 hours at room temperature and normal lighting conditions. Paclitaxel is usually infused over 3 or 24 hours every 3 weeks. Experience with other schedules as brief as 1 hour and as long as 96 hours has also been reported (209–211). Due to paclitaxel's aqueous insolubility, it is formulated in Cremophor EL (polyoxyethylated castor oil) 50% and dehydrated alcohol 50%. Only glass or polyolefin containers and nitroglycerin tubing (polyethylene lined) are recommended for administration, since significant amounts of the plasticizer diethylhexylphthalate (DEHP) may be leached from PVC-containing tubing and plastic solution bags after contact with Cremophor EL. Upon preparation, solutions may show haziness, which is attributed to the formulation vehicle. Paclitaxel should be administered through an in-line filter not greater than 0.22 μm. No significant loss of potency has been noted following simulated delivery through intravenous tubing containing an in-line (0.22 μm) filter. In addition, the use of filter devices such as IVEX-2 filters, which incorporate short inlet and outlet PVC-coated tubing, has not resulted in significant leaching of DEHP. The feasibility of several portable infusion pumps and set-ups as well as administered practices has been recently substantiated (212).

The following premedication is recommended to reduce the incidence of hypersensitivity reactions (HSRs): dexamethasone 20 mg orally or intravenously 12 and 6 hours before treatment; diphenhydramine 50 mg intravenously 30 minutes before treatment; and a histamine H$_2$-antagonist such as cimetidine 300 mg, famotidine 20 mg, or ranitidine 150 mg intravenously 30 minutes before treatment.

The high molecular weight, bulky structure, and principal hepatic metabolism of the taxanes render them ideal candidates for intracavitary administration. The feasibility of administering paclitaxel intraperitoneally as a single dose every 3 weeks and weekly has been studied. Severe abdominal pain precludes the administration of paclitaxel doses above 125 mg/m^2 on a single-dosing schedule and weekly doses below 75 mg/m^2 are well tolerated; systemic toxicity is mild at doses less than 175 mg/m^2. Intraperitoneal drug concentrations are several orders of magnitude higher than levels required to induce pertinent microtubule effects in vitro. Paclitaxel concentrations of this magnitude are also maintained for several days, indicating that intraperitoneal clearance of drug is very slow. Biologically relevant paclitaxel concentrations are also readily achieved and sustained in the plasma for several days after treatment, which is encouraging, since achieving relevant systemic concentrations appears to be important for a drug to be advantageous when given intraperitoneally. Intrathecal administration has not been studied.

Dosage: Paclitaxel is usually administered at a dose of 175 mg/m^2 over 3 hours or 135 to 175 mg/m^2 over 24 hours every 3 weeks. Although higher paclitaxel doses have not been determined to be superior to lower doses, early phase II studies involving untreated or minimally pretreated patients were performed with higher paclitaxel doses, 250 mg/m^2 over 24 hours, which usually caused severe neutropenia and often required hematopoietic growth factors (see section on toxicity, hematologic). Traditionally, phase II studies of anticancer agents have not used doses that are likely to induce severe neutropenia, and a greater degree of myelosuppression has been accepted with the taxanes than has previously been accepted in the development of other anticancer drugs. Due to the limited supply of paclitaxel when broad phase II testing began, it was felt that using high starting doses would obviate repeating studies at high doses if results were equivocal with low starting doses. However, adequate dose-response studies have not been completed in most relevant tumor types. The following doses have been recommended on less orthodox schedules: (a) 200 mg/m^2 over 1 hour as either a single dose or divided into 3 consecutive daily doses every 3 weeks and (b) 140 mg/m^2 over 96 hours every 3 weeks.

Since patients with abnormal renal and hepatic functions were not eligible to participate in early trials of paclitaxel, only limited information is available about the pharmacologic behavior and toxicity of paclitaxel in patients with excretory organ dysfunction. Renal clearance accounts for a small proportion (<10%) of total clearance; thus dose modifications are not required in patients with severe renal dysfunction (55, 213, 214). The magnitude of excretion of both paclitaxel and metabolites into bile is similar to that of other anticancer agents, such as the vinca alkaloids, with which dose modifications are required for hepatic excretory dysfunction.

Preliminary data from a prospective evaluation of patients with hepatic dysfunction indicate that those with moderate elevations in serum concentrations of hepatocellular enzymes and/or bilirubin are more likely to develop severe myelosuppression than patients without hepatic dysfunction (215). Although official recommendations for dose reductions have not been formulated, it seems prudent to reduce paclitaxel doses by at least 50% in patients with moderate or severe hepatic excretory dysfunction (hyperbilirubinemia) or significant elevations in hepatocellular enzymes.

The severity of both hematologic and nonhematologic toxicities does not seem to be affected by age (216, 217); however, the pharmacologic behavior of paclitaxel in elderly patients has not been evaluated prospectively.

Pharmacology: In early studies of paclitaxel administered on prolonged (6- and 24-hour infusion) schedules, substantial interpatient variability was noted (218–222). Plasma drug disappearance was characterized by a linear biphasic process, and $T_{1/2\alpha}$ and $T_{1/2\beta}$ averaged 0.34 and 5.8 hours, respectively. Peak plasma concentrations on 3- to 96-hour schedules are in the range of levels capable of inducing significant biologic effects in vitro (>0.05 to 0.1 μM) (206–209, 218–222).

From a pharmacologic prospective, the results of a pivotal study of a 3-hour schedule in patients with advanced ovarian cancer and more recent trials in both adults and children indicate that the pharmacokinetic behavior of paclitaxel is nonlinear (206, 207, 223). Nonlinear pharmacokinetic behavior, particularly that due to nonlinear drug elimination, is typically more apparent with shorter infusion schedules, resulting in higher plasma concentrations that approach or exceed the K_ms of saturable elimination or distribution processes. A combination of saturable distribution and elimination appears to be responsible for paclitaxel's nonlinear pharmacokinetic behavior, with tissue distribution becoming effectively saturated at relatively lower drug concentrations (achieved with ≤175 mg/m² over 3-hour dosing schedules), compared with elimination processes (achieved with ≤175 mg/m² over 3-hour dosing schedules). This nonlinear pharmacokinetic profile may have important clinical implications. For example, dose escalation, especially on shorter administration schedules, may result in disproportionate increases in both AUC and peak plasma concentrations, as well as disproportionate increases in toxicity; whereas dose reductions may result in disproportionate decreases in AUC and/or C_{peak}, thereby possibly decreasing antitumor activity.

V_d values for paclitaxel are much larger than the volume of total body water, suggesting extensive binding of drug to plasma proteins and/or other tissue constituents, possibly tubulin. Indeed, plasma protein binding is extensive (>95%) (218, 220, 222). At clinically relevant concentrations (0.1 to 0.6 μM), protein binding is concentration independent, indicating nonspecific hydrophobic binding. Albumin and α1-acid glycoprotein contribute equally to the binding, with a minor contribution from lipoproteins (224). None of the drugs that are commonly administered with paclitaxel, such as ranitidine, dexamethasone, diphenhydramine, doxorubicin, 5-fluorouracil, and cisplatin, appear to alter protein binding (224). Despite extensive binding to plasma proteins, paclitaxel is readily eliminated from the plasma compartment, suggesting lower-affinity reversible binding. Drug binding to platelets is extensive and saturable, whereas binding to red blood cells is insignificant (225).

The tissue distribution of paclitaxel has not been extensively studied. Limited data indicate that biologically relevant drug concentrations (>0.1 μM) are achieved in third-space fluid collections such as ascites (220). The penetration of paclitaxel into the central nervous system, as manifested by detection in the cerebrospinal fluid, is negligible, which may explain paclitaxel's virtual lack of central nervous system toxicity (205, 226). Tissue distribution

studies in animals, using radiolabeled drug, have revealed high tissue:plasma concentration ratios in virtually all tissues except brain and testes, which are generally considered "tumor sanctuary" sites (227).

The principal mechanism of systemic clearance of paclitaxel is hepatic detoxification with subsequent biliary excretion of both parent compound and metabolites into the feces. Renal clearance contributes minimally to systemic clearance (<10%) (206, 218–222). Although low levels of metabolites have been found in the plasma of patients receiving brief infusions, extrahepatic excretion of metabolites contributes minimally to clearance. In contrast, high concentrations of paclitaxel and metabolites are excreted in the bile. In humans, 20% of an administered dose of paclitaxel is recovered as either paclitaxel or metabolites from bile collected for 24 hours after treatment (228). Since paclitaxel is widely distributed to peripheral compartments and biliary collections were not carried out for long periods following treatment in humans, it is conceivable that hepatic metabolism and biliary excretion account for a much greater share of total clearance. This is the case in rats, in which 98% of total radioactivity can be recovered from feces collected for 6 days following treatment with ^{14}C-paclitaxel (229). Preliminary studies in humans receiving radiolabeled drug also indicate that 71% of administered agent is excreted in the feces within 5 days following treatment (230).

The predominant human paclitaxel metabolites have intact side chains at taxane ring positions C-2 and C-13 and are hydroxylated derivatives. The major metabolite in human plasma and bile is 6-αhydroxpaclitaxel (206, 228, 230–234). All derivatives that have been identified possess much less cytotoxic activity against leukemia cell lines in vitro than paclitaxel, but some are as active as paclitaxel in stabilizing microtubules against disassembly in a cell-free system. Hepatic cytochrome P450 mixed-function oxidases play a major role in the metabolism of paclitaxel in humans (231–233). CYP3A isoforms are responsible for the formation of 6-αhydroxypaclitaxel, whereas CYP2C isoforms or other as yet unidentified isoforms may be responsible for the formation of minor metabolites.

Indications: Paclitaxel is currently approved in the United States and worldwide for the treatment of patients with epithelial ovarian cancer after failure of first-line or subsequent chemotherapy (176, 235). In the first-line treatment of patients with suboptimally debulked stages III and IV disease, the combination of paclitaxel and cisplatin results in better response rates and overall survival than combination chemotherapy with cyclophosphamide and cisplatin (236). In the United States, paclitaxel is also approved for the treatment of patients with metastatic breast cancer after failure of combination chemotherapy or relapse within 6 months of adjuvant chemotherapy (235, 237). Prior therapy should have included an anthracycline unless clinically contraindicated. The role of paclitaxel in the treatment of earlier stages of breast cancer is currently being evaluated (237). Paclitaxel has also demonstrated prominent activity in chemotherapy-naive patients with advanced small and non-small-cell lung, bladder, endometrial, esophageal, and head and neck carcinomas and Kaposi's sarcoma (176, 235). Significant activity has also been noted in previously treated patients with lymphoma and cisplatin-resistant testicular carcinoma (176, 235).

Toxicities

Hypersensitivity Reactions: The incidence of major HSRs in early phase I trials approached 25 to 30% (238, 239). Severe manifestations of HSRs include dyspnea with bronchospasm, urticaria, and hypotension. HSRs usually occur within 2 to 3 minutes after treatment and almost always occur within the first 10 minutes; most occurred after the first or second dose. Most major HSRs resolve completely after stopping treatment and occasionally after treatment with antihistamines, fluids, and vasopressors. Although minor reactions, such as flushing and rashes, have also been noted in as many as 40% of patients, minor HSRs do not portend the development of major reactions. Although HSRs may be caused by either paclitaxel itself or its Cremophor EL vehicle, the latter has been felt to be responsible, since it induces histamine release and similar manifestations in dogs, and other drugs formulated in it induce similar HSRs. Phase I development was completed using prolonged (24-hour) infusions and premedication with corticosteroids and histamine H_1- and H_2-antagonists (see section on administration), since similar regimens have proven effective in preventing repeated reactions to radiographic contrast agents that also cause histamine release. Although these measures are not fully protective, the incidence of major HSRs ranges from 1 to 3%. In an assessment of the relative safety and efficacy of two different paclitaxel schedules (24- vs. 3-hour) with standard premedication in women with recurrent or refractory ovarian cancer, the incidence of major HSRs was low and similar (2.1 vs. 1.0%) for 3 or 24 hours, respectively, with premedication (240). Patients who have major HSRs may be rechallenged with paclitaxel, which is administered at a substantially lower infusion rate and gradually increased after treatment with high doses of corticosteroids (dexamethasone 20 mg intravenously every 6 hours for 4 doses) without recurrence, although this approach is not always successful.

Hematologic: Neutropenia is the principal toxicity of paclitaxel. The onset is usually on day 8 to 10; recovery is typically complete by day 15 to 21; and the toxicity is not cumulative (239). At doses of 200 to 250 mg/m^2 given over 24 hours, granulocyte counts are frequently below 500/μL, even in untreated patients. This dose range was initially recommended for phase II studies because the duration of severe neutropenia (<500/μL) was usually short (<5 days) and treatment delays for unresolved toxicity were rare. Although the rate of febrile or infectious sequelae was originally reported to be low (<10% of courses) at these doses, relative to that of severe neutropenia, these complications were more common in later studies. Therefore, hematopoietic colony-stimulating factors are commonly used to prevent complications of neutropenia in trials of doses in this range. In most patients, particularly those who had received large doses of other chemotherapy agents previously, the maximum tolerated dose without hematopoietic colony-stimulating factors is 175 to 200 mg/m^2. A critical determinant of the severity of neutropenia is the length of time that plasma drug concentrations are maintained above biologically relevant levels (0.05 to 0.1 μMol/L), which may explain why neutropenia is more severe with longer infusions (206–208). This does not imply that shorter infusions should always be used, since the optimal dose and schedule have not been determined for most tumors. Notwithstanding these differences, the main clinical determinant of the severity of neutropenia is the extent of prior myelotoxic therapy. Severe thrombocytopenia and anemia are rare.

Neurotoxicity: A peripheral neuropathy characterized by sensory symptoms such as numbness and paresthesia in a glove-and-stocking distribution is the principal neurotoxic effect of paclitaxel (239, 241, 242). There is often symmetric distal loss of sensation carried by both large (proprioception, vibration) and small (temperature, pin-prick) fibers. Symptoms may begin as soon as 24 to 72 hours after treatment with higher doses (>250 mg/m^2), but usually occur only after multiple courses at 135 to 250 mg/m^2. Severe neurotoxicity precludes chronic treatment with paclitaxel doses above 250 mg/m^2 over 3 or 24 hours, but severe neurotoxicity is rare at conventional doses (<200 mg/m^2) even in patients who previously received other neurotoxic agents such as cisplatin.

The distal, symmetric, length-dependent neurologic deficits suggest that paclitaxel causes a sensory and motor axonal loss similar to the "dying-back" neuropathies that may have their origin in the cell body or in axonal transport, but a few patients have the simultaneous onset of symptoms in the arms and legs, involvement of the face (perioral numbness), the predominance of large fiber loss, and diffuse areflexia suggestive of a neuronopathy. Both types of neuropathy depend on the dose of paclitaxel or its combination with cisplatin (241, 242). Motor and autonomic dysfunction may also occur, especially at high doses and in patients with preexisting neuropathies caused by diabetes mellitus and alcoholism. In addition, optic nerve disturbances, characterized by scintillating scotomata, may occur (243). Transient myalgia, usually noted 2 to 5 days after therapy, is common at doses above 170 mg/m^2, and myopathy has been noted with high doses of paclitaxel (>250 mg/m^2) in combination with cisplatin (239, 241). Nonsteroidal antiinflammatory agents are of minimal use in palliating and preventing symptoms, and narcotics are usually administered prophylactically on days 2 to 5 post-treatment in patients who have been symptomatic. Antihistamines have also been reported to be useful in preventing acute myalgias (244).

Cardiac: Paclitaxel causes cardiac rhythm disturbances, but the importance of these effects is not known (239, 245, 246). The most common effect, a transient asymptomatic bradycardia, was noted in 29% of patients in one early trial. Isolated asymptomatic bradycardia without hemodynamic effects does not appear to be an indication for discontinuing paclitaxel. More important bradyarrhythmias, including Mobitz type I (Wenckebach syndrome), Mobitz type II, and third-degree heart block have also been noted, but the incidence in a large database was only 0.1% (245, 246). All events occurred in patients enrolled in trials that required continuous cardiac monitoring, indicating that second- and third-degree heart block is likely underreported, since continuous cardiac monitoring is not usually performed. Most documented episodes have been asymptomatic and reversible. Myocardial infarction, cardiac ischemia, atrial arrhythmias, and ventricular tachycardia have also been noted (245, 246). Whether there is a direct causal relationship between paclitaxel and ventricular and atrial tachycardias and ischemic events is uncertain. There is no evidence that paclitaxel induces cumulative toxicity nor that it augments the acute cardiac effects of the anthracyclines; however, the frequency of congestive cardiotoxicity in patients treated with paclitaxel and doxorubicin in one trial was higher than expected from the anthracycline alone (247). In patients treated with paclitaxel and an anthracycline, potential drug effects on ventricular function should be evaluated at lower cumulative anthracycline doses than might otherwise be used with anthracyclines alone.

Once cardiac effects were documented, eligibility in most early trials was restricted to patients with no history of cardiac disease. However, this broadly described population undoubtedly excludes many patients who might otherwise be good candidates for paclitaxel, and the precise risks for cardiotoxicity in this population is not known. Routine cardiac monitoring during paclitaxel therapy is not necessary, but is advisable for patients who may not be able to tolerate the drug's potential brady-arrhythmic effects, such as those with atrio-ventricular conduction defects or ventricular dysfunction.

Miscellaneous: Drug-related gastrointestinal effects such as vomiting and diarrhea are infrequent. Higher doses may cause mucositis, especially in patients with leukemia, who may be more prone to mucosal barrier breakdown, or in patients receiving 96-hour infusions (205, 209). Rare cases of neutropenic enterocolitis have also been noted, particularly in patients given high doses of paclitaxel in combination with doxorubicin and cyclophosphamide (248, 249). Like other anticancer agents, paclitaxel induces alopecia of the scalp, but all body hair is often lost with cumulative therapy. Inflammation may occur at the injection site, along the course of an injected vein, and in areas of previous drug extravasation, as well as inflammatory skin reactions over previously radiated sites (radiation recall). Amitriptyline 10–50 mg/day has been reported to be useful in ameliorating a syndrome of neuropathic pruritus associated with neuropathy in the distal extremities following treatment with 3-hour infusions of paclitaxel (250).

Docetaxel

Nomenclature and Structure

Generic name: docetaxel

Commercial names: Taxotere

Chemical name: 4-acetoxy-2α-benzoyloxy-5β,20-epoxy-1,7β,10β-trihydroxy-9-oxo-tax-11-ene-13α-yl-(2R,3S)-3-tert-butoxy-carbonylamino-2-hydroxy-3-phenylpropionate

Molecular weight: 807.9

Chemical formula $C_{43}H_{53}O_{14}N$

Availability: Although docetaxel has been recommended for approval for treating anthracycline-resistent breast cancer in the United States, it is currently available for investigational use as a concentrated sterile solution in a clear glass 15-mL vial. Each vial contains 2 mL of docetaxel at a concentration of 40 mg/mL in polysorbate 80. The contents of the ampule must be diluted before use with a solution of ethyl alcohol and water, which is packaged separately in a clear glass 15-mL solvent vial. The premix solution is prepared after the do-

cetaxel vials have reached room temperature for 5 minutes. With a syringe and needle, the entire contents of the solution vial is added to the drug vial to obtain 8 mL of premix solution containing 10 mg of docetaxel/mL. The mixture should be allowed to stand for 5 minutes and should be clear and homogeneous. Persistent foam after this time is normal.

Storage: Unopened vials of docetaxel should be refrigerated at 4°C (39°F). It is recommended that the vials be protected from light. The solvent vial can be stored at room temperature of 4°C (39°F).

Administration: The premix solution of docetaxel must be diluted in either 0.9% Sodium Chloride Injection, USP, or 5% Dextrose Injection, USP. The volume of the solution should be adjusted to achieve a final docetaxel concentration of 1 mg/mL or less in no less than 250 mL of infusate. Final solutions are stable at room temperature and normal lighting conditions for 8 hours. To minimize patient exposure to the plasticizer DEHP which may be leached from PVC-containing infusion sets, docetaxel should be mixed and administered through non-PVC-lined administration sets. Docetaxel is most commonly administered as a 1-hour intravenous infusion every 3 weeks. Despite the use of a polysorbate 80 formulation instead of Cremophor EL, which is used to formulate paclitaxel, a relatively high rate of HSRs, as well as a fluid retention syndrome, has led to the use of several premedication regimens, the most popular of which is dexamethasone 8 mg orally twice daily for 5 days starting 1 day before docetaxel, with or without both H_1- and H_2-histamine antagonists given intravenously 30 minutes before docetaxel (See section on paclitaxel administration) and methylprednisolone 40 mg given the day before, the day of, and the day after treatment with docetaxel.

Dosage: Although several administration schedules have been evaluated, docetaxel is most commonly administered intravenously at a dose of 100 mg/m^2 as a 1-hour infusion every 3 weeks. Another popular schedule uses 1-hour infusions of docetaxel 50 mg/m^2 on days 1 and 8 every 3 weeks. Lower doses of docetaxel (60 to 75 mg/m^2) as a 1-hour infusion may be associated with a lower incidence of both hematologic and nonhematologic toxicities; however, the relative therapeutic advantage of high versus low doses is not clear.

Docetaxel has not yet been rigorously evaluated in patients with excretory organ dysfunction; however, the principal role of the liver in drug metabolism and excretion, as well as preliminary results, indicate that dose modifications should be performed in such patients. The results of a study involving patients with liver metastases with and without elevations in plasma levels of hepatocellular enzymes and/or alkaline phosphatase indicate that docetaxel clearance is reduced, predisposing these patients to more severe neutropenia, mucositis, and rashes than patients with or without liver metastases and no liver function test abnormalities. Although specific recommendations for dosing modifications in patients with liver dysfunction have not yet been formulated, a review of population data of patients with normal serum bilirubin concentrations indicates that clearance is reduced by 27% in patients with SGOT and alkaline phosphatase concentrations above 2.5- and 1.5-fold the upper limits of normal. These patients are more susceptible to toxicity and therefore it seems prudent to reduce doses by 25% in such patients. In view of minimal renal excretion (<10%), modifications for renal dysfunction are not necessary (55).

Pharmacology: The pharmacologic behavior of docetaxel has been primarily studied using a single 1-hour every 3 weeks dosing schedule (251–256). The pharmacokinetic behavior of docetaxel on 1- or 2-hour schedules is linear at doses of 115 mg/m^2 or less and optimally fits a three-compartment model. $T_{1/2\gamma}$ values range from 11.4 to 13.6 hours. In an analysis of pooled pharmacokinetic data, using a population approach, an optimal three-compartment model generated the following parameter value estimates: $T_{1/2\gamma}$, 10.4 hours; clearance, 0.36 L/hr; and Vd_{ss}, 67.3 L/m^2 (257). Both V_d and clearance rate values are high, indicating extensive protein binding and/or drug distribution. Docetaxel binds rapidly and avidly to plasma proteins (>90%), especially to albumin α_1-acid glycoprotein, and lipoproteins. Peak plasma concentrations generally exceed levels required to induce relevant biologic effects in vitro.

There is limited information available about the distribution of docetaxel in humans. In rats and dogs, tissue distribution studies using ^{14}C-docetaxel have demonstrated a rapid initial distribution phase of plasma radioactivity, with an apparent $T_{1/2}$ of 10 minutes (258). In mice, autoradiographic studies indicate that docetaxel rapidly accumulates in almost all tissues except the central nervous system. Immediately after treatment, tissue uptake of radioactivity is highest in the liver, bile, and intestines, which is consistent with substantial hepatobiliary extraction and excretion. High levels of radioactivity are also found in the stomach, indicating the possibility of gastric excretion, as well as in the spleen, bone marrow, myocardium, skeletal muscles, and pancreas.

The metabolism and elimination profiles of docetaxel resemble those of paclitaxel. Urinary excretion accounts for a small percentage of docetaxel disposition in humans, averaging 2% in one study (259). In both dogs and mice treated with ^{14}C-docetaxel, fecal excretion of radioactivity accounts for 70 to 80% of drug disposition, whereas urinary excretion accounts for 10% or less (254, 260). In mice, 3% of the dose is excreted in the feces as the parent compound in the first 24 hours, and the excretion of three metabolites accounts for 75% of the administered dose. Similar profiles have been noted in humans treated with ^{14}C-docetaxel. Approximately 5% and 80% of the total radioactivity is recovered in the urine and feces, respectively, within 7 days of dosing, with most excretion occurring in the first 48 hours. Several metabolites have been detected in the bile and feces of both humans and rats, as well as in microsomal and liver perfusion studies. As with paclitaxel, the hepatic cytochrome P450 mixed-function oxidases are responsible for the bulk of drug metabolism, and CYP3A, CYP2B, and CYP1A isoforms may play major roles in biotransformation (260–263). The main metabolic pathway consists of successive oxidations of the tertiary butyl group on the side chain at the C-13 position of the taxane ring; all metabolites appear to maintain their 10-deacetylbaccatin III or 7-epi isomer structural backbones. These metabolites also seem to be much less active than docetaxel (261, 264).

Indications: Docetaxel has consistently demonstrated significant antitumor activity in patients with metastatic breast carcinoma as first-line or salvage treatment, previously treated ovarian carcinoma, and non-small-cell lung cancer as first-line therapy or in platinum-refractory disease (177). Approval has been recommended in the United States for treatment of patients with anthracycline-resistant breast cancer, and it is registered for breast and lung cancer therapy in many other countries. Impressive activity has also been preliminarily reported in patients with head and neck, bladder, pancreatic, and small cell lung carcinomas.

Toxicities

Hematologic: Neutropenia is the principal toxicity of docetaxel. At 100 mg/m^2 of docetaxel (1-hour schedule), neutrophil count nadirs are less than 500/μL in 50 to 80% of courses in previously untreated patients and 83% of courses in heavily pretreated patients (177, 265–268). Neutrophil nadirs occur usually on day 9 and recover generally by days 15 to 21. Neutropenia is not cumulative. Treatment delays due to incomplete resolution of hematologic toxicity are unusual. Febrile neutropenia requiring hospitalization and parenteral antibiotics has been reported in 11 to 14% of courses involving one-third or more of patients (266, 267). The severity of neutropenia does not seem to be related to the infusion duration, but there has been only limited experience with prolonged infusion schedules. Significant effects on platelets and red blood cells are uncommon.

Hypersensitivity: Although docetaxel is not formulated in Cremophor EL, both major and minor HSRs occurred in approximately 25% of patients receiving docetaxel without premedication in early developmental studies (177). These reactions are similar to HSRs induced by paclitaxel. Major HSRs, characterized by dyspnea, bronchospasm, and hypotension, usually occur during the first two courses and within minutes after the start of treatment. Symptoms generally resolve within 15 minutes after the cessation of treatment; however, treatment can usually be resumed without further consequence, occasionally after treatment with diphenhydramine. Most HSRs are minor and may be characterized by flushing, chest tightness, and low back pain. Both the incidence and the severity of HSRs appear to be reduced by several premedication regimens including: (*a*) dexamethasone 10 mg given orally 12 and 6 hours before treatment; (*b*) dexamethasone 8 mg given orally twice daily for 5 days beginning 1 day before treatment, given with or without H$_1$- and H$_2$-histamine antagonists 30 minutes before treatment; and (*c*) methylprednisolone 40 mg on the day before, the day of, and the day after docetaxel. Treatment should be discontinued immediately for severe HSRs and, possibly, moderate reactions. In addition, treatment with diphenhydramine 50 mg intravenously, or an equivalent H$_1$-histamine antagonist, and dexamethasone 10 mg intravenously have been recommended. Patients have been retreated successfully following the resolution of symptoms and premedication with dexamethasone 10 mg intravenously and/or diphenhydramine 10 mg intravenously 30 minutes before docetaxel. Mild manifestations have been managed by decreasing the rate of the docetaxel infusion until symptoms resolve.

Fluid Retention: Docetaxel induces a unique cumulative fluid-retention syndrome characterized by edema, weight gain, pleural effusions, and ascites (267–270). The etiology of this syndrome does not appear to be related to hypoalbuminemia or cardiac, renal, or hepatic dysfunction. Instead, docetaxel likely causes a capillary permeability abnormality. Plasma renin concentrations have also been elevated in some patients. In early studies that did not use prophylactic medications, fluid retention was not usually significant at cumulative docetaxel doses below 400 mg/m^2, but the incidence and severity increase sharply at cumulative doses above 400 mg/m^2, often resulting in the delay or termination of treatment. Both peripheral edema and third-space fluid collections usually resolve slowly after treatment is stopped. Aggressive and early treatment with diuretics is increasingly being used successfully to manage fluid retention. Preliminary studies also suggest that the incidence of fluid retention may be reduced by using lower single-treatment doses (<60 to 75 mg/m^2) or an alternate administration schedule (e.g., divided doses on days 1 and 8 every 3 weeks). Premedication with corticosteroids, with or without H$_1$- and H$_2$-histamine antagonists may reduce the incidence of fluid retention and increase the median number of courses before the onset of this toxicity. Several dosing schedules have been used successfully including: dexamethasone 8 mg orally twice daily for 5 days and methylprednisolone 40 mg/day for 3 consecutive days beginning 24 hours before docetaxel.

Dermatologic: Skin toxicity, typically characterized by an erythematous pruritic maculopapular rash that affects the forearms and hands, may occur in 50 to 75% of patients receiving docetaxel (265–268). Other cutaneous effects include superficial desquamation of the hands and feet and onycho-dystrophy characterized by brown discoloration, ridging, onycholysis, soreness, and brittleness of the fingernails. Docetaxel also induces palmar-plantar erythrodysthesia that may respond to pyridoxine or cooling (269, 270). The use of premedication may decrease the incidence of skin toxicity. Alopecia occurs in most patients. Drug extravasation may produce localized pain and discoloration without necrosis. Phlebitis has also been reported.

Neurologic: Mild-to-moderate peripheral neurotoxicity has been reported in approximately 40% of previously untreated patients in phase II studies (265–268). The peripheral neuropathy is similar to that induced by paclitaxel, predominately affecting large-fiber sensory function. Patients usually complain of paresthesias and numbness. Peripheral motor dysfunction resulting in extremity weakness may also occur. Patients who were previously treated with platinum compounds may be particularly susceptible to peripheral neurotoxicity, with the incidence approaching 74% in one trial (271). Nonetheless, severe toxicity has been unusual following repetitive treatment with single doses of 100 mg/m^2 or less, except in patients with antecedent disorders such as alcohol abuse (266). Transient myalgias are often noted in the peritreatment period.

Miscellaneous: Malaise or asthenia has been noted in most patients receiving docetaxel. It is typically mild to moderate; however, it can occasionally be severe enough to warrant dosage reduction or discontinuation of treatment. Cardiac conduction disturbances and ischemia have been noted in the peritreatment period, but there is no convincing evidence that directly links docetaxel to these episodes (265, 267). The incidence of stomatitis appears to be higher with docetaxel than with paclitaxel, particularly with prolonged infusions. Nausea, vomiting, and diarrhea occur, but severe gastrointestinal effects are rare.

Drug Interactions: The possibility of sequence-dependent interactions between the taxanes and other chemotherapy agents was studied as part of the effort to incorporate the taxanes into combination chemotherapy. The sequence of cisplatin followed by paclitaxel (24-hour schedule) induced more profound neutropenia than the reverse drug sequence in phase I stud-

ies, which could be explained by a 33% reduction in the clearance rate of paclitaxel following cisplatin (271). However, this sequence was also the suboptimal sequence in vitro with respect to cytotoxicity (272). The mechanisms for these sequence-dependent effects in vitro are not entirely clear; however, paclitaxel has been shown to inhibit the repair of cisplatin-DNA adducts (273). It is also possible that treatment with cisplatin before paclitaxel is antagonistic, since cisplatin inhibits cell-cycle progression in the G$_2$ phase, thereby preventing further progression into the mitotic phases, which may be the optimal period of cell sensitivity to the taxanes. The selection of the sequence of paclitaxel followed by cisplatin for subsequent clinical trials of the paclitaxel-cisplatin chemotherapy combination was based on these results. Although the mechanism for sequence-dependent pharmacologic interactions between paclitaxel and cisplatin is not known, one potential mechanism is the modulation of cytochrome P450–dependent paclitaxel-metabolizing enzymes by cisplatin (274). The ability to modulate cytochrome P450 mixed-function oxidases is not shared by all the platinum compounds; carboplatin does not appear to be capable of modulating P450 systems (274). In addition, the use of paclitaxel and carboplatin in combination, specifically with carboplatin following paclitaxel, has been noted by some investigators to result in significantly less thrombocytopenia than with carboplatin alone (275).

The potential for sequence-dependent interactions has also been studied during developmental studies of paclitaxel in combination with either doxorubicin or cyclophosphamide (249, 276, 277). Mucositis is more prominent when paclitaxel (24-hour infusion) is administered before doxorubicin than with the reverse sequence (276, 277). Pharmacologic studies suggest that the increased toxicity is due to a reduction in the clearance (32%) of doxorubicin when it is administered after paclitaxel (277). Based on these results and the lack of data demonstrating a superior drug sequence with respect to cytotoxicity, the sequence of doxorubicin followed by paclitaxel is being pursued. Similarly, hematologic toxicity has been more profound with the sequence of cyclophosphamide before paclitaxel (24-hour infusion) than with the reverse sequence (249). However, the mechanism for these differential effects is not clear, since neither pharmacologic nor cytotoxicity studies have demonstrated differences between the sequences. Although these studies may potentially be used as paradigms to assess other taxane-based chemotherapy combinations, it should be emphasized that sequence-dependent interactions have been noted only with prolonged paclitaxel infusions and not with short (e.g., 3-hour) schedules. Sequence-dependent effects have also not been observed with docetaxel-based drug combinations, in which docetaxel is administered as a 1-hour infusion (278).

Another source of drug interactions may be due to the effects of other classes of drugs on the metabolism of the taxanes. Various pharmacologic inducers of cytochrome P450 mixed-function oxidases, such as phenytoin and phenobarbital, accelerate the metabolism of both paclitaxel and docetaxel in human microsomal studies (231–233, 260–263). Preliminary clinical observations have also indicated the possibility of interactions between paclitaxel and inducers of cytochrome P450 enzymes. In pediatric patients, rapid drug clearance has been associated with the use of anticonvulsant agents (279). Similarly, plasma paclitaxel concentrations and toxicity were much lower than predicted in patients with malignant brain tumors treated with 96-hour infusions of paclitaxel, possibly due to the induction of taxane metabolism by the anticonvulsant agents (283). Conversely, many types of agents that can inhibit cytochrome P450 mixed-function oxidases interfere with the microsomal metabolism of both paclitaxel and docetaxel in vitro (231–233, 260–263). These include inhibitors of CYP3A isoforms, which are involved in paclitaxel's major metabolic pathway, and inhibitors of CYP2C isoforms such as orphenadrine, erythromycin, testosterone, and troleandomycin. Both ketoconazole and fluconazole have also been shown to inhibit the metabolism of paclitaxel in vitro (281).

There has also been concern that H_2-histamine antagonist premedications may be an important source of drug interactions. Use of these agents with the taxanes may produce variable pharmacologic and toxicologic effects, since these agents differentially inhibit cytochrome P450 metabolism, with cimetidine being the most potent inhibitor. However, H_2-histamine antagonists do not appear to alter the metabolism and pharmacologic disposition of the taxanes in vitro and in animals (281, 282).

In addition, the results of a clinical trial, in which patients were randomized to receive either cimetidine or famotidine premedication before their first course of paclitaxel and then crossed over to the alternate premedication during their second course, has failed to show significant toxicologic and pharmacologic differences between these H_2-histamine antagonists (283). In one recent study using human and rat liver slices and microsomes, quinidine, ketoconazole, dexamethasone, and Cremophor EL inhibited the microsomal metabolism of paclitaxel; however, the inhibitory concentrations of these agents exceed those achieved in the clinic (284). In contrast, paclitaxel metabolism was not altered by either cimetidine, dexamethasone, or diphenhydramine, drugs regularly coadministered with paclitaxel.

Estramustine

Estramustine, which consists of an estradiol molecule linked to a nor-nitrogen mustard through a carbamate ester group (Fig. 22.3), was synthesized in the mid-1960s as an alkylating agent specifically for the treatment of advanced prostate carcinoma. The estradiol portion of the molecule was designed to facilitate uptake by steroid receptors in malignant cells, followed by the intracellular release of the nitrogen mustard alkylating moiety. However, estramustine's antitumor activity is due to its effects on microtubule dynamics. In its proprietary form, the approved agent, estramustine phosphate, has a phosphate at the 17β position of the steroid D ring, which renders it more water soluble and, therefore, more feasible for clinical administration.

Nomenclature and Structure

Generic name: estramustine
Commercial name: Emcyt
Chemical name: Estra 1,3,5(10)-triene-3,17-diol(17β)-,3-[bis(2-chloroethyl)carbamate] 17-(dihydrogen phosphate), disodium salt, monohydrate.
Molecular weight: 582.4
Chemical formula: $C_{23}H_{30}Cl_2NNa_2O_6P$-$H_2O$

Availability: Estramustine is available as white opaque capsules, each containing estramustine phosphate sodium as the disodium salt monohydrate equivalent to 140 mg estramustine phosphate. A parenteral formulation is also available for investigational purposes.

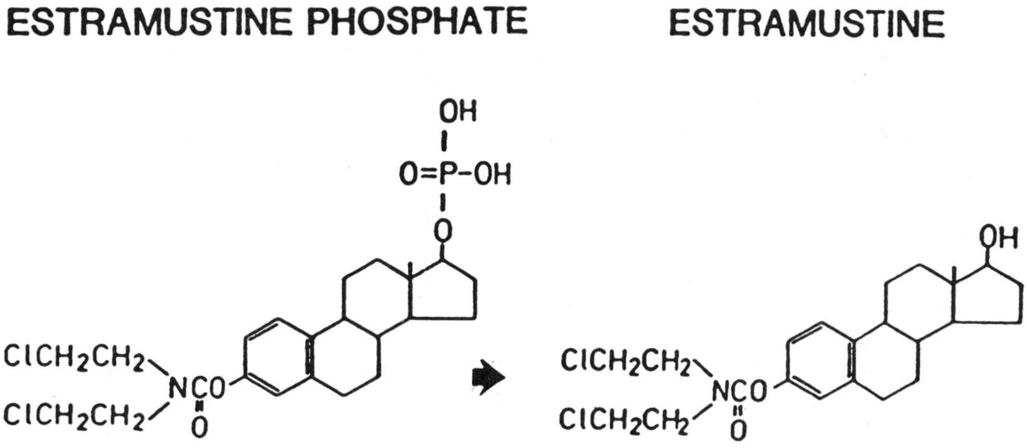

ESTRAMUSTINE PHOSPHATE   ESTRAMUSTINE

Figure 22.3.   Structures of estramustine phosphate and estramustine.

Storage: Estramustine should be refrigerated at 2 to 8°C (36 to 46°F). It should not be frozen. The medication should be stored in its original tightly closed light-resistant container. It should be stored away from moisture and direct light.

Administration: Estramustine is generally administered orally in 3 to 4 divided doses each day. It is recommended that patients take estramustine at least 1 hour before or 2 hours after meals. The agent should be swallowed with water. Milk and calcium-rich foods or drugs (e.g., calcium-containing antacids) should be avoided because of the possibility of salt formation (see section on drug interactions).

Dosage: The recommended daily dose is 14 mg/kg or one 140-mg capsule for each 10 kg (22 lb) of body weight, though most patients in studies in the United States have received daily doses of 10 to 16 mg/kg. Such doses have been given to some patients for more than 3 years.

Mechanism of Action: Several observations support the fact that estramustine is not active by virtue of hormonal mechanisms (285–289). First, although estrogens are released following treatment with estramustine, it is active in cell lines that lack estrogen receptors. Second, it inhibits the growth of tumors that are not responsive to estrogens. Finally, the binding of estramustine is not inhibited by 1000-fold excess concentrations of estradiol. Several other observations are not consistent with alkylating activity as its principal mechanism, including the drug's lack of alkylating activity in vitro at concentrations that induce cytotoxicity and the absence of direct DNA damage following treatment at lethal concentrations; noncovalent

binding of the drug; the reversibility of various effects; and the sensitivity of alkylating agent–resistant cells to estramustine. In addition, the principal clinical toxicities of estramustine are not characteristic of an alkylating agent (285, 286, 289).

The demonstration that estramustine produces metaphase arrest led to further evidence that the antineoplastic effects of the drug are mediated through their inhibitory and dissociative effects on microtubule structure and function (290, 291). Estramustine binds to and dissociates tau and high-molecular-weight MAPs, which results in the inhibition of microtubule assembly and the subsequent disassembly of microtubules (292–294). The agent has been demonstrated to bind with different affinities to MAPs isolated from various tumor cells and tissues. There is also evidence that estramustine directly interacts with tubulin (295).

Estramustine binds to specific proteins in tissues, commonly referred to as estramustine-binding protein (EMBP), which was originally isolated from prostate tissue. Similar proteins have been found in other tissues and tumors such as prostate adenocarcinoma and astrocytoma (296). There is also evidence that EMBP levels in prostate cancer are related to neither the androgen concentrations nor the androgen dependency of the tumors (297). Instead, EMBP levels correlated with the degree of tumor cell differentiation.

Estramustine also enhances the effects of radiation in vitro (298, 299). These radiation-enhancing effects are most prominent after prolonged treatment of cells with estramustine before irradiation and may be related to the degree of accumulation of cells in the G_2/M phase of the cell cycle as a result of estramustine (290).

Mechanisms of Resistance: The mechanisms for cellular resistance to estramustine are distinct from those that have been characterized for other antimicrotubule agents. Unlike typical drug resistance due to MDR, the degree of resistance for estramustine-resistant cells does not usually exceed 4- to 5-fold; MDR does not confer cross-resistance to other agents to which resistance is conferred by the MDR phenotype; and estramustine-resistance is not associated with increased Pgp mRNA or protein levels (286, 300–302). In fact, estramustine has been demonstrated to be a weak MDR-reversal agent (300–302). In addition, neither modified expression of glutathione S-transferase nor increased intracellular levels of glutathione appear to account for estramustine-resistance in vitro (286). The results of drug efflux studies indicate that some estramustine-resistant cells without increased levels of Pgp have altered patterns of drug extrusion (286).

Pharmacology: Both the pharmacologic and biologic half-lives of estramustine are long; terminal $T_{1/2}$s range from 20 to 24 hours following intravenous administration of radiolabeled estramustine phosphate (303). Immediately after injection, estramustine phosphate predominates in plasma; however, it is dephosphorylated to extramustine, so that the dephosphorylated compound is the predominant species at 4 hours posttreatment. Dephosphorylation occurs in the gastrointestinal tract, liver, and other phosphatase-rich tissues such as prostate. Peak plasma levels in multiple-dose studies with 600 mg/m² given 3 times daily have been 326 ng/mL for estromustine (the dephosphorylated estrone derivative), 82 ng/mL for estramustine phosphate, 36 ng/mL for estramustine, 162 ng/mL for estrone, and 17 ng/mL for estradiol (304).

The oral bioavailability of estramustine phosphate is approximately 75% (303, 305). It is excreted as metabolites of both the alkylating and estrogenic moieties into the bile, feces, and urine. Urinary excretion accounts for 23% of total drug disposition within 48 hours posttreatment (306). Only small quantities of unmetabolized drug are found, indicating that drug disposition is principally due to nonrenal mechanisms. The steroidal component of the molecule is conjugated, primarily in the liver, as the glucuronide and excreted into the bile, feces, and urine.

Indications: Estramustine phosphate is indicated in the palliative treatment of patients with metastatic and/or progressive carcinoma of the prostate (307, 308).

Toxicity

Gastrointestinal: At conventional doses, nausea and vomiting, which are usually transient and responsive to antiemetics, are the principal toxicities of the oral formulation of estramustine phosphate. Intractable vomiting that may require the termination of therapy is noted occasionally after 6 to 8 weeks of treatment. Diarrhea may occur in as many as 15 to 30% of patients.

Cardiovascular: Cardiovascular effects, which are potentially the most hazardous toxicities of estramustine phosphate, may occur in as many as 10% of patients who have not previously been treated with estrogens (289, 305–308). Patients with depressed cardiac function may develop worsening symptoms of congestive heart failure during treatment, most likely due to the salt-retaining effects of the estrogenic portion of the drug. Other rare cardiovascular complications include thromboembolism and cardiac ischemic and cerebrovascular events. Thus, patients with preexisting cardiac and cerebrovascular disease, as well as hypertension, should be monitored closely.

Endocrine: Gynecomastia and nipple tenderness are experienced by most patients, but these effects can be prevented by prophylactic breast irradiation.

Miscellaneous: Myelosuppression is uncommon. Other rare effects include liver function test abnormalities, fever, urticaria, and other rashes.

Drug Interactions: Drugs that reduce glutathione may enhance the activity of estramustine (308). In addition, the combination of estramustine and other antimicrotubule agents, including VBL and paclitaxel, may produce synergistic cytotoxicity in vitro (309, 310, 311).

As previously discussed (see administration), milk, dairy products, or calcium-rich food and medications (e.g., calcium-containing antacids) should not be taken with estramustine phosphate. Milk and calcium-containing products significantly decrease the rate and extent of drug absorption, presumably because of salt formation (312).

REFERENCES

1. Dustin P. Microtubules. 2nd ed. New York: Springer-Verlag, 1984.

2. Hyams JF, Lloyd CW. Microtubules. New York: Wiley-Liss, 1993.

3. Amos LA, King A. Arrangement of subunits in flagellar microtubules. J Cell Sci 1974;14:523–530.

4. Sullivan KF. Structure and utilization of tubulin isotypes. Annu Rev Cell Biol 1988;4:687–716.

5. Ludena RF. Are tubulin isotypes functionally significant? Mol Biol Cell 1983;4:445–457.

6. Olmsted JB. Microtubule-associated proteins. Annu Rev Cell Biol 1986;2:421–457.

7. Vallee RB, Bloom GS, Theurkauf WE. Microtubule associated proteins: subunits of the cytomatrix. J Cell Biol 1984;99:38s–44s.

8. Penningroth SM, Kirschner MW. Nucleotide binding and phosphorylation in microtubule assembly in vitro. J Mol Biol 1977;115:643–673.

9. Mitchison TJ. Localization of exchangeable GTP binding site at the plus end of microtubules. Science 1993;261:1044–1047.

10. Carlier M-F. Role of nucleotide hydrolysis in the polymerization of actin and tubulin. Cell Biophys 1988;12:105–112.

11. Erickson HP, O'Brien ET. Microtubule dynamic instability and GTP hydrolysis. Annu Rev Biophys Biomol Struct 1992;21:145–166.

12. Mitchison T, Krischner M. Dynamic instability of microtubule growth. Nature 1984;312:237–242.

13. Bruchovsky N, Owen AA, Becker AJ, Till JE. Effects of vinblastine on the proliferative capacity of L cells and their progress through the division cycle. Cancer Res 1965;25:1232–1237.

14. Schrek R, Stefani SS. Toxicity of microtubular drugs to leukemic lymphocytes. Exp Mol Pathol 1981; 34:369–378.

15. Strychmans PA, Lurie PM, Manaster J, et al. Mode of action of chemotherapy in vivo on human acute leukemia. II. vincristine. Eur J Cancer 1973;9:613–620.

16. Rosner F, Hirshaut Y, Grunwald HW, Dietrich, M. In vitro combination chemotherapy demonstrating potentiation of vincristine cytotoxicity by prednisone. Cancer Res 1975;35:700–705.

17. Himes RH. Interactions of the catharanthus (vinca) alkaloids with tubulin and microtubules. Pharmacol Ther 1991;51:256–267.

18. Jordan MA, Wilson L. Kinetic analysis of tubulin exchange at microtubule ends at low vinblastine concentrations. Biochemistry 1990;29:2730–2739.

19. Wilson L, Jordan MA, Morse A, Margolis RL. Interaction of vinblastine with steady-state microtubules in vitro. J Mol Biol 1982;159:125–149.

20. Jordan MA, Margolis RL, Himes RH, Wilson L. Identification of a distinct class of vinblastine binding sites on microtubules. J Mol Biol 1986;187:61–73.

21. Jordan MA, Thrower D, Wilson L. Mechanism of inhibition of cell proliferation by *Vinca* alkaloids. Cancer Res 1991;51:2212–2222.

22. Moscow JA, Cowan KH. Multidrug resistance. J Natl Cancer Inst 1988;80:14–20.

23. Beck WT, Mueller TJ, Tanzer LR. Altered cell surface membrane glycoproteins in vinca-alkaloid-resistant human leukemic lymphoblasts. Cancer Res 1979;39:2070–2076.

24. Cornwell MM, Tsuruo T, Gottesman MM, Pastan I. ATP-binding properties of P-glycoprotein from multidrug-resistant KB cells. FASEB J 1987;1:51–54.

25. Cornwell MM, Safa AR, Felsted RL, Gottesman MM, Pastan I. Membrane vesicles from multidrug-resistant human cancer cells contain a specific 150- to 170-kDa protein detected by photoaffinity labeling. Proc Natl Acad Sci USA 1986;83:3847–3850.

26. Safa AR, Glover CJ, Meyers MB, et al. Vinblastine photoaffinity labeling of a high molecular weight surface membrane glycoprotein specific for multidrug-resistant cells. J Biol Chem 1986;261:6137–6140.

27. Fojo AT, Ueda K, Slamon DJ, Poplack DG, Gottesman MM, Pastan I. Expression of a multidrug-resistance gene in human tumors and tissues. Proc Natl Acad Sci USA 1987;84:265–269.

28. Greenberger LM, Williams SS, Horwitz SB. Biosynthesis of heterogeneous forms of multidrug resistance associated glycoproteins. J Biol Chem 1987; 262:13685–13689.

29. Choi K, Chen C, Kriegler M, Roninson IB. An altered pattern of cross-resistance in multidrug-resistant human cells results from spontaneous mutations in the *mdr1* (P-glycoprotein) gene. Cell 1988;53:519–529.

30. Hamada H, Hagiwara KI, Nakajima T, Tsuruo T. Phosphorylation of the M_r 170,000 to 180,000 glycoprotein specific to multidrug-resistant tumor cells: effects of verapamil, trifluoroperazine, and phorbol esters. Cancer Res 1987;47:2860–2865.

31. Houghton JA, Houghton PJ, Hazelton BJ, Douglas EC. In situ selection of a human rhabdomyosarcoma resistant to vincristine with altered *alpha*-tubulins. Cancer Res 1985;45:2706–2712.

32. Minotti AM, Barlow SB, Cabral F. Resistance to antimitotic drugs in Chinese hamster ovary cells correlates with changes in the level of polymerized tubulin. J Biol Chem 1991;266:3987–3994.

33. Cabral FR, Brady RC, Schiber MJ. A mechanism of cellular resistance to drugs that interfere with microtubule assembly. Ann NY Acad Sci 1986;466:745–756.

34. Cabral FR, Barlow SB. Resistance to the antimitotic agents as genetic probes of microtubule structure and function. Pharmacol Ther 1991;52:159–171.

35. Donoso JA, Haskins KM, Himes RH. Effect of microtubule proteins on the interaction of vincristine with microtubules and tubulin. Cancer Res 1979; 39:1604–1610.

36. Bowman LC, Houghton JA, Houghton PJ. GTP influences the binding of vincristine in human tumor cytosols. Biochem Biophys Res Commun 1986;135:695–700.

37. Ferguson PJ, Cass CE. Differential cellular retention of vincristine and vinblastine by cultured human promyelocytic leukemia HL-60/C-1 cells: the basis differential toxicity. Cancer Res 1985;45:5480–5488.

38. Himes RH, Kersey RN, Heller-Bettinger I, Sampson FE. Action of the *Vinca* alkaloids vincristine and vinblastine, and desacetyl vinblastine amide on microtubules in vitro. Cancer Res 1976;36:3798–3802.

39. Houghton JA, Meyer WH, Houghton BJ. Scheduling of vincristine: drug accumulation and response of xenografts of childhood rhabdomyosarcoma determined by frequency of administration. Cancer Treat Rep 1987;71:717–721.

40. Jordan MA, Himes RH, Wilson L. Comparison

of the effects of vinblastine, vincristine, vindesine, and vinepidine on microtubule dynamics and cell proliferation in vitro. Cancer Res 1985;45:2741–2747.

41. Ferguson PJ, Philips JR, Seiner M, Cass CE. Biochemical effects of Navelbine on tubulin and associated proteins. Cancer Res 1984;44:3307–3312.

42. Gout PW, Wijcik LL, Beer CT. Differences between vinblastine and vincristine in distribution in the blood of rats and binding by platelets and malignant cells. Eur J Cancer 1978;14:1167–1178.

43. Lengsfeld AM, Dietrich J, Schultze-Maurer B. Accumulation and release of vinblastine and vincristine in HeLa cells: light microscopic, cinematographic, and biochemical study. Cancer Res 1982;42:3798–3805.

44. Gout PW, Noble RL, Bruchovsky N, Beer, CT. Vinblastine and vincristine—growth-inhibitory effects correlate with their retention by cultured Nb2 node lymphoma cells. Int J Cancer 1984;34:245–248.

45. Bowman LC, Houghton JA, Houghton PJ. Formation and stability of vincristine-tubulin complex in kidney cytosols. Role of GTP and GTP hydrolysis. Biochem Pharmacol 1988;37:1251–1257.

46. Houghton JA, Williams LG, Houghton PJ. Stability of vincristine complexes in cytosols derived from xenografts of human rhabdomyosarcoma and normal tissues of the mouse. Cancer Res 1985;45:3761–3767.

47. Dorr RT, Alberts DS. Vinca alkaloid skin toxicity: antidote and drug disposition studies in the mouse. J Natl Cancer Inst 1985;74:113–120.

48. Sulkes A, Collins JM. Reappraisal of some dosage adjustment guidelines. Cancer Treat Rep 1987;71:229–233.

49. Jackson DV. Periwinkle alkaloids II: vincristine. In: Lockich J, ed. Cancer chemotherapy by infusion. Chicago: Precept Press, 1987:181–199.

50. Jackson DV, Bender RA. Cytotoxic thresholds of vincristine in a murine and human leukemia cell line in vitro. Cancer Res 1979;39:4346–4349.

51. Pinkerton CR, McDermott B, Philip T, et al. Continuous vincristine infusion as part of a high dose chemoradiotherapy regimen: drug kinetics and toxicity. Cancer Chemother Pharmacol 1988;22:271–274.

52. Anderson H, Scarffe JH, Ranson M, et al. VAD chemotherapy as remission induction for multiple myeloma. Br J Cancer 1995;71:326–330.

53. Wilson WH, Bryant G, Bates S, et al. EPOCH chemotherapy: toxicity and efficacy in relapsed and refractory non-Hodgkin's lymphoma. J Clin Oncol 1993;11:1573–1582.

54. Van den Berg HW, Desai ZR, Wilson R, et al. The pharmacokinetics of vincristine in man: reduced drug clearance associated with raised serum alkaline phosphatase and dose-limiting elimination. Cancer Chemother Pharmacol 1982;8:215–219.

55. Kinzel PE, Dorr RT. Anticancer drug renal toxicity and elimination: dosing guidelines for altered renal function. Cancer Treat Rev 1995;21:33–64.

56. Bender RA, Castle MC, Margileth DA, Oliverio VT. The pharmacokinetics of [3H]-vincristine in man. Clin Pharmacol Ther 1977;22:430–438.

57. Nelson RL. The comparative clinical pharmacology and pharmacokinetics of vindesine, vincristine, and vinblastine in human patients with cancer. Med Pediatr Oncol 1982;10:115–127.

58. Nelson RL, Dyke RW, Root MA. Comparative pharmacokinetics of vindesine, vincristine, and vinblastine in patients with cancer. Cancer Treat Rev 1980;7(Suppl):17–14.

59. Rowinsky EK, Donehower RC. The clinical pharmacology and use of antimicrotubule agents in cancer chemotherapeutics. Pharmacol Ther 1991;52:35–84.

60. El Dareer SM, White VM, Chen FP, Mellett LB, Hill DL. Distribution and metabolism of vincristine in mice, rats, dogs and monkeys. Cancer Treat Rep 1977;61:1269–1277.

61. Castle MC, Margileth DA, Oliverio VT. Distribution and excretion of [3H]vincristine in the rat and the dog. Cancer Res 1976;36:3684–3689.

62. Sethi VS, Jackson DV, White DR, et al. Pharmacokinetics of vincristine sulfate in adult cancer patients. Cancer Res 1981;41:3551–3555.

63. Jackson DV, Castle MC, Poplack DG, Bender RA. Pharmacokinetics of vincristine in the cerebrospinal fluid of subhuman primates. Cancer Res 1980;40:722–724.

64. Jackson DV, Sethi VS, Spurr CL, McWhorter JM. Pharmacokinetics of vincristine in the cerebrospinal fluid of humans. Cancer Res 981;41:1466–1468.

65. Sethi VS, Castle MC, Surratt P, Jackson DV, Spurr CL. Isolation and partial characterization of human urinary metabolites of vincristine sulfate (abstract). Proc Am Assoc Cancer Res 1981;22:173.

66. Houghton JA, Williams LG, Torrance PM, Houghton PJ. Determinants of intrinsic sensitivity to vinca alkaloids in xenografts of pediatric rhabdomyosarcomas. Cancer Res 1984;44:582–590.

67. Jackson DV, Sethi VS, Spurr CL, et al. Pharmacokinetics of vincristine infusion. Cancer Treat Rep 1981;65:1043–1048.

68. Rogers GM, Ries CA. Long-term effectiveness of vincristine in the therapy of refractory autoimmune thrombocytopenia (letter). N Engl J Med 1980;303:585.

69. Gutterman LA, Stevenson TD. Treatment of thrombotic thrombocytopenia purpura with vincristine. JAMA 1982;247:1433–1436.

70. Bradley WG, Lassman LP, Pearce GW, Walton JN. The neuropathy of vincristine in man: clinical, electrophysiological and pathological studies. J Neurol Sci 1970;10:107–131.

71. Legha SS, Vincristine neurotoxicity. Pathophysiology and management. Med Toxicol 1986;1:421–427.

72. Tuxen MK, Hansen SW. Neurotoxicity secondary to antineoplastic drugs. Cancer Treat Rev 1994;20:191–214.

73. Miller BR. Neurotoxicity and vincristine (letter). JAMA 1985;253:2045.

74. Griffiths JD, Stark RJ, Ding JC, Cooper IA. Vincristine neurotoxicity in Charcot-Marie-Tooth syndrome. Med J Aust 1985;143:305–306.

75. McGuire SA, Gospe SM Jr, Dahl G. Acute vincristine neurotoxicity in the presence of hereditary motor and sensory neuropathy type I. Med Pediatr Oncol 1989;17:520–523.

76. Blain PG. Adverse effects of drugs on skeletal muscle. Adverse Drug React Bull 1984;104:384.

77. Donoso JA, Green LS, Heller-Bettinger E, Samson FE. Action of the vinca alkaloids vincristine, vinblastine, and desacetyl vinblastine amide on axonal fibrillar organelles in vitro. Cancer Res 1977;37:1401–1407.

78. Yousif H, Richardson SG, Saunders WA. Partially reversible nerve deafness due to vincristine. Postgrad Med J 1990;66:688–689.

79. Bird RL, Rohrbaugh TM, Raney B Jr, Norris D.

Transient cortical blindness secondary to vincristine therapy in children. Cancer 1983;47:37–40.

80. Ripps H, Mehaffey L 3d, Siegel IM, Niemeyer G. Vincristine-induced changes in the retina of the isolated arterially-perfused cat eye. Exp Eye Res 1989; 48:771–790.

81. Hironen HE, Saknu TT, Heinonen E, Antila KJ, Valimaki IA. Vincristine treatment of acute lymphoblastic leukemia induces transient autonomic cardioneuropathy. Cancer 1988;64:801–805.

82. Gottlieb RJ, Cuttner J. Vincristine-induced bladder atony. Cancer 1971;28:674–675.

83. Carmichael SM, Eagleton L, Ayers CR, Mohler D. Orthostatic hypotension during vincristine therapy. Arch Intern Med 1970;126:290–293.

84. Grush OC, Morgan SK. Folinic acid rescue for vincristine toxicity. Clin Toxicol 1979;14:71–78.

85. Jackson DV Jr, Pope EK, McMahan RA, et al. Clinical trial of pyridoxine to reduce vincristine neurotoxicity. J Neurooncol 1986;4:37–41.

86. Jackson DV Jr, McMahan RA, Pope EK, et al. Clinical trial of folinic acid to reduce vincristine neurotoxicity. Cancer Chemother Pharmacol 1986;17:281–284.

87. Jackson DV, Wells HB, Atkins JN, et al. Amelioration of vincristine neurotoxicity by glutamic acid. Am J Med 1988;84:1016–1022.

88. Sharma RK. Vincristine and gastrointestinal transit. Gastroenterology 1988;95:1435–1436.

89. Harris AC, Jackson JM. Lactulose in vincristine-induced constipation. Med J Aust 1972;2P:573.

90. Agosti A, Bertaccini G, Paulucci R, Zanella E. Caerulein treatment for paralytic ileus. Lancet 1971; 1:395.

91. Garewal HS, Dalton WS. Metoclopramide in vincristine-induced ileus. Cancer Treat Rep 1985; 69:1309–1311.

92. Jackson DV, Wu WC, Spurr CL. Treatment of vincristine-induced ileus with sincalide, a cholecystokinin analogue. Cancer Chemother Pharmacol 1982; 8:83–85.

93. Castle MC. Plant alkyloids: the vinca alkaloids. In: Woolley PV, ed. Cancer management in man: biological response modifiers, chemotherapy, antibiotics, hyperthermia, supporting measures. Dordrecht: Kluwer Academic Publishers, 1987:147–151.

94. Kantor AF, Greene MH, Boice JD, Fraumeni JF, Flannery JT. Are vinca alkaloids associated with myocardial infarction (letter)? Lancet 1981;1:1111.

95. Stuart MJ, Cuaso C, Miller M, Oski F. Syndrome of recurrent increased secretion of antidiuretic hormone following multiple doses of vincristine. Blood 1975;45:315–320.

96. Kaufman IA, Khung FH, Koenig HM, Giammona ST. Overdosage with vincristine. J Pediatr 1976; 89:671–674.

97. Bunn PA, Ford SS, Shackney SE. The effects of colcemid on hematopoiesis in the mouse. J Clin Invest 1975;58:1280–1286.

98. Bellone JD. Treatment of vincristine extravasation (letter). JAMA 1981;245:343.

99. Ishii E, Hara T, Mizuno Y, Ueda K. Vincristine-induced fever in children with leukemia and lymphoma. Cancer 1988;61:660–662.

100. Benvenuto JA, Anderson RW, Kerkoff K, et al. Stability and compatibility of antitumor agents in glass and plastic containers. Am J Hosp Pharm 1981; 38:1914–1918.

101. Keller JH, Ensminger WD. Stability of cancer chemotherapeutic agents in a totally implanted drug delivery system. Am J Hosp Pharm 1982;39:1321–1323.

102. Yap H-Y, Blumenschein GR, Keating MJ, Hortobagyi GN, Tashima CK, Loo TL. Vinblastine given as a continuous 5-day infusion in the treatment of refractory advanced breast cancer. Cancer Treat Rep 1982;64:279–283.

103. Zeffren J, Yagoda A, Kelsen D, Winn R. Phase I-II trial of 5-day continuous infusion of vinblastine sulfate. Anticancer Res 1984;4:411–414.

104. Ratain MJ, Vogelzang NJ. Phase I and pharmacological study of vinblastine by prolonged continuous infusion. Cancer Res 1986;46:4827–4830.

105. Steele WH, Barber HE, Dawson AA, King DJ, Petrie JC. Protein binding of prednisone and vinblastine in the serum of normal subjects. Br J Clin Pharmacol 1982;13:595–596.

106. Owellen RJ, Hartke CA, Hains FO. Pharmacokinetics and metabolism of vinblastine in humans. Cancer Res 1977;37:2597–2602.

107. Owellen RJ, Hartke CA. The pharmacokinetics of 4-acetyl tritium vinblastine in two patients. Cancer Res 1975;35:975–980.

108. Greenius HF, McIntyre RW, Beer CT. The preparation of vinblastine- 4-acetyl-t- and its distribution in the blood of rats. J Med Chem 1968;11:254–257.

109. Hebden HF, Hadfield JR, Beer CT. The binding of vinblastine by platelets in the rat. Cancer Res 1970;30:1417–1424.

110. Creasey WA, Scott AI, Wei CC, Kutcher J, Schwartz A, Marsh JC. Pharmacological studies with vinblastine in the dog. Cancer Res 1975;35:1116–1120.

111. Lu K, Yap HY, Watts S, Loo TL. Comparative clinical pharmacology of vinblastine (VBL) in patients with advanced breast cancer: single versus continuous infusion (abstract). Proc Am Assoc Cancer Res and ASCO 1979;20:371.

112. Einhorn LH, Donohue J. Cis-diamminedichloroplatinum, vinblastine and bleomycin combination chemotherapy in disseminated testicular cancer. Ann Intern Med 1977;87:293–298.

113. Williams SD, Birch R, Einhorn LH, Irwin L, Greco FA, Loehrer PJ. Disseminated germ cell tumors: chemotherapy with cisplatin plus bleomycin plus either vinblastine or etoposide. A trial of the Southeastern Cancer Study Group. N Engl J Med 1987;316:1435–1440.

114. Bonadonna G, Zucadi R, Monfardini S, DeLina M, Uslenghi G. Combination chemotherapy of Hodgkin's disease with Adriamycin, bleomycin, vinblastine and imidazole carboxamide versus MOPP. Cancer 1979;36:252–259.

115. Bonadonna G, Valagussa P, Santoro A. Alternating non-cross-resistant combination chemotherapy or MOPP in stage IV Hodgkin's disease. A report of 8-year results. Ann Intern Med 1986;104:739–746.

116. Klimo P, Connors JM. MOPP/ABV hybrid program: combination chemotherapy based on early introduction of seven effective drugs for advanced Hodgkin's disease. J Clin Oncol 1985;3:1170–1182.

117. Hammon CB, Borcet LG, Tyrey L, Creasman CD, Parker RT. Treatment of metastatic trophoblastic disease: good and poor prognosis. Am J Obstet Gynecol 1974;115:451–457.

118. Gomez GA, Sokal JE. Use of vinblastine in the terminal phase of chronic myelocytic leukemia. Cancer Treat Rep 1979;63:1385–1387.

119. Tucker SB, Winkelmann RK. Treatment of Kaposi sarcoma with vinblastine. Arch Dermatol 1976; 112:958–961.

120. Starling KA, Donaldson MH, Haggard ME, Vietti TJ, Sutow WW. Therapy of histiocytosis X with vincristine, vinblastine, and cyclophosphamide. Am J Dis Child 1972;123:105–110.

121. Sternberg CN, Yagoda A, Scher HI, Watson RC, Herr HW, Morse MJ. M-VAC (methotrexate, vinblastine, Adriamycin, and cisplatin) for advanced transitional cell carcinoma of the urothelium. J Urol 1988; 139:461–469.

122. Yap H-Y, Blumenschein GR, Keating MJ, Hortobagyi GN, Tashima CK, Loo TL. Vinblastine given as a continuous 5-day infusion in the treatment of refractory advanced breast cancer. Cancer Treat Rep 1982;64:279–283.

123. Zeffren J, Yagoda A, Kelsen D, Winn R. Phase I-II trial of 5-day continuous infusion of vinblastine sulfate. Anticancer Res 1984;4:411–414.

124. Schulman P, Budman DR, Vinciguerra V, Weiselberg L, Abrams S, Degman T. Phase II study of divided-dose vinblastine in non-small cell bronchogenia carcinoma. Cancer Treat Rep 1982;66:171–172.

125. Ahn YS, Byrnes JJ, Harrington WJ, Cayer ML, Smith DS, Brunskill DE. Treatment of idiopathic thrombocytopenic purpura with vinblastine-loaded platelets. N Engl J Med 1978;298:1101–1107.

126. Ahn YS, Harrington WJ, Mylvaganam R, Allen LM, Rall LM. Slow infusion of vinca alkaloids in the treatment of idiopathic thrombocytopenic purpura. Ann Intern Med 1984;100:192–196.

127. Subar M, Muggia FM. Apparent myocardial ischemia associated with vinblastine administration. Cancer Treat Rep 1986;70:690–691.

128. Teutsch C, Lipton A, Harvey HA. Raynaud's phenomenon as a side effect of chemotherapy with vinblastine and bleomycin for testicular carcinoma. Cancer Treat Rep 1977;61:925–926.

129. Hantel A, Rowinsky EK, Donehower RC. Nifedipine and oncologic Raynaud's phenomenon (letter). Ann Intern Med 1988;108:767.

130. Israel RH, Olson JP. Pulmonary edema associated with intravenous vinblastine (letter). JAMA 1978;240:1585.

131. Dyke RW. Acute bronchospasm after vinca alkaloids in patients previously treated with mitomycin (letter). N Engl J Med 1984;310:389.

132. Dorr RT, Jones SE. Inapparent infiltrations associated with vindesine administration. Med Pediatr Oncol 1979;6:285–288.

133. Ginsberg SJ, Comis RL, Fitzpatrick AV. Vinblastine and inappropriate ADH secretion (letter). N Engl J Med 1978;296:941.

134. Rowinsky EK, Noe DA, Lucas VS, et al. A phase I, pharmacokinetic and absolute bioavailability study of oral vinorelbine (Navelbine) in solid tumor patients. J Clin Oncol 1994;12:1754–1763.

135. Robieux I, Sorio R, Vitali V, et al. Pharmacokinetics of vinorelbine in breast cancer patients with liver metastases (abstract). Proc Am Soc Clin Oncol 1995;14:458.

136. Rahmani R, Zhou XJ. Pharmacokinetics and metabolism of vinca alkaloids. In: Workman P, Graham MA, eds. Cancer surveys, pharmacokinetics and cancer chemotherapy, vol 17. Plainview, NY: Cold Spring Harbor Laboratory Press, 1993:269–281.

137. Rahmani R, Bruno R, Iliadis A, et al. Clinical pharmacokinetics of the antitumor drug Navelbine (5'-noranhydrovinblastine). Cancer Res 1987;47:5796–5799.

138. Krikorian A, Rahmani R, Bromet M, Bore P, Cano JP. Pharmacokinetics and metabolism of Navelbine. Semin Oncol 1989;16(Suppl 4):21–25.

139. Bore P, Rahmani R, van Cantfort J, Focan C, Cano JP. Pharmacokinetics of a new anticancer drug Navelbine, in patients. Cancer Chemother Pharmacol 1987;23:247–251.

140. Jehl F, Quoix E, Monteil H, Pauli G, Krikorian A. Human pharmacokinetics of Navelbine (NAV), a new vinca alkaloid, as determined by high performance liquid chromatography (HPLC) (abstract). Proc Am Soc Clin Oncol 1990;9:252.

141. Jehl F, Quoix E, Leveque D, et al. Pharmacokinetics and preliminary metabolic fate of Navelbine in humans as determined by high performance liquid chromatography. Cancer Res 1991;51:2073–2076.

142. Urien S, Bree F, Breillout F, et al. Vinorelbine high-affinity binding to human platelets and lymphocytes: distribution in human blood. Cancer Chemother Pharmacol 1988;23:231–234.

143. Leveque D, Quoiz E, Dumont P, et al. Pulmonary distribution of vinorelbine in patients with non-small lung cancer. Cancer Chemother Pharmacol 1993;33:176–178.

144. Sahnoun Z, Durand A, Placid M, et al. Research of Navelbine metabolites in the patient using high performance liquid chromatography. Bull Cancer 1990;77:598.

145. Rahmani, R, Bore, P, Cano, JP, et al. Phase I trial of escalating doses of orally administered Navelbine. Part I—Pharmacokinetics (abstract). Proc Am Soc Clin Oncol 1989;8:74.

146. Cvitkovic E, Izzo J. The current and future place of vinorelbine in cancer therapy. Drugs 1992; 44(Suppl 2):36–45.

147. Binet S, Fellous A, Lataste H, Krikorian A, Couzinier JP, Meininger V. In situ analysis of the action of Navelbine on various types of microtubules using immunofluorescence. Semin Oncol 1989;16(Suppl 4):5–8.

148. Hohneker JA A summary of vinorelbine (Navelbine) safety data from North American clinical trials. Semin Oncol 1994;21(Suppl 10):42–47.

149. Le Chevalier T, Brisgand D, Douillard J-Y, et al. Randomized study of vinorelbine and cisplatin versus vindesine and cisplatin versus vinorelbine alone in non-small cell lung cancer: results of a European multicenter trial including 612 patients. J Clin Oncol 1994;12:360–367.

150. Nelson RI, Dyke RW, Root MA. Clinical pharmacokinetics of vindesine. Cancer Chem Pharm 1979; 2:243–246.

151. Culp HW, Daniels WD, McMahon RE. Disposition and tissue levels of [^{3}H]-vindesine in rats. Cancer Res 1977;37:3053–3056.

152. Rahmani R, Kleisbauer JP, Cano JP, Martin M, Barbet J. Clinical pharmacokinetics of vindesine infusion. Cancer Treat Rep 1985;69:839–844.

153. Jackson DV Jr. The periwinkle alkaloids. In: Lokich JJ, ed. Cancer chemotherapy by infusion. Chicago: Precept Press, 1990:155–175.

154. Jackson DV Jr, Sethi VS, Long TR, Muss HB, Spurr CL. Pharmacokinetics of vindesine bolus and

infusion. Cancer Chemother Pharmacol 1984;13:114–119.

155. Ohnuma T, Norton L, Andrejczuk A, Holland JF. Pharmacokinetics of vindesine given as an intravenous bolus and 24-hour infusion in humans. Cancer Res 1985;45:464–469.

156. Rahmani R, Martin M, Favre R, Cano J-P, Barbet J. Clinical pharmacokinetics of vindesine: repeated treatments by intravenous bolus injections. Eur J Cancer Clin Oncol 1984;20:1409–1417.

157. Gralla RJ, Casper ES, Kelsen DP, et al. Cisplatin and vindesine chemotherapy for advanced carcinoma of the lung: a randomized trial investigating two dosage schedules. Ann Intern Med 1981;95:414–420.

158. Zhou XJ, Zhou-Pan XR, Gauthier T, et al. Human liver microsomal cytochrome P450 3A isoenzymes mediated vindesine biotransformation: metabolic drug interactions. Biomed Pharmacol 1993;4:853–861.

159. Owellen RJ, Root MA, Hains FO. Pharmacokinetic of vindesine and vincristine in humans. Cancer Res 1977;37:2603–2607.

160. Kris MG, Gralla RJ, Kelsen DP, Casper ES, Burke MT, Fione JJ. Trial of vindesine plus mitomycin in stage-3 non-small cell lung cancer: a regimen for outpatient treatment. Chest 1985;87:368–372.

161. Mathe G, Misset JL, DeVassal F. Phase II clinical trial with vindesine for remission induction in acute leukemia, blastic crises of chronic myeloid leukemia, lymphosarcoma, and Hodgkin's disease: absence of cross-resistance with vincristine. Cancer Treat Rep 1978;62:1427–1433.

162. Smith IE, Hedley DW, Powles TJ, McElwain TJ. Vindesine—a phase II study in the treatment of breast carcinoma, malignant melanoma, and other tumors. Cancer Treat Rep 1978;62:1427–1433.

163. Ohnuma T, Holland JF, Andrejczuk A, Greenspan E. Initial clinical and pharmacological studies with vindesine (abstract). Proc Am Assoc Cancer Res 1978;19:129.

164. Bodey GP, Yap, H-Y, Yap B-S, Valdivieso M. Continuous infusion vindesine in solid tumors. Cancer Treat Rev 1980;7(Suppl):39–45.

165. Bolin R, Riva R, Albani R, et al. Decreased phenytoin level during antineoplastic therapy: a case report. Epilepsia 1983;24:75–78.

166. Jarosinski PF, Moscow JA, Alexander MS, Lesko LJ, Balis FM, Poplack DG. Altered phenytoin clearance during intensive chemotherapy for acute lymphoblastic leukemia. J Pediatr 1988;112:996–999.

167. Tobe SW, Siu LL, Jamal SA, Skorecki KL, Murphy GF, Warner E. Vinblastine and erythromycin: an unrecognized serious drug interaction. Cancer Chemother Pharmacol 1995;35:188–190.

168. Lena N, Imbert AM, Pignon T, et al. Methotrexate-vindesine association in the treatment of head and neck cancer. Influence of vindesine on methotrexate's pharmacokinetic behavior. Cancer Chemother Pharmacol 1984;12:120–124.

169. Bore P, Lena N, Imbert AM, et al. Methotrexate-vindesine association in head and neck cancer: modification of methotrexate's hydroxylation in the presence of vindesine. Cancer Chemother Pharmacol 1986;66:862–867.

170. Tubiana N, Lena N, Barbet J, et al. Methotrexate-vindesine association in leukemia: pharmacokinetic study. Med Oncol Tumor Pharmacother 1985; 2:99–102.

171. Bender RA, Bleyer WA, Frisby SA. Alteration of methotrexate uptake in human leukemia cells by other agents. Cancer Res 1975;35:1305–1308.

172. Zager RF, Frisby SA, Oliverio VT. The effects of antibiotics and cancer chemotherapeutic agents on the cellular transport and antitumor activity of methotrexate in L1210 murine leukemia. Cancer Res 1973; 33:1670–1676.

173. Bender RA, Nichols AP, Norton L, et al. Lack of therapeutic synergism of vincristine and methotrexate in L1210 murine leukemia in vivo. Cancer Treat Rep 1978;62:997–1003.

174. Yalowich JC. Effect of microtubule inhibition on etoposide accumulation and DNA damage in human K562 cells in vitro. Cancer Res 1987;47:1010–1015.

175. Samuels ML, Johnson DE, Holoye PY. Continuous intravenous bleomycin (NSC-125066) therapy with vinblastine (NSC-49842) in stage II testicular neoplasia. Cancer Chemother Rep 1975;59:563–570.

176. Rowinsky EK, Cazenave LA, Donehower RC. Taxol: a novel investigational antineoplastic agent. J Natl Cancer Inst 1990;82:1247–1259.

177. Verweij J, Clavel M, Chevalier B. Paclitaxel (Taxol) and docetaxel (Taxotere): not simply two of a kind. Ann Oncol 1994;5:495–505.

178. Kingston DGI, Samaranayake G, Ivey CA. The chemistry of Taxol, a clinically useful anticancer agent. J Nat Prod 1990;53:1–12.

179. Rao S, Horwitz SB, Ringel I. Direct photoaffinity labeling of tubulin with Taxol. J Natl Cancer Inst 1992;84:785–788.

180. Rao S, Krauss NE, Heerding JM, et al. 3'-(p-Azidobenzamido)taxol photolabels the N-terminal 31 amino acids of beta-tubulin. J Biol Chem 1994;269:3132–3134.

181. Wilson L, Miller HP, Farrell KW, Snyder KB, Thompson WC, Purich DL. Taxol stabilization of microtubules in vitro: dynamics of tubulin addition and loss at opposite microtubule ends. Biochemistry 1985; 24:5254–5262.

182. Schiff PB, Fant J, Horwitz SB. Promotion of microtubule assembly in vitro by Taxol. Nature 1979; 22:665–667.

183. Schiff PB, Horwitz SB. Taxol stabilizes microtubules in mouse fibroblast cells. Proc Natl Acad Sci USA 1980;77:1561–1565.

184. Parness J, Horwitz SB. Taxol binds to polymerized microtubules in vitro. J Cell Biol 1981; 91:479–487.

185. Manfredi JJ, Parness J, Horwitz SB. Taxol binds to cellular microtubules. J Cell Biol 1982;94:688–696.

186. Ringel I, Horwitz SB. Studies with RP56976 (Taxotere): a semisynthetic analogue of Taxol. J Natl Cancer Inst 1991;83:288–291.

187. Diaz JF, Andreu JM. Assembly of purified GDP-tubulin into microtubules into microtubules induced by Taxol and Taxotere: reversibility, ligand stoichiometry and competition. Biochemistry 1993; 32:2747–2755.

188. Bissery M-C, Guenard D, Gueritte-Voegelein F, Lavelle F. Experimental antitumor activity of Taxotere (RP 56976, NSC 628503), a Taxol analogue. Cancer Res 1991;51:4845–4852.

189. Rowinsky EK, Donehower RC, Jones RJ,

Tucker RW. Microtubule changes and cytotoxicity in leukemic cell lines treated with Taxol. Cancer Res 1988; 48:4093–4100.

190. De Brabander M, Geuens G, Nuydens R, Willebrords R, De Mey J. Taxol induces the assembly of free microtubules in living cells and blocks the organizing capacity of the centrosomes and kinetochores. Proc Natl Acad Sci USA 1981;78:5608–5612.

191. Jordan MA, Toso RJ, Thrower D, Wilson L. Mechanism of mitotic block and inhibition of cell proliferation by Taxol at low concentrations. Proc Natl Acad Sci USA 1993;90:9552–9556.

192. Jordan MA, Thrower D, Wilson L. Mechanism of inhibition of cell proliferation by *Vinca* alkaloids. Cancer Res 1991;51:2212–2222.

193. Donaldson KL, Gollsby G, Kiener PA, Wahl AF. Activation of $p34^{cdc2}$ coincident with Taxol-induced apoptosis. Cell Growth Differ 1994;5:1041–1050.

194. Tishler RB, Schiff PB, Geard CR, Hall EJ. Taxol: a novel radiation sensitizer. Int J Radiat Oncol Biol Phys 1992;22:613–617.

195. Tishler RB, Geard CR, Hall EJ, Schiff PB. Taxol sensitizes human astrocytoma cells to radiation. Cancer Res 1992;52:3495–3497.

196. Choy H, Rodrieguez F, Wilcox, Koester SK, Degen D. Radiation sensitizing effects of Taxotere (RP 56976) (abstract). Proc Am Assoc Cancer Res 1992; 33:500.

197. Cabral F, Wible L, Brenner S, Brinkley BR. Taxol-requiring mutants of Chinese hamster ovary cells with impaired mitotic spindle activity. J Cell Biol 1983;97:30–39.

198. Cabral FR. Isolation of Chinese hamster ovary cell mutants requiring the continuous presence of Taxol for cell division. J Biol Biol 1983;97:22–29.

199. Horwitz SB, Cohen D, Rao S, Ringel I, Shen H-J, Yang C-P. Taxol: mechanisms of action and resistance. Monog Natl Cancer Inst 1993;15:63–67.

200. Horwitz SB, Lothstein L, Mellado W, et al. Taxol: mechanisms of action and resistance. Ann NY Acad Sci 1986;466:733–744.

201. Lehnert M, Emerson S, Dalton W, de Giulie R, Salmon S. In vitro evaluation of chemosensitzers for clinical reversal of P-glycoprotein-associated Taxol resistance. Monogr Natl Cancer Inst 1993;15:63–67.

202. Woodcock DM, Jefferson S, Linsenmeyer ME. Reversal of the multidrug resistance phenotype with Cremophor EL, a common vehicle for water-insoluble vitamins and drugs. Cancer Res 1990;50:4199–4203.

203. Webster L, Linenmyer M, Millward M, Morton C, Bishop J, Woodcock D. Measurement of Cremophor EL following Taxol: plasma levels sufficient to reverse drug exclusion mediated by the multidrug-resistant phenotype. J Natl Cancer Inst 1993;85:1685–1690.

204. Seidman AD, Reichman BS, Crown JPA, et al. Paclitaxel as second and subsequent chemotherapy for metastatic breast cancer: activity independent of prior anthracycline response. J Clin Oncol 1995;13:1152–1159.

205. Rowinsky EK, Burke PJ, Karp JE, Tucker RW, Ettinger DS, Donehower RC. Phase I and pharmacodynamic study of Taxol in refractory adult acute leukemia. Cancer Res 1989;49:4640–4647.

206. Gianni L, Kearns C, Gianni A, et al. Nonlinear pharmacokinetics and metabolism of paclitaxel and its pharmacokinetic/pharmacodynamic relationships in humans. J Clin Oncol 1995;13:180–190.

207. Huizing MT, Keung ACF, Rosing H, et al. Pharmacokinetics of paclitaxel and metabolites in a randomized comparative study in platinum-pretreated ovarian cancer patients. J Clin Oncol 1993; 11:2127–2135.

208. Ohtsu T, Sasaki Y, Tamura T, et al. Clinical pharmacokinetics and pharmacodynamics of paclitaxel: a 3-hour infusion versus a 24-hour infusion. Clin Cancer Res 1995;1:599–606.

209. Wilson WH, Berg S, Bryant G, et al. Paclitaxel in doxorubicin-refractory or mitoxantrone-refractory breast cancer: a phase I/II trial of 96 hour infusion. J Clin Oncol 1994;12:1621–1629.

210. Hochhauser D, Seidman AD, Gollub M, et al. Efficacy of prolonged paclitaxel infusion after failure of prior short taxane infusion: a phase II and pharmacologic study in metastatic breast cancer. Proceedings of the 17th Annual San Antonio Breast Cancer Symposium (abstract). Breast Cancer Res Treat 1994; 32:24.

211. Hainsworth JD, Thompson DS, Greco FA. Paclitaxel by 1-hour infusion: an active drug in metastatic non-small cell lung cancer. J Clin Oncol 1995;13:1609–1614.

212. Goldspiel BR, Kohler D, Koustenis AG, et al. Paclitaxel administration using portable infusion pumps. J Clin Oncol 1993;11:2287–2288.

213. Schilder LE, Egorin ME, Zuhowski EG, et al. The pharmacokinetics of taxol in a dialysis patient (abstract). Proc Am Soc Clin Oncol 1994;13:136.

214. Fazeny B, Olsen SJ, Willey T, et al. Pharmacokinetic assessment of paclitaxel in an ovarian cancer patient on hemodialysis (abstract). Proc Am Soc Clin Oncol 1994;13:136.

215. Venock AP, Egorin M, Braun TD, et al. Paclitaxel (TAXOL) in patients with liver dysfunction (CALGB 9264) (abstract). Proc Am Soc Clin Oncol 1994; 13:139.

216. Zaheer W, Lichtman SM, DeMarco L, et al. The use of Taxol in elderly patients (abstract). Proc Am Soc Clin Oncol 1994;13:441.

217. Bicher A, Sarosy G, Kohn E, et al. Age does not influence Taxol dose intensity in recurrent carcinoma of the ovary. Cancer 1993;71(Suppl 2):594–600.

218. Longnecker SM, Donehower RC, Cates AE, et al. High performance liquid chromatographic assay for Taxol (NSC 125973) in human plasma and urine pharmacokinetics in a phase I trial. Cancer Treat Rep 1986; 71:53–59.

219. Grem JL, Tutsch KD, Simon KJ, et al. Phase I study of Taxol administered as a short iv infusion daily for 5 days. Cancer Treat Rep 1987;71:1179–1184.

220. Wiernik PH, Schwartz EL, Strauman JJ, et al. Phase I clinical and pharmacokinetic study of Taxol. Cancer Res 1987;47:2486–2493.

221. Wiernik PH, Schwartz EL, Einzig A, et al. Phase I trial of Taxol given as a 24-hour infusion every 21 days: responses observed in metastatic melanoma. J Clin Oncol 1987;5:1232–1239.

222. Brown T, Havlin K, Weiss G, et al. A phase I trial of Taxol given by 6-hour intravenous infusion. J Clin Oncol 1991;9:1261–1267.

223. Sonnichsen D, Hurwitz C, Pratt C, Relling MV. Saturable pharmacokinetics and paclitaxel phar-

macodynamics in children with solid tumors. J Clin Oncol 1994;12:532–538.

224. Kumar GN, Walle UK, Bhalla KN, Walle T. Binding of Taxol to human plasma, albumin, and alpha 1-acid glycoprotein. Res Commun Chem Pathol Pharmacol 1993;80:337–344.

225. Wild MD, Walle K, Walle T. Extensive and saturable accumulation of paclitaxel (Taxol) by the human platelet. Cancer Chemother Pharmacol 1995; 36:41–44.

226. Glantz MJ, Choy H, Kearns CM, et al. Paclitaxel disposition in plasma and central nervous systems of humans and rats with brain tumors. J Natl Cancer Inst 1995;87:1077–1081.

227. Lesser G, Grossman SA, Eller S, Rowinsky EK. The neural and extra-neural distribution of systemically administered [³H]paclitaxel in rats: a quantitative autoradiographic study. Cancer Chemother Pharmacol 1996; in press.

228. Monsarrat B, Alvinerie P, Dubois J, et al. Hepatic metabolism and biliary clearance of Taxol in rats and humans. Monogr Natl Cancer Inst 1993;15:39–46.

229. Gaver RC, Deeb G, Willey T, et al. The disposition of paclitaxel (Taxol) in the rat (abstract). Proc Am Assoc Cancer Res 1993;34:390.

230. Walle T, Walle UK, Kumar GN, Bhalla KN. Taxol metabolism and disposition in cancer patients. Drug Metab Dispos 1995;23:1–7.

231. Cresteil T, Monsarrat B, Alvinerie P, et al. Taxol metabolism by human liver microsomes: identification of cytochrome P450 isoenzymes involved in its biotransformation. Cancer Res 1994;54:386–392.

232. Harris JW, Rahman A, Kim B-R, Guengerich P, Collins JM. Metabolism of Taxol by human hepatic microsomes and liver slices: participation of cytochrome P450 3A4 and an unknown P450 enzyme. Cancer Res 1994:15:4026–4035.

233. Harris JW, Katki A, Anderson LW, et al. Isolation, structural determination, and biological activity of 6alpha-hydroxytaxol, the principal human metabolite of Taxol. J Med Chem 1994;37:706–709.

234. Monsarrat B, Mariel E, Crois S, et al. Taxol metabolism. Isolation and identification of three major metabolites in rat bile. Drug Metab Dispos 1990; 18:895–901.

235. Rowinsky EK, Donehower RC. Drug therapy: paclitaxel (Taxol). N Engl J Med 1995;332:1004–1114.

236. McGuire WP, Hoskins WJ, Brady MR, et al. Taxol and cisplatin (TP) improves outcome in advanced ovarian cancer (AOC) as compared to cytoxan and cisplatin (CP) (abstract). Proc Am Soc Clin Oncol 1995;14:275.

237. Seidman AD. The emerging role of paclitaxel in breast cancer therapy. Clin Cancer Res 1995;1:247–250.

238. Weiss R, Donehower RC, Wiernik PH, et al. Hypersensitivity reactions from Taxol. J Clin Oncol 1990;8:1263–1268.

239. Rowinsky EK, Eisenhauer EA, Chaudhry V, Arbuck SA, Donehower RC. Clinical toxicities encountered with Taxol. Semin Oncol 1993;20(Suppl 3):1–15.

240. Eisenhauer E, ten Bokkel Huinink W, Swenerton KD, et al. European-Canadian randomized trial of Taxol in relapsed ovarian cancer: high vs. low dose and long vs. short infusion. J Clin Oncol 1994;12:2654–2666.

241. Rowinsky EK, Chaudhry V, Cornblath DR, Donehower RC. The neurotoxicity of Taxol. Monogr Natl Cancer Inst 1993;15:107–115.

242. Chaudhry V, Rowinsky EK, Sartorius SE, Donehower RC, Cornblath DR. Peripheral neuropathy from Taxol and cisplatin combination chemotherapy: clinical and electrophysiological studies. Ann Neurol 1994;35:490–497.

243. Capri G, Munzone E, Tarenzi E, Fulgaro F, Gianni L. Optic nerve disturbances: a new form of paclitaxel neurotoxicity (letter). J Natl Cancer Inst 1994; 86:1099–1101.

244. Martoni A, Zamagni C, Gheka A, Pannuti F. Antihistamines in the treatment of Taxol-induced paroxystic pain syndrome. J Natl Cancer Inst 1993; 85:676–677.

245. Rowinsky EK, McGuire WP, Guarnieri T, Christian MA, Donehower RC. Cardiac disturbances during the administration of Taxol. J Clin Oncol 1991; 9:1704–1712.

246. Arbuck SG, Strauss H, Rowinsky EK, et al. A reassessment of the cardiac toxicity associated with Taxol. Monogr Natl Cancer Inst 1993;15:117–132.

247. Gianni L, Munzone E, Capri G, et al. Paclitaxel by 3-hour infusion in combination with bolus doxorubicin in women with untreated metastatic breast cancer: high antitumor efficacy and cardiac effects in a dosing-finding and sequence-finding study. J Clin Oncol 1995;13:2688–2699.

248. Pestalozzi BC, Sotos GA, Choyke PL, et al. Typhlitis resulting from treatment with Taxol and doxorubicin in patients with metastatic breast cancer. Cancer 1993;71:1797–1800.

249. Kennedy MJ, Armstrong D, Donehower R, et al. The hematologic toxicity of the Taxol/cytoxan doublet is sequence-dependent (abstract). Proc Am Soc Clin Oncol 1994;13:137.

250. Freilich RJ, Seidman AD. Pruritus caused by 3-hour infusions of high-dose paclitaxel and improvement with tricyclic antidepressants. J Natl Cancer Inst 1995;87:933–934.

251. Extra J-M, Rousseau F, Bruno R, Clavel M, Le Bail N, Marty M. Phase I and pharmacokinetic study of Taxotere (RP 56976; NSC 628503) given as a short intravenous infusion. Cancer Res 1993;53:1037–1042.

252. Pazdur R, Newman RA, Newman BM, et al. Phase I trial of Taxotere: five-day schedule. J Natl Cancer Inst 1992;84:1781–1788.

253. Bissett D, Setanoians A, Cassidy J, et al. Phase I and pharmacokinetic study of Taxotere (RP 56976) administered as a 24-hour infusion. Cancer Res 1993; 53:523–527.

254. Bruno R, Sanderink GJ. Pharmacokinetics and metabolism of Taxotere (docetaxel). In: Workman P, Graham MA, eds. Cancer surveys. Pharmacokinetics and cancer chemotherapy, vol. 17. Cold Spring Harbor, NY: Cold Spring Harbor Laboratory Press, 1993:305–313.

255. Eisenhauer E, ten Bokkel Huinink W, Swenerton KD, et al. European-Canadian randomized trial of Taxol in relapsed ovarian cancer: high vs. low dose and long vs. short infusion. J Clin Oncol 1994;12:2654–2666.

256. Kumar GN, Walle UK, Bhalla KN, Walle T. Binding of Taxol to human plasma, albumin, and alpha 1-acid glycoprotein. Res Commun Chem Pathol Pharmacol 1993;80:337–344.

257. Bruno R, Dorr MB, Montay G, et al. Design and implementation of population pharmacokinetic studies during the development of docetaxel (RP 56976), a new anticancer drug (abstract). Clin Pharmacol Ther 1994;55:161.

258. Marland M, Gaillard C, Sanderink G, et al. Kinetics, distribution, metabolism and excretion of radiolabelled Taxotere (^{14}C-RP 56976) in mice and dogs (abstract). Proc Am Assoc Cancer Res 1993;34:393.

259. Aapro MS, Zulian G, Alberto P, Bruno R, Oulid-Aissa D, Le Bail N. Phase I and pharmacokinetic study of RP 56976 in a new ethanol-free formulation of Taxotere (abstract). Ann Oncol 1992;3(Suppl 3):53.

260. Gaillard C, Monsarrat B, Vuilhorgne M, et al. Docetaxel (Taxotere) metabolism in the rat in vivo and in vitro (abstract). Proc Am Assoc Cancer Res 1994; 35:428.

261. Gires P, Gaillard C, Martin S, et al. [^{14}C]-Docetaxel (Taxotere) disposition in the isolated perfused rat liver and effect of enzyme induction (abstract). Eur J Drug Metab Pharmacokinet 1994;19(Suppl 2):29.

262. Marre F, De Sousa G, Placidi M, Fabre JL, Rahamani R. Elucidation of hepatic biotransformation of Taxotere using human "in vitro" models (abstract). Bull Cancer 1993;80:527.

263. Zhou-Pan XR, Marre F, Zhou XJ, Gauthier T, Placidi M, Rahmani R. Preliminary characterization of Taxotere metabolism using human liver microsomal fractions (abstract). Maimonide 1992;1:s23.

264. Commercon A, Bourzat JD, Bezard D, Vuilhorgne M. Partial synthesis of major human metabolites of docetaxel. Tetrahedron 1994;50:10289–10298.

265. Fosella FV, Lee JS, Murphy WK, et al. Phase II study of docetaxel for recurrent or metastatic non-small cell lung cancer. J Clin Oncol 1994;12:1238–1244.

266. Francis PA, Rigas JR, Kris MG, et al. Phase II trial of docetaxel in patients with stage III and IV non-small cell lung cancer. J Clin Oncol 1994;12:1232–1237.

267. Frances P, Schneider J, Hann L, et al. Phase II trial of docetaxel in patients with platinum-refractory advanced ovarian cancer. J Clin Oncol 1994;12:2201–2201.

268. Chevallier B, Fumoleau P, Kerbrat P, et al. Docetaxel is a major cytotoxic drug for the treatment of advanced breast cancer: a phase II trial of the Clinical Screening Cooperative Group of the European Organization for Research and Treatment of Cancer. J Clin Oncol 1995;13:314–322.

269. Vukeljia SJ, Baker WJ, Burris HA III, Keeling JH, Von Hoff D. Pyridoxine therapy for palmar-plantar erthrodysesthesia associated with Taxotere. J Natl Cancer Inst 1993;85:1432–1433.

270. Zimmerman GC, Keeling JH, Lowry M, Medina J, Von Hoff DD, Burris HA. Prevention of docetaxel-induced erythrodysthesia with local hypothermia (letter). J Natl Cancer Inst 1994;86:557.

271. Rowinsky EK, Gilbert M, McGuire WP, et al. Sequences of Taxol and cisplatin: a phase I and pharmacologic study. J Clin Oncol 1991;9:1692–1703.

272. Rowinsky EK, Citardi M, Noe DA, Donehower RC. Sequence-dependent cytotoxicity between cisplatin and the antimicrotubule agents Taxol and vincristine. J Cancer Res Clin Oncol 1993;119:737–743.

273. Parker RJ, Dabholkar MD, Lee K-B, Bostoick-Burton F, Reed E. Taxol effect on cisplatin sensitivity and cisplatin cellular accumulation in human ovarian cancer cells. Monogr Natl Cancer Inst 1993;15:83–88.

274. LeBlanc GA, Sundseth SS, Weber GF, et al. Platinum anticancer drugs modulate P-450 mRNA levels and differentially alter hepatic drug and steroid hormone metabolism in male and female rats. Cancer Res 1992;52:540–547.

275. Kerns CM, Belani CP, Erkmen K, et al. Reduced platelet toxicity with combination carboplatin and paclitaxel; pharmacodynamic modulation of carboplatin-associated thrombocytopenia (abstract). Proc Am Assoc Cancer Res 1995;14:170.

276. Sledge GW, Robert N, Goldstein LJ, et al. Phase I trial of Adriamycin and Taxol in metastic breast cancer (abstract). Eur J Cancer 1993;29A(Suppl 6):s81.

277. Holmes FA, Newman RA, Madden V, et al. Schedule dependent pharmacokinetics (PK) in a phase I trial of Taxol (T) and doxorubicin (D) as initial chemotherapy for metastatic breast cancer (abstract). Proc 8th NCI-EORTC Symposium on New Drugs in Cancer Therapy, Amsterdam, March 15–18, 1994:197.

278. Verweij J, Planting AST, Van der Berg MEL, et al. A phase I study of docetaxel (Taxotere) and cisplatin in patients with solid tumors (abstract). Proc Am Soc Clin Oncol 1994;13:148.

279. Hurwitz CA, Relling MV, Weitman SD, et al. Phase I trial of paclitaxel in children with refractory solid tumors: a Pediatric Oncology Group study. J Clin Oncol 1993;11:2324–2329.

280. Fettel MR, Grossman SA, Balmaceda C, et al. Clinical and pharmacological study of preirradiation Taxol administered as a 96-hour infusion in adults with newly diagnosed glioblastoma multiforme (abstract). Proc Am Soc Clin Oncol 1994;13:179.

281. Klecker RW, Jamis-Dow CA, Egorin MJ, et al. Effect of cimetidine, probenecid, and ketoconazole on the distribution, biliary secretion, and metabolism of ^{3}H-Taxol in the Sprague-Dawley rat. Drug Metab Dispos Biol Fate 1994;22:254–258.

282. Reed E, Sarosy G, Jamis-Dow C, et al. Cimetidine does not influence Taxol steady-state levels (abstract). Proc Am Assoc Cancer Res 1993;34:395.

283. Slichenmyer W, McGuire W, Rowinsky EK, Chen T-L, Rowinsky EK. Pretreatment H2 receptor antagonists that differ in P450 modulation activity: comparative effects on paclitaxel clearance rates. Cancer Chemother Pharmacol 1995;36:227–232.

284. Jamis-Dow CA, Klecker RW, Katki AG, Collins JM. Metabolism of Taxol by human and rat liver in vitro. A screen for drug interactions and interspecies differences. Cancer Chemother Pharmacol 1995; 36:107–114.

285. Tew KD. The mechanism of action of estramustine. Semin Oncol 1983;10:21–26.

286. Tew KD, Glusker JP, Hartley-Asp B, et al. Preclinical and clinical prospectives on the use of estramustine as an antimitotic drug. Pharmacol Ther 1992; 56:323–339.

287. Muntzing J, Jensen G, Hogberg B. Pilot study on the growth inhibition by estramustine phosphate (Estracyt) of rat mammary tumors sensitive and insensitive to oestrogens. Acta Pharmacol Toxicol 1979;44:1–6.

288. Petrow V, Padilla GM. Design of cytotoxic steroids for prostate cancer. Prostate 1986;9:169–182.

289. Benson R, Hartley-Asp B. Mechanisms of action and clinical uses of estramustine. Cancer Invest 1990;8:375–380.

290. Hartley-Asp B. Estramustine-induced mitotic arrest in two human prostatic carcinoma cell lines, DU 145 and PC-3. Prostate 1984;5:93–100.

291. Tew KD, Hartley-Asp B. Cytotoxic properties of estramustine unrelated to alkylating and steroid constituents. Urology 1984;23:28–33.

292. Friden B, Wallin M, Deinum J, Prasade V, Ludena R. Effect of estramustine phosphate on the assembly of trypsin-treated microtubules and microtubules reconstituted from purified tubulin with either tau, MAP-2 or the tubulin-binding fragment of MAP-2. Arch Biochem Biophys 1987;257:123–130.

293. Sterns ME, Tew KD. Estramustine binds MAP-2 to inhibit microtubule assembly in vitro. J Cell Sci 1988;89:331–342.

294. Wallin M, Deinum J, Friden B. Interaction of estramustine phosphate with microtubule-associated proteins. Fed Eur Biochem Soc Lett 1985;179:289–293.

295. Dahllof B, Billstrom A, Cabral F, Hartley-Asp B. Estramustine depolymerizes microtubules by binding to tubulin. Cancer Res 1993;53:4573–4581.

296. Bergenheim AT, Bjork P, Bergh J, von Schoultz E, Svedberg H, Henriksson R. Estramustine-binding protein and specific binding of the anti-mitotic compound estramustine in astrocytoma. Cancer Res 1994;54:4974–4979.

297. Shiina H, Sumi H, Ishibe T, Usua T. Study of estramustine binding protein; its relationship to androgen dependency and histological differentiation in human prostatic carcinoma tissue. Urol Int 1994;52:213–216.

298. Kim JH, Khil MS, Kim SH, Ryu S, Gabel M. Clinical and biological studies of estramustine phosphate as a novel radiation sensitizer. Int J Radiat Oncol Biol Phys 1994;29:555–557.

299. Yoshida D, Piepmeir J, Weinstein M. Estramustine sensitizes human glioblastoma cells to irradiation. Cancer Res 1994;54:1415–1417.

300. Speicher LA, Sheridan VR, Godwin AK, Tew KD. Resistance to the antimitotic drug estramustine is distinct from the multidrug resistant phenotype. Br J Cancer 1991;64:267–273.

301. Speicher LA, Barrone LR, Chapman AE, et al. P-glycoprotein binding and modulation of the multi-drug-resistant phenotype by estramustine. J Natl Cancer Inst 1994;86:688–694.

302. Yang CP, Shen HJ, Horwitz SB. Modulation of the function of P-glycoprotein by estramustine. J Natl Cancer Inst 1994;86:723–725.

303. Forshell GP, Muntzing J, Ek A, et al. The absorption, metabolism and excretion of Estracyt (NSC-89199) in patients with prostatic cancer. Invest Urol 1976;14:128–131.

304. Kirdini RY, Karr JP, Murphy GP, et al. Prostate cancer: plasma concentrations of estramustine and its metabolites. NY State J Med 1980;80:1390–1393.

305. Lundgren R, Sundin T, Leinstedt E, et al. Cardiovascular complications of estrogen therapy for non-disseminated prostatic carcinoma. Scand J Urol Nephrol 1986;20:101–109.

306. Kirdini RY, Muntzing J, Varkarakis MJ, et al. Studies on the antiprostatic action of Estracyt, a nitrogen mustard of estradiol. Cancer Res 1974;34:1025–1031.

307. Murphy GP, Slack NH, Mittelman A, et al. Experiences with estramustine phosphate (Estracyt, Emcyt) in prostate cancer. Semin Oncol 1983;10(Suppl 3):34–42.

308. Hoisaeter PA, Bakke A. Estramustine phosphate (Estracyt): experimental and clinical studies in Europe. Semin Oncol 1983;10:27–33.

309. Tew KD, Woodworth A, Stearns ME. Relationship of glutathione depletion and inhibition of glutathione-S-transferase activity to the antimitotic properties of estramustine. Cancer Treat Rep 1986;70:715–720.

310. VanBell SJP, Schalleier D, deWasch G, et al. Broad phase II study of the combination of two microtubular inhibitors: estramustine and vinblastine (abstract). Proc Am Soc Clin Oncol 1988;7:207.

311. Pierta KJ, Rodman B, Hussain M, et al. Phase II evaluation of oral estramustine and oral etoposide in hormone-refractory adenocarcinoma of the prostate 1994;12:2005–2012.

312. Gunnarsson PO, Davidsson T, Andersson S-B, et al. Impairment of estramustine phosphate absorption by concurrent intake of milk and food. Eur J Clin Pharmacol 1990;38:189–193.

23

DNA Topoisomerase Inhibitors

Part 1 ———————————————

DNA Topoisomerase I Inhibitors

Nasir Shahab and Michael C. Perry

With the discovery of the double helix structure of DNA, scientists began to wonder what makes these two super-coiled strands separate during replication, an event commonly observed under the light microscope during cell replication (1). Later it was discovered that the two strands were topographically linked and therefore cannot come apart without at least one transient break in one of the strands (2–3). Wang then found that cell extracts of *Escherichia coli* were capable of inducing coiling and relaxation of DNA (4–5). This protein, initially called ω protein, was renamed 8 years later as *E. coli*–DNA topoisomerase I (6). Later, a similar enzyme was discovered in mouse cell extracts (7). Gellert et al., in 1976, discovered another enzyme from *Escherichia coli* with effects opposite to those of *E. coli*–DNA topoisomerase I (13). The topoisomerases are thus classified into topoisomerase I and topoisomerase II, based on their ability to cleave one or two DNA strands, respectively. Both are nuclear enzymes responsible for controlling, maintaining and modifying the structure and function of DNA. To perform these functions, the topoisomerases induce transient breaks in one or both strands of DNA, thus allowing the other strand to pass through the cut, and then rejoin the nicked strand to the intact DNA (8–12).

Topoisomerase I, exemplified by *E. coli*–DNA topoisomerase I, catalyzes relaxation of negatively charged super-coiled DNA (5) and thus is involved in the repression and activation of transcription, being more abundant in the transcriptionally active regions of the nucleus. A remarkable feature of this enzyme is that it needs no cofactors (4). Topoisomerase II, exemplified by *E. coli*–DNA topoisomerase II, also is involved in the conversion of relaxed DNA into negatively

super-coiled DNA. In contrast to topoisomerase I, topoisomerase II depends on ATP hydrolysis (13). These two opposing effects are important for maintaining the structure of DNA.

CAMPTOTHECINS

Historical Perspective

Milan Potmesil in his review on camptothecin (41) has described the 38 years of research done with this agent. Camptothecin, an alkaloid, exists in the wood, bark, leaves and fruit of an oriental tree, *Camptothecin acuminata* (20). This compound has been used in traditional Chinese medicine for the treatment of various illnesses including tumors (21). Wall et al. (20) and Perdue (22) isolated this compound from *Camptothecin acuminata* in the 1960s. Camptothecin and its analogues were also found in other plant families (31–34). The National Cancer Institute (NCI) later tested an extract from *Camptothecin acuminata* and established its antitumor activity (35). Subsequent studies revealed that camptothecin reversibly inhibits DNA and that its cytotoxic effects are S-phase specific (23–29). Clinical studies with a water-soluble sodium salt of camptothecin prepared by NCI—CAM-Na$^+$ (NSC-100880)—were discontinued after phase I and II trials, as it became clear that NSC-100880 had severe hematologic (myelosuppressive) and nonhematologic side effects (hemorrhagic cystitis) (36–39), despite its antitumor activity. It then became obvious that the active part of the drug was not its sodium salt but the lactone-E ring of the camptothecin molecule (40). With the discovery of topoisomerase I as the primary target for camptothecin and analogues in the 1980s (44–47), and the fact that topoisomerases I were overexpressed in human colon cancer and other malignancies (48–49), two new synthetic analogues, 9 AC (NSC 603071) (50) and 10,11 MDC (51), and two semisynthetic compounds, topotecan (SK&F 104864, NSC 609699) and CPT 11 (Irinotecan) (42–43), were developed. These drugs are currently undergoing clinical trials in the U.S. All of them have a therapeutic index superior to that of the parent compound, camptothecin.

Mechanism of Action

Earlier experiments with camptothecins have shown that cell death requires ongoing DNA synthesis (52). During the cell cycle, topoisomerases form a covalent bond with DNA, called a cleavable complex (14). This results in the breakage of one or the other DNA strand via a nucleophilic attack of the phosphodiester bond in DNA, forming a phosphotyrosine covalent link concurrent with the nicked intermediates. The other complementary strand passes through the nick. Topoisomerase I is then released, and the nicked site resealed (14). The end result is the conversion of super-coiled DNA to a relaxed, covalently closed circular product. Topoisomerase inhibitors stabilize the cleavable complex, increasing its half-life by making it last for the duration of drug exposure (15). The result is an increased concentration of the cleavable complex (53), which interacts with the replication fork, converting the noncytotoxic reversible DNA lesion (the cleavable complex) into a cytotoxic lesion (a single-strand DNA break) (54). The final endpoint is the inhibition of DNA and RNA synthesis, leading to cell death and arrest of the cell cycle at the G_2 phase (16–19, 53). DNA breakage has been measured in vivo by detecting covalent topoisomerase DNA intermediates in the peripheral blood (55, 56).

Topotecan

Topotecan was identified as a water-soluble analogue of camptothecin by SK&F (42).

Nomenclature and Structure

Generic Name: Topotecan, SK&F 104864
Commercial Name: Hycamtin
Chemical Name: (S)-10-(dimethylamino) methyl-4-ethyl-4, 9-dihydroxy-1H-pyranol 3',4',6,7 indolizino <1,2-b>-quinoline-3-14-(4H,12H)-dione
Molecular Formula: $C_{23}H_{23}N_3O_5$
Molecular Weight: 421.453 (free base)

Availability: Topotecan is supplied in vials as a light yellow, lyophilized cake. Each lyophilized vial contains 5 mg of the free base. Topotecan is supplied as either an AA (unbuffered) or AC/AF formulation (buffered).

Storage: Topotecan vials of the AA formulation must be stored at 5°C in the dark until used.

Topotecan vials of the AC/AF-AA formulation must be stored between 15 and 30°C (59 to 86°F).

Administration

Intravenous Solution: Topotecan should be administered intravenously after dilution in 0.9% sodium chloride injection or 5% dextrose injection. Until specific compatibility data are available, mixing topotecan with other intravenous fluids or drugs is not recommended. Topotecan should not be diluted with buffered solutions because of solubility and stability considerations. The lyophilized formulation must be reconstituted with 2 mL of sterile water for injection prior to dilution with 0.9% sodium chloride injection or 5% dextrose injection. Because the lyophilized dosage form contains no antibacterial preservatives, it is advised that the reconstituted (undiluted) solution be discarded 24 hours after initial reconstruction.

The final concentrations of topotecan intravenous solutions should be 10 to 500 µ/ mL in 0.9% sodium chloride injection or 5% dextrose injection. The desired amount of drug should be added to an intravenous solution hang bag, mixed and delivered within 24 hours. The following sets are recommended for delivery: Sodium Set 2C5423S (Baxter) and IV Administration Set A V1230 from AVI, Inc.

Oral Solution AA formulation: Each 5-mg vial of lyophilized topotecan, AC/AF-AA formulation accommodates 10 mL. Each 5-mg vial of topotecan AA formulation should be reconstituted with 10 mL of 5% dextrose injection solution to give a 0.5% solution of the drug.

The required dose of reconstituted solution should be drawn from the vial. Each 3.0 mL contains 1.5 mg of topotecan. Withdraw 3.0 mL for each m^2 of body surface area (BSA). The dose is placed in a beaker containing 100 mL of dextrose injection solution. The patient should drink the entire contents of the beaker, ensuring that no residual liquid remains behind. After the patient has drunk the contents of the beaker, an additional 100 mL of 5% dextrose injection solution should be added to the beaker, and the patient should drink the contents, ensuring that no residual liquid remains behind.

AC/AF-AA formulation: Each 5 mg of lyophilized topotecan, AC/AF-AA formulation accommodates 5 mL. Each 5-mg vial of topotecan AC/AF-AA formulation should be reconstituted with 5 mL of dextrose injection solution to give a 1.0 mg/mL solution of the drug.

The required dose of reconstituted solution should be drawn from the vial. Each 1.0 mL contains 1.0 mg of topotecan. Withdraw 1.5 mL for each m² of BSA. The dose should be placed in a beaker containing 100 mL of 5% dextrose injection solution. The patient should drink the entire contents of the beaker, ensuring that no residual liquid remains behind. After the patient has drunk the contents of the beaker, an additional 100 mL of 5% dextrose injection solution should be added to the beaker and the patient should again drink the contents ensuring that no residual liquid remains behind.

Contraindications: Topotecan should not be administered to any individual with a known hypersensitivity to chemically related compounds.

Precautions: Due to lack of information, topotecan should not be used in children or pregnant or nursing women. The effect of topotecan on sperm is unknown, therefore, sexually active males should use effective contraception. Due to the potential myelosuppression, a complete blood count should be done at least weekly in all patients.

Pharmacokinetic: Topotecan is a semisynthetic water-soluble derivative of camptothecin and was designed to be more soluble at acidic pH (66). It is unstable in solution and undergoes spontaneous hydrolysis at physiologic pH to a less-active open-ring specie. The hydrolysis is pH dependent, with the equilibrium favoring the open ring form at a pH > 7.0 and the lactone form in acidic conditions (67). The form with antineoplastic activity is the closed lactone (66); therefore, infusions of topotecan should only be administered in solutions with a pH between 4.0 to 4.5.

Pharmacokinetic studies of topotecan have been performed in adults and pediatric patients but have been limited by the instability of the parent drug in solution (68–73). Less than 20% of the drug is protein bound. In all studies, topotecan was rapidly hydrolyzed in vivo to the open carboxylate form (59, 68–70, 72, 86, 87). Typically, 50% of the total drug exists as the hydroxy acid by the end of a brief infusion (59,

72, 86). By 30 minutes after administration, the ratio of open ring to lactone is approximately 2:1. This ratio increases to 4 to 5:1 over the next several hours (68, 59).

The half-life of the drug has ranged from 1.7 to 8 hours, depending upon the schedule. The longest half-life was seen with a 24-hour infusion repeated every 3 weeks (57–60, 62, 63, 65). The volume of distribution of the lactone at steady state (V_{dss}) is high (mean V_{dss}, 87.3 L/m²; range, 25.6 to 186 L/m²), suggesting wide distribution and or tissue sequestration (66).

Renal elimination appears to be the major route of excretion. The mean percentage of total drug excreted in the urine over 24 hours is 53% (range, 39 to 80%) (57, 59, 68). The clearance rate for topotecan lactone is 1220 mL/min/m², with a range of 300 to 4760 mL/min/m². The clearance rate for total topotecan (lactone and hydroxy acid) is 493 mL/min/m², with a range of 163 to 815 mL/min/m² (68). Concurrent sampling of plasma and bile in a patient with a biliary drainage catheter revealed that peak biliary levels were 1.5-fold higher than concurrent plasma levels, a result that is consistent with active biliary excretion of the drug (72). No metabolites have been identified in the plasma, urine, or bile, but thermospray mass spectrometry studies have suggested that demethylation of topotecan might occur (64).

Pharmacodynamic studies have suggested a relationship between the dose of topotecan administered and the percentage decrease in a patient's absolute neutrophil count (57, 59). Though the hydroxy acid form of the drug is less active than the lactone form (68), it has been suggested that the hydroxy acid form might significantly contribute to the myelosuppressive effects of topotecan, possibly by interconversion to the active lactone in vivo (84).

CSF penetration of camptothecin appears to be negligible, but the mean CSF penetration of topotecan exceeds 30% (67). In a study on nonhuman primates, CSF concentrations of topotecan peaked at 30 minutes and ranged from 0.044 to 0.074 µM for the lactone and 0.065 to 0.097 µM for the total drug. CSF disappearance paralleled that in plasma. The degree of CSF penetrance is due to lack of protein binding (67). This is in sharp contrast to camptothecin, which has negligible CSF penetration because 97% of the drug is protein bound.

Intrathecal studies performed in nonhuman primates (85) had shown a significant pharmacokinetic advantage over intravenous administration. Following intraventricular administration of 0.1 mg of topotecan, hydrolysis of the lactone form of topotecan in CSF was rapid, with greater than 50% conversion to the less active open-ring form within 90 minutes of administration. The mean peak levels of lactone and total drug in ventricular CSF were 83 ± 18 μM and 88 ± 25 μM, respectively. Lumbar topotecan concentration peaked 2 hours later at 0.98 μM for the lactone and 2.95 μM for the total drug. Elimination of lactone and total drug from CSF was rapid. The mean clearance of lactone was 0.075 mL/min (range, 0.076 to 0.121 mL/min) and of total drug was 0.043 mL/min (range 0.061 to 0.087 mL/min). The mean terminal half life was 1.3 hours (range, 1.1 to 1.6 hours) for the lactone and 1.8 hours (range, 1.2 to 2.6 hours) for the total drug. Plasma concentrations measured concurrently were below the lower limits of assay quantitation.

Drug Resistance: Several camptothecin resistant cell lines have been described (74–79). The major feature of these cell lines was reduced topoisomerase I activity. Differences in topoisomerase I sensitivity toward camptothecins were also observed. Acquisition of resistance has been shown to be associated at first with decrease of the cellular topoisomerase I activity and then with the presence of a camptothecin-resistant form of topoisomerase I. Both rearrangements and reduced transcription of topoisomerase I gene have been detected in the resistant gent (76, 80).

Clinical Indications: Topotecan is the first semisynthetic water-soluble topoisomerase I inhibitor to enter clinical trials in the United States in over 20 years. In vitro studies demonstrated significant antitumor activity against a wide variety of human cancer cell lines, including breast, lung, colorectal, renal, and ovarian cancers (59, 88, 97). A subset of tumors resistant to established drugs were found to be sensitive to topotecan (88).

Topotecan has been extensively studied in mice bearing transplantable tumors and has demonstrated remarkable antitumor activity against a variety of tumors (98). Among these tumor models, P388 leukemia was most sensitive to topotecan treatment, which produced long-term tumor-free survivors. When treatment was started early after intraperitoneal implantation of P388 leukemia, L1210 leukemia, Lewis lung Ca, and B16 melanoma, curative activity was demonstrated in each of these tumors (99, 100). Topotecan was also found to be active against human colon cancer, rhabdomyosarcoma, and osteosarcoma (101). Cures have been observed following topotecan in mice with rhabdomyosarcomas and osteosarcoma (101).

Clinical Trials: During phase I trials, responses to topotecan were variable: ovarian cancer (1 PR) (59); non-small-cell lung cancer (1 CR, 3 PRs) (59, 89); small cell lung cancer (1 PR) (89); esophageal cancer (1 PR) (60); colorectal cancer (1 PR) (63); and acute leukemia (3 CRs, 2 PRs) (92). There were minor responses in patients with renal cell, squamous cell skin, non-small-cell lung, and ovarian carcinomas (57, 59–60, 63–65, 69).

Phase II studies are in progress at different centers, using daily dosing for 5 days every 3 to 4 weeks. Despite good results in the phase I studies, data so far available have been rather disappointing. Topotecan was not effective against non-small-cell lung cancers (90). In this trial, a dose of 2 mg/m^2 was used for 5 days. Initially, 30 patients were to be enrolled, but due to lack of any response in the first 20 patients (no CR; no PR), further patient accrual was halted.

Similar results were observed in other phase II trials involving renal cell cancer, prostate cancer, and colorectal cancers (91). In a renal cell cancer phase II study performed at Memorial Sloan-Kettering Cancer Center, 15 newly diagnosed patients were treated with 1.5 mg/m^2 daily for 5 days every 4 weeks, but no major response was seen (93). Results from studies on prostate and colorectal cancers have also been unconvincing, with only 2 of 28 and 1 of 16 partial responders, respectively (30, 94). A study published from the M. D. Anderson Cancer Center also reported a lack of response to topotecan in 12 patients with chronic lymphocytic leukemia (96).

Promising results have only been achieved in small cell lung cancer and advanced ovarian epithelial cancers (81–82, 95). There are multicentric phase II studies in progress using topotecan as second-line treatment in patients with limited/extensive-stage small cell lung cancer. Data from two of these studies have been presented in abstract form. In one, of 57 evaluable patients (27 sensitive tumors and 30 refractory tumors), 4 CRs and 5 PRs were seen in sensitive tumors, and 1 CR and 2 PRs in the refractory tumors (81). In the other phase II trial, topotecan was evaluated in patients with extensive-stage small cell lung cancer, and a partial response of 30% (7 of 18 patients) was noted (82). In an open phase II trial of topotecan in resistant ovarian epithelial tumors, partial remissions were seen in 14% of patients, whereas 61% had stable disease (95).

Currently, a phase III trial is being conducted by SK&F comparing topotecan with CAV (cyclophosphamide, doxorubicin, and vincristine) chemotherapy as second-line treatment for relapsed small cell lung tumors.

Because of its substantial CSF penetration following intravenous administration and lack of systemic side effects after intrathecal administration, topotecan should be evaluated in patients with central nervous system tumors (67). Topotecan holds a great promise for such tumors.

Combination Regimens: An earlier study showed that cotreatment of V79 Chinese hamster lung fibroblasts with camptothecin and a topoisomerase II inhibitor, etoposide or amsacrine, resulted in less cell killing than with amsacrine or etoposide alone (102). Therefore, it was suggested that simultaneous treatment with camptothecin and a topoisomerase II inhibitor would not benefit the patients (83). These observations were confirmed with similar in vitro studies on human colon carcinoma treated simultaneously with camptothecin and etoposide (103). Later studies have shown that these two classes of drugs have additive effects if the two treatments are separated by 6 or more hours. Thus sequential drug administration was found to be important for synergistic or additive actions (102–104). There is increasing evidence that the use of a topoisomerase II inhibitor, such as novobiocin, in combination with topotecan may produce synergistic cytotoxicity (121). Recent results indicate that topotecan and the nucleoside analogue 5-azacytidine are synergistic in a number of model systems in vitro and in vivo (105)

Combination with Ionizing Radiation: Repair of DNA following radiation proceeds in two distinct phases (106, 109). At first, there is sealing of broken DNA strands and repair of base damage, i.e., restoration of DNA primary structure. In the second phase, there is regeneration of normal chromatin structure. Substantial evidence suggests that topoisomerases are involved in such repair (106–108, 110). Several studies have been done to elucidate the determinants of the interacting response to the combined treatment of camptothecin with ionizing radiation (111–117). Mattern et al. have defined the role of topotecan in inhibiting DNA repair and thus producing synergistic cell killing (110). Topotecan also increases cell radiosensitization and, therefore, reduces survival of the irradiated cells (113). Specifically, radiation and camptothecins applied concomitantly or in close temporal proximity interact with each other in a purely additive mode; when radiation was applied 2 hours or more prior to camptothecin treatment, the cytotoxicity was decreased (118). Enhanced cytotoxicity was noted when topotecan was present during the first 30 minutes after radiation. Others have found that administration of camptothecin concomitantly or immediately after radiation delays any additive or synergistic cytotoxicity because of a dramatic reduction in topoisomerase I activity due to down-regulation in irradiated cells (119). Another factor important in the camptothecin-radiation interaction is the drug concentration used (120).

Toxicities

Hematologic: Reversible myelosuppression has been the most common toxicity reported in all phase I studies in patients with solid tumors. Granulocytopenia, with or without thrombocytopenia, has been the dose-limiting side effect. Compared with single-bolus schedules, intermittent and continuous infusion schedules have profound neutropenia. On all schedules, granulocytopenia was brief and noncumulative. The onset of neutropenia is usually between days 8 and 10, with resolution in the vast majority of patients by day 21. The mean duration of neutropenia is 14 days. Granulocyte colony-stimulating factor (G-CSF) administration after topotecan does not decrease neutropenia, and a new dose-limiting toxicity, thrombocytopenia, has been noted. Mild-to-moderate anemia was reported in continuous infusion trials. It was more severe in trials in which topotecan was given weekly instead of every 3 to 4 weeks. The exact mechanism of anemia remains obscure.

Gastrointestinal: These usually are of mild intensity. Grade 1 to 2 nausea and vomiting have been consistently reported in all the trials and are easily controlled with standard antiemetics. Other minor symptoms reported include abdominal pain, anorexia, stomatitis, cheilitis, glossitis, and diarrhea.

Gastroesophageal reflux was reported in one trial.

Cardiovascular: These are usually rare and include tachycardia, hypertension, hypotension, and syncope. One episode of myocardial ischemia was reported in a single phase I trial.

Respiratory: Minor dyspnea, cough, epistaxis, hemoptysis, laryngitis, and sinusitis have been observed.

Central and Peripheral Nervous Systems: Peripheral neuropathy, paresthesia, hyperesthesia, headache, and involuntary muscular contractions have been reported. Transient CSF pleocytosis was observed in animal studies following intraventricular administration (85). No acute or chronic neurotoxicity was noted after intraventricular therapy (85).

Skin: Grade 2 to 3 alopecia has been a consistent finding in almost all the trials. Other rare side effects include seborrhea, dry skin, skin discoloration, and erythematous rash. Pruritus was also reported.

Renal: Rarely, renal function abnormalities, hematuria, pyuria, and dysuria are seen. There has been no case report of hemorrhagic cystitis, commonly seen with the parent compound, camptothecin. The absence of urothelial toxicity is notable. This may be due to the slow conversion of the topotecan lactone from the hydroxy form at urinary pH. Also, smaller drug doses are required for cytotoxicity when topotecan is administered as the lactone, and this form is more soluble than camptothecin (68).

Liver and Biliary System: Grade I or II elevation of liver enzymes (SGOT, SGPT, δ-glutamyl transferase, phosphatase, and bilirubin) have been reported in rare patients. Clinical jaundice has been reported very uncommonly.

Eye: Conjunctivitis and ocular pain are rare complaints.

Psychiatric: Mild anxiety, depression, and sleep disturbances have been seen occasionally.

REFERENCES

1. Watson JD, Crick FHC. Genetical implications of the structure of deoxyribonucleic acid. Nature 1953; 171:964–967.

2. Weil R, Vinograd J. The cyclic helix and cyclic coil forms of polyoma viral DNA. Proc Natl Acad Sci USA 1963;50:730–738.

3. Dulbecco R, Vogt M. Evidence for a ring structure of polyoma virus DNA. Proc Natl Acad Sci USA 1963;70:236–243.

4. Wang JC. Degree of superhelicity of covalently closed cyclic DNAs from *Escherichia coli*. J Mol Biol 1969;43:263–272.

5. Wang JC. Interaction between DNA and *Escherichia coli* protein omega. J Mol Biol 1971;55:523–533.

6. Wang JC, Liu LF. DNA topoisomerases: enzymes that catalyze the concreted breaking and rejoining of DNA back bone bonds. Molecular genetics, Part III. New York: Academic Press, 1979:65–88.

7. Champoux JJ, Dulbecco R. Activity from mammalian cells that untwists superhelical DNA—possible swivel for DNA replication. Proc Natl Acad Sci USA 1972;69:143–146.

8. Osheroff N, Zechiedrich E, Gale KC. Catalytic function of DNA topoisomerase II. Bioessays 1991; 13:269–275.

9. Wang JC. Type I DNA topoisomerases. In: Boyer P, ed. The enzymes. New York: Academic Press, 1981; 14:331–344.

10. Wang JC. DNA topoisomerases. Annu Rev Biochem 1985;54:665–697.

11. Liu LF, Liu CC, Alberts B. Type II DNA topoisomerases: enzymes that can unknot a topologically knotted DNA molecule via a reversible double strand break. Cell 1980;19:697–707.

12. Liu LF. DNA topoisomerases: enzymes that catalyse the breaking and rejoining of DNA. Crit Rev Biochem 1983;15:1–24.

13. Gellert M, Mizuuchi K, O'Dea MH, Nash HA. An enzyme that introduces superficial turns into DNA. Proc Natl Acad Sci USA 1976;73:3872–3876.

14. Nelson EM, Tewey KM, Liu LF. Mechanism of antitumor drug action: poisoning of mammalian DNA topoisomerase II on DNA by 4′-(9-acridinylamino)-methanesulfon-*m*-anisidide. Proc Natl Acad Sci USA 1984;81:1361–1365.

15. Pommier Y, Capranico G, Orr A, et al. Distribution of topoisomerase II cleavage sites in simian virus 40 DNA and the effects of drugs. J Mol Biol 1991; 222:909–924.

16. Hsiang YH, Lihou MG, Liu LF. Arrest of replication forks by drug stabilized topoisomerase I DNA cleavable complexes as a mechanism of cell killing by camptothecin. Cancer Res 1989;49:5077–5082.

17. Berger NA, Chatterjee S, Schmotzer JA, et al. Etoposide (VP 16-213) induced gene alterations: potential contribution to cell death. Proc Natl Acad Sci USA 1991;88:8740–8743.

18. Renault G, Malvy C, Venegas W, et al. In vivo exposure to four ellipticine derivatives with clumping and sister chromatid exchange in murine bone marrow cells. Toxicol Appl Pharmacol 1987;89:281–286.

19. Zhang H, D'Arpa P, Liu LF. A model for tumor cell killing by topoisomerase poisons. Cancer Cells 1990;2:23–27.

20. Wall ME, Wani MC, Cook CE, et al. Plant antitumor agents. I. The isolation and structure of camptothecin, a novel alkaloid leukemia and tumor inhibitor from *Camptotheca acuminata*. J Am Chem Soc 1966; 88:3888–3890.

21. Huang SY, ed. Seven hundred herbal prescriptions for cancer medicine treatment (in Chinese). Taipei, Chinese Republic: Bada Educational and Cultural Publishers, 1986.

22. Perdue RE Jr, Smith RL, Wall ME, et al. *Camptotheca acuminata* Decaisne (*Nyssaceae*), source of camptothecin, an antileukemoid alkaloid. Technical Bulletin 1415. Washington, DC: U.S. Department of Agriculture, Agricultural Research Service, April 1970.

23. Bosmann HB. Camptothecin inhibits macromolecular synthesis in mammalian cells but not in isolated mitochondria of *E. coli.* Biochem Biophys Res Commun 1970;41:1412–1420.

24. Horwitz SB, Chang C-K, Grollman AP. Studies on camptothecin. 1. Effects on nucleic acid and protein synthesis. Mol Pharmacol 1971;7:632–644.

25. Kessel D. Effects of camptothecins on RNA synthesis in leukemia L1210 cells. Biochim Biophys Acta 1971;246:225–232.

26. Wu RS, Kumar A, Warner JR. Ribosomal formation is blocked by camptothecin, a reversible inhibitor of RNA synthesis. Proc Natl Acad Sci USA 1971; 68:3009–3014.

27. Abelson HT, Penman S. Selective interruption of high molecular weight RNA synthesis in HeLa cells by camptothecin. Natl New Biol 1972;237:144–146.

28. Kessel D, Bosman HB, Lohr K. Camptothecin effects on DNA synthesis on murine leukemia cells. Biochim Biophys Acta 1972;269:210–216.

29. Horwitz MS, Horwitz SB. Intracellular degradation of HeLa and adenovirus type 2 DNA induced by camptothecin. Biochem Biophys Res Commun 1971; 45:723–727.

30. Giantonio BJ, Kosierowsky R, Ramsey HE, et al. Phase II study of topotecan for hormone refractory prostate cancer (abstract). Proc Am Soc Clin Oncol 1993;12:247.

31. Govindacharia TR, Viswanathan N. 9-Methoxycamptothecin. A new alkaloid from *Mappia foetida* miers. Ind J Chem 1972;10:453–454.

32. Govindacharia TR, Viswanath N. Alkaloids of *Mappia foetida*. Phytochemistry 1972;11:3529–3531.

33. Arisawa M, Gunasekara SP, Farnworth NR, et al. Plant anticancer agents. XXI Constituents of *Merrliodendron megacarpum*. Plant Med 1981;43:404–407.

34. Gunasekera SP, Badawi MM, Cordell GA, et al. Potential anticancer agents. X. Isolation of camptothecin and 9-methoxy-camptothecin from *Ervatamia heyeana.* J Nat Prod 1979;42:475–477.

35. Wall ME. Alkaloids with antitumor activity. In: Mothes K; Schreiber K, HR Schutte, eds. International symposium on biochemistry and physiology of the alkaloids (abstract). Berlin: Academie-Verlag, 1969:77.

36. Gottlieb JA, Guarino AM, Call JB, et al. Preliminary pharmacologic and clinical evaluation of camptothecin sodium (NSC-100880). Cancer Chemother Rep 1970;54:461–470.

37. Muggia FM, Creaven PJ, Hansen HH, et al. Phase I clinical trial of weekly and daily treatment with camptothecin (NSC 100880): correlation with preclinical studies. Cancer Chemother Rep 1972;56:515–521.

38. Moertel CG, Schutt AJ, Reitemeier RJ, et al. Phase II study of camptothecin (NSC 100880) in the treatment of advanced gastrointestinal cancer. Cancer Chemother Rep 1972;56:95–101.

39. Gottlieb JA, Leuce JK. Treatment of malignant melanoma with camptothecin. (NSC 100880). Cancer Chemother Rep 1972;56:103–105.

40. Danishefsky S, Quick J, Horwitz SB. Synthesis and biological activity in the camptothecin series. Tetrahedron Lett 1973;27:2525–2528.

41. Potmesil M. Camptothecins: from bench research to hospital wards. Cancer Res 1994;54:1431–1439.

42. Johnson RK, McCabe FL, Faucette LF, et al. SK&F 104864, a new water soluble analogue of camptothecin with broad spectrum activity in pre clinical tumor models (abstract). Proc Am Assoc Cancer Res 1989;30:623.

43. Miyasaka S, Sawada S, Nokata, et al. New camptothecin derivatives. Japan Kokai 1985;197:90.

44. Hsiang YH, Hertzberg R, Hecht S, et al. Camptothecin induces routine linked DNA breaks via mammalian DNA topoisomerase I. J Biol Chem 1985; 260:14873–14878.

45. Hsiang YH, Liu LF. Identification of mammalian topoisomerase I as an intracellular target of the anticancer drug camptothecin. Cancer Res 1988; 48:1722–1726.

46. Jaxel C, Kohn KW, Wani MC, et al. Structure-activity study of the actions of camptothecin derivatives on mammalian topoisomerase I. Evidence for a specific receptor site and for a relation to anti tumor activity. Cancer Res 1989;49:1465–1469.

47. Hsiang YH, Liu LF, Wall ME, et al. DNA topoisomerase I-mediated DNA cleavage and cytotoxicity of camptothecin analogs. Cancer Res 1989; 49:4385–4389.

48. Giovanella BC, Stehlin JS, Wall ME, et al. DNA topoisomerase I-targeted chemotherapy of human colon cancer in xenografts. Science 1989;246:1046–1048.

49. Potmesil M, Hsiang YH, Liu LF, et al. Resistance of human leukemic and normal lymphocytes to drug induced DNA cleavage and low levels of DNA topoisomerase II. Cancer Res 1988;48:3537–3543.

50. Wall ME, Wani MC, Natschke SM, et al. Plant antitumor agents. Isolation of 11-hydroxy camptothecin from *Camptotheca acuminata* Decne: total synthesis and biological activity. J Med Chem 1986;29:1553–1555.

51. Wani MC, Nicholas AW, Manikumar G, et al. Plant antitumor agents. Total synthesis and anti leukemic activity of ring A substituted camptothecin analogues. Structure-activity correlations. J Med Chem 1987;30:1774–1779.

52. D'Arpa P, Beardmore C, Liu LF. Involvement of nucleic acid synthesis in cell killing mechanisms of topoisomerase poisons. Cancer Res 1990;50:6919–6924.

53. Chen AY, Liu LF. DNA topoisomerases: essential enzymes and lethal targets. Annu Rev Pharmacol Toxicol 1994;34:191–218.

54. Zhang H, D'Arpa P, Liu LF. A model for tumor cell killing by topoisomerase poisons. Cancer Cells 1990;2:23–27.

55. Ellis A, Nowak B, Plunkett W, et al. Drug induced DNA-protein crosslinks in nonradiolabeled cells; potential application to patient material (abstract). Proc Am Assoc Cancer Res 1992;33:438.

56. Ellis A, Nowak B, Plunkett W, et al. Quantification of topoisomerase-DNA complexes in leukemia cells from patients undergoing therapy with a topoisomerase-directed agent. Cancer Chemother Pharmacol 1994;34:249–256.

57. Wall J, Burris H, Rodriguez G, et al. Phase I trial of topotecan (SK&F 104864) in patients with refractory solid tumors (abstract). Proc Am Soc Clin Oncol 1991; 10:98.

58. Eckardt J, Burris H, Kuhn J, et al. Phase I and

pharmacokinetic trial of continuous infusion topotecan in patients with refractory solid tumors (abstract). Proc Am Soc Clin Oncol 1992;11:138.

59. Rowinsky EK, Grochow LB, Hendricks CB, et al. Phase I and pharmacologic study of topotecan: a novel topoisomerase I inhibitor. J Clin Oncol 1992; 10:647–656.

60. Sirott MN, Saltz L, Young C, et al. Phase I trial and clinical pharmacologic study of intravenous topotecan (abstract). Proc Am Soc Clin Oncol 1991; 10:104.

61. Murphy B, Saltz L, Sirott M, et al. Granulocyte colony stimulating factor does not increase maximum tolerated dose in a phase I study of topotecan (abstract). Proc Am Soc Clin Oncol 1992;11:139.

62. Ten Bokkel Huinink WW, Rodenhuis S, Beijnen J, et al. Phase study of topoisomerase I inhibitor topotecan (SK&F 104864-A) (abstract). Proc Am Soc Clin Oncol 1992;11:110.

63. Haas NB, LaCreta FP, Walczak J, et al. Phase I/pharmacokinetic trial of topotecan on a weekly 24 hour infusional schedule (abstract). Proc Am Assoc Cancer Res 1992;33:523.

64. Recondo G, Abbruzzese J, Newman B, et al. Phase I trial of topotecan administered by a 24 hour infusion (abstract). Proc Am Assoc Cancer Res 1991; 32:206.

65. Cole D, Blaney S, Balis F, et al. A phase I and pharmacokinetic study of topotecan in pediatric patients (abstract). Proc Am Soc Clin Oncol 1992;11:116.

66. Burris HA, Rothenberg ML, Kuhn JG, et al. Clinical trials with the topoisomerase I inhibitors. Semin Oncol 1992;16:663–669.

67. Blaney MS, Cole DE, Balis FM, et al. Plasma and cerebrospinal fluid pharmacokinetic study of topotecan in non human primates. Cancer Res 1993;53:725–727.

68. Grochow LB, Rowinsky EK, Johnson R, et al. Pharmacokinetics and pharmacodynamics of topotecan in patients with advanced cancer. Drug metabolism and disposition. 1992;20:706–713.

69. Burris H, Kuhn J, Wall J, et al. Early clinical trials of topotecan, a new topoisomerase I inhibitor. Proc 7th NCI-EORTC symposium on new drugs in cancer therapy, Amsterdam, 1992:118.

70. Beijnen JH, Smith BR, Keijer WJ, et al. High performance liquid chromatographic analysis of the new anti tumor drug SK&F 104864-A (NSC 609699) in plasma. J Pharm Biomed Anal 1990;8:789–794.

71. Verwei J, Lund B, Planting AST, et al. Clinical studies with topotecan: the EORTC experience (abstract). Ann Oncol (Suppl) 1992;3:118.

72. Kuhn J, Burris S, Wall J, et al. Pharmacokinetics of the topoisomerase I inhibitor, SK&F 104864 (abstract). Proc Am Soc Clin Oncol 1990;9:70.

73. Reid JM, Burch PA, Benson LM, et al. Phase I and clinical and pharmacologic evaluation of topotecan administered by a 24 hour continuous infusion (abstract). Proc Am Assoc Cancer Res 1992;32:259.

74. Andoh T, Ishii K, Suzuki Y, et al. Characterization of a mammalian mutant with a camptothecin resistant DNA topoisomerase I (abstract). Proc Natl Acad Sci USA 1987;84:5565–5569.

75. Gupta RS, Gupta R, Eng B, et al. Camptothecin resistant mutants of Chinese hamster ovary cells containing a resistant form of topoisomerase I. Cancer Res 1988;48:6404–6410.

76. Eng WK, McCabe FL, Tan KB, et al. Development of a stable camptothecin resistant subline of P388 leukemia with reduced topoisomerase I content. Mol Pharmacol 1990;38:471–480.

77. Kanzawa F, Sugimoto Y, Minato K, et al. Establishment of a camptothecin analogue (CPT 11)-resistant cell line of human non-small cell lung cancer: characterization and mechanism of resistance. Cancer Res 1990;50:5919–5924.

78. Sugimoto Y, Tsukahara S, Oh-hara T, et al. Decreased expression of DNA topoisomerase I in camptothecin resistant tumor cell lines as determined by a monoclonal antibody. Cancer Res 1990;50:6925–6930.

79. Tanizawa A, Pommier Y. Topoisomerase I alteration in a camptothecin resistant cell line derived from Chinese hamster DC3F cells in culture. Cancer Res 1992;52:1845–1848.

80. Madelaine I, Prost S, Naudin A, et al. Sequential modifications of topoisomerase I activity in a camptothecin resistant cell line established by progressive adaptation. Biochem Pharmacol 1993;45:339–348.

81. Wanders J, Ardizzoni A, Hansen HH, et al. Phase II study of topotecan in refractory and sensitive SCLC (abstract). Proc Am Assoc Cancer Res 1995; 36:1415.

82. Schiller JH, Kim K, Johnson D. Phase II study of topotecan in extensive stage small cell lung cancer (abstract). Proc Am Soc Clin Oncol 1994;13:A1093.

83. Kaufmann SH. Antagonism between camptothecin and topoisomerase II directed chemotherapeutic agents in a human leukemia cell line. Cancer Res 1991; 51:1129–1136.

84. Slichenmyer WJ, Rowinsky EK, Donehower RC, et al. The current status of camptothecin analogues as anti-tumor agents. J Natl Cancer Inst 1993;85:271–291.

85. Blaney SM, Cole DE, Godwin K, et al. Intrathecal administration of topotecan in non-human primates. Cancer Chemother Pharmacol 1995;36:121–124.

86. Kuhn J, Burris S, Irvin R, et al. Pharmacokinetics of topotecan following a 30 minute infusion or 3 day continuous infusion. Proc 7th NCI-EORTC symposium on new drugs in cancer therapy, Amsterdam, 1992:83.

87. Staubus AE, Rutherford M, Snuffer P, et al. Kinetics of ring opening of camptothecin analogues and topotecan in plasma and whole blood (abstract). Proc Am Assoc Cancer Res 1992;33:351.

88. Burris HA, Hanauske AR, Johnson RK, et al. Activity of topotecan, a new topoisomerase inhibitor, against human tumor colony forming units in vitro. J Natl Cancer Inst 1992;84:1816–1820.

89. Verweij J, Lund B, Beynen J, et al. Clinical studies with topotecan: the EORTC experience. Proc 7th NCI-EORTC symposium on new drugs in cancer therapy, Amsterdam, 1992:180.

90. Lynch TJ, Kalish L, Strauss G, et al. Phase II study of topotecan in metastatic non small cell lung cancer. J Clin Oncol 1994;12:347–352.

91. Creemerst GJ, Lund B, Verweij J. Topoisomerase I inhibitors: topotecan and Irenotecan. Cancer Treat Rev 1994;20:73–96.

92. Beran M, O'Brien S, Estey E, et al. Topotecan in patients with refractory and relapsed acute leukemia. Proc. 4th conference on DNA topoisomerases in therapy. 1992:54.

93. Ilson D, Motzer RJ, O'Moore P, et al. A phase

II study of topotecan in advanced renal cell carcinoma (abstract). Proc Am Soc Clin Oncol 1993;12:248.

94. Verweij J, Wanders J, Calabresi F, et al. Phase II study with topotecan in colorectal cancer. Proc EORTC early drug development meeting, Rotterdam. 1993:31.

95. Kudel KA, Edwards C, Freedman R, et al. An open phase II study to evaluate the efficacy and toxicity of topotecan administered intravenously as 5 daily infusions every 21 days to women with advanced epithelial ovarian carcinoma (abstract). Proc Am Soc Clin Oncol 1993;12:259.

96. O'Brien S, Kantarjian H, Ellis A, et al. Topotecan in chronic lymphocytic leukemia. Cancer 1995; 75:1104–1108.

97. Sinha BK. Topoisomerase inhibitors: a review of their therapeutic potential in cancer. Drugs 1995; 49:11–19.

98. Houghton PJ, Cheshire PJ, Hallman JD II, et al. Efficacy of topoisomerase I inhibitors, topotecan and Irinotecan, administered at low dose levels in protracted schedules to mice bearing xenografts of human tumors. Cancer Chemother Pharmacol 1995;36:393–403.

99. Johnson RK, Hertzberg RP, Kingsbury WD, et al. Preclinical profile of SK&F 104864, a water soluble analogue of camptothecin. Proc 6th NCI-EORTC symposium on new drugs in cancer therapy. 1991.

100. Johnson RK, McCabe FL, Gallagher G, et al. Comparative efficacy of topotecan, irinotecan, camptothecin and 9 aminocamptothecin in preclinical tumor models. Proc 7th NCI-EORTC symposium on new drugs in cancer therapy, Amsterdam, 1992:85.

101. Houghton PJ, Cheshire PJ, Myers L, et al. Evaluation of 9 dimethyl amino methyl 10 hydroxy camptothecin (topotecan) against xenografts derived from adult and childhood tumors (abstract). Ann Oncol 1992;3(Suppl 1):84.

102. D'Arpa P, Beardmore C, Liu LF. Involvement of nucleic acid synthesis in cell killing mechanisms of topoisomerase poisons. Cancer Res 1990;50:6919–6924.

103. Bertrand R, O'Conner PM, Kerrigan D, et al. Sequential administration of camptothecin and etoposide circumvents the antagonistic cytotoxicity of simultaneous drug administration in slowly growing human colon carcinoma HT-29 cells. Eur J Cancer 1992; 28A:743–748.

104. Anzai H, Frost P, Abbruzzese JN. Synergistic cytotoxicity with combined inhibition of topoisomerase I and II (abstract). Proc Am Assoc Cancer Res 1992; 33:431.

105. Anzai H, Frost P, Abbruzzese JN. Synergistic cytotoxicity with 2'deoxy-5-azacytidine and topotecan in vitro and in vivo. Cancer Res 1992;52:2180–2185.

106. Mattern MR, Zwelling LA, Kerrigan DJ, et al. Reconstitution of higher order DNA structure following x radiation. Biochem Biophys Res Commun 1983; 112:1077–1084.

107. Tan KB, Mattern MR, Boyce RA, et al. Elevated topoisomerase II activity in nitrogen mustard-resistant human cells. Proc Natl Acad Sci USA 1987; 84:7667–7671.

108. Boothman DA, Trask DK, Pardee AB. Inhibition of potentially lethal damage repair in human tumor cells by β-lapachone, an activator of topoisomerase I. Cancer Res 1987;49:605–612.

109. Cook PR, Brazell IA. Detection and repair of single strand breaks in mammalian DNA. Nature 1976; 263:679–682.

110. Mattern MR, Hoffmann GA, McCabe FL. Synergistic cell killing by ionizing radiation and topoisomerase I inhibitor. Cancer Res 1991;51:5813–5816.

111. Musk SRR, Steel GG. The inhibition of cellular recovery in human tumor cells by inhibitors of topoisomerase I. Br J Cancer 1990;62:364–367.

112. Boothman DA, Wang M, Schea RA, et al. Posttreatment exposure to camptothecin unbalances the lethal effects of x-rays on radioresistant malignant melanoma cells. Int J Radiat Oncol Biol Phys 1992;24:939–948.

113. Boscia RE, Korbut T, Holden SA, et al. Interaction of topoisomerase I inhibitor with radiation in cis-diamminedichloroplatinum (II)-sensitive and -resistant cells in vitro and in the FSAIIC fibrosarcoma in vivo. Int J Cancer 1993;53:118–123.

114. Falk SJ, Smith PJ. DNA damaging and cell cycle effects of the topoisomerase I poison camptothecin in irradiated human cells. Int J Radiat Biol 1992;61:749–757.

115. Del Bino G, Bruno S, Yi PN, et al. Apoptotic cell death triggered by camptothecin or teniposide. The cell cycle specificity and effects of ionizing radiation. Cell Prolif 1992;25:537–548.

116. Gorczyca W, Gong J, Ardelt B, et al. The cell cycle related differences in susceptibility of HL-60 cells. Cancer Res 1993;53:3186–3192.

117. Panayotis P. Preclinical studies of water insoluble camptothecin congeners: cytotoxicity, development of resistance and combination treatments. Clin Cancer Res 1995;1:1235–1244.

118. Hennequin C, Giocanti N, Balosso J, et al. Interaction of ionizing radiation with the topoisomerase I poison camptothecin in growing V-79 and HeLa cells. Cancer Res 1994;54:1720–1728.

119. Boothman DA, Fukunaga N, Wang M. Down regulation of topoisomerase I in mammalian cells following ionizing radiation. Cancer Res 1994;54:4618–4626.

120. Pantazis P, Early JA, Mendoza JT, et al. Cytotoxic efficacy of 9-nitro camptothecin in the treatment of human malignant melanoma cells in vitro. Cancer Res 1994;54:771–776.

121. Schwartz GN, Teicher BA, Eder JP Jr, et al. Modulation of anti-tumor alkylating agents by novobiocin, topotecan and lonidamine (abstract). Cancer Chemother Pharmacol 1993;32:455–462.

Part 2 _____

DNA Topoisomerase II Inhibitors

Ross Donehower and Eric Rowinsky

EPIPODOPHYLLOTOXINS

Extracts of the roots and rhizomes of the May apple or mandrake plant, *Podophyllum peltatum*, have been used as cathartics, emetics, and anti-helminthics and for the treatment of condylomata acuminata. Podophyllotoxin, an antimitotic agent that binds to a site on tubulin distinct from that occupied by the vinca alkaloids, was identified as the main constituent possessing cytostatic activity as early as the 1940s, but early podophyllotoxin derivatives possessed a prohibitive degree of clinical toxicity. However, two glycosidic derivatives of podophyllotoxin, etoposide and teniposide, have demonstrated highly significant clinical activity against a wide variety of neoplasms including Hodgkin's and non-Hodgkin's lymphomas, germ cell malignancies, leukemias, and small cell lung carcinoma. These compounds have a complex structure consisting of a multiringed moiety, known as epipodophyllotoxin, linked to a sugar, glucopyranoside, by an ether linkage. The structures of etoposide and teniposide differ only by the substitution of a methyl group (etoposide) for the thenylidene (teniposide) on the glucopyranoside sugar (Fig. 23.1). However, these agents possess basic similarities in their pharmacologic characteristics, toxicities, and spectra of antineoplastic action.

1. Etoposide

Nomenclature and Structure

Generic Names: etoposide, VP-16, VP-16-213

Commercial Name: Vepesid

Chemical name: 4'-demethylepipodophyllotoxin 9-[4,6-O-(R)-ethylidene-β glucopyranoside]; 4'demethylepipodophyllotoxin-β-D-ethylidene glucoside

Molecular Weight: 588.6

Chemical Formula: $C_{29}H_{32}O_{13}$

Availability: Etoposide for injection is available in 5-mL (100-mg) multiple-dose vials. Each mL contains 20 mg etoposide, 650 mg polyethylene glycol 300, 80 mg polysorbate 80/Tween 80, 30 mg benzyl alcohol, 2 mg citric acid, and 30.5% (v/v) ethyl alcohol. The pH of the clear yellow solution is 3 to 4.

Etoposide is also available in 50- and 100-mg pink capsules for oral use. The vehicle of the liquid-filled, soft-gelatin capsule consists of citric acid, glycerin, purified water, and polyethylene glycol 400. The soft-gelatin capsules contain gelatin, glycerin, sorbitol, and purified water and parabens (ethyl and propyl), with an iron oxide and titanium dioxide dye system.

Storage: Unopened vials are stable for 24 months at room temperature (25°C). Vials that are diluted to a concentration of 0.2 or 0.4 mg/mL are stable for 96 and 48 hours, respectively, at room temperature (25°C) in glass and plastic containers under normal room fluorescent lighting conditions. At concentrations of 0.2 and 0.4 mg/mL in Ringer's injection, lactate, or mannitol 10% in glass or plastic containers under the same conditions, the solutions are stable for 96 and 48 hours. At 1 mg/mL and 2 mg/mL, crystallization occurs in 2 hours and 30

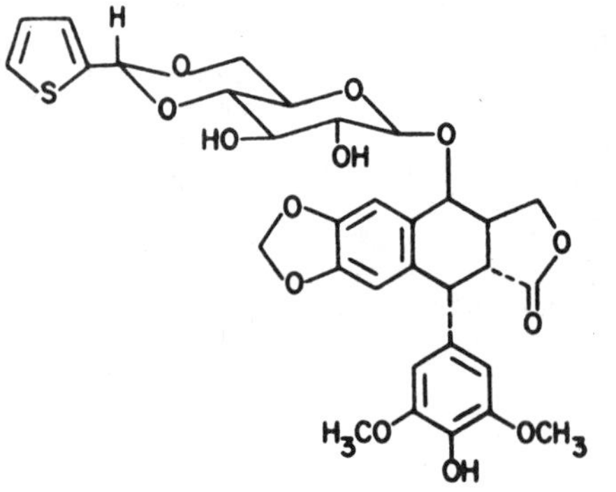

Teniposide (VM-26) 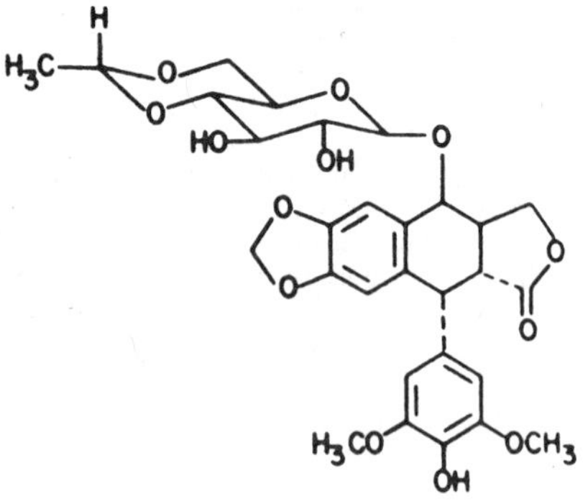   Etoposide (VP-16-213)

Figure 23.1.   Molecular structures of etoposide and teniposide.

minutes, respectively, in standard solution, or even sooner if the solution is stirred. The time to precipitation is highly unpredictable at concentrations above 0.4 mg/mL, and therefore, solutions with etoposide concentrations above 0.4 mg/mL are not recommended by the manufacturer for routine use. Etoposide concentrations of 0.6 mg/mL in 0.9% sodium chloride, 5% dextrose, or Ringer's lactate are stable for 8 hours.

Capsules must be stored under refrigeration at 2 to 8°C. The capsules are stable for 24 months under these conditions.

Administration: The parenteral formulation should be diluted to a final concentration of 0.2 or 0.4 mg/mL with either 5% dextrose or 0.9% sodium chloride, which is preferred. The agent should be infused intravenously over 30 to 60 minutes to avoid hypotension. Solutions with higher concentrations of etoposide (0.6 mg/mL) can generally be administered safely at a rate of 2.5 mL/min to patients receiving higher drug doses or to minimize the infusion of large volumes of fluid. Because of the poor solubility of etoposide in aqueous media, solutions should be monitored continuously for precipitation before and during administration (1, 2). Filter decomposition is not observed when solutions with etoposide concentrations of 0.1 to 0.4 mg/mL are passed through several commercially available filters, such as the 0.22-μm Millex-GS filter (3). In addition, significant drug loss due to binding to the filter does not occur when solutions with concentrations of 0.2 mg/mL are filtered over 6 hours through 0.22-μm cellulose ester membrane filters.

Etoposide is a vesicant, and care should be taken to avoid extravasation. Etoposide may also cause rashes after contact. Gloves for medical personnel are recommended during handling. In the event of skin or mucosal contact, the affected areas should be washed immediately with soap and water.

Intraperitoneal, intrapleural, and intrathecal routes of administration were considered to be contraindicated because of severe local inflammation and lethality in animal studies (4). However, several investigators have administered the drug intraperitoneally without severe local toxicities.

Blood counts should be checked prior to drug administration. Firm guidelines for dose modifications in patients with hepatic and renal dysfunction are not yet established; however, the primary renal pattern of elimination suggests that doses should be reduced for patients with severe renal dysfunction.

Mechanism of Action: Unlike the vinca alkaloids and the parent compound, podophyllotoxin, etoposide and teniposide do not inhibit microtubule assembly at clinically relevant concentrations. Instead, these agents induce an irreversible blockade of cells in the premitotic phases of the cell cycle, leading to accumulation of cells in the late S or G_2 phases (5, 6). Although the precise mechanisms of action for these compounds are not completely clear, cytotoxic effects appear to result from single- and double-strand breaks in DNA and DNA-protein cross-links. These effects are not induced when the drugs are incubated in vitro with purified DNA, which suggests that direct chemical cleavages in DNA are not occurring. The epipodophyllotoxins most likely exert their cytotoxic effects by interfering with the scission-reunion reaction of the enzyme topoisomerase II, by stabilizing the putative cleavable enzyme-DNA complex in a cleavable state (7). The enzyme then covalently binds to DNA, forming single-strand, protein-associated breaks. On a molar basis, teniposide is approximately 10-fold more effective than etoposide at inducing DNA strand breaks (8). Besides forming a cleavable complex, the epipodophyllotoxins inhibit the catalytic or "strand passing" activity of topoisomerase II that permits the enzyme to catenate DNA circles and disentangle topologically constrained DNA (9, 10).

Although the inhibitory effects of epidodophyllotoxins on the nuclear enzyme topoisomerase II appear to be primarily responsible for the induction of single-strand breaks, it has not been established that this mechanism accounts completely for the cytotoxic effects of these agents. It is also uncertain whether the inhibition of topoisomerase II–mediated activities accounts for the high frequency of sister chromatid exchanges, chromosomal aberrations, and mutagenic effects that are produced by the epipodophyllotoxins. DNA strand breaks can be detected at etoposide concentrations significantly below the levels required to affect cell kinetics and DNA synthesis (11). The inhibition of topoisomerase II is also quite reversible, and DNA strand breaks can be repaired rapidly after removal of epipodophyllotoxins (12, 13). Besides inhibiting topoisomerase II, these agents may exert cytotoxic actions after metabolic activation by peroxidases or other intracellular enzymes to form free radicals that bind directly to DNA in oxidation-reduction reactions (14, 15).

Etoposide is similar to its parent compound, podophyllotoxin, in that it also inhibits transport of nucleosides across the plasma membrane (16). The agent has been demonstrated to reversibly inhibit intracellular uptake of thymidine, uridine, adenosine, and guanine. The relevance of these effects to cytotoxicity is unknown, since animal cells can synthesize purines and pyrimidines, but these synthetic processes may be less efficient in neoplastic cells. It has been suggested that the ability of a drug to inhibit nucleoside transport may influence the efficacy of certain combinations of chemotherapeutic agents (17).

There appear to be several possible mechanisms of resistance to the cytotoxic effects of epipodophyllotoxins. In some cell lines, resistance is associated with decreased intracellular concentrations of etoposide and teniposide because of amplification of the multidrug resistance efflux pump, P-170 glycoprotein (18, 19). This mechanism is also reputed to be responsible for resistance to other classes of antineoplastic agents that are bulky, high-molecular-weight compounds, such as the antitumor antibiotics and the vinca alkaloids. Resistance to the epipodophyllotoxins may also be due to alterations in formation or repair of DNA strand breaks, low intracellular concentrations of topoisomerase II, or structural alterations of the enzyme, which may affect drug binding (20, 21). Cells that are resistant to etoposide have been fully cross-resistant to teniposide and vice versa in both in vitro and in vivo experimental systems, although several clinical reports suggest a lack of complete cross-resistance (22, 23).

Synergism between etoposide or teniposide and other antineoplastic agents has been evaluated in vitro. Etoposide has been demonstrated to be synergistic in vitro when combined with cytosine arabinoside, cyclophosphamide, carmustine, vincristine, cisplatin, hydroxyurea, and 5-fluorouracil (24–30). Teniposide has been shown to be synergistic in vitro with cytosine arabinoside, carmustine (BCNU), and hexamethylmelamine (24, 30, 31). In addition, the epipodophyllotoxins appear to be synergistic with methotrexate, and they enhance net cellular accumulation of methotrexate and methotrexate polyglutamates in vitro at clinically relevant concentrations (32). Etoposide-induced DNA damage and cy-

totoxicity are potentiated in vitro by the calcium channel antagonist verapamil (33, 34).

The cytotoxic effects of etoposide are markedly schedule dependent in animal models, and treatment with divided doses appears to result in better antineoplastic activity than single bolus doses. The life span of mice with L1210 leukemia implants increases with smaller and more frequent dosing intervals (35). For example, treatment intervals of 2 to 4 days are superior to treatment on day 1 only, daily treatment for 5 days, or treatment every 6 to 8 days. Similarly, divided-dosing schedules were superior to single-dosing schedules in randomized trials of etoposide in untreated patients with extensive small cell lung cancer (36, 37).

Pharmacology: In adults with normal renal and hepatic functions, etoposide's disposition in plasma is best described as a biphasic process, with a distribution half-life of approximately 1.5 hours and a terminal half-life that ranges from 3 to 11 hours, using high pressure liquid chromotography (HPLC) to measure drug concentrations (38). Maximal plasma levels and areas under the plasma concentration versus time curve (AUC) increase linearly with dose over a 100- to 600-mg/m^2 dose range (39). Mean peak plasma concentrations at etoposide's maximal tolerated single intravenous dose of 290 mg/m^2 are approximately 29 mg/mL (40). Etoposide does not accumulate in plasma following daily administration of 100 mg/m^2 for 5 consecutive days. In addition, plasma and renal clearances are independent of dose. Estimates of plasma clearance range from 16 ± 7 to 28.0 ± 9.7 mL/min/m^2 (40), while etoposide's urinary clearance ranges from 5.1 to 14.6 mL/min/m^2 and accounts for approximately 36% of the total disposition (39, 41). Using a two-compartment open model, the volume of distribution for etoposide at steady-state ranges from 7 to 17 L/m^2, which is equivalent to approximately 28% of body weight (42).

In mice, rats, and dogs, tissue distribution is greatest in the small intestine, kidneys, and liver, which reflects etoposide's primary biliary excretion as well as the 20 to 30% of the total dose that is eliminated in the urine (41). Following administration of radiolabeled etoposide to humans, 41.9 to 87.5% of the total radioactivity is recovered in the urine within 48 hours, with 66.8% in the form of unmetabolized drug. After an 80-mg/m^2 intravenous bolus, the mean urinary excretion over 48 hours is

39.8%, and fecal recovery ranges from 0 to 16% of administered radioactivity (42, 43). Only 6% or less of an intravenous dose is recovered in the bile as the parent compound. Thus, biliary excretion appears to be a minor route of drug elimination, and metabolism probably accounts for most of etoposide's nonrenal clearance in humans. In children, approximately 55% of a dose of etoposide is excreted in the urine over 24 hours, and the renal clearance, 7 to 10 mL/min/m^2, accounts for approximately 35% of total body clearance over a dose range of 80 to 600 mg/m^2. In one study of patients with hepatic and renal dysfunction, stepwise multiple linear regression analysis of patient-specific variables identified creatinine clearance and serum albumin as the best predictors of etoposide's systemic clearance, while hepatic function appeared to be an insignificant factor (44, 45). Recently, two groups of investigators demonstrated that there is no significant difference in the total clearance of etoposide between patients with obstructive jaundice and/or elevated plasma bilirubin levels and individuals with normal hepatic function (46, 47). One group found that patients with abnormally high bilirubin levels had a significantly higher fraction of etoposide in plasma that was not protein-bound, a significantly lower clearance of unbound etoposide, but a similar mean total etoposide clearance, compared with patients with normal liver function (46). In the other study, patients with both obstructive jaundice and normal hepatic function were found to have similar etoposide clearances, half-lives, and volumes of distribution (47). However, the magnitude of etoposide's renal clearance indicates that renal impairment would have a significant effect on etoposide disposition and that dose should be modified for patients with severe renal insufficiency.

Etoposide is metabolized by opening of its lactone ring, yielding its principal urinary metabolite, the hydroxy acid, 4'-demethylepipodophyllic acid-9-(4,6-O-ethylidene-β-D-glucopyranoside) (7, 42, 45, 48). A cis-lactone is also identifiable in plasma and urine (7, 38, 42, 45, 46). In addition, glucuronide and/or sulfate conjugates excreted in urine represent 5 to 22% of the total dose in humans (49–51). These metabolites do not have significant antineoplastic activity.

Etoposide is highly protein bound, with approximately 94% of total drug bound to serum proteins (42). However, the unbound fraction appears to be significantly greater in the plasma of cancer patients than in the plasma of normal volunteers (13.9 vs. 4.3%) (52). Etoposide does not penetrate effectively into the cerebrospinal fluid. For doses between 70 and 290 mg/m^2, low levels of radiolabeled etoposide (0.1 to 14.3% of simultaneous plasma levels) are detected in the cerebrospinal fluid from 2 to 54 hours after drug administration (41, 42). In two studies with high doses of etoposide (400 to 800 mg/m^2 and 900 to 2500 mg/m^2), cerebrospinal fluid concentrations were only 1.8 ± 1.7% of simultaneously measured plasma levels 12 hours postinfusion (39, 41, 42, 53).

After either intravenous or oral administration, peak plasma etoposide concentrations and AUC values exhibit marked intra- and interpatient variability, which confounds reliable estimates of absolute oral bioavailability (38, 54, 55). However, peak plasma levels and AUCs with the oral formulation are approximately 50% of identical parameters with parenteral routes of administration. Etoposide's overall bioavailability is approximately 50%, but it ranges from 25 to 75%. In addition, there is no evidence for a first-pass effect with etoposide or differences in metabolic and pharmacologic parameters between oral and parenteral routes of administration.

Indications: Etoposide is approved for use in refractory testicular carcinomas and small cell lung carcinomas. However, it is also very active in a wide range of other malignancies. The combination of cisplatin and etoposide with ifosfamide is potentially curative as second-line and third-line therapy, following relapse after cisplatin/velban-based therapies, and as first-line treatment in selected groups of patients with germ cell malignancies (46, 56–61). Adequate data on the use of oral etoposide in the treatment of testicular cancers are not available. Etoposide is probably the most active single agent against small cell lung carcinoma, and both oral and parenteral formulations are commonly incorporated into first-line combination chemotherapy regimens such as CAVE (with cyclophosphamide, doxorubicin, and vincristine), CAE (with cyclophosphamide and doxorubicin), with cisplatin, and with carboplatin and ifosfamide (48, 62–69). In addition, combinations of etoposide and cisplatin are active "salvage" regimens in previously treated patients with small cell lung cancer, although the impact on survival is limited (48, 62–69). Recently, prolonged daily oral administration of etoposide as a single agent for 21 days was also shown to be active in untreated and previously treated patients with small cell lung carcinoma (70–72).

Etoposide is also extremely active in non-Hodgkin's lymphomas and is commonly incorporated into aggressive "third-generation" regimens (e.g., ProMACE/MOPP [with methotrexate, doxorubicin, cyclophosphamide, prednisone, nitrogen mustard, vincristine, procarbazine], ProMACE/CytaBOM [with methotrexate, doxorubicin, cyclophosphamide, prednisone, cytarabine, bleomycin, vincristine]) for the primary treatment of non-Hodgkin's lymphomas (73, 74). In Hodgkin's disease, few studies of initial induction chemotherapy regimens that include etoposide have been evaluated, and a role for the agent has not yet been established. However, activity with combination chemotherapy regimens including etoposide has been demonstrated in patients who relapsed following first-line therapy (75). In addition, etoposide combined with ifosfamide is extremely active in gestational trophoblastic tumors and pediatric sarcomas, particularly Ewing's sarcoma (76–78). The agent has also been used in the treatment of refractory acute myelogenous leukemia, acute lymphoblastic leukemia, non-small-cell carcinoma of the lung, esophageal and gastric carcinomas, and Kaposi's sarcoma (48, 74–90). However, etoposide's ultimate role in the therapy of these malignancies remains to be defined. Little activity has been noted in adequate trials of etoposide in melanomas, sarcomas, and breast, bladder, cervix, colorectal, head and neck, and renal carcinomas (37, 42). Etoposide's activity in ovarian carcinomas appears to be limited when administered intravenously; however, it appears to be a promising agent when administered via the intraperitoneal route (91–96).

Dosage: Etoposide is rarely used as a single agent except in the treatment of Kaposi's sarcoma, where it has been employed intravenously in doses of 150 mg/m^2 per day for 3 days every 4 weeks. In general, the range of intravenous doses used in clinical trials is 50 to 150 mg/m^2 daily for 3 to 5 days every 3 to 4 weeks. In addition, etoposide is commonly administered on an alternate-day schedule, usually at intravenous doses of 100 to 125 mg/m^2 on days 1, 3, and 5. Myelosuppression is the dose-limiting toxicity of etoposide on a weekly bolus schedule, and safe doses range from 200 to 250

mg/m^2 (40, 45). Etoposide can also be administered safely as a continuous intravenous infusion over 3 and 5 days at 150 and 125 mg/m^2/day, respectively (48, 86, 87, 97, 98). Myelosuppression is also dose limiting on these continuous intravenous infusion schedules. In small cell lung carcinoma, the recommended oral dose of etoposide is twice the intravenous dose rounded to the nearest 50 mg. In addition, myelosuppression precludes dose escalation on a prolonged oral schedule of administration (daily for 21 days); the maximum tolerated dose is 50 mg/m^2/day for 21 days (69–80, 89).

Etoposide doses as high as 1500 mg/m^2 are associated with severe myelosuppression and tolerated without the need for autologous bone marrow rescue (100). However, mucositis and hepatotoxicity are dose-limiting nonhematologic effects of etoposide that preclude dose escalation above 2400 mg/m^2 (administered over 3 days) with autologous bone marrow rescue (101–103).

Toxicities: The following information on adverse reactions is based on a broad dose range of etoposide administered on both oral and intravenous schedules unless stated otherwise.

Hematologic: Myelosuppression is dose related and the major dose-limiting toxicity of etoposide. Granulocytopenia is common, with nadir granulocyte counts occurring 7 to 14 days after drug administration. Thrombocytopenia occurs less frequently, and nadir platelet counts are observed 9 to 16 days after the etoposide. Hematologic recovery is usually complete by day 20 after administration of standard dosages. Cumulative hematologic toxicity is unusual.

Gastrointestinal: Nausea and vomiting occur in approximately 30 to 40% of patients and are more frequently observed with oral than with intravenous administration. These toxicities are generally mild to moderate, and discontinuation of treatment because of adverse gastrointestinal effects is rarely required. Anorexia and diarrhea occur in less than 15% of patients. In addition, constipation, diarrhea, dysphagia, aftertaste, abdominal pain, stomatitis, and anorexia have been reported. Mucositis is a prominent toxicity at very high doses and appears to be the nonhematologic dose-limiting toxicity of etoposide (101–103).

Allergic: Etoposide induces transient hypotension following rapid intravenous administration, which usually responds to cessation of the infusion and administration of fluids or other appropriate supportive therapies (see Administration). When restarting the infusion, a slower infusion rate should be used. Anaphylactic-like symptoms, characterized by chills, fever, tachycardia, bronchospasm, and dyspnea, may be associated with hypotension and occur in approximately 0.7 to 2% of patients. These reactions are usually observed during or immediately after administration of etoposide and often respond promptly to the cessation of the infusion and administration of pressor agents, corticosteroids, antihistamines, or volume expanders.

Dermatologic: Reversible alopecia, sometimes progressing to total baldness, occurs in at least 8 to 20% of patients (41). Increased pigmentation, pruritus, and rare radiation recall dermatitis have been observed (104). Stevens-Johnson syndrome due to etoposide has also been reported (105).

Miscellaneous: Peripheral neuropathy is a rare toxicity of etoposide. Although several studies have demonstrated that this effect is more prevalent and severe in patients who have had prior VCR therapy, other investigations have shown the contrary (106–108). Acute central nervous system toxicity in patients with gliomas has also been reported with etoposide (104).

Reversible hepatotoxicity may be observed with very high doses of etoposide such as the doses that are used with autologous bone marrow rescue (101–103). Possible cardiac toxicity (e.g., myocardial infarction, congestive heart failure) has occurred in patients with preexisting coronary artery disease (110). In addition, acute respiratory insufficiency has been reported in a patient with lung cancer following combination treatment with mitomycin and etoposide (111). Therapy with etoposide has also been associated with the subsequent development of acute nonlymphocytic leukemia in a patient who had prior treatment with etoposide and cisplatin for small cell lung cancer (112).

2. Teniposide
Nomenclature and Structure
Generic Names: Teniposide, VM-26
Commercial Names: Vehem, Vumon
Chemical Name: 4'-demethylepipodophyl- lotoxin 9-[4,6-*O*)-2-thenylidene-β-D-gluco- pyranoside]; 4' - demethylepipodophyllo- toxin-β-D-thenylidene glucoside
Molecular Weight: 656.7
Chemical Formula: $C_{32}H_{32}O_{13}S$

Availability: Teniposide is available from the Bristol Myers Oncology Division as a nonaqueous solution in 5-mL ampules containing 50 mg (10 mg/mL) of teniposide, 300 mg *N,N*-dimethylacetamide, 2.5 g purified polyoxyethylated castor oil, maleic acid to adjust the pH to pH 5.1, and absolute alcohol to a volume of 5 mL.

Storage: Intact vials are stable for several years when stored at room temperature (25°C) and protected from light. Solutions of teniposide in plastic containers at concentrations of 100 µg/ mL in 0.9% sodium chloride or sterile water are stable for 8 hours, while solutions in glass containers are stable for 24 hours when the diluent is 0.9% sodium chloride (up to 400 µg/mL) or sterile water (up to 200 µ/mL). Solutions in plastic containers at 100 µg/mL in 5% dextrose precipitate within 4 hours at room temperature (25°C), while solutions in glass containers at this concentration are stable for 24 hours. Upon dilution, a slight opalescence may appear, owing to the surfactant that is present in the formulation.

Administration: Teniposide should be given by intravenous infusion only after it is diluted with either 5% dextrose or 0.9% sodium chloride to yield a final concentration as described above. Teniposide should never be administered by the intravenous push technique because it may induce severe hypotension that is probably due to its cremophor vehicle. The agent should be infused over at least 45 minutes to decrease the risk of hypotensive reactions.

Extravasation should be avoided. A 5- to 10-mL flush of normal saline before drug administration should be given before and after drug administration to assess venous patency and assure that all residual drug is washed from the tubing. Teniposide can also induce chemical phlebitis at the venous injection site and severe local reactions such as abdominal pain with intraperitoneal use. For this reason and because of delayed lethal toxicity with intraperitoneal administration in mice, the intraperitoneal route of delivery should be avoided until phase I studies are conducted.

Local bladder instillation of teniposide has been used in patients with superficial bladder malignancies (113). For these applications, 50 mg of teniposide was diluted in 30 mL of sterile water or 0.9% sodium chloride and administered over 1 hour. Approximately one-third of patients have developed severe chemical cystitis that tended to become progressively more severe with each successive course.

Mechanism of Action: The mechanisms of action and explanations for cellular resistance are similar for the epipodophyllotoxins teniposide and etoposide. These mechanisms are discussed in the preceding sections on etoposide.

Pharmacology: Instantaneous peak plasma concentrations of teniposide at its maximally tolerated intravenous dose of 67 mg/m^2 (weekly bolus) range from approximately 20 to 30 μg/mL (39, 42, 47). Teniposide's plasma disposition has been characterized as a biphasic process in some studies and as a triphasic process in others (38, 114–118). Therefore, reports of teniposide's elimination half-life vary according to the pharmacokinetic model that best fits the particular data: 6 to 10 hours in studies demonstrating biexponential decay, and between 20 hours and more than 48 hours in those demonstrating triphasic characteristics (37, 114). Differences in analytic methods and small sample sizes in most published studies may contribute to these discordant descriptions. A three-compartment model may indicate that teniposide could be excreted by the biliary route and then reabsorbed or that the drug may be distributed to an as yet undetermined "third" body compartment.

Teniposide's pharmacokinetic behavior has not differed significantly between children and adults (38, 45, 114). In a review of teniposide's pharmacologic characteristics, Clark and Slevin reported that teniposide's volume of distribution at steady state ranges from 8 to 30 L/m^2 in adults and 3 to 10 L/m^2 in children (38). The volume of distribution at steady state has been calculated to be approximately 28.5% of body weight, with a mean central compartment of 3.5 L (42, 43). Total plasma clearance has been 7 to 17 mL/min/m^2, and the drug's renal clearance has been reported to be less than that of etoposide, 1 to 3 mL/min/m^2. In recent studies using HPLC, urinary excretion of the parent compound appears to be approximately 4 to 14% of the administered dose, compared with a value of 45% using radiolabeled compound (42, 43, 115, 116). Biliary excretion accounts for 0 to 10% of the administered dose (42, 43).

Teniposide is more extensively metabolized than etoposide. Only 5 to 20% of the administered dose of teniposide is accounted for as unchanged drug, and information pertaining to the metabolism of teniposide is scant. Thus far, the hydroxy acid [4'-demethyl epipodophyllic acid-9-(4,6-O-ethylidene-β-D-glucopyranosine)] formed by opening of the lactone ring, the picro-lactone isomer, and aglycone glucuronide metabolites have been identified in plasma and urine (7, 38, 114, 117, 118). Only the aglycone has been demonstrated to possess anti-DNA activity (118).

Etoposide has a threefold increased plasma clearance and sixfold increased renal clearance over teniposide in humans. Teniposide's more complete metabolism and lower renal clearance appear to account for its slower elimination. In addition, another factor influencing teniposide's slower elimination rate may be its higher degree of protein binding (>99% for teniposide vs. 94% for etoposide) (119). These differences may also partially explain why the equitoxic dose ratio of etoposide to teniposide is approximately 4:1.

Only very low concentrations of teniposide, or none at all, are detectable in cerebrospinal fluid by HPLC or radiolabeled methods (114, 120, 121). Drug levels in cerebrospinal fluid are generally less than 1% of simultaneously measured plasma levels (42, 43, 116, 120). However, teniposide appears to penetrate more efficiently through the abnormal blood-brain barrier. In one report, the concentration of teniposide in the cerebrospinal fluid of a patient who had prior brain surgery and radiotherapy was 27% of simultaneously measured plasma concentrations (121). In addition, relatively high teniposide levels are obtained in primary CNS gliomas as well as in brain metastases. Very high drug levels were achieved in the brain tumor of a patient who was treated concurrently with glycerol, which was used to enhance drug penetration through the blood-brain barrier (122).

Indications: Adult trials have been conducted predominantly in lymphomas and brain tumors, and these studies show that teniposide is indeed an active antineoplastic agent (114, 123, 124). However, a major problem is the assessment of teniposide's activity relative to that of etoposide. Teniposide has been studied extensively in pediatric hematologic malignancies, and combinations with cytosine arabinoside appear to be highly effective in childhood acute lymphocytic leukemia (114, 125–128). This combination is apparently active as a salvage regimen after initial induction failure, as consolidation therapy after attaining remission status, and as part of the initial therapy of patients with poor prognostic factors. In adults with lymphomas, the cumulative single-agent response rates in pretreated patients have been 33% and 31% in Hodgkin's and non-Hodgkin's lymphomas, respectively (114, 129, 130). Treatment schemes employing combinations of teniposide, doxorubicin, bleomycin, and prednisone appear promising as active salvage therapy for Hodgkin's and non-Hodgkin's lymphomas. In addition, teniposide has antineoplastic activity in neuroblastoma, glioma, and small cell lung carcinoma (131–138). The agent is also active in bladder carcinomas when administered either parenterally or intravesicularly (113, 139). Tenoposide has been used successfully as induction therapy in familial erythrophagocytic lymphohistiocytosis, a rare, usually fatal disease of childhood characterized by fever, hepatosplenomegaly, pancytopenia, and nonmalignant lymphohistiocytic infiltration and erythrophagocytosis in reticuloendothelial organs (140).

Dosages: Optimal doses and schedules for teniposide remain unclear (114, 123, 124). Teniposide is generally administered at doses of 150 to 200 mg/m^2 twice weekly for 4 weeks in combination with other agents such as cytosine arabinoside for childhood or adult leukemias. For solid tumors, weekly doses of 60 to 90 mg/m^2 are used commonly, and more aggressive schedules employ doses up to 60 mg/m^2 daily for 5 days. The agent is also well tolerated as a continuous infusion for 5 days at daily doses of 60 mg/m^2 (89, 141).

Toxicities

Hematologic: Myelosuppression is the dose-limiting toxicity of teniposide. Leukopenia tends to predominate, although modest thrombocytopenia is also observed. Neither toxicity appears to be cumulative. The range for leukopenic nadirs is 3 to 14 days, but nadirs generally occur in approximately 7 to 10 days. Heavy prior treatment of marrow-bearing bones with irradiation and/or chemotherapy increases the risk of developing severe myelosuppression, and therefore, doses should be reduced in patients who have been heavily pretreated.

Gastrointestinal: Nausea and vomiting occur infrequently and are typically mild. Diarrhea occurs occasionally. Stomatitis is uncommon.

Miscellaneous: Hypotension observed following rapid administration of teniposide is probably due to the coinfusion of the polyoxyethylated castor oil diluent (142–144). When teniposide is infused over periods of 30 to 45 minutes or more, hypotension rarely develops. Fever, chills, bronchospasm, urticaria, and flushing may accompany hypotension. These toxic effects are usually self-limited and resolve with interruption of the infusion. Diphenhydramine and hydrocortisone have been given to ameliorate these reactions, with variable results. Delayed hypotension and cardiac toxicities have not been reported with teniposide. Pulmonary toxicity has also been described (140).

Reversible alopecia occurs in a minority of patients. Chemical phlebitis at the injection site is relatively common. Elevations of hepatic enzymes are rarely observed. Drug-induced peripheral neuropathy is usually of minor significance but may be more prevalent and severe in patients who have previously received VCR (141).

REFERENCES

1. Philips NC, Lauper RD. Review of etoposide. Clin Pharm 1983;2:112–119.

2. Trissel LA, ed. ASAP handbook on injectable drugs. 5th ed. Bethesda: American Society of Hospital Pharmacists, 1988.

3. McEvoy GK, ed. American Hospital Formulary Service drug information 87. Bethesda: American Society of Hospital Pharmacists, 1987.

4. Stahelin H. Delayed toxicity of epipodophyllotoxin derivatives (VM-26 and VP-16-213) due to a local effect. Eur J Cancer 1976;12:925–931.

5. Loike JD. VP16-213 and podophyllotoxin: a study on the relationship between chemical structure and biological activity. Cancer Chemother Pharmacol 1982;7:103–111.

6. Achterrath W, Niederle N, Raettig R, Hilgrad P. Etoposide—chemistry, preclinical and clinical pharmacology. Cancer Treat Rev 1982;9:(Suppl A):3–13.

7. van Maanen JMS, Retel J, de Vries J, Pinedo HM. Mechanism of action of antitumor drug etoposide: a review. J Natl Cancer Inst 1988;80:1526–1533.

8. Long BH, Brattain MG. The activity of etoposide (VP16-213) and teniposide (VM-26) against human lung tumor cells in vitro: cytotoxicity and DNA breakage. In: Issell BF, Muggia FM, Carter SK, eds. Etoposide (VP16): current status and new developments. New York: Academic Press, 1984:63–86.

9. Minocha A, Long BH. Inhibition of the DNA catenation activity by VP16-213 and VM26. Biochem Biophys Res Commun 1984;122:165–170.

10. Chen GL, Yang L, Rowe TC, Halligan BD,

Tewey KM, Liu LF. Nonintercalative antitumor drugs interfere with the breakage-reunion reaction of mammalian DNA topoisomerase II. J Biol Chem 1984; 259:13560–13566.

11. Kalwinsky DK, Look AT, Ducore J, Fridland A. Effects of the epipodyllotoxin VP-16-213 on cell cycle traverse, DNA synthesis, and DNA strand size in cultures of human leukemic lymphoblasts. Cancer Res 1983;43:1592–1597.

12. Long BH, Musial SF, Brattain MG. Single- and double-strand DNA breakage and repair in human lung adenocarcinoma cells exposed to etoposide and teniposide. Cancer Res 1985;45:3106–3112.

13. Long BH, Musial SF, Brittain MG. DNA breakage in human lung carcinoma cells and nuclei that are naturally sensitive or resistant to etoposide or teniposide. Cancer Res 1986;46:3809–3816.

14. Haim N, Roman J, Nemec J, Singha BK. Peroxidative free radical formation and o-demethylation of etoposide (VP-16) and teniposide (VM-26). Biochem Biophys Res Commun 1986;135:215–220.

15. Sinha BK, Trush MA, Kalyanaraman B. Free radical metabolism of VP-16 and inhibition of anthracycline-induced lipid peroxidation. Biochem Pharmacol 1983;32:3495–3498.

16. Loike JD, Horwitz SB. Effects of podophyllotoxin and VP-16-213 on microtubule assembly in vitro and nucleoside transport in HeLa cells. Biochemistry 1976;15:5435–5442.

17. Loike JD. VP16-213 and podophyllotoxin: a study on the relationship between chemical structure and biological activity. Cancer Chemother Pharmacol 1982;7:103–111.

18. Seeber S, Osieka R, Schmidt CG, Achterrath W, Crook ST. In vivo resistance towards anthracyclines, etoposide, and cis-diammine-dichloroplatin(II).Cancer Res 1982;42:4719–4725.

19. Pommier Y, Schwartz RE, Zwelling LA, et al. Reduced formation of protein-associated DNA strand breaks in Chinese hamster cells resistant to topoisomerase II inhibitors. Cancer Res 1986;46:611–616.

20. Pommier Y, Kerrigan D, Schwartz RE, Swack JA, McCurdy A. Altered DNA topoisomerase II activity in Chinese hamster cells resistant to topoisomerase II inhibitors. Cancer Res 1986;46:3075–3081.

21. Glisson B. Characterization of acquired epipodophyllotoxin-resistant Chinese hamster ovary cell line: loss of drug-stimulated DNA cleavage activity. Cancer Res 1986;46:1934–1938.

22. Bleyer WA, Krivit W, Chard RL Jr, Hammond D. Phase II study of VM-26 in acute leukemia, neuroblastoma and other childhood malignancies: a report from the Children's Cancer Study Group. Cancer Treat Rep 1979;63:977–981.

23. Gupta RS. Genetic, biochemical and cross resistance studies with mutants of Chinese hamster ovary cells resistant to the anticancer drugs VM-26 and VP16-213. Cancer Res 1983;43:1568–1574.

24. Rivera G, Avery T, Roberts D. Response of L1210 to combination of cytosine arabinoside and VM 26 or VP 16-213. Eur J Cancer 1975;11:639–647.

25. Dombernowsky P, Nissen NI. Schedule dependency of the antileukaemic activity of the podophyllotoxin-derivative VP 16-213 (NSC 141540) in L1210 leukemia. Acta Pathol Microbiol Immunol Scand 1973; 81:715–724.

26. Chiuten DF, Wodinsky I, Abraham D. Influence of treatment schedule on the toxicity and anti-tumour activity of mitotic inhibitors and semisynthetic podophyllotoxin derivatives (abstract). Proc Am Soc Clin Oncol 1979;20:402.

27. Burchenal JH, Lokys L, Turkevich J, Gale G. Rationale of combination chemotherapy. In: Prestayko A, Crooke ST, Carter SK, et al., eds. Cisplatin: current status and new developments. New York: Academic Press, 1980:113–124.

28. Damon LE, Cadman EC. Enhanced cytotoxicity of fluoropyrimidines by etoposide in L1210 cells (abstract). Proc Am Assoc Cancer Res 1986;27:180.

29. Ratain MJ, Schilsky RL, Wojack BR, Simon T, Senekjian EK, Vogelzang NJ. Hydroxyurea and etoposide: in vitro synergy and phase I clinical trial. J Natl Cancer Inst 1988;6:1412–1416.

30. Roberts D, Hillard S, Peck C. Sedimentation of DNA from L1210 cells after treatment with 4'demethylepipodophyllotoxin -9-(4,6-O-2-thenylidene-β-D-glucopyranoside) and 1-β-D-arabinofuranosyl-cytosine or both drugs. Cancer Res 1980;40:4225–4231.

31. Wampler GL, Carter WIT, Cambell ED. Combination chemotherapy with hexamethylmelamine in L1210 and P388 leukemias (abstract). Proc Am Assoc Cancer Res 1981;21:237.

32. Yalowich JC, Fry DW, Goldman ID. Teniposide (VM-26) and etoposide (VP-16-123)-induced augmentation of methotrexate transport and polyglutamation in Ehrlich ascites tumor cells in vitro. Cancer Res 1982; 42:3648–3653.

33. Yalowich JC, Ross WE. Verapamil-induced augmentation of etoposide accumulation of L1210 cells in vitro. Cancer Res 1985;45:1651–1656.

34. Yalowich JC, Ross WE. Potentiation of etoposide-induced DNA damage by calcium antagonists in L1210 cells in vitro. Cancer Res 1985;45:3360–3365.

35. Dombernowsky P, Nissen NI. Schedule dependency of the antileukemic activity of the podophyllotoxin-derivative VP 16-213 (NSC-141540) in L1210 leukemia. Acta Pathol Microbiol Scand 1973;81:715–724.

36. Slevin ML, Clark PL, Joel SP, et al. A randomized trial to evaluate the effects of schedule on the activity of etoposide in small-cell lung cancer. J Clin Oncol 1989;7:1333–1340.

37. Cavalli F, Sonntag RW, Jungi F. VP-16-213 monotherapy for remission induction of small-cell lung cancer: a randomized trial using three dosage regimens. Cancer Treat Rep 1978;62:473–475.

38. Clark PI, Slevin ML. The clinical pharmacology of etoposide and teniposide. Clin Pharm 1987;12:223–252.

39. Hande KR, Wedlund PJ, Noone RM, Wilkinson GR, Greco FA, Wolff SN. Pharmacokinetics of high-dose etoposide (VP-16-213) administered to cancer patients. Cancer Res 1984;44:379–382.

40. Muggia FM, Selawry OS, Hansen HH. Clinical studies with a new podophyllotoxin derivative, epipodophyllotoxin, 4'-demethyl-9-(4,6-O-2-thenylidene-β-D-glucopyranoside) (NSC-122819). Cancer Chemother Rep 1971;55:575–581.

41. Vespesid (etoposide [VP-16-213]) injection. Clinical experience overview. Bristol Myers, 1984.

42. Creaven PJ. The clinical pharmacology of VM26 and VP16-213: a brief overview. Cancer Chemother Pharmacol 1982;7:133–140.

43. Allen LM, Creaven PJ. Comparison of the hu-

man pharmacokinetics of VM-26 and VP-16, two antineoplastic epipodophyllotoxin glucopyranoside derivatives. Eur J Cancer 1975;11:697–707.

44. Arbuck SG, Douglas, HO, Crom WR, et al. Etoposide pharmacokinetics in patients with normal and abnormal organ functions. J Clin Oncol 1986;4:1690–1695.

45. Crom WR, Glynn-Barnhart AM, Rodman JH, Teresi ME, Kavanagh RE, Chistianson ML. Pharmacokinetics of anticancer drugs in children. Clin Pharm 1987;12:168–213.

46. Hande KR, Wolf SN, Greco FA, Hainsworth JD, Reed G, Johnson DH. Etoposide kinetics in patients with obstructive jaundice. J Clin Oncol 1990;8:1101–1108.

47. Stewart CF, Arbuck SG, Fleming RA, Evans WE. Changes in the clearance of total and unbound etoposide in patients with liver dysfunction. J Clin Oncol 1990;8:1874–1879.

48. O'Dwyer PJ, Leyland-Jones B, Alonso MT, Marsoni S, Wittes RE. Etoposide (VP-16-213). Current status of an active anticancer drug. N Engl J Med 1985; 31:692–700.

49. Evans WE, Sinkule JA, Crom WR, Dow L, Look AT, Rivera G. Pharmacokinetics of teniposide (VM26) and etoposide (VP16-213) in children with cancer. Cancer Chemother Pharmacol 1982;7:147–150.

50. Hande K, Bennett R, Hamilton R, Grote T, Branch R. Metabolism and excretion of etoposide in isolated, perfused rat liver models. Cancer Res 1988; 48:5692–5695.

51. Hande K, Anthony L, Hamilton R, Bennett R, Sweetman B, Branch R. Identification of etoposide glucuronide as a major metabolite of etoposide in the rat and rabbit. Cancer Res 1988;48:1829–1834.

52. Stewart CF, Pieper JA, Arbuck SG, Evans WE. Altered protein binding of etoposide in patients with cancer. Clin Pharmacol Ther 1989;45:49–55.

53. Postmus PE, Holthius JJ, Haaxma-Reiche H, et al. Penetration of VP 16-213 into cerebral spinal fluid after high dose intravenous administration. J Clin Oncol 1984;2:215–220.

54. Harvey VJ, Stein ML, Smithe MM, Johnston A, Wrigley PF. Variable bioavailability following repeated oral doses of etoposide. Eur J Cancer Clin Oncol 1985;21:1315–1319.

55. Smyth RD, Pfeffer M, Scalzo S, Comis RL. Bioavailability of etoposide (VP-16). Semin Oncol 1985; 12(Suppl 2):48–51.

56. Lederman GS, Garnick MB, Canellos GP, Richie JP. The treatment of metastatic germ-cell cancer with etoposide. J Clin Oncol 1983;1:706–709.

57. Loehrer PJ Sr, Lauer R, Roth BJ, Williams SD, Kalasinski LA, Einhorn LH. Salvage therapy in recurrent germ cell cancer: ifosfamide and cisplatin plus either vinblastine or etoposide. Ann Intern Med 1988; 109:540–546.

58. Williams SD, Einhorn LH. Etoposide salvage therapy for refractory germ cell tumors: an update. Cancer Treat Rev 1982;9(Suppl A):67–71.

59. Einhorn LH, Williams SD, Loehrer PJ, et al. Evaluation of optimal duration of chemotherapy in favorable-prognosis disseminated germ cell tumors: a Southeastern Cancer Study Group protocol. J Clin Oncol 1989;7:387–391.

60. Bosl GJ, Geller NL, Bajorin D, et al. A randomized trial of etoposide + cisplatin versus vinblastine + bleomycin + cisplatin + cyclophosphamide + dactinomycin in patients with good prognosis germ cell tumors. J Clin Oncol 1988;6:1231–1238.

61. Loehrer PJ Sr, Williams SD, Einhorn LH. Testicular cancer: the quest continues. J Natl Cancer Inst 1988;80:1373–1382.

62. Goodman GE, Miller TP, Manning MM, Davis SL, McMahon LJ. Treatment of small cell lung cancer with VP-16, vincristine, doxorubicin (Adriamycin), cyclophosphamide (EVAC), and high-dose chest radiotherapy. J Clin Oncol 1983;1:483–488.

63. Abeloff MD, Ettinger DS, Order SE, Khouri N, Mellits DE, Dorschell NT. Intensive induction chemotherapy in 54 patients with small cell carcinoma of the lung. Cancer Treat Rep 1981;65:639–645.

64. Sierocki JS, Hilaris BS, Hopfan S, et al. cis-dichlorodiammine platinum(II) and VP-16-213: an active induction regimen for small cell carcinoma of the lung. Cancer Treat Rep 1979;63:1593–1597.

65. Sierocki JS, Hilaris BS, Hopfan S, Martini N, Barton D, Golbey RB. Cisplatin and etoposide (VP-16) as a single regimen for small cell lung cancer. A phase II trial. Cancer 1989;63:638–642.

66. Einhorn LH. Initial therapy with cisplatin plus VP-16 in small-cell lung cancer. Semin Oncol 1986; 13(Suppl 3):5–9.

67. Loehrer PJ Sr, Einhorn LH, Greco FA. Cisplatin plus etoposide in small cell lung cancer. Semin Oncol 1988;15:2–8.

68. Comis RL. Oral etoposide in small-cell lung cancer. Semin Oncol 1986;13(Suppl 3):75–78.

69. Smith IE, Perren TJ, Ashley SA, et al. Carboplatin, etoposide, and ifosfamide as intensive chemotherapy for small-cell lung cancer. J Clin Oncol 1990;8:899–905.

70. Johnson DH, Greco FA, Strupp J, Hande KR, Hainsworth JD. Prolonged administration of oral etoposide in patients with relapsed or refractory small cell lung cancer: a phase II trial. J Clin Oncol 1990;8:1613–1617.

71. Slevin ML. Low-dose oral etoposide: a new role for an old drug. J Clin Oncol 1990;8:1607–1609.

72. Clark PI, Cottier B, Joel SP, Thompson PI, Slevin ML. Prolonged administration of single-agent oral etoposide in patients with untreated small cell lung cancer (SCLC) (abstract). Proc Am Soc Clin Oncol 1990;9:874.

73. Fisher R, DeVita VT Jr, Hubbard SM, et al. Diffuse aggressive lymphomas: increased survival after alternating flexible sequences of ProMACE and MOPP chemotherapy. Ann Intern Med 1983;98:304–309.

74. Longo D, DeVita V, Duffrey D, et al. Randomized trial of ProMACE-MOPP vs ProMACE-CytaBOM in stage II-IV aggressive non-Hodgkin's lymphoma (abstract). Proc Am Soc Clin Oncol 1987;6:206.

75. Tseng A Jr, Jacobs C, Coleman CN, Horning SJ, Lewis BJ, Rosenberg SA. Third-line chemotherapy for resistant Hodgkin's disease with lomustine, etoposide, and methotrexate. Cancer Treat Rep 1987;71:475–478.

76. Bolis G, Bonazzi C, Landoni F, et al. EMA/CO regimen in high-risk gestational trophoblastic tumor (GTT). Gynecol Oncol 1988;31:439–444.

77. Willemse PH, Aalders JG, Bouma J, Sleijfer DT. Chemotherapy-resistant gestational trophoblastic neoplasia treated successfully with cisplatin, etoposide, and bleomycin. Obstet Gynecol 1988;71:438–440.

78. Crist WM, Raney RB, Ragab A, et al. Intensive

chemotherapy including cisplatin with or without etoposide for children with soft-tissue sarcoma. Med Pediatr Oncol 1987;15:51–57.

79. Rosso R, Ardizzoni A, Salvati F, et al. Etoposide vs etoposide and cisplatin in the treatment of advanced non-small cell lung cancer; a FONICAP randomized study. Semin Oncol 1988;15(Suppl 7):49–55.

80. Malliard JA, Letendre L, Dalton RJ, et al. Phase I-II trial of VP-16 in the treatment of acute nonlymphocytic leukemia and blast crisis of chronic granulocytic leukemia. Med Pediatr Oncol 1986;14:306–309.

81. Nishikawa A, Nakamura Y, Nobori U, et al. Acute monocytic leukemia in children. Response to VP-16-213 as a single agent. Cancer 1988;60:2146–2149.

82. Ibrahim NK, Kouri FP, Salem PA. VP-16-based regimens in adult acute nonlymphoblastic leukemia. Oncology 1988;45:21–23.

83. Ho AD, Lipp T, Ehninger G, et al. Combination of mitoxantrone and etoposide in refractory acute myelogenous leukemia—an active and well-tolerated regimen. J Clin Oncol 1986;6:213–217.

84. Esumi N, Todo S, Arakawa S, Imashuka S. Etoposide and cytosine arabinoside combination chemotherapy for refractory acute lymphocytic leukemia in childhood. J Clin Oncol 1986;4:1089–1093.

85. Markowitz M, Metroka C, Moore A. VP 16-213 (etoposide) and bleomycin in the treatment of Kaposi's sarcoma (abstract). Proc Am Soc Clin Oncol 1984;3:58.

86. Goldberg RM, Jett JR, Therneau TM, et al. Bolus versus infusion regimens of etoposide and cisplatin in treatment of non-small cell lung cancer: a study of the North Central Cancer Treatment Group. J Natl Can Inst 1990;82:1899–1903.

87. Donehower RC. Evaluating cancer chemotherapy by infusion. J Natl Cancer Inst 1990;82:1867–1868.

88. Preusser P, Wilke H, Achterrath, et al. Phase II study with the combination etoposide, doxorubicin, and cisplatin in advanced measurable gastric cancer. J Clin Oncol 1989;7:1310–1317.

89. Sparano JA, Wiernik PH. Toxicity of etoposide, doxorubicin, and cisplatin in gastric cancer. J Clin Oncol 1990;8:938–939.

90. Ajani JA, Roth JA, Ryan B, et al. Evaluation of pre- and postoperative chemotherapy for resectable adenocarcinoma of the esophagus or gastroesophageal junction. J Clin Oncol 1990;8:1231–1238.

91. Harnett PR, Bell DR, Hillcoat BL, et al. Cisplatin plus VP 16-213 in advanced ovarian cancer. Gynecol Oncol 1988;30:159–162.

92. Chambers SK, Chambers JT, Kohorn EI, Schwartz PE. Etoposide (VP-16-213) plus cis-diamminedichloroplatinum as salvage therapy in advanced epithelial ovarian cancer. Gynecol Oncol 1987;27:233–240.

93. Zimm S, Cleary SM, Lucas WE, et al. Phase I/pharmacokinetic study of intraperitoneal cisplatin and etoposide (abstract). Cancer Res 1987;15:1712–1716.

94. Kuhnle H, Meerpohl HG, Lenaz L, et al. Etoposide in cisplatin-refractory ovarian cancer. Proc Am Soc Clin Oncol 1988;7:137.

95. Howell SB, Kirmani S, Lucas WE, et al. A phase II trial of intraperitoneal cisplatin and etoposide for primary treatment of ovarian epithelial cancer. J Clin Oncol 1990;8:137–145.

96. Reichman B, Markman M, Hakes T, et al. Intraperitoneal, cisplatin, and etoposide in the treatment of refractory recurrent ovarian carcinoma. J Clin Oncol 1989;7:1327–1332 and Proc Am Soc Clin Oncol 1988;7:135.

97. Bennett CL, Sinkule JA, Schilsky RL, Senekjian E, Choi KE. Phase I clinical and pharmacological study of 72-hour continuous infusion of etoposide in patients with advanced cancer. Cancer Res 1987;47:1952–1956.

98. Comis RL. The epipodophyllotoxins. In: Lokich J, ed. Cancer chemotherapy by infusion. 2nd ed. Chicago: Precept Press, 1990:240–252.

99. Hainsworth JD, Johnson DH, Frazier SR, Greco FA. Chronic daily administration of oral etoposide—a phase I trial. J Clin Oncol 1989;7:396–401.

100. Van Echo DA, Wiernik PH, Aisner J. High dose VP-16-213 for the treatment of patients with previously treated acute leukemia. Cancer Clin Trials 1980;3:325–328.

101. Wolfe SN, Fer MR, McKay CM, Hande KR, Hainsworth JD, Greco FA. High-dose VP-16-213 and autologous bone marrow transplantation for refractory malignancies: a phase I study. J Clin Oncol 1983;1:701–705.

102. Littlewood TJ, Spragg HP, Bentley DP. When is autologous bone marrow transplantation safe after high-dose treatment with etoposide? Clin Lab Haematol 1985;7:213–218.

103. Johnson DH, Greco FA, Wolfe SN. Etoposide-induced hepatic injury: a potential complication of high-dose therapy. Cancer Treat Rep 1983;67:1023–1024.

104. Fontana JA. Radiation recall associated with VP-16-213 therapy. Cancer Treat Rep 1979;63:224–225.

105. Jameson CH, Solanki DL. Stevens-Johnson syndrome associated with etoposide therapy. Cancer Treat Rep 1983;67:1050–1051.

106. Thant M, Hawley RJ, Smith MT, et al. Possible enhancement of vincristine neuropathy by VP-16-213. Cancer 1982;49:859–864.

107. Littlewood TJ, Bentley DP, McQueen IN. High dose etoposide does not cause peripheral neuropathy. Cancer Chemother Pharmacol 1987;19:180–181.

108. Jackson DV Jr, Wells HB, White DR, et al. Lack of potentiation of vincristine-induced neurotoxicity by VP-16-213. Am J Clin Oncol 1983;6:327–330.

109. Left RS, Thompson JM, Daly MB, et al. Acute neurological dysfunction after high-dose etoposide for malignant glioma. Cancer 1988;62:32–35.

110. Aisner J, Van Echo DA, Whitacre M, Wiernik PH. A phase I trial of continuous infusion VP16-213 (etoposide). Cancer Chemother Pharmacol 1982;7:157–160.

111. Rowinsky EK, Harwood KV, Ettinger DS. Sudden dyspnea occurring 24 hours after mitomycin plus etoposide combination therapy. Cancer Treat Rep 1987;71:103–104.

112. Ratain MJ, Kaminer LS, Bitran JD, et al. Acute nonlymphocytic leukemia following etoposide and cisplatin combination chemotherapy for advanced non-small cell carcinoma of the lung. Blood 1987;70:1412–1417.

113. Pavone-Macaluso M, Caramia G, Rizzo FP, Messana V. Preliminary evaluation of VM-26, a new epipodophyllotoxin derivative in the treatment of urogenital tumors. Eur Urol 1975;1:53–56.

114. O'Dwyer PJ, Alonso MT, Leyland-Jones B, Marsoni S. Teniposide: a review of 12 years of experience. Cancer Treat Rep 1984;68:1455–1464.

115. D'Incalci M, Rossi C, Sessa C, et al. Pharma-

cokinetics of teniposide in patients with ovarian cancer. Cancer Treat Rep 1985;69:73–77.

116. Holthuis JJ, de Vries LG, Postmus PE, et al. Pharmacokinetics of high-dose teniposide. Cancer Treat Rep 1987;71:599–604.

117. Rosse C, Zuchetti M, Sessa C, Urso R, Mangioni C, D'Incalci M. Pharmacokinetic study of VM-26 given as a prolonged i.v. infusion to ovarian cancer patients. Cancer Chemother Pharmacol 1984;13:211–214.

118. Evans WE, Sinkule JA, Crom WR, Dow L, Look AT, Rivera G. Pharmacokinetics of teniposide (VM-26) and etoposide (VP-16-213) in children with cancer. Cancer Chemother Pharmacol 1982;7:147–152.

119. Allen LM, Tejada F, Okonmah AD, Nordquist S. Combination chemotherapy of the epipodophyllotoxin derivatives, teniposide and etoposide. A pharmacodynamic rationale? Cancer Chemother Pharmacol 1982;7:151–156.

120. Sessa C, D'Incalci M, Farina P, et al. Pharmacokinetics of VM26 after 60 minutes or 24 hour infusion (abstract). Proc Am Assoc Cancer Res 1982;23:128.

121. Creaven PJ, Allen LM. PTG, a new anti-neoplastic epipodophyllotoxin. Clin Pharmacol Ther 1975; 18:221–226.

122. Stewart DJ, Richard MT, Hugenholtz H, Dennery J, Nundy D, Prior J. Penetration of teniposide (VM-26) into human intracerebral tumours. J Neurooncol 1984;2:315–324.

123. Macbeth FR. VM26: phase I and II studies. Cancer Chemother Pharmacol 1982;7:87–91.

124. Issell BF. The podophyllotoxin derivatives VP16-213 and VM26. Cancer Chemother Pharmacol 1982;7:73–80.

125. Grem JL, Hoth DF, Leyland-Jones B, King SA, Ungerleider RS, Wittes RE. Teniposide in the treatment of leukemia: a case study of conflicting priorities in the development of drugs for fatal diseases. J Clin Oncol 1988;2:351–379.

126. Rivera GK. The epipodophyllotoxin teniposide in therapy for childhood acute lymphocytic leukemia. J Clin Oncol 1988;6:191–193.

127. Linker CA, Levitt LJ, O'Donnell M, Ries CA, Forman SJ. Teniposide (VM-26) and ara-C in the treatment of adult acute lymphoblastic leukemia. Semin Oncol 1987;14(Suppl 1):78–85.

128. Rivera GK, Buchanana G, Boyett JM, et al. Intensive retreatment of acute lymphoblastic leukemia in first bone marrow relapse. A Pediatric Oncology Group study. N Engl J Med 1986;315:273–278.

129. Tseng A Jr, Jacobs C, Coleman CN, Horning SJ, Lewis BJ, Rosenberg SA. Treatment of refractory non-Hodgkin's lymphoma of unfavorable histology with teniposide, cytarabine, and cisplatin. Cancer Treat Rep 1987;71:645–647.

130. Grossberg H, Opfell R, Glick J, Bakemeir R, Schnetzer G III, Muggia F. Treatment of advanced refractory lymphoma with teniposide and lomustine. Cancer Treat Rep 1987;71:215–216.

131. Rivera G, Green A, Hayes A, Aurey T, Pratt C. Epipodophyllotoxin VM-26 in the treatment of childhood neuroblastoma. Cancer Treat Rep 1977; 61:1243–1248.

132. Hayes FA, Green AA, Casper J, Cornet J, Evans WE. Clinical evaluation of sequentially scheduled cisplatin and VM-26 in neuroblastoma: response and toxicity. Cancer 1981;48:1715–1718.

133. Sklansky BD, Mann-Kaplan RS, Reynolds AF, Rosenblum ML, Walker MD. 4'demethyl-epipodophyllotoxin-β-D-thenylidene-glucoside (PTG) in the treatment of malignant intracranial neoplasms. Cancer 1974;33:460–467.

134. Gerosa MA, DiStefano E, Oliva A. VM-26 monochemotherapy trial in the treatment of recurrent supratentorial gliomas: preliminary report. Surg Neurol 1981;15:128–134.

135. Kessinger A, Lemon HM, Foley JF. VM-26 as a second drug in the treatment of malignant gliomas. Cancer Treat Rep 1979;63:511–512.

136. Woods RL, Fox RM, Tattersall MH. Treatment of small cell bronchogenic carcinoma with VM-26. Cancer Treat Rep 1979;63:2011–2013.

137. Giaccone G, Donadio M, Bonardi G, Testore F, Calciati A. Teniposide in the treatment of small-cell lung cancer: the influence of prior chemotherapy. J Clin Oncol 1988;6:1264–1270.

138. Giaccone G, Donadio M, Bonardi G, Testore F, Calciati A. Teniposide (VM26): an effective treatment of brain metastases of small cell carcinoma of the lung. Eur J Clin Oncol 1988;24:629–631.

139. Oishi N, Berenberg J, Blumenstein BA, et al. Teniposide in metastatic renal and bladder cancer: a Southwest Oncology Group study. Cancer Treat Rep 1987;7:1307–1308.

140. Henter JI, Elinder G, Finkel Y, Soder O. Successful induction with chemotherapy including teniposide in familial erythrophagocytic lymphohistiocytosis. Lancet 1986;2:1402.

141. Booser DJ, Spitzer G, Chiuten DF, Valdivieso M. Epipodophyllotoxins VP-16-213 and VM-26: a phase I study of 5-day continuous intravenous infusion in bronchogenic carcinoma (abstract). Proc Am Assoc Cancer Res and Am Soc Clin Oncol 1981;22:508.

142. Carstensen H, Nolte H, Hertz H, Jensen T. Hypersensitivity reactions to teniposide in children. J Clin Oncol 1987;5:1491–1492.

143. Siddal SJ, Martin J, Nunn AJ. Anaphylactic reactions to teniposide. Lancet 1989;86340(1):394.

144. O'Dwyer PJ, King SA, Fortner CL, Leyland-Jones B. Hypersensitivity reactions to teniposide (VM-26): an analysis. J Clin Oncol 1986;4:1262–1269.

145. Commers JR, Foley JF. Pulmonary hyaline membrane disease occurring in the course of VM26 therapy. Cancer Treat Rep 1979;63:2009.

146. Griffiths JD, Start RJ, Ding JC, Cooper IA. Vincristine neurotoxicity enhanced in combination chemotherapy including both teniposide and vincristine. Cancer Treat Rep 1986;70:519–521.

24

Differentiation Agents

Raymond P. Warrell, Jr.

Observations that cytotoxic drug treatment has occasionally been associated with apparent differentiation of residual disease have caused persistent interest in the concept of "induced cytodifferentiation" as a method of cancer treatment. This chapter reviews those compounds that have been most clearly linked to differentiation (as opposed to immediate cytolysis) as a principal mechanism of action, and it focuses on drugs that are either widely available or currently undergoing clinical testing.

RETINOIDS

Dietary deficiencies of vitamin A (retinol) are associated with an increased cancer incidence, whereas retinol supplementation can reverse preneoplastic lesions in vitamin A–deficient animals (1, 2). Retinoids induce cellular differentiation and suppress proliferation or carcinogenesis in a number of cell lines and model systems (3–5). Consequently, retinoids have generated wide interest in use for both cancer treatment and prevention. Chemical structures of some therapeutically important retinoids are shown in Figure 24.1. All-*trans* retinoic acid (RA), 13-*cis* RA, and 9-*cis* RA are normally found in plasma in nanomolar concentrations (6). These "natural retinoids" are derived from intracellular oxidation of retinol that has been absorbed by the gastrointestinal tract. Conversely, exogenously administered retinoic acid probably enters the cell by diffusion, where it is bound by specific retinoic acid–binding proteins that serve both a sequestration function (regulating free intracytoplasmic concentrations) and a carrier function (delivering the compound to the endoplasmic reticulum for metabolic degradation) (7, 8) (Fig. 24.2).

The target of retinoid action is the cell nucleus, where these compounds bind either to retinoic acid receptors (RARs) (9–11) or to retinoid "X" receptors (RXRs) (12, 13). Retinoid receptors are part of a superfamily of nuclear proteins that includes receptors for thyroid hormone and vitamin D. Upon activation by their ligands, RAR/RAR homodimers or (more commonly) RAR/RXR heterodimers form and bind with high affinity to specific DNA segments within retinoid target genes, thereby regulating their transcription. A variety of downstream events then occur, including increased expression of transforming growth factor-β (14), a decrease in ornithine decarboxylase activity (14), and an increase in transglutaminase activity (15), which is linked to induction of programed cell death. The processes of retinoid-induced differentiation and inhibition of proliferation are not inextricably linked, and different signaling pathways, such as AP-1 activation (16), may be selectively targeted (17). Recently, two groups have shown that nonactivated retinoid receptors have important roles in silencing basal transcription of target genes via interaction with nuclear corepressor proteins (18, 19).

ALL-*TRANS* RETINOIC ACID

The clinical application of differentiation therapy has been most successful in the treatment of acute promyelocytic leukemia (APL) (20). All-*trans* RA induces complete remission in a very high proportion of patients with APL, and resistance to this agent in a previously untreated patient is exceedingly rare. Indeed, failure is almost always due to either early death (21–24) or misdiagnosis. In APL, reciprocal translocations between the long arms of chromosomes 15 and 17 result in fusion between a gene that encodes a specific retinoic acid receptor (RAR-α) and a gene known as *pml* (25). A fusion protein, PML/RAR-α, is then generated that blocks myeloid differentiation at the promyelocyte stage, and

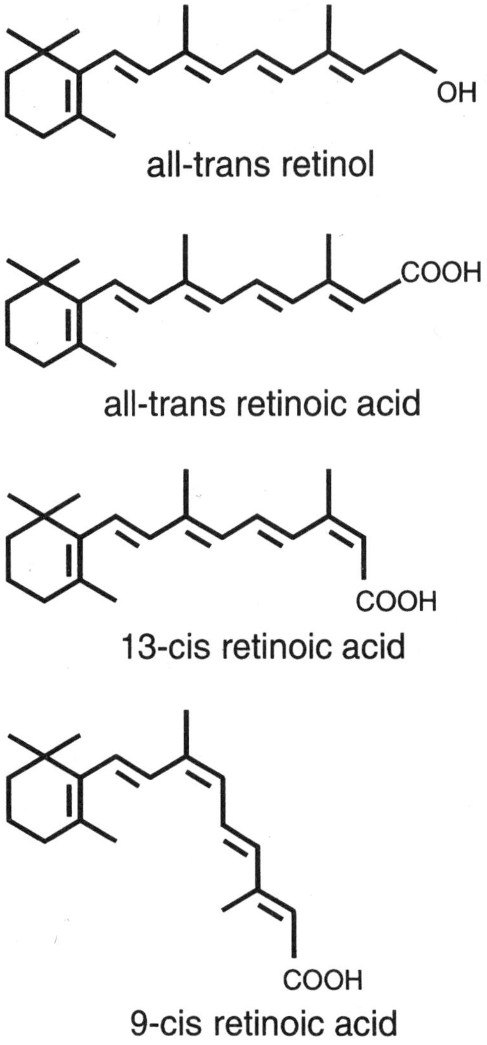

all-trans retinol

all-trans retinoic acid

13-cis retinoic acid

9-cis retinoic acid

Figure 24.1. Chemical structures of several clinically relevant retinoids.

this block appears to be overcome by exogenous provision of retinoic acid at pharmacologic concentrations. The mechanism(s) by which terminally differentiated cells are eliminated in vivo is not clear; however, experimental evidence suggests that programed cell death or apoptosis is initiated (26).

The clinical pharmacology of all-*trans* retinoic acid has proved to be unexpectedly different from that of other retinoids. The plasma half-life is relatively short (approximately 40 minutes) (27), and continuous treatment is associated with a progressive decrease in plasma drug concentrations (28, 29), possibly due to increased ex-

pression of cytoplasmic retinoic acid–binding proteins (30), induction of cytochrome P450 oxidases (31), and an increase in oxidative cofactors (32). Individuals vary widely in their native catabolic rates for this natural retinoid, such that some patients exhibit a very rapid catabolic phenotype prior to drug exposure (31). Trials of liposomally encapsulated all-*trans* RA have been initiated to test whether this formulation can attenuate the inducible catabolic activity (33).

Despite the high degree of initial activity, remissions induced by all-*trans* RA in patients with APL tend to be quite brief (3 to 5 months on average) (27). While resistance in cell lines has been associated with development of point mutations in RAR-α (34) or with altered expression of the PML/RAR-α protein (35), similar observations have not yet been made in samples derived from clinically resistant patients (29). Nonetheless, due to the relatively rapid emergence of resistance, most centers discontinue all-*trans* RA treatment shortly after complete remission has been achieved and then administer three cycles of anthracycline-based combination chemotherapy as "consolidation." These combined sequential treatment programs have yielded a highly significant increase in both relapse-free and overall survival in patients with APL (22–23, 36) (Fig. 24.3), and more than half of newly diagnosed patients are cured by these regimens. Regrettably, the high single-agent activity of all-*trans* RA observed in APL has not been replicated in other diseases, although minor activity has been reported in gliomas (37) and AIDS-related Kaposi's sarcoma (38).

13-*CIS* RETINOIC ACID

Of all retinoids, 13-*cis* retinoic acid has undergone the most extensive clinical examination. Nonetheless, the single-agent activity of this drug in patients with established cancer is quite limited. In the hematologic cancers, brief partial responses have been observed in patients with cutaneous T-cell lymphoma (39–42). Studies in patients with myelodysplastic syndromes (43–45) and chronic myelocytic leukemia (46) have yielded negative results. Among the solid tumors, disappointing results have been recorded in germ cell cancer and neuroblastoma (47–49), diseases in which cytotoxic drug treatment has been most commonly associated with cytodifferentiation. Negative results have also been recorded in carcinomas of the head and neck, lung, and bladder (50–52). Modest activity has been seen in patients with low-grade skin cancers, in-

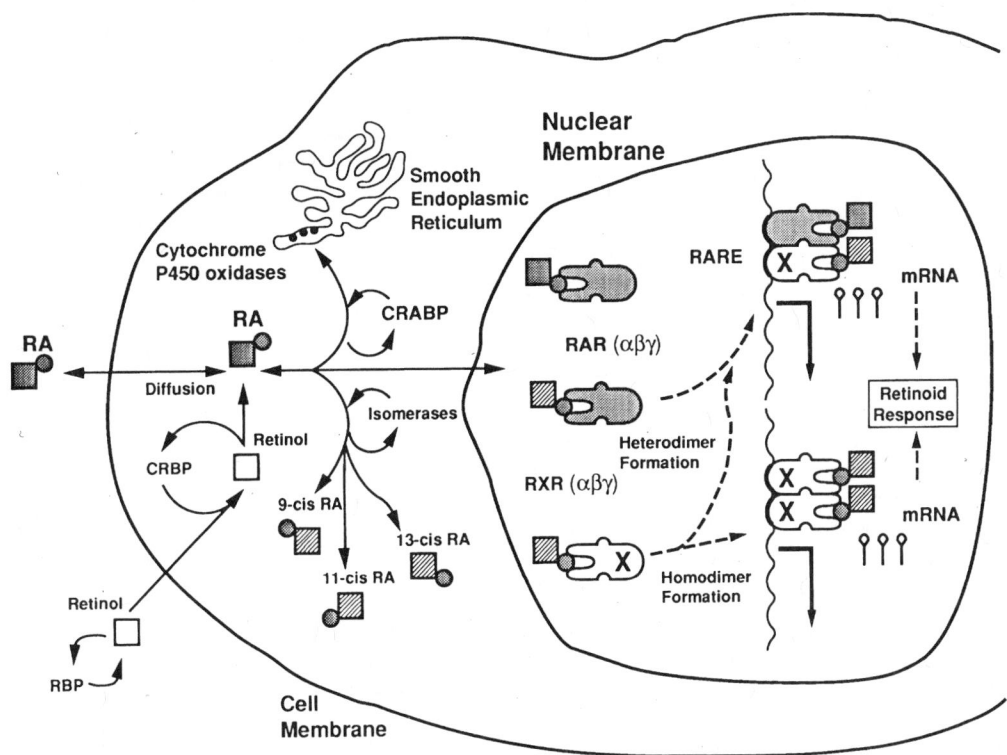

Figure 24.2. Metabolism of all-*trans* retinoic acid (RA). RA enters the cell by simple diffusion or by conversion from *retinol* (vitamin A) that has been absorbed from the gastrointestinal tract, bound in circulating form to retinol-binding proteins (*RBP*) and re-bound intracellularly to cellular retinol-binding proteins (*CRBP*). RA can be immediately metabolized upon binding to cellular retinoic acid–binding proteins (*CRABP*) and oxidized by *cytochrome P450 enzymes* located in *smooth endoplasmic reticulum*. Alternatively, RA (or its isomers) enter the cell nucleus and bind to retinoic acid receptors (*RARs*) or retinoid "X" receptors (*RXRs*). Upon dimerization of these receptors (i.e., formation of a RAR/RXR heterodimer or RXR/RXR homodimer), RA-activated receptors bind with high affinity to specific DNA segments (the retinoic acid response element (*RARE*)) and effect *mRNA* transcription. Ultimately, the retinoid response is mediated by primary target genes, by interference with other transcription factors, or by control of certain posttranscriptional actions. (Reprinted with permission from Warrell RP Jr, de Thé H, Wang Z-Y, Degos L. Acute promyelocytic leukemia. N Engl J Med 1993;329:177–189.)

cluding squamous cancers (53) and basal cell carcinomas (54), although a follow-up randomized study using a much lower dose did not confirm the latter activity (55).

The limited activity in advanced cancer has not diminished enthusiasm for exploration of 13-*cis* RA as a means of cancer prevention, either as primary prevention (to prevent an initial cancer) or secondary therapy (to reduce the risk of recurrence). Treatment with 13-*cis* RA (1 to 2 mg/kg/day for 3 months) in heavy tobacco users reverses oral leukoplakia (56), a known precursor of squamous carcinoma of the oral cavity. Since this dose causes considerable mucocutaneous toxicity, follow-up studies have used a high-dose

induction course followed by a lower dose (0.5 mg/kg/day) as maintenance (57). However, the duration of the clinical response is frequently brief, and most patients relapse if the drug is withdrawn. In an important preliminary study, adjuvant treatment with 13-*cis* RA (1 mg/kg/day) in patients who had undergone primary surgical excision and/or radiation treatment for head and neck cancer significantly reduced the incidence of second primary tumors of the aerodigestive tract (58). A large randomized multicenter study has been initiated to confirm these findings.

Despite the unimpressive single-agent data as primary anticancer treatment, 13-*cis* RA is being

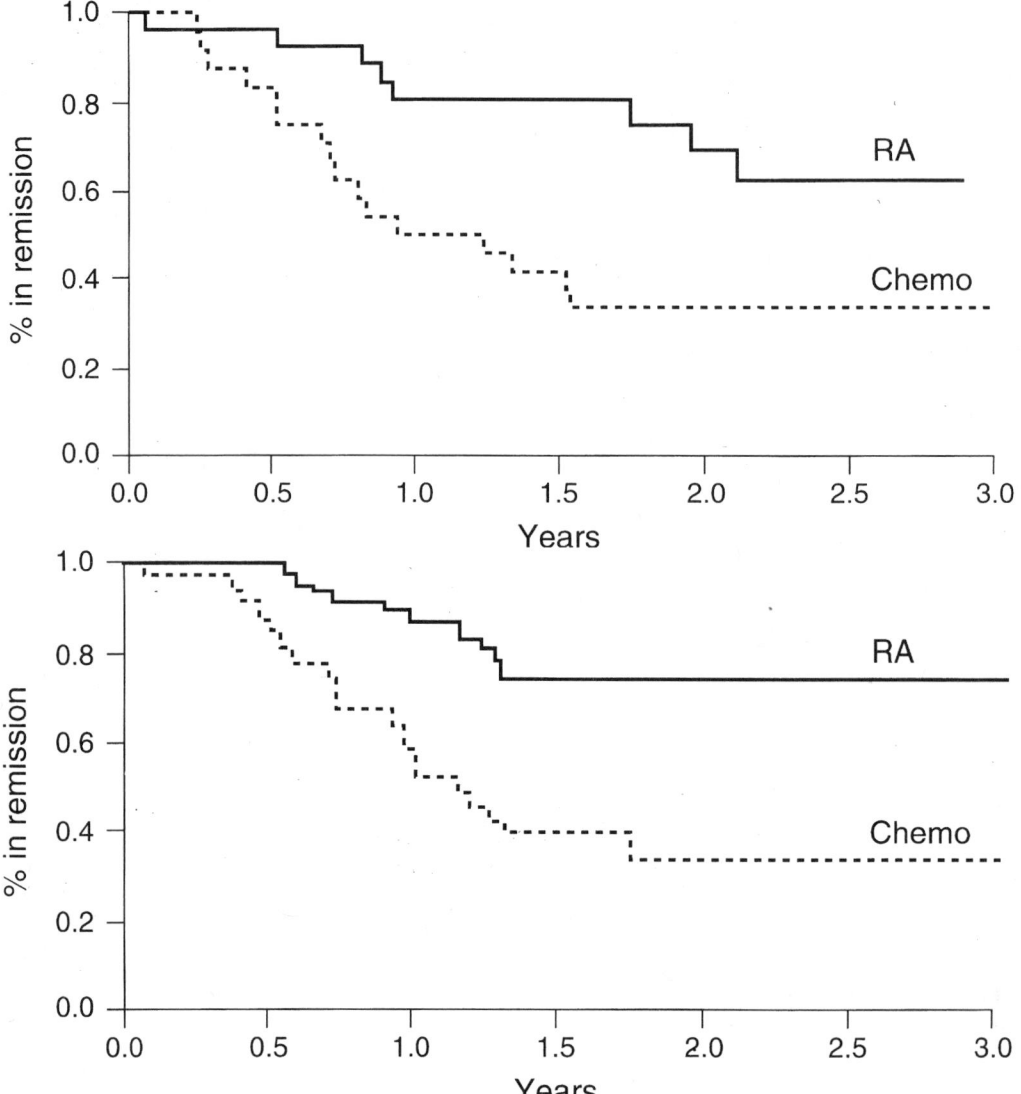

Figure 24.3.   Increase in relapse-free survival in patients with acute promyelocytic leukemia who underwent remission induction with all-*trans* retinoic acid followed by chemotherapy "consolidation," compared with control patients treated solely with chemotherapy. *Top panel,* the New York study compared with historic controls (22); *middle panel,* the European multicenter study compared with concurrently treated controls (24); *bottom panel,* the U.S. and Canadian Intergroup study (36) (kindly provided by M. Tallman).

explored in combination with other drugs, particularly α-interferon. Several in vitro studies have suggested that α-interferon and retinoids display unusual therapeutic synergy in killing various tumor cell lines (59, 60). Two studies (one each in squamous carcinomas of the skin and uterine cervix) revealed high activity for the combination of interferon plus 13-*cis* RA (61, 62), although the results in cervical cancer were not confirmed in later U.S. studies. Minimal activity

has been observed in melanoma (63), non-small-cell lung cancer (64–66), and head and neck cancer (67). Preliminary activity was observed for the combination in renal cell carcinoma (68), and confirmation of these results is being sought in a national randomized trial.

9-*CIS* RETINOIC ACID

The natural ligand for the retinoid "X" receptors (RXRs) is 9-*cis* RA, a naturally occurring iso-

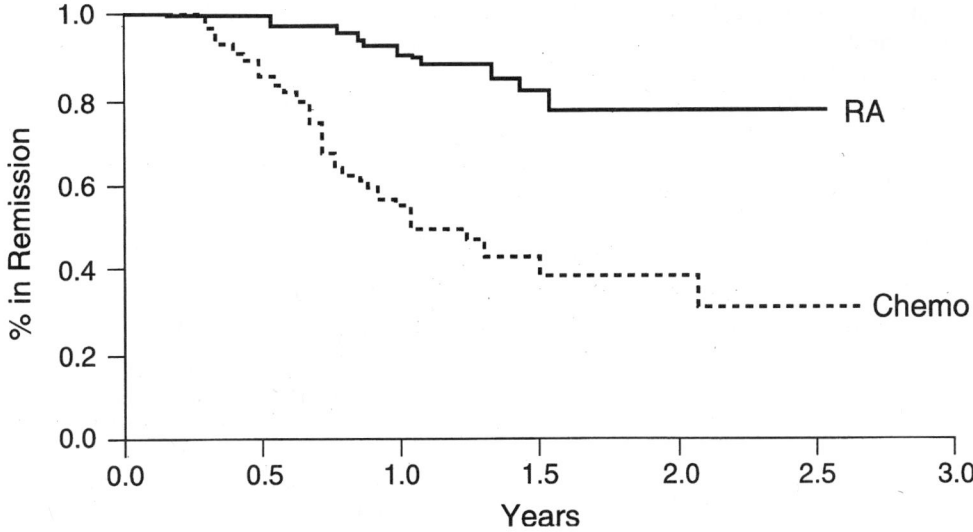

Figure 24.3. —*continued*

mer of all-*trans* RA (69, 70) (Fig. 24.1). Since 9-*cis* RA also binds to RARs, this pan-agonist effect suggested potentially more diverse biologic activity. To date, clinical trials of 9-*cis* RA have shown activity in APL that is comparable to that of all-*trans* RA (APL); however, the drug has not reversed clinically acquired retinoid resistance (71). The toxicity profiles of the two compounds are also quite similar (72). Current investigations are focused on kidney cancer and AIDS-related Kaposi's sarcoma.

SELECTIVE RETINOID RECEPTOR AGONISTS

Although 9-*cis* RA binds and activates both RARs and RXRs, novel agonists that are relatively receptor-specific for each family or for individual isoforms within the families have recently been synthesized (73, 74). LGD1069 (3-methyl TTNEB) is relatively RXR-specific and lacks significant binding to RARs. This drug appears to inhibit tumor growth by directly initiating programed cell death in certain cell lines (75). The toxicity profile for this drug also differs somewhat from that of the natural retinoids (76). Other synthetic retinoids, including pure RAR-agonists or ligands for RAR-β and RAR-γ, have also entered clinical trials (77, 78).

FENRETINIDE

Fenretinide (*N*-[4-hydroxyphenyl] retinamide; 4-HPR) has substantial chemopreventive activity against carcinomas of the breast, prostate, oral cavity, and bladder (79, 80); however, it does not bind any known retinoid receptor. A large Italian study showed that while fenretinide did not reduce the incidence of contralateral breast cancer (as prospectively specified), an unexpected reduction in ovarian carcinomas was observed (81). Unlike other retinoids, fenretinide lowers serum levels of retinol (82), which can result in nyctalopia (night blindness). This effect is ameliorated by interrupting daily dosing for 3 to 4 days per month.

Adverse Effects of Retinoids

Most retinoids share common side effects (Table 24.1). While these reactions are generally mild compared with those of most cytotoxic drugs, serious and occasionally fatal reactions have occurred, particularly in patients with APL. Moreover, while short-term therapy may be tolerable, retinoids used for cancer chemoprevention may entail indefinite—possibly lifelong— use; therefore, certain side effects, particularly metabolic complications, may assume increasing importance under those conditions.

Headache that occurs several hours after drug ingestion is the most common side effect of all-*trans* and 9-*cis* RA (20, 72, 83). This effect is less prominent with 13-*cis* RA, with which mucositis is the most common reaction. Although narcotics are occasionally required, mild analgesics generally control the headaches, and tolerance to this effect develops within the first

Table 24.1. Adverse Clinical Effects of the Retinoids

Skin/Mucous Membranes
  Skin dryness, itching, peeling
  Genital excoriations
  Angular cheilitis, lip cracking
  Skin/lymph node (especially tonsillar) infiltration with leukocytes

Neurologic
  Headache
  Intracranial hypertension ("pseudotumor cerebri")
  Night blindness[a]

Metabolic
  Hypertriglyceridemia
  Hypercholesterolemia
  Hypercalcemia

Hematologic[b]
  Leukocytosis
  Thrombosis

Gastrointestinal
  Hepatic toxicity (increased SGOT, alkaline phosphatase, bilirubin)

Cardiovascular[b]
  Congestive heart failure
  Fluid overload
  Lower extremity edema
  Episodic hypotension
  Weight gain
  Pericardial effusion

Pulmonary[b]
  Respiratory distress
  Pleural effusion
  Radiographic infiltrates

Musculoskeletal
  Bone pain
  Hyperostosis
  Myalgia

---

[a]Effect of fenretinide only.
[b]Occurs in patients with acute myelocytic leukemias only.

week of dosing. Pseudotumor cerebri has been documented in several patients (especially children) (84) who have required treatment with lumbar punctures and high-dose corticosteroids.

Dry skin, itching, flaking, nasal stuffiness, xerostomia, and cheilitis are relatively common with both all-*trans* and 13-*cis* RA. By contrast, 9-*cis* RA tends to induce more headache but fewer skin and mucous membrane reactions. Skin reactions are usually managed with topical lubricants and moisturizing agents; however, some patients, particularly patients receiving 13-*cis* RA, may require a decrease in the drug dose. Genital ulcerations have been observed with all-*trans* RA. Focally intense bone pain occurs in 10

to 20% of APL patients receiving all-*trans* RA (20), and narcotics may be required for relief. Although bone pain is less prominent with 13-*cis* RA, long-term treatment has been associated with the formation of bone spurs (85, 86). Hypercalcemia has been reported with all three isomers (72, 87, 88).

Hypertriglyceridemia occurs commonly during treatment with all-*trans* RA, 9-*cis* RA, 13-*cis* RA, and LGD1069 (89), but hypercholesterolemia is less striking (89). Cardiovascular consequences specifically related to hyperlipidemia have not yet been described, although acute pancreatitis has been reported (72). These complications may assume increasing importance as retinoids are used in more patients for extended periods. There are no data on the utility of specific hypolipidemic agents in ameliorating this effect. Hepatic toxicity (usually manifested by a transient increase in serum transaminases, alkaline phosphatase, or bilirubin) is a well-known side effect of all retinoids. Generally, this reaction occurs during the first several weeks of therapy and reverses after the drug is stopped. The use of all-*trans* RA in APL has been associated with thrombosis (90); however, this effect is probably related to the underlying coagulopathy of that disease rather than the drug, since thrombosis has not been reported in other diseases nor with other retinoids. Patients with APL may also experience severe sore throat and enlargement of Waldeyer's ring or cervical lymph nodes. This problem appears to be related to tissue infiltration with maturing myeloid cells, and it is dramatically responsive to corticosteroid therapy.

Like vitamin A (91), the natural retinoids are exceptionally potent teratogens. While this reaction is more important during treatment of nonmalignant conditions, diseases such as APL and breast cancer may occur in a relatively young age group, and a pregnancy test should be performed prior to treatment of any woman with child-bearing potential. The risk of fetal malformation (usually craniofacial abnormalities) appears to be highest in the first trimester and quite low in the third trimester (92–95).

Leukocytosis and the "Retinoic Acid Syndrome"

Leukocytosis (peripheral blood leukocytes $\geq$20,000 cells/mm^3) occurs in approximately one-half of APL patients treated with all-*trans* RA (89) who do not receive concurrent cytotoxic chemotherapy, and this finding is usually the first clinical indication of a biologic response. However, cytotoxic therapy specifically directed toward lowering the leukocyte count is not indicated in most patients. Such treatment can be hazardous, since even low-dose chemotherapy (hydroxyurea or cytosine arabinoside) can trigger the onset of a lethal coagulopathy (96). Two approaches have evolved to deal with this issue. The first (originating in the U.S.) is to administer full-dose chemotherapy early (e.g., within the first several days after starting retinoid treatment) only to patients who present with a high leukocyte count ($>10,000$ cells/mm^3) and simply observe all other patients irrespective of their leukocyte count (20–22, 96). The second approach (used in Europe) is to administer full-dose chemotherapy according to the rate of rise in the leukocyte count (24). Both approaches have yielded equivalent therapeutic results; however, the former approach appears to be associated with significantly lower morbidity and cost (97), since most patients do not require chemotherapy during induction.

Approximately 40% of patients with APL treated solely with all-*trans* RA experience the so-called retinoic acid syndrome. This disorder is characterized by high fever, respiratory distress, radiographic pulmonary infiltrates, weight gain, and pleural or pericardial effusions (98). This distinctive reaction, the most serious adverse effect of the drug, is caused by fluid retention and infiltration of myeloid cells into lungs, skin, muscle, kidney, and lymph nodes. Less commonly, the reaction can present as focally severe bone or muscle pain and fasciitis. Leukocytosis is frequently, but not invariably, associated with this syndrome, and about one-third of patients may have a normal or low blood leukocyte count (89, 98). Scrupulous avoidance of weight gain, elimination of intravenous fluids, aggressive use of diuretics if fluid retention is observed, and early recognition of other symptoms (especially unexplained fever or dyspnea) is critical. The appearance of these signs should prompt immediate steroid treatment without waiting for other diagnostic evaluation. Short courses of corticosteroids (dexamethasone 10 mg intravenously every 12 hours for 3 or more days) can reverse progression of the syndrome in most patients (96, 98). The illness can recur and additional or more prolonged corticosteroid therapy may be required. In a recent series, almost one-half of patients were treated, with almost complete protection from the syndrome and no important sequelae other than hyperglycemia

(96). Steroids also dramatically ameliorate many other features of retinoid toxicity in APL patients, including fever, bone pain, myalgia, and sore throat (with or without tonsillar enlargement).

VITAMIN D

"Deltanoids," such as 1,25-dihydroxyvitamin D_3, facilitate differentiation in a variety of cell types (99). Like the retinoids, the biologic effects of vitamin D are also mediated via nuclear receptors that have been identified in a variety of tissues, including myeloid cells and breast and colonic epithelium (100–102). Vitamin D decreases growth of leukemia, breast, colon, and prostate cancer cell lines (103–106), but these effects do not appear to be associated with cytodifferentiation. In HL60 cells, vitamin D induces differentiation into monocytes and macrophages (107) (unlike retinoids and dimethylsulfoxide (DMSO), which induce granulocytoid differentiation). Combinations of vitamin D with other differentiating agents such as retinoic acid are synergistic in some models (108, 109).

Several clinical responses were observed in an early study of patients with myelodysplastic syndromes who were treated with 1,25-dihydroxyvitamin D_3 at a dose of 2 mg/day, but intolerable hypercalcemia proved limiting (103). New analogues of vitamin D_3 that have recently entered clinical trials retain differentiating activity while causing minimal effects on calcium metabolism (109–112). One drug, calcipotriol, has been successfully used in several patients with skin recurrences of breast cancer (113) and cutaneous T-cell lymphoma (114).

Miscellaneous Agents

Butyric acid also induces erythroid differentiation in erythroleukemia cells, but high concentrations are required to reliably induce these effects (115). The rapid metabolism of sodium butyrate has precluded sustained achievement of therapeutic concentrations (116, 117); however, tributyrin, which yields three molecules of butyrate after hydrolysis, also has cytodifferentiating actions (118, 119). The relatively high butyrate concentrations that are achievable in the colon have suggested a use for butyrates as a chemoprevention strategy against colon cancer (120, 121). Phenylbutyrate also acts as a prodrug for phenylacetate (122), which promotes in vitro differentiation of certain cell lines (123, 124). Relatively high doses (250 to 550 mg/kg/day) have been used clinically (125), and early results suggest some activity in malignant gliomas (126) and prostate cancer (125).

Agents that increase intracellular levels of $3',5'$-cyclic adenosine monophosphate (cAMP) exert cytodifferentiating actions (127, 128). Although this action is not very potent by itself, these agents cause marked synergistic effects when used in combination with other drugs such as retinoids. Chemical analogues of cyclic-AMP, including dibutyryl-cyclic AMP and 8-Br-cyclic AMP, have been synthesized (128, 129), and several of these agents have been proposed for clinical use (130).

While numerous cytotoxic drugs have been proposed as differentiating agents, particularly when used at sublethal concentrations, convincing evidence that the differentiating effect is clinically relevant has not been obtained (131–133).

REFERENCES

1. Kark JD, Smith AH, Hames CG. Serum vitamin A (retinol) and cancer incidence in Evans County, Georgia. J Natl Cancer Inst 1981;66:7–16.

2. Stinson SF, Reznik G, Donahoe R. Effect of three retinoids on tracheal carcinogenesis with *N*-methyl-*N*-nitrosourea in hamsters. J Natl Cancer Inst 1981; 66:947–951.

3. Moon RC, Mehta RG, Rao KVN. Retinoids and cancer in experimental animals. In: Sporn MB, Roberts AB, Goodman DS, eds. The retinoids. Orlando, FL: Academic Press, 1993:573–596.

4. Hong WK, Itri LM. Retinoids and human cancer. In: Sporn MB, Roberts AB, Goodman DS, eds. The retinoids. Orlando, FL: Academic Press, 1993:597–630.

5. Warrell RP Jr. Retinoids in cancer. In: ES Kimball, Immunopharmaceuticals. Boca Raton: CRC Press, 1995:101–134.

6. Blaner WS, Olson JS. Retinol and retinoic acid metabolism. In: Sporn MB, Roberts AB, Goodman DS, eds. The retinoids. Orlando, FL: Academic Press, 1993:229–256.

7. Fiorella PD, Napoli JL. Expression of cellular retinoic acid binding protein (CRABP) in *Escherichia coli*: characterization and evidence that holo-CRABP is a substrate in retinoic acid metabolism. J Biol Chem 1991; 266:16572–16579.

8. Boylan JF, Gudas LJ. The level of CRABP-I expression influences the amounts and types of all-*trans* retinoic acid metabolites in F9 teratocarcinoma stem cells. J Biol Chem 1992;267:21486–21491.

9. Petkovich M, Brand NJ, Krust A, Chambon P. A human retinoic acid receptor which belongs to the family of nuclear receptors. Nature 1987;330:444–451.

10. Giguere V, Ong ES, Segui P, Evans RM. Identification of a receptor for the morphogen retinoic acid. Nature 1987;330:624–629.

11. Zelent A, Krust A, Petkovich M, Kastner P, Chambon P. Cloning of murine α and β retinoic acid receptors and a novel receptor γ predominantly expressed in skin. Nature 1989;339:714–717.

12. Mangelsdorf DJ, Ong ES, Dyck JA, Evans RM. Nuclear receptor that identifies a novel retinoic acid response pathway. Nature 1990;345:224–229.

13. Leid M, Kastner P, Lyons R, et al. Purification, cloning and RXR identity of the HeLa cell factor with which RAR or TR heterodimerize to bind DNA efficiently. Cell 1992;68:377–395.

14. Roberts AB, Sporn MB. Mechanistic interrelationships between two superfamilies: the steroid/retinoid receptors and transforming growth factor-β. Cancer Surv 1992;14:204–220.

15. Scott KFF, Meyskens FL Jr, Russell DH. Retinoids increase transglutaminase activity and inhibit ornithine decarboxylase activity in Chinese hamster ovary cells and in melanoma cells stimulated to differentiate. Proc Natl Acad Sci USA 1982;79:4093–4097.

16. Salbert G, Fanjul A, Piedrafita FJ, et al. Retinoic acid receptors and retinoid X receptor α—down-regulation of the transforming growth factor-β 1 promotor by antagonizing AP-1 activity. Mol Endocrinol 1993; 7:1347–1356.

17. Fanjul A, Dawson MI, Hobbs PD, et al. A new class of retinoids with selective activation of AP-1 inhibits proliferation. Nature 1994;372:107–111.

18. Horlein AJ, Naar AM, Heinzel T, et al. Ligand-independent repression by the thyroid hormone receptor mediated by a nuclear receptor co-repressor. Nature 1995;377:397–404.

19. Chen JD, Evans RM. A transcriptional co-repressor that interacts with nuclear hormone receptors. Nature 1995;377:454–457.

20. Warrell RP Jr, de Thé H, Wang Z-Y, Degos L. Acute promyelocytic leukemia. N Engl J Med 1993; 329:177–189.

21. Warrell RP Jr, Frankel SR, Miller WH Jr, et al. Differentiation therapy of acute promyelocytic leukemia with tretinoin (all-*trans* retinoic acid). N Engl J Med 1991;324:1385–1393.

22. Warrell RP Jr, Maslak P, Eardley A, Heller G, Miller WH Jr, Frankel SR. All-*trans* retinoic acid for treatment of acute promyelocytic leukemia: an update of the New York experience. Leukemia 1994;8:929–933.

23. Ohno R, Yoshida H, Fukutani H, et al. Multi-institutional study of all-*trans* retinoic acid as a differentiation therapy of refractory acute promyelocytic leukemia. Leukemia 1993;7:1722–1727.

24. Fenaux P, Le Dely MC, Castaigne S, et al. Effect of all-*trans* retinoic acid in newly diagnosed acute promyelocytic leukemia: results of a multicenter randomized trial. Blood 1993;82:3241–3249.

25. de Thé H, Chomienne C, Lanotte M, Degos L, Dejean A. The t(15;17) translocation of acute promyelocytic leukaemia fuses the retinoic acid receptor α gene to a novel transcribed locus. Nature 1990;347:558–561.

26. Martin S, Bradley J, Cotter T. HL-60 cells induced to differentiate towards neutrophils subsequently die via apoptosis. Clin Exp Immunol 1990; 79:448–453.

27. Muindi J, Frankel S, Huselton C, et al. Clinical pharmacology of oral all-*trans* retinoic acid in patients with acute promyelocytic leukemia. Cancer Res 1992; 52:2138–2142.

28. Muindi J, Frankel SR, Miller WH Jr, et al. Continuous treatment with all-*trans* retinoic acid results in a progressive decrease in plasma concentrations: im-

plications for relapse and retinoid "resistance" in acute promyelocytic leukemia. Blood 1992;79:299–303.

29. Warrell RP Jr. Acquired retinoid resistance in acute promyelocytic leukemia: new mechanisms, strategies, and implications. Blood 1993;82:1949–1953.

30. Delva L, Cornic M, Balitrand N, et al. Resistance to all-*trans* retinoic acid (ATRA) therapy in relapsing acute promyelocytic leukemia: study of in vitro ATRA sensitivity and cellular retinoic acid binding protein levels in leukemic cells. Blood 1993;82:2175–2181.

31. Rigas JR, Francis PA, Muindi JRF, et al. Constitutive variability in catabolism of the natural retinoid, all-*trans* retinoic acid, and its modulation by ketoconazole. J Natl Cancer Inst 1993;85:1921–1926.

32. Muindi JF, Young CW. Lipid hydroperoxides greatly increase the rate of oxidative catabolism of all-*trans* retinoic acid by human cell culture microsomes genetically enriched in specified cytochrome P-450 isoforms. Cancer Res 1993;53:1226–1229.

33. Mehta S, Sadeghi T, McQueen T, Lopez-Bernstein G. Liposomal encapsulation circumvents the hepatic clearance mechanisms of all-*trans* retinoic acid. Leuk Res 1994;18:587–596.

34. Robertson KA, Emami B, Collins SJ. Retinoic acid-resistant HL-60R cells harbor a point mutation in the retinoic acid receptor ligand-binding domain that confers dominant negative activity. Blood 1992; 80:1885–1889.

35. Dermine S, Grignani F, Clerici M, et al. Occurrence of resistance to retinoic acid in the acute promyelocytic cell line NB306 is associated with altered expression of the PML/RAR-α protein. Blood 1993; 82:1573–1577.

36. Tallman MS, Anderson J, Schiffer CA, et al. Phase III randomized study of all-*trans* retinoic acid (ATRA) vs daunorubicin (D) and cytosine arabinoside (A) as induction therapy and ATRA vs observation as maintenance therapy for patients with previously untreated acute promyelocytic leukemia (APL) (abstract). Blood (Suppl) 1995;86:125a.

37. Atiba J, Jamil S, Meyskens FJ, et al. Transretinoic acid (tRA) in the treatment of malignant gliomas (MG): a phase II study (abstract). Proc Am Soc Clin Oncol 1994;13:178.

38. Von Roenn J, von Gunten C, Mullane M, French S, Blough R, Benson AB III. All-transretinoic acid (TRA) in the treatment of AIDS-related Kaposi's sarcoma: a phase II Illinois Cancer Center study (abstract). Proc Am Soc Clin Oncol 1993;12:51.

39. Kessler JF, Jones SE, Levine N, Lynch PJ, Booth AR, Meyskens FR Jr. Isotretinoin and cutaneous helper T-cell lymphoma (mycosis fungoides). Arch Dermatol 1987;123:201–204.

40. Warrell RP Jr, Coonley CJ, Kempin SJ, et al. Isotretinoin in cutaneous T-cell lymphoma (letter). Lancet 1983;1:629.

41. Molin L, Thomsen K, Volden G, et al. Oral retinoids in mycosis fungoides and Sezary syndrome: a comparison of isotretinoin and etretinate. A study from the Scandinavian Mycosis Fungoides Group. Acta Derm Venereol (Stockh) 1987;67:232–236.

42. Neely SM, Mehlmauer M, Feinstein DI. The effect of isotretinoin in six patients with cutaneous T-cell lymphoma. Arch Intern Med 1987;147:529–531.

43. Greenberg BR, Durie BGM, Barnett TC, et al.

Phase I-II study of 13-*cis*-retinoic acid in myelodysplastic syndrome. Cancer Treat Rep 1985;69:1369–1374.

44. Picozzi VJ, Swanson GF, Morgan R, et al. 13-*Cis* retinoic acid treatment for myelodysplastic syndromes. J Clin Oncol 1986;4:589–595.

45. Koeffler HP, Heitjan D, Mertelsmann R, et al. Randomized study of 13-*cis* retinoic acid v placebo in the myelodysplastic disorders. Blood 1988;71:703–708.

46. Arlin ZA, Mertelsmann R, Berman E, et al. 13-*cis* retinoic acid does not increase the true response rate and the duration of true remission (induced by cytotoxic chemotherapy) in patients with chronic myelogenous leukemia. J Clin Oncol 1987;3:473–476.

47. Gold EJ, Bosl GJ, Itri LM. Phase II trial of 13-*cis* retinoic acid in patients with advanced nonseminomatous germ cell tumors. Cancer Treat Rep 1984; 68:1287–1288.

48. Finklestein JZ, Krailo MD, Lenarsky C, et al. 13-*cis* retinoic acid (NSC 122578) in the treatment of children with metastatic neuroblastoma unresponsive to conventional chemotherapy: report from the Children's Cancer Study Group. Med Pediatr Oncol 1992; 20:307–311.

49. Villablanca JG, Avramis VI, Khan AA, et al. Phase I trial of 13-*cis* retinoic acid in neuroblastoma patients following bone marrow transplantation (abstract). Proc Am Soc Clin Oncol 1992;11:A1263.

50. Lippman SM, Kessler JF, Al-Sarraf M, et al. Treatment of advanced squamous cell carcinoma of the head and neck with isotretinoin: a phase II randomized trial. Invest New Drugs 1988;6:13–17.

51. Grunberg S, Itri L. Phase II study of isotretinoin in the treatment of advanced non-small cell lung cancer. Cancer Treat Rep 1987;71:1097–1098.

52. Recondo G, Logothetis CJ, Hossan E, Sella A, et al. Results of the phase I trial combining 13-*cis*-retinoic acid with 5-fluorouracil, alpha interferon 2B in patients with chemotherapy refractory transitional cell carcinoma of the bladder (abstract). Proc Am Soc Clin Oncol 1991;10:A561.

53. Lippman SM, Meyskens FM Jr. Treatment of advanced squamous cell carcinoma of the skin with isotretinoin. Ann Intern Med 1987;107:499–501.

54. Peck GL, DiGiovanna JJ, Sarnoff DS, et al. Treatment and prevention of basal cell carcinoma with oral isotretinoin. J Am Acad Dermatol 1988;19:176–185.

55. Tangrea JA, Edwards BK, Taylor PR, et al. Long-term therapy with low-dose isotretinoin for prevention of basal cell carcinoma: a multicenter clinical trial. J Natl Cancer Inst 1992;84:328–332.

56. Hong WK, Endicott J, Itri LM, et al. 13-*Cis*-retinoic acid in the treatment of oral leukoplakia. N Engl J Med 1986;315:1501–1505.

57. Lippman SM, Batsakis JG, Toth BB, Weber RS, Lee JJ, et al. Comparison of low-dose isotretinoin with beta carotene to prevent oral carcinogenesis. N Engl J Med 1993;328:15–20.

58. Hong WK, Lippman SM, Itri LM, et al. Prevention of second primary tumors with isotretinoin in squamous cell carcinoma of the head and neck. N Engl J Med 1990;323:795–801.

59. Frey JR, Peck R, Bollag W. Antiproliferative activity of retinoids, interferon a and their combination in five human transformed cell lines. Cancer Lett 1991; 57:223–227.

60. Hemmi H, Breitman TR. Combinations of re-

combinant human interferons and retinoic acid synergistically induce differentiation of the human promyelocytic leukemia cell line HL-60. Blood 1987; 69:501–507.

61. Lippman SM, Kavanagh JJ, Paredes-Espinosa M, et al. 13-*Cis* retinoic acid plus interferon-alpha 2a: highly active systemic therapy for squamous cell carcinoma of the cervix. J Natl Cancer Inst 1992;84:241–245.

62. Lippman SM, Parkinson DR, Itri LM, et al. 13-*cis*-retinoic acid and interferon α-2a: effective combination therapy for advanced squamous cell carcinoma of the skin. J Natl Cancer Inst 1992;84:235–241.

63. Dhingra K, Papadopoulos N, Lippma, SM, et al. Phase II study of alpha-interferon and 13-*cis* retinoic acid in recurrent head and neck cancer. Invest New Drugs 1993;11:39–43.

64. Rinaldi DA, Lippman SM, Burris HA, et al. Phase II trial of 13-*cis* retinoic acid plus interferon-alpha-2a in patients with advanced squamous cell lung cancer. Anticancer Drugs 1993;4:33–36.

65. Athanasiadis I, Kies MS, Miller M, et al. Phase II study of all-*trans* retinoic acid and α interferon in patients with advanced non-small cell lung cancer. Clin Cancer Res 1995;1:973–979.

66. Arnold A, Ayong J, Douglas L, et al. Phase II trial of 13-*cis* retinoic acid plus interferon α in non small cell lung cancer. J Natl Cancer Inst 1994;86:306–309.

67. Voravud N, Lippman SM, Weber RS, et al. Phase I trial of 13-*cis* retinoic acid plus interferon-alpha in recurrent head and neck cancer. Invest New Drugs 1993;11:57–60.

68. Motzer RJ, Murray-Law T, Schwartz L, Fischer P, Scher HI. Antitumor activity of interferon alfa-2a (IFN-α) and 13-*cis* retinoic acid (C-RA) in patients with advanced renal cell carcinoma (RCC) (abstract). Proc Am Soc Clin Oncol 1994;13:232.

69. Heyman R, Mangelsdorf D, Dyck J, Stein RB, Eichele G, Evans RM. 9-*Cis* retinoic acid is a high affinity ligand for the retinoid X receptor. Cell 1992;68:397–406.

70. Levin AA, Sturzenbecker LJ, Kazmer S, et al. 9 *Cis* retinoic acid stereoisomer binds and activates the nuclear receptor RXR-α. Nature 1992;335:359–361.

71. Miller WH Jr, Jakubowski A, Benedetti F, et al. 9-*Cis* retinoic acid induces complete remission in acute promyelocytic leukemia but does not reverse clinically acquired resistance to all-*trans* retinoic acid. Blood 1995;85:3021–3027.

72. Miller VA, Rigas JR, Benedetti FM, Tong WP, Kris MG, Warrell RP Jr. Initial clinical trial of the retinoid receptor pan-agonist, 9-*cis* retinoic acid. Clin Cancer Res (in press).

73. Delescluse C, Cavey MT, Martin B, et al. Selective high affinity retinoic acid receptor α or β-γ ligands. Mol Pharmacol 1991;40:556–562.

74. Lehmann JM, Dawson MI, Hobbs PD, Husmann M, Pfahl M. Identification of retinoids with nuclear receptor subtype-selective activities. Cancer Res 1991;51:4804–4809.

75. Boehm MF, Zhang L, Zhi L, et al. Design and synthesis of potent retinoid X receptor selective ligands that induce apoptosis in leukemia cells. J Med Chem 1995;38:3146–3155.

76. Miller VA, Benedetti FM, Rigas JR, et al. Initial clinical study of a selective retinoid "X" receptor agonist (abstract). Proc Am Assoc Cancer Res 1995;36:242.

77. Boehm MF, Heyman RA, Patel S, Stein RB, Nagpal S. Retinoids: biological function and use in the treatment of dermatological diseases. Expert Opin Invest Drugs 1995;4:593–612.

78. Tohda S, Shudo K, Minden MD. The effects of retinoic acid analogues on the blast cells of acute myeloblastic leukemia in culture. Int J Oncol 1994;4:1311–1314.

79. Moon RC, Mehta RG. Chemoprevention of experimental carcinogenesis. Prev Med 1989;18:576–591.

80. Pienta KJ, Nguyen NM, Lehr JE. Treatment of prostate cancer in the rat with a synthetic retinoid fenretinide. Cancer Res 1993;53:224–226.

81. Costa A, Malone W, Perloff M, et al. Tolerability of the synthetic retinoid fenretinide (HPR). Eur J Clin Oncol 1989;25:805–808.

82. Formelli F, Clerici M, Campa T, et al. Five-year administration of fenretinide: pharmacokinetics and effects on plasma retinol concentrations. J Clin Oncol 1993;11:2036–2042.

83. Lee JS, Newman RA, Lippman SM, et al. Phase I evaluation of all-*trans* retinoic acid in adults with solid tumors. J Clin Oncol 1993;11:959–966.

84. Smith MA, Adamson PC, Balis FM, et al. Phase I and pharmacokinetic evaluation of all-*trans* retinoic acid in pediatric patients with cancer. J Clin Oncol 1992;10:1666–1673.

85. DiGiovanna J, Helfgott R, Gerber L, et al. Extraspinal tendon and ligament calcification associated with long-term therapy with etretinate. N Engl J Med 1986;315:1177–1182.

86. Kilcoyne R. Effects of retinoids on bone. J Am Acad Dermatol 1988;19:212–216.

87. Akiyama H, Nakamura N, Nagasaka S, Sakamaki H, Onozawa Y. Hypercalcaemia due to all-*trans* retinoic acid. Lancet 1992;339:308–309.

88. Niesvizky R, Siegel DS, Busquets X, et al. Hypercalcaemia and increased serum interleukin-6 levels induced by all-*trans* retinoic acid in patients with multiple myeloma. Br J Haematol 1995;89:217–218.

89. Frankel SR, Eardley A, Heller G, et al. All-*trans* retinoic acid for acute promyelocytic leukemia: results of the New York study. Ann Intern Med 1994;120:278–286.

90. Runde V, Aul C, Sudhoft T, Heyll A, Schneider W. Retinoic acid in the treatment of acute promyelocytic leukemia: inefficacy of the 13-*cis* isomer and induction of complete remission by the all-*trans* isomer complicated by thromboembolic events. Ann Hematol 1992;64:270–272.

91. Rothman KJ, Moore LL, Siinger MR, Nguyen U-SDT, Mannino S, Milunsky A. Teratogenicity of high vitamin A intake. N Engl J Med 1995;333:1369–1373.

92. Lammer EJ, Chen DT, Hoar RM, et al. Retinoic acid fetopathy. N Engl J Med 1985;313:837–841.

93. Dai WS, LaBraico JM, Stern RS. Epidemiology of isotretinoin exposure during pregnancy. J Am Acad Dermatol 1992;26:599–60.

94. Jick SS, Terris BZ, Jick H. First trimester topical tretinoin and congenital disorders. Lancet 1993; 341:1181–1182.

95. Stentoft J, Nielsen JL, Hvidman LE. All-*trans* retinoic acid in acute promyelocytic leukemia in late pregnancy. Leukemia 1994;8:1585–1588.

96. Vahdat L, Eardley A, Maslak P, Heller G, Scheinberg DA, Warrell RP Jr. Early mortality and the "retinoic acid syndrome" in acute promyelocytic leukemia: impact of leukocytosis, low-dose chemotherapy, PML/RAR-α isoform, and CD13 expression in patients treated with all-*trans* retinoic acid. Blood 1994; 84:3843–3849.

97. Eardley AM, Heller G, Warrell RP. Morbidity and costs of all-*trans* retinoic acid compared to standard chemotherapy for remission induction in acute promyelocytic leukemia. Leukemia 1994;8:934–939.

98. Frankel SR, Eardley A, Lauwers G, Weiss M, Warrell RP Jr. The "retinoic acid syndrome" in acute promyelocytic leukemia. Ann Intern Med 1992; 117:292–296.

99. Reichel H, Koeffler HP, Norman AW. The role of vitamin D endocrine system in health and disease. N Engl J Med 1989;320:980–991.

100. Kizaki M, Norman AW, Bishop JE, et al. 1,25-Dihydroxyvitamin D_3 receptor RNA: expression in hematopoietic cells. Blood 1991;77:1238–1247.

101. Meggouh F, Lointier P, Saez S. Sex steroid and 1,25-dihydroxyvitamin D_3 receptors in human colorectal adenocarcinoma and normal mucosa. Cancer Res 1991;51:1227–1233.

102. Eisman JA, Suva LJ, Sher E, et al. Frequency of 1,25-dihydroxyvitamin D_3 receptor in human breast cancer. Cancer Res 1981;41:5121–5124.

103. Koeffler HP, Hirji K, Itri L, et al. 1,25-Dihydroxyvitamin D_3: in vivo and in vitro effects on human preleukemic and leukemic cells. Cancer Treat Rep 1985;69:1399–1407.

104. Elstner E, Linker-Israeli M, Said J, et al. 20-Epivitamin D_3 analogues: a novel class of potent inhibitors of proliferation and inducers of differentiation of human breast cancer cell lines. Cancer Res 1995;55:2822–2830.

105. Wali RK, Bissonnette M, Khare S, Hart J, Sitrin MD, Brasitus TA. 1α,25-Dihydroxy-16-ene-23-yne-26,27-hexafluorocholecalciferol, a noncalcemic analogue of 1α,25-dihydroxyvitamin D_3, inhibits azoxymethane-induced colonic tumorigenesis. Cancer Res 1995;55:3050–3054.

106. Miller GJ, Stapleton GE, Hedlund TE, Moffatt KA. Vitamin D receptor expression 24-hydroxylase activity, and inhibition of growth by 1α,25-dihydroxyvitamin D_3 in seven human prostatic carcinoma cell lines. Clin Cancer Res 1995;1:997–1003.

107. Manglesdorf DJ, Koeffler HP, Donaldson CA, et al. 1,25-dihydroxyvitamin-D_3-induced differentiation in a human promyelocytic leukemia cell (HL-60): receptor-mediated maturation to macrophage-like cells. J Cell Biol 1984;98:391–398.

108. Doré BT, Uskokovic MR, Momparler RL. Increased sensitivity to a vitamin D_3 analog in HL-60 myeloid leukemic cells resistant to all-*trans* retinoic acid. Leukemia 1994;8:2179–2182.

109. Elstner E, Linker-Israeli M, Umiel T, et al. Synergistic induction of clonal proliferation and BCL-2, and induction of differentiation, BAX and apoptosis in APL cells (NB4) by combined treatment with a novel vitamin D_3 analog (KH 1060) and 9-*cis* retinoic acid (abstract). Blood (Suppl) 1995;38:435a.

110. Zhou J-Y, Norman AW, Lubbert ED, et al. Novel vitamin D analogues that modulate leukemic cell growth and differentiation with little effect on ei-

ther intestinal calcium absorption or bone calcium mobilization. Blood 1989;74:82–93.

111. Perlman K, Kutner A, Prahl J, et al. 24-Homologated 1,25-dihydroxyvitamin D_3 compounds: separation of calcium and cell differentiation activities. Biochemistry 1990;29:190–196.

112. Pakkala S, de Vos, S, Elstner E, et al. Antileukemic activities and effects on serum calcium of three novel vitamin D3 analogs (abstract). Blood (Suppl) 1993;82:255a.

113. Bower M, Colston KW, Stein RC, et al. Topical calcipotriol treatment in advanced breast cancer. Lancet 1991;337:701–702.

114. Scott-Mackie P, Hickish T, Mortimer P, Sloane J, Cunningham D. Calcipotriol and regression in T-cell lymphoma of skin (letter). Lancet 1993;342:172.

115. Augeron C, Laboisse CL. Emergence of permanently differentiated cell clones in a human colonic cancer cell line in culture after treatment with sodium butyrate. Cancer Res 1984;44:3961–3969.

116. Miller AA, Kurschel E, Osieka R, Schmidt CG. Clinical pharmacology of sodium butyrate in patients with acute leukemia. Eur J Clin Oncol 1987;23:1283–1287.

117. Daniel P, Brazier M, Cerutti, et al. Pharmacokinetic study of butyric acid administered as sodium and arginine butyrate salts. Clin Chim Acta 1989; 181:255–264.

118. Lea MA, Xiao Q, Sadukhan A, Sharma S, Newmark HL. Butyramide and monobutyrin: growth inhibitory and differentiating agents. Anticancer Res 1993;13:145–150.

119. Yuan Z, Eiseman J, Plaisance K, et al. Plasma pharmacokinetics (PK) of butyrate after the administration of tributyrin & Na butyrate to mice and rats (abstract). Proc Am Assoc Cancer Res 1995;36: 429.

120. Tanaka Y, Bush KK, Eguchi T, et al. Effects of 1,25-dihydroxyvitamin D_3 and its analogs on butyrate-induced differentiation of HT-29 human colonic carcinoma cells and on the reversal of the differentiated phenotype. Arch Biochem Biophys 1990;276:415–423.

121. Freeman JJ. Effects of differing concentrations of sodium butyrate on 1,2-dimethylhydrazine-induced rat intestine neoplasia. Gastroenterology 1986;91:596–602.

122. Samid D, Shack S, Sherman LT. Phenylacetate: a novel nontoxic inducer of tumor cell differentiation. Cancer Res 1992;52:1988–1992.

123. Samid D, Shack S, Myers CE. Selective growth arrest and phenotypic reversion of prostate cancer cells in vitro by nontoxic pharmacological concentrations of phenylacetate. J Clin Invest 1993;91:2288–2295.

124. Ram Z, Samid D, Walbridge S, et al. Growth inhibition, tumor maturation, and extended survival in experimental brain tumors in rats treated with phenylacetate. Cancer Res 1994;54:2923–2927.

125. Thibault A, Cooper MR, Figg WD, et al. A phase I and pharmacokinetic study of intravenous phenylacetate in patients with cancer. Cancer Res 1994; 54:1690–1694.

126. Samid D, Ram Z, Hudgins WR, et al. Selective activity of phenylacetate against malignant gliomas: resemblance to fetal brain damage in phenylketonuria. Cancer Res 1994;54:891–895.

127. Fontana J, Munoz M, Durham J. Potentiation

between intracellular cyclic-AMP-elevating agents and inducers of leukemic cell differentiation. Leuk Res 1985;9:1127–1132.

128. Cho-Chung YS. Role of cyclic AMP receptor proteins in growth, differentiation, and suppression of malignancy: new approaches to therapy. Cancer Res 1990;50:7093–7100.

129. Tagliaferri P, Katsaros D, Clair T, et al. Synergistic inhibition of growth of breast and colon human cancer cell lines by site-selective cyclic AMP analogues. Cancer Res 1988;48:1642–1650.

130. Cho-chung YS. Suppression of malignancy targeting cyclic AMP signal transducing proteins. Biochem Soc Trans 1992;20:425–429.

131. Cheson BD, Jasperse DM, Simon R, et al. A critical appraisal of low-dose cytosine arabinoside in patients with acute non-lymphocytic leukemia and myelodysplastic syndromes. J Clin Oncol 1986;4:1857–1864.

132. Degos L, Castaigne S, Tilly H, et al. Treatment of leukemia with low-dose ara-C: a study of 160 cases. Semin Oncol 1985;12(Suppl 3):196–199.

133. Ferrari AC, Waxman S. Differentiation agents in cancer therapy. In: Pinedo HM, Longo DL, Chabner BA, eds. Cancer chemotherapy and biological response modifiers annual 15. New York: Elsevier Science, 1994:337–366.

25

Hormones and Enzymes

Part 1

Hormonal Agents

Joseph Aisner, Robert J. Fram, Mario Eisenberger, and Joseph A. Fontana

Hormonal therapy is an important and effective means to treat many "hormonally sensitive" tumors such as cancers of the breast, endometrium, and prostate. These cancers can be effectively treated with hormonal maneuvers (i.e., ablative surgeries, hormone agonists, or antagonists), depending on clinical circumstances. Lymphoid leukemias, Hodgkin's and non-Hodgkin's lymphomas, myeloma, and other lymphoproliferative diseases are often treated with adrenocorticoid hormones as part of the therapy. In addition, hormonal therapies are sometimes applied therapeutically to other tumors such as ovarian cancer, renal carcinoma, and melanoma. Finally, some hormonal agents are used in supportive care for their "beneficial" side effects. Examples of such therapies include adrenocorticoids as antiemetics, androgens as anabolic agents, and progestins as appetite stimulants and anabolic agents.

One of the greatest difficulties in the use of hormonal therapies has been the inability to satisfactorily explain the mechanisms of action. Why, for example, do diametrically opposed actions such as an hormonal ablative drug or procedure and hormonal additive therapy both produce tumor regressions in the same setting? Recent advances in cellular and molecular biology have permitted the elucidation of many of the mechanisms by which hormones and hormone antagonists or agonists can regulate tumor growth. These mechanisms constitute a diverse spectrum of activities; however, many, if not all, of these agents first bind to a specific cell surface receptor. Interaction with and occupation of this receptor can inhibit either the production or the release of factors necessary for tumor growth, the induction of growth-inhibitory proteins, downregulation of specific receptors required for cellular proliferation, or the generation of DNA-binding proteins that inhibit oncogene expression with the subsequent cessation of cellular proliferation. This chapter reviews the hormonal agents commonly used for cancer, their applications, and their purported mechanisms of action. Specific therapy of the individual diseases and the hierarchy of the various treatment options are discussed in the chapters dealing with these tumors.

ADRENOCORTICOIDS

Adrenocorticoids (glucocorticoids) exert their biologic actions predominately through their binding to the glucocorticoid receptor (1–3). This receptor, which exists in the cytoplasm, requires ligand binding for its translocation to the nucleus and its subsequent homodimerization and binding to specific DNA sequence motifs located in the regulatory regions of a variety of genes. While the glucocorticoids can, through their nuclear receptor, stimulate gene transcription, the glucocorticoid receptor is capable of repressing gene expression (4, 5). Glucocorticoid-induced apoptosis and inhibition of cell proliferation are most likely mediated through transcriptional interference. Glucocorticoids can induce apoptosis in immature thymocytes and, at higher concentrations, in certain subsets of mature T cells (6). This inhibition of transcription appears to be mediated by the ability of the glucocorticoid receptor to inhibit AP-1 binding to its DNA consensus sequence (4). AP-1 is a nuclear transcription factor composed of homo- and heterodimers of the products of the *Jun* and *fos* protooncogenes (7). While the Jun proteins can dimerize with themselves, other Jun proteins, or any of the fos proteins, only the fos proteins can form heterodimers with the Jun proteins (8). These complexes, once formed, bind to the AP-1 consensus sequence, resulting in the activation of a number of genes (5). Recent studies indicate that AP-1 binding is necessary for the activation of a number of genes that play important roles in cell proliferation (9). AP-1-mediated activation of these genes most likely plays an essential role in the movement of cells along the cell cycle, specifically from G_r to the S phase. A number of investigators have shown that the glucocorticoid receptors inhibit AP-1 activation of genes by preventing AP-1 binding (5). In vitro experiments using purified glucocorticoid receptor and C-Jun proteins demonstrated that the glucocorticoid-mediated repression of AP-1 binding and subsequent gene activation is due to a direct interaction between the glucocorticoid receptor and C-Jun (4). Glucocorticoid-mediated inactivation of a number of essential genes, including the interleukin-2 gene whose activation appears to be essential for proliferation of a number of lymphoid subsets, is hypothesized to occur via inhibition of AP-1 binding (5). AP-1 mediator activation has been demonstrated for a number of genes, including the collagenase and stromelysin genes; AP-1 activation of the genes is also inhibited by glucocorticoids through its nuclear receptor (10–12).

The corticosteroids available for use include:

1. Generic name: cortisone acetate
   Trade names: various
   Chemical name: 21-(acetyloxy)-17-hydroxy-preg-4-ene-3,11,20-trione
   How available: tablets: 5, 10, and 25 mg; injectable: 25 and 50 mg
   Dosing: 25 to 300 mg/day according to disease or indications

2. Generic name: hydrocortisone
   Trade names: Cortef (Upjohn), Hydrocortone (MSD), others
   Chemical name: 21-(acetyloxy)-11β,17-dihydroxypreg-4-ene-3,20-dione
   How available: tablets: 5, 10, and 20 mg; injectable: 25 and 50 mg
   Dosing: 20 to 240 mg/day according to disease or indications

3. Generic name: prednisone
   Trade names: various
   Chemical name: 17α,21-dihydroxy-pregna-1,4-diene-3,11,20-trione
   How available: tablets: 1, 2.5, 5, 10, 20, 25, and 50 mg; solutions: 5 mg/5 mL
   Dosing: 5 to 100 mg/day according to disease or indications

4. Generic name: prednisolone
   Trade names: various
   Chemical name: 11β,17,21-trihydroxypregna-1,4-diene-3,20-dione
   How available: injectable: 20 mg/mL
   Dosing: 5 to 100 mg/day according to disease or indications

5. Generic name: methylprednisolone
   Trade names: Medrol (Upjohn), various
   Chemical name: 11β,17α,21-trihydroxy-6α-methyl-1,4-pregnadiene-3,20-dione
   How available: tablets: 2, 4, 8, 16, 24, and 32 mg; injectable: 20, 40, and 80 mg/mL
   Dosing: 4 to 200 mg/day depending on disease and indications

6. Generic name: dexamethasone
   Trade names: Decadron (MSD), various
   Chemical names: 9-fluoro-11β,17-dihydroxy-16α-methyl-21-pregna-1,4-diene-3,20-dione
   How available: tablets: 0.25, 0.5, 0.75, 1.0, 1.5, 2.0, 4.0, and 6.0 mg; elixir: 5 mg/5 ml; injectable: 16 mg/mL

Adrenocorticoids (corticosteroids) are important therapeutic agents in a diverse number of malignant diseases. They are a part of the primary modalities of treatment in acute lymphocytic leukemia, chronic lymphocytic leukemia, multiple myeloma, Waldenstrom's macroglobulinemia, and Hodgkin's and non-Hodgkin's lymphomas. In these diseases, the adrenocorticoids have been shown empirically to have single-agent antitumor activity, producing a reduction in the number of circulating tumor cells or a decrease in a measured parameter such as size or number of lymph nodes or concentrations of proteins (13, 14). There also appears to be some marginal activity against breast carcinoma (15). For the lymphocytic leukemias, these agents are usually part of combinations of agents that induce the killing or lysis of the malignant clone of cells. In addition, the adrenocorticoids may play a role in reducing antibody-mediated problems such as hemolytic anemia or immune thrombocytopenia (16). When used for these purposes, the corticosteroids are often given over prolonged periods in relatively low doses of 10 to 20 mg/day. For the Hodgkin's and non-Hodgkin's lymphomas, the adrenocorticoids are often part of the primary combination chemotherapy regimens and are usually used in pulsed high doses of 60 to 100 mg/m^2 of prednisone (or equivalents) daily for 7 to 14 days (17, 18). For plasma cell neoplasms, the adrenocorticoids, in addition to their possible antitumor activity (19), may increase the rate of protein degradation (20). Treatment of patients with metastatic prostate cancer with corticosteroids may result in symptomatic improvement and declines in PSA levels (21). The basis for these effects is not clear but may again be related to increased protein turnover.

Adrenocorticoids are often also used for their additional benefits. Pulsed high doses of glucocorticoids (e.g., 10 mg dexamethasone) have an antiemetic effect (22) and are often still included in combined antiemetic-agent regimens (23). Since these agents have considerable antitumor activity in the treatment of lymphomas, leukemias, and myeloma, their use as antiemetics in clinical trials should be considered with prudence, as their use could obscure the activity of other therapies. Recently the adrenocorticoids have been used to prevent allergic reactions to certain agents such as paclitaxel (24). Adrenocorticoids are also sometimes used for symptomatic management; for example, in the relief of intracerebral edema (25, 26), respiratory insufficiency from lymphangiitic lung metastases (26), hypercalcemia (26, 27), or bone pain from metastases (28).

ESTROGENS

Numerous elegant studies have demonstrated that estrogens stimulate the production of autocrine growth factors in breast carcinoma cells (29, 30). Whether the estrogen-mediated increases in these autocrine growth factors plays a role in estrogen stimulation of breast carcinoma growth is still debated (31). Other evidence suggests that estrogens directly stimulate proliferation by inducing transcription of the *c-fos* protooncogene (31). 17β-Estradiol is itself a poor mitogen; however, in combination with other growth factors such as insulin-like growth factor-1, there is a synergistic response, with a marked increase in proliferation as well as AP-1-mediated gene transcription in estrogen-receptor-positive breast carcinoma cell lines (31). Similar observations were made by Philips et al. (32), who found that 17β-estradiol markedly enhanced growth factor (i.e., epidermal growth factor or insulin-like growth factor-1)-mediated stimulation of AP-1-mediated gene transcription. In conditions in which growth factor–induced *c-fos* or *C-Jun* mRNA levels were unchanged by hormone treatment, the addition of antiestrogen inhibited this effect of 17β-estradiol (32). Thus, there appears to be a significant degree of "cross-talk" between the steroid receptors and the AP-1 family (33, 34). In the cases of insulin-like growth factor-1 and the epidermal growth factors, estradiol markedly enhanced their proliferative capacity and their enhancement of AP-1-mediated gene transcription. In addition, estradiol increased insulin-like growth factor-1 mRNA levels in a number of cell types (35); thus estradiol not only enhances insulin-like growth factor-1-mediated gene activation but also enhances insulin-like growth factor-1 levels.

Estrogens exert their proliferative action through their binding to the nuclear estrogen receptor (29). Previous studies suggested that the ligand-bound estrogen receptor exerts its action by binding to specific DNA sequences consisting of perfect palindromes separated by 3-base spacers (36). However, recent investigations suggest that the estrogen receptor may bind to a variety of imperfect palindromes in conjunction with adjacent SP-1 sites (37). In addition, the presence of accessory proteins that appear to be required in estrogen receptor-mediated transcription has been described (38).

Estrogens enhance breast carcinoma secretion of tissue plasminogen activator and other collagenolytic enzymes (39). These enzymes may enhance tumor progression by digesting surrounding basement membranes. Pharmacologic doses of estrogens inhibit breast carcinoma proliferation. The exact mechanism of this inhibition is unclear, but downregulation of estrogen receptor mRNA levels and subsequent protein levels remains a possibility.

The androgen dependence of cancer of the prostate has been recognized for many years since the description by Huggins and Hodges in 1941 of major clinical benefits associated with surgical castration or the administration of pharmacologic doses of estrogens (40). Since then, suppression of gonadal production of androgens has been established as the mainstay for the systemic treatment of patients with metastatic prostate carcinoma.

Over the past several years, much effort has been devoted to enhancing our knowledge about the endocrine control of prostatic cancer growth. In man, 90 to 95% of circulating testosterone is of gonadal origin, while only about 5 to 10% derives from the adrenal gland (41–43). The synthesis and release of gonadal testosterone is primarily regulated by the pituitary gonadotropin luteinizing hormone (LH) (41–43). Gonadal LH receptors directly mediate the production of testosterone by the testis (41–43).

Schally and coworkers identified and isolated a hypothalamic hormone, known as gonadotropin-hormone-releasing hormone (GNRH), which was shown to be directly responsible for the synthesis and release of the pituitary gonadotropins, LH and follicle-stimulating hormone (FSH) (44–50). Subsequent studies showed that GNRH and various analogues of the parent hormone could effectively modulate the pituitary secretion of FSH and LH and, consequently, the gonadal production of testosterone (44–50).

While the importance of gonadal testosterone in prostatic carcinoma growth is well established, the role of adrenal androgen precursors remains controversial (43). The adrenal gland produces substantial quantities of two androgenic precursors, androstenedione and dehydroepiandrosterone, both of which have relatively weak androgenic activity. However, they are readily transformed into testosterone. Circulating unbound testosterone diffuses into the prostatic cell and is converted by the enzyme 5-α-reductase to dihydrotestosterone (DHT). DHT is translocated into the nucleus, where it binds to specific cytosolic receptors and, subsequently, to nuclear chromatin (51). This activation or processing of the receptor results in the induction of specific proteins that may be essential for cellular proliferation. Androgens enhance the production and secretion of the potent growth factor transforming growth factor-α (TGF-α) in the androgen-dependent LNCAP prostatic carcinoma cell line (52, 53). Diethylstilbestrol (DES), the most commonly used estrogen, affects androgen metabolism by several different mechanisms. DES downregulates gonadal LH receptors, decreases the release of GNRH, and downregulates the pituitary GNRH receptors (54). Estrogens also increase the concentration of testosterone-binding globulin, which results in a decrease in the amount of circulating (active) free testosterone (55). Much interest has been focused on the direct effects of estrogens on prostatic cancer cells, and while estrogen cytosolic receptors have been identified, definitive evidence supporting a direct cytotoxic effect of estrogens is still lacking. Estrogens also stimulate the production of prolactin; however, this effect is of unknown clinical significance.

The estrogens available for use include:

1. Generic name: diethylstilbestrol
   Trade name: Diethylstilbestrol (Lilly), various
   Chemical name: 3,4-bis(p-hydroxyphenyl)-3-hexene;4,4'-dihydroxy-α,β-diethylstilbene
   How available: tablets: 1 and 5 mg; enteric coated: 0.25, 0.5, 1, and 5 mg
   Dosing: breast cancer: 5 mg t.i.d. or greater; prostate cancer: 1 to 3 mg daily

2. Generic: estradiol
   Trade names: Estinyl (Schering), Feminone (Upjohn)
   Chemical name: estra-1,3,5-triene-3,17β-diol
   How available: tablets: 0.02, 0.05, and 0.5 mg
   Dosing: breast cancer: 1 mg t.i.d. or greater; prostate cancer: 0.15 to 2 mg/day

3. Generic: conjugated estrogen
   Trade names: Premarin (Ayerst), various
   Chemical names: mixture of estrone, equilin, 17α-dihydroequilin, and 17α-estradiol
   How available: tablets: 0.625, 0.9, and 2.5 mg; injectable: 25 mg
   Dosing: breast cancer: 10 mg t.i.d. or greater; prostate cancer: 1.25 to 2.5 mg/day

4. Generic: esterified estrogens
   Trade names: Estratab (Reid); Menest (Beecham)
   Chemical names: mixture of natural estrogens
   How available: 0.3, 0.625, 1.25, and 2.5 mg
   Dosing: breast cancer: 10 mg t.i.d. or greater; prostate cancer: 1.25 to 2.5 mg/day

Estrogens in pharmacologic doses have found considerable utility in the treatment of metastatic breast and prostate cancer. For carcinoma of the breast, the frequency of response to estrogens and other hormonal manipulations is related to the biologic features of the disease and the patient (56). Numerous studies have demonstrated the predictive value of estrogen receptors in the cytosol of the tumor for response to hormonal therapy. The greatest predictive value is seen with negative (<10 pmol/mg) receptors, which correlates with a lack of response (57–59). Overall, about 30% of tumors in unselected postmenopausal women and about 50% of estrogen-receptor-positive tumors will respond to estrogen therapy, with a greater response seen in soft tissue disease (e.g., breast, skin, lymph nodes) than in visceral disease. Nodular lung metastases and pleural effusions often respond more like soft tissue disease than visceral disease, whereas liver metastases respond less often (56, 60, 61).

The use of estrogens is generally limited to postmenopausal women (62). DES is the most frequently used estrogen, and doses are started with 5 to 10 mg daily and escalated to tolerance. Most women find doses of 15 to 25 mg daily to be tolerable. There is, however, only minimal evidence of a dose-response phenomenon for the estrogens (63). Premarin (7.5 mg/day) and ethinyl estradiol (3 mg/day) are also sometimes used. Typically, responses tend to occur slowly, and a prolonged trial of therapy (8 to 12 weeks) is usually indicated in the absence of progressive disease. For this reason, women with estrogen-receptor-negative tumors, life-threatening visceral disease (visceral crisis), or rapidly progressive disease are usually not considered good candidates for a therapeutic trial of estrogens. In view of their toxicity profile, estrogens are usually reserved for second- or third-line treatments following antiestrogens, progestins, and aromatase inhibitors, although their response rate is as good as that of tamoxifen or other hormonal agents.

The most commonly used estrogen for prostate cancer is DES. Earlier studies conducted by the Veterans Administration Cooperative Urological Research Group (VACURG) indicated that doses of 1 mg and 5 mg of DES were equivalent in efficacy (and both were superior to placebo or 0.2 mg DES), but the incidence of cardiovascular side effects was significantly less with the lower dose (64). Side effects of DES include gynecomastia; other feminizing effects, such as changes in voice, body distribution of fat and hair; edema; thromboembolic phenomena (deep venous thrombophlebitis, pulmonary embolus); and cardiovascular problems (congestive heart failure, angina, acute myocardial infarction, and cerebral vascular accidents) (64). Because of these side effects, which are greatly enhanced in high-risk patients (age above 75 years, history of any cardiovascular or thromboembolic abnormalities), this drug has come under major criticism and disfavor from physicians caring for these patients. Subsequent studies with 1 mg of DES have shown that the suppression of testosterone is less sustained and predictable than with 2 or 3 mg/day (65). While the relative value of 1 mg versus 3 mg of DES remains unclear, the latter dose is more frequently used.

Estrogen administration in pharmacologic doses often produces anorexia, nausea and vomiting, enlargement and tenderness of breasts,

softening of skin, fluid retention, breakthrough bleeding, headaches, and pigmentation of areola and skin folds. The fluid retention can aggravate preexisting congestive heart failure. Occasionally, estrogen administration and, similarly, all other hormonal manipulations in patients with bone metastases will result in exacerbation of severe bone pain early in therapy, a so-called flare of disease (66, 67). This early exacerbation of symptoms is frequently followed by a subsequent response to continued therapy and disappears after 2 to 3 weeks of treatment. Similarly, hypercalcemia can be seen in the early phase of therapy and may be indicative of subsequent response (66–68).

PROGESTINS

Progestins produce a wide variety of effects on cellular differentiation and growth. The specific effect appears to depend on the cell type. Progestins have an indirect effect on tissue growth through their action on the hypothalamic-pituitary tract, resulting in the inhibition of gonadotropin-releasing hormone. In addition, progestins appear to have a direct effect on cellular proliferation, resulting in either stimulation or inhibition of growth, depending upon the growth conditions (69–72). The cellular effects of progestins appear to be mediated through the progesterone nuclear receptor, which is a member of the steroid-thyroid nuclear receptor superfamily (73). Two isoforms, PR-A and PR-B, of the progesterone nuclear receptor have been found (74). The progesterone-receptor complex modulates gene transcription by binding to specific DNA sequences located in the regulatory regions of genes. The binding of the progesterone receptor to these sequences requires ligand binding as well as homodimerization of the receptor (75). Ligand binding results in a conformational change in the receptor as well as its phosphorylation, which in turn results in gene transactivation (74). Recent analysis has demonstrated that the agonist-and-antagonist binding sites on the human progesterone receptor are distinct. Thus, the antiprogestins do not bind to the progestin binding site, but induce conformational changes by binding to a different region of the ligand-binding domain (75).

The progesterone receptor gene possesses an estrogen-response sequence in its promoter sequence. Estrogen is required for activation of the progesterone receptor gene (76). Recent studies utilizing breast carcinoma cell lines demonstrated more than a 90% reduction of progesterone receptor in the absence of estrogen. The addition of progestins to progesterone-receptor-positive human breast cancer cells in the presence of serum and estrogen results in growth inhibition, while the addition of progestins to the same breast carcinoma cells grown in the absence of estrogen results in growth stimulation (77, 78). Progestins, through the progesterone receptor, regulate the expression of a variety of genes. Interestingly, during progestin-induced growth inhibition of T47D cells, expression of the growth-stimulating growth factor TGF-α and the epidermal growth factor receptor were found (79–81). Whether these are compensatory mechanisms by which the cells attempt to override the progesterone-induced growth inhibition is not known. Jeng and Jordan (71) found that the addition of the progestin norethindrone to the human breast carcinoma cell line MCF-7 resulted in growth stimulation that was accompanied by a marked decrease in transforming growth factor β2 and β3 mRNA levels. Both the progestin stimulation of growth and inhibition of TGF-β2 and TGF-β3 mRNA levels were blocked by 4-hydroxytamoxifen. Recently, progestins were found to also interact with AP-1 complexes. The progestin medroxyprogesterone acetate (MPA) increased C-Jun mRNA levels, decreased Jun-B mRNA levels, and significantly decreased AP-1 activity during MPA-induced growth inhibition of T47D cells (82). Whether this is the mechanism by which MPA inhibits the growth of breast carcinoma cells is not known.

Hamburger et al. found that megestrol acetate increased the rate of adipogenic gene transcription (82). Megestrol acetate produced a dose-dependent increase in lipogenic enzymes in 3T3L1 cells. Several clinical studies likewise suggested that progestins may be useful in the treatment of cancer or AIDS cachexia (83, 84, 85). Conventional doses (160 mg/day) enhance weight gain in approximately one-third of the patients, and higher doses may be more effective. There appears to be a dose-response relationship, with increasing doses of megestrol acetate producing increasing weight gain.

The progestins available for use include:

1. Generic name: medroxyprogesterone acetate
   Trade names: Provera (Upjohn); various
   Chemical name: 17-hydroxy-6α-methylpreg-4-ene-3,20-dione
   How supplied: tablets: 2.5 and 10 mg; injectable (depo-provera): 100 mg/mL and 400 mg/mL
   Dosing: breast cancer: 400 mg/week; prostate cancer: 400 mg/week; endometrial cancer: 1 g/week

2. Generic name: hydroxyprogesterone caproate
   Trade names: Delalutin (Squibb); various
   Chemical name: 17-hydroxypreg-4-ene-3,20-dione
   How supplied: injectable: 125 mg/mL and 250 mg/mL
   Dosing: breast cancer: 400 mg/week; prostate cancer: 400 mg/week; endometrial cancer: 1 g/week.

3. Generic name: megestrol acetate
   Trade names: Megace (Bristol-Myers Laboratories)
   Chemical name: 17α-hydroxy-6-methylpregna-4,6-diene-3,20-dione acetate
   How available: tablets: 20 and 40 mg; oral suspension 40 mg/mL
   Dosing: breast cancer: 160 mg/day; prostate cancer: 160 mg/day; endometrial cancer: 160 mg/day; AIDS- or cancer-related cachexia: 800 mg/day

Progestins, particularly megestrol acetate (MA) and MPA, have found considerable utility in the treatment of breast and endometrial carcinoma (86–88). There have also been some reports of successful treatments of ovarian and prostatic carcinoma (89, 90). Although there are reports of antitumor activity in renal cell carcinoma, the effectiveness of progestins in renal carcinoma has not been substantiated. Finally, the progestins have been noted to increase appetite and produce weight gain (83). Randomized studies in AIDS and cancer cachexia have shown that MA can significantly improve appetite, increase weight, and improve the sense of well being (91–94). The studies in AIDS cachexia further demonstrated that this effect is related to dose and a dose of 800 mg/day appears to be more useful than lower doses (93, 94).

In breast cancer, the addition of various progestins has long been known to produce tumor regressions (95). Progestins appear to be approximately equivalent to the antiestrogen tamoxifen as the initial hormonal therapeutic maneuver and possess comparable activity as second-line treatment (96, 97). The progestins, however, appear to produce more weight gain than tamoxifen, which is used initially more often. Since many patients now receive tamoxifen as postoperative adjuvant treatment and pending further data on the forthcoming aromatase inhibitors, progestins should be considered the next step (depending upon tumor site) after the breast cancer has recurred following tamoxifen adjunctive therapy. The role of progestins as postoperative adjuvant treatment is not established. The conventional dose for the progestins is usually divided on a daily basis; however, the pharmacokinetics show a long half-life, and single daily dosing is adequate (98, 99). Several trials suggest a dose-response relationship in breast cancer for the progestins (100–102). However, a large randomized cooperative group trial of three different dose levels of MA failed to validate such a dose-response relationship (103).

Progestins have also been used in the treatment of malignant and premalignant endometrial diseases. Several studies have implied that the natural progression of adenomatous hyperplasia can be reversed by the use of progestins (104, 105). There is also a suggestion of a dose-response relationship for the treatment of advanced endometrial cancer (106, 107). Progestins have also have been advocated (108–110) as initial treatment, together with brachytherapy, for both operable and inoperable endometrial cancers. After the irradiation, the progestins are sometimes continued for prolonged periods (110). For recurrent or metastatic disease, progestins represent initial therapy and offer about a 30% probability of response with minimal side effects and a survival advantage compared with palliative irradiation alone (106–108, 111, 112).

In prostatic carcinoma, the progestins (particularly MA) appear to exert an antiandrogenic action. While the drug interferes with nuclear androgen binding, it also suppresses LH and testosterone (113). With prolonged treatment using standard doses, LH and testosterone suppression reverses with time (113). This reversal is considered a limitation of this drug and prompted investigators to use it in combination with low doses of estrogen (DES 0.5 mg/day), which resulted in more effective and sustained LH and testosterone suppression (114). In a relatively small randomized study, MA plus low-dose estrogen was shown to be comparable to high-dose DES (115); however, more data are needed with MA as first-line treatment. Its efficacy in patients failing first-line hormonal treatment is limited. The side effects of MA are feminization (less than with DES), weight gain, and somewhat less prominent cardiovascular problems than with estrogens. The conventional oral dose of MA for metastatic prostate cancer is 160 mg daily.

Progestins also have an inhibitory effect on ovarian cancer (116), and estrogen and progesterone receptors have been identified in these cancers (117). Progestins have been used alone in high doses (400 to 800 mg MA) and in combination with single-agent chemotherapy (118); however, their roles in recurrent disease and as part of initial therapy have yet to be defined.

Progestins have, in the past, been advocated for the treatment of renal cell carcinoma (119). Response rates as high at 16% were reported but have not been confirmed using modern response criteria. The subjective benefits of progestins such as an improved sense of well-being and improvement of appetite may have confounded the early assessment of their efficacy.

SURGICAL ABLATIVE THERAPIES

Castration, hypophysectomy, and adrenalectomy are the surgical approaches to modulating the hormonal environment. Some of the procedures such as orchiectomy for male breast cancer or prostate cancer and oophorectomy for breast cancer remain the most effective and definitive form of removing the source of gonadal hormones. Adrenalectomy and hypophysectomy, however, are much more difficult and morbid procedures. In the past, adrenalectomy and hypophysectomy for breast cancer produced reasonable responses in the setting of prior hormone responsiveness (56). The availability of medical adrenalectomy using aminoglutethimide plus hydrocortisone and the demonstration of its equivalence to surgical adrenalectomy (120), as well as other means for hormone suppression, have led to a virtual discontinuation of these procedures. Surgical castration, however, remains a highly effective and simple means of obtaining gonadal ablation.

For premenopausal women with advanced breast cancer, bilateral oophorectomy remains an important treatment step (56). Response frequency depends on hormone receptor status; response is seen in about 30% of unselected women and 50% or more of women with estrogen-receptor-positive tumors (56, 121, 122). The survival of women whose tumors respond to oophorectomy is longer than those whose tumors did not respond. Most importantly, oophorectomy can add a potential hormonal treatment step when used as the initial treatment for recurrent breast cancer in premenopausal women. At least for those women who respond, the use of oophorectomy can prolong the time of hormonal treatments. Although probably less effective because of dose and field considerations, castration can also be achieved with ovarian irradiation.

Adjuvant oophorectomy was first studied before the availability of estrogen receptors. Some of those studies suggested an increased disease-free period but no prolongation of overall survival (123–125). Information about potential hormonal responsiveness for subsequent therapy, however, is lost with adjuvant castration. Recently, the Early Breast Cancer Trialists presented an overview of randomized postoperative therapy studies (126). Their data suggest that adjuvant postoperative oophorectomy provides a survival benefit in premenopausal patients, and this effect is additive to adjuvant chemotherapy.

Surgical castration remains the preferred initial hormonal approach for male breast cancer (127). Surgical castration in the male produces a rapid decrease in circulating androgens to a level considered the baseline to which the other forms of gonadal androgen suppression for prostate cancer should be compared. This level is also known as the "castrate range" (usually reflecting serum testosterone levels of 50 mg/mL or less). Castrate testosterone levels are considered by many to be an effective state for optimal therapeutic benefits for both disseminated male breast cancer and prostate cancer. Following castration, both FSH and LH levels rise promptly. However, this finding is of unknown clinical significance and is probably insignificant.

The role of primary adrenal androgen suppression for prostate cancer remains unclear at this time. The vast majority of clinical trials dealing with the use of adrenalectomy, either medical or surgical, primarily involved patients with tumors that had failed primary gonadal ablation (128). In contrast to breast cancer, prostate cancer is largely unresponsive to second- and third-line endocrine manipulations, primarily because at this stage the tumor becomes largely independent of androgens. As a result, the role of adrenal androgen suppression has not undergone a fair testing as monotherapy. The superiority of combined androgen blockade employing an LHRH analogue and an antiandrogen over an LHRH analogue or orchiectomy in treating patients with metastatic disease remains controversial (see below).

ANTIESTROGENS

The estrogen receptor possesses two domains that appear to play a major role in gene transcription (129). These regions are located in the A/B and ligand-binding domains of the molecule and have been referred to as transactivating functions 1 and 2 (TAF1 and TAF2), respectively (129). Numerous antiestrogens have now been synthesized that inhibit estrogen receptor action and function as agonists or pure antagonists (130). Tamoxifen and 4-hydroxytamoxifen inhibit TAF2 function but can also serve as agonists through their activation of TAF1 function (129). In contrast, pure antagonists such as ICI 164,384 have been hypothesized to impair estrogen-receptor binding to DNA by inhibiting receptor dimerization or by some as-yet undescribed mechanism (131, 132).

Antiestrogens can inhibit cell proliferation through a variety of mechanisms. It has recently been shown that the antiestrogens can not only block estrogen-mediated stimulation of breast carcinoma cell growth, but they also can block growth factor–mediated proliferation (133). The antiestrogens tamoxifen and droloxirene inhibited both insulin-like growth factor-1 and epidermal growth factor-mediated proliferation of breast carcinoma cells (133). The mechanism by which the antiestrogens inhibit growth factor stimulation of breast carcinoma growth is unclear, since they do not inhibit either insulin-like growth factor-1 or epidermal growth factor–mediated stimulation of the nuclear transcription factors c-fos or c-myc (133).

Recent data from clinical trials suggest that the antiestrogen tamoxifen demonstrates efficacy that appears to be partially independent of the estrogen-receptor content of the primary tumor (126, 134). Since estrogen-receptor data may not fully predict which patients may respond to antiestrogen therapy, tamoxifen may possess an additional mechanism of action that is independent of the presence of a functional estrogen receptor. Tamoxifen induces the secretion of TGF-β in human breast carcinoma cell lines (135). TGF-β, in turn, inhibits the proliferation of these cell lines. In addition, tamoxifen induces the secretion of TGF-β in estrogen-receptor-negative human fetal fibroblasts (136). Recently Butta et al. (137). found that treatment of patients with tamoxifen resulted in enhanced secretion of TGF-β by the stromal fibroblasts surrounding the breast carcinoma cells. This tamoxifen-enhanced secretion of TGF-β was found in the stromal cells of both estrogen-reception-positive and estrogen-receptor-negative tumors.

Numerous investigations have been conducted on the mechanisms involved in the acquisition of tamoxifen resistance by breast carcinoma cells (138, 139). Osborne et al. demonstrated that tamoxifen resistance is often associated with altered tamoxifen pharmacology and perhaps the metabolism of tamoxifen to estrogenic forms (139). Another potential explanation derives from the observation that continued treatment with tamoxifen results in downregulation of the expression of the estrogen receptor (140)

The antiestrogen available for use is:

Generic name: tamoxifen

Trade name: Nolvadex (Zeneca Pharmaceuticals)

Chemical name: 2-[4-(1,2-diphenyl-1-butenyl) phenoxy]-N,N-dimethylethanamine 2-hydroxy-1,2,3-propanetricarboxylate (1:1)

How available: tablets: 10 mg

Dosing: 10 mg b.i.d.

With the discovery of antiestrogens, especially tamoxifen, a new and relatively nontoxic modality of therapy became available for estrogen-dependent tumors, specifically breast carcinoma (141). Several antiestrogens have been tested, including clomiphene citrate, nafoxidine, and tamoxifen (142). Only tamoxifen was found to have minimal toxicity, and it is now considered the first hormonal maneuver for postmenopausal women with advanced breast cancer (143, 144). The usual dose is 10 mg twice daily; higher doses add toxicity without convincingly increasing response frequency. The predictive value of estrogen-receptor proteins has added considerably to our treatment of breast cancer. Estrogen receptor (ER)-positive tumors respond with a frequency of 35 to 70% (depending on site of disease) while ER-negative tumors seldom respond (< 5%). Although response to tamoxifen has been seen in ER-negative tumors (routinely below 15%), tamoxifen is not recommended in this setting. Since the receptor proteins are thermolabile, there are false-negative ER determinations, which confuse the issue. The role of antiestrogens in premenopausal women is less well established (145), but there appears to be about the same frequency of response as with oophorectomy (146). In view of their competition with circulating estrogens, their use may be dependent on dose. Nevertheless, the data to support the use of tamoxifen use in this setting are not clear. Although responses to oophorectomy are seen after tamoxifen, responses to oophorectomy after tamoxifen failure (147) suggest that tamoxifen may be more appropriate as a second treatment after oophorectomy for premenopausal women, unless there is a compelling reason to avoid surgery.

Antiestrogens (particularly tamoxifen) increase the disease-free and overall survival when used as adjuvant treatment for postmenopausal women with ER-positive tumors. Recent studies also suggest that tamoxifen increases the disease-free survival of postmenopausal women with stage I, node-negative tumors, especially among women with ER-positive tumors (126). The metaanalysis overview by the Early Breast Cancer Trialists' Group, however, also suggested a strong benefit in overall survival (126). Despite the demonstrated positive effect of antiestrogens in these settings, the survival benefit is modest, and investigative therapies are clearly warranted. The use of antiestrogens as postoperative adjuvant treatment for postmenopausal women with ER-negative tumors has not been shown to improve disease-free or overall survival, and their use in this setting is thus not justified.

AROMATASE INHIBITORS

Aminoglutethimide (AG) blocks the conversion of cholesterol to Δ-5 pregnenolone by competitive inhibition of cytochrome P450. AG thus interferes with the enzyme desmolase, which promotes the cleavage of the cholesterol side chain (148). This inhibits the conversion to androgens. AG therefore acts at early steps in the inhibition of adrenal steroidogenesis, affecting the production of aldosterone, cortisol, and androgens. AG also blocks the aromatization of androgens to estrogens. The d-isomer of AG is a more potent aromatase inhibitor; the l-form is a more potent inhibitor of cholesterol cleavage (148). Side effects include nausea/vomiting, lethargy, ataxia, rash, thrombocytopenia (rare), and adrenal insufficiency. In contrast, type I aromatase inhibitors such as 4-hydroxyandrostenedione ((4-OHA), Fedrazole, and others not currently available in the U.S.) are more potent inhibitors than AG, may have milder side effects, and do not need corticosteroid replacement therapy. Thus, these compounds that block only the aromatization of androstenedione to estrogens may have a more important role in breast cancer than AG.

Some of the aromatase inhibitors such as AG produce the equivalent of a medical adrenalectomy, thereby inhibiting the formation of estrogens and androgens (120, 148, 149). These agents have therefore found considerable actual and potential use in the treatment of metastatic breast and prostate cancer. Other aromatase inhibitors such as 4-OHA produce a more defined block in the conversion of androgens to estrogens. Because there is no cleavage of the side chain, there is little block in the formation of glucocorticoids or mineralocorticoids; thus, these compounds have potential use even earlier in the hormonal selection process for breast cancer and possibly for endometrial cancer (140).

The aromatase inhibitor available for use is

Generic name: aminoglutethimide
Trade name: Cytadren (CIBA)
Chemical name: 3-(4-amino-phenyl)-3-ethyl-2,6-piperidinedione
How available: tablets: 250 mg
Dosing: 250 mg q.i.d.

Some authors have suggested that a dose of 250 mg twice a day reduces the incidence of side effects while largely conserving the activity of the AG. Prospective validation of these claims, however, is inadequate.

Aromatase inhibitors have a defined role in the treatment of breast cancer since AG has supplanted the use of surgical adrenalectomy or hypophysectomy (120, 149). Its role, in view of the toxicity spectrum, is as a second- or third-line treatment. Thus, it typically follows the use of tamoxifen and progestins. The usual dose is 250 mg four times a day. AG treatment requires steroid replacement, which is usually effectively accomplished with hydrocortisone (40 to 100 mg/day or its equivalent). Close monitoring for mineralocorticoid insufficiency is indicated, and although unlikely, supplementation may be necessary. Response, seen in 15 to 30% of women, tends to occur in the setting of response to prior hormonal therapy. Some observers feel that early discontinuation for rash is not warranted and that AG can be safely continued under observation (149). Recent studies have suggested that 4-OHA may produce a 40 to 50% response frequency when used earlier in the treatment schema (150). The reported toxicity was generally mild, and studies of 4-OHA and its newer analogues are under way to define its role in the

earlier treatment of breast cancer. This may be important since most patients are now receiving adjuvant tamoxifen. Newer 4-OHA derivatives and new discrete aromatase inhibitors are currently under active investigation.

The therapeutic benefits of AG in patients with progressive carcinoma of the prostate following gonadal suppression have been very modest, mostly subjective, and short-lived. This mostly symptomatic improvement, which has been reported in approximately 20% of the patients with advanced disease (151), may also be due to the effects of hydrocortisone, which is usually used in combination with AG to replace the depleted pool of glucocorticoids. AG causes a rapid drop in adrenal androgen levels (151). Its value as first-line treatment remains unestablished, and its use in combination with gonadal ablation has not yet been tested. As second-line treatment, AG has only modest efficacy and most likely does not affect survival in these patients. A common dose/schedule of AG is 250 mg four times a day initially for 2 weeks, followed by 500 mg/day thereafter, given with hydrocortisone and monitoring of electrolytes. New aromatase inhibitors are being evaluated and one, anastrozole (Arimidex), is now commercially available. The recommended dose is 1 mg once daily.

ANDROGENS

The mechanism by which large doses of androgens inhibit breast cancer is unclear, although there is both laboratory and clinical evidence that high doses of androgen inhibit gonadotropin-releasing hormone release and subsequent estrogen production. Androgens have been observed to bind to the estrogen receptor at concentrations approximately 1000-fold greater than estrogens (54, 152); under these conditions, androgens stimulate breast carcinoma proliferation (152, 153).

The androgens available for use include

1. Generic name: testosterone proprionate
   Trade names: Testosterone (Upjohn); various
   Chemical name: Δ^4-androstene-17β-proprionate-3-one
   How available: injectable: 25, 50, and 100 mg/mL
   Dosing: 50 to 100 mg i.m. three times a week

2. Generic name: methyltestosterone
   Trade names: Android (Brown); Metandren (CIBA); Oreton-methyl (Schering); various

Chemical name: 17β-hydroxy-17-methylan-drost-4-en-3-one
How available: tablets: 5, 10, and 25 mg
Dosing: 200 mg/day

3. Generic name: fluoxymesterone
   Trade names: Halotestin (Upjohn); Oratestryl (Squibb); various
   Chemical name: 9α-fluoro-11β,17β-dihy-droxy-17α-methyl-4-androsten-3-one
   How available: tablets: 2, 5, and 10 mg
   Dosing: 10 mg t.i.d.

4. Generic name: testolactone
   Trade name: Teslac (Squibb)
   Chemical name: 1,2,3,4,4α,4β,7,9,10,10α-decahydro-2hydroxy-2,4βdimethyl-7-oxo-1-phenanthrenepropionic acid lactone
   How available: tablets: 50 mg
   Dosing: 250 mg q.i.d.

Pharmacologic doses of androgens have been used as hormonal treatment for ER-positive breast carcinomas. The response to androgens is, at best, no better than that for estrogens and, in randomized trials, has been shown to be lower, with the added side effects of virilization (56). The facial hair, lowered voice, and clitoral enlargement can be disturbing. Thus, the androgens are less preferred than estrogens. The lower incidence of fluid retention could make these preferable in older women with congestive heart failure, however. When androgens are used, they tend to produce responses primarily in the setting of bone or soft tissue disease. The usual doses are: fluoxymesterone: 10 mg p.o. t.i.d., methyl testosterone: 200 mg every day orally, or testosterone propionate: 100 mg i.m. three times a week. Testolactone (100 mg three times a week i.m.) is similar to testosterone but may be less virilizing.

ANTIANDROGENS

Steroidal antiandrogens are usually progestational compounds that exert dual effects on the androgenic pathway. In addition to inhibition of nuclear androgen binding, steroidal antiandrogens suppress gonadotropin production via a negative biofeedback mechanism similar to that of estrogens and therefore suppress gonadal androgen production. Pure or nonsteroidal antiandrogens do not suppress gonadotropins and testosterone but are potent inhibitors of nuclear androgen binding. Studies monitoring hor-mones in normal volunteers and prostate cancer patients demonstrated that during the initial weeks of treatment with one such compound, flutamide, elevations (but still within the normal range) of testosterone and (to a lesser degree) LH occur (154). These hormonal changes usually stabilize with time and return to mean levels after several weeks. There is probably no clinical significance to the initial rise in testerone levels.

Antiandrogens have been used in the treatment of metastatic prostatic carcinoma. The antiandrogens produce most or all of their effects by inhibiting the nuclear binding of androgens (154). This mechanism is largely due to competitive inhibition of cytosolic DHT receptors (154). Less frequently, a "postreceptor" effect can be observed (146). Antiandrogens are divided into two large groups: steroidal and nonsteroidal (or pure) antiandrogens.

The antiandrogen (nonsteroidal) available for use is:

Generic name: flutamide
Trade name: Eulexin (Schering-Plough)
Chemical name: 2-methyl-N[4-nitro-3-(trifluoromethyl) phenyl] propranamide
How available: capsules: 125 mg
Dosing: 250 mg t.i.d.

Flutamide is a toluidine derivative supplied in oral form (154). The drug competes with DHT receptors and exerts its antitumor effects by suppressing nuclear androgen binding. Flutamide is well tolerated; side effects include diarrhea (10 to 15%), abdominal cramps, and discomfort that patients frequently describe as "gas pains." While flutamide as monotherapy has shown significant activity in previously untreated (with endocrine treatment) patients with prostate cancer, its relative value compared with estrogens, GNRH analogues, and orchiectomy remains unestablished. The drug is approved in the United States (1989) for combined use with GNRH analogues but also is used alone or in combination with finasteride, an inhibitor of 5α reductase, in men who wish to retain sexual potency (155). Current data suggest that the incidence of decreased libido and sexual impotence is significantly lower with flutamide monotherapy than with conventional forms of gonadal ablations.

Casodex is a new nonsteroidal antiandiogen that is active in patients with prostate cancer (156). This agent lacks the gastrointestinal toxicity associated with flutamide, and its prolonged half life (about 6 days) permits daily dosing (157). Its role in the treatment of patients with advanced disease is currently being evaluated in clinical trials (158).

LHRH ANALOGUES

GNRH analogues produce a medical form of castration, which may be reversible if applied for a limited time, usually less than 1 year. Most patients, however, because of their age or perhaps because of their underlying disease, have depressed baseline gonadal function. Thus, prolonged treatment for several months will most likely produce irreversible testosterone suppression. Treatment should continue permanently. The initial stimulatory phase (which in animals is associated with depletion of pituitary LH stores, suggesting an association between synthesis and release) may cause an initial flare of the disease in patients with disseminated prostatic cancer, manifested by increased bone pain (10 to 30%) and, less frequently, by increased urinary symptoms (159–161). The association between flare of disease and an increased incidence of neurologic complications, such as epidural cord compression, is unclear. However, because of the evidence suggesting that there may, in fact, be some clinical deterioration of the disease initially, this form of treatment should most likely not be offered to patients at high risk for known neurologic involvement. Contrary to the situation with breast cancer, the flare of clinical symptoms with GNRH treatment has not been shown to have any predictive value for a subsequent response to continued therapy. Synthesis of potent analogues of the naturally occurring GNRH introduced a new form of treatment for carcinoma of the prostate. The physiologic secretion of GNRH is pulsatile, and frequent low doses of this compound (or its analogue) activate the normal production and release of gonadotropins. Paradoxically, however, higher doses of GNRH given continuously cause inhibition of pituitary/gonadal function. With prolonged administration, following an initial rise in LH and testosterone, which lasts for approximately 7 days, there is a progressive decrease in the levels of these hormones, reaching nadirs after 4 weeks of continuous treatment (44).

The LHRH analogues available for use are:

1. Generic name: leuprolide acetate
   Trade name: Leupron (TAP Pharmaceuticals)
   Chemical name: 5-oxo-L-propyl-L-histidyl-L-

tryptophyl-L-seryl-L-tyrosyl-D-leucyl-L-leucyl-arginyl-N-ethyl-L-prolinamide acetate
   How available: injectable: aqueous: 1 mg/0.2 mL; depo: 7.5 mg/1 mL
   Dosing: s.c. 1 mg/day; i.m. 7.5 mg/month

2. Goserelin acetate implant
   Trade name: Zoladex
   Chemical name: pyro-Glu-His-Trp-Ser-Tyr-D-Ser (Bu$^+$)-Leu-Arg-Pro-Azgly-NH$_2$ acetate
   How available: injectable; implant: equivalent to 3 mg goserelin
   Dosing: administered subcutaneously every 28 days

The identification and chemical characterization of the naturally occurring GNRH in the hypothalamus by Schally et al. (44) opened a new avenue for the treatment of prostate carcinoma. Amino acid substitutions in various positions of the decapeptide result in compounds with 50 to 100 times the potency of the parent hormone. Leuprolide acetate (Lupron, TAP Pharmaceuticals, Chicago, IL) is the most developed GNRH analogue in the U.S. This drug was synthesized with substitutions in the position 6 and terminal amino acids. The drug is devoid of cardiovascular side effects and obviates the use of surgery for gonadal ablation; however, it requires continuous treatment. Leuprolide is given by daily subcutaneous injections (1 mg/day) or in a depo form (sustained release) at doses of 7.5 mg given monthly. The most prominent side effects are hot flashes (50 to 60%) and decrease in libido and impotence. Prospective randomized trials comparing leuprolide with 3 mg of DES have shown equivalence in efficacy but a significantly lower incidence of potentially serious cardiovascular side effects (161). More recent data demonstrate that GNRH analogues are as effective as surgical castration. Goserelin acetate, a new LHRH analogue, is (like leupron) equivalent to orchiectomy in terms of clinical responses in patients with advanced prostate cancer; it can be implanted subcutaneously on a monthly basis (162).

COMBINED ANDROGEN BLOCKADE FOR PATIENTS WITH ADVANCED PROSTATE CANCER

The role of combined androgen blockade in patients with metastatic prostate cancer remains controversial. The rationale for this approach was that significant levels of dihydrotestosterone were present in the prostate after gonadal ablation (114). Combined androgen blockade is directed at interfering with androgens synthesized by the adrenals as well as the testes. A randomized, double-blinded intergroup study sponsored by the National Cancer Institute demonstrated a significant increase in overall survival in patients who received leuprolide and flutamide, compared with leuprolide alone (163). While the increase in median survival was modest (about 7 months), a subpopulation of patients with good performance status and minimal disease appears to have a more dramatic improvement in survival. The statistical significance of this finding is unclear, however, because of sample size.

Further support for combined androgen blockade is provided by a trial undertaken by the European Organization for Research and Treatment of Cancer (EORTC). In this trial, patients with advanced disease were randomized to bilateral orchiectomy versus goserelin acetate and flutamide. A significant improvement in overall survival (about 7 months) was noted (164). A metaanalysis of seven trials with 1056 patients with advanced disease randomized to orchiectomy, with or without the antiandrogen nilutamide, also revealed a significantly increased percentage of patients with pain control and improvement in the odds ratio for progression of disease in those patients receiving combined androgen blockade (165). Although a 10% reduction in the annual odds ratio for death was noted in patients receiving nilutamide, this was not significant.

A follow-up study to the initial NCI-sponsored trial is under way in which patients with advanced disease receive orchiectomy with or without flutamide. This study, as well as a more extensive metaanalysis that includes trials that use flutamide as the antiandrogen, will clarify the role of combined androgen blockade in patients with advanced disease. The resolution of this issue is important, since combined androgen blockade is an expensive therapy. It is reasonable to consider this approach in patients with minimal disease and good performance status. The time of initiation, duration of this treatment, and whether such therapy can be given on an intermittent basis are not known. The impact of combined androgen blockade on survival also is unclear.

Another drug that produces both gonadal and adrenal inhibition is ketoconazole (KTZ). KTZ is a substituted imidazole, originally developed as an antifungal drug (166). When used in higher doses, KTZ produces both adrenal and gonadal suppression. In patients with previously untreated prostate cancer, KTZ causes a rapid decrease in circulating androgens and is associated with significant antitumor responses. Its relative value compared with standard gonadal ablation or combined endocrine approaches remains undefined, however. When used as a second-line endocrine manipulation, KTZ has shown little usefulness.

The agent available for use is:

Generic name: ketoconazole
Trade name: Nizoral (Janssen)
Chemical name: *cis*-1-acetyl-4-[4-[[2-(2,4-dichlorophenyl)-2-(1*H*-imidazol-1-ylmethyl)-1,3-dioxolan-4-yl]methoxyl]phenyl] piperazine
How available: tablets: 200 mg
Dosing: 400 mg t.i.d.

High doses of KTZ have been shown to inhibit gonadal and adrenal steroidogenesis by disrupting the P450-dependent enzyme system, especially C17–20 lysate (166). Clinical data demonstrate that KTZ causes a rapid decrease (90%) of testosterone and adrenal androgen precursors (70%) and is associated with clinical benefits in patients with previously untreated (endocrine treatment) disease. KTZ results in modest benefit to patients with previously treated disease. It is often used in clinical settings in which a rapid decline in testosterone is required, such as in patients with cord compression. The most common side effects are nausea/vomiting and elevation of liver enzymes. The recommended dose/ schedule of ketoconazole for the treatment of cancer of the prostate is 400 mg orally three times daily, with 40 to 100 mg of hydrocortisone replacement given in divided doses at 8 AM, 4 PM, and 8 PM. Lower doses of KTZ have also been given (200 mg t.i.d.); however, the endocrine effects at this dose are most likely suboptimal.

References

1. Green S, Chambon P. Nuclear receptors enhance our understanding of transcription regulation. Trends Genet 1988;4:309–314.

2. Evans RM. The steroid and thyroid hormone receptor family. Science 1988;240:889–895.

3. Beato M. Gene regulation by steroid hormones. Cell 1989;56:335–344.

4. Yang-Yen HF, Chambard JC, Sun Y-L, et al. Transcriptional interference between C-Jun and the glucocorticoid receptor: mutual inhibition of DNA

binding due to direct protein-protein interaction. Cell 1990;62:1205–1221.

5. Saatcioglu F, Helmberg A, Karin M. Modulation of immune function interference between nuclear receptors and AP-1. Fundam Clin Immunol 1994;2:2–11.

6. Galili U. Glucocorticoid-induced cytolysis of human normal and malignant lymphocytes. J Steroid Biochem 1983;19:483–490.

7. Angel P, Karen M. The role of Jun. Fos and the AP-1 complex in cell proliferation and transformation. Biochim Biophys Acta 1991;1072:129–157.

8. Smeal T, Angel P, Mern J, et al. Different requirements for mutation of Jun, Jun and Jun, Fos complexes. Genes Dev 1989;3:2091–2100.

9. Paedee A. GI events and regulation of cell proliferation. Science 1989;246:603–611.

10. Frisch SM, Ruley HE. Transcription from the stromelysin promotion is induced for interleukin 1 and repressed by dexamethasone. J Biol Chem 1987; 262:3335–3342.

11. Offringa R, Smis AM, Houweling A, et al. Similar effects of adenovirus EIA and glucocorticoid hormones on the expression of the metalloprotease stromelysin. Nucl Acids Res 1986;16:10974–10983.

12. Brinckerhoff CE, Plucinska IM, Sheldon LA, O'Connor GT. Half life of synovial cell collagenase mRNA is modulated by phorbol myristate acetate but not by all transretinoic acid or dexamethasone. Biochemistry 1986;25:6378–6384.

13. Hall TC, Choi OS, Abadi A, et al. High-dose corticoid therapy in Hodgkin's disease and other lymphomas. Ann Intern Med 1967;66:1144–1150.

14. Alexanian R, Haut A, Talley RW, et al. Treatment for multiple myeloma: combination chemotherapy with different melphalan dose regimens. Coop Study Adult Div South West Childrens Cancer Study Group (SWCCSG). JAMA 1969;208:1680–1684.

15. Dao TL, Tan E, Brooks V. A comparative evaluation of adrenalectomy and cortisone in the treatment of advanced mammary cancer. CA 1961;14: 1259–1265.

16. Cidlowski JA, Schwartzman RA. Corticosteroids. In: Holland JF, Frei E, Bast RC Jr, Kufe DW, Morton DL, Weichselbaum RR, eds. Cancer medicine. 3rd ed. Philadelphia: Lea & Febiger 1993;845–857.

17. Coltman CA. Chemotherapy of advanced Hodgkin's disease. Semin Oncol 1980;7:155–173.

18. Schein PS, Chabner BA, Canellos GP, et al. Potential for prolonged disease-free survival following combination chemotherapy of non-Hodgkin's lymphoma. Blood 1972;43:31–38.

19. Salmon SE, Shadduck RK, Schilling A. Intermittent high-dose prednisone (NSC-10023) therapy for multiple myeloma. Cancer Chemother Rep 1967; 51:179–187.

20. Bergsagel DE. Plasma cell myeloma: an interpretive review. Cancer 1972;30:1588–1594.

21. Tannock IF, Gospodarowicz M, McAkin W, et al. Treatment of metastatic prostate cancer with low dose prednisone: evaluation of pain and quality of life as pragmatic indices of response. J Clin Oncol 1989; 7:590–597.

22. Cassileth PA, Lusk EJ, Torri S, et al. Antiemetic efficacy of dexamethasone therapy in patients receiving cancer chemotherapy. Arch Intern Med 1983; 143:1347–1349.

23. Bruera ED, Roca E, Cedaro L, et al. Improved control of chemotherapy-induced emesis by the addition of dexamethasone to metoclopramide in patients resistant to metoclopramide. Cancer Treat Rep 1983; 67:381–383.

24. Wiernik PH, Schwartz EL, Strauman, et al. Phase I clinical and pharmacokinetic study of taxol. Cancer Res 1987;47:2486–2493.

25. Weissman DE. Glucocorticoid treatment for brain metastases and epidural spinal cord compression: a review. J Clin Oncol 1988;6:543–548.

26. Brennan MJ. Corticosteroids in the treatment of solid tumors. Med Clin North Am 1973;57:1225–1239.

27. Steward AF. Therapy of malignancy associated hypercalcemia. Am J Med 1983;74:475–480.

28. Foley K. Management of cancer pain. In: DeVita VT, Hellman S, Rosenberg S, eds. Cancer: principles and practice of oncology. 4th ed. Philadelphia: JB Lippincott, 1993:2417–2448.

29. Dickson RB, Lippman ME. Estrogenic regulation of growth and polypeptide growth factor secretion in human breast carcinoma. Endocr Rev 1987;8:29–43.

30. Lippman ME, Dickson RB, Gelmann EP, et al. Growth regulation of human breast carcinoma occurs through regulated growth factor secretion. J Cell Biochem 1987;35:1–16.

31. VanderBurg B, deGroot RP, Isbrucker L, et al. Direct stimulation by estrogen of growth factor signal transduction pathways in human breast cancer cells. J Steroid Biochem Mol Biol 1992;43:111–115.

32. Philips A, Chalbas D, Rochefort H. Estradiol increases and antiestrogen antagonizes growth factor-induced activator protein-1 activity in MCF-7 breast cancer cells without affecting C-FOS and C-Jun synthesis. J Biol Chem 1993;268:14103–14108.

33. Miner JN, Diamond MI, Yamamoto KR. Joints in the regulatory lattice: composite regulation by steroid receptor-AP1 complexes. Cell Growth Differ 1991; 2:525–530.

34. Schule R, Evans RM. Cross-coupling of signal transduction pathways: zinc finger meets leucine zipper. Trends Genet 1991;7:377–381.

35. Umayahara Y, Kawamori R, Watada H, et al. Estrogen regulation of the insulin-like growth factor 1 gene transcription involves an AP-1 enhancer. J Biol Chem 1994;269:16433–16442.

36. Mader S, Kumar V, deVernevil H, Chambon P. Three amino acids of the estrogen receptor are essential to its ability to distinguish an estrogen from a glucocorticoid responsive element. Nature 1989;338:271–274.

37. Krishnan V, Wang S, Safe S. Estrogen receptor-SP1 complexes mediate estrogen-induced cathepsin O gene expression in MCF-7 human breast cancer cells. J Biol Chem 1994;269:15912–15917.

38. Halachmi S, Marden E, Martin G, et al. Estrogen receptor associated proteins possible mediators of hormone induced transcription. Science 1994; 264:1455–1458.

39. Butler B, Kirland WL, Jorgenson TL. Induction of plasminogen activator by estrogen in a human breast cancer cell line (MCF-7). Biochem Biophys Res Commun 1979:90:1328–1334.

40. Huggins C, Hodges CV. Studies in prostatic cancer. I. The effect of castration estrogens and androgen injections on serum phosphatases in metastatic carcinoma of the prostate. Cancer Res 1941;1:293–297.

41. Horton RJ. Androgen hormones and prehor-

mones in young and elderly men. In: Grayhack JT, Wilson JD, Scherbenske MJ, eds. Benign prostatic hyperplasia. Proceedings of a workshop sponsored by the Kidney Disease and Urology Program of the NIAMDD. Washington, DC: U.S. Government Printing Office, 1976:183–188.

42. Lipsett MB. Steroid secretion by the human testes. In: Rosenberg E, Paulson CA, eds. The human testes. New York: Plenum Press 1979:407–421.

43. Sandberg AA. Endocrine control and physiology of the prostate. Prostate 1980;1:169–184.

44. Schally AV, Comaru-Schally AM, Redding TW. Antitumor effects of analogues of hypothalamic hormones in endocrine-dependent cancers (41797). Proc Soc Exp Biol Med 1984;175:259–281.

45. Schally AV, Kastin AJ, Arimura A. FSH-releasing hormone and LH-releasing hormone. Vitam Horm 1972;30:83–164.

46. Schally AV, Arimura A, Coy DH. Recent approaches to fertility control based on derivatives of LH-RH. Vitam Horm 1980;38:257–323.

47. Monahan MW, Amoss MS, Anderson HA, Vale W. Synthetic analog of the hypothalamic luteinizing hormone releasing factor with increased agonist or antagonist properties. Biochemistry 1973;12:4616–4620.

48. Coy DH, Vilchez-Martinez JA, Loy EJ, Schally AV. Analog of luteinizing hormone-releasing hormone with increased biological activity produced by D-amino acid substitutes in position 6. J Med Chem 1976; 19:423–428.

49. Peets EA, Henson MF, Neri R. On the mechanism of the antiandrogen action of flutamide in the rat. Endocrinology 1974;94:532–540.

50. Fujino M, Kobayashi S, Obayashi M, et al. Structure-activity relationships in the C-terminal part of luteinizing hormone releasing hormone (LHRH). Biochem Biophys Res Commun 1972;49:863–869.

51. Walsh PC. Physiologic basis for hormonal therapy in carcinoma of the prostate. Urol Clin North Am 1975;2:125–140.

52. Knabbe C, Kellner U, Schmahl M, Voigt KD. Suramin inhibits growth of human prostate carcinoma cells by inactivation of growth factor action (abstract). Proc Am Assoc Cancer Res 1980;30:295.

53. Schuurmans ALG, Bolt J, Berns PMJJ, Mulder E. Androgen receptor mediated regulation of growth and epidermal growth factor receptor level in the human prostate tumor cell LNCaP. In: Bresciani F, King RJB, Lippman ME, Raynaud JP, eds. Progress in cancer research and therapy. New York: Raven Press 1988:154–157.

54. Hsueh AJW, Dufau ML, Catt KJ. Direct inhibitory effect of estrogen on Leydig cell function of hypophysectomized rats. Endocrinology 1978;103:1096–1102.

55. Seftel AD, Spirnan JP, Resnick MJ. Hormonal therapy for advanced prostatic carcinoma. J Surg Oncol 1989;1(Suppl):14–20.

56. Kennedy BJ. Hormonal therapies in breast cancer. Semin Oncol 1974;1:119–130.

57. McGuire WL, Clark GM, Hubay CA, et al. Role of steroid hormone receptors as prognostic factors in primary breast cancer. NCI Monogr 1986;1:19–33.

58. Paridaens R, Sylvester RJ, Ferrazi E, et al. Clinical significance of the quantitative assessment of estrogen receptors in advanced breast cancer. Cancer 1980;46:2889–2895.

59. Lippman ME, Allegra JC. Estrogen receptor and endocrine therapy of breast cancer. N Engl J Med 1978;299:930–933.

60. Cutler S. Classification of extent of disease in breast cancer. Semin Oncol 1974;1:91–96.

61. Henderson IC, Cannelos GP. Cancer of the breast: the past decade. N Engl J Med 1980;302:17–30, 78–90.

62. Kennedy BJ. Massive estrogen administration in premenopausal women with metastatic breast cancer. Cancer 1962;15:641–648.

63. Carter AC, Sedransk N, Kelley RM, et al. Diethylstilbestrol: recommended dosages for different categories of breast cancer patients. JAMA 1977;237:2079–2085.

64. Byar DP. The Veterans Administration Cooperative Urological Research Group's studies of cancer of the prostate. Cancer 1973;32(5):1126–1130.

65. Schearer RJ, Hendry WF, Sommerville IF, et al. Plasma testosterone: an accurate monitor of hormone treatment in prostatic cancer. Br J Urol 1973;45:668–677.

66. Eisenberger M, O'Dwyer PF, Friedman M. Gonadotropin hormone releasing hormone: a new therapeutic approach for the treatment of prostate cancer. J Clin Oncol 1986;4:414–424.

67. Clarysse A. Hormone-induced tumor flare. Eur J Clin Oncol 1985;21:545–548.

68. Henderson IC. Treatment of metastases. In: Harris JR, Hellman S, Henderson IC, Kinne DW, eds. Breast diseases. Philadelphia: JB Lippincott 1987:398–428.

69. Hall TC, Dedrick MM, Nevinny HB. Prognostic value of hormonally induced hypercalcemia in breast cancer. Cancer Chemother Rep 1963;30:21–26.

70. VanderBurg B, Kalkhoven E, Isbrucker L, deLaat SW. Effects of progestins on the proliferation of estrogen-dependent human breast cancer cells under growth defined conditions. J Steroid Biochem Mol Biol 1992;42:457–465.

71. Jeng MH, Jordan VC. Growth stimulation and differential regulation of transforming growth factor-α1 (TGFα1), TGFα2, and TGFα3 messenger RNA levels by norethindrone in MCF-7 human breast cancer cells. Mol Endocrinol 1991;5:1120–1128.

72. Alkhalaf M, Murphy LC. Regulation of C-Jun and Jun-B by progestins in T47D human breast cancer cells. Mol Endocrinol 1992;6:1625–1633.

73. Beato M. Gene regulation by steroid hormones. Cell 1989;56:335–344.

74. Beck CA, Weigel NL, Edwards DP. Effects of hormone and cellular modulators of protein phosphorylation of human progesterone receptors. Mol Endocrinol 1992;6:607–620.

75. Tsai M-J, O'Malley BW. Molecular mechanisms of action of steroid/thyroid superfamily members. Annu Rev Biochem 1994;63:451–486.

76. Horwitz KB, McGuire WL. Estrogen control of progesterone receptor in human breast cancer: correlation with nuclear processing of estrogen receptor. J Biol Chem 1978;253:2223–2228.

77. Hissom JR, Moore MR. Progestin effects on the growth in the human breast cancer cell line T-47D—possible therapeutic implications. Biochem Biophys Res Commun 1987;145:706–711.

78. Vignon F, Bardon S, Chalbos D, Rochefort H. Antiestrogenic effect of R5020, a synthetic progestin in

human breast cancer cells in culture. J Clin Endocrinol Metab 1983;56:1124–1130.

79. Murphy LC, Murphy LJ, Dubin D, Bell GI, Shin RPC. Expression of the gene encoding epidermal growth factor in human breast cancer cells. Regulation by progestins. Cancer Res 1988;48:4555–4560.

80. Murphy LC, Murphy LJ, Shiu RPC. Progestin regulation of EGF-reception mRNA accumulation in T47D human breast cancer cells. Biochem Biophys Res Commun 1988;156:192–195.

81. Muphy LC, Dotzliu H. Regulation of transforming growth factor alpha and transforming growth factor-beta mRNA abundance in T47D human breast cancer cells. Mol Endocrinol 1989;3:611–617.

82. Hamburger AW, Parnes H, Gordan GB, et al. Megestrol acetate-induced differentiation of 3t3-L1 adipocytes in-vitro. Semin Oncol 1988;12(Suppl 1):76–78.

83. Aisner J, Tcheckmedyian NS, Tait N, et al. Studies of high dose megestrol acetate: potential applications to cachexia. Semin Oncol 1988;12(Suppl 1):68–75.

84. Van Roenn JH, Murphy RL, Weber KM, et al. Megestrol acetate for treatment of cachexia associated with human immunodeficiency virus (HIV) infection. Ann Intern Med 1988;109:840–841.

85. Lelli G, Angelli B, Giambiasi ME, et al. The anabolic effect of high dose medroxyprogesterone acetate in oncology. Pharmacol Res Comm 1983;15:561–568.

86. Sedlacek SM. An overview of megestrol acetate for the treatment of advanced breast cancer. Semin Oncol 1988;15(Suppl 1):3–13.

87. Wentz WB. Progestin therapy in lesions of the endometrium. Semin Oncol 1985;12(Suppl 1):23–27.

88. Caneta R, Florentine S, Hunter H, et al. Megestrol acetate. Cancer Treat Rev 1983;10:141–157.

89. Bonomi P, Pessis D, Bunting N, et al. Megestrol acetate used as primary hormonal therapy in stage D prostatic cancer. Semin Oncol 1985;12(Suppl 1):36–39.

90. Geisler HE. The use of high-dose megestrol acetate in the treatment of ovarian adenocarcinoma. Semin Oncol 1985;12(Suppl 1):20–22.

91. Tchekmedyian NS, Tait N, Moody M, et al. Megestrol acetate in cancer anorexia and weight loss. Cancer 1992;69:1268–1274.

92. Loprenzi CL, Ellison NM, Schaid DJ, et al. Controlled trial of megestrol acetate for the treatment of cancer anorexia and cachexia. J Natl Cancer Inst 1990;82:1127–1132.

93. Von Roenn JH, Armstrong D, Kotler DP, et al. Megestrol acetate in patients with AIDS-related cachexia. Ann Intern Med 1994;121:393–399.

94. Oster MH, Enders SR, Samuels SJ, et al. Megestrol acetate in patients with AIDS and cachexia. Ann Intern Med 1994;121:400–408.

95. Stoll BA. Progestin therapy of breast cancer: comparison of agents. Br Med J 1967;3:338–341.

96. Ettinger DS, Allegra J, Bertino LR, et al. Megestrol acetate versus tamoxifen in advanced breast cancer: correlation of hormone receptors and response. Semin Oncol 1986;13(Suppl 4):9–14.

97. Johnson PA, Muss H, Bonomi P, et al. Megestrol acetate as primary therapy for advanced breast cancer. Semin Oncol 1988;(Suppl 1):34–37.

98. Carpenter JT, Peterson L. Use of megestrol acetate in advanced breast cancer on a single-daily-dose schedule. Semin Oncol 1985;(Suppl 1):40–42.

99. Camaggi CM, Strocchi E, Giovannini M, et al. Medroxyprogesterone acetate (MAP) plasma levels after multiple high dose administration in advanced cancer patients. Cancer Chemother Pharmacol 1983;11:19–22.

100. Pannuti F, Martoni A. Di Marco AR, et al. Prospective, randomized clinical trial of two different high dosages of medroxyprogesterone acetate in the treatment of metastatic breast cancer. Eur J Cancer 1979;15:593–601.

101. Muss HB, Case LD, Capizzi RL, Cooper MR, Cruz J, et al. High- versus standard-dose megestrol acetate in women with advanced breast cancer. A phase III trial of the Piedmont Oncology Association. J Clin Oncol 1990;8:1797–1805.

102. Alexieva-Figusch J, Blankenstein MA, Hop WCJ, et al. Treatment of metastatic breast cancer patients with different dosages of megestrol acetate: dose relations, metabolic and endocrine effects. Eur J Cancer Clin Oncol 1984;20:33–40.

103. Abrams JS, Cirrincione C, Aisner J, et al. A phase III trial of megestrol acetate (MA) in metastatic breast cancer (MBC) (abstract). Proc Am Soc Clin Oncol 1992;11:56.

104. Wentz WB. Progestin therapy in endometrial hyperplasia. Gynecol Oncol 1974;2:362–367.

105. Steiner GJ, Kistner RW, Craig JM. Histological effects of progestins on hyperplasia and carcinoma in-situ of the endometrium: further observations. Metabolism 1965;14:356–386.

106. Geisler HE. The use of megestrol acetate in the treatment of advanced malignant lesions of the endometrium. Gynecol Oncol 1973;1:340–344.

107. Bonte J, Decoster MJ, Ide P, et al. Hormonoprophylaxis and hormonotherapy in the treatment of endometrial adenocarcinoma by means of medroxyprogesterone acetate. Gynecol Oncol 1978;6:60–75.

108. Malkasian GD Jr, Decker DG, Mussey E, et al. Progestogen treatment of recurrent endometrial carcinoma. Am J Obstet Gynecol 1971;110:15–21.

109. Beck RP. Experience in treating two-hundred and eighty-eight patients with endometrial carcinoma from 1968 to 1972. Am J Obstet Gynecol 1979;133:260–267.

110. Wentz WB. Progestin therapy in lesions of the endometrium. Semin Oncol 1985;12(Suppl 1):23–27.

111. Karlstedt K. Progesterone treatment for local recurrence and metastases in carcinoma corpus uteri. Acta Radiol (Stockh) 1971;10:187–192.

112. Wait RB. Megestrol acetate in the management of advanced endometrial carcinoma. Obstet Gynecol 1973;41:129–136.

113. Geller J, Albert JD. Comparison of various hormonal therapies for prostatic carcinoma. Semin Oncol 1983;10(Suppl 4):34–41.

114. Geller J, Albert J, Yen SSC, et al. Medical castration of males with megestrol acetate and small doses of diethylstilbestrol. J Clin Endocrinol Metab 1981;52(3):576–580.

115. Geller J. Rationale for blockade of adrenal as well as testicular androgens in the treatment of advanced prostate cancer. Semin Oncol 1985;12(Suppl 1):28–35.

116. Kottmeier HL. Carcinoma of the female genitalia. Baltimore: Williams & Wilkins, 1953.

117. Galli MC, DeGiovanni C, Nicoletti G, et al. The occurrence of multiple steroid hormone receptors in

disease-free and neoplastic human ovary. Cancer 1981; 41:1297–1302.

118. Geisler HE. The use of high-dose megestrol acetate in the treatment of ovarian adenocarcinoma. Semin Oncol 1985;12(Suppl 1):20–22.

119. Bloom HJG. Medroxyprogesterone acetate (Provera) in the treatment of metastatic renal cancer. Br J Cancer 1971;25:250–265.

120. Santen RJ, Worgul TJ, Samojlik E, et al. Randomized trial comparing surgical adrenalectomy with aminoglutethimide plus hydrocortisone in women with advanced breast cancer. N Engl J Med 1981; 305:545–551.

121. Schweitzer RJ. Oophorectomy/adrenalectomy. Cancer 1980;46:1061–1065.

122. Puga FJ, Welch JS, Bisel HF. Therapeutic oophorectomy in disseminated carcinoma of the breast. Arch Surg 1976;111:877–880.

123. Radvin RG, Lewison EF, Slack NH, et al. Results of a clinical trial concerning the worth of prophylactic oophorectomy for breast cancer. Surg Gynecol Obstet 1970;131:1055–1064.

124. Kennedy BJ, Fortuny IE. Therapeutic castration in the treatment of advanced breast cancer. Cancer 1964;17:1197–1202.

125. Meakin JW, Allt WEC, Beale FA, et al. Ovarian irradiation and prednisone following surgery for carcinoma of the breast. In: Salmon SE, Jones SE, eds. Adjuvant therapy of cancer. 1st ed. Amsterdam: North-Holland Press, 1977:95–100.

126. Early Breast Cancer Trialists Collaborative Group. Systemic or Immune Therapy: 133 randomized trials involving 31,000 recurrences and 24,000 deaths among 75,000 women. Lancet 339;1992:1–15, 71–85.

127. Kraybill WG, Kaufman R, Kinne D. Treatment of advanced male breast cancer. Cancer 1981;47:2185–2189.

128. Smith JA Jr. New methods of endocrine treatment of prostatic cancer. J Urol 1987;137:1–10.

129. Gronemeyer H. Transcription activation for estrogen and progesterone receptors. Annu Rev Gev Genet 1991;25:89–123.

130. Lerner LJ, Jordan VC. Development of antiestrogens and their use in breast cancer: eighth Cain memorial aware lecture. Cancer Res 1990;50:4177–4189.

131. Fawell SE, White R, Hoare S, et al. Inhibition of estrogen reception—DNA binding by the "pure" antiestrogen ICI 164,384 appears to be mediated by impaired receptor dimerization. Proc Natl Acad Sci USA 1990;87–6883–6887.

132. Ylikomi T, Bocquel MT, Berry M, et al. Cooperation of protosignals for nuclear accumulation of estrogen and progesterone receptors. EMBO 1992; 11:3681–3694.

133. Wosikowsui K, Kung W, Hasmonn M, et al. Inhibition of growth factor activated proliferation by anti-estrogens and effects on early gene expression by MCF-7 cells. Int J Cancer 1993;53:290–297.

134. Nolvadex Adjuvant Trial Organization. Controlled trial of tamoxifen as a single adjuvant agent in the management of early breast cancer. Br J Cancer 1988;37:608–611.

135. Knabbe C, Lippman ME, Wakefield LM, et al. Evidence that TGF-α is a hormonally regulated negative growth factor in human breast cancer. Cells 1984; 48:417–428.

136. Colletta AA, Wakefield LM, Howell FV, et al. Antiestrogens induce the secretion of active TGF-α from human fetal fibroblasts. Br J Cancer 1990;62:405–409.

137. Butta A, MacLennan K, Flandurn KC, et al. Induction of transforming growth factor α1 in human breast cancer in vivo following tamoxifen treatment. Cancer Res 1992;52:4261–4264.

138. Katzenellenbogen BS. Antiestrogen resistance: mechanisms by which breast cancer cells undermine the effectiveness of endocrine therapy. J Natl Cancer Inst 1991;83:1434–1435.

139. Osborne CK, Coronado E, Allfred DC, et al. Acquired tamoxifen resistance: correlation with reduced breast tumor levels of tamoxifen and isomerization of trans-4-hydroxytamoxifen. J Natl Cancer Inst 1991;83:1477–1482.

140. Wright PS, Cross-Doersen DE, Chmielewski PA, et al. m-RNA levels in tumor xenografts with quantitative audioradiography and in-situ hybridization. FASEB J 1995;9:279–283.

141. Jordan VC. Antiestrogenic and antitumor properties of tamoxifen in laboratory animals. Cancer Treat Rep 1976;60:1409–1414.

142. Tagnon HJ. Antiestrogens in the treatment of breast cancer. Cancer 1977;39:2959–2964.

143. Kiang DT, Kennedy BJ. Tamoxifen (antiestrogen) therapy in advanced breast cancer. Ann Intern Med 1977;87:687–690.

144. Mouridsen H, Palshof T, Patterson J, et al. Tamoxifen in advanced breast cancer. Cancer Treat Rev 1978;5:131–141.

145. Ingle JN, Krook JE, Green SJ, et al. Randomized trial of bilateral oophorectomy versus tamoxifen in premenopausal women with metastatic breast cancer. J Clin Oncol 1986;4:178–186.

146. Planting AS, Alexieva-Figusch J, Blonk van der Ivijst J, et al. Tamoxifen therapy in premenopausal women with metastatic breast cancer. Cancer Treat Rep 1985;69:363–385.

147. Kalman AM, Thompson T, Vogel CL. Response to oophorectomy after tamoxifen failure in premenopausal breast cancer. Cancer Treat Rep 1982; 66:1867–1868.

148. Brodie AMH. Aromatase inhibition and its pharmacological implications. Biochem Pharmacol 1985;34:3213–3219.

149. Santen RJ, Lipton A, Harvey H, et al. Use of aminoglutethimide and hydrocortisone as a 'medical adrenalectomy' for treatment of breast carcinoma. Prog Clin Cancer 1982;8:245–265.

150. Coombes RC, Goss P, Dowsett M, et al. 4-Hydroxyandrostenedione in treatment of postmenopausal patients with advanced breast cancer. Lancet 1984;2:1237–1239.

151. Havlin KA, Trump DL. Aminoglutethimide: theoretical considerations and clinical results in advanced prostate cancer. Cancer Treat Res 1988;39:83–96.

152. Zava DT, McGuire WL. Androgen action through estrogen receptor in a human breast cancer cell line. Endocrinology 1978;103:624–631.

153. Lippman M, Bolan G, Huff K. The effects of androgens and antiestrogens on hormone responsive breast cancer in long term tissue culture. Cancer Res 1976;36:4610–4618.

154. Neri R, Kassem N. Biological and clinical

properties of antiandrogens. Prog Cancer Res Ther 1984;31:507–518.

155. Fleshner N, Trachtenberg J. Novel androgen ablation in advanced prostatic carcinoma with minimal side effects (abstract). J Urol 1993;149(Suppl):258A.

156. Newling DWW for the Casodex Study Group. The response of advanced prostate cancer to a new non-steroidal antiandrogen: results of a multicenter open phase II study of casodex. Eur Urol 1990;18(3 Suppl):18–21.

157. Blackledge G. Casodex—mechanisms of action and opportunities for usage. Cancer Suppl 1993; 72:3830–3833.

158. Kaisary AV. Current clinical studies with a new non-steroidal antiandrogen, Casodex. Prostate Suppl 1994;5:27–33.

159. Sandow J. Clinical application of LHRH and its analogues. Clin Endocrinol 1983;18:571–592.

160. Clayton RN, Catt KJ. Gonadotropin-releasing hormone receptors: characterization, physiological regulation, and relationship to reproductive function. Endocrinol Rev 1981;2:186–203.

161. The Leuprolide Study Group. Leuprolide versus diethylstilbestrol for metastatic prostate cancer. N Engl J Med 1984;311(20):1281–1286.

162. Griffiths K, Eaton CL, Harper ME, et al. Hormonal treatment of advanced disease: some newer aspects. Semin Oncol 1994;21:672–687.

163. Crawford ED, Eisenberger MA, McCleod D, et al. Leuprolide with and without flutamide: a controlled double blind clinical trial. N Engl J Med 1989; 321(6):419–424.

164. Dennis LJ, Whelan P, Carneiro de Moura JL, et al. Goserelin acetate and flutamide versus bilateral orchiectomy: a phase III EORTC trial (30853). Urology 1993;42:119–130.

165. Bertagna C, De Gery A, Hucher M, et al. Efficacy of the combination of nilutamide plus orchiectomy in patients with metastatic prostatic cancer. A meta-analysis of seven randomized double-blind trials (1056 patients). Br J Urol 1994;73:396–402.

166. Trump DC, Havlin K, Messing E, et al. High dose ketoconazole in advanced hormone-refractory prostate cancer: endocrinologic and clinical effects. J Clin Oncol 1989;7:1093–1098.

Part 2 _____

L-Asparaginase

Alan P. Lyss

NOMENCLATURE

Generic name: L-asparaginase

Sources: *Escherichia coli* L-asparaginase (EC 3.5.1.1, NSC-109229); *Erwinia carotovora* L-asparaginase (NSC-106977); Polyethylene glycol (PEG)–modified *E. coli* L-asparaginase.

Commercial names: Elspar (*E. coli* L-asparaginase), Oncaspar (PEG-L-asparaginase).

Chemical name: L-asparaginase

Antitumor Activity

The single clinical indication for use of L-asparaginase is in the induction therapy of acute lymphoblastic leukemia (ALL). L-asparaginase as a single agent has yielded complete remission (CR) rates of 50 to 60% in ALL patients (1, 2). But remissions tend to be short-lived when L-asparaginase is continued as a single agent, with median remission durations of only 1 to 8 months. Therefore, this agent is usually used in combination with other antileukemic drugs (3). Among patients who experience a relapse, 30 to 50% of prior L-asparaginase responders will obtain a CR to reinduction therapy (2).

L-Asparaginase has minor activity against other hematologic malignancies (e.g., acute non-lymphocytic leukemia, blast crisis of chronic myelogenous leukemia) and no activity against a variety of solid tumors (2).

Mechanism of Action

In 1953 it was appreciated that guinea pig serum had antitumor activity, which was especially marked in the therapy of ALL and which was shown to reside in the enzyme L-asparaginase. Discovery of *E. coli* L-asparaginase resulted in the availability of large quantities of the enzyme and allowed the mechanism of action, pharmacology, and clinical usefulness of L-asparaginase to be studied further (1).

L-Asparaginase hydrolyzes L-asparagine to aspartic acid and ammonia, which results in a cellular deficiency of L-asparagine. Normal human cells and resistant tumor cells have high levels of asparagine synthetase, which allows them to synthesize additional L-asparaginase endogenously. Sensitive tumor cells lack asparagine synthetase and, therefore, require exogenous sources of L-asparagine. Treatment of sensitive tumors with L-asparaginase results in rapid inhibition of protein synthesis and delayed inhibition of DNA and RNA synthesis. As sensitive tumor cells become resistant to the drug, they develop high levels of asparagine synthetase and, therefore, the capability to synthesize L-asparagine from endogenous sources. Unfortunately, various measurements of in vitro effects of asparagine deprivation and in vivo measurement of asparagine synthetase and L-asparagine levels have failed to predict ultimate clinical response to therapy with L-asparaginase (2, 4).

Pharmacology

The volume of distribution for L-asparaginase is slightly greater than plasma volume, and there is indirect evidence that the drug may be sequestered within organs such as the liver. L-Asparaginase does not cross the blood-brain barrier, although responses in central nervous system leukemia have been described (2), possibly due to depletion of the CSF of L-asparagine that is derived from the circulating pool (5). The half-life after intravenous injection of *E. coli* L-asparaginase is 8 to 30 hours (1). Plasma half-life is shorter for *Erwinia* L-asparaginase and considerably longer for PEG L-asparaginase (5.73 ± 3.24 days) (6). Plasma levels after intramuscular injection are approximately 10 to 50% of those achieved after intravenous administration (2, 7). *E. coli* L-asparaginase may be detectable in plasma for 3 weeks after high doses, and PEG L-asparaginase may be detectable after standard doses for more than 26 days. In hypersensitive individuals, plasma clearance of L-asparaginase may be greatly accelerated (6, 7).

Availability and Storage

L-Asparaginase is supplied in 10-mL sterile vials that contain 10,000 IU of asparaginase and 80 mg mannitol in a white lyophilized powder or plug with no preservatives. The drug may be given either intravenously or intramuscularly. Vials should be stored at 2 to 8°C.

Preparation and Use

For intravenous use, each vial should be reconstituted with 5 mL of sterile water for injection or sodium chloride injection. This solution should be stored at 2 to 8°C and should be given within 8 hours following reconstitution.

For intramuscular use, each vial should be reconstituted with 2 mL sodium chloride injection and should be administered within 8 hours and only if clear. The reconstituted drug should be stored at 2 to 8°C until administration.

Administration

When administered by intravenous infusion, the reconstituted vials should be diluted with isotonic solutions of sodium chloride injection or 5% dextrose injection. If a small number of gelatinous fiberlike particles are noted after standing, filtration through a 5.0 micron filter during administration will remove the particles with no loss in potency. When administered intravenously, the drug should be given over no less than 30 minutes through the side arm of an infusion of 0.9% normal saline solution (NS) or D5W.

For intramuscular administration, the volume given at a single injection site should be limited to 2 mL. If more than 2 mL is required, a greater number of injection sites should be used.

Dosage

The usual doses of *E. coli* or *Erwinia* L-asparaginase in the induction therapy of ALL are 6000 IU/m² every other day for 3 to 4 weeks or daily doses of 1,000 to 20,000 IU/m² for 10 to 20 days (7). For PEG L-asparaginase, standard doses are 2000 to 2500 IU/m² every 14 days (9). As noted above, L-asparaginase is almost never used as a single agent for induction of remission in these patients and is most commonly used in regimens that employ vincristine, prednisone, and other agents.

Side Effects and Toxicities

In general, the toxic effects of L-asparaginase are due to hypersensitivity reactions and to the inhibitory effects of the drug on protein synthesis. This agent is not cytotoxic to bone marrow stem cells, oral and gastrointestinal tract mucosa, or hair follicles (2). Side effects are generally worse in adults than in children (3), may be dose-related (2, 8), and are usually reversible after discontinuation of therapy (2).

Hypersensitivity phenomena, including fever, dermatoses (especially urticaria), dyspnea, hypotension, agitation, and epigastric pain, are seen in 25% of patients and may not occur with continuation of therapy (2).

Anaphylaxis occurs in approximately 10% of patients and is more common with intravenous than with intramuscular administration and with intermittent (weekly or monthly) than with continuous (daily or thrice weekly) schedules. Skin testing is not helpful in determining risk of anaphylaxis, but the appearance of passive hemagglutinating antibody titers plus rapid plasma clearance of L-asparaginase may have prognostic utility (2). Patients who have received prior *E. coli* L-asparaginase should be treated with *Erwinia* L-asparaginase or PEG L-asparaginase if reinduction courses are required after an initial relapse (3, 9).

General malaise, anorexia, mild nausea, and vomiting are commonly observed during therapy and may result in weight loss in 25% of patients. Liver enzyme abnormalities are common, may correlate with hepatic steatosis upon histologic examination of the liver, and are transient, disappearing after treatment has been discontinued (1). Severe hepatotoxicity is seen in less than 5% of cases. Similarly, mild changes in renal function are common (34%) but result in acute renal failure (apart from renal failure due to rapid tumor lysis) in only 1% of cases (3). Severe transient hyperlipidemia has been described, but it is asymptomatic, nonprogressive after therapy is stopped, and requires no modification of treatment (10).

Effects of L-asparaginase on the pancreas are protean. Nonketotic hyperglycemia has been observed and has been associated with decreased levels of insulin. The hyperglycemia is easily controlled with exogenous insulin and disappears after therapy with L-asparaginase has been discontinued (1). Hypoamylasemia is common and is associated with clinical evidence of pancreatitis in 7% of patients (1, 3). Pancreatic toxicity is dose related and necessitates cessation of therapy (1).

L-Asparaginase causes predictable and very common effects on hemostatic factors, with reductions in fibrinogen and other clotting factors (factors IX and XI, antithrombin III, proteins C and S, histidine-rich glycoprotein, and α_2-macroglobulin) and fibrinolytic enzymes (plasminogen and α_2-antiplasmin) in 60 to 100% of treated patients (3, 8). Clinical bleeding is observed in less than 1% of patients, however, despite continuation of therapy with L-asparaginase.

Thrombotic and hemorrhagic events most commonly affect the central nervous system (CNS) and are approximately equally frequent, with cortical infarction, capsular infarction, intracerebral hemorrhage, hemorrhagic infarction, and cerebral venous and dural sinus thrombosis described (8). Symptoms may include headache, alterations in mental status, seizures, hemiparesis, and/or vomiting. Therapy for thrombotic and hemorrhagic events has varied, but the outcome of CNS events has been generally good, with 63% of pediatric patients recovering from neurologic deficits, and only 12% dying of neurologic causes (8). Second neurologic events have not been described in patients who required additional therapy with L-asparaginase, although some patients were preventatively treated with fresh frozen plasma infusions on the days of L-asparaginase therapy when retreatment was instituted (8).

CNS symptoms that were unassociated with cerebrovascular complications of L-asparaginase have been noted and include hallucinations, "fugue states," and inappropriate behavior. Diffuse slowing on electroencephalography has been described. These CNS effects have improved with discontinuation of therapy (1).

REFERENCES

1. Whitecar JP, Bodey GP, Harris JE, et al. L-Asparaginase. N Engl J Med 1970;282:732–734.
2. Capizzi RL, Bertino JR, Handschumacher RE. L-Asparaginase. Annu Rev Med 1970;21:433–442.
3. Investigational Drug Branch (Cancer Therapy Evaluation Program, National Cancer Institute). Guidelines for the use of L-asparaginase (EC-2, NSC-109229) and (Erwinia, NSC-106977). May 1978.
4. Capizzi RL, Bertino JR, Skeel RT, et al. L-Asparaginase. Ann Intern Med 1971;74:893–901.
5. Dibenedetto SP, Di Cataldo A, Ragusa R, Meli C, Lo Nigro L. Levels of L-asparagine in CSF after intramuscular administration of asparaginase from Erwinia in children with acute lymphoblastic leukemia. J Clin Oncol 1995;13:339–344.
6. Asselin BL, Whitin JC, Coppola DJ, Rupp IP, Sallan SE, Cohen HJ. Comparative pharmacokinetic studies of three asparaginase preparations. J Clin Oncol 1993;11:1780–1786.
7. Chabner BA, Myers CE. Clinical pharmacology of cancer chemotherapy. In: DeVita VT, Hellman S, Rosenberg SA, eds. Cancer: principles and practice of oncology. 3rd ed. Philadelphia: JB Lippincott, 1989:349–395.
8. Feinberg WM, Swanson MR. Cerebrovascular complications of L-asparaginase therapy. Neurology 1988;38:127–133.
9. Ettinger LJ, Kurtzberg J, Voute PA, Jurgens H, Halpern SL. An open-label, multicenter study of polyethylene glycol-l-asparaginase for the treatment of acute lymnphoblastic leukemia. Cancer 1995;75:1176–1181.
10. Steinherz PG. Transient severe hyperlipidemia in patients with acute lymphoblastic leukemia treated with prednisone and asparaginase. Cancer 1994;74:3234–3239.

26

Investigational Drugs

Daniel R. Budman and Stuart M. Lichtman

The hope for the eventual cure of malignancy rests with the development of safer agents with enhanced antitumor spectrums. As the effort to develop such agents spans many continents and innumerable laboratories, a review of new agents entering into clinical trials and other substances still under investigation can only be an overview that rapidly becomes dated. In addition, many pharmaceutical companies are becoming active in this area, leading to a plethora of unique substances in preclinical testing.

A variety of substances are currently being evaluated in the clinic (Table 26.1), and a profusion of biologic agents have been developed since the last issue of this text. Many of these agents are the result of maturing recombinant technology and therefore offer the advantage of being able to be produced in large quantities. Other biologic substances such as immunotoxins may be of value for in vivo treatment and also for in vitro purging of bone marrow contaminated with small numbers of neoplastic cells. First- and second-generation immunotoxins are currently being evaluated at several centers, and the ability to humanize these agents has made them more attractive. The ability, with emerging molecular biologic techniques, to make fusion proteins with antibodies or growth factor agonists is an exciting development for new approaches in the clinic (1). A variant of this scheme, involving the linking of a drug-activating enzyme to a specific monoclonal antibody to enhance specificity of the cytotoxic action (ADEPT), is also under active study (2, 3). In the ADEPT system, prodrugs are administered that are specifically activated by the modified monoclonal antibody, thus leading to a high microenvironment of cytotoxic drug (4).

Likewise, maturational agents (especially for myelodysplasia and for promyelocytic leukemia) and chemopreventive substances (including retinoids) remain under active study (5). In an analogous manner, numerous agents are approaching clinical trial that act on the controls of cell division (6, 7). The EORTC (European Organization for Research and Treatment of Cancer) has specifically targeted agents that interfere with cell cycle control as a high priority area for drug development (8). These agents (Table 26.2) may offer unique methods for controlling neoplastic growth. For example, the various isoforms of protein kinase C are believed to play a pivotal role in cellular proliferation. Signal transduction inhibitors may offer a entirely different approach to the treatment of neoplastic disease (9, 10). These substances demonstrate antitumor activity.

Antisense oligonucleotides are being pursued as both antiviral and antineoplastic agents and may thus offer a unique modality of treatment (9, 10). The efforts to introduce tumor suppressor genes into laboratory model systems to turn off uncontrolled growth may eventually reach clinical trial (11). As most patients die from the consequences of disseminated disease, inhibitors of metastatic potential have also received attention lately (12, 13). Investigators have also followed up leads in tumor-induced neovascularization. Inhibitors of angiogenesis, which are just being understood, have recently entered the clinic for evaluation in Kaposi's sarcoma and may also play a major role in the control of other solid tumors (12, 13). The ability of molecular genetics to modify growth factors by selected amino acid substitutions and thus make antagonists of function also offers exciting avenues for future therapeutic advances.

The field of photodynamic therapy, using an agent that concentrates in tumor tissue which is then activated by light, remains under intense study in numerous countries, with several agents in clinical trials, and many more in pre-

Table 26.1. New Agents in Clinical Trials

Classical cytotoxics (analogues/novel compounds)
Biochemical modulators of cytotoxic drug metabolism
Lipid encapsulation of cytotoxic compounds
Modulators of toxicity
Inhibitors of cellular repair mechanisms
Inhibitors of angiogenesis
Inhibitors of drug resistance
Maturational substances
Chemopreventive substances
Biologics
   Growth factors
   White cell response modifiers
   Immunotoxins
   Fusion proteins
Antiemetics
Inhibitors of bone reabsorption

Table 26.2. Agents Approaching Clinical Trials

Analogues of growth factors
Antisense oligodeoxynucleotides
Cytotoxics
   Analogues of existing compounds
   Novel substances
Fusion proteins
Inhibitors of metastatic potential
Signal transduction inhibitors
Bioactive peptides (combinatorial chemistry)

clinical testing. Radiation sensitizers exploiting the hypoxic environs of solid tumors ("bioreductive therapy") offer new avenues of tumor control (14–16).

Since the last edition of this text, the paradigm for drug discovery has been shifting from intensive structure-function analysis of a few candidate molecules to combinatorial chemistry, which allows the generation of up to 10^{11} molecules, selection of the molecule of interest, and generation of large quantities of the agent (17–20). These new techniques allow the generation of diverse molecules at reasonable cost and have the ability to isolate substances with high affinities for a target such as an enzyme or a receptor. This technique has been mainly applied to the generation of polypeptides, and these discoveries will eventually impinge on many areas of medicine. Interesting oligonucleotides can also be prepared with this technique, allowing new approaches using the power of molecular biology (19). Most of the results of these new approaches with combinatorial chemistry remain proprietary at the time of this assessment but are expected to have a major impact on the management of malignant disease.

This review deals with the more mundane classical cytotoxic agents, modifiers of drug toxicity, inhibitors of cellular repair, maturational agents, angiogenesis agents, and antagonists of endocrine action, which represent the majority of preclinical and clinical investigative work at the present time. These areas of intense research are more mature and will, in the immediate future, more directly affect the clinically oriented physician. Several additional materials are of use to the research physician: (*a*) for in vitro studies of standard and some experimental agents, the reviews of Dr. Andrew G. Bosanquet are slightly dated but remain invaluable for defining stability and compatibility (21); (*b*) for investigational agents sponsored by the National Cancer Institute, the Pharmaceutical Resources Branch publishes a comprehensive yearly compendium of investigational agents, describing their structures, manner of preparation of the clinical material, solution preparation, storage, and stability of each agent (22); (*c*) for investigational agents sponsored by the EORTC, their New Drug Office is of great value (23); and (*d*) for investigational agents sponsored by the pharmaceutical industry, a clinical brochure is on file with the FDA and is available to appropriate investigators.

The development of a new anticancer agent should follow the criteria in Table 26.3. A new drug is virtually useless if the compound cannot be extracted in sufficient quantities from natural sources or synthesized in bulk. Small molecules or amino acid structures that can be produced by bioengineering are obviously preferable to complex polycyclic structures. Shelf stability is a major concern when distribution of a potent

Table 26.3. Characteristics of an Ideal New Agent

Easily formulated
Long shelf life stability
Water soluble; light stable
Stable in intravenous solutions
Wide antitumor spectrum
Nonmutagenic; nonteratogenic
Enhanced therapeutic index
Bioavailable by the oral route
Able to penetrate the CNS
Minimal schedule dependency

drug to many parts of the world is undertaken. For commercial applications of a given agent, stability is of great concern, as storage conditions may not always follow strict pharmaceutical guidelines. Insufficient solubility of a drug has inhibited the development of scores of agents that could not be given in a clinically relevant amount of fluid. On the other hand, lipophilicity may be useful for the penetration of cell membranes and the central nervous system (CNS). Structure-function analysis of anticancer compounds usually indicates that a combination of water solubility and some lipophilicity is desirable. Lack of schedule dependency, which allows outpatient treatment in times of shrinking economic support for inpatient services, is also a concern. With the development of long-term survivors of neoplasia after drug treatment, the problems of the carcinogenicity, teratogenicity, and induction of sterility must be addressed (24, 25). Finally, even the huge cost of drug development must be considered (26), with the sponsorship of the National Cancer Institute (NCI) and the EORTC accelerating agents that otherwise would not reach the clinic in a timely fashion.

Investigational agents may arise from a variety of sources, as discussed in the chapter on antineoplastic drug development (Chapter 2). However, many of the currently available investigational anticancer agents are based upon analogue development. This pathway has been very successful in related pharmaceutical fields such as antibiotics, antihypertensives, and psychotropics. Much of the drug methodology from these fields can be adopted to antineoplastic drug development (Table 26.4), with the caveat that demonstration of superiority of the analogue over the parent compound can be very difficult. Thousands of analogues of each major class of anticancer drug have been prepared, of

Table 26.4. Rationale for Analogue Development

Known antitumor activity in parent compound
Basic analytic techniques for pharmacology already exist for the patent compound
Production methodology for basic structure known
Ability to compare chemical structure—function of the congeners with parent drug
Possibility of enhanced antitumor spectrum
Possibility of different pharmacokinetic profile
Possibility of reduced or absent side effects

which only a handful actually survive to be tested in the clinic.

This review of new agents covers only information available in the public domain as the result of meeting presentations and publications. As such, some of the information about some of the newer agents remains fragmentary, and the physician should always contact the pharmaceutical sponsor for more detailed information. When possible, each drug has been grouped by putative mechanism of action.

ALKYL-LYSOPHOSPHOLIPIDS

The alkyl-lysophospholipids, a class of surface-membrane-active substances, have not shown as much promise as expected, because of systemic toxicity when administered parenterally. However, they are of interest, as their mechanisms of action may include interference with cell signal message transduction (27), production of interleukin-2 (IL-2), macrophage activation, enhancement of cytotoxic effect by classical agents (28), and membrane peroxidation (29). Blocking of cells in G_1 and G_2 phases of the cell cycle, suggesting discrete mechanisms of inhibition, has been reported (30). These agents inhibit protein kinase C signal transduction and prevent binding of the tumor-promoting substances, phorbol esters, to HL-60 cells in vitro (31). The alkyl-phosphocholines of this group are also known to inhibit phospholipase C and phospholipase D, suggesting additional mechanisms of action (32, 33). In addition, cell culture experiments have demonstrated reduced binding of epidermal growth factor receptors in the presence of these drugs, leading to inhibition of growth in MCF-7 and ZR-75-1 hormone-dependent breast cancer lines (34). Apoptosis is induced in human leukemic cell lines by exposure to these compounds over 24 hours (35).

Compounds of this class have detergent characteristics, and structure-function studies have noted that antitumor properties correlate with the ether-linked aliphatic side chain in the sn-1 position of glycerol (36). A long alkyl chain with a polar head group is a necessary requirement for antitumor effect (37). Current structural data suggest that a 16- to 18-carbon chain at the sn-1 position with a substitution at sn-2 gives the best therapeutic index in vitro (38).

However, cell lines can differ significantly in their sensitivity to these agents and may even show growth stimulatory effects at low concentrations of these agents (39). In addition, the cell growth conditions may modify the results. For example, analogues of this class of agents were found to inhibit tumor cells in suspension but not in cluster formation in soft agar (40). The incorporation of these drugs into liposomes has enhanced their antitumor activity, thus suggesting their reevaluation in systemic treatment of malignant disease (41). In xenograft models, human estrogen-receptor-negative breast tumors were sensitive, while receptor-positive tumors were not, and incorporation into liposomes reduced toxicity (42). The mechanism of this differential cytotoxic effect remains unknown but suggests that entry criteria in future human trials may influence response rate.

ET-18-OCH₃ (1-O-octadecyl-2–O-methyl-rac-glycero-3-phosphocholine) causes an increase in membrane fluidity, is active in human xenografts, and must be bound to albumin prior to infusion, to prevent hemolysis (36). This drug had major toxicity when studied in man, with pulmonary edema and hepatotoxicity reported. An oral preparation was also poorly tolerated (43). Recent work has concentrated on the use of this agent in in vitro purging of malignant cells, with particular emphasis on leukemia (44). Early clinical trials have suggested benefit with this approach (45).

HEXADECYLPHOSPHOCHOLINE (Miltefosine; D 18506; NSC-605583) is active in preclinical screens (46) and in topical administration in breast cancer (47). In animal models, miltefosine is very active against *Leishmania*, suggesting additional uses for the drug (48). This agent is active in methylnitrosourea-induced rat breast carcinoma, with marked differences of cytotoxicity measured by the type of growth system used (49). In vitro, the parent compound was found to be more active than the metabolites (50). No receptor mechanism has been identified as necessary for cellular uptake of this compound (51). As with other members of this class, this drug has several other functions, including an stimulatory effect on hematopoietic cytokines (52). In the rat, this compound accumulated in the kidney and tumor tissue (53).

Clinical studies with this agent have been under way in Europe for several years. A phase I study of the oral formulation revealed dose-limiting nausea/vomiting and nephrotoxicity with suggested phase II dosing of 150 mg/day in divided doses (54). Retinal changes that are reversible have been noted in patients evaluated 2 months after initiation of this drug, which may portend a major difficulty in using this agent

(55). The oral schedule has been studied in colorectal carcinoma, producing nephrotoxicity, nausea/vomiting, leukocytosis, and thrombocytosis, with only minor activity (56). Cutaneous studies have continued with an overview of 412 patients with breast cancer treated in a variety of trials showing a major response rate of 27% (57). In cutaneous lymphoma, this drug has shown major activity, with major response rates around 50% in two studies at different institutions (58, 59). Histologically complete remissions were uncommon (58). Side effects of the topical application of this drug included pruritus in approximately one-third of patients, erythemia, xerodermia, exfoliation, paresthesia, and local pain (57). A heterocyclic analogue of miltefosine, OMPEP (octadecyl-[2-(*N*-methylpiperidino) ethyl]-phosphate), has shown a better therapeutic index in preclinical testing, with marked activity in rat mammary carcinoma (60).

ILMOFOSINE (BM41-440; 1-hexadecylthio-2-methoxymethyl-rac-glycero-3-phosphocholine; NSC 601679) was found to be one of the most potent compounds of this class and was studied in the human tumor stem cell assay showing activity at 10 μg/mL against lung carcinomas, gastrointestinal carcinomas, ovarian tumors, and hypernephromas (61). In vitro, this compound was found to downregulate cdc2 kinase activity and cause a cell cycle arrest in G_2 (62). The drug inhibits protein kinase C and interferes with the expression of the oncogene *c-fos* (27). In murine models, a dose-dependent suppression of tumor growth was noted. The drug can be administered orally (63). The drug as been studied in humans on two schedules: (*a*) a single- or multiple-dose oral administration on 1 day, and (*b*) a daily oral treatment for 8 weeks (64). A coated-film tablet was felt to slightly lessen nausea and vomiting. The maximum tolerated dose (MTD), defined by nausea, vomiting, and diarrhea, occurred at 7 mg/kg in the single-dose study. On the multiple-day schedule, the MTD was felt to be above 5 mg/kg/day with phase II doses at that level (64). A multicenter phase II study in metastatic carcinoma, including a variety of tumor types, reported no activity when the drug was administered orally at a dosage of 150–300 mg/day. Severe nausea/vomiting and loss of appetite occurred in two-thirds of patients (65). A new phase I study of this drug by the intravenous route has been reported with antitumor activity in non-small-cell lung cancer, ovarian carcinoma, and hypernephroma (66). Four intravenous schedules have been evaluated: (*a*) a single bolus every 28 days, (b) a 5-day schedule every 28 days, (c) a 120-hour continuous schedule every 21 days, and (d) a 7- and 10-day continuous infusion every 28 days. Dose-limiting toxicity in the single bolus schedule was hemolysis; the prolonged infusions gave hepatic, renal, and pulmonary toxicity (66). The 120-hour schedule has been adopted for the phase II trials in the United States.

ALKYLATORS

Research interest in this area of cytotoxic therapy has lessened with the concern about secondary malignancies and the lack of apparent benefit of newer compounds over established agents. Several drugs remain in experimental evaluation, but whether or not these agents will reach commercial approval for widespread use remains in doubt. Of this group, the DTIC analogues have generated the most interest in the United States.

ACNU (Nimustine; 3-((4-amino-2-methyl-5-pyrimidinyl)methyl)-1(2-chloroethyl)-1-nitrosourea hydrochloride; NSC-245382) is a water-soluble nitrosourea that advanced to clinical studies on the basis of its preclinical screen (67, 68) and its ability to cross the blood-brain barrier. Its major mode of action seems to be alkylation of DNA with minor carbamoylating function. In tissue culture, ACNU is unstable (69), with its cytotoxic action a function of the concentration of the drug over time (AUC) and of the speed of decomposition of parent compound (69). Resistance to the drug seems to be mediated by O^6-methyl-guanine-DNA methyltransferase (MGMT) (70). Unfortunately, in a male Wistar rat screen, ACNU is carcinogenic, as are other nitrosoureas (71). This drug has been best studied in Japan, with the dose-limiting toxicity of myelosuppression occurring at weeks 5 to 6 posttreatment (72). The MTD was 101.8 to 135.7 mg/m² as an intravenous bolus. As it can act as a radiation sensitizer, the Japanese investigators have given ACNU as a weekly bolus (30 mg/m² × 4) with standard radiation therapy to patients with nonsmall carcinoma of the lung. In a randomized study, a statistically higher complete response (CR) rate was noted in the arm receiving ACNU, although median survival in this arm was only 6 weeks longer than in the control. ACNU has been given at 100 mg/m² every 6 weeks in patients with refractory small cell carcinoma of the lung. All patients had been heavily pretreated with chemotherapy. The total response rate was 9% (13% in patients not previously exposed to CCNU). Major toxicities were leukopenia (median nadir, 2,500/μL) and thrombocytopenia (median nadir, 47,000/μL). Nausea and vomiting were also seen in 50% of patients (73). An EORTC trial confirmed minimal activity in previously treated patients (74). The same every-6-week schedule has been evaluated in untreated patients with colorectal carcinoma. One of nine evaluable patients achieved a partial response (PR), with hematologic toxicity similar to that of the previously described trial (75). It has also been used in the treatment of acute leukemia (76).

CNS disease has been treated with this drug. In a long-term follow-up of patients with glioma treated by various regimens, the highest CR rate (23%) was in patients treated by interferon, ACNU, and radiotherapy (77). A benefit was seen in the treatment of intracerebral non-Hodgkin's lymphoma by intraarterial administration of ACNU at doses of 80 to 100 mg/m²/injection (78). ACNU has been given by the intraventricular and intrathecal routes in humans, based upon pharmacologic data in beagle and rat models (79, 80). However, the drug is rapidly cleared from the CSF (mean half-life, 27 ± 7.4 min), as it is from the plasma (mean half-life, 29 min), and thus would not be expected to adequately mix throughout the CSF (79). Intrathecal pharmacokinetics have been evaluated, showing a maximum concentration of 9.86 to 12.79 μg/mL; the AUC was 260.8 to 502.2 μg/min/mL (81).

BZQ (2,5-diaziridinyl-3,6-bis(2-hydroxyethylamino-1,4-benzoquinone; NSC-224070) is another of the hundreds of benzoquinone derivatives that have been prepared. This more hydrophilic analogue of AZQ showed preclinical activity against P388, L1210, B16 melanocarcinoma, and intracerebral tumors. MTD was determined to be 33 mg/m², with a recommended phase II dose of 25 mg/m² given as an intravenous infusion. Nausea, vomiting, and anemia (mechanism not specified) were felt to be dose-limiting toxicities. Partial responses were seen in Hodgkin's and non-Hodgkin's lymphoma (82). This drug is potentially attractive, as it lacks the solubility problem of AZQ, penetrates the CNS (at least in animals), and is not myelosuppressive.

FOTEMUSTINE (S-10036; Servier 10036; diethyl-1-(3-(2-chloroethyl)-3-nitrosoureido)ethylphosphonate) is a nitrosourea analogue with a phosphonoalanine moiety, which is active against a large preclinical screen, has decreased mutagenicity, and has dose-limiting hematologic toxicity in animals (83). The drug does display the solubility problem of the classical nitrosoureas, must be dissolved in ethanol, and then administered in 5% glucose as a 1-hour intravenous infusion. In solution, it is stable for at least 4 hours. A phase I trial in France giving fotemustine on days 1, 8, 15, and 22, with a 4-week observation time posttreatment, revealed dose-limiting side effects to be thrombocytopenia at or above 100 mg/m^2/week. Myelosuppression was evidenced by a thrombocytopenic nadir at day 35 (duration, days 22–47) and a leukopenic nadir at day 42 (duration, days 36–47). Other toxicities were dose-related nausea and vomiting (above 125 mg/m^2/week) and occasional transient liver function abnormalities (83). Pharmacokinetics of fotemustine are limited to eight solid tumor patients, with the plasma drug levels determined by high-pressure liquid chromatography (HPLC). High intrapatient and interpatient variations in pharmacokinetic parameters were noted. Plasma half-life was 21 minutes, but clearance varied from 1 to 170 L/hr (84). A phase I trial in hematologic malignancies with a weekly × 3 induction schedule of fotemustine, followed by a once-every-3-week maintenance schedule, showed identical dose-limiting toxicities as indicated above. Responses were seen in Hodgkin's disease, non-Hodgkin's lymphoma, and chronic lymphocytic leukemia (85).

Experience with this agent is rapidly developing, with several phase II studies completed. The agent, given at 100 mg/m^2/week × 3 to 4, has a 27% response rate in malignant melanoma and is active in both previously treated and untreated patients (86). This study was expanded to 153 patients, giving a major response rate of 24%; the major toxicities were thrombocytopenia and leukopenia (87). It has activity in treating cerebral metastases with a 22.2% response rate (88).

The combination of fotemustine and dacarbazine (DTIC) has been studied in metastatic disease. Dacarabazine was administered 3 hours prior to fotemustine, to deplete cells of the DNA repair enzyme O^6-alkyltransferase activity, which may mediate nitrosourea resistance. There was a 33% response, with a 50% complete response of lung metastases (89). Acute lung toxicity is occasionally seen (90). A 26% response was also observed with this combination with the main side effects of thrombocytopenia and nausea (91). Increasing the DTIC dose does not appear to affect response but does increase hematologic toxicity (92).

This agent has also been used to treat gliomas, with a major response rate of 24% in recurrent disease (93). Fotemustine has been combined with radiation to treat newly diagnosed patients with gliomas, with acceptable toxicity (94). In recurrent disease, an objective response rate of 26.3% was observed. There was also a 16.7% response in brain metastases from non-small-cell lung cancer and 24.3% from melanoma (95).

No responses were seen in renal cell cancer refractory to immunotherapy (96). Fotemustine-5-fluorouracil (5-FU) combinations have been evaluated in vitro (97), and a sarcoma trial has been reported (98).

This drug has been used as a substitute for BCNU in an autologous marrow transplant program. Pharmacokinetics of these high dosages (150 mg/m^2/day × 2 and 300 mg/m^2/day × 1) showed a large interpatient difference, with AUC (total drug exposure in the serum) not related to dose. The plasma half-life was short (23 ± 10 min), with a tremendous variability in clearance (99).

Activity in non-small-cell lung cancer has also been observed. A response rate of 11% in previously treated and 26% in untreated patients was demonstrated (100). Another trial, using 100 mg/m^2 on days 1 and 8, had a 13.5% response rate (101). The cisplatin-fotemustine combination had a 23% response with acceptable toxicity (102).

Obviously, this drug will only be of use if it can be shown to have less toxicity than the traditional nitrosoureas, as it seems to have the same spectrum of activity in man. A model to predict hematologic toxicity is being developed with tumor type, age, and previous therapy (103).

HEPSULFAM (1,7-heptanediol disulfamate; NSC-329680) is an alkylating agent with structural similarities to busulfan that has activity in cell lines resistant to the latter agent. The drug causes DNA cross-strand linking and protein-DNA cross-linking. In preclinical studies, it causes thrombocytopenia and has activity in solid human tumor xenografts and human tumor cell lines (104–106).

MAFOSFAMIDE (ASTA Z 7557; MAFO; mafosfamide-cyclohexamine; cis-4-sulfoethyl-thio-cyclophosphamide; (2-(bis-(2-chloroethyl))-amino-cis-4-((2-sulfoethyl)-thio)-tetrahydro-2-H-1,3,2 oxaza-phosphorine-r-2-oxide cyclohexylamine salt; NSC-345842) is a member of the oxazaphosphorine group of alkylators and is related to cyclophosphamide. This class of drugs has been an area of active investigation for decades by Astra Pharma AG and has one of the broadest antitumor spectrums in man (107). Cyclophosphamide undergoes biotransformation into the reactive species, 4-hydroxy-cyclophosphamide (4-hydroxy-CP) in the liver. 4-hydroxy-CP and its hydrolysis product, phosphoramide mustard, are believed to be responsible for many of the biologic effects of this group of compounds. However, 4-hydroxy-CP is unstable, even at reduced temperatures (108). More stable derivatives such as 4-hydroperoxy-CP (4-HC) have been synthesized and are used for in vitro marrow purging (109). Mafosfamide was synthesized as a cyclophosphamide analogue in which an activated oxazaphosphorine would be stable in a solid state, water soluble, stable for 2 hours in solution, and capable of rapid hydrolysis to 4-hydroxy-CP (108). Mafosfamide may have potential synergism with other anticancer agents that activate the apoptotic cascade (110). This agent also has immunomodulatory activity at doses lower than used in classical cytotoxic therapy (111, 112). In animal systems, low doses of mafosfamide allowed expression of antitumor responses (113) and interfered with suppressor lymphocyte function (114).

As an antineoplastic agent, mafosfamide in man has an MTD of 1000 mg/m^2 given as a slow intravenous infusion over 2 to 3 hours (115). Severe side effects of pain in the injected vein and the sensation of burning of the mucous membranes of the mouth, nose, and throat led to abandonment of this agent as a classical cytotoxic (115). Unfortunately, even low doses of this drug in man (25 mg/m^2 i.v.) have resulted in venous irritation (112). Dose-related nausea (at or above 800 mg/m^2) and conjunctival irritation were other side effects. Minor leukocyte depression at days 14 to 16 occurred at the high-dose levels (115). The pain in the vein was felt to be a result of endothelial exposure to active alkylating metabolites; coinfusion of mesna prevented this symptom (107). Using this admixture (mesna 9 mg/mL with mafosfamide 6 mg/mL), the MTD was 3000 mg/m^2 (107).

However, the major use of this compound lies in in vitro marrow purging (116, 117). Successful transplantation after mafosfamide purging has been seen in non-Hodgkin's lymphoma (118), acute leukemia (119), and myelodysplastic syndromes (120). Mafosfamide-treated bone marrow may have a role to play in autologous transplantation for Philadelphia-positive chronic myelogenous leukemia (121–123).

MITOLACTOL (Dibromodulcitol; galactitol; DBD; NSC-104800) is an alkylating hexitol given orally. Enthusiasm for this agent in the United States has waned after an initial flurry of interest in breast and gynecologic malignancies. European investigations with this agent have continued. A recent phase I study of the combination of mitolactol and 5-FU has indicated that 1500 mg/m^2 of DBD can be given on day 1 p.o. with 1000 mg/m^2 of 5-FU by intravenous infusion over 4 hours daily × 4. Leukopenia, nausea, and vomiting were present but not dose-limiting. Remarkably, one CR and two PRs were noted in six evaluable patients with cervical carcinoma (124). This agent has also been evaluated for future use as a topical agent in localized carcinoma of the cervix. In animals, topical vaginal application resulted in only 1% of the dose absorbed into the systemic circulation (125).

PCNU (1-(2-chloroethyl)-3-(2,6-dioxo-3-piperidyl)-1-nitrosourea; NSC-95466) is another of the nitrosourea analogues that have undergone phase II trials. This agent has high alkylating activity and low carbamoylating activity (126). It was very active in the animal tumor screens and showed a lack of schedule dependency. The drug suffers from a lack of easy solubility in water and must first be reconstituted in N,N-dimethylacetamide, with further dilution in propylene glycol. Cumulative myelosuppression, as is seen with other nitrosoureas, was noted (127). Thrombocytopenia is dose limiting. In phase II trials, PCNU was given at 75 to 100 mg/m^2 as an intravenous infusion every 6 weeks. A response rate of 16% in malignant melanoma was noted (128). PCNU has been studied in gliomas in a phase I intracarotid trial. Dosages between 60 and 110 mg/m^2 were administered, with thrombocytopenia, headaches, restlessness, orbital pain, and ipsilateral visual impairment as major toxicities. Not all of these toxicities were reversible. A major response rate of 44% in glioma was noted (129). This agent suffers the generic problem of many analogues in that its therapeutic index is not improved over that of the parent compound, which precludes major interest in its development (130, 131).

TCNU (LS 2667; 1-(2-chlorethyl)-3-(2-(dimethyl-amino-sulphonyl) ethyl)-1-nitrosourea; tauromustine; NSC-608678) has generated much interest in Europe on the basis of being a novel nitrosourea having an amino acid linked to its active structure. Taurine was chosen as a carrier of the nitrosourea on the basis of information that this amino acid interacted with membrane phospholipids and was carrier mediated. This agent also demonstrated greater hydrophilicity than the older nitrosoureas. The degradation rate of TCNU increases in buffered aqueous solutions at pH above 4 (132).

In preclinical tumor screens, this agent was active against nitrosourea-resistant tumors and demonstrated greater antitumor activity than previous nitrosoureas (133, 134). Animal toxicology studies indicated that this agent may be less hepatotoxic than lomustine (CCNU) (134). However, TCNU is a marrow stem cell poison in mice, analogous to the classical nitrosoureas, and can cause chromosomal aberrations (135, 136). The metabolites of this compound formed by successive demethylation (LS 2724 and LS 2715) also damage marrow cells (137).

In a human small-cell xenograft, TCNU was curative. The activity inversely correlated with the amount of O^6-alkyl-guanine transferase (Mer-cell line) (138). The amount of this DNA-repair enzyme had been shown previously to be important in the cytotoxic action of nitrosoureas (139), which indicated that TCNU shared a common mechanism with other drugs of this class. The mode of action of this agent appeared to be cross-linking of DNA. Two major phase I trials have been completed. In the trial in the United Kingdom (140), dosages from 10 to 150 mg/m^2 p.o. once every 6 weeks were evaluated, with dose-limiting toxicity of thrombocytopenia (nadir, weeks 3 to 5). Leukopenia sometimes persisted for up to 8 weeks posttreatment. Cumulative hematopoietic toxicity was noted. In addition, nausea and vomiting were dose related, occurring at dosages above 70 mg/m^2. Pharmacokinetics were described by a biphasic decay with a terminal half-life of 60 minutes.

Major antitumor responses were seen in small cell carcinoma of the lung, squamous cell carcinoma of the lung, melanoma, hypernephroma, and gastric cancer. Only the melanoma patients had received previous chemotherapy (140). The Finsen Institute study (141) noted the cumulative marrow-suppressive properties of this drug, with thrombocytopenia and leukopenia being most common. Transient liver function abnormalities, diaphoresis, and tumor pain were other common findings. Doses from 20 to 170 mg/m^2 given once every 4 to 6 weeks were studied. Significant antitumor activity was noted in non-small-cell carcinoma of the lung. Pharmacokinetic studies pooled from the two institutions show a biphasic decay at higher doses and cir-

culating parent compound in the blood for up to 8 hours. The terminal half-life was 57 ± 22 minutes, with peak plasma values at 38 ± 22 minutes after oral administration.

Of interest for future possible pharmacodynamic control studies, the degree of thrombocytopenia could be correlated with the maximal concentration of the drug in the plasma (C_{max}) or the AUC (142). A formula to optimize the drug dose based upon height, weight, and platelet count has been developed (143). Phase II trials of TCNU given as a single oral dose of 130 to 150 mg/m^2 every 4 to 5 weeks have shown activity in chemotherapy-naive patients with non-small-cell lung carcinoma (144). Delayed cumulative thrombocytopenia (especially after three or more treatment cycles) and nausea and vomiting were significant problems. Transient hepatotoxicity was also noted (144). In previously treated patients with breast cancer, a response rate of 7% was obtained. Hematologic toxicity and virtually universal nausea and vomiting were major problems at drug dosages of 90 mg/m^2 in heavily pretreated and 110 mg/m^2 in minimally pretreated patients (145).

TCNU has been given to patients undergoing craniotomy for gliomas. In contrast to some of the previously described agents, TCNU achieves significant levels in the CNS (146). The major problem for the further development of this compound is the cumulative thrombocytopenia and pervasive nausea and vomiting seen as side effects. Analogues of this agent may therefore be of more use. Its activity in lung carcinoma is of great interest.

TCNU has been evaluated in colorectal cancers (147). 5-FU causes alterations in the pharmacokinetic profile of TCNU. Simultaneous administration of these two drugs or pretreatment with 5-FU decreases the plasma levels of TCNU by a factor of 2.5 to 3 over those obtained when TCNU was given alone (148). Synergism was observed when 5-FU was given after TCNU (149). A phase I trial determined a weekly oral dose of TCNU 40 mg/m^2, weeks 1 through 4, in combination with 400 mg/m^2 5-FU and 80 mg/m^2 leucovorin, once a week, weeks 1 through 8 (150).

CYSTEMUSTINE, a new chloro-2-ethyl nitrosourea derivative, has undergone clinical trials. Its major side effects were neutropenia and thrombocytopenia. No activity was observed in metastatic colorectal cancer, with minimal activity in other solid tumors (151–153). Increased activity was seen in glioma patients (153). In a phase II melanoma trial, increased activity was seen with increasing the dose from 60 to 90 mg/m² every 2 weeks (154).

TEMOZOLOMIDE (CCRG 81045; M & B 39831; 8-carbamoyl-3-methyl-imidazo (5,1-D)-1,2,3,5-tetrazin-4(3H)-one; NSC-362856) is an analogue of dacarbazine (DTIC) developed to spontaneously hydrolyze into the active metabolite MTIC (5-(3-methyltriazen-1-yl) imidazole-4-carboxamide), which is believed to be responsible for the antitumor effect. It is believed to be a DNA-methylating agent (155). In mice, the enzymatic conversion of DTIC into MTIC is efficient and rapid. By contrast, in man, DTIC is poorly converted into MTIC. Temozolomide is nonenzymatically converted into MTIC and has broad preclinical antitumor activity, particularly in brain tumors. The drug may be synergistic with other nitrosoureas (156, 157). The degree of antitumor effect correlates with the amount of MTIC generated and cumulative depletion of O^6-alkylguanine-DNA-alkyltransferase (ATase) (158–160). In human plasma, the compound is unstable, with a half-life of 24 minutes. In addition, a DTIC-resistant L1210 cell line is also resistant to this compound (156). This cell line has high levels of O^6-methylguanine-DNA methyltransferase, suggesting a mode of resistance similar to nitrosourea resistance (161).

The drug has been studied in a phase I trial in humans (162). It is dissolved in dimethyl sulfoxide (DMSO) (163) and given in normal saline over 1 hour (164). The compound can also be given by mouth, as it is virtually completely absorbed (163). Pharmacokinetic studies have suggested a possible enterohepatic circulation with a terminal plasma half-life of 1.8 hours (164). The discordance between the in vitro half-life and the in vivo half-life is not explained. Minor tumor responses have been seen (163). The drug may have activity in primary brain tumors (165). The phase I studies showed dose-limiting myelosuppression (155). No clinical responses were seen in a single-dose schedule repeated every 4 weeks, but when the dose was given over 5 days, responses were seen in melanoma, mycosis fungoides, and astrocytoma. The recommended phase II dose is 150 mg/m² p.o. for 5 days with dose escalations (155). A phase I study in children was done using a single oral dose on a daily × 5 schedule (166). After doses of 100 to 215 mg/m², peak plasma concentrations of 3.3 to 15.3 µg/mL were achieved.

Plasma clearance was related to body size, and lower interpatient variability was observed when values were adjusted to weight rather than surface area (166).

CB 10-277 (1-p-carboxyl-3,3-dimethylphenyl-triazene) is a phenyl dimethyltriazene DTIC analogue that, like dacarbazine, requires metabolic activation to its corresponding monomethyl species for antitumor activity (167). In preclinical models, its spectrum and level of activity were similar to those of dacarbazine. A phase I trial of short infusions showed the dose-limiting toxicity to be nausea and vomiting, which occurred in 80% of evaluable courses at 900 mg/m². Another common side effect was flushing (75% of courses). Responses occurred in melanoma, sarcoma, and carcinoid tumors. The AUC increased linearly with dose. Metabolism was evidenced by the presence of the monomethyl species (167). Responses were observed in patients with the highest leukocyte O^6-methyldeoxyguanosine levels and depletion of O^6-alkylguanine-DNA-alkyltransferase. The formation of the former compound in DNA is a critical cytotoxic event, while the formation of the latter can confer resistance to these agents (168, 169). In a phase I 24-hour continuous infusion trial, the dose-limiting toxicity was myelosuppression. The monomethyl metabolite AUC and the associated myelosuppression were more favorable than in the short infusion trial. The recommended phase II dose was 12,000 mg/m² (170). A phase II trial in this dose unfortunately did not show any significant activity (171).

EO9 ([3-hydroxy-5-aziridinyl-1-methyl-2-(1H-indole-4,7-dione)-propenol]; NSC 382459) is a compound in a series of novel and fully synthetic bioreductive alkylating agents (172). Bioreductive drugs undergo metabolic reduction to generate cytotoxic metabolites. This process is facilitated by the bioreductive enzymes and the lower oxygen conditions present in solid tumors, compared with normal tissue (14). Reduction in pH decreases the chemical stability and increases the cytotoxicity of EO9 (172). Although structurally similar to mitomycin C, preliminary in vitro evaluation of EO9 suggests that it has a different antitumor profile (172). It exerts significant antitumor effect against solid tumor cell lines, with minimal effects against leukemia models (172). The enzyme DT-diaphorase (DTD) may have a prominent role of in the activation of EO9. A direct correlation between DTD activity and tumor sensitivity to EO9 has been demonstrated in human colon carcinoma cell lines (172). An extremely fast excretion ($t_{(1/2)} = 1.9$ min) has been demonstrated, which is related to its rapid metabolic reduction rate (173). A limited-sampling model has been developed (174). A phase I study showed no significant toxicity up to 15 mg/m^2 (175).

KW-2149, 7-*N*-((2-([2-(γ-L-glutamylamino) ethyl]dithio)ethyl) mitomycin C is an analogue of mitomycin C and has in vitro activity against various tumors (176, 177), with possibly less bone marrow toxicity (178). The drug has some activity against mitomycin C–resistant tumors that are deficient in DT-diaphorase (176). The unchanged drug disappears rapidly, with a half-life of 9.7 minutes. Radiolabeled compound was excreted in mouse urine (33%) and feces (58%) within 144 hours. Tumor concentrations were lower than those of plasma or blood, with the lowest in the brain (179). The metabolites M-16 and M-18 do not significantly contribute to the drug's activity (180).

ANTIANDROGENS

The antiandrogen class of agents has been expanding with the realization that prostate cancer is becoming a greater public health problem as the population ages and that palliative therapy can be effectively accomplished with hormonal manipulation, including antagonism of the androgen receptor mechanism (181). Use of these agents as monotherapy has been well tolerated, with a maximum rise of baseline testosterone levels of 50% at 1 month after initiation of treatment in the absence of a luteinizing hormone–releasing hormone (LH/RH) agonist (182). These agents offer an excellent quality of life, as their side effects are usually minor, and they are often combined with an LH/RH agonist to offer "total androgen blockade" (183).

CASODEX (ICI 176334) is an oral antiandrogen in clinical trials that was found nontoxic at dosages from 10 to 150 mg/day, with a dose-response curve demonstrating that 28% of the lowest dose resulted in responses in prostatic carcinoma, with a 68% response at the highest dose level (184). Current recommended dosages are 150 mg/day (185). Breast swelling and/or "hot flushes" were seen in approximately one-third of patients; other toxicities were exceedingly rare (186). Monotherapy is equivalent to that of other drugs of this class (187). Endocrinologic evaluation of this agent revealed that se-

rum gonadotropin levels rise (LH, 100%; FSH, 7%) after treatment, with the total circulating testosterone level rising 66%. Estradiol levels also rose (188). The drug has just become commercially available in the United States (1996).

NILUTAMIDE (Anandron; RU 23908; 5,5-dimethyl-3(4-nitro-3(trifluoromethyl)phenyl)-2,4-imidazolidinedione) is a nonsteroidal antiandrogen that interferes with the androgen receptor but causes a compensatory rise in plasma androgen levels. In animals, bioavailability by the oral route is 70%, leading to an oral formulation for human trials. Pharmacokinetic studies have shown that 49 to 78% of the drug in the form of metabolites is excreted in the urine, a steady-state plasma level is reached after 2 weeks of twice-daily dosing, and chronic administration delays clearance of the drug (189). This drug has been found to rarely cause hepatotoxicity in man (190), and its toxic mechanism has been investigated in rat hepatocytes. Nilutamide is metabolized by the P450 system to a reactive intermediate forming superoxides with oxygen. In the animal model system, glutathione is depleted, leading to oxidative damage to key cellular proteins. This toxic effect could be prevented by increasing dietary thiols in the form of L-cystine (191). Other adverse events observed in man include difficulty with visual adaptation to darkness, transaminitis, and rare pulmonary toxicity (192). In the case of pulmonary toxicity, one large report indicated that patients were treated a mean of 113 days (range, 10 to 225), receiving 150 mg/day of the drug, with total cumulative exposure of 21.8 g (range, 3 to 38 g) (193). Clinical findings included bilateral infiltrates, a restrictive lung pattern on pulmonary functions, lymphocytosis on bronchoalveolar lavage, and reduced oxygen tension, with reversal after the drug was stopped (193). This drug also causes a mild increase in circulating hemoglobin (194).

New data have been emerging regarding the use of this agent as part of a total androgen-blockade treatment of metastatic prostate cancer. In a large European trial, patients were randomized to nilutamide with orchiectomy versus orchiectomy alone. The combination gave a 6.1-month advantage in time to progression and a similar advantage in survival, which were statistically significant (195). An overview analysis of seven randomized trials involving 1191 patients demonstrated the superiority of this drug (50% major response rate) with surgical castration over orchiectomy alone (196). As such, these trials are similar to the North American trials of LH/RH agonists with antiandrogens in metastatic prostate cancer giving "total androgen blockade."

ANTIANGIOGENESIS

Angiogenesis, the formation of new blood vessels, occurs in both normal and pathologic processes. New blood vessel growth occurs normally in ovulation, corpus luteum formation, placental development, wound healing, and exercised muscle (197). Angiogenesis is also associated with pathologic conditions such as tumors, psoriasis, arthritis, inflammation, and ocular disease (197). It has been postulated that tumor growth is angiogenesis dependent, with ample indirect and direct evidence (198, 199). Microvessel count is a good prognostic indicator and may be a useful predictor for the mode of recurrence in gastric carcinoma (200). Therapy using tumor vasculature as a target for therapy is being explored (201).

AGM-1470 (angiogenesis modulator 1470; TNP-470) inhibits proliferation and migration of capillary endothelial cells and inhibits angiogenesis in the chick embryo. It is derived from a family of compounds that are analogues of fumagillin, a naturally secreted antibiotic of *Aspergillus fumigatus fresenius* (199, 202). The compound can enhance B-cell proliferation (203) and inhibit angiogenesis and the growth of some tumors (204, 205). It has recently entered phase I trials (203). Other "antibiotic" angiogenesis inhibitors include herbimycin (206), epoenmycin, erbstatin, and staurosporine (199, 207). Staurosporine is also a potent inhibitor of protein kinases (207).

α_{2a}-*INTERFERON* has antiangiogenic properties (199). Patients with pulmonary capillary hemangiomatosis and systemic hemangiomatosis have been successfully treated (199, 208).

CARBOXYAMINOIMIDAZOLE (CAI; NSC 609974) is a novel inhibitor of signal transduction that inhibits bFGF (fibroblast growth factor)-stimulated endothelial cell proliferation, neural tube formation in vitro, and angiogenesis in the chick embryo chorioallantoic membrane (199). CAI causes inhibition of stimulated calcium influx and inhibits proliferation and migration in vitro and growth and dissemination in human cancer xenografts in vivo (209). It is currently being evaluated in clinical trials (210–213). A phase I study under way noted nausea, vomiting, and neurotoxicity as significant side effects (213). An analysis of CAI metabolites has been reported (212).

CT-2584 (1-(11-dodecylamino-10-hydroxyundecyl)-3,7-dimethylxanthine methanesulfonate) suppresses the production of a number of phosphatidic acid species involved in intracellular signaling as well as acid species critical to tumor cell survival. It suppresses tumor-induced angiogenesis and inhibits matrix metalloproteinase-9 synthesis (214).

THALIDOMIDE is a teratogen that was associated with severe limb defects and other anomalies in babies (199). Orally administered, thalidomide inhibits angiogenesis induced by bFGF in the rabbit cornea (199, 215).

GM 6001 (*N*-[2*R*-2-(hydroxyamidocarbonylmethyl)-4-methylpentanoyl)]-L-tryptophan methylamide) is a matrix metalloprotease inhibitor with antiangiogenic properties (197).

Inhibitors of collagenase have been thought to be antiangiogenic. Minocycline, a semisynthetic tetracycline antibiotic, decreases tumor-induced angiogenesis (216).

DS 4152 is a novel angiogenesis inhibitor isolated from a low-molecular-weight fraction of a sulfated polysaccharide produced by the bacterium *Arthrobacter* (217). It is thought to act by inhibition of the binding of FGF proteins to the endothelial cells. Early phase I data showed some coagulation abnormalities (217). A phase I trial in AIDS-related Kaposi's sarcoma is being conducted (218). Antiangiogenic effects of the quinoline-3-carboxamide linomide have been demonstrated in preclinical models (219).

ANTIESTROGENS

The development of antiestrogens has accelerated by the pharmaceutical industry with the realization of the huge potential market for endocrine manipulation, in both the adjuvant and the metastatic disease settings. However, development of these compounds has been retarded by differing effects in various species and even differences in agonist and antagonist actions between tissues (220). Several of the new antiestrogens show cytostatic effects, even in estrogen-receptor-negative cell lines (221). These antiestrogens also interact with the classical multiple drug resistance protein, P-glycoprotein (222). This class of drugs also shows antiangiogenesis effects (223). In contrast to tamoxifen, two members of this group have not been shown to modify hepatic DNA in animals (224). Whether pure antiestrogens with no agonist activity offer a therapeutic advantage is also under evaluation (225).

DROLOXIFENE (3-hydroxytamoxifen) has recently been reviewed (226) and is in phase III trials in the United States. The drug binds to the estrogen receptor and an antiestrogen protein (antiestrogen binding site), with the presence of estradiol modifying the strength of the binding (227). Droloxifene binding to the estrogen receptor is an order of magnitude tighter than that of tamoxifen (226). This agent prevents insulin-like growth factor-1 (IGF-1) stimulation of MCF-7 cells and downregulates the number of receptors (228). Droloxifene induces the production of TGF-β, is more active than tamoxifen in cell lines, and does not modify DNA by adduct formation as does tamoxifen (229). This agent has membrane antioxidant effects (230). In phase I trials, daily oral drug dosage was studied from 20 to 300 mg, with nausea, fatigue, hot flashes, and one episode of venous thrombosis not dose related (231). Terminal half-life is 1.5 days, in contrast to the prolonged excretion of tamoxifen (226). Phase II trials in metastatic breast cancer confirmed activity, with the major response rate being dose related: 30% at 20 mg/day, 47% at 40 mg/day, and 44% at 100 mg/day (226). FSH and LH were suppressed at the two higher dosage levels. Toxicities paralleled the phase I experience. Other studies have noted that dosages up to 400 mg/day are tolerated, and cumulative toxicity has not been seen. Tumor flare is also very uncommon (226). This drug has definite activity in man, but whether it represents a therapeutic advance or just another analogue remains unclear.

IDOXIFENE (pyrrolidino-4-iodotamoxifen) is another antiestrogen in clinical trials that has been shown to interact with the P-glycoprotein of the multiple drug resistance phenotype and to inhibit calmodulin-dependent cyclic AMP phosphodiesterase. Synergism with cisplatin was seen in human ovarian carcinoma cell lines (232). Results of a phase I trial have been published. This drug has tighter binding to the estrogen receptor than does tamoxifen, twice the terminal half-life of tamoxifen in the rat, and lower agonist activity (233). In man, dosages from 10 to 60 mg/day by the oral route have given a terminal half-life of 23 days, with dose linearity in AUC. After ingestion, peak serum levels occurred at 2 to 8 hours, with steady-state concentrations reached at 6 to 12 weeks. Side effects were similar to those of tamoxifen, and antitumor activity was observed (233). Evaluation of a loading dose schedule is under way to shorten the time to reach steady-state.

ICI 182780 (7-[9-(4,4,5,5-pentafluoropentyl-sulfinyl) nonyl]estra-1,3,5(10)-triene-3,17-diol) is an analogue of estradiol, with no known agonist activity (234). In the mouse, the estrogen receptor remains in the cytoplasm when exposed to this agent (235). In vitro, this drug increases the turnover of the estrogen receptor protein (236). In a tamoxifen-resistant human breast cancer cell line (MCF-7/LCC2), ICI 182780 demonstrated cytostatic effects (237). In tamoxifen-resistant MCF-7 cells, ICI 182780 retained growth inhibition and was 150 to 1540 times more effective in a tamoxifen-sensitive cell line (238). This drug also inhibited the growth of human ovarian carcinoma cell lines in a xenograft model (239). The phase I experience in man investigated dosages of 6 or 18 mg for 7 days. Minor side effects, including headache, dyspepsia, vaginal spotting, facial swelling, and hyperglycemia, were noted but felt not to be drug related. Serum drug levels did not reach steady-state and showed variability between individuals (234). Recently, ICI 182780 has been claimed to be effective in human breast cancer resistant to tamoxifen (240), but this conclusion has been criticized on the basis that the patients were not proven to be truly resistant.

PANOMIFENE (PAN) is an antiestrogen undergoing trials in Hungary. Two doses, 12 and 120 mg, were studied. Terminal half-life was 69 hours. Prolactin levels decreased slightly after a single dose of PAN (241).

TOREMIFENE (Fc-1157A; NK622; 4-chloro-1,2-diphenyl-1-(4(2-(N,N-dimethylamino)ethoxy)phenyl)-1-butene) is an analogue of tamoxifen in which a chloride group is added, resulting in markedly less estrogenic activity in animals than with the parent compound (242, 243). This drug causes chromosomal damage through metabolism by the P450 cytochrome system but less so than tamoxifen (244). In tissue culture, this agent, at levels above concentrations showing classical estrogen-antagonist activity, showed activity against estrogen-receptor-negative cell lines (699). These findings were extended to an estrogen-negative mouse uterine sarcoma in vivo (245). Phase I studies have shown an antiestrogenic effect at 68 mg/day, with a paucity of side effects under 440 mg in short-term dosing. Another phase I trial in Europe found no differences in the hormonal effects of this agent at 60 and 300 mg/day (246). A phase I trial of high-dose toremifene, exploring dosages of 200 to 400 mg/m^2 per day by mouth, noted vomiting, disorientation, and hallucinations at the highest dose level. Reversible corneal pigmentation and classical antiestrogen side effects also occurred. Three metabolites were identified by HPLC (247).

Phase II studies of chronic dosing at 60 mg/day have shown a response comparable to that of tamoxifen (243, 248, 249). A randomized phase III trial of a small number of patients demonstrated statistically equivalent response between the two drugs as primary therapy and no response on a cross-over after failing the initial treatment (250). Side effects were mild and included nausea, hot flushes, and diaphoresis. At 200 mg/day, some patients failing tamoxifen responded (249, 251), but this could not be confirmed in subsequent trials with much larger numbers of patients (252, 253). Antitumor effect has been seen with this agent in a desmoid tumor not responding to tamoxifen (254). There seems to be no significant benefit with this agent over tamoxifen in the clinical management of breast cancer.

RU 58668 is a steroidal antiestrogen, similar to ICI 182780, which has pure antiestrogen effects in animals and has demonstrated a long-term regression in MCF-7 xenograft models. Further development is under way (255).

ANTITUMOR ANTIBIOTICS AND DNA INTERCALATORS

Nowhere in medical oncology have structure-function relationships been studied to such a degree as with anthracyclines and acridine derivatives. The ability to modify these molecules (256), the presence of cell lines with anthracycline resistance (257), and the improvement in the understanding of nucleic acid chemistry have led to specific modifications (258) of the parent molecule to enhance a given biologic effect. The new family of anthracyclines, characterized by a morpholino group, has original features such as direct covalent linking to DNA after cytochrome P450 activation (259). These molecules are active at 100-fold lower concentrations than the other anthracyclines currently available (259). The amount of information about these compounds is voluminous and can only be superficially discussed in this chapter. Most of these drugs have shown antitumor activity. Their ultimate clinical utility will depend on whether they offer a therapeutic advance over the available anthracyclines.

AMONAFIDE (nafidimide; benzisoquinolinedione, 5-amino-2-(2-(dimethyl-amine)ethyl)-1*H*-benz(de) - isoquinoline - 1,3(2*H*) - dione; NSC - 308847) is a novel synthetic agent that combines structural features of other cytotoxics and is believed to act as an intercalator of DNA (260). It is unstable in dextrose solutions. The drug is active in the preclinical tumor screen but shows cross-resistance in cell lines resistant to other DNA intercalators (261). In animal models, some schedule dependency was noted, perhaps due to rapid egress of the drug out of target cells. Pharmacokinetic studies in dogs revealed penetration of the CSF with levels approaching 30% of plasma, significant biliary excretion (17%), and at least three metabolites (262). Amonafide is metabolized to *N*-acetyl-amonafide, and noramonafide. A 2-compartment pharmacokinetic model has been developed. Acetylator phenotyping with caffeine can predict amonafide acetylator status (263).

Phase I studies of single intravenous infusion (264, 265), 24-hour continuous infusion (266), and daily × 5 schedules (261, 265) in solid tumor patients have been completed. One phase I trial of amonifide given over 2 hours daily × 5 has been completed in acute leukemia (267). On the single-dose schedule in patients with solid tumors, the MTD was 1104 (264) to 1125 mg/m^2 (265), with dose-limiting leukopenia. At doses above 519 mg/m^2, acute toxicities such as diaphoresis, flushing, headache, pain at the injection site, tinnitus, and vertigo were noted and could be lessened by prolonging the infusion to 2 hours. The 24-hour schedule noted the onset of leukopenia and thrombocytopenia at 600 mg/m^2 (266). The daily × 5 schedule has been examined in great detail and has been used in phase II trials. On this schedule, myelotoxicity at days 14 to 15 was dose limiting and occurred above 400 mg/m^2/day with significant interpatient variability (261). Recommended phase II dose schedules have been 220 mg/m^2/day × 5 (265) at one institution and 400 mg/m^2/day at another (261). Other toxic effects noted are phlebitis, rash, mild nausea and vomiting, minor alopecia, and rare stomatitis. Pharmacokinetic studies have shown a terminal half-life of 3.5 ± 1.9 hours, with a variable renal excretion from 5 to 45% of the dose in 24 hours (261). Several metabolites are present, and variability in metabolism may explain the broad range seen in myelotoxicity. In leukemia, this drug has been given over 2 to 4 hours daily

$\times$ 5 with an MTD at 1400 mg/m^2/day with significant antitumor effect (267). At the highest dosage level (1800 mg/m^2), rash and mucositis were dose-limiting (267). Activity in refractory leukemias (268, 269) and breast cancer has been reported (270).

Pharmacokinetic studies in the leukemia patients revealed that the AUC was not linearly related to dose at the high levels studied, and metabolic conversion into N-acetylamonafide may allow the metabolite plasma levels to exceed the plasma levels of the parent compound (271). In a phase II study of pancreatic cancer (given at 300 mg/m^2/day over 1 hour $\times$ 5), the amount of N-acetylamonafide correlated with hematologic toxicity (272). A limited-sampling model of two plasma determinations to define the AUC of the parent compound and the N-acetyl derivative has been developed (273, 274). A phase I study of amonafide dosing based on acetylator phenotype was performed (275). The recommended doses for further phase II testing were 250 and 375 mg/m^2. The increased toxicity of fast acetylators was confirmed.

A phase II trial in breast cancer at doses of 800 to 900 mg/m^2 showed a 25% response rate in untreated patients. The patients' acetylator phenotypes were not evaluated or used in dosing (276). Activity in other solid tumors is disappointing. No significant activity has been seen in hypernephroma, colon cancer, or non-small-cell lung cancer (277–279).

A new class of antitumor agents similar to amonafide was synthesized from anthracene. The compound with a 2-(dimethylamino)ethyl side chain, azonafide, has been studied further (280). It was active against ip P388 leukemia and subcutaneous B16 melanoma.

AMSACRINE (m-AMSA; acridinyl anisidide; 4'-(9-acridinylamino)methane-sulfon-*m*-anisidide; N-(4-(9-acridinylamino)-3-methoxy phenyl)-methane-sulfonamide; NSC-249992) has been in clinical trials for over a decade and remains investigational. It has been a disappointment in solid tumors but has been useful in acute leukemia. This drug is one of many acridine derivatives that have a broad antitumor activity in preclinical screens (281) with intercalative properties (282) causing DNA strand breaks and DNA-protein cross-linking. The drug is poorly soluble and is suspended in N,N-dimethylacetamide (DMA), which is added to 0.0353 M L-lactic acid. This drug is then diluted in 5% dextrose and is incompatible with saline solutions (283). On a single-dose schedule in solid tumor patients, the MTD was 160 mg/m^2 as a 60-minute infusion, with myelosuppression (nadir, days 10 to 15) dose-limiting (283). Serum terminal half-life was 2.5 hours (283).

Pharmacokinetics of amsacrine used in combination for treatment of acute leukemia have noted that renal excretion is of minor importance, but hepatic function is critical in elimination of the drug (284). In leukemia, phase I trials have explored numerous schedules, most notably, daily $\times$ 3 and daily $\times$ 5. Continuous infusion schedules for 5 days were ineffective and associated with hyperbilirubinemia (285). Responses in acute leukemia were dose dependent, with most responses at 200 mg/m^2/day $\times$ 5 (286). Myelosuppression, hyperbilirubinemia (in 25% of patients), and dose-limiting mucositis were prominent (286). Nausea, vomiting, alopecia, extravasation necrosis, phlebitis, and cardiac arrhythmias have been reported (287). Cardiac events such as ECG abnormalities (arrhythmia, prolongation of QT interval, ST-T wave changes, premature ventricular contractions, fibrillation), cardiac arrest, and congestive failure may be less common than with the anthracyclines (288). This drug has been used in patients with ventricular arrhythmias (289), and a low level of serum potassium has been claimed to be an inciting factor for toxicity (290). Hypomagnesemia during drug administration is associated with prolongation of the QTc interval and may contribute to the risk of cardiac arrhythmia (291).

The use of this agent in leukemia has been extensively reviewed (292). Used as a single agent, complete remission in advanced leukemia occurs in approximately 20% of patients (292). Combination therapy, such as amsacrine with high-dose cytosine arabinoside, has resulted in high remission rates (293). Amsacrine has been used in the treatment of refractory leukemia. In combination with intermediate- and high-dose cytosine arabinoside, a 41% complete response was seen in CML in accelerated phase and blast crisis (294). However, prolongation of survival was not demonstrated (294). A 48% CR in refractory AML patients treated in combination with intermediate cytosine arabinoside was seen (295).

MITONAFIDE (NSC-300288) is structurally related to amonafide. This drug demonstrates DNA intercalation in vitro. The drug is more water soluble than the related compound and had broad activity in the preclinical screens. A pharmacokinetic study of a 1-hour infusion showed a clearance of 69 L/hr/m^2. The clearance is due to the biotransformation of the drug to amonafide, N-acetyl-amonafide, and N-desmethyl-amonafide, which build up in the plasma (296). An early phase I trial of mitonafide as a daily infusion × 5 demonstrated the MTD to be 138.6 mg/m², with limiting toxicity of myelosuppression. Less common toxicities included mucositis, neurotoxicity, and vomiting. The study is still ongoing (297). Solid tumor trials have not shown any significant activity but did confirm CNS toxicity of the short infusion (298). A phase I trial of 120-hour infusion was performed with a suggested phase II dose of 170 mg/m² (299). This schedule prevented the CNS toxicity previously observed in 1-hour infusion schedules.

ACLARUBICIN (aclacinomycin A; 2-ethyl 1,2,3,4,6,11-hexahydro-2,5,7-trihydroxy-6,11-dioxo-4-((2,3,6-trideoxy-4-O-(2,6-dideoxy-4-O -(2-*trans*-tetrahydro-6-methyl-5-oxo-2H-py-ran-2-yl)-A-L-lyxo-hexopyranosyl-3-(dimethyl-amino)-A-L-lyxo-hexopyranosyl)oxy)-,methy-lester,(1R-(1α,2β,4β))-1-naphthacenecarboxylic acid, hydrochloride, dihydrate; NSC-208734) is an anthracycline analogue with substitutions on the chromophore and trisaccharides connected to the C-7 of the ring structure, leading to greater inhibition of RNA synthesis than DNA synthesis (class II anthracycline) (300). This drug has been studied in humans for over a decade, with its ultimate role in the treatment of neoplastic disease uncertain. Aclacinomycin A has been reported to be nonmutagenic in the Ames assay and the mammalian cell HGPRT mutagenesis assay (301). However, its derivative, N-demethyl-aclacinomycin A, is mutagenic (302). The drug is not stable in alkaline solutions and may precipitate in solutions containing preservatives. Numerous phase I trials have been carried out, including evaluation of the intraperitoneal route, resulting in chemical peritonitis at 75 mg in 2 L (303). The role of this agent in solid tumors has been disappointing, with myelosuppression, gastrointestinal distress, and occasional cardiac toxicity noted (304–306). No activity was seen in a metastatic breast cancer trial (307). Aclacinomycin A has shown antineoplastic action in acute myeloid leukemia on a schedule of 100 mg/m²/day × 3, with toxicities of nausea, vomiting, mucositis, diarrhea, myelosuppression, and minimal alopecia (308, 309). On a divided dose, given as rapid intravenous infusion daily for 10 days, the complete remission rate in acute myeloid leukemia was 34% (310). Most studies have noted a response rate in acute leukemia from 11 to 35%. Aclacinomycin A (60 mg/m²/

day × 5) with etoposide (100 mg/m²/day × 5) has been touted as an effective salvage treatment in relapsed or refractory acute myeloid leukemia, with a 34% complete remission rate (311). A small series of patients with myelodysplasia also benefited from this agent (312). The development of an enzyme immunoassay may offer the ability to pharmacodynamically modify dosing (313). Whether this agent offers any unique property over numerous other active agents in acute leukemia remains a major question for future development of this compound.

EPIRUBICIN (Pharmarubicin; EPI; 4'epi-DX; IMI 28; FI 7701; NSC 256942) is a stereoisomer of doxorubicin, differing only in the position of the hydroxyl group (equatorial) on the C-4' of the aminosugar (314). As this drug is commercially available in many countries and has been reviewed in depth (315–317), this discussion concentrates on new developments. The drug has progressed on the basis of having a spectrum of antitumor action equivalent to that of doxorubicin in humans, less acute toxicity (nausea, vomiting, and less myelosuppression on a equivalent milligram basis), and a higher total-allowed cumulative dose (1035 to 1234 mg/m² before the onset of congestive heart failure (315). To attain the equivalent biologic effect of doxorubicin in man, approximately 25% more EPI must be given, so that 85 to 90 mg/m² given once every 3 weeks is equivalent to 60 mg/m² of doxorubicin (316). Comparative pharmacology of EPI and doxorubicin was recently reported. Both drugs showed a triphasic plasma decay pattern, with the half-life of each phase shorter for EPI, and 12% of parent and fluorescent metabolites excreted in the urine (318). This study parallels older pharmacokinetic studies showing more rapid clearance of EPI than of doxorubicin. The minor steric change in the molecule results in major changes in metabolism of this anthracycline. Metabolic studies of EPI indicate that it is quickly biotransformed to epirubicinol, EPI-glucuronide (with an AUC twice the size of EPI), epirubinicinol-glucuronide, and aglycones. Doxorubicin is not subject to formation of 4'glucuronide metabolites (319). In an attempt to improve the therapeutic index, EPI has been given as a continuous infusion over 9 to 16 days (320) and 21 days (321). Dose-limiting toxicity was mucositis with occasional myelosuppression. Pharmacokinetic studies suggest a greater AUC of EPI by infusion than by bolus. Phase II infusion (through a central venous access line) of dosages of 8 mg/m²/day × 14 (320) or 6 mg/

m^2/day $\times$ 21 (321) were suggested. EPI has also been given on a weekly schedule $\times$ 3 every 4 weeks at doses ranging from 20 to 45 mg/m^2 (322).

Much recent interest has centered around giving high-dose anthracyclines to enhance therapeutic effect. Several studies have given EPI as a rapid single infusion once every 21 days with MTD at 150 to 180 mg/m^2. Myelosuppression was dose-limiting, with manageable nausea, vomiting, stomatitis, transient drug fever, and alopecia (323–328). Antitumor responses were noted in anthracycline-sensitive tumors and in non-small-cell lung cancer. At 120 mg/m^2, EPI has given a 48% major response in cervical carcinoma (329). EPI has also been given as a daily $\times$ 3 high-dose schedule, with the MTD at 55 mg/m^2/day (330).

IODO-DOXORUBICIN (4'-iodo-4'-deoxy-doxorubicin; 4'-I-DOX) is the result of replacing a hydroxyl moiety of the amino sugar of doxorubicin with iodine. This compound was less cardiotoxic than doxorubicin in the male Sprague-Dawley rat model (331). Plasma concentrations were best fitted to a three-compartment model with half-lives of 5.2 min, 0.79 hours, and 10.3 hours (332). The drug was metabolized extensively to a 13-dihydroderivative, 4'-iodo-4'-deoxy-doxorubicinol (332, 333). Myelosuppression could be predicted by measuring the AUCs of the drug and its metabolite. A correlation existed between the relative amount of metabolism and the reduction in neutrophils (334). The drug has reached early phase I trials as a 1-minute intravenous bolus every 2 weeks. Mild myelosuppression was seen at 50 mg/m^2, with preliminary pharmacologic measurements showing a triexponential decay (335). A phase II trial at 80 mg/m^2 every 3 weeks in untreated metastatic breast cancer had minimal clinical activity with a 14% response rate (336). No activity was seen in advanced colorectal cancer or non-small-cell lung cancer at the same dose (337, 338).

PIRARUBICIN (THP; THP-adriamycin; 4'-O-tetrahydropyranyladriamycin; 4'-O-tetrahydropyranyldoxorubicin) has been in clinical trials in Europe and Japan since 1982 and more recently in the United States. THP is a modification of doxorubicin on the aminosugar moiety, with the substitution of a tetrahydropyranyl group for the hydrogen at the 4' position. The drug has been developed on the basis of broad activity in preclinical tumor screens, less cardiotoxicity in hamsters and rats, and a more potent cytolytic effect than the parent compound (339). The compound, which is highly lipophilic, is taken up rapidly by both sensitive and resistant cells (340). Reconstitution in 0.9% NaCl was impossible, and storage beyond 5 days in 5% glucose resulted in degradation of the compound with the formation of doxorubicin (341). In mice, THP disappeared more rapidly from plasma than doxorubicin (339). Japanese researchers have determined the MTD on a single infusion schedule to be 54 to 66 mg/m^2. Their suggested phase II dosing schedules are (a) in leukemia, 15 to 20 mg/m^2/day for 3 to 5 days, (b) for lymphoma, 40 to 50 mg/m^2 once every 3 weeks, or (c) for lymphoma, 15 to 30 mg/m^2/week (342, 343). All schedules have shown activity, with toxic effects of myelosuppression, nausea, vomiting, stomatitis, alopecia, ECG changes, diarrhea, and malaise noted. Cardiac toxicity was noted in trials in Japan (344). Phase I studies have been confirmed in Europe and the United States. On a single rapid infusion every 3 to 4 weeks, THP was shown to have an MTD of 70 mg/m^2, with dose-limiting myelosuppression (345, 346). Pharmacokinetic studies on this schedule revealed a triphasic plasma decay curve with a terminal half-life of 23.6 $\pm$ 7.6 hours (346). THP was metabolized into adriamycinol, adriamycinone, THP-adriamycinol, and doxorubicin (less than 10% of total metabolites) (346). A decrease in cardiac ejection fraction correlated with cumulative drug dosing. A phase I weekly $\times$ 3 study in the United States reached an MTD of 25 mg/m^2/week, with limiting toxicity of neutropenia at week 4 (347). At the MTD, alopecia was uncommon and nausea mild. On this weekly schedule, THP disposition could be described by a three-phase decay with a terminal half-life of 19.3 $\pm$ 2.1 hours. Doxorubicin is a known metabolite and reached substantial levels 30 minutes following administration, in contrast to previous findings (347). European studies indicated that the chance of cardiac damage is low below a cumulative THP dose of 650 mg/m^2 but rises rapidly at 750 mg/m^2 (348).

A number of phase II trials have been reported. There is demonstrated activity in breast carcinoma (349, 350). Elderly patients with advanced breast cancer had a 25% response rate. Cardiac toxicity and mucositis were not observed (351). An analysis of phase II breast cancer data suggests that pirarubicin is as effective as other intercalating drugs and is better tolerated than doxorubicin, with less alopecia and cardiotoxicity seen (352). Single-agent trials in gynecologic tumors showed activity in untreated cervical carcinoma, with a 31% major response rate (19% PR/12% CR) (353). Activity was lower in endometrial cancer and negligible in ovarian cancer, where many patients had previously received anthracyclines (353). Of 27 chemotherapy-naive patients with head and neck cancer, 5 responded with acceptable toxicity (354). No activity was seen in second-line therapy (355). Single-agent activity of 10% was seen in bladder cancer (356). No efficacy was noted in renal and colon cancers and melanoma (357). A modest response rate of 12% was noted in first-line monotherapy for small cell lung cancer (358).

THP has been evaluated in combination with cisplatin in relapsed/resistant ovarian cancer. Responses were observed in the relapsed group, with myelosuppression being dose limiting (359).

Pharmacokinetic and pharmacodynamic advantages were demonstrated for pirarubicin over doxorubicin after intraarterial hepatic administration (IAH) in a rat model (360). Pirarubicin showed higher local tumor concentrations than doxorubicin. This may be helpful in cells partially resistant to anthracyclines (360). In a phase I trial of IAH, responses were seen in metastatic liver disease, with minimal systemic toxicity (361). No hepatobiliary or vascular toxicity was noted. The dose-limiting toxicity was granulocytopenia (361).

SM-5887 ((7S,9S)-9-acetyl-9-amino-7-((2deoxy-β-D-erythropentopyranosyl)oxy)7,8,9,10-tetrahydro-6,11-dihydroxy-5,12-naphthacenedionehydrochloride) is a new analogue of doxorubicin showing 1/10th the cardiotoxicity of the parent compound in animal models. In a phase I trial, the MTD was 130 mg/m^2, with dose-limiting toxicities of leukopenia and thrombocytopenia (nadir, day 12). Pharmacokinetics demonstrated a triphasic decay with a terminal half-life of 4.2 hours. The suggested phase II dose was 100 mg/m^2 by rapid intravenous infusion every 3 weeks (362).

QUINOCARMYCIN MONOCITRATE (KW 2152; NSC 604122) and its analogue DX-52-1 (NSC 607097) are in the quinocarmycin family of antibiotics derived from culture broths of *Streptomyces melanovinaceus*. These drugs were developed especially against melanomas. The NCI COMPARE program suggested that DNA interaction is a mechanism by which the drugs exert their effect. They have demonstrated excellent-to-good activity in five-stage subcutaneous implanted human melanoma xenograft models (363, 364). These drugs will be in clinical trials at the time of publication of this book.

MORPHOLINO ANTHRACYCLINES have generated much interest. They are very potent in vitro and have activity in some doxorubicin-resistant cell lines (365), and their poorly stable derivatives, cyano-morpholino anthracyclines, are extremely potent (in the nanomolar range) in resistant cells (366). Morpholino anthracyclines are also more lipophilic than the parent compound. They differ from doxorubicin in mechanism of action, pattern of resistance, and metabolism (367). They are metabolized primarily by the cytochrome P450/3A system (368). Doxorubicin is primarily an inhibitor of topoisomerase II; these compounds inhibit both topoisomerase I and II, resulting in predominantly single-strand DNA cleavage and, to a lesser extent, DNA breakage (367). DNA interstrand cross-links are observed after preincubation with human liver microsomes and NADPH (367, 368). Animal models demonstrate more cytotoxicity and less cardiac toxicity than with doxorubicin (369).

MX2 (KRN 8602; DRN 8602 3′-deamino-3′-morpholino-13-deoxy-10-hydroxycarminomycin) has reached clinical trials. This agent shows better antitumor effect in preclinical screens and less cardiotoxicity in the rabbit model than doxorubicin and is cytotoxic against doxorubicin-resistant cell lines (370). Phase I results indicated an MTD of 18 mg/m^2 given as an infusion daily × 3, with nausea, vomiting, and myelosuppression (both leukopenia and thrombocytopenia) as limiting toxic effects (371). The nadir of the white count occured at 2 weeks. The suggested phase II dosage is 15 mg/m^2 over 3 days (371). Pharmacokinetic studies of KRN 8602 were done on a single-dose schedule with the MTD of 30 mg/m^2 (372). A triphasic decay curve with terminal half-life of 5.9 ± 0.4 hours was found, with two metabolites of the parent drug detected in the plasma (372). Using a dose of 35 mg/m^2 every 3 weeks, 2 of 12 patients (including 1 CR) with metastatic breast cancer responded. There was grade 3/4 hematologic toxicity, grade 3 nausea and vomiting, but no alopecia (373). In a rat model, favorable pharmacokinetic parameters were noted after intracarotid and intravenous injection in the treatment of malignant gliomas and leptomeningeal disease (374, 375).

MMDX (3′-deamino-3′-(2-methoxy-4-morpholinyl)-doxorubicin; FCE 23762) is also being studied. It is an inhibitor of both topoisomerase I and II (367). The drug is activated in the liver to a 10-times more potent metabolite (MMDX+) that cross-links DNA. It is highly active against a panel of human leukemia and lymphoma cell lines (376). Reduced cardiotoxicity is also noted (369). A phase I study in solid tumors showed some regression, with a final recommended dose of 1.25 mg/m^2 (377). Corticosteroids do not seem to inhibit the antitumor effect (378).

ANTHRAPYRAZOLES

The anthrapyrazoles are DNA-binding anticancer agents with broad-spectrum preclinical activity and reduced potential for free radical generation, as compared with doxorubicin (379). At the molecular and cellular levels, anthrapyrazoles are potent topoisomerase II inhibitors (380). The drugs showed activity in the *ras* transgenic mice model to predict response in mammary carcinoma (381). Dose-limiting toxicity has been leukopenia, and promising activity has been seen in breast cancer (379). Studies will need to determine whether these compounds are truly less toxic than the available anthracyclines and whether they offer a significant therapeutic advantage.

LOSOXANTRONE (DuP 941; CI-941) and DuP 937 are two anthrapyrazoles undergoing investigation (380). The anthracyclines are limited in their effectiveness by cumulative cardiotoxicity. The toxicity has been attributed to redox reactions that generate free radicals (382). The anthrapyrazoles were developed to circumvent this toxicity (380). DuP 941 and DuP 937 were tested and compared with mitoxantrone and other topoisomerase II inhibitors. The anthrapyrazoles were found to be closely related to mitoxantrone in terms of spectrum of activity, with reduced cardiotoxicity (380). DuP 941 was studied in a phase I trial at doses of 5 to 55 mg/m^2. The dose limiting toxicity was leucopenia. There was a wide interpatient variation in the dose-AUC relationship. The recommended phase II dose was 50 mg/m^2 (383). A breast cancer trial demonstrated dose-limiting neutropenia and 2 of 136 patients with severely decreased left ventricular ejection fraction (384).

A phase I trial of DUP-937 used a weekly bolus schedule every 3 weeks (385). Doses ranged from 0.55 to 16 mg/m^2/week. The dose-limiting toxicity was neutropenia, and the MTD was 16 mg/m^2/week for 3 weeks. The mean AUC values increased with dose. Linear pharmacoki-

netics were observed, as total body clearance, half-life, and volume of distribution did not change with increasing dose (385).

PIROXANTRONE (oxantrazole; oxanthrazole; anthrapyrazole dihydrochloride; 5-((3-aminopropyl)amino) - 7,10-dihydroxy-2 - (2-((2-hydroxyethyl)anthra - (1,9-*cd*)pyrazol - 6(2*H*) - one dihydrochloride; NSC-349174) shares some of the chemical characteristics of CI-941 in that both were synthesized as anthrapyrazole derivatives to lessen free radical formation (386) seen with the anthracenedione class of drugs. This drug was active in the preclinical screens, was not schedule dependent, and was found to be unstable in animal and human plasma (387). This agent is also unstable in neutral and alkaline aqueous solutions (388). In the human tumor clonogenic assay, this agent was much more cytotoxic to tumor cells than to human bone marrow, implying a good therapeutic index (388). Piroxantrone causes DNA strand breaks and DNA-protein cross-linking, suggesting an interaction with topoisomerase II (387).

A phase I pharmacokinetic study showed linear elimination over a 4-fold dose range. A limited-sampling strategy has also been developed. The plasma elimination was biexponential, with a mean $t_{1/2}\alpha$ of 3.2 ± 2.7 min and a mean $t_{1/2}\beta$ of 82 ± 92 min. Clearance was 840 ± 230 mL/min/m^2 (389). Another phase I trial indicated that myelosuppression occurred at 68 mg/m^2 as a single dose every 21 days, with one patient having asymptomatic ventricular tachycardia (390). Terminal half-life of this agent was 15 to 30 minutes (391). A phase I trial with G-CSF was also conducted (392). Dose-limiting neutropenia occurred in 3 of 6 patients treated with 185 mg/m^2. When G-CSF was added, dose-limiting thrombocytopenia occurred at 445 mg/m^2; the MTD of piroxantrone with G-CSF was 335 mg/m^2. Seven patients developed symptomatic congestive heart failure at cumulative doses ranging from 855 to 2475 mg/m^2, and two died of cardiotoxicity. Six of the seven patients had previously received doxorubicin. Phase II trials are under way, with antitumor activity noted in breast carcinoma. A phase II trial in soft tissue sarcoma at 150 mg/m^2 showed no activity (393).

ANTIMETABOLITES

Pharmaceutical development of the antimetabolites has expanded with the realization that inhibition of certain key enzymes such as thymidylate synthase may lead to an effective tumoricidal agent with an enhanced therapeutic index (394). As a result, many pharmaceutical firms are pursuing compounds that interfere with this enzyme, based upon structure-function analysis. Several of these compounds become polyglutamated within cells, leading to prolonged retention in such cells. Other agents lack this ability to chemically bind to glutamic acid residues and thus efflux from cells. Many of these compounds, such as 5-FU combined with folinic acid, are orders of magnitude more active than traditional thymidylate synthase inhibitors (395). Renewed interest in other steps in the folic acid pathway has led to additional substances that interfere with specific enzymes such as glycineamide ribonucleotide transformylase (396). Additional antimetabolites, many of them analogues of existing agents, continue to be investigated, but many are of uncertain benefit. Many of the older drugs in this class of agents have been combined in attempts to cause antitumor effects by biochemical modulation of metabolic pathways, but this approach has not yet led to major advances. As such, most of the older agents will probably disappear from clinical investigation but may serve as the basis for new analogues.

ACIVICIN (AT-125; U-42126; a-amino-3-chloro-4,5-dihydro-5-isoxaoleacetic acid; NSC-163501) is a fermentation product with a steric structure similar to glutamine. This agent is an irreversible inhibitor of L-glutamine amidotransferase and also inhibits L-asparagine synthetase. This agent has been well studied over the last 15 years and was reviewed extensively several years ago (397). The drug is reconstituted and infused in normal saline. In murine models, this agent is an S-phase inhibitor with schedule dependency. It elevates uridine triphosphate (UTP) intracellular pools, decreases intracellular levels of cytosine triphosphate (CTP) and guanosine triphosphate (GTP), and decreases early de novo pyrimidine synthesis. Phase I trials defined neurotoxicity as dose limiting for rapid infusion administration. Acute neurotoxicity could be correlated with plasma levels above 2.5 μg/mL (398). When this agent was given as a 72-hour infusion in an attempt to minimize peak levels, acivicin plasma levels above 0.9 μg/mL for more than 16 hours caused toxicity (399). Common neurologic findings included lethargy, somnolence, anxiety, hallucinations, paranoid psychosis, vertigo, and ataxia (398).

A paucity of antitumor effects in man when acivicin was used as a single agent has led to the use of this drug as a modifier of biochemical function. Dipyridamole, which blocks nucleoside salvage, potentiates acivicin. A phase I study of the combination of acivicin and dipyridamole given as a 72-hour simultaneous infusion revealed gastrointestinal distress, vertigo, and orthostatic hypotension as dose-limiting toxicities (399). The MTDs were acivicin 60 mg/m^2/72 hours and dipyridamole 23.1 mg/kg/72 hours (399). Pharmacologic studies of this combination revealed inhibition of CTP synthetase with at least 30% reduction of intracellular CTP pools in lymphocytes (400). Acivicin has also been shown to potentiate the effects of 5-FU (401), leading to another attempt at biochemical modulation of antimetabolites. This drug seems to have very limited use in the treatment of human malignancies, despite its effects on perturbation of biochemical pathways. Recently, an Eastern Cooperative Oncology Group (ECOG) trial reported that continuous infusion of acivicin at 60 mg/m^2 over 72 hours, combined with etoposide and cisplatin, did not enhance the antitumor effects in a phase II trial in non-small-cell lung cancer (402). Unless this drug can show a beneficial modulation of another agent in man, it will be dropped from clinical study despite its interesting mechanism of action.

AG-331 (N^6-[4-(morpholinosulfonyl)benzyl]-N^6-methyl-2,6-diamino-benz-indole gluconate) is a thymidylate synthase inhibitor that cannot be polyglutamated (403). The drug is lipophilic and rapidly taken up into cells in culture, with rapid reduction of thymidine triphosphate pools. In rat hepatoma cells, this drug reduced incorporation of deoxyuridine into DNA and blocked cells in S phase. Higher concentrations of AG-331 seemed to exert other cytotoxic actions (404). The drug is active against leukemia and colon cancer cell lines and does not seem to be perturbed by the expression of MDR protein. An initial phase I trial administering this agent over 10 minutes in dosages ranging from 12.5 to 225 mg/m^2 revealed flushing, nausea, and vomiting at the higher dose levels. The terminal $t_{1/2}$ of the drug was 20 hours, with a dose-dependent reduction in clearance. In man, phase I trials of a 1-hour daily $\times$ 5 and continuous infusion daily $\times$ 5 are ongoing. Antitumor activity has not yet been described (403).

AG-337 (3,4-dihydro-2-amino-6-methyl-4-oxo-5-(4-pyridylthio)-quinazolone) is a rationally designed nonclassical thymidylate synthase inhibitor with marked schedule dependency in preclinical evaluation. In vitro, this drug had cytotoxic activity against HCT116 human colorectal cells and HeLa Bu25TK human cervical carcinoma cells (405). The drug has been evaluated in man as a 24-hour intravenous infusion at doses ranging from 75 to 1350 mg/m^2, with local venous toxicity (406). Initial findings revealed the terminal $t_{1/2}$ in plasma to be 134 minutes, with dose-related linearity in AUC. Urinary excretion was 17% of the administered dose (406). Above 600 mg/m^2, the same investigators have found nonlinear kinetics, with the plasma disappearance curve best described by a Michaelis-Menten plot, suggesting saturation of clearance mechanisms (407). A 5-day infusion study noted grade 3–4 toxicity at 1130 mg/m^2/day, with dose-limiting leukopenia, thrombocytopenia, and mucositis prominent at days 7 to 10. One patient with previous exposure to 5-FU with colorectal carcinoma achieved a partial remission. The suggested phase II dose is 1000 mg/m^2/day (408). An oral formulation is under development.

AZACYTIDINE (NSC-102816) is an analogue of cytidine that is metabolically converted to the triphosphate derivative. This 5-azacytidine triphosphate is incorporated into RNA and, to a lesser extent, into DNA. This agent also inhibits methylation of DNA. In mice, exposure to this agent induced a lupuslike syndrome with the major effect of this drug on CD4 T cells (409). Despite 25 years of clinical experience with this agent, it remains experimental in the United States. The drug's main therapeutic indication has been acute nonlymphocytic leukemia. As many other agents are more convenient, less mutagenic, more stable, and less toxic (hematopoietic, nausea, vomiting, liver abnormalities), 5-azacytidine's role in frank malignancy remains questionable. The drug has been reviewed but not recently (410). Recent studies of the combination of mitoxanthrone with azacytidine showed no benefit over monotherapy with mitoxanthrone in acute nonlymphocytic leukemia or in patients with blast crisis of chronic myelogenous leukemia (411, 412).

In contrast to acute leukemia or solid tumors, in the myelodysplastic states, this drug does seem to have value where classical chemotherapy has been of little utility. Azacytidine given as a continuous infusion at 75 mg/m^2 daily $\times$ 7 every 4 weeks showed trilineage improvement in hematopoeisis in patients with refractory anemia with excess blasts and refractory anemia with excess blasts in transformation. Median duration of the response was 14.7 months (413).

Additional studies including the use of this agent by the subcutaneous route are still under way.

5-AZA-2'-DEOXYCYTIDINE (5-aza-DCyd; DAC, Decitabine, Dezocitidine; NSC-127716) is a deoxycytidine analogue that must be metabolized to the triphosphate form prior to incorporation into DNA. In human chronic myelogenous leukemia cell lines, this drug is more cytotoxic than cytosine arabinoside (414). The drug is a strong inhibitor of DNA methylation and is S-phase specific (therefore schedule dependent) (415). In vitro, the inhibition of methylation has been associated with activation of gene expression and differentiation of leukemic cells (416). In the human monoblastic leukemia cell line U-937, DAC induces marked hypomethylation of DNA, with a reduction in *c-myc* transcripts that occurs within 24 hours of exposure (417). This agent has also shown cytotoxicity with arrest of cells in S and G_2+M phases of the cell cycle (418). Recent in vitro work suggested that this agent is synergistic both with other cytotoxics and with 1,25-dihydroxy-vitamin D_3 in reducing clonogenicity of HL-60 cells (419). In ovarian cell lines, this drug enhances the cytotoxic effects of cisplatin, suggesting a potential role in this carcinoma (420). DAC also upregulates the number of epidermal growth factor receptors in solid tumor cell lines in vitro and may therefore have a role in therapies exploiting this receptor (421). The drug is degraded by deamination, and recent inhibitors of cytidine deaminase have been described to prolong the effect of this drug (422). In the rat model, loss of deoxycytidine kinase is correlated with resistance to this agent (423). Pharmacokinetic studies in man have suggested a terminal plasma half-life of 15 to 20 minutes, with CSF levels approaching 20% of serum levels (424).

In xenografts of human head and neck cancer, this agent showed remarkable activity (425). However, an EORTC phase II trial in this tumor type in humans, using a 1-hour infusion every 7 hours $\times$ 3 and repeated after 5 weeks, showed a paucity of activity and significant myelosuppression, nausea, and vomiting (426). In the L1210 leukemia model and in P388, DAC has shown efficacy but schedule dependency leading to continuous infusion trials in leukemia (427). Like cytosine arabinoside, this agent has been administered as a continuous infusion for 2 to 5 days (416). A pilot study in 12 patients with acute nonlymphocytic leukemia explored this drug at 90 to 120 mg/m^2 as a 4-hour infusion 3 times a day for 3 days, repeated at 4 to 6 week intervals, with complete remissions in 3 patients and mild nonhematologic toxicity (428). In contrast, the EORTC studied this agent in combination with idarubicin and m-amsacrine and found severe toxicity, including diarrhea, peritonitis, cerebellar toxicity, hepatotoxicity, gastrointestinal bleeding, and prolonged myelosuppression (429). Whether the toxicities can be clinically manageable will most likely depend upon the schedule employed, as the EORTC study used a longer duration of treatment. Of concern, an early study in children suggested the rapid development of drug resistance (430).

Like azacytidine, DAC has been evaluated in myelodysplasia (refractory anemia with excess blasts), with 50% of patients showing evidence of an increase in platelets, neutrophils, and red cells in the peripheral blood. DAC given as three 4-hour infusions for 3 days (45 mg/m^2/day) or as a continuous 3-day infusion of 50 mg/m^2/day resulted in hematologic improvement without excessive toxicity (431).

5-BENZYLOXYBENZYLURACIL (BBU) may be in clinical trials by the time of the publication of this edition. The enzyme dihydropyrimidine dehydrogenase (DPD), known to be the rate-limiting step in 5-FU degradation, can be blocked by this agent. This substance is the most active inhibitor of dihydrouracil dehydrogenase known (K$_i$ = 30 nM) and markedly potentiates the antitumor activities of 5-FU in murine model systems, improving the therapeutic index by a factor of five. Therefore, this agent may be clinically useful both to enhance cytotoxic effect and to decrease host toxicities due to 5-FU catabolism (432).

BREQUINAR (DUP-785; Brequinar sodium; Breq; phenylquinoline; 6-fluoro-2-(2'-fluoro-1, 1'-biphenyl-4-yl)-3-methyl-4-quinoline; NSC-368390) is under active investigation as an immunosuppressant because of its novel structure (a substituted quinoline carboxylic acid), its broad antitumor spectrum in animal model systems, and its good solubility in aqueous solvents. In tissue culture, this agent must be continually present to exert a toxic effect and is antagonized by exogenous uridine or orotic acid (433). The drug's mechanism of action is through inhibition of the mitochondrial enzyme dihydroorotic acid dehydrogenase (433), required by the de novo pyrimidine synthetic pathway. The drug binding is unique to the mammalian enzyme and involves a site distinct from the dihydroorotate binding site (434). Marked schedule dependency

has been noted in vitro; removal of the drug after a 24-hour exposure or less leads to cell recovery (435). Cells accumulated in the S phase of the cell cycle and were irreversibly damaged if Breq was present for 48 hours (435). However, inhibition of this pyrimidine pathway synthetic enzyme did not correlate with antitumor effect in murine models of colon cancer, perhaps indicating that other mechanisms of action and resistance are important (436). In vivo studies did demonstrate that inhibition of the pyrimidine pathway with Breq leads to depletion of pyrimidine nucleosides in plasma (437) and in lymphocytes (438). This observation has led to the evaluation of Breq with 5-FU and with 5-FU with folinic acid in vitro in an attempt to modulate this pathway. Treatment with Breq led to greater formation of FdUMP but did not enhance the cytotoxicity of the combination of 5-FU with folinic acid, suggesting that this approach is probably not clinically useful (439).

Combination studies with other agents revealed additive or synergistic effects with alkylating agents, doxorubicin, and cisplatin in colon xenografts (440). Synergism has also been noted with dipyridamole and 5-FU in Colon 26 cells (441) but not in L1210 leukemia (442). In human xenografts in nude mice, drug levels in the colon tumors were found to be 19 to 41% of the serum level (442). Given on a 5-day schedule in xenografts of human tumors grown in nude mice, this drug was active in head and neck cancers, non-small-cell lung tumors, and small cell lung tumors (443). This drug (given at 10 mg/mL in saline over 10 to 120 min) has been studied on a variety of schedules because of its schedule dependency: weekly (444, 445), biweekly (444), every 3 weeks (446, 447), and every 5 days repeated every 28 days (448 to 450). Suggested 5-day-treatment phase II dosages are 250 mg/m^2/day for good-risk patients and 170 mg/m^2/day for previously treated patients (449). Pharmacokinetics of this agent in all the trials have indicated nonlinear relationships between administered dose and pharmacologic parameters, with a terminal t$_{1/2}$ of 4 to 7 hours. Terminal half-lives also increased with repetitive dosing on a daily × 5 schedule, which suggests saturation of clearance mechanisms (451). Large intrapatient and interpatient variations in pharmacokinetics have been noted and are believed to be due to pharmacogenetic differences in metabolism of this agent. A recent analysis of plasma binding has shown that Breq binds to albumin via both high-affinity and low-affinity binding sites, but these effects could not explain the degree of pharmacologic variation noted in the phase I trials (452). Toxicities in all the trials included nausea, vomiting, pain at the intravenous site (lessened with additional fluid administration), leukopenia, thrombocytopenia, hematuria, metallic taste, mucositis, rash, photosensitivity reactions, angioneurotic edema, and hyperpigmentation (453).

Phase II trials of this agent as monotherapy have been disappointing. Breq demonstrated a 12% partial response rate in previously treated advanced breast cancer (454), no response in gastrointestinal malignancy (455), no activity in melanoma (456), no activity in head and neck cancer (457), and minimal activity in lung cancer (458). This drug would probably be dropped from further development except for its unique potential as an immunosuppressant in transplantation, as it can be administered orally and has shown synergistic effects with other immunosuppressants in preclinical models (459, 460). Therefore, further development of this drug is expected.

DMDC (1-[2-deoxy-2-methylene—D-erythropentofuranosyl] cytosine dihydrate) inhibits both DNA polymerase and ribonucleotide reductase. In human xenografts in nude mice, this agent exhibited broad antitumor activity against stomach, colon, pancreas, lung, renal, esophageal, and testis cancers (461). In vitro experimentation suggested the value of combining this agent with cisplatin (462). The drug has entered phase I evaluation in Japan, but results have not yet been reported (463).

DOXIFLURIDINE (5'dFUrd; 5'-FUR; 5'-deoxy-5-fluorouridine; RO 21-9738) is a prodrug of 5-FU, with a higher therapeutic index in some animal systems (464). The oral route has been evaluated in xenograft model systems, with schedule-dependent effects and a higher therapeutic index than 5-FU (465). The clinical development of this compound by the intravenous route has been retarded by cardiotoxicity (most noted at total dosages above 15 g/m^2), neurologic dysfunction, diarrhea, and mucositis (466, 467). Cardiotoxicity also occurs with 5-FU but is less frequent (468). The drug was infused in 5% dextrose solutions, but an oral 200-mg capsule is currently being evaluated with less toxicity (469). Pharmacokinetic studies, including the use of nuclear magnetic resonance (NMR) with 19F-labeled drug, have shown the presence of parent compound, 5-FU, 5,6-dihydrofluorouracil, and 5-fluoro-β-alanine (FBAL) in the plasma of patients (470). A conjugate of FBAL can be detected in the bile (less than 0.8% of injected fluorinated material injected) (471).

Classical pharmacokinetics of this drug given by rapid intravenous infusion revealed nonlinear pharmacokinetics (with saturable metabolism) and a terminal half-life from 16 to 28 minutes (472). In an attempt to ameliorate toxicity and increase therapeutic benefit, 5'd-FUR has been given as a continuous infusion of 750 mg/m^2/day for 3 months. In a small number of patients studied, approximately one-third of colorectal tumor patients showed a major response, with hand-foot syndrome as the major toxicity (473). This study contrasts with a larger randomized trial that gave this agent over 5 days with a low response rate in untreated colorectal patients, which suggests that schedule may be very important in man (474). In an unusual phase I trial, this agent was given as a 5-day intravenous course with dose escalations increased stepwise every day. Mucositis, thrombocytopenia, somnolence, fevers, nausea, and rashes were noted; one patient with nasopharyngeal carcinoma achieved a complete remission (475). Interferon has been combined with 5-FU in the treatment of gastrointestinal malignancy. In a similar manner, the intravenous preparation of doxifluridine given weekly has been combined with α_{2a}-interferon (3 million units, 3 times weekly) with dosages up to 5 g/m^2 without severe toxicity (476). The role of folinic acid with this agent remains unknown, but the combination of 5-FU with folinic acid did not show antitumor activity in doxifluridine failures (477).

Oral administration is more convenient, and a phase I trial showed dose-limiting toxicity of diarrhea at 1500 mg/day for treatment durations longer than 27 days (478). In divided doses (3 times a day), oral administration of this drug mimicked an infusion with bioavailability of 40 to 60% of parenteral use (469). Renal excretion became more important as the dose was escalated (4% at 400 mg/m^2/day to 17% at 1000 mg/m^2/day) (479). Oral doxifluridine has been evaluated with standard radiation therapy to the pelvis as a potential radiation sensitizer. Maximum tolerated dose of this bimodality therapy was judged to be 1000 mg/day, with nausea/vomiting and diarrhea as the most common side effects (480). A trial of oral doxifluridine with cisplatin resulted in a high response rate in untreated gastric cancer (481). This drug has also been evaluated with prednimustine and idarubicin as an oral treatment for breast cancer, with activity in small numbers of patients (482). At the present time, it remains unclear what the role of this agent will be in cancer chemotherapy, and additional oral analogues of 5-FU such as col-pecitabine remain under development.

EDATREXATE (10-EDAM; CGP 30694; 10-ethyl-10-deaza-aminopterin), an analogue of methotrexate, inhibits the target enzyme dihydrofolate reductase to the same extent as the parent compound but also shows increased transport into malignant cells and enhanced polyglutamation (thus preventing egress) (483). After an exhaustive structure-function analysis of antifols, the compound was synthesized to enhance uptake and is active in human xenografts (483, 484). 10-EDAM is more active in many preclinical tumor models than is methotrexate (485). The enhanced therapeutic index is believed to be due to increased uptake of this drug and poly-glutamylation leading to reduced efflux. The influx was found to display saturable kinetics (486). The drug demonstrates less inhibition of thymidylate synthase than does methotrexate (486). In tissue culture, 10-EDAM showed schedule dependency, with the level of drug within cell lines correlating with the extent of tumor inhibition (487). In vitro evaluation of human squamous carcinoma cell lines from patients with head and neck cancers indicated cytotoxic activity by 10-EDAM in cells partially resistant to methotrexate (488). One mechanism of resistance to this agent involves a structural change in the carrier molecule, leading to impaired transport into cells (489).

A phase I trial of this agent on either a weekly × 3 schedule or a continuous weekly schedule revealed dose-limiting toxicities of diarrhea, rash, leukopenia, and thrombocytopenia. Pharmacokinetic studies of these patients showed a triphasic plasma decay curve with terminal half-life of 7 to 11.9 hours (487, 490). Between 13 and 55% of the drug is cleared by the kidneys (with 88% of the drug excreted by this route within 4 hours of treatment). Two metabolites, 7-hydroxy-10-EDAM and 10-ethyl-10-deaza-2,4-diamino-pteroic acid, can be detected. Suggested phase II doses in adults are 100 mg/m^2 intravenously weekly × 3 (with a 2-week rest) or 80 mg/m^2 weekly (490). A phase I trial in children revealed hematologic toxicity with the MTD at 100 mg/m^2/week × 3 (491). Recently, cytotoxic synergy was found in vitro when this agent was administered prior to paclitaxel. A phase I study in man is ongoing with dose levels of 10-EDAM starting at 180 to 240 mg/m^2 and paclitaxel given

as a 3-hour infusion at 175 mg/m^2 24 hours later (492).

Phase II trials on a weekly schedule have shown a 32% major response rate in untreated non-small-cell lung cancer (493), but this high response could not be confirmed in a recent European study (494). In head and neck squamous cell carcinoma, a major response rate of 27% was obtained with 10-EDAM, which was equivalent to that with methotrexate (495). This agent is inactive in melanoma (496). Serious grade 3–4 toxicity was seen at 80 mg/m^2/week, with little antitumor activity in patients with pancreatic cancer (497). 10-EDAM has been incorporated into a non-small-cell lung carcinoma protocol (mitomycin, vinblastine, 10-EDAM), with a major response rate of 60%, and also with cisplatin and with cyclophosphamide, demonstrating a high response rate (486). This agent has also demonstrated activity in non-Hodgkin's lymphoma and minor activity in breast carcinoma (486).

Toxicities with this agent have been nausea, vomiting, stomatitis, fatigue, leukopenia, thrombocytopenia, liver function abnormalities, and rashes. This agent has demonstrated significant antitumor activity in human malignancy, but whether it offers an advance over older agents remains unclear.

5-ETHYNYLURACIL (776C85) inhibits the major degradative enzyme for 5-FU (dihydropyrimidine dehydrogenase; DPD) and thus shares a mechanism of action with 5-benzyloxybenzyluracil (discussed above). DPD-deficient patients are known to be hypersensitive to fluoropyrimidines. This agent is an irreversible inhibitor of DPD and is absorbed by the oral route. In CD-1 rats, this drug inhibited the enzyme at the microgram dose level (498). Ethynyluracil administered orally at 3.7 mg/m^2 completely blocks leukocyte DPD in man 1 hour after administration. The level of the enzyme at 24 hours is only 5% of baseline. The terminal half-life of this substance in a phase I study was 4 ± 2 hours. In the presence of both ethynyluracil and 5-FU, the terminal half-live of 5-FU to was prolonged 4.7 hours. In the presence of both this agent and 5-FU, plasma uracil concentrations were several times those seen with 776C85 alone. Suggested phase II dosing is a fixed dose of 10 mg per day by the oral route. Antitumor effects were not reported (407).

FAZARABINE (ara-AC; 1-D-arabinofuranosyl-5-azacytosine; NSC-281272) is a synthetic congener of both azacytosine and arabinosyl cytosine (ara-C), being unstable in aqueous solutions with the opening of the triazine ring. Ara-AC is phosphorylated by deoxycytidine kinase, as is ara-C, and eventually metabolized to the triphosphate form (499). Hence, cells lacking deoxycytidine kinase are resistant to both ara-C and ara-AC. Ara-AC is poorly metabolized by cytidine deaminase, unlike ara-C (500). Ara-AC is incorporated into DNA and inhibits DNA synthesis with much less effect on RNA and protein synthesis (501). This drug does not have a major effect on methylation of DNA, as does azacytidine, and does not seem to cause DNA strand breakage (502). Schedule dependency has been noted in vitro and in L1210 leukemia in mice (499). Intrathecal studies of this agent in nonhuman primates indicated a biphasic disappearance curve, high peak CSF drug concentrations, and absence of neurotoxicity (503). Phase I studies identified granulocytopenia as the limiting toxicity in adults (504) and children (505). Antitumor effects in man have been disappointing, with no activity against solid tumors and significant myelosuppression. In vitro evaluation of this agent for the treatment of acute myelogenous leukemia suggested no advantage over cytosine arabinoside (506). Synergy has been noted in vitro between this agent and cisplatin, but whether or not this drug will prove to be useful in combination therapy remains in doubt (507).

GEMCITABINE (LY 188011; 2'-2'-difluorodeoxycytidine; dFdC), a pyrimidine antagonist, is cell-cycle specific, inhibits DNA and RNA viruses, and has broad activity in preclinical tumor screens (508). Both antitumor effect and toxicity (mainly myelosuppression in animal systems) are schedule dependent (509). DFdC acts as a prodrug and must be converted intracellularly to the 5'-triphosphate nucleotide (dFdCTP) to exert its effect (509). Recent studies have noted that the triphosphate is incorporated into DNA and slows DNA elongation in intact cells (510). In cell lines, there may be a 4-fold difference in incorporation of the active form into DNA, and lesser amounts are also incorporated into RNA (509). Incorporation into DNA is both time and concentration dependent, while incorporation into RNA is contingent upon drug concentration. The major effects of this agent are on DNA (509). dFdCTP is poorly excreted from cells ($t_{1/2}$ is 3.3 hours at low levels of the drug in vitro) and binds to deoxycytidine monophosphate deaminase, preventing degradation of dFdCTP (511). In CEM cells, dCMP pools are depleted, and dFdCTP is incorporated into DNA (511). In human pancreatic xenografts, this agent demonstrated modest antitumor activity (512). Gemcitabine was more active than mitomycin C in lung and colorectal xenografts (513) and active on a weekly schedule against sarcoma and ovarian carcinoma xenografts in nude mice (514). In dogs, mice, and rats, this agent was deaminated and primarily eliminated in the urine (515).

This drug has been recently reviewed and may become commercially available by the time this edition is published (516). The drug has been studied on a variety of schedules: (*a*) single infusion every 2 weeks (508), (*b*) once weekly × 3 every 4 weeks (511), (*c*) twice weekly over 30 minutes for 3 consecutive weeks every 4 weeks (517), and (*d*) daily × 5 over 30 minutes every 3 weeks (518). Toxicities include thrombocytopenia, fatigue, malaise, fever, rash, a flulike syndrome, nausea, and vomiting. Thrombocytopenia was more prominent when the drug was infused over 30 minutes than when administered rapidly over 5 minutes (517). In a small number of patients, toxicities seemed to be more prominent on the daily × 5 schedule (519) than on the single infusion every 2 weeks or the twice-weekly schedule. Doses of drug on the weekly schedule were not limiting at 350 mg/m² (511); with the twice-weekly schedule, the MTD was 65 mg/m², with thrombocytopenia as the limiting toxicity (517).

This drug is active in a wide variety of human malignancies. Given as a 30-minute infusion at 1000 to 1250 mg/m²/week × 3 every 4 weeks, myelosuppression was seen in only 18% of cycles, with a 27% major response rate in untreated small cell lung cancer. The median duration of response was 12.5 weeks, with 63% of patients responding to salvage therapy (520). A similar dose and schedule in non-small-cell lung cancer resulted in a 20% major response rate with mild toxicity (521). Given at slightly higher dosages, other investigators also noted a 20% major response rate in non-small-cell lung cancer, with toxicities of edema, asthenia, and malaise (522). Antitumor responses have been noted in bladder cancer (523), in ovarian carcinoma refractory to cisplatin (524), 11% activity in pancreatic cancer (525), and 13% activity in head and neck cancer (526), with no activity seen in melanoma (527), gastric cancer (528), colorectal carcinoma (529), and hypernephroma (530). Significant side effects seen in the phase II experience included fatigue, liver function abnormalities, thrombocytosis, nausea/vomiting, and a flulike syndrome. Two patients with hypernephroma developed bronchospasm and dyspnea after receiving this agent (530). At the present time, the weekly administration schedule is preferred (531). The use of this agent in combination therapies needs to be explored, especially in lung and ovarian carcinoma (532).

FOSTEABINE (1-arabinofuranosylcytosine-5'-stearylphosphate; YNK 01) is a prodrug of cytosine arabinoside by virtue of its stearylphosphate residue. It had previously been shown to cause intravascular hemolysis when given parenterally. A phase I trial of this agent with oral dosages from 100 to 600 mg daily for 14 days revealed a one-compartment model with a $t_{(1/2)}$ of 9.4 hours and a suggestion of nonlinear kinetics for dose compared with AUC in small numbers of patients. Approximately 16% of the prodrug is believed to be absorbed, but radiolabeled studies have not been reported. Since cytosine arabinoside is degraded into uracil arabinoside (ara-U), presumably the prolonged detection of ara-U indicates prolonged levels of cytosine arabinoside (533).

LOMETREXOL (DDATHF; ICI D1694; 6R-5,10-dideazatetrahydrofolic acid) binds tightly to glycinamide ribonucleotide formyltransferase (an enzyme in the folic acid pathway) and requires polyglutamation (534). Inhibition of thymidylate synthase has been suggested as an additional step (535). It is related to an older agent, CB3717, which caused unpredictable toxicity (536). Analogues of this compound (LY 254155, LY 222306) have been described that are only monoglutamated and have activity in preclinical models resistant to DDATHF (534). Lometrexol demonstrated schedule-dependent cytotoxicity against the WiDr colonic cancer cell line (537). Similar dose and schedule changes were noted in the human ovarian cancer cell line SW626, with folic acid rescue ineffective 48 hours after DDATHF exposure (538). This agent has been compared in vitro with several of the new thymidylate synthase inhibitors such as BW1843U89 and found to be less active (395). Whether this finding has clinical significance is unknown. Preclinical animal toxicology suggested limiting side effects of neutropenia and mucositis (536). In contrast, the original drug with this mechanism of action, CB 3717, had shown renal toxicity (539). A phase I trial of this agent has been reported with dosages of 3 mg/m², 4.5 mg/m², and 6 mg/m² given on a weekly basis × 3 followed by a 2-week rest period. Thrombocytopenia was dose limiting, and cumulative toxicity was noted at the highest dose

level. Folinic acid seemed to be effective in shortening toxicity. A partial response in non-small-cell lung cancer was noted (540). Other phase I trials have noted side effects of arthalgia, malaise, nausea, and elevated liver function tests (536). Phase II studies are under way, and early reports have suggested a 27% response in colorectal cancer (541).

LY231514 has only fragmentary information published about its characteristics at the present time. This thymidylate synthase inhibitor demonstrates significant activity against human colon xenografts and has preclinical toxicology of vomiting, mucositis, weight loss, and myelosuppression. Early phase I data on a daily × 5 schedule giving this agent as a 10-minute infusion studied dosages of 0.2 to 0.52 mg/m², with nausea/vomiting, rash, somnolence, diarrhea, and stomatitis noted (542). Additional phase I information and early phase II data should be available soon.

PALA (N-(phosphonacetyl)-L-aspartate; NSC-22131), another drug with an uncertain future, may survive on its ability to modulate pyrimidine biosynthesis and enhance the effects of other antitumor agents such as 5-FU. PALA has been a disappointment as a single agent in humans. The compound is reconstituted in 5% glucose or 0.9% saline and is stable in solution for at least 14 days. This drug was rationally synthesized to tightly bind to aspartate carbamoyltransferase (ACTase) and thus block de novo pyrimidine biosynthesis (543). Uridine antagonizes PALA's antitumor effect. The drug has been reviewed in detail (543). In humans, a dose of 250 mg/m² was associated with modulation of the pyrimidine pathway (544). By itself, the drug has limiting toxicities of dermatitis, diarrhea, mucositis (5 to 10 days posttreatment), nausea, vomiting, paresthesias, and rarely seizures (543). PALA has been combined with dipyridamole with dose-limiting effects of diarrhea and abdominal pain (545), with L-alanosine (NSC-153353) in malignant melanoma (erythema, hemorrhagic blistering, and renal failure noted) (546), with 5-FU in pancreatic cancer (having a response rate of 14%) (547), with 5-FU in colorectal tumors (548), and with methotrexate, 5-FU, and folinic acid in colorectal cancers (549).

More recent studies of this agent have looked at high-dose 5-FU (2600 mg/m² over 24 hours given weekly with PALA, with dose-limiting diarrhea (550), or the addition of PALA to infusional 5-FU and folinic acid (551), PALA with infusional 5-FU and high-dose folinic acid (552), and PALA with 5-FU and radiation (553). Inhibition of the target enzyme, aspartate carbamoyltransferase, by PALA was transient in these studies (552). Demonstration that PALA improves the therapeutic index of other anticancer drugs is lacking at this time. A formulation of PALA in a liposome has been described with increased antitumor effects in vitro, but clinical studies have not been reported (554).

PIRITREXIM (BW 301U; PTX; 2,4-diamino-6-(2,5-dimethoxybenzyl)-5-methylpyrido (2,3-D)-pyrimidine) is another nonclassical antifol (based upon diaminopyrimidine) with lipophilic properties. PTX is a potent inhibitor of the target enzyme dihydrofolate reductase (DHFR) but does not inhibit histamine *N*-methyltransferase or diamine oxidase as did the original drug of this series, metoprine (555). As many of the original toxic effects of metoprine were felt to be histamine-mediated, antifols were discarded if they inhibited histamine metabolism. PTX rapidly enters sarcoma 180 cells in vitro by a simple diffusion process and does not require the reduced folate carrier (555). Unlike several of the other antifols, PTX does not inhibit thymidylate synthetase (555). This agent is not polyglutamated, and thus, toxicity can be reversed with short rescue courses of calcium leucovorin (folinic acid) (556). The drug has shown activity against some methotrexate-resistant cell lines. However, resistance has been described that involves both MDR and nonclassical mechanisms (557). In animals, the level of this drug in tissues was one order of magnitude higher than in plasma, rapid penetration into the CNS occurred, and oral bioavailability was 64% (556). Besides antitumor activity, PTX has shown extraordinary ability to inhibit the growth of *Pneumocystis carinii* and *Toxoplasma gondii*. This effect was due to inhibition of the parasites' DHFR enzymes by PTX. Sulfadiazine and PTX in combination showed synergism against these organisms (558). Hence, this agent may also prove useful in the treatment of opportunistic infections in the immunocompromised host. Initial phase I studies in cancer patients were done by a daily × 5 schedule by both the intravenous (in 5% dextrose) and oral routes. The MTD of the intravenous route occurred at 170 mg/m² day × 5, with toxicities of rashes, mucositis, phlebitis (which seemed to be related to the concentration of PTX infused–less at 0.144 mg/mL), leukopenia (at day 8), and thrombocytopenia (559). In man, PTX is 87 to 96% protein-bound, with a terminal plasma half-life of 3.1 to 5.3 hours. Hepatic dysfunction prolongs the excretion of this agent (559). Suggested phase II dosing by the intravenous route is 150 mg/m²/day × 5 in 1500 mL 5% dextrose over 6 hours (559).

Oral studies of this agent on the 5-day schedule revealed an MTD of 480 mg/m²/day, with the above toxicities plus nausea and vomiting. A divided-dose schedule lessened the GI toxicity (559). Administration of PTX on an oral 21-day schedule resulted in the above toxicities, liver function abnormalities, and diarrhea (560). Major antitumor responses were noted in bladder carcinoma progressing on M-VAC (561) and melanoma (560). This activity in urothelial carcinoma has been confirmed by a phase II trial administering the drug at 25 mg three times a day for 5 days in chemotherapy-naive patients. A response rate of 38% with a median response duration of 22 weeks and myelosuppression were noted (562). One patient was subsequently described as having an interstitial pneumonitis believed to be due to this drug (563). Additional phase II studies of this agent by the oral route have shown a major response rate of 26% in malignant melanoma (25 mg p.o. t.i.d. for 5 days every week × 3 with dosage escalation, repeated every month) (564), no significant responses in non-small-cell lung carcinoma using a 5-day schedule (565), and a 27% major response in squamous cell carcinoma of the head and neck with an oral 5-day schedule every 2 weeks (566). At the present time, it is unclear whether this antifol offers any advantage in therapy.

PT 523 (N-(4-amino-4-deoxypteroyl)-Nδ-hemiphthaloyl-L-ornithine) is an antifol that cannot be polyglutamated. In tissue culture, this agent was more active than methotrexate at nanomolar levels against H 35 rat hepatoma. Cell lines resistant to methotrexate on the basis of transport mutation or increased dihydrofolate reductase were resistant to this agent (567). This drug is believed to share the reduced folate carrier mechanism for uptake (568). Leucovorin antagonized the cytotoxic effects (567). PT 523 may be in clinical trials soon.

S-1 is an oral 5-FU agent that is currently undergoing trials in Japan. The drug is a combination of tegafur, 5-chloro-2,4-dihydroxypyridine (CDHP), and potassium oxonate. CDHP inhibits the catabolic enzyme for 5-FU, DPD, while oxonate inhibits pyrimidine phosphoribosyl-transferase (569). In xenografts, S-1 is more active than UFT. The drug has been studied as a single dose, daily as a single dose for 28 days with a 2-week rest, and daily as a twice a day administration for 28 days with a 2-week rest. Dose-limiting toxicity was leukopenia with mild diarrhea and stomatitis. Suggested phase II dosing is 75 mg twice a day (570).

TNP-351 (*N*-[4-[3-(2,4-diamino-7*H*-pyrrolo [2,3 - *d*] pyrimidin - 5 - yl) propyl]benzoyl - L-glutamic acid) is rapidly absorbed by cells and polyglutamated, with activity in preclinical screens in both leukemias and solid tumors. The drug inhibits an enzyme in folate metabolism, aminoimidazole carboxamide ribonucleotide transformylase (571), and recently was introduced into phase I trials in Japan (572). Clinical information is not yet available (463).

TOMUDEX (ZD 1694; ICI D1694; *N*-95-[*N*-(3,4-dihydro-2-methyl-4-oxoquinazolin-6-ylmethyl) - *N* - methylamino] - 2 - thenoyl) - L - glutamic acid) is an analogue of the thymidylate synthase inhibitor CB3717, with replacement of the *p*-aminobenzoate ring with a thiophene structure. This agent is rapidly taken up by cells by the reduced folate carrier and then polyglutamated (573). The polyglutamation seems to be necessary for cytotoxic function; its cytocidal ability increases with the number of glutamate residues added (574). Resistance occurs when the carrier mechanism is not functional. Phase I trials of a rapid intravenous infusion every 3 weeks explored dosages of 0.1 to 3.5 mg/m^2, with toxic effects above 1.6 mg/m^2. Toxicities were significant and numerous, including malaise, diarrhea, transaminitis, nausea/vomiting, leukopenia, drug fever, rash, and thrombocytopenia. Pharmacokinetic studies demonstrated a linear dose–AUC relationship and a terminal half-life of 50 to 100 hours. Suggested phase II dosage was 3 mg/m^2 (575). The American phase I trial differed slightly in its findings; the MTD was 4.5 mg/m^2 rather than 3.5 mg/m^2, and malaise with fever was more prominent (576). Both trials noted neutropenia as the dose-limiting toxicity. Whether these differences represent different pharmacogenetic parameters or undetermined drug interactions remains unknown. One phase II trial in 65 patients with colorectal carcinoma (41 evaluable at time of report) noted a 27% response rate. Grade 3–4 leukopenia occurred in 11%; vomiting, 12%; transaminitis, 6%; diarrhea, 12%; and fatigue, 5% of patients (577). Similar toxicities were seen in breast cancer patients, with a major response rate of 25% (578). At the present time, more information is needed to determine whether or not this agent offers any clinical advantages over standard therapeutics.

UFT is a combination of tegafur (1-(2-tetra hy-drofuryl)-5-fluorouracil) and uracil that can be given orally and is designed to maintain higher levels of 5-FU in the patient. Uracil is used to slow the metabolism of 5-FU. In a murine model system, UFT reduced intracellular dTTP pools for an extended time, suggesting a prolonged effect on thymidine synthase (579). Tegafur is a 5-FU prodrug that is available for oral administration in many countries but has never received FDA approval in the United States. Recent information suggests that UFT's absorption is lessened after gastrectomy, returning to baseline values at 3 months (580). Work on this combination has continued in Japan and was recently summarized (581). A randomized trial in man suggested that UFT, given at 300 to 400 mg/day for 2 years, was statistically better than observation (26% recurrence vs. 43%) in the management of surgically treated superficial bladder carcinoma (582). UFT has been combined with vinblastine and doxorubicin as adjuvant treatment for renal cell carcinoma in a single-arm trial suggesting benefit over historic controls (583). This agent has also been combined with folinic acid given by infusion, with dose-limiting toxicities of stomatitis and diarrhea (584). A phase II trial of UFT with oral leucovorin (UFT 300 to 350 mg/m^2/day with folinic acid 150 mg/day) resulted in a 42% major response rate in colorectal carcinoma with the most significant side effect of diarrhea (585). The advantage of this therapy is the oral route, but no prospective trial comparing this combination with 5-FU and leucovorin has been reported. Further studies are obviously warranted to determine whether or not UFT may be of value. With the advent of DPD inhibitors and higher-affinity thymidylate synthase inhibitors, the long-term future of this agent remains in doubt.

ANTIPROGESTINS

The development of this class of agents, first discovered over a decade ago, has been clouded by the political fight to restrict these drugs because of their use as abortifacients. As a result, clinical research in malignant disease has been painfully slow. Hormonal therapy has been the mainstay of much of the palliative treatment of malignant disease and also has been of use in the adjuvant setting for breast cancer. Since these agents offer a unique mode of action, they may offer new insights into therapy of neoplasia. Many compounds of this class have been developed, including RU 486, ZK 98299, ZK 98734,

Org 31719, Org 31806, and onapristone. ZK 98734 (lilopristone) is another antiprogestin structurally related to RU 486. Org 31710 and 31806 are more specific antiprogestins with a paucity of other endocrine effects (586). Antiprogestins have been evaluated in breast cancer cell lines, with evidence of growth inhibition of progesterone-receptor-positive cells in the presence of estrogen. In the absence of estrogen, this result was lost (587). In the DMBA rat model of breast cancer, these agents were marginally better than antiestrogens, but they showed significant antitumor activity when combined with antiestrogens (587). Pure antiestrogens (ICI 164384) combined with a potent antiprogestin, onapristone, show significant effects against several breast cancer tumor model systems (588). In tissue culture, onapristone enhances the apoptotic properties of vitamin D in MCF-7 cells (589). Another area of research is meningioma, which has been shown to express progesterone receptors and increased growth during pregnancy (590).

MIFEPRISTONE (RU 486; 11-[4-(dimethylamino)phenyl - 17 - hydroxy - 17 - (1 - propynyl)-11,17)-estra-4,9-dien-3-one) has been under development for many years in the endocrinologic and reproductive communities and is the best known antiprogestins in the United States because of coverage in the press. Depending upon the assay conditions, the drug can show either agonist or antagonist activity (591). Effects on progestin function in man can be seen at dosages as low as 0.1 mg/kg. As with most of these agents, the drug also displays antiglucocorticoid activity. At dosages of 1 to 2 mg/kg, this endocrinologic effect is seen inconsistently (592). However, at doses of 4 mg/kg and above, increases in secreted ACTH and cortisol in man suggest interference with the hypothalamic axis. A clinical addisonian syndrome after treatment with RU 486 has been extremely rare, even on a long-term chronic schedule, but when present is more apt to be seen at 200 to 400 mg/day (591). This agent has been studied in T-47D breast cancer cells, with the drug causing a drop of cells in cycle accompanied by a drop in *c-myc* expression (593). Antiprogestins seem to operate through the A isoform of the progesterone receptor by downregulating estrogen-receptor-induced gene transcription (594). This agent also reverses classical multidrug resistance but is not as effective as agents such as verapamil (595). RU 486 in tissue culture experiments of meningioma cells reduces the mitogenic effects of epidermal growth factor (590). Mifepristone reduced the growth of

meningioma xenografts in nude mice independent of progesterone receptor, suggesting that alternate mechanisms for antitumor effect may be present (596). RU 486 was also shown to enhance natural killer function in human peripheral leukocytes.

The pharmacology of this agent has been investigated for its endocrinologic effects. Oral absorption of RU 486 is high, but because of a first-pass metabolism by the liver, bioavailability is 40%. In man, unlike other species, this drug binds to a plasma glycoprotein (orosomucoid), which maintains drug levels for a prolonged period (591). At 50 mg dosage, the terminal half-life is 20 to 25 hours. Most of the drug and its metabolites are excreted in the feces (591). Initial experiments in metastatic breast cancer in humans have shown activity on a chronic daily dose schedule of 200 to 400 mg. At 200 mg/day, shrinkage of meningioma has been noted. The drug has been used in paraneoplastic Cushing's syndrome and has been suggested as potentially useful in steroid myopathy (591). Classical phase II trials in malignant disease are ongoing in several countries.

AROMATASE INHIBITORS

Aromatase inhibitors have continued to receive intense activity from synthetic chemists; 15 agents were listed as under evaluation in a recent review of the field (597). Therefore, this commentary can only be an overview of some of these agents under development. Drugs of this class have been divided into two groups based upon their mechanisms of action: (*a*) competitive inhibitors, and (*b*) suicide inhibitors (598). The former compounds do not damage the target enzyme, while the latter cause irreversible damage by covalent binding. Some investigators have further subdivided these drugs into steroidal and nonsteroidal classes based upon their structures (597).

ARIMIDEX (ZD1033; ICI D1033; 2,2'[5–1H-1,2,4-triazole-1-ylmethyl)-1,3-phenylene] bis(2-methylpropiononitrile)) inhibits placental aromatase in nanomolar concentrations of drug, was active orally in preclinical models, and is metabolized with urinary clearance. Only a minor amount of the parent compound (less than 10%) is cleared by the kidney (599). The drug is selective for the aromatase. Phase I studies in man have evaluated dosages from 0.1 to 60 mg as a single dose and as chronic dosing. A dose of 1 mg was the minimum threshold needed to reduce circulating estradiol to below the limits of detection at 24 hours. The serum half-life of this drug was 38 to 61 hours, with peak concentrations of drug reached within 2 hours after ingestion. Side effects were minor, and the suggested phase II dose is 1 mg/day (599). It has just been commercially released.

EXEMESTANE (FCE 24304; 6-methylenandrosta-1,4-diene-3,17-dione), a suicide inhibitor, causes irreversible damage to placental aromatase with no effect on 5-reductase or desmolase, thus showing high specificity (600). This drug did exhibit minor binding to the androgen receptor (600). A recent analogue of this agent, FCE 27993, that completely lacks this androgen effect has been described (601). FCE 27993 is effective in rat models of breast cancer and has been studied in a phase I trial in dosages ranging from 0.5 to 800 mg (598). The minimum threshold for consistent biologic effect on an oral dosing scheme was 25 mg, with maximal effect of suppressing circulating estrogens seen at 3 days posttreatment. No effect was seen on plasma cortisol or aldosterone levels (602). Plasma levels of exemestane were nondetectable by 24 hours after a single dose. Transient eosinophilia was also noted (602). A similar phase I trial evaluating dosages from 5 to 600 mg in postmenopausal women with breast cancer noted a lower threshold for biologic effects (5 mg/day), a 33% major response rate, and minor side effects of vertigo, headache, hot flushes, and nausea (603).

FADROZOLE (fadrozole hydrochloride; CGS 16849A; (tetrahydroimidazopyridine; 4-(5,6,7,8-tetrahydroimidazol(1,5)-pyridin-5-yl)-benzonitrile monohydrochloride) is a nonsteroidal aromatase inhibitor active orally. It belongs to the competitive inhibitor class of aromatase inhibitors and binds to the heme group on the enzyme (604). Compared with aminoglutethimide, fadrozole inhibition of this enzyme in vitro is 400 times higher and in vivo is 1000 times higher (605). However, the drug is not specific for this enzyme and also inhibits 11-hydroxylase and corticosterone methyl oxidase, leading to inhibition of cortisol and aldosterone formation (597). In the DMDA mammary tumor model, this agent lowers plasma estrogen levels, raises luteinizing hormone (LH) levels, and causes regression of the tumors. Administration of exogenous estrogen antagonizes the effect (606). Phase I data suggested that maximal biochemical inhibition occurs at 2 mg/day, with inhibition of C_{18}- and C_{21}-hydroxylases at 4 to 16 mg/day. Reduction of circulating estrogen levels has been seen within 5 hours of administration (607). Adrenal cortical function as measured by an ACTH challenge is blunted and, as expected, is seen as the dose increases (604). Postural hypotension was seen at the highest dosage (608). Antitumor effect has been seen in man at doses of 0.9 mg/day (609). Phase II trials have confirmed antitumor activity in metastatic breast cancer at dosages from 1–2 mg orally twice a day (610). Phase III trials are in progress in Europe and the United States.

LETROZOLE (CGS 20267; 4,4'-(1H-1,2,4-triazol-1-yl-methylene)-bis-benzonitrile) is a nonsteroidal inhibitor with eight times the potency of fadrazole (597). It is more specific, does not affect aldosterone or cortisol synthesis, and is orally active in preclinical models. Like many agents in this class, it is active in rat breast carcinoma models (598). In humans, letrozole suppressed circulating estradiol and estrone levels within 24 hours after an oral dose of 0.1 mg (604). Letrozole was studied at dosages from 0.1 to 5 mg/day, and at all levels, suppression of the aromatase was noted. Unlike fadrazole, letrozole did not blunt the ACTH stimulation of cortisol release. No significant side effects were noted (604). In a European phase II in patients with breast cancer, a daily oral dose of 0.5 mg gave a major response rate of 36% and minor toxicity, including one case of a flulike syndrome (611). This agent is in clinical trials.

ROGLETIMIDE (Pyridoglutethimide; 3-ethyl-3-(4-pyridyl) piperidine-2,6-dione) is a nonsteroidal aromatase inhibitor developed as an analogue of aminogluthemide. This drug is less potent than aminogluthemide (597). Suppression of circulating estrogens in man occurs at dosages above 200 mg twice a day, with side effects of nausea, lethargy, fatigue, vertigo, and hot flushes (598). Recent data suggest that this drug may enhance clearance of estrone as part of its actions (612).

VOROZOLE (R 83842; dextroenantiomer R83842; 6[(4-chlorophenyl)(1H-1,2,4-triazol-1-yl) methyl]-1-H-benzotriazole) is the active form of the racemic mixture of this drug, formerly referred to as R 76713 (vorozole racemate). The drug is the (+)-S-isomer and is a nonsteroidal compound with activity in the nanomolar range against aromatase (613). The drug did not show other endocrinologic effects and was active in the rat model (613). Vorozole has been studied in a dosage range from 1 to 5 mg/day, with a minor reduction in circulating cortisol seen at the highest dose level and a major response rate of

33% in this study (614). Side effects were minor and included headache and nausea. One patient with a history of thyrotoxicosis had thyroid enlargement without change in TSH (614). A phase II trial with estrogen-receptor-positive tumors, using a daily dose of 2.5 mg in postmenopausal patients with breast cancer, reported a 10% major response rate, with allergic skin reactions and gastrointestinal side effects (610). The drug remains under active evaluation.

TOPOISOMERASE I INHIBITORS

Topoisomerase I is the enzyme that relaxes supercoiled DNA by creating transient single-strand breaks through which another DNA strand can pass during DNA replication, RNA transcription, and other DNA functions (615). The breaks are resealed by the topoisomerase enzyme (615). Topoisomerase inhibitors stabilize the covalent complex between topoisomerase I and DNA, resulting in enzyme-linked DNA single-strand breaks that cannot be religated in the presence of the drug, leading to cytotoxicity (615).

Camptothecins

The camptothecins are anticancer drugs with a unique mechanism of action. They poison eukaryotic DNA topoisomerase I (616). The parent drug, sodium camptothecin, demonstrated objective antineoplastic activity, but development was limited because of unpredictable myelosuppression, gastrointestinal toxicity, and hemorrhagic cystitis (615). The design of camptothecin analogues has focused on substitutions in the A ring of the molecule to enhance aqueous solubility and increase antitumor activity (617).

Two water-soluble derivatives have been synthesized and are undergoing clinical trials, topotecan (TPT)[9(dimethylamino)methyl-10-hydroxycamptothecin (NSC609699)] and CPT-11 [7-ethyl-10-[4-(1-piperidino)-1-piperidino]carbonyloxycamptothecin, irinotecan, (NSC616348)] (618). A derivative that is not water soluble, 9-aminocamptothecin, is entering clinical trials because of activity in solid tumor xenografts (616).

In phase I trials of topoisomerase I inhibitors, the compounds were significantly more effective as a continuous exposure than as a 1-hour exposure (619). The dose-limiting toxicities differed; for topotecan, they were neutropenia and thrombocytopenia; for CPT-11, diarrhea; and for intoplicine, hepatotoxicity.

9-AMINOCAMPTOTHECIN (NSC603071) has significant preclinical activity in solid tumors (616, 620, 621). In mice, plasma levels remained above 13.3 nM, the lower limit of quantitation, for only 6 hours (617). The plasma profile of the intact lactone form of the drug demonstrated biexponential decay (617). The 9-amino substituent profoundly diminished the apparent extent of tissue distribution, effecting an enhanced rate of elimination, $t_{(1/2)}$ of 1.4 hours (617). In general, substitution at the 9 or 10 positions with amino, halogeno, or hydroxyl groups in compounds with 20S configurations results in enhanced topoisomerase I inhibition (622). 9-Aminocamptothecin had activity in chlorambucil-resistant chronic lymphocytic leukemia cell lines (623). Cultured cells that overexpress P-glycoprotein can develop some level of cross-resistance to the topoisomerase I inhibitors (624). The 9-aminocamptothecin can be converted in vivo from the 9-nitro derivative. This may have economic and clinical implications (625, 626). This drug is in phase I trials in the United States.

TOPOTECAN (TPT)[9(dimethylamino)methyl-10-hydroxycamptothecin, SK & F 104864, hycamptamine, NSC609699] has been extensively evaluated. It differs from the parent compound by the presence of a basic side chain (615), which results in greater water solubility. The drug has activity in resistant cell lines (615). Topotecan is reversibly hydrolyzed in a pH-dependent reaction in aqueous solutions to the ring-open hydroxy acid (627). The disposition of the closed-ring lactone and the hydroxy acid has been studied (627). Topotecan is partially hydrolyzed prior to administration in parenteral solutions. Renal clearance accounts for 30% of the drug elimination. The relationship between topotecan dose and myelotoxicity is well fit by a sigmoidal E_{max} model, as is the relationship between total topotecan AUC and myelotoxicity (627, 628). A limited-sampling model has been developed (629). The drug is schedule dependent (630, 631). It has a short half-life in plasma, with a plasma elimination showing a mean $t_{1/2}$ of 3.5 hours. As a 24-hour infusion, dose-limiting neutropenia occurred at doses of 1.75 mg/m^2/week (630). Pharmacodynamic analysis showed that the pharmacokinetic parameters of both the lactone and total drug were positively correlated with bone marrow toxicity (630). Pharmacokinetic modeling has described clearance from plasma and cerebrospinal fluid (632). Pharmacokinetic analysis showed a half-life of 3 hours with significant renal elimination and substantial biliary concentration (633).

In a phase I trial, the drug was given as a 30-minute infusion daily × 5 days every 3 weeks. The MTD was 1.5–2.0 mg/m²/day, with dose-limiting neutropenia. Further dose escalation has been attempted with growth factors (634, 635). A phase I trial of a 21-day continuous low-dose infusion has been reported. The DLT was myelosuppression, with thrombocytopenia greater than neutropenia. The MTD was 0.53 mg/m². Objective responses were seen in ovarian cancer, breast cancer, renal cancer, and non-small-cell lung cancer (636). Three- and 5-day continuous infusion schedules have also been evaluated (637), as well as an every-21-day bolus schedule (638).

The drug has shown promising antileukemic effects (634, 639, 640). The phase I study defined an MTD of 10 mg/m² by continuous infusion over 5 days every 3 to 4 weeks in patients with refractory or relapsed acute leuekmia (639). Phase I trials have shown responses in refractory ovarian cancer and non-small-cell lung cancer (641).

Activity has been seen against pediatric and adult CNS tumor xenografts (642). In a pediatric phase I trial, the recommended dose was 1.0 mg/m²/day for 3 days as a constant intravenous infusion followed by G-CSF for 14 days every 21 days (643). A relationship between systemic exposure to topotecan and myelosuppression was demonstrated (644). The possibility of individualized topotecan administration schedules has been suggested (644). A 24-hour pediatric continuous infusion trial recommended a starting dose of 5.5 mg/m² (615). Additional responses in phase I trials included non-small-cell lung cancer, ovarian cancer, small cell lung cancer, colon cancer, esophageal cancer, neuroblastoma, AML, and CML (633).

A phase II trial of 20 untreated patients with metastatic NSCLC has been performed at a dose of 2 mg/m² for 5 days every 21 days. No clinical responses were observed despite high-grade neutropenia (645). However, other investigators have noted activity in both small cell and non-small-cell lung cancer and ovarian cancer (646). Combination trials have been suggested by computer modeling (647).

CPT-11 [7-ethyl-10-[4-(1-piperidino)-1-piperidino]carbonyloxycamptothecin, irinotecan, (NSC 616348)] has been extensively evaluated. The major metabolite is 7-ethyl-10-hydroxycamptothecin (SN-38) (648). When given as a 90-minute infusion every 3 weeks, an MTD of 240 mg/m² was defined. Dose escalation is limited by an acute treatment-related syndrome of flushing, warmth, nausea, vomiting, and diarrhea. Anorexia, weight loss, and neutropenia also occur (634). Responses have been seen in refractory colorectal cancer, non-small-cell lung cancer, lymphoma, ovarian cancer, head and neck cancer, pancreatic cancer, and breast cancer (641).

A phase I trial of CPT-11 with etoposide (a topoisomerase II inhibitor) at 80 mg/m² on days 1, 3, and 5 with G-CSF in advanced lung cancer has been reported (648). The MTD was 90 mg/m² over 90 minutes weekly. The response rates for small cell and non-small-cell lung cancers were 58% and 22%, respectively (648). The recommended dose of CPT-11 is 80 mg/m². A high-dose (>350 mg/m²) regimen was analyzed. A non-dose-dependent diarrhea and a cholinergic syndrome affected nearly all patients. The MTD was 750 mg/m² (649). A phase II trial in colon cancer showed activity at 350 mg/m² every 3 weeks, which is felt to be the optimal schedule (650–652).

GG211 is a water-soluble camptothecin undergoing phase I trials. It has been studied from doses of 0.25 to 2.0 mg/m²/day as a 72-hour infusion. The steady-state concentration increases linearly with dose. Terminal half-life was 8.5 ± 3.4 hours. MTD is expected to be 1.9 mg/m²/day, with neutropenia as the dose-limiting toxicity (653).

GI147211C, a water-soluble camptothecin analogue, has shown preclinical activity in a number of xenograft models (654). This drug may be taken to clinical trials.

INTOPLICINE (RP 60475; NSC 645008) is an antitumor derivative in the 7*H*-benzo[e]pyrido[4,3-b]indole series. It strongly binds DNA and thereby increases the length of linear DNA (655). These properties are consistent with DNA unwinding. Intoplicine was found to be a dual topoisomerase I and II inhibitor, which is critical for the antitumor activity of this series of compounds (655). Intoplicine might circumvent topoisomerase I and II–mediated resistance by poisoning both enzymes simultaneously (656). The drug has shown greater cytotoxicity with solid-tumor cells (657). Activity was seen against breast, non-small-cell lung, and ovarian cancer colony-forming units. It was felt that plasma levels of 10 μg/mL would be required to demonstrate significant activity (658). The drug was found to be schedule dependent (657). Pharmacokinetic studies showed extensive drug binding to red blood cells. A plasma $t_{(1/2)}$ in excess of 40 hours was observed. The DLT was hepatocellular damage occurring at doses of 336 mg/m²/day and higher (659). In a 24-hour infusion, the elimination half-lives in whole blood and plasma are 171 and 89 hours, respectively. Sixty percent of the drug is excreted unchanged in the feces, and only 10% in the urine (660).

LIPOSOMAL PREPARATIONS

The use of liposomes to carry lipid-soluble agents to target tissue, change the pharmacokinetics of the antitumor substance, modify the toxicity of the treatment, and change dosing schedule is under development. It has been the subject of a number of reviews (661–663). Most applications of liposomes attempt to change tissue distribution and various pharmacokinetic parameters of the chemotherapy to increase the therapeutic index of the drugs (663). Early studies with liposomes showed uptake predominantly into cells of the reticuloendothelial system, with liver and spleen being responsible for clearance of the drug from the circulation. There was no evidence of tumor localization. (663). Liposomes can now be designed rationally, resulting in nonreactive liposomes (Sls) (664). Because of their reduced recognition by the body, they have been referred to as "stealth liposomes" (664).

ANNAMYCIN (4-demethoxy-2'-iodo-3'-hydroxy-4'-epidoxorubicin) is a lipophilic anthracycline antibiotic that has shown partial lack of cross-resistance with doxorubicin in vitro. A lyophilized liposomal formulation has been developed for clinical trials (665). The liposomal carrier increased plasma levels, enhanced tumor activity, and decreased its vesicant properties (665).

DAUNORUBICIN has shown activity in AIDS-related Kaposi's sarcoma. Twenty-five patients were treated with liposomal daunorubicin at a dose of 40 mg/m² every 2 weeks. In 24 evaluable patients, there were 2 CRs and 13 PRs. Responses were seen in doxorubicin-resistant patients. Improvement in quality-of-life measures was noted, with minimal toxicity. Myelosuppression was the commonest toxicity (666). A phase I/II trial showed improved pharmacokinetic profiles over free daunorubicin. The drug was well tolerated and showed a 55% response rate at doses of 50 and 60 mg/m². The median survival was 9 months (667).

Single-agent high-dose liposomal daunorubicin showed no activity in non-small-cell lung cancer (668). A phase II study in breast cancer at 100 mg/m² every 3 weeks showed some responses and minimal toxicity. Further dose escalations are planned (669).

DOXORUBICIN. In preclinical studies, a doxorubicin liposome formulation containing polyethylene-glycol (Doxil) showed a long circulation time in plasma, enhanced accumulation in tumors, and a superior therapeutic activity over free drug (670). Most of the administered dose was cleared from the plasma in 45 hours. Nearly 100% of the drug detected in plasma was encapsulated (670). The pharmacokinetics followed a pattern dictated by the liposome carrier (670).

Activity of liposomal doxorubicin has been seen in AIDS-related Kaposi's sarcoma (KS). In one trial, 16 patients were treated at 20 mg/m² every 2 or 3 weeks; 11 patients had a partial remission. The median duration of response was 14 weeks. Myelosuppression was the most common toxicity, with other side effects considered mild (671). Three patients with KS responded with moderate leukopenia (672). Thirty-four patients were treated at a dose of 20 mg/m² every 3 weeks with a 73.5% response rate. Responses lasted a median of 9 weeks (673). A phase I trial of liposome-encapsulated doxorubicin in egg PC/chol liposomes with a diameter of less than 1 μm has been reported (674).

PLATINUM. Cis-bis-neodecanoato-*trans-R,R*-1,2-diaminocyclohexane platinum(II) (L-NDDP) is a lipophilic cisplatin derivative that has been formulated entrapped in multilamellar liposomes composed of dimyristoylphosphatidyl choline and dimyristoylphosphatidyl glycerol (675). Reproducible batches can be produced which would be available for future clinical trials (675). The pharmacokinetics of L-NDDP and cisplatin were studied in the rat (676). Prolongation of the mean retention time of L-NDDP in the peritoneum was achieved after intraperitoneal administration. Kidney platinum levels were lower in rats receiving L-NDDP than in those receiving cisplatin administered by either the intraperitoneal or intravenous route. L-NDDP has enhanced efficacy in malignancies confined to the peritoneal cavity (676).

TLC D-99. Preclinical toxicology studies of liposome-encapsulated doxorubicin (TLC D-99) showed the encapsulated compound to be less toxic than free doxorubicin (677). The only significant side effect was fever. The empty liposomes showed no toxicity. The organ toxicities seen were qualitatively similar to those of the free drug, but less severe (677). A phase I trial showed that leukopenia was dose limiting, with the MTD 90 mg/m^2 every 3 weeks (678). No organ toxicity was noted. The drug produced less nausea, vomiting, and stomatitis than would be expected with free doxorubicin (678).

VINCRISTINE exposure has been enhanced by increasing the circulation longevity by liposomal incorporation (679). The incorporation of the ganglioside GM1 increased circulation longevity (679, 680). The vincristine-encapsulation procedure has been modified, which enhances drug retention (679). These two approaches are synergistic and increase the circulation half-life of vincristine from 1 hour to more than 12 hours. This chemical change has enhanced the activity against the murine P388 lymphocytic leukemia model (679). More cures were noted in the mouse mammary carcinoma (681). A phase I study at doses starting at 0.5 mg/m^2 has been reported in solid tumors (680).

MONOCLONAL ANTIBODY COC166–9 against ovarian cancer was conjugated with Adriamycin or cisplatin and entrapped in liposomes as immunochemical-liposomes MLA and MLP (682). MLA had activity on SKOV3 (ovarian cancer cell line) growth inhibition (682).

NOVEL COMPOUNDS

A large variety of compounds are under development in an attempt to exploit unique characteristics of tumors, such as their hypoxic environment, abnormal blood vessel formation, presence of resistance mechanisms, and differential sensitivity to toxic damage. As with other areas of drug development, combinatorial chemistry may have a profound effect on drug development in the above areas. Many of these compounds will fail to demonstrate sufficient activity for incorporation into standard therapy but offer unique approaches. The diligent reader will note that many of the compounds listed in this section in the prior edition are no longer discussed, and a host of new agents are under study.

AMIFOSTINE (WR 2721; ethyol; gammaphos; YM-08310; S-2-(3-aminopropylamino) ethyl-phosphoro-thionic acid; NSC 296961) was originally developed as a radiation protector in the hopes of increasing the therapeutic index in man (683). Aminothiol compounds interact with reactive intermediates and free radicals to prevent chemical damage to DNA. This drug was quickly shown to reduce DNA cross-linking by alkylating agents (684), and it selectively protects

normal tissue more than neoplastic tissue (685). Hence, major emphasis was placed on developing this agent to protect normal tissue against the effects of cytotoxics. Studies suggest that normal tissues take up this agent by facilitated diffusion, while neoplastic cells only concentrate the drug by passive diffusion. In the microenvironment of the cell, amifostine (a prodrug) is converted by dephosphorylation to WR 1065, which is the active agent. A low pH, such as found in tumors, and poor vascularity reduce the amount of active drug reaching tumor tissue, thus adding to the differential effects. This compound also inhibits parathyroid hormone (PTH) secretion and inhibits nephrocalcinosis in a rat model (686). Amifostine has been given at dosages from 740 to 910 mg/m^2 by intravenous infusion, with major toxicities of nausea, vomiting, transient hypotension, and transient hypocalcemia (687). The active metabolite, WR 1065, is believed to be responsible for the hypotension. The parent drug is rapidly cleared from the plasma (within 6 minutes) in man and persists in tissue for 30 to 180 minutes in animals (688).

As this drug has been under development for more than a decade, a large amount of data has evolved. Although a radioprotector in preclinical models, amifostine given at 75 mg/m^2/day as a 5-minute infusion with a total cumulative dose of 1300 mg/m^2 (range 280–3700 mg/m^2) did not protect against radiation side effects in patients with cervical cancer (689). This drug did seem to allow a greater carboplatin dose (400–500 mg/m^2) to be administered when two infusions of amifostine at 740 mg/m^2 were given over 15 minutes at the time of chemotherapy treatment. No change in carboplatin pharmacokinetics was noted (690).

This study was followed by an EORTC phase I trial of three doses of amifostine with a 15-minute infusion of carboplatin, demonstrating an ability to give larger amounts of cytotoxic agent. Side effects, including severe nausea/vomiting and hypotension, were significant, resulting in a reduction of the amifostine dose from 910 to 740 mg/m^2 (691). These investigators did find changes in terminal half-life and AUC of ultra-filterable platinum (691). The platinum drugs are not rapidly inactivated by amifostine or its metabolite. These results thus imply that a combination treatment with amifostine and a platinum compound will not reduce antitumor efficacy (692). This drug did show a protective role in the use of cyclophosphamide (688) and prevention of cisplatin nephrotoxicity (692). Less hematotoxicity was found on two sequential trials of amifostine with either carboplatin or cisplatin, without affecting platinum-DNA adduct formation in normal buccal cells (693). Combined with mitomycin, amifostine reduced the degree of thrombocytopenia (694). The drug also seems to offer protection to normal stem cells in marrow purged ex vivo with 4-hydroperoxycyclophosphamide, leading to more rapid engraftment after autologous transplantation (695). The role of this drug in preventing secondary malignancies needs to be defined.

BATIMASTAT (BB-94; [4-*N*-hydroxyamino)-2*R*-isobutyl-3*S*-(thienyl-thiomethyl) succinyl]-L-phenylalanine-*N*-methylamide) was developed to be an analogue of the substrate for metalloproteinase, because activation of this enzyme is believed to be involved in metastatic progression. In mice, concentrations of this agent were determined by bioassay to effect a plasma level 10-fold greater than the IC_{50} needed to inhibit collagenase. In a xenograft model of colon carcinoma, chronic intraperitoneal dosing with BB-94 reduced the size of the primary lesion and the number and location of metastases (696). In an ovarian xenograft model, this agent caused resolution of ascites and prolongation of survival (697). An early phase I trial in man has been reported with dosing at 150 mg/m^2 by the intraperitoneal route. No significant side effects were noted with BB-94 levels maintained in the plasma over 21 days at therapeutic levels (698).

BUTHIONINE SULFOXIMINE (L-BSO; buthionine-(*SR*)-sulfoximine; NSC 326231) is an irreversible inhibitor of γ-glutamylcysteine synthetase. In tissue culture, BSO can lower glutathione levels to 10% of control (699). As discussed in the chapter on drug resistance, glutathione is believed to be involved in one of the mechanisms of resistance used by cells to prevent irreversible damage induced by alkylating agents, doxorubicin, and radiation (700–703). BSO is active orally in mice (699). Reduction of glutathione by BSO in L1210 leukemia cells caused enhanced DNA-DNA cross-linking in the presence of melphalan (704). In vitro, human non-small-cell lung cancer (SW-1573), ovarian carcinoma, and breast carcinoma (MCF-7) cell lines in the presence of BSO were twice as sensitive to cytotoxic agents (705). Human gastric cancer xenografts demonstrated increased sensitivity to cisplatin after treatment with BSO (706). Clonogenicity was reduced by BSO in melanoma cells (707). In marked contrast, treatment of the breast carcinoma cell line MCF-7 with BSO

increased resistance to paclitaxel, suggesting that glutathione depletion may have many roles (708).

BSO may also have a differential effect in mice in that bone marrow may be more resistant to its glutathione-depleting action than are most other organs (709). This area remains controversial, as other studies have noted 83% depletion of glutathione levels in marrow and only 40% depletion in lung tissue (710). However, despite a 90% reduction of glutathione levels in tumor cells by BSO in a mouse leukemia model, the therapeutic index was not improved (709). The administration of BSO to nude mice bearing human solid tumor xenografts did show enhanced therapeutic index (711). In the B-16 melanoma model, the effect of BSO could be correlated with cellular glutathione peroxidase activity, and the combination of this agent with melphalan showed a synergistic effect (712). Of great interest, in tissue culture, human myeloma cells were very sensitive to BSO (713). In addition, the choice of alkylating agent administered may be critical, as unexpected toxicities were seen in mice treated with BSO and cyclophosphamide (714).

Phase I studies of BSO have been reported; a recent evaluation of BSO as an infusion over 30 minutes every 12 hours for a total of 6–10 doses demonstrated side effects of nausea/vomiting. Glutathione, as measured in circulating leukocytes, was maximally depleted after 6 doses, with a non-dose-dependent decrease in glutathione level (715). Plasma half-life of this agent was less than 2 hours with doses between 1.5 and 13.1 g/m^2 (715). Investigators have suggested a prolonged infusion of BSO, based upon animal models (716).

CARDIOXANE (ICRF-187; dexrazoxan; AD 529; Zinerard; (4,4' - (- 1 - methyl - 1,2 - ethane-diyl)bis-(+)-2,6-piperazinedione; NSC-169780) is the (+) enantiomer of ICRF-159, with greater solubility than the racemic mixture (ICRF-159). This agent is usually stored under refrigeration and administered in 5% dextrose (717). As a single agent, it has been studied on a variety of schedules: days 1 to 3, 48-hour continuous infusion, days 1 to 5, and weekly. Dose-limiting toxicities of leukopenia and thrombocytopenia were seen in adults in most trials (718–720) and hepatic function abnormalities in children (721) and in adults on a once-weekly × 4 schedule every 6 weeks (722). In the weekly study, the MTD was 3.8 g/m^2/week. The terminal half-life of this agent was 3.2 ± 0.9 hours (722). The drug had marginal antitumor activity as a single agent but was able to inhibit free radical formation by doxorubicin in perfused rat hearts (723). In dogs, this agent had a cardioprotective role in preventing anthracycline damage (724). Timing of administration was important, with concurrent use better than sequential administration of drugs (725). Modulation of anthracycline toxicity was also seen in spontaneously hypertensive rats (726, 727). However, recent in vitro work suggests that this agent inhibits the single-strand breaks caused by topoisomerase II–dependent cytotoxic agents. Nontoxic doses of cardioxane could also inhibit cytotoxicity in vitro seen with etoposide and daunorubicin (728). These results were tested in other animals (729), leading to a clinical trial in humans (729, 730). A phase I trial of cardioxane with epirubicin, cyclophosphamide, and 5-FU encountered significant hematologic toxicity and localized vascular toxicity believed to be due to the ICRF-187 (731). Pharmacologic evaluation of this study revealed no change in the anthracycline parameters, with a 30% increase in cardioxane terminal half-life when epirubicin was administered at 100 mg/m^2 (732). The use of GM-CSF did not prevent hematologic toxicity of cardioxane with doxorubicin doses above 72 mg/m^2, suggesting that the cytotoxic agent and its putative protector might interact adversely in the bone marrow (733). No perturbation of doxorubicin pharmacology by cardioxane was identified (734). Because of concerns about toxicity of this agent in combination with anthracyclines and because cardioxane may interfere with antitumor efficacy, this drug has just been licensed in the States after many years of evaluation.

CM 101 (GBS toxin) is an interesting polysaccharide with a unique mode of action. In mice, this agent causes an inflammation of the tumor neovasculature. A phase I study in man has studied doses from 7.5 to 37.5 µg/kg as a 15-minute infusion on days 1, 3, and 5. Leukopenia, fever, chills, and liberation of TNF have been documented, with two regressions noted—one in a patient with duodenal carcinoma and another in a patient with Kaposi's sarcoma. No delayed or chronic toxicities have been noted (735).

CYCLOCREATINE (AM 285; 1-carboxymethyl-2-iminoimidazolidine) was developed to be an analogue of the substrate for the enzyme creatine kinase, which is overexpressed in many tumors (736). This drug is phosphorylated by the enzyme and is believed to interfere with ATP generation (737). Cytotoxicity by this agent is mainly in the S phase of the cell cycle and is believed to interfere with cellular energy homeostasis (736). Cells expressing high levels of creatine kinase are more sensitive to cyclocreatine (738). This agent seems to also potentiate cytotoxic effects in xenografts (738). In a human colony-forming system, this drug was active in the millimolar range (737). Infusion schedules of cyclocreatine have been studied in the rat, with suggestion of earlier uptake of drug by tumor than by host tissue (739). A phase I study in man, administering this drug over 3 hours, noted fluid retention, but the evaluation of the drug was still in progress (740).

DEXNIGULDIPINE (R-NG) is a dihydropyridine able to antagonize the classical multiple drug resistance pump. The drug also affects protein C kinase (741). The drug has been studied as a phase I agent in acute leukemia at doses from 1250 to 2250 mg/day orally, with toxicities of vertigo, hypotension, tachycardia, bradycardia, and hypocalcemia noted. Refractory patients demonstrated a meaningful remission of 24% when classical induction therapy was combined with this agent (742). This drug has been studied in myeloma patients at a dose of 2.5 g/day orally for 8 days with VAD (vincristine, doxorubicin, dexamethasone) or VECD (vincristine, epirubicin, cyclophosphamide, dexamethasone), with some activity seen in refractory patients (743). Dexverapamil, an isomer of the racemic verapamil, is under similar evaluation (744).

EFLORNITHINE (DMFO; α-difluoromethylornithine) was developed as an irreversible inhibitor of ornithine decarboxylase, leading to a decrease in intracellular putrescine and spermidine levels (745). This decrease in polyamines was paralleled by a rise in the enzyme S-adenosylmethionine carboxylase. Purine and pyrimidine ribonucleotide pools were also increased (745). The drug can be given orally in divided dosages up to 10 g/day, with toxicities of nausea, vomiting, diarrhea, thrombocytopenia, and transient hearing loss. This drug has been disappointing as a cytotoxic but is believed to have chemopreventative properties. One recent trial suggested that chronic oral dosing had significant activity in anaplastic gliomas and needs confirmation (746). In mice, DMFO delayed the appearance of secondary tumors after radiation (747). Gastric tumors were prevented when DMFO was administered with a carcinogen in a rat model (748). Antimetastatic effects have also been seen in rodent systems (749). Chronic oral dosing in animals on a daily schedule for a year revealed dose-dependent toxicities to be conjunctivitis, hyperkeratosis, weight loss, dermatitis, liver necrosis, and gastric inflammation (750). Phase I trials for chemoprevention have been presented. An examination of dosages between 200 and 1600 mg/m^2/day revealed dose-limiting side effects of decreased auditory acuity, diarrhea, fatigue, joint pain, insomnia, and rash, with linear pharmacokinetics (751). A phase I trial using inhibition of the target enzyme ornithine decarboxylase as an endpoint suggested a phase II chemopreventive dose of 500 mg/m^2 (752).

DMP 840 ((R,R) 2,2'-[1,2 ethanediylbis[imino (1 - methyl - 2,1 - ethane - diyl)] - bis {5 - nitro - 1H benz[de]-isoquinoline-1,3-2H) dione} dimethanesulfonate; NSC D640430) is an analogue of a compound discovered as an inhibitor of protein kinase, which demonstrated antitumor activity (753). The drug binds to G-C bases in DNA with high affinity and is believed to be an intercalcator. In tissue culture, DMP 840 is active at nanomolar concentrations against both resting and growing cells. The drug does demonstrate some activity against classical multiple-drug-resistant (MDR-1) cell lines. Single-strand breaks in DNA and inhibition of thymidine and uridine incorporation into nucleic acids were observed in vitro (754). The drug is soluble at 3 mg/mL (755). Of note, this agent demonstrates minimal cytotoxic effect against murine tumor lines (P388, L1210) in mice as measured by prolongation of survival. In xenograft models, this agent was curative in MX-1 mammary carcinoma and demonstrated schedule dependence, with daily × 9 dosing giving optimal results. Oral administration was inferior to intravenous. Antitumor activity was dose dependent, with little effect below 2 mg/kg in this system (753). In xenografts of colon cancer and rhabdomyosarcoma, DMP 840 showed marked antitumor activity and was non-cross-resistant with vincristine (755). A phase I study in man has reported a short infusion schedule daily × 5, with dose-limiting neutropenia and significant venous irritation requiring central access. Heavily pretreated patients had an MTD of 10.8 mg/m^2; minimally treated patients had an MTD of 14 mg/m^2. Other side effects noted were malaise, fatigue, mucositis, pruritus, and hypersensitivity vasculitis. Recommended phase II dosing is 10.8 mg/m^2 (756).

ETANIDAZOLE, a less lipophilic analogue of misonidazole, is amply discussed in the radiation therapy literature. As hypoxic cell sensitizers are being studied with alkylating agents, this drug was evaluated in a phase I trial with cyclophosphamide and carboplatin. Etanidazole was administered as two doses 90 minutes apart immediately prior to the chemotherapy. The initial dose level was associated with neuropathy and possible perturbation of carboplatin pharmacokinetics (757). Further clinical studies are in progress.

FARANOX is a chloroethylaminophenylacetic acid derivative undergoing trials in Lithuania. Information is fragmentary. Phase I evaluation established a safe oral dose of 90 to 120 mg/m^2. A phase II trial of 188 patients with diverse histologies revealed a major response rate of 35 to 40% in melanoma and 42% in lymphoma. Combination trials with other cytotoxics demonstrated a slightly higher response rate in melanoma (758).

GOSSYPOL, derived from cottonseed oil, has been used as a contraceptive agent in China. The compound is active against a variety of cell lines, is active in the Dunning prostate cancer rat model, and affects cells at a variety of levels (759). The drug is active in prostate cancer cell lines and in the MAT-LyLu rat model. Initial studies in humans by the oral route in dosages from 30 to 70 mg/day suggested chronic dosing of 30 mg/day. Toxicities include xerostomia, transaminitis, xeroderma, fatigue, nausea/vomiting, ileus, and hair loss (759). Trials in metastatic prostate carcinoma are expected.

KW-2189, a derivative of duocarmycin B_2, is an antitumor antibiotic that binds to the minor groove of DNA and alkylates adenine. The drug is metabolized by an esterase to a more toxic form (DU-86) and is active in a variety of xenograft models. A phase I trial in Japan has studied doses from 0.1 to 0.4 mg/m^2 as a single intravenous infusion, with dose-limiting toxicities of leukopenia and thrombocytopenia that occurred 5 weeks and 4 weeks posttreatment, respectively. The terminal half-life of the parent compound was 0.65 to 1.26 hours, with the metabolite undetectable 1 hour posttreatment. Clinical development continues (760).

LIBLOMYCIN (NK313) is a bleomycin analogue developed in Japan with decreased pulmonary toxicity in animal models. The drug has a bulky lipophilic group at its amino terminus. The MTD in humans is 140 mg/m^2 as a 15-minute intravenous infusion weekly × 4, with dose-limiting myelosuppression. Other toxicities noted were nausea, vomiting, transient liver function abnormalities, and transient rises in BUN, but no pulmonary toxicity (761). A phase II trial in previously treated lymphoma patients has been reported, using a dose of 80 to 100 mg/ m^2/week × 4. One out of 4 patients with Hodgkin's disease showed a major response, with a variety of major responses in non-Hodgkin's lymphomas, lasting from 4 to 13 weeks. Responses occurred rapidly (at a mean of 14 days), with toxicities of leukopenia, nausea/vomiting, hair loss, transient increases in SGOT and SGPT, and drug fever. Eleven patients had CO_2 diffusing capacity done, and 6 showed no apparent drop in function (762). The role of this agent in the treatment of malignant disease remains uncertain, as it does not represent a major therapeutic advance at this time.

LONIDAMINE (LND; 1-(2,4-dichlorobenzyl)-1-H-indazol-3-carboxylic acid) is an orally active drug that has been undergoing phase II trials in the United States and Europe for many years. It has not been able to achieve licensing status in the United States. The drug interferes with mitochondrial function by inhibiting hexokinase (763, 764). In addition, the drug induces morphologic changes in both mitochondrial and cell membranes. The drug is usually used as a radiation sensitizer but has additional properties in its own right. In vitro, LND enhances the uptake of doxorubicin into Ehrlich ascites tumor (765) by changing membrane permeability (766). In preclinical models, addition of LND to a topoisomerase II inhibitor enhanced the effects of added alkylators (767). In ovarian carcinoma cell lines, LND enhanced the cytotoxic effects of cisplatin in both sensitive (A2780) and resistant (A2780/cp8) lines, with evidence of stabilizing the block in S/G_2 of the cell cycle (768). This drug had minimal activity in human small cell lung carcinoma cells (769). Phase I studies demonstrated myalgia, somnolence, and hyperesthesia of the skin (770). Plasma half-life of the drug is 2.5 to 11.7 hours. Phase II trials have noted, in addition, nausea, photophobia, testicular pain, and ototoxicity. Myelosuppression was not seen. Occasional responses have been seen in small cell lung carcinoma (771) and breast carcinoma (772) at escalating doses from 60 to 450 mg/m^2/day. LND is not very effective as monotherapy for malignancy, and the phase II trials were disappointing. Prednisone (5 mg b.i.d.) has been used to symptomatically relieve complaints of myalgia.

Lonidamine, combined with radiation, has prolonged survival in squamous cell lung carcinoma (dose, 150 mg p.o. t.i.d.) (773) and offers a survival benefit for lung cancer patients treated with chemotherapy, radiation, and LND (774). However, these results could not be confirmed by a randomized phase III trial (775). Use of this agent with MACC (methotrexate, doxorubicin, cyclophosphamide, and lomustine) was well tolerated in patients with non-small-cell lung cancer but was of questionable benefit (776). A recent trial of this agent with radiation in the treatment of brain metastases gave marginal improvement over historic controls (777). Prolongation of survival in squamous cell carcinoma of the head and neck has been seen when LND is added to radiation therapy with enhanced local control (778). Benefit has also been seen in the treatment of head and neck carcinoma with methotrexate and LND, with side effects of testicular pain (21%) and myalgia (31%) (779). This drug may prove to be useful in head and neck tumors.

MGBG (methyl-GAG; mitoguazone; methylglyoxal bis(guanylhydrazone; NSC-32946) is a drug that does not seem to die gracefully and every decade seems to be "rediscovered." The drug inhibits polyamine biosynthesis by interfering with S-adenosylmethione decarboxylase. Previous studies had discarded this agent as too toxic because of problems with myelosuppression and mucositis. More recent evidence suggests that the drug has a terminal half-life of 100 hours. The drug and the new phase II evaluations have recently been reviewed (780). Significant activity has been demonstrated in AIDS-related lymphoma, administering this agent at 600 mg/m^2 on days 1 and 8 and then every 2 weeks. No significant myelosuppression was reported, but lethargy, nausea/vomiting, transient somnolence, and paresthesia were noted (780)

PENCLOMEDINE (PEN; NSC 338720) is a picoline derivative undergoing phase I trials as a 1-hour infusion on a daily × 5 schedule every 28 days. The drug is relatively insoluble and must be dissolved in a vehicle containing soybean oil and egg white. The mechanism of action is unknown, but suggested actions include alkylation. Dose levels from 50 to 350 mg/m^2/day have been studied, with neurotoxicity noted at the higher levels, including one case of ataxia that was believed to be secondary to cerebellar dysfunction. Nausea has also been noted. A significant response occurred in a patient with ovarian carcinoma. No drug accumulation was noted, and the terminal half-life was 18.4 hours (781).

PHENYLACETATE, a metabolite of phenyl-alanine, causes a cytotoxic effect on chronic lymphocytic leukemia cells in culture. The mechanism of action is believed to be depletion of glutamine, with formation of cytoplasmic vacuoles in a dose- and time-dependent manner (782). This agent induced differentiation and slowed tumor growth in a brain tumor model of 9L gliosarcoma in Fischer 344 rats (783). Changes were analogous to biochemical changes seen in phenylketonuria, with a decline of cholesterol synthesis in the malignant cells (784). In vitro, this agent has a chemopreventive action and is synergistic with lovastatin (785). In hormone-resistant prostate cell lines, phenylacetate demonstrated growth inhibition and was synergistic in causing growth inhibition in the presence of suramin (786). A phase I trial has been described with nonlinear pharmacokinetics and dose-limiting toxicity of CNS depression. The drug was metabolized to phenylacetylglutamine and excreted by the urinary tract. Because of problems with dosing, the authors suggested the use of adaptive feedback control to keep phenylacetate plasma concentrations between 200 and 300 μg/mL (787).

PSC-833, a nonimmunosuppressive derivative of cyclosporin D, is nonnephrotoxic and has been undergoing trials to reverse classical multiple-drug resistance on the basis of in vitro data and previous studies with cyclosporin A. A phase I study of PSC-833 with etoposide revealed that the etoposide pharmacokinetics were modified with an increase in AUC; this was associated with enhanced toxicity (788). A dose of 6.6 mg/kg/day achieved plasma PSC-833 concentrations of 1000 to 2000 ng/mL, the level needed in vitro to inhibit the MDR pump. Dose-limiting CNS toxicity occurred at or above 12 mg/kg/day of this drug. In combination with etoposide, toxicities included myelosuppression, thrombocytopenia, and reversible hyperbilirubinemia (788). Similar findings have been reported in an additional phase I study of these two drugs, with one patient in addition demonstrating grade 3 pulmonary toxicity (789). Whether this agent will modulate MDR enough to be clinically useful and not just manifest antitumor activity by increasing the AUC of the cytotoxic agent remains to be determined.

S 9788 (bismethane sulphonate salt of 6-[4-(2,2-di(4-fluorophenyl)-ethylamino)-1-piperidinyl]-*N*,*N*′-di-2-propenyl-1,3,5-trazine-2,4-diamine) is a triazinoaminopiperidine analogue undergoing trials in France in an attempt to reverse classical multiple drug resistance. This drug did not reverse resistance in cell lines not overexpressing the P-glycoprotein (790). In vitro, the drug does have cytotoxic activity against a variety of cell lines in addition to its resistance-modulating effects. (790). The drug is dissimilar to other MDR-reversal agents but does have a lipophilic structure with a planar aromatic ring. In some cell lines, this agent is much more potent than verapamil and is more active if given after the cytotoxic drug rather than before. In the case of doxorubicin, micromolar quantities of S 9788 blocked egress of the cytotoxic agent from cells (791). Another mode of action may be by redistributing the doxorubicin that is taken up into cells (792). Duration of exposure to S 9788 correlated with the degree of reversal of MDR drug resistance seen in cell lines, and S 9788 was active at clinically achievable levels of 1 μM (793). As a phase I trial by itself, the drug demonstrated hypotension, bradycardia, and atrioventricular block as dose-limiting toxicities when used as a 30-minute infusion. On a more complex 4.5-hour infusion schedule, S 9788 showed dose-related increases in plasma concentrations and some activity in non-Hodgkin's lymphoma when combined with cytotoxic agents (794).

SR-2508 (*N*-(2-hydroxyethyl)-2-nitro-1*H*-imidazole-1-acetamide) is another misonidazole analogue that has undergone phase I evaluation with cyclophosphamide. The drug did not change the pharmacokinetics of cyclophosphamide or its metabolites (795).

TIRAPAZAMINE (Tira; SR 4233; WIN 59075; 3-amino-1,2,4-benzotriazine-1,4-di-*N*-oxide; NSC 130181) is a bioreductive compound with selective toxicity against hypoxic cells. Additional drugs of this class have been recently characterized (796). In the mouse, extensive bioreduction occurs, with the production of intermediates SR 4317 and SR 4233 and eventual formation of a glucuronide. Pharmacokinetics were linear with dose (797). With radiation, this agent increases the destruction of hypoxic tumor without enhancing the effect on normal tissue (798). Recent studies have suggested that this agent is not working as a radiation sensitizer but as an additive cytotoxic (799). In a model mouse tumor, treatment with SR 4233 prior to cisplatin enhanced the therapeutic index without affecting renal or hematopoietic function (800). This drug did not show a significant benefit in a mouse model of photodynamic therapy (801). In T-cell lymphoma xenografts, tirapazamine enhanced the effect of radiolabeled antibody, suggesting a possible new direction in the ongoing monoclonal therapy of lymphomas in man (802).

A phase I study on a 3 times a week schedule with standard radiation therapy noted toxicity of muscle cramping that was not dose related. Quinine sulfate was able to minimize this problem. Additional toxicities included nausea/vomiting and diffuse rash (803). Muscle cramping was found to be common, independent of the schedule of the drug and whether or not radiation was also included. Creatine phosphokinase was elevated in some patients, as were cardiac isoenzymes in one case (804). A possible explanation for this toxicity is that this agent uncouples oxidative phosphorylation, leading to ATP depletion in sensitive cells (805). A phase I study of tirapazamine with cisplatin is under way with Tira (130 to 260 mg/m^2 given prior to the platinum (75 mg/m^2). There was no evidence of a pharmacologic drug interaction, and major toxicity was nausea and vomiting (806). As a single agent, an MTD of 450 mg/m^2 was seen, with reversible tinnitus and deafness that was most pronounced in patients previously treated with cisplatin (807).

SWAINSONINE, an indolizidine alkaloid, blocks polysaccharide metabolism and inhibits Golgi-mannosidase II, causing a reduction in invasive potential. These changes in vitro are associated with an upregulation of metalloproteinase expression (808). In mice, this compound shows a wide tissue distribution with little or no protein binding. The highest levels of swainsonine were found in the bladder, kidney, and thymus (809). Human tumor xenografts in mice were inhibited by this drug. A phase I study in man has administered this agent as a continuous infusion over 5 days with dose levels from 50 to 550 µg/kg/day studied. Swainosine has a 12-hour terminal half-life, and cellular targets were saturated at 150 µg/kg/day. Antitumor effects were noted in a patient with a head and neck carcinoma. Toxicities included edema, liver function abnormalities, and hyperamylasemia without symptoms of pancreatitis. Dyspnea was also reported (810). As target enzymes were exposed to serum concentrations 100 to 400 times higher than their IC$_{50}$ (811), toxicity may be reduced by more conservative dosing.

TETRAHYDROURIDINE (THU) was origi-nally studied in humans over 10 years ago (812). This agent inhibits cytidine/deoxycytidine deaminase, thus preventing the biodegradation of ara-C. With the recent interest in high-dose ara-C in acute leukemia, THU has been restudied as a 3-hour coinfusion with ara-C (813). In solid tumor patients, high doses of THU (350 mg/m^2) with conventional dosages of ara-C (100 mg/m^2) resulted in peak plasma levels equivalent to those with 1000 mg/m^2 of ara-C. Degradation of ara-C into ara-U (1-D-arabino-furanosyluracil) was inhibited, with a change in the plasma disposition curve to monophasic and a substantial increase in the AUC. Major toxicities were myelosuppression, nausea, and vomiting (813). This drug combination has been tested in refractory leukemia with two dose levels of ara-C (100 and 200 mg/m^2) and one of THU (350 mg/m^2). More responses were seen at the higher ara-C dose. Toxicities were similar to those of high-dose ara-C except that cerebellar toxicity was absent (814). Evaluation of THU with ara-C via the intrathecal route in monkeys found prolonged CSF levels of ara-C (815). There has been little interest in this compound since the last edition, but the realization that several of the newer antimetabolites are deaminated may revive interest in this drug.

WIN 33377 (N-[1-(2-diethylamino ethylamino)-9-oxo-9-H-thioxanthen-4-yl] methane sulfonamide) is a hycanthone derivative with broad preclinical activity. The mechanism of action is unknown, but inhibition of DNA synthesis has been observed. A single-dose schedule in man has studied dosages from 33 to 335 mg/m^2 with minor toxicity to date. Pharmacokinetic parameters were linear and dose dependent (816). A daily × 5 phase I schedule over 2 hours studied 4.8 to 89 mg/m^2/day, with ventricular arrhythmia as the dose-limiting toxicity. The agent is now being studied on a 24-hour infusion schedule (817).

HEAVY METALS

PLATINUM COMPOUNDS. The success of cisplatin and carboplatin in clinical cancer therapy has stimulated pharmaceutical chemists to examine and synthesize innumerable new agents, which have subsequently passed through clinical testing. The number of platinum analogues continues to expand. Mechanisms of reducing cisplatin toxicity, particularly nephrotoxicity, by various compounds are being evaluated with mixed results (818, 819). Emergence of resistance to cisplatin appears to be a major prognostic factor indicating outcome in otherwise sensitive malignancies such as testicular and ovarian cancers (820). A dosing plateau is apparent, even in sensitive tumor types, beyond which additional dose escalations do not increase response (820). Causes of resistance include decreased drug accumulation, increased detoxification, increased repair of DNA-platinum adducts, and increased tolerance of DNA lesions (820, 821). Clinical trials are being developed involving protection of specific toxicities, decreasing intracellular glutathione (by buthionine sulfoximine; BSO) (822), decreasing DNA repair, and introducing new analogues (820).

Platinum complexes based on the 1,2-diaminocyclohexane carrier ligand (DACH complexes), such as Ormaplatin and Oxaliplatin, entered clinical trials on the basis of their ability to overcome cisplatin resistance (823). These drugs have been limited by neurotoxicity (824, 825). Another class, the ammine/amine platinum (IV)dicarboxylates, circumvent resistance mediated at the plasma membrane. An example is the orally administered drug JM216 (823, 826, 827).

Classical structure-activity relationships state that platinum-based coordination complexes of transplatin, the *trans* isomer of cisplatin, is inactive. However, the development of active isomers may yet be another way of overcoming resistance (823). Extensive reviews of new platinum complexes are available (828–831), and the development of newer agents is under way (831).

CYCLOPLATAM (amine(cyclopentylamino)-S-(-)malatoplatinum (II)) is a mixed-amine platinum analogue with markedly enhanced aqueous solubility (300 mg/mL) that demonstrated a better preclinical screen activity than carboplatin and cisplatin and is not nephrotoxic (832). It is currently undergoing development (833). A 58% response rate at a dose of 100 mg/m^2 was seen in advanced ovarian cancer without oto- or neurotoxicity (834).

DWA2114R (2-aminomethylpyrrolidine-(1,1-cyclobutanedicarboxylato)-platinum) is similar in structure to carboplatin (835) and was developed as a result of screening platinum analogues against the resistant tumor line colon 26 (836). In the preclinical screen, it shared antitumor activity with carboplatin and was not nephrotoxic (837). A phase I study of a single dose given over 20 minutes revealed the MTD to be 1000 mg/m^2, with dose-limiting leukopenia. Nausea, vomiting, and anorexia were mild. Renal damage was not seen. Antitumor activity in testicular carcinoma was noted (838). A 1-hour infusion resulted in an MTD of 700 mg/m^2. Mild nephrotoxicity and hepatotoxicity with no ototoxicity were seen. The recommended phase II dose was 600 mg/m^2 every 2 to 3 weeks (839). Pharmacokinetic studies indicated a triphasic decay curve with a terminal half-life of 22 hours. Total platinum showed a biphasic decay, and the AUC depended on the dose (839). Forty-two to 100% of the platinum was excreted in the urine (838, 839). Development of this compound continues.

JM 216 [AF-bis(aceto)-B-ammine-CD-dichloro-E-cyclohexylamine platinum (IV)] is an oral platinum compound with good bioavailability, low emetogenic potential, and spectrum similar to that of carboplatin (840). A phase I trial showed that oral absorption was saturable at 300 mg/m^2. An MTD was not reached. There was a correlation between myelosuppression and total platinum plasma concentration (C_{max}) on day 5 (on a daily × 5 schedule) (840). An oral schedule of a single dose every 21 days without hydration is under way (841). Toxicity includes delayed emesis and minimal thrombocytopenia, no nephrotoxicity or neurotoxicity (829).

OXALIPLATIN, a platinum complex based on the 1,2-diaminocyclohexane moiety, has entered clinical trials on the basis of overcoming acquired cisplatinum resistance (823). It is an *l*-isomer of a *trans* 1,2-DACH compound (829). The pharmacokinetics of oxaliplatin (1R,2R-diaminocyclohexane)oxalatoplatinum(II) (1-OHP, NSC 266046) have been studied in rabbits (842). Tissue platinum levels at 24 hours postinjection were lower in the organs examined (including kidney and liver) than with cisplatin. Plasma levels of the unchanged species and filterable platinum for 1-OHP declined more rapidly than for cisplatin. The protein binding of 1-OHP was greater than that of cisplatin. The renal clearance for both the unchanged species and filterable platinum was 2-fold greater than that for cisplatin (842). There was dose-limiting toxicity of peripheral sensory neuropathy (824). Neuropathy developed during infusion at dosages above 135 mg/m^2, which was exacerbated by touching cold surfaces or liquids and resolved within 7 days. Patients receiving 4 courses or more developed a severe sensory neuropathy that persisted up to 6 months (824, 829). Grade 2/3 neurologic toxicity occurred in 44% of patients, of whom 74% had complete reversal within 5 months (843, 844). Doses of 130 mg/m^2 by various routes did not require any specific precaution (845). Single-agent activity in refractory colon cancer has been seen (846). A high-dose folinic acid, 5-FU, and oxaliplatin regimen showed a 46% response in previously treated metastatic colon cancer (847).

LOBAPLATIN (1,2-diamminomethyl-cyclobutane-platinum (II)-lactate) (D-19466) is a cisplatin analogue developed with reduced toxicity compared with cisplatin and carboplatin. Pharmacokinetic analysis of lobaplatin showed a short plasma half-life and rapid urinary excretion (848). A phase I trial using a 72-hour continuous infusion has been conducted (849). The dose-limiting toxicity was thrombocytopenia. The recommended phase II dose was 45 mg/m^2 over 72 hour every 4 weeks (849). No relationship was detected between the percentage decrease in platelet or leukocyte count and the creatinine clearance in the 11 patients studied (849). Activity in ovarian cancer patients previously treated with platinum compounds was observed (849–851). A phase II study in head and neck cancer showed limited efficacy (10% RR) in previously untreated patients (852).

Other Platinum Compounds

One of the first *trans*-platinum compounds (*trans*-ammine (cyclohexylaminedichlorodihydroxo) platinum (IV) (JM355) showing antitumor activity is undergoing development to circumvent cross-resistance to cisplatin (823). TRK-710 (1-1,2-diaminocyclhexane)Pt(II)(α-acetyl-γ-methyltetronate) is an analogue currently in phase I study in Japan (853).

CI-973 ([SP-4-3-(*R*)]-[1,1-cyclobutanedicarboxylato(2-)](2-methyl-1,4-butanediamine-*N,N'*) platinum; CI-973, NK121) is a cisplatin analogue that is not cross-resistant with cisplatin (854). It has activity against preclinical tumor models analogous to that of cisplatin, with additional activity against tumors with acquired cisplatin resistance (854). CI-973 has dose-limiting leukopenia that is short-lived, minor thrombocytopenia, and reduced nephrotoxicity, gastrointestinal toxicity, and ototoxicity, compared with currently available drugs (829, 854)

TITANIUM. Titanocenedichloride (MKT 4) is an antineoplastic metal complex with activity in experimental tumors (855). The organ toxicity in animal studies was low, with no severe nephrotoxicity or myelotoxicity (855–857). In drug-resistant ovarian cancer cell lines, MKT 4 showed no cross-resistance to cisplatin or doxorubicin (855, 858). In vitro activity was seen in human

renal cell carcinoma (859). The drug is in human trials in Germany, with nephrotoxicity seen.

PODOPHYLLOTOXIN AND UNUSUAL TOPOISOMERASE II INHIBITORS

ETOPOSIDE PHOSPHATE (Etopophos) is one of a series of derivatives of the parent drug etoposide. This drug should be commercially available at the time of publication of this edition. Unlike the parent compound, etoposide phosphate is water soluble. Etoposide is relatively insoluble in aqueous solutions and is formulated in polysorbate 80, polyethylene glycol, and alcohol (860). Allergic phenomena and hypotension have been observed at conventional doses, necessitating slow infusion of this agent. More extreme toxicities occur with the high-dose schedules used for transplantation (860).

The drug has been studied using various schedules. In a day 1, 3, 5 schedule of doses ranging 50 to 150 mg/m^2 over 30-minutes infusion, no measurable etoposide phosphate was detected in plasma by 15 to 60 minutes after the end of the infusion (861). The mean half life ranged from 5.5 to 9.3 hours. The pharmacokinetics of etoposide were linear over the range studied, with dose-limiting toxicity of myelosuppression (861). A similar schedule with a 5-min infusion at doses of 50 to 200 mg/m^2 showed leukopenia occurring at doses above 75 mg/m^2, with a nadir count between days 15 and 19 posttreatment. The MTD was between 175 and 200 mg/m^2 (860). The pharmacokinetics of etoposide phosphate showed a peak plasma concentration at 5 minutes, with a t$_{1/2}$ of 7 minutes. Etoposide reached a peak concentration at 7 to 8 minutes with a t$_{1/2}$ of 6 to 9 hours (860). Both etoposide phosphate and etoposide showed dose-related linear increases in maximum plasma concentration (C$_{max}$) and AUC (860). High-dose studies useful in the transplant setting over 2 hours daily × 2 have been reported and demonstrate linear pharmacokinetics (862). A phase I study of oral etoposide phosphate used a schedule of daily × 5 every 3 weeks (863). Etoposide phosphate was not detected in plasma after administration. The relative bioavailability of etoposide after oral etoposide phosphate was 76 ± 27%, with a range of 37 to 144% (863).

FOSTRIECIN is an antitumor antibiotic with in vitro effects that include topoisomerase II inhibition (864). A phase I study demonstrated mild and reversible liver function abnormalities.

Pharmacokinetics at 38 mg/m² showed a plasma clearance of 200 to 400 mL/min, a short elimination half-life, and no evidence of saturable metabolism (864).

IST-622 (6-*O*-(3-ethoxypropionyl)-3′,4′-*O*-exo-benzylidenenchartreusin) is a new synthetic derivative of chartreusin. At high concentration, it is also a topoisomerase I inhibitor (865). Following oral administration, antitumor effects were seen in various mouse tumors such as P388, L1210 leukemia, B16 melanoma, Lewis lung carcinoma, Colon 26 and Colon 38 adenocarcinomas, and M5076 reticulum-cell sarcoma (866). The drug is well absorbed from small intestine and is now undergoing phase I trials in Japan (865, 867).

NK611, a podophyllotoxin-derivative dimethylaminoetoposide, has been studied in cell lines (868). A high-performance liquid chromatographic assay for the compound has been developed, and the drug has been assessed in a phase I study of both an oral and intravenous dose of this agent in man (869). This drug is undergoing additional phase I trials (870, 871). Mean urinary recovery of unchanged NK and its metabolites was 16.3% and 12.%, respectively (871). An MTD of 120 mg/m² has been defined with dose-limiting neutropenia (870).

PROTEIN SYNTHESIS INHIBITORS

Most currently available agents used in the clinic interfere with either nucleic acid metabolism or cell division. In the past, protein synthesis inhibitors were too nonspecific to be of use in the treatment of malignant disease and therefore did not offer a therapeutic advantage. Only L-asparaginase has survived development, and it has a very limited role. However, there has been new interest in this area as the mechanism of action differs from that of the traditional agents. Whether any of these agents will prove clinically useful remains unknown.

GIROLINE (RP 49532A; (15,25)-3-amino-1-[4-(2-amino-1*H*-imizadoyl)]-2-chloropropanol 2HCL), a compound isolated from a marine sponge, has activity against doxorubicin-resistant cell lines. Preclinical toxicology revealed major toxic effects to be hepatic, muscle, and testicular. A phase I trial of this agent given as a 24-hour infusion in dosages ranging from 3 to 15 mg/m² showed dose-limiting toxicity of hypotension with shock that was delayed and slowly reversible. Asthenia, nausea/vomiting, prolongation of the prothrombin and partial

thromboplastin times, erythema, and myalgia were also noted (872). A phase I trial of this agent over 1-hour revealed dose-limiting toxicity to be hypotension (873). This agent has been dropped from further clinical development but may serve as the basis of analogues.

ZILASCORB (5,6-benzylidene-D1-ascorbic acid) is a reversible protein synthesis inhibitor with activity in xenograft models. It is metabolized to hippuric acid, which does not have cytostatic activity (874). Information about this agent remains fragmentary, but it is now in phase II trials, and responses have been reported in ovarian, pancreatic, and colorectal carcinoma patients (875). The agent has been formulated in an oral form and is absorbed when gastric acid is inhibited (875). Further studies are under way.

RETINOIDS

Retinoids are natural derivatives of vitamin A that act as regulators of physiologic processes, including vision and morphogenesis (876). Vitamin A and some of its analogues, the retinoids, are established modulators of cell proliferation and differentiation in vivo and in vitro (5, 876, 877). Recent clinical trials have demonstrated the efficacy of retinoids in the prevention and treatment of cancer (877–880).

Most functions of the retinoids are mediated by the oxidized product of retinol, all-*trans* retinoic acid (RA) (876). This can be further converted by intracellular isomerases to 9-*cis* RA, 11-*cis* RA, or 13-*cis* RA (876). Two types of nuclear retinoid receptors, RARs and RXRs, have been identified (877). The RARs bind all-*trans*-RA and 9-*cis*-RA, and the RXRs bind 9-*cis* RA selectively (877). Both RXRs and RARs can bind a variety of synthetic retinoids, some of which exhibit different degrees of receptor selectivity (877).

There are numerous synthetic retinoids undergoing preclinical investigations. TTAB [4-(5,6,7,8-tetrahydro-5,5,8,8,-tetramethyl-2-anthracenyl)benzoid acid] and TTNN [6-(5,6,7,8-tetrahydro-5,5,8,8-tetramethyl-2-naphtalenyl)-2-naphthalenecarboxylic acid] bind preferentially to RARs, and two retinoids (SR11203 and SR11217) bind preferentially to RXRs (877). The combination of SR11217 and TTNN or TTAB and IFN-α resulted in 90% inhibition of growth of ME180 cervical cancer cells (877).

ALL-TRANS *RETINOIC ACID* (ATRA) has had the most success in oncologic practice. It has shown a high degree of activity in acute promyelocytic leukemia (876, 881, 882) and it induces complete remission in a high proportion of patients. Remissions tend to be brief, and patients show resistance to further treatment (881–885). The action of ATRA depends on the presence of the PML/RAR-α fusion protein (876). Complications can include the "RA syndrome," which resembles a "capillary leak syndrome" (876, 886). Serial pharmacokinetic studies show that continuous daily ATRA treatment is associated with a decline in plasma drug concentration (887). The metabolism of the drug is upregulated within days of beginning therapy. Studies using P450 inhibitors such as ketoconazole and the development of retinoids with different pharmacokinetic properties are under way (887). It has just been released commercially.

13-CIS-RETINOIC ACID has also been evaluated in chemoprevention trials. It was studied in a 1-year trial to prevent the incidence of new cancers in patients previously treated for squamous cell carcinoma of the head and neck. New tumors developed in 4% of the treated patients, compared with 24% in the placebo arm (888). Activity is seen in early-stage cutaneous T-cell lymphoma (876). In contrast, in myelodysplasia, this drug did not demonstrate meaningful activity when studied in a double-blind, placebo-controlled trial (889). 13-Cis-retinoic acid had previously shown a chemoprotective effect in experimental models of bladder carcinoma. As with many human trials, this drug demonstrated unacceptable mucocutaneous toxicity in the chemopreventive trials for bladder cancer (876). A synthetic retinoid, etretinate, at 50 mg/day was also reported to be active in preventing recurrence of bladder cancer. However, these findings could not be confirmed in subsequent trials (876). Hence, the role of this agent is modest.

FENRETINIDE has demonstrated chemopreventive properties against carcinogen-induced rodent mammary cancer (890). The combination of tamoxifen and fenretinide is more effective than tamoxifen or fenretinide alone in the prevention of the rat mammary cancer (890). This compound shows a preferential accumulation in breast instead of liver tissue. Studies are under way in the prevention of breast cancer, basal cell carcinoma, and recurrences of leukoplakia (891). A phase I trial showed that the combination is nontoxic, and phase III trials are ongoing (890).

4-HPR (N-(4-hydroxyphenyl)retinamide) is a synthetic derivative of retinoic acid. It does not accumulate in the liver and shows only mild toxicity (892). The compound induces apoptosis at a pharmacologically relevant level in human neuroblastoma cells (892). This drug has entered clinical trials.

RO-40-8757 is a third-generation retinoid that shows greater antiproliferative activity than 13-cis or all-trans retinoic acid against breast, cervical, lung, and colorectal cancer cell lines (893). The dose-limiting toxicity is vomiting (893).

INHIBITORS OF CELL SIGNAL TRANSDUCTION

The rapid development in understanding the mechanisms of cell-cycle control and the role of external signal agonists affecting cell growth is expected to have a profound effect on the agents used in the clinic. The National Cancer Institute has targeted development of protein-tyrosine kinase inhibitors based upon the known structure of naturally occurring inhibitors (894). Early structures such as herbimycin A have been shown to selectively inhibit the in vitro growth of Philadelphia chromosome–positive chronic myelogenous leukemia cells and Philadelphia chromosome–positive acute lymphatic leukemia cells by interfering with tyrosine kinase (206). The involvement of isoprenoids, unsaturated lipids, in signal transduction is also an area of potential drug development (895). At the present time, the reported compounds remain limited and are mainly in preclinical testing. The EORTC has targeted for further research compounds that interfere with cell-cycle signals. Of interest, cytotoxics such as the topoisomerase inhibitor fostriecin may also interfere with protein phosphatase 1 and 2A needed for preventing early entry into mitosis, thus offering new leads for drug development (896). A phase I trial of fostriecin did not yield an MTD. A transient reversible hepatitis was seen during the first 10 days of treatment (897). In vitro data suggest that both activation and inhibition of various pathways of signal transduction can change the sensitivity of target cells to chemotherapeutic agents (898). Therefore, these agents may eventually find a role in combination with classical cytotoxic agents. The agents currently in trial are relatively nonselective, so major efforts are currently being made to enhance the specificity of these substances. Combinatorial chemistry, discussed earlier, may find great utility in drug development in this area.

BOMBESIN ANTAGONISTS include agents such as RC-3095 (D-tri[6],Leu[13],(CH$_2$NH)Leu[14] bombesin), and several variants that are short polypeptides were synthesized to specifically block the receptor. Gastrin-releasing peptide, the mammalian form of bombesin, is present in many solid tumors and acts as an autocrine factor. A review of this literature is beyond the scope of this review. Bombesin antagonists have blocked the growth of human small cell lung cancer, breast cancer (899), colon cancer, pancreatic cancer, and prostate cancer cell lines (900). Chronic administration of RC-3095 in Hs746T human gastric cancer xenografts inhibited the tumor's growth and specifically antagonized the binding of bombesin (900). Similar findings have been noted with other human tumor xenografts. In the MCF-7 breast cancer xenografts, RC-3095 also downregulated the binding capacity of epidermal growth factor receptors in the tumors (899). Similar downregulation of epidermal growth factor receptors was seen in a hamster pancreatic cancer model (901). In the Dunning rat R-3327H prostate cancer model, the combination of RC-3095 with an LH/RH agonist enhanced the antitumor effect and increased apoptosis in the tumor (902). Human trials and preclinical toxicology have not been described to date. Analogous development is in progress with gastrin antagonists (903) and neuropeptide antagonists in small cell lung cancer (904). Cholecystokinin receptor antagonists such as MK-329 have been taken into clinical trial in pancreatic cancer without evidence of benefit (905).

CYCLIN INHIBITORS are attractive, as these molecules play an essential role in cell-cycle function. Several agents have been described that inhibit cyclin function, including butyrolactone I (inhibits cdc2 and cdc2 kinase) (906); the purines N^6-dimethylaminopurine, N^6-(δ 2-isopentenyl)adenine, and 2-(2-hydroxyethylamino)-6-benzylamino-9-methyl purine (olomoucine) inhibit the p34cdc2/cyclin B kinase, which is essential for cell-cycle regulation (907). Pharmaceutical companies with combinatorial chemistry programs are targeting this area. Further development is anticipated.

PROTEIN KINASE INHIBITORS are an active area of pharmaceutical development, and early drugs in clinical trial are discussed below. Drugs of this class may have utility in both malignant and nonmalignant disease (such as psoriasis and atherosclerosis) (908, 909). Even agents that seem to be chemopreventive, such as genistein, have been shown to interfere with tyrosine kinase and arrest cells in culture at the G_2-M boundary (910). However, genistin does not show selectivity against malignant cells (206). Agents that affect calmodulin, such as dexniguldipine hydrochloride (B859-35), have also been reported to inhibit protein kinase (741). At least some of these agents are believed to compete for the ATP-binding site on the tyrosine kinase (206).

One of the most active compounds yet discovered is PD 153035, a specific tyrosine kinase inhibitor that can inhibit epidermal growth factor (EGF) kinase at picomolar concentrations with no effect on kinases associated with platelet-derived growth factor, fibroblast growth factor receptor, colony-stimulating factor-1 (CSF-1) receptor, or the insulin receptor. Of interest, this heterocyclic compound inhibited the tyrosine kinase associated with Erb-B_2 and caused a reversion of morphology of EGF-transformed fibroblasts (911). This compound offers the advantages of high specificity, high binding, and the lack of a protein structure, in contrast to the ongoing trials of antibodies to the growth factor receptors.

BRYOSTATIN (Bryostatin 1; NSC 339555), a macrocyclic lactone isolated from a marine organism, perturbs protein kinase C, either as an activator or an inhibitor, depending upon the conditions. This agent has been found to inhibit tumor promotion (912) and had antitumor activity in preclinical screens (913). This agent also inhibited the growth and cloning efficiency of acute myelogenous leukemia cells. In tissue culture, bryostatin 1 enhanced ara-C formation into ara-CTP and demonstrated a selective effect on leukemic cells, which was not universal. Ara-C incorporation into DNA was also enhanced in several specimens from leukemic patients (914). Scheduling bryostatin prior to vincristine was found to be markedly synergistic, with long-term survivals in a murine model of macroglobulinemia (915). Bryostatin has a variety of biologic effects, including differentiation in some cell lines, enhancement of cytokine effect, degranulation of neutrophils, platelet aggregation, and stimulation of release of other tissue factors (916).

Phase I trials of this agent in man have been reported. Bryostatin was studied as a 1-hour infusion every 2 weeks in dosages from 5 to 65 µg/m², with myalgia being dose-limiting. Cellulitis and thrombosis occurred at the injection site. Some of these local effects may have been due to the ethanol used as a vehicle. Mild fatigue and hypotension were also noted. Decreases in platelet count and leukocyte count occurred within 24 hours. Suggested phase II dosages were 35 to 50

$\mu g/m^2$ (917). These authors also evaluated a weekly schedule with infusion of the drug over 24 hours, using a different formulation of the drug. Dose-limiting toxicity was myalgia with suggested phase II dosing at 25 $\mu g/m^2$/week. Il-6 and TNF plasma levels were not affected by the treatment, and one patient with ovarian carcinoma achieved a partial remission (918). In contrast, a Cancer Research Campaign Phase I trial on a variety of schedules noted a rise in TNF and IL-6 levels following treatment. Dose-related myalgia 2 to 3 days after treatment appeared to be cumulative. Phlebitis was not a major problem with the nonalcoholic formulation. Of the eight melanoma patients disease treated, two achieved partial remissions (10+ months, and 6 weeks) (919). Obviously, further work with this agent, both as a single drug on a variety of schedules and as an enhancer of chemotherapeutic effect, is anticipated.

8-CHLORO-cAMP (8-chloroadenosine 3',5'-cyclic monophosphate, 8-chloro-cyclic adenosine monophosphate) is believed to regulate the levels of the regulatory isoforms RI and RII, which are subunits of cyclic-AMP-dependent protein kinase. In tissue culture, this agent inhibited glioma cell lines at micromolar dosages without causing differentiation (920). This biologic effect occurred at dosages not inhibiting normal rat astrocytes, implying a role for this agent in primary brain tumors. The metabolite of this agent, 8-chloroadenosine, was more active than the parent compound in a dye-exclusion cytotoxic assay, suggesting an alternate mechanism of action (921). In a pancreatic cell line, 8-chloro-cAMP showed dose-dependent growth inhibition without affecting the receptor of IGF-1 (insulin-like growth factor-1) or the receptor for EGF (epidermal growth factor) (922). In leukemic blast cells from patients, 8-chloro-cAMP reduced the clonigenic potential of the cells, with suggested maturational effects in 4 out of 6 samples studied (923). HPLC analysis of the clinically used drug revealed purity of 95 to 99%, with variation by lot (924). Early results of a phase I trial have noted mild hypercalcemia that resolves after treatment and reversible minor increases in serum creatinine. When given on a 5-day infusion schedule, one minor response was noted (925). A more complete phase I study of continuous intravenous infusion for 5 days a week for 2 weeks with 1-week rest has been reported in 17 patients. Dose levels from 0.01 to 0.25 mg/kg/hour were evaluated, with dose-limiting renal failure at 0.2 mg/kg/hour and

above. Tolerable levels achieved plasma concentrations that were inhibitory in vitro. The suggested phase II dose was 0.125 mg/kg/hour (926).

7-HYDROXYSTAUROSPORINE (UCN-01) is a derivative of the protein kinase C inhibitor staurosporine, which is used in laboratory evaluation of signal transduction. The drug is active in the A498 renal carcinoma model in the nanomolar dose range. In vitro, the drug causes apoptosis and also affects cyclin kinases. The parent compound inhibits thymocyte proliferation (927). UCN-01 has shown preclinical activity and is being evaluated for eventual clinical testing. In human plasma, the drug is degraded into an unknown metabolite. In a mouse model, no parent drug was recovered in the urine, and oral absorption was poor (13%). Subcutaneous dosing is suggested for human trials, which will start in 1995 (928).

L86-8275 was discussed in the New Strategies and Targets Symposia at the 1995 American Association of Cancer Research meeting, but little written information is available at the time of this review. The drug, under development at the National Cancer Institute, is a flavonoid derivative showing inhibition of protein kinase C at nanomolar dosages, which also causes inhibition of cyclin kinases. In tissue culture, cells accumulate in G_1 and G_2. Phase I trials are evaluating a 72-hour schedule.

PENTOSAN POLYSULFATE (PPS), a polyanionic mucopolysaccharide with anticoagulant properties, inhibits tumor growth in xenograft models. In xenografts, PPS blocked the autocrine function of heparin-binding growth factors but did not affect growth mechanisms in soft agar that did not depend upon these factors (929). PPS inhibits protein tyrosine kinases from the Jurkat lymphocyte line and a rat lung tissue in a concentration-dependent manner. In addition, the drug inhibits a variety of serine/threonine kinases (930). PPS has been used as an antithrombotic agent but has also been noted to occasionally cause thrombocytopenia (931). This drug inhibits heparin-binding growth factors at levels of 0.1 $\mu g/mL$ of plasma, and affects the APTT at levels of 1 $\mu g/mL$ of plasma (932). In patients treated with PPS at 15 mg/m^2 subcutaneously, inhibitory effects of patient serum on growth factors persisted 4 hours after administration (932). Another charged polysaccharide, D-gluco-D-galactan (DS-4152), has been recently described to bind growth factors in vitro (933).

SURAMIN (moranyl; Bayer 305; germanin;

Fourneau 309; sym - bis(*m* - aminobenzoyl - *m* - amino-*p*-methylbenzoyl-1-naphthylamino-4,6,8 trisulfonate carbamide; NSC-34936) is a polysulfonated naphthylurea (molecular weight, 1429) used in the treatment of trypanosomiasis for over 60 years. As an anticancer drug, it has recently been extensively reviewed (934). Modern studies have indicated that this agent can block the action of mammalian DNA primase, DNA polymerase, reverse transcriptase, and *E. coli* RNA polymerase (935). Very recent studies have indicated that suramin inhibits calcium- and phospholipid-dependent protein kinase C in a dose-dependent manner (936). However, in prostate cancer cell lines, suramin increased tyrosine phosphorylation, suggesting other mechanisms of action (937). Additional evidence suggesting alternate modes of action comes from in vitro studies of the breast cancer cell line MCF-7, in which suramin causes accumulation in the G_2/M phase of the cell cycle. The authors suggested that this phenomenon could be exploited with cell-cycle-specific drugs or radiation (938).

Early studies found that the drug blocks the action of autocrines (939) and showed a concentration-dependent inhibition of non-small-cell lung cancer cell lines (940). As can be seen from the above, the mechanism of action of this agent probably involves several different discrete sites. In vitro, this agent inhibited cell proliferation of 8 of 10 lymphoid lines at a concentration of 200 µg/mL and caused thymic atrophy in mice (941).

This drug has completed phase I trials in humans with the intent to achieve a steady-state serum level of 250 to 300 µg/mL through a variety of dosing schedules. The terminal half-life of this agent is very long (45 to 55 days), making repetitive dosing difficult. The best evaluated schedule was 350 mg/m²/day as a continuous infusion for 3 weeks. Plasma levels of the drug were monitored twice a week. Despite these measures, toxicities were substantial, with proteinuria, approximate doubling of serum creatinine levels, photophobia, tearing, blurring of vision, vortex keratopathy (reversible), coagulopathy with bleeding, reversible elevation of serum transaminases, leukopenia, thrombocytopenia, adrenal insufficiency, and a Guillain-Barré-like syndrome. Antitumor responses were seen in adrenal carcinoma, hypernephroma, and T-cell leukemia-lymphoma. Antitumor activity correlated with development of coagulopathy (939). The coagulopathy was studied in three patients, with findings of elevation of circulating heparin sulfate and dermatan sulfate (942). Pharmacokinetics in cancer patients have suggested a large variation in parameters, thus requiring close monitoring of the plasma level of the drug to adjust dosing (943). Peak blood levels of suramin could be correlated with the development of neurotoxicity. Plasma peak levels below 300 µg/mL did not result in neuropathy, while levels above 400 µg/mL resulted in 100% of patients showing this toxicity (943). The neuropathy could be debilitating and did not respond to plasmapheresis or steroid therapy (944).

In an effort to make this drug more manageable, alternate dosing schemes have been investigated. Investigators in the Netherlands have used a loading schedule of 600 mg/m² as a 24-hour infusion followed by a 6-hour weekly treatment. A Bayesian estimation allowed the investigators to maintain the plasma level of suramin between 150 and 300 µg/mL (945). Studies at the University of Maryland used short intermittent dosing with pharmacologic monitoring. Patients received a test dose of 200 mg to determine their individual disposition curve of the drug, followed by Bayesian estimation to maintain plasma concentrations below the toxic level (946). Estimates of the central compartment allowed dosing to be within target concentrations in 85% of treatments (947). The dose-limiting toxicities were fatigue, lethargy, diminished renal function, and neuropathy. Responses were noted in hormone-refractory prostate cancer (946).

Early phase II studies have shown antitumor responses at a plasma drug levels above 200 µg/mL in adrenal carcinoma, hypernephroma, and high-grade lymphoma (948). The major utility of this drug seems to be in hormone-refractory prostate carcinoma, and phase III trials are ongoing. Because of the risk of adrenal insufficiency, replacement corticosteroids should be administered with this drug. Additional toxicities have recently been reported, including hypophosphatemia due to a Fanconi's syndrome, mitochondrial myopathy with decreased cytochrome c oxidase (949), coagulopathy, thrombocytopenia, allergic skin reactions (950), and acute renal failure (951). A high incidence of postoperative morbidity including hemorrhage, delayed wound healing, and bowel dysmotility led investigators to suggest that surgical procedures be limited within 1 month of treatment (952).

TYRPHOSTIN DERIVATIVES are low-molecular-weight inhibitors of tyrosine kinase activity that are being developed as specific inhibitors of signal pathways and as potential antitumor agents (908). These molecules can discriminate between EGFR (epidermal growth factor receptor) kinase and Erb-B$_2$ kinase and can inhibit cell growth in vitro (953). Investigators in this area have postulated that "cocktails" of these agents will be developed to inhibit several specific pathways at the same time (908). Numerous compounds have been developed, with AG1296 reversibly inhibiting human platelet-derived growth-factor-receptor proliferation (954), and additional compounds blocking other steps in the signaling process (955). Preclinical toxicology has not been reported.

SPINDLE INHIBITORS

Much interest in cytotoxic agents that interfere with the mitotic apparatus of cells has developed over the past several years with the realization these agents offer a broad spectrum of antitumor activity and reversible toxicity (956). Since the last edition of this text, two agents of this group, paclitaxel and vinorelbine, have received approval by the FDA for use in the United States, and a third, docetaxel, is commercially available in Europe. This third agent will probably also soon become available in the United States. Within the last several years, the National Cancer Institute Drug Evaluation Program has identified 32 compounds with 19 distinct chemical structures that interfere with mitotic function; these agents offer leads for new drugs of this class (957). Biochemistry of the tubulin molecule has clarified the binding sites for drugs and also allowed more rational drug design. In addition, liposomes have been developed to prolong the serum half-life of vincristine (681).

CI 980 (*S*-(-) ethyl 5-amino 1,2-dihydro-2-methyl-3-phenylpyrido[3,4-b]pyrazin-7-ylcarbamate; NSC 613862) is one of the isomers of an older formulation (NSC 370147) that inhibits the formation of microtubules and leads to depolymerization of already assembled microtubules. Drugs of this class were originally synthesized to interfere with folic acid metabolism but were found to inhibit mitosis by binding to the colchicine-binding site on microtubules (958). This drug is active in the nanomolar range in tissue culture and demonstrated irreversible effects against leukemic cells (958). The drug demonstrates activity in vinca-resistant cell lines, has a long half-life in mice, and is easily detectable by HPLC (959). In mice, CI 980 displayed vesicant

activity but less than the vinca alkaloids (960). Recent results in man revealed dose-limiting neurotoxicity including coma in the phase I trial and transient decline in cognitive function in 67% of study subjects when the drug was administered at 13.5 mg/m^2 over 72 hours as part of a phase II trial (961).

ECTEINASCIDIN 743 (ET743) is a tetrahydroisoquinoline alkaloid expected to be in phase I trials during 1996. In preclinical studies, no schedule dependency was noted, and the drug is believed to be an inhibitor of tubulin function. It is active against murine tumors such as P388 and B16 melanoma and extremely active against human xenograft tumor MX-1. Leukopenia was the main toxicity in dogs (962).

E7010 (*N*-[2-4-hydroxyphenyl) amino]-3-pyridinyl] - 4 - methoxybenzesulfonamide) inhibits tubulin polymerization. This agent displayed a broad antitumor activity in preclinical screens and could be given orally. Of interest, E7010 was active against vincristine-resistant P388 cells, against cisplatin-resistant P388, and 5-fluorouracil-resistant P388. In xenograft models, this drug was active against human breast, colorectal, gastric, and lung tumors. In vinca-sensitive tumors, E7010 demonstrated superior activity (963). In a phase I study, dose-limiting toxicity occurred at 480 mg/m^2 by the oral route with the appearance of paresthesia. Nausea and vomiting were also noted. Antitumor activity was seen in a case of uterine sarcoma. Further studies are evaluating a daily × 5 schedule (964).

LU 103793 (*N,N*-dimethyl-L-valyl-L-valyl-*N*-methyl-L-prolyl-L-proline benzylamide) is a dolastatin 15 derivative active against preclinical models of P388, MX-1, KB3–1, and a variety of human tumors refractory to doxorubicin, paclitaxel, vinblastine, or cisplatin. The drug is water soluble and active in tissue culture in the nanomolar range (965). In a human tumor clonagenic assay system, the drug is active at the 0.1 µg/mL level (966). Of note, the classically multiple-drug-resistant cell line P388/ADR is resistant to this drug. This drug is believed to affect microtubule assembly, as it blocks cells in G$_2$/M and inhibits in vitro purified brain microtubule polymerization (965). In xenograft model systems, the drug displayed schedule-dependent effects, with a multiple-dose treatment most effective (967). This agent is in phase I trials in Europe and the United States.

RHIZOXIN, a macrocyclic lactone with a structure similar to maytansine, is an order of magnitude more active than vincristine in cell lines (968). The compound binds to tubulin and is active in both vincristine- and doxorubicin-resistant cell lines (969). In vitro, the drug is active at nanomolar concentrations (970) and has activity in human tumor xenograft models including breast cancer, lung cancer, and melanoma. No cross-resistance with cisplatin or etoposide could be demonstrated (970). Resistance was correlated with amino acid changes in tubulin (971). Schedule dependency was also found (972). Phase I studies in Europe have determined the maximum tolerated dose to be 2.6 mg/m^2, with a suggested phase II dose of 2.0 mg/m^2. Major toxicities are mucositis, diarrhea, and leukopenia (968).

VINXALTINE (S 12363) was recently reviewed (968). This agent is a substituted vinca alkaloid with a valine substitution on the C23 of the vindoline ring to enhance lipophilicity. It shared the expected toxicities of vincas, having a maximum tolerated dose of 0.40 mg/m^2 given intravenously weekly, with a t$_{1/2}$ of 12 hours. An every-other-week dosing schedule revealed a maximum tolerated dose of 0.6 mg/m^2. Although antitumor responses were noted, the advantage of this agent has not been evident, and its future remains in doubt at present (968).

1069C85 (methyl N-[6-(3,4,6-trimethoxybenzyloxy) imidazo (1,2b)-pyridazin-2yl] carbamate) is a novel substance that binds to tubulin at the colchicine-binding site, with activity against drug-resistant cell lines. 1069C85 is active in nanomolar concentrations. This drug is an order of magnitude more toxic to cell lines than doxorubicin and could be given orally in preclinical models with a bioavailability of 20% (973). The drug has entered phase I trials (973).

REFERENCES

1. Kihara A, Pastan I. Cytotoxic activity of chimeric toxins containing the epidermal growth factor-like domain of heregulins fused to PE38KDEL, a truncated recombinant form of *Pseudomonas* exotoxin. Cancer Res 1995;55:71–77.

2. Mauger AB, Burke PJ, Somani HH, Fiedlos F, Knox RJ. Self-immolative prodrugs: candidates for antibody-directed enzyme prodrug therapy in conjunction with a nitroreductase enzyme. J Med Chem 1994; 37:3452–3458.

3. Bagshawe KD. Antibody-directed enzyme prodrug therapy (ADEPT). Adv Pharmacol 1993;24:99–121.

4. Rodrigues ML, Presta LG, Kotts CE, et al. Development of a humanized disulfide-stabilized anti-p185HER2 Fv-b-lactamase fusion protein for activation of a cephalosporin doxorubicin prodrug. Cancer Res 1995;55:63–70.

5. McBurney MW, Costa S, Pratt MAC. Retinoids and cancer: a basis for differentiation therapy. Cancer Invest 1993;11:590–598.

6. Levitzki A. Signal-transduction therapy. A novel approach to disease management. Eur J Biochem 1994; 226:1–13.

7. Stancovski I, Peles E, Ben Levy R, Lemprecht R, Kelman Z, Goldman-Michael R. Signal transduction by the neu/erB-2 receptor: a potential target for anti-tumor therapy. J Steroid Biochem Mol Biol 1992;43:95–103.

8. Hendriks HR, Connors TA, Lobbezoo MW, Meijer L. Mechanism-based screening using cell cycle control targets: limitations and expectations. Ann Oncol 1994;5(Suppl 5):100a.

9. Nishizuka Y. Studies and prospectives of the protein kinase C family for cellular regulation. Cancer 1989;63:1892–1903.

10. Basu A. The potential of protein kinase C as a target for anticancer treatment. Pharmacol Ther 1993; 59:257–280.

11. Fujiwara T, Grimm EA, Roth JA. Gene therapeutics and gene therapy for cancer. Curr Opin Oncol 1994;6:96–105.

12. Kohn EC. Development and prevention of metastasis. Anticancer Res 1993;13:2553–2559.

13. Duffy MJ. Inhibiting tissue invasion and metastasis as targets for cancer therapy. Biotherapy 1992; 4:45–52.

14. Workman P, Stratford IJ. The experimental development of bioreductive drugs and their role in cancer therapy. Cancer Metastasis Rev 1993;12:73–82.

15. Stratford IJ. Bioreductive drugs in cancer therapy. BJR Suppl 1992;24:128–136.

16. Chaplin DJ. Bioreductive therapy. Int J Radiat Oncol Biol Phys 1992;22:685–687.

17. Gallop MA, Barrett RW, Dower WJ, Fodor SPA, Gordon EM. Applications of combinatorial technologies to drug discovery. 1. Background and peptide combinatorial libraries. J Med Chem 1994;37:1233–1251.

18. Kenan DJ, Tsai DE, Keene JD. Exploring molecular diversity with combinatorial shape libraries. Trends Biochem Sci 1994;19:57–64.

19. Ecker DJ, Vickers TA, Hanecak R, Driver V, Anderson K. Rational screening of oligonucleotide combinatorial libraries for drug discovery. Nucleic Acids Res 1993;21:1853–1856.

20. Houghten RA. Combinatorial libraries. Finding the needle in the haystack. Curr Biol 1994;4:564–567.

21. Bosanquet AG. Review stability of solutions of antineoplastic agents during preparation and storage for in vitro assays. Cancer Chemother Pharmacol 1989; 23:197–207.

22. Copies NCI. Copies of NCI investigational drug—pharmaceutical data can be obtained from the Pharmaceutical Resource Branch, National Cancer Institute, Executive Plaza North, Bethesda, MD, 1995.

23. EORTC. New Drug Development Office, Free University Hospital, Gebouw Zuid, Amstelveenseweg 601, 1081 JC Amsterdam, The Netherlands, 1995.

24. Rieche K. Carcinogenicity of antineoplastic agents in man. Cancer Treat Rev 1984;11:39–67.

25. Kaldor J, Day NE, Hemminki K. Quantifying the carcinogenicity of antineoplastic drugs. Eur J Cancer 1984;24:703–711.

26. Dimasi JA. Cost of new drug development (abstract). Clin Pharmacol Ther 1989;45:126a.

27. Uberall F, Kampfer S, Schubert C, Doppler W, Grunicke HH. Role of protein kinase C in *ras*-mediated *fos*-expression. Adv Enzyme Regul 1994;34:257–268.

28. Grunicke H, Hofmann J, Utz I, Uberall F. Role of protein kinases in antitumor drug resistance. Ann Hematol 1994;69(Suppl 1):s1–s6.

29. Wagner BA, Buettner GR, Burns CP. Membrane peroxidative damage enhancement by the ether lipid class of antineoplastic agents. Cancer Res 1992; 52:6045–6051.

30. Sidoti C, Principe P, Vandamme B, Broquet C, Braquet P. Cytostatic activity of new synthetic anti-tumor aza-alkyllysophospholipds. Int J Cancer 1992; 51:712–717.

31. van Blitterswijk WJ, van der Bend RL, Kramer IM, Verhoeven AJ, Hilkmann H, de Widt J. A metabolite of an antineoplastic ether phospholipid may inhibit transmembrane signalling via protein kinase C. Lipids 1987;22:842–846.

32. Eibl H, Unger C. From (ether)-lysolecithins to alkylphosphocholines: new and selective antitumor drugs. Sixth NCI-EORTC Symposium on New Drugs for Cancer Therapy 1989;44:67a.

33. Pawelczyk T, Lowenstein JM. Inhibition of phospholipase C delta by hexadecylphosphorylcholine and lysophospholipids with antitumor activity. Biochem Pharmacol 1993;45:493–497.

34. Kosano H, Takatani O. Reduction of epidermal growth factor binding in human breast cancer cell lines by an alkyl-lysophospholipid. Cancer Res 1988; 48:6033–6036.

35. Diomede L, Piovani B, Re F, et al. The induction of apoptosis is a common feature of the cytotoxic action of ether-linked glycerophospholipids in human leukemia cells. Int J Cancer 1994;57:645–649.

36. Burns CP. Membranes and cancer chemotherapy. Cancer Invest 1988;6:439–451.

37. Unger C, Damenz W, Kim DJ, et al. Hexadecylphosphocholine: studies on the antineoplastic activity in vitro and in vivo. Fourth European Conference on Clinical Oncology and Cancer Nursing 1987; 4:67a.

38. Vogler WR, Olson AC, Hajdu J, Shoji M, Raynor R, Kuo JF. Structure-function relationships of alkyl-lysophospholipid analogs in selective antitumor activity. Lipids 1993;28:511–5116.

39. Sobottka SB, Berger MR, Eibl H. Structure-activity relationships for four anti-cancer alkylphosphocholine derivatives in vitro and in vivo. Int J Cancer 1993;53:418–425.

40. Langen P, Maurer HR, Brachwitz H, Eckert K, Veit A, Vollgraf C. Cytostatic effects of various phospholipid analogues on different cells in vitro. Anticancer Res 1992;12:2109–2112.

41. Zeisig R, Jungmann S, Arndt D, Schutt A, Nissen E. Antineoplastic activity in vitro of free and liposomal alkylphosphocholines. Anti-Cancer Drugs 1993;4:57–64.

42. Fichtner I, Zeisig R, Naundorf H, et al. Antineoplastic activity of alkylphosphocholines (APC) in human breast carcinomas in vivo and in vitro; use of liposomes. Breast Cancer Res Treat 1994;32:269–279.

43. Berdel WE, Fink U, Rastetter J. Clinical phase I pilot study of the alkyl lysophospholipid derivative ET-18-OCH3. Lipids 1987;22:967–969.

44. Mollinedo F, Martinez-Dalmau R, Modolell M. Early and selective induction of apoptosis in human leukemia cells by the alkyl-lysophospholipid ET-18-OCH3. Biochem Biophys Res Commun 1993;192:603–609.

45. Vogler WR, Berdel WE. Autologous bone marrow transplantation with alkyl-lysophospholipid-purged marrow. J Hematother 1993;2:93–102.

46. Hilgard P, Stekar J, Harleman JH, et al. Hexadecylphosphocholine-an alkylphosphocholine with major preclinical antitumor activity. Sixth NCI-EORTC Symposium on New Drugs for Cancer Therapy 1989; 4:22a.

47. Unger C, Breiser A, Nagel GA, Peuckert M, Eibl H. Phase I trial of topically applied hexadecylphosphocholine. Sixth NCI-EORTC Symposium on New Drugs for Cancer Therapy 1989;4:107a.

48. Kuhlencord A, Maniera T, Eibl H, Unger C. Hexadecylphosphocholine: oral treatment of visceral leishmaniasis in mice. Antimicrob Agents Chemother 1992;36:1630–1634.

49. Berger MR, Betsch B, Gebelein M, Amtmann E, Heyl P, Scherf HR. Hexadecylphosphocholine differs from conventional cytostatic agents. J Cancer Res Clin Oncol 1993;119:541–548.

50. Ries UJ, Fleer EA, Breiser A, et al. In vitro and in vivo antitumoral activity of alkylphosphonates. Eur J Cancer 1992;29A:96–101.

51. Fleer EA, Berkovic D, Eibl H, Unger C. Investigations on the cellular uptake of hexadecylphosphocholine. Lipids 1993;28:731–736.

52. Vehmeyer K, Liersch T, Eibl H, Unger C. Hexadecylphosphocholine amplifies the effect of granulocyte colony-stimulating factor on differentiating hematopoietic progenitor cells. Prog Exp Tumor Res 1992;34:69–76.

53. Kotting J, Berger MR, Unger C, Eibl H. Alkylphosphocholines: influence of structural variation on biodistribution at antineoplastically active concentrations. Cancer Chemother Pharmacol 1992;30:105–112.

54. Verweij J, van der burg M, Stoter G. A dose-finding study of miltefosine (hexadecylphosphocholine) in patients with metastatic solid tumors. J Cancer Res Clin Oncol 1992;118:606–608.

55. Theischen M, Bornfeld N, Becher R, Kellner U, Wessing A. Hexadecylphosphocholine may produce reversible functional defects of the retinal pigment epithelium. Ger J Ophthalmol 1993;2:113–115.

56. Planting AS, Stoter G, Verweij J. Phase II study of daily oral miltefosine (hexadecylphosphocholine) in advanced colorectal cancer. Eur J Cancer 1993; 29A:518–519.

57. Ten Bokkel Huinink W, Olavel M, Oad-Cl-Mawia N, et al. Skin-metastatic breast cancer: overview analysis of clinical phase II trial on topical treatment with miltefosine. Breast Cancer Res Treat 1994; 32(Suppl):35a.

58. Dummer R, Krasovec M, Roger J, Sindermann H, Burg G. Topical administration of hexadecylphosphocholine in patients with cutaneous lymphomas: results of a phase I/II study. J Am Acad Dermatol 1993; 29:963–970.

59. Jorg B, Kerl H, Thiers BH, Brocker EB, Burg G. Therapeutic approaches in cutaneous lymphoma. Dermatol Clin 1994;12:433–441.

60. Stekar J, Hilgard P, Voegeli R, et al. Antineoplastic activity and tolerability of a novel heterocyclic

alkylphospholipid, D-20133. Cancer Chemother Pharmacol 1993;32:437–444.

61. Hermann DB, Neumann HA. Cytotoxic activity of the thioether phospholipid analogue BM 41.440 in primary human tumor cultures. Lipids 1987;22:955–957.

62. Hofmann J, O'Connor PM, Jackman J, et al. The protein kinase C inhibitor ilmofosine (BM 41 440) arrests cells in G2 phase and suppressed CDC2 kinase activation through a mechanism different from that of DNA damaging agents. Biochem Biophys Res Commun 1994;199:937–943.

63. Herrmann DB, Pahlke W, Munder PG, Bicker U. Antineoplastic and antimetastatic activity of the thioether phospholipid ilmofosine (BM 41.440) in vivo. Proc AACR 1988;29:1317a.

64. Herrmann DBJ, Neumann HA, Berdel WE, et al. Phase I trial of the thioether phospholipid analogue BM 41.440 in cancer patients. Lipids 1987;22:962–966.

65. Winkelmann M, Ebeling K, Strohmeyer G, et al. Treatment results of the thioether lipid ilmofosine in patients with malignant tumours. J Cancer Res Clin Oncol 1992;118:405–407.

66. Rodriguez G, Wall J, Burris H, et al. Results of phase I clinical trials with ilmofosine in patients with solid tumors. Ann Oncol 1994;5(Suppl 5):137a.

67. Shimizu F, Arakawa M. Antitumor activity of 3-((4-amino-2-methyl-5-pyrimidinyl) methyl)-1-(2-chloroethyl)-1-nitrosourea hydrochloride in a variety of experimental tumors. Gann 1978;69:545–548.

68. Inoue K, Fujimoto S, Ogawa M. Comparison of antitumor activities of nitrosourea derivatives against mammary breast carcinomas (MX-1) in nude mice. Gann 1980;71:686–691.

69. Ozawa S, Sugiyama Y, Mitsuhashi Y, Kobaashi T, Inaba M. Cell killing action of cell cyclep phase-nonspecific antitumor agents is dependent on concentration-time product. Cancer Chemother Pharmacol 1988; 21:185–190.

70. Chen JM, Zhang YP, Sui L, Moschel RC, Ikenaga M. Modulation of O^6-methylguanine-DNA methyltransferase-mediated 1-[(4-amino-2-methyl-5-pyrimidinyl)methyl]-3-(2-chloroethyl)-3-nitrosourea resistance by O6-benzylguanine in vitro and in vivo. Anticancer Res 1993;13:801–805.

71. Berger MR, Petru E, Schmahl D. Carcinogenicity of 1-(4-amino-2-methylpyrimidine-5-yl)-methyl-3-(2-chloroethyl)-3-nitrosourea hydrochloride and three related N-nitroso derivatives following repeated intravenous administration to male Wistar rats. Oncology 1988;45:127–133.

72. Japan Radiation-ACNU Study Group. A randomized prospective study of radiation versus radiation plus ACNU in operable non-small cell carcinoma of the lung. Cancer 1989;63:249–254.

73. Joss RA, Siegenthaler P, Ludwig C, Alberto P, Castiglione MM, Cavalli F. Phase II trial of Nimustine (ACNU; 3-((4-amino-2-methyl-5-pyrimidinyl) methyl)-1-(2-chloroethyl)-1-nitrosourea hydrochloride) in patients with small cell carcinoma of the lung after failure on combination chemotherapy. Invest New Drugs 1989;4:175–179.

74. Planting AS, Splinter TA, Ardizzoni A, et al. Phase II study of ACNU as second-line treatment in small-cell lung cancer. EORTC Lung Cancer Cooperative Group. Cancer Chemother Pharmacol 1992; 29:409–411.

75. Haasjes JG, Planting AST, Van der Burg MEL, et al. Phase II trial of ACNU in colorectal cancer. Sixth NCI-EORTC Symposium on New Drugs for Cancer Therapy 1989;4:345a.

76. Ikuta K, Fujioka K, Sumita H, et al. High-dose busulfan, VP-16 and ACNU therapy with stem cell transplantation for the treatment of children with acute leukemia. Rinsho Ketsueki 1993;34:636–642.

77. Yoshida J, Kajita Y, Wakabayashi T, Sugita K. Long-term follow-up results of 175 patients with malignant glioma: importance of radical tumour resection and postoperative adjuvant therapy with interferon, ACNU and radiation. Acta Neurochir 1994;127:55–59.

78. Yamasaki T, Kikuchi H, Shima N, Paine JT, Moritake K, Yamabe H. Chemotherapeutic effects of intra-arterial administration of ACNU in primary intracerebral non-Hodgkin's lymphoma. Surg Neurol 1993;40:383–389.

79. Levin VA, Chamberlain M, Silver P, Rodriguez L, Prados M. Phase I/II study of intraventricular and intrathecal ACNU for leptomeningeal neoplasia. Cancer Chemother Pharmacol 1989;23:301–307.

80. Yoshida TK, Beuls E, Shimizu K, Koulousakis A, Sturm V. Intrathecal chemotherapy with ACNU for meningeal gliomatosis. Br J Cancer 1992;66:999–1004.

81. Kochi M, Kuratsu J, Mihara Y, et al. Ventriculolumbar perfusion 3-[(4-amino-2-methyl-5-pyrimidinyl)methyl]-1-(2-chloroethyl)-1-nitrosourea hydrochloride. Neurosurgery 1993;33:817–823.

82. Gilby ED, Green JA. Phase I study of the potential antineoplastic compound BZQ (2,5-diaziridinyl-3,6-bis(2-hydroxyethylamino-1,4 benzoquinone) NSC 224070. Sixth NCI-EORTC Symposium on New Drugs for Cancer Therapy 1989;4:421a.

83. Khayat D, Lokiec F, Bizzari JP, et al. Phase I clinical study of the new amino acid-linked nitrosourea, S 10036, administered on a weekly schedule. Cancer Res 1987;47:6782–6785.

84. Lokiec F, Santoni J, Khayat D, et al. Clinical application of the pharmacokinetic study of the nitrosourea fotemustine (S 10036). Second International Congress on Neo-Adjuvant Chemotherapy 1988;2:33a.

85. Jacquillat C, Khayat D, Weil M, Bizzari JP. Clinical phase I-II study of the nitrosourea Servier 10036 (fotemustine) in hematological malignancies. Fourth European Conference on Clinical Oncology and Cancer Nursing 1987;4:83a.

86. Khayat D, Bizzari JP, Frenay M, et al. Interim report of phase II study of new nitrosourea S 10036 in disseminated melanoma. J Natl Cancer Inst 1988; 80:1407–1408.

87. Jacquillat C, Khayat D, Banzet P, et al. Final report of the phase II study of the nitrosourea fotemustine (S 10036) in 153 patients with disseminated malignant melanoma (DMM) including brain metastases. Proc AACR 1989;30:1088a.

88. Merimsky O, Chaitchik S. Fotemustine-dacarbazine combinations in the treatment of metastatic melanoma (letter). Eur J Cancer 1993;29A:481–482.

89. Aamdal S, Gerard B, Bohman T, D'Incalci M. Sequential administration of dacarbazine and fotemustine in patients with disseminated malignant melanoma—an effective combination with unexpected toxicity. Eur J Cancer 1992;28:447–450.

90. Gerard B, Aamdal S, Lee SM, et al. Activity and unexpected lung toxicity of the sequential administration of two alkylating agents—dacarbazine and fote-

mustine—in patients with melanoma. Eur J Cancer 1993;29A:711–719.

91. Binder M, Winkler A, Dorffner R, Glebowski E, Wolff K, Pehamberger J. Fotemustine plus dacarbazine in advanced stage III malignant melanoma. Eur J Cancer 1992;28A:1814–1816.

92. Lee SM, Margison GP, Woodcock AA, Thatcher N. Sequential administration of varying doses of dacarbazine and fotemustine in advanced malignant melanoma. Br J Cancer 1993;67:1356–1360.

93. Namer M, Bourdin S, Poisson M, et al. Fotemustine (S 10036) in the treatment of the malignant gliomas in adults. Sixth NCI-EORTC Symposium on New Drugs for Cancer Therapy 1989;4:331a.

94. Bourdin S, Juin P, Hery M, et al. Combination of fotemustine (S 10036) and radiotherapy in malignant gliomas: report of the French Multicentric Study. Proc AACR 1989;30:1089a.

95. Khayat D, Giroux B, Berille J, et al. Fotemustine in the treatment of brain primary tumors and metastases. Cancer Invest 1994;12:414–420.

96. Lasset C, Merrouche Y, Negrier S, et al. Phase II study of fotemustine as second-line treatment after failure of immunotherapy in metastatic renal cell carcinoma. Cancer Chemother Pharmacol 1993;32:329–331.

97. Fischel JL, Formento P, Berlion M, et al. Cytotoxic effects of the combination of a new nitrosourea, fotemustine, combined with 5-fluorouracil and folinic acid depend on the sequence of their administration. Bull Cancer 1992;79:81–90.

98. Kerbrat P, Somers R, Verweij J, et al. Phase II study of fotemustine in advanced soft tissue sarcomas. A trial of EORTC Soft Tissue and Bone Sarcoma Group. Eur J Cancer 1992;29A:143–144.

99. Rigal-Huguet F, Giroux B, Lokiec F, Gaspard MH, Attal M, Pris J. High-dose S 10036 (Fotemustine) in a combination regimen with autologous bone marrow transplantation (ABMT): pharmacokinetics (PK) and tolerance (abstract). Sixth NCI-EORTC Symposium on New Drugs for Cancer Therapy 1989;4:446a.

100. Pujol JL, Monnier A, Berille J, et al. Phase II study of nitrosourea fotemustine as single-drug chemotherapy in poor-prognosis non-small-cell lung cancer. Br J Cancer 1994;69:1136–1140.

101. Rudd R, Allen R, Berille J, Spiro SG, Trask C, Souhami RL. Phase II study of fotemustine in untreated inoperable non-small-cell lung cancer. Cancer Chemother Pharmacol 1994;34:444–446.

102. Riviere A, Le Cesne A, Berille J, Baio S, Le Chevalier T. Cisplatin-fotemustine combination in operable non-small cell lung cancer: preliminary report of a French multicentre phase II trial. Eur J Cancer 1994;30A:587–590.

103. Raymond E, Haon C, Coste M, Boaziz C, Giroux B. Multifactorial analysis of fotemustine toxicity using the logistic regression method (abstract). Fifth International Congress of Anti-Cancer Chemotherapy 1995;101a.

104. Berger DP, Winterhalter BR, Dengler WA, Fiebig HH. Preclinical activity of hepsulfam and busulfan in sold tumor xenografts and human bone marrow. Anti-Cancer Drugs 1992;3:531–539.

105. Marshall MV, Marshall MH, Degen DR, et al. In vitro cytotoxicity of hepsulfam against human tumor cell lines and primary human tumor colony forming units. Stem Cells 1993;11:62–69.

106. Winton EF, Srinivasiah J, Kim BK, et al. Effect of recombinant human interleukin-6 (rhIL-6) and rhIL-3 on hematopoietic regeneration as demonstrated in a nonhuman primate chemotherapy model. Blood 1994; 84:65–73.

107. Brock N, Hilgard P, Peukert M, Pohl J, Sindermann H. Basic and new developments in the field of oxazaphosphorines. Cancer Invest 1988;6:513–532.

108. Niemeyer U, Engel J, Scheffler G, Molge K, Sauerbier D, Weigert W. Chemical characterization of ASTA Z 7557 (INN mafosfamide, cis-4-sulfoethylthio-cyclophosphamide), a stable derivative of 4-hydroxy-cyclophosphamide. Invest New Drugs 1984;2:133–139.

109. Auber ML, Horwitz LJ, Blaauw A, et al. Evaluation of drugs for elimination of leukemic cells from the bone marrow of patients with acute leukemia. Blood 1988;71:166–172.

110. Davidoff AN, Mendelow BV. Cell-cycle disruptins and apoptosis induced by the cyclophosphamide derivative mafosfamide. Exp Hematol 1993; 21:922–927.

111. Pohl J, Reissmann T, Voegeli R. Oxazaphosphorine effects in L 5222 rat leukemia. Methods Findings Exp Clin Pharmacol 1987;9:589–594.

112. Stahl M, Schober C, Schmidt S, et al. Pilot study with low dose mafosfamide in patients with progressive, metastatic renal cell carcinoma (RCC). Sixth NCI-EORTC Symposium on New Drugs for Cancer Therapy 1989;4:76a.

113. Skorski T, Kawalec M. New application of a stabilized active cyclophosphamide derivative (Mafosfamide, ASTA Z 7654)-immunogenic properties of lymphatic leukemia L 1210 cells treated in vitro with the drug. Invest New Drugs 1987;5:167–169.

114. Hilgard P, Pohl J, Stekar J, Voegeli R. Oxazaphosphorines as biological response modifiers—experimental and clinical perspectives. Cancer Treat Rev 1985;12:155–167.

115. Bruntsch U, Groos G, Hiller TA, Wandt H, Tigges FJ, Gallmeier WM. Phase I study of mafosfamide-cyclohexylamine (ASTA Z-7557, NSC 345842) and limited phase I data on mafosfamide-lysine. Invest New Drugs 1985;3:293–296.

116. Herve P, Plouvier CE, Flesch M, Tamayo E, Leconte des Floris R, Peters A. Autologous bone marrow transplantation for acute leukemia using transplant chemopurified with a metabolite of oxazaphosphorines (ASTA Z 7557, INN mafosfamide). First clinical results. Invest New Drugs 1984;2:245–252.

117. Murgo AJ, Weinberger BB. Pharmacological bone marrow purging in autologous transplantation: focus on the cyclophosphamide derivatives. Crit Rev Oncol Hematol 1993;14:41–60.

118. Gorin NC, Coiffier B, Hayat M, et al. Recombinant human granulocyte-macrophage colony-stimulating factor after high dose chemotherapy and autologous bone marrow transplantation with unpurged and purged marrow in non-Hodgkin's lymphoma: a double-blind placebo-controlled trial. Blood 1992; 80:1149–1157.

119. Laporte JP, Douay L, Lopez M, et al. One hundred twenty-five adult patients with primary acute leukemia autografted with marrow purged by mafosfamide: a 10-year single institution experience. Blood 1994;84:3810–3818.

120. Laporte JP, Isnard F, Lesage S, et al. Autologous bone marrow transplantation with marrow

purged by mafosfamide in seven patients with myelo-dysplastic syndromes in transformation (AML-MDS): a pilot trial. Leukemia 1993;7:2030–2033.

121. Carlo-Stella C, Mangoni L, Piovani G, Garau D, Almici C, Rizzoli V. Biological and chemical selection of Ph-negative clones. Stem Cells 1993;11(Suppl 3):77–82.

122. Rizzoli V, Magnoni L, Almici C, Caramatti C, Dotti GP, Carlo-Stella C. Autologous transplantation for chronic myelogenous leukemia with mafosfamide-treated marrow. Stem Cells 1993;11(Suppl 3):25–30.

123. Skorski T, Nieborowskia-Skorska M, Barletta C, et al. Highly efficient elimination of Philadelphia leukemic cells by exposure to bcr/abl antisense oligodeoxynucleotides combined with mafosfamide. J Clin Invest 1993;92:194–202.

124. Telekes A, Kerpel-Fronius S, Borsi M, Hernadi Z, Rado J, Eckhardt S. Human tolerance study of dibromodulcitol (DBD, Mitolactol) and 5-fluorouracil (5-FU) combination. Fourth European Conference on Clinical Oncology and Cancer Nursing 1987;4:84a.

125. Sebestyen JK, Institoris L, Pethes G. Absorption and metabolism of dibromodulcitol after intravaginal administration in rats. Sixth NCI-EORTC Symposium on New Drugs for Cancer Therapy 1989;4:101a.

126. Montgomery JA, McCaleb GS, Johnston TP. Inhibition of solid tumors by nitrosoureas. I. Lewis lung carcinoma. J Med Chem 1977;20:291–295.

127. Stewart DL, Benjamin RS, Leavens M, Valdiviesco M, Burgess MA, Bodey GP. Phase I trial and pharmacology of 1-(2,6-dioxo-3-piperidyl)-1-nitrosourea (NSC 95466) in adults with solid tumors. Cancer Res 1980;40:3750–3754.

128. Earhart RH, Muggia FM, Golumb FM. Phase II trial of PCNU in advanced malignant melanoma: an Eastern Cooperative Oncology Group pilot study. Invest New Drugs 1985;3:297–301.

129. Stewart DJ, Grahovac Z, Russel NA, et al. Phase I study of intracarotid PCNU. J Neurooncol 1987;5:245–250.

130. Dinapoli RP, Brown LD, Arusell RM, et al. Phase III comparative evaluation of PCNU and carmustine with radiation therapy for high-grade glioma. J Clin Oncol 1993;11:1316–1321.

131. Shapiro WR. Chemotherapy of malignant gliomas: studies of the BTCG. Rev Neurol 1992;148:428–434.

132. Loftsson T, Baldvinsdottir J. Degradation of tauromustine (TCNU) in aqueous solutions. Acta Pharm Nord 1992;4:129–132.

133. Bibby MC, Double JA, Morris CM. Anti-tumor activity of TCNU in a panel of transplantable murine colon tumors. Eur J Cancer Clin Oncol 1988;24:1361–1364.

134. Hartley-Asp B, Christensson PI, Gunnarsson K, et al. Anti-tumor, toxicological and pharmacokinetic properties of a novel taurine-based nitrosourea (TCNU). Invest New Drugs 1988;6:19–30.

135. Molineux G, Schofield R, Testa NG. Haematopoietic effects of TCNU in mice. Cancer Treat Rep 1987;71:837–841.

136. Hartley-Asp B. Genotoxicity of tauromustine, a new water soluble taurine-based nitrosourea. I. Mutagenic and clastogenic activity of tauromustine in vitro. Mutagenesis 1992;7:427–431.

137. Matthew A, Bibby MC, Double JA, Crawford SM. Anti-tumor activity and bone marrow toxicity of the TCNU metabolites, LS2724 and LS2715. Sixth NCI-EORTC Symposium on New Drugs for Cancer Therapy 1989;4:406a.

138. Fergusson RJ, Anderson LE, Macpherson JS, Robbins P, Smyth JF. Activity of a new nitrosourea (TCNU) in human lung cancer xenografts. Br J Cancer 1988;57:339–342.

139. D'Incalci M, Citti L, Taverna P, Catapano CV. Importance of the DNA repair enzyme O^6-alkylguanine alkyltransferase (AT) in cancer chemotherapy. Cancer Treat Rev 1988;15:279–292.

140. Smyth JF, Macpherson JS, Warrington PS, et al. Phase I study of TCNU, a novel nitrosourea. Eur J Cancer Clin Oncol 1987;12:1837–1843.

141. Vibe-Petersen J, Bork E, Moller H, Hansen H. A phase I clinical evaluation of 1-(2-chloroethyl)-3-(2-(dimethylaminosulphonyl)ethyl)-1-nitrosourea (TCNU). Eur J Cancer Clin Oncol 1987;12:1837–1843.

142. Gunnarsson PO, Vibe-Petersen J, Macpherson JS, et al. Pharmacokinetics of tauromustine in cancer patients. Phase I studies. Cancer Chemother Pharmacol 1989;23:176–180.

143. Van Glabbeke M, Renard J, Smyth J, Gundersen S, Dombernowsky P, Cavalli F. Optimal dose of tauromustine (TCNU): a retrospective analysis of the phase II studies conducted by the EOTC Early Clinical Trials Cooperative Group (ECTG). Sixth NCI-EORTC Symposium on New Drugs for Cancer Therapy 1989; 4:335a.

144. Vibe-Petersen J, Bach F, Gersel-Pedersen A, Smyth J, Hansen HH. A phase II trial of TCNU in patients with squamous cell, adeno- and large cell carcinoma of the lung. Fourth European Conference on Clinical Oncology and Cancer Nursing 1987;4:1a.

145. Dombernowsky P, Clavel M, Smyth JF, Renard J, Pinedo H. Phase II study of TCNU (LS 2667) in advanced breast cancer. Fourth European Conference on Clinical Oncology and Cancer Nursing 1987;4:141a.

146. Smyth JF, Macpherson JS, Whittle IR, Miller JD. Disposition of TCNU in human brain tumors. Proc AACR 1988;29:775a.

147. Singh G, Graffner HO, Milsom JW, Chaudry IH. Tauromustine is more effective than conventional chemotherapy in the treatment of colonic tumors. Dis Colon Rectum 1993;36:394–399.

148. Hill SR, Bibby MC. 5-Fluorouracil causes alterations in the pharmacokinetic profile of tauromustine in NMRI mice. Cancer Chemother Pharmacol 1994;34:57–62.

149. Hill SR, Pollard LA, Bibby MC. Sequence-dependent activity of 5-fluorouracil plus tauromustine in a transplantable well-differentiated murine colon adenocarcinoma. Anticancer Res 1992;12:2169–2175.

150. Taal BG, ten Bokkel Huinink WW, Rodenhuis S. Combination chemotherapy with tauromustine (TCNU), 5-fluorouracil and leucovorin in advanced colorectal carcinoma: a dose-finding study. Ann Oncol 1993;4:81–82.

151. Kerbrat P, Adenis A, Rebattu P, et al. Phase II study of cystemustine in metastatic colorectal carcinoma. A trial of the EORTC Clinical Screening Group. Eur J Cancer 1993;29A:1597–1599.

152. Mathe G, Misset JL, Triana BK, Godeneche D, Madelmont JC, Meyniel G. Phase I trial of cystemustine, a new cysteamine (2-chloroethyl) nitrosourea: an

intrapatient escalation scheme. Drugs Exp Clin Res 1992;18:155–158.

153. Chollet P, Adenis A, Chauvergne J, et al. Results of two phase II trials with cystemustine in five different tumoral localizations. Ann Oncol 1994; 5(Suppl 5):144a.

154. Chollet P, Adenis A, Chauvergne J, et al. Results of two phase II trials with cystemustine in advanced malignant melanoma. Ann Oncol 1994;5(Suppl 5):144a.

155. Newlands ES. Current development of temozolomide. Ann Oncol 1994;5(Suppl 5):119a.

156. Stevens MFG, Hickman JA, Langdon SP, et al. Antitumor activity and pharmacokinetics in mice of 8-carbamoyl-3-methyl-imidazo (5,1-d)-1,2,3,5 tetrazin-4(3H)-one (CCRG 81045; M & B 39831), a novel drug with potential as an alternative to dacarbazine. Cancer Res 1987;47:5846–5852.

157. Plowman J, Waud WR, Koutsoukos AD, Rubinstein LV, Moore TD, Grever MR. Preclinical antitumor activity of temozolomide in mice: efficacy against human brain tumor xenografts and synergism with 1,3-bis(2-chloroethyl)-1-nitrosourea. Cancer Res 1994;54:3793–3799.

158. Tsang LIH, Gescher A, Slack JA. A comparative investigation of the in vitro disposition and cytotoxicity of temozolomide and dacarbazine. Sixth NCI-EORTC Symposium on New Drugs for Cancer Therapy 1989;4:420a.

159. Lee SM, Thatcher N, Crowther D, Margison GP. Inactivation of O6-alkylguanine-DNA alkyltransferase in human peripheral blood mononuclear cells by temozolomide. Br J Cancer 1994;69:452–456.

160. Gander M, Leyvraz S, Perey L, et al. O6-alyl-guanine-DNA alkyltransferase depletion induced by temozolomide: a mechanism of interest for an association with a nitrosourea. Ann Oncol 1994;5(Suppl 5):86a.

161. Catapano CV, Broggini M, Erba E, et al. In vitro and in vivo methazolastone-induced DNA damage and repair in L-1210 leukemia sensitive and resistant to chloroethylnitrosoureas. Cancer Res 1987;47:4884–4889.

162. Baer JC, Freeman AA, Newlands ES, Watson AJ, Rafferty JA, Margison GP. Depletion of O6-alkylguanine-DNA alkyltransferase correlates with potentiation of temozolomide and CCNU toxicity in human tumour cells. Br J Cancer 1993;67:1299–1302.

163. Newlands ES, Slack J, Blackledge G, et al. Phase I trial of Temozolomide (CCRG81045; M & B 29831; NSC 362856). Sixth NCI-EORTC Symposium on New Drugs for Cancer Therapy 1989;4:491a.

164. Slack JA, Newlands ES, Blackledge GRP, et al. Phase I clinical pharmacokinetics of Temozolomide (CCRC81045;C 362856). Proc AACR 1989;30:993a.

165. O'Reilly SM, Newlands ES, Glaser MG, et al. Temozolomide: a new oral cytotoxic chemotherapeutic agent with promising activity against primary brain tumours. Eur J Cancer 1993;29A:940–942.

166. Ames MM, Reid JM, Stevens DC, Rhodes WL, Nicholson S, Reamn G. Temozolomide (TEM) pharmacokinetics in the Children's Cancer Study Group Phase I trial of TEM administrated as a single oral dose on a daily × 5 schedule. Proc AACR 1995;36:236.

167. Foster BJ, Newell DR, Carmichael J, et al. Preclinical, phase I and pharmacokinetic studies with the dimethyl phenyltriazene CB10–277. Br J Cancer 1993; 67:362–368.

168. Lee SM, O'Connor PJ, Thatcher N, Crowther D, Margison GP, Cooper DP. Relationships between the formation of O6-methyldeoxyguanosine by 1-p-carboxyl-3,3-dimethylphenyltriazene in DNA and O6-alkylguanine-DNA alkyltransferase in human peripheral leukocytes. Cancer Res 1994;54:4072–4076.

169. Lee SM, Thatcher N, Crowther D, Margison GP. In vivo depletion of O6-alkylguanine-DNA-alkyltransferase in lymphocytes and melanoma of patients with CB 10-277, a new DTIC analogue. Cancer Chemother Pharmacol 1992;31:240–246.

170. Foster BJ, Newell DR, Gumbrell LA, Jenns KE, Calvert AH. Phase I trial with pharmacokinetics of CB10-277 given by 24 hours continuous infusion. Br J Cancer 1993;67:369–373.

171. Bleehen NM, Calvert AH, Lee SM, et al. A Cancer Research Campaign (CRC) phase II trial of CB10-277 given by 24 hour infusion for malignant melanoma. Br J Cancer 1994;70:775–777.

172. Hendriks HR, Pizao PE, Berger DP, et al. EO9: a novel bioreductive alkylating indoloquinone with preferential solid tumour activity and lack of bone marrow toxicity in preclinical models. Eur J Cancer 1993;29A:897–906.

173. Workman P, Binger M, Kooistra KL. Pharmacokinetics, distribution, and metabolism of the novel bioreductive alkylating indoloquinone EO9 in rodents. Int J Radiat Oncol Biol Phys 1992;22:713–716.

174. McLeod A, Setanoians A, Aamdal S, Lund B, Graham MA. Phase I pharmacokinetics of bioreductive alkylating drug EO9. Ann Oncol 1994;5(Suppl 5):170a.

175. Lund B, Aamdal S, Koier I. Phase I study of the bioreductive indoloquinone EO9. Ann Oncol 1994; 5(Suppl 5):136a.

176. Lee JH, Naito M, Tsuruo T. Nonenzymatic reductive activation of 7-N-((2-([2-(γ-L-glutamyla-mino)ethyl]dithio)ethyl))mitomycin C by thiol molecules: a novel mitomycin C derivative effective on mitomycin C-resistant tumor cells. Cancer Res 1994; 54:2398–2402.

177. Dirix LY, Gheuens EE, van der Heyden S, van Oosterom AT, De Bruijn EA. Cytotoxic activity of 7-N-2((2-(-γ-L-glutamylamino)-ethyl)dithio)ethyl)-mitomycin C and metabolites in cell lines with different resistance patterns. Anti-Cancer Drugs 1994;5:343–354.

178. Ashizawa T, Okabe M, Gomi K, Hirata T. Reduced bone marrow toxicity of KW-2149, a mitomycin C derivative, in mice. Anti-Cancer Drugs 1993;4:181–188.

179. Kobayashi S, Ushiki J, Takai K, et al. Disposition and metabolism of KW-2149, a novel anticancer agent. Cancer Chemother Pharmacol 1993;32:143–150.

180. Gomi K, Ashizawa T, Okamoto A, Okabe M. Characteristics of antitumor activities of M-16 and M-18, major metabolites of a new mitomycin C derivative KW-2149 in mice. Fifth International Congress of Anti-Cancer Chemotherapy 1995;198a.

181. McLeod DG. Antiandrogenic drugs. Cancer 1993;71(3 Suppl):1046–1049.

182. Decensi A, Torrisi R, Fontana V, et al. Long-term endocrine effects of administration of either a non-steroidal antiandrogen or a luteinizing hormone-releasing hormone agonist in men with prostate cancer. Acta Endocrinol 1993;129:315–321.

183. Soloway MS, Matzkin H. Antiandrogenic agents as monotherapy in advanced prostatic carcinoma. Cancer 1993;71 (3 Suppl):1083–1088.

184. Kasimis B, Soloway M, Kreis W, et al. Casodex (ICI 176,334) therapy in patients with advanced prostate cancer: results of a phase II study. Proc Am Soc Clin Oncol 1989;8:518a.

185. Kaisary AV. Current clinical studies with a new nonsteroidal antiandrogen, Casodex. Prostate Suppl 1994;5:27–33.

186. Soloway MS, Kasimis B, Smith JA, et al. Efficacy and safety of the nonsteroidal antiandrogen casodex in the treatment of advanced prostate cancer. American Urological Association annual meeting 1989, 707a.

187. Tyrrell CJ. Casodex: a pure non-steroidal antiandrogen used as monotherapy in advanced prostate cancer. Prostate Suppl 1992;4:97–104.

188. Verhelst J, Denis L, Van Vliet P, et al. Endocrine profiles during administration of the new nonsteroidal anti-androgen Casodex in prostate cancer. Clin Endocrinol 1994;41:525–530.

189. Pendyala L, Creaven PJ, Huben R, Tremblay D, Bertagna C. Pharmacokinetics of anadron in patients with advanced carcinoma of the prostate. Cancer Chemother Pharmacol 1988;21:73–76.

190. Pescatore P, Hammel P, Durand F, et al. Fatal fulminant hepatitis induced by nilutamide (Anandron). Gastroenterol Clin Biol 1993;17:499–501.

191. Fau D, Berson A, Eugene D, Fromenty B, Fisch C, Pessayre D. Mechanism for the hepatotoxicity of the antiandrogen, nilutamide. Evidence suggesting that redox cycling of this nitroaromatic drug leads to oxidative stress in isolated hepatocytes. J Pharmacol Exp Ther 1992;263:69–77.

192. Harris MG, Coleman SG, Faulds D, Chrisp P. Nilutamide. A review of its pharmacodynamic and pharmacokinetic properties. Drugs Aging 1993;3:9–25.

193. Pfitzenmeyer P, Foucher P, Piard F, et al. Nilutamide pneumonitis: a report on eight patients. Thorax 1992;47:622–627.

194. Decensi A, Torrisi R, Fontana V. Stimulation of erythropoiesis by the non-steroidal anti-androgen nilutamide in men with prostate cancer: evidence for an agonistic effect? Br J Cancer 1994;69:617–619.

195. Janknegt RA. Total androgen blockade with the use of orchiectomy and nilutamide (Anandron) or placebo as treatment of metastatic prostate cancer. Anandron International Study Group. Cancer 1993;72 (12 Suppl):3874–3877.

196. Bertagna C, De Gery A, Hucher M, Francois JP, Zanirato J. Efficacy of the combination of nilutamide plus orchiectomy in patients with metastatic prostatic cancer. A meta-analysis of seven randomized double-blind trials (1056 patients). Br J Urol 1994; 73:396–402.

197. Galardy RE, Grobelny D, Foellmer HG, Fernandez LA. Inhibition of angiogenesis by the matrix metalloprotease inhibitor N-[2R-2-(hydroxyamidocarbonymethyl)-4-methylpentanoyl)]-L-tryptophan methylamide. Cancer Res 1994;54:4715–4718.

198. Folkman J. What is the evidence that tumors are angiogenesis dependent? J Natl Cancer Inst 1990; 82:4–6.

199. Folkman J. Tumor angiogenesis. In: Mendelsohn J, Howley PM, Israel MA, Liotta LA, eds. The molecular basis of cancer. Philadelphia: WB Saunders, 1995:206–232.

200. Maeda K, Chung Y-S, Takatsuka S, et al. Tumor angiogenesis as a predictor of recurrence in gastric carcinoma. J Clin Oncol 1995;13:477–481.

201. Bicknell R. Vascular targeting and the inhibition of angiogenesis. Ann Oncol 1994;5(Suppl 4):45–50.

202. Ingber D, Fujita T, Kishimoto S, et al. Synthetic analogues of fumagillin that inhibit angiogenesis and suppress tumour growth. Nature 1990;348:555–557.

203. Antoine N, Bours V, Heinren E, Simar LJ, Castronovo V. Stimulation of human B-lymphocyte proliferation by AGM-1470, a potent inhibitor of angiogenesis. J Natl Cancer Inst 1995;87:136–139.

204. Yamaoka M, Yamamoto T, Ikeyama S, et al. Angiogenesis inhibitor TNP-470 (AGM-1470) potently inhibits the tumor growth of hormone-independent human breast and prostate carcinoma cell lines. Cancer Res 1993;53:5233–5236.

205. Yamaoka M, Yamamoto T, Masaki T, et al. Inhibition of tumor growth and metastasis of rodent tumors by the angiogenesis inhibitor o-(chloroacetyl-carbamoyl) fumagillol (TNP-470; AGM-1470). Cancer Res 1993;53:4262–4267.

206. Okabe M, Kawamura K, Miyagishima T, et al. Effect of herbimycin A, an inhibitor of tyrosine kinase, on protein tyrosine kinase activity and phosphotyrosyl proteins of Ph1-positive leukemia cells. Leuk Res 1994; 18:213–220.

207. Oikawa T, Shimamura M, Ashino H, et al. Inhibition of angiogenesis by staurosporine, a potent protein kinase inhibitor. J Antibiot 1992;45:1155–1160.

208. Ezekowitz RA, Mulliken JB, Folkman J. Interferon alfa-2a therapy for life-threatening hemangiomas of infancy. N Engl J Med 1992;326:1456–1463.

209. Cole K, Kohn E. Calcium-mediated signal transduction: biology, biochemistry, and therapy. Cancer Metastasis Rev 1994;13:31–44.

210. Teicher BA, Holden SA, Chen YN, Ara G, Korbut TT, Northey D. CAI: effects on cytotoxic therapies in vitro and in vivo. Cancer Chemother Pharmacol 1994;34:515–521.

211. Figg WD, Cole EA, Reed E, et al. Pharmacokinetics of CAI following multiple day dosing. Proc AACR 1995;36:235a.

212. Soltis M, Cole K, Yeh H, Jacobs W, Kohn E. Human CAI metabolites: isolation, identification, and characterization. Proc AACR 1995;36:238.

213. Tutsch K, Arzoomanian R, Alberti D, et al. Phase I and pharmacokinetic study of oral carboxyamidotriazole (CAI). Proc AACR 1995;36:238.

214. Singer JW, Rice GC, Burstein S, Bianco JA. CT-2584, a novel synthetic compound that alters phospholipid metabolism, is selectively cytotoxic to tumor cells and inhibits matrix metalloproteinase 9 synthesis and tumor-induced angiogenesis. Ann Oncol 1995;5(Suppl 5):127a.

215. D'Amato RJ, Loughnan MS, Flynn E, Folkman J. Thalidomide is an inhibitor of angiogenesis. Proc Natl Acad Sci USA 1994;91:4082–4085.

216. Tamargo RJ, Bok RA, Brem H. Angiogenesis inhibition by minocycline. Cancer Res 1991;51:672–675.

217. Eckhardt G, Burris H III, Eckardt S, et al. Initial phase I assessment of the novel angiogenesis inhibitor DS4152. Ann Oncol 1994;5(Suppl 5):72a.

218. Gill PS, Kidane S, Tulpule A, Espina BM, Masuo K, Sobel RS. A phase I study of DS-4152, a novel

angiogenesis inhibitor in the treatment of AIDS-related Kaposi's sarcoma. Ann Oncol 1994;5(Suppl 5):101a.

219. Vukanovic J, Passaniti A, Hirata T, Traystman RJ, Hartley-Asp B, Isaacs JT. Antiangiogenic effects of the quinoline-3-carboxamide linomide. Cancer Res 1993;1833–1837.

220. Kangas L. Agonistic and antagonistic effects of antiestrogens in different target organs. Acta Oncol 1992;31:143–146.

221. Coradini D, Biffi A, Cappelletti V, Di Fronzo G. Activity of tamoxifen and new antiestrogens on estrogen receptor positive and negative breast cancer cells. Anticancer Res 1994;14:1059–1064.

222. Rao US, Fine RL, Scarborough GA. Antiestrogens and steroid hormones: substrates of the human P-glycoprotein. Biochem Pharmacol 1994;48:287–292.

223. Gagliardi A, Collins DC. Inhibition of angiogenesis by antiestrogens. Cancer Res 1993;53:533–535.

224. White IN, de Matteis F, Davies A, et al. Genotoxic potential of tamoxifen and analogues in female Fischer F344/n rats, DBA/2 and C57BL/6 mice and in human MCL-5 cells. Carcinogenesis 1992;13:197–203.

225. Wakeling AE. The future of new pure antiestrogens in clinical breast cancer. Breast Cancer Res Treat 1993;25:1–9.

226. Rauschning W, Pritchard KI. Droloxifene, a new antiestrogen: its role in metastatic breast cancer. Breast Cancer Res Treat 1994;31:83–94.

227. Kawamura I, Lacey E, Tanaka Y, Nishigaki F, Manda T, Shimomura K. Binding sites of droloxifene in the cytosol of 7,12-dimethylbenz[a]anthracene-induced rat mammary tumor cells. Jpn J Cancer Res 1994; 85:639–644.

228. Kawamura I, Lacey E, Mizota T, et al. The effect of droloxifene on the insulin-like growth factor-I-stimulated growth of breast cancer cells. Anticancer Res 1994;14:427–431.

229. Hasmann M, Rattel B, Loser R. Preclinical data for Droloxifene. Cancer Lett 1994;84:101–116.

230. Wiseman H, Smith C, Halliwell B, Cannon M, Arnstein HR, Lennard MS. Droloxifene (3-hydroxytamoxifen) has membrane antioxidant ability: potential relevance to its mechanism of therapeutic action in breast cancer. Cancer Lett 1992;66:61–68.

231. Buzdar AU, Kau S, Hortobagyi GN, et al. Phase I trial of droloxifene in patients with metastatic breast cancer. Cancer Chemother Pharmacol 1994; 34:313–316.

232. Sharp SY, Rowlands MG, Jarman M, Kelland LR. Effects of a new antiestrogen, idoxifene, on cisplatin- and doxorubicin-sensitive and -resistant human ovarian carcinoma cell lines. Br J Cancer 1994;70:409–414.

233. Coombes RC, Haynes BP, Dowsett M, et al. Idoxifene: report of a phase I study in patients with metastatic breast cancer. Cancer Res 1995;55:1070–1074.

234. Wakeling AE, Dukes M, Bowler J. A potent pure antioestrogen with clinical potential. Cancer Res 1991;51:3867–3873.

235. Dauvois S, White R, Parker MG. The antiestrogen ICI 182780 disrupts estrogen receptor nucleocytoplasmic shuttling. J Cell Sci 1993;106:1377–1388.

236. Parker MG. Action of "pure" antiestrogens in inhibiting estrogen receptor action. Breast Cancer Res Treat 1993;26:131–137.

237. Coopman P, Garcia M, Brunner N, Derocq D, Clarke R, Rochefort H. Anti-proliferative and anti-estrogenic effects of ICI 164,384 and ICI 182,780 in 4-OH-tamoxifen-resistant human breast cancer cells. Int J Cancer 1994;56:295–300.

238. Hu XF, Veroni M, De Luise M, et al. Circumvention of tamoxifen resistance by the pure anti-estrogen ICI 182,780. Int J Cancer 1993;55:873–876.

239. Langdon SP, Crew AJ, Ritchie AA, et al. Growth inhibition of oestrogen receptor-positive human ovarian carcinoma by anti-oestrogens in vitro in a xenograft model. Eur J Cancer 1994;30A:682–686.

240. Howell A, DeFriend D, Robertson J, Blamey R, Walton P. Response to a specific antioestrogen (ICI 182780) in tamoxifen-resistant breast cancer. Lancet 1995;345:29–30.

241. Erdelyi-Toth V, Szamel I, Gyergyay F, Pap E, Kralovanszky J. Pharmacokinetic profile and endocrine effects of panomifene according to a phase IA study. Ann Oncol 1994;5(Suppl 5):177a.

242. Litherland S, Jackson I. Antioestrogens in the management of hormone-dependent cancer. Cancer Treat Rev 1988;15:183–194.

243. Kallio S, Kngas L, Blanco G, et al. A new triphenylethylene compound, Fc-1157a. I. Hormonal effects. Cancer Chemother Pharmacol 1986;17:103–108.

244. Styles JA, Davies A, Lim CK, et al. Genotoxicity of tamoxifen, tamoxifen epoxide and toremifene in human lymphoblastoid cells containing human cytochrome P450s. Carcinogenesis 1994;15:5–9.

245. Kangas L, Nieminen AL, Blanco G, et al. A new triphenylethylene compound, Fc-1157a. II. Antitumor effects. Cancer Chemother Pharmacol 1986; 17:109–113.

246. Szamel I, Hindy I, Vincze B, Eckhardt S, Kangas L, Hajba A. Influence of toremifene on the endocrine regulation in breast cancer patients. Eur J Cancer 1994;30A:154–158.

247. Bishop J, Murray R, Webster L, et al. Phase I clinical and pharmacokinetics study of high-dose toremifene in postmenopausal patients with advanced breast cancer. Cancer Chemother Pharmacol 1992; 30:174–178.

248. Valavaara R, Pyrhonen S, Heikkinen M, et al. Toremifene, a new antiestrogenic compound for the treatment of advanced breast cancer. Phase II study. Eur J Cancer Clin Oncol 1988;24:785–790.

249. Modig H, Nilsson I, Westman G. Toremifene, a new antiestrogen—results of treatment in patients with breast cancer. Sixth NCI-EORTC Symposium on New Drugs for Cancer Therapy 1989;4:313.

250. Stenbygaard LE, Herrstedt J, Thomsen JF, Svendsen KR, Engelhom SA, Dombernowsky P. Toremifene and tamoxifen in advanced breast cancer—a double-blind cross-over trial. Breast Cancer Res Treat 1993;25:57–63.

251. Ebbs SR, Roberts JV, Wilson AJ, Baum M. Elucidating the action of the antioestrogen? Response to toremifene (Fc-1157a) therapy in tamoxifen failed patients. Br J Cancer 1987;56:860.

252. Vogel CL, Shemano I, Schoenfelder J, Gams RA, Green MR. Multicenter phase II efficacy trial of toremifene in tamoxifen-refractory patients with advanced breast cancer. J Clin Oncol 1993;11:345–350.

253. Pyrhonen S, Valavaara R, Vuorinen J, Hajba A. High dose toremifene in advanced breast cancer resistant to or relapsed during tamoxifen treatment. Breast Cancer Res Treat 1994;29:223–228.

254. Wilson AJ, Baum M, Singh L, Kangas L. Antioestrogen therapy of pure mesenchymal tumor (letter). Lancet 1987;1:508.

255. Van de Velde P, Nique F, Bouchoux F, et al. RU 58,668, a new pure antiestrogen inducing a regression of human mammary carcinoma implanted in nude mice. J Steroid Biochem Mol Biol 1994;48:187–196.

256. Arcamone F. Chemical approaches to anticancer drug development. Cancer Treat Rep 1988;15:65–68.

257. Hill BT, Denis LY, Li XT, Whelan RDH. Identification of anthracycline analogues with enhanced cytotoxicity and lack of cross-resistance to adriamycin using a series of mammalian cell lines in vitro. Cancer Chemother Pharmacol 1985;14:194–201.

258. Capranico G, De Isabella P, Penco S, Tinelli S, Zunino F. Role of DNA breakage in cytotoxicity of doxorubicin, 9-deoxydoxorubicin, and 4-demethyl-6-deoxydoxorubicin in murine leukemia P 388 cells. Cancer Res 1989;49:2022–2027.

259. Robert J, Gianni L. Pharmacokinetics and metabolism of anthracyclines. Cancer Surv 1993;17:219–252.

260. Brana MF, Castellano JM, Roldan CM, et al. Synthesis and mode(s) of action of a new series of imide derivatives of 3-nitro-1,8-naphthalic acid. Cancer Chemother Pharmacol 1980;4:61–66.

261. Legha SS, Ring S, Raber M, Felder TB, Newman RA, Krakoff IH. Phase I clinical investigation of benzisoquinolinedione. Cancer Treat Rep 1987;71:1165–1169.

262. Lu K, McLean MA, Vestal ML, Newman RA. Pharmacokinetics of amonifide in dogs. Cancer Chemother Pharmacol 1988;21:134–138.

263. Kreis W, Budman DR, Allen SL, et al. Clinical pharmacokinetics of amonafide (NSC 308847) in 51 patients. Proc AACR 1992;33:260a.

264. Saez R, Craig J, Weiss G, et al. Phase I clinical trial of amonafide. Proc Am Soc Clin Oncol 1988;7:225a.

265. Leiby JM, Malspeis L, Staubus AE, Kraut EH, Grever MR. Amonifide (NSC 308847). A clinical phase I study of two schedules of administration. Proc AACR 1988;29:1103a.

266. Richardson RL, Schutt AJ, O'Connell MJ, Creagan ET. Phase I study of amonifide (A) (NSC-308847) given by 24 hour continuous intravenous infusion (24H-CIV) every 4 weeks. Proc Am Soc Clin Oncol 1987;6:135a.

267. O'Brian S, Keating M, Benvenuto JA, Kantarjian H, Estey E, McCredie K. Phase I clinical investigation of benzisoquinolinedione (Amonifide) in leukemia. Proc AACR 1989;30:1061a.

268. Allen SL, Budman DR, Fusco D, et al. Phase I trial of amonafide + cytosine arabinoside for poor risk acute leukemias. Proc AACR 1994;35:225a.

269. Allen SL, Budman DR, Fusco D, et al. Phase I trial of amonafide for refractory, relapsed or 2° acute leukemias and blast crisis of chronic myelogenous leukemia. Proc Am Soc Clin Oncol 1992;11:276a.

270. Allen SL, Ratain M, Korzun AH, et al. Phase II study of amonafide in previously treated metastatic breast cancer (CALGB 8841). Proc AACR 1991;32:183a.

271. Felder TB, Benvenuto JA, Andersson BS, Newman RA. Disposition of amonifide in adults with acute leukemia. Proc AACR 1988;29:742a.

272. Ratain MJ, Choi KE, Liebner MA, Grayhack J, Foody N, Schilsky RL. Phase II and pharmacodynamic study of amonafide (BIDA) in advanced pancreatic cancer. Sixth NCI-EORTC Symposium on New Drugs for Cancer Therapy 1989;4:326a.

273. Ratain MJ, Staubus AE, Schilsky RL, Malspeis L. Limited sampling models for amonafide pharmacokinetics. Proc AACR 1988;29:766a.

274. Ratain MJ, Rosner G, Allen SL. Population pharmacodynamic study of amonafide: a Cancer and Leukemia Group B study. J Clin Oncol 1995;13:741–747.

275. Ratain MJ, Mick R, Berezin F, et al. Phase I study of amonafide dosing based on acetylator phenotype. Cancer Res 1993;53:2304–2308.

276. Kornek G, Raderer M, Depisch D, et al. Amonafide as first-line chemotherapy for metastatic breast cancer. Eur J Cancer 1994;30A:398–400.

277. Higano CS, Craig J, Goodman P, et al. A phase II trial of amonafide in advanced renal cell cancer. Proc Am Soc Clin Oncol 1989;8:574a.

278. Marschke RFJ, Wieand HS, O'Connell MJ, et al. Advanced colorectal adenocarcinoma: treatment with amonafide (letter). J Natl Cancer Inst 1994;86:944–945.

279. Gesme DHJ, Jett JR, Schreffler DD, et al. A randomized phase II trial of amonafide or trimetrexate in patients with advanced non-small cell lung cancer. A trial of the North Central Cancer Treatment Group. Cancer 1993;71:2723–2726.

280. Sami SM, Dorr RT, Alberts DS, Remers WA. 2-substituted 1,2-dihydro-3H-dibenz[de,h]isoquinoline-1,3-diones. J Med Chem 1993;36:765–770.

281. Cain BF, Atwell GJ. The experimental antitumor properties of three congeners of the acridylmethanesulphonanilide (AMSA) series. Eur J Cancer 1974;10:539–549.

282. Waring MJ. DNA-binding characteristics of the acridinylmethane-sulphonanilide drugs: comparison with antitumor properties. Eur J Cancer 1976;12:995–1001.

283. Von Hoff DD, Howser D, Gormley P, et al. Phase I study of methanesulfonamide, N-(4-(9-acridinylamino)-3-methoxyphenyl)-(m-AMSA) using a single-dose schedule. Cancer Treat Rep 1978;62:1421–1426.

284. Jurlina JL, Varcoe AR, Paxton JW. Pharmacokinetics of amsacrine in patients receiving combination chemotherapy for treatment of acute myelogenous leukemia. Cancer Chemother Pharmacol 1985;14:21–25.

285. Estey EH, Keating MJ, McCredie KB, Freireich EJ. Continuous-infusion amsacrine in patients with refractory acute myelogenous leukemia. Cancer Treat Rep 1987;71:1113–1114.

286. Arlin ZA, Sklaroff RB, Gee TS, et al. Phase I and II trial of 4'-(9-acridinylamino)methanesulfon-m-anisidide in patients with acute leukemia. Cancer Res 1980;40:3304–3306.

287. Weiss RB, Charles LMJ, Macdonald JS. M-AMSA: an exciting new drug in the National Cancer Institute Drug Development Program. Cancer Clin Trials 1980;3:203–209.

288. Weiss RB, Grillo-Lopez AJ, Marsoni S, Posada JGJ, Hess F, Ross BJ. Amsacrine-associated cardiotoxicity: an analysis of 82 cases. J Clin Oncol 1986;4:918–928.

289. Puccio CA, Feldman EJ, Arlin ZA. Amsacrine

is safe in patients with ventricular ectopy. Am J Hematol 1988;28:197–198.

290. Feldman EJ, Arlin ZA, Sullivan P, Engelking C. Preventing amsacrine-induced cardiac arrhythmias (letter). J Clin Oncol 1987;5:2014.

291. Seymour JF. Induction of hypomagnesemia. Am J Hematol 1993;42:262–267.

292. Cassileth PA, Gale RP. Amsacrine: a review. Leuk Res 1986;10:1257–1265.

293. Arlin ZA, Feldman E, Kempin S, et al. Amsacrine with high-dose cytarabine is highly effective therapy for refractory and relapsed acute lymphoblastic leukemia in adults. Blood 1988;72:433–435.

294. Bauduer F, Delmer A, Blanc MC, et al. Treatment of chronic myelogenous leukemia in blast crisis and in accelerated phase with high- or intermediate-dose cytosine arabinoside and amsacrine. Leuk Lymphoma 1993;10:195–200.

295. Jehn U, Heinemann V. Phase II study for treatment of refractory acute leukemia with intermediate-dose cytosine arabinoside and amsacrine. Anticancer Res 1993;13:379–381.

296. Brode E, Poveda Velasco A, Diaz-Rubio E, Rossell Costa R, Benavides Fissure A. Pharmacokinetic characterization of mitonafide in man. Methods Findings Exp Clin Pharmacol 1992;14:131–140.

297. Poveda A, Herranz C, Martin M, Schlick E. Phase I study of mitonafide in solid tumors. Sixth NCI-EORTC Symposium on New Drugs for Cancer Therapy 1989;4:413a.

298. Llombart M, Poveda A, Forner E, et al. Phase I study of mitonafide in solid tumors. Invest New Drugs 1992;10:177–181.

299. Rosell R, Carles J, Abad A, et al. Phase I study of mitonafide in 120 hour continuous infusion in non-small cell lung cancer. Invest New Drugs 1992;10:171–175.

300. Dodion P, Egorin MJ, Riggs CEJ, Ferraro T, Tamburini JM, Bachur NR. Comparative purine metabolism and disposition of class II anthracycline antibiotics. Cancer Chemother Pharmacol 1985;15:153–160.

301. Steinheider G, Westendorf J, Marquadt H. Induction of chromosomal aberrations by the anthracycline antitumor antibiotics N,N-dimethyldaunomycin and aclacinomycin A. Experimentia 1987;43:586–588.

302. Umezawa K, Haresaku M, Muramatsu M, Matsushima T. Mutagenicity of anthracycline glycosides and bleomycins in salmonella assay system. Biomed Pharmacother 1987;41:214–218.

303. Kerr JG, Archer S, DeAngelis C, Farrell S, Hanna S, McKee J. Phase I and pharmacokinetic study of high volume intraperitoneal aclacinomycin-A (aclarubicin). Invest New Drugs 1987;5:171–176.

304. Forastiere AA, Budman DR, Richards FII, Aisner J, Weinberg V, Wood WC. Phase II trial of aclarubicin in advanced breast cancer: a Cancer and Leukemia Group B study. Cancer Treat Rep 1983;67:1137–1138.

305. Pazdur R, Samson MK, Baker LH. Aclacinomycin A. Phase II evaluation in advanced soft tissue sarcoma. Am J Clin Oncol 1987;10:237–239.

306. Pazdur R, Samson MK, Baker LH. Aclacinomycin A. Phase II evaluation in bronchogenic squamous-cell carcinoma. Am J Clin Oncol 1987;10:234–236.

307. Natale RB, Cody RL, Simon MS, Wheeler RH. An in vivo and in vitro trial of aclarubicin in metastatic breast cancer: a novel approach to the study of analogs. Cancer Chemother Pharmacol 1993;31:485–488.

308. Case DCJ, Ervin TJ, Boyd MA, Bove LG, Sonneborn HL, Paul SD. Phase II study of aclarubicin in acute myelogenous leukemia. Am J Clin Oncol 1987; 10:523–526.

309. Majima H, Ohta K. Clinical studies of aclacinomycin A (ACM). Biomed Pharmacother 1987; 41:233–237.

310. Machover D, Gastiaburu J, Delgado M, et al. Phase I-II study of aclarubicin for treatment of acute myeloid leukemia. Eur J Haematol 1987;47:33–42.

311. Rowe JM, Chang AY, Bennett JM. Aclacinomycin A and etoposide (VP 16-213): an effective regimen in previously treated patients with refractory acute myelogenous leukemia. Blood 1988;71:992–996.

312. Shibuya T, Morioka E, Taniguchi S, Ohhara N, Okamura S, Niho Y. Treatment of four patients with myelodysplastic syndrome with a small dose of aclacinomycin-A. Leuk Res 1987;11:851–854.

313. Sohda M, Fujiwara K, Saikusa H, et al. Sensitive enzyme immunoassay for the quantification of aclacinomycin-A using β-D-galactosidase as a label. Cancer Chemother Pharmacol 1985;14:53–58.

314. Ganzina F. 4'Epi-doxorubicin, a new analogue of doxorubicin: a preliminary overview of preclinical and clinical data. Cancer Treat Rev 1983;10:1–22.

315. Weiss RB, Sarosy G, Clagett-Carr K, Russo M, Leyland-Jones B. Review. Anthracycline analogs: the past, present, and future. Cancer Chemother Pharmacol 1986;18:185–197.

316. Young CW, Raymond V. Clinical assessment of the structure-activity relationship of anthracyclines and related synthetic derivatives. Cancer Treat Rep 1986;70:51–63.

317. Cersosimo RJ, Hong WK. Epirubicin: a review of the pharmacology, clinical activity, and adverse effects of an Adriamycin analogue. J Clin Oncol 1986; 4:425–439.

318. Camaggi CM, Comparsi R, Strocchi E, Testoni F, Angelelli B, Pannuti F. Epirubicin and doxorubicin comparative metabolism and pharmacokinetics. A cross-over study. Cancer Chemother Pharmacol 1988; 21:221–228.

319. Mross K, van der Vijgh WJF, Gall H, Boven E, Pinedo HM. Pharmacokinetics and metabolism of epidoxorubicin and doxorubicin in humans. J Clin Oncol 1988;6:517–526.

320. Weiss AJ, Oldham FB. Phase I evaluation of epirubicin (Pharmarubicin) given by continuous infusion. Proc Am Soc Clin Oncol 1987;6:557a.

321. de Vries EGE, Greidanus J, Mulder NH, et al. A phase I and pharmacokinetic study with 21-day continuous infusion of epirubicin. J Clin Oncol 1987; 5:1445–1451.

322. Snyder R, Bishop J, Brodie G, et al. Phase I study of epirubicin given on a weekly schedule. Cancer Treat Rep 1987;71:273–276.

323. Karp D, Colajori E, Karpovsky B, et al. A phase I trial of high dose epirubicin (EPI) in advanced cancer. Proc Am Soc Clin Oncol 1989;8:325a.

324. Martoni A, Melotti B, Guaraldi M, Piana E, Pacciarini MA, Pannuti F. A phase I study of high dose epirubicin. Sixth NCI-EORTC Symposium on New Drugs for Cancer Therapy 1989;4:174a.

325. Holdener EE, Jungi WJ, Fiebig HH, et al. Phase

I study of high-dose epirubicin in nonsmall cell lung cancer (NSCLC). Proc Am Soc Clin Oncol 1988;7:806a.

326. Blackstein M, Wilson K, Meharchand J, Shepherd F, Fontaine B, Lassus M. Phase I study of epirubicin in metastatic breast cancer. Proc Am Soc Clin Oncol 1988;7:87a.

327. Case CDJ, Gams R, Ervin TJ, Boyd MA, Oldham FB. Phase I-II trial of high-dose epirubicin in patients with lymphoma. Cancer Res 1987;47:6393–6396.

328. Walde D, Case A, Lassus M, Bettello P. High dose epirubicin in previously untreated patients (PT) with advanced metastatic cancer: a phase I study. Proc Am Soc Clin Oncol 1988;7:280a.

329. Wong LC, Choy DTK, Ngan HYS, Sham JST, Ma HK. 4-epidoxorubicin in recurrent cervical cancer. Cancer 1989;89:1279–1282.

330. Feld R, Wierzbicki R, Walde D, et al. High dose epirubicin (E) given as a daily × 3 schedule in patients (PTS) with untreated extensive non-small cell lung cancer (NSCLC). A phase I-II study. Proc AACR 1988;29:826a.

331. Podesta A, Della Torre P, Pinciroli G, Iatropoulos MJ, Brughera M, Mazue G. Evaluation of 4'-iodo-4'-deoxydoxorubicin-induced cardiotoxicity in two experimental rat models. Toxicol Pathol 1994; 22:68–71.

332. Robert J, Armand JP, Huet S, Klink-Alakl M, Recondo G, Hurteloup P. Pharmacokinetics and metabolism of 4'-iodo'4'-deoxy-doxorubicin. J Clin Oncol 1992;10:1183–1190.

333. Twelves CJ, Dobbs NA, Lawrence M, Summerhayes M, Rubens RD. Clinical pharmacology of iododoxorubicin in a phase II study of advanced breast cancer. Ann Oncol 1994;5(Suppl 5):146a.

334. Mross K, Mayer U, Zeller W, Becker K, Hossfeld DK. Pharmacodynamic and pharmacokinetic aspects of iodo-doxorubicin. Oncol Res 1992;4:227–231.

335. Mross K, Langenbuch T, Burk K, Kaplan E, Hossfeld DK. Phase I study of iodo-doxorubicin (4'-I-Dox) in solid tumors in man. Proc Am Soc Clin Oncol 1989;8:304a.

336. Twelves CJ, Dobbs NA, Lawrence MA, et al. Iododoxorubicin in advanced breast cancer: a phase II evaluation of clinical activity, pharmacology and quality of life. Br J Cancer 1994;69:726–731.

337. Villar-Grimalt A, Aranada E, Massutit B, et al. Phase II study with iododoxorubicin in measurable advanced colorectal adenocarcinoma. Effective rescue using weekly high-dose 5-fluorouracil (WFU). Spanish Cooperative Group for Gastrointestinal Tumor Therapy (TTD), Work Group of SEOM (Spanish Medical Oncology Society). Tumori 1994;80:124–127.

338. Sorensen JB, Stenbygaard L, Drivsholm L, Dombernowsky P, Hansen HH. Phase II study of 4'-iodo-4'-deoxydoxorubicin in non-resectable non-small-cell lung cancer. Cancer Chemother Pharmacol 1993;32:399–402.

339. Iguchi H, Tone H, Ishikura T, Takeuchi T, Umezawa H. Pharmacokinetics and disposition of 4'-O-tetrahydropyranyladriamycin in mice by HPLC analysis. Cancer Chemother Pharmacol 1985;15:132–140.

340. Fiallo M, Laigle A, Borrel MN, Garnier-Suillerot A. Accumulation of degradation products of doxorubicin and pirarubicin formed in cell culture medium within sensitive and resistant cells. Biochem Pharmacol 1993;45:659–665.

341. Dine T, Cazin JC, Gressier B, et al. Stability

and compatibility of four anthracyclines: doxorubicin, epirubicin, daunorubicin and pirarubicin with PVC infusion bags. Pharm Weekbl Sci 1992;14:365–369.

342. Yamada K, Shirakawa S, Ohno R, et al. A phase II study of (2''R)-4'-O-tetrahydropyranyladriamycin (THP) in hematological malignancies. Invest New Drugs 1987;5:299–305.

343. Ohno R, Kimura K, Amaki I, et al. Treatment of acute leukemia and malignant lymphoma with (2''R)-4'-O-tetrahydropyranyl-adriamycin. Cancer Chemother Pharmacol 1987;20:230–234.

344. Majima H. Cardiac toxicity in patients treated with (2''R)-4-tetra-hydropyranyladriamycin (THP-ADM), preliminary report. Proc Am Soc Clin Oncol 1987;6:74a.

345. Miller AA, Scheulen ME, Kleeberg UR, Seeber S, Schmidt CG. Phase I study of pirarubicin. J Cancer Res Clin Oncol 1988;114:91–94.

346. Sridhar KS, Samy TSA, Agarwal RP, et al. Phase I study of 4'-O-tetrahydropyranyladriamycin. Proc AACR 1988;29:736a.

347. Raber MN, Newman RA, Lu K, et al. Phase I clinical trial and pharmacokinetic evaluation of 4'-O-tetrahydropyranyladriamycin (THP-adriamycin). Cancer Chemother Pharmacol 1989;23:311–315.

348. Herait P, Poutignat N, Schneider M, Brienza S, Misset JL, Mathe G. Cardiac tolerance of 4'-O-tetrahydropyranyladriamycin (THP-ADM; 1609 RB). Updated results. Sixth NCI-EORTC Symposium on New Drugs for Cancer Therapy 1989;4:184a.

349. Dorval T, Extra JM, Spielmann M, et al. THP-adriamycin (T) (1609 RB) in advanced breast cancer (BC)—compiled data from three phase II studies. Proc Am Soc Clin Oncol 1989;8:208a.

350. Scheithauer W, Samonigg H, Depisch D, et al. Activity of 4'-O-tetrahydropyranyladriamycin (pirarubicin; THP) in metastatic breast cancer—a phase II study. Proc Am Soc Clin Oncol 1989;8:117a.

351. Chevallier B, Mignot L, Delozier T, Morvan F, Ferme C, Herait P. Phase II study of tetrahydropyranyl adriamycin (pirarubicin) in elderly patients with advanced breast cancer. Am J Clin Oncol 1992;15:395–398.

352. Herait P, Poutignat N, Marty M, Bugat R. Early assessment of a new anticancer drug analogue—are the historical comparisons obsolete? The French experience with pirarubicin. Eur J Cancer 1992;28A:1670–1676.

353. Chauvergne J, Fumoleau P, Cappelaere P, et al. Phase II study of pirarubicin (THP) in patients with cervical, endometrial and ovarian cancer: study of the Clinical Screening Group of the European Organization for Research and Treatment of Cancer (EORTC). Eur J Cancer 1993;29A:350–354.

354. Sridhar KS, Hussein AM, Benedetto P, Ardalan B, Savaraj N, Richman SP. Phase II trial of 4'-O-tetrahydropyranyladriamycin (pirarubicin) in head and neck carcinoam. Cancer 1992;70:1591–1597.

355. De Mulder PH, Cappelaere P, Cognetti F, et al. A phase II study of pirarubicin in patients with advanced recurrent head and neck squamous cell carcinoma. Cancer Chemother Pharmacol 1994;33:438–440.

356. Mahjoubi M, Kattan J, Ghosn M, Droz JP, Philippot I, Herait P. Phase II trial of pirarubicin in the treatment of advanced bladder cancer. Invest New Drugs 1992;10:317–321.

357. Roche H, Guiochet N, Kerbrat P, et al. Phase

II trials of tetrahydropyranyl-adriamycin (Pirarubicin) on renal and colon carcinoma, melanoma, and soft tissue sarcoma. Am J Clin Oncol 1993;16:137–139.

358. Kleisbauer JP, Taytard A, Balmes P, et al. A phase II trial of pirarubicin in untreated disseminated small cell lung cancer. A cooperative study of the French Pneumo-Cancerology Group. Rev Mal Respir 1992;9:179–184.

359. du Bois A, Meerpohl HG, Madjar H, et al. Phase II study of pirarubicin combined with cisplatin in recurrent ovarian cancer. J Cancer Res Clin Oncol 1994;120:173–178.

360. Munck JN, Riggi M, Rougier P, et al. Pharmacokinetic and pharmacodynamic advantages of pirarubicin over adriamycin after intraarterial hepatic administration in the rabbit VX2 tumor model. Cancer Res 1993;53:1550–1554.

361. Munck JN, Rougier P, Chabot GG, et al. Phase I and pharmacological study of intra-arterial hepatic administration of pirarubicin in patients with advanced hepatic metastases. Eur J Cancer 1994;30A:289–294.

362. Ogawa M, Inoue K, Horikoshi N, et al. Phase I trial of a new anthracycline compound, SM-5887. Proc Am Soc Clin Oncol 1988;7:206a.

363. Plowman J, Dykes DJ, Narayanan VL, et al. Efficacy of the quinocarmycins KW2152 and DX-521-1 against human melanoma lines growing in culture and in mice. Cancer Res 1995;55:862–867.

364. Boyd MR, Paull KD. Some practical considerations and applications of the National Cancer Institute in vitro anticancer drug discovery screen. Drug Devel Res 1995;34:91–109.

365. Streeter DG, Johl JS, Gordon GR, Peters JH. Uptake and retention of morpholinyl anthracyclines by adriamycin-sensitive and -resistant P 388 cells. Cancer Chemother Pharmacol 1986;16:247–252.

366. Scudder SA, Brown JM, Sikic BI. DNA crosslinking and cytotoxicity of the alkylating cyanomorpholino derivative of doxorubicin in multidrug resistant cells. J Natl Cancer Inst 1988;80:1294–1298.

367. Lau DH, Duran GE, Lewis AD, Sikic BI. Metabolic conversion of methoxymorpholino doxorubicin: from a DNA strand breaker to a DNA cross-linker. Br J Cancer 1994;70:79–84.

368. Lewis AD, Lau DH, Duran GE, Wolf CR, Sikic BI. Role of cytochrome P-450 from the human CYP3A gene family in the potentiation of morpholino doxorubicin by human liver microsomes. Cancer Res 1992; 52:4379–4384.

369. Danesi R, Agen C, Grandi M, Nardini V, Bevilacqua G, Del Tacca M. 3'-Deamino-3'-(2-methoxy-4-morpholinyl)-doxorubicin (FCE 23762): a new anthracycline derivative with enhanced cytotoxicity and reduced cardiotoxicity. Eur J Cancer 1993;29A:1560–1565.

370. Watanabe M, Komeshima N, Nakajima S, Tsuruo T. MX2, a morpholino anthracycline, as a new antitumor agent against drug-sensitive and multi-drug resistant human and murine tumor cells. Cancer Res 1988;48:6653–6657.

371. Ogawa M, Tabata M, Horikoshi N, et al. Phase I trial of 3'-deamino-3'-morpholino-13-deoxy-10-hydroxycarminomycin hydrochloride (KRN-8602). Proc Am Soc Clin Oncol 1989;8:238a.

372. Majima H. Phase I clinical and pharmacokinetic study of KRN 8602. Proc Am Soc Clin Oncol 1989; 8:245a.

373. Watanabe T, Narabayashi M, Haga S, et al. MX2; 3'-deamino-3'-morpholino-13-deoxy-10-hydroxycarminomycin (KRN8602) in refractory metastatic breast cancer; results of a preliminary phase II trial. Jpn J Clin Oncol 1993;23:246–249.

374. Yamamoto H, Arita N, Ohnishi T, et al. Pharmacokinetics of MX2, a new morpholino anthracycline, in CSF following intravenous injection. Gan To Kagaku Ryoho 1993;20:1227–1230.

375. Kiya K, Ogasawara H, Fujita H, et al. Pharmacokinetics and antitumor activity of MX2, a new morpholino anthracycline in brain tumor intracerbral transplanted in rats. Gan To Kagaku Ryoho 1993; 20:631–635.

376. Kuhl JS, Duran GE, Chao NJ, Sikic BI. Effects of the methoxymorpholino derivative of doxorubicin and its bioactivated form versus doxorubicin on human leukemia and lymphoma cell lines and normal bone marrow. Cancer Chemother Pharmacol 1993; 33:10–16.

377. Vasey PA, Bissett D, Cassidy J, Kaye SB. Methoxymorpholinyl-doxorubicin (FCE 23762)—clinical phase I study in adults with refractory solid tumours. Ann Oncol 1994;5(Suppl 5):139a.

378. Georni MC, Ripamonti M, Marsiglio A. Pretreatment with dexamethasone does not interfere with the antitumor activity of FCE 23762 on mice bearing P388/DX leukemia. Proc AACR 1995;36:2133.

379. Judson IR. The anthrapyrazoles: a new class of compounds with clinical activity in breast cancer. Semin Oncol 1992;19:687–694.

380. Leteurtre F, Kohlhagen G, Paull K, Pommier Y. Topoisomerase II inhibition and cytotoxicity of the anthrapyrazoles DuP 937 and DuP 941 (losoxantrone) in the National Cancer Institute Preclinical Antitumor Drug Discovery Screen. J Natl Cancer Inst 1994; 86:1239–1244.

381. Dexter DL, Diamond M, Creveling J, Chen SF. Chemotherapy of mammary carcinomas arising in ras transgenic mice. Invest New Drugs 1993;11:161–168.

382. Myers CE. Anthracyclines. Cancer Chemother Biol Response Modif 1992;13:45–52.

383. Foster BJ, Newell DR, Graham MA, et al. Phase I trial of the anthrapyrazole CI-941: prospective evaluation of a pharmacokinetically guided dose-escalation. Eur J Cancer 1992;28:463–469.

384. Barbu M, Azarnia N, Calvert H. The safety profile of losoxantrone (DUP 941), a new anthrapyrazole administered on a q3w schedule in patients with advanced breast cancer. Ann Oncol 1994;5(Suppl 5):144a.

385. Belanger K, Jolivet J, Maroun J, et al. Phase I pharmacokinetic study of DUP-937, a new anthrapyrazole. Invest New Drugs 1993;11:301–308.

386. Fry DW, Boritzki TJ, Besserer JA, Jackson RC. In vitro DNA strand scission and inhibition of nucleic acid synthesis in L 1210 leukemia cells by a new class of DNA complexes, the anthra-(1,9-cd) pyrazol-6(2H)-ones (anthrapyrazones). Biochem Pharmacol 1985; 34:3499–3508.

387. Frank SK, Mathiesen DA, Szurszewski M, Kuffel MJ, Ames MM. Preclinical pharmacology of the anthrapyrazole analog oxantrazole (NSC-349174, Piroxantrone). Cancer Chemother Pharmacol 1989; 23:213–218.

388. Winterhalter BR, Fiebig HH, Berger DP, Widmer KH, Lohr GW. High antitumor activity of oxanthrazole: a new anthrapyrazole in a combined in vitro

and in vivo test procedure with human tumor xenografts. Sixth NCI-EORTC Symposium on New Drugs for Cancer Therapy 1989;4:181a.

389. Berg SL, Savarese DM, Balis FM, et al. Pharamcokinetics of piroxantrone in a phase I trial of piroxantrone and granulocyte-colony stimulating factor. Cancer Res 1993;53:2587–2590.

390. Hantel A, Noe DA, Grochow LB, et al. A phase I and pharmacokinetic study of oxantrazole (OAZ). Proc Am Soc Clin Oncol 1988;7:253a.

391. Ames MM, Loprinzi CL. Preliminary pharmacologic and toxicologic data from a phase I clinical trial of oxantrazole incorporating a pharmacologically guided dose-escalation scheme. Proc AACR 1988; 29:778a.

392. Savarese DM, Denicoff AM, Berg SL, et al. Phase I study of high-dose piroxantrone with granulocyte colony-stimulating factor. J Clin Oncol 1993; 11:1795–1803.

393. Zalupski MM, Benedetti J, Balcerzak SP, et al. Phase II trial of piroxantrone for advanced or metastatic soft tissue sarcoma. A Southwest Oncology Group study. Invest New Drugs 1993;11:337–341.

394. van der Wilt CL, Peters GJ. New targets for pyrimidine antimetabolites in the treatment of solid tumors. 1: Thymidylate synthase. Pharm World Sci 1994; 16:84–103.

395. Erlichman C, Mitrovski B. Comparative cytotoxicity of folate-based inhibitors of thymidylate synthase and 5-fluorouracil ± leucovorin in MGH-U1 cells. Cancer Chemother Pharmacol 1994;34:51–56.

396. Taylor EC. Design and synthesis of inhibitors of folate-dependent enzymes as antitumor agents. Adv Exp Med Biol 1993;338:387–408.

397. O'Dwyer PJ, Alonso MT, Leyland-Jones B. Acivicin: a new glutamine antagonist in clinical trials (review article). J Clin Oncol 1984;2:1064–1071.

398. Earhart RH, Koeller JM, Davis TE, et al. Phase I trial and pharmacokinetics of Acivicin administered by 72-hour infusion. Cancer Treat Rep 1983;67:683–692.

399. Willson JK, Fischer PH, Tutsch K, et al. Phase I clinical trial of a combination of dipyridamole and Acivicin based upon inhibition of nucleoside salvage. Cancer Res 1988;48:5585–5590.

400. Fischer PH, Willson JK, Risueno C, et al. Biochemical assessment of the effects of Acivicin and dipyridamole given as a continuous 72-hour intravenous infusion. Cancer Res 1988;48:5591–5596.

401. Ardalan B, Chandrasekaran B, Hrishikeshavan HJ. Biochemical mechanisms for the scheduled synergism of (aS,5S)-2-amino-3-chloro-4,5-dihydro-5-isoxazolacetic acid and 5-fluorouracil in P388 leukemia. Cancer Chemother Pharmacol 1985;15:44–48.

402. Bonomi P, Finkelstein D, Chang A. Phase II trial of acivicin versus etoposide-cisplatin in non-small cell lung cancer. An Eastern Cooperative Oncology Group study. Am J Clin Oncol 1994;17:215–217.

403. Clendeninn NJ, Peterkin JJ, Webber S, et al. AG-331, a "non-classical" lipophilic thymidylate synthase inhibitor for the treatment of solid tumors. Ann Oncol 1994;5(Suppl 5):133a.

404. O'Connor BM, Webber S, Jackson RC, Galivan J, Rhee MS. Biological activity of a novel rationally designed lipophilic thymidylate synthase inhibitor. Cancer Chemother Pharmacol 1994;34:225–229.

405. Calvete JA, Balmanno K, Taylor GA, et al. Pre-

clinical and clinical studies of prolonged administration of the novel thymidylate synthase inhibitor, AG337. Ann Oncol 1994;5(Suppl 5):134a.

406. Rafi I, Taylor GA, Balmanno K, et al. A phase I study of the novel antifolate 3,4-dihydro-2-amino-6-methyl-4-oxo-5-(4-pyridythio)- quinazolone dihydrochloride (AG337) given by a 24 hr. intravenous continuous infusion. Ann Oncol 1994;5(Suppl 5):131a.

407. Khor SP, Lucas S, Schilsky R, et al. A phase I/ pharmacokinetic study of 5-ethynyluracil plus 5-fluorouracil in cancer patients with solid tumors. Proc AACR 1995;36:241.

408. Rafi I, Taylor GA, Calvete JA, et al. A phase I clinical study of the novel antifolate AG337 given by a 5 day continuous infusion. Proc AACR 1995;36:240a.

409. Quddus J, Johnson KJ, Gavalchin J, et al. Treated activated CD4+ T cells with either of two distinct DNA methyltransferase inhibitors, 5-azacytidine or procainamide, is sufficient to cause a lupus-like disease in syngeneic mice. J Clin Invest 1993;92:38–53.

410. Glover AB, Leyland-Jones B, Chun HG, Davies B, Hoth DF. Azacytidine: 10 years later. Cancer Treat Rep 1987;71:737–746.

411. Goldberg J, Gryn J, Raza A, et al. Mitoxantrone and 5-azacytidine for refractory/relapsed ANLL or CML in blast crisis: a leukemia intergroup study. Am J Hematol 1993;43:286–290.

412. Dutcher JP, Eudey L, Wiernik PH, et al. Phase II study of mitoxantrone and 5-azacytidine for accelerated and blast crisis of chronic myelogenous leukemia: a study of the Eastern Cooperative Oncology Group. Leukemia 1992;6:770–775.

413. Silverman LR, Holland JF, Weinberg RS, et al. Effects of treatment with 5-azacytidine on the in vivo and in vitro hematopoiesis in patients with myelodysplastic syndromes. Leukemia 1993;7(Suppl 1):21–29.

414. Limonta M, Colombo T, Damia G, et al. Cytotoxic activity and mechanism of action of 5-aza-2'-deoxycytidine in human CML cells. Leuk Res 1993; 17:977–982.

415. Colombatti A, Attadia V, Zagonel V, Pinto A. 5-Aza-2'-deoxycytidine: from preclinical to clinical applications in leukemia. Sixth NCI-EORTC Symposium on New Drugs for Cancer Therapy 1989;4:460a.

416. de Vos D, Vrijhof WP. Dezocitidine (DAC): current status and future prospects. Sixth NCI-EORTC Symposium on New Drugs for Cancer Therapy 1989; 4:350a.

417. Attadia V. Effects of 5-aza-2'-deoxycytidine on differentiation and oncogene expression in the human monoblastic leukemia cell line U-937. Leukemia 1993;7(Suppl 1):9–16.

418. Levya A, Schwartsmann G, Boeije LCM, Pinedo HM, de Waal F. Growth inhibitor effects of 5-aza-2'-deoxycytidine in HL-60 promyelocytic leukemia cells resistant to differentiation induction. Biochem Biophys Res Commun 1986;141:629–635.

419. Momparler RL, Dore BT, Labiberte J, Momparler LF. Interaction of 5-aza-2'-deoxycytidine with amsacrine or 1,25-dihydroxyvitamin D3 on HL-60 myeloid leukemia cells and inhibitors of cytidine deaminase. Leukemia 1993;7(Suppl 1):17–20.

420. Lenzi R, Frost P, Abbruzzese JL. Modulation of cisplatin resistance by 2'-deoxy-5-azacytidine in human ovarian tumor cell lines. Anticancer Res 1994; 14:247–351.

421. Caraglia M, Pinto A, Correale P, et al. 5-aza-

2'-deoxycytidine induces growth inhibition and upregulation of epidermal growth factor receptor on human epithelial cancer cells. Ann Oncol 1994;5:269–276.

422. Laliberte J, Marquez VE, Momparler RL. Potent inhibitors for the deamination of cytosine arabinoside and 5-aza-2'-deoxycytidine by human cytidine deaminase. Cancer Chemother Pharmacol 1992;30:7–11.

423. Stegmann AP, Honders MW, Kester MG, Landegent JE, Willemze R. Role of deoxycytidine kinase in an in vitro model for ara C- and DAC-resistance: substrate-enzyme interactions with deoxycytidine, 1-β-D-arabinosylcytosine and 5-aza-2'-deoxycytidine. Leukemia 1993;7:1005–1011.

424. Momparler RL, Rivard GE, Gyger M. Clinical trial on 5-aza-2'-deoxycytidine in patients with acute leukemia. Pharmacol Ther 1985;30:277–286.

425. Braakhus BJM, van Dongen GAMS, van Walsum M, Leyva A, Snow GB. Preclincial antitumor activity of 5-aza-2'-deoxycytidine against human head and neck xenografts. Invest New Drugs 1988;6:299–304.

426. Abele R, Gundersen S, Smyth J, Bruntsch U, Pinedo HM. Phase II studies with 5-aza-2'deoxycytidine (DAC) in colorectal, head and neck (H + N), melanoma and renal carcinoma. Fourth European Conference on Clinical Oncology and Cancer Nursing 1987; 4:90a.

427. Driscoll JS, Johns DG, Plowman J. Comparison of activity of arabinosyl-5-azacytosine, arabinosyl cytosine, and 5-azacytidine against intracerebrally implanted L 1210 leukemia. Invest New Drugs 1985; 3:331–334.

428. Petti MC, Mandelli F, Zagonel V, et al. Pilot study of 5-aza-2'-deoxycytidine (Decitabine) in the treatment of poor prognosis acute myelogenous leukemia patients: preliminary results. Leukemia 1993; 7(Suppl 1):36–41.

429. Willemze R, Archimbaud E, Muus P. Preliminary results with 5'-aza-2'-deoxycytidine (DAC)-containing chemotherapy in patients with relapsed or refractory acute leukemia. The EORTC Leukemia Cooperative Group. Leukemia 1993;7(Suppl 1):49–50.

430. Rivard GE, Momparler RL, Demers J, et al. Phase I study of 5-aza-2'-deoxycytidine in children with acute leukemia. Leuk Res 1981;5:453–462.

431. Zagonel V, Lo Re G, Marotta G, et al. 5-aza-2'-deoxycytidine (Decitabine) induces trilineage response in unfavourable myelodysplastic syndromes. Leukemia 1993;7(Suppl 1):30–35.

432. Naguib FNM, Hao S-N, el Kouni MH. Potentiation of 5-fluorouracil efficacy by the dihydrouracil dehydrogenase inhibitor, 5-benzyloxybenzyluracil. Cancer Res 1994;54:5166–5170.

433. Peters GJ, Sharma SL, Laurensse E, Pinedo HM. Inhibition of pyrimidine de novo synthesis by DUP-785 (NSC 368390). Invest New Drugs 1987;5:235–244.

434. Chen SF, Perrella FW, Behrens DL, Papp LM. Inhibition of dihydroorate dehydrogenase activity by brequinar sodium. Cancer Res 1992;52:3521–3527.

435. Schwartzmann G, Peters GJ, Laurensse E, et al. DUP 785 (NSC 368390): schedule-dependency of growth-inhibitory and antipyrimidine effects. Biochem Pharmacol 1988;37:3257–3266.

436. Peters GJ, Boven E, Braahuis BJM, de Kant E, Kraal I, Pinedo HM. Is in vitro sensitivity to Brequin sodium DUP-785 (NSC 368390) related to the activity and inhibition of dihydroorate dehydrogenase? Sixth NCI-EORTC Symposium on New Drugs for Cancer Therapy 1989;4:139a.

437. Peters GJ, Laurensse E, Sharma SL, Leyva A, Pinedo HM. In vitro and in vivo antipyrimidine activity of DUP-785 (NSC 368390). Proc AACR 1987; 28:1310a.

438. Peters GJ, Nadal JC, Schwartsmann G, Laurensse E, Pinedo HM. Effects of pyrimidine metabolism in patients treated with DUP-785 in a phase I trial. Fourth European Conference on Clinical Oncology and Cancer Nursing 1987;4:80a.

439. Chen TL, Erlichman C. Biochemical modulation of 5-fluorouracil with or without leucovorin by a low dose of brequinar in MGH-U1 cells. Cancer Chemother Pharmacol 1992;30:370–376.

440. Dexter dL, Dusak BA, Forbes M. Combination studies with Brequinar sodium (DUP 785) and selected anticancer drugs against experimental tumors. Proc AACR 1988;29:1326a.

441. Peters GJ, Kraal I, Nadal JC, Pinedo HM. In vitro and in vivo studies on several combinations with Brequinar sodium (DUP-785; NSC 368390). Sixth NCI-EORTC Symposium on New Drugs for Cancer Therapy 1989;4:117a.

442. Shen HS, Chen SF, Behrens DL, Whitney CC, Dexter DL, Frobes M. Distribution of the novel anticancer drug candidate Brequinar sodium (DUP-785; NSC 368390) into normal and tumor tissues of nude mice bearing human colon carcinoma xenografts. Cancer Chemother Pharmacol 1988;22:183–186.

443. Boven E, Winograd B, Berger DP, et al. Phase II preclinical drug screening in human tumor xenografts: a first European multicenter collaborative study. Cancer Res 1992;52:5940–5947.

444. Bork E, Hansen HH. Phase I clinical and pharmacokinetic studies of DUP-785 (NSC 368390) using a weekly and biweekly schedule. Proc AACR 1988; 29:910a.

445. Currie VE, O'Hehir MA, Baltzer L, Slavik WM, Bertino JR. Phase I trial of DUP 785 given on a single weekly intravenous dosing schedule. Proc Am Soc Clin Oncol 1988;7:293a.

446. Schwartsmann G, ten Bokkel Huinink WW, Dodion P. Phase I study of DUP-785 (NSC 368390) in solid tumors. Proc Am Soc Clin Oncol 1987;6:158a.

447. Joggi J, Schwartsmann G, ten Bokkel Huinink WW, et al. Phase I study of DUP-785 (NSC 368390) in solid tumors. Proc AACR 1988;29:909a.

448. Artega C, Brown T, Kuhn J, et al. Phase I clinical trial of DUP-785 (Brequinar sodium, C 368390). Proc Am Soc Clin Oncol 1988;7:228a.

449. De Forni M, Armand JP, Fontana X, et al. Phase I DUP-785 (NSC 368390) as short iv 5 days schedule in advanced malignancies. Proc AACR 1989; 30:964a.

450. Donehower R, Vito B, Noe D, et al. Phase I and pharmacokinetic study of Brequinar (Breq; DUP 785). Proc Am Soc Clin Oncol 1988;7:249a.

451. de Forni M, Chabot GG, Armand JP, et al. Phase I and pharmacokinetic study of brequinar (DUP 785; NSC 368390) in cancer patients. Eur J Cancer 1993; 29A:983–988.

452. King S-YP, Agra AM, Shen H-SL, et al. Protein binding of brequinar in the plasma of healthy donors and cancer patients and analysis of the relationship be-

tween protein binding and pharmacokinetics in cancer patients. Cancer Chemother Pharmacol 1994;35:101–108.

453. Schwartsmann G, Bork E, Vermorken JB, et al. Mucocutaneous side effects of Brequinar sodium. Cancer 1989;63:243–248.

454. Cody R, Stewart D, De Forni M, et al. Multicenter phase II study of brequinar sodium in patients with advanced breast cancer. Am J Clin Oncol 1993;16:526–538.

455. Moore M, Maroun J, Robert F, et al. Multicenter phase II study of brequinar sodium in patients with advanced gastrointestinal cancer. Invest New Drugs 1993;11:61–65.

456. Natale R, Wheeler R, Moore M, et al. Multicenter phase II study of brequinar sodium in patients with advanced melanoma. Ann Oncol 1992;3:659–660.

457. Urba S, Doroshow J, Cripps C, et al. Multicenter phase II trial of brequinar sodium in patients with advanced squamous carcinoma of the head and neck. Cancer Chemother Pharmacol 1992;31:167–169.

458. Maroun J, Ruckdeschel J, Natale R, et al. Multicenter phase II study of brequinar sodium in patients with advanced lung cancer. Cancer Chemother Pharmacol 1993;32:64–66.

459. Kahan BD, Chou T, Tejpal N, Wang M, Chee C, Stepkowski S. Synergistic effects of cyclosporin analogs-A, D, G, IMM-125—with rapamycin and/or brequinar. Transplant Proc 1994;26:3021–3024.

460. Makowska L, Sher LS, Cramer DV. The development of Brequinar as an immunosuppressive drug for transplantation. Immunol Rev 1993;136:51–70.

461. Fujita F, Fujita M, Fujita M, et al. Antitumor activity of DMDC, 1-[2-deoxy-2-methylene-β-D-erythropentofuranosyl] cytosine dihydrate, on human tumor xenografts I. Proc AACR 1993;34:2468a.

462. Fujita F, Fujita M, Sakamoto Y, Taguchi T. Antitumor effect of DMDC, 1-[2-deoxy-2-methylene-β-D-erythropentofuranosyl] cytosine dihydrate, on human tumor xenografts II. Proc AACR 1993;34:2469a.

463. Tsukagoshi S. Development of antimetabolites, II. Gan To Kagaku Ryoho 1993;20:19–26.

464. Peters GJ, Braakhuis BJM, de Bruijn EA, Laurensse EJ, van Walsum M, Pinedo HM. Enhanced therapeutic efficacy of 5'deoxy-5-fluorouridine in 5-fluorouracil resistant head and neck tumors in relation to 5-fluorouracil metabolising enzymes. Br J Cancer 1989;59:327–334.

465. De Cesare M, Pratesi G, De Braud F, Zunino F, Stampino CG. Remarkable antitumor activity of 5'-deoxy-5-fluorouridine in human colorectal tumor xenografts. Anticancer Res 1994;14:549–554.

466. Fossa SD, Dahl O, Hoel R, Heier M, Loeb M. Doxifluridine (5'-FUrd) in patients with advanced colorectal carcinoma. Cancer Chemother Pharmacol 1985;15:161–163.

467. Alberto P, Mermillod B, Germano G, et al. A randomized comparison of doxifluridine and fluorouracil in colorectal carcinoma. Eur J Cancer Clin Oncol 1988;24:559–563.

468. Collins C, Weiden PL. Cardiotoxicity of 5-fluorouracil. Cancer Treat Rep 1987;71:733–736.

469. Van Oosterom AT, de Pooter CHM, Tjaden UR, de Bruijn EA. Doxifluorouridine capsules for continuous site specific delivery of fluorouracil. Proc AACR 1989;30:1135a.

470. Malet-Martino MC, Martino R, Lopez A, et al. New approach to metabolism of 5'-deoxy-5-fluorouridine in humans with fluorine-19 NMR. Cancer Chemother Pharmacol 1984;13:31–35.

471. Martino R, Bernadou J, Malet-Martino MC, Roche H, Armand JP. Excretion of doxifluridine catabolites in human bile assessed by 19F NMR spectrometry. Biomed Pharmacother 1987;41:104–106.

472. Scaaf LJ, Dobbs BR, Edwards IR, Perrier DG. The pharmacokinetics of doxifluridine and 5-fluorouracil after single intravenous infusions of doxifluridine to patients with colorectal cancer. Eur J Clin Pharmacol 1988;34:439–443.

473. Schuster D, Heim ME, Linder-Ciccolunghi S, Queisser W. Phase II clinical study of doxifluridine (5'DFUR). 24 hr intravenous infusion in advanced colorectal cancer. Proc AACR 1987;28:801a.

474. Bajetta E, Colleoni M, Rosso R, et al. Prospective randomised trial comparing fluorouracil versus doxifluridine for the treatment of advanced colorectal cancer. Eur J Cancer 1993;29A:1658–1663.

475. Oliver IN, Reece PA, Morris PG, et al. Phase I pharmacokinetic study of doxifluridine given by five day stepped dose infusion. Sixth NCI-EORTC Symposium on New Drugs for Cancer Therapy 1989;4:122a.

476. Antimi M, Majoli L, Minelli M, Stampino CG, Pandolfi A, Papa G. A phase I safety study of doxifluridine and interferon-alpha-2a in patients with advanced neoplastic disease. Tumori 1993;79:336–339.

477. Colleoni M, Bajetta E, de Braud F, Zilembo N, Nole F, Nelli P. Reversal of resistance to doxifluridine and fluororuracil in metastatic colorectal cancer: the role of high-dose folinic acid. Tumori 1992;78:258–261.

478. Alberto P, Righetti A, Decoster G, Abele R, Holdener EE. Phase I trial of doxifluridine (DFUR). Proc Am Soc Clin Oncol 1988;7:241a.

479. de Pooter CHM, Van Oosterom AT, Tjaden UR, de Bruijn EA. Influence of renal function in oral dFUrd treatment. Sixth NCI-EORTC Symposium on New Drugs for Cancer Therapy 1989;4:130a.

480. Spagnesi S, Ducci F, Laddaga M, et al. A phase I-II study of oral doxifluridine plus radiotherapy in radiosensitive tumors of the pelvic region. Tumori 1993;79:250–253.

481. Koizumi W, Kurihara M, Sasai T, et al. A phase II study of combination therapy with 5'-deoxy-5-fluorouridine and cisplatin in the treatment of advanced gastric cancer with primary foci. Cancer 1993;72:658–662.

482. Alberto P. Phase II study of an oral combination of doxifluridine, prednimustine and idarubicin (FUPRIDA) for first line treatment of advanced breast cancer. Ann Oncol 1993;4:423–425.

483. Sirotnak FM, Schmid FA, Samuels LL, DeGraw JI. 10-Ethyl-10-deaza-aminopterin: structural design and biochemical, pharmacologic, and antitumor properties. Monogr Natl Cancer Inst 1987;5:127–131.

484. Fry DW, Jackson RC. Biological and biochemical properties of new anticancer folate antagonists. Cancer Metastasis Rev 1987;5:251–270.

485. Sirotnak FM, Degraw JI, Schmid FA, Goutas LJ, Moccio DM. New folate analogs of the 10-deaza-aminopterin series. Cancer Chemother Pharmacol 1984;12:26–30.

486. Grant SC, Kris MG, Young CW, Sirontak FM. Edatrexate, an antifolate with antitumor activity: a review. Cancer Invest 1993;11:36–45.

487. Braakhuis BJ, Jansen G, Noordhuis P, Kegel A, Peters GJ. Importance of pharmacodynamics in the in vitro antiproliferative activity of the antifolates methotrexate and 10-ethyl-10-deazaaminopterin against human head and neck squamous cell carcinoma. Biochem Pharmacol 1993;46:2155–2161.

488. van der Laan BF, Jansen G, Kathmann GA, Westerhof GR, Schornagel JH, Hordijk GJ. In vitro activity of novel antifolates against human squamous carcinoma cell lines of the head and neck with inherent resistance to methotrexate. Int J Cancer 1992;51:909–914.

489. Matherly LH, Angeles SM, McGuire JJ. Determinants of the disparate antitumor activities of (6R)-5,10-dideaza-5,6,7,8-tetrahydrofolate and methotrexate toward human lymphoblastic leukemia cells, characterized by severely impaired antifolate membrane transport. Biochem Pharmacol 1993;46:2185–2195.

490. Kris MG, Kinahan JJ, Gralla RJ, et al. Phase I trial and clinical pharmacological evaluation of 10-ethyl-10-deazaaminopterin in adult patients with advanced cancer. Cancer Res 1988;48:5573–5579.

491. Tan C, Meyers P, Steinherz P, Wollner N, Mondora A, Young CW. Phase I clinical and pharmacologic study of 10-ethyl-10-daza-aminopterin (10-EDAM) in children with advanced cancer. Proc AACR 1988;29:914a.

492. Fennelly D, Gilewski T, Hudis C, et al. Phase I trial of sequential edatrexate (etx) followed by paclitaxel (ptx); a design based upon in vitro synergy in patients with advanced breast cancer. Proc AACR 1995;36:247.

493. Shum KY, Kris MG, Gralla RJ, Burke MT, Marks LD, Heelan RT. Phase II study of 10-ethyl-10-deaza-aminopterin in patients with stage III and IV non-small cell lung cancer. J Clin Oncol 1988;6:446–450.

494. Souhami R, Rudd RM, Spiro SG, Allen R, Lamond P, Harper PG. Phase II study of Edatrexate in stage III and IV non-small-cell lung cancer. Cancer Chemother Pharmacol 1992;30:465–468.

495. Schornegel J, Cappelaere P, Vemorken J, Snow G. A randomized phase II study of 10-ethyl-deaza-aminopterin (10-EDAM) and methotrexate in advanced head and neck squamous cell carcinoma (AHNC). An EORTC study. Proc Am Soc Clin Oncol 1989;8:679a.

496. Verma S, Quirt IC, Eisenhauer EA, et al. A phase II study of weekly edatrexate (10-EDAM) in metastatic melanoma. A National Cancer Institute of Canada Clinical Trials Group study. Ann Oncol 1993;4:254–255.

497. Moore DFJ, Pazdur R, Abbruzzese JL, et al. Phase II trial of edatrexate in patients with advanced pancreatic adenocarcinoma. Ann Oncol 1994;5:286–287.

498. Lambe CU, Donell BB, Shockcor J, Nelson DJ. 5-Fluorouracil catabolism in rats is decreased by 5-ethynyluracil (776C85), an inactivator of uracil reductase. Proc AACR 1995;36:2165a.

499. Grem JL, Shoemaker DD, Hoth DF, et al. Arabinosyl-5-azacytosine: a novel nucleoside entering clinical trials. Invest New Drugs 1987;5:315–328.

500. Heideman RL, Balis FM, McCully C, Poplack DG. Preclinical pharmacology of arabinosyl-5-azacytosine in nonhuman primates. Cancer Res 1988;48:4294–4298.

501. Townsend A, Leclerc JM, Dutschman G, Cooney D, Cheng YC. Metabolism of 1-β-D-arabinosyl-5-azacytosine and incorporation into DNA of human T-lymphoblastic cells (Molt-4). Cancer Res 1985;45:3522–3528.

502. Glazer RJ, Knode MC. 1-β-D-Arabinosyl-5-azacytosine: cytocidal activity and effects on the synthesis and methylation of DNA in human colon carcinoma cells. Mol Pharmacol 1984;26:381–387.

503. Heideman RL, McCully C, Balis FM, Poplack DG. Cerebrospinal fluid pharmacokinetics and toxicology of intraventricular and intrathecal arabinosyl-5-azacytosine (fazarabine, NSC 281272) in the nonhuman primate. Invest New Drugs 1993;11:135–140.

504. Amato R, Ho D, Schmidt S, Krakoff IH, Raber M. Phase I trial of a 72-h continuous-infusion schedule of fazarabine. Cancer Chemother Pharmacol 1992;30:321–324.

505. Bernstein ML, Whitehead VM, Grier H, et al. A phase I trial of fazarabine in refractory pediatric solid tumors. A Pediatric Oncology Group study. Invest New Drugs 1993;11:309–312.

506. Yang GS, McCulloch EA. A comparison of the lethal effects in culture of cytosine arabinoside and arabinofuranosyl-5-azacytosine acting on the blast cells to acute myeloblastic leukemia. Hematol Pathol 1992;6:125–130.

507. Abbruzzese JL, Frost P. Studies on the mechanism of the synergistic interaction between 2'-deoxy-5-azacytidine and cisplatin. Cancer Chemother Pharmacol 1992;30:31–36.

508. Clavel MD, Guastalla JP, Peters GG, Leyva A. Phase I study of LY 188011, 2'-2'-difluorodeoxycytidine. Sixth NCI-EORTC Symposium on New Drugs for Cancer Therapy 1989;4:124a.

509. Ruiz van Haperen VW, Veerman G, Vermorken JB, Peters GJ. 2',2'-difluoro-deoxycytidine (gemcitabine) incorporation into RNA and DNA of tumour cell lines. Biochem Pharmacol 1993;46:762–766.

510. Ross DD, Cuddy DP. Molecular effects of 2',2'-difluorodeoxycytidine (Gemcitabine) on DNA replication in intact HL-60 cells. Biochem Pharmacol 1994;48:1619–1630.

511. Weeks A, Abbruzzese J, Gravel D, et al. Phase I clinical and pharmacology study of difluorodeoxycytidine. Proc AACR 1989;30:1085a.

512. Schultz RM, Merriman RL, Toth JE, et al. Evaluation of new anticancer agents against the MIA PaCa-2 and PANC-1 human pancreatic carcinoma xenografts. Oncol Res 1993;5:223–228.

513. Fujita M, Fujita F, Inaba H, Taguchi T. Antitumor activity of LY 188011, a new deoxycytidine analog, against human cancers xenografted into nude mice. Gan To Kagaku Ryoho 1994;21:517–523.

514. Boven E, Schipper H, Erkelens CA, Hatty SA, Pinedo HM. The influence of the schedule and the dose of gemcitabine on the anti-tumour efficacy in experimental human cancer. Br J Cancer 1993;68:52–56.

515. Shipley LA, Brown TJ, Cornpropst JD, Hamilton M, Daniels WD, Culp HW. Metabolism and disposition of gemcitabine, and oncolytic deoxycytidine

analog, in mice, rats, and dogs. Drug Metab Dispos Biol Fate Chem 1992;20:849–855.

516. Lund B, Kristjansen PE, Hansen HH. Clinical and preclinical activity of 2′,2′-difluorodeoxycytidine. Cancer Treat Rev 1993;19:45–55.

517. Poplin EA, Corbett T, Flaherty L, et al. Difluorodeoxycytidine (dFdC)-gemcitabine: a phase I study. Invest New Drugs 1992;10:165–170.

518. O'Rourke TJ, Brown TD, Havlin K, et al. Phase I clinical trial of gemcitabine given as an intravenous bolus on 5 consecutive days (letter). Eur J Cancer 1994; 30A:417–418.

519. O'Rourke T, Brown T, Havlin K, et al. Phase I trial and immunologic assessment of difluorodeoxycytidine. Proc Am Soc Clin Oncol 1989;8:320a.

520. Cormier Y, Eisenhauer E, Muldal A, et al. Gemcitabine is an active new agent in previously untreated extensive small cell lung cancer (SCLC). A study of the National Cancer Institute of Canada Clinical Trials Group. Ann Oncol 1994;5:283–285.

521. Anderson H, Lund B, Bach F, Thatcher N, Walling J, Hansen HH. Single-agent activity of weekly gemcitabine in advanced non-small-cell lung cancer: a phase II study. J Clin Oncol 1994;12:1821–1826.

522. Abratt RP, Bezwoda WR, Falkson G, Goedhals L, Hackling D, Rugg TA. Efficacy and safety profile of gemcitabine in non-small-cell lung cancer: a phase II study. J Clin Oncol 1994;12:1535–1540.

523. Pollera CF, Ceribelli A, Crecco M, Calabresi F. Weekly gemcitabine in advanced bladder cancer: a preliminary report from a phase I study. Ann Oncol 1994;5:182–184.

524. Lund B, Hansen OP, Theilade K, Hansen M, Neijt JP. Phase II study of gemcitabine (2′,2′-difluorodeoxycytidine) in previously treated ovarian cancer patients. J Natl Cancer Inst 1994;86:1530–1533.

525. Casper ES, Green MR, Kelsen DP, et al. Phase II trial of gemcitabine (2′,2′-difluorodeoxycytidine) in patients with adenocarcinoma of the pancreas. Invest New Drugs 1994;12:29–34.

526. Catimel G, Vermorken JB, Clavel M, et al. A phase II study of Gemcitabine (LY 188011) in patients with advanced squamous cell carcinoma of the head and neck. Ann Oncol 1994;5:543–547.

527. Sessa C, Aamdai S, Wolff I, et al. Gemcitabine in patients with advanced malignant melanoma or gastric cancer: phase II studies of the EORTC Early Clinical Trials Group. Ann Oncol 1994;5:471–472.

528. Christman K, Kelsen D, Saltz L, Tarassoff PG. Phase II trial of gemcitabine in patients with advanced gastric cancer. Cancer 1994;73:5–7.

529. Moore DFJ, Pazdur R, Daugherty K, Tarassoff P, Abbruzzese JL. Phase II study of gemcitabine in advanced colorectal adenocarcinoma. Invest New Drugs 1992;10:323–325.

530. Mertens WC, Eisenhauer EA, Moore M, et al. Gemcitabine in advanced renal cell carcinoma. A phase II study of the National Cancer Institute of Canada Clinical Trials Group. Ann Oncol 1993;4: 331–332.

531. Kaye SB. Gemcitabine: current status of phase I and II trials (editorial). J Clin Oncol 1994;12:1527–1531.

532. Lilenbaum RC, Green MR. Novel chemotherapeutic agents in the treatment of non-small-cell lung cancer. J Clin Oncol 1993;11:391–402.

533. Braess J, Ramsauer B, Hiddemann W, et al.

Pharmacokinetics of YNK01 (fosteabine)—the oral derivative of cytosine arabinoside. Ann Oncol 1994; 5(Suppl 5):173a.

534. Habeck LL, Leitner TA, Shackelford KA, et al. A novel class of monoglutamated antifolates exhibits tight-binding inhibition of human glycinamide ribonucleotide formyltransferase and potent activity against solid tumors. Cancer Res 1994;54:1021–1026.

535. Mitrovski B, Pressacco J, Mandelbaum S, Erlichman C. Biochemical effects of folate-based inhibitors of thymidylate synthase in MGH-U1 cells. Cancer Chemother Pharmacol 1994;35:109–114.

536. Cassidy J, Kaye SB. New drugs in clinical development in Europe. Hematol Oncol Clin North Am 1994;8:289–303.

537. Smith SG, Lheman NL, Moran RG. Cytotoxicity of antifolate inhibitors of thymidylate and purine synthesis to WiDr colonic carcinoma cells. Cancer Res 1993;53:5697–5706.

538. Erba E, Sen S, Sessa C, Vikhanskaya FL, D'Incalci M. Mechanism of cytotoxicity of 5,10-dideazatetrahydrofolic acid in human ovarian carcinoma cells in vitro and modulation of the drug activity by folic or folinic acid. Br J Cancer 1994;69:205–211.

539. Clarke SJ, Jackman AL, Judson IR. The history of the development and clinical use of CB 3717 and ICI D1694. Adv Exp Med Biol 1993;339:277–287.

540. Ray MS, Muggia FM, Leichman CG, et al. Phase I study of (6R)-5,10-dideazatetrahydrofolate: a folate antimetabolite inhibitory to de novo purine synthesis. J Natl Cancer Inst 1993;95:1154–1159.

541. Nord LD, Martin DS. Enhancement of thymidylate synthase inhibition. Curr Opin Oncol 1993; 5:1017–1022.

542. Vasey PA, Calvert AH, Kaye SB, Cassidy J. Clinical phase I study of LY231514 (an inhibitor of thymidylate synthase) using a daily ×5 q21 schedule. Ann Oncol 1994;5(Suppl 5):131a.

543. Grem JL, King SA, O'Dwyer PJ, Leyland-Jones B. Biochemistry and clinical activity of N-(phosphonacetyl)-L-aspartate: a review. Cancer Res 1988;48:4441–4454.

544. Casper ES, Vale K, Williams L, Martin DS, Young CW. Phase I and clinical pharmacological evaluation of biochemical modulation of 5-fluorouracil with N-(phosphonacetyl)-L-aspartic acid. Cancer Res 1983;43:2324–2329.

545. Markman M, Chan TC, Cleary S, Howell SB. Phase I trial of combination therapy of cancer with N-(phosphonacetyl)-L-aspartic acid and dipyridamole. Cancer Chemother Pharmacol 1987;99:80–83.

546. Morton RF, Creagan ET, Cullinan SA. Phase II studies of single-agent cimetidine and the combination N-(phosphonacetyl)-L-aspartate (NSC-224131) plus L-alanosine (NSC-153353) in advanced malignant melanoma. J Clin Oncol 1987;5:1078–1082.

547. Rosvold E, Schilder R, Walczak J, et al. Phase II trial of PALA in combination with 5-fluorouracil in advanced pancreatic cancer. Cancer Chemother Pharmacol 1992;29:305–308.

548. Ardalan B, Singh G, Silberman H. A randomized phase I and II study of short-term infusion of high-dose fluorouracil with or without N-(phosphonacetyl)-L-aspartic acid in patients with advanced pancreatic and colorectal cancers. J Clin Oncol 1988; 6:1053–1058.

549. Kemeny N, Reichman B, Gordon C, et al.

Phase I trial of N-(phosphonacetyl)-L-aspartate (PALA), methotrexate (MTX), 5-fluorouracil (FU), and leucovorin (LV) in advanced colorectal cancer. Proc AACR 1987;28:743a.

550. Haas NB, Hines JB, Hudes GR, Johnston N, Ozols RF, O'Dwyer PJ. Phase I trial of 5-fluorouracil by 24-hour infusion weekly. Invest New Drugs 1993; 11:181–185.

551. Jodrell DI, Oster W, Kerr DJ, et al. A phase I-II study of N-(phosphonacetyl)-L-aspartic acid (PALA) added to 5-fluorouracil and folinic acid in advanced colorectal cancer. Eur J Cancer 1994;30A:950–955.

552. Grem JL, McAtee N, Steinberg SM, et al. A phase I study of continuous infusion 5-fluorouracil plus calcium leucovorin in combination with N-(phosphonacetyl)-L-aspartate in metastatic gastrointestinal adenocarcinoma. Cancer Res 1993;53:4828–4836.

553. Ardalan B, Ucar A, Reddy R, et al. Phase I trial of low dose N-(phosphonacetyl)-L-aspartic acid and high dose 5-fluorouracil administered concomitantly with radiation therapy for unresectable localized adenocarcinoma of the pancreas. Cancer 1994;74:1869–1873.

554. Sharma A, Straubinger NL, Straubinger RM. Modulation of human ovarian tumor cell sensitivity to N-(phosphonacetyl)-L-aspartate (PALA) by liposome drug carriers. Pharm Res 1993;10:1434–1441.

555. Duch DS, Edelstein MP, Bowers SW, Nichol CA. Biochemical and chemotherapeutic studies on 2,4-diamino-6-(2,5-dimethoxybenzyl)-5-methyl-pyrido (2,3-d)pyrimidine (BW 301U), a novel lipid-soluble inhibitor of dihydrofolate reductase. Cancer Res 1982; 42:3987–3994.

556. Sigel CW, Macklin AW, Woolley JLJ, et al. Preclinical biochemical pharmacology and toxicology of Piritrexim, a lipophilic inhibitor of dihydrofolate reductase. Monogr Natl Cancer Inst 1987;5:111–120.

557. Assaraf YG, Borgnia MJ. Differential reversal of lipophilic antifolate resistance in mammalian cells with modulators of the multidrug resistance phenotype. Anti-Cancer Drugs 1993;4:395–406.

558. Kovacs JA, Alloegra CJ, Swan JC, et al. Potent antipneumocystis and antitoxoplasma activities of Piritrexim, a lipid-soluble antifolate. Antimicrob Agents Chemother 1988;32:43–443.

559. Laszlo J, Brenchman WDJ, Morgan E, et al. Initial studies of Piritrexim. Monogr Natl Cancer Inst 1987;5:121–125.

560. Feun LG, Clendeninn NJ, Savaraj N, et al. Phase I trial of Piritrexim (BW301, PTX) capsules using prolonged, low-dose administration. Proc AACR 1988; 29:903a.

561. Feun LG, Savaraj N, Benedetto P, Waldman S, Collier M, Clendeninn NJ. Oral piritrexim in advanced bladder cancer: an effective drug after progression on MVAC chemotherapy? Am J Clin Oncol 1994;17:448–451.

562. de Wit R, Kaye SB, Roberts JT, Stoter G, Scott J, Verweij J. Oral piritrexim, an effective treatment for metastatic urothelial cancer. Br J Cancer 1993;67:388–390.

563. de Wit R, Verweij J, Slingerland R, Stoter G. Piritrexim-induced pulmonary toxicity. Am J Clin Oncol 1993;16:146–148.

564. Feun LG, Robinson WA, Savaraj N, Hanlon J, Collier M, Clendeninn NJ. Phase II trial of Piritrexim (BW 301, PTX) capsules in metastatic melanoma (MM) using prolonged low-dose administration. Proc AACR 1989;30:1087a.

565. Kris MG, Gralla RJ, Burke MT, et al. Phase II trial of oral Piritrexim (BW301U) in patients with stage III non-small cell lung cancer. Cancer Treat Rep 1987; 71:763–764.

566. Uen WC, Huang AT, Clendeninn NJ, Craig J, Spaulding M. Phase II Piritrexim study in squamous head and neck cancer. Proc AACR 1988;29:827a.

567. Rhee MS, Galivan J, Wright JE, Rosowsky A. Biochemical studies of PT523, a potent nonpolyglutamatable antifolate, in cultured cells. Mol Pharmacol 1994;45:783–791.

568. Rosowsky A, Bader H, Wright JE, Keyomarsi K, Matherly LH. Synthesis and biological activity of N o-hemiphthaloyl-α,o-diaminoalkanoic acid analogues of aminopterin and 3'5-dichloroaminopterin. J Med Chem 1994;37:2167–2174.

569. Uchida J, Takechi T, Nakano K, et al. Preclinical studies of S-1, a new oral tegafur plus two modulators. Proc AACR 1995;36:2423a.

570. Taguchi T. Clinical trial phase I study of S-1 a new oral pyrimidine fluoride anticancer drug. Fifth International Congress of Anti-Cancer Chemotherapy 1995;:118a.

571. Itoh F, Russello O, Akimoto H, Beardsley GP. Novel pyrrolo[2,3-d]pyrimidine antifolate TNP-351: cytotoxic effect on methotrexate-resistant CCRF-CEM cells and inhibition of transformylases of de novo purine biosynthesis. Cancer Chemother Pharmacol 1994; 34:273–279.

572. Yoshimura A. New analogues of methotrexate. Gan To Kagaku Ryoho 1992;19:2133–2139.

573. Jackman AL, Taylor GA, Gibson W, et al. ICI D 1694, a quinazoline antifolate thymidylate synthase inhibitor that is a potent inhibitor of L1210 tumor cell growth in vitro and in vivo: a new agent for clinical study. Cancer Res 1991;51:5579–5586.

574. Jackman AL. Tomudex (ZD D1694), a clinically active quinazoline-based thymidylate synthase inhibitor. Ann Oncol 1994;5(Suppl 5):122a.

575. Clarke SJ, Ward J, de Boer M, et al. Phase I study of the new thymidylate synthase inhibitor tomudex (ZD1694) in patients with advanced malignancy. Ann Oncol 1994;5(Suppl 5):132a.

576. Sorensen JM, Jordan E, Grem JL, et al. Phase I trial of ZD1694 (Tomudex), a direct inhibitor of thymidylate synthase. Ann Oncol 1994;5(Suppl 5):132a.

577. Zalcberg J, Cunningham D, Van Cutsem E, et al. Good antitumour activity of the new thymidylate synthase inhibitor Tomudex (ZD1694) in colorectal cancer. Ann Oncol 1994;5(Suppl 5):133a.

578. Smith IE, Spielman M, Bonneterre J, et al. Tomudex (ZD1694), a new thymidylate synthase inhibitor with antitumour activity in breast cancer. Ann Oncol 1994;5(Suppl 5):132a.

579. Kakito H, Ohkubo T, Kagawa Y, et al. Effects of 5-fluorouracil and a combination of tegafur and uracil (UFT) on nucleotide metabolism in L1210 ascites tumor. Cancer Invest 1993;11:530–533.

580. Maehara Y, Takeuchi H, Oshiro T, et al. Effect of gastrectomy on the pharmacokinetics of tegafur, uracil, and 5-fluorouracil after oral administration of a 1:4 tegafur and uracil combination. Cancer Chemother Pharmacol 1994;33:445–449.

581. Kurihara M. Clinical experience with UFT in Japan. Adv Exp Med Biol 1993;339:243–251.

582. Kubota Y, Hosaka M, Fukushima S, Kondo I. Prophylactic oral UFT therapy for superficial bladder cancer. Cancer 1993;71:1842–1845.

583. Masuda F, Nakada J, Kondo I, Furuta N. Adjuvant chemotherapy with vinblastine, adriamycin, and UFT for renal-cell carcinoma. Cancer Chemother Pharmacol 1992;30:477–479.

584. Gonzalez Baron M, Feliu J, Ordonez A, et al. Phase I study of UFT plus leucovorin in advanced colorectal cancer: a double modulation proposal. Anticancer Res 1993;13:759–762.

585. Pazdur R, Lassere Y, Rhodes V, et al. Phase II trial of uracil and tegafur plus oral leucovorin: an effective oral regimen in the treatment of metastatic colorectal carcinoma. J Clin Oncol 1994;12:2296–2300.

586. Kloosterboer HJ, Deckers GH, Schoonen WG. Pharmacology of two new very selective antiprogestogens: org 31710 and Org 31806. Hum Reprod 1994;9(Suppl 1):47–52.

587. Klijn JG, Setyono-Han B, Sander HJ, et al. Preclinical and clinical treatment of breast cancer with antiprogestins. Hum Reprod 1994;9(Suppl 1):181–189.

588. Nishino Y, Schneider MR, Michna H. Enhancement of the antitumor efficacy of the antiprogestin, onapristone, by combination with the antiestrogen, ICI 164384. J Cancer Res Clin Oncol 1994;120:298–302.

589. Narvaez CJ, Welsh JE. Induction of apoptosis by vitamin D in MCF-7 cells is potentiated by the antiprogestin onapristone. Proc AACR 1995;36:416a.

590. Koper JW, Lamberts SW. Meningiomas, epidermal growth factor and progesterone. Hum Reprod 1994;9(Suppl 1):190–194.

591. Spitz IM, Bardin CW. Clinical pharmacology of RU 486–an antiprogestin and antiglucocorticoid. Contraception 1993;48:403–444.

592. Murphy AA, Castellano PZ. RU486: pharmacology and potential use in the treatment of endometriosis and leiomyomata uteri. Curr Opin Obstet Gynecol 1994;6:269–278.

593. Musgrove EA, Sutherland RL. Effects of the progestin antagonist RU 486 on T-47D breast cancer cell cycle kinetics and cell cycle regulatory genes. Biochem Biophys Res Commun 1993;195:1184–1190.

594. McDonnell DP, Goldman ME. RU486 exerts antiestrogenic activities through a novel progesterone receptor A form-mediated mechanism. J Biol Chem 1994;269:11945–11949.

595. Gruol DJ, Zee MC, Trotter J, Bourgeois S. Reversal of multidrug resistance by RU 486. Cancer Res 1994;54:3088–3091.

596. Matsuda Y, Kawamotot K, Kiya K, Kurisu K, Sugiyama K, Uozumi T. Antitumor effects of antiprogesterones on human meningioma cells in vitro and in vivo. J Neurosurg 1994;80:527–534.

597. Masamura S, Adlercreutz H, Harvey H, et al. Aromatase inhibitor development for treatment of breast cancer. Breast Cancer Res Treat 1994;33:19–26.

598. Goss PE, Gwyn KMEH. Current perspectives on aromatase inhibitors in breast cancer. J Clin Oncol 1994;12:2460–2470.

599. Plourde PV, Dyroff M, Dukes M. Arimidex: a potent and selective fourth-generation aromatase inhibitor. Breast Cancer Res Treat 1994;30:103–111.

600. di Salle E, Ornati G, Giudici D, Lassus M, Evans TR, Coombes RC. Exemestane (FCE 24304), a new steroidal aromatase inhibitor. J Steroid Biochem Mol Biol 1992;43:137–143.

601. Di Salle E, Briatico G, Giudici D, et al. Novel aromatase and 5 alpha-reductase inhibitors. J Steroid Biochem Mol Biol 1994;49:289–294.

602. Evans TR, Di Salle E, Ornati G, et al. Phase I and endocrine study of exemestrane (FCE 24304), a new aromatase inhibitor, in postmenopausal women. Cancer Res 1992;52:5933–5939.

603. Lemmens J, Paridaens R, Thomas J, Wildiers J. Phase I study of exemestane (FCE 24304), a new aromatase inhibitor, in metastatic breast cancer (MBC). Ann Oncol 1994;5(Suppl 5):134a.

604. Demers LM. Effects of fadrozole (CGS 16949A) and letrozole (CGS 20267) on the inhibition of aromatase activity in breast cancer patients. Breast Cancer Res Treat 1994;30:95–102.

605. Cavalli F, Beretta K, Willems Y, Brunner KW, Nadjafi C, Sessa C. Phase I-II study in postmenopausal patients (pts) with advanced breast cancer of CGS 16949A: a new, highly potent and selective aromatase inhibitor. Proc Am Soc Clin Oncol 1988;7:84a.

606. Schieweck K, Bhatnagar AS, Matter A. Antagonism by estradiol of the anti-tumor effect of the aromatase inhibitor CGS 16949A in DMBA-induced mammary tumors. Proc AACR 1988;29:968a.

607. Nomura Y, Abe O, Tominaga T, et al. Phase I study of CGS16949A—a new aromatase inhibitor. Comparative Study Group for CGS16949A. Gan To Kagaku Ryoho 1994;21:189–197.

608. Lipton A, Harvey HA, Demers LM, et al. A phase I trial of CGS 16949A—a new aromatase inhibitor. Proc Am Soc Clin Oncol 1989;8:72a.

609. Hoffken K, Kolbel M, Hayungs J, et al. Phase I study on the new aromatase inhibitor CGS 16 949A in breast cancer patients. Proc Am Soc Clin Oncol 1989; 8:200a.

610. Goss PE, Clark R, Ambus U, et al. Phase II study of vorozole (R 83 842) a new aromatase inhibitor in postmenopausal women with advanced breast cancer. Breast Cancer Res Treat 1994;32(Suppl):67a.

611. Cocconi G, Bisagni G, Ceci G, et al. CGS 20267 a new oral aromatase inhibitor: phase I study in postmenopausal advanced breast cancer patients. Ann Oncol 1994;5(Suppl 5):135a.

612. Fox K, Glick J, Schultz C, et al. Rogletimide (ROG) may increase the clearance of estrone sulfate in postmenopausal females when administered as therapy for advanced metastatic breast cancer. Breast Cancer Res Treat 1994;32(Suppl):67a.

613. Wouters W, Van Ginckel R, Krekels M, Bowden C, De Coster R. Pharmacology of vorozole. J Steroid Biochem Mol Biol 1993;44:617–621.

614. Johnston SRD, Smith IE, Doody D, Jacobs S, Robertshaw H, Dowsett M. Clinical and endocrine effects of the oral aromatase inhibitor vorozole in postmenopausal patients with advanced breast cancer. Cancer Res 1994;54:5875–5881.

615. Blaney SM, Balis FM, Cole DE, et al. Pediatric phase I trial and pharmacokinetic study of topotecan administered as a 24-hour continuous infusion. Cancer Res 1993;53:1032–1036.

616. Tanizawa A, Fujimori A, Fujimori Y, Pommier Y. Comparison of topoisomerase I inhibition, DNA damage, and cytoxicity of camptothecin derivatives presently in clinical trials. J Natl Cancer Inst 1994; 86:836–842.

617. Supko JG, Malspeis L. Pharmacokinetics of the 9-amino and 10,11-methylenedioxy derivatives

of camptothecin in mice. Cancer Res 1993;53:3062–3069.

618. Slichenmyer WJ, Rowinsky EK, Donehower RC, et al. The current status of camptothecin analogues as anticancer agents. J Natl Cancer Inst 1993;85:271–287.

619. Von Hoff DD, Burris HA III, Eckardt J, et al. Preclinical and phase I trials of topoisomerase I inhibitors. Cancer Chemother Pharmacol 1994;34(Suppl):s41–S45.

620. Chiou T-J, Ren Q-F, Grem JL. Potentiation of 9-aminocamptothecin cytotoxicity by interferon α. Proc AACR 1995;36:446a.

621. Pantazis P, Kozielski AJ, Mendoza JT, Early JA, Hinz HR, Giovanella BC. Camptothecin derivatives induce regression of human ovarian carcinomas grown in nude mice and distinguish between non-tumorigenic and tumorigenic cells in vitro. Int J Cancer 1993;53:863–871.

622. Wall ME, Wani MC, Nicholas AW, et al. Plant antitumor agents. 30. Synthesis and structure activity of novel camptothecin analogs. J Med Chem 1993; 36:2689–2700.

623. Silber R, Degar B, Costin D, et al. Chemosensitivity of lymphocytes from patients with B-cell chronic lymphocytic leukemia to chlorambucil, fludarabine, and camptothecin analogs. Blood 1994;84:3440–3446.

624. Mattern MR, Hofman GA, Polsky RM, Funk LR, McCabe LR, Johnson RK. In vitro and in vivo effects of clinically important camptothecin analogues on multidrug-resistant cells. Oncol Res 1993; 5:467–474.

625. Pantazis P, Harris N, Hinz H, Giovanella B. Conversion of 9-nitrocamptothecin to 9-aminocamptothecin by human, dog, and mouse cells in vivo and in vitro. Proc AACR 1995;36:447a.

626. Hinz HR, Harris NJ, Natelson EA, Giovanella BC. Pharmacokinetics of the in vivo and in vitro conversion of 9-nitro-20(S)-camptothecin to 9-amino-20(S)-camptothecin in humans, dogs, and mice. Cancer Res 1994;54:3096–3100.

627. Grochow LB, Rowinsky EK, Johnson R, et al. Pharmacokinetics and pharmacodynamics of topotecan in patients with advanced cancer. Drug Metab Dispos Biol Fate Chem 1992;20:706–713.

628. van Warmerdam LJC, Verweij J, Schellens JHM, et al. Pharmacokinetics and pharmacodynamics of topotecan administered daily for 5 days every 3 weeks. Cancer Chemother Pharmacol 1995;35:237–245.

629. van Warmerdam LJ, Verweij J, Rosing H, Schellens JH, Maes RA, Beijnen JH. Limited sampling models for topotecan pharmacokinetics. Ann Oncol 1994;5:259–264.

630. Haas NB, La Creta FP, Walczak J, et al. Phase I/pharmacokinetic study of topotecan by 24-hour continuous infusion weekly. Cancer Res 1994;54:1220–1226.

631. O'Dwyer PJ, LaCreta FP, Haas NB, et al. Clinical, pharmacokinetic and biologic studies of topotecan. Cancer Chemother Pharmacol 1994; 34(Suppl):s46–S52.

632. Sung C, Blaney SM, Cole DE, Balis FM, Dedrick RL. A pharmacokinetic model of topotecan clearance from plasma and cerebrospinal fluid. Cancer Res 1994;54:5118–5122.

633. Burris H, Fields S, Kuhn J, Eckardt J, von Hoff D. Current directions in the development of topotecan. Ann Oncol 1994;5(Suppl 5):162a.

634. Slichenmyer WJ, Rowinsky EK, Grochow LB, Kaufman SH, Donehower RC. Camptothecin analogues: studies from the Johns Hopkins Oncology Center. Cancer Chemother Pharmacol 1994;34(Suppl):s53–S57.

635. Verweij J, Lund B, Beijnen J, et al. Phase I and pharmacokinetics study of topotecan, a new topoisomerase I inhibitor. Ann Oncol 1993;4:673–678.

636. Hochster H, Liebes L, Speyer J, et al. Phase I trial of low-dose continuous topotecan infusion in patients with cancer: an active and well-tolerated regimen. J Clin Oncol 1994;12:553–559.

637. Burris HA III, Awada A, Kuhn JG, et al. Phase I and pharmacokinetic studies of topotecan administered as a 72 or 120 h continuous infusion. Anti-Cancer Drugs 1994;5:394–402.

638. Wall JG, Burris HA III, Von Hoff DD, et al. A phase I clinical and pharmacokinetic study of the topoisomerase I inhibitor topotecan (SK&F 104864) given as an intravenous bolus every 21 days. Anti-Cancer Drugs 1992;3:337–345.

639. Kantarjian HM, Beran M, Ellis A, et al. Phase I study of Topotecan, a new topoisomerase I inhibitor, in patients with refractory or relapsed acute leukemia. Blood 1993;81:1146–1151.

640. Rowinsky EK, Adjei A, Donehower RC, et al. Phase I and pharmacodynamic study of the topoisomerase I inhibitor topotecan in patients with refractory acute leukemia. J Clin Oncol 1994;12:2193–2203.

641. Burris HA III, Rothenberg ML, Kuhn JG, Von Hoff DD. Clinical trials with the topoisomerase I inhibitors. Semin Oncol 1992;19:663–669.

642. Friedman HS, Houghton PJ, Schold SC, Keir S, Bigner DD. Activity of 9-dimethylaminomethyl-10-hydroxycamptothecin against pediatric and adult central nervous system tumor xenografts. Cancer Chemother Pharmacol 1994;34:171–174.

643. Pratt CB, Stewart C, Santana VM, et al. Phase I study of topotecan for pediatric patients with malignant solid tumors. J Clin Oncol 1994;12:539–543.

644. Stewart CF, Baker SD, Heideman RL, Jones D, Crom WR, Pratt CB. Clinical pharmacodynamics of continuous infusion topotecan in children: systemic exposure predicts hematologic toxicity. J Clin Oncol 1994;12:1946–1954.

645. Lynch TJJ, Kalish L, Strauss G, et al. Phase II study of topotecan in metastatic non-small-cell lung cancer. J Clin Oncol 1994;12:347–352.

646. Burris H, Fields S, Kuhn J, Eckardt J, Von Hoff D. Current directions in the development of topotecan. Sixth NCI-EORTC Symposium on New Drugs for Cancer Therapy 1995;162a.

647. Chou TC, Motzer RJ, Tong Y, Bosl GJ. Computerized quantitation of synergism and antagonism of taxol, topotecan, and cisplatin against human teratocarcinoma cell growth: a rational approach to clinical protocol design. J Natl Cancer Inst 1994;86:1517–1524.

648. Masuda N, Fukuoka M, Kudoh S, et al. Phase I and pharmacologic study of irinotecan and etoposide with recombinant human granulocyte colony-stimulating factor support for advanced lung cancer. J Clin Oncol 1994;12:1833–1841.

649. Armand JP, Abigerges D, Chabot GG, et al. High dose intensity of CPT-11 administered as single

dose every 3 weeks: the Institut Gustave Roussy experience. Ann Oncol 1994;5(Suppl 5):189a.

650. Armand JP. CPT-11: the choice of its optimal schedule. Fifth International Congress of Anti-Cancer Chemotherapy 1995;s77.

651. Herait P. CPT-11: future directions. Fifth International Congress of Anti-Cancer Chemotherapy 1995;s774.

652. Bugat R, Rougier P, Brunet P, et al. Clinical efficacy of CPT-11 in patients with inoperable advanced colorectal cancer: results of a multicenter open phase II study. Fifth International Congress of Anti-Cancer Chemotherapy 1995;s775.

653. Kunka R, O'Dwyer P, Cassidy J, et al. Pharmacokinetics and dynamics of GG211, a new topoisomerase I inhibitor, during a 72 hour continuous infusion. Proc AACR 1995;36:234a.

654. Emerson DL, McIntyre G, Luzzio MJ, Wissel PS. Pre-clinical anti-tumor activity of a novel water-soluble camptothecin analog, (GI147211C). Ann Oncol 1994;5(Suppl 5):185a.

655. Riou JF, Fosse P, Nguyen CH, et al. Intoplicine (RP 60475) and its derivatives, a new class of antitumor agents inhibiting both topoisomerase I and II activities. Cancer Res 1993;53:5987–5993.

656. Poddevin B, Riou JF, Lavelle F, Pommier Y. Dual topoisomerase I and II inhibition by intoplicine (RP-60475), a new antitumor agent in early clinical trials. Mol Pharmacol 1993;44:767–774.

657. Bissery MC, Nguyen CH, Bisagni E, Vrignaud P, Lavelle F. Antitumor activity of intoplicine (RP 60475, NSC 645008), a new benzo-pyrido-indole: evaluation against solid tumors and leukemias in mice. Invest New Drugs 1993;11:263–277.

658. Eckardt JR, Burris HA III, Kuhn JG, et al. Activity of intoplicine (RP60475), a new DNA topoisomerase I and II inhibitor, against human tumor colony-forming units in vitro. J Natl Cancer Inst 1994;86:30–33.

659. Pazdur R, Newman RA, Minor T, et al. Phase I clinical trial of intoplicine (RP60475F): 72-hour infusion repeated every 21 days. Ann Oncol 1994;5(Suppl 5):189a.

660. van Gijn R, Kuijs S, Dubbelman AC, et al. Pharmacokinetics of intoplicine (RP60475F) given as a 24-h continuous infusion in a phase I study. Ann Oncol 1994;5(Suppl 5):189a.

661. Sugarman SM, Perez-Soler R. Liposomes in the treatment of malignancy: a clinical perspective. Crit Rev Oncol Hematol 1992;12:231–242.

662. Perez-Soler R. Liposomes as carriers of antitumor agents toward a clinical reality. Cancer Treat Rev 1989;16:67.

663. Gabizon AA. Liposomal anthracyclines. Hematol Oncol Clin North Am 1994;8:431–450.

664. Lasic DD, Paphadjopoulos D. Liposomes revisited. Science 1995;267:1275–1276.

665. Perez-Soler R, Zou Y, Ling Y-H, Priebe W. Preclinical studies with the lipophilic and non cross-resistant anthracycline annamycin (ANN) formulated in a liposomal carrier. Ann Oncol 1994;5(Suppl 5):96a.

666. Presant CA, Scolaro M, Kennedy P, et al. Liposomal daunorubicin treatment of HIV-associated Kaposi's sarcoma. Lancet 1993;341:1242–1243.

667. Gill PS, Espina BM, Muggia F, et al. Phase I/II clinical and pharmacokinetic evaluation of liposomal daunorubicin. J Clin Oncol 1995;13:996–1003.

668. Gatzemeier U, Neuhauss R, Schluter I, Nuyts GD, Eestermans GH. Single agent, high dose DaunoXome for the treatment of stage IIIB and IV non small cell lung cancer (NSCLC): a phase II pilot trial. Fifth International Congress of Anti-Cancer Chemotherapy 1995;:200a.

669. Erdkamp FLG, Hupperets PSGJ, Ten Bokkel Huinink WW, Nuyts GD, Eestermans GH. Phase II study of liposomal encapsulated daunorubicin (DaunoXome) in advanced breast cancer. Ann Oncol 1995;5(Suppl 5):212a.

670. Gabizon A, Catane R, Uziely B, et al. Prolonged circulation time and enhanced accumulation in malignant exudates of doxorubicin encapsulated in polyethylene-glycol coated liposomes. Cancer Res 1994;54:987–992.

671. Simpson JK, Miller RF, Spittle MF. Liposomal doxorubicin for treatment of AIDS-related Kaposi's sarcoma. Clin Oncol 1993;5:372–374.

672. Wagner D, Kern WV, Kern P. Liposomal doxorubicin in AIDS-related Kaposi's sarcoma: long term experiences. Clin Invest 1994;72:417–423.

673. Harrison M, Tomlinson D, Stewart S. Liposomal-entrapped doxorubicin: an active agent in AIDS-related Kaposi's sarcoma. J Clin Oncol 1995;13:914–920.

674. Conley BA, Egorin MJ, Whitacre MY, Carter DC, Zuhowski EG, Van Echo DA. Phase I and pharmacokinetic trial of liposome-encapsulated doxorubicin. Cancer Chemother Pharmacol 1993;33:107–112.

675. Perez-Soler R, Francis K, al-Baker S, Pilkiewicz F, Khokhar AR. Preparation and characterization of liposomes containing a lipophilic cisplatin derivative for clinical use. J Microencapsul 1994;11:41–54.

676. Vadiei K, Siddik ZH, Khokhar A, al-Baker S, Sampedro F, Perez-Soler R. Pharmacokinetics of liposome-entrapped cis-bis-neodecanoato-trans-R,R-1,2-diaminocyclohexane platinum(II) and cisplatin given iv and ip in the rat. Cancer Chemother Pharmacol 1992; 30:365–369.

677. Kanter PM, Bullard GA, Pilkiewicz FG, Mayer LD, Cullis PR, Pavelic ZP. Preclinical toxicology study of liposome encapsulated doxorubicin (TLC D-99): comparison with doxorubicin and empty liposomes in mice and dogs. In Vivo 1993;7:85–95.

678. Cowens JW, Creaven PJ, Greco WR, et al. Initial clinical (phase I) trial of TLC D-99 (doxorubicin encapsulated in liposomes). Cancer Res 1993;53:2796–2802.

679. Boman NL, Masin D, Mayer LD, Cullis PR, Bally M. Liposomal vincristine which exhibits increased drug retention and increased circulation longevity cures mice bearing P388 tumors. Cancer Res 1994;54:2830–2833.

680. Gelmon K, Mayer L, Bally M, Embree L, Goldie J. Phase I study of vincristine sulfate liposome injection and strategies for improving the liposome vincristine preparation. Ann Oncol 1994;5(Suppl 5):140a.

681. Vaage J, Donovan D, Mayhew E, Uster P, Woodle M. Therapy of mouse mammary carcinomas with vincristine and doxorubicin encapsulated in sterically stabilized liposomes. Int J Cancer 1993;54:959–964.

682. Qian HN, Li WJ. Target therapy of ovarian carcinoma by monoclonal antibodies bearing chemical drugs entrapped in liposomes. Chin Med J 1993; 106:343–347.

683. Klingerman MM, Shaw MT, Slavik M, Yuhas JM. Phase I clinical studies with WR-2721. Cancer Clin Trials 1980;3:217–221.

684. DeNeve WJ, Evertt CK, Suminski JE, Valeriota FA. Influence of WR2721 on DNA cross-linking by nitrogen mustard in normal mouse bone marrow and leukemia cells in vitro. Cancer Res 1988;48:6002–6005.

685. Yuhas JM, Spellman JM, Culo F. The role of WR-2721 in radiotherapy and/or chemotherapy. Cancer Clin Trials 1980;3:211–216.

686. Hirschel-Scholz S, Caverzasio J, Bonjour JP. Prevention of parathyroid hormone-dependent nephrocalcinosis by chronic administration of the organic phosphorothioate WR-2721. Calcif Tissue Int 1987; 40:103–108.

687. Schein PS. WR-2721: a novel chemotherapy and radiation therapy protecting agent. Cancer Invest 1988;6:38a.

688. Capizzi RL, Scheffler BJ, Schein PS. Amifostine-mediated protection of normal bone marrow from cytotoxic chemotherapy. Cancer 1993;72 (11 Suppl):3495–3501.

689. Mitsuhashi N, Takahashi I, Takahashi M, Hayakawa K, Niibe H. Clinical study of radioprotective effects of amifostine (YM-08310, WR-2721) on long-term outcome for patients with cervical cancer. Int J Radiat Oncol Biol Phys 1993;26:407–411.

690. Budd GT, Ganapathi R, Bauer L, et al. Phase I study of WR-2721 and carboplatin. Eur J Cancer 1993; 29A:1122–1127.

691. Vermorken JB, Punt CJA, Eeltink CM, et al. Phase I trial of carboplatin and amifostine (WR-2721). Proc AACR 1995;36:240.

692. Treskes M, van der Vijgh WJF. WR2721 as a modulator of cisplatin- and carboplatin-induced side effects in comparison with other chemoprotective agents: a molecular approach. Cancer Chemother Pharmacol 1993;33:93–106.

693. Delaflor-Weiss E, Blommaert F, Gill I, Muggia FM, Kortes V, Den Engelese L. Amifostine (WR2721) protects from bone marrow toxicity of combination of cisplatin (P) and carboplatin (C) without decreasing platinum-DNA adduct formation. Ann Oncol 1994; 5(Suppl 5):125a.

694. Poplin EA, Lo Russo P, Lokich JJ, et al. Randomized clinical trial of mitomycin-C with or without pretreatment with WR-2721 in patients with advanced colorectal cancer. Cancer Chemother Pharmacol 1994; 33:415–419.

695. Shpall EJ, Stemmer SM, Hami L, et al. Amifostine (WR-2721) shortens the engraftment period of 4-hydroxyperoxycyclophosphamide-purged bone marrow in breast cancer patients receiving high dose chemotherapy with autologous bone marrow support. Blood 1994;83:3132–3137.

696. Wang X, Fu X, Brown PD, Crimmin MJ, Hoffman RM. Matrix metalloproteinase inhibitor BB-94 (Batimastat) inhibits human colon tumor growth and spread in a patient-like orthotopic mode in nude mice. Cancer Res 1994;54:4726–4728.

697. Davies B, Brown PD, East N, Crimmin MJ, Balkwill FR. A synthetic matrix metalloproteinase inhibitor decreases tumor burden and prolongs survival of mice bearing human ovarian carcinoma xenografts. Cancer Res 1993;53:2087–2091.

698. Beattie GJ, Young HA, Smyth JF. Phase I study of intra-peritoneal metallo-proteinase inhibitor BB94 with malignant ascites. Ann Oncol 1994;5(Suppl 5):72a.

699. Ozols RF, Masuda H, Hamilton TC. Mechanisms of cross-resistance between radiation and antineoplastic drugs. Monogr Natl Cancer Inst 1988;6:159–165.

700. Mitchell JB, Russo A. The role of glutathione in radiation and drug induced cytotoxicity. Br J Cancer 1987;8(Suppl):96–104.

701. Fojo A, Hamilton TC, Young RC, Ozols RF. Multidrug resistance in ovarian cancer. Cancer 1987; 60(Suppl 8):2075–2080.

702. Edwards PG. Evidence that glutathione may determine the differential cell-cycle phase toxicity of a platinum (IV) antitumor agent. J Natl Cancer Inst 1980; 80:734–738.

703. Lai GM, Ozols RF, Young RC, Hamilton TC. Effect of glutathione on DNA repair in cisplatin-resistant human ovarian cancer cell lines. J Natl Cancer Inst 1989;81:535–539.

704. Dorr RT. Reduced thiol content in L1210 cells treated with BSO increases DNA crosslinking by melphalan. Biochem Biophys Res Commun 1987;144:47–52.

705. Mans DR, Schuurhuis GJ, Treskes M, et al. Modulation by D,L-buthionine-S,R-sulphoximine of etoposide cytotoxicity on human nonsmall cell lung, ovarian and breast carcinoma cell lines. Eur J Cancer 1992;28A:1447–1452.

706. Saikawa Y, Kubota T, Kuo TH, et al. Enhancement of antitumor activity of cisplatin on human gastric cancer cells in vitro and in vivo by buthionine sulfoximine. Jpn J Cancer Res 1993;84:787–793.

707. Revesz L, Edgren MR, Wainson AA. Selective toxicity of buthionine sulfoximine (BSO) to melanoma cells in vitro and in vivo. Int J Radiat Oncol Biol Phys 1994;29:403–406.

708. Liebmann JE, Hahn SM, Cook JA, Lipschultz C, Mitchell JB, Kaufman DC. Glutathione depletion by L-buthionine sulfoximine antagonizes taxol cytotoxicity. Cancer Res 1993;53:2066–2070.

709. Kramer RA, Greene K, Ahmad S, Vistica DT. Chemosensitization of L-phenylalanine mustard by the thiol modulating agent buthionine sulfoximine. Cancer Res 1987;47:1593–1597.

710. Lee FY, Allalunis-Turner MJ, Siemann DW. Depletion of tumor versus normal tissue glutathione by buthionine sulfoximine. Br J Cancer 1987;56:33–38.

711. Ozols RF, Louie KG, Plowman J, et al. Enhanced melphalan cytotoxicity in human ovarian cancer in vitro and in tumor-bearing nude mice by buthionine sulfoximine depletion of glutathione. Biochem Pharmacol 1987;36:147–153.

712. Prezioso JA, Fitz Gerald GB, Wick MM. Melanoma cytotoxicity of buthionine sulfoximine (BSO) alone and in combination with 3,4-dihydroxybenzylamine and melphalan. J Invest Dermatol 1992;99:289–293.

713. Dorr RT, Liddil JD, Soble MJ. Cytotoxic effects of glutathione synthesis inhibition by L-buthionine-(SR)-sulfoximine on human and murine tumor cells. Invest New Drugs 1986;3:305–313.

714. Soble MJ, Dorr RT. Lack of enhanced myelotoxicity with buthionine sulfoximine and suflhydryl-dependent anticancer agents in mice. Res Commun Chem Pathol Pharmacol 1987;55:161–180.

715. Bailey HH, Mulcahy RT, Tutsch KD, et al.

Phase I clinical trial of intravenous L-buthionine sulfoximine and melphalan: an attempt at modulation of glutathione. J Clin Oncol 1994;12:194–205.

716. Malaker K, Hurwitz SJ, Bump EA, et al. Pharmacodynamics of prolonged treatment with L,S-buthionine sulfoximine. Int J Radiat Oncol Biol Phys 1994; 29:407–412.

717. Beijnen JH, van Gijn R. Chemical stability of the cardioprotective agent ICRF-187 in infusion fluids. J Parenter Sci Technol 1993;47:166–171.

718. Von Hoff DD, Howser D, Lewis BJ, Holcenberg J, Weiss RB, Young RC. Phase I study of ICRF-187 using a daily for 3 days schedule. Cancer Treat Rep 1981;65:249–252.

719. Koeller JM, Earhart RH, Davis HL. Phase I trial of ICRF-187 by 48-hour continuous infusion. Cancer Treat Rep 1981;65:459–463.

720. Liesmann J, Belt R, Haas C, Hoogstraten B. Phase I evaluation of ICRF-187 (NSC-169780) in patients with advanced malignancy. Cancer 1981; 47:1959–1962.

721. Holcenberg JS, Tutsch KD, Earhart RH, et al. Phase I study of ICRF-187 in pediatric cancer patients and comparison of its pharmacokinetics in children and adults. Cancer Treat Rep 1986;70:703–709.

722. Vogel CL, Gorowski E, Davila E, et al. Phase I clinical trial and pharmacokinetics of weekly ICRF-187 (NSC 169780) infusion in patients with solid tumors. Invest New Drugs 1987;5:187–198.

723. Rajagopalan S, Politi PM, Sinha BK, Myers CE. Adriamycin-induced free radical formation in the perfused rat heart: implications for cardiotoxicity. Cancer Res 1988;48:4766–4769.

724. Herman EH, Ferrans VJ, Youngs RS, Hamlin RL. Effect of pretreatment with ICRF-187 on the total cumulative dose of doxorubicin tolerated by beagle dogs. Cancer Res 1988;48:6918–6925.

725. Herman EH, Ferans VJ. Timing of treatment with ICRF-187 and its effect on chronic doxorubicin cardiotoxicity. Cancer Chemother Pharmacol 1993; 32:445–449.

726. Herman EJ, el Hage A, Ferrans VJ. Protective effect of ICRF-187 on doxorubicin-induced cardiac and renal toxicity in spontaneously hypertensive (SHR) and normotensive (WKY) rats. Toxicol Appl Pharmacol 1988;92:42–53.

727. Dardir M, Herman EH, Ferrans VJ. Effects of ICRF-187 on the cardiac and renal toxicity of epirubicin in spontaneously hypertensive rats. Cancer Chemother Pharmacol 1989;23:269–275.

728. Sehested J, Jensen PB, Sorensen BS, Holm B, Friche E, Demant EJ. Antagonist effect of the cardioprotector (+)-1,2-bis(3,5-dioxopiperazinyl-1-yl)propane (ICRF-187) on DNA breaks and cytotoxicity induced by the topoisomerase II directed drugs daunorubicin and etoposide (VP-16). Biochem Pharmacol 1993;46:389–393.

729. Green MD. Rationale and strategy for prevention of anthracycline cardiotoxicity with bisdioxopiperazine, ICRF-187. Pathol Biol 1987;35:49–53.

730. Speyer JL, Green MD, Kramer E, et al. Protective effect of the bispiperazinedione ICRF-187 against doxorubicin-induced cardiac toxicity in women with advanced breast cancer. N Engl J Med 1988;319:745–752.

731. Sorensen B, Bastholt L, Mirza MR, et al. The cardioprotector ADR-529 and high-dose epirubicin given in combination with cyclophosphamide, 5-fluorouracil, and tamoxifen: a phase I study in metastatic breast cancer. Cancer Chemother Pharmacol 1994; 34:439–443.

732. Jakobsen P, Sorensen B, Bastholt L, et al. The pharmacokinetics of high-dose epirubicin and of the cardioprotector ADR-529 given together with cyclophosphamide, 5-fluorouracil, and tamoxifen in metastatic breast-cancer patients. Cancer Chemother Pharmacol 1994;35:45–52.

733. Walsh C, Blum RH, Oratz R, Goldenberg A, Downey A, Speyer JL. Phase I study of doxorubicin, ICRF-187 and granulocyte/macrophage-colony-stimulating factor. J Cancer Res Clin Oncol 1992;118:61–66.

734. Hochster H, Liebes L, Wadler S, et al. Pharmacokinetics of the cardioprotector ADR-529 (ICRF-187) in escalating doses combined with fixed-dose doxorubicin. J Natl Cancer Inst 1992;84:1725–1730.

735. Hellerqvist CG, DeVore RF, Sundell HW, et al. Early results of a phase I trial of CM101 in cancer patients. Proc AACR 1995;36:224a.

736. Martin KJ, Winslow ER, Kaddurah-Daouk R. Cell cycle studies of cyclocreatine, a new anticancer agent. Cancer Res 1994;54:5160–5165.

737. Martin KJ, Chen S-F, Clark GM, et al. Evaluation of creatine analogues as a new class of anticancer agents using freshly explanted human tumor cells. J Natl Cancer Inst 1994;86:608–613.

738. Martin KJ, Winslow ER, O'Keefe M, et al. AM285 (cyclocreatine): single agent and combination therapy against SCLC, colon and prostate tumors. Fifth International Congress of Anti-Cancer Chemotherapy 1995;:116a.

739. Schimmel L, Riera T, Kaddurah-Daouk R. Accumulation, depletion and antitumor activity of cyclocreatine administered via different schedules and routes. Fifth International Congress of Anti-Cancer Chemotherapy 1995;:281a.

740. Staddon A, Henry D, Ferraresi R, Bonnem EM. A phase I study of AM 285 (cyclocreatine) in patients with refractory/relapsing tumors. Fifth International Congress of Anti-Cancer Chemotherapy 1995;150a.

741. Schuller HM, Orloff M, Reznik GK. Inhibition of protein-kinase-C-dependent cell proliferation of human lung cancer cell lines by the dihydropyridine dexniguldipine. J Cancer Res Clin Oncol 1994;120:354–358.

742. Scheulen ME, Meusers P, Schroder J, et al. Phase I/II trial of additive dexniguldipine (hADM) in acute myeloid leukemia (AML) refractory to previous daunorubicin and high dose cytarabine (hAD). Proc AACR 1995;36:203.

743. Reiter WW, Ludescher C, Wormann B, et al. A phase II trial with dexniguldipine, a new multidrug resistance modulator, in combination with VAD or VECD in patients with refractory anemia. Ann Oncol 1994;5(Suppl 5):160a.

744. Kornek G, Raderer M, Funovics J, et al. Dexverapamil (DVPM), epirubicin (EPI) plus GmCSF in advanced pancreatic cancer: phase I/II study. Ann Oncol 1994;5(Suppl 5):159a.

745. Porter CW, Janne J. Modulation of antineoplastic drug action by inhibitors of polyamine biosynthesis. In: McCann PP, Pegg AE, Sjoerdsma A, eds. Inhibition of polyamine metabolism. Orlando: Academic Press, 1987:213–248.

746. Levin VA, Prados MD, Yung WK, Gleason MJ, Ictech S, Malec M. Treatment of recurrent gliomas with eflornithine. J Natl Cancer Inst 1992;84:1432–1437.

747. Ootsuyama A, Tanooka H. Effect of an inhibitor of tumor promotion, α-difluoromethylornithine, on tumor induction by repeated beta irradiation in mice. Jpn J Cancer Res 1993;84:34–36.

748. Lehnert T, Buhl K, Ivankovic S. Inhibition of gastric tumorigenesis by α-difluoromethylornithine in rats treated with N-methyl-N'-nitro-N-nitrosoguanidine. J Cancer Res Clin Oncol 1993;119:594–598.

749. Sanborn G, Niederkorn J, Kan-Mitchell J, Albert D. Prevention of metastasis of intraocular melanoma in mice treated with difluoromethylornithine. Graefes Arch Clin Exp Ophthalmol 1992;230:72–77.

750. Crowell JA, Goldenthal EI, Kelloff GJ, Malone WF, Boone CW. Chronic toxicity studies of the potential cancer preventive 2-(difluoromethyl)-di-ornithine. Fundam Appl Toxicol 1994;22:341–354.

751. Creaven PJ, Pendyala L, Petrelli NJ. Evaluation of α-difluoromethylornithine as a potential chemopreventive agent: tolerance to daily oral administration in humans. Cancer Epidemiol Biomarkers Prev 1993;2:243–247.

752. Love RR, Carbone PP, Verma AK, et al. Randomized phase I chemoprevention dose-seeking study of α-difluoromethylornithine. J Natl Cancer Inst 1993; 85:732–737.

753. McRipley RJ, Burns-Horwitz PE, Czerniak PM, et al. Efficacy of DMP 840: a novel bis-naphthalimide cytotoxic agent with human solid tumor xenograft selectivity. Cancer Res 1994;54:159–164.

754. Kirshenbaum MR, Chen S-F, Behrens CH, et al. (R,R)-2,2'-[ethanediylbis[imino(1-methyl-2,1-ethanediyl)]] - bis[5 - nitro - 1H - benz[de]isoquinoline - 1,3 - (2H)-dione] dimethanesulfonate (DMP 840), a novel bis-naphthalimide with potent nonselective tumoricidal activity in vitro. Cancer Res 1994;54:2199–2206.

755. Houghton PJ, Cheshire PJ, Hallman JC III, et al. Evaluation of a novel bis-naphthalimide anticancer agent, DMP 840, against human xenografts derived from adult, juvenile, and pediatric cancers. Cancer Chemother Pharmacol 1994;33:265–272.

756. Cobb P, Kuhn J, Finizio M, et al. Phase I trial of a new bis-naphthalimide, DMP 840, given on a daily × 5 schedule every 28 days. Ann Oncol 1994;5(Suppl 5):137a.

757. Shulman LN, Buswell L, Goodman H, et al. Phase I pharmacokinetic study of the hypoxic cell sensitizer etanidazole with carboplatin and cyclophosphamide in the treatment of advanced ovarian cancer. Int J Radiat Oncol Biol Phys 1994;29:545–548.

758. Breivis P, Didziapetriene J. Faranox—a new antitumour agent. Fifth International Congress of Anti-Cancer Chemotherapy 1995;275a.

759. Naik HR, Petrylak D, Yagoda A, Lehr JE, Ahktar A, Pienta KJ. Preclinical studies of gossypol in prostate carcinoma. Int J Oncol 1995;6:209–213.

760. Niitani H, Horikoshi N, Hasegawa K, Fukuoka M, Kudoh S, Hino M. Phase I study of KW-2189, a derivative of new anticancer antibiotic duocarmycin. Proc AACR 1995;36:243a.

761. Ariyoshi Y, Ota K, Suzuki A, et al. Phase I study of Libomycin (NK313). Proc Am Soc Clin Oncol 1989;8:287a.

762. Yoshida T, Ogawa M, Ota K, et al. Phase II study of NK313 in malignant lymphomas: an NK313 Malignant Lymphoma Study Group trial. Cancer Chemother Pharmacol 1993;31:445–448.

763. Floridi A, Paggi MG, D'Atri S, et al. Effect of lonidamine on the metabolism of Ehrlich ascites tumor cells. Cancer Res 1981;41:4661–4666.

764. Floridi A, Paggi MG, D'Atri S, et al. Lonidamine, a selective inhibitor of aerobic glycolysis of murine tumor cells. J Natl Cancer Inst 1981;66:497–499.

765. Floridi A, Gamacurta A, Bagnato A, Bianchi C, Paggi MG. Modulation of adriamycin uptake by lonidamine in Ehrlich ascites tumor cells. Exp Mol Pathol 1988;49:421–431.

766. Floridi A, Bianchi C, Bagnato A, et al. Lonidamine-induced outer membrane permeability and susceptibility of mitochondria to inhibition by adriamycin. Anticancer Res 1987;7:1149–1152.

767. Schwartz GN, Teicher BA, Eder JPJ, et al. Modulation of antitumor alkylating agents by novobiocin, topotecan, and lonidamine. Cancer Chemother Pharmacol 1993;32:455–462.

768. Silvestrini R, Zaffaroni N, Villa R, Orlandi L, Costa A. Enhancement of cisplatin activity by lonidamine in human ovarian cancer cells. Int J Cancer 1992; 52:813–817.

769. Kiura K, Ohnoshi T, Ueoka H, et al. An adriamycin-resistant subline is more sensitive than the parent human small cell lung cancer cell line to lonidamine. Anticancer Drug Des 1992;7:463–470.

770. Band PR, Deschamps M, Besner JG, et al. Phase I toxicologic study of lonidamine in cancer patients. Oncology 1984;41(Suppl 1):56–59.

771. Murray N, Shah A, Band P. Phase II study of lonidamine in patients with small cell carcinoma of the lung. Cancer Treat Rep 1987;71:1283–1284.

772. Band PR, Maroun J, Pritchard K, et al. Phase II study of lonidamine in patients with metastatic breast cancer: a National Cancer Institute of Canada Clinical Trials Group study. Cancer Treat Rep 1986; 70:1305–1310.

773. Privitera G, Ciottoli GB, Patane C, et al. Phase II double-blind randomized study of lonidamine and radiotherapy in epidermoid carcinoma of the lung. Radiother Oncol 1987;10:285–290.

774. Filipazzi V, Cattaneo MT, Rho B, et al. Cisplatin plus epirubicin and etoposide followed by irradiation plus lonidamine in stage III nonsmall cell lung cancer. Oncology 1993;50:10–13.

775. Scarantino CW, McCunniff AJ, Evans G, Young CW, Paggiarino DA. A prospective randomized comparison of radiation therapy plus lonidamine versus radiation therapy plus placebo as initial treatment of clinically localized but nonresectable nonsmall cell lung cancer. Int J Radiat Oncol Biol Phys 1994;29:999–1004.

776. Buccheri G, Ferrigno D, Rosso A. A phase II study of methotrexate, doxorubicin, cyclophosphamide, and lomustine chemotherapy and lonidamine in advanced non-small cell lung cancer. Cancer 1993; 72:1564–1572.

777. Stewart DJ, Eapen L, Girard A, Verma S, Genest P, Evans WK. Phase II study of lonidamine plus radiotherapy in the treatment of brain metastases. J Neurooncol 1993;15:19–22.

778. Magno L, Terraneo F, Bertoni F, et al. Double-

blind randomized study of lonidamine and radiotherapy in head and neck cancer. Int J Radiat Oncol Biol Phys 1994;29:45–55.

779. Colella E, Merlano M, Blengio F, et al. Randomized phase II study of methotrexate (MTX) versus methotrexate plus lonidamine (MTX + LND) in recurrent and/or metastatic carcinoma of the head and neck. Eur J Cancer 1994;30A:928–930.

780. Von Hoff DD. MGBG: teaching an old drug new tricks. Ann Oncol 1994;6:487–493.

781. Berlin J, Stewart J, Tutsch K, et al. Phase I and pharmacokinetic trial of penclomedine (NSC 338720). Proc AACR 1995;36:238a.

782. Call TG, Stenson MJ, Witzig.TE. Effects of phenylacetate on cells from patients with B-chronic lymphocytic leukemia. Leuk Lymphoma 1994;14:145–149.

783. Ram Z, Samid D, Walbridge S, et al. Growth inhibition, tumor maturation, and extended survival in experimental tumors in rats with phenylacetate. Cancer Res 1994;54:2923–2927.

784. Samid D, Ram Z, Hudgins WR, et al. Selective activity of phenylacetate against malignant gliomas: resemblance to fetal brain damage in phenylketonuria. Cancer Res 1994;54:891–895.

785. Samid D, Hudgins WR, Shack S, et al. Phenylacetate: exploring new targets for cancer intervention. Ann Oncol 1994;5(Suppl 5):150a.

786. Samid D, Shack S, Myers CE. Selective growth arrest and phenotypic reversion of prostate cancer cells in vitro by nontoxic pharmacological concentrations of phenylacetate. J Clin Invest 1993;91:2288–2295.

787. Thibault A, Cooper MR, Figg WD, et al. A phase I and pharmacokinetic study of intravenous phenylacetate in patients with cancer. Cancer Res 1994; 54:1690–1694.

788. Boote DJ, Dennis IF, Twentyman PR, et al. A phase I study of intravenous SDZ PSC-833 in combination with etoposide in patients with advanced cancer. Ann Oncol 1994;5(Suppl 5):159a.

789. Fisher GA, Hausdorff J, Collins H, et al. Phase I clinical trial of etoposide with PSC833, a potent inhibitor of multidrug resistance (MDR). Ann Oncol 1994;5(Suppl 5):158.

790. Hill BT, van der Graaf WT, Hosking LK, de Vries EG, Mulder NH, Whelan RD. Evaluation of S9788 as a potential modulator of drug resistance against human tumour sublines expressing differing resistance mechanisms in vitro. Int J Cancer 1993; 55:330–337.

791. Julia AM, Roche H, Berlion M, et al. Multidrug resistance circumvention by a new triazinoaminopiperidine derivative S9788 in vitro: definition of the optimal schedule and comparison with verapamil. Br J Cancer 1994;69:868–874.

792. Huet S, Chapey C, Robert J. Reversal of multidrug resistance by a new lipophilic cationic molecule, S9788. Comparison with 11 other MDR-modulating agents in a model of doxorubicin-resistant rat glioblastoma cells. Eur J Cancer 1993;29A:1377–1383.

793. Perez V, Pierre A, Leonce S, Anstett M, Atassi G. Effect of duration of exposure to S9788, cyclosporin A or verapamil on sensitivity of multidrug resistant cells to vincristine or doxorubicin. Anticancer Res 1993; 13:985–990.

794. Rossi JF, Sarkany M, Khayat D, et al. Phase I

trial of S9788. A multidrug resistance (MDR) modulator as a 4.5 hour fractionated infusion. Fifth International Congress of Anti-Cancer Chemotherapy 1995; 159a.

795. Chan KK, Hong PS, Tutsch K, Trump DL. Clinical pharmacokinetics of cyclophosphamide and metabolites with and without SR-2508. Cancer Res 1994;54:6421–6429.

796. Minchinton AI, Lemmon MJ, Tracy M, et al. Second-generation of 1,2,4-benzotriazine 1,4-di-N-oxide bioreductive anti-tumor agents: pharmacology and activity in vitro and in vivo. Int J Radiat Oncol Biol Phys 1992;22:701–705.

797. Walton MI, Workman P. Pharmacokinetics and bioreductive metabolism of the novel benzotriazine di-N-oxide hypoxic cell cytotoxin tirapazamine (WIN 59075; SR 4233; NSC 130181) in mice. J Pharmacol Exp Ther 1993;265:938–947.

798. Brown JM. SR 4233 (tirapazamine): a new anticancer drug exploiting hypoxia in solid tumors. Br J Cancer 1993;67:1163–1170.

799. Lambin P, Guichard M, Chavaudra N, Malaise EP. The effect of the hypoxic cell drug SR-4233 alone or combined with the ionizing radiations on two human tumor cell lines having different radiosensitivity. Radiother Oncol 1992;24:201–204.

800. Dorie MJ, Brown JM Tumor-specific, schedule-dependent interaction between tirapazamine (SR 4233) and cisplatin. Cancer Res 1993;53:4633–4636.

801. Baas P, Oppelaar H, Stavenuiter M, van Zandwijk N, Stewart FA. Interaction of the bioreductive drug SR 4233 and photodynamic therapy using photofrin in a mouse tumor model. Int J Radiat Oncol Biol Phys 1993;27:665–670.

802. Wilder RB, McGann JK, Sutherland WR, et al. The hypoxic cytotoxic SR 4233 increases the effectiveness of radioimmunotherapy in mice with human non-Hodgkin's lymphoma xenografts. Int J Radiat Oncol Biol Phys 1994;28:119–126.

803. Coleman CN, Buswell L, Riese N, et al. A phase I study of multiple dose tirapazamine (Tira, SR4233) given concurrently with radiation therapy (RT). Fifth International Congress of Anti-Cancer Chemotherapy 1995:115a.

804. Doherty N, Hancoock SL, Kaye S, et al. Muscle cramping in phase I clinical trials of tirapazamine (SR 4233) with and without radiation. Int J Radiat Oncol Biol Phys 1994;29:379–382.

805. Ara G, Coleman CN, Teicher BA. SR-4233 (Tirapazamine) acts as an uncoupler of oxidative phosphorylation in human MCF-7 breast carcinoma cells. Cancer Lett 1994;85:195–203.

806. O'Dwyer PJ, Kilpatrick D, Langer C, et al. Phase I and pharmacokinetic study of cisplatin in combination with the hypoxic cell bioreductive agent tirapazamine (WIN 59075 SR 4233). Fifth International Congress of Anti-Cancer Chemotherapy 1995;130a.

807. Senan S, Rampling R, Wilson P, et al. Phase I and pharmacokinetic study of tirapazamine (SR4233), a highly selective hypoxic cell cytotoxin. Ann Oncol 1994;5(Suppl 5):135a.

808. Korczak B, Dennis JW. Inhibition of N-linked oligosaccharide processing in tumor cells is associated with enhanced tissue inhibitor of metalloproteinases (TIMP) gene expression. Int J Cancer 1993;53:634–639.

809. Bowen D, Adir J, White SL, Bowen CD, Mat-

sumoto K, Olden K. A preliminary pharmacokinetic evaluation of the antimetastatic immunomodulator swainsonine: clinical and toxic implications. Anticancer Res 1993;13:841–844.

810. Goss PE, Baptiste J, Fernandes B, Baker M, Dennis JW. A phase I study of swainsonine in patients with advanced malignancies. Cancer Res 1994; 54:1450–1457.

811. Baptista JA, Goss P, Nghiem M, Krepinsky JJ, Baker M, Dennis JW. Measuring swainsonine in serum of cancer patients: phase I clinical trial. Clin Chem 1994;40:426–430.

812. Wong PP, Currie VE, Mackey RW, et al. Phase I evaluation of tetrahydrouridine combined with cytosine arabinoside. Cancer Treat Rep 1979;63:1245–1249.

813. Kreis W, Chan K, Budman DR, et al. Effect of tetrahydrouridine on the clinical pharmacology of 1-B-D-arabinofuranosylcytosine when both drugs are coinfused over three hours. Cancer Res 1988;48:1337–1342.

814. Kreis W, Budman DR, Allen S, et al. Phase I-II study and clinical pharmacology for the combination of ara-C plus tetrahydrouridine (THU) in relapsed/refractory leukemia. Proc AACR 1989;30:1056a.

815. Poplack DG, Riccardi R. Pharmacologic approaches to the treatment of central nervous system malignancy. Dev Oncol 1987;44:137–156.

816. LoRusso PM, Graham MA, Purvis J, et al. Phase I pharmacokinetic study of the novel antitumor agent WIN 33377. Proc AACR 1995;36:238a.

817. Schilder RJ, DeMaria D, Purvis J, et al. Phase I pharmacokinetic study of the novel thioxantone antitumor agent WIN 33377 on a five daily dose schedule. Proc AACR 1995;36:240a.

818. Pinzani V, Bressolle F, Haug IJ, Galtier M, Blayac JP, Balmès P. Cisplatin-induced renal toxicity and toxicity-modulating strategies: a review. Cancer Chemother Pharmacol 1994;35:1–9.

819. Gandara DR, Nahhas WA, Adelson MD, et al. Randomized placebo-controlled multicenter evaluation of diethyldithiocarbamate for chemoprotection against cisplatin induced toxicities. J Clin Oncol 1995; 13:490–496.

820. Muggia FM, Los G. Platinum resistance: laboratory findings and clinical implications. Stem Cells 1993;11:182–193.

821. Mellish KJ, Kelland LR. Mechanisms of acquired resistance to the orally active platinum-based anticancer drug bis-aceto-amine-dichloro-cyclohexylamine platinum (IV) (JM216) in two human ovarian carcinoma cell lines. Cancer Res 1995;54:6194–6200.

822. Meijer C, Mulder NH, Timmer-Bosscha H, Sluiter WJ, Meersma GJ, de Vries EG. Relationship of cellular glutathione to the cytotoxicity and resistance of seven platinum compounds. Cancer Res 1992; 52:6885–6889.

823. Kelland LR, Barnard CFJ, Mellish KJ, et al. A novel trans-platinum coordination complex possessing in vitro and in vivo antitumor activity. Cancer Res 1994;54:5618–5622.

824. Extra JM, Espie M, Calvo M, Ferme C, Mignot L, Marty M. Phase I study of oxaliplatin in patients with advanced cancer. Cancer Chemother Pharmacol 1990;25:299–303.

825. Schilder RJ, LaCreta FP, Perez RP, et al. Phase I and pharmacokinetic study of Ormaplatin (Tetrapla-

tin, NSC 363812) administered on a day 1 and day 8 schedule. Cancer Res 1994;54:709–717.

826. Mellish KJ, Kelland LR, Harrap KR. In vitro platinum drug chemosensitivity of intrinsic and acquired cisplatin-resistant human cervical carcinoma cell lines. Br J Cancer 1993;68:240–250.

827. Loh SY, Mistry P, Kelland LR, Abel G, Harrap KR. Reduced drug accumulation as a major mechanism of acquired resistance to cisplatin in a human ovarian carcinoma cell line: circumvention studies using novel platinum (II) and (IV) ammine/amine complexes. Br J Cancer 1992;66:1109–1115.

828. Christian MC. The current status of new platinum analogs. Semin Oncol 1992;19:720–733.

829. Weiss RB, Christian MC. New cisplatin analogues in development. A review. Drugs 1993;46:360–377.

830. Kelland LR. New platinum antitumor complexes. Crit Rev Oncol Hematol 1993;3:191–219.

831. Farrell N. Nonclassical platinum antitumor agents: perspectives for design and development of new drugs complementary to cisplatin. Cancer Invest 1993;11:578–589.

832. Gorbunova VA, Smirnova NB, Orel NF, Konovalova AL, Singin AS. A phase I and pharmacokinetic trial of cycloplatam in patients with refractory solid tumors. Ann Oncol 1994;5(Suppl 5):126a.

833. Presnov MA, Konovalova AL. Cycloplatam and Oxoplatin—the new antitumor platinum compounds of the second generation. Arch Geschwulstforsch 1988;58:43–49.

834. Gorbunova VA, Smirnova NB, Orel NF. Phase II of cycloplatam in advanced ovarian carcinoma. Fifth International Congress of Anti-Cancer Chemotherapy 1995;232a.

835. Ota K. New platinum derivatives in Japan. Int Cong Ser 1987;776:329–338.

836. Koizumi M, Honda M, Morikawa K, et al. Antitumor activity of a new platinum cytostatic, DWA2114R. Dev Oncol 1988;54:695–699.

837. Majima H, Kinoshita H. Clinical pharmacokinetics of (R)-(-)-1,1-cyclobutane-dicarboxylato-(2-aminomethylpyrrolidine) platinum (II) (DWA2114R). Dev Oncol 1988;54:491–498.

838. Majima H, Ohta K. Phase I and clinical pharmacokinetic studies of DWA2114R. Proc Am Soc Clin Oncol 1988;7:219a.

839. Niitani H, Fukuoka M, Furusawa M, et al. A phase I study on a weekly schedule of DWA2114R. Gan To Kagaku Ryoho 1992;19:1027–1032.

840. Judson I, McKeage M, Raynaud F, et al. A phase I trial of the oral platinum anticancer drug JM 216 [AF-bis(acetato)-B-ammine-CD-dichloro-E-cyclohexylamine platinum (IV)]. Ann Oncol 1994;5(Suppl 5):126a.

841. McKeage MJ, Mistry P, Ward J, Boxall FE, Loh S. Phase I study of orally administered ammine diacetodichloro (cyclohexylamine)platinum (Pt) (IV) (po JM216). Proc Am Soc Clin Oncol 1993;12:130a.

842. Kizu R, Higashi S, Kidani Y, Miyazaki M. Pharmacokinetics of (1R, 2R-diaminocyclohexane) oxalatoplatinum(II) in comparison with cisplatin following a single intravenous injection in rabbits. Cancer Chemother Pharmacol 1993;31:475–480.

843. Brienza S, Gastiaburu J, Cvitkovic E, et al. Clinical characteristics and reversiblity of neurological

signs after long term oxaliplatin (L-OHP-Transplatin) therapy. Ann Oncol 1994;5(Suppl 5):128a.

844. Brienza S, Fandi A, Hugret F, et al. Neurotoxicity of long term oxaliplatin therapy. Proc AACR 1993; 34:406a.

845. Krikorian A, Vignoud J, Brienza S, Itzhaki M. Oxaliplatin (L-OHP): global safety. Fifth International Congress of Anti-Cancer Chemotherapy 1995;257a.

846. Diaz-Rubio E, Marty M, Extra JM, et al. Multicentric phase II study with oxaliplatin (L-OHP) in 5-FU refractory patients with advanced colorectal cancer. Fifth International Congress of Anti-Cancer Chemotherapy 1995;161a.

847. de Gramont A, Tournigand C, Louvet C, et al. High-dose folinic acid, 5-fluorouracil 48h infusion and oxaliplatin in metastatic colorectal cancer. Fifth International Congress of Anti-Cancer Chemotherapy 1995; 114a.

848. Mross K, Meyberg L, Fiebig H, et al. Pharmacokinetics of the platinum derivate D-19466. Eur J Cancer 1991;52:s197.

849. Gietema JA, Guchelaaer H-J, deVries EGE, Aulenbacher P, Sleijfer DT, Mulder NH. A phase I study of lobaplatin (D-19466) administered by 72h continuous infusion. Anti-Cancer Drugs 1993;4:51–55.

850. Gietema JA, de Vries EG, Sleijfer DT, et al. A phase I study of 1,2-diamminomethyl-cyclobutane-platinum(II)-lactate (D-19466; lobaplatin) administered daily for 5 days. Br J Cancer 1993;67:396–401.

851. Gietema JA, Cats A, Guchelaar HJ, et al. A phase II study with lobaplatin (D-19466) in patients with relapsed ovarian cancer. Ann Oncol 1994;5(Suppl 5):128a.

852. Degardin M, de Forni M, Chevallier B, et al. Phase II study of lobaplatin in head and neck cancer (HNC). Ann Oncol 1994;5(Suppl 5):126a.

853. Inoue S, Mizuno S. Cytometric characterization of cisplatin and a new platinum analog, TRK-710. Fifth International Congress of Anti-Cancer Chemotherapy 1995;214a.

854. Elliott WL, Roberts BJ, Howard CT, Leopold WR III. Chemotherapy with [SP-4–3-(R)]-[1,1-cyclobutanedicarboxylato(2-)](2-methyl-1,4-butanediamine-N,N') platinum (CI-973, NK121) in combination with standard agents against murine tumors in vivo. Cancer Res 1994;54:4412–4418.

855. Kurbacher CM, Mallmann P, Kurbacher JA, et al. In vitro activity of titaneocenedichloride versus cisplatin and doxorubicin in primary and recurrent epithelial ovarian cancer. Anticancer Res 1994;14:1961–1966.

856. Koepf-Maier P, Gerlach S. Pattern of toxicity by titanocene dichloride in mice. Blood and urine chemical parameters. J Cancer Res Clin Oncol 1986; 111:243–247.

857. Koepf-Maier P, Gerlach S. Pattern of toxicity by titanocene dichloride in mice. Hematologic parameters. Anticancer Res 1986;6:235–240.

858. Harstrick A, Schmoll HJ, Sass G, Poliwoda H, Rustum Y. Titanocenedichloride activity in cisplatin and doxorubicin-resistant human ovarian carcinoma cell lines. Eur J Cancer 1993;29A:1000–1002.

859. Kurbacher CM, Nagel W, Mallmann P, et al. In vitro activity of titanocenedichloride in human renal cell carcinoma compared to conventional antineoplastic agents. Anticancer Res 1994;14:1529–1533.

860. Budman DR, Igwemezie LN, Kaul S, et al. Phase I evaluation of a water-soluble etoposide prodrug, etoposide phosphate, given as a 5-minute infusion on days 1, 3, and 5 in patients with solid tumors. J Clin Oncol 1994;12:1902–1909.

861. Fields SZ, Igwemezie LN, Kaul S, et al. Phase I study of etoposide phosphate (etopophos) as a 30-minute infusion on days 1, 3, and 5. Clin Cancer Res 1995;1:105–111.

862. Kreis W, Budman DR, Fields SZ, Hock K, Schacter LP. Pharmacologic evaluation of high dose etoposide phosphate with G-CSF administered as a 2 hour infusion daily × 2 in patients with solid tumors. Proc AACR 1995;36:233a.

863. Sessa C, Zucchetti M, Cerny T, et al. Phase I clinical and pharmacokinetic study of oral etoposide phosphate. J Clin Oncol 1995;13:200–209.

864. Moore MJ, Erlichman C, Pillon L, Manzo J, Thiessen JJ, Eisenhauer A. A phase I study of fostriecin in a daily × 5 schedule. Proc AACR 1995;36:239.

865. Furue H. Topoisomerase inhibitors in Japan. Gan To Kagaku Ryoho 1993;20:42–49.

866. Tashiro T, Kon K, Yamamoto M, Yamada N, Tsuruo T, Tsukagoshi S. Antitumor effects of IST-622, a novel synthetic derivative of chartreusin, against murine and human tumor lines following oral administration. Cancer Chemother Pharmacol 1994;34:287–292.

867. Hino M, Niitani H. DNA topoisomerase inhibitor. Nippon Rinsho 1993;51:3291–3300.

868. Takigawa N, Ohnoshi T, Ueoka H, et al. In vitro comparison of podophyllotoxin analogues; etoposide, teniposide and NK 611 using human lung cancer cell lines. Gan To Kagaku Ryoho 1993;20:473–477.

869. Zucchetti M, De Fusco M, Sessa C, Frohlich A, Reichert S, D'Incalci M. High-performance liquid chromatographic assay for the determination of the novel podophyllotoxin derivative dimethylaminoetoposide (NK611) in human plasma. J Chromatogr Biomed Appl 1994;654:97–102.

870. Schilling T, Mross K, Berdel WR, et al. Phase I clinical and pharmacokinetic trial of the podophyllotoxin derivative NK611. Ann Oncol 1994;5(Suppl 5):193a.

871. Fukuoka M, Takada M, Negoro S, Furuse K, Niitani H. Phase I and pharmacokinetic study of NK611 (dimethylaminoetoposide): daily 1-hour intravenous infusion for 5 days—Cooperative Study Group of NK611 in Japan. Ann Oncol 1994;5(Suppl 5):193a.

872. Catimel G, Coquart R, Guastalla JP, et al. Phase I study of RP 49532A, a new protein-synthesis inhibitor, in patients with advanced refractory solid tumors. Cancer Chemother Pharmacol 1995;35:246–248.

873. Alakl M, Armand JP, Gandia D, et al. Phase I and pharmacokinetics of RP 49532: giroline in cancer patients. Proc AACR 1991;10:310.

874. Bibow K, Jonsson G, Larsen R, Solheim E, Ramdahl T, Dornish JM. In vivo metabolism of zilascorb(2H). Ann Oncol 1994;5(Suppl 5):178a.

875. Klem B, Bibow K, Ramdahl T, Boyce M, Osmundsen K. The bioavailability of zilascorb(2H) is increased by concurrent administration of a gastric acid inhibitor. Ann Oncol 1994;5(Suppl 5):177a.

876. Warrell RPJ. Applications for retinoids in cancer therapy. Semin Hematol 1994;31(Suppl 5):1–13.

877. Lotan R, Dawson MI, Zou C-C, Jong L, Lotan

D, Zou C-P. Enhanced efficacy of combinations of retinoic acid- and retinoid X receptor-selective retinoids and α-interferon in inhibition of cervical carcinoma cell proliferation. Cancer Res 1995;55:232–236.

878. Bollag W, Holdener EF. Retinoids in cancer prevention and therapy. Ann Oncol 1992;3:513–526.

879. Hong WK, Itri LM. Retinoids and human cancer. In: Sporn MB, Roberts AB, Goodman DS, eds. The retinoids. New York: Raven Press, 1994:597–658.

880. Smith MA, Parkinson DR, Cheson BD, Friedman MA. Retinoids in cancer therapy. J Clin Oncol 1992;10:839–864.

881. Tallman MS All-*trans*-retinoic acid in acute promyelocytic leukemia and its potential in other hematologic malignancies. Semin Hematol 1994;31(Suppl 5):38–48.

882. Warrell RPJ, de Thé H, Wang ZY, et al. Acute promyelocytic leukemia. N Engl J Med 1993;329:177–189.

883. Castaigne S, Chomienne C, Daniel MT, et al. All-*trans*-retinoic acid as a differentiation therapy for acute promyelocytic leukemia. I. Clinical results. Blood 1990;76:1704–1709.

884. Muindi JR, Frankel SR, Huselton C, et al. Clinical pharmacology of oral all-*trans* retinoic acid in patients with acute promyelocytic leukemia. Cancer Res 1992;52:2138–2142.

885. Chen ZX, Xue YQ, Zhang R, et al. A clinical and experimental study on all-*trans* retinoic acid-treated acute promyelocytic leukemia patients. Blood 1991;78:1413–1419.

886. Frankel SR, Eardley A, Lauwers G, et al. The "retinoic acid syndrome" in acute promyelocytic leukemia. Ann Intern Med 1992;117:292–296.

887. Adamson PC. Pharmacokinetics of all-*trans*-retinoic acid: clinical implications in acute promyelocytic leukemia. Semin Hematol 1994;31(Suppl 5):14–17.

888. Benner SE, Lippman SM, Hong WK. Retinoid chemoprevention of second primary tumors. Semin Hematol 1994;31(Suppl 5):26–30.

889. Koeffler HP, Keitjan D, Mertelsmann R, et al. Randomized study of 13-*cis*-retinoic acid v placebo in the myelodysplastic disorders. Blood 1988;71:703–708.

890. Cobleigh MA, Dowlatshahi K, Deutsch TA, et al. Phase I/II trial of tamoxifen with or without fenretinide, an analog of vitamin A, in women with metastatic breast cancer. J Clin Oncol 1993;11:474–477.

891. Costa A, Formelli F, Chiesa F, Decensi A, De Palo G, Veronesi U. Prospects of chemoprevention of human cancers with the synthetic retinoid fenretinide. Cancer Res 1994;54(Suppl 7):2032s–2037s.

892. Mariotti A, Marcora E, Bunone G, et al. N-(4-hydroxyphenyl)retinamide: a potent inducer of apoptosis in human neuroblastoma cells. J Natl Cancer Inst 1994;86:1245–1247.

893. Arnold A, Hirte H, Kowaleski B, et al. A phase I trial of the arotinoid RO 40–8757 in patients with solid tumors. Ann Oncol 1994;5(Suppl 5):148a.

894. Burke TRJ. Protein-tyrosine kinases: potential targets for anticancer drug development. Stem Cells 1994;12:1–6.

895. Inglese J, Koch WJ, Caron MG, Lefkowitz RJ. Isoprenylation in regulation of signal transduction by G-protein-coupled receptor kinases. Nature 1992; 359:147–150.

896. Roberge M, Tudan C, Hung SMF, Harder KW, Jirik FR, Anderson H. Antitumor drug fostriecin inhibits the mitotic entry checkpoint and protein phosphatases 1 and 2A. Cancer Res 1995;54:6115–6121.

897. Moore MJ, Erlichman C, Pillon L, Thiessen JJ, Eisenhauer E. A phase I clinical and pharmacokinetic study of fostriecin in a daily × 5 schedule. Ann Oncol 1994;5(Suppl 5):188a.

898. Christen RD, Isonishi S, Jones JA, et al. Signaling and drug sensitivity. Cancer Metastasis Rev 1994;13:175–189.

899. Yano T, Pinski J, Groot K, Schally AV. Stimulation by bombesin and inhibition by bombesin/gastrin-releasing peptide antagonist RC-3095 of human breast cancer cell lines. Cancer Res 1992;52:4545–4547.

900. Qin Y, Halmos G, Cai R-Y, Szoke B, Ertl T, Schally AV. Bombesin antagonists inhibit in vitro and in vivo growth of human gastric cancer and binding of bombesin to its receptors. Cancer Res Clin Oncol 1994;120:519–528.

901. Szepeshazi K, Schally AV, Groot K, Halmos G. Effect of bombesin, gastrin-releasing peptide (GRP)(14–27) and bombesin/GRP receptor antagonist RC-3095 on growth of nitrosoamine-induced pancreatic cancers in hamsters. Int J Cancer 1993;54:282–289.

902. Pinski J, Halmos G, Szepeshazi K, Schally AV. Antagonists of bombesin/gastrin-releasing peptides as adjuncts to agonists of luteinizing hormone-releasing hormone in the treatment of experimental prostate cancer. Cancer 1993;72:3263–3270.

903. Watson SA, Steele RJ. Gastrin antagonists in the treatment of gastric cancer. Anti-Cancer Drugs 1993;4:599–604.

904. Langdon S, Sethi T, Ritchie A, Muir M, Smyth J, Rozengurt E. Broad spectrum neuropeptide antagonists inhibit the growth of small cell lung cancer in vivo. Cancer Res 1992;52:4554–4557.

905. Abbruzzese JL, Gholson CF, Daugherty K, et al. A pilot clinical trial of the cholecystokinin receptor antagonist MK-329 in patients with advanced pancreatic cancer. Pancreas 1992;72:165–171.

906. Kitagawa M, Okabe T, Ogino H, et al. Butyrolactone I, a selective inhibitor of cdk2 and cdc2 kinase. Oncogene 1993;8:2425–2432.

907. Vesely J, Havlicek L, Strnad M, et al. Inhibition of cyclin-dependent kinases by purine analogues. Eur J Biochem 1994;224:771–786.

908. Levitzki A. Tyrphostins: tyrosine kinase blockers as novel antiproliferative agents and dissectors of signal transduction. FASEB J 1992;6:3275–3282.

909. Levitzki A, Gazit A. Tyrosine kinase inhibition: an approach to drug development. Science 1995; 267:1782–1788.

910. Matsukawa Y, Marui N, Sakai T, et al. Genistein arrests cell cycle progression at G2-M. Cancer Res 1993;93:1328–1331.

911. Fry DW, Kraker AJ, McMichael A, et al. A specific inhibitor of the epidermal growth factor receptor tyrosine kinase. Science 1994;265:1093–1095.

912. Hennings H, Blumberg PM, Pettit GR, et al. Bryostatin 1, an activator of protein kinase C, inhibits tumor promotion by phorbol esters in SENCAR mouse skin. Carcinogenesis 1987;8:1343–1346.

913. Hornung RL, Pearson JW, Beckwith M, et al. Preclinical evaluation of bryostatin as an anticancer agent against several murine tumor cell lines: in vitro versus in vivo activity. Cancer Res 1992;52:101–107.

914. Grant S, Jarvis WD, Turner AJ, Wallace HJ, Pettit GR. Effects of brystatin 1 and rGM-CSF on the metabolism of 1-β-D-arabinofuranosylcytosine in human leukaemic myeloblasts. Br J Haematol 1992; 82:522–528.

915. Mohammad RM, al-Katib A, Pettit GR, Sensenbrenner LL. Successful treatment of human Waldenstrom's macroglobulinemia with combination biological and chemotherapy agents. Cancer Res 1994; 54:165–168.

916. Kraft AS. Bryostatin 1: will the oceans provide a cancer cure? J Natl Cancer Inst 1993;85:1790–1792.

917. Prendiville J, Crowther D, Thatcher N, et al. A phase I study of intravenous bryostatin 1 in patients with advanced cancer. Br J Cancer 1993;68:418–424.

918. Jayson GC, Prendiville JA, Crowther D, et al. A phase I trial of bryostatin 1 in advanced cancer. Ann Oncol 1994;5(Suppl 5):139a.

919. Philip PA, Rea D, Thavasu P, et al. Phase I study of bryostatin 1: assessment of interleukin-6 and tumor necrosis factor alpha induction in vivo. The Cancer Res Campaign Phase I Committee. J Natl Cancer Inst 1993;85:1812–1818.

920. Langeveld CH, Jongenelen CA, Heimans JJ, Stoof JC. 8-Chloro-cyclic adenosine monophosphate, a novel cyclic AMP analog that inhibits human glioma cell growth in concentrations that do not induce differentiation. Exp Neurol 1992;117:196–203.

921. Langeveld CH, Jongenelen CA, Heimans JJ, Stoof JC. Growth inhibition of human glioma cells induced by 8-chloroadenosine, an active metabolite of 8-chloro cyclic adenosine 3':5'-monophosphate. Cancer Res 1992;52:3994–3999.

922. Ohmura E, Wakai K, Isozaki O, et al. Inhibition of human pancreatic cancer cell (MIA PaCa-2) growth by cholera toxin and 8-chloro-cAMP in vitro. Br J Cancer 1993;67:279–283.

923. Pinto A, Aldinucci D, Gattei V, et al. Inhibition of the self-renewal capacity of blast progenitors from acute myeloblastic leukemia patients by site-selective 8-chloroadenosine 3'-5'cyclic monophosphate. Proc Natl Acad Sci USA 1992;89:8884–8888.

924. Cummings J, Leonard RCF, Miller WR. Preclinical pharmaceutical analysis and preliminary clinical pharmacokinetics of the signal transduction pathway modulator, 8-ClcAMP. Ann Oncol 1994;5(Suppl 5):178a.

925. Harris AL, Salisbury AJ, Talbot DC, Cho-Chung YS, Long L, Miki K. Phase I study of 8-chloro cAMP. Ann Oncol 1994;5(Suppl 5):138a.

926. Tortora G, Ciardiello F, Pepe S, et al. Phase I clinical study with 8-chloro-cAMP and evaluation of immunological effects in cancer patients. Clin Cancer Res 1995;1:377–384.

927. Zilberman Y, Gutman Y. Multiple effects of staurosporine, a kinase inhibitor, on thymocyte functions. Comparison with the effect of tyrosine kinase inhibitors. Biochem Pharmacol 1992;44:1563–1568.

928. Hill DL, Tillery KF, Rose LM, Posey CF. Disposition in mice of 7-hydroxystaurosporine, a protein kinase inhibitor with antitumor activity. Cancer Chemother Pharmacol 1994;35:89–92.

929. Zugmaier G, Lippman ME, Wellstein A. Inhibition by pentosan polysulfate (PPS) of heparin-binding growth factors released from tumor cells and blockage by PPS of tumor growth in animals. J Natl Cancer Inst 1992;84:1716–1724.

930. Srivastava AK, Sekaly RP, Chiasson JL. Pentosan polysulfate, a potent anti HIV and anti tumor agent, inhibits protein serine/threonine and tyrosine kinases. Mol Cell Biochem 1993;120:127–133.

931. Tardy-Boncet B, Tardy B, Grelac F, et al. Pentosan polysulfate-induced thrombocytopenia and thrombosis. Am J Hematol 1994;45:252–257.

932. Parker BW, Swain SM, Zugmaier G, De Lap RL, Lippman ME, Wellstein A. Detectable inhibition of heparin-binding growth factor activity in sera from patients treated with pentosan polysulfate. J Natl Cancer Inst 1993;85:1068–1073.

933. Nakayama Y, Iwahana M, Sakamoto N, Tanaka NG, Osada Y. Inhibitory effects of a bacteria-derived sulfated polysaccharide against basic fibroblast growth factor-induced endothelial cell growth and chemotaxis. J Cell Physiol 1993;154:1–6.

934. Eisenberger MA, Reyno LM. Suramin. Cancer Treat Rev 1994;20:259–273.

935. Ono K, Nakane H, Fukushima M. Differential inhibition of various deoxyribonucleic and ribonucleic acid polymerases by suramin. Eur J Biochem 1988; 172:349–353.

936. Lopez-Lopez R, Langeveld CH, Pizao PE, et al. Effect of suramin on adenylate cyclase and protein kinase C. Anticancer Drug Des 1994;9:279–290.

937. Sartor O, McLellan CA, Myers CE, Borner MM. Suramin rapidly alters cellular tyrosine phosphorylation in prostate cancer cell lines. J Clin Invest 1992;90:2166–2174.

938. Foekens JA, Sieuwerts AM, Stuurman-Smeets EM, Peters HA, Klijn JG. Effects of suramin on cell-cycle kinetics of MCF-7 human breast cancer cells in vitro. Br J Cancer 1993;67:232–236.

939. Stein CA, LaRocca RV, Thomas R, McAtee N, Myers CE. Suramin: an anticancer drug with a unique mechanism of action. J Clin Oncol 1989;7:499–508.

940. Bergh J. Suramin is a potent inhibitor of cell proliferation in human non-small cell lung cancer lines. Proc Am Soc Clin Oncol 1989;8:214a.

941. Spigelman Z, Dowers A, Kennedy S, et al. Antiproliferative effects of suramin on lymphoid cells. Cancer Res 1987;47:4694–4698.

942. Horne MK, Stein CA, LaRocca RV, Myers CE. Circulating glycosaminoglycan anticoagulants associated with suramin treatment. Blood 1988;71:273–279.

943. Cooper M, LaRocca R, Stein C, Myers CE. Pharmacokinetic monitoring is necessary for the safe use of suramin as an anticancer drug. Proc AACR 1989; 30:963.

944. LaRocca R, Stein C, Myers C, Dalakas M, McAtee N. Suramin induced acute polyneuropathy. Proc Am Soc Clin Oncol 1989;8:227.

945. van Rijswijk RE, van Loenen AC, Wagstaff J, et al. Suramin: rapid loading and weekly maintenance regimens for cancer patients. J Clin Oncol 1992; 10:1789–1794.

946. Eisenberger MA, Reyno LM, Jodrell DI, et al. Suramin, an active drug for prostate cancer: interim observations in a phase I trial. J Natl Cancer Inst 1993; 85:594–597.

947. Jodrell DI, Reyno LM, Sridhara R, et al. Suramin: development of a population pharmacokinetic model and its use with intermittent short infusions to control plasma drug concentrations in patients with prostate cancer. J Clin Oncol 1994;12:166–175.

948. Myers CE, Stein C, LaRocca R, Cooper M, Cas-

sidy J, McAtee N. Suramin: an antagonist of heparin-binding tumor growth factors with activity against a broad spectrum of human tumors. Proc Am Soc Clin Oncol 1989;8:256.

949. Rago RP, Miles JM, Sufit RL, Spriggs DR, Wilding G. Suramin-induced weakness from hypophosphatemia and mitochondrial myopathy. Association of suramin with mitochondrial toxicity in humans. Cancer 1994;73:1954–1959.

950. Arit W, Reincke M, Siekmann L, Winkelmann W, Allolio B. Suramin in adrenocortical cancer: limited efficacy and serious toxicity. Clin Endocrinol 1994; 41:299–307.

951. Figg WD, Cooper MR, Thibault A, et al. Acute renal toxicity associated with suramin in the treatment of prostate cancer. Cancer 1994;74:1612–1614.

952. Cole DJ, Ettinghausen SE, Pass HI, et al. Postoperative complications in patients receiving suramin therapy. Surgery 1994;116:90–95.

953. Gazit A, Osherov N, Posner I, Bar-Sinai A, Gilon C, Levitzki A. Tyrphostins. 3. Structure-activity relationship studies of α-substituted benzylidenemalononitrile 5-S-aryltyrphostins. J Med Chem 1993;36:3556–3564.

954. Kovalenko M, Gazit A, Böhmer A, et al. Selective platelet-derived growth factor receptor kinase blockers reverse sis-transformation. Cancer Res 1994; 54:6106–6114.

955. Osherov N, Gazit A, Gilon C, Levitzki A. Selective inhibition of the epidermal growth factor and HER2/neu receptors by tyrphostins. J Biol Chem 1993; 268:11134–11142.

956. Hamel E. Natural products which interact with tubulin in the vinca domain: maytansine, rhizoxin, phomopsin A, dolastins 10 and 15 and halichondrin B. Pharmacol Ther 1992;55:31–51.

957. Paull KD, Lin CM, Malspeis L, Hamel E. Identification of novel antimitotic agents acting at the tubulin level by computer-assisted evaluation of differential cytotoxicity data. Cancer Res 1992;52:3893–3900.

958. de Ines C, Leynadier D, Barasoain I, et al. Inhibition of microtubules and cell cycle arrest by a new 1-deaza-7,8-dihydropteridine antitumor drug, CI 980, and by its chiral isomer, NSC 613863. Cancer Res 1994; 54:75–84.

959. Raynaud F, Walton M, Judson I. High-performance liquid chromatographic assay for the measurement of the novel microtubule inhibitor 1069C85 in biological tissues and fluids. J Chromatogr 1993; 622:243–248.

960. MacDonald JR, Pegg DG. Extravasation injury potential of CI-980, a novel synthetic mitotic inhibitor. Cancer Chemother Pharmacol 1993;32:365–367.

961. Gelke CK, Meyers CA, Kudelka AP, et al. Neurotoxicity of CI-980. Proc AACR 1995;36:242a.

962. Rinehart KL, Gravalos LG, Faircloth G, Jimeno J. ET743: preclinical antitumor development of a marine derived natural product. Proc AACR 1995;36:390a.

963. Koyanagi N, Nagasu T, Fujita F, et al. In vivo tumor growth inhibition produced by a novel sulfonamide, E7010, against rodent and human tumors. Cancer Res 1994;54:1702–1706.

964. Tsukagoshi S, Niitani H, Furue H, Taguchi T, Koyanagi N, Kitoh K. A novel tubulin-interacting agent, E7010—its antitumour efficacies and the current clinical status. Ann Oncol 1994;5(Suppl 5):200a.

965. Cocchiaro C, Nelson C, de Arruda M, et al. In vitro cytotoxicity and mechanism of action of LU103793. Proc AACR 1995;36:391a.

966. Calero-Villalona M, Degen D, Barlozzari T, Von Hoff D. LU103793: evaluation by human tumor clonogenic assay of a novel dolastatin. Proc AACR 1995;36:394a.

967. Smith P, Nelson C, Spiegelman M, Robinson S, Barlozzari T. In vivo anti-tumor activity of LU103793: evidence for schedule dependency in MX-1, KB3–1 and P388 tumor models. Proc AACR 1995; 36:394a.

968. Budman DR. New vinca alkaloids and related compounds (review). Semin Oncol 1992;19:639–645.

969. Fox BW. Current results with rhizoxin: the evaluation of a clinical and a basic scientist. Ann Oncol 1992;3:707–709.

970. Takigawa N, Ohnoshi T, Ueoka H, et al. Assessment of antitumor activity rhizoxin for human lung cancer cell lines: a potent new drug for drug-resistant lung cancer. Gan To Kagaku Ryoho 1993; 20:1221–1226.

971. Takahashi M, Matsumoto S, Iwasaki S, et al. Molecular basis for determining the sensitivity of eucaryotes to the antimitotic drug rhizoxin. Mol & Gen Genet 1990;222:169–175.

972. Hendriks HR, Plowman J, Berger DP, et al. Preclinical antitumour activity and animal toxicology studies of rhizoxin, a novel tubulin-interacting agent. Ann Oncol 1992;3:755–763.

973. Raynaud FI, Kelland LR, Walton MI, Judson IR. Preclinical pharmacology of 1069C85, a novel tubulin binder. Cancer Chemother Pharmacol 1994; 35:169–173.

Section Three

Management of Drug Toxicity

27

Hematologic Complications of Cancer Chemotherapy

H. Clark Hoagland and Dennis A. Gastineau

The spectrum of chemotherapeutic agents for neoplasia has continued to expand. As these new agents become available, the hematologic toxicities of these agents become evident. The possibility of a cure or prolonged remission for many hematologic neoplasms has increased significantly with new agents and new combinations of chemotherapeutic agents. Since cytotoxic drugs are not tumor specific, those cells in the body that are normally in active division and replication are severely affected by a cancer-therapeutic compound.

The organ most consistently and frequently affected by cancer chemotherapeutic agents is the bone marrow and, secondarily, the peripheral blood cells (1). The suppression of the stem cells in the marrow or the interference with the active proliferation of a particular cell line is predictable, based on the chemotherapeutic agent being used. The depression of peripheral blood cell lines guides the physician in determining the tolerable dose, the use of drug combinations, the mode of administration, and the frequency of administration of a particular agent or combination of agents.

The bone marrow contains the precursor populations (multipotent stem cells) for all major blood components—namely, erythrocytes, leukocytes, platelets, lymphocytes, and plasma cells. The kinetics of a particular cell line affected by a given drug determine the severity of the depression of that cell line (2, 3). For example, the depression of red blood cells, giving rise to anemia, occurs much more slowly than drug-induced leukopenia (neutropenia) because of the difference in the half-lives of the mature cells of these two cell lines. When one compares the half-

life of the red cell (approximately 120 days) with the half-life of platelets (5 to 7 days) and with the half-life of granulocytes (6 to 8 hours), it is evident why the latter two are more frequently involved in earlier and more severe suppression by chemotherapy.

If a particular agent predominantly affects the stem cells rather than cells in specific phases of the cell cycle, then all cell lines will be suppressed. Very few classes of chemotherapeutic agents, however, selectively depress the stem cell (1). Examples of these agents are the general group of nitrosoureas (carmustine and lomustine). Other classes of agents, mainly the cell-cycle agents that are not specifically phase selective (such as the anthracyclines and certain alkylators, e.g., busulfan), may cause slightly more delayed suppression of bone marrow cells and longer recoveries than phase-specific agents such as the antimetabolites and vinca alkaloids.

The degree of cytopenia induced by a particular agent will also be determined by multiple factors involving the host that specifically affect the cellularity of the bone marrow compartment (3) (Table 27.1). These factors include (a) the age of the patient (the younger patient has a much more cellular marrow with a decreased percentage of fat and, therefore, is more tolerant of a given dose of drug than is the elderly patient); (b) the degree of bone marrow reserve in relation to the amount of involvement by a particular neoplastic process (fibrosis and tumor cells including leukemic cells); (c) the degree of compromise by previous chemotherapy or radiation therapy, or both; (d) the nutritional status of the patient (the greater the negative nitrogen balance with its associated loss of weight, the less the

Table 27.1. Factors Altering Drug Pharmacokinetics and Subsequent Hematotoxicity

Compliance in taking the drug
Variability of drug absorption
Active gastrointestinal disease (e.g., sprue, lymphoma)
Previous surgery or radiation
Concurrent medications that inhibit absorption (e.g., antacids)
Altered protein binding in plasma
Compartmental fluid excess (e.g., ascites, pleural effusion—methotrexate)
Alterations in drug metabolism
  Genetic enzyme alterations
  Age of patient
  Liver disease
  Enzyme changes due to drugs (e.g., phenobarbital)
Factors affecting drug excretion
  Liver disease
  Renal disease
  Effusions or ascites

tolerance); and (e) the ability of the liver or kidneys to metabolize and/or excrete the compound (3, 4).

Recent evidence suggests that the use of certain biologic modifiers such as granulocyte-monocyte colony-stimulating factor (GM-CSF) or granulocyte colony-stimulating factor (G-CSF) may be able to shorten the duration of cytopenias associated with chemotherapy. This is accomplished by enhancing the stem cell's ability to differentiate and more rapidly recover from the chemotherapeutic insult by the various agents known to cause myelosuppression (5–9).

Because of the differences in the peripheral blood half-lives of leukocytes and platelets, drugs that induce myelosuppression result in leukopenia first, followed by thrombocytopenia. Generally, leukopenia is more severe than thrombocytopenia. Ifosfamide, a structural analogue of cyclophosphamide, an alkylating agent, has a dose-limiting toxicity of leukopenia much more than thrombocytopenia (10). Rarely, thrombocytopenia is the predominant dose-limiting cytopenia, and platelets may be the cell line that is the slowest to recover after bone marrow suppression.

Nitrosoureas typically produce a late and often severe thrombocytopenia that occurs 4 to 6 weeks after the administration of the agent (11–14). Thrombocytopenia may occur after recovery from leukopenia and may persist for 1 to 2 weeks after the nadir occurs. Severe bone marrow hy-

poplasia may be seen after administration of busulfan (3, 11). This is not necessarily a predictable suppression, and the bone marrow hypoplasia and peripheral thrombocytopenia and leukopenia may be severe and prolonged, persisting for several months. Thrombocytopenia may persist long after the granulocyte count has returned to near normal values and is the last to recover after the administration of busulfan. This phenomenon is not common for other alkylating agents and is often predictable.

Another unusual manifestation after bone marrow suppression is the pattern of recovery following the use of cytosine arabinoside, especially in patients with acute leukemia (3, 11). After severe hypoplasia has resulted from the administration of this agent, it is not unusual to see a transient blastemia (circulating myeloblasts) for a period of 1 to 7 days. This does not necessarily indicate continued activity of the leukemic process and is merely a part of the recovery after the use of this antipyrimidine compound. Continued observation will demonstrate the prompt disappearance of these blasts from the peripheral blood. At the time of this blastemia, if a bone marrow specimen is obtained, in addition to severe hypoplasia, islands of reactive normal myelopoiesis can be found, again indicating recovery rather than persistence of the leukemic process. In those situations in which the blasts of the leukemic process contain Auer rods, none of these cytoplasmic lysosomal inclusions will be seen in the circulating transient blastemia, again indicating that this is a normal recovery from cytosine arabinoside.

Very few cancer chemotherapy drugs are truly nonmyelosuppressive. The only agents known to be completely nontoxic to normal bone marrow are the steroidal hormones (an exception is tamoxifen, which rarely causes leukopenia and thrombocytopenia). However, agents such as bleomycin, vincristine, and L-asparaginase generally do not cause bone marrow suppression (15–18). However, exceptions to this occur when specific organ involvement, such as hepatic decompensation, may not allow for appropriate catabolism of a given agent, thereby causing excessive and prolonged blood levels of the active drug or metabolite. Vincristine in the presence of liver disease is a typical example of such a situation. L-Asparaginase, while being nonmyelosuppressive, does produce significant hematologic toxicity because of its effect on protein anabolism in the liver, with a resultant decrease in the production of coagulation factors, specifically the vitamin K–dependent factors, factor V (parahemophilic factor, labile factor, or proaccelerin), and fibrinogen (17).

Sideroblastic anemia as an early manifestation of the myelodysplastic process (preleukemic process) may develop 1 to 10 years following the administration of chemotherapy, especially alkylators in conjunction with radiation therapy. Although rarely seen with isolated alkylator therapy, it may occur. The sideroblastic anemia, although similar to the idiopathic condition, may be the preceding event to acute nonlymphocytic leukemia. Certain cytogenetic abnormalities are characteristic of the acquired defects secondary to chemotherapy, and when found, they help to substantiate the relationship between the chemotherapeutic agent and the secondary bone marrow dysplastic process. These include changes of 5q-, 7q-, −5, −7, +8, and 9; 11 translocation (19).

MECHANISM AND DURATION OF MYELOSUPPRESSION

In general, if one can identify the mode of action of a specific cancer chemotherapeutic agent

Table 27.2. Cell Cycle Activity of Chemotherapeutic Agents

I. Cycle-active phase-specific agents	Ref.	II. Cycle-active phase-nonspecific agents	Ref.
G_1-phase specific	31	Alkylating agents	
Steroids		Busulfan	
L-Asparaginase		Chlorambucil	
Diglycoaldehyde		Cyclophosphamide	
S-phase specific		Nitrogen mustard	
Antimetabolites		Phenylalanine mustard (L-PAM)	
Antifolates		Ifosfamide	10
Methotrexate	23, 24	Antibiotic-type agents	
Baker's antifol (triazinate)		Anthracyclines	43–45, 54
Antipyrimidines		Daunorubicin	
Azacytidine	35, 36	Doxorubicin (Adriamycin)	
Cytarabine		Rubidazone	
Fluorouracil	37	Dactinomycin	
Antipurines		Mithramycin	
Mercaptopurine		Mitomycin C (Mutamycin)	46
Thioguanine		Nitrosoureas	
Steroids (?)		Carmustine (BCNU)	47
Cyclophosphamide (?)	38, 39	Lomustine (CCNU)	48
Miscellaneous		Semustine (Methyl-CCNU)	
Hydroxyurea		Miscellaneous	
Procarbazine		Cisplatin	
Diglycoaldehyde		Dacarbazine (DTIC)	49
G_2-phase specific		Chlorozotocin (DCNU)	
Bleomycin	40	Streptozotocin	
M-AMSA	41	Carboplatin	
Razoxane (ICRF)			
M-phase specific			
Vinca alkaloids			
Vincristine			
Vinblastine			
Epipodophyllotoxins	42		
Etoposide (VP-16-213)			
Teniposide (VM-26)			
Rozoxane (ICRF)			
G_0-phase specific			
Alkylators (mustard-type)			
Busulfan			
Nitrogen mustard			
Phenylalanine mustard (L-PAM)			

(i.e., where it exerts its maximal activity in the cell cycle), then one can predict not only the rapidity with which myelosuppression will ensue but also the duration of the myelosuppression. Obviously, there are exceptions to this generalization. Table 27.2 offers a guideline to the specific location of activity of most of the available and commonly used agents. Agents that are specifically cell-cycle active and phase specific produce a fairly rapid cytopenia (most notably, granulocytopenia followed by thrombocytopenia). Recovery seems to be quicker, especially from agents that are active in S phase (DNA synthesis phase) and M phase (mitosis). Agents that are cycle active but not phase specific show an intermediate-type pattern. Agents that tend to be noncycle active or exert their effect in cells in G_0 or in the resting phase have the greatest delay in causing myelosuppression and the most protracted depression of myeloid elements. The last-mentioned group of agents tends to affect the stem cells before specific delineation in erythropoiesis, granulopoiesis, or megakaryopoiesis.

Not every chemotherapeutic agent can be completely classified by its activity in one or another phase of the cell cycle, and therefore, it becomes difficult to use this as the sole guide for predicting the character and degree of myelosuppression. Combining chemotherapeutic agents may change the toxicity pattern of each, and the myelosuppression is not predictable by simply adding the known toxicity profiles. Therefore, the type of agent, the dose, and the route of administration will determine the degree of myelosuppression, the time to the nadir, and the expected duration of suppression. Table 27.3 broadly categorizes those agents that cause myelosuppression with subsequent recovery.

To avoid undue and severe prolongation of myelosuppression, it is essential to know which organ is primarily responsible for activating, metabolizing, or eliminating the chemotherapeutic agent. If the liver is damaged by tumor, ethanol or other toxins, or infection, it may be unable to activate certain compounds (e.g., cyclophosphamide) or to metabolize and excrete others (e.g., the anthracyclines). Therefore, monitoring of hepatic enzymes, the serum glutamic oxaloacetic transaminase (SGOT), alkaline phosphatase, and bilirubin, is essential to prevent severe toxicity. Drug doses must be altered accordingly. Like-

Table 27.3. Drug Class or Compound and Degree and Duration of Myelosuppression (1, 2)

Drug or Drug Class	Degree of Suppression[a]	Nadir of Myelosuppression (days)	Duration of Marrow Recovery (days)
Anthracycline	III	6–13	21–24
Vinca alkaloids	I–II	4–9	7–21
Mustard alkylator			
Nitrogen mustard	III	7–14	28
Antifolates	III	7–14	14–21
Antipyrimidines	III	7–14	22–24
Antipurines	II	7–14	14–21
Podophyllotoxins	II	5–15	22–28
Alkylators	II	10–21	18–40
Nitrosoureas	III	26–60	35–85
Miscellaneous[b]			
Busulfan	III	11–30	24–54
Carboplatin	III	16	21–25
Cisplatin	II	14	21
Dacarbazine	III	21–28	28–35
Hydroxyurea	II	7	14–21
Mithramycin	I	5–10	10–18
Mitomycin	II	28–42	42–56
Procarbazine	II	25–36	35–50
Rozoxane (ICRF)	II	11–16	12–25

[a]I, mild; II, moderate; III, severe (based on common dose schedules).
[b]Agents differing from their class of compounds.

Table 27.4. Sites of Excretion, Metabolism, or Inactivation of Chemotherapeutic Agents

Liver	Kidney
M-AMSA	Alkylators
Anthracyclines	Antipurines
Antipurines	Azacytidine
Azathioprine	Bleomycin
Corticosteroids	Carboplatin
Cyclophosphamide	Chlorozotocin
Cytosine arabinoside	Cyclophosphamide
DTIC	Cytosine arabinoside
Dactinomycin	Etoposide
Fluorouracil	Hydroxyurea
Hexamethylmelamine	Methotrexate
Mitomycin C	Nitrosoureas
Vinblastine	Procarbazine
Vincristine	Streptozotocin

wise, renal impairment and insufficiency will prolong the plasma half-life and clearance of the chemotherapeutic agent or its active metabolite. This is especially true of such agents as the nitrosoureas, methotrexate, and other antimetabolites. Table 27.4 gives a simplified overview of some of the pathways of excretion, metabolism, and inactivation.

Certain enzyme levels may be decreased or may be kinetically abnormal, a change that will prolong the plasma clearance of the active fraction of a given chemotherapeutic agent. Cytidine deaminase, which inactivates cytosine arabinoside, and xanthine oxidase, which metabolizes mercaptopurine, are two typical examples of enzymes that produce this type of potential problem. At present, these changes are difficult to determine and are primarily research endeavors that are not used clinically in everyday practice.

ANEMIA AND RED CELL CHANGES

Severe anemia is generally not a significant problem with the antineoplastic agents currently in use. Although the stem cells and red cell precursors may be affected to the same degree as the precursors of granulopoiesis and megakaryopoiesis, the long half-life of red cells makes a serious decrease in hemoglobin level less apparent than the decrease of elements with much shorter half-lives. Nonetheless, striking changes can occur in the bone marrow after administration of many of the antimetabolites, as these are especially active in altering the production of DNA synthesis in the developing erythroblasts (20, 21). The most pronounced changes have been seen after the use of folic acid antagonists (methotrexate and trimetrexate) (22, 23), although similar changes have been seen with the antipyrimidines and antipurines as well as with some of the alkylating agents. Because these are cell-cycle-phase-specific agents inhibiting the production of DNA, nuclear development lags behind cytoplasmic maturation, with resultant findings indistinguishable from those changes seen in vitamin B_{12} or folate deficiency. However, if the levels of these two vitamins are measured in the plasma or red cells, they will be found to be perfectly normal, excluding a nutritional or metabolic deficiency that may be exaggerating the changes seen in the red cell precursors.

Macrocytosis in the peripheral blood is likewise a manifestation of the megaloblastic or megaloblastoid changes demonstrated in the bone marrow after the use of these agents. The finding of oval macrocytes in association with hypersegmented polymorphonuclear leukocytes and giant bands, however, is not nearly as common as that seen with true vitamin B_{12} or folic acid deficiency. The red cells tend to be round rather than oval but are clearly macrocytic, and the calculated or measured indices always delineate true macrocytosis of the circulating mature nonnucleated erythrocyte.

A striking peripheral macrocytosis with an exceedingly high mean corpuscular volume is a frequent finding in patients who are receiving continuous therapy with hydroxyurea (24). Such changes are not fully explained just by interference with DNA production, because the degree of megaloblastic change seen in the bone marrow does not correlate with the level of the mean corpuscular volume measured in the peripheral blood. Likewise, these patients do not have evidence of vitamin B_{12} or folate deficiency. Hydroxyurea acts as an inhibitor of the conversion of ribonucleotides to the corresponding deoxy forms, and this is the main reason for the extreme macrocytosis (25). Mean corpuscular volumes above 115 μm^3 are commonly seen in patients taking hydroxyurea on a daily basis.

TAXOL

Paclitaxel (Taxol) has demonstrated activity in several solid tumors, including non-small-cell lung cancer and ovarian cancer. It acts as a tubulin polymerization enhancer and has myelosuppression as a major side effect, but in addition, severe mucositis occurs that is not abrogated by the shortening of the neutropenic phase. In addition, recently Cavalleti and colleagues (26) reported significant peripheral neuropathy in patients previously treated with cisplatin. The neuropathy was a distal, symmetric sensory polyneuropathy. This side effect may be more prominent in patients treated previously with neurotoxic drugs. The primary toxicity is myelosuppression, with dose limitation at about 60% that of nonhematologic toxicity (mucositis).

COMBINATION OF CHEMOTHERAPY AND RADIATION

The effect of combining multiagent chemotherapy and radiation therapy markedly increases the hematologic toxicity, with a nearly tenfold increase in interruption of therapy in patients treated with craniospinal radiation following system chemotherapy (27). The addition of radiation to any chemotherapeutic regimen will cause more rapid and dramatic reductions of platelets and white cells during the radiation than when radiation is used alone.

HEMOLYTIC UREMIC SYNDROME

The complex of microangiopathic hemolytic anemia, thrombocytopenia, and renal dysfunction has been recognized in a small subset of patients with malignancies treated with chemotherapeutic drugs. Although most frequently seen in childhood, it has been noted with increasing frequency in patients receiving mitomycin as a single agent or in combination with other therapeutic modalities (28, 29). Coagulation profiles have been examined on numerous patients, and with rare exception, all have been found to be within normal limits except for isolated thrombocytopenia, which at times can be severe. Bone marrow examinations have been performed to rule out chemotherapy-induced myelosuppression as well as bone marrow involvement from the neoplastic process. In one recently reported study, mitomycin C was part of the treatment regimen in 84 of 85 patients identified (29). In all but nine of these patients, a cumulative dose of more than 60 mg of mitomycin C had been administered. The apparent risk of developing this syndrome after the administration of mitomycin C is between 4 and 15%. The syndrome carries with it a high mortality, as over 50% of patients demonstrated to have the syndrome died. Conventional treatment has been unsatisfactory. More recently, the use of staphylococcal protein A (SPA) immunophoresis has shown some promise in reversing the renal dysfunction as well as the thrombocytopenia (30).

COAGULATION DEFECTS

Although direct suppression of the bone marrow as the result of cancer chemotherapy most commonly leads to thrombocytopenia, sometimes with serious consequences, other effects of cancer chemotherapy on the coagulation factors may eventuate in clinical bleeding. Patients receiving mithramycin therapy may rarely develop minor coagulation abnormalities with a mild bleeding diathesis, primarily mucosal in origin (such as epistaxis), associated with acquired platelet dysfunction (31). Mithramycin produces abnormally prolonged bleeding times, as well as abnormal platelet aggregation with adenosine diphosphate (ADP) and epinephrine and absence of a platelet aggregation response to collagen. This entire process occurs in the absence of thrombocytopenia. Total platelet levels of ADP are likewise reduced. These abnormalities are completely reversible when the drug is discontinued.

The most noticeable coagulation effects from chemotherapy result from the use of L-asparaginase, and in many studies this has been shown to be a decreased synthesis rather than an accelerated consumption or degradation of the fibrinogen molecule (17, 18, 30, 32). When tests of the coagulation schema have been obtained, prolongations of the prothrombin time, partial thromboplastin time, and thrombin time have all been ascribed to the decrease in fibrinogen. Monitoring of specific factor assays, however, reveals that those factors produced by the liver under the influence of vitamin K may be suppressed during the administration of L-asparaginase. This is not unexpected because L-asparaginase has a widespread effect on protein synthesis in general, and many plasmatic factors are depressed during the administration of this drug. Although suppression of fibrinogen production is seen in 70% of patients treated with L-asparaginase, actual bleeding episodes are rare as a direct result of the decreased production of the coagulation proteins made by the liver. Likewise, this does not seem to be dose dependent, and the factors may return to normal levels with continued administration of the drug. Thrombotic events, including stroke, have been seen with high dose L-asparaginase.

MANAGEMENT OF DRUG-INDUCED MYELOSUPPRESSION

Anemia

Rarely is anemia severe enough to require transfusion therapy in patients receiving antineoplastic agents. If the hemoglobin level decreases below 9 or 10 g/dL, one needs to exclude other causes such as hemolysis, blood loss, or other factors that might be influencing the level of circulating hemoglobin. Attributing an anemia of this severity or greater merely to drug-induced myelosuppression may overlook other treatable and potentially correctable causes of the anemia. When the level of hemoglobin is not commensurate with the patient's activities, or when the anemia is symptomatic, packed red blood cells should be administered. Leukocyte-poor packed cells or frozen red blood cells are reserved for those patients with frequent allergic reactions, fever, and chills or those who have demonstrable leukoagglutinins in their serum because of previous blood product exposure and the subsequent development of leukocyte or platelet antibodies. The use of leukocyte filters reduces anti-HLA antibody formation when used prior to immunization. Ninety-four to 97% of leukocytes can be removed. The remaining level is below the immunizing level and that level producing febrile transfusion reactions. It is possible that this may prevent cytomegalovirus (CMV) transmission as well.

Erythropoietin (EPO) (50 to 150 units/kg) is effective in the treatment of chemotherapy-associated anemia and may decrease the number of red cell transfusions required.

Thrombocytopenia

Clinically significant thrombocytopenia with severe bleeding is likewise an infrequent complication of cancer chemotherapy, especially if care is taken in selecting the drug or combination of drugs and the correct dosages, based on the age of the patient, previous radiation therapy to significant areas of active bone marrow production, and previous drug therapy. The patient's nutritional status will affect the response to the chemotherapeutic agents. Patients in severe negative nitrogen balance tolerate drugs less well than do patients in positive nitrogen balance, even in the absence of significant weight loss.

Transient but significantly decreased platelet counts secondary to chemotherapeutic agents may be managed by the administration of low doses of corticosteroids (i.e., prednisone 5 to 10 mg b.i.d.), if treatment is deemed necessary, during the short duration of the nadir of the drug-induced thrombocytopenia. If, however, the patient manifests easy bruising and active bleeding other than petechiae, the use of platelet concentrates may be required until recovery from myelosuppression is observed.

Refractoriness to platelet transfusions (defined as a rise of <10,000 platelets/μL 1 hour after transfusion) may be delayed or prevented by the use of leukocyte-reduced products at the onset of therapy. Patients who have not been previously sensitized to foreign platelet antigens or in whom platelets have been given in the past during periods of active immunosuppression (either by the disease or by the drugs utilized for the disease) can be given random donor platelets.

When the patient is refractory to random donor platelets, then the use of single donor platelets obtained by plateletpheresis is indicated. HLA-matching of the recipient and donor may be effective if HLA-antibodies are demonstrated on a frozen lymphocyte antibody panel. Finally, some patients may be refractory to all platelet transfusions without a clear cause (HLA antibodies, sepsis). The equivalent of 6 units of random donor platelets may be obtained from a single matched source and given every day or every other day to maintain adequate hemostasis until the patient's own platelet count can recover from the myelosuppression.

Granulocytopenia

The major consequence of granulocytopenia is the increased risk of a severe infection or the accentuation or aggravation of an already existing infectious process. If the nadir of the absolute granulocytopenia is 1000 leukocytes/mm^3 or greater, the chance of developing a significant infection is small (50, 51, 55, 56). However, the lower the nadir below 1000 leukocytes/mm^3, the greater the incidence of infection developing, especially if the nadir persists for longer than 7 to 10 days. Several studies have shown that patients with absolute granulocyte counts below 500/mm^3 for 5 days or longer have a significant chance of developing a serious bacterial infection (33). If the leukocyte count decreases below 1000/mm^3, and especially if the absolute granulocyte count is less than 500/mm^3, one has to be very suspicious of any febrile manifestation. A patient who experiences chills and subsequent temperature spikes to greater than 38.5°C should have appropriate cultures drawn from the blood, orifices, and possible infection sites, with rapid institution of broad-spectrum bactericidal antibiotic coverage. To wait for culture results or other clinical clues regarding a toxic patient is unnecessarily subjecting the patient to possible severe morbidity and mortality.

Currently, several drug programs have been suggested as providing excellent broad-spectrum bactericidal coverage. The particular combination of antibiotics used depends on the nosocomial infections found in a given hospital setting. The combination of vancomycin and ceftazidime is an excellent program when *Staphylococcus epidermidis* is a predominant organism and has been widely used. However, with the emergence of vancomycin resistance, the empiric use of vancomycin at first fever is no longer recommended. Its use in documented infections or with fever unresponsive to initial therapy remains acceptable. If there is clinical suspicion of a gram-negative or anaerobic infection secondary to a ruptured viscus, then the addition of clindamycin might be indicated until definitive results of cultures have been obtained.

More recently, consideration has been given to the use of prophylactic antibiotics since the combination of trimethoprim and sulfamethoxasole (Bactrim, Septra) has become available. The new generation of quinolones has been effective in reducing the days of fever and number of documented infections, although resistance development remains a concern. This new class of antibiotics has broad-spectrum bactericidal activity and in some institutions has been used as a single agent in patients with granulocytopenia and fever, although combination with rifampin is generally considered superior.

Reverse isolation has not been efficacious in the prevention of infection in the granulocytopenic patient. The use of protected environments such as the laminar-airflow rooms, along with gut sterilization utilizing nonabsorbable antibiotics such as gentamicin, vancomycin, and nystatin, reduced the frequency of severe septic episodes in all patients undergoing ablative therapy. The overall results, however, have not been encouraging enough to justify using such measures with every patient, as improvements in complete remission and long-term survival have not been established (52, 53, 56).

When antibiotics fail to control fever in a clinically septic patient after appropriate 48- to 72-hour coverage or when there is further clinical deterioration despite antibiotic therapy, the addition of amphotericin has been clinically useful in allowing time for recovery of the neutrophil count. The use of prophylactic fluconazole in bone marrow transplant patients has dramatically reduced the number of fungal infections in our unit as elsewhere, but there remains concern for development of resistant strains of fungi.

CYTOKINES IN CHEMOTHERAPY

In the past 10 years, the biology of growth factors has increased the intensity of chemotherapy previously limited by hematopoietic toxicity. Monocytes, endothelial cells, and T cells produce cytokines (57) capable of reducing the total time of neutropenia induced by chemotherapy, febrile days, and total days of hospitalization. The combination of cytokines that stimulate pluripotent stem cells (the interleukins IL-1, IL-3, IL-6), myeloid progenitors (IL-3, GM-CSF), and committed progenitors (EPO, G-CSF, GM-CSF) raised the hope that chemotherapy-induced neutropenia could be nearly abrogated. Although nonhematopoietic toxicity still limits doses to just 30 to 50% above the previous hematopoietic toxic limiting levels, the increased intensity is hoped to increase tumor response rates and overall survival.

The first approved drug for supporting myelopoiesis was G-CSF, demonstrated to reduce the total days of neutropenia, days of fever, and days of intravenous antibiotic use when given immediately after chemotherapy in cycle 1 (58). Other approved growth factors include recombinant GM-CSF and EPO. rGM-CSF has been shown to reduce the days of neutropenia, days of antibiotic use, length of hospital stay, and incidence of culture-positive infections in ABMT for lymphoid malignancies (59). However, another study in small cell carcinoma of the lung showed only a decrease in the days of neutropenia, but no effect upon febrile days or antibiotic use (60), and a multicenter study from Germany (61) failed to show an effect of G-CSF upon the use of intravenous antibiotics and days of hospitalization, although fewer days of febrile neutropenia were again noted. EPO, released initially upon data in patients with renal failure, has been shown to reduce transfusion requirements in patients receiving cisplatin and in patients with multiple myeloma (62).

The use of cytokines in established neutropenia is more controversial, and although many authors advocate the use of cytokines, the American Society of Clinical Oncology (ASCO) has published recommendations for the use of colony-stimulating factors (63). These guidelines recommend that growth factors be used prophylactically only when the expected incidence of febrile neutropenia exceeds 40%, and primarily when there has been a documented occurrence in a previous cycle of therapy. The guidelines suggest that most patients developing neutropenia after standard chemotherapy do not benefit from the use of cytokines.

A randomized trial in the Eastern Cooperative Oncology Group is under way to help further define the status of growth factors in established neutropenia. Current clinical use of growth factors according to supportive care guidelines at Mayo Rochester conform to the ASCO recommendations. Although thrombopoietin has now been characterized, the protein is not yet available for large-scale clinical trials. Thrombocytopenia remains the major dose-limiting hematologic toxicity for most regimens (64). Hematopoietic growth factors allow increases of chemotherapy doses of 30 to 40%, after which the nonhematologic toxicities become dose limiting.

HIV EFFECTS ON TOXICITY

Patients with HIV disease have a high incidence of toxicities from chemotherapy, because of associated treatments such as the retroviral drugs compounding the cytopenias, suppression of marrow by HIV, and HIV-associated infections (66). Long-term survivors have been reported, but as rare exceptions (67).

CONCLUSION

Myelosuppression, including leukopenia, neutropenia, thrombocytopenia, and rarely anemia induced by cancer chemotherapeutic agents, is generally reversible, and with dose management and the use of cytokines, these drugs may be used without undue morbidity. Physicians responsible for administering aggressive cancer chemotherapy need know the biologic characteristics of normal myeloid cells as well as the site of action and mode of action of the agents being used to combat the neoplasia. Severe life-threatening problems can usually be avoided through knowledge of the idiosyncrasies of chemotherapeutic agents. With the new advances in antibiotic development, development of cytokine therapy, and knowledge of cancer chemotherapy pharmacology, these agents may be used in increased doses for more effective outcomes.

REFERENCES

1. Von Hoff DD, 2nd ed. Cancer chemotherapy handbook. Norwalk, CT: Appleton & Lange, 1994.
2. Henderson ES. The granulocytopenic effects of cancer chemotherapeutic agents. In: Dimitrov NV, Nodine JH, eds. Drugs and hematologic reactions. New York: Grune & Stratton, 1974:207–221.
3. Creaven PJ, Mihich E. The clinical toxicity of anticancer drugs and its prediction. Semin Oncol 1977; 4:147–163.
4. Dewys WD, Begg C, Lavin P, et al. Prognostic effect of weight loss prior to chemotherapy in cancer patients. Am J Med 1980;69:491–497.
5. Monsoy RL, Skelly RR, Mac Vittie TJ, et al. The effect of recombinant GM-CSF on recovery of monkeys transplanted with autologous bone marrow. Blood 1987;70:1696–1699.
6. Gabrilove JL, Jakubowski A, Scher H, et al. The effect of granulocyte colony stimulating factor on neutropenia and associated morbidity of chemotherapy for transitional cell carcinoma of the urethelium. N Engl J Med 1988;318:1414–1422.
7. Bronchurd MH, Scharffe JH, Thatcher N, et al. A phase I/II study of recombinant granulocyte stimulating factor in patients receiving intensive chemotherapy for small cell lung cancer. Br J Cancer 1986; 56:808–813.
8. Morstyn G, Souza L, Keech J, et al. Effect of granulocyte colony stimulating factor on neutropenia induced by cytotoxic chemotherapy. Lancet 1988;1:1667–1671.
9. Antman K, Griffin J, Elias A, et al. Use of rGM-CSF to ameliorate chemotherapy-induced myelosuppression in sarcoma patients (abstract). Blood 1987; 70(Suppl 1):373.
10. Sarosy G. Ifosfamide—pharmacologic overview. Semin Oncol 1989;16:2–8.
11. Chabner BA, Myers CE, Coleman CN, et al. The clinical pharmacology of antineoplastic agents. N Engl J Med 1975;292:1107–1113, 1159–1168.
12. Cancer chemotherapy. Med Lett Drugs Ther 1976;18:109–116.
13. Schein PS, Bull JM, Doukak D, et al. Sensitivity of human and murine hematopoietic precursor cells to 2-[3-(2-chloroethyl)-3-nitrosoureido]-D-glucopyranose 1,3-bis(2-chloroethyl)-1-nitrosourea. Cancer Res 1978; 38:257–260.
14. Wasserman TH, Slavik M, Carter SK. Clinical comparison of the nitrosoureas. Cancer 1975;36:1258–1268.
15. Bennett JM, Reich SD. Bleomycin. Ann Intern Med 1979;90:945–948.
16. Blum RH, Carter SK, Agre K. A clinical review of bleomycin: a new antineoplastic agent. Cancer 1973; 31:903–914.
17. Whitecar JP Jr, Bodey GP, Harris JE, et al. L-Asparaginase. N Engl J Med 1970;282:732–734.
18. Ramsay NKC, Coccia PF, Krivit W, et al. The effect of L-asparaginase on plasma coagulation factors in acute lymphoblastic leukemia. Cancer 1977;40:1398–1401.
19. Dewald GW, Noel P, Dahl RJ, Spurbeck J. Chro-

mosome abnormalities in malignant hematologic disorders. Mayo Clin Proc 1985;60:657–689.

20. McGrath BP, Ibels LS, Raik E, et al. Erythroid toxicity of azathioprine: macrocytosis and selective marrow hypoplasia. Q J Med 1975;44:57–63.

21. Van Dyk JJ, Falkson HC, van der Merwe AM, et al. Unexpected toxicity in patients treated with iphosphamide. Cancer Res 1972;32:921–924.

22. Frei E III, Jaffe N, Tattersall MHN, et al. New approaches to cancer chemotherapy with methotrexate. N Engl J Med 1975;292:846–851.

23. Weinstein GD. Methotrexate. Ann Intern Med 1977;86:199–204.

24. Kennedy BJ. Hydroxyurea therapy in chronic myelogenous leukemia. Cancer 1972;29:1052–1056.

25. Bhuyan BK, Scheidt LG, Fraser TJ. Cell cycle phase specificity of antitumor agents. Cancer Res 1972; 32:298–407.

26. Cavalleti G, Bogliun G, Marzorati L, et al. Peripheral neurotoxicity of taxol in patients previously treated with cisplatin. Cancer 1995;75:1141–1150.

27. Marks LB, Cuthbertson D, Freidman HS. Hematologic toxicity during craniospinal irradiation: the impact of prior chemotherapy. Med Pediatr Oncol 1995;25:45–51.

28. Pavy MD, Wiely EL, Abeloff MD. Hemolytic uremic syndrome associated with mitomycin therapy. Cancer Treat Rep 1982;66:457–461.

29. Rothschild N, Erickson B, Sisk R, et al. Cancer associated hemolytic uremic syndrome: analysis of 85 cases from a national registry. J Clin Oncol 1989;7:781–789.

30. Capizzi RL, Bertino JR, Skeel TR, et al. L-Asparaginase: clinical, biochemical, pharmacological, and immunological studies. Ann Intern Med 1971; 74:893–901.

31. Ahr DJ, Scialla SJ, Kimball DB Jr. Acquired platelet dysfunction following mithramycin therapy. Cancer 1978;41:448–454.

32. Haskell CM, Canellos GP, Leventhal BG, et al. L-Asparaginase: therapeutic and toxic effects in patients with neoplastic disease. N Engl J Med 1969; 281:1028–1034.

33. Rodriguez V, Bodey GP, Freireich EF, et al. Randomized trial of protected environment-prophylactic antibodies in 145 adults with acute leukemia. Medicine (Baltimore) 1978;57:253–266.

34. Bodey GP, Rodriguez V, Chang H-Y, et al. Fever and infection in leukemic patients: a study of 494 consecutive patients. Cancer 1978;41:1610–1622.

35. Von Hoff DD, Slavik M, Muggia FM. 2-Azacytidine: a new anticancer drug with effectiveness in acute myelogenous leukemia. Ann Intern Med 1976; 85:237–245.

36. Karon M, Sieger L, Leimbrock S, et al. 5-Azacytidine: a new active agent for the treatment of acute leukemia. Blood 1973;42:359–365.

37. Kaufman S. 5-Fluorouracil in the treatment of gastrointestinal neoplasia. N Engl J Med 1973;288:199–201.

38. Gershwin ME, Goetzl EF, Steinberg AD. Cyclophosphamide: use in practice. Ann Intern Med 1974; 80:531–540.

39. Baran DT, Griner PF, Klemperer MR. Recovery from aplastic anemia after treatment with cyclophosphamide. N Engl J Med 1976;295:1522–1523.

40. Yagoda A, Mukherji B, Young C, et al. Bleo-

mycin, an antitumor antibiotic: clinical experience in 274 patients. Ann Intern Med 1972;77:861–870.

41. Issell BF. Amsacrine (AMSA). Cancer Treat Rev 1980;7:73–83.

42. Mathé G, Schwarzenberg L, Pouillart P, et al. Two epipodophyllotoxin derivatives, VM 26 and VP 16213, in the treatment of leukemias, hematosarcomas, and lymphomas. Cancer 1974;34:985–992.

43. Tan C, Tasaka H, Yu K-P, et al. Daunomycin, an antitumor antibiotic, in the treatment of neoplastic disease: clinical evaluation with specific reference to childhood leukemia. Cancer 1967;20:333–353.

44. Benjamin RS, Wiernik PH, Bachur NR. Adriamycin chemotherapy—efficacy, safety, and pharmacologic basis of an intermittent single high-dosage schedule. Cancer 1974;33:19–27.

45. Blum RH, Carter SK. Adriamycin: a new anticancer drug with significant clinical activity. Ann Intern Med 1974;80:249–259.

46. Crooke ST, Bradner WT, Mitomycin C: a review. Cancer Treat Rev 1976;3:121–139.

47. Young RC, DeVita VT Jr, Serpick AA, et al. Treatment of advanced Hodgkin's disease with [1,3 bis(2-chloroethyl)-1-nitrosourea] BCNU. N Engl J Med 1971;285:475–479.

48. Wasserman TH, Slavik M, Carter SK. Methyl-CCNU in clinical cancer therapy. Cancer Treat Rev 1974;1:251–269.

49. Loo TL, Householder GE, Gerulath AH, et al. Mechanism of action and pharmacology studies with DTIC (NSC-45388). Cancer Treat Rep 1976;60:149–152.

50. Klastersky J. The use of synergistic combinations of antibiotics in patients with haematological diseases. Clin Haematol 1976;5:361–377.

51. McCredie KB, Hester JP. White blood cell transfusions in the management of infections in neutropenic patients. Clin Haematol 1976;5:379–394.

52. Bodey GP, Rodriguez V. Protected environment-prophylactic antibiotic programmes: microbiological studies. Clin Haematol 1976;5:395–408.

53. Levine AS. Protected environment-prophylactic antibiotic programmes: clinical studies. Clin Haematol 1976;5:409–424.

54. Speth AL, Minderman H, Haanen C, et al. Idarubicin vs daunorubicin: preclinical and clinical pharmacokinetic studies. Semin Oncol 1989;17:2–9.

55. Rodriguez V, Bodey GP. Antibacterial therapy: special considerations in neutropenic patients. Clin Haematol 1976;5:347–360.

56. Bodey GP, Rodriguez V, Cabanillas F, et al. Protected environment-prophylactic antibiotic program for malignant lymphoma: randomized trial during chemotherapy to induce remission. Am J Med 1979; 66:74–81.

57. Dinarello CA, Mier JW. Lymphokines. N Engl J Med 1987;317:940–945.

58. Crawford J, Ozer H, Stoller R, et al. Reduction by granulocyte colony-stimulating factor of fever and neutropenia induced by chemotherapy in patients with small-cell lung cancer (r-met HuG-CSF). N Engl J Med 1991;325:164–170.

59. Nemunaitis J, Rabinowe SN, Singer JW, et al. Recombinant granulocyte-macrophage colony-stimulating factor after autologous bone marrow transplantation for lymphoid cancer. N Engl J Med 1991; 324:1773–1778.

60. Hamm JT, Schiller JH, Oken MM, et al. Gran-

ulocyte-macrophage colony-stimulating factor (GM-CSF) in small cell carcinoma of the lung (SCCL): preliminary analysis of a randomized controlled trial (abstract). Proc Am Soc Clin Oncol 1991;10:255a.

61. Schmitz N, Dreger P, Zander AR, Ehninger G, et al. Results of a randomized, controlled multicentre study of recombinant human granulocyte colony-stimulating factor (Filgrastim) in patients with Hodgkin's disease and non-Hodgkin's lymphoma undergoing autologous bone marrow transplantation. Bone Marrow Transplant 1995;15:261–266.

62. Case DC Jr, Bukowski RM, Carey RW, et al. Recombinant human erythropoietin therapy for anemic cancer patients on combination therapy. J Natl Cancer Inst 1993;85:801–806.

63. American Society of Clinical Oncology. Recommendations for the use of hematopoietic colony-stimulating factors: evidence-based clinical practice guidelines. J Clin Oncol 1996;14:1957–1960.

64. Sternberg CN, de Mulder PH, van Oosterom AT, et al. Escalated M-VAC chemotherapy and recombinant human granulocyte-macrophage colony-stimulating factor (rhGM-CSF). Ann Oncol 1993;4:403–407.

65. Vose J, Armitage JO. Clinical applications of hematopoietic growth factors. J Clin Oncol 1995;13:1023–1035.

66. Imrie KR, Sawka CA, Kutas G, et al. HIV-associated lymphoma of the gastrointestinal tract: the University of Toronto AIDS-Lymphoma Study Group experience. Leuk Lymphoma 1995;16(3–4):343–349.

67. Greenberg AL, Droller DG. Successful treatment of a patient with seropositive human immunodeficiency virus with high risk Burkitt's leukemia. Cancer 1994;74:1261–1264.

28

Oral Toxicity

Douglas E. Peterson and Mark M. Schubert

The oral cavity can be profoundly affected by cytotoxic chemotherapy used for treatment of cancer patients. Complications arising in the oral cavity often have a marked influence on the overall course of these individuals. Multiple reasons account for these outcomes. First, normal oral labial and buccal mucosa has a turnover rate of approximately 5 to 16 days (1) and is thus at high risk for the cytotoxic effects of antineoplastic agents (2, 3). Second, many oral diseases are chronic and asymptomatic until late in their progression. Patients are often unaware of the diseases and do not seek dental care; thus, oral disease is common and is frequently encountered in chemotherapy patients. Third, the oral cavity in most adult patients harbors an extensive microbial flora that is commonly altered in a setting of prolonged neutropenia (4). This newly acquired flora can cause systemic infection.

This chapter reviews the normal anatomy of oral structures most frequently affected by chemotherapy, followed by discussion of the etiology, diagnosis, and management of relevant oral lesions (Table 28.1). Since patients undergoing treatment for acute leukemia are typically at extreme risk for oral complications, they serve as the reference population unless otherwise noted.

NORMAL ANATOMY

The dentition and its supporting structures represent a complex, dynamic relationship. Teeth are suspended in a stroma of connective tissue that both supplies vasculature to the dental pulp and supports the teeth during function. This connective tissue, the periodontal ligament, extends chiefly from the cementum of teeth to alveolar bone. The space superior to the ligament between the tooth and the inner aspect of the free gingiva is called the periodontal sulcus; sulcular epithelium is normally nonkeratinized and nonulcerated.

Gingival mucosa can be directly examined by the clinician. This mucosa terminates in a free edge surrounding the inferior margin of the clinical crowns of the teeth. The tissue is normally pale pink, with stipling evident. The alveolar mucosa covers the alveolar bony processes of both dental arches. In health, the junction of the gingival mucosa and alveolar mucosa is usually sharply delineated by a scalloped border, the mucogingival junction.

Mucosa lining the cheeks and lips of the oral cavity consists of nonkeratinized epithelium containing both minor salivary glands (chiefly mucous in character), and ectopic sebaceous glands in the anterior one-third of the mouth. Normally, the mucosa has a smooth, moist appearance, with a pink hue.

Dental pulp consists of a highly vascular connective tissue. Its components include a gelatinous ground substance, cellular elements, terminal blood vessels, nerves, and collagen. Its primary function is dentin formation during organogenesis; it normally retains its ability to sense hot and cold stimuli (usually interpreted as an uncomfortable sensation) throughout most of its life. The pulp communicates with the marrow spaces of the bone, chiefly through the foramen.

DIRECT STOMATOTOXIC EFFECTS

Mucositis

Cytotoxic effects of chemotherapy upon replicating oral mucosal cells can result in severe oral mucositis (5, 6). This lesion represents significant compromise of normal oral functions; these processes include clearance of oral microorganisms through shedding of the surface layer, and provision of a chemical barrier that

Table 28.1. Common Complications of Chemotherapy

Problem	Time Seen Following Chemotherapy	Clinical Signs and Symptoms	Laboratory Findings	Treatment	Course
Mucositis and ulceration	5–16 days after initiation of chemotherapy	Broad, shallow or deep ulceration on mucosa Poorly defined borders May be hemorrhagic Mucosal erythema Distinct ovoid deep ulcerations with white necrotic centers and dense surrounding band of erythema May involve keratinized tissue	Microbial pathogens may be present	Palliation-viscous Xylocaine (Astra); Benadryl (Parke-Davis) and Kaopectate (Upjohn); dyclonine hydrochloride or cocaine rinses. Benzocaine in Orabase (Hoyt) for discrete lesions; systemic analgesics; ice chips If secondary infection, parenteral antibiotics to cover gram (−) organisms in addition to conventional gram (+) flora If hemorrhage, topical thrombin Soft, bland diet as tolerated	Resolves following cessation of chemotherapy
Xerostomia	Variable	Dry mouth Thick ropy saliva Dysgeusia Difficulty with speech and nutrition	Noncontributory	Lemon drops (artificial sweeteners) (used only for acute management) Lemon glycerine swabs Sugarless gum Ice chips Saliva substitute Fluoride (Fl⁻) rinses; nonacidulated Fl⁻ rinse every day Sialogogues; pilocarpine bethanechol	Resolves following cessation of chemotherapy
"Odontogenic" pain of neurotoxic origin	During course of neurotoxic agent (i.e., vincristine)	Spontaneous, constant, dental pain often mimicking pulpitis Difficult to localize May be bilateral Afebrile No swelling, lymphadenopathy, significant caries, or periodontitis	Noncontributory, rule out temporomandibular joint dysfunction or pulpal pathoses	Systemic pain medications if needed	Resolves following discontinuation of neurotoxic agent
Angular cheilitis	Variable, incidence increases with xerostomia	Cracking, bleeding, possible exudate and pain in corner of mouth	Smear will likely demonstrate fungi if *Candida* spp. present	Check occlusal vertical dimension Mycolog (Squibb) ointment K-Y Jelly (Johnson & Johnson)	Observe for secondary infection
Acute necrotizing ulcerative gingivitis (ANUG)	Variable, may be unrelated to chemotherapy, but incidence increases with neutropenia	Gingival pain and bleeding Fever Lymphadenopathy Gingival necrosis with punched out papillae Fetor oris	May see leukocytosis if no myelosuppression Fusospirochetal smear (+)	Parenteral antibiotics, penicillin drug of choice; oral debridement	Resolves following appropriate therapy in 7–10 days

Table 28.1—*continued*

Problem	Time Seen Following Chemotherapy	Clinical Signs and Symptoms	Laboratory Findings	Treatment	Course
Moniliasis	Variable, more likely with prolonged neutropenia, antibiotics, or steroid use	White curds, plaques ulcerations Mildly painful Affects buccal and palatal mucosa most frequently Corners of mouth may be affected, especially in edentulous patients (*see* Angular cheilitis)	Neutropenia, (+) smear for *Candida* spp. Positive barium swallow with esophageal involvement (rule out false negative)	Clotrimazole troches Nystatin ointment Amphotericin B if esophageal or systemic involvement suspected	Resolves with antifungal therapy or with marrow recovery
Herpes labialis	Variable	Crops of vesicular lesions approximating the mucocutaneous junction; frequently extraoral	Increased nuclear/cytoplasmic ratio Viral inclusion bodies Seropositive if immunocompetent	Keep dry if exudate present; Prevention-keep lubricated; often secondary infection in neutropenic host. Topical therapy with neosporin Acyclovir (Burroughs/Wellcome)	10–14 days, depending on host resistance
Salivary gland infection	Variable, most common in debilitated patient with diminished oral intake and dehydration	Swelling (may be unilateral or bilateral) Pain Suppuration from duct when no myelosuppression Xerostomia Fever	Variable, (+) bacterial or viral cultures, cytomegalovirus common	Antibiotics (parenteral) to cover *Staphylococcus* spp. if bacterial Rehydrate Watch for possible airway obstruction	Resolution depends on host status and treatment
Odontogenic infection	Variable	May present with fever of unknown origin, pain, lymphadenopathy Swelling not a consistent finding with neutropenia May be subclinical until neutropenia develops	Neutropenia Blood culture may be (+)	Parenteral broad-spectrum antibiotics to cover for opportunistic organisms and normal flora Pulpal therapy or extraction in presence of adequate cell counts (polymorphonuclear leukocyte >1000/mm³ and platelets >40,000/mm³)	Variable; depends on organism, hematologic status, extent of infection
Mucosal bleeding	10–14 days	Hematoma or bleeding, especially from mucosal sites commonly traumatized In case of neutropenic patient, likely chance of secondary infection Possible sublingual or pharyngeal extension airway obstruction	Thrombocytopenia Blast crisis with functional decrease in platelets	Remove partial and full dentures Eliminate orthodontic bands or retainers Cover for secondary infection Topically applied epinephrine or cocaine	Resolves with increased platelets Resolving hematoma may extrude granulation plug from healing base; do not disturb

Table 28.1—*continued*

Problem	Time Seen Following Chemotherapy	Clinical Signs and Symptoms	Laboratory Findings	Treatment	Course
Gingival bleeding	Variable, typically 10–14 days after initiation of chemotherapy	Marginal hemorrhage from gingiva May be spontaneous if platelets <40,000/mm³ May be presenting sign	Thrombocytopenia	Platelets Topical thrombin solution-soaked 2×2s Topically applied epinephrine or cocaine Aminocaproic acid Microfibrillar collagen Undisturbed clot Pressure therapy Discontinue mechanical hygiene	Resolves as platelets increase

Modified from Lockhart PB. Dental management of patients receiving chemotherapy. In: Peterson DE, Sonis ST, eds. Oral complications of cancer chemotherapy. The Hague; Martinus Nijhoff, 1983:125–127. With permission.

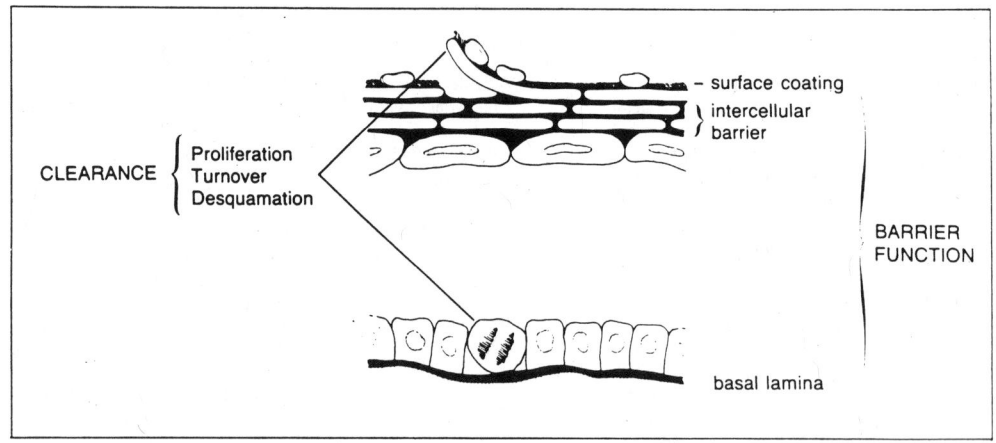

Figure 28.1.   Protective functions in oral epithelium are primarily achieved through clearance of surface cells, an intercellular permeability barrier, and a differentially permeable basal lamina. (Reprinted with permission from Squier CA. Barrier functions of oral epithelia. In: Mackenzie IC, Squier CA, Dabelsteen E, eds. Oral mucosal diseases: biology, etiology and therapy. Copenhagen: Lædgeforeningens Forlag, 1987:7–9.)

limits penetration of compounds into the epithelium (1) (Fig. 28.1). In addition, mucosal immune components, including T cells, B cells, and mast cells (7), can be substantially reduced in number and function.

In the initial clinical stages of mucositis, the patient experiences a mucosal "burning" sensation within 1 week of administration of the drugs; the mucosa may appear erythematous. The lesion then typically ulcerates within 5 days, with ulcerations subsequently becoming confluent (Fig. 28.2A). Histologic changes associated with these clinical findings most commonly include collagen degeneration and epithelial atrophy (8). Once ulcerated, the oral mucosa can be-

come secondarily infected when the patient is granulocytopenic. Thus, drug-induced mucositis represents a potential portal of entry for systemic infection.

Drugs typically causing oral mucositis include methotrexate, doxorubicin (Adriamycin), 5-fluorouracil, busulfan, and bleomycin. Patients who experience mucositis during one course of chemotherapy often experience mucositis of similar extent and location during subsequent courses of the same regimen. The lesions typically last for 10 to 14 days after cessation of chemotherapy (Fig. 28.2B). Sites most commonly involved include the tongue and buccal/labial mucosa; heavily keratinized surfaces such as

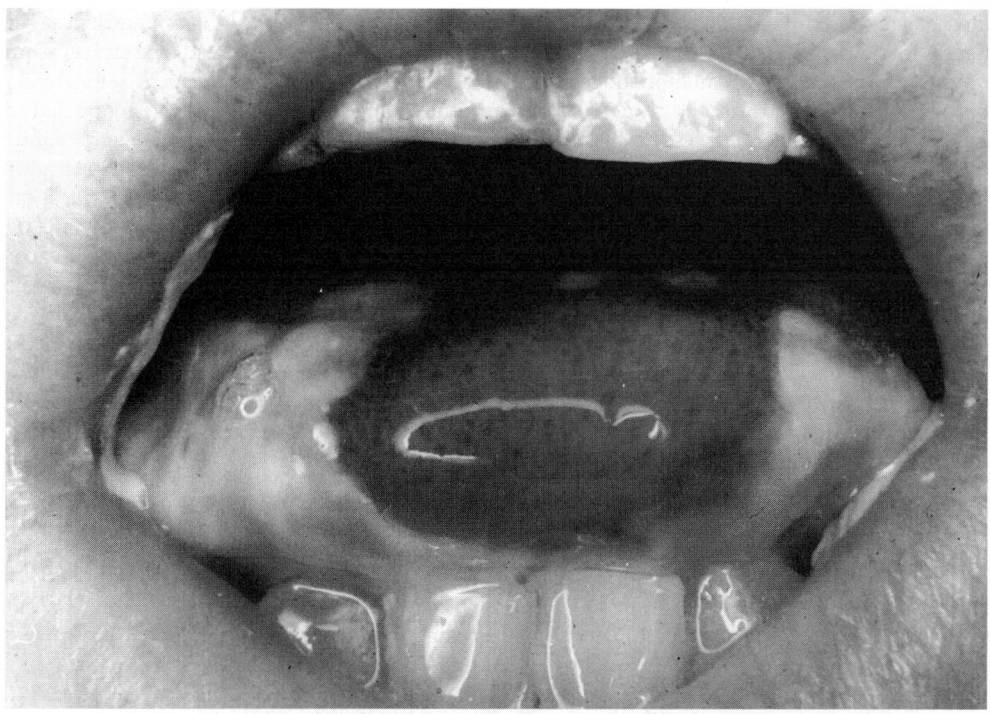

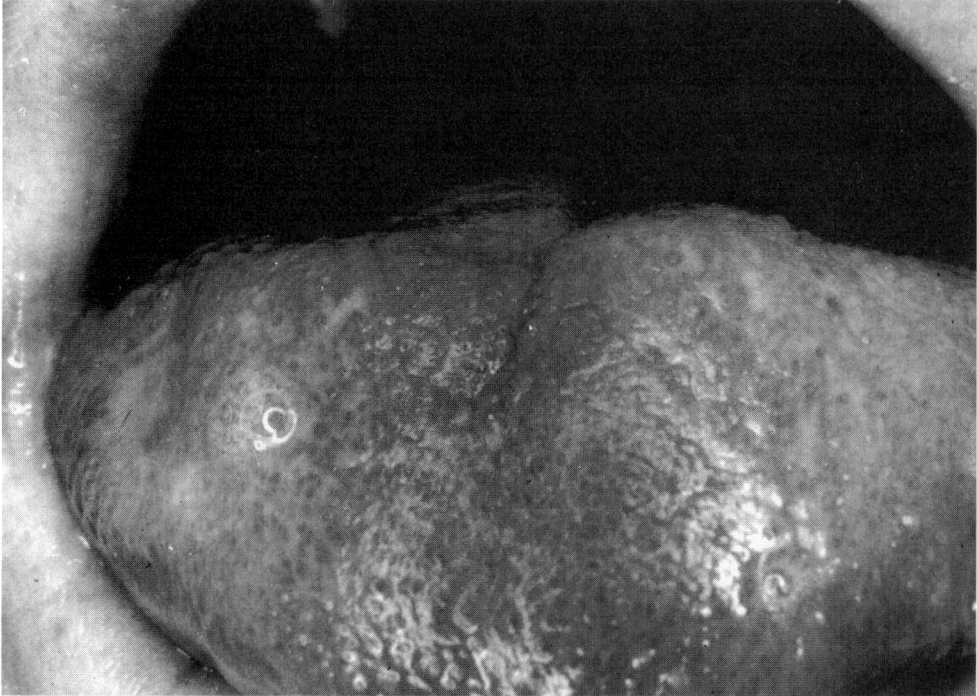

Figure 28.2.   Oral mucositis. A. This lesion demonstrates the result of intense, direct stomatotoxic effects on the oral mucosa in a cancer patient receiving 5-fluorouracil for metastatic breast carcinoma. The chemotherapy was discontinued 1 week earlier. Note the extensive, confluent pseudomembranous ulcerations. **B.** Ulcerative component of mucositis in same patient resolved approximately 21 days after discontinuation of chemotherapy. Substantial dorsal tongue architectural changes remain; moderate dysgeusia is present.

hard palate and attached gingiva are infrequently involved.

While direct toxicity of chemotherapy is the primary cause of mucositis, the clinical expression of mucositis generally results from additional damage caused by a number of factors. The influence of indigenous normal oral flora on mucositis has not been clearly delineated; however, it has been implicated for a number of years as a contributing factor (9–14). Steps to improve oral hygiene have been associated with reduction of mucositis severity, presumably by reducing the level of oral microbial carriage. Oral infections caused by pathogens acquired during hospitalization and immunosuppression can also influence the clinical presentation of mucositis.

Oral mucosal tissues are less able to resist and repair damage caused by normal oral function, because of chemotherapy-associated toxicity to proliferating epithelial cells. Oral functions such as eating, talking, and mouth breathing can thus accentuate mucositis. Emesis also can increase mucositis severity; potential for damage to oral mucosa exists when exposed to acidic gastric fluid. Vigorous tongue movements during vomiting can result in significant irritation to the less well keratinized lateral and ventral tongue surfaces.

Given these multiple factors associated with oral mucositis, adequate management of the lesion can be difficult for both physician and patient. Unfortunately, there has been little prospective study as to prevention of the disorder. Thus, technology does not currently exist to directly prevent chemotherapy damage to oral mucosa and salivary glands. Therapy currently remains primarily focused on symptom palliation.

Protocols to manage mucositis should specifically address efficacy, patient acceptance, and appropriate dosing. A "stepped" approach is typically used, with progression from one level to the next as follows:

1. Bland rinses (e.g., normal saline, sodium bicarbonate)
2. Coating agents (e.g., antacid solutions, milk of magnesia)
3. Water-soluble lubricants, including artificial salivas for xerostomia
4. Topical anesthetics (e.g., lidocaine, benzocaine, dyclonine)
5. Antihistamines (e.g., diphenhydramine)

Topical, focal application of anesthetic agents is preferred over widespread oral topical administration; this approach may reduce the uncomfortable effects associated with generalized oral mucosal anesthesia. However, ulcerative mucositis may become extensive and involve multiple oral sites. In these instances, topical rinses such as viscous Xylocaine (Astra), Kaopectate (Upjohn) mixed with Benadryl (Parke-Davis), or Tessalon Perles (Scherer) may be used to palliate pain. Milk of magnesia should not be used to prolong the contact of the anesthetic agent with the ulcerated surface, since it can cause dehydration of mucosa and further exacerbate the lesion.

These topical approaches, combined as needed with systemic analgesics and narcotics (e.g., Dilaudid or morphine sulfate by bolus or drip), are typically useful in controlling pain associated with ulcerative oral mucositis. The patient should be reassured that healing should occur, beginning approximately 2 weeks after cessation of cytotoxic agents. In addition, hematologic recovery should increase the likelihood of resolution of secondary infections that may have developed during the ulcerative, neutropenic phase.

A review of studies examining efficacy of selected oral rinses in reducing severity of oral mucositis and associated secondary infection is presented later in this chapter. In addition, laboratory and clinical investigators are currently studying new strategies to prevent this lesion; technologies associated with low-dose helium-neon laser (15) or cytokines such as epidermal growth factor (16) and transforming growth factor β3 (17) are being analyzed. Successes with these and related approaches would represent a substantial improvement in controlling the direct and indirect sequelae of this lesion.

Nutrition in the oral mucositis patient is also an important concern. Pain and bleeding associated with oral mucositis can severely alter normal eating patterns of the patient, resulting in weight loss and malnutrition. Ideally, voluntary dietary intake should be encouraged; however, this can be difficult in practice. The following guidelines can be used to mitigate these difficulties (18):

1. Eat a bland diet, avoiding spiced, acidic, or salted foods.
2. Avoid foods with coarse texture, using blenderized foods if necessary.

3. Avoid extremely hot or cold foods.
4. Supply added calories and nutrients by drinking shakes prepared with nutritional supplements or ice cream.
5. Rinse mouth with a topical anesthetic prior to eating a soft diet if oral intake is painful. Caution in mastication is essential.
6. Chew sugar-free gum or sugar-free hard candy to stimulate saliva if xerostomia is a problem.
7. Use nasogastric or nasoduodenal tube feedings, or total parenteral nutrition if necessary.
8. Use antiemetics if indicated.

Levels of intervention are also influenced by the degree of neutropenia (e.g., absolute neutrophil count (ANC) $<1000/mm^3$ ("neutropenic diet"); ANC $<500/mm^3$ ("low microbial diet")). In general, the food choices are not different between these two clasifications; however, food preparation techniques are different. A specific difference between the two regimens is that the low microbial diet allows only bottled juices, while the neutropenic diet allows foil-covered juices.

Salivary Gland Dysfunction

Saliva normally provides critically protective functions for oral tissues, including both mucosal lubrication and delivery of an array of antimicrobial factors including salivary mucins, secretory IgA, lactoferrin, and transferrin (5). By comparison, quantitative/qualitative compromise in salivary secretion exacerbates the clinical course of myelosuppressed cancer patients with chemotherapy-induced oral mucositis.

Few studies have systematically investigated salivary gland dysfunction in chemotherapy patients (19–22); most trials have investigated salivary gland abnormalities in patients receiving upper mantle radiation or bone marrow transplantation (BMT) (23, 24). One must distinguish between (a) primary compromise of saliva production and secretion caused by the cytoreductive agents and (b) other covariates that contribute to compromised saliva-oral tissue interactions. For example, anticholinergic drugs used to control nausea can reduce saliva output, while conditions such as mouth breathing or oxygen support can have a desiccating effect on oral mucosa. Conversely, dysphagia can lead to pooling of oral secretions. These conditions, as well as true salivary gland dysfunction, typically lead to a profound change in patterns of microbial colonization and oral disease.

Histopathologic studies of minor salivary gland histopathology have revealed predominant changes within 3 weeks following chemotherapy; ductal dilation and acinar degeneration have been documented as prominent changes (8). These lesions generally resolve during the several weeks following cessation of chemotherapy, with minimal or no residual sequelae. Thus, unlike high-dose upper mantle radiation effects on salivary tissue, chemotherapy-associated salivary gland injury is usually transient and reversible. Relative to BMT conditioning regimens, chemotherapy with or without total lymph node irradiation does not induce irreversible damage to the parotid gland; however, total body irradiation can cause lasting reduction in glandular secretion (25, 26).

Flow rate and sialochemical analyses have demonstrated a considerable range of salivary changes during periods of chemotherapy administration. The disparate results likely stem from differing chemotherapy protocols used across the studies; thus, the drugs might have affected salivary function to different degrees (20–22). For example, one study of outpatients receiving cancer chemotherapy reported decreased whole saliva flow rates, amylase, and IgA levels, but increased lysozyme (21). In contrast, a study of inpatients receiving cancer chemotherapy revealed no significant changes in salivary flow rates, pH, or protein (19). Similarly, another study demonstrated no change in flow rate or potassium levels but detected significant reductions in sodium and protein for resting and stimulated parotid and submandibular/sublingual glands (22).

Strategies incorporating oral antimicrobial prophylactic rinses (e.g., gentamicin, vancomycin, nystatin) during periods of profound myelosuppression are generally effective in reducing the risk of oral mucosal infection when ulceration and compromised immunity exists. As such, reversible changes associated with xerostomia primarily evoke patient discomfort and impaired function rather than substantial increase in risk for infection. Xerostomia can impair mastication and speech and can exacerbate oral mucositis and angular cheilitis. Dysgeusia may develop following both altered taste bud function (27) and increased xerostomia.

Changes in salivary function can thus potentially occur during chemotherapy; they do not, however, appear to have significant long-term effects on oral health. Exceptions may include salivary changes in those patients receiving chemotherapy plus irradiation as part of conditioning regimens for BMT (24). Radiation in this setting can also compromise growth and development of the craniofacial complex in children, mediated in part through growth hormone deficiency (see below; 28–30).

Effective management of xerostomia can enhance the patient's overall status during the acute phase of cancer management. Typically, frequent oral rinses with sterile water or saline can be of benefit, as can salivary stimulants such as sugarless gum. Sodium bicarbonate, a mucolytic emollient, can be useful when saliva becomes viscous. Diets high in water content (e.g., Jello; General Foods Corp.) should be encouraged. Commercially available artificial saliva substitutes (e.g., Xero-lube; Scherer) may be used; however, these products are not designed to reconstitute all components (e.g., antimicrobial proteins) found in normal saliva. Pilocarpine hydrochloride, recently approved for use in head and neck cancer patients experiencing chronic radiation-induced xerostomia, is not routinely indicated in the chemotherapy patient with transient xerostomia. Dry or cracked lips occurring secondary to xerostomia should be gently cleaned every 2 to 4 hours with gauze and coated with K-Y jelly (Johnson & Johnson). Patients will often describe considerable relief from xerostomia through prompt, topical, palliative efforts to restore moisture to the oral cavity.

Some chemotherapy patients may complain of drooling and apparent sialorrhea rather than oral dryness. Rather than increased salivary output, these patients typically have difficulty in managing salivary secretions because of painful mucositis and attendant dysphagia. Palliative efforts, including frequent intraoral suction and bicarbonate rinses, should be implemented. In addition, drugs with antisialogogue activity such as antihistamines (e.g., diphenhydramine), tricyclic antidepressants (e.g., amitriptyline), or atropine sulfate can be considered if no cardiac or other contraindications exist.

Neurotoxicity

Chemotherapy can cause severe, deep-seated, throbbing mandibular or maxillary pain in some patients (3). The vinca alkaloids (e.g., vincristine and vinblastine) are most commonly associated with this disorder. Diagnosis is typically established by exclusion of more obvious causes, such as carious involvement of the dental pulp with resultant pulpitis and necrosis. Often bilateral, drug-induced neurotoxicity can be very uncomfortable to the patient; codeine-containing analgesics may be useful in controlling pain. Fortunately, the neurotoxicity is transient and subsides shortly after cessation of chemotherapy.

Dentinal hypersensitivity can be associated with chemotherapy administration and is usually reported as a generalized increased sensitivity to hot and cold. These sensitivities usually resolve after therapy is discontinued. Topical brush-on fluorides and desensitizing toothpastes can ameliorate symptoms in many cases.

Stress-associated temporomandibular joint neuromuscular dysfunction may be present in selected cases; masticatory muscle palpation tenderness and pain radiating to the ear are hallmark findings. Increased clenching and/or bruxing are the most common causes and usually emerge in a setting of sleep dysfunction, increased stress, and, less frequently, medication reactions. The short-term use of muscle relaxants or anxiety-reducing agents plus physical therapy (moist heat applications) will often resolve these symptoms. Occlusal splints may be indicated for patients to use while sleeping, to reduce clenching/bruxing tendencies.

Chemotherapy patients often report an alteration in taste during cancer therapy. Although the symptom persists for several weeks, it typically resolves in the months after discontinuation of the drugs. The taste-receptor cell has a turnover rate of approximately 10 days and can regenerate if not irreversibly damaged (31, 32). The chemotherapeutic effect is thus reversible, unlike similar symptoms in many head and neck cancer patients receiving high-dose radiation to salivary glands.

Despite the frequent clinical occurrences, few studies document types and degrees of chemosensory dysfunction associated with cancer chemotherapy (33). The contribution of olfaction to the reported experience of taste also needs to be considered when assessing patients. Other covariates include the patient's tasting of chemotherapy agents (diffusion into the oral cavity, or "venous taste phenomena") and changes in olfaction that alter taste experience (34). Conditioned aversions to foods in association with chemotherapy-induced nausea upon eating can also be misinterpreted as taste abnormalities.

Dentoalveolar Abnormalities

Cancer chemotherapy may have potentially significant effects on dental and alveolar growth and development in long-term survivors of childhood cancer (35, 36). Effects of chemotherapy on maturing teeth appear to be similar to, but less severe than, those reported in irradiated patients (35–40). Changes include enamel/dentinal hypoplasia or agenesis, which apparently results from direct damage to ameloblasts and odontoblasts. Damage to developing teeth by chemotherapy is most pronounced when drugs are administered to patients under 5 years of age. In addition, dental abnormalities in young children are more severe if cranial irradiation (e.g., >2400 cGy as treatment for acute lymphoblastic leukemia) is used (28). Alterations manifest as shortened tapered roots, microdontia, and incomplete enamel formation have also been circumstantially associated with chemotherapy.

Eruption patterns for affected teeth may also be delayed. Significant changes in normal dental functional capacity are not prominent; however, it is unclear whether long-term prognosis for these teeth is altered or if the teeth exhibit atypical responses to routine dental treatment, including orthodontic interventions.

INDIRECT STOMATOTOXIC EFFECTS

Oral Mucosal Infection

Although chemotherapy-induced oral mucositis predisposes to systemic infection, deleterious microfloral shifts can occur in the absence of clinically documented mucosal ulceration. The dynamics of systemic infection of oral origin in myelosuppressed cancer patients have shifted considerably during the past 25 years. For example, data published in the late 1960s demonstrated a shift to primarily gram-negative enteric bacilli (GNB) colonizing the oropharynx in hospitalized patients (41); the oral flora changed from chiefly aerobic and anaerobic gram-positive cocci and bacilli to a flora in which gram-negative organisms predominated. In the 1970s, microbial surveillance cultural studies in acute nonlymphocytic leukemia (ANLL) patients revealed that multiple pathogens could be acquired while the patient was hospitalized. Common pathogens included *Pseudomonas aeruginosa*, *Staphylococcus aureus*, and *Escherichia coli* (42–45).

A number of ecologic pressures have caused this profile to change during the past decade. As a new generation of antibiotics and biologic response modifiers have been used in clinical practice, the microfloral shifts in myelosuppressed cancer patients have been directed to more gram-positive infections, with a decrease in gram-negative infections (46–50). In addition, broad-spectrum antibiotic therapy has promoted shifts to more resistant bacteria or to fungi such as *Candida* spp. and *Torulopsis glabrata* (44). Whether gram-negative or -positive in origin, most infections in the compromised host continue to be caused by organisms colonizing at or near the site of infection (46, 47, 51).

Infection prevention remains a critical issue in chemotherapy patients. Multiple topical and systemic approaches have been used to prevent mucosal infection in the granulocytopenic cancer patient; key interventions are listed in Table 28.2 (52). These strategies have either been shown to be effective in controlled studies or are justifiable empirically; cooked foods of low microbial content to reduce acquisition of new organisms is an example of this latter category. Several of these approaches continue to be used in combination; for example, rates of acquisition of nosocomial organisms can be affected by the various protocols for gastrointestinal decontamination currently in use. Active immunization and granulocyte transfusions have not generally proven to be effective in humans. However, substantial advances in cytokine technology, including granulocyte colony-stimulating factor (G-CSF) and granulocyte-macrophage colony-stimulating factor (GM)-CSF, continue to portend success in enhancing host defenses compromised by cancer chemotherapy (53, 54).

Table 28.2. Strategies for Mucosal Infection Prevention in Granulocytopenic Cancer Patients

Reduction in mechanical and thermal trauma
Reduction in acquisition of new organisms
Gastrointestinal decontamination
Selective decontamination/colonization preservation
Protected environments and other isolation techniques
Antifungal prophylaxis
Antiviral prophylaxis
Cytokines (eg., granulocyte/macrophage colony-
   stimulating factor)
Passive immunization
Active immunization (Questionable efficacy)

From Peterson DE. Pretreatment strategies for infection prevention in chemotherapy patients. NCI Monogr 1990;9:61–71.

The risk of infection in the immunocompromised patient increases as the degree and duration of suppression increase. However, alterations in specific immune constituents will largely dictate the nature of infection. Neutropenia continues to be identified as the primary risk factor predisposing to infection in cancer patients (46, 47). The most significant increases in risk occur when the neutrophil count decreases to less than $1000/mm^3$.

In principle, topical delivery of antimicrobial agents to alimentary tract mucosa is superior to systemic administration relative to degree of side effects. Thus, various topical oral microbials have been used for prevention or treatment of chemotherapy-induced oral mucositis and associated infection, with varying degrees of success. Historically, studies of either 0.12% or 0.2% chlorhexidine have produced mixed results regarding efficacy. The drug has been reported to reduce severity and/or duration of mucositis in cancer patients (55, 56). McGaw and Belch, in a double-blind, placebo-controlled prophylactic trial, reported reduced mucositis scores during remission induction; they suggested that 0.1% chlorhexidine mouth rinses may be of value in the prevention of oral candidiasis in myelosuppressed leukemic patients (57). In 1988, Ferretti et al. reported effective prophylaxis of oral mucositis and candidiasis with 0.12% chlorhexidine rinses in 51 BMT patients (56). This study was also a double-blind, prospective, placebo-controlled trial.

In contrast, a subsequent study by Weisdorf et al. in 100 BMT recipients did not reveal similar results (58); in this study, however, prophylactic acyclovir was not routinely used, and compliance with scheduled chlorhexidine doses was only 71.8%. A recent study by Foote et al., using a human model of radiation-induced oral mucositis, reported a trend toward increased mucositis and toxicity (e.g., mouthwash-induced discomfort, dysgeusia, and staining of dentition) in patients randomized to receive chlorhexidine rinse containing 12% alcohol vehicle (59). There is need to investigate whether similar effects occur in patients undergoing chemotherapy, without bone marrow or peripheral blood stem cell rescue.

During the past 5 years, there have been few substantial studies of topical oral rinses other than chlorhexidine. Benzydamine hydrochloride (60), beta-carotene (61), and allopurinol (62) have previously and preliminarily been reported to be effective in reducing the incidence of chemotherapy- and/or radiation-induced oral mucositis (Table 28.3). Larger prospective, double-blind, placebo-controlled trials should be considered for these drugs. In contrast, several studies have demonstrated that oral sucralfate suspension is not effective in the prevention and treatment of oral mucositis in either pediatric patients receiving chemotherapy for newly diagnosed ANLL (63) or patients receiving high-dose radiation (64, 65).

As discussed above, infection of the ulcerated tissue can readily occur. *Candida albicans* is a common cause of superficial fungal infections of alimentary mucosa, including the oral cavity (46, 66) (Fig. 28.3). Fortunately, many of these pathoses can be prevented by intensive infection prevention strategies such as described above. In addition, the lesions often respond well to topical or systemic antifungal therapy when such therapy is instituted promptly. However, systemic candidal infections can occur in the patient

Table 28.3. Historical Perspective: Reduction in Incidence and/or Severity of Oral Mucositis

Investigators	Patient Population	Intervention
Prada and Chiesa (1987)	Head and neck cancer $(N = 36)^a$	Benzydamine hydrochloride
Mills (1988)	Oral squamous cell carcinoma $(N = 20)^b$	Beta-carotene[c]
Shenep et al. (1988)	Acute nonlymphocytic leukemia $(N = 48)$	Sucralfate[d]
Tsavaris et al. (1988)	Gastrointestinal cancer $(N = 16)$	Allopurinol[e]

[a]Peterson DE. Pretreatment strategies for infection prevention in chemotherapy patients. NCI Monogr 1990;9:61–71.
[b]Chemotherapy and/or radiotherapy patients.
[c]Nonblinded, randomized trial.
[d]Limited efficacy in prevention and treatment of oral mucositis in children/adolescents.
[e]Open label, noncontrolled trial.

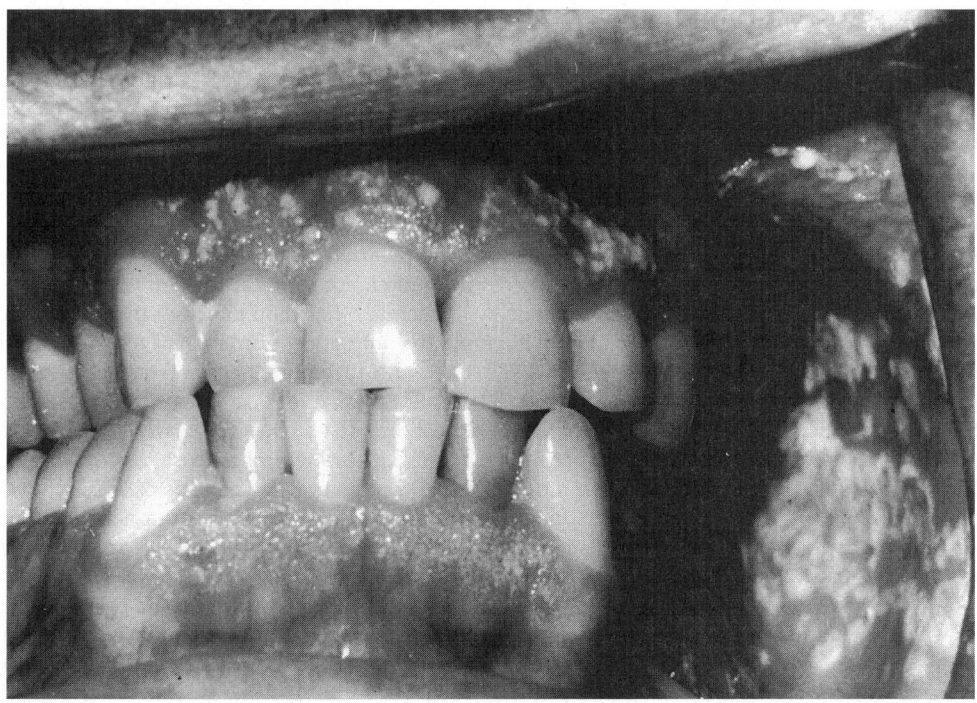

Figure 28.3.   Pseudomembranous candidiasis in an allogeneic bone marrow transplant patient with compromised salivary gland function secondary to chronic graft-versus-host disease. The quantitative/qualitative changes in saliva associated with acinar and ductal fibrosis provided a setting for emergence of *Candida albicans*.

with chemotherapy-induced myelosuppression and can present a diagnostic dilemma to the clinician. There are no pathognomonic signs or symptoms of disseminated candidiasis; the clinician must thus maintain a high index of suspicion in the immunocompromised cancer patient who has fever nonresponsive to antibiotics, regardless of presence or absence of obvious mucosal lesions. Other findings consistent with disseminated candidiasis include acute tachycardia, tachypnea, and hypotension, and/or a gradual worsening of the clinical condition. Unfortunately, reliable serologic assays to detect fungemia do not exist; blood specimens are culture positive in only 30 to 50% of patients with disseminated infection (47).

The most frequent sites of oral candidiasis are the tongue, the mucosa (palatal, buccal, gingival), and the lip commissures. The infection can produce considerable mucosal pain. The clinical appearance of oral candidiasis is varied but is typically described as raised, white, "curdy-looking" lesions (67). The lesions tend to have a firm yellow-white center with varying degrees of marginal erythema. Ulceration is often present

beneath the pseudomembrane, thus providing a portal of entry for systemic dissemination. Because of the invasive nature of the active portion of the infection, biopsy may be required to establish definitive diagnosis of these lesions, because of the high rate of false-negative surface cultures; however, this approach may not be appropriate for the profoundly suppressed patient.

Strategies for fungal prophylaxis remain controversial. While topical clotrimazole historically has shown efficacy in renal transplant recipients and patients with solid malignant tumors (68), its efficacy in leukemic patients is less clear. Nystatin oral rinse (swish and swallow regimens) can be painful when mucositis is present and can cause nausea and vomiting when swallowed. Triazole antifungal agents continue to be evaluated.

Amphotericin B typically produces effective infection resolution in patients with relatively intact neutrophil function; however, significant neutropenia is associated with impaired infection response rates. Fluconazole has been reported to significantly reduce fungal infections in BMT patients (69), but treatment of disseminated candidal infections with this agent requires further investigation. Approaches to the therapy of candidiasis are summarized in Table 28.1.

Viral infections following chemotherapy or BMT can also cause considerable oral disease (70, 71). These infections, particularly in BMT patients, are predominately caused by herpes simplex virus (HSV), varicella zoster virus, and cytomegalovirus (CMV) (46, 47). As with drug-induced mucositis, oropharyngeal viral infection can both cause substantial patient discomfort and interfere with normal oral function. HSV-induced mucositis is similar in clinical appearance to the mucositis that develops secondary to direct stomatotoxic effects of either induction drugs or conditioning chemoirradiation regimens used prior to BMT. Severe pain is a predominant feature, and narcotic pain control is often required.

Early recognition of HSV infection is important, since the infection can often be successfully managed with acyclovir (71). The risk for such reactivation appears to be considerably higher in BMT patients than in patients receiving induction chemotherapy. In this context, we retrospectively analyzed factors associated with acute oropharyngeal HSV infection in 627 patients who had undergone allogeneic BMT for leukemia, lymphoma, or aplastic anemia (72); 233 (37%) of the patients developed HSV infection; all but 2 were seropositive for HSV prior to transplant. Sixty-two percent of seropositive patients had at least one episode of HSV reactivation during the first 100 days following transplant. Other factors that placed patients at increased risk for HSV infection were a pretransplant diagnosis of leukemia, being in remission at the time of transplant, and/or having been conditioned for transplant with chemoradiotherapy.

Patients identified to be at risk for HSV mucosal infection may benefit from acyclovir prophylaxis; many centers use serum HSV titers above 1:8 or 1:16 as levels above which low-dose oral acyclovir (e.g., two 200-mg tablets every 4 hours, five times daily) should be administered. Dosing can be switched to the parenteral route if the patient is unable to continue enteral administration due to nausea or oral/esophageal ulcerative mucositis developing secondary to chemotherapy.

Over the past several years, CMV has been increasingly recognized as a cause of oral lesions in immunosuppressed patients (73–75). The clinical appearance is nonspecific; laboratory testing is necessary for diagnosis. Surface swab cultures may not be reliable, possibly because the virus tends to infect endothelial cells and fibroblasts with resulting low levels of free virus (74). The development of immunohistochemical stains for CMV has significantly improved the ability to diagnose this disease (75). Ganciclovir is the drug of choice for treatment.

Factors other than marrow suppression, hospitalization, and antimicrobial use can contribute to the development of oral infections. For example, removable prostheses can increase risk of infection in two ways (2). First, ill-fitting appliances can abrade oral mucosa, already compromised by the cytotoxic effects of chemotherapy; this mechanical irritation can exacerbate mucosal ulceration. Second, appliances soaked in denture cups containing water or selected denture disinfectants can readily become colonized with a variety of pathogens, including *P. aeruginosa*, *E. coli*, *Enterobacter* spp., *S. aureus*, *Klebsiella* spp., *T. glabrata* and *C. albicans*. Careful attention to denture adaptation and soaking solutions is therefore mandatory for infection prevention; with proper care, the beneficial effects of enhanced appearance, nutrition, and self-image can often be preserved for the chemotherapy patient by permitting restricted denture use during chemotherapy (18).

Dental Pulpal/Periapical Infection

Prevention or treatment of dental pulpal/periapical infections is also important (2). These infections are most commonly associated with extensive dental caries, a bacterial infection (Fig. 28.4). Conversely, noninfectious osseous periapical processes, such as leukemic infiltrates contiguous to dental root apices, can mimic acute infection (4).

Acute pulpal/periapical infections occur considerably less frequently than other acute oral infections in chemotherapy patients; few studies have analyzed risk for, or causative organisms associated with, the pulpal/periapical pathoses. A recent retrospective study of 276 BMT patients, in whom 23 postendodontic periapical radiolucencies were documented in 23 patients, provides additional insights into this issue (76). Neither increased systemic infection (febrile neutropenic days) nor incidence and type of oral infectious complications were significantly different between those patients, with or without

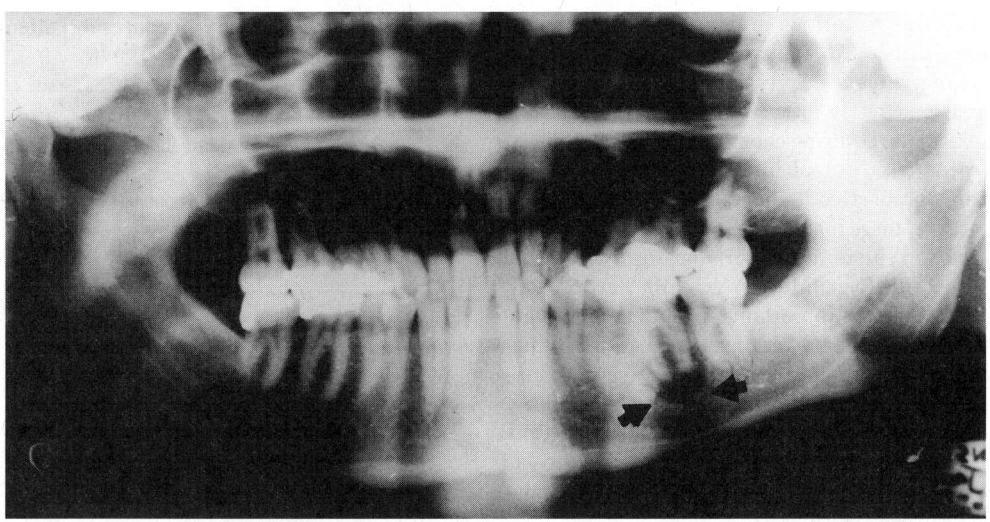

Figure 28.4.   Roentgenograph of periapical pathosis associated with mandibular left first molar (*arrows*). This acute nonlymphocytic leukemic patient was granulocytopenic and febrile (38.3°C) at admission and complained of intense pain in this region. This acute infection should be treated by either dental extraction (if appropriate) or endodontic therapy (root canal) in a setting of broad-spectrum antibiotics.

osseous lesions. The data suggest that nontreatment of asymptomatic postendodontic periapical radiolucencies does not increase incidence of infectious complications during BMT.

Empiric guidelines for prevention of pulpal and periapical infections during myelosuppression have been used in many cancer centers during the past decade (Table 28.4) (52). Given the success of these guidelines on patient management, it is important that each patient scheduled to receive myelosuppressive chemotherapy undergo oral evaluation well before the period of myelosuppression whenever possible. Careful attention should be directed to extensive carious lesions and/or periapical pathoses, in addition to oral mucosal and/or periodontal lesions.

Documentation of pulpal disease can be typically established with thorough history, clinical examination, and radiographs. Thermal testing may also be of value; lingering pain (>30 seconds) following administration of hot/cold stimuli is suggestive of irreversible pulpitis. Traditional diagnostic approaches are thus used to determine pulpal status, with the exception of percussion in the granulocytopenic patient. Pulpal therapy before initiation of chemotherapy may be indicated, based on the testing. Most pulpal interventions can successfully reduce risk of infectious flare during myelosupppression, with the exception of management of acutely infected pulpal tissue. This latter lesion, most com-

Table 28.4. Empiric Guidelines for Endodontic Care in Patients Scheduled to Receive Myelosuppressive Chemotherapy

Diagnosis	Management
Reversible pulpitis	Caries control
Irreversible pulpitis	Initial biomechanical preparation of canal(s); temporary double closure
Necrotic pulp with chronic periapical pathosis	No endodontic treatment unless patient has 7 days from completion of endodontic therapy to onset of myelosuppression (<1000 granulocytes/ mm^3)
Necrotic pulp with acute periapical infection	Endodontic therapy or extraction, depending on systemic status of patient and scheduling of chemotherapy

From Peterson DE. Pretreatment strategies for infection prevention in chemotherapy patients. NCI Monogr 1990;9:61–71.

monly due to carious involvement of the pulp, can be difficult to manage if the patient is experiencing myelosuppression due to marrow disease.

Patients requiring chemotherapy occasionally present with pulpal infections associated with nonrestorable teeth that should be extracted; however, there may not be sufficient time for the extraction site to heal before the onset of myelosuppression (e.g., <1000 ANC/mm^3). Appropriate treatment is important, since pathogens can readily disseminate because of direct communication of the dental pulp with the systemic circulation. Judicious management may call for pulpal therapy to eliminate the acute infection prior to neutropenia; the extraction can then be performed when the patient's hematologic status returns to normal.

On occasion, however, extractions for reasons of severe pulpal or periodontal infection must be performed prior to chemotherapy. To this end, two studies have contributed to the development of an effective clinical protocol. One study examined 28 consecutive ANLL patients with indications for dental extractions that included severe periodontal disease and/or evidence of pulpal necrosis with resultant pathosis (77). The criteria for severe periodontal disease were a periodontal pocket more than 6 mm apical to the cemento-enamel junction (determined by periodontal probing) or radiographic evidence of extensive dissolution of alveolar bone. Similarly, both clinical and radiographic data were used to document pulpal necrosis and resultant periapical conditions. Positive clinical findings included sensitivity to percussion in a setting of more than 2000 granulocytes/mm^3 and/or lack of response to an electrical pulp tester. Radiographic data included evidence of dissolution of lamina dura consistent with periapical pathosis.

Specific surgical guidelines were used. The extraction was as atraumatic as possible and included alveolectomies as necessary to achieve primary closure with multiple interrupted sutures. When possible, the extraction was performed at least 10 days prior to the patient's granulocyte count becoming less than 500/mm^3; i.e., the extraction must have occurred 3 to 4 days before the start of most chemotherapeutic protocols. If this interval could not be obtained, extractions were usually delayed until the granulocyte count had increased to the required level after discontinuation of chemotherapy. No hemostatic packing agents were used within extraction sites. If the platelet count was less than

Table 28.5. Oral Surgical Procedures in Patients with Acute Nonlymphocytic Leukemia

	Patient Status		
		Admitted for Treatment	
	Complete Remission	Granulocytes >2000/mm^3	Granulocytes ≤2000/mm^3
Number of patients	8	5	15
Extractions	40	22	57
Mean/patient	5	4.4	3.8
Surgical extractions	2	8	3
Alveolectomies	9	1	7
Complications	1	0	0

From Overholser CD, Peterson DE, Bergman SA, Williams LT. Dental extractions in patients with acute nonlymphocytic leukemia. J Oral Maxillofac Surg 1982;40:296–298. With permission.

40,000/mm^3, random donor or histocompatibility-matched platelets (as available) were transfused ½ hour before surgery in an attempt to obtain platelet increments of 40,000/mm^3 or greater at time of surgery. If the absolute granulocyte count was less than 2000/mm^3 on the day of extractions, a prophylactic antibiotic regimen of ticarcillin (75 mg/kg intravenously, ½ hour preoperatively, repeated 6 hours postoperatively) and amikacin (150 mg/m^2 intravenously, ½ hour preoperatively, repeated 6 hours postoperatively) was used.

One hundred nineteen extractions were performed. All patients were monitored postoperatively for complications that included bleeding and/or acute infections, to an endpoint of either disease remission or patient death. No significant clinical adverse sequelae occurred, including wound breakdown or infection (Table 28.5). The outcomes were comparable to those occurring in nonleukemic patients. While other centers may use variations of these guidelines, this approach has been successful in our institutions. It thus appears that with adherence to proper technique, extractions prior to chemotherapy can be safely performed in these patients. This conclusion has been supported by a subsequent independent investigation of Williford et al. (78).

Periodontal Infection

Most adults in this country have some degree of periodontal disease (gingivitis and/or periodontitis). This disease principally reflects the inflammatory response to bacteria that colonize the surface of the tooth contiguous to gingiva,

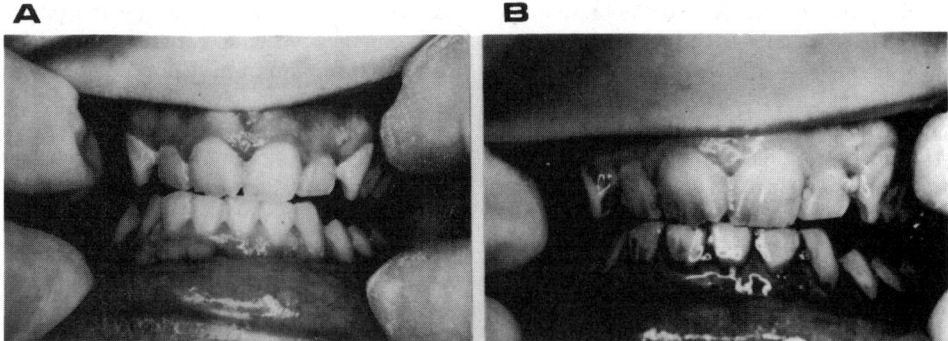

Figure 28.5.   Visualization of plaque, a soft adhesive bacterial product that is a primary etiologic factor in periodontal disease. A. Using clinical examination, the plaque level is difficult to assess. **B.** Using an erythrosine dye that stains plaque, a high level of plaque is noted. This patient has poor oral hygiene with associated gingival inflammation. Such deposits on a patient experiencing prolonged, profound myelosuppressive chemotherapy may promote acute periodontal infection and/or mucositis. (From Peterson DE. Dental care. In: Wiernik PH, ed. Supportive care of the cancer patient. Mt. Kisco, NY: Futura, 1983:145–171. With permission.)

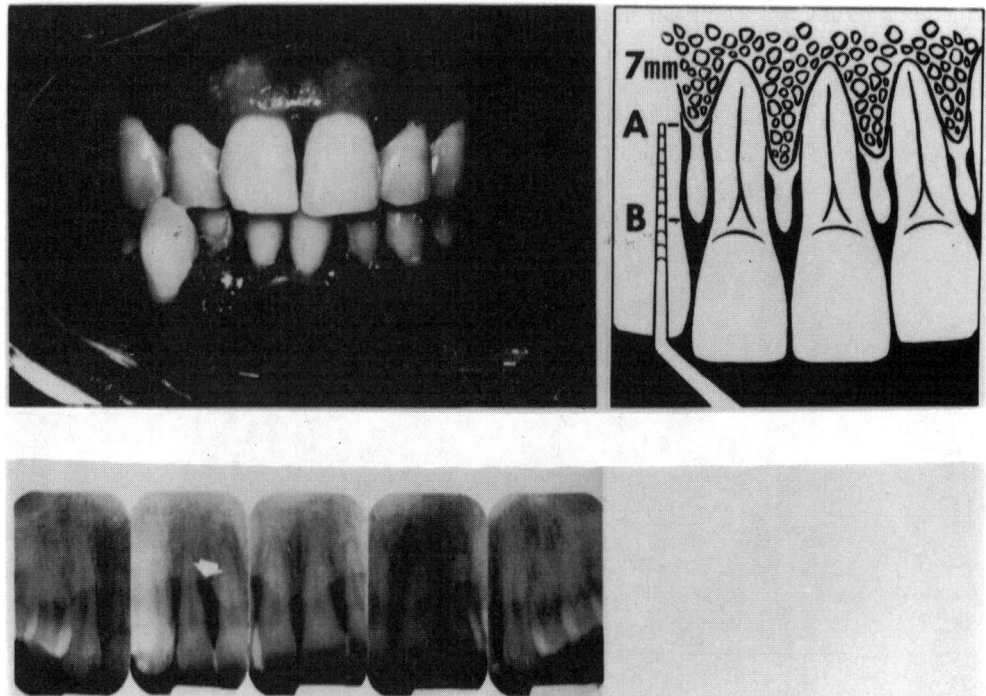

Figure 28.6.   Schematic, radiographic, and clinical appearance of periodontal disease in a patient with acute nonlymphocytic leukemia presenting for remission induction therapy. Oral examination revealed chronic, severe asymptomatic periodontal disease, including 7-mm periodontal pockets (A–B). This chronic oral infection can become acute during subsequent myelosuppressive therapy. (From Peterson DE. Dental care. In: Wiernik PH, ed. Supportive care of the cancer patient. Mt. Kisco, NY: Futura, 1983:145–171. With permission.)

metabolize local nutrients, and elaborate toxins that eventually penetrate the epithelium of the gingival sulcus (Fig. 28.5). Ulceration of the epithelium lining the space between the tooth and gingiva results in a gingival pocket. In the early stages of periodontitis, the connective tissue attachment is lost near the crown of the tooth and the pocket epithelium begins to migrate apically along the root surface. At this stage, a periodontal pocket is recognized (Fig. 28.6). In periodontitis, unlike gingivitis, inflammation affects supporting bone. Alteration in bone homeostasis occurs with a net loss of bony support that, when advanced, is characterized by mobility and eventual loss of the teeth.

Gingivitis and periodontitis can thus be characterized as an inflammatory response to metabolites of a mixed infection established on the tooth surface. The principal clinical sign is bleeding through ulcerated epithelium, the total surface area of which can become several square centimeters as the periodontal pockets deepen. It is usually chronic and asymptomatic; the patient is thus often unaware of the presence of periodontal disease. Pain, mobility, and abscess formation typically occur only late in periodon-

tal disease progression, causing the patient to seek emergency dental care. Thus, many adult patients presenting for chemotherapeutic management of cancer have some degree of periodontal disease.

Patterns of periodontal disease can be altered specifically in patients with hematologic malignancies. Occasionally, the newly diagnosed leukemic patient will present with an acutely infected infiltrate of the gingiva (Fig. 28.7). The engorged tissue is usually friable and edematous; maintaining optimal oral hygiene becomes very difficult. Once chemotherapy is initiated, however, enough resolution generally occurs to permit more comprehensive hygiene care. By comparison, the effects of intensive chemotherapy on alveolar bone do not appear to be of high clinical significance; reports of chemotherapy-associated osseous destruction are infrequent (79).

Chemotherapy patients with chronic periodontal disease may develop acute periodontal infections with associated systemic sequelae during granulocytopenia (Fig. 28.8). Beginning in the late 1970s, there have been several studies identifying the periodontium and/or dentition as sources for acute, systemic infection in cancer

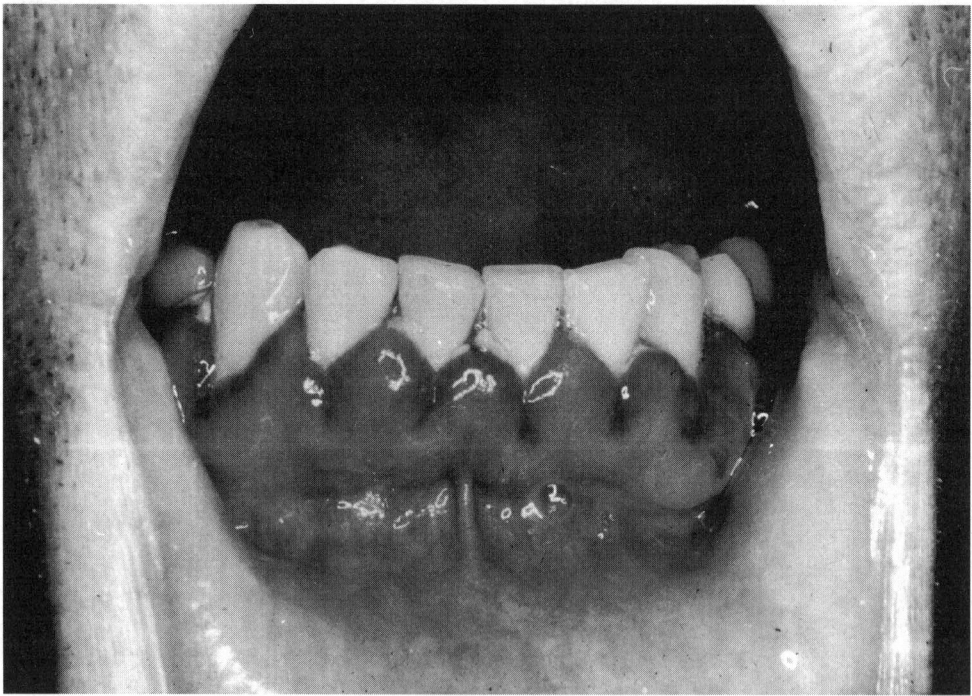

Figure 28.7.   Gingival leukemic infiltrate. This lesion results in pseudopocket formation, making thorough oral hygiene measures difficult. Partial resolution of such infiltrates often occurs following initiation of remission induction therapy.

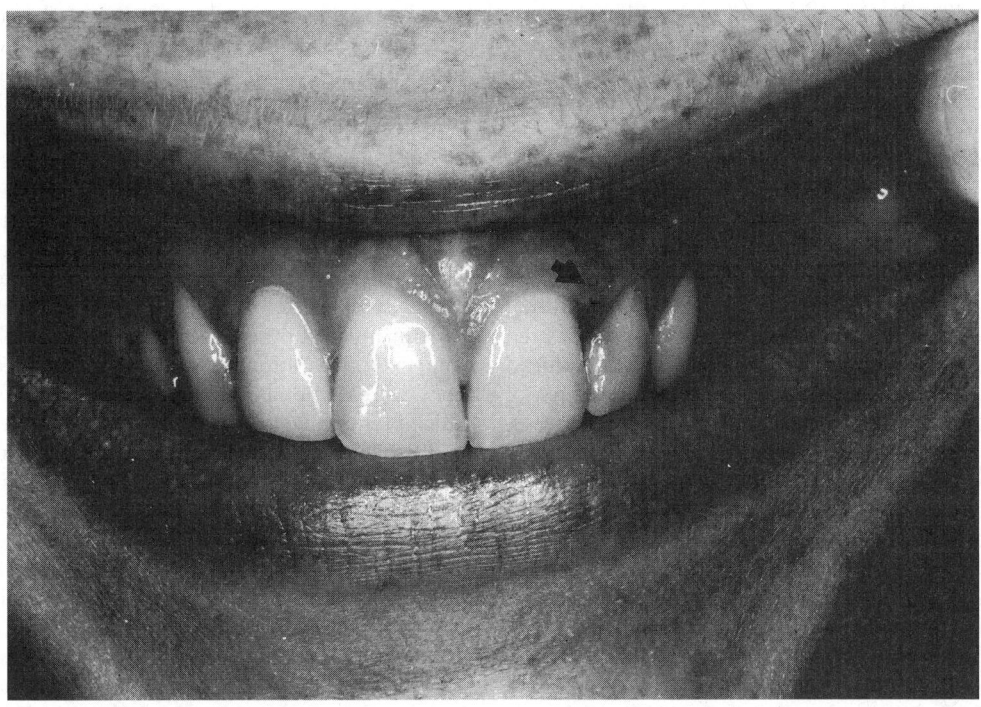

Figure 28.8.   Acute periodontal infection in a patient with acute myelogenous leukemia 15 days after initiation of anthracycline-cytosine arabinoside combination therapy. The patient complained of intense pain in the maxillary incisor region (*arrow*) and became febrile (38.3°C) shortly thereafter. No other source of infection was clinically documented. Granulocyte count was <%100/mm³; minimal acute inflammatory signs were present.

Table 28.6. Historic Perspective: Reduction in Incidence and/or Severity of Dental/Periodontal Infection

Investigators	Patient Population	Intervention
Lindquist et al. (1978)	Breast carcinoma ($N = 17$)	Dental plaque evaluations
Beck (1979)	Chemotherapy ($N = 47$)	Toothbrushing, Cepacol mouthwash, Vaseline
Daeffler (1980)	Cancer patients (n/a)	Survey and literature review
Greenberg et al. (1982)	Acute nonlymphocytic leukemia ($N = 33$)[a]	Prechemotherapy dental treatment
Hickey et al. (1982)	Testicular carcinoma ($N = 21$)	Prechemotherapy dental treatment +/− water lavage
Wright et al. (1985)	Cancer patients ($N > 2950$)[b]	Oral disease prevention program

From Peterson DE. Pretreatment strategies for infection prevention in chemotherapy patients. NCI Monogr 1990;9:61–71.
[a]9 patients on "initial study"; 24 patients on "modified study."
[b]Noncontrolled clinical trial.

patients (52) (Table 28.6). Lindquist et al. evaluated 17 breast carcinoma patients receiving chemotherapy and related dental plaque levels to incidence and duration of "stomatitis" during granulocytopenia (9). Patients with no measurable dental plaque developed less severe stomatitis for a shorter duration; however, no statistical analyses for levels of significance were presented. Greenberg et al. reported that the oral cavity (most frequently the periodontium) was the likely source for 7 of 12 episodes of septicemia in 33 ANLL patients; the authors concluded that potential oral sources of bacteremia should be eliminated prior to chemotherapy for acute leukemia (80). Hickey et al. reported that selected prechemotherapy dental treatment, including dental scaling and oral hygiene instructions, resulted in less severe stomatitis in a study of 21 testicular carcinoma patients; however, the statistical analyses did not include levels of significance of difference between those patients receiving prechemotherapy dental care and those who did not receive such prophylactic measures (14). Wright et al. summarized their experience using an oral disease prevention program in more than 2950 cancer patients receiving radiation and/or chemotherapy; they concluded that a variety of potential oral sequelae associated with cancer therapy can be prevented, reduced in severity, or alleviated (81). The approach of thorough prechemotherapy periodontal assessment and therapy is thus dramatically opposed to the removal of all teeth in leukemic patients in remission (82); this latter philosophy, proposed in 1976, is no longer advocated.

One study in 1982 reported that approximately 25% of all acute infections experienced by ANLL patients during induction arise in a site of preexistent periodontal disease (Fig. 28.8) (83). However, infection prevention approaches adopted since that time have substantially reduced this incidence; acute periodontal flares are currently an infrequent occurrence in myelosuppressed cancer patients.

These infections, although not common, can contribute to complexity of patient management. The lesions are often subtle in presentation and may remain undetected unless the oral tissues are thoroughly examined. As with other acute infections in the myelosuppressed patient (46, 47, 84, 85), acute periodontal infections often present with minimal signs of inflammation. In addition, extensive ulceration that may be present is not directly observable, yet may represent a source for disseminated infection by organisms such as *C. albicans*.

Studies of the periodontium as a locus of acute infection during myelosuppression thus continue to be relevant to contemporary clinical issues addressing oral lesions in chemotherapy patients. Historically, surveillance cultures of gingival tissue have constituted the primary experimental evidence demonstrating succession of GNB in the mouth during immunosuppression (86). This procedure entails streak inoculation of selective agar with cotton swabs of the attached gingivae. However, acute periodontal infections are not equivalent to mucositis, which results from the direct, stomatotoxic effects of cytotoxic drugs. Acute periodontal lesions should be viewed as an indirect result of reduction in

host defenses occurring in a setting of chronic, preexistent periodontal disease. Thus, culturing of mucosa or attached gingiva may potentially lead to inaccurate data when the subgingival site is the primary site of acute infection.

Studies in the later 1980s thus specifically examined subgingival sites versus attached gingiva. In 1986, one study investigated the possibility that the magnitude of the quantitative microbial load at the sample site was associated positively or negatively with a shift in level of GNB in myelosuppressed cancer patients (87). Data from both supra- and subgingival specimens were combined in this determination, in which predominant flora at time of admission to the hospital and at midpoint of myelosuppressive chemotherapy were compared. In general, no significant interpopulation differences were identified when ANLL pre- and midchemotherapy values were compared with the same small cell lung carcinoma (SCC) values; the singular exception was that total colony-forming units in oral rinse specimens from ANLL prechemotherapy patients were significantly lower than those in SCC prechemotherapy oral rinses ((34 ± 43) × 10^4 vs. (234 ± 215) × 10^4; $p = .02$). Midchemotherapy GNB shifts tended to occur at sites where the total cultivated microflora decreased relative to prechemotherapy levels. Large intersubject variations were observed, reflecting high standard deviations typical of oral culture findings when individual sites are analyzed. None of these patients developed an acute periodontal infection.

Specific oral sites thus showed quantitative and proportional increases in normally nonindigenous facultative GNB during myelosuppressive regimens in fewer than half the ANLL and SCC cancer patients. All oral sites were typically colonized by these bacteria in affected patients, but most sites did not harbor the organisms before chemotherapy. Antibiotic administration and reductions in levels of indigenous microflora may have contributed to the succession of coliforms. In ANLL patients, nonpathogenic *Pseudomonas* spp. were the most commonly recovered isolates, but pathogenic species were also detected.

Sources of GNB are both endogenous and exogenous. Exogenous sources include food, water, hands of hospital personnel, sinks, and hospital apparatus such as respirators. The use of stringent infection control measures, however, has markedly reduced the acquisition and prevalence of infections caused by exogenous pathogenic GNB and other microorganisms (46, 47). The indigenous alimentary tract flora, including the periodontal flora, may provide colonization resistance to potential pathogens; strategies to preserve alimentary tract anaerobes have been incorporated into clinical practice at selected centers (52). This model remains controversial, and further basic and applied research is indicated.

A companion study to the 1986 study cited above examined the specific relationship of periodontal disease to qualitative and proportional shifts in the oral microflora of 21 ANLL patients (7 males and 14 females; mean age, 51.0 years; range, 25 to 81 years) observed during standardized myelosuppressive regimens (Table 28.7) (88). Supra- and subgingival microbial plaque specimens were individually collected from two contralateral molar sites in each participant at hospital admission (day 1) and during the point of maximal myelosuppression (day 14). Periodontal disease indices obtained at day 1 included site-specific measures of attachment loss and clinical assessment of disease status. Using a residualized change score analysis, periodontal disease status and attachment loss were positively correlated with increases in proportional recovery of Staphylococcus spp. from supragingival sites and total yeast from supra- and subgingival sites. When age-related covariation in microbial shifts was controlled in the analysis, periodontal disease status and attachment loss demonstrated no significant correlation with increases in total yeast at supragingival sites.

These findings suggest that periodontal disease may contribute to patterns of oral microbial successions during cancer chemotherapy. In particular, attachment loss and periodontal disease classification at hospital admission were correlated with shifts in several pathogens midchemotherapy. Higher site-specific levels of attachment loss and more severe clinical assessments of periodontal disease status were associated with increases in proportional recoveries of both Staphylococcus and yeast species within supragingival and/or subgingival plaque specimens. Enteric bacilli and staphylococci were presumed to be members of the plaque ecosystem because of their frequent and high-level occurrence in both supra- and subgingival samples of individual teeth that were sampled separately.

The above studies documented periodontal flora in patients who did not progress to acute periodontal infection during myelosuppression. To examine the nature of systemic infection of periodontal origin in comparable patients, subgingival microbial flora associated with 27 acute exacerbations of preexistent periodontal disease in 24 patients with chemotherapy-induced myelosuppression was examined (89). All but two acute periodontal infections developed during low granulocyte levels (<1000/mm³). Suspected pathogens were detected in high concentrations in subgingival plaque specimens in 17 episodes of acute periodontal infection; a single pathogen was recovered in 10 acute infections, and more than 1 pathogen was recovered in 7 acute infections. S. epidermidis, C. albicans, S. aureus, and P.

Table 28.7. Relative Distribution of Indigenous and Acquired Bacteria before and during Myelosuppressive Chemotherapy in Patients with Acute Nonlymphocytic Leukemia[a]

Microflora	Supragingival Plaque		Subgingival Plaque	
	Prechemotherapy	Midchemotherapy	Prechemotherapy	Midchemotherapy
Gram-negative enteric bacilli	2.1 ± 1.7*	16.6 ± 7.4	3.1 ± 2.7*	14.4 ± 7.5
Fusobacterium nucleatum	4.2 ± 1.6	11.4 ± 7.2	7.2 ± 3.9	12.5 ± 7.6
Black-pig. Bacteroides sp.	0.1 ± 0.1	0.3 ± 0.3	0.9 ± 0.8	1.4 ± 1.4
Lactobacillus sp.	1.1 ± 0.6	2.7 ± 2.3	0.3 ± 0.1*	9.4 ± 5.3
Staphylococcus sp.	0.0 ± 0.0*	3.2 ± 1.9	0.0 ± 0.0*	3.5 ± 2.5
Pseudomonas aeruginosa	0.3 ± 0.3	0.2 ± 0.2	0.3 ± 0.2	0.0 ± 0.0
Neisseria sp.	5.9 ± 3.3	12.0 ± 6.7	9.8 ± 4.6	17.2 ± 6.5
Streptococcus mutans	1.0 ± 0.7	2.2 ± 1.6	0.6 ± 0.5	0.1 ± 0.1
Veillonella sp.	19.9 ± 4.0	15.5 ± 6.6	21.1 ± 5.6	23.2 ± 6.8
Total yeast	0.4 ± 0.4	0.5 ± 0.3	0.1 ± 0.0*	0.6 ± 0.4

From Reynolds MA, Minah GE, Peterson DE et al. Periodontal disease and oral microbial successions during myelosuppressive cancer chemotherapy. J Clin Periodontal 1989;16:185–189. With permission.
[a]Values reported are the mean ± SE percent total viable count (TVC). $N = 21$. Asterisks indicate prechemotherapy and midchemotherapy differences ($p \leq .10$) using a one-way analysis of covariance with repeated measures, controlling for differences related to antibiotic administration and hygiene protocol. Pretreatment TVC of Staphylococcus spp. was 0.002 ± 0.002.

aeruginosa predominated, with combinations of these detected in some patients. Concomitant bacteremias developed in two of these patients. The subgingival microflora associated with 10 acute periodontal infections was characterized by predominately indigenous microorganisms, which in nine episodes were in abnormal proportions, compared with microbial profiles in noncancer patients with similar degrees of periodontal disease. Thus, pathogens typically associated with infections in myelosuppressed cancer patients, as well as indigenous oral flora, can be associated with acute periodontal infections during granulocytopenia.

The microbiologic findings described in the studies above collectively emphasize the importance of the periodontium as a nidus for infection in neutropenic patients. Such infection may be associated with either pathogens or increased numbers of indigenous oral bacteria. Management of acute periodontal infections includes culturing and both local and systemic therapy. To assure accurate microbiologic documentation, a subgingival specimen should be collected from the infected site by gently placing a collection instrument (e.g., sterile paper point or periodontal file) into the pocket and withdrawing a specimen under nitrogen gas flow (85% nitrogen; 10% hydrogen; 5% carbon dioxide) (90). Care must be exerted in specimen collection and processing under anaerobic conditions to maximize the representative nature of the specimen. Broad-spectrum antibiotic therapy should be considered while culture results are pending. Local therapy consists of irrigation with effervescent agents (e.g., Glyoxide, Marion Laboratories), which are toxic to anaerobic bacteria normally colonizing the periodontal pocket, as well as supervised gentle mechanical plaque removal (dental brushing and flossing). The efficacy of chlorhexidine in treating these infections has not been thoroughly studied.

The issue of the risk of dental scaling and prophylaxis in patients in whom profound myelosuppression will occur within 2 weeks of the oral procedure has been raised in the literature on an ongoing basis (52). For example, some investigators have maintained that performing the procedure in advance of myelosuppression could (*a*) lead to a salutary reduction in microbial flora that could otherwise cause periodontal infection with systemic dissemination, (*b*) enhance healing of chronically infected periodontal tissues, and (*c*) reduce the incidence of fevers of unknown origin. Conversely, some clinicians have re-

mained concerned that such interventions may increase risk for oral complications with potential systemic significance.

To more fully examine this controversy, the impact of a noninvasive oral examination versus invasive oral interventions (periodontal probing, dental scaling) prior to chemotherapy on subsequent development of fever and/or bacteremia in the granulocytopenic cancer patient was investigated (91). Hospital records were reviewed for 100 patients who had been assigned to receive either the noninvasive or invasive procedures. Patients in the latter group who had fewer than 2000 granulocytes/mm^3 had received prophylactic broad-spectrum antibiotics 1 hour prior to the oral procedure and 6 hours after the initial dose. Temperature values immediately before and up to 48 hours after the oral intervention were noted and occurrence of fever and/or bacteremia documented for each group. There was no statistically significant difference in incidence of fever and/or bacteremia between the two groups of patients. Although periodontal probing and dental scaling are procedures that invade mucosal barriers, such interventions did not appear to significantly affect the incidence of fever or bacteremia among persons in this study.

Mucosal Hemorrhage and Anemia

Spontaneous gingival bleeding can be a primary early clinical indicator of impaired bone marrow function due to neoplastic involvement (4). As described above, most adults in this country have some degree of periodontal disease. Chronic trauma associated with normal functions of the oral cavity can also induce minor hemorrhage, which prompts the patient to seek professional care.

Disease- or chemotherapy-associated thrombocytopenia can thus result in bleeding. Spontaneous palatal petechiae are often observed when the platelet level is below 50,000 to 60,000/mm^3; spontaneous gingival oozing is common when the platelet count is below 15,000/mm^3. Patients who do not perform thorough oral hygiene care while undergoing myeloablative regimens are more prone to gingival hemorrhage, since plaque can readily form and exacerbate periodontal ulceration existent prior to myelosuppression.

Oral hemorrhage associated with thrombocytopenia is rarely a debilitating complication, although its occurrence can be frustrating to the patient. Gauze soaked in topical thrombin can be used as needed and is usually successful in reducing oozing. Platelet transfusions are usually not required, except for patients whose platelet counts are profoundly suppressed, resulting in hemodynamically significant bleeding episodes.

Anemia can be manifested in the oral cavity as well. Typical changes include pallor of the oral mucosa as well as atrophic glossitis that can usually be managed palliatively until the underlying erythrocyte abnormality is corrected.

Bone Marrow/Peripheral Blood Stem Cell Transplantation

Oral complications associated with BMT or PBSCT can be similar to those noted in patients undergoing high-dose chemotherapy without marrow rescue. Thus, chemotherapy and chemoradiotherapy conditioning regimens can cause significant oral toxicity (92). The risks associated with ulcerative mucositis, xerostomia, and oral infections are substantial until the oral mucosa heals (e.g., 18 to 28 days post-BMT) and neutrophil counts are sustained above $500/mm^3$. The risk of oral infection slowly declines during this period, although oral candidiasis and reactivation of HSV can occur in susceptible patients. Oral bleeding, especially that associated with mucositis, can be a clinical problem until mucosal healing has occurred and platelet counts can be continually maintained above approximately 20,000 to $30,000/mm^3$.

In general, the severity of mucositis depends primarily on the type of conditioning regimen used, although oral tissues in different transplant cohorts (i.e., autologous PBSCT; allogeneic related or unrelated BMT; syngeneic transplantation) may recover at slightly different rates. While healing appears to partially depend on rate of engraftment (especially neutrophils), the slower recovery rates in allogeneic patients (versus autologous/syngeneic patients) are clearly related to emergence of acute graft-versus-host disease (GVHD) in the allogeneic cohort. Oral acute GVHD can become apparent as early as 18 to 21 days posttransplant and is characterized by mucosal erythema, atrophy, ulceration, and hyperkeratotic striae and plaques. Topical steroid rinses, creams, and gels can help reduce symptoms and promote healing of ulcerations.

Oral infection profiles in BMT patients are similar to those seen in immunosuppressed patients receiving chemotherapy without transplant. In the 1980s and early 1990s, pseudomembranous candidiasis was common; fortunately, use of prophylactic fluconazole during the past several years is reducing the incidence of oral and associated disseminated candidal infection. Reactivation of HSV and CMV is noted in the early period post-BMT; however, prophylaxis with acyclovir for HSV and ganciclovir for CMV has proven to significantly reduce infection. The risk of oral bacterial infection has been reduced over the past 10 years in the setting of increasingly sophisticated oral hygiene protocols as well as improved bacterial prophylaxis and treatment interventions. Opportunistic gram-negative pathogens such as *P. aeruginosa*, *Neisseria* spp., and *E. coli*, as well as gram-positive cocci such as staphylococci and streptococci, however, remain of substantial concern.

Chronic GVHD is the most significant late oral complication seen in allogeneic BMT recipients. Its clinical presentation is similar to that seen in acute GVHD, with mucosal erythema, atrophy, and oral lichen planus–like lesions as classic components. GVHD can damage major and minor salivary glands, with resulting xerostomia and mucocoeles involving minor salivary gland tissue.

SUMMARY

The oral cavity is highly susceptible to the direct and indirect toxic effects of cancer chemotherapy. Oral complications in the myelosuppressed cancer patient can have a profound influence on the outcome of cancer treatment. Oral care should be both preventive and therapeutic as indicated to minimize risk for oral and associated systemic complications. Future research should be targeted at technology development to reduce the incidence and severity of oral mucositis, as well as improved infection prevention, detection, and treatment.

REFERENCES

1. Squier CA. Barrier functions of oral epithelia. In: Mackenzie IC, Squier CA, Dabelsteen E, eds. Oral mucosal diseases: biology, etiology, and therapy. Copenhagen: Lædgeforeningens Forlag, 1987:7–9.

2. Peterson DE. Oral complications associated with hematologic neoplasms and their treatment. In: Peterson DE, Elias EG, Sonis ST, eds. Head and neck management of the cancer patient. Boston: Martinus Nijhoff, 1986:351–361.

3. Peterson DE, D'Ambrosio JA. Diagnosis and management of acute and chronic oral complications of nonsurgical cancer therapies. Dent Clin North Am 1992;36:945–966.

4. Peterson DE, D'Ambrosio JA. Nonsurgical management of head and neck cancer patients. Dent Clin North Am 1994;38:425–445.

5. Peterson DE. Oral toxicity of chemotherapeutic agents. Semin Oncol 1992;19:478–491.

6. Sonis ST, Clark J. Prevention and management of oral mucositis induced by antineoplastic therapy. Oncology 1991;5:11–18.

6a. Rosenberg SW. The Sonis/Clark article reviewed. Oncology 1991;18–22.

7. Challacombe SJ. Tissue immune systems and mucosal diseases. In: Mackenzie IC, Squier CA, Dabelsteen E, eds. Oral mucosal diseases: biology, etiology and therapy. Copenhagen, Lædgeforeningens Forlag, 1987:36.

8. Lockhart PB, Sonis ST. Alterations in the oral mucosa caused by chemotherapeutic agents. J Dermatol Surg Oncol 1981;7:1019–1025.

9. Lindquist SF, Hickey AJ, Drane JB. Effect of oral hygiene on stomatitis in patients receiving cancer chemotherapy. J Prosthet Dent 1978;40:312–314.

10. Beck S. Impact of a systematic oral care protocol on stomatitis after chemotherapy. Cancer Nurs 1979; 3:185–199.

11. Daeffler R. Oral hygiene measures for patients with cancer (I). Cancer Nurs 1980;3:347–356.

12. Daeffler R. Oral hygiene measures for patients with cancer (II). Cancer Nurs 1980;3:427–432.

13. Daeffler R. Oral hygiene measures for patients with cancer (III). Cancer Nurs 1981;4:29–35.

14. Hickey AJ, Toth BB, Lindquist SB. Effect of intravenous hyperalimentation and oral care on the development of oral stomatitis during cancer chemotherapy. J Prosthet Dent 1982;47:188–193.

15. Ciais G, Namer M, Schneider M, et al. La laserthérapie dans la prévention et le traitement des mucites liées à la chimiothérapie anticancéreuse. Bull Cancer 1992;79:183–191.

16. Sonis ST, Costa JW, Evitts SM, Lindquist LE, Nicolson M. Effect of epidermal growth factor on ulcerative mucositis in hamsters that receive cancer chemotherapy. Oral Surg Oral Med Oral Pathol 1992; 74:749–755.

17. Sonis ST, Lindquist L, Van Vugt A, et al. Prevention of chemotherapy-induced ulcerative mucositis by transforming growth factor β3. Cancer Res 1994; 54:1135–1138.

18. Williams LT, O'Dwyer JL. Guidelines for oral hygiene, denture care and nutrition in patients with oral complications. In: Peterson DE, Sonis ST, eds. Oral complications of cancer chemotherapy. The Hague: Martinus Nijhoff, 1983:151–167.

19. Schubert MM, Izutsu KT. Iatrogenic causes of salivary gland dysfunction. J Dent Res 1987;66:680–688.

20. Schum CA, Izutsu KT, Molbo DM, Truelove EL, Gallucci B. Changes in salivary buffer capacity in patients undergoing cancer chemotherapy. J Oral Med. 1979;34:76–80.

21. Main BE, Calman KC, Ferguson MM, et al. The effect of cytotoxic therapy on saliva and oral flora. Oral Surg Oral Med Oral Pathol 1984;58:545–548.

22. Baum BJ, Bodner L, Box PC, Izutsu KT, Pizzo PA, Wright WE. Therapy-induced dysfunction of salivary glands: implications for oral health. Spec Care Dent 1985;(Nov–Dec):274–277.

23. Izutsu KT, Truelove EL, Bleyer WA, Anderson WM, Schubert MM, Rice JC. Whole saliva albumin as an indicator of stomatitis in cancer therapy patients. Cancer 1981;48:1450–1454.

24. Schubert MM, Sullivan KM, Truelove EL. Head and neck complications of bone marrow transplantation. In: Peterson DE, Elias EG, Sonis ST, eds. Head and neck management of the cancer patient. Boston: Martinus Nijhoff, 1986:401–427.

25. Jones LR, Toth BB, Keene HJ. Effects of total body irradiation on salivary gland function and caries-associated oral microflora in bone marrow transplant patients. Oral Surg Oral Med Oral Pathol 1992;73:670–676.

26. Chaushu G, Itzkovitz-Chaushu S, Yefenof E, Slavin S, Or R, Garfunkel AA. A longitudinal follow-up of salivary secretion in bone marrow transplant patients. Oral Surg Oral Med Oral Pathol Oral Radiol Endod 1995;79:164–169.

27. State FA, Hamed MS, Bondok AA. Effect of vincristine on the histological structure of taste buds. Acta Anat 1977;99:445–449.

28. Fayle SA, Curzon ME. Oral complications in pediatric oncology patients. Pediatr Dent 1991;13:289–295.

29. Williams MC, Martin MV. A longitudinal study of the effects on the oral mucosa of treatment for childhood leukaemia. Int J Paediatr Dent 1992;2:73–79.

30. Fleming P. Dental management of the pediatric oncology patient. Curr Opin Dent 1991;1:577–582.

31. Bartoshuk LM, Desnoyers S, Hudson C, et al. Tasting on localized areas. NY Acad Sci 1987;510:166–168.

32. Beidler LM, Smallman RL. Renewal of cells within taste buds. J Cell Biol 1965;263–272.

33. Bartoshuk LM. Chemosensory alterations and cancer therapies. NCI Monogr 1990;9:179–184.

34. Fetting JH, Wilcox PM, Sheidler VR, et al. Tastes associated with parenteral chemotherapy for breast cancer. Cancer Treat Rep 1985;69:1249–1251.

35. Jaffe N, Toth BB, Hoar RE, Ried HL, Sullivan MP, McNeese MD. Dental and maxillofacial abnormalities in long-term survivors of childhood cancer: effects of treatment with chemotherapy and radiation to the head and neck. Pediatrics 1984;73:816–823.

36. Rosenberg SW, Kolodney H, Wong GY, Murphy ML. Altered dental root development in long-term survivors of pediatric acute lymphoblastic leukemia. Cancer 1987;59:1640–1648.

37. Beumer J III, Curtis T, Harrison RE. Radiation therapy of the oral cavity: sequelae and management, parts 1 and 2. Head Neck Surg 1979;1:301–312, 392–408.

38. Burke FJT, Fram JW. The effect of irradiation on developing teeth. Oral Surg Oral Med Oral Pathol 1979;47:11–13.

39. Dahllöf G, Barr M, Blome P, et al. Disturbances in dental development after total body irradiation in bone marrow transplant recipients. Oral Surg Oral Med Oral Pathol 1988;65:41–44.

40. Dahllöf G, Heimdahl A, Blome P, Lönnquist B, Ringdén O. Oral condition in children treated with bone marrow transplantation. Bone Marrow Transplant 1988;3:43–51.

41. Johanson WG, Pierce AK, Sanford JP. Changing pharyngeal bacterial flora of hospitalized patients: emergence of gram-negative bacilli. N Engl J Med 1969; 281:1137–1140.

42. Wade JC. Principles of infection management. In: Peterson DE, Elias EG, Sonis ST, eds. Head and neck management of the cancer patient. Boston: Martinus Nijhoff, 1986:141–159.

43. Klastersky J. Infections in patients with cancer:

prevention. In: Moossa AR, Robson MC, Schimpff SC, eds. Comprehensive textbook of oncology. 2nd ed. Baltimore: Williams & Wilkins, 1991:1749–1753.

44. Schimpff SC. Infections in patients with cancer: overview and epidemiology. In: Moossa AR, Robson MC, Schimpff SC, eds. Comprehensive textbook of oncology. 2nd ed. Baltimore: Williams & Wilkins, 1991:1720–1732.

45. Valenti WM, Trudell RG, Bentley DW. Factors predisposing to oropharyngeal colonization with gram-negative bacilli in the aged. N Engl J Med 1978; 298:1108–1111.

46. Pizzo PA, Meyers J, Freifeld AG, Walsh T. Infections in the cancer patient. In: DeVita Vt, Hellman S, Rosenberg SA, eds. Cancer: principles and practice of oncology. 4th ed. Philadelphia: JB Lippincott, 1993:2292–2337.

47. Rolston KVI, Bodey GP. Infections in patients with cancer. In: Holland JF, Frei E, Bast RC, Kufe DW, Morton DL, Weichselbaum RR, eds. Cancer medicine. 3rd ed. Philadelphia: Lea & Febiger, 1993:2416–2441.

48. Weisman SJ, Scoopo FJ, Johnson GM, et al. Septicemia in pediatric oncology patients: the significance of viridans streptococcal infections. J Clin Oncol 1990; 8:453–459.

49. Wingard JR. Infectious and noninfectious systemic consequences. NCI Monogr 1990;9:21–26.

50. Donnally JP. Viridans streptococci and allogeneic bone marrow transplant recipients. Doctoral thesis. University of Nijmegen, The Netherlands, 1993.

51. Schimpff SC, Young VM, Greene WH, Vermeulen GD, Moody MR, Wiernik PH. Origin of infection in acute nonlymphocytic leukemia: significance of hospital acquisition of potential pathogens. Ann Intern Med 1972;77:707–714.

52. Peterson DE. Pretreatment strategies for infection prevention in chemotherapy patients. NCI Monogr 1990;9:61–71.

53. Gabrilove JL. Treatment of iatrogenic and disease-related neutropenia by recombinant human granulocyte colony stimulating factor. Presented at: Oral complications of cancer therapies: diagnosis, prevention and treatment. National Institutes of Health Consensus Development Conference, April 17–19, 1989.

54. Canellos GP, Demetri GD. Myelosuppression and "conventional" chemotherapy: what price, what benefit? J Clin Oncol 1992;11:1–2.

55. Ferretti GA, Hansen IA, Whittenbury K, Brown AT, Lillich TT, Ash RC. Therapeutic use of chlorhexidine in bone marrow transplant patients: case studies. Oral Surg Oral Med Oral Pathol 1987;63:683–687.

56. Ferretti GA, Ash RC, Brown AT, Parr MD, Romond EH, Lillich TT. Control of oral mucositis and candidiasis in marrow transplantation: a prospective, double-blind trial of chlorhexidine digluconate oral rinse. Bone Marrow Transplant 1988;3:483–493.

57. McGaw WT, Belch A. Oral complications of acute leukemia: prophylactic impact of a chlorhexidine mouth rinse regimen. Oral Surg Oral Med Oral Pathol 1985;60:275–280.

58. Weisdorf DJ, Bostrom B, Raether D, et al. Oropharyngeal mucositis complicating bone marrow transplantation: prognostic factors and the effect of chlorhexidine mouth rinse. Bone Marrow Transplant 1989;4:89–95.

59. Foote RL, Loprinzi CL, Frank AR, et al. Randomized trial of a chlorhexidine mouthwash for alleviation of radiation-induced mucositis. J Clin Oncol 1994;12:2630–2633.

60. Prada A, Chiesa F. Effects of benzydamine on the oral mucositis during antineoplastic radiotherapy and/or intra-arterial chemotherapy. Int J Tissue React 1987;9:115–119.

61. Mills EED. The modifying effect of beta-carotene on radiation and chemotherapy induced oral mucositis. Br J Cancer 1988;57:416–417.

62. Tsavaris N, Caragiauris P, Kosmidis P. Reduction of oral toxicity of 5-fluorouracil by allopurinol mouthwashes. Eur J Surg Oncol 1988;14:405–406.

63. Shenep JL, Kalwinsky DK, Hutson PR, et al. Efficacy of oral sucralfate suspension in prevention and treatment of chemotherapy-induced mucositis. J Pediatr 1988;113:758–763.

64. Barker G, Loftus L, Cuddy P, Barker B. The effects of sucralfate suspension and diphenhydramine syrup plus kaolin-pectin on radiotherapy-induced mucositis. Oral Surg Oral Med Oral Pathol 1991;71:288–293.

65. Epstein JB, Wong FLW. The efficacy of sucralfate suspension in the prevention of oral mucositis due to radiation therapy. Int J Radiat Oncol Biol Phys 28 1994:693–698.

66. Epstein JB, Vickars L, Spinelli J, Reece D. Efficacy of chlorhexidine and nystatin rinses in prevention of oral complications in leukemia and bone marrow transplantation. Oral Surg Oral Med Oral Pathol 1992; 73:682–689.

67. Peterson DE. Oral candidiasis. Clin Ger Med 1992;3:513–527.

68. Owens NJ, Nightingale CH, Schweizer RT, Schauer PK, Dekker PT, Quintiliani R. Prophylaxis of oral candidiasis with clotrimazole troches. Arch Intern Med 1984;144:290–293.

69. Goodman JL, Drew JW, Greenfield RA, et al. A controlled trial of fluconazole to prevent fungal infections in patients undergoing bone marrow transplantation. N Engl J Med 1992;326:845–851.

70. Saral R. Management of acute viral infections. NCI Monogr 1990;9:107–110.

71. Bustamante CI, Wade JC. Herpes simplex virus infection in the immuno-compromised cancer patient. J Clin Oncol 1991;9:1903–1915.

72. Schubert MM, Peterson DE, Flournoy N, Meyers JD, Truelove EL. Oral and pharyngeal herpes simplex infection after allogeneic bone marrow transplantation: analysis of factors associated with infection. Oral Surg Oral Med Oral Pathol 1990;70:286–293.

73. Schubert MM. Oral manifestations of viral infections in immunocompromised patients. Curr Opin Dent 1991;1:384–397.

74. Schubert MM, Epstein JB, Lloid ME, Cooney E. Oral infections due to cytomegalovirus in immunocompromised patients. J Oral Pathol Med 1993;22:268–273.

75. Lloid ME, Schubert MM, Myerson D, et al. Cytomegalovirus infection of the tongue following marrow transplantation. Bone Marrow Transplant 1994; 14:99–104.

76. Peters E, Monopoli, Woo SB, Sonis S. Assessment of the need for treatment of postendodontic asymptomatic periapical radiolucencies in bone marrow transplant patients. Oral Surg Oral Med Oral Pathol 1993;76:45–48.

77. Overholser CD, Peterson DE, Bergman SA, Williams LT. Dental extractions in patients with acute non-

lymphocytic leukemia. J Oral Maxillofac Surg 1982; 40:296–298.

78. Williford SK, Salisbury PK, Peacock JE, et al. The safety of dental extractions in patients with hematologic malignancies. J Clin Oncol 1989;7:798–802.

79. Stansbury DM, Peterson DE, Suzuki JB. Rapidly progressive acute periodontal infection in a patient with acute leukemia. J Periodontol 1988;59:544–547.

80. Greenberg MS, Cohen SG, McKitrick JC, Cassileth PA. The oral flora as a source of septicemia in patients with acute leukemia. Oral Surg 1982;53:32–36.

81. Wright WE, Haller JM, Harlow SA, Pizzo PA. An oral disease prevention program for patients receiving radiation and chemotherapy. J Am Dent Assoc 1985;110:43–47.

82. Chapman RM, Crosby WH. Elective dental extractions in leukemia (letter). N Engl J Med 1976; 295:114.

83. Overholser CD, Peterson DE, Williams LT, Schimpff SC. Periodontal infection in patients with acute nonlymphocytic leukemia: prevalence of acute exacerbations. Arch Intern Med 1982;142:551–554.

84. Bodey GP, Buckley M, Sathe YS, Freireich EJ. Quantitative relationships between circulating leukocytes and infection in patients with acute leukemia. Ann Intern Med 1966;64:328–340.

85. Sickles EA, Greene WH, Wiernik PH. Clinical presentation of infection in granulocytopenic patients. Arch Intern Med 1975;135:715–719.

86. Newman KA, Schimpff SC, Young VM, Wiernik PH. Lessons learned from surveillance cultures in patients with acute nonlymphocytic leukemia. Am J Med 1981;70:423–431.

87. Minah GE, Rednor JL, Peterson DE, Overholser CD, DePaola LG, Suzuki JB. Oral succession of gram-negative bacilli in myelosuppressed cancer patients. J Clin Microbiol 1986;24:210–213.

88. Reynolds MA, Minah GE, Peterson DE, et al. Periodontal disease and oral microbial successions during myelosuppressive cancer chemotherapy. J Clin Periodontol 1989;16:185–189.

89. Peterson DE, Minah GE, Overholser CD, et al. Microbiology of acute periodontal infection in myelosuppressed cancer patients. J Clin Oncol 1987;5:1461–1468.

90. Aranki A, Syed SA, Kenney EB, et al. Isolation of anaerobic bacteria from human gingiva and mouse cecum by means of simplified glove box procedure. Appl Microbiol 1969;17:568–576.

91. Weikel DS, Peterson DE, Rubinstein LE, Metzger-Samuels C, Overholser CD. Incidence of fever following invasive oral interventions in the myelosuppressed cancer patient. Cancer Nurs 1989;12:265–270.

92. Schubert MM. Oro-pharyngeal mucositis. In: Atkinson K, ed. Clinical bone marrow transplantation. Cambridge: Cambridge University Press, 1994:378–384.

29

Dermatologic Toxicity

Antoinette F. Hood

Many adverse reactions to chemotherapeutic agents are manifested in rapidly proliferating tissues such as the mucous membranes, skin, hair, and nails. Although these reactions are rarely life threatening, they may elicit significant disfigurement and patient concern. Occasionally, cutaneous complications are the rate-limiting factor in the administration of antineoplastic medications. The incidence of cutaneous toxicity is quite variable; some reactions such as alopecia and stomatitis are clearly dose dependent, while others such as acral erythema and hyperpigmentation occur unpredictably.

Evaluating an oncology patient with a cutaneous eruption may be challenging for the clinician. In addition to the underlying neoplasia, which itself may produce paraneoplastic manifestations, the patient is almost always on multiple medications. In this setting, it may be very difficult to determine the precise role played by an individual medication in the causation of a specific reaction. In evaluating a patient suspected of having a reaction to a medication, attention must be given to (a) timing (duration between administration of various medications and onset of the eruption); (b) morphology of the cutaneous eruption; (c) associated clinical and laboratory findings, such as fever and neutropenia; (d) supportive evidence from biopsy; and (e) documentation of similar occurrences in the literature.

In this chapter the various dermatologic toxicities of specific medications are discussed. Tables 29.1 to 29.9 provide an overview of the different types of cutaneous complications that are seen, with a listing of the drugs causing these reactions. Because it occurs so commonly with antineoplastic medications, alopecia is discussed in some detail.

Alopecia

Alopecia associated with chemotherapeutic agents is directly related to the cytotoxic effect of the drugs on the rapidly proliferating cell population in the hair matrix. Cytotoxic drugs produce partial or complete inhibition of mitoses and impaired metabolic processes in the hair matrix. This results in either a thin, weakened hair shaft or complete failure to form a hair. The thinned hair shaft is susceptible to fracture, and even mild trauma such as normal hair grooming will result in hair breakage and hair loss. Alopecia caused by mitotic inhibition affects only actively growing anagen hairs, which account for approximately 85% of the scalp hairs. Chemotherapeutic agents therefore produce an "anagen effluvium." Anagen effluvium is diffuse but may be initially incomplete. (Fig. 29.1) Repetitive exposure to cytotoxic chemicals will result in complete loss of scalp hair. Other terminal hair fol-

Table 29.1. Chemotherapeutic Agents Producing Stomatitis

Actinomycin D
Bleomycin
Cyclophosphamide
Daunorubicin
Doxorubicin
5-Fluorouracil
Interleukin-2
Mercaptopurine
Methotrexate
Mithramycin
Nitrosoureas
Procarbazine
Vinblastine
Vincristine

Table 29.2. Chemotherapeutic Drugs Implicated in the Production of Alopecia

Amsacrine
Bleomycin
Cyclophosphamide
Cytarabine
Dactinomycin
Daunorubicin
Dacarbazine
Doxorubicin
Etoposide
5-Fluorouracil
Hydroxyurea
Ifosfamide
Interleukin-2
Methotrexate
Nitrosoureas
Procarbazine
Vinblastine
Vincristine

Table 29.3. Drugs Producing Tissue Injury

Drugs Producing Phlebitis	Drugs Producing Chemical Cellulitis
Actinomycin D	Actinomycin D
Amsacrine	Bleomycin
Carmustine	Cisplatin
Dacarbazine	Dacarbazine
Daunorubicin	Daunorubicin
Doxorubicin	Doxorubicin
Mechlorethamine	5-Fluorouracil
Mitomycin	Mechlorethamine
Mitoxantrone	Methotrexate
Vinblastine	Mithramycin
	Mitomycin
	Mitoxantrone
	Streptozotocin
	Vinblastine
	Vincristine

licles such as those of eyebrows and eyelashes, beard, axillary hair, and pubic hair are variably affected, depending on the rate of hair matrix mitoses, the percentage of hairs in anagen, and the dose of the drug.

Hair loss is noticable 1 to 2 weeks after chemotherapy is administered and becomes most apparent 1 to 2 months later. Alopecia induced by chemotherapeutic agents is dose dependent and is reversible upon cessation of the medication. Occasionally, during prolonged cycles of chemotherapy, hair will regrow, but the hair is usually thinner than before chemotherapy was instigated. For unknown reasons, hair regrowth following chemotherapy may be associated with change in color or texture (1, 2).

Because of the psychologic stress produced by chemotherapy-induced alopecia, consider-

Table 29.4. Chemotherapeutic Agents Associated with Hypersensitivity Reactions

Amsacrine
Asparaginase
Bleomycin
Chlorambucil
Cisplatin
Cyclophosphamide
Daunorubicin
Doxorubicin
Etoposide
Mechlorethamine
Melphalan
Methotrexate
Procarbazine
Thio-TEPA

Table 29.5. Chemotherapeutic Agents Associated with Hyperpigmentation

Skin (localized hyperpigmentation)
  Bleomycin
  Cyclophosphamide
  Doxorubicin
  5-Fluorouracil
  Ifosfamide
  Triethylenethiophosphoramide (thio-TEPA)
Skin (diffuse hyperpigmentation)
  Cyclophosphamide
  Hydroxyurea
  Methotrexate
Mucous membranes
  Busulfan
  Cyclophosphamide
  Doxorubicin
  5-Fluorouracil
Nails
  Bleomycin
  Cyclophosphamide
  Daunorubicin
  Doxorubicin
  5-Fluorouracil
  Hydroxyurea
Hair
  Methotrexate
Teeth
  Cyclophosphamide

able effort has been directed toward diminishing or inhibiting this reaction. The onset of scalp hair loss may be delayed with the use of scalp hypothermia or scalp tourniquets; however these products are *not* recommended for patients with leukemia or in those who are at risk of scalp metastasis. Recent studies have shown that the use of IMUVERT (a membrane vesicle–ribosome preparation from a bacterium) either partially or completely reverses the alopecia effects of several chemotherapeutic agents in a rodent model (3).

The reader is referred to several chapters in this book that provide detailed information about hypersensitivity and extravasation reactions and oral complications of chemotherapeutic agents and to several reviews on mucocutaneous complications of chemotherapy (4, 5).

Table 29.6. Chemotherapeutic Agents That Interact with Radiation (X-Ray Radiation and UV Light)

Radiation enhancement
   Actinomycin
   Bleomycin
   Doxorubicin
   Etoposide
   5-Fluorouracil
   Hydroxyurea
   Interferons
   Methotrexate
Radiation recall
   Actinomycin D
   Doxorubicin
Photosensitivity
   Dacarbazine
   5-Fluorouracil
   Methotrexate
   Mitomycin
   Vinblastine
Reactivation of UV light-induced erythema
   Methotrexate

Table 29.7. Chemotherapeutic Drugs Causing Inflammation of Seborrheic or Actinic Keratoses

Actinomycin D
Cisplatin
Cytarabine
Dacarbazine
Doxorubicin
5-Fluorouracil
Pentostatin

Table 29.8. Acral Erythema/Erythrodysesthesia

Bleomycin
Cytarabine
Doxorubicin
5-Fluorouracil
Methotrexate
Thio-TEPA

Table 29.9. Miscellaneous Reactions

Raynaud's phenomenon and scleroderma-like changes
   Bleomycin
   Vincristine
   Vinblastine
Hypertrichosis
   Cyclosporine
Folliculitis
   Actinomycin D
   Methotrexate
Localized urticaria at the site of injection
   Doxorubicin
Neutrophilic eccrine hidradenitis
   Bleomycin
   Cytarabine
   Bleomycin
Vasculitis
   Cytarabine
   Hydroxyurea
   Methotrexate

ALKYLATING AGENTS

Alkylating agents frequently produce mucocutaneous reactions. Many of the reported complications are abnormalities of pigmentation, particularly patterned hyperpigmentation (6) (Fig. 29.2) or IgE-mediated hypersensitivity reactions (urticaria, angioedema, and anaphylaxis).

Cyclophosphamide

Alopecia is a common, dose-related complication of cyclophosphamide chemotherapy. More than 50% of patients receiving intensive or prolonged therapy with cyclophosphamide experience alopecia. It is particularly frequent when the cumulative dose exceeds 5 g. The alopecia is usually reversible when therapy is discontinued, but as mentioned above, the new hair may be quite different in texture or color. *Stomatitis* and mucosal ulcerations may be seen in

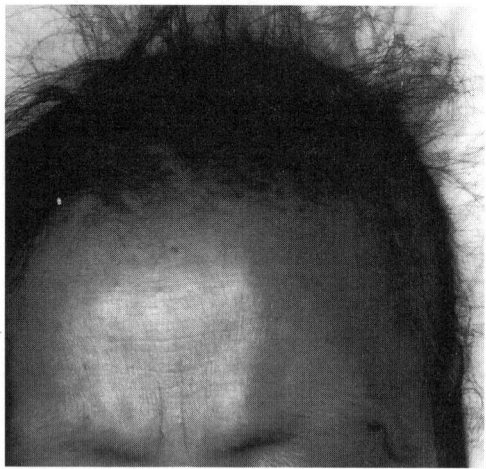

Figure 29.1.   Anagen effluvium.

association with cyclophosphamide administration; however, the frequency of this complication is lower than with other therapeutic agents. There are many reports of *altered pigmentation* associated with cyclophosphamide administration. Generalized hyperpigmentation of the skin and mucous membranes has been described, as has hyperpigmentation limited to the nails, palms and soles, or teeth. Nail hyperpigmentation typically occurs as either transverse or horizontal bands. The color abnormality initially appears at the proximal portion of the nail and grows distally over a 6-month period (7). Hypopigmentation of the nails occurs in horizontal bands, which may be multiple if chemotherapy is administered in cycles (8) (Fig. 29.3).

Hypersensitivity reactions such as urticaria and anaphylaxis have been reported in a few instances. In one patient, recurrent urticaria was associated with repetitive administrations of cyclophosphamide. Serum samples contained homocytotropic antibody activity of the IgE type (9). Another patient, with a history of hypersensitivity to mechlorethamine, developed angioedema after having been given cyclophosphamide. This reaction suggests cross-sensitivity among the alkylating agents (10).

Mechlorethamine

Topical mechlorethamine is associated with allergic and irritant *contact dermatitis* and local *hyperpigmentation*. *Anaphylactic reactions* have been occasionally reported. Systemic administration of this drug may also be associated with hypersensitivity reactions such as *angioedema*

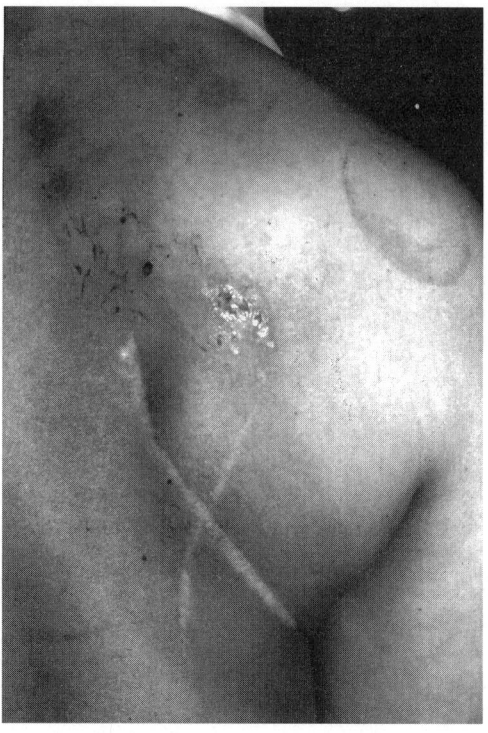

Figure 29.2.   Patterned hyperpigmentation occurring under occlusive dressings in a patient on combination chemotherapy that includes cyclophosphamide.

and *pruritus*. Cross-sensitivity with cyclophosphamide has been reported (10).

Chlorambucil

Cutaneous reactions to chlorambucil are uncommon. Two patients with generalized urticaria and periorbital edema have been reported (11).

Melphalan

Mucocutaneous reactions to melphalan are infrequent. Hypersensitivity reactions such as *pruritus, urticaria, angioedema* and *anaphylaxis* occur in approximately 4% of individuals receiving this drug (12).

Regional perfusion of melphalan has been associated with bullous reactions, desquamation, and cutaneous necrosis.

Busulfan

Hyperpigmentation is commonly seen in association with busulfan administration. The pigmentation is typically widespread but generally spares the palmar creases and the mucous mem-

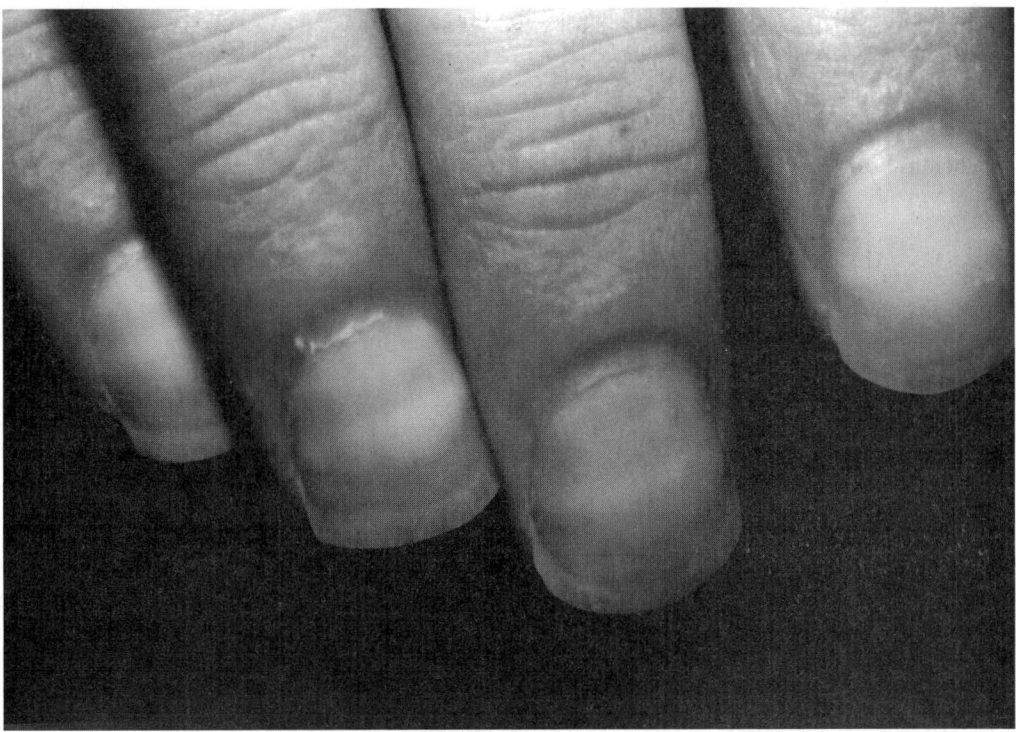

Figure 29.3.   White transverse bands of the nails.

branes. Biopsy of hyperpigmented skin shows increased melanin in the basal layer but no increase in the number of melanocytes. Hyperpigmentation has also been reported in association with alopecia, anhidrosis, glossitis, and porphyria cutanea tarda.

Acute febrile neutrophilic dermatosis manifested by erythematous, edematous plaques, bullae, and a cutaneous biopsy that showed diffuse infiltration of neutrophils, has been seen in one patient (13).

Distinctive *histopathologic changes* are seen in cutaneous biopsy specimens from patients receiving busulfan (14). These changes, which occur in the keratinocytes, are seen 15 to 45 days after administration of the drug. The changes include nuclear enlargement, alteration of nuclear contours and chromatin patterns, and development of abundant pale eosinophilic cytoplasm. Similar cytopathic changes have been observed in other organs including the lung, bladder, and cervix.

Triethylenethiophosphoramide (thio-TEPA)

Patterned *hyperpigmentation* has been described in patients receiving high-dose intrave-

nous thio-TEPA and cyclophosphamide for the treatment of metastatic breast adenocarcinoma (15). The hyperpigmentation was localized to areas that were occluded by bandages or monitors. The pigmentary changes were usually not preceded by significant erythema or desquamation. Thio-TEPA levels measured in adhesive bandages and gauze containing sweat were higher than the plasma concentrations of the drug. This suggests that thio-TEPA is secreted in sweat and may be concentrated under occlusive bandages. Hyperpigmentation is thought to result from a direct toxic effect of the chemical on the melanocytes in the basal layer of the epidermis.

Dacarbazine

Photosensitivity (16), alopecia, facial flushing, chemical cellulitis, chemical phlebitis, and inflammation of actinic keratoses have all been described in association with dacarbazine administration.

Carmustine (BCNU)

Mucocutaneous adverse reactions include *alopecia, stomatitis*, pain, and *phlebitis* at the site of injection. Topical contact with the medication may induce *hyperpigmentation*.

Streptozocin

Chemical cellulitis has been described in association with streptozocin.

ANTIMETABOLITES

Mucocutaneous reactions such as stomatitis and alopecia are frequently observed after administration of antimetabolites. Other reactions include hyperpigmentation, interactions with radiation, acral erythema, and neutrophilic hidradenitis.

Methotrexate

The buccal mucosa is particularly vulnerable to the toxic effects of methotrexate, and *stomatitis* is frequently reported. The severity of mucositis is related to the dose and frequency of administration; severe stomatitis is occasionally a rate-limiting factor in the administration of the medication.

Alopecia may occur following methotrexate administration. Hair regrowth always occurs after discontinuation of the medication. If repetitive cycles of medicine are given, regrowth may occur during subsequent cycles.

The development of *erythema*, particularly in pressure areas such as the elbows, palms, soles, and the intertriginous areas, has been reported following methotrexate administration. The erythema is followed by desquamation. Following pulse administration of high-dose methotrexate, subepidermal bullae may form, with subsequent focal loss of the epidermis.

Two to 3 days after methotrexate is given, patients may develop ill-defined *macular or papular erythematous eruptions*. These reactions typically occur following the first treatment course. Resolution of the eruption occurs within 2 weeks.

If methotrexate is given within 3 weeks of radiation therapy, a *radiation therapy recall phenomenon* may occur. The reaction is usually limited to the site of irradiation and is occasionally severe, with necrosis and ulceration of the epidermis (17).

Photosensitivity and phototoxic reactions may occur after exposure to sunlight that normally does not produce a sunburn effect.

An uncommon *photoreactivation phenomenon* has been described. In this situation, a patient is initially exposed to ultraviolet light and develops mild erythema. If high-dose methotrexate is given within 2 to 5 days of the ultraviolet light, the patient develops a severe sunburn reaction (erythema and blisters) in the exposed areas (18).

Widespread cutaneous *hyperpigmentation* may follow a course of methotrexate. One patient was described who developed hyperpigmented bands in scalp hair following sequential courses of methotrexate chemotherapy, the so-called flag sign (19).

Other uncommon mucocutaneous complications associated with methotrexate include urticaria, anaphylaxis, vasculitis, chemical cellulitis, and exacerbation of acne vulgaris.

5-Fluorouracil (5-FU)

Stomatitis and alopecia occur in association with systemic administration of 5-FU. Diffuse erythema, scaling, desquamation, and bulla formation were reported in 13% of patients receiving 5-fluorouracil in one study (20).

Infrequently reported reactions include erythema and ulcers in areas previously irradiated, exacerbation of seborrheic dermatitis, severe xerosis, and fissuring of the palms and soles.

A frequent complication of systemic 5-FU administration is *photosensitivity*. Up to 57% of patients in one series developed marked erythema in sun-exposed areas after exposure to doses of sunlight that normally would not produce a sunburn effect (21). Repetitive episodes of plaque-type *polymorphous light eruption* was described in one patient who received multiple courses of systemic 5-fluorouracil (21).

Patients receiving 5-FU frequently develop *hyperpigmentation*. The hyperpigmentation may be diffuse and widespread, limited to radiation portal sites, or present over veins used for drug infusions.

Nail changes that have been described in patients on 5-FU include hyperpigmentation of the nails (diffuse hyperpigmentation or transverse bands of hyperpigmentation), onycholysis, onychoschizia, and ridge formation.

In patients with actinically damaged skin, *inflammation and subsequent disappearance of actinic keratoses* typically occurs in association with 5-FU (22). Other complications include *acral erythema* and *chemical cellulitis* at sites of drug extravasation.

Although hypersensitivity reactions to 5-FU are uncommon, if patients have been previously treated with topical 5-FU, systemic administration of the drug may result in a papular pruritic erythematous eruption localized to areas of prior topical therapy (23).

Cytarabine (ara-C)

Alopecia is often associated with cytarabine therapy.

Palmar-plantar erythrodysesthesia (acral erythema) syndrome was initially described in patients receiving high-dose ara-C (24). This reaction is characterized by tender erythema of the palms and soles, which may progress to vesiculation and desquamation (Fig. 29.4). *Neutrophilic eccrine hidradenitis* is manifested by tender papules and plaques that may occur anywhere on the skin surface (25). Diagnosis is confirmed with a biopsy of the skin. The lesions spontaneously resolve within a week.

Other cutaneous complications of ara-C chemotherapy include *vasculitis* (26), *inflammation of actinic keratoses*, and a peculiar syndrome characterized by fever, arthralgias, conjunctivitis, and a diffuse erythematous eruption. This eruption begins within 24 hours of drug administration and may be completely prevented by premedication by corticosteroids (7, 27).

6-Mercaptopurine and 6-Thioguanine

Both 6-mercaptopurine and 6-thioguanine may produce mucositis; 6-thioguanine has been associated with inflammation of preexisting actinic keratoses. Otherwise, neither is commonly associated with mucocutaneous reactions.

ANTIBIOTICS

Mucocutaneous reactions to the antibiotics include alopecia, mucositis, chemical cellulitis, hyperpigmentation, and radiation interactions, among others.

Bleomycin

High concentrations of bleomycin are found in the skin; as a result, cutaneous reactions occur frequently. Up to 40% of patients develop *stomatitis* and *alopecia*.

Erythrodysesthesia of the palms and soles (*acral erythema*) has been reported. Erythema occurring over pressure areas, particularly the elbows, scapulae, scrotum, and vulva, has been described; occasionally the erythema progresses to ulceration. *Radiation recall* localized to sites of prior irradiation has been noted.

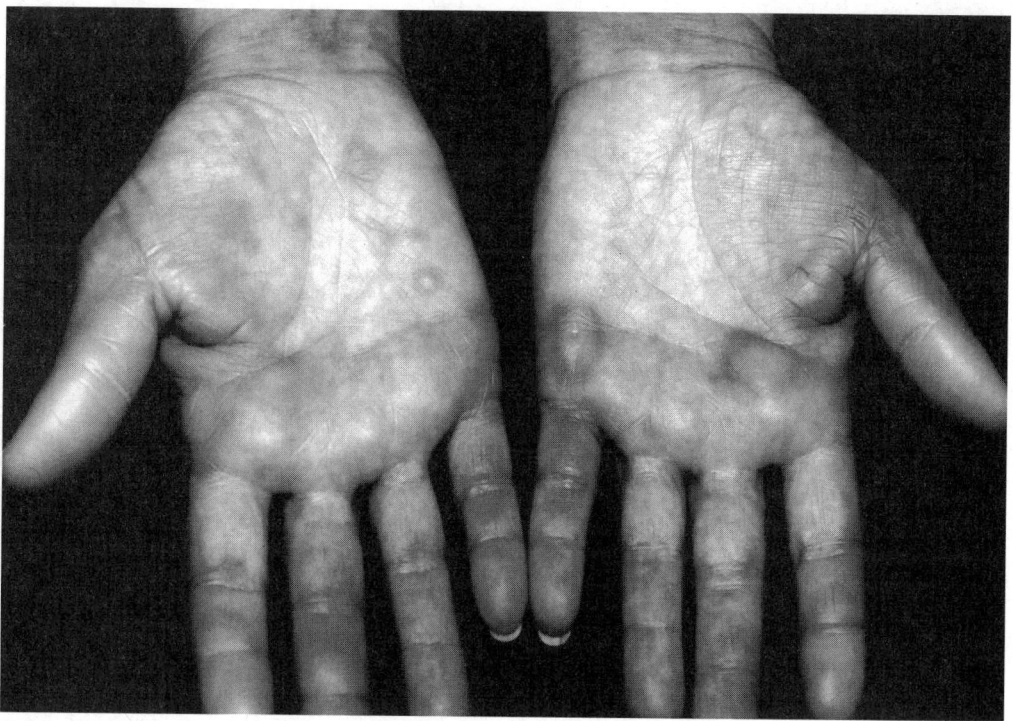

Figure 29.4.   Acral erythema associated with cytarabine.

A peculiar reaction characterized by *infiltrative nodules and plaques on the hands* following administration of bleomycin has been described. Although these lesions resolve after the medicine has been discontinued, one patient subsequently developed gangrene of the fingertips.

Hyperpigmentation commonly occurs with bleomycin therapy. The hyperpigmentation may be generalized or localized to pressure areas or to the fingernails. A very unusual patterned hyperpigmentation, known as *"flagellate"* hyperpigmentation, seems to be unique to bleomycin therapy (28) (Fig. 29.5). This hyperpigmentation has been experimentally induced by rubbing the skin during intravenous administration of bleomycin (29). It has been hypothesized that the vasodilation induced by vigorous rubbing or scratching results in an increase in local concentration of bleomycin and subsequent melanogenesis.

Other mucocutaneous reactions associated with bleomycin include *Raynaud's phenomenon* (30), penile calcification (31), onychodystrophy, neutrophilic hidradenitis, radiation enhancement, hypersensitivity reaction, and chemical cellulitis.

Actinomycin D

Mucositis and *transient alopecia* commonly occur in association with actinomycin D.

Radiation-associated reactions have been described in association with actinomycin D. *Radiation enhancement* occurs when actinomycin D is given simultaneously with radiation therapy. This combination results in more severe erythema at the radiation site than would be expected with radiation alone (32). *Radiation recall* occurs in patients who have received radiation therapy in the distant past and subsequently develop erythema at the site of irradiation when actinomycin D is administered (33). This reaction may occur many months after the initial radiation therapy is given.

A peculiar *acneform eruption* may occur shortly after systemic administration of actinomycin D. This reaction is characterized by erythema of the face and upper trunk and an explosive appearance of papules and pustules (34).

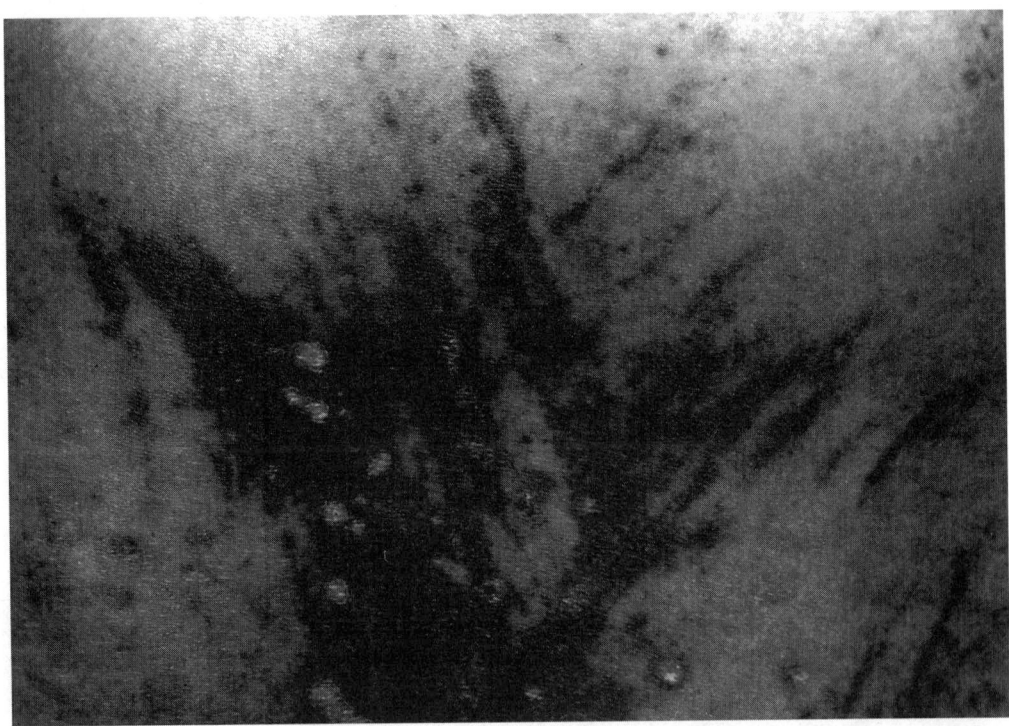

Figure 29.5.   Hyperpigmentation associated with bleomycin. Linearity is due to scratching while or shortly after medication is being administered.

Sterile intrafollicular pustules are seen microscopically. The rash resolves spontaneously within 2 weeks. Its clinical importance is that it is frequently confused with septic embolic phenomena.

Patients may develop a *macular and papular erythematous eruption* that begins on the face or abdomen and then generalizes. This eruption may be accompanied by fever and lethargy (35). The rash resolves within 2 weeks and may recur with subsequent courses of medication.

Other cutaneous reactions associated with this medication include inflammation of actinic keratoses, chemical phlebitis, chemical cellulitis, and erythema multiforme.

Doxorubicin

Alopecia, usually severe, occurs in most patients who receive doxorubicin. In addition to loss of scalp hair, patients may note loss of axillary and pubic hair. Stomatitis occurs in a high percentage of patients receiving doxorubicin. This complication appears to be a function of dose schedule and can be reduced by increasing the intervals between administration of the medicine.

Hyperpigmentation, particularly of the nails, is seen frequently in association with doxorubicin (Fig. 29.6). Pigmentary changes occur more frequently in dark-complexioned individuals. In addition to nail plate hyperpigmentation, pigmentary changes have been described on the palmar creases, palms and soles, dorsa of the knuckles, buccal mucosa, and tongue.

Doxorubicin is a potent vesicant and as such may produce severe *chemical cellulitis* when inadvertent extravasation occurs. Chemical cellulitis and ulceration may be followed by a peculiar *tissue recall phenomenon* characterized by recurrence of pain, erythema, and tissue necrosis at the site of earlier cellulitis (36). A similar recall reaction has been reported following phlebitis (37).

Radiation enhancement and radiation recall may occur after administration of doxorubicin. Radiation recall reactions occur more frequently if there was a preceding radiation dermatitis and may rarely occur as late as 15 years after the initial radiation (38, 39). *Hypersensitivity reactions*, ranging from urticaria at the site of injection to generalized urticaria and angioedema, may occur in association with doxorubicin administration. The *localization of urticaria* to skin in the im-

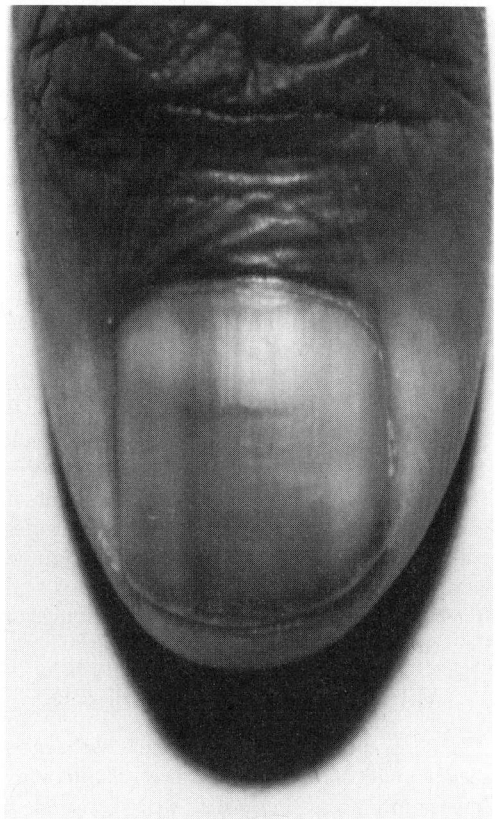

Figure 29.6.   Vertical streaking hyperpigmentation of the nail.

mediate vicinity of the intravenous injection may occur in up to 3% of patients receiving doxorubicin infusion (40). This peculiar localized reaction (*a*) may occur the first time the drug is administered, (*b*) is not prevented by premedication with antihistamine, and (*c*) does not always occur with subsequent infusion. These observations suggest a nonallergic mechanism; however, an episode of anaphylaxis was reported following a localized urticarial flare (41).

Other mucocutaneous toxicities seen with doxorubicin administration include palmarplantar erythrodysesthesia syndrome and inflammation of the actinic keratoses.

Daunorubicin

Severe mucositis is commonly associated with daunorubicin administration. Other mucocutaneous reactions are not common but include hyperpigmentation of the nails and skin, alopecia, chemical cellulitis, and generalized and localized (at the injection site) urticarial reactions.

Mithramycin

Mucositis occurs in up to 15% of patients receiving mithramycin. *Chemical cellulitis* may occur at sites of mithramycin extravasation. Generalized cutaneous *hyperpigmentation* may occur. *Toxic epidermal necrolysis* has been described in association with mithramycin administration; one of the patients with toxic epidermal necrolysis died (42).

There is an eruption that is peculiar to mithramycin. This reaction begins with macular erythema on the face and neck and progresses to deep erythema and coarsening of facial features. This was described in up to 35% of patients in one series (43). The eruption gradually fades, with residual desquamation and hyperpigmentation. Other patients have been described with transient and discrete erythematous papules on the head and upper trunk (44).

Mitomycin C and Mitoxantrone

Mitomycin C and mitoxantrone have been associated with *phlebitis* and *chemical cellulitis* at extravasation sites. *Stomatitis, hyperpigmentation, photosensitivity,* and a pruritic *vesicular eruption* have also been described in association with mitomycin C (5).

VINCA ALKALOIDS

Vincristine

Complications of vincristine therapy include reversible *alopecia, chemical cellulitis, stomatitis, and inflammation of actinic keratoses.*

Vinblastine

Alopecia, stomatitis, chemical phlebitis, and *chemical cellulitis* have been reported following vinblastine administration. *Photosensitivity* to short-wave ultraviolet light (UVB) is well documented in the literature (45). Patients receiving vinblastine should be warned about photosensitivity, and appropriate sunscreen preparations should be generously applied if ultraviolet light exposure is anticipated.

ENZYMES

L-Asparaginase

L-Asparaginase has a high frequency of *hypersensitivity reactions* (46). Urticaria is the most common cutaneous manifestation of hypersensitivity to L-asparaginase; other reported reactions include dyspnea, hypotension, serum sickness–like reactions, and anaphylaxis. Generalized and localized "rashes" as well as pruritus and peripheral edema have also been associated with L-asparaginase administration.

MISCELLANEOUS CHEMOTHERAPEUTIC AGENTS

Procarbazine

Mucocutaneous reactions to procarbazine are not common; however, alopecia, mucositis, and erythematous macular and papular eruptions have been described. Urticaria occurs occasionally (47).

Hydroxyurea

Most of the mucocutaneous reactions associated with hydroxyurea have occurred in patients on long-term maintenance therapy. Adverse reactions in these patients include *alopecia, hyperpigmentation, onychodystrophy,* and *lichen planus–like skin lesions* (48). *Palpable purpura with histologic evidence of leukocytoclastic vasculitis* has been described in several patients receiving hydroxyurea. Other skin changes include dermatomyositis-like lesions, palmar-plantar erythrodysesthesia syndrome, a fixed drug eruption, and radiation enhancement.

Amsacrine

Mucocutaneous reactions to amsacrine include stomatitis, alopecia, chemical phlebitis, and hypersensitivity reactions.

Cisplatin

Administration of cisplatin has been associated with inflammation of preexisting actinic keratoses, chemical cellulitis, and hypersensitivity reactions.

Etoposide (VP-16)

Administration of etoposide has been associated with a patchy and diffuse erythematous eruption. Although the clinical manifestations are relatively nonspecific, a biopsy of the skin will show very distinctive cytologic changes in the keratinocytes. Scattered enlarged, ballooned keratinocytes are present, with haphazardly distributed chromatin. These "starburst cells" have also been seen in epidermis that was topically treated with podophyllin, a chemically related medication (49).

Other mucocutaneous reactions include alopecia, radiation recall, and hypersensitivity reactions.

Pentostatin

Pentostatin has been associated with inflammation of preexisting actinic keratoses.

Hexamethylene Bisacetamide

One patient receiving hexamethylene bisacetamide developed palpable purpura of the lower extremities. Biopsy revealed histologic changes typical of leukocytoclastic *vasculitis*, and immunofluorescence studies revealed deposition of immunoglobulin and complement in the dermal vasculature, suggesting an immune complex–mediated reaction (50).

Interleukin 2 (IL-2)

Capillary leak syndrome characterized by peripheral and central edema is a common complication of IL-2 therapy. Some of these patients develop persistent macular erythema with associated pruritus and burning sensations. This reaction is typically localized to the head and neck region. Eruptions resolve with desquamation following the discontinuance of medication (51).

Other mucocutaneous complications include stomatitis, alopecia, superficial ulcerations, erosions in surgical scars, erythema nodosum, and exacerbation of psoriasis.

Interferons

Cutaneous reactions to interferons are common and include alopecia, pruritus, nonspecific dermatitis, and transient eruptions (52). Local erythematous reactions at the site of injection have also been reported. Additional cutaneous reactions include radiation enhancement, reactivation of herpes simplex virus infection, exacerbation of psoriasis, and increased growth of eyelashes.

Cyclosporine

Folliculitis and *hypertrichosis* have been reported in association with cyclosporine administration. The hypertrichosis may be of lanugo or terminal hairs and typically occurs within the first 6 months of therapy. It resolves with dis-continuation of the medication (53). Gingival hyperplasia similar to that seen with patients taking phenytoin has been reported in up to 25% of patients receiving cyclosporine (54).

CONCLUSION

The administration of chemotherapeutic agents is frequently associated with mucocutaneous complications. Although these reactions are rarely life threatening, they may be physically and psychologically debilitating. Awareness of and sensitivity to these reactions is an important aspect of medical care for these patients.

REFERENCES

1. Wall RL, Conrad FG. Cyclophosphamide therapy. Arch Intern Med 1961;108:456–482.
2. Keidan SE. Actinomycin D in the treatment of carcinoma in children. Br J Surg 1966;53:614–618.
3. Hussein AM. Chemotherapy-induced alopecia: new developments. South Med J 1993;86:489–496.
4. Bronner AK, Hood AF. Cutaneous complications of chemotherapeutic agents. J Am Acad Dermatol 1983;9:645–663.
5. Kerker BJ, Hood AF. Chemotherapy-induced cutaneous reactions. Semin Dermatol 1989;8:173–181.
6. Singal R, Tunnessen WW, Wiley JM, Hood AF. Discrete pigmentation after chemotherapy. Pediatr Dermatol 1991;8:231–235.
7. Shah SS, Rybak ME, Griffin TW. The cytarabine syndrome in an adult. Cancer Treat Rep 1983;67:405–406.
8. James WD, Odom RB. Chemotherapy induced traverse white lines in the fingernails. Arch Dermatol 1983;119:334–335.
9. Lakin JD, Cahill RA. Generalized urticaria to cyclophosphamide: type I hypersensitivity to an immunosuppresive agent. J Allergy Clin Immunol 1976;58:160–171.
10. Ross WE, Chabner BA. Allergic reactions to cyclophosphamide in a mechlorethamine-sensitive patient. Cancer Treat Rep 1977;61:495–496.
11. Millard LG, Rajah SM. Cutaneous reaction to chlorambucil (letter). Arch Dermatol 1977;113:1298.
12. Cornwell GG, et al. Hypersensitivity reactions to IV melphalan during treatment of multiple myeloma. Cancer and Leukemia Group B experience. Cancer Treat Rep 1979;63:399–403.
13. Dosik H, Hurwitz DJ, Rosner F, Schwartz JM, et al. Bullous eruption and elevated leukocyte alkaline phosphatase in the course of busulfan-treated chronic granulocytic leukemia. Blood 1970;35:543–547.
14. Hymes SR, et al. Cutaneous busulfan effect in patients receiving bone marrow transplantation. J Cutan Pathol 1985;12:125–129.
15. Horn TD, Beveridge RA, Egorin MJ, Abeloff MD, Hood AF. Observations and proposed mechanism of N,N′,N″-triethylenethiophosphoramide (thio-TEPA)-induced hyperpigmentation. Arch Dermatol 1989;125:524–527.
16. Yung CW, Winston EM, Lorincz AL, et al. Da-

carbazine-induced photosensitivity. J Am Acad Dermatol 1981;4:541–543.

17. Kim YH, Aye MS, Fayos JV, et al. Radiation necrosis of the scalp: a complication of cranial irradiation and methotrexate. Radiology 1977;124:813–814.

18. Korossy KS, Hood AF. Methotrexate reactivation of sunburn reaction. Arch Dermatol 1981;117:310–311.

19. Wheeland RG, Burgdorf WHC, Humphrey GB. The flag sign of chemotherapy. Cancer 1963;51:1356–1358.

20. Kennedy BJ, Theologides A. The role of 5-fluorouracil in malignant disease. Ann Intern Med 1961;55:719–730.

21. Falkson G, Schultz EJ. Skin changes in patients treated with 5-fluorouracil. Br J Dermatol 1962;74:229–236.

22. Johnson TM, Rapini RP, Duvic M. Inflammation of actinic keratoses from systemic chemotherapy. J Am Acad Dermatol 1987;17:192–197.

23. Bernstein T. Skin reactions to 5-fluorouracil. N Engl J Med 1977;297:337–338.

24. Burgdorf WHC, Gilmore WA, Garick RG. Peculiar acral erythema secondary to high-dose chemotherapy for acute myelogenous leukemia. Ann Intern Med 1982;97:61–62.

25. Flynn TC, Harrist TJ, Murphy GF, Loss RW, Moschella SL. Neutrophilic eccrine hidradenitis. A distinctive rash associated with cytarabine therapy and acute leukemia. J Am Acad Dermatol 1984;11:584–590.

26. Hippe E, Jonsson V, Schroder HD, et al. Ara-C vasculitis (letter). Eur J Dermatol 1988;41:96.

27. Castleberry RP, Crist WB, Holbrook T. The cytosine arabinoside (Ara-C) syndrome. Med Pediatr Oncol 1981;9:257–264.

28. Cohen IS, Master MB, O'Keefe EV, et al. Cutaneous toxicity of bleomycin therapy. Arch Dermatol 1973;107:553–555.

29. Guillet G, Guillet MH, deMeaux H, Gauthier Y, Sureve-Baseille JE, Geniaux M, Orreteguy C. Cutaneous pigmented stripes and bleomycin treatment. Arch Dermatol 1986;122:381–382.

30. Rothberg H. Raynaud's phenomenon after vinblastine-bleomycin chemotherapy. Cancer Treat Rep 1978;62:569–570.

31. Ihde DC, Gormley PE, Francis RS, De Vita VT, et al. Reversible penile calcifications associated with bleomycin (NSC-125066)-induced pulmonary toxicity. Cancer Chemother Rep 1975;59:1039–1041.

32. Frei E III. The clinical use of actinomycin. Cancer Chemother Rep 1974;58:49–54.

33. D'Angio GJ, Farber S, Maddock CL, et al. Potentiation of x-ray effects by actinomycin D. Radiology 1959;73:175–177.

34. Epstein EH, Lutzner MH. Folliculitis induced by actinomycin D. N Engl J Med 1969;281:1094–1096.

35. Cassady JR, Mayer G, Jaffe N, Filler RM, et al. Fever, lethergy and rash complicating treatment for Wilms' tumor—a new syndrome? Radiology 1975;115:171–174.

36. Cohen SC, DiBella NJ, Michalak JL. Recall injury from Adriamycin. Ann Intern Med 1975;83:232.

37. Baer D, Wilkinson LS. Daunomycin, Adriamycin and recall effect. Ann Intern Med 1976;85:259–260.

38. Burdon J, Bell R, Sullivan J, Henderson M, et al. Adriamycin-induced recall phenomenon 15 years after radiotherapy (letter). JAMA 1978;10:931.

39. Donaldson SS, Glick JM, Wilbur JR. Adriamycin activating a recall phenomenon after radiation therapy. Ann Intern Med 1974;81:407–408.

40. Vogelzang NJ. "Adriamycin flare." A skin reaction resembling extravasation. Cancer Treat Rep 1979;63:2067–2069.

41. Etcubanas E, Wilbur JR. Uncommon side effects of Adriamycin chemotherapy. Cancer 1974;58:757–758.

42. Purpora D, Ahern MJ, Silverman M, et al. Toxic epidermal necrolysis after mithramycin (letter). N Engl J Med 1978;299:1412.

43. Kennedy BJ. Metabolic and toxic effects of mithramycin during tumor therapy. Am J Med 1970;49:494–503.

44. Koons CR, et al. Clinical studies of mithramycin in patients with embryonal cancer. Bull Johns Hopkins Hosp 1966;118:462–475.

45. Breza TS, Helprin KM, Taylor JR, et al. Photosensitivity reaction to vinblastine. Arch Dermatol 1975;111:1168–1170.

46. Weiss RB, Bruno S. Hypersensitivity reactions to cancer chemotherapeutic agents. Ann Intern Med 1981;94:66–72.

47. Glovsky MM, Braunwald J, Opelz G, Alenty A, et al. Hypersensitivity to procarbazine associated with angioedema, urticaria and low serum complement activity. J Allergy Clin Immunol 1976;57:134–140.

48. Kennedy BJ, Smith LR, Goltz RW. Skin changes secondary to hydroxyurea therapy. Arch Dermatol 1975;111:183–187.

49. Yokel BK, Friedman KJ, Farmer DR, Hood AF, et al. Cutaneous pathology following etoposide therapy. J Cutan Pathol 1987;14:326–330.

50. Rowinsky EK, McGuire WP, Anhalt GJ, Ettinger DS, Donehower RC, et al. Hexamethylene bisacetamide-induced cutaneous vasculitis. Cancer Treat Rep 1987;71:471–474.

51. Gaspari AA, Lotze MT, Rosenberg SA, et al. Dermatologic changes associated with interleukin-2 administration. JAMA 1987;258:1624–1629.

52. Spiegel RJ. Intron A (interferon alfa-2b): clinical overview and future directions 1986. Semin Oncol 1986;13:89–101.

53. Wyscoki GP, Daley TD. Hypertrichosis in patients receiving cyclosporine therapy. Clin Exp Dermatol 1987;12:191–196.

54. Daley TD, Wysocki GP, Day C, et al. Clinical and pharmacological correlations in cyclosporine A-induced gingival hyperplasia. Oral Surg Oral Med Oral Pathol 1986;62:417–421.

30

Extravasation

Gerald H. Clamon

The accidental extravasation of chemotherapeutic agents during intravenous administration has been reported in approximately 0.1 to 6% of patients (1, 2). Cancer patients may be more prone to drug extravasation because of multiple venipunctures, phlebitis limiting future sites of venous access, lymphedema due to prior surgery, and generalized debility. The consequences of extravasation can vary from mild erythema and discomfort to severe pain, tissue necrosis, skin ulceration, and invasion of deep structures such as tendons or joints. Factors affecting the degree of tissue damage include the vesicant nature of the extravasated drug, the concentration of the extravasated agent, the volume infiltrated into the tissues, the site of infiltration (i.e., dorsum of the hand vs. antecubital fossa vs. forearm), and possibly the subsequent management by the physician or nurse. Other local reactions that do not involve drug extravasation also occur. Local phlebitis is common with nitrogen mustard (mechlorethamine), with BCNU (carmustine) because of its diluent, and with bisantrene because of its insolubility (3). Hypersensitivity reactions, often called flare reactions, with erythema and urticaria along the course of the vein, can occur with anthracyclines such as doxorubicin (Adriamycin), daunorubicin, and aclarubicin (4). Unfortunately, these are among the drugs that may give the most severe extravasation reactions, and a very careful and cautious approach must be taken to any local reaction due to these agents.

The time course of the injury after drug extravasation varies. With the most toxic agents, such as anthracyclines, nitrogen mustard, and the vinca alkaloids, the injury often comes on gradually. With the anthracyclines, a stinging type of pain is often felt during the extravasation. Over 7 to 10 days, erythema, heat, and pain develop, followed by progression to ulceration.

The ulceration may then enlarge for 2 to 3 months (5). The edges are often red and painful, and the lesions may have a yellow necrotic base that will not heal spontaneously (4, 6). Full-thickness skin necrosis may occur, and if the ulcer is over tendons or neurovascular structures, these tissues may also undergo necrosis. The tissues are thin over the dorsum of the hand, at the antecubital fossa, and over the flexor surface of the wrist, and damage to the underlying tendons and nerves may lead to joint contractures and chronic damage. In the absence of surgical intervention, many of the deep and painful lesions will never heal (7). The occurrence of pain during administration of a vesicant drug should be an alert that extravasation may have occurred, even if there is no visual evidence present. Agents that can cause skin ulceration are listed in Table 30.1.

MECHANISMS OF TISSUE INJURY

Several mechanisms have been proposed for the severe damage caused by anthracyclines such as doxorubicin and its analogues. These agents lead to the development of free radicals that are toxic to the tissues. The ability of these agents to bind to DNA further impedes the ability of the damaged tissues to heal. Studies have shown that doxorubicin is retained in the extravasated area for months (8). It has been hypothesized that DNA-doxorubicin complexes are released from dead cells and taken up by adjacent cells by endocytosis. This sets up a continuing cycle of doxorubicin damage. Such retention and recirculation of the doxorubicin suggests that early surgical excision may be valuable in preventing further spread of injury.

Histologic studies of chemotherapy-induced ulcers in man have been carried out 2 to 3 months after extravasation (5, 7, 9). Blood vessels

Table 30.1. Antineoplastic Agents Associated with Extravasation Injury

Agents Which May Cause Skin Ulceration
  Doxorubicin
  Daunorubicin
  Idarubicin
  Mitoxantrone
  Mithramycin
  Actinomycin D
  Bleomycin
  Mitomycin
  Melphalan
  Streptozotocin
  Nitrogen mustard
  BCNU
  Vinblastine
  Vincristine
  Vindesine
  Vinorelbine
  VP-16
  Cisplatin
  Taxol
Experimental agents
  m-Amsa (amsacrine)
  Bisantrene
  Mitoguazone
  Aclacinomycin
  Epirubicin
  Triglycidylurazol
  4-Hydroxyanisole
  Amonafide
  Didemnin B
  Elsamicin

in the ulcer are damaged, but at the margins, the blood vessels are viable. Inflammatory cells are rarely present, which suggests that the use of steroids to reduce "inflammation" would not be effective therapy. Dimethyl sulfoxide (DMSO) and α-tocopherol are antioxidants that might neutralize free radicals formed by anthracyclines. These agents appear to be active antidotes in some animal models and in some clinical trials in humans.

The application of cold may slow drug diffusion throughout the tissues, prevent drug uptake into cells, and thereby interrupt the cycle of damage. Both in small animals and in humans, the application of cold seems to reliably decrease injury and ulceration due to doxorubicin extravasation.

While numerous other agents have been proposed, their lack of efficacy as antidotes in small animal trials has obviated their use in human clinical trials. Among the many agents tested were hydrocortisone, bicarbonate, isoproterenol, glutathione, L-carnitine, benzoic acid, coenzyme Q, deferoxamine, dopamine, human serum albumin, iron dextran, and N-acetylcysteine (10, 11).

DHM3 (bi (3,5-dimethyl-5-hydroxymethyl-2-oxomorpholin-3-yl) is a radical dimer that reacts with doxorubicin to form deoxydoxorubicin aglycone. This inactivates the anthracycline. In a pig model, it was highly effective in reducing the size of ulcers induced by intradermal doxorubicin (12).

ANIMAL MODELS

Extravasation injury due to anthracyclines and other chemotherapeutic drugs has been studied in the rat, the mouse, and the pig. Rodent skin may be a less appropriate model than pig skin for the study of extravasation in humans. Rodent skin differs from human skin in that rodents have a thin vascular muscle layer fixed to the skin (13). Because of the greater vascularity, anthracycline injury in rodents is less apt to progress to ulceration. Intradermal injection is required to induce ulceration in most animal models. Most human accidental extravasations are likely subcutaneous. In animal models, intradermal injection is necessary to cause ulceration; subcutaneous injection causes minimal lesions. Increasing the dose of doxorubicin concentration and/or the volume injected causes larger ulcers with longer times to healing. Concentrations below 0.01 to 0.2 mg/mL injected intradermally will not cause severe ulceration, and concentrations below 0.25 mg/mL injected subcutaneously will not produce severe damage (14, 15). Studies in rats given intradermal doxorubicin, actinomycin D, mitomycin, or BCNU, and then either potential antidotes or surgical excision of the damaged area, showed superior healing with surgical excision. Early surgical excision followed by a reexcision of nonviable tissue 1 week later led to the best healing (16). With doxorubicin injury in rats, neither hydrocortisone, propranolol, or isoproterenol were of benefit. At increasing doses of DMSO and α-tocopherol, doxorubicin injury was alleviated in rats (17). Similarly, DMSO and α-tocopherol are effective in reducing mitomycin- and actinomycin D–induced damage in rats. DMSO and α-tocopherol did not help with BCNU dermal injury.

In a mouse model, the addition of cold to the extravasated area reduced doxorubicin injury; heat to the area exacerbated the extent of damage

(18). In a mouse model, DMSO and α-tocopherol were not able to reduce doxorubicin injury (19).

At least three trials in pigs gave mixed results for DMSO as an antidote for doxorubicin injury. In one trial, cooling the area reduced doxorubicin damage, but DMSO was of no benefit (20). However, in a second trial using pigs, DMSO was effective, and in a third trial, the results with DMSO were equivocal (10, 11). Hyaluronidase has been reported to decrease vinca alkaloid injury in a mouse model. Simple dilution with normal saline was also effective in reducing vinca injury (21). Mild skin heating alone also reduced vinca alkaloid ulceration significantly, whereas cooling exacerbated vinca alkaloid extravasation injury. Thiosulfate has been demonstrated in an animal model to reduce injury due to nitrogen mustard (22).

CLINICAL TRIALS

Most trials in humans involve the management of doxorubicin extravasation. Once extravasation has occurred, aspiration of any free drug via the intravenous cannula *before it is removed* may reduce the extent of injury. At the M. D. Anderson Hospital, Larson reported on 50 consecutive cases of drug extravasation involving doxorubicin or vincristine, which were managed uniformly (2). The extremity was placed in a sling, and the patient was instructed to apply ice for 20 minutes four times a day for 3 days. The patient then reported to a surgeon for evaluation. If the patient had persistent pain or evidence of progressive necrosis, a wide local excision was performed. Often the wound needed to be covered with a biologic covering and later skin grafted. Using cold packs without injections of antidotes, only 12 of 50 patients required surgery. Early surgery in cases of extravasation reduced the extent of later injury in 40 patients with extravasation (16). However, even with surgery, residual damage has frequently been noted in patients with drug administered near the elbow, the wrist, or the back of the hand.

The role of antidotes in extravasation injury is not entirely clear. Although bicarbonate has been reported as helpful in one case of doxorubicin extravasation (23), bicarbonate itself may cause tissue necrosis (24). Studies with bicarbonate and doxorubicin in vitro suggest that the combination might increase cytotoxocity and damage (25). There has been no proven benefit from steroids, and no other antidotes appear particularly promising in animal studies, with the exception of DMSO and DHM3. DMSO, with or without other agents, seems the most promising antidote at this time.

In one of the more carefully managed trials, Olver et al. treated 20 patients with an anthracycline extravasation with topical 99% DMSO (26). Patients with doxorubicin (18 cases) or daunorubicin (2 cases) extravasation presented with swelling in the area of extravasation (17 patients), erythema (15 patients), or pain (12 patients). They received DMSO to an area twice the size of the drug injury every 6 hours for 14 days. The drug was allowed to dry from the skin. Due to early deaths, only 16 of the 20 patients could be followed for 3 months. However, ulceration did not develop, and surgery was not required in any patient. In a recent trial, DMSO applied every 8 hours for 7 days was effective in preventing ulceration in 51 of 52 patients with extravasation due to doxorubicin, epirubicin, mitoxantrone, or mitomycin (27). Other trials of DMSO in combination with other techniques such as DMSO, ice, bicarbonate, and dexamethasone, DMSO and α-tocopherol, or ice, glucocorticoid, and DMSO have been successful as well (28–30).

Other nonsurgical techniques have been reported to reduce doxorubicin injury. Injection of saline into the area of the extravasation along with application of topical corticosteroids as well as oral steroids or oral nonsteroidal antiinflammatory agents was reported to avoid surgery in 37 of 40 patients (31). Patients received 20 mL of saline for injuries in the wrist area, 40 mL for lesions on the dorsum of the hand, and 60–90 mL for forearm or antecubital fossa extravasation. Thiosulfate (2%) has also been infiltrated into areas of extravasation and reported to reduce injury from doxorubicin, epirubicin, vinblastine, or mitomycin C. In comparison with a group of patients treated with hydrocortisone and dexamethasone, patients receiving thiosulfate therapy healed extravasation injuries in 5 days, versus 21 days for the steroid therapy (32).

Mitomycin has been reported to cause severe, chronic, painful ulceration, similar to that of doxorubicin, when extravasated. Although wide local excision has been recommended, in two cases local injection of pyridoxine ameliorated damage due to mitomycin extravasation (33). These investigators suggest infiltration with a volume approximately equal to that of the extravasated mitomycin.

Although vinca drugs are reported to cause injury requiring surgery for painful nonhealing ulcers, it is not clear from clinical case reports what the optimum management should be. Based upon animal data, the manufacturer recommends local injection of hyaluronidase and heat to the area. Hyaluronidase (Wyeth) comes in a 300-unit vial to which 1 to 2 mL of normal saline is added. The area of extravasation is to be "liberally" injected (34, 35).

Thiosulfate is suggested as the antidote for nitrogen mustard extravasation. Clear clinical reports on the effectiveness of such thiosulfate injections are not available. The recommended antidote for nitrogen mustard has been to prepare a ⅙-M solution of sodium thiosulfate. This is prepared by mixing 4 mL of a 10% sodium thiosulfate solution with 6 mL of sterile water for injection (34). The thiosulfate is injected into the extravasation site in excess of the amount of mustard extravasated.

Taxol-induced skin injury secondary to extravasation has been reported (36). These injuries were noted 2 to 7 days after the injection of the Taxol and healed with conservative therapy. However, a more extensive infiltration around an Infusaport caused a necrotic ulcer that required skin grafting in one individual.

After any drug extravasation, if a patient has persistent pain after a 2 to 3 day trial of conservative management, surgical consultation should be obtained (37–41). Earlier excision may facilitate healing and avoid a more prolonged course of pain. To completely remove all tissues infiltrated by anthracyclines, some surgeons have suggested exposing the wound to ultraviolet light. The natural fluorescent properties of doxorubicin allow detection of the extent of its spread (5, 42, 43). Advocates of surgical intervention emphasize that delay in treatment of severe extravasations is more apt to leave the patient with permanent functional impairment. Extravasation into the hand or antecubital fossa is more apt to result in loss of forearm or hand function (43). Mitomycin may be similarly detected if 100 mg of fluorescein is administered intravenously and the wound then exposed to UV light (44).

PREVENTION

Prevention of extravasation is the optimum management. Administration of chemotherapy by experienced individuals is a must. The site of administration should be in the proximal forearm in a large-bore, easily visualized vein. When venous access is a problem, those patients still needing therapy with a vesicant agent should have a central line such as a Hickman line or an Infusaport. Chemotherapy should not be given distal to a recent site of venipuncture, or extravasation might occur where the vein was recently penetrated. Flexible catheters, rather than rigid needles, are less likely to pierce the vein, particularly if they are to be left for any length of time. The site should be carefully watched during administration, and the patient should be advised to speak up if any pain occurs during administration. The infusion should be stopped immediately if there is any suggestion or question of extravasation. Furthermore, agents not previously thought to be vesicants, such as mitoxantrone, have later proved capable of severe injury (45). All extravasation incidents should be observed, and adequate follow-up planned.

REFERENCES

1. Cox K, Stuart-Harris R, Abdini G, Grygiel J, Raghavan D. The management of cytotoxic-drug extravasation: guide-lines drawn up by a working party for the Clinical Oncological Society of Australia. Med J Aust 1988;148:185–189.

2. Larson DL. Treatment of tissue extravasation by antitumor agents. Cancer 1982;49:1796–1799.

3. Harwood KV, Aisner J. Treatment of chemotherapy extravasation: current status. Cancer Treat Rep 1984;68:939–945.

4. Banerjee A, Brotherston TM, Lamberty BGH, Campbell RC. Cancer chemotherapy agent-induced perivenous extravasation injuries. Postgrad Med J 1987;63:5–9.

5. Rudolph R, Larson DL. Etiology and treatment of chemotherapeutic agent extravasation injuries: a review. J Clin Oncol 1987;5:1116–1126.

6. Rudolph R, Stein RS, Patillo R. Skin ulcers due to Adriamycin. Cancer 1976;38:1087–1094.

7. Reilly JJ, Neifeld JP, Rosenberg SA. Clinical course and management of accidental adriamycin extravasation. Cancer 1977;40:2053–2056.

8. Garnick M, Israel M, Khetarpal V, Luce J. Persistence of anthracycline levels following dermal and subcutaneous adriamycin extravasation (abstract). Proc Am Assoc Cancer Res 1981;22:173.

9. Luedke DW, Kennedy PS, Rietschel RL. Histopathogenesis of skin and subcutaneous injury caused by Adriamycin. Plast Reconstr Surg 1979;63:463–465.

10. Okano T, Ohnuma T, Efremidis A, Holland JF. Doxorubicin-induced skin ulcer in the piglet. Cancer Treat Rep 1983;67:1075–1078.

11. Desai MH, Teres D. Prevention of doxorubicin-induced skin ulcers in the rat and pig with dimethyl sulfoxide (DMSO). Cancer Treat Rep 1982;66:1371–1374.

12. Averbuch SD, Gaudiano G, Koch TH, Bachur NR. Doxorubicin-induced skin necrosis in the swine model: protection with a novel radical dimer. J Clin Oncol 1986;4:88–94.

13. Dorr RT, Alberts DS, Chen HSG. Experimental

model of doxorubicin extravasation in the mouse. J Pharmacol Methods 1980;4:321–334.

14. Rudolph R, Suzuki M, Luce JK. Experimental skin necrosis produced by Adriamycin. Cancer Treat Rep 1979;63:529–537.

15. Cohen MH. Amelioration of Adriamycin skin necrosis: an experimental study. Cancer Treat Rep 1979;63:1003–1004.

16. Loth TS, Eversmann WW. Treatment methods for extravasation of chemotherapeutic agents: a comparative study. J Hand Surg 1986;11A:338–396.

17. Svingen BA, Powis G, Appel PL, Scott M. Protection against adriamycin-induced skin necrosis in the rat by dimethyl sulfoxide and α-tocopherol. Cancer Res 1981;41:3395–3399.

18. Dorr RT, Alberts DS, Stone A. Cold protection and heat enhancement of doxorubicin skin toxicity in the mouse. Cancer Treat Rep 1985;69:431–437.

19. Dorr RT, Alberts DS. Failure of DMSO and vitamin E to prevent doxorubicin skin ulceration in the mouse. Cancer Treat Rep 1983;67:499–501.

20. Harwood KV, Bachur N. Evaluation of dimethyl sulfoxide and local cooling as antidotes for doxorubicin extravasation in a pig model. Oncol Nurs Forum 1987;14:39–44.

21. Dorr RT, Alberts DS. Vinca alkaloid skin toxicity: antidote and drug disposition studies in the mouse. J Natl Cancer Inst 1985;74:113–120.

22. Dorr RT, Soble M, Alberts DS. Efficacy of sodium thiosulfate as a local antidote to mechlorethamine skin toxicity in the mouse. Cancer Chemother Pharmacol 1988;22:299–302.

23. Zweig JI, Kabakow B. An apparently effective counter measure for doxorubicin extravasation (letter). JAMA 1978;239:2116.

24. Gaze NR. Tissue necrosis caused by commonly used intravenous infusions. Lancet 1978;2:417–419.

25. Kappel B, Hindenburg AA, Taub RN. Treatment of anthracycline extravasation—a warning against the use of sodium bicarbonate. J Clin Oncol 1987;5:825–826.

26. Olver IN, Aisner J, Hament A, Buchanan L, Bishop JF, Kaplan RS. A prospective study of topical dimethyl sulfoxide for treating anthracycline extravasation. J Clin Oncol 1988;6:1732–1735.

27. Bertelli G, Dini d Forno G, Gozza A, Silvestro S, Venturini M, Rosso R, Pronzato P. Clinical results with antidotes to vesicant chemotherapy extravasations (abstract). Proc ASCO 1994;13:468.

28. Ludwig CV, Stoll HR, Obrist R, Obrecht JP. Prevention of cytotoxic drug induced skin ulcers with dimethyl sulfoxide (DMSO) and α-tocopherole. Eur J Cancer Clin Oncol 1987;23:327–329.

29. Lawrence JH, Walsh D, Zapotowski KA, Denham A, Goodnight SH, Gandara DR. Topical dimeth-

ylsulfoxide may prevent tissue damage from anthracycline extravasation. Cancer Chemother Pharmacol 1989;23:316–318.

30. Nobbs P, Barr RD. Soft-tissue injury caused by antineoplastic drugs is inhibited by topical dimethyl sulphoxide and alpha tocopherol. Br J Cancer 1983;48:873–876.

31. Scuderi N, Onesti MG. Antitumor agents: extravasation, management and surgical treatment. Ann Plastic Surg 1994;32:39–44.

32. Tsavaris NB, Komitsopoulou P, Karagiaouris P, Loukatou P, Tzannou I, Mylonakis N, Kosmidis P. Prevention of tissue necrosis due to accidental extravasation of cytostatic drugs by a conservative approach. Cancer Chemother Pharmacol 1992;30:330–333.

33. Rentschler R, Wilbur D. Pyridoxine: a potential local antidote for mitomycin-c extravasation. J Surg Oncol 1988;37:269–271.

34. Parashos PJ. A rational approach for the management of tissue extravasation due to antineoplastic drugs. MicroLink Update 1986;2:13–15.

35. Bellone JD. Treatment of vincristine extravasation (letter). JAMA 1981;245:343.

36. Ajani JA, Dodd LG, Daugherty K, Warkentin D, Ilson DH. Taxol-induced soft tissue injury secondary to extravasation: characterization by histopathology and clinical course. J Natl Cancer Inst 1994;86:51–53.

37. Loth TS. Minimal surgical debridement for the treatment of chemotherapeutic agent-induced skin extravasations. Cancer Treat Rep 1986;70:401–404.

38. Preuss P, Partoft S. Cytostatic extravasations. Ann Plast Surg 1987;19:323–327.

39. Rudolph R. Ulcers of the hand and wrist caused by doxorubicin hydrochloride. Orthop Rev 1978;7:93–95.

40. Ignoffo RJ, Friedman MA. Therapy of local toxicities caused by extravasation of cancer chemotherapeutic drugs. Cancer Treat Rep 1980;7:17–27.

41. Bowers DG Jr, Lynch JB. Adriamycin extravasation. Plast Reconstr Surg 1978;61:86–92.

42. Duray PH, Cuono CB, Madri K. Demonstration of cutaneous doxorubicin extravasation by rhodamine filtered fluorescence microscopy. J Surg Oncol 1986;31:21–25.

43. Andersson AP, Dahlstrom KK. Clinical results after doxorubicin extravasation treated with excision guided by fluorescence microscopy. Eur J Cancer 1993;29A:1712–1714.

44. Argenta LC, Manders EK. Mitomycin C extravasation injuries. Cancer 1983;51:1080–1082.

45. Peters FTM, Beijnen JH, Huinink WWB. Mitoxantrone extravasation injury. Cancer Treat Rep 1987;71:992–993.

31

Hypersensitivity Reactions

Raymond B. Weiss

Nearly all of the available chemotherapeutic agents can produce hypersensitivity reactions (HSRs) in at least an occasional patient, and some cause reactions in 5 to 10% of patients receiving the drug. There are now three agents (L-asparaginase, paclitaxel, and docetaxel) for which HSRs are frequent enough to be a major form of treatment-limiting toxicity.

The observation and reporting of HSRs from such drugs has spurred development of means to ameliorate or prevent this form of toxicity. For example, a new chemically modified form of L-asparaginase (pegaspargase) was developed specifically to circumvent the HSRs and other toxicities of this cytotoxic enzyme. It was approved for marketing in 1994. Another example is the now standard process of premedication with corticosteroids and antihistamines to decrease the incidence and severity of HSRs from paclitaxel.

This chapter delineates the chemotherapeutic agents that produce HSRs, the type of reaction, the clinical manifestations, and the mechanism (if identified). In addition, recommendations are provided on means of preventing or minimizing such reactions and evaluating them. The term *hypersensitivity reaction* will apply to any drug-related episode with manifestations of any of the four major types of drug-induced allergy. It does not imply that all such reactions are mediated immunologically by antibody or sensitized lymphocytes.

The mechanism of such reactions remains unknown for most of the chemotherapeutic agents. Although many HSRs from cytotoxic agents are probably immunologically mediated, there are other possible mechanisms for type I, or immediate, reactions. Some chemotherapeutic agents appear to degranulate mast cells and basophils through a direct effect on the cell surface, thus releasing histamine and other vasoactive substances. Direct degranulation also results from use of meperidine, morphine, codeine, curare, hydralazine, and radiopaque dyes. Some agents may activate the alternative complement pathway, also resulting in release of vasoactive substances from mast cells. Such events are not mediated by IgE and are termed *anaphylactoid reactions*. Anaphylactic reactions are, by definition, mediated by IgE (or sometimes IgG or IgM) and imply prior exposure to the drug or a similar antigen. Angioedema and urticaria occasionally result from stressful situations, and thus a neural mechanism for vasoactive mediator release exists. It is not known whether any such instances have occurred in conjunction with cytotoxic drug administration. In the case of bleomycin, the rare acute reactions appear to result from direct pyrogen release from leukocytes, and no immunologic mediators are involved.

Hypersensitivity reactions are generally divided into four types originally defined by Gell and Coombs (1). Table 31.1 lists these types and summarizes the mechanisms by which they are produced.

L-ASPARAGINASE

L-Asparaginase remains the antitumor drug most likely to cause HSRs. HSRs are the principal treatment-limiting side effect, occurring in a consistent 10 to 25% of patients receiving this drug as part of combination therapeutic regimens (2–4). This high rate of HSRs is undoubtedly related to the fact that L-asparaginase is a polypeptide of bacterial origin that can stimulate production of IgE or other antibodies. These immunoglobulins can then mediate an acute anaphylactic reaction.

The clinical manifestations of L-asparaginase hypersensitivity are usually those of type I reactions (Table 31.1). Full anaphylaxis, with shock

Table 31.1. Types of Hypersensitivity Reactions [Gell and Coombs Classification (1)]

Type	Major Signs and Symptoms	Mechanism
I	Urticaria, angioedema, rash, bronchospasm, abdominal cramping, extremity pain, agitation and anxiety, hypotension	Antigen interaction with IgE bound to mast cell membrane causes degranulation Drug binding to mast cell surface causes degranulation Activation of classic or alternative complement pathways produces anaphylatoxins Neurogenic release of vasoactive substances
II	Hemolytic anemia	Antibody reacts with cell-bound antigen and activates complement
III	Deposition of immune complexes in tissues results in various forms of tissue injury	Antigen-antibody complexes form intravascularly and deposit in or on tissues
IV	Contact dermatitis, granuloma formation, homograft rejection	Sensitized T lymphocytes react with antigen and release lymphokines

and loss of consciousness and occasionally death, has occurred. Evans et al. (2) studied 36 patients with L-asparaginase reactions. Sixteen (44%) patients had severe reactions that included the presence of respiratory distress and/or hypotension with a decrease in systolic blood pressure of more than 20 mm Hg (i.e., anaphylaxis). The other patients also had type I reactions but without hypotension (2).

A number of factors enhance the risk of L-asparaginase-induced HSRs (Table 31.2). Most reactions will occur within the first 11 doses of the drug (5). Immunogenicity with this drug can be long-lasting, at least 3 years after initial drug exposure (6).

L-Asparaginase is rarely used as a single agent and is most often administered concurrently with, or sequentially to, vincristine-prednisone and perhaps other agents. Use in such combination regimens seems to reduce the frequency of reactions. Intramuscular administration also appears to reduce the frequency of anaphylaxis (7, 8), but milder type I reactions still occur up to several hours after treatment (9).

The basis for the observation that intramuscular administration of drug reduces the frequency and severity of HSRs, or in some cases delays their onset, is uncertain. A reasonable explanation is the fact that the pharmacokinetics of the intramuscular route differ from those of the intravenous route. Maximal drug absorption takes place 10 to 24 hours after intramuscular administration, and peak plasma levels are lower than with the intravenous route (10). However, when a drug dose as high as 25,000 international units/m^2 is used, the peak plasma

Table 31.2. Factors That Increase Risk of L-Asparaginase Hypersensitivity

History of atopy or allergy
Prior drug exposure (weeks to even several years previously)
Infrequent drug administration (e.g., weekly intervals)
Intravenous administration
Use without concomitant prednisone, 6-mercaptopurine, and/or vincristine
High drug doses

level may be high enough to counteract any advantage of intramuscular administration, thus explaining why a 19% and 25% rate of systemic HSRs, respectively, occurred in two studies (3, 11), despite intramuscular L-asparaginase injection and concomitant use of vincristine and prednisone.

The mechanism of L-asparaginase-induced HSRs is not completely understood. Khan and Hill (12) provided good evidence that IgE mediates the reaction in at least some cases. In five patients who experienced an HSR, the reactivity was mediated by a skin-sensitizing IgE, as demonstrated by skin testing and Prausnitz-Kustner reaction studies (12). More recently, Fabry et al. (13) showed that patients sustaining HSRs had evidence of complement activation, with elevated levels of the C3 split product, C3d. These investigators suggested that IgG or IgM immune complexes initiate the complement activation process and thus mediate the reactivity.

Despite various attempts to detect reactivity before a dose of L-asparaginase is administered, there is no reliable way to determine which patients will sustain an HSR. Intradermal skin testing can give both false-negative and false-positive results. Test doses of small amounts of drug are also valueless. In one study (2), an intravenous test dose rarely produced a reaction and was falsely negative in most patients who developed an HSR. Unfortunately, one must approach each dose of L-asparaginase to be administered as the one that could incite a serious HSR and be prepared to quickly reverse any reaction with appropriate medication. This means that antianaphylaxis medication should be close at hand, and the patient should be observed for reactions during the hour after each dose injection. Intramuscular drug administration is preferable, when feasible, to minimize the risk of anaphylaxis.

When an HSR to the *Escherichia coli* derivative occurs, the *Erwinia chrysanthemia* derivative (previous species name was *carotovora*) can be used as a substitute with equal antitumor efficacy. *E. coli*–type L-asparaginase has been marketed for over 15 years, but the *Erwinia* derivative is still not commercially available in the United States. However, the Food and Drug Administration (FDA) has authorized its distribution by the sponsor, Speywood Pharmaceuticals Ltd., on an individual basis for those patients who have an HSR to the *E. coli* form of the drug.

Cross-reactivity between these two agents was originally reported to be rare (14). A patient who was reactive to one derivative was unlikely to react to the other derivative. However, three studies (3, 5, 10) have shown that up to 25% of patients who react to *E. coli* L-asparaginase will cross-react to the *Erwinia* derivative. Precautions for HSRs must be taken when administering the substitute form of L-asparaginase, because not only might cross-reactivity produce another HSR from the first dose, but also new antibodies to the substitute might develop just as readily as they did to the original form of the drug.

Although *Erwinia*-derived drug is an excellent and inexpensive substitute for the *E. coli* product, patients can still suffer HSRs from it. Another (but more expensive) alternative to use when an HSR occurs is pegaspargase. This compound is a covalent conjugate of *E. coli* L-asparaginase with molecules of monomethoxypolyethylene glycol (PEG). To more effectively circumvent the disadvantage of HSRs and to prolong blood levels of this drug, Abuchowski et al. (15) modified L-asparaginase with PEG at a site not involved with the antitumor activity,

based on the observation that polymer conjugation to proteins could decrease their immunogenicity and extend plasma half-life. This agent showed good antitumor activity in animal tumors compared with that of the native asparaginase (16). It was approved by the FDA for marketing in 1994, to be used for patients who develop an HSR to the native form of this drug. Administration of pegaspargase is more convenient for the patient because doses are given less frequently and in smaller volumes. Unfortunately, patients may also develop an HSR to pegaspargase (17, 18), but the reactions are rarely more than grade 1.

TAXOIDS

Paclitaxel and Docetaxel

Paclitaxel was approved for marketing in 1992 and is now one of the most widely used drugs in clinical oncology. HSRs were a major toxicity in the initial clinical trials and an obstacle to further study of this agent in the 1980s. Measures were then taken to prevent or minimize HSRs from this drug. Nevertheless, severe reactions can still occur at a rate of approximately 2%, with mild reactions (usually mild rashes or flushing) occurring in up to 40% of patients (19, 20).

Weiss et al. (21) collected 27 cases of definite HSRs from paclitaxel. Forty-one percent of these patients developed hypotension as part of the HSR, often with a diastolic pressure of zero. Rashes and dyspnea/bronchospasm occurred in about 75% of the patients. One patient had a fatal cardiorespiratory arrest.

Most (80%) of the patients had the HSR develop within 10 minutes of initiating the drug, after only a few milligrams had been infused. Only one patient sustained an HSR from a drug dose other than the first or second; half occurred with the first treatment. There are no known risk factors.

To prevent or ameliorate these HSRs, investigators prolonged the drug infusion time to 6 or 24 hours and used a three-drug prophylactic regimen (Table 31.3) consisting of an antihistamine, a corticosteroid, and an H-2 receptor antagonist. This prophylactic therapy does not fully prevent severe HSRs, but the reported current 2% rate of severe reactions provides good evidence that it reduces the risk of such problems. The infusion duration was lengthened at the same time as the premedication regimen was implemented, making it impossible to determine which new mea-

Table 31.3. Prophylaxis of Hypersensitivity Reactions from Antitumor Drugs

Premedication

20 mg dexamethasone orally 12 and 6 hours before treatment and 20 mg i.v. just before administration of the antitumor drug

50 mg diphenhydramine orally and i.v. in same schedule as the dexamethasone

150 mg ranitidine (or 300 mg cimetidine) i.v. 30 minutes before administration of the antitumor agent; as a substitute, consider 25 mg ephedrine sulfate orally 1 hour before treatment unless unstable angina or hypertension necessitates withholding it

Treatment setup

Intravenous access must be established

Blood pressure monitoring is available

Epinephrine and i.v. diphenhydramine are readily available in case of a reaction

Observe the patient for an HSR up to 2 hours afterward

---

sure reduced the risk of HSRs. Thus, shorter infusion times were clinically tested and compared with the 24-hour schedule, some in a randomized prospective fashion (19). Such trials have now demonstrated that the risk of an HSR is no greater with a 3-hour infusion (19), or even a 1-hour infusion, of paclitaxel (22).

The cause of these reactions has been suggested to be the drug excipient Cremophor EL, which must be used to maintain the solubility of paclitaxel (21). The high frequency of hypotension and its rapid onset clinically are consistent with Cremophor effects noted in dogs, in which Cremophor and its fatty acid constituents induced histamine release and hypotension within 10 minutes of administration (23). The mechanism is unknown, but the clinical features and the fact that HSRs have occurred so often with the first paclitaxel dose suggest a nonimmunologic anaphylactoid reaction. On the other hand, Cremophor EL may have been falsely implicated as the cause, because the paclitaxel analogue docetaxel has a different excipient (Tween 80), and it produces HSRs at a rate similar to that of paclitaxel. It appears that either the two taxoids themselves are the cause or Cremophor EL and Tween 80 are equally capable of initiating HSRs.

Paclitaxel is an effective antitumor agent for a variety of cancers, and the question arises whether it can be safely administered again after an HSR occurrence. The patient may have experienced the reaction from the first dose of this drug, and if it cannot be given again, the patient may lose an opportunity to have a beneficial antitumor response. Peereboom et al. (24). evaluated the risk of further problems in eight patients who had developed severe manifestations of HSRs from paclitaxel. The patients all had more intensive premedication dosing, and the drug infusion rate was reduced to 10 or 25% of the usual rate for the first several hours. Five of these patients had no further HSR manifestations, and the other three had only minor symptoms (24). However, there are anecdotal reports (25, 26) from others who have tried the same approach with less success.

Docetaxel is a semisynthetic analogue of paclitaxel, derived from the needles of the European yew tree (*Taxus baccata*). It was available only for investigational purposes, but a New Drug Application for marketing was approved in May 1996 by the FDA. Its spectrum of antitumor activity is similar to that of paclitaxel, but there are differences in toxicity (27). One toxicity where there is similarity is HSRs.

When docetaxel was first evaluated in clinical trials, it was assumed that premedication to prevent HSRs was unnecessary because the excipient was Tween 80, not Cremophor EL. Cremophor was believed to be the culprit in HSRs from paclitaxel, and because docetaxel was not formulated with Cremophor, such reactions were considered unlikely. That assumption has now been proven incorrect, because docetaxel can initiate HSRs with approximately the same frequency and same manifestations as those with paclitaxel (28–29). Most of these reactions have occurred with the first or second dose of docetaxel (27), much like those from paclitaxel. When HSRs became a treatment-limiting toxicity with this drug, premedication regimens similar to those used with paclitaxel were implemented, but they have had variable success in reducing the incidence and severity of such reactions (31, 32).

A problem from this drug that has turned out to be a chronic treatment-limiting toxicity is the development of peripheral edema, pleural effusions, and ascites, with occasional progression to anasarca. It commonly develops after about five cycles of docetaxel, with no resolution unless the drug is discontinued. The etiology of this fluid-accumulation syndrome is unknown. It is unlikely to be a manifestation of HSR, but attempts have been made to decrease its incidence and severity with corticosteroid premedication, as with acute HSR prophylaxis regimens (31). Some success has been achieved in reducing the frequency of such toxicity, but drug discontinuation is still often necessary.

Another acute and common toxicity from this drug is the development of erythematous or edematous skin plaques that begin on the extremities and may spread to the trunk (33). These lesions begin within a few days after drug administration and may be pruritic. They probably are more a manifestation of direct skin toxicity from docetaxel, rather than an HSR. However, there may be some overlap of the manifestations of this skin toxicity and a type I reaction. Treatment has been topical steroids (33).

ELLIPTINIUM

Elliptinium is classified as investigational in the United States but is marketed in some European countries for the treatment of breast cancer. It represents a new class of synthetic compounds whose parent structure was derived from a plant called ochrosia. HSRs in the form of type II reactions have been a major toxicity problem.

Criel et al. (34) first observed intravascular hemolysis induced by this drug, which occasionally resulted in renal failure. Subsequent studies indicated that hemolytic anemia could occur in up to 7% of patients treated with elliptinium (35). The manifestations of these HSRs have been hypotension, flank pain, dyspnea, restlessness, rigors, decrease in serum hemoglobin, and hemoglobinuria (black urine). Other laboratory abnormalities such as decrease in serum haptoglobin, rise in serum bilirubin, and free hemoglobin in the plasma have been observed.

Type II HSRs can result in hemolysis through the development of antidrug antibodies that react with antigen fixed to red cell surfaces. This binding initiates the sequence of complement activation, finally resulting in red cell lysis. Type II reactions induced by antitumor drugs are rare (36), and elliptinium is the only drug that causes this problem with any frequency. An IgM antibody mediates the reaction (34), and it agglutinates normal red cells only in the presence of elliptinium. The antibody appears in 20 to 40% of patients receiving weekly drug administration, and as many as two-thirds of patients with such antibody develop hemolysis. Patients without antibody do not develop clinical evidence of hemolysis. Since weekly drug administration appeared to induce antibody formation and cause

the high rate of hemolytic episodes, a different dosing schedule of treatment, daily for 3 days every 3 weeks, was devised with serial prospective testing for the presence of antibody (37–39). If the antibody titer reaches 1:32, the drug should be discontinued. The titers will decline in a few weeks, and no hemolysis should occur. However, deaths have been reported from hemolysis despite the absence of antielliptinium antibodies (40).

In addition to causing the more common type II reactions, elliptinium also appears to cause type I reactions. Dyspnea, hypotension, tachycardia, and chest pain have occasionally occurred in the absence of intravascular hemolysis (41). These problems quickly subsided when the drug infusion was stopped. Prolonging drug infusion to 3 or more hours seemed to reduce the severity of these abnormalities.

Alberici et al. (42) have attempted to identify the immunogenic determinant of elliptinium. They demonstrated that the quaternary ammonium–containing ring in the elliptinium structure plays a major role in antigenicity, but the haptogenic mechanism is still not known.

EPIPODOPHYLLOTOXINS: TENIPOSIDE AND ETOPOSIDE

Both teniposide and etoposide are semisynthetic derivatives of podophyllotoxin, which is extracted from the root of the May apple plant. Their antitumor efficacy spectra are similar, although teniposide is used mostly for pediatric malignancies and etoposide is used for cancers in adults. Teniposide has been in clinical use for 25 years, and HSRs have long been recognized as one of its toxicities. In the past 15 years, HSRs have also been reported from etoposide, but perhaps with a lower frequency.

Teniposide causes HSRs in approximately 6% of patients overall (43). However, the incidence of reactions in patients with neuroblastoma is much higher, up to 13% (43–45). Why patients with craniospinal tumors or neuroblastoma are more likely to have HSRs from teniposide is unknown. As O'Dwyer et al. (43) point out, it is not a drug-dose relationship, because higher doses are used for treatment of lymphoid malignancies. Neuroblastomas produce excess catecholamines, and these vasoactive substances may provide a milieu in which HSRs from teniposide are more likely. However, this disease specificity may be more apparent than real, because Kellie et al. (46) observed a reaction rate of 41% in a group of patients with acute leukemia who were treated with teniposide. Many of these reactions were grade 1 in severity and may have been ignored or not reported in other studies of this drug. In addition, unusually high cumulative teniposide doses were administered. In this study, the reactions became more common as the cumulative teniposide drug increased. It is therefore probable that the apparent disease specificity would disappear if the total drug courses and patient monitoring were equivalent in all studies of teniposide.

Reactions may occur from any teniposide dose, including the first one. In fact, a large fraction (32%) of patients in the series collected by O'Dwyer et al. (43) reacted with their initial exposure to teniposide. The timing of the reaction can be either after only a few milligrams of drug have been infused or up to several hours after drug administration. HSR manifestations from teniposide have included dyspnea and wheezing, hypotension or hypertension, urticaria, pruritus, angioedema, facial flushing, and rash (43, 45). No deaths have been reported. There are no known risk factors for sustaining a reaction, and few patients have any history of allergy. Severe hypotension (presumably due to an HSR) has occurred even when teniposide is administered via the intraperitoneal route (47).

Etoposide has also been clearly demonstrated to cause HSRs (48–50), but the incidence of this toxicity is difficult to determine because of the anecdotal nature of these reports. Such isolated instances suggest a lower risk of HSRs from etoposide than from teniposide. This fact may be due to either underreporting or a truly lower incidence. Although underreporting could account for a part of the lower number of cases, HSRs do not occur at an incidence of up to 20%, as has been observed in some series of patients treated with teniposide (51). The only study providing comparative data regarding the incidence of HSRs from these two agents is that of Kellie et al. (46), and reactions of all grades from etoposide were less frequent. A reasonable estimate of the overall incidence with etoposide is 1 to 3%, although in one report (52) the incidence reached a high of 51%. The clinical manifestations of these HSRs are similar to those from teniposide. Most reactions have occurred from the first or second etoposide doses (48, 49, 52).

The mechanism of these type I reactions from the epipodophyllotoxins is not known, but it is unlikely to be IgE-mediated because of the frequency of reactions from the first drug exposure. Equally unknown is the reason for the slightly lower incidence of reactions from etoposide. Since there is only a minor difference in chemical structure between the two congeners, this difference is unlikely to be the explanation. Moreover, despite the number of reported cases of HSRs from intravenous etoposide, there have been no published reports of reactions from the marketed oral formulation of etoposide. In fact, one patient who had an immediate reaction to the first dose of intravenous etoposide tolerated oral administration of the drug without problems. One possible reason for a difference in the two analogues is that teniposide might produce a reactive metabolite in higher concentration than etoposide does. Another possible explanation is the difference in formulation of the two drugs: teniposide is formulated with Cremophor EL and etoposide with Tween 80 and benzyl alcohol. Cremophor could be the inducer of the teniposide-related reactions, as might be the case with paclitaxel. However, Nolte et al. (54) attempted to implicate Cremophor by studying in vitro histamine release from both teniposide and Cremophor, and only teniposide degranulated basophils. Moreover, this effect was dose dependent and not IgE mediated.

Whether the excipient Tween 80 (or the benzyl alcohol) is the HSR inducer for parenteral etoposide is not known. The oral etoposide capsules contain citric acid, glycerin, and polyethylene glycol but not Tween 80.

Rechallenge with teniposide has been attempted (usually after antihistamine and corticosteroid premedication) with some success, thus allowing further drug administration (56). In some cases, decreasing the infusion rate of either teniposide or etoposide also aids in reducing further HSRs (43, 55). Etoposide can also be substituted for teniposide, with no cross-reactivity in most cases (45). However, at least two patients (45) have also reacted to etoposide. These facts give some insight into the mechanism of reactions. In some cases, substitution of the congener results in cross-reactivity, so the inciting agent must be the chemotherapeutic agent, not the excipient. In other cases, without cross-reactivity, the reverse may be true; the excipient (Cremophor EL) may be the offending agent.

In one case, a rare type II hemolytic reaction was reported secondary to teniposide (56). A drug-dependent IgG was found to mediate the reaction. Despite an incidence as high as 13% for type I HSRs due to teniposide, only this single case of type II reaction has been published.

CISPLATIN AND CARBOPLATIN

Cisplatin reactions have been reported since the initial clinical use of this drug in the early 1970s (57). There has never been a reliable determination of the incidence of cisplatin-induced reactions, but the reported rates of this toxicity seem to be lower in the past 15 years than in the 1970s. For example, in a study reported in 1979 (58), the rate of HSRs was 20% of patients, and in another study, reported in 1978 (59), the rate was 14%. No reports of patient series treated more recently have rates anywhere near these levels. There are several possible reasons for this change. One reason is that antiemetics are liberally prescribed as premedication for any patient receiving cisplatin, and dexamethasone and diphenhydramine are often used for this purpose, perhaps suppressing any HSR while minimizing vomiting. Another reason is that no patient in the study by Gralla et al. (60), which had a 6% rate of reactions, developed hypersensitivity before receiving six or more doses of cisplatin. Cisplatin is usually given for fewer cycles nowadays, and immunogenic reactivity may not have time to develop. If the number of cisplatin cycles exceeds six, the risk of reaction may rise. Whatever the reason, the frequency of HSRs from cisplatin is much lower than it used to be and has now become almost an anecdotal occurrence.

Intravenous cisplatin can cause HSRs, and so can drug instilled intravesically for bladder cancer. The incidence of these latter reactions is much higher than that with intravenous administration. In a study of intravesical cisplatin use by Blumenreich et al. (61), 5 of 24 patients had drug-related rashes, and another patient had a severe anaphylactic reaction, for an overall incidence of HSRs reaching 20%. Denis (62) reported that 7 (10.4%) of 67 patients sustained anaphylactic reactions from intravesical cisplatin. The minimum number of repetitive drug instillations before a reaction occurred was eight, given over 4 months. There was an incidence of 14% among those patients who received a minimum of 4 months of treatment. These data support the hypothesis that a certain minimum number of cisplatin courses (six or more) is necessary to induce reactivity.

From the above data, one could conclude that cisplatin administered intravesically (presumably involving systemic drug absorption) is more allergenic than that given intravenously, but there is no logical explanation for such a difference. One possible reason is that this route of drug administration results in an unusually high number of drug exposures compared with the number of exposures with drug given intravenously. Another is that antiemesis premedication would not be routinely used with cisplatin administered in this fashion. Studies of cisplatin administered intrapleurally or intraperitoneally have not shown a correspondingly high incidence of HSRs (63). It is puzzling that cisplatin administered in the bladder is systemically allergenic, whereas drug administered in body cavities (presumably with no less total drug absorption) is not, but again the reason may be that fewer cycles of drug are given into body cavities than intravesically.

The manifestations of the type I HSRs to cisplatin, whatever the route of administration, are anxiety, pruritus, cough, dyspnea, diaphoresis, angioedema, vomiting, bronchospasm, rashes and urticaria, and hypotension. Prompt administration of corticosteroids and antihistamines usually effectively aborts any reaction. A single death has been reported (64) from a cisplatin-induced HSR, but this patient may represent a very unusual platinum sensitivity. She previously had a seizure from carboplatin, so when cisplatin was to be given as a substitute, she was heavily premedicated against having an HSR. She had one anyway, despite receiving only a very small cisplatin dose.

The mechanism of cisplatin-related type I reactions has been investigated in only a few patients (57, 65, 66). Khan et al. (57), demonstrated that at least one case of cisplatin-induced reaction was mediated by IgE. In contrast, Wiesenfeld et al. (65) studied a patient who sustained a reaction for evidence of IgE-mediated reactivity and found none. Goldberg et al. (66) skin tested two patients after reactions to cisplatin, and both had skin reactivity to the drug, whereas six control patients who also received cisplatin therapy did not.

When analyzing a patient who sustains an HSR, apparently from an antitumor agent, one must always consider the possibility that the drug formulation product (the excipient) or other drugs administered concurrently are the allergens, not the antitumor agent. In the case of cisplatin, other agents, such as antiemetics and diuretics, are frequently administered with it. Mannitol, by itself, has apparently caused HSRs in rare instances (67). One patient (68) clearly had an HSR to mannitol (given to promote osmotic diuresis) administered just before cisplatin was to be given. It is possible that some of the reported HSRs ascribed to cisplatin have been due to mannitol administered as an osmotic diuretic with the cisplatin.

Type II reactions with hemolytic anemia have been reported in a few patients treated with cisplatin (69–71). These cases of hemolysis were proven to be due to cisplatin by appropriate laboratory tests (direct antiglobulin testing using polyspecific and monospecific reagents) and the recurrence of hemolysis with drug rechallenge. However, one must be cautious in ascribing possible hemolytic episodes to the presence of cisplatin-induced antibodies. Zeger et al. (72) have shown that cisplatin can cause a nonimmunologic binding to red cell membranes and gamma globulins, thus giving a false-positive direct antiglobulin test even in the absence of any hemolysis, as occurred in at least one patient (69). Anemia is a common toxicity from cisplatin, especially if it is administered repetitively, and transfusions may be required. However, this anemia is related to both the chronic myelotoxic effect of cisplatin and an erythropoietin deficiency from renal tubular damage by the drug. In only rare instances is it due to hemolysis, but a sudden decrease in hematocrit when using cisplatin should raise suspicion of a type II reaction. Appropriate studies should then be performed to evaluate this possibility.

Analogues of cisplatin with nearly equivalent antitumor efficacy and lower rates of nephrotoxicity have been under wide clinical test, and one, carboplatin, is now marketed. A number of anecdotal reports of carboplatin-induced HSRs have been published in the past few years (73–78). Only the report by Hendrick et al. (74) provides any data regarding the frequency of such reactions. These authors observed 16 patients with HSRs from carboplatin "out of over 200 patients" treated with this drug. With this information, the incidence seems to be in the 6–8% range. Whether this is more or less than occurs with its analogue cisplatin is impossible to determine. However, there is no reason to expect that one analogue would produce such reactions more often than the other. Two patients have been reported who had a type I HSR to cisplatin and then developed a similar reaction to carboplatin (73, 79), and one patient (80) reacted first

to carboplatin and then to cisplatin used as substitute therapy. Clearly, there is a risk of cross-reactivity from these analogues when one is substituted for the other. In addition, several of the reported patients (75–77) had been treated with cisplatin previously and then, after receiving only a few doses of carboplatin, developed an HSR to it. These patients were probably sensitized to the cisplatin, and only a few doses of carboplatin were necessary to precipitate a reaction.

The mechanism of reaction to carboplatin has been studied by allergists in one case (77). The patient had skin-test reactivity to both carboplatin, which precipitated the reaction, and to cisplatin, which she had received previously. For technical reasons, these investigators were unable to test for specific IgE, but the patient did have a high level of IgE a month after the HSR, which fell to normal 3 months later.

PROCARBAZINE

Procarbazine has been known to produce HSRs since its initial clinical use in the early 1960s (81). The most common manifestation of reaction is an erythematous maculopapular rash, but urticaria and angioedema have also been observed (82). The incidence of such type I reactions has never been well documented. The anecdotal nature of these HSR reports suggests that they are uncommon, but Andersen and Videbaek (83) observed 12 cases of HSR (17.6%) in 68 patients receiving procarbazine. Sandberg-Wollheim et al. (84) reported skin reactions in 20 (11.7%) of 171 patients treated with procarbazine, and Coyle et al. (85) saw 8 (35%) of 23 patients with symptoms and signs of hypersensitivity from procarbazine.

The skin manifestations are most often diffuse, pruritic, maculopapular rashes, but urticaria has also been reported. Other drug eruptions have been toxic epidermal necrolysis (86) and fixed drug eruptions (87).

Procarbazine can also produce rare instances of pulmonary toxicity with features of type III reactions (85, 88–91). These patients have interstitial pneumonitis and eosinophilia in the peripheral blood and/or lung biopsy specimen, and they improve with procarbazine withdrawal and corticosteroid therapy. High fever and arthralgias have also been observed (85, 88, 91).

The mechanism(s) of these HSRs from procarbazine has been poorly studied and is not known. Only two patients have been studied in detail in an attempt to define a mechanism. One patient (82) was found to have a low complement level, due possibly to depletion of complement fragments from release of anaphylotoxins or formation of immune complexes. The other patient (87) clearly had a fixed-drug skin eruption, but the pathogenesis of such reactions has not been determined. Skin patch testing with procarbazine in this patient was nonreactive (87). However, this sort of test is not necessarily reliable, because the HSRs may be due to a procarbazine metabolite and not the parent compound.

Some patients have been clearly shown to be reactive to only procarbazine and not the other drugs (both chemotherapeutic agents and drugs such as allopurinol) commonly used with procarbazine (58). Many of the reported patients have been rechallenged with procarbazine after suspension of treatment and resolution of the symptoms (82, 83, 87, 88), and their HSR manifestations promptly recurred. Two patients who were rechallenged had severe reactions (85). One patient (90) was rechallenged twice with procarbazine and had a recurrence of pneumonitis each time. It appears that procarbazine cannot be safely readministered, even with use of concomitant steroids and antihistamines to minimize further HSRs. Most patients receive procarbazine in the mechlorethamine, vincristine, procarbazine, and prednisone (MOPP) regimen for Hodgkin's disease and are already receiving prednisone as part of the chemotherapeutic regimen; HSRs to procarbazine still occur, despite the steroid. The only apparent means of preventing such reactions, once they develop, is to discontinue the procarbazine permanently.

CYTARABINE (CYTOSINE ARABINOSIDE)

Although cytarabine has been in clinical use for 30 years, HSRs have only recently been observed with more than anecdotal frequency. This change may be due to the fact that the cytarabine doses now being widely used are 10 to 15 times higher than those used prior to the 1980s. Four distinct forms of HSRs to this drug have now been recorded.

The first form of HSR is type I, with dyspnea, chest pain, fever, maculopapular rash, urticaria, and hypotension (92–95). The most common manifestation of reaction has been rash, but anaphylaxis with hypotension to shock levels has occurred in a few patients (89, 95). The mechanism of type I reactions has been studied in three patients (92, 94, 95), and the evidence implied that the reactions were mediated by IgE.

Another acute reaction induced by this drug has been called the "cytarabine syndrome" by Castleberry et al. (93). This type of reaction was first reported in 1971 (96) and was characterized by high fever, rigors, diaphoresis, myalgia, arthralgia, and maculopapular rash after each cytarabine dose in one patient. Other patients (97) have been reported to develop similar acute reactions, with one having hypotension reaching shock level and requiring vasopressor support (98). This cytarabine syndrome may or may not be a form of HSR. Williams and Larson (98) suggested that this was a form of HSR because of the presence of circulating immune complexes in their patient (perhaps a type III reaction?). However, no studies have been done to investigate this possibility. One patient (96) had intradermal skin tests, and he did not have a reaction. Although an immunologic basis for the manifestations of the "cytarabine syndrome" is possible, a more likely mechanism is direct cytarabine toxicities with no mediation by antibodies.

The frequency of this acute reaction varies from isolated case reports to as high as 33% (93) of patients treated with cytarabine. It is probably more common than the rare instance for which a case report is published. Patients with acute leukemia have leukopenia and often become septic with associated fever, myalgia, diaphoresis, rigors, and even hypotension. When such symptoms occur, they are probably often ascribed to sepsis, and the possibility of a cytarabine toxicity may not be appreciated.

The type I reactions described from cytarabine can be initiated by moderate or high doses of drug. However, a third type of reaction induced by cytarabine seems to be generally dose related. First described by Burgdorf et al. (99), this reaction is characterized by intense, often painful, erythema of the palms and soles, with later development of bullae and desquamation (100–105). Dysesthesias often herald the onset of the erythema, and the edema may be marked enough to limit finger motion. The erythema begins a median of 6 days after initiating cytarabine therapy. Some patients also have fever, facial edema and erythema, and/or erythematous maculopapular rashes characteristic of a type I reaction (100, 103, 104). In most cases, only the hands are involved, but this exanthem has also been described as involving only the ears (106). The skin usually heals without scarring, and patients have been treated with cytarabine again without recurrence of this toxicity (102). Steroids have been used to hasten resolution of this skin reaction (107).

The incidence of this palmar-plantar reaction has varied from 14 to 33% of patients treated with cytarabine doses of 1000 mg/m^2 or more (100, 105), especially if eight or more doses at this level have been administered. Some patients treated with conventional cytarabine doses of 100 mg/m2 have also developed this acral erythema (102–104). The incidence at this lower drug dose level is not defined, but it is much lower than at high doses.

Skin biopsies from the site of the reaction have been obtained from some patients (100, 102, 103). The histologic abnormalities are nonspecific and are typical of drug-induced skin eruptions.

The mechanism of these skin reactions involving primarily the palms and soles is not known. It may be a vasculitis that peculiarly involves certain small peripheral blood vessels, due possibly to a type III reaction. However, the relationship to drug dose is more indicative of a direct cytotoxicity to skin and subcutaneous tissues. In addition, this phenomenon is not limited to patients receiving cytarabine. It has also been observed in patients receiving doxorubicin, hydroxyurea, cyclophosphamide, and 6-mercaptopurine (108, 109).

The fourth type of cytarabine-induced reaction is a dermatosis termed *neutrophilic eccrine hidradenitis*, in which histologically there is a marked accumulation of neutrophils around the dermal sweat glands, (110, 111). The skin lesions are erythematous plaques or nodules that may be tender and are not pruritic. The mechanism of this apparent drug-induced problem is not known. Flynn et al. (111) suggested that this is a form of an HSR, but it is more likely a variant of the direct cytotoxic effect cytarabine can have on skin tissues. Although the first reported cases (109, 110) were patients being treated with cytarabine, the existence of another case (112) related to other antitumor agents suggests that its genesis is not limited to cytarabine.

and bronchospasm, and sometimes hypotension. Such reactions have even occurred when doxorubicin was administered intravesically (118), presumably due to systemic drug absorption. Other anthracyclines have also induced such generalized reactions (119, 120), but neither the intravenous nor the oral formulations of idarubicin have been reported to induce a type I reaction. Cross-reactivity between anthracyclines (daunorubicin and doxorubicin) has been documented in one case (117). Since the chemical structure of the various anthracycline analogues is very similar, cross-reactivity is likely to occur.

Doxorubicin can also cause erythema, pruritus, and urticaria localized at, or adjacent to, the drug injection site (121, 122). This phenomenon is referred to as a "flare" reaction. Although it can raise concern that the drug was extravasated or that more serious allergy manifestations will develop, it does not seem to progress to a generalized HSR, and it is not due to anthracycline extravasation. It is usually transient and will disappear without treatment. Further drug can be given later without concern for more serious problems because the reactions often do not recur, and if they do, they are not more intense or generalized. To obviate the concern about a worse reaction, one can administer premedication with antihistamines and corticosteroids, which will prevent further problems. Doxorubicin analogues such as zorubicin (rubidazone), aclarubicin, idarubicin, and epirubicin are also known (120, 123–125) to produce such "flare" reactions, and other anthracyclines will presumably be recognized to do so as they are introduced to clinical use.

The mechanism of the type I generalized reactions due to any of the anthracyclines has not been investigated. Although the cytotoxic antibiotic is undoubtedly the initiator of these HSRs, the drug manufacturer has recommended reconstitution of the dessicated doxorubicin with saline (instead of distilled water) to reduce the frequency of the localized "flare" reactions. However, Solimando and Wilson (114) demonstrated that systemic type I HSRs are not inhibited by use of saline reconstitution.

ANTHRACYCLINE ANTIBIOTICS

Both daunorubicin and doxorubicin have occasionally produced severe and generalized type I reactions (113–117). These HSRs are characterized by urticaria, pruritus, angioedema, dyspnea

CYCLOPHOSPHAMIDE AND IFOSFAMIDE

Although cyclophosphamide is immunosuppressive, it can cause antibody-mediated type I reactions (including anaphylaxis and shock) in rare instances (126–132). Some of these reactions were reproduced on rechallenge with the drug. HSRs have occurred from both oral and intravenous administration of cyclophosphamide. Cross-reactivity with other alkylating agents is variable. Some patients reactive to cyclophosphamide have tolerated chlorambucil as a substitute without further reactions (132), but at least one (133) did not. Another patient was treated with ifosfamide and did not cross-react (129). The alkylating agents have similar chemical structures. Why cross-reactivity does not occur more often is unclear, particularly in the case of the two analogues, cyclophosphamide and ifosfamide.

The mechanism of cyclophosphamide HSRs appears to be IgE-mediated, based on studies in a few patients (126, 128, 130, 134). Lakin and Cahill (126) demonstrated skin reactivity and serum-specific IgE to cyclophosphamide, but others (128, 131, 134) have found that cyclophosphamide metabolites can be the antigenic determinant rather than the parent compound. Cyclophosphamide must be activated in the liver, so the fact that a reaction develops up to 16 hours after drug administration (131) is consistent with the fact a metabolite can be the antigen rather than parent drug.

The paradox of an immunosuppressive agent stimulating IgE production may be explained by the fact that in animals this drug can potentiate IgE synthesis (132). Drug inhibition of T-suppressor-cell activity on IgE B cells enhances the activity of the B cells, and more IgE is produced. Thus, the immunogenicity of an agent with otherwise low reactivity may be actually promoted in some patients.

Ifosfamide is a cyclophosphamide analogue that has a similar spectrum of antitumor activity. It causes more chemical cystitis than cyclophosphamide, and it can only be used in conjunction with mesna, which reduces the incidence of cystitis. Type I reactions have been reported (135, 136) when ifosfamide and mesna were used together. Both drugs were given together, as they must be to minimize cystitis toxicity, so it is not possible to know which agent caused the reaction. Use of mesna with cyclophosphamide has also caused acute HSRs (137, 138); however, rechallenge with mesna alone implicated it as the allergen, and skin reactivity was positive for mesna in five patients so tested (137). This reactivity was postulated to be an example of a fixed drug eruption, rather than an IgE-mediated one (137).

MISCELLANEOUS ALKYLATING AGENTS

Melphalan produces HSRs when administered orally (139) or intravenously (140), with the intravenous route being much more likely to cause reactions. While the oral form has produced only a few isolated instances of HSRs, intravenous melphalan produced serious reactions in 2.4 and 4.8%, respectively, of two large series of patients with myeloma (140, 141). All of these reactions occurred after at least 2 prior doses of melphalan and up to 28 doses. In one of these studies (141), different groups of patients were also treated with intravenous melphalan plus other cytotoxic agents. It is surprising that none of these other patients sustained HSRs. Cyclophosphamide has been used as a substitute for melphalan after a reaction, with no cross-reactivity occurring (141).

It is unclear why melphalan administered intravenously is so much more allergenic than it is given orally. Two cases have even been reported (140, 142) in which the patient was reactive to intravenous drug but not to the oral form. Melphalan has variable absorption orally, but lower drug absorption cannot be the whole explanation. A possible allergen could be the excipient used in formulation of the intravenous drug, but melphalan is dissolved only in 10% ethanol and is mixed with normal saline for injection. No studies of the mechanism have been performed. The fact that all reported patients had previous exposure to melphalan before developing a reaction (rather than the HSR occurring with the first dose) suggests an immunologic basis, perhaps IgE-mediated. A fact supporting this possibility is the absence of reported reactions to parenteral melphalan when it is used in the isolated-limb perfusion technique for treatment of melanoma metastases in extremities. The drug is used only once in such treatment.

Reports of HSRs to other alkylating agents have been limited to a few isolated cases. Chlorambucil has produced both severe skin reactions of the erythema multiforme type and type I reactions (143–146). One case involved not only acute HSR symptoms but also evidence of hemolysis (146). These patients all had rechallenge with chlorambucil and reacted again, usually more severely. Several were treated with other alkylators and had no cross-reactivity (143). Isolated instances of acute HSRs to intravenous mechlorethamine (147) and thiotepa given intravesically (148) have been observed.

METHOTREXATE AND TRIMETREXATE

Both low-dose (oral or intravenous) and high-dose methotrexate can cause occasional instances of type I HSRs (149–155). They are often more intense when the drug is used in high doses. The mechanism for these reactions has not been elucidated, but Vega et al. (153) evaluated a patient with various allergy and skin tests. The results suggested that the HSR in their patient was IgE mediated. It is known that methotrexate itself is the allergen, because one case (154) has been studied carefully to show that the HSR was produced by methotrexate itself and not the benzyl alcohol used as a preservative.

Methotrexate also occasionally produces pneumonitis with features suggestive of type III hypersensitivity (156, 157), including blood and/or lung eosinophilia, bilateral hilar adenopathy, sudden onset with no relation to drug dose or treatment duration, concomitant rashes and pleural effusions, and rapid resolution upon drug withdrawal or steroid treatment. The increased numbers of lymphocytes in alveolar lavage specimens from reactive patients (158), suggests an immunologic mechanism. However, many patients with pneumonitis do not have further reactions, despite methotrexate rechallenge, so the issue is unclear. In addition, corticosteroids generally reverse the reaction, but occasionally, the pneumonitis is fatal despite use of steroids (159).

Trimetrexate is an antifolate analogue of methotrexate. It too can occasionally induce generalized type I HSRs (160). Three patients had a reaction after the first dose of trimetrexate, including one who had anaphylaxis and hypotension. None of these patients had prior exposure to antifolate drugs, and rechallenge with trimetrexate in four patients caused repeat reactions.

A more common form of reaction with trimetrexate is an erythematous papular eruption that can be generalized or limited to the head, extremities, or chest (161). This sort of reaction typically occurs a few days after receiving trimetrexate and can occur from a patient's first exposure to an antifol. The reaction seems to be a direct epidermal toxicity rather than one mediated by antibody or anaphylotoxins.

Methotrexate rarely can also cause severe degrees of a similar direct epidermal toxicity. This problem is characterized by an erythematous desquamating or vesicular-bullous eruption that can be localized to the distal extremities or be generalized (162, 163). These skin reactions appear to be related to high doses or altered renal clearance of methotrexate.

Another form of methotrexate toxicity suggestive of a type III reaction is cutaneous vasculitis. Marks et al. (164) briefly described eight patients who developed discrete purpuric skin lesions, apparently induced by methotrexate. The lesions disappeared when methotrexate was discontinued and recurred with methotrexate rechallenge. No studies to define the mechanism were performed.

5-FLUOROURACIL

Rare instances of type I HSRs have been reported secondary to 5-fluorouracil (5-FU) (165–167). Two patients had a severe hypotensive episode, and the other had angioedema. Rechallenge with 5-FU in the latter patient caused a repetition of the reaction. None of these patients had any studies performed to determine the mechanism of reaction, although one patient had skin testing with 5-FU and was nonreactive (166). 5-FU also causes a palmar-plantar dermatitis similar to that with cytarabine (168–171). This condition begins with hand-foot paresthesias and progresses to erythema, swelling, and desquamation. The reaction occurs with high frequency (up to 30%) in patients receiving continuous infusion 5-FU (169) and only very rarely (140) in patients who receive the drug in an intermittent bolus schedule. Patients who have an underlying skin disorder may be more prone to developing such reactions (173). The mechanism of these reactions is unknown, but it appears not to be immunologically mediated and is probably a direct epidermal injury effect. A mechanism of direct skin toxicity is further supported by the fact that pyridoxine helps resolve it (174).

MITOXANTRONE

A few isolated instances of HSRs from mitoxantrone have been reported, including one patient who developed shock (175, 176). One patient (175) was rechallenged with the drug and had a similar reaction. Two patients had an erythematous rash secondary to mitoxantrone. No studies were done on these patients to determine the mechanism.

MITOMYCIN

Mitomycin is administered primarily intravenously but is also instilled intravescially as a treatment for bladder cancer. Rare instances of reactions from both routes of administration have been reported (177–183). Although the intravenous route is used more often than the intravesical one, the latter seems to result in more HSRs (up to 9% of patients receiving drug via this route) (182). This fact is surprising, because pharmacokinetic studies of mitomycin instilled intravesically indicate very little systemic drug absorption from the bladder ("well below the threshold for toxicity") (184). Generalized pruritus and erythematous rashes (but sometimes involving only the palms and soles), angioedema, and fever have been reported. Most patients have received more than five bladder instillations of mitomycin before reactions occur. Desquamation often ensues as the rashes resolve, especially those involving the palms and soles.

Nissenkorn et al. (179) asked the reacting patients to wash their hands carefully after voiding following the drug instillation, based on their hypothesis that the reaction might be a topical drug effect in the form of a contact dermatitis. Hand washing seemed to prevent recurrence of the palmar reactions in two patients, but one patient had repeated generalized rashes with each drug instillation, despite precautionary measures to avoid skin contact with drug-contaminated urine. Intradermal or patch skin testing in patients with such reactions was positive in all instances, whereas normal controls were not reactive (179, 180, 183).

Mitomycin hypersensitivity seems to be a type IV form of HSR. It develops through drug contact on the bladder epithelium and is not caused by drug contamination on skin surfaces. It is probably not an IgE-mediated phenomenon.

BLEOMYCIN

Occasional severe hyperpyrexic (fevers $\geq 40°$ C) episodes occur from bleomycin (185–189). Some of these reactions cause hypotension and initiate disseminated intravascular coagulation with a fatal outcome. They occur most often in patients with lymphoma and are not dose related; they have occurred from as little as 1 unit of drug or after as much as 60 units cumulative dose. Although these episodes have been termed a form of anaphylactic reaction (187), they are not. They are caused by the direct release of pyrogenic cytokines (190) in rare, unusually sensitive individuals. A few rare instances of reactions more suggestive of type I HSRs have also been reported (191, 192). One patient developed

marked angioedema and eosinophilia, but the reaction occurred 2 days after the patient received the first bleomycin dose, making it unlikely to be an immunologically based reaction. Two patients had urticaria. The mechanism of these reactions is unknown.

VINCA ALKALOIDS

HSRs to the vinca alkaloids are almost unknown. No well-documented reports of HSRs caused by one of the three marketed vinca drugs (vincristine, vinblastine, or vinorelbine) have been published. An acute toxicity of vinblastine that might be confused with an HSR can occur when mitomycin and vinblastine are administered simultaneously (193, 194). This phenomenon is characterized by acute onset of dyspnea within several hours of receiving these two drugs. No other pulmonary symptom (e.g., cough, chest pain, sputum production) occurs. Chest x-rays usually show new diffuse infiltrates, but occasional patients have no new findings (194). It has been observed from use of combinations of mitomycin plus vinblastine, vindesine, or vinorelbine but not vincristine (193, 194). It has not occurred from a vinca alkaloid alone, so some sort of interaction between mitomycin and a vinca agent must produce the fulminant dyspnea. Rechallenge with the same drug combination in two patients precipitated the same symptoms again (194). The mechanism is not known, but it is unlikely to be an immunologically mediated toxicity.

MISCELLANEOUS CYTOTOXIC AGENTS

A single case of a type I reaction to dacarbazine has been published (195). The reaction was reproduced with drug rechallenge, but no studies were performed to define its mechanism.

Hydroxyurea can rarely initiate hyperpyrexia that has been termed an HSR (196, 197). The fever may reach 41°C and be accompanied by rigors and sweats. Discontinuation of therapy allows the fever to regress, and rechallenge with the drug causes its prompt return (196, 197). No type I HSRs have been reported from hydroxyurea.

Pentostatin is an antibiotic, and like any other antibiotic, it can initiate HSRs. O'Dwyer et al. (198) collected five cases of HSRs from this drug, characterized by pruritus, fever, erythematous rash, edema, and eosinophilia. Rechallenge in three patients produced recurrence of the same symptoms in all of them (198). No investigations were performed to define the mechanism.

Diaziquone has caused similar type I HSRs, with bronchospasm, rash, urticaria, and hypotension (typical type I HSR manifestations) in 1 to 3% of patients treated (199, 200). The mechanism of these reactions has also not been investigated, but the excipient, dimethylacetamide (rather than the diaziquone), has been suggested (199) as the possible allergen.

A number of drugs that have been evaluated in clinical trials in the past decade but have now disappeared because of inactivity against human cancers, have produced HSRs in a few patients. Two (didemnin and echinomycin) were formulated with Cremophor EL, which may have been the reason for the acute reactions (201, 202). Even in phase II trials with small numbers of patients, these two agents produced HSRs with type I manifestations at a rate of approximately 10%. Some of these reactions occurred on the first dose, much as occurs with paclitaxel.

ALDESLEUKIN

Aldesleukin (interleukin-2) has rarely been reported to produce manifestations of type I HSR (203). Rechallenge produced the same symptoms and signs again. The mechanism of this reaction is unknown.

Aldesleukin can also sensitize patients to iodine-containing radiocontrast dyes, thus precipitating type I reactions when such contrast material is used for diagnostic x-rays (204, 205). This sensitization has been reported to occur in up to 28% of patients (205). The reactions can occur when aldesleukin is being administered concurrently to use of the radiographic dye or when the dye is used several weeks after administration of this drug.

ANCILLARY DRUGS

Filgrastim and sargramostim are two granulocyte-stimulating agents in wide use for myelosuppression support during cancer chemotherapy. Both agents have produced type I HSRs (206–208). In one study (208), sargramostim caused HSRs in 9 of 81 patients treated on a clinical trial involving dose-intensive chemotherapy. Antiemetics (e.g., ondansetron), often used in conjunction with antitumor agents, may also cause HSRs (209) and cause confusion regarding whether it is the antiemetic or the antitumor drug that is the cause of any reaction occurring. Even the corticosteroid dexamethasone, also used as an antiemetic, has been reported to be

the apparent cause of an HSR (210). It is important to exclude such ancillary drugs used with antitumor agents as the cause when an HSR occurs with cancer chemotherapy. If the ancillary drug being used can be isolated as the cause, the antitumor drug is exonerated, and therapy with it can continue. In addition, the offending drug might have an effective substitute, so that therapy could continue. An example is substituting the alternative white cell growth factor when an HSR occurs to one of them. It appears that there is a lack of cross-reactivity between these two agents. One patient who reacted to sargramostim had no reaction to filgrastim when it was used as a substitute (207).

PREVENTION AND EVALUATION OF REACTIONS

If a patient develops an HSR to any antitumor drug, treatment (depending on the type and severity of the reaction) is usually stopped. It is logical to ask if the drug can be used again. A blanket answer cannot be provided because it depends on the drug, the cancer being treated, and the severity of the reaction. Any patient who has a severe type I reaction resulting in significant hypotension (i.e., "anaphylaxis") probably should not be treated with that agent again unless special circumstances dictate otherwise. If a suitable analogue or another drug in the same chemical class is available, it could be substituted in hopes that cross-reactivity will not occur.

If the reaction is moderate, reuse of the drug may be possible if it is preceded by methods to prevent or minimize HSR recurrences. Greenberger et al. (211, 212) have demonstrated that use of pretreatment antihistamines and corticosteroids will reduce the incidence and severity of type I reactions caused by radiographic contrast agents. Such reactions are examples of a nonantibody-mediated release of vasoactive substances (i.e., an anaphylactoid reaction). Pretreatment administration of prednisone and diphenhydramine resulted in a marked decrease in the frequency and severity of such reactions (211, 212). Ephedrine may add an additional measure of protection against such anaphylactoid reactions (213). Weiss et al. (21) have adapted these premedication recommendations for use in prevention of HSRs related to paclitaxel. The same premedications and schedule (Table 31.3) can be used to prevent or minimize second reactions after a patient has demonstrated reactivity to a previous dose of a particular drug or for drugs known to have a propensity to precipitate an HSR (e.g., docetaxel).

As has been indicated throughout this chapter, only in scattered instances has the mechanism of HSRs from antitumor drug been investigated. Such an investigation is important for several reasons. First, there may be benefits to the patient from an evaluation of the cause of a reaction. These benefits might include desensitization of the offending drug so the patient could continue receiving a necessary agent or even ruling out a true HSR in favor of a side effect or toxic reaction. The patient would then not be given another drug of the same class with similar toxic effects. In addition, there are potential advantages for developing chemotherapeutic agents by evaluating HSRs, such as structurally altering an immunogenic compound to produce an equally effective but less allergenic drug. This is exactly what has been achieved with pegaspargase (18).

The first step in evaluating an adverse reaction to an antitumor agent involves deciding whether or not the reaction was a true HSR or, more correctly, whether the reaction was caused by immunologic reactivity to the substance. This determination is often the most difficult part of the analysis because many toxic reactions can mimic immunologic reactivity through direct release of mediators. Several factors can help indicate whether a reaction might have an immunologic basis. First, immunologic reactions usually require a prior exposure; one must be sensitized before becoming **hyper**sensitized. This prior sensitization could occur during an earlier course of a drug or during the same period of administration if the agent is given over a sufficiently long time (probably more than 1 week). In addition, certain symptom complexes are more diagnostic of immunologically mediated disorders. These include urticaria, angioedema, bronchospasm (wheezing), laryngospasm, cytopenias, arthritis, mucositis, vasculitic syndromes, and vesicular dermatitis. A lack of any of these symptoms or an adverse reaction to an agent soon after the first dose makes it less likely that the patient had an immunologically mediated HSR.

Another factor that may help clarify the cause of an adverse reaction in some individuals is their prior allergic history. This is especially true in questions of IgE-mediated reactions, in which patients who tend to form an IgE antibody response to a drug also tend to form them to other antigens such as seasonal pollens. Thus, suspicion that a patient might have had an IgE-me-

diated reaction to an antitumor agent may be heightened if the patient has a prior history of IgE-mediated allergic disease.

While the aforementioned clues serve to direct the clinician to investigate the etiology of a suspected HSR, the only way to determine the exact cause is to evaluate the patient's specific immune reactivity to the suspected agent. In this respect, it is helpful to use the patient's symptoms as a guide to the appropriate laboratory evaluation of a possible HSR. The proper methods for use in evaluating the mechanism of an HSR are beyond the scope of this chapter, and consultation with an allergist-immunologist is recommended.

Many chemotherapeutic agents are formulated with compounds that stabilize or solubilize the active drug and are widely used in the pharmaceutical industry for this purpose. One particular point to keep in mind is that the drug formulation product (excipient) (Table 31.4) or other drugs administered concurrently with the antitumor drug, and not the antitumor drug itself, may be the cause of an HSR. Cremophor EL is thought (21) to play a role in the etiology of the HSRs occurring with paclitaxel administration. Polysorbate 80 (Tween 80) can cause histamine release in dogs, with resultant hypotension, and degranulation of isolated rat mast cells (214). It could be the cause of HSRs occurring from docetaxel. Thus, whenever evaluating the cause of a suspected drug reaction, any diluents or excipients involved should be ruled out as the initiator of the reaction. A good example of the results of such efforts is provided by Wilson et al. (215). Cytarabine preserved with benzyl alcohol caused an HSR that was later proven to be due to the benzyl alcohol and not the antitumor agent. Moreover, later treatment in the same patient with vincristine and heparin, both preserved with benzyl alcohol, also caused HSRs. Since most reports of HSRs to cancer chemotherapeutic agents have not even attempted to rule out the excipient as the cause of the reaction, it is unknown how many reported reactions

Table 31.4. Excipients for Antitumor Drugs with Potential for Causing Hypersensitivity Reactions

Benzyl alcohol
Cremophor EL
Dimethylacetamide
Mannitol
Parabens
Polysorbate 80 (Tween 80)

have falsely implicated the antitumor drug. The same is true of any drugs administered concomitantly, such as mesna, WBC growth factors, or mannitol, which may cause (68, 138, 206, 207) HSRs that occur in conjunction with use of an antitumor agent.

SUMMARY

The list of chemotherapeutic agents that can induce HSRs (Table 31.5) is long and covers most such agents in clinical use. The only antitumor drugs not yet reported in at least one case to cause an HSR are the nitrosoureas (carmustine, lomustine, etc.), altretamine, and dactinomycin. Certain antitumor agents (e.g., the taxoids docetaxel and paclitaxel, L-asparaginase, mitomycin used intravesically) produce HSRs with sufficient frequency to require special precautions with their use. Other drugs (e.g., dacarbazine) have been reported only extremely rarely to cause such toxicity. As new antitumor agents enter clinical trials, most cause at least an isolated instance of such reactions. Unfortunately, the

Table 31.5. Cancer Chemotherapeutic Agents Causing Hypersensitivity Reactions

Drug	Type of Reaction	Frequency	Probable Mechanism of Reaction
1. L-Asparaginase	Type I	10 to 25%	IgE; IgG, complement?
2. Paclitaxel	Type I	Up to 10% without premedications (2% with premedication)	Nonspecific release of vasoactive substances?
3. Docetaxel	Type I	Same as paclitaxel	Nonspecific release of vasoactive substances?
4. Elliptinium	Type II	Up to 10% (depending on administration schedule)	IgM
	Type I	Case reports	Unknown
5. Teniposide	Type I	5 to 15%	Nonspecific release?
6. Cisplatin	Type I	Intravesically: up to 20%; intravenously: 1% (higher after >6 doses)	IgE; nonspecific release?
7. Procarbazine	Type 1	Up to 15%	Unknown
	Type III	Case reports	Immune complexes?
8. Carboplatin	Type I	Up to 8% IgE	?
9. Intravenous melphalan	Type I	2 to 5%	Unknown
10. Mechlorethamine			
Topical	Type IV	10 to 20%	T-cell sensitization
Intravenous	Type I	Case reports	Unknown
11. Anthracycline antibiotics	Type I	Varies depending on anthracycline (<1% to 5%)	Unknown (nonspecific release)
12. Diaziquone	Type I	1 to 3%	Unknown
13. Etoposide	Type I	1 to 3%	IgE or nonspecific release?
14. Methotrexate	Type I	Case reports	Unknown
	Type III	Case reports	Immune complexes
	Type II	Case reports	IgG
15. Trimetrexate	Type I	Case reports	Unknown
16. Cytarabine	Type I	Case reports	IgE
	Rashes	5 to 30% (depending on dose)	Direct skin toxicity?
17. Cyclophosphamide	Type I	Case reports	IgE (reactive to a metabolite)
18. Ifosfamide	Type I	Case reports	Unknown
19. Pentostatin	Type I	Case reports	Unknown
20. Chlorambucil	Type I	Case reports	Unknown
21. 5-Fluorouracil	Type I	Case reports	Unknown
22. Mitoxantrone	Type I	Case reports	Unknown
23. Mitomycin	Type I or III?	Case reports	Unknown
	Type IV	Up to 10% intravesically	Contact dermatitis
24. Bleomycin	Type I	Case reports	Unknown
25. Aldesleukin	Type I	Case reports	Unknown
26. Dacarbazine	Type I	Case reports	Unknown

mechanism of HSRs remains unknown and inadequately investigated for most such drugs.

REFERENCES

1. Gell PHG, Coombs RRA. Clinical aspects of imunology. Oxford: Blackwell Scientific Publications, 1975.

2. Evans WE, Tsiatis A, Rivera G, et al. Anaphylactoid reactions to *Escherichia coli* and *Erwinia* asparaginase in children with leukemia and lymphoma. Cancer 1982;49:1378–1983.

3. Clavell LA, Gelber RA, Cohen HJ, et al. Fouragent induction and intensive asparaginase therapy for treatment of childhood acute lymphocytic leukemia. N Engl J Med 1986;315:657–663.

4. Rausen AR, Gludewell O, Holland JF, et al. Superiority of L-asparaginase combination chemotherapy in advanced acute lymphocytic leukemia of childhood. Randomized comparative trial of combination versus solo therapy. Cancer Clin Trials 1979;1:137–144.

5. Billett AL, Carls A, Gelber RD, Sallan SE. Allergic reactions to *Erwinia* asparaginase in children with acute lymphoblastic leukemia who had previous allergic reactions to *Escherichia coli* asparaginase. Cancer 1992;70:201–206.

6. Albo V, Miller D, Leuken S, Hammond D, Sather H: Toxicity experience with a second course of E. coli L-asparaginase (L-asp) therapy 3 years after induction course in children with acute lymphoblastic leukemia (ALL) in continuous remission (abstract). Proc Am Soc Clin Oncol 1982;2:68.

7. Nesbit M, Chard R, Evans A, Karon M, Hammond GD, for the Children's Cancer Study Group. Evaluation of intramuscular versus intravenous administration of L-asparaginase in childhood leukemia. Am J Pediatr Hematol Oncol 1979;1:9–13.

8. Harris RE, McCallister JA, Provisor DS, et al. Methotrexate/L-asperaginase combination chemotherapy for patients with acute leukemia in relapse: a study of 36 children. Cancer 1980;46:2004–2008

9. Spiegel RJ, Echelberger CK, Poplack DG. Delayed allergic reactions following intramuscular L-asparaginase. Med Pediatr Oncol 1980;8:123–125.

10. Ho DHW, Yap HY, Brown N, et al. Clinical pharmacology of intramuscularly administered L-asparaginase. J Clin Pharmacol 1981;21:72–78.

11. Land VJ, Shuster JJ, Pullen J, et al. Unexpectedly high incidence of alergic reactions with high dose (HD) weekly asparaginase (ASP) consolidation (cons) therapy (Rx) in children with newly diagnosed non-T, non-B acute lymphoblastic leukemia (ALL): a Pediatric Oncology Group (POG) study (abstract). Proc Am Soc Clin Oncol 1989;8:215.

12. Khan A, Hill JM. Atopic hypersensitivity to L-asparaginase. Resistance to immunosuppression. Int Arch Allergy 1971;40:463–469.

13. Fabry U, Korholz D, Jurgens H, Gobel U, Wahn V. Anaphylaxis to L-asparaginase during treatment for acute lymphoblastic leukemia in children—evidence of a complement-mediated mechanism. Pediatr Res 1985; 19:400–408.

14. Ohnuma T, Holland JF, Meyer P. *Erwinia carotovora* asparaginase in patients with prior anaphylaxis to asparaginase from *E. coli*. Cancer 1972;30:376–381.

15. Abuchowski A, van Es T, Palczuk NC, et al. Treatment of L5178Y tumor-bearing BDF1 mice

16. Teske E, Rutteman GR, van Heerde P. Misdorp W. Polyethylene glycol-L-asparaginase versus native L-asparaginase in canine non-Hodgkin's lyhmphoma. Eur J Cancer 1990;26:891–895.

17. Ho DH, Brown NS, Yen A, et al. Clinical pharmacology of polyethylene glycol-L-asparaginase. Drug Metab Disp 1986;14:349–352.

18. Abshire T, Pollock B, Billett A, Bradley P, Buchanan G. Weekly polyethylene glycol conjugated (PEG) L-asparaginase (asp) produces superior induction remission rates in childhood relapsed acute lymphoblastic leukemia (rALL): a Pediatric Oncology Group (POG) study 9310 (abstract). Proc Am Soc Clin Oncol 1995;14:344.

19. Eisenhauer EA, ten Bokkel Huinick WW, Swenerton KD, et al. European-Canadian randomized trial of paclitaxel in relapsed ovarian cancer: high-dose versus low-dose and long versus short influsion. J Clin Oncol 1994;12:2654–2666.

20. Onetto N, Canetta R, Winograd B, et al. Overview of taxol safety. Monogr Natl Cancer Inst 1993; 15:131–139.

21. Weiss RB, Donehower RH, Weirnik PH, et al. Hypersensitivity reactions from taxol. J Clin Oncol 1990;8:1263–1268.

22. Hainsworth JD, Greco FA. Paclitaxel administered by 1-hour infusion. Preliminary results of a phase I/II trial comparing two schedules. Cancer 1994; 74:1377–1382.

23. Lorenz W, Reimann H-J, Schmal A, Dormann P, Schwarz B, Neugebauer E. Histamine release in dogs by Cremophor EL and its derivatives: oxethylated oleic acid is the most effective constitutent. Agents Actions 977;7:63–67.

24. Peereboom DM, Donehower RC, Eisenhauer EA, et al. Successful re-treatment with taxol after major hypersensitivity reactions. J Clin Oncol 1993;11:885–890.

25. Laskin MS, Lucchesi KJ, Morgan M. Paclitaxel rechallenge failure after a major hypersensitivity reaction. J Clin Oncol 1993;11:2456–2457.

26. Del Priore G, Smith P, Warshal DP, Dubeshter B, Angel C. Paclitaxel-associated hypersensitivity reaction despite high-dose steroids and prolonged infusions. Gynecol Oncol 1995;56:316–318.

27. Verweij J, Clavel M, Chevalier B. Paclitaxel (Taxol) and docetaxel (Taxotere): not simply two of a kind. Ann Oncol 1995;5:495–505.

28. Piccart MJ, Core M. ten Bokkel Huinink W, van Oosterom A, et al. Docetaxel: an active new drug for treatment of advanced epithelial ovarian cancer. J Natl Cancer Inst 1995;87:676–681.

29. Burris H, Irvin R, Kuhn J, et al. Phase I clinical trial of taxotere administered as either a 2-hour or 6-hour intravenous infusion. J Clin Oncol 1993;11:950–958.

30. Chevallier B, Fumoleau P, Kerbrat P, et al. Docetaxel is a major cytotoxic drug for the treatment of advanced breast cancer: a phase II trial of the Clinical Screening Cooperative Group of the European Organization for Research and Treatment of Cancer. J Clin Oncol 1995;13:314–322.

31. Schrijvers D, Wanders J, Dirix L, et al. Coping with toxicities of docetaxel (Taxotere). Ann Oncol 1993; 4:610–611.

32. Mertens WC, Eisenhauer EA, Jolivet J, Ernst S, Moore M, Muldal A. Docetaxel in advanced renal carcinoma. Ann Oncol 1994;5:185–187.

33. Zimmerman GC, Keeling JH, Burris HA, et al. Acute cutaneous reactions to docetaxel, a new chemotherapeutic agent. Arch Dermatol 1995;131:202–206.

34. Criel AM, Hidajat M, Clarysse A, Verwilghen RL. Drug dependent red cell antibodies and intravascular haemolysis occurring in patients treated with 9 hydroxy-methyl-ellipticinium. Br J Haemtol 1980; 46:549–556.

35. Caillé P, Mondesir JM, Droz JP, et al. Phase II trial of elliptinium in advanced renal cell carcinoma. Cancer Treat Rep 1985;69:901–902.

36. Doll DC, Weiss RB. Hemolytic anemia associated with antineoplastic agents. Cancer Treat Rep 1985; 69:8777–782.

37. Mondesir J-M, Bidart J-M, Goodman A, et al. Drug-induced antibodies during a 2-N-methyl-9-hydroxyellipticinium acetate (NSC-264137) treatment: schedule dependency and relationship to hemolysis. J Clin Oncol 1985;3:735–740.

38. Buzdar AU, Esparza L, Hortobagyi GN, et al. Elliptinium acetate in treatment of advanced breast cancer—a phase II study. Oncology 1990;47:101–104.

39. Rouesse J, Spielmann M, Turpin F, Le Chevalier T, Azab M, Mondesir JM. Phase II study of elliptinium acetate salvage treatment of advanced breast cancer. Eur J Cancer 1993;29A:856–859.

40. Treat J, Greenspan A, Rahman A, McCabe MS, Byrne PJ. Elliptinium: phase II study in advanced measurable breast cancer. Invest New Drugs 1989;7:231–234.

41. Clarysse A, Brugarolas A, Siegenthaler P, et al. Phase II study of 9-hydroxy-2N-methyl-ellipticinium acetate. Eur J Cancer Clin Oncol 1984;20:243–247.

42. Alberici GF, Fellous R, Bidart J-M, et al. Human antibodies to the antineoplastic drug elliptinium: characterization and structure-activity relationships. J Allergy Clin Immuno 1986;77:624–630.

43. O'Dwyer PJ, King SA, Fortner CL, Leyland-Jones B. Hypersensitivity reactions to teniposide (VM-26): an analysis. J Clin Oncol 1986;4:1262–1269.

44. Hayes FA, Abromowitch M, Green AA. Allergic reactions to teniposide in patients with neuroblastoma and lymphoid malignancies. Cancer Treat Rep 1985;69:439–441.

45. Carstensen H, Nolte H, Hertz H, Jensen T. Hypersensitivity reactions to teniposide in children. J Clin Oncol 1987;5:1491–1942.

46. Kellie SJ, Crist WM, Pui C-H, et al. Hypersensitivity reactions to epipodophyllotoxins in children with acute lymphoblastic leukemia. Cancer 1991; 67:1070–1075.

47. Canal P, Dugot R, Chatelut E, et al. Phase I/pharmacokinetic study of intraperitoneal teniposide (VM 266). Eur J Cancer Clin Oncol 1989;25:815–820.

48. O'Dwyer PJ, Weiss RB. Hypersensitivity reactions induced by etopside. Cancer Treat Rep 1985; 68:959–961.

49. Ogle KM, Kennedy BJ. Hypersensitivity reactions to etoposide. A case report and review of the literature. Am J Clin Oncol 1988;11:663–665.

50. de Souza P, Friedlander M, Wilde C, Kirsten F, Ryan M. Hypersensitivity reactions to etoposide. A report of three cases and review of the literature. Am J Clin Oncol (CCT) 1994;17:387–389.

51. Dahl GV, Rivera K, Look AT, et al. Teniposide plus cytarabine improves outcome in childhood acute lymphocytic leukemia presenting with a leukocyte count ≥100 × 10^9/L. J Clin Oncol 1987;5:1015–1021.

52. Hudson MM, Weinstein HJ, Donalson SS, et al. Acute hypersensitivity reactions to etoposide in a VEPA regimen for Hodgkin's diseae. J Clin Oncol 1993; 11:1080–1084.

53. Siderov J, Zalcberg J. Safe administration of oral etoposide after hypersensitivity reaction to intravenous etoposide. Anti-Cancer Drugs 1994;5:602–603.

54. Nolte H, Cartensen H, Hertz H. VM-26 (teniposide)-induced hypersensitivity and degranulation of basophils in children. Am J Pediatr Hematol Oncol 1988;10:308–312.

55. Sutherland CM, Loutfi A. Unusual reaction to VP-16-213 and avoidance by prolonged infusion. Cancer Treat Rep 1982;66:409.

56. Habibi B, Lopez M, Serdaru M, et al. Immune hemolytic anemia and renal failure due to teniposide. N Engl J Med 1982;306:1091–1093.

57. Khan A, Hill JM, Grater W, Loeb E, MacLennan A, Hill N. Atopic hypersensitivity to cis-dichlorodiammineplatinum (II) and other platinum complexes. Cancer Res 1975;3:2766–2770.

58. Anderson T, Javadpour N. Schilsky R, Barlock A, Young RC. Chemotherapy for testicular cancer: current status of the National Cancer Institute combined modality trial. Cancer Treat Rep 1979;63:1687–1692.

59. Cheng E, Cvitkovic E, Wittes RE, Golbey RB. Germ cell tumors (II). VAB II in metastatic testicular cancer. Cancer 1978;42:2162–2168.

60. Gralla RJ, Casper ES, Kelsen DP, et al. Cisplatin and vindesine combination chemotherapy for advanced carcinoma of the lung: a randomized trial investigating two dosage schedules. Ann Intern Med 1981;95:414–420.

61. Blumenreich MS, Needles B, Yagoda A, Sogani P, Grabstald H, Whitmore WF. Intravesical cisplatin for superficial bladder tumors. Cancer 1982;50:863–865.

62. Denis L. Anaphylactic reactions to repeated intravesical instillation with cisplatin. Lancet 1983; 1:1378–1379.

63. Markman M. No increase in allergic reactions with intracavitary administration of cisplatin (letter). Lancet 1984;2:1164

64. Zweizig S, Roman LD, Muderspach LI. Death from anaphylaxis to cisplatin: a case report. Gynecol Oncol 1994;53:121–122.

65. Wiesenfeld M, Reinders E, Corder M, Yoo T-J, Dietz B. Lovett J. Successful retreatment with cis-dichlorodiammine-platinum (II) after apparent allergic reactions. Cancer Treat Rep 1979;63:219–221.

66. Goldberg A, Altaras MM, Mekori YA, Beyth Y, Confino-Cohen R. Anaphylaxis to cisplatin: diagnosis and value of pretreatment in prevention of recurrent allergic reactions. Ann Allergy 1994;73:271–272.

67. Lamb JD, Keogh JAM. Anaphylactoid reaction to mannitol. Can Anaesth Soc J 1979;26:435–436.

68. Ackland SP, Hillcoat BL. Immediate hypersensitivity to mannitol: a potential cause of apparent hypersensitivity to cisplatin. Cancer Treat Rep 1985; 69:562–563.

69. Getaz EP, Beckley S, Fitzpatrick J. Dozier A. Cisplatin-induced hemolysis. N Engl J Med 1980; 302:334–335.

70. Levi JA, Aroney RS, Dalley DN. Haemolytic anemia after cisplatin treatment. Br Med J 1981; 282:2003–2004.

71. Cinollo G, Dini G, Franchini E, Lanino E, Sindaco F, Garaventa A. Positive direct antiglobulin test in a pediatric patient following high-dose cisplatin. Cancer Chemother Pharmacol 1988;21:85–86.

72. Zeger G, Smith L, McQuiston D, Goldfinger D. Cisplatin-induced nonimmunologic adsorption of immunoglobulin by red cells. Transfusion 1988;28:493–495.

73. Allen JC, Walker R, Luks E, Jennings M, Barfoot S, Tan C. Carboplatin and recurrent childhood brain tumors. J Clin Oncol 1987;5:459–463.

74. Hendrick AM, Simmons D, Cantwell BMJ. Allergic reactions to carboplatin. Ann Oncol 1992;3:239–240.

75. Tonkin KS, Rubin P, Levin L. Carboplatin hypersensitivity: case reports and review of the literature. Eur J Cancer 1993;29A:1356–1357.

76. Planner RS, Weerasiri T, Timmins D, Grant P. Hypersensitivity reactions to carboplatin. J Natl Cancer Inst 1991;83:1763–1764.

77. Windom HH, McGuire WP, Hamilton RG, Adkinson NF. Anaphylaxis to carboplatin—a new platinum chemotherapeutic agent. J Allergy Clin Immunol 1992;90:681–683.

78. Weidmann B, Mulleneisen N, Bojko P, Niederle N. Hypersensitivity reactions to carboplatin. Report of two patients, review of the literature, and discussion of diagnostic procedures and management. Cancer 1994;73:2217–2222.

79. Bacha DM, Caparros-Sison B, Allen JA, Walker R, Tan CTC. Phase I study of carboplatin (CBDCA) in children with cancer. Cancer Treat Rep 1986;70:865–869.

80. Shlebak AA, Clark PI, Green JA. Hypersensitivity and cross-reactivity to cisplatin and analogues. Cancer Chemother Pharmacol 1995;35:349–351.

81. Brunner KW, Young CW. A methylhydrazine derivative in Hodgkin's disease and other malignant neoplasms. An Intern Med 1965;63:69–86.

82. Glovsky MM, Braunwald J, Opelz G, Alenty A. Hypersensitivity to procarbazine associated with angioedema, urticaria, and low serum complement activity. J Allergy Clin Immunol 1976;57:134–140.

83. Andersen E, Videbaek A. Procarbazine-induced skin reactions in Hodgkin's disease and other malignant lymphomas. Scand J Haematol 1980;24:149–151.

84. Sandberg-Wollheim M, Malmstron P, Stromblad L-G, et al. A randomized study of chemotherapy with procarbazine, vincristine, and lomustine with and without radiation therapy for astrocytoma grades 3 and/or 4. Cancer 1991;68:22–29.

85. Coyle T, Bushunow P, Winfield J. Wright J, Graziano S. Hypersensitivity reactions to procarbazine with mechlorethamine, vincristine, and procarbazine chemotherapy in the treatment of glioma. Cancer 1992; 69:2532–2540.

86. Eyre HJ, Quagliana JM, Eltringham JR, et al. Randomized comparisons of radiotherapy and CCNU versus radiotherapy, CCNU plus procarbazine for the treatment of malignant gliomas following surgery. J Neurooncol 1983;1:171–177.

87. Giguere JK, Douglas DM, Lupton GP, Baker JR, Weiss RB. Procarbazine hypersensitivity manifested as a fixed drug eruption. Med Pediatr Oncol 1988;16:378–380.

88. Lokich JJ, Moloney WC. Allergic reaction to procarbazine. Clin Pharmacol Ther 1972;13:573–574.

89. Jones SE, Moore M, Blank N, Castellino RA. Hypersensitivity to procarbazine (Matulane) manifested by fever and pleuropulmonary reaction. Cancer 1972;29:498–500.

90. Ecker MD, Jay B, Keohane MF. Procarbazine lung. Am J Roentgenol 1987;131:527–528.

91. Lewis LD. Procarbazine associated alveolitis. Thorax 1984;39:206–207.

92. Rassiga AL, Schwartz HJ, Forman WB, Crum Ed. Cytarabine-induced anaphylaxis. Demonstration of antibody and successful desensitization. Arch Intern Med 1980;140:425–426.

93. Castleberry RP, Crist WM, Holbrook T, Malluh A, Gaddy D. The cytosine arabinoside (Ara-C) syndrome. Med Pediatr Oncol 1989;9:257–264.

94. Markman M, Howell SB, King M, Pfeifle C, Wasserman SI. Anaphylactic reaction to cytarabine: in vitro evidence that the response is immunoglobulin E mediated. Med Pediatr Oncol 1984;12:201–203.

95. Berkowtiz FE, Wehde S, Ngwenya ET, Greeff M, Wadee AA, Rabson AR. Anaphylactic shock due to cytarabine in a leukemic child. Am J Dis Child 1987; 141:1000–1001.

96. Burke PJ, Owens AH. Attempted recruitment of leukemic myeloblasts to proliferative activity by sequential drug treatment. Cancer 1971;28:830–936.

97. Manoharan A. The cytarabine syndrome in adults. Aust NZ J Med 1985;15:451–452.

98. Williams SF, Larson RA. Hypersensitivity reaction to high-dose cytarabine. Br J Haematol 1989; 73:274–275.

99. Burgdorf WH, Gilmore WA, Ganick RG. Peculiar acral erythema secondary to high-dose chemotherapy for acute myelogenous leukemia. Ann Intern Med 1982;97:61–62.

100. Herzig RH, Wolff SN, Lazarus HM, Phillips GL, Karanes PC, Herzig GP. High-dose cytosine arabinoside therapy for refractory leukemia. Blood 1983; 62:361–369.

101. Baer MR, King LE, Wolff SN. Palmar-plantar erythrodysesthesia and cytarabine (letter). Ann Intern Med 1985;102:556.

102. Shall L, Lucas GS, Whittaker JA, Holt PJA. Painful red hands: a side-effect of leukaemia therapy. Br J Dermatol 1988;119:249–253.

103. Levine LE, Medenica MM, Lorincz AL, Soltani K, Raab B, Ma A. Distinctive acral erythma occurring during therapy for severe myelogenous leukemia. Arch Dermatol 1985;121:101–104.

104. Cordonnier C, Roujeau JC, Vernant JP, Matheron S, Ganem G. Cancer chemotherapy and acral erythema (letter). Ann Intern Med 1982;97:783.

105. Peters WG, Willemze R. Palmar-plantar skin changes and cytarabine (letter). Ann Intern Med 1985; 103:805.

106. Krulder JWM, Vlasveld LT, Willemze R. Erythema and swelling of ears after treatment with cytarabine for leukemia. Eur J Cancer 1990;26:649–650.

107. Brown J, Burck K, Black D, Collins C. Treat-

ment of cytarabine acral erythema with corticosteroids. J Am Acad Dermatol 1991;24(part 1):1023–1025.

108. Baack BR, Burgdorf WHC. Chemotherapy-induced acral erythema. J Am Acad Dermatol 1991; 24:457–461.

109. Jones AP, Crawford SM. Anthracycline-induced toxicity affecting palmar and plantar skin. Br J Cancer 1989;59:814.

110. Harrist TJ, Fine JD, Berman RS, Murphy GF, Mihm MC. Neutrophilic eccrine hidradenitis. A distinctive type of neutrophilic dermatosis associated with myelogenous leukemia and chemotherapy. Arch Dermatol 1982;118:263–266.

111. Flynn TC, Harrist TJ, Murphy GF, Loss RW, Moschella SL. Neutrophilic eccrine hidradenitis: a distinctive rash associated with cytarabine therapy and acute leukemia. J Am Acad Dermatol 1984;11:584–590.

112. Beutner KR, Packman CH, Markowitch W. Neutrophilic eccrine hidradenitis associated with Hodgkin's disease and chemotherapy. Arch Dermatol 1986;122:809–811.

113. Arnold DJ, Stafford CT. Systemic allergic reaction to adriamycin. Cancer Treat Rep 1979;63:150–151.

114. Solimando DA, Wilson JP. Doxorubicin-induced hypersensitivity reactions. Drug Intell Clin Pharm 1984;18:808–811.

115. Collins JA. Hypersensitivity reaction to doxorubicin. Drug Intell Clin Pharm 1984;18:402–403.

116. Freeman AI. Clinical note. Allergic reaction to daunorubicin. Cancer Chemother Rep (part 1) 1970; 54:475–476.

117. Crowther D, Powles RL, Bateman CJT, et al. Management of adult acute myelogenous leukaemia. Br Med J 1973;1:131–137.

118. Crawford ED, McKenzie D, Mansson W, et al. Adverse reactions to the intravesical administration of doxorubicin hydrochloride: report of 6 cases. J Urol 1986;136:668–669.

119. Bickers J, Benjamin R, Wilson H, Eyre H, Hewlett J, McCredie K. Rubidazone in adults with previously treated acute leukemia and blast cell phase of chronic myelocytic leukemia: a Southwest Oncology Group study. Cancer Treat Rep 1981;65:427–430.

120. Tan CTC, Mitta SK, Steinherz L, Miller DR. Phase I trial of rubidazone (NSC 164011) in children with cancer. Med Pediatr Oncol 1981;9:347–353.

121. Etcubanas E, Wilbur JR. Uncommon side effects of adriamycin (NSC-123127). Cancer Chemother Rep (part 1) 1974;58:757–758.

122. Vogelzang NJ. "Adriamycin flare": a skin reaction resembling extravasation. Cancer Treat Rep 1979;63:2067–2069.

123. Glass E. Aclacinomycin A flare. Cancer Treat Rep 1982;66:1983.

124. Berman E, Wittes RE, Leyland-Jones B, et al. Phase I and clinical pharmacology studies of intravenous and oral administration of 4-demethoxydaunorubicin in patients with advanced cancer. Cancer Res 1983;43:6096–6101.

125. Cassidy J, Rankin EM. Hypersensitivity reaction to epirubicin. Med Oncol Tumor Pharmacother 1989;6:297–298.

126. Lakin JD. Cahill RA. Generalized urticaria to cyclophosphamide: type I hypersensitivity to an immunosuppressive agent. J Allergy Clin Immunol 1976; 58:160–171.

127. Ross WE, Chabner BA. Allergic reaction to cyclophosphamide in a mechlorethamine-sensitive patient. Cancer Treat Rep 1977;61:495–496.

128. Knysak DJ, McLean JA, Solomon WR, Fox DA, McCune WJ. Immediate hypersensitivity reaction to cyclophosphamide. Arthritis Rheum 1994;37:1101–1104.

129. Salles G, Thierry V, Archimbaud E. Anaphylactoid reaction with bronchospasm following intravenous cyclophosphamide administration. Ann Hematol 1991;62:74–75.

130. Kim HC, Kesarwala HH, Colvin M, Saidi P. Hypersensitivity reaction to a metabolite of cyclophosphamide. J Allergy Clin Immunol 1985;76:591–594.

131. Popescu NA, Sheehan MG, Kouides PA, et al. Allergic reactions to cyclophosphamide: delayed clinical expression associated with positive immediate skin tests to drug metabolites in five patients (abstract). J Allergy Clin Immunol 1995;95:288.

132. Krutchik AN, Buzdar AU, Tashima CK. Cyclophosphamide-induced urticaria: occurrence in a patient with no cross-sensitivity to chlorambucil. Arch Intern Med 1978;138:1725–1726.

133. Kritharides L, Lawrie K, Varigos GA. Cyclophosphamide hypersensitivity and cross-reactivity with chlorambucil. Cancer Treat Rep 1987;71:1323–1324.

134. Cromar BW, Colvin M, Casale TB. Validity of skin tests to cyclophosphamide and metablites. J Allergy Clin Immunol 1991;88:965–967.

135. Case D, Anderson J, Ervin T, Gottlieb A. Phase II trial of ifosfamide and mesna in previously treated patients with non-Hodgkin's lymphoma: Cancer and Leukemia Group B study 8552. Med Pediatr Oncol 1988;16:182–186.

136. Pratt CB, Sandlund JT, Meyer WH, Cain AM. Mesna-induced urticaria. Drug Intell Clin Pharm 1988; 22:913–914.

137. Zonzits E, Aberer W, Tappeiner G. Drug eruptions from mesna. Arch Dermatol 1992;128:80–82.

138. Seidel A, Andrassy K, Ritz E, Kasser U, Lemmel E-M. Allergic reactions to mesna (letter). Lancet 1991;338:381.

139. Lawrence BV, Harvey HA, Lipton A. Anaphylaxis due to oral melphalan. Cancer Treat Rep 1980; 64:731–732.

140. Cornwell GG, Pajak TF, McIntyre OR. Hypersensitivity reactions to IV melphalan during treatment of multiple myeloma: Cancer and Leukemia Group B experience. Cancer Treat Rep 1979;63:399–403.

141. Cooper MR, McIntyre OR, Propert KJ, et al. Single sequential and multiple alkylating agent therapy for multiple myeloma: a CALGB study. J Clin Oncol 1986;4:1331–1339.

142. Bleichner F, Mende S. Allergische reaktion auf melphalan (letter). Onkologie 1986;5:195.

143. Hitchins RN, Hocker GA, Thomson DB. Chlorambucil allergy—a series of three cases. Aust NZ J Med 1987;17:600–602.

144. Barone C, Cassano A, Astone A. Toxic epidermal necrolysis during chlorambucil therapy in chronic lymphocytic leukaemia. Eur J Cancer 1990;26:1262.

145. Zervas J, Karkantaris CH, Kapiri E, Theocharis S, Konstantopoulos K. Allergic reaction to chlorambucil in chronic lymphocytic leukaemia: case report. Leuk Res 1992;16:329–330.

146. Thompson-Moya L, Martin T, Heuft H-G,

Neubauer A, Herrmann R. Case report: allergic reaction with immune hemolytic anemia resulting from chlorambucil. Am J Hematol 1989;32:230–231.

147. Wilson KS, Alexander S. Hypesensitivity to mechlorethamine (letter). Ann Intern Med 1981;94:823.

148. Veenema RJ, Dean AL, Uson AC, Roberts M, Longo F. Thiotepa bladder instillations; therpy and prophylaxis for superficial bladder tumors. J Urol 1969; 101:711–715.

149. Paradis L, Des Roches A, Paradis J, Shultz Y. Methotrexate allergy: a case report (abstract). J Allergy Clin Immunol 1995;95(part 2):289.

150. Klimo P, Ibrahim E. Anaphylactic reaction to methotrexate in high doses as adjuvant treatment of osteogenic sarcoma (letter). Cancer Treat Rep 1981; 65:725.

151. Bokemeyer C, Schmoll H-J, Schoffski P, Scholltissek M, Poliwoda H. A case of hypersensitivity reaction to high dose methotrexzte (HD-MTX) (abstract). Ann Oncol 1992;3(Suppl 5):171.

152. Recker DP, Minor JR, Miller FW, Successful prevention of an anaphylactoid reaction to high-dose methotrexate (letter). DICP Ann Pharmacother 1989; 23:1032.

153. Vega A, Cabanas R, Contreras J, et al. Anaphylaxis to methotrexate: a possible IgE-mediated mechanism. J Allergy Clin Immunol 1994;94:268–270.

154. Gluck-Kuyt I, Irwin LE. Anaphylactic reaction to high-dose methotrexate. Cancer Treat Rep 1979; 63:797–798.

155. Cohn JR, Cohn JB, Fellin F, Cantor R. Systemic anaphylaxis from low dose methotrexate. Ann Allergy 1993;70:384–385.

156. Sostman HD, Matthay RA, Putman CE, et al. Methotrexate-induced pneumonitis. Medicine 1976; 55:371–388.

157. Searles G, McKendry RJR. Methotrexate pneumonitis in rheumatoid arthritis: potential risk factors. Four case reports and a review of the literature. J Rheumatol 1987;14:1164–1171.

158. White DA, Rankin JA, Stover DE, Gellene RA, Gupta S. Methotrexate pneumonitis. Bronchoalveolar lavage findings suggest an immunologic disorder. Am Rev Resp Dis 1989;139:18–21.

159. Newman ED, Harrington TM. Fatal methotrexate pneumonitis in rheumatoid arthritis. Arthritis Rheum 1988;31:1585–1586.

160. Grem JL, King SA, Costanza ME, Brown TD. Hypersensitivity reactions to trimetrexate. Invest New Drugs 1990;8:211–214.

161. Weiss RB, James WD, Major WB, Porter MB, Allegra CJ, Curt GA. Skin reactions induced by trimetrexate, an analog of methotrexate. Invest New Drugs 1986;4:159–163.

162. Haim N, Kedar A, Robinson E. Methotrexate-related deaths in patients previously treated with cis-diamminedichloride platinum. Cancer Chemother Pharmacol 1984;13:223–225.

163. Doyle LA, Berg C, Bottino G, Chabner B. Erythema and desquamation after high-dose methotrexate. Ann Intern Med 1983;98:611–612.

164. Marks CR, Willkens RF, Wilske KR, Brown PB. Small-vessel vasculitis and methotrexate (letter). Ann Intern Med 1984;100:916.

165. DeBeer R, Kabakow B. Anaphylactoid reaction. Associated with intravenous administration of 5-fluorouracil. NY State J Med 1979;79:1750–1751.

166. Sridhar KS. Allergic reaction to 5-fluorouracil infusion. Cancer 1986;58:862–864.

167. Santos AM, Medina FS. Anaphylactic reaction following iv administration of fluorouracil (letter). Cancer Treat Rep 1986;70:1346.

168. Lokich JJ, Moore C. Chemotherapy-associated palmar-plantar erythrodysesthesia syndrome. Ann Intern Med 1984;101:798–800.

169. Cantrell JE, Hart RD, Taylor RF, Harvey JH. Pilot trial of prolonged continuous-infusion 5-fluorouracil and weekly cisplatin in advanced colorectal cancer. Cancer Treat Rep 1987;71:615–618.

170. Bellmunt J, Navarro M, Hidalgo R, Sole LA. Palmar-plantar erythrodysesthesia syndrome associated with short-term continuous infusion (5 days) of 5-fluorouracil. Tumori 1988;74:329–331.

171. Comandone A, Bretti S, La Grotta G, et al. Palmar-plantar erythrodysesthesia syndrome associated with 5-fluorouracil treatment. Anticancer Res 1993; 13:1781–1784.

172. Atkins JN. Fluorouracil and the palmar-plantar erythrodysesthesia syndrome (letter). Ann Intern Med 1985;102:419.

173. Vukelja SJ, James WD, Weiss RB. Severe dermatologic toxicity from 5-fluorouracil in the presence of seborrheic dermatitis. Int J Dermatol 1989;28:353–354.

174. Fabian CJ, Molina R, Slavik M, Dahlberg S, Giri S,Stephens R. Pyridoxine therapy for palmar-plantar erythrodysesthesia associated with continuous 5-fluorouracil infusion. Invest New Drugs 1990; 8:57–63.

175. Taylor WB, Cantwell BMJ, Roberts JT, Harris AL. Allergic reactions to mitoxantrone (letter). Lancet 1986;1:1439.

176. Anderson KC, Cohen GI, Garnick MB. Phase II trial of mitoxantrone. Cancer Treat Rep 1982; 66:1929–1931.

177. Ritch PS, Louie AC. Skin rash following therapy with mitomycin C. Cancer 1984;54:32–33.

178. Cheirsilpa A, Leelasethakul S, Auethaveekiat V, et al. High-dose mitomycin C: activity in hepatocellular carcinoma. Cancer Chemother Pharmacol 1989; 24:50–53.

179. Nissenkorn I, Herrod H, Soloway MS. Side effects associated with intravesical mitomycin C. J Urol 1981;126:596–597.

180. Colver GB, Inglis JA, McVittie E, Spencer M-J, Tolley DA, Hunter JAA. Dermatitis due to intravesical mitomycin C: a delayed-type hypersensitivity reaction? Br J Dermatol 1990;122:217–224.

181. Arregui MA, Aguirre A, Gil N, Goday J, Raton JA. Dermatitis due to mitomycin C bladder instillations: study of 2 cases. Contact Dermatitis 191;24:368–370.

182. De Groot AC, Conemans JMH. Systemic allergic contact dermatitis from intravesical instillation of the antitumor antibiotic mitomycin C. Contact Dermatitis 1991;24:201–209.

183. Vidal C, de la Fuente R, Gonzalez Quintela A. Three cases of allergic dermatitis due to intravesical mitomycin C. Dermatology 1992;184:208–209.

184. Dalton JT, Guillaume Wientjes M, Badalament RA, Drago JR, Au JL-S. Pharmacokinetics of intravesical mitomycin C in superficial bladder cancer patients. Cancer Res 1991;51:5144–5152.

185. Carter JJ, McLaughlin ML, Bern MM. Bleo-

mycin-induced fatal hyperpyrexia. Am J Med 1983; 74:523–525.

186. Ma DDF, Isbister JP. Cytotoxic-induced fulminant hyperpyrexia. Cancer 1980;45:2249–2251.

187. Inbar MJ, Baratz M, Figer A, et al. Idiosyncratic reaction to bleomycin in an epithelial tumor. Cancer Chemother Pharmacol 1984;13:71–72.

188. Rosenfelt F, Palmer J, Weinstein I, Rosenbloom B. A fatal hyperpyrexial respone to bleomycin following prior therapy: a case report and literature review. Yale J Biol Med 1982;55:529–531.

189. Leung W-H, Johnson YNL, Chan T-K, Kumana CR. Fulminant hyperpyrexia induced by bleomycin. Postgrad Med J 1989;65:417–419.

190. Dinarello CA, Ward SB, Wolff SM. Pyrogenic properties of bleomycin (NSC-125066). Cancer Chemother Rep 1973;57:393–398.

191. Trope C, Johnsson J-E, Larsson G, Simonsen E. Bleomycin alone or combined with mitomycin C in treatment of advanced or recurrent squamous cell carcinoma of the vulva. Cancer Treat Rep 1980;64:639–642.

192. Kansur T, Little D, Tavassoli M. Fulminant and fatal angioedema caused by bleomycin treatment. Arch Intern Med 1984;144:2267.

193. Dyke RW. Acute bronchospasm after a vinca alkaloid in patients previously treated with mitomycin (letter). N Engl J Med 1984;310:389.

194. Rivera MP, Kris MG, Gralla RJ, White DA. Syndrome of acute dyspnea related to combined mitomycin plus vinca alkaloid chemotherapy. Am J Clin Oncol (CCT) 1995;18:245–250.

195. Abhyankar S, Rao S, Pollio L, Miller ST. Anaphylactic shock due to dacarbazine (NSC 45388) (letter). Am J Dis Child 1988;142:918.

196. Jacobs P, Wood L, Foster J. Hydroxyurea hypersensitivity reaction (letter). S Afr Med J 1989;75:506.

197. Bauman JL, Shulruff S, Hasegawa GR, Roden R, Hartsough N, Bauernfeind RA. Fever caused by hydroxyurea. Arch Intern Med 1981;141:260–261.

198. O'Dwyer PJ, King SA, Eisenhauer E, Grem JL, Hoth DF. Hypersensitivity reactions to deoxycoformycin. Cancer Chemother Pharmacol 1988;23:173–175.

199. Posada JG, O'Dwyer PJ, Hoth DF. Anaphylactic reactions to diaziquone. Cancer Treat Rep 1984; 68:1215–1217.

200. Tilchen EJ, Fleming T, Mills G, et al. Phase II evaluation of diaziquone in pancreatic carcinoma: a Southwest Oncology Group study. Cancer Treat Rep 1987;71:1309–1310.

201. Weiss RB, Peterson BL, Allen SL, Browning SM, Duggan DB, Schiffer CA. A phase II trial of didemnin B in myeloma. A Cancer and Leukemia Group B (CALGB) study. Invest New Drugs 1994;12:41–43.

202. Marshall ME, Wolf MK, Crawford ED, et al.

Phase II trial of echinomycin for the treatment of advanced renal cell carcinoma. A Southwest Oncology Group study. Invest New Drugs 1993;11:207–209.

203. Baars JW, Wagstaff J, Hack CE, Wolbink G-J, Eerenberg-Belmer AJM, Pinedo HM. Angioneurotic oedema and urticaria during therapy with interleukin-2 (IL-2). Ann Ocol 1992;3:243–244.

204. Heinzer H, Huland E, Huland H. Adverse reaction to contrast material in a patient treated with local interleukin-2 (letter). AJR 1992;158:1407.

205. Zukiwski AS, David CL, Coan J, Wallace S, Gutterman JU, Mavligit GM. Increased incidence of hypersensitivity to iodine-containing radiographic contrast media after interleukin-2 administration. Cancer 1990;65:1521–1524.

206. Jaiyesimi I, Giralt SS, Wood J. Subcutaneous granulocyte colony-stimulating factor and acute anaphylaxis (letter). N Engl J Med 1991;325:587.

207. Engler RJM, Weiss RB. Recombinant human granulocyte-macrophage colony-stimulating factor (GM-CSF) as a cause of anaphylaxis (abstract). J Allergy Clin Immunol 1995;95:283.

208. O'Shaughnessy JA, Denicoff AM, Venzon DJ, et al. A dose intensity study of FLAC (5-fluorouracil, leucovorin, doxorubicin, cyclophosphamide) chemotherapy and Escherichia coli-derived granulocyte-macrophage colony-stimulating factor (GM-CSF) in advanced breast cancer patients. Ann Oncol 1994;5:709–716.

209. Chen M, Tanner A, Gallo-Torres H. Anaphylactoid-anaphylactic reactions associated with ondansetron. Ann Intern Med 1993;119:862.

210. Chan ATC, O'Brien MER. Hypersensitivity to dexamethasone (letter). Br Med J 1993;306:109.

211. Greenberger PA, Patterson R, Simon R, et al. Pretreatment of high-risk patients requiring radiographic contrast media studies. J Allergy Clin Immunol 1981;67:185–187.

212. Greenberger PA, Halwig JM, Patterson R, Wallemark CB. Emergency administration of radiocontrast media in high-risk patients. J Allergy Clin Immunol 1986;77:630–634.

213. Greenberger PA, Patterson R, Tapio CM. Prophylaxis against repeated radiocontrast media reactions in 857 cases. Adverse experience with cimetidine and safety of β-adrenergic antagonists. Arch Intern Med 1985;145:2197–2200.

214. Masini E, Planchenault J, Pezziardi F, Gautier P, Gagnol JP. Histamine-releasing properties of polysorbate 80 in vitro and in vivo: correlation with its hypotensive action in the dog. Agents Actions 1985; 16:470–477.

215. Wilson JP, Solimando DA, Edwards MS. Parenteral benzyl alcohol-induced hypersensitivity reaction. Drug Intell Clin Pharm 1986;20:689–691.

32

Ocular Side Effects of Chemotherapy

Linda J. Burns

The increased use of chemotherapeutic agents for hematologic and oncologic diseases, combined with longer patient survival, has led to a higher incidence and recognition of ophthalmologic side effects. Although such side effects are relatively uncommon, they may be quite disabling, and blindness may occur (1–5). Therefore, the clinician must be aware of the ocular side effects of chemotherapeutic agents, inform the patient of potential risks, and perform an appropriate baseline ophthalmologic examination prior to the initiation of therapy. This chapter reviews the clinical manifestations and pathophysiology associated with ocular toxicity of common chemotherapeutic agents.

ALKYLATING AGENTS

Busulfan

Busulfan is primarily used in schedules of oral administration for the treatment of chronic myelogenous leukemia (CML). This agent has been found to produce cataracts in experimental animals. When rats were fed busulfan at 1 to 2.5 mg/kg/day, anterior and posterior subcapsular cataracts developed after 4 to 5 weeks (6). The development of cataracts in patients taking busulfan was first reported in 1969 (7). Of 19 patients with CML receiving chronic oral busulfan, 6 had lentricular opacity and 2 had definite posterior subcapsular cataracts. The patients with busulfan-related lens toxicity had received drug treatment for a mean of 113.5 months for those with cataracts and 27.2 months for those with early lens changes. Patients without lens toxicity had received treatment for a mean of 12 months. There was no age difference between the groups. Lens changes due solely to CML were not noted.

Other groups have since reported patients who developed cataracts taking 1 to 6 mg/day of busulfan over at least 4 years (8–10).

The mechanism of busulfan-induced cataract formation is not known. Drug-induced damage to the lens may be a consequence of a direct toxic effect on the proliferating lens epithelial cells (6, 11). Pathologic examination of the lenses extracted from patients reveals hydropic swelling of lens fibers, vacuole formation, cortical liquification, and posterior migration of lens epithelial cells (12). These pathologic changes are similar to those noted in cataracts extracted from patients treated with steroids and in cataracts secondary to old age (13, 14).

In addition to cataract formation, one case of a sicca syndrome in a patient with CML treated with busulfan has been reported (10). The patient, a 52-year-old woman, developed bilateral cataracts following 5 years of busulfan therapy. Three years later, severe xerostomia and keratitis sicca developed, with progression to blindness.

Chlorambucil

Chlorambucil is given orally and is a convenient alkylating agent for the treatment of malignancies requiring long-term management such as chronic lymphocytic leukemia, nodular lymphomas, and multiple myeloma. Ocular toxicity is rare. Keratitis has been noted (15), and in one case, diplopia, bilateral edema, and retinal hemorrhages have been reported (16).

Cisplatin

Cisplatin was the first heavy metal compound used as a cancer chemotherapeutic agent. Cisplatin entered into clinical trials in 1971 and since then has become established as a highly effective drug for treating ovarian carcinomas, testicular tumors, and head and neck cancers.

Several cases of ophthalmologic toxicity have been reported in association with intravenous administration of this drug, including papilledema (17), unilateral retrobulbar neuritis (17), bilateral retrobulbar neuritis (18), bilateral optic nerve swelling (19), optic neuritis (20), transient cortical blindness (21, 22), and transient left homonymous hemianopsia (23).

Recently, retinal toxicity was described in patients who received intravenous high-dose cisplatin 200 mg/m^2 in 5 divided daily doses over 2 to 4 cycles as therapy for refractory or newly diagnosed ovarian carcinoma (24). Of 13 patients, 8 developed symptoms of blurred vision, and 3 also developed altered color perception. Blurred vision developed gradually after the third or fourth cycle of therapy and was not improved by the use of previously adequate corrective lenses. Symptoms of altered color vision generally presented as a loss of color discrimination and saturation, particularly on the blue-yellow axis. Visual symptoms progressed with the administration of additional cisplatin. Off therapy, blurred vision gradually and completely resolved, but altered color vision persisted for up to 16 months. On funduscopic examination, an irregular pigmentation of the macular area was found in 6 of 13 patients. The optic discs were normal. Anatomically, visual dysfunction was localized to the retina by changes on the electroretinogram characteristic of dysfunction of the cone-mediated system of the retina.

Intraarterial administration of cisplatin is an area of investigation for regionally confirmed tumors of the head and neck. Intracarotid artery bolus infusion of cisplatin 60 to 100 mg/m^2 has been reported to result in mild blurring of vision or permanent ipsilateral blindness secondary to retinal damage (25). Ocular toxicity has also limited the use of intraarterial chemotherapy in patients with intracranial tumors. Visual loss was accompanied by a pigmentary retinopathy in patients following intracarotid bolus infusion of 200 mg of cisplatin alone or with carmustine (BCNU) in 8 of 11 patients treated for recurrent malignant gliomas (26). Three of 41 intracarotid infusions of cisplatin in patients with malignant glioma resulted in ocular toxicity, either periorbital pain or thrombosis of the central retinal artery (27). Retrobulbar neuritis accompanied in-

traarterial administration of cisplatin 50 mg/m^2/day as a 24-hour continuous infusion with 5-fluorodeoxyuridine (28). In contrast, infusion of cisplatin via the supraophthalmic portion of the carotid artery protected the ipsilateral eye from damage in 13 patients with recurrent malignant glioma (29).

The mechanism of ophthalmologic toxicity secondary to cisplatin has not been established. Other metals including gold, lead, mercury, and thallium are also known to cause papilledema and retrobulbar neuritis (18, 30). It is not known if these metals have a direct toxic effect on nerve fibers or if a vascular disturbance leads to optic nerve inflammation.

Cyclophosphamide

Cyclophosphamide is an alkylating agent commonly used in oral and intravenous forms for many hematologic and neoplastic diseases. Single doses of cyclophosphamide given at 40 to 80 mg/kg intravenously to dogs or rhesus monkeys were not associated with clinical or pathologic eye changes (31). Doses of 250 mg/kg injected subcutaneously in rats caused inflammation of the ciliary body and processes (32). The first report of ophthalmologic toxicity in humans was by Kende et al. in 1979 (33). Twenty-nine children with a variety of childhood tumors were given cyclophosphamide 750 mg/m^2 by intravenous push on alternate days for a total of 5 doses. Five patients complained of blurring of vision. Two of these patients noted visual blurring within minutes following drug administration, and the other three patients, 24 hours following administration. In all cases, symptoms completely reversed, with reversal occurring within 1 hour in three patients, 3 days in one patient, and 2 weeks in one patient. In addition, several cases of blepharoconjunctivitis associated with use of cyclophosphamide have been reported to the National Registry of Drug-Induced Ocular Side Effects (4).

Nitrogen Mustard

Nitrogen mustard, or mechlorethamine, was the first alkylating agent to receive clinical trial. It is primarily used in the treatment of patients with Hodgkin's disease. Given intravenously, nitrogen mustard has never been reported to have ocular side effects. Following intracarotid injection, three patients with brain tumors developed severe necrotizing uveitis in the ipsilateral eye (34).

Nitrosoureas

The nitrosoureas (bis-chloronitrosourea, BCNU; lomustine, CCNU; methyl-CCNU) are clinically reactive against the lymphomas, malignant melanomas, brain neoplasms, and gastrointestinal carcinomas. In dogs, BCNU injected via the carotid artery at doses of 2 to 4 mg/kg resulted in corneal opacity and blindness in three of four animals (35). However, intracarotid injection of 1 to 20 mg/kg BCNU for 4 weeks in rhesus monkeys resulted in no ophthalmic lesions (36).

The ocular side effects of nitrosoureas in humans are not well established. Lokich et al. reported in 1974 that 2 of 31 patients treated with oral methyl-CCNU 150 to 200 mg/m^2 and intravenous doxorubicin 40 to 90 mg/m^2 developed transient visual blurring and loss of depth perception 1 week following therapy (37). There were no detectable physical abnormalities of the lens or retina. Bilateral optic neuroretinitis was reported in a man with multiple myeloma, 8 days following chemotherapy with BCNU 50 mg intravenously, cyclophosphamide 650 mg intravenously, procarbazine 100 mg orally on days 1 to 4, and prednisolone 40 mg orally four times daily on days 1 to 4 (38). Louie et al. summarized several other cases of nitrosourea-induced retinopathy including progressive blindness and diplopia, recurrent blurred vision and retrobulbar pain, optic atrophy and blindness, retinopathy with exudates and hemorrhages, and normal visual acuity, but with small vessel leaks per fluorescein angiography (39). Of more than 200 patients studied on Brain Tumor Study Group protocols using nitrosoureas, only 1 case of a possible ocular side effect was reported (39).

Intracarotid infusion of BCNU for treatment of intracranial tumors has been reported to result in both transient and permanent ophthalmic complications felt to reflect both immediate vascular injury within the distribution of the ophthalmic artery and chronic ocular ischemia (40). Seven of 10 patients treated with intraarterial carotid infusions of BCNU to a minimum dose of 450 mg/m^2 in two treatments developed decreased vision on the side of infusion at a mean of 6 weeks following treatment (41). In three of these patients, the visual loss progressed to the absence of light perception. Funduscopic exam-

ination revealed arterial narrowing, nerve fiber-layer infarcts, and intraretinal hemorrhages.

More recently, greater numbers of patients have been treated with intracarotid infusions of either BCNU (42) or BCNU alternating with cisplatin (43). Seventy-nine patients with recurrent brain tumors were treated by Watne et al. with multiple cycles of internal carotid injections of 160 mg of BCNU; patients also received intravenous vincristine and oral procarbazine (42). The most prominent side effects were eye pain during the BCNU infusion (in 178 of 236 courses) and transient conjunctival edema (25 courses). Rogers et al. entered 43 patients with recurrent malignant glioma in a trial of alternating courses of intracarotid infusion of BCNU (2 doses, 300 to 400 mg each) and cisplatin (2 doses, 150 to 200 mg each) at 4- to 6-week intervals (43). Before each treatment, all patients underwent fundu-scopic examinations, and 40 patients underwent complete ophthalmologic examinations. Ice was routinely applied to the ipsilateral eye during BCNU infusion. In 14 patients, eye pain mandated a decreased rate of infusion. The eye pain usually resolved within 10–20 minutes of stopping the infusion. Sixteen patients experienced other types of ocular toxicity, including retinal vascular occlusive phenomena (13 patients), reduced visual acuity (12 patients, of whom 6 were blind), disc edema (6 patients), retinal pigment epithelial changes (6 patients), and central retinal artery occlusion and macular edema (2 patients). In seven patients, the ocular toxicity occurred abruptly 7 to 10 days after the first course of BCNU or cisplatin. It was unclear if the retinal vascular and optic nerve toxicity was due to BCNU, cisplatin, or both. Retinal pigment epithelial changes have not been reported secondary to BCNU and most likely were due to cisplatin. Supraophthalmic infusion of BCNU, instead of intracarotid perfusion, has been reported to protect the eye from toxicity (29).

BCNU has also been used in high-dose chemotherapy regimens in conjunction with autologous bone marrow transplantation. Two such case reports are in the literature (41, 44). Shingleton et al. described ocular toxicity in 2 of 50 patients who received 800 mg/m^2 of BCNU with bone marrow rescue (41). Each developed bilateral nerve fiber-layer infarcts. Six patients with colorectal cancer who received BCNU 450 mg/m^2, mitomycin 25 mg/m^2 with lonidamine all developed qualitative and quantitative changes in the tear films, leading to mild transient damage to the corneal and conjunctival epithelium (44).

ANTIBIOTICS

Doxorubicin (Adriamycin)

Doxorubicin is an anthracycline antibiotic with a wide spectrum of activity. Ocular side effects are quite rare, with some patients reporting conjunctivitis (15, 45). Increased lacrimation may occur 5 to 15 days after a single dose (46).

Mithramycin

Mithramycin is an antibiotic that has antitumor activity against testicular carcinoma but also has a specific hypocalcemic effect that is valuable in the treatment of malignant hypercalcemia. No ocular side effects have been reported from mithramycin use, although a periorbital pallor may occur (15).

Mitomycin C

Mitomycin C is used primarily in the treatment of gastrointestinal carcinoma. Intravenous use of this drug has been associated with blurring of vision (15). Mitomycin C has also been used at high doses in conjunction with BCNU as cytoreductive chemotherapy for bone marrow transplantation in six patients, with mild changes in the quality and quantity of tear films noted in all patients (44).

ANTIMETABOLITES

Cytosine Arabinoside

Cytosine arabinoside has potent clinical activity against acute myeloblastic leukemia and lesser activity against the blastic crisis of CML and acute lymphoblastic leukemia. It has also recently been used in high doses for refractory leukemia (47–49) and as part of a salvage chemotherapy regimen for lymphoma (50).

Cytosine arabinoside causes retinal dysplasia in rats treated in the postnatal period (51–53). In humans, low doses of cytosine arabinoside have not been reported to have ocular side effects. High doses of the drug, however, have been reported to result in corneal toxicity. Three patients with leukemia who received 3 g/m^2 intravenously every 12 hours for 4 to 5 days developed ocular pain, tearing, foreign body sensation, photophobia, and blurred vision (47).

These patients all had bilateral conjunctival hyperemia and fine corneal epithelial capacities. The symptoms disappeared without treatment in 1 week. When 3 g/m^2 of cytosine arabinoside was infused intravenously every 12 hours for 2 to 6 days, 27 of 57 patients with refractory acute leukemia developed ophthalmologic toxicity (48). Conjunctivitis and photophobia began 4 to 8 days after initiation of therapy and lasted from 2 to 9 days. The incidence of side effects increased with increasing duration of therapy. Use of glucocorticoid eye drops (0.1% dexamethasone, 2 drops each eye every 6 to 8 hours) before the first dose of cytosine arabinoside ameliorated or prevented the conjunctivitis and photophobia. Slit-lamp examination revealed corneal damage similar to that observed with excessive ultraviolet light exposure. In another phase I-II study of high-dose cytosine arabinoside in 64 patients with refractory leukemia, 20% of patients developed mild to moderate conjunctivitis and photophobia (49). All patients received prophylactic glucocorticoid eye drops. More recently, Higa et al. has reported that artificial tears are as effective as glucocorticoid drops and that eye drops likely decrease toxicity by diluting intraocular concentrations of the drug (54).

Conjunctivitis is also part of a syndrome noted by Castleberry et al. in 1981 (55). Six patients receiving cytosine arabinoside intravenously at 100 to 150 mg/m^2 developed fever, myalgias, bone pain, and occasionally chest pain, maculopapular rash, and conjunctivitis. The symptoms all occurred within 6 to 12 hours of drug infusion.

The mechanism of the ocular toxicity of cytosine arabinoside is unclear. It has been suggested that the ocular damage may result from inhibition of corneal epithelial DNA synthesis and that repeated administration of high doses of cytosine arabinoside might result in drug levels sufficiently high to continuously suppress synthesis of corneal epithelial DNA (56).

5-Fluorouracil

5-Fluorouracil has antitumor activity against many types of solid tumors, including breast, colon, and ovarian carcinomas. Topical preparations of 5-fluorouracil, when applied near the eye, are associated with eyelid inflammation, circumorbital edema, conjunctival irritation, and corneal erosions (57–59). Systemic use of this drug has been shown to cause acute and chronic conjunctivitis that may lead to tear-duct stenosis and ectropion of the lower lids (60–64).

Hamersly et al. first reported in 1973 that 16 of 46 patients treated with weekly injections of 5-fluorouracil complained of eye symptoms (60). The most frequent symptom was excess tearing in 14 patients, with 7 complaints of eye irritation, 5 of reddening of the eyes, and blurring of vision in 2 patients. The eye symptoms gradually appeared after initiation of treatment and resolved 1 to 2 weeks after the drug was discontinued. Complete eye examinations in three patients showed no abnormalities other than a positive Schirmer test. Twenty-five percent of patients receiving intravenous 5-fluorouracil in combination with cyclophosphamide and methotrexate as therapy for breast carcinoma were reported to have developed a burning sensation in the conjunctiva associated with redness of the mucosa and lacrimation (61).

5-Fluorouracil-induced dermatitis of the eyelids was considered the cause of four cases of epiphora due to bilateral cicatricial ectropion in recipients of prolonged systemic treatment with 5-fluorouracil (62). In two patients, surgical repair of the ectropion was unsuccessful in relieving conjunctival symptoms while 5-fluorouracil was continued. Six cases of 5-fluorouracil-associated conjunctival erythema and chronic increase in lacrimation were reported by Haidak et al. (63). Only one patient's symptoms improved after 2 to 3 weeks off therapy. One patient had fibrosis of the lacrimal sac. Four additional cases of epiphora associated with prolonged administration of 5-fluorouracil were subsequently reported (64). All four patients exhibited punctal stenosis, and in three, canalicular stenosis could also be demonstrated. Silastic tube intubation of the lacrimal systems resulted in symptomatic improvement.

In eight patients receiving 5-fluorouracil for carcinoma of the colon, the drug was found only in the patients with excess lacrimation, with peak concentration in the tears occurring 15 minutes after intravenous drug administration (65). It was suggested that 5-fluorouracil causes local irritation of the lacrimal gland, resulting in the appearance of the drug in tears and subsequent tear-duct fibrosis.

Cyclophosphamide, methotrexate, and 5-fluorouracil (CMF) is a combination chemotherapy regimen used in breast cancer. Ocular toxicity is a frequent sequela from CMF chemotherapy, and symptoms usually consist of conjunctivitis with mild to marked tearing, ocular pruritus, and/or burning (66, 67). Symptoms typically begin 11–17 days after starting a cycle of CMF and last for 10–15 days (67). The specific agents responsible for the ocular irritation have not been clearly identified. Of the three drugs in the CMF regimen, 5-fluorouracil has most commonly been associated with ocular irritation. No effective treatment for CMF-induced ocular toxicity has been well established, although both cromolyn eye drops (68) and cryotherapy (69) have been reported as being potentially beneficial for 5-fluorouracil associated conjunctivitis.

A complete eye and lacrimal system examination should therefore be performed on all patients receiving 5-fluorouracil who note ocular inflammation or tearing. It has been recommended that if 5-fluorouracil treatment is nearly complete, a trial of topical antibiotic-steroids to decrease inflammation may be warranted. If further 5-fluorouracil therapy is necessary, patients could be considered for silastic tubing intubation of the lacrimal system (64).

5-Fluorouracil may also potentiate radiation effects on the eye. When combined therapy of surgery, radiotherapy, and regional chemotherapy of 5-fluorouracil infusion through the superficial temporal artery was used in 68 cases of carcinoma of the paranasal sinuses, 9 of 57 patients developed impaired vision (70). Of these nine patients, four had decreased vision, and five patients had complete visual loss. There is one report of 5-fluorouracil given intraarterially concurrently with radiation therapy which resulted in 4 of 23 patients developing blindness (71). In 1976, Chan and Shukorsky reported a comparative study of 40 patients with malignant tumors of the nasal cavity and paranasal sinuses (72); 22 received radiotherapy of 6000 rads over 6 weeks, and 18 received radiation plus intraarterial 5-fluorouracil. The incidence of eye toxicity, including blindness, cataracts, corneal lesions, and chronic conjunctivitis, was significantly higher in those who received combination therapy. The incidence of total blindness at 3 years was four times more frequent in the group receiving 5-fluorouracil. Over 50% of patients receiving 5-fluorouracil developed a clinically significant cataract, compared with 10% of patients treated with radiation alone. All patients receiving 5-fluorouracil developed corneal lesions, and 75% developed chronic conjunctivitis, compared with 15% and 25%, respectively, of patients treated only with radiation.

Methotrexate

Methotrexate is a folic acid antagonist that has therapeutic activity in breast cancer, choriocarcinoma, osteogenic sarcoma, acute leukemia, and non-Hodgkin's lymphoma. Ocular side effects such as conjunctivitis, increased lacrimation, blurring of vision, photophobia, and ocular pain may occur in 25% of patients who receive systemic methotrexate (4, 15). Ocular toxicity has been commonly reported in patients receiving high-dose methotrexate therapy. Conjunctivitis occurred in seven patients receiving methotrexate 120 to 600 mg/m^2 intravenously every 2 weeks without leucovorin rescue (73). Four of 13 patients receiving intermittent high-dose methotrexate therapy of 30 to mg/kg infused intravenously over 6 hours with leucovorin rescue developed recurrent ocular symptoms 2 to 7 days following chemotherapy (74). The symptoms consisted of burning, blurring of vision, pruritus, and dryness. Three of the four symptomatic patients had unremarkable ophthalmologic examinations at the time of methotrexate infusion except for decreased reflex production of tears in two patients. Symptoms were partially relieved in two patients with methylcellulose eye drops. All patients had cessation of symptoms when methotrexate therapy was discontinued. Analysis of methotrexate levels in tears of both symptomatic and asymptomatic patients revealed levels similar to those achieved in the plasma. One symptomatic patient had acidic tears, and it was suggested that this patient's symptoms may have been secondary to precipitation of methotrexate in the conjunctival sac.

There are two reports of optic nerve atrophy involving four patients with acute lymphoblastic leukemia who received systemic methotrexate along with intrathecal cytosine arabinoside and 2400 rads of total brain irradiation as part of induction chemotherapy (75, 76). Because this dose of radiation is below that associated with neurotoxicity, it is possible that blindness resulted from potentiation of radiation toxicity to the optic chiasm by systemic or intrathecal chemotherapy.

Methotrexate is also one of three drugs in a commonly used combination chemotherapy regimen for breast cancer, CMF. Conjunctivitis is a common sequela of CML chemotherapy (66, 67). Although of the three drugs, 5-fluorouracil is the one most commonly associated with ocular irritation, methotrexate may play an active role in the development of CMF-induced symptoms.

HORMONAL AGENTS

Corticosteroids

Corticosteroids are frequently used both as single agents and as components of combination chemotherapy for a wide spectrum of hematologic and neoplastic disorders. Administration of corticosteroids systemically or topically may result in glaucoma or increased intraocular pressure secondary to a decrease in aqueous outflow (77–80). However, the most commonly recognized ophthalmologic side effect of corticosteroid use is the development of posterior subcapsular cataracts.

Since 1960, the relationship between systemic corticosteroids and the formation of posterior subcapsular cataracts has been generally accepted (81). Most reports describe the development of cataracts in patients who received steroids for nonmalignant conditions, including rheumatic diseases (81) and the nephrotic syndrome (82, 83), and following renal transplantation (79, 80, 84). Cataracts have occurred in approximately 22% of reported patients receiving steroids for nonmalignant illnesses (85).

It is not clear if the incidence of cataract formation is correlated with dosage and duration of steroid treatment or if younger patients are more prone to develop cataracts at lower doses and within a shorter time period than older patients. Black et al. found that the dosage and duration of steroid therapy was proportional to the development of cataracts in 44 predominantly adult patients with rheumatoid arthritis (81). In 693 patients of various ages treated with steroids for nonmalignant diseases, treatment for longer than 1 year and a daily dose greater than 10 mg of prednisone or equivalent were risk factors for development of cataracts (86). In children receiving steroids for the nephrotic syndrome, there was an overall incidence of 28.5% of cataract development but a 75% incidence in children treated for more than 2 years (82). Cataracts developed in 36% of children who received more than 10 mg of prednisone for more than 6 months following renal transplantation (84). However, in 1977 Forman et al. reported that total corticosteroid dose and duration of therapy were not critical factors in the development of cataracts in 39 nephrotic children and suggested that there is an individual susceptibility to cataract inducibility by steroids (83). Most recently, Limaye et al. have reported no statistical correlation between total dose of steroids and cataract formation in 45 patients between the ages of 11 months and 27 years with the nephrotic syndrome (87).

Cataract formation has been recently reported in survivors of treatment for acute lymphocytic leukemia (88). Of 82 survivors, all patients had completed or nearly completed a 25 to 31 month protocol that included either 3.4 or 10.2 $g/m^2/$ year of systemic prednisone and cranial irradiation (1800 to 2800 rads). The only ocular morbidity attributed to treatment included cataracts, which occurred in 52% of patients and were felt to be due primarily to the systemic corticosteroid administration.

Cataracts that result from corticosteroid use rarely cause visual impairment (85, 88). A history of insignificant photophobia or increase in glare may be obtained. Once cataracts form, they are usually stable in development with cessation of therapy. However, small numbers of patients have demonstrated cataract reversal (83), whereas others have shown progressive changes following reduction of dosage or discontinuation of steroids (89).

The pathology of steroid-related cataracts is similar to that of busulfan- or age-related cataracts (14, 90). A number of factors may be involved in the mechanism of corticosteroid-induced cataract formation, including inhibition of the sodium-potassium ATP'ase pump mechanism (85), binding of corticosteroids to lens proteins with alteration in the native configuration of the lens crystallins (91), and oxidation of protein groups with aggregation of lens crystallins (85).

Tamoxifen

Tamoxifen is a nonsteroidal antiestrogen used primarily in the treatment of breast carcinoma. Ophthalmologic side effects were previously thought to be uncommon, with ocular toxicity reported in eight patients prior to 1992. Four patients who received high doses of tamoxifen, 120 to 160 mg twice daily for more than 1 year, developed ocular manifestations of superficial corneal opacities, decreased visual acuity, and retinopathy (92). Funduscopic examination revealed white refractile opacities within the retina in the paramacular area with macular edema. Visual loss was progressive in at least two patients. An additional patient developed a similar retinopathy after receiving a total dose of 90 g of tamoxifen over 16 months (93). Ocular toxicity of tamoxifen was attributed to the use of high dosages, as 19 patients treated with tamoxifen at a

maximum dose of 40 mg daily for periods of 3 months to 4 years had no ocular side effects (94).

However, ocular toxicity with standard oral-dose therapy was reported in three patients. Two patients who received 30 mg daily of tamoxifen for either 9 or 14 months developed retinopathy with transitory visual impairment (95). A 57-year-old woman treated with 30 to 40 mg of tamoxifen a day orally for 7 months developed bilateral optic neuritis (96). The optic neuritis regressed when tamoxifen was discontinued. A 42-year-old woman developed bilateral optic disc swelling, retinal hemorrhages, and visual impairment 3 weeks after starting treatment with 10 mg of tamoxifen twice daily (97). The ocular findings resolved completely with discontinuation of tamoxifen.

In 1992, Pavlidis et al. reported the results of a prospective investigation of the incidence and course of ocular toxicity after low-dose tamoxifen treatment in cancer patients (98). Sixty-three patients could be analyzed. All patients received tamoxifen at a dose of 20 mg daily for a median duration of 25 months (range, 6 to 51 months). Total median tamoxifen dose was 14.4 g (range, 3.6 to 30 g). All patients received an initial ophthalmologic examination and follow-up examinations at 6-month intervals. Four of the 63 patients (6.3%) developed ocular toxicity 10, 27, 31, and 35 months after the initiation of tamoxifen, with total doses of 6.0, 16.2, 18.6, and 21.0 g, respectively. All four patients had decreased visual acuity of different degrees as well as retinopathy, consisting of bilateral macular edema and yellow-white dots in the paramacular and fovea areas. One patient had subepithelial corneal opacities just below the visual axis.

Following withdrawal of tamoxifen, visual acuity completely recovered in the patients who were treated for 10 and 27 months. The patient treated for 31 months had minimal residual impairment. The patient treated for 35 months had improved visual acuity to pretreatment levels. Although macular edema regressed in all patients, the refractile retinal opacities did not regress. The authors concluded that even low-dose tamoxifen treatment can induce ocular toxicity, that long-term administration of tamoxifen is a prerequisite, and that most toxicity is reversible after tamoxifen discontinuation.

The mechanism of tamoxifen ocular toxicity is unknown. Pathologically, the lesions have been confined to the nerve fibers and inner plexiform layers of the retina. The lesions are most numerous in the paramacular area, and electron microscopy demonstrates features suggestive of axonal degeneration (99).

PLANT ALKALOIDS

Vinblastine and Vincristine

The vinca alkaloids include two widely used cancer chemotherapeutic agents, vinblastine and vincristine. These drugs are used for the treatment of lymphomas, acute leukemia, and solid tumors in children, with the dose-limiting side effect of these agents being neurologic toxicity. The most common toxic manifestation is a mixed sensory-motor neuropathy (100).

Twenty of 40 patients treated with vincristine or vinblastine for leukemia or other malignancies developed ocular signs of toxicity (101). Fourteen of the 20 patients developed ptosis, 13 had recti and oblique muscle paresis, 6 developed lagophthalmos associated with seventh nerve palsy, and 2 had corneal hyposthesia. The total dose of drug given and duration of treatment to time of onset of ocular toxicity were 2.6 to 136 mg over a mean of 10 weeks (range, 2 to 44 weeks). In three patients, ocular findings were the first evidence of vincristine toxic side effects. The ocular symptoms improved or resolved in 15 of 20 patients when the vincristine dosage was lowered or the drug discontinued. Of 107 patients with leukemia who did not receive vincristine chemotherapy, 9 patients had ocular muscle paresis, and lagophthalmos was seen in 3 patients.

In a study of 50 children and adults with acute leukemia receiving vincristine 2 mg/m^2 intravenously every 10 to 14 days in combination with prednisone, methotrexate, and 6-mercaptopurine, cranial nerve palsies attributed to vincristine toxicity were a late manifestation of neuropathy in 5 patients (102). Bilateral ptosis, the most frequent manifestation, was observed in four children and one adult. Three patients complained of diplopia, photophobia, and difficulty in focusing on both distant and near objects. All patients had antecedent peripheral muscle weakness. Improvement with discontinuation of therapy was noted within 2 to 6 weeks, with complete recovery within 4 months.

In addition to cranial nerve palsies, vincristine was reported to have caused optic neuropathy in three patients (103, 104). One patient with Hodgkin's disease complained of blurred vision and at autopsy had optic neuropathy (103). The other two cases were in children with acute leu-

kemia. Vision improved after discontinuation of the vincristine (104). There is also one case report of a patient who developed bilateral optic atrophy and blindness (105). The patient, an 18-year-old man with poorly differentiated diffuse lymphocytic lymphoma, received vincristine 2 mg intravenously, cyclophosphamide 600 mg orally for 5 days, and prednisone 100 mg orally daily for 5 days. The second course was given after 10 days, and subsequent courses at 3-week intervals. The patient complained of blurred vision following the fifth course and became blind following the sixth course. He remained completely blind 6 months following discontinuation of vincristine.

Three children with malignancies developed transient cortical blindness while receiving vincristine as part of their chemotherapy regimen (106). The patients all had reactions after the first, second, or third dose, with doses ranging from 1.5 to 2.0 mg/m^2. In all cases, the blindness completely resolved. One patient received additional vincristine at a standard dose and had a life-threatening reaction and recurrent transient blindness.

One patient was reported who developed night blindness following combination chemotherapy that included vincristine for therapy of malignant melanoma (107). An extensive routine ophthalmologic examination was unrevealing, and color vision was normal. The functional abnormality appeared to affect both cone-mediated and rod-mediated mechanisms.

Injecting vincristine directly into the vitreous body of rats results in arrest of cell division in metaphase in lens epithelium (89) and in disappearance of microtubules, formation of crystalloid inclusions, and impairment of axonal transport (108). Optic neuropathy has not been reported in experimental animals given vincristine systemically (103). The blood-retinal barrier probably protects the eye from vincristine administered systemically, and it has been suggested that ocular toxicity occurs when this barrier is compromised, either by a drug in the therapeutic regimen or by the disease process itself (107).

MISCELLANEOUS DRUGS

Allopurinol

Allopurinol is a xanthine oxidase inhibitor given to patients receiving chemotherapy, to prevent hyperuricemia. There were 30 cases of suspected allopurinol-induced cortical and subcapsular cataracts reported to the National Registry of Drug Induced Ocular Side Effects as of 1982 (109). There is also evidence, via phosphorescence emission peaks, that allopurinol is photobound in the human lens and is cataractogenic in patients in whom photobinding has occurred (110, 111). However, two subsequent clinical studies found no evidence that allopurinol use increases the risk of cataract formation (112, 113). Clair et al. identified 51 allopurinol users with a mean of 6.9 years of allopurinol use and compared their lenses with those of 76 patients who did not use allopurinol (113). Medical records were reviewed or prospective ophthalmologic examinations were performed. There was no evidence of an increased risk for cataract formation among users of allopurinol. Therefore, the causal relationship for allopurinol use and cataract formation remains unclear. In addition, there is an incidence of less than 1% of optic neuritis, macular retinitis, iritis, conjunctivitis, and amblyopia in patients taking allopurinol (114). Again, the causal relationship is unknown.

Cyclosporine

Cyclosporine is an immunosuppressive drug widely used in recipients of bone marrow and solid organ transplants. The clinical spectrum of cyclosporine neurotoxicity includes blurred vision. Cortical blindness, a rare complication, has been reported in 10 patients (115). Magnetic resonance imaging demonstrated either diffuse white-matter high signals or focal cortical and white-matter lesions, reversible in all cases. EEGs showed nonspecific slowing and dysrhythmia, but no epileptiform activity, and the spinal fluid analysis was normal in all patients. The mechanisms of cyclosporine toxicity manifested as cortical blindness and the reason for the selective vulnerability of the occipital cortex are unknown.

2'-Deoxycoformycin

2'-deoxycoformycin (pentostatin) is a potent inhibitor of adenosine deaminase. It is presently being used in clinical trials for treatment of patients with hairy cell leukemia (116) and refractory lymphoid malignancies (117). The ocular side effects of 2'-deoxycoformycin are conjunctivitis 116–120) and keratitis (121). Conjunctivitis is usually mild to moderate and transient (116–120). Of 23 patients with hairy cell leukemia

treated with 2 to 4 mg/m^2 intravenously on a biweekly schedule, 6 developed a mild conjunctivitis (116). Three of 17 patients with refractory lymphoid malignancies treated with 2'-deoxycoformycin developed moderately severe keratitis (121). Two patients had received 5 mg/m^2 daily for 5 days, but 1 patient developed symptoms after 3 doses given on a twice-weekly schedule. Slit-lamp examination showed bilateral keratitis morphologically indistinguishable from the dendritic ulceration of herpetic keratitis. Symptoms subsided in a week, with corneal healing over 14 to 21 days.

Interferon

Recombinant interferon has been used for the treatment of hairy cell leukemia, CML, and non-Hodgkin's lymphoma. Only rarely have visual disturbances or conjunctivitis been reported (114). One patient showed evidence of rejection of a corneal transplant after 2 weeks of interferon therapy at a dose of 2×10^6 units/m^2 three times per week (122). The rejection episode ceased with interruption of interferon therapy for 1 week and administration of prednisone ophthalmic drops.

Mitotane

Mitotane is an oral chemotherapeutic agent best known by its trivial name, o,p'-DDD, whose biochemical mechanism of action is unknown. Mitotane is used in the treatment of inoperable adrenal cortical carcinoma of both functional and nonfunctional types. Infrequently occurring ocular side effects include subcapsular cataracts and toxic retinopathy with papilledema, retinal hemorrhages, and edema (123).

Paclitaxel

Paclitaxel is approved for the treatment of refractory ovarian and breast cancer. Two instances of ocular toxicity associated with paclitaxel have been described. Capri et al. reported visual disturbances and neurologic findings consistent with optic nerve toxicity in patients with relapsed breast cancer during an ongoing trial of paclitaxel administered at the dose of either 125 mg/m^2 or 225 mg/m^2 every 3 weeks by 3-hour infusion (124). Nine (19%) of 47 patients (3 treated with 195 mg/m^2 and 6 with 235 mg/m^2 of paclitaxel noted scintillating scotoma in the visual fields of both eyes at the end of the drug

Table 32.1. Ocular Toxicity Associated with Chemotherapeutic Agents

Drug	Clinical Features	References
Alkylating agents		
Busulfan	Anterior and posterior cataracts	(7–10)
	Sicca syndrome	(10)
Chlorambucil	Keratitis	(15)
	Diplopia, retinal hemorrhages	(16)
Cisplatin		
Intravenous	Papilledema; retrobulbar and optic neuritis	(17–20)
	Transient cortical blindness	(21–22)
	Transient homonymous hemianopsia	(23)
	Blurred vision, altered color perception	(24)
Intraarterial	Blurred vision, permanent blindness	(25–27)
Cyclophosphamide	Blurred vision	(33)
	Blepharoconjunctivitis	(4)
Nitrogen mustard	Necrotizing uveitis	(34)
Nitrosoureas		
Intravenous	Blurred vision	(37–39)
Intraarterial	Eye pain, conjunctival edema, decreased vision	(40–43)
Antibiotics		
Doxorubicin	Conjunctivitis	(15)
	Increased lacrimation	(46)
Mithramycin	Periorbital pallor	(15)
Mitomycin C	Blurred vision	(15)
Antimetabolites		
Cytosine arabinoside	Conjunctivitis, photophobia	(47–49, 50)
5-Fluorouracil		
Intravenous	Conjunctivitis, tear duct stenosis, ectropion of lower lid	(60–64)
With radiation	Visual loss, conjunctivitis, corneal lesions	(70–72)
Methotrexate	Conjunctivitis, blurred vision, photophobia	(4, 15, 73, 74)
Hormonal agents		
Corticosteroids	Glaucoma, increased intraocular pressure	(77–80)
	Posterior subcapsular cataracts	(79–89)
Tamoxifen	Retinopathy, optic neuritis, decreased visual acuity	(92–98)
Plant alkaloids		
Vinblastine and vincristine	Cranial nerve palsies	(101, 102)
	Optic neuropathy, blindness	(103–105)
	Transient cortical blindness	(106)
	Night blindness	(107)
Miscellaneous agents		
Allopurinol	Cataracts	(109–113)
	Optic neuritis, iritis, conjunctivitis	(114)
Cyclosporine	Blurred vision, cortical blindness	(115)
2'-Deoxycoformycin	Conjunctivitis	(116–120)
	Keratitis	(121)
Interferon	Conjunctivitis	(114)
	Corneal transplant rejection	(122)
Mitotone	Subcapsular cataracts, retinopathy	(123)
Paclitaxel	Optic neuritis	(124)
	Photopsia	(125)
Procarbazine	Papilledema, retinopathy	(114)

infusion). The scotoma always spontaneously resolved and did not necessarily recur with the subsequent drug administration. Three of the nine patients also noted a subjective reduction of vision. The cranial nerves were not involved in any of the three patients. For the duration of follow-up of these 3 patients, the visual symptoms did not improve. Neurophysiologic assessment of the optic pathways in these 3 patients excluded an involvement of the retina and suggested damage to the optic nerve.

Seidman et al. reported that 6 of 25 patients receiving paclitaxel at doses of 250 to 275 mg/m^2 as a 3-hour infusion experienced photopsia, described as flashing lights across the entire visual field, usually beginning during the final 30 minutes of drug infusion, with a duration of 15 minutes to 3 hours (125). The photopsia recurred with rechallenge at the same or slightly reduced dose (250 to 275 mg/m^2) without any apparent chronic sequelae. Symptoms did not occur at doses below 250 mg/m^2. One patient had diastolic hypertension associated with the visual symptoms, and both resolved with treatment with sublingual nifedipine. The pathophysiologic mechanism underlying the photopsia was unclear, although the possibility of a vascular etiology was suggested.

Procarbazine

Procarbazine is a hydrazine derivative antineoplastic agent useful in combination with other drugs in the treatment of Hodgkin's disease. Use of procarbazine is rarely associated with retinal hemorrhage, papilledema, photophobia, diplopia, and inability to focus (114).

CONCLUSION

As reviewed in this chapter, ocular toxicity is a relative uncommon, but potentially serious, side effect of cancer chemotherapy (Table 32.1). With some drugs, a direct causal relationship has not yet been demonstrated or the use of combination therapy has made identification of the agent responsible for the ocular side effect impossible. Ocular toxicity may be reversible if the side effect is recognized early and the offending drug dosage decreased or the drug discontinued. Therefore, clinicians and oncology nurses (126) must be aware of potential ocular toxicities of chemotherapeutic agents and include the possibility of a chemotherapeutic-induced ophthalmologic disorder in a patient who develops an ocular problem during therapy.

REFERENCES

1. Griffin JD, Garnick MB. Eye toxicity of cancer chemotherapy: a review of the literature. Cancer 1981; 48:1539–1549.
2. Visel M, Oster MW. Ocular side effects of cancer chemotherapy. Cancer 1982;49:1999–2002.
3. Oster MW. Ocular side effects of cancer chemotherapy. In: Perry MC, Yarbro JW, eds. Toxicity of chemotherapy. Orlando, FL: Grune & Stratton, 1984:181–197.
4. Fraunfelder FT, Meyer SM. Ocular toxicity of antineoplastic agents. Am Acad Ophthalmol 1983;90:1–3.
5. Imperia PS, Lazarus HM, Lass JH. Ocular complications of systemic cancer chemotherapy. Surv Ophthamol 1989;34:209–230.
6. Grimes P, von Sallman L, Frichette A. Influence of Myleran on cell proliferation in the lens epithelium. Invest Ophthalmol 1964;3:566–576.
7. Podos SM, Canellos GP. Lens changes in chronic granulocytic leukemia. Am J Ophthalmol 1969;68:500–504.
8. Ravindranathan MP, Paul VJ, Kuriakose ET. Cataract after busulfan treatment. Br Med J 1972;1:218–219.
9. Dahlgren S, Holm G, Svanborg N, Watz R. Clinical and morphological side-effects of busulfan (Myleran) treatment. Acta Med Scand 1972;192:129–135.
10. Sidi Y, Douer D, Pinkhas J. Sicca syndrome in a patient with toxic reaction to busulfan. JAMA 1977; 238:1951.
11. Grimes T, von Sallman L. Interference with cell proliferation and induction of polyploidy in rat lens epithelium during prolonged Myleran treatment. Exp Cell Res 1966;42:265–273.
12. Hamming N, Apple D, Goldberg M. Histopathology and ultrastructure of busulfan-induced cataracts. Graefes Arch Clin Exp Ophthalmol 1976; 200:139–147.
13. Eshaghian J, Streeten BW. Human posterior subcapsular cataract: an ultrastructural study of the posteriorly migrating cells. Arch Ophthalmol 1980; 98:134–143.
14. Griener JV, Chylack CT. Posterior subcapsular cataracts: histopathology of steroid-associated cataracts. Arch Ophthalmol 1979;97:135–136.
15. Fraunfelder FT. Drug-induced ocular side effects and drug interactions. 2nd ed. Philadelphia: Lea & Febiger 1982:316–332.
16. Bregeat M, Hermans R. Oedeme papillaire spontanement criable aucous d'un traitement par le chlorambucil. Bull Soc Belge Ophtalmol 1972; 1960:567–569.
17. Ostrow S, Hahn D, Wiernik PH, Richards RD. Ophthalmologic toxicity after cis-dichlorodiammine platinum (II) therapy. Cancer Treat Rep 1978;62:1591–1593.
18. Becher R, Schutt P, Osieka R, Schmidt CG. Peripheral neuropathy and ophthalmologic toxicity after treatment with cis-dichloroaminoplatinum II. J Cancer Res Clin Oncol 1980;96:219–221.
19. Walsh TJ, Clark AW, Parhad IM, Green WR. Neurotoxic effects of cisplatin therapy. Arch Neurol 1982;39:719–720.
20. Bosl GJ, Lage PH, Fraley EE, et al. Vinblastine, bleomycin and cis-diamminedichloroplatinum in the treatment of advanced testicular carcinoma. Am J Med 1980;68:492–496.

21. Berman I, Mann M. Seizures and transient cortical blindness associated with *cis*-platinumdiammine-dichloride therapy in a 30 year old man. Cancer 1980; 45:764–766.

22. Pippitt CH, Muss HB, Homesley HD, Jobson VW. Cisplatin-associated cortical blindness. Gynecol Oncol 1981;12:253–255.

23. Cohen RJ, Cuneo RA, Cruciger MP, Jackman AE. Transient left homonymous hemianopsia and encephalopathy following treatment of testicular carcinoma with cisplatinum, vinblastine, and bleomycin. J Clin Oncol 1983;1:392–393.

24. Wilding G, Caruso R, Lawrence TS, et al. Retinal toxicity after high-dose cisplatin therapy. J Clin Oncol 1985;3:1683–1689.

25. Stewart DJ, Wallace S, Feun L, et al. A phase I study of intracarotid artery infusion of *cis*-diamminedichloroplatinum (II) in patients with recurrent malignant intracerebral tumors. Cancer Res 1982;42:2059–2062.

26. Miller DF, Bay JW, Lederman RJ, Purvis JD, Rogers LR, Tomsak RL. Ocular and orbital toxicity following intracarotid injection of BCNU (carmustine) and cisplatinum for malignant gliomas. Ophthalmology 1985;92:402–406.

27. Calvo FA, Dy C, Henriquez I, Hidalgo V, Bilbao I, Santos M. Postoperative radical radiotherapy with concurrent weekly intra-arterial *cis*-platinum for treatment of malignant glioma: a pilot study. Radiother Oncol 1989;14:83–88.

28. Urba S, Forastiere AA. Retrobulbar neuritis in a patient treated with intraarterial cisplatin for head and neck cancer. Cancer 1988;62:2094–2097.

29. Kapp JP, Vance RB. Supraophthalmic carotid infusion for recurrent glioma. J Neurooncol 1985;3:5–11.

30. Grant WM. Toxicology of the eye. 3rd ed. Springfield, IL: Charles C Thomas, 1986:467–468, 550–557, 586–588, 896–901.

31. Lee C-C, Castles TR, Kintner LD. Single-dose toxicity of cyclophosphamide (NSC-26271) in dogs and monkeys. Cancer Chemother Rep 1973;4:51–76.

32. Levine S, Sowinski R. Cyclitis produced in rats by cyclophosphamide. Invest Ophthalmol 1974;13:697–699.

33. Kende G, Sirkin SR, Thomas PRM, Freeman AI. Blurring of vision—a previously undescribed complication of cyclophosphamide therapy. Cancer 1979;44:69–71.

34. Anderson B, Anderson B. Necrotizing uveitis incident to perfusion of intracranial malignancies with nitrogen mustard and related compounds. Trans Am Ophthalmol Soc 1960;58:95–104.

35. DeWys WD, Fowler EH. Report of vasculitis and blindness after intracarotid injection of 1,3-bis (2-chloroethyl)-1-nitrosourea (BCNU; NSC-409962) in dogs. Cancer Chemother Rep 1973;57:33–40.

36. Crafts DC, Levin VA, Nielsen S. Intracarotid BCNU (NSC-409962): a toxicity study in six rhesus monkeys. Cancer Treat Rep 1976;60:541–545.

37. Lokich JJ, Skarin AT, Frei E. 1,-(2-chloroethyl)-3-cyclohexyl-1-nitrosourea (methyl CCNU) and Adriamycin combination therapy. Cancer 1974;34:1593–1597.

38. McLennan R, Taylor HR. Optic neuroretinitis

in association with BCNU and procarbazine therapy. Med Pediatr Oncol 1978;4:43–48.

39. Louie AC, Turrisi AT, Muggia FM, Bono VH Jr. Letter to the editor. Med Pediatr Oncol 1978;5:245–247.

40. Grimson BS, Mahaley MS Jr, Dubey HD, Dudka L. Ophthalmic and central nervous system complications following intracarotid BCNU (carmustine). J Clin Neuro Ophthalmol 1981;1:261–264.

41. Shingleton BJ, Bienfang DC, Albert DM, Ensminger WD, Greenberg HS. Ocular toxicity associated with high dose carmustine. Arch Ophthalmol 1982;100:1766–1772.

42. Watne K, Hannisdal E, Nome O, Hager B, Hirschberg H. Combined intra-arterial and systemic chemotherapy for recurrent malignant brain tumors. Neurosurgery 1992;30:223–227.

43. Rogers LR, Purvis JB, Lederman RJ, et al. Alternating sequential intracarotid BCNU and cisplatin in recurrent malignant glioma. Cancer 1991;68:15–21.

44. Cruciani F, Tamanti N, Abdolrahiumzadeh S, Francei F, Gabrieli CB. Ocular toxicity of systemic chemotherapy with megadoses of carmustine and mitomycin. Ann Ophthalmol 1994;26:97–100.

45. Curran CF, Luce JK. Ocular adverse reactions associated with Adriamycin (doxorubicin). Am J Ophthalmol 1989;108:709–711.

46. Blum RH. An overview of studies with Adriamycin (NSC-123127) in the United States. Cancer Chemother Rep 1975;6:247–251.

47. Hopen G, Mondino BJ, Johnson BL, Chervenick PA. Corneal toxicity with systemic cytarabine. Am J Ophthalmol 1981;91:500–504.

48. Herzig RH, Wolff SN, Lazarus HM, Phillips GL, Karanes C, Herzig GP. High-dose cytosine arabinoside therapy for refractory leukemia. Blood 1983;62:361–369.

49. Kantarjian HM, Estey EH, Plunkett W, et al. Phase I–II clinical and pharmacologic studies of high dose cytosine arabinoside in refractory leukemia. Am J Med 1986;81:387–394.

50. Velasquez WS, Cabanillas F, Salvador P, et al. Effective salvage therapy for lymphoma with cisplatin in combination with high-dose Ara-C and dexamethasone (DHAP). Blood 1988;71:117–122.

51. Shimada M, Wakaizumi S, Kasubuchi Y, Kusunoki T, Nakamura T. Cytosine arabinoside and rosette formation in mouse retina. Nature 1973;246:151–152.

52. Shimada M, Wakaizumi S, Kusunoki T. Developmental abnormality of the retina caused by postnatal administration of cytosine arabinoside. Biol Neonate 1975;26:359–366.

53. Percy DH, Danylchuk KD. Experimental retinal dysplasia due to cytosine arabinoside. Invest Ophthalmol Visual Sci 1977;16:353–364.

54. Higa GM, Gockerman JP, Hunt AL, Jones MR, Horne BJ. The use of prophylactic eye drops during high-dose cytosine arabinoside therapy. Cancer 1991;68:1691–1693.

55. Castleberry RP, Crist WM, Holbrook T, Malluh A, Gaddy D. The cytosine arabinoside (ara-C) syndrome. Med Pediatr Oncol 1981;9:257–264.

56. Ritch PS, Hansen RM, Heuer DK. Ocular toxicity from high-dose cytosine arabinoside. Cancer 1983;51:430–432.

57. Dillaha CJ, Jansen GT, Honeycutt WM, Brad-

ford AC. Selective cytotoxic effect of topical 5-fluoro-uracil. Arch Dermatol 1963;88:247–256.

58. Dillaha CJ, Jansen GT, Honeycutt WM, Holt GA. Further studies with topical 5-fluorouracil. Arch Dermatol 1965;92:410–417.

59. Williams AC, Klein E. Experiences with local chemotherapy and immunotherapy in pre-malignant and malignant skin lesions. Cancer 1970;25:450–462.

60. Hamersly J, Luce JK, Florentz TR, Burkholder MM, Pepper JJ. Excessive lacrimation from fluorouracil treatment. JAMA 1973;225:747–748.

61. Bonadonna G, Brusamolino E, Valagussa P, et al. Combination chemotherapy as an adjuvant treatment in operable breast cancer. N Engl J Med 1976; 294:405–410.

62. Straus DJ, Mausolf FA, Ellerby RA, McCracken JD. Cicatricial ectropion secondary to 5-fluorouracil therapy. Med Pediatr Oncol 1977;3:15–19.

63. Haidak DJ, Hurwitz B, Yeung KY. Tear-duct fibrosis (dacryostenosis) due to 5-fluorouracil. Ann Intern Med 1978;88:657.

64. Caravella LP, Burns JA, Zangmeister M. Punctal-canalicular stenosis related to systemic fluorouracil therapy. Arch Ophthalmol 1981;99:284–286.

65. Christophidis N, Vajda FJE, Lucas I, Louis WJ. Ocular side effects with 5-fluorouracil. Aust NZ J Med 1979;9:143–144.

66. Bonadonna G, Valagussa P. Current status of adjuvant chemotherapy for breast cancer. Semin Oncol 1987;15:8–22.

67. Loprinzi CL, Love RR, Garrity JA, Ames MM. Cyclophosphamide, methotrexate, and 5-fluorouracil (CMF)-induced ocular toxicity. Cancer Invest 1990; 8:459–465.

68. Cohen JM. Cromolyn for chemotherapy conjunctivitis. J Clin Oncol 1985;3:1690.

69. Loprinzi CL, Wender DB, Veeder MH, et al. Inhibition of 5-fluorouracil-induced ocular irritation by ocular ice packs. Cancer 1994;74:945–948.

70. Sato Y, Morita M, Takahashi H-O, Watanabe N, Kirikae I. Combined surgery, radiotherapy, and regional chemotherapy in carcinoma of the paranasal sinuses. Cancer 1970;25:571–579.

71. Goepfert H, Jesse R, Lindberg R. Arterial infusion and radiation therapy in the treatment of advanced cancer of the nasal cavity and paranasal sinuses. Am J Surg 1973;126:464–468.

72. Chan RC, Shukorsky LJ. Effects of irradiation on the eye. Radiology 1976;120:673–675.

73. Hansen HH, Selawry OS, Holland JF, McCall CB. The variability of individual tolerance to methotrexate in cancer patients. Br J Cancer 1971;25:298–305.

74. Doroshow JH, Locker GY, Gaasterland DE, Hubbard SP, Young RC, Myers CE. Ocular irritation from high-dose methotrexate therapy: pharmacokinetics of drug in the tear film. Cancer 1981;48:2158–2162.

75. Fishman ML, Bean SC, Cogan DG. Optic atrophy following prophylactic chemotherapy and cranial radiation for acute lymphocytic leukemia. Am J Ophthalmol 1976;82:571–576.

76. Margileth DA, Poplack DG, Pizzo PA, Leventhal BG. Blindness during remission in two patients with acute lymphoblastic leukemia. Cancer 1977; 39:58–61.

77. Schwartz B. The response of ocular pressure to corticosteroids. Int Ophthalmol Clin 1966;6:929–989.

78. Goldman H. Cortisone glaucoma. Int Ophthalmol Clin 1966;6:991–1003.

79. Porter R, Crombie AL, Gardner PS, Uldall RP. Incidence of ocular complications in patients undergoing renal transplantation. Br Med J 1972;3:133–136.

80. Ticho V, Durst A, Licht A, Berkowitz S. Steroid-induced glaucoma and cataract in renal transplant recipients. Israel J Med Sci 1977;13:871–874.

81. Black RL, Olgesby RB, von Sallmann L, Bunim JJ. Posterior subcapsular cataracts induced by corticosteroids in patients with rheumatic diseases treated with corticosteroids. Arch Ophthalmol 1961;66:625–630.

82. Kobayashi Y, Akaishi K, Nishio T, Kobayashi Y, Kimura Y, Nagata M. Posterior subcapsular cataract in nephrotic children receiving steroid therapy. Am J Dis Child 1974;128:671–673.

83. Forman AR, Loreto JA, Tina LU. Reversibility of corticosteroid-associated cataracts in children with the nephrotic syndrome. Am J Ophthalmol 1977;84:75–78.

84. Fine RN, Korsch BM, Brennan LP, et al. Renal transplantation in young children. Am J Surg 1973; 125:559–569.

85. Urban RC Jr, Cotlier E. Corticosteroid-induced cataracts. Surv Ophthalmol 1986;31:102–110.

86. Spaeth GL, von Sallman L. Corticosteroids and cataracts. Int Ophthalmol Clin 1966;6:915–929.

87. Limaye SR, Pillai S, Tina LU. Relationship of steroid dose to degree of posterior subcapsular cataracts in nephrotic syndrome. Ann Ophthalmol 1988; 20:225–227.

88. Hoover DL, Smith LEH, Turner SJ, Gelber RD, Sallan SE. Ophthalmic evaluation of survivors of acute lymphoblastic leukemia. Ophthalmology 1988;95:151–155.

89. Crews SJ. Posterior subcapsular lens opacities in patients on long-term corticosteroid therapy. Br Med J 1963;1:1644–1647.

90. Streeten BW, Eshaghian J. Human posterior subcapsular cataract. Arch Ophthalmol 1978;96:1653–1658.

91. Ono S, Hirano H, Obra K. Presence of cortisol-binding protein in the lens. Ophthalmic Res 1972; 3:233–240.

92. Kaiser-Kupfer MI, Lippman ME. Tamoxifen retinopathy. Cancer Treat Rep 1978;62:315–320.

93. McKeown CA, Swartz M, Blom J, Maggiano JM. Tamoxifen retinopathy. Br J Ophthalmol 1981; 65:177–179.

94. Beck M, Mills PV. Ocular assessment of patients treated with tamoxifen. Cancer Treat Rep 1979; 63:1833–1834.

95. Vinding T, Nielsen NV. Retinopathy caused by treatment with tamoxifen in low dosage. Acta Ophthalmol 1983;61:45–50.

96. Pugesgaard T, Von Eyben FE. Bilateral optic neuritis evolved during tamoxifen treatment. Cancer 1986;58:383–386.

97. Ashford AR, Donev I, Tiwari RP, Garrett TJ. Reversible ocular toxicity related to tamoxifen therapy. Cancer 1988;61:33–35.

98. Pavlidis NA, Petris C, Briassoulis E, et al. Clear evidence that long-term, low-dose tamoxifen treatment can induce ocular toxicity. Cancer 1992;69:2961–2964.

99. Kaiser-Kupfer MI, Kupfer C, Rodrigues MM. Tamoxifen retinopathy: 1. A clinicopathologic report. Ophthalmology 1981;88:89–93.

100. Rosenthal S, Kaufman S. Vincristine neurotoxicity. Ann Intern Med 1974;80:733–737.

101. Albert DM, Wong VG, Henderson ES. Ocular complications of vincristine therapy. Arch Ophthalmol 1967;78:709–713.

102. Sandler SG, Tobin W, Denderson ES. Vincristine-induced neuropathy: a clinical study of fifty leukemic patients. Neurology 1969;19:367–374.

103. Sanderson PA, Kuwabara T, Cogan DG. Optic neuropathy presumably caused by vincristine therapy. Am J Ophthalmol 1976;81:146–150.

104. Norton SW, Stockman JA III. Unilateral optic neuropathy following vincristine chemotherapy. J Pediatr Ophthalmol Strabismus 1979;16:190–193.

105. Awidi AS. Blindness and vincristine. Ann Intern Med 1980;93:781.

106. Byrd RL, Rohrbaugh TM, Raney RB Jr, Norris DG. Transient cortical blindness secondary to vincristine therapy in childhood malignancies. Cancer 1981; 47:37–40.

107. Ripps H, Carr RE, Siegel IM, Greenstein VC. Functional abnormalities in vincristine-induced night blindness. Invest Ophthalmol Vis Sci 1984;25:787–794.

108. Hansson H-A. Retinal changes induced by treatment with vincristine and vinblastine. Doc Ophthalmol 1972;31:65–87.

109. Fraunfelder FT, Hanna C, Dreis MW, Cosgrove KW. Cataracts associated with allopurinol therapy. Am J Ophthalmol 1982;94:137–140.

110. Lerman S, McGaw JM, Gardner K. Allopurinol therapy and cataractogenesis in humans. Am J Ophthalmol 1982;94:141–146.

111. Lerman S, Megaw J. Further studies on allopurinol therapy and human cataractogenesis. Am J Ophthalmol 1984;97:205–209.

112. Jick H, Brandt DE. Allopurinol and cataracts. Am J Ophthalmol 1984;98:355–358.

113. Clair WK, Chylack LT, Cook EF, Goldman L. Allopurinol use and the risk of cataract formation. Br J Ophthalmol 1989;73:173–176.

114. Physicians' Desk Reference. 43rd ed. Oradell, NJ: Medical Economics, 1989:814, 1739, 1751, 1936.

115. Ghalie R, Fitzsimmons WE, Bennett D, Kaiser H. Cortical blindness: a rare complication of cyclosporine therapy. Bone Marrow Transplant 1990;6:147–149.

116. Kraut EH, Bouroncle BA, Grever MR. Pentostatin in the treatment of advanced hairy cell leukemia. J Clin Oncol 1989;7:168–172.

117. O'Dwyer PJ, Wagner B, Leyland-Jones B, Wittes R, Cheson BD, Hoth DF. 2'-Deoxycoformycin (pentostatin) for lymphoid malignancies. Ann Intern Med 1988;108:733–743.

118. Grever MR, Siaw MFE, Jacob WF et al. The biochemical and clinical consequences of 2'-deoxycoformycin in refractory lymphoproliferative malignancy. Blood 1981;57:406–416.

119. Major PP, Agarwal RP, Kufe DW. Clinical pharmacology of deoxycoformycin. Blood 1981;58:91–96.

120. Kefford RF, Fox RM. Deoxycoformycin-induced response in chronic lymphocytic leukaemia: deoxycoformycin toxicity in non-replicating lymphocytes. Br J Haematol 1982;50:627–636.

121. Spiers ASD, Ruckdeschel JC, Horton J. Effectiveness of pentostatin (2'-deoxycoformycin) in refractory lymphoid neoplasms. Scand J Haematol 1984; 32:130–134.

122. Jacobs AD, Champlin RE, Golde DW. Recombinant α-2-interferon for hairy cell leukemia. Blood 1985;65:1017–1020.

123. Hoffman DL, Mattox VR. Treatment of adrenocortical carcinoma with o,p'-DDD. Med Clin North Am 1972;56:999–1012.

124. Capri G, Nunzone E, Tarenzi E, et al. Optic nerve disturbances: a new form of paclitaxel neurotoxicity. J Natl Cancer Inst 1994;86:1099–1100.

125. Seidman AD, Barrett S. Photopsia during 3-hour paclitaxel administration at doses ≥250 mg/m². J Clin Oncol 1994;12:1737–1738.

126. Cloutier AO. Ocular side effects of chemotherapy: nursing management. Oncol Nurs Forum 1992;19:1251–1259.

33

Cardiotoxicity of Chemotherapeutic Drugs

Michael S. Ewer and Robert S. Benjamin

Drug therapies used for the treatment of patients with cancer may damage a number of organs and organ systems. Among those most frequently damaged are tissues with rapid cell turnover, such as the hemopoietic system, the gastrointestinal tract, and the genitourinary tract. The heart, made up of tissue without rapid cell turnover, and therefore incapable of rapid recovery, is only occasionally affected by chemotherapy. Because the cardiac effects of such therapy may be disabling or life threatening and, therefore, may necessitate a major modification of treatment, cardiac toxicity of antimalignant therapy is of special interest. While in some instances the effects of chemotherapeutic drugs on the heart are self-limited and readily reversible with the withdrawal of the offending agent, in others, the damage may be devastating, progressive, irreversible, and ultimately fatal. Some forms of cardiotoxicity are poorly predictable; they may affect patients without warning, sometimes during the first exposure. In other settings, the toxicity is well defined and readily predictable, in that most patients react in a similar fashion. Finally, despite the predictable toxicity of some drugs, there is considerable variation in the exposure needed to achieve similar levels of tissue damage. Some drugs are toxic by themselves, but their toxicity may be potentiated when they are used in combination with specific other agents, the combination being more toxic than the sum of the toxicities of the individual components; other combinations of drugs may offer protection from toxic effects.

As it is often necessary to achieve the greatest antitumor potential of a drug while keeping end-organ toxicity at an acceptable level and because of the considerable variation in the toxic effects

of some of these drugs on end-organ function, the evaluation and treatment of patients treated with toxic drugs often must be individualized. Most cardiotoxic drugs can be grouped according to their cardiac effect: those that produce a decrease in myocardial contractility or relaxation; those that cause or exacerbate ischemia; and those that affect the cardiac conduction system, resulting in dysrhythmias or blocks (Table 33.1). The cardiotoxicities of antineoplastic drugs, the evaluation of patients treated with such agents, and the prevention of cardiac end-organ damage are the focus of this chapter, which is modified from a more comprehensive evaluation of the cardiac complications of cancer and its treatment (1).

AGENTS WITH MYOCARDIAL DEPRESSANT ACTIVITY

Several antineoplastic agents have been implicated as causative agents in cardiomyopathies. The anthracyclines have received most attention, but other anthraquinones are also associated with myopathy. Adriamycin, the most widely used agent in this group, has been extensively studied and serves as a model for anthracycline-associated and related cardiomyopathies (2–12).

Anthracyclines and Other Anthraquinones

The anthracyclines are a class of red-pigmented antibiotics (rhodomycins) isolated from a soil bacillus, the actinomycete *Streptomyces*. They are polycyclic aromatic compounds, more specifically, planar cyclic chromophores, all of

Table 33.1. Antineoplastic Drugs Associated with Cardiotoxicity

---

Drugs associated with myocardial depression
  Anthracyclines
    Doxorubicin (Adriamycin)
    THP Adriamycin (Pirarubicin)
    Idarubicin
    Epirubicin
    Daunorubicin
  Other anthraquinones
    Mitoxantrone
    Toxicity intensifiers
      Cyclophosphamide
      Mitomycin C
      Etoposide
      Melphalan
      Vincristine
      Bleomycin
    Toxicity inhibitors
      Dexrazoxane (Zinocard, ICRF-187)
  Other agents associated with myocardial depression
    Cyclophosphamide
    Alpha-interferon
Antineoplastic agents associated with ischemia
  5-Fluorouracil (5-FU)
  Vinblastine
  Vincristine
  Bleomycin
  Cisplatin
  Biological response modifiers such as Interleukin-2
Antineoplastic agents associated with hypotension
  Interleukin-2
  Homoharringtonine
Miscellaneous agents with known or suspected cardiac toxicity
  Paclitaxel (Taxol)
  Bleomycin
  Actinomycin D
  Mitomycin C
  Alkylating agents
    Cyclophosphamide
    Ifosfamide

---

which contain a B ring quinone as a common feature, linked to one or more sugars (13). Their antitumor effect is felt to result primarily from intercalation into the DNA of actively cycling cells, with subsequent blockage of DNA synthesis and cell death (14). It is increasingly felt that a major mechanism of action is direct DNA damage, mediated through inhibition of topoisomerase II, but it is also apparent that Adriamycin has multiple additional potential mechanisms of action: inhibition of topoisomerase I, helicases, and a number of additional enzyme systems as well as free radical formation and inhibition of tumor

angiogenesis (15–29). All of the anthracyclines and other anthraquinones cause myelosuppression and varying degrees of alopecia, mucositis, and a cumulative dose-related cardiotoxicity (30).

ADRIAMYCIN

Adriamycin is one of the most widely used antineoplastic agents. Its effectiveness is in part limited by the cumulative dose-related cardiotoxicity, which usually occurs late during a course of treatment or may present months or years after the completion of therapy. An early form of toxicity, sometimes occurring within hours of drug administration and consisting primarily of supraventricular tachydysrhythmias and ventricular ectopy, has been reported. Early Adriamycin toxicity may also present as a myopericarditis, which may progress to significant cardiac dysfunction within a few weeks of the first administration of the drug (6). Electrocardiographic changes consisting of ST segment and T wave changes or other abnormalities may also be seen (2, 3). Early toxicity is more likely to be observed in elderly patients or in patients who have received large single doses of the drug. Such changes are usually transient and are not cumulative dose related (3, 31). Rhythm disturbances are the most common cardiac manifestation during infusion of Adriamycin; some studies suggest that dysrhythmias occur in a large percentage of patients treated with bolus administration schedules (32, 33). Such dysrhythmias usually are not life threatening and do not represent a contraindication for continued use of Adriamycin. Furthermore, many of the dysrhythmias attributed to anthracyclines may represent preexisting conditions, according to a study using pretreatment Holter monitoring prior to anthracycline therapy (34). Sudden death following Adriamycin administration has been reported but is extremely rare (32). The mechanism of cardiac damage in patients with early toxicity is uncertain; treatment is usually not indicated or consists of supportive measures.

Of much greater clinical importance is late or chronic Adriamycin-associated cardiomyopathy, which is slowly progressive, potentially irreversible, and life threatening. This complication is related to cumulative dose, but it follows a hyperbolic curve rather than being a linear relationship. When the cumulative dose is below 400 mg/m^2, cardiomyopathy is unusual. Its incidence increases more rapidly, however, as the cumulative dose approaches, and then exceeds,

550 mg/m^2 with the usual rapid infusion schedule of drug administration (2, 5, 11). Cardiomyopathy may occur at lower doses when other drugs are used concomitantly (see below). Initially described as refractory to supportive therapy, irreversible, and invariably fatal, Adriamycin-induced cardiomyopathy is now recognized as not being uniformly progressive; anthracycline-associated cardiac dysfunction does respond to supportive care regimens (11, 35, 36).

The pathogenesis of Adriamycin-associated cardiomyopathy has not been fully elucidated, and the exact mechanism of cardiotoxicity in patients treated with doxorubicin and related drugs as well as the sequence of events that leads to cardiac dysfunction are still under investigation. It appears that Adriamycin causes myocyte damage by a mechanism at least somewhat different from those involved in the destruction of tumor cells, although there are conflicting preclinical data (see discussion of cardiac protectors, below) (29). Direct damage to membrane lipids appears to be responsible, at least in part. Indirect damage through oxygen free radicals that affect calcium transport and eventually depress myocardial function also plays a role and may be more important (37, 38). The almost total absence of catalase and superoxide dismutase within cardiac muscle makes it very difficult to counteract free radical production through the normal scavenger mechanisms (39). There is increasing evidence that the generation of the oxygen free radicals is mediated through a doxorubicin-iron complex (40). Adriamycin undergoes extensive metabolism (41). Adriamycinol, one of its principal metabolites, has been found to have a greater effect on the calcium pump of the sarcoplasmatic reticulum than does the parent Adriamycin, which raises the possibility that the antitumor effect, presumed by many to be mediated by the parent compound, may be distinct from the cardiotoxic effect (42). Furthermore, there is evidence that secondary alcohol metabolites may mediate the Fe(II)-induced cardiac damage (43).

Adriamycin cardiomyopathy may become manifest months and even years after successful completion of a course of chemotherapy at or near the maximum tolerated dose (44). As a greater number of patients treated with Adriamycin are cured, and therefore survive for long periods of time following their chemotherapy, some who have significant, but subclinical, cardiac damage may experience additional stresses that are poorly tolerated, and which then result in symptomatic cardiac dysfunction months or years following the initial cardiac insult (45).

The effect of Adriamycin exposure on the genesis of coronary artery disease, myocardial infarction, and other cardiac injuries that occur with aging is unknown. In one review, 12 of 43 patients with Adriamycin-induced cardiomyopathy died because of progressive cardiac dysfunction (35). Fatal cardiomyopathy is unusual, however, when the drug is given as a 48- to 96-hour infusion. Even when diagnosed within 4 weeks of drug administration, only 2 of 22 patients who had clinical evidence of congestive heart failure succumbed to their cardiac complication (36).

Clinical Manifestations of Adriamycin Toxicity

Adriamycin produces a cardiomyopathy clinically indistinguishable from other forms of congestive heart failure. Clinically, cardiac dysfunction may be left-sided or biventricular; the cardiac damage is diffuse histologically (see below). Patients may be asymptomatic in the early stages and may exhibit only minimal signs of cardiac dysfunction. One of the first signs of cardiac abnormality, and one that is occasionally overlooked, is a resting tachycardia in patients with a previously normal resting heart rate. Nonproductive cough and neck vein distention may be present. As the abnormalities progress, patients experience increasing degrees of dyspnea; dyspnea at rest is a poor prognostic sign. Congestive heart failure may be precipitated by stresses, including volume overload, surgery or other trauma, general anesthesia, alcohol abuse, anemia, pregnancy, cachexia, hypoproteinemia, or infection (9, 45–47).

Cardiac examination of a patient with fully developed myopathy often reveals a diastolic (S3) gallop, an enlarged area of cardiac dullness, an exaggerated increase in cardiac rate with minimal exertion, and, when pulmonary congestion ensues, diffuse rales. Hepatomegaly may be present. The chest roentgenogram shows nonspecific findings of increased cardiac silhouette size and engorged vasculature. Various degrees of pleural effusion may be seen. The electrocardiogram also demonstrates nonspecific findings; as with congestive heart failure of other etiologies, decrease in the mean QRS voltage of the standard leads has been reported (48). The importance of this finding is diminished because of the many other conditions commonly encountered in cancer patients that also decrease the mean QRS voltage, such as pleural or pericardial effusions, chronic lung disease, and anasarca (11).

The left ventricular ejection fraction (defined as the ratio of the quantity of blood in the left ventricle before the onset of, and at the end of, systole), which can be derived from echocardiographic or nuclear studies or by other methods, is the most frequently used parameter for following the cardiac status in patients receiving Adriamycin or a related agent (49). Despite the limitations of these studies, most patients receiving anthracyclines can be followed safely with the use of noninvasively derived estimates of the left ventricular ejection fraction. Nuclear imaging techniques also provide important information concerning both systolic and diastolic cardiac function and thus may be useful to accurately and reproducibly follow patients through their courses of chemotherapy. A few centers make extensive use of the first-pass study, whereby a bolus of isotope is followed as it passes through the heart, thus identifying changes in chamber dimensions during the cardiac cycle. Left ventricular and right ventricular ejection fractions may be calculated accurately from these data (50).

The most widely used nuclear technique for estimating cardiac function is the cardiac blood pool scan, a method extensively used and studied in evaluating patients receiving Adriamycin or other cardiotoxic agents. The technique requires electrocardiographic gating and an acquisition time of several minutes during which data are accumulated in a computer memory bank. These data can then be manipulated to provide an estimation of ejection fraction, information regarding wall motion symmetry, and parameters of cardiac relaxation (diastolic function). Because of the long acquisition time and the required gating, patients with cardiac rhythm disturbances and patients who cannot lie motionless are better studied with ultrasonic or first-pass techniques.

Echocardiographic measurements of cardiac function are often used to evaluate patients receiving Adriamycin. Fractional shortening, circumferential shortening, and systolic time intervals may be calculated but offer no clinical advantage over the more commonly used ejection fraction. Changes in diastolic function as an early sign of cardiotoxicity are being studied; following changes in parameters of diastolic function following doxorubicin may hold promise but have not yet been shown to have clear advantages over the commonly used ejection fractions (51). Echocardiography is generally preferred over nuclear studies in pediatric patients and those with dysrhythmias.

The generally employed studies of myocardial function have suboptimal predictive value. At low cumulative doses of a regimen with dose-related toxicity, false-positive results may far exceed true-positive evidence of cardiac dysfunction. Failure to recognize this phenomenon may result in overuse of expensive functional tests and limit the use of potentially important therapy because of the fear of cardiotoxicity.

Cardiac Biopsy

Evaluation of structural changes in myocardial tissue obtained by cardiac biopsy from patients treated with anthracyclines provides vital information concerning the toxicity of Adriamycin and related compounds (10, 52–54). Studying biopsy material offers the best clinical measure of cardiac damage and, in selected patients, provides essential information needed to arrive at a decision as to whether or not to continue or terminate chemotherapy using cardiotoxic drugs.

The procedure for obtaining myocardial tissue originated in Japan, where it was introduced in the early 1960s (55). The technique was later modified by investigators at Stanford University, where the original work describing the structural changes associated with Adriamycin was undertaken (53, 54, 56). Most laboratories obtain myocardial tissue from the right ventricle. The bioptome is an instrument about 16 inches in length with a scissors-like handle at one end connected to a biting jaw at the other. During the procedure, the bioptome is positioned at the apex of the right ventricle, and specimens are taken from the lower portion of the septum; entry is either via the right internal jugular vein or the femoral vein. Several small tissue specimens (usually three, but the number may vary according to the size of the individual specimens) measuring 2 to 3 mm in diameter are obtained and placed in 5% buffered glutaraldehyde solution for fixation. The procedure usually takes about 15 minutes and is routinely performed on an outpatient basis. Patients report little or no sensation during tissue removal. Major complications are rare but include cardiac tamponade from perforation of the free right ventricular wall with the bioptome, pericarditis, dysrhythmia, vagal stimulation with hypotension and bradycardia, and local problems associated with the venous access site. In a series of 1350 procedures, cardiac perforation with tamponade occurred in less than 0.6% of the patients. Minor problems were seen in 0.8% (57).

Billingham described distinctive ultrastructural changes in patients with Adriamycin cardiomyopathy: vacuolization due to distention of the sarcoplasmic reticulum, and myofibrillar dropout. In more severe cases, there is actual necrosis. Cardiac biopsy specimens are therefore graded according to their ultrastructural changes as seen by electron microscopy; light microscopy is rarely useful (53, 54, 58, 59). The original Billingham grading system ranged from grade 0 (no evidence of anthracycline damage) to grade 3 (severe changes affecting the majority of cells), with grade 2 constituting intermediate damage (53). Later modifications to the scale by Billingham divided grade 2 into two subgroups, 2-A and 2-B (60). The grading system was also modified by Mackay et al., whereby the intermediate grades of 0.5 and 1.5 were added; grade 3 changes are rarely seen with careful dose limitation or continuous infusion schedules (8, 59). The Mackay grading system is semiquantitative, with both the degree and the extent of the abnormalities contributing to the final grade. It is not unusual to find completely normal myocardium next to tissue demonstrating marked abnormalities, even though they occur on adjacent electron-microscopic grids; thus, adequate specimens are essential to grade the tissue properly. A tissue grade of 0 is applied to specimens in which myocardial fibers appear normal, while higher grades show progressively increasing changes of dilation of the sarcoplasmic reticulum, myofibrillar dropout, and necrosis.

The biopsy grade is the single most sensitive parameter in assessing the degree of myocardial damage due to anthracyclines, but it does not take other causes of cardiac damage into account. Other forms of damage may be seen in the cancer patient, and so a combination of functional tests (ejection fraction) and morphologic studies (biopsy grade) offers the best guide for following patients receiving unusually high cumulative dosages of these drugs or patients with multifactorial myocardial dysfunction (8, 10, 61).

Patients who have received 200 to 400 mg/m^2 of Adriamycin by standard schedules, who do not have a history of heart disease, and are without risk factors for toxicity demonstrate a median biopsy grade of 1, a level not usually associated with clinical cardiac symptoms; patients who have received 400 to 500 mg/m^2 have

a median biopsy grade of 1.5; while those who have received more than 500 mg/m^2 have a median biopsy grade of 2 or higher (10). This dose/biopsy-grade relationship establishes the fact that morphologic changes in the myocardium are detectable at doses unlikely to be associated with clinically evident cardiac dysfunction. In addition, a high-grade cardiac biopsy ($\geq$1.5) predicts a high risk of developing congestive heart failure with continued drug administration (10). Thus, the biopsy grade establishes a cardiac damage scale with which to measure the degree of damage to the heart of an individual patient, but which also provides a damage scale on which the cardiotoxic effects of other anthracyclines or of different dosage schedules can be measured and compared. The cardiac damage scale has allowed a comparison of extended-dose (continuous infusion) schedules with standard infusion administration, as well as comparisons of other anthracyclines (epirubicin) or anthraquinones (mitoxantrone) with each other and with Adriamycin (62–64). Such comparisons have contributed significantly to our understanding of the relative cardiotoxicities of different drugs and various administration schedules (Table 33.2).

Risk Factors for Anthracycline-Associated Cardiac Dysfunction

Several groups of patients appear to be at greater risk of developing cardiac dysfunction at relatively low doses of anthracyclines. Extremes of age are an established risk factor for greater toxicity, and careful attention to monitoring is essential in both the pediatric and geriatric populations (5, 61, 65–68). Some forms of underlying heart disease predispose patients to increased damage (61, 68, 69). Evidence suggests that the common denominator may be increased left ventricular wall tension. Frequently encountered entities that fall into this category include conditions with gradients across the left ventricular outflow tract such as aortic stenosis, systemic hypertension, or cardiomyopathies of all types, including hypertrophic cardiomyopathy. A recent report suggests that female gender may also be a risk factor for Adriamycin cardiotoxicity when initial treatment is given during childhood (70). In contrast, no such relationship was noted in the large prognostic factor study of Von Hoff et al., although patients of all ages were evaluated in that study (68). Ischemic heart disease not associated with myopathy may add some risk in that the increased metabolic needs associated with

Table 33.2. Comparision of Relative Toxicities of Different Cardiotoxic Drugs and Dosage Schedules[a]

Drug	Schedule	Relative Myelosuppressive Potency of Single Dose Compared with Doxorubicin Administered by Standard Schedule	Approximate Relative Cardiotoxicity[b]	Cardiotoxicity Index Compared with Doxorubicin Administered by Standard Schedule[c]	Recommended Maximum Dose[d] (mg/m²)
Doxorubicin	Rapid infusion	1	1	1	400
Doxorubicin	Weekly	1	0.7	0.7	550
Doxorubicin	24-hr infusion	1	0.62	0.62	550
Doxorubicin	48-hr infusion	1	0.57	0.57	625[d]
Doxorubicin	96-hr infusion	1	0.5	0.5	800–1,000[d]
Epirubicin	Rapid infusion	0.67	0.66	0.44	900
Mitoxantrone	Rapid infusion	5	0.5	2.5	160
Daunorubicin	Rapid infusion	0.67	0.75[e]	0.5[e]	800[e]
Idarubicin	Rapid infusion	5	0.53	2.67	150
Pirarubicin	Rapid infusion	1	0.62	0.62	650[e]
Doxorubicin + Dexrazoxane	Rapid infusion	1[e]	0.5[e]	0.5[e]	800–1,000[e]
Doxorubicin 300 mg/m² + Dexrazoxane	Rapid infusion	1[e]	0.73[e]	0.73[e]	550[e]

[a]From Holland JF, Frei E III, Bast RC Jr, et al. Cancer Medicine. 4th ed. Baltimore: Williams & Wilkins, 1996. With permission.
[b]Factor by which the cardiotoxic effects of the cumulative dose of rapid infusion doxorubicin can be compared with the cumulative dose of the agent, combination and schedule listed, when given at an equivalent myelosuppressive dose. Dose producing clinically significant congestive heart failure in 5% of patients.
[c]Derived by dividing 400 mg/m², the recommended maximum dose of rapid infusion doxorubicin, by the recommended maximum dose for the agent in question. The Cardiotoxicity Index represents a factor with which to multiply the cumulative dose of a drug administered to obtain an approximation of toxicity that might be expected had the resultant amount of doxorubicin been given by rapid infusion. For example, if a cumulative dose of 120 mg/m² mitoxantrone had been administered, the patient would be expected to demonstrate cardiac damage approximately equal to 300 mg/m² doxorubicin given by rapid infusion ($120 \times 2.5 = 300$). This value is useful when changing from one cardiotoxic regimen to another. When the sum of the products of the indices and the cumulative doses administered exceeds 400, the risk of clinically significant cardiotoxicity exceeds 5%.
[d]Less toxic by endomyocardial biopsy.
[e]Inadequate data.

chemotherapy may offset a precarious balance between oxygen supply and demand. Anthracyclines and related agents are not known to cause primary myocardial ischemia.

Irradiation through portals that include the heart is a well-documented risk factor for developing cardiomyopathy at lower cumulative doses of Adriamycin. Patients with prior cardiac radiation require close monitoring and a reduction of cumulative dose (53, 68). Malnutrition, at least in children, has also been reported to potentiate Adriamycin cardiotoxicity (71).

A number of other antineoplastic drugs have also been associated with increased Adriamycin toxicity. Cyclophosphamide is the most extensively studied, and its compounding effect on Adriamycin toxicity is of particular clinical importance because the drugs are often used together. While there is evidence both for and against additional clinical cardiac toxicity of Adriamycin and cyclophosphamide in combination, cyclophosphamide at high doses is known to be cardiotoxic, and the combination is definitely more cardiotoxic in a monkey model (5, 72). Actinomycin D, mithramycin, mitomycin C, etoposide, melphalan, vincristine, bleomycin, and dacarbazine all reportedly increase Adriamycin toxicity, but the evidence for all but mitomycin C has not been persuasive (73–76). On the other hand, mitomycin C appears to add substantially to Adriamycin toxicity, even when given after the completion of Adriamycin therapy (77). Other anthracyclines and related agents such as mitoxantrone (an anthraquinone), demonstrate intrinsic cardiac toxicity that is additive (see below) (62, 78).

Schedule Dependency

Decreased anthracycline cardiotoxicity can be achieved through modification of the dose schedule. The initial suggestions by Weiss et al. were viewed with skepticism, primarily because the endpoint, clinical congestive heart failure attributed to Adriamycin, was vague (79). Despite confirmation of their findings by Chlebowski et al., it was not until the large review of approximately 4000 patients by Von Hoff and colleagues that statistically significant, decreased cardiac toxicity of weekly administration was acknowledged (66, 80). The review encompassed a number of studies that analyzed the relationship between the cumulative incidence of heart failure and cumulative dose. The weekly schedule allowed approximately 200 mg/m^2 of additional Adriamycin to be given above the amount usually tolerated with the standard (rapid infusion, 21- to 28-day cycle). No such benefit was detected when the drug was given by a three-consecutive-day schedule.

Subsequently, in studies of 100 and 146 patients, highly significant decreases in cardiac toxicity were noted on cardiac biopsies with weekly Adriamycin schedules (81, 82). In one study, it was estimated that patients treated with weekly Adriamycin could receive an additional 168 mg/m^2 (81). The most plausible interpretation of the data was that Adriamycin cardiotoxicity is related to peak plasma levels. The best way to decrease peak levels is to prolong infusion time. Thus, a series of trials of continuous infusion Adriamycin was initiated at The University of Texas M. D. Anderson Cancer Center using infusion times of 24 to 96 hours and measuring cardiotoxicity by endomyocardial biopsy (7, 36, 52, 64, 83–85). Patients treated with continuous infusions had a significantly lower incidence of high-grade endomyocardial pathologic changes on biopsy, despite significantly higher cumulative doses. Antitumor activity in patients with breast cancer or sarcoma was comparable to activity in historic controls (84, 85).

Randomized studies in patients with soft tissue sarcomas and osteosarcoma confirmed equivalent antitumor activity of continuous infusion and bolus administration (86, 87). Similar activity has been noted in other cancers, but for-

mal trials demonstrating the point have not been carried out. The longer the infusion duration, the less the observed cardiac toxicity (Table 33.2) (10, 36). Twenty-four-hour infusions are similar to weekly administration and permit the administration of an additional 150 to 200 mg/m^2 of doxorubicin with equivalent cardiotoxicity. Longer infusions allow still more doxorubicin to be administered before similar degrees of toxicity are seen. With 48-hour infusions, 600 to 650 mg/m^2 can be given, and with 96-hour infusions, 800 to 1000 mg/m^2 can be given with less cardiotoxicity than is seen with 450 mg/m^2 of rapid-infusion doxorubicin (10). The cardiotoxicity of prolonged (30 to 90 days) continuous infusions has not been well defined. Infusions shorter than 48 hours should be avoided unless mucositis limits adequate dosage. The inconvenience of the portable infusion pumps and indwelling catheters that are required for continuous-infusion doxorubicin protocols have contributed to the reluctance of many clinicians to use such schedules. Many oncologists continue to use conventional, less cumbersome schedules or less toxic analogues.

Cardiac Protectors

Many compounds have been studied to evaluate possible protection of the myocardium from anthracycline-associated cardiotoxicity. Initially, free-radical scavengers were tried; however, vitamin E (α-tocopherol) did not offer clinically useful protection in human subjects, nor was N-acetylcysteine useful (88, 89).

The most interesting agent to protect patients from the cardiotoxic effects of Adriamycin is the iron chelator dexrazoxane (Zinocard, ICRF-187), an agent from the group of bisdiketopiperazines. In a study of 92 patients randomized to receive an Adriamycin-containing regimen (50 mg/m^2 Adriamycin with 500 mg/m^2 cyclophosphamide and 500 mg/m^2 fluorouracil given every 21 days) or the same regimen together with dexrazoxane, the investigators found a significant decrease in cardiotoxic effects as determined by ejection fractions, biopsy grades, and clinical signs or symptoms of cardiac dysfunction (12, 90). Other toxicities and antitumor effects were unaffected.

Subsequent studies, while confirming the cardioprotective activity of dexrazoxane, indicated a possible decrease in antitumor effect as well. One explanation for this unexpected result comes from a preclinical study that indicated a decrease in cytotoxicity and topoisomerase II—

mediated DNA breaks when dexrazoxane was given with anthracyclines (29). There was no suggestion of diminished clinical antineoplastic activity when dexrazoxane was given to patients who had already received 300 mg/m^2 Adriamycin (personal communication, Dr. Sunil Gupta, Medical Director, Pharmacia Inc., Columbus, Ohio).

It is difficult to compare the relative benefits of dexrazoxane given with conventional-dose Adriamycin with those of continuous-infusion Adriamycin without dexrazoxane. Preliminary data, however, suggest that dexrazoxane offers cardiac protection equivalent to that of the 96-hour continuous-infusion Adriamycin schedule. The cardioprotective activity of dexrazoxane additionally offers promise that other drugs may also selectively diminish cardiac toxicity. The drug has recently been approved in the United States for patients who have previously received at least 300 mg/m^2 of Adriamycin and who are to receive additional treatment with that drug. The use of dexrazoxane in pediatric patients or in patients considered for retreatment after initial primary or adjuvant treatment is under consideration. The ultimate role of dexrazoxane in preventing Adriamycin cardiotoxicity has not been defined and will require further studies.

Cardiac Monitoring of Patients Receiving Doxorubicin

Most patients undergoing treatment for cancer can tolerate at least some Adriamycin. Patients with significant cardiomyopathy or patients who have experienced cardiotoxicity from anthracyclines or related drugs are the major exceptions. Patients being evaluated for Adriamycin therapy are screened, starting with a complete medical history and physical examination. Initial laboratory studies include a chest roentgenogram and a determination of ejection fraction.

Patients with risk factors for early toxicity should be monitored closely from the outset, with a follow-up examination and determination of left ventricular function after every one or two cycles. Patients without risk factors should be reassessed after receiving a cumulative dose of 300 to 350 mg/m^2 by standard infusion or its equivalent by a less cardiotoxic schedule (Table 33.2) and after each two cycles thereafter only if continuation of doxorubicin beyond the doses recommended in Table 33.2 is deemed critical from an oncologic point of view. The most important aspect, however, is keeping track of cumulative dose, since within this dose range, the risk of heart failure is 5% or less in the absence of other cardiac risk factors.

Patients who continue to have an ejection fraction of 60% or more generally tolerate their next cycle of Adriamycin well, while patients with ejection fractions of 45% or less are at considerably increased risk (10). Patients with intermediate ejection fractions that have not changed from baseline and who have received bolus equivalents of less than 400 mg/m^2 generally can continue with the next cycle of Adriamycin-containing chemotherapy. Patients with intermediate ejection fractions that have shown a decrease from the baseline or patients who have received more than 400 mg/m^2 (standard schedule) should be considered for alternate therapy with a noncardiotoxic regimen or evaluation with cardiac biopsy if further anthracycline therapy is necessary. Exercise testing in patients with intermediate ejection fractions is not useful in predicting future cardiotoxicity (91). For patients who continue their treatment above cumulative dosages of 400 mg/m^2 of Adriamycin and who have intermediate ejection fractions, reevaluation of the ejection fraction prior to every cycle and of the biopsy grade prior to every second cycle is appropriate. A biopsy grade of 1.5 is a contraindication to continued anthracycline treatment (10).

OTHER ANTHRACYCLINES AND ANTHRAQUINONES

Clinically, the cumulative dose-related cardiotoxicity of daunorubicin, idarubicin, epirubicin, pirarubicin, and mitoxantrone is identical to that seen with Adriamycin. The cumulative dosage likely to cause cardiotoxicity, however, is different for each agent; none has been studied as extensively as has Adriamycin.

Based on data derived from ejection fractions and from cardiac biopsy specimens, at equivalent oncologic dosages, epirubicin demonstrates a small but statistically significant decrease in cardiac toxicity, compared with Adriamycin given by rapid infusion (Table 33.2) (63, 92). It is similar to weekly Adriamycin but is considerably more toxic than Adriamycin administered by 96-hour continuous infusion (63). Mitoxantrone, an anthraquinone, demonstrates cardiotoxicity almost identical to that of 96-hour continuous infusion Adriamycin (62, 93). Idarubicin is the least studied commercially available anthracycline, since it is used only in the treatment of leukemia. Preliminary data suggest that 150 mg/m^2 intravenously is a safe cumulative dose for patients without previous anthracycline exposure (94). THP Adriamycin (pirarubicin), a doxorubicin analogue, is used in Japan and France; preliminary data suggest that it may have significantly less cardiotoxicity than Adriamycin given by standard infusion schedules (95).

Crossing over from one agent to another does not offer protection, and considerable care must be exercised when offering a new cardiotoxic treatment to a patient who has been previously treated with other cardiotoxic regimens. The best approach to prescribing cardiotoxic agents in sequence is to calculate the percentage of the maximum cumulative dose already used (Table 33.2) and subtract from 100% to estimate the percentage of the maximum cumulative dose of the second agent that is unlikely to cause permanent cardiac damage.

TREATMENT

The most important treatment consideration in managing patients with anthracycline-associated cardiac dysfunction is the avoidance of additional cardiotoxic regimens. Once established, cardiac dysfunction resulting from cardiotoxic therapies differs little from other forms of cardiomyopathy and is usually treated according to similar guidelines. Mild left ventricular dysfunction, with or without obvious fluid retention, can be managed with diuretics and salt restriction; some patients can be treated with alternate-day diuretic therapy alone (furosemide 20 to 40 mg orally). When more serious cardiac dysfunction is present, agents to reduce afterload, such as captopril (6.25 to 25 mg three times daily) or enalapril (5 to 20 mg two times daily), are useful and often result in subjective as well as objective improvement. Digitalis preparations (digoxin 0.125 to 0.25 mg daily, titrated to a serum digoxin level of 1.4 to 1.7) improve cardiac contractility and may be added to the regimen either before or following afterload-reducing agents. The success of treatment depends, in part, upon the interval between administration of the drug and the diagnosis of cardiac dysfunction. It is also related to administration schedule. If heart failure occurs less than 4 weeks from the last Adriamycin dose, it is much more likely to be fatal (5).

When the cardiac dysfunction is moderate or severe or associated with left ventricular dilation, or when persistent cardiac dysrhythmias are present, anticoagulation (warfarin sodium titrated to maintain the prothrombin time at about 1.5 times control) or antiplatelet therapy (enteric-coated aspirin, 300 mg daily) should be considered. In cases of severe cardiac dysfunction, bed rest and oxygen may be required. In selected cases, admission to an intensive care unit for intravenous vasopressor agents may be helpful. There is no specific therapy for chemotherapy-related cardiomyopathy. In selected patients who have achieved oncologic stability or cure, cardiac transplantation may be considered for the treatment of end-stage anthracycline-associated cardiomyopathy (96).

Other Drugs with Myocardial Depressant Activity

Significant decreases in myocardial function are occasionally noted with other agents. α-Interferon has been associated with a dramatic decrease in ejection fraction (97). The mechanism is unknown; patients surviving the initial episode usually go on to recover cardiac function. One reported case of interferon cardiotoxicity could be interpreted as indicating that interferon may provoke functional deterioration in a patient with asymptomatic Adriamycin cardiomyopathy (98). We, too, have observed such a case.

ANTINEOPLASTIC AGENTS ASSOCIATED WITH MYOCARDIAL ISCHEMIA

A number of agents have the potential for causing myocardial ischemia, with or without frank myocardial infarction. The agent most extensively studied that demonstrates this effect is 5-fluorouracil (5-FU) (99, 100). The ischemic events are seen more frequently when the agent is administered in combination with cisplatin. Isolated reports of myocardial ischemia have also appeared following the administration of vinblastine, vincristine, bleomycin, cisplatin, and biologic-response modifiers such as interleukin-2 (101). The wide spectrum of ischemic responses suggests that such phenomena occur more frequently than is generally appreciated.

Electrocardiographic change of a nonspecific variety may be seen in nearly half the patients treated with 5-FU, and as many as 16% show electrocardiographic evidence of ischemia (ST segment depression or elevation, or changes suggesting myocardial infarction) (100). Many of these patients have underlying coronary artery disease, suggesting that preexisting coronary artery abnormalities may augment the ischemic potential of 5-FU. The mechanism of ischemia is uncertain, but coronary artery vasoactivity or spasm probably plays a role; prevention by a calcium channel blocker has been reported (102). Selected patients may be treated with intravenous nitroglycerin or intravenous diltiazem during the administration of 5-FU, to reduce the risk of myocardial ischemia or infarction.

In patients with fixed arteriosclerotic lesions and an inability to increase their oxygen supply, high-output states may also result in myocardial ischemia. Ischemia may also result from fever often produced by biologicals (e.g., the interferons or interleukins) and from hyperthyroidism. Tumor necrosis factor has been associated with a hypercoagulable state, suggesting a possible alternate mechanism, vascular occlusion, in patients being treated with cytokines and other biologicals.

Patients showing evidence of myocardial ischemia, regardless of mechanism, should be observed closely for rhythm abnormalities; the level of observation and intervention should depend on the overall prognosis. Individuals with known preexisting coronary artery disease can be placed on a calcium channel–blocking agent (diltiazem 60 mg given orally three times a day) or a long-acting nitrate to help reduce the likelihood of developing exacerbations of angina. Controlled underlying ischemia or evidence of ischemia associated with antineoplastic therapy should not be considered an absolute contraindication for further treatment with the implicated agent or agents.

ANTINEOPLASTIC AGENTS ASSOCIATED WITH HYPOTENSION

Many patients develop some degree of hypotension as a consequence of their chemotherapy. The most frequent cause is volume depletion, often as a result of nausea and vomiting. Other causes of hypotension related to chemotherapy are decreased cardiac output, loss of vascular tone, and increased permeability of the small vessels and capillaries (capillary leak). Most instances of hypotension in patients receiving chemotherapy are transient phenomena that can be managed with careful monitoring and administration of fluids or vasopressor agents. Rare instances of profound hypotension have been reported and may be life threatening.

Interleukin-2 is associated with significant hypotension, frequently requiring pressor agents; the phenomenon is usually transient. Interleukin-2-related myocardial ischemia, the exact mechanism of which has not yet been determined, is possibly related to the hypotension, though a direct toxic effect has not been excluded. Interleukin-2 is also associated with an increased incidence of supraventricular dysrhythmia (103, 104).

Homoharringtonine, an investigational agent used in the treatment of leukemias, is associated with dose-related, sometimes severe, hypotension that is seen immediately following intravenous administration of the drug (105). Intravenous epinephrine has been helpful in stabilizing patients in this setting.

MISCELLANEOUS AGENTS WITH KNOWN OR SUSPECTED CARDIOTOXICITY

PACLITAXEL

Considerable interest has surrounded the possible cardiac effects of the recently approved agent paclitaxel. Asymptomatic bradycardia has occurred in 29% of patients who were treated with maximum tolerated doses of paclitaxel, and more severe rhythm abnormalities have been reported, but usually on patients with underlying cardiac abnormalities or in the presence of electrolyte imbalance, and usually detected only with continuous electrocardiographic monitoring (106). After several studies requiring such monitoring, it was concluded that serious cardiac problems are rare with the use of this agent, and most patients can be treated without special monitoring (107, 108). Patients with significant underlying cardiac disease, however, have been excluded from most paclitaxel trials. The safety of this drug in patients with significant preexisting heart problems has, therefore, not yet been defined.

BLEOMYCIN

Bleomycin is an antitumor antibiotic unrelated to the anthracyclines and is most commonly used in treating lymphomas and testicular cancers. Its primary toxicity is pulmonary. It has been associated with at least four episodes of severe pericarditis, although its etiologic role is at best speculative, as the patients all received concomitant combination chemotherapy or had received mediastinal irradiation (109, 110). White et al. reported a small series of patients who experienced an acute chest pain syndrome during infusions of bleomycin (111). The 10 patients experienced retrosternal pressure and pain and/or pleuritic pain. About half the time, there were modest ECG changes, although one patient experienced diffuse ST-segment elevation, suggesting pericarditis. There were no long-term sequelae.

MITOMYCIN C

Cardiac damage from mitomycin C when given alone is rare but real; moreover, this agent clearly enhances the cardiotoxicity of anthracyclines (77, 112).

Alkylating Agents

CYCLOPHOSPHAMIDE

Cyclophosphamide is an alkylating agent, widely used both orally and intravenously. It has essentially no cardiac side effects at standard doses. However, there are occasional reports of cardiotoxicity when the drug is given at very high doses such as those used in preparation for a bone marrow transplant. Toxicity has ranged from minor, transient ECG changes and asymptomatic elevation of cardiac enzymes at a total dose of 100 mg/kg (2.5 g/m^2) to fatality at high doses. An unusual form of cardiac damage is associated with high-dose cyclophosphamide administration; when severe, the damage takes the form of a hemorrhagic myocarditis (72). The process is often acute, is related to the dose/course (usually $\geq$4.5 g/m^2) rather than the cumulative dose, and is associated with decreased ejection fractions and mean QRS voltage. While severe hemorrhagic myocarditis may be fatal, milder presentations may be asymptomatic and reversible (113). Treatment is supportive.

IFOSFAMIDE

Ifosfamide is a potent alkylating agent currently most used in treating sarcomas, testicular cancer, lymphomas, and gynecologic malignancies. Its primary toxicity is hemorrhagic cystitis, which can be largely eliminated by concomitant administration of the uroprotectant mesna; with mesna, its dose-limiting toxicities are nephrotoxicity and central neurotoxicity. Because of its structural similarity to cyclophosphamide, there is a theoretical possibility of cardiotoxicity, especially at high doses. Animal studies have shown that on a milligram-to-milligram basis, ifosfamide may cause more acute cardiac depression than cyclophosphamide (114).

Several human studies have reported congestive heart failure associated with ifosfamide administration, although it is not clear that ifosfamide was causally related to the heart failure (115,

116). A report of severe reversible cardiac dysfunction from high-dose ifosfamide concludes, "high-dose ifosfamide should be added to the list of antineoplastic therapies associated with major cardiac complications" (117). In that report, largely reversible cardiac dysfunction and clinical congestive heart failure was noted in 9 of 52 patients (53 treatment regimens) in the setting of a bone marrow transplant protocol with multiple agents; prior Adriamycin therapy; intensive hydration; a greater than 50% increase in serum creatinine in 8 of the 9, with significant renal insufficiency in 4 of the 9; and no mention of the confounding effects of sepsis. Despite the authors' contentions, our own extensive experience suggests that clinically significant cardiac dysfunction cannot be attributed directly to ifosfamide (118–120).

Because ifosfamide is frequently administered with Adriamycin, however, especially in treating sarcomas, the theoretical potential for increased cardiotoxicity of this regimen over treatment with Adriamycin alone should be kept in mind. Increased cardiac toxicity has not yet been reported, despite the frequent combination of these drugs (121–124). In a randomized study comparing Adriamycin and dacarbazine with the same two drugs plus ifosfamide in 339 eligible patients with sarcomas, the only two cases of congestive heart failure were on the arm without ifosfamide (121).

References

1. Ewer M, Benjamin R. Cardiac complications. In: Holland J, Frei E III, Bast R Jr, Kufe D, Morton D, Weischselbaum R, eds. Cancer medicine. Philadelphia: Lea & Febiger, in press.

2. Lefrak E, Pitha J, Rosenheim S, et al. A clinicopathologic analysis of adriamycin cardiotoxicity. Cancer 1973;32:302–314.

3. Blum R, Carter S. Adriamycin, a new anticancer drug with significant clinical activity. Ann Intern Med 1974;80:249–259.

4. Bonadonna G, Beretta G, Tancini G, et al. Adriamycin (NSC-123127) studies at the Istituto Nazionale Tumori, Milan. Cancer Chemother Rep 1975;6:231–245.

5. Minow R, Benjamin R, Lee E, et al. Adriamycin cardiomyopathy—risk factors. Cancer 1977;39:1397–1402.

6. Bristow M, Thompson P, Martin R, et al. Early anthracycline cardiotoxicity. Am J Med 1978;65:823–832.

7. Benjamin R, Legha S, Valdivieso M, et al. Reduction of Adriamycin cardiac toxicity by schedule manipulation. In: Muggia F, Young C, Carter S, eds. Anthracycline antibiotics in cancer therapy. The Hague: Martinus Nijhoff, 1982:352–357.

8. Ewer M, Ali M, Mackay B, et al. A comparison of cardiac biopsy grades and ejection fraction estima-

tions in patients receiving Adriamycin. J Clin Oncol 1984;2:112–117.

9. Mortensen S, Aabo K, Jonsson T, et al. Clinical and non-invasive assessment of anthracycline cardiotoxicity: perspectives on myocardial protection. Int J Clin Pharmacol Res 1986;6:137–150.

10. Benjamin R, Chawla S, Ewer M, et al. Adriamycin cardiac toxicity—an assessment of approaches to cardiac monitoring and cardioprotection. In: Hacker M, Lazo J, Tritton T, eds. Organ directed toxicities of anticancer drugs. Boston: Martinus Nijhoff, 1988:41–55.

11. Ali M, Ewer M. Cardiovascular problems in the patient with cancer: effects of chemotherapy. Prim Care Cancer 1989;9:29–32.

12. Speyer J, Green M, Kramer E, et al. Protective effect of the bispiperazinedione ICRF-187 against doxorubicin-induced cardiac toxicity in women with advanced breast cancer. N Engl J Med 1988;319:745–752.

13. Ghione M. Development of adriamycin (NSC-123127). Cancer Chemother Rep 1975;6:83–89.

14. Di Marco A. Adriamycin (NSC-123127): mode and mechanism of action. Cancer Chemother Rep 1975;6:91–106.

15. Lown J. Anthracycline and anthraquinone anticancer agents: current status and recent developments. Pharmacol Ther 1993;60:285–214.

16. Capranico G, Gutelli E, Zunino F. Change of the sequence specificity of daunorubicin-stimulated topoisomerase II DNA cleavage by epimerization of the amino group of the sugar moiety. Cancer Res 1995;55:312–317.

17. Skladanowski A, Konopa J. Interstrand DNA crosslinking induced by anthracyclines in tumor cells. Biochem Pharmacol 1994;47:2269–2278.

18. Skladanowski A, Konopa J. Relevance of interstrand DNA crosslinking induced by anthracyclines for their biological activity. Biochem Pharmacol 1994;47:2279–2287.

19. Bonner J, Liengswangwong V. Topoisomerase II-independent doxorubicin-induced cytotoxicity in an extremely doxorubicin-resistant cell line. Biochem Biopsy Res Commun 1994;198:582–589.

20. Zwelling L, Bales E, Altschuler E, et al. Circumvention of resistance by doxorubicin, but not by idarubicin, in a human leukemia cell line containing an intercalator-resistant form of topoisomerase II: evidence for a non-topoisomerase II-mediated mechanism of doxorubicin cytotoxicity. Biochem Pharmacol 1993;45:516–520.

21. Crow R, Crothers D. Inhibition of topoisomerase I by anthracycline antibiotics: evidence for general inhibition of topoisomerase I by DNA-binding agents. J Med Chem 1994;37:3191–3194.

22. Maragoudakis M, Peristeris P, Missirlis E, et al. Inhibition of angiogenesis by anthracyclines and titanocene dichloride. Ann NY Acad Sci 1994;732:280–293.

23. Bachur N, Yu F, Johnson R, et al. Helicase inhibition by anthracycline anticancer agents. Mol Pharmacol 1992;41:993–998.

24. Tanaka M, Yoshida S. Mechanism of the inhibition of calf thymus DNA polymerases alpha and beta by daunomycin and adriamycin. J Biochem 1980;87:911–918.

25. Montecucco A, Lestingi M, Rossignol J, et al. Lack of discrimination between DNA ligases I and III by two classes of inhibitors, anthracyclines and distamycins. Biochem Pharmacol 1993;45:1536–1539.

26. Look M, Musche E. Lipid peroxides in the polychemotherapy of cancer patients. Chemotherapy 1994;40:8–15.

27. Praet M, Ruysschaert J. In-vivo and in-vitro mitochondrial membrane damages induced in mice by adriamycin and derivatives. Biochim Biophys Acta 1993;1149:79–85.

28. Grataroli R, Leonardi J, Chautan M, et al. Effect of anthracyclines on phospholipase A1 activity and prostaglandin E2 production in rat gastric mucosa. Biochem Pharmacol 1993;46:349–355.

29. Sehested M, Jensen P, Sorensen B, et al. Antagonistic effect of the cardioprotector (+)-1,2-bis (3,5-dioxopiperazinyl-1-yl)propane (ICRF-187) on DNA breaks and cytotoxicity induced by topoisomerase II directed drugs daunorubicin and etoposide (VP-16). Biochem Pharmacol 1993;46:389–393.

30. Benjamin R. A practical approach to adriamycin (NSC 123127) toxicology. Cancer Chemother Rep 1975;6:191–194.

31. Weaver S, Fulkerson P, Lewis RP, et al. A paucity of chronic electrocardiographic changes with adriamycin therapy. J Electrocardiology 1978;11:233–238.

32. Wortman J, Lucas V, Schuster E, et al. Sudden death during doxorubicin administration. Cancer 1979;44:1588–1591.

33. Signori E, Guevarra D. Evaluation of cardiac arrhythmias by 24-hour Holter monitoring during adriamycin administration (abstract). Proc Am Assoc Cancer Res 1981;22:355.

34. de Planque M, Beukers A, Benraadt T, et al. Occurrence of rhythm and conduction disturbances before, during, and after anthracycline (abstract). Proc Am Soc Clin Oncol 1985;4:25.

35. Haq M, Legha S, Choksi J, et al. Doxorubicin-induced congestive heart failure in adults. Cancer 1985;56:1361–1365.

36. Benjamin R, Chawla S, Hortobagyi G, et al. Continuous-infusion adriamycin. In: Rosenthal C, Rotman M, eds. Clinical applications of continuous infusion chemotherapy and concomitant radiation therapy. New York: Plenum Press, 1986:19–25.

37. Myers C, McGuire W, Liss R, et al. Adriamycin: the role of lipid peroxidation in cardiac toxicity and tumor response. Science 1977;197:165–167.

38. Doroshow J. Role of reactive oxygen production in doxorubicin cardiac toxicity. In: Hacker M, Lazo J, Tritton T, eds. Organ directed toxicities of anticancer drugs. Boston: Martinus Nijhoff, 1988:31–40.

39. Doroshow J, Locker G, Myers C. Enzymatic defenses of the mouse heart against reactive oxygen metabolites: alterations produced by doxorubicin. J Clin Invest 1980;65:128–135.

40. Myers C. Role of iron in anthracycline action. In: Hacker M, Lazo J, Tritton T, eds. Organ directed toxicities of anticancer drugs. Boston: Martinus Nijhoff, 1988:17–30.

41. Bachur N. Adriamycin (NSC-123127) pharmacology. Cancer Chemother Rep 1975;6:153–158.

42. Olson R, Mushlin P, Brenner D, et al. Doxorubicin cardiotoxicity may be caused by its metabolite, doxorubicinol. Proc Natl Acad Sci USA 1988;85:3585–3589.

43. Minotti G, Cavaliere A, Mordente A, et al. Sec-

ondary alcohol metabolites mediate iron delocalization in cytosolic fractions of myocardial biopsies exposed to anticancer anthracyclines. Novel linkage between anthracycline metabolism and iron-induced cardiotoxicity. J Clin Invest 1995;95:1595–1605.

44. Steinherz L, Steinherz P, Tan C. Cardiac failure and dysrhythmias 6–19 years after anthracycline therapy: a series of 15 patients. Med Pediatr Oncol 1995; 24:352–361.

45. Ali M, Ewer M, Gibbs H, et al. Late doxorubicin-associated cardiotoxicity in children: the possible role of intercurrent viral infection. Cancer 1994;74:182–188.

46. Ferrans V. Overview of cardiac pathology in relation to anthracycline cardiotoxicity. Cancer Treat Rep 1978;62:955–961.

47. Aabo K, Mortsensen S, Jonsson T, et al. Acute cardiac failure from doxorubicin cardiotoxicity provoked in relation to second-look laparotomy. Cancer Treat Rep 1985;69:730–731.

48. Minow R, Benjamin R, Lee E, et al. QRS voltage change with Adriamycin administration. Cancer Treat Rep 1978;62:931–934.

49. Alexander J, Dainiak N, Berger H, et al. Serial assessment of doxorubicin cardiotoxicity with quantitative radionuclide angiocardiography. N Engl J Med 1979;300:278–283.

50. Dymond D, Elliot A, Stone D. Factors that affect the reproducibility of measurements of left ventricular function from first-pass radionuclide ventriculograms. Circulation 1982;65:311–322.

51. Ewer M, Ali M, Gibbs H, et al. Cardiac diastolic function in pediatric patients receiving doxorubicin. Acta Oncol 1994;33:645–649.

52. Benjamin R, Ewer M, MacKay B, et al. An endomyocardial biopsy study of anthracycline-induced cardiomyopathy—detection, reversibility, and potential amelioration (abstract). Proc AACR/ASCO 1979; 20:372.

53. Billingham M, Bristow M, Glastein E, et al. Adriamycin cardiotoxicity: endomyocardial biopsy evidence of enhancement by irradiation. Am J Surg Pathol 1977;1:17–23.

54. Billingham M, Mason J, Bristow M, et al. Anthracycline cardiomyopathy monitored by morphologic changes. Cancer Treat Rep 1978;62:865–872.

55. Sakakibara SS. Endomyocardial biopsy. Jpn Heart J 1962;3:537–543.

56. Mason J. Techniques for right and left ventricular endomyocardial biopsy. Am J Cardiol 1978; 41:887–892.

57. Ewer M, Carrasco C, MacKay B, et al. Cardiac biopsy procedures at a cancer center (abstract). Proc Am Soc Clin Oncol 1991;10:336.

58. Mackay B, Keyes L, Benjamin R, et al. Cardiac biopsy. Tex Soc Electron Microsc J 1980;11:7–15.

59. Mackay B, Ewer M, Carrasco C, et al. Assessment of anthracycline cardiomyopathy by endomyocardial biopsy. Ultrastruct Pathol 1994;18:203–211.

60. Billingham M. Role of endomyocardial biopsy in diagnosis and treatment of heart disease. In: Silver M, ed. Cardiovascular pathology. New York: Churchill Livingstone, 1991:1465–1468.

61. Bristow M, Mason J, Billingham M, et al. Doxorubicin cardiomyopathy: evaluation by phonocardiography, endomyocardial biopsy, and cardiac catheterization. Ann Intern Med 1978;88:168–175.

62. Benjamin R, Chawla S, Ewer M, et al. Evaluation of mitoxantrone cardiac toxicity by nuclear angiography and endomyocardial biopsy: an update. Invest New Drug 1985;3:117–121.

63. Chawla S, Benjamin R, Hortobagyi G, et al. Decreased cardiotoxicity of 96 hour continuous infusion adriamycin compared with epirubicin (abstract). Proc Am Soc Clin Oncol 1986;5:44.

64. Legha S, Benjamin R, Mackay B, et al. Reduction of doxorubicin cardiotoxicity by prolonged continuous intravenous infusion. Ann Intern Med 1982; 96:133–139.

65. Ramos A, Meyer R, Korfhagen J, et al. Echocardiographic evaluation of adriamycin cardiotoxicity in children. Cancer Treat Rep 1976;60:1281–1284.

66. Von Hoff D, Rozencweig M, Layard M, et al. Daunomycin-induced cardiotoxicity in children and adults: a review of 110 cases. Am J Med 1977;62:200–208.

67. Pratt C, Ransom J, Evans W. Age-related adriamycin cardiotoxicity in children. Cancer Treat Rep 1978;62:1381–1385.

68. Von Hoff D, Layard M, Basa P, et al. Risk factors for doxorubicin-induced congestive heart failure. Ann Intern Med 1979;91:710–717.

69. Minow R, Benjamin R, Gottlieb J. Adriamycin (NSC 123127) cardiomyopathy–an overview with determination of risk factors. Cancer Chemother Rep 1975;6:195–201.

70. Lipshultz S, Lipsitz S, Mone S, et al. Female sex and higher drug dose as risk factors for late cardiotoxic effects of doxorubicin therapy for childhood cancer. N Engl J Med 1995;332:1738–1743.

71. Obama M, Cangir A, Van Eys J. Nutritional status and anthracycline cardiotoxicity in children. South Med J 1983;76:577–578.

72. Appelbaum F, Strauchen J, Graw R, Jr, et al. Acute lethal carditis caused by high-dose combination chemotherapy. A unique clinical and pathological entity. Lancet 1976;1:58–62.

73. Mosijczuk A, Ruymann F, Mease A, et al. Anthracycline cardiomyopathy in children: report of two cases. Cancer 1979;44:1582–1587.

74. Bitran J. Doxorubicin cardiotoxicity and melphalan. Ann Intern Med 1981;95:243–244.

75. Praga C, Beretta G, Vigo P, et al. Adriamycin cardiotoxicity: a survey of 1273 patients. Cancer Treat Rep 1979;63:827–834.

76. Beretta G, Villani F. Cardiomyopathy in adults after combination adriamycin and DTIC. Cancer Treat Rep 1980;64:353.

77. Buzdar A, Legha S, Tashima C, et al. Adriamycin and mitomycin C: possible synergistic cardiotoxicity. Cancer Treat Rep 1978;62:1005–1008.

78. Schell F, Yap H, Blumenschein G, et al. Potential cardiotoxicity with mitoxantrone. Cancer Treat Rep 1982;66:1641–1643.

79. Weiss A, Metter G, Fletcher W, et al. Studies on Adriamycin using a weekly regimen demonstrating its clinical effectiveness and lack of cardiac toxicity. Cancer Treat Rep 1976;60:813–822.

80. Chlebowski R, Paroly W, Pugh R, et al. Adriamycin given as a weekly schedule without a loading course: clinically effective with reduced incidence of cardiotoxicity. Cancer Treat Rep 1980;64: 47–51.

81. Torti F, Bristow M, Howes A, et al. Reduced

cardiotoxicity of doxorubicin delivered on a weekly schedule. Assessment by endomyocardial biopsy. Ann Intern Med 1983;99:745–749.

82. Valdivieso M, Burgess M, Ewer M, et al. Increased therapeutic index of weekly doxorubicin in the therapy of non-small cell lung cancer: a prospective randomized study. J Clin Oncol 1984;2:207–214.

83. Legha S, Benjamin R, Mackay B, et al. Adriamycin therapy by continuous intravenous infusion in patients with metastatic breast cancer. Cancer 1982; 49:1762–1766.

84. Benjamin R, Yap B. Infusion chemotherapy for soft tissue sarcomas. In: Baker L, ed. Soft tissue sarcoma. The Hague: Martinus Nijhoff, 1983:109–115.

85. Hortobagyi G, Frye D, Buzdar A, et al. Decreased cardiac toxicity of doxorubicin administered by continuous intravenous infusion in combination chemotherapy for metastatic breast carcinoma. Cancer 1989;63:37–45.

86. Zalupski M, Metch B, Balcerzak S, et al. Phase III comparison of doxorubicin and dacarbazine given by bolus versus infusion in patients with soft-tissue sarcomas: a Southwest Oncology Group study. J Natl Cancer Inst 1991;83:926–932.

87. Bielack S, Bieling P, Fuchs N, et al. Can doxorubicin administration be altered from "bolus" to continuous infusion without compromising antineoplastic efficacy (abstract 0772). 5th Intl Cong Anti-Cancer Chemotherapy 1995;5:167.

88. Legha S, Wang Y, Mackay B, et al. Clinical and pharmacologic investigation of the effects of α-tocopherol on adriamycin cardiotoxicity. Ann NY Acad Sci 1982;393:411–417.

89. Myers C, Bonow R, Palmeri S, et al. A randomized controlled trial assessing the prevention of doxorubicin cardiomyopathy by N-acetylcysteine. Semin Oncol 1983;10:53–55.

90. Speyer J, Green M, Zeleniuch-Jacquotte A, et al. ICRF-187 permits longer treatment with doxorubicin in women with breast cancer. J Clin Oncol 1992;10:117–127.

91. Ewer M, Ali M, Chawla S, et al. A comparison of resting and exercise ejection fractions with cardiac biopsy grades in patients receiving adriamycin (abstract). Proc Am Soc Clin Oncol 1985;4:27.

92. Jain K, Casper E, Geller N, et al. A prospective randomized comparison of epirubicin and doxorubicin in patients with advanced breast cancer. J Clin Oncol 1985;3:818–826.

93. Allegra J, Woodcock T, Woolf S, et al. A randomized trial comparing mitoxantrone with doxorubicin in patients with stage IV breast cancer. Invest New Drugs 1985;3:153–161.

94. Anderlini P, Benjamin RS, Wong FC, et al. Idarubicin cardiotoxicity: a retrospective study in acute myeloid leukemia and myelodysplasia. J Clin Oncol 1995;13:2827–2834.

95. Benjamin R, Fenoglio C, Hortobagyi G, et al. Cardiotoxicity of pirarubicin (abstract). Proc Am Assoc Cancer Res 1990;31:178.

96. Armitage JM, Kormor R, Griffith B, et al. Heart transplantation in patients with malignant disease. J Heart Transplant 1990;9:627–629.

97. Crum E. Biological-response modifier-induced emergencies. Semin Oncol 1989;16:579–587.

98. Zimmerman S, Adkins D, Graham M, et al. Irreversible, severe congestive cardiomyopathy occurring in association with interferon alpha therapy. Cancer Biother 1994;9:291–299.

99. Mancuso L, Bondi F, Marchi S, et al. Cardiac toxicity of 5-fluorouracil. Report of a case of spontaneous angina. Tumori 1986;72:121–124.

100. Ewer M, Benjamin R, Hong W, et al. Electrocardiographic changes in patients receiving chemotherapy with 5-fluorouracil and cisplatinum with and without diethyldithiocarbamate (abstract). Proc 15th Intl Cong Chemo 1987:203.

101. Ognibene F, Rosenberg S, Lotze M, et al. Interleukin-2 administration causes reversible hemodynamic changes and left ventricular dysfunction similar to those seen in septic shock. Chest 1988;94:750–754.

102. Oleksowicz L, Bruckner H. Prophylaxis of 5-fluorouracil induced coronary vasospasm with calcium channel blockers. Am J Med 1988;85:750–751.

103. Lee R, Lotze M, Skibber J, et al. Cardiorespiratory effects of immunotherapy with interleukin-2. J Clin Oncol 1989;7:7–20.

104. Margolin K, Rayner A, Hawkins M, et al. Interleukin-2 and lymphokine-activated killer cell therapy of solid tumors: analysis of toxicity and management guidelines. J Clin Oncol 1989;7:486–498.

105. Legha S, Keating M, Pickett S, et al. Phase I clinical investigation of homoharringtonine (NSC 141633). Cancer Treat Rep 1984;68:1085–1091.

106. Rowinsky E, McGuire W, Guarnieri T, et al. Cardiac disturbances during the administration of Taxol. J Clin Oncol 1991;9:1704–1712.

107. Rowinsky E, Eisenhauer E, Chaudhry V, et al. Clinical toxicities encountered with paclitaxel (TAXOL). Semin Oncol 1993;20:1–15.

108. Gibbs H, Ewer M, Holmes F, et al. Cardiac monitoring during administration of Taxol-doxorubicin chemotherapy in patients with metastatic breast cancer: a preliminary report (abstract). Proc Am Soc Clin Oncol 1992;11:87.

109. Durkin W, Pugh R, Solomon J, et al. Treatment of advanced lymphomas with bleomycin (NSC-125066). Oncology 1976;33:140–145.

110. Mosende C, Gutierrez M, Caparros B, et al. Combination chemotherapy with bleomycin, cyclophosphamide and dactinomycin for the treatment of osteogenic sarcoma. Cancer 1977;40:2779–2786.

111. White D, Schwartzberg L, Kris M, et al. Acute chest pain syndrome during bleomycin infusions. Cancer 1987;59:1582–1585.

112. Ravrym M. Cardiotoxicity of mitomycin C in man and animals (letter). Cancer Treat Rep 1979; 63:555.

113. Gottdiener J, Appelbaum F, Ferrans V, et al. Cardiotoxicity associated with high dose cyclophosphamide therapy. Arch Intern Med 1981;141:758–763.

114. Herman E, Mhatre R, Warardekar V, et al. Comparison of the cardiovascular action of NSC-109,724 (ifosphamide) and cyclophosphamide. Toxicol Appl Pharmacol 1978;23:178–190.

115. Einhorn L. VP 16 plus ifosphamide plus cisplatin as salvage therapy in refractory testicular cancer. Cancer Chemother Pharmacol 1986;18:45S–50S.

116. Klein H, Wickramanayake P, Coerper C, et al. High-dose ifosphamide and mesna as continuous infusion over five days–a phase I/II trial. Cancer Treat Rep 1983;10:167–173.

117. Quezado Z, Wilson W, Cummion R, et al. High-dose ifosfamide is associated with severe, re-

versible cardiac dysfunction. Ann Intern Med 1993; 118:31–36.

118. Benjamin RS, Legha SS, Patel SR, et al. Single-agent ifosfamide studies in sarcomas of soft tissue and bone: the M. D. Anderson experience. Cancer Chemother Pharmacol 1993;31(Suppl 2):s174–179.

119. Patel S, Vadhan-Raj S, Trevino C, et al. Phase II study of high dose ifosfamide (HDI) + G-CSF in patients (PTS) with malignant bone tumors (BT) and metastatic soft-tissue sarcomas (STS) (abstract). Proc Am Soc Clin Oncol 1992;11:413.

120. Patel S, Hays C, Papadopoulos N, et al. Pilot study of high-dose ifosfamide (HDI) + G-CSF in patients with bone and soft-tissue sarcomas (abstract). Proc Am Soc Clin Oncol 1995;14:515.

121. Antman K, Crowley J, Balcerzak S, et al. An intergroup phase III randomized study of doxorubicin and dacarbazine with or without ifosfamide and mesna in advanced soft tissue and bone sarcomas. J Clin Oncol 1993;11(7):1276–1285.

122. Bramwell V, Quirt I, Warr D, et al. Combination chemotherapy with doxorubicin, dacarbazine, and ifosfamide in advanced adult soft tissue sarcoma. J Natl Cancer Inst 1989;81:1496–1499.

123. Elias A, Ryan L, Sulkes A, et al. Response to mesna, doxorubicin, ifosfamide, and dacarbazine in 108 patients with metastatic or unresectable sarcoma and no prior chemotherapy. J Clin Oncol 1989;7:1208–1216.

124. Elias A, Ryan L, Alsner J, et al. Mesna, doxorubicin, ifosfamide, dacarbazine (MAID) regimen for adults with advanced sarcoma. Semin Oncol 1990; 17:41–49.

34

Pulmonary Toxicity of Chemotherapeutic Drugs

David W. Koh and Mario Castro

The correlation between chemotherapeutic medications for malignancy and pulmonary toxicity has been known for decades. Advances in the chemotherapeutic armamentarium have enabled patients to live longer, yet the "double-edged sword" of chemotherapy toxicity has limited our ability to dramatically improve outcome in many malignancies. As the list of chemotherapeutic agents grows, so does the list of those agents causing lung injury (Table 34.1) (1–3). The clinician administering chemotherapy must be aware of the potential for significant morbidity and mortality from the pulmonary toxicity induced by these agents.

Evaluation of a chemotherapy patient who presents with pulmonary infiltrates represents a challenge for the clinician. Pulmonary infiltrates in an immunocompromised host can represent infection, metastatic disease, recurrence of the primary cancer, or pulmonary toxicity secondary to the chemotherapy itself. There are reports that two or more of the aforementioned etiologies of pulmonary disease occur in 5 to 20% of patients receiving chemotherapy (4). Therefore, even if there is a suspicion of chemotherapy-induced pulmonary toxicity, other sources of pulmonary disease must be evaluated. Currently, the diagnosis of pulmonary toxicity from chemotherapy lies in the exclusion of other factors.

The clinician should be alerted to the diagnosis of drug-induced lung injury when there is a history of drug exposure, subjective complaints (shortness of breath, nonproductive cough, fever), and objective evidence of a significant deterioration from baseline (pulmonary function tests, arterial blood gases, radiographs). This chapter provides an overview of the incidence of lung injury with certain well-known

agents, an insight into the pathogenesis of those agents for which the mechanism has been elucidated, the common and sometimes unusual clinical presentations of pulmonary toxicity, the effect on outcome from the underlying drug toxicity, and potential treatment modalities for the most commonly used chemotherapeutic agents.

INCIDENCE

The overall incidence of pulmonary disease caused by chemotherapeutic agents in a recent series was 20% (3). Of course, the incidence for each drug varies significantly. Bleomycin (5), nitrosoureas (6), mitomycin (7), busulfan (8), ara-C (9), interleukin-2 (10), and methotrexate (11) commonly have an association with pulmonary toxicity. However, many other antineoplastic agents are associated with pulmonary damage (Table 34.1). Predicting pulmonary toxicity from chemotherapeutic agents is complicated by the differing mechanisms of toxicity. Some agents, such as methotrexate, can produce an idiosyncratic reaction such as hypersensitivity pneumonitis (8, 11). Other agents, such as bleomycin, have a much more predictable incidence depending on the dose (8). Depending on the definition of drug-induced lung toxicity, reports of the specific incidences for various agents vary from series to series. Unfortunately, using current modalities of diagnosis, including lung biopsy, pulmonary function testing, and clinical presentation, there are no specific markers of toxicity. Complicating the issue further is the frequent use of combination therapy, including multiagent chemotherapy, radiation therapy, and high concentrations of oxygen, making it extremely difficult to identify a specific agent.

Table 34.1. Chemotherapeutic Agents Associated with Pulmonary Toxicity

Cytotoxic antibiotics	*Plant alkaloids*
Bleomycin	Vincristine
Peplomycin	Vinblastine
Liblomycin	Vindesine
Mitomycin C	Teniposide (VM-26)
Doxorubicin	Etoposide (VP-16)
Nitrosoureas	*Miscellaneous cytotoxics*
BCNU	Procarbazine
(carmustine)	Taxol
Methyl-CCNU	L-Asparaginase
(semustine)	
CCNU (lomustine)	
Alkylating agents	*Biologic response modifiers*
Busulfan	Interleukin-2
Cyclophosphamide	Granulocyte-macrophage
Ifosfamide	colony-stimulating factor
Melphalan	(GM-CSF)
Chlorambucil	Interferon—α, γ
	Bacillus-Calmette-Guerin
	(BCG)
Antimetabolites	
Methotrexate	
Azathioprine	
Cytarabine (ara-C)	
Fludarabine	

PATHOGENESIS

The elucidation of the pathogenesis of toxicity from antineoplastic medications is mostly derived from animal experimentation. Tracheal instillation of bleomycin into rats, a common technique for looking at injury patterns, has become a model of pulmonary fibrosis. Unfortunately, these mechanisms may not apply to humans, and well-defined pulmonary toxicity (based on histologic confirmation) in clinical trials is lacking. The following is a general overview of the potential mechanisms of drug-induced injury to the lung. There appear to be four common mechanisms of injury to the lungs: imbalance of the oxidant-antioxidant system, direct cytotoxic injury to the lung parenchymal cells, capillary leak syndrome, and a hypersensitivity reaction (Figure 34.1).

Damage from oxygen free radicals is one mechanism of tissue injury from chemotherapeutic agents. The oxidant molecules include superoxide anion (O_2^-), hydrogen peroxide (H_2O_2), hydroxyl radical (OH^-), singlet oxygen ($^1O_2$), and hypochlorous acid (HOCl). Injuries from these free radicals are prevented by anti-oxidants such as superoxide dismutase (SOD), glutathione peroxidase, catalase, ceruloplasmin, and α-tocopherol (vitamin E). The theory is that certain cytotoxic agents (bleomycin and cyclophosphamide) cause an imbalance by creating more oxidants or by reducing the antioxidants (BCNU and cyclophosphamide) (2). Thus, the normal antioxidant protective mechanisms available to scavenge oxygen radicals are overwhelmed, leading to an inflammatory, and subsequently fibrotic, reaction.

Given the nature of the medications, cytotoxic agents can directly injure alveolar endothelial cells and cause type I epithelial cell necrosis (12). For example, bleomycin toxicity is likely related to lack of an enzyme in the lung that inactivates bleomycin, allowing accumulation of intracellular bleomycin. Then, depending on the state of proliferation of the cell, DNA damage ensues, causing atypical metaplastic changes in the nuclei of type I and II cells (13).

Once cellular injury occurs, changes take place in the underlying lung matrix. There is a fine balance of collagen synthesis and breakdown in the lung. Increased collagen deposition can result in severe irreversible pulmonary fibrosis. Certain drugs such as bleomycin have been shown to stimulate fibroblast proliferation and directly increase collagen deposition (14, 15). Furthermore, the destruction of the lung parenchyma and the ensuing inflammatory process can activate neoproduction of elastin by actin-expressing smooth muscle cells, resulting in pulmonary fibrosis (16).

The capillary leak syndrome, or noncardiogenic pulmonary edema, is rare (2). Several agents, given either orally, intravenously, or intrathecally, can cause this response (Table 34.2) (3). The mechanism is unclear but is likely related to damage to the pulmonary endothelium by these agents. Mitomycin C, in particular, has a propensity to produce this reaction as part of the hemolytic uremic syndrome. Recent evidence suggests that mitomycin-induced lung injury may be the result of oxygen free radicals effect on the endothelium (17).

Pulmonary toxicity from some antineoplastic medications may represent an immunologic response such as that seen with drug hypersensitivity. Chemotherapeutic agents may stimulate the production of certain mediators (chemokines) responsible for attracting various inflammatory cells that then mediate this immunologic response. For example, bronchoalveolar lavage in patients with bleomycin-induced pulmonary

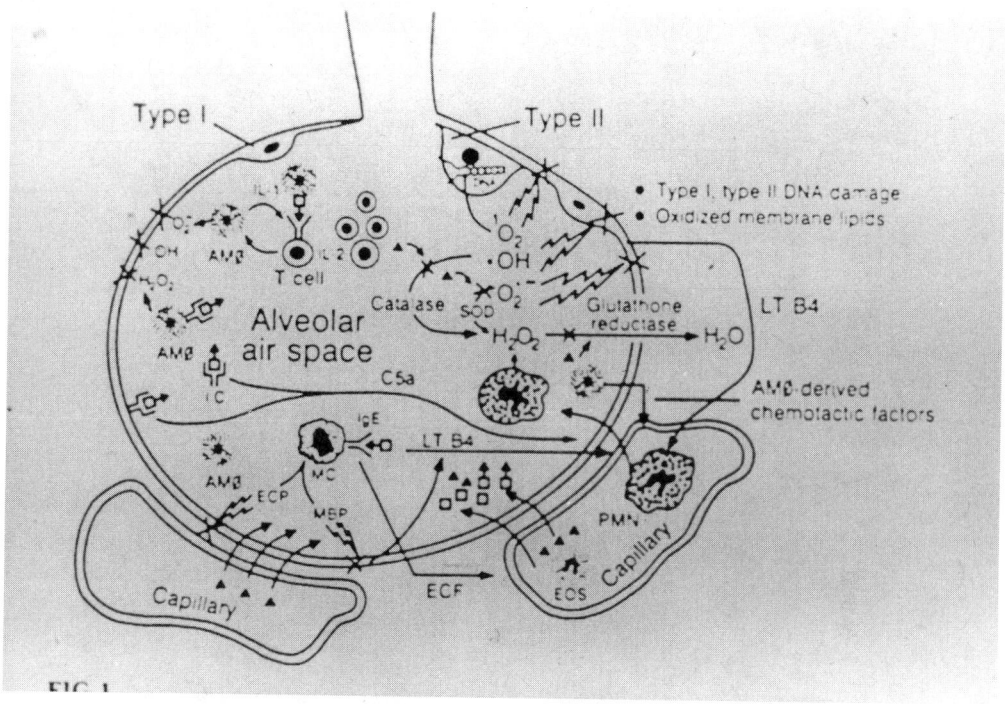

Figure 34.1.   Pathogenesis of chemotherapy-induced pulmonary toxicity. *IL-1*, interleukin 1; *IL-2*, interleukin 2; *AMϕ*, alveolar macrophage; *IC*, immune complex; *MC*, mast cell; *MBP*, major basic protein; *ECP*, eosinophil cationic protein; *ECF*, eosinophil chemotactic factor; *LTB4*, leukotriene B4; *EOS*, eosinophil; *PMN*, polymorphonuclear cell; SOD, superoxide dismutase. The *closed triangles* indicate the drug or drug metabolite (hapten); the *open squares* indicate the conjugate; and the *crossed lines* indicate injury to the alveolar capillary membrane and type I cells. (Reprinted with permission from Pisani RJ, Rosenow EC. Drug-induced pulmonary disease. In: Simmons DH, Tierney DF, eds. Current pulmonology, vol. 13. Philadelphia: Mosby Yearbook, 1992:311–348. With permission.)

toxicity demonstrates an increase in the number of neutrophils and lymphocytes (18, 19). Lymphocytes and macrophages may then in turn recognize the chemotherapeutic agent as a foreign antigen and elicit a hypersensitivity reaction. Agents known to cause a hypersensitivity pneumonitis with peripheral eosinophilia include bleomycin (20), methotrexate (11), and procarbazine (21, 22).

PATHOLOGY

The common pathologic finding in most chemotherapy-induced pulmonary toxicity is diffuse alveolar damage (Fig. 34.2). The changes seen include endothelial cell damage, disruption of the type I pneumocytes, and reactive changes from the type II pneumocytes. The reaction of the type II cells may cause the nuclei to look atypical. Nuclear changes can be so dramatic that the cells look malignant (3). The direct cytotoxic changes start as endothelial blebs in the alveolar capillaries associated with interstitial

Table 34.2. Chemotherapeutic Agents Known to Cause Noncardiogenic Pulmonary Edema

Cytarabine (ara-C) (9)
Methotrexate (248)
Cyclophosphamide (183)
Teniposide (VM-26) (249)
Mitomycin C (114)
Bleomycin ± oxygen (82)
Tumor necrosis factor (animal model) (250)
Interleukin-2 (10, 226)

edema (13). As the lesions progress, electron microscopy demonstrates a decrease in the number of type I pneumocytes and a proliferation of type II pneumocytes (8). The final pathway in some cases includes pulmonary fibrosis. Most of the cells seen in the alveoli and interstitium are mononuclear. A lymphocytic predominance occurs in the bronchoalveolar lavage fluid when diffuse alveolar damage is present. The impor-

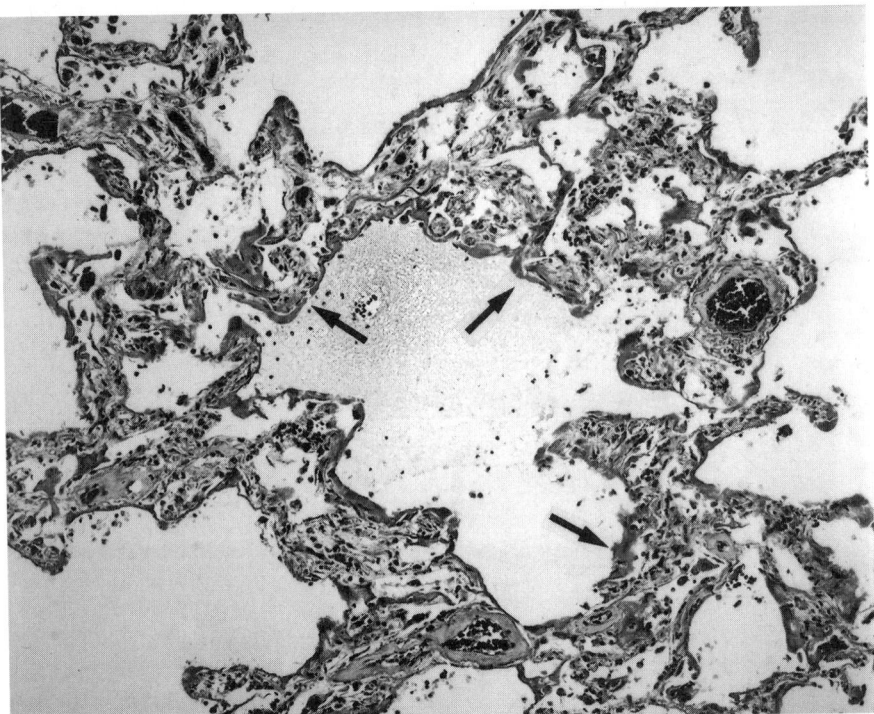

Figure 34.2.   Mitomycin C toxicity manifests as diffuse alveolar damage. The alveolar spaces are lined by hyaline membranes (*arrows*), and the interstitium is widened by a combination of edema and chronic inflammation (hematoxylin and eosin stain).

Table 34.3. Chemotherapeutically Induced Pulmonary Toxicity Presenting as Acute Respiratory Insufficiency

Bleomycin ± oxygen ± radiation (79, 82)
Mitomycin C (hemolytic uremic syndrome) (114)
Procarbazine
Methotrexate
Interleukin-2 (226)
Tumor necrosis factor (251)
Ara-C (212)
Interferon-α (252)
Doxorubicin radiotherapy (134)

Table 34.4. Chemotherapeutic Agents Associated with Bronchiolitis Obliterans

Bleomycin (253, 254)
Cyclophosphamide (255)
Methotrexate (201)
Procarbazine (256)
Mitomycin C (3)

tant exception to this occurs during a hypersensitivity pneumonitis when eosinophils infiltrate the interstitium and alveoli.

CLINICAL FEATURES

The clinical presentation varies according to the mechanism of injury from the antineoplastic agent. In general, patients complain of a nonproductive cough, fever, and dyspnea. However, the clinical spectrum can be insidious, starting with a mild cough and low-grade fever. Pulmonary injury may present acutely with respiratory insufficiency (Table 34.3) and the adult respiratory distress syndrome (ARDS) (Table 34.2). Weight loss is common (3). Other unique presentations of chemotherapy-induced pulmonary toxicity include: bronchospasm, pleural effusion, bronchiolitis obliterans (Table 34.4), pulmonary veno-occlusive disease (Table 34.5), "sarcoidosis," pulmonary alveolar proteinosis, pneumothorax, and pulmonary hemorrhage (3). Given the lack of specificity of clinical presentation, the clinician must factor in concomitant risk factors and objective data.

The associated risk factors tend to occur more frequently with particular agents (Table 34.6). The antineoplastic medications that are more often associated with lung injury include bleomycin, mitomycin C, BCNU, ara-C, methotrexate and interleukin-2. There is consensus that using combinations of bleomycin, cyclophosphamide, carmustine, methotrexate, or mitomycin C in a multidrug regimen increases the risk for pulmonary toxicity (23–27).

Bleomycin produces little myelosuppression, though it does appear to produce a more toxic effect on the lungs with increasing age of the patient (8) (Table 34.6). The incidence of pulmonary toxicity from bleomycin is relatively constant until above the age of 70 (28). Therefore, all patients, regardless of age, should be followed carefully for pulmonary toxicity.

Given the patient population, many have received prior, concomitant, or subsequent radiation therapy in addition to chemotherapy (Table 34.6). The incidence of complications from radiation depends substantially on the dose, the amount of lung tissue irradiated, and the specific chemotherapeutic agent used. For example, thoracic radiation for lung or breast cancer has a 10% risk of producing complications (29). Acute complications include radiation pneumonitis at 6 to 12 weeks postradiation, while long-term toxicity may be manifested as pulmonary fibrosis at 6 months to years after the irradiation (29). A total dose of 5000 rads to a 100 cm^2 area of lung or whole lung irradiation of 2500 rads leads to an approximate 50% incidence of acute or chronic pulmonary disease (30). Therefore, it is plausible that pulmonary damage from γ-irradiation predisposes patients to chemotherapy-induced pneumonitis. However, only bleomycin, busulfan, cyclophosphamide, and mitomycin C have demonstrated this association (2, 31).

High FiO_2 by itself can generate reactive oxygen species that, in turn, cause a cascade of damage to the alveoli and lung parenchyma (32). Alternatively, some chemotherapeutic agents induce pulmonary injury via release of oxygen free radicals. Therefore, it is not surprising that oxygen therapy may act in a synergistic manner with chemotherapeutic agents to injure the lung (Table 34.6). Agents thought to propagate lung injury with high FiO_2 include bleomycin (33), cyclophosphamide (33), mitomycin C(34), and BCNU (35).

Concomitant illnesses may predispose the patient to drug-induced toxicity (Table 34.6). Patients with sarcoidosis and leukemia appear to be at increased risk of pulmonary hemorrhage (36). Tobacco use appears to sensitize lung tissue to the effects of chemotherapy. In one study,

Table 34.5. Chemotherapeutic Agents Associated with Pulmonary Venoocclusive Disease (PVOD)

Bleomycin (257)
Mitomycin C (258)
BCNU (259)
Etoposide (VP-16) (3)
Cyclophosphamide (3)

Table 34.6. Risk Factors for Development of Chemotherapeutically Induced Pulmonary Toxicity

Risk Factor	Agent Implicated
Cumulative dose	Bleomycin (8), busulfan (8), carmustine (6, 143), interleukin-2 (232)
Age	Bleomycin (8)
Concurrent or previous radiotherapy	Bleomycin (79, 81), busulfan (170), mitomycin (7), cyclophosphamide (31), doxorubicin (131, 133–135), actinomycin D (132, 139, 140)
Oxygen therapy	Bleomycin (33, 82, 260, 261), cyclophosphamide (33), mitomycin (34)
Combination chemotherapy	Bleomycin (25, 86), carmustine (24), mitomycin (27), cyclophosphamide (25, 26, 86), methotrexate (26)
Preexisting lung disease	
COPD/Tobacco use	Carmustine (6), interleukin-2 (232)
Lymphoma	Bleomycin (28)
Sarcoidosis, leukemia (36)	

Modified with permission from Cooper JAD, White DA, Matthay RA. Drug-induced pulmonary disease. Part 1: cytotoxic drugs. Am Rev Respir Dis 1986;133:324.

BCNU toxicity appeared more frequently in patients with preexisting lung disease and tobacco use (6). Further evidence is provided by retrospective analysis of a study in which the combination of bleomycin, vinblastine, and cisplatin was given against germ cell tumors (37). Before therapy, the mean diffusion capacity (DL_{CO}) in nonsmokers was 88% of predicted and in smokers, 79%. After treatment, the DL_{CO}s dropped to 85% and 72%, respectively. The drop in DL_{CO} was statistically significant in the smokers; it was not in the nonsmokers, though clinical correlation with actual pulmonary toxicity was not reported in this subgroup nor in a previous study (38).

DIAGNOSIS

Although there may be clinical suspicion, arriving at a presumptive diagnosis is usually difficult. Chest radiographs have both a low specificity and sensitivity when used to evaluate drug-induced pulmonary disease. The typical radiographic presentation of bibasilar reticular-nodular infiltrates appears 6 weeks to 3 months after treatment (39) (Fig. 34.3A and B). Pleural effusions are uncommon but associated with some chemotherapeutic agents (Table 34.7) (31). Hypersensitivity pneumonitis most often presents as a diffuse acinar infiltrate; pleural effusions are more common in this setting (2). Most of the findings on computed tomography (CT) of the chest consist of scattered, predominantly peripheral and ill-defined opacities (40), though findings consistent with cardiogenic or noncardiogenic pulmonary edema can also be seen. CT of the chest (41, 42) and gallium-67 lung scans (43) have more sensitivity than chest radiographs but are not diagnostic of chemotherapy-induced toxicity. CT of the chest has not proven as sensitive as following DL_{CO} for detecting potential early pulmonary toxicity. In one study, CT of the chest was abnormal in only 65% of patients with chemotherapy-induced pulmonary toxicity, while all patients had some reduction in DL_{CO} (40). Another study reported only a 38% incidence of abnormalities on CT of the chest (42).

Pulmonary function tests may provide useful markers for heralding pulmonary toxicity. The most sensitive component of pulmonary function testing is the DL_{CO}, which may decrease prior to clinical symptoms or radiographic changes of pulmonary toxicity (44). Measurement of airflows and lung volumes are often not

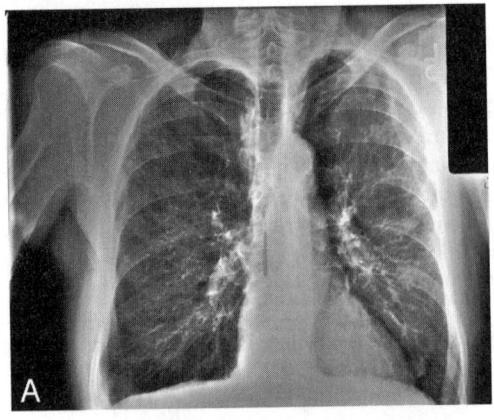

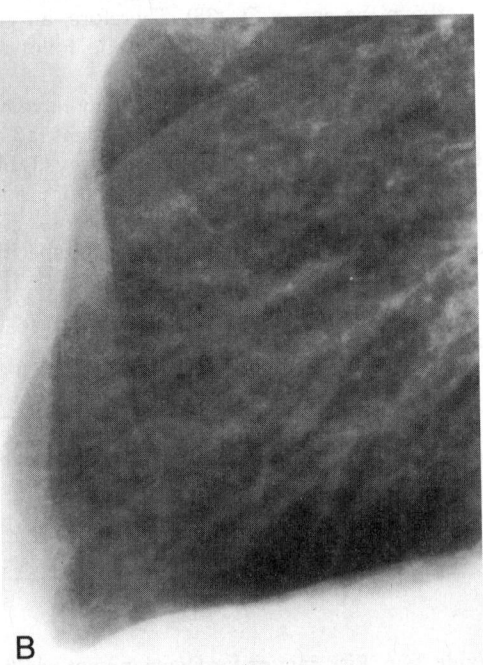

Figure 34.3. Chest radiograph of patient with mitomycin C pulmonary toxicity demonstrating (**A**) bilateral interstitial infiltrates with a predominance in the lower lungs and (**B**) septal lines.

sensitive enough to detect toxicity prior to clinical onset. Currently, serial measurements of DL_{CO} prior to initial therapy and subsequent cycles of chemotherapy appears to be the most effective way of screening for pulmonary toxicity when using certain agents, as discussed later. In general, a decline in the DL_{CO} of more than 25% from baseline is considered a significant change. In addition, when abnormal prior to treatment,

Table 34.7. Chemotherapeutic Agents Associated with Pleural Effusion

---

Mitomycin C (119, 122, 262)
Methotrexate
Granulocyte-macrophage colony-stimulating factor
(GM-CSF) (263)
Interleukin-2 (226)
Bleomycin (20)
Cytarabine (ara-C) (212)
Doxorubicin (131)
Fludarabine (221)
Procarbazine (21)
Melphalan (264)

---

measurement of DL_{CO} and room air blood gases may group patients into a high-risk category. Patients who have an alveolar-arterial O_2 difference of more than 30 mm Hg or a DL_{CO} less than 60% of that predicted prior to bone marrow transplantation have a higher mortality (45). In this patient population, it is important to keep in mind that the DL_{CO} should be corrected for the patient's hemoglobin level, as anemia significantly reduces the DL_{CO}. Furthermore, in a patient with reduced lung volumes (e.g., due to previous lung surgery or restrictive lung disease), the DL_{CO} should be corrected for the appropiate alveolar volume.

Fiberoptic bronchoscopy is useful in certain circumstances: (*a*) to exclude infectious etiologies, by either bronchoalveolar lavage or quantitative cultures from protected-brush specimens; (*b*) to obtain tissue for diagnosis, by either transbronchial lung biopsy or transbronchial needle aspirate; or (*c*) to point to a specific diagnosis; for example, eosinophilia in the bronchoalveolar lavage fluid may suggest the diagnosis of hypersensitivity pneumonitis. However, transbronchial biopsy specimens often do not show pathognomonic changes to conclusively confirm or exclude the diagnosis of drug-induced pulmonary toxicity. This likely reflects the small tissue sample that is obtained by transbronchial biopsies and the nonspecific pathologic features of chemotherapy-induced lung injury. Open lung biopsy, especially with the advent of video-assisted thoracoscopy, provides more lung tissue and therefore a better appreciation for generalized architectural changes. However, open lung biopsy places patients at greater risk, and the results may not affect clinical management (46, 47).

The treatment of pulmonary toxicity from chemotherapeutic agents depends on the specific agent and is discussed in detail below. In general, depending upon the severity of the toxicity, supportive therapy with oxygen, diuretics, bronchodilators, vasopressors, and artificial ventilation is provided as required. In most cases, the offending agent is removed, though in certain circumstances the drug may be continued with careful follow-up, as with methotrexate. Following discontinuation of the drug, many clinicians administer corticosteroids, depending upon the likelihood of response. The determinants of response include the specific offending agent, the duration of toxicity, the underlying immune competence and health of the individual, and the specific manifestation of toxicity (end-stage fibrosis from bleomycin is not likely to respond). The response to therapy is quite varied. In some instances, the response is quite dramatic, with complete resolution of clinical symptoms, radiographic abnormalities, and pulmonary function testing; in others, there is no response, and unfortunately, patients progress to death.

The second part of this chapter discusses the specific chemotherapeutic agents that are known to cause pulmonary toxicity (Table 34.1). The discussion of these agents follows, with classification into various groups by mechanism of action. Some agents in each category are not discussed because they lack an association with pulmonary toxicity. Newer agents are continuously added to this list as our experience with their usage and toxicity increases.

CYTOTOXIC ANTIBIOTICS

Bleomycin

Bleomycin is a cytotoxic antibiotic derived from *Streptomyces verticillus* (48). Its primary use is against squamous cell carcinomas of various organs, lymphomas, and testicular cancer (49, 50). Since the first clinical trials, there was documentation of its pulmonary toxicity and its low incidence of myelosuppression (51). Therefore, bleomycin's limitation rests in its propensity to cause lung injury with increasing doses. There is such predictability of pulmonary toxicity that it is used as a model of pneumonitis evolving to pulmonary fibrosis in many animal models.

There are many reasons why bleomycin has such a propensity to cause pulmonary injury. Most studies have been done on animal models though, based on clinical experience, they are also likely to be applicable to humans. Bleomycin preferentially concentrates in the lung and skin because those organs lack an enzyme, bleomycin A_2 hydrolase, which breaks bleomycin down (51, 52). Bleomycin A_2 hydrolase is an aminopeptidase that slowly inactivates bleomycin (53). The gene for bleomycin A_2 hydrolase has been cloned, and the tumor's resistance to bleomycin may be related to its ability to interact with this gene (54, 55). The type II pneumocyte is particularly susceptible to damage from bleomycin because it has a relative deficiency of bleomycin A_2 hydrolase (56). This supports the theory that bleomycin A_2 hydrolase is important in determining the pulmonary toxicity of bleomycin.

Another explanation for bleomycin's ability to injure the lung is based on the interaction of oxygen and bleomycin, leading to an imbalance of the oxidant/antioxidant system. Support for this theory comes from in vitro studies. Bleomycin becomes activated when it complexes with ferrous ions and oxygen to generate free radicals (57, 58). The radicals then preferentially cleave DNA at G-C and G-T sequences (59). Further evidence of the synergistic effect of oxygen and bleomycin is provided by experiments demonstrating decreased toxicity from bleomycin in

a hypoxic environment (60). Finally, SOD, an antioxidant, lessens the cytotoxicity induced by bleomycin in cell cultures (61). The concentration of SOD in patient's blood is inversely proportional to the cytotoxic effect of bleomycin by a chromosomal assay (62).

Bleomycin, by itself, appears to have the ability to stimulate the production of cytokines that may add to the cascade of destruction and inflammation (50). Bronchoalveolar lavage in patients with bleomycin-induced pulmonary toxicity demonstrates an increased number of neutrophils and lymphocytes (18, 19). It is thought that the bleomycin then causes release of superoxides from the neutrophils, though the role of these inflammatory cells in bleomycin toxicity is unclear (63).

Pathologic changes in the lung from bleomycin-induced toxicity follow a characteristic pattern (Fig. 34.4). In the first several days, there is tissue inflammation and edema. Along with type I pneumocyte injury, there is endothelial destruction and edema of the vasculature (13). This may account for the reduction in the DL_{CO} seen on pulmonary function testing (2). The disrupted type I cells die, and migration of the hy-

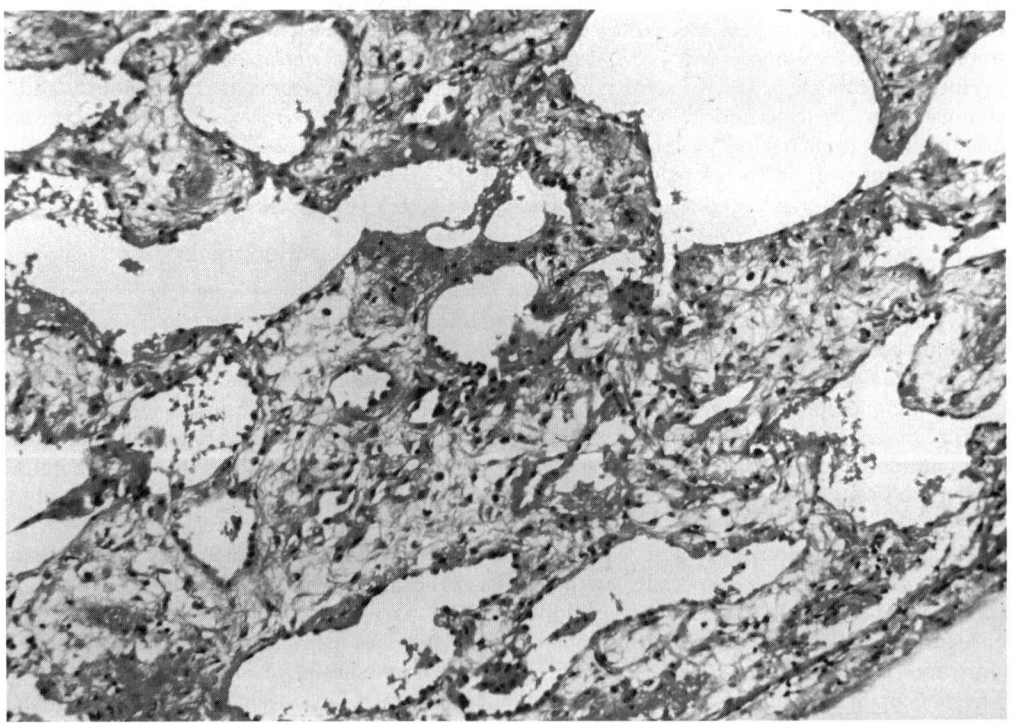

Figure 34.4. Histology of advanced bleomycin-induced lung injury with extensive interstitial fibrosis and a nonspecific interstitial pneumonitis.

perplastic and dysplastic type II cells takes place (12, 31). This marked atypia of the type II cell is felt by some pathologists to be quite characteristic of the cytotoxic changes induced by chemotherapy. Furthermore, there is alveolar hemorrhage as inflammatory cells infiltrate into the alveolar walls and airspaces (64). Cell destruction initiates chemotaxis of inflammatory cells such as lymphocytes, plasma cells, and macrophages by the fourth week (13). Many of these features give the histologic appearance of desquamative interstitial pneumonitis (DIP) and usual interstitial pneumonitis (UIP) (65).

This marked inflammatory reaction can then attract fibroblasts and other cells, leading to deposition of fibrin and collagen in the interstitium. The fibroblasts are exposed to a number of mediators, including transforming growth factor-β (TGF-β) and platelet-derived growth factor (PDGF), from the resident cells (18). TGF-β is a potent stimulus of type I and III collagen gene expression and production (66). PDGF is a potent chemokine and stimulator of connective tissue cells (67, 68). In animal models of bleomycin, both of these mediators have been demonstrated

to be important in the development of pulmonary fibrosis. This inflammatory process can also activate neoproduction of elastin by actin-expressing smooth muscle cells, resulting in pulmonary fibrosis (16). Once the pulmonary fibrosis occurs, the process is usually irreversible (Fig. 34.5).

There are essentially three patterns of clinical presentations from bleomycin-induced pulmonary toxicity: chronic progressive pulmonary fibrosis, hypersensitivity pneumonitis, and bronchiolitis obliterans organizing pneumonia (BOOP). Dyspnea usually ensues, along with hypoxemia, as pulmonary involvement progresses to chronic pulmonary fibrosis. Fever is probably more common with the less prevalent bleomycin-induced hypersensitivity pneumonitis than with chronic pulmonary fibrosis. Physical examination will reveal the typical fine bibasilar "velcro" rales.

Descriptions of BOOP associated with bleomycin, a unique manifestation of this drug, have surfaced in the last decade (69–71). Histologically, BOOP is characterized by organizing pneumonitis and plugs of fibrous tissue in the

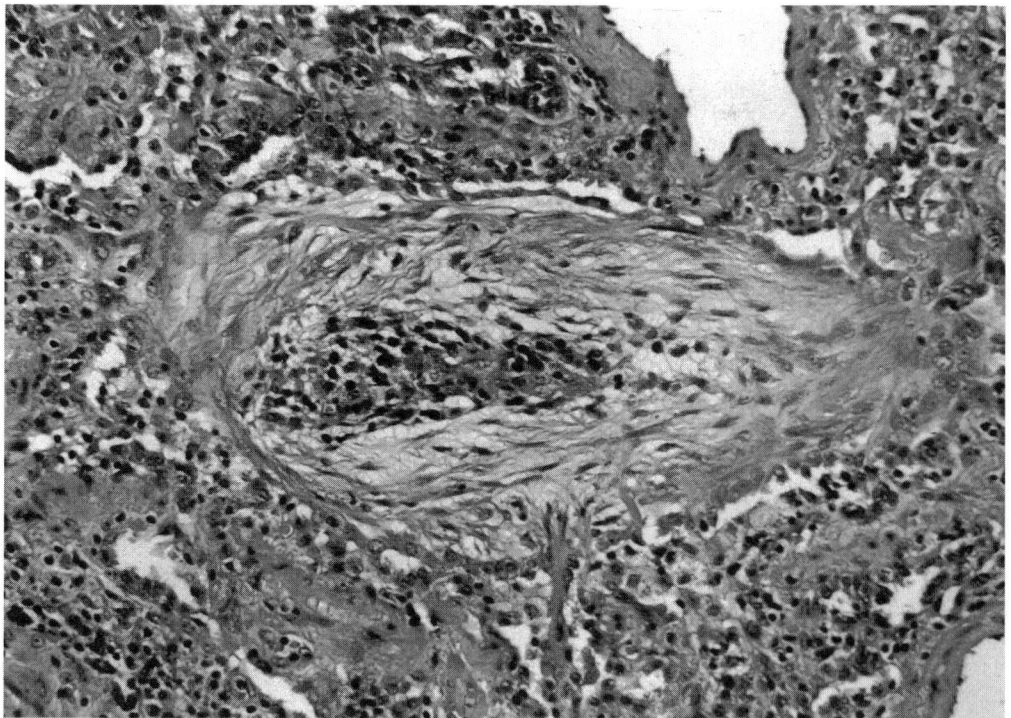

Figure 34.5. Drug-induced bronchiolitis obliterans organizing pneumonitis demonstrating the lumen of an alveolar duct plugged with organizing fibroblastic tissue. The nearby alveolar septa are expanded by fibrosis and a lymphocytic infiltrate.

small airways (Fig. 34.5). The recognition of BOOP is clinically relevant because the nodular infiltrates of BOOP can mimic metastatic disease (Figs. 34.6 and 34.7A) (69, 70).

A recent review of the literature demonstrated a 1 to 2% incidence of autopsy-proven lethal pulmonary toxicity from bleomycin, while 2 to 3% experienced nonlethal pulmonary fibrosis (50). Using frequent surveillance, the overall incidence of pulmonary toxicity is 10% for bleomycin (28), though the literature reports an incidence of 2 to 46% (72). The wide range of reported toxicity most likely stems from the lack of consistent criteria used to define direct pulmonary toxicity from bleomycin.

The associated risk factors for bleomycin-induced pulmonary toxicity have been extensively evaluated, more so than for any other drug (Table 34.6). Probably the most significant risk factor is total dose of the medication. Ginsberg et al. reanalyzed previous articles and found that the overall risk of pulmonary toxicity increased from 10 to 30% as the total bleomycin dose increased to more than 450 to 500 units (8). With the higher doses, the mortality also increased to 5% (73, 74). Although higher cumulative doses predict a higher risk for pulmonary toxicity, sporadic cases have occurred with lower doses (75). Administration of bleomycin within the last 6 months predisposes the patient to increased risk of pulmonary toxicity during the reintroduction of bleomycin (76). Bleomycin's prolonged accumulation in tissue probably accounts for this effect.

Older patients, especially those over 70 years, have a predilection for developing pulmonary toxicity (49, 77, 78). In one study, younger patients appeared to tolerate higher doses of bleomycin, though there was a 10% incidence of pulmonary toxicity in patients with a mean age of 24 years (79). Younger individuals still demonstrate the dose-dependent effect of bleomycin on pulmonary toxicity, and clinicians should be vigilant for the development of toxicity, despite the patient's age.

The synergistic effect of radiation and bleomycin may be manifested as pulmonary toxicity in two forms. The first occurs when bleomycin is given prior to radiotherapy. Apparently, bleomycin sensitizes the tissue to radiation therapy. In one study, no one who received under 3000 rads developed clinical signs and symptoms of pulmonary toxicity (80). However, 44% of patients who received 5000 to 6000 rads with bleomycin developed pulmonary infiltrates (80). This incidence is higher than the expected rates seen with radiation therapy alone. Of the patients developing pulmonary complications, half of them died of respiratory failure (80). None of these patients came close to receiving high doses (>450 to 500 U) of bleomycin. Another study of small cell carcinoma patients treated with radiation and bleomycin produced similar results (81). The second form of toxicity occurs in patients who have had prior radiation therapy. Patients who received radiation therapy within the past year have a 42% risk of developing pulmonary toxicity, compared with 4% in those who did not receive prior radiation therapy (79).

Another synergistic risk factor with bleomycin-induced pulmonary toxicity is high concentrations of inhaled oxygen. Noncardiogenic pulmonary edema developed within 18 to 48 hours of exposure to high FiO_2 in patients with a history of bleomycin administration in the prior 6 to 12 months (82, 83). High concentrations of oxygen corresponded to an average FiO_2 of 0.39, and low concentrations to an average FiO_2 of 0.24 in the earlier study (82). Some advocate the prophylactic administration of glucocorticoids in patients with a history of bleomycin exposure who are exposed to an FiO_2 greater than 0.30 (84). The anesthesiologist and other physicians taking care of patients with a recent history of bleomycin exposure should give oxygen cautiously and sparingly if at all possible.

Concomitant use of other antineoplastic medication with bleomycin increases the incidence of pulmonary toxicity. Several studies using combination chemotherapy with BACOP (bleomycin, Adriamycin, cyclophosphamide, vincristine, and prednisone) (85, 86), COP-bleo (cyclophosphamide, vincristine, prednisone, and bleomycin) (87), and M-BACOD (methotrexate, bleomycin, Adriamycin, cyclophosphamide, vincristine, and dexamethasone) (25) have demonstrated this association. The incidence of pulmonary toxicity was 9% using lower doses of bleomycin (10 $U/m^2/day$ for 4 days) in one study (87), compared with 33% using higher doses of bleomycin (15 $U/m^2/day$ for 2 days) in another (85). With reduction of the bleomycin dose, there was a significant decline in pulmonary toxicity. The authors felt that the cyclophosphamide increased the propensity of bleomycin to cause lung toxicity.

The underlying disease may affect the potential of bleomycin to induce lung injury. For example, bleomycin appear to have more toxic effects on the lung when used in lymphoma patients (28). However, this may reflect the accumulation of bleomycin in areas of lymphomatous infiltration in the lungs.

Since the kidneys are the primary route of bleomycin excretion, renal impairment increases the risk of bleomycin toxicity. The $t_{1/2}$ of bleomycin does not become affected until the creatinine clearance is less than 25 to 35 mL/min (18). Often, the bleomycin-induced pulmonary toxicity occurs in the setting of combination chemotherapy with other nephrotoxic agents such as cisplatin (88–90).

A single high dose of bleomycin causes an anaphylactic reaction in about 6% of patients (28). Some advocate using continuous intravenous administration at a low rate to alleviate this problem. Continuous administration of bleomycin may result in a lower incidence of pulmonary toxicity and better activity against the cancer (91, 92). However, others argue that the incidence of pulmonary toxicity is similar regardless of the mode of delivery (93).

No diagnostic test exists that will firmly establish the diagnosis of bleomycin-induced pulmonary toxicity. This ambiguity accounts for the wide variations (2 to 46%) in reported frequencies of toxicities in earlier studies (72). Often, upon analyzing the clinical and objective data and assessing the potential risk factors for a specific patient, the diagnosis is made by exclusion. In particular, one needs to exclude infection, metastatic disease, cardiogenic pulmonary edema, or reactions to other treatments (i.e., other medications or radiation).

The chest radiographic pattern of bleomycin-induced pulmonary toxicity is a bibasilar reticular pattern (Fig. 34.8). Less frequently, one can see an alveolar pattern, especially in severe disease or with hypersensitivity reactions (20, 94). Multiple nodular infiltrates due to bleomycin toxicity, which histologically are BOOP, can mimic metastatic disease (Figs. 34.6 and 7A) (69, 70). Radiographic studies, especially CT of the chest, have facilitated the clinical recognition of

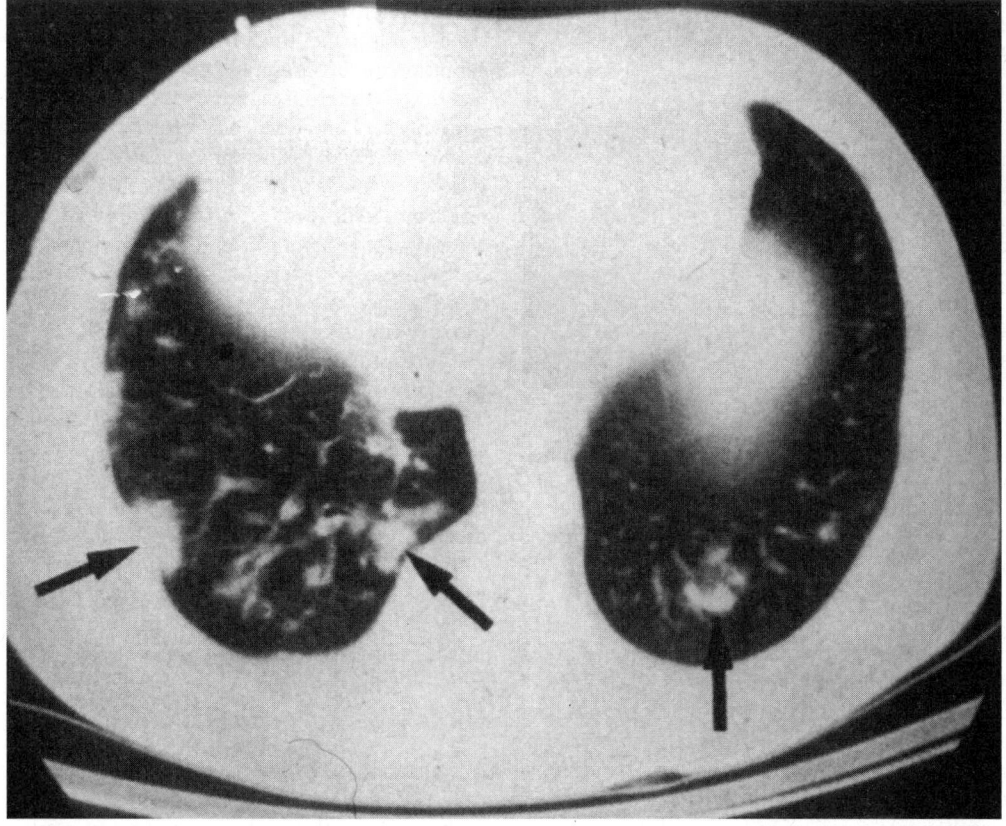

Figure 34.6. Computed tomography of bleomycin pulmonary toxicity demonstrating alveolar nodular infiltrates in a patient with a seminoma; histologically, these areas demonstrate bronchiolitis obliterans organizing pneumonitis.

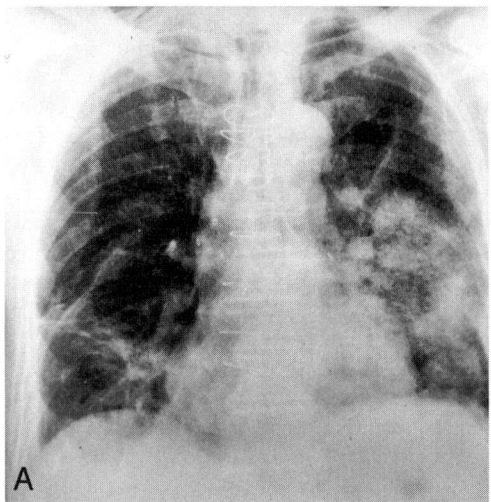

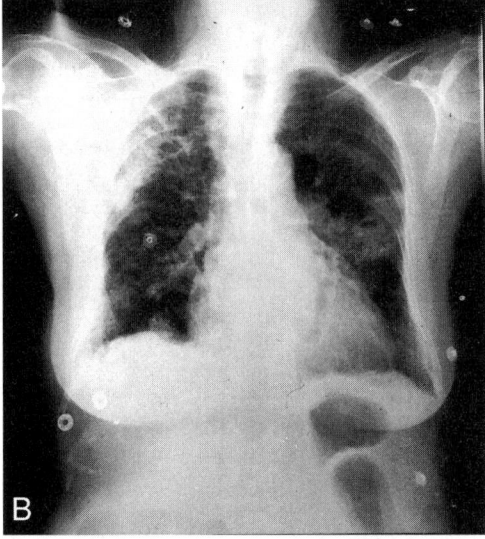

Figure 34.7. Chest radiographs of patients with different radiographic presentations of bronchiolitis obliterans organizing pneumonitis. A. Multiple nodular infiltrates, which may be difficult at times to distinguish from metastatic disease. **B.** Bilateral interstitial infiltrates and an area of consolidation in the right upper lung.

BOOP, reflecting the increased sensitivity of CT over chest radiographs (Fig. 34.6). Only 15% of CT-documented infiltrates are present on routine chest x-ray (42). However, the chest radiograph may help to serve as a baseline, since most reversible disease will resolve over 6 to 12 months (95).

Pulmonary function testing, especially the DL_{CO}, has been particular helpful in alerting the clinician to the potential of pulmonary toxicity from bleomycin. A progressive fall in DL_{CO} often precedes the onset of clinical symptoms (44, 95). Obtaining a baseline measurement of DL_{CO} and subsequent readings prior to further chemotherapy helps to screen for toxicity while being noninvasive and relatively inexpensive. Indeed several studies support the use of DL_{CO} as part of routine evaluation (44, 50, 92). Because of the poor specificity of DL_{CO}, others recommend the use of screening DL_{CO} only in patients with risk factors (96). In one study, the practice of discontinuing bleomycin once the DL_{CO} dropped 25% from the initial value decreased the pulmonary toxicity from 7% to 0.06% (1 in 153 patients) (37). Therefore, it would seem prudent that if the DL_{CO} falls more than 25% from the initial baseline value, the clinician be aware of the possibility of pulmonary toxicity from bleomycin and consider switching to alternative therapy (97).

Early detection and cessation of bleomycin is the most effective way of treating pulmonary toxicity. Corticosteroid therapy has been shown to be most effective in the setting of hypersensitivity pneumonitis (20). Documentation of corticosteroids benefiting the more prevalent presentation of progressive pulmonary fibrosis is lacking. Numerous animal studies reveal an equivocal role for corticosteroids demonstrating a decrease in collagen synthesis. However, there is no decrease in overall inflammation and damage from bleomycin with the administration of steroids (18). Some case reports suggest that high-dose corticosteroids (1 g of methylprednisolone a day) may have a role in treating pulmonary fibrosis from bleomycin (84, 98, 99).

Once pulmonary toxicity occurs, the overall mortality approaches 50% (5). Most of the fatalities are in a group of patients with the following clinical features: pO$_2$ below 55 mm Hg, consolidated infiltrates on chest radiographs, and severe dyspnea (50, 79). Controlled clinical trials evaluating prophylactic corticosteroids in the setting of exposure to high concentrations of oxygen in patients exposed to bleomycin and the use of high-dose corticosteroids to treat bleomycin pulmonary toxicity are needed.

Peplomycin

Peplomycin is structurally similar to bleomycin except for a substitution at the terminal amine moiety. It was developed in the hopes of retaining the antitumor activity of bleomycin without the effects of pulmonary toxicity. In fact,

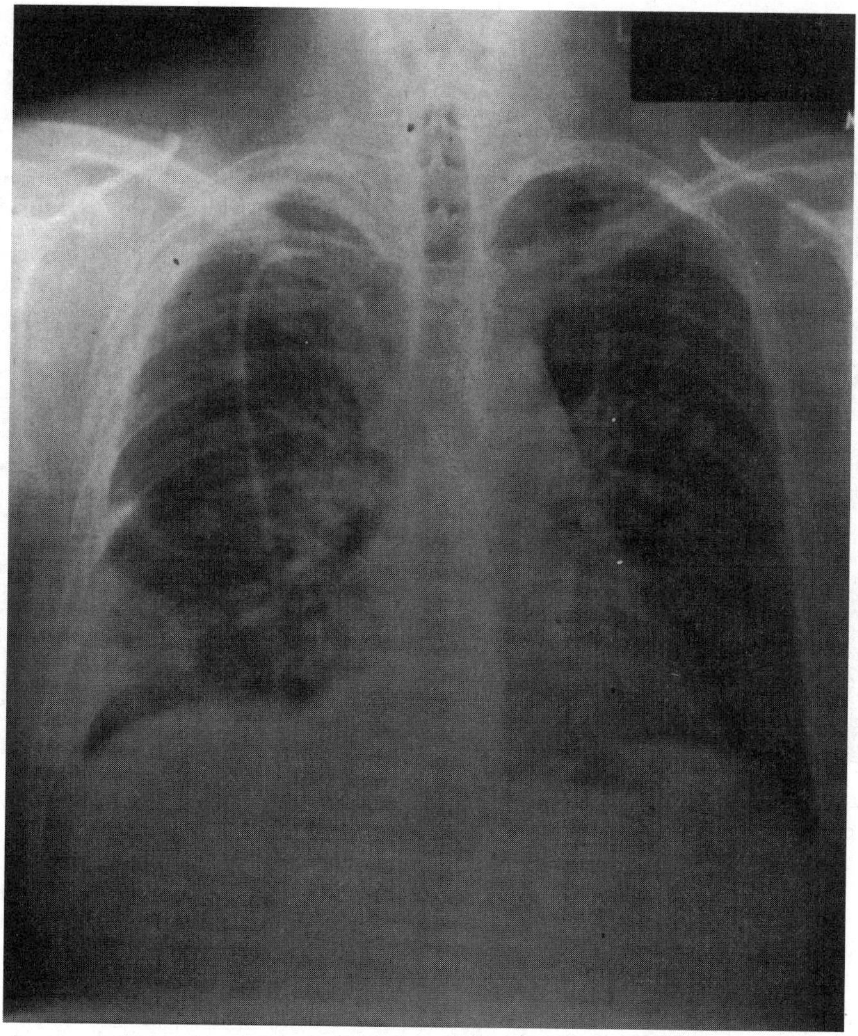

Figure 34.8. Chest radiograph of a patient with bleomycin-induced pulmonary toxicity demonstrating a bibasilar reticular pattern and an alveolar infiltrate at the right base.

initial trials demonstrated that peplomycin had an equal or stronger antitumor effect and similar tissue distribution (100, 101). One study demonstrated a 100% increase in survival in mice by combining bleomycin and peplomycin at 1/6th the optimal dose (102).

Unfortunately, the pulmonary toxicity from peplomycin is similar to that of bleomycin, except that hypersensitivity pneumonitis has not been seen. Peplomycin demonstrates a dose-dependent lung injury pattern. At doses of 10 mg/m^2 and 15 mg/m^2 twice weekly (range, 190 to 350 mg), pulmonary toxicity occurred in 50% of patients, as evidenced by a fall in pulmonary function; 75% of the patients with a decline in

pulmonary function had a fatal outcome. However, no pulmonary toxicities were noted at doses of 5 mg/m^2 (103). In a phase II trial (median dose, 160 mg), only 1 of 21 patients experienced clinical symptoms and a fall in lung function (104).

Pathologically, the pulmonary fibrosis is similar to bleomycin manifesting as usual interstitial pneumonitis (65). High concentrations of oxygen (105) and pretreatment with radiotherapy (31) also increase the risk of pulmonary toxicity from peplomycin. Combination protocols using cisplatin or carboplatin show that peplomycin may have less pulmonary toxicity than bleomycin (106, 107).

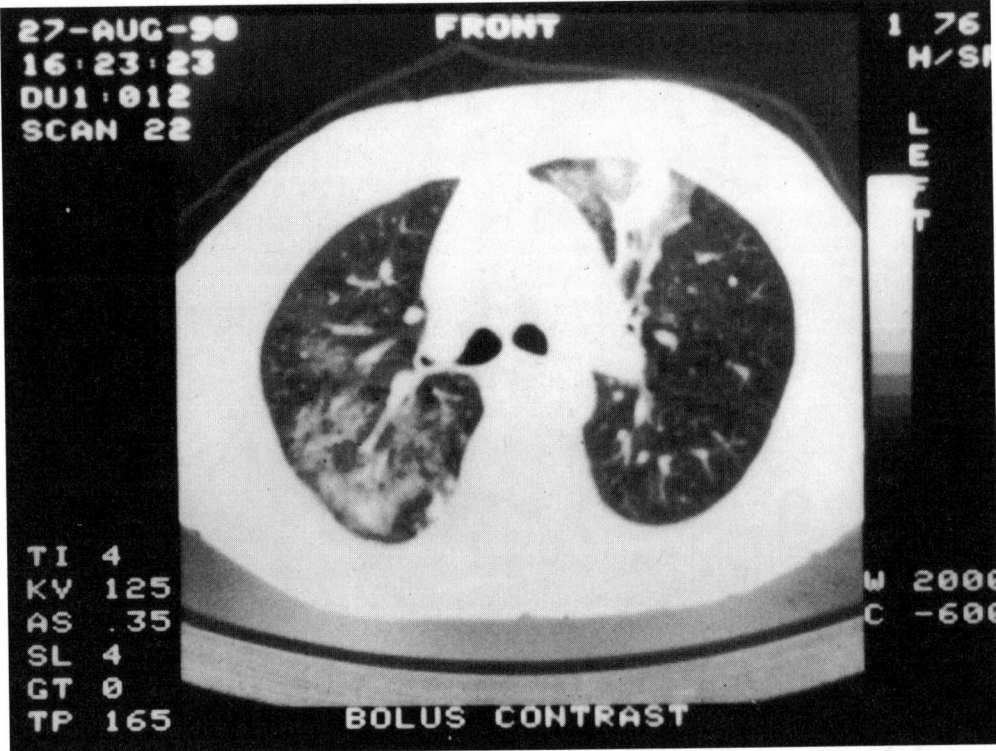

Figure 34.9. Computed tomography of bronchiolitis obliterans organizing pneumonitis demonstrating bilateral patchy airspace opacities.

Liblomycin

Liblomycin (NK313), a bleomycin analogue with a lipophilic group at the amino-terminal end, appears to have better efficacy with certain cancers (leukemia, Ehrlich carcinoma, and hepatoma) in animals (108). In both phase I and phase II studies, there were no pulmonary toxicities (109, 110).

Tallysomycin

Tallysomycin appears to be more potent with some tumors than bleomycin. However, it is also 2 to 3 times more potent in causing pulmonary toxicity in animal studies (101). There was a 10% incidence of pulmonary toxicity during the phase I trial (111).

Mitomycin C

Mitomycin C is a chemotherapeutic agent that has been used in the treatment of various solid tumors, including breast, gastrointestinal tract, and non-small-cell lung cancers (112, 113). A variety of toxicities have been described as a result of mitomycin C, including hemolytic uremic syndrome, and renal, cardiac, and pulmonary toxicity (2, 7, 8, 114–120). Pulmonary toxicity from this agent was first described in 1971 by Simasoto et al. (117). Since then, over 79 patients have been described who developed pulmonary toxicity from mitomycin C, usually in combination with other agents (113, 120–122).

Pulmonary toxicity from mitomycin C has been reported to occur in 3 to 12% of patients (119–121, 123). The clinical presentation of mitomycin C pulmonary toxicity is similar to that seen in other cytotoxic drug reactions. Typically, patients present with a nonproductive cough, dyspnea, and fatigue. Histologic findings are similar to those from other cytotoxic agents, including marked atypia of the type II pneumocyte; however, alveolar septal edema and mononuclear cell interstitial infiltrates are more marked (119) (Fig. 34.2). Chest radiographs typically demonstrate a diffuse reticular pattern, with or without nodularity, and pleural effusions are not uncommon (2) (Fig. 34.3). Two unusual presentations of mitomycin-induced pulmonary toxicity are noncardiogenic pulmonary edema, associated with the hemolytic uremia syndrome (Fig. 34.10), and acute bronchospasm in patients receiving both mitomycin C and vinca alkaloids (27, 112, 114, 115, 118, 122, 124, 125).

Recent evidence suggests that mitomycin-induced lung injury may involve endothelial injury by oxygen free radicals (17, 113). Pathologically, a thrombotic microangiopathy has been described in patients treated with mitomycin C, in which fibrin and platelet thrombi have been noted in the pulmonary arterioles and capillaries (126) (Fig. 34.10). This particular effect on the pulmonary vasculature may explain why the DL$_{CO}$ is so often reduced in patients receiving this agent.

The utility of pulmonary function studies in mitomycin C–induced pulmonary toxicity was recently evaluated. Castro et al. prospectively followed 40 patients who received mitomycin alone or in combination with vinblastine and cisplatin (122). They found a high incidence of decline in DL$_{CO}$ (>20% decline from baseline) in 28% of the patients after only three cycles of chemotherapy. The average decline in DL$_{CO}$ was 14 ± 3.3%. Mitomycin C–induced pulmonary tox-

icity was found in 5% of their patients *without* a premonitory decline in DL$_{CO}$. Previous reports of pulmonary function testing in patients with pulmonary toxicity induced by mitomycin C have predominantly noted the presence of hypoxemia, a restrictive defect, and an abnormal DL$_{CO}$ (121, 123, 127, 128). Verweij et al. prospectively studied 37 patients receiving mitomycin C, alone or in combination, for the development of pulmonary toxicity (121). The DL$_{CO}$ decreased from a baseline of 75 ± 12% to 64 ± 10% in the 20 patients who received doses up to 30 mg/m^2 of mitomycin C, though no patient developed pulmonary toxicity.

Corticosteroid therapy has been reported to be highly effective in patients who develop mitomycin C pulmonary toxicity (7, 119, 122, 128). One author hypothesizes that the effectiveness of corticosteroids in the prophylaxis and treatment of mitomycin C pulmonary toxicity may be due to its "global anti-inflammatory effect," and paradoxically, this may diminish mitomycin C's antineoplastic effect (113). Recently, a study of prophylactic dexamethasone prior to mitomycin C administration reported a 3.5% (2 of 57 patients) incidence of pulmonary toxicity attribut-

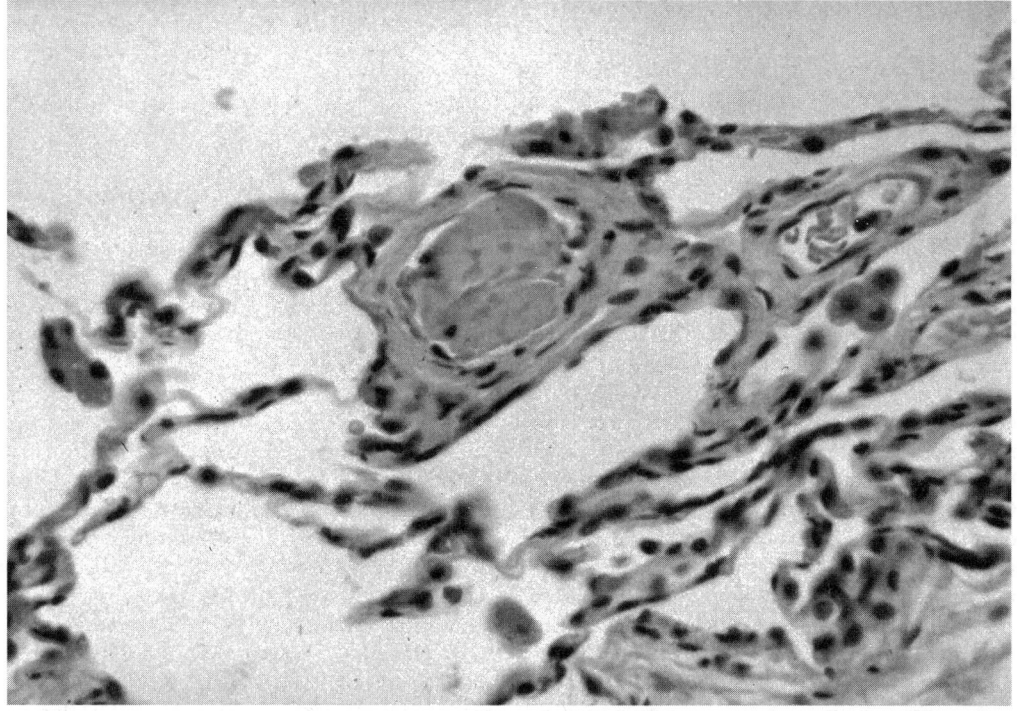

Figure 34.10.   Mitomycin C toxicity manifest as hemolytic uremic syndrome in a patient with colon carcinoma who received 2 months of adjuvant mitomycin C and 5-fluorouracil. Histology demonstrates intimal hyperplasia of the arterioles, intracapillary thrombi, and prominent nuclear atypia of the capillary cells and type II pneumocytes.

able to this agent (129). The authors concluded that the use of mitomycin C (8 mg/m^2) with prior administration of corticosteroids is a useful and safe addition to chemotherapy regimens in the treatment of non-small-cell lung cancer. Of note, the prophylactic corticosteroid was not randomized, and therefore, whether the efficacy of the chemotherapy is compromised is unknown. There are no objective data that show that corticosteroids interfere with the antineoplastic effect of mitomycin C.

ANTHRACYCLINES

Doxorubicin

Doxorubicin, an anthracycline, is a product of *Streptomyces peucetius*. It has been in clinical use since the late 1960s (130). Its major side effects are bone marrow suppression and cardiac toxicity. Pulmonary toxicity is usually only seen in the setting of radiation therapy (Table 34.6). Patients present with a nonproductive cough and rapidly progressive dyspnea (131). Two types of radiation pneumonitis occur more rapidly and frequently after administration of doxorubicin: acute inflammatory pneumonitis (occurs 1 to 2 months after radiation) and chronic fibrosing pneumonitis (occurs several months after radiation). Chest radiographs usually reflect signs of nonspecific pulmonary fibrosis, and 50% have pleural effusions without necessarily having cardiac insufficiency (131).

Doxorubicin appears to potentiate pulmonary damage from radiation therapy (132, 133). One trial gave a treatment protocol of doxorubicin (40 mg/m^2), cyclophosphamide (1500 mg/m^2), and vincristine (2 mg) with radiation therapy (134); 26 of the 71 patients (37%) showed evidence of pulmonary disease. Eleven of these patients were strongly suspected of having radiation pneumonitis, and seven subsequently died of respiratory failure. Postmortem examination revealed findings consistent with radiation pneumonitis, including the lung opposite the radiation site. Even at low dose (10 mg/m^2), doxorubicin has radiation-sensitizing effects in vitro (135). In one trial, doxorubicin was given in combination with other chemotherapeutic agents (methotrexate, cyclophosphamide, mitomycin C, bleomycin, or CCNU), 1 month after completion of the irradiation (131). Over 50% of these patients developed radiation pneumonitis, and 25% ultimately died of respiratory insufficiency. The authors felt that doxorubicin had predisposed the patients to pneumonitis.

There is little knowledge of the pathogenesis of doxorubicin-induced radiation pneumonitis. However, once this syndrome develops, the prognosis is poor. There are few therapeutic options available except corticosteroids at high doses (1 mg/kg/day) early in the development of pneumonitis (136, 137).

Epirubicin

Epirubicin, which differs only in the 4'-OH position from doxorubicin, may confer less toxicity and better clearance from tissue, while having the same tumor-killing ability (138). It is unclear if this will reduce the incidence of radiation pneumonitis.

ACTINOMYCIN D

Like doxorubicin, actinomycin D is from *S. peucetius*. Actinomycin D also seems to increase the risk of radiation pneumonitis (Table 34.6) (139). Patients have an increased risk of radiation pneumonitis up to 1 year after the administration of actinomycin D (132, 140). There may also be a sensitizing effect to Adriamycin. In a case report by Cassady et al., a patient who had prior radiation therapy and actinomycin D developed pneumonitis 10 days after receiving Adriamycin (132). In another case report, a post–actinomycin D/radiation therapy patient developed pneumonitis 24 hours after receiving Adriamycin (137).

NEOCARZINOSTATIN

Neocarzinostatin is an investigational polypeptide antineoplastic antibiotic that has a low incidence of pulmonary toxicity. There appear to be only two published cases of pulmonary toxicity (141, 142).

ALKYLATING AGENTS

Nitrosoureas

The nitrosoureas are a class of agents that have the capabilities of alkylating and carbamylating cells. They are used in the treatment of various neoplasms including lymphoma, malignant melanoma, and especially intracranial tumors (gliomas) because of their ability to cross the blood-brain barrier (143, 144). The nitrosoureas include BCNU (carmustine), CCNU (lomustine), methyl CCNU (semustine), chlorozotocin, and streptozotocin. All have been associated with pulmonary toxicity (145–147) except streptozotocin. The following discussion concentrates on BCNU, since this is the best studied and documented.

BCNU (Carmustine)

The pathogenesis of BCNU-induced pulmonary toxicity is similar to that of bleomycin, although the precise mechanism is not known. One proposed mechanism is a reduction in the antioxidant, glutathione reductase, resulting in increased levels of free radicals, such as H_2O_2 and lipid peroxides (148, 149). The incidence of pulmonary toxicity from BCNU varies from 1 to 50% (6, 24, 150). The acute phase of pulmonary toxicity from BCNU demonstrates type II pneumocyte hyperplasia and interstitial thickening, as a result of mononuclear cell infiltrates, with minimal fibrosis. The late phase demonstrates normal alveoli interspersed with focal areas of interstitial fibrosis, elastosis, prominent fibroblasts, and focal lymphocytic infiltrates (151). The pulmonary arteries hypertrophy, and the pulmonary veins have intimal fibrosis. These changes are most notable in the apices with subpleural fibrosis and are less prominent in the bases (151). Electron microscopy shows loss of the type I pneumocytes, with a bare basement membrane and endothelial damage (150). The predominance in the upper lobes may be related to the younger age of the patients receiving BCNU, as there is an increase in perfusion to the upper lobes in children (152, 153).

BCNU-induced pulmonary toxicity is similar to that of bleomycin except for two unique clinical presentations. First, the effects of pulmonary toxicity may not present for many years after treatment (up to 17 years, with most presenting within 1 to 4 years (6)). Second, the infiltrates are seen preferentially in the upper zones of the lungs (150). Patients may also present with a rapid fulminant course similar to noncardiogenic pulmonary edema (154). Fever is more prominent in the setting of BCNU and cyclophosphamide toxicity (155). Pneumothorax has also been reported with BCNU-induced fibrosis and can be bilateral (156).

BCNU-induced pulmonary toxicity demonstrates a dose-dependent relationship (Table 34.6). A cumulative dose of 1200 to 1500 mg/m² has been associated with a 50% incidence of recipients developing pulmonary toxicity (6, 143). In bone marrow transplant patients, high-dose BCNU (1200 mg/m²) has been associated with a 9.5% incidence of fatal interstitial pneumonitis (157). O'Driscoll et al. recently reported on long-term follow-up of 17 of 31 children who received BCNU and survived their cancers. All but four received a cumulative dose of BCNU above 1300 mg/m². All of them had pulmonary function and radiographic abnormalities after 17 years (150).

Combination chemotherapy with cyclophosphamide may increase the incidence of pulmonary toxicity (24). The incidence with this combination reaches 30 to 50% (155, 158). The mean time of onset is 48 ± 14 days after initiation with high-dose consolidation chemotherapy (155). The incidence of pulmonary toxicity appears to correlate with higher serum levels of BCNU and not cyclophosphamide, leading most to believe that the toxicity is secondary to BCNU (158). In bone marrow transplant patients, low-dose BCNU (600 mg/m²), when combined with cyclophosphamide and cisplatin in one series, resulted in fatal interstitial pneumonitis in 2 of 22 patients (159).

Preexisting lung disease (especially if secondary to smoking) and a tobacco history of more than 10 cigarettes/day may increase the incidence of BCNU-induced pulmonary injury (6, 160). Younger age (31–50 years old) has also been reported to increase the likelihood of developing pulmonary toxicity, but this is likely due to the higher dose of BCNU they received (8).

Pulmonary function testing consistently demonstrates a reduced DL_{CO} and forced vital capacity in patients with biopsy-proven pulmonary fibrosis even if asymptomatic (150). The chest radiograph may show any of the following: diffuse interstitial infiltrates, diffuse alveolar infiltrates, pleural effusions or fibrosis, hilar/mediastinal adenopathy, or localized pulmonary consolidation (153). The chest CT localizes these lesions with more sensitivity. However, the chest CT may be normal, even in the setting of decreased pulmonary function and biopsy-proven pulmonary fibrosis (153).

Administration of corticosteroids does not prevent BCNU-induced pulmonary toxicity (6, 150). In fact, many patients are already on corticosteroids because of central nervous system tumors. Long-term steroids may be of benefit when the pulmonary toxicity is from a combination of cyclophosphamide and BCNU (155, 158).

Mortality from BCNU-induced pulmonary toxicity ranges from 15 to 35% (6, 150). Pulmonary function abnormalities do not resolve. The time course to pulmonary fibrosis can be from several months up to 17 years. Although mortality with the combination of BCNU and cyclophosphamide approaches 30%, the survivors do actually improve clinically and symptomatically with steroids (155).

Busulfan

Busulfan is an alkylsulfonate useful for my-eloproliferative disorders such as chronic gran-ulocytic leukemia or in induction regimens for bone marrow transplantation (144). In 1961, bu-sulfan was one of the first cytotoxic agents re-ported to be associated with pulmonary toxicity (161). The incidence of clinical pulmonary tox-icity is often quoted at 2 to 4%, but histologically, the incidence is as high as 46% (2, 8, 73, 120). The onset of busulfan-induced toxicity symptoms be-gins from 6 weeks to 10 years following the ini-tiation of therapy, with most presenting within 3.5 years (3, 8). Symptoms include dyspnea, dry cough, weakness, weight loss, and fever over weeks to months (8, 162).

The alkylating agents appear to have direct cytotoxic effects causing epithelial cell loss, but the exact mechanism has not been elucidated (163). Epithelial cells are extremely sensitive to busulfan, making the epithelial cells in the lung, uterine cervix, and urinary tract vulnerable (164). The pathology of busulfan-induced pul-monary toxicity demonstrates malignant-ap-pearing epithelial cells, desquamation of type II pneumocytes, mononuclear cell infiltration, and proliferation of fibroblasts, with resultant fibro-sis (162). Pulmonary ossification (165), pulmo-nary alveolar proteinosis (166), and alveolar cell carcinomas (167) have also been associated with busulfan.

The dosage of busulfan is a significant risk factor for busulfan-induced toxicity (Table 34.6). Patients who receive a total dose of more than 500 mg appear to have a higher incidence of pul-monary toxicity (8). The concomitant use of other chemotherapeutic agents (168, 169) or radiation therapy (170) may predispose to pulmonary tox-icity at lower doses of busulfan.

Pulmonary function testing with DL_{CO} and chest radiographs are not good markers for im-pending pulmonary toxicity from busulfan (120). This may be related to the lower incidence of toxicity in these studies using small doses of bu-sulfan (500 mg). Once pulmonary fibrosis devel-ops, the chest radiograph often demonstrates bilateral alveolar infiltrates due to type II pneumocyte desquamation and alveolar protein-osis (Fig. 34.11) (162). Pulmonary function test-ing demonstrates a restrictive pattern, and hy-poxemia is usually present (166).

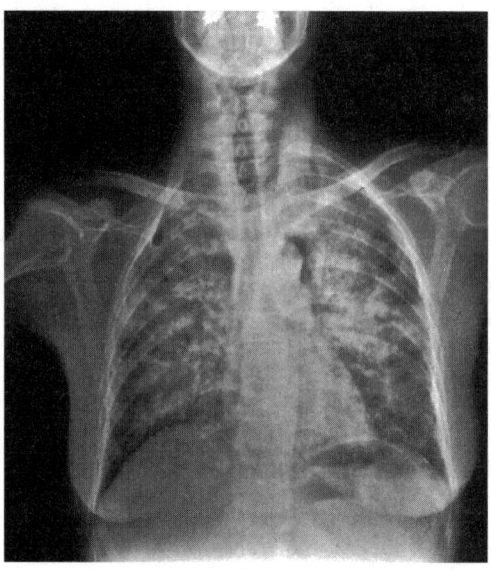

Figure 34.11. Patient with chronic granulocytic leu-kemia treated for 1 month with busulfan and interferon presenting with progressive dyspnea and cough. Chest radiograph demonstrates extensive bilateral alveolar in-filtrates; histologically, this represents alveolar proteino-sis and type II cell desquamation.

Withdrawal of the medication should be prompt once there are pulmonary symptoms (8). No controlled trials have shown corticosteroid therapy to decrease mortality, although there are a few anecdotal case reports of steroid respon-siveness (120). As long as the patient has no con-traindications, a trial course of high-dose ste-roids is recommended for quicker symptomatic relief (8). The overall prognosis is poor once pul-monary toxicity develops, with a mean survival after diagnosis of 5 months (2). Mortality has been reported from 50 to 80% (3, 120).

Cyclophosphamide

Cyclophosphamide is a nitrogen mustard that obtains its activity by cleavage of a cyclic phos-phamide group (144). There are well docu-mented reports of cyclophosphamide causing pulmonary toxicity since the first reported case in 1967 in a patient with Hodgkin's disease (171). Most of the documented cases have involved the use of other agents, such as vincristine, metho-trexate, BCNU, and thoracic irradiation, which may have contributed to the lung injury (84, 120). However, cyclophosphamide also induces pulmonary toxicity when administered for non-malignant diseases (172–174). The incidence of cyclophosphamide-induced pulmonary toxicity is probably 1%, with occasional clustering of reported cases (2).

The exact mechanism involved in cyclophosphamide-induced pulmonary toxicity is unclear. Cyclophosphamide is metabolized by lung supernatant, producing 4-hydroxycyclophosphamide, acrolein, and phosphoramide mustard (175). At this point, it is unclear if 4-hydroxycyclophosphamide induces lung injury. Both cyclophosphamide and phosphoramide mustard cause an imbalance of the oxidant/antioxidant system, predisposing the lung to oxidant injury (176, 177). Acrolein appears to exert its toxic effect by decreasing the microsomal enzyme activity in the lung (175). Another possible mechanism of cyclophosphamide toxicity could be the upregulation of T lymphocytes, causing pulmonary fibrosis via activation of the inflammatory system (178).

Associated risk factors for pulmonary toxicity include radiation therapy, (possibly) high FiO_2, and combination chemotherapy (Table 34.6). Cyclophosphamide may potentiate the effect of radiation, especially when high doses of cyclophosphamide in the range of 160 to 200 mg/kg are given (120, 179). When radiation, BCNU, and cyclophosphamide are given together, the incidence of pulmonary toxicity increases to 39% (155). In rats, 100% oxygen for 4 days induced fatal pulmonary damage when given after cyclophosphamide (180). However, there have not been human clinical trials to support this association.

Combination chemotherapy with cyclophosphamide as part of a protocol increases the incidence of pulmonary toxicity. In one study, six different high-dose chemotherapy protocols without radiation were reviewed. Out of 178 patients, there were 4 cases of interstitial pneumonitis, 5 cases of noncardiogenic pulmonary edema, 2 cases of pulmonary hemorrhage, and 24 patients with a significant drop in DL_{CO} (>25%) (181). The 24 patients with decreased DL_{CO} all received cyclophosphamide. The four patients with interstitial pneumonitis received both cyclophosphamide and relatively low doses of BCNU. Cyclophosphamide predisposes the lung to damage when used with BCNU (24). Four of the patients with noncardiogenic pulmonary edema received cyclophosphamide. High-dose cyclophosphamide (range of 50 to 120 mg/kg/day for 4 days) predisposed patients in another study to develop alveolar hemorrhage (182). There is one reported case of cyclophosphamide alone inducing noncardiogenic pulmonary edema (183). Therefore, it appears that

cyclophosphamide has a direct role in causing lung injury, but it also subjects the lung to damage by other chemotherapeutic agents.

Patients with cyclophosphamide-induced pulmonary toxicity usually present with a nonproductive cough, dyspnea, and fever (>50%) 2 weeks (range, 2 weeks to 13 years) after the initiation of treatment (2). On physical examination, there are fine inspiratory crackles (8). Radiographic changes consist mostly of bibasilar infiltrates, but diffuse infiltrates (183) and focal infiltrates (120) have been described.

Discontinuation of the cyclophosphamide is the primary treatment, as no specific therapy exists. There have been anecdotal cases of improvement of symptoms with corticosteroids, though deaths still occur (73). Approximately 60% of patients with cyclophosphamide-induced toxicity will recover from their acute pneumonitis (2).

Chlorambucil

Chlorambucil, a nitrogen mustard, is a phenylbutyric acid derivative of mechlorethamine used mainly in the treatment of chronic lymphocytic leukemia and other lymphoproliferative disorders (144). Since its introduction in 1955, over a dozen reports have documented chlorambucil-induced pulmonary fibrosis (184–192). Given its long history of use and the paucity of published reports of pulmonary toxicity, its incidence is probably less than 1% (2). A cumulative dose above 2000 mg and reexposure to chlorambucil seem to predispose patients to a greater incidence of pulmonary toxicity (184). Administration of fludarabine phosphate may potentiate the effects of chlorambucil.

The time interval from the initiation of chlorambucil and clinical presentation of toxicity is several days to 72 months (191). Patients with chlorambucil-induced pulmonary toxicity present with a nonproductive cough, dyspnea, fatigue, weakness, and weight loss over a 2 to 3 week period (73). Besides withdrawing chlorambucil, steroids may be of benefit (190). One study reported that 7 of 17 patients survived with chlorambucil-induced pulmonary fibrosis. Five of the survivors received steroids, compared with only 3 of the 10 patients who died (191).

Melphalan

Melphalan, like chlorambucil, is a synthetic derivative of mechlorethamine (144). There are very few reported cases of pulmonary toxicity from melphalan, and none since 1980 (120). However, Taetle et al. suggest that as many as

50% of patients may have histopathologic changes (atypical epithelial cell proliferation without pneumonitis) that are not clinically evident (193).

ANTIMETABOLITES

Methotrexate

Methotrexate is a folate antagonist that causes a deficiency of folate coenzymes, inhibiting cell reproduction (144). Since the first reported case of methotrexate-associated pneumonitis in 1969 (194), there have been numerous reports of pulmonary toxicity during its use for cancer and inflammatory disorders. Methotrexate-induced pneumonitis is unique because of its low mortality. The incidence of methotrexate-induced pulmonary toxicity is variable, ranging from 0 to 12% (11, 195, 196). There appear to be no associated risks with age, dose, length of therapy, radiation therapy, or gender of the patient (11). Patients with rheumatologic disorders may be more prone to methotrexate-induced pulmonary injury (196). Methotrexate given daily or weekly predisposes the lung to more toxicity than does giving it every 2 to 4 weeks (8).

Methotrexate accumulates preferentially in the lungs, but the mechanism of injury is unclear (197). The atypical cellular changes seen with cytotoxic agents are not seen with methotrexate (3). There are several different theories as to how methotrexate causes pulmonary injury. The first theory is that methotrexate initiates an immunologic reaction. Support for this theory comes from cases of hypersensitivity pneumonitis with eosinophilia and fever that respond to corticosteroids (8). Bronchoalveolar lavage reveals a lymphocyte predominance with an increase in helper T cells (198, 199) or an increase in suppressor T cells (200). There have also been reports of granulomatous formations with giant cells (11) and bronchiolitis obliterans (201), which may further support the immunologic theory. Alternatively, methotrexate-induced injury may be related to direct cytotoxic effects on the lung, as cessation of the drug has been known to resolve the pneumonitis (11, 202).

Another intriguing aspect of methotrexate-induced toxicity is that the drug can be reintroduced without recurrence of pneumonitis. It is also unclear why there are clusters of reported cases as high as 12%, even with low-dose methotrexate (196). This suggests that there needs to be an immunologic trigger present in addition to the methotrexate to initiate the pneumonitis. Some have speculated that the trigger is an impurity in the preparation, an environmental substance, or an infectious agent such as a virus (74).

There are several different clinical presentations, depending on the type of reaction the patient is experiencing. These may include acute pneumonitis (the most common), chemical pleuritis, chronic progressive pulmonary fibrosis, and noncardiogenic pulmonary edema (203, 204). The usual presentation is that of acute pneumonitis with symptoms of fever, malaise, myalgias, headache, peripheral eosinophilia (40%), rash (17%), nonproductive cough, and dyspnea within several weeks of starting therapy (8, 11, 120). Chemical pleuritis occurs in 9%, presenting as sudden-onset pleuritic chest pain lasting 3 to 5 days (205). The chronic progressive pulmonary fibrosis is more insidious and may not appear until years after the administration of methotrexate (120). The noncardiogenic pulmonary edema has been seen after intrathecal injections of methotrexate, which may be related to a neurohormonal response (203, 204).

Radiographic changes include a bibasilar reticulonodular appearance similar to that in other pneumonitis (11) (Fig. 34.12). However, there are descriptions of acinar infiltrates (206), hilar adenopathy (8, 11), and pleural effusions (205). Pulmonary function testing demonstrates a restrictive pattern with a decreased DL_{CO} once the disease is clinically evident and, therefore, is not predictive of toxicity (207).

Steroids probably hasten the recovery (208) and may decrease mortality (8). Resolution of symptoms does occur without the administration of steroids (11). Unique to methotrexate pneumonitis is the low overall mortality of 1% (2), although chronic progressive pulmonary fibrosis in the elderly carries a very poor prognosis (73).

Azathioprine and 6-Mercaptopurine

6-Mercaptopurine (6-MP) and the closely related compound azathioprine have had rare case reports of pneumonitis since they were first used in 1953 and 1963, respectively (209). In the literature, there have been only three cases of 6-MP-induced pneumonitis (73) and three cases of azathioprine-induced pneumonitis (2). The use of intravenous 6-MP appears to be gaining interest again, and it remains to be seen if there will be more reports of 6-MP-induced pneumonitis (210).

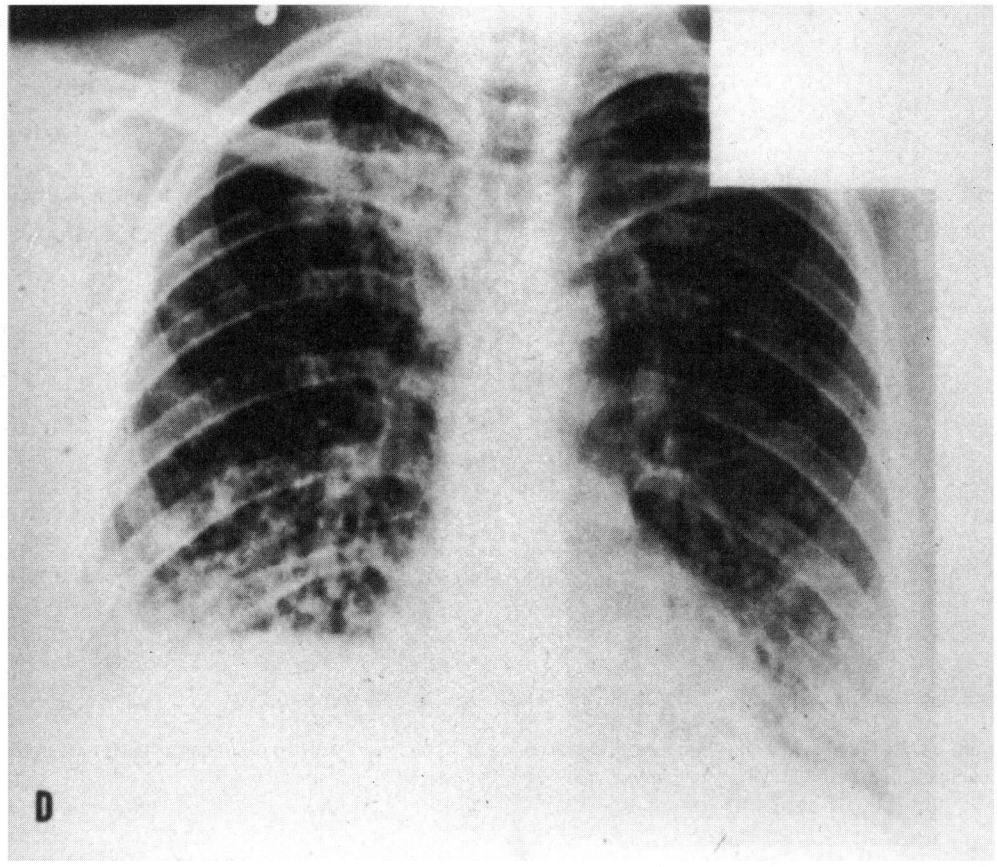

Figure 34.12. Chest radiograph of patient with methotrexate-induced pulmonary toxicity demonstrating bilateral interstitial infiltrates with a basilar predominance.

Cytarabine (Ara-C)

Cytarabine (ara-C) is a synthetic analogue of deoxycytidine and has activity against acute leukemia (211). Ara-C was not recognized as a significant cause of pulmonary toxicity until 1981. Haupt et al. demonstrated a significantly higher frequency of unexplained pulmonary edema in a retrospective study (9). Since then, ara-C has been documented as a cause of noncardiogenic pulmonary edema in many other studies (212–215). The reported incidence of toxicity ranges from 4 to 28% (214–216).

The pathogenesis of ara-C-produced noncardiogenic pulmonary edema is not well understood. It is speculated that the interference of DNA synthesis by ara-C or the lysis products from the leukemic cells may impair or injure cell wall function of the pneumocytes and capillary endothelium. This, in turn, causes increased permeability, which results in pulmonary edema

(217). On autopsy, the lungs are filled with proteinaceous fluid in the alveoli and interstitium (9) (Fig. 34.13).

Symptoms of fever, dry cough, and dyspnea usually develop during treatment (2 to 20 days) (212, 214) but may not occur for up to 27 days after treatment (9). Radiographically, there is a bibasilar interstitial pattern that progresses to an alveolar pattern over 3 to 7 days (218).

Reported risk factors for ara-C toxicity include the dose and *Streptococcus* viridans bacteremia. One study noted a sharp increase in the incidence of subacute pulmonary failure when patients were given high-dose ara-C (3 g/m^2) for 9 days (212). However, other studies have not found a correlation with dosage (9, 214). *Streptococcus* viridans septicemia may precede the clinical presentation of noncardiogenic pulmonary edema. One report found that 8 of 12 patients with pulmonary failure due to ara-C had

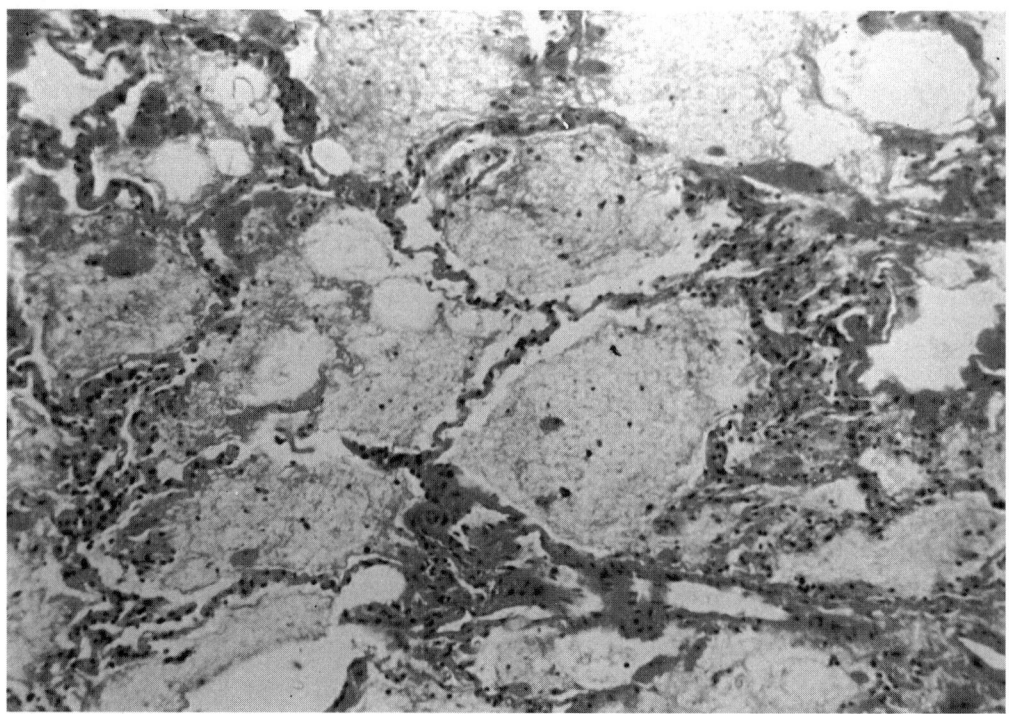

Figure 34.13. Histology of ara-C-induced noncardiogenic pulmonary edema demonstrating marked intraalveolar proteinaceous material with minimal parenchymal abnormalities and no cellular atypia.

a preceding episode of *Streptococcus* viridans septicemia (214). Another report made similar observations (219).

High-dose corticosteroids appear to help resolve symptoms and radiographic abnormalities (9, 214, 219). The mortality ranges from 1 to 50% (197, 215). If there is suspicion of *Streptococcus viridans* septicemia, appropriate antibiotics must be started immediately.

Fludarabine Phosphate

Fludarabine phosphate, a derivative of vidarabine (ara-A), is used against lymphoid malignancies. There have been six cases of pulmonary toxicity associated with fludarabine phosphate, although these patients also received chlorambucil (220). One patient appeared to have a hypersensitivity pneumonitis by transbronchial biopsy; the another had fibrosing pneumonitis on open lung biopsy (221). It remains to be seen if fludarabine phosphate by itself can cause pulmonary toxicity or if it only potentiates the effects of chorambucil.

Interleukin-2

Interleukin-2 (IL-2) is given alone or in combination with autologous lymphokine-activated killer cells (LAK) (222), interferon-α (INF-α), (223) or tissue necrosis factor (TNF) (224) in a variety of cancers, but primarily for metastatic melanoma and metastatic renal cell carcinoma. The incidence of pulmonary edema from capillary leak syndrome depends upon the dose, route of administration, and concomitant administration of LAK, INF-α, or TNF, ranging from 0 to 100% (10, 225). The side effects are considerable, with the most devastating being a capillary leak syndrome and cardiovascular collapse (226).

IL-2 probably exerts its effects by activating lymphocytes and starting the cascade of cellular mediators which have inflammatory and vasoactive properties. IL-2 activated lymphocytes cause increased permeability of the endothelial cells in vitro (10). This permeability is blocked when lymphocyte-depleted mice are given IL-2 or when steroids are administered prior to IL-2

(227, 228). Pathologically, there is a marked mononuclear cell infiltrate in the interstitium and perivascular areas (229).

The clinical presentation of IL-2 toxicity consists of hypotension, fever, dyspnea, anorexia, fever, rash, and mucositis (230). Fever and hypotension are the most common symptoms, occurring 90 to 100% of the time (231). Symptoms usually occur during or immediately after the administration of IL-2 because of its short $t_{1/2}$ life of 1 hour (231).

Associated risk factors for IL-2 pulmonary toxicity include dose, concomitant therapy, and preexisting lung disease (Table 34.6). High-dose, bolus infusions of IL-2 (600,000 u/kg every 8 hours, days 1 to 5 and 12 to 16 for 28 doses) produced a 66% incidence of radiographic abnormalities in contrast to only 14% when similar doses were given by continuous infusion (232). These results are supported by others who found an incidence of pulmonary edema of 50% with high-dose bolus infusion (233) compared with 10% by low-dose continuous infusion (231). Inhalation and low-dose continuous infusion of IL-2 for treatment of pulmonary metastasis resulted in adequate regression of the metastatic lesions with no episodes of pulmonary edema (225, 234). It is even more impressive that no patients showed symptomatic evidence of pulmonary edema, since pulmonary metastasis is one of the risk factors for development of capillary leak syndrome (235). Concomitant administration of LAK has been shown to increase the incidence of pulmonary edema (222, 232). The mechanism is still unclear, but interferon-α and TNF appear to increase the toxic effects of IL-2 as well (223, 224). A pretreatment FEV_1 of less than 3 L was correlated with a higher incidence of pulmonary edema induced by IL-2 (232).

Chest radiographs reveal pleural effusions (52%), diffuse infiltrates (41%), and focal infiltrates (22%), of which 77% resolve within 4 weeks of therapy (232). In the same study, radiographic abnormalities were not seen in 21% of patients with clinically evident pulmonary edema. On the other hand, radiographic abnormalities were seen in 20% of asymptomatic patients. Therefore, chest radiographs are neither sensitive nor specific for detecting IL-2 pulmonary toxicity. All parameters of pulmonary function testing (FVC, FEV_1, TLC, PaO_2) decrease after every administration of IL-2, again reflecting the high incidence of subclinical disease (222).

Cessation of IL-2 and supportive care with pressors, oxygen, and at times intubation usually result in quick resolution of symptoms. The combination of low-dose cyclophosphamide and decreasing the IL-2 dose may decrease the incidence of pulmonary edema (236). Despite the high incidence of significant pulmonary toxicity from IL-2, mortality rates from IL-2 are around 2% (31, 230).

Paclitaxel (Taxol)

Paclitaxel has been in use since 1983 for a variety of cancers including ovarian, breast, lung, and head and neck cancers (237). Paclitaxel causes a severe hypersensitivity in some patients, which may be associated with bronchospasm (237). There are two cases of pulmonary compromise secondary to paclitaxel. The first report consisted of shortness of breath and bronchospasm (238), and the second involved a women who developed fatal lipid embolism to the lungs 12 hours after receiving paclitaxel (239).

VINCA ALKALOIDS

Vinblastine and vindesine are vinca alkaloids used to treat lymphoma, and breast, lung, and ovarian cancer (240). These antimicrotubular agents rarely cause toxicity to the lungs by themselves (241). However, in combination with mitomycin, they may predispose the lungs to injury. The incidence of toxicity ranges from 3 to 39% (27, 124, 242, 243). A severe inflammatory reaction is seen, with marked interstitial infiltration by mononuclear and polymorphynuclear cells. Alveolar cells become hyperplastic and dysplastic, with evidence of alveolar edema. Mild fibrosis along with possible early granulomas can also be seen (241, 242, 244).

Interestingly, vinca alkaloid–induced pulmonary toxicity presents with obstructive airways disease instead of a restrictive process as seen with other cytotoxic agents (27, 124, 125). Patients usually present within 1 to 5 hours of administration of the vinca alkaloid, with complaints of dyspnea and even wheezing. The presentation can be more chronic and insidious (27). Pulmonary function testing documents mild obstructive abnormalities (which may be secondary to tobacco use) with worsening after the administration of vinca alkaloids (27). Chest radiographs may reveal bilateral diffuse interstitial infiltrates (27). There has been one report of vindesine possibly causing an interstitial pneumonitis in a patient who also received radiation (241). Most of the reports are in cases in which mitomycin C has been given before or concomitantly with a vinca alkaloid. Prior smoking may be a risk factor for toxicity (27, 125, 244).

Most of the patients received supportive care with bronchodilators, corticosteroids, theophylline, and ventilatory support if needed. The mortality has been reported to be as high as 40 to 55% once the pulmonary infiltrates develop (27, 242).

PROCARBAZINE

Procarbazine has been reported to cause a hypersensitivity reaction with pulmonary infiltrates and eosinophilia (21, 245, 246). These reactions usually occur within hours of giving procarbazine and resolve with steroid therapy. Often other chemotherapeutic agents are being administered, such as those in the MOPP program. Lung biopsy reveals a mononuclear and eosinophilic infiltration, which suggests a hypersensitivity reaction (21). In addition, there has been a report of a late-onset pneumonitis (3 days after procarbazine was given), which responded within 24 hours after steroids were given (247).

CONCLUSION

The pulmonary toxicity from chemotherapeutic agents is a substantial challenge for the practicing clinician administering these agents. Targeting chemotherapeutic regimens to deliver specific antineoplastic activity without causing harm has long been a challenge. Improved markers predicting toxicity from chemotherapeutic agents are needed (2). Clearly, pulmonary function and radiographic studies are suboptimal in predicting pulmonary toxicity from most agents. Potential markers for pulmonary toxicity include (a) reduced levels of specific enzymes that are protective against the cytotoxic effects of antineoplastic agents, such as bleomycin hydroxylase A_2 (51, 52); (b) an imbalance of oxidants/antioxidants leading to damage by oxygen radicals, such as deficiency of glutathione reductase (148, 149) or SOD (61, 62); or (c) release of cellular mediators indicative of inflammation and tissue remodeling, such as PDGF or TGF-β (18).

Treatment of chemotherapeutically induced pulmonary toxicity is often unsuccessful, with progressive pulmonary fibrosis ensuing. Innovations in delivery systems, gene therapy, and monoclonal antibodies have made substantial progress and, one hopes, will improve our success in both targeting chemotherapy to neoplastic cells and treating or preventing toxicity from these agents. However, with increasing numbers of chemotherapeutic agents being used and improving survival, one would expect to see an increasing incidence of pulmonary toxicity. The clinician must be knowledgeable about these potential toxicities, their prevention, and treatment.

ACKNOWLEDGMENTS

The authors would like to thank Beverly A. McDonald for her assistance in the preparation of this manuscript and Randy A. Brown, M.D., for his thoughtful comments in reviewing the manuscript.

REFERENCES

1. Rosenow EC. The spectrum of drug-induced pulmonary disease. Ann Intern Med 1972;77:977–991.
2. Cooper JAD, White DA, Matthay RA. Drug-induced pulmonary disease. Part 1: cytoxic drugs. Am Rev Respir Dis 1986;133:321–340.
3. Rosenow EC. Drug-induced pulmonary disease. Toledo: Mosby-Year Book, 1994:255–310. (Bone R, ed. Disease-a-month; vol 5)
4. Cockerill F, Wilson W, Carpenter H, et al. Open lung biopsy in immunocompromised patients. Arch Intern Med 1985;145:1398–1404.
5. Comis RL. Bleomycin pulmonary toxicity, In: Crooke ST, Umezawa H, eds. Bleomycin. New York: Academic Press, 1978:279–291.
6. Aronin P, Mahaley M, Rudnick S, et al. Prediction of BCNU pulmonary toxicity in patients with malignant gliomas. An assessment of risk factor. N Engl J Med 1980;303:183–191.
7. Buzdar A, Legha S, MA L, Tashima C, Hortobagyi GN, Blumenschein GR. Pulmonary toxicity of mitomycin. Cancer 1980;45:236–244.
8. Ginsberg SJ, Comis RL. The pulmonary toxicity of antineoplastic agents. Semin Oncol 1982;9:34–51.
9. Haupt H, Hutchins G, Moore G. Ara-C lung: noncardiogenic pulmonary edema complicating cytosine arabinoside therapy of leukemia. Am J Med 1981; 70:256–261.
10. Glauser F, De Blois G, Bechard D, Fowler A, Merchant R, Fairman R. Review: cardiopulmonary toxicity of adoptive immunotherapy. Am J Med Sci 1988; 296:406–412.
11. Sostman H, Matthay R, Puman C, Smith G. Methotrexate-induced pneumonitis. Medicine 1976; 55:371–388.
12. Aso Y, Yoneda K, Kikkawa Y. Morphologic and biochemical study of pulmonary changes induced by bleomycin in mice. Lab Invest 1976;35:558–568.
13. Adamson I, Bowden D. The pathogenesis of bleomycin-induced pulmonary damage in mice. Am J Pathol 1974;77:185–197.
14. Otsuka K, Murota S, Mori Y. Stimulatory effect of bleomycin on the synthesis of acid glycosaminoglycans in cultured fibroblasts derived from rat granuloma. Biochim Biophys Acta 1976;444:359–368.

15. Clark JG, Kostal KM, Marino BA. An alveolar macrophage product increases fibroblast prostaglandin E_2 and cyclic adenosine monophosphate and suppresses fibroblast proliferation and collagen production. J Clin Invest 1983;72:2082–2091.

16. Crouch E. Pathobiology of pulmonary fibrosis. Am J Physiol 1990;259:L159–L184.

17. Pritsos CA, Sartorelli AC. Generation of reactive oxygen radicals through bioactivation of mitomycin antibiotics. Cancer Res 1986;436:3528–3532.

18. Hay J, Shazeidi, Laurent G. Mechanisms of bleomycin-induced lung damage. Arch Toxicol 1991; 65(2):81–94.

19. White DA, Kris MG, Stover DE. Bronchoalveolar lavage cell populations in bleomycin lung toxicity. Thorax 1987;42:551–552.

20. Holoye P, Luna M, MacKay B, Bedrossian C. Bleomycin hypersensitivity pneumonitis. Ann Intern Med 1978;88:47–49.

21. Jones S, Moore M, Blank N, Castellino R. Hypersensitivity to procarbazine manifested by fever and pleuropulmonary reaction. Cancer 1972;29:498–500.

22. Garbes I, Henderson E, Gomez G, Bakshi S, Parhasarathy K, Castillo N. Procarbazine-induced interstitial pneumonitis with a normal chest x-ray: a case report. Med Pediatr Oncol 1986;14:238–241.

23. Skarin A, Lokich J, Goodman R, et al. Combined intensive chemotherapy and radiotherapy in oat cell carcinoma of the lung (abstract). Proc Am Soc Clin Oncol 1975;16:264.

24. Durant J, Norgard M, Murad T, Bartolucci A, Langford K. Pulmonary toxicity associated with bis-chloroethylnitrosourea (BCNU). Ann Intern Med 1979; 90:191–194.

25. Bauer K, Skarin A, Balikian J, Garnick M, Rosenthal D, Canellos G. Pulmonary complications associated with combination chemotherapy programs containing bleomycin. Am J Med 1983;74:557–563.

26. White D, Orenstein M, Godwin T, Stover D. Chemotherapy-associated pulmonary toxic reactions during treatment for breast cancer. Arch Intern Med 1984;144:953–956.

27. Luedke D, McLaughlin TT, Daugahday C, et al. Mitomycin C and vindesine associated pulmonary toxicity with variable clinical expression. Cancer 1985; 55:542–545.

28. Blum R, Carter SK, Agre K, et al. A clinical review of bleomycin. Cancer 1973;31:903–914.

29. Gross N. Pulmonary effects of radiation therapy. Ann Intern Med 1977;86:81–92.

30. Wesselius L. Pulmonary complications of cancer therapy. Compr Ther 1992;18:17–20.

31. Kreisman H, Wolkove N. Pulmonary toxicity of antineoplastic therapy. In: Perry MC, ed. The chemotherapy sourcebook. 1st ed. Williams & Wilkins, 1992:598–619.

32. Doelman C, Bast A. Oxygen radicals in lung pathology. Free Radical Biol Med 1990;9(5):381–400.

33. Hakkinen P, Whiteley J, Witschi H. Hyperoxia, but not thoracic x-irradiation, potentiates bleomycin and cyclophosphomide-induced lung damage in mice. Am Rev Respir Dis 1982;126:281–285.

34. Franklin R, Buroker TR, Vaishampayan W, et al. Combined therapies in esophageal squamous cell cancer (abstract). Proc Am Assoc Cancer Res 1979; 20:223.

35. Kehrer J, Paraidathathu T. Enhanced oxygen toxicity following treatment with 1,3-bis(2-chloroethyl)-1-nitrosourea. Fundam Appl Toxicol 1984; 4:760–767.

36. Williams B, Francis A, Durrant S. Simultaneous presentation of sarcoidosis and acute myeloid leukemia: predisposition to pulmonary hemorrhage. J Clin Pathol 1994;47:672–673.

37. Hansen S. Late-effects after treatment for germ-cell cancer with cisplatin, vinblastine, and bleomycin. Dan Med Bull 1992;39(5):391–399.

38. Boyer M, Raghavan D, Harris P, et al. Lack of late toxicity in patients treated with cisplatin-containing combination chemotherapy for metastatic testicular cancer. J Clin Oncol 1990;8:21–26.

39. Horowitz A, Friedman M, Smith J, et al. The pulmonary changes of bleomycin toxicity. Radiology 1973;106:65–68.

40. Patz E, Peters W, Goodman P. Pulmonary drug toxicity following high-dose chemotherapy with autologous bone marrow transplantation: CT findings in 20 cases. J Thorac Imag 1994;9:129–134.

41. Padley S, Adler B, Hansell D, Müller N. High-resolution computed tomography of drug-induced lung disease. Clin Radiol 1992;46:232–236.

42. Bellamy E, Husband J, Blaquiere R, et al. Bleomycin-related lung damage: CT evidence. Radiology 1985;156:155–158.

43. Moinuddin M. Radionuclide scanning in the detection of drug-induced lung disorders. J Thorac Imag 1991;6(1):62–67.

44. Comis R, Kuppinger M, Ginsberg S. Role of single breath carbon monoxide diffusing capacity in monitoring the pulmonary effects of bleomycin in germ tumor cell patients. Cancer Res 1979;39:5076–5080.

45. Crawford S, Fisher L. Predictive value of pulmonary function tests before marrow transplantation. Chest 1992;101(5):1257–1264.

46. Canham I, Kennedy T, Merrick T. Unexplained pulmonary infiltrates in the compromised patient. An invasive investigation in a consecutive series. Cancer 1983;52:325–329.

47. McKenna R, Mountain C, McMurtrey M. Open lung biopsy in immuno-compromised patients. Chest 1984;86:671–674.

48. Umezawa H, Maeda K, Takeuchi T, Okami Y. New antibiotics, bleomycin A and B. Cancer 1966; 19:201–209.

49. Yogada A, Mukherji B, Young C, et al. Bleomycin, an antitumor antibiotic: clinical experience in 274 patients. Ann Intern Med 1972;77:861–870.

50. Comis R. Bleomycin pulmonary toxicity: current status and future directions. Semin Oncol 1992; 19(2 Suppl 5):64–70.

51. Ichikawa T, Nakano I, Hirokawa I. Bleomycin treatment of the tumors of penis and scrotum. J Urol 1969;102:699–707.

52. Umezawa H, Hori S, Sawa T, Yoshioka T, Takauchi T. A bleomycin inactivating enzyme in mouse tissue. J Antibiot 1974;27:419–424.

53. Ohnuma T, Holland J, Masuda H, Waligunda J, Goldberg G. Microbiological assay of bleomycin: inactivation, tissue distribution and clearance. Cancer 1974;33:1230–1238.

54. Sebti S, Mignano J, Jani J, et al. Bleomycin hydrolase: molecular cloning, sequencing, and biochem-

ical studies reveal membership in the cysteine protein-ase family. Biochemistry 1989;28:6544–6548.

55. Sebti S, Jani J, Mistry J, et al. Metabolic inacti-vation: a mechanism of human tumor resistance to bleomycin. Cancer Res 1991;51:227–232.

56. Lazo J, Merrill W, Pham E, Lynch T, Mc Callis-ter J, Ingbar D. Bleomycin hydrolase activity in pul-monary cells. J Pharmacol Exp Ther 1984;231:583–588.

57. Sausville E, Stein R, Peisach J, Horwitz S. Prop-erties and products of the degradation of DNA by bleo-mycin and iron (II). Biochemistry 1978;17:2746–2754.

58. Martin WI, Kachel D. Bleomycin-induced pul-monary endothelial cell injury: evidence for the role of iron-catalyzed toxic oxygen-derived species. J Lab Clin Med 1987;110:153–158.

59. Mirabelli CA, Ting A, Huang CH, Mong S, Crooke ST. Bleomycin and talisomycin sequence spe-cific strand scission of DNA: a mechanism of double strand cleavage. Cancer Res 1982;42:2779–2785.

60. Berend N. Protective effect of hypoxia on bleo-mycin lung toxicity in the rat. Am Rev Respir Dis 1984; 130:307–308.

61. Cunningham M, Ringrose P, Lokesh B. Inhibi-tion of the genotoxicity of bleomycin by superoxide dismutase. Mutat Res 1984;135:199–202.

62. Larramendy ML, Bianchi MS, Padron J. Corre-lation between the anti-oxidant enzyme activities of blood fractions and the yield of bleomycin-induced chromosome damage. Mutat Res 1989;214:129–136.

63. Cutroneo KR, Sterling KMJ. The biochemical and molecular basis of bleomycin-induced pulmonary fibrosis. Focus Pulmon Pharmacol Toxicol 1988;1:1–22.

64. Thrall R, McCormick J, Jack R, McReynolds R, Ward P. Bleomycin induced pulmonary fibrosis in rats. Am J Pathol 1979;95:117–130.

65. Lehne G, Lote G. Pulmonary toxicity of cyto-toxic and immunosuppressive agents. Acta Oncol 1990;29:113–124.

66. Rossi P, Karsenty G, Roberts AB, Roche NS, Sporn MB, de Crombrugghe B. A nuclear factor 1 bind-ing site mediated the transcriptional activation of a type I collagen promoter by TGFbeta. Cell 1988;52:405–414.

67. Grotendorst GR, Seppa HEJ, Kleinman HK, Martin GR. Attachment of smooth muscle cells to col-lagen and their migration toward platelet-derived growth factor. Proc Natl Acad Sci USA 1981;78:3669–3672.

68. Seppa H, Grotendorst G, Seppa S, Schiffmann E, Martin GR. Platelet-derived growth factor is che-motactic for fibroblasts. J Cell Biol 1982;92:584–588.

69. Cohen M, Austin J, Smith-Vaniz A, et al. Nod-ular bleomycin toxicity. Am J Clin Pathol 1989;92:101–104.

70. Santrach P, Askin F, Wells R, et al. Nodular form of bleomycin-related pulmonary injury in pa-tients with osteogenic sarcoma. Cancer 1989;164:806–811.

71. Dineen M, Englander L, Huben R, et al. Bleo-mycin-induced nodular pulmonary fibrosis masquer-ading as metastatic testicular cancer. J Urol 1986; 136:473–475.

72. De Lena M, Guzzon A, Monfardini S, Bona-donna G. Clinical, radiologic and histopathologic stud-ies on pulmonary toxicity induced by treatment with bleomycin. Cancer 1972;56:343–355.

73. Collis C. Lung damage from cytotoxic drugs. Cancer Chemother Pharmacol 1980;4:17–27.

74. Wilson J. Pulmonary toxicity of antineoplastic drugs. Cancer Treat 1978;62:2008–2013.

75. Iacovino J, Leitner J, Abbas A, Lokich J, Snider G. Fatal pulmonary reaction from low doses of bleo-mycin. An idiosyncratic tissue response. JAMA 1976; 235:1253–1255.

76. Crooke S, Einhorn L, Comis R, et al. The effects of prior exposure to bleomycin on the incidence of pul-monary toxicities. Med Pediatr Oncol 1978;5:93–98.

77. Mathe G, for the Clinical Screening Coopera-tive Group of the European Organization for Research on the Treatment of Cancer. Study of the clinical effi-cacy of bleomycin in human cancer. Br Med J 1970; 2:643–645.

78. Halman K, Bleehan N, Brewin T. Clinical stud-ies with bleomycin. Br Med J 1972;4:635–638.

79. Samuels M, Johnson D, Holoye P, Lanzotti V. Large-dose bleomycin therapy and pulmonary toxic-ity. A possible role of prior radiotherapy. JAMA 1976; 235:117–120.

80. Nygaard K, Smith-Erichsen N, Hatlevoll R, Ref-sum S. Pulmonary complications after bleomycin, ir-radiation and surgery for esophageal cancer. Cancer 1978;41:17–22.

81. Einhorn L, Krause M, Hornback N, et al. En-hanced pulmonary toxicity with bleomycin and radio-therapy in oat cell lung cancer. Cancer 1976;37:2414–2416.

82. Goldiner P, Carlon G, Cvitkovic E, Schweizer O, Howland W. Factors influencing postoperative morbidity and mortality in patients treated with bleo-mycin. Br Med J 1978;1:1664–1667.

83. Ingrassia TI, Ryu, JH, Trastek, VF, et al. Oxygen exacerbates bleomycin pulmonary toxicity. Mayo Clin Proc 1991;66:173–178.

84. Gilson A, Sahn S. Reactivation of bleomycin lung toxicity following oxygen administration. Chest 1985;88:304–306.

85. Schein P, De Vita V, Hubbard S, et al. Bleo-mycin, adriamycin, cyclophosphamide, vincristine, and prednisone (BACOP). Ann Intern Med 1976; 85:417–422.

86. Skarin A, Rosenthal D, Maloney W. The treat-ment of advanced non-Hodgkin's lymphoma (NHL) with bleomycin, adriamycin, cyclophosphamide, vin-cristine and prednisone. Blood 1977;49:759–770.

87. Coltman CA Jr, Luce JK, McKelvey EM, et al. Chemotherapy of non-Hodgkin's lymphoma: 10 years experience in the Southwest Oncology Group. Cancer Treat Rep 1977;61:1067–1078.

88. Bennett W, Pastore L, Houghton D. Fatal pul-monary bleomycin toxicity in cisplatinum-induced acute renal failure. Cancer Treat Rep 1980;64:921–924.

89. Perry D, Weiss R, Taylor H. Enhanced bleo-mycin toxicity during acute renal failure. Cancer Treat Rep 1982;66:592–593.

90. Dalgleish A, Woods R, Levi J. Bleomycin pul-monary toxicity: its relationship to renal dysfunction. Med Pediatr Oncol 1984;12:313–317.

91. Siki B, Collins J, Mimnaugh E, Gram T. Im-proved therapeutic index of bleomycin when admin-istered by continuous infusion in mice. Cancer Treat Rep 1978;62:2011–2017.

92. Cooper K, Hong W. Prospective study of the

pulmonary toxicity of continuously infused bleomycin. Cancer Treat Rep 1981;65:419–425.

93. Krakoff I, Cvitkovic E, Currie V, Yeh S, La Monte C. Clinical pharmacologic and therapeutic studies of bleomycin given by continuous infusion. Cancer 1977;40:2027–2037.

94. White DA, Stover DE. Severe bleomycin-induced pneumonitis: clinical features and response to corticosteroids. Chest 1984;86:723–728.

95. Van Barneveld R, Sleijfer D, VanDer Mark T, et al. Natural course of bleomycin-induced pneumonitis. A follow-up study. Am Rev Respir Dis 1987;135:48–51.

96. Lucraft H, Wilkinson P, Stretton T, Read G. Role of pulmonary function tests in the prevention of bleomycin pulmonary toxicity during chemotherapy for metastatic testicular teratoma. Eur J Cancer Clin Oncol 1982;18:133–139.

97. Wolkowicz J, Sturgeon MB, Rawji M, et al. Bleomycin-induced pulmonary function abnormalities. Chest 1992;101:97–101.

98. Harmann L, Frytak S, Richardson R, Coles D, Cupps R. Life threatening bleomycin pulmonary toxicity with ultimate reversibility. Chest 1990;98:497–499.

99. Maher J, Daly P. Severe bleomycin lung toxicity: reversal with high dose corticosteroids. Thorax 1993;48:92–94.

100. Matsuda A. Fundamental studies on a new antitumor antibiotic peplomycin. Prostate 1981;1(Suppl):119–123.

101. Sikic B, Siddik Z, Gram T. Relative pulmonary toxicity and antitumor effects of two new bleomycin analogs, peplomycin and tallysomycin A. Cancer Treat Reports 1980;64(4–5):659–667.

102. Muller W, Zahn R, Maidhof A, Schroder H, Backmann M, Umezawa H. Synergistic effect of peplomycin in combination with bleomycin on L5178y mouse lymphoma cells in vivo. J Antibiot 1984;37(3):239–243.

103. Sorensen P, Rorth M, Hansen H. Phase I evaluation of peplomycin with special reference to pulmonary toxicity. Eur J Cancer Clin Oncol 1983;19(3):319–325.

104. Sorensen P, Rorth M, Hansen H, Dombernowsky P, Host H. A phase II trial of peplomycin in squamous cell carcinoma of the lung. Eur J Cancer Clin Oncol 1983;19(1):25–27.

105. Ekimoto H, Takada K, Takahashi K, Matsuda A, Takita T, Umezawa H. Effect of oxygen concentration on pulmonary fibrosis caused by peplomycin in mice. J Antibiot 1984;37(6):659–663.

106. Hirabayashi K, Okada E. Combination chemotherapy with 254-S, ifosfamide, and peplomycin for advanced or recurrent cervical cancer. Cancer 1993;71(9):2769–2775.

107. Shimamoto T, Tateyama H, Kohso T, Hamada M. Neoadjuvant chemotherapy using a platinum, vincristine and peplomycin combination in patients with carcinoma of the uterine cervix. Asia Oceania J Obstet Gynecol 1993;19(3):261–269.

108. Takahshi K, Ekimoto H, Minamide S, et al. Liblomycin, a new analogue of bleomycin. Cancer Treat Rev 1987;14:169.

109. Yoshida T, Ogawa M, Ota K, et al. Phase II study of NK313 in malignant lymphomas: an NK313 Malignant Lymphoma Study Group trial. Cancer Chemother Pharmacol 1993;31:445–448.

110. Ariyoshi Y, Ota K, Suzuki A, et al. Phase I study of liblomycin (NK313) (abstract). Proc Am Soc Clin Oncol 1989;8:287.

111. Paolozzi F, Gaver R, Newman N, et al. Phase I trial of tallysomycin S10b, a bleomycin analog. Invest New Drugs 1990;8:171–180.

112. Samson MK, Comis RL, Baker LH, Ginsberg S, Fraile RJ, Crooke ST. Mitomycin-C in advanced adenocarcinoma and large cell carcinoma of the lung. Cancer Treat Rep 1978;62:163–165.

113. Spain R. The case for mitomycin in non-small cell lung cancer. Oncology 1993;50(1):35–52.

114. Sheldon R, Slaughter D. A syndrome of microangiopathic hemolytic anemia, renal impairment, and pulmonary edema in chemotherapy-treated patients with adenocarcinoma. Cancer 1986;58:1428–1436.

115. Lesesne JB, Rothschild N, Erickson B, et al. Cancer associated hemolytic-uremic syndrome: analysis of 85 cases from a national registry. J Clin Oncol 1989;7:781–789.

116. Buzdar AU, Legha SS, Tashima CK, et al. Adriamycin and mitomycin-C: possible synergistic cardiotoxicity. Cancer Treat Rep 1970;62:1005–1008.

117. Simasoto Y, Baba K, Watanabe S. Pulmonary lesions produced by antitumor drugs. Studies on autopsy cases. Jpn J Cancer Clin 1971;17:21–34.

118. Verweij J, van der Burg MEL, Pinedo HM. Mitomycin-C induced hemolytic uremic syndrome. Six case reports and review of the literature on renal, pulmonary and cardiac side effects of the drug. Radiother Oncol 1987;8:33–41.

119. Orwoll ES, Kiessling PJ, Patterson JR. Interstitial pneumonia from mitomycin. Ann Intern Med 1978;89:352–355.

120. Twohig K, Matthay R. Pulmonary effects of cytotoxic agents other than bleomycin. Clin Chest Med 1990;11(1):31–54.

121. Verweij J, van Zanten T, Souren T, Golding R, Pinedo HM. Prospective study on the dose relationship of mitomycin C-induced interstitial pneumonitis. Cancer 1987;60:756–761.

122. Castro M, Veeder M, Mailliard JA, Tazelaar HD, Jett J. A prospective study of pulmonary toxicity in patients receiving mitomycin. Chest 1996, in press.

123. Gunstream S, Seidenfeld J, Sobonya R, McMahon L. Mitomycin-associated lung disease. Cancer Treat Rep 1983;67:301–304.

124. Kris M, Pablo D, Gralla R, Burke M, Prestifilippo J, Lewin D. Dyspnea following vinblastine or vindesine administration in patients receiving mitomycin plus vinca alkaloid combination therapy. Cancer Treat Rep 1984;68:1029–1031.

125. Rao S, Ramaswamy G, Levin M, et al. Fatal acute respiratory failure after vinblastine-mitomycin therapy in lung carcinoma. Arch Intern Med 1985;145:1905–1907.

126. Murgo AJ. Thrombotic microangiopathy in the cancer patient including those induced by chemotherapeutic agents. Semin Hematol 1987;24:161–177.

127. Kuebler JP, Chang AYC, Pandya KJ, Tormey DC, Isreal B. Pulmonary toxicity associated with a mitomycin-C containing regimen (abstract). Clin Res 1982;30:859A.

128. Chang AY, Kuebler JP, Pandya KJ, Israel RH, Marshall BC, Tormey DC. Pulmonary toxicity induced

by mitomycin C is highly responsive to glucocorticoids. Cancer 1986;57:2285–2290.

129. Gralla RJ, Bolton JS, Clark RA, Lang AC. Mitomycin in non-small cell lung cancer (NSCLC): does pulmonary toxicity limit its use (abstract)? Proc Am Soc Clin Oncol 1992;11:292A.

130. Bonadonna G, Monfardini S, de Lena M, Fossati-Bellani F. Clinical evaluation of Adriamycin, a new antitumour antibiotic. Br Med J 1969;3:503–506.

131. Verschoore J, Lagrange J, Boublil J, et al. Pulmonary toxicity of combination of low-dose doxorubicin and irradiation for inoperable lung cancer. Radiother Oncol 1987;9:281–288.

132. Cassady J, Richter M, Piro A, Jaffe N. Radiation-adriamycin interactions: preliminary clinical observations. Cancer 1975;36:946–949.

133. Philips T, Fu K. The interaction of drug and radiation on normal tissues. Int J Radiat Oncol Biol Phys 1978;4:59–64.

134. Johnson R, Brereton H, Kent C. "Total" therapy for small cell carcinoma of the lung. Ann Thorac Surg 1978;25:510–515.

135. Bistrovic M, Nagy B, Maricic Z, Kolaric K. Interaction of adriamycin and radiation in combined treatment on mouse L-cells. Eur J Cancer 1978;14:411–414.

136. Rosiello R, Merrill WW. Radiation-induced lung damage. Clin Chest Med 1990;11:65–71.

137. McInerney D, Bullimore J. Reactivation of radiation pneumonitis by adriamycin. Br J Radiology 1977;50:224–227.

138. Launchbury A, Habboubi N. Epirubicin and doxorubicin: a comparison of their characteristics, therapeutic activity and toxicity. Cancer Treat Rev 1993;19:197–228.

139. Wara W, Philips T, Margolis L, Smith V. Radiation pneumonitis: a new approach to the derivation of time-dose factors. Cancer 1973;32:547–552.

140. Braun S, DoPico G, Olson C, Caldwell W. Low-dose radiation pneumonitis. Cancer 1975;35:1322–1324.

141. Selzar S, Griffin T, D'Orsi C, et al. Pulmonary reaction associated with neocarzinostatin therapy. Cancer Treat Rep 1978;6:1271–1272.

142. Calvo D, Legha S, McKelvey E, et al. Zenostatin-related pulmonary toxicity. Cancer Treat Rep 1981;65:165–167.

143. Weiss R, Poster D, Penta J. The nitrosoureas and pulmonary toxicity. Cancer Treat Rev 1981;8:111–125.

144. Calabresi P, Parks RJ. Chemotherapy of neoplastic diseases. In: Gilman A, Goodman LS, Rall TW, et al., eds. The pharmacological basis of therapeutics. New York: MacMillan 1985:1240–1307.

145. Ahlgren J, Smith F, Kerwin D, Sikic B, Weiner J, Schein P. Pulmonary disease as a complication of chlorozotocin chemotherapy. Cancer Treat Rep 1981;65:223–229.

146. Cordonnier C, Vernant J-P, Mital P, Lange F, Bernaudin J-F, Rochant H. Pulmonary fibrosis subsequent to high doses of CCNU for chronic leukemia. Cancer 1983;51:1814–1818.

147. Lee W, Moore R, Wampler G. Interstitial pulmonary fibrosis as a complication of prolonged methyl-CCNU therapy. Cancer Treat Rep 1978;62:1355–1358.

148. Arrick BA, Nathan CF. Glutathione metabolism as a determinant of therapeutic efficacy: a review. Cancer Res 1984;44:4224–4232.

149. Smith AC, Boyd MR. Preferential effects of 1,3-bis(2-chloroethyl)-1-nitrosureas (BCNU) on pulmonary glutathione reductase and glutathione/glutathione disulfide rations: possible implications for lung toxicity. J Pharmacol Exp Ther 1984;229:658–663.

150. O'Driscoll B, Hasleton P, Taylor P, Poulter L, Gattamaneni H, Woodcock A. Active lung fibrosis up to 17 years after chemotherapy with carmustine (BCNU) in childhood. N Engl J Med 1990;323(6):378–382.

151. Hasleton P, O'Driscoll B, Lynch P, et al. Late BNCU lung: a light and ultrastructural study on the delayed effect of BCNU on the lung parachyma. J Pathol 1991;164:31–36.

152. Bhuyan U, Peters AM, Gordon I, Davies H, Helms P. Effect of posture on regional ventilation in children and adults. Thorax 1989;44:480–484.

153. Taylor P, O'Driscoll B, Gattaneni H, Woodcock A. Chronic lung fibrosis following carmustine (BCNU) chemotherapy: radiological features. Clin Radiol 1991;44:299–301.

154. Patten G, Billi J, Rotman H. Rapidly progressive fatal pulmonary fibrosis induced by carmustine. JAMA 1980;244:687–688.

155. Todd N, Peters W, Ost A, Roggli V, Piantadosi C. Pulmonary drug toxicity in patients with primary breast cancer treated with high-dose combination chemotherapy and autologous bone marrow transplantation. Am Rev Resp Dis 1993;147:1264–1270.

156. Holoye P, Jenkins D, Greenberg S. Pulmonary toxicity in long-term administration of BCNU. Cancer Treat Rep 1976;60:1691–1694.

157. Phillips GL, Fay JW, Herzig GP, et al. Intensive 1,3-bis(2-chloroethyl)-1-nitrosourea (BCNU), NSC #4366650 and cryopreserved autologous marrow transplantation for refractory cancer. A phase I-II study. Cancer 1983;52:1792–1802.

158. Jones R, Matthes S, Dufton C, et al. Pharmacokinetic/pharmacodynamic interactions of intensive cyclophosphamide, cisplatin, and BCNU in patients with breast cancer. Breast Cancer Res Treat 1993;26:S-11–S-17.

159. Peters WP, Shpall EJ, Jones RB, et al. High-dose combination alkylating agents with bone marrow support as initial treatment for metastatic breast cancer. J Clin Oncol 1988;6:1368–1376.

160. Limper A, McDonald J. Delayed pulmonary fibrosis after nitrosourea therapy. N Engl J Med 1990;323(6):407–409.

161. Oliner H, Schwartz R, Rubio F, Dameshek W. Interstitial pulmonary fibrosis following busulfan therapy. Am J Med 1961;31:134–139.

162. Burns W, McFarland W, Matthew M. Busulfan-induced pulmonary disease. Report of a case and review of the literature. Am Rev Respir Dis 1970;101:408–413.

163. Littler W, Kay J, Hasleton P, Heath D. Busulfan lung. Thorax 1969;24:639–655.

164. Koss L, Melamed M, Mayer K. The effect of busulfan on human epithelia. Am J Clin Pathol 1965;44:385–397.

165. Kuplic J, Higley C, Niewoehner D. Pulmonary ossification associated with long-term busulfan therapy in chronic myeloid leukemia. Am Rev Respir Dis 1972;106:759–762.

166. Aymard J, Gyger M, Lavallee R, Legresley L, Desy M. A case of pulmonary alveolar proteinosis complicating chronic myelogenous leukemia. A peculiar pathologic aspect of busulfan lung? Cancer 1984; 53:954–956.

167. Min K-W, Gyorkey F. Interstitial pulmonary fibrosis, atypical epithelial changes and bronchiolar cell carcinoma following busulfan therapy. Cancer 1968;22:1027–1032.

168. Hawkins D, Sanders S, MacDonald F, Drage C. Pulmonary toxicity recurring after a six week course of busulfan therapy and after subsequent therapy with uracil mustard. Chest 1978;73:415–416.

169. Schallier D, Impens N, Warson F, Van Belle S, De Wasch G. Additive pulmonary toxicity with melphalan and busulfan therapy. Chest 1983;84:492–493.

170. Soble A, Perry H. Fatal radiation pneumonia following subclinical busulfan injury. AJR 1977;128:15–18.

171. Andre R, Rochant H, Dreyfus B, et al. Fibrose interstitielle diffuse du poumon au cours d'une maladie de Hodgkin traitee par des doses elevees d'endoxan. Bull Soc Med Hop (Paris) 1967;118(1):1133–1141.

172. Stentoft J. Progressive pulmonary fibrosis complicating cyclophosphamide therapy. Acta Med Scand 1987;221:403–407.

173. Burke DA, Stoddart JC, Ward MK, Simpson CG. Fatal pulmonary fibrosis occurring during treatment with cyclophosphamide. Br Med J 1982;285:696.

174. Mark G, Lehimgar-Zadeh A, Ragsdale B. Cyclophosphamide pneumonitis. Thorax 1978;33:89–93.

175. Patel J. Metabolism and pulmonary toxicity of cyclophosphamide. Pharmacol Ther 1990;47:137–146.

176. Gurtoo H, Hipkens J, Sharma S. Role of glutathione in the metabolism-dependent toxicity and chemotherapy of cyclophosphamide. Cancer Res 1981; 41:3584–3591.

177. Patel J, Block E. Cyclophosphamide-induced depression of the antioxidant defuse mechanisms of the lung. Exp Lung Res 1985;8:153–165.

178. Schrier D, Phan S. Modulation of bleomycin-induced pulmonary fibrosis in the BALB/C mouse by cyclophosphamide-sensitive T cells. Am J Pathol 1984; 116:270–278.

179. Trask C, Joannides T, Harper P, et al. Radiation-induced lung fibrosis after treatment of small cell carcinoma of the lung with very high-dose cyclophosphamide. Cancer 1985;55:57–60.

180. Patel J, Block E, Hood C. Biochemical indices of cyclophosphamide-induced lung injury. Toxic Appl Pharmacol 1984;76:128–138.

181. Seiden M, Elias A, Ayash L, et al. Pulmonary toxicity associated with high dose chemotherapy in the treatment of solid tumors with autologous marrow transplant: an analysis of four chemotherapy regimens. Bone Marrow Transplant 1992;10:57–63.

182. Slavin R, Millan J, Mullins G. Pathology of high dose intermittent cyclophosphamide therapy. Hum Pathol 1975;6:693–709.

183. Maxwell I. Reversible pulmonary edema following cyclophosphamide treatment. JAMA 1974; 229:137–138.

184. Carr MJ. Chlorambucil induced pulmonary fibrosis: report of a case and review. Va Med 1986; 113:677–680.

185. Godard P, Marty J, Michel F. Interstitial pneumonia and chlorambucil. Chest 1979;76:471–473.

186. Refvem O. Fatal intraalveolar and interstitial lung fibrosis in chlorambucil-treated chronic lymphocytic leukemia. Mt Sinai J Med 1977;44:847–851.

187. Cole S, Myers T, Klatsky A. Pulmonary disease with chlorambucil therapy. Cancer 1978;41:455–459.

188. Lane S, Besa E, Justh G, et al. Fatal interstitial lung disease following high dose chlorambucil therapy (abstract). Proc Am Soc Clin Oncol 1979;20:313.

189. Rubio F. Possible pulmonary effects of aklylating agents. N Engl J Med 1972;287:1150–1151.

190. Rose MS. Busulphan toxicity syndrome caused by chlorambucil. Br Med J 1975;2:123.

191. Mohr M, Kingreen D, Rühl, Huhn D. Interstitial lung disease—an underdiagnosed side effect of chlorambucil? Ann Hematol 1993;67:305–307.

192. Giles F, Smith M, Goldstone A. Chlorambucil lung toxicity. Acta Haematol 1990;83:156–158.

193. Taetle R, Dickman P, Feldman P. Pulmonary histopathologic changes associated with melphalan therapy. Cancer 1978;42:1239–1245.

194. Acute Leukemia Group B. Acute lymphocytic leukemia in children. JAMA 1969;207:923–928.

195. Furst D, Erikson N, Clute L, Koehnke R, Burmeister L, Kohler J. Adverse experience with methotrexate during 176 weeks of a longterm prospective trial in patients with rheumatoid arthritis. J Rheumatol 1990;17:1628–1635.

196. Hargreaves M, Mowat A, Benson M. Acute pneumonitis associated with low dose methotrexate treatment for rheumatoid arthritis: report of five cases and review of published reports. Thorax 1992;47:628–633.

197. Anderson L, Collins G, Ojima Y. A study of the distribution of methotrexate in human tissues and tumours. Cancer Res 1970;30:1344–1348.

198. Hirata T, Nagai S, Oshima S, Izumi T. Comparative study of T-cell subsets in BAL fluid in patients with hypersensitivity pneumonitis and sarcoidosis (abstract). Chest 1982;82(Suppl):232.

199. White D, Rankin J, Stover D, et al. Methotrexate pneumonitis. Bronchoalveolar lavage findings suggest an immunologic disorder. Am Rev Respir Dis 1989;139:18–21.

200. Akoun G, Mayaud C, Touboul J, Denis M, Milleron B, Perrot J. Use of bronchoalveolar lavage in the evaluation of methotrexate lung disease. Thorax 1987; 42:652–655.

201. Bedrossian C, Miller W, Luna M. Methotrexate-induced diffuse interstitial pulmonary fibrosis. South Med J 1979;72:313–318.

202. Clarysse A, Cathey W, Cartwright G, Wintrobe M. Pulmonary disease complicating intermittent therapy with methotrexate. JAMA 1969;209:1861–1864.

203. Berstein M, Sobel D, Wimmer R. Non-cardiogenic pulmonary edema following injection of methotrexate into the cerebrospinal fluid. Cancer 1982; 50:866–868.

204. Hamous J, Guffy M, Aschenbrener C. Fatal acute respiratory failure following intrathecal methotrexate administration. Cancer Treat Rep 1983;67:1025–1026.

205. Urban C, Nirenberg A, Caparros B, Anac S, Cacavio A, Rosen G. Chemical pleuritis as the cause of

acute chest pain following high-dose methotrexate treatment. Cancer 1983;51:34–37.

206. Everts C, Westcott J, Bragg D. Methotrexate therapy and pulmonary disease. Radiology 1973; 107:539–543.

207. Wall M, Wohl M, Jaffe N. Lung function in adolescents receiving high dose methotrexate. Pediatrics 1979;63:741–746.

208. Zusman J, Frentz J, Waring W. Rapid resolution of "methotrexate lung" with preoperative steroids (abstract). Proc Am Assoc Cancer Res and Am Soc Clin Oncol 1979;20:412.

209. Lennard L. The clinical pharmacology of 6-mercaptopurine. Eur J Clin Pharmacol 1992;43:329–339.

210. Pinkel D. Intravenous mercaptopurine: life begins at 40. J Clin Oncol 1993;11(9):1826–1831.

211. Stentoft J. The toxicity of cytarabine. Drug Safety 1990;5(1):7–27.

212. Anderson D, Cogan B, Keating M, Estey E, McCredie K, et al. Subacute pulmonary failure complicating therapy with high-dose ara-C in acute leukemia. Cancer 1985;56:2181–2184.

213. Donehower R, Karp J, Burke P. Pharmacology and toxicity of high-dose cytarabine by 72-hour continuous infusion. Cancer Treat Rep 1986;70:1059–1065.

214. Peters W, Willemze R, Colly L, Guiot H. Side effects of intermediate- and high-dose cytosine arabinoside in the treatment of refractory or relapsed acute leukaemia and non-Hodgkin's lymphoma. Neth J Med 1987;30:64–74.

215. Jehn U, Goldel N, Rienmüller R, Wilmanns W. Non-cardiogenic pulmonary edema complicating intermediate and high-dose ara-C treatment for relapsed acute leukemia. Med Oncol Tumor Pharmacother 1988;5:41–47.

216. Jehn U, Heinemann V. Phase II—study of treatment of refractory acute leukemia with intermediate-dose cytosine arabinoside and amsacrine. Anticancer Res 1993;13:379–382.

217. Aronchick J, Gefter W. Drug-induced pulmonary disease: an update. J Thorac Imag 1991;6:19–29.

218. Tjon A, Tham R, Peters W, de Bruine F, Willemze R. Pulmonary complications of cytosine arabinoside therapy: radiographic findings. AJR 1987; 149:23–27.

219. Dybedal I, Lamvik J. Respiratory insufficiency in acute leukemia following treatment with cytosine arabinoside and septicemia with streptococcus viridans. Eur J Haematol 1989;42(4):405–406.

220. Chun H, Leyland-Jones B, Cheson B. Fludarabine phosphate: a synthetic purine antimetabolite with significant activity against lymphoid malignancies. J Clin Oncol 1991;9(1):175–188.

221. Hurst P, Habib M, Garewal H, et al. Pulmonary toxicity associated with fludarabine monophosphate. Invest New Drug 1987;5:207–210.

222. Villlani F, Gallimberti M, Rizzi M, Manzi R. Pulmonary toxicity of recombinant interleukin-2 plus lymphokine-activated killer cell therapy. Eur Respir J 1993;6:828–833.

223. Schantz S, Dimery I, Lippman S, Clayman G, Pellegrino C, Morice R. A phase II study of interleukin-2 and interferon-alpha in head and neck cancer. Invest New Drugs 1992;10:217–223.

224. Negrier M, Pourreau C, Palmer P, et al. Phase I trial of recombinant interleukin-2 followed by recombinant tumor necrosis factor in patients with metastatic cancer. J Immunol 1992;11:93–102.

225. Huland E, Huland H, Heinzer H. Interleukin-2 by inhalation: local therapy for metastatic renal cell carcinoma. J Urol 1992;147:344–348.

226. Lee R, Lotze M, Skibber J, et al. Cardiorespiratory effects of immunotherapy with interleukin-2. J Clin Oncol 1989;7:7–20.

227. Rosenstein M, Ettinghausen S, Rosenberg S. Extravasation of intravascular fluid mediated by the systemic administration of recombinant interleukin-2. J Immunol 1986;137:1735–1742.

228. Papa J, Vetto J, Ettinghausen S, Mule J, Rosenberg S. Effects of corticosteroids on the antitumor activity of lymphokine-activated killer cells and IL-2 in mice. Cancer Res 1986;46:5618–5623.

229. Glauser F, DeBlois G, Bechard D, et al. A comparison of the cardiopulmonary effects of continuous versus bolus infusion of recombinant interleukin-2 in sheep. Cancer Res 1988;48:2221–2225.

230. Dillman R, Church C, Oldham R, West W, Schwartzberg L, Birch R. Inpatient continuous-infusion interleukin-2 in 788 patients with cancer. Cancer 1993;71:2358–2370.

231. Ardizzoni A, Bonavia M, Viale M, et al. Biologic and clinical effects of continuous infusion interleukin-2 in patients with non-small cell lung cancer. Cancer 1994;73:1353–1360.

232. Vogelzang P, Bloom S, Mier J, Atkins M. Chest roentgenographic abnormalities in IL-2 recipients: incidence and correlation with clinical paramters. Chest 1992;101:746–752.

233. Mann H, Ward J, Samlowdki W. Vascular leak syndrome associated with interleukin-2: chest radiographic manifestations. Radiology 1990;176:191–194.

234. Huland E, Heinzer H, Huland H. Inhaled interleukin-2 in combination with low-dose systemic interleukin-2 and interferon alpha in patients with pulmonary metastatic renal-cell carcinoma: effectiveness and toxicity of mainly local treatment. J Cancer Res Clin Oncol 1994;120(4):221–228.

235. West W, Tawer K, Yannelli J, et al. Constant continuous infusion recombinant interleukin-2 in adoptive immunotherapy of advanced cancer. N Engl J Med 1987;316:898–905.

236. Mitchell M, Kempf R, Harel W. Effectiveness and tolerability of low-dose intravenous interleukin-2 in disseminated melanoma. J Clin Oncol 1988;6:409–424.

237. Rowinsky E, Eisengauer E, Chaudhry V, Arbuck S, Donehower R. Clinical toxicities encountered with paclitaxel (Taxol). Semin Oncol 1993;20(4):1–15.

238. Rowinsky E, Burke P, Karp J, et al. Phase I and pharmacodynamic study of taxol in refractory acute leukemias. Cancer Res 1989;49:4640–4647.

239. Brandwein M, Rosen M, Harpaz N, et al. Fatal pulmonary lipid embolism associated with taxol therapy. Mt Sinai J Med 1988;55:187–189.

240. Rowinsky E, Donehower R. The clinical pharmacology and use of antimicrotubule agents in cancer chemotherapeutics. Pharmacol Ther 1991;52:35–84.

241. Bott S, Stewart F, Prince-Fiocco M. Interstitial lung disease associated with vindesine and radiation therapy for carcinoma of the lung. South Med J 1986; 79:894–896.

242. Ozols R, Hogan W, Ostchega Y, Young R. MVP (mitomycin, vinblastine and progesterone): a sec-

ond-line regimen in ovarian cancer with a high incidence of pulmonary toxicity. Cancer Treat Rep 1983; 67:721–722.

243. Hoelzer K, Harrison B, Suedke S, et al. Vinblastine-associated pulmonary toxicity in patients receiving combination therapy with mitomycin and cisplatin. Drug Intell Clin Pharm 1986;20:287–289.

244. Konits P, Aisner J, Sutherland J, Wiernik P. Possible pulmonary toxicity secondary to vinblastine. Cancer 1982;50:2771–2774.

245. Garbes I, Henderson E, Gomez G, Bakshi S, Parthasarathy K, Castillo N. Procarbazine-induced interstitial pneumonitis with a normal chest x-ray: a case report. Med Pediatr Oncol 1986;14:238–241.

246. Ecker M, May B, Keohane M. Procarbazine lung. AJR 1978;131:527–528.

247. Brooks BJ Jr, Hendler N, Alvarez S, Ancalmo N, Grinton S. Delayed life-threatening pneumonitis secondary to procarbazine. Am J Clin Oncol 1990; 12(3):244–246.

248. Lascari AD, Strano AJ, Johnson WW, Collins JG. Methotrexate-induced sudden fatal pulmonary reaction. Cancer 1977;40:1393–1397.

249. Commers J, Foley J. Pulmonary hyaline membrane disease occurring in the course of VM-26 therapy. Cancer Treat Rep 1979;63:2093–2095.

250. Hocking DC, Phillips PG, Ferro TJ, Johnson A. Mechanism of pulmonary edema induced by tumor necrosis factor-alpha. Circ Res 1990;67:68–77.

251. Demetri GD, Spriggs DR, Sherman ML, Arthur KA, Imamura K, Kufe DW. A phase I trial of recombinant human tumor necrosis factor and interferon-gamma: effects of combination cytokine administration in vivo. J Clin Oncol 1989;7:1545–1553.

252. Stevenson HC, Ochs JJ, Halverson L, Oldham RK, Sherwin SA, Foon KA. Recombinant alpha interferon in retreatment of two patients with pulmonary lymphoma: dramatic responses with resolution of pulmonary complications. Am J Med 1984;77:355–358.

253. Collins JF, Orozco CR, McCullough B, Coalson JJ, Johanson WG. Pulmonary fibrosis with small airway disease: a model in nonhuman primates. Exp Lung Res 1982;3:91–108.

254. Glasier CM, Siegel MJ. Multiple pulmonary nodules: unusual manifestation of bleomycin toxicity. Am J Radiol 1981;137:155–156.

255. Topilo AA, Rothenberg SP, Cottrell TS. Interstitial pneumonia after prolonged treatment with cyclophosphamide. Am Rev Respir Dis 1973;108:114–117.

256. Horton LW, Chappell AG, Powell DEB. Diffuse interstitial pulmonary fibrosis complicating Hodgkin's disease. Br J Dis Chest 1977;71:44–48.

257. Rose AG. Pulmonary veno-occlusive disease due to bleomycin therapy for lymphoma. S Afr Med 1983;64:636–638.

258. Knight BK, Rose AG. Pulmonary veno-occlusive disease after chemotherapy. Thorax 1985;40:874–875.

259. Lombard CM, Churg A, Winokur S. Pulmonary veno-occlusive disease after chemotherapy. Chest 1987;92:871–876.

260. Rinaldo J, Goldstein R, Snider G. Modification of oxygen toxicity after lung injury by bleomycin in hamsters. Am Rev Respir Dis 1982;126:1030–1033.

261. Tryka AF, Godleski JJ, Brain JD. Differences in effects of immediate and delayed hyperoxia exposure on bleomycin-induced pulmonary injury. Cancer Treat Rep 1984;68:759–764.

262. Cantrell JE, Phillips TM, Schein PS. Carcinoma-associated hemolytic-uremic syndrome: a complication of mitomycin C chemotherapy. J Clin Oncol 1985;3:723–734.

263. Shogan JE, Brandt SJ, Jones RB, et al. Toxicity from recombinant human granulocyte-macrophage colony stimulating factor (rHuGM-CSF) after high dose chemotherapy and autologous bone marrow transplant (ABMT) (abstract). Proc AACR 1988; 29:53.

264. Major PP, Laurin S, Bettez P. Pulmonary fibrosis following therapy with melphalan: report of two cases. Can Med Assoc J 1980;123:197–202.

35

Gastrointestinal Toxicity of Chemotherapeutic Agents

William F. Maule

Gastrointestinal tract dysfunction in patients receiving chemotherapy for malignant disease promotes malnutrition, accelerates weight loss, exacerbates fluid and electrolyte imbalance, and may lead to reduced doses of potentially life-extending therapy. This chapter reviews the most important syndromes of gastrointestinal toxicity, outlines other causes for similar symptoms in patients receiving chemotherapy, reviews standard approaches to symptom relief, and outlines potential alternative approaches.

MUCOSAL INFLAMMATION

Toxic effects of antineoplastic chemotherapy on replicating cells of the gastrointestinal tract produce mucosal cell death and loss of functional epithelium. The clinical manifestations are dictated by the level of the gut that is most affected. The antimetabolites, the antitumor antibiotics, and the vinca alkaloids are most closely associated with luminal side effects, but inflammation, superficial erosion, and ulceration through mucosa have been noted with a variety of other agents. The pathology of the syndrome was best characterized (1) in patients who received cystosine-arabinoside (ara-C). The initial lesion is a sloughing of the epithelium with replacement of specialized glandular elements by undifferentiated stem cells. Scattered islands of regenerating glands separated by abnormal mucosa characterize the second stage of the process, which is followed by complete healing within 7 to 10 days. Asymptomatic submucosal bleeding may occur, or there may be a frank hemorrhage into the gut lumen revealed as hematemesis,

melena, mucoid, or bloody stools. In the small intestine, necrosis is more severe in villus tips than in mucosal crypts.

Oropharynx

Painful erythema and ulceration of the oropharynx following chemotherapy compromise nutrient intake and increases the risk of systemic infection. Symptoms are potentiated by prior or current radiation therapy, oropharyngeal malignancy, oral/dental infection, and the severity and duration of neutropenia (2). Concurrent oral candidiasis, de novo bacterial infection of the oropharynx, extension of bacterial periodontal disease, or infection with cytomegalovirus or herpesvirus may obscure the diagnosis.

Inflammation occurs because of direct effects of chemotherapy on the mucosal cells and because neutropenia predisposes to infection from oral flora. The duration and severity of symptoms follow the course of myelosuppression, starting before leukocyte nadir and continuing until neutrophil recovery. The dual effects of chemotherapy suggest specific approaches to therapy.

Sucralfate, an aluminum salt of sucrose, binds to inflamed tissue in the ulcer craters of patients with peptic ulcer disease. The precise mechanism of healing is unknown. Forty-eight children who were receiving induction therapy for acute nonlymphocytic leukemia received either sulcralfate suspension (75 mg/kg/day in 4 doses) or a similar tasting placebo at the initiation of chemotherapy (3). Because of the inconvenience and discomfort of repeated oral dosing, a difference of 40% or more in outcome was required to reject the hypothesis that sucralfate was no more effective than placebo. However, no statistically significant differences in symptom score, oral intake, weight loss, or oral infections were noted between the two groups of patients. In a different approach, which addressed the effects of neutropenia (4), 17 children were treated with granulocyte-macrophage colony-stimulating factor (GM-CSF) after induction chemotherapy (with or without total body irradiation) for leukemia. Although the duration and severity of neutropenia were markedly reduced by GM-CSF, there was no consistent reduction in mucositis compared with historic controls.

There are scant placebo-controlled data showing benefit from any agent used to prevent mucositis; similarly, only limited uncontrolled data demonstrate efficacy for dinoprostone (prostaglandin E$_2$), silver nitrate, beta-carotene, pentoxifylline, or triple-antibiotic lozenges (5). However, when patients were interviewed by a dental hygienist and an oncology nurse prior to initiation of chemotherapy and were trained in specific tasks to reduce oral trauma and oral colonization (special toothbrushes, frequent saline rinses, avoidance of medications with potential to induce mucosal trauma) the incidence of severe mucositis occurring during 1100 cycles of chemotherapy was reduced from over 10% to less than 2% (6).

Esophagus

Mucositis involving the gastroesophageal junction or distal esophagus is most likely to be mistaken for gastroesophageal reflux disease (GERD). GERD (7) is typically diagnosed when patients complain of postprandial retrosternal burning that ascends from the abdomen to the chest. Waterbrash (a sense of fluid entering the posterior hypopharynx) and worsening of symptoms with recumbent posture are common. Dysphagia from mucosal inflammation and stricture may occur in a minority of sever cases. Successful therapy includes behavioral measures such as weight loss in the obese, avoiding bed for at least 4 hours after eating, sleeping with the head of the bed elevated, and proscription of tobacco, alcohol, fatty foods, or foods that produce symptoms. Antacids, histamine-receptor antagonists, and proton-pump inhibitors (see below) are used to neutralize or reduce production of gastric acid. Sucralfate binds to inflamed mucosa and promotes healing. Cisapride and metoclopramide may accelerate gastric emptying of food

and acid. All are rational forms of therapy in chemotherapy-induced disease, since stomach acid is likely to exacerbate inflamed epithelium, induce stricturing, and increase the risk of hemorrhage.

Symptoms of esophageal mucositis may also be confused with *Candida* esophagitis, cytomegalovirus esophagitis, or esophagitis from herpesvirus. Endoscopic examination with biopsies and/or brushings is diagnostic and well tolerated, even by neutropenic, thrombocytopenic hosts (8).

Barrett's esophagus, a relatively unusual sequela of GERD, occurs when chronic regurgitation of gastric acid destroys the squamous epithelium of the lower esophagus, and the mucosal stem cell regenerates gastric columnar epithelium in its place (9). Infrequently, the regenerated epithelium resembles intestinal mucosa and presents an increased risk for adenocarcinoma (10). In one series, 9 of 16 women (11) treated for breast cancer developed endoscopic and pathologic evidence for Barrett's esophagus after 6 courses of adjuvant chemotherapy. Although pretreatment endoscopy was normal in all 16, columnar epithelium was found from 3 to 9 cm above the esophageal sphincter 1 month after the last course of cytoxan (CTX), methotrexate (MTX), and fluorouracil (5-FU). Three of the nine patients had intestinal metaplasia. The authors hypothesized that esophageal inflammation due to the chemotherapy regimen destroyed the native squamous epithelium and that it was replaced by columnar cells. However, when 15 other women were treated with a similar regimen (12) and underwent endoscopy 11 months after the last cycle, none had Barrett's esophagus, even though 12 had oral mucositis, diarrhea or odynophagia during therapy.

Similarly, when 18 women with advanced breast cancer treated with CTX, MTX, 5-FU, vincristine (VCR), *cis*-platinum (DDP), and doxorubicin (DOX) were examined after 6 courses of therapy, none had Barrett's, even though 15 of 18 had symptomatic mucositis during therapy (13). In the same study, 20 men treated with six cycles of CTX, VCR, and bleomycin (BLE) underwent endoscopy after therapy. Only 1 of 20 had Barrett's epithelium, and he had reported chronic heartburn and esophageal reflux symptoms prior to therapy. Thus, despite the earlier report, it is clear that chemotherapy that produces mucositis or mucositis, reflux, and vomiting of gastric contents does not consistently induce Barrett's epithelium.

Stomach and Duodenum

Direct infusion of antimetabolites into the liver via the hepatic artery is effective because most of the blood supply to normal liver is provided by the portal vein, while the hepatic artery is the main source for hepatic neoplasms. Hepatic artery infusions permit larger doses of drug to be delivered to target lesions, while most of the active agent is extracted from plasma by the liver before it enters the peripheral circulation. To minimize loss of the active drug into the celiac circulation, catheter placement includes ligation of arteries that arise from the common hepatic artery distal to the catheter. These vessels perfuse the distal stomach and duodenum (14).

Hepatic artery infusion of 5-FU, fluorodeoxyuridine (FUDR), mitomycin-C (MMC), or MTX may produce inflammation of the stomach and duodenum as well as gastric (15) and duodenal ulcer (16) in 15 to 25% of patients. The inflammation may occur early in the course of therapy or after several cycles. Symptoms usually respond to dose reduction or termination of the infusions. A potentially reversible syndrome resembling sclerosing cholangitis occurs in 10% of patients (14), usually after several cycles of therapy. Patients with inflammation or ulcer of the foregut present with pain, nausea, vomiting, bleeding, or perforation; those with cholangitis complain of nausea, vomiting, and jaundice and have abnormal liver chemistries. Some have speculated that the inflammation and ulceration are due to ischemic changes following arterial ligation. However, the arterial supply to the stomach includes three separate sources, and it is unusually resistant to ischemic damage (17). In addition, the ischemia hypothesis does not explain why symptoms and signs of inflammation usually subside when the infusions are decreased or halted. Finally, biopsy specimens from chemotherapy-associated ulcers do not demonstrate characteristic ischemic necrosis. Biopsy specimens may have bizarre-appearing cells with neoplastic features. These changes are reversible and disappear with healing (15, 18). *Helicobacter pylori*, the etiologic agent of peptic ulcer disease (19), has not been detected in chemotherapy-associated ulcers (15). Inflammation and ulceration associated with hepatic artery infusions of chemotherapy probably result from toxicity to proximal gut epithelium and represent another facet of the mucositis syndrome.

Acid peptic disease of the stomach and duo-

Table 35.1. Medications Used to Control Acid-Peptic Diseases

Medication	Oral Dose	Intravenous Dose	Cost[a] 24 hours (i.v.)[b]/1Month (p.o.)
Histamine receptor antagonists			
Cimetidine Tagamet	400 mg b.i.d. or 800 mg q.h.s.	300 mg q6h	12.25 / 92.60
Raniditine Zantac	150 mg b.i.d. or 300 mg q.h.s.	300 mg/24h	10.14 / 90.06
Famotidine Pepsid	20 mg b.i.d. or 40 mg q.h.s.	40 mg/24h	7.19 / 89.33
Nizatidine Axid	150 mg b.i.d. or 300 mg q.h.s.	none	NA / 92.31
Sucralfate Carafate	1000 mg q.i.d.	none	NA / 88.30
Misoprostol Cytotec	200 μg b.i.d.	none	NA / 85.20
Omeprazol Prilosec	20 mg q.d.	none	NA / 109.90
Prokinetic agents			
Metoclopramide Reglan	10 mg q.i.d.	10 mg q.i.d.	8.87 / 74.40
Cisapride Propulsid	10 mg q.i.d.	none	NA / 82.80

[a]Average wholesale cost, Baton Rouge, LA, September 1995.
[b]Does not include cost of administration.

denum produces cycles of daily epigastric burning, worse when the stomach is empty, relieved by food or antacids, with recurrence within an hour or two after eating (20). Nocturnal pain awakening patients from sleep is a typical feature of the syndrome and helps differentiate it from functional dyspepsia (21). Histamine-receptor antagonists (22), proton-pump inhibitors (23), sucralfate (24), or high-potency antacids reliably relieve pain and promote healing. Treatment of hepatic artery–related ulceration requires decreasing or discontinuing the agent and initiating acid-suppression therapy to mitigate symptoms and lessen the risk of bleeding, obstruction, or perforation (25, 26, 27). Table 35.1 shows medications currently used to treat acid peptic disease. If patients are able to take medications orally, no advantage accrues to parenteral administration. Misoprostol, a prostaglandin E_1 analogue that has been shown to be effective in preventing ulcers from nonsteroidal antiinflammatory drugs (NSAIDs) (28), is ineffective for ulceration associated with hepatic artery catheters (29).

Older patients are more likely to present with complication of chronic peptic ulcer disease, such as bleeding, perforation, or obstruction (30), as the first clinical manifestation of the disease. Perforation of the stomach or duodenum has been reported in four previously asymptomatic patients treated with systemic dexamethasone and 5-FU or DDP (31). Perforations were ascribed to the corticosteroid, but in every case, patients were receiving sulindac for pain relief. The role of corticosteroids in ulcer development is controversial (32), but NSAIDs have long been associated with asymptomatic ulcer disease, especially in women and the elderly (33).

Perforation from peptic ulcer has typically been treated successfully by operation. Recently, treatment with nasogastric suction, acid suppression, and broad-spectrum antibiotics has been reported to be as efficacious as surgery in a large controlled trial from Hong Kong (34). Although medical therapy is not recommended for cancer patients in whom operation is reasonable, it may offer an alternative for those patients with widely disseminated disease or may serve as a temporizing measure for patients with severe but transient myelosuppression.

Small Bowel

At least 7 L of fluid and electrolytes are circulated through the gastrointestinal tract proxi-

mal to the ileocecal valve every 24 hours. Obligate oropharyngeal, gastric, duodenal, pancreatic, and biliary secretions account for 80% of the luminal volume and occur regardless of oral intake. Most absorption of nutrients occurs in the duodenum and proximal jejunum, while the distal small bowel primarily reabsorbs electrolytes, bile salts, and water. Less than 1 L of ileal effluent enters the colon daily, and at least 80% (mostly water, bicarbonate, and potassium) is reabsorbed by colonic mucosa. In the small bowel, secretion occurs in epithelial crypts, absorption in villi. Clinically important diarrhea may result when the balance between secretion and absorption is impaired; gut motility plays a minor role (35). If the distal jejunum and ileum have impaired resorption, large volumes of fluid and electrolytes can enter the colon and overwhelm its absorptive capabilities. Conversely, injury to colon mucosa generally results in relatively small volume diarrhea, since a relatively small solute and volume load enters the large bowel.

Oral and parenteral therapy with antimetabolites causes diarrhea. Life-threatening fluid and electrolyte imbalance, bleeding, and death have been reported (36). The etiology of the symptoms is not totally clear, but they probably result from direct epithelial damage to mucosal cells, analogous to the mucositis described above. Chemotherapy-induced diarrhea from the small bowel is primarily an inflammatory syndrome; symptomatic malabsorption is unusual. To determine the cause of growth retardation and weight loss during treatment for acute lymphocytic leukemia, 16 children (37) had serial anthropomorphic studies, fecal fat and volume determinations, hydrogen breath analysis for measurement of lactose malabsorption, and serum and urine analysis following d-xylose ingestion, to test for the development of malabsorption while receiving MTX or DOX + MTX for maintenance of remission. Sustained anorexia was not found, and there was no clinical evidence of malabsorption. Transient malabsorption of d-xylose and lactose was found, which normalized quickly after treatment.

Similarly, when 27 adults being treated for both solid tumors and hematologic malignancies with oral and intravenous chemotherapy underwent hydrogen breath tests for lactose malabsorption, 14 were abnormal, but only 3 had cramping or diarrhea with lactose challenge during the test (38). Finally, when small bowel morphology, symptoms, and disaccharidase enzyme activity were measured in patients being treated for disseminated melanoma with bleomycin, dacarbazine, vindesine, and dactinomycin, no consistent relationships were noted between symptoms, enzyme activity, and mucosal microscopy (39).

Chemotherapy-associated large-volume diarrhea, with or without periumbilical cramping, and unaccompanied by fever, bleeding, or symptoms of bowel obstruction is likely due to small bowel mucosal toxicity. Other considerations include food poisoning with toxigenic *Staphylococcus aureus*, *Clostridium perfringens*, *Bacillus cereus*, or enterotoxigenic *Escherichia coli*; parasitic infestations by *Giardia*, *Cryptosporidia*, or *Isospora belli*; and rotavirus or Norwalk virus infection (40). Celiac sprue may become symptomatic in previously compensated patients who have had malignancy-associated stomach or proximal bowel surgery (41). Similarly, bile salt malabsorption can be "unmasked" by small bowel resection in patients who were previously asymptomatic. Bacterial overgrowth with pain and diarrhea has been described in elderly patients with no predisposing anatomic defects (42).

Therapy of large-volume diarrhea consists initially of fluid and electrolyte replacement with iso-osmolar oral fluids. Resuscitation fluids should contain glucose to drive active resorption of sodium and decrease stool volume. An effective outpatient rehydration regimen includes ¾ tsp of table salt, 1 tsp of baking soda, 4 tbsp of granulated sugar, and 1 cup of orange juice added to 1 L of tap water (40). Plain water, tea, and carbonated beverages should not be used because none contain appreciable amounts of sodium, potassium, or bicarbonate. Commercial electrolyte solutions offer no advantage to the above regimen. Opiates (paregoric) or synthetic analogues such as codeine (43) or loperamide (44) inhibit secretion in crypt cells and stimulate absorption in the villi of damaged mucosa. Intravenous octreotide, a synthetic 8-amino acid analogue of somatostatin, cures refractory diarrhea associated with 5-FU toxicity in over 80% of patients (45). In a separate study (46), 40 patients with 5-FU-associated diarrhea who failed outpatient therapy with oral fluids and a restricted diet were admitted to hospital and randomly assigned to subcutaneous octreotide (500 units three times/day) or loperamide (4 mg orally, three times/day). Sixteen of 20 treated with octreotide had complete resolution of diarrhea within a mean of 3.4 days, while only 6 of 20 patients treated with loperamide resolved

within 6.1 days. Unfortunately, the expense of octreotide therapy ($700/2500 units) prevents routine use in patients with mild or moderate symptoms.

Colon

Colonic bacteria (10^{12}/cm (3)) include over 400 species, are predominantly (>99%) anaerobes, and account for one-third of dry stool weight (47). Typhlitis, localized cecal inflammation with invasion by colonic bacteria, occurs in more than 10% of patients who die while being treated for acute leukemia (48) and has been reported following a variety of chemotherapeutic regimens (49–52). Although typhlitis has been reported in patients with cyclic neutropenia in the absence of chemotherapy, a likely explanation for the syndrome in patients receiving chemotherapy is direct mucosal inflammation followed by invasion by colonic bacteria. Fever and right lower quadrant abdominal pain occurring during severe (<500 leukocytes/mm^3) neutropenia are the most common presentation. Abdominal tenderness is inconstantly reported, and stool may be normal, mucoid, or frankly bloody. When more than the cecum is involved, the syndrome is called neutropenic enterocolitis (50). Stool cultures are uniformly negative for enteric pathogens or *Clostridium difficile* enterotoxin.

The differential diagnosis should include appendicitis or diverticular abscess when symptoms are localized and inflammatory or infectious colitis if diarrhea is present. *Salmonella*, *Shigella*, *Campylobacter*, *Yersinia* (53), and pseudomembranous colitis (54) secondary to *C. difficile* enterotoxin can be eliminated from consideration by stool culture and toxin assay. When diarrhea is accompanied by azotemia and elevated creatinine levels, infection with toxigenic *E. coli* serotype 0157:H7 (55) should be considered (most hospital laboratories do not serotype *E. coli* cultured from stool). Fresh stool specimens and pinch biopsies of rectal and sigmoid mucosa may be safely obtained during symptom-limited flexible sigmoidoscopy. Mucosal swabs of the rectum to stain with methylene blue for fecal leukocytes, a simple and specific test for inflammatory diarrhea, have limited usefulness in neutropenic hosts. Pseudomembranous colitis from *C. difficile* is an important hospital-acquired infection (56), is endemic in nursing home patients, and occurs in patients being treated with chemotherapy, even in the absence of antibiotic exposure (57). Transient colitis syndrome (58), idiopathic ulcerative colitis (UC), and microscopic or collagenous colitis (59, 60) can usually be eliminated from consideration by rectal biopsy. NSAIDs are increasingly being identified as uncommon sources of localized or diffuse ulceration in colon as well as in the upper gastrointestinal tract (61, 62).

Pathologic examination of operative specimens in patients with typhlitis or neutropenic enterocolitis demonstrates denuded colonic mucosa with localized or diffuse ulceration that may penetrate to the muscularis propria. The pathology is similar to severe colitis from bacterial infection or UC. Initial reports recommended laparotomy for patients with neutropenic enterocolitis, even profoundly myelosuppressed patients, because of the prohibitive mortality with medical therapy. However, more recent series document improvement with nonsurgical regimens (52).

Reports of "toxic megacolon," a term appropriated from the UC literature, imply that a different approach is required when the colon diameter exceeds 7 cm on plain films of the abdomen (63). In UC (64), pain, fever above 38.5°C, abdominal tenderness, more than 10 bloody stools/day, and signs of systemic toxicity define fulminant colitis or, formerly, toxic megacolon. Fulminant colitis has been associated with a variety of bacterial pathogens, including *Salmonella*, *Shigella*, and *Campylobacter*, and with *C. difficile*-associated diarrhea. The syndrome may be precipitated by opiates, antibiotics, barium-enhanced x-ray examinations, metabolic derangements, or colonoscopy in patients with underlying bowel inflammation. Plain x-rays of the abdomen may demonstrate thickened colon valvulae with shaggy mucosa indicative of diffuse edema and ulceration.

Previously, the diameter of the colon on plain films was felt to have diagnostic and prognostic significance, but it is now generally accepted that severe colitis is defined by the degree of systemic toxicity and the penetration of inflammatory cells into the muscularis propria of the bowel, not by colonic diameter (64, 65). When the muscular layers of the bowel are involved with an inflammatory process, coordinated peristalsis is impaired. Bacterial digestion of fecal contents produces carbon dioxide which, when combined with swallowed nitrogen from ambient air, distends the paralyzed gut. Therapy (65) includes nasogastric suction, bowel rest, intravenous hyperalimentation, and electrolyte replacement,

with special attention to potassium, phosphate, calcium, and magnesium. Broad-spectrum antibiotics with anaerobic as well as aerobic efficacy are indicated, and consultation from a general surgeon should be considered. Serial examinations of the abdomen, preferably by the same physician, and repeated plain film x-rays are required to monitor response to therapy. In UC careful, repeated, examinations are necessary because treatment with steroids may prevent the usual response to peritoneal irritation and conceal a perforation. In neutropenic enterocolitis, an inadequate leukocyte response may also prevent stimulation of protective reflexes. Patients who fail to improve over 2 to 3 days, with or without an increase in bowel diameter, are likely to have inflammation of the muscularis propria and an increased risk of perforation, septic shock, and death. Progression of symptoms often occurs simultaneously with a decrease in the frequency of stooling because peristalsis has stopped. Anecdotal reports of neutropenic enterocolitis have emphasized the diagnostic efficacy of barium enema, contrast-enhanced computed axial tomography, and attempted colonoscopy. Since bacterial, amoebic, and pseudomembranous enterocolitis can only be proved by stool examination or culture and because abdominal ultrasound has high sensitivity and specificity (66) for appendicitis or abscess, procedures that have been shown to precipitate severe colitis should be avoided.

CONSTIPATION

Constipation may be defined as fewer than 1 stool/week or the presence of scybalous subjectively inadequate stools. Constipation is ubiquitous in elderly populations (67). In patients undergoing chemotherapy, the vinca alkaloids may produce constipation concurrent with, or well after, the conclusion of chemotherapy. In addition, treatment with opiates for pain relief dramatically alters fluid absorption from the small bowel and promotes constipation (see above). Other medications including calcium channel antagonists; anticholinergics (antipsychotics, antidepressants), cations (iron, calcium, or aluminum-containing antacids), anticonvulsants, and anti-Parkinson's medications decrease stool frequency. Inactivity because of weakness, pain, or concurrent medical problems such as stroke, angina, or Parkinson's disease contribute to constipation as does the hypercalcemia of malignancy, hypokalemia, or hypomagnesemia. Intestinal pseudoobstruction, an uncommon paraneoplastic syndrome most associated with squamous cell carcinoma of the lung, may present as constipation with bloating, abdominal pain, nausea, and vomiting. Therapy is problematic (68, 69).

Dietary fiber supplementation or bulk-forming psyllium (66) may improve symptoms, but patients who require narcotic analgesics or who have neurotoxic constipation from VCR may require cathartics to improve transit. Lactulose, a nonabsorbable disaccharide, promotes osmotic diarrhea and is effective. Sorbitol syrup is a less expensive alternative with equal efficacy (70). Warm tap water or saline enemata may be effective for patients with distal obstipation from analgesics, but soapsuds enemas should be avoided because of the risk of inflammatory colitis (71). Stool softeners have no proven efficacy, despite proprietary claims to the contrary.

NAUSEA AND VOMITING

When the intent of chemotherapy is to eradicate a malignancy, chemotherapy-induced nausea and vomiting may limit the dose of potentially life-saving treatment: when chemotherapy is being used for incurable disease, significant side effects detract from palliation and, by promoting malnutrition and fluid and electrolyte losses, may shorten life. Patients have repeatedly reported that nausea and vomiting are the most distressing side effects of systemic chemotherapy. Women, younger patients, and patients without prior alcohol use are at higher risk for chemotherapy-induced symptoms (72–74). Medications that produce the most severe emetogenic reactions (Table 35.2) are generally not those that produce the inflammatory syndromes described above.

The physiology of nausea and emesis has been clearly elucidated (72, 75). The vomiting center (VC) in the lateral medullary redicular formation is the final common pathway for stimuli that elicit vomiting. Stimulation of the VC arises in the chemoreceptor trigger zone (CTZ) of the area postrema in the medulla. Other input arises in the pharynx and gastrointestinal tract via the vagus nerve and sacral parasympathetic fibers, the vestibular apparatus via the eighth cranial nerve, and from higher brainstem and cortical centers. The CTZ lies outside the blood-brain barrier and samples emetogenic toxins in the plasma and cerebrospinal fluid. Neurotransmission within the CTZ depends upon type 1 (H1) histamine receptors, type 2 (D2) dopamine receptors, and type 3 (5HT3) serotonin receptors. H1 receptors mediate motion-induced symptoms and probably do not affect responses to chemotherapy. Medications (Table 35.3) that block D2 receptors (phenothiazines, metoclopramide, butyrophenones) prevent or reduce the emetic response to low or moderately emetogenic chemotherapy. High-dose regimens of antidopaminergic medications are frequently associated with intolerable extrapyramidal side effects and drowsiness, which may be alleviated or prevented with concurrent administration of anticholinergics (scopolamine) or antihistamines (diphenhydramine). Serotonin-receptor antagonists (ondansetron, granisetron), especially when combined with high-potency synthetic corticosteroids (dexamethasone), have improved efficacy against moderately emetogenic and highly emetogenic regimens. Antiserotonergic medications have minimal side effects. Cannabinoids (nabilone) and benzodiazepines (lorazepam, alprazolam) may be useful adjunctive medications and probably serve by mediating inputs from limbic or cortical centers. Dysphoric reactions limit general use of cannabinoids, and drowsiness and respiratory depression may be associated with benzodiazepines.

As chemotherapy regimens have become more intensive, combinations of antiemetic agents have evolved to suppress more severe and long-lasting symptoms (Table 35.3). Nevertheless, high-dose DDP and CTX remain refractory to all but the most intensive therapy and are also associated with "delayed" nausea and vomiting, in which symptoms reoccur more than 24

Table 35.2. Emetogenic Potential of Chemotherapeutic Medications Ranked from Most to Least Emetogenic

Cisplatin	Etoposide
Dacarbazine	Mitomycin
Dactinomycin	Methotrexate
Cyclophosphamide	Fluorouracil
Lomustine	Hydroxyurea
Carboplatin	Bleomycin
Doxorubicin	Vinblastine
Daunorubicin	Vincristine
Cytarabine	Chlorambucil
Procarbazine	

Adapted from Dieh V, Marty M. Efficacy and safety of antiemetics. Cancer Treat Rev 1994;20:379–392.

Table 35.3. Doses in Selected Antiemetic Regimens

Regimen Rectal	Initial Dose	Cost[a] p.o. / i.v. / p.r.
Moderately emetogenic chemotherapy		
Prochlorperazine	5–10 mg p.o.	.87 / 6.93 / 2.85
Compazine	5–10 mg i.v.	
	25-mg rectal suppository	
Thiethylperazine	10 mg p.o.	.73 / 4.15 / NA
Torecan	10 mg i.m.	
Dexamethasone	10 mg i.v.	NA / 11.36 / NA
Decadron		
Dronabinol	10 mg p.o.	12.86 / NA / NA
Marinol		
Ondansetron	8 mg p.o., 10 mg i.v.	18.03 / 116.51 / NA
Zofran		
Highly emetogenic chemotherapy		
Dexamethasone	20 mg IV plus	NA / 22.72 / NA
Metoclopramide	3 mg/kg body weight i.v.[b]	NA / 42.04 / NA
	q2h × 2 plus	
Diphenhydramine	25–50 mg i.v.	NA / 8.94 / NA
Benadryl	q2h × 2 plus	
Lorazepam	1–2 mg i.v.	NA / 12.67 / NA
Ativan		
or		
Dexamethasone	20 mg i.v. plus	NA / 22.72 / NA
Ondansetron	32 mg i.v. (divided doses)	NA / 196.66 / NA

Adapted from Grunberg SM, Hesketh PJ. Control of chemotherapy-induced emesis. N Engl J Med 1993;329:1790–1796.
[a]Average wholesale cost, Baton Rouge, LA, September 1995.
[b]60-kg patient.

hours after administration (76). It is not clear that delayed vomiting represents a qualitatively different process, but medications that are effective for the initial management of emesis are less effective at preventing delayed symptoms (77, 78).

A second syndrome, anticipatory nausea and vomiting, occurs after the initial cycle of chemotherapy but prior to follow-up cycles. Symptoms may be elicited by the sight, sound, or smell of stimuli that the patient associates with the administration of chemotherapy. The probability of anticipatory nausea and vomiting increases with the more emetogenic medications and with multiple cycles of therapy (74). Initially, symptoms may be elicited only by specific stimuli such as the room or persons who administered the therapy; however, with repeated episodes, more and more stimuli separate from the therapeutic environment may become capable of eliciting the response. Psychosocial models have been proposed (79) to account for the behavior, but the most parsimonious explanation is that anticipatory nausea and vomiting is a classically conditioned autonomic response to the pairing of a noxious unconditioned stimulus (chemother-apy) with a previously innocuous environment. The close pairing of these events in spatial and temporal contiguity results in the innocuous stimuli acquiring properties of the emetogenic chemotherapy (80). The phenomena of stimulus generalization, in which events distant from chemotherapy acquire power to elicit symptoms, are particularly prevalent in classical conditioning using noxious stimuli.

By definition, those operations that prevent the association of stimuli, such as successful treatment of nausea and vomiting in the initial presentation, will prevent anticipatory responses. Other strategies that prevent the association should decrease or abolish the conditioned response, and benzodiazepines, including alprazolam and lorazepam (72), have been shown to ameliorate symptoms. Midazolam, another benzodiazepine, reliably produces amnesia for events occurring during conscious sedation for invasive gastrointestinal or pulmonary procedures. Although respiratory depression is a potential side effect of midazolam, it is reversible with intravenous flumazanil without diminishing the amnestic effect. Controlled trials to evaluate the efficacy of midazolam versus other benzodiazepines for the control of anticipatory nausea and vomiting are warranted.

The particular juxtaposition of the symptoms of chemotherapy-associated nausea and vomiting with the administration of medications makes confusion with other causes of nausea and vomiting unlikely. However, increased intracranial pressure from infections or mass lesions; metabolic disturbances, especially fever, acidosis, hypercalcemia, and hyperkalemia; obstruction, pseudoobstruction or paresis of the gastrointestinal tract from medications or diabetes should be considered if symptoms fail to respond to proven therapy.

REFERENCES

1. Slavin RE, Dias MA, Sarol R. Cytosine arabinoside induced gastrointestinal toxic alterations in sequential chemotherapeutic protocols. Cancer 1978; 42:1747–1759.

2. Peterson DE. Oral toxicity of chemotherapeutic agents. Semin Oncol 1992;19:478–491.

3. Shenep JL, Kalwinsky KD, Hutson PR, George SL, Dodge RK, Blankenship KR, Thornton D. Efficacy of oral sucralfate suspension in prevention and treatment of chemotherapy-induced mucositis. J Pediatr 1988;113:758–763.

4. Gordon B, Spadinger A, Hodges E, Ruby E, Stanley R, Coccia P. Effect of granulocyte-macrophage colony-stimulating factor on oral mucositis after hematopoietic stem-cell transplantation. J Clin Oncol 1994; 12:1917–1922.

5. Verdi CJ. Cancer therapy and oral mucositis: an appraisal of drug prophylaxis. Drug Safety 1993;9:185–195.

6. Graham KM, Pecoraro DA, Ventura JM, Meyer CC. Reducing the incidence of stomatitis using a quality assessment and improvement approach. Cancer Nurs 1993;16:117–122.

7. Mittal RK. Gastroesophageal reflux disease: is it primarily a motility disorder? Semin Gastrointest Dis 1992;3:129–139.

8. Baehr PH, Mcdonald GB. Esophageal infections: risk factors, presentation, diagnosis and treatment. Gastroenterology 1994;106:509–532.

9. Spechler SJ, Goyal RK, eds. Barrett's esophagus: pathophysiology, diagnosis, and management. New York: Elsevier, 1985.

10. Dent J, Bremner CG, Collen MJ, Haggitt RC, Spechler SJ. Barrett's oesophagus. J Gastroenterol Hepatol 1991;6:1–22.

11. Sartori S, Nielsen I, Indelli M, Trevisani L, Pazzi P, Grandi E. Barrett esophagus after chemotherapy with cyclophosphamide, methotrexate and 5-fluorouracil (CMF): an iatrogenic injury? Ann Intern Med 1991;114:210–211.

12. Peters FTM, Sleijfer D, Gustaaf W, Kleibeuker JH. Is chemotherapy associated with development of Barrett's esophagus? Dig Dis Sci 1993;38:923–936.

13. Herrera JL, Uzei C, Martino R, Cooke C, DiPalma JA. Barrett's esophagus: lack of association with

14. Kemeny N, Daly J, Reichman B, Geller N, Botet J, Oderman P. Intrahepatic or systemic infusion of fluorodeoxyuridine in patients with liver metastases from colorectal carcinoma. Ann Intern Med 1987;107:459–465.

15. Doria MI, Doria LK, Faintuch J, Levin B. Gastric mucosal injury after hepatic arterial infusion chemotherapy with floxuridine. Cancer 1994;73:2042–2047.

16. Goldin E, Peretz T, Libson E. Giant duodenal ulcer: the hepatic intra-arterial chemotherapy variant. Postgrad Med J 1988;64:431–433.

17. Reinus JF, Brandt LJ, Boley S. Ischemic diseases of the bowel. Gastroenterol Clin North Am 1990; 19:319–343.

18. Kwee WS, Wils JA, Schlangen J, Nuyens CM, Arends JW. Gastric epithelial atypia complicating hepatic arterial infusion chemotherapy. Histopathology 1994;24:151–154.

19. NIH Consensus Development Panel on *Helicobacter pylori* in Peptic Ulcer Disease. *Helicobacter pylori* in peptic ulcer disease. JAMA 1994;272:65–69.

20. Kurata J. Epidemiology: peptic ulcer risk factors. Semin Gastrointest Dis 1993;4:2–12.

21. Talley NJ, Phillips SJ. Non-ulcer dyspepsia: potential causes and pathophysiology. Ann Intern Med 1988;108:865–879.

22. Feldman M, Burton ME. Histamine$_2$-receptor antagonists: standard therapy for acid-peptic diseases. N Engl J Med 1990;323:1672–1680, 1749–1755.

23. Maton PN. Omeprazole. N Engl J Med 1991; 324:965–975.

24. McCarthy DM. Sucralfate. N Engl J Med 1991; 325:1017–1025.

25. Peterson WL, Richardson CT. Sustained fasting achlorhydria: a comparison of medical regimens. Gastroenterology 1985;88:666–669.

26. Ballesteros A, Hogan DL, Koss MA, Isenberg JI. Bolus or intravenous infusion of ranitidine: effects on gastric pH and acid secretion. Ann Intern Med 1990; 112:334–339.

27. Laine L, Peterson WL. Bleeding peptic ulcer. N Engl J Med 1994;331:717–727.

28. Graham DY, White RH, Moreland LW, Schubert TT, Katz R, et al. and the Misoprostol Study Group. Duodenal and gastric ulcer prevention with misoprostol in arthritis patients taking NSAIDS. Ann Intern Med 1993;119:257–262.

29. Mavligit G, Faintuch J, Levin B, Wallace S, Charnsangavej C, Carrasco C, Patt Y. Gastroduodenal mucosal injury during hepatic arterial infusions of chemotherapeutic agents: lack of protection by prostaglandin E_1 analogue. Gastroenterology 1987;92:566–569.

30. Cryer B, Feldman M. Pepetic ulcer disease in the elderly. Semin Gastrointest Dis 1994;5:166–178.

31. Liaw CC, Huang J, Wang HM, Wang CH. Spontaneous gastroduodenal perforation in patients with cancer receiving chemotherapy and steroids. Cancer 1993;72:1382–1385.

32. Lewis JH. Gastrointestinal injury due to medicinal agents. Am J Gastroenterol 1986;81:819–834.

33. Gabriel SE, Jaakkimainen L, Bombardier C. Risk for serious gastrointestinal complications related to use of nonsteroidal anti-inflammatory drugs: a meta-analyusis. Ann Intern Med 1991;115:787–796.

adjuvant chemotherapy for localized breast carcinoma. Gastrointest Endosc 1992;38:551–553.

34. Crofts TJ, Park KGM, Steele RJC, Chung SSC, Li AKC. A randomized trial of nonoperative treatment for perforated peptic ulcer. N Engl J Med 1989;320:970–973.

35. Turnberg LA, ed. Absorption and malabsorption. Semin Gastrointest Dis 1992;3:177–243.

36. Grem JL, Shoemaker DD, Petrelli NJ. Severe and fatal toxic effect observed in treatment with high and low dose leucovorin plus 5-fluorouracil for colorectal carcinoma. Cancer Treat Rep 1987;71:1122–1125.

37. Halton J, Atkinson SA, Bradley C, Dawson S, Barr RD. Acute lymphoid leukemia: no evidence of consistent chemotherapy-induced intestinal malabsorption. Am J Pediatr Hematol Oncol 1993;15:271–276.

38. Parnes HL, Fung E, Schiffer CA. Chemotherapy-induced lactose intolerance in adults. Cancer 1994; 74:1629–1633.

39. Smit JM, Mulder N, Sleijfer DT, Bouman JG, Koudstall J, Elema JD, Seeger W. Gastrointestinal toxicity of chemotherapy and the influence of hyperalimentation. Cancer 1986;58:1990–1994.

40. Guerrant RL, Bobak DA. Bacterial and protozoal gastroenteritis. N Engl J Med 1991;325:327–340.

41. Trier JS. Celiac sprue. N Engl J Med 1991; 325:1709–1719.

42. Montgomery RT, Haeney MR, Ross IN, Sammons HG, Barford AV, et al. The ageing gut: a study of intestinal absorption in relation to nutrition in the elderly. Q J Med 1978;47:197–211.

43. Schiller LR, Davis GR, Santa Ana CA, Morawski SG, Fordtran JS. Studies of the mechanism of the antidiarrheal effect of codeine. J Clin Invest 1982; 70:999–1008.

44. Schiller LR, Santa Ana CA, Morawski SG, Fordtran JS. Mechanism of the antidiarrheal effect of loperamide. Gastroenterology 1984;86:1475–1480.

45. Petrelli NJ, Rodriquez-Bigas M, Rustum Y, Herrera L, Creaven P. Bowel rest, intravenous hydration, and continuous high-dose infusion of octreotide acetate for the treatment of chemotherapy-induced diarrhea in patients with colorectal carcinoma. Cancer 1993;72:1543–1546.

46. Gebbia V, Carreca I, Testa A, Valenza R, Curto G, et al. Subcutaneous octreotide versus oral loperamide in the treatment of diarrhea following chemotherapy. Anti-Cancer Drugs 1993;4:443–445.

47. Simon GL, Gorbach SL. Intestinal flora in health and disease. Gastroenterology 1984;86:174–183.

48. Kunkel JM, Rosenthal D. Management of the ileocecal syndrome: neutropenic enterocolitic. Dis Colon Rectum 1986;29:196–199.

49. Stellato TA, Shenk RR. Gastrointestinal emergencies in the oncology patient. Semin Oncol 1989; 16:521–531.

50. Beadle GF. Acute ileotyphlitis as a complication of cytotoxic drug treatment of a non-seminomatous germ cell tumor of the testis. Aust NZ J Med 1990; 20:594–595.

51. Petruzzelli GJ, Johnson JT, deVries EJ. Neutropenic enterocolitis: a new complication of head and neck cancer chemotherapy. Arch Otolaryngol Head Neck Surg 1990;116:209–211.

52. Pestalozzi BC, Sotos GA, Choyke PL, Fisherman JS, Cowan KH, O'Shaughnessy JA. Typhlitis resulting from treatment with Taxol and doxorubicin in patients with metastatic breast cancer. Cancer 1993; 71:1797–1800.

53. Cover TL, Aber RC. *Yersinia enterocolitica.* N Engl J Med 1989;321:16–24.

54. Bartlett JG, Chang TW, Gurwith M, Gorbach SL, Onderdonk AB. Antibiotic-associated pseudomembranous colitis due to toxin-producing clostridia. N Engl J Med 1978;298:531–534.

55. Boyce TG, Swerdlow DL, Griffin PM. *Escherichia coli* 0157:H7 and the hemolytic uremic syndrome. N Engl J Med 1995;333:364–368.

56. McFarland LV, Mulligan ME, Kwok RYY, Stamm WE. Nosocomial acquisition of *Clostridium difficile* infection. N Engl J Med 1989;320:204–210.

57. Anand A, Glatt AE. *Clostridium difficile* infection associated with antineoplastic chemotherapy: a review. Clin Infect Dis 1993;17:109–113.

58. Nostrant TT, Kumar NB, Appelman HD. Histopathology differentiates acute self limited colitis from ulcerative colitis. Gastroenterology 1987;92:318–328.

59. Rams H, Rogers AI, Ghandur-Mnaymneh L. Collagenous colitis. Ann Intern Med 1987;106:108–113.

60. Giardiello FM. A review of atypical colitides: collagenous and lymphocytic colitis. Prog Inflammatory Bowel Dis 1993;14:1–4.

61. Gibson GR, Whitacre EB, Ricotti CA. Colitis induced by nonsteroidal anti-inflammatory drugs: a report of four cases and a review of the literature. Arch Intern Med 1992;152:625–632.

62. Fortson WC, Tedesco FJ. Drug-induced colitis: a review. Am J Gastroenterol 1984;79:878–883.

63. Wodzinski MA, Snowden JA, Reilly JT. Toxic megacolon complicating chemotherapy for acute myeloid leukemia. Postgrad Med J 1994;70:921–923.

64. Present DH. Toxic megacolon: is there a superior approach to management? In: Barkin JS, Rogers AI, eds. Difficult decisions in digestive diseases. Chicago: Year Book Medical Publishers, 1989.

65. Buckell NA, Williams GT, Bartram CI, Lennard-Jones JE. Depth of ulceration in acute colitis: correlation with outcome and clinical and radiologic features. Gastroenterology 1980;79:19–25.

66. Mueller PR, vanSonnenberg E. Interventional radiology in the chest and abdomen. N Engl J Med 1990;322:1364–1371.

67. Wald A. Constipation and fecal incontinence in the elderly. Semin Gastrointest Dis 1994;5:179–188.

68. Colemont LJ, Camilleri M. Chronic intestinal pseudoobstruction: diagnosis and treatment. Mayo Clin Proc 1989;64:60–70.

69. Camilleri M, Malagelada JR, Abell TL, Brown ML, Hench V, Zinsmeister AR. Effect of six weeks of treatment with cisapride in gastroparesis and intestinal pseudoobstruction. Gastroenterology 1989;96:704–712.

70. Lederle FA, Busch DL, Mattox KM, West MJ, Aske DM. Cost-effective treatment of constipation in the elderly: a randomized double-blind comparison of sorbitol and lactulose. Am J Med 1990;89:597–601.

71. Pike BF, Phillippi PJ, Lawson EH. Soap colitis. N Engl J Med 1971;285:217–218.

72. Grunberg SM, Hesketh PJ. Control of chemotherapy-induced emesis. N Engl J Med 1993;329:1790–1796.

73. Diehl V, Marty M. Efficacy and safety of antiemetics. Cancer Treat Rev 1994;20:379–392.

74. Grunberg S, Leonard RFC, Smyth J, Selby P, Soukop M, eds. Chemotherapy induced emesis: a review of aetiology, mechanisms, methodology and prospects for clinical management. Br J Cancer Suppl 1992;19:S1–S76.

75. Malagelada J, Camilleri M. Unexplained vomiting: a diagnostic challenge. Ann Intern Med 1984; 101:211–218.

76. Kris MG, Gralla RJ, Clark RA, Tyson LB, O'Connell JP, Wertheim MS, Kelsen DP. Incidence course and severity of delayed nausea and vomiting following the administration of high-dose cisplatin. J Clin Oncol 1985;3:1379–1384.

77. Kris MG, Gralla RJ, Tyson LB, Clark RA, Cirrincione C, Groshen S. Controlling delayed vomiting: double-blind, randomized trial comparing placebo, dexamethasone alone, and metoclopramide plus dexamethasone in patients receiving cisplatin. J Clin Oncol 1989;7:108–114.

78. The Italian Group for Antiemetic Research. Dexamethasone, granisetron or both for the prevention of nausea and vomiting during chemotherapy for cancer. N Engl J Med 1995;332:1–5.

79. Razavi D, Delvaux N, Farvacques C, De Brier F, Van Heer C, et al. Prevention of adjustment disorders and anticipatory nausea secondary to adjuvant chemotherapy: a double-blind, placebo-controlled study assessing the usefulness of alprazolam. J Clin Oncol 1993;11:1384–1390.

80. Kimble GA. Hilgard and Marquis' conditioning and learning. New York: Appleton Century Crofts, 1961.

36

Hepatotoxicity of Chemotherapeutic Agents

Paul D. King and Michael C. Perry

Abnormal liver function in a patient receiving cancer chemotherapy evokes an imposing differential diagnosis. Recognizing that problems arise in cancer chemotherapy when pretreatment liver function is abnormal, when drugs that possess known hepatic toxicity are to be given, or as a result of tumor or immunosuppression, guides identification of the underlying cause. Commonly used tests of liver function (Table 36.1) and liver biopsy can further narrow the differential diagnosis by characterizing the pattern of abnormalities; many diseases, infections, and toxins cause a predictable pattern of injury.

Most hepatotoxic drug reactions are idiosyncratic, occurring because of either hypersensitivity mechanisms or host metabolic idiosyncrasy (1). The clinician must always consider that liver injury is due to an idiosyncratic drug reaction, especially in a setting such as an oncology service where patients typically receive many drugs. However, chemotherapeutic agents often possess predictable, dose-dependent ("direct") hepatotoxicity. Standard criteria for the recognition of drug-induced liver disorders (2) and for grading of chemotherapy hepatotoxicity (3) have been established, but most reports of drug hepatotoxicity do not use such guidelines. This chapter addresses the spectrum of hepatotoxic effects of chemotherapeutic agents. Other reviews have recently been published (4–8).

Besides drug reactions, there are multiple potential causes of abnormal liver tests that may be important in the population being considered for chemotherapy (Table 36.2). Cancer patients may have known or occult hepatic metastases or portal vein thrombosis. Paraneoplastic cholestasis, a rare syndrome most commonly associated with renal cell carcinoma (Stauffer's syndrome), has also been reported with other tumors (Table 36.3). Fulminant hepatic failure (9) or hepatic rupture (10) may complicate liver metastases. Virtually all patients have been exposed to hepatotoxins, including other medications, alcohol, and chemicals, and many will receive blood products during surgery or chemotherapy. Patients may have other coexisting medical conditions that affect the liver or, because of their immunocompromised state, be prone to infectious complications, including viral and fungal (11) hepatitis. Baseline evaluation of patients about to undergo chemotherapy should therefore always include liver tests. Hepatic imaging, typically a computer assisted tomography (CT) scan if not already done as part of staging, is done as clinically indicated. Noninvasive dynamic tests of liver function such as the MEGX test correlate with liver histology (12) and survival in cirrhosis (13), but their role in predicting hepatotoxicity is not yet established.

Assessment of liver function prior to chemotherapy (5) helps identify underlying liver disease and aids in the choice of drug and dose.

Table 36.1. Liver Functions and Tests

Function	Test
Bile secretion	Serum bilirubin
Protein synthesis	Serum albumin
Intermediary metabolism	BUN, blood ammonia
Clotting factors	Fibrinogen level
Detoxification	MEGX test (12)
Iron storage	Serum ferritin
Copper storage	Ceruloplasmin level
Vitamin storage	Prothrombin time
Glycogen storage	Serum glucose, liver biopsy

Table 36.2. Potential Causes of Hepatic Abnormalities in Cancer Patients

Direct effects of the tumor
  Hepatic metastases
  Portal vein thrombosis
Indirect effects of the tumor
  Paraneoplastic syndromes (Stauffer's syndrome)
  Infiltration with amyloid or light-chain deposits
Preexisting liver disease
Chemotherapeutic drugs
Other hepatotoxic medications
Coexisting medical conditions
Infections

Table 36.3. Tumors Associated with Paraneoplastic Cholestasis

Renal cell carcinoma (211)
Medullary thyroid cancer (212)
Renal sarcoma (213)
Hodgkin's disease (214)
Non-Hodgkin's lymphoma (215)
Gastrointestinal carcinoma (216)
Prostate carcinoma (217)
Schwannoma (218)

Periodic reevaluation of liver function is also indicated to detect the evolution of hepatic dysfunction. If liver tests are abnormal, the etiology must be defined as clearly as possible; liver biopsy may be required. The distinction between a drug-induced and a disease-induced abnormality is clearly important in the patient's management (14).

Chemotherapy has been reported to reactivate chronic hepatitis B virus infection, possibly because of an increase in viral synthesis during immunosuppression followed by a rebound in the host's immune responses to the infection when therapy is discontinued (15). This has occurred even after low-dose pulse methotrexate therapy (16) and in several reported cases was fatal (17, 18). Immunosuppression also results in increased viremia in hepatitis C virus infection, which can also rarely lead to severe hepatitis (19).

SINGLE CHEMOTHERAPEUTIC AGENTS

Hepatotoxic reactions to chemotherapeutic drugs may occur in a variety of patterns, including parenchymal cell injury with fatty change, hepatocellular necrosis, or fibrosis; ductular injury with cholestasis; vascular lesions such as peliosis hepatis or venoocclusive disease (VOD); and hepatic neoplasms (7, 20). Hepatocellular injury is the most common pattern. As direct hepatotoxins, most chemotherapeutic drugs can be expected to cause a predictable pattern of injury.

Alkylating Agents

The alkylating agents include the nitrogen mustards, ethylenemines, alkylsulfonates, nitrosoureas, and triazenes. Four nitrogen mustards are currently used in therapy: mechlorethamine, cyclophosphamide, melphalan, and chlorambucil.

Mechlorethamine, given intravenously, rapidly undergoes chemical transformation and combines with either body water or reactive compounds. Hepatic metabolism is not considered important, and nitrogen mustard does not cause hepatic abnormalities (20), presumably because of its rapid degradation.

In an attempt to achieve greater selectivity for neoplastic tissues, the chemical structure of mechlorethamine was modified, resulting in cyclophosphamide. The liver mixed-function oxidase system converts cyclophosphamide to 4-hydroxycyclophosphamide, which is in equilibrium with its acyclic tautomeric form, aldophosphamide. In cells susceptible to cytolysis, nonenzymatic cleavage of aldophosphamide yields phosphoramide mustard and acrolein. These two compounds are highly cytotoxic and may represent active forms of the drug.

In spite of its requirement for hepatic metabolism for activity, cyclophosphamide is an uncommon hepatic toxin, and only a few reports of elevated hepatic enzymes are attributed to the drug (22–26). This effect is likely due to an idiosyncratic reaction rather than direct toxicity. Diffuse hepatocellular destruction was noted on biopsy of one patient (25), and another demonstrated massive hepatic necrosis (22).

When used to treat vasculitis, cyclophosphamide has been associated with liver damage when its administration was preceded by azathioprine (27). Biopsy in three of the four patients in this report showed liver cell necrosis. In two patients, cyclophosphamide had previously been given without antecedent azathioprine, and hepatic injury had not been seen, suggesting an apparent interaction of the two drugs to cause liver cell necrosis.

Melphalan is rapidly hydrolyzed in plasma, and approximately 15% is excreted unchanged in the urine. At usual doses, it is not associated with hepatotoxicity, but it does produce transient abnormalities in liver function tests at the high doses used in autologous bone marrow transplantation (28, 29).

Chlorambucil, also a nitrogen mustard derivative, was linked to the development of liver damage in 6 patients from an autopsy series of 181 patients with leukemia or lymphoma (30). Two patients had postnecrotic cirrhosis, and a third had areas of fibrosis. Variable degrees of centrilobular or periportal liver degeneration and necrosis were seen. Bile thrombi were seen, usually in central areas, but occasionally midzonal or periportal in location. All six patients were jaundiced, and chlorambucil was implicated as the principal cause in three. All patients in this series had abnormal liver function tests. In another reported case, idiosyncratic hepatotoxicity and a rash developed; rechallenge produced the same reaction (31). This drug must be considered a rare cause of liver dysfunction.

Busulfan is the only alkylsulfonate currently used, primarily for the myeloproliferative disorders. After administration, the drug is rapidly cleared from the blood, and almost all labeled busulfan is excreted in the urine as methanesulfonic acid. Hepatic metabolism is apparently not important. In standard doses, busulfan rarely causes hepatic dysfunction but has been linked to at least one case of cholestatic hepatitis (32); another case of cholestasis (33) occurred in a patient in blast crisis who also had leukemic infiltration of the liver.

As a group, the alkylating agents are seldom implicated as hepatotoxins and, with the possible exception of cyclophosphamide, can be given in the face of altered liver function with relative safety.

Nitrosoureas

The nitrosoureas include carmustine (BCNU), lomustine (CCNU), streptozotocin, and the investigational agents chlorozotocin and methyl CCNU. They seem capable of functioning as both alkylating and carbamoylating agents. BCNU also depletes hepatic stores of glutathione (34), which may increase the risk of oxidant injury from other sources. BCNU-induced liver abnormalities have been reported in up to 26% of patients (35), from 6 to 127 days following treatment. Elevations of serum aminotransferases, alkaline phosphatase, and/or bilirubin are usually mild and revert to normal over a brief period, although fatalities have been reported. The effects of CCNU are similar (36).

Streptozotocin-induced hepatotoxicity is manifest primarily as aminotransferase elevations and occurs in 15 to 67% of patients (37, 38). These changes appear a few days to weeks after treatment and rapidly revert to normal without the production of symptoms or the development of chronic changes.

Antimetabolites

The antimetabolites currently in clinical use include cytosine arabinoside, 5-fluorouracil, 6-mercaptopurine, azathioprine, 6-thioguanine, and methotrexate.

Cytosine arabinoside (ara-C) is currently the mainstay of treatment of acute myelogenous leukemia and its variants. It differs from the naturally occurring pyrimidine, cytidine, in that arabinoside replaces ribose as the sugar moiety attached to the pyrimidine base. Intracellularly, ara-C is metabolized in three successive phosphorylation reactions to the triphosphate derivative ara-CTP, which inhibits DNA synthesis both by inhibition of DNA polymerase and by misincorporation into the DNA molecule. Its effects are thus limited to cells actively synthesizing DNA.

In an early series using ara-C, abnormal liver function tests were reported in 37 of 85 leukemic patients (39), but many had liver function abnormalities prior to treatment, confounding factors such as sepsis or hemolysis, or resolution of biochemical abnormalities despite continuation of therapy. No definite evidence of hepatotoxicity could be found. Ever since, establishing the drug as a hepatotoxin has been especially difficult, since leukemic patients have frequently received transfusions, are subject to infections, are on multiple medications, and are not candidates for liver biopsy because of their usual thrombocytopenia. In patients in whom biopsies have been possible, drug-induced intrahepatic cholestasis has been demonstrated (40, 41). Although 24 of 27 leukemic patients given high-dose ara-C by continuous infusion over 72 hours developed abnormal liver tests (42), the effects are reversible and not dose limiting (42, 43, 44).

5-Fluorouracil (5-FU) is used in the treatment of breast cancer, head and neck cancer, lung cancer, and gastrointestinal cancers. When given intravenously, 5-FU is metabolized by anabolism in tissues to its active form, 5-fluoro-2-deoxyuridine-5-monophosphate, which inhibits thymidylate synthetase. The drug is also catabolized, primarily in the liver, as dihydrouracil dehydrogenase reduces the pyrimidine ring. The reduced compound is then cleaved to α-fluoro-β-alanine, ammonia, urea, and carbon dioxide, as in the degradation of uracil. Both the toxicity and the antitumor effect are potentiated if catabolism is blocked by dihydrouracil dehydrogenase inhibition. Approximately 15% of the administered drug is excreted in the urine unchanged. Although the liver plays a key role in its catabolism, 5-FU has not been reported to cause liver damage when given orally, and only rare reports of possible hepatotoxicity have been noted when the drug is given intravenously (45).

When the 5-FU metabolite fluorodeoxyuridine (FUDR, floxuridine) is given intraarterially by implantable pump for hepatic metastases from colorectal carcinoma, new toxicities become apparent (46). There are two major pictures: (*a*) chemical hepatitis with rises in aminotransferases, alkaline phosphatase, and serum bilirubin and (*b*) stricture of the intrahepatic or extrahepatic bile ducts, accompanied by elevated alkaline phosphatase and bilirubin levels (47–49). Toxicity appears to be both time and dose dependent. With rare exceptions, the hepatitis picture usually improves with the temporary cessation of chemotherapy, but the development of secondary sclerosing cholangitis is irreversible (50, 51). Two patterns of sclerosis may be seen, a diffuse pattern and the diffuse pattern plus short segments of tight stricture, usually located in the proximal bile ducts (52). Compared with conventional intravenous 5-FU therapy, intraarterial FUDR offers a higher response rate, but at the cost of increased liver toxicity (53, 54).

The purine analogue 6-mercaptopurine (6-MP) is used chiefly in the maintenance therapy of acute lymphocytic leukemia. When activated by hypoxanthine-guanine phosphoribosyl transferase to the monophosphate nucleotide, the drug inhibits de novo purine synthesis. Phosphorylation to the triphosphate permits incorporation into DNA. The drug is metabolized by xanthine oxidase to 6-thiouric acid.

Hepatotoxicity induced by 6-MP may occur in a variety of settings, especially when the dose of the drug exceeds the usual daily dose of 2 mg/kg, and may present as either hepatocellular or cholestatic liver disease (55, 56). Preclinical animal studies noted the development of hepatic necrosis in mice and rats (57), and shortly after its introduction, 6-MP was incriminated in the development of jaundice (58). Biopsy revealed bland cholestasis, with minimal hepatic necrosis but significant cytologic atypia and disorganized hepatic cords (59), a picture confirmed on multiple occasions (60). Stopping the drug was followed by resolution of the jaundice.

6-MP may also produce a hepatocellular injury pattern (56). Serum bilirubin levels are usually between 3 and 7 mg/dL, with moderate elevations in aminotransferases and alkaline phosphatase. Most episodes of jaundice occur more than 30 days after the initiation of therapy. Changing the route of administration from oral to intravenous did not alter the production of hepatotoxicity, as 14 of 40 patients developed AST or ALT values above 150 U/L (61). It has been suggested that there is a direct toxic effect of the drug, because rechallenge after discontinuation of the drug does not necessarily shorten the latent period, and systemic manifestations of hypersensitivity such as rash, arthralgias, and eosinophilia are not usually present (56). However, in a series of 396 patients treated an average of 60 months with 1.5 mg/kg/day of 6-MP for refractory inflammatory bowel disease, hepatitis occurred in only 1 patient, and liver biopsy suggested hypersensitivity (62).

Azathioprine (AZ), the nitroimidazole derivative of 6-MP, is used for the prevention of solid organ transplant rejection and in the management of patients with autoimmune diseases such as autoimmune hepatitis and inflammatory bowel disease (63). Like 6-MP, AZ induces liver toxicity (8). Hepatotoxicity is seen chemically as increased serum bilirubin and alkaline phosphatase levels with moderate elevations in aminotransferases and histologically as cholestasis with variable parenchymal cell necrosis.

Most reports of AZ hepatic toxicity have been in the renal transplant population, which has a high incidence of viral hepatitis, causing some observers to doubt the hepatotoxic potential of AZ. In some renal transplant patients, liver abnormalities progressed when AZ was stopped; in others, they improved even though the drug was continued or the patient was rechallenged. A prospective study of patients with psoriasis who were receiving AZ did not show deterioration of liver function (64). AZ is probably hepatotoxic, but compared with 6-MP, its effects are less frequent, milder, and less dose dependent. It has been speculated that patients who develop hepatotoxicity are those who convert AZ into 6-MP at an unusually rapid rate (8), an example of host metabolic idiosyncrasy.

A prospective study of psoriatic patients receiving AZ did not reveal deterioration of liver function tests (64), but a retrospective review of patients with neuromuscular disease found a 9% incidence of hepatotoxicity (65). In another report, 3 of 25 patients with rheumatoid arthritis developed fever, chills, rash, and hepatotoxicity (66). There is also a report of AZ toxicity documented by both histopathology and rechallenge (67). A patient receiving high doses of AZ for an autoimmune neurologic disorder developed rapidly progressive and fatal sclerosing hepatitis (68).

Several renal transplant patients have developed hepatic VOD after immunosuppressive therapy with AZ (69, 70). The clinical presentation varied from a mild viral-like syndrome to rapidly fulminant liver failure and death, with severe progressive portal hypertension in some patients. An association has been reported with cytomegalovirus infections, but not with AZ dose, type or duration of transplant, or the type of underlying kidney disease (70).

6-Thioguanine, another antipurine, has been implicated in the production of hepatic VOD (71–74) and in a single case of peliosis hepatis (75). An early report (76) described jaundice among the adverse reactions.

The folic acid analogue, methotrexate (MTX), is often a component of combination chemotherapy programs for breast cancer, head and neck cancer, gestational trophoblastic disease, acute lymphoblastic leukemia, and non-Hodgkin's lymphomas. In high doses, it is a key component of therapy for osteosarcoma. It is also used to treat a variety of nonmalignant diseases, including psoriasis, psoriatic arthritis, and rheumatoid arthritis.

MTX binds tightly to dihydrofolate reductase, blocking the reduction of dihydrofolate to its active form, tetrahydrofolic acid. Tetrahydrofolic acid is essential for the one-carbon transfer reactions required for the synthesis of thymidylate, a precursor to DNA, and the purines adenosine and guanosine, precursors of both DNA and RNA.

In standard doses, MTX is excreted unchanged in the urine. In high doses, it is partially metabolized by the liver to 7-hydroxymethotrexate, which is also slightly soluble in acid solution (77). When used in high doses with leucovorin "rescue," MTX diffuses into both normal and malignant cells. Leucovorin enters normal cells, blocking the effects of MTX.

When MTX was used for maintenance therapy in children with acute leukemia, it led to the development of hepatic cirrhosis and fibrosis (78–80). Fatty change, focal hepatitis, or portal fibrosis in previously untreated patients made the evaluation of MTX's role in the production of hepatotoxicity difficult.

Elevations of aminotransferases and serum lactate dehydrogenase (LDH) are quite common following high-dose MTX therapy, with an incidence of 14.1% in one report of treatment of gestational trophoblastic disease (81). The enzymes rise with each course and are higher in patients treated with a daily schedule than in those treated on an intermittent schedule. These abnormalities resolve within 1 month after the cessation of therapy. High-dose MTX therapy results in acute aminotransferase elevation that is transient, reversible, and, at least in children, does not result in chronic liver disease (82).

The role of chronic MTX therapy, such as that used in the treatment of psoriasis or rheumatoid arthritis (RA), in the production of hepatotoxicity is much less clear. Patients who take daily oral MTX are reported to develop fibrosis or cirrhosis more than twice as frequently as those who take the drug intermittently parenterally (83). Given continuously by mouth, MTX hepatotoxicity increases with the length of therapy or cumulative dose. Patients with RA or psoriasis who received cumulative doses of less than 2 g of MTX had a low incidence of hepatotoxicity, even though the average duration of therapy ranged from 28 to 48 months (84–86). This suggests that for the development of toxicity, cumulative dose is more important than duration of therapy. Age, obesity, decreased renal function, diabetes mellitus, and alcohol consumption have also been associated with an increased risk of toxicity (87). The combination of MTX and salicylates greatly increased the frequency of abnormal liver enzyme values (88).

Although some studies of sequential liver biopsy specimens in RA patients treated with MTX did not show fibrosis or cirrhosis on light microscopy (89), others found significant worsening of hepatic histologic grade, with the common development of hepatic fibrosis (87). However, hepatic histologic abnormalities occurred very commonly in RA patients who had *not* received MTX (90), and electron microscopic analysis of sequential biopsy samples found minimal hepatic ultrastructural changes not felt to be clinically significant (91). Hepatic fibrosis tends to regress when therapy is discontinued (92). Cirrhosis is quite uncommon in RA patients treated with MTX (87). An American College of

Rheumatology committee has recommended that liver tests and hepatitis B and C serologies be performed prior to starting treatment with MTX (92). A pretreatment liver biopsy is recommended only in patients with a history of excessive alcohol use, abnormal baseline AST values, or chronic hepatitis B or C infection. Liver tests are monitored every 4 to 8 weeks, and liver biopsy is suggested if persistently abnormal values are seen. For RA patients without other risk factors for liver disease (such as alcohol use), routine liver biopsies during MTX therapy yield little useful information (93). In general, the risk: benefit ratio of long-term, low-dose oral MTX for rheumatic diseases seems acceptable (94–96). In the setting of psoriasis, MTX toxicity is of more concern. Cases of liver failure due to chronic MTX therapy are well documented (97). Cirrhosis is a serious complication, affecting up to 24% of psoriatic patients treated with oral MTX for 5 years (98). Liver biopsy is recommended after a 1.5 g cumulative dose in patients with psoriasis (99).

There are two case reports of the development of hepatocellular carcinoma following MTX-induced fibrosis: in a child with acute lymphoblastic leukemia and in a patient heterozygous for α-1-antitrypsin deficiency, raising the additional question of long-term carcinogenesis with the use of this agent (100, 101).

Antitumor Antibiotics

The antitumor antibiotics include doxorubicin, daunorubicin, mitoxantrone, bleomycin, mitomycin, mithramycin (plicamycin), and dactinomycin. Doxorubicin, an anthracycline antibiotic, acts through DNA intercalation, alteration of membrane function, and free radical formation (4). It is extensively metabolized in the liver, and liver antioxidant capacity, including that provided by glutathione production, may protect against free radical injury (34). Therefore, dose reductions must be made for altered hepatic function. Doxorubicin has been reported to cause hepatic damage in only one series (102). Six patients with acute lymphoblastic leukemia were treated with induction therapy using vincristine, prednisone, and doxorubicin. Shortly after administration, increases in AST, ALT, and bilirubin were seen, with focal infiltration by inflammatory cells and steatosis on liver biopsies. This was considered an idiosyncratic reaction.

Mitoxantrone, an anthraquinone antibiotic,

may have a lower incidence of serious toxicities than other anthracycline anticancer drugs (103). When used in leukemic patients, the drug has produced transient elevations in AST and ALT levels (104).

Bleomycin is composed of several polypeptides and exerts its effect by single-strand scission of DNA, which may lead to breakage of double-stranded DNA. Because it does not cause myelosuppression, it is often used in combination with other chemotherapeutic agents for lymphomas, testicular carcinomas, and various squamous carcinomas. Bleomycin is excreted in the urine and inactivated by an aminopeptidase present in many tissues, including liver. The lungs and skin lack this aminopeptidase and are thus susceptible to injury from bleomycin. Most human studies have found a very low incidence of liver dysfunction; a review of more than 1000 patients treated with bleomycin concluded that hepatic toxicity was not consistently reported, nor could it be specifically ascribed to bleomycin (105).

Mitomycin is an antitumor antibiotic but acts as an alkylating agent, primarily by inhibiting DNA synthesis. The metabolism of the drug is unclear, but it is found in high concentrations in the bile. Since urinary excretion cannot account for its rapid clearance, it has been suggested that mitomycin is cleared from the serum by metabolism (106). Although mitomycin has a broad spectrum of antitumor activity, it has a low level of efficacy. The article that reported abnormalities in liver function tests did not discuss the patients' clinical states (107).

Plicamycin (mithramycin) is the most hepatotoxic chemotherapeutic agent commercially available (108, 109). With the discovery of less toxic and more effective drugs, it is now rarely used except for the treatment of tumor hypercalcemia refractory to other therapy. The drug binds to DNA and is a potent inhibitor of RNA transcription from DNA. Subsequent reduction in messenger RNA synthesis brings a secondary inhibition of the production of enzymes. Plicamycin could thus block the production of many intracellular enzyme systems necessary for normal hepatic function.

Elevations of aminotransferases (often to enormous levels) and LDH occur in virtually 100% of patients treated with plicamycin. Milder elevations in alkaline phosphatase occur, but serum bilirubin is usually normal. These changes begin on the day of drug administration, peak on the second day, and return to normal by 4 to 21 days after treatment. Liver biopsy shows centrilobular hepatocellular necrosis. Coagulation factors II, V, VII, and X, some of which are synthesized by the liver, are depressed. Since the drug may produce significant thrombocytopenia, the combination may result in an unusual bleeding diathesis. The toxicity can be reduced by a reduction in drug dose. Changing the administration of the drug to an alternate-day schedule decreases toxicity and, in animal studies, was more effective (110). A review of patients treated with low-dose plicamycin for hypercalcemia revealed a 16% incidence of mild reversible hepatic dysfunction (111).

Liver toxicity from dactinomycin is seen as occasional instances of transient AST elevations in children who have previously received radiotherapy with fields involving the liver. Since dactinomycin is known to produce a "recall reaction" in tissues previously radiated, it is possible that its administration reactivates prior radiation damage to the liver. The administration of chemotherapy following hepatic radiation has been marked by greater than anticipated leukopenia and thrombocytopenia, suggesting that radiation-induced hepatic toxicity prolongs excretion and thus toxicity of the drug (112).

The National Wilms' Tumor Study Group has reported severe hepatic toxicity, in the form of VOD in four of five patients, when single-dose dactinomycin was used with vincristine (113). The authors emphasized the importance of other potential contributing factors, such as the use of halogenated hydrocarbon inhalational anesthetic agents. The United Kingdom Children's Cancer Study Group's Wilm's tumor trial also reported hepatotoxicity associated with pulsed dactinomycin (114). However, their frequency was lower than that reported from the United States, and they suggested that dactinomycin-related liver toxicity is dose related. VOD has been documented in Wilm's tumor patients treated with vincristine and conventional 5-day divided-dose dactinomycin (115).

A syndrome of hepatopathy-thrombocytopenia (HTS) has also been reported in Wilm's patients (116). HTS was noted in 5 of 355 (1.4%) patients treated with combination chemotherapy but was not seen in 146 patients who received only vincristine. Moderate increases in ALT and AST values were seen, with prolonged prothrombin times. Two patients developed jaundice and ascites. The syndrome occurred within 10 weeks of diagnosis, lasted an average of 12 days, and resolved with supportive therapy. Hepatic VOD was believed to be the cause.

Spindle Inhibitors

The spindle inhibitor vincristine is excreted primarily by the liver but has seldom been implicated as a hepatotoxin. It has produced hepatotoxicity when used in combination with radiation (see below). Transient aminotransferase elevations, confirmed on rechallenge, have also been reported in a single case (117).

Etoposide (VP 16-213) is excreted primarily in the bile but is not usually considered hepatotoxic at standard doses (118). A recent report, however, identified three patients who experienced severe hepatocellular injury at standard doses (119). At high doses, etoposide has induced hyperbilirubinemia, elevated aminotransferases, and elevated alkaline phosphatase activity approximately 3 weeks after administration (120, 121). These cleared over 12 weeks without sequelae. Elevated serum bilirubin levels have been correlated with subsequent leukopenia (122).

Paclitaxel (Taxol) and docetaxel (Taxotere) are members of the newest class of spindle inhibitors. They work by a different mechanism, binding to microtubules rather than to tubulin dimers. Both are extensively excreted by the liver, and caution is warranted in patients with liver impairment (see below). With paclitaxel, elevation from baseline hepatic functions (bilirubin, 8%; alkaline phosphatase, 23%; transaminase, 33%) were seen in 4 to 17% of patients treated with doses of less than 190 mg/m^2 and in 16 to 37% of patients treated at higher doses (123).

Miscellaneous Agents

Cisplatin is a rare cause of hepatic toxicity (steatosis and cholestasis) at standard doses (124), but minor AST elevations are not uncommon (125). At high doses, it has been reported to produce abnormal liver tests, especially AST and ALT (126). The authors suggested that cisplatin-induced acute hepatic injury is dose related.

Carboplatin is a cisplatin derivative developed to meet the need for a platinum compound with a better therapeutic index. A case of carboplatin-induced liver failure has been reported (127). A case of autopsy-documented hepatic VOD has been reported in a patient who received high-dose carboplatin and etoposide (128). Although multiple other medications were given as well, the potential role of carboplatin in the production of liver disease deserves mention.

Escherichia coli L-asparaginase (L-Asp) hydrolyzes L-asparagine in serum. Depletion of this nonessential amino acid results in death of acute lymphoblastic leukemia cells, which cannot synthesize it. Hepatic toxicity is quite frequent with L-Asp. The mechanism is uncertain, but probably involves impaired protein synthesis from asparagine depletion. Liver steatosis, likely from decreased lipoprotein synthesis, is found at autopsy in 42 to 87% (129–131). Decreased serum levels of albumin, ceruloplasmin, haptoglobin, transferrin, and γ-globulins, as well as decreased levels of coagulation factors II, VII, IX, X, and fibrinogen (129), are common. The partial thromboplastin time rises progressively. Moderate elevations of aminotransferase, bilirubin, and alkaline phosphatase also occur. Hyperammonemia may occur as asparagine is broken down. These common changes with L-Asp are usually mild and reversible.

Procarbazine, initially synthesized as a monoamine oxidase inhibitor, was later found to have activity in Hodgkin's disease, non-Hodgkin's lymphomas, small cell lung cancer, and melanoma. The drug is well absorbed orally and is partially excreted in the urine. Most of the drug is rapidly converted to azo-procarbazine by erythrocyte and hepatic microsomal enzymes. From this point on, its metabolism is not clearly defined, and several possible pathways exist. Modification of the dosage in the face of hepatic dysfunction is probably advisable (132). Procarbazine has been implicated as a cause of granulomatous hepatitis (133).

Hydroxyurea was noted to produce "liver toxicity" that was not further characterized in one patient in a phase I study, with no mention of hepatotoxicity since (134). One case report describes hydroxyurea-induced hypersensitivity hepatitis with recurrence upon rechallenge (135). A review article (7) lists hydroxyurea as a cause for peliosis hepatis, but the original citation is not given.

There have been several reports of hepatic vascular toxicity in patients with melanoma treated with single-agent dacarbazine (DTIC) (136–141). Clinical findings include acute hepatic failure, shock, and death within a few days after the onset of the syndrome (136). Pathologically, the process involves small and medium-sized veins, but unlike classic nonthrombotic VOD, acute thrombotic occlusions are seen. Eosinophilia and eosinophilic infiltrates are frequently present, suggesting an allergic idiosyncratic mechanism (136, 137). Such toxicity may be more frequent than commonly thought.

Biologic Response Modifiers

Recombinant α-interferon is used in the treatment of hairy cell leukemia, multiple myeloma, non-Hodgkin's lymphomas, AIDS-related Kaposi's sarcoma, and myeloproliferative disorders. Its use is often accompanied by an increase in aminotransferases, which clears with discontinuation of therapy (142, 143). At high doses, hepatotoxicity may be dose limiting (140, 144). Paradoxically, the drug is used to treat chronic viral hepatitis with reversal of abnormal liver tests (145).

Interleukin-2 (IL-2) is used in the therapy of renal cell carcinoma and melanoma. Many patients undergoing therapy with IL-2 experience elevations of serum bilirubin in the 2 to 7 mg/dL range due to intrahepatic cholestasis (146). Elevations of AST, ALT, and alkaline phosphatase and hypoalbuminemia and prolonged prothrombin times are also frequent. The mechanism is unknown, and reversal usually occurs within several days after the cessation of therapy.

Hormones

Although many new agents are now available, androgens are still used in the hormonal manipulation of breast cancer and carry the risk of intrahepatic biliary stasis (147). The chronic use of any 17-alkyl androgen has the potential for the development of hepatic adenocarcinomas (148, 149).

Cholestatic hepatitis, likely idiosyncratic, has been reported following the use of the antiandrogen flutamide for prostate cancer (150) and megestrol acetate (151) and tamoxifen therapy for breast cancer (152).

Hepatic Venoocclusive Disease

Autologous bone marrow transplantation (ABMT), which commonly uses very high doses of chemotherapeutic agents, and combination chemotherapy may result in hepatotoxicity (Table 36.4). VOD, a nonthrombotic obliteration of small intrahepatic veins by loose connective tissue (153), frequently occurs in the setting of ABMT (154). In a Memorial Sloan-Kettering Can-

Table 36.4. Chemotherapeutic Agents Producing Venoocclusive Disease

---

At conventional doses
  Azathioprine
  Cytosine arabinoside
  Dacarbazine
  6-Mercaptopurine
  6-Thioguanine

Autologous bone marrow transplantation
  Busulfan
  Cyclophosphamide
  Carmustine (BCNU)
  Lomustine (CCNU)
  Mitomycin C
  BCNU and etoposide

---

cer Center study, 46 of 180 consecutive patients (26%) developed jaundice with a bilirubin above 4 mg/dL. The major cause of the elevated bilirubin was VOD, which was seen in 22 of the 180 patients (12%). The venous occlusion may progress to fatal hepatocellular necrosis. The presenting symptoms of VOD are sudden abdominal pain, rapidly accumulating ascites, and hepatomegaly. It is assumed that injury to the endothelium of these vessels secondary to unknown processes initiates the process of subintimal fibroplasia. The resultant vascular engorgement causes hepatomegaly and ascites. The acute phase is characterized by marked centrilobular hemorrhage and hepatocellular necrosis. If the acute phase does not reverse, the veins undergo progressive fibrosis, and atrophy of centrilobular hepatocytes occurs (153). Therapy is largely supportive and consists mainly of salt and fluid restriction.

In the setting of ABMT, graft-versus-host disease may be associated with VOD, but most cases of VOD are likely drug induced. Although occasionally seen with single-agent DTIC (136–139, 155, 156), 6-thioguanine (71), following renal transplantation and AZ therapy (70) or following ABVD (doxorubicin (Adriamycin), bleomycin, vinblastine, dacarbazine) chemotherapy for Hodgkin's disease (157, 158), most cases of VOD have followed high-dose chemotherapy in preparation for ABMT (159–163). In ABMT, the incidence approaches 20%, with mortality ranging from 7 to 50% (153). VOD associated with 6-thioguanine may be reversible upon discontinuation of the drug (71, 73). Indeed, such hepatotoxicity may be the dose-limiting toxicity of preparatory regimens for ABMT (164). Thus, less-toxic regimens or agents that could prevent VOD are needed. In regard to the latter, pretreatment with glutathione monoethyl ester has been reported to protect the liver in an animal model treated with high doses of alkylating agents (165).

The chemotherapeutic agents involved in VOD have included alkylating agents, antimetabolites, and various combinations, typically drugs that undergo some sort of hepatic metabolism (153, 166–170). High-dose cyclophosphamide chemotherapy, alone or with other agents, in preparation for ABMT, has caused hepatic VOD (153, 164). Busulfan at doses of 16 mg/kg or higher may produce hepatic VOD in about 20% of adult patients and up to 5% of children undergoing bone marrow transplantation (171, 168). Busulfan clearance occurs more rapidly in children than in adults, accounting for the difference in rates (172). Dimethyl busulfan is also frequently implicated (173).

ABMT regimens may produce hepatotoxicity without VOD, as was the case when high doses of both BCNU and etoposide were used to treat high-grade gliomas (174). Two of four patients in this report developed ascites, hyperbilirubinemia, and thrombocytopenia and died; a third had transient ascites.

COMBINATION CHEMOTHERAPY

The increasing use of combination chemotherapy has produced new evidence of hepatotoxicity, and more instances can be anticipated in the future. Combination chemotherapy uses several chemotherapeutic agents, each with a different mechanism of action and toxicity profile. Along with the potential for greater tumor kill, however, the possibility for enhanced toxicity occurs. The addition of 6-MP to doxorubicin (Adriamycin) to treat refractory leukemic patients produced an example of this phenomenon (175). Hyperbilirubinemia and elevated levels of AST and alkaline phosphatase increased with each course and returned to normal between treatments. Liver tissue at autopsy showed intrahepatic cholestasis, hepatocellular necrosis, leukemic infiltration, or fatty change. The investigators felt that the intracellular accumulation of doxorubicin may have potentiated the hepatotoxic effects of 6-MP.

An uncommon form of hepatic disease, nodular regenerative hyperplasia (NRH), was observed in patients with chronic granulocytic leukemia treated with the combination of busulfan and 6-thioguanine (176). NRH is characterized by diffuse nodules of regenerative hepato-cytes, without the fibrous septa of cirrhosis, and there is no progression to cirrhosis. The syndrome may be clinically silent or progress, as in the cases reported, to portal hypertension. As in VOD, the initiating injury is believed to be vascular, in this case to the portal vein branches (177).

Many of the agents used in the treatment of acute lymphoblastic leukemia are potential hepatotoxins, but there have been few instances of documented hepatotoxicity. This may be related to the means of detection used; although light mi-croscopic changes were minimal, electron microscopic examination of liver biopsy specimens from children given MTX and 6-MP showed significant abnormalities in all patients (178). In another study, liver biopsy specimens from children receiving maintenance therapy with 6-MP and MTX revealed mild inflammatory and fatty changes in many, and early portal fibrosis in 3 of 16 biopsies after more than 2 years of therapy (179). Interpretation of reported cases has been complicated by the fact that children who present at an older age and require more transfusions are more likely to develop increased ALT values in a pattern consistent with acute or chronic non-A, non-B hepatitis (180). The availability of hepatitis C testing should help resolve this problem.

Adjuvant chemotherapy for breast cancer with cyclophosphamide, MTX, and 5-FU has produced both abnormal liver function tests and focal defects on radionuclide scans (181). Liver biopsy specimens showed severe local inflammation. A larger study using cyclophosphamide and 5-FU, with doxorubicin replacing MTX as adjuvant therapy, found that 77% of patients developed liver function abnormalities (182). These abnormalities appeared within the first 3 months of therapy and normalized in 90% within a year of cessation of treatment. A cholestatic hepatitis picture was seen in a patient receiving ftorafur, doxorubicin, and cyclophosphamide (183). In this setting, liver biopsy may be necessary to exclude tumor metastases and confirm the impression of drug-induced changes.

Hepar lobatum, previously seen almost exclusively with healed or tertiary syphilis, has also been described in association with combination chemotherapy for breast cancer (184).

While the addition of 5-iodo-2'deoxyuridine to 5-FU did not increase hepatotoxicity, the addition of leucovorin produced greater toxicity than FUDR alone (185). In the adjuvant setting, intrahepatic 5-FU and mitomycin combined with hepatic irradiation produced elevations in liver enzymes and chronic liver damage with one death (186). The combination of N-phosphon-acetyl-L-aspartate (PALA) and 5-FU caused transient hepatic abnormalities in 15 of 17 patients, with ascites, hyperbilirubinemia, and hypoalbuminemia (187).

The combination of 5-FU and levamisole, used as adjuvant therapy for resected stage III colon cancer, also carries the potential for hepatotoxicity. In a series of 1025 patients treated in a randomized trial of observation alone, levamisole, or the combination of 5-FU and levamisole, 39.6% of patients receiving both drugs showed laboratory abnormalities consistent with hepatic toxicity (188). Elevations of alkaline phosphatase were most common, followed by elevations of transaminases or serum bilirubin. These changes were asymptomatic and resolved when therapy was stopped. They were occasionally associated with rises in carcinoembryonic antigen (CEA) or with fatty liver on CT scan or liver biopsy. The pattern of abnormal liver function tests and abnormal CT scan may lead the unwary to inappropriately conclude that the patient's disease is progressing.

Reversible hepatic steatosis was seen in approximately 30% of patients with metastatic colorectal cancer treated with the combination of α_2-interferon and 5-FU (189). The changes all reversed with the cessation of therapy, but recognition of this condition is essential to avoid an erroneous label of progressive disease.

Apparently otherwise tolerable doses of irradiation can induce severe injury when combined with chemotherapeutic agents that in themselves are also unlikely to produce toxicity. Vincristine produced severe hepatic toxicity when given in conjunction with abdominal radiation therapy for lymphoma (190). The radiation encompassed the entire liver to total doses of 1500 to 2500 rads and was given with monthly vincristine. Ten of 35 patients developed severe toxicity (AST greater than 3 times normal, clinical evidence of liver failure), and there was a death from hepatitis and thrombocytopenia. Another nine patients had moderate toxicity. The investigators postulated that radiation delayed the transit of vincristine through the liver and its excretion into bile. Another case of fatal acute radiation hepatitis occurred in a patient with non-Hodgkin's lymphoma, who had received abdominal irradiation (2250 rads to the liver) and vincristine (191). A similar phenomenon has been described with radiation and doxorubicin (192).

Many drugs without antineoplastic effects may cause hepatotoxicity. Intensive chemotherapy has been implicated in the development of fatal hepatic necrosis following haloalkane anesthesia (193). Allopurinol, commonly given with chemotherapy to prevent uric acid nephropathy and secondary gout, has also been linked to fulminant hepatic failure, presumably due to a hypersensitivity reaction (194, 195). There is also a report of allopurinol hepatotoxicity possibly potentiated by an interaction with tamoxifen (196). Several cases of fatal, massive hepatic necrosis and others of liver damage have been attributed to ketoconazole, the oral therapy for systemic fungal infections (197–199). These are also thought to be idiosyncratic reactions. Fluconazole may cause hepatitis but has been reported to cause abnormal liver enzymes without significant liver biopsy changes (200). The antiemetic ondansetron has been implicated in hepatocellular injury and jaundice (201). The current popularity of "alternative" medicines has led to the recognition of "herbal hepatitis" (202). Specific inquiry about such nonstandard agents is particularly important when hepatotoxicity occurs in the outpatient setting. Hepatitis has also been attributed to granulocyte colony-stimulating factor (G-CSF) (203), and CSF-secreting tumors may cause paraneoplastic hepatitis (204).

Finally, a syndrome of hyperammonemia has been reported in patients who have received high-dose combination chemotherapy for hematologic neoplasms (205, 206). This syndrome is characterized by progressive mental status changes, respiratory alkalosis, and markedly elevated plasma ammonium levels. Mildly elevated liver tests have been seen in some patients, but the etiology of this is not clear (205).

DOSE MODIFICATIONS WITH ALTERED HEPATIC FUNCTION

Although extensive guidelines have been published for the use of drugs in renal failure, few guidelines exist for the use of drugs when hepatic function is altered. The physician must often choose both drug and dose empirically. Table 36.5 outlines a dose modification scheme. Clearly, known hepatotoxic drugs must be avoided in the setting of abnormal liver function.

Doxorubicin (Adriamycin) is rapidly cleared from the plasma and slowly excreted in the urine and bile, with its predominant metabolism in the liver. Most of the drug is excreted through the bile, with up to 50% of the drug recoverable in the bile or feces in 7 days. Impaired liver function delays excretion and eventually results in increased accumulation in plasma and tissues. Reducing the amount of doxorubicin administered decreases the effective product of concentration and time ($C \times T$) to values similar to those of patients with normal liver function receiving higher doses. Attempts have been made to correlate altered liver function tests with plasma levels, but only an elevated serum bilirubin has been uniformly associated with abnormal doxorubicin pharmacokinetics. It has been suggested that a caveat be attached to dose modification: "Whenever the need for rapid antitumor effect is overwhelming, full dose Adriamycin should be given to patients with normal bilirubin" (207). The goal is to select a dose of doxorubicin capable of reducing the white blood cell count to approximately 1000 cells/mm^3 at the nadir of the drug effect, 10 to 14 days posttreatment.

Daunorubicin, an anthracycline antibiotic structurally very similar to doxorubicin, is used in the treatment of acute granulocytic leukemia, usually with ara-C. The manufacturer suggests that the dose be reduced 25% for a serum bili-

Table 36.5. Dose Modification with Hepatic Dysfunction—If on the Day of Therapy Give the Following % of Drug (See Text for Paclitaxel Modification)

Bilirubin	SGOT	Adriamycin	Daunorubicin	Vinblastine Vincristine VP-16	Cyclophosphamide Methotrexate	5-FU
<1.5	<60	100%	100%	100%	100%	100%
1.5–3.0	60–180	50%	75%	50%	100%	100%
3.1–5.0	>180	25%	50%	Omit	75%	100%
5.0		Omit	Omit	Omit	Omit	Omit

rubin between 1.2 and 3 mg/dL and 50% for a serum bilirubin above 3 mg/dL.

Both vincristine and vinblastine are excreted primarily by the liver into the bile, with less than 5% of radioactively labeled vincristine appearing in the urine. Toxicity increases in the presence of hyperbilirubinemia, presumably related to the metabolism of the drugs. Since assay methods for blood levels of these drugs have only recently become available, there are few data available regarding drug distribution and metabolism. At this time, there is no clear relationship between any degree of alteration of any liver function test and a suggested dose reduction. Many oncologists reduce the dose of either drug by 50% if the serum bilirubin is between 1.5 and 3 mg/dL or the AST is between 60 and 180 IU/L. If the bilirubin exceeds 3 or the AST exceeds 180 IU/L, the drug is not given.

Van den Berg and colleagues, using a radioimmunoassay for vincristine, found an 11-fold range of dose-corrected area under the plasma concentration versus time values ($AUC_{0-\infty}$) (208). Patients with raised serum alkaline phosphatase levels had elevated AUC values, suggesting that elimination of the drug was impaired when the serum alkaline phosphatase was raised. The authors recommended that reductions be made in the calculated dose of vincristine when serum alkaline phosphatase values are elevated, even when bilirubin and aminotransferase values are normal (209).

Examining paclitaxel in patients with liver dysfunction, Venook et al. found that dose-limiting toxicity, defined as an absolute granulocyte count (ANC) below 550/μL, lasting more than 3 days; grade 3 stomatitis lasting more than 3 days; or other grade 4 toxicity, was related to both dose and bilirubin level (210). They suggested that patients with AST levels more than twice normal and bilirubins of 1.5 mg/dL or less could receive paclitaxel at a dose of less than 135 mg/m^2, those with bilirubins of 1.6–3.0 mg/dL could receive 75 mg/m^2 or less, and those with bilirubins above 3 mg/dL could receive 50 mg/m^2.

REFERENCES

1. Lee WM. Drug-induced hepatotoxicity. N Engl J Med 1995;333:1118–1127.
2. Benichou C. Criteria of drug-induced liver disorders: report of an international consensus meeting. J Hepatol 1990;11:272–276.
3. Oken MM, Creech RH, Tormey DC, Horton J. Toxicity and response criteria of the Eastern Cooper-

ative Oncology Group. Am J Clin Oncol 1982;5:649–655.
4. Sznol M, Ohnuma T, Holland JF. Hepatic toxicity of drugs used for hematologic neoplasia. Semin Liver Dis 1987;7:237–256.
5. Perry MC. Chemotherapeutic agents and hepatotoxicity. Semin Oncol 1992;19:551–565.
6. Zimmerman HJ. Hepatotoxic effects of oncotherapeutic agents. In: Popper H, Schaffner F, eds. Progress in liver diseases, vol 8. Orlando: Grune & Stratton, 1986;621–642.
7. McDonald GB, Tirumali N. Intestinal and liver toxicity of antineoplastic drugs. West J Med 1984;140:250–259.
8. Menard DB, Gisselbrecht C, Marty M, Reyes F, Dhumeaux D. Antineoplastic agents and the liver. Gastroenterology 1980;78:142–164.
9. Harrison HB, Middleton HM, Crosby JH, et al. Fulminant hepatic failure: an unusual presentation of metastatic liver disease. Gastroenterology 1981;80:820–825.
10. Schoedel KE, Dekker A. Hemoperitoneum in the setting of metastatic cancer to the liver. A report of two cases with a review of the literature. Dig Dis Sci 1992;37:153–154.
11. Thaler M, Pastakia B, Shawker TH, et al. Hepatic candidiasis in cancer patients: the evolving picture of the syndrome. Ann Intern Med 1988;108:88–100.
12. Shiffman ML, Luketic VA, Sanyal AJ, et al. Hepatic lidocaine metabolism and liver histology in patients with chronic hepatitis and cirrhosis. Hepatology 1994;19:933–940.
13. Oellerich M, Burdelski M, Lautz HU, et al. Predictors of one-year pretransplant survival in patients with cirrhosis. Hepatology 1991;14:1029–1034.
14. Armitage JO, Burns CP, Kent TH. Liver disease complicating the management of acute leukemia during remission. Cancer 1978;41:737–742.
15. Hoofnagle JH, Dusheiko GM, Schafer DF, et al. Reactivation of chronic hepatitis B virus infection by cancer chemotherapy. Ann Intern Med 1982;96:447–449.
16. Flowers MA, Heathcote J, Wanless IR, et al. Fulminant hepatitis as a consequence of reactivation of hepatitis B virus infection after discontinuation of low-dose methotrexate therapy. Ann Intern Med 1990;112:381–382.
17. Thung SN, Gerber MA, Klion F, Gilbert H. Massive hepatic necrosis after chemotherapy withdrawal in a hepatitis B virus carrier. Arch Intern Med 1985;145:1313–1314.
18. Galbraith RM, Eddleston ALWF, Williams R, et al. Fulminant hepatic failure in leukemia and choriocarcinoma related to withdrawal of cytotoxic drug therapy. Lancet 1975;2:528.
19. Lim LH, Lau GKK, Davis GL, et al. Cholestatic hepatitis leading to hepatic failure in a patient with organ-transmitted hepatitis C virus infection. Gastroenterology 1994;106:248–251.
20. DeSmet VJ. Drug-induced liver disease: pathogenetic mechanisms and histopathological lesions. Eur J Med 1993;2:36–47.
21. Zimmerman HJ, Alpert HK, Howe J. The effect of nitrogen mustard (bis-B-chlorethylamine) on liver function and structure in patients with neoplastic disease. J Lab Clin Med 1952;40:387–389.

22. Aubrey DA. Massive hepatic necrosis after cyclophosphamide. Br Med J 1970;3:588.

23. Walters D, Robinson RG, Dick-Smith JB, Corrigan AB, Webb J. Poor response in two cases of juvenile rheumatoid arthritis to treatment with cyclophosphamide. Med J Aust 1972;2:1070.

24. Bacon AM, Rosenberg SA. Cyclophosphamide hepatotoxicity in a patient with systemic lupus erythematosus. Ann Intern Med 1982;97:62–63.

25. Goldberg JW, Lidsky MD. Cyclophosphamide-associated hepatotoxicity. South Med J 1985;78:222–223.

26. Snyder LS, Heigh RL, Anderson ML. Cyclophosphamide-induced hepatotoxicity in a patient with Wegener's granulomatosis. Mayo Clin Proc 1993; 68:1203–1204.

27. Shaunak S, Munro JM, Weinbren K, Walport MJ, Cox TM. Cyclophosphamide-induced liver necrosis: a possible interaction with azathioprine. Q J Med, New Series 1988;252:309–317.

28. Lazarus HM, Herzig RH, Graham-Pole J, et al. Intensive melphalan chemotherapy and cryopreserved autologous bone marrow transplantation in the treatment of refractory cancer. J Clin Oncol 1983;1:359–367.

29. Leff RS, Thompson JU, Johnson DB, et al. Phase II trial of high dose melphalan and autologous bone marrow transplantation for metastatic colon carcinoma. J Clin Oncol 1986;4:1586–1591.

30. Amromin GD, Delman RM, Shanbran E. Liver damage after chemotherapy for leukemia and lymphoma. Gastroenterology 1962;42:401–410.

31. Koler RD, Forsgren AL. Hepatotoxicity due to chlorambucil. Report of a case. JAMA 1958;167:316–317.

32. Morris LE, Guthrie TH. Busulfan-induced hepatitis. Am J Gastroenterol 1988;83:682–683.

33. Underwood JCE, Shahani RT, Blackburn EK. Jaundice after treatment of leukemia with busulfan. Br Med J 1971;1:556–557.

34. Meredith MJ, Reed DJ. Depletion in vitro of mitochondrial glutathione in rat hepatocytes and enhancement of lipid peroxidation by Adriamycin and 1,3-bis(2-chloroethyl)-1-nitrosurea (BCNU). Biochem Pharmacol 1983;32:1383–1388.

35. De Vita VT, Carbone PP, Owens AH Jr, Gold GI, Krant MJ, Edmonson J. Clinical trials with 1,3-bis (2-chloroethyl)-1-nitrosourea, NSC-409962. Cancer Res 1965;25:1876–1881.

36. Hoogstraten B, Gottlieb JA, Cadili E, Tucker WG, Talley RW, Haut A. CCNU (1,[2-chloroethyl]-3-cyclohexyl-1 nitrosourea, NSC-79037) in the treatment of cancer. Cancer 1973;32:38–43.

37. Broder LE, Carter SK. Pancreatic islet cell carcinoma II: results of therapy with streptozotocin in 52 patients. Ann Intern Med 1973;79:108–118.

38. Schein PS, O'Connell MJ, Blom J, et al. Clinical antitumor activity and toxicity of streptozotocin (NSC-85998). Cancer 1974;34:993–1000.

39. Ellison RR, Holland JF, Weil M, et al. Arabinosyl cytosine: a useful agent in the treatment of acute leukemia in adults. Blood 1968;32:507–523.

40. Pizzuto J, Aviles A, Ramos E, Cervera J, Aguirre J. Cytosine arabinoside induced liver damage: histopathologic demonstration. Med Pediatr Oncol 1983;11:287–290.

41. George CB, Mansour RP, Redmond J, Gandara DR. Hepatic dysfunction and jaundice following high-dose cytosine arabinoside. Cancer 1984;54:2360–2362.

42. Donehower RC, Karp JE, Burke PJ. Pharmacology and toxicity of high-dose cytarabine by 72-hour continuous infusion. Cancer Treat Rep 1986;70:1059–1065.

43. Kremer WB. Cytabarine. Ann Intern Med 1975; 82:684–688.

44. Kantarjian HM, Estey EH, Plunkett W, Keating MJ, Walters RS, et al. Clinical studies: phase I-II clinical and pharmacologic studies of high-dose cytosine arabinoside in refractory leukemia. Am J Med 1986; 81:387–394.

45. Bateman JR, Pugh RP, Cassidy FR, Marshall GJ, Irwin LE. 5-Fluorouracil given once weekly: comparison of intravenous and oral administration. Cancer 1971;28:907–913.

46. Hohn D, Melnick J, Stagg R, et al. Biliary sclerosis in patients receiving hepatic arterial infusions of floxuridine. J Clin Oncol 1985;3:98–102.

47. Doria MI Jr, Shepard KV, Levin B, Riddell RH. Liver pathology following hepatic arterial infusion chemotherapy: hepatic toxicity with FUDR. Cancer 1986;58:855–861.

48. Kemeny N, Daly J, Reichman B, Geller N, Botet J, Oderman P. Intrahepatic or systemic infusion of fluorodeoxyuridine in patients with liver metastases from colorectal carcinoma. Ann Intern Med 1987;107:459–465.

49. Chang AE, Schneider PD, Sugarbaker PH, Simpson C, Culnane M, Steinberg S. A prospective randomized trial of regional versus systemic continuous 5-fluorodeoxyuridine chemotherapy in the treatment of colorectal liver metastases. Ann Surg 1987;206:685–693.

50. Pettavel J, Gardiol D, Bergier N, Schnyder P. Fatal liver cirrhosis associated with long-term arterial infusion of floxuridine. Lancet 1986:1162–1163.

51. Shepard KV, Levin B, Karl RC, et al. Therapy for metastatic colorectal cancer with hepatic artery infusion chemotherapy using a subcutaneous implanted pump. J Clin Oncol 1985;3:161–169.

52. Niederhuber JE, Grochow LB. Status of infusion chemotherapy for the treatment of liver metastases. Princ Pract Oncol Updates 1989;3:1–9.

53. Hohn D, Stagg RJ, Friedman MA, et al. A randomized trial of continuous intravenous versus hepatic intraarterial floxuridine in patients with colorectal cancer metastatic to the liver: the Northern California Oncology Group trial. J Clin Oncol 1989:7:1646–1654.

54. Martin JK, O'Connell MJ, Wieand HS, et al, Intra-arterial floxuridine vs systemic fluorouracil for hepatic metastases from colorectal cancer: a randomized trial. Arch Surg 1990;125:1022–1027.

55. Einhorn M, Davidson I. Hepatotoxicity of mercaptopurine. JAMA 1964;188:802–806.

56. Shorey J, Schenker S, Suki WN, Combes B. Hepatotoxicity of mercaptopurine. Arch Intern Med 1968; 122:54–58.

57. Phillips FS, Sternberg SS, Hamilton L, Clarke DA. The toxic effects of 6-mercaptopurine and related compounds. Ann NY Acad Sci 1957;60:283–296.

58. Farber S. Summary of experience with 6-mercaptopurine. Ann NY Acad Sci 1954;60:412–414.

59. McIlvanie SK, MacCarthy JD. Hepatitis in as-

sociation with prolonged 6-mercaptopurine therapy. Blood 1959;14:80–90.

60. Clark PA, Hsia YE, Huntsman RG. Toxic complications of treatment with 6-mercaptopurine. Two cases with hepatic necrosis and intestinal ulceration. Br Med J 1960;1:393–395.

61. Adamson PC, Zimm S, Ragab AH, et al. A phase II trial of continuous-infusion 6-mercaptopurine for childhood solid tumors. Cancer Chemother Pharmacol 1990;26:343–344.

62. Present DH, Meltzer SJ, Krumholz MP, Wolke A, et al. 6-Mercaptopurine in the management of inflammatory bowel disease: short- and long-term toxicity. Ann Intern Med 1989;111:641–649.

63. Rosman M, Bertino JR. Azathioprine. Ann Intern Med 1973;79:694–700.

64. DuVivier A, Munro DD, Verboy J. Treatment of psoriasis with azathioprine. Br Med J 1974;1:49–51.

65. Kissel JT, Levy RJ, Mendell JR, Griggs RC. Azathioprine toxicity in neuromuscular disease. Neurology 1986;36:35–39.

66. Jeurissen MEC, Boerbooms AMT, van de Putte LBA, Kruijsen MWM. Azathioprine induced fever, chills, rash, and hepatotoxicity in rheumatoid arthritis. Ann Rheum Dis 1990;49:25–27.

67. Small P, Lichter M. Probable azathioprine hepatotoxicity: a case report. Ann Allergy 1989;62:518–520.

68. Barrowman JA, Kutty PK, RA MU, Huang SN. Sclerosing hepatitis and azathioprine (letter). Dig Dis Sci 1986;31:221–222.

69. Marubbio AT, Danielson B. Hepatic veno-occlusive disease in a renal transplant patient receiving azathioprine. Gastroenterology 1975;69:739–743.

70. Read AE, Wiesner RH, LaBrecque DR, et al. Hepatic veno-occlusive disease associated with renal transplantation and azathioprine therapy. Ann Intern Med 1986;104:651–655.

71. Gill RA, Onstad GR, Cardamone JM, Maneval DC, Sumner HW. Hepatic veno-occlusive disease caused by 6-thioguanine. Ann Intern Med 1982;96:58–60.

72. Satti MB, Weinbren K, Gordon-Smith EC. 6-Thioguanine as a cause of toxic veno-occlusive disease of the liver. J Clin Pathol 1982;35:1086–1091.

73. Krivoy N, Raz R, Carter A, Alroy G. Reversible hepatic veno-occlusive disease and 6-thioguanine (letter). Ann Intern Med 1982;96:788.

74. Griner PF, Elbad AWA, Packman CH. Veno-occlusive disease of the liver after chemotherapy of acute leukemia. Ann Intern Med 1976;85:578–582.

75. Larrey D, Freneaux E, Berson A, et al. Case report: peliosis hepatis induced by 6-thioguanine administration. Gut 1988;29:1265–1269.

76. Council on Drugs. Evaluation of two antineoplastic agents: pipobroman (Vercyte) and thioguanine. JAMA 1967;200:139–140.

77. Leme PR, Creaven PJ, Allen LM, Berman M. Kinetic model for the disposition and metabolism of moderate and high-dose methotrexate (NSC 740) in man. Cancer Chemother Rep 1975;59:811–817.

78. Colsky J, Greenspan EM, Warren TN. Hepatic fibrosis in children with acute leukemia after therapy with folic acid antagonists. Arch Pathol Lab Med 1955;59:198–206.

79. McIntosh S, Davidson DL, O'Brien RT, Pearson HA. Methotrexate hepatotoxicity in children with leukemia. J Pediatr 1977;90:1019–1021.

80. Hutter RVP, Shipkey FH, Tan CTC, Murphy ML, Chowdhury M. Hepatic fibrosis in children with acute leukemia: a complication of therapy. Cancer 1960;13:288–307.

81. Berkowitz RS, Goldstein DP, Bernstein MR. Ten year's experience with methotrexate and folinic acid as primary therapy for gestational trophoblastic disease. Gynecol Oncol 1986;23:111–118.

82. Weber BL, Tanyer G, Poplack DG, et al. Transient acute hepatotoxicity of high-dose methotrexate therapy during childhood. NCI Monogr 1987;5:207–212.

83. Podurgiel BJ, McGill DB, Ludwig J, Taylor WF, Muller SA. Liver injury associated with methotrexate therapy for psoriasis. Mayo Clin Proc 1973;48:787–792.

84. MacKenzie AH. Hepatotoxicity of prolonged methotrexate therapy for rheumatoid arthritis. Cleve Clin Q 1985;52:129–135.

85. Tolman KG, Clegg DO, Lee RG, Ward JR. Methotrexate and the liver. J Rheumatol 1985;12:29–34.

86. Warin AP, Landells JW, Leveae GM, Baker H. A prospective study of the effects of weekly oral methotrexate on liver biopsy. Br J Dermatol 1975;93:321–322.

87. Kremer JM, Lee RG, Tolman KG. Liver histology in rheumatoid arthritis patients receiving long-term methotrexate therapy: a prospective study with baseline and sequential biopsy samples. Arthritis Rheum 1989;32:121–127.

88. Fries JF, Singh G, Lenert L, Furst DE. Aspirin, hydroxychloroquine, and hepatic enzyme abnormalities with methotrexate in rheumatoid arthritis. Arthritis Rheum 1990;33:1611–1619.

89. Weinblatt ME, Trentham DE, Fraser PA, et al. Long-term prospective trial of low-dose methotrexate in rheumatoid arthritis. Arthritis Rheum 1988;31:167–175.

90. Rau R, Karger T, Herborn G, Frenzel H. Liver biopsy findings in patients with rheumatoid arthritis undergoing long term treatment with methotrexate. J Rheumatol 1989;16:489–493.

91. Kremer JM, Kaye GL. Electron microscopic analysis of sequential liver biopsy samples from patients with rheumatoid arthritis. Arthritis Rheum 1989;32:1202–1213.

92. Kremer JM, Alarcon GS, Lightfoot RW Jr, et al. Methotrexate for rheumatoid arthritis. Suggested guidelines for monitoring liver toxicity. Arthritis Rheum 1994;7:316–328.

93. Bridges SL, Alarcon GS, Koopman WJ. Methotrexate-induced liver abnormalities in rheumatoid arthritis (editorial). J Rheumatol 1989;16:1180–1183.

94. Lanse SB, Arnold GL, Gowans JDC, Kaplan MM. Low incidence of hepatotoxicity associated with long-term, low-dose oral methotrexate in treatment of refractory psoriasis, psoriatic arthritis, and rheumatoid arthritis: an acceptable risk/benefit ratio. Dig Dis Sci 1985;30:104–109.

95. Kaplan MM. Methotrexate hepatotoxicity and the premature reporting of Mark Twain's death: both greatly exaggerated (editorial). Hepatology 1990;12:784–786.

96. Lewis JH, Schiff E. Methotrexate-induced chronic liver injury: guidelines for detection and prevention. Am J Gastroenterol 1988;83:1337–1345.

97. Gilbert SC, Klintmalm G, Mentor A, et al. Methotrexate-induced cirrhosis requiring liver transplantation in three patients with psoriasis: a word of caution

in light of the expanding use of this 'steroid sparing' agent. Arch Intern Med 1990;150:889–891.

98. Zachariae H, Kragballe K, Søgaard H. Methotrexate induced liver cirrhosis. Studies including serial liver biopsies during continued treatment. Br J Dermatol 1980;102:407–412.

99. Roenigk HH, Auerbach R, Maibach HI, et al. Methotrexate in psoriasis: revised guidelines. J Am Acad Dermatol 1988;19:145–156.

100. Ruymann FB, Mosijczuk A, Sayers RJ. Hepatoma in a child with methotrexate-induced hepatic fibrosis. JAMA 1977;238:2631–2633.

101. Fried M, Kalra J, Ilardi C, Sawitsky A. Hepatocellular carcinoma in a long-term survivor of acute lymphocytic leukemia. Cancer 1987;60:2548–2552.

102. Aviles A, Herrera J, Ramos E, Ambriz R, Aguirre J, Pizzuto J. Hepatic injury during doxorubicin therapy. Arch Pathol Lab Med 1984;108:912–913.

103. Shenkenberg TD, Von Hoff DD. Mitoxantrone: a new anticancer drug with significant clinical activity. Ann Intern Med 1986;105:67–81.

104. Paciucci PA, Sklarin NT. Mitoxantrone and hepatic toxicity (letter). Ann Intern Med 1986;105:805–806.

105. Blum RH, Carter SK, Agre K. A clinical review of bleomycin. A new antineoplastic agent. Cancer 1973;31:903–914.

106. Crooke ST, Bradner WT. Mitomycin C: a review. Cancer Treat Rev 1976;3:121–139.

107. Robert J, Barbier P, Manaster J, Jacobs E. Hepatotoxicity of cytostatic drugs evaluated by liver function tests and appearance of jaundice. Digestion 1968;1:229–232.

108. Brown JH, Kennedy BJ. Mithramycin in the treatment of disseminated testicular neoplasms. N Engl J Med 1965;272:111–118.

109. Kennedy BJ. Metabolic and toxic effects of mithramycin during tumor therapy. Am J Med 1970;49:494–503.

110. Yarbro JW, Kennedy BJ. A comparison of the rate of recovery from inhibition of RNA synthesis in mouse liver and transplantable glioma. Cancer Res 1967;27:1779–1782.

111. Green L, Donehower RC. Hepatic toxicity of low doses of mithramycin in hypercalcemia. Cancer Treat Rep 1984;68:1379–1381.

112. Tefft M, Traggis D, Filler RM. Liver irradiation in children: acute changes with transient leukopenia and thrombocytopenia. Am J Roentgenol Radiat Ther Nucl Med 1969;106:750–765.

113. Green DM, Finklestein JZ, Norkool P, D'Angio GJ. Severe hepatic toxicity after treatment with single-dose dactinomycin and vincristine. Cancer 1988;62:270–273.

114. Pritchard J, Raine J, Wallendszus K. Hepatotoxicity of actinomycin-D. Lancet 1989;1:168.

115. Bjork O, Eklof O, Willi U, Ahstrom L. Venoocclusive disease and peliosis of the liver complicating the course of Wilms' tumor. Acta Radiol Diagn 1985;26:589–597.

116. Raine J, Bowman A, Wallendszus K, et al. Hepatopathy-thrombocytopenia syndrome–a complication of dactinomycin therapy for Wilm's tumor. A report from the United Kingdom Children's Cancer Study Group. J Clin Oncol 1991;9:268–273.

117. El Saghir NS, Hawkins KA. Hepatotoxicity following vincristine therapy. Cancer 1984;54:2006–2008.

118. Issell BF, Crooke ST. Etoposide (VP-16-213). Cancer Treat Rev 1979;6:107–124.

119. Tran A, Housset C, Boboc B, et al. Etoposide (VP-16-213) induced hepatitis. Report of three cases following standard-dose treatments. J Hepatol 1991;12:36–39.

120. Johnson DH, Greco FA, Wolff SN. Etoposide-induced hepatic injury: a potential complication of high-dose therapy. Cancer Treat Rep 1983;67:1023–1024.

121. Chan HY, Meyers FJ, Lewis JP. High-dose VP-16 with intermediate dose cytosine arabinoside in the treatment of relapsed acute nonlymphocytic leukemia. Cancer Chemother Pharmacol 1987;20:265–266.

122. Perry MC, Moertel CG, Schutt AJ, et al. Phase II studies of dianhydrogalactitol and VP-16-213. Cancer Treat Rep 1976;60:1247–1250.

123. Huizing MT, Sewberath Misser VH, Pieters RC, ten Bokkel Huinik WW, Veenhof CHN, et al. Taxanes: a new class of antitumor agents. Cancer Invest 1995;13:381–404.

124. Cavalli F, Tschopp L, Sonntag RW, Zimmerman A. A case of liver toxicity following cis-diammine dichloroplatinum (II) treatment. Cancer Treat Rep 1978;62:2125–2126.

125. Hill JM, Loeb E, MacLellan A, Hill NO, Khan A, King JJ. Clinical studies of platinum coordination compounds in the treatment of various malignant diseases. Cancer Chemother Rep 1975;59:647–659.

126. Pollera CF, Ameglio F, Nardi M, Vitelli G, Marolla P. Cisplatin-induced hepatic toxicity (letter). J Clin Oncol 1987;5:318–319.

127. Hruban RH, Sternberg SS, Meyers P, Fleisher M, Menendez-Botet C, Boitnott JK. Fatal thrombocytopenia and liver failure associated with carboplatin therapy. Cancer Invest 1991;9:263–268.

128. Christian MC. Two toxicities associated with carboplatin use: a. gross hematuria b. hepatic venoocclusive disease. Bethesda, MD: Department of Health & Human Services bulletin, National Institutes of Health, National Cancer Institute, 1989.

129. Haskell CM, Canellos GP, Leventhal BG, et al. L-Asparaginase: therapeutic and toxic effects in patients with neoplastic disease. N Engl J Med 1969;281:1028–1034.

130. Capizzi RL, Bertino JR, Handschumacher RE. L-Asparaginase. Annu Rev Med 1970;21:433–444.

131. Oettgen HF, Stephenson PA, Schwartz MK, et al. Toxicity of E. coli L-asparaginase in man. Cancer 1970;25:253–278.

132. Chabner BA, Myers CE. Clinical pharmacology of cancer chemotherapy. In: DeVita VT Jr, Hellman S, Rosenberg SA, eds. Cancer: principles and practice of oncology. 3rd ed. Philadelphia: JB Lippincott, 1989:349–393.

133. McMaster KR, Hennigar GR. Drug-induced granulomatous hepatitis. Lab Invest 1981;44:61–73.

134. Thurman WG, Bloedow C, Howe CD, et al. A phase I study of hydroxyurea. Cancer Chemother Rep 1963;29:103–107.

135. Heddle R, Calvert AF. Hydroxyurea induced hepatitis. Med J Aust 1980;1:121.

136. Ceci G, Bella M, Melissari M, Gabrielli M, Bocchi P, Cocconi G. Fatal hepatic vascular toxicity of DTIC. Cancer 1988;61:1988–1991.

137. McClay E, Lusch CJ, Mastrangelo MJ. Allergy-induced hepatic toxicity associated with dacarbazine (letter). Cancer Treat Rep 1987;71:219–220.

138. Erichsen C, Jonsson R. Veno-occlusive liver disease after dacarbazine therapy (DTIC) for melanoma. J Surg Oncol 1984;27:268–270.

139. Asbury RF, Rosenthal SN, Descalzi ME, Ratcliffe RL, Arseneau JC. Hepatic veno-occlusive disease due to DTIC. Cancer 1980;45:2670–2674.

140. Golberg RM, Ayoob M, Sigals R, et al. Phase I-II trial of lymphoblastoid interferon in metastatic malignant melanoma. Cancer Treat Rep 1985;69:813–816.

141. Greenstone MA, Dowd PM, Mikhailidis DP, Scheuer PJ. Hepatic vascular lesions associated with dacarbazine treatment. Br Med J 1981;282:1744–1745.

142. Kirkwood JM, Ernstoff MS. Interferons in the treatment of human cancer. J Clin Oncol 1986;4:336–352.

143. Quesada JR, Talpaz M, Rios A, et al. Clinical toxicity of interferons in cancer patients. J Clin Oncol 1986;4:234–243.

144. Figlin RA, DeKernion JB, Maldazys J, et al. Clinical and phase I-II studies: treatment of renal cell carcinoma with alpha (human leucocyte) interferon and vinblastine in combination. Cancer Treat Rep 1985;69:263–267.

145. Korenman A, Baker B, Waggoner J, et al. Long-term remission of chronic hepatitis B after alpha-interferon therapy. Ann Intern Med 1991;114:629–634.

146. Fisher B, Keenan AM, Garra BS, et al. Interleukin-2 induces profound reversible cholestasis: a detailed analysis in treated cancer patients. J Clin Oncol 1989;7:1852–1862.

147. Werner SC, Hanger FM, Kritzler R. Jaundice during methyl testosterone therapy. Am J Med 1950;8:325.

148. Bernstein MS, Hunter RL, Hachnin S. Hepatoma and peliosis hepatitis in Fanconi's anemia. N Engl J Med 1971;284:1135–1136.

149. Henderson JT, Richmond J, Sumerling MD. Androgenic-anabolic steroid therapy and hepatocellular carcinoma. Lancet 1973;1:934.

150. Rosman AS, Frissora-Rodeo C, Marshall AT, et al. Cholestatic hepatitis following flutamide. Dig Dis Sci 1993;38:1756–1759.

151. Foitl DR, Hyman G, Lefkowitch JH. Jaundice and intrahepatic cholestasis following high-dose megestrol acetate for breast cancer. Cancer 1989;63:438–439.

152. Pinto HC, Baptista A, Camilo ME, deCosta EB, Valente A, DeMoura MC. Tamoxifen-associated steatohepatitis—report of 3 cases. J Hepatol 1995;23:95–97.

153. Rollins BJ. Hepatic veno-occlusive disease. Am J Med 1986;81:297–306.

154. Wasserheit C, Acaba L, Gulati S. Abnormal liver function in patients undergoing autologous bone marrow transplantation for hematological malignancies. Cancer Invest 1995;13:347–354.

155. Sutherland CM, Krementz ET. Hepatic toxicity of DTIC. Cancer Treat Rep 1981;65:321–322.

156. Lacroix WF, Runne U, Hauk H, Doepfmer K, Groth W, Wacker D. Acute liver dystrophy with thrombosis of hepatic veins: a fatal complication of dacarbazine treatment. Cancer Treat Rep 1983;67:779–784.

157. Joensuu H, Soderstrom K, Nikkanen V. Fatal necrosis of the liver during ABVD chemotherapy for Hodgkin's disease. Cancer 1986;58:1437–1440.

158. Houghton AN, Shafi N, Rickles FR. Acute hepatic vein thrombosis occurring during therapy for Hodgkin's disease. Cancer 1979;44:2324–2329.

159. McIntyre RE, Magidson JG, Austin GE, Gale RP. Fatal veno-occlusive disease of the liver following high-dose 1,3-bis (2-chloroethyl)-1-nitrosourea (BCNU) and autologous bone marrow transplantation. Am J Clin Pathol 1981;75:614–617.

160. Lazarus HM, Gottfried MR, Herzig RH, et al. Veno-occlusive disease of the liver after high-dose mitomycin C therapy and autologous bone marrow transplantation. Cancer 1982;49:1789–1795.

161. Beschorner WE, Pino J, Boitnott JK, Tutschka PJ, Santos GW. Pathology of the liver with bone marrow transplantation. Am J Pathol 1980;99:369–386.

162. Woods WG, Dehner LP, Nesbit ME, et al. Fatal veno-occlusive disease of the liver following high dose chemotherapy, irradiation and bone marrow transplantation. Am J Med 1980;68:285–290.

163. Siegel R, Greenough T, Antman K, et al. Hepatic veno-occlusive disease (VOD) in autologous bone marrow transplantation (BMT) (abstract). Proc Am Soc Clin Oncol 1987;6:154.

164. Antman K, Eder JP, Elias A, et al. High-dose alkylating agent preparative regimen with autologous bone marrow support: the Dana-Farber Cancer Institute/Beth Israel Hospital experience. Cancer Treat Rep 1987;71:119–125.

165. Teicher BA, Crawford JM, Holden SA, et al. Glutathione monoethyl ester can selectively protect liver from high dose BCNU or cyclophosphamide. Cancer 1988;62:1275–1281.

166. Lehrner LM, Enck RE. Hepatic-vein thrombosis after chemotherapy for histiocytoma (letter). Ann Intern Med 1978;88:575–576.

167. Ayash LJ, Hunt M, Antman KH, et al. Hepatic venoocclusive disease in autologous bone marrow transplantation of solid tumors and lymphomas. J Clin Oncol 1990;8:1699–1706.

168. Vassal G, Hartmann O, Benhamou E. Busulfan and veno-occlusive disease of the liver. Ann Intern Med 1990;112:881.

169. Shulman HM, McDonald GB, Matthews D, et al. An analysis of hepatic veno-occlusive disease and centrilobular hepatic degeneration following bone marrow transplantation. Gastroenterology 1980;79:1178–1191.

170. Gottfried MR, Sudilovsky O. Hepatic veno-occlusive disease after high-dose mitomycin and autologous bone marrow transplantation. Hum Pathol 1982;13:646–650.

171. Grochow LB, Jones RJ, Brundett RB, et al. Pharmacokinetics of busulfan: correlation with veno-occlusive disease in patients undergoing bone marrow transplantation. Cancer Chemother Pharmacol 1989;25:55–61.

172. Vassal G, Gouyette A, Hartmann E, Pico JL, Lemerle J. Pharmacokinetics of high-dose busulfan in children. Cancer Chemother Pharmacol 1989;24:386–390.

173. Shulman HM, McDonald GB, Matthews D, Doney KC, Kopecky KJ, Gauvreau JM, Thomas ED. An analysis of hepatic venocclusive disease and centrilobular hepatic degeneration following bone marrow transplantation. Gastroenterology 1980;79:1178–1191.

174. Wolff S. High-dose carmustine and high-dose etoposide: a treatment regimen resulting in enhanced hepatic toxicity. Cancer Treat Rep 1986;70:1464–1465.

175. Minow RA, Stern MH, Casey JH, Rodriquez V, Luna MA. Clinco-pathologic correlation of liver damage in patients treated with 6-mercaptopurine and adriamycin. Cancer 1976;38:1524–1528.

176. Key NS, Kelly PMA, Emerson PM, Chapman RWG, Allan NC, McGee JO. Oesophageal varices associated with busulphan-thioguanine therapy for chronic myeloid leukaemia. Lancet 1987;1050–1052.

177. Wanless IR, Godwin TA, Allen F, et al. Nodular regenerative hyperplasia of the liver in hematological disorders: a possible response to obliterative portal venopathy. A morphometric study of nine cases with a hypothesis on the pathogenesis. Medicine 1980; 59:367–379.

178. Harb JM, Kamen BA, Werlin SL, et al. Hepatic ultrastructure in leukemic children treated with methotrexate and 6-mercaptopurine. Am J Pediatr Hematol Oncol 1983;5:323–331.

179. Topley JM, Benson J, Squier MV, Chessells JM. Hepatotoxicity in the treatment of acute lymphoblastic leukaemia. Med Pediatr Oncol 1979;7:393–399.

180. Hetherington ML, Buchanan GR. Elevated serum transaminase values during therapy for acute lymphoblastic leukemia correlate with prior blood transfusion. Cancer 1988;62:1614–1618.

181. Vaughan WP, Wilcox PM, Alderson PO, Ettinger DS, Abeloff MD. Hepatic toxicity of adjuvant chemotherapy for carcinoma of the breast. Med Pediatr Oncol 1979;7:351–359.

182. Larroquette CA, Hortobagyi GN, Buzdar AU, Holmes FA. Subclinical hepatic toxicity during chemotherapy for breast cancer. JAMA 1986;256:2988–2990.

183. Patakfalvi A, Gelencser E, Sipos J. Drug hepatitis of cholestatic type in association with a fac-regimen for breast cancer. Acta Med Hung 1987;44:377–385.

184. Qizilbash A, Kontozoglou T, Sianos J, et al. Hepar lobatum associated with chemotherapy and metastatic breast cancer. Arch Pathol Lab Med 1987; 111:58–61.

185. Remick SC, Benson AB III, Weese JL, et al. Phase I trial of hepatic artery infusion of 5-iodo-2′-deoxyuridine and 5-fluorouracil in patients with advanced hepatic malignancy: biochemically based chemotherapy. Cancer Res 1989;49:6437–6442.

186. McCracken JD, Weatherall TJ, Oishi N, Janaki L, Boyer C. Adjuvant intrahepatic chemotherapy with mitomycin and 5-FU combined with hepatic irradiation in high-risk patients with carcinoma of the colon: a Southwest Oncology Group phase II pilot study. Cancer Treat Rep 1985;69:129–131.

187. Kemeny N, Seiter K, Martin D, et al. A new syndrome: ascites, hyperbilirubinemia, and hypoalbuminemia after biochemical modulation of fluorouracil with N-phosphonacetyl-L-aspartate (PALA). Ann Intern Med 1991;115:946–951.

188. Moertel CG, Fleming TR, MacDonald JS, Haller DG, Laurie JA. Hepatic toxicity associated with fluorouracil plus levamisole adjuvant therapy. J Clin Oncol 1993;11:2386–2390.

189. Sorenson P, Edal AL, Madsen EL, Fenger C, Poulsen MC, Petersen OF. Reversible hepatic steatosis in patients treated with interferon alfa-2a and 5-fluorouracil. Cancer 1995;75:2592–2596.

190. Glicksman AS, Grunwald HW. Vincristine enhanced hepatic radiation toxicity. Personal communication.

191. Hansen MM, Ranek L, Walbom S, Nissen NI. Fatal hepatitis following irradiation and vincristine. Acta Med Scand 1982;212:171–174.

192. Kun LE, Camitta BM. Hepatopathy following irradiation and Adriamycin. Cancer 1978;42:81–84.

193. Spiegel RJ, Pizzo PA, Fantone JC, Zimmerman HJ. Fatal necrosis after high-dose chemotherapy following haloalkane anesthesia. Cancer Treat Rep 1980; 64:1023–1029.

194. Raper R, Ibels L, Lauer C, Barnes P, Lunzer M. Fulminant hepatic failure due to allopurinol. NZ Med J 1984;14:63–65.

195. Ohsawa T, Ohtsubo M. Hepatitis associated with allopurinol. Drug Intell Clin Pharm 1985;19:431–433.

196. Shah KA, Levin J, Rosen N, Greenwald E, Zumoff B. Allopurinol hepatotoxicity potentiated by tamoxifen. NY State J Med 1982:1745–1746.

197. Heiberg JK, Svejgaard E. Toxic hepatitis during ketoconazole treatment. Br Med J 1981;283:825.

198. MacNair AL, Gascoigne E, Heap J, Schuermans V, Symoens J. Hepatitis and ketoconazole therapy. Br Med J 1981;283:1058.

199. Firebrace DAJ. (letter) Br Med J 1981;283:1058–1059.

200. Trujillo MA, Galgiani JN, Sampliner RE. Evaluation of hepatic injury arising during fluconazole therapy. Arch Intern Med 1994;154:102–104.

201. Verrill M, Judson I. Jaundice with ondansetron. Lancet 1994;344:190–191.

202. Gordon DW, Rosenthal G, Hart J, Sirota R, Baker AL. Chaparral ingestion. The broadening spectrum of liver injury caused by herbal medications. JAMA 1995;273:489–490.

203. Günther G, Mauz-Körholz C, Körholz D, Burdach S. G-CSF and liver toxicity in a patient with neuroblastoma. Lancet 1992;340:1352.

204. Suzuki A, Takahashi T. Liver damage in patients with colony-stimulating-factor producing tumors. Am J Med 1993;94:125–132.

205. Mitchell RB, Wagner JE, Karp JE, et al. Syndrome of idiopathic hyperammonemia after high-dose chemotherapy: review of nine cases. Am J Med 1988; 85:662–667.

206. Watson AJ, Chambers T, Karp JE, et al. Transient idiopathic hyperammonemia in adults. Lancet 1985;2:1271–1274.

207. Benjamin RS. A practical approach to Adriamycin (NSC-123127) toxicology. Cancer Chemother Rep 1975;6:191–194.

208. Van den Berg HW, Desai ZR, Wilson R, et al. The pharmacokinetics of vincristine in man: reduced drug clearance associated with raised serum alkaline phosphatase and dose-limited elimination. Cancer Chemother Pharmacol 1982;8:215–219.

209. Desai ZR, Van den Berg HW, Bridges JM, et al. Can severe vincristine neurotoxicity be prevented? Cancer Chemother Pharmacol 1982;8:211–214.

210. Venook A, Egorin M, Brown TD, Batist G, Budman DR, et al. Paclitaxel (Taxol) in patients with liver dysfunction (abstract). Proc Am Soc Clin Oncol 1994;350:139.

211. Strickland RC, Schenker S. The nephrogenic hepatic dysfunction syndrome: a review. Dig Dis 1977; 22:49–55.

212. Tiede DJ, Tefferi A, Kochhar R, et al. Paraneoplastic cholestasis and hypercoagulability associated with medullary thyroid carcinoma. Cancer 1994; 73:702–705.

213. Sharara AI, Panella TJ, Fitz JG. Paraneoplastic hepatopathy associated with soft tissue sarcoma. Gastroenterology 1992;103:330–332.

214. Perrera DR, Greene ML, Fenster LF. Cholestasis associated with extrabiliary Hodgkin's disease. Gastroenterology 1974;67:680–685.

215. Watterson J, Priest JR. Jaundice as a paraneoplastic phenomenon in a T-cell lymphoma. Gastroenterology 1989;97:1319–1322.

216. Abels JC, Rekers PE, Binkley GE, Pack GT, Rhoads CP. Metabolic studies in patients with cancer of the gastrointestinal tract. II. Hepatic dysfunction. Ann Intern Med 1942;16:221–240.

217. De la Tassa M, Conzález IC, Fernandez ML, Egocheaga AA, Toraño MA. Colestasis y carcinoma de próstata. Descripción de un caso y revisión de las colestasis paraneoplásicas. Med Clin (Barc) 1991;96:22–25.

218. Henderson AR, Grace DM. Liver-originating isoenzymes of alkaline phosphatase in the serum: a paraneoplastic manifestation of a malignant schwannoma of the sciatic nerve. J Clin Pathol 1976;29:237–240.

37

Renal and Electrolyte Abnormalities Due to Chemotherapy

William P. Patterson and Garry P. Reams

The kidney is an important organ involved in the excretion of both exogenous and endogenous substances. Some chemotherapeutic agents are metabolized by the kidney, and others are excreted either as metabolites or as unchanged compounds. Many anticancer drugs are nephrotoxic, causing either acute or chronic renal failure (e.g., cisplatin) or a specific renal lesion (e.g., ifosfamide). Some agents are not usually nephrotoxic, but may become so under certain circumstances. In the presence of renal insufficiency, other drugs excreted by the kidney may accumulate and exert more significant toxicity than usual. Finally, any chemotherapeutic agent may induce renal failure, acid/base disorders, or electrolyte abnormalities as a result of a dramatic response to therapy, as characterized by the rapid tumor lysis syndrome or by acute uric acid nephropathy.

This chapter discusses basic renal physiology as it applies to chemotherapeutic agents and the current methods of assessing kidney function. Chemotherapeutic agents that are known to be nephrotoxic are presented in detail individually, and the basis of the nephrotoxicity, the means to prevent and manage the side effects, and current experimental approaches to lessen toxicity are discussed. Finally, a schedule of dose modifications for commonly used chemotherapy drugs in the presence of renal insufficiency is presented.

RENAL PHYSIOLOGY

Most chemical compounds taken into the body are metabolized first, with urinary or bili-

ary excretion. Renal dysfunction can modify the normal pathway of drug metabolism and excretion in two ways: (*a*) the rate of drug biotransformation may be altered and/or (*b*) the excretion of metabolites may be impaired. The retention of drug metabolite in patients can lead to several difficulties. It the metabolites are pharmacologically active, then the duration of effect of a drug will be prolonged. If the drug metabolites are pharmacologically inactive, the metabolite as well as the drug are measured, and patients will appear to be resistant to a drug when plasma levels are deemed "adequate."

Excretion of Drugs

The main processes by which the kidney handles chemical compounds include filtration and active and passive transport (1). The determinants of the filtration of a drug across the glomerulus include (*a*) molecular size, (*b*) protein binding, (*c*) glomerular integrity, and (*d*) nephron number.

Drugs with a large volume of distribution are not subject to filtration, since very little of the drug is present in the plasma at any one time (1). The amount of drug actually filtered and excreted depends upon renal blood flow and the rate of nonrenal metabolism and excretion (1). In addition, the rate of urine flow affects drug elimination. A dilute urine favors excretion, and an increase in urine flow rate allows less time for reabsorption to occur (1). Once a drug gains access to the tubular fluid through the glomerulus or proximal tubule, it may be passively reabsorbed by the more distal sites in the nephron. Urinary pH can affect the state of ionization of the molecule and, consequently, can determine the reabsorption of a drug (1). In general, un-ionized drugs will be reabsorbed, and ionized drugs will be excreted. Other variables in renal disease that may affect a drug's pharmacokinetics include (a) variable absorption due to edema (2), nausea, or delayed gastric emptying (3); (b) alterations in serum albumin or albumin binding due to uremia (1); or (c) alteration of liver metabolism due to uremia (4, 5).

CLINICAL ASSESSMENT

An accurate assessment of renal function is helpful not only in selecting appropriate drug dosage and in identifying patients at high risk of developing renal dysfunction but also in identifying nephrotoxicity from chemotherapeutic agents. These agents may not only diminish glomerular filtration rate (GRF) but may also cause proximal and/or distal tubular dysfunction. Renal function assessment, therefore, should be directed not only at determining GFR but also at evaluating proximal and distal tubular function.

Glomerular Filtration Rate

An ideal marker for glomerular filtration should be metabolically inert and nontoxic and should not alter renal function. Furthermore, it should be freely filtrable, not bound to plasma proteins or blood cells, and, of course, it should neither be reabsorbed nor secreted by the renal tubules.

Inulin, a fructose polysaccharide derived from dahlia roots and Jerusalem artichokes, is filtered but neither reabsorbed nor secreted, and its clearance is equal to the GFR (6, 7). Creatinine is filtered and secreted by the kidney. There is no net tubular reabsorption, and, therefore, the endogenous creatinine clearance technique is not a true measurement of GFR (6). Nonetheless, the endogenous creatinine clearance is the usual technique employed by physicians as a clinical measurement of GFR. However, the magnitude of the disparity between creatinine and inulin clearance is not generally appreciated because of the contribution of tubular secretion of creatinine to the total endogenous creatinine clearance and the effects of renal insufficiency on the tubular secretion of creatinine (8, 9). In individuals with normal renal function, the creatinine clearance is not significantly different from the inulin clearance. The creatinine:inulin clearance ratio rises as inulin clearance decreases; thus, as the inulin clearance declines, the creatinine clearance progressively overestimates the actual GFR (8–10).

Serum creatinine concentration is determined by (a) the volume of creatinine distribution, (b) the rate of production (related to muscle mass), (c) the rate of excretion, and (d) the noncreatinine chromogen contribution. The significance of the noncreatinine chromogen component is inversely proportional to the actual serum creatinine concentration (8, 11–13). In subjects with "normal" serum creatinine levels, the contribution of noncreatinine chromogen to the total serum creatinine concentration is significant. The amount of noncreatinine chromogen present in different subjects is both unpredictable and unrelated to the amount of creatinine present (12, 13). Plasma creatinine, regardless of the method employed to determine its concentration, is of limited value in predicting either the level of endogenous creatinine clearance or the level of inulin clearance. Significant increases in plasma creatinine do not occur until the creatinine clearance is below 70 mL/min/1.73 m^2 or the inulin clearance is below 50 mL/min/1.73 m^2.

Some authors have advocated that changes in the reciprocal of the serum creatinine or changes in the logarithm of the serum creatinine versus time are sensitive indices of deterioration of renal function (14, 15). In early renal disease, however, GFR can decrease substantially without changes in serum creatinine. In late renal disease, furthermore, serum creatinine may rise disproportionately as GFR falls. At extremely low GFRs (inulin clearance less than 20 mL/min), tubular secretion of creatinine appears to be progressively impaired. The importance of an accurate measurement of GFR may be questioned when a low GFR exists, because although fractional creatinine clearance may be high, the absolute difference between creatinine clearance and GFR, in terms of mL/min, is small (16). However, small differences in GFR may markedly influence decisions. In early renal disease, when the physician wishes to follow its progression, an accurate measurement of GFR is clearly necessary to avoid being lulled into a false sense of security by a "normal" endogenous creatinine clearance.

While inulin clearance is an impractical technique for determining GFR, creatinine clearance is potentially inaccurate, particularly in patients with renal dysfunction. Presently, however, radioactive tracers are used to accurately and efficiently determine GFRs. The clearance of radioactive tracers correlates well with that of inulin and can be performed in several hours (17). However, caution should be exerted, since the GFR determined by standard clearance technique of radioisotopes differs from the GFR calculated from disappearance curves of radioisotopes (18). The radioisotopes available for GFR determinants are ^{51}Cr-labeled EDTA (ethylenediaminetetraacetic acid), ^{99m}Tc-labeled DTPA (diethylenetriamine pentaacetic acid), and iodine-labeled diatrizoate and iothalamate.

Proximal and Distal Tubular Function

Proximal tubular dysfunction is a constellation of renal defects, most commonly including glucosuria, aminoaciduria, proteinuria, and hypophosphatemia (19). Reabsorption of salt and water may be unimpaired. This process may be first recognized with abnormalities on urine dipstick tests. Distal tubular dysfunction may also occur. Clinically this condition may be characterized by polyuria and renal tubular acidosis (20).

URIC ACID NEPHROPATHY

Uric acid is filtered by the glomeruli and reabsorbed and secreted by the tubules. As the principal end product of purine metabolism, its excretion may increase significantly in some malignancies or in response to therapy. Its highest concentration occurs in the distal tubule, the area of the kidney responsible for acidification of urine. Urate has decreased solubility in an acid medium, which accounts for the renal lesion in acute uric acid nephropathy. Acute uric acid nephropathy develops when urate production and excretion exceeds the solubility in the distal tubule and collecting ducts. Spontaneous hyperuricemia and nephropathy may occur with some hematologic malignancies but is rare with solid tumors (21). Large cell lymphomas, Burkitt's lymphoma, and the acute leukemias are the cancers most commonly associated with spontaneous urate nephropathy, with lymphomas causing this condition more frequently than leukemias (21).

The more common situation is the development of acute urate nephropathy in the presence of response to chemotherapy or radiotherapy (22). Patients whose cancers have a high cell turnover rate, such as bulky responsive tumors, aggressive hematologic cancers, small cell lung cancer, and testicular cancer, are at greater risk,

although this was not a problem in the original cisplatin study (23). (Of note, in acute leukemia the height of the blast count does not correlate with the risk of urate nephropathy (22).) The lesion seen in the kidney is that of urate crystals loosely formed in the distal tubule and collecting ducts. If treated appropriately, the abnormalities are reversible, with improvement in renal function. Urate calculi are rare, as the exposure to high urate levels is brief, but calculi can develop with chronic hyperuricemia, as observed in myeloproliferative syndromes (21, 24). The clinical presentation of acute uric acid nephropathy is that of uremia, namely, nausea, emesis, malaise, anorexia, and oliguria (21). Flank pain and hematuria are rare, as nephrolithiasis is uncommon. Other causes of acute renal failure cannot be differentiated from urate nephropathy by serum creatinine, urea nitrogen, or uric acid levels (25). Serum phosphate levels may be elevated and may be associated with hypocalcemia, particularly with rapid tumor lysis (21). Urate crystals may be present in the urine, but their absence does not rule out the diagnosis, as the crystalluria may be seen only acutely (21). A urinary urate:creatinine ratio above one on a random sample is specific for the diagnosis (25).

Prevention and, if necessary, early treatment are the primary aspects of the management of urate nephropathy, with prevention being the more important. Patients at significant risk for hyperuricemia require

1. Hydration to maintain a urinary output above 3 L daily (>100 mL/hr) (21, 22, 26).
2. Urinary alkalinization to keep urine pH above 7.0 (100 mEq/m^2 daily) (21, 22).
3. Allopurinol, 600 mg daily for 2 to 3 days, then 300 mg orally daily

It is best if these measures can be initiated at least 48 hours prior to chemotherapy. Should hyperuricemia develop, prompt recognition and institution of therapy are necessary to prevent acute renal failure. If oliguria has not developed, then the above measures may be adequate to reverse the abnormalities. Allopurinol may be given intravenously or orally; therapeutic levels of its active metabolite, oxypurinol, are attained within minutes by the intravenous route and within 1 to 3 hours orally (27). In the presence of anuria or oliguria, it is necessary to exclude ureteral obstruction before assuming urate nephropathy is the etiology. This is best done by ultrasound, to avoid nephrotoxic contrast media. Once hydronephrosis is ruled out, then urinary flow must be established by hydration and furosemide. If diuresis does not occur within a few hours, then dialysis should be initiated (21). Hemodialysis is preferred, as it is more effective than peritoneal dialysis in lowering total body urate (21).

There are potential complications to the measures taken to prevent hyperuricemia. Fluid overload can occur and requires close attention to input and output. Alkalinization may cause metabolic alkalosis and associated hypokalemia (21, 22). Allopurinol, an inhibitor of xanthine oxidase, may increase xanthine levels and cause xanthine crystals to form in an acid urine (28). Oxypurinol, the active metabolite of allopurinol, may form crystals in high-dose allopurinol administration with oliguria (29); thus, the dose of allopurinol must be reduced in the presence of renal failure. Finally, rare cases of interstitial nephritis and renal failure have been related to allopurinol. The clinical picture is one of eosinophilia and exfoliative dermatitis. Management requires discontinuation of the drug and administration of corticosteroids (30).

RAPID TUMOR LYSIS SYNDROME

The rapid tumor lysis syndrome is characterized by massive cell death due to therapy in extremely sensitive tumors, resulting in severe, life-threatening metabolic derangements. These include hyperkalemia, hyperphosphatemia, hypocalcemia, and hyperuricemia. As a consequence of the urate level and the electrolyte abnormalities, acute renal failure, cardiac arrhythmias, and sudden death may ensue (31). Potassium and phosphate are released from the dying cells, with hypocalcemia as a result of the hyperphosphatemia (31–33).

The tumors most commonly associated with the rapid tumor lysis syndrome are Burkitt's and undifferentiated lymphomas and acute lymphoblastic leukemia (31, 32, 34). It occurs less commonly in other non-Hodgkin's lymphomas, myeloproliferative syndromes, and rarely in solid tumors, except in small cell lung cancer (35–37). An association exists between the degree of elevation of the serum lactic dehydrogenase level and the development of the syndrome (31, 34). In addition, the presence of renal insufficiency or hyperuricemia increases the risk of the rapid tumor lysis syndrome (31, 34), although it may occur with normal renal function (34). The clinical

manifestations include tetany, malaise, symptoms of uremia, and the above laboratory derangements occurring within 24 to 48 hours after the initiation of chemotherapy. Other abnormalities include prolongation of the QT interval, soft tissue deposition of calcium salts, and progressive azotemia (31, 33).

Prophylaxis is the key; adequate hydration, urinary alkalinization, and the use of allopurinol are appropriate and should be initiated at least 12, and preferably 24, hours prior to therapy. If the patient develops the syndrome, the following aggressive steps are required to prevent further morbidity or mortality:

1. Intravenous hydration to maintain urinary output, if possible, of 100 mL/hr.
2. Urinary alkalinization to maintain urinary pH at 7 or above, generally 100 mEq/m² daily of sodium bicarbonate.
3. Allopurinol, 600 mg per day initially.
4. Hemodialysis is indicated if hyperkalemia (>6 mEq/L), hyperphosphatemia (>10 mg/dL), hyperuricemia (>10 mg/dL), acidosis, volume overload, symptomatic hypocalcemia, or a serum creatinine level above 10 mg/dL develops (31).

Therapy, including diuresis, must be continued for at least 5 days, as the tumor lysis is generally limited (31, 34). Complications of therapy for this condition include volume overload, the toxicity of allopurinol, and metabolic alkalosis with potential exacerbation of symptomatic hypocalcemia (31, 34). During the initial management of the patient at risk, it is important to monitor serum electrolytes, calcium, phosphorus, BUN, and creatinine every 6 to 8 hours for 48 hours.

NEPHROTOXIC CHEMOTHERAPEUTIC AGENTS

Cisplatin

Cisplatin is a heavy metal complex that has revolutionized the treatment of many human cancers (23, 38–40), but dose-limiting nephrotoxicity is a major stumbling block in its use (41, 42). The types of renal and electrolyte disorders associated with cisplatin administration have been well characterized, and both acute and chronic forms of renal injury have been described (43–46). An acute form of renal failure occurs primarily in patients who have not received adequate hydration during therapy. It consists of azotemia, a rising serum creatinine level, and, in experimental animals, an oliguric phase preceding polyuria. In addition, subtle changes in renal function occur without overt renal insufficiency, consisting of decreased effective renal plasma flow (47) and tubular dysfunction despite aggressive hydration (48). Early tubular damage (i.e., within 1 to 3 hours after cisplatin administration) has been demonstrated by measurement of urinary β_2-microglobulin, a sensitive indicator of proximal tubular injury (49).

The chronic lesion has become of greater concern in recent years as many patients have been cured or placed into long-term remission from their cancers because of cisplatin treatment. This lesion consists of a decrease in GFR (50) ranging from a mean of 12 to 23% (51–53). This decrease persisted and was only partially reversible (51, 53) when followed up to 8 years following therapy (51). These abnormalities are not necessarily characterized by a remarkable increase in serum creatinine level or decrease in creatinine clearance and are better identified by sensitive measures of renal function such as radioisotope clearance. Cumulative renal tubular damage due to cisplatin has been demonstrated by increased urinary excretion of tubular enzymes such as alanine aminopeptidase (54) and β_2-microglobulin (55). The proximal tubular enzyme elevations appeared to correlate well with urinary excretion of protein, magnesium, and a decrease in proximal tubular salt and water reabsorption (55). These findings point to proximal tubular injury, but distal functioning may be altered as well (55, 56).

Unusual manifestations of cisplatin toxicity to the kidney have been described. One case of hemolytic uremic syndrome was reported in a 14-year-old female after 8 months of bleomycin, dacarbazine, and cisplatin therapy (57). She had abrupt onset of hypertension and declining creatinine clearance. Another series described the development of hypertension in 6 of 34 males after 6 courses of cisplatin, vinblastine, and bleomycin for germ cell tumors (51). There was no correlation between the risk of hypertension and the degree of renal dysfunction as measured by ^{51}Cr-EDTA clearance (51). Vascular ischemic events without hypertension have been reported in cisplatin-based regimens for germ cell cancer (58); these patients also received bleomycin. The relationship, if any, of the vascular injury and the development of hypertension is not known.

Cisplatin also induces several electrolyte dis-

orders, the most prominent and well-described being hypomagnesemia (59–63). This abnormality is characterized by a decreased serum magnesium, which is symptomatic in 1 to 10% of patients (62, 63). Symptoms include dizziness, muscle weakness, tetany, paresthesias, and tremulousness (62). One patient was reported with seizures due to cisplatin-induced hypomagnesemia (64). This disorder appears to be dose related (61, 62) but can occur after a single treatment (65); in one series, hypomagnesemia developed after a median cisplatin dose of 120 mg (59). The magnesium deficit requires replacement with oral magnesium, and patients have persistent renal losses of magnesium despite decreased serum magnesium levels for months or even years after they complete cisplatin therapy (60). Seventy-one patients receiving high-dose intracavitary cisplatin with systemically administered sodium thiosulfate were evaluated for decreased serum magnesium levels; 8% of those with initially normal levels became hypomagnesemic. Of 21 patients with initial hypomagnesemia, 33% returned to normal values following therapy (66); 67% remained hypomagnesemic. In addition to evaluating serum magnesium levels, a number of studies have reported defects in calcium homeostasis due to cisplatin therapy (63, 67, 68). Some patients develop hypocalciuria (68), even when serum magnesium levels are normal. Hypocalcemia appears to develop in those with the most severe renal magnesium wasting and the greatest hypomagnesemia (67).

The hypomagnesemia results from a proximal tubular defect, interfering with magnesium reabsorption and thus increasing fractional excretion (61, 64) of the cation. Although conclusive evidence is lacking, a similar defect may have caused cisplatin-related hypocalciuria (68) in patients who had persistent renal magnesium wasting years after therapy. The authors hypothesized a lesion in the distal convoluted tubule.

Cisplatin is occasionally associated with a defect in sodium and water handling by the kidney, with some patients developing hyponatremia (69, 70). In one series (70), 10% of patients developed urinary sodium wasting and orthostatic hypotension. Six of seven patients were hyponatremic. Both plasma renin activity and serum aldosterone levels were decreased. Serum vasopressin levels and vasopressin suppression by hydration were normal, suggesting that this defect was not due to inappropriate antidiuretic hormone excess (70). One study evaluating renal sodium and water handling in 15 men receiving standard-dose cisplatin therapy for testicular cancer demonstrated no defects in sodium or water handling (71). Case reports have suggested otherwise (69, 72), although one patient so described (72) had a malignant CNS tumor.

The mechanism of cisplatin nephrotoxicity is an area of intense investigation. Morphologic damage is greatest in the renal tubules, with the greatest concentration of platinum in the straight segment of the proximal tubule (73, 74). Using radioactive platinum, it was demonstrated that platinum is uniformly distributed throughout the kidney within 5 minutes (75), with the greatest platinum density after 24 hours in the juxtamedullary and outer stripe region (73) (i.e., the area of the proximal tubules). On a subcellular level, the highest concentrations of platinum are in the microsomal fractions of liver and kidney (76), with high concentrations in the mitochondria as well. Reversible changes in mitochondrial respiration and calcium accumulation occur with cisplatin administration and accompany mitochondrial swelling and morphologic aberrations (77).

Platinum binds readily to plasma proteins (73), and the reactive species, the free molecule, is filtered at the glomerulus (73). Bound platinum can potentially react with strong nucleophiles (78); the significance of this is unknown. In one animal study, renal protein platinum binding was studied in guinea pigs sensitive and resistant to cisplatin toxicity. Subcellular platinum was evenly distributed between mitochondria, microsomes, and cytosol in both groups, but the sensitive animals had significantly more platinum bound to cytosolic proteins (79). Long-term studies in rats 15 months after platinum administration revealed atrophic and hyperplastic proximal tubules. One month after platinum therapy, elevated platinum levels were seen in the cortex and in the outer and inner stripe regions (80). The proximal tubule is damaged by cisplatin as documented by morphologic data (73), increased excretion of proximal tubular enzymes (54, 81–83), and autoradiographic concentration of radioactive platinum in the proximal renal tubular regions (73, 75).

The toxicity of cisplatin appears to be related to the unbound plasma compound; thus, pharmacokinetic monitoring could be valuable (84). Acute nephrotoxicity correlates with elevated 5-minute plasma concentrations (85). Creatinine clearance is a poor predictor of platinum disposition (86), but peak free levels of platinum correlate significantly with a decline in creatinine clearance after four cycles of cisplatin therapy (86). With repeated courses, there is a reduced clearance of free platinum (87). Tubular transport of cisplatin metabolites is probably involved in the compound's nephrotoxicity (88, 89).

Prediction of cisplatin nephrotoxicity prior to initiation of cisplatin therapy would be a useful tool in preventing renal damage. Creatinine clearance and blood urea nitrogen are poor predictors (86, 87). Age appears not to be predictive of nephrotoxicity, with the elderly at no increased risk (90), although children may be at less risk than adults. Routine laboratory tests are not helpful, except in one study that suggested hyperuricemia and hypoalbuminemia predispose to nephrotoxicity in patients receiving cisplatin (91).

Prevention of cisplatin nephrotoxicity primarily involves sodium chloride hydration. This standard prophylaxis usually consists of giving 2 to 3 L of normal saline over 8 to 12 hours on the day of cisplatin administration, using various schedules (45, 92, 93). Originally it was thought that the chloride anion was important in preventing nephrotoxicity; however, the mechanism of the protection is not known (94–96). Investigators have attempted to avoid nephrotoxicity in patients receiving high doses of cisplatin by using 3% normal saline (95–97). It is unclear if this adds further protection from high doses of cisplatin, but some studies have suggested that cisplatin in 3% saline may have a decreased antitumor effect in animals (98, 99); this has not been studied in humans. In one study of high-dose cisplatin, nephrotoxicity was avoided by intense hydration with 7 L of 0.9% NaCl infusions daily (100). One small study demonstrated that high-dose (60 mg/m^2 for 3 consecutive days) cisplatin in the outpatient clinic was associated with significant toxicity and, thus, not recommended (101). Older patients tolerate hypertonic saline (102), which does not alter cisplatin pharmacokinetics (103).

Intravenous thiol compounds have been used in situations in which high doses of intraperitoneal or intrapleural cisplatin are given (94, 104, 105). The most commonly used compound, sodium thiosulfate, cannot be given concurrently with intravenous cisplatin, as it is believed the thiol will inactivate the cisplatin (45, 106). One animal study demonstrated that intravenous sodium thiosulfate did not increase the therapeutic index of cisplatin (107). However, experiments suggest that sodium thiosulfate is concentrated in the renal tubules and does not change cisplatin pharmacokinetics when given intravenously (104). Intravenous thiosulfate has protected against high-dose intraarterial cisplatin nephrotoxicity when used in hepatic malignancies (108). The current practice is to use intravenous sodium thiosulfate when high-dose intraperitoneal or intrapleural cisplatin is administered.

Other investigators have examined the use of continuous infusion cisplatin to improve efficacy and lessen toxicity (109, 110). Nephrotoxicity as well as other nonrenal side effects decreased (109, 110) if adequate hydration was provided with at least 3 L of normal saline daily. A phase I trial demonstrated that up to 25 mg/m² of cisplatin daily for 5 days could be given with minimal side effects (110). Pharmacokinetic studies demonstrated lower free platinum levels, lower drug exposure, and decreased renal excretion (111), along with subclinical evidence of proximal tubular injury (112). While one study suggested less hypomagnesemia (109), another demonstrated more with continuous infusion in a nonrandomized, two-arm comparison with bolus cisplatin (112).

Management of cisplatin nephrotoxicity requires that either the drug be discontinued, the dosage be reduced substantially, or another drug be substituted (113, 114). Obviously, this is not compatible with treatment of the primary tumor, as there is a dose-response relationship in the use of cisplatin. Dialysis is not effective in treatment of the acute renal failure induced by cisplatin (115). A prospective trial of magnesium supplementation demonstrated less nephrotoxicity if prophylactic magnesium was given, both intravenously and orally, than when no supplements were received (116). Prevention of cisplatin nephrotoxicity through the use of carboplatin and other platinum analogues is being investigated (113, 114). Carboplatin does not exhibit nephrotoxicity and may be preferable to cisplatin in certain situations.

Cisplatin has been used in patients with ureteral obstruction due to tumor mass (117). If the tumor was responsive to cisplatin, there was an improvement in creatinine clearance. Currently, in tumors that are known to be responsive, carboplatin has been substituted for cisplatin in patients with ureteral obstruction. A small number of case reports describe the use of cisplatin in patients with single kidneys, and according to these reports, these patients have suffered no unusual or unexpected adverse effects (118).

In one animal study, rats were exposed to a nephrotoxic dose of radiation therapy and then were administered cisplatin. These animals did not suffer any immediate ill effects, although over time they developed more significant renal failure due to the radiation nephritis combined with the nephrotoxic effects of the cisplatin (119). This study may have relevance to patients who receive abdominal radiation therapy and systemic cisplatin. Three patients who received whole-body hyperthermia along with 60 to 80 mg/m² of cisplatin developed elevated serum creatinine levels (2.7 to 13.6 mg/dL) soon after therapy (120). The pharmacokinetics of cisplatin were not changed, and the mechanism of renal injury was not elucidated (120).

Numerous studies have examined the nephrotoxicity of cisplatin in combination with aminoglycosides, mostly in animal models (121–123). In all studies, nephrotoxicity was greater with the combination of cisplatin and aminoglycosides. In humans, reports of greater toxicity exist when aminoglycosides are combined with cisplatin, although this is generally mild (124). However, one report described acute renal failure following the combined use of gentamicin, cephalothin, and cisplatin (125).

When cisplatin is combined with other chemotherapeutic agents, the nephrotoxicity of both agents may be altered. Methotrexate decreases renal platinum excretion but (with the exception of increasing area under the curve values) does not alter platinum pharmacokinetics (126). On the other hand, concomitant or prior cisplatin administration increases the systemic and renal toxicity of methotrexate (127–129). Prior cisplatin therapy places patients at risk for renal tubular damage from ifosfamide (130). In mice, less toxicity and better tumor kill was seen when 5-fluorouracil preceded cisplatin than when cisplatin preceded 5-flurouracil (131).

Numerous agents have been tried in experimental animal systems to prevent cisplatin nephrotoxicity, including buthionine sulfoximine (132), nifedipine (133), sodium 2-mercaptoethane sulfonate (mesna) (134–136), fosfomycin (136), atrial natriuretic factors (137), metallothionein synthesis induction (138, 139), diethyldithiocarbamate (140), and indazolone carboxilic acid (141). Oral amifostine (WR2721) has been approved by the FDA for prevention of cisplatin nephrotoxicity; the compound protects against myelosuppression, nephrotoxicity, neurotoxicity, and ototoxicity (134). Studies in humans have suggested that some compounds may be beneficial in decreasing the risk of nephrotoxicity, including reduced glutathione (142), captopril (143, 144), and verapamil (145), but this study examined decreases in GFR and effective renal plasma flow after one course only. Another study suggested no benefit with verapamil after four courses of cisplatin (146). Finally, fosfomycin reduces nephrotoxicity (147), particularly in the proximal tubule (136).

Nitrosoureas

Streptozotocin, a nitrosourea, is used primarily to treat pancreatic islet cell tumors (148, 149). The principal toxicity of streptozotocin in the kidney involves the renal tubule, where tubulointerstitial nephritis and tubular atrophy occur (150). This lesion may be manifested by proximal tubule defects including hypokalemia, proximal renal tubular acidosis, and a Fanconi-like syndrome. Nephrotoxicity is not dose related but is rare at streptozotocin doses of less than 1 to 1.5 g/m^2 week. Some renal toxicity occurs in most patients and requires close monitoring of serum creatinine, bicarbonate, potassium, and urinary pH, protein, and glucose levels, although serious or fatal renal failure is uncommon (151). Patients who develop an elevation of serum creatinine level that subsequently returns to normal should probably not receive further streptozotocin. Streptozotocin renal failure can be severe (151), requiring dialysis or causing fatality. Affected patients can develop uric acid nephrolithiasis, as the drug is uricosuric (152). One report described successful management of streptozotocin-induced renal impairment in a patient receiving further streptozotocin by forced diuresis with normal saline (8 L in 6 to 8 hours) and furosemide (153). In one patient, indomethacin reversed streptozotocin-induced nephrogenic diabetes insipidus (154).

The other two commercially available nitrosoureas, lomustine (CCNU) and carmustine (BCNU), are chemically related and cause delayed renal failure that shares some similarities to that of streptozotocin (155). Glomerular and tubular lesions occur with glomerular basement membrane splitting and microaneurysm formation (156). Unfortunately, the renal failure due to these agents may develop as a late complication of their use, occurring months to years following therapy. These patients develop azotemia and proteinuria followed by progressive renal failure, often requiring dialysis (45). The incidence of renal failure appears to increase dramatically after a total dose of nitrosourea of 1500 mg/m^2, and renal failure has been described in patients who received as little as 1000 mg/m^2. The outlook for patients who develop renal abnormalities is unpredictable, and a significant number of patients require dialysis.

Antitumor Antibiotics

The antitumor antibiotic mitomycin C has been associated with a syndrome of renal failure and microangiopathic hemolytic anemia that most commonly occurs after at least 6 months of therapy but may occur much earlier. It appears in up to 20% of patients receiving total doses of 100 mg or more (157). It is characterized by the abrupt onset of a microangiopathic hemolytic anemia with schistocytes, increased fibrin degradation products, thrombocytopenia, and renal abnormalities consisting of azotemia, proteinuria, and hematuria. In addition, the patients are usually hypertensive. The renal failure is generally reversible (157). The kidneys reveal glomerular and arteriolar necrosis, "onion-skinning," and fibrin deposition in capillary walls (158). The lesion appears to be a drug-induced vasculitis.

Another antitumor antibiotic, mithramycin, may cause renal failure in up to 40% of patients. This appears to be related to the cumulative doses in patients who receive 25 to 50 μg/kg daily for 5 consecutive days. It occurs less frequently on an alternate-day schedule (159). The lesion in the kidney reveals necrosis of both proximal and distal renal tubules.

Ifosfamide

Ifosfamide has recently been released for the management of refractory testicular cancer, cervical cancer, malignant lymphomas, and metastatic sarcomas (160). The drug has two described genitourinary toxicities. The first is hematuria (160), which is a significant problem and requires the use of the uroprotective compound, mesna (160–162). Most patients who receive ifosfamide develop microscopic hematuria, and a significant number of patients develop gross hematuria (160, 161). This hematuria may be severe enough to require modification of dose or discontinuation of the drug.

The second renal toxicity of ifosfamide consists of a proximal tubular defect, a Fanconi-like syndrome (163, 164). Originally, this abnormality was reported in patients who received high doses of bolus ifosfamide; thus, the administration of this drug was changed to a split, fractionated dose (164). However, a number of publications have described a Fanconi-like syndrome that may occur during the course of fractionated-dose ifosfamide administration (163, 164). This syndrome appears to be reversible, but in one investigator's experience (WPP, unpublished observation), the patient eventually developed renal failure requiring dialysis.

Mesna does not appear to protect against the proximal tubular abnormality induced by ifosfamide (165, 166). To prevent hematuria, mesna is given at 20% of the ifosfamide dose prior to, and every 4 hours after, ifosfamide for 3 to 5 doses (160). A false-positive reaction for ketones can occur due to mesna (167).

Methotrexate

The antimetabolite methotrexate is not normally toxic to the kidneys, although 90% of the drug is excreted unchanged in the urine (168). When given in high doses, however, methotrexate may precipitate in the renal tubules and collecting ducts because the the high concentration exceeds the solubility of methotrexate at pH 5.0 (168). The nephrotoxicity of methotrexate is related to this precipitation. A clinical study in patients receiving high-dose methotrexate concluded that (a) high doses of the drug cause a decrease in GFR to a mean of 93% of baseline in patients without toxicity and to a mean of 61% in those with systemic methotrexate toxicity; (b) urinary alkalinization, with adequate hydration, does not alter plasma methotrexate decay; and (c) monitoring serum creatinine and methotrexate levels to provide adequate rescue lessens systemic toxicity, even in the presence of methotrexate-induced renal failure (169).

Renal excretion of methotrexate is a complex process involving glomerular filtration and tubular reabsorption and secretion. High-dose methotrexate may inhibit active secretion (170). There is considerable intra- and interpatient variation in methotrexate clearance, so characterization of a particular patient's pharmacokinetic profile is difficult (170). It is clear that the length of exposure correlates with toxicity; thus, given the variable clearance of methotrexate, it is important to closely monitor serum creatinine and methotrexate levels during high-dose therapy (169, 170). Patients who receive high-dose methotrexate may develop renal failure if precautions are not taken, including brisk diuresis and alkalinization of the urine. In general, ade-

quate sodium bicarbonate is given intravenously to keep the urinary pH above 7, and it is reasonable to delay high-dose methotrexate therapy until this degree of alkalinization is attained (168). Some physicians use acetazolamide to maintain urinary bicarbonate excretion; however, this has not been shown to be necessary if adequate sodium bicarbonate is administered intravenously to maintain urinary pH above 7.

In the presence of renal insufficiency or failure, methotrexate excretion is decreased significantly, and patients may suffer greater bone marrow suppression and gastrointestinal side effects because of prolonged exposure to high serum methotrexate levels. Patients with ileal conduits may experience increased methotrexate toxicity (171), particularly if the creatinine clearance is low. If renal failure is induced by methotrexate, then the patient may be managed conservatively unless uremia or electrolyte disorders develop, which may necessitate dialysis. The drug itself is not readily dialyzable. Methotrexate-induced renal failure generally resolves within 2 to 3 weeks of drug withdrawal (172, 173).

Methotrexate toxicity can be potentiated by other antineoplastic agents. Cisplatin may alter methotrexate pharmacokinetics (127, 129) and enhance methotrexate toxicity (127, 174). Renal impairment has been reported in three patients receiving procarbazine followed immediately by methotrexate (175). The mechanism of this interaction is unclear.

Cyclophosphamide

Cyclophosphamide induces two abnormalities in the genitourinary system. The first and most common is hemorrhagic cystitis (176–180), which appears to be related to metabolites of the parent compound and can occur in up to 10% of patients receiving intermittent or chronic low-dose cyclophosphamide and in up to 40% of those who receive cyclophosphamide during bone marrow transplantation. This complication may be manifest by a range of abnormalities, from microscopic hematuria to grossly bloody urine. Prevention consists of frequent voiding and vigorous hydration, especially in patients who receive oral, low-dose, prolonged cyclophosphamide.

A review of 100 patients who developed hemorrhagic cystitis due to cyclophosphamide revealed several points (179). Intravenous therapy and treatment in children produced cystitis at lower doses and at lower cumulative doses. These patients had symptoms of gross hematuria (78%), dysuria (45%), and microscopic hematuria (93%). Bladder cancer developed in 5 of the 100 affected patients. Symptoms persisted for 1 week to 1 year in 40 patients; 16 subjects were symptomatic for 2 to 8 years; and 21 patients had a recurrence of symptoms 3 months to 10 years after drug use was discontinued. Gas gangrene has been described as a complication of cyclophosphamide-induced cystitis (181).

Treatment of cystitis due to cyclophosphamide involves hydration and withdrawal of the drug (180, 182). If this is unsuccessful, then a large-bore bladder catheter (to prevent clot obstruction) is inserted and saline irrigation is done (180). Cystoscopy and fulguration may be required next (180, 182). If hemorrhage persists, continuous silver nitrate irrigation may be attempted. Other agents that may be instilled include ϵ-aminocaproic acid (180), prostaglandins E_2 (183) and $F_{2\alpha}$ (184), vitamin E (180), and formalin (180, 185). Formalin may have significant side effects, such as fibrosis, chemical cystitis, renal papillary necrosis, anuria due to reflux, and (rarely) death (180). Therefore, reflux should be ruled out first and then 1 to 4% solutions employed, with no more than 15 cm of water pressure for 20 minutes, without catheter clamping, using Trendelenburg positioning (186).

Agents to prevent the hemorrhagic cystitis are under investigation. A compound used to prevent ifosfamide cystitis, mesna, has been evaluated in prevention of cystitis from cyclophosphamide. A prospective randomized study of forced diuresis versus mesna in bone marrow transplant patients receiving high doses of cyclophosphamide demonstrated significantly less macroscopic hematuria with mesna (187). The investigators noted no difference in lymphopenia between the two groups, but six of seven graft failures were in the mesna-treated patients. Other reports document the efficacy of mesna in preventing cyclophosphamide cystitis in small groups of patients (188, 189). No human data exist regarding the influence of mesna on cyclophosphamide activity, but one animal study of intraperitoneal mesna and mafosfamide (an active metabolite of cyclophosphamide) demonstrated decreased systemic toxicity and decreased antitumor efficacy (190). Given biologic and pharmacokinetic variables, this observation may or may not extend to humans.

Other experimental measures to protect against cyclophosphamide cystitis have included the administration of reduced glutathione (191), misoprostol (192) (a synthetic prostaglandin), N-acetylcysteine (193), prostaglandins (194), sucralfate (195), and oral sodium pentosanpolysulfate (196), a heparin analogue. Continuous infusion cyclophosphamide, 350 mg/m^2/day for 5 days, was not associated with significant cystitis in one study (197).

The importance of preventing cyclophosphamide cystitis lies in the association between cyclophosphamide cystitis and bladder cancer. Almost 50 cases of bladder cancer following cyclophosphamide therapy have been reported (198–200). These patients generally have received chronic therapy and have often been given a cumulative cyclophosphamide dose of more than 100 g (198, 199). The subjects did not necessarily suffer previous hemorrhagic cystitis (199, 201). Upper urinary tract malignancies presumed to be due to cyclophosphamide have been reported (200), with five cases now in the literature.

The second abnormality due to cyclophosphamide consists of an antidiuretic-hormone-like excess syndrome (202–205). This generally occurs in patients who receive very high doses of cyclophosphamide, although reports document it in patients who received moderate-dose cyclophosphamide (206). It consists of decreased urinary output, hyponatremia, and inappropriate urinary osmolality in the face of decreased serum osmolality. This syndrome generally resolves within 24 hours after discontinuation of the drug; if water restriction is required, cystitis may be a significant complication. One paper suggests using mesna to prevent hemorrhagic cystitis (207) in this situation. One case of transient nephrogenic diabetes insipidus has been reported after high-dose cyclophosphamide therapy for bone marrow transplantation (208).

Vincristine

Vincristine has been associated with a picture similar to that of the syndrome of inappropriate antidiuretic hormone (209–212). This consists of hyponatremia and an inappropriate urinary osmolality in the face of a decreased serum osmolality. Generally, these abnormalities are associated with the neurologic side effects of vincristine.

Bleomycin

While bleomycin does not cause renal toxicity, it is important to remember that the compound is excreted primarily by the kidneys, and therefore, dosage must be adjusted in the presence of renal insufficiency or failure. Specific recommendations are discussed in the section on dose modifications at the end of the chapter.

Investigational and Miscellaneous Agents

The investigational drug 5-azacytidine is used in management of relapsed acute nonlymphocytic leukemia and is undergoing trials in patients with myelodysplastic syndromes. The drug has been implicated in the development of a proximal tubular defect described as either a complete or partial Fanconi-like syndrome (213). It is not known whether this is reversible, and the management of this defect consists of maintaining a normal acid-base balance and careful monitoring and replacement of abnormal electrolytes, particularly phosphate and potassium.

Pentostatin (2'-deoxycoformycin) is active in

the treatment of hairy cell leukemia (214, 215). Phase I studies of doses up to 1 mg/kg for 3 to 5 days demonstrated nephrotoxicity manifested by a rising serum creatinine level. The complication was usually reversible after discontinuation of the drug (216, 217). Lower doses (4 mg/m^2 for 3 days) are better tolerated.

The investigational nitrosoureas, methyl-CCNU and chlorozotocin, have toxicities similar to those of the other nitrosoureas (155, 218, 219). These compounds cause a progressive chronic nephropathy, which is delayed in onset, irreversible, and characterized by a gradually increasing serum creatinine level, proteinuria, enzymuria, and a decrease in urinary concentrating ability (218, 219). It is difficult to determine which of these two drugs is more nephrotoxic; in animals equimolar doses of chlorozotocin are associated with greater renal damage (218). Review of a large series of patients with methyl-CCNU nephrotoxicity revealed a high risk of severe renal injury with cumulative doses exceeding 1200 mg/m^2 (219).

Interleukin-2 (IL-2) is being used in the treatment of various malignancies. Renal abnormalities of prerenal azotemia and serum creatinine elevations with oliguria are common at moderate doses (1 to 10 million units/m^2) and very frequent at high doses (>10 million units/m^2) (220, 221). Investigations into the common toxicities of fluid retention, azotemia, and hypophosphatemia suggested the mechanisms to be an increase in vascular permeability, an induction of a respiratory alkalosis with intracellular shift of phosphate, and increased renal phosphorus reabsorption (222).

Renal and urinary toxicities have been reported from α (available) and γ (investigational) interferons. These are uncommon and consist of proteinuria and azotemia; they resolve upon drug discontinuation (223).

Table 37.1 Chemotherapeutic Drugs Not Requiring Dose Modification in Renal Failure

No dose modification in renal failure

Actinomycin D	Etoposide
Busulfan	5-Fluorouracil
Carboplatin	Melphalan
Chlorambucil	Mitoxantrone
Cytosine arabinoside	Vinblastine
Doxorubicin (Adriamycin)	Vincristine

No dose modification, but closer monitoring in renal failure[a]

Dacarbazine (DTIC)	6-Mercaptopurine
Daunorubicin	Procarbazine
Hydroxyurea	6-Thioguanine

[a]Serial evaluation for proteinuria or azotemia as the drug has significant renal excretion or is given in high doses.

Table 37.2 Chemotherapeutics Requiring Dose Modification in Renal Failure: Suggested Percentage Dose for GFR

Drug	>60 mL/min	30–60 mL/min	10–30 mL/min	<10 mL/min
Bleomycin	NC	75	75	50
Cisplatin	NC	50	omit	omit
Cyclophosphamide	NC	NC	NC[a]	50
Methotrexate	NC	50	omit	omit
Mithramycin	NC	75	75	50
Mitomycin	NC	75	75	50
Nitrosoureas	NC	omit	omit	omit

[a]NC, no change.

DOSE MODIFICATIONS

In the presence of renal insufficiency, some drugs require dose modification. Two references (224, 225) present this information in greater detail. One paper suggests a decrease in most drugs (224); those that may need only minimal adjustment in this reference may only require more careful monitoring rather than a decrease. Tables 37.1 and 37.2 summarize the data.

REFERENCES

1. Reed WE, Sabatini S. The use of drugs in renal failure. Semin Nephrol 1986;6:259–295.
2. Muther RS, Bennett WM. Drug metabolism in renal failure. In: Brenner BM, Stein JH, eds. Chronic renal failure. New York: Churchill Livingstone, 1981:287–323.
3. McNamee PT, Moore GW, McGeown MG, et al. Gastric emptying in chronic renal failure. Br Med J 1985;292:310–311.
4. Reidenberg MM. The biotransformation of drugs in renal failure. Am J Med 1977;62:482–485.
5. Gibson TP. Renal disease and drug metabolism: an overview. Am J Kidney Dis 1986;8:7–17.
6. Pitts RF. Clearance and rate of glomerular filtration. In: Physiology of the kidney and body fluids. Chicago: Year Book, 1968:62–70.
7. Smith H. Clearance involving tubular excretion: endogenous creatinine chromagen clearance. In: The kidney: structure and function. New York: Oxford, 1951:190–194.
8. Bauer JH, Brooks CS, Burch RN. Clinical appraisal of creatinine clearance as a measure of glomerular filtration rate. Am J Kidney Dis 1982;2:337–346.
9. Bauer JH, Brooks CS, Burch RN. Renal function studies in man with advanced renal insufficiency. Am J Kidney Dis 1982;2:30–35.
10. Kim KE, Onesti G, Ramirez O, et al. Creatinine clearance in renal disease: a reappraisal. Br Med J 1969;4:11–14.
11. Rapoport A, Husdan H. Endogenous creatinine clearance and serum creatinine in the clinical assessment of kidney function. Can Med Assoc J 1968;99:149–156.
12. Doolan PD, Alpen EL, Theil GB. A clinical appraisal of the plasma concentration and endogenous clearance of creatinine. Am J Med 1962;32:65–79.
13. Healy JK. Clinical assessment of glomerular filtration rate by different forms of creatinine clearance and a modified phenosulphophthalein excretion tests. Am J Med 1968;44:348–350.
14. Mitch WE, Walsen M, Buffington GA, et al. A simple method of estimating progression of chronic renal failure. Lancet 1976;2:1326–1328.
15. Rutherford WE, Blandin J, Miller JP, et al. Chronic progressive renal disease: rate of change of serum creatinine concentration. Kidney Int 1977;11:62–70.
16. Tobias GT, McLaughlin RF, Hopper J. Endogenous creatinine clearance. N Engl J Med 1962;266:317–323.
17. Barbour GL, Crumb CK, Boyd CM, Reeves RD,
Rastogi SP, Patterson RM. Comparison of inulin, iotholomate, and ^{99}Tc-DTPA for measurement of glomerular filtration rate. J Nucl Med 1976;17:317–320.
18. Reams GP, Singh A, Logan W, Holmes RA, Bauer JH. Total and split renal function in patients with renovascular hypertension: effects of angiotensin-converting enzyme inhibition. J Clin Hypertens 1987;3:153–163.
19. Cogan MG. Disorders of proximal nephron function. Am J Med 1982;72:275–288.
20. Sebastion A, Hulter HN, Kurtz I, Maher T, Schambelan M. Disorders of distal nephron function. Am J Med 1982;72:289–306.
21. Perry MC, Hoagland HC, Wagoner RD. Uric acid nephropathy. JAMA 1976;236:961–962.
22. Garnick MB, Mayer RJ. Acute renal failure associated with neoplastic disease and its treatment. Semin Oncol 1978;5:156–165.
23. Einhorn L, Donohue JP. Cis-diamminedichloroplatinum, vinblastine, and bleomycin combination chemotherapy in disseminated testicular cancer. Ann Intern Med 1977;87:293–298.
24. Robinson RR, Yarger WE. Acute uric acid nephropathy. Arch Intern Med 1977;137:839–840.
25. Kelton J, Kelley WN, Holmes EW. A rapid method for the diagnosis of acute uric acid nephropathy. Arch Intern Med 1978;138:612–615.
26. Holland P, Holland NH. Prevention and management of acute hyperuricemia in childhood leukemia. J Pediatr 1968;72:358–366.
27. Hande K, Reed E, Chabner B. Allopurinol kinetics. Clin Pharmacol Ther 1978;23:598–605.
28. Albin A, Stephens BG, Hirata T, et al. Nephropathy, xanthinuria, or orotic aciduria complicating Burkitt's lymphoma treated with chemotherapy and allopurinol. Metabolism 1972;21:771–778.
29. Stote RM, Smith LH, Dubb JW, et al. Oxypurinol nephrolithiasis in regional enteritis secondary to allopurinol therapy. Ann Intern Med 1980;92:384–385.
30. Gelbart DR, Weinstein AB, Fajardo LF. Allopurinol induced interstitial nephritis. Ann Intern Med 1977;86:197–198.
31. Cohen LF, Balow JE, Magrath IT, et al. Acute tumor lysis syndrome. Am J Med 1980;68:486–491.
32. Arsenau JC, Bagley CM, Anderson T, et al. Hyperkalemia, a sequel to chemotherapy of Burkitt's lymphoma. Lancet 1973;1:10–14.
33. Brereton HD, Anderson T, Johnson RE, et al. Hyperphosphatemia and hypocalcemia in Burkitt's lymphoma. Arch Intern Med 1975;135:307–309.
34. Tsokos GC, Balow JE, Spiegel RJ, et al. Renal and metabolic complications of undifferentiated and lymphoblastic lymphomas. Medicine 1981;60:218–229.
35. Bell R, Forbes IK, Sullivan JR, et al. Complications of tumor overkill when associated with high dose methotrexate therapy. Clin Exp Pharmcol Physiol 1979;5(Suppl):47–55.
36. Cervantes F, Ribera JM, Granena A, et al. Tumor lysis syndrome with hypocalcemia in accelerated chronic granulocytic leukemia. Acta Haematol 1982;68:157–159.
37. Vogelzang NJ, Nelimark RA, Nath KA. Tumor lysis syndrome after induction chemotherapy of small cell bronchogenic carcinoma. JAMA 1983;249:513–514.
38. Young RC, VonHoff DD, Gormley P, et al. Cis-dichlorodiammineplatinum (II) for the treatment of

advanced ovarian cancer. Cancer Treat Rep 1979; 63:1539–1544.

39. Wittes RE, Cvitkovic E, Shah J, Gerold F, Strong E. *Cis*-dichlorodiammine platinum (II) in the treatment of epidermoid carcinoma of the head and neck. Cancer Treat Rep 1977;61:359–366.

40. Yagoda A, Watson R, Gonzalez-Vitale L, Grasstald H, Whitmore W. *Cis*-dichlorodiammine platinum (II) in advanced bladder cancer. Cancer Treat Rep 1976; 60:917–923.

41. Higby DJ, Wallace HJ, Holland JF. *Cis*-diamminedichloroplatinum (II) (NSC-119875): a phase I study. Cancer Chemother Rep 1973;57:459–463.

42. Talley RW, O'Bryan RM, Gutterman JV, et al. Clinical evaluation of toxic effects of *cis*-diamminedichloroplatinum (NSC-119875) phase I clinical study. Cancer Chemother Rep 1973;57:465–471.

43. Loeher PJ, Einhorn LH. Cisplatin. Ann Intern Med 1984;100:704–713.

44. Safirstein R, Winston J, Goldstein M, Moel D, Dikman S, Guttenplan J. Cisplatin nephrotoxicity. Am J Kidney Dis 1986;8:356–357.

45. Ries F, Klastersky J. Nephrotoxicity induced by cancer chemotherapy with special emphasis on cisplatin toxicity. Am J Kidney Dis 1986;8:368–379.

46. Roth BJ, Einhorn LH, Greist A. Long-term complications of cisplatin-based chemotherapy for testis cancer. Semin Oncol 1988;15:345–350.

47. Offerman JJG, Meijer S, Sleijfer DT, et al. Acute effects of *cis*-diamminedichloroplatinum (CDDP) on renal function. Cancer Chemother Pharmacol 1984; 12:36–38.

48. Groth S, Nielsen H, Sorensen JB, Christensen AB, Pedersen AG, Rorth M. Acute and long-term nephrotoxicity of *cis*-platinum in man. Cancer Chemother Pharmacol 1986;17:191–196.

49. de Gislain C, Dumas M, d'Athis P, Lautissier JL, Escousse A, Guerrin J. Urinary β_2-microglobulin: early indicator of high dose *cis*diamminedichloroplatinum nephrotoxicity? Influence of furosemide. Cancer Chemother Pharmacol 1986;18:276–279.

50. Dentino M, Luft FC, Yum MN, Williams SD, Einhorn LH. Long term effects of cisdiamminedichloride platinum (CDDP) on renal function and structure in man. Cancer 1978;41:1274–1281.

51. Hansen SW, Groth S, Daugaard G, Rossing N, Rorth M. Long-term effects on renal function and blood pressure of treatment with cisplatin, vinblastine, and bleomycin in patients with germ cell cancer. J Clin Oncol 1988;6:1728–1731.

52. Fjeldborg P, Sorensen J, Helkjaer P. The long-term effect of cisplatin on renal function. Cancer 1986; 58:2214–2217.

53. Macleod PM, Tyrell CJ, Keeling DH. The effect of cisplatin on renal function in patients with testicular tumours. Clin Radiology 1988;39:190–192.

54. Goren MP, Wright RK, Horowitz ME. Cumulative renal tubular damage associated with cisplatin nephrotoxicity. Cancer Chemother Pharmacol 1986; 18:69–73.

55. Daugaard G, Abildgaard U, Holstein-Rathlou NH, Bruunshuus I, Bucher D, Leyssac PP. Renal tubular function in patients treated with high dose cisplatin. Clin Pharmacol Ther 1988;44:164–172.

56. Swainson CP, Colls BM, Fitzharris BM. *Cis*-platinum and distal renal tubule toxicity. NZ Med J 1985;98:375–378.

57. Weinblatt ME, Kahn E, Scimeca PG, Kochen JA. Hemolytic uremic syndrome associated with cisplatin therapy. Am J Pediatr Hematol Oncol 1987;9:295–298.

58. Doll DC, List AF, Greco FA, Hainsworth JD, Hande KR, Johnson DH. Acute vascular ischemic events after cisplatin-based combination chemotherapy for germ-cell tumors of the testis. Ann Intern Med 1986;105:48–51.

59. Schilsky RL, Anderson T. Hypomagnesemia and renal magnesium wasting in patients receiving cisplatin. Ann Intern Med 1979;90:929–931.

60. Schilsky RL, Barlock A, Ozols RF. Persistent hypomagnesemia following *cis*-platin chemotherapy for testicular cancer. Cancer Treat Rep 1982;66:1767–1769.

61. Lam M, Adelstein DJ. Hypomagnesemia and renal magnesium wasting in patients treated with cisplatin. Am J Kidney Dis 1986;8:164–169.

62. Bell DR, Woods RL, Levi AJ. *Cis*-diamminedichloroplatinum-induced hypomagnesemia and renal magnesium wasting. Eur J Cancer Clin Oncol 1985; 21:287–290.

63. Giaccone G, Donadio M, Ferrati P, et al. Disorders of serum electrolytes and renal function in patients treated with *cis*-platinum on an outpatient basis. Eur J Cancer Clin Oncol 1985;21:433–437.

64. Bellin SL, Selim M. Cisplatin-induced hypomagnesemia with seizures: a case report and review of the literature. Gynecol Oncol 1988;30:104–113.

65. Bitran JD, Desser RK, Billings AA, et al. Acute nephrotoxicity following *cis*-dichlorodiammineplatinum. Cancer 1982;49:1784–1788.

66. Markman M, Cleary S, Howell SB. Hypomagnesemia following high-dose intracavitary cisplatin with systemically administered sodium thiosulfate. Am J Clin Oncol 1986;9:440–443.

67. Stewart AF, Keating T, Schwartz PE. Magnesium homeostasis following chemotherapy with cisplatin: a prospective study. Am J Obstet Gynecol 1985; 153:660–665.

68. Mavichak V, Coppin CML, Wong NLM, Dirks JH, Walker V, Sutton RAL. Renal magnesium wasting and hypocalciuria in chronic cisplatinum nephropathy in man. Clin Sci 1988;75:203–207.

69. Lammers PJ, White L, Ettinger LJ. *Cis*-platinum-induced renal sodium wasting. Med Pediatr Oncol 1984;12:343–346.

70. Hutchison FN, Perez EA, Gandara DR, Lawrence HJ, Kaysen GA. Renal salt wasting in patients treated with cisplatin. Ann Intern Med 1988;108:21–25.

71. Daugaard G, Strandgaard S, Holstein-Rathlou NH, et al. The renal handling of sodium and water is not affected by the standard-dose cisplatin treatment for testicular cancer. Scand J Clin Lab Invest 1987; 47:455–459.

72. Ritch PS. *Cis*-dichlorodiammineplatinum II-induced syndrome of inappropriate secretion of antidiuretic hormone. Cancer 1988;61:448–450.

73. Safirstein R, Winston J, Moel D, Dikman S, Guttenplan J. Cisplatin nephrotoxicity: insights into mechanism. Int J Androl 1987;10:325–346.

74. Stewart DJ, Mikhael NZ, Nanji AA, et al. Renal and hepatic concentrations of platinum: relationship to cisplatin time, dose, and nephrotoxicity. J Clin Oncol 1985;3:1251–1256.

75. Ewen C, Perera A, Hendry JH, McAuliffe CA, Sharma H, Fox BW. An autoradiographic study of the intrarenal localisation and retention of cisplatin, iproplatin and paraplatin. Cancer Chemother Pharmacol 1988;22:241–245.

76. Litterst CL. Cisplatinum: a review, with special reference to cellular and molecular interactions. Agents Action 1984;15:520–524.

77. Gordon JA, Gattone VH. II. Mitochondrial alterations in cisplatin-induced renal failure. Am J Physiol 1986;250:f991–998.

78. Hegedus L, van der Vijgh WJF, Klein I, Kerpel-Fronius S, Pinedo HM. Chemical reactivity of cisplatin bound to human plasma proteins. Cancer Chemother Pharmacol 1987;20:211–212.

79. Litterest CL, Schweitzer VG. Covalent binding of platinum to renal protein from sensitive and resistant guinea pigs treated with cisplatin: possible role in nephrotoxicity. Res Commun Chem Pathol Pharmacol 1988;61:35–47.

80. Dobyan DC. Long-term consequences of cis-platinum-induced renal injury: a structural and functional study. Anat Rec 1985;212:239–245.

81. Gordon JA, Gattone VH II, Schoolworth AC. α-Glutamyl transpeptidase excretion in cisplatin-induced acute renal failure. Am J Kidney Dis 1986;8:18–25.

82. Nekulova M, Mechl Z, Kerpel-Fronius S, Skalkova D, Sopkova B. The excretion of urinary enzymes, proteins and creatinine in patients receiving cisplatinum. Neoplasma 1987;34:183–188.

83. Daugaard G, Abildgaard U, Holstein-Rathlou NH, Amtorp O, Leyssac PP. Effect of cisplatin on renal haemodynamics and tubular function in the dog kidney. Int J Androl 1987;10:347–351.

84. Fournier C, Vennin P, Hecquet B. Correlation between free platinum AUC and total platinum measurement 24h after i.v. bolus injection of cisplatin in humans. Cancer Chemother Pharmacol 1988;21:75–77.

85. Kelsen DP, Alcock N, Young CW. Cisplatin nephrotoxicity—correlation with plasma platinum concentrations. Am J Clin Oncol 1985;8:77–80.

86. Reece PA, Stafford I, Russell J, Khan M, Gill PG. Creatinine clearance as a predictor of ultrafilterable platinum disposition in cancer patients treated with cisplatin: relationship between peak ultrafilterable platinum plasma levels and nephrotoxicity. J Clin Oncol 1987;5:304–309.

87. Reece PA, Stafford I, Russell J, Gill PG. Reduced ability to clear ultrafilterable platinum with repeated courses of cisplatin. J Clin Oncol 1986;4:1392–2398.

88. Daley-Yates PT, McBrien DCH. The renal fractional clearance of platinum antitumor compounds in relation to nephrotoxicity. Biochem Pharamcol 1985; 34:1423–1428.

89. Daley-Yates PT, McBrien DCH. Cisplatin metabolites in plasma, a study of their pharmacokinetics and importance in the nephrotoxic and antitumor activity of cisplatin. Biochem Pharmacol 1984;33:3063–3070.

90. Hrushesky WJ, Shimp W, Kennedy BJ. Lack of age-dependent cisplatin nephrotoxicity. Am J Med 1984;76:579–584.

91. Nanji AA, Stewart DJ, Mikhael NZ. Hyperuricemia and hypoalbuminemia predispose to cisplatin-induced nephrotoxicity. Cancer Chemother Pharmacol 1986;17:274–276.

92. Finley RS, Fortner CL, Grove WR. Cisplatin nephrotoxicity: a summary of preventative interventions. Drug Intell Clin Pharm 1985;19:362–367.

93. Brock J, Alberts DS. Safe, rapid administration of cisplatin in the outpatient clinic. Cancer Treat Rep 1986;70:1409–1414.

94. Fuks JZ, Wadler S, Wiernik PH. Phase I and II agents in cancer therapy: two cisplatin analogues and high-dose cisplatin in hypertonic saline or with thiosulfate protection. J Clin Pharmacol 1987;27:357–365.

95. Ozols RF, Corden BJ, Jacob J, Wesley MN, Ostchega Y, Young RC. High-dose cisplatin in hypertonic saline. Ann Intern Med 1984;100:19–24.

96. Ozols RF, Ostchega Y, Myers CE, Young RC. High-dose cisplatin in hypertonic saline in refractory ovarian cancer. J Clin Oncol 1985;3:1246–1250.

97. Daugaard G, Rossing N, Rorth M. Effects of cisplatin on different measures of glomerular function in the human kidney with special emphasis on high dose. Cancer Chemother Pharmacol 1988;21:163–167.

98. Aamdal S, Fodstad O, Kaalhus O. Reduced antineoplastic activity in mice of cisplatin administered with high salt concentration in the vehicle. J Natl Cancer Inst 1984;73:743–751.

99. Aamdal S, Fodstad O, Storeng R, Pihl A. Reduced antitumor activity of cis-platin after concurrent intravenous administration of thiosulfate. Proc Am Assoc Cancer Res 1986;27:292.

100. Hall KS, Fossa SD, Aas M. High-dose cis-platinum combination chemotherapy in advanced nonseminomatous malignant germ cell tumors with emphasis on nephrotoxicity. Cancer Chemother Pharmacol 1986;18:74–77.

101. Merlano M, Grimaldi A, Brunetti I, Modenesi M, Accomando E, Rosso R. High-dose cisplatin in the outpatient clinic: a feasibility study. Tumori 1987; 73:341–344.

102. Bajorin D, Bosl GJ, Fein R. Phase I trial of escalating doses of cisplatin in hypertonic saline. J Clin Oncol 1987;5:1589–1593.

103. Bajorin DF, Bosl GJ, Alcock NW, Niedzwiecki D, Gallina E, Shurgot B. Pharmacokinetics of cis-diamminedichloroplatinum(II) after administration in hypertonic saline. Cancer Res 1986;46:5969–5972.

104. Pfeifle CE, Howell SB, Felthouse RD, et al. High-dose cisplatin with sodium thiosulfate protection. J Clin Oncol 1985;3:237–244.

105. Markman M, Clearly S, Howell SB. Nephrotoxicity of high-dose intracavitary cisplatin with thiosulfate protection. Eur J Cancer Clin Oncol 1985; 21:1015–1018.

106. Aamdal S, Fodstad O, Pihl A. Some procedures to reduce cisplatinum toxicity reduce antitumor activity. Cancer Treat Rev 1987;14:389–395.

107. Aamdal S, Fodstad O, Pihl A. Sodium thiosulfate fails to increase the therapeutic index of intravenously administered cis-diamminedichloroplatinum (II) in mice bearing murine and human tumors. Cancer Chemother Pharmacol 1988;21:129–133.

108. Abe R, Akiyoshi T, Koba F, Tsuji H, Baba T. 'Two-route chemotherapy' using intra-arterial cisplatin and intravenous sodium thiosulfate, its neutralizing agent, for hepatic malignancies. Eur J Cancer Clin Oncol 1988;24:1671–1674.

109. Salem P, Khalyl M, Jabboury K, Hashimi L. Cis-diamminedichloroplatinum (II) by 5-day continuous infusion. Cancer 1984;53:837–840.

110. Posner MR, Ferrari L, Belliveau JF, et al. A phase I trial of continuous infusion cisplatin. Cancer 1987;59:15–18.

111. Belliveau JF, Posner MR, Ferrari L, et al. Cisplatin administered as a continuous 5-day infusion: plasma platinum levels and urine platinum excretion. Cancer Treat Rep 1986;70:1215–1217.

112. Forastiere AA, Belliveau JF, Goren MP, Vogel WC, Posner MR, O'Leary GP. Pharmacokinetic and toxicity evaluation of five-day continuous infusion versus intermittent bolus cis-diamminedichloroplatinum(II) in head and neck cancer patients. Cancer Res 1988;48:3869–3874.

113. Von Hoff DD. Whither carboplatin?—a replacement for or an alternative to cisplatin? J Clin Oncol 1987;5:169–171.

114. Pendyala L, Madajewicz S, Lele SB, Arbuck SG, Creaven PJ. Evaluation of the nephrotoxicity of iproplatin (CHIP) in comparison to cisplatin by the measurement of urinary enzymes. Cancer Chemother Pharmacol 1985;15:203–207.

115. Brivet F, Pavlovitch J-M, Gouyette A, Cerrina M-L, Tchernia G, Dormont J. Inefficiency of early prophylactic hemodialysis in cis-platinum overdose. Cancer Chemother Pharmacol 1986;18:183–184.

116. Willox JC, McAllister EJ, Sangster G, Kaye SB. Effects of magnesium supplementation on testicular cancer patients receiving cis-platin: a randomised trial. Br J Cancer 1986;54:19–23.

117. Barton C, Duchesne G, Williams M, Fisher C, Horwich A. The impact of hydronephrosis on renal function in patients treated with cisplatin-based chemotherapy for metastatic nonseminomatous germ cell tumors. Cancer 1988;62:1439–1443.

118. Hrushesky WJM, Borch R, Levi F. A circadian time dependence of cisplatin urinary pharmacokinetics. Clin Pharmacol Ther 1982;32:330–339.

119. Moulder JE, Holcenberg JS, Kamen BA, Cheng M, Fish BL. Renal irradiation and the pharmacology and toxicity of methotrexate and cisplatinum. Int J Radiat Oncol Biol Phys 1986;12:1415–1418.

120. Gerad H, Egorin MJ, Whitacre M, Van Echo DA, Aisner J. Renal failure and platinum pharmacokinetics in three patients treated with cis-diamminedichloroplatinum(II) and whole-body hyperthermia. Cancer Chemother Pharmacol 1983;11:162–166.

121. Kawamura J, Soeda A, Yoshia O. Nephrotoxicity of cis-diamminedichloroplatinum (II) (cis-platinum) and the additive effects of antibiotics: morphological and functional observation in rats. Toxicol Appl Pharmacol 1981;38:535–541.

122. Bregman CL, Williams PD. Comparative nephrotoxicity of carboplatin and cisplatin in combination with tobramycin. Cancer Chemother Pharmacol 1986;18:117–123.

123. Jongejan HTM, Provoost AP, Molenaar JC. Potentiation of cis-diamminedichloroplatinum nephrotoxicity by amikacin in rats. Cancer Chemother Pharmacol 1988;22:178–180.

124. Haas A, Anderson L, Lad T. The influence of aminoglycosides on the nephrotoxicity of cis-diamminedichloroplatinum in cancer patients. J Infect Dis 1983;147:363.

125. Gonzalez-Vitale JC, Hayes DM, Cvitkovic E, Sternberg SS. Acute renal failure after cis-dichlorodiammineplatinum (II) and gentamicin-cephalothin therapies. Cancer Treat Rep 1978;62:693–698.

126. Preiss R, Brovtsyn VK, Perevodchikova NI, et al. Effect of methotrexate and the pharmacokinetics and renal excretion of cisplatin. Eur J Clin Pharmacol 1988;34:139–144.

127. Milano G, Thyss A, Renee N, et al. Altered pharmacokinetics and clinical consequences of low dose methotrexate plus cisplatin in the treatment of advanced head and neck cancer. Eur J Clin Oncol 1986;22:843–847.

128. Goren MP, Wright RK, Horowitz ME, Meyer WH. Enhancement of methotrexate nephrotoxicity after cisplatin therapy. Cancer 1986;58:2617–2621.

129. Crom WR, Pratt CB, Green AA, et al. The effect of prior cisplatin therapy on the pharmacokinetics of high-dose methotrexate. J Clin Oncol 1984;2:655–661.

130. Goren MP, Wright RK, Pratt CB, et al. Potentiation of ifosfamide neurotoxicity, hematotoxicity, and tubular nephrotoxocity by prior cis-diamminedichloroplatinum(II) therapy. Cancer Res 1987;47:1457–1460.

131. Pratesi G, Gianni L, Manzotti C, Zunino F. Sequence dependence of the antitumor and toxic effects of 5-fluorouracil and cis-diamminedichloroplatinum combination on primary colon tumors in mice. Cancer Chemother Pharmacol 1988;21:237–240.

132. Mayer RD, Kan-ei L, Cockett ATK. Inhibition of cisplatin-induced nephrotoxicity in rats by buthionine sufoximine, a glutathione synthesis inhibitor. Cancer Chemother Pharmacol 1987;20:207–210.

133. Deray G, Dubois M, Beaufils H, et al. Effects of nifedipine on cisplatinum-induced nephrotoxicity in rats. Clin Nephrol 1988;30:146–150.

134. Millar BC, Siddik ZH, Millar JL, Jinks S. Mesna does not reduce cisplatin induced nephrotoxicity in the rat. Cancer Chemother Pharmacol 1985;15:307–309.

135. Kempf SR, Ivankovic S. Nephrotoxicity and carcinogenic risk of cis-platin (CDDP) prevented by sodium 2-mercaptoethanesulfonate (mesna): experimental results. Cancer Treat Rev 1987;14:365–372.

136. Wagner T, Kreft B, Bohlmann G, Schwieder G. Effects of fosfomycin, mesna, and sodium thiosulfate on the toxicity and antitumor activity of cisplatin. Cancer Res Clin Oncol 1988;114:497–501.

137. Capasso G, Anastasio P, Giordano D, Albarano L, De Santo NG. Beneficial effects of atrial natriuretic factor on cisplatin-induced acute renal failure in the rat. Am J Nephrol 1987;7:228–234.

138. Naganuma A, Satoh M, Imura N. Prevention of lethal and renal toxicity of cis-diamminedichloro platinum(II) by induction of metallothionein synthesis without compromising its antitumor activity in mice. Cancer Res 1987;47:983–987.

139. Satoh M, Naganuma A, Imura N. Metallothionein induction prevents toxic side effects of cisplatin and Adriamycin used in combination. Cancer Chemother Pharmacol 1988;21:176–178.

140. Qazi R, Chang AYC, Borch RF, et al. Phase I clinical and pharmacokinetic study of diethyldithiocarbamate as a chemoprotector from toxic effects of cisplatin. J Natl Cancer Inst 1988;80:1486–1488.

141. Radacic M, Boranic M, Skaric D, et al. Reduction of cis-dichlorodiammine(II) caused nephrotoxicity by indazolone carboxilic acid. Oncol 1987;44:34–37.

142. Oriana S, Bohm S, Spatti G, Zunino F, Di Re F. A preliminary clinical experience with reduced glu-

tathione as protector against cisplatin-toxicity. Tumori 1987;73:337–340.

143. Offerman JJ, Sleijfer DT, Mulder NH, Meijer S, Koops HS, Donker AJM. The effect of captopril on renal function in patients during the first cis-diamminedichloroplatinum II infusion. Cancer Chemother Pharmacol 1985;14:262–264.

144. Offerman JJG, Mulder NH, Sleijfer DT et al. Influence of captopril on cis-diamminedichloroplatinum-induced renal injury. Am J Nephrol 1985;5:433–436.

145. Sleijfer DT, Offerman JJG, Mulder NH, et al. The protective potential of the combination of verapamil and cimetidine on cisplatin-induced nephrotoxicity in man. Cancer 1987;60:2823–2828.

146. Offerman JJG, Meijer S, Sleijfer DT, et al. The influence of verapamil on renal function in patients treated with cisplatin. Clin Nephrol 1985;24:249–255.

147. Umeki S, Watanabe M, Yagi S, Soejima R. Supplemental fosfomycin and/or steroids that reduce cisplatin-induced nephrotoxicity. Am J Med Sci 1988; 295:6–10.

148. Broder LE, Carter SK. Pancreatic islet cell carcinoma. II. results of therapy with streptozotocin in 52 patients. Ann Intern Med 1973;79:108–118.

149. Moertel CG, Hanley JA, Johnson LA. Streptozotocin alone compared with streptozotocin plus fluorouracil in the treatment of advanced islet cell carcinoma. N Engl J Med 1980;303:1189–1194.

150. Meyerowitz RL, Sartiano GP, Cavallo T. Nephrotoxic and cytoproliferative effects of streptozotocin. Cancer 1976;38:1550–1555.

151. Sadoff L. Nephrotoxocity of streptozotocin (NSC85998). Cancer Chemother Rep 1979;54:457–459.

152. Hricik DE, Goldsmith GH. Uric acid nephrolithiasis and acute renal failure secondary to streptozotocin nephrotoxicity. Am J Med 1988;84:153–156.

153. Tobin MV, Warenius HM, Morris AI. Forced diuresis to reduce nephrotoxicity of streptozotocin in the treatment of advanced metastatic insulinoma. Br Med J 1987;294:1128.

154. Delaney V, de Pertuz Y, Nixon D, Bourke E. Indomethacin in streptozotocin-induced nephrogenic diabetes insipidus. Am J Kidney Dis 1987;9:79–83.

155. Schaeppi U, Fleischman RW, Phelan RS, et al. CCNU (NSC 79037): preclinical toxicologic evaluation of a single intravenous infusion in dogs and monkeys. Cancer Chemother Rep 1974;5:53–64.

156. Tuttle SE, Sharma HM, Bay WH, Hebert LA. Glomerular basement membrane splitting and microaneurysm formation associated with nitrosourea therapy. Am J Nephrol 1985;5:388–394.

157. Glaubiger D, Ramu A. Antitumor antibiotics. In: Chabner B, ed. Pharmacologic principles of cancer treatment. Philadelphia: WB Saunders, 1982:409–410.

158. Hanna WT, Krauss S, Regester RF, et al. Renal disease after mitomycin C therapy. Cancer 1981; 48:2583–2588.

159. Kennedy BJ. Mithramycin therapy in advanced testicular neoplasms. Cancer 1970;26:755–766.

160. Zalupski M, Baker LH. Ifosfamide. J Natl Cancer Inst 1988;80:556–566.

161. Shaw IC. Mesna and oxazaphosphorine cancer chemotherapy. Cancer Treat Rev 1987;14:359–364.

162. Sakurai M, Saijo N, Shinkai T, et al. The protective effect of 2-mercapto-ethane sulfonate (MESNA)

on hemorrhagic cystitis induced by high-dose ifosfamide treatment tested by a randomized crossover trial. Jpn J Clin Oncol 1986;16:153–156.

163. Goren MP, Wright RK, Horowitz ME, Pratt CB. Ifosfamide-induced subclinical tubular nephrotoxicity despite mesna. Cancer Treat Rep 1987;71:127–130.

164. Patterson WP, Khojasteh A. Ifosfamide-induced renal tubular defects. Cancer 1989;63:649–651.

165. Sangster G, Kaye SB, Calman KC, Dalton JF. Failure of 2-mercaptoethane sulphonate sodium (mesna) to protect against ifosfamide nephrotoxicity. Eur J Cancer Clin Oncol 1984;20:435–436.

166. Hilgard P, Burke H. Sodium-2-mercaptoethane sulfonate (MESNA) and ifosfamide nephrotoxicity. Eur J Cancer Clin Oncol 1984;20:1451–1452.

167. Klein HO, Wickramanayake PD, Coerper CL, Christian E, Pohl J, Brock N. High dose ifosfamide and mesna as continuous infusion over 5 days—a phase I/II trial. Cancer Treat Rev 1983;10(Suppl A):167–173.

168. Schilsky RL. Renal and metabolic toxicities of cancer treatment. In: Perry MC, Yarbro JW, eds. Toxicity of chemotherapy. Orlando, FL: Grune & Stratton, 1984:325–326.

169. Abelson HT, Fosburg MT, Beardsley GP, et al. Methotrexate-induced renal impairment: clinical studies and rescue from systemic toxicity with high-dose leucovorin and thymidine. J Clin Oncol 1983;3:208–216.

170. Winograd B, Lippens RJJ, Oosterbaan MJM, Dirks MJM, Vree TB, van der Klein E. Renal excretion and pharmacokinetics of methotrexate and 7-hydroxymethotrexate following a 24-hr high dose infusion of methotrexate in children. Eur J Clin Pharmacol 1986; 30:231–238.

171. Bowyer GW, Davies TW. Methotrexate toxicity associated with an ileal conduit. Br J Urol 1987; 60:592.

172. Ahmad S, Shen F, Bleyer WA. Methotrexate-induced renal failure and ineffectiveness of peritoneal dialysis. Arch Intern Med 1978;138:1146–1147.

173. Hande KR, Balow JE, Drake JC, et al. Methotrexate and hemodialysis. Ann Intern Med 1977; 87:495–496.

174. Haim N, Kedar A, Robinson E. Methotrexate-related deaths in patients previously treated with cis-diamminedichloride platinum. Cancer Chemother Pharmacol 1984;13:223–225.

175. Price P, Thompson H, Bessell EM, Bloom HJG. Renal impairment following the combined use of high-dose methotrexate and procarbazine. Cancer Chemother Pharmacol 1988;21:265–267.

176. Johnson WW, Meadows DC. Urinary bladder fibrosis and telangiectasia associated with long-term cyclophosphamide therapy. N Engl J Med 1971; 284:290–294.

177. Philips FS, Sternberg SS, Cronin AP, et al. Cyclophosphamide and urinary bladder toxicity. Cancer Res 1961;21:1577–1589.

178. Rubin JS, Rubin RT. Cyclophosphamide hemorrhagic cystitis. J Urol 1966;96:313–316.

179. Stillwell TJ, Benson RC. Cyclophosphamide-induced hemorrhagic cystitis. Cancer 1988;61:451–457.

180. Klein FA, Smith MJV. Urinary complications of cyclophosphamide therapy: etiology, prevention, and management. South Med J 1983;76:1413–1416.

181. Galloway NTM. Gas gangrene of the bladder

complicating cyclophosphamide cystitis. Br J Urol 1984;56:100–101.

182. Jerkins GR, Noe HN, Hill D. Treatment of complication of cyclophosphamide cystitis. J Urol 1988;139:923–925.

183. Mohiuddin J, Prentice HG, Schey S, Blacklock H, Dandona P. Treatment of cyclophosphamide-induced cystitis with prostaglandin E2l. Ann Intern Med 1984;101(1):142.

184. Shurafa M, Shumaker E, Cronin S. Prostaglandin F2-alpha bladder irrigation for control of intractable cyclophosphamide-induced hemorrhagic cystitis. J Urol 1987;137:1230–1231.

185. Garat JM, Martinez E, Aragona F. Open instillation of formalin for cyclophosphamide-induced hemorrhagic cystitis in a child. Eur Urol 1985;11:192–194.

186. Fair WR. Formalin in the treatment of massive bladder hemorrhages: techniques, and complications. Urology 1974;3:573–576.

187. Hows JM, Mehta A, Ward L, et al. Comparison of mesna with forced diuresis to prevent cyclophosphamide induced haemorrhagic cystitis in marrow transplantation: a prospective randomised study. Br J Cancer 1984;50:753–756.

188. Finn GP, Sidau RNB. Protecting the bladder from cyclophosphamide with mesna. N Engl J Med 1986;314:61.

189. Ehrlich RM, Freedman A, Goldsobel AB, Stiehm ER. The use of sodium 2-mercaptoethane sulfonate to prevent cyclophosphamide cystitis. J Urol 1984;131:960–962.

190. Wagner T, Zink M, Schwieder G. Influence of mesna and cysteine on the systemic toxicity and therapeutic efficacy of activated cyclophosphamide. J Cancer Res Clin Oncol 1987;113:160–165.

191. Odoardo T, Cavelletti E, Besati A, et al. Prevention of cyclophosphamide-induced urotoxicity by reduced glutathione and its effect on acute toxicity and antitumor activity of the alkalating agent. Cancer Chemother Pharmacol 1985;14:188–193.

192. Gray KJ, Engelmann UH, Johnson EH, Fishman IJ. Evaluation of misoprostol cytoprotection of the bladder with cyclophosphamide (Cytoxan) therapy. J Urol 1986;136:497–500.

193. Primack A. Amelioration of cyclophosphamide-induced cystitis. J Natl Cancer Inst 1971;47:223–227.

194. Ueda S, Yoshida M, Yano S, et al. Comparison of the effects of primary prostaglandins on isolated human urinary bladder. J Urol 1985;133:114–117.

195. Stillwell TJ, Benson RC. Cyclophosphamide-induced hemorrhagic cystitis. Cancer 1988;61:451–457.

196. Parsons CL. Successful management of radiation cystitis with sodium pentosanpolysulfate. J Urol 1986;136:813–814.

197. Tchekmedyian NS, Egorin MJ, Cohen BE, et al. Phase I clinical and pharmacokinetic study of cyclophosphamide administered by five-day continuous infusion. Cancer Chemother Pharmacol 1986;18:33–38.

198. Brade W, Seeber S, Herdrich K. Comparative activity of ifosfamide and cyclophosphamide. Cancer Chemother Pharmacol 1986;18:S1–S9.

199. Samra Y, Hertz M, Lindner A. urinary bladder tumors following cyclophosphamide therapy: a report of two cases with a review of the literature. Med Pediatr Oncol 1985;13:86–91.

200. Brenner DW, Schellhammer PF. Upper tract urothelial malignancy after cyclophosphamide therapy: a case report and literature review. J Urol 1987; 137:1226–1227.

201. Pedersen-Bjergaard J, Ersboll J, Hansen VL, et al. Carcinoma of the urinary bladder after treatment with cyclophosphamide for non-Hodgkin's lymphoma. N Engl J Med 1988;318:1028–1032.

202. DeFronzo RA, Colvin OM, Braine H, et al. Cyclophosphamide and the kidney. Cancer. 1974;33:483–491.

203. DeFronzo RA, Braine H, Colvin OM, et al. Water intoxication in man after cyclophosphamide therapy. Ann Intern Med 1973;178:861–869.

204. Harlow PJ, DeClerck YA, Shore NA, et al. Fatal case of inappropriate ADH secretion induced by cyclophosphamide therapy. Cancer 1979;44:896–898.

205. Steele TH, Serpick AA, Block JB. Antidiuretic response to cyclophosphamide in man. J Pharmacol Exp Ther 1973;185:245–253.

206. Bressler RB, Huston DP. Water intoxication following moderate-dose intravenous cyclophosphamide. Arch Intern Med 1985;145:548–549.

207. Haas A, Chin T, Stiehm ER. Cyclophosphamide-induced water intoxication: treatment with fluid restriction and 2-mercaptoethane sulfonate. Am J Dis Child 1986;140:1094–1095.

208. Finn G, Denning D. Transient nephrogenic diabetes insipidus following high-dose cyclophosphamide chemotherapy and autologous bone marrow transplantation. Cancer Treat Rep 1987;71:220–221.

209. Cutting HO. Inappropriate secretion of antidiuretic hormone secondary to vincristine therapy. Am J Med 1971;51:269–271.

210. Fine RN, Clarke RR, Shore NA. Hyponatremia and vincristine therapy. Am J Dis Child 1966;112:256–259.

211. Slater LM, Wainer RA, Serpick AA. Vincristine neurotoxicity with hyponatremia. Cancer 1969; 23:122–125.

212. Suskind RM, Brusilow SW, Zehr J. Syndrome of inappropriate secretion of antidiurectic hormone produced by vincristine toxicity. J Pediatr 1972;81:90–92.

213. Petersen BA, Collins AJ, Vogelzang NJ et al. 5-Azacytidine and renal tubular dysfunction. Blood 1981;57:182–185.

214. Quesada JR. Treatment of hairy cell leukemia. N Engl J Med 1984;311:412.

215. Spiers ASD, Parekh SJ, Bishop MB. Hairy cell leukemia: induction of complete remission with pentostatin (2'-deoxycoformycin). J Clin Oncol 1984; 2:1336–1342.

216. Major PP, Agarwall RP, Kufe DW. Clinical pharmacology of pentostatin. Blood 1981;58:91–96.

217. Poplack DG, Sallan SE, Rivera G, et al. Phase I study of pentostatin in acute lymphoblastic leukemia. Cancer Res 1981;41:3343–3346.

218. Kramer RA, Boyd MR, Dees JH. Comparative nephrotoxicity of 1-(2-chloroethyl)-3-(trans-4-methyl cyclohexyl)-4-nitrosourea (MeCCNU) and chlorozotocin: functional-structural correlations in the Fischer 344 rat. Toxicol Appl Pharmacol 1986;82:540–550.

219. Weiss RB, Posada JG, Kramer RA, Boyd MR. Nephrotoxicity of semustine. Cancer Treat Rep 1983; 67:1105–1112.

220. West WH, Tauer KW, Yannelli JR, et al. Constant infusion recombinant interleukin-2 in adoptive immunotherapy of advanced cancer. N Engl J Med 1987;316:898–905.

221. Rosenberg SA, Lotze MT, Muul LM, et al. A progress report on the treatment of 157 patients with advanced cancer using lymphokine-activiated killer cells and interleukin-2 or high-dose interleukin-2 alone. N Engl J Med 1987;316:889–897.

222. Kozeny GA, Nicholas JD, Creekmore S, et al. Effects of interleukin-2 immunotherapy on renal function. J Clin Oncol 1988;6:1170–1176.

223. Krown SE. Interferon and interferon inducers in cancer treatment. Semin Oncol 1986;13:207–217.

224. Shinn AF, Rutkowski D, Wilner FM, Morita Y. Dosage modifications of cancer chemotherapeutic agents in renal failure. Drug Intell Clin Pharm 1977; 11:140–141.

225. Powis G. Effect of human renal and hepatic disease on the pharmacokinetics of anticancer drugs. Cancer Treat Rev 1982;9:85–124.

38

Neurotoxicity of Chemotherapeutic Agents

David R. Macdonald

Not uncommonly, damage to the nervous system occurs as a complication of antineoplastic therapy. Neurotoxicity may follow treatment with radiation therapy, chemotherapy, biologic response modifiers, or combination therapy. No portion of the nervous system is immune from potential damage. Neurologic toxicity may occur as an uncommon and unexpected complication of treatment or may occur as a known and well-recognized complication of treatment. In the latter instance, neurologic toxicity may be the dose-limiting factor that prevents the more aggressive use of that form of treatment. With the increasing use of multimodality therapy, dose-intensive therapy, and experimental therapy, the incidence of neurologic toxicity from antineoplastic therapy continues to rise. Damage to the nervous system may follow treatment of either tumors involving the nervous system or systemic cancer. The neurologic complications of antineoplastic therapy may occur as a *direct* result of damage to the nervous system (when the agent itself is toxic to the nervous system) or from *indirect* damage to the nervous system (such as meningitis that occurs as a complication of severe myelosuppression from chemotherapy).

Distinguishing chemotherapy drug-related problems from other metastatic or nonmetastatic neurologic complications of cancer is sometimes difficult. Serious neurotoxicity may require discontinuation of the chemotherapeutic agent and thus may limit the use of a potentially effective drug. Direct toxicity to the peripheral nervous system may be acceptable, if it is reversible and not severe (vincristine neuropathy). Significant central nervous system toxicity usually requires discontinuation if irreversible. Indirect neurotoxicity may be reversible if the end-organ failure is

reversible (drug-induced hepatic or renal failure) or may be irreversible (intracranial hemorrhage from thrombocytopenia).

The central and peripheral nervous systems are protected against potentially neurotoxic effects of chemotherapeutic agents because:

The dose-limiting toxicity of most chemotherapy agents is due to effects on rapidly growing tissues such as bone marrow or GI tract (unlike the nervous system) and occur at doses below those that affect the nervous system.

Most chemotherapeutic agents that are water soluble and relatively large molecules are effectively excluded from entry to the nervous system by the blood-brain barrier and blood-nerve barriers, if intact.

Significant neurologic toxicity generally results in the exclusion of the drug from widespread use.

New developments in cancer chemotherapy have resulted in an increase in clinically important neurotoxicity due to several factors:

Some new chemotherapeutic agents are sufficiently effective in the treatment of certain systemic cancers that their associated neurotoxicity has been considered acceptable (e.g., cisplatin, paclitaxel).

Multiagent chemotherapeutic regimens may increase neurotoxicity because of additive or synergistic effects.

Multimodality therapy that combines chemotherapy with radiation therapy or immunotherapy may increase neurotoxicity (e.g., methotrexate and cranial radiotherapy).

Innovative methods of drug administration may produce increased neurotoxicity. High-dose therapy (e.g., high-dose cytosine arabinoside, high-dose BCNU (carmustine) with autologous bone marrow transplant, high-dose methotrexate with folinic acid rescue, or high-dose chemotherapy with granulocyte or granulocyte/macrophage colony-stimulating factor therapy to promote bone marrow recovery) may now be possible, as previously dose-limiting systemic toxicities can be prevented, leading to new or increased neurotoxicity. Direct administration of drugs to the nervous system, such as intrathecal chemotherapy, intracarotid chemotherapy, osmotic opening of the blood-brain barrier, or direct intracranial intratumoral therapy, may also increase neurotoxicity.

New chemotherapeutic agents in early stages of clinical trials testing may be found to have neurotoxicities not suspected in preclinical testing.

Some new chemotherapeutic agents have been selected for testing against brain tumors because they cause neurologic toxicity, implying penetration through the blood-brain barrier (e.g., spirohydantoin mustard, acivicin-AT 125, fludarabine).

The causes of neurologic symptoms in patients on chemotherapy are classified in Table 38.1. The major neurologic toxicities of the commonly used chemotherapeutic agents and promising

Table 38.1. Cause of Neurologic Symptoms in Patients on Chemotherapy

Direct neurotoxicity from chemotherapy

Indirect neurotoxicity from chemotherapy
  Metabolic encephalopathy
  Coagulopathy, with hemorrhage
  Myelosuppression, with CNS infection
  Psychologic effects

Unrelated to chemotherapy
  Neurologic side effects of concurrent drugs
  Neurologic complications of cancer
    Primary or metastatic tumors
    Metabolic encephalopathy
    CNS infections
    Vascular disorders (hemorrhage, infarction)
    Complications of radiotherapy
    Paraneoplastic syndrome
    Psychologic effects

Coincidental neurologic disorders

Table 38.2. Neurologic Syndromes in Patients on Chemotherapy[a]

Encephalopathy
  Asparaginase
  Carmustine (HD, IA)
  Cisplatin
  Corticosteroids
  Cytarabine (HD, IT)
  Fludarabine (HD)
  5-Fluorouracil (± levamisole)
  Etoposide (HD)
  Ifosfamide
  Interferon
  Interleukin-2
  Methotrexate (HD, IA, IT)
  Procarbazine
  Retinoic acid
  Tamoxifen
  Thiotepa (HD)
  Vincristine

Cerebellar dysfunction
  Cytarabine (HD)
  5-Fluorouracil

Myelopathy
  Cytarabine (IT)
  Methotrexate (IT)
  Thiotepa (IT)
  Vincristine (IT)

Peripheral neuropathy/myopathy
  Cisplatin
  Corticosteroids
  Cytarabine
  Docetaxel
  Etoposide
  Paclitaxel
  Procarbazine
  Suramin
  Vincristine
  Vinorelbine

[a]HD, high dose; IA, intraarterial; IT, intrathecal.

new chemotherapeutic agents currently under investigational study are listed in Tables 38.2 and 38.3. The major systemic toxicities of these agents are discussed elsewhere in this book. Several detailed reviews of the neurologic complications of cancer chemotherapy are available (1–8). The neurotoxicity of several selected agents is briefly discussed in this section.

METHOTREXATE

Methotrexate is a chemotherapeutic agent widely used in the treatment of gestational choriocarcinoma, epidermal carcinomas of the head and neck, lymphoma, and lung cancer. It is also

Table 38.3. Neurotoxicity of Chemotherapeutic Agents

Agent	Neurotoxicity
Alkylating agents	
Chlorambucil (Leukeran) (180)	Seizures, encephalopathy (rare; with overdose)
Cyclophosphamide (Cytoxan, CTX) (7, 8)	SIADH (rare)
Ifosfamide (8, 157–165)	Encephalopathy: confusion, lethargy, coma, psychosis, seizures (common with high-dose, reversible), ataxia, cranial neuropathies, peripheral neuropathy (uncommon)
Melphalan (Alkeran, L-PAM, L-phenylalanine mustard)	None known
Nitrogen mustard (mechlorethamine) (7, 8, 181)	IV (usual dose): none IV (high-dose, for bone marrow transplantation): headache, hallucinations, encephalopathy, seizures Intracarotid: cerebral edema, necrosis, demyelination
Thio-TEPA (182)	Intrathecal: chemical meningitis, myelopathy (uncommon)
Antimetabolites	
Cytarabine (Ara-C, cytosine arabinoside) (14, 53–61)	IV (usual-dose): none IV (high-dose): encephalopathy—confusion, obtundation, seizures, leukoencephalopathy, cerebellar dysfunction—ataxia, dysmetria, (dose related, ?reversible), peripheral neuropathy Intrathecal: myelopathy (?uncommon), leukoencephalopathy (?uncommon), aseptic meningitis (uncommon)
Fludarabine (2-F-Ara-AMP) (191, 192)	Encephalopathy—headache, obtundation, coma, seizures, visual loss, cortical blindness Spastic/flaccid paralysis; progressive, may be fatal (dose related—common at high dose, uncommon at low dose)
5-Fluorouracil (5-FU) (1–8, 38–52)	Cerebellar dysfunction (ataxia, dysmetria, dysarthria), encephalopathy (uncommon), diplopia, peripheral neuropathy (rare)
Methotrexate (MTX) (1–37)	Oral: none IV (usual dose): none IV (high-dose): acute encephalopathy—seizures, confusion, hemiparesis, coma (transient, reversible); leukoencephalopathy—mineralizing microangiopathy, seizures, hemiparesis, dementia, cortical atrophy (delayed progressive) Intrathecal: chemical meningitis—fever, headache, stiff neck, CSF leukocytosis (acute, transient), myelopathy, paraplegia; leukoencephalopathy—seizures, hemiplegia, dementia, calcification (delayed, progressive) Neurotoxicity exacerbated by cranial radiotherapy Possible increased neurotoxicity after blood-brain barrier modification
Plant alkaloids	
Etoposide (epipodophyllotoxin, VP-16) (183)	Peripheral neuropathy (uncommon at usual doses, may exacerbate neuropathy of vincristine, cisplastin) Encephalopathy (confusion, somnolence, seizures; at high doses for brain tumor)
Paclitaxel (Taxol; also docetaxel, Taxotere)	Peripheral neuropathy (dose-related; distal sensory loss, itching; motor weakness, autonomic neuropathy, less common; reversible), myalgias, arthralgias, ocular toxicity (uncommon)
Vinblastine (Velban, VLB)	Mild neurotoxicity, similar to vincristine, at high doses or with other neurotoxic agents
Vincristine (Oncovin, VCR) (1–8, 62–69)	Peripheral neuropathy (areflexia, distal sensory loss, motor weakness, foot drop (1–5, atrophy) Autonomic neuropathy (ileus, constipation, impotence, urinary retention, postural hypotension) Muscle pain (jaw, legs)

Table 38.3—*continued*

Agent	Neurotoxicity
Vincristine (Oncovin, VCR) (1–8, 62–69) —*continued*	Cranial neuropathy (optic atrophy, diplopia, VI palsy, VII palsy, etc) Central (seizures, SIADH) (Above toxicities dose related, reversible) **Fatal ascending myelopathy and encephalopathy after intrathecal injection**
Vindesine (diacetyl vinblastine amide sulfate) (2, 7, 8)	Similar to vincristine
Antibiotics	
Doxorubicin (Adriamycin and other anthracycline antibiotics— daunorubicin, epirubicin, mitoxantrone) (7, 35, 184)	IV (usual dose): none **Intrathecal: severe (?fatal) myelopathy, encephalopathy** Cerebral damage—after intracarotid injection following osmotic blood-brain barrier modification Anterior horn cell loss after experimental injection into peripheral nerve
Miscellaneous	
Amsacrine (m-AMSA) (185–186)	Encephalopathy—headache, confusion, dizziness, seizures (uncommon) Peripheral neuropathy (?)
L-**Asparaginase** (2, 3, 7, 8, 187)	Encephalopathy (delirium, coma, seizures; reversible; usual doses—up to 15%; high doses—up to 60%) Intracranial hemorrhage or infarction (due to coagulopathy)
Carboplatin (Parplatin) (103–105)	Minimal neurotoxicity (ototoxicity, peripheral neuropathy) at usual doses
Cisplatin (Platinol, DDP) (2–8, 35, 73–102)	Ototoxicity (high frequency, progressive, ?reversible; exacerbated by cranial RT, especially in children) Peripheral neuropathy (dose related, cumulative, reversible; distal, symmetric, predominantly large fiber, sensory—paresthesias, vibration and proprioception loss; relative sparing pin, temperature; reduced reflexes; mild weakness; autonomic neuropathy) Encephalopathy (confusion, seizures; may be due to electrolyte disturbance) Cerebral herniation (acute cerebral deterioration, headache, hemiparesis, coma, seizures—may be related to overhydration, increased cerebral edema, electrolyte disturbance, seizures—in patients with large intracranial tumors) Retinopathy (?) Cranial neuropathy (?)
Mitotane (*o, p'*-DDD) (188)	Encephalopathy (mild, common)—lethargy, somnolence, vertigo, generalized weakness, headache, visual disturbances, depression; retinopathy
Procarbazine (PCZ, Natulan) (2–8)	Oral (usual dose, 150–300 mg/day): minimal neurotoxicity High dose oral, or IV or IA: encephalopathy (drowsiness, confusion, coma), peripheral neuropathy (distal symmetric polyneuropathy)
Nitrosoureas	
BCNU (carmustine) (2, 8, 106–120)	IV (usual dose, 200 mg/m^2 or 80 mg/m^2/day × 3 days): none IV (high dose): encephalopathy, confusion, seizures Intracarotid: severe local pain during infusion (face, eye, head), eye toxicity (retinopathy, blindness, necrosis) Encephalopathy, seizures, hemiparesis (may mimic or exacerbate radiation necrosis)
CCNU (lomustine) (112)	Oral (usual dose): visual loss (rare)

Table 38.3.—*continued*

Agent	Neurotoxicity
Investigational agents	
Acivicin (AT-125) (189)	Encephalopathy—headache, confusion, ataxia, delirium, aphasia, hallucinations (reversible)
Diaziquone (AZQ) (92)	None known
Hexamethylmelamine (HMM) (193–195)	Encephalopathy—confusion, ataxia, hallucinations, depression
	Parkinsonism (uncommon)
	Peripheral neuropathy (common, sensorimotor)
Mitoguazone (methyl-GAG, MGBG) (196)	Myalgias (may be severe)
	Myopathy—muscle weakness, tenderness (reversible)
PALA (*N*-phosphonoacetyl-L-asparate) (40, 197)	Encephalopathy—confusion, lethargy, delirium, hallucinations, seizures, generalized weakness
	Perioral numbness
Spiromustine (spirohydantoin mustard) (198–199)	Encephalopathy—confusion, lethargy, hallucinations, tremor, myoclonus
	Mydriasis
	(?Anticholinergic effect—neurotoxicity reduced by physostigmine)
Suramin (93, 176–179)	Sensorimotor demyelinating polyneuropathy (acute, areflexic flaccid weakness; bulbar, respiratory involvement; reversible; related to plasma level)
Thymidine (TdR) (39, 200)	Encephalopathy—headache, confusion, hallucinations, seizures
	Cerebellar dysfunction—dizziness, tremor, ataxia
	Neurotoxicity increased when given with 5-fluorouracil
Hormonal agents	
Corticosteroids (dexamethasone, prednisone, etc.) (5, 8, 121–134)	Proximal myopathy (may be severe)
	Mood alterations—euphoria, depression
	Psychosis
	Insomnia
	Tremor
	Epidural lipomatosis—with cord compression (rare)
	Pseudorheumatism (muscle aches, joint pains, on steroid taper or withdrawal)
	Altered phenytoin blood levels
Tamoxifen (Nolvadex) (201–203)	Headache
	Retinopathy (uncommon)
	Encephalopathy—confusion, lethargy (uncommon)
Biologic response modifiers	
Interferon (41, 135–145)	Headache
	Encephalopathy—confusion, lethargy, hallucinations, seizures (rare)
	Peripheral neuropathy (uncommon)
Interleukin-2 (IL-2) (141, 146–154)	Headache
	Encephalopathy (confusion, coma, seizures)
	Aseptic meningitis
	Increased intracranial pressure, cerebral edema—after intracerebral IL-2
Radiation sensitizers	
Bromodeoxyuridine (BUdR) (also: FUdR, IUdR) (204–205)	IV—? increased risk of cerebral radiation necrosis (theoretical)
	Intracarotid—stroke, TIA, ? increased risk of cerebral radiation necrosis (theoretical)
Misonidazole (also: metronidazole, etanidazole) (206–210)	Peripheral neuropathy—distal, symmetric, sensory>motor, polyneuropathy (common, dose related, dose limiting, reversible)
	Ototoxicity (uncommon)
	Encephalopathy (rare)

used in maintenance chemotherapy for childhood leukemia (both systemically and intrathecally) and in high dose with leucovorin rescue for osteogenic sarcoma and primary central nervous system lymphoma. Its principal mode of action is as a competitive inhibitor of the enzyme dihydrofolate reductase, leading to the inhibition of DNA, RNA and protein synthesis by limiting the availability of reduced folates. The principal systemic toxicities include nausea, vomiting, diarrhea, mucositis, myelosuppression, renal failure, hepatotoxicity, pulmonary toxicity, and alopecia. These toxicities are dose related, and at least some are preventable with folinic acid (leucovorin) rescue.

Methotrexate has little or no neurotoxicity when used orally or intravenously in usual doses. High-dose intravenous use (usually over 1 g/m^2) is occasionally followed by an acute encephalopathy with seizures, confusion, hemiparesis, and coma. The encephalopathy is usually transient and reversible. It typically occurs after several courses of high-dose methotrexate and may not recur on subsequent courses (9). A progressive leukoencephalopathy, characterized clinically by progressive personality and intellectual decline, dementia, hemiparesis, and sometimes seizures, and pathologically by cortical atrophy, cerebral necrosis, and mineralizing microangiopathy, may follow high-dose intravenous methotrexate. The risk of leukoencephalopathy is increased with increasing cumulative doses of methotrexate and by concurrent cranial radiotherapy (10, 11). There is no known treatment for methotrexate-induced leukoencephalopathy.

Intrathecal methotrexate, given either by lumbar puncture or by intraventricular injection via an Ommaya reservoir, is used in the treatment of leptomeningeal metastases from leukemia, lymphoma, or solid tumors and in the prophylaxis of meningeal leukemia. Acutely, intrathecal methotrexate may cause a chemical meningitis with fever, headache, nuchal rigidity, and cerebrospinal fluid (CSF) leukocytosis. This is uncommon, usually occurs within hours of the injection, and resolves spontaneously. Aminophylline may help relieve severe acute intrathecal methotrexate neurotoxicity (12). Bacterial contamination resulting in meningitis is the principal differential diagnosis. Intrathecal methotrexate may occasionally produce a myelopathy with paraplegia or a cauda equina syndrome. Intrathecal agents must be prepared in sterile preservative-free solutions, as the bacteriostatic agents

used as preservatives in multiuse vials are neurotoxic (13, 14). A progressive leukoencephalopathy may also follow intrathecal methotrexate (Figs. 38.1 and 38.2). The risk of leukoencephalopathy is increased with increasing total dose of methotrexate, with concurrent cranial or craniospinal radiotherapy (especially in young children), and when methotrexate is used as treatment for meningeal tumor rather than for prophylaxis (10, 15–18). Prolonged elevation of CSF methotrexate levels may predispose to the development of methotrexate leukoencephalopathy. Intraventricular injection is thus hazardous if there is an obstructive hydrocephalus. Localized leukoencephalopathy has been reported following injection into an Ommaya reservoir

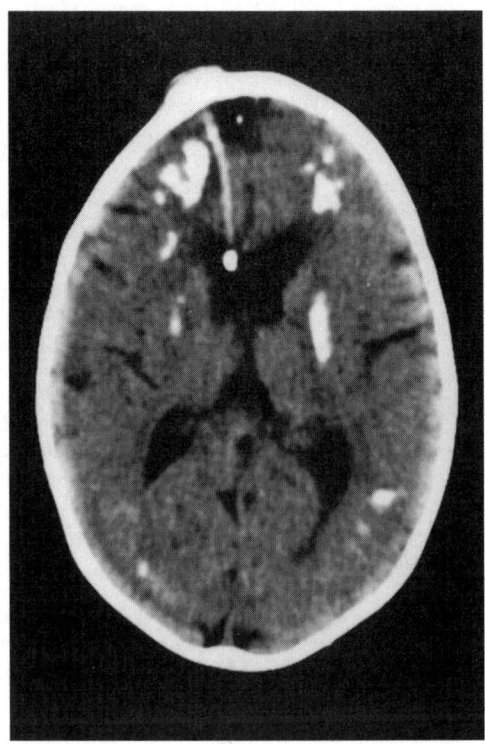

Figure 38.1.   A 3 ½-year-old boy with acute lymphoblastic leukemia since age 7 months, treated with systemic chemotherapy, cranial radiotherapy, and intraventricular methotrexate and cytarabine for several CNS recurrences; history of seizures and slowed speech and intellectual development. Noncontrast cranial CT scan shows multifocal intracerebral calcifications involving grey-white matter junction areas and basal ganglia, mild cortical atrophy, and ventricular dilation, consistent with mineralizing microangiopathy. A ventricular catheter from the Ommaya reservoir is seen entering the right lateral ventricle.

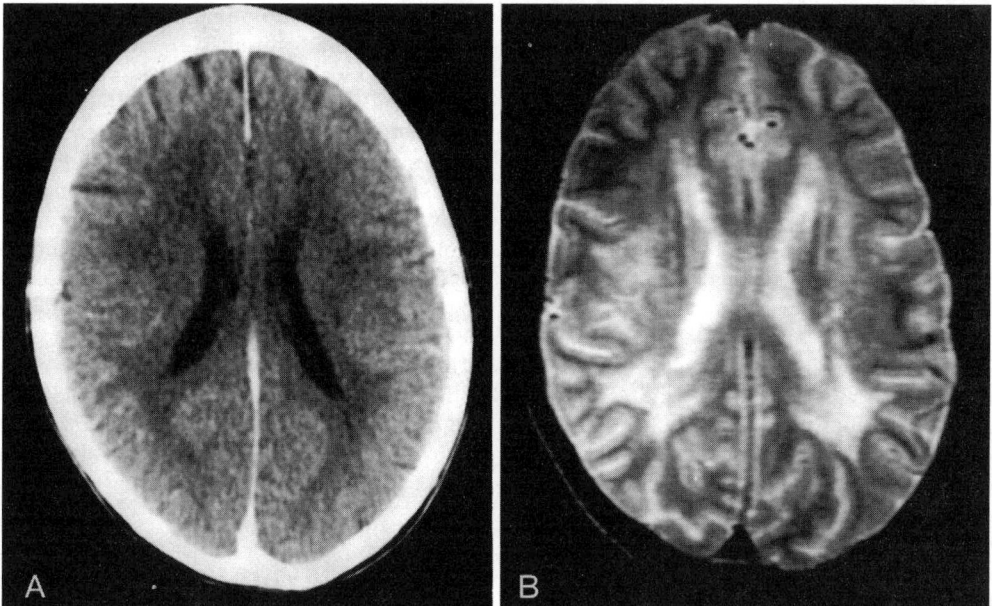

Figure 38.2. A 24-year-old man with acute lymphoblastic leukemia since age 6 years, treated with systemic chemotherapy and cranial radiotherapy plus intrathecal methotrexate for several CNS recurrences; history of seizures and mild memory and cognitive impairment. **A.** Noncontrast cranial CT scan demonstrating diffuse white matter hypodensity, mild cortical atrophy, and ventricular dilation, consistent with leukoencephalopathy. **B.** T2-weighted MRI (TR 2000, TE 70) demonstrating markedly increased signal from periventricular, biparietal-occipital, and right frontoparietal subcortical white matter areas, consistent with leukoencephalopathy.

when the ventricular catheter is malpositioned and does not enter the lateral ventricle (19, 20).

The long-term consequences of prophylactic or symptomatic treatment of childhood leukemia include behavioral disturbances, poor school performance, memory loss, intellectual decline, growth retardation, hormonal disturbances, and abnormal CT or MRI scans (cerebral atrophy, ventricular dilation, white matter changes, intracerebral calcifications). Although cranial or craniospinal radiation therapy may account for most of these complications, intrathecal methotrexate alone may produce some of the intellectual and behavioral problems or exacerbate those produced by radiotherapy (10, 15, 21–26).

Accidental intrathecal methotrexate overdose may produce an ascending myelopathy and necrotizing leukoencephalopathy. Doses of 50 mg or less probably produce few serious sequelae. Moderate overdose, in the 50 to 100 mg range, may produce an acute chemical meningitis unless early intervention with CSF drainage is undertaken. Massive overdose, over 500 mg, will cause myelopathy and encephalopathy, which

may be fatal. Rapid, aggressive treatment with CSF drainage, ventriculolumbar perfusion, high-dose leucovorin rescue, alkaline diuresis, intensive systemic support, and possibly intrathecal carboxypeptidase-G2 may allow survival and recovery of neurologic function (27–31).

Osmotic blood-brain barrier modification, temporarily opening the blood-brain barrier by intracarotid injection of hyperosmolar mannitol, has been proposed as a mechanism to increase the delivery of water-soluble compounds (normally excluded by the intact blood-brain barrier) to improve the treatment of brain tumors. Methotrexate is the most common chemotherapeutic agent administered following osmotic blood-brain barrier disruption. Headache, increased neurologic deficits, and seizures have been reported in patients following this therapy. These symptoms may be due to an increase in local cerebral edema. The toxicities generally have been transient and reversible. Recently, concern has been expressed that osmotic blood-brain barrier modification followed by methotrexate chemotherapy may increase the delivery of methotrexate to the normal brain distant from tumor more than to the tumor itself, possibly increasing the risk of methotrexate encephalopathy in normal brain distant from tumor (32–37).

5-FLUOROURACIL

5-Fluorouracil (5-FU) is a fluorine-substituted analogue of the pyrimidine uracil. Its primary mechanism of action is inhibition of the enzyme thymidylate synthetase; this reduces thymidine monophosphate formation and thus blocks DNA synthesis. It is also incorporated into RNA. It is cell-cycle specific in that it is selectively toxic to proliferating cells but is not phase specific. 5-FU is usually administered intravenously, either by bolus or by prolonged infusion, but is also sometimes given by intraarterial injection, direct injection into body cavities, and topically. It readily enters the CSF. 5-FU is used alone against adenocarcinomas of the colon and rectum and in combination with other agents against carcinoma of the breast, stomach, pancreas, and liver. Combinations of 5-FU plus allopurinol, α-interferon, cisplatin, folinic acid, levamisole, PALA (N-phosphonoacetyl-L-aspartic acid) or thymidine are under investigation, especially in colorectal carcinoma. Combinations of 5-FU and levamisole are commonly used as adjuvant treatment for colorectal carcinoma, and 5-FU plus folinic acid (leucovorin) as treatment for metastatic colorectal carcinoma. The major systemic toxicities of 5-FU include alopecia, diarrhea, nausea and vomiting, mucositis, and myelosuppression. The systemic toxicities are reduced somewhat by prolonged infusions or allopurinol and increased by bolus administration or combination therapy (7, 38–42).

The major neurotoxicity of 5-FU is an acute cerebellar dysfunction characterized by the rapid onset of gait ataxia, limb incoordination, dysarthria, and nystagmus; diplopia is occasionally present. A more diffuse encephalopathy, with headache, confusion, disorientation, lethargy, and seizures sometimes is seen. Peripheral neuropathy is rare and may be confused with palmar-plantar erythrodysesthesia. The neurotoxic effects are probably dose and schedule related and reversible with drug withdrawal or dose reduction. Neurotoxicity is reported in up to 5% of patients receiving 5-FU alone. Patients with abnormalities of pyrimidine metabolism, such as dihydropyrimidine dehydrogenase deficiency, may be at high risk for 5-FU neurotoxicity. The neurotoxicity of 5-FU may be potentiated by concomitant administration with α-interferon, cisplatin, folinic acid, PALA, or thymidine. It is not prevented by allopurinol but possibly is by thiamine. An inflammatory multifocal leukoencephalopathy, resembling multiple sclerosis and sometimes misdiagnosed as brain metastases, may develop during 5-FU plus levamisole therapy (Fig. 38.3); it usually resolves with drug withdrawal or corticosteroid therapy; cranial radiotherapy may exacerbate the neurotoxicity. A similar syndrome may occur following levamisole alone. The mechanism of 5-FU neurotoxicity is unknown, but conversion of 5-FU to fluorocitrate in the CNS with subsequent inhibition of the Krebs tricarboxylic acid cycle has been postulated (7, 8, 38–52). 5-FU analogues such as fotofur and carmofur may also cause neurotoxicity such as encephalopathy and ataxia (8).

CYTARABINE

Cytarabine (Ara-C, cytosine arabinoside) is an analogue of the pyrimidine compound cytidine. It acts primarily as an inhibitor of DNA polymerase but also by incorporation into DNA, resulting in the production of abnormal DNA. Cytarabine is used primarily in the chemotherapy of leukemia and lymphomas, often in combination with other agents. Recently it has been used in a high dose (2 or 3 g/m^2 each 12 hours for several days) in the treatment of resistant leukemias and lymphomas and primary central nervous system lymphoma. The principal systemic toxicities include nausea, vomiting, diarrhea, and myelosuppression (which may be severe). Cytarabine is also used intrathecally in the treatment or prophylaxis of meningeal leukemia or lymphoma. A slow-release form of cytarabine (DTC 101) in which cytarabine is encapsulated in Depo-Foam (microscopic particles of nonconcentric chambers of lipid bilayer membrane) is under investigation for intrathecal treatment of carcinomatous meningitis (7, 53, 54).

Cytarabine has little or no neurotoxicity following usual intravenous doses. Following high-dose intravenous therapy, encephalopathy (confusion, obtundation, seizures, and coma), leukoencephalopathy, cerebellar dysfunction (ataxia and dysmetria), and sometimes peripheral neuropathy have been reported. These neurotoxicities are dose and schedule related. Increasing dose, over 18 g/m^2/course, results in an increasing frequency of neurotoxicity. Older patients and those with abnormal renal or hepatic function are more susceptible to neurotox-

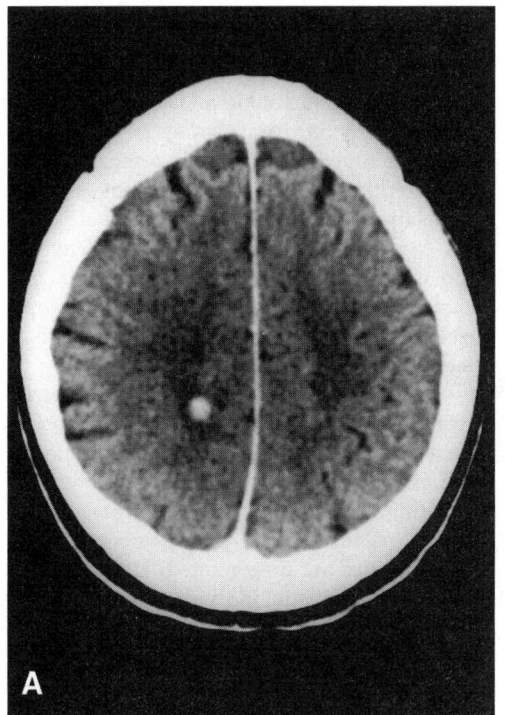

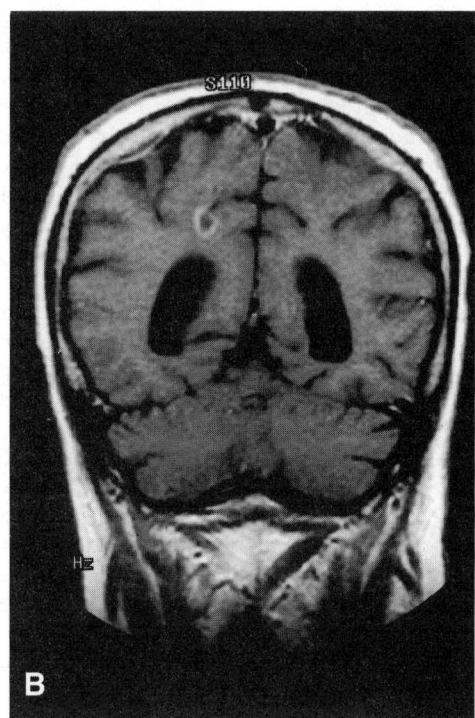

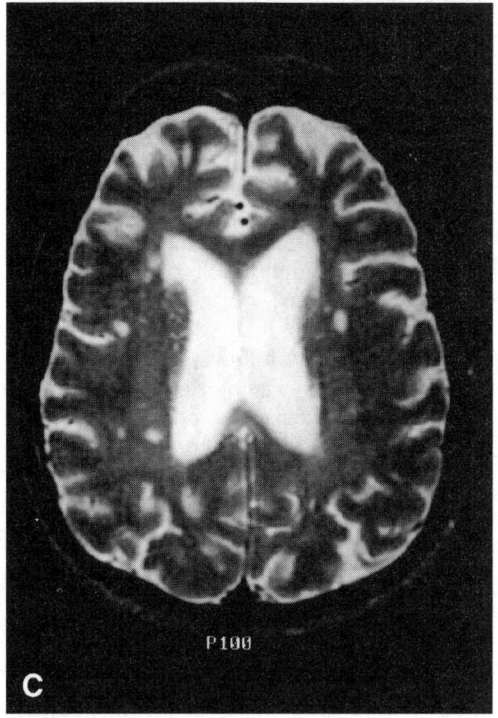

Figure 38.3. Multifocal inflammatory leukoencephalopathy secondary to 5-fluorouracil plus levamisole chemotherapy given as adjuvant treatment of colon carcinoma in 54-year-old man. A. Contrast-enhanced cranial CT scan demonstrating an enhancing lesion in the right parietal area. **B.** T1-weighted coronal gadolinium-enhanced MRI demonstrating a ring-enhancing right parietal lesion. **C.** T2-weighted axial cranial MRI demonstrating multiple areas of increased signal intensity in the periventricular white matter region.

icity. Patients with multiple risk factors may have up to a 30% incidence of neurotoxicity. The risk seems higher in subsequent than initial courses of therapy. The neurologic symptoms often develop several days after the start of therapy and may be heralded by the development of nystagmus, allowing treatment to be stopped; however, some patients seem to develop the full neurotoxic syndrome abruptly. Once the drug is stopped, the neurologic symptoms seem to resolve, at least partially, in some but not all patients. Fatalities have been reported. Purkinje cell loss in the cerebellum has been found in some patients. Following intrathecal or intraventricular injection, an aseptic meningitis may occasionally be seen. The encapsulated intrathecal cytarabine preparation (DTC 101) may produce somewhat more meningeal irritation than standard cytarabine, but this can usually be prevented by concurrent oral corticosteroids. A myelopathy with paraplegia or cauda equina syndrome has been reported following intrathecal injection via lumbar puncture. In some cases the toxicity was attributed to the use of a preservative-containing solution for preparation, but in other cases the myelopathy seemed directly due to cytarabine. A leukoencephalopathy has also been reported. Concurrent cranial radiotherapy may increase the risk of neurotoxicity with cytarabine (7, 14, 53–61).

VINCRISTINE

Vincristine (Oncovin, VCR), a plant alkaloid derived from the periwinkle plant, is a widely used chemotherapeutic agent. It acts as a mitotic inhibitor by interfering with the function of microtubules, especially the mitotic spindle, resulting in mitotic arrest. Because of its relative lack of myelosuppression, vincristine is used in combination with other chemotherapeutic agents in the treatment of many tumors, including leukemias, lymphomas (as part of the MOPP (mechlorethamine, vincristine, procarbazine, prednisone) and CHOP (cyclophosphamide, doxorubicin, vincristine, prednisone) regimens), and breast carcinoma (as part of the CMFVP (cyclophosphamide, methotrexate, fluorouracil, vincristine, prednisone) regimen). Vincristine is a strong vesicant, producing local skin ulceration if extravasation occurs during intravenous injection. Little nausea, vomiting, or mucositis occurs. Myelosuppression is mild. Constipation may occur. Hyponatremia can be seen from a syndrome of inappropriate antidiuretic hormone secretion (SIADH).

The dose-limiting toxicity of vincristine is the development of peripheral neuropathy. This characteristically begins with loss of the deep tendon reflex at the ankle and may progress to complete areflexia, distal symmetric sensory loss (pin and temperature more than vibration and proprioception), motor weakness, foot drop, and muscle atrophy. An autonomic neuropathy with ileus, constipation, impotence, urinary retention, or postural hypotension may occur. Cranial neuropathies including optic neuropathy, diplopia, facial palsies, and vocal cord paralysis have occasionally occurred. Muscle pain involving the jaw or legs may occasionally acutely develop following an injection. The discomfort may last for several hours or several days and sometimes is sufficiently severe to require a dose reduction or discontinuation of vincristine. Central neurotoxicity with seizures and SIADH is uncommon. All these toxicities are dose related, although there is high variability in individual susceptibility. The neurotoxicities are usually reversible. Patients with a preexisting neuropathy (diabetic, familial—such as Charot-Marie-Tooth disease, compressive, or nutritional) may develop a severe neuropathy after vincristine. Previous or concurrent therapy with other neuropathy-inducing chemotherapeutic agents (e.g., cisplatin, paclitaxel) may exacerbate the neuropathy. The neurotoxicity is attributed to the inhibition of axoplasmic transport by the action of vincristine on axonal microtubules (1–8, 62–64).

A *fatal ascending myelopathy and encephalopathy* has occurred after the accidental intrathecal injection of vincristine. Despite aggressive support and vigorous attempts at CSF lavage, an ascending flaccid paralysis and progressive encephalopathy leading to brain death has occurred almost universally following intrathecal vincristine injection. Postmortem studies have shown severe, extensive axonal loss, demyelination, and necrosis. The intrathecal injection of vincristine and probably any of the related vinca alkaloids (vinblastine, vindesine, vinorelbine) or the epipodophyllotoxins (etoposide (VP-16) and teniposide (VM-26)) must be avoided (65).

The coadministration of oral glutamic acid has been reported to reduce somewhat the peripheral neuropathy produced by weekly intravenous vincristine. The mechanism of action of glutamic acid in reducing vincristine neurotoxicity is unknown, and the eventual clinical role of glutamic acid remains to be determined. Survival following inadvertent intrathecal injection of vincristine has been reported in a patient treated with immediate CSF drainage, ventriculolumbar perfusion with 2.5% fresh frozen plasma in lactated Ringer's solution, and intravenous glutamic acid (66, 67). Other agents reported to prevent or reduce vincristine neurotoxicity include insulin-like growth factor-I and the ACTH (4-9) analogue, ORG 2766 (68, 69).

Other vinca alkaloids, such as vindesine, vinblastine, and vinorelbine (Navelbine), seem to cause less neurotoxicity than vincristine, although (like vincristine) concurrent or sequential treatment with other neurotoxic agents (e.g., cisplatin, paclitaxel) may produce more severe neuropathy (70–72).

CISPLATIN

Cisplatin (Platinol, DDP) is a chemotherapeutic agent with a wide spectrum of activity. The mechanism of action has not been clearly defined, but cisplatin likely acts by binding to DNA and can form interstrand cross-links, interfering with DNA synthesis and transcription. Cisplatin is highly effective against testicular tumors and ovarian carcinoma. It is also active against head and neck cancer, bladder cancer, and small cell carcinoma of lung. It has activity against primary brain tumors (malignant gliomas, medulloblastoma) as well. The major systemic toxicities include nausea and vomiting (which may be severe), renal failure (usually preventable with adequate intravenous hydration), and electrolyte disturbances (including hyponatremia, hypocalcemia, and hypomagnesemia). Myelosuppression is relatively mild except at high doses. Doses of 60 to 100 mg/m^2/course are typical, but doses up to 200 mg/m^2 have been given with aggressive support (7).

Neurotoxicity from cisplatin is common and dose limiting. Ototoxicity, characterized by a progressive high-frequency sensorineural hearing loss and tinnitus, likely due to a direct action of cisplatin on the cochlea, is common. It is dose related, exacerbated by concurrent cranial radiotherapy, and worse in children. The reversibility is questionable (8, 73–76). Vestibular toxicity, with vertigo, nystagmus, or ataxia, is less common. The dose-limiting neurotoxicity is peripheral neuropathy. The distal, symmetric, predominantly large-fiber, sensory polyneuropathy, producing paresthesias, vibratory, and proprio-

ceptive loss with relative sparing of pin and temperature sensation, is dose related and cumulative (total dose usually over 300 to 600 mg/m^2). The deep tendon reflexes are reduced, Lhermitte's sign is common, mild weakness may occur, and autonomic neuropathy has been reported. The proprioceptive loss may cause a sensory ataxia. Symptoms may begin or progress even after cisplatin has been discontinued. Electrophysiologic studies show a sensory axonal neuropathy. Pathologic studies reveal axonal loss and secondary demyelination of peripheral nerves and ventral nerve roots, with secondary degeneration of the dorsal columns of the spinal cord; the primary site of damage is probably the dorsal root ganglion neurons. The neuropathy tends to recover slowly over months. Concurrent treatment with vincristine, etoposide (VP-16), or paclitaxel may exacerbate the neuropathy (77–86). Several agents, including amifostine (WR2721), the ACTH (4-9) analogue ORG 2766, neurotrophins, reduced glutathione, insulin-like growth factor-I, and nerve growth factor, have been reported protective against cisplatin-induced neurotoxicity (87–96).

An encephalopathy with confusion and seizures can occur, especially with high doses, but it may be due to cisplatin-induced fluid and electrolyte disturbances. Cerebral herniation with severe headache, increasing hemiparesis, acute cerebral deterioration, seizures, coma, and death has been reported in patients with large intracranial tumors. It may be related to overhydration and electrolyte disturbances producing increased cerebral edema and seizures. Pretreatment with corticosteroids to control cerebral edema and the prevention of fluid and electrolyte disturbances may prevent the development of this complication. High-dose cisplatin therapy for patients with large cerebral tumors (such as glioblastoma) must be considered hazardous. Retinopathy, cranial neuropathy, and cortical blindness have occasionally been reported following cisplatin therapy. Intracarotid administration of cisplatin may increase the risk of encephalopathy and cranial neuropathy, including optic neuropathy and ototoxicity (35, 97–102).

Carboplatin, an analogue of cisplatin that causes less nausea, vomiting, and nephrotoxicity but more myelosuppression than cisplatin, usually produces much less neurotoxicity as well. Ototoxicity has been reported in children following intravenous carboplatin for recurrent brain tumor (most of whom had prior cranial radiotherapy) and following intraarterial carboplatin with osmotic blood-brain barrier disruption (103–105).

NITROSOUREAS

The nitrosoureas include BCNU (carmustine), CCNU (lomustine), and methyl-CCNU (semustine) as well as several new investigational agents such as PCNU and ACNU. All have similar actions and toxicities. They act predominantly as alkylating agents, binding to DNA, but may produce interstrand and intrastrand crosslinks as well as carbamoylated proteins. BCNU is a mild vesicant. It may produce local discomfort in the vein during infusion, at least partly as it generally is dissolved in alcohol then diluted for infusion. Nausea and vomiting (which may be severe but usually is short-lived) are common. Myelosuppression is delayed and cumulative. Nadir blood counts occur 4 to 5 weeks following treatment, and the degree of myelosuppression increases with subsequent courses of therapy. Pulmonary fibrosis is a serious late complication. It occurs in less than 5% of patients with cumulative total doses of BCNU below 1400 mg/m^2, but the risk increases rapidly with higher doses. Pulmonary failure may occur. Restrictive lung disease may follow craniospinal radiation with or without nitrosourea chemotherapy. Renal insufficiency is a late cumulative dose-related complication as well. Hepatotoxicity is uncommon (7, 8, 106–108).

BCNU (and other nitrosoureas) have little neurotoxicity at the usual intravenous doses (200 mg/m^2 or 80 mg/m^2/day $\times$ 3 days). High-dose (600 to 800 mg/m^2 or more) intravenous BCNU with autologous bone marrow transplantation has produced an encephalopathy with confusion and seizures (109–110). The intracarotid injection of BCNU (usually 100 to 200 mg/m^2) will produce severe local pain in the ipsilateral face, eye, and head during infusion. Severe eye toxicity with retinopathy, blindness, or ocular necrosis has been reported (111). Eye toxicity may be preventable by intracarotid infusions above the level of the ophthalmic artery. Ocular toxicity has been reported with oral CCNU and concurrent cranial radiation therapy (112). A severe ipsilateral encephalopathy with seizures, hemiparesis, progressive neurologic deficits, and cerebral necrosis has followed intracarotid BCNU. The pathology is similar to that of radiation necrosis. Concurrent cranial radiotherapy and intracarotid BCNU chemotherapy may in-

crease the risk of neurotoxicity (113–115). At least some of the neurotoxicity may be explained by a streaming effect that may occur, with intracarotid injections leading to unpredictable variability in drug delivery to the various distal branches of the carotid artery and thus unequal drug concentrations, with extreme drug levels in branches where the drug has channeled and subtherapeutic levels in other vessels. Various techniques are under development to prevent drug streaming (116, 117). Possible heterogeneity of local drug delivery is a problem for any regional chemotherapeutic approach (such as intracarotid chemotherapy). It is not a problem with intravenous or oral chemotherapy.

The local administration of BCNU or other nitrosoureas directly into brain tumors, by either direct infusion or implanted drug permeated wafers, may sometimes cause a local reaction ranging from brain edema to necrosis (118–120).

CORTICOSTEROIDS

Adrenal corticosteroids, such as dexamethasone (Decadron) and prednisone, are widely used in oncology. In hematologic malignancies (leukemias and lymphomas), corticosteroids are used for a direct lymphocytolytic effect. In neurooncology, the corticosteroids, especially dexamethasone, are used to reduce increased intracranial pressure and control cerebral edema associated with primary and metastatic brain tumor and to control spinal cord edema from epidural metastases or other causes of spinal cord compression. High-dose corticosteroids also have an antiemetic effect and are used as part of many antiemetic regimens to control nausea and vomiting produced by other chemotherapeutic agents. Corticosteroids may produce an extensive variety of systemic toxicities including cushingoid features, truncal obesity, hyperglycemia, opportunistic infections (especially oral candidiasis), electrolyte disturbances, hypertension, gastrointestinal bleeding, capillary fragility with easy bruising, osteoporosis (with increased risk of fracture), aseptic bone necrosis, peripheral edema, impaired wound healing, glaucoma, and cataracts (5, 7, 8, 121).

A variety of neurologic toxicities may be produced by corticosteroids. The risk of toxicity is increased by increased doses of the agent, increased duration of therapy, and individual susceptibility. The frequency of steroid-induced side effects varies considerably from series to series. Up to 50% of patients in some series are reported to experience at least one steroid-induced toxicity, including neurotoxicity. The most common neurotoxicity is a proximal myopathy (5, 8, 122–129). It may be so severe that some patients cannot stand, walk, or lift their arms. Occasionally, respiratory function can be compromised. Mood alterations, either euphoria or depression, are common. Euphoria, improved sense of well-being, and improved appetite may be produced with the introduction of steroid therapy or an increased dose of corticosteroids. Insomnia and other sleep disturbances are common. Steroid psychosis is uncommon (130). Tremor, especially a fine-action tremor, is common at high doses. Epidural lipomatosis (increased deposition of fat in the spinal epidural space, resulting in spinal cord compression) is a rare complication of high-dose steroid therapy (131). Most of the neurotoxicities are dose related and reversible with reduction in the steroid dose. Some toxicities, however, such as depression, anorexia, and pseudorheumatism (muscle aches and joint pains), are produced by rapid steroid taper (132). In addition, in patients with brain tumor, recurrence of cerebral edema with increased intracranial pressure and increasing focal deficits can occur if steroids are withdrawn too rapidly, before the tumor is controlled by other therapies.

Drug interactions between dexamethasone and phenytoin (and perhaps other anticonvulsants) may result in reduced bioavailability of dexamethasone (causing increased cerebral edema in brain tumor patients when phenytoin is started) or altered phenytoin blood levels (causing toxicity if dexamethasone is reduced and seizures if dexamethasone is increased) (133, 134).

BIOLOGIC RESPONSE MODIFIERS

The biologic response modifiers are a variety of naturally occurring compounds that in physiologic dose control or modify a number of biologic responses in health and disease, including immunity; blood cell differentiation, proliferation, and activation; and responses to fever and infection. The biologic response modifiers currently in clinical or investigational use include the interferons (α, β, γ), interleukin-2, tissue necrosis factor, and the colony-stimulating factors such as erythropoietin, granulocyte colony-stimulating factor (G-CSF), and granulocyte/macrophage colony-stimulating factor (GM-CSF). Most of these are now produced by recombinant DNA

technology, and some of the side effects that occurred due to impurities in earlier naturally produced compounds are now reduced. Therapeutically, the biologic response modifiers are often used in high doses, sometimes several orders of magnitude higher than are needed to produce their physiologic actions.

α-Interferon is used therapeutically in the treatment of several leukemias (especially hairy cell leukemia) and has been used against multiple myeloma, lymphoma, melanoma, renal cell carcinoma, brain tumor, and a variety of viral diseases (including AIDS). It is given by injection, either alone or in combination with other chemotherapeutic agents or biologic response modifiers. Common systemic toxicities include fever, chills, nausea, fatigue, malaise, anorexia, myalgias, myelosuppression, and occasionally hepatotoxicity (135–140). These are dose and schedule related. Neurologic symptoms may occur in over one-third of patients treated but are severe in less than 10%. An acute and reversible neurotoxicity generally occurs only at high doses and includes headache and encephalopathy (confusion, lethargy, hallucination, and rarely seizures). Tolerance may develop with ongoing treatment. Preexisting brain metastases, primary brain tumor, other organic brain abnormalities, and increasing age may predispose patients to neurotoxicity. Paresthesias and a mild distal sensorimotor peripheral neuropathy are sometimes seen. A delayed, progressive, chronic neurotoxicity with neuropsychiatric disturbances (depression, anxiety, hallucinations), memory loss, visual-perceptual disturbances, and parkinsonism, sometimes accompanied by white matter changes on CT or MRI, is occasionally seen (41, 141–145).

Interleukin-2 (IL-2) has received considerable recent publicity. It is administered alone or in conjunction with lymphokine-activated killer cells (LAK cells), tumor-infiltrating lymphocytes (TILs), or other agents. It is thought to act primarily by activation of the immune system, although it may have some direct cytotoxicity. The systemic toxicities are extensive, are often severe, and may require intensive care. Reported toxicities include fever, chills, generalized malaise, fatigue, anorexia, diarrhea, nausea and vomiting, myelosuppression, a capillary leak syndrome (pulmonary edema, hypotension, and fluid retention), renal failure, cardiac arrhythmias, electrolyte imbalance, superficial phlebitis, and skin infections at the injection sites. A variety of neurotoxicities have been reported. Most are dose and schedule related and reversible. Headache, agitation, and mild encephalopathy (disorientation, confusion) are common. More severe encephalopathy (including delirium, delusions, seizures, and coma) and transient focal neurologic deficits mimicking transient ischemic attacks have been reported. The onset of neurologic symptoms may be delayed several days after onset of therapy and may last more than 1 week following the end of therapy. An aseptic meningitis may occur following intracranial injection. Intracerebral injection of IL-2 into brain tumors has produced increased intracranial pressure and increased neurologic deficits, presumably by increasing local cerebral edema. Dementia has been seen following intraventricular IL-2 therapy (141, 146–154).

Cyclosporine has been used to prevent graft rejection after transplantation. It is being investigated as a modifier of p-glycoprotein-induced multidrug resistance. Neurologic toxicities include cortical blindness, encephalopathy, seizures, and demyelinating polyneuropathy (155, 156).

OTHER AGENTS

Ifosfamide

Ifosfamide, an analogue of cyclophosphamide in the nitrogen mustard family of alkylating agents, is widely used against sarcomas in adults and children; carcinomas of bladder, cervix, testicle, and lung; and brain tumors such as medulloblastoma. It is typically given with mesna, a uroprotective agent, to prevent hemorrhagic cystitis. Ifosfamide must be activated by hepatic metabolism into its active form; one byproduct, acrolein, is responsible for the hemorrhagic cystitis. Other systemic toxicities include myelosuppression, renal toxicity, alopecia, and nausea with vomiting (157, 158).

Neurotoxicity, characterized by encephalopathy, seizures, cerebellar dysfunction, parkinsonism and other extrapyramidal signs, delirium, and sometimes coma, is a dose limiting effect of ifosfamide, occurring in up to 30% of patients on this drug. The onset is typically within 24 hours of the start of ifosfamide infusion but may be delayed several days. The neurotoxicity usually clears within 3 to 4 days of stopping the drug, but persistent symptoms and death have been reported. Significant encephalopathy usually requires a dose reduction, although some patients have been successfully re-challenged at the same dose without recurrence. Methylene blue and diazepam have been reported to reverse the encephalopathy. Peripheral neuropathy has also been reported.

Ifosfamide neurotoxicity is dose and schedule dependent. High doses (especially over 5 g/m^2/ day), rapid infusions, prolonged infusions, renal or hepatic impairment, low serum albumin or calcium levels, underlying brain dysfunction, prior cisplatin therapy, and concurrent phenobarbital therapy may predispose to ifosfamide neurotoxicity. The mechanism of neurotoxicity is unknown but may be due to chloroacetaldehyde, a neurotoxic metabolite of ifosfamide (8, 158–165).

Paclitaxel

Paclitaxel (Taxol), originally derived from the bark of the Pacific yew tree, and docetaxel (Taxotere), a derivative of paclitaxel, are taxane chemotherapeutic agents with activity against ovarian, breast, lung, head and neck, bladder, and testicular cancers and possibly malignant gliomas. Paclitaxel promotes the polymerization of tubulin, leading to stabilization and dysfunction of microtubules, causing cell arrest in the G$_2$ and mitotic phases of the cell cycle (which may account for its radiotherapy sensitization properties) as well as cell death.

Paclitaxel is usually administered as a 3- or 24-hour intravenous infusion. Myelosuppression (especially neutropenia) is dose limiting. Other systemic toxicities include hypersensitivity reactions during infusions (attributed to the cremophor vehicle and preventable by premedication with corticosteroids and histamine H$_1$ and H$_2$ antagonists), cardiac toxicity, mucositis, nail changes, and alopecia (166).

Paclitaxel neurotoxicity may be dose limiting. Most common is a distal, symmetric, predominantly sensory polyneuropathy causing distal loss of both large-fiber (vibration and proprioception) and small-fiber (pin and temperature) sensation. Distal itching sensation may be a prominent manifestation of the sensory peripheral neuropathy. Arthralgias and myalgias may also develop. An ocular toxicity characterized by flashing lights has also been reported. Electrophysiologic tests suggest an axonopathy or possibly sensory neuronopathy and not demyelination as the mechanism of the neurotoxicity. A motor neuropathy, which is sometimes proximal, and autonomic neuropathy are less common. The neuropathy is individual dose dependent, developing in up to 60% of patients with breast cancer treated at high dose (over 250 mg/m²) but less common following conventional doses (135 or 175 mg/m²); it is also probably cumulative dose dependent, becoming more common and more severe with increasing total dose. The onset of neuropathic symptoms is usually several days after the paclitaxel infusion but may follow high doses within 24 hours. The neuropathic symptoms are usually reversible after paclitaxel is stopped, but recovery may be prolonged. Preexisting neuropathic conditions such as diabetes mellitus or alcoholism may increase the risk of neurotoxicity. Concurrent therapy with paclitaxel and other neurotoxic chemotherapeutic agents such as cisplatin may produce more severe neurotoxicity (86, 166–172). Nerve growth factor and other neuroprotective agents such as amifostine are under investigation as possible preventative treatments for paclitaxel-induced neurotoxicity (173).

Docetaxel (Taxotere) has a mechanism of action similar to that of paclitaxel and produces a similar spectrum of neurotoxic effects, especially a sensory-motor peripheral neuropathy that is dose dependent and may be severe and disabling at high dose levels (174, 175).

Suramin

Suramin, a polysulfonated naphthylurea, initially developed as an antiparasite agent against African trypanosomiasis, is an active agent against hormone-refractory prostate cancer and is under investigation in non-Hodgkin's lymphoma, adrenocortical and other cancers, and AIDS. Its mechanism of action is unclear but may relate to inhibition of several growth factors and intracellular second-messenger enzyme systems. Systemic toxicities include coagulopathy, adrenal insufficiency, and malaise. The dose-limiting toxicity is a sensorimotor demyelinating polyneuropathy resembling acute Guillain-Barré syndrome, characterized by a severe areflexic flaccid paralysis, often involving proximal and distal muscles, sometimes with bulbar and respiratory involvement requiring ventilatory support. Sensory and autonomic symptoms are common. The neuropathy is reversible with appropriate support. The neuropathy is correlated with the maximum plasma suramin level, with an estimated 40% risk of neurotoxicity with suramin plasma concentrations over 350 µg/mL,

and with the duration of elevated suramin levels. Pharmacokinetic monitoring may help prevent suramin neurotoxicity. Nerve growth factor may also prevent suramin-induced neuropathy (93, 176–179).

References

1. Weiss HD, Walker MD, Wiernik PH. Neurotoxicity of commonly used antineoplastic agents. N Engl J Med 1974;291:75–81,172–133.

2. Young DF, Posner JB. Nervous system toxicity of the chemotherapeutic agents. In: Vinken PJ, Bruyn GW, Klawans HL, eds. Handbook of clinical neurology. Amsterdam: North-Holland, 1980;39:91–129.

3. Kaplan RS, Wiernik PH. Neurotoxicity of antineoplastic drugs. Semin Oncol 1982;9:103–130.

4. Macdonald DR. Neurologic complications of chemotherapy. Neurol Clin 1991;9:955–967.

5. Rottenberg DA, ed. Neurological complications of cancer treatment. Boston: Butterworth-Heinman, 1991.

6. Tuxen MK, Hansen SW. Neurotoxicity secondary to antineoplastic drugs. Cancer Treat Rev 1994; 20:191–214.

7. Pratt WB, Ruddon RW, Ensminger WD, Maybaum J. The anticancer drugs. 2nd ed. New York: Oxford University Press, 1994.

8. Posner JB. Neurologic complications of cancer. Philadelphia: FA Davis, 1995.

9. Walker RW, Allen JC, Rosen G, et al. Transient cerebral dysfunction secondary to high-dose methotrexate. J Clin Oncol 1986;4:1845–1850.

10. Bleyer WA, Griffin TW. White matter necrosis, mineralizing microangiopathy, and intellectual abilities in survivors of childhood leukemia: associations with central nervous system irradiation and methotrexate therapy. In: Gilbert HA, Kagan AR, eds. Radiation damage to the nervous system. New York: Raven Press, 1980:155–174.

11. Allen JC, Rosen G, Mehta BM, Horten B. Leukoencephalopathy following high-dose IV methotrexate chemotherapy with leucovorin rescue. Cancer Treat Rep 1980;64:1261–1273.

12. Bernini JC, Fort DW, Greiner JC, et al. Aminophylline for methotrexate-induced neurotoxicity. Lancet 1995;345:544–547.

13. Gagliano RG, Costanzi JJ. Paraplegia following intrathecal methotrexate. Report of a case and review of the literature. Cancer 1976;37:1663–1668.

14. Hahn AF, Feasby TE, Gilbert JJ. Paraparesis following intrathecal chemotherapy. Neurology 1983; 33:1032–1038.

15. Poplack DG, Brouwers P. Adverse sequelae of central nervous system therapy. Clin Oncol 1985; 4:263–285.

16. Cruz-Sanchez FF, Artigas J, Cervos-Navarro J, et al. Brain lesions following combined treatment with methotrexate and craniospinal irradiation. J Neurooncol 1991;10:165–171.

17. Bleyer WA, Drake JC, Chabner BA. Neurotoxicity and elevated cerebrospinal-fluid methotrexate concentration in meningeal leukemia. N Engl J Med 1973;289:770–773.

18. Shapiro WR, Chernik NL, Posner JB. Necrotizing encephalopathy following intraventricular instillation of methotrexate. Arch Neurol 1973;28:96–102.

19. Lemann W, Wiley RG, Posner JB. Leukoencephalopathy complicating intraventricular catheters: clinical, radiographic and pathologic study of 10 cases. J Neurooncol 1988;6:67–74.

20. de Waal P, Algra PR, Heimans JJ, et al. Methotrexate induced brain necrosis and severe leukoencephalopathy due to disconnection of an Ommaya device. J Neurooncol 1993;15:269–273.

21. Riccardi R, Brouwers P, DiChiro G, Poplack DG. Abnormal computed tomography brain scans in children with acute lymphoblastic leukemia: serial long-term follow-up. J Clin Oncol 1985;3:12–18.

22. Ebner F, Ranner G, Slavc J, et al. MR findings in methotrexate-induced CNS abnormalities. AJNR 1989;10:959–964.

23. Mulhern RK, Ochs J. Fairclough D, et al. Intellectual and academic achievement status after CNS relapse: a retrospective analysis of 40 children treated for acute lymphoblastic leukemia. J Clin Oncol 1987;5:933–940.

24. Mulhern RK, Wasserman AL, Fairclough D, Ochs J. Memory function in disease-free survivors of childhood acute lymphocytic leukemia given CNS prophylaxis with or without 1800 cGy cranial irradiation. J Clin Oncol 1988;6:315–320.

25. Ochs J, Mulhern R, Fairclough D, et al. Comparison of neuropsychologic functioning and clinical indicators of neurotoxicity in long-term survivors of childhood leukemia given cranial radiation or parenteral methotrexate: a prospective study. J Clin Oncol 1991;9:145–151.

26. Butler RW, Hill JM, Steinherz PG, et al. Neuropsychologic effects of cranial irradiation, intrathecal methotrexate, and systemic methotrexate in childhood cancer. J Clin Oncol 1994;12:2621–2629.

27. Addiego JE Jr, Ridgway D, Bleyer WA. The acute management of intrathecal methotrexate overdose: pharmacologic rationale and guidelines. J Pediatr 1981;98:825–828.

28. Ettinger LJ. Pharmacokinetics and biochemical effects of a fatal intrathecal methotrexate overdose. Cancer 1982;50:444–450.

29. Spiegel RJ, Cooper PR, Blum RH, et al. Treatment of massive intrathecal methotrexate overdose by ventriculolumbar perfusion. N Engl J Med 1984; 311:386–388.

30. Jakobson AM, Kreuger A, Mortimer O, et al. Cerebrospinal fluid exchange after intrathecal methotrexate overdose. A report of two cases. Acta Paediatr 1992;81:359–361.

31. Adamson PC, Balis FM, McCully CL, et al. Rescue of experimental intrathecal methotrexate overdose with carboxypeptidase-G2. J Clin Oncol 1991;9:670–674.

32. Neuwelt EA, Howieson J, Frenkel EP, et al. Therapeutic efficacy of multiagent chemotherapy with drug delivery enhancement by blood-brain barrier modification in glioblastoma. Neurosurgery 1986; 19:573–582.

33. Neuwelt EA, Goldman DL, Dahlborg SA, et al. Primary CNS lymphoma treated with osmotic blood-brain barrier disruption: prolonged survival and preservation of cognitive function. J Clin Oncol 1991; 9:1580–1590.

34. Gumerlock MK, Belshe BD, Madsen R, Watts C. Osmotic blood-brain barrier disruption and chemotherapy in the treatment of high grade malignant glioma: patient series and literature review. J Neurooncol 1992;12:33–46.

35. Neuwelt EA, Glasberg M, Frenkel E, Barnett P. Neurotoxicity of chemotherapeutic agents after blood-brain barrier modification: neuropathological studies. Ann Neurol 1983;14:316–324.

36. Warnke PC, Blasberg RG, Groothuis DR. The effect of hyperosmotic blood-brain barrier disruption on blood-to-tissue transport in ENU-induced gliomas. Ann Neurol 1987;22:300–305.

37. Shapiro WR, Voorhies RM, Hiesiger EM, et al. Pharmacokinetics of tumor cell exposure to [14-C]-methotrexate after intracarotid administration without and with hyperosmotic opening of the blood-brain and blood-tumor barriers in rat brain tumors: a quantitative autoradiography study. Cancer Res 1988;48:694–701.

38. Bruckner H, Glass LL, Chesser MR, McKenna A, Holland JF. Leucovorin's (LV) dose-dependent effect on high-dose (HD) every two week 5-fluorouracil's (5-FU) neurotoxicity (NT) and efficacy against colorectal cancer (abstract). Proc Am Soc Clin Oncol 1989; 8:465.

39. Buroker TR, Moertel CG, Fleming TR, et al. A controlled evaluation of recent approaches to biochemical modulation or enhancement of 5-fluorouracil therapy in colorectal carcinoma. J Clin Oncol 1985;31:1624–1631.

40. Muggia FM, Camacho FJ, Kaplan BH, et al. Weekly 5-fluorouracil combined with PALA: toxic and therapeutic effects in colorectal cancer. Cancer Treat Rep 1967;71:253–256.

41. Kemeny N, Younes A. Alfa-2a interferon and 5-fluorouracil for advanced colorectal carcinoma: the Memorial Sloan-Kettering experience. Semin Oncol 1992;19(Suppl 3):171–175.

42. Woolley PV, Ayoob MJ, Smith FP, et al. A controlled trial of the effect of 4-hydroxypyrazolopyrimidine (allopurinol) on the toxicity of a single bolus dose of 5-fluorouracil. J Clin Oncol 1985;3:103–109.

43. Riehl JB, Brown WJ. Acute cerebellar syndrome secondary to 5-FU therapy. Neurology 1964;14:961–967.

44. Moertel CG, Reitemeier RJ, Bolton CF, Shorter RG. Cerebellar ataxia associated with fluorinated pyrimidine therapy. Cancer Chemother Rep 1964;41:15–18.

45. Curran CF, Luce JK. Fluorouracil and palmar-plantar erythrodysesthesia. Letter to the editor. Ann Intern Med 1989;111:858.

46. Harris BE, Carpenter JT, Diasio RB. Severe 5-fluorouracil toxicity secondary to dihydropyrimidine dehydrogenase deficiency. A potentially more common pharmacogenetic syndrome. Cancer 1991;68:499–501.

47. Amin G, Shahinian H, Miller D, et al. Severe neurotoxicity following 5-fluorouracil (FUra) chemotherapy in patients with dihydropyrimidine dehydrogenase (DPD) deficiency (abstract). Proc Am Soc Clin Oncol 1995;14:A361.

48. Hook CC, Kimmel DW, Kvols LK, et al. Multifocal inflammatory leukoencephalopathy with 5-fluorouracil and levamisole. Ann Neurol 1992;31:262–267.

49. Chen TC, Hinton DR, Leichman L, et al. Mul-

tifocal inflammatory leukoencephalopathy associated with levamisole and 5-fluorouracil: case report. Neurosurgery 1994;35:1138–1143.

50. Kimmel DW, Wijdicks EFM, Rodriguez M. Multifocal inflammatory leukoencephalopathy associated with levamisole therapy. Neurology 1995;45:374–376.

51. Koenig H, Patel A. Biochemical basis for fluorouracil neurotoxicity. The role of Krebs cycle inhibition by fluoroacetate. Arch Neurol 1970;23:155–160.

52. Moore DH, Fowler WC, Crumpler LS. 5-Fluorouracil neurotoxicity. Gynecol Oncol 1990;36:152–154.

53. Chamberlain MC, Khatibi S, Kim JC, et al. Treatment of leptomeningeal metastasis with intraventricular administration of depot cytarabine (DTC 101). A phase I study. Arch Neurol 1993;50:261–264.

54. Kim S, Chatelut E, Kim JC, et al. Extended CSF cytarabine exposure following intrathecal administration of DTC 101. J Clin Oncol 1993;11:2186–2193.

55. Herzig RH, Hines JD, Herzig GP, et al. Cerebellar toxicity with high-dose cytosine arabinoside. J Clin Oncol 1987;5:927–932.

56. Baker WJ, Royer GL Jr, Weiss RB. Cytarabine and neurologic toxicity. J Clin Oncol 1991;9:679–693.

57. Rubin EH, Andersen JW, Berg DT, et al. Risk factors for high-dose cytarabine neurotoxicity: an analysis of a Cancer and Leukemia Group B trial in patients with acute myeloid leukemia. J Clin Oncol 1992; 10:948–953.

58. Winkelman MD, Hines JD. Cerebellar degeneration caused by high-dose cytosine arabinoside. A clinicopathologic study. Ann Neurol 1983;14:246–250.

59. Hwang T-L, Yung WKA, Estey EH, Fields WS. Central nervous system toxicity with high-dose Ara-C. Neurology 1985;35:1475–1479.

60. Breuer AC, Pitman WS, Dawson DM, Schoene WC. Paraparesis following intrathecal cytosine arabinoside. A case report with neuropathologic findings. Cancer 1977;40:2817–2822.

61. Resar LMS, Phillips PC, Kastan MB, et al. Acute neurotoxicity after intrathecal cytosine arabinoside in two adolescents with acute lymphoblastic leukemia of B-cell type. Cancer 1993;71:117–123.

62. Sandler SG, Tobin W, Henderson ES. Vincristine-induced neuropathy: a clinical study of fifty leukemic patients. Neurology 1969;19:367–374.

63. Casey EG, Jellife AM, LeQuesne M, Millett YC. Vincristine neuropathy: clinical and electrophysiological observations. Brain 1973;96:69–86.

64. McGuire SA, Gospe SM Jr, Dahl G. Acute vincristine neurotoxicity in the presence of hereditary motor and sensory neuropathy type I. Med Pediatr Oncol 1989;17:520–523.

65. Williams ME, Walker AN, Bracikowski JP, et al. Ascending myeloencephalopathy due to intrathecal vincristine sulfate. A fatal chemotherapeutic error. Cancer 1983;51:2041–2047.

66. Dyke RW. Treatment of inadvertent intrathecal injection of vincristine. N Engl J Med 1989;32:1270–1271.

67. Jackson DV, Wells HB, Atkins JN, et al. Amelioration of vincristine neurotoxicity by glutamic acid. Am J Med 1988;84:1016–1022.

68. Strong DB, Wenk ML, Contreras PC. Effects of insulin-like growth factor-I on the neurotoxicity and efficacy of antineoplastic agents (abstract). Proc Am Assoc Cancer Res 1994;35:A1921.

69. van Kooten B, van Diemen HAM, Groenhout KM, et al. A pilot study on the influence of a corticotropin (4–9) analogue on vinca alkaloid-induced neuropathy. Arch Neurol 1992;49:1027–1031.

70. Hohneker JA. A summary of vinorelbine (Navelbine) safety data from North American clinical trials. Semin Oncol 1994;21(Suppl 10):42–47.

71. Le Chevalier T, Brisgand D, Douillard J-Y, et al. Randomized study of vinorelbine and cisplatin versus vindesine and cisplatin versus vinorelbine alone in advanced non-small-cell lung cancer: results of a European multicenter trial including 612 patients. J Clin Oncol 1994;12:360–367.

72. Fazeny B, Zifko U, Meryn S, et al. Navelbine-induced neurotoxicity in patients with advanced breast cancer pretreated with paclitaxel (abstract). Proc Am Soc Clin Oncol 1994;13:A29.

73. Feun LG, Stewart DJ, Maor M, et al. A pilot study of cis-diamminedichloroplatinum and radiation therapy in patients with high grade astrocytomas. J Neurooncol 1983;1:109–113.

74. Granowetter L, Rosenstock JC, Packer RJ. Enhanced cis-platinum neurotoxicity in pediatric patients with brain tumors. J Neurooncol 1983;1:293–297.

75. Schaefer SD, Post JD, Close LG, Wright CG. Ototoxicity of low- and moderate-dose cisplatin. Cancer 1985;56:1934–1939.

76. Cohen BH, Zweidler P, Goldwein JW, et al. Ototoxic effect of cisplatin in children with brain tumors. Pediatr Neurosurg 1990–91;16:292–296.

77. Roelofs RI, Hrushesky W, Rogin J, Rosenberg L. Peripheral sensory neuropathy and cisplatin chemotherapy. Neurology 1984;34:934–938.

78. van der Hoop RG, van der Burg MEL, ten Bokkel Huinink WW, et al. Incidence of neuropathy in 395 patients with ovarian cancer treated with or without cisplatin. Cancer 1990;66:1697–1702.

79. Cavaletti G, Marzorati L, Boglium G, et al. Cisplatin-induced peripheral neurotoxicity is dependent on total-dose intensity and single-dose intensity. Cancer 1992;69:203–207.

80. Gregg RW, Molepo JM, Monpetit VJA, et al. Cisplatin neurotoxicity: the relationship between dosage, time, and platinum concentration in neurologic tissues, and morphologic evidence of toxicity. J Clin Oncol 1992;10:795–803.

81. Thompson SW, Davis LE, Kornfeld M, et al. Cisplatin neuropathy. Clinical electrophysiologic, morphologic, and toxicologic studies. Cancer 1984; 54:1269–1275.

82. Riggs JE, Ashraf M, Snyder RD, et al. Prospective nerve conduction studies in cisplatin therapy. Ann Neurol 1988;23:92–94.

83. Boogerd W, ten Bokkel Huinink WW, Dalesio O, et al. Cisplatin induced neuropathy: central, peripheral and autonomic nerve involvement. J Neurooncol 1990;9:255–263.

84. Mollman JE, Hogan WM, Glover DJ, McCluskey LF. Unusual presentation of cis-platinum neuropathy. Neurology 1988;38:488–490.

85. Siegal T, Haim N. Cisplatin-induced peripheral neuropathy. Frequent off-therapy deterioration, demyelinating syndromes, and muscle cramps. Cancer 1990;66:1117–1123.

86. McGuire WP, Hoskins WJ, Brady MF, et al. Cyclophosphamide and cisplatin compared with pacli-

taxel and cisplatin in patients with stage III and stage IV ovarian cancer. N Engl J Med 1996;334:1–6.

87. Mollman JE, Glover DJ, Hogan WM, Furman RE. Cisplatin neuropathy. Risk factors, prognosis, and protection by WR-2721. Cancer 1988;61:2192–2195.

88. Mollman JE. Cisplatin neurotoxicity. N Engl J Med 1990;322:126–127.

89. Capizzi RL. Protection of normal tissues from the cytotoxic effects of chemotherapy by amifostine (Ethyol): clinical experiences. Semin Oncol 1994; 21(Suppl 11):8–15.

90. Alberts DS, Noel JK. Cisplatin-associated neurotoxicity: can it be prevented? Anticancer Drugs 1995; 6:369–383.

91. van der Hoop RG, Vecht CJ, van der Burg MEL, et al. Prevention of cisplatin neurotoxicity with an ACTH (4-9) analogue in patients with ovarian cancer. N Engl J Med 1990;322:89–94.

92. Apfel SC, Arezzo JC, Lipson L, et al. Nerve growth factor prevents experimental cisplatin neuropathy. Ann Neurol 1992;31:76–80.

93. Windebank AJ, Smith AG, Russell JW. The effect of nerve growth factor, ciliary neurotrophic factor, and ACTH analogs on cisplatin neurotoxicity in vitro. Neurology 1994;44:488–494.

94. Gao W-Q, Dybdal N, Shinsky N, et al. Neurotrophin-3 reverses experimental cisplatin-induced peripheral sensory neuropathy. Ann Neurol 1995;38:30–37.

95. Cascinu S, Cordella L, Del Ferro E, et al. Neuroprotective effect of reduced glutathione on cisplatin-based chemotherapy in advanced gastric cancer: a randomized double-blind placebo-controlled trial. J Clin Oncol 1995;13:26–32.

96. Contreras PC, Steffler C, Gruner JA, et al. Insulin-like growth factor-I prevents the peripheral neuropathy induced by paclitaxel, cisplatin, and vincristine. Ann Neurol 1995;38:315–316.

97. Walker RW, Cairncross JG, Posner JB. Cerebral herniation in patients receiving cisplatin. J Neurooncol 1988;6:61–65.

98. Cohen RJ, Cuneo RA, Cruciger MP, et al. Transient left homonymous hemianopsia and encephalopathy following treatment of testicular carcinoma with cisplatinum, vinblastine, and bleomycin. J Clin Oncol 1983;1:392–393.

99. Kupersmith MJ, Frohman LP, Choi IS, et al. Visual system toxicity following intra-arterial chemotherapy. Neurology 1988;38:284–289.

100. Mahaley MS, Hipp SW, Dropcho EJ, et al. Intracarotid cisplatin chemotherapy for recurrent gliomas. J Neurosurg 1989;70:371–378.

101. Newton HB, Page MA, Junck L, Greenberg HS. Intra-arterial cisplatin for the treatment of malignant gliomas. J Neurooncol 1989;7:39–45.

102. Maiese K, Walker RW, Gargan R, Victor JD. Intra-arterial cisplatin-associated optic and otic toxicity. Arch Neurol 1992;49:83–86.

103. Allen JC, Walker R, Luks E, et al. Carboplatin and recurrent childhood brain tumors. J Clin Oncol 1987;5:459–463.

104. Gaynon PS, Ettinger LJ, Baum ES, et al. Carboplatin in childhood brain tumors. A Children's Cancer Study Group phase II trial. Cancer 1990;66:2465–2469.

105. Williams PC, Henner WD, Roman-Goldstein S, et al. Toxicity and efficacy of carboplatin and eto-poside in conjunction with disruption of the blood-brain tumor barrier in the treatment of intracranial neoplasms. Neurosurgery 1995;37:17–28.

106. Aronin PA, Mahaley MS Jr, Rudnick SA, et al. Prediction of BCNU pulmonary toxicity in patients with malignant gliomas. An assessment of risk factors. N Engl J Med 1980;303:183–188.

107. O'Driscoll BR, Haselton PS, Taylor PM, et al. Active lung fibrosis up to 17 years after chemotherapy with carmustine (BCNU) in childhood. N Engl J Med 1990;323:378–382.

108. Jakacki RI, Schramm CM, Donahue BR, et al. Restrictive lung disease following treatment for malignant brain tumors: a potential late effect of craniospinal irradiation. J Clin Oncol 1995;13:1478–1485.

109. Burger PC, Kamenar E, Schold SC, et al. Encephalomyelopathy following high-dose BCNU therapy. Cancer 1981;48:1318–1327.

110. Phillips GL, Wolff SN, Fay JW, et al. Intensive 1, 3-bis (2-chloroethyl)-1-nitrosourea (BCNU) monochemotherapy and autologous marrow transplantation for malignant glioma. J Clin Oncol 1986;4:639–645.

111. Kupersmith MJ, Frohman LP, Choi IS, et al. Visual system toxicity following intra-arterial chemotherapy. Neurology 1988;38:284–289.

112. Wilson WB, Perez GM, Kleinschmidt-DeMasters BK. Sudden onset of blindness in patients treated with oral CCNU and low-dose cranial irradiation. Cancer 1987;59:901–907.

113. Mahaley MS Jr, Whaley RA, Blue M, Bertsch L. Central neurotoxicity following intracarotid BCNU chemotherapy for malignant gliomas. J Neurooncol 1986;3:297–314.

114. Shapiro WR, Green SB. Re-evaluating the efficacy of intra-arterial BCNU. J Neurosurg 1987;66:313–315.

115. Rosenblum MK, Delattre J-Y, Walker RW, et al. Fatal necrotizing encephalopathy complicating treatment of malignant gliomas with intra-arterial BCNU and irradiation: a pathological study. J Neurooncol 1989;7:269–281.

116. Blacklock JB, Wright DC, Dedrick RL, et al. Drug streaming during intra-arterial chemotherapy. J Neurosurg 1986;64:284–291.

117. Saris SC, Shook DR, Blasberg RG, et al. Carotid artery mixing with diastole-phased pulsed drug infusion. J Neurosurg 1987;67:721–725.

118. Yamashima T, Yamashita J, Shoin K. Neurotoxicity of local administration of two nitrosoureas in malignant gliomas. Neurosurgery 1990;26:794–800.

119. Brem H, Mahaley MS Jr, Vick NA, et al. Interstitial chemotherapy with drug polymer implants for the treatment of recurrent gliomas. J Neurosurg 1991; 74:441–446.

120. Brem H, Tamargo RJ, Olivi A, et al. Biodegradable polymers for controlled delivery of chemotherapy with and without radiation therapy in the monkey brain. J Neurosurg 1994;80:283–290.

121. Bluming AZ, Zeegen PL. Cataracts induced by intermittent Decadron used as an antiemetic. J Clin Oncol 1986;4:221–223.

122. Lane RJ, Mastaglia FL. Drug-induced myopathies in man. Lancet 1978;2:562–566.

123. Weissman DE, Duffner D, Vogel V, Abeloff MD. Corticosteroid toxicity in neuro-oncology patients. J Neurooncol 1987;5:125–128.

124. Weissman DE. Glucocorticoid treatment for

brain metastases and epidural spinal cord compression: a review. J Clin Oncol 1988;6:543–551.

125. Vick NA. Letter to the editor. J Neurooncol 1987;6:199.

126. Taylor LP, Posner JB. Steroid myopathy in cancer patients treated with dexamethasone. Neurology 1989;39(Suppl 1):129.

127. Dropcho EJ, Soong S-J. Steroid-induced weakness in patients with primary brain tumors. Neurology 1991;41:1235–1239.

128. DeAngelis LM, Gnecco C, Taylor L, et al. Evolution of neuropathy and myopathy during intensive vincristine/corticosteroid chemotherapy for non-Hodgkin's lymphoma. Cancer 1991;67:2241–2246.

129. Heimdal K, Hirschberg H, Stettebo H, et al. High incidence of serious side effects of high-dose dexamethasone treatment in patients with epidural spinal cord compression. J Neurooncol 1992;12:141–144.

130. Stiefel FC, Breitbart WS, Holland JC. Corticosteroids in cancer: neuropsychiatric complications. Cancer Invest 1989;7:479–491.

131. Haddad SF, Hitchon PW, Godersky JC. Idiopathic and glucocorticoid-induced spinal epidural lipomatosis. J Neurosurg 1991;74:38–42.

132. Rotstein J, Good RA. Steroid pseudorheumatism. Arch Intern Med 1957;99:545–555.

133. Chalk JB, Ridgeway K, Brophy T, Yelland JO, Eadic MJ. Phenytoin impairs the bioavailability of dexamethasone in neurological and neurosurgical patients. J Neurol Neurosurg Psychiatry 1984;47:1087–1090.

134. Lachner TE. Interaction of dexamethasone with phenytoin. Pharmacotherapy 1991;11:344–347.

135. Kirkwood JM, Ernstoff MS. Interferons in the treatment of human cancer. J Clin Oncol 1984;2:336–352.

136. Mahaley MS Jr, Urso MB, Whaley RA, et al. Immunobiology of primary intracranial tumors. Part 10: therapeutic efficacy of interferon in the treatment of recurrent gliomas. J Neurosurg 1985;63:719–725.

137. Quesada JR, Talpaz M, Rios A, Kurzrock R, Gutterman JU. Clinical toxicity of interferons in cancer patients: a review. J Clin Oncol 1986;4:234–243.

138. Spiegel R. The alpha interferons: clinical overview. Semin Oncol 1987;14(Suppl 2):1–12.

139. Figlin RA. Biotherapy with interferon—1988. Semin Oncol 1988;15(Suppl 6):3–9.

140. Krown SE. Approaches to interferon combination therapy in the treatment of AIDS. Semin Oncol 1990;17(Suppl 1):11–15.

141. Triozzi PL, Kinney P, Rinehart JJ. Central nervous system toxicity of biological response modifiers. Ann NY Acad Sci 1990;594:347–354.

142. Rohatiner AZS, Prior PF, Burton AC, et al. Central nervous system toxicity of interferon. Br J Cancer 1983;47:419–422.

143. Meyers CA, Scheibel RS, Forman AD. Persistent neurotoxicity of systemically administered interferon-alpha. Neurology 1991;41:672–676.

144. Meyers CA, Obbens EAMT, Scheibel RS, Moser RP. Neurotoxicity of intraventriculatory administered alpha-interferon for leptomeningeal disease. Cancer 1991;68:88–92.

145. Pavol MA, Meyers CA, Rexer JL, et al. Pattern of neurobehavioral deficits associated with interferon alfa therapy for leukemia. Neurology 1995;45:947–950.

146. Rosenberg SA, Lotze MT, Muul LM, et al. A progress report on the treatment of 157 patients with advanced cancer using lymphokine-activated killer cells and interleukin-2 or high-dose interleukin-2 alone. N Engl J Med 1987;316:889–897.

147. Merchant RE, Grant AJ, Merchant LH, Young HF. Adoptive immunotherapy for recurrent glioblastoma multiforme using lymphokine activated killer cells and recombinant interleukin-2. Cancer 1988; 62:665–671.

148. Parkinson DR. Interleukin-2 in cancer therapy. Semin Oncol 1988;15(Suppl 6):10–26.

149. Demicoff KD, Rubinow DR, Papa MZ, et al. The neuropsychiatric effects of interleukin-2/lymphokine activated killer cell treatment. Ann Intern Med 1987;107:293–300.

150. Bernard JT, Ameriso S, Kempf RA, et al. Transient focal neurologic deficits complicating interleukin-2 therapy. Neurology 1990;40:154–155.

151. Merrill JE. Interleukin-2 effects in the central nervous system. Ann NY Acad Sci 1990;594:188–199.

152. Siegel JP, Puri RK. Interleukin-2 toxicity. J Clin Oncol 1991;9:694–704.

153. Meyers CA, Yung WKA. Delayed neurotoxicity of intraventricular interleukin-2: a case report. J Neurooncol 1993;15:265–267.

154. Forman AD. Neurologic complications of cytokine therapy. Oncology 1994;8:105–110.

155. Rubin AM, Kang H. Cerebral blindness and encephalopathy with cyclosporin A toxicity. Neurology 1987;37:1072–1076.

156. Walker RW, Brochstein JA. Neurologic complications of immunosuppressive agents. Neurol Clin 1988;6:261–278.

157. Zalupski M, Baker LH. Ifosfamide. J Natl Cancer Inst 1988;80:556–566.

158. Fields KK, Elfenbein GJ, Lazarus HM, et al. Maximum tolerated doses of ifosfamide, carboplatin, and etoposide given over 6 days followed by autologous stem-cell rescue: toxicity profile. J Clin Oncol 1995;13:323–332.

159. Pratt CB, Green AA, Horowitz ME, et al. Central nervous system toxicity following the treatment of pediatric patients with ifosfamide/mesna. J Clin Oncol 1986;4:1253–1261.

160. Watkin SW, Husband DJ, Green JA, et al. Ifosfamide encephalopathy: a reappraisal. Eur J Cancer Clin Oncol 1989;25:1303–1310.

161. Anderson NR, Tandon DS. Ifosfamide extrapyramidal neurotoxicity. Cancer 1991;68:72–75.

162. Miller LJ, Eaton VE. Ifosfamide-induced neurotoxicity: a case report and review of the literature. Ann Pharmacother 1992;26:183–187.

163. Simonian NA, Gilliam FG, Chiappa KH. Ifosfamide causes a diazepam-sensitive encephalopathy. Neurology 1993;43:2700–2702.

164. Kupfer A, Aeschlimann C, Wermuth B, et al. Prophylaxis and reversal of ifosfamide encephalopathy with methylene-blue. Lancet 1994;343:763–764.

165. Patel SR, Forman AD, Benjamin RS. High-dose ifosfamide-induced exacerbation of peripheral neuropathy. J Natl Cancer Inst 1994;86:305–306.

166. Rowinsky EK, Donehower RC. Paclitaxel (Taxol). N Engl J Med 1995;332:1004–1014.

167. Rowinsky EK, Chaudhry V, Cornblath DR, Donehower RC. Neurotoxicity of Taxol. Monogr Natl Cancer Inst 1993;15:107–115.

168. Postma TJ, Vermorken JB, Liefting AJ, et al. Paclitaxel-induced neuropathy. Ann Oncol 1995;6:489–494.

169. Capri G, Munzone E, Tarenzi E, et al. Optic nerve disturbances: a new form of paclitaxel neurotoxicity. J Natl Cancer Inst 1994;86:1099–1101.

170. Seidman AD, Barrett S, Canezo S. Photopsia during 3-hour paclitaxel administration at doses >250 mg/m². J Clin Oncol 1994;12:1741–1742.

171. Rowinsky EK, Chaudhry V, Forastiere AA, et al. Phase I and pharmacologic study of paclitaxel and cisplatin with granulocyte colony-stimulating factor: neuromuscular toxicity is dose-limiting. J Clin Oncol 1993;11:2010–2020.

172. Chaudhry V, Rowinsky EK, Sartorius SE, et al. Peripheral neuropathy from Taxol and cisplatin combination chemotherapy: clinical and electrophysiological studies. Ann Neurol 1994;35:304–311.

173. Apfel SC, Lipton RB, Arezzo JC, Kessler JA. Nerve growth factor prevents toxic neuropathy in mice. Ann Neurol 1991;29:87–90.

174. Hilkens PHE, Verweij J, Stoter G, et al. Peripheral neurotoxicity induced by docetaxel. Neurology 1996;46:104–108.

175. New PZ, Jackson CE, Rinaldi D, et al. Peripheral neuropathy secondary to docetaxel (Taxotere). Neurology 1996;46:108–111.

176. La Rocca RV, Meer J, Gilliatt RW, et al. Suramin-induced polyneuropathy. Neurology 1990;40:954–960.

177. Bitton RJ, Figg WO, Venzon DJ, et al. Pharmacologic variables associated with the development of neurologic toxicity in patients treated with suramin. J Clin Oncol 1995;13:2223–2229.

178. Reyno LM, Egorin MJ, Eisenberger MA, et al. Development and validation of a pharmacokinetically based fixed dosing scheme for suramin. J Clin Oncol 1995;13:2187–2195.

179. Russell JW, Windebank AJ, Podratz JL. Role of nerve growth factor in suramin neurotoxicity studied in vitro. Ann Neurol 1994;36:221–228.

180. Byrne TN Jr, Mosely TAE, Finer MA. Myoclonic seizures following chlorambucil overdose. Ann Neurol 1981;9:191–194.

181. Sullivan KM, Storb R, Shulman HM, et al. Immediate and delayed neurotoxicity after mechlorethamine preparation for bone marrow transplantation. Ann Intern Med 1982;97:182–189.

182. Gutin PH, Levi JA, Wiernik PH, Walker MD. Treatment of malignant meningeal disease with intrathecal thioTEPA: a phase II study. Cancer Treat Rep 1977;61:885–887.

183. Leff RS, Thompson JM, Daly MB, et al. Acute neurologic dysfunction after high-dose etoposide therapy for malignant glioma. Cancer 1988;62:32–35.

184. Siegal T, Melamed E, Sandbank U, Cantane R. Early and delayed neurotoxicity of mitoxantrone and doxorubicin following subarachnoid injection. J Neurooncol 1988;6:135–140.

185. Issel BF. Amsacrine (AMSA). Cancer Treat Rev 1980;7:73–83.

186. Mittelman A, Arlin ZA. AMSA-induced seizures in patients with hypokalemia. Cancer Treat Rep 1983;67:102–103.

187. Feinberg WM, Swenson MR. Cerebrovascular complication of L-asparaginase therapy. Neurology 1988;38:127–133.

188. Gutierrez ML, Crooke ST. Mitotane (o,p'-DDD). Cancer Treat Rev 1980;7:49–55.

189. O'Dwyer PJ, Alonso MT, Leyland-Jones B. Acivicin: a new glutamine antagonist in clinical trails. J Clin Oncol 1984;2:1064–1071.

190. Schold SC, Mahaley MS, Vick NA, et al. Phase II diaziquone-based chemotherapy trials in patients with anaplastic supratentorial astrocytic neoplasms. J Clin Oncol 1987;5:464–471.

191. Chun HG, Leyland-Jones BR, Caryk SM, Hoth DF. Central nervous system toxicity of fludarabine phosphate. Cancer Treat Rep 1986;70:1225–1228.

192. Warrell RP, Berman E. Phase I and II study of fludarabine phosphate in leukemia: therapeutic efficacy with delayed central nervous system toxicity. J Clin Oncol 1986;4:74–79.

193. Johnson BL, Fisher RI, Bender RA, DeVita VT Jr, Chabner BA, Young RC. Hexamethylmelamine in alkylating agent-resistant ovarian carcinoma. Cancer 1978;42:2157–2161.

194. Wharton JT, Rutledge F, Smith JP, Herson J, Hodge MP. Hexamethylmelamine: an evaluation of its role in the treatment of ovarian cancer. Am J Obstet Gynecol 1979;133:833–844.

195. Manetta A, MacNeill C, Lyter JA, et al. Hexamethylmelamine as a second-line agent in ovarian cancer. Gynecol Oncol 1990;36:93–96.

196. Warrell RP, Burchenal JH. Methylglyoxalbis(guanylhydrazone) (methyl-GAG): current status and future prospects. J Clin Oncol 1983;1:52–65.

197. Wiley RG, Gralla RJ, Casper ES, Kemeny N. Neurotoxicity of the pyrimidine synthesis inhibitor N-phosphonoacetyl-L-aspartate. Ann Neurol 1982;12:175–183.

198. Brown TD, Ettinger DS, Donehower RC. A phase I trial of spirohydantoin mustard (NSC 172112) in patients with advanced cancer. J Clin Oncol 1986;4:1270–1276.

199. Pazdur R, Redman BG, Corbett T, et al. Phase I trial of spiromustine (NSC 172112) and evaluation of toxicity and schedule in a murine model. Cancer Res 1987;47:4213–4217.

200. Lynch G, Kemeny N, Chun H, et al. Phase I evaluation and pharmacokinetic study of weekly IV thymidine and 5-FU in patients with advance colorectal carinoma. Cancer Treat Rep 1985;69:179–184.

201. Ashford AR, Donev I, Tiwari RP, Garrett TJ. Reversible ocular toxicity related to tamoxifen therapy. Cancer 1988;61:33–35.

202. Pavlidis NA, Petris C, Briassoulis E, et al. Clear evidence that long-term low-dose tamoxifen treatment can induce ocular toxicity. A prospective study of 63 patients. Cancer 1992;69:2961–2964.

203. Pluss JL, DiBella NJ. Reversible central nervous system dysfunction due to tamoxifen in a patient with breast cancer. Ann Intern Med 1984;101:652.

204. Kinsella TJ, Mitchell JB, Russo A, et al. Continuous intravenous infusions of bromodeoxyuridine as a clinical radiosensitizer. J Clin Oncol 1984;2:1144–1150.

205. Greenberg HS, Chandler WF, Diaz RF, et al. Intra-arterial bromodeoxyuridine radiosensitization and radiation in treatment of malignant astrocytomas. J Neurosurg 1988;69:500–505.

206. Gutin PH, Wara WM, Phillips TL, Wilson CB. Hypoxic cell radiosensitizers in the treatment of malignant brain tumors. Neurosurgery 1980;6:567–576.

207. Melgaard B, Hansen HS, Kamieniecka Z, et al. Misonidazole neuropathy: a clinical, electrophysiological, and histological study. Ann Neurol 1982;12:10–17.

208. Melgaard B, Kohler O, Sand Hansen H, et al. Misonidazole neuropathy. A prospective study. J Neurooncol 1988;6:227–230.

209. Kun LE, Ho K-C, Moulder JE. Fatal misonidazole-induced encephalopathy. An RTOG case report. Cancer 1982;49:423–426.

210. Riese NE, Loeffler JS, Wen P, et al. A phase I study of etanidazole and radiotherapy in malignant glioma. Int J Radiat Oncol Biol Phys 1994;29:617–620.

39

Vascular Toxicity

Donald C. Doll and John W. Yarbro

Thrombotic events are well-known complications of cancer. In fact, venous thrombosis, especially if recurrent, should alert one to consider an underlying neoplasm (1). During the past decade, it has become increasingly apparent that the administration of chemotherapy or hormonotherapy may be associated with vascular toxicity (2, 3). Such vascular toxicity encompasses a heterogenous group of disorders, ranging from asymptomatic phlebitis to potentially lethal syndromes such as hepatic venoocclusive disease or thrombotic microangiopathic syndrome. However, the precise pathogenesis of these toxic effects has not been elucidated, and it is not clear whether such events are caused by the antineoplastic agents themselves or by the underlying neoplasms. This chapter reviews various syndromes of vascular toxicity reported to be associated with chemo/hormonotherapy (Table 39.1) and discusses putative pathogenic mechanisms.

PULMONARY VENOOCCLUSIVE DISEASE

Pulmonary venoocclusive disease (PVOD) is an uncommon cause of pulmonary hypertension usually diagnosed by lung biopsy or at autopsy (4). Typical histologic findings of this disorder include occlusion or narrowing of pulmonary veins and venules by loose to paucicellular fibrous material, or less often, collagen-rich connective tissue (4). Although the pathogenesis of PVOD is not clear, exposure to inhaled toxins, respiratory infections, immunologic disorders, and a genetic predisposition have been proposed (4–6). Several cases of PVOD associated with chemotherapy have been described (7–10).

The clinical scenario of PVOD consists of increasing dyspnea, hypoxia, respiratory failure, and pulmonary hypertension, which may cul-

minate in death. Although there are only a few anecdotal reports of PVOD associated with chemotherapy, such findings may be related to a failure to recognize this complication and/or underutilization of elastic tissue stains on histologic examinations.

Rose (7) reported two patients with lymphoma treated with bleomycin and prednisone who were noted at autopsy to have PVOD. Joselson and Warnock (8) described a case of PVOD in a patient with cervical carcinoma who had been treated with bleomycin, mitomycin, and cisplatin. Each patient had evidence of pulmonary interstitial fibrosis at autopsy, and the investigators stressed the importance of using elastic tissue stains to improve the accuracy of the pathologic diagnosis. Waldhorn et al. (9) documented PVOD associated with microangiopathic hemolytic anemia after treatment with 5-fluorouracil, mitomycin, and Adriamycin for gastric cancer, although no autopsy findings of interstitial lung disease or microangiopathic blood changes were observed. In addition, Lombard et al. (10) reported PVOD in two patients after carmustine (BCNU) therapy for malignant gliomas and in one patient following radiation and mechlorethamine, vincristine, procarbazine, and prednisone (MOPP) and cyclophosphamide, vincristine, procarbazine, and prednisone (COPP) chemotherapy for Hodgkin's disease. PVOD has also been reported in a patient with untreated Hodgkin's disease (11) and after preparative regimens for bone marrow transplantation (BMT) (12, 13).

There is no standard effective therapy for PVOD (5). If a diagnosis is established antemortem, the offending drug should be discontinued. Azathioprine, by suppressing autoimmune vasculitis, has been effective in an isolated (not related to chemotherapy) case of PVOD (14). In ad-

Table 39.1. Vascular Complications Reported to be Associated with Antineoplastic Agents

Complications	Drug
Pulmonary venoocclusive disease	Bleomycin
	Mitomycin
	BCNU
Hepatic venoocclusive disease	Cyclophosphamide, BCNU, cisplatin
	Cyclophosphamide, busulfan
	Cyclophosphamide, total body irradiation
	Cyclophosphamide, high-dose cytosine arabinoside
	Dacarbazine
	Urethane
	Azathioprine
	Dactinomycin
	BCNU
	Etoposide
	Mitomycin
	6-Thioguanine
Budd-Chiari syndrome	Dacarbazine
	6-Thioguanine
	Cytosine arabinoside
	Methotrexate
Raynaud's phenomenon	Cisplatin-based chemotherapy
	Bleomycin
	Bleomycin and vinca alkaloid
	Bleomycin, cisplatin, vinca alkaloid
	Bleomycin, doxorubicin and vinblastine
Myocardial infarction and ischemia	Vinca alkaloids
	Vinblastine, bleomycin
	Cisplatin, bleomycin, vinca alkaloid
	Cisplatin, cyclophosphamide, doxorubicin
	Etoposide
	5-Fluorouracil
	Cisplatin, bleomycin, etoposide
Thrombotic microangiopathy	Mitomycin
	Cisplatin
	Carboplatin
	Bleomycin-based chemotherapy
Thrombosis and thromboembolic events	Cyclophosphamide, methotrexate, 5-fluorouracil ± vincristine, prednisone, doxorubicin, tamoxifen
	Cisplatin, vinblastine, bleomycin ± 5-fluorouracil, methotrexate, etoposide
	Paclitaxel
Hypotension	Etoposide
	Tenoposide
	Dacarbazine
	Homoharringtonine
	Vincristine
	BCNU
Hypertension	Cisplatin
	Cisplatin, vinblastine, bleomycin
	Mitomycin
	Procarbazine
Acral erythema	Cytosine arabinoside
	Hydroxyurea
	Protracted infusion of 5-fluorouracil or doxorubicin
	Methotrexate
	Mercaptopurine
	Etoposide

Table 39.1.— (Continued)

Complications	Drug
Leukocytoclastic vasculitis	Hydroxyurea
	Busulfan
	Methotrexate
	Hexamethylene bisacetamide
Retinal toxicity	BCNU (carotid infusion)
	Cisplatin (carotid infusion and intravenous high dose)
	Carboplatin

Adapted from Doll DC, Yarbro JW. Vascular toxicity associated with chemotherapy. Semin Oncol 1992;19:580–596.

dition, decreased pulmonary artery pressure after hydralazine therapy was helpful in one patient (11).

HEPATIC VENOOCCLUSIVE DISEASE

Hepatic venoocclusive disease (HVOD) is a nonthrombotic obliteration of the small intrahepatic branches of the hepatic veins by collagenous and reticular intimal thickening (15–17). By comparison, thrombotic occlusion of the large hepatic veins has been used to define the Budd-Chiari syndrome (15, 18). However, the clinical and pathologic findings may overlap in these syndromes, and distinctions may thus be superfluous. Major causes of HVOD are irradiation (19) and toxic pyrrolizidine alkaloids (16). Several chemotherapeutic agents, including urethane (20), 6-thioguanine (21–23), cytosine arabinoside (24, 25), BCNU (26), busulfan (27), dimethyl-busulfan (28), mitomycin C (29, 30), cyclophosphamide (28), dacarbazine (31), azathioprine (32, 33), and dactinomycin (34, 36) have been implicated in HVOD.

Regarding dactinomycin, there is a higher incidence of hepatic toxicity with the higher single-dose schedule than with divided doses (35). Isolated thrombocytopenia after dactinomycin may be a risk factor for subsequent development of full-blown HVOD (36). In several cases, combination chemotherapy has been administered as preparatory regimens for BMT (13, 23, 24, 26, 30, 31). Indeed, essentially all preparative regimens have been implicated in HVOD, and HVOD is now a major early complication of BMT (37).

In an early study at the University of Washington, in 255 consecutive patients undergoing BMT, the incidence of HVOD was 21% (38). However, HVOD subsequently developed in 109 of 355 consecutive patients (54%) undergoing BMT at their institution (39). Fifty-four patients had severe HVOD and 136 had mild or moderate HVOD. Factors predictive of severe HVOD included vancomycin treatment during cytoreductive therapy, elevated transaminase levels before transplantation, cytoreductive therapy with a high-dose regimen, acyclovir therapy before transplantation, mismatched or unrelated donor marrow, and prior radiation to the abdomen (39). The use of methotrexate for graft-versus-host disease prophylaxis (40), increased plasma levels of busulfan (41), low protein C levels before transplantation (42), and hepatitis C virus infection (43) have also been implicated as risk factors for HVOD. Despite these observations, no clinical factor is definitely predictive of HVOD in an individual patient.

Johns Hopkins investigators also reported HVOD in approximately 20% of their BMT patients (44). They noted this complication only with preparative regimens that used either busulfan or BCNU in combination with cyclophosphamide.

In contrast (38, 44), the Dana Farber group described HVOD in only 12 of 291 (4.1%) patients undergoing autologous BMT (45). In their study, evidence of metastatic liver disease was the only pretreatment factor predictive of HVOD. No individual preparative agent had a significant effect on the development of HVOD. A single 2-hour infusion of BCNU led to a higher frequency of HVOD than the same dose administered in a fractionated schedule.

Recently, Ansher et al. (46) reported that measuring plasma levels of transforming growth factor-β (TGF-β) may be worthwhile as a screening test for the development of HVOD or idiopathic interstitial pneumonitis associated with high-dose chemotherapy and BMT in patients with breast cancer. These investigators showed that the predictive value for the development of either condition was 90% or more when pretransplantation TGF-β levels were more than two standard deviations above the mean established in the control subjects. However, they found no relationship between plasma TGF-β levels and HVOD in patients with leukemia and lymphoma who were treated in a similar manner (47). Hence the role, if any, of TGF-β as a screening test for HVOD has not yet been determined. Also, elevated levels of tumor necrosis factor-α as a predictive test for HVOD needs confirmation (47a).

Clinically, HVOD may appear as weight gain, ascites, painful hepatomegaly, and elevated liver function tests. Persistent thrombocytopenia and refractoriness to platelet transfusions may be an early sign of HVOD (48). The diagnosis may be established by percutaneous or transvenous liver biopsy (15). Hepatic phlebography may be of benefit, because the large hepatic veins are replaced by fine and tortuous hepatic vessels. HVOD may vary from mild and reversible to life-threatening and lethal (49). Bearman et al. (50) developed a mathematical model for predicting fatal outcome after BMT, based on serum bilirubin and weight gain from day 7 before transplantation through day 16 after transplantation. This model may be useful when deciding potential therapeutic interventions for HVOD. Another mode of monitoring HVOD after BMT might be the serum concentration of an aminopeptide of type III procollagen (51, 52). Elevated serum concentration of this factor may identify patients who later develop HVOD. In addition, an increased level of type III procollagen may be helpful in the diagnosis of HVOD and may be used to monitor disease activity (51).

Because severe HVOD is lethal in most patients, interventions would be most welcome. In this regard, continuous low-dose heparin (52, 53), pentoxifylline (54–56), and prostaglandin E$_1$ (57, 58), have all been used as prophylaxis for HVOD. Unfortunately, none of these agents has been shown to be definitely effective in the prevention of HVOD after BMT.

Except for supportive care, there is no standard effective therapy for HVOD. Treatment for severe HVOD with recombinant human tissue plasminogen activator has produced conflicting results (59–61). Further studies of tissue plasminogen activator and similar agents are necessary before any definitive conclusions can be drawn.

Occlusion of the large hepatic veins, manifested clinically as the Budd-Chiari syndrome, has been reported in association with several chemotherapeutic agents. Dacarbazine, alone (62, 63) and in combination with other cytotoxic drugs (64, 65), and 6-thioguanine plus cytosine arabinoside (66) or methotrexate (67) have been described. Scintiscan of the liver in Budd-Chiari syndrome may show caudate sparing and may be helpful in the diagnosis of this condition (68).

Fatal hepatic necrosis with widespread thrombotic occlusion of the small hepatic veins has been observed in patients treated with dacarbazine (69–73). This disorder usually occurs during the second cycle of treatment and is characterized by the sudden onset of nausea, vomiting, and right upper quadrant pain progressing rapidly to circulatory shock and death (70–73).

RAYNAUD'S PHENOMENON

Raynaud's phenomenon is characterized by transient episodes of vasoconstriction accompanied by changes in color of the affected digits. Exposure to cold or emotional stress are common precipitating factors for vasospastic attacks. Raynaud's phenomenon has been documented following the administration of bleomycin alone (74–76) and bleomycin in combinations: bleomycin and a vinca alkaloid (77–83); bleomycin, cisplatin, and a vinca alkaloid (77, 82–95); bleomycin, etoposide, and cisplatin (96); and bleomycin, doxorubicin, and vincristine (97, 98). In addition, Raynaud's phenomenon and digital vasculitis have been reported with interferon therapy (99) and tamoxifen (100).

Vogelzang et al. (77) initially noted Raynaud's phenomenon in 21% of patients with testicular cancer treated with vinblastine and bleomycin and in 41% of patients also treated with cisplatin. Symptoms of painful digital ischemia on cold exposure were present in all 22 patients and occurred a mean of 10 months after the initiation of chemotherapy. Raynaud's phenomenon was usually chronic, persisting for 5 or more years. Although 50% of the patients had clinical improvement over time, 12 patients had lifestyle changes because of intractable digital ischemia. Arteriograms in two of the patients revealed diffuse arterial narrowing consistent with vasculitis or arteritis (77).

Subsequent reports by others noted Raynaud's phenomenon or persistent digital cold sensitivity following cisplatin, bleomycin, and velban in 2.6% to 49% of patients (82, 87, 91–95). Every reported patient with Raynaud's phenomenon has been treated with bleomycin, either alone or in combination regimens. This strongly suggests that bleomycin is the primary drug responsible for this disorder. In some patients, Raynaud's phenomenon is of minor or no clinical concern; in others, it is a severe debilitating chronic problem. Rarely, it may progress to digital gangrene (97, 97a, 98, 98a, 100) that may require amputation (98, 98a).

There are few data regarding the management of therapy-related Raynaud's phenomenon. Topical nitroglycerin and oral tolazaline hydrochloride were of no value in two patients (77). Nifedipine or other calcium channel blockers might be of benefit in some patients (101–103). A decision to discontinue chemotherapy should depend on the severity of the complaints and the type and curability of the tumor being treated.

MYOCARDIAL ISCHEMIA AND INFARCTION

Acute myocardial infarction has been reported to occur in association with vinca alkaloids (104–106); etoposide (107–108); cisplatin (109); vinblastine and bleomycin (110–111); vinblastine, bleomycin, and cisplatin (112–115); cisplatin, cyclophosphamide, and Adriamycin (116); cisplatin, etoposide, and bleomycin (117); and combination chemotherapy for Hodgkin's disease (118). Mediastinal irradiation (107, 116, 119), preexisting coronary artery disease (108, 112), smoking (111), and age greater than 40 years (113) were coexisting factors in some patients. Several patients had no known risk factors for heart disease and had normal coronary angiograms (110, 113, 115, 116, 118). Three patients had a prior history of Raynaud's phenomenon (11–115), and in one patient, ergonovine maleate precipitated diffuse coronary spasm and chest pain (115). In another case, coronary artery occlusion by fibrous intimal proliferation was demonstrated at autopsy (114). These results should be tempered by the data of the Testicular Cancer Intergroup Study (120). They found no greater risk of major cardiovascular complications in patients treated with cisplatin-based chemotherapy for testicular cancer than in an untreated control group.

Cardiac ischemia has been reported in association with vinca alkaloids (121–123), cisplatin (124), cyclophosphamide (125), and bleomycin infusions (126). Of note is the increasing number of reports of cardiac toxicity associated with 5-fluorouracil (127–150). Such toxicity has ranged from asymptomatic electrocardiographic changes to angina pectoris and myocardial infarction with cardiogenic shock and death. In one prospective study of 367 patients treated with continuous infusion of 5-fluorouracil, the incidence of cardiac toxicity was 7.6% (148). Although the mechanism is unknown, these events appear to be more likely when fluorouracil is administered at a high dose by continuous infusion in the presence of preexisting coronary artery disease (146–148). In some cases, prophylaxis with calcium channel blockers was effective in preventing angina (137–140). Physicians should be aware of the potential cardiotoxic properties of fluorouracil, and treatment should be discontinued immediately if coronary symptoms develop.

THROMBOTIC MICROANGIOPATHIC SYNDROME

A thrombotic microangiopathic syndrome characterized by microangiopathic hemolytic anemia, thrombocytopenia, and renal insufficiency has been reported after treatment with chemotherapeutic agents (151). Mitomycin, the most common drug causing this condition, has accounted for at least 150 published cases (152–196). Approximately 90% of patients have had adenocarcinomas, with breast, colorectal, and gastric cancers being most frequent (196). The median age of patients with mitomycin-induced thrombotic microangiopathy is 52 years, with the range of 21 to 86 years (151).

Clinically, virtually all patients have the triad of anemia, thrombocytopenia, and renal dysfunction (196). The anemia is usually severe, and the peripheral blood film reveals schistocytes and helmet cells typical of microangiopathic hemolysis. Most patients show no evidence of consumptive coagulopathy. Less common features include hematuria, congestive heart failure, pulmonary edema, proteinuria, interstitial pneumonitis, rash, fever, hypertension, neurologic changes, and pericarditis (152–196). Most patients with this syndrome have expired of renal failure within a few months after the diagnosis was established (196).

The cardinal histologic features in patients have been abnormalities in the renal vasculature. The principal light microscopic findings have been fibrin deposition and endothelial proliferation of the glomerular capillaries and afferent arterioles. In addition, glomerular basement membrane thickening or glomerular infarcts and necrosis have been described (153, 154, 156, 162–164, 169–171, 175, 182, 184, 187–189, 191, 192, 195). Electron microscopy reveals marked expansion of the glomerular subendothelial space with electron-lucent material. Similar histologic findings have been noted in patients with nephrotoxicity (but without thrombotic microangiopathy) associated with mitomycin (153, 197–200). Histologic findings observed in the mitomycin-associated microangiopathy syndrome are similar to those reported in hemolytic uremic syndrome and thrombotic thrombocytopenic purpura (200).

The incidence of mitomycin-associated thrombotic microangiopathy has been variable. Of 281 patients treated with mitomycin and 5-fluorouracil by the British Stomach Cancer Group (173), 24 (8.5%) developed this complication. In addition, 32 other patients (11.4%) experienced renal insufficiency. None of the 130 placebo-treated controls developed this syndrome, and only 4 had renal insufficiency (173). Hanna et al. (153) reported renal dysfunction in 14 of 143 patients (9.8%) treated with mitomycin and 5-fluorouracil, 2 of whom had evidence of microangiopathy. Death from renal failure occurred in 9 of the 14 patients. Pavy et al. (162) documented renal insufficiency in 4 of 94 patients (4.2%) treated with mitomycin, 2 of whom had microangiopathic hemolysis with renal failure. Valavaara and Nordman (185) observed renal toxicity in 10 of 118 patients (8.5%) treated with mitomycin, 5 of whom had microangiopathic hemolytic anemia. These results suggest that there may be two types of mitomycin-induced renal disorders: (a) a mild-to-severe renal insufficiency without microangiopathic hemolytic anemia and (b) renal failure as part of a more generalized thrombotic microangiopathic syndrome.

The onset of thrombotic microangiopathy associated with mitomycin is usually within 4 to 9 weeks from the last dose of chemotherapy, although it may occur, on occasion, 4 to 15 months after discontinuation of treatment (157, 161, 164, 174, 180, 196). It appears that this complication is dose related, with most patients having received a cumulative dose of mitomycin greater than 60 mg (196). Clinicians should be aware of the fact that the syndrome may develop at any time while the patient is receiving mitomycin and for months after treatment is discontinued. In general, corticosteroids, antiplatelet agents, and red blood cell transfusions have been ineffective as treatment of thrombotic microangiopathic syndrome. In fact, red blood cell transfusions may exacerbate renal failure and microangiopathic hemolysis and may precipitate acute pulmonary edema (156, 161, 163, 166, 169,

171, 181, 183, 188). Hence, red blood cell transfusions should be used with caution. Such progression after blood transfusions may be caused by activation of intravascular clotting (201). Plasma exchange or plasmapheresis in combination with other therapeutic modalities has been used in several patients (152, 165, 166, 170, 172, 186–189, 202). Although hemolytic anemia improved in some patients, renal failure was usually progressive and required maintenance dialysis. Cyclophosphamide, vincristine, and azathioprine have been tried in a few cases (186, 203, 204). Recently, protein A immunoadsorption of plasma has been used in the treatment of chemotherapy-associated microangiopathy syndrome (205, 206). Response to therapy was observed in 25 of 55 patients, with an estimated 1-year survival of 61% in responders. Clinical responses were correlated with normalization of serum levels of circulating immune complexes and complement components C3c and C4. This new modality may be the preferred treatment in patients with chemotherapy-induced thrombotic microangiopathic syndrome.

Thrombotic microangiopathy has also been described with other types of chemotherapy, including cisplatin and bleomycin regimens (207–213), carboplatin (214), and following combination chemotherapy for lymphoma (213, 215, 216) and acute leukemia (217). The clinical course is similar to that described with mitomycin.

THROMBOSIS AND THROMBOEMBOLIC COMPLICATIONS

The relationship between cancer and a hypercoagulable state has been well recognized for over a century (218). Chemo- or hormonotherapy may also be associated with thromboembolic phenomena, including venous and arterial thrombosis, cerebrovascular accidents, pulmonary embolism, and intestinal infarction (2, 3). Such complications have been described primarily with combination chemotherapy regimens for the treatment of head and neck cancer (207, 219, 220), germ cell tumors of the testis (113, 115, 221–223), lymphoma (225–228), and breast cancer (229–241).

Kukla et al. (219) reported five patients with squamous cell carcinoma of the head and neck who developed cerebrovascular accidents associated with cisplatin-based chemotherapy. Each of the patients was at least 50 years old, and three had a prior history of heart disease or stroke.

Licciardello et al. (207) described acute cerebrovascular events in two patients with head and neck cancer after administration of cisplatin and bleomycin or vindesine. Pretreatment levels of von Willebrand factor antigen (vWFAg) were elevated in each patient who developed acute strokes and showed further elevation after the administration of chemotherapy. On the other hand, none of 11 patients with normal pretreatment vWFAg levels experienced thrombotic events. Fallon et al. (220) documented 21 vascular complications during 400 cycles of cisplatin-based neoadjuvant chemotherapy for advanced squamous cell carcinoma of the head and neck. Every patient with these complications had at least two risk factors for cardiovascular disease.

Pulmonary emboli, deep venous thrombosis, cerebrovascular accidents, and mesenteric infarction have been documented during cisplatin combination chemotherapy for testicular cancer (113, 115, 117, 221–223). Ten of 52 (19%) newly diagnosed patients with germ cell tumors treated with cisplatin combinations by Cantwell et al. (223) had vascular events (3 arterial and 7 venous or pulmonary). These investigators noted a higher frequency of retroperitoneal metastases in patients with vascular complications than in those without such metastases. As mentioned above, however, the Testicular Cancer Intergroup Study (120) found no increased risk of cardiovascular events in patients with testicular cancer treated with cisplatin-based chemotherapy. Nonetheless, many patients who have testicular cancer are young and have no risk factors for vascular disease. Hence, one should at least be cognizant of potential vascular complications occurring during or shortly after treatment.

Lynch et al. (224) described two cases of myocardial infarction, one case of fatal pulmonary embolism, and one case of cerebrovascular accident following treatment with cisplatin, etoposide, and 5-fluorouracil infusion for non-small-cell lung cancer. Although each patient had risk factors for vascular disease, the authors suggested that the chemotherapy itself may have been a major factor in the thrombotic events.

Mortimer et al. (109) documented seven thromboembolic disorders during 57 cycles of intraarterial cisplatin and radiation therapy for primary brain tumors. Thrombotic disorders included pulmonary embolism, deep vein thrombosis, myocardial infarction, septic phlebitis, and hemorrhagic infarction.

There have been several reports of arterial and venous thrombosis in patients with breast cancer treated with chemotherapy protocols based on cyclophosphamide, methotrexate, 5-fluorouracil regimens, with or without vincristine, prednisone, tamoxifen, and doxorubicin (229, 232–241). Weiss et al. (229) initially documented a 5% incidence of thrombosis in 433 postmastectomy breast cancer patients treated with adjuvant chemotherapy. These investigators subsequently reported arterial thrombosis in 13 of 1014 (1.3%) patients with stage II or III breast cancer treated with combination chemotherapy. These results have been confirmed by others (232–238, 240, 241). The Eastern Cooperative Oncology Group (ECOG) (235) noted a frequency of venous and arterial thrombosis of 5.4% among 2352 patients treated with adjuvant chemotherapy or chemotherapy plus tamoxifen compared with 321 patients (1.6%, $p = .0002$) who were observed without treatment. The European Organization for Research and Treatment of Breast Cancer (240) reported thromboembolic events in 27 of 1292 patients (2.1%) assigned to chemotherapy compared with 10 of 1332 patients (0.8%) on an observation arm ($p = .004$). The Southwest Oncology Group also noted an increased incidence of thromboembolic complications in breast cancer patients treated with combination chemotherapy and tamoxifen (238). (Of note, the thrombotic events in all of the aforementioned studies always occurred while the patients were being treated with chemotherapy, with or without hormone therapy.) Very low dose warfarin may prevent such vascular complications in breast cancer patients who are receiving chemotherapy (241).

In addition, thromboses and thromboembolic phenomena have been described in patients undergoing chemotherapy for lymphoma (225–228), prostate cancer (242), osteogenic sarcoma (243), and esophageal cancer (244). Paclitaxel (245), α-interferon (246), and colony-stimulating factors (247–249) have also been implicated as causative factors in thrombotic events. Finally, although it has been suggested that tamoxifen is a risk factor for thromboembolic disease (234, 250), Rutguist and Mattson (251) found no increase in thrombotic events among breast cancer patients treated with tamoxifen alone or in combination with chemotherapy, compared with a no-treatment control arm.

HYPOTENSION AND HYPERTENSION

Hypotension associated with chemotherapy may be due to additives present in the pharmaceutical preparation, rapid infusion of the drug, or alterations of the autonomic nervous system, or it may be part of a hypersensitivity reaction. Rapid infusion of etoposide (252) or teniposide (253) may cause hypotension. Infusion over 30 to 60 minutes is usually not associated with this problem. It has been suggested that the diluent or other additives may cause the hypotension associated with etoposide (254).

Hypotension may be a dose-limiting complication associated with high-dose dacarbazine (255), high-dose BCNU (256), and homoharringtonine (257, 259). Citric acid present in the pharmaceutical preparation may cause the hypotension that occurs with dacarbazine (255). Although orthostatic hypotension is a well-known complication of vincristine (260, 261), it is uncommon, with an incidence of only 4% (1 of 26 patients) in a prospective study (261). Such hypotension may be due to drug-induced impairment in norepinephrine secretion (260) or may represent a neurotoxic reaction (261).

Sustained hypertension has been reported after intraarterial cisplatin (262). In addition, accelerated hypertension was noted in a patient following treatment with cisplatin, vinblastine, and bleomycin (263). Renal biopsy revealed narrowing of the interlobular arteries and fibrin thrombosis of the afferent arterioles. Hypertension has been documented in 16 to 17% of testicular cancer patients treated with cisplatin, bleomycin, and vinblastine (264, 295).

Hypertension may also develop in patients receiving procarbazine after ingestion of foods with a high tyramine content (265), as part of a hypersensitivity reaction to chemotherapy (266, 267), and as a manifestation of the thrombotic microangiopathy syndrome (151).

ACRAL ERYTHEMA

Acral erythema is a distinct entity characterized by a painful, sharply demarcated, and intense erythema of the palms, fingers, and soles of the feet that is followed by bullae formation, desquamation, and healing (268). High-dose cytosine arabinoside (268–271), standard-dose cytosine arabinoside (271), hydroxyurea (272), fluorouracil (especially prolonged and continuous infusions) (273–278), methotrexate (279), mercaptopurine (280), high-dose etoposide (281), and combination chemotherapy (269, 282) have all been reported to cause acral erythema. The pain associated with this disorder may be so intense that intravenous narcotics are necessary for relief. Pain may be worsened by cyclosporine in-

fusions (268) and may be alleviated by pyridoxine (267). Nicotine patches may act as prophylaxis for 5-fluorouracil-associated dermatitis (283).

LEUKOCYTOCLASTIC VASCULITIS

Leukocytoclastic vasculitis is a disorder of small cutaneous vessels with typical histologic features of fibrinoid degeneration and destruction of the blood vessel wall, with predominantly neutrophilic infiltration into the vessel wall perivascular region, hemorrhage, and leukocytoclasis (284). Palpable purpura of the lower extremities is the most common manifestation, but urticarial, infarctive, ulcerative, or livedoid lesions, nodules, vesicles, pustules, or bullae may be evident in affected patients (284). Leukocytoclastic vasculitis has been associated with the use of hydroxyurea (269), methotrexate (285–287), busulfan (269), and hexamethylene bisacetamide (288). Such vasculitis is probably due to a hypersensitivity reaction (267).

RETINAL TOXICITY

Retinal toxicity, manifested by unilateral fundal hemorrhages and exudates, was reported by Greenberg et al. (289) in four of six patients after intraarterial BCNU chemotherapy for malignant brain tumors. Three of the four patients developed blindness. Fluorescein angiography disclosed an arterial phase leak consistent with a toxic retinal vasculitis in two patients. Corneal opacities and blindness were previously observed in laboratory animals after intracarotid BCNU (290).

Bernauer et al. (291) documented an ocular microvasculopathy in 13 of 127 patients (10%) after BMT. All patients had cotton-wool spots in the fundus of both eyes, and three patients had bilateral optic-disc edema. The authors attributed these ischemic lesions to cyclosporine and total body irradiation.

Optic neuropathy, maculopathy, blurred vision, and altered color perception have been reported in association with high-dose intravenous cisplatin (292), intracarotid infusion of cisplatin (293), and carboplatin (294). Ophthalmologic examination is warranted in patients undergoing treatment with these agents if ocular complaints are noted.

PATHOGENESIS

The precise pathogenesis of vascular disorders associated with antineoplastic agents is not clear, and the role of specific drugs in the development of all of these phenomena is speculative. Nevertheless, there are several putative mechanisms.

One possible mechanism is endothelial cell damage secondary to antineoplastic agents and/or one of their metabolites (295, 296). In this regard, bleomycin causes a direct toxic effect on endothelial cells, capillaries, and small arterioles (297). Histologic studies of tumor specimens obtained after bleomycin have shown endothelial lesions ranging from vacuolization to detachment and necrosis (297). Further, bleomycin stimulates collagen production and fibroblast proliferation in vitro, and scleroderma has been reported after bleomycin treatment (298–300). Nitrosoureas, vincristine, doxorubicin, cyclophosphamide, and mitomycin may induce endothelial cell alterations in animal models and in vitro–cultured endothelial cells (296, 301, 302). Endothelial cell injury may be associated with abnormalities of von Willebrand factor (vWF), and increased vWF activity has been reported in patients with drug-associated vascular complications (207, 303). Moreover, increases in serum angiotensin-converting enzyme activity (304, 305) and endothelin (306, 307) may be secondary to endothelial cell injury and have been reported in animals treated with nitrosoureas (304) and bleomycin (305).

Drug-induced perturbation of the clotting cascade or platelet activation is another possible mechanism. Bleomycin (308), cisplatin (309), and high-dose chemotherapy (310) may induce platelet activation and aggregation. Cisplatin may produce such an effect via monocyte procoagulant activity (309). Antineoplastic agents may reduce fibrinolytic activity (311), increase fibrinopeptide A levels (312, 313), decrease thrombin time and partial thromboplastin time (314), and reduce levels of proteins C and S (315–318). Furthermore, tamoxifen may decrease antithrombin III levels (319–322), although this may not be clinically significant (321, 322). Such alterations in the coagulation system could induce a hypercoagulable state and initiate thrombosis.

An abnormality in the cytokine network is another possible factor. Tumor necrosis factor-α is known to downregulate thrombomodulin, prostaglandins E_1 and E_2, and protein S and upregulate cellular adhesion molecules and platelet-derived growth factor, producing a procoagulant effect (323, 324). Overexpression of tumor necrosis factor-α messenger RNA has been reported in peripheral mononuclear cells in the posttransplantation state (325). An abnormality of this cytokine or others (46) may be a causative factor in HVOD.

Hypomagnesemia may be involved in the development of vasospastic disorders (112). Hypomagnesemia, a common toxicity of cisplatin, occurs in 75 to 87% of patients (112, 326). Magnesium has a major role in the maintenance of vascular smooth muscle tone (327, 328), and magnesium deficiency has been observed to produce coronary artery spasm in dogs (327). Raynaud's phenomenon has been documented in patients who did not receive cisplatin, however (74–83). Finally, the idea of an abnormality in the sympathetic nervous system should be entertained. Autonomic neuropathy has been reported after treatment with cisplatin alone (329); cisplatin, vinblastine, and bleomycin (330); and vinca alkaloids (331–334). Autonomic dysfunction, in particular enhanced α-adrenergic tone, may potentiate arterial vasospasm. These observations suggest that multiple pathogenic mechanisms may be acting in concert and that the response of the host to both the cancer and its treatment may be central to our understanding of these heterogenous vascular events.

ACKNOWLEDGMENT

We are grateful to Jackie Rahmer for expert secretarial assistance.

REFERENCES

1. Prandoni P, Lensing AWA, Buller HR, et al. Deep-vein thrombosis and the incidence of subsequent symptomatic cancer. N Engl J Med 1992;327:1128–1133.

2. Doll DC, Yarbro JW. Vascular toxicity associated with antineoplastic agents. Semin Oncol 1992;19:580–596.

3. Doll DC, Yarbro JW. Vascular toxicity associated with chemotherapy and hormonotherapy. Curr Opin Oncol 1994;6:345–350.

4. Wagevoort CA. Pulmonary veno-occlusive disease. Entity or syndrome? Chest 1976;69:82–86.

5. Thadany V, Burrow C, Whitaker W, et al. Pulmonary veno-occlusive disease. Q J Med 1975;44:133–159.

6. Corrin G, Spencer H, Turner-Warwich M, et al. Pulmonary veno-occlusion—an immune complex disease? Virchows Arch [A] 1974;364:81–91.

7. Rose AG. Pulmonary veno-occlusive disease due to bleomycin therapy for lymphoma. S Afr Med J 1983; 64:636–638.

8. Joselson R, Warnock M. Pulmonary veno-occlusive disease after chemotherapy. Hum Pathol 1983; 13:88–91.

9. Waldhorn RE, Tsou E, Smith FP, et al. Pulmonary veno-occlusive disease associated with microangiopathic hemolytic anemia and chemotherapy of gastric adenocarcinoma. Med Pediatr Oncol 1984;12:394–396.

10. Lombard CM, Churg A, Winokur S. Pulmonary veno-occlusive disease following therapy for malignant neoplasms. Chest 1987;92:871–876.

11. Capewell SJ, Wright AJ, Ellis DA. Pulmonary veno-occlusive disease in association with Hodgkin's disease. Thorax 1984;39:554–555.

12. Troussard X, Bernaudin JF, Cordonnier C, et al. Pulmonary veno-occlusive disease after bone marrow transplantation. Thorax 1984;39:956–957.

13. Giralt SA, LeMaistre CF, Vriesendorp HM, et al. Etoposide, cyclophosphamide, total body in irradiation, and allogenic bone marrow transplantation for hematologic malignancies. J Clin Oncol 1990;12:1923–1930.

14. Sanderson JE, Spiro SG, Hendry AT, et al. A case of pulmonary veno-occlusive disease responding to treatment with azathioprine. Thorax 1977;32:140–148.

15. Zafrani S, Pinaudeau Y, Dhumeaux D. Drug-induced vascular lesions of the liver. Arch Intern Med 1983;143:495–502.

16. Bras G, Jelliffe DB, Stuart KL. Veno-occlusive disease of liver with non-portal type of cirrhosis occurring in Jamaica. Arch Pathol Lab Med 1954;57:285–300.

17. Rollins BJ. Hepatic veno-occlusive disease. Am J Med 1986;81:297–306.

18. Ledwig J, Hashimoto E, McGill DB. Classification of hepatic venous outflow obstruction: ambiguous terminology of the Budd-Chiari syndrome. Mayo Clin Proc 1990;65:51–55.

19. Reed GB Jr, Cox AJ Jr. The human liver after radiation injury: a form of veno-occlusive disease. Am J Pathol 1966;48:597–611.

20. Brodsky I, Johnson H, Killmann SA, et al. Fibrosis of central and hepatic veins, and perisinusoidal spaces of the liver following prolonged administration of urethane. Am J Med 1961;30:976–980.

21. Griner PF, Elbadawi A, Packman CH. Veno-occlusive disease of the liver after chemotherapy of acute leukemia: report of two cases. Ann Intern Med 1976;85:578–582.

22. Gill RA, Onstad GR, Cardamone JM, et al. Hepatic veno-occlusive disease caused by 6-thioguanine. Ann Intern Med 1982;96:58–60.

23. Sloane JP, Farthing MJG, Powles PL. Histopathological changes in the liver after allogeneic bone marrow transplantation. J Clin Pathol 1980;33:344–348.

24. Woods WG, Dehner LP, Nesbit ME, et al. Fatal veno-occlusive disease of the liver following high dose chemotherapy, irradiation and bone marrow transplantation. Am J Med 1980;68:285–290.

25. Burkhardt A, Kloppel G. Unusual obliterative disease of the hepatic veins in an infant. Virchows Arch [A] 1977;375:225–232.

26. McIntyre RE, Magidson JG, Austin GE, et al. Fatal veno-occlusive disease of the liver following high-dose 1,3-bis (2-chloroethyl)-1-nitrosourea (BCNU) and autologous bone marrow transplantation. Am J Clin Pathol 1981;75:614–617.

27. Vassal G, Hartmann O, Benhamon E. Busulfan and veno-occlusive disease of the liver (letter). Ann Intern Med 1990;112:881.

28. Shulman HM, McDonald GB, Matthews D, et al. An analysis of hepatic veno-occlusive disease and centrilobular hepatic degeneration following bone marrow transplantation. Cancer 1982;79:1178–1191.

29. Lazarus HM, Gottfried MR, Herzig RH, et al. Veno-occlusive disease of the liver after high-dose mitomycin C therapy and autologous bone marrow transplantation. Cancer 1982;49:1789–1795.

30. Gottfried MR, Sudilovsky O. Hepatic veno-occlusive disease after high-dose mitomycin C and autologous bone marrow transplantation therapy. Hum Pathol 1982;13:646–650.

31. Erichsen C, Jonsson PE. Veno-occlusive liver disease after dacarbazine therapy (DTIC) for melanoma. J Surg Oncol 1984;27:268–270.

32. Marubbio AT, Danielson B. Hepatic veno-occlusive disease in a renal transplant patient receiving azathioprine. Gastroenterology 1975;69:739–743.

33. Read AE, Wiesner RH, LaBrecque DR, et al. Hepatic veno-occlusive disease associated with renal transplantation and azathioprine therapy. Ann Intern Med 1986;104:651–655.

34. Green DM, Finkelstein JZ, Norkool P, et al. Severe hepatic toxicity after treatment with single-dose dactinomycin and vincristine. Cancer 1988;62:270–273.

35. Green DM, Norkool P, Breslow NE, et al. Severe hepatic toxicity after treatment with vincristine and dactinomycin using single-dose or divided-dose schedules: a report from the National Wilm's Tumor Study. J Clin Oncol 1990;8:1525–1530.

36. Raine J, Bowman A, Wallendszusk, et al. Hepatopathy-thrombocytopenia syndrome—a complication of dactinomycin therapy for Wilm's tumor. A report from the United Kingdom Children's Cancer Study Group. J Clin Oncol 1991;9:268–273.

37. Bearman SI. The syndrome of hepatic veno-occlusive disease after marrow transplantation. Blood 1995;85:3005–3020.

38. McDonald GB, Sharma P, Matthews DE, et al. Veno-occlusive disease of the liver after bone marrow transplantation: diagnosis, incidence, and predisposing factors. Hepatology 1984;4:116–122.

39. McDonald GB, Hinds MS, Fisher LD, et al. Veno-occlusive disease of the liver and multiorgan failure after bone marrow transplantation: a cohort study of 355 patients. Ann Intern Med 1993;118:255–267.

40. Essel JH, Thompson JM, Harman GS, et al. Increase in veno-occlusive disease of the liver associated with methotrexate use for graft-versus-host disease prophylaxis in patients receiving busulfan/cyclophosphamide. Blood 1992;79:2784–2788.

41. Grochow LB, Jones RJ, Brundett RB, et al. Pharmacokinetics of busulfan: correlation with veno-occlusive disease in patients undergoing bone marrow transplantation. Cancer Chemother Pharmacol 1989;25:55–61.

42. Faioni E, Krachmalnicoff A, Bearman SI, et al. Naturally occurring anticoagulants and bone marrow transplantation: plasma protein C predicts the development of veno-occlusive disease of the liver. Blood 1993;81:3458–3462.

43. Frikhofen N, Wiesneth M, Jainta C, et al. Hepatitis C virus infection is a risk factor for liver failure from veno-occlusive disease after bone marrow transplantation. Blood 1994;83:1998–2004.

44. Beschorner WE, Pino J, Boitnott JK, et al. Pathology of the liver with bone marrow transplantation: effects of busulfan, carmustine, acute graft-versus-host disease, and cytomegalovirus infection. Am J Pathol 1980;99:369–386.

45. Ayash LJ, Hunt M, Antman K, et al. Throm-

bocytopenia in veno-occlusive disease in autologous bone marrow transplantation of solid tumors and lymphomas. J Clin Oncol 1990;8:1699–1706.

46. Anscher MS, Peters WP, Reisenbichler H, Petros WP, Jirtle RL. Transforming growth factor B as a predictor of liver and lung fibrosis after autologous bone marrow transplantation for advanced breast cancer. N Engl J Med 1993;328:1592–1598.

47. Murase T, Jirtle RL, McDonald GB. Transforming growth factor β plasma concentrations in patients with leukemia and lymphoma receiving chemoradiotherapy and marrow transplantation (letter). Blood 1994;83:2383–2384.

47a. Gugliotta L, Catani L, Vianelli N, et al. High plasma levels of tumor necrosis factor-alpha may be predictive of veno-occlusive disease in bone marrow transplantation (letter). Blood 1994;83:2385–2386.

48. Rio B, Andreu G, Nicod A, et al. Thrombocytopenia in veno-occlusive disease after bone marrow transplantation or chemotherapy. Blood 1986;67:1773–1776.

49. Blostein MD, Paltiel OB, Thibaeelt A, Rybka WB. A comparison of clinical criteria for the diagnosis of veno-occlusive disease of the liver after bone marrow transplantation. Bone Marrow Transplant 1992; 10:439–443.

50. Bearman SI, Anderson GL, Mori M, Hinds MS, Shulman HM, McDonald GB. Veno-occlusive disease of the liver: development of a model for predicting fatal outcome after marrow transplantation. J Clin Oncol 1993;11:1729–1736.

51. Eltani M, Trivedi P, Hobbs JR, et al. Monitoring of veno-occlusive disease after bone marrow transplantation by serum aminopropeptide of type III procollagen. Lancet 1993;342:518–521.

52. Attal M, Huguet F, Rubie H, et al. Prevention of hepatic veno-occlusive disease after bone marrow transplantation by continuous infusion of low-dose heparin: a prospective, randomized trial. Blood 1992; 79:2834–2840.

52a. Heikinheimo M, Halila R, Fasth JA. Serum procollagen type II is an early and sensitive marker for veno-occlusive disease of the liver in children undergoing bone marrow transplantation. Blood 1994; 83:3036–3040.

53. Cahn JY, Flesch M, Brion A, et al. Prevention of veno-occlusive disease of the liver after bone marrow transplantation: heparin or no heparin? Blood 1992; 80:2149–2150.

54. Bianco JA, Appelbaum FR, Nemunaitis J, et al. Phase I-II trial of pentoxifylline for the prevention of transplant-related toxicities following bone marrow transplantation. Blood 1991;78:1205–1211.

55. Clift RA, Bianco JA, Appelbaum FR, et al. A randomized controlled trial of pentoxifylline for the prevention of regimen-related toxicities in patients undergoing allogeneic marrow transplantation. Blood 1993;82:2025–2030.

56. Attal M, Huguet F, Rubie H, et al. Prevention of regimen-related toxicities after bone marrow transplantation by pentoxifylline: a prospective, randomized trial. Blood 1993;82:732–736.

57. Bearman SI, Shen DD, Hinds MS, Hill HA, McDonald GB. A phase I/II study of prostaglandin E₁ for the prevention of hepatic veno-occlusive disease after bone marrow transplantation. Br J Haematol 1993; 84:727–730.

58. Gluckman E, Jolivet I, Scrobohaci ML, et al. Use of prostaglandin E₁ for prevention of liver veno-occlusive disease in leukemic patients treated by allogeneic bone marrow transplantation. Br J Haematol 1990; 74:277–281.

59. Bearman SI, Shuhart MC, Hinds MS, McDonald GB. Recombinant human tissue plasminogen activator for the treatment of established severe veno-occlusive disease of the liver after bone marrow transplantation. Blood 1992;80:2458–2462.

60. Rostic G, Bandini G, Belardinelli A, et al. Alteplase for hepatic veno-occlusive disease after bone marrow transplantation. Lancet 1992;339:1481–1482.

61. Ringden O, Wennberg L, Ericzon BG, et al. Alteplase for veno-occlusive disease after bone marrow transplantation. Lancet 1992;340:546–547.

62. Greenstone MA, Dowd PM, Mikhailidis DP, et al. Hepatic vascular lesions associated with dacarbazine treatment. Br Med J 1981;282:1744–1745.

63. Asbury RF, Rosenthal SN, Descalzi ME, et al. Hepatic veno-occlusive disease due to DTIC. Cancer 1980;45:2670–2674.

64. Houghton AN, Shafi N, Rickles FR. Acute hepatic vein thrombosis occurring during therapy for Hodgkin's disease. A case report. Cancer 1979;44:2324–2329.

65. Lehrner IM, Enck RE. Hepatic vein thrombosis after chemotherapy for histiocytoma (letter). Ann Intern Med 1977;88:575–576.

66. Wasser JS, Coleman M. Leukemia chemotherapy and centrilobular hepatic necrosis (letter). Ann Intern Med 1977;86:508–509.

67. Krivoy N, Raz R, Carter A, et al. Reversible hepatic veno-occlusive disease and 6-thioguanine (letter). Ann Intern Med 1982;96:788.

68. Meindok H, Langer B. Liver scan in Budd-Chiari syndrome. J Nucl Med 1976;17:365–368.

69. Frosch PJ, Czarnetzki BM, Macher E, et al. Hepatic failure in a patient treated with dacarbazine (DTIC) for malignant melanoma. J Cancer Res Clin Oncol 1979;95:281–286.

70. Feaux de Lacroix W, Runne U, Hauk H, et al. Acute liver dystrophy with thrombosis of hepatic veins: a fatal complication of dacarbazine treatment. Cancer Treat Rep 1983;67:779–784.

71. Joensuu H, Soderstrom K-O, Mikkanen V. Fatal necrosis of the liver during ABVD chemotherapy for Hodgkin's disease. A case report. Cancer 1986;58:1437–1440.

72. McClay E, Lusch CJ, Mastrangelo MJ. Allergy-induced hepatic toxicity associated with dacarbazine (letter). Cancer Treat Rep 1987;71:219–220.

73. Ceci G, Bella M, Melissani M, et al. Fatal hepatic vascular toxicity of DTIC: is it really a rare event? Cancer 1988;61:1988–1991.

74. Sundstrup B. Raynaud's phenomenon after bleomycin treatment (letter). Med J Aust 1978;2:266.

75. Adoue D, Arlet P. Bleomycin and Raynaud's phenomenon (letter). Ann Intern Med 1984;100:770.

76. Malcom D. Bleomycin-induced injury to the hands. J Med Soc NJ 1978;75:314–316.

77. Vogelzang NJ, Bosl GJ, Johnson K, et al. Raynaud's phenomenon: a common toxicity after combination chemotherapy for testicular cancer. Ann Intern Med 1981;95:288–292.

78. Teutsch C, Lipton A, Harvey HA. Raynaud's phenomenon as a side effect of chemotherapy with

vinblastine and bleomycin for testicular cancer. Cancer Treat Rep 1977;61:925–926.

79. Rothberg H. Raynaud's phenomenon after vinblastine-bleomycin chemotherapy (letter). Cancer Treat Rep 1978;62:569–570.

80. Soble AR. Chronic bleomycin-associated Raynaud's phenomenon (letter). Cancer Treat Rep 1978; 62:570.

81. Chernicoff DP, Bukowski RM, Young JR. Raynaud's phenomenon after bleomycin treatment (letter). Cancer Treat Rep 1978;62:570–571.

82. Schulen ME, Schmidt CG. Raynaud's phenomenon and cancer chemotherapy (letter). Ann Intern Med 1982;96:256.

83. Paty JG Jr, Ruffner BW. Bleomycin-vinblastine associated Raynaud's phenomenon (letter). J Rheumatol 1980;7:927–928.

84. Vogelzang NJ. Raynaud's phenomenon and cancer chemotherapy (letter). Ann Intern Med 1982; 96:256.

85. Grau JJ, Grau M, Milla A, et al. Cancer chemotherapy and Raynaud's phenomenon (letter). Ann Intern Med 1983;98:258.

86. Dunlop PR, Hendy-Ibbs PM. Raynaud's phenomenon and cryoglobulinemia during chemotherapy for testicular cancer (letter). Cancer Treat Rep 1983; 67:317–318.

87. Garnick MB, Canellos GP, Richie JP. Treatment and surgical staging of testicular and primary extragonadal germ cell cancer. JAMA 1983;250:1733–1741.

88. Kukla LJ, Burrows D, Bressler L, et al. Bleomycin-induced Raynaud's phenomenon (letter). Arch Dermatol 1981;117:604.

89. Bostrom B, Woods WG, Ramsay NKL, et al. Cisplatin, vinblastine, and bleomycin (CVP) therapy for relapsed disseminated neuroblastoma. Cancer Treat Rep 1984;68:1157–1158.

90. Fossa SD, Aass N, Kaalhus O, et al. Long term survival and morbidity in patients with metastatic malignant germ cell tumors treated with cisplatin-based combination chemotherapy. Cancer 1986;58:2600–2605.

91. Stefenelli T, Kuzmits R, Ulrich W, et al. Acute vascular toxicity after combination chemotherapy with cisplatin, vinblastine, and bleomycin for testicular cancer. Eur Heart J 1988;9:552–556.

92. Hansen SW, Olsen N. Raynaud's phenomenon in patients treated with cisplatin, vinblastine, and bleomycin for germ cell cancer: measurement of vasoconstrictor response to cold. J Clin Oncol 1989;7:940–942.

93. Boyer M, Raghaven D. Intensive late toxicity assessment program for patients treated for metastatic germ cell tumors with cisplatin-containing combination chemotherapy (abstract). Proc Am Soc Clin Oncol 1989;8:142.

94. Roth BJ, Greist A, Kubilis PS, et al. Cisplatin-based combination chemotherapy for disseminated germ cell tumors: long term follow-up. J Clin Oncol 1988;6:1239–1247.

95. Stoter G, Koopman A, Vendrick CPJ, et al. Ten year survival and later sequelae in testicular cnacer patients treated with cisplatin, vinblastine, and bleomycin. J Clin Oncol 1989;7:1099–1104.

96. Brada M, Horwich A, Peckham MJ. Treatment of favorable-prognosis non-seminomatous testicular germ cell tumors with etoposide, cisplatin, and reduced dose of bleomycin. Cancer Treat Rep 1987; 71:655–656.

97. Cohen IS, Mosher MB, O'Keefe EJ, et al. Cutaneous toxicity of bleomycin therapy. Arch Dermatol 1973;107:553–555.

97a. Von Gunten CF, Roth EL, Ronn JHV. Raynaud's phenomenon in three patients with acquired immune deficiency syndrome related-Kaposi's sarcoma treated with bleomycin. Cancer 1993;72:2004–2006.

98. Elomaa I, Pajunen M, Virkkunen P. Raynaud's phenomenon progressing to gangrene after vincristine and bleomycin therapy. Acta Med Scand 1984;216:323–326.

98a. Fertakos RJ, Mintzer DM. Digital gangrene following chemotherapy for AIDS-related Kaposi's sarcoma. Am J Med 1992;93:581–582.

99. Reid TJ III, Lombardo FA, Redmond J III, Hammond SL, Coffey JA, Oxen H. Digital vasculitis associated with interferon therapy. Am J Med 1992;92:702–703.

100. Goffin E, Angangio R, Shapiro LM, Lockwood LM. Digital gangrene following chemotherapy (letter). Am J Med 1994;96:571.

101. Malamet R, Wise RA, Ettinger WH, et al. Nifedipine in the treatment of Raynaud's phenomenon: evidence for inhibition of platelet activation. Am J Med 1985;78:602–608.

102. Rodenheffer RJ, Rommer JA, Wigley F, et al. Controlled double-blind trial of nifedipine in the treatment of Raynaud's phenomenon. N Engl J Med 1983; 308:880–883.

103. Hantel A, Rowinsky EK, Donehower RC. Nifedipine and oncologic Raynaud's phenomenon (letter). Ann Intern Med 1988;108:767.

104. Mandel EM, Lewinski U, Djaldetti M. Vincristine-induced myocardial infarction. Cancer 1975; 30:1979–1982.

105. Somers G, Abramow M, Wittek M, et al. Myocardial infarction: a complication of vincristine treatment? (Letter) Lancet 1976;2:690.

106. Lejonc JL, Vernant JP, Macquin I, et al. Myocardial infarction following vinblastine treatment (letter). Lancet 1980;2:692.

107. Schechter JP, Jones SE. Myocardial infarction in a 27 year old woman: possible complication of treatment with VP-16-213 (NSC-141540), mediastinal irradiation, or both (letter). Cancer Chemother Rep 1975; 59:887–888.

108. Aisner J, Van Echo DA, Whitacre M, et al. A phase I trial of continuous infusion VP-16-213 (etoposide). Cancer Chemother Pharmacol 1982;7:157–160.

109. Mortimer JE, Crowley J, Eyre H, Weiden P, Eltringham J, Stuckey WJ. A phase II randomized study comparing sequential and combined intra-arterial cisplatin and radiation therapy for primary brain tumors. Cancer 1992;69:1220–1223.

110. Ricci JA, Goldstein L. Coronary artery disease in the presence of bleomycin therapy (letter). Cancer Treat Rep 1982;66:410.

111. Vogelzang NJ, Frenning DH, Kennedy BJ. Coronary artery disease after treatment with bleomycin and vinblastine (letter). Cancer Treat Rep 1980; 53:1159–1160.

112. Vogelzang NJ, Torkelson JL, Kennedy BJ. Hypomagnesemia, renal dysfunction, and Raynaud's

phenomenon in patients treated with cisplatin, vinblastine and bleomycin. Cancer 1985;56:2765–2770.

113. Samuels BL, Vogelzang NJ, Kennedy BJ. Severe vascular toxicity associated with vinblastine, bleomycin and cisplatin chemotherapy. Cancer Chemother Pharmacol 1987;19:253–256.

114. Bodensteiner DC. Fatal coronary artery fibrosis after treatment with bleomycin, vinblastine, and cisplatin. South Med J 1981;74:898–899.

115. Doll DC, List AF, Greco FA, et al. Acute arterial ischemic events following cisplatin-based combination chemotherapy for germ cell tumors of the testis. Ann Intern Med 1986;105:48–51.

116. Talcott JA, Herman TS. Acute ischemic vascular events and cisplatin (letter). Ann Intern Med 1987;107:121–122.

117. Icli F, Karaoguz H, Dincol D, Demirkazik A, Gunel N, Karaoguz R, Unen A. Severe vascular toxicity associated with cisplatin-based chemotherapy. Cancer 1993;72:587–593.

118. House KW, Simon SR, Pugh RP. Chemotherapy-induced myocardial infarction in a young man with Hodgkin's disease. Clin Cardiol 1992;15:122–125.

119. Boiven JF, Hutchinson GB, Lubin JH, Mauch P. Coronary artery disease mortality in patients treated for Hodgkin's disease. Cancer 1992;69:1241–1247.

120. Nichols CR, Roth BJ, Williams SD, et al. No evidence of acute cardiovascular complications of chemotherapy for testicular cancer: an analysis of the Testicular Cancer Intergroup Study. J Clin Oncol 1992; 10:760–765.

121. Yancey RS, Talpaz M. Vindesine-associated angina and ECG changes (letter). Cancer Treat Rep 1982;66:587–588.

122. Dexeus F, Logothetis CJ, Samuels ML, et al. Continuous infusion of vinblastine for advanced hormone refractory prostate cancer. Cancer Treat Rep 1985;69:885–886.

123. Subar M, Muggia FM. Apparent myocardial ischemia associated with vinblastine administration (letter). Cancer Treat Rep 1986;690–691.

124. Tonirotti M, Riumdi R, Pulici S, et al. Ischemic cardiomyopathy from cis-diammine dichloroplatinum (CDDP). Tumori 1984;70:235–236.

125. Shachor J, Beker B, Geffen Y, et al. Acute ECG change during cyclophosphamide infusion in a patient with bronchogenic carcinoma (letter). Cancer Treat Rep 1985;69:734–735.

126. White DA, Schwartzberg LS, Kris MG, et al. Acute chest pain syndrome during bleomycin infusions. Cancer 1987;59:1582–1585.

127. Leone B, Rabinovitch M, Ferrari CR, et al. Cardiotoxicity as a result of 5-fluorouracil therapy. Tumori 1985;71:55–57.

128. Sanani S, Spaulding M, Masud AR, et al. 5-FU cardiotoxicity. Cancer Treat Rep 1981;65:1123–1125.

129. Labianca R, Beretta G, Clerici M, et al. Cardiotoxicity of 5-fluorouracil: a study of 1083 patients. Tumori 1982;68:505–510.

130. Pottage A, Holt S, Ludgate S, et al. Fluorouracil cardiotoxicity. Br Med J 1978;1:547.

131. Freeman N, Costanza M. 5-fluorouracil associated cardiotoxicity. Cancer 1988;61:36–45.

132. Gradishar W, Vokes E, Schilsky R, et al. Vascular events in patients receiving high-dose infusional 5-fluorouracil based chemotherapy: the University of Chicago experience. Med Pediatr Oncol 1991;19:8–15.

133. Vorbiof DA. Cardiotoxicity of 5-fluorouracil. S Afr Med J 1982;61:635–637.

134. Dent RG, McColl I. 5-fluorouracil and angina (letter). Lancet 1975;1:347–348.

135. Stevenson DL, Mikhaikidis DP, Gillet DS. Cardiotoxicity of 5-fluorouracil (letter). Lancet 1977;2:406–407.

136. Soukop M, McVie JG, Calman KC. 5-fluorouracil cardiotoxicity. Br Med J 1978;1:1422.

137. Kleiman NA, Lehane DE, Geyer E, et al. Prinzmetal's angina during 5-fluorouracil chemotherapy. Am J Med 1987;82:566–568.

138. Gammuci T, Zampa G. Cardiotoxicity of 5-FU. Tumori 1979;65:487–495.

139. Umsawasdi T, Sawarnkatata P. Cardiotoxicity of 5-fluorouracil. Cancer Chemother Rep 1975;59:1051–1053.

140. Oleksowiez L, Bruckner HW. Prophaylaxis of 5-fluorouracil induced coronary vasospasm with calcium channel blockers. Am J Med 1988;85:750–751.

141. Chaudary S, Song SYK, Jaski BE. Profound, yet reversible, heart failure secondary to 5-fluorouracil. Am J Med 1988;85:454–456.

142. Collins C, Weiden PL. Cardiotoxicity of 5-fluorouracil. Cancer Treat Rep 1987;71:733–736.

143. Rezkalla S, Kloner RA, Ensley J, et al. Continuous ambulatory ECG monitoring during fluorouracil therapy: a prospective study. J Clin Oncol 1989;7:509–514.

144. Patel B, Kloner RA, Ensley J, et al. 5-fluorouracil cardiotoxicity: left ventricular dysfunction and effects of coronary dilators. Am J Med Sci 1987; 294:238–243.

145. Jakubowski AA, Kemeny N. Hypotension as a manifestation of cardiotoxicity in three patients receiving cisplatin and 5-fluorouracil. Cancer 1988; 62:266–269.

146. Robben NC, Pippas AW, Moore JO. The syndrome of 5-fluorouracil cardiotoxicity: an elusive cardiopathy. Cancer 1993;71:493–509.

147. Schooben C, Papageorgiou E, Harstick A, et al. Cardiotoxicity of 5-fluorouracil in combination with folinic acid in patients with gastrointestinal cancer. Cancer 1993;72:2242–2247.

148. De Forni M, Makt-Martino MC, Jaillais P, et al. Cardiotoxicity of high dose continuous infusion fluorouracil: a prospective clinical study. J Clin Oncol 1992;10:1795–1801.

149. Anderson MR, Lokich JJ, Moore C. The syndrome of 5-fluorouracil cardiotoxicity: an elusive cardiopathy. Cancer 1993;72:2287–2288.

150. Forastiere AA, Metch B, Schuller DE, et al. Comparison of cisplatin plus fluorouracil and carboplatin plus fluorouracil versus methotrexate in advanced squamous cell carcinoma of the head and neck: a Southwest Oncology Group Study. J Clin Oncol 1992; 10:1245–1251.

151. Murgo AJ. Thrombotic microangiopathy in the cancer patient including those induced by chemotherapeutic agents. Semin Hematol 1987;24:161–177.

152. Gulati SC, Sordillo P, Kempin S, et al. Microangiopathic hemolytic anemia observed after treatment of epidermoid carcinoma with mitomycin C and 5-fluorouracil. Cancer 1980;45:2252–2257.

153. Hanna WT, Krauss S, Regester RF, et al. Renal disease after mitomycin C therapy. Cancer 1981; 48:2583–2588.

154. Harden E, Lucas VS, Proia A, et al. Hemolytic uremic syndrome during therapy with mitomycin C (MMC) plus 5-fluorouracil (5-FU) (abstract). Proc Am Soc Clin Oncol 1982;1:93.

155. Horne MK III, Cooper B. Microangiopathic hemolytic anemia with metastatic adenocarcinoma: response to chemotherapy. South Med J 1982;75:503–504.

156. Jones BG, Newman CE, Fielding JW, et al. Intravascular hemolysis and renal impairment after blood transfusion in two patients on long-term 5-fluorouracil and mitomycin C. Lancet 1980;1:1275–1277.

157. Karlin DA, Stroehlein JR. Rash, nephritis, hypertension, and hemolysis in patients on 5-fluorouracil, doxorubicin, and mitomycin C (letter). Lancet 1980;2:534–535.

158. Krauss S, Sonoda T, Solomon A. Treatment of advanced gastrointestinal cancer with 5-fluorouracil and mitomycin C. Cancer 1974;1598–1603.

159. Kressel BR, Ryan KP, Kuong AT, et al. Microangiopathic hemolytic anemia, thrombocytopenia, and renal failure in patients treated for adenocarcinoma. Cancer 1981;48:1734–1745.

160. Laffay DL, Tubbs RR, Valenzuela R, et al. Chronic glomerular microangiopathy and metastatic carcinoma. Hum Pathol 1979;10:433–438.

161. Lempert KD. Hemolysis and renal impairment syndrome in patients on 5-fluorouracil and mitomycin C (letter). Lancet 1980;2:369–370.

162. Pavy MD, Wiley EL, Abeloff MD. Hemolytic uremic syndrome associated with mitomycin therapy. Cancer Treat Rep 1982;66:457–461.

163. Rabadi SJ, Khandekar JD, Miller HJ. Mitomycin-induced hemolytic uremic syndrome: case presentation and review of the literature. Cancer Treat Rep 1982;66:1244–1247.

164. Rumpf KW, Rieger J, Landkisch PG, et al. Mitomycin-induced hemolysis and renal failure (letter). Lancet 1980;2:1037–1038.

165. Bruntsch U, Froos G, Tigges FJ, et al. Microangiopathic hemolytic anemia, a frequent complication of mitomycin therapy in cancer patients. Eur J Clin Oncol 1984;20:905–909.

166. Zimmerman S, Smith FP, Phillips TM, et al. Gastric carcinoma and thrombotic thrombocytopenic purpura: association with plasma immune complex concentration. Br Med J 1982;284:1432–1434.

167. Perry DJ. Reversible microangiopathic hemolytic anemia after mitomycin C. Cancer Chemother Pharmacol 1983;10:223.

168. Lyman NW, Michaelson R, Viscuso RL, et al. Mitomycin-induced hemolytic uremic syndrome. Successful treatment with corticosteroids and intense plasma exchange. Arch Intern Med 1983;143:1617–1618.

169. Grocker J, Jones EL. Hemolytic-uremic syndrome complicating long term mitomycin C and 5-fluorouracil therapy for gastric carcinoma. J Clin Pathol 1983;36:24–29.

170. Cantrell JE Jr, Phillips TM, Schein PS. Carcinoma-associated hemolytic-uremic syndrome: a complication of mitomycin C chemotherapy. J Clin Oncol 1985;3:723–734.

171. Jolivet J, Giroux L, Laurin S, et al. Microangiopathic hemolytic anemia, renal failure, and noncardiogenic pulmonary edema: a chemotherapy induced syndrome. Cancer Treat Rep 1983;67:429–434.

172. Tannock IF. Methotrexate and mitomycin for patients with metastatic transitional cell carcinoma of the urinary tract. Cancer Treat Rep 1983;61:503–504.

173. Fielding JWL, Fagg SL, Jones BG, et al. An interim report of a prospective, randomized, controlled study of adjuvant chemotherapy in operable gastric cancer: British Stomach Cancer Group. World J Surg 1983;7:390–399.

174. Laufman L, Courter S, Pritchard J. Fatal mitomycin C (MMC) syndrome heralded by pulmonary symptoms (abstract). Proc Am Soc Clin Oncol 1983;2:197.

175. Ravikumar TS, Sibley R, Reed K, et al. Renal toxicity of mitomycin C. Am J Clin Oncol 1984;7:279–285.

176. Loprinzi CL. Mitomycin C-induced pulmonary and renal toxicities. Wis Med J 1984;83:16–17.

177. Ito S, Hirono S. Two cases of microangiopathic hemolytic anemia caused by anticancer drugs which showed rapid improvement after adminstration of aspirin and dipyridamole. Rinsho Ketsueki 1982;23:730–735.

178. Jao W, Manaligod Jr. Renal disease associated with mitomycin therapy. Ultrastruct Pathol 1983;5:83–88.

179. Boven E, Pindeo HM. Mitomycin C. Interstitial pneumonitis and hemolytic uraemic syndrome. Neth J Med 1983;26:153–156.

180. Khojasteh A, Reynolds RD, Garcia AR, et al. Hemolytic uremic-like syndrome following a single dose of mitomycin C (abstract). Proc Am Soc Clin Oncol 1984;3:4.

181. Van Speeuwel JP, Hemrika MH, Dammaat CEM, et al. Letter to the editor (letter). Neth J Med 1983;26:287–288.

182. Peterson KB, Smith WE. Mitomycin induced hemolytic uremic syndrome. Samaritan Med 1984;2:17–20.

183. Simon P, Herve JP, Ramee MP, et al. La nephrotoxicite de la mitomycin C. Trois nouvelles observations et revue de la litterature. Nephrologie 1982;3:152–157.

184. Willie GR, Levy SM, Michaels RE, et al. Hemolytic uremic syndrome in a patient receiving mitomycin C and 5-fluorouracil. Henry Ford Hosp Med J 1983;31:104–109.

185. Valavaara R, Nordman E. Renal complications of mitomycin C therapy with special references to the total dose. Cancer 1985;55:47–50.

186. Hug V, Burgess A, Blumenschein G, et al. Effect of cyclophosphamide on the mitomycin-based syndrome of thrombotic thrombocytopenic purpura (letter). Cancer Treat Rep 1985;69:565–566.

187. Price TM, Murge AJ, Keveney JJ, et al. Renal failure and hemolytic anemia associated with mitomycin C: a case report. Cancer 1985;55:51–56.

188. Verwey J, Boven E, Van Der Muelen J, et al. Recovery from mitomycin C induced hemolytic uremic syndrome: a case report. Cancer 1984;54:2878–2881.

189. Garibotto G, Acquarone N, Saffioti S, et al. Successful treatment of mitomycin C associated hemolytic uremic syndrome by plasmapheresis. Nephron 1989;51:409–412.

190. Fields SM, Lindley CM. Thrombotic microangiopathy associated with chemotherapy: a case report and review of the literature. DICP 1989;23:582–588.

191. Sheldon R, Slaughter D. A syndrome of mi-

croangiopathic hemolytic anemia, renal impairment, and pulmonary edema in chemotherapy-treated patients with adenocarcinoma. Cancer 1986;58:1428–1436.

192. Hostetter AL, Tubbs RR, Ziegler T, et al. Chronic glomerular microangiopathy complicating metastatic carcinoma. Hum Pathol 1987;18:342–348.

193. Verwey J, Vries JD, Pinedo HM. Mitomycin C induced renal toxicity, a dose dependent side effect? Eur J Cancer Clin Oncol 1987;23:195–199.

194. Mergenthaler HG, Binsack T, Wilmanns W. Carcinoma associated hemolytic-uremic syndrome in a patient receiving 5-fluorouracil-adriamycin-mitomycin C combination chemotherapy. Oncology 1988; 45:11–14.

195. McCarthy JT, Staats BA. Pulmonary hypertension, hemolytic anemia, and renal failure: a mitomycin associated syndrome. Chest 1986;89:608–611.

196. Lessesne JB, Rothschild N, Erickson B, et al. Cancer associated hemolytic uremic syndrome: analysis of 85 cases from a national registry. J Clin Oncol 1989;7:781–789.

197. Liu KM, Mittelman A, Sproul EE, et al. Renal toxicity in man treated with mitomycin C. Cancer 1971; 28:1314–1320.

198. Weiss RB, Poster DS. The renal toxicity of cancer chemotherapeutic agents. Cancer Treat Rev 1982; 9:37–56.

199. Hamner RW, Verani R, Weinman EJ. Mitomycin associated renal failure. Case report and review. Arch Intern Med 1983;143:803–807.

200. Morel-Maroger L. Nephrology forum: adult hemolytic uremic syndrome. Kidney Int 1980;18:125–134.

201. Agnelli G, Gresele P, Nenci GG. Clotting activation after blood transfusion in patients reveiving 5-fluorouracil and mitomycin C treatment (letter). Cancer Chemother Pharmacol 1981;5:205–206.

202. Chow S, Roscoe J, Cattran DC. Plasmapheresis and antiplatelet agents in the treatment of the hemolytic uremic syndrome to mitomycin. Am J Kidney Dis 1986;7:407–412.

203. Grem JL, Merritt JA, Carbone PP. Treatment of mitomycin associated microangiopathic hemolytic anemia with vincristine. Arch Intern Med 1986; 146:566–568.

204. Zimmerman SE, Smith FP, Phillips TM, et al. Gastric carcinoma and thrombotic thrombocytopenic purpura: association with plasma immune complex concentrations. Br Med J 1982;284:1432–1434.

205. Korec S, Schein PS, Smith FP, et al. Treatment of cancer associated hemolytic uremic syndrome with staphylococcal protein A immunoperfusion. J Clin Oncol 1986;4:210–215.

206. Snyder HW Jr, Mittleman A, Oral A, et al. Treatment of cancer chemotherapy associated thrombocytopenia purpura/hemolytic uremic syndrome by protein A immunoadsorption of plasma. Cancer 1993; 71:1882–1892.

207. Licciardello J, Moake J, Rudy C, et al. Elevated plasma von Willebrand factor levels and arterial occlusive complications associated with cisplatin-based chemotherapy. Oncology 1985;42:296–300.

208. Jackson AM, Rose BD, Graff LG, et al. Thrombotic microangiopathy and renal failure associated with antineoplastic chemotherapy. Ann Intern Med 1984;101:41–44.

209. Desablens B, Fievet P, Pruna A, et al. Hemolytic-uremic syndrome after cancer chemotherapy without mitomycin C. Nephron 1986;42:340–344.

210. Van De Meer J, De Vries EGE, Vriesendorp R, et al. Hemolytic uremic syndrome in a patient on cisplatin, vinblastine, and bleomycin. J Cancer Res Clin Oncol 1985;110:119–122.

211. Gradishar WJ, Vokes EE, Mi K, et al. Chemotherapy related hemolytic-uremic syndrome after the treatment of head and neck cancer. A case report. Cancer 1990;66:1914–1918.

212. Watson PR, Githrie TH Jr, Caruana RJ. Cisplatin-associated hemolytic uremic syndrome: successful treatment with staphylococcal protein A column. Cancer 1989;64:1400–1403.

213. Coates AS, Childs A, Cox K, et al. Severe vascular adverse effects with thrombocytopenia and renal failure following emetogenic chemotherapy and ondansetron. Ann Oncol 1992;3:773–774.

214. Walker RW, Rosenblum MK, Kempin SJ, et al. Carboplatin-associated thrombotic microangiopathic hemolytic anemia. Cancer 1989;64:1017–1020.

215. Case records—MGH. Case 16-1988. N Engl J Med 1988;318:1047–1057.

216. Carey RW, Harris N. Thrombotic microangiopathy in three patients with cured lymphoma. Cancer 1989;63:1393–1397.

217. Byrnes JJ, Baquerizo H, Gonzalez M, et al. Thrombotic thrombocytopenic purpura subsequent to acute myelogenous chemotherapy. Am J Hematol 1986;21:299–304.

218. Sack GH, Levin J, Bell WR. Trousseau's syndrome and other manifestations of chronic disseminated coagulopathy in patients with neoplasms: clinical, pathophysiologic and therapeutic features. Medicine 1977;56:1–37.

219. Kukla LJ, McGuire WP, Lad T, et al. Acute vascular episode associated with therapy for carcinoma of the upper aerodigestive tract with bleomycin, vincristine, and cisplatin. Cancer Treat Rep 1982; 66:369–370.

220. Fallon B, Clark J, Frei E. Vascular complications during cisplatin-bleomycin-methotrexate and cisplatin 5-FU in induction chemotherapy for advanced stage III and IV squamous cell carcinoma of the head and neck (abstract). Proc Am Soc Clin Oncol 1986; 5:134.

221. Cantwell BMJ, Manniz KA, Roberts JT, et al. Thromboembolic events during combination chemotherapy for germ cell malignancy (letter). Lancet 1988; 2:1086–1087.

222. Hall MR, Richards MA, Harper PG. Thromboembolic events during combination chemotherapy for germ cell malignancy (letter). Lancet 1986;2:1259.

223. Lederman GS, Garnick MB. Pulmonary emboli as a complication of germ cell cancer treatment. J Urol 1987;137:1236–1237.

224. Lynch TJ Jr, Kass F, Kalish LA, et al. Cisplatin, 5-fluorouracil, and etoposide for advanced non-small lung cancer. Cancer 1993;71:2953–2957.

225. Seiffer EJ, Young RC, Longo DL. Deep venous thrombosis during therapy for Hodgkin's disease. Cancer Treat Rep 1985;69:1011–1013.

226. Clarke CS, Otridge BW, Carney DN. Thromboembolism. A complication of weekly chemotherapy in the treatment of non-Hodgkin's lymphoma. Cancer 1990;66:2027–2030.

227. Cantwell BMJ, Carmichael J, Ghani SE, et al. Thromboses and thromboemboli in patients with lymphoma during cytotoxic chemotherapy. Br Med J 1988; 2:179–180.

228. Miller TP, Dahlberg S, Weich JK, et al. Unfavorable histologies of non-Hodgkin's lymphoma treated with Pro-MACE-Cyta BOM: a groupwide Southwest Oncology Group Study. J Clin Oncol 1990; 8:1951–1958.

229. Weiss RB, Tormey DC, Holland JF, et al. Venous thrombosis during multimodal treatment of primary breast carcinoma. Cancer Treat Rep 1981;65:677–679.

230. Booth BW, Weiss RB. Venous thrombosis during adjuvant chemotherapy (letter). N Engl J Med 1981; 305:168.

231. Manni A, Trujillo JE, Pearson OH. Sequential use of endocrine therapy and chemotherapy for metastatic breast cancer: effects on survival. Cancer Treat Rep 1980;64:111–116.

232. Goodnough LT, Saito H, Manni A, et al. Increased incidence of thromboembolism in stage IV breast cancer patients treated with a five-drug chemotherapy regimen. A study of 159 patients. Cancer 1984;54:1264–1268.

233. Levine MN, Gent M, Hirsh J, et al. The thrombogenic effect of anticancer drug therapy in women with stage II breast cancer. N Engl J Med 1988;318:404–407.

234. Saphner T, Tormey DC, Gray R. Venous and arterial thrombosis in patients who received adjuvant therapy for breast cancer. J Clin Oncol 1991;9:286–294.

235. Fisher B, Redmond C, Wickerham DL, et al. Doxorubicin-containing regimens for the treatment of stage II breast cancer: the National Surgical Adjuvant Breast and Bowel Project experience. J Clin Oncol 1989; 7:572–582.

236. Pritchard KI, Pater J, Paul N, et al. Thromboembolic complications related to chemotherapy in a National Institute of Canada randomized trial for tamoxifen versus tamoxifen plus chemotherapy in postmenopausal women with axillary node positive receptor positive breast cancer (abstract). Proc Am Soc Clin Oncol 1989;8:25.

237. Wall JG, Weiss RB, Norton L, et al. Arterial thrombosis associated with adjuvant chemotherapy for breast carcinoma: a Cancer and Leukemia Group B Study. Am J Med 1989;87:1455–1466.

238. Rivkin SE, Green S, Metch B, et al. Adjuvant CMFVP versus tamoxifen versus concurrent CMFVP and tamoxifen for postmenopausal, node-positive, and estrogen receptor-positive breast cancer patients: a Southwest Oncology Group Study. J Clin Oncol 1994; 12:2078–2085.

239. Theodossiou C, Kroog G, Ettinghausen S, Tolcher A, Cowan K, O'Shaughnessy J. Acute arterial thrombosis in a patient with breast cancer after chemotherapy with 5-fluorouracil, doxorubicin, leucovorin, cyclophosphamide, and interleukin-3. Cancer 1994;74:2808–2810.

240. Clahsen PC, Van De Velde CJH, Julien JP, et al. Thromboembolic complications after perioperative chemotherapy in women with early breast cancer: a European Organization for Research and Treatment of Cancer Breast Cancer Cooperative Group study. J Clin Oncol 1994;12:1266–1271.

241. Levine M, Hirsh J, Gent M, et al. Double-blind randomized trial of very-low-dose warfarin for prevention of thromboembolism in stage IV breast cancer. Lancet 1994;343:886–889.

242. Kasimis BS, Spiers ASD. Thrombotic complications in patients with advanced prostatic cancer treated with chemotherapy (letter). Lancet 1979;1:159.

243. Del Prado PF, Meana JA, Carrion JR. Acute cerebrovascular accident after treatment with cisplatin. Acta Oncol 1992;31:593–595.

244. Gandia D, Spielman M, Kac J, Elias D, Girinsky T, Fuillot T, Rougier P. Cerebrovascular accident associated with chemotherapy for oesophageal carcinoma. Eur J Cancer 1992;28:245.

245. Sevelda P, Mayerhofer K, Obermain A, Stolzlechner J, Kurz C. Thrombosis with paclitaxel (letter). Lancet 1994;343:727.

246. Becker JC, Winkler B, Klingert S, Brocker EB. Antiphospholipid syndrome associated with immunotherapy for patients with melanoma. Cancer 1994; 73:1621–1624.

247. Conti JA, Scher HI. Acute arterial thrombosis after escalated-dose methotrexate, vinblastine, doxorubicin, and cisplatin chemotherapy with recombinant granulocyte colony-stimulating factor. Cancer 1992; 70:2699–2702.

248. Antman KS, Griffin JD, Elias A, et al. Effect of recombinant human granulocyte-macrophage colony-stimulating factor on chemotherapy-induced myelosuppression. N Engl J Med 1988;319:593–598.

249. Stephens LC, Haire WD, Pokorny KS, Kessinger A, Kotulak G. Granulocyte macrophage colony stimulating factor: high incidence of apheresis catheter thrombosis during stem cell collection. Bone Marrow Transplant 1993;11:57–59.

250. Fisher B, Costantino J, Redmond C, et al. A randomized clinical trial evaluating tamoxifen in the treatment of patients with node-negative breast cancer who have estrogen-receptor positive tumors. N Engl J Med 1989;320:479–484.

251. Rutqvist LE, Mattson A. Cardiac and thromboembolic morbidity among postmenopausal women with early stage breast cancer in a randomized trial of adjuvant tamoxifen. J Natl Cancer Inst 1993;85:1398–1406.

252. Issell BF, Crooke ST. Etoposide (VP-16-213). Cancer Treat Rev 1979;6:107–124.

253. O'Dwyer PJ, Alonso MT, Leland-Jones B, et al. Teniposide: a review of 12 years of experience. Cancer Treat Rep 1984;68:1455–1466.

254. Antman KH, Mayer RJ, Frei E III. Vascular, hormonal, teratogenic and miscellaneous toxicities of chemotherapeutic agents. In: Perry MC, Yarbro JW, eds. Toxicity of chemotherapy. Philadelphia: Grune & Stratton, 1984:521–538.

255. Buesa JM, Garcia M, Valle M, et al. Phase I trial of intermittent high-dose dacarbazine. Cancer Treat Rep 1984;68:499–504.

256. Henner WD, Peters WP, Eder JP, et al. Pharmacokinetics and immediate effects of high-dose carmustine in man. Cancer Treat Rep 1986;70:877–880.

257. Legha SS, Keating M, Picket S, et al. Phase I clinical investigation of homoharringtonine. Cancer Treat Rep 1984;68:1085–1091.

258. Neidhart JA, Young DC, Derocher D, et al. Phase I trial of homoharringtonine. Cancer Treat Rep 1983;67:801–804.

259. Warnell RP Jr, Coonley CJ, Gee TS. Homohar-

ringtonine: an effective new drug for remission induction in refractory non-lymphoblastic leukemia. J Clin Oncol 1985;3:617–621.

260. Carmichael SM, Eagleton L, Ayers CR, et al. Orthostatic hypotension during vincristine therapy. Arch Intern Med 1970;126:290–293.

261. DiBella NJ. Vincristine-induced orthostatic hypotension: a prospective clinical study (letter). Cancer Treat Rep 1980;64:359–360.

262. Kletzel M, Jaffe N. Systemic hypertension: a complication of intraarterial *cis*-diamminedichloroplatinum (II) infusion. Cancer 1981;47:245–247.

263. Harrell RM, Sibley R, Vogelzang NJ. Renal vascular lesion after chemotherapy with vinblastine, bleomycin, and cisplatin. Am J Med 1982;73:429–433.

264. Hansen SW, Groth S, Dauguard G, et al. Long-term effects on renal function and blood pressure of treatment with cisplatin, vinblastine, and bleomycin in patients with germ cell cancer. J Clin Oncol 1988; 6:1728–1731.

265. Spivack SD. Procarbazine. Ann Intern Med 1974;81:795–800.

266. O'Dwyer PJ, Weiss RB. Hypersensitivity reactions induced by etoposide. Cancer Treat Rep 1984; 68:959–961.

267. Weiss RB. Hypersensitivity reactions to cancer chemotherapy. In: Perry MC, Yarbro JW, eds. Toxicity of chemotherapy. Philadelphia: Grune & Stratton, 1984:101–123.

268. Kampmann KK, Graves T, Rogers SD. Acral erythema secondary to high-dose cytosine arabinoside with pain worsened by cyclosporine infusions. Cancer 1989;63:2482–2485.

269. Burgdorf WC, Gilmore WA, Ganick RG. Peculiar acral erythema secondary to high-dose chemotherapy for acute myelogenous leukemia. Ann Intern Med 1982;97:61–62.

270. Baer MR, King LE, Wolff SN. Palmar-plantar erythrodysesthesia and cytarabine (letter). Ann Intern Med 1985;102:556.

271. Cornonnier C, Roujeau JC, Vernant JP, et al. Cancer chemotherapy and acral erythema (letter). Ann Intern Med 1982;97:785.

272. Silver FS, Espinoza LR, Hartmann RC. Acral erythema and hydroxyurea (letter). Ann Intern Med 1983;98:675.

273. Lokich JJ, Moore C. Chemotherapy-associated palmar-plantar erythrodysesthesia syndrome. Ann Intern Med 1984;101:798–799.

274. Feldman LD, Ajani JA. Fluorouracil-associated dermatitis of the hands and feet. JAMA 1985; 254:3479.

275. Curran CF, Luce JF. Fluorouracil and palmar-plantar erythrodysesthesia (letter). Ann Intern Med 1989;111:858.

276. Vukelja SJ, Lanbando FA, James WD, et al. Pyridoxine for the palmar-plantar erythrodysesthesia syndrome (letter). Ann Intern Med 1989;111:688–689.

277. Bellmunt J, Mavarno M, Hidalgo R, et al. Palmar-plantar erythrodysesthesia syndrome associated with short-term continuous infusion (5 days) of 5-fluorouracil. Tumori 1988;74:329–331.

278. Atkins JK. Fluorouracil and the palmar-plantar erythrodysesthesia syndrome (letter). Ann Intern Med 1985;102:419.

279. Doyle LA, Berg C, Bottino G, et al. Erythema

and desquamation after high-dose methotrexate. Ann Intern Med 1983;98:611–612.

280. Cox GJ, Robertson DB. Toxic erythema of palms and soles associated with high dose mercaptopurine chemotherapy. Arch Dermatol 1986;122:1413–1414.

281. Murphy CP, Harden EA, Herzig RH. Dose related cutaneous toxicities with etoposide. Cancer 1993; 71:153–155.

282. Burke MC, Bernhard JD, Michelson AD. Chemotherapy induced painful acral erythema in childhood: Burgdorf's reaction. Am J Pediatr Hematol 1989; 11:44–45.

283. Kingsley EC. 5-Fluorouracil dermatitis prophylaxis with a nicotine patch (letter). Ann Intern Med 1994;120:8135.

284. Gibson LE. Cutaneous vasculitis: approach to diagnosis and systemic associations. Mayo Clin Proc 1990;65:221–229.

285. Fonderila CG, Milone GA, Parlovsky S. Cutaneous vasculitis after intermediate dose of methotrexate. Br J Haematol 1989;72:591–592.

286. Navarro M, Pedragosa R, Lafuerza A, et al. Leukocytoclastic vasculitis after high dose methotrexate (letter). Ann Intern Med 1986;105:471–472.

287. Marks CR, Willkins RF, Wilske KR, et al. Small-vessel vasculitis and methotrexate (letter). Ann Intern Med 1984;100:916.

288. Rowinsky EK, McGuire WO, Anhalt GJ, et al. Hexamethylene bisacetamide-induced cutaneous vasculitis. Cancer Treat Rep 1987;71:471–474.

289. Greenberg HS, Ensminer WE, Seeger JF, et al. Intraarterial BCNU chemotherapy for the treatment of malignant gliomas of the central nervous system: a preliminary report. Cancer Treat Rep 1981;65:803–810.

290. DeWys WD, Fowler ED. Report of vasculitis and blindness after intracarotid injection of 1,3-bis (2-chloroethyl)-1-nitrosourea (BCNU: NSC-409962) in dogs. Cancer Chemother Rep 1973;57:33–40.

291. Bernauer W, Gratwohl A, Keller A, Daicker B. Microvasculopathy in the ocular fundus after bone marrow transplantation. Ann Intern Med 1992; 116:956–957.

292. Wilding G, Caruso R, Lawrence TS, et al. Retinal toxicity after high-dose cisplatin therapy. J Clin Oncol 1985;3:1683–1685.

293. Feun LG, Wallace S, Stewart DJ, et al. Intracarotid infusion of *cis*-diamminedichloro-platinum in the treatment of recurrent malignant brain tumors. Cancer 1984;54:794–799.

294. Rankin EM, Pitts JF. Ophthalmic toxicity during carboplatin therapy. Ann Oncol 1993;4:337–338.

295. Lazo JS. Endothelial injury caused by antineoplastic agents. Biochem Pharmacol 1986;35:1912–1923.

296. Nicholson GL, Custead SE. Effects of chemotherapeutic drugs on platelet and metastatic tumor cell-endothelial cell interactions as a model for assessing vascular endothelial integrity. Cancer Res 1985; 45:331–336.

297. Adamson IYR, Bowden DH. The pathogenesis of bleomycin-induced pulmonary fibrosis in mice. Am J Pathol 1974;77:185–198.

298. Otsuka K, Murota SI, Mori Y. Stimulatory effect of bleomycin on the hyaluronic acid synthetase in cultured fibroblasts. Biochem Pharmacol 1978;27:1551–1554.

299. Finch WF, Rodan GP, Buckingham RB, et al.

Bleomycin-induced scleroderma. J Rheumatol 1980; 7:651–659.

300. Mosekey PL, Hemken C, Hunninghake GW. Augmentation of fibroblast proliferation by bleomycin. J Clin Invest 1986;78:1150–1154.

301. Gould VE, Miller J. Sclerosing alveolitis induced by cyclophosphamide: ultrastructural observations on alveolar injury and repair. Am J Pathol 1975; 81:513–530.

302. Cattell V. Mitomycin induced hemolytic uremic kidney: an experimental model in the rat. Am J Pathol 1985;121:88–95.

303. Charba D, Moake JL, Harris MA, Hester JP. Abnormalities of von Willebrand factor multimers in drug-associated thrombotic microangiopathies. Am J Hematol 1993;42:268–277.

304. Smith AC, Boyd MR. Effects of BCNU on pulmonary and serum angiotensin converting enzyme activity in rats. Biochem Pharmacol 1983;32:3719–3722.

305. Lazo JS. Angiotensin converting enzyme activity in mice after subacute bleomycin administration. Toxicol Appl Pharmacol 1981;59:395–404.

306. Lerman A, Hildebrand FL Jr, Margulies KB, et al. Endothelin. A new cardiovascular regulatory peptide. Mayo Clin Proc 1990;65:1441–1455.

307. Kanno K, Hirata Y, Emori T, et al. Endothelin and Raynaud's phenomenon. Am J Med 1991;90:130–132.

308. Gobel U, Ebell W, Jurgens H, et al. Coagulation changes following bleomycin treatment in animals (abstract). Proc Am Soc Clin Oncol 1983;2:39.

309. Yen T, Walsh JD, Pejler G, Berndt MC, Geczy CL. Cisplatin-induced platelet activation requires mononuclear cells: role of GMP-140 and modulation of procoagulant activity. Br J Haematol 1993;83:259–269.

310. Panella TJ, Peters W, White JG, et al. Platelets acquire a secretion defect after high dose chemotherapy. Cancer 1990;65:1711–1716.

311. Ruiz MA, Marugan I, Estelles P, et al. The influence of chemotherapy on the plasmatic coagulation and fibrinolytic system in lung cancer patients (abstract). Thromb Haemost 1987;58:110.

312. Edwards RL, Klaus M, Matthews E, et al. Heparin abolishes the chemotherapy induced increase in plasma fibrinopeptide A levels. Am J Med 1990;89:25–28.

313. Kuzel T, Exparaz B, Green D, et al. Thrombogenicity of intravenous 5-fluorouracil alone or in combination with cisplatin. Cancer 1990;65:885–889.

314. Canobbio L, Fassio T, Ardizzoni A, et al. Hypercoagulable state induced by cytostatic drugs in stage II breast cancer patients. Cancer 1986;54:1032–1036.

315. Conard J, Horellou MH, Van Dreden P, et al. Decrease in protein C in L-asparaginase-treated patients (letter). Br J Haematol 1985;59:725–727.

316. Rogers JS II, Murgo AJ, Fantana JA, et al. Chemotherapy for breast cancer decreases plasma protein C and protein S. J Clin Oncol 1988;6:276–281.

317. Feffer SE, Carmosino LS, Fox RL. Acquired protein C deficiency in patients with breast cancer receiving cyclophosphamide, methotrexate, and 5-fluorouracil. Cancer 1989;63:1303–1307.

318. Gordo BG, Haire WD, Patton DF, Munno PJ, Reed EL. Thrombotic complications of BMT: association with protein C deficiency. Bone Marrow Transplant 1993;11:61–65.

319. Enck RE, Rios CN. Tamoxifen treatment of metastatic breast cancer and antithrombin III levels. Cancer 1984;53:2607–2609.

320. Jordan VC, Fritz NF, Tormey DC. Long term adjuvant therapy with tamoxifen and effects on sex hormone binding globulin and antithrombin III. Cancer Res 1987;45:4517–4519.

321. Jones AL, Powles TJ, Trelearen JG, et al. Haemostatic changes and thromboembolic risk during tamoxifen therapy in normal women. Br J Cancer 1992; 66:744–747.

322. Love RR, Surawicz TS, Williams EL. Antithrombin III level, fibrinogen level, and platelet count changes with adjuvant tamoxifen therapy. Arch Intern Med 1992;152:317–320.

323. Jaattela M. Biologic activities and mechanisms of action of tumor necrosis factor-alpha/cachexin. Lab Invest 1991;64:724–742.

324. Bevilacqua MP, Pober JS, Majeau GR, Fiers W, Cotran RS, Fimbrone MA Jr. Recombinant tumor necrosis factor induces procoagulant activity in cultured human vascular endothelium: characterization and comparison with the actions of interleukin I. Proc Natl Acad Sci USA 1986;83:4533–4537.

325. Tanaka J, Imamura M, Kasai M, et al. Rapid analysis of tumor necrosis factor-alpha mRNA expression during veno-occlusive disease of the liver after allogeneic bone marrow transplantation. Transplantation 1993;55:430–433.

326. Schilsky RL, Anderson T. Hypomagnesemia and renal magnesium wasting in patients receiving cisplatin. Ann Intern Med 1979;90:929–931.

327. Turlapaty PDMV, Altur BM. Magnesium deficiency produces spasms of coronary arteries: relationship to etiology of sudden death ischemic heart disease. Science 1980;280:198–200.

328. Altura BM, Altura BT, Gebrewold A. Magnesium deficiency and hypertension: correlation between magnesium-deficient diets and microcirculatory changes in situ. Science 1984;223:1315–1317.

329. Rosenfield CS, Broder LE. Cisplatin-induced autonomic neuropathy. Cancer Treat Rep 1984;68:659–660.

330. Hansen SW. Autonomic neuropathy after treatment with cisplatin, vinblastine, and bleomycin for germ cell cancer. Br Med J 1990;300:511–512.

331. Carmichael SM, Eagleton L, Ayers CR, et al. Orthostatic hypotension during vincristine therapy. Arch Intern Med 1970;126:290–293.

332. Dibella NJ. Vincristine-induced orthostatic hypotension: a prospective clinical study. Cancer Treat Rep 1980;64:359–360.

333. Roca E, Bruera E, Politi PM, et al. Vinca alkaloid-induced cardiovascular autonomic neuropathy. Cancer Treat Rep 1985;69:149–151.

334. Hivornen HE, Salmi TT, Heinonen E, et al. Vincristine treatment of acute lymphoblastic leukemia induces transient autonomic cardioneuropathy. Cancer 1989;64:801–805.

40

Second Malignancies after Chemotherapy

John D. Boice, Jr., and Donna A. Shriner

Several decades ago, MOPP (mechlorethamine-vincristine-procarbazine-prednisone) was first used to effectively treat Hodgkin's disease patients. Today, multidrug regimens are available to treat practically all forms of cancer. These curative therapies, however, can result in long-term complications, the most serious being the heightened risk of developing a new cancer. Most, if not all, alkylating agents are leukemogenic, with the level of risk related to the cumulative dosage administered and the duration of treatment (1). Certain cytostatic drugs that target DNA-topoisomerase II, such as the epipodophyllotoxins, induce secondary leukemias, most often when combined with alkylating agents or cisplatin. Anthracyclines that inhibit topoisomerase-II may also be leukemogenic, again in the presence of alkylating agents. Other forms of chemotherapeutic agents, such as the antimetabolites, do not appear to be carcinogenic (Table 40.1).

The following sections focus on relatively large analytic studies of patients treated with chemotherapy that have provided information on the risk of secondary cancer. While case reports have been important in identifying possible hazards and in guiding research, they are not covered in this review, nor are hormonal therapies such as tamoxifen.

LEUKEMIA AFTER CHEMOTHERAPY

By far the most frequently reported cancer following chemotherapy is leukemia and the associated myelodysplastic syndromes (MDS). The risk of acute nonlymphocytic leukemia (ANLL) has been documented following alkylating agent treatment of Hodgkin's disease (2–22), multiple myeloma (23–27), non-Hodgkin's lymphoma (NHL) (28–35), breast cancer (36–41), ovarian cancer (41–45), lung cancer (46–51), testicular cancer (52–62), various childhood cancers (63–72), gastrointestinal cancer (73–75), brain cancer (76), and polycythemia vera (77).

The magnitude of risk can be expressed in several ways, including relative risk, absolute risk (excess risk), or cumulative probability (actuarial risk). A relative risk (RR) represents the observed number of leukemia cases divided by an expected number usually based on disease rates in the general population. The range of reported relative risks for leukemia following chemotherapy is quite wide, between 2- and 100-fold, depending on the disease being treated and the intensity of treatment. However, because leukemia is rare, absolute risks and cumulative probabilities are often used to indicate population impact. For example, a relative risk of two for leukemia associated with cyclophosphamide therapy for breast cancer would correspond to an excess of about five leukemias in 10,000 patients over a 10-year period (36). The cumulative probability of ANLL at 10 years is about 0.7% after treatment for breast cancer (37) but between 2 and 10% after treatment for Hodgkin's disease (2). In some clinical centers, perhaps 10 to 20% of newly diagnosed leukemias are therapy related (78).

The risk of ANLL after chemotherapy depends on many factors, including the drug or drugs administered, duration of treatment, cumulative dose, dose intensity, age of the patient, and (possibly) radiotherapy. Risk estimates also differ by whether the MDS are included. Like secondary ANLL, these preleukemic conditions are frequently fatal (79, 79a).

Table 40.1. Carcinogenicity of Anticancer Drugs

Drug	Classification[a]		References
	Human Carcinogen	Animal Carcinogen	
Alkylating agents			
Busulfan (Myleran)	+++	+	(1, 49)
Carmustine (BCNU)	++	+++	(1, 76)
Chlorambucil (Leukeran)	+++	+++	(1, 3, 5, 29, 42, 44, 77, 145)
Chlornaphazine	+++	+	(1, 129)
Cisplatin	++	+++	1, 141)
Cyclophosphamide (Cytoxan)	+++	+++	(1, 29, 36, 44, 49, 124, 127, 147)
Dacarbazine (DTIC)	+	+++	(1)
Ifosfamide	ND	+	(1)
Lomustine (CCNU)	++	+++	(1, 6, 9)
Mechlorethamine (nitrogen mustard)	++	+++	(1, 2, 9, 10)
Melphalan (phenylalanine mustard/Alkeran)	+++	+++	(1, 25, 36, 39, 44)
Mitomycin C	+	+++	(1)
Prednimustine	++	+/−	(29, 116)
Procarbazine	++	+++	(1, 5)
Semustine (methyl-CCNU)	+++	+	(1, 73, 74)
Thiotepa	+++	+++	(1, 42)
Treosulphan	+++	ND	(1, 42, 45)
Uracil mustard	+	+++	(1)
Antimetabolites			
5-Fluorouracil (5-FU)	−−	−−	(1)
6-Mercaptopurine (6-MP)	−−	−−	(1)
Methotrexate	−−	−−	(1, 80)
Mitotic inhibitors			
Vinblastine	+/−	−−	(1, 5)
Vincristine	−−	−−	(1)
DNA intercalation			
Dactinomycin (Actinomycin D)	−−	+	(1)
DNA strand breakage			
Bleomycin	−−	−−	(1)
DNA intercalation & DNA-topoisomerase II inhibition[b]			
Doxorubicin (Adriamycin)	+/−	+++	(1, 15, 83, 91)
Epirubicin (4'-epidoxorubicin)	+/−	−−	(84, 91)
Mitoxanthrone	+/−	−−	(91)
DNA-Topoisomerase II inhibition[b]			
Etoposide (VP-16)	+/−	−−	(9, 60, 66, 69)
Teniposide (VM-26)	+/−	−−	(91)
Razoxane	+/−	−−	(91, 142, 143)

[a] +++ Carcinogenic; ++ probably carcinogenic; + possibly carcinogenic; −− not known to be carcinogenic; +/− uncertain due to limited, inadequate, or inconsistent data; ND no data (1).
[b] For practical purposes, these anticancer drugs could be classified as human leukemogens; however, the leukemogenic effect is most notably apparent in the presence of an alkylating agent or cisplatin therapy.

Chemotherapeutic agents act by several mechanisms including DNA alkylation, mitotic inhibition, cellular metabolism interference, DNA intercalation, and DNA-topoisomerase II inhibition. The alkylating agents bind covalently to DNA and have been convincingly linked to leukemia in many studies of patient populations. It appears that some alkylating agents are less leukemogenic than others, e.g., cyclophosphamide appears to be less leukemogenic than melphalan (25, 44). Some combination chemotherapy might also be less leukemogenic than others, e.g., ABVD (doxorubicin-bleomycin-vinblastine-dacarbazine) appears to be less leukemogenic than MOPP (mechlorethamine-vincristine-procarbazine-prednisone) (2, 5). The antimetabolites, such as methotrexate (80) and 5-fluorouracil (73, 75), do not appear to carry a detectable risk of leukemia. The mitotic inhibitors, vinblastine and vincristine, probably are not leukemogenic, although a recent study suggested a possible risk for vinblastine (5). There is increasing evidence that the epipodophyllotoxins, etoposide and teniposide, increase the risk of leukemia either directly or in combination with other chemical agents (81, 82). The epipodophyllotoxins bind directly to the enzyme DNA-topoisomerase II leading to chromosome breakage and cell death. The anthracyclines, such as doxorubicin, also inhibit DNA-topoisomerase II and may cause leukemia in combination with alkylating agents (83, 84).

It is difficult, if not impossible, to disentangle the separate effects of cumulative dose, dose intensity, and duration of administration, since these measures are so intercorrelated; e.g., patients receiving large cumulative exposures usually have long durations of treatment. Dose-response relationships, however, have been reported among patients given alkylating agents for Hodgkin's disease (3, 20), breast cancer (36), gastrointestinal cancer (74), non-Hodgkin's lymphoma (29, 32), ovarian cancer (42, 44, 85), and childhood cancer (15). Duration of treatment has been proposed as an additional factor, with continuous exposure of stem cells to a stream of cytotoxic agents possibly enhancing the progression of a transformed cell (25). Recently, treatment for breast cancer with short-duration, high-dose, high-intensity cyclophosphamide, standard-dose doxorubicin, and granulocyte colony-stimulating factor has been implicated in the occurrence of excess leukemias of short latency (86).

The effect of gender and age on future ANLL risk is unclear. A few series have indicated that women may be at higher risk than men for second cancer development (87, 88), but this is not seen in other series (3). Age at treatment may be important, with risk generally increasing with increasing age at treatment (2). Chemotherapy for childhood cancer also appears to carry a high risk of leukemia (15), with adolescents at higher risk than younger patients (88).

Because radiotherapy is often given in combination with chemotherapy, it is important to learn whether the two modalities together might enhance the leukemogenic action of either modality alone. One large-scale study of breast cancer patients suggested a possible interaction between radiation and chemotherapy (36), but such an interaction is not generally seen in Hodgkin's disease patients (8). Radiotherapy is often given in high doses to small volumes of tissue, resulting more in cellular killing than in cellular transformation (89, 90). The leukemogenic effect of radiotherapy is generally much lower than that observed following alkylating agents.

Excess leukemias occur soon after the cessation of chemotherapy. The risk remains high for perhaps 10 years and then decreases in both relative and absolute terms (2). Cytogenetic studies have been valuable in defining the characteristics of drug-induced leukemias. The alkylating agents can cause the loss of whole chromosomes 5 and 7 or large segments of their long arms (91). Until recently, the alkylating agents have been implicated as the major actors in therapy-related leukemia development. Now it appears that certain cytostatic drugs that do not react directly with DNA but that target DNA-topoisomerase II can also result in secondary leukemias, especially when given in combination with alkylating agents or cisplatin. Such drugs include etoposide, teniposide, doxorubicin, 4'-epidoxorubicin, mitoxanthrone, and razoxane (91). Epipodophyllotoxin therapy has also been linked to balanced rearrangements of chromosome bands 11q23 and 21q22 (82, 91, 92). Chromosomal changes may present as early indicators of a developing ANLL.

Hodgkin's Disease

The treatment of Hodgkin's disease with supervoltage x-rays and combination chemotherapy is one of the great triumphs of modern cancer therapy. Forty years ago, the diagnosis of Hodgkin's disease meant nearly certain death within a few years; today, patients can be cured. This phenomenal success, however, has resulted in long-term complications of clinical importance, the most serious being second cancer development (93, 94). There are more studies describing the risk of ANLL following Hodgkin's disease than following any other cancer (Table 40.2). Several large series of many thousands of patients report over 100 secondary leukemias (3–5).

PERIOD OF RISK

Somewhat similar to the pattern of risk seen for radiation-induced leukemias, excess ANLL

Table 40.2. Acute Leukemia following Hodgkin's Disease

Study[a]	Number of Patients	Observed Leukemias	Relative Risk	Actuarial Risk (%/years)
IARC (3)	29,552	163	9.0	—[b]
IDHD (4)	12,411	158	27.5	2.4/20 years
Canada/US (5)	9,280	122	23.9	—
BNLI (6, 7)	2,846	16	16.2	1.4/15 years
Netherlands (8, 9)	1,939	31	34.7	4.0/15 years
UICC (10)	1,681	18	64.0	2.3/10 years
Stanford (11)	1,507	28	66.0	4.2/10 years
Milan (12)	1,329	19	—	3.6/10 years
Oslo (13)	1,152	9	24.3	—
LESG (14, 15)	1,036	12	89.0	4.2/20 years
Houston (16)	1,013	14	?	?
Gustave Roussy (17)	892	8	27.6	1.7/15 years
CALGB (18)	798	10	133	4.0/10 years
SWOG (19)	659	21	—	6.2/10 years
Denmark (20)	391	17	—	9.9/10 years
NCI (21)	473	9	—	6.0/10 years (est)
NCI (22)	192	7	95.7	10.0/10 years

[a]These institutions are not all independent series. For example, the International Database on Hodgkin's Disease (IDHD) also includes data from the British National Lymphoma Investigation (BNLI).
[b]—not reported.

following chemotherapy usually occurs from 3 to 10 years after initial treatment. In several small series, the risk of ANLL returned to near normal levels after about 10 years from the last cycle of chemotherapy (11, 20, 22). However, in the three largest series, ANLL risk remained significantly elevated for more than 10 years after treatment, although lower than in earlier time periods (3–5). Differences in studies might be related to different follow-up periods, inclusion of MDS, definition of start of follow-up, and the way salvage therapy, which can occur years later, was handled. For follow-up periods of 15 years, the overall relative risk of ANLL is of the order of 20-fold, and the cumulative risk, 4%, although for some intensively treated patients, the relative risk can approach 100-fold, and the cumulative risk, 10% (20, 22).

TYPE OF CHEMOTHERAPEUTIC AGENT

Combination chemotherapy, particularly MOPP (mechlorethamine-vincristine-procarbazine-prednisone), has been convincingly linked to secondary leukemias. There is mounting evidence that mechlorethamine (nitrogen mustard) is the most potent leukemogen of the four agents (2), although procarbazine is also a leukemogen in animals (1). Mechlorethamine was the strongest predictor of leukemia risk in most (3, 4, 9),

but not all (5), studies. ABVD (doxorubicin-bleomycin-vinblastine-dacarbazine) appears to be less leukemogenic than MOPP (12, 95), with the relative risks recently estimated as 1.5 and 5.9, respectively (5). Among 12,411 patients in the International Database on Hodgkin's Disease, a relative risk of 17 was linked to MOPP combination chemotherapy (4). MVPP (mechlorethamine-vinblastine-procarbazine-prednisone) has been reported to increase leukemia 7.2-fold (5). The PAVe regimen (procarbazine-melphalan-vinblastine) appears less leukemogenic with oral melphalan replacing mechlorethamine (11, 96). It is promising to note that the chemotherapy regimens introduced in the 1980s appear to carry a lower risk of leukemia than earlier drug therapies (8).

Procarbazine has generally not been related to high rates of leukemia (2, 9), although one recent study reports a 4.5-fold elevation (5). In contrast to studies of patients enrolled in clinical trials, it may be difficult in hospital-based studies to completely capture all chemotherapeutic treatments, especially salvage therapies that occur many years after initial treatment and for which high leukemia risks have been reported (6, 9, 21).

Because patients with Hodgkin's disease can be treated with combinations of drugs and may receive additional cytostatic chemicals for relapse, it is difficult to attribute independent effects to individual drugs. Nonetheless, increased ANLL has been ascribed to mechlorethamine (9); lomustine (CCNU) (6, 9); chlorambucil (3, 5); procarbazine (5); vinblastine (5); mechlorethamine and procarbazine combined (3); cyclophosphamide and teniposide combined (9); and cyclophosphamide and procarbazine combined (3).

DOSE RESPONSE

Cumulative dose is directly related to risk of therapy-induced leukemia. Patients intensively treated with alkylating agents are at high risk, especially those who receive additional salvage therapy for relapse or prolonged maintenance with MOPP (4, 6, 21). Further, the number of cycles or treatments received is directly related to ANLL risk (3, 6, 9). Attempts have been made to correlate risk of ANLL with measures of cumulative dose, and it is clear that the higher the dose, the higher the risk (9, 10, 15, 20, 97). Although quantitative data are sparse, a relative risk of 10 was reported following 60 mg/m^2 of mechlorethamine in the Union International Contra Cancer (UICC) series, compared with 0 mg/m^2 (10). In the Netherlands, a relative risk of 10 was linked to 100 mg, which reached a relative risk of 84 at about 220 mg (9). If a body surface area of 1.8 m^2 is assumed for patients in the Netherlands (9), then a relative risk of 10 would occur at approximately 56 mg/m^2, surprisingly close to the UICC value. Similar estimates for mechlorethamine (in mg/m^2) can be obtained from a smaller study of NHL patients (29). A 10-fold risk has also been reported following a median dose of 8070 mg of lomustine (CCNU) (9).

RADIOTHERAPY IMPACT

Radiation of sufficient dose can cause leukemia, but at the high localized therapeutic doses received by most patients with cancer, the energy deposited within relatively small tissue volumes appears to result more in cellular killing than cellular transformation, and radiogenic leukemias are rare (15, 89, 90). Radiotherapy alone has been linked to secondary leukemias in Hodgkin's disease in only a few series (3, 11). Whether radiotherapy, involved-field or subtotal nodal, can enhance or add to the risk of leukemia from chemotherapy alone is not entirely clear, but the enhancement, if any, appears small. Enhanced risk with extensive radiotherapy has been suggested in a few small series (12, 21, 22,

98) and one large one (4). The most recent evidence from several large studies, however, indicates that extensive radiotherapy and chemotherapy are associated with a leukemia risk that is similar to that observed from chemotherapy alone (3, 5, 6, 9).

OTHER FACTORS

Age at treatment has been consistently found to modify the leukemogenic effect of chemotherapy, with treatment over the age of 40 years carrying a higher risk, perhaps 4-fold higher, than treatment at a younger age (4, 9, 11, 12, 20). High risks, however, have also been recorded following treatment of childhood Hodgkin's disease (15), with the suggestion that adolescent exposure was riskier than exposure at younger ages (88). Females have been reported to be at a higher risk of secondary leukemia in a few series (7, 87), but not in others (3, 4, 10, 97).

SURVIVAL

Secondary leukemias following curative therapy for Hodgkin's disease are refractory to treatment and uniformly fatal, with a median survival of only 2 to 3 months (4, 12). The impact of leukemia deaths on overall mortality in Hodgkin's disease patients is on the order of 4% of all deaths (2).

Multiple Myeloma

Patients treated with alkylating agents for multiple myeloma are at high risk of developing acute leukemia (Table 40.3). Actuarial risks as high as 17% at 50 months have been reported (27). Treatments have involved melphalan, prednisone, procarbazine, vincristine, carmustine (BCNU), and cyclophosphamide in combination or in sequence (25–27). Median durations of treatment of 55 months are possible (23, 24). A clinical trial investigation of 648 patients found that the risk of acute leukemia or MDS was directly related to the duration of treatment with melphalan, that the highest risk occurred within 3 years of the last treatment, and that melphalan was more leukemogenic than cyclophosphamide (25). Patients with multiple myeloma develop leukemia in the absence of any therapy (27a), suggesting a predisposition unrelated to treatment as well as the possibility that multiple myeloma patients are more susceptible than other patients to the leukemogenic effects of cytotoxic drugs.

Table 40.3. Acute Leukemia following Multiple Myeloma and Non-Hodgkin's Lymphoma

Study	Number of Patients	Observed Leukemias and MDS	Relative Risk	Actuarial Risk (%/years)
Multiple myeloma				
Mayo Clinic (23, 24)	928	19	—[a]	9.2/10 years
MRC (25)	648	12		10/8 years
Houston (26)	476	12	100	—/9 years
Canada (27)	364	14	230	17.4/5 years
Non-Hodgkin's lymphoma				
Travis (28, 29)	11,386	35	1.8–13.4	<1/20 years
Ontario (30)	3,021	8	6.9	<1/16 years
Duke (31)	686	9	8.3	3.8/10 years
NCI (32)	517	9	105	7.9/24 years
UKCCSG (33)	261	6	—	~5/7 years
RPMI (34)	117	5	341	—
Denmark (35)	602	9	—	6.3/7 years

[a]— Not reported.

Non-Hodgkin's Lymphoma

Chemotherapy has increased ANLL among patients treated for NHL but not to the extent seen in patients treated for Hodgkin's disease (Table 40.3). Risks in different series reflect differences in the extent of chemotherapy given. For example, in a general population series, nearly 40% of patients did not receive chemotherapy (28, 29).

In an international cancer registry study, 35 leukemias occurred in 11,386 NHL patients, and the actuarial risk at 20 years was less than 1%, reflecting the high proportion of patients not given alkylating agents (28, 29). The risk associated with individual drugs was estimated for chlorambucil (RR = 2.4; mean dose, 6.5 g), cyclophosphamide (RR = 1.8; mean dose, 27.5 g), prednimustine (RR = 13.4; mean dose, 38.3 g), and mechlorethamine combined with procarbazine (RR = 12.6; mean doses, 195 mg and 15.9 g, respectively). Prednimustine is the C-21 prednisolone ester of chlorambucil. Again, cyclophosphamide carried a lower risk than other alkylating agents. Treatment with the epipodophyllotoxins, doxorubicin, or bleomycin was not associated with an increased ANLL risk. Radiotherapy did not increase the risk or enhance the leukemogenic effect of chemotherapy. Dose-response relationships were apparent for chlorambucil and prednimustine, based on cumulative dose or duration. A 6-month regimen of cyclophosphamide might result in about four excess leukemias in 10,000 patients followed for 10 years (29).

Intensively treated NHL patients (33, 35) and those given hemi- or total-body irradiation (32, 34) have much higher leukemia risks than those seen in other studies (29, 30). The effect of radiotherapy is noteworthy in that the low-dose, fractionated, whole-body exposures would be less likely to result in the same cell-killing effect seen following more conventional radiotherapy. Although cyclophosphamide was considered to produce secondary leukemias at the same magnitude of risk as other alkylating agents in one study (35), the nine ANLL patients also received chlorambucil or combination chemotherapy in addition to cyclophosphamide, so that individual drug effects would be difficult to discern.

Chronic Lymphocytic Leukemia

Although patients with chronic lymphocytic leukemia (CLL) are at increased risk of developing a second malignancy, cancer registry studies have not reported increases, possibly due to incomplete reporting practices (99). The evidence that chemotherapy increases the risk of leukemia in CLL patients comes mainly from case reports (100–106). Leukemia, however, can occur after CLL in the absence of treatment. One hospital series reported three ANLL/MDS diagnoses in 1374 patients, which was close to the number expected (107). The drug regimens and doses administered to CLL patients may be less intense than those used for other lymphoproliferative disorders.

Breast Cancer

An international case-control study of 82,700 breast cancer patients reported 90 cases of secondary leukemia and a relative risk of 10 associated with chemotherapy with alkylating agents (36) (Table 40.4). Chest wall radiotherapy was linked to a 2.4-fold risk and appeared to enhance the leukemogenic effect of chemotherapy (RR = 17.4). Cyclophosphamide was 10 times less leukemogenic than melphalan (RR = 3.1 vs. 31.4). Dose-response relationships were found for both melphalan and cyclophosphamide in terms of cumulative dose and duration of treatment. There was little evidence for a risk from cyclophosphamide at doses below 20 g. No increased risk was seen for treatments with fluorouracil, methotrexate, prednisone, doxorubicin, or vincristine. The leukemia risk was highest among current or recently treated patients (<3 years) and declined thereafter to low levels at 7 to 10 years.

In a large clinical trial series (38), the risk of melphalan-induced leukemia was similar to that reported in the international case-control study (36). Among 5299 breast cancer patients treated with adjuvant melphalan, 34 developed ANLL/MDS (RR = 24.0). The actuarial risk at 10 years was 1.7%, somewhat higher than the 0.7% reported following chemotherapy in a large U.S. cancer registry series (37). The excess risk of ANLL following chemotherapy for breast cancer is on the order of 5.8 cases per 10,000 women per year (37).

A large case-control series from Germany reported a relative risk of 2.7, based on 52 leukemia cases following treatment with cyclophosphamide (40). Risk increased with increasing cumulative dose, reaching 7-fold for doses above 30 g. The actuarial risk of 0.3% for leukemia at 10 years was substantially less than the 1.7% estimated by Fisher et al. (38) for adjuvant melphalan therapy. Cyclophosphamide-methotrexate-5-fluorouracil (CMF)-based adjuvant chemotherapy was also linked to a low risk among 2465 patients in Milan (39). Several small series report no leukemia risk following CMF (108, 109) or CAF (cyclophosphamide-doxorubicin-5-fluorouracil) (110).

There may be a very high risk of ANLL/MDS associated with mitolactol (dibromodulcitol) in patients with metastatic breast cancer (111, 112). Among 1092 patients, 28 ANLL cases occurred following a median dose of 12.8 g. It has also been proposed that doxorubicin used in the treatment of advanced-stage breast cancer is leukemogenic, especially when combined with cisplatin or alkylating agents (83). Doxorubicin is a DNA-topoisomerase II inhibitor and, similar to the leukemias seen following therapy with the epipodophyllotoxins, balanced chromosomal translocations were observed at 11q23. The number of leukemias, however, was only five.

A randomized trial in Canada reported four leukemias following high-dose 4'-epidoxorubi-

Table 40.4. Acute Leukemia following Breast Cancer and Ovarian Cancer

Study	Number of Patients	Observed Leukemias and MDS	Relative Risk	Actuarial Risk (%/years)
Breast cancer				
Curtis (36)[a]	82,700	90	10.0	—[b]
SEER (37)[a]	13,734	24	11.5	0.7/10 years
NSABP (38)	5,299	34	24.0	1.7/10 years
Milan (39)	2,465	3	2.3	0.2/15 years
Germany (40)	—	52	2.7	0.3/10 years
SWOG (41)	2,638	6	—	—
Ovarian cancer				
IARC (42)	99,113	114	12	—
SGO (43)	5,455	13	21.0	—
Greene (44)	3,363	35	93	8.5/10 years
Denmark (45)	553	8	175	7.6/5 years
Germany (41)	—	9	14.6	—

[a]Some overlap.
[b]— Not reported.

cin and cyclophosphamide (84). Three cases occurred within 18 months of randomization, and the characteristic 11q23 translocation abnormality was noted in one case. Other small series of breast cancer patients have not noted excess leukemias (113, 114), and few cases of leukemia have been reported following doxorubicin and cyclophosphamide combinations for breast cancer (110, 115). Nonetheless, these reports raise concern about high-dose anthracycline and cyclophosphamide combinations for patients in the adjuvant setting.

A series from Denmark reports five leukemias among 71 patients with advanced breast cancer treated with prednimustine, methotrexate, 5-fluorouracil, mitoxantrone, and tamoxifen (116). The authors conclude that prednimustine, a chlorambucil derivative, was the most likely culprit and caution against the use of such intense combination chemotherapy with alkylating agents in potentially curable patients. A portion of the high risk in this series was possibly attributable to the advanced age of the patients treated (mean, 61 years) and the intense cytogenetic screening of all patients who developed a refractory cytopenia.

Among 2548 women receiving higher than standard doses of cyclophosphamide and standard doses of doxorubicin to prevent recurrence of breast cancer, five cases of acute myeloid leukemia developed within 2 years (86). All women had also received a blood growth factor (granulocyte colony-stimulating factor, G-CSF). The expected number of ANLL cases in a general population of 2500 women followed for 2 years would be about 0.35. Assuming that a 10,000 mg cumulative dose of cyclophosphamide would double this risk (36), less than one ANLL case would still be expected. The five observed cases in such a short time raise concern that high-intensity regimens coupled with growth factor rescue may be more leukemogenic than standard treatments. All women were over the age of 50 years.

Ovarian Cancer

Early studies of patients with Hodgkin's disease or multiple myeloma treated with alkylating agents observed high risks of secondary leukemia; however, it was unclear whether leukemia might be part of the natural history of these lymphoproliferative disorders or whether patients with these conditions might be especially sensitive to the leukemogenic effect of chemical agents. Thus, it was noteworthy in 1977, when Reimer et al. (43) reported an increase in leukemia (13 observed vs. 0.62 expected) among 5455 ovarian cancer patients (Table 40.4). Since ovarian cancer rarely involves the bone marrow, the excess leukemias were ascribed to the alkylating agent therapy received, including melphalan, chlorambucil, cyclophosphamide, thiotepa, and uracil mustard. Historic data on 6596 women treated prior to the era of chemotherapy revealed no leukemia increase.

Combining data from five randomized clinical trials and two large cancer centers, Greene et al. (44) convincingly linked secondary leukemia to chemotherapy among 3363 women with ovarian cancer. Melphalan was found to be two to three times more leukemogenic than cyclophosphamide. A risk for chlorambucil had previously been reported (85). The actuarial risk at 10 years for alkylating agent therapy was 8.5%. Dose-response relationships were apparent for melphalan, cyclophosphamide, and chlorambucil (44, 85). The risk of ANLL was highest 5 to 6 years after therapy began and declined thereafter. Risk was highest shortly after chemotherapy had ceased. The drug-related leukemias were refractory to treatment, and all women died shortly after diagnosis (median, 2 months). Radiotherapy neither increased the risk of leukemia nor enhanced the leukemogenic effect of chemotherapy. The leukemogenic risk following melphalan for ovarian cancer appeared much higher than that seen following melphalan for breast cancer (39), but this difference could be attributable to differences in dose. Women in the breast cancer clinical trials uniformly received a cumulative dose of 600 mg of melphalan, whereas the excess leukemias in the ovarian cancer trials occurred among the women who received the highest doses (median 965 mg, ranging up to 9652 mg). The clinical trial series are important because they are much less susceptible to biases possible in other types of analytic or observational studies.

The largest study to date involved 99,113 survivors of ovarian cancer, among whom 114 leukemias developed (42). The relative risk associated with chemotherapy was 12, and radiotherapy neither increased the risk nor enhanced the effect of chemotherapy. Risk was greatest 4 to 5 years after treatment began and within the first year after treatment stopped. Risk decreased with time since last treatment. Dose-response trends were seen for chlorambucil, cyclophosphamide, melphalan, thiotepa, and treosulfan.

Doxorubicin and cisplatin combined also increased the occurrence of leukemia. Melphalan and chlorambucil were the most potent leukemogens, followed by thiotepa, with cyclophosphamide and treosulfan being the weakest.

Eight leukemias occurred against 0.04 expected following treosulfan (dihydroxybusulfan) treatment of 553 women with cancer of the ovary in Denmark (45). In Germany, cyclophosphamide for ovarian cancer was linked to a 14.6-fold risk of leukemia in a case-control investigation based on nine cases (40). Melphalan caused four excess leukemias in a series of 474 patients in Sweden (117). Cisplatin, etoposide, and bleomycin adjuvant therapy among 93 women may have caused the one case of acute myelomonocytic leukemia that occurred 22 months after diagnosis (118).

Lung Cancer

Chemotherapeutic agents frequently used to treat small cell lung cancer (SCLC) include cyclophosphamide, doxorubicin, etoposide, cisplatin, lomustine (CCNU), procarbazine, and vincristine. Secondary leukemias are noted after treatment with nitrosoureas, procarbazine, or alkylating agents administered for prolonged periods of time (Table 40.5). Small studies of intensively treated patients with SCLC report very large relative risks, 77 to 316, but are based on only a few leukemia cases (47, 48, 50). Actuarial risks as high as 44% at 2.5 years have also been reported, based on four leukemias among 119 patients (51). Although the risks are high, the total number of reports in the literature is modest and will likely decrease in the future, given that fewer cycles of chemotherapy are now recommended, and a marked reduction in the use of nitrosoureas and procarbazine has occurred (119). In a large cancer registry study, 16 leukemias occurred among 23,757 patients, and the relative risk associated with chemotherapy was 5.5 (46).

Busulfan was implicated in four acute leukemias occurring in 243 lung cancer patients treated within a clinical trial, whereas no leukemias occurred among similar numbers of lung cancer patients given cyclophosphamide (49). Procarbazine, cyclophosphamide, and nitrosoureas were believed to cause three leukemias among 158 patients treated at Stanford (50). Cyclophosphamide, doxorubicin, and vincristine (CAV), with or without etoposide, given to 377 patients with SCLC apparently caused two leukemias in one series (48).

Six acute leukemias and MDS occurred among 796 patients in Denmark treated with lomustine (CCNU), cyclophosphamide, and etoposide (47). High-dose etoposide and cisplatin were suggested as the cause of a new clinical syndrome, distinct from the secondary leuke-

Table 40.5. Acute Leukemia following Lung Cancer and Testicular Cancer

Study	Number of Patients	Observed Leukemias and MDS	Relative Risk	Actuarial Risk (%/years)
Lung cancer				
SEER (46)	23,757	16	6.3	—[a]
Denmark (47)	796	6	77	14/4 years
Vanderbilt (48)	377	2	154	1.9/7 years
England (49)	243	4	—	—
Stanford (50)	158	3	316	25/3.1 years
Chicago (51)	119	4	—	44/2.5 years
Testicular cancer				
IARC (52)	17,730	9	2.0	—
SEER (53)	9,739	14	6.3	—
ICRF (54)	2,013	22	2.5	—
Netherlands (55)	1,909	4	5.1	—
Lit. review (56)	1,868	11	—	0.6/5 years
England (57)	636	6	—	—
Indiana (58)	538	2	—	—
New York (59)	343	2	—	—
Denmark (60)	212	5	336	4.7/5.7 years
Germany (61, 62)	128	1	30–35	0.8/4.5 years

[a]— Not reported.

mias caused by alkylating agents, where four leukemias occurred among 199 patients with non-small-cell lung cancer (51). The median cumulative doses of etoposide and cisplatin were 6795 and 355 mg/m^2, respectively. The etoposide-related leukemias tend to occur early, involve 11q23 abnormalities, and have a reasonable prognosis.

Testicular Cancer

Leukemia occurs after testicular cancer in the absence of chemotherapy, as noted in several large-scale population-based studies (52–54, 120). Interestingly, testicular cancer is also increased following leukemia (121), and it has been postulated that leukemia may be part of the natural history of certain germ cell cancers (122). Thus, an association between secondary leukemias and chemotherapy for testicular cancer is not as strongly established as for other cancers.

There is suggestive evidence that intensive etoposide treatment, which began in 1983, coupled with cisplatin or alkylating agents is highly leukemogenic. In Denmark, patients who received more than 2 g/m^2 of etoposide were at high risk for leukemias that occurred early and showed abnormalities in 11q23 (60). Other series of more standard (lower) doses generally fail to reproduce such high risks (61, 62).

Differences in risk in various studies (Table 40.5) clearly reflect differences in the extent of multiagent chemotherapy. The high risk seen in Denmark (60) was concentrated among patients given very high doses of etoposide (>2 g) and perhaps reflected an interaction with cisplatin (61). Except for the population-based series, no

study reports more than six cases of acute leukemia. A literature review of 1868 patients with cancer of the testes given less than 2 g of etoposide computed the 5-year actuarial risk to be 0.6% (56).

Childhood Cancer

Children treated for a diverse set of cancers are at risk of developing chemotherapy-related leukemia (14, 146) (Table 40.6). Among 9170 children treated at Late Effects Study Group (LESG) centers, 22 leukemias developed, for a relative risk of 14 and an actuarial risk of 0.8% at 20 years (15). A dose response was seen for alkylating agent therapy, with risk reaching over 20-fold in the highest dose category. High-dose doxorubicin was related to a 4.9-fold risk, and doxorubicin appeared to enhance the leukemogenic effect of alkylating agents (15). Children with acute lymphocytic leukemia appear to be at high risk of ANLL if treated with epipodophyllotoxins (69, 72) but not otherwise (65). Etoposide has also been reported to increase the risk of ANLL in children treated for rhabdomyosarcoma (66, 123, 124). High risks of ANLL follow alkylating agent therapy for childhood Hodgkin's disease (15, 97). Relatively low risks of secondary leukemias among 30,880 children treated in the Nordic countries may be the result of less aggressive therapies (63). Epipodophyllotoxins were linked to secondary leukemias in a large series in England, especially in combination with alkylating agents (64). In one study, the schedule of drug administration appeared to be more important than the cumulative dose of etoposide and teniposide (69). Other intercalating topoisomerase II

Table 40.6. Acute Leukemia following Childhood Cancer

Study	Initial Childhood Cancer	Number of Patients	Observed Leukemias and MDS	Relative Risk	Actuarial Risk (%/years)
Nordic countries (63)	All cancers	30,880	15	2.8	—[a]
Britain (64)	All cancers	16,422	22	8	0.2/5 years
CCSG (65)	Acute lymphoid leukemia	9,720	2	—	—
LESG (14, 15)	All cancers	9,170	22	14	0.8/20 years
IRS (66)	Rhabdomyosarcoma	1,062	5	~7	—
St. Jude (67, 69)	Acute lymphoid leukemia	734	21	—	3.8/6 years
St. Jude (68)	All solid tumors	3,365	12	—	—
Gustave Roussy (70, 71)	All cancers	634	2	9	0.8/25 years
Texas (72)	Acute lymphoid leukemia	205	10	—	5.9/4 years

[a]—— Not reported.

inhibitors (doxorubicin, dactinomycin) may cause secondary ANLL in combination with alkylating agents and radiotherapy (69a).

Other Conditions

Two sets of randomized trials have provided information on the risk of acute leukemia associated with specific chemotherapeutic agents: methyl-CCNU (semustine) in the treatment of gastrointestinal cancer (73, 74) and chlorambucil in the treatment of polycythemia vera (77) (Table 40.7. Among 3633 patients with gastrointestinal cancer, 14 leukemias occurred in 2067 patients given semustine, whereas only 1 occurred in 1566 patients given other therapies (73). A dose response was later reported, confirming the leukemogenicity of this nitrosourea (74). Among 431 patients with polycythemia vera, acute leukemia developed in 1 of 134 (0.7%) treated with phlebotomy only, 9 of 156 (5.8%) treated with radioactive ^{32}P, and 16 of 141 (11.3%) treated with chlorambucil (77). BCNU was linked to ANLL in a small clinical trial series of patients with brain cancer (76). Methotrexate for gestational trophoblastic cancers did not increase the

risk of leukemia (80), nor did 5-fluorouracil and low-dose thiotepa in colorectal cancer patients (73, 75). Chemotherapy for some nonneoplastic conditions, such as cyclophosphamide for rheumatoid arthritis, has been linked to excessive leukemia (124a).

BLADDER CANCER AFTER CHEMOTHERAPY

Bladder cancer can occur after intensive treatment with cyclophosphamide (Table 40.8), often in conjunction with hemorrhagic cystitis (124a–129). In a large international study, 31 bladder cancers developed among 6171 2-year survivors of NHL (127). A 4.5-fold risk of bladder cancer was linked to cyclophosphamide therapy, and there was evidence of a dose response. For cumulative doses of cyclophosphamide of less than 20 g, 20 to 49 g, and 50 g or more, the relative risks of bladder cancer were 2.4, 6.0, and 14.5, respectively. Radiotherapy did not enhance the carcinogenic effect of cyclophosphamide, and kidney cancer was not linked to cyclophosphamide treatment. At cumulative doses of 50 g or more, about seven excess bladder cancers might

Table 40.7. Acute Leukemia after Chemotherapy for Various Disease

Study	Condition	Number of Patients	Observed Leukemias and MDS	Relative Risk	Actuarial Risk (%/years)
NCI Trials (73, 74)	Gastrointestinal cancer	3,633	15	12.4	4/6 years
VA (75)	Colorectal cancer	1,613	4	1.0	——[a]
NCI (76)	Brain cancer	1,628	2	24.6	——[c]
PVSG (77)	Polycythemia vera	141	16	13.5	~25/8 years
London (80)	Gestational trophoblastic tumors	457	1	~1.	0/7.8 years

[a]——[c] Not reported.

Table 40.8. Bladder Cancer after Chemotherapy for Various Conditions

Study	Condition	Number of Patients	Observed Leukemias and MDS	Relative Risk	Actuarial Risk (%/years)
SEER (125)	Non-Hodgkin's lymphoma	17,261	42	1.7	——[c]
Denmark (126)	Non-Hodgkin's lymphoma	471[a]	7	6.8	10.7/12 years
Travis (127)	Non-Hodgkin's lymphoma	6,171[a]	31	4.5	——
Baker (124a)	Rheumatoid arthritis	119[a]	6	——	——
Kinlen (128)	Rheumatoid arthritis	416[a]	5	10.0	——
Thiede (129)	Polycythemia vera	61[b]	10	——	——

[a]Treated with cyclophosphamide.
[b]Treated with chlornaphazine.
[c]—— Not reported.

occur among 100 patients followed for 15 years. Bladder cancer does not appear to be increased among patients with NHL not given cyclophosphamide (125, 130).

A high risk (RR = 6.8) of bladder cancer was associated with cyclophosphamide in a Danish series of 471 NHL patients given relatively high cumulative doses of 83 to 129 g (126). Intensive treatment of patients with rheumatoid arthritis and other conditions has also been found to elevate bladder cancer risk (124a, 128).

In Denmark, 10 bladder cancers developed in 61 patients treated with chlornaphazine for polycythemia vera (129). The bladder cancers occurred between 3 and 10 years after treatment. Chlornaphazine is a chemical analogue of 2-naphthylamine, another human bladder carcinogen (1).

NON-HODGKIN'S LYMPHOMA AFTER CHEMOTHERAPY

Patients treated for Hodgkin's disease are at high risk of developing NHL (Table 40.9), although a relationship with chemotherapy is not apparent (6). The range of relative and actuarial risks, however, is similar to those seen for ANLL. The increase in NHL is likely related to the immune status of patients, since excess NHL can occur in immunocompromised individuals following renal (130a), cardiac (131), and bone marrow transplantation (132). NHL also occurs in excess among patients treated with immunosuppressive drugs such as cyclophosphamide and among patients with immunodeficiency disorders (128, 133). There is little evidence that radiotherapy alone increases the risk of NHL in any series (134).

OTHER TUMORS

If the late effects of chemotherapy paralleled those after radiotherapy (135), enormous increases in solid cancers would have been expected. It is thus noteworthy that high risks of drug-related solid cancers among long-term survivors of cancer have not been seen in several large-scale studies of Hodgkin's disease patients intensively treated with chemotherapy (4, 5, 52). Although survivors of cancer are at risk for developing second malignancies for a variety of reasons (136), chemotherapy has been implicated for only a few sites: bladder cancer following cyclophosphamide (127) and chlornaphazine (129) and perhaps bone cancer following alkylating agent therapy (137). Among 9170 children with cancer, the actuarial risk of developing a bone cancer at 20 years was 2.8%, and the relative risk was 133. A case-control analysis of 64 bone cancers within this cohort found a 4.7-fold risk for alkylating agents after adjusting for radiotherapy, and there was evidence of a dose response. The most common chemotherapeutic agents were cyclophosphamide, triethylenemelamine, and chlorambucil. A recent study of Hodgkin's disease patients also found an association between chemotherapy and cancers of the bones, joints, articular cartilage, and soft tissues, based on a total of 24 cases (5).

For other solid cancers, there are as yet no clear patterns arising. Kidney cancer was not linked to chemotherapy in an analytic study of patients with NHL (127). Secondary lung cancer has been suggested as an outcome of chemotherapy for Hodgkin's disease in some studies (6, 138) but not others (5). The carcinogenic effect of radiotherapy in producing breast cancer might have been potentiated by chemotherapy

Table 40.9. Non-Hodgkin's Lymphoma (NHL) after Treatment for Hodgkin's Disease

Study	Number of Patients	Observed NHL	Relative Risk	Actuarial Risk (%/years)
IARC (52)	28,462	24	3.0	—[a]
IDHD (4)	12,411	106	32.0	3.2/20 years
Canada/US (5)	9,280	35	5.6	——
BNLI (6, 7)	2,846	17	16.8	1.5/15 years
Netherlands (8)	1,939	23	20.6	4.1/20 years
Stanford (11, 144)	1,507	9	18.0	1.6/15 years
Milan (12)	1,329	6	——	1.3/10 years
Gustave Roussy (17)	892	8	50.0	2.0/15 years

[a]—— Not reported.

in one series of Hodgkin's disease patients (139). Thyroid cancer has not been linked to chemotherapy, even in childhood (140). In a recent large-scale investigation of Hodgkin's disease patients, the relative risk of all solid cancers after any chemotherapy was 1.4 (5). Secondary cancers of the oral cavity and the digestive organs were linked to chemotherapy (5). A modest risk of 1.8-fold for female genital cancer was also associated with chemotherapy for Hodgkin's disease (5). The number of drug combinations in some series, over 200 in one study (5), and the effect of radiotherapy, coupled with genetic factors, environmental agents, and long latency, have made it difficult to link secondary solid cancers with prior chemotherapy.

SUMMARY

Chemotherapy, especially with the alkylating agents, can cause leukemia and myelodysplastic syndromes. Chromosomes 5 and 7 often display cytogenetic defects associated with alkylating agent–induced leukemias. Excess leukemias occur shortly after chemotherapy ceases, and treatment of these secondary leukemias is very disappointing. Risk decreases with time but is still elevated among 10-year survivors. There is some indication that the more modern treatment regimens, with fewer cycles and less use of nitrosoureas, procarbazine, and melphalan, might result in fewer secondary leukemias without sacrificing therapeutic benefit. Recently, the epipodophyllotoxins, in combination with alkylating agents or cisplatin, have been linked to increases in secondary leukemias that have a rapid onset and 11q23 abnormalities. These secondary leukemias also appear more responsive to treatment than those induced by alkylating agents. A recent concern is whether very high doses of alkylating agents over very short durations might be especially leukemogenic. Radiotherapy produces many fewer secondary leukemias than chemotherapy, and there is only weak evidence for any interaction between radiotherapy and chemotherapy.

Except for cancers of the bladder and perhaps bone, there are few solid cancers convincingly linked to chemotherapy. Studies of long-term survivors of Hodgkin's disease have not linked high overall risks of secondary solid cancers to chemotherapy.

Chemotherapy has increased the life span of many patients, but the adverse effects, the most serious being the development of a new cancer, must be carefully weighed against the therapeutic benefit. Caution should be exercised when considering alkylating agents for cancer patients at low risk for relapse and, especially, in the treatment of nonmalignant diseases such as rheumatoid arthritis. The increased use of adjuvant chemotherapy in patients with localized disease has heightened the need for careful risk-benefit evaluations for individual patients.

Focused case-control (or case-cohort) studies with detailed information on drug and radiation dose are needed to quantify the level of solid cancer risk attributable to combined modality therapy. Molecular forensics might also be applied to link specific changes in DNA to specific treatments, such as the possibility that a unique p53 mutational spectra might occur in bladder cancers following cyclophosphamide. The role of radiotherapy, immune dysfunction, host, and life-style factors in modulating chemotherapy risks should also be further elucidated. Finally, future studies should include potential biologic markers of risk in order to better predict those likely to develop a new cancer.

References

1. IARC (International Agency for Research on Cancer). IARC monographs on the evaluation of carcinogenic risks to humans, vol. 50, Pharmaceutical drugs. Lyon: IARC, 1990.
2. Henry-Amar M, Dietrich P-Y. Acute leukemia after treatment of Hodgkin's disease. Hematol Oncol Clin North Am 1993;7:369–387.
3. Kaldor JM, Day NE, Clarke EA, et al. Leukemia following Hodgkin's disease. N Engl J Med 1990;322:7–13.
4. Henry-Amar M. Second cancer after the treatment for Hodgkin's disease: a report from the International Database on Hodgkin's Disease. Ann Oncol 1992;4:117–128.
5. Boivin JF, Hutchison GB, Zauber AG, et al. Incidence of second cancers in patients treated for Hodgkin's disease. J Natl Cancer Inst 1995;87:732–741.
6. Swerdlow AJ, Douglas AJ, Hudson GV, Hudson BV, Bennett MH, MacLennan KA. Risk of second primary cancers after Hodgkin's disease by type of treatment: analysis of 2846 patients in the British National Lymphoma Investigation. Br Med J 1992;304:1137–1143.
7. Swerdlow AJ, Douglas AJ, Hudson GV, et al. Risk of second primary cancer after Hodgkin's disease in patients in the British National Lymphoma Investigation: relationship to host factors, histology and stage of Hodgkin's disease, and splenectomy. Br Med J 1993;68:1006–1011.
8. van Leeuwen FE, Klokman WJ, Hagenbeek A, et al. Second cancer risk following Hodgkin's disease: a 20-year follow-up study. J Clin Oncol 1994;12:312–325.

9. van Leeuwen FE, Chorus AM, van den Belt-Dusebout AW, et al. Leukemia risk following Hodgkin's disease: relation to cumulative dose of alkylating agents, treatment with teniposide combinations, numbers of episodes of chemotherapy, and bone marrow damage. J Clin Oncol 1994;12:1063–1073.

10. van der Velden JW, van Putten WL, Guinee VF, et al. Subsequent development of acute non-lymphocytic leukemia in patients treated for Hodgkin's disease. Int J Cancer 1988;42:252–255.

11. Tucker MA, Coleman CN, Cox RS, Varghese A, Rosenberg SA. Risk of second cancers after treatment for Hodgkin's disease. N Engl J Med 1988;318:76–81.

12. Valagussa P, Santoro A, Fossati-Bellani F, Banfi A, Bonadonna G. Second acute leukemia and other malignancies following treatment for Hodgkin's disease. J Clin Oncol 1986;4:830–837.

13. Abrahamsen JF, Andersen A, Hannisdal E, et al. Second malignancies after treatment of Hodgkin's disease: the influence of treatment, follow-up time, and age. J Clin Oncol 1993;11:255–261.

14. Tucker MA, Meadows AT, Boice JD Jr, Hoover RN, Fraumeni JF Jr. Cancer risk following treatment of childhood cancer. In: Boice JD Jr, Fraumeni JF Jr, eds. Radiation carcinogenesis, epidemiology and biological significance. New York: Raven Press, 1984:211–224.

15. Tucker MA, Meadows AT, Boice JD Jr, et al. Leukemia after therapy with alkylating agents for childhood cancer. J Natl Cancer Inst 1987;78:459–464.

16. Rodriguez MA, Fuller LM, Zimmerman SO, et al. Hodgkin's disease: study of treatment intensities and incidences of second malignancies. Ann Oncol 1993;4:125–131.

17. Dietrich PY, Henry-Amar M, Cosset JM, Bodis S, Bosq J, Hayat M. Second primary cancers in patients continuously disease-free from Hodgkin's disease: a protective role for the spleen? Blood 1994;84:1209–1215.

18. Glicksman AS, Pajak TF, Gottlieb A, Nissen N, Stutzman L, Cooper MR. Second malignant neoplasms in patients successfully treated for Hodgkin's disease: a Cancer and Leukemia Group B study. Cancer Treat Rep 1982;66:1035–1044.

19. Coltman CA Jr, Dixon DO. Second malignancies complicating Hodgkin's disease: a Southwest Oncology Group 10-year followup. Cancer Treat Rep 1982;66:1023–1033.

20. Pedersen-Bjergaard J, Larsen SO, Struck J, et al. Risk of therapy-related leukaemia and preleukaemia after Hodgkin's disease. Relation to age, cumulative dose of alkylating agents, and time from chemotherapy. Lancet 1987;2:83–88.

21. Tester WJ, Kinsella TJ, Waller B, et al. Second malignant neoplasms complicating Hodgkin's disease: the National Cancer Institute experience. J Clin Oncol 1984;2:762–769.

22. Blayney DW, Longo DL, Young RC, et al. Decreasing risk of leukemia with prolonged follow-up after chemotherapy and radiotherapy for Hodgkin's disease. N Engl J Med 1987;316:710–714.

23. Kyle RA, Pierre RV, Bayrd ED. Multiple myeloma and acute myelomonocytic leukemia. N Engl J Med 1970;283:1121–1125.

24. Kyle RA, Gertz MA. Second malignancies after chemotherapy. In Perry MC, ed. The chemotherapy sourcebook. Baltimore: Williams & Wilkins, 1992.

25. Cuzick J, Erskine S, Edelman D, Galton DA. A comparison of the incidence of the myelodysplastic syndrome and acute myeloid leukaemia following melphalan and cyclophosphamide treatment for myelomatosis. A report to the Medical Research Council's working party on leukaemia in adults. Br J Cancer 1987;55:523–529.

26. Gonzalez F, Trujillo JM, Alexanian R. Acute leukemia in multiple myeloma. Ann Intern Med 1977; 86:440–443.

27. Bergsagel DE, Bailey AJ, Langley GR, MacDonald RN, White DF, Miller AB. The chemotherapy of plasma-cell myeloma and the incidence of acute leukemia. N Engl J Med 1979;301:743–748.

27a. Bergsagel DE. Plasma cell neoplasms and acute leukaemia. Clin Haematol 1982;11:221–234.

28. Travis LB, Curtis RE, Glimelius B, et al. Second cancers among long-term survivors of non-Hodgkin's lymphoma. J Natl Cancer Inst 1993;85:1932–1937.

29. Travis LB, Curtis RE, Stovall M, et al. Risk of leukemia following treatment for non-Hodgkin's lymphoma. J Natl Cancer Inst 1994;86:1450–1457.

30. Lishner M, Slingerland J, Barr J, Panzarella T, Degendorfer P, Sotcliffe S. Second malignant neoplasms in patients with non-Hodgkin's lymphoma. Hematol Oncol 1991;9:169–179.

31. Lavey RS, Eby NL, Prosnitz LR. Impact on second malignancy risk of the combined use of radiation and chemotherapy for lymphomas. Cancer 1990;66:80–88.

32. Greene MH, Young RC, Merrill JM, DeVita VT. Evidence of a treatment dose-response in acute non-lymphocytic leukemias which occur after therapy of non-Hodgkin's lymphoma. Cancer Res 1983;43:1891–1898.

33. Ingram L, Mott MG, Mann JR, Raafat F, Darbyshire PJ, Morris-Jones PH. Second malignancies in children treated for non-Hodgkin's lymphoma and T-cell leukaemia with the UKCCSG regimens. Br J Cancer 1987;55:463–466.

34. Gomez GA, Aggarwal KK, Han T. Post-therapeutic acute malignant myeloproliferative syndrome and acute nonlymphocytic leukemia in non-Hodgkin's lymphoma. Cancer 1982;50:2285–2288.

35. Pedersen-Bjergaard J, Ersboll J, Sorensen HM, et al. Risk of acute nonlymphocytic leukemia and preleukemia in patients treated with cyclophosphamide for non-Hodgkin's lymphomas. Comparison with results obtained in patients treated for Hodgkin's disease and ovarian carcinoma with other alkylating agents. Ann Intern Med 1985;103:195–200.

36. Curtis RE, Boice JD Jr, Stovall M, et al. Risk of leukemia after chemotherapy and radiation treatment for breast cancer. N Engl J Med 1992;326:1745–1751.

37. Curtis RE, Boice JD Jr, Moloney WC, Ries LG, Flannery JT. Leukemia following chemotherapy for breast cancer. Cancer Res 1990;50:2741–2746.

38. Fisher B, Rockette H, Fisher ER, Wickerham DL, Redmond C, Brown A. Leukemia in breast cancer patients following adjuvant chemotherapy or post-operative radiation: the NSABP experience. J Clin Oncol 1985;3:1640–1658.

39. Valagussa P, Moliterni A, Terenziani M, Zambetti M, Bonadonna G. Second malignancies following CMF-based adjuvant chemotherapy in resectable breast cancer. Ann Oncol 1994;5:803–808.

40. Haas JF, Kittelmann B, Mehnert WH, et al. Risk of leukaemia in ovarian tumour and breast cancer patients following treatment by cyclophosphamide. Br J Cancer 1987;55:213–218.

41. Tallman MS, Gray R, Bennett JM, et al. Leukemogenic potential of adjuvant chemotherapy for early-stage breast cancer: the Eastern Cooperative Oncology Group experience. J Clin Oncol 1995;13:1557–1563.

42. Kaldor JM, Day NE, Pettersson F, et al. Leukemia following chemotherapy for ovarian cancer. N Engl J Med 1990;322:1–6.

43. Reimer RR, Hoover R, Fraumeni JF Jr, Young RC. Acute leukemia after alkylating-agent therapy of ovarian cancer. N Engl J Med 1977;297:177–181.

44. Greene MH, Harris EL, Gershenson DM, et al. Melphalan may be a more potent leukemogen than cyclophosphamide. Ann Intern Med 1986;105:360–367.

45. Pedersen-Bjergaard J, Nissen NI, Sorensen HM, et al. Acute non-lymphocytic leukemia in patients with ovarian carcinoma following long-term treatment with Treosulfan (=dihydroxybusulfan). Cancer 1980;45:19–29.

46. Travis LB, Curtis RE, Hankey BF, Fraumeni JF Jr. Acute nonlymphocytic leukemia after small-cell lung cancer. J Clin Oncol 1993;11:586–587.

47. Pedersen-Bjergaard J, Osterlind K, Hansen M, Philip P, Pedersen AG, Hansen HH. Acute nonlymphocytic leukemia, preleukemia, and solid tumors following intensive chemotherapy of small cell carcinoma of the lung. Blood 1985;66:1393–1397.

48. Johnson DH, Porter LL, List AF, Hande KR, Hainsworth JD, Greco FA. Acute nonlymphocytic leukemia after treatment of small cell lung cancer. Am J Med 1986;81:962–968.

49. Stott H, Fox W, Girling DJ, Stephens RJ, Galton DA. Acute leukaemia after busulphan. Br Med J 1977; 2:1513–1517.

50. Chak LY, Sikic BI, Tucker MA, Horns RC Jr, Cox RS. Increased incidence of acute nonlymphocytic leukemia following therapy in patients with small cell carcinoma of the lung. J Clin Oncol 1984;2:385–390.

51. Ratain MJ, Kaminer LS, Bitran JD, et al. Acute nonlymphocytic leukemia following etoposide and cisplatin combination chemotherapy for advanced non-small-cell carcinoma of the lung. Blood 1987;70:1412–1417.

52. Kaldor JM, Day NE, Band P, et al. Second malignancies following testicular cancer, ovarian cancer, and Hodgkin's disease: an international collaborative study among cancer registries. Int J Cancer 1987; 39:571–585.

53. Travis LB, Curtis RE, Hankey BF. Second malignancies after testicular cancer. J Clin Oncol 1995; 13:533–534.

54. Coleman MP, Bell CM, Fraser P. Second primary malignancy after Hodgkin's disease, ovarian cancer, and cancer of the testis: a population-based cohort study. Br J Cancer 1987;56:349–355.

55. van Leeuwen FE, Stiggelbout AM, van den Belt-Dusebout AW, et al. Second cancer risk following testicular cancer: a follow-up study of 1,909 patients. J Clin Oncol 1993;11:415–424.

56. Bokemeyer C, Schmoll HJ. Treatment of testicular cancer and the development of secondary malignancies. J Clin Oncol 1995;13:283–292.

57. Boshoff CH, Begent RHJ, Oliver RTD, et al. Secondary tumours following etoposide containing therapy for germ cell cancer (abstract 767). Proc Am Soc Clin Oncol 1994;13:245.

58. Nichols CR, Breeden ES, Loehrer PJ, Williams SD, Einhorn LH. Secondary leukemia associated with a conventional dose of etoposide: review of serial germ cell tumor protocols. J Natl Cancer Inst 1993;85:36–40.

59. Bajorin DF, Sarosdy MF, Pfister DG, et al. Randomized trial of etoposide and cisplatin versus etoposide and carboplatin in patients with good-risk germ cell tumors: a multiinstitutional study. J Clin Oncol 1993;11:598–606.

60. Pedersen-Bjergaard J, Daugaard G, Hansen SW, Philip P, Larsen SO, Rorth M. Increased risk of myelodysplasia and leukaemia after etoposide, cisplatin, and bleomycin for germ-cell tumours. Lancet 1991;338:359–363.

61. Bokemeyer C, Schmoll HJ. Secondary neoplasms following treatment of malignant germ cell tumors. J Clin Oncol 1993;11:1703–1709.

62. Bokemeyer C, Schmoll HJ, Kuczyk M, Beyer J, Siegert W. Risk of secondary leukemia following high cumulative doses of etoposide during chemotherapy for testicular cancer. J Natl Cancer Inst 1995;87: 58–59.

63. Olsen JH, Garwicz S, Hertz H, et al. Second malignant neoplasms after cancer in childhood or adolescence. Nordic Society of Paediatric Haematology and Oncology Association of the Nordic Cancer Registries. Br Med J 1993;307:1030–1036.

64. Hawkins MM, Wilson LM, Stovall MA, et al. Epipodophyllotoxins, alkylating agents, and radiation and risk of secondary leukaemia after childhood cancer. Br Med J 1992;304:951–958.

65. Neglia JP, Meadows AT, Robison LL, et al. Second neoplasms after acute lymphoblastic leukemia in childhood. N Engl J Med 1991;325:1330–1336.

66. Heyn R, Khan F, Ensign LG, et al. Acute myeloid leukemia in patients treated for rhabdomyosarcoma with cyclophosphamide and low-dose etoposide on Intergroup Rhabdomyosarcoma Study III: an interim report. Med Pediatr Oncol 1994;23:99–106.

67. Pui CH, Behm FG, Raimondi SC, et al. Secondary acute myeloid leukemia in children treated for acute lymphoid leukemia. N Engl J Med 1989;321:136–142.

68. Pui CH, Hancock ML, Raimondi SC, et al. Myeloid neoplasia in children treated for solid tumours. Lancet 1990;336:417–421.

69. Pui CH, Ribeiro RC, Hancock ML, et al. Acute myeloid leukemia in children treated with epipodophyllotoxins for acute lymphoblastic leukemia. N Engl J Med 1991;325:1682–1687.

69a. Sandoval C, Pui CH, Bowman LC, et al. Secondary acute myeloid leukemia in children previously treated with alkylating agents, intercalating topoisomerase II inhibitors, and irradiation. J Clin Oncol 1993; 11:1039–1045.

70. de Vathaire F, Schweisguth O, Rodary C, et al. Long-term risk of a second malignant neoplasm after a cancer in childhood. Br J Cancer 1989;59:448–452.

71. de Vathaire F, Francois P, Hill C, et al. Role of radiotherapy and chemotherapy in the risk of second malignant neoplasms after cancer in childhood. Br J Cancer 1989;59:792–796.

72. Winick NJ, McKenna RW, Shuster JJ, et al. Secondary acute myeloid leukemia in children with acute lymphoblastic leukemia treated with etoposide. J Clin Oncol 1993;11:209–217.

73. Boice JD Jr, Greene MH, Killen JY Jr, et al. Leukemia and preleukemia after adjuvant treatment of gastrointestinal cancer with semustine (methyl-CCNU). N Engl J Med 1983;309:1079–1084.

74. Boice JD, Greene MH, Killen JY Jr, et al. Leukemia after adjuvant chemotherapy with semustine (methyl-CCNU)—evidence of a dose-response effect. N Engl J Med 1986;314:119–120.

75. Boice JD, Greene MH, Keehn RJ, Higgins GA, Fraumeni JF Jr. Late effects of low-dose adjuvant chemotherapy in colorectal cancer. J Natl Cancer Inst 1980; 64:501–511.

76. Greene MH, Boice JD Jr, Strike TA. Carmustine as a cause of acute nonlymphocytic leukemia. N Engl J Med 1985;313:579.

77. Berk PD, Goldberg JD, Silverstein MN, et al. Increased incidence of acute leukemia in polycythemia vera associated with chlorambucil therapy. N Engl J Med 1981;304:441–447.

78. Pedersen-Bjergaard J. Radiotherapy- and chemotherapy-induced myelodysplasia and acute myeloid leukemia. A review. Leuk Res 1992;16:61–65.

79. Bennett JM, Moloney WC, Greene MH, Boice JD Jr. Acute myeloid leukemia and other myelopathic disorders following treatment with alkylating agents. Hematol Pathol 1987;1:99–104.

79a. Rosenbloom B, Schreck R, Koeffler HP. Therapy-related myelodysplastic syndromes. Hematol Oncol Clin North Am 1992;6:707–722.

80. Rustin GJ, Rustin F, Dent J, Booth M, Salt S, Bagshawe KD. No increase in second tumors after cytotoxic chemotherapy for gestational trophoblastic tumors. N Engl J Med 1983;308:473–476.

81. Kumar L. Epipodophyllotoxins and secondary leukaemia. Lancet 1993;342:819–820.

82. Ross JA, Potter JD, Robison LL. Infant leukemia, topoisomerase II inhibitors, and the MLL gene. J Natl Cancer Inst 1994;86:1678–1680.

83. Pedersen-Bjergaard J, Sigsgaard TC, Nielsen D, et al. Acute monocytic or myelomonocytic leukemia with balanced chromosome translocations to band 11q23 after therapy with 4-epi-doxorubicin and cisplatin or cyclophosphamide for breast cancer. J Clin Oncol 1992;10:1444–1451.

84. Shepherd L, Ottaway J, Myles J, Levine M. Therapy-related leukemia associated with high-dose 4-epi-doxorubicin and cyclophosphamide used as adjuvant chemotherapy for breast cancer. J Clin Oncol 1994;12:2514–2515.

85. Greene MH, Boice JD Jr, Greer BE, Blessing JA, Dembo AJ. Acute nonlymphocytic leukemia after therapy with alkylating agents for ovarian cancer: a study of five randomized clinical trials. N Engl J Med 1982; 307:1416–1421.

86. Goldberg KB, Goldberg P, eds. Secondary AML in high-dose chemotrial cause for careful monitoring, NCI says. Cancer Lett 1994;20:1–4.

87. Tarbell NJ, Gelber RD, Weinstein HJ, Mauch P. Sex differences in risk of second malignant tumours after Hodgkin's disease in childhood. Lancet 1993; 341:1428–1432.

88. Beaty O 3rd, Hudson MM, Greenwald C, et al. Subsequent malignancies in children and adolescents after treatment for Hodgkin's disease. J Clin Oncol 1995;13:603–609.

89. Boice JD Jr, Blettner M, Kleinerman RA, et al. Radiation dose and leukemia risk in patients treated for cancer of the cervix. J Natl Cancer Inst 1987; 79:1295–1311.

90. Curtis RE, Boice JD Jr, Stovall M, et al. Relationship of leukemia risk to radiation dose following cancer of the uterine corpus. J Natl Cancer Inst 1994; 86:1315–1324.

91. Pedersen-Bjergaard J, Rowley JD. The balanced and the unbalanced chromosome aberrations of acute myeloid leukemia may develop in different ways and may contribute differently to malignant transformation. Blood 1994;83:2780–2786.

92. Pedersen-Bjergaard J, Johansson B, Philip P. Translocation (3;21) (q26;2) in therapy-related myelodysplasia following drugs targeting DNA-topoisomerase II combined with alkylating agents, and in myeloproliferative disorders undergoing spontaneous leukemic transformation. Cancer Genet Cytogenet 1994;76:50–55.

93. Boice JD Jr. Second cancer after Hodgkin's disease—the price of success (editorial)? J Natl Cancer Inst 1993;85:4–5.

94. Boice JD Jr, Travis LB. Body wars: effect of friendly fire (cancer therapy) (editorial). J Natl Cancer Inst 1995;87:705–706.

95. Valagussa P, Santoro A, Fossati-Bellani F, Franchi F, Banfi A, Bonadonna G. Absence of treatment-induced second cancers after ABVD in Hodgkin's disease. Blood 1982;59:488–494.

96. Rosenberg SA, Kaplan HS. The evolution and summary results of the Stanford randomized clinical trials of the management of Hodgkin's disease: 1962–1984. Int J Radiat Oncol Biol Phys 1985;11:5–22.

97. Meadows AT, Obringer AC, Marrero O, et al. Second malignant neoplasms following childhood Hodgkin's disease: treatment and splenectomy as risk factors. Med Pediatr Oncol 1989;17:477–484.

98. Andrieu JM, Ifrah N, Payen C, Fermanian J, Coscas Y, Flandrin G. Increased risk of secondary acute nonlymphocytic leukemia after extended-field radiation therapy combined with MOPP chemotherapy for Hodgkin's disease. J Clin Oncol 1990;8:1148–1154.

99. Travis LB, Curtis RE, Hankey BF, Fraumeni JF Jr. Second cancers in patients with chronic lymphocytic leukemia. J Natl Cancer Inst 1992;84:1422–1427.

100. Roberts PD, Forster PM. Chronic lymphocytic leukaemia associated with acute myelomonocytic leukaemia. Br J Haematol 1973;25:203–206.

101. Zarrabi MH, Grunwald HW, Rosner F. Chronic lymphocytic leukemia terminating in acute leukemia. Arch Intern Med 1977;137:1059–1064.

102. Frenkel EP, Ligler FS, Graham MS, Hernandez JA, Kettman JR Jr, Smith RG. Acute lymphocytic leukemic transformation of chronic lymphocytic leukemia: substantiation by flow cytometry. Am J Hematol 1981;10:391–398.

103. Manoharan A, Catovsky D, Clein P, et al. Simultaneous or spontaneous occurrence of lympho- and myeloproliferative disorders: a report of four cases. Br J Haematol 1981;48:111–116.

104. Stern N, Shemesh J, Ramot B. Chronic lymphatic leukemia terminating in acute myeloid leukemia: review of the literature. Cancer 1981;47:1849–1851.

105. Wallis JP, Joyner MV. Acute myeloid leukaemia developing in a patient with longstanding untreated chronic lymphocytic leukaemia. Acta Haematol 1986;75:229–231.

106. Bracey AW, Maddox AM, Immken L, Hsu SM, Marks ME. Coexistence of myelodysplastic syndrome and untreated chronic lymphocytic leukemia with development of acute myeloid leukemia immediately after treatment of chronic lymphocytic leukemia. Am J Hematol 1989;30:174–180.

107. Robertson LE, Estey E, Kantarjian H, et al. Therapy-related leukemia and myelodysplastic syndrome in chronic lymphocytic leukemia. Leukemia 1994;8:2047–2051.

108. Valagussa P, Tancini G, Bonadonna G. Second malignancies after CMF for resectable breast cancer. J Clin Oncol 1987;5:1138–1142.

109. Arriagada R, Rutqvist LE. Adjuvant chemotherapy in early breast cancer and incidence of new primary malignancies. Lancet 1991;338:535–538.

110. Herring MK, Buzdar AU, Smith TL, et al. Second neoplasms after adjuvant chemotherapy for operable breast cancer. Am J Clin Oncol 1986;9:269–275.

111. Falkson G, Gelman RS, Dreicer R, et al. Myelodysplastic syndrome and acute nonlymphocytic leukemia secondary to mitolactol treatment in patients with breast cancer. J Clin Oncol 1989;7:1252–1259.

112. Bennett JM, Troxel AB, Gelman R, et al. Myelodysplastic syndrome and acute myeloid leukemia secondary to mitolactol treatment in patients with breast cancer. J Clin Oncol 1994;12:874–875.

113. Riggi M, Riva A. Therapy-related leukemia: what is the role of 4-epi-doxorubicin? J Clin Oncol 1993;11:1430–1431.

114. Marty M. Epirubicin and the risk of leukemia: not substantiated? International Collaborative Cancer Group Steering Committee. J Clin Oncol 1993;11:1431–1433.

115. Buzdar A, Iwaniec J, Kau S, et al. Secondary leukemia following adjuvant doxorubicin-containing chemotherapy for stage II or III breast cancer (abstract 112). Proc Am Soc Clin Oncol 1991;10:59.

116. Andersson M, Philip P, Pedersen-Bjergaard J. High risk of therapy-related leukemia and preleukemia after therapy with prednimustine, methotrexate, 5-fluorouracil, mitoxantrone, and tamoxifen for advanced breast cancer. Cancer 1990;65:2460–2464.

117. Einhorn N. Acute leukemia after chemotherapy (melphalan). Cancer 1978;41:444–447.

118. Williams S, Blessing JA, Liao SY, Ball M, Hanjani P. Adjuvant therapy of ovarian germ cell tumors with cisplatin, etoposide, and bleomycin: a trial of the Gynecologic Oncology Group. J Clin Oncol 1994; 12:701–706.

119. Ihde DC, Tucker MA. Second primary malignancies in small-cell lung cancer: a major consequence of modest success (editorial). J Clin Oncol 1992; 10:1511–1513.

120. Kleinerman RA, Liebermann JV, Li FP. Second cancer following cancer of the male genital system in Connecticut, 1935–82. Natl Cancer Inst Monogr 1985; 68:139–147.

121. Greene MH, Wilson J. Second cancer following lymphatic and hematopoietic cancers in Connecticut, 1935–82. Natl Cancer Inst Monogr 1985;68:191–217.

122. Nichols CR, Roth BJ, Heerema N, Griep J, Tricot G. Hematologic neoplasia associated with primary mediastinal germ-cell tumors. N Engl J Med 1990; 322:1425–1429.

123. Smith MA, Rubinstein L, Cazenave L, et al. Report of the Cancer Therapy Evaluation Program monitoring plan for secondary acute myeloid leukemia following treatment with epipodophyllotoxins. J Natl Cancer Inst 1993;85:554–558.

124. Smith MA, Rubinstein L, Ungerleider RS. Therapy-related acute myeloid leukemia following treatment with epipodophyllotoxins: estimating the risks. Med Pediatr Oncol 1994;23:86–98.

124a. Baker GL, Kahl LE, Zee BC, Stolzer BL, Agarwal AK, Medsger TA Jr. Malignancy following treatment of rheumatoid arthritis with cyclophosphamide. Long-term case-control follow-up study. Am J Med 1987;83:1–9.

125. Travis LB, Curtis RE, Boice JD Jr, Fraumeni JF Jr. Bladder cancer after chemotherapy for non-Hodgkin's lymphoma. N Engl J Med 1989;321:544–545.

126. Pedersen-Bjergaard J, Ersboll J, Hansen VL, et al. Carcinoma of the urinary bladder after treatment with cyclophosphamide for non-Hodgkin's lymphoma. N Engl J Med 1988;318:1028–1032.

127. Travis LB, Curtis RE, Glimelius B, et al. Bladder and kidney cancer following cyclophosphamide therapy for non-Hodgkin's lymphoma. J Natl Cancer Inst 1995;87:524–530.

128. Kinlen LJ. Incidence of cancer in rheumatoid arthritis and other disorders after immunosuppressive treatment. Am J Med 1985;78:44–49.

129. Thiede T, Christensen BC. Bladder tumours induced by chlornaphazine. A five-year follow-up study of chlornaphazine-treated patients with polycythaemia. Acta Med Scand 1969;185:133–137.

130. Travis LB, Curtis RE, Boice JD Jr, Hankey BF, Fraumeni JF Jr. Second cancers following non-Hodgkin's lymphoma. Cancer 1991;67:2002–2009.

130a. Birkeland SA, Storm HH, Lamm LU, et al. Cancer risk after renal transplantation in the Nordic countries, 1964–1986. Int J Cancer 1995;60:183–189.

131. Cleary ML, Sklar J. Lymphoproliferative disorders in cardiac transplant recipients are multiclonal lymphomas. Lancet 1984;2:489–493.

132. Witherspoon RP, Fisher LD, Schoch G, et al. Secondary cancers after bone marrow transplantation for leukemia or aplastic anemia. N Engl J Med 1989; 321:784–789.

133. Kinlen LJ. Immunosuppression and cancer. IARC Sci Publ 1992;116:237–253.

134. Boice JD Jr. Radiation and non-Hodgkin's lymphoma. Cancer Res 1992;52:5489s–5491s.

135. Boice JD Jr, Land CE, Preston D. Ionizing radiation. In: Schottenfeld D, Fraumeni JF Jr, eds. Cancer epidemiology and prevention. New York: Oxford University Press, in press.

136. Boice JD Jr, Storm HH, Curtis RE, et al. Introduction to the study of multiple primary cancers. Natl Cancer Inst Monogr 1985;68:3–9.

137. Tucker MA, D'Angio GJ, Boice JD Jr, et al. Bone sarcomas linked to radiotherapy and chemotherapy in children. N Engl J Med 1987;317:588–593.

138. Kaldor JM, Day NE, Bell J, et al. Lung cancer following Hodgkin's disease: a case-control study. Int J Cancer 1992;52:677–681.

139. Hancock SL, Tucker MA, Hoppe RT. Breast

cancer after treatment of Hodgkin's disease. J Natl Cancer Inst 1993;85:25–31.

140. Tucker MA, Jones PH, Boice JD Jr, et al. Therapeutic radiation at a young age is linked to secondary thyroid cancer. The Late Effects Study Group. Cancer Res 1991;51:2885–2888.

141. Greene MH. Is cisplatin a human carcinogen? J Natl Cancer Inst 1992;84:306–312.

142. Bhavnani M, Wolstenholme RJ. Razoxane and acute promyelocytic leukaemia. Lancet 1987;2:1085.

143. Bhavnani M, Azzawi SA, Yin JA, Lucas GS. Therapy-related acute promyelocytic leukaemia. Br J Haematol 1994;86:231–232.

144. Krikorian JG, Burke JS, Rosenberg SA, Kaplan HS. Occurrence of non-Hodgkin's lymphoma after therapy for Hodgkin's disease. N Engl J Med 1979; 300:452–458.

145. Lerner HJ. Acute myelogenous leukemia in patients receiving chlorambucil as long-term adjuvant chemotherapy for stage II breast cancer. Cancer Treat Rep 1978;62:1135–1138.

146. Robison LL, Mertens A. Second tumors after treatment of childhood malignancies. Hematol Oncol Clin North Am 1993;7:401–415.

147. Wheeler GE. Cyclophosphamide-associated leukemia in Wegener's granulomatosis. Ann Intern Med 1981;94:361–362.

41

Chemotherapy in Pregnancy

Donald C. Doll and John W. Yarbro

The simultaneous occurrence of cancer and pregnancy is uncommon, with a reported incidence of approximately 0.1% (1). Nevertheless, cancer is a primary cause of death in women of childbearing age (2). The predominant malignancies complicating pregnancy are those of the breast and gynecologic system, leukemia, lymphoma, melanoma, thyroid carcinoma, and colorectal carcinoma (3–6). Although a state of immunologic tolerance occurs with pregnancy (7), there is no evidence of an increased incidence of cancer in pregnant patients. However, whether pregnancy adversely influences the prognosis or biology of maternal cancer (and vice versa) continues to be an unsettled issue (8–12).

On the other hand, the immediate and delayed effects of diagnostic and therapeutic measures may be potentially deleterious to the fetus. It is well recognized that cytotoxic drugs, particularly folic acid antagonists administered during the first trimester of pregnancy, are associated with a significant risk of abortion and/or teratogenesis. However, delay or modification of cancer therapy to assure the birth of a healthy infant could adversely affect maternal prognosis. Thus, the decision to initiate chemotherapy in a pregnant patient is usually a difficult one for all involved and may be complicated by ethical and religious beliefs. With the increasing trend for women to delay childbearing, the concurrence of cancer and pregnancy may increase in the future, and the progress in both curative cancer chemotherapy and obstetric and neonatal care will only increase the difficulty of the decision to use chemotherapy.

PHARMACOLOGY DURING PREGNANCY

Pharmacokinetics may be altered by physiologic changes that occur during pregnancy. The stomach empties more slowly, and there is a decrease in gastrointestinal motility (13, 14), which could affect the rate and completeness of drug absorption. Although drug absorption is not appreciably changed until late in pregnancy, it is possible that the vinca alkaloids may induce autonomic neuropathy and perhaps alter absorption (15).

In pregnancy, there is a considerable increase in total body water, and plasma volume increases by approximately 50% (16), resulting in a larger dilutional space for water-soluble drugs. The albumin concentration decreases, and plasma proteins are increased. Chemotherapeutic agents must compete for binding sites on albumin and other plasma proteins. Such changes affect drug distribution, and hence plasma drug concentration, and are likely to be greatest for drugs of low lipid solubility that are tightly bound to plasma proteins (17). An increased distribution volume will decrease the peak concentration of a drug following bolus administration, and the half-life will be longer unless drug metabolism or excretion is also increased (18). Thus the concentration × time relationship may be altered; this association is particularly important for antineoplastic drugs, since both toxicity and therapeutic efficacy depend upon it (18). Whether the amniotic fluid functions as a pharmacologic third space is not known, but this would be relevant to methotrexate, where distribution into a third space such as pleural or ascitic fluid delays elimination and may increase toxicity (19).

Furthermore, hepatic oxidation by the mixed-function oxidase system is more rapid during pregnancy, and there are increases in renal plasma flow, glomerular filtration rate, and creatinine clearance (20). Such changes could lead to an increased clearance of drugs from the body. Given the altered physiologic state of pregnancy, there are inadequate pharmacokinetic studies to assess whether present dosages of antineoplastic agents used in the nonpregnant women are appropriate in pregnancy. It is unlikely that such data will ever become available. In its absence, we must assume that drug doses used in the nonpregnant state are adequate in pregnancy.

PLACENTAL TRANSFER AND FETAL PHARMACOKINETICS

The placenta is the portal of entry for drugs to the fetus. Drug characteristics that enhance transport across the placenta include a low molecular weight, a high lipid solubility, nonionization, and loose binding to plasma proteins (18, 19). Except for high-molecular-weight proteins, such as L-asparaginase or α-interferon, most antineoplastic agents possess these qualities and thus cross the placenta, enter the fetal circulation, and are then subject to the same pharmacokinetic principles as before placental transfer, but on a much smaller scale. However, since the multidrug resistant (MDR) P-glycoprotein has been described in the gravid endometrium (21), it may provide a natural fetal barrier for certain antineoplastic agents, such as the vinca alkaloids and the anthracycline antibiotics. This may be relevant to the treatment of acute leukemia in pregnancy, where such drugs have been used throughout gestation, and perhaps MDR protein may prevent in utero exposure of drugs to the fetus.

The immature fetal liver is capable of metabolizing a large number of substrates by oxidation, and the fetal kidney may be involved in drug elimination. It should be emphasized that a drug excreted into the amniotic fluid may be ingested by the fetus and reabsorbed from the gastrointestinal tract, potentially increasing any adverse effect on the fetus of drugs such as the antimetabolites, which are excreted in active form. In contrast, some agents (e.g., nitrogen mustards) are utilized and bound to tissue with essentially no active drug or metabolites excreted. Because movement of drug molecules is bidirectional, the placenta is also a route of drug elimination, and in fact, the placenta is the primary portal of exit of waste products and toxins from the fetus. Transplacental passage of antineoplastic agents has been reported in association with doxorubicin (22) and cisplatin (23, 24).

At birth, the ability of the neonate to metabolize and excrete many drugs is underdeveloped. Therefore, chemotherapy administered shortly before birth may be particularly hazardous because of delayed metabolism and excretion in the neonate when placental excretion can no longer occur.

ADVERSE EFFECTS OF ANTINEOPLASTIC AGENTS ON THE FETUS AND NEONATE

Cytotoxic drugs produce their effects predominantly on rapidly dividing cells, and thus fetal exposure may be associated with immediate and delayed deleterious effects (Table 41.1). The timing of such exposure is critical. Drugs administered in the first week after conception probably produce an "all or nothing" phenomenon, that is, a spontaneous abortion or a normal fetus. During the first trimester, when organogenesis occurs, drugs can produce congenital malformations and/or result in abortion (25). In the second and third trimesters, drugs do not cause significant malformations, but they may impair fetal growth and development. In particular, neuronal growth in the brain continues during this period, and damage after the first trimester can produce microcephaly, mental retardation, and impaired learning.

Teratogenicity

The teratogenic and mutagenic potential of chemotherapeutic agents has been well documented in animals (22–28), but extrapolation of data from animals to human organogenesis is dangerous because of differences in species susceptibility (29). For instance, many drugs that

Table 41.1. Adverse Effects of Antineoplastic Agents on the Fetus and Neonate

Immediate
  Spontaneous abortion
  Teratogenesis
  Organ toxicity
  Premature birth
  Low birth weight
Delayed[a]
  Carcinogenesis
  Sterility
  Retarded physical and/or mental growth and
    development
  Mutation
  Teratogenic in second generations

[a]Potential long-term complications of in utero exposure to antineoplastic agents.

produce defects in animals appear to be harmless to the human embryo (e.g., aspirin). Conversely, the absence of teratogenicity in animals is no guarantee of safety in man (e.g., thalidomide).

Multiple factors influence the probability of teratogenesis. As noted above, the timing of exposure is critical; several investigators have confirmed the observation that the phase of embryonic organogenesis in the first trimester is the critical period for teratogenesis (30–37). Nonetheless, the risk appears to be significantly lower than is commonly appreciated, probably because drug doses, frequency of administration, and duration of exposure are important variables. To be teratogenic, it appears that the dose must lie within a narrow range between that which causes death of the fetus and that which has no discernible effect. Synergistic teratogenic interactions may occur with combination chemotherapy (36, 37) or when chemotherapy is combined with radiotherapy (38–40). Individual and genetic susceptibility may also be important variables (26).

Table 41.2 shows data regarding fetal malformations associated with the use of chemotherapy during the first trimester (41–46). Such data have been reviewed by us (41, 42) and most recently by Wiebe and Sipila (43). In addition, a case report of multiple congenital anomalies associated with the sequential administration of 6-mercaptopurine and busulfan in the first trimester has been described (38). It is apparent, then, that a number of antineoplastic agents—given alone or in combination—may be teratogenetic when administered early in pregnancy. This interpretation should be tempered by the fact that the overall incidence of major congenital malformations is about 3% of all births (50), and the incidence of minor malformations may be as high as 9%. Furthermore, in several reported cases of congenital malformations, the mothers were also treated with radiation (38–40, 51, 52), which is well recognized as a potent teratogen in humans and animals (53).

The folic acid antagonists aminopterin and methotrexate have been more frequently reported than any other agent to be associated with fetal abnormalities when given during the first trimester (41, 42). Indeed, a syndrome of congenital anomalies has been recognized, the "aminopterin syndrome," with the most consistent anomaly being cranial dysostosis (i.e., delay of ossification of the bones of the calvarium) (54). Hypertelorism, a wide nasal bridge, anomalies

Table 41.2. Chemotherapy during First Trimester of Pregnancy

Class	Number of Exposed Patients	Number of Fetal Malformations
Alkylating agents		
Busulfan	24	2
Chlorambucil	6	1
Cyclophosphamide	7	3
Nitrogen mustard	6	0
Triethylenemelamine	4	0
Antimetabolites		
Aminopterin	52	10
Methotrexate	9	3
6-Mercaptopurine	20	0
Cytarabine	1	1
5-Fluorouracil	1	1
Hydroxyurea	3	0
Plant alkaloids		
Vinblastine	14	1
Antibiotics		
Daunorubicin	1	0
Miscellaneous		
Procarbazine	1	1
Amsacrine	1	1
Cisplatin	1	0
Total	151	24(15%)
Combinations	52	8(15%)

Data from Doll DC, Ringenberg QS, Yarbro JW. Management of cancer during pregnancy. Arch Intern Med 1988;148:2058–2064; Doll DC, Ringenberg QS, Yarbro JW. Antineoplastic agents and pregnancy. Semin Oncol 1989;16:337–346; and references 43–49.

of the external ears, and micrognathia may also be present. Intelligence may range from normal to below normal with poor speech development. Several of the infants have had limb deformities, and most of the abortuses and infants who died shortly after birth have cerebral anomalies. Recently, Kozlowski et al. (49) reported eight women experiencing 10 pregnancies after low-dose methotrexate exposure during the first trimester for treatment of rheumatic disease. The outcome of pregnancies included five full-term babies, three spontaneous abortions, and two elective abortions. All offspring were normal, with no abnormalities noted at a mean age of 11.5 years. Such findings suggest that methotrexate is not always teratogenic when given in the first trimester. Other antimetabolites have rarely been associated with fetal malformations. An isolated case of 5-fluorouracil-associated congenital abnormality also received radiotherapy (52). Of 20 patients exposed to 6-mercaptopurine alone, no fetal anomalies were documented (41,

42). Thus, if chemotherapy must be given, the folic acid antagonists should be avoided. On the other hand, the folate acid antagonist, methotrexate, has been used recently as a pharmacologic treatment for ectopic and cervical pregnancies, with a very high success rate (55, 56).

Alkylating agents appear to be less potent teratogens than antimetabolites, with six cases of fetal malformations reported among patients at risk (41, 42). Four of these six mothers had also received radiation therapy. In contrast to methotrexate, alkylating agents are frequently key ingredients in curative or significantly palliative therapeutic regimens.

Although vinblastine is highly teratogenic in animal models (57), there has been only one reported abnormality observed in the offspring of 14 women treated with vinblastine in the first trimester (41, 42). Therefore, the use of vinblastine in the first trimester may be relatively safe. There are no data on the closely related vinca alkaloid, vincristine. The vinca alkaloids, like the alkylating agents, are frequently included in curative regimens.

As depicted in Table 41.2, the apparent rate of fetal malformations associated with combination chemotherapy is similar to that observed with single agents (8 of 52 cases (15%) vs. 24 of 151 cases (15%)). If one excludes the folate antagonists and concomitant use of radiation, then the incidence for single agents declines to 6%. Of note, five of the eight malformations seen with combination regimens were in patients who received procarbazine, a primary agent in the MOPP (mechlorethamine, vincristine, procarbazine, prednisone) regimen for Hodgkin's disease. In addition, one fetus who was exposed to procarbazine alone also had congenital malformations. Definitive conclusions regarding the use of combination chemotherapy in the first trimester are hampered by the paucity of cases and the variability of the individual regimens. Nevertheless, as shown in Table 41.2, several reports document the delivery of normal infants exposed to antineoplastic agents in the first trimester. Indeed, Blatt et al. (32) reported eight normal babies of women who had been treated with various combinations in the first trimester. Aviles and Niz (58) reported 11 normal infants following intensive chemotherapy for acute leukemia in the first trimester. Long-term follow-up of children in the latter study revealed normal growth and development.

In contrast to these findings in the first tri-

mester of pregnancy, there is no evidence of an increased risk of teratogenicity associated with the administration of cytotoxic drugs in the second and third trimesters (30–36, 43, 46–48, 59–62). As shown in Table 41.3, of 166 cases treated with chemotherapy during the last two trimesters of pregnancy, there was 1 reported case of trisomy C following cytarabine and 6-thioguanine administration (63); 1 infant with multiple anomalies following third trimester exposure to busulfan (64); 1 neonate with adherence of the iris to the cornea following treatment with daunorubicin, 6-thioguanine, and cytosine arabinoside (65); and 1 infant with gaps and ring chromosomes following treatment with combination chemotherapy for acute leukemia (66). Since treatment was given after fetal organogenesis, it is possible that these anomalies were the result of chance occurrence. However, one should not assume that such exposure to antineoplastic agents is definitely safe, because exposure to drugs in utero may potentially have delayed adverse effects later in life.

A report by Russell et al. (67) described two neonates with birth defects born to women whose spouses had been treated prior to conception with combination chemotherapy for acute leukemia. Four other men receiving chemotherapy at the time of insemination have fathered normal offspring (32).

Other modes of therapy, including α-interferon (44, 68–70), all trans-retinoic acid (71), and topical and intravaginal 5-fluorouracil (72, 73)

Table 41.3. Chemotherapy during Second and Third Trimesters of Pregnancy

Class	Number of Exposed Patients	Number of Fetal Malformations
Alkylating agents	26	1
Antimetabolites	38	0
Antibiotics	1	0
Plant alkaloids	6	0
Combinations	95	1[a]
	166	2 (1.2%)

Data from Doll DC, Ringenberg QS, Yarbro JW. Management of cancer during pregnancy. Arch Intern Med 1988;148:2058–2064; Doll DC, Ringenberg QS, Yarbro JW. Antineoplastic agents and pregnancy. Semin Oncol 1989;16:337–346; and references 30–36, 43, 46–49, and 59–62.
[a]One case of trisomy C following cytarabine and 6-thioguanine was reported. Autopsy revealed no congenital malformation. One case of chromosomal gaps and rings in a phenotypic normal infant was noted following intensive antileukemic therapy.

have been used in pregnancy without any adverse effects. Also, a case of Goldenhar's syndrome has been reported in association with tamoxifen administration throughout gestation (74). More data are needed on such therapies before any conclusions can be made regarding their use in pregnancy.

In addition to teratogenicity, other immediate demonstrable effects of antineoplastic agents on the fetus include low birth weight, intrauterine growth retardation, spontaneous abortion, premature birth, and major organ toxicity. For example, Nicholson (31) reported that 40% of exposed fetuses were of low birth weight; such infants are at risk for developmental handicaps (75). Sutcliffe (76) enumerated 82 spontaneous and therapeutic abortions among 218 pregnancies associated with cytotoxic drugs. A stillborn fetus with diffuse myocardial necrosis after in utero exposure to daunorubicin has been reported (77).

POSTNATAL CARE AND FOLLOW-UP

Labor should be induced or cesarian section performed when maternal blood counts and performance are optimal and are not compromised due to cancer therapy (76). Neonatal cytopenias have been reported secondary to exposure to cancer chemotherapy (65, 78), and cyclophosphamide has produced neutropenia and thrombocytopenia in a breast-fed infant (79).

Little is known about the possible delayed effects of exposure to antineoplastic agents in utero. Major areas of concern include physical and/or mental development, infertility, carcinogenesis, and second-generation teratogenesis. Studies conducted on children exposed to folic acid antagonists in the first trimester suggest that some individuals will have impaired growth and mental development (54). Of 50 children born to women who were receiving treatment for leukemia or lymphoma, 48 (92%) of the 50 children are alive and well, with follow-up extending to 19 years (58, 65, 80). Of the 50 children, 21 were exposed during the first trimester. Of these, one child was found to have multiple congenital anomalies and diminished intellect and later developed a neuroblastoma and papillary thyroid carcinoma (65). Two other infants, appearing normal at birth, died within 3 months from septicemia and gastroenteritis, respectively. Of 24 fetuses delivered from mothers who were treated for Hodgkin's disease during pregnancy

at the Mayo Clinic, there was one degenerated fetus, one child with Down's syndrome, and one twin who died 48 hours postdelivery. Long-term follow-up of the other 21 children was not provided (81).

Antineoplastic agents can induce gonadal dysfunction via cytotoxic effects in germinal cells (82), and ovarian failure in long-term survivors of childhood malignancy has been described (83). In this regard, a large retrospective cohort study of fertility in 2283 survivors of cancer during childhood demonstrated that previous therapy with nonalkylating agents resulted in no apparent decrease in fertility in either sex, while prior exposure to alkylating agents reduced fertility by 33% (84). However, the decrease in fertility associated with alkylating agent therapy was noted only in men.

Transplacental carcinogenesis is well documented in animal studies, and the time of greatest susceptibility appears to be near the end of gestation (85). For instance, an increased incidence of pulmonary adenomas occurs in mice exposed to urethane in utero (86), and pregnant rats exposed to nitrosoureas during the latter half of gestation have a high incidence of neurogenic tumors in the offspring (87). Secondary malignancy is a well-recognized complication of antineoplastic agents (88), and an increase in mutations in lymphocytes (89) and chromosomal aberrations (90) have been reported in humans. The long-term effects of such derangements may not be demonstrable until later life or subsequent generations (91).

RECOMMENDATIONS

Pregnancy associated with cancer is rather uncommon, but the decision to initiate chemotherapy in such patients may be difficult for those involved, because of the possible deleterious effects on the offspring. When cure is a realistic goal, therapy should not be modified in such a way as to compromise that goal. On the other hand, when there is no hope for cure or even significant palliation, the primary goals should become protection of the fetus from the potential harmful effects of chemotherapy and delivery of a healthy infant.

Therapeutic decisions *must* be individualized. These decisions might best be facilitated by a multidisciplinary team, including the patient's family physician, obstetrician, oncologist, pediatrician, neonatologist, and other ancillary consultants. One member of the team should act as a spokesperson when communicating with the family and mother. Such interaction should begin as soon as the patient is initially diagnosed as having cancer.

During the first trimester, chemotherapeutic agents should be avoided, if possible. If this option is not feasible, then one needs to decide whether treatment can safely be postponed until the second trimester or later. There are essentially no data regarding the pharmacokinetics of antineoplastic agents in pregnancy, and until such studies are available, we must use established chemotherapeutic regimens. There are several tumors seen during pregnancy in which chemotherapy may increase the cure rate: breast cancer, leukemia, lymphoma, and ovarian cancer. If treatment must be given during the first trimester, folate antagonists should be avoided. There are no curative regimens requiring these agents for which a therapeutically equivalent substitute is lacking. When patients also receiving radiotherapy are excluded, there are only 2 cases of malformation in 50 patients receiving alkylating agents, so alkylating agents given alone may be relatively safe. Except for ovarian cancer, however, there are no curative regimens using single alkylating agents. The use of vinblastine in the first trimester also appears to be relatively safe, with only 1 reported case of malformation among 14 patients at risk. Thus, this agent might be considered in the pregnant Hodgkin's patient who requires chemotherapy during the first trimester (92). Five of the eight malformations seen with combination regimens were in patients who received procarbazine; therefore, combination regimens using this agent should be avoided.

Single and combination chemotherapy may be administered in the second and third trimester with a low risk of teratogenicity. Nonetheless, the least teratogenic regimens should be selected. The mother and family should be informed of the potential early and delayed effects of antineoplastic agents.

Delivery should be planned when maternal blood counts are optimal. A complete blood count should be obtained on the newborn, and examination for congenital malformations and organ dysfunction should be performed. Breastfeeding is contraindicated, as antineoplastic agents administered systemically may reach significant levels in milk (79, 93–98).

A national registry has been established at the University of Pittsburgh Genetics Institute for the effects of chemotherapy on the fetus as well as long-term follow-up of individuals exposed to chemotherapy in utero. Information from this database can be obtained by calling (412)-641-4168 (99). Such information may eventually reveal which agents are safest during pregnancy, what gestational age is the most vulnerable to teratogenic effects, and what the long-term effects of in utero exposure to antineoplastic agents may be.

ACKNOWLEDGMENT

We are grateful to Jackie Rahmer for expert secretarial support.

REFERENCES

1. Potter JF, Schoeneman M. Metastasis of maternal cancer to the placenta and fetus. Cancer 1979;25:380–388.
2. Silverberg E, Lubera J. Cancer statistics, 1989. CA 1989;39:3–20.
3. Barber HRK, Brunschwig A. Gynecologic cancer complicating pregnancy. Am J Obstet Gynecol 1963; 85:156–164.
4. Lutz MH, Underwood PB Jr, Rozier JC, et al. Genital malignancy in pregnancy. Am J Obstet Gynceol 1977;129:536–542.
5. Betson JR, Golden ML. Cancer and pregnancy. Am J Obstet Gynecol 1961;81:718–728.
6. Haas JF. Pregnancy in association with a newly diagnosed cancer: a population-based epidemiologic assessment. Int J Cancer 1984;34:229–235.
7. Gleicher N, Seigel I. Common denominators of pregnancy and malignancy. Prog Clin Biol Res 1981; 70:339–353.
8. Mackie RM, Bufaline R, Morabito A, Sutherland C, Cascinelli N. Lack of effect of pregnancy on outcome of melanoma. Lancet 1991;337:653–655.
9. Petrek JA, Dukoff R, Rogatko A. Prognosis of pregnancy-associated breast cancer. Cancer 1991; 67:869–872.
10. Clark RM, Chua T. Breast cancer and pregnancy: the ultimate challenge. Clin Oncol 1989;1:11–18.
11. Guinee VF, Olsson H, Moller T, et al. Effect of pregnancy on prognosis for young women with breast cancer. Lancet 1994;343:1587–1589.
12. Heres P, Wiltink J, Cuesta MA, et al. Colon carcinoma during pregnancy: a lethal coincidence. Eur J Obstet Gynecol Reprod Biol 1993;98:149–152.
13. Davison JS, Davison MC, Hay DM. Gastric emptying time in late pregnancy and labour. J Obstet Gynaecol Br Commonw 1970;77:37–41.
14. Parry E, Shields R, Turnbull AC. Transit time in the small intestine in pregnancy. J Obstet Gynaecol Br Commonw 1970;77:900–901.
15. Mitchell EP, Schein PS. Gastrointestinal toxicity of chemotherapeutic agents. In: Perry MC, Yarbro JW, eds. Toxicity of chemotherapy. Orlando, FL: Grune & Stratton 1984:269–296.
16. Pirani BBK, Campbell DM, MacGillivray I.

Plasma volume in normal first pregnancy. J Obstet Gynaecol Br Commonw 1973;80:884–887.

17. Mucklow JC. The fate of drugs in pregnancy. Clin Obstet Gynecol 1986;13:161–175.

18. Powis G. Anticancer drug pharmacodynamics. Cancer Chemother Pharmacol 1985;14:177–183.

19. Wan SH, Huffman DH, Azarnoff DL et al. Effect of route of administration and effusions on methotrexate pharmacokinetics. Cancer Res 1974;34:3487–3491.

20. Redmond GP. Physiological changes during pregnancy and their implications for pharmacological treatment. Clin Invest Med 1985;8:317–322.

21. Anceci RJ, Croop JM, Horitz SB, Housman D. The gene encoding multidrug resistance is induced and expressed at high levels during pregnancy in the secretory epithelium of the uterus. Proc Natl Acad Sci USA 1988;85:4350–4354.

22. Karp GI, von Oeyen P, Valone F, et al. Doxorubicin in pregnancy: possible transplacental passage. Cancer Treat Rep 1983;67:773–777.

23. Henderson CE, Elia G, Garfinkel D, et al. Platinum chemotherapy during pregnancy for serous cystadenocarcinoma of the ovary. Gynecol Oncol 1993; 49:92–97.

24. Shamkhani H, Anderson LM, Henderson CE, et al. DNA adducts in women and patas monkey: maternal and fetal tissues induced by platinum drug chemotherapy. Reprod Toxicol 1994;8:207–216.

25. Beeley L. Adverse effects of drugs in the first trimester of pregnancy. Clin Obstet Gynecol 1986; 13:177–195.

26. Cahen RL. Experimental and clinical chemoteratogenesis. Adv Pharmacol 1966;4:263–349.

27. Chaube S, Murphy ML. The teratogenic effects of the recent drugs active in cancer chemotherapy. Adv Teratol 1968;3:181–237.

28. Sieber SM, Adamson RH. Toxicity of antineoplastic agents in man: chromosomal aberrations, antifertility effects, congenital malformations and carcinogenic potential. Adv Cancer Res 1975;22:57–155.

29. Brent RL. Evaluating the alleged teratogenicity of environmental agents. Clin Perinatol 1986;13:609–613.

30. Sokal JE, Lessman EM. Effects of cancer chemotherapeutic agents on the human fetus. JAMA 1960; 172:1765–1771.

31. Nicholson HO. Cytotoxic drugs in pregnancy. J Obstet Gynaecol Br Commonw 1968;75:307–312.

32. Blatt J, Mulvihill JJ, Ziegler JL, Young RC, Poplack DG. Pregnancy outcome following cancer chemotherapy. Am J Med 1980;69:828–832.

33. Sweet DL Jr, Kinzie J. Consequences of radiotherapy and antineoplastic therapy for the fetus. J Reprod Med 1976;17:241–246.

34. Barber HRK. Fetal and neonatal effects of cytotoxic agents. Obstet Gynecol 1981;58:41S–47S.

35. Gilliland J, Weinstein L. The effects of cancer chemotherapeutic agents on the developing fetus. Obstet Gynecol Surv 1983;38:6–13.

36. Antman KH, Mayer RJ, Frei E. Vascular, hormonal, teratogenic and miscellaneous toxicities of chemotherapeutic agents. In: Perry MC, Yarbro JW, eds. Toxicity of chemotherapy. Orlando, FL: Grune & Stratton 1984:521–538.

37. Mulvihill JJ, McKeen EA, Rosner F, Zarrabi MH. Pregnancy outcome in cancer patients. Cancer 1987;60:1143–1150.

38. Diamond I, Anderson MM, McCreadie SR. Transplacental transmission of busulfan (Myleran) in a mother with leukemia. Production of fetal malformations and cytomegaly. Pediatrics 1960;25:85–90.

39. Toledo TM, Harper RC, Moser RH. Fetal effects during cyclophosphamide and irradiation therapy. Ann Intern Med 1971;74:87–91.

40. Abramovici A, Shaklai M, Pinkhas J. Myeloschisis in a six week embryo of a leukemic woman treated with busulfan. Teratology 1978;18:241–246.

41. Doll DC, Ringenberg QS, Yarbro JW. Management of cancer during pregnancy. Arch Intern Med 1988;148:2058–2064.

42. Doll DC, Ringenberg QS, Yarbro JW. Antineoplastic agents and pregnancy. Semin Oncol 1989; 16:337–346.

43. Wiebe VJ, Sipila EH. Pharmacology of antineoplastic agents in pregnancy. Crit Rev Oncol Hematol 1994;16:75–112.

44. Delmer A, Rio B, Bauduer F, Ajchenbaum F, Marie J-P, Zittoun R. Pregnancy during myelosuppressive treatment for chronic myelogenous leukemia. Br J Haematol 1992;82:783–784.

45. Patel M, Dukes IAF, Hull JC. Use of hydroxyurea in chronic myeloid leukemia during pregnancy: a case report. Am J Obstet Gynecol 1991;165:565–566.

46. Zemlickis D, Lishner M, Degendorfor P, Panzarella T, Sutcliffe SB, Koren G. Fetal outcome after in utero exposure to cancer chemotherapy. Arch Intern Med 1992;152:573–576.

47. Feldkamp M, Carey JC. Clinical teratology counseling and consultation case report: low dose methotrexate exposure in the early weeks of pregnancy. Teratology 1993;47:553–559.

48. Zuazu J, Julia A, Sierra J, et al. Pregnancy outcome in hematologic malignancies. Cancer 1991; 67:703–709.

49. Kozlowski RD, Steinbrunner JV, Mackenzie AH, Clough JD, Wilke WS, Segal AM. Outcome of first-trimester exposure to low-dose methotrexate in eight patients with rheumatic disease. Am J Med 1990;8:589–592.

50. Kalter H, Warkany J. Congenital malformations. N Engl J Med 1983;308:424–431, 491–497.

51. Greenberg LH, Tanaka KR. Congenital anomalies probably induced by cyclophosphamide. JAMA 1964;188:423–426.

52. Stephens JD, Golbus MS, Miller TR, et al. Multiple congenital anomalies in a fetus exposed to 5-fluorouracil during the first trimester. Am J Obstet Gynecol 1980;137:747–749.

53. Brent RL. The effects of embryonic and fetal exposure to x-ray, microwaves, and ultrasound. Clin Perinatol 1986;13:615–648.

54. Warkany J. Aminopterin and methotrexate: folic acid deficiency. Teratology 1978;17:353–358.

55. Goldenberg M, Biden D, Admon D, Mashiach S, Oelsner G. Methotrexate therapy of tubal pregnancy. Hum Reprod 1993;8:660–666.

56. Marcovici I, Rosenzweif BA, Brill AI, Khan M, Scommegna A. Cervical pregnancy: case reports and a current literature review. Obstet Gynecol Surv 1994; 49:49–55.

57. Ferm VJ. Congenital malformation in hamster

embryos after treatment with vinblastine and vincristine. Science 1963;141:426.

58. Aviles A, Niz J. Long-term follow-up of children born to mothers with acute leukemia during pregnancy. Med Pediatr Oncol 1988;16:3–6.

59. Nantel S, Parboosingh V, Poon M-C. Treatment of an aggressive non-Hodgkin's lymphoma during pregnancy with MACOP-B chemotherapy. Med Pediatr Oncol 1990;18:143–145.

60. King LA, Nevin PC, Williams PP, Carson LF. Treatment of advanced epithelial ovarian carcinoma in pregnancy with cisplatin-based chemotherapy. Gynecol Oncol 1991;41:78–80.

61. Willemse PHB, van der Silde R, Sleilfer DT. Combination chemotherapy and radiation for stage IV breast cancer during pregnancy. Gynecol Oncol 1990; 36:281–284.

62. Dreicer R, Love RR. High total dose 5-fluorouracil treatment during pregnancy. Wis Med J 1991; 90:582–583.

63. Maurer LH, Forcier RJ, McIntyre OR. Fetal group C trisomy after cytosine arabinoside and thioguanine (letter). Ann Intern Med 1971;75:809–810.

64. Boros SJ, Reynolds JW. Intrauterine growth retardation following third trimester exposure to busulfan. Am J Obstet Gynecol 1977;129:111–112.

65. Reynosa E, Shepherd F, Messner H, Farquharson HA, Garvey MB, Baker MA. Acute leukemia in pregnancy: the Toronto Leukemia Study Group experience with long-term follow-up of children exposed in utero to chemotherapeutic agents. J Clin Oncol 1987; 5:1098–1106.

66. Schleuning M, Clemm C. Chromosomal aberrations in a newborn whose mother received cytotoxic treatment during pregnancy. N Engl J Med 1987; 317:1666–1667.

67. Russell JA, Powles RL, Oliver RTD. Conception and congenital abnormalities after chemotherapy of acute myelogenous leukemia in two men. Br Med J 1976;1:1508.

68. Vianelli M, Gugliotta L, Tura S, Bovicelli L, Rizzo N, Gabrielli A. Interferon-alpha 2a treatment in a pregnant woman with essential thrombocythemia. Blood 1994;83:874–875.

69. Baer MR, Ozer H, Foon KA. Interferon-alpha therapy during pregnancy in chronic myelogenous leukemia and hairy cell leukemia. Br J Haematol 1992; 81:167–169.

70. Reichel RP, Linkesch W, Schetitska D. Therapy with reconbinant interferon alpha-2c during unexpected pregnancy in a patient with chronic myeloid leukemia. Br J Haematol 1992;82:472–478.

71. Harrison P, Chipping P, Fothergill GA. Successful use of all-*trans* retinoic acid in acute promyelocytic leukemia presenting during the second trimester of pregnancy. Br J Haematol 1994;86:681–682.

72. Le L, Pizzutic DJ, Greenberg M, Reid R. Accidental use of low-dose 5-fluorouracil in pregnancy. J Reprod Med 1991;36:872–874.

73. Kopelman JN, Miyazawa K. Inadvertent 5-fluorouracil treatment in early pregnancy: a report of three cases. Reprod Toxicol 1990;4:233–235.

74. Cullins SL, Pridjian G, Sutherland CM. Goldenhar's syndrome associated with tamoxifen given to the mother during gestation. JAMA 1994;271:1905–1906.

75. McCormick MC. The contribution of low birth weight to infant mortality and childhood morbidity. N Engl J Med 1985;312:82–90.

76. Sutcliffe SB. Treatment of neoplastic disease during pregnancy: maternal and fetal effects. Clin Invest Med 1985;8:333–338.

77. Schaison G, Jacquillat C, Auclerc G, et al. Les fisques foetoembryonnaines des chimiotherapies. Bull Cancer 1979;66:165–170.

78. Okun DB, Groncy PK, Sieger L, Tanaka KR. Acute leukemia in pregnancy: transient neonatal myelosuppression after combination chemotherapy in the mother. Med Pediatr Oncol 1979;7:315–319.

79. Durodola JI. Administration of cyclophosphamide during late pregnancy and early lactation: a case report. J Natl Med Assoc 1979;71:165–166.

80. Aviles A, Maqueo-Diaz JC, Talavera A, Guzmaio R, Garcia EL. Growth and development of children of mothers treated with chemotherapy during pregnancy: current status of 43 children. Am J Hematol 1991;36:243–248.

81. Habermann T, Earle J, Johansen K, et al. Synchronous presentation of Hodgkin's disease and pregnancy (abstract 1294). Proc Am Soc Clin Oncol 1993; 12:380.

82. Schilsky RL, Sherins RJ. Gonadal dysfunction. In: DeVita VT, Hellman S, Rosenberg SA, eds. Cancer: principles and practice of oncology. Philadelphia: JB Lippincott 1985:2032–2039.

83. Stillman RJ, Schinfeld JS, Schiff I, et al. Ovarian failure in long-term survivors of childhood malignancy. Am J Obstet Gynecol 1981;139:62–66.

84. Byrne J, Mulvihill JJ, Myers MH, et al. Effects of treatment on fertility in long-term survivors of childhood or adolescent cancer. N Engl J Med 1987; 317:1315–1321.

85. Rice JM. An overview of transplacental carcinogenesis. Teratology 1973;8:113–126.

86. Shimkin MB. Pulmonary tumors in experimental animals. Adv Cancer Res 1955;3:223–267.

87. Druckrey H, Ivankovic S, Preussmann R. Teratogenic and carcinogenic effects in the offspring after single injections of ethylnitrosourea to pregnant rats. Nature 1966;210:1378–1379.

88. Kyle RA. Second malignancies associated with chemotherapy. In: Perry MC, Yarbro JW, eds. Toxicity of chemotherapy. Orlando, FL: Grune & Stratton 1984:479–506.

89. Dempsey JL, Seshadri RS, Morley AA. Increased mutation frequency following treatment with cancer chemotherapy. Cancer Res 1985;45:2873–2877.

90. Shaw MW. Human chromosome damage by chemical agents. Annu Rev Med 1970;21:409–432.

91. Bender RA, Young RL. Effects of cancer treatment on individual and generational genetics. Semin Oncol 1978;5:47–56.

92. Ward FT, Weiss RB. Lymphoma and pregnancy. Semin Oncol 1989;16:397–409.

93. Sylvester RK, Lobell M, Teresi ME, Brundage D, Bubowy R. Excretion of hydroxyurea into milk. Cancer 1987;60:2177–2178.

94. Johns DG, Rutherford LD, Leighton PC, Vogel CL. Secretion of methotrexate into human milk. Am J Obstet Gynecol 1972;112:978–980.

95. Wiernik PH, Duncan JH. Cyclophosphamide in human milk (letter). Lancet 1971;1:912.

96. Egan PC, Constanza ME, Dodion P, Egorin MJ, Bachur NR. Doxorubicin and cisplatin excretion into human milk. Cancer Treat Rep 1985;69:1387–1389.

97. Amato D, Niblett JS. Neutropenia from cyclophosphamide in breast milk. Med J Aust 1977;1:383–384.

98. Ben-Baruch G, Menczer J, Goshen R, Kaufman B, Gorodetsky R. Cisplatin excretion in human milk. J Natl Cancer Inst 1992;84:451–452.

99. Randall T. National registry seeks scarce data on pregnancy outcome during chemotherapy. JAMA 1993;269:323.

42

Gonadal Complications and Teratogenicity of Cancer Therapy

Catherine E. Klein

Prior to the remarkable advances made in the past 40 years revolutionizing the treatment of such cancers as pediatric sarcomas and leukemias, high-grade lymphomas, Hodgkin's disease, and testis tumors, few cancer patients survived long enough for the devastating long-term complications of therapy to be of particular concern. Many young patients are now cured of these diseases, and as they reach adulthood, they must face not only the temporary, but the permanent, alterations in gonadal function that are now recognized as among the most prevalent side effects of cancer therapy. Thus, many young women must experience symptoms of premature gonadal failure, including menopause, sterility, and presumably the accelerated osteoporosis and coronary atherosclerosis associated with estrogen deprivation. Male survivors of cancer are routinely oligoazoospermic and infertile. Those patients who retain fertility are faced with real concerns regarding the risk of complicated pregnancies, birth defects, intellectual development, and future cancer risk in their offspring, should they choose to conceive.

While many questions remain, recognition of these complications has led to better documentation of risk factors and their frequency, more effective counseling both pre- and posttherapy, and new strategies to ameliorate or prevent some of the toxicities through hormonal manipulation, selection of alternative treatments, or pretreatment cryopreservation of germ cells. Obviously, the detrimental effect of cancer therapy on the fertility of surviving patients is not limited to the side effects of chemotherapy. The tumor itself may impinge on the gonads. Surgery may remove or significantly impair the function of reproductive structures, as is typical for young men with testicular cancer who undergo retroperitoneal lymph node dissection or men whose prostate cancer is treated with orchiectomy. Radiation therapy has long been recognized as a sterilizing and mutagenic force. Finally, the psychosocial aspects of cancer recovery often leave profound alterations in libido and sexuality, and this is a poorly understood area that deserves more attention.

THE HYPOTHALAMIC-PITUITARY-GONADAL AXIS

Regulation of both the germ cell and the endocrine function of the gonadal axis begins at the level of the hypothalamus (Fig. 42.1), where neurosecretory cells synthesize and release gonadotropin-releasing hormone (GnRH) in a pulsatile fashion into the hypothalamohypophysial-portal circulation. Gonadotrophs in the anterior pituitary, in turn, respond by synthesizing and releasing the gonadotropins, follicle-stimulating hormone (FSH) and luteinizing hormone (LH), which ultimately control gonadal function. In women, ovarian follicles are stimulated by FSH to grow and mature, while LH stimulates ovulation and corpus luteum formation. This is recognized clinically with normal menstrual cycling and appropriate levels of LH, FSH, estrogen, and progesterone. In normal men, FSH initiates, and testosterone sustains, spermatogenesis. LH controls androgen synthesis by the testicular Leydig

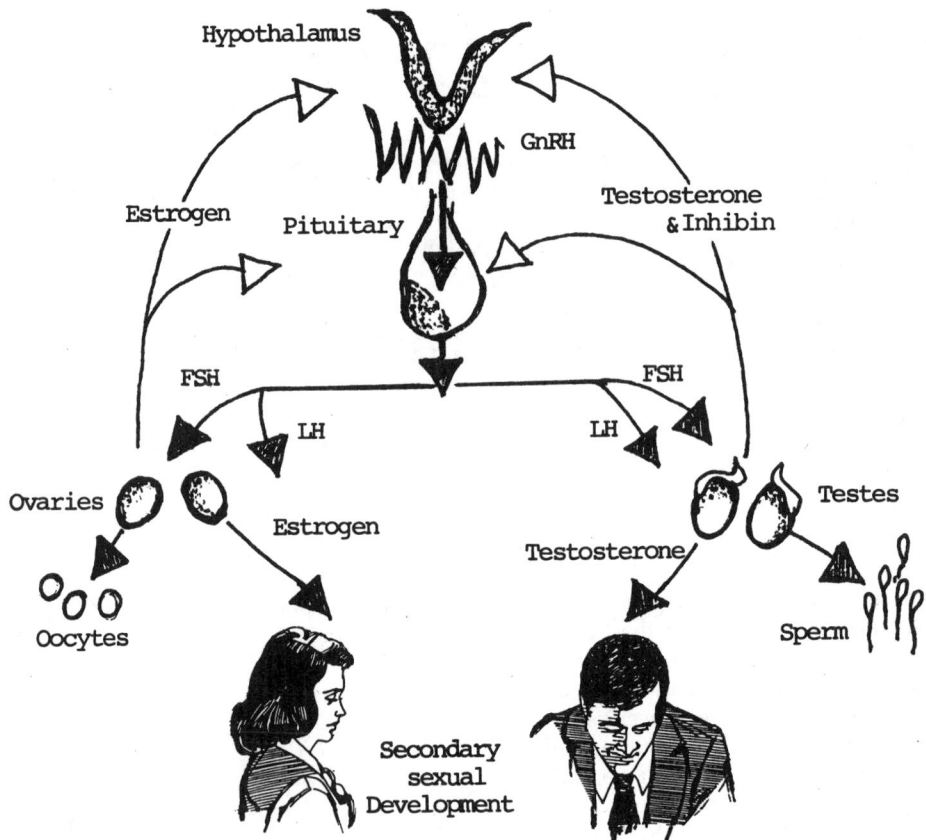

Figure 42.1.   The hypothalamic, pituitary, gonadal axis. The secretion of gonadotropin-releasing hormone (GnRH) from cells in the hypothalamus controls the pulsatile release of LH and FSH from the pituitary gland. These, in turn, regulate gamete production and sex steroid biosynthesis at the gonadal level. Feedback of sex steroids occurs at both the pituitary and hypothalamic levels.

cells (1). In both men and women, gonadal failure results in increased LH, from loss of the negative feedback of estrogen at the hypothalamus and pituitary in women, and decreases in both androgen and estrogen feedback in men (2). In response to decreased levels of sex steroids as well as the loss of inhibin, FSH levels are also elevated following gonadal damage. Particularly in women, a period of partial functioning may precede frank ovarian failure. This is characterized by sporadic, irregular menstrual cycling, with generally diminished estrogen and progesterone levels and correspondingly elevated gonadotropins. Women may conceive, however, during the normal ovulatory cycles. In men, spermatogenesis declines, but in the absence of extreme gonadal compromise, endocrine function is generally preserved, albeit at the expense of elevated LH and FSH. In both genders, germinal function may not be damaged in parallel

with endocrine function, so that FSH and LH elevations may be somewhat asynchronous. Nevertheless, the hallmark of primary gonadal failure from any cause is some pattern of elevation of gonadotropin levels, and this is the usual state in postpubertal patients receiving substantial doses of antineoplastic agents.

HISTORIC BACKGROUND

The effects of radiation and cytotoxic agents on gonadal functions have been recognized for much of this century. The radiosensitivity of the testes was noted in animals as early as 1903 and was repeatedly confirmed over the next 50 years (3, 4). Atomic Energy Commission studies of normal men, completed in the 1960s, confirmed the extraordinary sensitivity of spermatogonia to as little as 10 rads of x-irradiation, approximately three times less than the dose required in mice to produce equivalent damage (5). Following a single dose of 500 rads to the testicle, 50% of men are rendered permanently sterile. Oocytes, while more resistant, nevertheless demonstrate a dose-dependent sensitivity to irradiation, and at reproducible radiation doses, women experience permanent sterility and premature menopause at a frequency that increases with age. As in testicular radiation, a single dose of 500 rads to the ovaries is associated with predictable amenorrhea that persists for up to 18 months, and essentially all women over the age of 40 are rendered permanently infertile (6). More recently, secondary infertility has been reported in association with radiation administered to the hypothalamus or pituitary in conjunction with therapy for intracranial neoplasms (7). It is important to bear in mind the extreme sensitivity of the human gonad to the sterilizing effects of radiotherapy, as many of the studies from which the risk of infertility from cancer therapy is derived are confounded by the coadministration of x-ray therapy with the drugs discussed below.

Initial reports concerning the detrimental effects of chemotherapy on human male reproductive function appeared somewhat after the radiation toxicity was recognized (8), but by the 1940s, case reports had been confirmed by a pathologic study of the testes obtained from 30 men who received nitrogen mustard. Twenty-seven of these men had significant testicular atrophy and absent spermatogenesis (9). The first convincing report of menstrual irregularities or amenorrhea in women in association with cancer therapy appeared in 1956 (10), when Louis et al. reported four of four young women treated with busulfan for chronic myelogenous leukemia (CML) who developed menopausal symptoms within 3 months of starting therapy. Ovarian and endometrial histology were consistent with primary ovarian failure. Shortly thereafter, other alkylating agents, including nitrogen mustard, chlorambucil, and cyclophosphamide, when given in sufficient doses, were recognized to do the same (11–13). A variety of other chemotherapeutic agents of varying classes have subsequently been added to the list of presumed, or possible, ovarian toxins (Table 42.1). Many other commonly used drugs, however, have poorly documented effects on gonadal function in either men or women, and much of what is known has been inferred from more-recently published series documenting frequent ovarian failure or impaired spermatogenesis in association with combination chemotherapy for diseases with

Table 42.1. Relative Risks of Diminished Germ Cell Function Associated with Common Chemotherapeutic Agents

	Males	Females
Common	Cyclophosphamide	Busulfan
	Nitrogen mustard	Melphalan
	Procarbazine	Cyclophosphamide
	Nitrosoureas	Nitrosoureas
	Chlorambucil	
Possible	Vinblastine	Cisplatin
	Corticosteroids	Chlorambucil
	Cisplatin	Hydroxyurea
		Actinomycin D
		Vinblastine
		Etoposide
		Tamoxifen
Rare	Vincristine	Methotrexate
	6-Mercaptopurine	Doxorubicin
	Doxorubicin	Dacarbazine
	Methotrexate	Bleomycin
	5-FU	Vincristine
		5-FU
No data	Navelbine	Taxol
	Interferon	Navelbine
		Interferon

extended survival: Hodgkin's disease, breast cancer, and acute lymphocytic leukemia (14–19). Thus, the sensitivity of dividing germ cells to chemotherapeutic agents or to radiotherapy has been recognized from the very onset of their use, but until recently, the frequency and severity of toxicity were considered somewhat irrelevant and were poorly appreciated.

PRECLINICAL STUDIES

Although the effects of chemotherapy and radiotherapy on gonadal function have been extensively documented in humans, a number of preclinical models have been useful in better defining the nature and the mechanism of germ cell damage and in developing potential methods of circumventing these problems. Most animal studies have evaluated alkylating agents in male rodents and found that they produce marked inhibition of DNA synthesis in the differentiating spermatogonia, while relatively sparing the slowly dividing stem spermatogonia (20–22). Similar findings, again limited to the alkylating agents, have been reported in dogs and monkeys (23, 24). Within the post-stem-cell spermatogonial population, however, there appears to be a distinct species-specific and drug-specific variation in susceptibility. Whether this differential sensitivity with the stage of spermatogenesis is also characteristic of human males has been difficult to establish.

Few animal studies evaluating ovarian function have been published, as there are no well-accepted, reliable animal models for drug-induced female infertility (25). In female rats, alkylating agents appear to selectively target the medium and large follicles. Once the animal has become hypogonadal, the compensatory pituitary increases in gonadotropins may recruit the relatively resistant small follicles into the more sensitive pool, thereby aggravating the damage (26).

In most animal systems, male infertility is reversible. In contrast to other alkylators, however, chronic procarbazine administration can produce permanent sterility in male rodents (20). The very high frequency of long-term infertility seen in survivors of Hodgkin's disease treated with nitrogen mustard, vincristine, procarbazine, and prednisone (MOPP) or other procarbazine-containing combinations suggests that procarbazine may be significantly more toxic than other alkylating drugs in humans as well. Less is known about other classes of drugs; most have not been well studied in animals. In a cross-sectional study on the effects of doxorubicin, cytosine arabinoside, bleomycin, cyclophosphamide, hydroxyurea, vinblastine, and vincristine given as single injections to male mice, doxorubicin appeared to be the most toxic to stem cells (27). Presumably because of their relative specificity for S-phase, the antimetabolites, even when used in high dose, have not been associated with long-term gonadal damage.

CHEMOTHERAPY EFFECTS IN BOYS

In contrast to the early reports of profound gonadal damage with elevated gonadotropins and diminished spermatogenesis in adult men who had received nitrogen mustard therapy, reports of chemotherapy administered to prepubertal and pubertal boys suggested a relative resistance of the less mature testicle to drug-induced effects. This assumption was predicated on the finding of relatively normal LH and FSH levels in these posttherapy young patients. However, since those earliest reports, a number of histologic studies have been published, all of which demonstrated significant structural damage to the testicle, even in young boys.

While levels of LH, FSH, and serum testosterone following chemotherapy in prepubertal boys may be normal, testicular biopsies from boys receiving combination therapy for acute lymphoblastic leukemia or Hodgkin's disease commonly show seminiferous tubular damage and interstitial fibrosis (28, 29). Consistent with the normal hormone panels, the vast majority of postchemotherapy boys progress normally through puberty, only rarely needing androgen supplementation. Even when testicular biopsy shows that fewer than 50% of seminiferous tubules contain identifiable spermatogonia, more than 90% of prepubertal or pubertal boys demonstrate normal basal and stimulated hormone panels (30).

Perhaps a better reflection of the major disruption of seminiferous tubular histology, however, is the relatively high incidence of significant reproductive dysfunction as measured by subsequent sperm counts and motility assessments. Although the exact frequencies reported vary widely (30–32), it is clear that the immature male gonad is at major risk of permanent damage affecting the ultimate fertility of the patient. The frequency of normal sperm counts in series of pubertal or prepubertal patients treated with single-agent cyclophosphamide, for example, even years after therapy, has been reported to range between 0 and 100% (33, 34). A review of oral cyclophosphamide administered in cumulative doses of 0.7 to 52 g revealed gonadal damage in 10 of 63 (16%) prepubertal boys, while 10 of 15 (67%) pubertal boys had evidence of gonadal dysfunction (35).

Other drugs have been associated with similar long-term outcome. Chlorambucil given alone or in combination with prednisone and azathioprine for the treatment of renal disease in patients ranging from 6 to 15 years of age produced azoospermia in 17 of 21 patients for 3 to 11 years after cessation of treatment (36). Nitrosoureas used for childhood brain tumors have associated testicular failure (37). As Leydig cell dysfunction is only rarely documented, prepubertal damage to spermatogenesis can only be assessed with testicular biopsy or long-term follow-up of fertility, and it is possible that much of the difference in testicular susceptibility to chemotherapeutic agents previously attributed to pubertal stage may actually represent inappropriate assessment.

The other major factor that appears to determine the degree of damage to testicular function among prepubertal boys treated with cytotoxic chemotherapy is the cumulative dose of the drug administered, a relationship especially clear for the alkylating agents. A large metaanalysis of 30 studies comprising 456 patients treated with cyclophosphamide (either alone or in combination with other cytotoxic agents) or prednisone for renal disease, Hodgkin's disease, or leukemia, with no confounding exposure to either abdominal or gonadal radiation, found that the cumulative dose of cyclophosphamide had a profound effect on spermatogenesis assessed after reaching sexual maturity. While less than 10% of prepubertal boys who received under 400 mg/kg cyclophosphamide total dose demonstrated gonadal dysfunction, the incidence rose to 30% in those who received 400 to 500 mg/kg or more than 500 mg/kg (38). Likewise, the pubertal stage again exerted an independent, significant influence on the incidence of dysfunction, which varied between 0 and 24% in prepubertal boys and climbed to 68 to 95% in sexually mature adults. In many small series, a confounding effect of nutritional status can be shown to play an important role in determining the recovery and ultimate outcome of the spermatogenic epithelium in prepubertal boys who receive chemotherapy. Nevertheless, dose and maturational stage of the testicle appear to be the major determinants of the degree of damage to spermatogenesis, while the hormone axes remain relatively intact (39).

MOPP chemotherapy given to boys frequently produces significant impairment in subsequent spermatogenesis, which has been reported to last for years (32, 40). Remission induction for childhood acute leukemia with combinations including methotrexate, cytosine arabinoside, and vincristine, seems to exert a more readily reversible impact on spermatogenesis in boys (30). Prednisone, when used in adults, is associated with reversible oligospermia, but no information in available for children. Unfortunately, there are many poorly understood exceptions to these general trends, and reliable predictions for any given patient are impossible. Assumptions cannot be made that even minimal doses of chemotherapy given to prepubertal children will not result in permanent sterility, and short of testicular biopsy, there remains no good measure of gonadal damage until seminal analyses at puberty can be assessed (40).

As in therapy with single agents, Leydig cell function in prepubertal males seems to be somewhat more resistant to multiagent chemotherapy than does the germinal epithelial function. Gynecomastia associated with elevated FSH and LH levels was reported in 9 of 13 pubertal boys

receiving MOPP treatment (41). However, among 4 prepubertal boys who received the same four-drug regimen, all had normal basal and stimulated gonadotropin tests (32). Impaired spermatogenesis lasting years could be documented in most of these studies. Similarly, only 2 of 44 boys who recovered from acute lymphoblastic leukemia therapy had abnormal testosterone responses to human chorionic gonadotropin (HCG) challenge, and gonadotropin secretion was normal in 29 of 32 patients studied (31). A more recent report of 40 men treated for childhood Hodgkin's disease found that 26 of 28 who had received chemotherapy had elevated gonadotropin levels but normal serum testosterone and secondary sexual characteristics. Eleven of 13 tested were azoospermic. These changes persisted up to 17 years after treatment (42).

In sum, these data indicate that the seminiferous tubules of prepubertal boys are damaged by alkylating agents or combination chemotherapy, generally in an age- and dose-dependent manner, but that the endocrine secretory pathways of prepubertal and pubertal boys function relatively normally following chemotherapy for childhood cancer. Assessment is difficult, and absolute predictions are impossible.

CHEMOTHERAPY EFFECTS IN ADULT MEN

As single agents, the alkylating drugs have been widely recognized to produce some damage to the seminiferous epithelium. The duration and extent of the damage appear to be related to the age of the patient and the amount of the drug received, much as is observed in children. Cyclophosphamide administered in total doses of 9 g results in azoospermia in all men but is generally reversible with total doses as high as 18 g (43), although full recovery may take up to 3 to 4 years. Doses of chlorambucil as low as 400 mg have been associated with azoospermia in some men. Recovery may be prolonged and is probably related to total dose. Cheviakoff et al. reported that following a mean dose of 1464 mg, evidence of recovery may appear about 40 months after cessation of therapy (44). As in animals, procarbazine appears to be the single most toxic chemotherapeutic agent to the adult male gonad. While no studies of this drug as a single agent are available, inference can be drawn from multiple studies in Hodgkin's disease, in which patients received combination chemotherapy, either with or without procarbazine. Nineteen of 19 patients in one study treated with cyclophosphamide, vincristine, procarbazine, and prednisone (COPP) remained oligospermic 11 years after therapy, whereas 7 of 10 treated with COP and no procarbazine had return of spermatogenesis within 3 years (18, 45).

Methotrexate appears to exert minimal long-term testicular toxicity. Even when given over extended periods of time, only minor alterations in spermatogenesis can be documented, and these resolve within the first few weeks after therapy is stopped. Following high-dose therapy, oligospermia may be somewhat more common and protracted, with a reported incidence of 50% (46). Recovery within 1 to 2 years is anticipated. Little information is available with which to assess the potential gonadal toxicity of either single-agent vincristine or vinblastine. The slightly lower incidence of male infertility with the MOPP combination than with MVPP (with vinblastine substituted for vincristine), when used for the treatment of advanced Hodgkin's disease, suggests that vincristine may be slightly less toxic than vinblastine (47). While studies of

single-agent Adriamycin are also not available, it appears to have minimal long-term effect when used in combination therapy that does not include cyclophosphamide. When used with cyclophosphamide, however, it appears to augment the toxicity of that drug (48). No information on navelbine has been published.

An often-overlooked suppression of spermatogenesis occurs in association with corticosteroid administration. Within a month of beginning moderate-dose prednisone, profound oligospermia with additional sperm dysmotility is seen in most men. Reversibility is the rule (49).

With increasing numbers of long-term cancer survivors following treatment with curative combination chemotherapy, multiple reports have documented permanent infertility among patients with Hodgkin's disease, non-Hodgkin's lymphomas, seminomas, and the nonseminomatous testicular cancers (Table 42.2). For incompletely understood reasons, even prior to therapy, as many as 30% of young men presenting with Hodgkin's disease are oligospermic,

Table 42.2. Gonadal Effects of Combination Chemotherapy in Males

Disease	Regimen[a]	N	Azoospermia	%	Reference
Hodgkin's	ChlVPP	13	11	87	42
	MOPP	11	8	73	56
		6	5	83	45
		25	22	88	41
		21	18	86	55
	ABVD	13	0	0	54
	MVPP	64	54	84	51
		14	14	100	50
		41	36	88	59
		49	42	86	52
		33	33	100	60
Non-Hodgkin's	COPP	3	2	67	18
		4	00	00	45
	VAPEC-B	14	2	14	67
Testis cancer	PVB	28	4	14	61
		25	7	28	70
	PVB ± Dox	7	0	0	66
		6	1	17	65
		23	9	39	67
Leukemia	Multiple drugs	10	0	0	60
		4	3	75	59
Sarcoma	Dox + multiple drugs	32	2	6	68
	Dox, CPA, MTX + RT	26	17	65	46

[a]Abbreviations: MOPP, nitrogen mustard, vincristine, procarbazine, prednisone; MVPP, nitrogen mustard, vinblastine, procarbazine, prednisone; COPP, cyclophosphamide, vincristine, procarbazine, prednisone; TVPP, thiotepa, vincristine, procarbazine, prednisone; ChlVPP, chlorambucil, vinblastine, procarbazine, prednisone; CMF, cyclophosphamide, methotrexate, 5-fluorouracil; ABVD, doxorubicin, bleomycin, vinblastine, dacarbazine; PVB, cisplatin, vinblastine, bleomycin; dox, doxorubicin; CPA, cyclophosphamide; MTX, methotrexate; P, cisplatin; VCR, vincristine; bleo, bleomycin; ACTD, actinomycin D; VP-16, etoposide; l-PAM, l-phenylalanine mustard; mito, mitomycin; 5-FU, 5-fluorouracil; Vlb, vinblastine; VAPEC-B, vincristine, cyclophosphamide, doxorubicin, etoposide, bleomycin, prednisone.

and disorders of sperm motility and morphology are probably even more common (50, 51). This phenomenon appears poorly correlated with stage or extent of disease or with the age of the patient. Despite frequently elevated gonadotropin levels and abnormal testicular histology, return of normal function is anticipated when treatment is completed without gonadotoxic therapy. This observation significantly confounds the interpretation of posttherapy studies. In a prospective study of 37 men receiving the MVPP combination, 12 had low sperm counts before beginning treatment, but 14 of 14 studied after 2 cycles were azoospermic. Twenty-seven of 27 remained azoospermic in the first 12 months after treatment (52). In general, following therapy for Hodgkin's disease when MOPP-like regimens (nitrogen mustard, vincristine/vinblastine, procarbazine, and prednisone) are used, evidence of deficient spermatogenesis appears early in therapy, and infertility is universal by the third cycle. Following completion of treatment, the recovery rate remains very poor. Retrospective analyses of men off therapy for more than 2 years suggest that only 5 to 15% ever regain effective spermatogenesis (35). MOPP may be associated with slightly better recovery rates than MVPP, although there are no direct comparisons available. In contrast to the effect on spermatogenesis, Leydig cell function, while frequently impaired, seems well compensated; despite elevated gonadotropin levels and low-normal serum testosterone levels in most treated adults, few if any of these men require androgen replacement (40, 45). Occasional men develop gynecomastia (53).

Recent reports from a randomized prospective study comparing MOPP chemotherapy with the ABVD regimen (doxorubicin, bleomycin, vinblastine, and dactinomycin) for the treatment of advanced Hodgkin's disease provide convincing evidence that the latter combination produces less gonadal toxicity in both men and women (54, 55). Since it is equally efficacious in the induction of long-term remissions, ABVD should be the treatment of choice in men who are concerned about preservation of reproductive potential. Few studies are available with which to evaluate other combinations used more commonly in the treatment of non-Hodgkin's lymphomas. Scattered small reports suggest that the cyclophosphamide, vincristine, and prednisone (CVP) regimen without the procarbazine may be less toxic than MOPP or COPP (45, 56). A recent analysis of 14 men treated with VAPEC-B (doxorubicin, etoposide, vincristine, cyclophosphamide, and bleomycin) for either Hodgkin's disease or non-Hodgkin's lymphoma suggests that this may be an efficacious, relatively nontoxic regimen (57).

Evaluation of combination therapy for the induction of remission for acute leukemias is available largely for children and adolescents. Few series of adults have provided enough long-term survivors for adequate follow-up. Nevertheless, it appears that adult survivors of leukemia may fare somewhat better than their Hodgkin's counterparts, provided abdominal or testicular irradiation has not been used (58, 59). For example, Kreuser et al. found that 10 of 10 patients, 14 to 38 years old, treated for acute leukemia, demonstrated recovery of spermatogenesis by the second year of maintenance therapy (60).

Young men presenting with testis tumors are even more likely to demonstrate evidence of spermatogenic dysfunction at diagnosis than are young Hodgkin's disease patients. In a prospective series of 41 patients, Drasga et al. reported that 77% were oligoazoospermic and 17% azoospermic at initial presentation, leaving only 6% with adequate sperm counts with which to undertake cryopreservation (61). Other studies have reported oligospermia in up to 95% of newly diagnosed patients, an incidence far higher than is seen in either Hodgkin's disease or other disseminated cancers (50, 62). Abnormalities of sperm motility are even more common. Pretreatment testicular histology reflects these statistics and demonstrates spermatogenic arrest, hyalinized tubules, or totally absent tubules with only viable Sertoli cells evident (63). The etiology of this phenomenon is unknown, but some relationship to elevated HCG or the increased local heat from the tumor has been proposed.

After 2 months of therapy with cisplatin, vinblastine, and bleomycin, with or without doxorubicin, 94% of young men in Drasga's study were azoospermic. Patients completing therapy with either VAB or PVB demonstrate severe oligospermia in 75–100% of instances, and elevations of FSH are common (61, 64). However, in contrast to the MOPP-treated Hodgkin's patients, most studies show a time-dependent recovery of spermatogenesis with nearly 50% of patients recovering some sperm production after two years, and most patients within three years. Disorders of sperm motility may linger considerably longer (65–67). Testosterone levels are usually normal.

Both abdominal x-ray therapy, which is associated with almost 100% azoospermia, and retroperitoneal lymph node dissection (RPLND), which effects ejaculatory function, significantly decrease the likelihood of fertility in survivors of testis tumors (64). Modifications in surgical technique in recent years have significantly decreased the incidence of retrograde ejaculation following RPLND.

Less well studied are the male survivors of other tumor types. Shamberger et al. reported that 3 of 5 patients who had received adjuvant doxorubicin-based therapy for sarcoma recovered normal sperm counts, although concomitant radiation to the abdomen and pelvis or thigh and even more distant sites reduced the recovery rate substantially in 20 other patients studied (46). A similar study by Meistrich et al. estimated that 28% of men recovered adequate sperm counts after doxorubicin-based adjuvant treatment for osteosarcoma (68). Occasionally, elderly men with various forms of cancer develop gynecomastia as a result of cancer therapy, due to imbalance of testosterone and estrogens.

In summary, a substantial portion of adult men with Hodgkin's disease or testicular tumors are subfertile prior to any therapy. The older MOPP-like regimens for Hodgkin's disease produce uniform azoospermia that is permanent in more than 85% of patients, but newer regimens are considerably better tolerated and appear equally therapeutic. Most patients treated for testis cancer will become significantly oligospermic during therapy but recover spermatogenesis within 1 to 2 years of completing chemotherapy. Sperm motility and ejaculate volume may be more permanently altered, and the ultimate fertility rates are also affected if surgery or radiation therapy are part of the treatment strategy (69–72).

CHEMOTHERAPY EFFECTS IN PREPUBERTAL GIRLS

Careful studies of the gonadal effects of chemotherapy administered to prepubertal girls are unavailable, but what is published suggests variable ovarian toxicity, depending to some extent on the drug, its dose, and the duration of therapy. Unfortunately, much of the published information comes from studies on survivors of childhood leukemias and brain tumors, for which cranial radiation is part of the therapy, making hypothalamic disorders more difficult to exclude. Actual ovarian biopsies have been performed only rarely. Histologically, prepubertal ovaries appear to be significantly damaged by cancer chemotherapy. Follicular maturation arrest, stromal fibrosis, and partially depleted ova populations have all been reported following single-agent cyclophosphamide as well as cytosine arabinoside–based leukemic therapy (73, 74). As in boys, however, the histologic consequences of chemotherapeutic agents on the female gonad are not usually mirrored in recognizable alterations of the hormonal axes. Most of these young women have normal levels of gonadotropins and estrogens, and puberty progresses normally. Single-agent cyclophosphamide, for example, often given for nonmalignant disease, only rarely causes either delay in puberty or permanent sterility (75, 76). Most girls treated with procarbazine or nitrosoureas for brain tumors show biochemical evidence of primary ovarian dysfunction, but essentially all enter and progress normally through puberty. Clayton et al. have described 13 girls treated with a nitrosourea and procarbazine who also received craniospinal irradiation (77). Nine of these girls had abnormalities of FSH secretion. The ovarian dose of radiation was felt to be beneath the threshold for gonadal compromise. Over a period of years, apparently normal ovarian function resumed, and initially elevated gonadotropins returned to baseline in most of these women.

Little is reported about the gonadal toxicity suffered by girls treated for lymphomas, but 80% of those surviving combination therapy for acute lymphoblastic leukemia also proceed normally through puberty, and one study has suggested that despite evidence for primary gonadal damage, menarche may actually appear prematurely (78). Occasional reports of histologic evidence of ovarian destruction in association with antileukemic therapy including L-asparaginase or cytosine arabinoside suggest that in some instances, these drugs are potential toxins (79). Unfortunately, long-term follow-up of these patients, with fertility rates and menstrual status determined 10 to 20 years later, will be necessary to fully evaluate the ultimate effect of chemotherapy given to prepubertal and adolescent girls.

CHEMOTHERAPY EFFECTS IN ADULT WOMEN

Because the human ovary is relatively inaccessible to biopsy, the effects of antineoplastic agents on the female gonad are generally inferred from a variety of surrogate markers, including the incidence of amenorrhea (both acute and chronic), the serum hormone panels, and the long-term fertility rates and outcomes as measures of ovarian function. Rare autopsy or biopsy series have been reported in women treated with cyclophosphamide for nonneoplastic diseases (12, 13) or with multiagent therapy for malignancy. These studies consistently describe complete absence of ova and follicles with tunica albugineal thickening and stromal hyalinization (12, 13, 80). One autopsy series of patients treated for acute leukemia showed no difference in the number of primary follicles, but secondary follicles were markedly depleted (74). Clinically, women receiving these agents variably develop signs and symptoms of primary ovarian failure: vaginal dryness with dyspareunia, endometrial hypoplasia, decreased libido, hot flashes, oligomenorrhea evolving into amenorrhea, and low circulating levels of estrogens, with compensatory elevations of the gonadotropins, FSH and LH (81, 82).

As in adult men, alkylating agents are the most reliably gonadotoxic of chemotherapeutic agents in common clinical usage today. The precise frequency of permanent amenorrhea and infertility depends on a number of factors, but very early in the history of these drugs it was recognized that the effect was dose dependent: amenorrhea occurred sooner, lasted longer, and remained permanent more commonly as higher doses were administered. Concomitant radiation exposure and the age of the patient at the time therapy was administered were important covariables in the outcome. Continued drug administration after the onset of amenorrhea significantly increased the likelihood of its becoming permanent.

Alkylating agents are not only highly gonadotoxic but are strongly associated with mutagenesis and teratogenesis as well. Nitrogen mustard appears to be the most toxic, but few studies are available describing its effects when used as a single agent. Cyclophosphamide is the alkylating drug with the best-documented ovarian toxicity. An early report by Miller (12) described an adolescent girl treated with a total dose of 1.38 g/kg of cyclophosphamide administered over about 2½ years. Ovarian histology at autopsy showed complete destruction of ovarian structure, with no ova and no follicles evident. Subsequent series report amenorrhea in 50 to 75% of women treated with cyclophosphamide, often within a month of starting therapy (83–85). There is, however, a striking age-related susceptibility. In one study, the total dose of cyclophosphamide received before the onset of amenorrhea in women over 40 years was 5.2 g; in patients 30 to 39 years of age, the dose was 9.3 g; and for women 20 to 29 years of age, 20.4 g was administered before amenorrhea developed. Menses returned in 50% of those under 40 (16). This reversibility of amenorrhea has also been well-established and may be more common in association with cyclophosphamide than with other alkylating drugs. For women under the age of 40, return of menstrual function seems closely correlated with the dose of cyclophosphamide administered after the cessation of menses (15). This same study suggested a race-specific variation in sensitivity.

L-Phenylalanine mustard used as adjuvant chemotherapy for women with premenopausal breast cancer is associated with significant and age-related loss of ovarian function. In one of the earlier National Surgical Adjuvant Breast and Bowel Program (NSABP) studies, 73% of the women between the ages of 40 and 49, but only 22% of the women under the age of 39 developed amenorrhea; elevated LH and FSH levels appeared only in the older age group (86). Busulfan and chlorambucil as single agents have associated well-documented ovarian toxicity that is age related and dose related (87, 88). Freckman et al. reported that an average total dose of 525 to 750 mg/m^2 of chlorambucil resulted in "castration" in women treated for metastatic breast cancer (88).

Small series of patients treated with high-dose methotrexate, usually as adjuvant therapy for sarcomas, report that amenorrhea even during therapy is uncommon and that serum gonadotropins remain normal during and following therapy (46). Given in low dose to women with gestational trophoblastic tumors, methotrexate appears to exert no significant toxicity. Fluorouracil, Adriamycin, L-PAM, and bleomycin as single agents are probably also well tolerated. Fluorouracil added to L-PAM in the adjuvant treatment of breast cancer, appears to add no significant toxicity over L-PAM alone (86). Few data are available for etoposide, but some ovarian dysfunction was reported among women receiving the drug for gestational tumors (89). Vincristine and vinblastine likewise appear to be infrequent, reversible causes of amenorrhea (15, 90). Reliable information concerning Taxol or navelbine is also not available.

The nonsteroidal antiestrogen tamoxifen, although not as well characterized, appears to exert an estrogenic effect with significant elevations of serum estradiol levels associated with inappropriately modest decreases in gonadotropins in both premenopausal and postmenopausal women treated for breast cancer. Menstrual irregularities are common among the former, but the incidence of persistent amenorrhea is unclear (91). Reliable information about the ovarian effects of biologic response modifiers is unavailable.

As in men, the largest data sets concerning chemotherapeutic effects on gonadal function relate to combination chemotherapy, particularly for Hodgkin's disease (Table 42.3). As most of the women treated for this disease are of potential childbearing age, infertility following therapy has received considerable attention. The reported incidence of amenorrhea in various series of women treated with MOPP, MVPP, or COPP for Hodgkin's disease ranges from 15 to 80%, with a median of about 50% (15–19, 54, 92–95). Combined therapy, which includes pelvic radiation, obviously increases the rate of infertility. Interestingly, most studies show that about two-thirds of women develop amenorrhea during therapy, while the remainder develop it slowly

over the next several years. Even women treated in their teenage years have a high likelihood of experiencing premature menopause in their thirties, suggesting that damage incurred at the time of therapy may not be reversible. The extent to which the dose administered alters the incidence of ovarian failure is unclear. In at least one study, there appeared to be no difference between women receiving three cycles of MOPP and those receiving six (96). Age at the time of treatment, however, has repeatedly been shown to be an important variable affecting the incidence and time of onset of permanent amenorrhea.

The rapidity of onset of amenorrhea is clearly age related. Patients under the age of 40 may show signs of slowly progressing ovarian failure over a period of several years, while older women are essentially all menopausal within a year of the completion of therapy. In general, patients over the age of 25 may expect a rate of amenorrhea between 60 and 100%. This typically begins during therapy, and menses do not reappear. In women under the age of 25 when therapy is initiated, ovarian failure is reported in 5 to 30%, and menses cease gradually over the several months to several years following treatment. Even younger women should anticipate a greater than 50% likelihood of premature meno-

Table 42.3. Gonadal Effects of Combination Chemotherapy in Females

Disease	Regimen[a]	N	Amenorrhea	%	Reference
Ovary	P, VCR, MTX, Bleo, ACTD, VP-16	17	1	6	102
	VCR, ACTD, CPA	40	3	8	90
Breast	l-PAM ± 5-FU	37	8	21	86
		59	43	72	
	CMF	14	12	85	107
	CPA	18	15	83	16
	Mito	15	4	26	16
	5-FU	21	2	9	16
Hodgkin's	VLB, Bleo, MTX, + IFRT	15	1	6	15
	MVPP	44	17	38	30
		28	10	36	92
	MOPP	68	16	24	14
	COPP	14	8	57	18
	TVPP	34	32	94	93
	MOPP ± RT	24	11	46	94
	ABVD	24	0	0	54

[a]Abbreviations: MOPP, nitrogen mustard, vincristine, procarbazine, prednisone; MVPP, nitrogen mustard, vinblastine, procarbazine, prednisone; COPP, cyclophosphamide, vincristine, procarbazine, prednisone; TVPP, thiotepa, vincristine, procarbazine, prednisone; ChlVPP, chlorambucil, vinblastine, procarbazine, prednisone; CMF, cyclophosphamide, methotrexate, 5-fluorouracil; ABVD, doxorubicin, bleomycin, vinblastine, dacarbazine; PVB, cisplatin, vinblastine, bleomycin; dox, doxorubicin; CPA, cyclophosphamide; MTX, methotrexate; P, cisplatin; VCR, vincristine; bleo, bleomycin; ACTD, actinomycin D; VP-16, etoposide; l-PAM, l-phenylalanine mustard; mito, mitomycin; 5-FU, 5-fluorouracil; Vlb, vinblastine; VAPEC-B, vincristine, cyclophosphamide, doxorubicin, etoposide, bleomycin, prednisone.

pause within 5 to 10 years of therapy (97). Conclusive data evaluating the actual fertility rates in young women who may have preserved menstrual function but who are developing premature ovarian failure are unavailable. The conception rate in this group is probably somewhere under 50%. Preliminary reports suggest that the alternative regimen (ABVD) for the treatment of Hodgkin's disease may have lower rates of prolonged amenorrhea (55). Women receiving MACOP-B for aggressive lymphomas appear, in small series, to maintain fertility (98).

Other forms of combination chemotherapy for ovarian germ cell tumors and some sarcomas have provided additional information on post-chemotherapy reproductive potential. Women receiving cisplatin-containing therapy for germ cell tumors typically become amenorrheic during treatment, but over 90% resume menstruation within a few months after completing treatment (89, 99–104). It has been suggested that when treatment for gestational tumors includes methotrexate with an additional three or more other drugs, fertility is lower than with methotrexate and only two other drugs. In particular, the addition of either vincristine or actinomycin D appears to be associated with increased infertility (105). Among women with breast cancer, who may have age-related decreased reproductive potential to begin with (106), 80% receiving CMF (cyclophosphamide, methotrexate, and 5-fluorouracil) as surgical adjuvant therapy become menopausal within 10 months of beginning therapy (107, 108). Those given doxorubicin and cyclophosphamide usually become anovulatory within 3 months, or sooner if they are perimenopausal (109).

FERTILITY FOLLOWING HIGH-DOSE CHEMOTHERAPY

Increasing numbers of young patients are undergoing bone marrow transplantation following high-dose, ablative chemotherapy, but few carefully conducted studies are available with which to assess their likelihood of retaining fertility (110). Many published reports of young women conceiving and delivering normal children attest to the possibility of normal ovarian function following high-intensity therapy, but few document the total number of women treated or desiring fertility with which to evaluate the probability of such function. Little information on hormone levels or long-term follow-up has been published, and even fewer data

are available for men. Follow-up of 187 young women previously treated with bone marrow transplantation for either aplastic anemia or leukemia found the same age-dependent effect of cyclophosphamide as is seen in lower-dose therapies (111). Fertility rates among young women transplanted for aplastic anemia appear overall to be higher than those for leukemia patients, and in particular, women under age 26 years of age at the time of therapy were much more likely to do well. The addition of total body irradiation (TBI) had a significant, independent negative impact on residual ovarian function. No woman over the age of 25 had return of menstrual function if TBI was added to the conditioning regimen. Graft-vs-host disease prophylaxis with either methotrexate or cyclosporine was not associated with diminished likelihood of normal ovarian function. One recent report evaluated 30 women who had survived at least 18 months following bone marrow transplantation for acute leukemia. Of the 10 who had received only one transplant, 4 developed ovarian failure, 6 resumed spontaneous menstrual cycling, and 5 of those 6 became pregnant. Of the three pregnancies allowed to go to term, all produced a normal infant (112). Other studies have confirmed that TBI in addition to chemotherapy is a major risk factor for infertility (111). No reliable studies document the status of fertility in young men following high-dose ablative chemotherapy.

PROTECTIVE MEASURES

Protection in Men

Most reported data suggest that the gonadotoxic effects of chemotherapy are most pronounced in adult males, where spermatogenesis reflects a relatively brisk mitotic rate. It would appear that the prepubertal gonad of either sex or the adult female ovary, where the rate of germ cell mitosis may be somewhat more indolent, are probably relatively more resistant to the long-term damage associated with these agents. While there are significant exceptions to this principle, such a differential susceptibility is consistent with the notion that most chemotherapeutic agents affect the most rapidly dividing malignant as well as normal cells. In turn, this observation has led to the hypothesis that if spermatogenesis could be temporarily halted, perhaps by hormonal manipulation, the ultimate damage to germinal cell populations might be lessened (113).

A number of animal studies and initial trials

in humans have been performed to test this hypothesis. Reversible suppression of spermatogenesis has been documented both in humans and laboratory animals with administration of several GnRH analogues, androgens, and glucocorticoids. Both GnRH analogues and sex steroids have been administered in the prechemotherapy setting, and while the rate of spermatogenesis can be decreased, a protective effect has not been unequivocally documented. On one hand, some success has been reported in rats, dogs, and primates, particularly for procarbazine-induced damage, but other studies have failed to demonstrate protection, and isolated studies have occasionally shown increased damage from such manipulation (23, 114–122). Similarly, human trials to preserve fertility in men receiving combination therapy for Hodgkin's disease have been disappointing. Two attempts using GnRH analogues were unsuccessful (123, 124), and at the present time, preservation of fertility by hormonal manipulation remains unproven. For men who desire fertility following combination chemotherapy for advanced Hodgkin's disease, the ABVD regimen is clearly preferable to MOPP (55).

An interesting alternative approach to testicular protection has been explored in rats. The antioxidants ascorbate and N-acetylcysteine were administered to prevent the bioactivation of procarbazine to its spermatotoxic radicals. Compared with control animals given procarbazine and no protection, experimental groups receiving either antioxidant agent demonstrated significant reduction in postprocarbazine oligospermia (125).

For men anticipating gonadotoxic anticancer therapy, the best alternative to in vivo protection is semen cryopreservation. Because of the high prevalence of abnormal pretherapy semen analyses discussed above, many young men have been considered inappropriate candidates for this technique, but recently, successful impregnation has been achieved following artificial insemination using semen with quite low sperm counts and poor sperm motility (126, 127). This requires careful endocrinologically monitored timing with the woman's ovulation and impeccable technique in freezing, storing, and thawing semen specimens, but when these requirements are met, the technique may be effective in 40 to 45% of cases (127). Additionally, in vitro fertilization and subsequent implantation has been successful in cases with even lower sperm counts

and motility (128–130). Despite these encouraging reports, many centers report that the overall success rate among men who elect to preserve semen may be somewhat limited and perhaps is influenced by factors other than semen quality (131, 132). In one series from Memorial Sloan-Kettering Cancer Center, 48 of 69 men who had banked sperm were located, at a median of 27 months posttreatment, and only 11 had attempted to use their sperm for artificial insemination. Of these, only 3 had achieved successful pregnancies (126).

Recent very preliminary studies of testicular circulatory isolation suggests that this mechanical procedure is protective in a rat model and is feasible for clinical trials in humans (133).

Gonadal shielding remains the mainstay of protection from therapeutic radiation and should be provided in any combined-therapy approach.

Protection in Women

Analogous to the hypothesis in men, it has been proposed that suppression of ovarian ovulatory function by oral contraceptives or GnRH analogues might offer gonadal protection to cycling women anticipating potentially sterilizing radiation or chemotherapy. Occasional protection from both radiation- and chemotherapy-induced ovarian damage has been seen in some animal models (26, 113, 134). However, initial human trials encompassing small numbers of women have yielded conflicting results. The most promising report is that of Chapman and Sutcliffe, who administered oral contraceptives to young women anticipating MVPP therapy for Hodgkin's disease. At a mean follow-up of 26 months after treatment, resumption of normal menses was evident in five of the six women treated (135). Waxman et al., in an effort to downregulate the ovary, studied eight young women with Hodgkin's disease treated for 1 week with the GnRH analogue buserelin prior to the initiation of MVPP. They were unable to show any differences in amenorrhea or menopausal symptoms between controls and the treatment group (124), and after 3 years of follow-up, half of the pretreated women remained amenorrheic. It may be argued that the short pretreatment interval may compromise the protective effect of ovarian suppression, but often the initiation of cancer therapy is undertaken urgently, precluding more lengthy delay.

With the increasing availability and refinement of the techniques of in vitro fertilization, this option should be considered for women of childbearing age wishing to retain fertility after cancer chemotherapy. The induction of multiple follicles and subsequent cryopreservation of the retrieved oocytes has become a feasible pre-chemotherapy consideration for women anticipating cytotoxic therapy. Although most reports of successful pregnancies with this technique describe women with premature ovarian failure from a variety of non-cancer-related causes, Sauer et al. reported a young woman, amenorrheic following therapy for Hodgkin's disease, who was impregnated with a donor ovum recovered after insemination and uterine lavage (136). Offspring following in vitro fertilization appear to be normal.

For patients undergoing pelvic radiation therapy as part of the treatment program, oophoropexy can be undertaken. Generally, this is accomplished at the time of exploratory or staging laparotomy and moves the ovaries either medially behind the uterine fundus or laterally out of the radiation port. Radiation exposure is decreased by about 90%, and hormonal function is preserved in 55 to 95% of patients. Unfortunately, fertility is still somewhat compromised, possibly because of the abnormal tuboovarian anatomy or the unavoidable radiation scatter. In a study of 22 patients with Hodgkin's disease who had undergone oophoropexy, 1 of 2 receiving paraaortic radiotherapy and 2 of 12 receiving inverted-Y radiotherapy subsequently became pregnant (137, 138). In a study of 134 women who had undergone ovarian transposition, 126 of whom received radiation therapy, a total ovarian dose of 5 Gy was statistically associated with ovarian failure (138). Specific ovarian shielding may be useful in some cases.

Considerable debate has existed regarding the advisability of pregnancy for cancer survivors, particularly among physicians treating women with breast cancer, as the hormonal nature of this tumor has specific implications vis-a-vis pregnancy. Several large series report the survival of women treated for breast cancer who subsequently became pregnant (139–141). Their cancer-related prognosis does not seem to be affected by their pregnancies. The ideal timing of such pregnancies is somewhat less clear, and many physicians advise an initial 1- to 2-year disease-free interval.

OUTCOME OF PREGNANCY FOLLOWING CHEMOTHERAPY

For patients whose fertility is spared and for whom parenthood is anticipated, the concerns regarding teratogenic and mutagenic effects of chemotherapy become important (see Chapter 41 also). Teratogenesis refers to the specific morphologic changes produced in the fetus exposed to the drugs in utero. Mutagenesis is the induction of genetic alterations expressed in future generations. To assess the latter, a number of retrospective series have recently evaluated the outcome of pregnancy in women treated with chemotherapeutic agents as children or young adults, who completed therapy and then became pregnant (Table 42.4). Li et al. have published one of the largest series of offspring of patients treated as children for a variety of cancers.

Table 42.4. Selected Series of Pregnancies in Cancer Survivors

| Author | Parents | | Pregnancies | | | | | |
	M	F	Total	Abs[a]	Anomalies	Preterm	Normal	Ref
Holmes	29	19	93	11	8	1	76	(144)
Holmes								
Rustin		216	374	90	8		267	(105)
Li	62	84	286	45	8		236	(163)
Mulvihill		40	55	10	5	11	38	(148)
Green	25	35	202	33	5	13	158	(174)
Lacher		12	16	4	0		12	(93)
Aisner	29	34	84	16	2		66	(175)
Salooja[b]		5	5	2	0		3	(112)
Senturia	96				9		87	(146)

[a]Number of abortions, including spontaneous abortions, therapeutic abortions, and stillbirths.
[b]Series of bone marrow/high-intensity therapy recipients.

In a total of 286 subsequent pregnancies, they found no detectable increase in congenital anomalies, and chromosomal analysis was normal in 23 of 24 children tested (142). Women treated for trophoblastic tumors likewise appear to have pregnancies associated with no increased risk of congenital anomalies, spontaneous abortion, or neonatal mortality (105, 143). The incidence of chromosomal abnormalities was only 0.7% in the study group and compared favorably with the 1.6% incidence in the control group. With considerable follow-up, the offspring were developing normally, both physically and intellectually.

Pregnancies in women treated for Hodgkin's disease also appear to produce normal offspring. Holmes and Holmes compared the 93 pregnancies in their chemotherapy-treated patients with 288 sibling-control pregnancies. Overall, they could detect no difference between the groups in adverse outcomes of pregnancy, although when the subgroup who received both radiation and chemotherapy was analyzed separately, it appeared that combined treatment produced more spontaneous abortions in wives of male patients and that female patients were slightly more likely to produce abnormal offspring than were control women (144).

Fewer studies of fathers surviving cancer chemotherapy are available, and there has been some suggestion that among men with germ cell tumors, there is an excess of congenital anomalies and chromosomal abnormalities in the patients themselves (145). Nevertheless, there appear to be no excess anomalies detected in their offspring (146). When large series are combined, nearly 1400 live-born children have been reported to have an incidence of congenital defects approaching 4%. This incidence is no different than that seen in the general population, and the vast majority of these anomalies reflect the common, nongenetic abnormalities seen in the population at large (147, 148).

More subtle alterations in growth, development, and intellectual achievement have required longer-term follow-up for adequate assessment, but information to date suggests that offspring conceived following chemotherapy physically grow and mature appropriately and that their school performance is probably normal. Whether these children themselves are at an increased risk for germ-line alterations conferring an oncogenic potential is unclear. In addressing the question of cancer risk among these children, a National Cancer Institute study of offspring of cancer survivors found a slight, statistically insignificant excess of cancers in study children, compared with offspring of sibling-matched controls (0.3 vs. 0.23%). These numbers are not significantly different from those expected in the general population. When the children were analyzed by age and sex, however, it appeared that there was an excess of cancers diagnosed in male offspring under age five. Five cancers were detected in this group, with 1.7 expected (149). Some of these cancers potentially represented familial clustering of known hereditary cancers, i.e., retinoblastoma and Wilms' tumor.

Both men and women should be strongly counseled to avoid pregnancy during active cancer treatment, when the risks of both teratogenesis and mutagenesis are highest. Increasing literature is available concerning the management of women who conceive during active cancer treatment or who are pregnant when therapy is initiated. The specific risks and the magnitude of those risks to the fetus exposed in utero to chemotherapy agents depend not only on its gestational age but also on the specific drug and the dose administered. In general, the risks are highest in association with first trimester exposure, but even in this situation, the recommendation of therapeutic abortion is controversial and often unnecessary.

Aminopterin, one of the earliest folic acid antagonists, was consistently associated with major teratogenic effects. Presumably this drug, like folic acid, is concentrated in the amniotic fluid and, when administered during the first trimester, is associated with nearly universal, major fetal abnormalities, often of the CNS (150). No folate antagonist should be administered during the first trimester, but thereafter they appear to be safe. Other antimetabolites have rarely been associated with congenital abnormalities. First trimester exposure to 5-fluorouracil, cyclophosphamide, busulfan, and chlorambucil has been associated with low-birth-weight infants and other abnormalities on rare occasion (150–152). Vinblastine is teratogenic in animals but has only rarely been associated with malformations in humans. Fetal myocardial necrosis has been reported following maternal administration of anthracyclines (153). Cis-retinoic acid is among the most teratogenic of agents. Its associated embryopathy was reported by Lammer et al., who described 36 pregnancies in which 8 spontaneous abortions occurred, and an additional 5 had at least one major malformation. This estimated 26-fold excess in major malformations was comparable to that associated with thalidomide (154).

Whether multidrug combination therapy as administered for Hodgkin's disease, leukemia, or breast cancer adjuvant therapy significantly increases the risk to an exposed fetus is uncertain. Case reports and small series indicate that exposure in the second and third trimesters is associated with minimal risk to the fetus and that long-term development of these offspring is normal (155–159). In individuals with more indolent disease, diagnostic procedures and therapy may be safely delayed until later in pregnancy without adversely affecting the outcome of either the cancer or the pregnancy (160). Abdominal radiation should be avoided. One study of 16 children exposed to maternal antileukemic therapy could detect no difference in peripheral blood, bone marrow, cytogenetics, physical examination, neurologic assessment, school performance, or intelligence testing, compared with sibling controls (161). Nonteratogenic effects including low birth weight, intrauterine growth retardation, and more subtle developmental abnormalities remain to be defined. In utero exposure to diethylstilbestrol has been linked to the development of clear cell carcinomas in the female offspring of these women, but additional incontrovertible documentation of carcinogenesis from in utero exposure to chemotherapy is lacking. No information is available on the reproductive potential of these children.

Chemotherapy-related pancytopenia in the mother at the time of delivery has been reported to be associated with normal postpartum counts in the infant (162). Vaginal delivery has been uncomplicated in several of these cases.

PSYCHOSOCIAL ISSUES

Disfigurement, loss of fertility, anxiety about birth defects, sexual performance, and recurrence of tumor all significantly affect not only the single patient facing dating and mate selection issues but also the married patient in a stable relationship. In this latter group, the separation rate may be four times that of the general population (163–168). While many of the consequences of anticancer therapy can be effectively treated (estrogen replacement, reconstructive surgery), many cannot. Oncologists must be acutely aware of these issues, recognize them

early, and provide effective counseling to prevent additional major morbidity in these patients and allow them to feel open and hopeful regarding their problems. Excellent reviews are available for the interested reader seeking further information (169–171).

Anderson has proposed a model for physician assessment of sexual functioning, helping the provider to recognize and address many issues before they arise (170). Specific inquiry and careful documentation of current and prior sexual functioning, including frequency of activity, libido, arousal, orgasm, and sensation of resolution allow the health professional to readily define new and disabling cancer-therapy-related dysfunction and initiate appropriate therapy.

REFERENCES

1. Hazum E, Conn PM. Molecular mechanism of gonadotropin releasing hormone (GnRH) action. I. The GnRH receptor. Endocr Rev 1988;9:379–386.
2. Gooren K. Androgens and estrogens in their negative feedback action in the hypothalamo-pituitary-testis axis: site of action and evidence of their interaction. J Steroid Biochem 1989;33:757–761.
3. Albers-Schonberg. Uber eine bisher unbekannte Wirkung der Rontgenstrahlen auf den Organismus der Tiere. Muench Med Wochenschr 1903;50:1859.
4. Oakberg EF. Sensitivity and time of degeneration of spermatogenic cells irradiated in various stages of maturation in the mouse. Radiation Res 1955;2:389.
5. Clifton DK, Bremner WJ. The effect of testicular x-irradiation on spermatogenesis in man: a comparison with the mouse. J Androl 1983;4:387–392.
6. Jacox HW. Recovery following human ovum irradiation. Radiology 1939;32:538–545.
7. Rappaport R, Brauner R, Czernichow P. Effect of hypothalamic and pituitary irradiation on pubertal development in children with cranial tumours. J Clin Endocrinol Metabol 1982;54:1164–1168.
8. Spitz S. The histological effects of nitrogen mustards on human tumors and tissues. Cancer 1948;1:383–398.
9. Gilman A. The initial clinical trial of nitrogen mustard. Am J Surg 1963;105:574–578.
10. Louis J, Limarzi LR, Best WR. Treatment of chronic granulocytic leukemia with Myleran. Arch Intern Med 1956;97:299–307.
11. Ezdinli EZ, Stutzman L. Chlorambucil therapy for lymphomas and chronic lymphocytic leukemia. JAMA 1965;191:100–106.
12. Miller JJ, Williams GF, Leissring JC. Multiple late complications of therapy with cyclophosphamide including ovarian destruction. Am J Med 1971;50:530–535.
13. Sobrinho LG, Levine RA, Deconti RC. Amenorrhea in patients with Hodgkin's disease treated with antineoplastic agents. Am J Obstet Gynecol 1971;109:135–139.
14. Andrieu JM, Ochoa-Molina ME. Menstrual cycle, pregnancies and offspring before and after MOPP

therapy for Hodgkin's disease. Cancer 1983;52:435–438.

15. Horning SJ, Hoppe RT, Hancock SL, Rosenberg SA. Vinblastine, bleomycin, and methotrexate: an effective adjuvant in favorable Hodgkin's disease. J Clin Oncol 1988;6:1822–1831.

16. Koyama H, Wada T, Nishizawa Y, Iwanaga T, Aoki Y, et al. Cyclophosphamide-induced ovarian failure and its therapeutic significance in patients with breast cancer. Cancer 1977;39:1403–1409.

17. Koziner B, Myers J, Cirrincione C, et al. Treatment of stages I and II Hodgkin's disease with three different therapeutic modalities. Am J Med 1986; 80:1067–1078.

18. Kreuser ED, Ziros N, Hetzel WD, Heimple H. Reproductive and endocrine gonadal capacity in patients treated with COPP chemotherapy for Hodgkin's disease. J Cancer Res Clin Oncol 1987;113:260–266.

19. Whitehead E, Shalet SM, Blackledge G, Todd I, Crowther D, Beardwell CG. The effect of combination chemotherapy on ovarian function in women treated for Hodgkin's disease. Cancer 1983;52:988–993.

20. Gould SF, Powell D, Nett T, Glode LM. A rat model for chemotherapy-induced male infertility. Arch Androl 1983;11:141–150.

21. Lee I, Dixon R. Antineoplastic drug effects on spermatogenesis studied by velocity sedimentation cell separation. Toxicol Appl Pharmacol 1972;23:20–41.

22. Karashima T, Zalatnai A, Schally AV. Protective effects of analogs of luteinizing hormone-releasing hormone against chemotherapy-induced testicular damage in rats. Proc Natl Acad Sci USA 1988;85:2329–2333.

23. Goodpasture JC, Bergstrom K, Vickery BH. Potentiation of the gonadotoxicity of Cytoxan in the dog by adjuvant treatment with a luteinizing hormone-releasing hormone agonist. Cancer Res 1988;48:2174–2178.

24. Meistrich ML. Critical components of testicular function and sensitivity to disruption. Biol Reprod 1986;34:17–28.

25. Hirshfield AN. Histologic assessment of follicular development and its applicability to risk assessment. Reprod Toxicol 1987;1:71–79.

26. Ataya KM, McKanna JA, Weintraub AM, Clark MR, LeMaire WJ. A luteinizing hormone-releasing hormone agonist for the prevention of chemotherapy-induced ovarian follicular loss in rats. Cancer Res 1985; 45:3651–3656.

27. Lu CC, Meistrich ML. Cytotoxic effects of chemotherapeutic drugs on mouse testis cells. Cancer Res 1979;39:3575–3582.

28. Rapola J, Koskimies O, Huttenen NP, Floman P, Vilska J, Hallman N. Cyclophosphamide and the pubertal testis. Lancet 1973;1:98–99.

29. Uderzo C, Locasciulli A, Mazorati R. Correlation of gonadal function with histology of testicular biopsies at treatment discontinuation in childhood acute leukemia. Med Pediatr Oncol 1984;12:97–100.

30. Shalet SM, Hann IM, Lendon M, Jones PH, Beardwell CG. Testicular function after combination chemotherapy in childhood for acute lymphoblastic leukaemia. Arch Dis Child 1981;56:275–278.

31. Lendon M, Palmer MK, Hann IM, Shalet SM, Jones PH. Testicular histology after combination chemotherapy in childhood for acute lymphoblastic leukemia. Lancet 1978;2:439–441.

32. Whitehead E, Shalet SM, Jones PH, Beardwell CG, Deakin DP. Gonadal function after combination chemotherapy for Hodgkin's disease in childhood. Arch Dis Child 1982;47:287–291.

33. Watson AR, Rance CP, Bain J. Long-term effects of cyclophosphamide on testicular function. Br Med J 1985;291:1457–1460.

34. Hsu AC, Folami AO, Bain J, Rance CP. Gonadal dysfunction in males treated with cyclophosphamide for nephrotic syndrome. Fertil Steril 1979;31:173–177.

35. Chapman RM. Gonadal injury resulting from chemotherapy. Am J Ind Med 1983;4:149–161.

36. Guesry P, Lenoir G, Broyer M. Gonadal effects of chlorambucil given to prepubertal and pubertal boys for nephrotic syndrome. J Pediatr 1978;92:299–303.

37. Ahmed SR, Shalet SM, Campbell RHA, Deakin DP. Primary gonadal damage following treatment of brain tumors in childhood. J Pediatr 1983;103:562–565.

38. Rivkees SA, Crawford JD. The relationship of gonadal activity and chemotherapy-induced gonadal damage. JAMA 1988;259:2123–2125.

39. Matus-Ridley M, Nicosia SV, Meadows AT. Gonadal effects of cancer therapy in boys. Cancer 1985; 55:2353–2363.

40. Aubier F, Flamant F, Caillaud JM, Chaussain JM, Lemerle J. Male gonadal function after chemotherapy for solid tumors in childhood. J Clin Oncol 1989; 7:304–309.

41. Sherins RJ, Olweny CLM., Ziegler JL. Gynecomastia and gonadal dysfunction in adolescent boys treated with combination chemotherapy for Hodgkin's disease. N Engl J Med 1978;299:12–16.

42. Shafford EA, Kingston JE, Malpas JS, Plowman J, Pritchard J, Savage MO, Eden OB. Testicular function following the treatment of Hodgkin's disease in childhood. Br J Cancer 1993;68:1199–1204.

43. Buchanan JD, Fairley KF, Barrie JU. Return of spermatogenesis after stopping cyclophosphamide therapy. Lancet 1975;2:156–157.

44. Cheviakoff S, Calamera JC, Morgenfeld M, Mancini RE. Recovery of spermatogenesis in patients with lymphoma after treatment with chlorambucil. J Reprod Fertil 1973;33:155–157.

45. Roeser HP, Stocks AE, Smith AJ. Testicular damage due to cytotoxic drugs and recovery after cessation of therapy. Aust NZ J Med 1978;8:250–254.

46. Shamberger RC, Sherins RJ, Rosenberg SA. The effects of postoperative adjuvant chemotherapy and radiotherapy on testicular function in men undergoing treatment for soft tissue sarcoma. Cancer 1981;47:2368–2374.

47. da Cunha MF, Meistrich ML, Fuller LM, et al. Recovery of spermatogenesis after treatment for Hodgkin's disease: limiting dose of MOPP chemotherapy. J Clin Oncol 1984;2(6):571–577.

48. Fossa SD, Klepp O, Aakvaag A, Molne K. Testicular function after combined chemotherapy for metastatic testicular cancer. Int J Androl 1980;3:59–65.

49. Mancini RE, Lavieri JC, Muller F, Andrada JA, Saranceni DJ. Effect of prednisolone upon normal and pathologic human spermatogenesis. Fertil Steril 1966; 17:500–513.

50. Chapman RM, Sutcliffe SB, Malpas JS. Male gonadal dysfunction in Hodgkin's disease. A prospective study. JAMA 1981;245:1323–1328.

51. Chapman RM, Sutcliffe SB, Reis LH, Edwards

CRW, Malpas JS. Cyclical combination chemotherapy and gonadal function, retrospective study in males. Lancet 1979;1:285–289.

52. Whitehead E, Shalet SM, Blackledge G, Todd I, Crowther D, Beardwell CG. The effects of Hodgkin's disease and combination chemotherapy on gonadal function in the adult male. Cancer 1982;49:418–422.

53. Friedman NM, Plymate SR. Leydig cell dysfunction and gynaecomastia in adult males treated with alkylating agents. Clin Endocrinol 1980;12:553–556.

54. Santoro A, Bonadonna G, Valagussa P, et al. Long-term results of combined chemotherapy-radiotherapy approach in Hodgkin's disease: superiority of ABVD plus radiotherapy versus MOPP plus radiotherapy. J Clin Oncol 1987;5:27–37.

55. Viviani S, Santoro A, Ragni G, Bonfante V, Bestetti O, Bonadonna G. Gonadal toxicity after combination chemotherapy for Hodgkin's disease. Comparative results of MOPP vs ABVD. Eur J Cancer Clin Oncol 1985;21:601–605.

56. Sherins RJ, DeVita VT. Effect of drug treatment for lymphoma on male reproductive capacity. Ann Intern Med 1973;79:216–220.

57. Radford JA, Clark S, Crowther D, Shalet SM. Male fertility after VAPEC-B chemotherapy for Hodgkin's disease and non-Hodgkin's lymphoma. Br J Cancer 1994;69:379–381.

58. Evenson DP, Arlin Z, Welt S. Male reproductive capacity may recover following drug treatment with the L-10 protocol for acute lymphocytic leukemia. Cancer 1984;53:30–36.

59. Waxman JHX, Terry Y, Rees LH. Gonadal function in men treated for acute leukaemia. Br Med J 1983; 287:1093.

60. Kreuser ED, Hetzel WD, Wolfgang H, Hoelzer D, Kurrle E, Xiros N, Heimple H. Reproductive and endocrine gonadal functions in adults following multidrug chemotherapy for acute lymphoblastic or undifferentiated leukemia. J Clin Oncol 1988;6:588–595.

61. Drasga RE, Einhorn LH, Williams SD, Patel DN, Stevens EE. Fertility after chemotherapy for testicular cancer. J Clin Oncol 1983;1:179–183.

62. Vigersyy RA, Chapman RM, Berenberg J, Glass AR. Testicular dysfunction in untreated Hodgkin's disease. Am J Med 1982;73:482–486.

63. Berthelsen JG, Skakkebaek NE. Gonadal function in men with testicular cancer. Fertil Steril 1983; 39:68–75.

64. Fossa SD, Ous S, Abyholm T, Norman N, Loeb M. Post treatment fertility in patients with testicular cancer. II. Influence of cis-platin-based combination chemotherapy and of retroperitoneal surgery on hormone and sperm cell production. Br J Urol 1985; 57:210–214.

65. Johnson DH, Hainsworth JD, Linde RB, Greco FA. Testicular function following combination chemotherapy with cis-platin, vinblastine, and bleomycin. Med Pediatr Oncol 1984;12:233–238.

66. Kreuser ED, Harsch U, Hetzel WD, Schreml W. Chronic gonadal toxicity in patients with testicular cancer after chemotherapy. Eur J Cancer Clin Oncol 1986;22:289–294.

67. Hansen PV, Trykker H, Helkjaer PE, Andersen J. Testicular function in patients with testicular cancer treated with orchiectomy alone or orchiectomy plus cisplatin-based chemotherapy. J Natl Cancer Inst 1989; 81:1246–1250.

68. Meistrich ML, Chawla SP, Cunha MF, Johnson SL, Plager C, et al. Recovery of sperm production after chemotherapy for osteosarcoma. Cancer 1989;63:2115–2123.

69. Nijman JM, Koops HS, Oldhoff J. Sexual function after bilateral retroperitoneal lymph node dissection for non-seminomatous testicular cancer. Arch Androl 1987;18:255–267.

70. Nijman JM, Schraffordt Koops H, Kremer H, Sleijfer DT. Gonadal function after surgery and chemotherapy in men with stage II and III nonseminomatous testicular tumors. J Clin Oncol 1987;5:651–666.

71. Nijman JM, Schraffordt Koops H, Kremer J. Fertility and hormonal function in patients with a nonseminomatous tumor of the testis. Arch Androl 1985; 14:239–246.

72. Roth J, Einhorn LH, Greist A. Long-term complications of cisplatin-based chemotherapy for testis cancer. Semin Oncol 1988;15:345–350.

73. Miller JJ, Williams GF, Lessing JC. Multiple late complications of therapy with cyclophosphamide including ovarian destruction. Am J Med 1971;50:530–535.

74. Himelstein-Braw R, Peters H, Faber M. Morphologic study of the ovaries of leukaemic children. Br J Cancer 1978;38:82–87.

75. Lentz RD, Bergstein J, Steffes MW. Postpubertal evaluation of gonadal function following cyclophosphamide therapy before and during puberty. J Pediatr 1977;91:385–394.

76. Pennisi TAJ, Grushkin CM, Lieberman E. Gonadal function in children with nephrosis treated with cyclophosphamide. Am J Dis Child 1975;129:315–318.

77. Clayton PE, Shalet SM, Price DA, Jones PHM. Ovarian function following chemotherapy for childhood brain tumors. Med Pediatr Oncol 1989;17:92–96.

78. Quigley C, Cowell C, Jimenez M, et al. Normal or early development of puberty despite gonadal damage in children treated for acute lymphocytic leukemia. N Engl J Med 1989;321:143–151.

79. Himelstein-Braw R, Peters H, Faber M. Morphologic study of the ovaries of leukaemic children. Br J Cancer 1978;38:82–87.

80. Chapman RM, Rees LH, Sutcliffe SB, Edwards CRW, Malpas JS. Cyclical combination chemotherapy and gonadal function. Lancet 1979;1:285–289.

81. Chapman RM, Sutcliffe SB, Malpas JS. Cytotoxic-induced ovarian failure in women with Hodgkin's disease: I. Hormone function. JAMA 1979; 242:1877–1881.

82. Warne GL, Fairley KF, Hobbs JB, Martin FIR. Cyclophosphamide-induced ovarian failure. N Engl J Med 1973;298:1159–1162.

83. Qureshi MSA, Pennington JH, Goldsmity HJ, Cox PE. Cyclophosphamide therapy and sterility. Lancet 1972;1:1290–1291.

84. Schilsky RL, Lewis BJ, Sherins RJ. Gonadal dysfunction in patients receiving chemotherapy for cancer. Ann Intern Med 1980;93:109–114.

85. Uldall PR, Kerr DNS, Tacchi D. Sterility and cyclophosphamide. Lancet 1972;1:693–694.

86. Fisher B, Sherman B, Rockette H. L-Phenylalanine mustard in the management of premenopausal patients with primary breast cancer. Cancer 1979; 44:847–857.

87. Belohorsky B, Sirack J, Sandor L, Klauber E. Comments on the development of amenorrhea caused by Myleran in cases of chronic myelosis. Neoplasma 1960;7(4):397–403.

88. Freckman HA, Fry HL, Mendez ML, Maurer ER. Chlorambucil-prednisolone therapy for disseminated breast cancer. JAMA 1965;191:100–106.

89. Choo YC, Chan SWY, Wong LC, Ma HK. Ovarian dysfunction in patients with gestational trophoblastic neoplasm treated with short intensive courses of etoposide. Cancer 1985;55:2348–2352.

90. Gershenson DM. Menstrual and reproductive function after treatment with combination chemotherapy for malignant ovarian germ cell tumors. J Clin Oncol 1988;6:270–275.

91. Buckley MMT, Goa KL. Tamoxifen, a reappraisal of its pharmacodynamic and pharmacokinetic properties and therapeutic use. Drugs 1989;37:451–490.

92. King DJ, Ratcliffe MA, Dawson AA, Bennett B, MacGregor E. Fertility in young men and women after treatment for lymphoma: a population study. J Clin Pathol 1985;38:1247–1251.

93. Lacher MJ, Toner K. Pregnancies and menstrual function before and after combined radiation and chemotherapy for Hodgkin's disease. Cancer Invest 1986;4:93–100.

94. Schilsky RL, Sherins RJ, Hubbard SM, Wesley MN, Young RC, DeVita VT. Long-term follow-up of ovarian function in women treated with MOPP chemotherapy for Hodgkin's disease. Am J Med 1981; 71:552–556.

95. Horning SJ, Hoppe RT, Kaplan HS, Rosenberg SA. Female reproductive potential after treatment for Hodgkin's disease. N Engl J Med 1981;304:1377–1382.

96. Sherins RJ, Winokur S, DeVita VT Jr, Vaitukaitis J. Surprisingly high risk of functional castration in women receiving chemotherapy for lymphoma. Clin Res 1975;23:343A.

97. Waxman JHX, Terry YA, Wrigley PFM, Malpas JS, Besser GM, Lister TA. Gonadal function in Hodgkin's disease: long-term follow-up of chemotherapy. Br Med J 1982;285:1612–1613.

98. Muller U, Stahel RA. Gonadal function after MACOP-B or VACOP-B with or without dose intensification and ABMT in young patients with aggressive non-Hodgkin's lymphoma. Ann Oncol 1993;4:399–402.

99. Davis TE, Loprinzi CL, Buchler DA. Combination chemotherapy with cisplatin, vinblastine, and bleomycin for endodermal sinus tumors of the ovary. Gyn Oncol 1984;19:46–52.

100. Fossa SD, Aass N, Kaalhus O, Klepp O, Tveter K. Long-term survival and morbidity in patients with metastatic germ cell tumors treated with cisplatin-based combination chemotherapy. Cancer 1986; 58:2600–2605.

101. Marchetti M, Romagnolo C. Fertility after ovarian cancer treatment. Eur J Gynaecol Oncol 1992; 13:498–501.

102. Pektasides D, Rustin GJS, Mewlands ES, Begent RHJ, Bagshawe KD. Fertility after chemotherapy for ovarian germ cell tumours. Br J Obstet Gynaecol 1987;94:477–479.

103. Pfleiderer A. Therapy of ovarian malignant germ cell tumors and granulosa tumors. Int J Gynecol Pathol 1993;12:162–165.

104. Long L, Jaing P, Wang XP, Zhao TJ. Treatment of ovarian malignant germ cell tumors with preservation of fertility. Chin Med J (Engl Ed) 1993:106:303–306.

105. Rustin GJS, Booth M, Dent J, Salt S, Rustin F, Bagshawe KD. Pregnancy after cytotoxic chemotherapy for gestational trophoblastic tumours. Br Med J 1984;288:103–106.

106. Gratterola R. The premenopausal endometrial pattern in women with breast cancer. Cancer 1964; 17:1119.

107. Dnistrian AM, Schwartz MK, Frecchia AA. Endocrine consequences of CMF adjuvant therapy in premenopausal and postmenopausal breast cancer patients. Cancer 1983;51:803–807.

108. Samaan NA, DeAsis DN, Bugdar AO. Pituitary-ovarian function in breast cancer patients on adjuvant chemoimmunotherapy. Cancer 1987;41:2082–2087.

109. Schulz K, Schmidt-Rhode P, Weymar P, Kunzig H-J, Geiger W. The effect of combination chemotherapy on ovarian, hypothalamic and pituitary function in patients with breast cancer. Arch Gynaecol 1979;227:293–301.

110. Goldman JM. Bone marrow transplantation for chronic myeloid leukaemia. Hematol Oncol 1987; 5:265–279.

111. Sanders JE, Buckner CD, Amos D, et al. Ovarian function following marrow transplantation for aplastic anemia or leukemia. J Clin Oncol 1988;6:813–818.

112. Salooja N, Chatterjee R, McMillan AK, et al. Successful pregnancies in women following single autotransplantation for acute myeloid leukemia with a chemotherapy ablation protocol. Bone Marrow Transplant 1994;13:431–435.

113. Glode LM, Robinson J, Gould SF. Protection from cyclophosphamide-induced testicular damage with an analogue of gonadotropin-releasing hormone. Lancet 1981;1:1132–1134.

114. Delic JI, Bush C, Peckham MJ. Protection from procarbazine-induced damage of spermatogenesis in the rat by androgen. Cancer Res 1986;46:1909–1914.

115. Delic JI, Harwood JR, Stanley JA. Time dependence for the protective effect of androgen from procarbazine-induced damage to rat spermatogenesis. Cancer Res 1987;47:1344–1347.

116. Glode LM, Shannon JM, Nett T. Protection of rat spermatogenic epithelium from damage induced by procarbazine chemotherapy. Br J Cancer 1990; 62:61–64.

117. Lewis RW, Dowling KJ, Schally AV. D-Tryptophan-6 analog of luteinizing hormone-releasing hormone as a protective agent against testicular damage caused by cyclophosphamide in baboons. Proc Natl Acad Sci USA 1985;82:2977–2979.

118. Pogach LM, Lee Y, Gould S, Giglio W, Huan HFS. Partial prevention of procarbazine induced germinal cell aplasia in rats by sequential GnRH antagonist and testosterone administration. Cancer Res 1988; 48:4354–4360.

119. Schally AV, Paz-Bouza JI, Schlosser JV, Karashima T, Debeljuk L, Gandle B, Sampson M. Protective effects of analogs of luteinizing hormone-releasing hormone against x-radiation-induced testicular damage in rats. Proc Natl Acad Sci USA 1987;84:851–855.

120. Ataya K, Ramahi-Ataya A. Reproductive performance of female rats treated with cyclophospha-

mide and/or LHRH agonist. Reprod Toxicol 1993; 7:229–235.

121. da Cunha MF, Meistrich ML, Nader S. Absence of testicular protection by a gonadotropin-releasing hormone analogue against cyclophosphamide-induced testicular cytotoxicity in the mouse. Cancer Res 1987;47:1093–1097.

122. Morris ID, Shalet SM. Endocrine-mediated protection from cytotoxic-induced testicular damage. J Endocrinol 1989;120:7–9.

123. Johnson DH, Line R, Hainsworth JD, et al. Effects of luteinizing hormone releasing hormone agonist given during combination chemotherapy on post-therapy fertility in male patients with lymphoma: preliminary observations. Blood 1985;65:832–836.

124. Waxman JH, Ahmed R, Smith D, et al. Failure to preserve fertility in patients with Hodgkin's disease. Cancer Chemother Pharmacol 1987;19:159–162.

125. Horstman MG, Meadows GG, Yost GS. Separate mechanisms for procarbazine spermatotoxicity and anticancer activity. Cancer Res 1987;47:1547–1550.

126. Redman JR, Bajorunas DR, Goldstein MC, et al. Semen cryopreservation and artificial insemination for Hodgkin's disease. J Clin Oncol 1987;5:233–238.

127. Scammell GE, Stedronska J, Edmonds DK, White N, Hendry WF, Jeffcoate SL. Cryopreservation of semen in men with testicular tumors or Hodgkin's disease: results of artificial insemination of their partners. Lancet 1985;2:31–32.

128. Davis OK, Graf MJ, Bedford JM. Pregnancy achieved through in vitro fertilization with cryopreserved semen from a man with Hodgkin's lymphoma. Fertil Steril 1990;53:377–378.

129. Rowland GF, Cohen J, Steptoe PC, Hewitt J. Pregnancy following in vitro fertilization using cryopreserved semen from a man with testicular teratoma. Urology 1985;26:33–36.

130. Tournaye H, Camus M, Bollen N, Wisanto A. In vitro fertilization techniques with frozen-thawed sperm: a method for preserving the progenitive potential of Hodgkin's patients. Fertil Steril 1991;55:443–445.

131. Reed E, Sanger WG, Armitage JO. Results of semen cryopreservation in young men with testicular carcinoma and lymphoma. J Clin Oncol 1986;4:537–539.

132. Rhodes EA, Hoffman DJ, Kaempfer SH. Ten years of experience with semen cryopreservation by cancer patients: follow-up and clinical considerations. Fertil Steril 1985;44:512–516.

133. Gibbons JJ, Parra RO, Andriole GL, Johnson FE. Testicular circulatory isolation: a phase I study. Surg Oncol 1992;1:413–416.

134. Jarrell J, YoungLai EV, McMahon A, Barr R, O'Connell G, Belbeck L. Effects of ionizing radiation and pretreatment with [D-Leu6,des-GlyIO] luteinizing hormone-releasing hormone ethylamide on developing rat ovarian follicles. Cancer Res 1987;47:5005–5008.

135. Chapman R, Sutcliffe SB. Protection of ovarian function by oral contraceptives in women receiving chemotherapy for Hodgkin's disease. Blood 1981; 58:849–851.

136. Sauer MV, Guidice L, Macaso TM. Pregnancy following nonsurgical donor ovum transfer to a functionally agonadal woman. Fertil Steril 1987;48:324–325.

137. Gabriel D, Bernard S, Lambert, Croom RD. Oophoropexy and the management of Hodgkin's disease. Arch Surg 1986;121:1083–1085.

138. Haie-Meder C, Mlika-Cabanne N, Michel G, et al. Radiotherapy after ovarian transposition: ovarian function and fertility preservation. Int J Radiat Oncol Biol Phys 1993;25:419–424.

139. Cooper DR, Butterfield J. Pregnancy subsequent to mastectomy for cancer of the breast. Ann Surg 1970;171:429–433.

140. Donegan WL. Breast cancer and pregnancy. Obstet Gynecol 1977;50:244–252.

141. Rissaner PM. Carcinoma of the breast during pregnancy and lactation. Br J Cancer 1968;22:663–668.

142. Li FP, Fine W, Jaffe N. Offspring of patients treated for cancer in childhood. J Natl Cancer Inst 1979; 62:1193–1197.

143. Song HZ, Wu P, Wang Y, Yang X, Dong S. Pregnancy outcomes after successful chemotherapy for choriocarcinoma and invasive mole: long term follow-up. Am J Obstet Gynecol 1988;158:538–545.

144. Holmes GE, Holmes FF. Pregnancy outcome of patients treated for Hodgkin's disease. Cancer 1978; 41:1317–1322.

145. Dexeus FH, Logothetis CJ, Chong C, Sella A, Ogden S. Genetic abnormalities in men with germ cell tumors. J Urol 1988;140:80–84.

146. Senturia YD, Peckham CS. Children fathered by men treated with chemotherapy for testicular cancer. Eur J Cancer 1990;26:429–432.

147. Byrne J, Mulvihill JJ, Myers MH, et al. Effects of treatment on fertility in long-term survivors of childhood or adolescent cancer. N Engl J Med 1987; 317:1315–1321.

148. Mulvihill JJ, McKeen EA, Rosner F, Zarrabi MH. Pregnancy outcome in cancer patients. Cancer 1987;60:1143–1150.

149. Mulvihill JJ, Connelly RR, Austin DF, et al. Cancer in offspring of long-term survivors of childhood and adolescent cancer. Lancet 1987;2:813–817.

150. Nicholson HO. Cytotoxic drugs in pregnancy. J Obstet Gynaecol Br Commonw 1968;75:307–312.

151. Jacobs C, Donaldson SC, Rosenberg SA. Management of the pregnant patient with Hodgkin's disease. Ann Intern Med 1981;95:669–675.

152. Stephens JD, Globus MS, Miller TR. Multiple congenital anomalies in a fetus exposed to 5-FU during the first trimester. Am J Obstet Gynecol 1980;137:747–749.

153. Turchi JJ, Villasis C. Anthracyclines in the treatment of malignancy in pregnancy. Cancer 1988; 61:435–440.

154. Lammer EJ, Chen DT, Hoar RM. Retinoic acid embryopathy. N Engl J Med 1985;313:837–841.

155. Blatt J, Mulvihill JJ, Ziegler JL, Young RC, Poplack DG. Pregnancy outcome following cancer chemotherapy. Am J Med 1980;69:828–832.

156. Doll DC, Ringenberg S, Yarbro JW. Management of cancer during pregnancy. Arch Intern Med 1988;148:2058–2064.

157. Garrett MJ. Teratogenic effects of combination chemotherapy (letter). Ann Intern Med 1974;80:667.

158. Reynoso EE, Shepherd FA, Messner HA, Farquarson HA, Garvey MB, Baker MA. Acute leukemia during pregnancy: the Toronto Leukemia Study Group experience with long-term follow-up of children exposed in utero to chemotherapeutic agents. J Clin Oncol 1987;5:1098–1106.

159. Schipira DS, Chudley AE. Successful pregnancy following continuous treatment with combina-

tion chemotherapy before conception and throughout pregnancy. Cancer 1984;54:800–803.

160. Nisce LZ, Tome MA, He S, Lee BJ, Kutcher GJ. Management of coexisting Hodgkin's disease and pregnancy. Am J Clin Oncol 1986;9(2):146–151.

161. Aviles A, Niz J. Long-term follow-up of children born to mothers with acute leukemia during pregnancy. Med Pediatr Oncol 1988;16:3–6.

162. Meador JM, Armentrout SA, Slater LM. Third trimester chemotherapy and neonatal hematopoiesis. Cancer Chemother Pharmacol 1987;19:177–179.

163. Li FP, Gimbrere K, Gelber RD, et al. Outcome of pregnancy in survivors of Wilms' tumor. JAMA 1987;257:216–219.

164. Andersen BL. How cancer affects sexual functioning. Oncology 1990;4:81–88.

165. Qureshi MSA, Pennington JH, Goldsmith HJ, Cox PE. Cyclophosphamide therapy and sterility. Lancet 1972;2:1290–1291.

166. Gritz ER, Wellisch DK, Wang H, Siau J, Landsverk JA, Cosgrove MD. Long-term effects of testicular cancer on sexual functioning in married couples. Cancer 1989;64:1560–1567.

167. Madorsky ML, Ashmalla MG, Schusler I. Post-prostatectomy impotence. J Urol 1976;115:401–403.

168. Maguire GP, Lee EG, Bevington DJ. Psychiatric problems in the first year after mastectomy. Br Med J 1978;1:963–965.

169. Morris T, Greer HS, White P. Psychological and social adjustment to mastectomy: a two-year follow-up study. Cancer 1977;40:2381–2387.

170. Andersen BL. Sexual functioning morbidity among cancer survivors. Cancer 1985;55:1835–1842.

171. Auchincloss SS. Sexual dysfunction in cancer patients: issues in evaluation and treatment. In: Holland JC, Rowland JH, eds. Handbook of psychooncology: psychological care of the patient with cancer. New York: Oxford University Press, 1989:383–413.

172. Rieker PP, Fitzgerald EM, Kalish L, et al. Psychosocial factors, curative therapies, and behavioral outcomes. Cancer 1989;64:2399–2407.

173. Green DM, Zevon MA, Lowrie G, Seigelstein N, Hall B. Congenital anomalies in children of patients who received chemotherapy for cancer in childhood and adolescence. N Engl J Med 1991;325:141–146.

174. Aisner J, Wiernik PH, Pearl P. Pregnancy outcome in patients treated for Hodgkin's disease. J Clin Oncol 1993;11:507–512.

43

Toxicity of Biologic Response Modifiers

Ernest C. Borden, Jeffrey Crawford, Alan Cross, Robert O. Dillman, Marc Ernstoff, Michael J. Hawkins, and Meyer Heyman

Molecular biology has brought advances to human medicine for which applications in oncology have been at the cutting edge. Early promises of immunotherapeutic approaches to human malignancy have been realized with demonstration of tumor regression as a result of administration of lymphokines produced by recombinant DNA technology. These molecules are potent modifiers of cellular function. They are active in vitro in the pM range. They have pleiotropic effects on normal, in addition to malignant, cell function. It is thus not surprising that being physiologic regulators, side effects have been observed. Side effects, such as have occurred with interleukin-2 (IL-2) and tumor necrosis factor (TNF), may limit reaching doses for optimal therapeutic efficacy. On balance, however, clinical benefits from biological response modifiers (BRMs) far outweigh toxicities.

Lymphokines, which act as BRMs, augment the host immune system by enhancing effector cell number, cytotoxicity, antigen recognition, and production of other cytokines. They may also have direct cytostatic or cytotoxic effects that may make tumor cells more susceptible to cytotoxicity of effector cells or cytotoxic agents. Cytokines that stimulate and modulate normal tissue proliferation may increase the ability of the host to tolerate damage from cytotoxic molecules. Further, monoclonal antibodies have been licensed for clinical use for both imaging and therapeutic purposes. The purpose of this review is to provide information regarding the nature and management of side effects of BRMs including interferons (IFNs), IL-2, TNF, the hematopoietic growth factors, erythropoietin (EPO), and monoclonal antibodies.

INTERFERONS

Interferons may be the most potent biologic regulators currently used in medicine for therapeutic purposes; the possible exception to this statement are glucocorticoids. Interferons for the most part, however, are safe drugs to use (1). Individual IFN types (IFN-α, IFN-β, IFN-γ) cause similar, though somewhat differing toxicities. Toxicity is, for the most part, dose related and includes effects on a wide array of organ systems (1–3).

Flulike symptoms, the most common acute toxicity, are seen in virtually all patients. Flulike symptoms begin about 4 to 6 hours following a dose and include fever, headache, chills, or rigors, myalgias, low backache, arthralgias, fatigue, and malaise. Rigors appear more frequently in patients treated with IFN-γ (4–5). Acute flulike symptoms can be partially blocked with the use of acetaminophen. Aspirin at a dose of 600 mg four times daily was found ineffective in ameliorating the myalgias, nausea, fever, and anorexia attendant upon treatment with IFN. Indomethacin is effective in the prevention of IFN-induced febrile reactions (rarely dose limiting) but like aspirin has little or no effect on the incidence of major constitutional complaints. Prednisone, by contrast, may be effective in abrogating these flulike symptoms, but its overall effect on immune response remains to be clarified. A tachyphylaxis occurs, and the severity of these acute symptoms decreases with repeated administration of the cytokine.

A small randomized study evaluating the effects of acetaminophen, indomethacin, and dexamethasone on IFN-γ suggested that prophylactic use of acetaminophen for IFN-induced malaise appeared as good as the other agents. Patients may continue to have malaise, chills, fever, headache, myalgias, and arthralgias during continuous treatment schedules with IFN-γ. Chronically, patients may continue to have low-grade temperature elevations and with the decrease in appetite associated with IFN-γ develop subclinical dehydration that contributes to the malaise. Vigorous fluid intake by mouth usually improves the tolerance of the agent. Occasionally, intravenous hydration as an outpatient may be warranted.

Gastrointestinal symptoms are seen in as high as 50% of individuals. The most common complaint is anorexia. Stomatitis is unusual. Slight elevation in liver transaminases is common, but frank hepatitis and liver failure are rare. Although hyperbilirubinemia has been reported, it is uncommon, and the physician should consider other causes.

Fatigue may reflect a central nervous system toxicity and is common, particularly in older patients. It may be disabling with IFN-α, but is less severe with IFN-β (6). Slight confusion and minimal-to-severe depression, including stupor and coma, may occasionally occur. These effects are reversible, but stupor and coma may take as long as 3 to 4 weeks to recover. Generalized diffuse slowing on the EEG is seen in these patients. Patients can also complain of irritability, loss of libido, insomnia, and an overall increase in anxiety. Visual abnormalities include blurred vision, dry eyes, photophobia, and, rarely, retinal hemorrhages. Peripheral neuropathy is also uncommon. Recurrence of migraine headaches has been reported as well.

The most common cardiac toxicity is sinus tachycardia. More serious cardiovascular toxicity (<50% of patients) includes supraventricular tachyarrhythmias, which may be controlled with β-blockers or calcium channel blockers. Ventricular arrhythmias are uncommon. Cardiac toxicity is usually seen at dosages of over 10 Mu/day in older patients (>70 years) and in patients with underlying heart disease.

Hematologic abnormalities commonly occur with IFNs and are usually characterized by leukoneutropenia. It is uncommon to see infectious complications from the fall in white blood cell count. Bone marrow evaluations in patients being treated with IFN-α have shown the bone marrow to be cellular, with an apparent block in maturation. There is a decrease in colony forming units of the granulocyte and granulocyte-macrophage lineage. In general, white blood cell counts return within a few days to 1 week. Nadir white blood cell counts can be seen as early as 4 days or as late as 2 weeks following the start of continuous-dose treatments. Thrombocytopenia occasionally occurs, particularly in those patients with impaired marrow function.

Renal abnormalities are rare and have included an increase in protein excretion and the development of partially reversible nephrotic syndrome and renal failure. Other metabolic abnormalities associated with high-dose IFN-α treatment have included hypocalcemia, hyperkalemia, and transient elevations in creatinine and urea nitrogen.

Skin reactions include dryness and pruritis. As with other cytokines, patients can be taught to self-administer subcutaneous injections similar to the use of insulin. Local reactions at the injection site are unusual with IFN-α, but can be mild (erythema) to severe (local necrosis) with IFN-β. Hair thinning is also seen, but frank alopecia is exceedingly rare.

No therapeutic interventions have been identified that will circumvent the chronic toxicities. If severe or disabling, IFN doses should be withheld (sometimes for 2 to 3 weeks), with resumption at a 50% dose reduction.

INTERLEUKIN 2

IL-2 used at high doses is the only agent currently approved by the FDA for the treatment of patients with advanced renal cell carcinoma. Intravenous administration of high doses of IL-2 results in a marked reduction of peripheral vascular resistance and clinically significant hypotension. With repeated administration, capillary permeability increases and requires aggressive use of fluids to prevent hypotension. Because of these toxicities, treatment with high-dose IL-2 requires in-hospital monitoring, usually in an intensive care unit. Hence, high-dose IL-2 is generally offered only to fully ambulatory patients with completely normal cardiac, renal and pulmonary function.

Three reviews have discussed in detail toxicities and the management of patients treated with high doses of IL-2 (7–9). Patients with atherosclerotic cardiovascular disease or who were heavy smokers were usually not considered candidates for high-dose IL-2. The primary physiologic event following bolus intravenous-injection IL-2 is decreased peripheral vascular resistance within 2 to 4 hours of drug administration, resulting in hypotension and increased cardiac output. Because capillary permeability increases during treatment with IL-2, intravenous fluids are used judiciously even at the beginning of therapy, and pressors such as dopamine and/or phenylephrine are often required. As the IL-2 effects reverse and the blood pressure stabilizes, the pressor infusion rate is gradually decreased. If, at the time of the next injection the need for pressors is low, the next dose of IL-2 is given. If, however, pressor usage is already close to maximal, the next dose of IL-2 is held.

The clinical changes that occur in patients over 5 days of high dose IL-2 treatment have followed a typical pattern. Pulmonary infiltrates and blood oxygen desaturation develop secondary to increased capillary permeability and increase in reliance on pressors (instead of fluid) to support the blood pressure. Hypotension and decreased intravascular volume reduce renal blood flow and glomerular filtration, resulting in prerenal azotemia. Treatment is discontinued when pressor support is maximal and decreasing renal (cr $\geq$ 4.5 mg/dL) and pulmonary function (O_2 saturation with 2 L nasal $O_2 \leq 90\%$) prevent continued fluid administration. Low-dose dopamine was administered in some patients to increase renal blood flow, but this approach has not been studied in a systematic manner. Upon discontinuation of IL-2, the physiologic changes associated with IL-2 administration rapidly reverse. However, despite stopping IL-2, some patients with pulmonary infiltrates develop a more severe form of lung damage that resemble adult respiratory distress syndrome and require more prolonged hospitalization.

Hematologic toxicity includes anemia, lymphopenia with rebound lymphocytosis, eosinophilia, and thrombocytopenia and has not been overly problematic. Although granulocytopenia occurs only occasionally and is usually mild and transient, 10 to 30% of patients treated with IL-2 develop bacterial infections, most commonly from *Staphylococcus aureus* and *Staphylococcus epidermidis*. While the possible reasons for a high incidence of sepsis in patients receiving an intensive treatment regimen are numerous, a contributing factor may be an IL-2-induced defect in granulocyte chemotaxis and Fc receptor expression. Many of the IL-2 treatment-related deaths occurred in patients who became septic toward the end of their treatment. Randomized trials have since documented the benefit of prophylactic antibiotics in preventing sepsis during administration of IL-2 (10).

Other IL-2 toxicities have typically not been life threatening. Fever and chills have been almost universal, occurring 2 to 4 hours after the dose and usually controlled with acetaminophen and NSAIDs, although cases of malignant hypothermia have been reported. With repeated dosing fatigue, myalgias, and anthralgias have become more pronounced and may reduce compliance with chronic-dosing regimens. Gastrointestinal toxicity manifested by nausea, vomiting, diarrhea, and/or mucositis have occurred frequently in patients receiving high-dose IL-2. More severe complications such as bowel hemorrhage, infarction, and perforation have also been reported but much less frequently. Concomitant administration of NSAIDs may have predisposed patients to gastritis and peptic ulcer disease. Hyperbilirubinemia, typically ranging between 2 to 7 mg/dL, occurs commonly and is due to intrahepatic cholestasis. Modest elevations of hepatic transaminases and alkaline phosphatase and minor evidence of liver dysfunction (elevated prothrombin time and decreased serum albumin) occur in conjunction with the hyperbilirubinemia. However, all evidence of liver dysfunction typically resolves within several days of stopping high-dose IL-2 and there has been no convincing evidence for hepatic necrosis or permanent damage.

Not surprisingly, diseases possibly mediated by immunologic processes, including thyroiditis, psoriasis, polymyositis/dermatomyositis, erythema nodosum, and a fatal case of pemphigus vulgaris, have been reported to occur or be exacerbated in patients being treated with IL-2. Macular erythematous rashes, most prominent on the head and neck and associated with burning and pruritis, occur commonly and at times progress to generalized erythroderma and desquamation.

Neurologic complications of high-dose IL-2 include agitation, paranoia, somnolence, hallucinations, seizures, and occasionally coma. Severe mental changes have occurred and, unlike other toxicities, often progress for a few days after stopping IL-2. Therefore, IL-2 should be discontinued at the first sign of neurologic toxicity and not resumed until mentation has returned to the patient's pretreatment baseline.

Patients with intolerable toxicity should not receive further treatment with high-dose IL-2 unless there is clear demonstration of a significant antitumor effect. In the absence of such evidence patients are generally not considered for further therapy if the following toxicities were encountered:

Cardiovascular: Sustained ventricular tachycardia ($\geq$ 5 beats); cardiac rhythm disturbances not controlled or unresponsive to management; recurrent chest pain with ECG changes, documented angina or myocardial infarction; or pericardial tamponade

Central nervous system: Coma or toxic psychosis lasting more than 48 hours

Gastrointestinal: Bowel ischemia, perforation, or GI bleeding requiring surgery

Pulmonary: Any condition requiring intubation for longer than 72 hours after stopping IL-2 (e.g., ARDS, respiratory failure, obstruction)

Renal: Renal dysfunction requiring dialysis for longer than 72 hours after stopping IL-2

Side effects from IL-2 are dose related. Lower subcutaneous doses are being investigated and are better tolerated. The constellation of side effects from subcutaneous administration are qualitatively similar to that of high-dose intravenous administration, but quantitatively much less severe. Local injection-site erythema may occur.

TUMOR NECROSIS FACTOR

Over a century ago, William Coley observed that tumors regressed following the injection of cultures of bacteria into patients with cancer. These efforts were not continued because of the toxicities of the regimen as well as the inconsistent response of these tumors. Subsequent availability as a purified recombinant protein led to the re-evaluation of tumor necrosis factor as a treatment for cancer. Preclinical data suggest that recombinant TNF-α has antitumor activity when injected directly into tumors or when given systemically. The antitumor effect of this cytokine may in part be related not so much to its direct toxicity to neoplasms, but rather, to endothelial activation and vascular damage resulting in hemorrhagic necrosis of the tumor, which is rich in new vascular supply. TNF-α may also recruit and activate neutrophils that participate in the inflammatory response, leading to necrosis of the tumor, perhaps through the release of granular enzymes such as elastase as well as the elaboration of reactive oxygen intermediates.

TNF-α has been administered to human volunteers both as part of phase I studies for possible cancer immunotherapy and to study the physiologic effects of TNF in man. In phase I-II trials for use in patients with cancer, TNF-α was tolerated at doses of up to 50 to 200 μ/m^2 (11–13). When further studies were initiated to assess the efficacy of TNF-α, however, large doses were required for a measurable antitumor effect, and these doses approached lethal levels when given systemically. Significant side effects observed were severe hypotension, thromboembolic pneumonia, cardiopulmonary dysfunction, and central nervous system impairment. In one study, severe hypophosphatemia was noted that resulted in significant, right-sided myocardial dysfunction after a dose of 175 $\mu g/m^2/day$ for 5 days. Many of these adverse effects were similar to the clinical events associated with sepsis, which given the important role of TNF-α in sepsis, was not unanticipated.

Experimental studies have found it possible to separate the antitumor and toxic properties of TNF (14). Given the rather narrow therapeutic/toxic ratio of TNF, other strategies that combine TNF with other modalities have been initiated. With the recognition that high levels of TNF-α are required locally around the tumor for a prolonged period of time for consistent antitumor effect, regional rather than systemic therapy is being investigated to minimize toxicity and to maximize the exposure of the tumor to TNF-α. In one study of 22 patients with chemotherapy-resistant metastases to the liver, TNF-α was given at doses up to 150 $\mu g/m^2/day$ by continuous 5-day infusion through hepatic arterial catheters. A clinical antitumor effect was noted in 2 of 14 patients, and in 7 of 14 patients decreases in carcinoembryonic antigen levels of more than 25% were observed (15). More commonly, TNF-α has been administered via isolation perfusion of the limbs of patients with melanoma or sarcoma. Since the initial patient had severe hypotension and renal failure despite its local administration, subsequent patients receive a continuous infusion of dopamine at the outset of the isolated limb perfusion and for 72 hours. With this prophylaxis as well as hyperhydration, the high doses of TNF-α used in this study were administered with acceptable toxicity (16).

HEMATOPOIETIC GROWTH FACTORS G-CSF AND GM-CSE

Hematopoietic growth factors can profoundly influence hematopoiesis that has been altered either by disease or chemotherapy. G-CSF is a relatively lineage-specific molecule that stimulates the proliferation and differentiation of myeloid precursors to become neutrophils and also enhances the function of these neutrophils. In addition, G-CSF promotes the release of progenitor cells from the bone marrow into the peripheral circulation. While GM-CSF shares some of the effects that G-CSF has on later stages of neutrophil differentiation, it does not appear to have the same effects on early myeloid stem cells that G-CSF has. On the other hand, GM-CSF does have clear multilineage effects at the level of the multipotential progenitor cells, and it can enhance the development of erythroid progenitors and megakaryocyte progenitors. Furthermore, GM-CSF has effects on the more mature granulocyte-marophage progenitors to lead to enhanced production of both eosinophils and monocytes. Despite these differences in biology, both cytokines have had their major clinical use in the treatment or prophylaxis of neutropenic states (17–21).

While CSFs have been used in the management of neutropenia secondary to bone marrow failure or myelodysplastic syndromes, the response has been variable, and the clinical benefits from long-term use in this patient population are unclear. The largest experience within clinical trials and in clinical practice with the CSFs involves the administration of CSFs to aid in hematopoietic reconstitution following myelosuppressive treatments.

Existing clinical data suggest that starting G- or GM-CSF between 24 and 72 hours after chemotherapy may provide optimal neutrophil recovery. While continuing the CSF until the postnadir neutrophil recovery exceeds 10,000 cells/mm^3 has been shown to be safe and effective, a shorter duration of administration sufficient to achieve adequate clinical neutrophil recovery may be a reasonable alternative and may result in a modest shortening in the duration of treatment and significant cost savings. The guidelines for dosing suggest that G-CSF should be dosed at 5 μg/kg/day and GM-CSF at 250 μg/m^2/day. While both of these agents can be administered subcutaneously or intravenously, subcutaneous administration is generally preferable. In addition, available data suggest that rounding the dose to the nearest vial size may enhance both patient convenience and reduce costs. The use of higher doses of CSFs is not generally warranted, although data are emerging with mobilization of progenitor cells suggesting that a higher dose of 10 μg/kg of G-CSF is more effective (19).

The predominant side effect associated with the administration of G-CSF has been medullary bone pain. The incidence varies between 15 and 40% of patients and seems to be higher at higher doses of G-CSF. The onset of pain can be at any point during treatment, but it most commonly occurs prior to the onset of neutrophil recovery. Infrequent side effects include exacerbations of preexisting inflammatory conditions, particularly eczema, psoriasis, and other dermatitis, rare allergic reactions, and the development of acute neutrophilic dermatosis (Sweet syndrome). Injection-site reactions or fever related to G-CSF are quite rare. Therefore, in a febrile patient receiving G-CSF, one should consider other causes of fever, particularly infection. In the pediatric population with chronic continuous administration, alopecia and splenomegaly have been described (21).

Toxicities for GM-CSF include injection-site reactions, rash, fever, edema, fatigue, paresthesias, anorexia, diarrhea, and bone pain. In early trials using higher doses, additional cardiac effects were seen, including pericarditis, atrial fibrillation, pleural effusion, thrombotic events, and the capillary leak syndrome. Furthermore, a first-dose reaction has been described consisting of transient flushing, tachycardia, hypotension, musculoskeletal pain, dyspnea, nausea, rigors, and leg spasms. All of these side effects have been less commonly described when GM-CSF has been used at lower more conventional CSF doses and may be less common with the glycosylated form of GM-CSF, currently in clinical use.

Although it would appear from the literature that GM-CSF has a broader range of toxicities than G-CSF, it is not clear whether the side effects of G- or GM-CSF differ markedly when administered at conventional doses, because of a lack of comparative trials (17–21). The most common clinical distinction between the two remains the higher incidence of grade I or II fever with GM-CSF. Guidelines about the equivalency of the available recombinant preparations of G-CSF and GM-CSF cannot be proposed at this time because of the lack of large-scale perspective comparative trials evaluating both the toxicities and the relative efficacies of these two CSFs. Until these such studies are performed, the ASCO Ad Hoc Colony Stimulating Factor Guideline Expert Panel recommends that each cytokine be used for the specific indication based on the strength of evidence available from individual clinical trials (17).

ERYTHROPOIETIN

Rigorous trials have demonstrated the efficacy of EPO in increasing hematocrit and decreasing transfusion requirements in patients with renal failure on chronic dialysis, solid tumors, and hematologic malignancies. EPO has been administered with very few adverse effects to patients with many different types of malignancies (22–25). Although, as expected, peak plasma levels are higher following intravenous injections, lower but more sustained levels are obtained with subcutaneous injection because of slow continuous absorption from the injection sites, resulting in a relatively greater degree of erythroid stimulation (23).

The use of EPO in dialysis-dependent renal failure has been associated with the development of hypertension in approximately one-third of treated individuals (22, 23). Indeed, 3 to 5% of patients with chronic renal failure treated with EPO have developed hypertensive encephalopathy and seizures. Most of these episodes, however, occurred early in treatment, during periods of rapid hemodynamic change. Decreasing the dose or discontinuing EPO with vigorous antihypertensive therapy decreases the risk of hypertensive crisis. The pathophysiology of EPO-induced hypertension has been the subject of recent reviews (22–26). Although the precise cause of EPO-induced hypertension in patients with chronic renal failure has not been clarified, the frequent development of hypertension appears to be unique to patients with chronic renal failure, since hypertension has rarely been seen in other populations treated with EPO, including normal volunteers, patients with AIDS, those with rheumatoid arthritis, autologous blood donors, or cancer patients (23, 26, 27, 28). However, particular attention should be paid to those cancer patients with preexisting hypertension and renal insufficiency, who may be at increased risk for precipitous increase in blood pressure coincident with the rise in hematocrit.

Although disturbances of the coagulation and fibrinolytic pathway have been reported in individual patients receiving EPO, no consistent or reproducible pattern has been described (26). Moreover, there has been no evidence of any increased incidence of small or large vessel thrombosis, such as stroke, myocardial infarction, or peripheral arterial thrombosis in EPO-treated patients, including those with underlying diabetes mellitus (26). Although anecdotal reports of deep vein and vascular access thrombosis have been described in patients with cancer receiving EPO, only a total of eight incidents of thrombosis were seen among 153 patients in a randomized trial of EPO in cancer patients receiving chemotherapy. These events were evenly distributed between the EPO and placebo groups. Thus, there is little evidence that EPO produces a significant thrombotic risk either in patients on chronic hemodialysis or those with malignancy who are receiving chemotherapy. The routine use of aspirin or other prophylactic anticoagulation in cancer patients who are to receive EPO is, therefore unwarranted and potentially dangerous, considering the frequent coexistence of thrombocytopenia and abnormal tumor vasculature.

Approximately 5% of patients with chronic renal failure who receive EPO intravenously develop a flulike syndrome consisting of low-grade fever, myalgia, bone pain, and diaphoresis beginning 2 hours after administration and persisting for approximately 12 hours. The administration of antiinflammatory drugs has resulted in remission of these symptoms after 2 weeks of treatment. The incidence of this flulike illness among patients with AIDS, chronic inflammatory disorders (rheumatoid arthritis), and cancer has not been specifically reported, but appears not to be a major obstacle to therapy in these groups of patients receiving EPO (22, 29).

Approximately one-third of patients with chronic renal failure who have received erythropoietin subcutaneously have reported pain at the injection site. This has been attributed to the acid pH (6.9) of the EPO solution, to which citric acid has been added as a preservative. Amelioration of this pain by adding lidocaine to the diluent used with the EPO has recently been reported (30).

Rare patients will become sensitized to the serum albumin used in the diluent and develop IgE serum antibodies or a rash at the injection site. Since the molecular structure of the recombinant product is identical to the naturally occurring hormone, no IgG antibody has been detected either in patients or normal volunteers receiving EPO. Unlike G-CSF and GM-CSF, which may induce proliferation of leukemic blasts, no tumors have been described that bear EPO receptors, with the exception of the blasts of erythroleukemia. Moreover, there has been no in vitro evidence of stimulation of solid tumor growth by EPO (27).

MONOCLONAL ANTIBODIES

The toxicities and side effects associated with monoclonal antibody administration may be categorized as allergic or nonallergic. Adverse events have included fever, rigors/chills, sweats, maculopapular erythematous rash, urticaria, pruritis, edema, hypotension, headache, nausea, vomiting, diarrhea, fatigue, elevated hepatic transaminases, throat tightness, pain, thrombocytopenia, dyspnea, bronchospasm, anaphylactic shock, and even death. However, adverse events vary greatly, depending on the nature of the antibody (mouse or human), the distribution of the target antigen on normal tissues, and whether or not the antibody reacts with circulating cells (31).

Allergic reactions may be classified as acute or delayed. Because most of the initial monoclonal antibodies were mouse proteins, there was great concern that infusion of the these products would be associated with acute anaphylactoid reactions. Fortunately, such complications have been uncommon and have been extremely rare with human or humanized antibodies, such as chimeric antibodies that contain mostly human constant immunoglobulin and only mouse variable-region protein or only the idiotypic determinants of a selected mouse antibody (31, 32). Patients with a known history of allergic reaction to rodents or their byproducts have typically been excluded from trials of mouse antibodies. Acute allergic reactions have included anaphylactic shock, less severe anaphylactoid reactions such as bronchospasm, dyspnea, and tachycardia, and generalized pruritis and urticaria. The more severe reactions can be successfully managed with epinephrine. The dermatologic symptoms may be seen as part of a full anaphylactic reaction with laryngeal edema, hypotension, and bronchospasm, or alone. Pruritus and urticaria alone typically resolve without treatment, but may be responsive to diphenhydramine or epinephrine. Premedication with steroids and/or diphenhydramine does not appreciably affect the frequency of the side effects. Fever, sweats, chills, nausea, and prostration may be a manifestation of a mild acute allergic reaction, but this complex of symptoms is much more commonly associated with a direct antibody/antigen reaction with circulating cells, as discussed below.

Because of the anticipated production of human antimouse antibodies (HAMA) in response to murine antibody immunoglobulin exposure, there was concern that delayed reactions such as serum sickness would be a significant problem following infusion of murine monoclonal antibodies. Furtunately, immune-complex complications related to HAMA have been uncommon (31). Classic serum sickness has been seen 2 to 3 weeks following exposure to moderate and high doses of murine antibodies. A typical symptom complex includes fever, malaise, arthralgias/arthritis, myalgias, maculopapular erythematous rash, and fatigue. Proteinuria has been rarely observed in these few patients, and renal insufficiency is extremely rare. Serum sickness can be managed with nonsteroidal antiinflammatory agents, and corticosteroids in more severe cases.

The most antibody-specific adverse events associated with infusions of monoclonal antibodies are related to antibody binding to the target antigen. These include direct effects on tumor and nontumor cells that express the antigen and indirect effects mediated by the secondary release of various cytokines as a result of antibody binding to the target antigen or formation of immune complexes with circulating soluble agents (33). The most predictable symptom complex has been seen in association with monoclonal antibody binding to circulating cells, especially B or T lymphocytes, granulocytes, or leukemia cells. The typical symptom complex includes fever, chills, sweats, prostration, nausea, and sometimes dyspnea and hypotension, which occur within a matter of hours after the antibody is initiated. Studies with radiolabeled cells have shown that once antibody binds to circulating cells, they are removed in the reticuloendothelial system, including the lung, liver, and spleen. When large numbers of cells are removed in the lungs, this may be associated with dyspnea and hypotension. For this reason, when it is known that an antibody will react with circulating cells, the initial infusion rate is slow, and high-dose bolus administration is avoided. Many of the symptoms related to the removal of circulating target cells are probably secondary to the release of various cytokines such as interleukins and interferons. Nearly all patients who have received antilymphocyte and/or antigranulocyte antibodies have experienced such side effects if they had levels of circulating target cells at the time of infusion, and no high titers of endogenous antimouse antibodies to block the effect. The presence of antimouse antibodies actually prevents many of these side effects by altering the pharmacology and bioavailability of the monoclonal antibody, which limits binding to the target antigen. Corticosteroids typically will prevent such reactions, but acetaminophen and diphenhydramine have little prophylactic benefit.

Adverse events may also be seen because of direct effects on noncancerous tissue that also expresses the target antigen. This has been especially true for antibodies that cross-react with adenocarcinomas and cells of the gastrointestinal tract (34). Such antibodies have been associated with a high frequency of diarrhea, nausea and vomiting, abdominal pain, and even large and/ or small bowel mucosal damage in some patients. Other antibodies that are known to cross-react with antigens on neural tissue have been associated with specific pain syndromes in some patients. Cross-reactivity with normal tissue antigens is particularly a concern when antibodies are conjugated to cytotoxic substances such as radioisotopes, chemotherapy agents, or natural toxins. The incidence of gastrointestinal toxicity is greater when antibodies are conjugated to a cytotoxic agent than with administration of the naked antibody. Another adenocarcinoma antibody that cross-reacts with antigens on neural sheaths produced unacceptable neurotoxicity when conjugated to the A chain of the natural toxin, ricin.

In some instances, monoclonal antibodies are given to patients who are known to have free or soluble circulating antigen. Examples include the circulating idiotype in lymphoma, carcinoembryonic antigen (CEA), or prostrate-specific antigen (PSA). Only rarely have symptoms have been noted in the presence of the immune complexes formed by the binding of antibody to circulating antigen, probably because of the small size of such complexes, since the monoclonal antibody binds to only one determinant on the circulating antigen. For this reason, the presence of circulating antigen is not a contraindication to antibody treatment, although the binding to soluble antigen greatly alters the pharmacokinetics of the antibody. However, acute arthralgias, myalgias, nerve palsies, fever, and rashes have occasionally been seen in this setting and attributed to the acute immune complex formation.

One adverse event that theoretically could be a problem with a cytotoxic antibody preparation is that of tumor lysis syndrome. This has not been described with any of the antibody preparations tested to date, and therefore prehydration, mannitol, and allopurinol prophylaxis are not routinely administered.

CONCLUSION

As summarized in this chapter, BRMs affect a wide array of organ systems. Applications in toxicities from administration of biologicals are, for the most part, a direct function of dose and schedule. The mechanisms of antitumor action differ from those of other treatment modalities. The potential for benefits from combined modality approaches thus are substantial. Combining BRMs concomitantly with other therapies will yield a different spectrum of side effects. The next decade should witness continued expansion of clinical application of BRMs not only in malignancies, but also in other human disease syndromes. Understanding mechanisms underlying not only therapeutic action but also side effects should markedly enhance clinical applications.

REFERENCES

1. Quesada JR, Talpez M, Rios A, et al. Clinical toxicity of interferons in cancer patients: a review. J Clin Oncol 1986;4:234–243.
2. Borden EC. Interferons. In: Cancer medicine. 4th ed. James Holland, ed. Baltimore: Williams & Wilkins, 1996, in press.
3. Goldstein D, Laszlo J. Interferon therapy in cancer: from imagination to interferon. Cancer Res 1986; 46:4315–4329.
4. Ernstoff MS, Trautman T, Kirkwood JM, Davis CA, Reich S. et al. A randomized phase I/II study of continuous versus bolus infusion of recombinant interferon gamma in patients with metastatic melanoma. J Clin Oncol 1987;5:1804–1810.
5. Schiller JH, Storer B, Paulnock DM, Brown RR, Datta SP, et al. A direct comparison of biological response modulation and clinical side effects by interferon-beta ser, interferon-gamma, or the combination of interferons beta ser and gamma in humans. J Clin Invest 1990;86:1211–1221.
6. Carlin JM, Borden EC, Sondel PM, Byrne GI. Interferon-induced indoleamine 2,3-dioxygenase activity in human mononuclear phagocytes. J Leukocyte Biol 1989;45:29–34.
7. Lee RE, Lotze MT, Skibber JM, et al. Cardiorespiratory effects of immunotherapy with interleukin-2. J Clin Oncol 1989;7:7–20.
8. Margolin KA, Rayner AA, Hawkins MJ, et al. Interleukin-2 and lymphokine-activated killer cell therapy of solid tumors: analysis of toxicity and management guidelines. J Clin Oncol 1989;7:486–498.
9. Siegel JP, Puri RK. Interleukin-2 toxicity. J Clin Oncol 1991;9:694–704.
10. Bock SN, Lee RE, Fisher B, et al. A prospective randomized trial evaluating prophylactic antibiotics to prevent triple-lumen catheter-related sepsis in patients treated with immunotherapy. J Clin Oncol 1990;8:161–169.
11. Budd GT, Green S, Baker LH, Hersh EP, Weick

JK, Osborne CK. A Southwest Oncology Group phase II trial of recombinant tumor necrosis factor in metastatic breast cancer. Cancer 1991;68:1694–1695.

12. Van der Poll T, Buller HR, ten Cate JW. Effect of tumor necrosis factor in normal subjects. N Engl J Med 1990;323:1350–1351.

13. del Giglio A, Zukiwski AA, Ali MK, Mavligit GM. Severe symptomatic dose-limiting hypophosphatemia induced by hepatic arterial infusion of recombinant tumor necrosis factor in patients with liver metastases. Cancer 1991;67:2459–2461.

14. Takahashi N, Brouckaert P, Fiers W. Induction of tolerance allows separation of lethal and antitumor activities of tumor necrosis factor in mice. Cancer Res 1991;51:2366–2372.

15. Mavligit GM, Zukiwski AA, Charnsangavej C, Carrasco CH, Wallace S, Gutterman JU. Regional biologic therapy: hepatic arterial infusion of recombinant human tumor necrosis factor in patients with liver metastases. Cancer 1992;69:557–561.

16. Lienard D, Ewalenko P, Delmotte J, Renard N, Lejeune FJ. High dose recombinant tumor necrosis factor alpha in combination with interferon gamma and melphalan in isolation perfusion of the limbs for melanoma and sarcoma. J Clin Oncol 1992;10(1):52–60.

17. American Society of Clinical Oncology. American Society of Clinical Oncology recommendations for the use of hematopoietic colony-stimulating factors: evidence based clincal practical guidelines. J Clin Oncol 1994;12:2471–2508.

18. Crawford J, Ozer H, Stoller R, et al. Reduction by granulocyte colony-stimulating factor of fever and neutropenia induced by chemotherapy in patients with small cell lung cancer (rmetHuG-CSF). N Engl J Med 1991;325:164–170.

19. Lee ME, Crawford J. Delivery of high dose chemotherapy with recombinant human granulocyte colony stimulating factor support. In: Armitage JO, Antman KH, eds. High dose cancer therapy. 2nd ed. Baltimore: Williams & Wilkins, 1995:342–371.

20. Scheding S, Brugger W, Mertelsmann RH, Kanz L. Granulocyte-macrophage colony stimulating factor. In: Armitage JO, Antman KH, eds. High dose cancer therapy. 2nd ed. Baltimore: Williams & Wilkins, 1995:319–341.

21. Petros WP, Peters WP. Colony stimulating factors. In: Chabner B, Longo D, eds. Cancer chemotherapy. 2nd ed. Philadelphia: Lippincott-Raven Press, 1995:639–654.

22. Gimenez LF, Scheel PH. Clinical application of recombinant erythropoietin in renal dialysis patients. Hematol Oncol Clin North Am 1994;8(5):913–926.

23. Erslev AJ. Erythropoietin. N Engl J Med 1991; 324(19):1339–1344.

24. Case DC, Bukowski RM, Carey RW, et al. Recombinant human erythropoietin therapy for anemic cancer patients on combination chemotherapy. J Natl Cancer Inst 1993;85:801–806.

25. Henry DH, Abels RI. Recombinant human erythropoietin in the treatment of cancer and chemotherapy induced anemia: results of double-blind and open label follow-up studies. Semin Oncol 1994; 21(2):21–28.

26. Singbartl G. Adverse events of erythropoietin in long-term and in acute/short term treatment. Clin Invest 1994;72:S36–S43.

27. Miller CB. The use of erythropoietin in cancer patients. Hematol Oncol Ann 1994;2(4):288–296.

28. Henry DH. Clinical application of recombinant erythropoietin in anemic cancer patients. Hematol Oncol Clin North Am 1994;8(5):961–973.

29. Means RT Jr. Clinical application of recombinant erythropoietin in the anemnia of chronic disease. Hematol Oncol Clin North Am 1994;8(5):933–944.

30. Alon US, Allen S, Rameriz Z, et al. Lidocaine for the alleviation of pain associated with subcutaneous erythropoietin injection. J Am Soc Nephrol 1994; 5:1161–1162.

31. Dillman RO, Beauregard JC, Jamieson M, Amox D, Halpert SE. Toxicities associated with monoclonal antibody infusions in cancer patients. Mol Biother 1988;1:81–85.

32. Maloney DG, Liles TM, Czerwinski DK, Waldichuk C, Rosenberg J, Grillo-Lopez A, Levy R. Phase I clinical trial using escalating single-dose infusion of chimeric anti-CD20 monoclonal antibody (IDEC-C2B8) in patients with recurrent B cell lymphoma. Blood 1994;84:2457–2466.

33. Vadhan-Raj S, Cordon-Cardo C, Carswell E, Mintzer D, Dantis L, et al. Phase I trial of a mouse monoclonal antibody against GD3 ganglioside in patients with melanoma: induction of inflammatory responses at tumor sites. J Clin Oncol 1988;10:1636–1648.

34. Mellstedt H, Frodin JE, Masucci G, Ragnhammar P, Fagerberg J, et al. The therapeutic use of monoclonal antibodies in colorectal carcinoma. Semin Oncol 1991;18:462–477.

Section Four

Combination Chemotherapy Programs

44

Chemotherapy Programs

Victoria J. Dorr, Debra Morris, and Mary Lorber

This chapter is to provide a reference for the chemotherapy programs cited elsewhere in this text and currently in use. Also included are references considered to be of either historic importance or of potential importance as second-line chemotherapy. No attempt has been made to be encyclopedic, and the choice of regimens must, therefore, be considered arbitrary. The reader is cautioned to review the cited articles to confirm doses and schedules and for specifics regarding patient selection, dose adjustments, and other modifications.

BREAST CARCINOMA

AC (Adjuvant)

Doxorubicin (Adriamycin)	60 mg/m^2 i.v. day 1
Cyclophosphamide	600 mg/m^2 i.v. day 1
*Repeat every 21 days for 4 cycles	

Source: Fisher B, Brown AM, Dimitrov NV, et al. Two months of Adriamycin-cyclophosphamide with and without interval reinduction therapy compared with six months of cyclophosphamide, methotrexate and 5-fluorouracil in positive-node breast cancer patients with tamoxifen-nonresponsive tumors: results from NSABP B-15. J Clin Oncol 1990;8:1483–1496.

Or

Doxorubicin (Adriamycin)	30 mg/m^2 i.v. day 1
Cyclophosphamide	150 mg/m^2 p.o. days 3–6
*Repeat every 21 days	

Source: Brooks RJ, Jones SE, Salmon SE, et al. Adjuvant chemotherapy of axillary node-negative carcinoma of the breast using doxorubicin and cyclophosphamide. NCI Monogr 1986;1:135–137.

CAF (Adjuvant or Metastatic)

Cyclophosphamide	500 mg/m^2 i.v. day 1
Doxorubicin (Adriamycin)	50 mg/m^2 i.v. day 1
5-Fluorouracil	500 mg/m^2 i.v. day 1
*Repeat cycle every 21 days	

Source: Smalley RV, Carpenter J, Bartolucci A, Vogel C, Krauss S. A comparison of cyclophosphamide, Adriamycin, 5-fluorouracil (CAF) and cyclophosphamide, methotrexate, 5-fluorouracil, vincristine, prednisone (CMFVP) in patients with metastatic breast cancer: a Southeastern Cancer Study Group project. Cancer 1977;40(2):625–632.

Or

Cyclophosphamide	100 mg/m^2/day p.o. days 1–14
Doxorubicin (Adriamycin)	30 mg/m^2 i.v. days 1 and 8
5-Fluorouracil	500 mg/m^2 i.v. days 1 and 8
*Repeat every 28 days	

Source: Aisner J, Weinberg V, Perloff M, et al. Chemotherapy versus chemoimmunotherapy (CAF v CAFVP v CMF ± MER) for metastatic carcinoma of the breast: a CALGB study. J Clin Oncol 1987;5:1523–1533.

CFP (Adjuvant)

Cyclophosphamide	150 mg/m²/day i.v. days 1–5
5-Fluorouracil	300 mg/m²/day i.v. days 1–5
Prednisone	10 mg/m²/day p.o. days 1–7

*Repeat every 28 days

Source: Ingle JN, Everson LK, Wieand HS, et al. Randomized trial to evaluate the addition of tamoxifen to cyclophosphamide, 5-fluorouracil, prednisone adjuvant therapy in premenopausal women with node-positive breast cancer. Cancer 1989;63:1257–1264.

CMF (Adjuvant or Metastatic)

Below age 60:

Cyclophosphamide	100 mg/m²/day p.o. days 1–14
Methotrexate	40 mg/m² i.v. days 1 and 8
5-Fluorouracil	600 mg/m² i.v. days 1 and 8

Above age 60:

Cyclophosphamide	100 mg/m²/day p.o. days 1–14
Methotrexate	30 mg/m² i.v. days 1 and 8
5-Fluorouracil	400 mg/m² i.v. days 1 and 8

*Repeat every 28 days for 6 cycles

Source: Bonadonna G, Brusamolino E, Valagussa P, et al. Combination chemotherapy as an adjuvant treatment in operable breast cancer. N Engl J Med 1976;294:405–410.

CMFP (Adjuvant and Metastatic)

Cyclophosphamide	100 mg/m² p.o. days 1–14
Methotrexate	40 mg/m² i.v. days 1 and 8
5-Fluorouracil	600 mg/m² i.v. days 1 and 8
Prednisone	20 mg p.o. q.i.d. days 1–7

*Repeat every 28 days

Note: For women over age 65 the following substitutions are recommended:

Methotrexate	30 mg/m² i.v. day 1, 8
5-Fluorouracil	400 mg/m² i.v. day 1, 8

Source: Marschke RF Jr, Ingle JN, Schaid DJ, et al. Randomized clinical trial of CFP versus CMFP in women with metastatic breast cancer. Cancer 1989;63(10):1931–1937.

CNF (Metastatic)

Cyclophosphamide	500 mg/m² i.v. day 1
Mitoxantrone	10 mg/m² i.v. day 1
5-Fluorouracil	500 mg/m² i.v. day 1

*Repeat every 21 days

Source: Bennett JM, Muss HB, Doroshow JH, et al. A randomized multicenter trial comparing mitoxantrone, cyclophosphamide, and fluorouracil with doxorubicin, cyclophosphamide, and fluorouracil in the therapy of metastatic breast carcinoma. J Clin Oncol 1988;6(10):1611–1620.

Cooper Regimen (Adjuvant)

5-Fluorouracil	12 mg/kg/week × 8 weeks i.v., then every other week for 7 months
Methotrexate	0.7 mg/kg/week × 8 weeks i.v., then every other week for 7 months
Vincristine	0.035 mg/kg/week × 5 weeks i.v., then once a month
Cyclophosphamide	2 mg/kg/day p.o. × 9 months

Prednisone   0.75 mg/kg/day p.o. × 10 days, then ½ above daily ×
                                                                       10 days, then ¼ above daily × 10 days, then 5 mg/
                                                                       day × 20 days, then discontinue

Source: Cooper RG, Holland JF, Glidewell O. Adjuvant therapy of breast cancer. Cancer 1979;
44:793–798.

Docetaxel (Taxotere) (Metastatic)

Taxotere   100 mg/m^2 i.v. over 1 hour day 1
*Repeat every 21 days

Source: Ravdin P, Valero V, Burris H 3rd, Von Hoff DD, Hortobagyi G. Docetaxel (Taxotere)
therapy in anthracycline/anthracenedione or paclitaxel resistant metastatic breast cancer (RMBC)
(abstract). Proc Annu Meet Am Soc Clin Oncol 1995;14:A77.

DVM (Metastatic)

Doxorubicin   50 mg/m^2 i.v. days 1 and 28
Vincristine   1 mg/m^2 i.v. days 1 and 28
Mitomycin C   10 mg/m^2 i.v. day 1
*Repeat every 8 weeks

Source: Ingle JN, Mailliard JA, Schaid DJ, et al. Randomized trial of doxorubicin alone or combined
with vincristine and mitomycin C in women with metastatic breast cancer. Am J Clin Oncol 1989;
12(6):474–480.

FAC (Adjuvant or Metastatic)

5-Fluorouracil   500 mg/m^2 i.v. days 1 and 5
Doxorubicin   50 mg/m^2 i.v. day 1 by continuous infusion (CI) over
                                                                       48–96 hours.
Cyclophosphamide   500 mg/m^2 i.v. day 1
*Repeat every 21 days

Source: Hortobagyi GN, Frye D, Buzdar AU, et al. Decreased cardiac toxicity of doxorubicin administered by continuous intravenous infusion in combination chemotherapy for metastatic breast
carcinoma. Cancer 1989;63(1):37–45.

M-VAC (Metastatic)

Methotrexate   30 mg/m^2 i.v. days 1, 15, 22
Vinblastine   3 mg/m^2 i.v. days 2, 15, 22
Doxorubicin (Adriamycin)   30 mg/m^2 i.v. day 2
Cisplatin   70 mg/m^2 i.v. day 2
*Repeat every 28 days

Source: Langer CJ, Catalano R, Weiner LM, et al. Phase II evaluation of methotrexate, vinblastine,
doxorubicin, and cisplatin (M-VAC) in advanced, measurable breast carcinoma. Cancer Invest
1995;13(2):150–159.

NFL

Mitoxantrone (Novantrone)   12 mg/m^2 i.v. day 1
5-Fluorouracil   350 mg/m^2/day i.v. days 1–3
Leucovorin   300 mg/day i.v. days 1–3 (given 1 hour prior to 5-FU)
*Repeat every 21 days

Source: Hainsworth JD, Andrews MB, Johnson DH, Grecco FA. Mitoxantrone, fluorouracil, and
high dose leucovorin: an effective, well-tolerated regimen for metastatic breast cancer. J Clin Oncol
1991;9:1731–1736.

Paclitaxel (Taxol) (Metastatic)

Paclitaxel   175 mg/m^2 i.v. over 3 hours day 1

*Premedicate with Decadron 20 mg p.o. 6 and 12 hours prior to paclitaxel; diphenhydramine 50 mg i.v. 30–60 minutes prior to paclitaxel; and cimetidine 300 mg or ranitidine 50 mg i.v. 30–60 min prior to paclitaxel.

*Repeat every 21 days

Source: Gelmon K, Nabholtz JM, Bontenbal M, et al. Randomized trial of two doses of paclitaxel in metastatic breast cancer after failure of standard therapy (abstract). Ann Oncol 1994;198(Suppl 5):198(Abstract 493).

VAM (Metastatic)

Vinblastine   6 mg/m^2 i.v. days 1 and 28
Adriamycin   30 mg/m^2 i.v. days 1 and 28
Mitomycin C   10 mg/m^2 i.v. day 1

*Repeat every 8 weeks

Source: Shipp SK, Muss HB, Westrick MA, et al. Vincristine, doxorubicin and mitomycin (VAM) in patients with advanced breast cancer previously treated with cyclophosphamide, methotrexate and fluorouracil (CMF). A clinical trial of the Piedmont Oncology Association (POA). Cancer Chemother Pharmacol 1983;11(2):130–133.

VATH (Metastatic)

Vinblastine   4.5 mg/m^2 i.v. day 1
Doxorubicin (Adriamycin)   45 mg/m^2 i.v. day 1
Thiotepa   12 mg/m^2 i.v. day 1
Fluoxymesterone (Halotestin)   10 mg/m^2 p.o. t.i.d.

*Repeat every 21–28 days

Source: Hart RD, Perloff M, Holland JF. One day VATH (vinblastine, Adriamycin, thiotepa, and Halotestin) therapy for advanced breast cancer refractory to prior chemotherapy. Cancer 1981; 48:1522–1527.

VD (Metastatic)

Vinorelbine (Navelbine)   25 mg/m^2 i.v. day 1 and 8
Doxorubicin   50 mg/m^2 i.v. day 1

*Repeat every 21 days

Source: Hochster HS. Combined doxorubicin/vinorelbine (Navelbine) therapy in the treatment of advanced breast cancer. Semin Oncol 1995;22(2 Suppl 5):55–59, discussion 59–60.

Vinblastine and Mitomycin C (Metastatic)

First 2 cycles:
    Mitomycin C   10 mg/m^2 i.v. days 1 and 28
    Vinblastine   5 mg/m^2 i.v. days 1, 14, 28, 42
Subsequent cycles:
    Mitomycin C   10 mg/m^2 i.v. day 1
    Vinblastine   5 mg/m^2 i.v. days 1 and 21

*Repeat every 6 to 8 weeks

Source: Garewal HS, Brooks RJ, Jones SE, Miller TP. Treatment of advanced breast cancer with mitomycin C combined with vinblastine or vindesine. J Clin Oncol 1983;1:772–775.

Vinorelbine (Navelbine) (Metastatic)

Vinorelbine   30 mg/m^2 i.v. days 1, 8, 15, 22

*Repeat every 28 days

Source: Fumoleau P, Delozier T, Extra JM, Canobbio L, Delgado FM, Hurteloup P. Vinorelbine (Navelbine) in the treatment of breast cancer: the European experience. Semin Oncol 1995;22(2 Suppl 5):22–28; discussion 28–29.

CARCINOMA OF UNKNOWN PRIMARY SITE

BEP

Cisplatin	20 mg/m^2/day i.v.p.b. days 1–5
Etoposide	100 mg/m^2/day i.v.p.b. days 1–5
Bleomycin	30 u i.v. day 1

*Repeat cycle every 21 days

Source: Hainsworth JD, Johnson DH, Grecco FA. Cisplatin-based combination chemotherapy in the treatment of poorly differentiated carcinoma and poorly differentiated adenocarcinoma of unknown primary site. Results of a 12-year experience. J Clin Oncol 1992;10:912–922.

ICE (mini)

Ifosfamide	1000 mg/m^2 i.v. day 1, hr 0–1
Mesna	333 mg/m^2 i.v. day 1, 30 min before ifosfamide, then 4 and 8 hr after ifosfamide
Etoposide	150 mg/m^2 i.v. over 11 hr, day 1, hr 1–11
Carboplatin	200 mg/m^2 i.v. day 1, hr 11–12
Etoposide	150 mg/m^2 i.v. over 11 hr, day 1, hr 12–24

*Entire 24-hr cycle is repeated on day 2, for total administration time of 48 hr
*This 48-hr cycle is repeated every 28 days

Source: Fields KK, Zorsky PE, Hiemenz JW, Kronish LE, Elfenbein GJ. Ifosfamide, carboplatin, and etoposide: a new regimen with a broad spectrum of activity. J Clin Oncol 1994;12:544–552.

ENDOCRINE TUMORS

Adrenal Gland Neoplasm

Cisplatin and Etoposide

Cisplatin	25 mg/m^2/day i.v. days 1–3
Etoposide	100 mg/m^2/day i.v. days 1–3

*Repeat every 21–28 days

Source: Burgess MA, Legha SS, Sellin RV. Chemotherapy with cisplatin and etoposide (VP-16) for patients with advanced adrenal cortical-carcinoma (abstract). Proc Annu Meet Am Soc Clin Oncol 1993;12:Abstract 544.

Mitotane (*o,p'*-DDD)

Mitotane	2–10 g/day p.o. in three to four divided doses

*Recommend glucocorticoid and mineralocorticoid replacement

Source: Luton JP, Cerdas S, Billaud L, et al. Clinical features of adrenocortical carcinoma, prognostic factors, and the effect of mitotane therapy. N Engl J Med 1990;322(17):1195–1201.

Malignant Carcinoid Tumor

Interferon

Interferon-α	6×10^6 IU i.m. daily for 8 weeks then 6×10^6 IU i.m. 3 times weekly

Source: Bajetta E, Zilembo N, di Bartolomeo M, et al. Treatment of metastatic carcinoids and other neuroendocrine tumors with recombinant interferon-alpha-2a. A study by the Italian Trials in Medical Oncology group. Cancer 1993;72:3099–3105.

Octreotide

Octreotide	150–500 μg s.q. t.i.d. (titrate dose)

Source: Moertel CG. An odyssey in the land of small tumors. J Clin Oncol 1987;5:1503–1522.

Pancreatic Endocrine Tumors

Interferon

Interferon-α 6×10^6 IU i.m. daily for 8 weeks then
                                        6×10^6 IU i.m. 3 times weekly

Source: Bajetta E, Zilembo N, di Bartolomeo M, et al. Treatment of metastatic carcinoids and other neuroendocrine tumors with recombinant interferon-alpha-2a. A study by the Italian Trials in Medical Oncology group. Cancer 1993;72:3099–3105.

Octreotide

Octreotide   50 μg s.q. initial test dose day 1 then
                                        150–250 μg s.q. t.i.d.

Source: Saltz L, Trochanowski B, Buckley M, et al. Octreotide as an antineoplastic agent in the treatment of functional and nonfunctional neuroendocrine tumors. Cancer 1993;72:244–248.

Streptozocin and Doxorubicin

Streptozocin   500 mg/m^2/day i.v. days 1–5
Doxorubicin   50 mg/m^2 i.v. days 1, 22
*Repeat every 6 weeks

Source: Moertel CG, Lefkopulo M, Lipsitz S, Hahn RG, Klassen D. Streptozocin-doxorubicin, streptozocin-fluorouracil or chlorozotocin in the treatment of advanced islet-cell carcinoma. N Engl J Med 1992;326:519–523.

Streptozocin and 5-Fluorouracil

Streptozocin   500 mg/m^2/day i.v. days 1–5
5-Fluorouracil   400 mg/m^2/day i.v. days 1–5
*Repeat every 6 weeks

Source: Moertel CG, Hanley JA, Johnson LA. Streptozocin alone compared with streptozocin plus fluorouracil in the treatment of advanced islet-cell carcinoma. N Engl J Med 1980;303:1189–1194.

Pheochromocytoma

CVD

Cyclophosphamide   750 mg/m^2 i.v. day 1
Vincristine   1.4 mg/m^2 i.v. day 1
Dacarbazine   600 mg/m^2 i.v. days 1 and 2
*Repeat every 21 days

Source: Averbuch SD, Steakley CS, Young RC, et al. Malignant pheochromocytoma: effective treatment with a combination of cyclophosphamide, vincristine, and dacarbazine. Ann Intern Med 1988;109:267–273.

Pituitary adenomas

Octreotide

Octreotide   50–100 μg s.q. b.i.d. or t.i.d. (titrate dose)

Source: Chanson P, Weintraub BD, Harris AG. Octreotide therapy for thyroid-stimulating hormone-secreting pituitary adenomas: a follow-up of 52 patients. Ann Intern Med 1993;119:236–240.

Thyroid Cancer

Doxorubicin

Doxorubicin   60 mg/m^2 i.v. day 1
*Repeat every 21 days

Source: Shimaoka K, Schoenfeld DA, DeWys WD, et al. A randomized trial of doxorubicin versus doxorubicin plus cisplatin in patients with advanced thyroid carcinoma. Cancer 1985;566:2155–2160.

Doxorubicin and Cisplatin

Doxorubicin	60 mg/m^2 i.v. day 1
Cisplatin	40 mg/m^2 i.v. day 1

*Repeat every 21 days

Source: Shimaoka K, Schoenfeld DA, DeWys WD, et al. A randomized trial of doxorubicin versus doxorubicin plus cisplatin in patients with advanced thyroid carcinoma. Cancer 1985;566:2155–2160.

GASTROINTESTINAL

Anal Cancer

5-FU/MMC

5-Fluorouracil	750 mg/m^2/day i.v. days 1–5 and 29–33
Mitomycin C	15 mg/m^2 i.v. day 1
Radiotherapy	45 Gy over 5 weeks (1.8 Gy/day)

*After a rest period of 6 weeks a boost of 15–20 Gy was given if partial or complete response
*Surgical resection was performed in the case of residual disease or no response

Source: Roelofsen F, Bosset JF, Eschwege F, Pfeiffer M, Van Glabbeke M, Bartelink H. Concomitant radiotherapy and chemotherapy superior to radiotherapy alone in the treatment of locally advanced anal cancer. Results of a phase III randomized trial of the EORTC Radiotherapy and Gastrointestinal Cooperative Groups (abstract). Proc Annu Meet Am Soc Clin Oncol 1995;14:A454.

Or

5-Fluorouracil	1000 mg/m^2/day i.v. days 1–4 and 29–32
Mitomycin C	10 mg/m^2 i.v. days 1 and 29
Radiotherapy	45 Gy over 5 weeks (1.8 Gy/day)

*Patients with residual tumor at biopsy 6 weeks after treatment received salvage CT-RT including cisplatin

Source: Flam MS, John M, Pajak T, et al. Radiation (RT) and 5-fluorouracil (5FU) vs radiation, 5FU, mitomycin-c (MMC) in the treatment of anal carcinoma: results of a phase III randomized RTOG/ECOG intergroup trial (abstract). Proc Annu Meet Am Soc Clin Oncol 1995;14:A443.

5-FU-MMC

5-Fluorouracil	1000 mg/m^2 CI i.v. days 1–4 and 29–32
Mitomycin	15 mg/m^2 i.v. push day 1
Radiation therapy	3000 cGy (200 cGy/day) days 1–5, 8–12, and 15–19

*Surgery was performed 4–6 weeks after completion of XRT

Source: Nigro ND, Seydel HG, Considine B, Vaitkevicus VK, Leichman L, Kinzie JJ. Combined preoperative radiation and chemotherapy for squamous cell carcinoma of the anal canal. Cancer 1983;51:1826–1829.

Biliary Tract Cancer

FAM

5-Fluorouracil	600 mg/m^2 i.v. push days 1, 8, 29, and 36
Doxorubicin	30 mg/m^2 i.v. push days 1 and 29
Mitomycin	10 mg/m^2 i.v. push day 1

*Repeat cycle every 8 weeks

Source: Harvey JH, Smith FP, Schein PS. 5-Fluorouracil, mitomycin, and doxorubicin (FAM) in carcinoma of the biliary tract. J Clin Oncol 1984;2:1245–1248.

Colorectal Cancer

ADJUVANT THERAPY
5-FU-Levamisole

5-Fluorouracil	450 mg/m^2/day i.v. push days 1–5, then; 3 weeks later, 450 mg/m^2 weekly × 48 weeks
Levamisole	50 mg p.o. every 8 hours daily × days 1–3 every 14 days × 52 weeks

Source: Moertel CG, Fleming TR, MacDonald JS, et al. Levamisole and fluorouracil for adjuvant therapy of resected colon carcinoma. N Engl J Med 1990;322:352–358.

Low-Dose Leucovorin/5-FU

5-Fluorouracil	425 mg/m^2/day i.v. days 1–5
Leucovorin	20 mg/m^2/day i.v. days 1–5

*Repeat every 4–5 weeks × 6 months; leucovorin administered prior to 5-FU

Source: O'Connell MJ, Malliard J, MacDonald J, et al. An intergroup trial of intensive course 5-FU and low dose leucovorin as surgical adjuvant therapy for high risk colon cancer (abstract). Proc Am Soc Clin Oncol 1993;12:Abstract 190.

High-Dose Leucovorin and 5-FU

5-Fluorouracil	370–400 mg/m^2/day i.v. days 1–5
Leucovorin	200 mg/m^2/day i.v. day 1–5

*Repeat every 5 weeks; leucovorin administered prior to 5-FU

Source: Zaniboni A, Erlichman C, Seitz JF, et al. FUFA increases disease-free survival (DFS) in resected B$_2$, C colon cancer (CC abstract). Proc Am Soc Clin Oncol 1993;12:Abstract191.

Weekly Fluorouracil plus High-Dose Leucovorin

5-Fluorouracil	500 mg/m^2 i.v. day 1, weeks 1–6
Leucovorin	500 mg/m^2 i.v. day 1, weeks 1–6

*Repeat every 8 weeks; leucovorin administered prior to 5-FU

Source: Wolmark N, Rockette H, Fisher B, et al. The benefit of leucovorin-modulated fluorouracil as postoperative adjuvant therapy for primary colon cancer: results from the National Surgical Adjuvant Breast and Bowel Project protocol C-03. J Clin Oncol 1993;11:1879–1887.

5-FU/XRT (Rectal)

5-Fluorouracil	500 mg/m^2/day i.v. days 1–5, 36–40
	225 mg/m^2 CI i.v. days 56–96
	450 mg/m^2/day i.v. days 120–124, 134–138, 169–173
Radiation therapy	4500 cGy in 180 cGy fractions daily × 6 weeks, start day 56

Source: O'Connell MJ, Martensen JA, Wieand US, et al. Improved adjuvant therapy for rectal cancer by combining protracted infusion fluorouracil with radiation therapy after curative surgery. N Engl J Med 1994;331:502–507.

METASTATIC DISEASE
FUCI

5-Fluorouracil	300 mg/m^2/day by continuous i.v. infusion

*Continued until progression or toxicity

Source: Lokich JA, Ahlgren JD, Gullo JJ, et al. A prospective randomized comparison of continuous infusion fluorouracil with a conventional bolus schedule in metastatic colorectal carcinoma: a Mid-Atlantic Oncology Program study. J Clin Oncol 1989;7:425–432.

Intraarterial FUDR/5-FU-Leucovorin

FUDR	0.2 mg/kg/day via hepatic artery catheter days 1–14
5-Fluorouracil	425 mg/m^2/day i.v. days 22–26
Leucovorin	20 mg/m^2/day i.v. days 22–26

*Repeat every 5 weeks

Source: O'Connell M, Mailliard J, Nagorney D, Fitzgibbons R, Bernath A, Wieand H. Sequential intrahepatic 5-fluorodeoxyuridine (FUDR) and systemic 5-fluorouracil (5FU) + leucovorin (LV) in patients with metastatic colorectal cancer (CRC) confined to the liver (abstract). Proc Annu Meet Am Soc Clin Oncol 1994;13:A662.

5-FU-Leucovorin (Low Dose)

5-Fluorouracil	425 mg/m^2 i.v. daily × 5 days
Leucovorin	20 mg/m^2 i.v. daily × 5 days

*Repeat cycle every 4 to 5 weeks; administer leucovorin immediately prior to 5-FU

Source: Buroker TR, O'Connell MJ, Wieand HS, et al. Randomized comparison of two schedules of fluorouracil and leucovorin in the treatment of advanced colorectal cancer. J Clin Oncol 1994; 12:14–20.

5-FU-Leucovorin (High Dose)

5-Fluorouracil	600 mg/m^2 i.v. day 1 weekly × 6
Leucovorin	500 mg/m^2 i.v. day 1 weekly × 6

*Repeat cycle following 2-week rest period; administer 5-FU 1 hr after initiating leucovorin infusion

Source: Buroker TR, O'Connell MJ, Wieand HS, et al. Randomized comparison of two schedules of fluorouracil and leucovorin in the treatment of advanced colorectal cancer. J Clin Oncol 1994; 12:14–20.

MFL

Methotrexate	250 mg/m^2 i.v. day 1, hr 0–2
5-Fluorouracil	500 mg/m^2 i.v. push day 1, hr 3 and 23
Leucovorin	15 mg/m^2 i.v. push × 1 on hr 24, then 15 mg/m^2 p.o. q 6 hr × 7

*Alkalinize urine to pH of 8.0 prior to administration of MTX
*Repeat every 2 weeks × 8, every 3 weeks × 2, every 4 weeks × 2

Source: Glimelius B. Biochemical modulation of 5-fluorouracil: a randomized comparison of sequential methotrexate, 5-fluorouracil and leucovorin versus sequential 5-fluorouracil and leucovorin in patients with advanced symptomatic colorectal cancer. The Nordic Gastrointestinal Adjuvant Tumor Therapy Group. Ann of Oncol 1993;4(3):235–240.

Esophageal Cancer

FU-MMC

Radiation therapy	200 cGy/d (maximum 6000 cGy over 6 to 7 weeks) start day 1
5-Fluorouracil	1000 mg/m^2/day CI i.v. days 2–5 and 29–32
Mitomycin	10 mg/m^2 i.v. day 2

Source: Coia LR, Paul AR, Engstrom PF. Combined radiation and chemotherapy as primary management of adenocarcinoma of the esophagus and gastroesophageal junction. Cancer 1988;61:643–649.

FU-PT-XRT (Wayne State)

5-Fluorouracil	1000 mg/m^2 CI i.v. days 1–4
Cisplatin	75 mg/m^2 i.v. day 1
Radiation therapy	50 Gy over 5 weeks

*Chemotherapy given weeks 1, 5, 8, 11

Source: Herskovic A, Martz K, al-Sarraf M, et al. Combined chemotherapy and radiotherapy compared with radiotherapy alone in patients with cancer of the esophagus. N Engl J Med 1992; 326:1593–1598.

FU-PB-MMC

Cisplatin	100 mg/m^2 i.v. days 1 and 29
5-Fluorouracil	1000 mg/m^2 CI i.v. days 1–4 and 29–32
Mitomycin	10 mg/m^2 i.v. day 57
Bleomycin	20 U/day CI i.v. days 57–60, and 78–81
Radiation therapy	200 cGy/day (maximum 5000 cGy) days 1–5, 8–12, 15–19, 99–103, and 106–110

Source: Leichman L, Herskovic A, Leichman CG, et al. Nonoperative therapy for squamous-cell cancer of the esophagus. J Clin Oncol 1987;5(3):365–370.

Paclitaxel

Paclitaxel (Taxol)	250 mg/m^2 i.v. over 24 hours day 1

*Repeat every 21 days
*Granulocyte colony-stimulating factor was used to prevent neutropenia

Source: Ajani JA, Ilson DH, Daugherty K, Kelsen DP. Paclitaxel in the treatment of carcinoma of the esophagus. Semin Oncol 1995;22(3 Suppl 6):35–40.

TCF

Paclitaxel (Taxol)	175 mg/m^2 i.v. over 3 hr day 1
Cisplatin	20 mg/m^2/day i.v. day 1–5
5-Fluorouracil	750 mg/m^2/day i.v. day 1–5

*Repeat every 28 days

Source: Ajani JA, Ilson D, Bhalla K, et al. Taxol, cisplatin, and 5-FU (TCF): a multi-institutional phase II study in patients with carcinoma of the esophagus (abstract). Proc Annu Meet Am Soc Clin Oncol 1995;14:Abstract 489

Gastric Cancer

EAP

Etoposide	120 mg/m^2 i.v. days 4–6
Doxorubicin	20 mg/m^2 i.v. push days 1 and 7
Cisplatin	40 mg/m^2 i.v. days 2 and 8

*Repeat cycle every 3 to 4 weeks.

Source: Wilke M, Preusser P, Fink U, et al. Preoperative chemotherapy in locally advanced and nonresectable gastric cancer: a phase II study with etoposide, doxorubicin, and cisplatin. J Clin Oncol 1989;7:1318–1326.

ELF

Etoposide	120 mg/m^2/day i.v. days 1–3
Leucovorin	300 mg/m^2 i.v. days 1–3
5-Fluorouracil	500 mg/m^2 i.v. push day 1–3

*Repeat every 21 days

Source: Wilke H, Preusser P, Stahl M, et al. Etoposide, folinic acid, and 5-fluorouracil in carboplatin-pretreated patients with advanced gastric cancer. Cancer Chemother Pharm 1991;29:83–84.

FAM

5-Fluorouracil	600 mg/m^2 i.v. push days 1, 8, 29, and 36
Doxorubicin	30 mg/m^2 i.v. push days 1 and 29
Mitomycin	10 mg/m^2 i.v. push day 1

*Repeat cycle every 8 weeks

Source: MacDonald JS, Schein PS, Woolley PV, et al. 5-Fluorouracil, doxorubicin, and mitomycin (FAM) combination chemotherapy for advanced gastric cancer. Ann Intern Med 1980;93:533–536.

FAMTX

5-Fluorouracil	1500 mg/m^2 i.v. day 1 (1 hr after MTX)
Doxorubicin	30 mg/m^2 i.v. day 15
Methotrexate (MTX)	1500 mg/m^2 i.v. day 1
Leucovorin	15 mg/m^2 p.o. q 6h × 12 (start 24 hr after MTX)

*Hydrate and alkalinize urine prior to MTX
*Repeat every 28 days

Source: Wils JA, Klein HO, Wagener DJ, et al. Sequential high-dose methotrexate and fluorouracil combined with doxorubicin—a step ahead in the treatment of advanced gastric cancer: A trial of the European Organization for Research and Treatment of Cancer Gastrointestinal Tract Cooperative Group. J Clin Oncol 1991;9:827–831.

FAP

5-Fluorouracil	300 mg/m^2 i.v. push days 1–5
Doxorubicin	40 mg/m^2 i.v. push day 1
Cisplatin	60 mg/m^2 i.v. day 1

*Cycle repeated every 5 weeks

Source: Cullinan SA, Moertel CG, Wieand HS, et al. Controlled evaluation of three drug combination regimens versus fluorouracil alone for the therapy of advanced gastric cancer. North Central Cancer Treatment Group. J Clin Oncol 1994;12:412–416.

5-FU

5-Fluorouracil	500 mg/m^2/day i.v. days 1–5

*Repeat every 28 days

Source: Cullinan SA, Moertel CG, Wieand HS, et al. Controlled evaluation of three drug combination regimens versus fluorouracil alone for the therapy of advanced gastric cancer. North Central Cancer Treatment Group. J Clin Oncol 1994;12:412–416.

Pancreatic Cancer

FAM

5-Fluorouracil	600 mg/m^2 i.v. push days 1, 8, 29, and 36
Doxorubicin	30 mg/m^2 i.v. push days 1 and 29
Mitomycin	10 mg/m^2 i.v. push day 1

*Repeat cycle every 8 weeks

Source: Leonard RC, Cull A, Stewart ME, Knowles G, Carter DC, Palmer KR. Chemotherapy for pancreatic cancer significantly prolongs survival and quality of life is unimpaired. Br J Cancer 1992;65:8.

Gemcitabine

Gemcitabine	1000 mg/m^2 i.v. weekly for 7 weeks, then 1 week rest, then 1000 mg/m^2 i.v. weekly for 3 weeks, then 1 week rest

*Repeat 3 week cycle every 28 days

Source: Rothenberg ML, Burris HA 3rd, Andersen JS, et al. Gemcitabine: effective palliative therapy for pancreas cancer patients failing 5-FU (abstract). Proc Annu Meet Am Soc Clin Oncol 1995; 14:A470.

SMF

Steptozocin	1000 mg/m^2 i.v. days 1, 8, 29, and 36
5-Fluorouracil	600 mg/m^2 i.v. push days 1, 8, 29, and 36
Mitomycin C	10 mg/m^2 i.v. push day 1

Source: Bukowsi RM, Balcerzak SP, O'Bryan RM, Bonnet JD, Chen TT. Randomized trial of 5-fluorouracil and mitomycin C with or without streptozocin for advanced pancreatic cancer. A Southwest Oncology Group study. Cancer 1983;52:1577–1582.

GENITOURINARY

Bladder Cancer

CISCA

Cyclophosphamide	650 mg/m^2 i.v. day 1
Doxorubicin	50 mg/m^2 i.v. day 1
Cisplatin	100 mg/m^2 i.v. day 2

*Repeat every 21–28 days

Source: Sternberg JJ, Bracken RB, Handel PB, Johnson DE. Combination chemotherapy (CISCA) for advanced urinary tract carcinoma: a preliminary report. JAMA 1977;238:2282–2287.

CMV

Cisplatin	100 mg/m^2 i.v. day 2 (give 12 hours after methotrexate)
Methotrexate	30 mg/m^2 i.v. days 1, 8
Vinblastine	4 mg/m^2 i.v. days 1, 8

*Repeat every 21 days

Source: Harker WG, Meyers FJ, Freiha FS, et al. Cisplatin, methotrexate, and vinblastine (CMV): an effective chemotherapy regimen for metastatic transitional cell carcinoma of the urinary tract: a Northern California Oncology Group study. J Clin Oncol 1985;3:1463–1470.

Gemcitabine

Gemcitabine	1200 mg/m^2/day i.v. days 1, 8, 15

*Repeat every 28 days

Source: Stadler W, Kuzel T, Raghaven D, et al. A phase II study of gemcitabine in the treatment of patients with advanced transitional cell carcinoma (abstract 638). J Clin Oncol Proc ACSO 1995; 14:241.

MVAC

Methotrexate	30 mg/m^2 i.v. days 1, 15, 22
Vinblastine	3 mg/m^2 i.v. days 2, 15, 22
Doxorubicin	30 mg/m^2 i.v. day 2
Cisplatin	70 mg/m^2 i.v. day 2

*Repeat every 28 days

Source: Sternberg CH, Yagoda A, Scher HI, et al. Preliminary results of M-VAC (methotrexate, vinblastine, doxorubicin, and cisplatin) for transitional cell carcinoma of the urothelium. J Urol 1985;133:403–407.

Paclitaxel

Paclitaxel (Taxol)	250 mg/m^2 i.v. over 24 hours day 1

*Repeat every 21 days
*Recombinant human granulocyte colony-stimulating factor (rhG-CSF) was given at 5 μg/kg/ day s.q. for at least 10 days each cycle

*Premedicate with Decadron 20 mg p.o. 6 and 12 hours prior to paclitaxel; diphenhydramine 50 mg i.v. 30–60 minutes prior to paclitaxel; and cimetidine 300 mg or ranitidine 50 mg i.v. 30–60 min prior to paclitaxel

Source: Roth BJ, Dreicer R, Einhorn LH, et al. Significant activity of paclitaxel in advanced transitional-cell carcinoma of the urothelium: a phase II trial of the Eastern Cooperative Oncology Group. J Clin Oncol 1994;12:2264–2270.

VIG

Vinblastine	0.11 mg/kg/day i.v. days 1, 2
Ifosfamide	1200 mg/m^2/day i.v. days 1–5
Gallium nitrate	300 mg/m^2/day i.v. CI days 1–5
Calcitriol	0.5 μg/day p.o. days -3 to 5

*Repeat every 21 days.
*Recombinant human granulocyte colony-stimulating factor (rhG-CSF) was given at 5 μg/kg/day s.q. days 7–16

Source: Einhorn LH, Roth BJ, Ansari R, Dreicer R, Gonin R, Loehrer PJ. Phase II trial of vinblastine, ifosfamide, and gallium combination chemotherapy in metastatic urothelial carcinoma. J Clin Oncol 1994;12:2271–2276.

Prostate Cancer

Cyclophosphamide (Oral)

Cyclophosphamide	150 mg p.o. daily days 1–14

*Repeat every 28 days

Source: Raghavan D, Cox K, Pearson BS, et al. Oral cyclophosphamide for the management of hormone-refractory prostate cancer. Br J Urol 1993;72:625–628.

Estramustine

Estramustine	14 mg/kg/day p.o. in 3 or 4 divided doses

Source: Murphy GP, Slack NH, Mittelman A. Use of estramustine phosphate in prostate cancer by the National Prostatic Cancer Project and by Roswell Park Memorial Institute. Urol 1984; 23(Suppl):54–63.

Estramustine plus Vinblastine

Estramustine phosphate	600 mg/m^2/day p.o. days 1–42
Vinblastine	4 mg/m^2/day i.v. weekly $\times$ 6

*Repeat every 8 weeks

Source: Hudes G, Greenburg R, Krigel RL, et al. Phase II study of estramustine and vinblastine, two microtubule inhibitors, in hormone-refractory prostate cancer. J Clin Oncol 1992;11:1754–1761.

MP

Mitoxantrone	12 mg/m^2 i.v. day 1
Prednisone	5 mg p.o. b.i.d.

*Repeat every 21 days

Source: Tannock I, Osaha D, Ernst S, et al. Chemotherapy with mitoxantrone (M) and prednisone (P) palliates patients with hormone-resistant prostate cancer (HRPC). Results of a randomized Canadian trial (abstract A653). Proc Am Soc Oncol 1995;14:245.

Renal Cell Carcinoma

Interferon-α

Interferon	5–15 $\times$ 10^6 IU s.q. or i.m. daily or 3–5 times a week

Source: Tsavaris N, Mylonakis N, Bacoyiannis C, Tsoutsos H, Karabelis A, Kosmidis P. Treatment of renal cell carcinoma with escalating doses of alpha-interferon. Chemotherapy 1993;39:361–366.

Circadian or Constant-Infusion FUDR

Floxuridine (FUDR)   0.15 mg/kg/day continuous infusion i.v. or
                                        0.25 mg/kg/day via hepatic artery days 1–14
*For Circadian: 68% of dose between 1500–2100 hr + 15% between 2100–0300 hr + 2% between
0300–0900 hr + 15% between 0900–1500 hr
*Repeat every 28 days

Source: Hrushesky WJM, von Roemling R, Lanning RM, et al. Circadian-shaped infusions of
floxuridine for progressive metastatic renal cell carcinoma. J Clin Oncol 1990;8:1504–1513.

High-Dose IL-2

Interleukin-2   600,000 or 720,000 IU/kg i.v. q8h up to 14 doses or
                                        when toxicity develops
*Repeat cycle in 7–10 days; this course can be repeated every 12 weeks
*Discontinue therapy for hypotension requiring pressor support, oliguria unresponsive to fluid
and diuretics, respiratory distress, cardiac arrythmias, mental confusion

Source: Parkinson DR, Sznol M. High-dose interleukin-2 in the therapy of metastatic renal-cell
carcinoma. Semin Oncol 1995;22:61–66.

Low-Dose IL-2

Interleukin-2 3×10^6 IU s.q. b.i.d. days 1–5 weekly for 6 weeks

Source: Stadler WM, Vogelzang NJ. Low-dose interleukin-2 in the treatment of metastatic renal-
cell carcinoma. Semin Oncol 1995;22:67–73.

IL-2/IFN-α/5-FU

Interleukin-2 20×10^6 IU/m^2 s.q. 3 days 1, 3, 5 weeks 1, 4
                                        5×10^6 IU/m^2 s.q. 3 days 1, 3, 5 weeks 2, 3
Interferon-α 6×10^6 IU/m^2 s.q. day 1 weeks 1, 4
                                        5×10^6 IU/m^2 s.q. days 1, 3, 5 weeks 2, 3
                                        9×10^6 IU/m^2 s.q. days 1, 3, 5 weeks 5–8
5-Fluorouracil   750 mg/m^2 i.v. day 1 weeks 5–8
*Repeat every 2 months

Source: Atzpodien J, Kirchner H, Hanninen EL, Deckert M, Fenner M, Poliwoda H. Interleukin-2
in combination with interferon-α and 5-fluorouracil for metastatic renal cell cancer. Eur J Cancer
1993;29A(Suppl 5):6–8.

IFN/IL-2

Interferon-α 9×10^6 IU s.q. days 1, 4 weekly, weeks 1–4
Interleukin-2 12×10^6 IU/day s.q. day 1–4 weekly, weeks 1–4
*Repeat every 6 weeks

Source: Voglezang NJ, Lipton A, Figlin RA. Subcutaneous interleukin-2 plus interferon alpha-2a
in metastatic renal cancer: An outpatient multicenter trial. J Clin Oncol 1993;11:1809–1816.

Testicular Cancer

BEP

Bleomycin   30 U i.v. days 2, 9, 16
Etoposide   100 mg/m^2/day i.v. days 1–5
Cisplatin   20 mg/m^2/day i.v. days 1–5
*Repeat every 21 days

Source: Williams SD, Birch R, Einhorn LH, et al. Disseminated germ cell tumors: chemotherapy
with cisplatin plus bleomycin plus either vinblastine or etoposide. A trial of the Southeastern
Cancer Study Group. N Engl J Med 1987;316:1435–1440.

EP

Cisplatin	20 mg/m^2/day i.v. days 1–5
Etoposide	100 mg/m^2/day i.v. days 1–5

*Repeat every 21 days

Source: Motzer RJ, Sheinfeld J, Mazumdar M, et al. Etoposide and cisplatin adjuvant therapy for patients with pathologic stage II germ cell tumors. J Clin Oncol 1995;13:2700–2704.

PVB

Cisplatin	20 mg/m^2/day i.v. days 1–5
Vinblastine	0.15 mg/kg i.v. days 1, 2
Bleomycin	30 U i.v. days 2, 9, 16

*Repeat every 21 days

Source: Einhorn LH, Donohue J. Cis-dichlorodiammineplatinum, vinblastine and bleomycin combination chemotherapy in disseminated testicular cancer. Ann Intern Med 1977;87:293–298.

VAB-6

Vinblastine	4 mg/m^2 i.v. day 1
Dactinomycin	1 mg/m^2 i.v. day 1
Bleomycin	30 U i.v. push day 1 then 20 U/m^2/day i.v. CI days 1–3
Cisplatin	120 mg/m^2 i.v. day 4
Cyclophosphamide	600 mg/m^2 i.v. day 1

*Repeat every 21 days

Source: Vugrin D, Herr HW, Whitmore WF, Sogani PC, Golbey RB. VAB-6 combination chemotherapy in disseminated cancer of the testis. Ann Intern Med 1981;95:59–61.

VelP (Salvage)

Vinblastine	0.11 mg/kg i.v. days 1, 2
Ifosfamide	1200 mg/m^2/day i.v. days 1–5
Cisplatin	20 mg/m^2/day i.v. days 1–5

*Repeat every 21 days

Source: Motzer RJ, Geller NL, Tan CCY, et al. Salvage chemotherapy for patients with germ cell tumors. The Memorial Sloan Kettering Cancer Center experience (1979–1989) Cancer 1991; 67:1305–1310.

VIP (Salvage)

Etoposide (VP-16)	100 mg/m^2/day i.v. days 1–5
Ifosfamide	1200 mg/m^2/day i.v. days 1–5
Cisplatin	20 mg/m^2/day i.v. days 1–5

*Repeat every 21 days

Source: Harstrick A, Schmall HJ, Wilke H, et al. Cisplatin, etoposide, and ifosfamide salvage therapy for refractory or relapsing germ cell carcinoma. J Clin Oncol 1991;9:1549–1555.

GYNECOLOGICAL CANCER

Cervical Cancer

BIP

Bleomycin	30 units/m^2 i.v. over 24 hours day 1
Ifosfamide	5000 mg/m^2 i.v. over 24 hours day 2
Mesna	6000 mg/m^2 i.v. over 36 hours day 2
Cisplatin	50 mg/m^2 i.v. day 2

*Repeat every 21 days

Source: Buxton EJ, Meanwell CA, Hilton C, et al. Combination bleomycin, ifosfamide, and cisplatin chemotherapy in cervical cancer. J Natl Cancer Inst 1989;81:359–361.

BOMP

Bleomycin	10 U i.m. days 1, 8, 15, 22
Vincristine	1 mg/m^2 i.v. days 1, 8, 22, 29
Mitomycin C	10 mg/m^2 i.v. day 1
Cisplatin	50 mg/m^2 i.v. days 1, 22

*Repeat every 6 weeks

Source: Vogl SE, Moukhtar M, Calanoy A, Greenwald EH, Kaplan BH. Chemotherapy for advanced cervical cancer with bleomycin, vincristine, mitomycin C, and *cis*-diamminedichloroplatinum (BOMP). Cancer Treat Rep 1980;64:1005–1007.

Endometrial Cancer

AC

Doxorubicin	60 mg/m^2 i.v. day 1
Cyclophosphamide	500 mg/m^2 i.v. day 1

*Repeat every 21 days

Source: Thigpen JT, Blessing JA, DiSaia PJ, Yordan E, Carson LF, Evers C. A randomized comparison of doxorubicin alone versus doxorubicin plus cyclophosphamide in the management of advanced recurrent endometrial carcinoma: a Gynecological Oncology Group study. J Clin Oncol 1994;12:1408–1414.

MCA

Megestrol	80 mg p.o. t.i.d.
Doxorubicin	40 mg/m^2 i.v. day 1
Cyclophosphamide	400 mg/m^2 i.v. day 1

*Repeat every 28 days

Source: Horton J, Elson P, Gordon P, Hahn R, Creech R. Combination chemotherapy for advanced endometrial cancer. An evaluation of three regimens. Cancer 1982;49:2441–2445.

MVAC

Methotrexate	30 mg/m^2 i.v. days 1, 15, 22
Vinblastine	3 mg/m^2 i.v. days 2, 15, 22
Doxorubicin	30 mg/m^2 i.v. day 2
Cisplatin	70 mg/m^2 i.v. day 2

*Repeat every 28 days

Source: Long HJ 3rd, Langdon RM Jr, Cha SS, et al. Phase II trial of methotrexate, vinblastine, doxorubicin, and cisplatin in advanced/recurrent endometrial carcinoma. Gynecol Oncol 1995; 58:240–243.

PA

Cisplatin	50 mg/m^2 i.v. day 1
Doxorubicin	50 mg/m^2 i.v. day 1

*Repeat every 21 days

Source: Deppe G, Malviya VK, Malone JM, Christensen CW, Saunders D. Treatment of recurrent and metastatic endometrial carcinoma with cisplatin and doxorubicin. Eur J Gynaecol Oncol 1994; 15:263–266.

PAC

Cisplatin	50 mg/m^2 i.v. day 1
Doxorubicin	50 mg/m^2 i.v. day 1
Cyclophosphamide	500 mg/m^2 i.v. day 1

*Repeat every 28 days

Source: Burke TW, Gershenson DM, Morris M, et al. Postoperative adjuvant cisplatin, doxorubicin, and cyclophosphamide (PAC) chemotherapy in women with high-risk endometrial carcinoma. Gynecol Oncol 1994;55:47–50.

VFP

Etoposide (VP-16)	80 mg/m^2/day i.v. days 1–3
5-Fluorouracil	600 mg/m^2/day i.v. days 1–3
Cisplatin	35 mg/m^2/day i.v. days 1–3

*Repeat every 28 days

Source: Paraiso D, Dorval T, Boufessa F, et al. Phase II study of VP-16-213(VP), 5-fluorouracil (5FU) and cisplatin (CDDP) for patients (PTS) with metastatic endometrial carcinoma (abstract A711). Proc Annu Meet Am Soc Clin Oncol 1992;11.

Gestational Trophoblastic Neoplasm

EMA/CO (High-Risk Disease)

Etoposide (VP-16)	100 mg/m^2/day i.v. days 1, 2
Methotrexate	100 mg/m^2 i.v. bolus day 1, then 200 mg/m^2 i.v. by 12 hour infusion
Leucovorin	15 mg p.o. q12h days 2, 3 (start 24 hours after methotrexate started)
Actinomycin D	0.5 mg/day i.v. days 1, 2
Cyclophosphamide	600 mg/m^2 i.v. day 8
Vincristine	1 mg/m^2 i.v. day 8 (max 2 mg)

*Repeat every 14 days

Source: Newlands ES, Bagshawe KD, Begent RH, Rustin GJ, Holden L. Results with the EMA/CA (etoposide, methotrexate, actinomycin D, cyclophosphamide, vincristine) regimen in high risk gestational trophoblastic tumors, 1979 to 1989. Br J Obstet Gynaecol 1991;98:550–557.

MAC III (High-Risk Disease)

Methotrexate	1 mg/kg/day i.m. days 1, 3, 5, 7
Leucovorin	0.1 mg/kg/day i.m. or p.o. days 2, 4, 6, 8
Actinomycin D	12 μg/kg/day i.v. days 1–5
Cyclophosphamide	3 mg/kg/day i.v. days 1–5

*Repeat every 21 days

Source: Berkowitz RS, Goldstein DP, Bernstein MR. Modified triple chemotherapy in the management of high-risk metastatic gestational trophoblastic tumors. Gynecol Oncol 1984;19:173–181.

Methotrexate (Low-Risk Disease)

Methotrexate	1 mg/kg/day i.m. days 1, 3, 5, 7
Leucovorin	0.1 mg/kg/day i.m. or p.o. days 2, 4, 6, 8

*Repeat every 14 days until serum hCG ≤ 5 mIU/mL, then give one additional cycle
*If hCG does not fall by 1 log at day 14 increase doses by 50%; if no response after 2 cycles, the patient should be switched to:

Actinomycin D	12–15 μg/kg/day i.v. days 1–5

*Repeat every 2 weeks

Source: Berkowitz RS, Goldstein DP, Bernstein MR. Ten year's experience with methotrexate and folinic acid as primary therapy for gestational trophoblastic disease. Gynecol Oncol 1986;23:111–118.

Weekly Methotrexate (Low-Risk Disease)

Methotrexate   40 mg/m² i.v. day 1
*Repeat every 7 days until 3 normal consecutive weekly serum hCG

Source: Gleeson NC, Finan MA, Fiorica JV, Robert WS, Hoffman MS, Wilson J. Nonmetastatic gestational trophoblastic disease. Weekly methotrexate compared with 8-day methotrexate-folinic acid. Eur J Gynaecol Oncol 1993;14:461–465.

Ovarian Cancer

BEP (Germ Cell Tumor)

Bleomycin   30 U i.v. days 2, 9, 16
Etoposide   100 mg/m²/day i.v. days 1–5
Cisplatin   20 mg/m²/day i.v. days 1–5
*Repeat every 21 days

Source: Williams SD. Treatment of germ cell tumors of the ovary. Semin Oncol 1991;18:292–296.

CarboC

Carboplatin   300 mg/m² i.v. day 1
Cyclophosphamide   600 mg/m² i.v. day 1
*Repeat every 21 days

Source: Swerenton K, Jeffrey J, Stuart G, et al. Cisplatin-cyclophosphamide versus carboplatin-cyclophosphamide in advance ovarian cancer: a randomized phase III study of the National Cancer Institute of Canada Clinical Trials Group. J Clin Oncol 1992;10:718–726.

CC

Cisplatin   75 mg/m² i.v. day 1
Cyclophosphamide   600 mg/m² i.v. day 1
*Repeat every 21 days

Source: Swerenton K, Jeffrey J, Stuart G, et al. Cisplatin-cyclophosphamide versus carboplatin-cyclophosphamide in advance ovarian cancer: a randomized phase III study of the National Cancer Institute of Canada Clinical Trials group. J Clin Oncol 1992;10:718–726.

CIS/TAX

Cisplatin   75 mg/m² i.v. day 2
Taxol (paclitaxel)   135 mg/m² i.v. over 24 hours day 1
*Repeat every 21 days
*Premedicate with Decadron 20 mg p.o. 6 and 12 hours prior to paclitaxel; diphenhydramine 50 mg i.v. 30–60 minutes prior to paclitaxel; and cimetidine 300 mg or ranitidine 50 mg i.v. 30–60 min prior to paclitaxel

Source: McGuire WP, Hoskins WJ, Brady MF, et al. Cyclophosphamide and cisplatin compared with paclitaxel and cisplatin in patients with stage III and stage IV ovarian cancer. N Engl J Med 1996;334:1–6.

H-CAP

Hexamethylmelamine   150 mg/m²/day p.o. days 1–14
Cyclophosphamide   350 mg/m² i.v. days 1, 8
Doxorubicin   20 mg/m² i.v. days 1, 8
Cisplatin   60 mg/m² i.v. days 1, 8
*Repeat every 4 weeks

Source: Grecco FA, Johnson DH, Hainsworth JD. A comparison of hexamethylmelamine (Altretamine), cyclophosphamide, doxorubicin, and cisplatin (H-CAP) vs. cyclophosphamide, doxorubicin, cisplatin (CAP) in advanced ovarian cancer. Cancer Treat Rev 1991;18(Suppl A):47–55.

Hexa-CAF

Hexamethylmelamine	150 mg/m^2/day p.o. days 1–14
Cyclophosphamide	150 mg/m^2/day p.o. days 1–14
Methotrexate	40 mg/m^2 i.v. days 1 and 8
5-Fluorouracil	600 mg/m^2 i.v. days 1 and 8

*Repeat every 28 days

Source: Young RC, Chabner BA, Hubbard SP. Advanced ovarian adenocarcinoma: a prospective clinical trial of melphalan (L-PAM) versus combination chemotherapy. N Engl J Med 1978; 299:1261–1266.

Hexalen

Hexamethylmelamine	65 mg/m^2/day p.o. q.i.d. days 1–14

*Repeat every 28 days

Source: Rustin G, Crawford M, Lambert J, Ledermann J, Burnett R. Phase 2 trial of oral hexalen inpatients with ovarian carcinoma relapsing in more than 6 months after initial chemotherapy. Br J Cancer 1994;69(Suppl 21):13.

PAC-I

Cisplatin (platinum)	50 mg/m^2 i.v. day 1
Doxorubicin (Adriamycin)	50 mg/m^2 i.v. day 1
Cyclophosphamide	750 mg/m^2 i.v. day 1

*Repeat every 3 weeks

Source: Ehrlich CE, Einhorn L, Williams SD, Morgan J. Chemotherapy for stage III–IV epithelial ovarian cancer with *cis*-dichlorodiammineplatinum (II), Adriamycin, and cyclophosphamide. A preliminary report. Cancer Treat Rep. 1979;63:281–288.

Taxol

Paclitaxel (Taxol)	175 mg/m^2 i.v. over 3 hours day 1

*Repeat every 21 days

*Premedicate with Decadron 20 mg p.o. 6 and 12 hours prior to paclitaxel; diphenhydramine 50 mg i.v. 30–60 minutes prior to paclitaxel; and cimetidine 300 mg or ranitidine 50 mg i.v. 30–60 min prior to paclitaxel

Source: Eisenhauer EA, ten Bokkel Huinink WW, Swenerton KD, et al. European-Canadian randomized trial of paclitaxel in relapsed ovarian cancer: high-dose versus low-dose and log versus short infusion. J Clin Oncol 1994;12:2654–2666.

HEAD AND NECK CANCER

CF

Cisplatin	100 mg/m^2 i.v. day 1
5-Fluorouracil	1000 mg/m^2/day on days 1–5 by continuous i.v. infusion

*Repeat every 21–28 days for 3 cycles

Source: Martin M, Malaurie E, Michel Langlet P, et al. A randomized prospective study of cisplatin and 5-FU as neoadjuvant chemotherapy in head and neck cancer: a final report (abstract). Proc Annu Meet Am Assoc Cancer Res 1995;14:A843.

Docetaxel

Taxotere (docetaxel)	100 mg/m^2 i.v. over 1 hr day 1

*Repeat every 21 days

Source: Dreyfuss A, Posner M, Clark J, et al. Docetaxel (TXTR): an active drug against squamous cell carcinoma of the head and neck (SCCHN) (abstract). Proc Annu Meet Am Soc Clin Oncol 1995;14:A875.

MVAC

Methotrexate	30 mg/m^2 i.v. day 1
Vinblastine	3 mg/m^2 i.v. day 1
Doxorubicin	30 mg/m^2 i.v. day 2
Cisplatin	70 mg/m^2 i.v. day 2

*Repeat every 4 weeks
*GM-CSF was given at 5 μg/kg/day s.q. days 3–14

Source: Degardin M, Cappelaere P, Caty A, Lefebvre JL. M-VAC chemotherapy (methotrexate, vinblastine, doxorubicin, cisplatin) and GM-CSF in advanced, recurrent and/or metastatic squamous cell carcinoma of head and neck (SCCHN): phase II study—preliminary results (abstract). Proc Annu Meet Am Assoc Cancer Res 1995;14:A865.

Paclitaxel

Taxol (paclitaxel)	250 mg/m^2 i.v. day 1 over 24 hours

*Repeat every 21 days
*Granulocyte colony-stimulating factor was used to prevent neutropenia
*Premedicate with Decadron 20 mg p.o. 6 and 12 hours prior to paclitaxel; diphenhydramine 50 mg i.v. 30–60 minutes prior to paclitaxel; and cimetidine 300 mg or ranitidine 50 mg i.v. 30–60 min prior to paclitaxel

Source: Forastiere AA. Current and future trials of Taxol (paclitaxel) in head and neck cancer. Ann Oncol 1994;5(Suppl 6):S51–54.

PFL

Cisplatin	100 mg/m^2 i.v. day 1
5-Fluorouracil	800 mg/m^2/day continuous i.v. infusion days 1–5
Leucovorin	50 mg/m^2/day p.o. q 6h days 1–5.

*Repeat every 21 days

Source: Vokes EE, Schilsky RL, Weichselbaum RR, et al. Cisplatin, 5-fluorouracil, and high-dose oral leucovorin for advanced head and neck cancer. Cancer 1989;63(6 Suppl):1048–1053.

VP

Navelbine (vinorelbine)	25 mg/m^2 i.v. days 1, 8
Cisplatin	80 mg/m^2 i.v. day 1

*Repeat every 3 weeks

Source: Gebbia V, Testa A, Di Gregorio C, et al. Vinorelbine plus cisplatin in recurrent or previously untreated unresectable squamous cell carcinoma of the head and neck. Am J Clin Oncol 1995; 18(4):293–296.

LEUKEMIA

Acute Lymphocytic Leukemia

ALL, (Childhood, Standard Risk)
Induction

Prednisone	40 mg/m^2/day p.o. days 1–29 (max 60 mg/day)
Vincristine	1.5 mg/m^2 i.v. days 1, 8, 15, 22 (max 2 mg/day)
L-Asparaginase	6000 IU/m^2/day 3 times weekly for 6 doses

Triple Intrathecal Therapy (TIT)   Day 0, 22, 29, 35, then every 2 months

Methotrexate	15 mg i.t.
Hydrocortisone	50 mg i.t.
Cytarabine	50 mg i.t.

CNS Consolidation

6-Mercaptopurine   75 mg/m^2/day p.o. days 29–43

Continuation

Methotrexate   1 gm/m^2 i.v. over 24 hours on week 7; at 12 hours start
                                    cytarabine
Cytarabine   1 gm/m^2 i.v. over 24 hours on weeks 7, 19, 31, 43, 55, 67
Methotrexate   20 mg/m^2 i.m. weekly, weeks 10–17, 22–29, 34–41, 46–
                                    53, 58–65, 70–156
6-Mercaptopurine   75 mg/m^2 p.o. daily, weeks 10–17, 22–29, 34–41, 46–53,
                                    58–65, 70–156
Vincristine   1.5 mg/m^2 i.v. days 1 and 8, weeks 8, 17, 25, 41, 57 (max
                                    2 mg/day)
Prednisone   40 mg/m^2 p.o. days 1–7 weeks 8, 17, 25, 41, 57 (max 60
                                    mg/day)

Source: Land VJ, Shuster JJ, Crist WM, et al. Comparison of two schedules of intermediate-dose
methotrexate and cytarabine consolidation therapy for childhood B-precursor cell acute lymphoblastic leukemia: a Pediatric Oncology Group study. J Clin Oncol 1994;12:1939–1945.

ALL, Adult

L-10

Prednisone   60 mg/m^2 p.o. daily × 35 days, then taper
Vincristine   1.5–2.0 mg/m^2 i.v. days 1, 7, 14, 21, and 28
Cyclophosphamide   600–1000 mg/m^2 i.v. day 1 (optional)
Adriamycin   20 mg/m^2 i.v. days 15, 16, and 17
Methotrexate   6 mg/m^2 i.v. days 3, 4, 9, 10, 34, and 35
Cyclophosphamide   600 mg/m^2 i.v. day 35
Adriamycin   30 mg/m^2 i.v. day 35

Source: Schauer P, Arlin ZA, Mertelsmann R, et al. Treatment of acute lymphoblastic leukemia in
adults: result of the L-10 and L-10m protocols. J Clin Oncol 1983;1:462–470.

ALL, Adult

Induction Therapy

Daunorubicin   50 mg/m^2/day i.v. days 1–3
Vincristine   2 mg/m^2 days 1, 8, 15, and 22
Prednisone   60 mg/m^2 p.o. days 1–28
L-Asparaginase   6000 units/m^2 i.m. days 17–28
If BM on day 14 has residual leukemia:
Daunorubicin   50 mg/m^2 i.v. day 15
If BM on day 28 has residual leukemia:
Daunorubicin   50 mg/m^2 i.v. days 29 and 30
Vincristine   2 mg i.v. days 29 and 36
Prednisone   60 mg/m^2 p.o. days 29–42
L-Asparaginase   6000 units/m^2 i.m. days 29–35

Consolidation Therapy

Treatment A (cycles 1, 3, 5, and 7)
Daunorubicin   50 mg/m^2 i.v. days 1 and 2
Vincristine   2 mg i.v. days 1 and 8
Prednisone   60 mg/m^2 p.o. days 1–14
L-Asparaginase   12,000 units i.m. days 2, 4, 7, 9, 11, and 14
Treatment B (cycles 2, 4, 6, 8)
Teniposide   165 mg/m^2 i.v. days 1, 4, 8, and 11
Cytarabine   300 mg/m^2 i.v. days 1, 4, 8, and 11

Treatment (cycle 9)

Methotrexate	690 mg/m^2 i.v. over 42 hours
Leucovorin	15 mg/m^2 i.v. every 6 hours × 12 doses beginning at 42 hours

Maintenance Therapy

Methotrexate	20 mg/m^2 p.o. weekly
6-Mercaptopurine	75 mg/m^2 p.o. daily

*Continue for 30 months of complete response

CNS Prophylaxis

Initiated within 1 week of CR:

Cranial irradiation	1800 cGy in 10 fractions over 12–14 days
Methotrexate	12 mg i.t. weekly for 6 weeks

Patients with CNS involvement at diagnosis:
Begin weekly intrathecal methotrexate during induction chemotherapy:

Methotrexate	12 mg i.t. weekly for 10 doses
Radiation therapy	2800 cGy

Source: Linker CA, Levitt LJ, O'Donnell M, Forman SJ, Ries CA. Treatment of adult acute lymphoblastic leukemia with intensive cyclical chemotherapy: a follow-up report. Blood 1991;78:2814–2822.

Or

Course I: Induction (4 weeks)

Cyclophosphamide*	1200 mg/m^2 i.v. day 1
Daunorubicin*	45 mg/m^2/day i.v. days 1, 2, 3
Vincristine	2 mg i.v. days 1, 8, 15, 22
Prednisone*	60 mg/m^2/day p.o. or i.v. days 1–21
L-Asparaginase	6000 IU/m^2 s.q. days 5, 8, 11, 15, 18, 22

*For patients ≥ 60 years old:

Cyclophosphamide	800 mg/m^2 i.v. day 1
Daunorubicin	30 mg/m^2 i.v. days 1, 2, 3
Prednisone	60 mg/m^2/day p.o. or i.v. days 1–7

Course II: Early intensification (4 weeks, repeat once)

Intrathecal methotrexate	15 mg i.t. day 1
Cyclophosphamide	1000 mg/m^2 i.v. day 1
6-Mercaptopurine	60 mg/m^2/day p.o. days 1–14
Cytarabine	75 mg/m^2/day s.q. days 1–4, 8–11
Vincristine	2 mg i.v. days 15, 22
L-Asparaginase	6000 IU/m^2 s.q. days 15, 18, 22, 25

Course III: CNS prophylaxis and interim maintenance (12 weeks)

Cranial irradiation	2400 cGy days 1–12
Intrathecal methotrexate	15 mg i.t. days 1, 8, 15, 22, 29
6-Mercaptopurine	60 mg/m^2/day p.o. days 1–70
Methotrexate	20 mg/m^2 p.o. days 36, 43, 50, 57, 64

Course IV: Late intensification (8 weeks)

Doxorubicin	30 mg/m^2 i.v. days 1, 8, 15
Vincristine	2 mg i.v. days 1, 8, 15
Dexamethasone	10 mg/m^2/day p.o. days 1–14
Cyclophosphamide	1000 mg/m^2 i.v. day 29
6-Thioguanine	60 mg/m^2/day p.o. days 29–42
Cytarabine	75 mg/m^2/day s.q. days 29–32, 36–39

Course V: Prolonged maintenance (until 24 months from diagnosis)

Vincristine	2 mg i.v. day 1 of every 4 weeks
Prednisone	60 mg/m^2/day p.o. days 1–5 of every 4 weeks
Methotrexate	20 mg/m^2 p.o. days 1, 8, 15, 22
6-Mercaptopurine	60 mg/m^2/day p.o. days 1–28

Source: Larson RA, Dodge RK, Burns CP, Lee EJ, Stone RM, et al. A five-drug regimen with intensive consolidation for adults with acute lymphoblastic leukemia: Cancer and Leukemia Group B study 8811. Blood 1995;85:2025–2037.

Acute Myelogenous Leukemia

7 + 3 (Ara-C/Daunorubicin)

Cytarabine	100 mg/m^2 CI i.v. days 1–7
Daunorubicin	45 mg/m^2 i.v. days 1, 2, and 3

*Bone marrow on day 14; if blasts, repeat induction; if aplastic repeat bone marrow weekly until remission or treatment failure documented
*Consolidation: repeat doses above with cytarabine for 5 days and daunorubicin for 2 days
*Consolidation begins when ANC > 1500 and platelets > 100,000

Source: Yates JW, Wallace HJ Jr, Ellison RR, Holland JF. Cytosine arabinoside and daunorubicin therapy in acute nonlymphocytic leukemia. Cancer Chemother Rep 1973;57:485–488.

7 + 3 + 3 (Ara-C/Daunorubicin)

Induction

Daunorubicin	45 mg/m^2/day i.v. days 1–3
Cytarabine	100 mg/m^2/day i.v. CI days 1–7
	2000 mg/m^2 q12h days 8–10

Consolidation
Cycles 1 and 3

Daunorubicin	60 mg/m^2 i.v. days 1, 2
Cytarabine	200 mg/m^2 i.v. CI days 1–5

Cycle 2

Cytarabine	2000 mg/m^2 q12h i.v. days 1–3
Etoposide	100 mg/m^2 i.v. days 4, 5

*Patients were offered either autologous or allogeneic bone marrow transplant in first remission

Source: Mitus J, Miller KB, Schenkein DP, et al. Improved survival for patients with acute myelogenous leukemia. J Clin Oncol 1995;13:560–569.

Ara-C/Idarubicin

Cytarabine	100 mg/m^2/day CI i.v. days 1–7
Idarubicin	12 mg/m^2/day i.v. days 1–3

Consolidation

Cytarabine	100 mg/m^2 q12h days 1–5
Idarubicin	15 mg/m^2 i.v. day 1
Thioguanine	100 mg/m^2 p.o. q12h days 1–5

Source: Vogler WR, Velez-Garcia E, Omura G, Remey M. A phase three trial comparing daunorubicin or idarubicin combined with cytosine arabinoside in acute myelogenous leukemia. Semin Oncol 1989;16(Suppl 2):21–24.

ATRA (Acute Promyelocytic Leukemia only)

All *trans*-retinoic acid	22.5 mg/m^2/day p.o. q12h until CR or for 90 days, then
Cytarabine	200 mg/m^2/day CI i.v. days 1–7
Daunorubicin	60 mg/m^2/day i.v. days 1–3

Consolidation

Cytarabine	1000 mg/m^2 i.v. q12h days 1–4
Daunorubicin	45 mg/m^2/day i.v. days 1–3

*Note: WBC may increase with ATRA therapy

Source: Fenaux P, DeLey MC, Castaigne S, et al. Effect of all *trans* retinoic acid in newly diagnosed acute promyelocytic leukemia. Results of a multicenter randomized trial. European APL 91 Group. Blood 1993;82:3241–3249.

DAT

Induction

Daunorubicin	60 mg/m^2 i.v. days 5, 6, and 7
Cytarabine (Ara-C)	100 mg/m^2 i.v. over 30 min b.i.d. × days 1–7
6-Thioguanine	100 mg/m^2 p.o. every 12 hours days 1–7

Consolidation therapy

Two cycles of cytarabine (Ara-C) and thioguanine every 12 hours for 5 days followed by a single injection of daunorubicin; consolidation cycles were given at 21-day intervals

CNS therapy

Prophylactic 2400-cGy cranial irradiation; cytarabine, 100 mg/m^2 intrathecal divided into 5 doses

Maintenance therapy

Monthly 5-day cycles of cytarabine-thioguanine alternating with a single dose of daunorubicin

Source: Gale RP, Cline MJ. High remission-induction rate in acute myeloid leukemia. Lancet 1977; 1:497–499.

DCT

Induction

Daunorubicin	60 mg/m^2 i.v. days 1–3
Cytarabine	200 mg/m^2/day on days 1–5 by continuous i.v. infusion
Thioguanine	100 mg/m^2 p.o. q12h days 1–5

Maintenance Therapy

Methotrexate	20 mg/m^2 p.o. weekly
6-Mercaptopurine	75 mg/m^2 p.o. daily

**Continue for 30 months of complete response

CNS Prophylaxis

Initiated within 1 week of CR:

1800 cGy of cranial radiation in 10 fractions over 12–14 days

6 weekly doses of 12 mg Methotrexate IT

Patients with CNS involvement at diagnosis: begin weekly intrathecal methotrexate during induction chemotherapy:

Methotrexate	12 mg i.t. weekly for 10 doses
Radiation therapy	2800 cGy

Source: Linker CA, Levitt LJ, O'Donnell M, Forman SJ, Ries CA. Treatment of adult acute lymphoblastic leukemia with intensive cyclical chemotherapy: a follow-up report. Blood 78:2814–2822.

HiDAC Consolidation

Cytarabine	3000 mg/m^2 i.v. q12h days 1, 3, 5

**Repeat every 28 days for 4 courses

**Initial induction chemotherapy was performed with 7 + 3 as above

Source: Mayer RJ, Davis RB, Schiffer CA, et al. Intensive postremission chemotherapy in adults with acute myelogenous leukemia. Cancer and Leukemia Group B. N Engl J Med 1994;331:896–903.

Chronic Lymphocytic Leukemia

2-CdA

Cladaribine   0.09 mg/kg/day CI i.v. days 1–7
*Repeat every 4 weeks

Source: Saven A, Lemon RH, Kosty M, Beutler E, Piro LD. 2-Chlorodeoxyadenosine activity in patients with untreated chronic lymphocytic leukemia. J Clin Oncol 1995;13:590–594.

Pulse CP

Chlorambucil   30 mg/m^2 p.o. day 1
Prednisone   80 mg p.o. days 1–5
*Repeat every 4 weeks

Source: Raphael B, Andersen JW, Silber R, et al. Comparison of chlorambucil and prednisone versus cyclophosphamide, vincristine, and prednisone as initial treatment for chronic lymphocytic leukemia: long-term follow-up of an Eastern Cooperative Oncology Group randomized clinical trial. J Clin Oncol 1991;9:770–776.

Fludarabine/Prednisone

Fludarabine   30 mg/m^2/day i.v. days 1–5
Prednisone   30 mg/m^2/day p.o. days 1–5
*Repeat every 4 weeks

Source: O'Brien S, Kantarjian H, Beron M, et al. Results of fludarabine and prednisone therapy in 264 patients with chronic lymphocytic leukemia with multivariate analysis-derived prognostic model for response to treatment. Blood 1993;82:1695–1700.

Chronic Myelogenous Leukemia

Hydrea

Hydrea   40 mg/kg/day p.o. daily

Source: Hehlmann R, Heimpel H, Hasford J, et al. Randomized comparison of interferon-α with busulfan and Hydrea in chronic myelogenous leukemia. Blood 1994;12:4064–4077.

Interferon

Interferon-α 5×10^6 IU/m^2 s.q. daily
*Treatment was given at maximal tolerated dose to maintain WBC of 2×10^9 to 4×10^9/L and to reach hematologic remission

Source: Hehlmann R, Heimpel H, Hasford J, et al. Randomized comparison of interferon-α with busulfan and Hydrea in chronic myelogenous leukemia. Blood 1994;12:4064–4077.

Hairy Cell Leukemia

2-CdA

Cladaribine   0.09 mg/kg/day CI i.v. days 1–7

Source: Tallman MS, Hakimian D, Variakojis D, et al. A single cycle of 2-chlorodeoxyadenosine results in complete remission in the majority of patients with hairy cell leukemia. Blood 1992; 80:2203–2209.

LUNG CANCER

Non-Small-Cell Lung Cancer

CaN

Carboplatin   300 mg/m^2 i.v. day 1
Navelbine (vinorelbine)   25 mg/m^2 i.v. day 1
*Repeat every 28 days

Source: Masotti A, Borzellino G, Zannini G, Laterza E, Ricci F, Morandini G. Efficacy and toxicity of vinorelbine-carboplatin combination in the treatment of advanced adenocarcinoma or large-cell carcinoma of the lung. Tumori 1995;81(2):112–116.

CAP

Cyclophosphamide	400 mg/m^2 i.v. day 2
Doxorubicin (Adriamycin)	40 mg/m^2 i.v. day 1
Platinum (cisplatin)	60 mg/m^2 i.v. day 1

*Repeat every 28 days

Source: Eagan RT, Frytak S, Creagan ET, Ingle JN, Kvols LK, Coles DT. Phase II trial of cyclophosphamide, Adriamycin, and *cis*-dichlorodiammineplatinum by infusion in patients with adenocarcinoma and large cell carcinoma of the lung. Cancer Treat Rep 1979;63:1589–1591.

CaT

Carboplatin	7.5 AUC i.v. day 1 after Taxol
Paclitaxel (Taxol)	175 mg/m^2 i.v. day 1 over 1 hour

*Repeat every 21 days
*Granulocyte colony-stimulating support was used
*If absolute neutrophil count > 500 and platelet > 50,000, Taxol was increased by 35 mg/m^2/cycle (max 280 mg/m^2)

Source: Langer CJ, Leighton JC, Comis RL, et al. Paclitaxel by 24- or 1-hour infusion in combination with carboplatin in advanced non-small cell lung cancer: the Fox Chase Cancer Center experience. Semin Oncol 1995;22(4 Suppl 9):18–29.

Oral CE

Etoposide	50 mg/m^2/day p.o. days 1–14
Cyclophosphamide	50 mg/m^2/day p.o. days 14–28

*Repeat every 28 days

Source: Grunberg SM, Crowley J, Livingston R, et al. Extended administration of oral etoposide and oral cyclophosphamide for the treatment of advanced non-small-cell lung cancer: a Southwest Oncology Group study. J Clin Oncol 1993;11:1598–1601.

ICE

Ifosfamide	1800 mg/m^2/day i.v. days 1–5
Mesna	1200 mg/m^2/day i.v. days 1–5
Cisplatin	20 mg/m^2/day i.v. days 1–5
Etoposide	100 mg/m^2/day i.v. days 1–5

*Repeat every 28 days

Source: Erkisi M, Doran F, Burgut R, Kocabas A. A randomized trial of two cisplatin-containing regimens in patients with stage III-B and IV non-small cell lung cancer. Lung Cancer 1995;12:237–246.

MVP

Mitomycin C	8 mg/m^2 i.v. day 1
Vinblastine	6 mg/m^2 i.v. days 1, 22
Cisplatin	50 mg/m^2 i.v. days 1, 22

*Repeat every 6 weeks

Source: Ellis PA, Nicolson MC, Tait D, Smith IE. MVP with moderate dose cisplatin: a pragmatic and effective chemotherapy for symptom relief in non-small cell lung cancer (abstract). Br J Cancer 1994;69(Suppl 21):14.

Navelbine (Vinorelbine)

Vinorelbine	25 mg/m^2 i.v. day 1 weekly

Source: Furuse K, Kubota K, Kawahara M, et al. A phase II study of vinorelbine, a new derivative of vinca alkaloid, for previously untreated advanced non-small cell lung cancer. Japan Vinorelbine Lung Cancer Study Group. Lung Cancer 1994;11(5–6):385–391.

Small Cell Lung Cancer

ACE

Doxorubicin	45 mg/m^2 i.v. day 1
Cyclophosphamide	1000 mg/m^2 i.v. day 1
Etoposide	50 mg/m^2 i.v. days 1–5

*Repeat every 21–28 days

Source: Aisner J, Whitacre M, Abrams J, Propert K. Doxorubicin, cyclophosphamide, etoposide and platinum, doxorubicin, cyclophosphamide and etoposide for small-cell carcinoma of the lung. Semin Oncol 1986;13(3 Suppl 3):54–62.

CAV

Cyclophosphamide	1000 mg/m^2 i.v. day 1
Doxorubicin (Adriamycin)	50 mg/m^2 i.v. day 1
Vincristine	1.4 mg/m^2 (max 2 mg) i.v. day 1

*Repeat every 21 days

Source: Comis RL. Clinical trials of cyclophosphamide, etoposide, and vincristine in the treatment of small-cell lung cancer. Semin Oncol 1986;13:40–44.

CAVE

Cyclophosphamide	1000 mg/m^2 i.v. day 1
Doxorubicin (Adriamycin)	50 mg/m^2 i.v. day 1
Vincristine	2 mg i.v. day 1
Etoposide	100 mg/m^2 i.v. day 1

*Repeat every 3 weeks

Source: Tummarello D, Graziano F, Mari D, et al. Small cell lung cancer (SCLC): a randomized trial of cyclophosphamide, Adriamycin, vincristine plus etoposide (CAV-E) or teniposide (CAV-T) as induction treatment, followed in complete responders by alpha-interferon or no treatment, as maintenance therapy. Anticancer Res 1994;14(5B):2221–2227.

CAV/PE

PE

Cisplatin	60 mg/m^2 i.v. day 1
Etoposide	120 mg/m^2 IVPB days 1–3

CAV

Cyclophosphamide	600 mg/m^2 i.v. day 1
Doxorubicin	50 mg/m^2 IVP day 1
Vincristine	2 mg IVP day 1
Radiation therapy	5000 cGy in 25 fractions over 5 weeks

*Alternate PE and CAV every 21 days
*Repeat cycles for a total of 6 courses

Source: Souhami RL, Rudd R, Ruiz de Elvira MC, et al. Randomized trial comparing weekly versus 3-week chemotherapy in small cell lung cancer. J Clin Oncol 1994;12:1806–1813.

CEV

Cyclophosphamide	1000 mg/m^2 i.v. day 1
Etoposide	50 mg/m^2 i.v. day 1, then
	100 mg/m^2/day p.o. days 2–5

Vincristine   1.4 mg/m^2 i.v. day 1 (max 2 mg)
*Repeat every 21 days

Source: Comis RL. Clinical trials of cyclophosphamide, etoposide, and vincristine in the treatment of small-cell lung cancer. Semin Oncol 1986;13:40–44.

CODE

Cisplatin	25 mg/m^2 i.v. day 1 weekly × 9 weeks
Vincristine	1 mg/m^2 i.v. day 1 on weeks 1, 2, 4, 6 and 8
Doxorubicin	40 mg/m^2 IVP day 1, weeks 1, 3, 5, 7, 9
Etoposide	80 mg/m^2 i.v. day 1, weeks 1, 3, 5, 7, 9
	80 mg/m^2 p.o. days 2–3 on weeks 1, 3, 5, 7, 9

Patients with CR to continue with thoracic radiotherapy

Source: Murray N, Shah A, Osoba D, et al. Intensive weekly chemotherapy for the treatment of extensive stage small cell lung cancer. J Clin Oncol 1991;9:1632–1638.

ICE

Ifosfamide	3750 mg/m^2 CI i.v. over 24 h day 1
Mesna	5065 mg/m^2 CI i.v. start 15 min before ifosfamide, continue until 12 hr after ifosfamide
Carboplatin	300 mg/m^2 i.v. day 1
Etoposide	50 mg/day p.o. × 14 days, start day 1

*Repeat every 28 days for 6 to 8 cycles

Source: Wolff AC, Ettinger DS, Neuberg D, et al. Phase II study of ifosfamide, carboplatin, and oral etoposide for extensive disease small cell lung cancer. J Clin Oncol 1995;13:1615–1622.

PACE

Cisplatin	20 mg/m^2 i.v. days 1–5
Doxorubicin	45 mg/m^2 i.v. day 1
Cyclophosphamide	800 mg/m^2 i.v. day 1
Etoposide	50 mg/m^2 i.v. days 1–5

*Repeat every 21–28 days

Source: Aisner J, Whitacre M, Abrams J, Propert K. Doxorubicin, cyclophosphamide, etoposide and platinum, doxorubicin, cyclophosphamide and etoposide for small-cell carcinoma of the lung. Semin Oncol 1986;13(3 Suppl 3):54–62.

VP16/Cisplatin

Cisplatin	25 mg/m^2/day i.v. days 1–3
Etoposide	100 mg/m^2/day i.v. days 1–3

*Repeat every 21 days

Source: Loehrer PJ Sr, Einhorn LH, Grecco FA, et al. Cisplat plus etoposide in small cell lung cancer. Semin Oncol 1988;15(Suppl 3):2–8.

LYMPHOMA

Hodgkin's Disease

ABVD

Doxorubicin (Adriamycin)	25 mg/m^2 i.v. days 1 and 15
Bleomycin	10 units/m^2 i.v. days 1 and 15
Vinblastine	6 mg/m^2 i.v. days 1 and 15
Dacarbazine (DTIC)	150 mg/m^2/day i.v. days 1–5

*Repeat every 28 days
*Dacarbazine can also be given as 375 mg/m^2 i.v. days 1 and 15

Source: Bonadonna G, Zucali R, Monfardini S, DeLena M, Uslenghi C. Combination chemotherapy of Hodgkin's disease with Adriamycin, bleomycin, vinblastine, and imidazole carboxamide vs MOPP. Cancer 1975;36:252–259.

B-CAVe

Bleomycin	5 units/m^2 i.v. days 1, 28, 35
Lomustine (CCNU)	100 mg/m^2 p.o. days 1, 28
Doxorubicin	60 mg/m^2 i.v. days 1, 28
Vinblastine	5 mg/m^2 i.v. days 1, 28

*Repeat every 8 weeks

Source: Harker GW, Kushlan P, Rosenberg SA. Combination chemotherapy for advanced Hodgkin's disease after failure of MOPP: ABVD and B-CAVe. Ann Intern Med 1984;101:440–446.

BVCPP

BCNU	100 mg/m^2 i.v. day 1
Cyclophosphamide	600 mg/m^2 i.v. day 1
Vinblastine	5 mg/m^2 i.v. day 1
Procarbazine	50 mg/m^2 day 1 p.o.; 100 mg/m^2 p.o. days 2–10
Prednisone	60 mg/m^2 p.o. days 1–10

*Repeat every 28 days

Source: Bakemeier RF, Anderson JR, Castello WM, et al. BCVPP chemotherapy for advanced Hodgkin's disease: evidence for greater duration of complete remission, greater survival and less toxicity than with a MOPP regimen. Ann Intern Med 1984;101:447–456.

ChlVPP

Chlorambucil	6 mg/m^2 p.o. days 1–14 (dose not to exceed 10 mg)
Vinblastine	6 mg/m^2 i.v. days 1–8 (max 10 mg per single dose)
Procarbazine	100 mg/m^2 p.o. days 1–14 (dose not to exceed 150 mg p.o./day)
Prednisone	40 mg p.o. days 1–14

*Repeat every 28 days

Source: Selby P, Milan PS, Meldrum M, Mansi J, et al. Chl/VPP combination chemotherapy for Hodgkin's disease: long term results. Br J Cancer 1990;62:279–285.

C-MOPP

Cyclophosphamide	650 mg/m^2 days i.v. 1 and 8
Vincristine (Oncovin)	1.4 mg/m^2 i.v. days 1 and 8
Procarbazine	100 mg/m^2 p.o. days 1 to 14
Prednisone	40 mg/m^2 p.o. days 1 to 14

*Prednisone is used only in first and fourth courses
*Repeat every 28 days

Source: DeVita VT Jr, Serpick AA, Carbone PP. Combination chemotherapy in the treatment of advanced Hodgkin's disease. Ann Intern Med 1970;73:881–895.

MOPP

Nitrogen mustard	6 mg/m^2 i.v. days 1 and 8
Vincristine (Oncovin)	1.4 mg/m^2 i.v. days 1 and 8
Procarbazine	100 mg/m^2 p.o. days 1 to 14
Prednisone	40 mg/m^2 p.o. days 1 to 14

*Prednisone in the original report was given only in cycles 1 and 4; it is now given with all cycles
*Repeat every 28 days

Source: DeVita VT Jr, Serpick AA, Carbone PP. Combination chemotherapy in the treatment of advanced Hodgkin's disease. Ann Intern Med 1970;73:881–895.

MOPP/ABV Hybrid

Mechlorethamine	6 mg/m^2 i.v. day 1
Vincristine	1.4 mg/m^2 i.v. day 1 (max 2 mg)
Procarbazine	100 mg/m^2 p.o. days 1–7
Prednisone	40 mg/m^2 p.o. days 1–14
Doxorubicin	35 mg/m^2 i.v. day 8
Bleomycin	10 units/m^2 i.v. day 8, preceded by hydrocortisone 100 mg i.v.
Vinblastine	6 mg/m^2 i.v. day 8

*Repeat every 28 days
*If intractable chemical phlebitis develops 600 mg/m^2 of i.v. cyclophosphamide is substituted.

Source: Conners JM, Klimo P. MOPP/ABV hybrid chemotherapy for advanced Hodgkin's disease. Semin Hematol 1987;24:35–40.

MVPP

Nitrogen mustard	6 mg/m^2 i.v. days 1 and 8
Vinblastine	6 mg/m^2 i.v. days 1 and 8
Procarbazine	100 mg/m^2 p.o. days 1 and 14
Prednisone	40 mg/m^2 p.o. days 1 to 14

*Repeat every 28 days

Source: Nicholson WM, Beard MEJ, Crowther D, et al. Combination chemotherapy in generalized Hodgkin's disease. Br Med J 1970;3:7–10.

MVVPP

Nitrogen mustard	0.4 mg/m^2 i.v. day 1
Vincristine	1.4 mg/m^2 i.v. days 1, 8, and 15
Vinblastine	6 mg/m^2 i.v. days 22, 29, and 36
Procarbazine	100 mg/m^2 days 22–43
Prednisone	40 mg/m^2 p.o. days 1 to 21, then taper off over 2 weeks, omit from courses 2 and 4

*Repeat every 56 days for 3 courses

Source: Prosnitz LR, Farber LR, Fischer JJ, Bertino JR, Fischer DB. Long-term remissions with combined modality therapy for advanced Hodgkin's disease. Cancer 1976;37:2826–2833.

SALVAGE TREATMENTS
ABDIC

Doxorubicin (Adriamycin)	45 mg/m^2 i.v. day 1
Bleomycin	5 U/m^2 i.v. days 1 and 5
Dacarbazine (DTIC)	200 mg/m^2 i.v. days 1–5
CCNU	50 mg/m^2 p.o. day 1
Prednisone	40 mg/m^2 p.o. days 1–5

*Repeat every 28 days

Source: Tannie N, Hagemeister F, Velasquez W, Cabanillas F. Long-term follow-up with ABDIC salvage chemotherapy of MOPP-resistant Hodgkin's disease. J Clin Oncol 1983;1:432–439.

Dexa-BEAM

Dexamethasone	8 mg every 8 hours p.o. days 1–10
Carmustine	60 mg/m^2 i.v. day 2
Etoposide	75 mg/m^2/day i.v. days 4–7
Cytarabine	100 mg/m^2/day i.v. every 12 hours days 4–7
Melphalan	20 mg/m^2 i.v. day 3

*Repeat every 28 days

Source: Pfrundschuh MG, Rueffer U, Lathan B, Schmitz N, et al. Dexa-BEAM in patients with Hodgkin's disease refractory to multi-drug chemotherapy regimens: a trial of the German Hodgkin's Disease Study Group. J Clin Oncol 1994;12:580–586.

Mini-BEAM

BCNU	60 mg/m² i.v. day 1
Etoposide	75 mg/m² i.v. days 2–5
Cytarabine	100 mg/m² i.v. q12h days 2–5
Melphalan	30 mg/m² i.v. on day 6

*Repeat every 4–6 weeks

Source: Colwill R, Crump M, Couture F, et al. Mini BEAM as salvage therapy for relapsed or refractory Hodgkin's disease before intensive therapy and autologous bone marrow transplant. J Clin Oncol 1995;13:396–402.

CBVD

CCNU	120 mg/m² p.o. day 1
Bleomycin	15 U i.v. days 1 and 22
Vinblastine	6 mg/m² i.v. days 1 and 22
Dexamethasone	3 mg/m² p.o. days 1–21

*Repeat every 6 weeks

Source: Weiss J, Van Roemeling R, Peters HD, et al. Chemotherapy in pretreated Hodgkin's disease with lomustine, bleomycin, vinblastine, and dexamethasone. Dtsch Med Wochenschr 1983; 108:1428–1432.

CEP

CCNU	80 mg/m² p.o. day 1
Etoposide (VP-16)	100 mg/m²/day p.o. days 1–5
Prednimustine	60 mg/m²/day p.o. days 1–5

*Repeat every 28 days

Source: Santoro A, Viviani S, Valaqussa P, Bontante V, Bonadonna G. CCNU, etoposide, and prednimustine (EP) in refractory Hodgkin's disease. Semin Oncol 1986;13:23–26.

CEVD

CCNU	80 mg/m² p.o. day 1
Etoposide (VP-16)	120 mg/m²/day p.o. days 1–5 and 22–26 (60 mg/m² i.v.)
Vindesine	3 mg/m² p.o. on days 1 and 22
Dexamethasone	3 mg/m²/day p.o. on days 1–8
	1.5 mg/m²/day p.o. on days 9–26

*Repeat every 42 days

Source: Pfreundschuh MG, Schoppe WD, Fuchs R, Pflüger KH, Loeffter M, Diehl V. Lomustine, etoposide, vindesine, and dexamethasone (LEVD) in Hodgkin's lymphoma refractory to cyclophosphamide, vincristine, procarbazine, and prednisone (COPP) and doxorubicin, bleomycin, vinblastine, and dacarbazine (ABVD): a multicenter trial of the German Hodgkin's Study Group. Cancer Treat Rep 1987;71:1203–1207.

EVA

Etoposide (VP-16)	200 mg/m²/day p.o. days 1–5
Vincristine	2 mg i.v. day 1
Adriamycin	50 mg/m² i.v. day 2

*Repeat every 21–28 days

Source: Richards MA, Waxman JH, Man T, et al. EVA treatment for recurrent or unresponsive Hodgkin's disease. Cancer Chemother Pharmacol 1986;18:51–53.

EVAP

Etoposide	120 mg/m^2 i.v. days 1, 8, and 15
Vinblastine	4 mg/m^2 i.v. days 1, 8, and 15
Cytarabine	30 mg/m^2 i.v. days 1, 8, and 15
Cisplatin	40 mg/m^2 i.v. days 1, 8, and 15

*Repeat every 4 weeks

Source: Longo DL. The use of chemotherapy in the treatment of Hodgkin's disease. Semin Oncol 1990;17:716–735.

PCVP

Vinblastine	3 mg/m^2 i.v. day 1 every 2 weeks
Procarbazine	70 mg/m^2 p.o. every other day
Cyclophosphamide	70 mg/m^2 p.o. every other day
Prednisone	8 mg/m^2 p.o. every other day

*Therapy lasts for 1 year

Source: Mandelli F, Cimino G, Mauro FR, et al. Prognosis and management of patients affected by multi pre-treated Hodgkin's disease. Haematologia 1986;71:205–208.

VABCD

Vinblastine	6 mg/m^2 i.v. days 1, 22
Doxorubicin (Adriamycin)	400 mg/m^2 i.v. days 1, 22
Dacarbazine	800 mg/m^2 i.v. days 1, 22
CCNU	80 mg/m^2 p.o. day 1 every 6 weeks
Bleomycin	15 units i.v. days 1, 8, 15, 22, 29, 35

*Repeat every 6 weeks

Source: Einhorn LH, Williams SD, Stevens EE, Bond WH, Chenoweth L. Treatment of MOPP-refractory Hodgkin's disease with vinblastine, doxorubicin, bleomycin, CCNU, and dacarbazine. Cancer 1983;51(8):1348–1352.

Non-Hodgkin's Lymphoma

BACOP

Bleomycin	5 units/m^2 i.v. days 15 and 22
Doxorubicin (Adriamycin)	25 mg/m^2 i.v. days 1 and 8
Cyclophosphamide	650 mg/m^2 i.v. days 1 and 8
Vincristine (Oncovin)	1.4 mg/m^2 i.v. days 1 and 8
Prednisone	60 mg/m^2/day p.o. days 15–28

*Repeat every 28 days

Source: Schein PS, DeVita VT Jr, Hubbard S. Bleomycin, Adriamycin, cyclophosphamide, vincristine, and prednisone (BACOP) combination chemotherapy in the treatment of advanced histiocytic lymphoma. Ann Intern Med 1976;85:417–422.

CHOP

Cyclophosphamide (Cytoxan)	750 mg/m^2 i.v. day 1
Doxorubicin	50 mg/m^2 i.v. day 1
Vincristine (Oncovin)	1.4 mg/m^2 i.v. day 1 (max 2 mg)
Prednisone	100 mg p.o. days 1 to 5

*Repeat every 21 days

Source: McKelvey EM, Gottlieb JA, Wilson HE. Hydroxydaunomycin (Adriamycin) combination chemotherapy in malignant lymphoma. Cancer 1976;38:1484–1493.

CHOP-BLEO

Cyclophosphamide	750 mg/m^2 i.v. day 1
Doxorubicin	50 mg/m^2 i.v. day 1

Vincristine (Oncovin)	2 mg i.v. days 1 and 5
Prednisone	100 mg p.o. days 1 to 5
Bleomycin	15 units i.v. days 1 to 5
*Repeat every 21 or 28 days	

Source: Rodriguez V, Cabanillas F, Burgess M. Combination chemotherapy (CHOP-Bleo) in advanced (non-Hodgkin's) malignant lymphoma. Blood 1977;49:325–333.

C-MOPP

Cyclophosphamide	650 mg/m^2 i.v. days 1 and 8
Vincristine (Oncovin)	1.4 mg/m^2 i.v. days 1 and 8
Procarbazine	100 mg/m^2 p.o. days 1 to 14
Prednisone	40 mg/m^2 p.o. days 1 to 14
*Repeat every 28 days	

Note: Prednisone is used only in the first and fourth cycle.

Source: DeVita VT Jr, Canellos GP, Chabner B, Schein P, Hubbard SP, Young RC. Advanced diffuse histiocytic lymphoma, a potentially curable disease. Results with combination chemotherapy. Lancet 1975;1:248–250.

COD-BLAM IV

Cyclophosphamide	350 mg/m^2 i.v. day 1 (escalated 50 mg per course)
Adriamycin	35 mg/m^2 i.v. day 1 (escalated 5 mg per course)
Vincristine	1 mg/m^2 i.v. (max 2 mg) by 24 hr infusion days 1, 2
Bleomycin	4 units/m^2 i.v. bolus day 1 then 4 units/m^2 24 hr infusion × 5 days
Dexamethasone	10 mg/m^2 i.v. daily × 5 days
Procarbazine	100 mg/m^2 daily p.o. × 5 days
*Repeat every 21 days × 4	

At cycle 5:

Adriamycin	90 mg/m^2 i.v. day 1
Vincristine	1 mg/m^2 (max 2 mg) i.v. day 1
Dexamethasone	10 mg/m^2 p.o. × 5 days

For cycles 7 through 12: (MACE)

Methotrexate	120 mg/m^2 i.v. day 1 followed by citrovorum factor
Cytarabine	250 mg/m^2 i.v. day 1
Citrovorum factor	25 mg/m^2/day q 6h for 4 doses, starting 24 hr after methotrexate
Etoposide	100 mg/m^2 i.v. day 1

Source: Coleman M, Armitage JO, Gaynor M, et al. The COP-BLAM programs: evolving chemotherapy concepts in large cell lymphoma. Semin Hematol 1988;25(Suppl 2):23–33.

COMLA

Cyclophosphamide	1500 mg/m^2 i.v. day 1
Vincristine (Oncovin)	1.4 mg/m^2 i.v. days 1, 8, and 15
Methotrexate	120 mg/m^2 i.v. days 22, 29, 36, 43, 50, 57, 64, 71
Leucovorin	25 mg/m^2 p.o. q 6h × 4 doses; start 24 hr after methotrexate
Cytarabine	300 mg/m^2 i.v. days 22, 29, 36, 43, 50, 57, 64, and 71
*Repeat every 85 days	

Source: Berd D, Cornog J, DeConti RC, Levitt M, Bertino J. Long-term remission in diffuse histiocytic lymphoma treated with combination sequential chemotherapy. Cancer 1975;35:1050–1054.

COP

Cyclophosphamide	800 mg/m^2 i.v. day 1
Vincristine	2 mg i.v. day 1
Prednisone	60 mg/m^2/day p.o. days 1–5 then taper over 3 days
*Repeat day 14	

Source: Luce JK, Gamble JF, Wilson HE. Combined cyclophosphamide, vincristine, and prednisone therapy of malignant lymphoma. Cancer 1971;28:306–317.

COPP

Cyclophosphamide	600 mg/m^2 i.v. days 1 and 8
Vincristine (Oncovin)	1.4 mg/m^2 i.v. days 1 and 8
Procarbazine	100 mg/m^2 i.v. days 1–10
Prednisone	40 mg/m^2 i.v. days 1–14
*Repeat every 28 days	

Source: Stein RS, Moran EM, Desser RK. Combination chemotherapy of lymphomas other than Hodgkin's disease. Ann Intern Med 1974;81:601–609.

CVP

Cyclophosphamide	400 mg/m^2 p.o. days 1–5
Vincristine	1.4 mg/m^2 i.v. day 1
Prednisone	100 mg/m^2 p.o. days 1–5
*Repeat every 21 days	

Source: Bagley CM Jr, DeVita VT Jr, Berard CW, Canellos GP. Advanced lymphosarcoma: intensive cyclical combination chemotherapy with cyclophosphamide, vincristine, and prednisone. Ann Intern Med 1972;76:227–234.

DHAP

Dexamethasone	40 mg/day i.v. days 1–4
Cytarabine	2000 mg/m^2 q 12h × 2 day 2
Cisplatin	100 mg/m^2 i.v. CI day 1 over 24 hours
*Repeat every 21 days	

Source: Cabanillas F, Velasquez WS, McLaughlin P. Results of recent salvage chemotherapy regimens for lymphoma and Hodgkin's disease. Semin Hematol 1988;25(Suppl 2):47–50.

DICE

Dexamethasone	10 mg i.v. q 6h days 1–14
Ifosfamide	1000 mg/m^2 (max 1750 mg) i.v. days 1–14
Cisplatin	25 mg/m^2 i.v. days 1–4
Etoposide	100 mg/m^2 i.v. days 1–4
Mesna	200 mg/m^2 i.v. 1 hr prior to ifosfamide
	900 mg/m^2 24 hr i.v. and continue for 12 hr after last dose of ifosfamide

*Repeat every 21 days

Source: Goss PE, Shepherd FA, Scott JG, et al. Dexamethasone/ifosfamide/cisplatin/etoposide (DICE) as therapy for patients with advanced refractory non-Hodgkin's lymphoma: preliminary report of a phase II study. Ann Oncol 1991;2(Suppl 1):43–46.

ESHAP

Etoposide	40 mg/m^2/day i.v. days 1–4
Methyl prednisone	500 mg/day i.v. days 1–5
High-dose cytarabine	2000 mg/m^2 i.v. day 5 after cisplatin
Cisplatin	25 mg/m^2/day CI i.v. days 1–4
*Repeat every 21–28 days	

Source: Velasquez WS, McLaughlin P, Tucker S, et al. ESHAP—an effective chemotherapy regimen in refractory and relapsing lymphoma: a 4-year follow-up study. J Clin Oncol 1994;12:1169–1176.

HOP

Hydroxydaunorubicin (Adriamycin)	80 mg/m^2 i.v. day 1
Vincristine	1.4 mg/m^2 i.v. day 1 (max 2 mg)
Prednisone	100 mg p.o. days 1 to 5

*Repeat every 21 days

Source: McKelvey EM, Gottlieb JA, Wilson HE. Hydroxydaunomycin (Adriamycin) combination chemotherapy in malignant lymphoma. Cancer 1976;38:1484–1493.

ICE

Ifosfamide	1000 mg/m^2 over 1 hr days 1 and 2 (hr 0–1)
Etoposide	150 mg/m^2 i.v. over 11 hr days 1 and 2 (hr 1–11)
Carboplatin	200 mg/m^2 i.v. over 1 hr days 1 and 2 (hr 11–12)
Etoposide	150 mg/m^2 i.v. over 11 hr days 1 and 2 (hr 12–24)
Mesna	333 mg/m^2 i.v. 30 min prior to ifosfamide, repeat at 4 and 8 hr after each dose of ifosfamide

*Repeat every 28 days

Source: Fields KK, Zorsky PE, Hiemenz JW, Kronish LE, Elfenbein GJ. Ifosfamide, carboplatin, and etoposide: a new regimen with a broad spectrum of activity. J Clin Oncol 1994;12:544–552.

IMVP-16

Ifosfamide	1000 mg/m^2 continuous i.v. infusion over 24 hr, days 1–5
Mesna uroprotection	200 mg/m^2 bolus i.v. prior to ifosfamide, then 1000 mg/m^2 continuous infusion with ifosfamide, then 200 mg/m^2 i.v. over 12 hr post ifosfamide infusion
Methotrexate	30 mg/m^2 i.v. days 3 and 10
Etoposide	100 mg/m^2 i.v. days 1–3

*Repeat every 21–28 days

Source: Cabanillas F, Burgess MA, Bodey GP, Freireich EJ. Sequential chemotherapy and late intensification for malignant lymphomas of aggressive histologic type. Am J Med 1983;74:382–388.

MACOP-B

Methotrexate	400 mg/m^2 i.v. day 1 weeks 2, 6, and 10
Leucovorin rescue	15 mg p.o. q6h × 6 (24 hr after methotrexate)
Doxorubicin	50 mg/m^2 i.v. day 1 weeks 1, 3, 5, 7, 9, and 11
Cyclophosphamide	350 mg/m^2 i.v. day 1 weeks 1, 3, 5, 7, 9, and 11
Vincristine	1.4 mg/m^2 i.v. day 1 weeks 2, 4, 6, 8, 10, and 12
Bleomycin	10 units/m^2 i.v. day 1 weeks 4, 8, and 12
Prednisone	75 mg p.o. daily; dose tapered over the last 15 days
TMP/SMX	2 tablets p.o. twice daily throughout
Ketoconazole	200 mg p.o. once daily throughout

Source: Connors JM, Klimo P. MACOP-B chemotherapy for the treatment of diffuse large cell lymphoma: 1985 update. In: Skarin AT, ed. Update on treatment for diffuse large cell lymphoma. New York: John Wiley & Sons 1986:37–43.

m-BACOD

Methotrexate	200 mg/m^2 i.v. days 8 and 15
Calcium leucovorin rescue	10 mg/m^2 p.o. every 6 hr × 8 doses beginning 24 hr after each methotrexate dose
Bleomycin	4 units/m^2 i.v. day 1

Doxorubicin	45 mg/m^2 i.v. day 1
Cyclophosphamide	600 mg/m^2 i.v. day 1
Vincristine	1 mg/m^2 i.v. day 1 (max 2 mg)
Dexamethasone	6 mg/m^2 p.o. days 1–5.

*Repeat every 21 days

Source: Shipp MA, Harrington DP, Klatt MM, et al. Identification of major prognostic subgroups of patients with large cell lymphoma treated with m-BACOD or M-BACOD. Ann Intern Med 1986; 104:757–765.

M-BACOD

Methotrexate	3000 mg/m^2 i.v. days 8 and 15 with leucovorin rescue
Calcium leucovorin rescue	10 mg/m^2 p.o. q6h × 8 doses beginning 24 hr after each methotrexate dose
Bleomycin	4 units/m^2 i.v. day 1
Doxorubicin	45 mg/m^2 i.v. day 1
Cyclophosphamide	600 mg/m^2 i.v. day 1
Vincristine	1 mg/m^2 i.v. day 1
Dexamethasone	6 mg/m^2 p.o. days 1–5

*Repeat every 21 days

Source: Shipp MA, Harrington DP, Klatt MM, et al. Identification of major prognostic subgroups of patients with large cell lymphoma treated with m-BACOD or M-BACOD. Ann Intern Med 1986; 104:757–765.

MIME

Mesna	1330 mg/m^2/day i.v. on days 1–3
	500 mg p.o. 4 hr after the ifosfamide dose days 1–3
Ifosfamide	1330 mg/m^2/day i.v. days 1–3
Mitoxantrone	8 mg/m^2 i.v. day 1
Etoposide	65 mg/m^2/day i.v. days 1–3

*Repeat every 3 weeks for 6 courses then start ESHAP regime

Source: Cabinillas F. Experience with salvage regimens at MD Anderson Hospital. Ann Oncol 1991;2(Suppl 1):31–32.

ProMACE-CytaBOM

Cyclophosphamide	650 mg/m^2 i.v. push day 1
Doxorubicin	25 mg/m^2 i.v. push day 1
Etoposide (VP-16)	120 mg/m^2 i.v. infused slowly over 60 min, day 1
Prednisone	60 mg/m^2 p.o. days 1–14
Cytarabine	300 mg/m^2 i.v. push day 8
Bleomycin	5 units/m^2 i.v. push day 8
Vincristine	1.4 mg/m^2 i.v. push day 8
Methotrexate	120 mg/m^2 i.v. push day 8
Leucovorin rescue	25 mg/m^2 p.o. q6h × 6 day 9
TMP/SMX DS	1 tab p.o. b.i.d. day 1–21

*Repeat every 21 days

Note: Regimen is administered for a minimum of six cycles and should be given for two additional cycles after a clinical complete remission; no therapy is given on day 15; the cycle restarts on day 22

Source: Fisher RI, DeVita VT Jr, Hubbard SM, et al. Randomized trial of ProMACE-MOPP vs ProMACE-CytaBOM in previously untreated, advanced stage, diffuse aggressive lymphomas (abstract). Proc Am Soc Clin Oncol 1984;3:242.

MELANOMA

Adjuvant α-Interferon

Interferon-α_{2a} 3×10^6 U s.q. three times a week
*Continue for 3 years

Source: Cascinelli N. Evaluation of efficacy of adjuvant rIFNα 2A in melanoma patients with regional node metastases (abstract). Proc Am Soc Clin Oncol 1995;15:Abstract 1296.

Or

Interferon α_{2b} 20×10^6 U/m^2 i.v. 5 times weekly for 4 weeks, then
                               10×10^6 U/m^2 s.q. 3 times weekly $\times$ 48 weeks

Source: Kirkwood JM, Strawdeman MH, Ernstoff MS, et al. Interferon alfa-2b adjuvant therapy of high risk resected cutaneous melanoma: The Eastern Cooperative Group trial EST 1684. J Clin Oncol 1996;14:7–17.

DCBT

Dacarbazine   220 mg/m^2/day i.v. days 1–3 and 22–24
Cisplatin   25 mg/m^2/day i.v. day 1–3 and 22–24
Carmustine (BCNU)   150 mg/m^2 i.v. day 1
Tamoxifen   10 mg p.o. b.i.d. starting day 4
*Repeat every 6 weeks

Source: Lattanzi SC, Tosteson T, Maurer LH, et al. Dacarbazine (D), cisplatin (C), and carmustine (B) $\pm$ tamoxifen (T), in the treatment of patients (pts) with metastatic melanoma (MM): results of 5-yr follow-up (abstract). Proc Annu Meet Am Soc Clin Oncol 1993;12:Abstract 1333.

Docetaxel (Taxotere)

Docetaxel   100 mg/m^2 i.v. day 1
*Repeat every 21 days

Source: Aamdal S, Wollf I, Kaplan S, et al. Docetaxel (Taxotere) in advanced malignant melanoma: a phase II study of the EORTC Early Clinical Trials Group. Eur J Cancer 1994;30A:1061–1064.

IFN/IL-2

α-Interferon 6×10^6 U/m^2 s.q. days 1, 4
IL-2 7.8×10^6 U/m^2 CI i.v. days 1–4
*Repeat every 14 days

Source: Kruit WH, Goey SH, Calabresi F, et al. Final report of a phase II study of interleukin 2 and interferon alpha inpatients with metastatic melanoma. Br J Cancer 1995;71:1319–1321.

VBD

Vinblastine   6 mg/m^2 i.v. days 1 and 2
Bleomycin   15 units/m^2 i.v. CI days 1–5
Cisplatin   50 mg/m^2 i.v. day 5
*Repeat every 28 days

Source: Luikart SD, Kennealey GT, Kirkwood JM. Randomized phase III trial of vinblastine, bleomycin, and *cis*-dichlorodiammine-platinum versus dacarbazine in malignant melanoma. J Clin Oncol 1984;2:164–168.

CVD

Vinblastine   1.6 mg/m^2/day i.v. days 1–5
Dacarbazine   800 mg/m^2 i.v. day 1
Cisplatin   20 mg/m^2/day i.v. days 2–5
*Repeat every 21–28 days

Source: Legha SS, Ring S, Papadopoulos N, Plager C, Chawla S, Benjamin R. A prospective evaluation of a triple-drug regimen containing cisplatin, vinblastine, and dacarbazine (CVD) for metastatic melanoma. Cancer 1989;64(10):2024–2029.

MULTIPLE MYELOMA

ABCM

Adriamycin	30 mg/m^2 i.v. day 1
Carmustine (BCNU)	30 mg/m^2 i.v. day 1
Cyclophosphamide	100 mg/m^2/day p.o. days 22–25
Melphalan	6 mg/m^2/day p.o. days 22–25

*Repeat every 6 weeks

Source: MacLennan ICM, Chapman C, Dunn J, Kelly K. Combined chemotherapy with ABCM versus melphalan for treatment of myelomatosis. Lancet 1992;339:200–205.

BCAP

Carmustine (BCNU)	50 mg/m^2 i.v. day 1
Cyclophosphamide	200 mg/m^2 i.v. day 1
Doxorubicin (Adriamycin)	20 mg/m^2 i.v. day 2
Prednisone	60 mg/day p.o. days 1–5

*Repeat every 28 days

Source: Presant CA, Klahr C. Adriamycin, 1,3-bis (2-chloroethyl)-1-nitrosurea (BCNU, NSC #409962), cyclophosphamide plus prednisone (ABC-P) in melphalan resistant multiple myeloma. Cancer 1978;42:1222–1227.

Cyclophosphamide and Prednisone

Cyclophosphamide	150–250 mg/m^2 (500 mg max) i.v. or p.o. weekly
Prednisone	100 mg p.o. alternate days

Source: Wilson K, Shelley W, Belch A, et al. Weekly cyclophosphamide and alternate-day prednisone: an effective secondary therapy in multiple myeloma. Cancer Treat Rep 1987;71:981–982.

Dexa-BEAM

Dexamethasone	8 mg every 8 hours p.o. days 1–10
Carmustine	60 mg/m^2 i.v. day 2
Etoposide	75 mg/m^2/day i.v. days 4–7
Cytarabine	100 mg/m^2/day i.v. q12h days 4–7
Melphalan	20 mg/m^2 i.v. day 3

*Repeat every 28 days

Source: Pfrundschuh MG, Rueffer U, Lathan B, Schmitz N, et al. Dexa-BEAM in patients with Hodgkin's disease refractory to multi-drug chemotherapy regimens: a trial of the German Hodgkin's Disease Study Group. J Clin Oncol 1994;12:580–586.

Dexamethasone—High-Dose

Dexamethasone	40 mg p.o. days 1–4, 9–12, 17–20

*Repeat every 28 days

Source: Alexanian R, Barlogie B, Dixon D. High-dose glucocorticoid treatment of resistant myeloma. Ann Intern Med 1986;105:8–11.

M2

Vincristine	0.03 mg/kg i.v. day 1
Carmustine (BCNU)	0.5 mg/kg i.v. day 1
Cyclophosphamide	10 mg/kg i.v. day 1
Melphalan	0.25 mg/kg p.o. for 4 days or 0.1 mg/kg for 7–10 days

| Prednisone | 1.0 mg/kg/day p.o. for 7 days, taper after 1st week, discontinue on day 21 |

*Repeat every 35 days

Source: Case DC Jr, Lee BJ III, Clarkson BD. Improved survival times in multiple myeloma treated with melphalan, prednisone, cyclophosphamide, vincristine, and BCNU: M-2 protocol. Am J Med 1977;63:897–903.

Melphalan and Prednisone

| Melphalan | 9 mg/m^2 p.o. days 1–4 |
| Prednisone | 40 mg/m^2 p.o. t.i.d. days 1–4 |

*Repeat every 4 weeks

Source: Durie BGM, Dixon B, Carter S, et al. Improved survival duration with combination chemotherapy induction for multiple myeloma: a Southwest Oncology Group study. J Clin Oncol 1986;4:1127–1137.

VAD

Vincristine	0.4 mg/day CI i.v. days 1–4
Adriamycin	9 mg/m^2/day CI i.v. days 1–4
Dexamethasone	40 mg p.o. days 1–4, 9–12, 17–20

*Repeat every 28 days

Source: Barlogie B, Smith L, Alexanian R. Effective treatment of advanced multiple myeloma refractory to alkylating agents. N Engl J Med 1984;310:1353–1356.

VMCP-VCAP

VMCP

Vincristine	1 mg/m^2 i.v. day 1 (max 1.5 mg)
Melphalan	6 mg/m^2/day p.o. days 1–4
Cyclophosphamide	125 mg/m^2/day p.o. days 1–4
Prednisone	60 mg/m^2/day p.o. days 1–4

VCAP

Vincristine	1 mg/m^2 i.v. day 1 (max 1.5 mg)
Cyclophosphamide	125 mg/m^2/day p.o. days 1–4
Adriamycin	30 mg/m^2/day i.v. day 1
Prednisone	60 mg/m^2/day p.o. days 1–4

*Alternate VMCP with VCAP every 3 weeks for 6–12 months

Source: Salmon SE, Haut A, Bonnet JD, et al. Alternating combination chemotherapy and levamisole improves survival in multiple myeloma: a Southwest Oncology Group Study. J Clin Oncol 1983;1:453–461.

VMCP-VBAP

VMCP as above

VBAP

Vincristine	1 mg/m^2 i.v. day 1 (max 1.5 mg)
Carmustine (BCNU)	30 mg/m^2 i.v. day 1
Doxorubicin	30 mg/m^2 i.v. day 1
Prednisone	60 mg/m^2 p.o. days 1–4

*Repeat VMCP every 3 weeks for 3 cycles followed by VBAP for 3 cycles

Source: Salmon SE, Haut A, Bonnet JD, et al. Alternating combination chemotherapy and levamisole improves survival in multiple myeloma: a Southwest Oncology Group study. J Clin Oncol 1983;1:453–461.

NEUROLOGIC MALIGNANCIES

BCNU

Carmustine (BCNU)   200 mg/m^2 i.v. day 1
*Repeat every 6–8 weeks

Source: Levin VA, Silver P, Hannigan J, et al. Superiority of post-radiotherapy adjuvant chemotherapy with CCNU, procarbazine, and vincristine (PCV) over BCNU for anaplastic gliomas: NGOG 6g61 final report. Int J Radiat Oncol Biol Phys 1990;18(2):321–324.

PCV

Procarbazine   60 mg/m^2/day p.o. days 1–14
CCNU   110 mg/m^2 p.o. day 1
Vincristine   1.4 mg/m^2 i.v. days 8, 29 (max 2 mg)
*Repeat every 6–8 weeks

Source: Levin VA, Silver P, Hannigan J, et al. Superiority of post-radiotherapy adjuvant chemotherapy with CCNU, procarbazine, and vincristine (PCV) over BCNU for anaplastic gliomas: NGOG 6g61 final report. Int J Radiat Oncol Biol Phys 1990;18(2):321–324.

PEDIATRIC SOLID TUMORS

Ewing's Sarcoma

Alternating cycles of VAdCA + I/E

VAdCA
Vincristine   1.5 mg/m^2 i.v. day 1
Adriamycin (Doxorubicin)   75 mg/m^2 i.v. day 1 (STOP at a cumulative dose of 375
                                             mg/m^2 and substitute actinomycin)
Actinomycin (after max Adria)   1.25 mg/m^2 i.v. day 1
Cyclophosphamide   1200 mg/m^2 i.v. day 1
Mesna   360 mg/m^2 i.v. with Cytoxan, then at hr 1–4 by CI i.v.,
                                             then at hr 4, 7, 10

I/E
Ifosfamide   1800 mg/m^2/day i.v. days 1–5
Etoposide   100 mg/m^2/day i.v. days 1–5
Mesna   400 mg/m^2/day with ifosfamide, immediately after, and
                                             then q2h × 7 doses
*Repeat alternate cycles of VAdCA and IE every 3 weeks

Source: Grier H, Krailo M, Link M, et al. Improved outcome in nonmetastatic Ewing's sarcoma (EWS) and PNET of bone with the addition of ifosfamide (I) and etoposide (E) to vincristine (V), Adriamycin (Ad), cyclophosphamide (C), and actinomycin (A): a Children's Cancer Group (CCG) and Pediatric Oncology Group (POG) report (abstract). Proc Annu Meet Am Soc Clin Oncol 1994; 13:A1443.

Neuroblastoma

AC

Doxorubicin (Adriamycin)   35 mg/m^2 i.v. day 8
Cyclophosphamide   150 mg/m^2/day p.o. days 1–7
*Repeat every 21–28 days for 5 courses

Source: Nitschke R, Smith EI, Altshuler G, et al. Postoperative treatment of nonmetastatic visible residual neuroblastoma: a Pediatric Oncology Group study. J Clin Oncol 1991;9:1181–1188.

Cisplatin and Tenoposide

Cisplatin	90 mg/m^2 i.v. day 1
Tenoposide	100 mg/m^2 i.v. day 3
*Repeat every 21–28 days	

Source: Castleberry RP, Schuster JJ, Altshuler G, et al. Infants with neuroblastoma and regional lymph node metastases have a favorable outlook after limited postoperative chemotherapy: a Pediatric Oncology Group study. J Clin Oncol 1992;10:1299–1304.

SARCOMA

Osteosarcoma

Weekly High-Dose Methotrexate and Doxorubicin

HDMTX

Vincristine	2.0 mg/m^2 i.v. (2 mg max) day 1
Methotrexate	7500 mg/m^2 i.v. day 1 (30 min after VCR)
Calcium leucovorin	15 mg/m^2 i.v. q3h × 8 doses (2 hr after MTX) then 15 mg/m^2 p.o. q6h × 8 doses

HDMTX-Dox

HDMTX as above plus

Doxorubicin	75 mg/m^2 i.v. CI over 72 hr on day 6 (450 mg/m^2 max)

*HDMTX q week × 4 then HDMTX-Dox q 3 weeks × 6 then HDMTX q week × 4 then HDMTX-Dox q 3 weeks × 6 then HDMTX q week × 4

Source: Goorin AM, Perez-Atayde A, Gebhardt M, et al. Weekly high-dose methotrexate and doxorubicin for osteosarcoma: the Dana-Farber Cancer Institute/the Children's Hospital—Study III. J Clin Oncol 1987;5(8):1178–1184.

T-10

Preoperative

Methotrexate	8–12 g/m^2 i.v. weekly × 4
Calcium leucovorin rescue	15 mg/m^2 i.v. or p.o. q6h for at least 10 doses beginning 24 hr after MTX; monitor MTX levels

Postresection (BCD)

Bleomycin	15 units/m^2 i.v. days 1, 2
Cyclophosphamide	600 mg/m^2 i.v. days 1, 2
Actinomycin D	600 mcg/m^2 i.v. days 1, 2

then

Methotrexate	8–12 g/m^2 i.v. day 1 at weeks 9, 10, 14, 15
Calcium leucovorin rescue	15 mg/m^2 i.v. or p.o. q6h for at least 10 doses beginning 24 hr after MTX; monitor MTX levels
Doxorubicin	30 mg/m^2 i.v. days 1, 2 week 11

Maintenance (3 weeks later):
Grade 1–2 with Response

Doxorubicin	30 mg/m^2 i.v. days 1, 22
Cisplatin	120 mg/m^2 i.v. days 1, 22
BCD as above	Day 42

*Repeat maintenance cycle for total of 3 courses

Grade 3–4

Bleomycin	15 units/m^2 i.v. days 1, 2
Cyclophosphamide	600 mg/m^2 i.v. days 1, 2
Actinomycin D	600 μg/m^2 i.v. days 1, 2

then

Methotrexate	8–12 g/m^2 i.v. day 1 at weeks 9, 10, 14, 15
Calcium leucovorin rescue	15 mg/m^2 i.v. or p.o. q6h for at least 10 doses beginning 24 hr after MTX; monitor MTX levels
Doxorubicin	30 mg/m^2 i.v. days 1, 2 week 11

*Repeat maintenance for 4 courses

Source: Rosen G, Caparros B, Huvos A, et al. Preoperative chemotherapy for osteogenic sarcoma: selection of postoperative adjuvant chemotherapy based on the response of the primary tumor to preoperative chemotherapy. Cancer 1982;49:1221–1230.

Soft Tissue Sarcomas

ADIC

Doxorubicin (Adriamycin)	90 mg/m^2 i.v. CI over 96 hours
Dacarbazine	900 mg/m^2 i.v. CI over 96 hours

*Repeat every 21 days

Source: Zalupski M, Metch B, Balcerzak S, et al. Phase III comparison of doxorubicin and dacarbazine given by bolus versus infusion in patients with soft-tissue sarcomas: a Southwest Oncology Group Study. J Natl Cancer Inst 1991;83:920–926.

CYVADIC

Cyclophosphamide	500 mg/m^2 i.v. day 1
Vincristine	1.4 mg/m^2 i.v. day 1
Doxorubicin	50 mg/m^2 i.v. day 1
Dacarbazine	400 mg/m^2/day i.v. days 1–3

*Repeat every 21 days

Source: Bramwell V, Rouesse J, Steward W, et al. Adjuvant CYVADIC chemotherapy for adult soft tissue sarcoma—reduced local recurrence but no improvement in survival: a study of the European Organization for Research and Treatment of Cancer Soft Tissue and Bone Sarcoma Group. J Clin Oncol 1994;12(6):1137–1149.

Doxorubicin

Doxorubicin	75 mg/m^2 i.v. day 1

Repeat every 21 days

Source: Santoro A, Tursz T, Mouridsen H, et al. Doxorubicin versus CYVADIC versus doxorubicin plus ifosfamide in first-line treatment of advanced soft tissue sarcomas: a randomized study of the European Organization for Research and Treatment of Cancer Soft Tissue and Bone Sarcoma Group. J Clin Oncol 1995;13(7):1537–1545.

MAID

Mesna	2500 mg/m^2/day i.v. CI days 1–4
Doxorubicin (Adriamycin)	20 mg/m^2/day i.v. days 1–3
Ifosfamide	2500 mg/m^2/day i.v. days 1–3
DTIC	300 mg/m^2/day i.v. days 1–3

*Repeat every 21 days

Source: Elias AB, Ryan L, Aisner J, Antman KH. Mesna, ifosfamide, dacarbazine (MAID) regimen for adults with advanced sarcoma. Semin Oncol 1990;17(2 Suppl 4):41–49.

Pulse VAC

Vincristine	2 mg/m^2 i.v. weekly × 12 (max 2 mg/week)
Actinomycin D	0.075 mg/kg i.v. CI over 5 days every 3 months × 5 courses (max 0.5 mg/day)
Cyclophosphamide	10 mg/kg/day for 7 days i.v. or p.o. every 6 weeks

Source: Wilbur JR, Suton WW, Sullivan MD, Gottlieb J. Chemotherapy of sarcomas. Cancer 1975; 36:765–769.

Standard VAC

Vincristine	2 mg/m² i.v. weekly × 12 (max 2 mg/week)
Actinomycin D	0.075 mg/kg i.v. CI over 5 days every 3 months × 5 courses (max 0.5 mg/day)
Cyclophosphamide	2.5 mg/kg/day p.o. × 2 years

Source: Wilbur JR, Suton WW, Sullivan MD, Gottlieb J. Chemotherapy of sarcomas. Cancer 1975; 36:765–769.

Section Five

Drug Administration

45

Central Venous Access for Chemotherapy

Steven B. Standiford

HISTORY

The development of reliable techniques for access to the bloodstream has changed the face of oncology practice. Previously, aggressive therapy was accompanied by the discomforts of repeated venipuncture and by the risks of extravasation of vesicants, sclerosis of peripheral veins, and at times inability to establish needed venous access. Although first described in 1956 (1), the use of the central veins for the infusion of fluids did not become popularized until the development of total parenteral nutrition by Dudrick in 1968 (2). Broviac, in 1973, developed a silicone catheter that was tunneled from the site of insertion into the central circulation to a distant site (3). This catheter also had a felt cuff that was placed within this subcutaneous tunnel; the ingrowth of fibrous tissue into the felt cuff served to isolate potential infection from the skin from access into the bloodstream. This catheter was initially used primarily for intravenous nutrition. In 1979, Hickman made modifications to this catheter, allowing a larger lumen, and described its use in patients undergoing bone marrow transplantation (4). Use of these devices in oncology patients with venous access problems became more common.

These devices did not gain universal acceptance because of the inconvenience associated with an external catheter, with the need for daily flushing, frequent dressing changes, and some activity restrictions. In 1982, Niedenhuber described a modification of access to the central circulation, in which the entire device was implanted under the skin and accessed by direct puncture of a silicone diaphragm (5). Once the insertion site had healed, no dressing was needed, intermittent puncture of the diaphragm allowed the device to be accessed only when needed, and cancer patients were able to have a convenient method for receiving fluids, blood products, and medications, with no limitation on daily activities. Modifications continue to be developed in devices of this sort, allowing multiple lumens for simultaneous administration of incompatible fluids, and different shapes providing greater ease of cannulation and greater patient comfort. These advances have removed the difficulties and discomforts of venipuncture from the problems endured by cancer patients and have greatly improved quality of life for those patients.

PATIENT SELECTION

Every cancer patient who will receive intravenous chemotherapy, fluids, frequent blood products, or intravenous medications or who will require frequent blood tests to follow disease and potential toxicities of therapy should be evaluated to determine if insertion of a venous access device would be appropriate or beneficial.

Not every patient shows sufficient need. Some, undergoing therapies of short duration with few anticipated complications, will be well served by intermittent peripheral venipuncture. The potential need for an access device should be determined very early in the course of evaluation and initial treatment. Although these devices are easily inserted in the outpatient setting with local anesthesia, thought should be given to the potential need for such a device if a patient is undergoing a diagnostic or therapeutic procedure under general or local anesthesia. Patient comfort and expense can be minimized by a single trip to the operating room where several procedures are performed. Factors to be considered to determine whether a patient may benefit from insertion of such a device are listed in Table 45.1.

A chemotherapy course that extends over several months is often complicated by the development of limited peripheral veins for access, especially if sclerosing agents are used. Similarly, treatment regimens that include many individual days of therapy are better tolerated with placement of a reliable access device. Highly toxic regimens with anticipated neutropenia, anemia, and thrombocytopenia and risk of infections requiring frequent blood testing, blood and platelet transfusions, and systemic antibiotic administration, will certainly be more tolerable for the patient if frequent, and often uncomfortable, venipuncture is not an anticipated event. Not all patients have large superficial veins that lend themselves to easy venipuncture. In the pediatric population, chemotherapy courses are frequently prolonged; this, coupled with the anxiety associated with "needles" in children, makes consideration of a venous access device essential in this age group. Even in the adult population, some patients are sufficiently uncomfortable undergoing venipuncture that a single event to place an access device is far preferable to the anxiety over each planned treatment or blood test.

I consider placement of a venous access device to be essential at the time of diagnosis in a new acute leukemic patient. No matter how healthy the patient may appear at presentation, the large number of medications, fluids, and blood products administered, as well as the number of blood tests required, dictates the obvious need for such a device. Concerns over thrombocytopenia at presentation should not prevent proceeding with insertion under the

cover of platelet transfusions if needed. Thrombocytopenia can be anticipated to worsen during initial therapy and may make placement of a device later in the treatment course riskier.

Patients who will require only a short course of intermittent infusion, with low anticipated fluid requirements, who can be anticipated to have only short-lived neutropenia, can easily be managed by peripheral intravenous catheter use and direct antecubital venipuncture. Adjuvant therapy of breast cancer using only four cycles of doxorubicin and cyclophosphamide on a 3-week schedule will require only four infusion sessions over 9 weeks. Unless other factors are involved, the discomfort and cost of placing and removing a device will not be offset by the convenience of having a device used so little. Breast cancer patients who will receive other agents and schedules, such as six cycles of cyclophosphamide, 5-fluorouracil, and either methotrexate or doxorubicin, administered on days 1 and 8 of a 4-week cycle, will require 12 sessions of drug infusion, with associated more frequent blood drawing, and are good candidates for placement of a long-term device. Patients with lung cancer or colorectal cancer can similarly be anticipated to require enough infusion sessions and blood tests to be well served by placement of a device.

At the University of Missouri/Ellis Fischel Cancer Center, a standard evaluation is performed for every consultation received by the Division of Surgical Oncology, to assess what device would be most appropriate. The consultation form used in this evaluation is shown in Figure 45.1.

DEVICE OVERVIEW

Table 45.2 describes the most commonly used types of venous access devices. Each is available from a variety of manufacturers under differing brand names, with potential advantages and disadvantages over others of the same type. Selection of a particular model is usually dictated by surgeon preference, device availability, and cost. Photographs of various devices included here are meant to demonstrate the basic characteristics of each class of device, rather than to point out specific features unique to that manufacturer's device.

Peripherally inserted central catheters (PICC lines) (Fig. 45.2) are small polyethylene or silicone catheters inserted through an antecubital or arm vein (usually the basilic vein) and threaded into the central circulation. The catheter is measured and trimmed to an appropriate length

Table 45.1. Considerations in Determining the Need for a Venous Access Device

Planned duration of treatment

Planned agents, especially vesicant use

Planned treatment schedule (continuous, daily intermittent, or less frequent drug administration)

Need for support with fluids, blood products, antibiotics, and other medications

Anticipated frequency of blood tests

Status of peripheral venipuncture sites

Tolerance of venipunctures—especially in the pediatric population, but also in many adults

Diagnosis

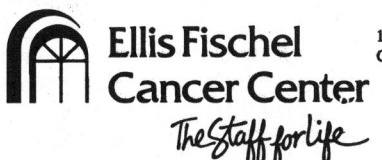

115 Business Loop 70 West
Columbia, MO 65203-3299

**Request for Venous Access Device
Consultation/Referral**

TO: DIVISION OF SURGICAL ONCOLOGY   DATE:

CONSULT NEEDED WITHIN _____day(s)   CLINIC DATE/TIME_____
                                                     INPATIENT? ROOM #_____
PATIENT DIAGNOSIS _____

PERTINENT CLINICAL DATA (please include specific regimen planned):

INSERTION DATE PREFERENCE:

PRIOR DEVICE?   PRIOR PROBLEMS?

HAS PATIENT, OR WILL PATIENT, RECEIVE RADIATION TO THE CHEST?

VASCULAR ACCESS DEVICE PREFERENCE:

    PICC   ___ single lumen   Implanted Port ___ single
                  ___ double lumen   ___ dual

    Percutaneous ___ single lumen   Tunnelled   ___ single
                  ___ double lumen   ___ dual
                  ___ triple lumen   ___ triple

    No preference ___

SURGEON PREFERENCE?   ___ yes Dr. _____
                        ___ no

Requesting Resident Physician _____Requesting Attending Physician_____
****
CONSULTANT RECOMMENDATION: _____

_____

_____

PLAN:_____

_____

_____

    LEVEL 1   LEVEL II   LEVEL III   LEVEL IV   LEVEL V

Date_____   Time_____   _____
                              Consultant Signature

Figure 45.1.   Venous access device consultation form—University of Missouri/Ellis Fischel Cancer Center.

prior to insertion. The connecting hub and a short length of catheter exit along the arm and are covered with a protective dressing. These devices are convenient for short-term courses of treatment, either by intermittent or continuous infusion. They do, however, require a fair amount of maintenance by the patient or caregivers, including daily or twice-daily flushes, weekly dressings, and some protection of the arm and catheter to prevent excessive motion or breakage. These devices can be inserted at the bedside or in the clinic and are the least expensive to buy and insert.

Peripherally inserted implantable ports use a silicone catheter similar to a PICC line, again inserted from a peripheral vein in the arm and threaded into the central circulation. Rather than having a catheter exit the skin, a small incision is made, and a small subcutaneous pocket is fashioned to hold a small port with a silicone diaphragm. Once healed, the device needs no special dressing except when cannulated. Flushes are needed monthly in an unused device, and some limitation of arm motion is frequently needed as well. As with peripherally inserted central catheters, these devices can be inserted at the bedside or in the clinic, with minimal local anesthesia, and are proving to be quite low in cost.

Both peripherally inserted devices are useful for intermittent or continuous infusions; however, the small lumen size of the catheter precludes using the devices for blood drawing. The commonest problems with the devices are occlusion (19%) (6); superficial phlebitis along the catheter (11%) (7), not always requiring device removal; and inability to thread the catheter to an appropriate central vein (6%) (6). The cost of these devices and their insertion is lower than that for direct central access devices.

Nontunneled central venous catheters (Fig.

Table 45.2. Types of Central Venous Access Devices

Peripherally inserted central catheter (PICC line)
Peripherally inserted implantable port
Nontunneled central venous catheter
Tunneled central venous catheter
Implantable central venous access port

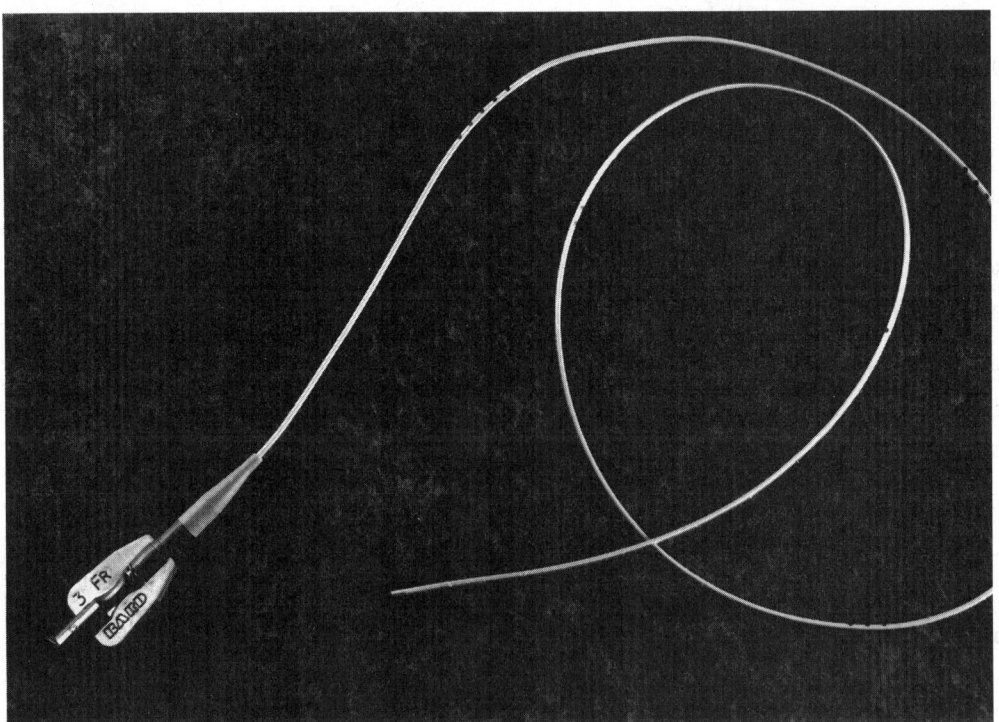

Figure 45.2.   Peripherally inserted central catheter (PICC). (Photograph courtesy of Bard Access Systems, Salt Lake City, UT.)

45.3), usually inserted percutaneously via the subclavian, internal jugular, or external jugular vein, have advantages and disadvantages similar to those of PICC lines in terms of durability, maintenance needs, and ease of insertion in a bedside or clinic setting. However, the shorter, larger-diameter catheter frequently allows blood drawing through it, and the placement of the device exiting in the low neck or in the infraclavicular space is often more comfortable for the patient requiring longer-term access. Insertion carries a small risk of pneumothorax, hemothorax, thoracic duct injury, arterial puncture, and rarely malposition of the catheter. Risk of subsequent dislodgment of the catheter is always a concern, requiring careful dressing techniques to maintain the catheter in place.

Tunneled central venous catheters (Fig. 45.4) are inserted either percutaneously into the subclavian vein, by direct cutdown into the cephalic vein at the shoulder or the facial vein in the neck, or by either cutdown or percutaneous approach into the internal or external jugular vein. Use of any of these devices through alternate routes, such as groin or leg veins, is discussed below. The Dacron felt cuff on these catheters is placed subcutaneously, within the tunnel from insertion site to vein entry. The fibrous ingrowth into this cuff prevents outside infection from reaching the bloodstream and also prevents accidental dislodgment of the catheter. These devices can be used for drawing blood as well as for infusion of medication, fluids, and blood products. Requirements for daily flushing are similar to those with any of the external catheters; however, an exit site dressing is not required after several weeks because of the fibrous ingrowth into the cuff.

Implantable subcutaneous venous access ports are the most convenient for the patient; however, insertion requires the most intervention (Fig. 45.5). The catheter is connected to a port that is buried in the subcutaneous space of the trunk. No dressing is required, except when the device is cannulated, and monthly flushing of an unused device is all that is required. The device is cannulated percutaneously by a noncoring needle placed through the silicone diaphragm.

DEVICE SELECTION

The single-lumen implantable venous access port is the mainstay of outpatient chemotherapy. The convenience of a device located over the trunk rather than in the arm, with minimal main-

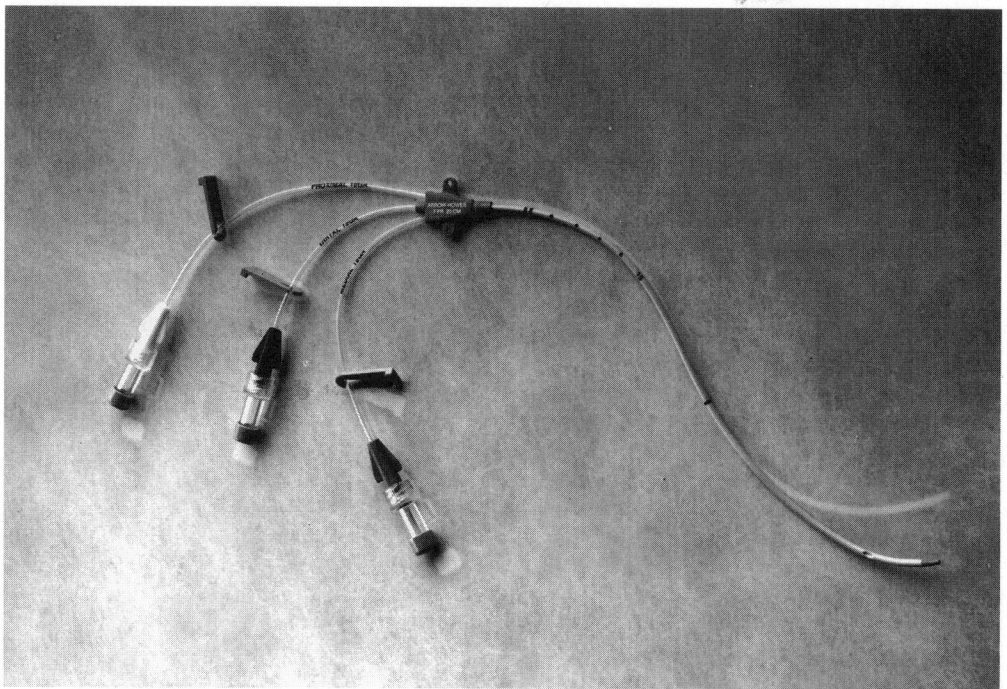

Figure 45.3.   Triple-lumen central venous catheter. (Photograph courtesy of Arrow International, Inc., Reading, PA.)

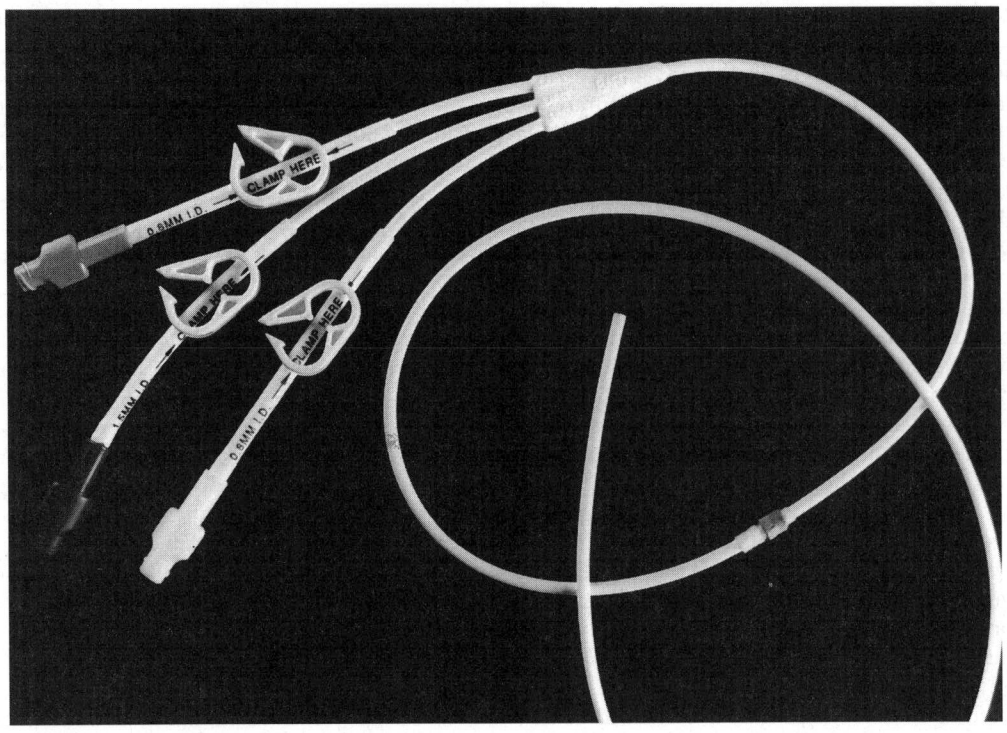

Figure 45.4.   Tunneled central venous catheter. (Photograph courtesy of Bard Access Systems, Salt Lake City, UT.)

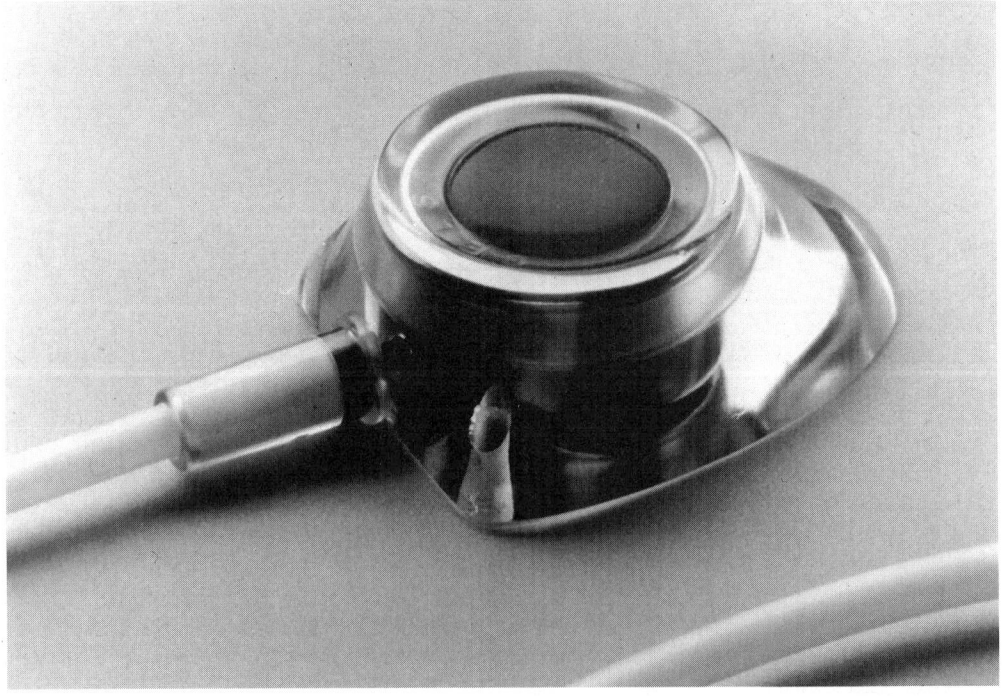

Figure 45.5.   Subcutaneous venous access port. (Photograph courtesy of B. Braun Medical, Inc., Bethlehem, PA.)

tenance requirements, which can be easily and reliably inserted and remain relatively inconspicuous is apparent. Removal of these devices is not complicated once planned therapies are completed, or they may be left in place for ease of blood drawing at follow-up visits. It is perhaps easier to discuss the situations in which another device may better serve the patient's needs.

Patients who will be receiving long-term continuous infusions, such as total parenteral nutrition or long low-dose 5-fluorouracil, often are best managed with a tunneled central venous catheter. These avoid the need to have a noncoring needle continuously in the device, which can lead to skin irritation and may eliminate the advantage of having a device that is buried below the skin and is intended to have no exposure to the outside world. In addition, patients expected to self-administer medications and fluids at home may benefit from the ease of an external hub connection.

Recent reviews from the M. D. Anderson Cancer Center have indicated that silicone nontunneled percutaneous catheters can be satisfactorily used for intermittent infusional therapy, with a low incidence of device failure, low rates of infection, and good patient acceptance (8). Economic analysis comparing the use of these devices with use of implanted ports showed the nontunneled catheter to be more cost-effective for at least 6 months, beyond which time the routine maintenance expenses of the catheters begin to exceed the higher initial insertion costs of the implantable ports. Patient convenience and acceptance of an external catheter, however, must be considered. Unfortunately, other cost issues must be considered as well. The cost of implanting a port may be associated with lower out-of-pocket expenses than percutaneous catheters, as some third-party payers do not reimburse for the cost of the dressings and flush solutions.

Shorter-term needs are often well served by a PICC line, provided that there is not a need for frequent venipuncture for blood studies. The peripherally inserted implantable port may serve as an alternative to avoid an external catheter or for slightly longer planned periods of therapy.

Dexterity, visual impairments, and support availability are additional factors to consider in device selection. Maintenance of external catheters, whether tunneled or not, may be compromised if visual or dexterity impairments preclude seeing or manipulating syringes and tubing safely and easily.

Infirm patients with limited home support may also be better served by an implantable device, as there is not a need for training a caregiver in daily maintenance routines. Mentally impaired patients, whether from degenerative diseases or psychiatric illness, must be assessed to determine if the catheter is at risk for dislodgment or damage because of an inability to understand or recall the safety issues associated with external catheters.

As stated above, acute leukemia is an indication for insertion of a tunneled catheter, usually one with at least two lumens. This group benefits so much from reliable access that such a catheter should be inserted as soon as possible after diagnosis. The ease of removal of one of these devices is also a consideration, as these patients will often develop refractory infections, which may be related to device colonization and may require device removal to make or exclude this diagnosis.

SITE SELECTION

After determination of the need for long-term venous access and selection of an appropriate device, the proposed site of insertion must be chosen. James (7) demonstrated that when placing peripherally inserted central catheters, the greatest success with placement into the central circulation occurred when the left cephalic vein was used. The more gentle curve that the left subclavian vein follows as it joins the internal jugular vein and then the superior vena cava probably allows the most direct route for these small catheters. Consideration of the patient's dominant hand is also needed; the discomfort from having a device on the more active (dominant) side may decrease tolerance of the device.

Central devices (tunneled or nontunneled catheters and venous access ports) can be inserted either percutaneously or via direct venous cutdown. Potential sites for either technique are listed in Table 45.3.

When inserting any of the central devices, site selection is again influenced by the dominant hand. Professions and hobbies should also be considered; a hunter may prefer to have the device situated on the side opposite where a gun butt rests while shooting. Prior surgery or radiotherapy in the area must also be considered. It is preferable, although not mandatory, to use the contralateral side following mastectomy or breast conservation surgery. Radiation fields, from breast cancer, lung cancer, head and neck

Table 45.3. Sites and Approaches for Central Venous Access

Percutaneous	Direct cutdown	Either
Subclavian vein, infraclavicular approach	Cephalic vein (deltopectoral groove)	Internal jugular vein
Subclavian vein, supraclavicular approach	Facial vein	External jugular vein
	Saphenous vein	Femoral vein
	Other retroperitoneal or intrathoracic sites	

cancer, or mediastinal tumors, should be avoided, if possible, because of the higher risk of wound problems in a radiated field.

The experience of the surgeon is also important. Many surgeons are most comfortable with the percutaneous infraclavicular approach to the subclavian vein. A surgeon should only place a device through an approach that he or she is comfortable with.

Comorbid conditions must be considered as well; a patient who is unable to lie flat because of dyspnea is not a candidate for any of the percutaneous approaches to catheter insertion and must be managed by direct venous cutdown. Prior catheterization by any site does not preclude using that site again; however, a site that had a satisfactory device which was removed after completion of planned therapies is preferable to a site that was complicated by thrombosis or catheter malposition.

Most commonly, vein branches leading to the superior vena cava are chosen. There has been historic concern that infradiaphragmatic approaches will be associated with an increased risk of thrombosis or device failure. Willard (9) has demonstrated that there is no increased risk of device occlusion, venous thrombosis, or infection when alternate routes such as the proximal saphenous vein, femoral vein, or gonadal vein are used. However, the subcutaneous port, or the exit site of the catheter, will be in a less comfortable location when an infradiaphragmatic entry site is used, as pants, belts, and undergarments may rub at the site, or the site may be in constant motion near the proximal thigh.

USUAL APPROACHES

The approach to the vein site for insertion of tunneled catheters, nontunneled catheters, or implantable central venous access ports, is quite similar. Insertion of these devices differs in how the exit site or implantation site is approached. These devices are usually inserted in a minor surgery room, although nontunneled catheters are easily inserted at the bedside with appropriate sterile barrier precautions. The need for monitoring is at the discretion of the surgeon inserting the device and involves whether intravenous sedation is used. Routine sterile skin preparation and surgical draping are performed, with a wide enough field selected to allow access to the anterior chest, infraclavicular region, deltopectoral groove, and up to the midneck. With this wide field available, one insertion site can be abandoned and another approached without a need for redraping. Local infiltration anesthesia is used. Landmarks are identified, and subclavian or internal jugular vein venipuncture is performed. A guide wire is passed through the needle, and a small stab wound is made at the wire insertion site.

When placing an implantable port, a transverse incision is made on the anterior chest wall at a satisfactory location for placement. Consideration of necklines of clothing and position of brassiere straps helps choose an appropriate site. A subcutaneous pocket is fashioned. Ideally, in a thin patient, this plane is just above the pectoralis major fascia; however, the plane may need to be more superficial in obese or large-breasted patients. The port is flushed with heparinized saline solution (100 units/mL) and placed into the subcutaneous pocket. Tacking sutures may be used to anchor the port to the underlying tissues to prevent flipping or motion of the port. A subcutaneous tunnel is created between the port site and the site of insertion of the guide wire, by use of a hemostat, a small probe, or one of the tunneling devices often supplied with the access port. The catheter is brought through this tunnel and exits adjacent to the guide wire. The catheter length is then measured. If the catheter is placed above the skin, following a straight line from the insertion site to the sternal notch and then to the angle of Louis, and cut at that length, a final catheter position low in the superior vena cava can be anticipated. A two-piece dilator and peel-away sheath is passed over the guide wire, and the wire and dilator are removed. The catheter is inserted through the sheath into the central circulation and stabilized while an assistant peels apart the sheath and removes it. The port is aspirated until good blood return is obtained and then reflushed with at least 5 mL of heparinized saline. Some surgeons will check the guide wire and catheter positions with intraoperative fluoroscopy. I find that with experience, correct catheter position can be anticipated, and confirmation of satisfactory placement at this time by a portable chest x-ray usually suffices. Placement at the level of the low superior vena cava or into the right atrium is preferred, to prevent venous thrombosis. Stanislav et al. reported no thromboses in 50 patients with catheters in the right atrium or low superior vena cava; 8 of 63 catheters above this level led to venous thrombosis (10). The wounds are closed with subcuticular absorbable suture. A chest x-ray is performed to confirm catheter position and to look for complications of insertion such as pneumothorax, hemothorax, or extrapleural hematoma. A noncoring needle may be left in place through the skin at this time, if use of the device for chemotherapy is planned for that day.

When inserting a tunneled catheter, a short stab wound is made at the planned site of catheter exit. In addition to cosmetic and comfort considerations as described for port sites, the exit site of an external catheter must be located to facilitate care of the catheter and site by the patient. A subcutaneous tunnel is fashioned by use of a hemostat, probe, or tunneling device, and the catheter is brought to the guide wire insertion site. The Dacron cuff should be placed 3 cm from the exit site. The catheter is then measured, trimmed, and inserted into the central circulation as described above. Satisfactory placement is confirmed with a radiologic study. Aspiration of blood from each lumen of the catheter confirms patency and adequate function, and each lumen is flushed with heparinized saline solution. The insertion site is closed with subcuticular absorbable suture, securing the catheter to the exit site with a nylon suture to stabilize the catheter until fibrous growth into the Dacron cuff protects from dislodgment; application of an occlusive dressing completes the procedure.

Nontunneled catheters do not require use of a two-piece sheath for insertion into the circulation. A dilator, supplied with the catheter, is passed over the guide wire to open the tract and then removed, leaving the guide wire in situ. The catheter is trimmed to an appropriate length and passed over the guide wire, taking care to back the guide wire out of the vein so that its end extends out the end of the catheter before passing the catheter forward. The catheter is advanced and the guide wire removed. Patency is confirmed by aspiration and flushing, and the catheter is secured to the skin with a nylon suture. An occlusive dressing is applied, and the position of the catheter confirmed with a chest x-ray.

UNUSUAL APPROACHES

At times, device placement through the usual routes via veins of the upper chest or neck is not possible. Superior vena caval thrombosis, extensive chest wall or neck disease, or planned surgery in the region may preclude using any approach leading to catheter position in the superior vena cava. The approach to the central circulation is then mandated through less commonly used veins of the retroperitoneum or lower extremity. Cutdown under local anesthesia of the saphenous vein in the proximal thigh, with the catheter threaded into the inferior vena cava, is an easy and safe approach (11). When using an implanted port or a tunneled catheter, the device can either be placed on the lower abdominal wall or in the lateral thigh. The inconvenience of these placement sites is the major disadvantage to this approach to a consistent and reliable vein for access. Less commonly, a direct percutaneous puncture can be made to the femoral vein (9). This site is commonly 2 to 3 cm higher than a saphenous vein approach and is subject to kinking by thigh flexion. An alternate route using the inferior epigastric vein, approached just before confluence with the external iliac vein, as described by Mahear (12), has the advantage of keeping the catheter above the inguinal ligament, reducing risk of catheter kinking.

Other approaches to the inferior vena cava are infrequently used because of the need for a general anesthetic for insertion. Through a retroperitoneal approach, the gonadal veins, or a direct approach to the inferior vena cava (13), or through a lumbar vein (14) can be used. Catheters or ports are then usually tunneled to the lower abdomen, although some surgeons prefer to tunnel toward the lower chest wall, where the stability of the rib cage provides a firmer base to allow easy cannulation of a port.

A percutaneous approach to the inferior vena

cava in the paralumbar region has also been described. The author has not used this technique; however, a report by Denny et al. (15) indicates that it is a safe and reliable route. A preplacement CT scan helps in deciding angle and position for needle placement, which is usually at the L2-L3 level in the right parasternal region. The device is then tunneled to the anterior trunk as with other approaches.

Transthoracic or transmediastinal approaches to the superior vena cava or right atrium are also described, though infrequently used. Again, each of these approaches require general anesthesia. Oram-Smith et al. describe an anterior mediastinotomy through the right third intercostal space, with placement of a purse-string suture on the right atrial appendage and catheter placement through that purse string (16). Another approach is through a right axillary thoracotomy, with placement of the catheter through the azygos vein or directly in the superior vena cava (17).

No large series has been published using any of these alternate techniques for central venous access. There seems to be no increased risk of thrombosis of the great veins with these approaches. Small series reports have indicated that these approaches are acceptable, reliable alternatives when traditional approaches are not available. Through the use of one of these approaches, long-term, convenient venous access can be established in any patient to allow anticancer or supportive therapies to be administered.

COMPLICATIONS

Complications of central venous access for cancer therapy include complications of placement, thrombosis, device malfunction, and infection. Complications of placement have been described above and should be familiar to any surgeon placing these devices. Pneumothorax or hemothorax should be handled by either close observation or tube thoracostomy; rarely will operative intervention be required for control of hemorrhage. Thoracic duct injury from left subclavian or internal jugular approaches may resolve without intervention but may require removal of the device to allow the duct injury to close.

Probably the most common and least reported complication of tunneled or nontunneled catheters is accidental displacement or removal.

With a portion of the device left dangling from the trunk, catheters or their connecting tubing can become tangled in clothing, apparatus, or even arms or legs and can be pulled back or out unwittingly. The only treatment for this is prevention, with adequate precautions and patient education.

Bruising or hematoma over the site of an access port following local trauma usually results only in mild swelling or tenderness at the site. This may be significant enough to require use of peripheral access for several days. Rarely does enough blood accumulate in the pocket to require aspiration. Close observation of the site is important to watch for signs of an infected hematoma, which would require device removal.

Thrombosis of any of these devices or of the associated great vein must be diagnosed and treated in a timely manner, to restore function and prevent development or progression of venous thrombosis. Thrombotic complications are manifested either by inability to infuse or withdraw through the device or by signs and symptoms of venous thrombosis in the region. Thrombosis can result from any of a number of causes, including human error in maintaining the device, pinching or crimping at the level where the catheter passes under the clavicle and over the first rib, hypercoagulable states, development of a fibrin sheath about the intravascular portion of the catheter, or thrombosis of the vessel surrounding the catheter tip.

Management of thrombosis depends on the type of device and the cause. A simple percutaneous line may be best managed by removal of the device; however, the patient should be evaluated to confirm that there are not signs of venous thrombosis of the central venous circulation. These findings may be subtle, with venous plethora of the chest or neck, mild edema, or a subjective complaint of neck swelling or dysphagia. With any suspicion of thrombosis, evaluation with Doppler ultrasound studies or venography should be performed. If no thrombosis is found, the device may be removed and a new device replaced without further intervention. However, if thrombosis is identified, systemic anticoagulation is mandatory to prevent further thrombosis. If access has been a problem in this patient and it is not anticipated that other easy sites are available for device placement, the device should be approached as described below for the more long-term devices.

Simple thrombosis of an access port or a tunneled catheter can often be managed by thrombolysis of the catheter with urokinase. A commercially available kit, Abbokinase Open-Cath (Abbott Labs, Inc.), delivers 5000 international units of urokinase to be instilled into a thrombosed device. The solution is left in situ for 5 to 30 minutes, with aspiration at 5-minute intervals to determine if the clot has been lysed. A second instillation may be needed. Catheter salvage of 77% with a single instillation is reported (18). With this system, many catheters can be salvaged that would otherwise have to be removed.

Development of a fibrin sheath may be the limiting event in the life span of venous access devices. Any foreign body will incite some reaction from the body and deposition of fibrin to attempt to isolate the foreign material. The intensity of this reaction varies from patient to patient. However, unless a device is in continuous use, it can be anticipated that some degree of deposition will occur around it. The first evidence of development of a fibrin sheath is inability to withdraw blood from a device (19). When occlusion to withdrawal occurs or when an established device is occluded to injection and aspiration, no central thrombosis can be identified, and the device cannot be salvaged with conventional thrombolytics, the development of a fibrin sheath can be presumed. At times, the sheath will be apparent on a contrast study performed for thrombosis. This catheter should be considered to have a short life span remaining, although repeated attempts to restore patency (which may be due to thrombosis) should be made with subsequent occlusions, especially if the planned course of treatment is nearly complete.

Device occlusion due to anatomic factors, such as kinks of the catheter in the subcutaneous tissues, may be correctable with local exploration of the tract. If a catheter has migrated or kinked in the central circulation, interventional radiologic techniques can be used to reposition the catheter tip and salvage the device (20). Kinking as the catheter passes below the clavicle and over the first rib, however, probably cannot be corrected. In fact, these catheters are prone to break at that point, which may lead to catheter embolism (21). If a ''pinch-off sign'' is noted in studies of an occluded catheter, great care must be taken to remove the catheter to prevent breakage. The catheter should be inspected on withdrawal to confirm that no breakage has occurred. Pinching at this level can perhaps be prevented by adequately dilating the tract that the catheter passes through on insertion and not attempting to pass a catheter through an introducer sheath that is too tight.

Hypercoagulable states are associated with many neoplastic conditions. Unfortunately, these patients are often those most benefited by long-term access devices. In addition, the only manifestation of the hypercoagulable state may be thrombosis of the access device. In 1990, Bern et al. published the results of a prospective randomized trial placing patients with access ports on either low-dose warfarin (1 mg daily) or placebo (22). Subjects were followed with noninvasive studies of thrombosis of the great veins. Nearly 40% of the control group developed catheter-associated thrombosis (most asymptomatic), whereas less than 10% of treated patients developed thrombosis. Very low dose warfarin prevented venous thrombosis and device failure, with no changes in coagulation parameters and no increase in complications (22). These data certainly support placing patients at a slightly increased risk for thrombosis on very low dose warfarin while a venous access device is in place. Some physicians have argued that all patients should be on this regimen; however, factors such as cost, compliance, and significance of occult thrombosis (since nearly 10% of the treated group developed evidence of thrombosis without symptoms) must be considered.

Great vein thromboses associated with central venous catheters account for 40% of upper extremity thromboses. These are often asymptomatic, although they can be associated with symptomatic or fatal pulmonary embolism (23, 24). Development of neck or arm pain, venous plethora, jugular venous distension, or arm or neck swelling should lead to subsequent investigations to determine if thrombosis is present. Duplex Doppler scanning (25), venography (26), or CT scanning (27) all can establish the diagnosis and determine the extent of the thrombosis. Contrast studies performed through the device can determine if the device itself is patent and if there is significant thrombosis proximal to the catheter tip, but they cannot determine the distal extent or degree of collateral flow.

Treatment of great vein occlusion due to central catheter thrombosis includes extremity elevation and adequate analgesia while other treatments are considered. It is not clear whether removal of the catheter is mandatory. Reports describing successful treatment with thrombolytics and anticoagulants with the catheter remaining in place (28) indicate that catheter removal may not be necessary. Successful treatment of the thrombosis with systemic anticoagulation has long been the standard therapy for upper extremity thromboses of any etiology. Recent development of thrombolytic agents has added an additional treatment option. When thrombolytic therapy is instituted within 1 week of symptoms, 90% of patients achieve successful clot dissolution. If, however, thrombolytic therapy is not instituted until more than a week after symptoms appear, only 56% are successfully treated in this manner. Thrombolytic therapy was initially given systemically, with the attendant risks of hemorrhagic complications. Local urokinase therapy administered through a peripheral vein distal to the thrombosis, at 1/50th the dose administered systemically, has the same success rate as systemic thrombolysis, without the risks of bleeding.

Infection remains the most significant complication of venous access. Many of these patients can be expected to develop neutropenia and other immune suppression because of their antineoplastic therapies or underlying disease. Rates of infectious complications for these devices are reported to range from 3 to 60% (29). Infection related to these devices must be promptly recognized and appropriately treated; on the other hand, a patient with a venous access device and evidence of systemic infection must also be evaluated for other, equally serious, infectious sources.

Infection related to a venous access device can occur at three levels, and their treatments differ. Tunneled catheters can develop infection at the site of exit from the skin. These exit site infections are manifested by local tenderness, induration, and erythema at the site of catheter exit without evidence of systemic infection. These are most commonly due to *Staphylococcus epidermidis* infection (30, 31). Often, the catheter can be managed with thorough local care and appropriate antibiotics. The catheter can be used during this episode, although consideration should be given to holding cytotoxic therapies until the infection has cleared, to avoid the risk of worsening the infection as neutropenia develops. Should systemic signs of infection develop, the catheter should be considered condemned and should be removed.

Infection involving the tunnel (in tunneled catheters) or the pocket (in implanted ports) indicates a more serious infection. These present with evidence of infection running along the course of the device toward the site of insertion into the central circulation. Erythema and tenderness are almost always present, and further evidence of cellulitis may also be seen. Systemic signs of infection are frequently seen. These devices must be removed, any associated abscess drained, necrotic tissue debrided, and systemic antibiotics started. These infections, although they can be severe, are rarely uncontrollable.

Line sepsis, or catheter-related sepsis, is the most serious complication of indwelling venous access devices. It is manifested by systemic signs of sepsis without associated evidence of involvement of the site or tract of the device. It is usually a diagnosis of exclusion, once other potential sources of sepsis are eliminated, or of retrospect, as the diagnosis is often made after the device is removed and cultured.

Line sepsis usually presents as fever without other complaints. It can occur at any time in a patient with an indwelling central catheter, whether or not the patient is neutropenic at the time. Reports of incidence of line sepsis in children indicate that only 48% of catheter infections occur during neutropenia (32) and that the relative risk of developing bacteremia during neutropenia only increases to 1.56 in the presence of an indwelling catheter (33). Blood cultures, obtained through the venous access device and through a peripheral stick, can be compared by semi-quantitative techniques to diagnose catheter-related sepsis. If the number of colony-forming units (CFUs) per milliliter in bacterial culture of an aspirate from the central venous device is at least five times the number from a peripheral blood culture, or if the total number of CFUs per mL from the central culture exceeds 100/mL, culture of a removed device tip will confirm infection of the catheter (34, 35).

The bacteriology of central venous catheter infection shows that infection is most commonly due to gram-positive organism. Coagulase-negative staphylococci are most commonly found in line sepsis. *Staphylococcus aureus* is the next most common, followed by gram-negative organisms (35). Infection by fungi, especially *Candida* species, is also a large problem in this population (36), with a mortality rate of 52%. The treatment of fungal infection requires a different and more intensive approach, as outlined below.

Catheter removal is not absolutely necessary in the usual circumstances of catheter sepsis. When the diagnosis of line sepsis is suspected, cultures should be obtained, appropriate studies

Table 45.4. Conditions to Consider Removal of Venous Access Device in Line Sepsis

Not responding to antibiotic therapy
Deterioration after initial response to antibiotic therapy
Positive follow-up line cultures
Recurrent line sepsis
History of device malfunction
Course of therapy complete or nearly complete
Fungal sepsis

to exclude other sources of sepsis performed, and broad-spectrum antibiotics should be started. The coverage of these antibiotics should certainly include coagulase-positive and -negative staphylococci, based on local institutional sensitivity profiles, and gram-negative (enteric) bacteria as well. The usual antibiotic course is 10 to 14 days, with follow-up cultures obtained to confirm bacteriologic clearance. The catheter may be left in place in initial or uncomplicated infections (34, 35). If the patient is neutropenic, antibiotic therapy should continue longer than this if the neutropenia has not resolved. Conditions under which device removal should be considered are listed in Table 45.4.

An important group in whom catheter removal should be considered is those with fungal sepsis related to line infection. In a review of 21 children with *Candida* line sepsis, fungemia persisted in only 2 of 13 who had lines removed; whereas, 6 of 8 whose lines were left in place were able to clear their fungemia (37). Of these eight, seven required catheter removal within 2 weeks, for persistent or recurrent sepsis or catheter malfunction. The only fungal sepsis-related deaths in this series were in children whose catheters were left in place. The identification of fungal line sepsis should be treated by line removal and aggressive antifungal antibiotic therapy (38). Clearance of fungemia can be anticipated within 24 hours of line removal.

SUMMARY

The quality of life for the cancer patient receiving chemotherapy can be greatly improved by appropriate assessment of needs for venous access and careful attention to the use of venous access devices. A comprehensive approach utilizing the skills of a surgeon, medical oncologist, oncology nurse, and specialty support from the disciplines of radiology and infectious disease is crucial for the safe placement and management of the venous access needs of this population.

REFERENCES

1. Kerri-Szantu M. The subclavian vein, a constant and convenient intravenous injection site. Arch Surg 1956;72:179–181.
2. Dudrick SJ, Wilmore DW, Vars HM, et al. Long term total parenteral nutrition with growth, development, and positive nitrogen balance. Surgery 1968; 64:134–142.
3. Broviac JW, Cole JJ, Scribner BH. A silicone rubber right atrial catheter for prolonged parenteral alimentation. Surg Gynecol Obstet 1973;136:602–606.
4. Hickman RO, Buckner CD, Clift RA, et al. A modified right atrial catheter for access to the venous system in marrow transplant recipients. Surg Gynecol Obstet 1979;148:871–875.
5. Niederhuber JE, Ensminger W, Gyres JW, et al. Totally implanted venous and arterial access system to replace external catheters in cancer treatment. Surgery 1982;92:706–712.
6. Winters V, Peters B, Coila S, et al. A trial with a new peripheral implanted vascular access device. Oncol Nurs Forum 1990;17:891–896.
7. James L, Bledsoe L, Hadaway LC. A retrospective look at tip location and complications of peripherally inserted central catheter lines. J Intraven Nurs 1993;16:104–109.
8. McCready D, Broadwater R, Ross M, et al. A case-control comparison of durability and cost between implanted reservoir and percutaneous catheters in cancer patients. J Surg Res 1991;51:377–381.
9. Willard W, Coit D, Lucas A, Groeger JS. Long-term vascular access via the inferior vena cava. J Surg Oncol 1991;46:162–166.
10. Stanislav GV, Fitzgibbons RJ, Bailey RT, et al. Reliability of implantable central venous access devices in patients with cancer. Arch Surg 1991;122:1280–1283.
11. Curtas S, Bonaventura M, Megrid M. Cannulation of inferior vena cava for long-term central venous access. Surg Gynecol Obstet 1989;168:121–124.
12. Mahear J. A technique for the positioning of central venous catheters in patients with thrombosis of the superior vena cava. Surg Gynecol Obstet 1983; 156:659–660.
13. Coit D, Turnbill A. Long-term central venous access through the gonadal vein. Surg Gynecol Obstet 1992;175:362–364.
14. Boddie A. Translumbar catheterization at the inferior vena cava for long-term vascular access. Surg Gynecol Obstet 1989;168:55–56.
15. Denny D, Greendwood L, Morse S, et al. Inferior vena cava: translumbar catheterization for central venous access. Radiology 1989;170:1013–1014.
16. Oram-Smith J, Mullen J, Harken A, et al. Direct right atrial catheterization for total parenteral nutrition. Surgery 1977;83:274–276.
17. Malt R, Kempster M. Direct azygos vein and superior vena cava cannulation for parenteral nutrition. J Parenter Enter Nutr 1983;7:580–581.
18. Hurtubise M, Bottino J, Lawson M, et al. Restoring patency of occluded central venous catheters. Arch Surg 1980;115:212–213.
19. Peters W, Bush W. The development of fibrin sheath on indwelling venous catheters. Surg Gynecol Obstet 1973;137:43–47.
20. Cassidy F. Zajko A, Bron K, et al. Noninfectious

complications of long-term central venous catheters; radiologic evaluation and management. Am J Radiol 1987;149:671–675.

21. Aitken D, Minton J. The "pinch-off sign": a warning of impending problems with permanent subclavian catheters. Am J Surg 1984;148:633.

22. Bern M, Lokich J, Wallach S, et al. Very low-dose warfarin can prevent thrombosis in central venous catheters: a randomized prospective trial. Ann Intern Med 1990;112:413–428.

23. Leiby J, Purcell H, DeMaria J, et al. Pulmonary embolism as a result of Hickman catheter-related thrombosis. Am J Med 1989;86:228–231.

24. Kaye G, Smith D, Johnston D. Fatal right ventricular thrombus secondary to Hickman catheterisation. Br J Clin Pathol 1990;11:780–781.

25. Falk R, Smith D. Thrombosis of upper extremity thoracic veins: diagnosis with duplex doppler sonography. Am J Radiol 1987;149:677–682.

26. Wechsler R, Spirn P, Conant E, et al. Thrombosis and infection caused by thoracic venous catheters: pathogenesis and imaging findings. Am J Radiol 1993;160:467–471.

27. Mori H, Fukuda T, Isomoto L, et al. CT diagnosis of catheter-induced septic thrombus of vena cava. J Comput Assist Tomogr 1990;14:236–238.

28. Fraschini G, Jadeja J, Lawson M, et al. Local infusion of urokinase for the lysis of thrombosis associated with permanent central venous catheters in cancer patients. J Clin Oncol 1987;5:672–678.

29. Alexander H. Infectious complications associated with long-term venous access devices: etiology, diagnosis, treatment, and prophylaxis. In: Vascular access in the cancer patient: devices, insertion techniques,

maintenance, and prevention in management of complications. Philadelphia: JB Lippincott, 1994:113.

30. Schuman E, Winters V, Gross G, Hayes J. Management of Hickman catheter sepsis. Am J Surg 1985; 149:627–628.

31. Harvey M, Trent R, Joshua D, et al. Complications associated with indwelling venous Hickman catheters in patients with hematologic disorders. Aust NZ J Med 1986;16:211–215.

32. Viscoli C. Aspects of infections in children with cancer. Recent Results Cancer Res 1988;108:71–81.

33. Van Hoff J, Bery A, Seashore J. The effect of right atrial catheters on infectious complications of chemotherapy in children. J Clin Oncol 1990;8:1255–1262.

34. Flynn P, Shenep J, Stokes D, Barrett F. In situ management of confirmed central venous catheter-related bacteremia. Pediatr Infect Dis J 1987;6:729–734.

35. Benezra D, Kiehn T, Gold J, et al. Prospective study of infections in indwelling central venous catheters using quantitative blood cultures. Am J Med 1988;85:495–498.

36. Lecciones J, Lee J, Navarro E, et al. Vascular catheter-associated fungemia in patients with cancer: analysis of 155 episodes. Clin Infect Dis 1992;114:875–883.

37. Eppes S, Troutman J, Gutman L. Outcome of treatment of candidemia in children whose central catheters were removed or retained. Pediatr Infect Dis 1989;8:99–104.

38. Fraser V, Jones M, Dunkel J, et al. Candidemia in a tertiary care hospital: epidemiology, risk factors, and predictors of mortality. Clin Infect Dis 1992; 15:414–421.

46

Safe Handling of Cytotoxic Drugs

Bruce R. Harrison

To begin this discussion, a definition of "cytotoxic drugs" seems in order. A number of terms have been used in the literature over the years: antineoplastic, cytotoxic, cytostatic, hazardous, or chemotherapeutic, along with drugs, agents, or chemicals. These refer to a group of toxic, therefore hazardous, chemicals that are approved for use as drugs to treat cancer primarily because of their cytotoxic properties. Very recently, the Occupational Safety and Health Administration (OSHA) and others (1–4) have begun to use the term "hazardous drug" to include the usual antineoplastic drugs as well as other cytotoxic drugs that are not used to treat cancer or other toxic drugs that are not cytotoxic. Hazardous drug products are those that would cause some harm to handlers during distribution and use if the handlers become exposed to the drug (2). For purposes of this discussion, these terms "hazardous drug" and "cytotoxic" or "antineoplastic" drug are used interchangeably except where specifically noted.

Twenty-five years ago, the question of risk from handling antineoplastic drugs was first raised (5). In the late 1970s and early 1980s, data began to appear in the literature (reviewed below) suggesting that healthcare professionals were being exposed to antineoplastic drugs in the typical work setting. The first recommendations for the safe handling of these drugs were published about this time, primarily in Scandinavia (6–9). This trend continued as various professional groups and institutions recognized this potential occupational hazard and published recommendations in several venues including nursing (10–12), pharmacy (13–18), medicine (19, 20), and occupational/public health (21–25). Maturing steadily, these recommendations culminated, in the United States, with the OSHA procedures that were published in early 1986 (26).

Over the past 5 years, refinement and development of safety measures for handling hazardous drugs continued (27–31). In 1990, the American Society of Health-System Pharmacists (formerly the American Society of Hospital Pharmacists) revised its "Technical Assistance Bulletin on Handling Cytotoxic and Hazardous Drugs." This remains one of the best sources for information on developing safety guidelines (4). OSHA has recently issued new guidelines for its personnel conducting on-site inspections of hospitals (1). It is these standards that institutions in the United States must meet.

The Joint Commission Accreditation of Healthcare Organizations (JCAHO) has no specific requirements for handling of antineoplastic drugs incorporated in its "Comprehensive Accreditation Manual for Hospitals" (32); however, in the section on managing the environment of care there are standards regarding the development of departmental safety plans and management of hazardous materials and wastes (see standards EC.1.2.1 and EC.1.2.3).

In late 1980, meaningful studies and pertinent references were few. Fifteen years later there is an almost unmanageable amount of material to assess. Despite the volume of literature, there are still gaps in our knowledge of the levels of exposure in various occupational settings and of the risks associated with this exposure. Data from properly designed epidemiologic studies will be necessary to fill these gaps. However, there are sufficient data available on the chemical properties and health effects of these drugs, the potential for acute or chronic environmental exposure to these drugs, and the appropriate procedures and equipment necessary to afford protection to workers from these drugs. In other words, there is sufficient reason for concern, and there is sufficient information available upon which to base sound occupational safety decisions.

This chapter discusses some of the new data available on the acute and chronic chemical properties of antineoplastic drugs, their mutagenic and carcinogenic potential, the level of environmental contamination in the work place, an assessment of the risk associated with anticipated exposure, and general recommendations for safe handling of these drugs.

A PROBLEM OF SAFETY

Safety in the work place is simply the prevention of injury by control of the environment and the use of proper work methods. This simple but far-reaching definition refers to safe ways of doing everything from lifting patients to crossing the street. In this case we are attempting to describe safe methods of handling a group of chemicals referred to as antineoplastic (hazardous) drugs. All of the principles, procedures, and equipment discussed in this chapter should make up part of an overall safety program for your hospital, pharmacy, clinic, or private oncologist's office.

All of the 40 or so antineoplastic agents and the 20 or so other hazardous drugs listed in any standard formulary are medicines approved for use in humans by the Food and Drug Administration. When used in accordance with the official package insert, these drugs are considered "safe." In the past, many health care professionals had been lulled into a sense of false security, assuming that these "drugs" were generally safe. However, it is now more broadly recognized that these drugs are chemicals and, as such, have a variety of properties other than therapeutic ones. Some of these properties may include mutagenicity and carcinogenicity (discussed below) but also caustic and irritant effects on the skin, eyes, and mucous membranes.

Toxic Effects on the Skin

Mechlorethamine, perhaps better known as nitrogen mustard, is the prototypic acutely hazardous antineoplastic drug. This alkylating agent, a relative of the sulfur mustards used during World War I, is a potent irritant and blistering agent. Spills on the skin can cause chemical burns (6), and inhalation of vapor can cause severe irritation of nasal and bronchial mucous membranes and the eyes (33, 34). The official package insert (33) gives an adequate description of the potential effects of inadvertent occupational exposure and outlines specific methods of handling and detoxification. This product's outer packaging also displays a warning label containing emergency handling and detoxification information. This is the only one of the antineoplastic drug products that provides such a complete and bold warning.

A number of other chemotherapy drugs have known topical effects. As early as 1966, carmustine (BCNU) was reported to cause inflammation and hyperpigmentation of the skin following inadvertent exposure during preparation or administration (35, 36). Nava et al. (37) also reported similar skin changes in 7 of 16 technicians and manual workers employed in the synthesis and packaging of carmustine and busulfan. Three nurses engaged in administration of carmustine were also included in this report. Doxorubicin was noted to cause contact dermatitis in a laboratory worker (38). Fluorouracil also has well-known topical irritant effects (39) and can cause definite morphologic changes in the epidermis of normal skin during chronic topical application (40).

Other more anecdotal reports of topical effects secondary to handling of antineoplastic drugs include heavy nosebleeds and a pruritic eczematous rash on the face and hands of an oncology nurse (these reactions cleared when she stopped handling cytostatic drugs) (41), skin irritation from an accidental spill of cyclophosphamide (42), and tingling of the mouth and nose during mixing of the investigational agents acridinyl anisidide (m-AMSA) and PCNU (both of these agents contain N,N-dimethylacetamide as diluents) (43). Crudi (44) reported nasal mucosal sores, skin pigmentation changes, and itching of the face, hands and arms when mixing chemotherapy agents.

A number of antineoplastic drugs are known to cause soft-tissue necrosis or cellulitis if extravasated during intravenous administration (45, 46). Accidental injection during the mixing or administration of these agents may lead to significant injury. Duvall and Baumann (47) described an "unusual accident" involving a needlestick injury from mitomycin to a patient during chemotherapy administration. This apparently innocent needle "prick" injury progressed to cellulitis with vesicular eruptions followed by sloughing of skin and formation of a 1.5 by 2 cm ulcer. This patient ultimately required debridement and split-thickness skin graft operation. Dorr (48) described a needlestick injury caused by vindesine. This incident occurred in the volar aspect of the wrist of a pharmacy technician who accidentally "bumped" into a needle and a syringe containing a 5-mg/mL solution of vindesine. The technician delayed reporting this "slight jab of the needle" because the apparent exposure was minimal. It was sufficient, however, to produce a 1 by 2 cm mildly painful lesion with central blanching and erythematous borders. This lesion took approximately 3 weeks to resolve. These accidents should serve to remind practitioners that incidental needle injuries involving antineoplastic drugs are not to be taken lightly. Injection is one of the routes of exposure for toxic or hazardous substances, and in this case, an acute ulcerative skin lesion may result. Prompt medical attention should be sought following any on-the-job needlestick. Treatment should conform to the conservative management currently recommended for extravasation of chemotherapy drugs (45, 49).

Ocular Toxicity

Injury to the eye can occur from accidental exposure in occupational settings. In 1976, Gundersen (6) presented three cases of conjunctival irritation and excessive lacrimation in nurses handling methotrexate. Others have complained of dryness, grittiness, and soreness associated with administering cytotoxic agents (50). There was no history of overt exposure to the eye in these cases. However, surveys conducted by Crudi et al. (51) and Valanis et al. (52) reported no increased incidence of eye problems.

Doxorubicin has been implicated as causing intraocular damage after accidental instillation during mixing of the drug (53). Symptoms included burning and lacrimation followed by edema of the upper lid, conjunctival injection, photophobia, and foreign-body sensation. Examination revealed a cellular infiltrate of the cornea and punctate epithelial keratopathy. Most symptoms resolved within a week with topical steroid treatment.

Fluorouracil is another antimetabolite known to cause epiphora, tear-duct fibrosis, and other ocular effects in patients receiving this drug (54–57). Haidak et al. (55) demonstrated fluorouracil in the tears of patients with symptoms at concentrations of 16.1 to 23.8 μg/mL 15 minutes after intravenous dosage. This was similar to the corresponding plasma concentrations. They postulated that local irritation of the lacrimal duct might be responsible for the symptoms observed. Shapiro et al. (58) demonstrated similar toxic effects in the ocular surface epithelium of rabbits. It is likely that accidental instillation of fluorouracil solution (pH 9, 643 mOsm/kg H_2O) into the eye could cause irritation or lacrimation (59).

Cytarabine is an antimetabolite cancer drug previously tested as an antiviral agent in the treatment of herpetic keratitis. Kaufman et al. (60), in experiments in normal human volunteers and rabbits, demonstrated reversible corneal toxicity characterized by opacities and punctate staining of the epithelium or frank corneal ulceration and iritis. Cytarabine was shown to inhibit corneal epithelial DNA synthesis, which the authors believe led to the corneal toxicity. Elliott and Schut (61) found similar results in their experiments on the eyes of monkeys, rabbits, and humans. Corneal toxicity following high-dose, systemic cytarabine for the treatment of acute leukemias has also been reported. Hopen et al. (62) described three cases of corneal toxicity that consisted of ocular pain, tearing, foreign-body sensation, photophobia, and blurred vision. Corneal changes resembled those from topical administration described above. A literature review revealed no reports of occupational exposure to the eye; however, in view of the above reported characteristic ocular toxicities, precautions should be taken to avoid eye contact with solutions of cytarabine.

Vinblastine is an antimitotic that can cause serious corneal injury following accidental splash injuries. Four cases have been reported in the literature (63–66), each of which produced a similar keratopathy and slow healing. In 1978, McLendon and Bron (66) described a physician who accidentally sprayed approximately 1 mL of vinblastine solution (1 mg/mL) in his face. In spite of irrigation, conjunctival redness and halos around lights developed bilaterally within 24 hours. Examination on the second day revealed bilateral conjunctival injection, diffuse right cystic epithelial keratopathy, combined discrete and confluent punctate epithelial keratopathy, punctate epithelial erosions, and epithelial microcysts. During the first week after injury, the patient experienced blepharospasm, photophobia, epiphora, lid swelling, and loss of visual acuity on the right. Most corneal changes improved over a period of 6 weeks on topical steroid therapy. Visual acuity returned to normal by 10 weeks, but some corneal changes on the left remained. Both Cordier and Mendelsohn (64) and, independently, McLendon and Bron (66) confirmed these toxic reactions experimentally on the corneas of rabbits.

Obviously, severe ocular toxicities can result from the accidental or careless splash or spray of several antineoplastic drugs. In addition to the agents reviewed above, other antineoplastic drugs may be likely to cause ocular injuries. Etoposide and carmustine contain hydroalcoholic diluents, 30.5% v/v and 10% v/v, respectively, and teniposide and paclitaxel contain the solvent cremophor as well as alcohol (67). Other investigational chemotherapy agents such as amsacrine (m-AMSA) and diaziquone (AZQ) contain caustic diluents such as N,N-dimethylacetamide (67). Any of these may cause ocular irritation or damage on their own. Additionally, the direct cytotoxic action of any of the antineoplastic drugs may induce corneal changes (in a manner similar to that for cytarabine discussed above).

In general, the most common toxic eye injuries are caused by accidental splashing of chemicals into the eyes (68). Initial treatment involves vigorous irrigation with water or saline for 15 to 30 minutes. During and following emergency medical treatment, prolonged irrigation with saline for 1 to 2 hours has proven to be beneficial (68, 69). Emergency eyewash facilities should be available in all antineoplastic drug preparation areas and preferably in administration areas as well. Protective eyewear should be worn any time these agents are handled outside a containment hood.

Systemic Effects?

Numerous anecdotal reports have appeared in the nursing and pharmacy literature suggesting that systemic absorption of antineoplastic drugs was occurring during their preparation or administration. Gundersen (6), in 1976, reported asthmalike respiratory symptoms and urticarial rashes in two nurses who prepared and administered drugs in a chemotherapy department. One of the two experienced relief from these symptoms by wearing a mask and preparing cyclophosphamide and methotrexate in front of an open window. In 1980, Crudi (44) described a variety of potential systemic side effects in a group of five nurses and five students in an outpatient chemotherapy unit (one nurse from the inpatient unit). These symptoms included lightheadedness, dizziness, nausea, vomiting, flulike

syndrome, and headache. Ladik et al. (70), also in 1980, described several pharmacists on her staff who complained of lightheadedness, dizziness, and facial flushing while preparing dacarbazine and cisplatin admixtures. After moving chemotherapy drug preparation from a horizontal-laminar-flow hood to a bacteriologic glove box, no further incidents were reported.

A series of well-documented reactions to m-AMSA was reported by Reynolds et al. (71) in 1982. In this report, nine pharmacists, pharmacy technicians, or nurses developed urticarial rash, nausea and vomiting, lightheadedness, epigastric pain, headache, or malaise while preparing this drug in horizontal-laminar-flow hoods. The reactions were fairly similar in these personnel working in three separate hospitals. The symptoms developed within a few minutes to 4 hours following the preparation of AMSA. One technician developed the same symptom of urticarial rash on three separate occasions. The addition of gloves or gloves, gown, and mask did not prevent this reaction. This series of reactions in multiple personnel prompted a recommendation that vertical-flow-containment hoods be used for preparation of the drug. No additional reactions were seen during a 3-month observation following the equipment change.

Another well-documented series of cases was reported in 1983 by Sotaniemi et al. (72). Three consecutive head nurses on an oncology unit developed liver disease, each after years of exposure to antineoplastic drugs. The number of drugs handled ranged from 500 to 600 solutions prepared per year. Multiple liver biopsies in all three nurses documented portal hepatitis with piecemeal necrosis in one and hepatic fibrosis and fat accumulation in two of the nurses. In the absence of other drug or alcohol use or other etiologic factors, the authors concluded that these manifestations were consistent with a causative connection between cytotoxic drug exposure and liver injury.

Case reports describing occupational exposure to antineoplastic drugs continue to appear in the literature (59, 73, 74). The use of these anecdotal case reports can be counterproductive to proper scientific inquiry and sound medical decision making. This is especially true when there are no control cases or other points of reference or when emotional issues or elements of personal behavior are involved. Caution is always advised when interpreting such reports. However, when a series of cases is well documented, as in the cases reported by Sotaniemi et al. (72)

or when an event can be documented repeatedly in the same individual or group, more credence can be given to the report. The cases presented above have not proved that occupational exposure to antineoplastic drugs caused systemic effects. It is apparent now, however, that they did serve to heighten awareness of the potential hazards of this group of agents and stimulated additional research on the questions they raised.

A stronger suggestion of systemic effects was noted by Valanis et al. (52, 75) in two controlled surveys. In one, a group of nurses handled antineoplastic drugs with only a modest amount of protection (75), and in the other, a group of pharmacists and pharmacy technicians (52), most used containment hoods and gloves when preparing drugs. Compared with controls, small but significant increases in the occurrence of acute symptoms were found. These included chronic throat irritation and diarrhea in the pharmacy group and dizziness, headache, eye irritation, chronic cough, sore throat, and nausea and vomiting in the nursing group. The use of control groups in these studies and the large sample size in the pharmacy study lends a great deal more credibility to the notion of systemic side effects caused by routine exposure to antineoplastic agents.

Allergic Reactions

Allergic reactions are well known in occupational settings involving the handling of pharmaceuticals (37, 76–79). Eleven of 18 workers involved in the production of melphalan and lympholysin experienced various allergic disorders including asthma, eczematous dermatitis, urticaria, vasomotor rhinitis, and sinusitis (37). Several antineoplastic drugs, including L-asparaginase, teniposide, bleomycin, and cisplatin are known allergens in patients receiving them (80). Mechlorethamine is a potent sensitizer in patients receiving topical treatment with this drug (81, 82). One pharmacist reported developing sensitization to mechlorethamine following repeated exposure during preparation of solutions and ointments for topical administration (Payne JT, personal communication, 1983). Significant exposure to these agents during preparation or administration may lead to sensitization or the development of asthmalike symptoms or urticarial rash such as those described in the reports above.

Soluble platinum salts have been implicated in causing occupational illness in chemists and factory workers. Clinical manifestations included rhinitis, conjunctivitis, asthma, urticaria, and contact dermatitis (83–86). The incidence of platinum sensitivity in some settings has been shown to be very high (60%). Development of sensitivity is related primarily to repeated exposures, but atopy is a predisposing factor.

Cisplatin, carboplatin, and iproplatin are soluble platinum salts but are not included in the above-cited reports of occupational illness. However, both cisplatin and carboplatin are well known to cause allergic reactions in patients receiving long-term treatment (87–89).

OSHA has published guidelines for handling these platinum compounds (90). The recommendations include provisions for containment, ventilation, the use of gloves, and personal protective clothing and environmental monitoring. OSHA restricts occupational exposure to platinum salts to 2 μg/m^3 in an 8-hour work period.

CARCINOGENICITY

The ability of some anticancer drugs to induce tumors is well established. As early as 1935, Haddow (91) recognized the paradoxical property of several carcinogenic polycyclic hydrocarbons to inhibit the growth of experimental animal tumors. Further work by Haddow and others confirmed the tumorigenicity of many early anticancer drugs, including the nitrogen mustards still used today.

Most antineoplastic drugs approved for use today have been tested for carcinogenicity in various animal models (92–100). The methods, dosages, and routes of administration used in these studies varied. Schmahl and Habs (101), however, concluded that despite the different methods used, the results of these studies were "relatively uniform and meaningful." Others have reviewed experimental carcinogenesis of antitumor drugs (102–104) and also have concluded that alkylating antitumor agents have a strong carcinogenic potential. Table 46.1 lists the antineoplastic drugs that have been found to be carcinogenic in animals.

Carcinogenesis in Man

Chemical carcinogenesis in humans is also a well-established phenomenon (105, 106). Both the International Agency for Research on Cancer (IARC) (107–111) and the National Toxicology Program (NTP) (112) have published lists of known or suspected human carcinogens (Table 46.2). The NTP criteria for classifying an agent

Table 46.1. Summary of Experimental Carcinogenic, Mutagenic, Chromosomal, Teratogenic, and Spermatotoxic Effects of Commercially Available Antineoplastic Drugs

Drug[a]	Carcinogenicity[b]	Mutagenicity[c]	Micronucleus Assay[d]	Sister-Chromatid Exchanges[e]	Teratogenicity[f]	Spermatotoxicity[g]
Altretamine	ND[h]	ND	ND	ND	+	ND
Asparaginase	ND	−	ND	ND	+	ND
Azacytidine	+	±	ND	±	+	ND
Azathioprine	±	−	+	±	+	ND
Bleomycin	ND	±	−	±	ND	+
Busulfan	±	±	+	+	+	+
Carboplatin	ND	±	+	+	+	ND
Carmustine	+	+	ND	+	+	+
Chlorambucil	+	+	ND	+	+	+
Cisplatin	+	+	+	+	±	+
Cladribine	ND	ND	ND	ND	ND	ND
Cyclophosphamide	+	+	+	+	+	+
Cytarabine	−	±	+	±	+	+
Dacarbazine	+	+	ND	±	+	ND
Dactinomycin	±	±	−	±	+	+
Daunorubicin	+	+	ND	+	+	+
Doxorubicin	+	+	+	+	+	+
Etoposide	ND	+	ND	+	+	ND
Estramustine	ND	ND	ND	ND	+	ND
Floxuridine	ND	±	ND	±	+	ND
Fludarabine	ND	+	+	ND	ND	ND
Fluorouracil	ND	−	+	−	+	+
Hydroxyurea	ND	±	−	±	+	+
Idarubicin	ND	+	ND	ND	ND	ND
Ifosfamide	±	+	+	ND	+	ND
Lomustine	+	+	ND	+	+	+
Mechlorethamine	+	+	+	+	+	+
Melphalan	+	+	ND	+	+[i]	ND
Mercaptopurine	±	±	+	±	+	−
Methotrexate	−	±	+	±	+	+
Mitomycin	+	±	+	+	+	+
Mitoxantrone	ND	+	ND	ND	ND	ND
Paclitaxel	ND	+	+	ND	ND	+
Pentostatin	ND	ND	ND	ND	±	ND
Procarbazine	+	+	+	+	+	+
Streptozocin	+	+	ND	ND	+	ND
Teniposide	ND	+	ND	+	+	ND
Thioguanine	ND	ND	ND	ND	+	ND
Thiotepa	+	+	+	+	+	+
Uracil mustard	+	+	ND	ND	ND	ND
Vinblastine	−	±	+	ND	+	+
Vincristine	−	±	+	±	+	+
Vinorelbine	ND	ND	ND	ND	ND	ND

[a]Generic name.
[b]Data summarized from references 92–100.
[c]Data summarized from references 98–100 and 160–175.
[d]Data summarized from references 98–100, 146, 181, and 182.
[e]Data summarized from references 98–100, 143, 149, 184 and 186–191.
[f]Data summarized from references 170, 173 and 202–206.
[g]Data summarized from references 212–216.
[h]ND, no data in sources used or insufficient data.
[i]The racemic mixture dl-sarcolysin was used in this study (203). Melphalan is l-sarcolysin.

Table 46.2. Substances or Groups of Substances and Medical Treatments That Are Known to Be Carcinogenic in Humans

Aflatoxins
4-Aminobiphenyl
Analgesic mixtures containing phenacetin[a]
Arsenic and certain arsenic compounds
Asbestos
Azathioprine[a]
Benzene
Benzidine
Bis(chloromethyl)ether and technical grade chloromethyl methyl ether
1,4-Butanediol dimethylsulfonate (Myleran)[a]
Certain combined chemotherapy for lymphomas[a]
Chlorambucil[b]
1-(2-Chloroethyl)-3-(4-methylcyclohexyl)-1-nitrosourea (MeCCNU)[a]
Chromium and certain chromium compounds
Conjugated estrogens[a]
Cyclophosphamide[a]
Diethylstilbestrol[a]
Erionite
Melphalan[a]
Methoxsalen with ultraviolet A therapy (PUVA)[a]
Mustard gas
2-Naphthylamine
Radon
Thorium dioxide
Vinyl chloride

From U.S. Department of Health and Human Services, Public Health Service, National Toxicology Program. Seventh annual report on carcinogens, 1994.
[a]Currently used as a drug.

as a "known carcinogen" require sufficient evidence from human studies to indicate a causal relationship between exposure to the substance and human cancer. Substances "which may reasonably be anticipated to be carcinogenic" are defined as those for which there is limited evidence of carcinogenicity in humans or sufficient evidence of carcinogenicity in experimental animals (112). IARC has published similar criteria (107). Table 46.3 lists common antineoplastic drugs that are suspected or likely to be carcinogenic in humans. Although both of these agencies have included several antineoplastic drugs in the category of "known human carcinogen," none are regulated by OSHA.

Documentation of the carcinogenicity in humans comes primarily from clinical observations of induced or second malignancies in cancer patients or patients with noncancerous diseases who are treated with antineoplastic drugs. These observations are in the form of case reports and retrospective analyses of clinical trials. One of the earliest and perhaps best known of this type of report was by Theide et al. (113) in 1964. They found that chlornaphazine, an alkylating agent, induced bladder cancer in patients receiving treatment for polycythemia vera. Similarly, cyclophosphamide was shown to cause a ninefold increase in bladder cancer in patients treated for nonuroepithelial tumors (114).

Chlornaphazine was withdrawn from the market in 1963 because of its carcinogenic property. Chemically, chlornaphazine is a nitrogen mustard that is biotransformed into the known carcinogen, β-naphthylamine. A close look at chlornaphazine's structure-activity relationships and degradation pathway might have entirely prevented these cytostatically induced tumors (115).

The classic example of a clinical trial in which a "side effect" of secondary cancer occurred was described by Berk et al. (116) in 1981. This study was designed to determine the most effective treatment for polycythemia vera by comparing the standard therapy, phlebotomy, with oral chlorambucil therapy or radioactive phosphorus (^{32}P). A total of 431 eligible patients were randomized to receive one of these therapies. After a median follow-up of more than 6 years, there was no significant difference in survival among the groups. However, the chlorambucil-treated group had a 13-fold increase in the incidence of

Table 46.3. Other Antineoplastic Drugs That Are Suspected Human Carcinogens

Drug[a]	Agency
Azacytidine	IARC 2A[b]
Bleomycin	IARC 2B
Carmustine	NTP[c], IARC 2A
Cisplatin	NTP, IARC 2A
Dacarbazine	NTP, IARC 2B
Daunorubicin	IARC 2B
Doxorubicin	NTP, IARC 2A
Lomustine	NTP, IARC 2A
Mechlorethamine	NTP, IARC 2A
Mitomycin	IARC 2B
Procarbazine	NTP, IARC 2A
Streptozocin	NTP, IARC 2B
Thiotepa	NTP, IARC 1
Uracil mustard	IARC 2B

[a]Generic name.
[b]International Agency for Research on Cancer; 1, known human carcinogen; 2A, probable human carcinogen; 2B, possible human carcinogen (111).
[c]National Toxicology Program; substances that may reasonably be anticipated to be (human) carcinogens (112).

acute leukemias, compared with the phlebotomy treatment group.

A number of case studies and reviews have been published on the incidence of secondary cancers, usually acute leukemias, in Hodgkin's disease (117–122), multiple myeloma (123), ovarian carcinoma (124–130), and breast carcinoma (127, 128, 131, 132). Coupled with studies in nonmalignant diseases, such as rheumatoid arthritis (133–135), and in other solid tumors (136, 137), the literature strongly suggests that prolonged exposure to alkylating drugs increases the incidence of acute leukemias and other tumors (138, 139). A likely addition to this list are the epipodophyllotoxins and other topoisomerase-II inhibitors (140).

From the data presented above, it seems clear that some alkylating antitumor drugs are carcinogenic or leukemogenic in humans. This evidence supports the conjecture made by Cronkite (141) over 30 years ago: "Any drug or chemical capable of inducing bone marrow damage must be assumed to be potentially a leukemogen." However, as he pointed out, much additional data and analysis was needed to adequately assess the risk associated with exposure to these or other agents. With each passing year, more data have become available that can be applied to such an assessment.

MUTAGENESIS

A mutation is a permanent transmissible change in the genetic material, often in a single gene. If such a change occurs in somatic cells, a cancer may develop; if gonadal cells are affected, the progeny will carry the mutation. Expression of a mutation in gonadal cells varies from lethality, which gives rise to dead offspring, to those affecting morphologic characteristics, such as a change in color, and to those that cause physical or mental defects (142).

Mutations can be classified by analysis of the inherited material for chromosomal aberrations or drastic rearrangement of the base-pair sequences of DNA. Point mutations, or single base-pair changes in DNA, may also occur. These are usually recessive, causing little or no effect at the time of induction. Drastic changes in chromosomal material in a cell may lead to altered growth or cell death, the lethal expression referred to above (142).

Many methods are available to test or monitor for mutagenicity or genotoxicity. Some of the typical testing systems used include reverse mutation systems, micronuclei in lymphocytes, and chromosomal breakage or aberrations. Large numbers of chemicals found in our everyday environment have been shown to be mutagenic using one or more of these systems. Some of these include nitrites and nitrates used widely in meat processing (143), some insecticides and herbicides (143), cigarette smoke (144, 145), and a large number of drugs (143, 146), including caffeine (143, 147) and the antineoplastic drugs. All of these tests, as well as a host of other tests for genotoxicity, have been advocated as short-term screening tests for carcinogens and for monitoring genotoxicity in the occupational environment (143, 148–150). They also have been used in a variety of occupational settings as a screen for exposure to mutagens (151–158). More germane to this discussion, measuring urine mutagenicity and clastogenic changes in lymphocytes in personnel occupationally exposed to anticancer drugs has been suggested (159). The sections below discuss in greater detail the use of these nonspecific methods of monitoring exposure to mutagens.

The Ames Test

Reverse mutation systems use specially designed mutated strains of bacteria to measure reversion back to wild type. The best known of these tests is the *Salmonella*/mammalian-microsome mutagenicity test or "Ames test" (148), which is useful in screening for different kinds of point mutations. Briefly, this is a relatively simple and sensitive bacterial test in which chemicals are tested on petri dishes using specially constructed mutant strains of *Salmonella typhimurium*. These strains lack the ability to synthesize histidine, an essential metabolite, and were selected for their sensitivity and specificity in being reverted from requiring histidine back to prototrophy (able to produce their own histidine) by a wide variety of mutagens (Fig. 46.1). Many carcinogenic and noncarcinogenic chemicals have been tested in this system, which has shown a high correlation (85%) of the carcinogens being detected as mutagens (148). Thus, there is a high probability that chemicals found to be mutagenic in this test will also be carcinogenic.

Many of the antineoplastic drugs have been shown to be mutagenic in the Ames test or similar test systems using *Escherichia coli* or by ob-

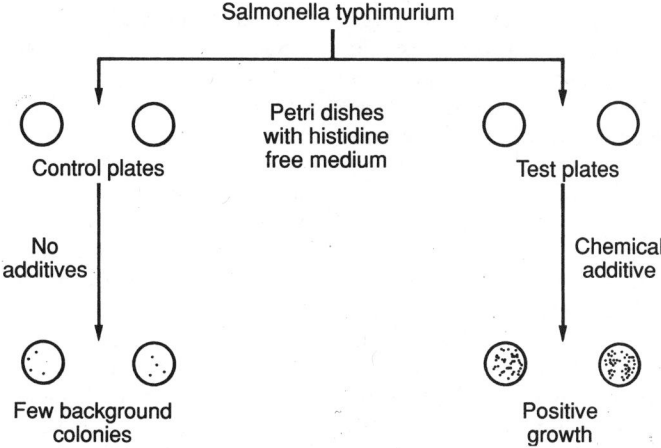

Figure 46.1. Schema showing simplified Ames test. Specially constructed strains of *Salmonella typhimurium* possess a selected mutation that prevents them from producing their own histidine. These bacteria are cultured in petri dishes on histidine-free media. A suspected carcinogenic chemical is added to the test plate (*right arm*). Compounds capable of inducing mutations cause a reversion back to the wild-type, or prototrophic state, allowing colony growth. Few colonies grow on the control plates. Colony growth on the test plates is compared with that on the control plates. Results are usually reported as a ratio of revertant colonies on the test plate to the background colonies on the control plate.

servation of chromosomal damage in mammalian cells (160–175). Table 46.1 lists the antineoplastic drugs that have been shown to be mutagenic in these bacterial test systems.

The Ames mutagenicity assay system, as described above, or the more sensitive bacterial fluctuation test (a variation of the Ames test in which the bacteria are grown in liquid culture media rather than on culture plates) (154) has been used to detect mutagens in the urine of test animals (168, 175) and patients receiving antineoplastic drugs (176–178). Urine mutagenicity testing of personnel handling antineoplastic drugs has been used frequently to screen groups of health professionals for exposure to mutagens. The details of these studies are discussed below.

The Micronucleus Assay

The micronucleus assay can detect cellular exposure to both spindle poisons and clastogenic agents. Micronuclei arise from chromosome fragments or whole chromosomes that do not adhere to the mitotic spindle during a mitotic cycle and are excluded from the nucleus. These cytoplasmic chromatin masses are easily identified under a microscope as small round bodies of nuclear material adjacent to the main nucleus. Compared with traditional metaphase analysis,

micronucleus determination is relatively simple and quick to score and is a sensitive indicator of both chromosomal aberrations and loss of chromosomes (146, 179, 180).

The micronucleus assay has been used to screen large numbers of chemicals, including many antineoplastic drugs, for clastogenic activity (98–100, 146, 181, 182). Analysis of micronucleus formation has been used in the work place to screen for cytogenetic damage (150, 179, 180, 183) This assay has also been used to screen potentially exposed health care workers, usually in conjunction with other screening tests discussed below.

Sister-Chromatid Exchange

The use of induced sister-chromatid exchanges (SCEs) is considered to be the simplest and most sensitive mammalian system to test for the genetic effects of mutagenic or carcinogenic chemicals. SCEs can be induced at lower concentrations than those normally found in chromosomal aberration studies, and this technique is recommended for detecting DNA-damaging chemicals (149, 184).

Briefly, this process involves culturing mammalian cells, usually human lymphocytes, in the presence of bromodeoxyuridine. The bromodeoxyuridine is incorporated into chromosomes that have sister chromatids, and after two cycles of DNA replication, the chromosomes contain one chromatid unifilarly substituted and one bifilarly substituted with this compound. These chromatids are then differentially stained with a combined Giesma/fluorescent dye, which allows direct visualization of SCEs, or the reciprocal interchange of DNA between chromatids, in metaphase chromosomes (149, 185).

Carrano et al. (185) described a linear relationship between SCEs and mutations as a function of dose in Chinese hamster ovary cells exposed to chemicals known to interact with DNA. Hundreds of chemicals have been studied experimentally for their ability to induce SCEs (143). Antineoplastic drugs have also been tested extensively in this system (98–100, 143, 149, 184, 186–191). Table 46.1 lists the antineoplastic drugs that have been shown experimentally to increase SCEs.

As with the Ames test, analysis of SCE frequencies has been used as a screening test for occupational exposure to genotoxic agents (143, 150, 152). Patients treated with cytostatic agents have been shown to have increased SCE (189, 192–198). Raposa (184) reviewed these data and concluded that SCE is a useful technique for monitoring exposure to known mutagenic and carcinogenic chemicals, including antineoplastic agents. He noted that several of these drugs, cyclophosphamide, lomustine, doxorubicin, busulfan, mitomycin, thiotepa, and chlorambucil, are potent inducers of SCE. Others, such as 5-fluorouracil, bleomycin, vincristine, dacarbazine, dactinomycin, 6-thioguanine, methotrexate, and cytarabine, do not readily increase SCEs in patients. In Table 46.1, many of the latter group have been designated as ±, which indicates that both positive and negative studies were found. However, most of the positive results were only weakly positive compared with potent inducers of SCE.

Of greater interest, SCE frequencies have been used to monitor health professionals for potential occupational exposure to antineoplastic drugs. Details of these studies are discussed below.

TERATOGENICITY AND SPERMATOTOXIC EFFECTS

Teratogenic effects are those that induce a congenital malformation, or a structural abnormality that develops during the prenatal period. A structural abnormality may result from a mutation in the germ cell or from interference with developmental differentiation processes. A teratogenic agent can induce interference with development by the death of a cell population or by significantly reducing the number of cells differentiating, or cells may survive but are prevented from differentiating. This interference may affect any cellular process from DNA replication through translation or may induce alteration of cellular components, cell membranes, or extracellular products (199–201).

Many antineoplastic agents have been implicated in causing teratogenic effects in animals (170, 173, 202–206). Table 46.1 summarizes these results. Proving teratogenic effects in humans has been somewhat more difficult. Despite a number of case reports and case series documenting abnormalities in the offspring of patients receiving antineoplastic drug treatment (extensively reviewed by Schardein (202)), apparently normal deliveries predominate after single-agent treatment (207, 208) as well as after full-course combination chemotherapy (209, 210). Even more difficult to evaluate are expected second-generation effects from fetal exposure prior to the 5th and 6th months of development (211).

Spermatotoxic effects from exposure to antineoplastic agents are well documented in experimental animals (212–216). Table 46.1 summarizes the agents causing these effects. Azoospermia, oligospermia, decreased sperm motility, and chromosomal aberrations have been found in patients receiving chemotherapy (217–220). In the adult male, spermatogenesis is a continuous process that can be affected by many exogenous factors including occupational exposure to chemicals (211, 221–223) and metals (224, 225). Spermatotoxicity secondary to occupational exposure to antineoplastic drugs has not been studied; however, if systemic absorption occurs, some effect on spermatogenesis can be expected. Just as adrenocortical suppression or hypoglycemia has been reported in pharmaceutical manufacturing workers (226, 227), low-level chronic exposure to agents such as cyclophosphamide may affect spermatogenesis or pregnancy outcome or may induce teratogenic effects (212, 219). Until definitive studies have been completed, appropriate precautions should be used when handling antineoplastic agents. As has been recommended for females (1, 4), males planning families should be temporarily reassigned to other duties.

EVIDENCE OF EXPOSURE

Reviewing the data presented thus far, antineoplastic drugs have mutagenic properties in bacteria and cultured mammalian cells in vitro, can cause chromosomal damage in cultured human lymphocytes, can induce malformations in offspring of test animals given these agents, and can damage or kill sperm in experimental or clinical settings. Furthermore, many, especially the alkylating agents, cause tumors in test animals, and several are known or strongly suspected to cause cancer in humans when given in therapeutic doses. These properties would generally cause one to institute common-sense safety precautions when handling these chemicals (and, indeed, this has been the case, as is discussed in more detail below).

In terms of quantifying the risk of occupational exposure, however, these data serve only as a hazard identification or hazard assessment. To assess risk and, subsequently, the level and type of safety procedures and equipment necessary to avoid that risk, an exposure assessment is necessary. If there is no exposure, obviously there is no risk to employees regardless of the potency of the carcinogen considered. If there is no exposure, then the level and types of precautions necessary are minimal (105).

Occupational exposure to antineoplastic drugs may occur not only during preparation, administration, handling of patient excreta, or handling of contaminated waste materials but also during drug delivery, storage of bulk supplies or wastes, or during inventory. Potential routes for entry into the systemic circulation include inhalation, injection, ingestion, and absorption. There are limited data on which of these routes is most important. Many authors have suggested inhalation, which may seem the most logical route, but some recent data would seem to support ingestion as the primary route. Skin absorption may be a significant factor as well; some antineoplastic drugs are well known to pass through the skin. It seems more likely that entry results from a combination of these routes.

Chemical contamination of surfaces and room air during solution and feed preparation and other mixing and weighing procedures has been well described (228–233). Kleinberg and Quinn (234) detected small amounts of 5-fluorouracil in the downstream airflow of a horizontal-laminar-flow hood. In the 1980s, ambient monitoring was used to evaluate contamination in clinics or pharmacies preparing antineoplastic drugs (235–237). Although small amounts of 5-fluorouracil and cyclophosphamide were found in clinic areas by Neal et al. (235), few precautions and no containment hoods were used at the time of this early study. Neither McDiarmid et al. (236) nor Pyy et al. (237) were able to demonstrate either fluorouracil or cyclophosphamide, respectively, in hospital pharmacy drug preparation areas where containment hoods were being used. More recent studies, however, have detected small amounts of cyclophosphamide and methotrexate in isolated samples (238–240), while Sessink et al. (241) found no cyclophosphamide, fluorouracil, or methotrexate in a hospital pharmacy preparation area in which a containment hood was in use. In manufacturing areas (237, 242), however, much higher levels were found in many of the areas. Aerosolization or droplet contamination during simulated mixing procedures involving vials also has been shown (243–246). Tablet trituration may also cause aerosol formation. Both Dorr and Alberts (247) and Shahsavarani et al. (248) found local environmental contamination following experimental trituration of tablets.

Absorption of chemicals through the skin has been found to be quite variable (249) and probably more dependent on the location than skin thickness (250). Carmustine, applied topically for the treatment of mycosis fungoides, was absorbed; between 5 and 28% of the applied dose was recovered in the urine of patients treated with this drug (251). Cyclophosphamide also has been shown to be absorbed through the skin of patient volunteers (252). Dorr and Alberts (247), using human skin in a standard in vitro transdermal drug penetration model, were not able to demonstrate absorption of daunorubicin, vincristine, vinblastine, or melphalan. One of three samples of doxorubicin demonstrated dermal penetration on the order of 0.009%. Their conclusion was that dermal absorption is not an important route of entry for these drugs.

The amount of systemic exposure in the occupational setting is, intuitively, far less than that received by patients during treatment. However, in the occupational setting, personnel may be exposed to multiple agents for long periods. Thus, measurement of low levels of the various antineoplastic drugs, or a surrogate for them, becomes important in assessing exposure.

In 1970, Ng (5) was the first to publish his concerns about occupational exposure to potentially hazardous cytotoxic drugs. During the

1970s, a few additional reports were published expressing concerns about potential hazards (6, 41, 253, 254). It was during this period that a group of occupational health scientists from the Finnish Institute of Occupational Health began investigations to determine the level of exposure to cytotoxic drugs in occupational settings. Beginning with this study, the evidence that currently documents occupational exposure is reviewed below.

Urine Mutagenicity Screening

Falck et al. (255) studied mutagenic activity in urine concentrates of patients on chemotherapy, nurses who administered these drugs, and an unexposed group of psychologists and office clerks. The screening test used was the bacterial fluctuation test referred to above, with strains of tryptophan-dependent *E. coli* and the histidine auxotrophic *S. typhimurium*. Urine from the nurses was collected on Thursday afternoons of a regular work week and on Monday mornings after a work-free weekend. The results showed a statistically significant increase in urine mutagenicity of the nurses over that of the controls. In a less well known continuation of this study, Vainio et al. (154) reported a decrease in the urine mutagenicity of these nurses as improvements in working conditions were made over a 2-year period (e.g., the use of personal protective clothing and containment hoods). As they concluded, these studies showed the utility of biologic monitoring for exposure to genotoxic agents.

This first study spawned many similar investigations. From 1979 to 1995, at least 30 studies were published that used urine mutagenicity screening in potentially exposed hospital or industry personnel (154, 255–284). Table 46.4 contains a summary of these studies.

Positive urine mutagenesis was reported in nine of these studies, involving a total of 175 personnel. No significant increase in urine mutagenicity was found in 19 studies (at least two other studies were inconclusive). A number of methodologic problems, including questionable sensitivity at low exposure doses, have been identified with the use of the Ames or fluctuation tests for screening urine concentrates (145, 177, 262, 264, 265, 268, 269, 284, 285). Additionally, in 8 of these 19 studies, negative results should be expected, since appropriate safety precautions were in force (256, 259, 260, 266, 268, 273, 277, 281) or the quantities of test-sensitive drug handled were relatively low (259, 264–266, 271, 277, 280).

In the study reported by Staiano et al. (256), for instance, six of the pharmacists studied prepared drugs in a vertical-laminar-flow containment hood. The negative results confirmed that the safety measures employed were effective in reducing exposure below the level of detection via the Ames test. Two other pharmacists from another hospital were also tested in this study. They prepared antineoplastic drugs in a horizontal-laminar-flow hood and used only aseptic technique as a precautionary measure (286, 287). No increase in urine mutagenicity was found in these two pharmacists. This author agrees with Wilson and Solimando (287) that sound aseptic technique in informed individuals is an important safety measure and probably contributed to the negative results in this case. However, it is more likely that the timing of urine sample collection was a major factor contributing to the negative results. A single urine sample was obtained 48 hours after a single 4- to 6-hour exposure and compared with samples taken 48 hours before and at the time of exposure. It is unlikely that mutagens would have been detected using this methodology (178).

Gibson et al. (265) questioned the sensitivity of the bacterial mutagenicity assay for detecting occupational exposure in health care personnel in settings where the doses handled are relatively low. The two nurses in this study handled only seven and three cytotoxic agents over 6- and 8-day periods, respectively. Other negative studies reported 11 infusions per week (271) and 12 to 15 solutions per week (277). While these figures may represent a typical workload in some practices, they are far less than the average 165 doses per week (prepared and administered) reported to Valanis and Shortridge (288) by nurses working in physicians' offices or the 239 genotoxic doses prepared in 1 week by a subject from the study by Anderson et al. (178, 258). Rogers (289) found that nurses who handled a greater number of cytotoxic drugs were more likely to have mutagenic urine.

Several studies used various "before and after" designs to strengthen the statements that could be made regarding the results (154, 255, 258, 273, 275, 282). Among these is the particularly well designed study by Anderson et al. (258) and its companion report by Nguyen et al. (178).

In this study, six pharmacists or technicians prepared between 12 and 90 cytotoxic drugs per

Table 46.4. Summary of Controlled Biologic Monitoring Studies of Personnel Handling Antineoplastic Drugs

Author (Reference)	Exposed Subjects	Test	Results	Work Conditions/Precautions
Falck et al., 1979 (255)	7 RN	UM	+	Prepare and administer; no precautions; 7/7 positive subjects (see Vainio et al. (154))
Norppa et al., 1980 (290)	20 RN	SCE	+	Preparation daily; precautions not specified
Waksvik et al., 1981 (291)	10 RN	SCE	+	Preparation: avg 2150 hr exposure; gloves, masks, some fume hoods
		CA	+	Preparation: avg 2150 hr exposure; gloves, masks, some fume hoods
	11RN	SCE	−	Preparation: avg 1078 hr exposure; gloves, masks, some fume hoods
		CA	−	Preparation: avg 1078 hr exposure; gloves, masks, some fume hoods
Staiano et al., 1981 (256)	6 RPh	UM	−	Prepare only; vertical hood, gloves
	2 RPh			Horizontal hood, aseptic technique
Bos et al., 1982 (257)	29 RN, 3 other	UM	+[a]	Prepare and administer; precautions not stated
Anderson et al., 1982 (258)	6 RPh/tech	UM	+	Prepare only; horizontal hood, no precautions (before)
	4 RPh/tech	UM	−	Prepare only; vertical hood (after)
Jagun et al., 1982 (315)	15 RN	TE	+	Handling conditions not specified; gloves (80%)
Kolmodin-Hedman et al., 1983 (259)	5 RN	UM	+	Prepare and administer; daily handling, no precautions
		SCE	−	Prepare and administer; daily handling, no precautions
	5 RN	UM	−	Prepare and administer; infrequent handling; gloves, gowns, masks, glasses, safety cabinet
		SCE	−	Prepare and administer; infrequent handling; gloves, gowns, masks, glasses, safety cabinet
	5 RN	UM	−	Prepare and administer; gloves, gowns, masks, glasses, safety cabinet
	3 RPh/tech	UM	+	Prepare only; no precautions
	7 RPh/tech	UM	−	Prepare only; gloves, gowns, masks, glasses, safety cabinet
Ratcliffe, 1983 (260)	10 RN	UM	−	Prepare and administer; 7/10 vertical hood, gloves
	11 RPh/tech	UM	−	Prepare only; 9/11 vertical hood, gloves
Rorth et al., 1983 (261)	13 RN	UM	−	Prepare and administer; gloves, gowns, safety cabinet
Gibson et al., 1983 (262)	7 RN	UM	I	Prepare and administer; gloves, gown, mask
Hoffman, 1983 (263)	10 RN	UM	−	Administer only; optional use of gloves
Stiller et al., 1983 (292)	5 RN	SCE	−	Prepare only; gloves
		CA	−	Prepare only; gloves
	4 MD	SCE	−	Prepare only; gloves, protective glasses
		CA	−	Prepare only; gloves, protective glasses
Chrysostomou et al., 1984 (320)	19 RN	MF	+	Administer and some prepare; gloves, masks to prepare
	5 RPh	MF	+	Prepare only; vertical flow hood
Vainio et al., 1984 (154)	7 RN	UM	+	Prepare and administer; gloves, mask, hood (unspecified) 3/7 positive subjects (same group as Falck et al. (218))
Venitt et al., 1984 (264)	2 RPh	UM	−	Prepare only; gloves, gown, mask, horizontal hood
	8 RN	UM	−	Administer only; gloves, gown, masks, goggles

Table 46.4—*continued*. Summary of Controlled Biologic Monitoring Studies of Personnel Handling Antineoplastic Drugs

Author (Reference)	Exposed Subjects	Test	Results	Work Conditions/Precautions
Nava et al., 1984 (37)	16 Workers (manufacturing)	CA	+	Synthesis and packaging of alkylating drugs; no environmental or personal precautions
Nikula et al., 1984 (305)	11 RN	CA	+	Prepare and administer; gloves, masks, fume hood × 1 year
Gibson et al., 1984 (265)	2 RN	UM	−	Administer only; no precautions
Barale et al., 1985 (266)	21 RN	UM	−	Prepare and administer; optional gloves, mask
		SCE	−	Prepare and administer; optional gloves, mask
Cloak et al., 1985 (267)	10 RN	UM	−	Administer only; no precautions
	3 RN	UM	−	Prepare and administer; gloves on open counter
	7 LVN/aide	UM	−	Disposed of excreta; no precautions
Everson et al., 1985 (268)	10 RN	UM	−	Prepare only; vertical hood, gloves
	9 RN	UM	−	Prepare only; vertical hood, gloves
	4 RN	UM	−	Prepare and administer; horizontal hood, gloves
	3 Tech	UM	−	Prepare only; horizontal hood, gloves
Benhamou et al., 1986 (269)	30 RN	UM	+	Prepare and administer; no precautions
1988 (304)		SCE	−	Prepare and administer; no precautions
		CA	−	Prepare and administer; no precautions
Friederich et al., 1986 (270)	24 RN	UM	−	Prepare and administer; gloves in 11/24
Jordan et al., 1986 (293)	18 RN	SCE	−	Prepare and administer; no precautions
Stucker et al., 1986 (271)	17 RN	UM	+	Prepare and administer; no precautions
		SCE	−	Prepare and administer; no precautions
		CA	−	Prepare and administer; no precautions
Pohlova et al., 1986 (272)	38 Chemists/plant workers	UM	+	Precautions not specified
		SCE	+	Precautions not specified
		CA	+	Precautions not specified
Conner et al., 1986 (273)	6 RPh	UM	−	Prepare only; vertical hood, gloves, gown
Bayhan et al., 1987 (316)	13 RN	TE	+	Administer only; no precautions
Penin et al., 1987 (294)	13 RN	SCE	+	Prepare and administer; some gloves, masks, no hoods
Rogers and Emmett, 1987 (274)	59 RN	UM	+	Administer only 31/59; Prepare and administer 28/59; <20% gloves, gowns, masks; no hoods
Burgaz et al., 1988 (317)	10 RN	TE	−	Administer only; gloves (30%)
Caudell et al., 1988 (275)	8 RN	UM	I	Administer only; no precautions
Ferguson et al., 1988 (295)	6 RPh	SCE	+	Prepare only; gloves, vertical-flow hood
		CA	−	Prepare only; gloves, vertical-flow hood
		MN	−	Prepare only; gloves, vertical-flow hood
Sorsa et al., 1988 (276)	17 Manufacturing	UM	−	Precautions not specified
		SCE	−	Precautions not specified
		CA	−	Precautions not specified
		MN	−	Precautions not specified
	25 Production	UM	−	Precautions not specified
		SCE	−	Precautions not specified
		CA	−	Precautions not specified
		MN	−	Precautions not specified
	47 RN/RPh	UM	−	Handling conditions/precautions not specified
		SCE	−	Handling conditions/precautions not specified
Poyen et al., 1988 (277)	29 RN	UM	−	Prepare and administer; gloves, masks, vertical hood 62%; no precautions, 17%
	18 RN	UM	−	Disposed of excreta; precautions not specified
Clonfero et al., 1989 (278)	9 RN	UM	+	Prepare and administer; precautions not specified

Table 46.4—continued. Summary of Controlled Biologic Monitoring Studies of Personnel Handling Antineoplastic Drugs

Author (Reference)	Exposed Subjects	Test	Results	Work Conditions/Precautions
Elliott et al., 1990 (279)	6 RPh	UM	−	Prepare only; precautions not specified
		SCE	−	Prepare only; precautions not specified
Ferguson et al., 1990 (318)	24 RN	MN	−	Handling conditions/precautions not specified
	10 RPh	MN	−	Prepare only; gloves, vertical flow hood?
Krepinsky et al., 1990 (280)	10 RN	UM	−	Prepare and administer; gloves, gowns, masks, no hood
		SCE	−	Prepare and administer; gloves, gowns, masks, no hood
		CA	−	Prepare and administer; gloves, gowns, masks, no hood
Medkova 1990 (306)	23 RN	CA	+	Prepare and administer; full protective clothing (not specified, safety cabinet with exhaust)
	7 MD	CA	+	Administer only; full protective clothing (not specified)
	10 other	CA	−	Handling contaminated laundry, general cleaning; full protective clothing (not specified)
Oestreicher et al., 1990 (296)	8 RN	SCE	−	Prepare and administer; safety cover × 3–4 months
		CA	+	Prepare and administer; safety cover × 3–4 months
	8 RPh	SCE	−	Prepare only; gloves, vertical flow hood
		CA	−	Prepare only; gloves, vertical flow hood
Sarto et al., 1990 (297)	12 RN	SCE	−	Preparation; gloves, masks, horizontal hood?
		CA	−	Preparation; gloves, masks, horizontal hood?
		TE	+	Preparation; gloves, masks, horizontal hood?
Cooke et al., 1991 (307)	11 RN	CA	−	Administer only; gloves, masks
	50 RPh	CA	−	Prepare only; vertical flow hood
Guinee et al., 1991 (281)	15 Pharm Tech	UM	−	Prepare only; gloves, gowns, vertical flow hood
		SCE	−	Prepare only; gloves, gowns, vertical flow hood
		CA	−	Prepare only; gloves, gowns, vertical flow hood
Milkovic-Kraus and Horvat, 1991 (298)	42 RN	SCE	+	Daily exposure (not specified); no precautions
		CA	+	Daily exposure (not specified); no precautions
Sardas et al., 1991 (299)	23 RN	SCE	+	Handling conditions not specified; no precautions
Thiringer et al., 1991 (282)	60 RN	UM	+	Prepare and administer; gloves, some masks, safety hood
		SCE	+	Prepare and administer; gloves, some masks, safety hood
		MN	−	Prepare and administer; gloves, some masks, safety hood
		TE	−	Prepare and administer; gloves, some masks, safety hood
Goloni-Bertollo et al., 1992 (300)	15 RN	SCE	+	Prepare on open counter; gloves, gowns and masks (53%)
		CA	+	Prepare and administer; gloves, some masks, safety hood
Jung et al., 1992 (301)	9 RPh	SCE	−	Prepare only; gloves, gowns, masks, vertical flow hood
		CA	−	Prepare only; gloves, gowns, masks, vertical flow hood

Table 46.4—*continued.* **Summary of Controlled Biologic Monitoring Studies of Personnel Handling Antineoplastic Drugs**

Author (Reference)	Exposed Subjects	Test	Results	Work Conditions/Precautions
Gorecka and Gorski 1993 (302)	37 RN	SCE	−	Handling conditions/precautions not specified
Grummet et al., 1993 (308)	106 RN/MD	CA	+	Prepare and administer; no hoods, personal precautions not specified
Reitz et al., 1993 (309)	27 RN/MD	CA	+	10 MD administer, 17 RN prepare; precautions not specified
Anwar et al., 1994 (312)	20 RN	CA	+	Handling conditions not specified; no precautions
		MN	+	Handling conditions not specified; no precautions
Dubeau et al., 1994 (321)	11 RN, RPh, Tech	MF	+	Prepare only; gloves, vertical-flow hood
Machado-Santelli et al., 1994 (319)	25 RN	MN	+	Prepare only; gloves (84%), masks (76%), no hoods
Newman et al., 1994 (283)	24 RN	UM	−	Prepare and administer (70%); administer only (30%)
				Gloves (65%), rare gowns, masks, glasses, hoods
		TE	−	Gloves (65%), rare gowns, masks, glasses, hoods
Roth et al., 1994 (303)	6 RPh	SCE	−	Prepare only; gloves, gowns, masks, vertical-flow hood
		CA	−	Prepare only; gloves, gowns, masks, vertical-flow hood
		MN	−	Prepare only; gloves, gowns, masks, vertical-flow hood
Sessink et al., 1994 (310)	17 RN/Pharm Tech	CA	+	(Dutch) Prepare and administer; most gloves, gowns, masks; vertical-flow hoods
	11 RN/other	CA	−	(Czech) Prepare and administer; most gloves, gowns, masks; vertical-flow hoods
Fuchs et al., 1995 (311)	10 RN	CA	+	Prepare with no precautions
	81 RN	CA	−	Prepare only?; gloves (90%), masks (55%), vertical-flow hood

[a]Smokers only.
Key: UM, urine mutagenicity; SCE, sister-chromatid exchange; CA, chromosome aberrations; MN, micronucleus test; TE, thioether excretion; MF, mutation frequency; RN, registered nurse; RPh, registered pharmacist; MD, medical doctor; LVN, licensed vocational nurse; Tech, technician; I, inconclusive.

day during a 5-day work week. No special precautions were used at the time, and all drugs were mixed in an open-faced horizontal-laminar-flow unit. Eight consecutive 24-hour urine collections were obtained from these individuals and three controls (administrative staff pharmacists who were not exposed to cytotoxic drugs). The urine concentrates were tested for the presence of mutagens via the Ames mutagenicity test. Results from the initial urine collections demonstrated a significant increase in urinary mutagens in all six experimental subjects. Repetition of this procedure in two subjects wearing a respiratory mask and in two others wearing disposable gloves yielded similar results. In a third method of intervention, use of a class II biologic safety cabinet plus gloving, no substantial increase in urine mutagenicity was found in four subjects (four of the original six subjects).

This study is important in several respects: (*a*) the longitudinal design ensured that the excretion of urinary mutagens would not be missed due to the variable pharmacodynamic properties of these drugs; (*b*) in contrast to some other studies using the Ames test, the potential exposure in this study was relatively high; (*c*) the use of various safety measures following the initial positive results confirmed that controlled ventilation is important in reducing exposure (in this case at least to the limits of detectability); and (d) Connor et al. (273) conducted a follow-up study using the same methods, which confirmed negative urine mutagenicity in a similar group of six pharmacists working in a class II biologic safety cabinet and wearing gloves and gown.

Although there are design limitations in some of the studies reviewed here and some methodologic problems in others, it is clear from several well-designed positive studies that occupational exposure to antineoplastic drugs does occur in some settings. It is clear, also, that institution of various safety measures, such as the use of vertical-flow containment hoods and gloves, does reduce this exposure.

Despite the many problems cited above, urine mutagenicity tests remain a viable choice for biomonitoring groups of health care professionals, not individuals, who are potentially exposed to antineoplastic drugs. Thiringer et al. (282) note that because of increased variability introduced by confounding factors such as diet, medication use, smoking status, age, and sex, the optimal design should be a matched study for at least smoking habits, age, and sex. The results of these studies should be interpreted with full knowledge of the utility and limitations inherent in this method. For example, urine mutagenicity reflects recent exposure to genotoxic substances as opposed to long-term, cumulative effects. Because of low sensitivity, negative results should not be construed or advertised to mean that no exposure has occurred. As found in many recent biologic monitoring studies, urine mutagenicity is often combined with other screening methods to optimize detection of exposure to genotoxic substances. Several of these methods are discussed below.

Sister-Chromatid Exchange

In 1980 Norppa and other investigators (290) from the Finnish Institute of Occupational Health reported a significant increase in the frequency of SCEs in a group of 20 nurses working in oncology units. These nurses had daily or almost daily contact with various cytotoxic drugs and prepared between 10 and 50 doses per day. Waksvik et al. (291) found small but significant increases in chromosome gaps as well as SCEs in a group of 10 nurses with a history of longterm handling of cytotoxic drugs. The average estimated time of drug handling was 2150 hours. In a second group of 11 oncology nurses with an average of 1078 hours of exposure, no increase

in these parameters was found, compared with those of office personnel.

SCE has been used as a biologic monitoring methodology in at least 24 controlled studies of workers handling cytotoxic drugs (259, 266, 271, 272, 276, 279–282, 290–304). Table 46.4 summarizes these studies along with studies using other methodologies. Only five use SCE alone; most studies combined SCE with one or more other screening methods. Ten studies showed an increase in SCEs. Two of these were in manufacturing settings (272, 276), where larger amounts of cytotoxic drugs would be expected. However, the details of the amounts of drugs handled were not given.

As found in the urine mutagenicity studies, some of the negative SCE results should be expected because of the routine use of vertical-flow containment hoods and personal protective gear (281, 296, 301, 303) or relatively low exposure (266, 271, 280, 292). In the otherwise well designed study by Krepinsky et al. (280), the amount of drug handled during the 1-week study period was well documented but was only on the order of milligrams for most of the ten "exposed" nurses. Making a simple conversion to the usual dose of each drug, an average of approximately five doses per week was prepared by each member of this group. If this figure is doubled to include administration of each of the preparations by the same nurse, ten doses handled per week is still a very low potential exposure for this study group, as discussed in the section above. This likely contributed to the negative results reported in this study.

In the study by Barale et al. (266), the total amount of cytotoxic drug handled by each "exposed" participant, classified as either an alkylating agent, antimetabolite, or vinca alkaloid, was listed as total grams over the 2-week study period. While seven of them handled large amounts of drug, over 1000 g total for one participant, many were exposed to very little drug. Five of the 21 handled less than 20 g, and two handled only 2 g during the entire 2-week period. If these five and their matched control are eliminated from the data, the exposed group shows a significant increase in SCEs over the control group by either a t test or the Wilcoxon signed ranks test.

Interpretation of analyses of confounding variables in small data sets is difficult at best. However, all studies should provide data that quantitate the potential exposure of the study group. This should be done in terms of doses or preparations per week (or other time period) and whether these doses are prepared only, administered only, or both prepared and administered. A nurse who prepares a cytotoxic drug and also administers it to the patient has twice the exposure potential of a pharmacist who only prepares the same dose and drug or the nurse who only administers it. Data of this type are missing in 4 of the 24 SCE studies reviewed.

Other Biologic Indicators of Exposure

Cytogenetic analysis for chromosomal abnormalities (CAs) in the form of chromatid or chromosome breaks, gaps, translocations, or dicentrics also has been a much used method of biologic monitoring in health care and manufacturing workers. Table 46.4 displays 24 controlled studies that used this method (37, 271, 272, 276, 280, 281, 291, 292, 295–298, 300, 301, 303–312). Often, analysis for CAs was done in conjunction with other methodologies. Only one-third of these studies used CA as the sole method of screening. Thirteen of these studies reported significant increases in CAs over those of controls.

Urinary thioether excretion has been used to monitor potential exposure to alkylating agents in several occupational groups (313, 314). Jagun et al. (315) found a significant increase in urinary thioether excretion in 15 nurses who regularly handled cytotoxic drugs (at least 10 doses per week), and Bayhan et al. (316) also found a significantly increased level in 13 nurses working on an intravenous therapy team who used no precautions, compared with 26 sex-matched office workers. Sarto et al. (297) reported increased urinary thioethers in 12 exposed nurses who used "complete protective measures." Three other studies, however, found no significant increase (282, 283, 317). Burgaz et al. (317) showed a positive, but not statistically significant, trend in a group of 10 nurses who took only minimum precautions, and Thiringer et al. (282) found no increase in 60 oncology nurses who used safety hoods and gloves, compared with 60 matched controls.

Sorsa et al. (276) reported micronuclei in cytokinesis-blocked peripheral blood lymphocytes as an indicator of occupational exposure in hospital or manufacturing workers handling cytotoxic drugs. This was done in conjunction with monitoring of SCEs, CAs, and urine mutagenicity. A positive trend was noted for the manufacturing workers. Several other recent studies have used screening for micronuclei in groups of po-

tentially exposed health care workers (282, 295, 303, 312, 318, 319). Only two of these studies reported an increase in micronuclei in the exposed groups (312, 318); in both, however, few or no precautions were used. In three of the negative studies (282, 295, 303), exposed personnel used vertical-flow containment hoods and gloves for protection.

An infrequently reported method of assessing genotoxic damage, mutation frequency, was used in two studies of health care workers handling antineoplastic drugs (320, 321). In both studies the nurses and pharmacists used protective measures, but in both, significantly more mutations were detected than in controls matched for age, sex, and smoking. In both studies the increase in mutation frequency was related to the length of exposure.

Although not a usual method of biologic monitoring for exposure to genotoxic agents, several researchers have studied immune function as an indirect indicator of exposure. Lassila et al. (322) measured immune function in 10 exposed nurses and 10 controls and found no significant differences. Jochimsen et al. (323) monitored several hematologic parameters before and after prednisolone stimulation in 18 oncology nurses and 18 nurses who had never handled antineoplastic drugs. There was no significant difference between the two groups, either before or after the stimulation test. Dubeau et al. (321), however, reported a decrease in lymphocyte populations and clonal potential of T cells in a group of health care workers exposed to antineoplastic drugs. They concluded that alterations in the immune system provide essential information regarding exposure to genotoxic agents and that biologic monitoring in exposed populations should include immune system assessment.

In summary, 58 controlled studies using various biologic monitoring methods in potentially exposed health care workers, are summarized in Table 46.4. Of these, 31 reported a significant increase in evidence of genotoxicity in at least one monitored group, compared with controls. Conversely, 37 studies reported negative results in at least one monitored group. Formal metaanalysis of these studies would be difficult because of the wide variety of biologic monitoring and statistical methods used, as well as the lack of complete data on handling conditions and the type of precautions used by the "exposed" participants. Despite the variation in results, a number of well-designed studies show that systemic exposure of health care workers handling antineoplastic drugs did occur. Further, these studies confirmed that the use of standard safety techniques, such as the use of personal protective clothing and vertical-flow containment hoods, reduced this exposure.

Teratogenicity as Evidence of Exposure

Evidence for significant occupational exposure to antineoplastic drugs resulting in increased untoward pregnancy outcomes has been reported in several epidemiologic studies (274, 324–331). Two well-designed studies from the Finnish Institute of Occupational Health used national registries to identify cases among nurses. In the study by Hemminki et al. (324), a significant increase in the number of malformations was found in nurses who handled cytotoxic drugs at least weekly during pregnancy (odds ratio, 4.7; 95% confidence limits, 1.2–18.1). Selevan et al. (325) found a significant increase in fetal loss in nurses occupationally exposed to antineoplastic drugs during the first trimester of pregnancy (odds ratio, 2.30; 95% confidence interval, 1.20–4.39).

In an unrelated study, Rogers and Emmett (274) surveyed nurses from a professional society and from private oncologists' offices and clinics in the Baltimore area. The unexposed control group consisted of community health nurses. Each subject was asked to complete a pregnancy history. The results showed a significant increase in the number of untoward pregnancy outcomes (odds ratio, 2.5; $p \le .04$).

In a well-designed study by Stucker et al. (327), the frequency of spontaneous abortion among nurses handling antineoplastic drugs was significantly greater than that among controls (risk ratio, 2.2; 95% confidence interval, 1.2–4.1). Saurel-Cubizolles et al. (330) reported an increase in ectopic pregnancy in a group of women handling antineoplastic drugs in 18 hospitals in Paris (odds ratio, 10; 95% confidence interval, 2.1–56.2).

In another case-control study from the Finnish Institute of Occupational Health, Taskinen et al. (326) did not find an increase in spontaneous abortions among women working in various occupations within the pharmaceutical industry in general. This included pharmacists but only a small number of subjects exposed to antineoplastic drugs. In a Danish cohort study, Skov et al. (329) found no association between nurses potentially exposed during pregnancy and the incidence of miscarriages, malformations, or low birth weight. Stucker et al. (331) likewise found no significant decrease in the birth weight of offspring born to nurses exposed to antineoplastic drugs during or before pregnancy.

Results from these epidemiologic studies and from the animal and patient studies cited previously support the contention that occupational exposure to antineoplastic drugs during pregnancy increases the risk of fetal loss and malformations. Implicit in this assessment is systemic absorption of these drugs during preparation and administration. Other occupational exposures, such as organic solvents, anesthetic gases, or ethylene oxide, also have been associated with increased risk of untoward pregnancy outcome (332, 333).

In view of these potential toxic effects to the fetus, most guidelines (1) allow female employees who are pregnant or are planning a pregnancy to choose whether to prepare or administer cytotoxic drugs. This is best accomplished by allowing reassignment to areas where exposure is unlikely.

Direct Chemical Evidence of Exposure

The biologic monitoring methods presented above provide indirect evidence of exposure; that is, the effect observed is the result of the presence of a chemical (or antineoplastic drug) in the system of the subject. Such is the case when CAs or increased SCEs are noted in cells or urinary mutagens are obtained from a subject exposed to an alkylating chemical. These genotoxic changes are not specific to any antineoplastic drug or drugs but may be due to a variety of chemical exposures including smoking, working in chemical laboratories, handling insecticides, or taking a variety of drugs. Methods that directly measure a particular cytotoxic agent would provide substantial validation of occupational exposure.

A variety of methods for chemical analysis of antineoplastic drugs has been used (334). Although some of these methods are time consuming and/or expensive to perform, many are sufficiently sensitive to be used in detecting the low levels expected as a result of occupational exposure. Sensitive gas chromatography and high-performance liquid chromatography methods have been developed in recent years (238, 252, 335). A number of studies published in recent years have used these methods to investigate the extent of systemic exposure.

Using gas chromatographic methods, Hirst et al. (252) first reported detecting cyclophosphamide in the urine of two outpatient clinic nurses. The drug solutions were prepared and administered in the usual manner in an open room with no special ventilation. Neither of the nurses wore protective clothing. The daily exposure was low to moderate, ranging from 800 mg to 5.2 g. Small quantities of cyclophosphamide ranging from 0.35 to 9.08 μg were found in eight (32%) urine samples obtained on work days when this drug was handled.

In another study, hospital workers preparing and administering cyclophosphamide provided a single 24-hour urine sample starting on the 4th day of a full work week. A record was kept of all preparation and administration procedures. All of the 20 subjects claimed to have worn at least gloves during the observation period. Small quantities of cyclophosphamide, ranging from 0.7 to 2.5 μg/24 hours, were found in the urine of five of these nurses. Of interest, all five of these subjects were smokers, leading the authors to speculate that a finger-shunt effect may play a role (336). This mechanism was also suggested by Bos et al. (257) when they found increased urinary mutagens in smokers exposed to antineoplastic drugs but not in the nonsmoking exposed group.

Sessink et al. have published a series of studies (238, 240, 241, 310) using similar gas chromatography/mass spectrometry methods, which clearly document the presence of cyclophosphamide in the urine of pharmacy technicians (240, 241, 310), nurses (241, 310), and others (310). Small quantities, ranging from 0.04 to 19.4 μg/24 hours, were found not only in individuals directly involved in preparation or administration of cyclophosphamide but in technicians and nurses working indirectly with this agent (i.e., labeling and delivery). This suggests that exposure occurred via sources other than direct handling. In view of the data discussed earlier that documented surface contamination in pharmacy preparation and clinic administration areas, a likely source for the systemic cyclophosphamide found in these studies was contact with contaminated surfaces (310). Ingestion, therefore, was the most likely route of entry.

Ensslin et al. (337) also reported cyclophosphamide in 12 of 31 urine samples obtained from 21 nurses, pharmacists, or pharmacy technicians preparing antineoplastic drugs using standard safety precautions, a vertical-flow safety cabinet, and gloves. Amounts detected in this study ranged from 3.48 to 38.23 μg/24 hours. Van Kan et al. (338) reported finding no cyclophosphamide in the urine of five pharmacy technicians preparing drug using stringent safety precautions.

In other studies of this nature, Johnson and Gross (339) found no methotrexate in either the blood or urine of 14 nurses in an ambulatory patient care setting, although some of the subjects handled moderate amounts of methotrexate with no precautions other than gloves. Guinee et al. (281) likewise found no methotrexate in the urine of 15 pharmacy technicians preparing moderate amounts of antineoplastic drugs using full safety precautions. No methotrexate was detected by Friederich et al. (270) in blood samples of four oncology nurses who used no precautions. While developing a new high-performance liquid chromatography assay for methotrexate, Mader et al. (335) noted drug in urine samples of nurses handling high-dose (up to 20 g per dose) methotrexate.

Venitt et al. (264) used flameless atomic absorption spectrophotometry to screen for the presence of platinum in urine from a group of nurses and pharmacists handling several platinum-containing agents. All participants wore gloves, masks, clean-room clothing or plastic aprons, and goggles (nurses only). No increase in urinary platinum was found compared with unexposed controls. Patients receiving cisplatin had significant levels of platinum in their urine. Neither Friederich et al. (270) nor Clonfero et al. (278) were able to detect urinary platinum in oncology nurses. A new voltammetric detection method for urinary platinum, tested by Ensslin et al. (340), was found to be very sensitive (picogram range) and much cheaper than other reported methods. In this study, 2 of 21 hospital workers who handled cisplatin and carboplatin using standard safety precautions had elevated urinary platinum levels.

Although urinary platinum now appears to be a viable alternative for monitoring occupational exposure, there are some study design considerations. Single urine samples obtained at the end of a work week or on the same day as exposure may have missed the peak excretion period of cisplatin. Animal pharmacology studies with radiolabeled platinum show that retention varies with the route of administration (i.e., intravenous vs. oral vs. inhalation) (341, 342). However, a urinary platinum excretion study of workers handling catalytic material showed an increase in the excretion of platinum at the end of a work week (343). A longitudinal study design would clarify the excretion pattern in exposed hospital workers. Additionally, although platinum may not be a "normal urinary constituent in healthy people" (264, 344), there is evidence of significant levels of platinum in the tissues of the normal population (345). Background urinary platinum levels may confound efforts to determine low-level exposure; matched control groups should be used whenever possible.

It is clear from the results of the studies cited above that low-level systemic exposure to cyclophosphamide, methotrexate, and cisplatin can occur during routine handling, and of particular concern, whether or not safety precautions are used. Although confirmatory studies using other antineoplastic agents would be ideal, it can be theorized that experiments with other cytotoxic drugs handled using similar procedures and conditions would yield similar results. In view of the limited sensitivity of some biologic screening tests, such as the urine mutagenicity assay, direct chemical analyses should be used in their stead (270), especially in exposed groups using standard safety precautions.

QUANTITATIVE RISK ASSESSMENT

The first two steps of a quantitative risk assessment (QRA) have been discussed: the hazard identification and the exposure assessment. Hazard identification involves a qualitative evaluation of the available information regarding the ability of a particular substance to induce carcinogenic effects and the importance of these data to humans. The exposure assessment defines the amount of a substance that comes into contact, or may come into contact, with human populations (105). In both cases, the data are somewhat limited, which makes proceeding to the third step even more difficult.

In viewing the hazard posed from occupational exposure to cytotoxic drugs, much information from long-term animal bioassays suggests that these agents are indeed carcinogenic. Additionally, the genotoxic effects on a variety of bacterial, animal, and human cell types are well documented. More convincingly, numerous case series and follow-up reports on clinical trials of patients exposed to long-term, therapeutic doses of these agents document significant increases in the occurrence of malignancies, usually leukemias. However, most of these reports fall short of the epidemiologic studies necessary to determine the incidence rates of these induced cancers. Further, there are no epidemiologic studies looking at the incidence of cancer in the occupationally exposed populations.

The exposure assessment suffers from a similar lack of information regarding human exposure. Limited ambient monitoring has demonstrated low-level contamination of air in occupational settings where antineoplastic drugs are handled. However, only a few agents have been tested, and the types of work conditions were limited. There are fairly convincing data from urinary mutagenicity and cytogenic monitoring studies that show that exposure does occur in the typical work place; however, these data are not sufficient to apply to a dose-response assessment. There is further evidence of systemic exposure in the form of direct chemical analyses of urine of exposed nurses and hospital workers and epidemiologic studies of the teratogenic effects of these drugs in nurses exposed during pregnancy. Obviously, far more environmental and personnel monitoring will be necessary to fully characterize exposure to cytotoxic drugs in all populations affected.

The third step in QRA is the hazard, or dose-response, assessment (105, 346). This is an attempt to quantitatively define the response associated with a particular dose of the carcinogen in question. Data for this assessment usually come from human exposures or long-term animal bioassays. Estimating the response that occurs at the low levels of exposure requires some form of mathematic low-dose extrapolation procedure (347, 348).

In the case of the dose-response assessment for antineoplastic drugs, the poor data discussed above make such an assessment very difficult. None of the standard models used for risk estimation, such as the one-hit or linear model or the log-probit model, can be used. However, given the constraints and estimates below, some examples of possible dose-response curves for estimating the risk of exposure to low-doses of cyclophosphamide are presented in Figure 46.2.

For purposes of this exercise, several clinical trials, which documented the induction of leukemias or other cancers following long-term, low-dose alkylating agents, were used to estimate an average total exposure dose in these patients (114, 116, 124–130, 134, 135, 349). There were many deficiencies in these data. Often, data on total dose, latency, or duration of therapy were not given. Not only did the amount and duration of treatment vary from study to study, different drugs were used, making a conversion

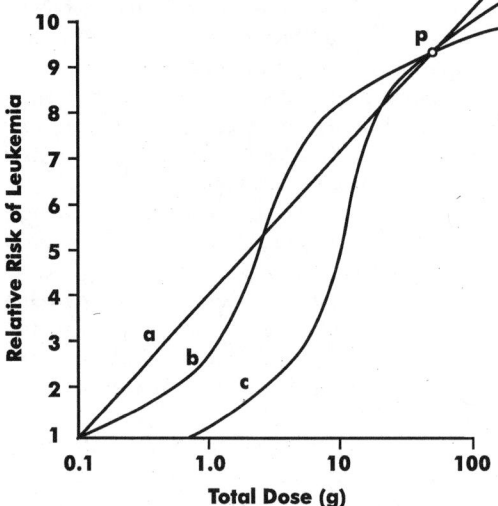

Figure 46.2.   Example dose-response curves for estimating the relative risk of leukemia from occupational exposure to cyclophosphamide. Point *P* was estimated from (*a*) the average total dose received by patients for treatment of various malignant and nonmalignant disorders who later developed a second malignancy (leukemia) and (*b*) the average relative risk of developing leukemia reported for these patients. See text for further discussion.

to a common alkylating agent necessary. For purposes of this discussion, doses of chlorambucil or melphalan were converted to therapeutically equivalent doses of cyclophosphamide. However, as discussed by Kaldor et al. (130) and Green et al. (350), these drugs probably do not share equal leukemogenic potential. This total patient exposure dose was then related to an average relative risk of developing leukemia as reported in many of these studies. (The reported relative risk in studies with melphalan or chlorambucil was divided by three) (130). These two averages are plotted at point *P* on the graph in Figure 46.2.

An estimate of low-dose occupational exposure to cyclophosphamide was made from projections of the data presented in the several studies discussed above in which cyclophosphamide was found in the urine of health care workers (240, 241, 252, 310, 336, 337). A moderately high level of handling was assumed: 3 to 5 doses or 3 to 4 g of cyclophosphamide per day. The daily exposure dose was estimated to be approximately 650 μg. This exposure was then assumed to occur daily, 5 days a week, for 3.5 years, resulting in an estimated occupational exposure

dose. This duration of exposure was chosen because it is similar to the average duration of treatment in the clinical trials above.

The predictions below are based on a moderate daily exposure to cyclophosphamide. It would be easy to find examples of individuals exposed to twice as much cyclophosphamide on a daily basis. Also, many nurses and pharmacists working today may have had 5, 10, or even 20 years of exposure. How such an increase in exposure duration affects these predictions is uncertain.

Figure 46.2 shows three possible curves: *a*, a straight-line projection from the average total exposure dose/risk through the no-risk (relative risk of 1) no-dose point; *b*, a sigmoid dose-response curve, often postulated to be the true shape of a dose-response curve (351); and *c*, a curvilinear dose-response curve depicting the possibility of a threshold dose.

Using the estimated occupational exposure dose of 0.57 g of cyclophosphamide, the relative risk of developing leukemia can be estimated for each of these curves. This crude estimation procedure predicts relative risks of approximately 3 and 2 for curves *a* and *b*, respectively. There would be no increased risk predicted for this dose level using curve *c*, which demonstrates a threshold dose or dose below which no response is seen (in this example, 0.7 g).

This discussion has focused on cyclophosphamide for several reasons: it is one of the most commonly used antineoplastic and immunosuppressive agents, tens of thousands of patients have received this drug as a single agent, and there are exposure data available for this drug and few others. Obviously, a variety of cytotoxic drugs are handled during treatment of cancer patients; for each of these there is a dose-response curve with its attendant risk. It is not known whether these risks are additive or not. The intensity of exposure has not been addressed, nor has the latency of tumor induction. While the time to tumor induction for the index studies cited above averaged 5.4 years, there is no information regarding the latent period following low-dose occupational exposure to cytotoxic drugs. All of these issues must be addressed and appropriate data collected before the QRA can be completed.

The example dose-response curves presented above have been constructed for discussion purposes only and were not calculated from standard modeling procedures. However, the resulting estimates of relative risk for developing leukemia are similar to the risks of developing leukemias or other cancers reported in a number of epidemiologic studies in occupationally exposed populations (352–357). To establish the true range of relative risk from handling cytotoxic drugs, epidemiologic studies of occupationally exposed workers must be conducted. Until such studies are completed, the QRA will remain incomplete and the level of risk a matter of speculation.

SAFE HANDLING OF CYTOTOXIC AGENTS

As the potential hazards associated with the handling of cytotoxic drugs were first recognized, it became clear that there was no formal estimate of the risk on which to base safe handling practices. It is common practice in such cases, where there is controversy or a lack of information, to develop policy that covers the possibility of significant hazard. Most early guidelines were developed in this vein, guided by the conservative philosophy found in published recommendations for handling known carcinogens in the laboratory (358–360). Indeed, most of the general recommendations for handling antineoplastic drugs published in the United States were adapted from these or similar policies (15, 361).

Formal guidelines were first published in Sweden (7, 41) in 1978 and in Norway (6, 8, 9) in 1979. These were followed by recommendations published by professional pharmacy societies in Australia (13) and Canada (14) in 1980 and 1981. Although local policy was being developed in Great Britain (42, 254, 362) and the United States (10, 15–18, 361, 363) during this period, it was not until 1983 in Great Britain (364–365) and 1986 in the U.S. (26) that government-supported guidelines were published. In addition to the recommendations from various disciplines summarized in the introduction, scores of guidelines and policy statements, too numerous to mention here, have been published in the U.S. since 1982.

In spite of the large number of published guidelines from diverse sources, the basis of the recommendations is similar throughout. All require specific operational and personnel practices designed to reduce individual exposure. These include the use of protective clothing and gloves, control of the environment, and proper storage and disposal of cytotoxic agents. Other requirements include routine medical surveillance, employee education and training programs, emergency procedures for spills or acute

exposures, and defining the overall responsibility for the safety program. The goal of all of the guidelines is to protect the employee from unnecessary risk by reducing exposure to the lowest practically achievable level.

Most of the recently published guidelines provide an adequate framework from which one can develop local policy. However, as mentioned in the introduction, the OSHA guidelines (1) should be used as the rule. The referenced technical manual is used as a guide by OSHA inspectors during a site visit to individual hospitals, clinics, or pharmacies, and the institutions are held to the provisions therein. (Regulatory backing for OSHA activities regarding cytotoxic drugs can be found in the OSHA General Industry Standards 29 CFR 1910.132, subpart I, Personal Protective Equipment.) Likewise, the JCAHO requirements for departmental safety plans and education of the employee working in any hazardous setting should be consulted when developing local policy.

The appendix that accompanies this chapter contains an example of basic guidelines for handling antineoplastic drugs in a hospital setting. These can be altered easily to accommodate other needs. The "Technical Assistance Bulletin on Handling Cytotoxic and Hazardous Drugs," from the American Society of Health-System Pharmacists (4), provides a very detailed and helpful set of recommendations for anyone currently preparing or updating local policy. Some aspects of these guidelines are discussed below.

Disposal of Cytotoxic Wastes

Disposal of hazardous wastes is a broad and complicated subject, encompassing a morass of Environmental Protection Agency (EPA) (366), state, and local regulations. Few articles on this subject have appeared in the literature in recent years (367–374). Most recommendations for handling cytotoxic drugs have some discussion of disposal (27).

Research reports from the Environmental Control and Research Program of the National Cancer Institute (375–377) and others (247, 378, 379) have provided detailed methods for chemical deactivation of many commercially available antineoplastic drugs. A careful reading of these reviews and reports will provide a sound basis for making local policy decisions on disposal of cytotoxic drugs.

An excellent general reference, which addresses all aspects of disposal of chemicals from identification and classification to incineration, is the National Academy of Sciences' *Prudent Practices for Disposal of Chemicals from Laboratories* (380). This book provides a common-sense approach to disposing of chemicals, which is adapted easily to the hospital setting.

A number of issues must be addressed when developing disposal guidelines. Seven of the currently available antineoplastic drugs, chlorambucil, cyclophosphamide, daunorubicin, melphalan, mitomycin, streptozocin, and uracil mustard, appear on the EPA hazardous waste list (U-list, as opposed to the P-list or acutely hazardous wastes) and therefore are subject to regulation. However, by virtue of the properties of toxicity, carcinogenicity, mutagenicity, or teratogenicity, which most of the cytotoxic agents possess, all of these agents should be considered hazardous wastes (381).

A waste generator is considered a conditionally exempt small-quantity generator if it generates no more than 100 kg of hazardous waste per month. This exemption allows the generator to treat or dispose of hazardous waste in an on-site facility or ensure its delivery to an off-site facility for disposal. Hazardous waste may be accumulated on-site up to 1000 kg prior to becoming subject to full regulation. The small-quantity generator is exempt from the registration, manifesting, and record-keeping requirements if the waste is treated or disposed of on-site (382).

The choice of on-site or off-site disposal is of major concern. The cost of storing hazardous wastes on-site can be prohibitive, if not in terms of dollars, in terms of the space, security, and record keeping required. Likewise, transporting waste via a licensed waste hauler to a hazardous waste landfill or disposal plant is very costly. On-site disposal may be via chemical deactivation (see references above), release into the sanitary sewer (370, 380), or incineration (1, 380). Each of these has inherent advantages and disadvantages, equipment costs, or regulatory restrictions associated with it (369). The most frequently recommended method for hospitals has been high-temperature incineration. The standard medical-pathologic incinerator typically found in the hospital setting does not routinely achieve the temperatures necessary to completely degrade organic compounds (approximately 1000°C). In addition, although such an incinerator may have a state permit for operation, it is unlikely that the permit allows incineration of hazardous wastes.

Finally, the EPA regulations do not consider empty containers to be hazardous wastes. An empty container is defined as one that contains no more than 3% by weight of the total capacity of the container (383). A glass vial, for instance, that contains more than this amount, must be considered hazardous waste along with its contents. The weight of many discarded glass vials may make up as much as one-third of the weight of chemotherapy waste in an average pharmacy (384). Local policy should address procedures for routinely separating nonempty cytotoxic drug vials from other waste; these must then be handled as hazardous waste. The empty containers and other trace-contaminated waste may be handled as regulated medical waste and incinerated as indicated above.

Personal Protective Gloves

The use of protective gloves is an essential safety requirement when handling any potentially harmful chemical. Current guidelines recommend double surgical-quality latex rubber disposable gloves with extra-long cuffs when handling antineoplastic drugs. This recommendation, however, should not be taken too strictly. Glove selection should be based on a number of factors including permeation properties, thickness, method of manufacture, and dexterity. No protective glove material is impermeable. Any glove product selected is permeable to some extent by every liquid chemical given enough time (385). However, glove materials can be chosen that afford the wearer adequate protection for a given task.

Permeation across a glove membrane is thought to be a three-step process: (a) the challenging chemical dissolves in the outer surface of the membrane, (b) the chemical diffuses through the membrane, and (c) the chemical reaches the inside surface of the membrane and is removed. The diffusion step depends upon the solubility of the chemical in the glove material. Other factors that affect the permeation rate include the thickness of the membrane and the concentration gradient (385, 386).

Both latex rubber and polyvinyl chloride (PVC) provide adequate protection against water-based solutions (387, 388). These same polymers, however, provide little or no protection against many organic solvents (387–389). Since most commercially available antineoplastic drugs are dilute aqueous solutions, both latex rubber and PVC gloves should provide a reasonable barrier to these solutions. Conversely, non-water-soluble drugs in special vehicles, such as carmustine, etoposide, or paclitaxel, may permeate the glove membrane more readily.

Several studies of these two and other glove materials found this to be the case (240, 259, 390–398). Both Slevin et al. (392) and Stoikes et al. (394) demonstrated permeation of microgram quantities of several antineoplastic drugs across membranes of both latex rubber and PVC after a 1-hour exposure. The studies by Connor (391, 398) and Laidlaw (393) and their colleagues at the University of Texas Health Science Center at Houston also showed glove permeation by several cytotoxic agents. Their studies are notable for demonstrating universal penetration of thin PVC glove material by the 20 agents tested. This reinforces the need to purchase high-quality, thick PVC gloves if this glove material is chosen.

Concentration versus time plots from some of these studies (391, 393–397) showed that small quantities of carmustine, thiotepa, fluorouracil, mitoxantrone, and methotrexate had permeated the glove material by 5 to 60 minutes after exposure. Drug permeation increased significantly over 60- to 90-minute test periods. These data suggest that gloves should be worn no more than 30 minutes to protect the worker from an undetected spill. Employee training should emphasize that no matter which glove is being used, they are disposable and should be discarded whenever a splash or spill is suspected or after 30 minutes of use.

Biologic Safety Cabinets

Yodaiken and Bennett (26) considered the use of a biologic safety cabinet (BSC) an essential component of a safety program for handling antineoplastic drugs. Its use was suggested very early in the sequence of recommendations that has led to the current state of practice (254). Although use of a BSC has been consistently recommended, some controversy still exists about which type is most appropriate.

The National Sanitation Foundation standard no. 49 (399) describes the specifications and standards that apply to class II biohazard cabinetry, including types A, B1, B2, and B3. There are several reviews of the relative design features and use of these cabinets (400–403), including the excellent, in-depth review by Kruse et al. (403).

The BSC was designed to provide operator protection from hazardous biologic materials while also providing an aseptic work area. The type A hood should provide adequate protection

as long as the contaminants generated during mixing procedures behave as particles (400, 404–406). The original type B cabinet (now type B1) was also designed for use with volatile chemicals, but only this and the B2 cabinets provide protection from volatile chemicals (407). In the type B2 BSC, none of the cabinet airflow is recirculated through the work zone. The need for this extra protection must be assessed by the user. Services that handle large volumes of cytotoxic drugs, including investigational agents that require nonaqueous vehicles, or that are involved in research procedures in which cytotoxic agents are dissolved in organic solvents, should consider this added protection. This choice must be weighed against the added cost of installing the required external venting equipment and of exhausting conditioned building air to the outside.

Regardless of which cabinet is chosen, the importance of selection and development of good aseptic technique and procedural controls cannot be overemphasized. All of the class II cabinets are open systems; each has a front opening, usually 8 inches high, which allows operator access to the work surface. Improper technique, negligence, or faulty equipment can lead to escape of contaminants from the work zone. Employee training and routine monitoring of technique can help reduce the likelihood of these incidents. Employees must be made aware of the possibility of overt exposure while using a class II BSC.

Where concern for exposure of this kind is high, the use of a class III BSC (glovebox) (400, 403) or isolator (408, 409) may be considered. The class III BSCs are closed systems in which the work surface is accessed via glove ports, and items are passed in and out of the cabinet through an air lock. The class III BSC operates at a vacuum relative to the room and circulates high-energy particulate air (HEPA) filtered air through the work zone. When connected to an external exhaust, this BSC is recommended for handling chemical carcinogens.

An isolator is a totally enclosed ventilated work area in which positive pressure is maintained relative to room air. The large cabinet is made of class III PVC and contains a central half-suit and side-mounted glove ports similar to those of the glovebox described above. The half-suit allows the operator complete access to the work area while remaining physically isolated from the sterilized atmosphere within. The glove ports allow additional operators to assist in drug preparation, but the access is limited. The unit contains both supply and exhaust HEPA filters to maintain an aseptic atmosphere within the work area and to protect the outer environment from contamination with hazardous drugs. All items enter the work area through a sterilizing air lock. Routine sterilization of the isolator work surfaces and contents is accomplished with peracetic acid (408, 409). Although maintenance procedures for an isolator are rigorous, Larrouturou et al. (409) found that when long-term maintenance costs were considered, the isolator was less expensive than maintaining a class II BSC in an aseptic room.

Handling Oral Antineoplastic Drugs

Despite the general concerns regarding the safe handling of antineoplastic drugs, little has been written about proper handling of oral dosage forms. Intuitively, solid dosage forms seem to pose less threat than their liquid counterparts, usually containing relatively small amounts of drug compared with standard intravenous doses. However, as discussed above, several studies have shown local environmental contamination after crushing of tablets or during manufacturing or packaging operations (237, 247, 248, 276). If tablets are crushed or capsules emptied to facilitate administration to patients, exposure to tablet dust is possible. The few data available suggest that tablet dust is not likely to be inhaled (247, 248). The particles probably settle on, or are transferred to, flat surfaces, clothing, food or drink containers, and the hands and likely enter the body by ingestion.

A number of comments have appeared in the literature over the years encouraging proper handling of oral antineoplastic drugs (410–412). Some recommendations were included in general published guidelines (365, 413). However, as shown in a survey by Sauer et al. (414), use of protective equipment when handling oral antineoplastic drugs in institutional pharmacies was infrequent.

The ASHP Technical Assistance Bulletin on Handling Cytotoxic and Hazardous Drugs (4) provides some detail on handling oral dosages forms. These recommendations include proper identification and warning labels; use of gloves for routine handling; use of containment hoods, respiratory protection, and gloves and gowns during compounding procedures; proper cleaning of equipment used for counting, pouring, or compounding; and proper disposal of used or unusable oral dosage forms and contaminated supplies. Hazardous tablets or capsules should not be placed in automated counting or packaging machines. All policies and procedures in practices where oral medications are handled should contain guidelines such as these.

Other Hazardous Drugs

As mentioned, there are other toxic drugs that are not used in the treatment of cancer but, nonetheless, should be handled as hazardous drugs as described above. Table 46.5 lists some of the agents that have been classified by three agencies as toxic or potentially carcinogenic. Still other references could be used to designate additional nonantineoplastic agents as having teratogenic, allergenic, or other toxic properties. These agents, in addition to the usual antineoplastic drugs, should be considered for inclusion in the

Table 46.5. Other Potentially Hazardous Drugs That Should be Considered for Special Handling[a]

Drug[b]	Agency
Chloramphenicol	IARC 2A[c]
Coal tars	IARC 1
Cyclosporine	IARC 1
Epinephrine	EPA[d]
Ganciclovir	Ref. 1, 3
Hexachloraphene	EPA, IARC 3
Iron dextran	IARC 2B, NTP[e]
Metronidazole	IARC 2B, NTP
Paraldehyde	EPA
Pentamidine	Ref. 1
Phenacetin	EPA, IARC 2A, NTP
Phenazopyridine	IARC 2B, NTP
Phenoxybenzamine	IARC 2B, NTP
Phenytoin	IARC 2B, NTP
Propylthiouracil	IARC 2B, NTP
Reserpine	EPA, IARC 3, NTP
Ribavirin	Ref. 1, 3
Resorcinol	EPA
Saccharin	EPA
Selenium sulfide	EPA
Warfarin	EPA
Zidovudine	Ref. 1, 3

[a]Does not include anesthetics or hormones.
[b]Generic or common name.
[c]International Agency for Research on Cancer; 1, known human carcinogen; 2A, probable human carcinogen; 2B, possible human carcinogen; 3, not classified (111).
[d]Environmental Protection Agency acute or hazardous waste (381).
[e]National Toxicology Program; substances that may reasonably be anticipated to be (human) carcinogens (112).

policies and procedures for safe handling of all hazardous drugs (4). McDiarmid et al. (3) have discussed their experience in reviewing such agents at their institution.

CONCLUSIONS

Antineoplastic drugs are chemicals with a variety of hazardous properties. Several of these therapeutic agents can cause irritation or damage to the skin, eyes, or mucous membranes. Many have been shown to be mutagenic in bacteria or mammalian cells in culture. Long-term bioassays in animals have established that many alkylating agents and antitumor antibiotics are carcinogenic. Case series reports, retrospective analysis of clinical trials, and case-referent studies have shown alkylating agents to cause leukemias and other tumors in patients receiving these drugs for the treatment of malignant or nonmalignant conditions. Epidemiologic studies of nurses exposed to cytotoxic drugs during pregnancy found increased risk of malformations and fetal loss.

Using ambient monitoring, antineoplastic drugs have been demonstrated in the air of a horizontal-laminar-flow hood, clinic and pharmacy drug preparation areas, and in drug manufacturing and packaging areas. Biologic monitoring of chromosome aberrations, sister chromatid exchanges, and urinary mutagens has clearly related an increase in these markers with the handling of cytotoxic drugs. Direct chemical analysis of urine from nurses and pharmacists handling cyclophosphamide, methotrexate, and cisplatin found small but significant quantities following typical occupational exposure. The introduction of special techniques, personal protective clothing, and the use of a biologic safety cabinet has been associated with reduction of exposure. In spite of the information available regarding the potential risks of handling antineoplastic drugs, a formal assessment of risk is not feasible at this time. Additional long-term prospective epidemiologic studies are necessary to provide the data to complete this assessment. However, policies have been developed that are designed to eliminate potential risk associated with exposure to cytotoxic drugs. These handling guidelines follow routine common-sense safety procedures for handling any hazardous substance. The goal of these procedures is to reduce exposure to antineoplastic drugs to the lowest practicable level.

ACKNOWLEDGMENTS

The author thanks Kathryn S. Harrison, M.A., Melvin E. Liter, M.S., Pharm.D., Byron G. Peters, R.Ph., and Raymond J. Godefroid, R.Ph., for their review of this chapter, as well as Elisabeth Heiberg, M.D., H. Joachim Reimers, M.D., and Preben Bjerregaard, M.D. for their translations of the Norwegian, Swedish, German, and Danish, and Emily A. Dierker, Pharm.D., and Melissa Johnson, Pharm.D., for their assistance with literature review.

REFERENCES

1. Anon. Controlling occupational exposure to hazardous drugs. In: OSHA technical manual (OSHA instruction CPL 2–2.20B CH-4). Washington: Directorate of Technical Support, Occupational Safety and Health Administration; 1995:chap 21.

2. Myers CE, Zellmer WA, Friedman MK, et al. Development of a symbol for hazardous drug products. Pharmacopeial Forum 1994;20:8575–8578.

3. McDiarmid MA, Gurley HT, Arrington D. Pharmaceuticals as hospital hazards: managing the risks. J Occup Med 1991;33:155–158.

4. Anon. ASHP technical assistance bulletin on handling cytotoxic and hazardous drugs. Am J Hosp Pharm 1990;47:1033–1049.

5. Ng LM. Possible hazards of handling antineoplastic drugs (letter). Pediatrics 1970;46:648–649.

6. Gundersen S. Safety rules in preparation and infusion of cytostatic materials. Tidsskr Nor Laegeforen 1976;96:1388.

7. Hakansson L, Landersjo L. Instructions for handling and administration of cytostatics. Stockholm, Sweden: National Social Welfare Board, Department of Drugs, 1978.

8. Directorate of Labour Inspection. Guidelines concerning the handling of cytostatic agents. Oslo, Norway, 1980.

9. Eriksen IL. Handling of cytotoxic drugs: governmental regulations and practical solutions. Pharm Internat 1982g:264–267.

10. Oncology Nursing Society. Cancer chemotherapy guidelines and recommendations for nursing education and practice. Pittsburgh: Oncology Nursing Society, 1984.

11. Rubadue CL. Potential health hazards with antineoplastic drugs. Occup Health Nurs 1985;33:363–366.

12. Gullo SM. Safe handling of antineoplastic drugs: translating the recommendations into practice. Oncol Nurs Forum 1988;15:595–601.

13. Davis MR. Handling and preparation of cytotoxic drugs—minimising the risks. Aust J Hosp Pharm 1980;10:127–130.

14. Canadian Society of Hospital Pharmacists. Guidlelines for the handling of hazardous pharmaceuticals. Can J Hosp Pharm 1981;34:126–128.

15. Harrison BR. Developing guidelines for working with antineoplastic drugs. Am J Hosp Pharm 1981; 38:1686–1693.

16. Anon. Recommendations for handling cytotoxic agents. Providence: National Study Commission on Cytotoxic Exposure, 1982.

17. Stolar MH, Power LA, Viele CS. Safe handling of cytotoxic drugs in hospitals. Am J Hosp Pharm 1983; 40:1163–1171.

18. Anon. ASHP technical assistance bulletin on handling cytotoxic drugs in hospitals. Am J Hosp Pharm 1985;42:131–137.

19. Hillcoat BL, Levi J, Snyder R. Preparation and administration of antineoplastic agents. Med J Aust 1983;1:424–426.

20. Anon. Guidelines for handling parenteral antineoplastics. JAMA 1985;253:1590–1592.

21. Farrant E. Safe handling of cytotoxic drugs. Occup Health 1981ğ:402–405.

22. Vainio H. Inhalation anesthetics, anticancer drugs and sterilants as chemical hazards in hospitals. Scand J Work Environ Health 1982;8:94–107.

23. Stellman JM, Zoloth SR. Cancer chemotherapeutic agents as occupational hazards: a literature review. Cancer Invest 1986;4:127–135.

24. Rogers B. Health hazards to personnel handling antineoplastic agents. Occup Med State Art Rev 1987;2:513–525.

25. Widstrom J, Edling C. Antineoplastic agents. In: Burne OK, Edling C, eds. Occupational hazards in the health professions. Boca Raton, FL: CRC Press, 1989:131–139.

26. U.S. Department of Labor, Office of Occupational Medicine: Occupational Safety and Health Administration. Work practice guidelines for personnel dealing with cytotoxic (antineoplastic) drugs. Publ. no. 8-1.1, 1986.

27. Kaijser GP, Underberg WJM, Beijnen JH. The risks of handling cytotoxic drugs: II. Recommendations for working with cytotoxic drugs. Pharm Weekbl (Sci) 1990;12:228–235.

28. McDiarmid MA. Medical surveillance for antineoplastic-drug handlers. Am J Hosp Pharm 1990; 47:1061–1066.

29. Medkova J. Guidelines for and possibilities of safe handling of cytostatics. Acta Univ Palacki Olomuc 1991;130:333–339.

30. Mayer DK. Hazards of chemotherapy—implementing safe handling practices. Cancer (Suppl) 1992; 70:988–992.

31. Harrison BR. Safe handling of antineoplastic drugs. Top Hosp Pharm Manage 1994;14:1–10.

32. Joint Commission on Accreditation of Healthcare Organizations. 1996 Comprehensive accreditation manual for hospitals, 1994.

33. Merck & Co., Inc. Mechlorethamine (Mustargen) package insert. West Point, PA, September 1994.

34. Thestrup-Pedersen K, Christiansen JV, Zachariae H. Precautions for personnel applying topical nitrogen mustard to patients with mycosis fungoides. Dermatologica 1982;165:108–113.

35. Frost P, DeVita V. Pigmentation due to a new antitumor agent. Arch Dermatol 1966;94:265–268.

36. Gottlieb JA. Hazards of handling antineoplastic drugs (letter). Pediatrics 1971;47:480.

37. Nava C, Vangosa GB, Forni A. Pathological manifestations in workers engaged in the production or administration of cytotoxic drugs. Boll Chim Farm 1984;123:547–551.

38. Reich SD, Bachur NR. Contact dermatitis associated with Adriamycin and daunorubicin (letter). Cancer Chemother Rep 1975;59(part 1):677–678.

39. Clemmons DE, Aeling JL, Nuss DD. Dermatitis medicamentosa: a pitfall for the unwary. Arch Dermatol 1976;112:1178–1179.

40. Zelickson AS, Mottaz J, Weiss LW. Effects of topical fluorouracil on normal skin. Arch Dermatol 1975;111:1301–1306.

41. Johansson H. How hazardous are cytostatic agents to personnel? Vardfacket 1979;3(1):10–16.

42. Knowles RS, Virdin JE. Handling of injectable antineoplastic agents. Br J Med 1980;281:589–594.

43. Honda DH, Ignoffo RJ, Power LA. Safety consideration in the preparation of parenteral antineoplastics. CSHP Voice 1981;8:94–96.

44. Crudi CB. A compounding dilemma: I've kept the drug sterile but have I contaminated myself? (letter). NITA 1980;3:77–78.

45. Larson DL. What is the appropriate management of tissue extravasation by antitumor agents? Plast Reconstr Surg 1985;75:397–402.

46. Rudolph R, Larson DL. Etiology and treatment of chemotherapeutic agent extravasation injuries: a review. J Clin Oncol 1987;5:1116–1126.

47. Duvall E, Baumann B. An unusual accident during the administration of chemotherapy. Cancer Nurs 1980;3:305–306.

48. Dorr RT. Practical techniques for preparation and administration of cytotoxic agents. Presented at the symposium Practical approaches to safe handling of anticancer products. Mayaguez, Puerto Rico: Nov 2–5, 1983.

49. Dorr RT. Antidotes to vesicant chemotherapy extravasations. Blood Rev 1990;4:41–60.

50. McFarlane A. Ophthalmic problems in staff handling cytotoxic drugs (letter). Aust J Hosp Pharm 1986;16:145.

51. Crudi CB, Stephens BL, Maier P. Possible occupational hazards associated with the preparation/administration of antineoplastic agents. NITA 1982; 5:264–266.

52. Valanis BG, Vollmer WM, Labuhn KT, Glass AG. Association of antineoplastic drug handling with acute adverse effects in pharmacy personnel. Am J Hosp Pharm 1993;50:455–462.

53. Wertenbaker C. Intraocular inflammation from accidental instillation of doxorubicin. Cancer Treat Rep 1987;71:221–222.

54. Hamersley J, Luce JK, Florentz TR, et al. Excessive lacrimation from fluorouracil treatment (letter). JAMA 1973;225:747–748.

55. Haidak DJ, Hurwitz BS, Yeung KY. Tear-duct fibrosis (dacryostenosis) due to 5-fluorouracil (letter). Ann Intern Med 1978;88:657.

56. Christophidis N, Lucas I, Vajda FJE, Louis WJ. Lacrimation and 5-fluorouracil (letter). Ann Intern Med 1978;89:574.

57. Caravella LP, Burns JA, Zangmeister M. Punctal-canalicular stenosis related to systemic fluorouracil therapy. Arch Ophthalmol 1981;99:284–286.

58. Shapiro MS, Thoft RA, Friend J, et al. 5-Fluorouracil toxicity to the ocular surface epithelium. Invest Ophthalmol Vis Sci 1985;26:580–583.

59. Curran CF, Luce JK. Accidental acute exposure to fluorouracil. Oncol Nurs Forum 1989;16:468.

60. Kaufman HE, Capella JA, Maloney ED, et al. Corneal toxicity of cytosine arabinoside. Arch Ophthalmol 1964;72:535–540.

61. Elliott GA, Schut AL. Studies with cytarabine

in normal eyes of man, monkey, and rabbit. Am J Ophthalmol 1965;60:1074–1082.

62. Hopen G, Mondino BJ, Johnson BL, Chervenick PA. Corneal toxicity with systemic cytarabine. Am J Ophthalmol 1981;91:500–504.

63. Mosci L. Astigmatism against the rule in a case of burning of the cornea by vincaleukoblastine. Ann Ottalmol Clin Ocul 1967;93:94–100.

64. Cordier J, Mendelsohn P. Corneal ulceration from an antimitotic. Bull Soc Ophthalmol Fr 1970; 70:116–122.

65. Lisch K. Ophthalmic-pharmacologic complications. Klin Monatsbl Augenheilkd 1976;169:129–133.

66. McLendon BF, Bron AJ. Corneal toxicity from vinblastine solution. Br J Ophthalmol 1978;62:97–99.

67. Dorr RT, Von Hoff DD, eds. Cancer chemotherapy handbook. 2nd ed. Norwalk, CT: Appleton & Lange, 1993.

68. Teir H. Toxicologic effects on the eyes at work. Acta Ophthalmol (Copenh) 1984;161(Suppl):60–65.

69. Saari KM, Leinonen J, Aine E. Management of chemical eye injuries with prolonged irrigation. Acta Ophthalmol (Copenh) 1984;161(Suppl):52–59.

70. Ladik CF, Stoehr GP, Maurer MA. Precautionary measures in the preparation of antineoplastics (letter). Am J Hosp Pharm 1980;37:1184–1185.

71. Reynolds RD, Ignoffo R, Lawrence J, et al. Adverse reactions to AMSA in medical personnel (letter). Cancer Treat Rep 1982;66:1885.

72. Sotaniemi EA, Sutinen S, Arranto AJ, et al. Liver damage in nurses handling cytostatic agents. Acta Med Scand 1983;214:181–189.

73. McDiarmid M, Egan T. Acute occupational exposure to antineoplastic agents. J Occup Med 1988; 30:984–987.

74. Rodriquez P, Yap CY. Abnormal blood results found in pharmacists preparing cytotoxics (letter). Aust J Hosp Pharm 1991;21:39.

75. Valanis BG, Hertzberg V, Shortridge L. Antineoplastic drugs: handle with care. AAOHN J 1987; 35:487–492.

76. Conde-Salazar L, Guimaraens D, Romero L. Occupational contact dermatitis from cytosine arabinoside synthesis. Contact Dermatitis 1984;10:44–45.

77. Anon. Occupational exposures to formaldehyde in dialysis units. MMWR 1986;35:399–401.

78. Sargeni EV, Kirk GD. Establishing airborne exposure control limits in the pharmaceutical industry. Am Ind Hyg Assoc J 1988;49:309–313.

79. Ford MA, Cristea G, Robbins WD, et al. Delayed psyllium allergy in three nurses. Hosp Pharm 1992;27:1061–1062.

80. Weiss RB, Baker JR. Hypersensitivity reactions from antineoplastic agents. Cancer Metastasis Rev 1987;6:413–432.

81. Zackheim HS, Arnold JE, Farber EM, Cox AJ. Topical therapy of psoriasis with mechlorethamine. Arch Dermatol 1972;105:702–706.

82. Van Scott EJ, Kalmanson JD. Complete remissions of mycosis fungoides lymphoma induced by topical nitrogen mustard. Cancer 1973;32:18–30.

83. Pepys J. Allergy to platinum compounds. In: Grossblatt N, ed. Platinum group metals. Washington, DC: National Academy of Sciences, 1977:105–124.

84. Boggs PB. Platinum allergy. Cutis 1985;35:318–320.

85. Merget R, Schultze-Werninghaus G, Muthorst T, et al. Asthma due to the complex salts of platinum—a cross-sectional survey of workers in a platinum factory. Clin Allergy 1988;18:569–580.

86. Bolm-Audorff U, Bienfait HG, Burkhard J, et al. Prevalence of respiratory allergy in a platinum refinery. Int Arch Occup Environ Health 1992;64:257–260.

87. Goldberg A, Altaras MM, Mekori YA, et al. Anaphylaxis to cisplatin: diagnosis and value of pretreatments in prevention of recurrent allergic reactions. Ann Allergy 1994;73:271–272.

88. Shlebak AA, Clark PI, Green JA. Hypersensitivity and cross-reactivity to cisplatin and analogues. Cancer Chemother Pharmacol 1995;35:349–351.

89. Chang SM, Fryberger S, Crouse V, et al. Carboplatin hypersensitivity in children: a report of five patients with brain tumors. Cancer 1995;75:1171–1175.

90. National Institute for Occupational Safety and Health. U.S. Department of Health and Human Services. Occupational health guideline for soluble platinum salts (as platinum) 1978:1–5.

91. Haddow A. Influence of certain polycyclic hydrocarbons on the growth of the Jenson rat sarcoma (letter). Nature 1935;136:868–869.

92. Shimkin MB, Weisburger JH, Weisburger EK, et al. Bioassay of 29 alkylating chemicals by the pulmonary-tumor response in strain A mice. J Natl Cancer Inst 1966;36:915–935.

93. Stoner GD, Shimkin MB, Kniazeff AJ, et al. Test for carcinogenicity of food additives and chemotherapeutic agents by the pulmonary tumor response in strain A mice. Cancer Res 1973;33:3069–3085.

94. Weisburger JH, Griswold DP, Prejean JD, et al. The carcinogenic properties of some of the principal drugs used in clinical cancer chemotherapy. Recent Results Cancer Res 1975;52:1–17.

95. Weisburger EK. Bioassay program for carcinogenic hazards of cancer chemotherapeutic agents. Cancer 1977;40:1935–1949.

96. Leopold WR, Miller EC, Miller JA. Carcinogenicity of antitumor cis-platinum(II) coordination complexes in the mouse and rat. Cancer Res 1979;39:913–916.

97. Gold LS, Sawyer CB, Magaw R, et al. A carcinogenic potency database of the standardized results of animal bioassays. Environ Health Perspect 1984; 58:9–319.

98. Nesnow S, Argus M, Bergman H, et al. Chemical carcinogens: a review and analysis of the literature of selected chemicals and the establishment of the gene-tox carcinogen data base. Mutat Res 1986;185:1–195.

99. Cimino MC, Auletta AE. Availability of the GEN-TOX database on the National Library of Medicine TOXNET system (letter). Mutat Res 1993;297:97–99.

100. Chemical Carcinogenesis Research Information System. National Library of Medicine. Bethesda: U.S. Department of Health and Human Services, 1995.

101. Schmahl D, Habs M. Experimental carcinogenesis of antitumor drugs. Cancer Treat Rev 1978; 5:175–184.

102. Harris CC. The carcinogenicity of anticancer drugs: a hazard in man. Cancer 1976;37:1014–1023.

103. Lien EJ, Ou X. Carcinogenicity of some anticancer drugs—a survey. J Clin Hosp Pharm 1985; 10:223–242.

104. Litterst CL. Toxicity of antineoplastic drugs,

with special reference to teratogenesis, carcinogenesis, and the reproductive system. In: Haley TJ, Berndt WO, eds. Handbook of toxicology. Washington, DC: Hemisphere, 1987;8:310–363.

105. U.S. Interagency Staff Group on Carcinogens. Chemical carcinogens: a review of the science and its associated principles. Environ Health Perspect 1986; 67:210–282.

106. Shields PG, Harris CC. Principles of carcinogenesis: chemical. In: DeVita VT, Hellman S, Rosenberg SA, eds. Cancer: principles and practice of oncology. Philadelphia: JB Lippincott, 1993;200–212.

107. International Agency for Research on Cancer, World Health Organization. IARC monographs on the evaluation of the carcinogenic risk of chemicals to humans. Chemicals and industrial processes associated with cancer in humans. IARC Monogr 1979;(Suppl 1):1–70.

108. International Agency for Research on Cancer, World Health Organization. IARC monographs on the evaluation of the carcinogenic risk of chemicals to humans. Some antineoplastic and immunosupressive agents. IARC Monogr 1981;26:37–384.

109. International Agency for Research on Cancer, World Health Organization. IARC monographs on the evaluation of the carcinogenic risk of chemicals to humans. Genetic and related effects: an updating of selected IARC monographs from volumes 1 to 42. IARC Monogr 1987;(Suppl 6).

110. International Agency for Research on Cancer, World Health Organization. IARC monographs on the evaluation of carcinogenic risks to humans. Overall evaluation of carcinogenicity: an updating of IARC monographs volumes 1 to 42. IARC Monogr 1987; (Suppl 7).

111. International Agency for Research on Cancer, World Health Organization. IARC monographs on the evaluation of carcinogenic risks to humans. Pharmaceutical drugs. IARC Monogr 1990;50:26–136.

112. U.S. Department of Health and Human Services, Public Health Service, National Toxicology Program. Seventh annual report on carcinogens, 1994.

113. Thiede T, Chievitz E, Christensen BC. Chlornaphazine as a bladder carcinogen. Acta Med Scand 1964;175:721–725.

114. Fairchild WV, Spence R, Solomon HD, Gangai MP. The incidence of bladder cancer after cyclophosphamide therapy. J Urol 1979;122:163–164.

115. Schmahl D, Auer TR. Iatrogenic carcinogenesis. New York: Springer-Verlag, 1977:30–39.

116. Berk PD, Goldberg JD, Silverstein MN, et al. Increased incidence of acute leukemia in polycythemia vera associated with chlorambucil therapy. N Engl J Med 1981;304:441–447.

117. Rosner F, Grunwald H. Hodgkin's disease and acute leukemia. Am J Med 1975;58:339–353.

118. Brody RS, Schottenfeld D, Reid A. Multiple primary cancer risk after therapy for Hodgkin's disease. Cancer 1977;40:1917–1926.

119. Pedersen-Bjergaard J, Larsen SO. Incidence of acute nonlymphocytic leukemia, preleukemia, and acute myeloproliferative syndrome up to 10 years after treatment of Hodgkin's disease. N Engl J Med 1982; 307:965–971.

120. Kaldor LM, Day NE, Band P, et al. Second malignancies following testicular cancer, ovarian cancer and Hodgkin's disease: an international collaborative study among cancer registries. Int J Cancer 1987; 39:571–585.

121. Prior P, Pope DJ. Hodgkin's disease: subsequent primary cancers in relation to treatment. Br J Cancer 1988;58:512–517.

122. Kaldor JM, Day NE, Clarke EA, et al. Leukemia following Hodgkin's disease. N Engl J Med 1990; 322:7–13.

123. Rosner F, Grunwald H. Multiple myeloma terminating in acute leukemia. Am J Med 1974;57:927–939.

124. Reimer RR, Hoover R, Fraumeni JB, et al. Acute leukemia after alkylating-agent therapy of ovarian cancer. N Engl J Med 1977;297:177–181.

125. Greene MH, Boice JD, Greer BE, et al. Acute nonlymphocytic leukemia after therapy with alkylating agents for ovarian cancer. N Engl J Med 1982; 307:1416–1421.

126. De Gramont A, Remes P, Krulik M, et al. Acute leukemia after treatment for ovarian cancer. Oncology 1986;43:165–172.

127. Mehnert WH, Haas JF, Kittelmann B, et al. A case-control study of leukemia as a second primary malignancy following ovarian and breast neoplasms. IARC Sci Publ 1986;78:203–221.

128. Haas JF, Kittelmann B, Mehnert WH, et al. Risk of leukemia in ovarian tumor and breast cancer patients following treatment by cyclophosphamide. Br J Cancer 1987;55:213–218.

129. Prior P, Pope DJ. Subsequent primary cancers in relation to treatment of ovarian cancer. Br J Cancer 1989;59:453–459.

130. Kaldor JM, Day NE, Pettersson F, et al. Leukemia following chemotherapy for ovarian cancer. N Engl J Med 1990;322:1–6.

131. Lerner HJ. Acute myelogenous leukemia in patients receiving chlorambucil as long-term adjuvant chemotherapy for stage II breast cancer. Cancer Treat Rep 1978;62:1135–1138.

132. Rosner F, Carey RW, Zarrabi MH. Breast cancer and acute leukemia: report of 24 cases and a review of the literature. Am J Hematol 1978;4:151–172.

133. Kinlen LJ. Incidence of cancer in rheumatoid arthritis and other disorders after immunosuppressive treatment. Am J Med 1985;78:44–48.

134. Baker GL, Kahl LE, Zee BC, et al. Malignancy following treatment of rheumatoid arthritis with cyclophosphamide. Am J Med 1987;83:1–9.

135. Patapanian H, Graham S, Sambrook PN, et al. The oncogenicity of chlorambucil in rheumatoid arthritis. Br J Rheumatol 1988;27:44–47.

136. Stott H, Fox W, Girling DJ, et al. Acute leukaemia after busulphan. Br Med J 1977;2:1513–1517.

137. De Gramont A, Rioux E, Fortin P, Shields C. Acute leukemia secondary to lung cancer. Oncology 1985;42:107–111.

138. Rieche K. Carcinogenicity of antineoplastic agents in man. Cancer Treat Rev 1984;11:39–67.

139. Levine EG, Bloomfield CD. Leukemias and myelodysplastic syndromes secondary to drug, radiation, and environmental exposure. Semin Oncol 1992; 19:47–84.

140. Smith MA, Rubinstein L, Ungerleider RS. Therapy-related acute myeloid leukemia following treatment with epipodophyllotoxins: estimating the risks. Med Pediatr Oncol 1994;23:86–98.

141. Cronkite EP. Evidence for radiation and

chemicals as leukemic agents. Arch Environ Health 1961;3:297–303.

142. Malling HV. Chemical mutagens as a possible genetic hazard in human populations. Am Ind Hyg Assoc J 1970;31:657–666.

143. Abe S, Sasaki M. Sister chromatid exchange as an index of mutagenesis and/or carcinogenesis. In: Sandberg A, ed. Sister chromatid exchange. New York: Alan R Liss, 1982:461–514.

144. Lambert B, Lindblad A, Nordenskjold M, Werelius B. Increased frequency of sister chromatid exchanges in cigarette smokers. Hereditas 1978;88:147–149.

145. Kawano H, Inamasu T, Ishizawa M, et al. Mutagenicity of urine from young male smokers and non-smokers. Int Arch Occup Environ Health 1987;59:1–9.

146. Heddle JA, Hite M, Kirkhart B, et al. The induction of micronuclei as a measure of genotoxicity. A report of the U.S. Environmental Protection Agency Gene-Tox Program. Mutat Res 1983;123:61–118.

147. Nagao M, Takahashi Y, Yamanaka H, Sugimura T. Mutagens in coffee and tea. Mutat Res 1979; 68:101–106.

148. Ames BN, McCann J, Yamasaki E. Methods for detecting carcinogens and mutagens with the *Salmonella*/mammalian-microsome mutagenicity test. Mutat Res 1975;31:347–364.

149. Wolff S. Sister chromatid exchange: the most sensitive mammalian system for determining the effects of mutagenic carcinogens. In: Berg K, ed. Genetic damage in man caused by environmental agents. New York: Academic Press, 1979;229–246.

150. Sorsa M, Falck K, Norppa H, Vainio H. Monitoring genotoxicity in the occupational environment. Scand J Work Environ Health 1981;7(Suppl 4):61–65.

151. Funes-Cravioto F, Zapata-Gayon C, Kolmodin-Hedman B, et al. Chromosome aberrations and sister-chromatid exchange in workers in chemical laboratories and a rotoprinting factory and children of women laboratory workers. Lancet 1977;2:322–325.

152. Sandberg AA. Sister chromatid exchange in human states. In: Sandberg A, ed. Sister chromatid exchange. New York: Alan R Liss 1982:619–651.

153. Hogstedt B, Gullberg B, Hedner K, et al. Chromosome aberrations and micronuclei in bone marrow cells and peripheral blood lymphocytes in humans exposed to ethylene oxide. Hereditas 1983;98:105–113.

154. Vainio H, Falck K, Sorsa M. Mutagenicity in urine of workers occupationally exposed to mutagens and carcinogens. In: Aitio A, Riihimaki V, Vainio H, eds. Biological monitoring and health surveillance of workers exposed to chemicals. Washington, DC: Hemisphere, 1984:323–330.

155. Dolara P, Mazzoli S, Rosi D, et al. Exposure to carcinogenic chemicals and smoking increases urinary excretion of mutagens in humans. J Toxicol Environ Health 1981;8:95–103.

156. Pasquini R, Monarca S, Sforzolini GS, et al. Mutagens in urine of carbon electrode workers. Int Arch Occup Environ Health 1982;50:387–395.

157. Laires A, Borba H, Rueff J, et al. Urinary mutagenicity in occupational exposure to mineral oils and iron oxide particles. Carcinogenesis 1982;3:1077–1079.

158. Kriebel D, Commoner B, Bollinger D, et al. Detection of occupational exposure to genotoxic agents with a urinary mutagen assay. Mutat Res 1983;108:67–69.

159. Vainio H. Current trends in the biological monitoring of exposure to carcinogens. Scand J Work Environ Health 1985;11:1–6.

160. Holden HE, Ray VA, Wahrenburg MG, et al. Mutagenicity studies with 6-mercaptopurine. 1. Cytogenetic activity in vivo. Mutat Res 1973;20:257–263.

161. Hannan MA, Al-Dakan AA, Hussain SS, Amer MH. Mutagenicity of cisplatin and carboplatin used alone and in combination with four other anticancer drugs. Toxicology 1989;55:183–191.

162. Benedict WF, Banerjee A, Gardner A, Jones PA. Induction of morphological transformation in mouse CH3/10T1/2 clone 8 cells and chromosomal damage in hamster A(T1)C1-3 cells by cancer chemotherapeutic agents. Cancer Res 1977;37:2202–2208.

163. Benedict WF, Baker MS, Haroun L, et al. Mutagenicity of cancer chemotherapeutic agents in *Salmonella*/microsome test. Cancer Res 1977;37:2209–2213.

164. Matney TS, Nguyen TV, Connor TH, et al. Genotoxic classification of anticancer drugs. Teratogenesis Carcinog Mutagen 1985;5:319–328.

165. Matheson D, Brusick D, Carrano R. Comparison of the relative mutagenic activity for eight antineoplastic drugs in the Ames *Salmonella*/microsome and TK+/− mouse lymphoma assays. Drug Chem Toxicol 1978;1:277–304.

166. Seino Y, Nagao M, Yahagi T, et al. Mutagenicity of several classes of antitumor agents to *Salmonella typhimurium* TA98, TA100, and TA92. Cancer Res 1978; 38:2148–2156.

167. Gupta RS, Bromke A, Bryant DW, et al. Etoposide (VP16) and teniposide (VM26): novel anticancer drugs, strongly mutagenic in mammalian but not prokaryotic test systems. Mutagenesis 1987;2:179–186.

168. Pak K, Iwasaki T, Miyakawa M, et al. The mutagenic activity of anti-cancer drugs and the urine of rats given these drugs. Urol Res 1979;7:119–124.

169. Franza BR, Oeschger NS, Oeschger MP, et al. Mutagenic activity of nitrosourea antitumor agents. J Natl Cancer Inst 1980;65:149–154.

170. Hales B. Comparison of the mutagenicity and teratogenicity of cyclophosphamide and its active metabolites, 4-hydroxycyclophosphamide, phosphoramide mustard, and acrolein. Cancer Res 1982;42:3016–3021.

171. Marzin D, Jasmin C, Maral R, Mathe G. Mutagenicity of eight anthracycline derivatives in five strains of *Salmonella typhimurium*. Eur J Cancer Clin Oncol 1983;10:641–647.

172. Dickins M, Wright K, Phillips M, Todd N. Toxicity and mutagenicity of 6 anti-cancer drugs in Chinese hamster V-79 cells co-cultured with rat hepatocytes. Mutat Res 1985;157:189–197.

173. Manandhar M, Cheng M, Iatropoulos MJ, Noble JF. Genetic toxicity profile of the new antineoplastic drug mitoxantrone in the mammalian test systems. Arzneimittelforschung 1986;36:1375–1379.

174. DeMarini DM, Brock KH, Doerr CL, Moore MM. Mutagenicity and clastogenicity of teniposide (VM-26) in L5178Y/TK+/− − 3.7.2C mouse lymphoma cells. Mutat Res 1987;187:141–149.

175. Safirstein R, Daye M, Guttenplan JB. Mutagenic activity and identification of excreted platinum in human and rat urine and rat plasma after administration of cisplatin. Cancer Lett 1983;18:329–338.

176. Minnich V, Smith ME, Thompson D, Kornfeld

S. Detection of mutagenic activity in human urine using mutant strains of *Salmonella typhimurium*. Cancer 1976;38:1253–1258.

177. Tuffnell PG, Gannon MT, Dong A, et al. Limitations of urinary mutagen assays for monitoring occupational exposure to antineoplastic drugs. Am J Hosp Pharm 1986;43:344–348.

178. Nguyen TV, Theiss JC, Matney TS. Exposure of pharmacy personnel to mutagenic antineoplastic drugs. Cancer Res 1982;42:4792–4796.

179. Hogstedt B. Micronuclei in lymphocytes with preserved cytoplasm: a method for assessment of cytogenetic damage in man. Mutat Res 1984;130:63–72.

180. Fenech M, Morley AA. Cytokinesis-block micronucleus method in human lymphocytes: effect of in vivo ageing and low dose x-irradiation. Mutat Res 1986;161:193–198.

181. Tinwell H, Ashby J. Genetic toxicity and potential carcinogenicity of taxol. Carcinogenesis 1994; 15:1499–1501.

182. Pleskova I, Blasko M, Siracky J. Chromosomal aberrations, sister chromatid exchange (SCEs) and micronuclei induction with three platinum compounds (*cis*-DDP, CHIP, CBDCA) in V79 cells in vitro. Neoplasma 1984;31:655–659.

183. Yager JW, Sorsa M, Selvin M. Micronuclei in cytokinesis-blocked lymphocytes as an index of occupational exposure to alkylating cytostatic drugs. IARC Sci Publ 1988;89:213–216.

184. Raposa T. SCE and chemotherapy of non-cancerous and cancerous conditions. In: Sandberg A, ed. Sister chromatid exchange. New York: Alan R Liss, 1982:579–617.

185. Carrano AV, Thompson LH, Lindl PA, Minkler JL. Sister chromatid exchange as an indicator of mutagenesis. Nature 1978;271:551–553.

186. Nevstad NP. Sister chromatid exchanges and chromosomal aberrations induced in human lymphocytes by the cytostatic drug Adriamycin in vivo and in vitro. Mutat Res 1978;57:253–258.

187. Banerjee A, Benedict WF. Production of sister chromatid exchanges by various cancer chemotherapeutic agents. Cancer Res 1979;39:797–799.

188. Singh B, Gupta RS. Mutagenic responses of thirteen anticancer drugs on mutation induction at multiple genetic loci and on sister chromatid exchanges in Chinese hamster ovary cells. Cancer Res 1983;43:577–584.

189. Abe T, Tsuda S, Maekawa T, et al. Sister chromatid exchanges induced by cancer chemotherapeutic agents in vitro and in vivo: consideration of the hazard of drugs as possible mutagens and carcinogens causing second malignancies. Cancer Treat Rep 1985;69:505–514.

190. Chibber R, Ord MJ. The mutagenic and carcinogenic properties of three second generation antitumor platinum compounds: a comparison with cisplatin. Eur J Cancer Clin Oncol 1989;25:27–33.

191. Zhang S, Huang J, Chen P, Li C. Sister chromatid exchange and cell cycle patterns of normal human bone marrow cells after in vitro exposure to cytostatic drugs. Cancer Genet Cytogenet 1988;31:157–163.

192. Schinzel A, Schmid W. Lymphocyte chromosome studies in humans exposed to chemical mutagens: the validity of the method in 67 patients under cytostatic therapy. Mutat Res 1976;40:139–166.

193. Raposa T. Sister chromatid exchange studies for monitoring DNA damage and repair capacity after cytostatics in vitro and in lymphocytes of leukaemic patients under cytostatic therapy. Mutat Res 1978; 57:241–251.

194. Lambert B, Ringbord U, Harper E, Lindblad A. Sister chromatid exchanges in lymphocyte cultures of patients receiving chemotherapy for malignant disorders. Cancer Treat Rep 1978;62:1413–1419.

195. Musilova J, Michalova K, Urban J. Sister-chromatid exchanges and chromosomal breakage in patients treated with cytostatics. Mutat Res 1979;67:289–294.

196. Palmer RG, Dore CJ, Denman AM. Chlorambucil-induced chromosome damage to human lymphocytes is dose-dependent and cumulative. Lancet 1984;1:246–249.

197. Shinkai T, Saijo N, Eguchi K, et al. Cytogenetic effect of carboplatin on human lymphocytes. Cancer Chemother Pharmacol 1988;21:203–207.

198. Sardas S, Erdogan F, Sardas OS, et al. Sister chromatid exchange studies for monitoring DNA damage in lymphocytes of malignant lymphoma patients under cytostatic therapy. Anti-Cancer Drugs 1994; 5:487–489.

199. Neubert D. Teratogenicity: any relationship to carcinogenesis? In: Montesano R, Bartsch H, Tomatis L, eds. Molecular and cellular aspects of carcinogen screening tests. Lyon: International Agency for Research on Cancer, 1980:169–178.

200. Beckman DA, Brent RL. Mechanism of known environmental teratogens: drugs and chemicals. Clin Perinatol 1986;13:649–687.

201. Schardein JL. Principles of teratogenesis applicable to drug and chemical exposure. In: Schardein JL. Chemically induced birth defects. New York: Marcel Dekker, 1993:1–40.

202. Schardein JL. Cancer chemotherapeutic agents. In: Schardein JL. Chemically induced birth defects. New York: Marcel Dekker, 1993:457–508.

203. Aleksandrov VA. Characteristics of the pathogenic action of sarcolysin on the embryogeny of rats. Doklady Akademii Nauk SSSR 1966;171:746–749.

204. Sieber SM, Whang-Peng J, Botkin C, Knutsen T. Teratogenic and cytogenic effects of some plant-derived antitumor agents (vincristine, colchicine, maytansine, VP-16-213, and VM-26) in mice. Teratology 1978;18:31–48.

205. Kai S, Kohmura H, Ishikawa K, et al. Teratogenic effects of carboplatin, an oncostatic drug, administered during early organogenic period in rats. J Toxicol Sci 1989;14:115–130.

206. Airhart MJ, Robbins CM, Knudsen TB, et al. Occurrence of embryotoxicity in mouse embryos following in utero exposure to 2'-deoxycoformycin (pentostatin). Teratology 1993;47:17–27.

207. Sweet DL, Kinzie J. Consequences of radiotherapy and antineoplastic therapy for the fetus. J Reprod Med 1976;17:241–246.

208. Gililland J, Weinstein L. The effects of cancer chemotherapeutic agents on the developing fetus. Obstet Gynecol Surv 1983;38:6–13.

209. Mulvihill JJ, McKeen EA, Rosner F, Zarrabi MH. Pregnancy outcome in cancer patients. Cancer 1987;60:1143–1150.

210. Pizzuto J, Aviles A, Noriega L, et al. Treatment

of acute leukemia during pregnancy: presentation of nine cases. Cancer Treat Rep 1980;64:679–683.

211. Parvinen M, Lahdetie J. Biology and toxicology of spermatogenesis and oogenesis. In: Hemminki K, Sorsa M, Vainio H, eds. Occupational hazards and reproduction. New York: Hemisphere, 1985:3–15.

212. Lu CC, Meistrich ML. Cytotoxic effects of chemotherapeutic drugs on mouse testis cells. Cancer Res 1979;39:3575–3582.

213. Meistrich ML, Finch M, da Cunha MF, et al. Damaging effects of fourteen chemotherapeutic drugs on mouse testis cells. Cancer Res 1982;42:122–131.

214. Trasler JM, Hales BF, Robaire B. Chronic low-dose cyclophosphamide treatment of adult male rats: effect of fertility, pregnancy outcome and progeny. Biol Reprod 1986;34:275–283.

215. Ehling UH, Kratochvilova J, Lehmacher W, Neuhauser-Klaus A. Mutagenicity testing of vincristine sulfate in germ cells of male mice. Mutat Res 1988; 209:107–113.

216. Kadota T, Chikazawa H, Kondoh H, et al. Toxicity studies of paclitaxel. (II) One-month intermittent intravenous toxicity in rats. J Toxicol Sci 1994;19(Suppl 1):11–34.

217. Maguire LC, Dick FR, Sherman BM. The effects of anti-leukemic therapy on gonadal histology in adult males. Cancer 1981;48:1967–1971.

218. Shamberger RC, Sherins RJ, Rosenberg SA. The effects of postoperative adjuvant chemotherapy and radiotherapy on testicular function in men undergoing treatment for soft tissue sarcoma. Cancer 1981; 47:2368–2374.

219. Watson AR, Rance CP, Bain J. Long-term effects of cyclophosphamide on testicular function. Br Med J 1985;291:1457–1460.

220. Petersen PM, Hansen SW, Giwercman A, et al. Dose-dependent impairment of testicular function in patients treated with cisplatin-based chemotherapy for germ cell cancer. Ann Oncol 1994;5:355–358.

221. Dixon RL. Aspects of male reproductive toxicology. In: Hemminki K, Sorsa M, Vainio H, eds. Occupational hazards and reproduction. New York: Hemisphere, 1985:57–71.

222. Meistrich ML. Effects of chemotherapy and radiotherapy on spermatogenesis. Eur Urol 1993;23:136–142.

223. Veulemans H, Steeno O, Masschelein R, Groeseneken D. Exposure to ethylene glycol ethers and spermatogenic disorders in man: a case-control study. Br J Ind Med 1993;50:71–78.

224. Mortensen JT. Risk for reduced sperm quality among metal workers, with special reference to welders. Scand J Work Environ Health 1988;14:27–30.

225. Lerda D. Study of sperm characteristics in persons occupationally exposed to lead. Am J Ind Med 1992;22:567–571.

226. Newton RW, Browning MCK, Iqbal J, et al. Adrenocortical suppression in workers manufacturing synthetic glucocorticoids. Br Med J 1978;1:73–74.

227. Albert F, Bassani R, Coen D, Vismara A. Hypoglycaemia by inhalation (letter). Lancet 1993;342:47–48.

228. Sansone EB, Losikoff AM, Pendleton RA. Potential hazards from feeding test chemicals in carcinogen bioassay research. Toxicol Appl Pharmacol 1977; 39:435–450.

229. Sansone EB, Losikoff AM. A note on the chemical contamination resulting from the transfer of solid and liquid materials in hoods. Am Ind Hyg Assoc J 1977;38:489–491.

230. Sessink PJM, de Roos JH, Pierik FH, et al. Occupational exposure of animal caretakers to cyclophosphamide. J Occup Med 1993;35:47–52.

231. Sansone EB, Losikoff AM, Pendleton RA. Sources and dissemination of contamination in material handling operations. Am Ind Hyg Assoc J 1977; 38:433–442.

232. Hill RH, Gagnon YT, Teass AW. Evaluation and control of contamination in the preparation of analytical standard solutions of hazardous chemicals. Am Ind Hyg Assoc J 1978;39:157–160.

233. Sansone EB, Losikoff AM. Potential hazard associated with scraping preparative thin layer chromatography plates. Am Ind Hyg Assoc J 1979;40:543–545.

234. Kleinberg ML, Quinn MJ. Airborne drug levels in a laminar-flow hood. Am J Hosp Pharm 1981; 38:1301–1303.

235. Neal AD, Wadden RA, Chiou WL. Exposure of hospital workers to airborne antineoplastic agents. Am J Hosp Pharm 1983;40:597–601.

236. McDiarmid MA, Egan T, Furio M, et al. Sampling for airborne fluorouracil in hospital drug preparation area. Am J Hosp Pharm 1986;43:1942–1945.

237. Pyy L, Sorsa M, Hakala E. Ambient monitoring of cyclophosphamide in manufacture and hospitals. Am Ind Hyg Assoc J 1988;49:314–317.

238. Sessink PJM, Anzion RB, Van den Broeck PHH, Bos RP. Detection of contamination with antineoplastic agents in a hospital pharmacy department. Pharm Weekbl Sci 1992;14(1):16–22.

239. McDevitt JJ, Lees PSJ, McDiarmid MA. Exposure of hospital pharmacists and nurses to antineoplastic agents. J Occup Med 1993;35:57–60.

240. Sessink PJM, van de Kerkhof MCA, Anzion RBM, et al. Environmental contamination and assessment of exposure to antineoplastic agents by determination of cyclophosphamide in urine of exposed pharmacy technicians: is skin absorption an important exposure route? Arch Environ Health 1994;49:165–169.

241. Sessink PJM, Boer KA, Scheefals APH, et al. Occupational exposure to antineoplastic agents at several departments in a hospital: environmental contamination and excretion of cyclophosphamide and ifosfamide in urine of exposed workers. Int Arch Occup Environ Health 1992;64:105–112.

242. Sessink PMJ, Timmersmans JL, Anzion RBM, Bos RP. Assessment of occupational exposure of pharmaceutical plant workers to 5-fluorouracil: determination of a-fluoro-b-alanine in urine. J Occup Med 1994;36:79–83.

243. Hoy RH, Stump LM. Effect of an air-venting filter device on aerosol production from vials. Am J Hosp Pharm 1984;41:324–326.

244. Egan PC, Russell MR, Caliendo MA. Using fluorescence of antineoplastic agents to demonstrate proper handling technique (letter). Am J Hosp Pharm 1985;42:1271–1272.

245. Stellman JM. The spread of chemotherapeutic agents at work: assessment through simulation. Cancer Invest 1987;5:75–81.

246. Harrison BR, Godefroid RJ, Kavanaugh EA. Quality-assurance testing of staff pharmacists handling cytotoxic agents. Am J Health-Syst Pharm 1996; 53:402–407.

247. Dorr RT, Alberts DS. Topical absorption and inactivation of cytotoxic anticancer agents in vitro. Cancer (Suppl) 1992;70:983–987.

248. Shahsavarani S, Godefroid RJ, Harrison BR. Evaluation of occupational exposure to tablet trituration dust (abstract). 28th Annual ASHP midyear clinical meeting, Atlanta, GA, 1993 Dec 6.

249. Feldmann RJ, Maibach HI. Absorption of some organic compounds through the skin in man. J Invest Dermatol 1970;54:399–404.

250. Maibach HI, Feldmann RJ, Milby TH, et al. Regional variation in percutaneous penetration in man. Arch Environ Health 1971;23:208–211.

251. Zackheim HS, Feldmann RJ, Lindsay C, Maibach HI. Percutaneous absorption of 1,3-bis (2-chloroethyl)-1-nitrosourea (BCNU, carmustine) in mycosis fungoides. Br J Dermatol 1977;97:65–67.

252. Hirst M, Tse S, Mills DG, et al. Occupational exposure to cyclophosphamide. Lancet 1984;1:186–188.

253. Anon. Occupational hazards of cytostatic agents—hospital pharmacists' discussions. Pharm J 1977;(Oct 6):335.

254. Donner AL. Possible risks of working with antineoplastic drugs in horizontal laminar flow hoods (letter). Am J Hosp Pharm 1978;35:900.

255. Falck K, Grohn P, Sorsa M, et al. Mutagenicity in urine of nurses handling cytostatic drugs (letter). Lancet 1979;1(June 9):1250–1251.

256. Staiano N, Gallelli JF, Adamson RH, Thorgeirsson SS. Lack of mutagenic activity in urine from hospital pharmacists admixing antitumor drugs (letter). Lancet 1981;1:615–616.

257. Bos RP, Leenaars AO, Theuws JLG, et al. Mutagenicity of urine from nurses handling cytostatic drugs, influence of smoking. Int Arch Occup Environ Health 1982;50:359–369.

258. Anderson RW, Puckett WH, Dana WJ, et al. Risk of handling injectable antineoplastic agents. Am J Hosp Pharm 1982;39:1881–1887.

259. Kolmodin-Hedman B, Hartvig P, Sorsa M, Falck K. Occupational handling of cytostatic drugs. Arch Toxicol 1983;54:25–33.

260. Ratcliffe JM. Occupational exposure to cancer chemotherapeutic agents in pharmacists and nurses. National Institute of Occupational Safety and Health (Industry-Wide Study EP:80–41). Washington, DC: Government Printing Office, 1983.

261. Rorth M, Jorgensen J, Jorgensen V, et al. Mutagenicity in the urine of nurses in an oncological department. Ugeskr Laeger 1983;145:475–478.

262. Gibson JF, Baxter PJ, Hedworth-Whitty RB, Gompertz D. Urinary mutagenicity assays: a problem arising from the presence of histidine associated growth factors in XAD-2 prepared urine concentrates, with particular relevance to assays carried out using the bacterial fluctuation test. Carcinogenesis 1983; 4:1471–1476.

263. Hoffman DM. Lack of urine mutagenicity of nurses administering pharmacy prepared doses of antineoplastic agents. Am J IV Ther Clin Nutrit 1983; Sep:28–31.

264. Venitt S, Crifton-Sleigh C, Hunt J, et al. Monitoring exposure of nursing and pharmacy personnel to cytotoxic drugs: urinary mutation assays and urinary platinum as markers of absorption. Lancet 1984; 1:74–77.

265. Gibson JF, Gompertz D, Hedworth-Whitty RB. Mutagenicity of urine from nurses handling cytotoxic drugs. Lancet 1984;1:100–101.

266. Barale R, Sozzi G, Toniolo P, et al. Sister-chromatid exchanges in lymphocytes and mutagenicity in urine of nurses handling cytostatic drugs. Mutat Res 1985;157:235–240.

267. Cloak MM, Connor TH, Stevens KR, et al. Occupational exposure of nursing personnel to antineoplastic agents. Oncol Nurs Forum 1985;12:33–39.

268. Everson RB, Ratcliffe JM, Flack PM, et al. Detection of low levels of urinary mutagen excretion by chemotherapy workers which was not related to occupational drug exposures. Cancer Res 1985;45:6487–6497.

269. Benhamou S, Callais F, Sancho-Garnier H, et al. Mutagenicity in urine from nurses handling cytostatic agents. Eur J Cancer Clin Oncol 1986;22:1489–1493.

270. Friederich U, Molko F, Hofmann V, et al. Limitations of the Salmonella/mammalian microsome assay (Ames test) to determine occupational exposure to cytostatic drugs. Eur J Cancer Clin Oncol 1986;22:567–575.

271. Stucker I, Hirsch A, Doloy T, et al. Urine mutagenicity, chromosomal abnormalities and sister chromatid exchanges in lymphocytes of nurses handling cytostatic drugs. Int Arch Occup Environ Health 1986; 57:195–205.

272. Pohlova H, Cerna M, Rossner P. Chromosomal aberrations, SCE and urine mutagenicity in workers occupationally exposed to cytostatic drugs. Mutat Res 1986;174:213–217.

273. Connor TH, Theis JC, Anderson RW, et al. Reevaluation of urine mutagenicity of pharmacy personnel exposed to antineoplastic agents. Am J Hosp Pharm 1986;43:1236–1239.

274. Rogers B, Emmett EA. Handling antineoplastic agents: urine mutagenicity in nurses. Image J Nurs Sch 1987;19:108–113.

275. Caudell KA, Vredevoe DL, Dietrich MF, et al. Quantification of urinary mutagens in nurses during potential antineoplastic agent exposure—a pilot study with concurrent environmental and dietary control. Can Nurs 1988;11:41–50.

276. Sorsa M, Pyy L, Salomaa S, et al. Biological and environmental monitoring of occupational exposure to cyclophosphamide in industry and hospitals. Mutat Res 1988;204:465–479.

277. Poyen D, DeMeo MP, Botta A, et al. Handling of cytostatic drugs and urine mutagenesis. Int Arch Occup Environ Health 1988;61:183–188.

278. Clonfero E, Granella M, Gori GP, et al. Escrezione urinaria di mutageni e cisplatino nel personale infermieristico dei reparti di oncologia medica esposto a farmaci citostatici. Med Lav 1989;5:412–419.

279. Elliott G, Ferguson L, Everts R, Edwards R. Monitoring mutagenicity in urine and peripheral blood lymphocytes of pharmacists occupationally exposed to anticancer drugs. NZ Med J 1990;103:13–16.

280. Krepinsky A, Bryant DW, Davison L, et al. Comparison of three assays for genetic effects of antineoplastic drugs on cancer patients and their nurses. Environ Mol Mutagen 1990;15:83–92.

281. Guinee EP, Beuman GH, Hageman G, et al. Evaluation of genotoxic risk of handling cytostatic

drugs in clinical pharmacy practice. Pharm Weekbl Sci 1991;13:78–82.

282. Thiringer G, Granung G, Holmen A, et al. Comparison of methods for the biomonitoring of nurses handling antitumor drugs. Scand J Work Environ Health 1991;17:133–138.

283. Newman MA, Valanis BG, Schoeny RS, Hee SQ. Urinary biological monitoring markers of anticancer drug exposure in oncology nurses. Am J Public Health 1994;84:852–855.

284. Ong T, Stockhausen A, Adamo D, Whong W. The urine mutagenicity system: studies related to recovery, storage, and concentration procedures. Scand J Work Environ Health 1985;11:45–50.

285. Baker R, Arlauskas A, Bonin A, Angus D. Detection of mutagenic activity in human urine following fried pork or bacon meals. Cancer Lett 1982;16:81–89.

286. Wilson JP, Solimando DA. Antineoplastics: a safety hazard? (letter). Am J Hosp Pharm 1981;38:624.

287. Wilson JP, Solimando DA. Aseptic technique as a safety precaution in the preparation of antineoplastic agents. Hosp Pharm 1981;16:575–581.

288. Valanis B, Shortridge L. Self protective practices of nurses handling antineoplastic drugs. Oncol Nurs Forum 1987;14(3):23–27.

289. Rogers B. Work practices of nurses who handle antineoplastic agents. Am Assoc Occup Health Nurses J 1987;35:24–31.

290. Norppa H, Sorsa M, Vainio H, et al. Increased sister chromatid exchange frequencies in lymphocytes of nurses handling cytostatic drugs. Scand J Work Environ Health 1980;6:299–301.

291. Waksvik H, Klepp O, Brogger A. Chromosome analyses of nurses handling cytostatic agents. Cancer Treat Rep 1981;65:607–610.

292. Stiller A, Obe G, Pribilla W. No elevation of the frequencies of chromosomal alterations as a consequence of handling cytostatic drugs: analyses with peripheral blood and urine of hospital personnel. Mutat Res 1983;121:253–259.

293. Jordan DK, Jochimsen PR, Lachenbruch PA, Corder MP. Sister chromatid exchange analysis in nurses handling antineoplastic drugs. Cancer Invest 1986;4:101–107.

294. Penin IR, Goyanes UJ, Campos AC. Determinacion de las tasas de mutagenidad en diplomados en enfermeria manipuladores de citostaticos. Rev Assoc Esp Farm Hosp 1987;11:119–122.

295. Ferguson LR, Everts R, Robbie MA, et al. The use within New Zealand of cytogenic approaches to monitoring of hospital pharmacists for exposure to cytotoxic drugs: report of a pilot study in Auckland. Aust J Hosp Pharm 1988;18:228–233.

296. Oestreicher U, Stephan G, Glatzel M. Chromosome and SCE analysis in peripheral lymphocytes of persons occupationally exposed to cytostatic drugs handled with and without use of safety covers. Mutat Res 1990;242:271–277.

297. Sarto F, Trevisan A, Tomanin R, et al. Chromosomal aberrations, sister chromatid exchanges, and urinary thioethers in nurses handling antineoplastic drugs. Am J Ind Med 1990;18:689–695.

298. Milkovic-Kraus S, Horvat D. Chromosomal abnormalities among nurses occupationally exposed to antineoplastic drugs. Am J Ind Med 1991;19:771–774.

299. Sardas S, Gok S, Karakaya AE. Sister chromatid exchanges in lymphocytes of nurses handling antineoplastic drugs. Toxicol Lett 1991;55:311–315.

300. Goloni-Bertollo EM, Tajara EH, Manzato AJ, Varella-Garcia M. Sister chromatid exchanges and chromosome aberrations in lymphocytes of nurses handling antineoplastic drugs. Int J Cancer 1992; 50:341–344.

301. Jung D, Klein S, Fuchs J, et al. Gene monitoring of pharmaceutical staff preparing cytostatics. Krankenhauspharmazie 1992;13:101–104.

302. Gorecka D, Gorski T. The influence of cigarette smoking on sister chromatid exchange frequencies in peripheral lymphocytes among nurses handling cytostatic drugs. Pol J Occup Med Environ Health 1993;6:143–148.

303. Roth S, Norppa H, Jarventaus H, et al. Analysis of chromosomal aberrations, sister-chromatid exchanges and micronuclei in peripheral lymphocytes of pharmacists before and after working with cytostatic drugs. Mutat Res 1994;325:157–162.

304. Benhamou S, Pot-Deprun J, Sancho-Garnier H, Chouroulinkov I. Sister chromatid exchanges and chromosomal aberrations in lymphocytes of nurses handling cytostatic agents. Int J Cancer 1988;41:350–353.

305. Nikula E, Kiviniity K, Leisti J, et al. Chromosome aberrations in lymphocytes of nurses handling cytostatic agents. Scand J Work Environ Health 1984; 10(2):71–84.

306. Medkova J. Cytogenetic analysis of peripheral lymphocytes in occupationally exposed health personnel. Acta Univ Palacki Olomuc 1990;126:93–106.

307. Cooke J, Wiliams J, Morgan RJ, et al. Use of cytogenic methods to determine mutagenic changes in the blood of pharmacy personnel and nurses who handle cytotoxic agents. Am J Hosp Pharm 1991;48:1199–1205.

308. Grummt T, Grummt HJ, Schott G. Chromosomal aberrations in peripheral lymphocytes of nurses and physicians handling antineoplastic drugs. Mutat Res 1993;302:19–24.

309. Reitz M, Afghanyar S, Gutjahr P. Increasing rates of DNA single-strand breaks in lymphocytes of clinical personnel handling cytostatic drugs. J Cancer Res Clin Oncol 1993;119:237–242.

310. Sessink PJM, Cerna M, Rossner P, et al. Urinary cyclophosphamide excretion and chromosomal aberrations in peripheral blood lymphocytes after occupational exposure to antineoplastic agents. Mutat Res 1994;309:193–199.

311. Fuchs J, Hengstler JG, Jung D, et al. DNA damage in nurses handling antineoplastic agents. Mutat Res 1995;342:17–23.

312. Anwar WA, Salama SI, El Serafy MM, et al. Chromosomal aberrations and micronucleus frequency in nurses occupationally exposed to cytotoxic drugs. Mutagenesis 1994;9:315–317.

313. Van Doorn R, Leijdekkers CM, Bos RP, et al. Enhanced excretion of thioethers in urine of operators of chemical waste incinerators. Br J Ind Med 1981; 38:187–190.

314. Vainio H, Kilpikari I. Urinary thioether excretion as a biological parameter of chemical exposure. In: Aitio A, Riihimaki V, Vainio H, eds. Biological monitoring and surveillance of workers exposed to chemicals. Washington, DC: Hemisphere, 1984:247–252.

315. Jagun O, Ryan M, Waldron HA. Urinary thioether excretion in nurses handling cytotoxic drugs (letter). Lancet 1982;2(Aug 21):443–444.

316. Bayhan A, Burgaz S, Karakaya AE. Urinary thioether excretion in nurses at an oncologic department. J Clin Pharm Ther 1987;12:303–306.

317. Burgaz S, Ozdamar YN, Karakaya AE. A signal assay for the detection of genotoxic compounds: application on the urines of cancer patients on chemotherapy and nurses handling cytotoxic drugs. Hum Toxicol 1988;7:557–560.

318. Ferguson LR, Everts R, McKinnon HM, Gerred AJ. Monitoring of drug absorption by pharmacists and oncology nurses in four New Zealand hospitals using estimation of cytokinesis-blocked micronuclei: a follow-up study in Auckland. Aust J Hosp Pharm 1990; 20:212–217.

319. Machado-Santelli GM, Cerqueira EM, Oliveira CT, de Braganca Pereira CAA. Biomonitoring of nurses handling antineoplastic drugs. Mutat Res 1994; 322:203–208.

320. Chrysostomou A, Morley AA, Seshadri R. Mutation frequency in nurses and pharmacists working with cytotoxic drugs. Aust NZ J Med 1984;14:831–834.

321. Dubeau H, Zazi W, Baron C, Messing K. Effects of lymphocyte subpopulations on the clonal assay of HPRT mutants: occupational exposure to cytostatic drugs. Mutat Res 1994;321:147–157.

322. Lassila O, Toivanen A, Nordman E. Immune function in nurses handling cytostatic drugs (letter). Lancet 1980;2:482.

323. Jochimsen PR, Corder MP, Lachenbruch PA, Spaight ME. Preparation and administration of chemotherapy—haematological consequences for hospital-based nurses. Med Toxicol 1988;3:59–63.

324. Hemminki K, Kyyronen P, Lindbohm M. Spontaneous abortions and malformations in the offspring of nurses exposed to anaesthetic gases, cytostatic drugs, and other potential hazards in hospitals, based on registered information of outcome. J Epidemiol Community Health 1985;39:141–147.

325. Selevan SG, Lindbohm M, Hornung RW, Hemminki K. A study of occupational exposure to antineoplastic drugs and fetal loss in nurses. N Engl J Med 1985;313:1173–1178.

326. Taskinen H, Lindbohm ML, Hemminki K. Spontaneous abortions among women working in the pharmaceutical industry. Br J Ind Med 1986;43:199–205.

327. Stucker I, Calliard JF, Collin R, et al. Risk of spontaneous abortion among nurses handling antineoplastic drugs. Scand J Work Environ Health 1990; 16:102–107.

328. Medkova J. Analysis of the health condition of the children born to the personnel exposed to cytostatics at an oncology unit. Acta Univ Palacki Olomuc 1991;130:323–332.

329. Skov T, Maarup B, Olsen J, et al. Leukaemia and reproductive outcome among nurses handling antineoplastic drugs. Br J Ind Med 1992;49:855–861.

330. Saurel-Cubizolles MJ, Job-Spira N, Estryn-Behar M. Ectopic pregnancy and occupational exposure to antineoplastic drugs. Lancet 1993;341:1169–1171.

331. Stucker I, Mandereau L, Hemon D. Relationship between birthweight and occupational exposure to cytostatic drugs during or before pregnancy. Scand J Work Environ Health 1993;19:148–153.

332. Kline JK. Maternal occupation: effects on spontaneous abortions and malformations. Occup Med State Art Rev 1986;1:381–403.

333. Taskinen HK. Effects of parental occupational exposures on spontaneous abortion and congenital malformation. Scand J Work Environ Health 1990; 16:297–314.

334. Sorsa M, Hemminki K, Vainio H. Occupational exposure to anticancer drugs—potential and real hazards. Mutat Res 1985;154:135–149.

335. Mader RM, Rizovski B, Steger GG, Rainer H. Determination of methotrexate in human urine at nanomolar levels by high-performance liquid chromatography with column switching. J Chromatogr Biomed Appl 1993;613:311–316.

336. Evelo CTA, Bos RP, Peters JGP, Henderson PT. Urinary cyclophosphamide assay as a method for biological monitoring of occupational exposure to cyclophosphamide. Int Arch Occup Environ Health 1986; 58:151–155.

337. Ensslin AS, Stoll Y, Pethran A, et al. Biological monitoring of cyclophosphamide and ifosfamide in urine of hospital personnel occupationally exposed to cytostatic drugs. Occup Environ Med 1994;51:229–233.

338. van Kan HJM, Pelders MG, Simons KA. Controlling contamination with cytotoxic drugs in the hospital pharmacy department. Ziekenhuisfarmacie 1994; 10:89–91.

339. Johnson BL, Gross J. Handling methotrexate—a safety problem (letter)? Am J Nurs 1982;(Oct):1581.

340. Ensslin AS, Pethran A, Schierl R, Fruhmann G. Urinary platinum in hospital personnel occupationally exposed to platinum-containing antineoplastic drugs. Int Arch Occup Environ Health 1994;65:339–342.

341. Moore W, Hysell D, Hall L, et al. Preliminary studies on the toxicity and metabolism of palladium and platinum. Environ Health Perspect 1975;10:63–71.

342. Moore W, Malanchuk M, Crocker W, et al. Whole body retention in rats of different ^{191}Pt compounds following inhalation exposure. Environ Health Perspect 1975;12:35–39.

343. Adamson RH, Rosenberg B. Toxicology and pharmacology. In: Grossblatt N, ed. Platinum group metals. Washington, DC: National Academy of Sciences 1977:79–104.

344. Messerschmidt J, Alt F, Tolg G, et al. Adsorptive voltammetric procedure for the determination of platinum baseline levels in human body levels. Fresenius J Anal Chem 1992;343:391–394.

345. Hightower JW, Haensel V. Environmental considerations. In: Grossblatt N, ed. Platinum group metals. Washington, DC: National Academy of Sciences, 1977:125–164.

346. Samuels SW, Adamson RH. Quantitative risk assessment: report of the subcommittee on environmental carcinogenesis, National Cancer Advisory Board. J Natl Cancer Inst 1985;74:945–951.

347. Gaylor DW, Shapiro RE. Extrapolation and risk estimation for carcinogenesis. In: Mehlman MA, Shapiro RE, Blumenthal H, eds. Advances in modern toxicology: new concepts in safety evaluation (part 2). New York: Hemisphere, 1979;1:65–87.

348. Moolgavkar SH. A two-stage carcinogenesis

model for risk assessment. Cell Biol Toxicol 1989;5:445–460.

349. Baltus JAM, Boersma JW, Hartman AP, Vandenbroucke JP. The occurrence of malignancies in patients with rheumatoid arthritis treated with cyclophosphamide: a controlled retrospective follow-up. Ann Rheum Dis 1983;42:368–373.

350. Greene MH, Harris EL, Gershenson DM, et al. Melphalan may be a more potent leukemogen than cyclophosphamide. Ann Intern Med 1986;105:360–367.

351. Radomski JL. Evaluating the role of environmental chemicals in human cancer. In: Mehlman MA, Shapiro RE, Blumenthal H, eds. Advances in modern toxicology: new concepts in safety evaluation (part 2). New York: Hemisphere, 1979;1:27–43.

352. Li FP, Fraumeni JF, Mantel N, Miller RW. Cancer mortality among chemists. J Natl Cancer Inst 1969; 43:1159–1164.

353. Olin R. Leukemia and Hodgkin's disease among Swedish chemistry graduates (letter). Lancet 1976;2:916.

354. Vainio H. Is passive smoking increasing cancer risk? Scand J Work Environ Health 1987;13:193–196.

355. Olsson H, Brandt L. Risk of non-Hodgkins lymphoma among men occupationally exposed to organic solvents. Scand J Work Environ Health 1988; 14:246–251.

356. Reif JS, Pearce NE, Fraser J. Cancer risks among New Zealand meat workers. Scand J Work Environ Health 1989;15:24–29.

357. Alderson M. Occupational cancer. London: Butterworth, 1986.

358. National Cancer Institute. Safety standards for research involving chemical carcinogens. DHEW publ. no. (NIH) 76-900, June 1975.

359. Anon. Handling chemical carcinogens in the laboratory—problems of safety. Lyon: International Agency for Research on Cancer. IARC Sci Publ. no. 33, 1979.

360. National Institutes of Health. Guidelines for the laboratory use of chemical carcinogens. NIH publ. no. 1981;81–2385.

361. Zimmerman PF, Larsen RK, Barkley EW, Gallelli JF. Recommendations for the safe handling of injectable antineoplastic drug products. Am J Hosp Pharm 1981;38:1693–1695.

362. Goldberg LA. The preparation of cytotoxic drugs. Pharm J 1983;230:224–225.

363. Reich SD. Antineoplastic agents as potential carcinogens: are nurses and pharmacists at risk? Cancer Nurs 1981;4:500–502.

364. Health and Safety Executive. Precautions for the safe handling of cytotoxic drugs. London: Health and Safety Executive, 1983 (Guidance Note MS21).

365. Anon. Guidelines for the handling of cytotoxic drugs—working party report. Pharm J 1983(Feb 26); 230:231.

366. Environmental Protection Agency. Protection of environment. 40 Code of Federal Regulations, parts 260–280, July 1995.

367. Bacovsky R. Disposal of hazardous pharmaceuticals. Can J Hosp Pharm 1981;34:12–13.

368. Wilson SJ. Safe disposal of some commonly used injectable antineoplastic drugs. J Clin Hosp Pharm 1983;8:295–299.

369. Vaccari PL, Tonat K, DeChristoforo R, et al. Disposal of antineoplastic wastes at the National Institutes of Health. Am J Hosp Pharm 1984;41:87–93.

370. Richardson ML, Bowron JM. The fate of pharmaceutical chemicals in the aquatic environment. J Pharm Pharmacol 1985;37:1–12.

371. Harris J, Dodds LJ. Handling waste from patients receiving cytotoxic drugs. Pharm J 1985;235:289–291.

372. Goc A, Moody ML. Antineoplastic drug disposal. Ill Pharm 1985;47:17–19.

373. Johnson EG, Janosik JE. Manufacturers' recommendations for handling spilled antineoplastic agents. Am J Hosp Pharm 1989;46:318–319.

374. Jones P. Disposal of cytotoxics (letter). Pharm J 1989;242:56.

375. Castegnaro M, Adams J, Armour MA, et al., eds. Laboratory decontamination of carcinogens in laboratory wastes: some antineoplastic agents. IARC Sci Publ no. 73. Lyon: International Agency for Research on Cancer, 1985.

376. Lunn G, Sansone EB. Reductive destruction of dacarbazine, procarbazine hydrochloride, isoniazid, and iproniazid. Am J Hosp Pharm 1987;44:2519–2524.

377. Lunn G, Sansone EB, Andrews AW, Hellwig LC. Degradation and disposal of some antineoplastic drugs. J Pharm Sci 1989;78:652–659.

378. Benvenuto JA, Connor TH, Monteith DK, et al. Degradation and inactivation of antitumor drugs. J Pharm Sci 1993;82:988–991.

379. Wren AE, Melia CD, Garner ST, Denyer SP. Decontamination methods for cytotoxic drugs. 1. Use of a bioluminescent technique to monitor the inactivation of methotrexate with chlorine-based agents. J Clin Pharm Ther 1993;18:133–137.

380. Prudent practices for disposal of chemicals from laboratories. Washington, DC: National Academy Press, 1983.

381. Code of Federal Regulations. Title 40—Protection of the environment. Chap 1—Environmental Protection Agency. Part 261—Identification and listing of hazardous waste. Paragraphs 261.10–261.33, 1995.

382. Code of Federal Regulations. Title 40—Protection of the environment. Chap 1—Environmental Protection Agency. Part 261—Identification and listing of hazardous waste. Paragraph 261.5, 1995.

383. Code of Federal Regulations. Title 40—Protection of the environment. Chap 1—Environmental Protection Agency. Part 261—Identification and listing of hazardous waste. Paragraph 261.7, 1995.

384. Peters BG, Harrison BR. Assessment of chemotherapy wastes produced by two medical center pharmacies (abstract). American Society of Hospital Pharmacists annual meeting, Denver, CO, June 10, 1993.

385. Perkins JL. Chemical protective clothing: selection and use. Appl Ind Hyg 1987;2:222–230.

386. Crank J, Park GS. Methods of measurement. In: Crank J, Park GS, eds. Diffusion in polymers. New York: Academic Press, 1968:1–39.

387. McFee DR. How well do gloves protect hands against solvents? Am Soc Saf Eng J 1964;9(5):11–16.

388. Sansone EB, Tewari YB. The permeability of laboratory gloves to selected solvents. Am Ind Hyg Assoc J 1978;39:169–174.

389. Williams JR. Permeation of glove materials by

physiologically harmful chemicals. Am Ind Hyg Assoc J 1979;40:877–882.

390. Thomsen K, Mikkelsen HI. Protective capacity of gloves used for handling of nitrogen mustard. Contact Dermatitis 1975;1:268–269.

391. Connor TH, Laidlaw JL, Theiss JC, et al. Permeability of latex and polyvinyl chloride gloves to carmustine. Am J Hosp Pharm 1984;41:676–679.

392. Slevin ML, Ang LM, Johnston A, Turner P. The efficiency of protective gloves used in the handling of cytotoxic drugs. Cancer Chemother Pharmacol 1984; 12:151–153.

393. Laidlaw JA, Connor TH, Theiss JC, et al. Permeability of latex and polyvinyl chloride gloves to 20 antineoplastic drugs. Am J Hosp Pharm 1984;41:2618–2623.

394. Stoikes ME, Carlson JD, Farris FF, Walker PR. Permeability of latex and polyvinyl chloride gloves to fluorouracil and methotrexate. Am J Hosp Pharm 1987; 44:1341–1346.

395. Thomas PH, Fenton-May V. Protection offered by various gloves to carmustine exposure. Pharm J 1987;238:775–777.

396. Mader RM, Rizovski B, Steger GG, et al. Permeability of latex membranes to anti-cancer drugs. Int J Pharm 1991;68:151–156.

397. Dinter-Heidorn H, Carstens G. Comparative study on protective gloves for handling cytotoxic medicines: a model study with carmustine. Pharm Weekbl (Sci) 1992;14:180–184.

398. Connor TH. Permeability testing of glove materials for use with cancer chemotherapy drugs. Oncology 1995;52:256–259.

399. National Sanitation Foundation. Standard no. 49 for class II biohazard safety cabinetry. Ann Arbor, MI: National Sanitation Foundation, 1992.

400. Stuart DG, Greenier TJ, Rumery RA, Eagleson JM. Survey, use, and performance of biological safety cabinets. Am Ind Hyg Assoc J 1982;43:265–270.

401. Willcox GS, Mahoney CD, Welch DW, et al. A comparison of laminar airflow cabinetry. Cancer Chemother Update 1983;1(2):1–3.

402. Avis KE, Levchuk JW. Special considerations in the use of vertical laminar-flow workbenches. Am J Hosp Pharm 1984;41:81–87.

403. Kruse RH, Puckett WH, Richardson JH. Biological safety cabinetry. Clin Micro Rev 1991;4:207–241.

404. Coriell LL, McGarrity GJ. Biohazard hood to prevent infection during microbiological procedures. Appl Microbiol 1968;16:1895–1900.

405. Koesterer MG. Evaluation of vertical laminar-flow biological safety cabinets with uranine dye aerosol. Am Lab 1979;11:79–86.

406. Clark RP, Goff MR. The potassium iodide method for determining protection factors in open-fronted microbiological safety cabinets. J Appl Bacteriol 1981;51:439–460.

407. Stuart DG, First MW, Jones RL Jr, Eagleson JM Jr. Comparison of chemical vapor-handling by three types of class II biological safety cabinets. P&MC Forum 1983; March/April:16–24.

408. Favier M, Hansel S, Bressolle F. Preparing cytotoxic agents in an isolator. Am J Hosp Pharm 1993; 50:2335–2339.

409. Larrouturou P, Huchet J, Taugourdeau MC. Centralized preparation of hazardous drugs: choice between isolator and laminar airflow. Pharm Weekbl (Sci) 1992;14:88–92.

410. Challen RG. Handling and packaging of oral cytotoxic drugs (letter). Aust J Hosp Pharm 1983; 13:124.

411. Plumridge RJ, Batty KT. Handling oral cytotoxic drugs (letter). Aust J Hosp Pharm 1986;16:82.

412. Morris JT. Handling Cytotoxics (letter). Pharm J 1988;240:171–172.

413. Anon. Guidelines for pharmacists on cytotoxic medicines. NZ Pharm 1990;10(Jun):22–24.

414. Sauer KA, Coons SJ, Berger PK. Survey of training, handling practices, and risk perceptions of Kentucky pharmacists working with antineoplastic agents. Am J Hosp Pharm 1991;48:119–120.

Appendix: Handling of Antineoplastic and Hazardous Drugs: Hazardous Drug Safety and Health Plan

1. Purpose: to establish a policy for handling antineoplastic drugs within the medical center.

2. Policy: all services in the medical center that handle any hazardous drugs will establish a written policy outlining procedures for the safe transport, storage preparation, administration, and disposal of these agents.

a. Each service chief will submit his or her policy to the chief of staff for review.

b. Each service will establish a training program that will inform the employee of the following:

(1) The identity of the potentially hazardous materials used in the service

(2) Emergency procedures to be followed in the case of accidental exposure

(3) Potential health hazards and symptoms expected from exposure to these drugs

(4) Procedures for cleaning spills

(5) Who to notify in the event of an exposure or spill

(6) Who to notify for additional information on these chemicals

(7) Where to seek medical attention

c. Each service chief will submit the following records to the safety manager and the employee health unit. These records will be updated as necessary.

(1) A permanent record listing the names of employees preparing, administering, and/or disposing of hazardous drugs (high-risk employees)

(2) A record of all areas in these respective services where antineoplastic and hazardous agents are stored, prepared, administered, or destroyed.

3. Delegation of authority:

a. Chief, supply service will ensure the safe storage, transport, and disposal of all hazardous drugs that are received by this medical center through normal supply channels, that all are identified as potentially hazardous materials during their movement through the supply service, and that all supply service employees are aware of their hazardous properties and procedures for proper handling.

b. Chief, pharmacy service will ensure the safe storage, preparation, dispensing, and disposal of all hazardous drugs that are received from supply service or from other sources, that all pharmacy personnel required to handle or dispense these drugs are trained in the proper handling techniques, and that all antineoplastic drugs leaving the pharmacy are properly labeled.

c. Chief, nursing service will ensure the safe storage, administration, and disposal of hazardous drugs that are received from pharmacy service, and that all nursing personnel required to administer these drugs or care for patients receiving these drugs are trained in the proper handling techniques.

d. Chief, environmental management service will ensure that hazardous and antineoplastic drug wastes are safely transported to storage and disposal areas, that all service employees working in areas where these drugs are handled are aware of the potential hazard and are trained in the safe handling of these wastes, and will assist all using services in cleanup of spills.

e. Chief, engineering service will ensure that all engineering service employees involved with disposal of antineoplastic or hazardous drug wastes are aware of the potential hazard and are trained in the safe handling of these wastes; that these drug wastes are properly stored prior to on-site disposal; that these wastes are properly and safely incinerated in accordance with local, state, and Environmental Protection Agency (EPA) guidelines; and that all hazardous drug wastes to be disposed of by an outside firm are safely stored, properly labeled, manifested, and transported in accordance with state, EPA, and Department of Transportation regulations.

f. Safety manager will serve as the medical center hazardous drug officer and as such will monitor all affected services for compliance with the requirements of this memorandum; will establish contact with the responsible person in each service and establish a mechanism of reporting acute exposures, spills, and unsafe working conditions; and will investigate the circumstances surrounding each incident that results in employee exposure or in personal injury. The safety manager will report all accidents and records of service compliance to the safety committee.

4. Procedures:

a. Medical surveillance:

(1) Every employee determined to be at high risk will be given an appropriate physical examination by the Employee Health Unit. The purpose of this examination is to establish a baseline against which changes can be measured. These evaluations should be performed before job placement, periodically during employment, following acute exposure, and at the time of termination or transfer.

(2) All employees determined to be at high risk will be given an annual physical examination. These examinations will be designed to detect changes in general health and in specific areas vulnerable to exposure to chemicals such as the skin, buccal and nasal mucosal membranes, and the eyes. These examinations will include a history, physical examination, and laboratory assessment (CBC with differential, liver and renal function tests, and urinalysis).

(3) The employee will provide, as part of the history, a description of duties that involve hazardous drugs, the exposure level (usually in terms of drugs or doses handled per unit time), and the type of protective equipment routinely used.

(4) All employees acutely exposed to an antineoplastic drug will be examined and treated by the employee health unit. An assessment of the extent of exposure will be made. The physical examination should focus on exposed areas plus other vulnerable areas such as the eyes, mucous membranes, and respiratory tract.

(5) Service chiefs will ensure that all high-risk employees and other exposed employees report for the appropriate examination.

(6) Records, when established, will be maintained as a part of the employee health record.

b. Personnel practices:

(1) All employees handling antineoplastic drugs will wear personal protective clothing to include disposable gloves, disposable low-permeability fabric gown, and eye protection. Gowns will be closed in the front and will have long sleeves and tight-fitting cuffs at the wrists. Potentially contaminated clothing will be removed prior to leaving a work area.

(2) An NIOSH-approved dust/mist respirator or face mask will be worn when airborne particles or aerosols of antineoplastic drugs are generated during handling, unless proper ventilation (i.e., class II biologic safety cabinet) is available.

(3) There will be no eating, drinking, smoking, chewing of gum or tobacco, application of cosmetics, or storage of food in areas where antineoplastic drugs are used.

(4) All personnel will wash their hands immediately after completion of any procedures in which antineoplastic drugs have been used.

(5) In situations where splashes, sprays, or aerosols are anticipated, eye protection and a face shield should be worn.

(6) All personnel handling hazardous drugs will use correct work practices that reduce or eliminate spills and aerosol formation. These will include strict aseptic technique and use of negative pressure. Each employee will be able to demonstrate proper use of these techniques during periodic examinations.

(7) Mechanical pipetting aids will be used for all pipetting procedures. Oral pipetting is prohibited.

(8) Only employees who have received proper training will prepare or administer antineoplastic drugs. All services will document this training.

(7) Hazardous drug preparation and administration work load will be distributed among the trained personnel to minimize daily exposure.

(8) Employees will report all spills, exposures, or unsafe conditions to their supervisors.

(9) Employees who are pregnant, planning a pregnancy (male or female), breast-feeding, or who have a written statement from a physician that provides medical reasons why they should not be exposed to antineoplastic or other hazardous drugs will be offered work in other areas where this exposure is not likely. Each employee has the right to choose to accept this alternative worksite or not.

c. Operational practices:

(1) All areas where hazardous drugs are stored, prepared, or disposed of will be posted with signs bearing the "BIOHAZARD," "CANCER HAZARD," or "HAZARDOUS DRUG" symbol.

(2) Supervisors of all areas where these drugs are stored, prepared, or disposed of will designate personnel authorized entry to the area and post the area as "off limits" to patients and general employees.

(3) Preparation for clinical use will be conducted only in a class II biologic safety cabinet by properly trained personnel. These hoods will be marked as hazardous drug preparation areas. These hoods will meet the specifications of the National Sanitation Foundation standard no. 49 and will be certified at least every 6 months. These drugs will not be prepared in open environments such as clinics and nursing units. Clinical services requiring these drugs for their patients should contact pharmacy service.

(4) Only minimum working quantities of hazardous drugs will be stored in patient care and preparation areas.

(5) Syringes containing antineoplastic or hazardous agents, fluid bags to which they have been added, and dispensed oral dosage forms will be labeled "Hazardous drug: dispose of properly" or with some similar warning prior to dispensing.

(6) General housekeeping procedures will suppress the formation of aerosols by the use of a wet mop or a vacuum cleaner equipped with a HEPA filter or water trap. Dry sweeping or mopping is prohibited in areas where spills have occurred or in preparation or administration areas.

(7) Contaminated materials (i.e., syringes, gauze pads, gowns, gloves, etc.) will be discarded only in closed metal containers lined with 4-mil plastic bags. These will be labeled with "CAUTION: HAZARDOUS DRUG WASTES" or some similar warning. Needles, syringes and needles, or i.v. bags with sets and needles will be discarded in appropriate "sharps" containers that are puncture proof and have "tamper-proof" lids.

(8) Spills

(a) In the event of breakage of containers of powder, tablet, or liquid hazardous drugs, steps should be taken to prevent spread of the spill and to prevent other employees from coming into the contaminated area. Absorbent materials such as spill pillows or towels should be placed over and around the spill to prevent it from moving under cabinets or shelving units.

(b) Immediately put on personal protective clothing including heavy-duty gloves, respirator, gown, and eye protection.

(c) Absorb spill with chemical-spill pillows, gauze pads, paper towels, or plastic-backed absorbent pads. Wash contaminated surfaces with water and reabsorb. Place all contaminated materials in 4-mil plastic bags. Decontaminate area if a neutralizing agent is available. Wash all contaminated surfaces at least three times.

(d) Seal and double bag all contaminated materials. Mark as hazardous wastes. Contact housekeeping to remove waste and to terminally clean area.

(e) Personnel involved in the cleanup should wash all potentially exposed skin surfaces with soap and water.

(f) Notify the medical center safety manager of the spill.

(g) If the spill is a dry powder, cover with a generous supply of water-dampened absorbent towel or gauze.

(h) Broken glass should be handled only with heavy-duty gloves and disposal scoop, then placed in a cardboard or plastic container prior to disposal in hazardous waste bags or placed in a sharps container.

(9) Accidental exposure

(a) In the event of an accidental acute exposure, all exposed surfaces should be rinsed thoroughly with copious amounts of water. An emergency shower or eyewash will be available.

(b) If applicable, wash exposed surfaces with appropriate neutralizing solution, then wash thoroughly with soap and water.

(c) For eye exposure, immediately flood the affected eye with water or isotonic eyewash designated for that purpose, for at least 15 minutes. Seek medical attention immediately.

(d) Report exposure to supervisor.

(10) Environmental management employees will collect sharps containers when full and transport them to the secure holding area for incineration. Hazardous drug disposal bags or containers will not be left unattended but will be taken directly to the secure holding area and placed in the approved closed containers. Environmental management personnel will wear gloves when handling these containers. Isolation gowns, respirators, and eye protection will be worn when handling open bags or improperly sealed or broken containers.

(11) Trace amounts or empty containers of antineoplastic or hazardous drug wastes will be handled as regulated medical wastes and destroyed by incineration either on or off site. Engineering service personnel receiving these wastes for incineration will wear gloves

when handling bags or disposal containers. Disposable gowns, respirators, and eye protection will also be worn when handling open containers or improperly sealed or broken containers.

(12) Expired or contaminated antineoplastic drugs in large amounts, such as a half-full 100-mg vial or 250-ml i.v. bag of an antineoplastic drug solution, will be considered hazardous waste and must be labeled, manifested, and transported to a licensed hazardous waste disposal facility.

(13) Employees will wear personal protective clothing when handling urine, feces, or soiled linens or clothing of patients who have received hazardous drugs within the previous 48 hours. They will dispose of urine and feces carefully but in the usual manner. Contaminated linens and clothing will be placed and sealed in a water-soluble laundry bag (same procedure as for contaminated linens) and sent to laundry service for cleaning. Potentially contaminated garments will not be worn or transported outside the work area but placed in the appropriate containers.

(14) If a patient expires within 24 hours of receiving a hazardous drug, the mortuary staff will be informed of the potential for exposure to body fluids containing these drugs by the attending physician. This will be accomplished by marking the autopsy request form.

(15) During chemotherapy or hazardous drug therapy, and for 48 hours afterward, the patient's inpatient chart and room will be labeled "Chemotherapy patient" or with some similar warning to notify employees to take appropriate precautions.

47

Stability and Compatibility of Intravenous Oncology Drugs[a]

These tables are designed to provide information regarding the stability and compatibility of commercially available intravenous cytotoxic drugs.[a] The term *stability* refers to the length time during which at least 90 % of the drug remains chemically stable after recommended reconstitution. *Compatibility* refers to the stable admixture of one or more agents with a particular cytotoxic drug in a large-volume solution. The specific conditions of stability and compatibility are listed for each agent or admixture and are relevant only to administration solutions, not syringes or portable infusion devices. The compiled data were generated from information either submitted to the U.S. Food and Drug Administration, on file with the drug manufacturer, or published in the primary scientific literature.

The reader should be cautioned that the admixture of two agents outside the stated conditions (e.g., higher than published concentrations) cannot be inferred to be stable. Until scientific studies demonstrate that an admixture is stable in solution for a specific time and at specific concentrations, administration of each agent in a separate intravenous line or separated by an adequate flush is recommended.

The information contained in this guide is derived from a search of the primary literature compiled, reviewed, and approved by the editorial board of Medi-Span Knowledge Base Group of Burlingame, California. The scope of the literature evaluation conducted by Medi-Span Knowledge Base Group is designed to provide practical information to health care professionals.

This guide is intended to supplement the knowledge of nurses, pharmacists, and physicians regarding the stabilities and compatibilities of oncology drugs. This information is advisory only and is not intended to replace sound clinical judgment in the delivery of health care services.

Medi-Span Knowledge Base Group and Cetus Corporation disclaim all warranties, whether expressed or implied, including any warranty as to the quality, accuracy, or suitability of this information for any particular purpose.

Please consult complete prescribing information for any drug mentioned herein.

ACKNOWLEDGMENTS

Medi-Span Knowledge Base Group and Cetus Corporation wish to thank Peter J. Forni, Pharm.D., for his preparation of these tables, and Robert J. Ignoffo, Pharm.D., Clinical Professor, School of Pharmacy, University of California, San Francisco, for his review of these tables.

[a]Modified from Cetus Corporation.

Table 47.1. Reconstitution

Product	Constituting Solution	Amount/Vial	Constituting Volume	Final Concentration	Stability and Compatibility Comments
Aldesleukin (IL-2)	Water for injection	22 M IU (1.3 mg)	1.2 mL	18 M IU/mL (1.1 mg/mL)	Stable for 48 hours at 2° to 30°C. Do not use sodium chloride or bacteriostatic diluents. Do not shake; swirl gently.
Asparaginase	Sodium chloride 0.9%	10,000 IU	5 mL	2,000 IU/mL	Stable for 8 hours at 5°C. Keep refrigerated. May use a 5-micron filter. Do not shake vigorously.
	Water for injection	10,000 IU	5 mL	2,000 IU/mL	Stable for 8 hours at 5°C. Keep refrigerated. May use a 5-micron filter. Do not shake vigorously.
Azathioprine	Water for injection	100 mg	10 mL	10 mg/mL	Stable for 16 days at 20° to 25°C in fluorescent light. Refrigeration at 4°C may cause visible precipitate after 4 days. Incompatible with parabens.
Bleomycin	Dextrose 5%	15 units	5 mL	3 units/mL	Unstable. Greater than 10% loss within 24 hours at room temperature.
	Sodium chloride 0.9%	15 units	5 mL	3 units/mL	Manufacturer recommends that solution be used within 24 hours; however, other data show it to be stable for 4 weeks at 4°C.
Carboplatin	Dextrose 5%	50 mg	5 mL	10 mg/mL	Manufacturer recommends that solution be used within 8 hours; however, prefilled syringes show no loss in 5 days at 4°C, and 3% loss in 24 hours at 37°C.
	Dextrose 5%	150 mg	15 mL	10 mg/mL	Manufacturer recommends that solution be used within 8 hours; however, prefilled syringes show no loss in 5 days at 4°C, and 3% loss in 24 hours at 37°C.
	Dextrose 5%	450 mg	45 mL	10 mg/mL	Manufacturer recommends that solution be used within 8 hours; however, prefilled syringes show no loss in 5 days at 4°C, and 3% loss in 24 hours at 37°C.
	Sodium bicarbonate Sodium chloride 0.9%	150 mg 50 mg, 150 mg, 450 mg	21.6 mL 5 mL, 15 mL, 45 mL	7 mg/mL 10 mg/mL	Unstable. 13% loss within 24 hours at 27°C. Manufacturer recommends that solution be used within 8 hours; however, prefilled syringes show no loss in 5 days at 4°C, and 3% loss in 24 hours at 37°C.
	Sodium chloride 0.9% Water for injection	150 mg 50 mg, 150 mg, 450 mg	21.6 mL 5 mL, 15 mL, 45 mL	7 mg/mL 10 mg/mL	8% loss within 24 hours at 27°C. Manufacturer recommends that solution be used within 8 hours; however, prefilled syringes show no loss in 5 days at 4°C, and 3% loss in 24 hours at 37°C.

Drug	Diluent	Vial Size	Volume	Concentration	Stability
	Water for injection	50 mg	50 mL	1 mg/mL	Stable for 14 days at room temperature.
	Water for injection	150 mg	10 mL	15 mg/mL	Stable for 24 hours at 22° to 25°C.
	Water for injection	150 mg	21.6 mL	7 mg/mL	Stable for 7 days at 27°C.
Carmustine	Dehydrated alcohol & water	100 mg	3 mL & 27 mL	3.3 mg/mL	Dissolve in alcohol diluent, then add water. Stable for 8 hours at 25°C and for 24 hours at 4°C when protected from light.
	Dextrose 5%	100 mg	30 mL	3.3 mg/mL	Excluding alcohol diluent, drug is dissolved by heating to 60°C in a water bath for 5 minutes, with vigorous shaking 3 times. Stable for 24 hours at room temperature.
Cisplatin	Already in solution	50 mg, 100 mg	None	1 mg/mL	To manufacturer's expiration date on package when properly stored.
	Bacteriostatic water for injection	10 mg, 50 mg	10 mL, 50 mL	1 mg/mL	Stable for 72 hours at 25°C. Unstable at 4°C. Avoid aluminum needles (precipitates).
	Sodium chloride 0.9%	10 mg, 50 mg	10 mL, 50 mL	1 mg/mL	Stable for 22 months at 5°C in glass vials, but forms precipitate that requires sonication. Stable for 10 months at 40°C with no precipitate.
	Water for injection	10 mg, 50 mg	10 mL, 50 mL	1 mg/mL	Stable for 35 days at 30°C. Avoid aluminum needles (precipitates).
Cyclophosphamide	Bacteriostatic water with benzyl alcohol	500 mg	25 mL	20 mg/mL	Greater drug loss in 24 hours than with bacteriostatic water with parabens.
	Water for injection	100 mg, 200 mg, 500 mg, 1 g, 2 g	5–100 mL	20 mg/mL	Stable for 24 hours at 25°C and for 6 days at 5°C. Store below 30°C.
	Water for injection	500 mg	25 mL	20 mg/mL	In polypropylene syringes (B-D) with Luer-Loks, 3% loss in 4 weeks at 4°C and 10% loss in 11 weeks. Avoid freezing.
Cytarabine	Bacteriostatic water with benzyl alcohol	100 mg	5 mL	20 mg/mL	Stable for 48 hours at 15° to 30°C.
	Bacteriostatic water with benzyl alcohol	200 mg	10 mL	20 mg/mL	Stable for 48 hours at 15° to 30°C.
	Bacteriostatic water with benzyl alcohol	500 mg	10 mL	50 mg/mL	Stable for 48 hours at 15° to 30°C.
	Bacteriostatic water with benzyl alcohol	1 g, 2 g	10 mL, 20 mL	100 mg/mL	Stable for 48 hours at 15° to 30°C.
	Bacteriostatic water with benzyl alcohol	1 g	4 mL	250 mg/mL	Stable for 5 days at 30°C.

Table 47.1. *continued*

Product	Constituting Solution	Amount/Vial	Constituting Volume	Final Concentration	Stability and Compatibility Comments
	Sodium chloride 0.9%	100 mg	2 mL, 5 mL	50 mg/mL, 20 mg/mL	For intrathecal use. Manufacturer recommends that this unpreserved solution be used within 24 hours; however, it has been shown to be stable for 7 days at −10° to 22°C in plastic syringes.
	Water for injection	100 mg	5 mL	20 mg/mL	Stable for 48 hours at 15° to 30°C.
	Water for injection	500 mg	10 mL	50 mg/mL	Stable for 48 hours at 15° to 30°C.
	Water for injection	1 g, 2 g	10 mL, 20 mL	100 mg/mL	Stable for 48 hours at 15° to 30°C.
Dacarbazine	Water for injection	100 mg, 200 mg	9.9 mL, 19.7 mL	10 mg/mL	Stable for 72 hours at 4°C and for 8 hours at 25°C.
Dactinomycin	Water for injection	0.5 mg	1.1 mL	0.5 mg/mL	Use immediately. Do not use bacteriostatic diluents or cellulose ester membrane filters.
Daunorubicin	Water for injection	20 mg	4 mL	5 mg/mL	Stable for 4 days at 15° to 25°C.
Doxorubicin	Already in solution	10 mg, 20 mg, 50 mg, 200 mg	None	2 mg/mL	To manufacturer's expiration date on package when properly stored. Protect from light. Avoid aluminum needles (precipitates).
	Sodium chloride 0.9%	10 mg, 20 mg, 50 mg, 150 mg	5–75 mL	2 mg/mL	Stable for 7 days at 25°C and for 15 days at 5°C when protected from light. Avoid aluminum needles and bacteriostatic diluents (precipitates).
	Water for injection	10 mg, 20 mg, 50 mg, 150 mg	5–75 mL	2 mg/mL	Stable for 7 days at 25°C and for 15 days at 5°C when protected from light. Avoid aluminum needles and bacteriostatic diluents (precipitates).
Etoposide	Already in solution	100 mg	None	20 mg/mL	To manufacturer's expiration date on package when properly stored.
Filgrastim (G-CSF)	Already in solution	300 μg	1 mL	300 μg/mL	To manufacturer's expiration date on package when properly stored. Refrigerate; do not freeze. Allow to come to room temperature before injection. Avoid shaking. Discard any solution left in vial at room temperature for longer than 6 hours.

Drug	Diluent	Vial size	Volume to add	Concentration	Comments
	Already in solution	480 µg	1.6 mL	300 µg/mL	To manufacturer's expiration date on package when properly stored. Refrigerate; do not freeze. Allow to come to room temperature before injection. Avoid shaking. Discard any solution left in vial at room temperature for longer than 6 hours.
Floxuridine	Water for injection	500 mg	5 mL	100 mg/mL	Stable for 14 days at 2° to 8°C.
Fludarabine	Water for injection	50 mg	2 mL	25 mg/mL	Manufacturer recommends that this unpreserved solution be used within 8 hours; however, other data show it to be stable for 16 days at room temperature when not protected from light.
Fluorouracil	Already in solution	500 mg, 1 g, 2.5 g, 5 g	None	50 mg/mL	To manufacturer's expiration date on package when properly stored.
Idarubicin	Sodium chloride 0.9%	5 mg, 10 mg	5 mL, 10 mL	1 mg/mL	Stable for 72 hours at 25°C and for 7 days at 2° to 8°C. Avoid bacteriostatic diluents (precipitates).
Ifosfamide	Bacteriostatic water with benzyl alcohol	1 g	10 mL	100 mg/mL	Incompatible. Results in a turbid solution, which separates into 2 layers. Layers dissolve completely with no drug loss when diluted to 60 mg/mL or less.
	Bacteriostatic water for injection	1 g, 3 g	20 mL, 60 mL	50 mg/mL	Stable for 7 days at 30°C and for up to 6 weeks at 2° to 8°C.
	Sodium chloride 0.9%	1 g	12.5 mL	80 mg/mL	Stable for 9 days at 27° to 37°C when protected from light.
	Water for injection	1 g, 3 g	20 mL, 60 mL	50 mg/mL	Manufacturer recommends that this unpreserved solution be used within 6 hours; however, other data show it to be stable for 7 days at 25°C.
Leucovorin	Bacteriostatic water with benzyl alcohol	50 mg, 100 mg	5 mL, 10 mL	10 mg/mL	Stable for 7 days.
	Bacteriostatic water with benzyl alcohol	350 mg	17 mL	20 mg/mL	Stable for 7 days.
	Sterile water for injection	350 mg	17 mL	20 mg/mL	Solutions should be used immediately.
Mechlorethamine	Sodium chloride 0.9%	10 mg	10 mL	1 mg/mL	Unstable. Drug decomposes within 1 hour at 25°C. Use immediately. Use mild agitation to dissolve.
	Water for injection	10 mg	10 mL	1 mg/mL	Unstable. Drug decomposes within 1 hour at 25°C. Use immediately. Use mild agitation to dissolve.

Table 47.1. continued

Product	Constituting Solution	Amount/Vial	Constituting Volume	Final Concentration	Stability and Compatibility Comments
Mesna	Already in solution	200 mg, 400 mg, 1 g	None	100 mg/mL	To manufacturer's expiration date on package when properly stored.
Methotrexate	Already in solution	5 mg	None	2.5 mg/mL	To manufacturer's expiration date on package when properly stored.
	Already in solution	50 mg, 100 mg, 200 mg, 250 mg	None	25 mg/mL	To manufacturer's expiration date on package when properly stored.
	Dextrose 5% in sodium chloride 0.9%	20 mg, 25 mg, 50 mg, 100 mg, 250 mg	2–10 mL	10–25 mg/mL	Stable for 24 hours at 25°C.
	Dextrose 5% in water	20 mg, 25 mg, 50 mg, 100 mg, 250 mg	2–10 mL	10–25 mg/mL	Stable for 24 hours at 25°C.
	Sodium chloride 0.9%	20 mg, 25 mg, 50 mg, 100 mg, 250 mg	2–10 mL	2–125 mg/mL	Stable for 4 weeks at 25°C and for 3 months at 4°C when protected from light.
	Water for injection	20 mg, 25 mg, 50 mg, 100 mg, 250 mg	2–10 mL	2–125 mg/mL	Stable for 4 weeks at 25°C and for 3 months at 4°C when protected from light.
Mitomycin	Sodium chloride 0.9%	50 mg	50 mL	1 mg/mL	Incompatible. Precipitates or degrades within 4 days.
	Water for injection	5 mg, 20 mg, 40 mg	5–40 mL	0.5–1 mg/mL	Stable for 7 days at 25°C and for 14 days at 5°C. Use mild agitation to dissolve.
	Water for injection	30 mg	50 mL	0.6 mg/mL	Stable for 4 days at 4°C.
	Water for injection	30–40 mg	50 mL	0.6–0.8 mg/mL	Stable for 4 days at 25°C in glass or PVC containers when protected from light.
	Water for injection	40 mg	50 mL	0.8 mg/mL	Incompatible. Precipitates after 24 hours at 4°C.
	Water for injection	50 mg	50 mL	1 mg/mL	Incompatible. Precipitates or degrades within 4 days.
Mitoxantrone	Already in solution	20 mg	None	2 mg/mL[a]	To manufacturer's expiration date on package when properly stored. Refrigeration may cause precipitate, which will redissolve on warming. Not light-sensitive.[a] Dilute to at least 50 mL prior to administration.
	Already in solution	25 mg	None	2 mg/mL[a]	To manufacturer's expiration date on package when properly stored. Refrigeration may cause precipitate, which will redissolve on warming. Not light-sensitive.[a] Dilute to at least 50 mL prior to administration.

Drug	Reconstitution fluid	Amount	Diluent volume	Concentration	Stability
	Already in solution	30 mg	None	2 mg/mL[a]	To manufacturer's expiration date on package when properly stored. Refrigeration may cause precipitate, which will redissolve on warming. Not light-sensitive.[a] Dilute to at least 50 mL prior to administration.
Paclitaxel	Already in solution	30 mg	None	6 mg/mL[a]	To manufacturer's expiration date on package when properly stored. Refrigerate at 2° to 8°C. Freezing does not adversely affect the product.[a] Dilute to 0.3 to 1.2 mg/mL prior to administration.
Pentostatin	Water for injection	10 mg	5 mL	2 mg/mL	Manufacturer states that this unpreserved solution is stable for 8 hours at room temperature; however, other data suggest it is stable for 72 hours at room temperature.
Plicamycin	Water for injection	2500 µg	4.9 mL	500 µg/mL	Stable for 24 hours at 25°C and for 48 hours at 5°C. Use immediately. Use mild agitation to dissolve.
Sargramostim (GM-CSF)	Water for injection	250 µg	1 mL	250 µg/mL	Manufacturer recommends that this unpreserved solution be used within 6 hours; however, solution retains activity for 24 hours. Do not freeze.
	Water for injection	500 µg	1 mL	500 µg/mL	Manufacturer recommends that this unpreserved solution be used within 6 hours; however, solution retains activity for 24 hours. Do not freeze.
Streptozocin	Dextrose 5%	1 g	9.5 mL	100 mg/mL	Stable for 12 hours at 20°C when protected from light.
	Sodium chloride 0.9%	1 g	9.5 mL	100 mg/mL	Stable for 12 hours at 20°C when protected from light.
Thiotepa	Water for injection	15 mg	15 mL	10 mg/mL	Stable for 5 days at 5°C.
Vinblastine	Already in solution	10 mg	None	1 mg/mL	To manufacturer's expiration date on package when properly stored.
	Bacteriostatic sodium chloride 0.9%	10 mg	10 mL	1 mg/mL	Stable for 30 days at 5°C when protected from light. Unstable at 37°C in implantable pump.
	Sodium chloride 0.9%	10 mg	10 mL	1 mg/mL	Stable for 30 days at 5°C when protected from light.
Vincristine	Already in solution	1 mg, 2 mg, 5 mg	None	1 mg/mL	To manufacturer's expiration date on package when properly stored.

Table 47.2. Dilution of IV Fluids

Product	Diluting Solution	Final Solution Concentration	Container Type[a]	Stability and Compatibility Comments
Aldesleukin (IL-2)	Dextrose 5%	>5 µg/mL	G/P	Stable for 48 hours at 2° to 30°C. Avoid bacteriostatic water or sodium chloride 0.9%. Add albumin if concentration is less than 10 µg/mL. Do not freeze or use in-line filters.
Asparaginase	Dextrose 5%	200 IU/mL	G	Stable for 8 hours at 2° to 8°C. Do not use a 0.2-micron filter. May use a 5-micron filter. Administer over 30 minutes.
	Sodium chloride 0.9%	200 IU/mL	G	Stable for 8 hours at 2° to 8°C. Do not use a 0.2-micron filter. May use a 5-micron filter. Administer over 30 minutes.
Azathioprine	Dextrose 5%	2 mg/mL	P	Stable for 8 days at 25°C.
	Sodium chloride 0.45%	2 mg/mL	G/P	Stable for 16 days at 25°C.
	Sodium chloride 0.9%	2 mg/mL	P	Stable for 16 days at 25°C.
Bleomycin	Dextrose 5%	0.15–3 units/mL	G/P	Unstable. 10% loss in 10 hours and up to 16% loss in 24 hours at room temperature.
	Dextrose 5%	0.3 units/mL	B	Stable for 18 hours at 25°C.
	Dextrose 5%	0.3 units/mL	G	Stable for 24 hours at 25°C.
	Dextrose 5%	0.3 units/mL	P	Unstable. Drug decomposes within 1 hour at 25°C.
	Sodium chloride 0.9%	0.015 units/mL	G	Stable for 24 hours at 25°C and for 48 hours at 4°C.
	Sodium chloride 0.9%	0.015–0.03 units/mL	P	Stable for 4 days at 25°C and for 14 days at 4°C and 90 days at −15°C.
	Sodium chloride 0.9%	0.045 units/mL	G	Stable for 24 hours at 25°C and for 14 days at 4°C.
	Sodium chloride 0.9%	0.15 units/mL	P	Stable for 24 hours at 25°C and for 48 hours at 4°C.
	Sodium chloride 0.9%	0.3–3 units/mL	G/P	Stable for 24 hours at 23°C.
	Sodium chloride 0.9%	3 units/mL	G	Stable for 72 hours at 25°C.
Carboplatin	Dextrose 5%	0.5 mg/mL	G	Stable for 24 hours at 25°C.
	Dextrose 5%	2 mg/mL	G	Stable for 24 hours at 25°C.
	Dextrose 5% & sodium chloride 0.9%	1 mg/mL	G	4% loss in 24 hours at 25°C.
Carmustine	Dextrose 5%	0.1–1 mg/mL	G	Stable for 8 hours at 25°C and for 48 hours at 4°C when protected from light.

Drug	Solution	Concentration		Stability
	Dextrose 5%	1.25 mg/mL	G	Stable for 7 hours at 25°C when not protected from light.
	Dextrose 5%	1.25 mg/mL	P	Unstable. Drug decomposes within 1 hour at 25°C. Significant adsorption onto PVC.
	Dextrose 5%	1.25 mg/mL	B	Stable for 7 hours at 25°C when not protected from light.
	Sodium chloride 0.9%	0.1–1 mg/mL	G	Stable for 8 hours at 25°C and for 48 hours at 4°C when protected from light.
Cisplatin	Dextrose 5%	0.1 mg/mL	G	Unstable. Greater than 10% loss within 2 hours at 25°C. Avoid aluminum needles (precipitates).
	Dextrose 5% & sodium chloride 0.33%	0.05–0.2 mg/mL	G	With mannitol. Stable for 72 hours at 4° to 25°C. Avoid aluminum needles (precipitates).
	Dextrose 5% & sodium chloride 0.33%	0.05–0.2 mg/mL	G	With mannitol & potassium chloride 20 mEq. Stable for 72 hours at 4° to 25°C. Avoid aluminum needles (precipitates).
	Dextrose 5% & sodium chloride 0.45%	0.05–0.2 mg/mL	G	With mannitol. Stable for 72 hours at 4° to 25°C. Avoid aluminum needles (precipitates).
	Dextrose 5% & sodium chloride 0.45%	0.05–0.5 mg/mL	G/P	Stable for 24 hours at 25°C. Avoid aluminum needles (precipitates).
	Dextrose 5% & sodium chloride 0.9%	0.05–0.5 mg/mL	G	Stable for 24 hours at 25°C. Avoid aluminum needles (precipitates).
	Sodium bicarbonate 5%	0.05–0.2 mg/mL	G	Unstable. Precipitates within 8 hours at 25°C. Avoid aluminum needles (precipitates).
	Sodium chloride 0.1%	0.05–0.2 mg/mL	G	Unstable. Greater than 10% loss within 4 hours at 25°C. Avoid aluminum needles (precipitates).
	Sodium chloride 0.225%	0.05–0.2 mg/mL	G	Stable for 72 hours at 4° to 25°C. Avoid aluminum needles (precipitates).
	Sodium chloride 0.3%	0.05–0.2 mg/mL	G	Stable for 72 hours at 4° to 25°C. Avoid aluminum needles (precipitates).
	Sodium chloride 0.45%	0.05–0.5 mg/mL	G	Stable for 24 hours at 25°C. Avoid aluminum needles (precipitates).
	Sodium chloride 0.9%	0.05–0.5 mg/mL	G	Stable for 24 hours at 25°C. Avoid aluminum needles (precipitates).
	Sodium chloride 0.9%	0.1 mg/mL	B	Stable for 24 hours at 25°C. Avoid aluminum needles (precipitates).
	Water for injection	0.05–0.2 mg/mL	G	Unstable. Greater than 10% loss within 4 hours at 25°C. Avoid aluminum needles (precipitates).
	Water for injection	1 mg/mL	P/B	Stable for 35 days at 30°C. Avoid aluminum needles (precipitates).

Table 47.2. *continued*

Product	Diluting Solution	Final Solution Concentration	Container Type[a]	Stability and Compatibility Comments
Cyclophosphamide	Dextrose 5%	0.1–3.1 mg/mL	G	Stable for 8 hours at 27°C and for 6 days at 5°C.
	Dextrose 5%	6.6 mg/mL	G/P/B	Stable for 24 hours at 25°C.
	Dextrose 5%	6.7 mg/mL	G/B	Stable for 24 hours at 25°C.
	Dextrose 5% & sodium chloride 0.9%	0.1–3.1 mg/mL	G	Stable for 8 hours at 27°C and for 6 days at 5°C.
	Dextrose 5% in lactated Ringer's	Not stated	G	Stable for 24 hours at 27°C and for 6 days at 5°C.
	Dextrose 5% in Ringer's	Not stated	G	Stable for 24 hours at 27°C and for 6 days at 5°C.
	Lactated Ringer's	Not stated	G	Stable for 24 hours at 27°C and for 6 days at 5°C.
	Sodium chloride 0.45%	Not stated	G	Stable for 24 hours at 25°C and for 28 days at 5°C.
	Sodium chloride 0.9%	0.1–3.1 mg/mL	G	Stable for 8 hours at 27°C and for 6 days at 5°C.
	Sodium chloride 0.9%	4 mg/mL	G	Stable for 24 hours at room temperature and for 4 weeks when refrigerated.
	Sodium chloride 0.9%	4 mg/mL	P	Stable for 4 weeks at 4°C. 8% loss in 19 weeks at 4°C and at −20°C.
	Sodium lactate ⅙ molar	Not stated	G	Stable for 24 hours at 27°C and for 6 days at 5°C.
Cytarabine	Dextrose 5%	0.5–1.87 mg/mL	G/P	Stable for 8 days at 25°C. May use a 5-micron filter.
	Dextrose 5%	1.25 mg/mL & 25 mg/mL	E	5% loss in 28 days at 4° to 35°C.
	Dextrose 5%	8 mg/mL, 24 mg/mL, 32 mg/mL	G/P	Stable for 7 days at −20° to 25°C.
	Dextrose 5% & sodium chloride 0.9%	0.5 mg/mL	G/P	Stable for 8 days at 25°C. May use a 5-micron filter.
	Dextrose 5% in lactated Ringer's	0.5 mg/mL	G/P	Stable for 8 days at 25°C. May use a 5-micron filter.
	Lactated Ringer's	0.5 mg/mL	G/P	Stable for 24 hours at 5°C. May use a 5-micron filter.
	Sodium chloride 0.9%	0.5 mg/mL	G/P	Stable for 8 days at 25°C. May use a 5-micron filter.
	Sodium chloride 0.9%	1.25 mg/mL & 25 mg/mL	E	8% loss in 28 days at 4° to 35°C.
	Sodium chloride 0.9%	8 mg/mL, 24 mg/mL, 32 mg/mL	G/P	Stable for 7 days at −20° to 25°C.
Dacarbazine	Dextrose 5%	0.2–1.7 mg/mL	G/P/B	Stable for 8 hours at 25°C and for 24 hours at 4°C when protected from light.
	Sodium chloride 0.9%	0.2 mg/mL	G/P	Stable for 8 hours at 25°C and for 24 hours at 4°C when protected from light.

Drug	Diluent	Concentration		Stability
Dactinomycin	Dextrose 5%	9.8 mg/L	G/P	Stable for 24 hours at 25°C. Flush filter.
	Sodium chloride 0.9%	7.5 mg/L	B	Stable for 24 hours at 25°C. Flush filter.
	Sodium chloride 0.9%	9.8 mg/L	G/P	Stable for 24 hours at 25°C. Flush filter.
Daunorubicin	Dextrose 5%	0.02 mg/mL	G	Stable for 100 hours at 21°C when protected from light. Flush filter.
	Dextrose 5%	0.1 mg/mL	G	Stable for 4 weeks at 25°C when protected from light (less than 5% loss).
	Lactated Ringer's	0.02 mg/mL	G	Stable for 54 hours at 21°C when protected from light. Flush filter.
	Lactated Ringer's	0.1 mg/mL	G	Stable for 4 weeks at 25°C when protected from light (less than 5% loss).
	Normosol R	0.02 mg/mL	G	Stable for 95 hours at 21°C when protected from light. Flush filter.
	Sodium chloride 0.9%	0.02 mg/mL	G	Stable for 80 hours at 21°C when protected from light. Flush filter.
	Sodium chloride 0.9%	0.1 mg/mL	G	Stable for 4 weeks at 25°C when protected from light (less than 5% loss).
Doxorubicin	Dextrose 5%	0.01–0.18 mg/mL	G	Stable for 40 hours at 25°C. May use a 0.22-micron filter. Avoid aluminum needles (precipitates).
	Dextrose 5%	0.01–0.18 mg/mL	P/B	Stable for 48 hours at 25°C. May use a 0.22-micron filter. Avoid aluminum needles (precipitates).
	Dextrose 5%	0.1 mg/mL	G	Stable for 4 weeks at 25°C when protected from light.
	Dextrose 5%	0.5 mg/mL	E	Stable for 14 days at 4° to 35°C.
	Dextrose 5%	1.25 mg/mL	E	Stable for 14 days at 4° to 35°C.
	Lactated Ringer's	0.01–0.02 mg/mL	G	Stable for 48 hours at 25°C. May use a 0.22-micron filter. Avoid aluminum needles (precipitates).
	Normosol R (pH 7.4)	0.01–0.02 mg/mL	G	Stable for 40 hours at 25°C. May use a 0.02-micron filter. Avoid aluminum needles (precipitates).
	Sodium chloride 0.9%	0.01–0.02 mg/mL	G	Stable for 24 hours at 25°C. May use a 0.22-micron filter. Avoid aluminum needles (precipitates).
	Sodium chloride 0.9%	0.1 mg/mL	G	Stable for 6 days at 25°C when protected from light. Greater than 10% loss after 6 days.
	Sodium chloride 0.9%	0.5 mg/mL	E	Stable for 14 days at 4° to 35°C.
	Sodium chloride 0.9%	1.25 mg/mL	E	Stable for 28 days at 4° to 22°C.
Etoposide	Dextrose 5%	0.2 mg/mL	G/P	Stable for 4 days at 25°C.
	Dextrose 5%	0.4 mg/mL	G	Stable for 4 days at 21°C in both light and dark.
	Dextrose 5%	0.4 mg/mL	P	Stable for 48 hours at 25°C.
	Dextrose 5%	0.6 mg/mL	G/P	Stable for 8 hours at 25°C. May precipitate when concentration is greater than 0.4 mg/mL.
	Dextrose 5%	1 mg/mL	G/P	Stable for 2 hours at 25°C. May precipitate when concentration is greater than 0.4 mg/mL.

Table 47.2. *continued*

Product	Diluting Solution	Final Solution Concentration	Container Type[a]	Stability and Compatibility Comments
	Lactated Ringer's	0.2–0.4 mg/mL	G	Stable for 4 days at 21°C when not protected from light.
	Mannitol 10%	0.2–0.4 mg/mL	G/P	Stable for 8 hours at 25°C.
	Sodium chloride 0.9%	0.2 mg/mL	G/P	Stable for 4 days at 25°C.
	Sodium chloride 0.9%	0.4 mg/mL	G/P	Stable for 4 days at 21°C in both light and dark.
	Sodium chloride 0.9%	0.6 mg/mL	G/P	Stable for 8 hours at 25°C. May precipitate when concentration is greater than 0.4 mg/mL.
	Sodium chloride 0.9%	1 mg/mL	G/P	Stable for 2 hours at 25°C. May precipitate when concentration is greater than 0.4 mg/mL.
Filgrastim (G-CSF)	Dextrose 5%	2–15 µg/mL	G/P/B	Add albumin to a concentration of 2 mg/mL. Stable for 7 days at 2° to 8°C and at controlled room temperature of 15° to 30°C. Manufacturer recommends that this unpreserved solution be refrigerated, and used within 24 hours. Do not freeze.
	Dextrose 5%	>15 µg/mL	G/P/B	Stable for 7 days at 2° to 8°C and at controlled room temperature of 15° to 30°C. Manufacturer recommends that this unpreserved solution be refrigerated, and used within 24 hours.
Floxuridine	Dextrose 5%	0.5 mg/mL	G/P	Stable for 7 days at 25° to 37°C.
	Sodium chloride 0.9%	0.5 mg/mL	G/P	Stable for 7 days at 25° to 37°C.
Fludarabine	Dextrose 5%	0.04 mg/mL	G/P	Stable for 48 hours at 4° to 25°C.
	Sodium chloride 0.9%	0.04 mg/mL	G/P	Stable for 48 hours at 4° to 25°C.
Fluorouracil	Dextrose 5%	0.5 mg/mL	G/P	Stable for 72 hours at 25° to 37°C.
	Dextrose 5%	1.5 mg/mL	G/P	Stable for 8 weeks at room temperature in both light and dark.
	Dextrose 5%	8.3 mg/mL	B	Stable for 48 hours at 25°C when not protected from light.
	Dextrose 5%	8.3 mg/mL	G	Unstable. 10% loss in 7 hours at 25°C when not protected from light.
	Dextrose 5%	8.3 mg/mL	P	Stable for 43 hours at 25°C when not protected from light.
	Dextrose 5%	10 mg/mL	P	Stable for 7 days at 25°C and for 16 weeks at 5°C when protected from light.
	Dextrose 5%	10 mg/mL	E	Stable for 28 days at 4° to 35°C.
	Dextrose 5%	100 mg/mL	P	Stable for 7 days at 25°C and for 16 weeks at 5°C when protected from light.

	Solution	Concentration		Stability
	Dextrose 5% in lactated Ringer's	0.5 mg/mL	G/P	Stable for 24 hours at 5°C when protected from light.
	Sodium chloride 0.9%	0.5 mg/mL	G/P	Stable for 72 hours at 25° to 37°C.
	Sodium chloride 0.9%	1.5 mg/mL	G/P	Stable for 8 weeks at room temperature in both light and dark.
	Sodium chloride 0.9%	10 mg/mL	E	Stable for 28 days at 4° to 35°C.
	Total parenteral nutrition	1 mg/mL	Not stated	Stable for 48 hours at room temperature in ambient light.
Idarubicin	Dextrose 5%	0.01 mg/mL	G	Stable for 72 hours at room temperature when protected from light. Dilute solutions are light-sensitive and degrade in light exposure longer than 6 hours (10% loss). Drug is unstable in alkaline solutions.
	Dextrose 5%	0.1 mg/mL	G/P	Stable for 4 weeks at 25°C when protected from light.
	Dextrose 5% & sodium chloride 0.9%	0.01 mg/mL	G/P	Stable for 72 hours at 25°C when protected from light. 10% loss in 6 hours when not protected from light.
	Lactated Ringer's	0.1 mg/mL	G/P	Stable for 4 weeks at 25°C when protected from light.
	Sodium chloride 0.9%	0.01 mg/mL	G/P	Stable for 72 hours at 25°C when protected from light. 10% loss in 6 hours when not protected from light.
	Sodium chloride 0.9%	0.1 mg/mL	G/P	Stable for 4 weeks at 25°C when protected from light.
Ifosfamide	Dextrose 5%	0.6 mg/mL & 16 mg/mL	G/P	Stable for 7 days at room temperature and for 6 weeks at 4° to 8°C.
	Dextrose 5% & sodium chloride 0.9%	0.6 mg/mL & 16 mg/mL	G/P	Stable for 7 days at room temperature and for 6 weeks at 4° to 8°C.
	Lactated Ringer's	0.6 mg/mL & 16 mg/mL	G/P	Stable for 7 days at room temperature and for 6 weeks at 4° to 8°C.
	Sodium chloride 0.9%	0.6 mg/mL & 16 mg/mL	G/P	Stable for 7 days at room temperature and for 6 weeks at 4° to 8°C.
	Sodium chloride 0.9%	10 mg/mL	P	Stable for 8 days at 4° to 25°C.
	Sodium lactate ⅙ molar	0.6 mg/mL & 16 mg/mL	G/P	Stable for 7 days at room temperature and for 6 weeks at 4° to 8°C.
	Sterile water for injection in portable IV cassette	20 mg/mL, 40 mg/mL, 80 mg/mL	P	Stable for 8 days at 35°C.
Leucovorin	Dextrose 5%	0.91 mg/mL	G/P	Stable for 24 hours at room temperature.
	Dextrose 10%	0.05 mg/mL	G	Stable for 24 hours at room temperature when protected from light.
	Dextrose 10% & sodium chloride 0.9%	0.05 mg/mL	G	Stable for 24 hours at room temperature when protected from light.
	Lactated Ringer's	0.05 mg/mL	G	Stable for 24 hours at room temperature when protected from light.
Mechlorethamine	Not recommended	—	—	Unstable. Drug rapidly decomposes.

Table 47.2. *continued*

Product	Diluting Solution	Final Solution Concentration	Container Type[a]	Stability and Compatibility Comments
Mesna	Dextrose 5%	1 mg/mL	G	Stable for 24 hours at room temperature.
	Dextrose 5%	20 mg/mL	G	Stable for 48 hours at room temperature.
	Dextrose 5% & sodium chloride 0.45%	1 mg/mL	G	Stable for 72 hours at room temperature.
	Dextrose 5% & sodium chloride 0.45%	20 mg/mL	G	Stable for 48 hours at room temperature.
	Lactated Ringer's	1 mg/mL	G	Stable for 24 hours at room temperature.
	Sodium chloride 0.9%	1 mg/mL	G	Stable for 48 hours at room temperature.
Methotrexate	Dextrose 5%	0.96 mg/mL	G/P	Stable for 24 hours at 25°C.
	Dextrose 25% & amino acids 4.25%	0.05 mg/mL	G/P	Stable. No particulate matter in 24 hours at 5°C.
	Sodium bicarbonate 0.05 molar	2 mg/mL	G	Stable for 12 hours at room temperature when not protected from light.
Mitomycin	Dextrose 5%	0.02–0.4 mg/mL	G/P	Unstable. 10% loss in 1 to 2 hours at 25°C.
	Dextrose 5%	0.05 mg/mL	P	Unstable. 74% loss in 12 hours at 28°C.
	Lactated Ringer's	0.06–0.12 mg/mL	G	Stable for 24 hours at 25°C. May differ by formulation and buffering.
	Sodium chloride 0.9%	0.4 mg/mL	G/P	Stable for 24 hours at 25°C.
	Sodium chloride 0.9%	0.6 mg/mL	G/P	Stable for 7 days at 4°C when protected from light (6% to 8% loss).
	Sodium lactate	0.02–0.04 mg/mL	G	Stable for 24 hours at 25°C. May differ by formulation and buffering.
Mitoxantrone	Dextrose 5%	0.005 mg/mL	P	Stable for 48 hours at room temperature.
	Dextrose 5%	0.02–0.5 mg/mL	P	Stable for 7 days at room temperature and at 5°C. Not light-sensitive.
	Dextrose 5% & sodium chloride 0.9%	0.02–0.5 mg/mL	P	Stable for 7 days at room temperature and at 5°C. Not light-sensitive.
	Sodium chloride 0.9%	0.005 mg/mL	G	Stable for 48 hours at room temperature.
	Sodium chloride 0.9%	0.02–0.5 mg/mL	G	Stable for 48 hours at room temperature.
	Sodium chloride 0.9%	0.02–0.5 mg/mL	P	Stable for 7 days at room temperature and at 5°C. Not light-sensitive.
Paclitaxel	Dextrose 5% & sodium chloride 0.9%	0.3–1.2 mg/mL	G/B/L	Stable for 27 hours at 25°C when not protected from light. Solutions may show slight haziness with no significant loss of potency. May use a 0.22-micron filter. Should use non-PVC-containing administration sets (i.e., polyethylene) to minimize leaching.
Pentostalin	Dextrose 5%	0.02 mg/mL	G/P	Stable for 48 hours at 22° to 23°C and at pH 5.7; however, at a pH of less than 5, drug is unstable. Stable for 96 hours when refrigerated.
	Sodium chloride 0.9%	0.02 mg/mL	G/P	Stable for 48 hours at 22° to 23°C and for 96 hours when refrigerated.

Drug	Solution	Concentration	Container type	Comments
Plicamycin	Dextrose 5%	23.8 µg/mL	G/P	Stable for 24 hours at 25°C. Do not use a cellulose ester membrane filter.
	Dextrose 5%	45.5 µg/mL	B	Unstable. Drug decomposes at 25°C.
	Sodium chloride 0.9%	45.5 µg/mL	B	Stable for 24 hours at 25°C. Do not use a cellulose ester membrane filter.
	Sodium chloride 0.9%	45.5 µg/mL	G	Unstable. Drug decomposes within 1 hour at 25°C.
Sargramostim (GM-CSF)	Sodium chloride 0.9%	<10 µg/mL	P	Add 1 mg albumin per 1 mL sodium chloride 0.9% to prevent adsorption. Manufacturer recommends that this unpreserved solution be used within 6 hours. Do not freeze.
	Sodium chloride 0.9%	>10 µg/mL	P	Manufacturer recommends that this unpreserved solution be used within 6 hours. Do not freeze.
Streptozocin	Dextrose 5%	Not stated	G/P	Stable for 24 hours at 25°C and for 96 hours at 5°C when protected from light.
	Sodium chloride 0.9%	Not stated	G/P	Stable for 24 hours at 25°C and for 96 hours at 5°C when protected from light.
Thiotepa	Dextrose 5%	Not stated	G	Stable for 5 days at 5°C when protected from light.
	Dextrose 5% & sodium chloride 0.9%	Not stated	G	Stable for 5 days at 5°C when protected from light.
	Lactated Ringer's	Not stated	G	Stable for 5 days at 5°C when protected from light.
	Sodium chloride 0.9%	Not stated	G	Stable for 5 days at 5°C when protected from light.
Vinblastine	Dextrose 5%	0.02 mg/mL	G	Stable for 21 days at 4°C and at 25°C when protected from light.
	Dextrose 5%	0.17 mg/mL	G/P/B	Stable for 24 hours at 25°C when protected from light. May use a 0.22-micron filter.
	Lactated Ringer's	0.02 mg/mL	G	Stable for 21 days at 4°C and at 25°C when protected from light. May be frozen for 4 weeks at −20°C.
	Sodium chloride 0.9%	0.02 mg/mL	G	Stable for 21 days at 4°C and at 25°C when protected from light. May be frozen for 4 weeks at −20°C.
	Sodium chloride 0.9%	1 mg/mL	I	Unstable in infusaid 400. 24% loss in 24 hours at 37°C.
Vincristine	Dextrose 5%	0.0167–0.02 mg/mL	G/P	Stable for 24 hours at 25°C. Do not use a filter.
	Dextrose 5%	0.17 mg/mL	G/P	Stable for 24 hours at room temperature.
	Dextrose 5%	0.2 mg/mL	G	Stable for 21 days at 4°C and at 25°C when protected from light.
	Lactated Ringer's	0.02 mg/mL	G	Stable for 21 days at 4°C and at 25°C when protected from light.
	Sodium chloride 0.9%	0.02 mg/mL	G	Stable for 21 days at 4°C and at 25°C when protected from light.

aContainer type: **G**, glass; **P**, polyvinyl chloride; **B**, polypolefin; **E**, ethylene vinyl acetate pump; **I**, implantable pump; **L**, polypropylene.

Table 47.3. Oncology Product Compatibilities

| | | | | Part A: Oncology Product with Oncology Products | |
Oncology Product A	Oncology Product B	Condition[a]	Diluting Solution	Concentration of Products	Stability and Compatibility Comments
Bleomycin	Cisplatin	Y	Not applicable	3 units/mL & 1 mg/mL	No visible precipitate after sequential injection.
	Cisplatin & cytarabine	A	Sodium chloride 0.9%	0.12 units/mL & 0.2 mg/mL & 1.05 mg/mL	Stable for 24 hours at 25°C.
	Cyclophosphamide	Y	Not applicable	3 units/mL & 20 mg/mL	No visible precipitate after sequential injection.
	Cytarabine & cisplatin	A	Sodium chloride 0.9%	0.12 units/mL & 1.05 mg/mL & 0.2 mg/mL	Stable for 24 hours at 25°C.
	Doxorubicin	Y	Not applicable	3 units/mL & 2 mg/mL	No visible precipitate after sequential injection.
	Fludarabine	Y	Not applicable	1 unit/mL & 1 mg/mL	Physically compatible for 4 hours at room temperature in fluorescent light.
	Fluorouracil	A	Sodium chloride 0.9%	0.02–0.03 units/mL & 1 mg/mL	Stable for 7 days at 4°C. May adsorb onto plastic.
	Fluorouracil	Y	Not applicable	3 units/mL & 50 mg/mL	No visible precipitate after sequential injection.
	Methotrexate	A	Sodium chloride 0.9%	0.02–0.03 units/mL & 0.25–0.5 mg/mL	Unstable. Drug decomposes within 7 days at 4°C.
	Methotrexate	Y	Not applicable	3 units/mL & 25 mg/mL	No visible precipitate after sequential injection.
	Mitomycin	A	Sodium chloride 0.9%	0.02–0.03 units/mL & 0.01–0.05 mg/mL	Unstable. Drug decomposes within 7 days at 4°C.
	Mitomycin	Y	Not applicable	3 units/mL & 0.5 mg/mL	No visible precipitate after sequential injection.
	Vinblastine	A	Sodium chloride 0.9%	0.02–0.03 units/mL & 0.01–0.1 mg/mL	Stable for 7 days at 4°C. May adsorb onto plastic.
	Vinblastine	Y	Not applicable	3 units/mL & 1 mg/mL	No visible precipitate after sequential injection.
	Vincristine	A	Sodium chloride 0.9%	0.02–0.03 units/mL & 0.05–0.1 mg/mL	Stable for 7 days at 4°C. May adsorb onto plastic.
	Vincristine	Y	Not applicable	3 units/mL & 1 mg/mL	No visible precipitate after sequential injection.
Carboplatin	Fludarabine	Y	Dextrose 5%	1 mg/mL & 5 mg/mL	Physically compatible for 4 hours at room temperature in fluorescent light.
	Fluorouracil	A	Sterile water	1 mg/mL & 10 mg/mL	Unstable. Greater than 20% loss of carboplatin within 24 hours at room temperature.
	Ifosfamide	A	Sterile water	1 mg/mL & 1 mg/mL	Both drugs stable for 5 days at room temperature.
	Ifosfamide & etoposide	A	Sterile water	1 mg/mL & 2 mg/mL & 0.2 mg/mL	All drugs stable for 7 days at room temperature.
	Mesna	A	Sterile water	1 mg/mL & 1 mg/mL	Unstable. Greater than 10% loss of carboplatin within 24 hours at room temperature.

Carmustine	Cisplatin	A	See manufacturer's package inserts	1.4 mg/mL & 0.86 mg/mL	Both drugs stable for 3 hours at 23°C.
	Fludarabine	Y	Dextrose 5%	1.5 mg/mL & 1 mg/mL	Stable for 4 hours at room temperature in fluorescent light.
Cisplatin	Bleomycin & cytarabine	A	Sodium chloride 0.9%	0.2 mg/mL & 0.12 units/mL & 1.05 mg/mL	Stable for 24 hours at 25°C.
	Carmustine	A	Dextrose 5%	0.86 mg/mL & 1.4 mg/mL	Both drugs stable for 3 hours at 23°C.
	Carmustine	A	Sodium chloride 0.9%	0.86 mg/mL & 1.4 mg/mL	Both drugs stable for 3 hours at 23°C.
	Cyclophosphamide & etoposide	A/Y	Sodium chloride 0.9%	0.2 mg/mL & 2 mg/mL & 0.2 mg/mL	Stable for 7 days at room temperature.
	Cytarabine & bleomycin	A	Sodium chloride 0.9%	0.2 mg/mL & 1.05 mg/mL & 0.12 units/mL	Stable for 24 hours at 25°C.
	Etoposide	A	Dextrose 5% & sodium chloride 0.45%	0.2 mg/mL & 0.2–0.4 mg/mL	Stable for 24 hours at 25°C.
	Etoposide	A	Sodium chloride 0.9%	0.2 mg/mL & 0.2 mg/mL	Stable for 15 days at room temperature when protected from light.
	Etoposide	A	Sodium chloride 0.9%	0.2 mg/mL & 0.2–0.4 mg/mL	Stable for 24 hours at 25°C.
	Etoposide	A	Sodium chloride 0.9%	0.2 mg/mL & 0.4 mg/mL	Stable. 10% loss of etoposide within 7 days at room temperature.
	Etoposide	A	Sodium chloride 0.9%	10 mg/mL & 20 mg/mL	Both drugs stable for 7 days in PVC containers.
	Floxuridine	A	Sodium chloride 0.9%	0.5 mg/mL & 10 mg/mL	Physically compatible for 14 days when protected from light; however, a 13% loss and an 18% loss of floxuridine occur at 7 days and at 14 days, respectively.
	Floxuridine & leucovorin	A	Sodium chloride 0.9%	0.2 mg/mL & 0.7 mg/mL & 0.14 mg/mL	All drugs stable for 7 days.
	Fluorouracil	A	Sodium chloride 0.9%	0.2 mg/mL & 1 mg/mL	Unstable. 10% loss of cisplatin in 1.5 hours and 25% loss in 4 hours at 25°C in fluorescent light.
	Fluorouracil	Y	Not applicable	1 mg/mL & 50 mg/mL	No visible precipitate after sequential injection.
	Ifosfamide	A	Sodium chloride 0.9%	0.2 mg/mL & 20 mg/mL	Both drugs stable for 7 days at room temperature.
Cyclophosphamide	Bleomycin	Y	Not applicable	20 mg/mL & 3 units/mL	No visible precipitate after sequential injection.
	Cisplatin	Y	Not applicable	20 mg/mL & 1 mg/mL	No visible precipitate after sequential injection.
	Cisplatin & etoposide	A	Sodium chloride 0.9%	2 mg/mL & 0.2 mg/mL & 0.2 mg/mL	All drugs stable for 7 days at room temperature.
	Doxorubicin	A	Sodium chloride 0.9%	0.67 mg & 11.7 mg/mL	Both drugs stable for 7 days at 25°C.

Table 47.3. *continued*

Part A: Oncology Product with Oncology Products

Oncology Product A	Oncology Product B	Condition[a]	Diluting Solution	Concentration of Products	Stability and Compatibility Comments
	Doxorubicin	Y	Not applicable	20 mg/mL & 2 mg/mL	No visible precipitate after sequential injection.
	Fludarabine	Y	Dextrose 5%	10 mg/mL & 1 mg/mL	Physically compatible for 4 hours at room temperature in fluorescent light.
	Fluorouracil	A	Sodium chloride 0.9%	1.67 mg/mL & 8.3 mg/mL	Both drugs stable for 15 days at room temperature.
	Fluorouracil	Y	Not applicable	20 mg/mL & 50 mg/mL	No visible precipitate after sequential injection.
	Methotrexate	A	Sodium chloride 0.9%	1.67 mg/mL & 0.025 mg/mL	9.3% loss of cyclophosphamide along with a degradation product at 7 days at room temperature. Also, a pH change occurs from 6.30 to 4.57. No loss of methotrexate within 14 days.
	Methotrexate	Y	Not applicable	20 mg/mL & 25 mg/mL	No visible precipitate after sequential injection.
	Methotrexate & fluorouracil	A	Sodium chloride 0.9%	1.67 mg/mL & 0.025 mg/mL & 8.3 mg/mL	9.3% loss of cyclophosphamide within 7 days at room temperature; other drugs are stable.
	Mitomycin	Y	Not applicable	20 mg/mL & 0.5 mg/mL	No visible precipitate after sequential injection.
	Vinblastine	Y	Not applicable	20 mg/mL & 1 mg/mL	No visible precipitate after sequential injection.
	Vincristine	Y	Not applicable	20 mg/mL & 1 mg/mL	No visible precipitate after sequential injection.
Cytarabine	Bleomycin & cisplatin	A	Sodium chloride 0.9%	1.05 mg/mL & 0.12 units/mL & 0.2 mg/mL	Stable for 24 hours at 25°C.
	Cisplatin & bleomycin	A	Sodium chloride 0.9%	1.05 mg/mL & 0.2 mg/mL & 0.12 units/mL	Stable for 24 hours at 25°C.
	Daunorubicin & etoposide	A	Dextrose 5%	200 mg & 25 mg & 300 mg	All drugs stable for 72 hours at 20°C.
	Daunorubicin & etoposide	A	Sodium chloride 0.45%	200 mg & 25 mg & 300 mg	All drugs stable for 72 hours at 20°C.
	Etoposide & daunorubicin	A	Dextrose 5%	200 mg & 300 mg & 25 mg	All drugs stable for 72 hours at 20°C.
	Etoposide & daunorubicin	A	Sodium chloride 0.45%	200 mg & 300 mg & 25 mg	All drugs stable for 72 hours at 20°C.
	Fludarabine	Y	Dextrose 5%	50 mg/mL & 1 mg/mL	No visible precipitate at 4 hours at room temperature in fluorescent light.
	Fluorouracil	A	Dextrose 5%	0.4 mg/mL & 0.25 mg/mL	Both drugs stable for 8 hours at 25°C. No significant UV spectrum changes.
	Methotrexate	A	Dextrose 5%	0.4 mg/mL & 0.2 mg/mL	Both drugs stable for 8 hours at 25°C. No significant UV spectrum changes.
	Methotrexate	A	Dextrose 5%	30–50 mg/12 mL & 12 mg/12 mL	Hydrocortisone sodium succinate 15–25 mg/12 mL. All drugs stable for 24 hours at 25°C.
	Methotrexate	A	Elliot's B solution	30–50 mg/12 mL & 12 mg/12 mL	Hydrocortisone sodium succinate 15–25 mg/12 mL. All drugs stable for 10 hours at 25°C.

Drug	Second Drug		Solution	Concentration	Remarks
	Methotrexate	A	Lactated Ringer's	30–50 mg/12 mL & 12 mg/12 mL	Hydrocortisone sodium succinate 15–25 mg/12 mL. All drugs stable for 24 hours at 25°C.
	Methotrexate	A	Sodium chloride 0.9%	30–50 mg/12 mL & 12 mg/12 mL	Hydrocortisone sodium succinate 15–25 mg/12 mL. All drugs stable for 24 hours at 25°C.
	Vincristine	A	Dextrose 5%	0.016 mg/mL & 0.004 mg/mL	Both drugs stable for 8 hours at 25°C. No significant UV spectrum changes.
Daunorubicin	Cytarabine & etoposide	A	Dextrose 5%	25 mg & 200 mg & 300 mg	All drugs stable for 72 hours at 20°C.
	Cytarabine & etoposide	A	Sodium chloride 0.45%	25 mg & 200 mg & 300 mg	All drugs stable for 72 hours at 20°C.
	Etoposide & cytarabine	A	Dextrose 5%	25 mg & 300 mg & 200 mg	All drugs stable for 72 hours at 20°C.
	Etoposide & cytarabine	A	Sodium chloride 0.45%	25 mg & 300 mg & 200 mg	All drugs stable for 72 hours at 20°C.
	Fludarabine	Y	Dextrose 5%	2 mg/mL & 1 mg/mL	Incompatible. Slight haze forms at 4 hours at room temperature, visible in high-intensity light.
Doxorubicin	Bleomycin	Y	Not applicable	2 mg/mL & 3 units/mL	No visible precipitate after sequential injection.
	Cisplatin	Y	Not applicable	2 mg/mL & 1 mg/mL	No visible precipitate after sequential injection.
	Cyclophosphamide	Y	Not applicable	2 mg/mL & 20 mg/mL	No visible precipitate after sequential injection.
	Cyclophosphamide	A	Sodium chloride 0.9%	11.7 mg/mL & 0.67 mg/mL	Both drugs stable for 7 days at 25°C.
	Fludarabine	Y	Dextrose 5%	2 mg/mL & 1 mg/mL	Physically compatible for 4 hours at room temperature in fluorescent light.
	Fluorouracil	A	Dextrose 5%	0.01 mg/mL & 0.25 mg/mL	Incompatible. Precipitates and color changes.
	Fluorouracil	Y	Not applicable	2 mg/mL & 50 mg/mL	No visible precipitate after sequential injection.
	Methotrexate	Y	Not applicable	2 mg/mL & 25 mg/mL	No visible precipitate after sequential injection.
	Mitomycin	Y	Not applicable	2 mg/mL & 0.5 mg/mL	No visible precipitate after sequential injection.
	Vinblastine	A	Sodium chloride 0.9%	0.5–1.5 mg/mL & 0.075–0.15 mg/mL	May be stable for 10 days at 8° to 32°C; however, HPLC erratic.
	Vinblastine	Y	Not applicable	2 mg/mL & 1 mg/mL	No visible precipitate after sequential injection.
	Vincristine	A	Dextrose 2.5% & sodium chloride 0.45%	1.4 mg/mL & 0.033 mg/mL	Both drugs stable for 14 days at 25°C.
	Vincristine	A	Sodium chloride 0.9%	1.4 mg/mL & 0.033 mg/mL	Both drugs stable for 14 days at 25°C.
	Vincristine	A	Sodium chloride 0.45% & Ringer's	1.4 mg/mL & 0.033 mg/mL	Both drugs stable for 1 day and 7 days, respectively, at 25°C.
	Vincristine	Y	Not applicable	2 mg/mL & 1 mg/mL	No visible precipitate after sequential injection.
Etoposide	Cisplatin	A	Dextrose 5% & sodium chloride 0.45%	0.2 mg/mL & 0.2 mg/mL	Stable for 24 hours at 25°C.
	Cisplatin	A	Dextrose 5% & sodium chloride 0.45%	0.4 mg/mL & 0.2 mg/mL	Mannitol 1.875% & potassium chloride 0.02 mEq/mL. Stable for 24 hours at 25°C.
	Cisplatin	A	Sodium chloride 0.9%	0.2 mg/mL & 0.2 mg/mL	Both drugs stable for 15 days at room temperature when protected from light.

Table 47.3. *continued*

Part A: Oncology Product with Oncology Products

Oncology Product A	Oncology Product B	Condition[a]	Diluting Solution	Concentration of Products	Stability and Compatibility Comments
	Cisplatin	A	Sodium chloride 0.9%	0.2–0.4 mg/mL & 0.2 mg/mL	Stable for 24 hours at 25°C.
	Cisplatin	A	Sodium chloride 0.9%	0.4 mg/mL & 0.2 mg/mL	Both drugs stable for 7 days in PVC containers.
	Cisplatin	A	Sodium chloride 0.9%	0.4 mg/mL & 0.2 mg/mL	Physically compatible for 48 hours at 22°C in fluorescent light or in the dark.
	Cisplatin & cyclophosphamide	A	Sodium chloride 0.9%	0.2 mg/mL & 0.2 mg/mL & 2 mg/mL	All drugs stable for 7 days at room temperature.
	Cisplatin & floxuridine	A	Sodium chloride 0.9%	0.3 mg/mL & 0.2 mg/mL & 0.7 mg/mL	All drugs stable for 7 days at room temperature.
	Cytarabine & daunorubicin	A	Dextrose 5%	300 mg & 200 mg & 25 mg	All drugs stable for 72 hours at 20°C.
	Cytarabine & daunorubicin	A	Dextrose 5% & sodium chloride 0.45%	0.4 mg/mL & 0.267 mg/mL & 0.033 mg/mL	Physically compatible and stable for 72 hours at 20°C.
	Cytarabine & daunorubicin	A	Sodium chloride 0.45%	300 mg & 200 mg & 25 mg	All drugs stable for 72 hours at 20°C.
	Daunorubicin	A	Dextrose 5% & sodium chloride 0.45%	0.4 mg/mL & 0.033 mg/mL	Physically compatible and stable for 72 hours at 20°C.
	Daunorubicin & cytarabine	A	Dextrose 5%	300 mg & 25 mg & 200 mg	All drugs stable for 72 hours at 20°C.
	Daunorubicin & cytarabine	A	Sodium chloride 0.45%	300 mg & 25 mg & 200 mg	All drugs stable for 72 hours at 20°C.
	Fludarabine	Y	Dextrose 5%	0.4 mg/mL & 1 mg/mL	Physically compatible for 4 hours at room temperature in fluorescent light.
	Fluorouracil	A	Sodium chloride 0.9%	0.2 mg/mL & 10 mg/mL	Stable for 7 days at room temperature and for 1 day at 35°C.
	Ifosfamide	A	Sodium chloride 0.9%	0.2 mg/mL & 2 mg/mL	Stable for 7 days at room temperature.
	Ifosfamide & carboplatin	A	Sterile water	0.2 mg/mL & 2 mg/mL & 1 mg/mL	Stable for 5 days at room temperature.
	Ifosfamide & cisplatin	A	Sodium chloride 0.9%	0.2 mg/mL & 2 mg/mL & 0.2 mg/mL	Stable for 5 days at room temperature.
	Mitoxantrone	A	Sodium chloride 0.9%	0.5 mg/mL & 0.05 mg/mL	Stable for 22 hours at room temperature.
Floxuridine	Carboplatin	A	Sterile water	10 mg/mL & 1 mg/mL	Both drugs stable for 7 days at room temperature.
	Cisplatin	A	Sodium chloride 0.9%	10 mg/mL & 0.5 mg/mL	Physically compatible; however, a 13% loss of floxuridine occurs within 7 days.
	Cisplatin & etoposide	A	Sodium chloride 0.9%	0.7 mg/mL & 0.2 mg/mL & 0.3 mg/mL	All drugs stable for 7 days at room temperature.

Drug		Diluent	Concentration	Comments
Cisplatin & leucovorin	A	Sodium chloride 0.9%	0.7 mg/mL & 0.2 mg/mL & 0.14 mg/mL	All drugs stable for 7 days at room temperature.
Etoposide	A	Sodium chloride 0.9%	10 mg/mL & 0.2 mg/mL	Both drugs stable for 15 days at room temperature.
Fludarabine	Y	Dextrose 5%	3 mg/mL & 1 mg/mL	Physically compatible for 4 hours at room temperature in fluorescent light.
Fluorouracil	A	Sodium chloride 0.9%	10 mg/mL & 10 mg/mL	Both drugs stable for 15 days at room temperature.
Fluorouracil & leucovorin	A	Sodium chloride 0.9%	0.7 mg/mL & 5 mg/mL & 0.14 mg/mL	All drugs stable for 15 days at room temperature.
Leucovorin	A	Sodium chloride 0.9%	1 mg/mL & 0.03 mg/mL	Physically compatible and stable for 48 hours at 4°C and at 20°C. No loss of floxuridine and 10% loss of leucovorin within 48 hours at 40°C.
Fludarabine				
Bleomycin	Y	Dextrose 5% & sodium chloride 0.9%	1 mg/mL & 1 unit/mL	Physically compatible for 4 hours at room temperature in fluorescent light.
Carboplatin	Y	Dextrose 5%	1 mg/mL & 5 mg/mL	Physically compatible for 4 hours at room temperature in fluorescent light.
Carmustine	Y	Dextrose 5%	1 mg/mL & 15 mg/mL	Physically compatible for 4 hours at room temperature in fluorescent light.
Cisplatin	Y	Dextrose 5%	1 mg/mL & 1 mg/mL	Physically compatible for 4 hours at room temperature in fluorescent light.
Cyclophosphamide	Y	Dextrose 5%	1 mg/mL & 10 mg/mL	Physically compatible for 4 hours at room temperature in fluorescent light.
Cytarabine	Y	Dextrose 5%	1 mg/mL & 50 mg/mL	Physically compatible for 4 hours at room temperature in fluorescent light.
Dacarbazine	Y	Dextrose 5%	1 mg/mL & 4 mg/mL	Physically compatible for 4 hours at room temperature in fluorescent light.
Dactinomycin	Y	Dextrose 5%	1 mg/mL & 0.01 mg/mL	Physically compatible for 4 hours at room temperature in fluorescent light.
Daunorubicin	Y	Dextrose 5%	1 mg/mL & 2 mg/mL	Incompatible at 4 hours at room temperature in fluorescent light.
Doxorubicin	Y	Dextrose 5%	1 mg/mL & 2 mg/mL	Physically compatible for 4 hours at room temperature in fluorescent light.
Etoposide	Y	Dextrose 5%	1 mg/mL & 0.4 mg/mL	Physically compatible for 4 hours at room temperature in fluorescent light.
Floxuridine	Y	Dextrose 5%	1 mg/mL & 3 mg/mL	Physically compatible for 4 hours at room temperature in fluorescent light.
Fluorouracil	Y	Dextrose 5%	1 mg/mL & 16 mg/mL	Physically compatible for 4 hours at room temperature in fluorescent light.
Ifosfamide	Y	Dextrose 5%	1 mg/mL & 25 mg/mL	Physically compatible for 4 hours at room temperature in fluorescent light.

Table 47.3. *continued*

		Part A: Oncology Product with Oncology Products			
Oncology Product A	Oncology Product B	Condition[a]	Diluting Solution	Concentration of Products	Stability and Compatibility Comments
	Mechlorethamine	Y	Dextrose 5%	1 mg/mL & 1 mg/mL	Physically compatible for 4 hours at room temperature in fluorescent light.
	Mesna	Y	Dextrose 5%	1 mg/mL & 10 mg/mL	Physically compatible for 4 hours at room temperature in fluorescent light.
	Methotrexate	Y	Dextrose 5%	1 mg/mL & 15 mg/mL	Physically compatible for 4 hours at room temperature in fluorescent light.
	Mitoxantrone	Y	Dextrose 5%	1 mg/mL & 0.5 mg/mL	Physically compatible for 4 hours at room temperature in fluorescent light.
	Pentostatin	Y	Dextrose 5% & sodium chloride 0.9%	1 mg/mL & 0.4 mg/mL	Physically compatible for 4 hours at room temperature in fluorescent light.
	Vinblastine	Y	Dextrose 5%	1 mg/mL & 1 mg/mL	Physically compatible for 4 hours at room temperature in fluorescent light.
	Vincristine	Y	Dextrose 5%	1 mg/mL & 1 mg/mL	Physically compatible for 4 hours at room temperature in fluorescent light.
Fluorouracil	Bleomycin	A	Sodium chloride 0.9%	1 mg/mL & 0.02–0.03 units/mL	Stable for 7 days at 4°C. May adsorb onto plastic.
	Carboplatin	A	Sterile water	10 mg/mL & 1 mg/mL	Unstable. Greater than 20% loss of carboplatin within 24 hours at room temperature.
	Cisplatin	A	Sodium chloride 0.9%	1 mg/mL & 0.2 mg/mL	Unstable. Greater than 10% loss of cisplatin within 1.5 hours and 25% loss within 4 hours at 25°C in light or dark.
	Cisplatin	Y	Not applicable	50 mg/mL & 1 mg/mL	No visible precipitate after sequential injection.
	Cyclophosphamide	A	Sodium chloride 0.9%	8.3 mg/mL & 1.67 mg/mL	Both drugs stable for 15 days at room temperature.
	Cyclophosphamide	Y	Not applicable	50 mg/mL & 20 mg/mL	No visible precipitate after sequential injection.
	Cyclophosphamide & methotrexate	A	Sodium chloride 0.9%	8.3 mg/mL & 1.67 mg/mL & 0.025 mg/mL	9.3% loss of cyclophosphamide within 7 days at room temperature.
	Cytarabine	A	Dextrose 5%	0.25 mg/mL & 0.4 mg/mL	Both drugs stable for 8 hours at 25°C. No significant UV spectrum changes.
	Doxorubicin	A	Dextrose 5%	0.25 mg/mL & 0.01 mg/mL	Incompatible. Color changes to purple.
	Doxorubicin	Y	Not applicable	50 mg/mL & 2 mg/mL	No visible precipitate after sequential injection.
	Etoposide	A	Sodium chloride 0.9%	10 mg/mL & 0.2 mg/mL	Both drugs stable for 7 days at room temperature and for 1 day at 35°C.
	Floxuridine	A	Sodium chloride 0.9%	10 mg/mL & 10 mg/mL	Both drugs stable for 15 days at room temperature.

Floxuridine & leucovorin	A	Sodium chloride 0.9%	5 mg/mL & 0.7 mg/mL & 0.14 mg/mL	All drugs stable for 15 days at room temperature.
Ifosfamide	A	Sodium chloride 0.9%	10 mg/mL & 2 mg/mL	Both drugs stable for 5 days at room temperature.
Leucovorin	A	Sodium chloride 0.9%	10 mg/mL & 0.2 mg/mL	Both drugs stable for 15 days at room temperature when protected from light.
Leucovorin	Y	Not applicable	50 mg/mL & 10 mg/mL	No visible precipitate after sequential injection.
Methotrexate	A	Dextrose 5%	0.25 mg/mL & 0.2 mg/mL	Unstable. Both drugs decompose within 1 hour at 25°C. Altered UV spectrum.
Methotrexate	A	Fluorouracil (as diluent)	500 mg/10 mL & 50 mg/10 mL	Both drugs stable for 24 hours at 25°C.
Methotrexate	A	Sodium chloride 0.9%	10 mg/mL & 0.03 mg/mL	Both drugs stable for 15 days at room temperature.
Methotrexate	Y	Not applicable	50 mg/mL & 25 mg/mL	No visible precipitate after sequential injection.
Mitomycin	Y	Not applicable	50 mg/mL & 0.5 mg/mL	No visible precipitate after sequential injection.
Vinblastine	Y	Not applicable	50 mg/mL & 1 mg/mL	No visible precipitate after sequential injection.
Vincristine	A	Dextrose 5%	0.01 mg/mL & 0.004 mg/mL	Both drugs stable for 8 hours at 25°C. No UV spectrum changes.
Vincristine	Y	Not applicable	50 mg/mL & 1 mg/mL	No visible precipitate after sequential injection.
Ifosfamide				
Carboplatin	A	Sterile water	1 mg/mL & 1 mg/mL	Both drugs stable for 5 days at room temperature.
Carboplatin & etoposide	A	Sterile water	2 mg/mL & 1 mg/mL & 0.2 mg/mL	All drugs stable for 7 days at room temperature.
Cisplatin	A	Sodium chloride 0.9%	2 mg/mL & 0.2 mg/mL	Both drugs stable for 7 days at room temperature.
Cisplatin & etoposide	A	Sodium chloride 0.9%	2 mg/mL & 0.2 mg/mL & 0.2 mg/mL	All drugs stable for 5 days at room temperature.
Etoposide	A	Sodium chloride 0.9%	2 mg/mL & 0.2 mg/mL	Both drugs stable for 5 days at room temperature.
Fludarabine	Y	Dextrose 5%	25 mg/mL & 1 mg/mL	Physically compatible for 4 hours at room temperature in fluorescent light.
Fluorouracil	A	Sodium chloride 0.9%	2 mg/mL & 10 mg/mL	Both drugs stable for 5 days at room temperature.
Mesna	A	Dextrose 5%	0.6 mg/mL & 0.6 mg/mL	Both drugs stable for 24 hours at room temperature.
Mesna	A	Dextrose 5%	3.3 mg/mL & 3.3 mg/mL	Physically compatible and stable for 24 hours at 21°C in fluorescent light.
Mesna	A	Dextrose 5%	5 mg/mL & 5 mg/mL	Physically compatible and stable for 24 hours at 21°C in fluorescent light.
Mesna	A	Dextrose 5% & sodium chloride 0.45%	0.6 mg/mL & 0.6 mg/mL	Both drugs stable for 24 hours at room temperature.
Mesna	A	Lactated Ringer's	0.6 mg/mL & 0.6 mg/mL	Both drugs stable for 24 hours at room temperature.
Mesna	A	Lactated Ringer's	3.3 mg/mL & 3.3 mg/mL	Physically compatible and stable for 24 hours at 21°C in fluorescent light.

Table 47.3. *continued*

| | | | Part A: Oncology Product with Oncology Products | | |
Oncology Product A	Oncology Product B	Condition[a]	Diluting Solution	Concentration of Products	Stability and Compatibility Comments
	Mesna	A	Lactated Ringer's	5 mg/mL & 5 mg/mL	Physically compatible and stable for 24 hours at 21°C in fluorescent light.
	Mesna	A	Sodium chloride 0.9%	0.6 mg/mL & 0.5 mg/mL	Both drugs stable for 24 hours at room temperature.
	Mesna	A	Sodium chloride 0.9%	50 mg/mL & 40 mg/mL	Both drugs stable for 14 days at room temperature.
	Mesna	A	Sodium chloride 0.9%	83.3 mg/mL & 79 mg/mL	No loss of ifosfamide within 9 days at room temperature; however, a 7% loss occurs within 9 days at 37°C. Mesna not tested.
Leucovorin	Bleomycin	Y	Not applicable	10 mg/mL & 3 units/mL	No visible precipitate after sequential injection.
	Cisplatin	A	Sodium chloride 0.9%	0.14 mg/mL & 0.2 mg/mL	Both drugs stable for 15 days at room temperature when protected from light.
	Cisplatin	Y	Not applicable	10 mg/mL & 1 mg/mL	No visible precipitate after sequential injection.
	Cisplatin & floxuridine	A	Sodium chloride 0.9%	0.14 mg/mL & 0.2 mg/mL & 0.7 mg/mL	All drugs stable for 7 days at room temperature.
	Cyclophosphamide	Y	Not applicable	10 mg/mL & 20 mg/mL	No visible precipitate after sequential injection.
	Doxorubicin	Y	Not applicable	10 mg/mL & 2 mg/mL	No visible precipitate after sequential injection.
	Floxuridine	A	Sodium chloride 0.9%	0.03 mg/mL & 1 mg/mL	Physically compatible and stable for 48 hours at 4°C and 20°C. No loss of floxuridine and 10% loss of leucovorin within 48 hours at 40°C.
	Floxuridine	A	Sodium chloride 0.9%	0.2 mg/mL & 10 mg/mL	Both drugs stable for 15 days at room temperature when protected from light.
	Floxuridine	A	Sodium chloride 0.9%	0.24 mg/mL & 2 mg/mL	Physically compatible and stable for 48 hours at 4°C and at 20°C. No loss of floxuridine and 7% loss of leucovorin within 48 hours at 40°C.
	Floxuridine	A	Sodium chloride 0.9%	0.96 mg/mL & 4 mg/mL	Physically compatible and stable for 48 hours at 4°C, 20°C, and 40°C.
	Floxuridine & fluorouracil	A	Sodium chloride 0.9%	0.14 mg/mL & 0.7 mg/mL & 5 mg/mL	All drugs stable for 15 days at room temperature.
	Fluorouracil	A	Sodium chloride 0.9%	0.2 mg/mL & 10 mg/mL	Both drugs stable for 15 days at room temperature when protected from light.
	Fluorouracil	Y	Not applicable	10 mg/mL & 50 mg/mL	No visible precipitate after sequential injection.
	Methotrexate	Y	Not applicable	10 mg/mL & 25 mg/mL	No visible precipitate after sequential injection.
	Mitomycin	Y	Not applicable	10 mg/mL & 0.5 mg/mL	No visible precipitate after sequential injection.

	Vinblastine	Y	Not applicable	10 mg/mL & 1 mg/mL	No visible precipitate after sequential injection.
	Vincristine	Y	Not applicable	10 mg/mL & 1 mg/mL	No visible precipitate after sequential injection.
Mechlorethamine	Fludarabine	Y	Dextrose 5%	1 mg/mL & 1 mg/mL	Physically compatible for 4 hours at room temperature in fluorescent light.
Mesna	Carboplatin	A	Sterile water	1 mg/mL & 1 mg/mL	Unstable. Greater than 10% loss of carboplatin within 24 hours at room temperature.
	Cisplatin	A	Sodium chloride 0.9%	0.11 mg/mL & 0.067 mg/mL	Unstable. Weakly detectable cisplatin after 1 hour.
	Cisplatin	A	Sodium chloride 0.9%	3.3 mg/mL & 0.067 mg/mL	Unstable. No detectable cisplatin after 1 hour.
	Ifosfamide	A	Dextrose 5%	0.6 mg/mL & 0.6 mg/mL	Stable for 24 hours at room temperature.
	Ifosfamide	A	Dextrose 5% & lactated Ringer's	3.3 mg/mL & 5 mg/mL	Physically compatible for 24 hours at room temperature.
	Ifosfamide	A	Dextrose 5% & sodium chloride 0.9%	0.6 mg/mL & 0.6 mg/mL	Stable for 24 hours at room temperature in polyethylene containers.
	Ifosfamide	A	Lactated Ringer's	0.6 mg/mL & 0.6 mg/mL	Stable for 24 hours at room temperature.
	Ifosfamide	A	Sodium chloride 0.9%	0.6 mg/mL & 0.6 mg/mL	Stable for 24 hours at room temperature.
	Ifosfamide	A	Sodium chloride 0.9%	40 mg/mL & 50 mg/mL	Stable for 14 days at room temperature.
	Ifosfamide	A	Sodium chloride 0.9%	79 mg/mL & 83.3 mg/mL	No loss of ifosfamide within 9 days at room temperature; however, a 7% loss occurs within 9 days at 37°C. Mesna not tested.
Methotrexate	Bleomycin	A	Sodium chloride 0.9%	0.25–0.5 mg/mL & 0.02–0.03 units/mL	Unstable. Drug decomposes within 7 days at 4°C.
	Bleomycin	Y	Not applicable	25 mg/mL & 3 units/mL	No visible precipitate after sequential injection.
	Cisplatin	Y	Not applicable	25 mg/mL & 1 mg/mL	No visible precipitate after sequential injection.
	Cyclophosphamide	A	Sodium chloride 0.9%	0.025 mg/mL & 1.67 mg/mL	Less than 7% loss of cyclophosphamide within 14 days at room temperature.
	Cyclophosphamide & fluorouracil	A	Sodium chloride 0.9%	0.025 mg/mL & 1.67 mg/mL & 8.3 mg/mL	9.3% loss of cyclophosphamide within 7 days at room temperature.
	Cytarabine	A	Dextrose 5%	0.2 mg/mL & 0.4 mg/mL	Both drugs stable for 8 hours at 25°C. No UV spectrum changes.
	Cytarabine	A	Dextrose 5%	12 mg/12 mL & 30–50 mg/12 mL	Hydrocortisone sodium succinate 15–25 mg/12 mL. All drugs stable for 24 hours at 25°C.
	Cytarabine	A	Elliot's B solution	12 mg/12 mL & 30–50 mg/12 mL	Hydrocortisone sodium succinate 15–25 mg/12 mL. All drugs stable for 10 hours at 25°C.
	Cytarabine	A	Lactated Ringer's	12 mg/12 mL & 30–50 mg/12 mL	Hydrocortisone sodium succinate 15–25 mg/12 mL. All drugs stable for 24 hours at 25°C.
	Cytarabine	A	Sodium chloride 0.9%	12 mg/12 mL & 30–50 mg/12 mL	Hydrocortisone sodium succinate 15–25 mg/12 mL. All drugs stable for 24 hours at 25°C.

Table 47.3. continued

Oncology Product A	Oncology Product B	Condition[a]	Part A: Oncology Product with Oncology Products Diluting Solution	Concentration of Products	Stability and Compatibility Comments
	Doxorubicin	Y	Not applicable	25 mg/mL & 2 mg/mL	No visible precipitate after sequential injection.
	Fludarabine	Y	Dextrose 5%	15 mg/mL & 1 mg/mL	Physically compatible for 4 hours at room temperature in fluorescent light.
	Fluorouracil	A	Dextrose 5%	0.2 mg/mL & 0.25 mg/mL	Unstable. Both drugs decompose within 1 hour at 25°C. Altered UV spectrum.
	Fluorouracil	A	Fluorouracil (as diluent)	50 mg/10 mL & 500 mg/10 mL	Both drugs stable for 24 hours at 25°C.
	Fluorouracil	A	Sodium chloride 0.9%	0.03 mg/mL & 10 mg/mL	Both drugs stable for 15 days at room temperature.
	Leucovorin	Y	Not applicable	25 mg/mL & 10 mg/mL	No visible precipitate after sequential injection.
	Mitomycin	Y	Not applicable	25 mg/mL & 0.5 mg/mL	No visible precipitate after sequential injection.
	Vinblastine	Y	Not applicable	25 mg/mL & 1 mg/mL	No visible precipitate after sequential injection.
	Vincristine	A	Dextrose 5%	0.008–0.1 mg/mL & 0.004–0.01 mg/mL	Both drugs stable for 8 hours at 25°C. No UV spectrum changes.
	Vincristine	Y	Not applicable	25 mg/mL & 1 mg/mL	No visible precipitate after sequential injection.
Mitomycin	Bleomycin	A	Sodium chloride 0.9%	0.01 mg/mL & 0.02 units/mL	Unstable. 20% loss of bleomycin within 7 days at 4°C.
	Bleomycin	A	Sodium chloride 0.9%	0.01 mg/mL & 0.03 units/mL	Unstable. 20% loss of bleomycin within 7 days at 4°C.
	Bleomycin	A	Sodium chloride 0.9%	0.01–0.05 mg/mL & 0.02–0.03 units/mL	Unstable. Drug decomposes within 7 days at 4°C.
	Bleomycin	A	Sodium chloride 0.9%	0.05 mg/mL & 0.02 units/mL	Unstable. 52% loss of bleomycin within 7 days at 4°C.
	Bleomycin	A	Sodium chloride 0.9%	0.05 mg/mL & 0.03 units/mL	Unstable. 52% loss of bleomycin within 7 days at 4°C.
	Bleomycin	Y	Not applicable	0.5 mg/mL & 3 units/mL	No visible precipitate after sequential injection.
	Cisplatin	Y	Not applicable	0.5 mg/mL & 1 mg/mL	No visible precipitate after sequential injection.
	Cyclophosphamide	Y	Not applicable	0.5 mg/mL & 20 mg/mL	No visible precipitate after sequential injection.
	Doxorubicin	Y	Not applicable	0.5 mg/mL & 2 mg/mL	No visible precipitate after sequential injection.
	Fluorouracil	Y	Not applicable	0.5 mg/mL & 50 mg/mL	No visible precipitate after sequential injection.
	Leucovorin	Y	Not applicable	0.5 mg/mL & 10 mg/mL	No visible precipitate after sequential injection.
	Methotrexate	Y	Not applicable	0.5 mg/mL & 25 mg/mL	No visible precipitate after sequential injection.
	Vinblastine	Y	Not applicable	0.5 mg/mL & 1 mg/mL	No visible precipitate after sequential injection.
	Vincristine	Y	Not applicable	0.5 mg/mL & 1 mg/mL	No visible precipitate after sequential injection.

Drug		Solution	Concentration	Comments
Mitoxantrone	Y	Dextrose 5%	0.5 mg/mL & 1 mg/mL	Physically compatible for 4 hours at room temperature in fluorescent light.
Paclitaxel	Y	Dextrose 5%	1.2 mg/mL & 1 unit/mL	No precipitate or change in color or turbidity within 4 hours.
Bleomycin				
Carboplatin	Y	Dextrose 5%	1.2 mg/mL & 5 mg/mL	No visible precipitate after sequential injection.
Cisplatin	Y	Dextrose 5%	1.2 mg/mL & 1 mg/mL	No visible precipitate after sequential injection.
Cyclophosphamide	Y	Dextrose 5%	1.2 mg/mL & 10 mg/mL	No visible precipitate after sequential injection.
Cytarabine	Y	Dextrose 5%	1.2 mg/mL & 50 mg/mL	No visible precipitate after sequential injection.
Dacarbazine	Y	Dextrose 5%	1.2 mg/mL & 4 mg/mL	No precipitate or change in color or turbidity within 4 hours.
Doxorubicin	Y	Dextrose 5%	1.2 mg/mL & 2 mg/mL	No visible precipitate after sequential injection.
Etoposide	Y	Dextrose 5%	1.2 mg/mL & 0.4 mg/mL	No visible precipitate after sequential injection.
Floxuridine	Y	Dextrose 5%	1.2 mg/mL & 3 mg/mL	No precipitate or change in color or turbidity within 4 hours.
Fluorouracil	Y	Dextrose 5%	1.2 mg/mL & 16 mg/mL	No visible precipitate after sequential injection.
Ifosfamide	Y	Dextrose 5%	1.2 mg/mL & 25 mg/mL	No precipitate or change in color or turbidity within 4 hours.
Methotrexate	Y	Dextrose 5%	1.2 mg/mL & 15 mg/mL	No visible precipitate after sequential injection.
Mitoxantrone	Y	Dextrose 5%	1.2 mg/mL & 0.5 mg/mL	Incompatible. Decreased turbidity, below normal range.
Vinblastine	Y	Dextrose 5% & sodium chloride 0.9%	1.2 mg/mL & 0.12 mg/mL	No precipitate or change in color or turbidity within 4 hours.
Vincristine	Y	Dextrose 5%	1.2 mg/mL & 0.05 mg/mL	No precipitate or change in color or turbidity within 4 hours.
Sargramostim (GM-CSF)	Y	Sodium chloride 0.9%	10 µg/mL & 1 unit/mL	Physically compatible for 4 hours at 22°C in fluorescent light.
Bleomycin				
Carmustine	Y	Sodium chloride 0.9%	10 µg/mL & 1.5 mg/mL	Physically compatible for 4 hours at 22°C in fluorescent light.
Cisplatin	Y	Sodium chloride 0.9%	10 µg/mL & 1 mg/mL	Physically compatible for 4 hours at 22°C in fluorescent light.
Etoposide	Y	Sodium chloride 0.9%	10 µg/mL & 0.4 mg/mL	Physically compatible for 4 hours at 22°C in fluorescent light.
Fludarabine	Y	Sodium chloride 0.9%	10 µg/mL & 3 mg/mL	Physically compatible for 4 hours at 22°C in fluorescent light.
Fluorouracil	Y	Sodium chloride 0.9%	10 µg/mL & 16 mg/mL	Physically compatible for 4 hours at 22°C in fluorescent light.
Idarubicin	Y	Sodium chloride 0.9%	10 µg/mL & 0.5 mg/mL	Incompatible. Haze forms immediately.

Table 47.3. *continued*

Part A: Oncology Product with Oncology Products

Oncology Product A	Oncology Product B	Condition[a]	Diluting Solution	Concentration of Products	Stability and Compatibility Comments
	Ifosfamide	Y	Sodium chloride 0.9%	10 µg/mL & 25 mg/mL	Physically compatible for 4 hours at 22°C in fluorescent light.
	Mechlorethamine	Y	Sodium chloride 0.9%	10 µg/mL & 1 mg/mL	Physically compatible for 4 hours at 22°C in fluorescent light.
	Methotrexate	Y	Sodium chloride 0.9%	10 µg/mL & 15 mg/mL	Physically compatible for 4 hours at 22°C in fluorescent light.
	Mitomycin	Y	Sodium chloride 0.9%	10 µg/mL & 0.5 mg/mL	Incompatible. Haze forms within 30 minutes.
	Mitoxantrone	Y	Sodium chloride 0.9%	10 µg/mL & 0.5 mg/mL	Physically compatible for 4 hours at 22°C in fluorescent light.
	Pentostatin	Y	Sodium chloride 0.9%	10 µg/mL & 0.4 mg/mL	Physically compatible for 4 hours at 22°C in fluorescent light.
	Vinblastine	Y	Sodium chloride 0.9%	10 µg/mL & 0.12 mg/mL	Physically compatible for 4 hours at 22°C in fluorescent light.
	Vincristine	Y	Sodium chloride 0.9%	10 µg/mL & 0.05 mg/mL	Physically compatible for 4 hours at 22°C in fluorescent light.
Vinblastine	Bleomycin	A	Sodium chloride 0.9%	0.01–0.1 mg/mL & 0.02–0.03 units/mL	Stable for 7 days at 4°C. May adsorb onto plastic.
	Bleomycin	Y	Not applicable	1 mg/mL & 3 units/mL	No visible precipitate after sequential injection.
	Cisplatin	Y	Not applicable	1 mg/mL & 1 mg/mL	No visible precipitate after sequential injection.
	Cyclophosphamide	Y	Not applicable	1 mg/mL & 20 mg/mL	No visible precipitate after sequential injection.
	Doxorubicin	A	Sodium chloride 0.9%	0.075–0.15 mg/mL & 0.5–1.5 mg/mL	May be stable for 10 days at 8° to 32°C; however, HPLC erratic.
	Doxorubicin	Y	Not applicable	1 mg/mL & 2 mg/mL	No visible precipitate after sequential injection.
	Fludarabine	Y	Dextrose 5%	0.12 mg/mL & 1 mg/mL	Physically compatible for 4 hours at room temperature in fluorescent light.
	Leucovorin	Y	Not applicable	1 mg/mL & 10 mg/mL	No visible precipitate after sequential injection.
	Methotrexate	Y	Not applicable	1 mg/mL & 25 mg/mL	No visible precipitate after sequential injection.
	Mitomycin	Y	Not applicable	1 mg/mL & 0.5 mg/mL	No visible precipitate after sequential injection.
	Vincristine	Y	Not applicable	1 mg/mL & 1 mg/mL	No visible precipitate after sequential injection.
Vincristine	Bleomycin	A	Sodium chloride 0.9%	0.05–0.1 mg/mL & 0.02–0.03 units/mL	Stable for 7 days at 4°C. May adsorb onto plastic.
	Bleomycin	Y	Not applicable	1 mg/mL & 3 units/mL	No visible precipitate after sequential injection.

974

Other Product	Condition[a]	Diluting Solution	Concentration of Products	Stability and Compatibility Comments
Cisplatin	Y	Not applicable	1 mg/mL & 1 mg/mL	No visible precipitate after sequential injection.
Cyclophosphamide	Y	Not applicable	1 mg/mL & 20 mg/mL	No visible precipitate after sequential injection.
Cytarabine	A	Dextrose 5%	0.004 mg/mL & 0.016 mg/mL	Both drugs stable for 8 hours at 25°C. No significant UV spectrum changes.
Doxorubicin	A	Dextrose 2.5% & sodium chloride 0.45%	0.033 mg/mL & 1.4 mg/mL	Both drugs stable for 14 days at 25°C.
Doxorubicin	A	Sodium chloride 0.9%	0.033 mg/mL & 1.4 mg/mL	Both drugs stable for 14 days at 25°C.
Doxorubicin	A	Sodium chloride 0.45% & Ringer's	0.033 mg/mL & 1.4 mg/mL	Both drugs stable for 7 days and 1 day, respectively, at 25°C.
Doxorubicin	Y	Not applicable	1 mg/mL & 2 mg/mL	No visible precipitate after sequential injection.
Fludarabine	Y	Dextrose 5%	1 mg/mL & 1 mg/mL	Physically compatible for 4 hours at room temperature in fluorescent light.
Fluorouracil	A	Dextrose 5%	0.004 mg/mL & 0.01 mg/mL	Both drugs stable for 8 hours at 25°C. No UV spectrum changes.
Fluorouracil	Y	Not applicable	1 mg/mL & 50 mg/mL	No visible precipitate after sequential injection.
Leucovorin	Y	Not applicable	1 mg/mL & 10 mg/mL	No visible precipitate after sequential injection.
Methotrexate	A	Dextrose 5%	0.004–0.01 mg/mL & 0.008–0.1 mg/mL	Both drugs stable for 8 hours at 25°C. No UV spectrum changes.
Methotrexate	Y	Not applicable	1 mg/mL & 25 mg/mL	No visible precipitate after sequential injection.
Mitomycin	Y	Not applicable	1 mg/mL & 0.5 mg/mL	No visible precipitate after sequential injection.
Vinblastine	Y	Not applicable	1 mg/mL & 1 mg/mL	No visible precipitate after sequential injection.

Part B: Oncology Product with Other Products

Oncology Product	Other Product	Condition[a]	Diluting Solution	Concentration of Products	Stability and Compatibility Comments
Bleomycin	Amikacin sulfate	A	Sodium chloride 0.9%	0.02–0.03 units/mL & 1.25 mg/mL	Stable for 7 days at 4°C.
	Aminophylline	A	Sodium chloride 0.9%	0.02–0.03 units/mL & 0.25 mg/mL	Unstable. Drug decomposes within 7 days at 4°C.
	Ascorbic acid	A	Sodium chloride 0.9%	0.02–0.03 units/mL & 2.5–5 mg/mL	Unstable. Drug decomposes within 7 days at 4°C.
	Carbenicillin disodium	A	Sodium chloride 0.9%	0.02–0.03 units/mL & 4–12 mg/mL	Unstable. Drug decomposes within 7 days at 4°C.
	Cefazolin sodium	A	Sodium chloride 0.9%	0.02–0.03 units/mL & 1 mg/mL	Unstable. Drug decomposes within 7 days at 4°C.
	Cephalothin sodium	A	Sodium chloride 0.9%	0.02–0.03 units/mL & 2–5 mg/mL	Unstable. Drug decomposes within 7 days at 4°C.
	Cephapirin sodium	A	Sodium chloride 0.9%	0.02–0.03 units/mL & 3 mg/mL	Stable for 7 days at 4°C. May adsorb onto plastic.

Table 47.3. *continued*

Part B: Oncology Product with Other Products

Oncology Product	Other Product	Condition[a]	Diluting Solution	Concentration of Products	Stability and Compatibility Comments
	Dexamethasone sodium phosphate	A	Sodium chloride 0.9%	0.02–0.03 units/mL & 0.05 mg/mL	Stable for 7 days at 4°C. May adsorb onto plastic.
	Diazepam	A	Sodium chloride 0.9%	0.02–0.03 units/mL & 0.05–0.1 mg/mL	Incompatible.
	Diphenhydramine hydrochloride	A	Sodium chloride 0.9%	0.02–0.03 units/mL & 0.1 mg/mL	Stable for 7 days at 4°C. May adsorb onto plastic.
	Droperidol	Y	Not applicable	3 units/mL & 2.5 mg/mL	No visible precipitate after sequential injection.
	Gentamicin sulfate	A	Sodium chloride 0.9%	0.02–0.03 units/mL & 0.01–0.6 mg/mL	Stable for 7 days at 4°C. May adsorb onto plastic.
	Heparin sodium	A	Dextrose 5%	0.02–0.03 units/mL & 10–1,000 units/mL	Stable for 24 hours. May adsorb onto plastic.
	Heparin sodium	A	Sodium chloride 0.9%	0.02–0.03 units/mL & 10–200 units/mL	Stable for 7 days at 4°C. May adsorb onto plastic.
	Heparin sodium	Y	Not applicable	3 units/mL & 1000 units/mL	No visible precipitate after sequential injection.
	Hydrocortisone sodium phosphate	A	Sodium chloride 0.9%	0.02–0.03 units/mL & 0.1–2 mg/mL	Stable for 7 days at 4°C. May adsorb onto plastic.
	Hydrocortisone sodium succinate	A	Sodium chloride 0.9%	0.02–0.03 units/mL & 0.3–2.5 mg/mL	Unstable. Drug decomposes within 7 days at 4°C.
	Leucovorin calcium	Y	Not applicable	3 units/mL & 10 mg/mL	No visible precipitate after sequential injection.
	Metoclopramide hydrochloride	Y	Not applicable	3 units/mL & 5 mg/mL	No visible precipitate after sequential injection.
	Nafcillin sodium	A	Sodium chloride 0.9%	0.02–0.03 units/mL & 2.5 mg/mL	Unstable. Drug decomposes within 7 days at 4°C.
	Ondansetron hydrochloride	Y	Sodium chloride 0.9%	1 unit/mL & 1 mg/mL	Physically compatible for 4 hours at 22°C in fluorescent light.
	Penicillin G sodium	A	Sodium chloride 0.9%	0.02–0.03 units/mL & 2000–5000 units/mL	Unstable. Drug decomposes within 7 days at 4°C.
	Phenytoin sodium	A	Sodium chloride 0.9%	0.02–0.03 units/mL & 0.5 mg/mL	Stable for 7 days at 4°C. May adsorb onto plastic.
	Sargramostim	Y	Sodium chloride 0.9%	1 unit/mL & 10 μg/mL	Physically compatible for 4 hours at 22°C in fluorescent light.
	Streptomycin sulfate	A	Sodium chloride 0.9%	0.02–0.03 units/mL & 4 mg/mL	Stable for 7 days at 4°C. May adsorb onto plastic.
	Terbutaline sulfate	A	Sodium chloride 0.9%	0.02–0.03 units/mL & 0.0075 mg/mL	Unstable. Drug decomposes within 7 days at 4°C.

Drug	Additive		Solution	Concentration	Remarks
	Tobramycin sulfate	A	Sodium chloride 0.9%	0.02–0.03 units/mL & 0.5 mg/mL	Stable for 7 days at 4°C. May adsorb onto plastic.
Carboplatin	Ondansetron hydrochloride	Y	Sodium chloride 0.9%	0.18–9.9 µg/mL & 16–160 µg/mL	Physically compatible when carboplatin is administered over 10 to 60 minutes.
	Ondansetron hydrochloride	Y	Dextrose 5% & sodium chloride 0.9%	5 mg/mL & 1 mg/mL	Physically compatible when carboplatin is administered over 10 to 60 minutes.
	Sargramostim	Y	Sodium chloride 0.9%	5 mg/mL & 10 µg/mL	Physically compatible for 4 hours at 22°C in fluorescent light.
Carmustine	Ondansetron hydrochloride	Y	Dextrose 5% & sodium chloride 0.9%	1.5 mg/mL & 1 mg/mL	Physically compatible for 4 hours at 22°C in fluorescent light.
	Sargramostim	Y	Sodium chloride 0.9%	1.5 mg/mL & 10 µg/mL	Physically compatible for 4 hours at 22°C in fluorescent light.
	Sodium bicarbonate	A	Dextrose 5%	0.1 mg/mL & 0.1 mEq/mL	Unstable. Drug decomposes within 1 hour at 25°C.
	Sodium bicarbonate	A	Sodium chloride 0.9%	0.1 mg/mL & 0.1 mEq/mL	Unstable. Drug decomposes within 1 hour at 25°C.
Cisplatin	Droperidol	Y	Not applicable	2.5 mg/mL & 1 mg/mL	No visible precipitate after sequential injection.
	Furosemide	Y	Not applicable	1 mg/mL & 10 mg/mL	No visible precipitate after sequential injection.
	Heparin sodium	Y	Not applicable	1 mg/mL & 1,000 units/mL	No visible precipitate after sequential injection.
	Hydroxyzine hydrochloride	A	Sodium chloride 0.9%	0.2 mg/mL & 0.5 mg/mL	Physically compatible for 48 hours at room temperature in glass containers.
	Leucovorin calcium	A	Sodium chloride 0.9%	0.2 mg/mL & 0.14 mg/mL	Both drugs stable for 15 days at room temperature when protected from light.
	Leucovorin calcium	Y	Not applicable	1 mg/mL & 10 mg/mL	No visible precipitate after sequential injection.
	Magnesium sulfate	A	Dextrose 5% & sodium chloride 0.45%	0.05 mg/mL & 1 mg/mL	Physically compatible for 48 hours at 25°C and for 96 hours at 4°C in PVC containers.
	Magnesium sulfate	A	Dextrose 5% & sodium chloride 0.45%	0.2 mg/mL & 2 mg/mL	Physically compatible for 48 hours at 25°C and for 96 hours at 4°C in PVC containers.
	Mannitol	A	Dextrose 5% & sodium chloride 0.45%	0.05 mg/mL & 18.75 mg/mL	Physically compatible for 48 hours at 25°C and for 96 hours at 4°C in PVC containers.
	Mesna	A	Sodium chloride 0.9%	0.067 mg/mL & 0.11 mg/mL	Unstable. Weakly detectable cisplatin after 1 hour.
	Mesna	A	Sodium chloride 0.9%	0.067 mg/mL & 3.3 mg/mL	Unstable. No detectable cisplatin after 1 hour.
	Metoclopramide hydrochloride	Y	Not applicable	1 mg/mL & 5 mg/mL	No visible precipitate after sequential injection.
	Metoclopramide hydrochloride	A	See manufacturer's package insert	173 mg & 10–160 mg	Use immediately.
	Ondansetron hydrochloride	Y	Sodium chloride 0.9%	0.48 mg/mL & 16–160 µg/mL	Physically compatible when cisplatin is administered over 1 to 8 hours.

Table 47.3. *continued*

Oncology Product	Other Product	Condition[a]	Part B: Oncology Product with Other Products Diluting Solution	Concentration of Products	Stability and Compatibility Comments
	Ondansetron hydrochloride	Y	Sodium chloride 0.9%	1 mg/mL & 1 mg/mL	Physically compatible for 4 hours at 22°C in fluorescent light.
	Sargramostim	Y	Sodium chloride 0.9%	1 mg/mL & 10 µg/mL	Physically compatible for 4 hours at 22°C in fluorescent light.
Cyclophosphamide	Amikacin sulfate	Y	Dextrose 5%	20 mg/mL & 5 mg/mL	Physically compatible for 4 hours at 25°C in fluorescent light.
	Ampicillin sodium	Y	Dextrose 5%	20 mg/mL & 20 mg/mL	Physically compatible for 4 hours at 25°C in fluorescent light.
	Ampicillin sodium	Y	Sodium chloride 0.9%	20 mg/mL & 20 mg/mL	Physically compatible for 4 hours at 25°C in fluorescent light.
	Azlocillin sodium	Y	Dextrose 5%	20 mg/mL & 20 mg/mL	Physically compatible for 4 hours at 25°C in fluorescent light.
	Cefamandole nafate	Y	Dextrose 5%	20 mg/mL & 20 mg/mL	Physically compatible for 4 hours at 25°C in fluorescent light.
	Cefazolin sodium	Y	Dextrose 5%	20 mg/mL & 20 mg/mL	Physically compatible for 4 hours at 25°C in fluorescent light.
	Cefoperazone sodium	Y	Dextrose 5%	20 mg/mL & 20 mg/mL	Physically compatible for 4 hours at 25°C in fluorescent light.
	Ceforanide	Y	Dextrose 5%	20 mg/mL & 20 mg/mL	Physically compatible for 4 hours at 25°C in fluorescent light.
	Cefotaxime sodium	Y	Dextrose 5%	20 mg/mL & 20 mg/mL	Physically compatible for 4 hours at 25°C in fluorescent light.
	Cefoxitin sodium	Y	Dextrose 5%	20 mg/mL & 20 mg/mL	Physically compatible for 4 hours at 25°C in fluorescent light.
	Cefuroxime sodium	Y	Dextrose 5%	20 mg/mL & 30 mg/mL	Physically compatible for 4 hours at 25°C in fluorescent light.
	Cephalothin sodium	Y	Dextrose 5%	20 mg/mL & 20 mg/mL	Physically compatible for 4 hours at 25°C in fluorescent light.
	Cephapirin sodium	Y	Dextrose 5%	20 mg/mL & 20 mg/mL	Physically compatible for 4 hours at 25°C in fluorescent light.
	Chloramphenicol sodium succinate	Y	Dextrose 5%	20 mg/mL & 20 mg/mL	Physically compatible for 4 hours at 25°C in fluorescent light.
	Clindamycin phosphate	Y	Dextrose 5%	20 mg/mL & 12 mg/mL	Physically compatible for 4 hours at 25°C in fluorescent light.

Doxycycline hyclate	Y	Dextrose 5%	20 mg/mL & 1 mg/mL	Physically compatible for 4 hours at 25°C in fluorescent light.
Droperidol	Y	Not applicable	20 mg/mL & 2.5 mg/mL	No visible precipitate after sequential injection.
Erythromycin lactobionate	Y	Dextrose 5%	20 mg/mL & 5 mg/mL	Physically compatible for 4 hours at 25°C in fluorescent light.
Furosemide	Y	Not applicable	20 mg/mL & 10 mg/mL	No visible precipitate after sequential injection.
Gentamicin sulfate	Y	Dextrose 5%	20 mg/mL & 16 mg/mL	Physically compatible for 4 hours at 25°C in fluorescent light.
Heparin sodium	Y	Not applicable	20 mg/mL & 1000 units/mL	No visible precipitate after sequential injection.
Hydroxyzine hydrochloride	A	Dextrose 5%	1 mg/mL & 0.5 mg/mL	Physically compatible for 48 hours.
Kanamycin sulfate	Y	Dextrose 5%	20 mg/mL & 2.5 mg/mL	Physically compatible for 4 hours at 25°C in fluorescent light.
Leucovorin sodium	Y	Not applicable	20 mg/mL & 10 mg/mL	No visible precipitate after sequential injection.
Metoclopramide hydrochloride	Y	Not applicable	20 mg/mL & 5 mg/mL	No visible precipitate after sequential injection.
Metoclopramide hydrochloride	A	See manufacturer's package insert	560 mg & 10–160 mg	Physically compatible for 24 hours at 25°C.
Metronidazole	Y	Dextrose 5%	20 mg/mL & 5 mg/mL	Physically compatible for 4 hours at 25°C in fluorescent light.
Mezlocillin sodium	Y	Dextrose 5%	20 mg/mL & 80 mg/mL	Physically compatible for 4 hours at 25°C in fluorescent light.
Minocycline hydrochloride	Y	Dextrose 5%	20 mg/mL & 0.2 mg/mL	Physically compatible for 4 hours at 25°C in fluorescent light.
Moxalactam	Y	Dextrose 5%	20 mg/mL & 20 mg/mL	Physically compatible for 4 hours at 25°C in fluorescent light.
Nafcillin sodium	Y	Dextrose 5%	20 mg/mL & 20 mg/mL	Physically compatible for 4 hours at 25°C in fluorescent light.
Ondansetron hydrochloride	Y	Dextrose 5% & sodium chloride 0.9%	10 mg/mL & 1 mg/mL	Physically compatible for 4 hours at 25°C in fluorescent light.
Ondansetron hydrochloride	Y	Not applicable	20 mg/mL & 16–160 µg/mL	Physically compatible with cyclophosphamide as a 5-minute bolus.
Oxacillin sodium	Y	Dextrose 5%	20 mg/mL & 20 mg/mL	Physically compatible for 4 hours at 25°C in fluorescent light.
Penicillin G potassium	Y	Dextrose 5%	20 mg/mL & 100,000 units/mL	Physically compatible for 4 hours at 25°C in fluorescent light.
Piperacillin sodium	Y	Dextrose 5%	20 mg/mL & 60 mg/mL	Physically compatible for 4 hours at 25°C in fluorescent light.
Sargramostim	Y	Sodium chloride 0.9%	10 mg/mL & 10 µg/mL	Physically compatible for 4 hours at 22°C in fluorescent light.
Tetracycline hydrochloride	Y	Dextrose 5%	20 mg/mL & 2.5 mg/mL	Physically compatible for 4 hours at 25°C in fluorescent light.

Table 47.3. *continued*

Oncology Product	Other Product	Condition[a]	Diluting Solution	Concentration of Products	Stability and Compatibility Comments
				Part B: Oncology Product with Other Products	
	Ticarcillin disodium	Y	Dextrose 5%	20 mg/mL & 30 mg/mL	Physically compatible for 4 hours at 25°C in fluorescent light.
	Tobramycin sulfate	Y	Dextrose 5%	20 mg/mL & 0.8 mg/mL	Physically compatible for 4 hours at 25°C in fluorescent light.
	Trimethoprim/sulfamethoxazole	Y	Dextrose 5%	20 mg/mL & 0.8/4 mg/mL	Physically compatible for 4 hours at 25°C in fluorescent light.
	Vancomycin hydrochloride	Y	Dextrose 5%	20 mg/mL & 5 mg/mL	Physically compatible for 4 hours at 25°C in fluorescent light.
Cytarabine	Carbenicillin disodium	A	Dextrose5%	0.1 mg/mL & 0.6 mg/mL	Incompatible. Outside the pH range for carbenicillin.
	Cephalothin sodium	A	Dextrose 5%	0.8 mg/mL & 1 mg/mL	Both drugs stable for 8 hours at 25°C.
	Gentamicin sulfate	A	Dextrose 5%	0.1 mg/mL & 0.08 mg/mL	Physically compatible for 24 hours.
	Gentamicin sulfate	A	Dextrose 5%	0.3 mg/mL & 0.24 mg/mL	Incompatible.
	Heparin sodium	A	Dextrose 5% & sodium chloride 0.9%	0.5 mg/mL & 10–20 units/mL	Incompatible. Haze forms.
	Hydrocortisone sodium succinate	A	Dextrose 5% & sodium chloride 0.9%	0.36 mg/mL & 0.5 mg/mL	Physically compatible for 40 hours.
	Hydrocortisone sodium succinate	A	Ringer's	0.36 mg/mL & 0.5 mg/mL	Incompatible.
	Hydroxyzine hydrochloride	A	Dextrose 5%	1 mg/mL & 0.5 mg/mL	Physically compatible at 48 hours in glass containers.
	Insulin, regular	A	Dextrose 5%	0.1 mg/mL & 40 units/L	Incompatible. Fine precipitate.
	Insulin, regular	A	Dextrose 5%	0.5 mg/mL & 40 units/L	Incompatible. Fine precipitate.
	Methylprednisolone sodium succinate	A	Dextrose 5% & sodium chloride 0.9%	0.36 mg/mL & 0.25 mg/mL	Physically compatible for 24 hours.
	Methylprednisolone sodium succinate	A	Dextrose 10% & sodium chloride 0.9%	0.36 mg/mL & 0.25 mg/mL	Physically compatible for 24 hours.
	Methylprednisolone sodium succinate	A	Sodium chloride 0.9%	0.36 mg/mL & 0.25 mg/mL	Physically compatible for 24 hours.
	Methylprednisolone sodium succinate	A	Sodium lactate ⅙ molar	0.36 mg/mL & 0.25 mg/mL	Incompatible.
	Methylprednisolone sodium succinate	A	Ringer's	0.36 mg/mL & 0.25 mg/mL	Incompatible.
	Metoclopramide hydrochloride	A	See manufacturer's package inserts	50–500 mg & 10–160 mg	Physically compatible for 48 hours at 25°C.

980

Nafcillin sodium	A	Dextrose 5%	0.1 mg/mL & 4 mg/mL	Incompatible. Precipitates.
Ondansetron hydrochloride	Y	Sodium chloride 0.9%	50 mg/mL & 1 mg/mL	Physically compatible for 4 hours at 22°C in fluorescent light.
Oxacillin sodium	A	Dextrose 5%	0.1 mg/mL & 2 mg/mL	Incompatible. Outside the pH range for oxacillin.
Penicillin G sodium	A	Dextrose 5%	0.2 mg/mL & 2 MU/L	Incompatible. Outside the pH range for penicillin G sodium.
Potassium chloride	A	Dextrose 5% & sodium chloride 0.9%	0.17 mg/mL & 80 mEq/L	Physically compatible for 24 hours.
Potassium chloride	A	Dextrose 5% & sodium chloride 0.9%	2 mg/mL & 100 mEq/L	Physically compatible and stable for 8 days.
Prednisolone sodium phosphate	A	Dextrose 5%	0.4 mg/mL & 0.2 mg/mL	Both drugs stable for 8 hours at 25°C.
Sargramostim	Y	Sodium chloride 0.9%	50 mg/mL & 10 µg/mL	Physically compatible for 4 hours at 22°C in fluorescent light.
Sodium bicarbonate	A	Dextrose 5%	0.2–1 mg/mL & 0.05 mEq/mL	Stable for 7 days at 8°C and at 22°C in glass or PVC containers.
Sodium bicarbonate	A	Dextrose 5% & sodium chloride 0.225%	0.2–1 mg/mL & 0.05 mEq/mL	Stable for 7 days at 8°C and at 22°C in glass or PVC containers.
Dacarbazine				
Heparin sodium	A	Sodium chloride 0.9%	10 mg/mL & 100 units/mL	Incompatible. Precipitates in IV line.
Hydrocortisone sodium phosphate	A	Not stated	Not stated	Physically compatible.
Hydrocortisone sodium phosphate	A	Not stated	Not stated	Incompatible. Precipitates.
Lidocaine hydrochloride	A	Not stated	Not stated & 1% or 2%	Physically compatible.
Metoclopramide hydrochloride	A	See manufacturer's package inserts	140 mg & 10–160 mg	Physically compatible for 8 hours at 25°C.
Ondansetron hydrochloride	Y	Dextrose 5% & sodium chloride 0.9%	4 mg/mL & 1 mg/mL	Physically compatible for 4 hours at 22°C in fluorescent light.
Sargramostim	Y	Sodium chloride 0.9%	4 mg/mL & 10 µg/mL	Physically compatible for 4 hours at 22°C in fluorescent light.
Dactinomycin				
Ondansetron hydrochloride	Y	Dextrose 5% & sodium chloride 0.9%	0.01 mg/mL & 1 mg/mL	Physically compatible for 4 hours at 22°C in fluorescent light.
Sargramostim	Y	Sodium chloride 0.9%	0.01 mg/mL & 10 µg/mL	Physically compatible for 4 hours at 22°C in fluorescent light.
Daunorubicin				
Dexamethasone sodium phosphate	A	Not stated	Not stated	Incompatible. Precipitates.
Heparin sodium	A	Dextrose 5%	0.2 mg/mL & 4 units/mL	Incompatible.
Hydrocortisone sodium succinate	A	Dextrose 5%	0.2 mg/mL & 0.5 mg/mL	Physically compatible.
Ondansetron hydrochloride	Y	Dextrose 5% & sodium chloride 0.9%	2 mg/mL & 1 mg/mL	Physically compatible for 4 hours at 22°C in fluorescent light.

Table 47.3. continued

Oncology Product	Other Product	Condition[a]	Diluting Solution	Concentration of Products	Stability and Compatibility Comments
			Part B: Oncology Product with Other Products		
Doxorubicin	Aminophylline	A	Not stated	Not stated	Incompatible. Color change.
	Cephalothin sodium	A	Not stated	Not stated	Incompatible. Precipitates.
	Dexamethasone sodium phosphate	A	Not stated	Not stated	Incompatible. Precipitates.
	Diazepam	A	Not stated	Not stated	Incompatible. Precipitates.
	Droperidol	Y	Not applicable	2 mg/mL & 2.5 mg/mL	No visible precipitate after sequential injection.
	Furosemide	A	See manufacturer's package inserts	2 mg/mL & 10 mg/mL	Incompatible. Precipitates.
	Heparin sodium	A	See manufacturer's package inserts	2 mg/mL & 1000 units/mL	Incompatible. Precipitates.
	Hydrocortisone sodium succinate	A	Not stated	Not stated	Incompatible. Precipitates.
	Leucovorin calcium	Y	Not applicable	2 mg/mL & 10 mg/mL	No visible precipitate after sequential injection.
	Metoclopramide hydrochloride	A	See manufacturer's package inserts	103.8 mg & 10–160 mg	Physically compatible for 24 hours at 25°C.
	Ondansetron hydrochloride	Y	Sodium chloride 0.9%	2 mg/mL & 1 mg/mL	Physically compatible for 4 hours at 22°C in fluorescent light.
	Sargramostim	Y	Sodium chloride 0.9%	2 mg/mL & 10 µg/mL	Physically compatible for 4 hours at 22°C in fluorescent light.
Etoposide	Hydroxyzine hydrochloride	A	Dextrose 5%	1 mg/mL & 0.5 mg/mL	Physically compatible for 48 hours.
	Metoclopramide hydrochloride	A	See manufacturer's package inserts	86.5 mg & 10–160 mg	Physically compatible for 48 hours at 25°C.
	Morphine sulfate	A	Not stated	Not stated & 50 mg/mL	Stable for 24 hours.
	Ondansetron hydrochloride	Y	Dextrose 5% & sodium chloride 0.9%	0.4 mg/mL & 1 mg/mL	Physically compatible for 4 hours at 22°C in fluorescent light.
	Potassium chloride	A	Sodium chloride 0.9%	0.2–0.4 mg/mL & 0.04 mEq/mL	Physically compatible for 8 hours.
	Potassium chloride	A	Dextrose 5%	0.2–0.4 mg/mL & 0.04 mEq/mL	Physically compatible for 8 hours.
	Potassium chloride	A	Lactated Ringer's	0.2–0.4 mg/mL & 0.04 mEq/mL	Physically compatible for 8 hours.
	Potassium chloride	A	Mannitol 10%	0.2–0.4 mg/mL & 0.04 mEq/mL	Physically compatible for 8 hours.

Drug			Solution	Concentration	
	Sargramostim	Y	Sodium chloride 0.9%	0.4 mg/mL & 10 µg/mL	Physically compatible for 4 hours at room temperature in fluorescent light.
Floxuridine	Heparin sodium	A	Sodium chloride 0.9%	2.5–12 mg/mL & 200 units/mL	Stable for 4 days at 37°C.
	Ondansetron hydrochloride	Y	Dextrose 5% & sodium chloride 0.9%	3 mg/mL & 1 mg/mL	Physically compatible for 4 hours at 22°C in fluorescent light.
Fludarabine	Acyclovir sodium	Y	Dextrose 5%	1 mg/mL & 7 mg/mL	Physically incompatible at 4 hours. Darker color visible.
	Amikacin sulfate	Y	Dextrose 5%	1 mg/mL & 5 mg/mL	Physically compatible for 4 hours at room temperature in fluorescent light.
	Aminophylline	Y	Dextrose 5%	1 mg/mL & 2.5 mg/mL	Physically compatible for 4 hours at room temperature in fluorescent light.
	Amphotericin B	Y	Dextrose 5%	1 mg/mL & 0.6 mg/mL	Incompatible. Small amount of precipitate forms within 4 hours at room temperature in fluorescent light.
	Ampicillin sodium	Y	Dextrose 5% & sodium chloride 0.9%	1 mg/mL & 20 mg/mL	Physically compatible for 4 hours at room temperature in fluorescent light.
	Ampicillin sodium/sulbactam sodium	Y	Dextrose 5% & sodium chloride 0.9%	1 mg/mL & 20/10 mg/mL	Physically compatible for 4 hours at room temperature in fluorescent light.
	Aztreonam	Y	Dextrose 5%	1 mg/mL & 40 mg/mL	Physically compatible for 4 hours at room temperature in fluorescent light.
	Butorphanol tartrate	Y	Dextrose 5%	1 mg/mL & 0.04 mg/mL	Physically compatible for 4 hours at room temperature in fluorescent light.
	Cefazolin sodium	Y	Dextrose 5%	1 mg/mL & 20 mg/mL	Physically compatible for 4 hours at room temperature in fluorescent light.
	Cefoperazone sodium	Y	Dextrose 5%	1 mg/mL & 40 mg/mL	Physically compatible for 4 hours at room temperature in fluorescent light.
	Ceforanide	Y	Dextrose 5%	1 mg/mL & 20 mg/mL	Physically compatible for 4 hours at room temperature in fluorescent light.
	Cefotaxime sodium	Y	Dextrose 5%	1 mg/mL & 20 mg/mL	Physically compatible for 4 hours at room temperature in fluorescent light.
	Cefotetan disodium	Y	Dextrose 5%	1 mg/mL & 20 mg/mL	Physically compatible for 4 hours at room temperature in fluorescent light.
	Ceftazidime	Y	Dextrose 5%	1 mg/mL & 40 mg/mL	Physically compatible for 4 hours at room temperature in fluorescent light.
	Ceftizoxime sodium	Y	Dextrose 5%	1 mg/mL & 20 mg/mL	Physically compatible for 4 hours at room temperature in fluorescent light.

983

Table 47.3. *continued*

Oncology Product	Other Product	Condition[a]	Diluting Solution	Concentration of Products	Stability and Compatibility Comments
				Part B: Oncology Product with Other Products	
	Ceftriaxone sodium	Y	Dextrose 5%	1 mg/mL & 20 mg/mL	Physically compatible for 4 hours at room temperature in fluorescent light.
	Cefuroxime sodium	Y	Dextrose 5%	1 mg/mL & 30 mg/mL	Physically compatible for 4 hours at room temperature in fluorescent light.
	Chlorpromazine hydrochloride	Y	Dextrose 5%	1 mg/mL & 2 mg/mL	Incompatible. Haze forms within 30 minutes at room temperature in fluorescent light.
	Cimetidine hydrochloride	Y	Dextrose 5%	1 mg/mL & 12 mg/mL	Physically compatible for 4 hours at room temperature in fluorescent light.
	Clindamycin phosphate	Y	Dextrose 5%	1 mg/mL & 10 mg/mL	Physically compatible for 4 hours at room temperature in fluorescent light.
	Dexamethasone sodium phosphate	Y	Dextrose 5%	1 mg/mL & 1 mg/mL	Physically compatible for 4 hours at room temperature in fluorescent light.
	Diphenhydramine hydrochloride	Y	Dextrose 5%	1 mg/mL & 2 mg/mL	Physically compatible for 4 hours at room temperature in fluorescent light.
	Doxycycline hyclate	Y	Dextrose 5%	1 mg/mL & 1 mg/mL	Physically compatible for 4 hours at room temperature in fluorescent light.
	Droperidol	Y	Dextrose 5%	1 mg/mL & 0.4 mg/mL	Physically compatible for 4 hours at room temperature in fluorescent light.
	Famotidine	Y	Dextrose 5%	1 mg/mL & 2 mg/mL	Physically compatible for 4 hours at room temperature in fluorescent light.
	Fluconazole	Y	Dextrose 5%	1 mg/mL & 2 mg/mL	Physically compatible for 4 hours at room temperature in fluorescent light.
	Furosemide	Y	Dextrose 5%	1 mg/mL & 3 mg/mL	Physically compatible for 4 hours at room temperature in fluorescent light.
	Ganciclovir sodium	Y	Dextrose 5%	1 mg/mL & 20 mg/mL	Incompatible. Dark color forms within 4 hours at room temperature in fluorescent light.
	Haloperidol lactate	Y	Dextrose 5%	1 mg/mL & 0.2 mg/mL	Physically compatible for 4 hours at room temperature in fluorescent light.
	Heparin sodium	Y	Dextrose 5%	1 mg/mL & 40 units/mL	Physically compatible for 4 hours at room temperature in fluorescent light.
	Heparin sodium	Y	Dextrose 5%	1 mg/mL & 100 units/mL	Physically compatible for 4 hours at room temperature in fluorescent light.
	Heparin sodium	Y	Dextrose 5%	1 mg/mL & 1000 units/mL	Physically compatible for 4 hours at room temperature in fluorescent light.

Drug		Solution	Concentration	Comments
Sargramostim	Y	Sodium chloride 0.9%	3 mg/mL & 10 µg/mL	Physically compatible for 4 hours at 22°C in fluorescent light.
Zidovudine	Y	Dextrose 5%	1 mg/mL & 4 mg/mL	Physically compatible for 4 hours at room temperature in fluorescent light.
Fluorouracil				
Cephalothin sodium	A	Dextrose 5%	0.5 mg/mL & 1 mg/mL	Both drugs stable for 8 hours at 25°C. No UV spectrum changes.
Diazepam	A	Not stated	Not stated	Incompatible. Precipitates.
Droperidol	A	See manufacturer's package inserts	50 mg/mL & 2.5 mg/mL	Incompatible. Precipitates.
Droperidol	Y	Not applicable	50 mg/mL & 25 mg/mL	Incompatible. Precipitates immediately.
Furosemide	Y	Not applicable	50 mg/mL & 10 mg/mL	No visible precipitate after sequential injection.
Heparin sodium	Y	Not applicable	50 mg/mL & 1000 units/mL	No visible precipitate after sequential injection.
Hydrocortisone sodium succinate	Y	Lactated Ringer's	50 mg/mL & 10 mg/mL	Physically compatible for 4 hours at room temperature.
Leucovorin calcium	A	Sodium chloride 0.9%	10 mg/mL & 0.2 mg/mL	Stable for 15 days at room temperature when protected from light.
Mannitol	Y	Dextrose 5% & sodium chloride 0.45%	1 mg/mL & 200 mg/mL	No precipitate or color change after 24 hours.
Mannitol	Y	Dextrose 5% & sodium chloride 0.9%	1 mg/mL & 200 mg/mL	No precipitate or color change after 24 hours.
Mannitol	Y	Dextrose 5% & sodium chloride 0.45%	2 mg/mL & 200 mg/mL	No precipitate or color change after 24 hours.
Mannitol	Y	Dextrose 5% & sodium chloride 0.9%	2 mg/mL & 200 mg/mL	No precipitate or color change after 24 hours.
Metoclopramide hydrochloride	Y	Not applicable	50 mg/mL & 5 mg/mL	No visible precipitate after sequential injection.
Metoclopramide hydrochloride	A	See manufacturer's package inserts	840 mg & 10–160 mg	Incompatible.
Ondansetron hydrochloride	Y	Not applicable	<0.8 mg/mL & 16–160 µg/mL	Physically compatible when fluorouracil is administered at 20 mL/hour.
Ondansetron hydrochloride	Y	Dextrose 5% & sodium chloride 0.9%	16 mg/mL & 1 mg/mL	Incompatible. Precipitates immediately.
Potassium chloride	Y	Sodium chloride 0.9%	50 mg/mL & 40 mEq/L	Physically compatible for 4 hours at room temperature.
Prednisolone sodium phosphate	A	Dextrose 5%	0.25 mg/mL & 0.2 mg/mL	Both drugs stable for 8 hours at 25°C. No UV spectrum changes.
Sargramostim	Y	Sodium chloride 0.9%	16 mg/mL & 10 µg/mL	Physically compatible for 4 hours at 22°C in fluorescent light.
Vitamin B complex with vitamin C	Y	Sodium chloride 0.9%	50 mg/mL & 2 mg/mL	Physically compatible for 4 hours at room temperature.

Table 47.3. *continued*

| | | | | Part B: Oncology Product with Other Products | |
Oncology Product	Other Product	Condition[a]	Diluting Solution	Concentration of Products	Stability and Compatibility Comments
Idarubicin	Heparin sodium	A	Not stated	Not stated	Incompatible. Precipitates immediately.
	Sargramostim	Y	Sodium chloride 0.9%	0.5 mg/mL & 10 µg/mL	Incompatible. Haze forms immediately.
Ifosfamide	Ondansetron hydrochloride	Y	Dextrose 5% & Sodium chloride 0.9%	25 mg/mL & 1 mg/mL	Physically compatible for 4 hours at 22°C in fluorescent light.
	Sargramostim	Y	Sodium chloride 0.9%	25 mg/mL & 10 µg/mL	Physically compatible for 4 hours at 22°C in fluorescent light.
Leucovorin	Droperidol	Y	Not applicable	10 mg/mL & 2.5 mg/mL	Incompatible. Precipitates immediately.
	Fluconazole	Y	Not applicable	10 mg/mL & 2 mg/mL	Physically compatible for 24 hours at room temperature in fluorescent light.
	Foscarnet sodium	Y	Not applicable	10 mg/mL & 24 mg/mL	Incompatible. Cloudy yellow solution.
	Furosemide	Y	Not applicable	10 mg/mL & 10 mg/mL	No visible precipitate after sequential injection.
	Heparin sodium	Y	Not applicable	10 mg/mL & 1000 units/mL	No visible precipitate after sequential injection.
	Metoclopramide hydrochloride	Y	Not applicable	10 mg/mL & 5 units/mL	No visible precipitate after sequential injection.
Mechlorethamine	Methohexital sodium	A	Dextrose 5%	0.04 mg/mL & 2 mg/mL	Unstable. Drug decomposes within 3 hours.
	Methohexital sodium	A	Sodium chloride 0.9%	0.04 mg/mL & 2 mg/mL	Unstable. Drug decomposes within 3 hours.
	Ondansetron hydrochloride	Y	Sodium chloride 0.9%	1 mg/mL & 1 mg/mL	Physically compatible for 4 hours at 22°C in fluorescent light.
	Sargramostim	Y	Sodium chloride 0.9%	1 mg/mL & 10 µg/mL	Physically compatible for 4 hours at 22°C in fluorescent light.
Mesna	Hydroxyzine hydrochloride	A	Dextrose 5%	3 mg/mL & 0.5 mg/mL	Physically compatible for 48 hours.
	Ondansetron hydrochloride	Y	Dextrose 5% & sodium chloride 0.9%	10 mg/mL & 1 mg/mL	Physically compatible for 4 hours at 22°C in fluorescent light.
	Sargramostim	Y	Sodium chloride 0.9%	10 mg/mL & 10 µg/mL	Physically compatible for 4 hours at 22°C in fluorescent light.
Methotrexate	Cephalothin sodium	A	Dextrose 5%	0.4 mg/mL & 1 mg/mL	Both drugs stable for 8 hours at 25°C. No UV spectrum changes.
	Droperidol	A	See manufacturer's package inserts	25 mg/mL & 2.5 mg/mL	Incompatible. Precipitates.
	Furosemide	Y	Not applicable	25 mg/mL & 10 mg/mL	No visible precipitate after sequential injection.

Drug		Solution	Concentration	Remarks
	Heparin sodium	Y	Not applicable	25 mg/mL & 1000 units/mL	No visible precipitate after sequential injection.
	Hydroxyzine hydrochloride	A	Dextrose 5%	1 mg/mL & 0.5 mg/mL	Physically compatible at 48 hours.
	Hydroxyzine hydrochloride	A	Dextrose 5%	3 mg/mL & 0.5 mg/mL	Physically compatible at 48 hours.
	Leucovorin calcium	Y	Not applicable	25 mg/mL & 10 mg/mL	No visible precipitate after sequential injection.
	Metoclopramide hydrochloride	Y	Not applicable	25 mg/mL & 5 mg/mL	No visible precipitate after sequential injection.
	Metoclopramide hydrochloride	A	See manufacturer's package inserts	50–200 mg & 10–160 mg	Use immediately.
	Ondansetron hydrochloride	Y	Dextrose 5% & sodium chloride 0.9%	15 mg/mL & 1 mg/mL	Physically compatible for 4 hours at 22°C in fluorescent light.
	Prednisolone sodium phosphate	A	Dextrose 5%	0.2 mg/mL & 0.2 mg/mL	Unstable. Both drugs decompose within 1 hour at 25°C. UV spectrum changes.
	Sargramostim	Y	Sodium chloride 0.9%	15 mg/mL & 10 µg/mL	Physically compatible for 4 hours at 22°C in fluorescent light.
	Sodium bicarbonate	A	Dextrose 5%	0.75 mg/mL & 0.05 mEq/mL	Stable for 7 days at 5°C and for 72 hours at 25°C when exposed to light.
	Vancomycin hydrochloride	Y	Not applicable	Not stated & 0.51 mg/mL	Physically compatible for 1 hour during simultaneous infusion.
Mitomycin	Droperidol	Y	Not applicable	0.5 mg/mL & 2.5 mg/mL	No visible precipitate after sequential injection.
	Furosemide	Y	Not applicable	0.5 mg/mL & 10 mg/mL	No visible precipitate after sequential injection.
	Heparin sodium	Y	Not applicable	0.5 mg/mL & 1000 units/mL	No visible precipitate after sequential injection.
	Heparin sodium	A	Sodium chloride 0.9%	5–15 mg/30 mL & 1000–10,000 units/30 mL	Stable for 48 hours at 25°C.
	Leucovorin calcium	Y	Not applicable	0.5 mg/mL & 10 mg/mL	No visible precipitate after sequential injection.
	Ondansetron hydrochloride	Y	Sodium chloride 0.9%	0.5 mg/mL & 1 mg/mL	Physically compatible for 4 hours at 22°C in fluorescent light.
	Sargramostim	Y	Sodium chloride 0.9%	0.5 mg/mL & 10 µg/mL	Incompatible. Slight haze forms in 30 minutes.
Mitoxantrone	Hydrocortisone sodium phosphate	A	Dextrose 5%	0.05–0.2 mg/mL & 0.1–2 mg/mL	Incompatible. Blue precipitate forms in PVC containers.
	Hydrocortisone sodium phosphate	A	Dextrose 5%	0.05–0.2 mg/mL & 0.1–2 mg/mL	Physically compatible in glass containers.
	Hydrocortisone sodium phosphate	A	Sodium chloride 0.9%	0.05–0.2 mg/mL & 0.1–2 mg/mL	Physically compatible and stable for 24 hours at room temperature.
	Ondansetron hydrochloride	Y	Dextrose 5% & sodium chloride 0.9%	0.5 mg/mL & 1 mg/mL	Physically compatible for 4 hours at 22°C in fluorescent light.
	Sargramostim	Y	Sodium chloride 0.9%	0.5 mg/mL & 10 µg/mL	Physically compatible for 4 hours at 22°C in fluorescent light.

Table 47.3. *continued*

Oncology Product	Other Product	Condition[a]	Part B: Oncology Product with Other Products Diluting Solution	Concentration of Products	Stability and Compatibility Comments
Paclitaxel	Acyclovir sodium	Y	Dextrose 5%	1.2 mg/mL & 7 mg/mL	No precipitate or change in color or turbidity within 4 hours.
	Amikacin sulfate	Y	Dextrose 5%	1.2 mg/mL & 5 mg/mL	No precipitate or change in color or turbidity within 4 hours.
	Aminophylline	Y	Dextrose 5%	1.2 mg/mL & 2.5 mg/mL	No precipitate or change in color or turbidity within 4 hours.
	Amphotericin B	Y	Dextrose 5%	1.2 mg/mL & 0.6 mg/mL	Incompatible. Increased turbidity immediately.
	Ampicillin sodium/sulbactam sodium	Y	Dextrose 5% & sodium chloride 0.9%	1.2 mg/mL & 20/10 mg/mL	No precipitate or change in color or turbidity within 4 hours.
	Butorphanol tartrate	Y	Dextrose 5%	1.2 mg/mL & 0.04 mg/mL	No precipitate or change in color or turbidity within 4 hours.
	Calcium chloride	Y	Dextrose 5%	1.2 mg/mL & 20 mg/mL	No precipitate or change in color or turbidity within 4 hours.
	Ceforanide	Y	Dextrose 5%	1.2 mg/mL & 20 mg/mL	No precipitate or change in color or turbidity within 4 hours.
	Cefotetan disodium	Y	Dextrose 5%	1.2 mg/mL & 20 mg/mL	No precipitate or change in color or turbidity within 4 hours.
	Ceftazidime	Y	Dextrose 5%	1.2 mg/mL & 40 mg/mL	No precipitate or change in color or turbidity within 4 hours.
	Ceftriaxone sodium	Y	Dextrose 5%	1.2 mg/mL & 20 mg/mL	No precipitate or change in color or turbidity within 4 hours.
	Chlorpromazine hydrochloride	Y	Dextrose 5%	1.2 mg/mL & 2 mg/mL	Incompatible. Decreased turbidity, below normal range.
	Cimetidine hydrochloride	Y	Dextrose 5%	1.2 mg/mL & 12 mg/mL	No precipitate, color change, or gas production within 4 hours.
	Dexamethasone sodium phosphate	Y	Dextrose 5%	1.2 mg/mL & 1 mg/mL	No precipitate, color change, or gas production within 4 hours.
	Diphenhydramine hydrochloride	Y	Dextrose 5%	1.2 mg/mL & 2 mg/mL	No precipitate, color change, or gas production within 4 hours.
	Droperidol	Y	Dextrose 5%	1.2 mg/mL & 0.4 mg/mL	No precipitate or change in color or turbidity within 4 hours.
	Famotidine	Y	Dextrose 5%	1.2 mg/mL & 2 mg/mL	No precipitate or change in color or turbidity within 4 hours.
	Fluconazole	Y	Dextrose 5%	1.2 mg/mL & 2 mg/mL	No precipitate or change in color or turbidity within 4 hours.

988

Furosemide	Y	Dextrose 5%	1.2 mg/mL & 3 mg/mL	No precipitate or change in color or turbidity within 4 hours.
Ganciclovir sodium	Y	Dextrose 5%	1.2 mg/mL & 20 mg/mL	No precipitate or change in color or turbidity within 4 hours.
Gentamicin sulfate	Y	Dextrose 5%	1.2 mg/mL & 5 mg/mL	No precipitate or change in color or turbidity within 4 hours.
Haloperidol lactate	Y	Dextrose 5%	1.2 mg/mL & 0.2 mg/mL	No precipitate, color change, or gas production within 4 hours.
Heparin sodium	Y	Dextrose 5%	1.2 mg/mL & 100 units/mL	No precipitate or change in color or turbidity within 4 hours.
Hydrocortisone sodium phosphate	Y	Dextrose 5%	1.2 mg/mL & 1 mg/mL	No precipitate or change in color or turbidity within 4 hours.
Hydrocortisone sodium succinate	Y	Dextrose 5%	1.2 mg/mL & 1 mg/mL	Incompatible. Decreased turbidity, below normal range..
Hydromorphone hydrochloride	Y	Dextrose 5%	1.2 mg/mL & 0.5 mg/mL	No precipitate or change in color or turbidity within 4 hours.
Hydroxyzine hydrochloride	Y	Dextrose 5%	1.2 mg/mL & 4 mg/mL	Incompatible. Decreased turbidity, below normal range.
Lorazepam	Y	Dextrose 5%	1.2 mg/mL & 0.1 mg/mL	No precipitate, color change, or gas production within 4 hours.
Magnesium sulfate	Y	Dextrose 5%	1.2 mg/mL & 100 mg/mL	No precipitate or change in color or turbidity within 4 hours.
Mannitol	Y	Dextrose 5%	1.2 mg/mL & 150 mg/mL	No precipitate or change in color or turbidity within 4 hours.
Meperidine hydrochloride	Y	Dextrose 5%	1.2 mg/mL & 4 mg/mL	No precipitate or change in color or turbidity within 4 hours.
Mesna	Y	Dextrose 5%	1.2 mg/mL & 10 mg/mL	No precipitate or change in color or turbidity within 4 hours.
Methylprednisolone sodium succinate	Y	Dextrose 5%	1.2 mg/mL & 5 mg/mL	Incompatible. Decreased turbidity, below normal range.
Metoclopramide hydrochloride	Y	Dextrose 5%	1.2 mg/mL & 5 mg/mL	No precipitate or change in color or turbidity within 4 hours.
Morphine sulfate	Y	Dextrose 5%	1.2 mg/mL & 1 mg/mL	No precipitate or change in color or turbidity within 4 hours.
Nalbuphine hydrochloride	Y	Dextrose 5%	1.2 mg/mL & 10 mg/mL	No precipitate or change in color or turbidity within 4 hours.
Ondansetron hydrochloride	Y	Dextrose 5%	1.2 mg/mL & 0.5 mg/mL	No precipitate or change in color or turbidity within 4 hours.

Table 47.3. *continued*

Part B: Oncology Product with Other Products

Oncology Product	Other Product	Condition[a]	Diluting Solution	Concentration of Products	Stability and Compatibility Comments
	Pentostatin	Y	Dextrose 5% & sodium chloride 0.9%	1.2 mg/mL & 0.4 mg/mL	No precipitate or change in color or turbidity within 4 hours.
	Potassium chloride	Y	Dextrose 5%	1.2 mg/mL & 0.1 mEq/L	No precipitate or change in color or turbidity within 4 hours.
	Prochlorperazine/edisylate	Y	Dextrose 5%	1.2 mg/mL & 0.5 mg/mL	No precipitate, color change, or gas production within 4 hours.
	Ranitidine hydrochloride	Y	Dextrose 5%	1.2 mg/mL & 2 mg/mL	No precipitate, color change, or gas production within 4 hours.
	Sodium bicarbonate	Y	Dextrose 5%	1.2 mg/mL & 1 mEq/L	No precipitate or change in color or turbidity within 4 hours.
	Vancomycin hydrochloride	Y	Dextrose 5%	1.2 mg/mL & 10 mg/mL	No precipitate, color change, or gas production within 4 hours.
	Zidovudine	Y	Dextrose 5%	1.2 mg/mL & 4 mg/mL	No precipitate or change in color or turbidity within 4 hours.
Pentostatin	Ondansetron hydrochloride	Y	Sodium chloride 0.9%	0.4 mg/mL & 1 mg/mL	Physically compatible for 4 hours at 22°C in fluorescent light.
	Sargramostim	Y	Sodium chloride 0.9%	0.4 mg/mL & 10 μg/mL	Physically compatible for 4 hours at 22°C in fluorescent light.
Sargramostim (GM-CSF)	Acyclovir sodium	Y	Sodium chloride 0.9%	10 μg/mL & 7 mg/mL	Incompatible. White precipitate at 4 hours at room temperature in fluorescent light.
	Amikacin sulfate	Y	Sodium chloride 0.9%	10 μg/mL & 5 mg/mL	No visible precipitate at 4 hours at room temperature in fluorescent light.
	Aminophylline	Y	Sodium chloride 0.9%	10 μg/mL & 2.5 mg/mL	No visible precipitate at 4 hours at room temperature in fluorescent light.
	Amphotericin B	Y	Dextrose 5%	10 μg/mL & 0.6 mg/mL	Physically compatible for 4 hours at room temperature in fluorescent light.
	Amphotericin B	Y	Sodium chloride 0.9%	10 μg/mL & 0.6 mg/mL	Incompatible. Immediate yellow precipitate.
	Ampicillin sodium	Y	Sodium chloride 0.9%	10 μg/mL & 20 mg/mL	Incompatible. Precipitates at 4 hours at room temperature in fluorescent light.
	Ampicillin sodium/sulbactam sodium	Y	Sodium chloride 0.9%	10 μg/mL & 20/10 mg/mL	Incompatible. Precipitates in 4 hours at room temperature in fluorescent light.

Drug		Solution	Concentration	Observation
Aztreonam	Y	Sodium chloride 0.9%	10 µg/mL & 40 mg/mL	No visible precipitate at 4 hours at room temperature in fluorescent light.
Calcium gluconate	Y	Sodium chloride 0.9%	10 µg/mL & 40 mg/mL	No visible precipitate at 4 hours at room temperature in fluorescent light.
Cefazolin sodium	Y	Sodium chloride 0.9%	10 µg/mL & 20 mg/mL	No visible precipitate at 4 hours at room temperature in fluorescent light.
Cefonicid sodium	Y	Sodium chloride 0.9%	10 µg/mL & 20 mg/mL	Incompatible. Visible precipitate at 4 hours at room temperature in fluorescent light.
Cefoperazone sodium	Y	Sodium chloride 0.9%	10 µg/mL & 40 mg/mL	Incompatible. Slight haze forms immediately at room temperature in fluorescent light.
Ceforanide	Y	Sodium chloride 0.9%	10 µg/mL & 20 mg/mL	No visible precipitate at 4 hours at room temperature in fluorescent light.
Cefotaxime sodium	Y	Sodium chloride 0.9%	10 µg/mL & 20 mg/mL	No visible precipitate at 4 hours at room temperature in fluorescent light.
Cefotetan disodium	Y	Sodium chloride 0.9%	10 µg/mL & 20 mg/mL	No visible precipitate at 4 hours at room temperature in fluorescent light.
Ceftazidime	Y	Sodium chloride 0.9%	10 µg/mL & 40 mg/mL	Incompatible. Large visible particle at 4 hours at room temperature in fluorescent light.
Ceftriaxone sodium	Y	Sodium chloride 0.9%	10 µg/mL & 20 mg/mL	No visible precipitate at 4 hours at room temperature in fluorescent light.
Cefuroxime sodium	Y	Sodium chloride 0.9%	10 µg/mL & 30 mg/mL	No visible precipitate at 4 hours at room temperature in fluorescent light.
Chlorpromazine hydrochloride	Y	Sodium chloride 0.9%	10 µg/mL & 2 mg/mL	Incompatible. Slight haze forms immediately at room temperature in fluorescent light.
Clindamycin phosphate	Y	Sodium chloride 0.9%	10 µg/mL & 10 mg/mL	No visible precipitate at 4 hours at room temperature in fluorescent light.
Dexamethasone sodium phosphate	Y	Sodium chloride 0.9%	10 µg/mL & 1 mg/mL	No visible precipitate at 4 hours at room temperature in fluorescent light.
Diphenhydramine hydrochloride	Y	Sodium chloride 0.9%	10 µg/mL & 1 mg/mL	No visible precipitate at 4 hours at room temperature in fluorescent light.
Doxycycline hyclate	Y	Sodium chloride 0.9%	10 µg/mL & 1 mg/mL	No visible precipitate at 4 hours at room temperature in fluorescent light.
Droperidol	Y	Sodium chloride 0.9%	10 µg/mL & 0.4 mg/mL	No visible precipitate at 4 hours at room temperature in fluorescent light.
Famotidine	Y	Sodium chloride 0.9%	10 µg/mL & 2 mg/mL	No visible precipitate at 4 hours at room temperature in fluorescent light.
Fluconazole	Y	Sodium chloride 0.9%	10 µg/mL & 2 mg/mL	No visible precipitate at 4 hours at room temperature in fluorescent light.
Furosemide	Y	Sodium chloride 0.9%	10 µg/mL & 3 mg/mL	No visible precipitate at 4 hours at room temperature in fluorescent light.

Table 47.3. *continued*

| | | | Part B: Oncology Product with Other Products | | |
Oncology Product	Other Product	Condition[a]	Diluting Solution	Concentration of Products	Stability and Compatibility Comments
	Ganciclovir sodium	Y	Sodium chloride 0.9%	10 μg/mL & 20 mg/mL	Incompatible. Fine precipitate at 4 hours at room temperature in fluorescent light.
	Gentamicin sulfate	Y	Sodium chloride 0.9%	10 μg/mL & 5 mg/mL	No visible precipitate at 4 hours at room temperature in fluorescent light.
	Haloperidol lactate	Y	Sodium chloride 0.9%	10 μg/mL & 0.2 mg/mL	Incompatible. Fine precipitate at 4 hours at room temperature in fluorescent light.
	Heparin sodium	Y	Sodium chloride 0.9%	10 μg/mL & 100 units/mL	No visible precipitate at 4 hours at room temperature in fluorescent light.
	Hydrocortisone sodium phosphate	Y	Sodium chloride 0.9%	10 μg/mL & 1 mg/mL	Incompatible. Visible filamentous particle at 4 hours at room temperature in fluorescent light.
	Hydrocortisone sodium succinate	Y	Sodium chloride 0.9%	10 μg/mL & 1 mg/mL	Incompatible. Visible particles within 1 hour at room temperature in fluorescent light.
	Hydromorphone hydrochloride	Y	Sodium chloride 0.9%	10 μg/mL & 0.5 mg/mL	Incompatible. Visible particles within 30 minutes at room temperature in fluorescent light.
	Hydroxyzine hydrochloride	Y	Sodium chloride 0.9%	10 μg/mL & 4 mg/mL	Incompatible. Haze and particles within 4 hours at room temperature in fluorescent light.
	Imipenem-cilastatin sodium	Y	Sodium chloride 0.9%	10 μg/mL & 5 mg/mL	Incompatible. Visible precipitate within 4 hours at room temperature in fluorescent light.
	Lorazepam	Y	Sodium chloride 0.9%	10 μg/mL & 0.1 mg/mL	Incompatible. Bluish haze forms within 1 hour at room temperature in fluorescent light.
	Magnesium sulfate	Y	Sodium chloride 0.9%	10 μg/mL & 100 mg/mL	No visible precipitate at 4 hours at room temperature in fluorescent light.
	Mannitol	Y	Sodium chloride 0.9%	10 μg/mL & 150 mg/mL	No visible precipitate at 4 hours at room temperature in fluorescent light.
	Meperidine hydrochloride	Y	Sodium chloride 0.9%	10 μg/mL & 4 mg/mL	No visible precipitate at 4 hours at room temperature in fluorescent light.
	Mesna	Y	Sodium chloride 0.9%	10 μg/mL & 10 mg/mL	No visible precipitate at 4 hours at room temperature in fluorescent light.
	Methylprednisolone sodium succinate	Y	Sodium chloride 0.9%	10 μg/mL & 5 mg/mL	Incompatible. Visible particles within 4 hours at room temperature in fluorescent light.
	Metoclopramide hydrochloride	Y	Sodium chloride 0.9%	10 μg/mL & 5 mg/mL	No visible precipitate at 4 hours at room temperature in fluorescent light.
	Metronidazole	Y	Sodium chloride 0.9%	10 μg/mL & 5 mg/mL	No visible precipitate at 4 hours at room temperature in fluorescent light.

Mezlocillin sodium	Y	Sodium chloride 0.9%	10 μg/mL & 40 mg/mL	No visible precipitate at 4 hours at room temperature in fluorescent light.
Miconazole	Y	Sodium chloride 0.9%	10 μg/mL & 3.5 mg/mL	No visible precipitate at 4 hours at room temperature in fluorescent light.
Minocycline hydrochloride	Y	Sodium chloride 0.9%	10 μg/mL & 0.2 mg/mL	No visible precipitate at 4 hours at room temperature in fluorescent light.
Mitomycin	Y	Sodium chloride 0.9%	10 μg/mL & 0.5 mg/mL	Incompatible. Haze forms within 30 minutes at room temperature in fluorescent light.
Morphine sulfate	Y	Sodium chloride 0.9%	10 μg/mL & 1 mg/mL	Incompatible. Haze and precipitate form within 1 hour at room temperature in fluorescent light.
Nalbuphine hydrochloride	Y	Sodium chloride 0.9%	10 μg/mL & 10 mg/mL	Incompatible. Haze forms within 30 minutes and filaments form within 4 hours at room temperature in fluorescent light.
Netilmicin sulfate	Y	Sodium chloride 0.9%	10 μg/mL & 5 mg/mL	No visible precipitate at 4 hours at room temperature in fluorescent light.
Ondansetron hydrochloride	Y	Sodium chloride 0.9%	10 μg/mL & 0.5 mg/mL	Incompatible. Filamentous particles within 30 minutes at room temperature in fluorescent light.
Piperacillin sodium	Y	Sodium chloride 0.9%	10 μg/mL & 40 mg/mL	Incompatible. Precipitates at 4 hours at room temperature in fluorescent light.
Potassium chloride	Y	Sodium chloride 0.9%	10 μg/mL & 0.1 mEq/L	No visible precipitate at 4 hours at room temperature in fluorescent light.
Prochlorperazine edisylate	Y	Sodium chloride 0.9%	10 μg/mL & 0.5 mg/mL	No visible precipitate at 4 hours at room temperature in fluorescent light.
Promethazine hydrochloride	Y	Sodium chloride 0.9%	10 μg/mL & 2 mg/mL	No visible precipitate at 4 hours at room temperature in fluorescent light.
Ranitidine hydrochloride	Y	Sodium chloride 0.9%	10 μg/mL & 2 mg/mL	No visible precipitate at 4 hours at room temperature in fluorescent light.
Sodium bicarbonate	Y	Sodium chloride 0.9%	10 μg/mL & 1 mEq/L	Incompatible. Precipitates at 4 hours at room temperature in fluorescent light.
Tetracycline hydrochloride	Y	Sodium chloride 0.9%	10 μg/mL & 2.5 mg/mL	No visible precipitate at 4 hours at room temperature in fluorescent light.
Ticarcillin disodium	Y	Sodium chloride 0.9%	10 μg/mL & 30 mg/mL	No visible precipitate at 4 hours at room temperature in fluorescent light.
Ticarcillin disodium/clavulanate potassium	Y	Sodium chloride 0.9%	10 μg/mL & 31 mg/mL	No visible precipitate at 4 hours at room temperature in fluorescent light.
Tobramycin sulfate	Y	Sodium chloride 0.9%	10 μg/mL & 5 mg/mL	Incompatible. Precipitate and filaments form at 4 hours at room temperature in fluorescent light.
Trimethoprim/sulfamethoxazole	Y	Sodium chloride 0.9%	10 μg/mL & 0.8/4 mg/mL	No visible precipitate at 4 hours at room temperature in fluorescent light.

Table 47.3. *continued*

Oncology Product	Other Product	Condition[a]	Diluting Solution	Concentration of Products	Stability and Compatibility Comments
				Part B: Oncology Product with Other Products	
	Vancomycin hydrochloride	Y	Sodium chloride 0.9%	10 µg/mL & 10 mg/mL	No visible precipitate at 4 hours at room temperature in fluorescent light.
	Zidovudine	Y	Sodium chloride 0.9%	10 µg/mL & 4 mg/mL	No visible precipitate at 4 hours at room temperature in fluorescent light.
Vinblastine	Droperidol	Y	Not applicable	1 mg/mL & 2.5 mg/mL	No visible precipitate after sequential injection.
	Furosemide	A	See manufacturer's package inserts	1 mg/mL & 10 mg/mL	Incompatible. Precipitates.
	Furosemide	Y	Not applicable	1 mg/mL & 10 mg/mL	Incompatible. Precipitates immediately.
	Heparin sodium	A	Sodium chloride 0.9%	1 mg/mL & 200 units/mL	Unstable. Drug decomposes within 24 hours at 37°C.
	Heparin sodium	Y	Not applicable	1 mg/mL & 1000 units/mL	No visible precipitate after sequential injection.
	Leucovorin calcium	Y	Not applicable	1 mg/mL & 10 mg/mL	No visible precipitate after sequential injection.
	Metoclopramide hydrochloride	Y	Not applicable	1 mg/mL & 5 mg/mL	No visible precipitate after sequential injection.
	Metoclopramide hydrochloride	A	See manufacturer's package inserts	9.5 mg & 10–160 mg	Physically compatible for 48 hours at 25°C.
	Ondansetron hydrochloride	Y	Dextrose 5% & sodium chloride 0.9%	0.12 mg/mL & 1 mg/mL	Physically compatible for 4 hours at 22°C in fluorescent light.
	Sargramostim	Y	Sodium chloride 0.9%	0.12 mg/mL & 10 µg/mL	Physically compatible for 4 hours at 22°C in fluorescent light.
Vincristine	Droperidol	Y	Not applicable	1 mg/mL & 2.5 mg/mL	No visible precipitate after sequential injection.
	Furosemide	A	See manufacturer's package inserts	1 mg/mL & 10 mg/mL	Incompatible. Precipitates.
	Furosemide	Y	Not applicable	1 mg/mL & 10 mg/mL	Incompatible. Precipitates immediately.
	Heparin sodium	Y	Not applicable	1 mg/mL & 1000 units/mL	No visible precipitate after sequential injection.
	Leucovorin calcium	Y	Not applicable	1 mg/mL & 10 mg/mL	No visible precipitate after sequential injection.
	Metoclopramide hydrochloride	A	See manufacturer's package inserts	2.4 mg & 10–160 mg	Physically compatible for 48 hours at 25°C.
	Metoclopramide hydrochloride	Y	Not applicable	5 mg/mL & 1 mg/mL	No visible precipitate after sequential injection.
	Ondansetron hydrochloride	Y	Dextrose 5% & sodium chloride 0.9%	0.05 mg/mL & 1 mg/mL	Physically compatible for 4 hours at 22°C in fluorescent light.
	Sargramostim	Y	Sodium chloride 0.9%	0.05 mg/mL & 10 µg/mL	Physically compatible for 4 hours at 22°C in fluorescent light.

Condition: A, admixture (drugs are used as an admixture in the IV bag); Y, Y-site (drugs are combined at the Y-site in the IV line).

Table 47.4. References

PRODUCT	AUTHORS/TITLE/CITATION
Aldesleukin (IL-2)	**Cetus Oncology Corp. Proleukin package insert. September 1992.**
Asparaginase	**McEvoy GK, ed.** American hospital formulary: drug information 1993. Bethesda, Md: American Society of Hospital Pharmacists, 1992:524–526. **Physicians' Desk Reference.** 47th ed. Montvale, NJ: Medical Economics, 1993:1521–1523. **Vogenberg FR, Souney PF.** Stability guidelines for routinely refrigerated drug products. Am J Hosp Pharm 1983;40:101–102.
Azathioprine	**Johnson CA, Porter WA.** Compatibility of azathioprine sodium with intravenous fluids. Am J Hosp Pharm 1981;38:871–875. **Physicians' Desk Reference.** 47th ed. Montvale, NJ: Medical Economics, 1993:785–787.
Bleomycin	**Adams JA, Wilson JP, Sollmando DA.** Instability of bleomycin in plastic containers. Am J Hosp Pharm 1982;39:1636. **Benvenuto JA, Adams SC, Vyas HM, et al.** Pharmaceutical issues in infusion chemotherapy stability and compatibility. In: Lokich JJ, ed. Cancer chemotherapy by infusion. Chicago: Precept Press; 1987:101–113. **Benvenuto JA, Anderson RW, Kerkof K, et al.** Stability and compatibility of antitumor agents in glass and plastic containers. Am J Hosp Pharm 1981;38:1914–1918. **Bristol Laboratories (personal communications).** Arbus M, Assistant Director Medical Services, Oncology. February 11, 1988. **Butler LD, Munson JM, DeLuca PP.** Effect of inline filtration on the potency of low-dose drugs. Am J Hosp Pharm 1980;37:935–941. **Dorr RT, Peng Y-M, Alberts DS.** Bleomycin compatibility with selected intravenous medications. J Med 1982;13:121–130. **Joffe A.** Comment on handling of anticancer drugs. Drug Intell Clin Pharm 1984;18:417. **Koberda M, Zieske PA, Raghavan NV, Payton RJ.** Stability of bleomycin sulfate reconstituted in 5% dextrose injection or 0.9% sodium chloride injection stored in glass vials or polyvinyl chloride containers. Am J Hosp Pharm 1990;47:2528–2529. **Lokich JJ.** Combination chemotherapy and infusional schedules. In: Lokich JJ, ed. Cancer chemotherapy by infusion. Chicago: Precept Press; 1987:560–568. **Markman M, Cleary S, Lucas W, et al.** IP chemotherapy employing a regimen of cisplatin, cytarabine and bleomycin. Cancer Treat Rep 1986;70:755–760. **Physicians' Desk Reference.** 47th ed. Montvale, NJ: Medical Economics, 1993;742–743. **Trissel LA, Tramonte SM, Grilley BJ.** Visual compatibility of ondansetron hydrochloride with selected drugs during simulated Y-site injection. Am J Hosp Pharm 1991;48:988–992.
Carboplatin	**Flora KP, Greene RF, Jackson WE, et al.** Carboplatin. In: Flora C, ed. NCI investigational drugs: pharmaceutical data. Bethesda, MD: National Cancer Institute, 1990:29. **Fournier C, Hecquet B, Bastian G, Khayat D.** Modification of the physiochemical and pharmacologic properties of anticancer platinum compounds by commercial 5-fluorouracil formulations: a comparative study using cisplatin and carboplatin. Cancer Chemother Pharmacol 1992;29:461–466. **Lokich J, Anderson N, Bern M, et al.** Etoposide plus carboplatin admixture. Am J Clin Oncol (CCT) 1992;15:314–318. **Physicians' Desk Reference.** 47th ed. Montvale, NJ: Medical Economics, 1993;751–754. **Sewell GJ, Riley CM, Rowland CG.** The stability of carboplatin in ambulatory continuous infusion regimes. J Clin Pharm Ther 1987;12:427–432. **Trissel LA, Tramonte SM, Grilley BJ.** Visual compatibility of ondansetron hydrochloride with selected drugs during simulated Y-site injection. Am J Hosp Pharm 1991;48:988–992. **Williams DA.** Stability and compatibility of admixtures of antineoplastic drugs. In: Lokich JJ, ed. Cancer chemotherapy by infusion. Chicago: Precept Press, 1990:52–73.

Table 47.4. *continued*

PRODUCT	AUTHORS/TITLE/CITATION
Carmustine	**Benvenuto JA, Anderson RW, Kerkof K, et al.** Stability and compatibility of antitumor agents in glass and plastic containers. Am J Hosp Pharm 1981;38:1914–1918.
	Bristol Laboratories (personal communications). Arbus M, Assistant Director Medical Services, Oncology. February 11, 1988.
	Chan KK, Zackheim HS. Stability of nitrosourea solutions. Arch Dermatol 1973;107:298.
	Colvin M, Hartner J, Summerfield M. Stability of carmustine in the presence of sodium bicarbonate. Am J Hosp Pharm 1980;37:677–678.
	Davignon JP, Yang KW, Wood HB, et al. Formulation of three nitrosoureas for intravenous use. Cancer Chemother Rep part 3. 1973;4:7–11.
	Laskar PA, Ayers JW. Degradation of carmustine in aqueous media. J Pharm Sci 1977; 66:1073–1076.
	Levin VA, Levin EM. Dissolution and stability of carmustine in the absence of ethanol. Sel Cancer Ther 1989;5:33–35.
	Levin VA, Zackheim HS, Liu J, et al. Stability of carmustine for topical application. Arch Dermatol 1982;118:450–451.
	Physicians' Desk Reference. 47th ed. Montvale, NJ: Medical Economics, 1993:740–742.
	Tepe P, Hassenbusch SJ, Benoit R, Anderson JH. BCNU stability as a function of ethanol concentration and temperature. J Neurooncol 1991;10:121–127.
	Trissel LA, Kleinman LM, Davignon JP, et al. Investigational drug information. Drug Intell Clin Pharm 1976;10:48–49.
	Trissel LA, Tramonte SM, Grilley BJ. Visual compatibility of ondansetron hydrochloride with selected drugs during simulated Y-site injection. Am J Hosp Pharm 1991;48:988–992.
Cisplatin	**A.H. Robins.** Reglan injectable compatibility chart. May 1987.
	Bohart RD, Ogawa G. An observation on the stability of cis-dichlorodiammineplatinum (II): a caution regarding its administration. Cancer Treat Rep 1979;63:2117–2118.
	Bristol Laboratories (personal communications). Arbus M, Assistant Director Medical Services, Oncology. February 2, 1988.
	Cheung Y, Cradock JC, Vishnuvajjala BR, et al. Stability of cisplatin, iproplatin, carboplatin, and tetraplatin in commonly used intravenous solutions. Am J Hosp Pharm 1987;44:124–130.
	Earhart RH. Instability of cis-dichlorodiammineplatinum in dextrose solution. Cancer Treat Rep 1978;62(7):1105–1106.
	Fournier C, Hecquet B, Bastian G, Khayat D. Modification of the physiochemical and pharmacologic properties of anticancer platinum compounds by commercial 5-fluorouracil formulations: a comparative study using cisplatin and carboplatin. Cancer Chemother Pharmacol 1992;29:461–466.
	Greene RF, Chatterji DC, Hiranaka PK, et al. Stability of cisplatin in aqueous solution. Am J Hosp Pharm 1979;36:38–43.
	Hussain AA, Haddadin M, Iga K. Reaction of cis-platinum with sodium bisulfite. J Pharm Sci 1980;69(3):364–365.
	Kristjansson F, Sternson LA, Lindenbaum S. An investigation on possible oligomer formation in pharmaceutical formulations of cisplatin. Int J Pharm 1988;41:67–74.
	LaFollette JM, Arbus MH, Lauper RD. Stability of cisplatin admixtures in polyvinyl chloride bags. Am J Hosp Pharm 1985;42:2652.
	LeRoy AF. Some quantitative data on cis-dichlorodiammine-platinum (II) species in solution. Cancer Treat Rep 1979;63(2):231–233.
	Lokich J, Anderson N, Bern M, et al. Etoposide admixed with cisplatin. Cancer. 1989; 63:818–821.
	Mariani EP, Southard BJ, Woolever JT, et al. Physical compatibility and chemical stability of cisplatin in various diluents and in large-volume parenteral solutions. In: Prestayko AW, et al, eds. Cisplatin current status and new developments. New York: Academic Press; 1980:305–316.
	Markman M, Cleary S, Lucas W, et al. IP chemotherapy employing a regimen of cisplatin, cytarabine and bleomycin. Cancer Treat Rep 1986;70:755–760.

Table 47.4. *continued*

PRODUCT	AUTHORS/TITLE/CITATION
Cisplatin *cont.*	**Marquardt ED.** Visual compatibility of hydroxyzine hydrochloride with various antineoplastic agents. Am J Hosp Pharm 1988;45:2127. **Physicians' Desk Reference.** 47th ed. Montvale, NJ: Medical Economics, 1993:754–757. **Prestayko AW, Cadiz M, Crooke ST.** Incompatibility of aluminum-containing IV administration equipment with cis-dichlorodiammineplatinum (II) administration. Cancer Treat Rep 1979;63:2118–2119. **Stewart CF, Fleming RA.** Compatibility of cisplatin and fluorouracil in 0.9% sodium chloride injection. Am J Hosp Pharm 1990;47:1373–1377. **Trissel LA, Tramonte SM, Grilley BJ.** Visual compatibility of ondansetron hydrochloride with selected drugs during simulated Y-site injection. Am J Hosp Pharm 1991;48:988–992. **Vogenberg FR, Souney PF.** Stability guidelines for routinely refrigerated drug products. Am J Hosp Pharm 1983;40:101–102.
Cyclophosphamide	**A.H. Robins.** Reglan injectable compatibility chart. May 1987. **Athanikar N, Boyer B, Deamer R, et al.** Visual compatibility of 30 additives with a parenteral nutrient solution. Am J Hosp Pharm 1979;36:511–513. **Benvenuto JA, Anderson RW, Kerkof K, et al.** Stability and compatibility of antitumor agents in glass and plastic containers. Am J Hosp Pharm 1981;38:1914–1918. **Brooke D, Bequette RJ, Davis RE.** Chemical stability of cyclophosphamide in parenteral solutions. Am J Hosp Pharm 1973;30:134–137. **Brooke D, Scott JA, Bequette RJ.** Effect of briefly heating cyclophosphamide solutions. Am J Hosp Pharm 1975;32:44–45. **Galleli JF.** Stability studies of drugs in intravenous solutions. Part 1. Am J Hosp Pharm 1967;24:425–433. **Kirk B, Melia CD, Wilson JV, et al.** Clinical stability of cyclophosphamide injection. Br J Parenter Ther 1984;5:90–97. **Lokich J, Bern M. Anderson N, et al.** Cyclophosphamide, methotrexate, and 5-fluorouracil in a three-drug admixture. Cancer. 1989;63:822–824. **Marquardt ED.** Visual compatibility of hydroxyzine hydrochloride with various antineoplastic agents. Am J Hosp Pharm 1988;45:2127. **Physicians' Desk Reference.** 47th ed. Montvale, NJ: Medical Economics, 1993:744–745. **Trissel LA, Tramonte SM, Grilley BJ.** Visual compatibility of ondansetron hydrochloride with selected drugs during simulated Y-site injection. Am J Hosp Pharm 1991;48:988–992.
Cytarabine	**A.H. Robins.** Reglan injectable compatibility chart. May 1987. **Athanikar N, Boyer B, Deamer R, et al.** Visual compatibility of 30 additives with a parenteral nutrient solution. Am J Hosp Pharm 1979;36:511–513. **Benvenuto JA, Anderson RW, Kerkof K, et al.** Stability and compatibility of antitumor agents in glass and plastic containers. Am J Hosp Pharm 1981;38:1914–1918. **Cheung Y, Vishnuvajjala BR, Flora KP.** Stability of cytarabine, methotrexate sodium, and hydrocortisone sodium succinate admixtures. Am J Hosp Pharm 1984;41:1802–1806. **Cradock JC, Kleinman LM, Rahman A.** Evaluation of some pharmaceutical aspects of intrathecal methotrexate sodium, cytarabine and hydrocortisone sodium succinate. Am J Hosp Pharm 1978;35:402–406. **Ennis CE, Merritt RJ, Neff DN.** In vitro study of inline filtration of medications commonly administered to pediatric cancer patients. J Parenter Enter Nutr 1983;7:156–158. **Keller JH, Ensminger WD.** Stability of cancer chemotherapeutic agents in a totally implanted drug delivery system. Am J Hosp Pharm 1982;39:1321–1323. **Markman M, Cleary S, Lucas W, et al.** IP chemotherapy employing a regimen of cisplatin, cytarabine and bleomycin. Cancer Treat Rep 1986;70:755–760. **Marquardt ED.** Visual compatibility of hydroxyzine hydrochloride with various antineoplastic agents. Am J Hosp Pharm 1988;45:2127. **McRae MP, King JC.** Compatibility of antineoplastic, antibiotic and corticosteroid drugs in intravenous admixtures. Am J Hosp Pharm 1976;33:1010–1013.

Table 47.4. *continued*

PRODUCT	AUTHORS/TITLE/CITATION
Cytarabine *cont.*	**Munson JW, Kubiak EJ, Cohon MS.** Cytosine arabinoside stability in intravenous admixtures with sodium bicarbonate and in plastic syringes. Drug Intell Clin Pharm 1982;16:765–767. **Notari RE, Chin ML, Wittebort R.** Arabinosylcytosine stability in aqueous solutions: pH profile and shelflife predictions. J Pharm Sci 1872;61(8):1189–1196. **Physicians' Desk Reference.** 47th ed. Montvale, NJ: Medical Economics, 1993:2442–2444. **Robinson WA, Krebs LU.** The "real stuff" for intrathecal injection during leukemia therapy. Lancet. 1982;1:283. **Rochard EB, Barthes DMC, Courtois PY.** Stability of fluorouracil, cytarabine, or doxorubicin hydrochloride in ethylene vinylacetate portable infusion-pump reservoirs. Am J Hosp Pharm 1992;49:619–623. **Seargeant LE, Kobrinsky NL, Sus CJ, Nazeravich DR.** In vitro stability and compatibility of daunorubicin, cytarabine and etoposide. Cancer Treat Rep 1987;71:1189–1192. **Trissel LA.** Handbook of injectable drugs. 7th ed. Bethesda, MD: American Society of Hospital Pharmacists; 1992:267. **Trissel LA, Tramonte SM, Grilley BJ.** Visual compatibility of ondansetron hydrochloride with selected drugs during simulated Y-site injection. Am J Hosp Pharm 1991;48:988–992. **Wolfert RR, Cox RM.** Room temperature stability of drug products labeled for refrigerated storage. Am J Hosp Pharm 1975;32:585–587.
Dacarbazine	**A.H. Robins.** Reglan injectable compatibility chart. May 1987. **Benvenuto JA, Anderson RW, Kerkof K, et al.** Stability and compatibility of antitumor agents in glass and plastic containers. Am J Hosp Pharm 1981;38:1914–1918. **Dorr RT.** Incompatibilities with parenteral anticancer drugs. Am J IV Therapy 1979;6:42–52. **Kirk B.** The evaluation of high-protective giving set. The photosensitivity of intravenous dacarbazine solutions. Br J Parenter Ther 1987;8:78, 81–82, 85–86. **Nelson RW, Young R, Lamnin M.** Visual incompatibility of dacarbazine and heparin. Am J Hosp Pharm 1987;44:2028. **Physicians' Desk Reference.** 47th ed. Montvale, NJ: Medical Economics, 1993;1641–1642. **Trissel LA, Kleinman LM, Davignon JP, et al.** Investigational drug information. Drug Intell Clin Pharm 1976;10:48–49. **Trissel LA, Tramonte SM, Grilley BJ.** Visual compatibility of ondansetron hydrochloride with selected drugs during simulated Y-site injection. Am J Hosp Pharm 1991;48:988–992.
Dactinomycin	**Benvenuto JA, Anderson RW, Kerkof K, et al.** Stability and compatibility of antitumor agents in glass and plastic containers. Am J Hosp Pharm 1981;38:1914–1918. **Couvreur P, Kante B, Lenaerts V, et al.** Tissue distribution of antitumor drugs associated with polyalkylcyanoacrylate nanoparticles. J Pharm Sci 1980;69:199–202. **Ennis CE, Merritt RJ, Neff DN.** In vitro study of inline filtration of medications commonly administered to pediatric cancer patients. J Parenter Enter Nutr 1983;7:156–158. **Kanke M, Eubanks JL, DeLuca PP.** Binding of selected drugs to a treaed inline filter. Am J Hosp Pharm 1983;40:1323–1328. **Physicians' Desk Reference.** 47th ed. Montvale, NJ: Medical Economics, 1993:1491–1493. **Trissel LA, Tramonte SM, Grilley BJ.** Visual compatibility of ondansetron hydrochloride with selected drugs during simulated Y-site injection. Am J Hosp Pharm 1991;48:988–992.

Table 47.4. *continued*

PRODUCT	AUTHORS/TITLE/CITATION
Daunorubicin	**Dorr RT.** Incompatibilities with parenteral anticancer drugs. Am J IV Therapy 1979;6:45–52. **Pavlik EJ, Kenady DE, van Nagell JR, et al.** Properties of anticancer agents relevant to in vitro determinations of human tumor cell sensitivity. Cancer Chemother Pharmacol 1983;11:8–15. **Physicians' Desk Reference.** 47th ed. Montvale, NJ: Medical Economics, 1993:2555–2557. **Poochikian GK, Cradock JC, Flora KP.** Stability of anthracycline antitumor agents in four infusion fluids. Am J Hosp Pharm 1981;38:483–486. **Seargeant LE, Kobrinsky NL, Sus OJ, Nazeravich DR.** In vitro stability and compatibility of daunorubicin, cytarabine and etoposide. Cancer Treat Rep 1987;71:1189–1192. **Trissel LA, Kleinman LM, Davignon JP, et al.** Investigational drug information. Drug Intell Clin Pharm 1978;12:404–406. **Trissel LA, Tramonte SM, Grilley BJ.** Visual compatibility of ondansetron hydrochloride with selected drugs during simulated Y-site injection. Am J Hosp Pharm 1991;48:988–992.
Doxorubicin	**A.H. Robins.** Reglan injectable compatibility chart.May 1987. **Awang DVC, Graham KC.** Microwave thawing of frozen drug solutions. Am J Hosp Pharm 1987;44:2256. **Beijnen JH, Neef C, Meuwissen OJAT, et al.** Stability of intravenous admixtures of doxorubicin and vincristine. Am J Hosp Pharm 1986;43:3022–3027. **Benvenuto JA, Anderson RW, Kerkof K, et al.** Stability and compatibility of antitumor agents in glass and plastic containers. Am J Hosp Pharm 1981;38:1914–1918. **Cohen MH, Johnston-Early A, Hood MA.** Drug precipitation within IV tubing: a potential hazard of chemotherapy administration. Cancer Treat Rep 1985;69:1325–1326. **Dorr RT.** Incompatibilities with parenteral anticancer drugs. Am J IV Therapy 1979;6:42–52. **Ennis CE, Merritt RJ, Neff DN.** In vitro study of inline filtration of medications commonly administered to pediatric cancer patients. J Parenter Enter Nutr 1983;7:156–158. **Gardiner WA.** Possible incompatibility of doxorubicin hydrochloride with aluminum. Am J Hosp Pharm 1981;38:1276. **Hoffman DM, Grossano DD, Damin L, Woodcock TM.** Stability of refrigerated and frozen solutions of doxorubicin hydrochloride. Am J Hosp Pharm 1979;36:1536–1538. **Lokich JJ, Zipoli TE, Moore C, et al.** Doxorubicin/vinblastine and doxorubicin/cyclophosphamide combination chemotherapy by continuous infusion. Cancer. 1986;58:1020–1023. **Physicians' Desk Reference.** 47th ed. Montvale, NJ: Medical Economics, 1993:560–563. **Poochikian GK, Cradock JC, Flora KP.** Stability of anthracycline antitumor agents in four infusion fluids. Am J Hosp Pharm 1981;38:483–486. **Rochard EB, Barthes DMC, Courtois PY.** Stability of fluorouracil, cytarabine, or doxorubicin hydrochloride in ethylene vinylacetate portable infusion-pump reservoirs. Am J Hosp Pharm 1992;49:619–623. **Trissel LA, Tramonte SM, Grilley BJ.** Visual compatibility of ondansetron hydrochloride with selected drugs during simulated Y-site injection. Am J Hosp Pharm 1991;48:988–992. **Wood MJ, Irwin WJ, Scott DK.** Photodegradation of doxorubicin, daunorubicin, and epirubicin measured by high-performance liquid chromatography. J Clin Pharm Ther 1990;15:291–300.
Etoposide	**A.H. Robins.** Reglan injectable compatibility chart. May 1987. **Bjorkman S, Roth B.** Chemical compatibility of mitoxantrone and etoposide (VP-16). Acta Pharm Nord 1991;3:251. **Bristol Laboratories (personal communications).** Arbus M, Assistant Director Medical Services, Oncology. February 11, 1988. **Bristol-Myers Oncology Division (personal communications).** Arbus M, Assistant Director Medical Affairs, Oncology. April 10, 1989.

Table 47.4. *continued*

PRODUCT	AUTHORS/TITLE/CITATION
Etoposide *cont.*	**Lokich J. Anderson N, Bern M, et al.** Etoposide admixed with cisplatin. Cancer 1989; 63:818–821.
	Lokich J, Anderson N, Bern M, et al. Etoposide plus carboplatin admixture. Am J Clin Oncol (CCT). 1992;15:314–318.
	Marquardt ED. Visual compatibility of hydroxyzine hydrochloride with various antineoplastic agents. Am J Hosp Pharm 1988;45:2127.
	Phillips NC, Lauper RD. Review of etoposide. Clin Pharm 1983;2:112–119.
	Physicians' Desk Reference. 47th ed. Montvale, NJ: Medical Economics, 1993:758–760.
	Seargeant LE, Kobrinsky NL, Sus CJ, Nazeravich DR. In vitro stability and compatibility of daunorubicin, cytarabine and etoposide. Cancer Treat Rep 1987;71:1189–1192.
	Trissel LA, Tramonte SM, Grilley BJ. Visual compatibility of ondansetron hydrochloride with selected drugs during simulated Y-site injection. Am J Hosp Pharm 1991;48:988–992.
Filgrastim (G-CSF)	**Amgen Inc.** Neupogen product monograph. February 21, 1991.
	Amgen Inc. (personal communications). Flynn JT, Associate Manager, Professional Services. December 17, 1991.
	Physicians' Desk Reference. 47th ed. Montvale, NJ: Medical Economics, 1993:605–608.
Floxuridine	**Keller JH, Ensminger WD.** Stability of cancer chemotherapeutic agents in a totally implanted drug delivery system. Am J Hosp Pharm 1982;39:1321–1323.
	Physicians' Desk Reference. 47th ed. Montvale, NJ: Medical Economics, 1993:1980–1981.
	Roche Laboratories (personal communications). Akiyama C, Product Services Manager, Professional Services. February 23, 1988.
	Smith JA, Morris A, Duafala ME, et al. Stability of floxuridine and leucovorin calcium admixtures for intraperitoneal administration. Am J Hosp Pharm 1989;46:985–989.
	Trissel LA, Tramonte SM, Grilley BJ. Visual compatibility of ondansetron hydrochloride with selected drugs during simulated Y-site injection. Am J Hosp Pharm 1991;48:988–992.
Fludarabine	**Flora KP, Greene RF, Jackson WE, et al.** Fludarabine phosphate. In: Flora C, ed. NCI investigational drugs: pharmaceutical data. Bethesda, MD: National Cancer Institute; 1990:72.
	Physicians' Desk Reference. 47th ed. Montvale, NJ: Medical Economics, 1993:696–698.
	Trissel LA, Parks NPT, Santiago NM. Visual compatibility of fludarabine phosphate with antineoplastic drugs, anti-infectives, and other selected drugs during simulated Y-site injection. Am J Hosp Pharm 1991;48:2186–2189.
Fluorouracil	**A.H. Robins.** Reglan injectable compatibility chart. May 1987.
	Allen LV, Stiles ML. Compatibility of various admixtures with secondary additives at Y-injection sites of intravenous administration sets. Part 2. Am J Hosp Pharm 1961; 38:380–381.
	Athanikar N, Boyer B, Deamer R, et al. Visual compatibility of 30 additives with a parenteral nutrient solution. Am J Hosp Pharm 1979;36:511–513.
	Benvenuto JA, Anderson RW, Kerkof K, et al. Stability and compatibility of antitumor agents in glass and plastic containers. Am J Hosp Pharm 1981;38:1914–1918.
	Cohen MH, Johnston-Early A, Hood MA. Drug precipitation within IV tubing: a potential hazard of chemotherapy administration. Cancer Treat Rep 1985;69:1325–1326.
	Dorr RT. Incompatibilities with parenteral anticancer drugs. Am J IV Therapy 1979;6:42–52.
	Driessen O, de Vos D, Timmermans PJA. Adsorption of fluorouracil on glass surfaces. J Pharm Sci 1978;67(10):1494–1495.
	Fournier C, Hecquet B, Bastian G, Khayat D. Modification of the physiochemical and pharmacologic properties of anticancer platinum compounds by commercial 5-fluorouracil formulations: a comparative study using cisplatin and carboplatin. Cancer Chemother Pharmacol 1992;29:461–466.

Table 47.4. *continued*

PRODUCT	AUTHORS/TITLE/CITATION
Fluorouracil *cont.*	**Hardin TC, Clibon U, Page CP, et al.** Compatibility of 5-fluorouracil and total parenteral nutrition solutions. J Parenter Enter Nutr 1982;6(2):163–165. **King JC.** Letter. Am J Hosp Pharm 1978;35:18. **Kleinberg ML, Stauffer GL, Latiolais CJ.** Effect of microwave radiation on redissolving precipitated matter in fluorouracil injection. Am J Hosp Pharm 1980;37:678–679. **Kowaluk EA, Roberts MS, Blackburn HD, et al.** Interactions between drugs and polyvinyl chloride infusion bags. Am J Hosp Pharm 1981;38:1308–1314. **Kowaluk EA, Roberts MS, Polack AE.** Interactions between drugs and intravenous delivery systems. Am J Hosp Pharm 1982;39:460–467. **Lokich J, Bern M, Anderson N, et al.** Cyclophosphamide, methotrexate, and 5-fluorouracil in a three-drug admixture. Cancer. 1989;63:822–824. **McRae MP, King JC.** Compatibility of antineoplastic, antibiotic and corticosteroid drugs in intravenous admixtures. Am J Hosp Pharm 1976;33:1010–1013. **Morrison RA, Oseekey KB, Fung H.** 5-Fluorouracil and methotrexate sodium: an admixture incompatibility? Am J Hosp Pharm 1978;35:15, 18. **Physicians' Desk Reference.** 47th ed. Montvale, NJ: Medical Economics, 1993:1978–1980. **Quebbeman EJ, Hamid AAR, Hoffman NE, et al.** Stability of fluorouracil in plastic containers used for continuous infusion at home. Am J Hosp Pharm 1984;41:1153–1156. **Rochard EB, Barthes DMC, Courtois PY.** Stability of fluorouracil, cytarabine, or doxorubicin hydrochloride in ethylene vinylacetate portable infusion-pump reservoirs. Am J Hosp Pharm 1992;49:619–623. **Roche Laboratories (personal communications).** Akiyama C, Product Services Manager, Professional Services. February 23, 1988. **Stewart CF, Fleming RA.** Compatibility of cisplatin and fluorouracil in 0.9% sodium chloride injection. Am J Hosp Pharm 1990;47:1373–1377. **Trissel LA, Tramonte SM, Grilley BJ.** Visual compatibility of ondansetron hydrochloride with selected drugs during simulated Y-site injection. Am J Hosp Pharm 1991;48:988–992. **Woloschuk DMM, Wermeling JR, Pruemer JM.** Stability and compatibility of fluorouracil and mannitol during simulated Y-site administration. Am J Hosp Pharm 1991;48:2158–2160.
Idarubicin	**Adria Laboratories.** Hospital formulary product information. October 19, 1990. **Beijnen JH, Rosing H, deVries PA, Underberg WJM.** Stability of anthracycline antitumor agents in infusion fluids. J Parenter Sci Technol 1985;39:220–222. **Physicians' Desk Reference.** 47th ed. Montvale, NJ: Medical Economics, 1993:563–565.
Ifosfamide	**Behme RJ, Brooke D, Kensler TT, Scott JA.** Incompatibility of ifosfamide with benzyl-alcohol-preserved bacteriostatic water for injection. Am J Hosp Pharm 1988;45:627–628. **Munoz M, Girona V, Pujol M, et al.** Stability of ifosfamide in 0.9% sodium chloride solution or water for injection in a portable i.v. pump cassette. Am J Hosp Pharm 1992;49:1137–1139. **Physicians' Desk Reference.** 47th ed. Montvale, NJ: Medical Economics, 1993:745–747. **Radford JA, Margison JM, Swindell R, et al.** The stability of ifosfamide in aqueous solution and its suitability for continuous 7-day infusion of ambulatory pump. Cancer Chemother Pharmacol 1990;26:144–146. **Trissel LA, Tramonte SM, Grilley BJ.** Visual compatibility of ondansetron hydrochloride with selected drugs during simulated Y-site injection. Am J Hosp Pharm 1991;48:988–992.

Table 47.4. *continued*

PRODUCT	AUTHORS/TITLE/CITATION
Leucovorin	**Lor E, Sheybani T, Takagi J.** Visual compatibility of fluconazole with commonly used injectable drugs during simulated Y-site administration. Am J Hosp Pharm 1991;48:744–746.
	Lor E, Takagi J. Visual compatibility of foscarnet with other injectable drugs. Am J Hosp Pharm 1990;47:157–159.
	Physicians' Desk Reference. 47th ed. Montvale, NJ: Medical Economics, 1993:1238–1240.
	Smith JA, Morris A, Duafala ME, et al. Stability of floxuridine and leucovorin calcium admixtures for intraperitoneal administration. Am J Hosp Pharm 1989;46:985–989.
Mechlorethamine	**Physicians' Desk Reference.** 47th ed. Montvale, NJ: Medical Economics, 1993:1566–1568.
	Trissel LA, Tramonte SM, Grilley BJ. Visual compatibility of ondansetron hydrochloride with selected drugs during simulated Y-site injection. Am J Hosp Pharm 1991;48:988–992.
Mesna	**Bristol-Myers Oncology Division.** Mesnex (mesna) product monograph. June 1989.
	Marquardt ED. Visual compatibility of hydroxyzine hydrochloride with various antineoplastic agents. Am J Hosp Pharm 1988;45:2127.
	Physicians' Desk Reference. 47th ed. Montvale, NJ: Medical Economics, 1993:749.
	Trissel LA. Handbook of injectable drugs. 7th ed. Bethesda, MD: American Society of Hospital Pharmacists; 1992:568.
	Williams DA. Stability and compatibility of admixtures of antineoplastic drugs. In: Lokich JJ, ed. Cancer chemotherapy by infusion. Chicago: Precept Press; 52–73.
Methotrexate	**A.H. Robins.** Reglan injectable compatibility chart. May 1987.
	Bender JF, Grove WR, Fortner CL. High-dose methotrexate with folinic acid rescue. Am J Hosp Pharm 1977;34:961–965.
	Benvenuto JA, Anderson RW, Kerkof K, et al. Stability and compatibility of antitumor agents in glass and plastic containers. Am J Hosp Pharm 1981;38:1914–1918.
	Bristol Laboratories (personal communications). Arbus M, Assistant Director Medical Services, Oncology. February 11, 1988.
	Cheung Y, Vishnuvajjala BR, Flora KP. Stability of cytarabine, methotrexate sodium, and hydrocortisone sodium succinate admixtures. Am J Hosp Pharm 1984;41:1802–1806.
	Cohen MH, Johnston-Early A, Hood MA. Drug precipitation within IV tubing: a potential hazard of chemotherapy administration. Cancer Treat Rep 1985;69:1325–1326.
	Cradock JC, Kleinman LM, Rahman A. Evaluation of some pharmaceutical aspects of intrathecal methotrexate, cytarabine and hydrocortisone sodium succinate. Am J Hosp Pharm 1978;35:402–406.
	Dorr RT, Peng Y-M, Alberts DS. Bleomycin compatibility with selected intravenous medications. J Med 1982;13:121–130.
	Dutter MJ, Gallelli JF, Kleinman LM, et al. Intrathecal methotrexate. Lancet 1972;1:540.
	Lapidas B. Letter. Am J Hosp Pharm 1976;33:760.
	Lokich J, Bern M, Anderson N, et al. Cyclophosphamide, methotrexate, and 5-fluorouracil in a three-drug admixture. Cancer 1989;63:822–824.
	Marquardt ED. Visual compatibility of hydroxyzine hydrochloride with various antineoplastic agents. Am J Hosp Pharm 1988;45:2127.
	McRae MP, King JC. Compatibility of antineoplastic, antibiotic and corticosteroid drugs in intravenous admixtures. Am J Hosp Pharm 1976;33:1010–1013.
	Pelsor FR. Letter. Am J Hosp Pharm 1976;33:760.
	Physicians' Desk Reference. 47th ed. Montvale, NJ: Medical Economics, 1993:1245–1249.
	Robinson WA, Krebs LU. The "real stuff" for intrathecal injection during leukemia therapy. Lancet 1982;1:283.
	Seay R, Bostrom B. Apparent compatibility of methotrexate and vancomycin. Am J Hosp Pharm 1990;47:2656–2658.

Table 47.4. *continued*

PRODUCT	AUTHORS/TITLE/CITATION
Methotrexate *cont.*	**Shapiro WR, Young DF, Mehta BM.** Methotrexate: distribution in cerebrospinal fluid after intravenous, ventricular and lumbar injections. N Engl J Med 1975;293:161–165. **Trissel LA, Tramonte SM, Grilley BJ.** Visual compatibility of ondansetron hydrochloride with selected drugs during simulated Y-site injection. Am J Hosp Pharm 1991;48:988–992.
Mitomycin	**Beijnen JH, van Gijn R, Underberg WJM.** Chemical stability of the antitumor drug mitomycin C in solutions for intravesical instillation. J Parenter Sci Technol 1990; 44:332–335. **Benvenuto JA, Anderson RW, Kerkof K, et al.** Stability and compatibility of antitumor agents in glass and plastic containers. Am J Hosp Pharm 1981;38:1914–1918. **Bristol Laboratories (personal communications).** Arbus M, Assistant Director Medical Services, Oncology. February 11, 1988. **Dorr RT, Peng Y-M, Alberts DS.** Bleomycin compatibility with selected intravenous medications. J Med 1982;13:121–130. **Keller JH.** Stability of mitomycin admixtures. Am J Hosp Pharm 1986;43:59, 64. **Physicians' Desk Reference.** 47th ed. Montvale, NJ: Medical Economics, 1993;749–751. **Quebbeman EJ, Hoffman NE, Ausman RK, et al.** Stability of mitomycin admixtures. Am J Hosp Pharm 1985;42:1750–1754. **Trissel LA, Tramonte SM, Grilley BJ.** Visual compatibility of ondansetron hydrochloride with selected drugs during simulated Y-site injection. Am J Hosp Pharm 1991;48:988–992.
Mitoxantrone	**Bjorkman S, Roth B.** Chemical compatibility of mitoxantrone and etoposide (VP-16). Acta Pharm Nord 1991;3:251. **Physicians' Desk Reference.** 47th ed. Montvale, NJ: Medical Economics, 1993:1256–1257. **Trissel LA.** Handbook of Injectable Drugs. 7th ed. Bethesda, MD: American Society of Hospital Pharmacists; 1992:628. **Trissel LA, Tramonte SM, Grilley BJ.** Visual compatibility of ondansetron hydrochloride with selected drugs during simulated Y-site injection. Am J Hosp Pharm 1991;48:988–992.
Paclitaxel	**Trissel LA, Bready BB.** Turbidimetric assessment of the compatibility of taxol with selected other drugs during simulated Y-site injection. Am J Hosp Pharm 1992;49:1716–1719. **Trissel LA, Martinez JF.** Turbidimetric assessment of the compatibility of taxol with 42 other drugs during simulated Y-site injection. Am J Hosp Pharm 1993;50:300–304. **Waugh WN, Trissel LA, Stella VJ.** Stability, compatibility, and plasticizer extraction of taxol (NSC-125973) injection diluted in infusion solutions and stored in various containers. Am J Hosp Pharm 1991;48:1520–1524.
Pentostatin	**Al-Razzak LA, Benedetti AE, Waugh WN, Valentino JS.** Chemical stability of pentostatin (NSC-218321), a cytotoxic and immunosuppressant agent. Pharm Res 1990;7:452–460. **Flora KP, Greene RF, Jackson WE, et al.** Pentostatin. In: Flora C, ed. NCI investigational drugs: pharmaceutical data. Bethesda, MD: National Cancer Institute; 1990:129. **Physicians' Desk Reference.** 47th ed. Montvale, NJ: Medical Economics, 1993:1798–1800. **Trissel LA, Tramonte SM, Grilley BJ.** Visual compatibility of ondansetron hydrochloride with selected drugs during simulated Y-site injection. Am J Hosp Pharm 1991;48:988–992.
Plicamycin	**Physicians' Desk Reference.** 47th ed. Montvale, NJ: Medical Economics, 1993:1649–1651.

Table 47.4. *continued*

PRODUCT	AUTHORS/TITLE/CITATION
Sargramostim (GM-CSF)	**Immunex Corp.** Recombinant human GM-CSF: information on reconstitution, administration, and stability. 1990. **Physicians' Desk Reference.** 47th ed. Montvale, NJ: Medical Economics, 1993:1153–1156. **Trissel LA, Bready BB, Kwan JW, Santiago NM.** Visual compatibility of sargramostim with selected antineoplastic agents, anti-infectives, and other drugs during simulated Y-site injection. Am J Hosp Pharm 1992;49:402–406.
Streptozocin	**Physicians' Desk Reference.** 47th ed. Montvale, NJ: Medical Economics, 1993:2486–2487. **Trissel LA, Kleinman LM, Davignon JP, et al.** Investigational drug information. Drug Intell Clin Pharm 1978;12:404–406.
Thiotepa	**Physicians' Desk Reference.** 47th ed. Montvale, NJ: Medical Economics, 1993:1274.
Vinblastine	**A.H. Robins.** Reglan injectable compatibility chart. May 1987. **Benvenuto JA, Anderson RW, Kerkof K, et al.** Stability and compatibility of antitumor agents in glass and plastic containers. Am J Hosp Pharm 1981;38:1914–1918. **Black J, Buechter DD, Chinn JW, et al.** Studies on the stability of vinblastine sulfate in aqueous solution. J Pharm Sci 1988;77:630–634. **Butler LD, Munson JM, DeLuca PP.** Effect of inline filtration on the potency of low-dose drugs. Am J Hosp Pharm 1980;37:935–941. **Cohen MH, Johnston-Early A, Hood MA.** Drug precipitation within IV tubing: a potential hazard of chemotherapy administration. Cancer Treat Rep 1985;69:1325–1326. **Couvreur P, Kante B, Lenaerts V, et al.** Tissue distribution of antitumor drugs associated with polyalkylcyanoacrylate nanoparticles. J Pharm Sci 1980;69:199–202. **Keller JH, Ensminger WD.** Stability of cancer chemotherapeutic agents in a totally implanted drug delivery system Am J Hosp Pharm 1982;39:1321–1323. **Physicians' Desk Reference.** 47th ed. Montvale, NJ: Medical Economics, 1993:1343–1346. **Trissel LA, Tramonte SM, Grilley BJ.** Visual compatibility of ondansetron hydrochloride with selected drugs during simulated Y-site injection. Am J Hosp Pharm 1991;48:988–992. **Vogenberg FR, Souney PF.** Stability guidelines for routinely refrigerated drug products. Am J Hosp Pharm 1983;40:101–102. **Wolfert RR, Cox RM.** Room temperature stability of drug products labeled for refrigerated storage. Am J Hosp Pharm 1975;32:585–587.
Vincristine	**A.H. Robins.** Reglan injectable compatibility chart. May 1987. **Beijnen JH, Neef C, Meuwissen OJAT, et al.** Stability of intravenous admixtures of doxorubicin and vincristine. Am J Hosp Pharm 1986;43:3002–3027. **Beijnen JH, Vendrig DEMM, Underberg WJM.** Stability of vinca alkaloid anticancer drugs in three commonly used infusion fluids. J Parenter Sci Technol 1989;43:84–87. **Benvenuto JA.** Errors in oncologic agent stability study. Am J Hosp Pharm 1983;40:1628. **Benvenuto JA, Anderson RW, Kerkof K, et al.** Stability and compatibility of antitumor agents in glass and plastic containers. Am J Hosp Pharm 1981;38:1914–1918. **Butler LD, Munson JM, DeLuca PP.** Effect of inline filtration on the potency of low-dose drugs. Am J Hosp Pharm 1980;37:935–941. **Cohen MH, Johnston-Early A, Hood MA.** Drug precipitation within IV tubing: a potential hazard of chemotherapy administration. Cancer Treat Rep 1985;69:1325–1326. **Ennis CE, Merritt RJ, Neff DN.** In vitro study of inline filtration of medications commonly administered to pediatric cancer patients. J Parenter Enter Nutr 1983;7:156–158. **Kanke M, Eubanks JL, DeLuca PP.** Binding of selected drugs to a treated inline filter. Am J Hosp Pharm 1983;40:1323–1328. **McRae MP, King JC.** Compatibility of antineoplastic, antibiotic and corticosteroid drugs in intravenous admixtures. Am J Hosp Pharm 1976;33:1010–1013.

Table 47.4. *continued*

PRODUCT	AUTHORS/TITLE/CITATION
	Physicians' Desk Reference. 47th ed. Montvale, NJ: Medical Economics, 1993:1327–1328.
	Trissel LA, Tramonte SM, Grilley BJ. Visual compatibility of ondansetron hydrochloride with selected drugs during simulated Y-site injection. Am J Hosp Pharm 1991;48:988–992.
	Vogenberg FR, Souney PF. Stability guidelines for routinely refrigerated drug products. Am J Hosp Pharm 1983;40:101–102.
	Wolfert RR, Cox RM. Room temperature stability of drug products labeled for refrigerated storage. Am J Hosp Pharm 1975;32:585–587.

48

Patient Education

Mary H. Johnson and Verna A. Rhodes

In today's health care arena, patient education presents additional challenges. Patients with cancer and their family/friend support groups must solve myriad problems and symptoms that result from disease(s), treatment, and learning to live with pathologic condition(s). Appropriate patient education that provides proactive management of the symptoms experienced is of utmost importance to allay fears and to promote/enhance quality of life. In the United States, 85% of the estimated 1,252,000 new cases of cancer annually will receive antineoplastic treatment (i.e., surgery, radiation, chemotherapy, and/or a combination) (1). The increasing prevalence of cancer across the life span, especially beyond age 55 years, shortened hospital stays, and increased outpatient treatment have shifted the responsibility for symptom management to patients and their families. Chemotherapy agents are used as primary and adjunct treatment for most of this expanding number of new cancer cases. Most patients receiving chemotherapy will be treated in ambulatory care settings (e.g., offices, clinics, work place). Shortened hospital stays and the pronounced increase in outpatient antineoplastic treatments have limited the amount of time for patient preparation, education, and guidance. Yet, inherent in nursing is the responsibility to provide sufficient educational instruction, information, and materials to enable patients to perform adequate self-care (2). Self-care consists of activities initiated and performed by patients to maintain or improve their current health (3). Although important for all, these actions pertain particularly to an outpatient population (4–6).

DEMOGRAPHIC SOCIOECONOMIC FACTORS AFFECTING PATIENT EDUCATION

Changing demographic patterns in our country point to an increasing older population. Today, approximately 12.5% of the people are over 65 years of age. This represents a 22.3% increase in this population within the last decade. Projected percentage increases by the year 2025 for the following age groups are 65 to 74 years, 10.7%; 75 to 84 years, 5.9%; and 85 years and over, 2.1%. By the year 2030, 21% of the population, or almost 1 in 4, will be over 65 years of age (7). The number of people 85 years of age or over is increasing three to four times faster than any other age group. At present, 50% of all cancers occur after age 65; this percentage will rise as the number of elderly people increases (1, 5, 8). People 65 years and over may experience more than one cancer during their lifetime.

With this extended life span, functional capacities and needs vary widely within the 40-year span from 55 to 95 years of age. Neugarten refers to those aged 55 to 74 as "young-old" and to those 75 years of age or more as "old-old." The "healthy elderly" and the "frail elderly" are two other terms that are also used. This latter terminology, relating to functional abilities, is particularly useful from a health care perspective (11–15). As the number of centenarians increases, the age span for this single developmental stage (from 55 to over 100 years of age) approximates that of all others (from infancy through midadulthood). The goal of health care is to foster successful aging, as demonstrated by an ability to perform self-care and to adjust to the detrimental changes while continuing to grow and contribute to society (10, 12, 14, 16–17).

Persons age 55 years and older may still have children living at home. In addition, the household may have one or more dependent parents and/or grandparents in or outside the home. The expansion of employed adults within a single household and the diverse geographic locations of family or potential caregivers are among socioeconomic factors to be considered. These demographic changes have multiple implications for oncology nurses and necessitate a complete patient assessment.

PATIENT ASSESSMENT

Assessment provides information about the patient's ability to perform self-care before, during, and after therapy. This information is used as a basis for making nursing judgments and decisions affecting the patient's therapeutic self-care demand/need or a summation of action to be taken, work, and/or teaching to be done. An assessment of basic conditioning factors, including personal and sociocultural factors, patterns of living, health state, and developmental state, provides the foundation for building teaching strategies (3, 14, 18). This information is essential for effective education. Table 48.1 lists the basic conditioning factors (3). Educational needs may change during the course of cancer, so assessment and teaching must be an ongoing and dynamic process (20–21)

The information gained from the nursing assessment helps determine the nurse's role in patient education. A sample basic conditioning factor assessment (Table 48.2) follows the discussion of individual basic conditioning factors. Goals for education should be established with the patient and family. Teaching is easier if

Table 48.1. Basic Conditioning Factors

Sets of Basic Conditioning Factors (BCFs)

Personal and sociocultural (age, sex, family, social, cultural, etc.)

Pattern of living, including self-care practices that are an integral part of the pattern

Health state and health care systems (symptoms and actions taken in response to symptoms)

Development state and system, including self-management system and the ability to manage the system

the patient desires and expects to learn about anticipated treatment. Regardless of their degree of participation in the education process, patients will become immersed in the experience of living with the diagnosis of cancer and the effects of chemotherapy. Continued assessment of these experiences guides the patient educator in developing strategies to assist the patient in attaining an optimal quality of life.

Personal and Sociocultural Factors

An assessment of the patient's age, sex, family, and number of persons with whom the patient resides yields helpful information relevant to self-care and to possible patient education strategies. Whether or not the patient is employed and his/her occupation may influence self-care management. Tasks for each stage of life must also be considered in relation to the individual patient (see Table 48.3) (13, 15, 22, 23). An individual, comprehensive assessment is required because of the older population's diversified personal, psychologic, and sociocultural involvements. Regardless of age, attention must be given to the individual's social role, self-concept, and self-esteem. Signs of role strain (i.e., social isolation, decreased self-esteem, altered self-concept, and coping difficulties) may occur. There is a high potential for role change, particularly later in life and/or with changes in usual self-care abilities (3, 8–17, 20–24). Although the educational level attained is important in assessment, instructional methods depend on more than the number of years of formal schooling. Patients who cannot read or who have learning disabilities require special consideration (24, 27). These special situations are discussed later in the chapter.

The sociocultural orientation of the patient, including values and attitudes, are also assessed. The patient's value system may differ from that of the health care provider, and these differences must be respected. For example, self-help may not be valued by some cultures. Evidence of consistent attentiveness to self-care and potential health care needs by patient, family, and/or significant others and the ability to make judgments and carry out actions is important at all ages. Individuals who view self independently of others and as being of value are usually more motivated to accept and manage treatment regimens. Note patients' expressions about how they are affected by what they have been experiencing. Listen for statements about limitations in

Table 48.2. Example of an Assessment of the Basic Conditioning Factors

Personal and sociocultural

Age	35 years
Sex	Female
Family	Married (2nd marriage) with 2 daughters, 12 and 14, and a son 8 (daughter from first marriage); mother and father deceased, 2 sisters, 1 brother
Education level	College graduate
Occupation	Teacher
Religion	Methodist, attends regularly
Sociocultural orientation	Caucasian, middle class, raised in Midwest
Relevant life experience	Both parents died at an early age (with cancer before patient turned 30)
Social roles	Wife, mother, sister, breadwinner

Patterns of living

Living environment and family system	Lives with husband and children 100 miles from treatment center
Health habits (S-C practices)	Considers herself to have good body and oral hygiene; teeth are in good repair; overweight; doesn't exercise; sees dentist regularly; inconsistent with BSE; has not enrolled in cancer-screening program; sees doctor for routine yearly pap smear; and gets suntanned every summer
	Takes Tylenol for headaches; daily multiple vitamin; birth control pills
Support systems	Main source of support are close friends—husband does not cope well with problems; sisters are usually supportive but having difficulty dealing with patient's diagnosis; patient has always provided emotional support for the family
Preferred learning style	Is an avid reader; feels comfortable in groups but prefers reading and one-to-one demonstrations

Health state and health care systems

Present health state	Recently diagnosed with breast cancer; patient sought medical help after she discovered a breast lump while taking a shower; had mastectomy with reconstruction and is preparing to take adjuvant chemotherapy
Present health concerns	Treatment and duration, side effects of chemotherapy, prognosis, and financial concerns
Previous health concerns and self-care actions	3 normal pregnancies—only hospitalizations were for childbirth
Perception of health care	Views system as helpful—patient wants to be an informed consumer and involved in decision-making
Developmental state	Early adult transitions
Self-management system for care— physical, emotional, spiritual	Readily seeks medical advice when she has a problem; looks to close friends for emotional support; feels she has strong spiritual faith— does not seek counseling from minister

self-care activities and the amount of energy required for performance.

Relevant life experiences (e.g., other illnesses and/or hospitalizations) may reveal attitudes and values pertinent to the present illness. Patients often indicate how they have previously coped with various symptoms or state what teaching methods have been helpful in other situations. The life experiences of others who have had meaningful roles in their lives may also be influential.

Patterns of Living

Information is obtained about how the patient and family are coping with and responding to the diagnosis of cancer and the array of demands created by illness. The nurse also needs to understand the common coping patterns of significant others. Coping affects learning, and the acquisition of knowledge serves as a coping mechanism for some patients. Thus, teaching may alleviate anxiety caused by lack of knowl-

Table 48.3. Adult Developmental States—Task to Be Assessed

Stages	Tasks (Theorist)	Family Lifestyle—Tasks/Roles (Age Varies)
Departure from home Age 18–22	Intimacy vs. isolation (Erickson, Peck) Choose study/career/work Break psychologic ties Develop peer relationships Manage time/home	
Early adult Age 23–28	Select mate/marriage adjustments Parenting Launch occupational career ladder (Havinghurst) Start civic responsibility	Wife/husband Wife/mother Husband/father Infant (daughter and/or son)

Beginning the third decade
Age 29–34
	Early adult transition (Levinson)
	Settling down
	   Search for personal values
	   Reappraise relationships
		↓
		↓
		Daughter/sister
		Son/brother

Midlife evaluation Age 35–43	Reexamine marriage/work/child relationships Search for meaning Reevaluate personal priorities and values Relate to aging parents Adjust to single life Stress management	↓ ↓ ↓
Midlife revitalization Age 44–55	Generativity vs. stagnation/self-absorption (Erickson) Valuing wisdom vs. physical relationships (Peck) Emotional flexibility vs. emotional impoverishment Mental flexibility vs. mental rigidity Socializing vs. sexualizing relationships Launch teenage children Adjust to empty nest Adjust to realities of work (Havinghurst) Maturing relationship with spouse Adult social and civic responsibilities Adjusting to physiologic changes Developing leisure activities	 Wife, mother, grandmother Husband, father, grandfather ↓

	Varied Classification of Task (Theorist)	

	Ego integrity vs. despair (Erickson)
	
	Ego differentiation vs. work role preoccupation/
	  recognizing physical decline (Peck)
	Ego transcendence vs. ego preoccupation/
	  acceptance of one's own death without fear
		Widow/widower
		Wife, mother, grandmother
		Husband, father, grandfather
		↓
		
		↓

Elderly adult Age 55+	Adjusting to retirement, social role changes, health decline, death of spouse (Havinghurst) Establishing satisfactory living arrangements	↓ ↓
Preretirement Age 56–64	Midlife transition Payoff years (Levinson)	↓
Retirement Age 65+	Reassess finances Disengage from paid work Deeper personal relations Finance new leisure Adjust to health problems Adjust to loss of mate Manage stress accompanying change	Widow/widower Wife, mother, grandmother Great-grandmother Husband, father, grandfather, Great-grandfather ↓

Table 48.3—*continued*

Stages	Tasks (Theorist)		Family Lifestyle—Tasks/Roles (Age Varies)
	Varied Classification of Task (Theorist)		
Young old	Healthy old	90%	
Age 55–74 (Neugarten)	well	60%	↓
	moderately impaired	30%	
	or		
Old old			
Age 75+ (Neugarten)	Frail old	10%	Widow/widower
			Wife, mother, grandmother
			Great-grandmother,
			Great-great grandmother
			Husband, father, grandfather,
			Great-grandfather, Great-
			great-grandfather

edge. Patients experiencing anxiety who do not use learning as a coping strategy will require appropriate interventions to decrease anxiety before learning can take place.

The extent of the patient's involvement, as well as that of other family members within the larger context of community and neighborhood, is relevant in determining and evaluating the quality of self-care. It is important to appraise the influence of these patterns and structures on the development and adequacy of an individual's self-care ability. Family structure should be assessed for accessibility and willingness to help. Older patients may consider treatment choices and knowledge related to side effects of treatment and care to be the sole responsibility of the health care providers. In addition, there may be family problems that interfere with the patient's ability to concentrate on learning. The impact of illness on the financial status of the family should be estimated and addressed as needed (13, 17, 28).

Identification of key support persons and the nature of support derived from their social network may indicate gaps or weaknesses in the person's support system that, in turn, may suggest the need for intervention to promote social and emotional health and to assist with care. Social support reaffirms a person's sense of personal worth and is important in the adjustment to chronic disease. Mounting evidence shows that social support has a positive effect on health status, lessening the effects of psychosocial and physical stress on the individual by increasing coping ability. Both self-esteem and social support are indicators of positive lifestyle and self-care practices (29, 30). Social support facilitates

compliance (31). Family members or significant others need to be included in the teaching process and provided information about the patient's current status and expected progress. These strategies may assist them in being more supportive of the patient. Family and natural helping networks are essential sources of social support for the elderly; the trend toward varied geographic locations away from central family support systems may add to the care dilemma. Traditionally, women have been the caregivers; however, the changing roles of women in the work place and the expectations of formal organizations in providing solutions to the problems of the ill, the infirm, and particularly the elderly may present conflicts.

Teaching strategies are also used to support the patient's value system. Language barriers present an obvious challenge. Clarity of meaning must also be considered. Some commonly used words may have a different meaning for the patient than that intended by the nurse (or physician), and inappropriate information may be gained (4, 32–34).

Little is currently known about patient learning styles. One way to obtain this information is to ask patients, "How do you go about learning something new?" Patients may be more attentive to information about prognosis and treatment than to that about diagnostic tests (35). The educator builds on self-care measures that the patient identifies during assessment. Some concepts may need to be unlearned, and others relearned. For example, a patient who has always taken aspirin for fever will need to know that this is not appropriate while receiving chemotherapy.

Health State and Health Care System

Health care includes data about aspects of human structure, function, and symptomatology. The patient, family/significant others, nurses, physicians, other members of the health care team, and the medical record are sources of information. The health state assessment is evaluated in terms of normality by age group and/or degree and extent of pathology. Assessment of the patient's health belief system, health state, self-care actions, and perception of health care is a continuous process. Recent studies revealed that the reality of patients' experiences after treatment were not what they anticipated (36–38). The patient's physical symptoms must be considered in assessing readiness to learn. Symptoms such as pain or fatigue can be barriers to learning and may also affect retention. Although concentration is often considered to be a type of fatigue, Cimprich (39) reported the importance of assessing and differentiating between concentration and alertness (39). If physical symptoms are present, it will be helpful to know how the patient has dealt with them. Visual acuity, hearing loss, and use of certain medications can affect learning at any age but are more likely to be problems in the elderly. Previous experiences with the diagnosis and treatment of cancer may reveal useful information in understanding patients' fears and misconceptions. Most patients have some knowledge about cancer and chemotherapy, obtained from magazines, newspapers, television, and radio or from relatives or friends who have received chemotherapy. Cancer and its treatment continue to be equated with death, pain, alienation, helplessness, and hopelessness (40–43). The public considers chemotherapy to have more negative side effects than surgery or radiation therapy (44–46). In spite of advanced scientific progress, antineoplastic drugs are sometimes viewed as palliative at best, rather than curative. During the initial phase of diagnosis, patients need information to assist them in making decisions about treatment options. Patients in the throes of making major decisions are most vulnerable to promoters of questionable therapies (46). Informed consent is discussed later in the chapter.

Developmental State and System

In adulthood, major developmental tasks, as well as family life cycle roles, are determined within a social context by the interaction of individuals with their social systems (Table 48.3).

Although models for understanding adult development are based on the premise that adult development occurs in definable, predictable, and sequential patterns, the functional differentiation among the "healthy" and "frail" elderly is less determinable (13, 15, 23, 26). In addition, the actual timetable when certain tasks (e.g., marriage, parenting) occur may vary. Developmental state encompasses not only learning to live with oneself as one changes but learning to live in a particular way, dependent upon a set of values or as one's culture changes. For example, morale in older persons, as in younger individuals, is affected by socioeconomic status, educational level, and age-related role changes; however, health status is an important determinant of morale in older individuals. Hence, the nurse educator must be cognizant of the powerful psychologic impact of disease, particularly cancer, and attempt to minimize the negative psychologic effects of disease and dysfunction.

Patients undergoing antineoplastic therapy may offer verbal and nonverbal cues signifying spiritual needs that affect their ability to care for self. The patient's definition and perception of spirituality should be clarified. In an effort to assess and to develop plans to support or intervene with patients' spiritual needs, patient educators must first define their own personal perspective of spirituality. Spiritual beliefs range from Judeo-Christian and Moslem to secular humanism, Eastern mysticism, and occult views, among others. Religion is not synonymous with spirituality. Instead, religion is an organized expression of spirituality. The definition of spirituality varies (e.g., inner being, energy fields, eternal essence, oneness with nature and universe). Spirituality, particularly for the elderly, can be devoid of a religious context and simply be an affirmation of life or life lived fully (47). Spirituality also is considered a belief in something beyond the physical nature, a sense of a force beyond oneself, a life-giving and integrating energy. Concerns regarding the concepts of hope, courage, love, good, evil, et cetera universally evolve while living with this chronic disease (48). A survey of 76 health education professionals explored the meaning of spirituality and found that spirituality (*a*) is a unifying force, (*b*) provides meaning in life, (*c*) is a common bond between individuals, and (*d*) is based on individual perceptions, values, and faith. Patients may experience considerable distress, e.g., mental anguish or suffering (34) or spiritual distress regarding life forces or varied beliefs. Some patients are prone to rely on their religion in times of crises, while others may begin searching for spiritual truths and/or acknowledge their reliance on a higher power. The former individuals' spiritual distress is limited, compared with that of the latter group; yet, a positive outcome may result if the struggle brings a person to a deeper understanding of life and a deeper sense of peace, meaning, and purpose. If the struggle or distress leads the individual to feel abandoned, isolated, or without hope, it is a negative experience (47). Spiritual activities commonly used to cope with illness include praying, reading the Bible, talking to clergy, and receiving communion. Nurses need to support the patient's beliefs as a strength and resource, yet make it specific to that person's spiritual background (47–49). Raleigh studied 45 patients with cancer and 45 patients with chronic illnesses to identify sources of hope (50). The most commonly reported strategies that supported hope or raised hope were (a) getting busy doing something, (b) prayer or religious activities, (c) thinking about other things, and (d) talking to others. It behooves nurses caring for cancer patients to be cognizant of patients' use of spiritual coping strategies in an effort to improve their knowledge, interventions, and instruction to other health care providers (49, 51).

Family members and significant others are a part of the developmental system and a real presence in the life of the patient with cancer. The effect of social support on quality of life has been documented. In fact, "family" ranked first as a source supporting hope (50). A collaborative relationship between the health care team, the patient, and a supportive family and/or significant other is ideal. Unfortunately, some family systems may be a hindrance rather than a help in the self-care management of the person living with cancer, its chronicity, and its concomitant medical therapies. Innovative strategies may be required to help the patient and family support system not only meet new sets of demands that are not among their usual knowledge and skills but also reorder time, adjust to changes in the course of the disease, prevent social isolation, and normalize interactions with others. The self-management system depends not only on the knowledge of what to do but also on the ability to discriminate and to make judgments and decisions (40, 52–54).

CONCEPTUAL FRAMEWORK

Orem's self-care deficit theory of nursing provides the conceptual framework for this chapter.

It is one of several nursing theories that guide the nurse in planning and implementing patient care. The self-care deficit theory of nursing is based on the premise that all individuals are capable of self-care. The self-care act contains three elements: the capacity or potential for action (self-care agency), the demand or requisite for action (self-care demand), and the method or measure appropriate to meet the required action (3).

Patients with cancer experience many new demands or needs for self-care. Much of the care for this chronic multistage disease is in the home, which demands knowledge of not only what to do to prevent and/or manage symptoms but also what to report to the health care provider. For example, the experience of nausea, vomiting, and retching by the postchemotherapy patient produces new demands or needs for self-care actions (18, 41, 42, 52). The response to these new demands depends upon patients' knowledge of what to do when symptoms occur, their care capabilities, and their capacity to perform the needed self-care action (3, 18, 52–55). Two steps to assist the patient in achieving self-care for this or other demands are (a) identifying and prioritizing the unmet needs (deficits) and (b) selecting appropriate methods of assisting that overcome or compensate for those deficits.

Self-care agency refers to a set of human abilities for meeting self-care requisites such as acquiring knowledge, making decisions, and taking action for change. The patient's level of self-care agency is determined by a thorough assessment of the basic conditioning factors (Table 48.1). Self-care activities are defined as learned, deliberate behaviors on behalf of oneself (3, 18, 20, 53–55). All individuals require self-care agency in three major categories of demand: universal (i.e., air, food, water), developmental (i.e., maturation, prevention of deleterious effects related to development), and health deviation (i.e., self-care requisites arising from medical therapy). Self-care agency is stimulated when a patient experiences a therapeutic self-care demand. The phrase "therapeutic self-care demand" refers to sets of actions that are needed to perform or obtain specific elements of therapeutic care. Within an individual, the interaction of therapeutic self-care demand and self-care agency are crucial components of their self-care system (3, 18, 41, 52–56).

Self-care deficits occur when the person cannot engage in one or more required self-care activities. Patients with cancer may experience many therapeutic self-care demands for which they have inadequate self-care agency. Self-care deficits may be health-related or health-derived limitations that render an individual incapable of effective or complete self-care. This deficit state signals the need for nursing. The nurse's ability or power to act on behalf of the patient to compensate for this lack is then needed and is called nurse agency (Fig. 48.1). An important aspect of nursing agency, which is a part of the broader nursing system, is the ability of nurses to assess and provide care that compensates for or aids in meeting these self-care deficits. Nursing system is that continuing series of actions and knowledge-based judgments produced by nurses in a helping environment that includes both patient and nurse variables (3).

Figure 48.1. illustrates the theoretical integration of the elements of self-care and nursing agency. Methods of assisting patients include guiding, teaching, supporting, coaching, doing for, and providing a therapeutic environment. "Doing for" implies a passive recipient of care, focuses directly on the therapeutic self-care demand, and is wholly compensatory in nature. Other methods of assisting focus on facilitating and activating the patient's self-care agency (18, 41, 52–56) and are, therefore, only partially compensatory or supportive-educative in nature.

PATIENT EDUCATION TEACHING LEARNING CORRELATES

Patient education is an integral part of nursing care and may involve one or more methods of assisting (i.e., guidance, support, provision of a developmental environment, doing for, and teaching). Of these, teaching is a more restricted method of assisting that is prescribed when the patient is deficient in the skill or knowledge needed to care for self. It is an interactive process that can support the development of new knowledge and/or skills. Watson distinguishes teaching as a method of assisting patients to resume self-care (35). Patient teaching is more than merely conveying information to the patient or some unknown process of information synthesis occurring within the patient that results in an appropriate patient response (57–59). The nurse as teacher facilitates learning. The nurse must be knowledgeable about the disease and antici-

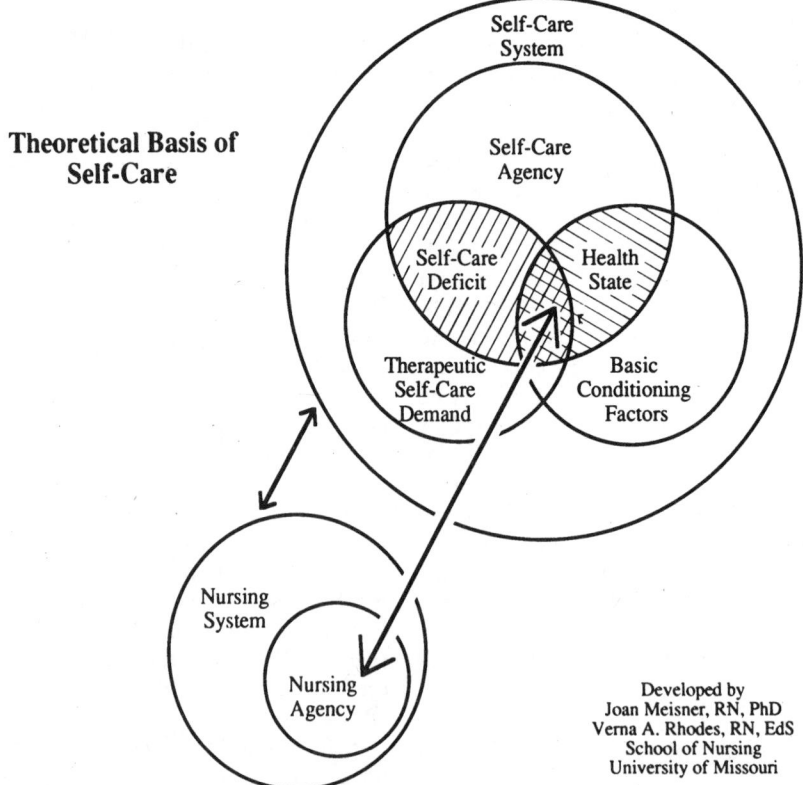

Figure 48.1.   Theoretical integration of the self-care component.

pated treatment to gain the trust and confidence of the patient as well as to devise an appropriate teaching plan. Additional requisites of nurse agency critical for the successful performance of this role are (*a*) realness or genuineness, (*b*) nonpossessive caring and prizing, (*c*) empathetic understanding, (*d*) trust and respect, and (*e*) sensitive and accurate listening (60–65).

Caring is the essence of nursing. This pivotal factor is essential for patient education and the teaching-learning process. Caring may encompass each of the additional requisites. Caring in a professional nurse-patient relationship has been referred to as "the direct or indirect nurturant and skillful activities, processes, and decisions related to assisting people to achieve or maintain health" (60, 62–65).

Proactive prophylactic strategies are essential; yet, the emotional and psychologic needs of patients and caregivers must be evaluated on an ongoing basis. A critical step in the development of an appropriate teaching plan is for the nurse educator to accurately assess and understand patients' perceptions of not only their condition and their learning needs but also the most important nurse caring behaviors. Current research suggests that patients appear to value nurses' instrumental or technical caring skills (e.g., knowing how to give shots, start intravenous fluids, manage equipment) more highly than nurses do. Conversely, nurses rank their expressive behaviors (e.g., listening, talking, psychosocial skills) higher (62–65). Nurses may be assuming a certain level of technical competence in their individual practice, while patients may not have that same assurance. Continued research is warranted to better understand the perceptions on the concept of care held by nurses and patients. While the specific components of caring and nurse caring behaviors lack scientific description and definition, caring is considered of utmost importance in the patient education/teaching-learning process.

Learning

Learning is a change in human disposition or capability that persists over time (16, 57–59, 66). In other words, learning is an associative process that takes place inside an organism but may also lead to an observable change in behavior. It is implied by a relatively permanent change in behavior. For example, the immunosuppressed patient who has overcome an infectious process now carefully monitors visitors for signs of infection. Principles of learning (Table 48.4) (16,

57–59, 66) need to be used in planning patient education.

The three domains of learning are cognitive, psychomotor, and affective. Each domain contains specific activities, which are listed (Table 48.5) in ascending order of complexity. Cognitive learning specifies processes primarily related to intellectual activities necessary for understanding diseases and treatment alternatives. Psychomotor learning leads to skilled physical movements such as those required for giving an injection, changing a dressing, and caring for a venous access catheter. Affective learning relates to the patient's feelings and attitudes regarding cancer diagnosis and treatment plan. Attitudes toward altered self-concept, diagnosis, and treatment plan are a part of the affective domain. These are developed and organized by learning and appear to be affected and amenable to change by a caring, empathetic nurse educator (Table 48.5) (57–59).

The learning process depends upon internal conditions (e.g., cognitive ability and readiness) as well as external events (e.g., the patient's environment). Instruction or teaching may be defined as those events external to the learner that are designed to promote learning. In other words, teaching is that part of the patient's external environment that directs, stimulates, encourages, and guides learning activities. Some of the characteristics of a good learning situation are listed in Table 48.6 (3, 11, 16, 57–59, 66).

Patient education is most effective and satisfactory when the patient feels a need for knowledge or skill. Voluntary participation and self-pacing are essential. Efficiency of performance must not be confused with power to learn. Adverse elementary or secondary school experiences may influence patients' attitudes and readiness for learning. Older adults may learn slowly because of preexisting and current disease (5). Loss of concentration can reduce the ability to retain important information or adhere to complex treatment regimens (39). Some may lack confidence in their ability to learn new material and adapt to new therapeutic self-care demands. The rate of learning is improved by motivation, and the nurse educator must use appropriate teaching methods, based upon an individual patient's assessment data (11, 12, 16, 67, 68).

ANALYSIS OF BCF ASSESSMENT FOR PLANNING PATIENT EDUCATION

The completed Basic Conditioning Factors (BCF) Assessment provides a database for all

Table 48.4. Principles of Learning

- Learning is individual.
  Each learner differs from another.
  Good teaching must consider the individual differences.
  How individuals learn may be more important than what they learn.
  The most enduring motivation for learning is internal motivation.
- Learning is possible for all ages in the absence of dementing disease.
  Teaching techniques/strategies should accommodate common age-related sensory changes, i.e., enlarged lettering for visuals, attention to enunciation, clarity, and volume of speech.
  The rate, speed, or pace of instruction should be slower for the older population.
- Learning is patterned.
  It has a system of organized and systematic responses at all stages of the learning process. The learner responds as a "whole person" in a unified manner to the "whole" situation.
  There is no typical personality of old age; instead, there is a continuity with previous patterns.
- Learning is active.
  It does not take place without activity by the learner.
  Adults are active processors of information (not sponges or receptacles into which knowledge is poured).
  What is learned will not depend on actual content only, but on what the patient already knows and on how the individual processes the information received.
- Learning is purposeful.
  Learning is effective to the degree to which it is directed by the learner toward the attainment of a worthwhile goal.
  Informed learning is most likely to occur when information is made meaningful to the patient.
  It is important to ascertain the patient's perceptions of the event. (How meaningful and/or important the situation is to his/her life may relate to how the patient handles the topic.) Level of instruction necessitates an evaluation of the patient's intellectual capabilities—too difficult, too easy.
  Patient education materials should be phrased between a sixth and eighth grade level.
- Learning is creative.
  It is the acquisition of knowledge, mastery of skills, the attainment of understanding, and, for the particular learner, is a new way of acting.
  Adults learn in a variety of patterns. Factors to be considered in selecting teaching techniques:
    Preferred learning style
    Learning patterns in use
    Characteristics of the learner (analyze: i.e., homemaker, professor, barber)
    Your own abilities
- Learning transfers.
  Transfer depends on understanding; understanding depends upon the discovery of essential relationships that have been generalized by the learner and deliberately applied to the solution of practical problems.

nursing. This chapter focuses primarily on the findings that enable the nurse educator to make judgments about the existing health care situation and decisions about what teaching can and must be done. A series of questions should be posed (3, 53, 54):

1. What actions are needed to perform self-care, i.e., what is the therapeutic self-care demand?
2. Does the patient have a deficit preventing self-care to meet the specific therapeutic self-care demand?
3. If so, what is it? and why does it exist? For example, Is there a lack of willingness to learn? Is there a learning disability? Does the patient have insufficient energy to accomplish a task even though the steps are well memorized and understood?
4. What family member/significant other can provide assistance without disrupting the patient's previously developed self-care capabilities?
5. What is the patient's potential for performing self-care at a future time? increasing or deepening self-care knowledge? fostering a desire to engage in self-care? consistently merging essential new and old self-care measures into the system of self-care and daily living?

The specific plan of instruction uses answers to these questions. Patients who have been included in the discussion of their therapeutic self-

Table 48.5. Learning Domains and Associated Activities for Patient Learning

Learning Domains	What the Nurse Can Do to Help Patients Learn

Cognitive domain
Fact learning (memorization)
  Repeat the facts
  Pay attention
  Intend to learn
  Make the new information meaningful
	Repeat information; ask patients to repeat information.
	Draw patients' attention, and emphasize what is important. Tell the patients you will ask them to repeat it. Reinforce attention on following visit and before discharge.
	Explain how and why the information must be learned.
	Use examples that are important and meaningful to the patients. Use analogies common to them. Ask patients to explain how the information related to their life, to previous experience, etc.

Concept learning (classification, i.e., putting things into categories according to establish criteria)
  Practice categorizing by guessing and receiving feedback
  Make the concept meaningful
  Differentiate this concept from similar concepts
	Give patients simple, clear examples and incorrect examples of the concepts. Allow patients to guess, i.e., "Yes, that is an example of infection" or "No."
	Give detailed feedback about why the response is correct or incorrect.
	Use examples that are important and meaningful to patients. Ask the patients to give examples of the concept in their life.
	Point out similarities and differences to like concepts during feedback. Given patients progressively more refined examples and give incorrect examples that are part of a similar category.

Principle (a comprehensive and fundamental law, doctrine or assumption)
Problem solving (application of rules in unique situations and setting)
  Restate the previously learned concepts needed to understand the rule.
  Put the rule together in own words.
  Demonstrate or describe instances in which the rule is applied.
  Use the rule to solve hypothetical self-care problems that are realistic to patient's own home situation.
	Be sure patients know the related concepts well.
	Give verbal instructions:
	1. State expected performance.
	2. Get patients to recall component concepts.
	3. Give verbal cues for the rules as a whole.
	4. Ask patients to demonstrate the rule.
	5. Ask patients to verbally state the rule (e.g., if white blood cells are mature and adequate in number, then they will fight infection).
	6. Give patients realistic situations that might occur at home and ask them to describe what they would do in the situation. If patients have difficulty solving the problem, give hints to the solution, but do not solve it for them.
	7. Provide positive reinforcement at each step in learning the rule and solving the problem.
	8. Space review of solving problem situations using the rule over time. Use simple situations first, then add complexity to the situation.

Psychomotor domain (Motor skill learning, i.e., activities that require coordinated muscular movement and practice) Memorize the steps in the procedure. Practice each subtask until smooth and correct. Put all subtasks together into entire procedure. Practice until correct and smooth. Continue to practice the skill until it is automatic, i.e., can be done without thinking about each step.	Acting for—doing for until skill learned. Break the procedure into small subtasks. Direct the patient's attention to each subtask and the sequence of tasks. Demonstrate the procedure as a whole and each subtask individually. Stay with patients while they perform each subtask. Verbally guide them through task. Do not allow errors to occur. If an error occurs, stop patients immediately and have them start that subtask from the beginning. Do not distract patients by explaining things during practice. Allow complete concentration on the task. Provide feedback at each step. Verbally guide patients as they link each subtask. Provide feedback. Again, do not allow errors to occur. Do not leave patients unattended to practice until they are performing the entire procedure without error.

Table 48.5—*continued*

Learning Domains	What the Nurse Can Do to Help Patients Learn
Affective domain (relating to, arising from, or influencing feelings or emotions; expressing emotions—deals with attitudes, values, and preferences Predisposition to act Interact with and observe the behavior of the model. Pay attention to the facts presented. Experience dissonance or discomfort if attitudes presented are inconsistent with previously held attitudes. Evaluate own belief system. Try new attitudes and act as if they were his own.	Make sure patients understand the concepts that are important in the attitude (e.g., cancer treatment with chemotherapy) Build up the model (person with desired attitude) as highly credible (e.g., the reach to recovery volunteer or a fellow ostomy patient). Provide patients with relevant facts related to the attitude (e.g., people with cancer can live normal lives). Provides patients with positive reinforcement as they try new or changed attitude.

Adapted and reprinted by permission from Watson, PM. Patient education: the adult with cancer. Nurs Clin North Am 1982;17(4).

care demands usually are motivated to learn. At this point, the patient is the key determinant of what the self-care task is and how it is to be learned.

Analysis for Learning Self-Care Task

Based on an analysis of the BCF assessment, the following questions must be addressed: What does the patient need to learn? What learning need(s) is the most urgent for self-care?

Select the first prioritized learning need or task. Break that learning task into minute logical segments. This task description or analysis lists all of the steps in a process in order of their occurrence (57).

Starting with the first prioritized written learning objective, ask yourself the following:

STATED TASKS

Query: "For the patient to do this, what does he or she have to do or know?"

RELATED SUBTASKS

Query: "For the patient to be able to do this, what subtask does he or she have to be able to do or know?"

RELATED SPECIFIC SUBTASKS

Query: "Is this behavioral segment already known by the patient?" If yes, use the prioritized learning objective as the first learning task in the sequence of steps. If no, continue to formulate additional enabling steps or objectives until you reach the knowledge level of the patient. In other words, how far the steps are broken down in a

task description depends upon the knowledge base of the patient. Task description is not designed to analyze prerequisite skills for a task but merely to list the steps of task performance in correct order (58).

After determining which tasks or steps the patient needs to know, take the first learning task stated as a specific outcome and determine appropriate learning strategies.

SPECIFIC LEARNING STRATEGIES FOR THE TASKS (TABLE 48.5)

Inquire: "What type of learning is this?" cognitive, psychomotor, or affective?

This step, determining the type of learning required by the task, is crucial for successful patient learning. Different learning styles are used to learn different material. As nursing students, the way one learned the names of the 206 bones in the human body (fact learning) differed from the way one learned to don sterile gloves (psychomotor learning). Furthermore, the ability to list the side effects of antineoplastic drugs (fact learning) was acquired differently from the ability to recognize that a platelet count of 20,000/mm^3 indicates possible bleeding problems (concept learning). These two examples still differ from how the nurse reaches a decision regarding the patient with a low platelet count who evidences bleeding gums (problem solving).

Using patient assessment data and following the above steps to classify the required type of learning, a prescription of specific teaching activities based upon educational research may be designed for the patient, matching the learning

Table 48.6. Desirable Characteristics for a Good Learning Situation

- Instructor helps the patients perceive their problem and direct their activities toward its solution and should assist the patient in understanding the goals of treatments.
  Discover what the patient wants from it.
- Physical environment that promotes comfort:
  Furniture should be appropriate for adult comfort.
  Varied room accessories may assist the oncology patient.
  Ventilation, heat, lighting, and outside noise should be controlled.
  A refreshment or "break" area is helpful in outpatient facilities.
- Active patient/family participation in the teaching/learning process.
- Teaching methods are planned in accordance with the patient's learning style. A variety of methods (e.g., learning by doing) may assist in learning.
- Use reinforcement by repetition.
  Repetition makes for good learning. Important parameters of reinforcement are schedules, amount, and delay of reinforcement.
  Performance generally increases as the amount of reward increases (e.g., if the use of a relaxation video enabled the patient to experience less nausea following chemotherapy, the intervention will likely by repeated). Yet, a patient who has experienced severe nausea and receive some relief may view the intervention more favorably than the patient who has experienced minimal nausea and receives "the same amount" of relief (i.e., the rule of marginal utility may exist).
  Rewards given shortly after the response or behavior are most effective.
- Positive reinforcement affects a wide array of behaviors and is of practical significance. Careful assessment of the individual patient is essential to identify the events that actually are rewarding. For instance, food may be a reward to one patient who had been "NPO" (nothing by mouth) for diagnostic tests, but may be revolting to another patient who has been "NPO," but is nauseated.
  Some people learn through praise, support, and encouragement, while others learn through threat, denial, and punishment. Whether we like it or not, the latter examples of negative reinforcement do control our behavior to a significant extent (e.g., legal system and even some religions).

---

specified in the objective with appropriate learning activities to produce that type of learning.

The last question in the series of steps is "From research and theory, what are the conditions that facilitate this type of learning in the learner, and/or in the learning situation?" (Tables 48.5 and 48.6).

Teaching Process

Today's dynamic patient population and health care system necessitate a variety of unique methods to meet pertinent patient outcomes. Due to shortened hospitalization, high technical performance is an expectation of patients and families and/or their caregivers. The complexity of maintaining optimal quality of life during treatment of oncologic diseases demands an increased volume of information on an ongoing basis. Among several teaching techniques, repetition is one of the keys to successful patient education. During the initial phase of diagnosis and at the beginning of treatment, teaching is aimed at helping patients understand their treat-

ment options. Teaching during this time usually results in short-term acquisition of facts and concepts (20). Repetition of the same message in various forms may be required to make new ideas concrete. As patients progress through treatment, they will need information and guidance in the incorporation of chemotherapy and its effects into their lives. Side effects and self-care measures need ongoing, consistent review. It is equally important to emphasize the positive aspects of chemotherapy and the goals of treatment.

If clinical trials are an option, informed consent is an issue of central importance. The patient needs to be well informed about any experimental portions of the treatments and any expectations of them as a participant (69). Assure patients that everything possible will be done to minimize side effects and that they will be given detailed information on how to deal with side effects that occur.

Informed consent is defined by the Department of Health and Human Services as the "knowing consent of an individual or his legally

Table 48.7. Teaching as a Method of Assisting Patients Receiving Antineoplastic Drugs

	Initial Phase	Treatment Phase
Stage of disease	Diagnosis and acute induction: initial treatment ("quick fix")	Remission: consolidation treatment or adjuvant therapy
Perception of patient	Patient sees threat to health state	Patient beginning to see health state returning to baseline
System of care (based on patient need)[a]	Wholly compensatory ⟶ Partially compensatory ⟶ Supportive (education)	
Focus	Facilitate diagnosis and treatment: enhance patient's strategies for coping with the physical and psychologic crisis	Patients assuming responsibility for self-care; problem-solving skills needed for self-care and coping
Methods of assisting	Doing for patient, establishing a protective environment, guidance, coaching, and some teaching	Teaching, coaching, support, guidance
Teaching	Teaching to have patient acquire enough understanding of disease and treatment to gain consent for treatment: cooperation with some participation in treatment program Teaching to alleviate anxiety when appropriate	Teaching to enable patient to retain knowledge and skill of self-care and to transfer to other settings such as home and work
Learning	Expect some things learned to be forgotten or repressed. Keep all information simple and concise; conserve patient's energy to cope with disease, treatment, and an interruption of lifestyle.	Expect patient to learn and take responsibility for own care. Build patient's expectations of same. Retention and transfer require repetition, reinforcement, and follow-up outside the acute care setting. Complexity and variations are built into the learning situations. The patient should be given practice in solving self-care problems that are likely to occur.

Adapted and reprinted by permission from Watson, PM. Patient education: the adult with cancer. Nurs Clin North Am 1982;17(4).
[a]Three systems of care: wholly compensatory—recipient patient is passive (no active role); partially compensatory—recipient patient and nurse each have responsibility for action dependent upon need; supportive-education—recipient patient agency is adequate for doing and learning self-care, but needs assistance and support.

authorized representative so situated as to be able to exercise free power of choice without inducement or any element of force, fraud, deceit, distress, or any other form of constraint or coercion" (70). Informed consent includes the following: the purpose of the study (clarifying that the study involves research), the procedures to be followed, the nature and extent of time commitment, the type of information to be obtained, a description of any possible physical and emotional discomfort (stating which risks are attributable to a specific drug(s) or procedure(s)), an explanation of medical treatments that may be available in case of injury, methods to ensure privacy and confidentiality, the names of people to contact for answers to questions about the study,

a statement that participation is voluntary and that nonparticipation or termination carries no penalty or loss of benefits to which the subject is otherwise entitled, a disclosure of any appropriate alterative procedures or courses of treatment that might be advantageous to the subject, and a description of possible gains of the research (69, 70). Most informed consent procedures are written at a highly technical level (71). Unfortunately, the language and readability of these documents have not been sufficiently simplified. Jubelirer reported that selected cooperative groups' consent forms required college-level reading comprehension. Similarly, these authors found the readability for Cancer and Leukemia Group B consent forms for protocols 9344, 9222,

9140, and 9331 was grade 14, except for the latter, which was grade 15. Therefore, educational responsibilities arising from the informed consent process include (a) interpreting the terminology of the consent form, (b) answering the patient's questions, (c) discussing long- and short-term medical risks and benefits, (d) discussing potential side effects, and (e) indicating interventions that can be used to alleviate or prevent them. Although studies of informed consent have documented patients' lack of knowledge after signing consent forms (72–74), they have not identified specific causes for this insufficient knowledge. The Patient's Bill of Rights gives the patient the right to the information in terms the patient can understand. This becomes crucial when patients are discharged "quicker and sicker." In spite of thorough explanations of informed consent, patients may be physically and/or emotionally unable to retain the explanation.

Evidence from cognitive psychology shows that people can remember approximately seven items of information at one time (75–76). Persons with cancer may be expected to recall even less information because of their physical and psychologic stress. Nurses should distinguish the information patients must be given to meet the legal, ethical, and educational requirements of informed consent and the information they need to cope with chemotherapy (42, 52). Informed consent can be regarded as part of a series of educational encounters (77). It is desirable to assure patients that side effects can generally be managed, but it is important to differentiate informed consent procedures from the procedures designed to prepare patients for chemotherapy. The latter should emphasize the minimal symptom experience pattern.

One of the greatest concerns of patients before they start chemotherapy is how the drugs will specifically affect them (41, 78). Given general information about antineoplastic agents and their potential side effects, they will be left wanting to know, or trying to imagine, what they as an individual will experience. This uncertainty can create anxiety. The following patient statements (41) reflect some of these feelings:

"Not knowing quite what to expect; lack of information."
"Being fearful and not knowing, even though they (health care workers) had gone through the routine and what they were going to do, still the wonder of (the subject) not absolutely knowing".

Until recently, preparatory information only included procedural information of specific events that would happen and behavioral instruction or actions the patient should take as a part of self-management (79, 80). Sensory information reflects the experience of an event, such as receiving chemotherapy, from the patient's point of view, as it describes in concrete sensory terms what patients can expect before, during, and after the treatment (79). Sensory information conveyed in a positive, unthreatening manner and given before the target event permits the formulation of a more effective mental schema. This enables the person to interpret incoming stimuli with new meaning and to draw from an existing repertoire of coping strategies. Thus, an accurate schema or image decreases ambiguity of the event, activates innate coping, and permits effective cognitive, rather than ineffective emotional, management of the threat. The patient's expectation of an experience and the actual experience have been shown to be related (36). Leventhal and Johnson reported that patients' expectations concerning sensations associated with stressful medical procedures differed from their sensory experiences (79). Preparation for stressful events can reduce symptom experience (occurrence and distress) and facilitate postoperative adaptation (14, 13–24). Rhodes et al. reported a statistically significant relationship ($p = .015$) between patients' expectations of symptom experience and their experience of symptom distress (36).

Preparatory sensory information including neutral descriptions of specific sensations to be experienced and realistic expectations help the patient to cope and to develop self-care behaviors more easily. The predominant pattern of symptom experience is used in the development of sensory and/or preparatory protocols (18, 41, 52, 56). In other words, if a patient is starting a chemotherapy regimen whose participants have experienced little or no nausea, then it is appropriate to give this factual information to prepare the (new) patient. The amount of factual information given will depend on what patients want to know and what they need to know to safely cope with chemotherapy. For example, if a treatment regimen consists of cisplatin and etoposide, it may not interest patients to know that cisplatin is the drug more likely to cause nausea and vomiting, but it is important to them (and for them) to know when this potential side effect might occur and how to manage it.

Identifying a time sequence in which side effects generally occur may allay anxiety. Patients may not feel so overwhelmed when they learn that not all side effects occur at once. It may also help them distinguish side effects of chemotherapy from other possible causes of similar symptoms. For example, nausea or vomiting experienced 10 days after receiving antineoplastic agents is not a typical side effect of the chemotherapy and another source should be sought. Side effects may be classified as immediate, early, delayed, and late (81). Immediate side effects, such as nausea or vomiting, occur within the first 24 hours. Stomatitis and alopecia, considered early side effects, have an onset of days to weeks. Delayed effects such as anemia and peripheral neuropathy occur within weeks to months. Late effects, such as second malignancies, may not appear until months or years later.

Discussing the practical aspects of receiving chemotherapy is also important to patients. Patients want to know: What is the procedure for administration of chemotherapy? Does the treatment hurt? Where am I taken for treatment? How long does a procedure last? How many treatments will I need? What arrangements for treatment do I make when bad weather interferes with transportation? They need some of this information to make plans, to modify their work schedules, or to find transportation to the treatment center, etc. These issues represent patients' attempts to develop a plan to incorporate chemotherapy treatments into their lives.

Patients may have difficulty knowing which symptoms to report and when to report them. Specific guidelines and instructions, such as those in Table 48.8, will help the patient make these decisions.

Selection of Patient Education Materials

Audiovisual materials are effective teaching tools. In this era of multimedia, the use of television and video as teaching aids can be valuable. It has been reported that video presentations alone are as effective as any other method of teaching, and videos are more effective than written information alone (82, 83). A variety of free audiovisual materials is available from the American Cancer Society and from pharmaceutical companies, in addition to those for rent or sale. All teaching materials, whether printed or audiovisual, are selected to augment and use the principle, "repetition makes for good learning."

The selection of teaching tools and methods is influenced by the individual patient assess-

ment. Health care professionals are challenged to select cost-effective, efficient methods of teaching that ensure sound learning. In most situations, a multidisciplinary approach is most effective. For example, a patient may view a video followed by a demonstration, with a return demonstration and written instructions to refer to at home.

A wide selection of patient education materials exists. Some references for individuals and families living with cancer are available without cost (Table 48.9) (84–89). Other sources of free materials include pharmaceutical companies.

Patient education materials need to be evaluated carefully, not only for accuracy and presentation of content, but also for reading level (Table 48.10). An estimated 23 million American adults are functionally illiterate and thus cannot comprehend the usual health care instructions. Research has demonstrated that the magnitude of the literacy dilemma in the United States cannot be determined by assessing years of education completed (90–92). In a recent survey of 127 patients, the median education was 10th grade, yet over 30% could not be expected to read at the 10th grade level (71). A sizable group of people with learning disabilities and an increasing elderly population with various types of learning impairments add to the difficulty of teaching patients with a literacy problem (9, 11, 16, 17, 27, 71). These individuals' reading, writing, listening, and speaking skills are not well developed, limiting the reality of self-care. The goal of the nurse educator is to have the patient process the message and decide to make a permanent behavioral change. Three factors interact at all educational levels to support comprehension: logic, language, and experience. To become part of an individual's self-care behavior, the suggested content must make sense to the patient, must fit in the individual's current lifestyle, must be achievable, and must be worth pursuing (i.e., time, energy, and money). These factors must be considered in attempting to increase a patient's competency in self-care and self-management of his or her health problems.

Several factors that affect readability are listed in Table 48.11 (93, 94). Although type size, writing style, and illustrations can be visually evaluated, teaching materials need to be tested for readability. Methods suggested to measure readability are the SMOG formula (93) and the FRY formula (94). Either of these two indices of readability will help determine the degree of difficulty in reading materials. Although the FRY

Table 48.8 Guidelines for Chemotherapy Patients

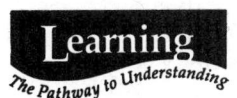

Chemotherapy Instruction Card

This card provides guidelines about when to call your doctor or nurse while you are taking chemotherapy.

How do I call my doctor or nurse?

If you experience any of the side effects listed on the back of this card, or if you have questions about your health or treatment, call the hospital where you had your treatment. Ask for your doctor or nurse by name, or ask for the doctor on call for oncology.

- ❏ Ellis Fischel Cancer Center .... (314) 882-2100
- ❏ University Hospital & Clinics .... (314) 882-4141
- ❏ Your doctor _____
- ❏ Your nurse _____

What drugs and treatments did I receive today?

You received the following chemotherapy drugs and treatments during this visit:

_____
_____
_____
_____

When should I call my doctor or nurse?

Call your doctor or nurse right away if you experience any of the following side effects:

- ❏ vomiting, or throwing up, for more than 2 days afer chemotherapy
- ❏ nausea, or upset stomach, that keeps you from eating or drinking for more than 2 days after chemotherapy
- ❏ 2 temperature readings of 100°F, or 37.8°C, or higher taken by mouth 4 hours apart
- ❏ sores in your mouth after chemotherapy that are painful and keep you from eating or drinking
- ❏ burning sensation, pain or blood when you urinate
- ❏ diarrhea or loose, watery bowel movements that last more than 2 days after chemotherapy
- ❏ new pain in any part of your body that lasts more than a day or that doesn't get better with pain medicine

After–treatment medicines

_____
_____
_____
_____

Developed by Mary Johnson, M.S., R.N., O.C.N.

Reviewed by the Patient Education Committee
The Staff for Life

10/13/94
Distribution #0293504

If you need ADA assistance, please call (314) 882-4997.

🖥 an equal opportunity employer

Ellis Fischel Cancer Center
The Staff for Life
115 Business Loop 70 West
Columbia, Missouri 65203
(314) 882-2100

University Hospital & Clinics
The Staff for Life
One Hospital Drive
Columbia, Missouri 65212
(314) 882-4141

© Copyright 1994 by the Curators of the University of Missouri, a Public Corporation.

---

formula takes a few minutes longer than the SMOG formula, it is considered to be more accurate (27, 95). The SMOG is quick, easy to perform, and predicts the grade-level difficulty of a passage within 1.5 grades with 68% accuracy (27). The name SMOG was selected to draw an analogy between an interference affecting readability and one affecting the atmosphere. The following procedure for the SMOG is included as an example:

1. Select 30 sentences: 10 consecutive sentences near the beginning, 10 consecutive sentences from the middle, and 10 consecutive sentences from the end.
2. Count the words, including repetitions, containing three or more syllables. Hyphenated words are considered one word. Pronounce words aloud and count syllables.
3. Calculate the grade level. Determine the nearest perfect square root of the total number of words of three or more syllables. Then, add 3 to the square root to define the grade level.

If readability is too high, comprehension is decreased, and recall will be sketchy and inaccurate. In addition, motivation for further instruction from printed sources is reduced.

Some people's optimal learning style includes comprehension from the spoken word. Cues not available in the written format (i.e., tone, stress of voice, action, or gesture) may be beneficial. Oral materials may be tested for comprehension level by converting a spoken or taped message

Table 48.9. Examples of Free Patient Education References

Title	Description of Content	Source
Chemotherapy and You—A Guide to Self-Help During Treatment	A 56-page booklet that answer questions about chemotherapy, and gives suggestions for dealing with side effects	National Cancer Institute
What Are Clinical Trials All About?	A 23-page booklet designed for patients who are considering participating in investigational cancer protocols; includes explanation of types of trials, informed consents, and questions to ask.	
Taking Time—Support for People with Cancer and the People Who Care for Them	A 68-page booklet written for people with cancer and their families; describes feelings and emotions and how others in similar situations have coped; suggests ways to share feelings, deal with friends, and solve problems	
Eating Hints—Recipes and Tips for Better Nutrition During Cancer Treatment	A 96-page booklet that describes various eating problems associated with cancer treatment and ways to deal with them; includes many simple recipes for nutritious foods	
Caring for the Patient with Cancer at Home	A 90-page booklet to provide general assistance in dealing with issues and problems associated with cancer; includes guidelines about when to notify the physician	American Cancer Society
Look Good . . . Feel Better	A 17-page booklet written for women with cancer receiving chemotherapy and/or radiation therapy; provides information on hair, skin, and nail care and makeup techniques	

Table 48.10. Samples of Same Content for Different Reading Levels

College reading level:
  If nausea, diarrhea, or other gastrointestinal disturbances persist for more than two days, contact your physician.
12th grade reading level:
  If you experience nausea, diarrhea, or other stomach or bowel problems for more than two days, contact your physician.
8th grade reading level:
  If you have nausea, loose bowel movements, or other stomach or bowel problems that last for two days, call your doctor.
4th grade reading level:
  If you have an upset stomach, loose bowel movements, or other problems that last for two days, call your doctor.

into written form and then applying a valid readability formula to the printed text. Audiotaped materials may be useful for some individuals; however, many patients with low literacy skills do not possess the language or thinking skills needed to process complex and abstract ideas in any form. Word recognition skills alone are insufficient; in fact, pictures and/or demonstrations may be needed. These issues represent the patients' attempt to develop a plan to incorporate chemotherapy treatments into their lives.

OUTCOMES, EVALUATION, AND DOCUMENTATION

Outcomes are resultant benefits to the patient and family from participating in patient education. Outcomes define the desired effect of teaching interventions on the patient's behavior. Outcome criteria are essential for evaluation. In 1982, the Oncology Nursing Society (ONS) published the original *Outcome Standards for Cancer Patient Education* (96, 97). The revised ONS standards indicate that the patient and family will possess sufficient knowledge and understanding about their disease and therapy for them to attain self-

Table 48.11. Factors Affecting Readability

Length of sentence
Vocabulary
   Multisyllable
   Technical words
Headings
Line width
Type size
Illustrations
Style of writing

management, participate in therapy, and experience optimal living (98).

Evaluation is the continuous assessment of the patient interventions, outcomes, and progress toward meeting established learning objectives. If the evaluation of patient education indicates that actual outcomes are not the same as desired outcomes, the nurse then evaluates each phase of the teaching process until reasons for the less than optimal outcomes can be identified. Further assessment and additional or remedial learning may be required.

Evaluation itself can be a learning experience for the patient by reinforcing positive behaviors and guiding the correction of misinformation or misunderstandings (99). There are several methods that can be used to gather information to evaluate learning, including patient-kept records or diaries, patient reports, questionnaires and/or interviews with patients and their families, questionnaires and/or interviews with staff, direct observation, oral or written tests, and research using statistical comparisons (100, 101). Regardless of which of the described methods are used, the patient needs to know how and when evaluation will be done. It is not always necessary to use the word "evaluation." For example, "Let's talk about how you're managing your chemotherapy. Then I will ask you some questions to see if I've explained things clearly." The most important concept of evaluation is that the person is more important than the performance or product (102, 103). Assist the patient in maintaining dignity and self-esteem throughout the evaluation.

Evaluation can also be a learning opportunity for the nurse educator. Feedback received from patients' progress or lack of progress helps the nurse to change the teaching approach or to consider alterative teaching strategies. Evaluation also adds to the nurse educator's existing knowledge base. Reporting the effectiveness of patient education may help to guide others in selecting teaching interventions and developing programs.

Documentation of patient education activities tells other members of the health care team what patients have learned, what needs to be learned, and what needs to be reviewed. Accurate documentation contributes to continuity of care, serves as a legal record of what the patient was taught, can be used for reimbursement, and helps satisfy accreditation standards.

Documentation of the patient's learning program is complete if it includes information provided to patients that assists them in making decisions about treatment options, information contributing to their exercise of self-care, information on how well the patient/family achieved the learning objectives, and their reaction to the learning situation and to the content being taught. Flow charts or checklists are easy to complete and are often used.

SUMMARY

Patient education is increasingly important for cancer patients (104, 105). Its aim is to promote a higher quality of life and cost-effective care. Patient education provides acquisition of knowledge and/or skills that enhance self-care and reduce disruption in daily functioning. Since the time frame available for such teaching is short, innovative, creative strategies are required for teaching self-care to individuals. Teaching strategies based upon the patient's BCFs and learning style will be most effective. Telephone and/or in-home visits for follow-up may be used in addition to traditional methods. Intellectual skills include discriminations, concepts, rules, and higher-order rules, each increasing in complexity. Cognitive strategies that necessitate the recall of intellectual skills and information are internally organized skills. The learner uses these cognitive strategies to manage his or her own processes of attending, learning, remembering, and thinking.

The learning of psychomotor skills is attended by the recall of directive routine that provides the sequence and pattern for the performance and often by recall of part-skills that are combined into the total motor act. Problem solving may be viewed as a process by which the learner discovers a combination of previously learned rules that can be applied to achieve a solution for a novel situation. These processes yield new learning for the patient. Appropriate patient education that provides proactive management of symptom experience may alleviate fears, enhance the quality of life, and be cost effective. Appropriate patient education is essential to enhance patients' quality of life and to reduce health care costs.

ACKNOWLEDGMENT

The authors wish to acknowledge R.W. McDaniel, Ph.D., R.N., Associate Professor, Sinclair School of Nursing, University of Missouri—Columbia, for her editorial assistance.

REFERENCES

1. Wingo PA, Bolden S, Tong T. Cancer statistics. CA 1995;45(1):8–30.

2. Hicks LL, Sallmeyer JM, Coleman JR. Role of the nurse in managed care. Washington, DC: American Nurses Publishing, 1993.

3. Orem DE. Nursing concepts of practice. 5th ed. St. Louis: Mosby-Year Book, 1995.

4. Rhodes VA, McDaniel RW. The management of symptom experience—introduction. Semin Oncol Nurs 1995;11(4):231.

5. Morra ME. Future trends in patient education. Semin Oncol Nurs 1991;7(2):143–145.

6. Schulmeister L. Establishing a cancer patient education system for ambulatory patients. Semin Oncol Nurs 1991;7(2):118–124.

7. U.S. Department of Commerce Economics and Statistics Administration, Bureau of the Census. Statistical abstract of the United States 1993 (abstract). 113th ed.

8. Goldsmith S. The US health care system in the year 2000. JAMA 1986;256:3371–3375.

9. Northrup B. Gray matters. Wall Street Journal 1987;Apr 24:33D–34D.

10. Frank-Stromberg M, Welch-McCaffrey D. Cancer in the elderly: introduction. Semin Oncol Nurs 1988;4(3):155.

11. Klevins C, ed. Materials and methods in adult education. Los Angeles: Klevins Publications, 1972:1151.

12. Madison MA, McConnell ES. Gerontological nursing: concepts and practice. Philadelphia: WB Saunders, 1988.

13. Neugarten BL. Middle age and aging. Chicago: University of Chicago Press, 1975:5–21, 93–98, 137–147, 163–177.

14. Sullivan T, Munroe DJ. A self-care practice theory of nursing the elderly. Educ Gerontol 1986;12:13.

15. Havinghurst RJ. Developmental tasks and education. New York: McKay Publishing, 1952.

16. Knowles MS. The adult learner: a neglected species. Houston: Gulf Publishing, 1978.

17. Welch-McCaffrey D. To teach or not to teach? Overcoming barriers to patient education in geriatric oncology. Oncol Nurs Forum l986;13(4):25–31.

18. Rhodes VA, Watson PM, Hanson B. Patients'

descriptions of the influence of tiredness and weakness on self-care abilities. Cancer Nurs 1987;11(3):186–194.

19. Blumberg BD, Gentry ED. Selecting a systematic approach for educating hospitalized cancer patients. Semin Oncol Nurs 1991;7(2):112–117.

20. Welch-McCaffrey D. Evolving patient education needs in cancer. Oncol Nurs Forum 1985;12(5):62–64.

21. Adams M. Information and education across the phases of cancer care. Semin Oncol Nurs 1991;7(2):105–111.

22. Peck RC. Psychological developments in the second half of life. In: Neugarten BL, ed. Middle age and aging. Chicago: University of Chicago Press, 1968.

23. Erikson EH. Adulthood. New York: WW Norton, 1978.

24. Butler RN, Lewis MI. Aging and mental health. St. Louis: CV Mosby, 1973.

25. Gray J. Education for health in old age. In: Gray J, ed. Prevention of disease in the elderly. London: Churchill Livingstone, 1985.

26. Wilson CM, Rimer BK, Bennet DJ, et al. Educating the older cancer patient: obstacles and opportunities. Health Educ Q 1984;10:76–87.

27. Doak CC, Doak LG, Root JH. Teaching patients with low literacy skills. Philadelphia: JB Lippincott, 1985.

28. Woods NF, Lewis FM, Ellison ES. Living with cancer. Cancer Nurs 1989;12(1):28–33.

29. Cobb S. Social support as a moderator of life stress. Psychosom Med 1976;38(5):300–314.

30. McNett SC. Social support, threat, and coping responses and effectiveness in the functionally disabled. Nurs Res 1987;36(2):98–103.

31. Muhlenkamp AF, Sayles JA. Self-esteem, social support, and positive health practices. Nurs Res 1986; 35(6):334–338.

32. Rhodes VA, Watson PM, Johnson MH. Development of reliable and valid measures of nausea and vomiting. Cancer Nurs 1984;7(1):33–41.

33. Rhodes VA, Watson PM, Johnson MH, Beck NC. Postchemotherapy symptom occurrence and distress. New York: Springer-Verlag, 1989.

34. Rhodes VA, Watson PM. Symptom distress—the concept: past and present. Semin Oncol Nurs 1989; 3(4):242–297.

35. Watson PM. Patent education: the adult with cancer. Nurs Clin North Am 1982;17(4):739–752.

36. Rhodes VA, Watson PM, McDaniel RW, Hanson BM, Johnson MH. Expectation and occurrence of postchemotherapy side effects: nausea and vomiting. Cancer Pract 1995;3(4):1–7.

37. Tierney A, Taylor J, Closs S. Knowledge, expectations, and experience of patients receiving chemotherapy for breast cancer. Scand J Caring Sci 1992; 6(2):75–80.

38. Andrykowski NA, Gregg ME. The role of psychological variables in postchemotherapy nausea: anxiety and expectation. Psychosom Med 1992;54:48–58.

39. Cimprich C. Symptom management: loss of concentration. Semin Oncol Nurs 1995;11(4):279–288.

40. Richardson JL, Marks G, Levine A. The influence of symptoms of disease and side effects of treatment on compliance with cancer therapy. J Clin Oncol 1988;6(11):1746–1752.

41. Rhodes VA, McDaniel RW, Hanson BM, John-

son MH. Sensory information from patients on selected antineoplastic chemotherapy. Cancer Nurs 1994; 17(1):45–51.

42. Rhodes VA, Johnson MH, McDaniel RW. Nausea, vomiting, and retching: management of the symptom experience. Semin Oncol Nurs 1995;11(4):256–265.

43. Barnes S, Thomas A. A modified cancer education program. Effect on cancer knowledge and beliefs of the elderly. Cancer Nurs 1990;13(1):48–55.

44. American Cancer Society. Public attitudes toward cancer and cancer tests. CA 1980;30:92–98.

45. American Cancer Society. Black Americans' attitudes toward cancer and cancer tests. CA 1981; 31:212–218.

46. Jarvis W. Helping your patients deal with questionable cancer treatments. CA 1986;36(5):293–301.

47. Fehring RJ, Rantz MJ. Spiritual distress. In: Maas M, Buckwalter KC, Hardy MA, eds. Nursing diagnosis and interventions for the elderly. Redwood City, CA: Addison Wesley, 1991:598–609.

48. Carson V. Spiritual dimensions of nursing practice. Philadelphia: WB Saunders, 1989.

49. Sodestrom KE, Martinson IM. Patients' spiritual coping strategies: a study of nurse and patient perspectives. Oncol Nurs Forum 1987;14(2):4146.

50. Raleigh EDH. Sources of hope in chronic illness. Oncol Nurs Forum 1992;19(3):443–448.

51. Kaye J, Robinson KM. Spirituality among caregivers. IMAGE: J Nurs Scholarship 1994;26(3):218–221.

52. Rhodes VA, Watson PM, Johnson M, Madden R, Beck NC. Patterns of nausea, vomiting, and distress in patients receiving antineoplastic drug protocols. Oncol Nurs Forum 1987;14(4):35–43.

53. Sullivan T. Self-care model for nursing. New directions for nursing in the 80's. Kansas City, MO: American Nurses' Association, 1980:57–68.

54. Villejo L, Meyers C. Brain function, learning styles, and cancer patient education. Semin Oncol Nurs 1991;7(2):97–104.

55. Strowig S. Patient education: a model for autonomous decision-making and deliberate action in diabetes self-management. Med Clin North Am 1982; 66(6)1293–1307.

56. McDaniel RW, Rhodes VA, Nelson RA, Hanson BM. Sensory perceptions of women receiving tamoxifen for breast cancer. Cancer Nurs 1995;18(3):215–221.

57. Gagne RM. The conditions of learning. 3rd ed. New York: Holt, Rinehart & Winston, 1977.

58. Travers EM. Essentials of learning. 4th ed. New York: Macmillan, 1977.

59. Logan FA, Gordon WC. Fundamentals of learning and motivation. Dubuque, IA: William C. Brown, 1981.

60. Leininger M. Caring: an essential human need. Proceedings of Three National Caring Conferences. Thorofare, NJ: Slack, 1981:13.

61. Blauvelt N, Brandt D, Simpson B, Stover D. Planning for cancer patient care and teaching to enhance the oncology product line. In: Engstrom PF, Anderson PN, Mortenson LE, eds. Advances in cancer control: cancer control research and the emergence of the oncology product line. New York: Alan R Liss, 1988:211–218.

62. Larson PJ. Important nurse caring behaviors perceived by patients with cancer. Oncol Nurs Forum 1984;2(6):46–50.

63. Larson PJ. Cancer nurses' perceptions of caring. Cancer Nurs 1986;9(2):86–91.

64. Mayer D. Cancer patients' and families' perceptions of nurse caring behaviors. Top Clin Nurs 1986; 8(2):63–69.

65. Mayer D. Oncology nurses' versus cancer patients' perceptions of nurse caring behaviors: a replication study. Oncol Nurs Forum 1987;14(3):48–52.

66. Heidgerken LE. Teaching in schools of nursing: principles and methods. Philadelphia: JB Lippincott, 1953.

67. Giloth BE. Promoting patient involvement: educational, organizational, and environmental strategies. Patient Educ Counseling. 1990;16(1):29–38.

68. Hiromoto BM, Dungan J. Contact learning for self-care activities. A protocol study among chemotherapy outpatients. Cancer Nurs 1991;14(3):148–154.

69. Rimer B, Jones WL, Keintz MK, Catalano RB, Engstrom PF. Informed consent: a crucial step in cancer patient education. Health Educ Q 1989; 10(Suppl):3042.

70. Department of Health and Human Services. Protection of human subjects: informed consent. Washington: Federal Register, January 27, 1982;Part IX.

71. Jubelirer SJ. Level of reading difficulty in educational pamphlets and informed consent documents for cancer patients. W Va Med J 1991:554–557.

72. Fernsler JI, Cannon CA. The whys of patient education. Semin Oncol Nurs 1991;7(2):79–86.

73. Muss H, White D, Michielutte R, et al. Written informed consent in patients with breast cancer. Cancer 1979;43:1549–1556.

74. Dodd M, Mood D. Chemotherapy: helping patients to know the drugs they are receiving and their possible side effects. Cancer Nurs 1981;4(4):311–318.

75. Miller GA. The magical number seven, plus or minus two: some limits on our capacity for processing information. Psychol Rev 1956;63(2):81–97.

76. Klatzky RL. Human memory: structures and processes. 2nd ed. San Francisco: WH Freeman, 1980.

77. Rimer B, Jones WL, Keintz MK, Engstrom PF, Catalano RB. Cancer patients' recall of important information. In: Engstrom PF, Anderson PN, Mortenson LE, eds. Advances in cancer control: epidemiology and research. New York: Alan R Liss, 1984:153–159.

78. Manson H, Manderino MA, Johnson MH. Chemotherapy: thoughts and images of patients with cancer. Oncol Nurs Forum 1993;20:527–531.

79. Leventhal H, Johnson JE. Laboratory and field experimentation: development of a theory of self-regulation. In: Woolridge PJ, Schmitt MH, Skipper JK, Leonard RC, eds. Behavioral science and nursing theory. St. Louis: CV Mosby, 1983.

80. Dodd M. Measuring informational intervention for chemotherapy knowledge and self-care behavior. Res Nurs Health 1984;7:43–50.

81. Perry MC, Yarbro JW. Complications of chemotherapy: an overview. In: Perry MC, Yarbro JW, eds. Toxicity of chemotherapy. Orlando, FL: Grune & Stratton, 1984:1–19.

82. Grassman D. Development of inpatient oncology educational and support programs. Oncol Nurs Forum 1993;20(4):669–676.

83. Nielson E, Sheppard MA. Television as a patient education tool. Patient Educ Council 1990;15:73–75.

84. U.S. Department of Health and Human Services. Eating hints: recipes and tips for better nutrition during cancer treatment (NIH publication no. 91-2079). Bethesda, MD: 1990.

85. Cosmetic, Toiletry, and Fragrance Association. Look good . . . feel better: caring for yourself inside and out. St. Louis: National Cosmetology Association, 1988.

86. American Cancer Society. Caring for the patient with cancer at home: a guide for patients and families (publication no. 88-100M-no. 4656-PS). New York, New York, 1990.

87. U.S. Department of Health and Human Services. What are clinical trials all about? A booklet for patients with cancer (NIH publication no. 90-2706). Bethesda, MD: 1989.

88. U.S. Department of Health and Human Services. Taking time: support for people with cancer and the people who care about them (NIH Publication No. 92–2059). Bethesda, MD: 1992.

89. U.S. Department of Health and Human Services. Chemotherapy and you: a guide to self-help during treatment (NIH Publication No. 94–1136). Bethesda, MD: 1992.

90. Stephens ST. Patient education materials: are they readable? Oncol Nurs Forum 1992;19(1):83–85.

91. Tucker T, Friedell G, Stallones L, et al. Cancer mortality in rural Appalachian Kentucky. 1988. Lexington: University of Kentucky.

92. Glazer-Waldman H, Hall K, Weiner M. Patient education in a public hospital. Nurs Res 1985;34:184–185.

93. McLaughlin G. SMOG—grading—a new readability formula. J Reading 1969;12:639–646.

94. Fry E. A readability formula that saves time. In: Harker WJ, ed. Classroom strategies for secondary reading. Newark, DE: International Reading Association, 1977:29–35.

95. Meade CD, Diekman J, Thornhill DG. Readability of American Cancer Society patient education literature. Oncol Nurs Forum 1992;19(1):51–55.

96. McNally J, Stair JC, Sommerville ET. Guidelines for cancer nursing practice. Philadelphia: Grune & Stratton, 1985.

97. American Nurses' Association and Oncology Nursing Society. Standards of oncology nursing practice. Kansas City, MO: ANA, 1987.

98. American Nurses' Association and Oncology Nursing Society. Standards for oncology nursing education: patient, family, and public. Kansas City, MO: ANA, 1989.

99. Turk DC, Salovey P, Lih, MD. Adherence. A cognitive behavioral perspective. In: Gerber KE, Nehemkis AM, eds. Compliance the dilemma of the chronically ill. New York: Springer Publishing, 1986:44–72.

100. Rankin S, Duffy K. Patient education: issues, principles, and guidelines. Philadelphia: JB Lippincott, 1983.

101. Frank-Stromberg M, Cohen R. Evaluating written patient education materials. Semin Oncol Nurs 1991;7(2):125–134.

102. Narrow B. Patient teaching in nursing practice: a patient and family-centered approach. New York: John Wiley, 1979.

103. Lipitz M, Bussigel M, Bannerman J, et al. What is wrong with patient education programs? Nurs Outlook 1990;38:184–189.

104. Rhodes VA, McDaniel RW, Johnson MH. Patient education—self-care guides. Semin Oncol Nurs 1995;11(4):298–305.

105. Johnson J, Blumberg B. A commentary on cancer patient education. Health Educ Q. 1987; 10(Suppl):718.

49

Nursing Implications in the Administration of Cancer Chemotherapy

Connie Henke Yarbro

The progress made in the past two decades in cancer chemotherapy has allowed cure and control of tumors previously refractory to treatment. Concurrently, there has been a major expansion in the role of the oncology nurse (1–10). Oncology nurses have had a substantial impact on the development, evaluation, and delivery of chemotherapeutic agents. Today, chemotherapy has become standard practice in outpatient and hospital settings, and oncology nurses have developed standards and guidelines to ensure safe and competent care for cancer patients receiving chemotherapeutic agents (11–20).

The complexity of the therapeutic regimens, the sophisticated care required to meet the special medical problems encountered, and the enormous need for psychosocial support and education of the cancer patient all place major responsibility on the nurse involved with the administration of combination chemotherapy. The role played by the nurse in the cancer care team is key. Close collaboration between the nurse and physician has a significant impact on the outcome of treatment. The nurse-patient relationship is critical to provide emotional support, patient education, precise compliance with complex regimens, and preventive interventions necessary to minimize morbidity. A high level of effective communication is necessary to exchange the patient care information essential to quality care. Nurse-to-nurse communication is also important, since patients may move from hospital to clinic to office to home while continuing adherence to a complex therapeutic regimen.

ROUTES OF THERAPY

Modern chemotherapy employs a variety of agents given by several different routes in multiple settings. The nurse must be familiar with all of these, since in most instances, it is the nurse who represents the final link between a complex therapeutic plan and the actual administration of the drugs to the patient. Oral medications continue to be essential in combination regimens, not only for supportive agents but for chemotherapeutic agents as well. For example, procarbazine and prednisone in the mechlorethamine, vincristine, procarbazine, prednisone (MOPP) regimen; cyclophosphamide in the cyclophosphamide, methotrexate, fluorouracil (CMF) regimen; and lomustine, semustine, 6-mercaptopurine, and methotrexate in a variety of regimens are routinely given orally. Other oral chemotherapeutic agents are etoposide, used in the treatment of small cell lung cancer (21), and hydroxyurea for chronic myelogenous leukemia (22).

Careful patient instruction and continuous reinforcement is necessary to avoid patient errors and/or noncompliance. Levine et al. (23) evaluated compliance with allopurinol and prednisone in a group of primarily indigent patients with newly diagnosed hematologic malignancies. Compliance with oral medications improved in the group receiving a variety of educational intervention strategies.

In some areas, special attention is mandatory. For example, after high-dose methotrexate, the accurate administration of oral leucovorin rescue is lifesaving. With medications of this importance, the nurse should physically place the medication in the patient's hands, repeat the physician's instructions to ensure patient understanding, provide a medication calendar that requires the patient to check off each dose taken, and follow up with a phone call to the patient's home. Relatives should be aware of the importance of this medication.

Parenteral routes of administration include subcutaneous, intramuscular, and a variety of intravenous techniques (push, sidearm, piggyback, and infusion). Vascular access catheters attached to a port or pump may also be used in the administration of parenteral chemotherapy. Direct or regional infusion into a body organ or cavity is also an option.

The intravenous route remains the major route of chemotherapy administration in spite of the many new methods, and it is the route of most concern for nurses on a day-to-day basis. This chapter deals primarily with this route.

Central venous and right atrial catheters are discussed elsewhere in this volume (Chapter 45). For practical purposes, they represent a modification of the ordinary intravenous route and are primarily indicated in patients requiring intensive chemotherapy, parenteral nutrition, continuous drug delivery, or long-term venous access or in patients with limited vascular access (24–30). Since these catheters are long-term devices, the patient's preference and personal situation should be considered prior to the selection of a specific vascular access device (VAD) (31). For example, some patients may not like the thought of a catheter exiting from the body, and such a device would interfere with their body image. On the other hand, some patients incur major anxiety with each venipuncture. Vocation may influence the choice: for example, patients who use their hands or arms as a part of their job may need a VAD to prevent any possible morbidity from extravasation. Thus, the nurse must be knowledgeable about the various VADs and consider the patient's preference and personal situation before a selection is made. In addition, the nurse must assess the patient's and family's willingness and ability to care for the catheter at home. Teaching specific techniques to the patient and family is an extremely important activity for the oncology nurse (27, 31–34).

Other routes of chemotherapy are less commonly used and are discussed elsewhere in this book. The intrathecal route is used primarily in acute lymphocytic leukemia to treat overt disease or for prophylaxis. It may be used to treat carcinomatous or lymphomatous meningitis. The agents involved are primarily methotrexate and cytosine arabinoside. A physician usually administers these agents, but the nurse plays a critical role. These patients may be receiving vincristine intravenously for treatment of their leukemia, often on the same visit during which the intrathecal medication is given. Inadvertent administration of vincristine into the spinal fluid has been reported and is a disastrous error since it leads to total paralysis and death (35).

Arterial infusions are increasingly used to achieve high concentrations of drug locally, especially in the liver. These applications are discussed in Chapter 16.

A number of special devices are increasingly used for the administration of chemotherapy, including implantable devices and ambulatory infusion pumps attached to central venous catheters. Because of the shift of health care delivery from the inpatient setting to the outpatient and home settings, ambulatory infusion pumps have become a popular and cost-effective means of providing long-term infusions. There are three types of ambulatory pump delivery systems available: peristaltic, syringe-driven, and elastomeric. Each provides unique advantages and disadvantages. Rapsilber and Camp-Sorrell (36) provide an excellent review of ambulatory infusion pumps. Table 49.1 lists the advantages and disadvantages of the three different types of ambulatory infusion pumps. Implantable pumps are available that can be programed with an external computer to regulate the rate and time of flow.

Major nursing responsibilities include patient and family teaching about the device and its management, loading and calibrating the pump (36–39), specific care associated with implantable devices (39–43), and preventing and identifying complications such as catheter occlusion, extravasation, and infection (44, 45).

PRETREATMENT ASSESSMENT

An outline of the essential pretreatment measures is shown in Table 49.2. Before treatment begins, the nurse must *independently* assess the patient's physical condition, emotional state, understanding of the status of his or her disease, and understanding of the proposed treatment. This assessment is essential to develop a specific plan of nursing care and to determine patient

Table 49.1. Advantages and Disadvantages of Different Types of Ambulatory Infusion Pumps

Type of Device	Advantages	Disadvantages
Syringe	Lightweight and portable Cost effective Ease of patient use Excellent for antibiotics and pain management No dose calculations Little or no maintenance Visual drug flow Alarms	Device can fracture and break if dropped Limited volumes Not for large-volume infusions Drug stability factor Requires adequate manual dexterity to work with syringe and tubing Free-flow risk
Elastomeric	Lightweight, portable, and concealable Ease of patient use Excellent for antibiotics No programing No maintenance Reservoir and tubing attached	Difficult to fill Admixture considerations Drug stability factor Calculate concentrations and volumes Limited infusion rates Not for large-volume infusions Reimbursement concerns Cost prohibitive in long-term therapies
Peristaltic	Provides intermittent and continuous infusions All types of infusion therapy Alarm systems Wide range of infusion rates and volumes	Requires programing Carrying pouch heavy when full Upstream occlusion Free-flow risk Labor intensive

From Rapsilber LM, Camp-Sorrell D. Ambulatory infusion pumps: application to oncology. Semin Oncol Nurs 1995;11:213–220. With permission.

educational needs. With the shift in the administration of cancer chemotherapy from the hospital to the outpatient clinic, the office, or the home, appropriate patient selection is an important part of this assessment. For example, performance status, ability for self-care, motivation, and adequate family support are essential elements to the success of outpatient chemotherapy (31, 46, 47). Furthermore, the nurse is often one of the few regular contacts that the patient has with the cancer care team and as such often becomes a major element in the patient's emotional support system. This role of the nurse is as important as the technical role usually emphasized. The nurse is not only the final link between the therapeutic plan and the patient but often the most important emotional link between the cancer care team and the patient.

Whether research or standard therapy is being given, informed consent is mandatory, since it represents the willing participation of the patient after the potential risks and benefits of a proposed therapy have been explained. For standard therapy, informed consent is often unwritten, although increasingly, written documentation is being used. For experimental therapy, a

Table 49.2. Pretreatment Measures for the Administration of Chemotherapy

1. Baseline assessment of history, diagnosis, current physical status, psychologic status and resources, treatment plan, and past experience with chemotherapy.
2. Verify that informed consent has been obtained.
3. Initiate necessary patient education.
4. Review for presence of significant laboratory data and for symptoms of toxicity.
5. Check physician's order for drug(s), dose, route, rate, and time of administration.
6. Verify the dosage of the drug calculation according to the patient's body surface area and any modifications of dose.
7. Administer antiemetics or other medications as ordered in preparation of chemotherapy.
8. Ensure that emergency drugs are available.
9. Verify patient identity (particularly crucial in outpatient settings where patients do not wear wrist bands).

carefully written document prepared especially for the specific protocol in use is universal. The nurse should be sure that the patient understands the nature of the treatment and its possible risks as well as treatment alternatives and has given informed consent. The nurse should also be sure that where applicable, written documentation is present in the chart. The *legal* responsibility for informed consent is placed on the physician, but the nurse shares the *moral and ethical* responsibility with the physician.

Upon completion of the initial patient assessment, the nurse should begin teaching the patient and family what to expect from the treatment procedure and the potential side effects. Patients who are informed and have been psychologically prepared for the stresses of chemotherapy are less depressed, experience fewer side effects, and show greater improvement and ability to cope (48).

Most of the intravenous chemotherapy given to oncology patients is administered by oncology-certified nurses; thus, these nurses must be knowledgeable about the diseases and monitoring parameters as well as the drugs. Before delivering chemotherapy, the nurse must determine that all necessary laboratory analyses have been obtained and are within normal limits. Diagnostic procedures that have been inadvertently omitted should be obtained before the initiation of chemotherapy (especially important for research protocols). This is particularly important for procedures documenting the size or extent of a lesion that might be used as an index of response to therapy. A review of drug allergies should be routine. In addition, the patient should be assessed for the presence of any complicating conditions or toxicities that could contraindicate or modify the administration of chemotherapy, i.e., poor dentition, stomatitis, bleeding, infection, or decreased deep tendon reflexes.

The physician's order or the drug prescription should be carefully checked to confirm that it is correct and in accordance with the protocol requirements. It is important for the nurse to recalculate the dose on the basis of the patient's current weight and height, since one of the most common errors of drug dosing arises from inaccurate calculation of a patient's body surface area, which may be done on one occasion and not checked thereafter. It is also important with some drugs to double check the cumulative total dose given; doxorubicin and daunorubicin are additive and cause cardiotoxicity, and bleomycin causes pulmonary toxicity. The nurse should also ascertain that any dosage modifications made are appropriate to the modifications specified by the protocol with regard to white blood count, platelet count, BUN and creatinine, and liver function tests.

Administration of antiemetics prior to chemotherapy administration is equally important. The development of the 5-HT3 antagonists (e.g., ondansetron, granisetron) has contributed greatly to our ability to effectively control nausea and vomiting (49, 50). There are a variety of antiemetic regimens for mild, moderate, or severe nausea and vomiting. A recent study by Hesketh et al. (51) reported that good antiemetic control can be obtained with a variety of chemotherapy regimens by adjusting the intravenous dose of ondansetron to the intrinsic emetogenicity of the chemotherapy regimen. A single intravenous dose of either 8, 24, or 32 mg of ondansetron combined with a single 20-mg intravenous dose of dexamethasone was used in this study. A more detailed discussion of the emetogenic potential of antineoplastic agents and antiemetic regimens appears elsewhere in this text. However, the oncology nurse must continuously monitor and evaluate the effectiveness of the antiemetics administered. Standard antiemetic protocols are useful guidelines for the oncology nurse.

Finally, the nurse should ensure that necessary emergency drugs are present and verify patient identity before proceeding with chemotherapy administration. The development of a protocol or process to guarantee that all the elements of a thorough and complete pretreatment evaluation are carried out will ensure a complete assessment. A number of assessment tools are available for gathering the information needed to develop specific nursing care plans (52, 53).

ADMINISTRATION OF CANCER CHEMOTHERAPY

In many institutions, the pharmacist is responsible for reconstitution and storage of drugs, but when the nurse must assume this responsibility, knowledge of the details of drug preparation, safe handling, and disposal is essential. The nurse must know or have readily available information on the interaction of drugs, stability of drugs in solution, diluents required, storage requirements, and available preparations. Attention must be given to drug incompatibilities, potentiation, synergism, and augmentation or diminution by other treatment modalities. Nurses are concerned about the issues of drug handling and disposal, and recommendations and guidelines have been developed (54–56). Institutions and oncology offices should adopt specific guidelines and policies for their personnel. These issues are dealt with in other sections of this volume. There is no substitute for skill in the careful technical administration of intravenous chemotherapy. Serious or life-threatening complications can be avoided if an organized process is carefully followed. Table 49.3 outlines the steps of such a structured approach. The available literature today provides the nurse with numerous guidelines for the administration of intravenous chemotherapy agents (6, 9–12, 16–20). In addition, there are several controversial issues that nurses must consider regarding the site of drug administration, size of needle to use, and method of drug sequencing. Table 49.4 outlines these controversial issues.

ACUTE COMPLICATIONS

There are numerous complications, both immediate and delayed, with which the nurse should be familiar, and these differ from one drug to another. The most dreaded immediate complication unique to chemotherapy is extravasation of a vesicant agent capable of producing tissue necrosis. The most extreme example of this phenomenon is doxorubicin extravasation, which may require major debridement, followed by skin grafting or extensive flap mobilization plastic surgery. The major vesicants are listed in Table 49.5. Although the literature has suggested many actions in the event of an extravasation, there are few carefully collected data documenting the best approach for treatment. Identification of patients at high risk for extravasation and prevention of the complication are the soundest approaches currently available (57). (See Chapter 30 for detailed discussion of extravasation.)

A number of drugs are local irritants because of their physical characteristics (Table 49.5). Some irritant drugs (e.g., doxorubicin) are also vesicants. Injection of these drugs into veins may result in disruption of the endothelial lining with thrombosis. This may limit long-term use. Dilution in free-flowing intravenous fluid will reduce damage to the endothelial lining. Large veins with a high blood flow are less likely to be damaged. Carmustine and dacarbazine are irritants that often cause local pain and discomfort along the venous pathway. These drugs should be administered through a free-flowing intravenous line. Alternating the drip rate or placing ice along the venous pathway above the insertion site may relieve discomfort. A local anesthetic (Xylocaine) has been administered intravenously prior to drug administration; however, no proof of efficacy is available regarding this method (6, 7, 12). Venous spasm may also occur if the drug

Table 49.3. Sequence of Events for the Administration of Chemotherapy Administration of Intravenous Medications

1. Vein selection: Select site for venipuncture by examining both arms to identify suitable veins. Begin distally and move proximally; e.g., begin at the dorsum of the hand rather than at the major veins of the antecubital fossa. If a vesicant is to be administered, a vein in the distal forearm should be selected to avoid sites where damage to underlying nerves or tendons could occur. Avoid a vein that has been used for venous access in the last 24 hours to prevent leakage. Avoid sclerosed or inflamed veins and extremities with compromised circulation (e.g., lymphedema from mastectomy, phlebitis, or immobilized fractures).

2. Selection of cannula depends on the purpose and duration of infusion, rate of flow, and the size and availability of the patient's veins. A butterfly or scalp-wing needle is suitable for short-term infusions. An intracatheter or over-the-needle catheter is ideal for longer infusions or caustic agents. (Other vascular access devices are discussed elsewhere in this volume.)

3. Place patient in comfortable position and prepare site according to institutional policy.

4. When the cannula has been successfully positioned, secure with tape, test the vein patency, and return blood flow with normal saline or 5% dextrose in water. Observe for swelling and redness, and solicit patient's feelings.

5. The cannula insertion site should be visible at all times to observe for vein irritation, allergic reactions, and local infiltration.

6. Administer antiemetics or other medications as ordered (e.g., hydration fluids for cisplatin, mesna prior to ifosfamide).

7. Administer chemotherapeutic agents as ordered. The sequence of drug administration is controversial. Some administer vesicants first, others administer these agents last or "sandwiched" between two nonvesicant drugs. Carmustine or dacarbazine, which cause pain and irritation upon administration, should be administered last.

8. For intravenous push or bolus injection, the drug may be injected directly through the cannula or through the sidearm or port of a free-flowing i.v. The drug(s) should be infused slowly with even pressure and blood return checked with every 3 to 5 mL of drug. Flush cannula and tubing between drugs and upon completion.

9. For drugs given by intravenous infusion or drip, the running infusion should be checked frequently and the treatment concluded with a saline flush.

10. If there is any doubt about the vein patency or drug infusion, discontinue immediately. Discontinue immediately if the patient reports any untoward symptoms.

11. After needle is removed, apply pressure to the injection site for 3 to 4 minutes, preferably with arm elevated to prevent hematoma.

12. Apply adhesive bandage or sterile dressing.

13. Document medications given, injection site, time, dose, and any unusual patient reactions.

14. Assess the patient's status and review instructions and care with the patient. For patients receiving their first treatment, it is good practice to call them the following day.

15. Dispose of equipment according to institutional policies.

Information from refs 6, 9–12, 16–20.

Table 49.4. Controversial Issues Regarding the Administration of Chemotherapeutic Agents

A. Use of the antecubital fossa for administering chemotherapeutic agents
   1. Favoring the use of the antecubital fossa
      a) Larger veins permit more rapid infusion/ administration of drugs.
      b) Larger veins permit potentially irritating chemotherapeutic agents to reach the general circulation sooner with less irritation to smaller veins.
   2. Avoiding the use of the antecubital fossa
      a) Arm mobility is restricted with a needle in place.
      b) The risk of extravasation is increased due to patient mobility (e.g., coughing, vomiting).
      c) Infiltration could cause extensive reconstruction efforts to be necessary with limited arm use during the healing process, resulting in increased morbidity and decreased function.
      d) Because of the subcutaneous tissues, early infiltration is more difficult to assess.
      e) Many chemotherapeutic agents are thought to cause venous thrombosis. Blood is usually drawn from the antecubital fossa. Fibrosed veins would make blood drawing more difficult.

B. Needle size
   1. Favoring the use of a larger gauge (e.g., #19 and #21 scalp-vein needles)
      a) Potentially irritating chemotherapeutic agents can reach the general circulation sooner, with less irritating effect on the peripheral veins.
      b) Drug administration time is decreased, which reduces the patient's exposure to a potentially stressful environment.
   2. Favoring the use of a small gauge (e.g., #23 and #25 scalp-vein needles)
      a) Smaller-gauge needles are less likely to puncture the wall of a small vein.
      b) Scar tissue may be formed with needle insertion; small-gauge needles cause less scar tissue formation.

   c) Less pain may be experienced by the patient during the insertion of a smaller-gauge needle.
   d) Increased blood flow around a smaller-bore needle increases dilution of the chemotherapeutic agent.
   e) Mechanical phlebitis may be minimized with a smaller-bore needle.
   f) Potential episodes of nausea and vomiting may be decreased by slow infusion of the chemotherapeutic agents.

C. Methods of drug sequencing
   1. Favoring the administration of vesicants first
      a) Vascular integrity decreases over time.
      b) The vein is most stable and less irritated at the initiation of the treatment.
      c) The initial assessment of vein patency is most accurate.
      d) The patient's awareness of symptomatic changes becomes less accurate over time.
   2. Favoring the administration of vesicants last
      a) Vesicants are irritating and may increase vein fragility.
      b) Venous spasm can occur at the beginning of intravenous "push" or bolus therapy, which the patient may report as painful; the nurse must decide if the complaint is spasm or infiltration.

D. Side-arm versus direct-push administration
   1. Favoring side-arm administration
      a) Freely running intravenous line allows maximal dilution of drugs that could be potentially irritating.
      b) Can more readily interrupt the administration of the drug while maintaining venous access.
   2. Favoring direct-push administration
      a) Integrity of the vein can be more easily assessed and the early signs of extravasation noted more easily.

From Cancer chemotherapy guidelines module II. Recommendations for nursing practice in the acute care setting; Cancer chemotherapy guidelines module III. Recommendations for nursing practice in the outpatient setting; Cancer chemotherapy guidelines module IV. Recommendations for nursing practice in the home care setting. Pittsburgh: Oncology Nursing Society, 1988. With permission.

is too cold or too concentrated. Nursing assessment of signs and symptoms of extravasation versus other reactions are outlined in Table 49.6. Fortunately, allergic and anaphylactic reactions are rarely encountered in chemotherapy, but as with any drug administration, the nurse must be aware of possible anaphylaxis and the management of this potentially fatal complication. Asparaginase, cisplatin, and bleomycin have been known to cause anaphylactic reactions. Patients should be observed carefully, and supportive equipment, medications, and management guidelines should be available (20).

ROLE OF NURSING IN THE MANAGEMENT OF CHEMOTHERAPEUTIC SIDE EFFECTS

A significant role of oncology nurses with chemotherapy administration is the alleviation of side effects that chemotherapy inevitably causes. There are numerous resources that describe specific nursing interventions for the many side effects of chemotherapy (13, 39, 57–61). This chapter does not describe all of the specific interventions but focuses on those in which nursing research has provided guidance and substantiation of efficacy. Oncology nurses have quantified distressing side effects of chemotherapy and developed strategies to relieve the side effects from a physical and psychosocial perspective in the three major areas of nausea and vomiting, stomatitis, and alopecia.

Nausea and Vomiting

Oncology nurses have studied the variables affecting nausea and vomiting (62–65) and developed reliable and valid measurement instruments (66, 67) that have allowed the further study of patterns of nausea and vomiting and effective nursing interventions (68, 69). Antiemetics have been the foundation for adequate treatment of nausea and vomiting. Until recently, most antiemetic therapy was empirical. It is probably fair to state that the advent of cisplatin and the severe nausea and vomiting associated with this agent initiated many of the antiemetic and combination antiemetic clinical trials. Thus, oncology nurses have undertaken studies that have attempted to find the most effective antiemetic agent for cancer patients receiving chemotherapeutic agents. Drugs that have been examined by oncology nurses include dexamethasone (70), droperidol (71, 72), metaclopromide (73), and numerous combination an-

Table 49.5. Vesicant and Irritant Chemotherapeutic Agents

Vesicants	Irritants
Dactinomycin	Carmustine
Daunomycin	Cisplatin
Doxorubicin	Dacarbazine
Estramustine	Etoposide
Mechlorethamine	5-Fluorouracil
Mitomycin C	Paclitaxel
Vinblastine	Plicamycin
Vincristine	Streptozocin
Vindesine	Teniposide
Vinorelbine	

Table 49.6. Nursing Assessment of Extravasation versus Other Reactions

Assessment Parameter	Extravasation		Irritation of the Vein	Flare Reaction
	Immediate Manifestations	Delayed Manifestations		
Pain	Severe pain or burning that lasts minutes or hours and eventually subsides; usually occurs while the drug is being given and around the needle site	Hours—48	Aching and tightness along the vein	No pain
Redness	Blotchy redness around the needle site; it is not always present at time of extravasation	Later occurrence	The full length of the vein may be reddened or darkened	Immediate blotches or streaks along the vein, which usually subside within 30 minutes with or without treatment
Ulceration	Develops insidiously; usually occurs 48–96 hours later	Later occurrence	Not usually	Not usually
Swelling	Severe swelling; usually occurs immediately	Hours—48	Not likely	Not likely; wheals may appear along vein line
Blood return	Inability to obtain blood return; presence-rate	Good blood return during drug administration	Usually	Usually
Other	Change in the quality of infusion	Local tingling and sensory deficits	—	Urticaria

From Cancer chemotherapy guidelines. Recommendations for the management of vesicant extravasation, hypersensitivity, and anaphylaxis. Pittsburgh: Oncology Nursing Society, 1992. With permission.

tiemetic regimens (74–76). Nonpharmacologic management of nausea and vomiting or behavioral interventions have been examined (77–81). Relaxation techniques have been useful adjuncts in minimizing nausea and vomiting or preventing anticipatory nausea and vomiting. Headley (82) reported that patients receiving chemother-apy in the evening reported less stress than patients treated in the morning.

Stomatitis

The prevention and treatment of stomatitis has also received attention by oncology nurses.

Table 49.7. Evaluation of Stomatitis/Mucositis and Nursing Guidelines

Grade	Description	Interventions
Grade 0	Normal moist mucosa without evidence of inflammation or ulceration	Assessment of mouth twice daily **Oral care regimen** after meals and bedtime: Patient should brush with soft toothbrush and nonabrasive toothpaste Floss q 24 hr with unwaxed dental floss (platelets permitting) Use Water-Pik on lowest setting Avoid commercial mouthwashes due to high alcohol content Rinse with salt/soda solution Avoid hydrogen peroxide for routine care Avoid lemon-glycerine swabs Remove dentures except at mealtime Avoid alcohol and tobacco
Grade 1	Mild mucosal reddening with one or two small ulcerations and minimal discomfort	Oral care regimen q 2 hr while awake and q 6 hr at night Floss if bleeding does not occur Lip lubricant PRN and artificial saliva Use mild analgesic q 3–4 hr Assess need for oral antifungal agent Avoid spicy, acidic, or crusty rough foods Encourage bland foods, high in protein
Grade 2	Moderate erythema with one or two mucosal ulcerations measuring >1 cm in diameter; moderate discomfort requiring local and systemic analgesia; patient able to eat and drink	Use analgesic mixture (swish and swallow) every 2–4 hr Monitor weight Institute nutritional program with >10% weight loss
Grade 3	Confluent ulcerations covering >25% of the oral mucosa; analgesics required; patient is able to take fluids only	Evaluate for infection Culture suspicious lesions Use soaked gauze or toothettes for cleaning Do not floss Alternate warm saline mouthwash with antibacterial or antifungal oral suspension q 2 hr while awake and q 4 hr at night
Grade 4	Severe discomfort due to multiple mucosal ulcerations covering >50% of the oral mucosa, complicated by bleeding; analgesics (morphine) required; patient is unable to eat or drink fluids	Lip lubricant q 2 hr Irrigate mouth with sodium bicarbonate solution followed by saline rinse if thick mucus and crusts are present Provide dietary supplements, enteral feedings, or i.v. fluids as necessary Local analgesics as ordered Systemic analgesics as ordered

Information taken from references 39, 57, 60, 84.

Beck (83) evaluated the effect of a systematic oral care protocol on the development of stomatitis in patients receiving chemotherapy. She reported significantly less stomatitis and fewer oral infections in those patients who received an oral care protocol. While oral care regimens may not prevent stomatitis, prophylactic oral care may minimize the mucosal breakdown, thus preventing serious infections and helping to maintain nutritional status (60). Oncology nurses must not only be aware of which drugs cause stomatitis but be able to evaluate the degrees of stomatitis, to provide the appropriate oral care regimens. Table 49.7 identifies the different grades of stomatitis/mucositis and appropriate nursing interventions (39, 57, 60, 84).

Alopecia

Although hair loss is not a life-threatening side effect of chemotherapy, alopecia is very distressing to many patients. Nursing studies have looked for ways to prevent or slow hair loss. Lovejoy (85) evaluated the effects of scalp ischemia on hair loss in patients receiving doxorubicin. The study subjects who received treatment with a special sphygmomanometer cuff placed around the head and inflated to 50 mm Hg above systolic pressure experienced less hair loss than the control subjects. Dean et al. (86) examined the effects of lowering scalp temperature on the degree of hair loss in patients receiving doxorubicin. With scalp temperatures of 23 to 24°C, hair loss was prevented in those patients who received 50 mg or less of doxorubicin. If the doses were greater than 60 mg, the scalp hypothermia was less effective.

Since the earlier studies, products have been developed to prevent alopecia by scalp icing, with varying results. In a controlled study by Kennedy et al. (87), the product studied was not effective in preventing or delaying alopecia. However, a similar study with a different scalp hypothermia product reported it as an effective method in preventing hair loss (88). Regardless of whether scalp hypothermia is used, early patient education is essential in preparation for hair loss, so that wigs and turbans will be available when needed (89).

CONCLUSION

Advances in chemotherapy and supportive care have dramatically increased patient survival and improved quality of life. These advances have also had a major impact on the responsibilities of nurses who are involved with chemotherapy. The nurse must not only assess the physical and emotional status of the patient and plan the nursing care to be followed during the course of treatment but also provide patient education, counseling, and emotional support throughout. Knowledge of drugs, their mode of action, and expected effects is essential. A skillful technique is required with the administration of these drugs. It is the responsibility of the oncology nurse to keep abreast of new and innovative treatment methods and supportive measures for patients receiving cancer chemotherapy and to contribute to the development of additional methods through participation in research. Nurses are the key to the safety and quality of life of patients receiving chemotherapy.

REFERENCES

1. Hubbard SM, DeVita V. Chemotherapy research nurse. Am J Nurs 1976;76:560–565.
2. Hubbard SM, Donehower MG. The nurse in a cancer research setting. Semin Oncol 1980;7:9–17.
3. Henke C. Emerging roles of the nurse in oncology. Semin Oncol 1980;7:4–8.
4. Yarbro CH. Nursing factors concerning the administration of intravenous anti-tumor chemotherapy. In: Tiffany R, ed. Cancer nursing update: proceedings of the 2nd International Cancer Nursing Conference. London: Baillière-Tindall, 1980:64–66.
5. Hubbard SM. Clinical research and cancer nursing. Oncol Nurs Forum 1981;8:17–23.
6. Yarbro CH. The role of the oncology nurse in cancer chemotherapy. In: Hellman K, Carter SK, eds. Fundamentals of cancer chemotherapy. New York: McGraw-Hill, 1987:379–386.
7. Lind J, Bush NJ. Nursing's role in chemotherapy administration. Semin Oncol Nurs 1987;3:83–86.
8. Hubbard SM. Reflections on the oncology nurse's role in cancer therapy: future challenges. Semin Oncol Nurs 1987;3:154–158.
9. Yarbro CH, Lind J. Nursing considerations in cancer chemotherapy. In: Carter S, Bakowski MT, Hellman K, eds. Chemotherapy of cancer. 3rd ed. New York: Churchill Livingstone, 1988:325–340.
10. Gallina EJ. Practical guide to chemotherapy administration for physicians and oncology nurses. In: DeVita V, Hellman S, Rosenberg SA, eds. Cancer: principles and practice of oncology. 4th ed. Philadelphia: JB Lippincott, 1993:2570–2580.
11. Reymann PE. Chemotherapy: principles of administration. In: Groenwald SL, Frogge MH, Goodman M, Yarbro CH, eds. Cancer nursing: principles and practice. 3rd ed. Boston: Jones and Bartlett, 1993:293–330.
12. Wujcik D. Chemotherapy administration. Cancer Nurs 1987;10:53–64.
13. McNally JM, Somerville ET, Miaskowski C, Rostad M, eds. Guidelines for cancer nursing practice. 2nd ed. Philadelphia: WB Saunders, 1991.
14. American Nurses' Association and Oncology Nursing Society. Standards of oncology nursing prac-

tice. Kansas City, MO: American Nurses' Association, 1987.

15. Oncology Nursing Society. Standards of advanced practice in oncology nursing. Pittsburgh: Oncology Nursing Society, 1990.

16. Cancer chemotherapy guidelines module I. Recommendations for cancer chemotherapy course content and clinical practicum. Pittsburgh: Oncology Nursing Society, 1988.

17. Cancer chemotherapy guidelines module II. Recommendations for nursing practice in the acute care setting. Pittsburgh: Oncology Nursing Society, 1988.

18. Cancer chemotherapy guidelines module III. Recommendations for nursing practice in the outpatient setting. Pittsburgh: Oncology Nursing Society, 1988.

19. Cancer chemotherapy guidelines module IV. Recommendations for nursing practice in the home care setting. Pittsburgh: Oncology Nursing Society, 1988.

20. Cancer chemotherapy guidelines. Recommendations for the management of vesicant extravasation, hypersensitivity and anaphylaxis. Pittsburgh: Oncology Nursing Society, 1992.

21. Comis RL. Oral etoposide in small-cell lung cancer. Semin Oncol 1986;13(Suppl):75–78.

22. Yarbro JW. Mechanism of action of hydroxyurea. Semin Oncol 1992;19(Suppl 9):1–10.

23. Levine AM, Richardson JL, Marks G, et al. Compliance with oral drug therapy in patients with hematologic malignancy. J Clin Oncol 1987;5:1469–1476.

24. Reed WP, Newman AK, DeJongh C, et al. Prolonged venous access for chemotherapy by means of the Hickman catheter. Cancer 1983;52:185–192.

25. Wagman LD, Kirkemo A, Johnston MR. Venous access: a prospective, randomized study of the Hickman catheter. Surgery 1984;95:303–308.

26. Raaf JH. Results from use of 826 vascular access devices in cancer patients. Cancer 1985;55:1312–1321.

27. Simon RC. Small-gauge central venous catheters and right atrial catheters. Semin Oncol Nurs 1987; 3:87–95.

28. Wickham R, Purl S, Welker D. Long-term central venous catheters: issues for care. Semin Oncol Nurs 1992;8:133–147.

29. Hadaway LC. Comparison of vascular access devices. Semin Oncol Nurs 1995;11:154–166.

30. Brant JM. The use of access devices in cancer pain control. Semin Oncol Nurs 1995;11:203–212.

31. Winslow MN, Trammell L, Camp-Sorrell D. Selection of vascular access devices and nursing care. Semin Oncol Nurs 1995;11:167–173.

32. Daeffler RJ, Lewinski J. Patient education: home care of the Hickman/Broviac catheter. Oncol Nurs Forum 1982;9:59–63.

33. Goodman MS, Wickham R. Venous access devices: an overview. Oncol Nurs Forum 1984;11:16–23.

34. McDermott MK. Patient education and compliance issues associated with access devices. Semin Oncol Nurs 1995;11:221–226.

35. Williams ME, Walker AN, Bracikowski JP, Garner L, Wilson KD, Carpenter JT. Ascending myeloencephalopathy due to intrathecal vincristine sulfate. Cancer 1983;51:2041–2047.

36. Rapsilber LM, Camp-Sorrell D. Ambulatory in-

fusion pumps: application to oncology. Semin Oncol Nurs 1995;11:213–220.

37. Mioduszewski J, Zarbo AG. Ambulatory infusion pumps: a practical view at an alternative approach. Semin Oncol Nurs 1987;3:106–111.

38. Culhane M, Jenkins J. The Auto-Syringe infusion pump: a patient's guide. Oncol Nurs Forum 1984; 11:87–91.

39. Tennebaum L. Cancer chemotherapy and biotherapy: a reference guide. 2nd ed. Philadelphia: WB Saunders, 1994.

40. Hagle ME. Implantable devices for chemotherapy: access and delivery. Semin Oncol Nurs 1987;3:96–105.

41. Almadrones L, Campana P, Dantis EC. Arterial, peritoneal, and intraventricular access devices. Semin Oncol Nurs 1995;11:194–202.

42. Esparza DM, Weyland B. Nursing care for the patient with an Ommaya reservoir. Oncol Nurs Forum 1982;9:17–20.

43. Roemeling R, MacDonald M, Langevin T, Buchwald H, Hrushesky WJM. Chemotherapy via implanted infusion pump: new perspectives for delivery of long-term continuous treatment. Oncol Nurs Forum 1986;13:17–24.

44. Rumsey KA, Richardson DK. Management of infection and occlusion associated with vascular access devices. Semin Oncol Nurs 1995;11:174–183.

45. Ingle RJ. Rare complications of vascular access devices. Semin Oncol Nurs 1995;11:184–193.

46. Miller SA. Considerations in the outpatient administration of cisplatin. Semin Oncol Nurs 1987; 3(Suppl):3–7.

47. Frogge MH. Practical considerations for administration of cisplatin in the outpatient setting. Semin Oncol Nurs 1987;3(Suppl):16–22.

48. Burish TG, Snyder SL, Jenkins RA. Preparing patients for cancer chemotherapy: effect of coping preparation and relaxation interventions. J Consult Clin Psychol 1991;59:518–525.

49. Kris MG. Ondansetron. A specific serotonin antagonist for the prevention of chemotherapy-induced vomiting. PPO Updates 1994;8(2):1–11.

50. Perez EA, Gandara DR. The clinical role of granisetron (Kytril) in the prevention of chemotherapy-induced emesis. Semin Oncol 1994;21(Suppl 5):15–21.

51. Hesketh PJ, Beck T, Uhlenhopp M, et al. Adjusting the dose of intravenous ondansetron plus dexamethasone to the emetogenic potential of the chemotherapy regimen. J Clin Oncol 1995;13:2117–2122.

52. Welch D, Follo J, Nelson E. The development of a specialized nursing assessment tool for cancer patients. Oncol Nurs Forum 1982;9:37–44.

53. Miakowski CA, Nielsen B. A cancer nursing assessment tool. Oncol Nurs Forum 1985;12:37–42.

54. Miller SA. Issues in cytotoxic drug handling safety. Semin Oncol Nurs 1987;3:133–141.

55. Stolar M, Power L, Viele C. Recommendations for handling cytotoxic drugs in hospitals. Am J Hosp Pharm 1983;40:1163–1171.

56. Office of Occupational Medicine. Work practice guidelines for personnel dealing with cytotoxic (antineoplastic) drugs. Occupational Safety and Health Administration, U.S. Dept. of Labor. Washington, DC: OSHA instruction publication 8-1.1, 1986.

57. Goodman M, Ladd LA, Purl S. Integumentary

and mucous membrane alterations. In: Groenwald SL, Frogge MH, Goodman M, Yarbro CH, eds. Cancer nursing: principles and practice. 3rd ed. Boston: Jones and Bartlett, 1993:734–799.

58. Camp-Sorrell D. Chemotherapy: toxicity management. In: Groenwald SL, Frogge MH, Goodman M, Yarbro CH, eds. Cancer nursing: principles and practice. 3rd ed. Boston: Jones and Bartlett, 1993:331–365.

59. Gross J, Johnson BL. Handbook of oncology nursing. Boston: Jones and Bartlett, 1994.

60. Goodman M. Managing the side effects of chemotherapy. Semin Oncol Nurs 1989;5(Suppl):29–52.

61. Groenwald SL, Frogge MH, Goodman M, Yarbro CH, eds. Cancer symptom management. Boston: Jones and Bartlett, 1996.

62. Scogna DM. Variables affecting nausea and vomiting. Oncol Nurs Forum 1977;4:5–7.

63. Kennedy M, Packard R, Grant MM, Padilla GV. Chemotherapy related nausea and vomiting: a survey to identify problems and interventions. Oncol Nurs Forum 1981;8:19–22.

64. Zook DJ, Yasko JM. Psychologic factors: their effect on nausea and vomiting experienced by clients receiving chemotherapy. Oncol Nurs Forum 1983; 10:76–81.

65. Rhodes VA, Watson PM, Johnson MH. Association of chemotherapy-related nausea and vomiting with pretreatment and posttreatment anxiety. Oncol Nurs Forum 1986;13:41–47.

66. McCorkle R, Young K. Development of a symptom distress scale. Cancer Nurs 1978;1:373–378.

67. Rhodes VA, Watson PM, Johnson MH. Development of reliable and valid measures of nausea and vomiting. Cancer Nurs 1984;7:33–41.

68. Rhodes VA, Watson PM, Johnson MH, et al. Patterns of nausea, vomiting, and distress in patients receiving antineoplastic drug protocols. Oncol Nurs Forum 1987;14:35–44.

69. Rhodes VA, Johnson MH, McDaniel RW. Nausea, vomiting, and retching: the management of the symptom experience. Semin Oncol Nurs, 1996;11:256–265.

70. Gathercole F, Connolly N, Birdsell J. The use of dexamethasone (Hexadrol) as an antiemetic in association with chemotherapy for neoplastic disease. Oncol Nurs Forum 1982;9:17–19.

71. Lamb HC, Cox FM. Clinical use of droperidol (Inapsine) in patients with chemotherapy induced nausea and vomiting. Oncol Nurs Forum 1982;9:23–25.

72. Berry-Opersteny D, Heusinkueld KB. Prophylactic antiemetics for chemotherapy-associated nausea and vomiting. Cancer Nurs 1983;6:117–123.

73. Daniels M, Belt RJ. High-dose metoclopramide as an antiemetic for patients receiving chemotherapy with cisplatinum. Oncol Nurs Forum 1982;9:20–22.

74. Clark RA, Tyson LB, Gralla RJ, Kris MG. Antiemetic therapy: management of chemotherapy-induced nausea and vomiting. Semin Oncol Nurs 1989; 5:53–57.

75. Tyson LB, Kris MG, Gralla RJ, et al. Double blind randomized trial for the control of delayed emesis: comparison of placebo vs dexamethasone vs metoclopramide plus dexamethasone (abstract). Proc Am Soc Clin Oncol 1987;6:267.

76. Simms SG, Rhodes VA, Madsen RW. Comparison of prochlorperazine and lorazepam antiemetic regimens in the control of postchemotherapy symptoms. Nurs Res 1993;42:234–239.

77. Cotanch PH. Relaxation training for control of nausea and vomiting in patients receiving chemotherapy. Cancer Nurs 1983;6:277–283.

78. Cotanch PH. Relaxation techniques as antiemetic therapy. In: Laszlo J, ed. Antiemetics and cancer chemotherapy. Baltimore: Williams & Wilkins, 1983:164–176.

79. Cotanch PH, Hockenberry M, Herman S. Self-hypnosis as antiemetic therapy in children receiving chemotherapy. Oncol Nurs Forum 1985;12:41–46.

80. Cotanch PH, Strum S. Progressive muscle relaxation as antiemetic therapy for cancer patients. Oncol Nurs Forum 1987;14:33–37.

81. Troesch LM, Rodehaver CB, Delaney EA, et al. The influence of guided imagery on chemotherapy-related nausea and vomiting. Oncol Nurs Forum 1993; 20:1179–1185.

82. Headley JA. The influence of administration time on chemotherapy-induced nausea and vomiting. Oncol Nurs Forum 1987;14:43–47.

83. Beck S. Impact of a systematic oral care protocol on stomatitis after chemotherapy. Cancer Nurs 1979; 2:185–199.

84. Dose AM. The symptom experience of mucositis, stomatitis, and xerostomia. Semin Oncol Nurs, 1996;11:248–255.

85. Lovejoy N. Preventing hair loss during Adriamycin therapy. Cancer Nurs 1979;2:117–122.

86. Dean JC, Salmon SE, Griffith KS. Prevention of doxorubicin-induced hair loss with scalp hypothermia. N Engl J Med 1979;301:1427–1429.

87. Kennedy M, Packard R, Grant M, Padilla GV, Presant C, Chillar R. The effects of using Chemocap on occurrence of chemotherapy-induced alopecia. Oncol Nurs Forum 1983;10:19–24.

88. Parker R. The effectiveness of scalp hypothermia in preventing cyclophosphamide induced alopecia. Oncol Nurs Forum 1987;14:49–53.

89. Pickard-Holley S. The symptom experience of alopecia. Semin Oncol Nurs, 1996;11:235–238.

Section Six

Current Therapy of Specific Solid Tumors

50

Chemotherapy of Melanoma

Faith E. Nathan, David Berd, Michael J. Mastrangelo

The patient with surgically incurable melanoma presents a vexing problem for the medical oncologist. Despite the fanfare surrounding biologic therapies, chemotherapy remains the mainstay of treatment for the physician in clinical practice. Although single agents at conventional doses produce bona fide remissions, these are infrequent. There have been many attempts to improve the modest therapeutic efficacy of these agents. Postsurgical adjuvant therapy has not been clearly proven to be of discernible benefit. Until recently, combinations of drugs yielded no real improvement over treatment with the individual components. The introduction of cisplatin and the move toward regional and systemic dose intensification have resulted in some promising regimens. This chapter reviews these various new approaches and from among them recommends what currently appear to be the most promising.

SINGLE-AGENT CHEMOTHERAPY

Not unexpectedly, chemotherapeutic agents were first used singly in the treatment of patients with surgically incurable melanoma. This literature has been exhaustively reviewed (1–5). The most active single agent for the treatment of metastatic melanoma is dimethyl-triazeno-imidazole-carboxamide (dacarbazine; DTIC), which produces an overall response rate of 20% (Table 50.1). Complete remissions are infrequent; however, the median duration of response approaches 1 year (9). Subcutaneous, lymph node, and pulmonary metastases are most likely to respond, whereas DTIC is essentially ineffective against brain metastases. The therapeutic efficacy of DTIC does not appear to be dose or schedule dependent in humans. Doses and schedules have varied widely and include 2 or

4.5 mg/kg/day × 10 days, 250 mg/m^2/day × 5 days, and 850 to 1000 mg/m^2/day × 1 dose. Treatment is repeated monthly. Hematologic toxicity is generally mild. Gastrointestinal toxicity (especially nausea and vomiting) varies directly with the intensity of the regimen, being most severe with the single infusion. Likewise, photosensitivity seems more common with large single doses. Thus, 3- or 5-day courses are reasonable compromises.

DTIC can cause mild disturbances in liver function chemistries (17). However, hepatic venoocclusive disease also may occur and result in acute hepatic failure that is often fatal (18, 19). Fortunately, this complication is rare. Although the pathogenesis of this phenomenon is uncertain, a drug reaction is suggested by its occurrence during a second or subsequent cycle of treatment and the associated eosinophilia.

The nitrosoureas (BCNU, CCNU, methyl-CCNU, chlorozotocin, fotemustine) are also active as single agents, with objective response rates ranging from 9 to 22%. Because of the lipid solubility of these compounds, it was hoped that they would be effective against brain metastases, but at conventional doses this is not the case. One exception may be fotemustine, a 2-chloroethyl-nitrosourea in which 1-amino-ethyl-phosphonic acid is grafted onto a nitrosourea molecule. In the French multicenter phase II study (30), 3 complete and 34 partial responses were seen among 153 evaluable patients, including 9 partial responses in 36 patients with cerebral metastases. In a smaller phase II study with 31 evaluable patients (31), 2 partial responses were observed among 10 patients with brain metastases. As with DTIC, subcutaneous, lymph node, and lung metastases are most responsive to the nitrosoureas. Median response duration varies from 2 to 6 months. By comparison with DTIC, hematologic toxicity is more severe and can be

Table 50.1. Single Agents Active in the Treatment of Metastatic Melanoma

Agent	Response rate (%) CR[a] + PR/total evaluable		References
Dacarbazine (DTIC)	371/1868	(20%)	(1, 6–16)
Nitrosoureas			
Carmustine (BCNU)	22/122	(18%)	(2)
Lomustine (CCNU)	35/270	(13%)	(2, 20, 21)
Semustine (methyl-CCNU)	54/347	(16%)	(2, 22–24)
Chlorozotocin	16/169	(9%)	(25–29)
Fotemustine	40/184	(22%)	(30, 31)
Vinca alkaloids			
Vincristine	6/52	(12%)	(32–37)
Vinblastine	8/62	(13%)	(38–47)
Vindesine	39/273	(14%)	(48–59)
Cisplatin (DDP)	17/114	(15%)	(60–64)
Taxol	12/73	(16%)	(66–68)
Taxotere	5/30	(17%)	(69)

[a]CR, complete response; PR, partial response.

prolonged. Gastrointestinal toxicity is modest. The oral nitrosoureas offer a major advantage in convenience of administration.

Of the vinca alkaloids, vindesine, a semisynthetic derivative of vinblastine, has been most extensively studied and produces an overall response rate of 14%. Antitumor activity appears to be schedule dependent: intermittent bolus therapy produced a 17% response rate (39/273) (49–56), whereas no responses were noted among 45 patients treated by continuous infusion (57–59). Toxicities are similar to those seen with other vinca alkaloids.

At doses ranging from 60 to 120 mg/m^2, cisplatin has produced objective remissions in 15% of patients. Although several complete responses have been noted, the median duration of response is only 3 months. Cisplatin has been disappointing as a single agent at conventional doses.

Taxol, a plant product isolated from the stem bark of the western yew (*Taxus brevifolia*), is the first of a new class of drugs, which mediates its antitumor effects by promoting and stabilizing the polymerization of microtubules (65). Three complete and nine partial responses were noted among 73 patients treated at a dose of at least 200 mg/m^2 as a 24-hour continuous infusion. Responses were noted in liver, lung, soft tissues, lymph nodes, and skin (66). One complete response exceeded 46 months in duration. Toxicities include neutropenia, peripheral neuropathy, and occasional acute hypersensitivity reactions (67, 68). Taxotere (docetaxel) is a semisynthetic taxoid synthesized from 10-deacetyl-baccatin III, a compound isolated from the needles of the Eu-

ropean yew. Like Taxol, it binds to and stabilizes microtubules, rendering them nonfunctional. Its activity against advanced melanoma has been investigated in a phase II trial by Aamdal et al. (69). Five partial responses were observed in 30 evaluable patients (17%). These were seen in soft tissue, lung, lymph nodes, skin, and liver. Observed toxicities were neutropenia, alopecia, malaise and fatigue, nausea and diarrhea, skin and sensory changes, and hypersensitivity reactions.

The interferons (α, β, and γ) are glycoproteins produced by a wide range of cells in response to various stimuli including viruses, double-stranded RNA, and mitogens. They perform immunoregulatory, antiviral, and antineoplastic functions. This latter effect appears to be mediated by an inhibition of cell proliferation, and for that reason, they are included with the chemotherapeutic agents. The α-interferons (both natural and recombinant) have been most frequently studied (Table 50.2). The intramuscular route has been employed most often. Schedules have included both daily and intermittent administration, and doses have ranged from 10^6 to 10^7 units. The overall response rate was 13.3% (55 of 414), with 5.1% of patients achieving complete remissions, which were often quite durable. Tumor regression has been noted with all routes, schedules, and doses; the available data do not permit the definition of the best regimen. A practical solution is 3 to 20 × 10^6 units (escalated as tolerated), three times a week until disease progression. The onset of tumor regression varied from one to several months. Remissions have also been noted with γ-interferon. Data

Table 50.2. Clinical Results with Interferons as Single Agents

Type	Investigators	Dose	Schedule	Route	PTS[a]	CR	PR	PR	MDR (Range)
α	Creagan et al. (70)	12×10^6 U/m²	TIW	i.m.	30	1	5	20%	7 mo (2–35+)
		50×10^6 U/M²			31	3	4	23%	6 mo (3–41+)
α	Hersey et al. (71)	$15–50 \times 10^6$ U/m²	TIW	i.m.	18	32	0	11%	(6, 12 mo)
					31	0	2	6%	
α	Legha et al. (72)	18×10^6 U	TIW	i.m.	35	0	3	9%	30 wk (27–88+)
		$3–36 \times 10^6$ U/m²							
α	Kuzmits et al. (73)	$5–30 \times 10^6$ U/m²	TIW	i.m.	11	1	0	9%	13+ mo
α	Elsasser-Beile et al. (74)	18×10^6 U	Daily	i.m.	30	3	0	10%	34 wk (24–50)
α	Krown et al. (75)	1×10^6 U	Daily	i.m.	16	0	0	6%	5 wk
		3×10^6 U			14	0	1	0%	—[b]
		9×10^6 U			14	0	0	0%	—
α	Lanthaler et al. (76)	2.5×10^6 U	Daily	i.m.	20	0	0	0%	—
α	Kirkwood et al. (77)	$3–100 \times 10^6$ U	Daily	i.m.	7	0	2	29%	3, 4 mo
				i.v.	16	2	0	13%	28+, 30+, mo
α	Coates et al. (78)	20×10^6 U/m²	Daily × 5 QOW	i.v.	15	0	0	0%	—
α	Dorval et al. (79, 80)	10×10^6 U/m²	TIW	s.c.	24	2	5	29%	3 mo (1–12.5)
α	Mughal et al. (81)	10^6 U/m²	TIW	s.c.	51	4	6	20%	—
α	Von Wussow et al. (82)	10^6 U	TIW	i.l.	51	3[c]	6[c]	18%	(2–20+ mo)
α	Haase et al. (83)	30–40 IU	Daily	i.v.	17	2	2	24%	7.5 mo (1.5–21+)
γ	Creagan et al. (84)	0.2–0.5 mg/m²	Daily	i.m.	28	0	3	11%	3.9+ mo (3.7–8.3)
γ	Ernstoff et al. (85)	3–3000 mg/m²	Daily × 14	i.v. (2 hr)	16	1	1	7%	6, 6 mo
			Daily × 14	i.v. (24 hr)	14				

[a]PTS, total evaluable patients; CR, complete response; PR, partial response; RR, overall response rate; MDR, median duration remission; U, units; TIW, three times per week; i.m., intramuscular; i.v., intravenous; QOW, every other week; s.c., subcutaneous; i.l., intralesional; IU, international units.
[b]No data.
[c]Systemic responses only.

Table 50.3. Single-Agent Treatment Regimens

Drug	Regimen	Adequate Trial[a]
Dacarbazine	250 mg/m² i.v.[b] daily × 5, q 4 wk	One 5-day course
Carmustine	100 mg/m² i.v. daily × 2, q 6 wk	One 2-day course
Lomustine	130 mg/m² p.o. once q 6 wk	One dose
Fotemustine	100 mg/m² i.v. weekly × 3, then q 3 wk after 4–5 wk interval	3 wk
Vincristine	1–2 mg/m² (not to exceed 2 mg/dose in the adult) i.v. weekly	4–6 wk
Vinblastine	0.1–0.2 mg/kg i.v. every 1 or 2 wk	4–6 wk
Vindesine	3–4 mg/m² i.v. bolus weekly	4–6 wk
Cisplatin	80–12 mg/m² i.v. q 3 wk	One dose
α-Interferon	10–20 × 10⁶ units i.m. TIW	4–8 wk
Taxol	250 mg/m² over 24 hours every 3 wk	6 wk
Taxotere	100 mg/m² i.v. every 3 weeks	6 wk

[a]With the exception of dacarbazine, a minimum adequate trial assumes that the drug has been administered to significant toxicity.
[b]i.v., intravenous; p.o., oral; i.m., intramuscular; TIW, three times per week.

with β-interferon as a single agent are meager. Attempts at combination therapy have included γ- and β-interferon (86); α-interferon with γ-interferon (87), DTIC (88), α-difluoromethylornithine (89), cimetidine (70, 90), or indomethacin (91); and β-interferon with DTIC and cimetidine (92). However, none of these combinations has better therapeutic efficacy than α-interferon alone.

In summary, there are a number of single agents that produce bona fide but infrequent remissions in patients with metastatic melanoma. These are listed along with suggested doses/schedules in Table 50.3. DTIC serves as the benchmark for comparisons. The oral nitrosoureas are convenient to administer, and fotemustine may be useful in the treatment of brain metastases. Cisplatin (conventional doses) and the vinca alkaloids are now most frequently used in combination regimens. The role of α-interferon continues to be debated. Some complete responses were noted at doses at which the common toxicities of fever, chills, and malaise were quite tolerable. Taxol and Taxotere are promising new drugs that await further study. However, the pace of development of new agents with greater antimelanoma activity has been slow. Betulinic acid, a pentacyclic triterpene extracted from the stem bark of *Ziziphus mauritiana* Lam (Rhamnaceae) appears to be selectively cytotoxic for human melanoma cells in vitro and in athymic nude mice (93). Perhaps this compound will emerge as a truly effective single agent in clinical trials. There have been many attempts by oncologists to improve the efficacy of currently available single agents including adjuvant use, combination regimens, dose intensification, and in vitro selection for chemosensitivity. These efforts are discussed below.

ADJUVANT CHEMOTHERAPY

The microstage of the primary tumor (by depth of invasion) and the extent of regional lymph node involvement allow the identification of patients at high risk for recurrence following definitive surgery. The definition of high risk varies but for stage I (local disease) includes Clark's level 3 or greater and Breslow thicknesses of 1.5 mm or more. Stage II (regional disease) and stage III (disseminated tumor) patients who are free of disease following surgery also have been placed in adjuvant trials. Most trials lack appropriate controls. Randomized prospective studies with an untreated control and at least one arm containing chemotherapy are summarized in Table 50.4. DTIC has been the agent studied most extensively. In the largest study, the World Health Organization (WHO) (95) randomized 761 evaluable patients, stage I (Clark's

Table 50.4. Randomized Prospective Trials of Adjuvant Chemotherapy

Investigator	Eligibility	No. of Patients	Arms	Results
				Median DFI
Hill et al. (94)	Stages I, II, III[a]	81	Control	73 wk
		84	DTIC[b]	40 wk
				% DF at 3 yr
Veronesi et al. (95)	Stage I, Clark 3–5	185	Control	30.4 ± 8.3
	Stage II	192	DTIC	37.2 ± 7.9
		203	BCG	34.8 ± 7.9
		181	DTIC + BCG	33.6 ± 7.9
				% DF at 5 yr
Lejeune et al. (96)	Stage I, Clark 3	96	Control	58
	(>1.5 mm), 4,	77	DTIC	50
	or 5	101	Levamisole	55
				Recurrences
Holterman et al.	Stages I, II	28	Control	9
Karakousis et al. (97, 98)		27	DTIC + Estracyt	8
		29	BCG	8
Quirt et al. (99)	Stage I, Clark 3–5	28	Control	No difference in
	Stage II	29	DTIC + BCG	DFI or survival
				Median DFI
Fisher et al. (100)	Stage I, Clark 4	41	Control	13 mo[c]
	(>2.25 mm), 5	40	Methyl-CCNU	30 mo[c]
	Stage II	42	BCG	13 mo
		43	BCG + TC	30 mo

[a]Stage I, local disease; stage II, regional disease; stage III disseminated disease.
[b]DTIC, dacarbazine; BCG, bacillus Calmette-Guerin; methyl-CCNU, semustine; TC, tumor cells; DFI, disease-free interval; DF, disease-free.
[c]$p = .068$.

level 3–5) or stage II, to surgery only, surgery plus DTIC, surgery plus bacillus Calmette-Guerin (BCG), or surgery plus DTIC plus BCG. Although the DTIC group fared better than the control, there was no statistically significant difference in survival. However, 540 patients would be required in each group to demonstrate statistical significance for a difference of this magnitude. Adjuvant DTIC seems worth reassessment. However, at least one death has been attributed to DTIC-induced hepatic venoocclusive disease. The data with methyl-CCNU are also interesting as the differences in median disease-free interval approach statistical significance ($p = .068$) (100). However, this agent is leukemogenic (101).

Levamisole is an anthelmintic drug reported to have immunomodulating activity, and for this reason, it has been extensively evaluated as a postsurgical adjuvant. It is approved as adjuvant therapy with 5-fluorouracil for patients with Dukes' C colon cancer, the only malignancy in which its use has led to improved survival. The mechanism of the apparent antitumor effect is unknown. Four randomized trials have reported results comparing levamisole with a surgery-only control arm (96, 102–103) as adjuvant therapy for melanoma (Table 50.5). Three studies (96, 102, 104) concluded that levamisole was not effective in increasing survival. In a trial in which the dose of levamisole was based on actual body

weight (103), the 5-year survival was 62% in the control group and 74% in the levamisole group ($p = .03$). The significance of this difference disappeared, however, when multifactorial analysis was performed.

α-Interferon is of some use in the treatment of metastatic melanoma, thus suggesting a possible role in the adjuvant setting. The results of several trials have been published (Table 50.6). Kokoschka et al. (105) evaluated the efficacy of α_{2b}-interferon in 135 stage I and II patients. No significant difference in overall survival was observed between the group that received interferon and the group that did not. WHO (106) conducted a randomized controlled trial in which 426 patients with pathologically documented lymph node metastases (419 also clinically positive) were randomized to interferon (218 patients) (3×10^6 U 3 times/week for 3 years) or surgery alone (208 patients). At a median follow-up of 19 months, the 2-year disease-free survival in the treated group was 46% and in the control group, 27% ($p = .01$). Subset analysis suggested an improved disease-free survival in men with increasing age and a decreasing survival in women with decreasing age, but this post hoc analysis was not planned in the study design, so its validity is questionable. A more recent analysis (107) with a median follow-up of 39 months showed that the disease-free survival of the interferon group had fallen to ap-

Table 50.5. Adjuvant Studies of Levamisole

Investigator	Eligibility	No. of Patients	Arms	Results[a]
				% DF at 5 yr[a]
Lejeune et al. (96)	Stage I, Clark 3 (>1.5 mm), 4, or 5	96	Control	58
		77	DTIC[b]	50
		101	Levamisole	55
				Recurrences
Loufi (102)	Stage I, Clark 3–5	73	Levamisole	22
		64	Control	17
				% 5-yr OS
Quirt (103)	Stage I, Clark (>0.75 mm), 4, 5 or satellite within 3 cm or intransit metastases, Stage II	137	Control	62
		136	BCG	59
		135	BCG + levamisole	65
		135	Levamisole	74
Spitler (104)	Clark 3–5 or cutaneous or subcutaneous or LN[c] recurrence	99	Control	No difference in survival
		104	Levamisole	

[a]DF, disease-free; OS, overall survival.
[b]DTIC, dacarbazine; BCG, bacillus Calmette-Guerin.
[c]LN, lymph nodes.

Table 50.6. Adjuvant Studies of Interferon

Reference	No. of Evaluable Patients	Dose	Difference from Control (*p* value)
Kokoschka (105)	~135	3 MU[a] SC t/i.w. × 3 mo, then 3 MU SC b.i.w. × 6 mo, then 2 MU SC b.i.w. × 10 mo	NS[b]
Cascinelli (106, 107)	426	3 MU SC t.i.w. × 3 yr	0.08[c]
Kirkwood (108)	262	20 MU/m²/d i.v. d 1–5 weekly × 4, then 10 MU/m²/d SC t.i.w. × 48 wk	Not stated

[a]MU, million units; SC, subcutaneously; t.i.w., three times weekly; b.i.w., two times weekly; i.v., intravenously; NS, not significant.
[b]Overall survival.
[c]Disease-free survival.

proximately 37% in the treated group (*p* = .08). The power of this study was inadequate to confirm the 10% difference between treated and control patients as statistically significant. Also of interest was the observation that the risk of recurrence increased when interferon treatment ceased at 3 years. Toxicity of this low-dose interferon regimen was minimal.

Preliminary results of an Eastern Cooperative Oncology Group (ECOG) trial (108) demonstrate an improved disease-free survival (DFS) in patients randomized to receive high-dose α-interferon (20 × 10⁶ U/m²/day i.v. daily for 5 days every week for 4 weeks followed by 10 × 10⁶ U/m²/day subcutaneously three times weekly for 48 weeks). At a median follow-up of 4.7 years, the DFS of the treated group is 38%, compared with 26% in the control group (109). Toxicity was significant; 66% of patients experienced grade 3 toxicity, 9% experienced grade 4 toxicity, and 2 deaths occurred. A detailed report is awaiting publication. These results led to the development of a 3-arm study in which high-risk patients are randomized to 1 year of high-dose α_{2b}-interferon, chronic low-dose interferon (3 × 10⁶/day three times weekly for 2 years), or observation. Although this trial is now closed to accrual, the results will not be available for some time.

The results obtained by Retsas et al. (110) using long-term vindesine treatment are of interest. The control group was concurrent, but allocation was not random. Both treatment and control groups were exhaustively analyzed for comparability. The disease-free interval, time to dissemination from lymph node metastases, survival following lymph node dissection, and overall survival were all significantly better (*p* = .0001, *p* < .001, *p* = .0227, *p* = .0095, respectively) in the vindesine-treated group. This observation is worthy of further testing in a randomized setting.

In summary, DTIC and α-interferon may each be of modest benefit in the adjuvant setting. Unfortunately, the trials were not of adequate power to confirm statistical significance of the differences observed. When treating stage I or stage II patients adjunctively, one risks injuring some individuals who were already cured by surgery. Thus, in the absence of an agent of demonstrated benefit, such individuals are best treated in a research setting. Stage III patients who have undergone resection of visceral metastases are at virtually 100% risk of recurrence and would be suitable subjects for future adjuvant trials. At present, clinical judgment must be exercised in subjecting any of these patients to an "off-protocol" course of chemotherapy with the hope of capitalizing on the "microscopic" nature of their residual disease.

COMBINATION CHEMOTHERAPY

A number of pharmacologic and biochemical rationales have been proposed as guidelines for the design of combination chemotherapy regimens. These range from the sequential inhibition of the production or action of an essential compound to the prevention of the emergence of drug resistance. In retrospect, no such hypotheses are apparent in the 45 combinations used to treat melanoma (presented in Tables 50.7–50.11). Instead, most of the reported regimens were devised empirically by combining whatever active agents were available. At conventional doses, DTIC is the most active single agent against melanoma. Is any combination that contains DTIC more active than DTIC alone? From Table 50.7 it can be seen that the two-drug regimens were not superior. If one specifically examines the fote-

Table 50.7. Combination Chemotherapy with Regimens Containing Dacarbazine (DTIC)

Regimens	Evaluable Patients	CR[a] and PR	Response Rate %	References
DTIC + VA	248	46	19	(111–116)
DTIC + NU	489	112	23	(12, 118–125)
DTIC + fotemustine	146	41	28	(122–125)
DTIC + DDP	104	23	22	(64, 126–129)
DTIC + Procarb	109	18	17	(6, 115)
DTIC + CTX	140	23	16	(116, 118, 130)
DTIC + Act D	139	26	19	(131–135)
DTIC + Anth	46	9	20	(119, 136)
DTIC + HU	28	5	19	(119)
DTIC + Cyclo	17	3	18	(137)
Totals	1320	265	20	
DTIC + VA + Anth	18	7	39	(114)
DTIC + VA + CTX	110	32	19	(13, 138, 139)
DTIC + VA + NU	901	220	24	(6, 7, 140–150)
DTIC + VA + DDP	255	81	32	(151–155)
DTIC + NU + Act D	91	24	26	(142, 156)
DTIC + NU + HU	331	80	24	(142, 146, 157, 158)
DTIC + DDP + Procarb	13	2	15	(127)
DTIC + DDP + NU	20	2	10	(169)
Totals	1739	448	26	
DTIC + NU + VA + HU	89	27	30	(157)
DTIC + NU + VA + Bleo	296	88	30	(159–165)
DTIC + NU + VA + Procarb	25	6	24	(166)
DTIC + NU + VA + Act D	57	14	25	(167, 168)
DTIC + NU + VA + Chl	121	27	22	(170)
DTIC + NU + DDP + TAM	440	177	40	(171–180)
Totals	1033	339	33	

[a]CR, complete response; PR, partial response; VA, vinca alkaloid; NU, nitrosourea; DDP, cisplatin; Procarb, procarbazine; CTX, cyclophosphamide; Act D, dactinomycin; Anth, Adriamycin or epirubicin; HU, hydroxyurea; Cyclo, cyclocytidine; Bleo, bleomycin; Chl, chlorpromazine; TAM, tamoxifen.

mustine-containing regimens, however, there is the suggestion of a modest improvement in activity (122–125). As with fotemustine used as a single agent, activity was noted on CNS metastases (123). The major toxicity was hematologic, although one case of fatal pulmonary toxicity was reported (125). This was felt to be due to a sequencing effect. Interestingly, at autopsy this patient was free of tumor.

The increment in antitumor effect of adding a third (+ 5%) or a fourth (+ 10%) drug clearly does not represent synergy and is not sufficient to warrant the resultant toxicity. However, if one examines the individual regimens, the four-drug combination of DTIC + BCNU + cisplatin + tamoxifen stands out from the rest, with an objective response rate of 40%. This regimen was designed by Del Prete et al. (171) who reported 4 complete and 7 partial remissions among 20

patients. Remissions were durable, and metastases in visceral sites regressed. McClay et al. while at Thomas Jefferson University (172) confirmed this report, noting 10 responses among 20 patients. Indeed, three of these patients subsequently achieved complete remission, two of whom were disease free 8 and 9 years after completing treatment. One patient relapsed in the brain; the other died of lung cancer, free of melanoma. Interestingly, the investigators noted a 30% incidence of deep venous thrombosis, which prompted them to delete tamoxifen from the regimen. Surprisingly, only 2 responses were noted in the next 20 patients treated with the three cytotoxic agents without tamoxifen. The Dartmouth group has had a similar experience, noting a 26% response rate among 19 patients treated with DTIC + BCNU + cisplatin, compared with a 50% response rate among 24 patients who received all four drugs (181). The Thomas Jefferson University group reinstated the tamoxifen, and to date, we have treated 147 patients with DTIC-BCNU-cisplatin and tamoxifen (178). The response rate is 40%, including 17 complete responses and 41 partial responses. Our results as well as those of others with this four-drug combination are shown on Table 50.8. Responses have been observed in all sites. The major toxicity we have observed is thrombocytopenia. Eleven percent of patients experienced nonfatal thromboembolism.

In view of the fact that tamoxifen by itself is virtually inactive against melanoma, the observations cited above suggest an indirect chemoenhancing effect. Hypothesizing that administration of tamoxifen at a high dose just before starting chemotherapy would provide high tumor cell concentrations and perhaps greater therapeutic efficacy, we initiated a trial in which patients received a 7-day loading dose of up to 160 mg/day of tamoxifen prior to each series of chemotherapy infusions (182). Patients receiving the 160-mg tamoxifen regimen had significantly more profound hematologic toxicity than another group previously treated with the same regimen of cytotoxic drugs but with low-dose tamoxifen (40 mg daily throughout). This escalation of hematologic toxicity again suggested a drug-tamoxifen interaction; however, there was no improvement in overall response rate.

The drug or drugs with which tamoxifen may be interacting have not been identified. In a randomized prospective trial, Cocconi et al. (221) observed 4 complete and 13 partial responses in

Table 50.8. Dacarbazine plus BCNU plus Cisplatin plus Tamoxifen Combination Chemotherapy in the Treatment of Metastatic Melanoma

Evaluable Patients	PR[a]	CR	% Responses	Reference
20	7	4	55	(171)
45	18	5	51	(173)
32	10	5	47	(174)
47	11	6	36	(175)
8	2	3	62	(176)
20	11	0	55	(177)
20	7	1	40	(178)
147	41	17	40	(179)
101	26	3	27	(180)
440	133 (30%)	44 (10%)	40	

[a]CR, complete response; PR, partial response.

52 patients treated with DTIC + tamoxifen (20 mg/m^2 p.o. daily) but only 3 complete and 3 partial responses in 60 patients treated with DTIC alone ($p = .03$). Since tamoxifen is inactive alone against melanoma, these data suggest an augmentation of the DTIC-mediated antitumor effect. In vitro data implicate cisplatin as a possible target for tamoxifen interaction (222). McClay et al. (223) treated 20 cisplatin-resistant patients with cisplatin and tamoxifen and observed 3 partial responses. They suggested that tamoxifen can overcome clinical resistance to cisplatin through a synergistic interaction, the mechanism of which they are currently investigating. However, our observation that short-course, high-dose tamoxifen significantly increased hematologic toxicity but not neurologic or renal toxicity suggests that BCNU is the major interactive partner, as cisplatin produces only minimal marrow toxicity. This conclusion is further supported by Buzaid et al. (224) who noted only three responses in 21 patients when BCNU was dropped from the regimen, despite the fact that the dose of cisplatin was doubled. In vitro data also suggest the nitrosoureas as a tamoxifen target. The combination of tamoxifen and fotemustine results in synergistic cytotoxicity (225).

Rusthoven et al. (180) have competed a well-designed, placebo-controlled randomized trial in which 97 patients received DTIC + BCNU + cisplatin, and 101 patients were treated with the same drugs plus tamoxifen (160 mg/day × 6 days loading regimen, followed by 40 mg/day maintenance). The results of this scientifically rigorous trial seemingly challenge the data cited above. Although the 21% response rate (6 CR, 14 PR) in the placebo group was similar to the combined Jefferson/Dartmouth experience of 18% in 39 patients, the addition of tamoxifen yielded only a 27% response rate (3 CR, 26 PR), and this increment was not statistically significant. This is in sharp contrast to the results obtained in multiple earlier phase II trials. What is equally disturbing is that despite the fact that dose intensity was equivalent in both arms, tamoxifen did not increase hematologic toxicity or the incidence of deep vein thrombosis (3 of 101 with, 6 of 97 without). Further, few menopausal symptoms were noted in the female patients. These observations suggest that the tamoxifen was virtually without biologic impact. Perhaps the results of the North Central Oncology Group trial will clarify these important issues.

Although cisplatin has demonstrated only minimal activity as a single agent (Table 50.1), is

Table 50.9. Combination Chemotherapy with Regimens Containing Platinum (DDP)

Regimens	Evaluable Patients	CR[a]	PR	Response Rate %	References
DDP + DTIC	104	4	19	22	(64, 126–127)
DDP + Ifosfamide	30	3	7	33	(183, 184)
DDP + VA	87	3	13	17	(185, 186)
DDP + Ara-C	46	2	7	20	(187, 188)
Totals	267	11	46	21	
DDP + DTIC + VA	255	18	63	32	(151–155)
DDP + DTIC + Procarb	13	0	2	15	(127)
DDP + DTIC + NU	20	1	1	10	(169)
DDP + Bleo + NU	25	0	12	48	(189)
DDP + Bleo + VA	204	11	43	26	(190–197)
Totals	517	30	121	29	
DDP + DTIC + NU + TAM	339	41	107	44	(171–180)

[a]CR, complete response; PR, partial response; DTIC, dacarbazine; VA, vinca alkaloid; Ara-C, cytosine arabinoside; Procarb, procarbazine; NU, nitrosourea; Bleo, bleomycin; TAM, tamoxifen.

it active in combinations other than the four-drug regimen described above? As can be seen from Table 50.9, only the three-drug combination of cisplatin, bleomycin, and lomustine (189) is of interest. Although a 48% response rate was noted, there were no complete remissions. Toxicity was substantial; three poor-performance-status patients died of septicemia during a period of chemotherapy-induced leukopenia. Further, this original report has not yet been confirmed.

The response of brain metastases to systemic chemotherapy is a rare event. Continuous infusion chemotherapy has generated considerable interest because of the theoretical advantage of prolonged drug exposure, and cisplatin administered in this fashion has gained favor because of decreased toxicity. Recent reports in which both cisplatin and BCNU given as continuous infusions, prior to external-beam radiotherapy, to treat primary brain tumors suggest improved efficacy in malignancies in which chemotherapy has had limited effectiveness. Response rates of over 50%, prior to radiotherapy, were reported in preliminary phase II studies (226, 227), and there is currently an ECOG study investigating this method. Adopting a similar regimen in the treatment of melanoma brain metastases may prove advantageous. The possibility of substituting fotemustine in the Dartmouth regimen is also of interest.

Are there regimens that contain neither DTIC nor cisplatin but which induce a significant percentage of complete responses? From Table 50.10, it is apparent that combinations of a nitrosourea and vinca alkaloid with or without bleomycin or procarbazine fall into this category. Overall response rates vary from 23 to 43%, and 30 to 50% of remissions are complete. These regimens warrant additional investigation. The vinca alkaloid (VA) + dactinomycin (Act D) + procarbazine regimen presented in Table 50.11 is also of interest in that it produces some complete remissions and has no drugs in common with the DTIC + BCNU + cisplatin + tamoxifen regimen.

The immunosuppressive effects of cancer chemotherapeutic agents are well known (228). Reasoning that the concomitant use of nonspecific immunostimulants such as BCG and other microbial products might reverse this immunosuppression and thus enhance the therapeutic efficacy of the chemotherapy, trials of combination regimens were initiated. Gutterman et al. (229) reported that DTIC + BCG produced a significantly higher response rate than that seen in a historic control group treated with DTIC alone. A similar beneficial effect could not be confirmed in randomized prospective trials (Table 50.12). Indeed, the more reasonable expectation that nonspecific immunostimulants would increase remission duration also was not fulfilled. More recently, it has been appreciated that chemotherapeutic agents could improve the action of biologicals by reducing tumor burden and/or potentiating the acquisition/expression of immunity by modulating regulatory mechanisms. Pretreatment with low-dose cyclophosphamide

Table 50.10. Combination Chemotherapy Regimens Containing a Nitrosourea (NU) as Most Active Component

Regimen	Evaluable Patients	CR[a]	PR	TR	Response Rate %	References
NU + VA	90	5	16	21	23	(198–201)
NU + CTX	40	?	?	4	10	(111, 202)
NU + DBD	26	0	1	1	4	(203)
NU + 6-TG	35	0	6	6	17	(204)
Totals	191	5	23	32	17	
NU + VA + Bleo	48	7	14	21	43	(205, 206)
NU + VA + Procarbazine	94	11	11	22	23	(207, 208)
NU + Caffeine + CHl	75	3	6	9	12	(209)
Totals	217	21	31	52	24	
NU + VA + Bleo + CTX	39	0	7	7	18	(214)
NU + VA + Procarbazine + CTX	12	22	2	4	33	(211)
Totals	51	2	9	11	22	

[a]CR, complete response; PR, partial response; TR, CR + PR; VA, vinca alkaloid; CTX, cyclophosphamide; DBD, dibromodulcitol; 6-TG, 6-thioguanine; Bleo, bleomycin; Chl, chlorpromazine.

Table 50.11. Miscellaneous Combination Chemotherapy Regimens

Regimen	Evaluable Patients	CR[a]	PR	TR	Response Rate %	References
5-FU + Procarb	19	2	3	7	37	(212)
VA + CTX	10	1	2	3	30	(213)
VA + Bleo	9	0	4	4	44	(191)
VA + Bleo + MTX	15	1	2	3	20	(214)
VA + CTX + Procarb	6	0	2	2	33	(213)
VA + Act D + Procarb	53	3	10	13	24	(215, 216)
Act D + HU + CTX	34	0	3	3	9	(217)
5-FU + MTX + CTX + VA	26	2	2	4	15	(218–220)

[a]CR, complete response; PR, partial response; TR, CR + PR; 5-FU, 5-fluorouracil; Procarb, procarbazine; VA, vinca alkaloid; CTX, cyclophosphamide; Bleo, bleomycin; MTX, methotrexate; Act D, dactinomycin; HU, hydroxyurea.

is being used to enhance the acquisition of immunity to melanoma vaccines and to facilitate the function of specifically cytotoxic killer cells (228). DTIC has been combined with interleukin-2 (IL-2) alone (234, 235) or with lymphokine-activated killer cells (236). High-dose cisplatin (150 mg/m^2) plus WR-2721 is being alternated with IL-2 (237). Interferon was added to a previously reported regimen consisting of bleomycin + vincristine + lomustine + DTIC (BOLD) (160–166), and a 62% response rate was reported (238). The overall response rate to BOLD is only 30% and to single-agent interferon 10–20%. An immunomodulatory potentiating effect of interferon on the chemotherapeutic agents was suggested. The most remarkable aspect of this study was the

50% response rate observed in patients with metastatic uveal melanoma. Interferon has been incorporated into other regimens as well, with response rates as noted in Table 50.13.

There are preclinical data to suggest that the sequential combination of IL-2 and DTIC has additive antitumor activity (248). Several clinical trials have combined IL-2 with one or more chemotherapeutic agents (Table 50.13). Richards et al. (245) integrated IL-2 and α-interferon between courses of DTIC + BCNU + cisplatin + tamoxifen and achieved a 100% objective response rate in nine patients. In a subsequent report of 36 evaluable patients (246), 24 objective responses (1 CR and 23 PRs) were observed. Following a second cycle of treatment, 9 of the PRs

Table 50.12. Randomized Trials of Chemotherapy with or without Nonspecific Immunostimulants in Patients with Disseminated Melanoma

	Chemotherapy	Chemoimmunotherapy		Significance
Costanzi et al. (158)				
Treatment	BHD[a]	BHD + BCG		
Response rate	29/82 (35%)	44/150 (29%)		NS
Presant et al. (230)				
Treatment	DTIC + CTX	DTIC + CTX + CP		
Response rate	5/29 (18%)	8/27 (29%)		NS
MDR (wk)	15.6	13		NS
MS (mo)	6.1	5.7		NS
Mastrangelo et al. (231)				
Treatment	MV	MV + BCG + TC		
Response rate	7/31 (23%)	6/31 (19%)		NS
MDR (wk)	6	8		NS
MS (mo)	6.5	8		NS
Kostinas et al. (216)				
Treatment	VAP	VAP + MER		
Response rate	8/40 (20%)	6/39 (15%)		NS
MS (mo)	5.5	6.5		NS
Clunie et al. (232)				
Treatment	DTIC 6/27	DTIC + CP		
Response rate	(22%)	6/22 (27%)		NS
MS (mo)	233	233		NS
Veronesi et al. (233)				
Treatment	DTIC	DTIC + BCG	DTIC + CP	NS
Response rate	19/76 (25%)	12/65 (19%)	12/55 (13%)	NS
MDR (wk)	4.5	5	5.5	NS
MS (mo)	9	6	8	NS

[a]BHD, BCNU + hydroxyurea + DTIC; BCG, bacillus Calmette-Guerin; NS, not statistically significant ($p > .05$); DTIC, dacarbazine; CTX, cyclophosphamide; CP, *Corynebacterium parvum*; MDR, median duration response; MS, median survival; MV, methyl-CCNU + vincristine; TC, allogeneic tumor cells; VAP, vinblastine + dactinomycin + procarbazine; MER, methanol extraction residue of BCG.

Table 50.13. Chemotherapy Regimens That Include Biologicals

Regimen	CR/PR[a]	Evaluable Patients	Response Rate (%)	References
IFN + DTIC + BLEO + VCR + CCNU	6/22	45	62	(238)
IFN + DTIC	12/4	60	53	(239)
IFN + DTIC	6/5	34	32	(240)
IL-2 + DTIC	1/6	32	22	(241)
IL-2 + DTIC + DDP	5/8	30	41	(242)
IL-2 + LAK + DTIC	2/5	27	26	(243)
IL-2 + DDP	3/5	20	44	(244)
IL-2 + IFN + DTIC + BCNU + DDP + TAM	12/21	45	73	(245, 246)
IL-2 + IFN + DTIC + BCNU + DDP	1/23	36	69	(177)
IL-2 + IFN + DTIC + CARBO	0/6	16	38	(247)

[a]CR, complete response; PR, partial response; IFN, α-interferon; DTIC, dacarbazine; Bleo, bleomycin; IL-2, VCR, vincristine; CCNU, lomustine; interleukin-2; DDP, cisplatin; LAK, lymphokine activated killer cells; BCNU, carmustine; TAM, tamoxifen; CARBO, carboplatin.

had achieved a complete response. The M. D. Anderson Cancer Center (249) has added IL-2 plus α-interferon to a combination chemotherapy regimen of cisplatin (C) + vinblastine (V) + DTIC (D) and achieved 27 complete remissions among 155 evaluable patients (17%). Remission duration ranged from 14+ to 55+ months, with 11 patients in unmaintained complete remission beyond 2 years. By comparison, only 16 of 285 patients (6%) treated with various DTIC-containing regimens (including 102 with CVD) achieved complete remission, and these were durable in only 4 patients. Although this biochemotherapy was quite toxic, no treatment-related deaths were reported.

The frequency, duration, and magnitude of tumor regression that we and others have observed from the combination of DTIC + BCNU + cisplatin + tamoxifen have been reproducible and lead us to recommend it as first-line treatment. Hematologic toxicity permitting, the VA + Act D + procarbazine regimen is worthy of consideration as second-line treatment because it has no drugs in common with the first-line regimen. The efficacy of combining chemotherapeutic agents and biologics is under continuing investigation. Durable complete remissions have been reported with cisplatin + vinblastine + DTIC + IL-2 + interferon; however, this observation awaits confirmation, and toxicity is substantial.

DOSE INTENSIFICATION

The demonstration of a log-linear dose-response curve for chemosensitive animal tumors (250) has generated interest in dose intensification as an approach to enhancing the efficacy of currently available chemotherapeutic agents. Indeed, for chemosensitive human tumors such as breast cancer, the rate of response is directly related to the intensity of treatment. Thus, it is quite reasonable to anticipate that further dose intensification might result in some cures. The question in melanoma is whether increasing the dose of a marginally effective drug will yield an increment in response sufficient to justify the added toxicity—an issue currently being explored through both systemic and regional dose intensification.

Systemic Dose Intensification

Cytotoxic agents that have myelosuppression as their predominant toxicity can be administered at increased dose with autologous bone marrow infusion used to ensure hematopoietic recovery (250). This approach has been explored with several agents, singly and in combination. The results are summarized in Table 50.14. The overall response rate of 54% is quite high, but the complete response rate was only 11%, and sustained complete remissions were rare. The patients included in these studies were largely heavily pretreated, had advanced disease, and were given high-dose therapy only once. However, in 17 patients who had not received prior chemotherapy, Antman et al. (261) were able to induce only 1 complete remission. It is of interest that regression of brain metastases has been seen with high-dose BCNU (255).

The toxicity of this approach is formidable. Despite marrow restoration, deaths due to sepsis are observed (258, 263). The use of hematopoietic growth factors could reduce hematologic toxicity (265) and may eventually obviate the need for bone marrow infusion. However, nonhematologic toxicities remain a serious problem. These include gastrointestinal toxicity with melphalan, hepatic venoocclusive disease with dacarbazine, and encephalomyelopathy, cardiac myonecrosis, and interstitial pneumonia with carmustine. These problems must be overcome before this approach can be extended to the treatment of postsurgical adjuvant patients. Several investigators have attempted high-dose systemic chemotherapy without autologous bone marrow rescue. Tchekmedyian et al. (266) noted 4 partial responses among 18 evaluable patients treated with vincristine (2 mg, days 1 and 8) and a dose of BCNU (750 mg/m^2) associated with reversible bone marrow toxicity and acceptable extramedullary toxicity. The number of treatment-related deaths (five) exceeded the number of responses. This regimen has no practical role in the treatment of melanoma.

Portlock et al. (267) administered high-dose cisplatin (50 mg/m^2/day) and DTIC (350 mg/m^2/day) concomitantly for 3 or 4 days. Because of profound toxicity, only 2 patients were treated with the 4-day regimen, whereas 11 patients tolerated the 3-day regimen. There were 4 complete and 6 partial responses among 13 evaluable patients. Remission durations for the complete responders ranged from 3+ to 27.5+ months. Partial remissions were of shorter duration (2+ to 6.5+ months), but at the time of their report, no patient had relapsed. The number of patients in this trial is too small to allow a conclusion regarding efficacy.

High-dose chemotherapy can also be used

Table 50.14. High-Dose Chemotherapy with Autologous Bone Marrow Rescue

		Response				
		Frequency				Duration (mo)
Investigators	Drug (Dose)	CR[a]	PR	PTS	RR	Median (Range)
Lazarus et al. (252)	MEL (180–225 mg/m^2)	6	6	20	60%	CR = 6 (4–14) PR = 2 (2–5)
McElwain et al. (253)	MEL (140 mg/m^2)	1	3	8	50%	CR = 4 PR = 2 (2–3)
McElwain et al. (254)	MEL (140 mg/m^2)	2	10	20	60%	CR = 5, 7 PR = 5 (4–11)[b]
Phillips et al. (255)	NU (1200 mg/m^2)	4	7	29	38%	CR = 12 (3–29+) CR + PR = 5.7 (1.5–29+)
Thomas et al. (256)	MEL (35–90 mg/m^2) NU (400–800 mg/m^2)	1	5	8	75%	CR = 10.5+ PR = 2.5 (1–5)
Ciobanu et al. (257)	NU (1050 mg/m^2) DDP (200 mg/m^2)	1	2	7	43%	CR = 3 PR = 1+, 5
Slease et al. (258)	CTX (160–200 mg/kg) NU (600–900 mg/m^2)	0	2	6	33%	PR = 2, 3
Eder et al. (259)	CTX (6 gm/m^2) TPS (180–900 mg/m^2)	0	2	4	50%	PR = ?
Wolff et al. (260)	TPA (180–1575 mg/m^2)	4	25	51	57%	3 (1–31+)
Antman et al. (261)	CTX (1500–7500 mg/m^2) DDP (75–180 mg/m^2) NU (150–750 mg/m^2)	1	10	17	65%	4.7 (1–23+)
Shea et al. (262)	CTX (1500–7500 mg/m^2) DDP (75–180 mg/m^2) NU (150–750 mg/m^2)	1	10	19	58%	4.7 (1–23)
Thatcher et al. (263)	DTIC + MEL (various)	5	11	27	59%	—
	DTIC + IFO (various)	0	2	10	20%	—
Moormeier et al. (264)[c]	CTX (7.5 g/m^2) TPA (675 mg/m^2) NU (150–750 mgm/m^2)	0	3	3	100%	PR = ?
Totals		26	98	229	54%	

[a]CR, complete response; PR, partial response; PTS, number of evaluable patients; PR, combined response rate; MEL, melphalan; NU, carmustine; DDP, cisplatin; CTX, cyclophosphamide; TPA, thiotepa; DTIC, dacarbazine; IFO, ifosfamide.
[b]Survival.
[c]Stem cell rescue.

systemically in combination with manipulations to protect or restore normal tissue function. The organic thiophosphate WR-2721 protects normal tissue from the cytotoxic effects of alkylating agents. Glover et al. (268, 269) used high-dose cisplatin (100 to 150 mg/m^2 as a single dose) in conjunction with WR-2721 (740 mg/m^2) to treat 58 patients. They noted 27 partial and 4 complete responses (53%). Of patients treated with 150 mg/m^2 of cisplatin, 69% responded (median remission duration, 7+ months). The major toxicity was neurologic. This regimen and the cisplatin + DTIC combination suggest that the responsiveness of melanoma to platinum is directly related to dose. Comparative studies will be required to determine if either high-dose regimen is better than the four-drug combination of DTIC + BCNU + cisplatin + tamoxifen.

Regional Therapy—Perfusion

Isolation perfusion of the extremities using chemotherapy was introduced in 1957 (270). Hyperthermia was added in the mid-1960s. This technique is widely used to treat intransit metastases and satellitosis in melanoma of the extremity. The results of several reported series are summarized in Table 50.15. The 65% overall response rate is excellent. What is even more impressive is the 44% complete response rate with many patients achieving permanent locoregional control. Hyperthermia adds significantly

Table 50.15. Extremity Perfusion for the Treatment of Inoperable Locoregional Metastases

Investigators	Hyperthermia	Drugs	PTS[a]	CR	PR	TR	PR
Hafström and Jönsson (271)	40–41°C 2 hr	L-PAM 0.45–0.9 mg/kg[b]	10	1	7	8	80%
Kroon et al. (272)	37–38°C	L-PAM 10–13 mg/L[c]	18	7	8	15	83%
Bulman and Jamieson (273)	37°C 70 min	L-PAM 1.5 mg/kg[b]	29	?	?	14	48%
Shiu et al. (274)	<38°C	HN$_2$ < 3 mg/kg[b]	10	2	0	2	20%
	38–41°C 1.5–3 hr	HN$_2$ 0.35–0.6 mg/kg[b]	19	6	6	12	63%
Golomb (275)	38 or 43°C 1.5–2 hr	L-PAM 1–2 mg/kg Act D 30–65 μg/kg Thiotepa 1–2 mg/kg alone or in combinations	44	10	22	32	72%
Vaglini et al. (276)	42.5–43°C 2.5 hr	L-PAM 1.5 mg/kg[b]	15	8	4	12	80%
Storm and Morton (277)	40–42°C 1 hr	L-PAM 1 mg/kg	26	21	0	21	81%
Aigner et al. (278)	40°C 1 hr	DTIC 73–133 mg/kg[d]		41	0	1	25%
Cox (279)	Normothermia	Thiotepa 1–1.8 mg/kg[b] or L-PAM 1.5–2 mg/kg[b]	19	9	0	9	47%
Minor et al. (280)	40–42°C 1 hr	L-PAM 0.75–1.5 mg/kg	22	18	4	22	100%
Coit et al. (281)	38–40.5°C 1 hr	Cisplatin 100–200 mg/m^2	7	2	0	0	29%
Liénard (283)	40°C 1.5 hr	rTNFα 4 mg L-PAM 10 mg/L[c]	29	26	3	29	100%
Totals			252	111	54	165	65%

[a]PTS, number of evaluable patients; CR, complete response; PR, partial response; TR, CR + PR; RR, response rate; L-PAM melphalan; HN$_2$, nitrogen mustard; Act D, dactinomycin; DTIC, dacarbazine; rTNFα, recombinant tumor necrosis factor alpha.
[b]Based on body weight.
[c]Based on extremity volume.
[d]Based on extremity weight.

to the toxicity (276), but from the data presented in Table 50.15, it is not possible to discern if this is essential for response. However, Stehlin et al. (282) reported a 76.7% 5-year survival in 30 patients treated with hyperthermic perfusion, compared with a 22.2% 5-year survival for 27 patients treated with normothermic techniques. Most studies have used parenteral melphalan. Our own experience suggests that nitrogen mustard is associated with increased tissue toxicity. A rationale for the regional use of dacarbazine is not apparent, since this drug requires activation by oxidative demethylation, which normally occurs in the liver. As expected, the response rate to DTIC has been low, although there was one complete regression of a solitary dermal satellite. The regional use of cisplatin deserves further study in view of the dose-response effect that has been demonstrated with systemic use. Recently,

tumor necrosis factor (TNF) has been incorporated into isolated limb perfusion regimens (283, 284). Response rates of over 90% have been reported. Systemic toxicity is of concern; 10% of patients experience severe hypotension (SBP< 80 mm Hg), and 16%, an ARDS-like syndrome (283). Although there have been no randomized prospective comparisons of systemic chemotherapy and regional hyperthermic perfusion, the latter procedure seems superior in achieving locoregional disease control and should be considered for intransit metastases and satellitosis in an extremity. Intralesional BCG is also a consideration for treatment of satellitosis confined to an extremity (4).

Hyperthermic perfusion has been used as an adjunct to surgery in the treatment of primary and/or regionally recurrent melanoma of an extremity. With two exceptions, these reports lack a randomized prospective surgery-alone control group and thus are difficult to interpret. Ghussen et al. (285) evaluated the effectiveness of regional hyperthermic (42°C) cytostatic (melphalan, 1 to 1.5 mg/kg body weight) perfusion (1 hour) in 107 patients with extremity melanoma: localized primary, 37; local recurrence or satellites, 37; intransit metastases, 4; positive regional nodes, 9; and intransit plus regional node metastases, 20. Patients were randomized to surgery alone or in conjunction with perfusion. Analysis 3.5 years after completion of patient entry showed 26 recurrences among 54 control patients and only 6 in 53 perfused patients ($p = .0001$). Five-year disease-free survival was 50% for the control group versus 90% for the perfused group ($p = .001$). Hafström et al. (286) randomized 69 patients to surgery (36 patients) or surgery plus regional hyperthermic perfusion (33 patients); 23 patients in the perfusion group and 30 in the control group experienced recurrences. The tumor-free survival was significantly better for the treated group (median, 17 months) than the control group (median, 10 months) ($p = .044$). There was no significant difference in overall survival between the groups. These results are sufficiently encouraging to justify further study. The final determination of clinical utility will require a careful analysis of morbidity, which can be considerable with regional perfusion.

Regional Therapy—Infusion

Arterial infusion is an alternative and potentially more versatile approach to regional dose intensification than perfusion but has been even less systematically studied. Published reports are summarized in Table 50.16. Some investigators used vascular occlusion to further enhance regional drug concentrations (tourniquet or embolization). Voigt and Loffler (296) found that cisplatin concentrations within the liver were significantly increased while systemic levels were reduced during transient angioocclusion with degradable starch microspheres. A variety of other drugs have also been tested. As mentioned above, the rationale for the nonhepatic regional infusion of dacarbazine is not readily apparent, as this drug requires activation by hepatic oxidative demethylation. Objective responses have been reported with other drugs, but direct comparison will be required to determine if these results are superior to those attainable with newer systemic therapies.

One notable exception appears to be the study of Mavligit et al. (294), who reported considerable success treating hepatic metastases from uveal melanoma with cisplatin and polyvinyl sponge particles. Hepatic metastases from uveal melanoma are virtually unresponsive to systemic therapy, and indeed, these investigators were unsuccessful with angioocclusion or cisplatin alone. Further study of this approach is warranted but will be hampered by the limited availability of the polyvinyl material (Ivalon) used to permanently occlude the hepatic microvasculature. Available data are insufficient at present to determine if similar results can be achieved by a degradable material such as gelatin microspheres. Our own experience has been disappointing. We treated 14 uveal melanoma patients with liver metastases by chemoembolization of the hepatic artery: 9, polyvinyl sponge; 3, gelfoam; 2, both. No objective responses were observed; however, eight patients had stable disease (297).

CHEMOSENSITIVITY TESTING

Currently available chemotherapies induce tumor regression with frequencies ranging from 12 to 50+%. Complete remissions are less common. Toxicity is variable but accompanies all regimens. A chemosensitivity assay capable of defining the responsiveness of a specific tumor to a spectrum of therapies would facilitate the more effective use of these therapies. Human melanoma can be grown in T-lymphocyte-deficient athymic nude mice—a model that serves as a reasonable clinical approximation. Using a panel of nine human melanoma cell lines, Bellet et al. (298, 299) demonstrated responses to chemotherapy similar to those observed clinically. Four cell lines were sensitive to dacarbazine, and three to carmustine. None responded to the clinically inactive drugs, doxorubicin (Adriamycin) and 5-azacytidine. This is a time-consuming and technically tedious system because the nude mice must be housed in a protected environment, and the growth rate of the tumors varies. Thus, chemosensitivity testing on an individual patient basis is impractical, and this model has not been studied prospectively. It could be used for the secondary screening of new agents prior to clinical trials (300).

A bilayer soft agar system developed by Hamburger and Salmon (301) allows the growth of human tumor stem cells including melanoma. This system has been adapted for in vitro chemosensitivity testing. Meyskens et al. (302) mea-

Table 50.16. Regional Arterial Infusion Therapy

Investigators	Treatment	Tumor sites	PTS[a]	Results
Oberfield and Sullivan (287)	FU or MTX Cl for 1–12 mo	Ext, pelvis H & N, liver	29	17 Responses (59%)
Bland et al. (288)	DDP 26.7 mg/m² per infusion with tourniquet outflow occlusion	Extremities	15	10 PR (66%)
Frost et al. (289)	DTIC, 800 mg/m² over 2–3 hr + DDP, 90 mg/m² every 4 wk	Extremity (8) Vulva (1)	9	1 CR, 2 PR (33%)
Calvo et al. (290)	DDP 75–150 mg/m² over 3–4 hr	Extremity (13) Liver (5), brain (1)	19	2 CR, 2 PR (21%)
Storm et al. (291)	DTIC, 250 mg/m² × 5 day DTIC + hyperthermia	Liver Liver	6 10	PR (17%) 1 CR, 2 PR (30%)
Gunderson et al. (292)	DTIC + radiation (36 Gy)	Leg	14	All lesions in radiated fields regressed
O'Keefe et al. (293)	DDP + gelatin sponge embolization inferior epigastric artery	Leg (2) Bladder (1)	3	1 Complete and 2 partial tumor necrosis
Mavligit et al. (294)	DDP (150 mg) + polyvinyl sponge	Liver	30	1 CR, 13 PR (47%), median survival 11 mo
Cantore et al. (295)	Carbo 300 mg/m² every 2 wk	Liver	8	3 PR

[a]PTS, number of evaluable patients; FU, fluorinated pyrimidine; MTX, methotrexate; CI, continuous infusion; DDP, cisplatin; DTIC, dacarbazine; Carbo, carboplatin; Ext, extremity; H & N, head and neck cancer; CR, complete response; PR, partial response.

sured the effect of nine chemotherapeutic agents singly on colony formation in soft agar from biopsy specimens from 50 patients with melanoma. Positive assays were obtained in only 19% of 200 in vitro trials. In 25 of 29 cases (86%), the soft agar assay correctly identified drugs to which the tumor was insensitive in vivo. Eight of 19 tumors (42%) sensitive in vitro were also sensitive in vivo. Schadendorf et al. (303) measured the effects of 10 agents on the ability to form tumor colonies from 26 biopsies of metastatic melanoma lesions from 19 patients. They retrospectively compared the in vitro results with the clinical responses of 11 patients. In 10 cases, in vitro testing correlated with clinical response in that the specimen was resistant in vitro, and the tumor was resistant in vivo. In one case of in vitro resistance, the patient had a mixed response to therapy. In three cases of in vitro sensitivity, a clinical response was observed to treatment, including one complete response. Our own unpublished experience has been less encouraging in that only 23 of 256 (9%) in vitro assays were positive, and of these 23, only 3 patients (13%) responded clinically. However, the assay correctly predicted clinical failure in 31 of 32 (97%) cases. Interest in chemosensitivity testing in melanoma has subse-quently waned, and in vitro screening has not become a standard component of melanoma chemotherapy.

CONCLUSIONS

Currently available single agents, when administered at conventional doses, produce clinically meaningful but infrequent remissions. Taxol and Taxotere are new agents that require further study. The newer high-dose and combination chemotherapy regimens appear to be bona fide improvements in the management of disseminated disease. Multiple phase II trials have demonstrated that the four-drug combination of DTIC + BCNU + cisplatin + tamoxifen produces durable remissions in 40 to 50% of patients treated and should be considered as first-line therapy. The M. D. Anderson Cancer Center group has used the regimen of cisplatin + vinblastine + DTIC + IL-2 + α-interferon to induce a significant number of durable complete remissions but with seemingly higher toxicity. High-dose platinum regimens also may be effective. Hepatic artery infusion of cisplatin and polyvinyl sponge particles may be the first useful treatment for hepatic metastases from uveal melanoma. Also, some success has also been noted in this disorder with systemically administered DTIC + CCNU + bleomycin + vincristine + interferon (238, 304). Regional hyperthermic perfusion can produce regression of inoperable dermal and subcutaneous metastases confined to an extremity. Fotemustine appears to have some efficacy against CNS metastases. Thus, although melanoma is not often curable with chemotherapy, the considered use of currently available regimens can induce clinically significant remissions and possibly prolong life.

SPECIFIC RECOMMENDATIONS

The specific recommendations for treatment that follow are based on the preceding assessment and our own clinical experience.

1. Disseminated melanoma excluding brain metastases

    First line: DTIC + BCNU + cisplatin + tamoxifen (171–183). It has been over 10 years since Del Prete and coworkers first reported results from this regimen, and with one exception, response rates have shown little variation over time. We endorse this regimen as initial treatment. A major advantage of this regimen is that it can be administered by oncologists in the community setting. The concomitant use of hematopoietic growth factors or peripheral blood stem cell support may improve patient tolerance of protracted therapy.

    Second line: α-interferon (70–85). The overall response rate to interferon is not impressive, but the apparent durability of complete responses makes it worthy of consideration.

    Third line: IL-2 (305). Although not discussed in this chapter as a single agent because of its status as a biologic agent, IL-2 may be considered if first- and second-line treatment fails. As with α-interferon, the overall response rate to IL-2 is not impressive, but responses may be durable. Lower-dose regimens are less effective than high-dose regimens, but the toxicity of the high-dose regimens is substantial.

    Fourth line: Patients who fail first- or second-line therapy or who are not candidates for IL-2, but have a good performance status, may be considered for investigational regimens. The early trials of Taxol (66–69) suggest activity, but it is still under investigation for the treatment of melanoma, so its true value remains to be defined. Alternatively, the vinca

alkaloid + dactinomycin + procarbazine (215, 216) regimen is attractive because it has no drugs in common with DTIC + BCNU + cisplatin + tamoxifen, and complete responses have been documented. However, toxicity is substantial.

2. Postsurgical adjuvant therapy

    Stage I (high-risk primary lesion) or stage II (four or fewer positive regional lymph nodes): In approaching this group, it must be remembered that many of these patients have already been cured surgically and that the benefit of adjuvant chemotherapy has not been demonstrated. Therefore, whenever possible, such patients should be considered for entry into clinical trials. The DTIC + BCNU + cisplatin + tamoxifen regimen should be considered for such a trial. Trials on the efficacy of interferon are ongoing, and interferon may be considered for use on an individual basis.

    Bulky stage II or stage III (disseminated) disease: Although clinically free of disease, these patients are at virtually 100% risk of recurrence. In an effort to capitalize on minimum residual disease status, consideration can be given to treating these patients for an arbitrary period such as 6 months (depending on tolerance) with either DTIC + BCNU + cisplatin + tamoxifen, a high-dose platinum regimen, or interferon. This is best done as part of a clinical trial. We are also testing active immunotherapy in this situation, and our initial results appear promising (306).

3. Regionally confined inoperable metastases

    (a) Extremity lesions (satellitosis only): intralesional Glaxo BCG may be of value in patients with purely intradermal disease (307). Subcutaneous and visceral disease is unlikely to respond. For intransit metastases unresponsive to systemic therapy, hyperthermic perfusion with melphalan (271–273, 276, 277, 280) may be tried. As an alternative, regional infusion with cisplatin can be considered (290). The role of TNF continues to be investigated.

    (b) Liver: Hepatic artery infusion of cisplatin with angioocclusion should be considered, preferably in the context of a clinical trial, especially for patients with uveal melanoma metastatic to the liver (294). Otherwise, the best treatment is systemic chemotherapy as described above.

    (c) Brain: This remains a formidable problem. High-dose BCNU could be considered as part of a clinical trial. Fotemustine is not approved for use in the United States. The administration of BCNU and cisplatin as continuous infusions may prove advantageous (226–227). Otherwise, conventional approaches such as surgery and radiation therapy must be used.

REFERENCES

1. Comis RL. DTIC (NSC-45388) in malignant melanoma: a perspective. Cancer Treat Rep 1976;60:165–176.

2. Ahmann DL. Nitrosoureas in the management of disseminated malignant melanoma. Cancer Treat Rep 1976;60:747–751.

3. Bellet RE, Mastrangelo MJ, Berd D, Lustbader E. Chemotherapy of metastatic melanoma. In: Clark WH Jr, Goldman LI, Mastrangelo MJ, eds. Human malignant melanoma. New York: Grune & Stratton 1978;325–354.

4. Mastrangelo MJ, Rosenberg SA, Baker AR, Katz HR. Cutaneous melanoma. In: DeVita VT Jr, Hellman S, Rosenberg SA, eds. Cancer: principles and practice of oncology. Philadelphia: JB Lippincott 1982:1124–1170.

5. Marsoni S, Hoth D, Simon R. Clinical drug development. An analysis of phase II trials 1970–1985. Cancer Treat Rep 1987;71:71–80.

6. Einhorn LH, Burgess MA, Vallejos C, et al. Prognostic correlations and response to treatment in advanced metastatic melanoma. Cancer Res 1974;34:1995–2004.

7. Carter RD, Krementz ET, Hill GJ II, et al. DTIC (NSC-45388) and combination therapy for melanoma. I. Studies with DTIC, BCNU, CCNU, vincristine, and hydroxyurea. Cancer Treat Rep 1976;60:601–609.

8. Carter SK, Friedman MA. 5-(3,3-dimethyl-1-triazeno) imidazole-4-carboxamide (DTIC, DIC, NSC-45388): a new anti-tumor agent with activity against malignant melanoma. Eur J Cancer 1972;8:85–92.

9. Bellet RE, Mastrangelo MJ, Laucius JF, Bodurtha AJ. Randomized prospective trial of DTIC (NSC-45388) alone versus BCNU (NSC-409962) plus vincristine (NSC-67574) in the treatment of metastatic malignant melanoma. Cancer Treat Rep 1976;60:595–600.

10. Ahmann DL, Hahn RG, Bisel HF. Clinical evaluation of 5-(3,3-dimethyl-1-triazeno) imidazole-4-carboxamide (NSC-45388), melphalan (NSC-8806) and hydroxyurea (NSC-32065) in the treatment of disseminated malignant melanoma. Cancer Chemother Rep 1972;56:369–372.

11. Costanzi JJ. DTIC (NSC-45388) studies in the Southwest Oncology Group. Cancer Treat Rep 1976;60:189–192.

12. Costanza ME, Nathanson L, Schoenfeld D, et al. Results with methyl-CCNU and DTIC in metastatic melanoma. Cancer 1977;40:1010–1015.

13. Pritchard KI, Quirt IC, Cowan DH, Osoba D, Kutas GJ. DTIC therapy in metastatic malignant melanoma: a simplified dose schedule. Cancer Treat Rep 1980;64:1123–1124.

14. Carbone PP, Costello W. Eastern Cooperative Oncology Group studies with DTIC (NSC-45388). Cancer Treat Rep 1976;60:193–198.

15. Salem PA, Sinno B, Hajj A, Kuzhaya S. High dose intermittent therapy with 5-(3,3 dimethyl-1-triazeno) imidazole-4-carboxamide (DTIC) in melanoma and other solid tumors (abstract). Proc Am Assoc Cancer Res 1976;17:116.

16. Thatcher N, Anderson H, James R, Craig P. DTIC by 24 hour infusion for metastatic melanoma (abstract). First Int Conf Skin Melanoma 1985;1:156.

17. Czarnetzki BM, Macher E. DTIC (dacarbazine) induced hepatic damage. Arch Dermatol Res 1981; 270:375–376.

18. McClay E, Lusch CJ, Mastrangelo MJ. Allergy-induced hepatic toxicity associated with dacarbazine (letter). Cancer Treat Rep 1987;71:219–220.

19. Ceci G, Balla M, Melissari M, Gabrielli M, Bocchi P, Cocconi G. Fatal hepatic vascular toxicity of DTIC. Is it really a rare event? Cancer 1988;61:1988–1991.

20. Beretta G, Pancera G, Locatelli C, Fraschini P. Lomustine (CCNU) and epirubicin (EPI) as alternative treatments to dacarbazine (DIC) for advanced malignant melanoma (abstract). First Int Conf Skin Melanoma 1985;1:148.

21. Wasserman TH, Slavik M, Carter SK. Review of CCNU in clinical cancer therapy. Cancer Treat Rev 1974;1:131–151.

22. Wasserman TH, Slavik M, Carter SK. Methyl-CCNU in clinical cancer therapy. Cancer Treat Rev 1974;1:251–259.

23. Bellet RE, Mastrangelo MJ, Berd D, Lustbader E. Randomized prospective phase III trial of methyl-CCNU (NSC-95441) alone versus methyl-CCNU plus vincristine (NSC-67574) in the treatment of patients with metastatic malignant melanoma (abstract). Proc Am Soc Clin Oncol 1977;18:284.

24. Gottlieb JA, McCredie KB, Hersh EM, Frei E III. Initial clinical studies with 1-2 (chloroethyl)-3-(4-methylcyclohexyl)-1-nitrosourea (methyl CCNU) (abstract). Proc Am Assoc Clin Res 1972;13:78.

25. Van Amburg AL, Presant CA, Burns D. Phase II study of chlorozotocin in malignant melanoma. A Southeastern Cancer Study Group report. Cancer Treat Rep 1982;66:1431–1433.

26. Hoth DF, Schein PS, Winokur S, et al. A phase II study of chlorozotocin in metastatic malignant melanoma. Cancer 1980;46:1544–1548.

27. Houghton AN, Camacho FJ, Gralla RJ, Wittes R. Phase II evaluation of chlorozotocin in patients with malignant melanoma. Cancer Treat Rep 1981;65:705–706.

28. Silver BA, Barlock AL, Lippman ME, Anderson T, Fisher RI. Phase II trial of chlorozotocin in malignant melanoma, breast cancer and other solid tumors. Cancer Treat Rep 1982;66:1229–1230.

29. Talley RW, Samson MK, Brownlee RW, Samhouri AM, Fraile RJ, Baker L. Phase II evaluation of chlorozotocin (NSC-178242) in advanced human cancer. Eur J Cancer 1981;17:337–343.

30. Jacquillat C, Khayat D, Banzet P, et al. Final report of the French multicenter phase II study of the nitrosourea fotemustine in 153 evaluable patients with disseminated malignant melanoma including patients with cerebral metastases. Cancer 1990;66:1873–1878.

31. Falkson CI, Falkson G, Falkson HC. Phase II trial of fotemustine in patients with metastatic malignant melanoma. Invest New Drugs 1994;12:251–254.

32. Costa G, Hreshchyshyn MM, Holland JF. Initial

clinical studies with vincristine. Cancer Chemother Rep 1962;24:39–44.

33. Holland JF, Scharlay C, Gailani S, et al. Vincristine treatment of advanced cancer: a cooperative study of 392 cases. Cancer Res 1973;33:1258–1264.

34. Gubisch NJ, Norena D, Perlia CP, Taylor SG III. Experience with vincristine in solid tumors. Cancer Chemother Rep 1963;32:19–22.

35. Shaw RK, Brunner JA. Clinical evaluation of vincristine (NSC-67574). Cancer Chemother Rep 1964; 42:45–48.

36. Reitmeier RJ, Moertel CG, Blackburn CM. Vincristine (NSC-67574) therapy of adult patients with solid tumors. Cancer Chemother Rep 1964;34:21–23.

37. Smart CR, Ottoman RE, Rochlin DB, Hornes J, Silva AR, Goepfert H. Clinical experience with vincristine (NSC-67574) in tumors of the central nervous system and other malignant diseases. Cancer Chemother Rep 1968;52:733–741.

38. Frei E, Franzino A, Shnider BI, et al. Clinical studies of vinblastine. Cancer Chemother Rep 1961; 12:125–129.

39. Armstrong JG, Dyke RW, Fouts PJ, Gahimer JE. Hodgkin's disease, carcinoma of the breast and other tumors treated with vinblastine sulfate. Cancer Chemother Rep 1962;18:49–71.

40. Acute Leukemia Group B, Eastern Cooperative Group. Neoplastic diseases. Treatment with vinblastine. Arch Intern Med 1965;111:846–852.

41. Bond WH, Rohn RJ, Bates LH, Hodes ME. Treatment of neoplastic diseases with an improved oral preparation of vinblastine sulfate. Cancer 1966; 19:213–219.

42. Hodes ME, Rohn RJ, Bond WH, Yardley JM, Corpening WS. Vincaleukoblastine. IV. A summary of two and one-half years experience in the use of vinblastine. Cancer Chemother Rep 1962;16:401–406.

43. Hill JM, Loeb E. Treatment of leukemia, lymphoma, and other malignant neoplasms with vinblastine. Cancer Chemother Rep 1961;15:41–61.

44. Falkson G, VanDyk JJ. The chemotherapy of malignant melanoma. S Afr Med J 1968;42:89–90.

45. Wright TL, Hurley J, Korst DR, et al. Vinblastine in neoplastic disease. Cancer Res 1963;23:169–179.

46. Smart CR, Rochlin DB, Nahum AM, Silva A, Wagner D. Clinical experience with vinblastine sulfate (NSC-49842) in squamous cell carcinoma and other malignancies. Cancer Chemother Rep 1964;34:31–45.

47. Bleehen NM, Jelliffee AM. Vinblastine sulphate in the treatment of malignant disease. Br J Cancer 1965; 19:268–273.

48. Currie VE, Wong PP, Krakoff IH, Young CW. Phase I trial of vindesine in patients with advanced cancer. Cancer Treat Rep 1978;62:1333–1336.

49. Camacho FJ, Young CW, Wittes RE. Phase II trial of vindesine in patients with malignant melanoma. Cancer Treat Rep 1980;64:179–181.

50. Retsas S, Newton KA, Westbury G. Vindesine as a single agent in the treatment of advanced malignant melanoma. Cancer Chemother Pharmacol 1979; 2:257–260.

51. Smith IE, Hedley DW, Powles TJ, McElwain TJ. Vindesine: a phase II study in the treatment of breast carcinoma, malignant melanoma and other solid tumors. Cancer Treat Rep 1978;62:1427–1433.

52. Quagliana JM, Stephens RL, Baker LH, Costanzi JJ. Vindesine in patients with metastatic malignant melanoma: a Southwest Oncology Group study. J Clin Oncol 1984;2:316–319.

53. Carmichael J, Atkinson RJ, Calman KC, Mackie RM, Naysmith AM, Smyth JF. A multicentre phase II trial of vindesine in malignant melanoma. Eur J Cancer Clin Oncol 1982;18:1293–1295.

54. Nelimark RA, Peterson BA, Vosika GJ, Conroy JA. Vindesine for metastatic malignant melanoma. A phase II trial. Am J Clin Oncol 1983;6:561–564.

55. Rumke P, Everall JD, Mulder JH, Rozencweig M, Czarnotzki B, Thomas D. EORTC phase II trial of vindesine in advanced melanoma (letter). Eur J Cancer Clin Oncol 1983;19:1173–1174.

56. Arseneau JC, Mellette SJ, Kuperminc M, Wolter J. Phase II study of vindesine in metastatic malignant melanoma (letter). Cancer Treat Rep 1981;65:355–356.

57. Wagstaff J, Anderson HA, Shiu W, Thatcher N. Phase II study of vindesine infusion in visceral metastatic malignant melanoma. Cancer Treat Rep 1983; 67:839–840.

58. Mayol XF, Beltran J, Rubio-Bazan R, Rifa J, Costa RR, Lopez JJL. Multicenter phase II trial with 5 day continuous infusion of vindesine in metastatic malignant melanoma. Cancer Treat Rep 1984;68:1199–1200.

59. DiBella NJ, Berris R, Garfield D, Fink K, Speer J, Sakamoto A. Vindesine in advanced breast cancer, lymphoma and melanoma. Invest New Drugs 1984; 2:323–328.

60. Chary KK, Higby DJ, Henderson ES, Swinerton KD. Phase I study of high-dose cis-dichlorodiammineplatinum (II) with forced diuresis. Cancer Treat Rep 1977;61:367–370.

61. Voigt H, Meigel WN, Meissner K, Mensing H, Medenwaldt B, Jensen G. Erfahrungen mit der hochdosierten cis-platin-therapie bein metastasierten malignen melanom. Onkologie 1982;3:120–129.

62. Al-Sarraf M, Fletcher W, Oishi N, et al. Cisplatin hydration with and without mannitol diuresis in refractory disseminated malignant melanoma: a Southwest Oncology Group study. Cancer Treat Rep 1982;66:31–35.

63. Mechl Z, Krejci P. Cis-diaminedichloroplatinum in the treatment of disseminated malignant melanoma. Neoplasma 1983;30:371–377.

64. Goodnight JE Jr, Moseley HS, Eilber FR, Sarna G, Morton DL. Cis-dichlorodiammineplatinum (II) alone and combined with DTIC for the treatment of disseminated malignant melanoma. Cancer Treat Rep 1979;63:2005–2007.

65. Scheff PB, Horwitz SB. Taxol stabilizes microtubules in mouse fibroblast cells. Proc Natl Acad Sci USA 1980;77:1561–1565.

66. Wiernik PH, Einzig AI. Taxol in malignant melanoma. NCI Monogr 1993;15:185–187.

67. Wiernik PH, Schwartz EL, Einzig A, Strauman J, Lipton RB, Dutcher JP. Phase I trial of Taxol given as a 24 hour infusion every 21 days: response observed in metastatic melanoma. J Clin Oncol 1987;8:1232–1239.

68. Einzig A, Trump DL, Sasloff J. Phase II pilot study of Taxol in patients with malignant melanoma (abstract). Proc Am Soc Clin Oncol 1988;7:249.

69. Aamdal S, Wolff I, Kaplan S, et al. Docetaxel (Taxotere) in advanced malignant melanoma. A phase II study of the EORTC Early Clinical Trials Group. Eur J Cancer 1994;30A:1061–1064.

70. Creagan ET, Ahmann DL, Frytak S, Long HJ, Chang MN, Itri L. Three consecutive phase II studies of recombinant interferon alfa-2a in advanced malignant melanoma. Updated analysis. Cancer 1987; 59(Suppl):638–646.

71. Hersey P, Hasic E, MacDonald M, et al. Effects of recombinant leukocyte interferon (rIFN-α A) on tumor growth and immune responses in patients with metastatic melanoma. Br J Cancer 1985;51:815–826.

72. Legha SS, Papadopoulos NEJ, Plager C, et al. Clinical evaluation of recombinant interferon alpha-2A (Roferon-A) in metastatic melanoma using two different schedules. J Clin Oncol 1987;5:1240–1246.

73. Kuzmits R, Kokoschka EM, Micksche M, Ludwig H, Flener R. Phase II results with recombinant interferons: renal cell carcinoma and malignant melanoma. Oncology 1985;42(Suppl 1):26–32.

74. Elsasser-Beile U, Drees N, Neumann HA, Schopf E. Phase II trial of recombinant leukocyte A interferon in advanced malignant melanoma. J Cancer Res Clin Oncol 1987;113:273–278.

75. Krown SE, Burk MW, Kirkwood JM, Kerr D, Morton DL, Oettgen HF. Human leukocyte (alpha) interferon in metastatic malignant melanoma: the American Cancer Society phase II trial. Cancer Treat Rep 1984;68:723–726.

76. Landthaler M, Geyer C, Papendick U, Braun-Falco O. α 2-Interferon treatment of metastasizing malignant melanoma. Dtsch Med Wochenschr 1987; 112:919–921.

77. Kirkwood JM, Ernstoff MS, Davis CA, Reiss M, Ferraresi R, Rudnick SA. Comparison of intramuscular and intravenous recombinant alpha-2 interferon in melanoma and other cancers. Ann Intern Med 1985; 103:32–36.

78. Coates A, Rallings M, Hersey P, Swanson C. Phase II study of recombinant α 2-interferon in advanced malignant melanoma. J Interferon Res 1986; 6:1–4.

79. Dorval T, Palangie T, Jouve M, et al. Clinical phase II trial of recombinant DNA interferon (interferon alpha 2b) in patients with metastatic melanoma. Cancer 1986;58:215–218.

80. Dorval T, Palangie T, Jouve M, et al. Treatment of metastatic malignant melanoma with recombinant interferon alfa 2b. Invest New Drugs 1987;5(Suppl):61–64.

81. Mughal TI, Robinson WA, Thomas MR, Spiegel RJ. Role of recombinant interferon alpha-2 in treatment of advanced malignant melanoma (abstract). Proc Am Soc Clin Oncol 1988;7:250.

82. Von Wussow P, Block B, Hartmann F, Deicher H. Intralesional interferon-alpha therapy in advanced malignant melanoma. Cancer 1988;61:1071–1074.

83. Haase KD, Lange OF, Scheef W. Interferon α treatment of metastasized malignant melanoma. Anticancer Res 1987;7:335–336.

84. Creagan ET, Ahmann DL, Long HJ, Frytak S, Sherwin SA, Chang MN. Phase II study of recombinant interferon-gamma in patients with disseminated malignant melanoma. Cancer Treat Rep 1987;71:843–844.

85. Ernstoff MS, Trautman T, Davis CA, et al. A randomized phase I/II study of continuous versus intermittent intravenous interferon gamma in patients with metastatic melanoma. J Clin Oncol 1987;5:1804–1810.

86. Schiller JH, Storer B, Bittner G, Willson JKV, Borden FC. Phase II trial of a combination of interferon β and interferon α in patients with advanced malignant melanoma. J Interferon Res 1988;8:581–589.

87. Creagan ET, Loprinzi CL, Ahmann DL, Schaid DJ. A phase I-II trial of the combination of recombinant leukocyte A interferon and recombinant human interferon-α in patients with metastatic malignant melanoma. Cancer 1988;62:2472–2474.

88. McLeod GRC, Thomson DB, Hersey P. Recombinant interferon alpha-2a in advanced malignant melanoma. A phase I-II study in combination with DTIC. Int J Cancer 1987;(Suppl 1):31–35.

89. Croghan MK, Booth A, Meyskens FL Jr. A phase I trial of recombinant interferon α and α-difluoromethylornithine in metastatic melanoma. J Biol Response Mod 1988;7:409–415.

90. Pehamberger H, Steiner A, Wolfe K. Recombinant leukocyte A interferon and cimetidine treatment in disseminated melanoma. Eur J Cancer Clin Oncol 1986;11:1407–1411.

91. Miller RL, Steis RG, Clark JW, et al. Randomized trial of recombinant α 2b-interferon with or without indomethacin in patients with metastatic malignant melanoma. Cancer Res 1989;49:1871–1876.

92. Abdi EA, McPherson TA, Tan YH. Combination of fibroblast interferon (HuIFNβ), carboxamide (DTIC), and cimetidine for advanced malignant melanoma. J Biol Response Mod 1986;5:423–428.

93. Pisha E, Gerhäuser C, Chai H, et al. Discovery of betulinic acid as a selective inhibitor of human melanoma that functions by induction of apoptosis (abstract). Presented at the 86th annual meeting Am Assoc Cancer Res 1995, March 21, Toronto.

94. Hill GJ II, Moss SE, Golomb FM, et al. DTIC and combination therapy for melanoma: III. DTIC (NSC 45388) surgical adjuvant study COG protocol 7040. Cancer 1981;47:2556–2562.

95. Veronesi U, Adamus J, Aubert C, et al. A randomized trial of adjuvant chemotherapy and immunotherapy in cutaneous melanoma. N Engl J Med 1982; 307:913–916.

96. Lejeune FJ, Macher E, Kleeberg U, et al. An assessment of DTIC versus levamisole as placebo in the treatment of high risk stage I patients after surgical removal of a primary melanoma of the skin. A phase III adjuvant study. EORTC protocol 18761. Eur J Cancer Clin Oncol 1988;24(Suppl 2):S81–S90.

97. Holtermann OA, Karakousis CP, Berger J, Constantine RI. Adjuvant therapy with DTIC and estracyt or BCG in malignant melanoma (abstract). Proc Am Soc Clin Oncol 1980;21:400.

98. Karakousis CP, Lopez R, Berger JL, Takita H, Friedman M, Holyoke ED. Feasibility of integration of modalities in melanomas and sarcomas. Am J Surg 1979;137:369–373.

99. Quirt IC, and National Cancer Institute of Canada Melanoma Study Group. Randomized controlled trial of adjuvant chemoimmunotherapy with DTIC and BCG after complete excision of primary melanoma with a poor prognosis or melanoma metastases. Can Med Assoc J 1983;128:929–933.

100. Fisher RI, Terry WD, Hodes RJ, et al. Adjuvant immunotherapy or chemotherapy for malignant melanoma. Surg Clin North Am 1981;61:1267–1277.

101. Shetty MR. Methyl CCNU therapy linked leukemia (letter). Cancer Chemother Pharmacol 1981; 6:199.

102. Loutfi A, Shakr A, Jerry M, Hanley J, Shibata H. Double blind randomized prospective trial of levamisole/placebo in stage I cutaneous malignant melanoma. Clin Invest Med 1987;10:325–328.

103. Quirt IC, Shelley WE, Pater JL, et al. Improved survival in patients with poor-prognosis malignant melanoma treated with adjuvant levamisole: a phase III study by the National Cancer Institute of Canada Clinical Trials Group. J Clin Oncol 1991;9:729–735.

104. Spitler LE. A randomized trial of levamisole versus placebo as adjuvant therapy in malignant melanoma. J Clin Oncol 1991;9:736–740.

105. Kokoschka EM, Trautinger F, Knobler RM, Pohl-Markl H, Misksche M. Long-term adjuvant therapy of high-risk malignant melanoma with interferon α2b. J Invest Dermatol 1990;95(Suppl):193S–197S.

106. Cascinelli N, Bufalino R, Morabito A, MacKie R. Results of adjuvant interferon study in WHO melanoma programme (letter). Lancet 1994;343:913.

107. Cascinelli N. Evaluation of efficacy of adjuvant rIFNα 2A in melanoma patients with regional node metastases (abstract). Proc Am Soc Clin Oncol 1995;14:410.

108. Kirkwood J, Hunt M, Smith T, Ernstoff M, Borden E, Blum R. A randomized controlled trial of high-dose ifn alfa-2b for high-risk melanoma: the ECOG trial EST-1684 (abstract). Proc Am Soc Clin Oncol 1993;12:390.

109. Kirkwood JM. Adjuvant therapy: from microbial immunostimulants to recombinant interferons. First Int Conf Adjuvant Therapy of Malignant Melanoma 1995;1:10.

110. Retsas S, Quigley M, Pectaside D, Macrae K, Henry K. Clinical and histologic involvement of regional lymph nodes in malignant melanoma: adjuvant vindesine improves survival. Cancer 1994;73:2119–2130.

111. Ahmann DL, Hahn RG, Bisel HF, Eagan RT, Edmonson JH. Comparative study of methyl-CCNU (NSC-95441) with cyclophosphamide (NSC-26271) and 5-(3,3-dimethyl-1-triazeno) imidazole-4-carboxamide (NSC-45388) with vincristine (NSC-67574) in patients with disseminated malignant melanoma. Cancer Chemother Rep 1975;59:451–453.

112. Ahmann DL, Hahn RG, Bisel HF. Evaluation of 1-(2-chloroethyl-3-4-methylcyclohexyl)-1-nitrosourea (methyl-CCNU, NSC 95441) versus combined imidazole carboxamide (NSC 45388) and vincristine (NSC 67574) in palliation of disseminated malignant melanoma. Cancer 1974;33:615–618.

113. Ahmann DL, Hahn RG, Bisel HF. A comparative study of 1-(2-chloroethyl)-3-cyclohexyl-1-nitrosourea (NSC 79037) and imidazole carboxamide (NSC 45388) with vincristine (NSC 67574) in the palliation of disseminated malignant melanoma. Cancer Res 1972;32:2432–2434.

114. Chauvergne J, Clavel B, Klein T, Pommatau E. Chemotherapy of malignant melanoma. Bull Cancer 1978;65:107–109.

115. Wittes RE, Wittes JT, Golbey RB. Combination chemotherapy in metastatic melanoma. A randomized study of three DTIC-containing combinations. Cancer 1978;41:415–421.

116. Retsas S, Athanasiou A, Flynn MD, Smith B, Newton KA, Westbury G. Combination chemotherapy with vindesine and DTIC in advanced malignant melanoma (abstract). Proc Am Soc Clin Oncol 1982;1:169.

117. Vorobiof DA, Sarli R, Falkson G. Combination chemotherapy with dacarbazine and vindesine in the treatment of metastatic malignant melanoma. Cancer Treat Rep 1986;70:927–928.

118. Costanza ME, Nathanson L, Lenhard R, et al. Therapy of malignant melanoma with an imidazole carboxamide and bis-chloroethyl nitrosourea. Cancer 1972;30:1457–1461.

119. Gerner RE, Moore GE, Dickey C. Combination chemotherapy in disseminated melanoma and other solid tumors in adults. Oncology 1975;31:22–30.

120. Joensuu H, Asola R, Minn H. Combination chemotherapy with dacarbazine and lomustine in disseminated malignant melanoma. Acta Radiol Oncol 1986;25:177–179.

121. Ahmann DL, Bisel HF, Edmonson JH, et al. Clinical comparison of Adriamycin and a combination of methyl-CCNU and imidazole carboxamide in disseminated malignant melanoma. Clin Pharmacol Ther 1976;19:821–824.

122. Avril MF, Bonneterre J, Delaunay M, et al. Combination chemotherapy of dacarbazine and fotemustine is disseminated malignant melanoma: experience of the French Study Group. Cancer Chemother Pharmacol 1990;27:81–84.

123. Avril MF, Bonneterre J, Cupissol D, et al. Fotemustine plus dacarbazine for malignant melanoma. Eur J Cancer 1992;28A:1807–1811.

124. Binder M, Winkler A, Dorffner R, Glebowski E, Wolff K, Pehamberger H. Fotemustine plus dacarbazine in advanced stage III malignant melanoma. Eur J Cancer 1992;28A:1814–1816.

125. Aamdal S, Gerard B, Bohman T, D'Incalci M. Malignant melanoma—an effective combination with unexpected toxicity. Eur J Cancer 1992;28:447–450.

126. Friedman MA, Kaufman DA, Williams JE, et al. Combined DTIC and cis-dichlorodiammineplatinum (II) therapy for patients with disseminated melanoma: a Northern California Oncology Group study. Cancer Treat Rep 1979;63:493–495.

127. Karakousis CP, Getaz EP, Bjornsson S, et al. Cis-dichlorodiammineplatinum (II) and DTIC in malignant melanoma. Cancer Treat Rep 1979;63:2009–2010.

128. Ahmann DL, Edmonson JH, Frytak S, Kvols LK, Bisel HF, Rubin J. Phase II study of ICRF-159 versus combination cis-dichlorodiammineplatinum (II) and DTIC in patients with disseminated malignant melanoma. Cancer Treat Rep 1978;62:151–153.

129. Oratz R, Speyer JL, Green M, Blum R, Wernz JC, Muggia FM. Treatment of metastatic melanoma with dacarbazine and cisplatin. Cancer Treat Rep 1987;71:877–878.

130. Presant CA, Bartolucci AA, Balch C, Troner M, Southeast Cancer Study Group. A randomized comparison of cyclophosphamide, DTIC with or without piperazinedione in metastatic malignant melanoma. Cancer 1982;49:1355–1357.

131. Gerner RE, Moore GE, Didolkar MS. Chemotherapy of disseminated malignant melanoma with dimethyl triazeno imidazole carboxamide and dactinomycin. Cancer 1973;32:756–760.

132. Samson MK, Baker LH, Talley RW, Fraile RJ, McDonald B. Phase I-II study of intermittent bolus administration of DTIC and actinomycin D in metastatic malignant melanoma. Cancer Treat Rep 1978;62:1223–1225.

133. Ramseur WL, Richards F II, Muss HB, et al. Chemoimmunotherapy for disseminated malignant melanoma: a prospective randomized study. Cancer Treat Rep 1978;62:1085–1087.

134. Halpern J, Catane R, Biran S, Fuks Z. DTIC and actinomycin D with and without *C. parvum* immunotherapy in advanced malignant melanoma. Tumori 1981;67:215–217.

135. Hochster H, Levin M, Speyer J, et al. Single dose dacarbazine and dactinomycin in advanced malignant melanoma. Cancer Treat Rep 1985;69:39–42.

136. Lopez M, Perno CF, DiLauro L, Papaldo P, Ganzina F, Barduagni A. Controlled study of DTIC versus DTIC plus epirubicin in metastatic malignant melanoma. Invest New Drugs 1984;2:319–322.

137. Samson MK, Baker LH, Izbicki RM, Ratanatharathorn V. Phase I-II study of DTIC and cyclocytidine in disseminated malignant melanoma. Cancer Treat Rep 1976;60:1369–1371.

138. Byrne MJ, Reynolds PM. Phase II study of cyclophosphamide, vincristine and DTIC + BCG in the treatment of malignant melanoma. Aust NZ J Med 1982;12:263–266.

139. Gardere S, Hussain S, Cowan DH. Treatment of metastatic malignant melanoma with a combination of 5-(3,3-dimethyl-1-triazeno) imidazole-4-carboxamide (NSC-45388), cyclophosphamide (NSC-26271), and vincristine (NSC-67574). Cancer Chemother Rep 1972; 56:357–361.

140. Beretta G, Bajetta E, Bonadonna G, Tancini G, Orefice S, Veronesi U. Polichemioterapia con 5-(3,3 dimetil-1-triazeno)-imidazole-4-carboxamide (DTIC; NSC-45388), 1,3-bis (2-cloroetil)-1-nitrosourea (BCNU; NSC-409962) e vincristina (NSC-67574) nel melanoma in fase metastatizzata. Tumori 1973;59:239–248.

141. Cohen SM, Greenspan EM, Ratner LH, Weiner MJ. Combination chemotherapy of malignant melanoma with imidazole carboxamide, BCNU and vincristine. Cancer 1977;39:41–44.

142. Beretta G, Bonadonna G, Cascinelli N, Morabito A, Veronesi U. Comparative evaluation of three combination regimens for advanced malignant melanoma: results of an international cooperative study. Cancer Treat Rep 1976;60:33–40.

143. Luce JK, Torin LB, Price H. Combination dimethyl triazeno imidazole carboxamide (NSC 45388; DIC), vincristine (NSC 67574; VCR) and 1,3-bis (2-chloroethyl)-1-nitrosourea (NSC 409962; BCNU) chemotherapy of disseminated malignant melanoma (abstract). Proc Am Assoc Cancer Res 1970;11:50.

144. Hill GJ II, Metter GE, Krementz ET, et al. DTIC and combination therapy for melanoma. II. Escalating schedules of DTIC with BCNU, CCNU and vincristine. Cancer Treat Rep 1979;63:1989–1992.

145. Hill GJ II, Krementz ET, Hill HZ. Dimethyl triazeno imidazole carboxamide and combination therapy for melanoma. IV. Late results after complete response to chemotherapy (Central Oncology Group protocols 7130, 7131 and 7131A). Cancer 1984;53:1299–1305.

146. Einhorn LH, Furnas B. Combination chemotherapy for disseminated malignant melanoma with DTIC, vincristine and methyl-CCNU. Cancer Treat Rep 1977;61:881–883.

147. McKelvey EM, Luce JK, Talley RW, Hersh EM, Hewlett JS, Moon TE. Combination chemotherapy with bis chloroethyl nitrosourea (BCNU), vincristine

and dimethyl triazeno imidazole carboxamide (DTIC) in disseminated malignant melanoma. Cancer 1977; 39:1–4.

148. Carmo-Pereira J, Costa FO, Pimentel P. Combination cytotoxic chemotherapy for metastatic cutaneous malignant melanoma with DTIC, BCNU and vincristine. Cancer Treat Rep 1976;60:1381–1383.

149. Kleeberg UR, Schreml W. Polychemotherapie des metastasierenden melanoms. Vincristin, carmustin, dacarbazin. Dtsch Med Wochenschr 1976;101:890–894.

150. Beretta G, Bonadonna G, Bajetta E, et al. Combination chemotherapy with DTIC (NSC-45388) in advanced malignant melanoma, soft tissue sarcomas and Hodgkin's disease. Cancer Treat Rep 1976;60:205–211.

151. Verschraegen CF, Kleeberg UR, Mulder J, et al. Combination of cisplatin, vindesine and dacarbazine in advanced malignant melanoma. A phase II study of the EORTC Malignant Melanoma Cooperative Group. Cancer 1988;62:1061–1065.

152. Carey RW, Anderson JR, Green M, Ellison RR, Nathanson L, Kennedy BJ. Treatment of metastatic malignant melanoma with vinblastine, dacarbazine and cisplatin: a report from the Cancer and Leukemia Group B. Cancer Treat Rep 1986;70:329–331.

153. Gundersen S. Dacarbazine, vindesine and cisplatin combination chemotherapy in advanced malignant melanoma. Cancer Treat Rep 1987;71:997–999.

154. Legha SS, Ring S, Papadopoulos N, et al. A prospective evaluation of a triple-drug regimen containing cisplatin, vinblastine and dacarbazine (CVD) for metastatic melanoma. Cancer 1989;63:2024–2029.

155. Pectasides D, Yianniotis H, Alevizakos N, et al. Treatment of metastatic malignant melanoma with dacarbazine, vindesine and cisplatin. Br J Cancer 1989; 60:627–629.

156. Samson MK, Baker LH, Cummings G, Talley RW, McDonald B, Bhathena DB. Clinical trial of chlorozotocin, DTIC and dactinomycin in metastatic malignant melanoma. Cancer Treat Rep 1982;66:371–373.

157. Costanzi JJ, Vaitkevicius VK, Quagliana JM, Hoogstraten B, Coltman CA Jr, Delaney FC. Combination chemotherapy for disseminated malignant melanoma. Cancer 1975;35:342–346.

158. Costanzi JJ, Al-Sarraf M, Groppe C, et al. Combination chemotherapy plus BCG in the treatment of disseminated malignant melanoma: a Southwest Oncology Group study. Med Pediatr Oncol 1982;10:251–258.

159. Cohen SM, Ohnuma T, Cheung T, Holland JF. Bleomycin, carmustine, vincristine and dacarbazine in patients with metastatic melanoma. Cancer Treat Rep 1983;67:947–948.

160. Seigler HF, Lucas VS, Pickett NJ, Huang AT. DTIC, CCNU, bleomycin and vincristine (BOLD) in metastatic melanoma. Cancer 1980;46:2346–2348.

161. York RM, Foltz A. Bleomycin, vincristine, lomustine and DTIC chemotherapy for metastatic melanoma. Cancer 1988;61:2183–2186.

162. Young DW, Lever RS, English JSC, Mackie RM. The use of BELD combination chemotherapy (bleomycin, vindesine, CCNU and DTIC) in advanced malignant melanoma. Cancer 1985;55:1879–1881.

163. Zacharias PM, for the Prudente Foundation Melanoma Study Group. Chemotherapy of disseminated melanoma with bleomycin, vincristine, CCNU and DTIC (BOLD regimen). Cancer 1989;63:1676–1680.

164. Jose DG, Minty CCJ, Hillcoat BL. Treatment of patients with disseminated malignant melanoma with bleomycin, oncovin, lomustine and DTIC (BOLD) (abstract). First Int Conf Skin Melanoma 1985;1:151.

165. Ceschia T, Cartei G, Clocchiatti L, et al. BELD polychemotherapy in advanced melanoma (abstract). Proc Sec Int Conf Melanoma, Venice, Italy, October 16–19, 1989;412.

166. Van Dyk JJ, Falkson G. A clinical trial of procarbazine plus vincristine plus bis-chloroethyl-nitrosourea plus imidazole carboxamide dimethyl triazeno in metastatic malignant melanoma. Med Pediatr Oncol 1975;1:107–111.

167. Creagan ET, Schutt AJ, Long HJ, Green SJ. Phase II study: the combination DTIC, BCNU, actinomycin D and vincristine in disseminated malignant melanoma. Med Pediatr Oncol 1986;14:86–87.

168. Mulder NH, Sleijfer DT, Smit JM, et al. Phase II study of bleomycin, actinomycin D, DTIC and vindesine in disseminated· malignant melanoma. Eur J Cancer Clin Oncol 1986;22:879–881.

169. McClay EF, Mastrangelo MJ, Sprandio JP, Bellet RE, Berd D. The importance of tamoxifen to a cisplatin-containing regimen in the treatment of metastatic melanoma. Cancer 1989;63:1292–1295.

170. McKelvey EM, Luce JK, Vaitkevicius VK, et al. Bis chloroethyl nitrosourea, vincristine, dimethyl triazeno imidazole carboxamide and chlorpromazine combination chemotherapy in disseminated malignant melanoma. Cancer 1977;39:5–10.

171. Del Prete SA, Maurer LH, O'Donnell J, Forcier RJ, Le Marbre P. Combination chemotherapy with cisplatin, carmustine, dacarbazine and tamoxifen in metastatic melanoma. Cancer Treat Rep 1984;68:1403–1405.

172. McClay E, Mastrangelo MJ, Bellet RE, Berd D. Combination chemo/hormonal therapy in the treatment of malignant melanoma. Cancer Treat Rep 1987; 71:465–469.

173. McClay EF, Mastrangelo MJ, Berd D, Bellet RE. Effective combination chemo/hormonal therapy for malignant melanoma: experience with three consecutive trials. Int J Cancer 1992;50:553–556.

174. Fierro MT, Bertero M, Novelli M, et al. Therapy for metastatic melanoma: effective combination of dacarbazine, carmustine, cisplatin and tamoxifen. Melanoma Res 1993;3:127–131.

175. Reintgen D, Saba H. Chemotherapy for stage 4 melanoma: a three-year experience with cisplatin, DTIC, BCNU, and tamoxifen. Semin Surg Oncol 1993; 9:251–255.

176. Crowell EBJ, Higa GM. The chemohormonal therapy of metastatic melanoma: possible benefit of tamoxifen. W Va Med J 1993;89:233–235.

177. Richards JM, Gilewski TA, Ramming K, Mitchel B, Doane L, Vogelzang NJ. Effective chemotherapy for melanoma after treatment with interleukin-2. Cancer 1992;69:427–429.

178. Berd D, Mastrangelo MJ. Combination chemotherapy of metastatic melanoma (letter). J Clin Oncol 1995;13:796.

179. Adlakha A, Robinson WA, Gonzalez R, Lamb MR, Ferguson J. Combination chemotherapy and tamoxifen in the treatment of disseminated malignant melanoma (abstract). Proc Sec Int Conf Melanoma, Venice, Italy, October 16–19, 1989;40.

180. Rusthoven J, Quirt I, Iscoe N, et al. A randomized trial comparing BCNU (B), dacarbazine (D), cisplatin (P) versus BDP and high-dose tamoxifen in the treatment of metastatic melanoma (abstract). Proc Am Soc Clin Oncol 1995;14:413.

181. Lattanzi SC, Tosteson T, Maurer LH, et al. Dacarbazine (S), cisplatin (C), and carmustine (B), and tamoxifen (T), in the treatment of patients (pts) with metastatic melanoma (MM): results of 5-year follow-up (abstract). Proc Am Soc Clin Oncol 1993;12:390.

182. Berd D, McLaughlin CJ, Hart E, et al. Short course, high-dose tamoxifen with cytotoxic chemotherapy for metastatic melanoma (abstract). Proc Am Soc Clin Oncol 1991;10:291.

183. Becher R, Seeber S, Schmidt CG. Combination chemotherapy with ifosfamide and cis-dichlorodiammineplatinum (II) in advanced malignant melanoma. J Cancer Res Clin Oncol 1980;97:301–306.

184. Berdel WE, Fink U, Emmerich B, et al. Chemotherapie maligner melanome mit cis-diaminodichloroplatinum und ifosfamid. Dtsch Med Wochenschr 1982;107:26–28.

185. Creagan ET, Ahmann DL, Schutt AS, Schaid DJ. Phase II study of the combination of vinblastine plus cisplatin administered by continuous 120-hour infusion for patients with advanced malignant melanoma. Cancer Treat Rep 1987;71:769–770.

186. Mulder JH, Dodion P, Cavalli F, et al. Cisplatin and vindesine combination chemotherapy in advanced malignant melanoma. An EORTC phase II study. Eur J Clin Oncol 1982;18:1297–1301.

187. Mulder NH, Sleijfer DT, Willemse PHB, Schraffordt Koops H, de Vries EGE. Carboplatin and Ara-C combination chemotherapy with activity in disseminated malignant melanoma (abstract). Proc Am Soc Clin Oncol 1989;8:286.

188. Bajetta E, Verusio C, Bonfante V, Bonadonna G. Cytarabine and cisplatin in advanced malignant melanoma. Cancer Treat Rep 1986;70:1441–1442.

189. Cohen SM, Ohnuma T, Ambinder EP, Holland JF. Lomustine, bleomycin and cisplatin in patients with metastatic malignant melanoma. Cancer Treat Rep 1986;70:688–689.

190. Creagan ET, Ahmann DL, Schutt AJ, Green SJ. Phase II study of the combination of vinblastine, bleomycin and cisplatin in advanced malignant melanoma. Cancer Treat Rep 1982;66:567–569.

191. Nathanson L, Wittenberg BK. Pilot study of vinblastine and bleomycin combinations in the treatment of metastatic melanoma. Cancer Treat Rep 1980; 64:133–137.

192. York RM, Lawson DH, McKay J. Treatment of metastatic malignant melanoma with vinblastine, bleomycin by infusion and cisplatin. Cancer 1983;52:2220–2222.

193. Nathanson L, Kaufman SD, Carey RW. Vinblastine, infusion bleomycin and cis-dichlorodiammineplatinum chemotherapy in metastatic melanoma. Cancer 1981;48:1290–1294.

194. Mechl Z, Nekulova M, Sopkova B, Kiss F. The VBD regimen (vinblastin-bleomycin-cisplatinum) with high doses of cisplatinum in the therapy of advanced malignant melanoma (abstract). Proc 13th Int Cong Chemother 1983; part 246:22–25.

195. Bajetta E, Rovej R, Buzzoni R, Vaglini M, Bonadonna G. Treatment of advanced malignant melanoma with vinblastine, bleomycin and cisplatin. Cancer Treat Rep 1982;66:1299–1302.

196. Richman SP, Woodcock TM, Kubota TT, Blumenreich MS, Gentile PS, Allegra JC. Phase II trial of vinblastine, bleomycin and cisplatin (VBP) followed by dacarbazine and mitolactol in metastatic melanoma. Cancer Treat Rep 1984;68:1395–1396.

197. Johnson DH, Presant C, Einhorn L, Bartolucci AA, Greco FA. Cisplatin, vinblastine and bleomycin in the treatment of metastatic melanoma: a phase II study of the Southeastern Cancer Study Group. Cancer Treat Rep 1985;69:821–824.

198. Moon JH, Gailani S, Cooper R, et al. Comparison of the combination of 1,3,-bis(2-chloroethyl)-1-nitrosourea (BCNU) and vincristine with two dose schedules of 5-(3,3-dimethyl-1-triazeno) imidazole 4-carboxamide (DTIC) in the treatment of disseminated malignant melanoma. Cancer 1975;35:368–371.

199. Stolinsky DC, Pugh RP, Bohannon RA, Bogdon DL, Bateman JR. Clinical trial of BCNU (NSC 409962) combined with vincristine (NSC 67574) in disseminated gastrointestinal cancer and other neoplasms. Cancer Chemother Rep 1974;58:947–950.

200. Moon JH. Combination chemotherapy in malignant melanoma. Cancer 1970;26:468–473.

201. Marsh JC, De Conti RC, Hubbard SP. Treatment of Hodgkin's disease and other cancers with 1,3-bis (2-chloroethyl)-1-nitrosourea (BCNU; NSC 409962). Cancer Chemother Rep 1971;55:599–606.

202. Murphy WK. Phase I-II study of combination chemotherapy with cyclophosphamide (CTX) and methyl CCNU (abstract). Proc Am Soc Clin Oncol 1975; 16:253.

203. Creagan ET, Ahmann DL, Schutt AJ, Green SJ. Phase II study of mitolactol and semustine combination chemotherapy for advanced malignant melanoma. Cancer Treat Rep 1982;66:1425–1426.

204. Morton RF, Creagan ET, Veeder MH, et al. Phase II study of the combination of carmustine and 6-thioguanine in advanced malignant melanoma. Cancer Treat Rep 1987;71:429–430.

205. De Wasch G, Bernheim J, Michel J, Lejeune F, Kemis Y. Combination chemotherapy with three marginally effective agents, CCNU, vincristine and bleomycin, in the treatment of stage III melanoma. Cancer Treat Rep 1976;60:1273–1276.

206. Everall JD, Dowd PM. Use of combination chemotherapy with CCNU, bleomycin and vincristine in the treatment of metastatic melanoma in patients resistant to DTIC therapy. Cancer Treat Rep 1979; 63:151–155.

207. Shelley W, Quirt I, Bodurtha A, et al. Lomustine, vincristine and procarbazine in the treatment of metastatic malignant melanoma. Cancer Treat Rep 1985;69:941–944.

208. Carmo-Pereira J, Costa FO, Pimentel P, Henriques E. Combination cytotoxic chemotherapy with CCNU, procarbazine and vincristine in disseminated cutaneous malignant melanoma: 3 years follow-up. Cancer Treat Rep 1980;64:143–145.

209. Cohen MH, Schoenfeld D, Wolter J. Randomized trial of chlorpromazine, caffeine and methyl CCNU in disseminated melanoma. Cancer Treat Rep 1980;64:151–153.

210. Livingston RB, Einhorn LH, Bodey GP, et al. COMB (cyclophosphamide, oncovin, methyl-CCNU and bleomycin). A four drug combination in solid tumors. Cancer 1975;36:327–332.

211. Green MR, Dillman RO, Horton C. Procarbazine, vincristine, CCNU and cyclophosphamide (POOCH) in the treatment of metastatic malignant melanoma. Cancer Treat Rep 1980;64:139–142.

212. Nordman EM, Mäntylä M. Treatment of metastatic melanoma with combined 5-fluorouracil and procarbazine. Cancer Treat Rep 1977;61:1709–1710.

213. Byrne MJ. Cyclophosphamide, vincristine and procarbazine in the treatment of malignant melanoma. Cancer 1976;38:1922–1924.

214. Porcile G, Musso M, Boccardo F, Rosso R, Santi L. Combination chemotherapy with vinblastine, bleomycin and methotrexate in DTIC-resistant metastatic melanoma. Tumori 1979;65:237–240.

215. Perlin E, Engler J, Reid JW, Lokey JL, Kostinas J. Treatment of malignant melanoma with vinblastine (NSC-49842), procarbazine (NSC-79213) and actinomycin D (NSC-3053). Cancer Chemother Rep 1975; 59:767–768.

216. Kostinas JE, Leone LA, Cuttner J, et al. Procarbazine, vinblastine and actinomycin D in stage III and IV melanoma with or without methanol-extracted residue of bacillus Calmette-Guerin. Cancer Treat Rep 1979;63:197–200.

217. Amato DA, Bruckner H, Guerry D IV, et al. Phase II evaluation of dibromodulcitol and actinomycin D, hydroxyurea and cyclophosphamide in previously untreated patients with malignant melanoma. Invest New Drugs 1987;5:293–297.

218. Hanham IWF, Newton KA, Westbury G. Seventy-five cases of solid tumors treated by a modified quadruple chemotherapy regimen. Br J Cancer 1971; 25:462–478.

219. Shnider BI, Baig M, Serpic A, Kayhoe DE. Combination chemotherapy with 5-fluorouracil, cyclophosphamide, vincristine and methotrexate. J Clin Pharmacol 1975;15:69–73.

220. Coltman C Jr, Costanzi JJ, Dudley GM III, Haut A, Lane M, Gehan EA. Further clinical studies of combination chemotherapy using cyclophosphamide, vincristine, methotrexate and 5-fluorouracil in solid tumors. Am J Med Sci 1971;261:73–78.

221. Cocconi G, Bella M, Calabresi F, et al. Treatment of metastatic malignant melanoma with dacarbazine plus tamoxifen. N Engl J Med 1992;327:516–523.

222. Hofmann J, Doppler W, Jakob A, et al. Enhancement of the anti-proliferative effect of cis-diamminedichloroplatinum (II) and nitrogen mustard by inhibitors of protein kinase C. Int J Cancer 1988;42:382–388.

223. McClay EF, McClay MET, Albright KD, et al. Tamoxifen modulation of cisplatin resistance in patients with metastatic melanoma: a biologically important observation. Cancer 1993;72:1914–1918.

224. Buzaid AC, Murren J, Durivage HJ. High-dose cisplatin with dacarbazine and tamoxifen in the treatment of metastatic melanoma. Cancer 1991;68:1238–1241.

225. Fischel JL, Barbé V, Berlon M, et al. Tamoxifen enhances the cytotoxic effects of the nitrosourea fotemustine. Results on human melanoma cell lines. Eur J Cancer 1993;29A:2269–2273.

226. Grossman SA, Wharam M, Sheidler V, et al. BCNU/cisplatin (B/C) followed by radiation in poor prognosis patients with high grade astrocytomas (HGA) (abstract). Proc Am Soc Clin Oncol 1992;11:149.

227. Gilbert MR, Lunsford LD, Kondziolka D, et al. A phase II trial of continuous infusion chemotherapy,

external beam radiotherapy and local boost radiotherapy for malignant melanoma (abstract). Proc Am Soc Clin Oncol 1993;12:176.

228. Ehrke MJ, Mihich E, Berd D, Mastrangelo MJ. Effects of anticancer drugs on the immune system in humans. Semin Oncol 1989;16:230–253.

229. Gutterman JU, Mavligit G, Gottlieb JA, et al. Chemoimmunotherapy of disseminated malignant melanoma with dimethyl triazeno imidazole carboxamide and bacillus Calmette-Guerin. N Engl J Med 1974;291:592–597.

230. Presant CA, Smalley R, Vogler WR. Southeast Cancer Study Group Therapy of metastatic malignant melanoma with cyclophosphamide plus DTIC with or without C. parvum (CP) (abstract). Proc Am Soc Clin Oncol 1977;18:283.

231. Mastrangelo MJ, Bellet RE, Berd D. A phase III comparison of methyl-CCNU + vincristine with or without BCG + allogeneic tumor cells in metastatic melanoma. Cancer Immunol Immunother 1978;6:231–236.

232. Clunie GJA, Gough IR, Dury M, Furnival CM, Bolton PM. A trial of imidazole carboxamide and Corynebacterium parvum in disseminated melanoma. Clinical and immunologic results. Cancer 1980;46:475–479.

233. Veronesi U, Aubert C, Bajetta E, et al. Controlled study with imidazole carboxamide (DTIC), DTIC + bacillus Calmette-Guerin (BCG), and DTIC + Corynebacterium parvum in advanced malignant melanoma. Tumori 1984;70:41–48.

234. Stoter G, Shiloni E, Gundersen S, et al. Alternating recombinant human interleukin-2 (rIL-2) and dacarbazine (DTIC) in metastatic melanoma (abstract). Proc Am Soc Clin Oncol 1989;8:281.

235. Papadopoulos NEJ, Howard J, Murray JL, et al. Phase I-II DTIC and interleukin 2 (IL2) trial for metastatic malignant melanoma (abstract). Proc Am Soc Clin Oncol 1989;8:290.

236. West W, Tauer K, Barth N, et al. Adoptive immunotherapy and sequential DTIC chemotherapy in metastatic melanoma (abstract). Proc Am Soc Clin Oncol 1989;8:281.

237. Atkins M, Demchak P, Mier J, Robert N, Gould J, Sznol M. Phase II study of alternating interleukin-2 (IL2) and cisplatin (cis DDP) with WR-2721 in metastatic melanoma (abstract). Proc Am Soc Clin Oncol 1989;8:287.

238. Pyrhönen S, Hahka-Kemppinen M, Muhonen T. A promising interferon plus four-drug chemotherapy regimen for metastatic melanoma. J Clin Oncol 1992;10:1919–1926.

239. Falkson CI, Falkson G, Falkson HC. Improved results with the addition of interferon alfa-2b to dacarbazine in the treatment of patients with metastatic malignant melanoma. J Clin Oncol 1991;9:1403–1408.

240. Ron IG, Inbar MJ, Gutman M, Merimsky O, Chaitchik S. Recombinant interferon alpha-2a in combination with dacarbazine in the treatment of metastatic malignant melanoma: analysis of long-term responding patients. Cancer Immunol Immunother 1993; 37:61–66.

241. Flaherty LE, Redman BG, Chabot GG, et al. A phase I-II study of dacarbazine in combination with outpatient interleukin-2 in metastatic malignant melanoma. Cancer 1990;65:2471–2477.

242. Flaherty LE, Robinson W, Redman BG, et al. A phase II study of dacarbazine and cisplatin in combination with outpatient administered interleukin-2 in metastatic malignant melanoma. Cancer 1993;71:3520–3525.

243. Dillman RO, Oldham R, Barth NM, et al. Recombinant interleukin-2 and adoptive immunotherapy with dacarbazine therapy in melanoma: a National Biotherapy Study Group trial. J Natl Cancer Inst 1990; 82:1345–1349.

244. Atkins M, Demchak P, Mier J, et al. Phase II study alternating interleukin-2 (IL-2) and cisplatin (CDDP) with WR-2721 in metastatic melanoma (abstract). Proc Am Soc Clin Oncol 1990;9:186.

245. Richards JM, Ramming K, Bitran JD, et al. Combination of chemotherapy and biological therapy for the treatment of melanoma (abstract). Clin Res 1990;38:844A.

246. Richards JM, Mehta N, Ramming K, Skosey P. Sequential chemoimmunotherapy in the treatment of metastatic melanoma. J Clin Oncol 1992;10:1338–1343.

247. Ron IG, Mordish Y, Eisenthal A, Skornick Y, Inbar MJ, Chaitchik S. A phase II study of combined administration of dacarbazine and carboplatin with home therapy of recombinant interleukin-2 and interferon alpha-2a in patients with advanced malignant melanoma. Cancer Immunol Immunother 1994;38:379–384.

248. LoRusso PM, Polin L, Ackerman SL, et al. Antitumor efficacy of interleukin-2 alone and in combination with chemotherapeutic agents in murine syngeneic solid tumor systems (abstract). Proc Am Assoc Cancer Res 1989;30:614.

249. Legha S, Ring S, Eton O, Plager C, Buzaid A, Papadopolous N. Durable complete responses (CR's) in metastatic melanoma treated with biochemotherapy using cisplatin + vinblastine + DTIC (CVD) and IL-2 and interferon-alpha (IFN α) (abstract). Proc Am Soc Clin Oncol 1995;14:412.

250. Frei E III, Canellos GP. Dose: a critical factor in cancer chemotherapy. Am J Med 1980;69:585–594.

251. Thomas ED. Marrow transplantation in malignant disease. J Clin Oncol 1983;1:517–531.

252. Lazarus HM, Herzig RH, Wolff SN, et al. Treatment of metastatic malignant melanoma with intensive melphalan and autologous bone marrow transplantation. Cancer Treat Rep 1985;69:473–477.

253. McElwain TJ, Hedley DW, Burton G, et al. Marrow autotransplantation accelerates haematological recovery in patients with malignant melanoma treated with high-dose melphalan. Br J Cancer 1979; 40:72–80.

254. McElwain TJ, Hedley DW, Gordon MY, Jarman M, Millar JL, Pritchard J. High dose melphalan and non-cryopreserved autologous bone marrow treatment of malignant melanoma and neuroblastoma. Exp Hematol 1979;7(Suppl 5):360–371.

255. Phillips GL, Fay JW, Herzig GP, et al. Intensive 1,3-bis (2-chloroethyl)-1-nitrosourea (BCNU), NSC 4366650 and cryopreserved autologous marrow transplantation for refractory cancer. A phase I-II study. Cancer 1983;52:1792–1802.

256. Thomas MR, Robinson WA, Hartmann D, Glode LM, Koppler H, Morton NJ. Treatment of advanced malignant melanoma with high dose chemotherapy and autologous bone marrow transplantation. Preliminary results. Am J Clin Oncol 1982;5:611–622.

257. Ciobanu N, Dutcher J, Gucalp R, et al. High dose chemotherapy with autologous bone marrow

transplantation (ABMT) for malignant melanoma after failure of interleukin-2 (IL2) and lymphokine activated killer (LAK) cells (abstract). Proc Am Soc Clin Oncol 1989;8:281.

258. Slease RB, Benear JB, Selby GB, et al. High dose combination alkylating agent therapy with autologous bone marrow rescue for refractory solid tumors. J Clin Oncol 1988;6:1314–1320.

259. Eder JP, Antman K, Elias A, et al. Cyclophosphamide and thiotepa with autologous bone marrow transplantation in patients with solid tumors. J Natl Cancer Inst 1988;80:1221–1226.

260. Wolff SN, Herzig RH, Fay JW, et al. High-dose thiotepa with autologous bone marrow transplantation for metastatic malignant melanoma: results of phase I-II studies of the North American Bone Marrow Transplantation Group. J Clin Oncol 1989;7:245–249.

261. Antman K, Eder JP, Elias A, et al. High-dose combination alkylating agent preparative regimen with autologous bone marrow support: the Dana Farber Cancer Institute/Beth Israel Hospital experience. Cancer Treat Rep 1987;71:119–125.

262. Shea TC, Antman KH, Eder PJ, et al. Malignant melanoma: treatment with high-dose combination alkylating agent chemotherapy and autologous bone marrow support. Arch Dermatol 1988;124:878–884.

263. Thatcher N, Lind M, Morgenstern G, et al. High-dose double alkylating agent chemotherapy with DTIC melphalan or ifosfamide and marrow rescue for metastatic malignant melanoma. Cancer 1989;63:1296–1302.

264. Moormeier JA, Williams SF, Kaminer LS, et al. High-dose tri-alkylator chemotherapy with autologous stem cell rescue in patients with refractory malignancies. J Natl Cancer Inst 1990;82:29–34.

265. Peters WP, Kurtzbers J, Atwater S, et al. Comparative effects of rHuG-CSF and rHuGM-CSF on hematopoietic reconstitution and granulocyte function following high dose chemotherapy and autologous bone marrow transplantation (ABMT) (abstract). Proc Am Soc Clin Oncol 1989;8:181.

266. Tchekmedyian NS, Tait N, Van Echo D, Aisner J. High-dose chemotherapy without autologous bone marrow transplant in melanoma. J Clin Oncol 1986;4:1811–1818.

267. Portlock C, Murren J, Buzaid A, Davis C, DeRosa W. High dose cisplatin (C) and dacarbazine (D) in metastatic melanoma (abstract). Proc Am Soc Clin Oncol 1989;8:284.

268. Glover D, Glick JH, Weiler C, Fox K, Guerry D. WR-2721 and high-dose cisplatin: an active combination in the treatment of metastatic melanoma. J Clin Oncol 1987;5:574–578.

269. Glover D, Glick J, Weiler C, Fox K, Grabelsky S, Guerry D. High dose *cis*-platinum (DDP) and WR-2721 (WR) in metastatic melanoma (abstract). Proc Am Soc Clin Oncol 1988;7:247.

270. Creech O, Krementz ET, Ryan RF, Winblad JN. Chemotherapy of cancer—regional perfusion utilizing an extracorporeal circuit. Ann Surg 1958; 148:616–632.

271. Hafström L, Jönsson P-E. Hyperthermic perfusion of recurrent malignant melanoma of the extremities. Acta Chir Scand 1980;146:313–318.

272. Kroon BBR, VanGeel AN, Benckhuijsen C,

Wieberdink J. Normothermic isolation perfusion with melphalan for advanced melanoma of the limbs. Anticancer Res 1987;7:441–442.

273. Bulman AS, Jamieson CW. Isolated limb perfusion with melphalan in the treatment of malignant melanoma. Br J Surg 1980;67:660–662.

274. Shiu MH, Knapper WH, Fortner JG, et al. Regional isolated limb perfusion of melanoma intransit metastases using mechlorethamine (nitrogen mustard). J Clin Oncol 1986;4:1819–1826.

275. Golomb FM. Perfusion of melanoma. Oncology 1972;26:197–205.

276. Vaglini M, Ammatuna M, Nava M, et al. Regional perfusion at high temperature in treatment of stage III A–III AB melanoma patients. Tumori 1983; 69:585–588.

277. Storm FK, Morton DL. Value of hyperthermic limb perfusion in advanced recurrent melanoma of the lower extremity. Am J Surg 1985;150:32–35.

278. Aigner K, Hild P, Breithaupt H, et al. Isolated extremity perfusion with DTIC. An experimental and clinical study. Anticancer Res 1983;3:87–94.

279. Cox KR. Survival after regional perfusion for limb melanoma. Aust NZ J Surg 1975;45:32–36.

280. Minor DR, Allen RE, Alberts D, Peng YM, Tardelli G, Hutchinson J. A clinical and pharmacokinetic study of isolated limb perfusion with heat and melphalan for melanoma. Cancer 1985;55:2638–2644.

281. Coit DG, Bajorin DF, Menendez-Botet C, et al. Phase I trial of hyperthermic isolation perfusion using cisplatin (CDDP) for metastatic intransit melanoma (abstract). Proc Am Soc Clin Oncol 1989;8:285.

282. Stehlin JS Jr, Giovanella BC, de Ipolyi PD, Muenz LR, Anderson RF. Results of hyperthermic perfusion for melanoma of the extremities. Surg Gynecol Obstet 1975;140:339–348.

283. Liénard D, Lejeune FJ, Ewalenko P. In transit metastases of malignant melanoma treated by high dose RTNF alpha in combination with interferon-gamma and melphalan in isolation perfusion. World J Surg 1992;16:234–240.

284. Lejeune F, Liénard D, Eggermont A, et al. Rationale for using TNFα and chemotherapy in regional therapy of melanoma. J Cell Biol 1994;56:52–61.

285. Ghussen F, Kruger I, Groth W, Stutzer H. The role of regional hyperthermic cytostatic perfusion in the treatment of extremity melanoma. Cancer 1988; 61:654–659.

286. Hafström L, Rudenstam CM, Bloomquist E, et al. Regional hyperthermic perfusion with melphalan after surgery for recurrent malignant melanoma of the extremities. J Clin Oncol 1991;9:2091–2094.

287. Oberfield RA, Sullivan RD. Prolonged and continuous regional arterial infusion chemotherapy in patients with melanoma. JAMA 1969;209:75–79.

288. Bland KI, Kimura AK, Brenne DE, et al. A phase II study of the efficacy of diamminedichloroplatinum (cisplatin) for the control of locally recurrent and intransit malignant melanoma of the extremities using tourniquet outflow-occlusion techniques. Ann Surg 1989;209:73–80.

289. Frost DB, Patt YZ, Mavligit G, Chuang VP, Wallace S. Arterial infusion of dacarbazine and cisplatin for recurrent regionally confined melanoma. Arch Surg 1985;120:478–480.

290. Calvo DB III, Patt YZ, Wallace S, et al. Phase

I-II trial of percutaneous intra-arterial *cis*-diammine-dichloroplatinum (II) for regionally confined malignancy. Cancer 1980;45:1278–1283.

291. Storm FK, Kaiser LR, Goodnight JE, et al. Thermochemotherapy for melanoma metastases in the liver. Cancer 1982;49:1243–1248.

292. Gundersen S, Hager B, Tausjo J. Radiation in combination with intra-arterial therapy with dacarbazine for metastatic malignant melanoma localized to a lower extremity. Cancer Treat Rep 1986;70:1015–1017.

293. O'Keefe F, Lorigan JG, Charnsangavej C, Carrasco CH, Richli WR, Wallace S. Chemotherapy and embolization via the inferior epigastric artery for the treatment of primary and metastatic cancer. Am J Radiol 1989;152:387–390.

294. Mavligit GM, Charnsangavej C, Carrasco CH, Patt YZ, Benjamin RS, Wallace S. Regression of ocular melanoma metastatic to the liver after hepatic arterial chemoembolization with cisplatin and polyvinyl sponge. JAMA 1988;260:974–976.

295. Cantore M, Fiorentini G, Altini E, et al. Intra-arterial hepatic carboplatin-based chemotherapy for ocular melanoma metastatic to the liver. Report of a phase II study. Tumori 1994;80:37–39.

296. Voigt H, Loffler T. Angioocclusive chemotherapy in melanoma: rationale and technical considerations. Anticancer Res 1987;7:443–444.

297. Sato T, Nathan FE, Berd D, Sullivan K, Mastrangelo MJ. Lack of effect from chemoembolization for liver metastases from uveal melanoma (abstract). Proc Am Soc Clin Oncol 1995;14:415.

298. Bellet RE, Danna V, Mastrangelo MJ, Berd D. Evaluation of a "nude" mouse–human tumor panel as a predictive secondary screen for cancer chemotherapeutic agents. J Natl Cancer Inst 1979;63:1185–1188.

299. Bellet RE, Danna V, Mastrangelo MJ, Eaton GJ, Berd D. Evaluation of the response of a panel of human melanoma tissue-cultured cell lines xenografted on nude mice to four anticancer drugs of known clinical activity. In: Proceedings of Third International Workshop on Nude Mice. New York: Gustav Fischer 1982:649–656.

300. Venditti J. Preclinical drug development, rationale and methods. Semin Oncol 1981;8:349–361.

301. Hamburger AW, Salmon SE. Primary bioassay of human tumor stem cells. Science 1977;197:461–463.

302. Meyskens FL Jr, Moon TE, Dana B, et al. Quantitation of drug sensitivity by human metastatic melanoma colony-forming units. Br J Cancer 1981;44:787–797.

303. Schadendorf D, Worm M, Algermissen B, et al. Chemosensitivity testing of human malignant melanoma: a retrospective analysis of clinical response and in vitro drug sensitivity. Cancer 1994;73:103–108.

304. Nathan FE, Sato T, Berd D, Mastrangelo MJ. BOLD + interferon: effective systemic therapy for metastatic uveal melanoma (abstract). Proc Am Soc Clin Oncol 1995;14:410.

305. Lotze MT, Rosenberg SA. Interleukin-2: clinical applications. In Davis VT, Hellman S, Rosenberg SA, eds. Biologic therapy of cancer. Philadelphia: JB Lippincott, 1991:159–177.

306. Berd D, Maguire HC Jr, Mastrangelo MJ. Treatment of human melanoma with a hapten-modified autologous vaccine. Ann NY Acad Sci 1993;690:147–152.

307. Bornstein RS, Mastrangelo MJ, Sulit H, et al. Immunotherapy of melanoma with intralesional BCG. NCI Monogr 1973;39:213–220.

51

Chemotherapy of Primary Brain Tumors

Roy A. Patchell

GENERAL ISSUES IN BRAIN TUMOR CHEMOTHERAPY

For over 40 years, chemotherapy has been used in the treatment of primary brain tumors; however, the results have been uniformly poor in all but a handful of tumor types. The use of chemotherapy for central nervous system tumors poses special problems not present in the treatment of nonneurologic cancers. There are at least four factors that make brain tumor treatment unusual, including (*a*) the lethality of relatively small tumor volumes, (*b*) the potential for serious brain edema, (*c*) low growth fractions in even the most malignant tumors, and (*d*) the presence of the blood-brain barrier (BBB) that restricts the entry of many chemotherapeutic agents into the brain.

The skull rigidity encloses the brain, and even moderate increases in intracranial volume are incompatible with life. Shapiro (1) has estimated that for primary brain tumors, a tumor of 100 g is fatal; 100 g is equivalent to about 1×10^{11} cells. The average brain tumor becomes symptomatic when its weight is between 30 and 60 g ($3-6 \times 10^{10}$ cells). Complete surgical resections are almost never possible in the treatment of most primary brain tumors. Extensive (but incomplete) resections leave behind at least 1 to 5 g of tumor ($1-5 \times 10^9$ cells). Modern external-beam radiation therapy can remove at most 2 logs of cells. If chemotherapy is to be effective, it must further reduce the tumor by 2 logs of cells to about 1×10^5 cells. (It is generally assumed that a tumor of 1×10^5 cells can be eliminated by the body's own immune system. (1)). Unfortunately, for most brain tumors, chemotherapy has not been able to bring about this reduction.

Even when large amounts of tumor are destroyed by radiation or chemotherapy, the brain is frequently unable to deal with the necrotic debris. The brain lacks lymphatics, and injury to intracranial structures usually produces cerebral edema. In addition, tumor blood vessels are usually incompletely formed and are prone to leak and produce edema. The edema itself occupies space and, at times, can be life threatening. Chemotherapeutic agents that produce or aggravate cerebral edema are not tolerated, and this reduces the number of agents available for brain tumor chemotherapy.

In addition to the mechanics of tumor reduction and cerebral edema, the growth characteristics of most primary brain tumors make successful chemotherapy difficult. Even the most aggressive glioblastomas have growth fractions of less than 50%, and in most neuroectodermal tumors, the growth fraction is much lower—in the range of 5 to 20% (2, 3). Since most chemotherapeutic agents available for brain tumors are given as intravenous infusions once every few weeks, cell-cycle-specific agents are less likely to be effective than cell-cycle-nonspecific agents.

The most serious limitation to brain tumor chemotherapy is the BBB. The BBB is a physiologic and pharmacologic barrier that is anatomically located in the tight junctions between capillary endothelial cells in the central nervous system (4). The BBB restricts the rate of passage of substances larger than 200 daltons (and also smaller ionized molecules). Most chemotherapeutic agents cross the BBB by simple diffusion. In 1962, Rall and Zubrod (5) stated the characteristics that were likely to allow diffusion across the BBB: (*a*) high lipid solubility, (*b*) low ionization, and (*c*) lack of protein binding.

The presence of the BBB is not absolute, and the BBB is usually disrupted in most brain tumors (6). The fact that there is a tumor "blush" during arteriography and that tumors demonstrate contrast enhancement with magnetic resonance imaging (MRI) and computerized tomographic (CT) scans, indicates that the BBB is not functioning normally in the area around tumors. However, the degree of BBB breakdown is variable, and in the area of brain adjacent to tumor, the BBB is relatively intact (7). Most early attempts at brain tumor chemotherapy used highly lipid-soluble drugs. More recent trials have experimented with water-soluble agents. Despite the incompleteness of the BBB, lipid-soluble agents appear to have the best penetration into brain tumors, and this fact severely restricts the number and type of chemotherapeutic agents that are likely to be effective in brain tumor chemotherapy.

Unfortunately, for almost all primary brain tumors, current chemotherapy has no or limited effectiveness. The standard treatment of most brain tumors is surgery followed by radiation therapy. Chemotherapy has not been shown unequivocally to increase survival for the most common tumor types.

CURRENT TREATMENT OF PRIMARY BRAIN TUMORS IN ADULTS

High-Grade Astrocytomas Including Glioblastoma Multiforme

GENERAL PRINCIPLES OF TREATMENT

High-grade gliomas are the most common type of primary brain tumor in adults and make up about half of all primary brain tumors. Several classification systems have been used to subdivide astrocytic tumors on the basis of histologic criteria. In the older Kernohan system (8), there are four grades of astrocytomas, with grades III and IV being considered high-grade astrocytomas. A newer system developed by Burger et al. (9) recognizes only three categories, with anaplastic astrocytomas and glioblastomas being considered high-grade tumors. The histologic grade is a significant prognostic factor. Even with the most advanced presently available treatment, the median survival of patients with glioblastomas is less than 1 year.

Surgery and postoperative radiation therapy are the principal treatments for high-grade astrocytomas. Surgery has several benefits, including establishing the diagnosis and reducing the tu-

mor mass. Studies by the Brain Tumor Study Group (BTSG) (now called the Brain Tumor Cooperative Group (BTCG) have shown that surgery by itself prolongs life a median of 14 weeks compared with no therapy (1, 10). In addition, aggressive resections appear to produce longer survivals than do biopsies or minimal resections (11–13). Postoperative radiation therapy, when given at doses of 6000 to 7000 cGy, produces a statistically significant increase in median survival to 36 weeks (10, 12, 13). The early studies used whole brain radiation therapy, but a later BTCG randomized trial (14) showed that reduced-dose whole brain radiation plus a coned-down boost to the tumor was equally effective.

CHEMOTHERAPY

Chemotherapy for brain tumors has been most extensively studied in the treatment of high-grade astrocytomas. To date, over 100 chemotherapeutic agents have been used in the treatment of high-grade astrocytomas (15–17). Much of the data on these agents come from small uncontrolled series or even individual case reports. Despite various claims of success, no agent has been unequivocally shown to be effective in clinical trials (17), although a large metaanalysis, analyzing the results of randomized trials from 1975 to 1989 (18), found that the addition of chemotherapy significantly increased the percentage of 1- and 2-year survivors. Of the drugs tested, the nitrosoureas, aziridinylbenzoquinone (AZQ), cisplatin, and procarbazine have shown the most promise against recurrent tumors (15–17).

Most small-scale studies have been performed in patients with recurrent tumors, while several large trials have used only adjuvant chemotherapy. A controversy exists about whether adjuvant chemotherapy really adds any benefit when compared with reserving chemotherapy for recurrent disease. Two trials, both performed by the European Organization for Research on Treatment of Cancer (EORTC), have examined the timing of chemotherapy in the treatment of high-grade gliomas. The first study (19) examined the advantages of lomustine (CCNU) given immediately after radiation therapy (adjuvant therapy) versus CCNU given only after tumor recurrence. The median survival of patients receiving adjuvant therapy was 43 weeks versus 63 weeks for patients treated at recurrence; this difference was not statistically significant. A second study (20) compared CCNU plus tenoposide (VM-26) given as either adjuvant therapy or only at recurrence. No significant difference was found between the two groups with regard to either time to progression or overall survival. The results of these two studies suggest that reserving therapy for recurrences may be as beneficial as adjuvant chemotherapy.

Since there have been several large-scale, prospective randomized trials published on the treatment of high-grade gliomas (21), the following discussion on the efficacy of adjuvant chemotherapy is confined to the results of randomized trials. The first phase III trial by the BTSG was a four-armed randomized study of 222 patients (13). This study showed that BCNU resulted in a slightly longer overall survival, with an increase in the percentage of 18-month survivors from 4% in patients treated with surgery plus radiation to 19% in patients treated with surgery and radiation plus BCNU. However, the increase in survival was not statistically significant. Two subsequent randomized studies also showed modest but statistically insignificant trends toward longer survival in patients treated with BCNU (10, 11). Procarbazine and streptozotocin were also found to have activity similar to that of BCNU, although with more toxicity (11, 12). In all cases, the drugs in the above-mentioned studies were given intravenously. These randomized trials indicate that BCNU is probably an active agent but that it has very limited effectiveness.

A controversy exists regarding the efficacy of multiagent chemotherapy regimens versus treatment with single agents. In a study published in 1989 (14), combination chemotherapy consisting of BCNU-procarbazine or BCNU-hydroxyurea-procarbazine-VM26 was compared with BCNU alone. There was no statistically significant difference among the groups, suggesting that combination chemotherapy therapy was no more effective than single-agent BCNU treatment.

In the treatment of anaplastic astrocytomas, there is some evidence to indicate that combination therapy may be superior to treatment with BCNU alone. Levin et al. (22) performed a study in which patients with high-grade astrocytomas were randomized following radiotherapy treatment to either intravenous BCNU or a multiagent regimen consisting of procarbazine, CCNU, and vincristine (PCV). Overall results showed an insignificant trend toward longer survival in the PCV group. However, a subgroup analysis of patients with anaplastic astrocytomas and Karnofsky performance scores over 70% found that patients treated with PCV survived almost twice as long as those treated with BCNU alone (151.1 vs. 82.1 weeks).

Due to the generally poor results achieved with conventional chemotherapy, attempts have been made to improve drug delivery. Alternative methods of drug delivery have consisted of intraarterial injections of drugs, manipulations of the BBB with osmotic agents, intratumoral chemotherapy, and high-dose therapy with bone marrow transplant.

Intraarterial therapy is theoretically well motivated in that the drug dose to the tumor is increased while the total dose delivered is usually less than with intravenous therapy (23). The technique is similar to that used for arteriography and involves the temporary placement of arterial catheters into the carotid or vertebral arteries. Over 25 intraarterial drugs have been investigated in the treatment of malignant gliomas (24). Drugs that have shown activity in phase II studies are BCNU, AZQ, and cisplatin (17, 24). However, up to 20% of patients have suffered serious complications including permanent ipsilateral blindness and late-onset leukoencephalopathy/dementia. The use of Millipore filters and selective catheterization above the level of the ophthalmic artery has reduced the number of ophthalmologic side effects (25, 26). A large randomized trial using intracarotid BCNU was published in 1992 by the BTCG (27). The study randomized 448 eligible patients to treatment with 200 mg/m^2 BCNU given every 8 weeks, either intravenously or intraarterially. (In addition, there was a second randomization that added intravenous 5-fluorouracil to half of the patients in each treatment arm.) Patients who received intraarterial BCNU had significantly shorter survival times than did the patients treated with intravenous drug. Analysis of the survival data showed that the inferior results with intraarterial BCNU were mainly due to poor outcomes in patients with anaplastic astrocytomas. In addition, intracarotid BCNU had substantial toxicity. Intraarterial chemotherapy for brain tumors has not been shown to be beneficial and has been largely abandoned.

Intratumoral injection of drugs is another novel attempt to increase the dose of chemotherapy to the tumor while reducing systemic exposure. Theoretically, very small doses into the tumor should produce a large concentration of drug in the tumor; as the drug diffuses out of the tumor, the amount reaching the systemic circulation should be small. The process should also avoid the restrictions of the BBB, since a vascular delivery route is not used. Early clinical studies involved the direct injection of various drugs into the tumor (24). Clinical trials have used implantable pumps to provide a continuous infusion of cisplatin (28). Modified Ommaya reservoirs have also been used to deliver continuous infusion (29). Too few patients have been treated so far to determine the efficacy of these techniques, although toxicity has been minimal.

Another attempt to deliver chemotherapy intratumorally has been the use of sustained-release biodegradable polymers that are surgically implanted directly into brain tumors or tumor cavities. To date, only the drug BCNU has been used in clinical studies. The implant procedure is a one-time event, and without a second major operation, the drug supply cannot be replenished. The polymers release BCNU for about 3 weeks before becoming inactive. Brem et al. (30) described a study of 21 patients who received up to 8 BCNU wafers for recurrent malignant gliomas. There was no apparent toxicity, and overall median survival was 48 weeks after implantation. Encouraged by these results, a randomized multicenter trial involving 222 patients was conducted (31). Patients with recurrent high-grade gliomas were treated with a second resection of tumor followed by implantation of either BCNU wafers or placebo wafers. Survival was significantly longer in the BCNU group than in the placebo group (median, 31 weeks vs. 23 weeks).

A different approach to increasing drug delivery to brain tumors is the transient disruption of the blood barrier (32). Mannitol is used to disrupt the BBB and allow a greater concentration of drug into the brain (and tumor). The mannitol is given intraarterially, and therefore, only the BBB in the specific arterial distribution is disrupted. Initial reports showed promise, but toxicity to normal brain has been a problem (33, 34). Subsequent laboratory investigations using quantitative autoradiography have shown that while the concentration of drug into tumor is increased, there is a disproportionally higher inflow of drug into normal brain (35). This technique has not been tested in a large clinical trial.

High-dose chemotherapy followed by autologous bone marrow transplantation has also been tried in an attempt to allow the delivery of higher doses of conventional intravenous chemotherapy. Since the main toxicity of BCNU is bone marrow suppression, this approach is theoretically promising (36, 37). Unfortunately, practical experience in several small phase II trials using BCNU (37–42) or VP-16 (43) has shown

the procedure to be toxic and to have no obvious effect on survival.

Low-Grade Astrocytomas

GENERAL PRINCIPLES OF TREATMENT

The overall prognosis for patients with low-grade gliomas is significantly better than with high-grade astrocytomas. The median survival for Kernohan grade I tumors is about 5 years. There is little doubt that surgery is useful therapy because it both makes the diagnosis and removes tumor. The role of radiotherapy, however, is less clear. Several retrospective studies have suggested that survival is increased when postsurgical radiotherapy is used. However, these studies suffer from patient selection bias, and there is other evidence to suggest that radiotherapy increases the rate of malignant transformation to high-grade tumors.

CHEMOTHERAPY

Because of the very low mitotic rate of these tumors, chemotherapy is almost never used in low-grade gliomas. Early trials using nitrosoureas as adjuvant therapy have shown no efficacy (15, 16). BCNU is known to produce tumors in animals, and converting a low-grade tumor to a higher-grade one is a possibility. At present, chemotherapy has no place in the initial management of low-grade astrocytomas in adults. However, when these tumors recur, they often show transformation to high-grade gliomas. In that case, chemotherapy with BCNU or other agents is likely to achieve results similar to those in the treatment of recurrent high-grade gliomas.

Oligodendrogliomas

GENERAL PRINCIPLES OF TREATMENT

Oligodendrogliomas are slow-growing tumors that occur primarily in the cerebral hemispheres; they account for about 5% of primary brain tumors. Pure oligodendrogliomas are usually "benign" and can sometimes be totally removed by surgery. In tumors that cannot be totally resected, the role of radiation therapy is controversial. Several retrospective reviews of large series of patients have suggested that survival is enhanced by postoperative radiotherapy (44, 45). However, these studies all suffer from patient selection bias and biased follow-up reporting. The actual benefit of radiation in the management of oligodendrogliomas is unknown.

CHEMOTHERAPY

The discovery that oligodendrogliomas are chemosensitive tumors is one of the few advances in brain tumor therapy in the last 20 years. Cairncross and Macdonald (47) initially showed that for histologically and clinically aggressive oligodendrogliomas, chemotherapy, consisting of procarbazine-CCNU-vincristine (PCV), produced responses in recurrent tumors and anaplastic oligodendrogliomas. The same chemotherapy regimen, given as adjuvant therapy before radiotherapy in patients with incomplete resections, has recently been shown to produce responses (47–49) in up to 70% of patients. PCV has also been shown to be effective in mixed oligoastrocytomas (50, 51) and in the treatment of nonanaplastic oligodendrogliomas (52). The high percentage of responses in these studies strongly suggests that oligodendrogliomas are sensitive to chemotherapy, and a randomized trial is under way.

Ependymomas

GENERAL PRINCIPLES OF TREATMENT

Ependymomas arise from ependymal cells that line the cerebrospinal fluid (CSF) pathways and the central canal of the spinal cord. Overall, about 70% of these tumors are found in the posterior fossa, and posterior fossa tumors are more common in children than adults. Surgical resection is the first step in treatment; however, due to the deep location of most of these tumors, surgical removal is frequently incomplete. Based on several retrospective studies (53–55), radiation therapy appears to increase survival. However, because ependymomas spread to involve the CSF in 8 to 30% of cases, the optimum size of radiation fields is controversial. The risk of CSF seeding is greatest in high-grade infratentorial tumors, and many investigators have recommended whole craniospinal axis radiation only in patients who have malignant cells in the CSF before treatment (56, 57) or in patients with high-grade infratentorial tumors even if the CSF is free from malignancy (53).

CHEMOTHERAPY

The use of chemotherapy in the treatment of ependymomas in adults has not been tested in a prospective randomized trial. For recurrent tumors, scant information is available. Nitrosoureas (58), mechlorethamine, vincristine, procarbazine, prednisone, and MOPP (mechlorethamine, vincristine, procarbazine, and prednisone) (59) have been tried in small numbers of patients with little success. Cisplatin has also been used in small numbers of patients, and several studies have shown responses of up to 50% (60, 61). In a phase II study (62), adjuvant chemotherapy consisting of CCNU-vincristine increased survival compared with historic controls. Adjuvant chemotherapy is also being examined in a randomized study by the Childrens' Cooperative Study Group (CCSG) comparing surgery plus radiation with surgery plus radiation plus CCNU-vincristine-prednisone.

Primary Central Nervous System Lymphoma (PCNSL)

GENERAL PRINCIPLES OF TREATMENT

PCNSLs (also known as microgliomas or reticulum cell sarcomas) are relatively rare and account for only 1 to 2% of all primary brain tumors. The tumors are more common in immunosuppressed individuals, especially in organ transplant recipients and in patients with the acquired immune deficiency syndrome (AIDS). The tumors are frequently multicentric and involve deep white matter. Surgery, other than biopsy to make the diagnosis, adds little to survival. Radiation therapy usually produces a dramatic response, but the tumors invariably recur. The median survival of patients treated with radiation is 12 to 18 months, with virtually no 5-year survivors (63). About 25% of patients with PCNSL have CSF seeding (64), and there have been reports of prolonged survival in small numbers of patients treated with whole craniospinal axis radiation (65–67).

CHEMOTHERAPY

No randomized trials have been reported in the treatment of PCNSLs. Several agents have been used in small series of patients, and methotrexate, cytarabine, procarbazine, CCNU, BCNU, and cyclophosphamide have shown activity when given as single-agent chemotherapy (63). In addition, about 40% of patients have partial or complete responses to corticosteroid treatment alone (64), although the effect is usually short lived. More durable responses in phase II trials have been achieved with combination chemotherapy regimens. DeAngelis et al. (68) gave preradiation intravenous and intrathecal methotrexate followed by postradiation high-dose cytarabine to 31 patients; the median survival was 41 months. However, not all trials have shown a clear benefit from chemotherapy. The

Radiation Therapy Oncology Group (RTOG) reported a study (69) containing 51 patients who received cyclophosphamide, doxorubicin, vincristine, and dexamethasone (CHOD) followed by radiotherapy. The median survival was only 12.8 months, and there was a substantial amount of delayed neurotoxicity.

A special situation exists in the treatment of organ transplant recipients who develop PCNSL (70). In these patients, the most likely cause of the tumor is an Epstein-Barr virus infection that results in a "benign" polyclonal lymphoproliferation. The suppressed immune systems of organ transplant recipients are unable to control the proliferation. Eventually a malignant clone is produced, and a lymphoma results. If the diagnosis of PCNSL is made early in the course (before the malignant clone is produced), treatment with reduction of immunosuppression and antiviral therapy may result in a complete remission of the PCNSL (71).

CHEMOTHERAPY OF PRIMARY BRAIN TUMORS THAT OCCUR PREDOMINANTLY IN CHILDREN

Brainstem Gliomas

GENERAL PRINCIPLES OF TREATMENT

Brainstem gliomas account for about 15% of all pediatric primary brain tumors. These tumors also occur in adults but constitute less than 5% of adult gliomas. The diagnosis is usually made on the basis of clinical presentation and characteristic findings on MRI scans. In the past, biopsy was occasionally performed to confirm the diagnosis; however, with recent improvements in posterior fossa imaging, tissue is now rarely obtained. Due to the location of these tumors, surgical removal is impossible, although tumors with an exophytic component may benefit from removal of the external part (72). Radiation therapy is the only treatment that has been shown to be of benefit. Unfortunately, even with high-dose radiation, the median survival is only 15 months, with about 20% of patients alive at 5 years (73).

CHEMOTHERAPY

Relatively few drugs have been used in the treatment of brainstem gliomas, and most studies have involved small numbers of patients. An additional problem has been the lack of histologic confirmation in most of the studies. Chemotherapy for recurrent tumors has not been effective. A review by Friedman and Oakes (60)

noted that the following drugs have been studied but found to be without substantial benefit: BCNU, CCNU, cisplatin, cyclophosphamide, dianhydrogalactitol, dibromodulcitol, methotrexate (intrathecally and low-dose intravenously), procarbazine, PCNU, AZQ, and combination therapies with COPP (cyclophosphamide-vincristine-procarbazine-prednisone). Carboplatin as single-agent therapy has recently been used without success (74). The only promising results with chemotherapy for recurrent tumors were early reports of high-dose cyclophosphamide (75) and high-dose methotrexate (76). Randomized trials using these agents have not been reported.

Adjuvant chemotherapy has been investigated in several studies by the CCSG. A randomized trial found no benefit from a combination of postradiation CCNU-vincristine-prednisone (77), while a nonrandomized study using preradiation 5-fluorouracil-CCNU plus hydroxyurea as a radiosensitizer failed to demonstrate any benefit from chemotherapy when compared with historic controls (72). To date, chemotherapy has not been of benefit in the treatment of brainstem gliomas.

Medulloblastoma

GENERAL PRINCIPLES OF TREATMENT

Medulloblastomas are the most common brain tumors in children and also occur occasionally in adults. Most medulloblastomas occur in the posterior fossa and have a strong tendency to spread in the CSF. Using both CSF cytology and myelography, evidence of leptomeningeal spread is present in about 30% of patients at diagnosis (78). Unlike most other brain tumors, extraneural metastases occur and are found in about 5% of patients.

Medulloblastomas are one of the few brain tumors in which substantial progress has been made, and this progress is directly attributable to advances in treatment. Surgery is the first treatment used, and there is a relationship between the extent of resection and subsequent survival (79). Unfortunately, all patients treated with surgery alone ultimately relapse, regardless of the degree of initial resection. Most of the dramatic increase in survival of medulloblastoma patients comes from improvements in radiation therapy. Radiation therapy typically consists of whole craniospinal axis radiation using 2500 to 3500 cGy, followed by a boost to the posterior fossa to bring the total tumor dose to 5000 to 5500 cGy. Known metastases in the CNS are treated with additional focal radiation to about 4000 cGy. The 5-year survival rate in patients aggressively treated with radiation therapy is 50 to 60% (80).

CHEMOTHERAPY

Currently, chemotherapy does not play a major role in the treatment of medulloblastoma. Many agents have been tried in small studies that have used clinical criteria (rather than radiologic or pathologic criteria) for assessing outcomes. Friedman and Oakes (46) listed over 20 drugs used as single-agent chemotherapy and more than a dozen combination regimens that have been used in the treatment of medulloblastoma. The most active single agents are cyclophosphamide, vincristine, cisplatin, and carboplatin. Combinations that have shown promise include procarbazine-CCNU-vincristine, cyclophosphamide-vincristine, and MOPP.

The usefulness of adjuvant chemotherapy has been examined in both phase II and phase III trials. The phase II trials have used small numbers of patients and are difficult to interpret (60). Two large randomized trials have been completed, and although not conclusive, both studies can be interpreted as showing some benefit for adjuvant chemotherapy. In a study (80, 81) with 287 patients, done by the International Society of Pediatric Oncology (SIOP), conventional surgery and radiation was compared with conventional surgery and radiation plus CCNU-vincristine. Although the chemotherapy arm produced consistently longer survivals, the overall difference was not statistically significant. However, subgroup analysis showed that chemotherapy produced significantly better results in patients with subtotal resections, involvement of the brainstem, those under 2 years of age, and those with advanced disease. A second randomized study by the CCSG compared surgery and radiation with surgery and radiation plus CCNU-vincristine-prednisone (81, 82). This study contained 198 patients, and a marginally significant survival advantage was found for patients with advanced disease, although overall survival was not significantly different.

Low-Grade Gliomas Including Cerebellar Astrocytomas and Chiasmatic/Hypothalamic Gliomas

GENERAL PRINCIPLES OF TREATMENT

Low-grade astrocytomas of the cerebral hemispheres are similar in presentation and management to those tumors found in adults, and will not be discussed separately. However, children also develop low-grade gliomas in the cerebellum and in the chiasmatic/hypothalamic region that do not resemble tumors found in adults.

Childhood cerebellar astrocytomas account for approximately 10% of pediatric brain tumors. The primary treatment is surgical removal, and with well-differentiated tumors, the median survival is longer than 18 years. The role of radiation therapy is controversial. For tumors that are incompletely removed or for clearly aggressive tumors, postoperative radiation therapy is occasionally used, but no definite benefit has been shown.

Gliomas of the optic chiasm and hypothalamic area usually occur in young children between 6 months and 3 years of age. These tumors can have a variable course; some behave like benign hamartoma-like tumors, while others are aggressive and rapidly expand to cause death (83). Surgery is useful, but complete resections are frequently impossible. Radiotherapy usually stabilizes disease, but as many as 50% of patients suffer recurrences (83). Radiation therapy, especially to the hypothalamic region, often causes intellectual impairment and is undesirable in young patients.

CHEMOTHERAPY

For cerebellar astrocytomas, chemotherapy has been used in a few patients with recurrent tumors; however, the numbers treated are too small to draw any conclusions. Drugs used include BCNU, CCNU, VP-16, BCNU-procarbazine, and BCNU-vincristine-methotrexate-prednisone (60). Due to the excellent prognosis of patients with cerebellar astrocytomas, adjuvant chemotherapy has not been used.

For gliomas of the optic chiasm/hypothalamic area, chemotherapy consisting of CCNU-vincristine, CCNU-vincristine-procarbazine, and cisplatin has been used for recurrent tumors, and some responses have been reported (83). For adjuvant therapy in aggressive tumors, Packer et al. (84) have reported success with a novel approach consisting of actinomycin D plus vincristine without prior or subsequent radiation therapy. With a median follow-up period of 4.3 years, 62.5% patients have remained disease free.

Supratentorial High-Grade Gliomas

GENERAL PRINCIPLES OF TREATMENT

The general principles of treatment for childhood supratentorial high-grade gliomas are similar to those in the adult, although the experience with pediatric tumors is less extensive. The usual initial treatment is maximum surgical resection. Radiotherapy is usually given after surgery; however, most tumors recur, and the median survival of children treated with surgery and radiation therapy is only 15 months (85).

CHEMOTHERAPY

Chemotherapy has a definite place in the management of pediatric high-grade gliomas. For recurrent tumors, several small phase II studies have been performed, and activity has been demonstrated for the nitrosoureas (86, 87). Drugs tested in small clinical trials but found to be of no or unclear benefit include cisplatin (88), carboplatin (89), CCNU-vincristine (90), COPP (91), MOPP (92), and "eight in one" (93).

Adjuvant chemotherapy consisting of CCNU-vincristine-prednisone given after surgery and radiation therapy has been tested in a phase III trial by the CCSG (94). Chemotherapy resulted in a statistically significant prolongation of both overall survival and disease-free survival. The 5-year survival rate was 42% for the chemotherapy group and only 10% in the control group. The 5-year disease-free survival rate was 45% in the chemotherapy group and 13% in the control group. These differences were still statistically significant even after major prognostic factors were taken into account. The results of this study are the best so far achieved in the treatment of high-grade gliomas, whether in children or adults. On the basis of these data, adjuvant chemotherapy should be used in all childhood supratentorial high-grade gliomas.

Central Nervous System Germ Cell Tumors

GENERAL PRINCIPLES OF TREATMENT

Pineal region tumors can conveniently be divided into germ cell tumors and non-germ-cell tumors. Tumors originating from germ cells include germinomas, embryonal cell carcinomas, teratomas, choriocarcinomas, and endodermal sinus tumors. Non-germ-cell tumors include true pineal tumors and other primary CNS tumors not considered germ cell tumors. Germ cell tumors of the CNS are not common and comprise only 3% of childhood brain tumors (95). Germinomas, the most common CNS germ cell tumor, account for about 60% of the total. Radiation therapy is the mainstay of treatment, and

the 5-year survival rate for histologically confirmed germinomas is 60 to 90% (96).

CHEMOTHERAPY

Recurrent tumors have been shown to be responsive to several chemotherapeutic agents including cyclophosphamide, cisplatin, cyclophosphamide-actinomycin D-vincristine-bleomycin, and etoposide (97–99).

Due to the relatively favorable prognosis of patients treated with radiation, adjuvant therapy per se has not been explored in series of patients. However, neoadjuvant (preradiation) chemotherapy has been tried in an attempt to decrease the radiation dose and field size. Allen, Kim, and Packer (100) reported a series of 11 germinomas treated with high-dose cyclophosphamide (1800 mg/m^2). Before radiation therapy, two courses of chemotherapy were given, and then patients were evaluated for completeness of response. In those patients who showed a complete response, the subsequent radiation dose was reduced to a mean tumor dose of 330 cGy and mean craniospinal dose of 2620 cGy. The full dose of radiation was given to patients who showed incomplete or no response to chemotherapy. Ten of the 11 germinoma patients had complete responses to chemotherapy. When the study was published in 1987, 10 of the 11 patients were still in continuous remission, with a median follow-up time of 47 months. Although the numbers involved in this study were small, it appears that neoadjuvant chemotherapy is effective and allows the use of a substantially reduced radiation dose without compromising long-term survival. A randomized trial of preradiation chemotherapy consisting of carboplatin, etoposide, and bleomycin is near completion (101).

SUMMARY

The value of chemotherapy for most brain tumors has not been established, and surgery and radiation therapy continue to be the mainstays of treatment. Progress has been made in the chemotherapy of specific tumor types, notably oligodendrogliomas and some pediatric brain tumors. Much of the research on chemotherapy of brain tumors has involved small clinical trials that have contained inadequate numbers of patients to determine the actual value of the agent studied. In the future, the most useful information is likely to come from large multicenter trials such as those currently being conducted by the BTCG and CCSG.

References

1. Shapiro WR. Treatment of neuroectodermal brain tumors. Ann Neurol 1982;12:231–237.

2. Hoshino T, Wilson CB. Review of basic concepts of cell kinetics as applied to brain tumors. J Neurosurg 1975;42:123–131.

3. Hoshino T, Nashima T, Cho KG, et al. S phase fraction of human brain tumors in situ measured by uptake of bromodeoxyuridine. Int J Cancer 1986; 38:369–374.

4. Reese TS, Karnofsky J. Fine structural localization of a blood-brain barrier to exogenous peroxidase. J Cell Biol 1967;34:207–217.

5. Rall DP, Zubrod CG. Mechanism of drug absorption and excretion. Passage of drugs in and out of the central nervous system. Annu Rev Pharmacol 1962; 2:109–128.

6. Long DM. Capillary ultrastructure and the blood-brain barrier in human malignant brain tumors. J Neurosurg 1970;32:127–144.

7. Levin VA, Freeman MA, Landahl HD. The permeability characteristics of brain adjacent to intracerebral rat tumors. Arch Neurol 1975;32:785–791.

8. Kernohan JW, Mabon RF, Svien HJ, Adson AW. A simplified classification of the gliomas. Mayo Clin Proc 1949;24:71–75.

9. Burger PC, Vogel FS, Green SB, et al. Glioblastoma multiforme and anaplastic astrocytoma: pathologic criteria and prognostic implications. Cancer 1985; 56:1106–1111.

10. Walker MD, Green SB, Byar DP, et al. Randomized comparisons of radiotherapy and nitrosoureas for the treatment of anaplastic astrocytomas: a cooperative clinical trial. N Engl J Med 1980;303:1323–1329.

11. Green SB, Byar DP, Strike TA, et al. Randomized comparisons of BCNU, streptozocin, radiosensitizer, and fractionation of radiotherapy in the postoperative treatment of malignant glioma (study 7702) (abstract). Proc Am Soc Clin Oncol 1984;3:260.

12. Green SB, Byar DP, Walker MD, et al. Comparisons of carmustine, procarbazine, and high-dose methylprednisolone as additions to surgery and radiotherapy for the treatment of malignant glioma. Cancer Treat Rep 1983;67:121–132.

13. Walker MD, Alexander E, Hunt WE, et al. Evaluation of BCNU and/or radiotherapy in the treatment of anaplastic gliomas. J Neurosurg 1978;49:333–343.

14. Shapiro WR, Green SB, Burger PC, et al. Randomized trial of three chemotherapy regimens and two radiotherapy regimens in postoperative treatment of malignant glioma. J Neurosurg 1989;71:1–9.

15. Shapiro WR, Ausman JI. The chemotherapy of brain tumors: a clinical and experimental review. In: Plum F, ed. Recent advances in neurology. Contemporary neurology series. Philadelphia: FA Davis, 1969:150–235.

16. Edwards MS, Levin VA, Wilson CB. Brain tumor chemotherapy: an evaluation of agents in current use for phase II and III trials. Cancer Treat Rep 1980; 64:1179–1205.

17. Kornblith PL, Walker M. Chemotherapy for malignant gliomas. J Neurosurg 1988;68:1–17.

18. Fine HA, Dear KBG, Loeffler JS, et al. Meta-analysis of radiation therapy with and without adjuvant chemotherapy for malignant gliomas in adults. Cancer 1993;71:2585–2597.

19. EORTC Brain Tumor Group. Effect of CCNU on survival rate, objective remission and duration of free interval in patients with malignant brain glioma—final evaluation. Eur J Cancer 1978;14:851–856.

20. EORTC Brain Tumor Group. Evaluation of CCNU, VM-26 plus CCNU, and procarbazine in supratentorial gliomas. J Neurosurg 1981;55:27–31.

21. Shapiro WR. Therapy of adult malignant brain tumors: what have the clinical trials taught us? Semin Oncol 1986;13:38–45.

22. Levin VA, Silver P, Hannigan J, et al. Superiority of postradiotherapy adjuvant chemotherapy with CCNU, procarbazine, and vincristine (PCV) over BCNU for anaplastic gliomas: NCO 6G61 final report. Int J Oncol Biol Phys 1990;18:321–324.

23. Hochberg FH, Pruitt AA, Beck DO, DeBrun G, Davis K. The rationale and methodology for intra-arterial chemotherapy with BCNU as treatment for glioblastoma. J Neurosurg 1985;63:876–880.

24. Stewart DJ. Novel modes of chemotherapy administration. Prog Exp Tumor Res 1984;28:32–50.

25. Vance RB, Kapp JP. Supraoptic carotid infusion with low dose cisplatin and BCNU for malignant glioma. J Neurooncol 1986;3:287–290.

26. Foo SH, Choi IS, Bernstein A, et al. Supraophthalmic intracarotid infusion of BCNU for malignant glioma. Neurology 1986;36:1437–1444.

27. Shapiro WR, Green SB, Burger PC, et al. A randomized comparison of intra-arterial versus intravenous BCNU, with or without intravenous 5-fluorouracil, for newly diagnosed patients with malignant gliomas. J Neurosurg 1992;76:772–781.

28. Bouvier G, Penn RD, Kroin JS, Beique R, Guerard MJ. Direct delivery of medication into brain tumor through multiple chronically implanted catheters. Neurosurgery 1987;20:286–291.

29. Patchell RA, Young AB, Ashton A. A phase I trial continuously infused intratumoral bleomycin for the treatment of recurrent glioblastoma multiforme (abstract). Neurology 1995;45(Suppl 4):A261.

30. Brem H, Mahaley S, Vick NA, et al. Interstitial chemotherapy with drug polymer implants for the treatment of recurrent gliomas. J Neurosurg 1991; 74:441–446.

31. Brem H, Piantadosi S, Burger PC, et al. Placebo-controlled trial of safety and efficacy of intraoperative controlled delivery by biodegradable polymers of chemotherapy for recurrent gliomas. Lancet 1995; 345:1008–1012.

32. Neuwelt EA, Diehl JT, Vu LH, et al. Monitoring of methotrexate delivery in patients with malignant brain tumors after osmotic blood-brain barrier disruption. Ann Intern Med 1981;94:449–454.

33. Neuwelt EA, Hill SA, Frenkel EP. Osmotic blood-brain barrier modification and combination chemotherapy. Neurosurgery 1984;15:362–366.

34. Neuwelt EA, Howieson J, Frenkel EP, et al. Therapeutic efficacy of multiagent chemotherapy with drug delivery enhancement by blood-brain barrier modification in glioblastoma. Neurosurgery 1986;19:573–582.

35. Hiesinger EM, Voorhies RM, Basler GA, et al. Opening the blood-brain and blood-tumor barriers in experimental rat brain tumors: the effect of intracarotid hyperosmolar mannitol on capillary permeability and blood flow. Ann Neurol 1986;19:50–59.

36. Kessinger A. High dose chemotherapy with au-

tologous bone marrow rescue for high grade gliomas of the brain: a potential for improvement in therapeutic results. Neurosurgery 1984;15:747–750.

37. Fine HA, Antman KH. High dose chemotherapy with autologous bone marrow transplantation for the treatment of high grade astrocytomas in adults: therapeutic rationale and clinical experience. Bone Marrow Transplant 1992;10:315–321.

38. Phillips GL, Wolff SN, Fay JW, et al. Intensive 1,3-bis(2-chloroethyl)-1-nitrosourea (BCNU) monotherapy and autologous marrow transplantation for malignant glioma. J Clin Oncol 1986;4:639–645.

39. Hochberg FH, Parker LM, Takvorian T, Canellos GP, Zervas NT. High-dose BCNU with autologous bone marrow rescue for recurrent glioblastoma multiforme. J Neurosurg 1981;54:455–460.

40. Wolff SN, Phillips GL, Herzig GP. High-dose carmustine with autologous bone marrow transplantation for the adjuvant treatment of high-grade gliomas of the central nervous system. Cancer Treat Rep 1987; 71:183–185.

41. Colombar P, Linassie C, Calais G, et al. High dose BCNU with autologous bone marrow transplantation (ABMT) and localized radiotherapy (RT) for patients (PTS) with astrocytomas grade III-IV (abstract). Proc Am Soc Clin Oncol 1991;10:128.

42. Biron P, Vial C, Cauvin F, et al. Strategy including surgery, high dose BCNU followed by ABMT and radiotherapy in supratentorial high grade astrocytomas—a report of 98 patients (pts). In Dicke KA, Armitage JO, Dicke-Evinger MJ, eds. Autologous bone marrow transplantation. Proceedings of the 5th International Symposium, Omaha NE, University of Nebraska Medical Center, 1991:637–642.

43. Giannone L, Wolff SN. Phase II treatment of central nervous system gliomas with high-dose etoposide and autologous bone marrow transplantation. Cancer Treat Rep 1987;71:759–761.

44. Roberts M, German WJ. A long term study of patients with oligodendrogliomas. Follow-up of 50 cases, including Dr. Harvey Cushing's series. J Neurosurg 1966;24:697–700.

45. Chui HW, Hazel JJ, Kim TH, et al. Oligodendrogliomas. Cancer 1980;45:1458–1466.

46. Cairncross JG, Macdonald DR. Successful chemotherapy for recurrent malignant oligodendroglioma. Ann Neurol 1988;23:360–364.

47. Macdonald DR, Cairncross JG. Chemotherapy as initial treatment for aggressive oligodendroglioma. Neurology (Suppl 1) 1989;39:261.

48. Macdonald DR, Gaspar LE, Cairncross JG. Successful chemotherapy for newly diagnosed aggressive oligodendrogliomas. Ann Neurol 1990;27:573–574.

49. Cairncross G, Macdonald D, Ludwin S, et al. Chemotherapy for anaplastic oligodendrogliomas. J Clin Oncol 1994;12:2013–2021.

50. Kryitsis AP, Yung WKA, Bruner J, et al. The treatment of anaplastic oligodendrogliomas and mixed gliomas. Neurosurgery 1993;32:365–371.

51. Glass J, Hochberg FH, Gruber ML, et al. The treatment of oligodendrogliomas and mixed oligodendrogliomas-astrocytomas with PCV chemotherapy. J Neurosurg 1992;76:741–745.

52. Mason WP, DeAngelis LM. Procarbazine, CCNU, and vincristine (PCV) chemotherapy (CT) for benign oligodendrogliomas (abstract). Neurology 1994;44(Suppl 2):a262–A263.

53. Chin HW, Maruyama Y, Markesbery WR, Young AB. Intracranial ependymoma. Cancer 1982; 49:2276–2280.

54. Mork SJ, Loken AC. Ependymoma: a follow-up study of 101 cases. Cancer 1977;40:907–915.

55. Salazar OM, Castro-Vita H, Van Houtte P, et al. Improved survival in cases of intracranial ependymoma after radiation therapy. J Neurosurg 1983; 59:652–659.

56. Kricheff II, Becker M, Schneck SA, Teveras JM. Intracranial ependymomas. A study of survival in 65 cases treated by surgery and irradiation. Am J Roentgenol Radium Ther Nucl Med 1964;91:167–175.

57. Barone BM, Elvidge AR. Ependymomas. A clinical survey. J Neurosurg 1970;33:428–438.

58. Shapiro WR. Chemotherapy of primary malignant brain tumors in children. Cancer 1975;35:975.

59. Cangir A, Ragab AH, Steuber P, Land VJ, Berry DH, Krischer JP. Combination chemotherapy with vincristine, procarbazine, prednisone with or without nitrogen mustard in children with recurrent brain tumors. Med Pediatr Oncol 1984;12:1–3.

60. Friedman HS, Oakes WJ. The chemotherapy of posterior fossa tumors in childhood. J Neurooncol 1987;5:217–229.

61. Walker RW, Allen JC. Cisplatin in the treatment of recurrent childhood primary brain tumors. J Clin Oncol 1988;6:62–66.

62. Bloom HJG. Intracranial tumors: response and resistance to therapeutic endeavors, 1970–1980. Int J Radiat Oncol Biol Phys 1982;8:1083–1113.

63. Freilich RJ, DeAngelis LM. Primary central nervous system lymphoma. Neurol Clin 1995;13:901–914.

64. Hochberg FH, Miller DC. Primary central nervous system lymphoma. J Neurosurg 1988;68:835–853.

65. Loeffler JS, Ervin TJ, Mauch P, et al. Primary lymphomas of the central nervous system: patterns of failure and factors that influence survival. J Clin Oncol 1985;3:490–494.

66. Rampen FHJ, van Andel JG, Sizoo W, et al. Radiation therapy in primary non-Hodgkin's lymphomas of the CNS. Eur J Cancer 1980;16:177–184.

67. Murray K, Kun L, Cox J. Primary malignant lymphoma of the central nervous system. J Neurosurg 1986;65:600–607.

68. DeAngelis LM, Yahalom J, Thaler HT, et al. Combined modality therapy for primary CNS lymphoma. J Clin Oncol 1992;10:635–643.

69. Schultz C, Scott C, Wasserman T, et al. Pre-radiation chemotherapy (CTX) with Cytoxan, Adriamycin, vincristine, and dexamethasone (CHOD) for primary central nervous system lymphomas (PCNSL): Initial report of the Radiation Therapy Oncology Group (RTOG) protocol 88-06 (abstract). Proc Am Soc Clin Oncol 1994;13:174.

70. Patchell RA. Primary central nervous system lymphoma in the transplant patient. Neurol Clin 1988; 6:297–303.

71. Starzl TE, Porter KA, Iwatsuki S, et al. Reversibility of lymphomas and lymphoproliferative lesions developing under cyclosporin-steroid therapy. Lancet 1984;1:583–587.

72. Hoffman HJ, Becker L, Craven MA. A clinically and pathologically distinct group of benign brain stem tumors. Neurosurgery 1980;7:243–248.

73. Bloom HJG, Walsh LS. Tumors of the central nervous system. In: Bloom HJG, Lemerle J, Neidhardt

MK, eds. Cancer in children, clinical management. New York: Springer Verlag, 1975:93–119.

74. Allen JC, Walker R, Luks E, Jennings M, Barfoot S, Tan C. Carboplatin and recurrent childhood brain tumors. J Clin Oncol 1987;5:459–463.

75. Allen JC, Helson L. High-dose cyclophosphamide chemotherapy for recurrent CNS tumors in children. J Neurosurg 1981;55:749–756.

76. Rosen G, Ghavimi F, Nirenberg A, Mosenda C, Mehta BM. High dose methotrexate with citrovorum factor rescue for the treatment of central nervous system tumors in children. Cancer Treat Rep 1977;61:681–690.

77. Jenkins RDT, Bosel C, Ertel I, et al. Brain-stem tumors in childhood: a prospective randomized trial of irradiation with and without adjuvant CCNU, VCR, and prednisone. J Neurosurg 1987;66:227–233.

78. Deutsch M. The impact of myelography on the treatment results for medulloblastoma. Int J Radiat Oncol Biol Phys 1984;10:999–1003.

79. Park TS, Hoffman HF, Hendrick EB, et al. Medulloblastoma: clinical presentation and management. J Neurosurg 1983;58:543–552.

80. Bloom HJG. Medulloblastoma in children: increasing survival rates and future prospects. Int J Radiat Oncol Biol Phys 1982;8:2023–2027.

81. Allen JC, Bloom J, Ertel I, et al. Brain tumors in children: current cooperative and institutional chemotherapy trials in newly diagnosed and recurrent disease. Semin Oncol 1986;13:110–122.

82. Evans AE. Therapeutic approaches to medulloblastoma and results: the trial of the Children's Cancer Study Group (CCSG) and the Radiation Therapy Oncology Group (RTOG). In: Bloom HJG, Piehler E, eds. Proceedings of the 13th international congress of chemotherapy. Symposium: chemotherapy for brain tumors in children. Vienna, 1983, SY 101, Part 208.

83. Packer RJ, Savino PJ, Bilaniuk L, et al. Chiasmatic gliomas of childhood: a reappraisal of natural history and effectiveness of cranial irradiation. Childs Brain 1983;10:393–403.

84. Packer RJ, Sutton LN, Bilaniuk LT, et al. Treatment of chiasmatic/hypothalamic gliomas of childhood with chemotherapy: an update. Ann Neurol 1988;23:79–85.

85. Phuphanich S, Edwards M, Levin V, et al. Supratentorial malignant gliomas of childhood: results of treatment with radiation therapy and chemotherapy. J Neurosurg 1984;60:495–499.

86. Fewer D, Wilson C, Boldrey E, et al. Phase II study of 1-(2-chlorethyl)-3-cyclohexyl-1-nitrosourea (CCNU: NSU 79037) in the treatment of brain tumors. Cancer Chemother Rep 1972;56:421–427.

87. Allen JC, Hancock C, Walker R, Tan C. PCNU and recurrent childhood tumors. J Neurooncol 1987; 5:241–244.

88. Sexauer CL, Khan A, Burger PC, et al. Cisplatin in recurrent pediatric brain tumors. Cancer 1985; 56:1497–1501.

89. Allen JC, Walker R, Luks E, et al. Carboplatin and recurrent childhood brain tumors. J Clin Oncol 1987;5:459–463.

90. Lefkowitz IB, Packer RJ, Sutton LN, et al. Results of treatment of children with recurrent gliomas with lomustine and vincristine. Cancer 1988;61:896–902.

91. Ettinger LJ, Sinniah D, Siegel SE, et al. Combination chemotherapy with cyclophosphamide, vincristine, procarbazine, and prednisone (COPP) in children with brain tumors. J Neurooncol 1985;3:263–269.

92. van Eys J, Baram TZ, Cangir A, Bruner JM, Martinez-Prieto J. Salvage chemotherapy for recurrent primary brain tumors in children. J Pediatr 1988; 113:601–606.

93. Pendergrass TW, Milstein JM, Geyer JR, et al. Eight drugs in one day chemotherapy in 107 children and rationale for preradiation chemotherapy. J Clin Oncol 1987;5:1221–1231.

94. Finlay JL, Goins SC. Brain tumors in children: III advances in chemotherapy. Am J Pediatr Hematol Oncol 1987;9:264–271.

95. Jennings MT, Gelman R, Hochberg F. Intracranial germ-cell tumors: natural history and pathogenesis. J Neurosurg 1985;63:155–167.

96. Sano K, Matsutani M. Pinealoma (germinoma) treated by direct surgery and postoperative irradiation. A long term follow-up. Childs Brain 1981;8:81–97.

97. Allen JC, Bosl G, Walker R. Chemotherapy trials in recurrent primary intracranial germ cell tumors. J Neurooncol 1985;3:147–152.

98. Calaminus G, Bamberg M, Baranzelli MC, et al. Intracranial germ cell tumors: a comprehensive update of the European data. Neuropediatrics 1994;25:26–32.

99. Kobayashi T, Yoshida J, Ishiyama J, et al. Combination chemotherapy with cisplatin and etoposide for malignant intracranial germ-cell tumors. J Neurosurg 1989;70:676–681.

100. Allen JC, Kim JH, Packer RJ. Neoadjuvant chemotherapy for newly diagnosed germ-cell tumors of the central nervous system. J Neurosurg 1987;67:65–70.

101. Finlay J, Walker R, Balmaceda C, et al. Chemotherapy without irradiation (XRT) for primary central nervous system (CNS) germ cell tumors (GCT): report of an international study (abstract). Proc Am Soc Clin Oncol 1992;11:150.

52
Head and Neck Cancer

Everett E. Vokes

Approximately 40,000 cases of head and neck cancer are diagnosed annually in the United States, representing about 5% of the total incidence of cancer (1). About one-third of these patients will present with early-stage disease (AJC stages I and II) (2), while two-thirds will present with locoregionally advanced disease. Distant disease is clinically seen in only about 20% of patients; however, autopsy series indicate a much higher incidence of systemic tumor dissemination (3, 4). Clinically, head and neck cancer represents a major source of morbidity, since major vital functions such as nutrition, respiration, and communication are affected. Most head and neck cancers are of squamous cell histology, and unless specified otherwise, all comments in this chapter are directed toward that histology.

Head and neck cancer is firmly associated with the risk factors of cigarette and alcohol abuse and, in particular, the combination of both (5, 6). This substance abuse can lead to significant comorbidity at the time of diagnosis, including cardiac, pulmonary, and hepatic diseases as well as malnutrition. These conditions frequently pose additional challenges to the treating physicians. Anatomically, head and neck cancer is a heterogeneous disease, since various sites can be affected. Some disease sites may have a different natural history than others; for example, laryngeal cancer has a better prognosis stage for stage than does cancer of the piriform sinus. However, due to the relatively low incidence of cancer in each of these anatomic subtypes and the similarity in their etiology, clinical history, and therapy, they are justly grouped together in most clinical trials.

STANDARD THERAPY

Standard therapy for head and neck cancer is based on surgery and radiotherapy as primary treatment modalities. This appropriately reflects the natural history of the disease with its locoregionally confined initial presentation and low incidence of distant metastases. Thus, local therapy modalities have been postulated to most likely result in cure or palliation.

Recent data suggest that chemotherapy can make a significant contribution to increase the efficacy of these local therapies in terms of increasing survival rates but also in terms of decreasing the extent to which mutilating surgery must be used. Treatment options and goals differ according to the stage of disease at the time of diagnosis.

Early-stage disease (T_1, T_2, N_0, M_0) is treated with curative intent, using single-modality therapy with surgery or radiotherapy (7, 8). The exact choice of modality depends on the available expertise at a given institution, the patient's general condition (operability), and the specific site of the tumor. A small lesion of the tongue might be treated more efficiently by local excision, thus avoiding a prolonged course of radiotherapy with its accompanying side effects of mucositis, loss of taste, and xerostomia. On the other hand, a small laryngeal lesion might be best treated with radiotherapy rather than laryngectomy, thus better preserving laryngeal function and reducing long-term morbidity. Newer surgical techniques, however, also allow the preservation of organ and organ function in this anatomic site and constitute an alternative treatment option. Since treatment alternatives exist that result in equivalent treatment outcome while resulting in differential short- and long-term toxicities, it is appropriate to discuss all options with the patient rather than simply offering the treatment favored by the individual physician seeing the patient first (usually the surgeon).

With this single-modality treatment approach, 60 to 90% of patients with early-stage disease will be free of disease at 2 to 5 years of follow-up and are considered cured of their primary malignancy. It is now clear, however, that these patients require close surveillance to monitor for the possible development of second malignancies, which occur at an annual incidence of 3 to 5%. These are etiologically explained by the high cumulative risk factor exposure of many patients, leading to "field carcinogenesis" (9).

Standard therapy for patients with locally or regionally advanced disease (T_3, T_4, and N_1 to N_3, M_0) usually consists of surgery followed by radiotherapy, or radiotherapy alone for inoperable patients or those with unresectable disease (an undefined entity). The use of chemotherapy in this setting can be increasingly justified and is discussed below. The goal of therapy for these patients is also cure. However, despite the apparent locoregional confinement of the disease and the use of two treatment modalities, cure will be achieved in only a minority of patients; generally, less than 30% of these patients are alive at 5 years of follow-up (7–13). The cause of death for the great majority of these patients is recurrent locoregional disease, indicating the inability of surgery and radiotherapy to completely eradicate regionally advanced cancer. This provides evidence that surgery does not eliminate all disease, even after "negative margins" have been achieved, and that at least some of the cells remaining must have intrinsic radiation resistance preventing the complete eradication of all tumor cells and leading to eventual (macroscopic) treatment failure.

A minority of patients also fail at distant sites, usually involving the lungs, bones, or liver. The patients that are cured again are at risk of developing second malignancies, i.e., lung or esophageal cancer (9, 14, 15), although that is less well studied in this group of patients.

Until recently, chemotherapy had a limited role in the standard care of head and neck cancer. Only patients presenting initially with clinically detectable distant disease or developing recurrent disease after prior local therapy were considered appropriate for primary chemotherapy (16, 17). In the setting of recurrent and/or metastatic disease, the treatment goals are the palliation of symptoms and prolongation of survival (18). Generally, 10 to 30% of patients with recurrent disease respond to chemotherapy; responses are usually partial and of only 3 to 6 months' duration. Furthermore, patients achieving partial response may derive benefit, since a

response may translate into relief of pain and other symptoms. However, definitive data regarding the impact of chemotherapy for recurrent disease on quality of life have not been generated to date. Regarding prolongation of life, only one study has been reported in which chemotherapy was compared with "best supportive care". This study suggested that a modest prolongation of life was indeed achieved and can serve to justify the continued exploration of chemotherapy in patients with recurrent disease.

The following describes in more detail the active single chemotherapy agents and their use in combination as defined in clinical trials of previously treated patients.

CHEMOTHERAPY FOR PATIENTS WITH RECURRENT OR METASTATIC HEAD AND NECK CANCER

Single Agents

Drugs with reproducible single-agent activity in previously treated patients are listed in Table 52.1.

Methotrexate, historically the most frequently used drug, remains a possible "standard" against which newer compounds can be evaluated (9, 15–18). In conventional doses, without the use of leucovorin rescue, partial response rates have averaged 10 to 30% and are of 2 to 4 months' duration (19–23). A standard treatment scheme consists of weekly doses of methotrexate, starting at 40 to 50 mg/m², with escalation in weekly increments of 10 mg/m² until grade 1 to 2 toxicity is observed. Myelosuppression and mucositis are frequently the dose-limiting tox-

Table 52.1. Active Chemotherapy Drugs in Head and Neck Cancer

Methotrexate
Cisplatin
Carboplatin
Bleomycin
5-Fluorouracil
Hydroxyurea
Mitomycin C
Cyclophosphamide
Doxorubicin
Ifosfamide
Paclitaxel
Docetaxel
Vinorelbine
Difluorodeoxycytidine

icities. The most recent experience with methotrexate as a single agent, however, clearly points out the limitations of this drug. In this large randomized multicenter study, methotrexate was compared with cisplatin/5-fluorouracil (5-FU) and carboplatin/5-FU. Responses to methotrexate were seen in only 10% of patients, and the median survival was 5.6 months (23).

Attempts at further increasing the efficacy of methotrexate through administration of higher doses with leucovorin rescue have been made. However, several randomized studies have failed to show consistently improved response rates or survival with the high-dose regimens, compared with conventional schedules (24–28), and toxicity was frequently more severe in patients treated with the high-dose regimens (23, 24, 28). Therefore, there is no role for high-dose methotrexate with leucovorin rescue in head and neck cancer.

Cisplatin is considered another standard agent in head and neck cancer. Response rates again range from 20 to 30% (29–31), with occasional patients achieving complete responses. Toxicities usually include nausea and vomiting, nephrotoxicity, ototoxicity, peripheral neuropathy, and mild myelosuppression. No clear dose-response curve for cisplatin has been demonstrated to date, with similar degrees of activity seen with doses ranging from 60 to 120 mg/m^2 (32). Veronesi et al. (33) directly compared cisplatin doses of 60 mg/m^2 and 120 mg/m^2, each administered every 3 weeks, and found no significant difference in response rates (10 vs. 18%) or survival. Pilot studies have further addressed the efficacy of very high dose cisplatin in head and neck cancer (34, 35) using schedules of 40 to 50 mg/m^2 for 5 days (total cycle dose, 200 mg/m^2) and achieving response rates of 46 and 73% in mixed groups of patients. In these trials, myelosuppression was more severe than with conventional-dose schedules; neuropathy and ototoxicity were also more severe. While the response rates achieved in these trials suggest that cisplatin in very high doses may have greater activity than at doses of 60 to 120 mg/m^2, no randomized trials have been conducted to confirm this impression. Two randomized studies have directly compared cisplatin with methotrexate. In both trials, response and survival rates were similar (36, 37) for the two drugs, indicating similar degrees of activity. However, investigators in Liverpool compared methotrexate, single-agent cisplatin, cisplatin/5-

FU, and cisplatin/methotrexate. In this study, cisplatin-containing chemotherapy was found to be superior to single-agent methotrexate (38).

Carboplatin, a cisplatin analogue, is less nephrotoxic and emetogenic than the parent compound, can be administered more easily, and can be given in the outpatient setting. It has also shown activity in head and neck cancer (23, 39, 40). Whether its activity is equal to that of cisplatin at equitoxic doses has not been established to date. A study comparing cisplatin/5-FU with carboplatin/5-FU (and methotrexate) suggested that the cisplatin-based combination might result in a higher response rate, although there was no difference in survival rates (23).

In summary, cisplatin has shown reproducible activity in patients with head and neck cancer and in direct randomized comparisons has been as active as methotrexate. Therefore, both of these agents are considered standard chemotherapy drugs in head and neck cancer.

Additional drugs with activity are listed in Table 52.1. 5-FU administered as an intravenous bolus was reported to have fairly low activity (15–18); some pilot data suggested that its activity may be substantially higher when administered as a 5-day continuous infusion every 3 weeks (41). However, a multiinstitutional study containing infusional 5-FU as a single agent in one study arm resulted in a response rate of 13%. Infusional 5-FU resulted in survival rates not significantly different from those achieved with single-agent cisplatin or the combination of the two drugs in this study, with a median of 5.7 months for the entire group (42).

Bleomycin, another active drug, has a partial response rate of approximately 20% (15–18). It was formerly incorporated into combination chemotherapy regimens because of its nonoverlapping toxicity spectrum but is now rarely used. A 39% response rate was reported for hydroxyurea, but the drug has been studied infrequently, both as a single agent or as part of combination chemotherapy regimens. Similarly, cyclophosphamide, doxorubicin, and mitomycin C have had inadequate study for a more precise assessment of their activity in this disease.

Several of the newer chemotherapy agents also have activity in head and neck cancer. Among the taxanes, paclitaxel has been studied in the phase II setting (43, 44). In a preliminary report, a response rate of 40% (12 of 30 patients) was reported. Phase II investigations of paclitaxel and cisplatin are currently in progress (43).

Similarly, docetaxel has been studied in a phase II study indicating activity in this disease (45).

Difluorodeoxycytidine (gemcitabine) also has single-agent activity, with a response rate of 13% (46). Like the taxanes, its administration in combination with cisplatin or carboplatin is being pursued. Finally, vinorelbine has been studied in a small European trial that indicated a response rate of approximately 20% as a single agent (47). Additional studies with this agent are currently in progress. The exact roles of these drugs as single agents or in combination with other drugs in the management of recurrent head and neck cancer remain to be established.

Combination Chemotherapy

Attempts at increasing the activity of available chemotherapeutic agents by using them in combination have had limited success to date in patients with recurrent and/or metastatic head and neck cancer.

No significant increase in response rates or survival was achieved when comparing single-agent cisplatin with the combination of cisplatin and methotrexate (48). A direct comparison of methotrexate with the combination of methotrexate, cisplatin, and bleomycin, conducted by the Eastern Cooperative Oncology Group, did result in statistically significantly improved response rates for the combination (48 vs. 35% overall response rates, and 16 vs. 8% complete response rates, respectively), with similar degrees of toxicity in both groups. Median survival, however, was only 5.6 months in both groups (49). Another study compared methotrexate, bleomycin, and hydroxyurea with a regimen consisting of these three drugs plus cisplatin. Here, the cisplatin-containing regimen was superior in overall and complete response rates, while survival was not noted to be different between the two study groups (50).

The combination of cisplatin and infusional 5-FU is frequently considered the most active available combination for head and neck cancer. Response rates in the recurrent disease setting have ranged from 20 to 70% (23, 42, 51–54).

The addition of leucovorin to the cisplatin/5-FU combination was investigated at the University of Chicago (55). A response rate of 56% was reported. Leucovorin has been shown to increase the cytotoxicity of 5-FU in vitro (56) and in randomized clinical studies in patients with metastatic colorectal cancer (57). A three-arm South-

west Oncology Group (SWOG) study compared single-agent methotrexate, cisplatin/5-FU, and carboplatin/5-FU (23). Patients treated with cisplatin and 5-FU had a significantly higher response rate than patients treated with methotrexate alone. There was no significant difference in survival. In another phase III study, cisplatin and 5-FU in combination resulted in a higher response rate than each drug given as single agents, without resulting in prolonged survival (42).

The addition of interferon to the cisplatin and 5-FU combination as a modulator has also been studied (58–60). Several phase II studies have been completed that suggest no major increase in response or survival rates. This question has been further addressed in a large multinational randomized study comparing cisplatin and 5-FU with cisplatin, 5-FU, and interferon. This study is closed to accrual, and early data should be available in the near future.

Browman and Cronin conducted a comprehensive analysis of these studies (18). They concluded that cisplatin-based combination therapy did result in higher response rates than other forms of chemotherapy for recurrent head and neck cancer, in particular, the combination of cisplatin and 5-FU. Regarding survival, it was felt that cisplatin was superior to methotrexate and that cisplatin/5-FU was the "best" available regimen.

From this experience with chemotherapy for patients with recurrent head and neck cancer several conclusions can currently be drawn:

1. Conventional-dose methotrexate and cisplatin continue to be the most active single agents, and partial response rates average 30%. Newer drugs with promising activity include the taxanes and gemcitabine. Investigations of topoisomerase I inhibitors are currently in progress.

2. Combination chemotherapy has resulted in slightly higher overall response rates but not in clinically meaningful prolongation of survival, while toxicity is increased.

3. Newer drugs and combinations, including that of cisplatin and Taxol, have shown promise in some pilot studies. It is hoped that these new combinations will result in increased survival rates in current and planned phase III studies.

4. Further research attempting to identify addi-

tional drugs and combinations with activity in this disease is needed.

In the 1980s, clinical research expanded to investigate chemotherapy in previously untreated patients with locally advanced disease (T_3, T_4, N_1 to N_3, but M_0). Exciting and at times controversial results have been achieved using neoadjuvant chemotherapy or concomitant chemoradiotherapy. The latter to some degree can now be considered "standard therapy" for unresectable disease.

INVESTIGATIONAL USES OF CHEMOTHERAPY

Neoadjuvant Chemotherapy

The concept of neoadjuvant chemotherapy has been extensively investigated in patients with head and neck cancer (9, 61–63). It involves the administration of a number of chemotherapy cycles to previously untreated patients with locally advanced head and neck cancer. Following chemotherapy, patients are reevaluated and assessed for response to chemotherapy and subsequently receive curative-intent surgery and/or radiotherapy, i.e., standard local therapy. From its very design, this requires a team approach and a prospective plan and timetable established at the time of initial diagnosis. Thus, patients are evaluated and treated by a group of physicians, including representatives from head and neck surgery, radiation oncology, medical oncology, dental care, and social support services.

The rationale for using chemotherapy prior to surgery and radiotherapy has been reviewed (9, 61–65) and includes better drug delivery to the tumor cell prior to the destruction of the local vasculature by surgery and radiation. It is also hoped that using chemotherapy earlier in the natural history of the disease will increase its efficacy because there are fewer drug-resistant cells. Also, if initial chemotherapy can decrease the size of the tumor, subsequent radiotherapy may have less bulky disease to treat locally and, therefore, might be more successful. Similarly, surgical margins are less likely to be involved with tumor. These factors may all contribute to improved locoregional tumor control. In addition, through its systemic activity, chemotherapy might succeed at eradicating microscopic distant metastases, which may be present in a substantial percentage of patients with advanced regional nodal disease at the time of diagnosis (3, 4).

The theoretical disadvantages of using neoadjuvant chemotherapy include the toxicity associated with the various chemotherapy regimens and the time required for its administration, resulting in a significant prolongation of the overall treatment time and, thus, in increased cost. There has also been concern that preoperative chemotherapy might result in a higher incidence of distant metastases (66). Finally, patients who fail to respond to chemotherapy and experience further tumor growth may lose their surgical treatment option and, thus, their chance for curative-intent therapy.

While the scientific foundation of neoadjuvant chemotherapy is speculative, its goals are clear. They include increased survival and preservation of organ function, i.e., less radical surgery.

Early clinical trials used one or two cycles of single-agent neoadjuvant chemotherapy, and their results seemed to support this concept. Using either methotrexate (67, 68) or cisplatin (30, 69), much higher response rates (50 to 70%) were achieved than were previously observed in patients with recurrent disease; in addition, complete responses (CRs) were seen.

Subsequent pilot studies used combination chemotherapy regimens. Hong et al. (70) reported a 76% overall response rate (20% CRs) following two cycles of the combination of cisplatin and infusional bleomycin. Spaulding et al. (71) reported an 80% overall response rate (30% CRs) to two cycles of cisplatin, vincristine, and bleomycin. A large study involving 114 patients treated with two cycles of neoadjuvant cisplatin, bleomycin, and methotrexate was published by Ervin et al. (72). The overall response rate in this trial was 78% (26% CRs). This study and others clearly demonstrated a survival advantage for patients achieving a CR, compared with patients achieving partial or no response. Patients achieving CR had a 3-year failure-free survival of 83%, compared with 44% for patients achieving a partial response (PR). This study did not include a control group, and it cannot be concluded that patients achieving a CR had a good survival rate as a consequence of chemotherapy; however, achieving a CR was clearly associated with a good prognosis and therefore can be considered an important prognostic factor.

The association of complete response with a good prognosis has also been demonstrated in several other pilot studies of neoadjuvant chemotherapy (73–75). Additional important prognostic factors have been identified: a good initial performance status, low nodal disease stage, and (in some studies) site of the primary disease (in particular nasopharyngeal cancer) have all been found to correlate with prolonged survival (70–77).

Al-Sarraf and his colleagues at Wayne State University investigated the use of three cycles of neoadjuvant cisplatin and a 5-day continuous infusion of 5-FU (Table 52.2). In this pilot study, 93% of patients responded, and 54% (33 of 61 patients) had a clinical complete response, indicating a high activity of this combination (73). Other investigators using cisplatin and 5-FU have since obtained similar data, with overall response rates ranging from 73 to 94%, and complete response rates from 23 to 54% (78–80). Patients achieving a clinical CR with this regimen again had a better prognosis than those achieving a lesser or no response. In addition, Al-Sarraf and his colleagues showed that patients attaining a histologic complete response (i.e., no residual tumor at subsequent surgery) had a better survival than those attaining a clinical complete response with residual microscopic disease evident at surgery (81). Finally, this group of investigators demonstrated that response to initial chemotherapy correlated with response to subsequent radiotherapy; only 1 of 18 patients who failed to respond to initial chemotherapy responded to subsequent radiotherapy, compared with 41 of 42 patients who achieved an initial response to chemotherapy (82).

Given these impressive response data, the cisplatin and 5-FU regimen has been a foundation for studies by other investigators. In particular, attempts have been concentrated on increasing the CR rate, since it is closely correlated with prognosis. These trials have included the administration of more than three cycles of neoadjuvant chemotherapy with cisplatin and 5-FU or the administration of cisplatin and 5-FU alternating with another regimen; however, the CR rate was not increased by increasing the number of neoadjuvant chemotherapy cycles or by using two alternating regimens (83, 84). Similarly, the addition of bleomycin (85) or methotrexate (75) or vinblastine (85) does not appear to have significantly increased the activity of cisplatin and 5-FU.

The addition of leucovorin as a biochemical modulator to cisplatin and 5-FU was also investigated. At our institution, two cycles of this regimen resulted in a 29% CR rate (86). Dreyfus et al. (87) reported a 66% CR rate using three cycles of a similar regimen.

In later studies at our institution, we also added interferon to this combination (PFL-interferon) (88). We reported a 51% complete response rate following three cycles of this regimen in a cohort of patients of whom over 90% had stage IV disease. Investigations of the newer chemotherapy drugs in this setting have recently been initiated.

What, then, have these pilot trials taught us about neoadjuvant chemotherapy for head and neck cancer?

1. High overall response rates, ranging from 80 to 100%, can be consistently achieved.
2. Complete responses can also be consistently achieved and range from 20 to 50%.
3. A complete response, and particularly a histologically confirmed complete response, correlates with good prognosis and subsequent response to radiotherapy.
4. The administration of standard local therapy is not compromised following neoadjuvant chemotherapy.

However, have the primary goals of improved overall survival and decreased morbidity been met? Although the response data to neoadjuvant chemotherapy and the survival data for patients achieving CR in many of these pilot studies were promising, the overall survival rates for most of these trials were disappointing. Two-year survival rates frequently range around 30 to 40% and are, therefore, within the range of survival rates reported from trials using surgery and radiotherapy only.

Several randomized studies have been conducted to fully investigate the impact of neoadjuvant chemotherapy on survival. These studies aimed at directly comparing the treatment outcome of standard therapy alone with that of neoadjuvant chemotherapy followed by standard therapy (89). Many randomized studies have been published; none of them have conclusively demonstrated a survival advantage for the chemotherapy-treated patients. However, critics have pointed out that most of these trials had flaws in their design (90–97). Most criticism has focused on the use of suboptimal chemotherapy in the experimental study arm. This included the use of single-agent methotrexate as neoadjuvant chemotherapy or the use of a single cycle of

Table 52.2. Randomized Trials of Induction and/or Adjuvant Chemotherapy[a]

Source (Ref)	Patients Analyzed	Drugs	Recent Response Rate to CT (CR)	Local Therapy	Outcome	Comments
Head and Neck Contracts (99)	443	Cisplatin, bleomycin; cisplatin also as "maintenance"	37 (3)	S/XRT	No significant difference in survival	Survival benefit for N_2 disease by subset analysis; decreased distant metastases with maintenance
Southwest Oncology (98)	158	Cisplatin, methotrexate, bleomycin, vincristine	70 (19)	S/XRT	No significant difference in survival	Induction CT; decreased distant metastases
VA Larynx Study (100)	332	Cisplatin, 5-FU	86 (31)	XRT vs. S/XRT	No significant difference in survival	Induction CT; decreased distant metastases
Intergroup (101)	448	Cisplatin, 5-FU	N/A (adjuvant)	S/XRT	No significant difference in survival	CT adjuvant to surgery prior to XRT; decreased incidence of distant metastases
Padua, Italy (102)	237	Cisplatin, 5-FU	80 (31)	S/XRT or XRT only	No significant difference in survival	Four cycles of CT; survival benefit for inoperable patients; reduced incidence of distant metastases

[a]Abbreviations: CR, complete response; N/A, not applicable; CT, chemotherapy; S/XRT indicates local therapy with surgery and/or radiotherapy.

neoadjuvant chemotherapy. Pilot studies have indicated that response rates increase with administration of combination chemotherapy and with up to three cycles of neoadjuvant chemotherapy; therefore, the CR rates in these studies, not surprisingly, are low. Other studies suffer from low patient entry numbers and thus may not have treated enough patients to show a survival difference. With few exceptions, these randomized trials have not been able to reproduce in their chemotherapy arm the response rates achieved in pilot studies of neoadjuvant chemotherapy using the combination of cisplatin and 5-FU. Another criticism is that some of these studies have included both resectable and unresectable patients or have given lower radiotherapy doses than those used for standard radiotherapy.

However, five large studies can be considered conclusive (98–102). All of these included the use of surgery and radiation therapy as part of the local therapy and enrolled sufficient patients to allow detection of smaller differences in survival. These studies are summarized in Table 52.3. Two of these studies (99, 101) largely administered the chemotherapy following local therapy (i.e., adjuvant chemotherapy), while three others (98, 100, 102) administered neoadjuvant chemotherapy as described above. In addition, three studies used the platinum/5-FU combination. Since this combination was long assumed to be the most active available regimen in head and neck oncology, these trials made important contributions by testing this combination in the phase III setting. The VA Larynx Study had organ preservation as an additional endpoint and is discussed below.

In analyzing these studies, it is remarkable that all five failed to achieve a significant difference in survival through the use of induction chemotherapy. The only exception here is the study of Paccagnella et al. (102), in which patients with unresectable disease had a superior survival if treated with induction chemotherapy followed by radiation rather than radiation therapy alone. However, this difference was statistically significant only by subset analysis. Another important observation from these five studies is that induction and/or adjuvant chemotherapy decreases the incidence of distant disease as the site of first failure. This, however, did not translate into improved survival, since distant failure is relatively rare compared with local failure. Unless chemotherapy can increase locoregional control, one should not expect to

see improved survival as a consequence of its use.

In reviewing these data, what conclusions regarding induction chemotherapy can be drawn?

1. Induction chemotherapy, including the combination of cisplatin and 5-FU, has failed to increase survival rates in patients with locoregionally advanced head and neck cancer.
2. Induction chemotherapy seems to have an impact on the systemic disease burden. However, decreasing metastatic disease will be important only *following* the identification of better locoregional therapy.
3. The possible interpretation of these findings is that sequential chemotherapy and radiation therapy are not non-cross-resistant (i.e., cells that survive the use of cisplatin-based induction chemotherapy are resistant to subsequent radiation therapy as well).
4. As a consequence of these findings, there is no role for induction therapy as a standard therapy in the typical patient with advanced head and neck cancer, with the notable exception of larynx cancer. Induction chemotherapy, however, remains a valuable tool for drug discovery. It will be of high priority to assess the taxanes, topoisomerase I inhibitors, and other new exciting drugs in this setting to optimally establish their response rates as single agents and in combination with other drugs.

The question of organ preservation has also gained increasing attention. Here, neoadjuvant chemotherapy is used primarily in an effort to permit less radical surgery. Preservation of the larynx or tongue are of highest clinical interest. Although closely linked to the question of whether induction chemotherapy can improve survival, an equal outcome in survival between two treatment groups might be acceptable if the group of patients receiving chemotherapy required less radical surgery. Pilot studies investigating organ preservation frequently focused on preservation of the larynx (103–105), since removal of the larynx is associated not only with the loss of natural speech but with additional functional, cosmetic, and psychologic defects and, thus, can have a severe impact on a patient's quality of life.

Given the knowledge that response to chemotherapy predicts subsequent response to radiotherapy, Jacobs et al. (103) designed a trial in

Table 52.3. Selected Randomized Trials of Radiotherapy versus Concomitant Chemoradiotherapy

Study	Drug	Patients Analyzed	Survival		Disease-Free Survival		Comments[a]
			Chemotherapy	Control	Chemotherapy	Control	
Shanta[111]	Bleomycin	107	59% (at 5 years)	23%	72% (at 5 years)	17%	Bleomycin administered in 3 doses and routes, no graphic survival analysis
Fu[112]	Bleomycin	104	43% (at 3 years, $p = .112$)	24%	31% (at 3 years, $p = .024$)	15%	Adjuvant CT with bleomycin and methotrexate on experimental arm
Lo[114]	5-FU	136	32% (at 5 years, $p < .05$)	14%	49% (at 2 years, $p < .5$)	18%	Bolus 5-FU
Browman[116]	5-FU	175	63% (at 2 years, $p = .08$)	50%	47% (at 2 years, $p = .06$)	30%	3-day infusional 5-FU
Haffty[112]	Mitomycin C (± coumarin)	113	56% (at 5 years, NS)	41%	67% (at 5 years, $p < .03$)	44%	Subgroup analysis of patients with resected head and neck cancer
Bachaud[126]	Cisplatin	83	75% (at 2 years, $p < .01$)	44%	65% (at 2 years, $p < .01$)	41%	Postoperative therapy, survival adjusted for "intercurrent disease"
Merlano[143]	Cisplatin, 5-FU	157	41% (at 3 years, $p < .05$)	23%	25% (at 3 years, $p = .009$)	7%	Chemotherapy given in rapid alternation with radiotherapy (not concomitant)

[a]CT, chemotherapy.

which 30 patients received three cycles of neoadjuvant chemotherapy followed by response evaluation and biopsy. Twelve patients had a histologic CR at the primary site and received subsequent local therapy consisting of radiotherapy only (modified neck dissection was performed in patients with neck node involvement). The relapse-free survival and overall survival for these 12 patients were 60% and 70%, respectively, at 2 years of follow-up, compared with 52% and 53%, respectively, for patients undergoing surgery. This small pilot trial suggested that in patients achieving CR with neoadjuvant chemotherapy, elimination of radical surgery may be feasible without compromising survival.

These observations led to the design of a randomized study conducted by the Veterans Administration Cooperative Study Program. Patients were randomized to receive standard therapy with laryngectomy followed by radiotherapy in the control arm or two cycles of neoadjuvant cisplatin and 5-FU in the experimental arm of the study. In this arm, partial and complete responders after two cycles received a third cycle followed by radiotherapy; patients having no response after two cycles or persistent disease after completion of radiotherapy received salvage laryngectomy. This study demonstrated that preservation of the larynx was feasible in 64% of patients receiving chemotherapy. Survival, on the other hand, did not differ in the two study arms and was 68% at 2 years on both study arms. These results were encouraging, as they showed the feasibility of substituting chemotherapy for radical surgery in most patients with advanced laryngeal cancer without compromising the chance of cure.

This trial has been criticized for the lack of a radiotherapy-alone control arm (106). It can be argued that larynx preservation can be achieved with radiation therapy alone, i.e., without induction chemotherapy. In that setting too, the use of surgery as a salvage procedure could be performed and is indeed a standard practice in some countries. Therefore, a current intergroup study in the United States randomizes patients to receive either radiotherapy alone, induction chemotherapy followed by radiation therapy as used in VA study, or radiotherapy with concomitant cisplatin as piloted by the Radiation Therapy Oncology Group (RTOG). Patients with stage T_4 (thyroid cartilage invasion) disease are excluded from this study, since it is felt that surgery is a necessary component of therapy for

these patients. So far, accrual to this study has been sluggish.

Concomitant Chemoradiotherapy

An alternative to the sequential use of chemotherapy followed by local therapy is the use of simultaneous, or concomitant, chemoradiotherapy. The rationale underlying the use of concomitant chemoradiotherapy is twofold:

1. Local antitumor activity of radiation may be enhanced by the simultaneous use of chemotherapeutic agents as radiation sensitizers. However, local toxicity to surrounding normal tissues in the head and neck, usually manifesting as mucositis, may also be increased. Possible mechanisms underlying radiosensitization have been reviewed (107–110).
2. The systemic activity of chemotherapy may eradicate distant micrometastases outside the irradiated field and thus may improve survival. Concomitant chemoradiotherapy is a valid concept in head and neck cancer on both accounts, since most patients fail locally, indicating a need for improved local control; however, a minority of patients also develop distant disease, which might be treated successfully with chemotherapy at the time of initial diagnosis.

Clinical trials testing this concept have been conducted since the 1960s. Earlier trials used a standard course of radiotherapy with intermittent administration of a single chemotherapy agent. More recently, studies have also used radiotherapy schedules with regular treatment interruptions, allowing the administration of more aggressive concomitant chemotherapy and subsequent recovery from toxicity during the treatment break.

In the initial trials, chemotherapy usually consisted of single agents frequently administered at low doses during a full course of conventional radiotherapy. Nevertheless, toxicities were frequently noted to be increased, while in many trials, the survival data were not impressive. Drugs used in these studies included methotrexate, bleomycin, 5-FU, hydroxyurea, mitomycin C, cisplatin, and carboplatin. Several randomized studies have published positive results, supporting the concept of concomitant chemoradiotherapy with single chemotherapy drugs (Table 52.4).

Table 52.4. Positive Randomized Trials of Concomitant Chemoradiotherapy

Author	Reference	No. of Patients	Drug	Outcome
Shanta and Krishnamurth	(111)	157	Bleomycin	Improved survival and disease-free survival with bleomycin
Fu et al.	(112)	104	Bleomycin	Improved disease-free survival with bleomycin
Lo et al.	(114)	151	5-FU	Improved survival and disease-free survival with 5-FU
Weissberg et al.	(121)	120	Mitomycin C	Improved disease-free survival with mitomycin C

Two positive trials used bleomycin as a radiosensitizer. Shanta and Krishnamurthi (111) reported a significant difference in initial response and in 5-year overall survival rates in patients treated with bleomycin and radiotherapy, compared with patients treated with radiotherapy alone. Fu et al. (112) have reported the long-term results of a Northern California Oncology Group trial. These investigators randomized patients with unresectable disease to standard radiotherapy or radiotherapy with concomitant bleomycin and additional cycles of methotrexate and bleomycin administered weekly for 16 weeks following completion of radiotherapy. In this trial, the locoregional complete response rates were 45% for standard therapy and 67% for the bleomycin-containing regimen. The relapse-free survival was 31% at 3 years in the chemotherapy-treated group, significantly higher than the 15% 3-year survival in the control group. A similar trend for overall survival was not statistically significant. This may, in part, have been due to the fairly low overall accrual to this study (104 patients). Acute toxicities were increased through the use of chemotherapy, but no increase in chronic toxicities was observed. These two randomized studies suggest a role for concomitant bleomycin and radiotherapy, although another randomized study (113) found no difference in treatment outcome but a significant increase in acute toxicities, especially mucositis.

5-FU was evaluated as a radiosensitizer in a randomized study reported by Lo et al. (114). Patients with unresectable head and neck cancer were randomized to receive either radiotherapy alone or radiotherapy with concomitant 5-FU administered on days 1 to 4 of radiotherapy and then on Mondays, Wednesdays, and Fridays of each week until the completion of radiation therapy. Local control and survival were improved for all patients in the concomitant therapy group. This difference in survival was statistically significant in patients with lesions in the oral cavity. The same trend for improved survival was seen in all anatomic subgroups included in the study (oral cavity, base of tongue, oropharynx), even though statistical significance was reached for one site only. Therefore, this study supports the use of 5-FU with radiotherapy.

In vitro studies have suggested that continuous exposure of cells to 5-FU optimizes radiation sensitization. Given the short half-life of 5-FU, this can be achieved in vivo only through the use of continuous intravenous infusion. The feasibility of this approach was demonstrated in phase I and phase II studies, both for 5-FU as a single agent and in combination with other drugs (115). Recently, Browman et al. (116) reported a randomized study using a 3-day continuous infusion of 5-FU at $1000 \text{ mg/m}^2/\text{day}$ given on weeks 1 and 4 of their full course of conventional irradiation therapy to patients with unresectable head and neck cancer. This study demonstrated a statistically significant improved complete response rate (68 vs. 56%). In addition, a trend toward improved survival was demonstrated (median, 33 vs. 25 months; $p = .08$). These studies together suggest a role for the use of 5-FU during radiation therapy with a goal of improving survival for patients with unresectable disease.

Mitomycin C is a bioreductive alkylating agent that preferentially kills oxygen-deficient cells (117, 118). Experiments in animal models have shown that a combination of radiation and mitomycin C can increase antitumor activity because mitomycin C kills hypoxic tumor cells that are not usually sensitive to radiotherapy (119, 120). Mitomycin C at 15 mg/m^2 given once or twice during a conventional course of radiation therapy has been studied at Yale University. A recent analysis of two randomized studies comparing radiation with radiation plus mitomycin-C (plus coumarin in the second study) included a total of 113 patients receiving postoperative therapy. This analysis suggested improved locoregional control, with no impact on the rate of distant metastases. There was a trend toward improved survival with chemotherapy. An earlier report of this study suggested a similar outcome difference for patients with unresectable disease (121, 122).

The use of bleomycin, 5-FU, and mitomycin C administered as single agents with concomitant radiotherapy is supported by these four positive randomized studies. Cisplatin has also been of interest as a radiosensitizer. Al-Sarraf et al. (123) published the results of an RTOG pilot study involving 124 patients with locally advanced inoperable head and neck cancer. Patients received three doses of cisplatin at 100 mg/m^2 intravenously every 21 days during radiotherapy. Sixty-nine percent had an initial clinical complete response, and the 1-year actuarial survival was 66%. Additional pilot studies using different cisplatin schedules have been conducted, although results have been less promising. A recent study using high-dose intra-arterial cisplatin with systemic thiosulfate protection has resulted in impressive early results. Nine of 22 patients achieved a CR, and 10 had a partial response, for an overall response rate of 86% (124).

Large randomized studies testing cisplatin with concomitant radiotherapy have not been published to date. Haselow et al. randomized patients to radiation therapy alone or radiation plus weekly doses of 20 mg/m^2 of cisplatin. This NCI-sponsored intergroup study was conducted in the early 1980s and, to date, has not been reported. An early analysis suggested no difference in outcome (125); however, the cisplatin dosing in this study was extremely conservative. In retrospect, it seems unclear what the investigators expected to accomplish with a maximum cisplatin dose of 160 mg/m^2. Preliminary data from a second study were reported from France. Bachaud et al. (126) compared standard postoperative radiation therapy with the same radiation therapy plus weekly doses of cisplatin at 50 mg. In a small study cohort of only 83 patients, the 2-year disease-free and overall survival rates were significantly improved in the cisplatin arm in a preliminary analysis. The 2-year survival rate was reported as "corrected for death from non-malignant disease" and was

75% for cisplatin/radiotherapy arm versus 44% for the control arm ($p < .05$). The locoregional failure rates were 41% in the chemotherapy arm and 21% in the radiotherapy arm ($p < .05$).

Altered-Schedule Chemoradiotherapy

In an effort to increase the efficacy and/or reduce the toxicity of chemoradiotherapy, treatment regimens have been designed that administer concomitant therapy with regularly scheduled treatment interruptions of both chemotherapy and radiotherapy, analogous to the customary administration of chemotherapy in cycles. It is hoped that these interruptions will allow normal tissues to recover from the treatment and also permit the administration of more effective chemotherapy with regard to the dose and the number of drugs. Most of these studies represent pilot projects.

O'Connor et al. (127) administered vincristine, bleomycin, and methotrexate with leucovorin rescue over 48 hours prior to and following a 2-week course of radiotherapy at 200 cGy per day. Patients received a total of three such cycles followed by surgical resection of persistent residual disease. The 5-year survival of 198 patients was 41% (including 28 patients who received salvage surgery for persistent or recurrent disease). The disease-free survival was 52% at 5 years. Although acute toxicities seemed increased, no significant increase in late toxicities was observed. No effect of the chemotherapy in reducing the incidence of distant metastases was apparent. Given these results, the authors designed a randomized trial comparing this regimen with neoadjuvant administration of the same drugs (128). The difference in disease-free survival between the two treatment arms was not statistically significant, although a trend favored the concomitant arm. This study continues, with the addition of a third arm of standard radiotherapy alone.

Additional trials using altered-schedule chemoradiotherapy have included continuous infusion 5-FU alone or in combination with other drugs. The first such trial was a phase I trial published by Byfield et al. (115), who administered escalating doses of a 5-day continuous infusion of 5-FU with concomitant radiotherapy for 4 days every other week to previously unirradiated patients with head and neck cancer. A total of five cycles (50 Gy) were administered to each patient, followed by additional radiation with external-beam boost, interstitial implant, or surgery. In this phase I trial, mucositis was found to correlate closely with the dose of 5-FU. Nine of 12 evaluable patients with stage IV disease and 1 of 2 evaluable patients with stage III disease achieved a CR (overall complete response rate, 67%). This trial demonstrated the feasibility of administering continuous infusion 5-FU with protracted radiotherapy to the head and neck.

Taylor et al. (129) expanded on this observation by adding cisplatin to infusional 5-FU and concomitant radiotherapy delivered every other week. These authors used 60 mg/m^2 of cisplatin with a 5-day continuous infusion of 5-FU at 800 mg/m^2/day. Severe mucositis and weight loss occurred in half of the patients. The response rate was 98%, with 55% complete responses. The median survival was 37 months. Of note, only 27% of their patients recurred locoregionally. Adelstein et al. piloted a regimen of cisplatin (75 mg/m^2) with a 4-day infusion of 5-FU (1000 mg/m^2/day) and concomitant radiotherapy to 30 Gy administered over 3 weeks (130). This was followed by a second chemotherapy cycle without radiation, surgery, and a second course of chemoradiotherapy, for a total radiation dose of 60 Gy. Mucositis and myelosuppression again were dose-limiting toxicities. The overall survival of 54 patients was 52%, and the disease-free survival, 70%. This regimen was further tested by the Eastern Cooperative Oncology Group (131). In 57 patients, the overall complete response rate was 77% after optional surgery. The actuarial 4-year disease-free and overall survival rates were 45% and 49%, respectively. Toxicity was significant, with a high incidence of enteral alimentation and severe neutropenia. Three toxic deaths were observed.

Wendt et al. (132) used twice-daily radiation with infusional 5-FU, augmented by leucovorin and cisplatin, divided into three treatment cycles. Of 59 patients, 81% achieved a complete response. Local control rate at 2 years was 92% for patients with stage III disease and 65% for those with stage IV; overall survival was projected at 52% at 2 years. A randomized study of this approach has been completed in Germany.

At the University of Chicago, we have studied alternate-week radiotherapy with concomitant continuous infusion 5-FU and daily hydroxyurea (FHX) (133). The choice of this combination of drugs was based on the known single-agent activity of both continuous infusion 5-FU and hydroxyurea in this disease as well as their known radiosensitizing potential. In addi-

tion, the two drugs have been shown in vitro to be synergistic (134). This phase I study identified the maximally tolerated doses of 5-FU and hydroxyurea. Of 15 evaluable patients with recurrent disease following prior local therapy, only 1 failed to respond. Of 17 evaluable patients without prior local therapy, 12 had a CR, with no patient developing recurrence in the irradiated field at short follow-up. Five patients had a PR. Moderate-to-severe mucositis and mild-to-moderate myelosuppression were seen. The high response rate achieved in patients being reirradiated suggested a possible value of this approach in patients with locoregional recurrence (instead of the traditional "chemotherapy alone" approach).

This concept has been pursued in additional studies at our institution that do indeed suggest that some patients treated in this fashion may be cured of locoregionally recurrent disease (135–137). The phase I/II data also suggested a possible benefit of using the FHX regimen in previously untreated patients. Several such studies have been initiated. The first study focused on patients with stage II and III disease (intermediate stage) (138). In a preliminary analysis of 32 patients, very high locoregional control and overall survival rates were documented. Indeed, only one patient failed within the radiation therapy field, while a second patient failed systemically. These data suggest that concomitant chemoradiotherapy may be useful in intermediate-stage disease, in which it might replace the use of surgery and improve locoregional control and survival data.

In patients with stage IV locoregionally advanced disease, we have conducted three feasibility studies that combine induction chemotherapy for systemic control (and organ preservation) with FHX chemoradiotherapy (139–141). These studies too suggest the feasibility and possible benefit from this approach. Most recently, we have reported on a study using three cycles of PFL-interferon followed by optional surgery and FHX chemoradiotherapy in 71 patients (140). The complete response rate to induction chemotherapy was 51%, organ preservation was achieved in all but 10 of 71 patients, and the 3-year survival rate in this cohort of stage IV patients was projected to be 60%. We are currently investigating a further intensified chemoradiotherapy program with the hope of preserving the activity of this overall approach while eliminating the need for induction chemotherapy.

Only two randomized studies comparing

chemoradiotherapy on an altered schedule with standard radiation therapy have been reported to date. Keane et al. (142) randomized 209 patients to radiation therapy (50 Gy and 20 fractions over 4 weeks) or split-course chemoradiotherapy using mitomycin-C and 5-FU with radiation therapy for two 14-day treatment cycles separated by a 2-week rest. This study used low doses of chemotherapy and low total doses of radiation therapy. Response and survival were similar in both treatment groups, with comparable toxicity. Given these findings, one might conclude that altered-schedule concomitant chemoradiotherapy is not effective. However, one might also conclude that the chemotherapy was able to offset the negative impact of the protraction of radiation in the experimental arm.

A second study was reported by Merlano et al. (143), who compared standard radiation therapy with an experimental approach using rapidly alternating chemoradiotherapy. Five daily doses of cisplatin and 5-FU 200 mg/m^2 both administered as brief intravenous infusions were followed by 2 weeks of radiation therapy; a total of three such cycles were administered. Survival was superior in the chemoradiotherapy group (41 vs. 23% at 3 years; $p<.05$). In addition, locoregional failures were more common in the radiation-only group. This study demonstrated a superior complete response rate, local control, and survival with rapidly alternating chemoradiotherapy. However, it has been criticized for the use of suboptimal radiation therapy in the control arm. Specifically, a mean dose of 62 Gy was reported for the control arm, although the intended dose was 65–75 Gy.

In conclusion, the above data suggest that concomitant chemoradiotherapy might be an acceptable standard therapy for patients with locoregionally advanced disease. Two trials using 5-FU both resulted in improved outcome, and additional data have been generated for mitomycin-C. The exact role of cisplatin or carboplatin in this setting remains to be determined. Furthermore, several of the newer drugs, including the taxanes, gemcitabine, and topoisomerase I inhibitors, are powerful radiation enhancers in preclinical models. Their integration into clinical concomitant-chemoradiotherapy schedules will be of high interest in the near future. Finally, altered-schedule intensive chemoradiotherapy has resulted in highly promising phase II data. Investigation of several of these regimens in large randomized studies will have high priority in the future. To date, randomized studies using this approach have suggested possible benefit in one case.

REFERENCES

1. Wingo PA, Tong T, Bolden S. Cancer statistics 1995. CA 1995;45:8–30.

2. American Joint Committee on Cancer. Manual for staging of cancer. 3rd ed. Philadelphia: JB Lippincott, 1988:27–68.

3. Kotwall C, Sako K, Razack MS, et al. Metastatic patterns in squamous cell cancer of the head and neck. Am J Surg 1987;154:439–442.

4. Zbaeren P, Lehmann W. Frequency and sites of distant metastases in head and neck squamous cell carcinoma. Arch Otolaryngol Head Neck Surg 1987; 113:662–664.

5. Rothman K, Keller A. The effect of joint exposure to alcohol and tobacco on risk of cancer of the mouth and pharynx. J Chron Dis 1972;113:711–716.

6. Decker J, Goldstein JC. Risk factors in head and neck cancer. N Engl J Med 1982;306:1151–1155.

7. Wenig BL. The role of surgery in head and neck cancer: standard care and new horizons. Semin Oncol 1994;21:289–295.

8. Sweeney PJ, Haraf DJ, Vokes EE, Dougherty M, Weichselbaum RR. Radiation therapy in head and neck cancer: indications and limitations. Semin Oncol 1994; 21:296–303.

9. Vokes EE, Weichselbaum RR, Lippman S, Hong WK. Head and neck cancer. N Engl J Med 1993; 328:184–194.

10. Marcial VA, Pajak TF, Kramer S, et al. Radiation Therapy Oncology Group (RTOG) studies in head and neck cancer. Semin Oncol 1988;15:39–60.

11. Cachin Y, Eschwege F. Combination of radiotherapy and surgery in the treatment of head and neck cancers. Cancer Treat Rev 1975;2:177–191.

12. Marcial VA, Pajak TF. Radiation therapy alone or in combination with surgery in head and neck cancer. Cancer 1985;55:2259–2265.

13. Mendenhall WM, Parsons JT, Amdur RJ, et al. Squamous cell carcinoma of the head and neck treated with radiation therapy. The impact of neck stage on local control. Int J Radiat Oncol Biol Phys 1988;14:249–252.

14. Hong WK, Lippman SM, Itri LM, et al. Prevention of second primary tumors with isotretinoin in squamous-cell carcinoma of the head and neck. N Engl J Med 1990;323:795–801.

15. Lippman SM, Batsakis JG, Toth BB, et al. Comparison of low-dose isotretinoin with beta carotene to prevent oral carcinogenesis. N Engl J Med 1993;328:15–20.

16. Mead GM, Jacobs C. Changing role of chemotherapy in treatment of head and neck cancer. Am J Med 1982;73:582–595.

17. Hong WK, Bromer R. Chemotherapy in head and neck cancer. N Engl J Med 1983;308:75–79.

18. Browman GP, Cronin L. Standard chemotherapy in squamous cell head and neck cancer: what we

have learned from randomized trials. Semin Oncol 1994;21:311–319.

19. Papac RJ, Jacobs EM, Foye LV, Donohue DM. Systemic therapy with amethopterin in squamous carcinoma of the head and neck. Cancer Chemother Rep 1963;32:47–54.

20. Lane M, Moore JE III, Levin H, Smith FE. Methotrexate therapy for squamous cell carcinoma of the head and neck. JAMA 1968;204:561–564.

21. Leone LA, Albala MM, Rege VB. Treatment of carcinoma of the head and neck with intravenous methotrexate. Cancer 1968;21:828–837.

22. Papac R, Minor DR, Rudnick S, Solomon LR, Capizzi RL. Controlled trial of methotrexate and bacillus Calmette-Guerin therapy for advanced head and neck cancer. Cancer Res 1973;38:3150–3153.

23. Forastiere AA, Metch B, Schuller DE, et al. Randomized comparison of cisplatin plus fluorouracil and carboplatin plus fluorouracil versus methotrexate in advanced squamous-cell carcinoma of the head and neck: a Southwest Oncology Group study. J Clin Oncol 1992;10:1245–1251.

24. Kirkwood JM, Canellos G, Pervin TJ, Pitman SW, Weichselbaum R, Miller D. Increased therapeutic index using moderate dose methotrexate and leucovorin twice weekly vs. weekly high dose methotrexate-leucovorin in patients with advanced squamous carcinoma of the head and neck. A safe new effective regimen. Cancer 1981;2414–2421.

25. Woods RL, Fox RM, Tattersall MHN. Methotrexate treatment of squamous cell head and neck cancers: dose resonse evaluation. Br Med J 1981;282:600–602.

26. Vogler WR, Jacobs J, Moffitt S, et al. Methotrexate therapy with or without citrovorum factor in carcinoma of the head and neck, breast and colon. Cancer Clin Trials 1979;2:227–236.

27. DeConti RC, Schoenfeld D. A randomized prospective comparison of intermittent methotrexate, methotrexate with leucovorin, and a methotrexate combination in head and neck cancer. Cancer 1981; 48:1061–1072.

28. Taylor SG IV, McGuire WP, Hauck WW, Showel JL, Lad TE. A randomized comparison of high-dose infusion methotrexate versus standard-dose weekly therapy in head and neck squamous cancer. J Clin Oncol 1984;2:1006–1011.

29. Wittes RE, Cvitkovic E, Shah J, Gerold FP, Strong EW. Cis-dichlorodiammineplatinum (II) in the treatment of epidermoid carcinoma of the head and neck. Cancer Treat Rep 1977;61:359–366.

30. Wittes R, Heller K, Randolph V, et al. Cis-dichlorodiammineplatinum (II)-based chemotherapy as initial treatment of advanced head and neck cancer. Cancer Treat Rep 1979;63:1533–1538.

31. Jacobs C, Bertino JR, Goffinet DR, Fee WE, Good RL. 24-hour infusion of cis-platinum in head and neck cancers. Cancer 1978;42:2135–2140.

32. Sako K, Razack MS, Kalnins I. Chemotherapy for advanced and recurrent squamous cell carcinoma of the head and neck with high and low dose cis-dichlorodiammineplatinum. Am J Surg 1978;136:529–533.

33. Veronesi A, Zagonel V, Tirelli U, et al. High-dose versus low-dose cisplatin in advanced head and neck squamous carcinoma: a randomized study. J Clin Oncol 1985;3:1105–1108.

34. Havlin KA, Kuhn JG, Myers JW, et al. High-dose cisplatin for locally advanced or metastatic head and neck cancer. Cancer 1989;63:423–427.

35. Forastiere AA, Takasugi BJ, Baker SR, Wolf GT, Kudla-Hatch V. High-dose cisplatin in advanced head and neck cancer. Cancer Chemother Pharmacol 1987; 19:155–158.

36. Hong WK, Schaefer S, Issell B, et al. A prospective randomized trial of methotrexate versus cisplatin in the treatment of recurrent squamous cell carcinoma of the head and neck. Cancer 1983;52:206–210.

37. Grose WE, Lehane DE, Dixon DO, Fletcher WS, Stuckey WJ. Comparison of methotrexate and cisplatin for patients with advanced squamous cell carcinoma of the head and neck region: a Southwest Oncology Group study. Cancer Treat Rep 1985;69:577–581.

38. Allison RS, Campbell JB, Dalby JE, Dorman EB, et al. A phase III randomised trial of cisplatinum, methotrextate, cisplatinum + methotrexate and cisplatinum + 5-FU in end stage squamous carcinoma of the head and neck. Br J Cancer 1990;61:311–315.

39. Aisner J, Sinibaldi V, Eisenberger M. Carboplatin in the treatment of squamous cell head and neck cancers. Semin Oncol 1992;19:60–65.

40. Zamboglou N, Schnabel T, Kolotas C, Achterrath W, Strehl H, et al. Carboplatin and radiotherapy in the treatment of head and neck cancer: six years' experience. Semin Oncol 1994;21:45–53.

41. Tapazoglou E, Kish J, Ensley J, Al-Sarraf M. The activity of a single-agent 5-fluorouracil infusion in advanced and recurrent head and neck cancer. Cancer 1986;57:1105–1109.

42. Jacobs C, Lyman G, Velez-Garcia E, et al. A phase III randomized study comparing cisplatin and fluorouracil as single agents and in combination for advanced squamous cell carcinoma of the head and neck. J Clin Oncol 1992;10:257–263.

43. Forastiere AA. Paclitaxel (Taxol) for the treatment of head and neck cancer. Semin Oncol 1994;21(5 Suppl 8):49–52.

44. Thornton D, Singh K, Putz B, Gams R, Schuller D, Smith R. A phase II trial of Taxol in squamous cell carcinoma of the head and neck (abstract 933). Proc Am Soc Clin Oncol 1994;13:288.

45. Catimel G, Verweij J, Mattijssen V, et al. Docetaxel (Taxotere): an active drug for the treatment of patients with advanced squamous cell carcinoma of the head and neck. Ann Oncol 1994;5(6):533–537.

46. Catimel G, Vermorken JB, Clavel M, de Mulder P, Judson I, et al. A phase II study of gemcitabine (LY 188011) in patients with advanced squamous cell carcinoma of the head and neck. Ann Oncol 1994;5(6):543–547.

47. Gebbia V, Testa A, Valenza R, Zerillo G, Restivo S, et al. A pilot study of vinorelbine on a weekly schedule in recurrent and/or metastatic squamous cell carcinoma of the head and neck. Eur J Cancer 1993; 29A:1358–1359.

48. Jacobs C, Meyers F, Hendrickson C, Kahler M, Carter S. A randomized phase III study of cisplatin with or without methotrexate for recurrent squamous cell carcinoma of the head and neck. Cancer 1983; 52:1563–1569.

49. Vogl SE, Schoenfeld DA, Kaplan BH, Lerner HJ, Engstrom PF, Horton J. A randomized prospective comparison of methotrexate with a combination of

methotrexate, bleomycin, and cisplatin in head and neck cancer. Cancer 1985;56:432–442.

50. Abele R, Honegger HP, Grossenbacher R, et al. A randomized study of methotrexate, bleomycin, hydroxyurea with versus without cisplatin in patients with previously untreated and recurrent squamous cell carcinoma of the head and neck. Eur J Cancer Clin Oncol 1987;23:47–53.

51. Kish JA, Weaver A, Jacobs J, et al. Cisplatin and 5-fluorouracil infusion in patients with recurrent and disseminated epidermoid cancer of the head and neck. Cancer 1984;53:1819–1824.

52. Rowland KM, Taylor SG, O'Donnel MR, et al. Cisplatin and 5-FU infusion chemotherapy in advanced recurrent cancer of the head and neck: an Eastern Cooperative Oncology Group pilot study. Cancer Treat Rep 1986;70:461–464.

53. Creagen E, Ingle J, Schutt A, et al. A phase II study of cisdiamine-dichloroplatinum and 5-fluorouracil in advanced upper aerodigestive neoplasms. Head Neck Surg 1984;7:1020–1023.

54. Choksi AJ, Hong WK, Dimery IW, et al. Continuous cisplatin (24-hour) and 5-fluorouracil (120-hour) infusion in recurrent head and neck squamous cell carcinoma. Cancer 1988;61:909–912.

55. Vokes EE, Choi KE, Schilsky RL, et al, Cisplatin, fluorouracil, and high dose leucovorin for recurrent or metastatic head and neck cancer. J Clin Oncol 1988; 6:618–626.

56. Houghton JA, Maroda SJ, Phillips JO, Houghton PJ. Biochemical determinants of responsiveness to 5-fluorouracil and its derivatives in xenographs of human colorectal adenocarcinomas in mice. Cancer Res 1987;41:144–149.

57. Erlichman C, Fine S, Wong A, et al. A randomized trial of fluorouracil and folinic acid in patients with metastatic colorectal carcinoma. J Clin Oncol 1988;6:469–475.

58. Bensmaine A, Azli N, Domenge C, et al. CDDP-5FU modulation by alpha IFN 2b (IFN) in metastatic and/or recurrent head and neck squamous cell carcinoma (HNSCC) (abstract 585). Ann Oncol 1992; 3(Suppl 5):153.

59. Hussain M, Benedetti J, Smith R, et al. Alpha interferon (aIFN) + 5-fluorouracil (5-FU) + cisplatin (CDD)) in advanced squamous cell carcinoma of the head and neck (SCCHN): a Southwest Oncology Group (SWOG) phase II trial (abstract 897). Proc Am Soc Clin Oncol 1994;13:279.

60. Arquette MA, Mortimer JE, Leohrer PJ, et al. A phase II Hoosier Oncology Group trial of interferon alpha-2b (IFN) added to cisplatin (CDDP) and 5-fluorouracil (FU) in recurrent or metastatic head and neck cancer (abstract 901). Proc Am Soc Clin Oncol 1994; 13:280.

61. Stupp R, Weichselbaum RR, Vokes EE. Combined modality therapy of head and neck cancer. Semin Oncol 1994;21:349–358.

62. Dimery IW, Hong WK. Overview of combined modality therapies for head and neck cancer. J Natl Cancer Inst 1993;85:95–111.

63. Rosenthal DI, Pisten DA, Glatstein E. A review of neoadjuvant chemotherapy for head and neck cancer: partially shrunken tumors may be both leaner and meaner. Int J Radiat Oncol Biol Phys 1993;28:315–320.

64. Van Putten LM. Experimental preoperative chemotherapy. In: Ragaz J, Bank PR, Goldie JH, eds. Recent results in cancer research; preoperative (neoadjuvant) chemotherapy. New York: Springer-Verlag, 1986:36–40.

65. Goldie JH, Coldman AJ. Theoretical considerations regarding the early use of adjuvant chemotherapy. In: Ragaz J, Bank PR, Goldie JH, eds. Recent results in cancer research: preoperative (neoadjuvant) chemotherapy. New York: Springer-Verlag, 1986:30–35.

66. Van Putten LM, Kram LKJ, Van Dierendonck HHC, et al. Enhancement by drugs of metastatic lung nodule formation after intravenous tumor cell injection. Int J Cancer 1975;15:588–595.

67. Tarpley JL, Chretien PB, Alexander JC, Hoye RC, Block JB, Ketcham AL. High dose methotrexate as a preoperative adjuvant in the treatment of epidermoid carcinoma of the head and neck. Am J Surg 1975; 130:25–29.

68. Pitman SW, Miller D, Weichselbaum R. Initial adjuvant therapy in advanced squamous cell carcinoma of the head and neck employing weekly high dose methotrexate with leucovorin rescue. Laryngoscope 1978;88:632–638.

69. Schaefer SD, Middleton R, Reisch J, et al. Cisplatinum induction chemotherapy in the multi-modality initial treatment of advanced stage IV carcinoma of the head and neck. Cancer 1983;51:2168–2174.

70. Hong WK, Shapshay SM, Bhutani R, et al. Induction chemotherapy in advanced squamous head and neck carcinoma with high-dose cis-platinum and bleomycin infusion. Cancer 1979;44:19–25.

71. Spaulding MB, Kahn A, De Los Santos R, Klotch D, Lore JM. Adjuvant chemotherapy in advanced head and neck cancer. An update. Am J Surg 1982;144:432–436.

72. Ervin TJ, Clark JR, Weichselbaum RR, et al. An analysis of induction and adjuvant chemotherapy in the multidisciplinary treatment of squamous-cell carcinoma of the head and neck. J Clin Oncol 1987;5:10–20.

73. Rooney M, Kish J, Jacobs J, et al. Improved complete response rate and survival in advanced head and neck cancer after three-course induction therapy with 120-hour 5-FU infusion and cisplatin. Cancer 1985; 55:1123–1128.

74. Kies MS, Gordon LI, Hauck WW, et al. Analysis of complete responders after initial treatment with chemotherapy in head and neck cancer. Otolaryngol Head Neck Surg 1985;93:199–205.

75. Vokes EE, Moran WJ, Mick R, Weichselbaum RR, Panje WR. Neoadjuvant and adjuvant methotrexate, cisplatin, and fluorouracil in multimodal therapy of head and neck cancer. J Clin Oncol 1989;7:838–845.

76. Mick R, Vokes EE, Weichselbaum RR, Panje WR. Prognostic factors in patients with advanced head and neck cancer undergoing multimodality therapy: the University of Chicago experience. Otolaryngol Head Neck Surg 1991;105:62–73.

77. Hill BT, Price LA, MacRae K. Importance of primary site in assessing chemotherapy response and 7-year survival data in advanced squamous-cell carcinomas of the head and neck treated with initial combination chemotherapy without cisplatin. J Clin Oncol 1986;4:1340–1347.

78. Choksi AJ, Dimery IW, Hong WK. Adjuvant chemotherapy of head and neck cancer: the past, the present, and the future. Semin Oncol 1988;15:45–59.

79. Thyss A, Schneider M, Santini J, et al. Induction chemotherapy with *cis*-platinum and 5-fluorouracil for squamous cell carcinoma of the head and neck. Br J Cancer 1986;54:755–760.

80. Vokes EE, Mick R, Lester EP, et al. Cisplatin and 5-fluorouracil does not yield long-term benefit in locally advanced head and neck cancer: results from a single institution. J Clin Oncol 1992;9:1376–1384.

81. Al-Kourainy K, Kish J, Ensley J, et al. Achievement of superior survival for histologically negative versus histologically positive clinically complete responders to cisplatin combination in patients with locally advanced head and neck cancer. Cancer 1987; 59:233–238.

82. Ensley JF, Jacobs JR, Weaver A, et al. Correlation between response to cisplatinum-combination chemotherapy and subsequent radiotherapy in previously untreated patients with advanced squamous cell cancers of the head and neck. Cancer 1984;54:811–814.

83. Ensley J, Kish J, Tapazoglou F, et al. An intensive, five course, alternating combination chemotherapy induction regimen used in patients with advanced, unresectable head and neck cancer. J Clin Oncol 1988; 6:1147–1153.

84. Vokes EE, Panje WR, Mick R, et al. A randomized study comparing 2 regimens of neoadjuvant and adjuvant chemotherapy in multimodal therapy for locally advanced head and neck cancer. Cancer 1990; 66:206–213.

85. Spaulding M, Ziegler P, Sundquist N, et al. Induction therapy in head and neck cancer. A comparison of two regimens. Cancer 1986;57:1110–1114.

86. Vokes EE, Schilsky RL, Weichselbaum RR, Kozloff M, Panje WR. Neoadjuvant cisplatin, fluorouracil and high-dose leucovorin for locally advanced head and neck cancer: a clinical and pharmacologic analysis. J Clin Oncol 1990;8:241–247.

87. Dreyfuss AI, Clark JR, Wright JE, et al. Continuous infusion high-dose leucovorin with 5-fluorouracil and cisplatin for untreated stage IV carcinoma of the head and neck. Ann Intern Med 1990;112:167–172.

88. Vokes EE, Ratain MJ, Mick R, et al. Cisplatin, fluorouracil, and leucovorin augmented by interferon alfa-2b in head and neck cancer: a clinical and pharmacologic analysis. J Clin Oncol 1993;11:360–368.

89. Tannock IF, Browman G. Lack of evidence for a role of chemotherapy in the routine management of locally advanced head and neck cancer. J Clin Oncol 1986;4:1121–1126.

90. Forastiere AA. Randomized trials of induction chemotherapy. A critical review. Hematol Oncol Clin North Am 1991;5:725–736.

91. Knowlton AH, Percapio B, Bobrow S, et al. Methotrexate and radiation therapy in the treatment of advanced head and neck tumors. Radiology 1975; 116:709–712.

92. Fazekas JT, Sommer C, Kramer S. Adjuvant intravenous methotrexate or definitive radiotherapy alone for advanced squamous cancers of the oral cavity, oropharynx, supraglottic larynx, or hypopharynx. Int J Radiat Oncol Biol Phys 1980;6:533–541.

93. Stell PM, Dalby JB, Strickland P, Fraser JG, Bradley PJ, Flood LM. Sequential chemotherapy and radiotherapy in advanced head and neck cancer. Clin Radiol 1983;34:463–467.

94. Stolwijk C, Wagener DJT, Van Den Broek P, et al. Randomized neo-adjuvant chemotherapy trial for advanced head and neck cancer. Neth J Med 1985; 28:347–351.

95. Holoye PY, Grossman TW, Toohill RJ, et al. Randomized study of adjuvant chemotherapy for head and neck cancer. Otolaryngol Head Neck Surg 1985; 93:712–717.

96. Toohill RJ, Anderson T, Byhardt RW, et al. Cisplatin and fluorouracil as neoadjuvant therapy in head and neck cancer. Arch Otolaryngol Head Neck Surg 1987;113:758–761.

97. Taylor SG, Applebaum E, Showel JL, et al. A randomized trial of adjuvant chemotherapy in head and neck cancer. J Clin Oncol 1985;3:672–679.

98. Schuller DE, Metch B, Mattox D, Stein DW, McCracken JD. Preoperative chemotherapy in advanced resectable head and neck cancer: final report of the Southwest Oncology Group. Laryngoscope 1988; 98:1205–1211.

99. Head and Neck Contracts Program. Adjuvant chemotherapy for advanced head and neck squamous carcinoma. Cancer 1987;60:301–311.

100. The Department of Veterans Affairs Laryngeal Cancer Study Group. Induction chemotherapy plus radiation compared with surgery plus radiation in patients with advanced laryngeal cancer. N Engl J Med 1991;324:1685–1690.

101. Laramore GE, Scott CB, Al-Sarraf M, et al. Adjuvant chemotherapy for resectable squamous cell carcinomas of the head and neck: report on intergroup study. Int J Radiat Oncol Biol Phys 1992;23:705–713.

102. Paccagnella A, Orlando A, Marchiori C, et al. Phase III trial of initial chemotherapy in stage III or IV head and neck cancers: a study by the Gruppo di Studio sui Tumori della Testa e del Collo. J Natl Cancer Inst 1994;86:265–272.

103. Jacobs C, Goffinet DR, Goffinet L, et al. Chemotherapy as a substitute for surgery in the treatment of advanced resectable head and neck cancer. Cancer 1987;60:1178–1183.

104. Pfister DG, Strong E, Harrison L, et al. Larynx preservation with combined chemotherapy and radiation therapy in advanced but resectable head and neck cancer. J Clin Oncol 1991;9:850–859.

105. Urba SG, Forastiere AA, Wolf GT, et al. Intensive induction chemotherapy and radiation for organ preservation in patients with advanced resectable head and neck carcinoma. J Clin Oncol 1994;12(5):946–953.

106. Tannock IF, Cummings BJ. Neoadjuvant chemotherapy in head and neck cancer: no way to preserve a larynx (letter). J Clin Oncol 1992;10:343–344.

107. Tannock IF, Rotin D. Keynote address: mechanisms of interaction between radiation and drugs with potential for improvements in therapy. NCI Monogr 1988;6:77–83.

108. Vokes EE, Weichselbaum RR. Concomitant chemoradiotherapy: rationale and clinical experience in patients with solid tumors. J Clin Oncol 1990;8:911–934.

109. Vokes EE. Interactions of chemotherapy and radiation. Semin Oncol 1993;20(1):70–79.

110. Steel GG, Peckham MJ. Exploitable mechanisms in combined radiotherapy-chemotherapy: the concept of additivity. Int J Radiat Oncol Biol Phys 1979; 5:85–91.

111. Shanta V, Krishnamurthi S. Combined bleomycin and radiotherapy in oral cancer. Clin Radiol 1980;31:617–620.

112. Fu KK, Phillips TL, Silverberg IY, et al. Combined radiotherapy and chemotherapy with bleomycin and methotrexate for advanced inoperable head and neck cancer: update of a Northern California Oncology Group randomized trial. J Clin Oncol 1987;5:1410–1418.

113. Cachin Y, Jortay A, Sancho H, et al. Preliminary results of a randomized EORTC study comparing radiotherapy and concomitant bleomycin to radiotherapy alone in epidermoid carcinomas of the oropharynx. Eur J Cancer 1977;13:1389–1395.

114. Lo TC, Wiley AL Jr, Ansfield FJ, et al. Combined radiation therapy and 5-fluorouracil for advanced squamous cell carcinoma of the oral cavity and oropharynx: a randomized study. Am J Roentgenol 1976;126:229–235.

115. Byfield JE, Sharp TR, Frankel SS, et al. Phase I and II trial of five-day infused 5-fluorouracil and radiation in advanced cancer of the head and neck. J Clin Oncol 1984;2:406–413.

116. Browman GP, Cripps C, Hodson DI, et al. Placebo-controlled randomized trial of infusional fluorouracil during standard radiotherapy in locally advanced head and neck cancer. J Clin Oncol 1994; 12:2648–2653.

117. Sartorelli AC. Therapeutic attack of hypoxic cells of solid tumors: presidential address. Cancer Res 1988;48:775–778.

118. Rockwell S, Kennedy KA, Sartorelli AC. Mitomycin-C as a prototype bioreductive alkylating agent: in vitro studies of metabolism and cytotoxicity. Int J Radiat Oncol Biol Phys 1982;8:753–755.

119. Rockwell S. Cytotoxicities of mitomycin-C and x-rays to aerobic and hypoxic cells in vitro. Int J Radiat Oncol Biol Phys 1982;8:1035–1039.

120. Rockwell S. Effects of mitomycin-C alone and in combination with x-rays on EMT_6 mouse mammary tumors in vivo. J Natl Cancer Inst 1983;71:765–771.

121. Weissberg JB, Son YH, Papac RJ. et al. Randomized clinical trial of mitomycin C as an adjunct to radiotherapy in head and neck cancer. Int J Radiat Oncol Biol Phys 1989;17:3–9.

122. Haffty BG, Son YH, Sasaki CT, et al. Mitomycin C as an adjunct to postoperative radiation therapy in squamous cell carcinoma of the head and neck: results from two randomized clinical trials. Int J Radiat Oncol Biol Phys 1993;24(2):241–250.

123. Al-Sarraf M, Pajak TF, Marcial VA, et al. Concurrent radiotherapy and chemotherapy with cisplatin in inoperable squamous cell carcinoma of the head and neck. Cancer 1987;59:259–265.

124. Robbins KT, Storniolo AM, Kerber C, et al. Phase I study of highly selective supradose cisplatin infusions for advanced head and neck cancer. J Clin Oncol 1994;12:2113–2020.

125. Haselow RE, Warshaw MG, Oken MM, et al. Radiation alone versus radiation plus weekly low-dose cis-platinum in unresectable cancer of the head and

neck. In: Fee WE Jr, Goepfert H, Johns ME, et al., eds. Head and neck cancer, vol 2. Philadelphia: BC Decker, 1990:279–281.

126. Bachaud J-M, David J-M, Boussin G, Daly N. Combined postoperative radiotherapy and weekly cisplatin infusion for locally advanced squamous cell carcinoma of the head and neck: preliminary report of a randomized trial. Int J Radiat Oncol Biol Phys 1991; 20:243–246.

127. O'Connor D, Clifford P, Edwards WG, et al. Long-term results of VBM and radiotherapy in advanced head and neck cancer. Int J Radiat Oncol Biol Phys 1982;8:1525–1531.

128. SECOG Clinical Trial Group. A randomized trial of combined multidrug chemotherapy and radiotherapy in advanced squamous cell carcinoma of the head and neck. Eur J Surg Oncol 1986;12:289–295.

129. Taylor SG IV, Murthy AK, Caldarelli DD, et al. Combined simultaneous cisplatin/fluorouracil chemotherapy and split course radiation in head and neck cancer. J Clin Oncol 1989;7:846–856.

130. Adelstein DJ, Sharah VM, Earle AS, et al. Chemoradiotherapy as initial management in patients with squamous cell carcinoma of the head and neck. Cancer Treat Rep 1986;70:761–767.

131. Adelstein DJ, Kalish LA, Adams GL, et al. Concurrent radiation therapy and chemotherapy for locally unresectable squamous cell head and neck cancer. An Eastern Cooperative Oncology Group pilot study. J Clin Oncol 1993;11:2136–2142.

132. Wendt TG, Hartenstein RC, Wustrow TPU, Lissner J. Cisplatin, fluorouracil with leucovorin calcium enhancement, and synchronous accelerated radiotherapy in the management of locally advanced head and neck cancer: a phase II study. J Clin Oncol 1989;7:471–476.

133. Vokes EE, Panje WR, Schilsky RL, et al. Hydroxyurea, fluorouracil, and concomitant radiotherapy in poor-prognosis head and neck cancer: a phase I-II study. J Clin Oncol 1989;7:761–768.

134. Moran RG, Danenberg PV, Heidelberger C. Therapeutic response of leukemic mice treated with fluorinated pyrimidines and inhibitors of deoxyuridylate synthesis. Biochem Pharmacol 1982;31:2929–2935.

135. Vokes EE, Haraf DJ, Weichselbaum RR, et al. Perspectives on combination chemotherapy with concomitant radiotherapy for poor prognosis head and neck cancer. Semin Oncol 1992;19:47–56.

136. Vokes EE, Haraf DJ, Mick R, et al. Intensified concomitant chemoradiotherapy with and without filgrastim for poor-prognosis head and neck cancer. J Clin Oncol 1994;12:2351–2359.

137. Haraf DJ, Vokes EE, Panje WR, Weichselbaum RR. Survival and analysis of failure following hydroxyurea, 5-fluorouracil and concomitant radiation therapy in poor prognosis head and neck cancer. Am J Clin Oncol 1991;14:419–426.

138. Vokes EE, Haraf DJ, Mick R, et al. Concomitant chemoradiotherapy for intermediate stage head and neck cancer (abstract). Proc Am Soc Clin Oncol 1994;13:282.

139. Vokes EE, Weichselbaum RR, Mick R, et al. Favorable long-term survival following induction chemotherapy with PFL and concomitant chemoradiotherapy for locally advanced head and neck cancer. J Natl Cancer Inst 1992;84:877–882.

140. Vokes EE, Kies M, Haraf DJ, et al. Induction chemotherapy followed by concomitant chemoradiotherapy for advanced head and neck cancer: impact on the natural history of the disease. J Clin Oncol 1995; 13:876–883.

141. Vokes EE, R Mick, Kies M, et al. Fluorouracil pharmacodynamics of induction chemotherapy in advanced head and neck cancer (abstract). Proc Am Soc Clin Oncol 1995;14:297.

142. Keane TJ, Cummings BJ, O'Sullivan B, et al. A randomized trial of radiation therapy compared to split course radiation therapy combined with mitomycin C and 5-fluorouracil as initial treatment for advanced laryngeal and hypopharyngeal squamous carcinoma. Int J Radiat Oncol Biol Phys 1993;25:613–618.

143. Merlano M, Vitale V, Rosso R, et al. Treatment of advanced squamous cell carcinoma of the head and neck with alternating chemotherapy and radiotherapy. N Engl J Med 1992;327:1115–1121.

53

Chemotherapy of Lung Cancer

Mohammad Jahanzeb and Daniel C. Ihde

Over the last five decades, the incidence of lung cancer has increased by epidemic proportions. In 1995, an estimated 169,900 cases of lung cancer will be diagnosed, resulting in 157,000 deaths (1). It is not only the leading cause of cancer death in both men and women, but it is also responsible for more U.S. cancer deaths than the second, third, and fourth greatest causes of cancer mortality (colorectal, breast, prostate) combined. The incidence is stable to decreasing in men but still rising in women, reflecting effects of changes in smoking patterns. Up to 85% of lung cancer is directly attributable to smoking and another 3% to secondhand smoking, according to a recent Surgeon General's report (2). Many patients present with metastatic disease, while others eventually develop distant spread requiring chemotherapy. More than a dozen "active" chemotherapeutic agents have been identified for the treatment of lung cancer, more than half of which have entered clinical trials in the last 6 to 7 years (3). This fact alone may point to a quickening pace of progress, although only modest improvements in the survival of all patients with lung cancer (currently 12 to 15% at 5 years) have been achieved.

Based on presentation, pattern of dissemination, rate of progression, likelihood of regression with chemotherapy, and prognosis, patients with primary lung cancer can be divided into two distinct groups: those who have small cell lung cancer (SCLC) and those who do not. SCLC, which comprises almost 20% of all cases of lung cancer, tends to disseminate early, progresses rapidly, and proves fatal in a matter of a few months in the absence of therapy, but is exquisitely sensitive to chemotherapy and radiotherapy (4). Cure rates are still low, as most responders relapse, and relapsed disease virtually always proves to be incurable.

The remaining (approximately 80%) histolo-gies of bronchogenic carcinoma constitute non-small-cell lung cancer (NSCLC) and principally consist of squamous cell carcinoma, adenocarcinoma, and large cell carcinoma. More than half of these patients have disease clinically confined to the chest at the time of presentation (5). Surgical resection alone can be curative in almost one-half of the earlier-stage patients (those with disease clinically confined within the pleural reflection) (6). Complete response to chemotherapy is rare in NSCLC patients, and partial responses are seen in much fewer than half the patients (7). Five-year survivors are rarely seen, even in the absence of therapy (5).

This chapter primarily focuses on the evolution and current role of chemotherapy in lung cancer, along with present and future research directions. The role of combined-modality therapy that does not include chemotherapy is only briefly discussed, as a detailed account is beyond the scope of this chapter.

CHEMOTHERAPY IN NSCLC

The approach to NSCLC is primarily surgical because such treatment can by itself cure almost one-half of early-stage patients (stages I and II) (6). Unfortunately, only 25 to 30% of patients belong to this group at the time of presentation (refer to Table 53.1 for staging system). Forty to 45% of patients have metastatic disease at the time of diagnosis, and 30 to 35% have regionally advanced (stage III) disease without distant metastases. Clearly an effective systemic therapy is needed to improve the cure rates. After three decades of therapeutic nihilism, there now seems to be at least a modest role for chemotherapy in prolonging survival as well as in the palliative management of ambulatory patients with NSCLC.

**Table 53.1. International (AJCC & UICC)[a]
Staging System for Lung Cancer**

T1	Tumor ≤3 cm without pleural or mainstem bronchus involvement
T2	Tumor >3 cm or involvement of mainstem bronchus ≥2 cm from carina, visceral pleural involvement, or lobar atelectasis
T3	Tumor with involvement of chest wall (including superior sulcus tumors), diaphragm, mediastinal pleura, pericardium, mainstem bronchus <2 cm from carina, or entire lung atelectasis
T4	Tumor with invasion of mediastinum, heart, great vessels, trachea, esophagus, vertebral body, carina or with a malignant pleural effusion
N0	No demonstrable metastasis to regional lymph nodes
N1	Ipsilateral hilar or peribronchial nodal involvement
N2	Metastasis to ipsilateral mediastinal or subcarinal lymph nodes
N3	Metastasis to contralateral mediastinal or hilar lymph nodes, or to ipsilateral or contralateral scalene or supraclavicular lymph nodes
M0	No (known) distant metastasis
M1	Distant metastasis present

Stage I	T1–2	N0	M0
Stage II	T1–2	N1	M0
Stage IIIa	T1–3	N2	M0
	T3	N0–2	M0
Stage IIIb	Any T	N3	M0
	T4	Any N	M0
Stage IV	Any T	Any N	M1

Modified from Mountain CF. A new international staging system for lung cancer. Chest 1986;89:225S–223S.
[a]AJCC, American Joint Commission on Cancer; UICC, Union Intérnationale Contre Cancer.

Historical Perspective

Mustard gas (sulfur mustard), used in the trench warfare of World War I, was the antecedent for water-soluble nitrogen mustards that were first used clinically in the 1940s for the treatment of NSCLC (8). Despite transient improvement in symptoms for some patients, no survival benefit was recorded. Large controlled trials of chemotherapy began in the latter half of the 1950s, when the Veterans Administration Surgical Oncology Group began a series of studies using alkylating agents, sometimes combined with hydroxyurea or methotrexate, in the adjuvant setting. These trials also failed to demonstrate a survival benefit (9). Cisplatin-based combinations then gained popularity as their apparently superior activity was documented.

Table 53.2. Commonly Used Effective Regimens in Non-Small-Cell Lung Cancer

Regimens shown to improve survival in controlled trials
PV

Cisplatin	100 mg/m² every 4 weeks
Vinblastine	5 mg/m² every week

PN

Cisplatin	120 mg/m² every 4–6 weeks
Vinorelbine (Navelbine)	30 mg/m² every week

Widely employed without proof of survival benefit
EP

Cisplatin	60–100 mg/m² every 4 weeks
Etoposide	120 mg/m² day 1–3 every 4 weeks

Since most chemotherapy is principally directed against disseminated cancer, whether apparent (macrometastatic) or potentially present (micrometastatic), we will discuss its role in patients with decreasing levels of tumor burden. Commonly used regimens in NSCLC are summarized in Table 53.2.

Chemotherapy for Metastatic NSCLC

Almost 45% of all cases of NSCLC have clinically detectable metastases at diagnosis. Metastatic NSCLC is virtually incurable. There are not even anecdotal reports of cure with chemotherapy alone in this setting. Several established agents show 15 to 20% response rates (RRs), and cisplatin-based combinations yield 20 to 40% RRs (7). Almost all of these responses are partial, as complete remissions are rare. Agents with documented activity, as defined by a single-agent RR of 15% or better, are cisplatin (and probably its analogue carboplatin), the vinca alkaloids vinblastine and vindesine, mitomycin, and ifosfamide. Alkylating agents and antimetabolites have displayed only infrequent activity (10). Etoposide, despite having single-agent activity below 15%, yields good responses in combination with cisplatin, perhaps due to synergistic activity (11).

Until recently there were no prospective randomized trials demonstrating a clear survival benefit of chemotherapy in metastatic NSCLC. Randomized studies that have shown such benefit have used cisplatin-based chemotherapy (12–14), although they are still outnumbered by negative studies (15–19). A literature review showed a 21% RR for single-agent cisplatin (20). The optimal dose of cisplatin is debatable, although no randomized trials show an advantage to giving more than 50 to 60 mg/m² of this drug and show higher doses to be more toxic (21, 22). In one study, response duration was better for the higher dose of cisplatin, but survival was better only among responders (23). Doses below 50 to 60 mg/m², however, may not be as effective. There is evidence that addition of cisplatin to a vinca alkaloid improves efficacy, but this has not been true for adding other drugs such as mitomycin (24, 25). A randomized Eastern Cooperative Oncology Group study demonstrated that single-agent carboplatin was superior to some cisplatin-based combinations with respect to survival, although response rates were low (26). Two-drug combinations of cisplatin with vinca alkaloids or etoposide generally yield nearly identical results in randomized trials and are better than treatment with etoposide or vinca alkaloid alone (27). A recent large three-arm randomized trial demonstrated better response rates and marginally better survival for a combination of cisplatin and vinorelbine than for vindesine and cisplatin, while the third arm, treatment with vinorelbine alone, was inferior in efficacy only to its combination with cisplatin and exhibited significantly less neurotoxicity than the cisplatin plus vindesine combination (28).

Is there a survival advantage to cisplatin-based chemotherapy? This question was recently addressed by a metaanalysis performed by the Non-Small Cell Lung Cancer Collaborators Group (29) (Table 53.3). Using updated individual patient data from 54 randomized clinical trials (RCTs) conducted in 1965 to 1991 and including more than 9000 patients, the group compared primary treatment alone with the same treatment in addition to cytotoxic chemotherapy. Analyses were carried out for two categories of chemotherapy: long-term alkylators ("old" chemotherapy) and cisplatin-based ("modern" chemotherapy) regimens. In patients with metastatic or locally advanced disease unsuitable for radiation, there were 11 RCTs involving 1190 patients. A pooled hazard ratio of 0.73 ($p = .00007$) was found in favor of cisplatin-based chemotherapy, translating into a 27% reduction in the rate of death, corresponding to an improvement in median survival from 6 months to 8 months and a 10% absolute improvement in 1-year survival. For long-term alkylators, a pooled hazard ratio of 1.26 ($p = .095$) suggested a relative detriment of chemotherapy equivalent to a 1-month reduction in median survival.

A retrospective analysis of over 2500 patients treated by Southwest Oncology Group (SWOG) also suggests that cisplatin-based chemotherapy plays a role in prolonging survival. Performance status, gender, and cisplatin use were found to be the major determinants of survival in this study (30).

Arguably, the best known among the randomized trials is the one conducted by the National Cancer Institute of Canada (NCIC) (12). In this study, patients were randomly assigned to best supportive care (BSC) or chemotherapy with either vindesine and cisplatin (Vds/P) or cyclophosphamide, doxorubicin, and cisplatin (CAP). The dose of cisplatin was different for the two regimens (120 mg/m² in Vds/P vs. 40 mg/m² in CAP). The median survival was 17 weeks for BSC, 24.7 weeks for CAP, and 32.6 weeks for Vds/P ($p = .01$). The response rates of Vds/P were also marginally better than those of CAP. It is not clear whether Vds/P was superior due to a higher dose of cisplatin or the addition of a vinca alkaloid. The survival benefit in this and other positive studies is modest enough that it

Table 53.3. Metaanalyses of Randomized Trials of Cisplatin-Based Chemotherapy in Non-Small-Cell Lung Cancer

Therapeutic Setting	No. Pts (No. Trials)	Relative Mortality Reduction	Absolute Benefit	*p* Value	Ref.
Palliative care in advanced disease	778 (8)	27%	10% at 1 year[a]	<.0001	(29)
Combined with RT in stage III	1780 (11)	13%	4% at 2 years	.01	(46)
Postsurgical adjuvant Rx	1062 (7)	13%	5% at 5 years	.12	(66)

[a]Median survival increased by 2 months.

has led opponents and proponents of palliative chemotherapy to refer to the same studies in support of their practice.

A unique feature of the NCIC study was a cost analysis (published subsequently) that showed CAP chemotherapy to be cheaper than BSC in terms of cost per patient ($7645 vs. $8594, respectively, in Canadian dollars) (31). This was due to extra costs for radiotherapy and increased costs of hospitalization for the BSC patients. Vds/P was the most expensive treatment ($12,232 per patient), perhaps due to the inpatient administration of cisplatin for this regimen. With outpatient cisplatin administration currently in vogue, the costs would be fairly comparable to CAP chemotherapy. Cost effectiveness (as measured by cost per year of life gained) figures were $14777 for Vds/P versus BSC and −$6171 for CAP versus BSC. Since CAP chemotherapy added to survival and saved expense compared with BSC, it can be concluded that this chemotherapy was the most cost-effective option on the basis of cost per day of life saved.

With the advent of better antiemetics and improvements in supportive care, cisplatin-based therapy is increasingly safer and better tolerated (32). Palliative chemotherapy with such regimens should be discussed with good-performance-status patients. A reasonable strategy is two to three cycles of chemotherapy followed by assessment of response, with additional therapy given only to patients with some evidence of tumor regression (whether or not criteria for partial response are satisfied). It saves patients with resistant disease from the unnecessary toxicity of further treatment with an ineffective regimen. Patients with poor performance status and more than minimal weight loss benefit only minimally if at all from chemotherapy, and the risk:benefit ratio of such treatment is markedly increased in such patients.

In discussing chemotherapy with eligible patients, it is important to highlight chances of response, symptomatic relief, and duration of response as well as the median length of survival extension of approximately 2 months. Patients can then make an educated decision, weighing these data against the toxicity, inconvenience, and expense of therapy.

Chemotherapy in Regionally Advanced/Inoperable NSCLC

Patients without overt distant metastases who cannot undergo a curative surgical resec-

tion due to regionally advanced disease have a dismal prognosis (33). In addition to their poor long-term survival, they often experience severe local symptoms. Response rates of chemotherapy are up to twice as high in this group of patients (50 to 60% for cisplatin-based chemotherapy) than in those with distant metastatic disease (34). In the U.S., chest irradiation alone has been the standard treatment for inoperable stage III NSCLC patients. The efficacy of chemotherapy may be better prior to the administration of irradiation or surgery. An initial response may facilitate subsequent local therapy by making radiotherapy more effective against less bulky disease or making a marginally resectable tumor resectable. Finally, one hopes that local shrinkage of tumor parallels eradication of distant micrometastases and thus provides an in vivo sensitivity assay for the overall effect of a chemotherapy regimen.

Chemotherapy with Radiation

Radiotherapy has been the standard treatment for inoperable stage III NSCLC. "Definitive" radiotherapy in doses of 6000 cGy and above achieves local control in more than half the patients but cures only 5 to 7% of them (6). Since the vast majority of inoperable stage III patients die of distant metastases, thoracic radiotherapy alone does not prolong the overall survival of this group of patients over that with minimal or no therapy in controlled studies (35). It is logical to add a systemic modality such as chemotherapy to attempt to improve these dismal results.

Several studies have compared radiotherapy alone with chemoradiotherapy sequentially or concurrently (36–44). Perhaps the most significant of the North American trials was conducted by the Cancer and Leukemia Group B (CALGB) (36). Some 155 evaluable patients with inoperable stage III NSCLC, good performance status (PS, 0 to 1), and less than 5% weight loss were randomly assigned to receive thoracic radiotherapy, 60 Gy over 6 weeks or the same radiotherapy preceded by cisplatin at 100 mg/m^2 on days 1 and 29 and vinblastine at 5 mg/m^2 on days 1, 8, 15, 22, and 29. Radiation was begun 3 weeks after the second dose of cisplatin in the chemotherapy group (day 50). Patients with malignant pleural effusions or involvement of supraclavicular lymph nodes were excluded, as they are recognized to have a very poor prognosis. Furthermore, pleural effusions cannot be comprehensively radiated to potentially curative doses. After a median follow-up of 34 months, median survival was 13.8 months for the combined modality arm and 9.7 months for the radiotherapy group ($p = .0066$). With 2 more years of follow-up, this difference was maintained, with only 7% survivors in the radiotherapy group, compared with 19% survival in the chemoradiotherapy arm (37). These results were confirmed in a subsequent three-arm Radiation Therapy Oncology Group (RTOG) trial that had similar entry criteria and added a third arm for hyperfractionated radiation to the two treatment arms of the CALGB study (38). Eligibility criteria were similar except that supraclavicular nodal metastases were permitted. Patients with inoperable stage II cancer were also eligible, although only 5% of the 452 evaluable patients were in this group. Median survivals were as follows: chemotherapy plus radiation, 13.8 months; hyperfractionated radiotherapy, 12.3 months; and standard radiation, 11.4 months. Survival in the chemotherapy plus radiation arm was significantly superior ($p = .03$).

Additionally, two European trials have shown similar results. French investigators treated 253 patients with locally advanced squamous cell or large cell lung carcinoma by randomizing them to receive thoracic radiotherapy (65 Gy in 26 fractions over 45 days) or the same radiotherapy sandwiched between 3 cycles each of pre- and postradiation chemotherapy with vindesine, cyclophosphamide, cisplatin, and lomustine (VCPC) (39). Two-year survival was 14% with radiotherapy alone and 21% with combined modality therapy, with these differences approaching statistical significance ($p = .08$). A subsequent communication with longer follow-up revealed a statistically significant difference in median survival (10 vs. 12 months, $p = .02$) (40).

An EORTC study compared split-course radiotherapy alone (30 Gy in 10 fractions over 2 weeks followed by a 3-week rest period before another 25 Gy in 10 fractions over 2 weeks) with the same radiotherapy with daily (6 mg/m^2) or weekly (30 mg/m^2) cisplatin (41). Some 331 patients with locally advanced inoperable NSCLC were randomly assigned to the three arms. Survival was significantly improved in the radiotherapy–daily cisplatin group compared with radiotherapy alone ($p = .009$). The respective 1-, 2-, and 3-year survival figures were 54%, 26%, and 16%, compared with 46%, 13%, and 2%. Survival in the radiotherapy–weekly cisplatin arm was

intermediate and not significantly different from either of the other two groups. More than 80% of patients receiving cisplatin experienced nausea and vomiting, and these side effects were severe in 27%.

The metaanalysis performed by the Non-Small Cell Lung Cancer Collaborators Group also analyzed survival in the locally advanced setting for patients receiving radiotherapy with or without chemotherapy (46). Trials that used chemotherapy as a radiosensitizer were excluded (Table 53.3). Analyses were again carried out for two different categories of chemotherapy: long-term alkylators ("old" chemotherapy) and cisplatin-based ("modern" chemotherapy) regimens. Twenty-two randomized trials involving 3033 patients were identified. Only two of the individual trials gave significantly better results in favor of chemotherapy in the conventional sense. The pooled hazard ratio (HR) for chemotherapy was 0.91 (95% CI, 0.84–0.98; $p = .01$) corresponding to a 3% absolute benefit in survival (from 16% to 19%) at 2 years. The HR for cisplatin-based chemotherapy was 0.87, yielding a survival benefit of 4% at 2 years. No clear benefit or detriment of long-term alkylators could be found in this particular setting (HR, 1.02; 95% CI, 0.86–1.20).

There are some negative studies as well, some of which can be criticized for inadequate power, using non-cisplatin-based chemotherapy, or omitting some prescribed therapy (42, 44, 45). It is reasonable to now consider two cycles of neoadjuvant therapy with cisplatin and vinblastine prior to radiotherapy as a standard treatment for locally advanced inoperable NSCLC against which newer therapies can be compared. This would of course apply only to patients similar to those enrolled in these trials, i.e., good-performance-status patients, with minimal or no weight loss, without malignant pleural effusions, and perhaps without supraclavicular lymph node metastases.

It is attractive to hypothesize that the results of combined modality therapy can be improved further by concurrent chemoradiotherapy with platinum compounds, as they possess radiosensitizing properties in addition to their systemic activity against NSCLC (47). A three-arm randomized RTOG trial is currently comparing the better arm of the CALGB study (cisplatin plus vinblastine followed by radiotherapy) with the same chemotherapy given concurrently with radiotherapy and a third arm of concurrent cisplatin, oral etoposide, and radiotherapy. CALGB has recently completed accrual on a randomized study designed to better their previous results by adding weekly carboplatin during radiotherapy and comparing it with radiotherapy alone after two cycles of cisplatin and vinblastine. The final results of this study are awaited.

Chemotherapy with Surgery

Neoadjuvant chemotherapy before surgery in NSCLC has some specific goals. These include increasing the resection rate, achieving better local control, and, most importantly, improving cure rates by eradicating micrometastases. There have been multiple phase II or "feasibility" studies looking at neoadjuvant chemotherapy or chemoradiotherapy prior to surgery in locally advanced NSCLC (48–53).

The main conclusions that can be drawn from such pilot studies are that this approach is feasible, that operative mortality is not increased due to prior chemotherapy, that in some studies 15 to 20% of patients achieve a pathologic complete remission, and that some patients will live long term. There was a poor correlation between radiographic and pathologic responses in these studies. In contrast to the large number of these pilot studies, only two randomized trials of neoadjuvant chemotherapy have been published (54, 55).

In a Spanish study, 60 eligible patients with stage IIIA NSCLC were randomly assigned to immediate surgery or three cycles of neoadjuvant chemotherapy with mitomycin, ifosfamide, and cisplatin followed by surgery (54). Approximately three-fourths of the patients underwent preoperative mediastinal staging. All patients received postoperative mediastinal radiation. Flow cytometery and K-*ras* oncogene analyses were also performed on tumors, although pathologic material was inadequate or unavailable for these tests in some patients. The trial was stopped prematurely, since prospectively specified early discontinuation criteria were fulfilled. There was an overwhelming improvement in median survival of the chemotherapy group (26 vs. 8 months, $p < .001$). The small sample size and poorer-than-expected survival of the control group diminish the generalizability of these results.

Another phase III randomized trial, also involving only 60 patients with stage IIIA NSCLC, was performed at M. D. Anderson Cancer Center (55). Patients received three cycles of preoperative chemotherapy with cyclophosphamide, cis-

platin, and etoposide or proceeded immediately to surgery. Identical postoperative chemotherapy was administered to those who responded to preoperative chemotherapy. No radiotherapy was given. This trial was also stopped early due to a significant survival advantage for the group receiving chemotherapy, with a 3-year survival of 56% versus 15% (median, 64 months vs. 11 months; logrank $p < .008$). There was significant myelosuppression observed with this chemotherapy; 80% of patients experienced severe neutropenia. This was also a small study with contamination of the groups with patients with more favorable T3N0 disease and relatively short follow-up.

There is clearly not sufficient evidence at present to change the standard of care in this stage of the disease. It is not unlikely that a survival benefit exists for chemotherapy with surgery, because it has been demonstrated in inoperable stage III and stage IV disease; the magnitude of this benefit, however, is much greater than expected and may be an artefact of the small numbers of patients enrolled in these studies. Furthermore, there are no reproducible criteria for "operable" or "potentially operable" NSCLC, since this assessment is left to the discretion of the thoracic surgeon. An NCI high-priority intergroup study is currently randomizing patients with pathologically proven N2 NSCLC to surgery or completion radiotherapy after neoadjuvant concurrent chemoradiotherapy with 2 cycles of cisplatin and etoposide. This trial will attempt to assess the benefit, if any, of surgery in patients with N2 disease.

Chemotherapy in Surgically Resected NSCLC

RATIONALE FOR ADJUVANT CHEMOTHERAPY

Trials of postoperative (adjuvant) chemotherapy are attractive because the pathologic stage is known for all patients. In addition, chemotherapy that is modestly active in the metastatic setting theoretically may be more efficacious when given to patients with minimal tumor burden. Response rates to the same chemotherapy are twice as high in the earlier stages of NSCLC than in stage IV disease. In one animal model of transplanted tumors, treatment prior to the development of visible nodules resulted in cure, but once such lesions were apparent, simple excision or chemotherapy alone failed to cure the disease

(56). A combination of the two modalities cured 50% of the animals. Unfortunately, human cancer is spontaneous, not transplanted and has doubled in size for perhaps many years (with the potential to develop increasing genetic abnormalities) before diagnosis.

Despite this appealing rationale and preclinical evidence, the most recent randomized trials of postoperative treatments employing "better" chemotherapy have shown marginal or no benefit in patients with NSCLC.

ADJUVANT CHEMOTHERAPY TRIALS WITH OR WITHOUT RADIATION

More than three decades ago, the Veterans Administration Surgical Oncology Group conducted a series of trials using alkylating agents alone or in combination with methotrexate or hydroxyurea that showed no survival benefit for chemotherapy (9, 57, 58). These trials have been criticized for using relatively inactive drugs and inadequate staging by current standards.

The next generation of adjuvant trials used cisplatin-based chemotherapy, still considered the most active combination regimens for NSCLC. The Lung Cancer Study Group (LCSG) completed three important trials of postoperative chemotherapy in NSCLC. Some 164 patients with locally advanced disease who had positive resection margins or tumor in the highest sampled mediastinal lymph node were randomized to receive postoperative radiotherapy (40 Gy split course to the mediastinum and the residual tumor site) or the same radiotherapy given concurrently with six cycles of CAP (cisplatin 40 mg/m², doxorubicin 40 mg/m², and cyclophosphamide 400 mg/m²) (59). Relatively fewer patients in the CAP group had nodal disease. Disease-free survival was superior in patients treated with chemotherapy (median, 8 vs. 14 months; $p = .004$), but overall survival was not significantly better (median, 13 vs. 20 months; $p = .133$).

In another trial, the same group of investigators compared immunotherapy with CAP chemotherapy after complete resection of stage II and IIIA NSCLC (60). This study randomized 141 patients with adenocarcinoma and large cell carcinoma to 6 cycles of CAP or a postoperative dose of intrapleural BCG (bacillus Calmette-Guerin) and 18 months of oral levamisole. Median time to recurrence was 7 months longer in the chemotherapy arm than with immunotherapy ($p = .018$). There was a borderline significant

improvement in survival of 7 months (median, 23 vs. 16 months; $p = .078$). Only 58% of the planned chemotherapy doses were delivered. Twelve of 62 eligible patients assigned to CAP did not receive any treatment.

Finally, the LCSG randomized 269 resected T2N0 (84%) or T1N1 (16%) patients to receive four cycles of CAP every 4 weeks or observation postoperatively (61). Survival was the same in the two arms after more than 6 years of follow-up. Compliance with chemotherapy was poor.

Although two of the above studies demonstrate some biological activity of chemotherapy in the postoperative adjuvant setting, no additional large American adjuvant trials have been completed.

A Finnish study involving 110 node-negative patients (T1-3N0), randomized them to six cycles of CAP chemotherapy or observation after a complete surgical resection (62). There was no significant difference in survival when the imbalance in surgical procedures was corrected (twice as many pneumonectomy patients in the observation group). A third of the patients received fewer than three cycles.

Two published randomized Japanese trials involving two to three cycles of adjuvant chemotherapy failed to show a survival benefit (63, 64). Most recently, a summary of another three-arm randomized trial from Japan became available (65). Some 310 evaluable patients were randomized to observation (control) or chemotherapy with either cisplatin plus vindesine plus UFT (a combination of ftorafur and uracil in a 1:4 molar ratio that is thought to result in increased levels of 5-FU in the tumor) or UFT alone. Five-year survival rates were 49%, 60.6%, and 64.1%, respectively (among three groups: $p = .043$).

It is possible that there is a survival benefit rendered by adjuvant therapy but it is too small to be detected by most of these trials. The metaanalysis performed by the Non-Small Cell Lung Cancer Collaborators Group also evaluated surgery (sometimes followed by chest irradiation) with or without postoperative chemotherapy in 14 randomized controlled trials involving almost 4000 patients (66). Seven of these trials used cisplatin-based regimens, and five used long-term alkylators (Table 53.2). Only three of these trials independently demonstrated statistically significant survival differences. The pooled hazard ratio (HR) for cisplatin-based trials was 0.87 (95% CI, 0.73–1.04; $p = .124$), demonstrating a nonsignificant 13% relative reduction in death rate for patients given chemotherapy. This translates into a 5% survival benefit at 5 years (from 47% to 52%). The pooled HR of long-term alkylators is 1.16 (CI, 1.05–1.25; $p = .004$), equivalent to a 16% relative detriment in the death rate and worsening of survival by 6% at 5 years.

These chemotherapy regimens were perhaps suboptimal, and the compliance with chemotherapy was sometimes poor. In breast cancer, substandard doses of chemotherapy compromise survival significantly compared with standard doses of the same chemotherapy (67). It is conceivable that delivering full doses of current optimal chemotherapy for an adequate number of cycles to most patients will prove more beneficial than substandard doses for 2 to 3 cycles given to fewer than two-thirds of the patients (as seen in some of the negative trials). An NCI intergroup high-priority protocol currently randomizes completely resected stage II and IIIA patients (with N1 or N2 disease) to radiotherapy alone (50.4 Gy/28 fractions/6 weeks) or identical radiotherapy and concurrent chemotherapy with cisplatin 60 mg/m² on day 1, and VP-16 120 mg/m² on days 1–3, beginning within 24 hours of radiotherapy, every 28 days for four cycles. Patients with mediastinal adenopathy above 1.5 cm currently require a preoperative mediastinoscopy. Patients are stratified by nodal status, histology, weight loss, and type of lymph node dissection. Accrual is brisk, but results will not be available for several years.

Novel Drugs in NSCLC

As mentioned above, until recently, only five drugs were known to have "activity" (15% response rate) in NSCLC. In the past few years, several new agents entering clinical trials have shown equal or higher response rates (Table 53.4). Camptothecins, taxanes, gemcitabine, vinorelbine, edatrexate, and high-dose epirubicin have been tested successfully in phase I and II trials, and some of these agents are now entering phase III testing or trials of combination therapy (68).

Taxanes (paclitaxel and docetaxel) mediate their cytotoxicity by promoting microtubular assembly and subsequent inhibition of disassembly, making the mitotic spindle extremely stable and arresting cells in the G_2 or M phase of the cell cycle. Paclitaxel (Taxol) is derived from the bark of the Pacific yew *Taxus brevifolia*, whereas the precursor of docetaxel (Taxotere), baccatin

Table 53.4. Newer Active Agents in NSCLC

Agent	RR
Paclitaxel	21–24%
Docetaxel	28–33%
Gemcitabine	20–70%
Edatrexate	10–30%
Irinotecan	20–32%
Vinorelbine	29–35%
Epirubicin[a]	19–36%
Topotecan	0–47%

Reprinted with permission from Jahanzeb M, Ihde DC. Role of adjuvant therapy in patients with surgically resected non-small cell lung cancer. Cancer Control 1994;1(5):471.
[a]High-dose.

III, is obtained from the needles of the European yew *Taxus baccata*.

Paclitaxel has been tested in phase II studies in NSCLC in doses of 200 to 250 mg/m² infused over 24 hours every 3 weeks, yielding 21 to 24% response rates in previously untreated patients (69, 70). Only occasional partial responses have been reported in patients who have failed or progressed after cisplatin-based therapy (71). Its main toxicities are myelosuppression and neuropathy. Other toxicities include stomatitis, diarrhea, bradycardia, other cardiac arrhythmias, myalgias, arthralgias, rash, alopecia, and occasional anaphylaxis (possibly related to the cremophor vehicle).

Docetaxel is a semisynthetic derivative of the parent compound. Dose-dependent neutropenia was the dose-limiting toxicity in phase I trials. In phase II trials, 60 to 100 mg/m² of docetaxel has been infused over 1 to 2 hours, yielding response rates of 21 to 33% in previously untreated patients and 21% in cisplatin-refractory patients (72–76). Significant side effects, in addition to myelosuppression, have been peripheral edema with or without pleural effusions, asthenia, dermatitis, and hypersensitivity. The incidence of edema, rash, and infusion-related reactions has been high, despite premedication with prednisone in some cases (77).

Vinorelbine (Navelbine), another antimitotic agent, is a semisynthetic vinca alkaloid that acts by depolymerizing microtubules, resulting in dissolution of the mitotic spindle (78). Modification in the catharenthine ring imparts certain pharmacologic properties to this drug, particularly a higher selectivity for the mitotic microtubules than for axonal microtubules, thereby improving its therapeutic index (79). It has been tested alone and in combinations in numerous phase I and II trials in addition to a large phase III randomized trial in NSCLC (28, 80–82). An initial phase II French study evaluated 78 previously untreated patients with inoperable NSCLC (81). Most of these patients had metastatic disease, although some patients with earlier stages were included. Vinorelbine was given at 30 mg/m^2 intravenously every week. A 29.4% partial response rate was observed. Grade 3 or 4 neutropenia was observed in 12.5% of patients, and two patients died of neutropenic sepsis. A multicenter phase II trial in the U.S. used oral vinorelbine to treat 156 evaluable patients with metastatic NSCLC and revealed a 12% response rate and an estimated median survival of 29 weeks (82). Significant gastrointestinal toxicity was seen in addition to myelosuppression.

After establishing vinorelbine's activity in NSCLC, a phase III randomized trial was carried out in Europe (28). This three-arm study randomized 612 previously untreated, inoperable NSCLC patients (56% with stage IV disease) to receive vinorelbine at 30 mg/m^2 weekly, either alone or in combination with cisplatin at 120 mg/m^2 every 4 to 6 weeks, or to a third arm combining the same dose and schedule of cisplatin with vindesine 3 mg/m^2 weekly. Responses in 569 evaluable patients were as follows: vinorelbine alone, 14%; vinorelbine plus cisplatin, 30%; and cisplatin plus vindesine, 19%. The corresponding median survivals were 31, 40, and 32 weeks, significantly favoring the cisplatin plus vinorelbine combination over vinorelbine alone. The incidence of grade 3 and 4 neutropenia was 52%, 78%, and 47%, respectively. Considerably more neurotoxicity occurred in the cisplatin plus vindesine arm than in the other two arms. There were two toxic deaths in each of the vinorelbine arms. Vinorelbine has recently been approved by the Food and Drug Administration in the United States for intravenous use in NSCLC.

Camptothecins (irinotecan (CPT-11), topotecan, and 9-aminocamptothecin) are derivatives of *Camptotheca accuminata* and belong to a unique class of drugs, the topoisomerase I inhibitors (83). Topoisomerase I is one of the critical nuclear enzymes required in resolving topologic problems in DNA (such as overwinding and underwinding) that normally arise during replication and transcription. Its inhibition by camptothecins causes single-stranded DNA breaks.

Irinotecan is a water-soluble compound that is converted to its active metabolite, SN-38, in vivo. Initial studies in Japan revealed activity in NSCLC. In a group of 72 previously untreated NSCLC patients with stage IIIB and IV disease, a 32% response rate was noted at a dose of 100 mg/m^2 every week (84). The median survival was 42 weeks. Grade 3 or 4 leukopenia was seen in 25% of patients, and diarrhea occurred in 21%. Combinations of this drug with cisplatin (85), etoposide, paclitaxel, cyclophosphamide, and doxorubicin are in different stages of development or execution.

Topotecan is another semisynthetic hydrophilic camptothecin analogue that in preliminary studies seems to be active against many malignancies. Phase I studies demonstrated leukopenia to be the dose-limiting toxicity. The addition of granulocyte-macrophage colony-stimulating factor (G-CSF) shortens the duration of neutropenia but does not allow dose escalation, as thrombocytopenia then becomes dose limiting (86). An intravenous bolus of 1.5 to 2 mg/m^2 daily for 5 days every 3 weeks was selected for initial phase II development. After initial evidence of activity, subsequent reports have been less encouraging, with response rates between 0 and 13% (87–89). Combinations with other agents such as paclitaxel, doxorubicin, and cisplatin are currently being evaluated (90, 91).

9-Aminocamptothecin is a newly formulated analogue of irinotecan. It has shown preliminary evidence of activity in NSCLC but is just entering clinical trials (92).

Edatrexate, a methotrexate analogue, blocks DNA synthesis by competing for the folate-binding site of the enzyme dihydrofolate reductase (DHFR), inhibiting the synthesis of nucleotides necessary for DNA replication. There is some evidence that edatrexate is preferentially taken up by tumor tissue and may have higher efficacy than methotrexate (93). In three phase II trials in NSCLC, response rates ranged between 10% and 32% at a dose of 80 mg/m^2/week (94–96). Mucositis was seen in most patients and was the dose-limiting toxicity. Myelosuppression was mild. Combinations with mitomycin and vinblastine as well as with cyclophosphamide and cisplatin have been evaluated (97, 98). Another combination with paclitaxel was investigated on the basis of data suggesting in vitro synergy of the two drugs (99).

Gemcitabine (deoxyfluorocytidine), another antimetabolite, is a fluorinated derivative of cytosine arabinoside with activity in solid tumors. After documenting in vitro activity (100), the initial maximal tolerated dose was determined to be 790 mg/m^2, although higher doses have been

Table 53.5. Influence of Modern Combination Chemotherapy on Survival among Patients with Small Cell Lung Cancer

	Survival	
Era	Limited Disease	Extensive Disease
Prechemotherapy		
Supportive care (median)	3 months	1.5 months
Surgery (5 year)	<1%	—
Radiotherapy (5 year)	1–3%	—
Chemotherapy		
Single agent (median)	6 months	4 months
Combination (median)	10–14 months	7–11 months
Combination (5 year)	2–8%	0–1%
Combination + XRT (median)	12–20 months	7–11 months
Combination + XRT (5 year)	6–15%	0–1%

Modified from Ihde DC. Drug therapy: chemotherapy of lung cancer. N Engl J Med 1992;327:1434. Reprinted by permission of the New England Journal of Medicine. Copyright 1992. Massachusetts Medical Society. All rights reserved.

used since without significant toxicities (101, 102). Myelosuppression (thrombocytopenia with relative sparing of granulocytes) and reversible liver toxicity have been dose limiting. Flulike symptoms were also commonly observed in addition to nausea, vomiting, peripheral edema, and rashes. Several phase II studies in NSCLC have consistently shown response rates above 20% (range, 21 to 24%) (101–103). Its relatively modest myelosuppression makes gemcitabine an attractive drug for use in drug combinations.

CHEMOTHERAPY IN SMALL CELL LUNG CANCER (SCLC)

Small cell lung cancer comprises 20% of lung cancer cases and is a distinct entity in terms of its clinical behavior, response to therapy, and prognosis (4). Stages I-IIIB are generally grouped together as "limited stage" in contrast to stage IV, which is termed "extensive." It is quite common, however, to include only patients with disease confined to one hemithorax and encompassable in one radiation port in the "limited" category. This definition of limited stage also excludes patients with malignant pleural effusions. With current standard staging techniques, 60 to 70% of SCLC patients have clinically detectable distant metastases at the time of presentation. Of the remaining patients, the vast majority have occult metastatic disease as evidenced in the past by the extremely high distant failure rate after local treatment alone (104). Chemotherapy is indicated in virtually all cases of SCLC (105). This particular tumor type is initially very sensitive

to chemotherapy, with overall response rates as high as 90% or more for those with limited-stage disease and 65 to 85% for extensive-disease patients (106). The corresponding complete response rates are 50 to 60% and 15 to 30%, respectively. Unfortunately, most responders relapse, and relapsed disease is virtually incurable. Although chemotherapy provides symptomatic relief in the vast majority of patients and results in a four- to fivefold increase in median survival compared with patients not receiving chemotherapy (Table 53.5), over 90% of patients eventually succumb to their disease (4).

Chemotherapy with Single Agents

Cyclophosphamide was the first agent shown to be efficacious in increasing survival in SCLC (10). Several other agents were subsequently found to be active. These include etoposide (VP-16) (107, 108), teniposide (VM-26) (109), doxorubicin (110), vincristine (111), carboplatin (112), hexamethylmelamine, mechlorethamine, procarbazine, lomustine, ifosfamide, and methotrexate (113). Cisplatin had lower response rates, perhaps because it was principally tested as a single agent in patients who had progressed on or after chemotherapy (113). In addition to having more resistant disease, such patients also tend to have poorer performance status and greater tumor burden. Carboplatin, a cisplatin analogue, produced objective responses in 18 of 30 patients (60%) (107) when given to previously untreated patients. Similarly, etoposide has a 40 to 80% response rate in previously untreated patients but only a 10 to 25% response rate as second-line therapy. The same is true of teniposide.

These observations stimulated discussion about the best way to test new agents in SCLC (113). A potentially active agent could be missed if tested in refractory patients. The concern that previously untreated patients could progress rapidly and never receive the chance to benefit from known active agents if initial use of a new experimental agent proved ineffective was addressed in a randomized trial by the Eastern Cooperative Oncology Group (114). The group did not find clear evidence of such detriment in this study involving 86 patients, provided standard combination chemotherapy was given to patients whose tumors progressed or were stable after one or two cycles, respectively, of the experimental drug.

Some investigators have also suggested testing experimental agents in relapsed patients who have enjoyed an unmaintained remission for more than 3 months, as they are much more likely to respond again (e.g., to cisplatin plus etoposide 50% of the time, even if this was their initial therapy) (115–117). Since second complete remissions are unlikely and cure almost impossible, these patients, who have generally lived beyond the expected median survival, are not deprived of potentially life-saving therapy by testing new agents. Another suggested strategy for new-drug evaluation is to lower the threshold of activity to a 10% response rate if a drug is tested in previously treated patients (113).

Combinations of active agents have been found more efficacious in producing tumor regression than single agents and have, in general, replaced single-agent therapy (118). Combination chemotherapy is mandatory for good-risk patients, for example, those with limited-stage disease and good performance status (approximately 25% of all SCLC patients belong to this group). There is still a role for single agents where excess toxicity of combination chemotherapy is anticipated without curative potential, for example, in treating extensive-disease patients who are elderly or any patient with poor performance status (the remaining 75% or so of SCLC patients). There is as yet no completed properly randomized trial comparing single-agent with combination chemotherapy in this latter group of patients.

Etoposide is arguably the most active agent in SCLC, yielding response rates as high as 80% in limited-stage disease. Given its efficacy and favorable toxicity profile, it seemed a logical drug to use as a single agent. With evidence sug-

gesting schedule dependency of etoposide (119) and availability of an oral formulation, a trial of daily oral etoposide was carried out in patients with relapsed disease (120). Responses were observed in 24% of the patients despite prior exposure to intravenous etoposide in most of these responders. A subsequent study demonstrated the efficacy of daily oral etoposide in a group of elderly patients (121). This regimen has not been compared directly with single-agent intravenous administration of etoposide. The combination of daily oral etoposide with cisplatin, when compared with intravenous etoposide with the same total cisplatin dose in a prospective, randomized trial in extensive-disease patients, showed no improvement in efficacy but an increase in fatal neutropenia (122).

Combination Chemotherapy

The superiority of combination chemotherapy over single agents in SCLC patients was demonstrated by randomized trials almost two decades ago. When two or three drug combinations of cyclophosphamide-containing chemotherapy were compared with cyclophosphamide alone, the response rates and survival were found to be superior for the combinations (118, 123–125). If combination chemotherapy is used in doses that produce only minimal myelosuppression, it is no more efficacious than single agents (126). Several uncontrolled studies have shown that high-dose cyclophosphamide can produce therapeutic results similar to those with standard combinations (127, 128). It is reasonable to conclude that the therapeutic results achieved depend on both the activity and dose of the agents used. Most combinations have included two to four drugs, as a higher number would necessitate greater dose reductions of individual drugs, which could compromise efficacy.

Alkylating agents such as cyclophosphamide and the nitrosoureas were initially the mainstay of therapy for SCLC and were often combined with vincristine and methotrexate (129, 130). Doxorubicin was added to the drug armamentarium as its activity became apparent. Its cumulative cardiotoxicity was realized later (131). Cyclophosphamide, doxorubicin, and vincristine (CAV) was the most frequently used North American drug regimen in the 1980s. With the advent of platinum compounds (cisplatin and later its analogue carboplatin), the cisplatin and etoposide combination (PE) became widely used. This combination was particularly attractive because of its tolerability with radiotherapy and because it had similar efficacy and less myelosuppression than CAV (132). The radiosensitizing properties of cisplatin are also attractive in the setting of combined-modality therapy (47).

In vitro studies have suggested synergy between cisplatin and etoposide, although it is questionable whether there is more than an additive effect clinically (11). The addition of etoposide to other active combinations in extensive-disease patients does not seem to improve their efficacy but adds more toxicity (133).

Carboplatin seems to have comparable efficacy and a different toxicity profile than cisplatin, with less nausea, vomiting, neurotoxicity, ototoxicity, and nephrotoxicity but more myelosuppression (134). Unlike cisplatin, it can be given without extensive intravenous hydration, which makes it attractive for outpatient administration. However, the new class of antiemetic agents (5-HT3 receptor blockers) has made cisplatin much more tolerable (32). Myelosuppression is usually the dose-limiting toxicity of most active agents except vincristine and, to a lesser extent, cisplatin.

Dose Intensity

In a comparison of two different dose levels of a combination of cyclophosphamide, methotrexate, and lomustine (CMC; 500/10/50 vs. 1000/15/100 mg/m^2), the higher-dose combination produced higher response rates and better survival (135). Most current chemotherapy programs produce moderately severe myelosuppression. Further dose escalation beyond these standard doses, with or without growth factor support, or even myeloablative doses with marrow rescue, have not been shown to improve survival to date (136–138). A randomized comparison of standard doses of cisplatin and etoposide with high or more toxic doses of the same agents failed to show a benefit (139). The same conclusion was reached after a randomized comparison of high-dose and conventional-dose regimens of cyclophosphamide, doxorubicin, and vincristine in two different studies (140, 141).

In one randomized trial, moderately intensive doses of cyclophosphamide, doxorubicin, and etoposide (CAE) were given with G-CSF support or placebo. Although G-CSF significantly decreased the incidence of febrile neutropenia and shortened the duration of neutropenia in the treatment group, life-threatening myelosuppression was still more common with these doses of chemotherapy than with the standard (but apparently no less efficacious) doses of CAV (136). CAE was also used in another European randomized trial with growth factors or placebo; twice as many dose reductions and febrile-neutropenic episodes were observed in the placebo group, without any significant differences in response rates or survival between the two groups (142). Before recommending routine administration of higher doses of chemotherapy necessitating growth factor support, increased efficacy of such regimens needs to be demonstrated.

Although multiple phase II trials of consolidation of initial chemotherapy remission with high-dose chemotherapy followed by autologous bone marrow transplantation (ABMT) have demonstrated conversions of partial remissions to complete remissions, no clear improvement in survival has occurred. One such trial prospectively enrolled 29 consecutive extensive-disease SCLC patients to receive late intensive combined-modality therapy (LICMRX) with ABMT if they achieved a good response to 12 weeks of conventional induction chemotherapy (138). Of the 10 patients found eligible for LICMRX after initial therapy, only 8 received it. Only one PR was converted to a CR, and there were no 2-year survivors, compared with 10% 2-year survival among 78 similar patients previously treated with similar induction therapy without subsequent LICMRX.

One randomized trial has compared consolidation chemotherapy with either one cycle of standard doses of cyclophosphamide, etoposide, and BCNU or myeloablative doses of these agents with ABMT after induction therapy (four cycles of cyclophosphamide, doxorubicin, methotrexate, and vincristine repeated every 3 weeks for three cycles, followed by prophylactic cranial irradiation, and then two more cycles of cisplatin and etoposide) (137). Although many partial remissions were converted to complete remissions with dose-intensive therapy and time to relapse was significantly delayed, no survival advantage was demonstrated.

A metaanalysis of patient outcomes in 60 published trials of different doses and schedules of CAV, PE, and CAE regimens likewise found no evidence of benefit with increased dose intensity of any of these regimens (143).

Alternating Chemotherapy

Because early emergence of resistant clones has been a widely accepted explanation for resistant relapse in the vast majority of SCLC patients responding to chemotherapy, a strategy to address this problem has been the focus of intense investigation. Using a mathematical model, Goldie and Coldman proposed that early use of as many drugs as possible by alternating mutually non-cross-resistant drugs might help circumvent this problem (144). A trial by the National Cancer Institute of Canada (NCIC) compared six cycles of CAV with six cycles of CAV and PE alternating with each other in extensive-disease SCLC patients. They found that the second regimen produced superior survival (median, 9.6 vs. 8.0 months; $p = .03$) (145). It is unclear whether this was due to the addition of etoposide/cisplatin or to the alternating schedule. When a subsequent trial in limited-stage patients compared six cycles of alternating CAV and PE with sequential administration of 3 cycles of CAV before 3 cycles of PE, no survival difference could be demonstrated (146). Later, two randomized three-arm studies compared CAV and PE with alternation of these two regimens and found no increase in efficacy with alternation overall, although a subset analysis of one study indicated benefit for the limited-stage-disease patients (132, 147). It is possible that including etoposide/cisplatin in the treatment of limited, but not extensive, disease patients is associated with improved survival, as demonstrated in an early randomized trial of the Southeastern Cancer Study Group that assigned patients to receive or not receive two cycles of cisplatin and etoposide if they responded to induction with six cycles of CAV (148).

The concept of alternating myelosuppressive and nonmyelosuppressive drugs in rapid succession with weekly chemotherapy has also been tested in SCLC. One such regimen (CODE) consists of cisplatin 25 mg/m² weekly for 9 weeks; vincristine 1 mg/m² in weeks 1, 2, 4, and 8; doxorubicin 25 mg/m² on day 1; and etoposide 80 mg/m²/day × 3 days in weeks 1, 3, 5, 7, and 9. It yielded a 61-week median survival for a favorable group of extensive-disease patients in a Canadian trial (149). Complete responders also received thoracic radiotherapy in this trial. A Japanese group was unable to reproduce these results and achieved a median survival of only 35 weeks (150). Subsequent addition of growth factors increased this figure to 59 weeks. The NCIC and the SWOG are currently comparing CODE with alternating CAV/PE in extensive-disease patients.

The SWOG tested a regimen of cyclophosphamide and doxorubicin in week 1; methotrexate, leucovorin, and vincristine in week 2; cisplatin and etoposide in week 3; and vincristine in week 4 for a total of 4 cycles in a group of 76 patients with limited or extensive disease, achieving a median survival of 16.6 months without using thoracic radiotherapy (151).

The first randomized comparison of weekly chemotherapy with standard 3-week (PE alternating with CAV every 3 weeks × 6 cycles vs. PE alternating with ifosfamide and doxorubicin every week × 12 weeks) chemotherapy revealed no benefit of the weekly treatment (152). A similar Belgian study reached the same conclusion (153).

The current standard of care is either four cycles of PE in standard doses or six cycles of PE alternating with CAV. Six cycles of CAV is also acceptable in extensive-disease patients. However, using an active and different regimen after disease progression rarely achieves a durable complete remission, indicating that in an important sense these regimens are not truly non-cross-resistant.

Almost all of the novel active drugs discussed in the NSCLC section (camptothecins, taxanes, vinorelbine, gemcitabine, edatrexate) are also active in SCLC in phase I/II trials, although there are even fewer available clinical data to comment on the possible clinical impact of these agents in this disease. Novel "doublets" of some of these drugs will be tested in extensive-stage SCLC patients by one cooperative group in the near future.

Optimal Duration of Chemotherapy

Prolonged administration of chemotherapy, sometimes for up to 2 years, has customarily been given in the past, but recent randomized trials have shown that this approach has no survival benefit (154, 155). Protracted treatment may increase the initial duration of response, but the increased toxicity of drug administration easily outweighs its benefits. Although relapsed disease is essentially incurable, selected patients have up to a 50% chance of responding again to combination chemotherapy with PE (115–117) or with single-agent etoposide (120, 121). Patients with a significant period of unmaintained remission (usually >3 months) have a much better chance of responding than those who relapse early or have primary refractory disease. It is therefore appropriate to discontinue chemotherapy after 4 to 6 cycles and resume at relapse if

Table 53.6. Commonly Used Effective Chemotherapy Regimens in Small Cell Lung Cancer[a]

Drug	Dose, Route and Day of Administration
PE	
Cisplatin	25 mg/m^2 i.v. days 1–3 or 80 mg/m^2 day 1
Etoposide	80–100 mg/m^2 i.v. days 1–3
CAV	
Cyclophosphamide	1000 mg/m^2 i.v. day 1
Doxorubicin	45 mg/m^2 i.v. day 1
Vincristine	2 mg i.v. day 1
CAE	
Cyclophosphamide	1000 mg/m^2 i.v. day 1
Doxorubicin	45 mg/m^2 i.v. day 1
Etoposide	50 mg/m^2 i.v. days 1–5
CAV and PE	
Alternating cycles of CAV and PE as above every 3 weeks	

Modified from: Brain MC, Carbone PP. Current therapy in hematology and oncology—3. St Louis: Mosby-Year Book 1988:214. With permission.
[a]Cycles repeated every 3 weeks.

possible. Commonly used chemotherapeutic regimens in SCLC are listed in Table 53.6.

Chemotherapy and Chest Irradiation

As with chemotherapy, SCLC patients are exquisitely sensitive to radiation; 70 to 90% of previously untreated thoracic tumors regress with this modality alone (156, 157). The high local failure rate after chemotherapy alone and the poor overall survival provided the impetus for combining thoracic radiotherapy (TRT) with chemotherapy to attempt to improve the therapeutic results. If early emergence of resistant tumor clones is a real problem, and these clonogens can then metastasize, it would be logical to expect better survival if the addition of another modality helps in their early eradication or minimizes their later development.

Several randomized trials of chemotherapy and TRT versus chemotherapy alone have documented the benefit of combined-modality therapy in extending survival in addition to improving local tumor control. Two metaanalyses were recently published combining data from all such controlled trials (158, 159). Only one of these, however, obtained individual patient data for analysis (158). TRT was found to render a modest survival advantage (3-year survival, 8.9 ±

0.9% vs. 14.3 ± 1.1%; $p = .001$) at the cost of a modest increase in toxicity. With cisplatin-based therapy currently in vogue and the availability of three-dimensional conformal treatment planning of radiotherapy, this toxicity should decrease further and perhaps improve the risk:benefit ratio to favor combined-modality therapy.

The optimal timing of initiation of TRT has not been resolved. A CALGB randomized trial involving 399 evaluable patients evaluated addition of thoracic irradiation with the first or fourth cycle of chemotherapy in limited-stage SCLC patients. A control arm of chemotherapy alone was also included (160). While both radiotherapy arms were found to be superior to chemotherapy alone in response and survival, there was a trend in favor of the program of late, as opposed to early, TRT. A randomized trial by the NCIC reported significantly improved local control and survival when TRT was started with the second cycle, compared with the sixth cycle, of an alternating regimen of six cycles of CAV/PE (161). Hyperfractionated radiotherapy with concurrent PE chemotherapy has shown promising results in phase II trials, but a randomized trial comparing it with conventional radiation did not show a benefit for this strategy (162). However, the two-year survival of more than 40% for both arms of this study was quite impressive for a cooperative group trial. Currently, standard treatment of limited-stage SCLC is to combine chemotherapy with TRT in all patients whose pulmonary function and performance status permit delivery of both modalities.

Prophylactic Cranial Irradiation

As the brain is a very common site of first recurrence from chemotherapy-induced response in SCLC, prophylactic cranial irradiation (PCI) has been advocated for patients who are complete responders to initial treatment (163). This approach clearly decreases relapses in the brain but has not been shown to improve survival, probably because of the systemic nature of the relapse manifesting itself in the brain first (164–169). In addition, documentation of late neuropsychiatric sequelae, possibly related to cranial irradiation, has dampened the enthusiasm for this approach (170). Many oncologists have evolved strong, but poorly justified, opinions about this strategy, making it difficult to carry out randomized trials. A recently published European multicenter randomized controlled trial of PCI (2400 cGy in eight fractions) involving 300 SCLC patients who had achieved a complete remission after induction chemotherapy, again revealed a significant decrease in brain and "brain-first" relapses without significant survival benefit ($p = .14$) (171). If the efficacy of chemotherapy is significantly improved in the future, PCI could potentially play an important role in improving survival.

Drug Resistance and Its Modulation

Recent evidence suggests that multiple-drug resistance (MDR) can be explained in many tumors on the basis of expression of a product of the *mdr-1* gene (172). This is a transmembrane glycoprotein (P-170) that actively transports a wide variety of substances from the intracellular compartment. It is abundantly expressed in normal tissues that may be exposed to potentially toxic substances (e.g., intestines, kidney) and may provide a natural protective mechanism against xenotoxins. In tumors, it serves to pump out chemotherapeutic agents, particularly those derived from biologic sources, despite wide variations in their chemical structure. It enhances efflux of drugs such as doxorubicin, etoposide, and the vinca alkaloids (173). SCLC has low levels of expression of *mdr*. A variety of agents have been found to have the ability to block this pump (e.g., verapamil, quinine, cyclosporin A, and cyclosporin D derivative PSC 833) and may eventually prove useful in circumventing this problem. However, this strategy would not address the multiple other mechanisms of resistance that malignant SCLC cells are likely to possess.

CHEMOPREVENTION

Since the vast majority of lung cancer patients are former or current smokers, second smoking-related malignancies, particularly NSCLC, are not uncommon in long-term survivors of SCLC (174, 175). In fact, 16% of such patients later died of NSCLC in one recently published study (175). As retinoids have shown promise in reducing the frequency of second primary cancers in patients with squamous cell carcinoma of head and neck (176) and resected stage I NSCLC (177), this approach with a placebo control is being investigated in patients with completely resected stage I NSCLC, and a trial in long-term survivors of SCLC is being organized.

FUTURE DIRECTIONS IN LUNG CANCER

Conventional chemotherapy has yielded poor response rates in NSCLC. These responses are usually partial and short-lived and render a modest survival advantage at best. The ongoing development of novel agents and their combinations with better response rates holds some promise for the future. These agents, when combined with older drugs, with each other, or with radiation and used in optimal schedules could significantly improve response rates, but the ultimate goal is to improve survival. Combinations of cisplatin and paclitaxel as well as cisplatin and vinorelbine are being tested against other cisplatin-based regimens. At least one cooperative group is planning to test cisplatin-based combinations of paclitaxel and vinorelbine with ifosfamide-based combinations of these drugs in stage IV NSCLC.

If increased efficacy of these regimens is suggested in advanced disease, they should be tested in the adjuvant setting, as more than half the patients resected with curative intent have micrometastases at the time of surgery.

We also clearly need new strategies to deal with SCLC, as optimizing the schedules of doses and fractionation of currently available chemotherapeutic agents and radiotherapy has achieved only modest gains in survival over the past decade. Novel active agents, such as the camptothecins and taxanes, and new analogues of older agents (e.g., vinorelbine, gemcitabine) may contribute to our armamentarium but are not expected to cure most of the patients.

SCLC is a largely preventable disease, as almost all cases are attributable to smoking. Besides cessation of smoking, which is perhaps the most effective way of reducing mortality from this disease (and from NSCLC), novel targets for chemotherapy need to be explored. Elucidation of the role of peptide growth hormones has led to strategies of intervention at several levels, including antisense strategies to block gene transcription or translation (178–180). Interfering with signal transduction is another approach under investigation. When scientifically appropriate, all of these techniques should undergo evaluation in the clinical setting.

SUMMARY

Lung cancer is the single greatest cause of cancer-related mortality in the United States. Despite significant improvements in therapeutic approaches, almost 9 out of 10 patients with this diagnosis still succumb to their disease. More than a dozen active chemotherapeutic agents that can predictably produce responses in lung cancer are either in use or under development.

However, there is no known curative chemo-therapeutic regimen for NSCLC to date. In fact, there is no single regimen that could be considered standard universally. All appropriate chemotherapy candidates should therefore be encouraged to enter clinical trials whenever possible. It is through such studies that some modest progress has been made. Chemotherapy has had an increasing role in the management of lung cancer over the last two to three decades. Besides being indicated in virtually all SCLC patients, it can now be considered standard therapy in selected patients with inoperable NSCLC, when combined with radiation, and can be considered as a single modality in good-risk patients with metastatic NSCLC.

REFERENCES

1. Wingo PA, Tong T, Bolden B. Cancer statistics 1995. CA: Cancer J Clin 1995;45(1):12–13.
2. Smoking and health in the Americas. A 1992 report of the Surgeon General, in collaboration with the Pan American Health Organization. U.S. Department of Health and Human Services, Public Health Service, Centers for Disease Control, National Center for Chronic Disease Prevention and Health Promotion, Office on Smoking and Health.
3. Lilenbaum RC, Green MR. Novel chemotherapeutic agents in the treatment of non-small-cell lung cancer. J Clin Oncol 1993;11:1391–1402.
4. Ihde DC. Drug therapy: chemotherapy of lung cancer. N Engl J Med 1992;327:1434–1441.
5. Mountain CF. A new international staging system for lung cancer. Chest 1986;89:225S–233S.
6. Ihde DC, Minna JD. Non-small cell lung cancer part II: treatment. Curr Probl Cancer 1991;15:109–154.
7. Gralla RJ, Kris MG. Chemotherapy in non-small cell lung cancer: results of recent trials. Semin Oncol 1988;15:2–5.
8. Lynch JP, Ware PF, Gaensler JP. Nitrogen mustard in the treatment of inoperable bronchogenic carcinoma. Surgery 1950;27:368–385.
9. Hughes FA, Higgins G. Veterans Administration surgical adjuvant lung cancer chemotherapy study: present status. J Thorac Cardiovasc Surg 1962;44:295–308.
10. Green RA, Humphrey E, Close H, et al. Alkylating agents in bronchogenic carcinoma. Am J Med 1969;46:516–525.
11. Schabel FM, Trader MW, Laster WR, et al. *Cis*-dichlorodiamine platinum (II). Combination chemotherapy and cross-resistance with tumors of mice. Cancer Treat Rep 1979;63:1459–1473.
12. Rapp E, Pater JL, Willan A, et al. Chemotherapy can prolong survival in patients with advanced non-small-cell lung cancer—report of a Canadian multicenter randomized trial. J Clin Oncol 1988;6:663–641.
13. Cartei G, Cartei F, Cantone A, et al. cisplatin-cyclophosphamide-mitomycin combination chemotherapy with supportive care versus supportive care alone for treatment of metastatic non-small cell lung cancer. J Natl Cancer Inst 1993;85:794–799.
14. Quoix E, Dietemann A, Charbonneau J, et al. Disseminated non small cell lung cancer (NSCLC): a randomised trial of chemotherapy (CT) versus palliative care (PC) (abstract). Lung Cancer 1988;4:a127.
15. Callerino R, Tummarello D, Guidi F, et al. A randomized trial of alternating chemotherapy versus best supportive care in advanced non-small cell lung cancer. J Clin Oncol 1991;9:1453–1461.
16. Woods RL, Williams CS, Page J, et al. A randomized trial of cisplatin and vindesine versus supportive care only in advanced non-small cell lung cancer. Br J Cancer 1990;61:608–611.
17. Tummarello D, Guidi F, Profiri E, et al. Chemotherapy vs. supportive care in advanced non-small cell lung cancer; a prospective randomized trial (abstract). Lung Cancer 1984:a127.
18. Kassa S, Lund E, Host H, et al. Combination chemotherapy versus symptomatic treatment in patients with non-small cell lung cancer; extensive disease (abstract). Proceedings of the 5th European Conference of Clinical Oncologists. 1989;ECCO-5:46.
19. Ganz PA, Figlin RA, Haskell CM. Supportive care versus supportive care and combination chemotherapy in metastatic non-small cell lung cancer. Cancer 1989;63:1271–1278.
20. Bunn PA Jr. The expanding role of cisplatin in the treatment of non-small-cell lung cancer. Semin Oncol 1989;16:10–21.
21. Klastersky J, Sculier JP, Ravez P, et al. A randomized study comparing a high and a standard dose of cisplatin in combination with etoposide in the treatment of advanced non-small-cell lung carcinoma. J Clin Oncol 1986;4:1780–1786.
22. Gandara DR, Crowley J, Livingston RB, et al. Evaluation of cisplatin intensity in metastatic non-small-cell lung cancer: a phase III study of the Southwest Oncology Group. J Clin Oncol 1993;11:873–878.
23. Gralla RJ, Casper ES, Kelsen DP, et al. Cisplatin and vindesine combination chemotherapy for advanced carcinoma of the lung: a randomized trial investigating two dosage schedules. Ann Intern Med 1981;95:414–420.
24. Elliott JA, Ahmedzai S, Hole D, et al. Vindesine and cisplatin combination chemotherapy compared with vindesine as a single agent in the management of non-small cell lung cancer: a randomized study. J Cancer Clin Oncol 1984;20:1025–1032.
25. Einhorn LH, Loehrer PJ, Williams SD, et al. Random prospective study of vindesine versus vindesine plus cisplatin plus mitomycin C in advanced non-small cell lung cancer. J Clin Oncol 1986;4:1037–1043.
26. Bonomi PD, Finkelstein DM, Ruckdeschel JC, et al. Combination chemotherapy versus carboplatin or iproplatin followed by combination chemotherapy in stage IV non-small cell lung cancer: an Eastern Cooperative Oncology Group study. In: Bunn PA Jr, Canetta R, Ozols RF, Rozencweig M, eds. Carboplatin (JM-8) current perspectives and future directions. Philadelphia: WB Saunders, 1990:307–316.
27. Bunn PA. The treatment of non-small cell lung cancer; current perspectives and controversies, future directions. Semin Oncol 1994;6:21(3 Suppl):49–59.
28. Le Chevalier T, Brisgand D, Douillard JY, et al. Randomized study of vinorelbine and cisplatin versus vindesine and cisplatin versus vinorelbine alone in advanced non-small-cell lung cancer: results of a Euro-

pean multicenter trial including 612 patients. J Clin Oncol 1994;12:360–367.

29. Stewart LA, Pignon J, Parmar MKB, Souhami R, et al. A meta-analysis using individual data patient from randomized clinical trials (RCTs) of chemotherapy (CT) in non-small-cell lung cancer (3) survival in the supportive care setting (abstract). Proc Am Soc Clin Oncol 1994;13:1118.

30. Albain KS, Crowley JJ, LeBlanc M, et al. Survival determinants in extensive-stage non-small-cell lung cancer; the Southwest Oncology Group experience. J Clin Oncol 1991;9:1618–1626.

31. Jaakkimainen L, Goodwin PJ, Pater J, Warde P, Murray N, Rapp E. Counting the costs of chemotherapy in a National Cancer Institute of Canada randomized trial in non-small-cell lung cancer. J Clin Oncol 1990;8:1301–1309.

32. Cubeddu LX, Hoffmann IS, Fuenmayer NT, et al. Efficacy of ondansetron (GR 38032F) and the role of serotonin in cisplatin induced nausea and vomiting. N Engl J Med 1990;322:810–816.

33. Martini N, Flehinger BJ. The role of surgery in N2 lung cancer. Surg Clin North Am 1987;67:1037–1049.

34. Kris MG, Gralla RJ, Wertheim MS, et al. Trial of the combination of mitomycin, vindesine, and cisplatin in patients with advanced non-small-cell lung cancer. Cancer Treat Rep 1986;70:1091–1096.

35. Johnson DH, Einhorn LH, Bartolucci A, et al. Thoracic radiotherapy does not prolong survival in patients with locally advanced, unresectable non-small cell lung cancer. Ann Intern Med 1990;113:33–38.

36. Dillman RO, Seagren SL, Propert KJ, et al. A randomized trial of induction chemotherapy plus high-dose radiation versus radiation alone in stage III non-small-cell lung cancer. N Engl J Med 1990;323:940–945.

37. Dillman RO, Seagren SL, Propert KJ, et al. A randomized trial of induction chemotherapy plus high-dose radiation versus radiation alone in stage III non-small-cell lung cancer (abstract). Proc Am Soc Clin Oncol 1993;12:1092.

38. Sause W, Scott C, Taylor S, et al. Radiation Therapy Oncology Group (RTOG) 88-08 and Eastern Cooperative Oncology Group (ECOG) 4588: preliminary results of a phase III trial in regionally advanced unresectable non-small-cell lung cancer. J Natl Cancer Inst 1995;87:198–205.

39. LeChevalier T, Arriagada R, Quoix E, et al. Radiotherapy alone versus combined chemotherapy and radiotherapy in non-resectable non-small-cell lung cancer: first analysis of a randomized trial in 353 patients. J Natl Cancer Inst 1991;83:417–423.

40. LeChevalier T, Arriagada R, Quoix E, et al. Radiotherapy alone versus combined chemotherapy and radiotherapy in non-resectable non-small-cell lung cancer (letter). J Natl Cancer Inst 1992;84:58.

41. Schaake-Koning C, van den Bogaert W, Dalesio O, et al. Effects of concomitant cisplatin and radiotherapy on inoperable non-small-cell lung cancer. N Engl J Med 1992;326:524–530.

42. Morton RF, Jett JR, McGinnis WL, et al. Thoracic radiation therapy alone compared with combined chemoradiotherapy for locally unresectable non-small cell lung cancer. A randomized, phase III trial. Ann Intern Med 1991;115:681–686.

43. Mattson K, Holsti LR. Holsti P, et al. Inoperable non-small cell lung cancer; radiation with or without chemotherapy. Eur J Cancer Clin Oncol 1988;24:477–482.

44. Trovo MG, Minatel E, Franchin G, et al. Radiotherapy (RT) versus RT enhanced by cisplatin (DDP) in stage III non-small cell lung cancer (NSCLC); randomized cooperative study (abstract). Lung Cancer 1991;7:162.

45. Ansari R, Tokars R, Fisher K, et al. A phase III study of thoracic irradiation with or without concomitant cisplatin in loco-regional unresectable non-small cell lung cancer (NSCLC): a Hoosier Oncology Group (HOG) protocol (abstract). Proc Am Soc Clin Oncol 1991;10:241.

46. Pignon J, Stewart L, Souhami R, et al. A meta-analysis using individual data patient from randomised clinical trials (RCTs) of chemotherapy (CT) in non-small-cell lung cancer (2) survival in the locally advanced (LA) setting (abstract). Proc Am Soc Clin Oncol 1994;13:1109.

47. Double EB. Keynote address: platinum-radiation interactions. NCI Monogr 1988;6:315–319.

48. Strauss GM, Langer MP, Elias AD, et al. Multimodality treatment of stage IIIA non-small-cell lung carcinoma: a critical review of the literature and strategies for future research. J Clin Oncol 1992;10:829–838.

49. Skarin A, Jockelson M, Sheldon T, et al. Neoadjuvant chemotherapy in marginally resectable stage III M$_0$ non-small cell lung cancer: long-term follow-up in 41 patients. J Surg Oncol 1989;40:266–274.

50. Gralla RJ. Preoperative and adjuvant chemotherapy in non-small cell lung cancer. Semin Oncol 1988;15:8–12.

51. Weiden PL, Piantadosi S. Preoperative chemotherapy (cisplatin and fluorouracil) and radiation therapy in stage III non-small-cell lung cancer: a phase II study of the Lung Cancer Study Group. J Natl Cancer Inst 1991;83:266–273.

52. Burkes RL, Ginsberg RJ, Shepherd FA, et al. Induction chemotherapy with mitomycin, vindesin and cisplatin for stage III unresectable non-small-cell lung cancer: results of the Toronto phase II trial. J Clin Oncol 1992;10:580–586.

53. Taylor SG IV, Trybula M, Bonomi PD, et al. Simultaneous cisplatin fluorouracil infusion and radiation followed by surgical resection in regionally localized stage III, non-small cell lung cancer. Ann Thorac Surg 1987;43:87–91.

54. Rosell R, Gomez-Codina J, Camps C, et al. A randomized trial comparing preoperative chemotherapy plus surgery with surgery alone in patients with non-small-cell lung cancer. N Engl J Med 1994;330:153–158.

55. Roth J, Fossella F, Komaki R, et al. A randomized trial comparing perioperative chemotherapy plus surgery with surgery alone in resected stage III non-small-cell lung cancer (abstract). Proc Am Soc Clin Oncol 1994;13:1106.

56. Humpherys SR, Karrer K. Relationship of dose schedules to the effectiveness of adjuvant chemotherapy. Cancer Chemother Rep 1970;54:379–397.

57. Shields TW, Robinette D, Keehn RJ. Bronchial carcinoma treated by adjuvant cancer chemotherapy. Arch Surg 1974;109:329–333.

58. Shields TW, Humphrey EW, Eastridge CE, et al. Adjuvant cancer chemotherapy after resection of carcinoma of the lung. Cancer 1977;40:2057–2062.

59. Lung Cancer Study Group. The benefit of adjuvant treatment for resected locally advanced non-small-cell lung cancer. J Clin Oncol 1988;6:9–17.

60. Holmes EC, Gail M. Surgical adjuvant therapy for stage II and stage III adenocarcinoma and large cell undifferentiated carcinoma. J Clin Oncol 1986;4:710–715.

61. Feld R, Rubinstein L, Thomas PA, et al. Adjuvant chemotherapy with cyclophosphamide, doxorubicin, and cisplatin in patients with completely resected stage I non-small-cell lung cancer. J Natl Cancer Inst 1993;85:299–306.

62. Niiraanen A, Niitamo-Korhonen S, Kouri M, et al. Adjuvant chemotherapy after radical surgery for non-small-cell lung cancer: a randomized study. J Clin Oncol 1992;10:1927–1932.

63. Ichinose Y, Hara N, Ohta M, et al. Postoperative adjuvant chemotherapy in non-small-cell lung cancer: prognostic value of DNA ploidy and postrecurrent survival. J Surg Oncol 1991;46:15–20.

64. Ohta M, Shimoyama M, Sawamura K, et al. Adjuvant chemotherapy for completely resected stage III non-small-cell lung cancer. J Thorac Cardiovasc Surg 1993;106:703–708.

65. Wada H, Hitomi S, Teramatsu T. Postoperative non-small cell lung cancer: a prospective randomized trial of cisplatin (P)-vindesine (VDS)-UFT vs UFT alone vs control (abstract). Proc Am Soc Clin Oncol 1994; 13:1084.

66. Stewart LA, Pignon JP, Arriagada R, et al. A meta-analysis using individual patient data from randomized clinical trials (RCTS) of chemotherapy (CT) in non-small-cell lung cancer (NSCLC): (1) survival in the surgical setting (abstract). Proc Am Soc Clin Oncol 1994;13:1117.

67. Wood WC, Budman DR, Korzun AH, et al. Dose and dose intensity of adjuvant chemotherapy for stage II, node-positive breast carcinoma. N Engl J Med 1994;330:1253–1259.

68. Feigal EG. New agents in non-small cell lung cancer. Cancer Control 1994;1:(5)474–484.

69. Chang A, Kim K, Glick J, Anderson T, Karp D, Johnson D. Phase II study of taxol in patients with stage IV non-small cell lung cancer (NSCLC); the Eastern Cooperative Oncology Group (ECOG) results (abstract). Proc Am Soc Clin Oncol 1992;11:981.

70. Murphy WK, Winn RJ, Fossella FV, et al. A phase II study of Taxol 9NSC 125973) in patients (pts) with non-small cell lung cancer (NSCLC) (abstract). Proc Am Soc Clin Oncol 1992;11:985.

71. Murphy WK, Winn RJ, Huber M, et al. Phase II study of Taxol (T) in patients (pt) with non-small cell lung cancer (NSCLC) who have failed platinum (P) containing chemotherapy (CTX) (abstract). Proc Am Soc Clin Oncol 1994;13:1224.

72. Cerny T, Wanders J, Kaplan S, et al. Taxotere is an active drug in non small cell lung (NSCLC) cancer: a phase II trial of the early clinical trials group (ECTG) (abstract). Proc Am Soc Clin Oncol 1993;12:1103.

73. Rigas JR, Francis PA, Kris MG, et al. Phase II trial of Taxotere in non-small cell lung cancer (NSCLC) (abstract). Proc Am Soc Clin Oncol 1993;12:1121.

74. Burris H, Eckardt J, Fields S, et al. Phase II trials of Taxotere in patients with non-small cell lung cancer (abstract). Proc Am Soc Clin Oncol 1993;12:1116.

75. Watanabe K, Yokoyama A, Furuse K, et al. Phase II trial of docetaxel in previously untreated non-small cell lung cancer (NSCLC) (abstract). Proc Am Soc Clin Oncol 1994;13:1095.

76. Fossella FV, Lee JS, Shin DM, et al. Taxotere (docetaxel DTXL), an active agent for platinum-refractory non-small cell lung cancer (NSCLC): preliminary report of a phase II study (abstract). Proc Am Soc Clin Oncol 1994;13:1115.

77. Miller VA, Rigas JR, Kris MG, et al. Phase II trial of docetaxel given at a dose of 75 mg/m^2 with prednisone premedication in non-small cell lung cancer (NSCLC) (abstract). Proc Am Soc Clin Oncol 1994; 13:1226.

78. Fellous A, Ohayon R, Vacassin T, et al. Biochemical effects of vinorelbine on tubulin and associated proteins. Semin Oncol 1989;16:9–14.

79. Nelson RL, Dyke RW, Root MA. Comparative pharmacokinetics of vindesine, vincristine and vinblastine in patients with cancer. Cancer Treat Rev 1980; 7(Suppl)17–24.

80. Rahmani R, Boré P, Cano JP, Herrera A, Krikorian A. Phase I trial of escalating doses or orally administered Navelbine (NVB): part I—pharmacokinetics (abstract). Proc Am Soc Clin Oncol 1989;8:289.

81. Depierre A, Lemarie E, Dabouis G, Garnier G, Jacoulet P, Dalphin JC. A phase II study of Navelbine (vinorelbine) in the treatment of non-small-cell lung cancer. Am J Clin Oncol 1991;14(2):115–119.

82. Vokes EE, Rosenberg R, Jahanzeb M, et al. Multicenter phase II study of weekly oral vinorelbine for stage IV non-small cell lung cancer. J Clin Oncol 1995; 13:637–644.

83. Hsiang YH, Hertzberg R, Hecht S, Liu LF. Camptothecin induces protein-linked DNA breaks via mammalian DNA topoisomerase I. J Biol Chem 1985; 260:14873–14878.

84. Fukuoka M, Negoro S, Niitani H, Taguchi T. A phase II study of a new camptothecin derivative, CPT-11 in previously untreated non-small cell lung cancer (NSCLC) (abstract). Proc Am Soc Clin Oncol 1990; 9:873.

85. Masuda N, Fukuoka M, Takada M, et al. CPT-11 dose in combination with cisplatin for advanced non-small cell lung cancer (abstract). Proc Am Soc Clin Oncol 1992;11:978.

86. Rowinsky E, Sartorius S, Grochow L, et al. Phase I and pharmacologic study of topotecan, an inhibitor of topoisomerase I, with granulocyte colony stimulating factor (G-CSF): toxicologic differences between concurrent and post-treatment G-CSF administration (abstract). Proc Am Soc Clin Oncol 1992;11:284.

87. Perez-Soler R, Glisson BS, Kane J, et al. Phase II study of topotecan in patients with non-small cell lung cancer (NSCLC) previously untreated (abstract). Proc Am Soc Clin Oncol 1994;13:1223.

88. Murphy B, Saltz L, Sirott M, et al. Granulocyte-colony stimulating factor (G-CSF) does not increase the maximum tolerated dose (MTD) in a phase I study of topotecan (T) (abstract). Proc Am Soc Clin Oncol 1992; 11:379.

89. Lynch, TJ Jr, Kalish L, Strauss G, et al. Phase II study of topotecan in metastatic non-small-cell lung cancer. J Clin Oncol 1994;12:347–352.

90. Lilenbaum RC, Rosner GL, Ratain MJ, et al. Phase I study of Taxol and topotecan in patients with advanced solid tumors (CALGB 9362) (abstract). Proc Am Soc Clin Oncol 1994;13:319.

91. Tolcher AW, O'Shaughnessy JA, Weiss RB, et

al. A phase I study of topotecan (a topoisomerase I inhibitor) in combination with doxorubicin (a topoisomerase II inhibitor) (abstract). Proc Am Soc Clin Oncol 1994;13:422.

92. Potmesil M, Canellakis ZN, Wall ME, et al. Pharmacokinetic studies of 9-amino-20 (S)-camptothecin (NSC 603071) and parent 20 (S)-camptothecin (NSC 94600): cellular partitioning (abstract). Proc of Am Assoc Cancer Res 1992;33:2586.

93. Sirotnak FM, DeGraw JI, Schmid FA, Goutas LJ, Moccio DM. New folate analogs of the 10-deaza-aminopterin series. Further evidence for markedly increased antitumor efficacy compared with methotrexate in ascitic and solid murine tumor models. Cancer Chemother Pharmacol 1984;12:26–30.

94. Shum KY, Kris MG, Gralla RJ, Burke MT, Marks LD, Heelan RT. Phase II study of 10-ethyl-10-deaza-aminopterin in patients with stage III and IV non-small-cell lung cancer. J Clin Oncol 1988;6:446–450.

95. Souhami RL, Rudd RM, Spiro SG, Allen R, et al. Phase II study of edatrexate in stage III and IV non-small-cell lung cancer. Cancer Chemother Pharmacol 1992;30:465–468.

96. Lee JS, Libshitz HI, Murphy WK, Jeffries D, Hong WK. Phase II study of 10-ethyl-10-deaza-aminopterin (10-EdAM; CGP 30 694) for stage IIIB or IV non-small cell lung cancer. Invest New Drugs 1990; 8:299–304.

97. Gralla RJ, Lee JS, Kris RL, et al. Multicenter, randomized trials comparing the combination of edatrexate, mitomycin and vinblastine (EMV) with mitomycin and vinblastine (MV) in 673 patients with stage III and IV non-small cell lung cancer (abstract). Proc Am Soc Clin Oncol 1994;13:1161.

98. Lee JS, Libshitz HI, Fossella FV, et al. Edatrexate improves the antitumor effects of cyclophosphamide and cisplatin against non-small cell lung cancer. Cancer 1991;68:959–964.

99. Fennelly DM, Rigas JR, Chou D, et al. Phase I trial of edatrexate plus paclitaxel using an administration schedule with demonstrated in vitro synergy (abstract). Proc Am Soc Clin Oncol 1994;13:1232.

100. Hertel LW, Boder GB, Kroin JS, et al. Evaluation of the antitumor activity of gemcitabine (2′,2′-difluoro-2′-deoxycytidine). Cancer Res 1990;50:4417–4422.

101. Abbruzzese JL, Grunewald R, Weeks EA, et al. A phase I clinical, plasma, and cellular pharmacology study of gemcitabine. J Clin Oncol 1991;9:491–498.

102. Abratt RP, Bezwoda WR, Falkson G, Goedhals L, et al. Efficacy and safety profile of gemcitabine in non-small-cell lung cancer: a phase II study. J Clin Oncol 1994;12:1535–1540.

103. Anderson H, Lund B, Bach F, Thatcher N, Walling J, Hansen HH. Single-agent activity of weekly gemcitabine in advanced non-small-cell lung cancer: a phase II study. J Clin Oncol 1994;12:1821–1826.

104. Mountain CF. Clinical biology of small cell carcinoma: relationship to surgical therapy. Semin Oncol 1978;5:272–279.

105. Ihde DC. Current status of therapy in small cell lung carcinoma. Cancer 1984;54:2722–2728.

106. Seifter EJ, Ihde DC. Therapy for small cell lung cancer: a perspective on two decades of clinical research. Semin Oncol 1988;15(3):278–299.

107. Pedersen AG, Hansen HH. Etoposide (VP-16) in the treatment of lung cancer. Cancer Treat Rev 1983; 10:245–264.

108. Cohen MH, Broder LE, Fossieck BE, Ihde DC, Minna JD. Phase II clinical trial of weekly administration of VP-16–213 in small cell bronchogenic carcinoma. Cancer Treat Rep 1977;61:489–490.

109. Pedersen AG, Bork E, Osterlind K, Dombernowsky P, Hansen HH. Phase II study of teniposide in small cell carcinoma of the lung. Cancer Treat Rep 1984;68:1289–1291.

110. Cortes EP, Takita H, Holland JF. Adriamycin in advanced bronchogenic carcinoma. Cancer 1974; 34:518–525.

111. Shaw RK, Bruner JA. Clinical evaluation of vincristine (NSC-67574). Cancer Chemother Rep 1964; 42:45–48.

112. Smith IE, Harland SJ, Robinson BA, et al. Carboplatin: a very active new cisplatin analog in the treatment of small cell lung cancer. Cancer Treat Rep 1985; 69:43–46.

113. Grant SC, Gralla RJ, Kris MG, Orazem J, Kitsis EA. Single-agent chemotherapy trials in small-cell lung cancer, 1970–1990: the case for studies in previously treated patients. J Clin Oncol 1992;10:484–498.

114. Ettinger DS, Finkelstein DM, Abeloff MD, et al. Justification for evaluating new anticancer drugs in selected untreated patients with extensive-stage small-cell lung cancer: an Eastern Cooperative Oncology Group randomized study. J Natl Cancer Inst 1992; 84(14):1077–1084.

115. Evans WK, Osaba D, Feld R, et al. Etoposide and cisplatin: an effective treatment for relapse in small cell lung cancer. J Clin Oncol 1985;3:65–71.

116. Einhorn LH, Williams SD, Loehrer PJ. Platinum (P) + VP-16 chemotherapy for refractory small cell lung carcinoma (abstract 689). Proc Am Assoc Cancer Res 1984;10:174.

117. Batist G, Carney DN, Cowna KH, et al. Etoposide and cisplatin in previously treated small cell lung cancer: clinical trial and in vitro correlates. J Clin Oncol 1986;4:982–986.

118. Lowenbraun S, Bartolucci A, Smalley RV, et al. The superiority of combination chemotherapy over single agent chemotherapy in small cell lung carcinoma. Cancer 1979;44:406–413.

119. Slevin ML, Clark PI, Joel SP, et al. An randomized trial to evaluate the effect of schedule on the activity of etoposide in small-cell lung cancer. J Clin Oncol 1989;7:1333–1340.

120. Einhorn LH, Pennington K, McClean J. Phase II trial of daily oral VP-16 in refractory small cell lung cancer: a Hoosier Oncology Group study. Semin Oncol 1990;17:32–35.

121. Johnson DH, Greco FA, Strupp J, Hande KR, Hainsworth JD. Prolonged administration of oral etoposide in patients with relapsed or refractory small-cell lung cancer: a phase II trial. J Clin Oncol 1990; 8:1613–1617.

122. Miller AA, Herndon J, Hollis D, et al. Phase III study of 21 day oral versus 3 day IV etoposide (E) in combination with IV cisplatin (C) in extensive small cell lung cancer: a Cancer and Leukemia Group B study (CALGB 9033) (abstract). Proc Am Soc Clin Oncol 1994;13:1074.

123. Carroll KB, Moussalli H, Brown D, Thatcher N. A comparison between a single agent short course chemotherapy regimen and a quadruple prolonged

course regimen for small-cell bronchogenic carcinoma of limited extent. Br J Dis Chest 1983;77:171–178.

124. Edmonson JH, Lagakos SW, Selawry OS, et al. Cyclophosphamide and CCNU in the treatment of inoperable small cell carcinoma and adenocarcinoma of the lung. Cancer Treat Rep 1976;60:925–932.

125. Aisner J, Alberto P, Bitran J, et al. Role of chemotherapy in small cell lung cancer: a consensus report of the International Association for the Study of Lung Cancer workshop. Cancer Treat Rep 1983;67:37–43.

126. Weiss RB. Small cell carcinoma of the lung: therapeutic management. Ann Intern Med 1975; 88:522–531.

127. Ettinger DS, Karp JE, Abeloff MD, Burke PJ, Braine HG. Intermittent high-dose cyclophosphamide chemotherapy for small cell carcinoma of the lung. Cancer Treat Rep 1978;62:413–424.

128. Souhami RL, Finn G, Gregory WM, et al. High-dose cyclophosphamide in small-cell carcinoma of the lung. J Clin Oncol 1985;3:958–963.

129. Eagan RT, Maurer LH, Forcier RJ, Tulloh M. Combination chemotherapy and radiation therapy in small cell carcinoma of the lung. Cancer 1973;32:371–379.

130. Nixon DW, Carey RW, Suit HD, Aisenberg AC. Combination chemotherapy in oat cell carcinoma of the lung. Cancer 1975;36:867–872.

131. Ferrans VJ. Anthracycline cardiotoxicity. Adv Exp Med Biol 1983;161:519–532.

132. Roth BJ, Johnson DH, Einhorn LH, et al. Randomized study of cyclophosphamide, doxorubicin, and vincristine versus etoposide and cisplatin versus alternation of these two regimens in extensive small-cell lung cancer: a phase III trial of the Southeastern Cancer Study Group. J Clin Oncol 1992;10:282–291.

133. Jackson VD, Zexan PJ, Caldwell RD, et al. VP-16-213 in combination chemotherapy with chest irradiation for small cell lung cancer: a randomized trial of Piedmont Oncology Association. J Clin Oncol 1984; 2:1343–1351.

134. Bunn PA Jr. Clinical experiences with carboplatin (paraplatin) in lung cancer. Semin Oncol 1992; 19:1–11.

135. Cohen MH, Creaven PJ, Fossieck BE Jr, et al. Intensive chemotherapy of small cell bronchogenic carcinoma. Cancer Treat Rep 1977;61:349–354.

136. Crawford J, Ozer H, Stoller R, et al. Reduction by granulocyte colony-stimulating factor of fever and neutropenia induced by chemotherapy in patients with small-cell lung cancer. N Engl J Med 1991; 325:164–170.

137. Humblet Y, Symann M, Bosly A, et al. Late intensification chemotherapy with autologous bone marrow transplantation in selected small-cell carcinoma of the lung: a randomized study. J Clin Oncol 1987;5:1864–1873.

138. Ihde DC, Deisseroth AB, Lichter AS, et al. Late intensive combined modality therapy followed by autologous bone marrow infusion in extensive-stage small-cell lung cancer. J Clin Oncol 1986;4:1443–1454.

139. Ihde DC, Mulshine JL, Kramer BS, et al. Prospective randomized comparison of high-dose and standard-dose etoposide and cisplatin chemotherapy in patients with extensive-stage small cell lung cancer. J Clin Oncol 1994;12:2022–2034.

140. Johnson DH, Einhorn LH, Birch R, et al. A randomized comparison of high-dose versus conventional-dose cyclophosphamide, doxorubicin and vincristine for extensive-stage small-cell lung cancer: a phase III trial of the Southeastern Cancer Study Group. J Clin Oncol 1987;5:1731–1738.

141. Figueredo AT, Hryniuk WM, Strautmanis I, Frank G, Rendell S. Co-trimoxazole prophylaxis during high-dose chemotherapy of small-cell lung cancer. J Clin Oncol 1985;3:54–64.

142. Trillet-Lenoir V, Green J, Manegold C, et al. Recombinant granulocyte colony stimulating factor reduces the infectious complications of cytotoxic chemotherapy. Eur J Cancer 1993;29A:319–324.

143. Klasa JR, Murray N, Coldman AJ. Dose intensity meta-analysis of chemotherapy regimens in small cell carcinoma of the lung. J Clin Oncol 1991;9:499–508.

144. Goldie JH, Coldman AJ, Gudauskas GA. Rationale for the use of alternating non-cross-resistant chemotherapy. Cancer Treat Rep 1982;66:439–449.

145. Evans WK, Feld R, Murray N, et al. Superiority of alternating non-cross-resistant chemotherapy in extensive small cell lung cancer. Ann Intern Med 1987;107:451–458.

146. Feld R, Evans WK, Coy P, et al. Canadian multicenter randomized trial comparing sequential and alternating administration of two non-cross-resistant chemotherapy combinations in patients with limited small-cell carcinoma of the lung. J Clin Oncol 1987; 5:1401–1409.

147. Fukuoka M, Furuse K, Saijo N, et al. Randomized trial of cyclophosphamide, doxorubicin, and vincristine versus cisplatin and etoposide versus alternation of these regimens in small-cell lung cancer. J Natl Cancer Inst 1991;83:855–861.

148. Einhorn LH, Crawford J, Birch R, et al. Cisplatin plus etoposide consolidation following cyclophosphamide, doxorubicin and vincristine in limited small-cell lung cancer. J Clin Oncol 1988;6:451–456.

149. Murray N, Shah A, Osoba D, et al. Intensive weekly chemotherapy for the treatment of extensive-stage small-cell lung cancer. J Clin Oncol 1991;9:1632–1638.

150. Fukuoka M, Takada M, Masuda N, et al. Dose intensive weekly chemotherapy (CT) with or without recombinant human granulocyte colony-stimulating factor (G-CSF) in extensive-stage (ES) small-cell lung cancer (SCLC) (abstract). Proc Am Soc Clin Oncol 1992; 11:967.

151. Taylor CW, Crowley J, Williamson SK, et al. Treatment of small-cell lung cancer with an alternating chemotherapy regimen given at weekly intervals: a Southwest Oncology Group pilot study. J Clin Oncol 1990;8:1811–1817.

152. Miles DW, Fogarty O, Ash CM, et al. Received dose-intensity: a randomized trial of weekly chemotherapy with and without granulocyte colony-stimulating factor in small-cell lung cancer. J Clin Oncol 1994;12:77–82.

153. Sculier JP, Paesmans M, Bureau G, et al. Multiple-drug weekly chemotherapy versus standard combination regimen in small-cell lung cancer: a phase III randomized study conducted by the European Lung Cancer Working Party. J Clin Oncol 1993;11:1858–1865.

154. Ettinger DS, Finkelstein DM, Abeloff MD, Ruckdeschel JC, Aisner SC, Eggleston JC. A randomized comparison of standard chemotherapy versus alternating chemotherapy and maintenance versus no

maintenance therapy for extensive-stage small-cell lung cancer: a phase III study of the Eastern Cooperative Oncology Group. J Clin Oncol 1990;8:230–240.

155. Bleehen NM, Fayers PM, Girling DJ, Stephens RJ. Controlled trial of twelve versus six courses of chemotherapy in the treatment of small-cell lung cancer. Br J Cancer 1989;59:584–590.

156. Perez CA, Krauss S, Bartolucci AA, et al. Thoracic and elective brain irradiation with concomitant or delayed multiagent chemotherapy in the treatment of localized small cell carcinoma of the lung: a randomized prospective study by the Southeastern Cancer Study Group. Cancer 1981;47:2407–2413.

157. Salazar OM, Rubin P, Brown JC, et al. Predictors of radiation response in lung cancer: a clinicopathobiological analysis. Cancer 1976;37:2636–2650.

158. Warde P, Payne D. Does thoracic irradiation improve survival and local control in limited-stage small-cell carcinoma of the lung? J Clin Oncol 1992; 6:890–895.

159. Pignon JP, Arriagada R, Ihde DC, et al. A meta-analysis of thoracic radiotherapy for small-cell lung cancer. N Engl J Med 1992;327:1618–1624.

160. Perry MC, Eaton WL, Propert KJ, et al. Chemotherapy with or without radiation therapy in limited stage small-cell carcinoma of the lung. N Engl J Med 1987;316:912–918.

161. Murray N, Coy P, Pater JL, et al. Importance of timing for thoracic irradiation in the combined modality treatment of limited-stage small-cell lung cancer. J Clin Oncol 1993;11:336–344.

162. Johnson DH, Kim K, Turrisi AT, et al. Cisplatin (P) & etoposide (E) + concurrent thoracic radiotherapy (TRT) administered once versus twice daily for limited-stage (LS) small cell lung cancer (SCLC): preliminary results of an intergroup trial (abstract). Proc Am Soc Clin Oncol 1994;13:1105.

163. Coy P, Hodson DI, Murray N, et al. Patterns of failure following loco-regional radiotherapy in the treatment of limited stage small cell lung cancer. Int J Radiat Oncol Biol Phys 1994;28:355–362.

164. Arriagada R, LeChevalier T, Borie F, et al. Prophylactic cranial irradiation for patients with small-cell lung cancer in complete remission. J Natl Cancer Inst 1995;87:183–190.

165. Maurer LH, Tulloh M, Weiss RB, et al. A randomized combined modality trial in small cell carcinoma of the lung. Comparison of combination chemotherapy-radiation therapy versus cyclophosphamide-radiation therapy effects of maintenance chemotherapy and prophylactic whole brain irradiation. Cancer 1980;45:30–39.

166. Beiler DD, Kane RC, Bernath AM, Cashdollar MR. Low dose elective brain irradiation in small cell carcinoma of the lung. Int J Radiat Oncol Biol Phys 1979;5:941–945.

167. Seydel HG, Creech R, Pagano M, et al. Combined modality treatment of regional small cell undifferentiated carcinoma of the lung: a cooperative study of the RTOG and ECOG. Int J Radiat Oncol Biol Phys 1983;9:1135–1141.

168. Aisner J, Whitacre M, Van Echo DA, Wiernik PH. Combination chemotherapy for small cell carcinoma of the lung: continuous versus alternating non-cross-resistant combinations. Cancer Treat Rep 1982; 66:221–230.

169. Niiranen A, Holsti P, Salmo M. Treatment of small cell lung cancer. Two-drug versus four-drug chemotherapy and loco-regional irradiation with or without prophylactic cranial irradiation. Acta Oncol 1989; 28:501–505.

170. Crossen JR, Garwood D, Glatstein E, Neuwelt EA. Neurobehavioral sequelae of cranial irradiation in adults: a review of radiation-induced encephalopathy. J Clin Oncol 1994;12:627–642.

171. Arriagada R, Le Chevalier T, Borie F, et al. Prophylactic cranial irradiation for patients with small-cell lung cancer in complete remission. J Natl Cancer Inst 1995;87:183–190.

172. Sikic BI. Modulation of multidrug resistance: at the threshold. J Clin Oncol 1993;11:1629–1635.

173. Goldstein LJ, Galski H, Fojo A, et al. Expression of a multidrug resistance gene in human cancers. J Natl Cancer Inst 1989;81:116–124.

174. Heyne KH, Lippman SM, Lee JJ, Lee JS, Hong WK. The incidence of second primary tumors in long-term survivors of small-cell lung cancer. J Clin Oncol 1992;10:1519–1524.

175. Johnson BE, Grayson J, Makuch RW, et al. Ten-year survival of patients with small-cell lung cancer treated with combination chemotherapy with or without irradiation. J Clin Oncol 1990;8:396–401.

176. Hong WK, Lippman SM, Itri LM, et al. Prevention of second primary tumors with isotretinoin in squamous-cell carcinoma of the head and neck. N Engl J Med 1990;323:795–801.

177. Pastorino U, Infante M, Maioli M, et al. Adjuvant treatment of stage I lung cancer with high dose vitamin A. J Clin Oncol 1993;11:1216–1222.

178. Lee M, Draoui M, Zia F, et al. Epidermal growth factor receptor monoclonal antibodies inhibit the growth of lung cancer lines. J Natl Cancer Inst Mongr 1992;13:117–123.

179. Garcia de Palazzo IE, Adams GP, Sundareshan P, et al. Expression of mutated epidermal growth factor receptor by non-small cell lung carcinomas. Cancer Res 1993;53:3217–3220.

180. Roth JA, Mukhopadhyay T, Tainsky MA, Fang K, Casson AG, Schneider PM. Molecular approaches to prevention and therapy of aerodigestive tract cancers. J Natl Cancer Inst Monogr 1992; 13:15–21.

54

Chemotherapy of Breast Cancer

Carl G. Kardinal and John T. Cole

With a better understanding of breast cancer biology, systemic therapy has been integrated into the multidisciplinary treatment of newly diagnosed disease. The recognition that breast cancer is frequently a systemic disease at diagnosis is a major conceptual change that has revolutionized our approach to this common malignancy. This conceptual change has provided the theoretic framework not only for systemic adjuvant therapy but also for breast-conserving surgery. Appropriately administered systemic therapy, in conjunction with conservative surgery and radiation, has improved the survival and decreased the morbidity of breast cancer patients, compared with radical surgery alone.

BREAST CANCER BIOLOGY

Henri Francois Le Dran (1685–1770), a French surgeon, proposed that breast cancer was a localized disease that spread to regional lymph nodes (RLNs) and that the only hope for cure was early surgery (1). Le Dran recognized that once a drop of "cancerous lymph" passed the adjacent lymph nodes, it contaminated the entire system. The concept that breast cancer was a localized disease that spread in an orderly fashion dominated cancer theory for the next 200 years.

The hypothesis that breast cancer is a localized disease was carried to its logical conclusion by William Stewart Halsted, who developed the radical mastectomy in 1890. The theoretical rationale for the radical mastectomy was based on an "orderliness" of tumor spread from the primary lesion in the breast to RLNs, followed ultimately by systemic metastases. The "proper" cancer operation consisted of removal of the primary tumor, RLNs, and pectoral muscles en

bloc. Radical cancer surgery based upon anatomic considerations remained unchallenged for over 75 years (2).

Changes in therapeutic principles depend upon changes in fundamental biologic principles. Without the proper theoretical framework, challenges to standard therapy cannot be made successfully. A major driving force behind challenging the fundamental principles of radical surgery through establishment of new concepts of breast cancer biology has been Bernard Fisher of the University of Pittsburgh. Fisher noted that the Halstedian theory of en bloc resection was based upon Virchow's proposal that RLNs are effective filters and barriers to tumor spread. In collaboration with his brother, Edwin Fisher, Bernard Fisher was able to demonstrate in the laboratory that RLNs were ineffective barriers to the passage of tumor cells and that hematogenous and lymphatic dissemination of tumor cells were of equal importance (3, 4). Fisher then proposed an *alternative hypothesis* of breast cancer biology (Table 54.1) and proceeded to verify the hypothesis through the clinical trials of the National Surgical Adjuvant Breast Project (NSABP) (2, 5–9).

Early NSABP trials confirmed the prognostic value of RLN involvement (10). These data and subsequent follow-up data confirmed that the natural history of breast cancer was directly related to the number of axillary nodes involved and that axillary nodal involvement was the single most important prognostic variable (Table 54.2, Fig. 54.1) (10–12). The prognostic value of axillary nodal involvement and the apparent lack of therapeutic value of axillary dissection confirmed that RLNs are ineffective tumor cell filters. Since 50% of patients are axillary node

Table 54.1. Two Divergent Hypotheses of Tumor Biology

Halstedian Hypothesis	The Fisher Alternative Hypothesis
Tumors spread in an orderly defined manner based upon mechanical considerations	No orderly pattern of tumor cell dissemination
Tumor cells traverse lymphatics to lymph nodes by direct extension, supporting en bloc dissection	Tumor cells traverse lymphatics by embolization, challenging the merit of en bloc dissection
The positive lymph node is an indicator of tumor spread and is the instigator of disease	The positive lymph node is an indicator of a host-tumor relationship that permits development of metastases rather than the instigator of distant disease
Regional lymph nodes are barriers to the passage of tumor cells	Regional lymph nodes are ineffective barriers to tumor cell spread
Regional lymph nodes are of anatomic importance	Regional lymph nodes are of biologic importance
The blood stream is of little significance as a route of tumor dissemination	The bloodstream is of considerable importance in tumor dissemination
A tumor is autonomous from its host	Complex host-tumor interrelationships affect every facet of the disease
Operable breast cancer is a local-regional disease	Operable breast cancer is a systemic disease
The extent and nuances of operation are the dominant factors influencing patient outcome	Variations in local-regional therapy are unlikely to substantially affect survival
No consideration is given to tumor multicentricity	Multicentric foci of tumor are not of necessity a precursor of clinical overt cancer

From Fisher B. Cancer surgery: a commentary. Cancer Treat Rep 1984;68(1):31–41.

Table 54.2. Treatment Failure After Standard Radical Mastectomy

		Percentage Treatment Failures			
	Number	18 Months	3 Years	5 Years	10 Years
All patients	370	19	—	39.7	49.5
Negative nodes	198	6	—	17.7	24.1
Positive nodes	172	35	—	71.0	76.1
Premenopausal					
Negative nodes	52	6	17	21.2	25.5
Positive nodes	60	50	61	70.0	76.3
1–3 nodes positive	24	13	—	45.8	56.6
≥4 nodes positive	36	64	82	86.1	88.9
Postmenopausal					
Negative nodes	146	8	15	16.4	23.6
Positive nodes	112	22	50	62.5	76.0
1–3 nodes positive	58	18	37	51.7	67.9
≥4 nodes positive	54	48	62	74.1	84.3

Data from Fisher B, Ravdin RG, Ausman RK, et al. Surgical adjuvant chemotherapy in cancer of the breast. Results of a decade of cooperative investigation. Ann Surg 1968;163:337–356; Fisher B, Slack N, Katrych D, et al. Ten year follow-up results of patients with carcinoma of the breast in a cooperative clinical trial evaluating surgical adjuvant chemotherapy. Surg Gynecol Obstet 1975; 140:528–534; and Fisher B, Bauer M, Wickerham L, et al. Relation of number of positive axillary nodes to the prognosis of patients with primary breast cancer. An NSABP update. Cancer 1983;52:1551–1557.

positive at diagnosis, micrometastases must be present in at least 50% of breast cancer patients or more at the time of initial presentation. These clinical data, in conjunction with the earlier laboratory data, further verified the alternative hypothesis.

The hypothesis that RLNs are not effective fil-ters was further tested in two surgical trials. If it is correct, more conservative operations should produce results equivalent to those of more radical surgery. Between August 1971 and August 1974, the NSABP conducted a clinical trial involving 1765 patients with clinical stage I or II breast cancer. Women with clinical stage I breast

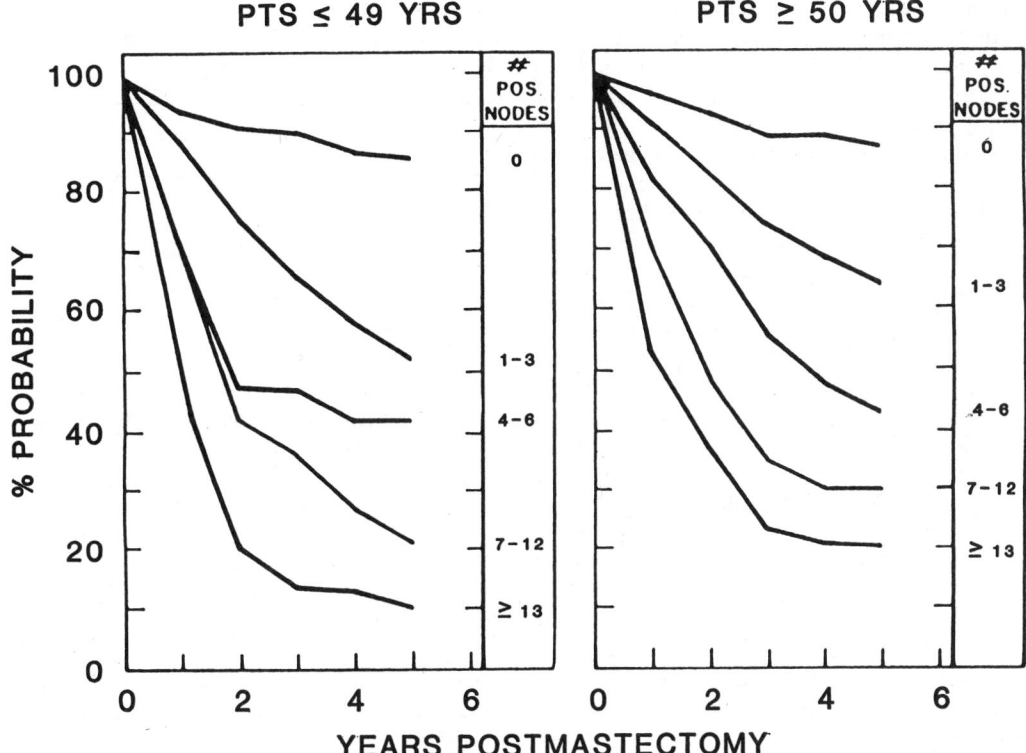

Figure 54.1. **Disease-free survival relative to age and number of positive axillary nodes for patients (*PTS*) ≤49 years and ≥50 years.** (From Fisher B, Bauer M, Wickerham L, Redmond CK, Fisher ER. Relation of number of positive axillary nodes to the prognosis of patients with primary breast cancer: an NSABP update. Cancer 1983;52:1551–1557. With permission.)

cancer (no palpable axillary adenopathy) were randomized to a standard Halsted radical mastectomy (RM) or to a total (simple) mastectomy (TM) with or without radiation. Clinical stage II patients (those with palpable axillary nodes) were randomized to RM or TM plus radiation. By stage, there no was no difference in disease-free or overall survival in any of the treatment groups (13).

Based upon the alternative hypothesis, the logical extension of this trial is that even more conservative breast-sparing operations should be equivalent to total mastectomy or the modified radical mastectomy (MRM). Between April 1976 and January 1984, the NSABP randomized 1855 women to an MRM or a segmental mastectomy (lumpectomy) with an axillary dissection (14). The data from this trial confirmed that women with primary breast tumors of 4 cm or less who were treated with a lumpectomy, axillary dissection, and primary breast irradiation had disease-free and overall survivals equivalent to those of women treated with MRM. Thus, the surgical principles of the alternative hypothesis

are sound. Despite the recent controversy regarding this trial, the data remain valid (15, 15a, 15b).

The other major principles of the alternative hypothesis—that there is no orderly pattern of tumor cell dissemination, that tumor cells traverse lymphatics by embolization, and that operable breast cancer is a systemic disease because of the presence of micrometastases at diagnosis—have also been tested. Numerous trials of systemic adjuvant chemotherapy and endocrine therapy have confirmed these principles by demonstrating improved disease-free and absolute survival in systemically treated patients (16, 17). The adjuvant therapy of breast cancer is discussed in more detail in the sections on stage I and stage II breast cancer.

Hormone Receptors

Breast cancer biology was further illuminated in the early 1970s by the description of the *estrogen receptor* and its relationship to response to endocrine therapy and to prognosis (18–22). It had been recognized for almost 100 years that some breast cancers are sex hormone dependent. On June 15, 1895, Beatson did the first bilateral oophorectomy for the treatment of advanced breast cancer. This was performed on a 33-year-old woman with locally recurrent breast cancer. Eight months following the oophorectomy, "all vestiges of the previous cancerous disease had disappeared" (23). Following Beatson's original report, oophorectomy became widely practiced but then was largely abandoned after only 10 years. The reasons why the procedure was abandoned are (*a*) the recognition that oophorectomy was not a curative procedure, as was originally thought by Beatson; (*b*) the lack of a sound therapeutic rationale; and (*c*) the risks of intra-abdominal surgery in the early 20th century. By 1905, a response rate to oophorectomy of 29.3% in premenopausal women with advanced breast cancer, with response durations of 6 to 12 months, had been confirmed (24). The procedure was abandoned as a failure despite the fact that this was the first effective systemic treatment for cancer of any type (25). It was not until the 1940s, when Charles Huggins described the hormonal responsiveness of prostatic cancer, that an interest in the hormonal treatment of breast cancer was resurrected (26–29). However, the same basic response rate of 20 to 30% to additive or ablative hormonal therapy and the same basic response duration of 6 to 12 months were again confirmed.

The pioneering work of Jensen and associates (18), McGuire and associates (21, 22), Wittliff (19), and DeSombre and associates (30) has established the relationship between responsiveness to additive or ablative forms of hormonal manipulation and the presence of the cytosol-binding protein for estrogen (ER) (Table 54.3). By restricting hormonal manipulation of patients whose tumors are ER positive (ER+; ≥10 fmol/mg protein), response rates to endocrine therapy can be increased from 25% in unselected cases to 55%. Interestingly, the response rates to additive (56%) and ablative (55%) hormonal therapy in ER+ cases are equivalent (Table 54.4). This reflects the fact that the most commonly used forms of hormonal therapy basically do the same thing, block the production or the action of estrogen. Responsiveness to hormonal therapy is directly related to the amount of ER present, as illustrated in Table 54.5 (31, 32).

Horwitz et al. (33) noted that the synthesis of progesterone receptor (PR) depends upon an intact cellular hormonal system. They then postu-

Table 54.3. Relationship Between Estrogen Receptor Status of Breast Cancer and Objective Response to Endocrine Therapy

	Responses/Total	
ER+		ER−
522/977 (53%)		36/567 (6%)

Modified from Wittliff JL. Steroid-hormone receptors in breast cancer. Cancer 1984;53:630–643.

Table 54.4. Relationship Between Estrogen Receptor Status and Response to Additive and Ablative Endocrine Therapy

	Responses/Total	
	ER+	ER−
Additive hormone treatment	59/105 (56%)	12/109 (11%)
Ablative endocrine therapy	59/107 (55%)	8/94 (8%)
Total	118/212 (56%)	20/203 (10%)

Modified from Wittliff JL: Steroid hormone receptors in breast cancer. Cancer 1984;54:630–643.

Table 54.5. Quantitation of ER and Response to Endocrine Therapy

ER (fmol/mg)	Primary Cancer (%)	Metastatic Biopsy (%)
0–10	9	8
10–50	50	40
100	83	61

Data from Allegra JC. Rational approaches to the hormonal treatment of breast cancer. Semin Oncol 1983;10 (Suppl 4):25–28; Osborne CK, Yochmowitz MG, Knight WA, McGuire WL. The value of estrogen and progesterone receptors in the treatment of breast cancer. Cancer 1980;46:2884–2888.

Table 54.6. Relationship Between Estrogen (ER) and Progesterone (PR) Receptor Status and Response to Endocrine Therapy

ER+ PR+	ER+ PR−	ER− PR−	ER± PR+
135/174 (78%)	55/164 (34%)	16/165 (10%)	5/11 (45%)

Modified from Wittliff JL: Steroid-hormone receptors in breast cancer. Cancer 1984;53:630–643.

lated that the presence of PR in addition to ER would further predict hormonal responsiveness. This has, indeed, proved to be the case; ER+ PR+ tumors yield a 78% rate of response to hormonal therapy (20) (Table 54.6). However, Bezwoda et al. have reported that response to tamoxifen correlated with the ER but not the PR level (34). Patients with an ER above 30 fmol/mg had a response rate to tamoxifen of 80%, regardless of PR.

The ER and PR content of a breast cancer is an important prognostic indicator as well as an indicator of response to endocrine therapy (35–41). Receptors correlate with cellular turnover rates, nuclear grade, and degree of histologic differentiation (42, 43). Receptors also correlate with disease-free interval (the time from diagnosis to documented recurrence), with receptor-positive patients having a significantly longer disease-free interval than receptor-negative patients (Fig. 54.2). This prolongation of disease-free interval is independent of menopausal status, tumor size, and nodal status (37). The prolonged disease-free interval of ER+ patients correlates well with the earlier clinical observa-

tion that patients with disease-free intervals of 2 years or longer are more likely to respond to hormonal therapy than are patients with shorter disease-free intervals. Interestingly, over the past two decades, the median level of ER has steadily increased from 14 fmol/mg in 1973 to 58 fmol/mg in 1992 (44). Over that same period, median tumor size at diagnosis has decreased, implying that smaller tumors have higher ER levels.

New considerations in breast cancer biology have focused on three major areas: growth factors, DNA flow cytometry, and oncogenes. The ultimate clinical relevance of these three areas has not yet been fully established, but it appears that each of these is aiding in the understanding of the natural history and behavior of breast cancers. New predictive prognostic variables will become of increasing importance in the management of stage I breast cancer, in which most patients are cured by local therapy alone.

Growth Factors

Several *growth factors* appear to have a role in the regulation of human breast cancer. These fac-

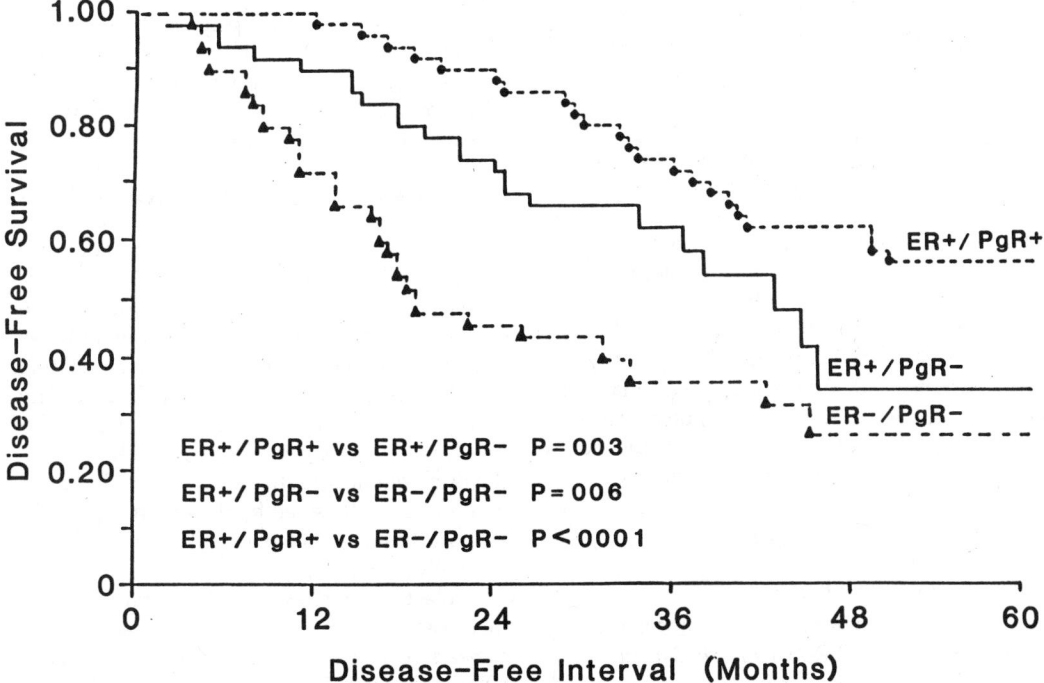

Figure 54.2.   Relationship between estrogen and progesterone receptor status and disease-free survival. Patients who were ER+ PgR+ (*n* = 104) had a significantly longer disease-free survival than patients who were ER+ PgR− (*n* = 39), or patients who were ER− PgR− (*n* = 40). (From Clark GM, McGuire WL, Hubay CA, et al. Progesterone receptors as a prognostic factor in stage II breast cancer. N Engl J Med 1983;309:1343–1347. With permission.)

tors may be either autocrine (autostimulatory) or paracrine (stimulatory to surrounding tissues such as connective tissue or vasculature) (45). It has also been demonstrated that in addition to ER and PR, breast cancer cells have receptors for multiple growth factors, such as epidermal growth factor, insulin-like growth factor I, somatostatin, prolactin, and luteinizing-hormone-releasing hormone (LHRH) (46–51). Other growth factors, such as platelet-derived growth factor and transforming growth factor-alpha (TGF-α), have a stimulatory effect on breast cancer tissue, while TGF-β has an inhibitory effect. There appears to be an inverse correlation between epidermal growth factor receptors and ER status, with ER-negative (ER−) tumors tending to have a higher level of epidermal growth factor receptor than ER+ tumors. Within the ER− group, tumors with higher levels of epidermal growth factor receptor tend to have a poorer prognosis. Inhibiting growth factors or blocking growth factor receptors may have therapeutic implications in the future.

DNA Flow Cytometry

DNA flow cytometric measurements of ploidy and the fraction of cells in the synthesis phase of the cell cycle (S-phase fraction) have been evaluated as prognostic factors in women with node-negative breast cancer (52). Approximately one-third to one-half of breast cancers have normal or *diploid* chromosomes; the remainder have excess or abnormal DNA (*aneuploid*). In retrospective studies, stage I patients with diploid tumors appear to have a better prognosis than those with aneuploid tumors. However, prospective studies have been unable to confirm a correlation between DNA index (ploidy) and any clinical variable, including time to recurrence and survival (53, 54). S-phase fraction may be an independent prognostic variable, but as yet, therapeutic decisions should not be based on S-phase fraction alone (55, 56).

Oncogenes

HER-2/*neu* ONCOGENE

Epidermal growth factor receptor is the gene product of the HER-2/*neu* (*erb* B$_2$) oncogene. Amplification of the HER-2/*neu* oncogene has been reported to be of prognostic importance in stage I and stage II breast cancer (57–59). In these studies, patients with higher levels of HER-2/neu protein had shorter disease-free intervals

and overall survival than patients with lower levels. HER-2/*neu* gene amplification may be an important independent prognostic variable. Higher levels of HER-2/neu protein have been found in ER− PR− tumors and in patients with more than three positive axillary nodes (60). However, these latter factors by themselves are poor prognostic signs.

p53 TUMOR SUPPRESSOR GENE

The *p53* tumor suppressor gene is linked to apoptosis (programed cell death). *p53* induces cell cycle–arresting factors and blocks cell entry into S phase. Loss of *p53* may therefore decrease the apoptotic potential of tumor cells (61). There appears to be an association between *p53* overexpression, tumor cell proliferation rate, and prognosis in node-negative breast cancer (62–64). However, Rosen and colleagues noted that *p53* (by immunohistochemical staining) was not a reliable prognostic indicator in node-negative breast cancer (65).

C-myc ONCOGENE

The c-*myc* oncogene is critical to the growth of human breast cancer cell lines and is directly regulated by estrogen in hormone-dependent breast cancer cells. c-*myc* amplification occurs in 20 to 30% of patients with breast cancer and has been associated with a poor prognosis (66, 67). These molecular biologic targets may be the future sites of cancer therapy.

ENDOCRINE THERAPY

The basis for the endocrine therapy of breast cancer is summarized in Figure 54.3 (68). *Estrogen* is a highly potent mammary mitogen; therefore, most forms of endocrine therapy for breast cancer are directed toward inhibiting, ablating, or otherwise interfering with estrogen activity. Estrogen is the major stimulus for the growth of hormone-dependent breast cancer. The ovary is the principle site of estrogen synthesis, but estrogen is also synthesized by the adrenal gland, by adipose tissue, and even by mammary tumors themselves (69, 70).

Prolactin is the next most important hormone in breast development and function. Prolactin appears to synergize with growth hormone to promote ductal development (71). Highly specific receptors for prolactin have been demonstrated in human mammary carcinoma (49, 72). The actual role of prolactin in human breast cancers is as yet undefined. However, since prolac-

The Endocrine Basis of Therapy

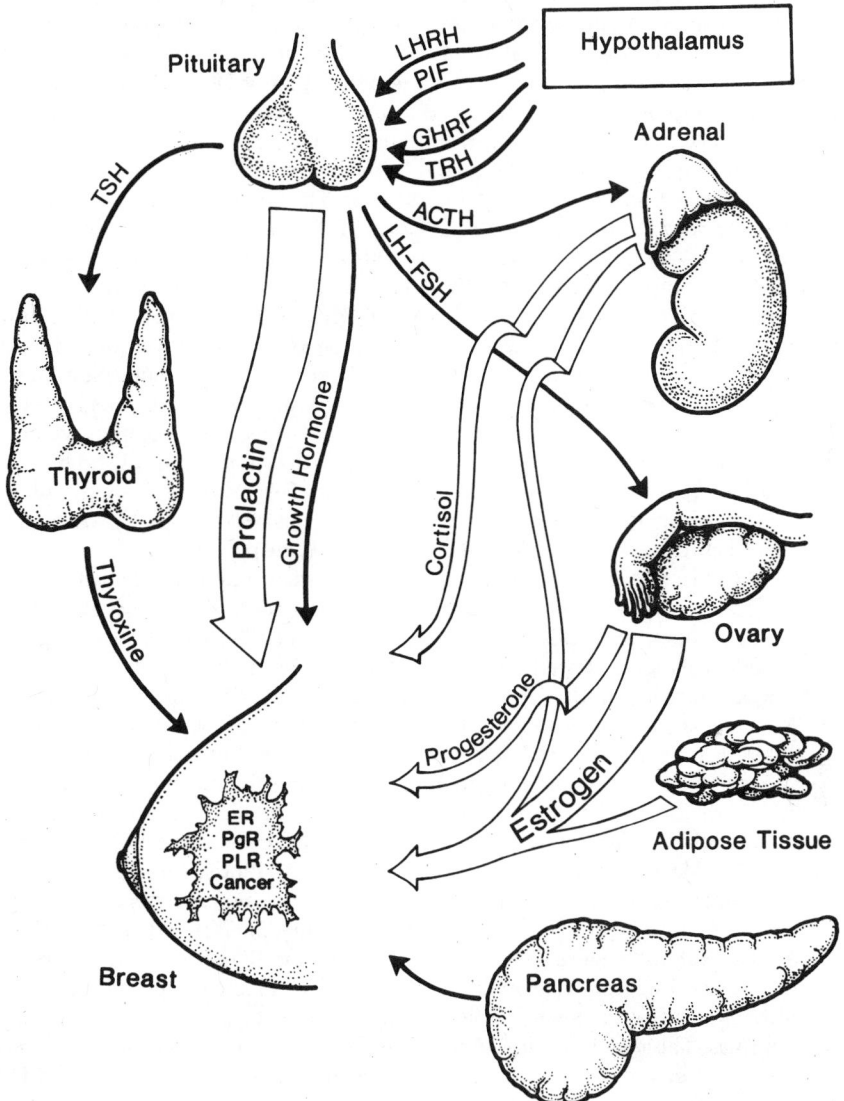

Figure 54.3.   The endocrine basis of breast cancer therapy. *Estrogen* and *prolactin* are the dominant mitogens to normal breast tissue. However, the role of prolactin in human breast cancer is not yet established. Ductal growth is promoted by estrogen in the presence of growth hormone; lobular development is promoted by prolactin and *progesterone*. Estrogen is synthesized not only in the *ovary* but also in *adrenal* and *adipose tissue*. The roles of *cortisol, thyroxine*, and insulin are permissive rather than regulatory. *LHRH*, luteinizing hormone releasing hormone; *PIF*, prolactin inhibitory factor; *GHRF*, growth hormone releasing factor; *TRH*, thyrotropin releasing hormone; *ACTH*, adrenocorticotropic hormone; *LH*, luteinizing hormone; *FSH*, follicle stimulating hormone; *TSH*, thyroid stimulating hormone; *ER*, estrogen receptor; *PgR*, progesterone receptor; *PLR*, prolactin receptor. (From Kardinal CG. Endocrine therapy of breast cancer. In: Donegan WL, Spratt JS, eds. Cancer of the breast. 4th ed. Philadelphia: WB Saunders, 1995:534–580. With permission.)

tin is a potent mammary mitogen, this hormone may be important in breast cancer growth and development.

Progesterone has no effect on the normal breast unless there is concomitant estrogen stimulation. Under these conditions, progesterone interacts with prolactin to promote lobuloalveolar development (73).

Enthusiasm regarding the endocrine therapy of breast cancer has been cyclic. The rapid rise and fall of use of the oophorectomy at the turn of the 20th century has already been discussed. There was a resurgence of interest in endocrine therapy from the 1940s through the 1960s, and several major breakthroughs occurred: (*a*) the full range of ablative therapy (oophorectomy, adrenalectomy, and hypophysectomy) was developed, and (*b*) additive hormonal therapy was initiated with high-dose estrogens, androgens, and progestins.

With the introduction of combination chemotherapy in the late 1960s and 1970s, endocrine therapy of breast cancer again fell out of favor (74, 75). Endocrine therapy was unreliable, yielding only a 20 to 30% objective response, and 6 to 8 weeks were required for the response to occur. With chemotherapy, objective responses occurred in 60 to 70% of patients treated, and the onset of action was relatively rapid.

In the 1980s, however, there was a strong resurgence of interest in endocrine therapy of breast cancer. Receptors for estrogen and progesterone and their role in predicting response to hormonal manipulation had been documented (Tables 54.4–54.6). Endocrine therapy could now be more specific, and higher response rates in selected cases could be anticipated. The introduction of tamoxifen, megestrol acetate, and the newer aromatase inhibitors relegated the more toxic androgens and estrogens to tertiary and quarternary roles. The major surgical ablative procedures of adrenalectomy and hypophysectomy are now of historic interest only. LHRH agonists have been synthesized and are being introduced into clinical practice (76). The era of hormonal therapy spawned in the 1980s will continue to mature in the 1990s (77).

Tamoxifen

Tamoxifen (Nolvadex) is currently the treatment of choice for postmenopausal women with hormonally responsive metastatic breast cancer. Tamoxifen has achieved this status because of its effectiveness (a 76% response rate in ER+ PR+ cases), safety, and favorable side-effect profile (78). A now classic Mayo Clinic trial compared diethylstilbestrol (DES), the previous hormonal agent of choice, with tamoxifen. This study confirmed an equivalent response rate and duration, but the toxicity of tamoxifen was considerably less than that of DES (79). Following this publication, DES was relegated to a tertiary role, and tamoxifen emerged as the primary agent for the initial treatment of hormonally responsive breast cancer. The response rates to tamoxifen in ER+ PR+, ER+ PR−, ER− PR+, and ER− PR− patients are essentially the same as those reported earlier (78%, 34%, 10%, and 45%, respectively (20)). However, Vogel et al. (80) reported a 25% response to tamoxifen in highly selected patients with "receptor-poor" metastatic breast cancer. They attributed this to false-negative receptor results and urged that receptor values be integrated with classical clinical and histopathologic variables. For example, patients with disease-free intervals of less than 2 years tend to be hormonally unresponsive.

Tamoxifen, a nonsteroidal antiestrogen structurally related to DES, is weakly estrogenic in castrated rats (81). This weak estrogenic activity of tamoxifen is both helpful and potentially harmful. Tamoxifen appears to protect against the development of *osteoporosis* in postmenopausal women but may promote bone loss in premenopausal women (82, 83, 83a). Tamoxifen exerts a favorable effect on plasma lipids and cardiovascular risk factors (84–87, 87a).

Tamoxifen binds reversibly with the estrogen receptor, forming an inert complex that blocks estrogen-mediated protein synthesis. Tamoxifen also has non-ER-dependent tumor-suppressive activity by enhancing the production of the inhibitory growth factor TGF-β and blocking the production of the enhancing growth factors IGF-I (insulin-like growth factor-I) and TGF-α (88–91). Tamoxifen is cytostatic rather than cytocidal and acts as a cell cycle inhibitor, with cells accumulating in the G_0 and G_1 phases (92, 93). In studies in rat mammary carcinoma, normal cell-cycling returns when the drug has been cleared from the system (94). The cytostatic action of tamoxifen and the potential reversibility of its effect have prompted prolonged use of this drug, especially in the adjuvant setting (95–97).

The toxicity of tamoxifen is usually minimal, but headaches, hot flashes, or both occur occasionally. Hot flashes can be particularly annoying and difficult to control; recommended treatments include vitamin E 800 units daily, transdermal clonidine, and Bellergal-S. Megestrol acetate 20 mg twice daily is effective in the treatment of hot flashes, but progestational agents do appear to alter tamoxifen metabolism (98–100). Reduced levels of antithrombin III have been reported (101, 102). However, there was no increased risk of thromboembolic events among 2365 postmenopausal women with early-stage breast cancer randomized to receive tamoxifen 40 mg daily versus no treatment (103). Of more concern have been the reports of endometrial cancer in women receiving long-term tamoxifen (104–106). More than 200 cases of endometrial cancer have been reported in women who are taking or have taken tamoxifen (107, 107a, 107b). The relative risk of developing endometrial cancer is from 2.5 to 6 times the baseline; that is, an increased risk from 1 case per 1000 per year to 2.5 to 6 cases per 1000 per year in women on long-term tamoxifen (Fig 54.4). Rutqvist et al. (108) have also reported an increased risk of colorectal and gastric cancers in women on long-term tamoxifen, but this needs to be verified. Tamoxifen is not associated with an increased risk of hepatocellular carcinoma.

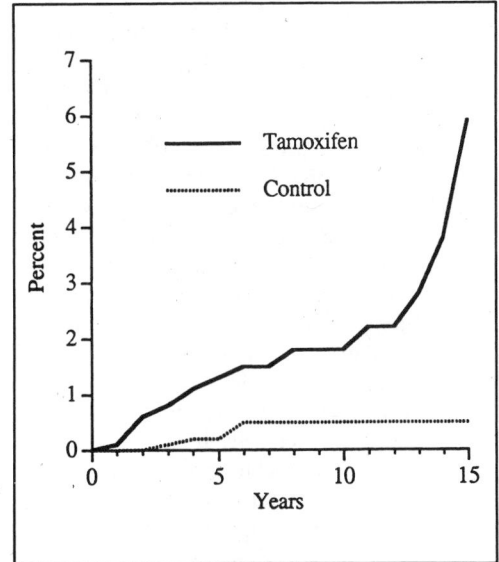

Figure 54.4. Cumulative incidence of endometrial cancer during follow-up by treatment group (tamoxifen vs. control) in the Stockholm trial. (From Rutqvist LE, Johansson H, Signomklao T, et al. Adjuvant tamoxifen therapy for early stage breast cancer and second primary malignancies. J Natl Cancer Inst 1995;87:645–651. With permission.)

TAMOXIFEN IN PREMENOPAUSAL WOMEN

For decades, *oophorectomy* was considered the treatment of choice for hormonally responsive breast cancer in premenopausal women (109, 110). Tamoxifen, however, has successfully challenged the traditional role of oophorectomy as primary therapy in this group of patients (111, 112). In randomized controlled trials involving over 200 patients, the response rates and durations of response associated with oophorectomy and tamoxifen are equivalent. In addition, prior response to tamoxifen may be a good predictor of response to subsequent oophorectomy (113, 114). This implies that tamoxifen should be used as primary therapy and oophorectomy restricted to patients who have responded previously to tamoxifen. Tamoxifen has emerged as the primary treatment of choice in premenopausal women as well as in postmenopausal women with hormonally responsive metastatic breast cancer.

TAMOXIFEN DOSE

In *postmenopausal* patients, tamoxifen does not have a significant dose-response curve. Responses to the standard dose of 20 mg daily are equivalent to responses to 40 mg daily, and doses up to 90 mg daily are no more effective. In *premenopausal* women, the usual recommended dose is still 20 mg daily; however, many studies cited previously have used 40 mg daily, and doses up to 120 mg daily have been evaluated (115). The higher doses are more effective in suppressing menses but are not more effective in inducing an antitumor response. Although tamoxifen is often prescribed as 10 mg twice daily, because of the long half-life of the drug, the same biologic effect can be achieved with a single daily dose of 20 mg (116).

TAMOXIFEN FLARE

Tamoxifen flare occurs in approximately 10% of cases (117). This curious phenomenon is characterized by increased bone or soft tissue pain and occasionally hypercalcemia. When a flare occurs, it develops in the first few weeks of therapy. Contrary to its manifestations, which may resemble progression, a flare generally heralds a response to treatment. Flares should be treated with analgesics or other symptomatic therapy, and full-dose tamoxifen should be continued. Brooks and Lippman (118) have proposed that the flare occurs because it requires several weeks for tamoxifen to reach therapeutic levels, and at lower concentrations the drug may be estrogenic and stimulatory. Legha et al. (119) noted *hypercalcemia* in 9 of 470 patients with metastatic breast cancer who were treated with tamoxifen. Mild hypercalcemia was not considered to be a reason for stopping tamoxifen and was treated with saline diuresis and oral phosphates. If hypercalcemia was severe ($\geq$15 mg/100 mL), a brief interruption of tamoxifen usually helped to control the hypercalcemia. Tamoxifen could be reinstituted within a few days. If hypercalcemia recurred, a small dose of prednisone, 10–30 mg daily, was found to be helpful.

Hormonal flares are by no means unique to tamoxifen and were described as "induced hypercalcemia" with high-dose DES by Hall et al. in 1963 (120). The same significance was noted; that is, hormonally induced hypercalcemia may indicate that the tumor has retained its hormonal responsiveness and that hormonal treatment should be continued. Hypercalcemia and pain flares have also been reported with megestrol acetate and, again, may herald a response (121).

TAMOXIFEN AS PRIMARY THERAPY

Tamoxifen has been evaluated as primary therapy for breast cancer in *elderly women* (122–124). A 27% complete remission rate and a 61% total objective response rate can be anticipated. Overall survival is the same as in elderly women treated with mastectomy; however, the local recurrence rate in tamoxifen-treated patients is higher. Surgery should be performed if at all possible, despite the age of the patient; however, in elderly patients who are poor surgical candidates because of intercurrent medical disease, tamoxifen alone may provide worthwhile palliation (125, 126).

Pure Antiestrogens

A series of new compounds with pure antiestrogenic properties are now entering clinical trials. These include ICI 164,384 and ICI 182,780, which are 17α alkysulfinyl derivatives of 17β-estradiol, droloxifene (3-OH tamoxifen), and toremifene, which is a triphenylethylene derivative structurally related to tamoxifen (127–132). Toremifene, the best studied of these drugs, causes growth inhibition of breast cancer cells by inducing some cells to undergo apoptosis and by inhibiting other cells from entering mitosis (133).

The pure antiestrogens may offer advantages and disadvantages compared with tamoxifen. The pure antiestrogens do not induce a tumor flare in patients with bone metastases and would not be anticipated to induce or stimulate occult endometrial cancers. However, in the absence of any estrogenic activity, the pure antiestrogens might be expected to accelerate the development of osteoporosis and induce atherosclerosis. These drugs may therefore be poor candidates for long-term adjuvant therapy or chemoprevention.

It had been hoped that patients with metastatic disease who have become refractory to tamoxifen would remain sensitive to the pure antiestrogens, but unfortunately, this is rarely the case. There is major cross-resistance between tamoxifen and toremifene (134).

The use of tamoxifen in the adjuvant setting in stage I and stage II breast cancer, as well as the potential use of tamoxifen as a chemopreventive agent in women at high risk of developing breast cancer, is discussed below.

Progestins

The progestational agents megestrol acetate (Megace) and medroxyprogesterone acetate (MPA, Provera) appear to have activity equivalent to that of tamoxifen in advanced, hormonally responsive breast cancer in postmenopausal women (135–138). However, progestins are generally relegated to a secondary role since the duration of response to initial tamoxifen is slightly greater than for megestrol (Fig. 54.5, *A* and *B*). Patients initially treated with tamoxifen who are crossed over to megestrol or MPA after treatment failure have a response rate of only 14 to 22%. Patients treated initially with MPA or megestrol who are subsequently treated with tamoxifen respond only 5 to 23% of the time. Clearly, better second-line hormonal therapy is needed. However, selected patients with non-life-threatening disease, such as bone metastasis, may respond to secondary or even tertiary forms of hormonal manipulation.

Progestins have a direct cytotoxic action on human breast cancer cells in long-term tissue culture but probably act in vivo as antiestrogenic compounds that inhibit estrogen-induced protein synthesis (139). Progestins may also act by the inhibition of autocrine growth factors (140).

The side effects of progestins are minimal but are slightly greater than those of tamoxifen. Progestins have a mild glucocorticoid action, and weight gain is a frequent problem. Johnson et al. (141) noted a 5% or greater increase in weight in 23% of breast cancer patients treated with progestins. The appetite-stimulating effect of pro-

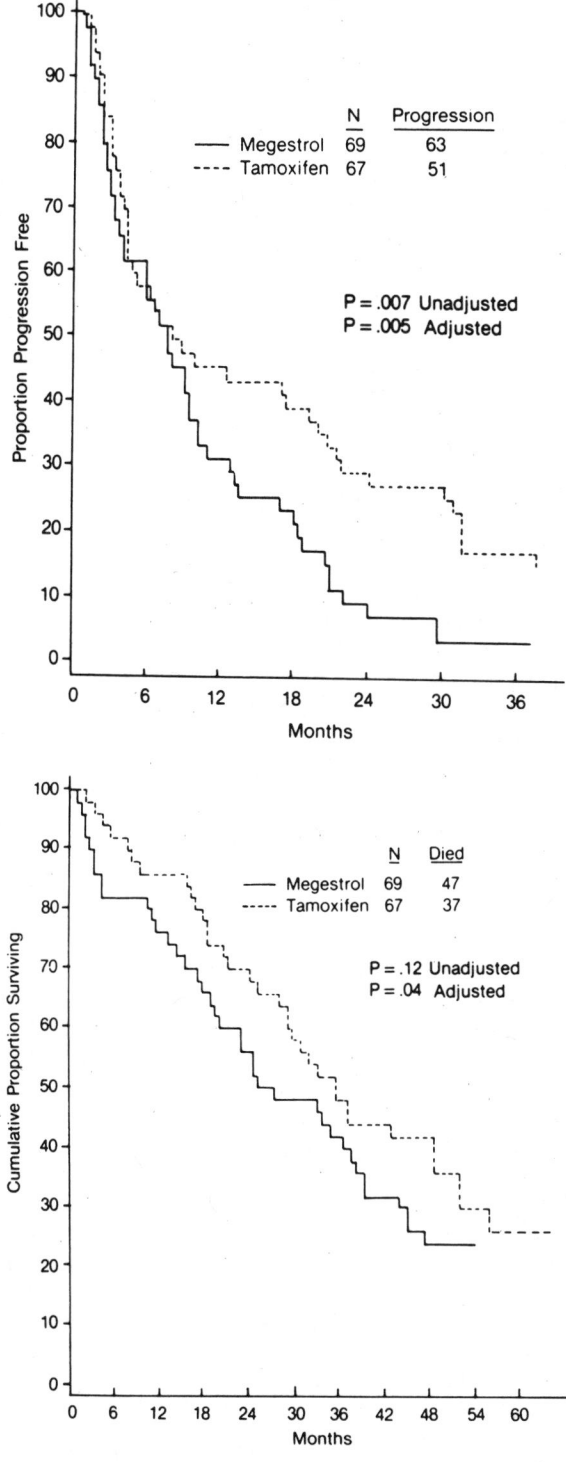

Figure 54.5.   A. Time to progression (months) for all patients for initial treatment (Kaplan-Meier). Adjusted *p* value determined using Cox proportional hazards model. **B.** Survival for all patients by initial treatment (Kaplan-Meier). Adjusted *p* value determined using Cox proportional hazards model. (From Muss HB, Wells HB, Paschold EH, et al. Megestrol acetate versus tamoxifen in advanced breast cancer: 5-year analysis—a phase III trial of the Piedmont Oncology Association. J Clin Oncol 1988;6:1098–1106. With permission.)

gestins is currently being exploited for the treatment of cancer anorexia and cachexia (142). The usual recommended dose of megestrol for this purpose is 800 mg daily, but doses as low as 160 mg daily may be beneficial.

The standard dosage for megestrol acetate for the treatment of advanced breast cancer is 160 mg daily as a single or divided dose and 500 mg three times weekly for MPA (143). Unlike tamoxifen, progestins have been thought to have a steep dose-response curve. MPA in doses of 1000 mg daily has been reported to yield a higher response than 500 mg three times weekly (144). The definitive dose-response trial of megestrol in metastatic breast cancer was performed by the Cancer and Leukemia Group B (145). A group of 368 women with metastatic breast cancer were randomized to receive 160 mg per day, 800 mg per day, or 1600 mg per day. Response rates were identical at the three dose levels (24%, 24%, and 28%, respectively). However, the response duration of the highest dose level was significantly shorter than that of the two lower dose levels (7.8 versus 13.9 and 14.2 months). The incidence of serious vascular complications, arterial thrombi, and pulmonary emboli was higher at the higher dose level. It can be safely concluded that there is no advantage to the high dose over the standard dose of 160 mg daily.

Aromatase Inhibitors

In postmenopausal and oophorectomized premenopausal women, estrogen production occurs in adrenal tissue, adipose tissue, and even breast cancer tissue and is mediated by the enzyme aromatase. This enzyme stimulates the conversion of androstenedione to estrone (69, 70). Inhibitors of the aromatase system have been under intense investigation since the 1960s (146).

Until recently, the only commercially available aromatase inhibitor was aminoglutethimide (AG). Postmenopausal women treated with AG have a 72% decline in their plasma estrone levels and an 85% decrease in their urinary estrone excretion over a 12-week period (147). AG is an active agent in postmenopausal women as well as oophorectomized premenopausal women with metastatic breast cancer (148, 149), and AG is equivalent to surgical adrenalectomy in the treatment of advanced breast cancer.

Since AG also blocks adrenal steroidogenesis, hydrocortisone replacement is required with standard-dose AG therapy. In addition, AG has a series of other undesirable side effects, such as lethargy in 48% of patients, rash in 33%, orthostatic hypotension in 20%, ataxia in 10%, and drug fever in 2.5%. Leukopenia, thrombocytopenia, and even pancytopenia may occur in up to 5% of patients (150). For these reasons, AG has never become a very popular drug.

Several new aromatase inhibitors, 4-hydroxyandrostenedione (4-OHA), letrozole (LGS 20267), fadrozole (CGS 16949A), anastrozole, and rogletimide are currently entering clinical trials (151–159, 159a, 159b). These drugs have the advantage that they are selective aromatase inhibitors that do not block adrenal steroidogenesis. Therefore, concurrent cortisol replacement is not required. The other undesirable side effects of AG are also greatly reduced. The main side effects of these new drugs are hot flashes in 28%, nausea and vomiting in 13%, and anorexia in 5%. No hematologic toxicity has been observed. Fadrozole, anastrozole, letrozole, and 4-OHA appear to be as active as AG in preliminary studies. Letrozole is active in doses ranging from 0.1 to 5 mg orally once daily; fadrozole is administered orally in doses of 1 to 4 mg daily; and 4-OHA is given intramuscularly in doses of 250 to 500 mg every 1 to 2 weeks.

The standard dose schedule of AG is 250 mg twice daily for 14 days, increasing to four times a day thereafter, plus hydrocortisone 20 to 30 mg daily in a single morning dose. Low-dose AG (250 mg twice daily), with or without hydrocortisone replacement, has been reported to be equivalent to standard-dose AG but with fewer side effects (160, 161). Anastrozole (Arimidex) is now commercially available. The recommended does is 1 mg daily as a single oral dose (161a).

Estrogens

Prior to the introduction of tamoxifen, DES, a synthetic estrogen, was the hormonal treatment of choice in postmenopausal women with advanced breast cancer (79, 162). The response rate to DES in patients with ER+ tumors is 63%. In general, the median duration of response to estrogen is 12 to 18 months, but responses of longer than 5 years have been documented. DES may be a better second-line hormonal agent than megestrol, but a comparative trial has not yet been conducted (163).

The mechanism by which estrogens act on metastatic breast cancer is unknown. Tumor cells that contain ER bind estrogens with greater affinity and specificity. High-dose estrogen by mass action is actually antiestrogenic.

The most commonly used estrogen is still DES in the dosage of 5 mg three times daily. Other estrogen preparations that have been used are ethinyl estradiol, 3 mg daily, and conjugated equine estrogens, 30 mg daily.

Nausea is a common early side effect of DES. This may be avoided by increasing the dose in a stepwise fashion, that is, starting with 5 mg daily for 5 to 7 days, increasing to 5 mg twice daily for an additional 5 to 7 days, and then giving the full dosage of 5 mg three times daily. Increased nipple, areolar, and axillary pigmentation is frequent. Fluid retention occurs in about one-third of patients and may aggravate or even precipitate congestive heart failure. The use of high-dose estrogens may be associated with thromboembolic phenomena.

Breakthrough or withdrawal uterine bleeding in postmenopausal women on estrogen therapy occurs in 40% of patients. This is usually of little clinical significance and responds to cessation of treatment or abates spontaneously with continued therapy, but if it persists, it may require further investigation. Persistent uterine bleeding associated with estrogen therapy may signal the presence of an endometrial carcinoma.

Patients who respond to estrogen therapy initially but in whom the disease progresses later may respond to the sudden withdrawal of estrogens. *Estrogen rebound regression* was originally described by Escher in 1949 and occurs in up to 32% of estrogen responders (164, 165). The duration of rebound regression is usually 3 to 10 months, but Nestro et al. (166) reported that the median duration is in excess of 18 months. *Tamoxifen withdrawal responses* have also been reported (167).

Androgens

Androgens were the first additive hormonal agents to prove useful in the treatment of metastatic breast cancer (168, 169). Androgens exert an antiestrogenic effect by complex interactions with three receptors: ER, PR, and androgen receptor (AR). Androgens compete with estradiol for the ER and can bind to PR. Since the dosage of androgen required to give an antiestrogenic effect is in the range to saturate the AR but is too low to saturate the ER, it has been postulated that the therapeutic effect is mediated via the AR. This is verified, at least to some degree, by the observation that in tissue culture of human

breast cancer, antiandrogens such as cyproterone inhibit the antiestrogenic effect of androgens (170).

Androgens exert desirable subjective hematopoietic and anabolic effects (162). Patients treated with androgens may experience an increased sense of well-being, pain relief, increased appetite, and weight gain.

The side effects of androgens are predominantly those associated with the physiologic effects of male hormones, that is, virilization with frontal baldness, plethora, acne, hirsutism, fluid retention, and less commonly, an increased libido and clitoral hypertrophy. The virilizing effects vary with the androgenic preparation used. They occur in more than 50% of patients treated with testosterone propionate, and in 35 to 40% of patients treated with fluoxymesterone. The virilizing and therapeutic effects of androgens appear to be inseparable. Androgens with a 17-α methyl substitution, such as fluoxymesterone and methyltestosterone, may cause reversible cholestatic jaundice and, rarely, a multifocal hepatocellular necrosis termed peliosis hepatis (171, 172). Large areas of cystic hemorrhagic necrosis of peliosis hepatis may cause an abnormal liver scan that can be confused with metastases. Patients with breast cancer may need to reduce their dosage of thyroid replacement medication during androgen therapy (173).

Fluoxymesterone (Halotestin) is the androgen of choice. The dosage for fluoxymesterone is 20 to 30 mg daily by mouth.

Adrenal Corticosteroids

Adrenal corticosteroids are widely used in the treatment of metastatic breast cancer, but objective data to support this use are sparse. Kelly (174) reported a brief objective response of 18% in patients with metastatic breast cancer. Despite this information, prednisone is commonly incorporated into combination chemotherapy regimens such as CMFVP, CMFP, CFP, and CAFVP (C, cyclophosphamide; M, methotrexate; F, 5-fluorouracil; V, vincristine; P, prednisone; A, Adriamycin). Prednisone used in combination with chemotherapy probably only contributes to the side effects of sodium and fluid retention, aggravation or precipitation of diabetes, hypertension, hypokalemia, muscle weakness, and defects in cell-mediated immunity.

Corticosteroids may be a useful adjunct in the management of patients with far-advanced metastatic disease, frequently causing euphoria, stimulating appetite, and decreasing pain (175). Subjective improvement occurs in as many as 75% of patients treated. Bruera et al. (176) reported a randomized double-blind study of methylprednisolone versus placebo in terminally ill cancer patients and confirmed these observations. Terminally ill cancer patients treated with 32 mg of methylprednisolone daily had less severe pain, increased appetite, and a better sense of well-being than placebo-treated controls.

Combination Hormonal Therapy

Numerous combinations of hormonal agents have been evaluated in the treatment of metastatic breast cancer: fluoxymesterone plus ethinyl estradiol, DES plus testosterone propionate, tamoxifen plus megestrol acetate, tamoxifen plus medroxyprogesterone acetate, tamoxifen plus DES, tamoxifen plus prednisone, tamoxifen plus AG, tamoxifen plus fluoxymesterone, medroxyprogesterone acetate plus AG, and ethinyl estradiol plus medroxyprogesterone acetate. The combinations failed to demonstrate an advantage over the use of single-agent hormonal therapy. This is what would be anticipated, because the mechanism of action of each of these agents is basically the same—inhibition of the synthesis or action of estrogen.

Newer Agents for Hormonal Manipulation

LHRH AGONISTS

In animals, chronic treatment with supraphysiologic doses of luteinizing hormone releasing hormone (LHRH) agonists causes (*a*) a decrease in gonadotrophin (FSH and LH) excretion, (*b*) a decrease in prolactin excretion, (*c*) a decrease in plasma sex steroid concentration, (*d*) a reduction in the weight of secondary sexual organs, and (*e*) an inhibition of the actions of the sex steroids at their target organs (177). LHRH analogues, therefore, act directly or indirectly on the pituitary, the gonads, and the target organs of the sex steroids. Schally et al. (76) have demonstrated significantly decreased tumor weight and volume in mouse and rat mammary cancers treated with D-Trp-LH-RH (decapeptyl). Currently, the LHRH analogues, buserelin, goserelin, decapeptyl, and leuprolide, are being evaluated in clinical trials in advanced breast cancer.

Goserelin (Zoladex), an LHRH agonist, was reported to yield a 45% objective response rate (10% complete response plus 35% partial response) in 134 premenopausal women with metastatic breast cancer (178). The highest response rates were seen in patients with local-regional metastases (62.5%) followed by osseous (46.7%), visceral (45%), and multiple sites (35.1%). Side effects included amenorrhea, vaginal spotting, and, infrequently, headache and sleep disturbances. Leuprolide was tested in 26 premenopausal women, with similar results (179). Attempts at total estrogen suppression with goserelin plus tamoxifen have been evaluated in premenopausal women with metastatic breast cancer. The combination appears to be more active than goserelin alone but has not been tested against tamoxifen alone (180, 181).

The Eastern Cooperative Oncology Group has conducted a phase II study of Zoladex in postmenopausal women (182). In ER+ patients, the response rate was only 11% (4 of 36 patients), and there were no responses in 16 ER− patients. Zoladex has now been approved for the treatment of metastatic breast cancer in ER+ premenopausal women in a dose of 3.6 mg subcutaneously once monthly.

SOMATOSTATIN

Somatostatin inhibits growth hormone release, prolactin secretion, insulin and glucagon release, and pentagastrin-induced gastric secretion (183). Somatostatin also inhibits other growth factors such as epidermal growth factor, insulin-like growth factor I (IGF-I), and transforming growth factor alpha (TGF-α). Somatostatin analogues possess significant antitumor activity in experimental tumors, including rat mammary carcinomas (183).

Somatostatin analogues may inhibit human breast cancers by reducing the release of growth hormone and prolactin and interfering with the action or secretion of endogenous growth factors (184). There may be a significant synergism between LHRH agonists and somatostatin analogues in the inhibition of tumor growth in experimental tumor models.

Since both somatostatin and tamoxifen inhibit growth factors, especially IGF-I, there has been considerable interest in evaluating this combination in breast cancer therapy (185). Preliminary data from the North Central Cancer Treatment Group (NCCTG) confirm that the combination is active and essentially nontoxic. However, clinical trials have been hampered by the lack of availability of a depot preparation. The only somatostatin analogue currently available is octreotide (Sandostatin), which has a very short circulatory half-life. This preparation must be administered by subcutaneous injection every 8 hours. It is hoped that a depot preparation will soon become available.

The next few years should be very productive ones in the area of breast cancer hormonal therapy. Newer agents promise to be of great clinical utility and low toxicity. The importance of hormonal therapy in the treatment of breast cancer cannot be overemphasized.

CYTOTOXIC CHEMOTHERAPY OF BREAST CANCER

The excitement generated by Richard Cooper's report in 1969 to the American Association of Cancer Research was tremendous (75). Cooper reported an 88% response (53 of 60 patients) to combination chemotherapy in hormone-resistant breast cancer. Cooper's regimen was CMFVP (C, cyclophosphamide; M, methotrexate; F, 5-fluorouracil; V, vincristine; P, prednisone). Following Cooper's report, clinical trials testing CMFVP and multiple variants of CMFVP were conducted (Table 54.7). Although none of these trials had a response rate of 88%, it was confirmed that in patients with metastatic breast cancer, combinations of cytotoxic drugs could produce an objective response rate in the range of 60%, with 10 to 15% complete responses, and a response duration of 8 to 12 months or more (186–196).

Combination chemotherapy was rapidly adopted as the treatment of choice for metastatic breast cancer because of its predictably high response rate and rapid onset of action. Conversely, hormonal therapy was relegated to a secondary or tertiary role, since response rates were low and unpredictable and the onset of response might take 6 to 8 weeks. By the late 1970s, it was felt that with more fine-tuning of the pharmacokinetics of chemotherapeutic agents and the integration of drug pharmacokinetics with cell-cycle kinetics, the potential for cytotoxic agents in breast cancer was almost limitless (197). The 1980s were foreseen as a period of great progress for breast cancer chemotherapy, but this did not happen. Promising new agents did not materialize, cell cycle kinetics proved to be of less importance clinically than in the laboratory, and new combinations of existing agents failed to produce an increasing response rate or duration of response. In short, the cytotoxic chemotherapy of breast cancer plateaued. With the exception of the taxanes and vinorelbine, the chemotherapeutic treatment of advanced breast cancer is essentially the same today as it was in 1979.

Single Agents in Breast Cancer

Breast cancer is responsive to all major classes of cytotoxic drugs: alkylating agents, antimetabolites, mitotic inhibitors, and the antitumor antibiotics. The available phase II data of single agent chemotherapy in advanced breast cancer are presented in Table 54.8. These data have been compiled from multiple phase II studies and should be interpreted as indicating the actual response rate rather than as absolute values. Presenting data in this manner entails many problems, since dosage levels or dosage schedules (infusion vs. intravenous push, single-day treatment vs. 5-day treatment schedules) may vary. More importantly, prior therapy and response criteria may not be specified (198–202).

As can be seen in Table 54.8, patients who have been treated previously with chemotherapy and those who have never been treated often show a marked difference in response rate for the same agent: 0 vs. 20% for ifosfamide, 6 vs. 38% for cisplatin, 28 vs. 52% for doxorubicin, and 13 vs. 31% for mitoxantrone. This tremendous discrepancy in responses may well mean that an active drug might be overlooked if it is tested only in previously treated patients. For this reason, and since none of the chemotherapeutic regimens are curative, it is perfectly justifiable to test new phase II agents in chemotherapy-naive patients.

Although several single agents have activity in breast cancer, in current clinical practice they are generally incorporated into combination chemotherapeutic regimens. Most of the single agents will not be discussed individually; however, a few deserve special consideration, particularly the anthracycline analogues, including the hydroxyquinone mitoxantrone; the taxanes; vinorelbine; and the antimetabolite 5-fluorouracil (5-FU). Renewed interest in 5-FU has been sparked by leucovorin modulation and by continuous infusion, an administration technique that has seemed to enhance activity.

ANTHRACYCLINE ANTIBIOTICS
Doxorubicin (Adriamycin)

Adriamycin remains the most active single agent in the treatment of breast cancer, although this position of prominence is currently being

Table 54.7. Variations of the Cooper CMFVP Regimen in Advanced Carcinoma of the Breast

Reference	Regimen[a]	Number Evaluable	Number Responding	Response Rate (%)	Medial Response Duration (months)
Cooper, 1969 (75)	CMFVP	60	53	88	—
Davis et al., 1974 (186)	CMFVP	74	31	42	7
CALGB[b] 1974 (187)	CMFVP	82	41	50	6
Ramirez et al., 1975 (188)	CMFVP	48	30	62	—
Brunner et al., 1975 (189)	CMFVP	91	45	49	8
WCSG[c] 1975 (190)	CMFPT$_3$	60	35	58	11
Ramirez et al., 1975 (188)	CMFV	52	23	44	—
Ahmann et al., 1975 (191)	CFVP	41	19	46	5
Canellos et al., 1976 (192)	CMFP	40	27	68	8
Ahmann et al., 1975 (191)	CFP	49	28	57	4
CALGB 1974 (187)	FVP	82	30	37	6
Brunner et al., 1975 (189)	CMV	46	15	33	8
Brunner et al., 1975 (189)	CMP	49	22	45	7
Canellos et al., 1976 (193)	CMF	93	49	53	6
Otis and Armentrout 1975 (194)	CMF	42	27	64	10
Creech et al., 1975 (195)	CMF	46	21	46	8
DeLena et al., 1975 (196)	CMF	41	27	66	4+
Total all Cooper variants		996	523	53	

Modified from Kardinal CG. Chemotherapy. In: Donegan WL, Spratt JS, eds. Cancer of the breast. 2nd ed. Philadelphia: WB Saunders, 1979;405–447.
[a]C, cyclophosphamide; M, methotrexate; F, 5-fluorouracil; V, vincristine; P, prednisone; T$_3$, triiodothyronine.
[b]Cancer and Leukemia Group B.
[c]Western Cancer Study Group.

challenged by paclitaxel. Doxorubicin produces a 52% objective response rate in previously untreated patients and 28% in patients who have had prior chemotherapy (Table 54.8). Doxorubicin has a series of undesirable side effects such as cardiac toxicity, almost universal alopecia, and marked corrosiveness if the drug infiltrates the skin. This has prompted the search for a less toxic, equipotent analogue and for methods to reduce the cardiac toxicity of doxorubicin.

Using the standard dosage schedule for doxorubicin of 50 to 75 mg/m^2 intravenously every 3 weeks, the incidence of cardiomyopathy increases dramatically once a cumulative dose of 450 mg/m^2 is exceeded. There have been three approaches to modifying the development of doxorubicin-induced cardiomyopathy: changing to a weekly dosage schedule, using a continuous-infusion technique, and the addition of bispiperazinedione (ICRF-187).

Weekly doxorubicin has been studied extensively by Torti et al. (203). Endomyocardial biopsies were performed in 98 patients receiving 60 mg/m^2 of doxorubicin every 3 weeks and in 27 patients receiving 20 mg/m^2 of doxorubicin once weekly. At equivalent cumulative doses of doxorubicin, the weekly schedule was associated with significantly less anthracycline-induced

Table 54.8. Compiled Phase II Data of Single Agent Chemotherapy in Advanced Breast Cancer

Agent	Number Evaluable	CR[a]	PR	$\dfrac{CR + PR}{EVAL} \times 100$
Alkylating agents				
Chlorambucil	54	0	11	20%
Cyclophosphamide	189	0	60	32%
Ifosfamide (prior chemo)	6	0	0	0
Ifosfamide (no prior chemo)	20	0	4	20%
L-PAM (melphalan)	75	0	17	23%
Nitrogen mustard	92	0	32	35%
Prednimustine (prior chemo)	32	0	10	31%
Prednimustine (no prior chemo)	18	4	7	61%
Thiotepa	162	0	38	23%
Drugs with alkylating-like activity				
BCNU[b]	76	0	16	21%
CCNU[c]	155	0	18	12%
Methyl-CCNU	82	0	3	4%
Carboplatin	14	0	0	0
Cisplatin (prior chemo)	80	1	4	6%
Cisplatin (no prior chemo)	50	13	6	38%
Dibromodulcitol	104	1	7	8%
MGBG[d]	96	1	6	7%
Streptonigrin	9	0	2	22%
Streptozotocin	19	0	0	0
Antimetabolites				
Arabinosyl cytosine	64	0	6	9%
5-Azacytidine	27	0	2	7%
Fludarabine	18	0	1	6%
5-Fluorouracil	1142	0	320	28%
5-FU (infusion)	166	2	43	27%
5-FU + leucovorin	228	6	62	30%
Ftorafur	31	2	16	58%
Methotrexate	259	0	87	34%
Triazinate	52	0	2	4%
Trimetrexate	40	0	3	8%
Mitotic inhibitors				
Vinblastine	95	0	19	20%
Vincristine	164	0	32	20%
Vindesine	141	1	28	21%
Vinorelbine (prior chemo)	67	3	21	36%
Vinorelbine (no prior chemo)	157	11	53	41%
Etoposide (VP-16)	234	2	17	8%
Teniposide (VM-26)	42	0	3	7%
Paclitaxel (prior chemo)	225	12	53	29%
Paclitaxel (no prior chemo)	51	5	25	59%
Antitumor antibiotics				
Anthracyclines				
Doxorubicin (prior chemo)	428	13	106	28%
Doxorubicin (no prior chemo)	92	3	45	52%
4′-Deoxydoxorubicin	27	0	1	4%
Epirubicin	140	6	41	34%
Idarubicin	130	6	42	37%
Menogaril	25	0	4	16%
Pirarubicin	71	4	18	31%
Rubidazone	88	1	4	6%
Hydroxyquinones				
Bisantrene	229	2	27	13%
Mitoxantrone (prior chemo)	411	6	48	13%
Mitoxantrone (no prior chemo)	217	13	55	31%

Table 54.8.—*continued*

Agent	Number Evaluable	CR[a]	PR	$\frac{CR + PR}{EVAL} \times 100$
Other				
Aclacinomycin-A	22	0	0	0
Bleomycin	22	0	1	5%
Mitomycin C	70	0	29	41%
Miscellaneous				
Alpha interferon-recombinant	76	0	2	3%
Hexamethylmelamine	39	0	11	28%
Spiromerganium	103	1	2	3%

Modified from Livingston RB, Carter SK. Single agents in cancer chemotherapy. New York: IFI Plenum, 1970; Anonymous. Compilation of phase II results with single antineoplastic agents (series). Cancer Treat Symp 1985;4:4; Gasparini G, Caffo O, Barni S, et al. Vinorelbine is an active antiproliferative agent in pretreated advanced breast cancer patients; a phase II study. J Clin Oncol 1994; 12(10):2094–2101; Fumoleau P, Delgado FM, Delozier T, et al. Phase II trial of weekly intravenous vinorelbine in first-line advanced breast cancer chemotherapy. J Clin Oncol 1993;11(7):1245–1252; Rowinsky EK, Donehower RC. Paclitaxel (Taxol) [published erratum appears in N Engl J Med 1995;333(1):75]. N Engl J Med 1995;332(15):1004–1014.
[a]CR, complete response; PR, partial response.
[b]BCNU, N, N-bis(2-chloroethyl)-N-nitrosourea.
[c]CCNU, N-(2-chlorethyl)-N'-cylohexyl-N-nitrosourea.
[d]MGBG, methylglyoxal bis(guanylhydrazone).

cardiac damage, as confirmed by biopsy ($p =$ .002). This response to weekly doxorubicin is equivalent to the every 3-week dose schedule (204).

Continuous-infusion doxorubicin in advanced breast cancer has been associated with less cardiotoxicity by the M. D. Anderson Cancer Center (205). Investigators there compared 48-hour (79 patients) and 96-hour (62 patients) continuous infusion with bolus intravenous administration (133 patients). No difference in response rate was observed. At cumulative doses of 450 mg/m^2 or higher, the frequency of clinical congestive heart failure decreased 75% in continuous infusion groups ($p = .004$). According to Legha (206), when doxorubicin is administered by 96-hour infusion, the risk of cardiac toxicity is almost negligible up to a cumulated dose level of 800 mg/m^2, but with 48-hour infusions, 600 mg/m^2 can be safely tolerated.

Bispiperazinedione (ICRF-187) has been reported to protect against doxorubicin-induced cardiac toxicity in women with advanced breast cancer (207). Cardiac toxicity was evaluated by clinical examination, by left ventricular ejection fraction measured by multigated nuclear scans, and by endomyocardial biopsy. A group of 92 women was randomized to receive 5-fluorouracil plus doxorubicin plus cyclophosphamide (FDC) or FDC plus ICRF-187. At equivalent cumulative doses of doxorubicin, the group receiving ICRF-187 had significantly less cardiac toxicity ($p=.001$) and no alteration in antitumor

effect. With the concurrent use of ICRF-187, doxorubicin doses up to 700 mg/m^2 appear to be well tolerated (208).

A series of *doxorubicin analogues* are currently under study in clinical trials: epirubicin, idarubicin, 4'-deoxydoxorubicin, pirarubicin, and rubidisone. Among these, the agent studied most extensively in breast cancer has been epirubicin.

Epirubicin

In a small series of previously untreated patients with breast cancer, epirubicin had a response rate of 67% (16 of 24 patients), which is equivalent to that of doxorubicin. However, this finding should be confirmed in a larger series (209). The advantage of epirubicin is that it is associated with less cardiac toxicity than doxorubicin and with decreased hepatic clearance, which means that the drug can be used in patients with advanced liver metastases (210). However, epirubicin has not been released for use in the United States, since it is felt that it does not have any true advantage over doxorubicin.

Mitoxantrone

Mitoxantrone is a synthetic hydroxyquinone related structurally to doxorubicin. Mitoxantrone is an active drug in breast cancer, as well as in acute leukemia and lymphoma (211). Clinically significant cardiac toxicity occurs in approximately 3% of patients receiving cumulative doses of 175 to 250 mg/m^2. Significant alopecia is much less frequent in patients treated with mitoxantrone than in those treated with doxorubicin, and it occurs in fewer than 10% of cases. Nausea and vomiting are uncommon. Mitoxantrone appears not to be a vesicant if it is infiltrated. The dose-limiting toxicity is myelosuppression, which may be prolonged. The current consensus is that mitoxantrone is an active drug in breast cancer which is less toxic than doxorubicin, but its response rate is approximately 10% less than that of doxorubicin (212–215). Mitoxantrone probably has a role in the treatment of frail elderly patients or patients with breast cancer who have an intercurrent medical illness (216–218). The dosage of mitoxantrone as a single agent is 10 to 14 mg/m^2 intravenously every 3 weeks.

TAXANES

The taxanes are novel antimicrotubule agents that have shown outstanding activity against breast cancer (218a). *Paclitaxel* (Taxol, Bristol Laboratories), a derivative from the bark of the western yew tree, *Taxus brevifolia*, has excellent single-agent activity in the advanced disease setting. Holmes et al. (219) administered paclitaxel to 25 patients, all of whom had previous chemotherapy, 11 for metastatic disease. Paclitaxel was given at a dose of 250 mg/m^2 by continuous infusion over 24 hours every 21 days. The overall response rate was 56%, with 2 complete remissions. Neutropenia was the dose-limiting effect, with a median granulocyte count of 100 to 200/mm^3 for most courses (219). Subsequently, Reichman and co-workers combined paclitaxel with G-CSF in an attempt to limit neutropenia. Paclitaxel was given at 250 mg/m^2 over 24 hours every 21 days, with G-CSF administered at 5 µg/kg/day on days 3 to 10. No patient had been previously treated with chemotherapy for metastatic disease. Twenty-six patients were evaluable for response; 62% responded, with 3 complete responses. Median time to response was 5 weeks (220).

A large Canadian and European trial has explored paclitaxel given as a 3-hour infusion at doses of 175 mg/m^2 and 135 mg/m^2. Seventy percent of the patients in this large study had previous chemotherapy for metastatic disease. In the 225 patients treated at the higher dose level (175 mg/m^2), there were 29% responders, with 5% complete responses. At the 135 mg/m^2 dose level, 22% of the 229 patients responded, with 2% being complete responses. Grade 4 neutropenia was seen in 18% of patients treated at 175 mg/m^2 and 12% of those treated at 135 mg/m^2.

Only one patient had febrile neutropenia (221). Based on this study, the current recommended single agent dose of paclitaxel is 175 mg/m^2 given over 3 hours every 21 days.

Paclitaxel appears to be active in patients previously treated with anthracyclines (222, 223, 223a). The duration of infusion appears to be important. A longer infusion time of 96 hours resulted in a 53% response rate in a group of 22 patients with anthracycline-refractory disease treated with a dose of 140 mg/m^2 (224). Paclitaxel is also being evaluated in combination with doxorubicin or with cisplatin (225–227, 227a).

The role of paclitaxel in the adjuvant setting is currently being evaluated in an intergroup study. The basic schema being investigated is four cycles of standard chemotherapy (Adriamycin plus cyclophosphamide) alone or followed by four cycles of paclitaxel. The NSABP is also evaluating the potential role of paclitaxel in the adjuvant setting.

Docetaxel (Taxotere, Rhône-Poulenc Rorer Pharmaceuticals) is a semisynthetic taxane that also appears to be very active in patients with advanced breast cancer (228). In a phase II study by Chevallier et al. (229) for the European Organization for Research and Treatment of Cancer (EORTC) using a docetaxel dose of 100 mg/m^2 given every 3 weeks as first line therapy in 35 patients with measurable disease, 68% of 31 evaluable patients responded. Half of the responses occurred after 11 weeks of treatment. Median time to progression was 37+ weeks, with a median survival of 16+ months. All patients experienced grade 3 or 4 neutropenia; however, no grade 3 or 4 infection was noted. Some degree of fluid retention occurred in 76% of patients, with 30% developing serous effusions. These problems led to treatment discontinuation in 70% of patients in this study. Phase II trials in the U.S. (230) and Canada (231, 231a) have yielded similar response rates at the 100 mg/m^2 dose level.

In an attempt to lessen toxicity, a subsequent EORTC study used a reduced dose of docetaxel of 75 mg/m^2 every 3 weeks. In 34 patients with no prior therapy for advanced disease, a 50% response rate was noted; however, toxicity was still significant, as 41% of patients went off study because of problems with fluid retention, and 74% developed grade 4 neutropenia (232). Fluid retention can be substantially reduced with dexamethasone, 8 mg twice daily for 4 days starting 1 day prior to docetaxel administration. An additional 2 days of dexamethasone, 4 mg twice daily, should also be given for a total of 6 days of treatment (232a).

Docetaxel appears to be active in patients refractory to anthracyclines. In a study of 33 evaluable anthracycline refractory patients from M. D. Anderson Cancer Center, a response rate of 55% was noted (233).

The taxanes are highly active agents in breast cancer therapy. Their exact role in breast cancer therapy is being actively investigated in both the adjuvant setting as well as for the treatment of metastatic disease. The major role of paclitaxel at the present time is in patients who have failed anthracycline (234).

VINORELBINE

Vinorelbine (Navelbine, Burroughs Wellcome) is a new vinca alkaloid that differs from vinblastine by virtue of a modification of the cantheranthine moiety (235). Vinorelbine is highly active as a single agent in previously untreated patients with advanced breast cancer. Fumoleau et al. (201) reported a response rate of 41% in 145 previously untreated patients at a dose of 30 mg/m^2/week, with 7% complete responses, quite similar to the results of other studies using vinorelbine as initial therapy (236, 237).

Combination therapy using vinorelbine with other drugs active against breast cancer has also been explored. The combination of vinorelbine and doxorubicin was given as initial therapy for advanced disease in 89 evaluable patients by Spielman et al. (238). Vinorelbine was given at 25 mg/m^2 days 1 and 8, while the doxorubicin was given at 50 mg/m^2 day 1 of each 3 week cycle. The overall response rate was 74%, with 21% complete responses. Neutropenia was the major toxicity, with 41% of patients experiencing grade 3 or 4 neutropenia; however, only 3% of cycles required hospitalization for febrile neutropenia. The combination of vinorelbine and doxorubicin gave an overall response rate of 54% in a U.S. multicenter trial by Hochster et al. (239). Combinations of vinorelbine with mitoxantrone or epirubicin also appear to be potentially useful (240, 241).

Vinorelbine plus mitomycin C has also been used in several different schemas. Scheithauer et al. (242) gave vinorelbine at 30 mg/m^2 every 3 weeks with mitomycin C 15 mg/m^2 every 6 weeks as second-line therapy and found an overall response rate of 35% in 34 evaluable patients. Hematologic toxicity was mild. A more intense vinorelbine plus mitomycin combination that used weekly vinorelbine at 30 mg/m^2/week for the first month, with half doses on days 8 and 22, together with mitomycin C at 8 mg/m^2 on day 1 and 29 then every 6 weeks, produced objective responses in 44% of anthracycline-refractory patients (243).

The lack of significant toxicity, other than self-limited and brief neutropenia and phlebitis, makes vinorelbine an attractive option in some patients with advanced breast cancer. The role of vinorelbine in the adjuvant setting has not been defined; however, NSABP is planning to evaluate vinorelbine in older women with node positive breast cancer.

5-FLUOROURACIL

5-FU was synthesized in 1957 as an antitumor agent by Heidelberger et al. at the University of Wisconsin and was rapidly introduced into clinical practice (244). As a single agent, 5-FU became the most commonly used nonhormonal drug in the treatment of advanced breast cancer (245). With the introduction of combination chemotherapy in the 1970s, 5-FU was incorporated into many commonly used regimens, including Cooper's original CMFVP.

5-FU Plus Leucovorin

There is now renewed interest in 5-FU since it has been demonstrated that leucovorin (LV) can potentiate 5-FU cytotoxicity. The major cytotoxic mechanism of 5-FU is the inhibition of DNA synthesis by binding to the enzyme thymidylate synthetase. This blocks the conversion of uridylate to thymidylate and thus blocks DNA synthesis. The degree of intracellular binding of the 5-FU metabolite, 5FdUMP, to thymidylate synthetase depends on the intracellular availability of methyl-tetrahydrofolate (mTHF). LV is converted intracellularly to mTHF. Therefore, the addition of LV increases the intracellular availability of mTHF and, in turn, enhances the inhibition of thymidylate synthetase (provided a series of complex conditions are met) (246). The proper conditions for LV enhancement of 5-FU are not met in all tumor systems but are met in colorectal cancers and probably also in breast cancer (247, 248).

When LV is administered with 5-FU, the toxicity is altered. At LV doses of 20 to 200 mg/m^2, with 5-FU (370 mg/m^2) given intravenously daily for 5 consecutive days, the major toxicity is stomatitis and mild diarrhea; approximately 20% of patients develop leukopenia with a white blood cell count of less than 2000/μL (247). When the dose of LV is increased to 500 mg/m² once weekly, some patients develop a profuse watery diarrhea that can result in severe dehydration and even renal failure. Great caution must be taken at these levels, and at the first sign of significant diarrhea, chemotherapy must be discontinued and fluid replacement initiated to prevent a possible catastrophe (249). Several clinical trials of 5-FU plus LV in previously treated patients with advanced breast cancer have now been reported. Swain et al. (250), using a 500 mg/m² dose of LV plus 5-FU, 375 mg/m² given daily for 5 consecutive days, noted a 24% objective response rate in 54 previously treated patients. Jabboury et al. (251), using LV 200 mg/m²/day over 30 minutes plus 5-FU, 200 mg/m²/day by continuous infusion for 5 to 12 days, reported a 60% response (12 of 20 patients) in patients previously treated with chemotherapy. Marini et al. (252), using LV, 200 mg/m²/day plus 5-FU, 370 mg/m² given immediately after the LV daily for 5 consecutive days, noted a 44% response (16 of 36 patients). The combination of 5-FU plus LV is also being incorporated into other breast cancer treatment regimens as is discussed in the section on combination chemotherapy.

Continuous Infusion of 5-FU

The continuous infusion of 5-FU was introduced by Lokich et al. (253) and appears to have utility in previously treated patients with advanced breast cancer. Jabboury et al. (254) evaluated 5-FU, 250 mg/m²/day, given by continuous infusion. The median duration of the infusion was 65 days, with a range of 19 to 508 days. Five of 32 patients responded. The main toxicities were stomatitis in 13 patients, the hand-foot syndrome (palmar-plantar erythrodysesthesia) in 6, and Coombs-positive hemolytic anemia in 2. Myelosuppression was uncommon. Using similar regimens, Hatfield et al. (255) reported a 28% response (7 of 25 patients), and Huan et al. (256) reported a 53% response (15 of 28 patients). 5-FU given by continuous infusion is feasible with ambulatory infusion pumps, but its role in the treatment of patients with metastatic breast cancer is yet to be defined (257).

Combination Chemotherapy

Since breast cancer responds to all of the major classes of chemotherapeutic agents, it is uniquely suited for combination chemotherapy. The use of combination chemotherapy has more than doubled the response rates of single agents. However, given the drugs currently available, the results of all commonly used combinations are more or less the same: a 60% objective response, with a 10 to 15% complete response and a response duration of 8 to 12 months. However, at times responses are dramatic, with decreased bone pain, improved performance status, increased appetite, and overall improvement in the quality of life. Bedridden patients may return to useful, productive lives, and responses may last for years rather than the median of 8 to 12 months.

A series of factors are predictive of a good response to chemotherapy: good performance status, a limited number of disease sites, response to prior hormonal therapy, and soft tissue–dominant metastases. Other factors are associated with a decreased probability of response: bone-dominant or liver-dominant metastases, prior chemotherapy, prior radiation therapy, and decreased lymphocyte counts. Menopausal status does not influence response to chemotherapy in patients with advanced breast cancer (258), and healthy patients over age 70 have been shown to not only tolerate but also respond to the commonly used chemotherapy regimens for metastatic disease (259, 260).

DNA flow cytometry and S-phase fraction have been reported to be predictive of response to cytotoxic drugs (261, 262). There seems to be a strong correlation between S-phase fraction and response to chemotherapy. In one series, all 12 patients with an S-phase fraction of 10% or more responded to treatment, and 6 of these responses were complete. DNA ploidy and histologic grade did not correlate with response (263).

FIRST-LINE CHEMOTHERAPY

First-line chemotherapeutic regimens for metastatic breast cancer have classically fallen into one of two overlapping categories: the Cooper CMFVP variants (Table 54.7) and the Adriamycin (doxorubicin)-based combinations. Each has had strong supporters, but it has been difficult to define which represents "standard" or "state-of-the-art" therapy. Currently, a series of new drugs, singly or in combination, are being evaluated as first-line agents. The role of these new agents (paclitaxel, vinorelbine, and mitoxantrone) will be defined over the next few years. The dosage schedules for commonly used first-line chemotherapy regimens are outlined in Tables 54.9 and 54.10 and in Chapter 44.

CMF Versus CAF

CMF (C, cyclophosphamide; M, methotrexate; F, 5-fluorouracil) is the active component of the original five-drug Cooper CMFVP regimen. CMF, CMFVP, and other variants have been tested extensively against CAF (A, Adriamycin/doxorubicin) and CAFVP. The Cancer and Leukemia Group B (CALGB) has conducted two such trials (266–267). In the first trial, CAFVP versus CMFVP was tested. The overall response rate for CAFVP was 71%, compared with 50% for CMFVP ($p = .002$), but the response duration and survival were equivalent.

Table 54.9. First-Line Non-Adriamycin Chemotherapy Regimens for Breast Cancer

1. CMFVP (Cancer and Leukemia Group B)
   Cyclophosphamide 100 mg/m² p.o. days 1–14
   Methotrexate 40 mg/m² i.v. days 1 and 8
   5-FU 500 mg/m² i.v. days 1 and 8
   Vincristine 1 mg/m² i.v. days 1 and 8
   Prednisone 40 mg/m² p.o. days 1–14
   No treatment days 15–28; repeat on a 28-day cycle
2. CMF (National Cancer Institute of Milan)
   Cyclophosphamide 100 mg/m² p.o. days 1–14
   Methotrexate 30–40* mg/m² i.v. days 1 and 8
   5-FU 400–600* mg/m² i.v. days 1 and 8
   No treatment days 15–28; repeat on a 28-day cycle
   *Lower dose level for patients ≥65 years old
3. CMF (National Cancer Institute of Milan)
   Cyclophosphamide 600 mg/m² i.v. day 1
   Methotrexate 40 mg/m² i.v. day 1
   5-FU 600 mg/m² i.v. day 1
   Cycle repeated every 21 days
4. CMFP (Eastern Cooperative Oncology Group)
   Cyclophosphamide 100 mg/m² p.o. days 1–14
   Methotrexate 30–40* mg/m² i.v. days 1 and 8
   5-FU 400–600* mg/m² i.v. days 1 and 8
   Prednisone 40 mg/m² p.o. days 1–14
   *Lower dose level given to patients ≥65 years old
5. CFP (Mayo Clinic)
   Cyclophosphamide 150 mg/m² i.v. daily × 5
   5-FU 300 mg/m² i.v. daily × 5
   Prednisone 30 mg/day for 14 days, then 20 mg/day for 7 days, and 10 mg/day thereafter
   5-day CF cycles repeated every 5 weeks

From Kardinal CG. Chemotherapy. In: Donegan WL, Spratt JS, eds. Cancer of the breast. 2nd ed. Philadelphia: WB Saunders, 1979;405–447; Bonadonna G, Zambetti M, Valagussa P. Sequential or alternating doxorubicin and CMF regimens in breast cancer with more than three positive nodes. Ten-year results. JAMA 1995;273(7):542–547.

Table 54.10. First-Line Adriamycin (Doxorubicin)-Containing Regimens for Breast Cancer[a]

1. AC (National Surgical Adjuvant Breast Project)
   Doxorubicin (Adriamycin) 60 mg/m² i.v. day 1
   Cyclophosphamide 600 mg/m² i.v. day 1
   Repeat every 21 days
2. CAF (Cancer and Leukemia Group B)
   Cyclophosphamide 100 mg/m² p.o. days 1–14
   Adriamycin 25 mg/m² i.v. days 1 and 8
   5-FU 500 mg/m² i.v. days 1 and 8
   No treatment days 15–18; repeat cycle every 28 days
3. CAF (Southeastern Cancer Study Group)
   Cyclophosphamide 500 mg/m² i.v. day 1
   Adriamycin 500 mg/m² i.v. day 1
   5-FU 500 mg/m² i.v. day 1
   Repeat cycle every 3 weeks
4. FAC (M. D. Anderson Cancer Center)
   5-FU 500 mg/m² i.v. days 1 and 8
   Adriamycin 50 mg/m² i.v. by continuous infusion over 48 to 96 hours
   Cyclophosphamide 500 mg/m² i.v. on day 1
   Repeat cycle every 28 days

Modified from Kardinal CG. Chemotherapy. In: Donegan WL, Spratt JS, eds. Cancer of the breast. 2nd ed. Philadelphia: WB Saunders, 1979;405–447; Fisher B, Brown AM, Dimitrov NV, et al. Two months of Adriamycin-cyclophosphamide with and without interval reinduction therapy compared with six months of cyclophosphamide, methotrexate and 5-fluorouracil in positive-node breast cancer patients with tamoxifen-nonresponsive tumors: results from NSABP B-15. J Clin Oncol 1990;8:1483–1496.
[a]The total comulative dose of Adriamycin in all regimens should not exceed 450 mg/m².

In the second CALGB trial, CMF versus CAF versus CAFVP was tested. This trial also tested nonspecific immunotherapy with the methanol extraction residue of bacillus Calmette-Guerin vaccine (MER). MER produced toxicity without apparent response or survival benefit and was dropped from the trial. The authors concluded that CAF and CAFVP were equivalent and that both were superior to CMF.

The Southeastern Cancer Study Group tested CAF versus CMFVP (268). The response rate for CAF was 55% and for CMFVP was 40% ($p = .01$), but again response duration and survival were the same. CAF probably has a slight advantage over CMF; however, the data are not compelling (269). The role of 5-FU in the CAF combination is being questioned, and the two drug AC combination is now in common use. With AC, greater dose intensity of Adriamycin and cyclophosphamide can be achieved with equivalent toxicity.

Mitoxantrone Combinations

The combination of mitoxantrone (Novantrone, N) with 5-FU and cyclophosphamide (CNF) was compared with CAF in three large clinical trials involving 526 chemotherapy-naive patients with metastatic breast cancer (270–272). Response rates for CNF were 29 to 46%, compared with 37 to 42% for CAF. There was no difference in median response duration or survival. Cardiac toxicity and alopecia were significantly lower in the CNF groups. The recommended dosage schedule for CNF is cyclophosphamide 500 mg/m² intravenously, mitoxantrone 10 mg/m² intravenously, and 5-FU 500 mg/m² intravenously on day 1 and repeated every 3 weeks. CNF may have a role as first-line therapy in patients with a poor performance status or intercurrent medical illness.

There has been considerable interest in the mitoxantrone (N), 5-FU (F), and leucovorin (L) combination; the NFL regimen. Response rates from 45 to 65% were reported in previously treated patients (273, 274). These reports prompted the NCCTG to perform a phase I–II trial of NFL using accelerated doses of mitoxantrone with G-CSF support. The NCCTG was not able to duplicate the response rate in previously treated patients, even when the dose of mitoxantrone had been doubled. Standard dose NFL (N, 12 mg/m² i.v. day 1; L, 300 mg total i.v. 1 hour before F, 350 mg/m² i.v., days 1, 2, and 3; repeated every 3 weeks), however, is well tolerated and may have a role as second-line therapy. NFL has also been evaluated as first-line therapy in metastatic breast cancer and appears to have a higher response rate and longer time to progression than CMF (275, 276). The exact role of mitoxantrone in the treatment of breast cancer is not yet fully defined.

Cisplatin Combinations

Cisplatin as a single agent has significant activity in previously untreated patients with metastatic breast cancer (Table 54.8). Cisplatin combinations have also been tested as first-line and second-line therapy. Several small clinical trials in previously untreated patients testing the *CAP* (P, cisplatin) regimens have been reported (277). The basic dosage schedule is as follows:

Cyclophosphamide, 400 mg/m² i.v. day 1
Doxorubicin, 40 mg/m² i.v. day 1
Cisplatin, 40 mg/m² i.v. day 1
(cycle repeated every 3–4 weeks)

Reported response rates were from 50 to 83%.

Two other cisplatin-based regimens have been tested as first-line chemotherapy in advanced breast cancer.

1. Cisplatin, 100 mg/m² day 1
   Etoposide, 100 mg/m² days 1, 2, 3
   (cycle repeated every 21 days)
2. MVAC
   Methotrexate, 30 mg/m² days 1, 15, 22
   Vinblastine, 3 mg/m² days 2, 15, 22
   Doxorubicin, 30 mg/m² day 2
   Cisplatin, 70 mg/m² day 2
   (cycle repeated every 28 days)

The combination of *cisplatin* and *etoposide* has been evaluated in previously treated as well as previously untreated patients. There was a 47% (24 of 51) response in previously untreated patients, with a response duration of 39 weeks (278). In previously treated patients, however, the response rate to cisplatin plus etoposide is in the range of 25% (11 of 44) to 38% (11 of 290 (279, 280). *MVAC* has been evaluated as first-line chemotherapy for metastatic breast cancer. Response rates from 63 to 83% have been reported, but with considerable toxicity (281, 282). Cisplatin combinations are active in metastatic breast cancer but are not more active than the more commonly used, less toxic CMF and CAF regimens. These regimens cannot be recommended with any degree of enthusiasm.

ALTERNATING NON-CROSS-RESISTANT CHEMOTHERAPY IN BREAST CANCER

Since breast cancer responds to all major classes of chemotherapeutic agents, it would seem to provide an ideal setting for alternating non-cross-resistant chemotherapy. Goldie and associates (283, 284) provided the theoretic and mathematical rationale for this approach to therapy, based on the observation that drug-resistant tumor cells emerge during cancer chemotherapy and constitute a formidable obstacle to achieving long-term remission or cure. Alternating the sequence of chemotherapeutic agents with different mechanisms of action should give the greatest tumor cell kill and prevent or delay the emergence of drug-resistant clones (283, 285).

Since doxorubicin is not cross-resistant with CMF, one might anticipate that regimens alternating CMF combinations with doxorubicin combinations would result in increased response rates and response durations. A large series of these trials is summarized in Table 54.11 (286–297). These trials showed marginally significant improvement in overall response with no improvement in survival. Alternating non-cross-resistant chemotherapy in metastatic breast cancer has not lived up to the theoretic expectations.

SECOND-LINE CHEMOTHERAPY

Many regimens have activity in metastatic breast cancer in patients previously treated with CMF/CMFVP or CAF (298). If the patient has not received an anthracycline as part of the first-line chemotherapeutic regimen, doxorubicin or mitoxantrone should be incorporated into the second-line program. If the patient has been treated with an anthracycline, paclitaxel and vinorelbine are emerging as the second-line treatments of choice. Infusion chemotherapy with 5-FU or 5-FU plus leucovorin could be considered; infusion vinblastine, a mitomycin C–containing

regimen, or possibly even a cisplatin-based combination could be used. Responses are often brief, and complete remissions are rare. Although many patients may obtain temporary palliation with second-line chemotherapy regimens, quality-of-life issues must be considered in patients with advanced cancer (299, 300). Clearly we need more effective, less toxic therapy. It cannot be too strongly emphasized that participation in clinical trials is the only means to that end.

Second-Line Doxorubicin Combinations

Doxorubicin as a single agent yields objective responses in 28% of patients previously treated with CMF/CMFVP. Doxorubicin has been evaluated in a variety of combinations in previously treated patients. *VATH* (vinblastine, Adriamycin, thiotepa, Halotestin) was one of the earliest regimens tested (301, 302). Halotestin (fluoxy-

Table 54.11. Randomized Trials Comparing a Single Regimen with Alternating Non-Cross-Resistant Regimens

| Regimen[a] | Number of Patients | Response Rate (%) | | Median Duration (months) | | Reference |
		PR + CR[b]	CR	Response	Survival	
CFP vs.	23	48	15	12	24	Ahmann et al., 1978 (287)
A/L-PAM	27	52	9	13	21	
CFP → A/L-PAM or	50	68+	10	16	22	
A/L-PAM ↔ CFP (2)						
CA vs.	26	50	12	10		Kennealey et al., 1978 (288)
CA ↔ MF (1)	22	55	32	10		
CAF vs.	46	63	13			Tormey et al., 1979 (289)
DAV ↔ CMF (3)	48	71	10			
CFP vs.	18	18	0	9	14	Nemoto et al., 1982 (290)
CA vs.	42	42	2	12	18	
CFP ↔ CA (1)	20	63++	0	11	19	
CMFP vs.	135	59	14	11	19	Tormey et al., 1983 (291)
CMFP ↔ AV (2)	176	58	14	10	16	
CAF vs.	66	29	2	8	15	Vogel et al., 1984 (292)
CAF ↔ CAMELEON (3)	91	17++	0	11+++	16	
CFP vs.	41	46	7		18	Creagan et al., 1984 (293)
CAP ↔ CFP (4)	45	49	4		11	
CMF ↔ A + Mito C (1)	28	67	46	14		Cruciani et al., 1987 (294)
CAF vs.	497	52	11		17	Aisner et al., 1995 (295)
VATH → CMFVP vs.		58	11		17	
VATH ↔ CMFVP (1)		52	12		17	
A → CMF (4)	44	77.5	29.5	28	22	Zambetti et al., 1995 (296)
MF ↔ CAV	41	68	12		13.7	Kiang et al., 1995 (297)

Modified from Henderson IC, Hayes DF, Come S, Harris JR, Canellos G. New agents and new medical treatments for advanced breast cancer. Semin Oncol 1987;14:34–64.
[a]Abbreviations: C, cyclophosphamide; A, doxorubicin; F, 5-fluorouracil; P, prednisone; L-PAM, L-phenylalanine mustard; M, methotrexate; D, dibromodulcitol; V, vincristine; CAMELEON, cytosine arabinoside, methotrexate, leucovorin rescue, vincristine; Mito C, Mitomycin C; VATH, vinblastine, Adriamycin, thiotepa, halotestin; (number) cycles before first crossover and/or number of cycles between each subsequent regimen alteration. +$p = .07$; ++$p = .025$; +++$p = .08$ (other differences not statistically significant)
[b]PR, partial rsponse; CR, complete response.

mesterone) was incorporated into the VATH regimen as a bone marrow stimulant. However, as an androgen, it yields a 20% objective response in unselected patients with metastatic breast cancer. A 52% objective response in 19 patients refractory to CMF/CMFVP was reported for the 5-day VATH regimen, and a 49% objective response was seen in 29 patients with the 1-day VATH regimen (Table 54.12).

Several other clinical trials have tested doxorubicin in combination with a vinca alkaloid in previously treated patients. Tannir et al. (303) from the M. D. Anderson Cancer Center reported a 43% response (18 of 42 patients) to sequential continuous *infusion doxorubicin and vinblastine* in patients previously treated with CMFVP. Doxorubicin (25 mg/m^2/day) was given as a continuous intravenous infusion for 2 days, followed by vinblastine, 1.4 mg/m^2/day for 4 days. The cycle was repeated every 3 weeks. The NCCTG randomized 173 previously treated patients to doxorubicin (D) versus *DVM* (doxorubicin, vincristine, mitomycin C) (304). The doxorubicin dose was 60 mg/m^2; the DVM dosage schema are in Table 54.12. There was an objective response of 24% (20 of 83 patients) to D and 37% (29 of 78 patients) to DVM ($p = .036$).

The *VAM* combination of vinblastine, Adriamycin, and mitomycin C has been tested in two clinical trials. Oster and Park from Columbia University evaluated 15 previously treated patients; 11 responded (3 complete responses, 8 partial responses) for a response rate of 73% (305). However, Luikart et al. (306) observed only a 33% response (9 of 27 patients, with 3 complete responses and 6 partial responses) to VAM. The VAM dosage schema are in Table 54.12.

It appears that the addition of a vinca alkaloid enhances the response to doxorubicin in previously treated patients. The vinca of choice is vinblastine because of its lack of neurotoxicity and its equivalent efficacy to vincristine in advanced breast cancer. Mitomycin C and thiotepa might enhance the response of the doxorubicin-vinblastine combination, but verifiable data are sparse.

Second-Line Vinblastine Combinations

In the management of previously treated patients with advanced breast cancer, *vinblastine* has assumed a prominent role that may not be totally justified. VATH and VAM have already been discussed (Table 54.12). *Vinblastine administered in continuous infusion* was reported to give

Table 54.12. Second-Line Chemotherapy Regimens for Advanced Breast Cancer

1. NFL (273)
   Mitoxantrone (Novantrone) 12 mg/m^2 i.v. day 1
   5-Fluorouracil 350 mg/m^2 i.v. days 1, 2, 3
   Leucovorin 300 mg (total dose) days 1, 2, 3 given 1 hour prior to the 5-FU
   Repeat every 21 days
2. Paclitaxel (Taxol) (221)
   175 mg/m^2 in 500 or 1000 ml 5% dextrose or 0.9% saline i.v. over 3 hours
   Use only glass bottles and polyethylene-lined administration sets
   Premedicate with:
   Dexamethasone 20 mg p.o. approximately 6 and 12 hours prior to Taxol
   Diphenhydramine 50 mg i.v. 30 to 60 minutes prior to Taxol
   Cimetidine 300 mg or ranitidine 50 mg i.v. 30 to 60 minutes prior to Taxol
   Repeat every 21 days
3. One-Day VATH (Cancer and Leukemia Group B)
   Vinblastin 4.5 mg/m^2 day 1
   Adriamycin 45 mg/m^2 day 1
   Thiotepa 12 mg/m^2 day 1
   Halotestin 10 mg p.o. t.i.d. continuously
   Repeat every 21 days
4. DVM (North Central Cancer Treatment Group)
   Doxorubicin 50 mg/m^2 days 1 and 28
   Vincristine 1 mg/m^2 days 1 and 28
   Mitomycin C 10 mg/m^2 day 1
   Repeat cycle every 8 weeks
5. VAM (Yale University)
   Vinblastine 6 mg/m^2 days 1 and 28
   Adriamycin 30 mg/m^2 days 1 and 28
   Mitomycin C 10 mg/m^2 day 1
   Repeat cycle every 8 weeks
6. Vinblastine + mitomycin C (University of Arizona)
   First two cycles:
   Mitomycin C 10 mg/m^2 i.v. days 1 and 28
   Vinblastine 5 mg/m^2 i.v. days 1, 14, 28, 42
   Subsequent cycles:
   Mitomycin C 10 mg/m^2 i.v. day 1
   Vinblastine 5 mg/m^2 days 1 and 21
   Repeat every 6 to 8 weeks

Modified from Kardinal CG. Chemotherapy. In: Donegan WL, Spratt JS, eds. Cancer of the breast, 2nd ed. Philadelphia: WB Saunders, 1979:405–447.

a 40% objective response (12 of 30 patients, with 1 complete response and 11 partial responses) in refractory advanced breast cancer (307). Vinblastine was administered as a 5-day continuous infusion at 1.4 to 2.0 mg/m^2/day. Myelosuppression was mild to moderate at doses between 1.4 and 1.8 mg/m^2, but it became severe at 2 mg/m^2. Two subsequent studies using 1.2 to 1.8 mg/

m² of vinblastine by continuous intravenous infusion have been reported (308, 309). No responses were observed in either (0 of 17 patients in the first trial, and 0 of 15 patients with measurable disease in the second trial). No responses (0 of 18) were observed in a trial of continuous infusion *vincristine* (310). The efficacy of continuous-infusion vinca alkaloids as single agents in advanced, previously treated breast cancer is questionable.

Vinblastine plus mitomycin C has been evaluated in several clinical trials in advanced, previously treated breast cancer. A 40% objective response rate (12 of 30 cases) was reported in a trial evaluating mitomycin C, 20 mg/m² given on day 1, and vinblastine, 0.15 mg/kg given on days 1 and 21. The cycles were repeated every 6 to 8 weeks (311). Similarly, a 32% response (7 of 22 patients) was noted in a second trial of mitomycin C and vinblastine (dosage schedule in Table 54.12) (312). However, only a 14% response to mitomycin C and vinblastine (3 of 22) was noted in a third reported trial (313). Mitomycin C plus vinblastine appears to be an active combination in advanced, refractory breast cancer. Median response durations, however, are relatively short, between 127 and 164 days for the trials reported above.

High-Dose Chemotherapy and Autologous Stem Cell Transplantation

Dose intensity has significant influence on the response rate and duration in the chemotherapy of metastatic breast cancer (314). The dose-response curves for cytotoxic drugs in animal tumor models are steep. However, for human breast cancer, dose-response data are largely retrospective (315). Based on the steep dose-intensity curves for many chemotherapeutic agents, it is hypothesized that increasingly higher doses should be associated with higher response rates and even potential cure in advanced breast cancer. A safe means of administration of potentially lethal doses of chemotherapy is needed to test this hypothesis. Autologous bone marrow transplant (ABMT), with or without peripheral stem cell support, is currently being tested as a technique for safely administering these dose levels. The transplant per se is not therapeutic but is a salvage technique for the administration of high-dose chemotherapy. Inherent in ABMT is the fact that the dose-limiting toxicity of the chemotherapeutic agent employed is myelosuppression. Toxicity to the gastrointestinal, cardiac,

neurologic, and other systems is not reduced by this technique.

Multiple alkylator regimens are generally using because of their steep dose-response curves and variable nonhematologic toxicities (316). In an early trial, Peters et al. (317) reported a 54% complete response rate using high-dose cyclophosphamide, cisplatin, and carmustine or melphalan as initial treatment of metastatic disease in 22 patients. Median survival was 10.1 months for the group as a whole. Autologous marrow support was given in this group of patients.

Similar results were noted by Williams et al. (318) also using a multiple alkylator regimen. Median survival of the 59 patients treated with two different induction regimens prior to high-dose alkylator therapy was 13.3 months. In a group of 62 patients treated at the Dana Farber Cancer Institute, 7 of 19 complete responders (37%) remained in remission at a median follow-up of 43 months (319).

Recent trials have used peripheral blood stem cells together with, or in lieu of, autologous marrow (320–322). The isolation of marrow or peripheral blood progenitor cells (CD34⁺) is being explored as a method of reducing contamination by residual breast cancer cells (323, 323a). Multiple cycles of dose-intensive therapy have also been shown to be feasible. At present, there are no results from randomized prospective trials comparing standard chemotherapy with high-dose therapy plus stem cell support in the advanced disease setting. The use of high-dose chemotherapy, with peripheral stem cell support or with autologous bone marrow support, for the treatment of metastatic breast cancer remains investigational and cannot be justified outside the setting of a controlled clinical trial.

Because of the encouraging results in the setting of advanced disease, high-dose alkylator therapy has been used in the high-risk adjuvant setting. Peters reported 102 patients with high-risk stage II or III breast cancer, defined as 10 or more involved axillary lymph nodes, who received induction chemotherapy with CAF, followed by high-dose therapy and autologous marrow support. Of the 85 evaluable patients, the estimated event-free survival was 72%, with a median follow-up of 2 years. This compared favorably with event-free survival rates of 30 to 38% in several previous CALGB trials using standard adjuvant chemotherapy (324). An intergroup trial is currently under way that randomizes patients with 10 or more nodes to standard adjuvant chemotherapy or to high-dose chemotherapy and ABMT with stem cell support. This trial should help establish whether there is a role for this more toxic and expensive therapy in the adjuvant setting.

Chemohormonal Therapy

The use of combined hormonal and cytotoxic drug therapy is based upon *three assumptions*: (a) breast cancers are heterogeneous, that is, composed of varying proportions of receptor-positive and receptor-negative cells; (b) there is a differential response between receptor-positive and receptor-negative cells to both chemotherapy and hormonal therapy; and (c) there is no antagonism of chemotherapy-induced cytotoxicity by hormonal agents or, conversely, no antagonism of the effects of hormonal therapy by chemotherapy. The first assumption appears to be true. If the latter two assumptions are true, the response rates for combined therapy should at least be additive.

With regard to the second assumption, estrogen receptor (ER) is strongly predictive of response to hormonal therapy; however, do ER+ and ER− tumors respond differently to cytotoxic chemotherapy? Retrospective data are conflicting. Lippman et al. (325) reported a 75% objective rate of response to cytotoxic chemotherapy in ER− patients but only a 12% response in ER+ patients. Kiang et al. (326) reported the opposite finding, an 86% response in ER+ patients and a 36% response in ER− patients. The CALGB performed a prospective randomized trial of CAF (C, cyclophosphamide; A, Adriamycin; F, 5-fluorouracil) chemotherapy. Patients were stratified by ER status. The response rates of ER+ and ER− patients to CAF were identical (56%). However, the time to treatment failure, response duration, and survival were significantly greater in ER+ patients than in ER− patients (Table 54.13) (327). This lack of a differential response of ER+ and ER− breast cancer to cytotoxic chemotherapy has been confirmed in a second prospective, randomized trial (328). This trial also noted that ER+ patients who responded to chemotherapy had a greater duration of response and survival than ER− patients. There is no differential response. Cytotoxic chemotherapy kills ER+ and ER− cells indiscriminately. At least with reference to ER+ cells, chemotherapy and hormonal therapy appear to be competing for the same cell population.

With regard to the third assumption, antagonism between the antiestrogenic drug tamoxi-

Table 54.13. Results of CAF-Treated Patients by ER Status

| | | Median (months) | | |
CR + PR/Total	TTF[a]	Response Duration	Survival
ER+: 15 + 17/57 (56%)	15.3	19.1	23.7
ER−: 9 + 33/75 (56%)	8.3	8.9	15.7
p values	.0061	.0015	.0058

[a]TTF = time to treatment failure

Modified from Kardinal CG, Perry MC, Korzun AH, Wood W. Lack of differential response of estrogen receptor positive (ER+) vs. ER negative (ER−) breast cancer to Cytoxan + Adriamycin + 5-fluorouracil (CAF) chemotherapy (abstract). Proc Am Soc Clin Oncol 1986;5:74.

fen and various chemotherapeutic agents has been demonstrated in human breast cancer cell lines in tissue culture (329). Since tamoxifen acts as a cell-cycle inhibitor arresting cells in G_1 and G_0, and since chemotherapeutic agents are most active in actively proliferating cell systems, the antagonism between tamoxifen and chemotherapy is not unexpected. The third assumption also appears to be invalid.

Several clinical trials have evaluated combination chemotherapy with and without tamoxifen. In the largest of these trials, conducted by the CALGB (330, 331), patients were stratified by ER status, dominant site of metastatic disease, menopausal status, and prior adjuvant chemotherapy. They were then randomized to CAF chemotherapy (as in Table 54.11), with or without tamoxifen 10 mg orally twice daily. A total of 474 patients were entered; less than 5% were ineligible or inevaluable. Regardless of ER status or menopausal status, the addition of tamoxifen conferred no significant advantage in response rate, response duration, time to treatment failure, or survival over CAF alone. The NCCTG, in a similar trial, was unable to demonstrate a difference in time to disease progression or survival by the addition of tamoxifen to CFP over CFP alone (332). These trials have confirmed that the mere addition of a hormonal agent (e.g., tamoxifen) to combination chemotherapy (e.g., CAF or CFP) adds nothing to the response rate or response duration, regardless of receptor status. This confirms in vivo results that chemotherapy kills breast cancer cells indiscriminately, regardless of receptor status. It also confirms that chemotherapy and hormonal therapy compete for the same pool of ER cells.

Estrogen recruitment (estrogen priming) of breast cancer cells prior to chemotherapy has been attempted to stimulate DNA synthesis, increase mitotic rate, and (it was hoped) increase sensitivity to chemotherapy. Allegra (333) treated 25 patients with tamoxifen (10 mg twice daily for 10 days) to induce cell synchronization, followed by Premarin (0.625 mg twice daily for 4 days) to recruit cells into DNA synthesis (*Premarin priming*). After the Premarin regimen, methotrexate (M) (200 mg/m² i.v.) was administered, followed 1 hour later by 600 mg/m² 5-FU (F); leucovorin rescue was started 24 hours after the M to F chemotherapy. There was a 72% overall response rate, with 56% complete responses, in the 25 patients. This has never been duplicated; in fact, Eisenhauer et al. (334), using the same regimen, reported only a 10% overall response, with 3% complete responses, in 30 patients. Estrogenic recruitment was tested in a randomized trial of 117 patients by Conte et al. (335). They tested CEF (cyclophosphamide, 600 mg/m²; epirubicin, 60 mg/m²; 5-FU, 600 mg/m²) versus DES-CEF (diethylstilbestrol). There was no significant difference in response rate or survival between the two treatment arms.

Two other large trials have evaluated estrogen recruitment. One tested CAF, with or without estrogenic recruitment, the other, CMF with or without DES. Neither trial demonstrated a benefit to estrogenic recruitment (336, 337).

Despite negative therapeutic results, chemohormonal trials have been helpful in promoting a better understanding of breast cancer biology. This is particularly true in the area of the chemosensitivity of receptor positive tumors, that is, the lack of differential response to chemotherapy between ER+ and ER− breast cancers. Also of importance is the recognition that chemotherapy and hormonal therapy, when used together, compete for the same pool of ER+ cells. Chemohormonal trials are important clinically, since they verify that receptor-positive breast cancer should be treated sequentially and not concurrently with hormonal therapy and chemotherapy. Advanced ER+ breast cancer should be treated initially with hormonal manipulation; at treatment failure, combination chemotherapy should be initiated. Hormonally responsive breast cancer may respond to secondary, tertiary, or even quaternary forms of endocrine manipulation before cytotoxic drugs are necessary. The exception to the rule is the ER+ patient with life-threatening metastatic disease; rapid chemotherapeutic action is necessary.

SYSTEMIC ADJUVANT THERAPY

The theoretic basis for systemic adjuvant therapy of operable breast cancer is the Fisher hypothesis outlined in Table 54.1. Primary breast cancer is frequently a systemic disease at diagnosis with occult micrometastases in bone marrow, lung, liver, or other sites. Two classic prognostic variables are predictive of recurrence: the presence or absence of axillary nodal metastases and the hormone receptor status of the primary tumor (Table 54.2; Figs. 54.1 and 54.2). In addition, S-phase fraction appears to be an independent prognostic variable. Many other prognostic variables such as HER-2/*neu* (*erb* B₂), ploidy, epidermal growth factor receptors, haptoglobin-related protein epitopes, nm23 RNA, *p53* tumor suppressor gene, and c-*myc* oncogene levels have all been evaluated as prognostic markers. None reliably isolates patients who do not require adjuvant therapy (52–67, 338, 339).

As prognostic variables become more reliable, it may be possible to restrict systemic adjuvant therapy to patients at greatest risk of recurrence. Currently, 75% of axillary node–positive patients and 25% of axillary node–negative patients will have recurrences and ultimately die of the disease. The converse is that 25% of axillary node-positive and 75% of node-negative patients are cured by local therapy alone. With more specific prognostic indicators, these patients could be saved the cost, side effects, and potential risks of adjuvant treatment (340).

Perioperative Adjuvant Trials

The first prospective, randomized breast cancer adjuvant therapy trial was conducted by the National Surgical Adjuvant Breast Project (NSABP) between April 1958 and October 1961. This initial trial, NSABP B-01, was designed to test the hypothesis that chemotherapy would cure patients by destroying tumor cells disseminated in the blood at the time of surgery. A total 826 patients were randomly assigned to *perioperative thiotepa* (TSPA) or placebo administered at the time of surgery and on each of the first 2 postoperative days. One subset of patients, premenopausal women with four or more positive nodes who received perioperative TSPA, had significantly greater 5- and 10-year survival (56.5 vs. 24.3%, 5-year; 24.8 vs. 13.5%, 10-year) than those who received placebo (10, 11, 341).

The Scandinavian Adjuvant Chemotherapy Group chaired by R. Nissen-Meyer randomized

1026 women (507 treated and 519 controls) to no treatment or to cyclophosphamide (5 mg/kg/day for 6 days, with the first injection immediately after wound closure). With 20-year follow-up, the relapse rate was 60.5% in the control group and 48% in the treatment group ($p<.001$) (342).

More recently, the Ludwig Breast Cancer Study Group evaluated the role of *perioperative chemotherapy* in node-positive breast cancer (343). The Ludwig Group randomized 1229 axillary node–positive women into three treatment groups. One group received a single course of perioperative intravenous CMF beginning 36 hours after mastectomy; a second group received six cycles of conventional CMF starting 25 to 32 days after surgery; the third group received both the perioperative cycle and the conventionally timed regimen. Tamoxifen was added to the conventionally timed regimen in postmenopausal women. At a median follow-up of 42 months, the disease-free survival was 40% for the single perioperative group, 62% for conventional CMF, and 60% for the combined program ($p<.0001$). These results are graphically illustrated in Figure 54.6. In stage II breast cancer, a single perioperative cycle of adjuvant CMF is significantly less effective than conventional CMF and does not contribute to the efficacy of conventional CMF when it is used in combination. There is an isolated report that in stage I breast cancer, a single perioperative cycle of CMF may improve disease-free survival (344). This remains to be verified. Perioperative chemotherapy, like ablative hormonal therapy, is largely of historic interest.

Adjuvant Therapy of Stage II Breast Cancer

From the data obtained from the perioperative trials, it became apparent that cancer cells disseminated at the time of the surgery were less important than established micrometastases. Breast cancer, particularly stage II and stage III, is a systemic disease, and both systemic and local therapy are required to eradicate the disease.

THE NSABP STUDIES

Between September 1972 and February 1975, the NSABP conducted a landmark clinical trial comparing L-phenylalanine mustard (L-PAM) or mephalan with placebo in 370 women with stage II breast cancer (341, 345). These patients were stratified by menopausal status (≤ 49 vs. ≥ 50 years of age) and by the number of positive axillary nodes (one to three vs. four or more). L-PAM was administered in a dose of 0.15 mg/kg/day for 5 consecutive days every 6 weeks for 2 years. This study demonstrated improvement in disease-free and absolute survival in women 49 years of age or younger. Premenopausal women with one to three, as well as those with four or more, positive nodes benefited, but the advantage was greater for women with fewer

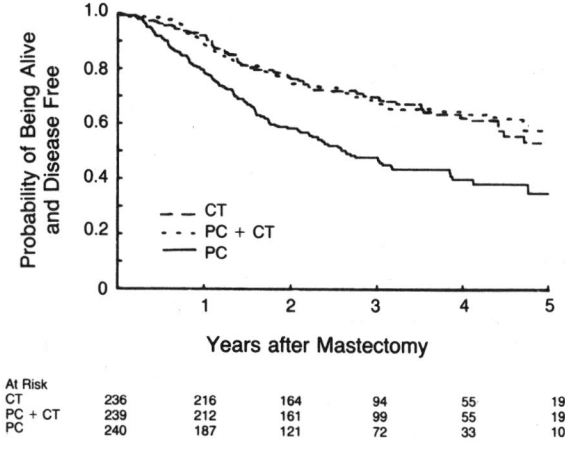

Figure 54.6. Disease-free survival according to treatment group among 715 premenopausal or perimenopausal patients with positive nodes at 42 months' median follow-up. *PC* denotes perioperative chemotherapy; *CT*, conventionally timed therapy. *"At risk"* refers to the number of patients being followed at the start of each year. Test for heterogeneity, $p<.0001$. Pairwise *p* values are as follows: $p<.0001$ (perioperative vs. conventionally timed), and p = .86 (perioperative + conventionally timed vs. conventionally timed). (From The Ludwig Breast Cancer Study Group. Combination adjuvant chemotherapy for node-positive breast cancer. Inadequacy of a single perioperative cycle. N Engl J Med 1988;319:677–683. With permission.).

than four positive nodes (Fig. 54.7). No advantage or disadvantage of L-PAM was observed in patients 50 years of age or older. This was the first large prospective randomized trial that confirmed the benefit of adjuvant systemic therapy in stage II breast cancer.

Based upon the data of the initial L-PAM trial, the NSABP conducted a series of clinical trials sequentially: P versus PF; PF versus PMF; and PF versus PAF (P, L-PAM; F, 5-FU; M, methotrexate; A, Adriamycin). The P versus PF trial was important because the addition of 5-FU to L-PAM increased disease-free survival in postmenopausal women with four or more positive nodes (341). The addition of methotrexate to PF (PF vs. PMF) failed to produce an advantage over PF in any menopausal or nodal subset. However, the addition of doxorubicin (Adriamycin) to PF (PAF) in receptor-negative, stage II breast cancer resulted in significantly better disease-free and absolute survival (346).

Following completion of the sequential L-PAM studies, the NSABP performed a series of trials evaluating AC (Adriamycin plus cyclophosphamide) as adjuvant treatment. The first of this series was NSABP B-15, which compared (*a*) four cycles of AC (A, 60 mg/m²; C, 600 mg/m²) intravenously every 3 weeks, with (*b*) six cycles of CMF, with (*c*) four cycles of AC followed by three cycles of CMF (265). This study was performed on 2194 receptor-negative, node-positive women. This study confirmed that AC × 4 given over a period of 2 months was equivalent to 6 months of CMF and that there was no advantage

to the addition of three cycles of CMF following AC × 4. Because of patient tolerance and the rapidity of the treatment, AC × 4 has become the adjuvant therapy of choice in many institutions.

The next NSABP AC trial was B-18, which compared AC × 4 preoperatively with AC × 4 postoperatively in women with palpable breast cancers (347). AC × 4 resulted in a more than 50% reduction in the size of the mass in 80% of 549 patients treated preoperatively. There are no data yet available on tumor response and final outcome or on overall disease-free survival of the groups treated pre- or postoperatively. However, even if there is no difference, tumor downstaging with preoperative therapy can clearly be performed. The B-18 trial as well as a recent British study confirmed that there is a reduction in the requirement for mastectomy after preoperative chemotherapy for primary breast cancer, i.e., a substantial proportion of patients with larger primaries can be treated with breast-conserving surgery (348, 349).

The NSABP then performed two studies (B-22 and B-25) evaluating AC dose intensity. In B-22 (350), standard-dose AC × 4 (A, 60 mg/m²; C, 600 mg/m²) was tested against two arms in which the dose of C was intensified (1200 mg/m² × 2 and 1200 mg/m² × 4). The dose of A was constant (60 mg/m² × 4). There was no difference in disease-free or absolute survival between the standard dose and intensified dose arms. In NSABP B-25, the dose of C was further augmented to 2400 mg/m² × 2 or × 4, with growth

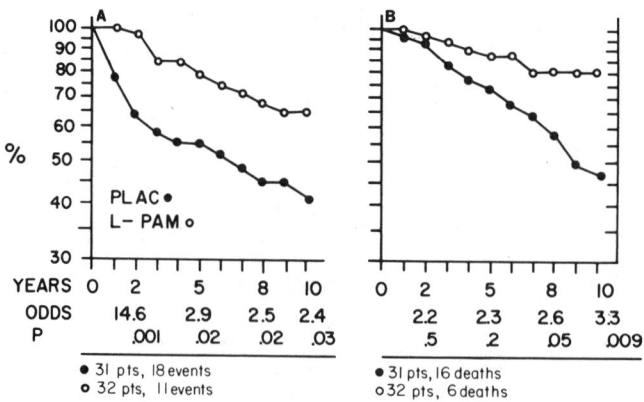

Figure 54.7.   Disease-free survival (A) and survival (B) of patients ≤49 years with 1–3 positive nodes. Cumulative odds ratios and cumulative *p* values demonstrate the benefit in this nodal group. NSABP B-05: *L-PAM* vs. placebo (*PLAC*) in stage II breast cancer. (From Fisher B, Redmond C, Fisher ER, Wolmark N. Systemic adjuvant therapy in treatment of primary operable breast cancer: National Surgical Adjuvant Breast and Bowel Project experience. NCI Monogr 1986;1:35–43. With permission.)

factor support. This trial has achieved its accrual goal, but no efficacy data are yet available. However, six cases of acute myelogenous leukemia have been reported among the 2548 participants in B-25 (351). The NSABP is closely monitoring this group of patients, as well as those enrolled on B-15 and B-22, to determine the actual risk of hematologic malignancies.

The NSABP adjuvant studies that have included tamoxifen are discussed below.

THE MILAN CANCER INSTITUTE TRIALS

In parallel with the NSABP studies, Bonadonna of the Instituto Nazionale Tumori of Milan initiated a series of clinical trials evaluating the three-drug combination CMF (cyclophosphamide, methotrexate, 5-FU; Table 54.9) in stage II breast cancer. The first of these trials was published in 1976, the 14-year follow-up data were published in 1989 (352, 353), and the 20-year follow-up was published in 1995 (354). Stratifications for menopausal status (pre- vs. post-) and axillary nodal status (1–3 vs. >3) were the same as those in the NSABP trial. A total of 386 patients were randomized, 207 to CMF and 179 as controls. All patients had a standard radical mastectomy. The results of the initial CMF trial with 20-year follow-up are illustrated in Figure 54.8 (354). As in the NSABP L-PAM study,

the greatest benefit was in premenopausal women with one to three positive nodes.

The second Milan Cancer Institute CMF trial tested 6 versus 12 treatment cycles. This study was designed empirically to test equivalency of response, with the hope that shorter treatment would be associated with fewer acute toxic reactions. Six months of CMF is equivalent to 12 months and may even have a slight advantage (Fig. 54.9). It appears that there is no benefit to prolonging the same drug combination beyond six cycles.

In an attempt to improve the disease-free and absolute survival of women at high risk of recurrence, Bonadonna et al. initiated a series of clinical trials evaluating sequential CMF and doxorubicin (264). The first of this series evaluated CMF versus CMF followed by doxorubicin. At 5 years, there was no difference in those with one to three positive nodes, but those with more than three positive nodes had significant improvement in both disease-free and absolute survival. To further refine and improve upon these data, they next tested four courses of doxorubicin (75 mg/m^2 every 3 weeks) followed by eight courses of CMF (C, 600 mg/m^2; M, 40 mg/m^2; F, 600 mg/m^2 every 3 weeks) [Dox →CMF] versus two course of CMF alternating with one course of doxorubicin for a total of 12 courses

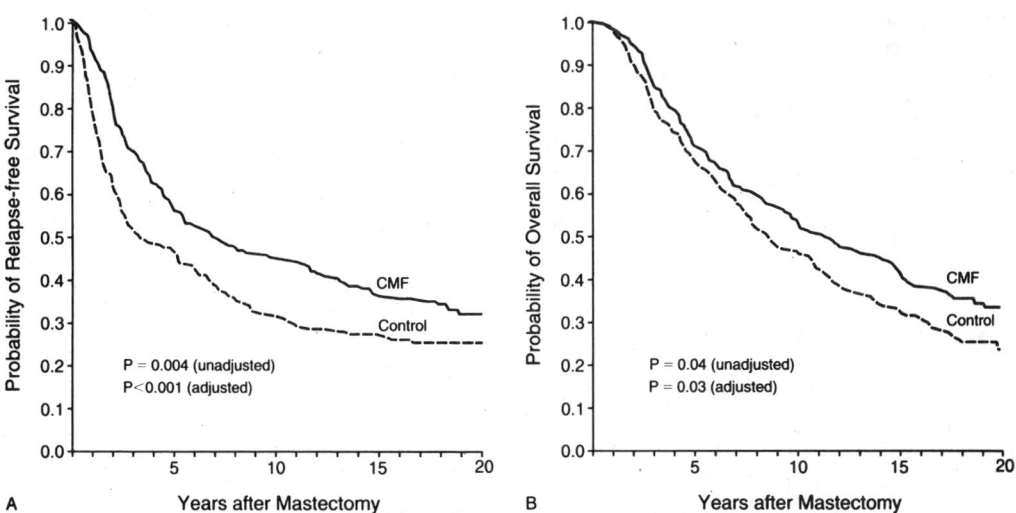

Figure 54.8. Relapse-free survival (A) and overall survival (B) according to treatment group. With respect to relapse-free survival, 48 of 179 patients in the control group were disease-free at 20 years, compared with 74 of 207 patients in the CMF group. With respect to overall survival, 44 of 179 patients in the control group were alive at 20 years, compared with 70 of 207 patients in the CMF group. (From Bonadonna G, Valagussa P, Moliterni A, et al. Adjuvant cyclophosphamide, methotrexate, and fluorouracil in node-positive breast cancer: the results of 20 years of follow-up. N Engl J Med 1995;332:901–906. With permission.)

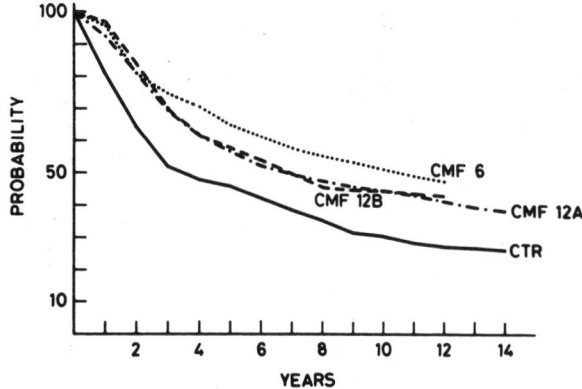

Figure 54.9. Second CMF program. Comparative relapse-free survival 12 years (*CMF 12B* vs. *CMF 6*) and consistency of treatment outcome compared with the first CMF program (*CMF 12A*). *CTR*, control. (From Bonadonna G. Conceptual and practical advances in the management of breast cancer. J Clin Oncol 1989;7(10):1380–1397. With permission.)

[CMF/Dox] in women with more than 3 positive nodes. There were 403 (of 405) evaluable patients. The results are graphically displayed in Figure 54.10. There was a clear advantage of the sequential regimen Dox → CMF over the alternating regimen CMF/Dox.

ADJUVANT CHEMOTHERAPY-INDUCED AMENORRHEA

The meta-analysis reported by the Early Breast Cancer Trialists' Collaborative Group (1992) seems to confirm or at least raise the question of benefit from adjuvant oophorectomy in premenopausal women. The question is: How much of the benefit gained from adjuvant chemotherapy in premenopausal women is through an endocrine effect? Many women receiving adjuvant chemotherapy become temporarily or permanently amenorrheic. Bianco et al. (1991), from the University of Naples, evaluated the prognostic role of drug-induced amenorrhea (DIA) on 221 premenopausal women treated with regimens containing adjuvant CMF (355). DIA, defined as cessation of menses for at least 3 months, occurred in 166 of 221 patients (75.1%). At a median follow-up of 69 months, patients who developed DIA had a significantly longer disease-free survival (Fig. 54.11) than those who did not. In this study, DIA as a prognostic variable was independent of age, number of involved nodes, and tumor size.

The Danish Breast Cooperative Group evaluated the effects of DIA in a group of 1032 pre- and perimenopausal women randomized to observation alone, cyclophosphamide monother-

apy, or CMF (356). CMF reduced relapse-free survival regardless of whether DIA was induced. However, cyclophosphamide alone only improved relapse-free survival in patients who developed DIA and had no effect in patients who retained normal menstrual function. In each of the studies reported, there is an inverse relationship between age and duration of treatment required to induce ovarian suppression (357). Amenorrhea is generally induced within 2 to 4 months in women over age 40. Younger women, aged 30 to 39, require higher cumulative doses to induce ovarian dysfunction, and women younger than age 30, as a rule, continue to menstruate with no major alterations in hormone levels despite adjuvant chemotherapy.

The NSABP reported a lack of association between disease-free survival and depressed ovarian function (358). In the NSABP series, improvement in disease-free survival was better in younger groups of women with a lower incidence of DIA. Bonadonna (1989) reported that women treated with CMF adjuvant chemotherapy who developed DIA and subsequently relapsed had the same response to therapeutic castration as those who did not develop DIA (353). Collectively, these data imply that the effect of adjuvant cytotoxic chemotherapy in premenopausal women who develop DIA is mediated through two mechanisms, endocrine ablation and a direct cytotoxic effect.

THE CALGB TRIALS

The Cancer and Leukemia Group B (CALGB) has performed several important adjuvant che-

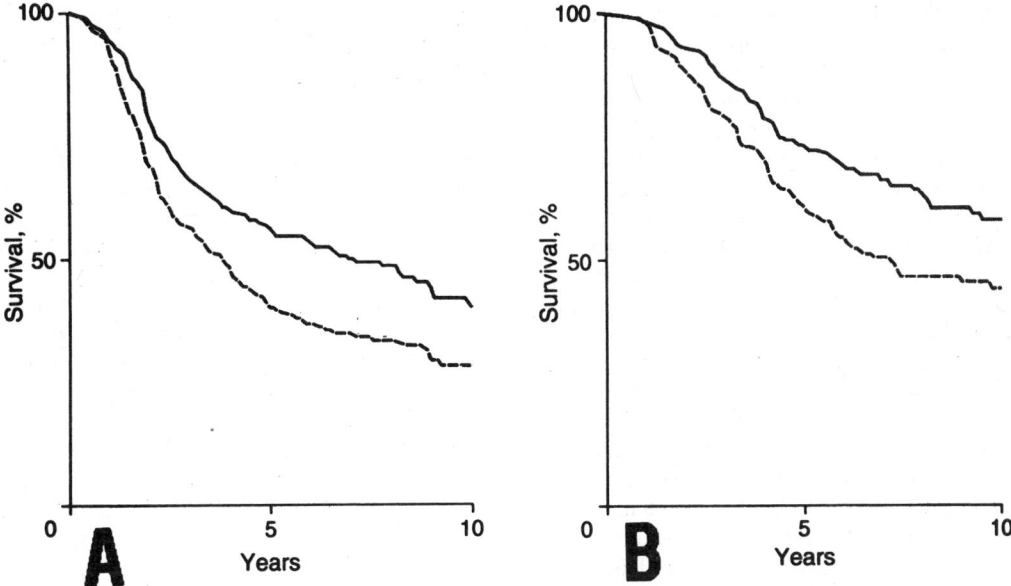

Figure 54.10. A. Comparative 10-year relapse-free survival in breast cancer with more than three positive nodes. *Solid line* indicates sequential administration of doxorubicin and a combination of cyclophosphamide, methotrexate, and fluorouracil (DOX→CMF) and *dashed line* indicates alternating administration (CMF/DOX). **B.** Comparative 10-year absolute survival in breast cancer with more than three positive nodes. *Solid line* indicates DOX→CMF and *dashed line* indicates CMF/DOX. (From Bonadonna G, Zambetti, Valagusa P. Sequential or alternating doxorubicin and CMF regimens in breast cancer with more than three positive nodes. Ten year results. JAMA 1995:273:542–547. With permission.)

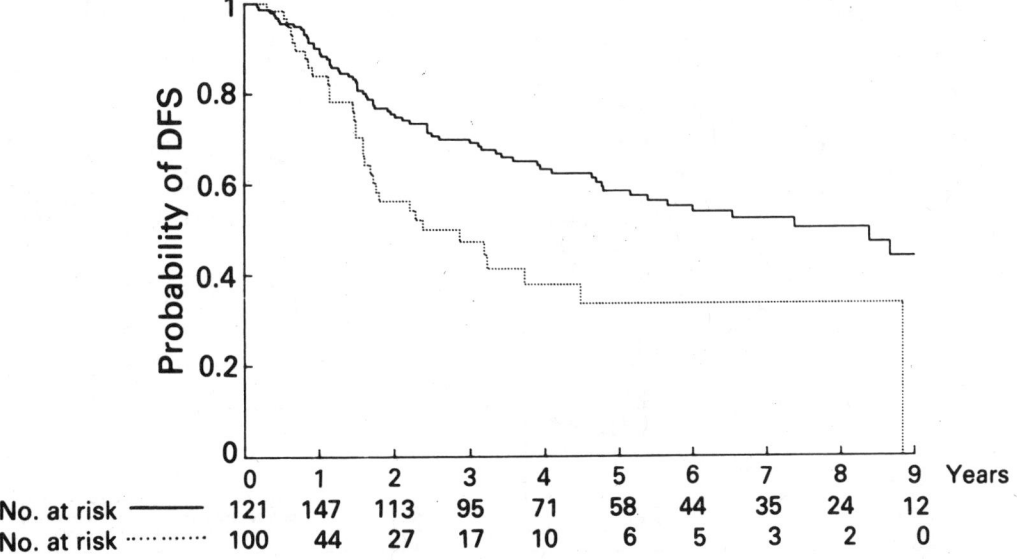

Figure 54.11.   Disease-free survival (*DFS*) curves for premenopausal women with drug-induced amenorrhea (DIA) (*solid line*) versus women who did not develop amenorrhea (*dashed line*) after receiving adjuvant chemotherapy, *p*<.001. (From Bianco AR, Del Mastro L, Gallo C, et al. Prognostic role of amenorrhea induced by adjuvant chemotherapy in premenopausal patients with early breast cancer. Br J Cancer 1991;63:799–803. With permission.)

motherapy trials in stage II breast cancer. The first was based on the clinical observations of Cooper and associates (359, 360), who empirically treated 100 women with primary breast cancer and four or more positive axillary nodes with 9 months of CMFVP (Table 54.9). Disease-free survival was 68% at 5 years. Since this was significantly greater than anticipated, the CALGB initiated a prospective, randomized trial comparing CMF with CMFVP (361). There were 772 evaluable patients. Patients were stratified by axillary nodal status (one to three vs. four or more), tumor size (<3 cm vs. 3 cm), and menopausal status (≤49 years of age vs. 50). Women with four or more positive axillary nodes who were treated with CMFVP had significantly greater disease-free survival than those treated with CMF (362). The improvement in disease-free survival was greater in postmenopausal than in premenopausal patients. CMF in women with one to three positive nodes was equivalent to CMFVP.

The second major CALGB adjuvant study analyzed 897 patients. This study tested CMFVP, but at two different dose intensities, for eight cycles followed by a second randomization to six additional cycles of CMFVP or VATH (Table

54.12). Disease-free survival was significantly superior in patients who were crossed over to VATH ($p=.01$). This was most marked in postmenopausal women with more than four positive nodes ($p = .02$) and in all patients with more than 10 positive nodes ($p = .006$) (363, 364). It was concluded that a second combination chemotherapy regimen, given after the tumor burden had been reduced by the initial chemotherapy, conveys a further cytocidal effect.

The CALGB has also tested the dose intensity of CAF (C, 300 mg/m²; A, 30 mg/m²; F, 300 mg/m² vs. C, 400 mg/m²; A, 40 mg/m²; F, 400 mg/m² vs. C, 600 mg/m²; A, 60 mg/m²; F, 600 mg/m²) in 1572 women with node-positive breast cancer (365). After a median follow-up of 3.4 years, the women treated with the high or moderate dose had significantly longer disease-free survival ($p<.001$) and survival ($p = .004$).

THE META-ANALYSIS

The Early Breast Cancer Trialists' Collaborative Group chaired by Richard Peto of Oxford reviewed 133 prospectively randomized trials of systemic adjuvant therapy in early breast cancer (17). These trials involved 75,000 women treated prior to 1985 with cytotoxic, hormonal, or im-

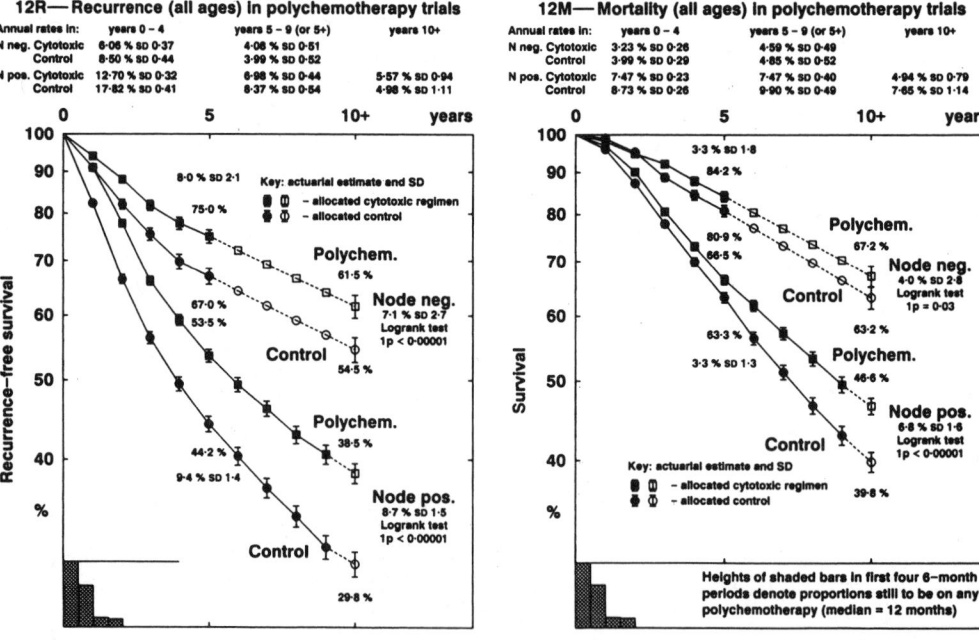

Figure 54.12. Ten-year outcome of adjuvant polychemotherapy trials, subdivided by nodal status. *12R*, recurrence (disease-free survival); *12M*, mortality. (From Early Breast Cancer Trialists' Collaborative Group. Systemic treatment of early breast cancer by hormonal, cytotoxic, or immune therapy: 133 randomised trials involving 31 000 recurrences and 24 000 deaths among 75 000 women. Lancet 1992;339:1–15,71–85. With permission.)

mune therapy. There were 31,000 recurrences and 24,000 deaths. A total of 11,000 women was enrolled in 31 randomized trials of long-term polychemotherapy versus no chemotherapy. There was significant improvement in both recurrence-free survival and absolute survival in patients treated with polychemotherapy (Fig. 54.12). The greatest benefit was noted in node-positive patients. The use of adjuvant chemotherapy in premenopausal women will reduce their annual odds of death by about 25% (366). A clear benefit from chemotherapy alone in postmenopausal women was more difficult to document in the meta-analysis. Of necessity, the meta-analysis involved a variety of chemotherapeutic regimens (CMF, AC, CMFV, CVF, CVM, CFP) given in different dose schedules and treatment duration. The results are therefore an indication of trends but nevertheless are very interesting.

Tamoxifen in the Adjuvant Setting

TAMOXIFEN ALONE IN NODE-NEGATIVE BREAST CANCER

In the Early Breast Cancer Trialists' Collaborative Group (1992) meta-analysis of 133 randomized trials of systemic adjuvant therapy for early breast cancer, 30,000 women were in tamoxifen trials (17). There were highly significant reductions in the annual rates of both recurrence (25%) and death (17%) in the tamoxifen-treated groups ($p<.00001$). There were no differences between different doses of tamoxifen (20, 30, or 40 mg per day). However, longer durations of tamoxifen therapy (2 to 5 years) were significantly more effective than shorter durations (<2 years). Of the 30,000 women in tamoxifen trials, nearly 13,000 had negative axillary lymph nodes. Tamoxifen in node-negative patients was associated with a significant reduction in relapse-free survival and overall survival for women of all ages (<50 and ≥50). In fact, the odds of death from any cause were reduced in women treated with tamoxifen. Data from the Early Breast Cancer Trialists' Collaborative Group in both node-positive and node-negative patients are graphically displayed in Figure 54.13. The data from several adjuvant tamoxifen trials in node-negative breast cancer are summarized in Table 54.14 (367–379).

NSABP trial B-14 is the only adjuvant trial designed specifically to evaluate tamoxifen in node-negative breast cancer. It is the largest trial ever performed in node-negative breast cancer,

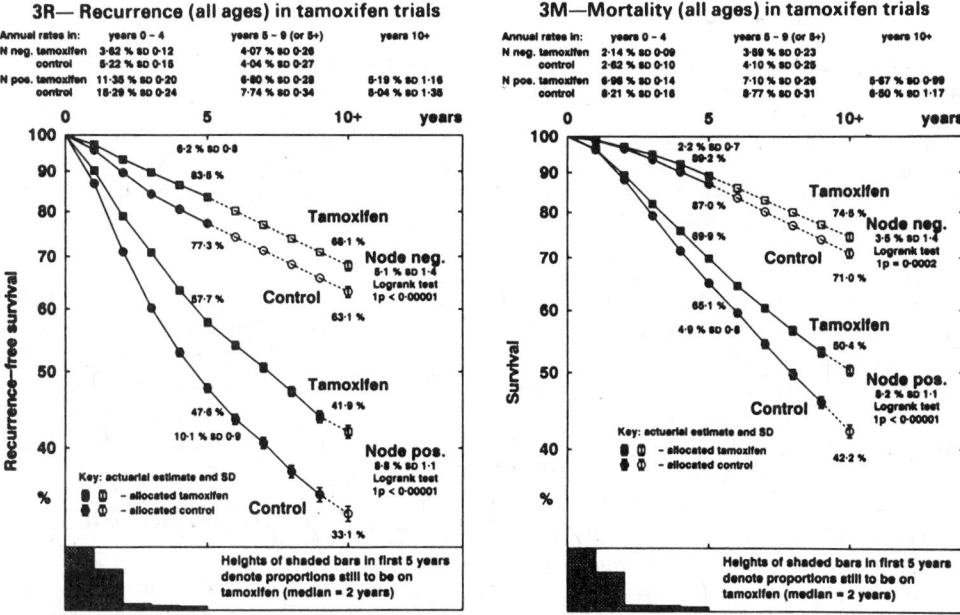

Figure 54.13.   Ten-year outcome of adjuvant tamoxifen trials, subdivided by nodal status. *3R,* recurrence (disease-free survival): *3M,* mortality. (From Early Breast Cancer Trialists' Collaborative Group. Systemic treatment of early breast cancer by hormonal, cytotoxic, or immune therapy: 133 randomised trials involving 31 000 recurrences and 24 000 deaths among 75 000 women. Lancet 1992;339:1–15,71–85. With permission.)

Table 54.14. Randomized Trials of Adjuvant Tamoxifen Alone (vs. Control) in Node-Negative Breast Cancer

Trial	Daily Dose (mg)	Duration of Therapy (years)	Premenstrual	Postmenstrual	Disease-Free Survival	Survival
NSABP B-14[a]	20	5 and 10	812	1832	$p < .0001$	$p \leq .05$
NATO[b]	20	2	0	604	$p \leq .05$	$p \leq .05$
Christie Hospital[c]	20	1	0	382	N.S.	N.S.
Stockholm[d]	40	2 and 5	0	696	$p < .01$ in ER+	N.S.
CRC[e]	20	2	316	571	$p \leq .05$	N.S.
Scottish[f]	20	5	212	539	$.05 < p < .1$	N.S.

Adapted from Love RR. Tamoxifen therapy in primary breast cancer. Biology, efficacy, and side effects. J Clin Oncol 1989;7:803.
[a]National Surgical Adjuvant Breast and Bowel Project (Fisher et al., 1989) (368).
[b]Nolvadex Adjuvant Trial Organization (Baum et al., 1983; 1985; 1988) (369–371).
[c]Ribiero & Palmer, 1983 (372); Ribiero & Swindell, 1985, 1988, (373, 374).
[d]Rutqvist et al., 1989 (375); Fornander et al., 1991 (376).
[e]Cancer Research Campaign (Abram et al., 1988) (377).
[f]Bartlett et al., 1987 (378); Stewart, 1992 (379).

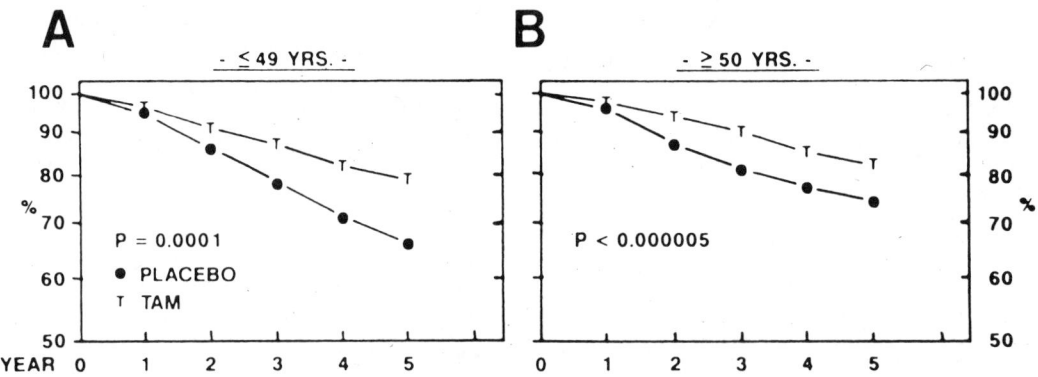

Figure 54.14.   Effect of tamoxifen (T) on disease-free survival related to age. A. Placebo: 438 patients, 111 events. Tamoxifen: 440 patients, 59 events (TAM = T = tamoxifen). **B.** Placebo: 988 patients, 207 events. Tamoxifen: 977 patients; 130 events. (From Fisher B, Wickerham DL, Redmond C. Recent developments in the systemic adjuvant therapy of breast cancer. Semin Oncol 1992;19:263–277. With permission.)

and the results from this trial are the basis for the tamoxifen chemoprevention trial in high-risk women (368, 380, 381). The NSABP conducted a prospective, randomized, double-blind, placebo-controlled trial of adjuvant tamoxifen (10 mg twice daily) in 2644 ER+ (≥10 fmol) patients with breast cancer and histologically negative axillary lymph nodes. There was a highly significant prolongation of disease-free survival in women treated with tamoxifen, compared with those receiving placebo (83% disease free at 4 years vs. 77% [$p<.00001$]), and there was a survival advantage in tamoxifen-treated postmenopausal women ($p = .02$) (382). Improved disease-free survival was observed in all subsets analyzed in the group treated with tamoxifen:

women ≤49 years of age, women ≥50 years of age; tumor size ≤2 cm, tumor size >2 cm; and tumors with ER 10 to 49 fmol, 50 to 99 fmol, and ≥100 fmol (Fig. 54.14). It is important to emphasize that women treated with tamoxifen had a significant reduction in the development of cancer of the opposite breast.

TAMOXIFEN ALONE IN STAGE II BREAST CANCER

The data from several trials of adjuvant tamoxifen alone are summarized in Table 54.15. Data from the Early Trialists' Collaborative Group in both node-positive and node-negative breast cancer are displayed in Figure 54.13. The first of the major tamoxifen adjuvant trials to

Table 54.15. Randomized Trials of Adjuvant Tamoxifen Alone (vs. Control) in Node-Positive Breast Cancer

Trial	Daily Dose (mg)	Duration of Therapy (years)	Premenstrual	Postmenstrual	Disease-Free Survival	Survival
NATO[a]	20	2	128	393	$p \le .05$	$p \le .05$
Christie Hospital[b]	20	1	0	206	$.05 < p < .1$	N.S.
Stockholm[c]	40	2	0	1407	$p \le .05$	N.S.
CRC[d]	20	2	140	232	$p < .01$	N.S.
Scottish[e]	20	5	0	456	$p \le .05$	$p \le .05$
Danish[f]	30	1	0	1650	$p < .05$	N.S.

Adapted from Love, RR. Tamoxifen therapy in primary breast cancer. Biology, efficacy, and side effects. J Clin Oncol 1989;7:803–815.
[a]Nolvadex Adjuvant Trial Organization (Baum et al., 1983; 1985; 1988) (369–371).
[b]Ribiero & Palmer, 1983 (372); Ribiero & Swindell, 1985, 1988 (373, 374).
[c]Rutqvist et al, 1989 (375); Fornander et al., 1991 (376).
[d]Cancer Research Campaign (Abram, 1988) (377).
[e]Bartlett et al., 1987 (378); Stewart, 1992 (379).
[f]Rose et al., 1985 (383).

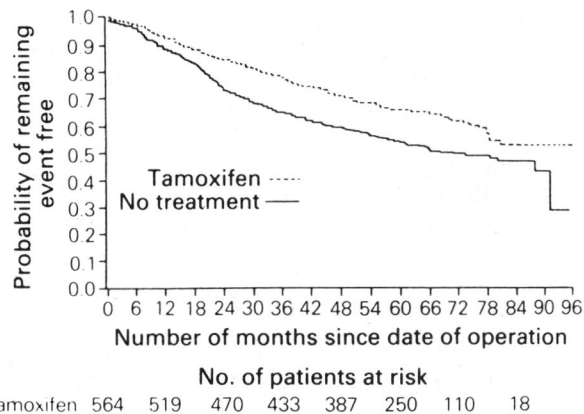

No. of patients at risk

Tamoxifen	564	519	470	433	387	250	110	18
No treatment	567	499	414	367	332	207	91	13

Figure 54.15. Event-free survival in stage II breast cancer. Tamoxifen vs. no treatment. Nolvadex Adjuvant Treatment Organization (NATO) trial. (From Baum M, Brinkley DM, Dossett JA, et al. Controlled trial of tamoxifen as a single adjuvant agent in the management of early breast cancer: analysis at eight years by 'Nolvadex' Adjuvant Trial Organisation. Br J Cancer 1988;57:608–611. With permission.)

confirm a survival advantage in patients treated with tamoxifen as a single agent was the Nolvadex Adjuvant Trial Organization (NATO) trial under the chairmanship of Prof. Michael Baum of King's College Hospital in London. The NATO trial consisted of 1285 patients aged 75 or younger. The study included premenopausal, node-positive patients as well as postmenopausal node-negative and node-positive patients (369–371). The patients were randomized to tamoxifen 10 mg twice daily for 2 years or to no further treatment. The results are displayed in Figure 54.15. The benefits of tamoxifen therapy in the NATO trial appear to be independent of menopausal, nodal, or ER status. However, in other large series, the benefit of tamoxifen was restricted to ER+ patients (113, 383–385).

ADJUVANT TAMOXIFEN PLUS CHEMOTHERAPY IN STAGE II BREAST CANCER

The early trials of combination therapy in the adjuvant setting were basically designed to determine whether the addition of tamoxifen to chemotherapy would enhance the effect of the chemotherapy. The NSABP performed the largest such study (386–388). In this study, 1891 women with primary operable breast cancer and positive axillary nodes were randomized to receive melphalan (L-PAM) and 5-fluorouracil (PF) or PF plus tamoxifen (PFT). The tamoxifen was administered as 10 mg twice daily for 2 years. The initial results of this trial are illustrated in Figure 54.16. Women aged 50 years or above derived a clear benefit from the addition of tamoxifen to PF, and this benefit increased with the level of both the ER and PgR. However, in women aged 49 years or below, the addition of tamoxifen provided no benefit, regardless of the ER or PgR level. Postmenopausal women treated with tamoxifen began to relapse in the third year, that is, 1 year after tamoxifen was discontinued. This prompted the NSABP to test whether women who are disease free at 2 years would benefit from an additional year of tamoxifen, and indeed they did (97) (Fig. 54.17). This is the first clinical trial to confirm Jordan's laboratory findings that tamoxifen is cytostatic rather than cytocidal, that discontinuation of tamoxifen will allow reactivation of latent tumor cells, and that prolonged tamoxifen therapy is of more benefit than shorter courses. Several other clinical trials have confirmed that short courses of tamoxifen (1 year) fail to enhance the effect of chemotherapy in either pre- or postmenopausal

women (389–393). The value of adding long-term (5 years) tamoxifen to chemotherapy in postmenopausal, node-positive women has been confirmed by the Eastern Cooperative Oncology Group (394, 395).

These studies have raised the obvious question: What is the optimal duration of tamoxifen therapy? The decision to treat for 5 years is arbitrary. The laboratory data would tend to support the use of tamoxifen indefinitely. The NSABP has evaluated 5 years versus 10 years of tamoxifen, and there was no advantage to continuing tamoxifen more than 5 years (385a)

In the trials of chemotherapy with or without tamoxifen the effect of tamoxifen alone cannot be evaluated. Given the beneficial effects of tamoxifen alone, particularly in postmenopausal women, reported in the European literature, one cannot help but wonder what, if any, additional effect is contributed by the chemotherapy. The definitive trial was performed by the NSABP (381, 396). The NSABP randomized 1124 eligible postmenopausal, receptor-positive, node-positive women to one of three treatment arms: tamoxifen alone for 5 years; tamoxifen for 5 years plus four cycles of Adriamycin (A) plus cyclophosphamide (C); and tamoxifen for 5 years plus a prolonged course of L-PAM (P) plus 5-fluorouracil (F), with or without Adriamycin (PF or

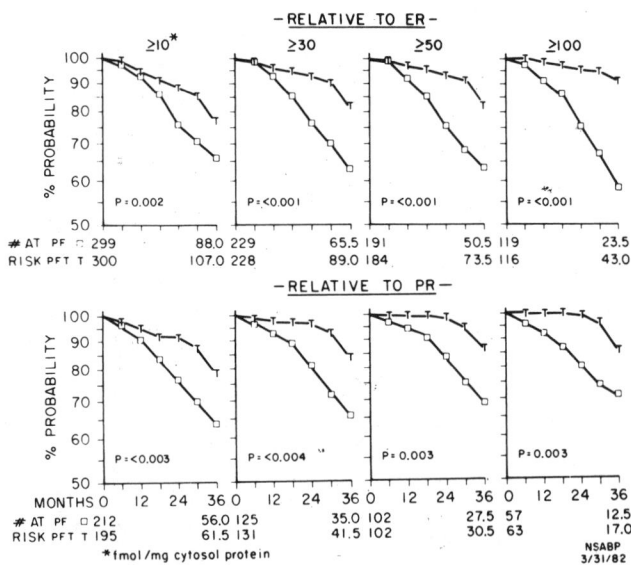

Figure 54.16. Disease-free survival of women ≥50 years of age with stage II breast cancer treated with PF vs. PFT (L-PAM + 5FU vs. L-PAM + 5FU + tamoxifen). Analysis relative to ER (estrogen receptor) and PR (progesterone receptor). (From Fisher B, Redmond C, Brown A, et al. Influence of tumor estrogen and progesterone receptor levels on the response to tamoxifen and chemotherapy in primary breast cancer. J Clin Oncol 1983;1(4):227–241. With permission.)

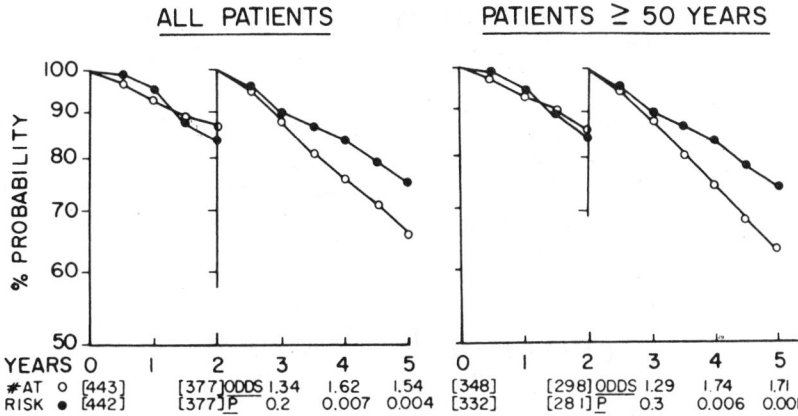

Figure 54.17.   Effect of an additional year of tamoxifen on the disease-free survival of patients who were free of disease 2 years after surgery. *Open circles* indicate women who received melphalan (L-PAM), fluorouracil, and tamoxifen alone, and *closed circles* indicate women who received this treatment plus an additional year of tamoxifen. (From Fisher B, Brown A, Wolmark N, et al. Prolonging tamoxifen therapy for primary breast cancer. Findings from the National Surgical Adjuvant Breast and Bowel Project clinical trial. Ann Intern Med 1987;106:649–654.)

PAF). The data from this trial confirm that the addition of chemotherapy (AC, PF, or PAF) clearly enhances the disease-free survival and overall survival in postmenopausal women treated with long-term tamoxifen. They also confirm that a short course of four cycles of AC is equivalent to longer-term chemotherapy with PF or PAF. The data for AC plus tamoxifen versus tamoxifen alone are shown in Figure 54.18.

The benefit of adding chemotherapy to tamoxifen in postmenopausal, node-positive women has been confirmed by Pearson et al. (397), the Italian Cooperative Group (GROCTA) (398), and the large meta-analysis performed by the Early Breast Cancer Trialists' Collaborative Group (16). The addition of CMF-based chemotherapy to tamoxifen has not been superior to tamoxifen alone in postmenopausal receptor-positive, node-positive breast cancer (399, 400). However, CMF-based chemotherapy alone has not been of proven efficacy in this group of patients.

Two important conclusions can be drawn from these studies: (*a*) Adriamycin-based chemotherapy significantly improves disease-free survival in node-positive, receptor-positive, tamoxifen-responsive women and (*b*) tamoxifen alone is not optimal treatment for node-positive, receptor-positive, postmenopausal women with breast cancer. However, tamoxifen alone retains an important role in the adjuvant therapy of older women with node-positive breast cancer (401).

Adjuvant Chemotherapy of Stage I Breast Cancer

The use of tamoxifen in node-negative breast cancer is discussed above. Adjuvant chemotherapy in stage I breast cancer is more controversial. Standard prognostic criteria are not sensitive and specific enough determinants in stage I breast cancer to identify those who clearly do not require adjuvant therapy. Overall, in up to 25 to 30% of stage I breast cancer patients the disease will recur and will ultimately prove fatal. The most reliable risk factor in predicting the probability of recurrence in operable breast cancer has been the status of the axillary lymph nodes. Determining the risk of recurrence in node-negative breast cancer has been considerably more difficult. Hormone receptor status has not been a consistently reliable prognostic indicator. A variety of other risk factors have been evaluated, such as *erb* B_2 (HER-2/*neu*) oncogene amplification (57, 402), cathepsin D (403), nm 23 RNA (343), haptoglobin-related protein (342), Ki 67 immunostaining (404), occult bone marrow micrometastases (405), and DNA ploidy and S-phase fraction (56, 406, 407). Elaborate schemata have been developed to try to integrate these various risk factors so that appropriate therapeutic decisions can be made in node-negative breast cancer (408, 409). This large series of potential prognostic factors has not produced reliable, reproducible data and should not yet be incorporated into the clinical decision-making

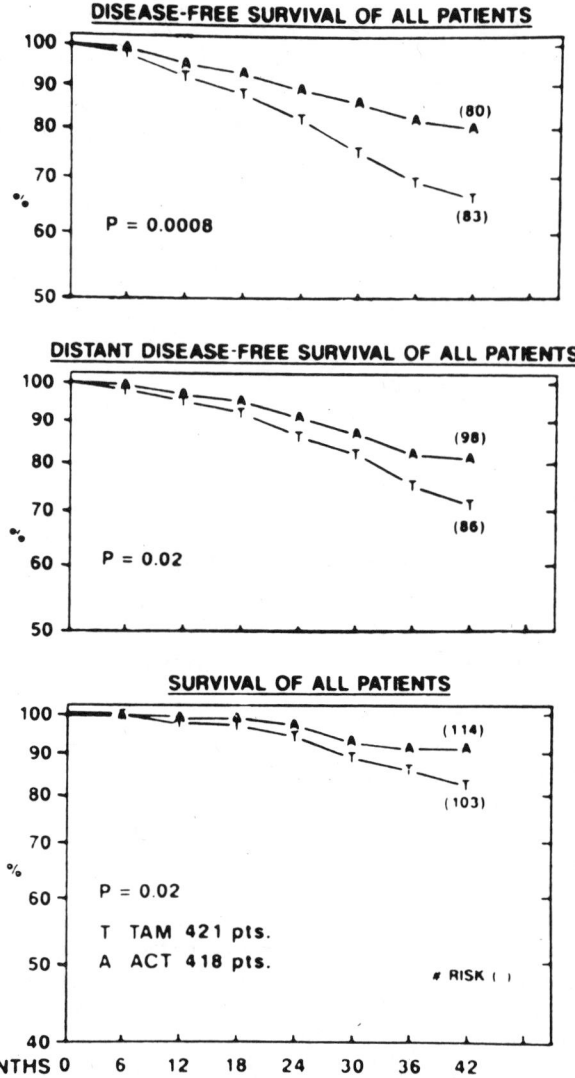

Figure 54.18.   Disease-free survival, distant disease-free survival, and survival of patients treated postoperatively with *ACT* (Adriamycin, Cytoxan, and tamoxifen) versus those receiving *TAM* (tamoxifen) alone. *A,* Adriamycin; *T,* tamoxifen. (From Fisher B, Wickerham DL, Redmond C. Recent developments in the systemic adjuvant therapy of breast cancer. Semin Oncol 1992;19:263–277.)

process. Currently, the only consistently reliable prognostic indicator in node-negative breast cancer is tumor size (410–415). Persons with tumors <1 cm in maximum diameter have a disease-free survival at 10 years of 92%; the disease-free survival at 10 years for tumors 1.0 to 1.9 cm is 78%, and for tumors ≥2 cm, 69%. Because of the good prognosis, node-negative patients with tumors less than 1 cm in diameter are not candidates for adjuvant therapy with cytotoxic drugs.

Several node-negative trials have been reported. These trials have altered the approach to stage I breast cancer, particularly in women whose tumors are 1 cm or more in diameter. Bonadonna evaluated six cycles of CMF versus an untreated control group in 90 node-negative, receptor-negative patients and reported a highly significant improvement in both disease-free and absolute survival with treatment (353). The NSABP analyzed 12 cycles of sequential methotrexate and 5-FU followed by leucovorin in 679 women with negative nodes and negative receptors (416, 417). Disease-free survival improved significantly in both premenopausal and postmenopausal women (Fig. 54.19). Finally, the Intergroup Study tested CMFP versus no treat-

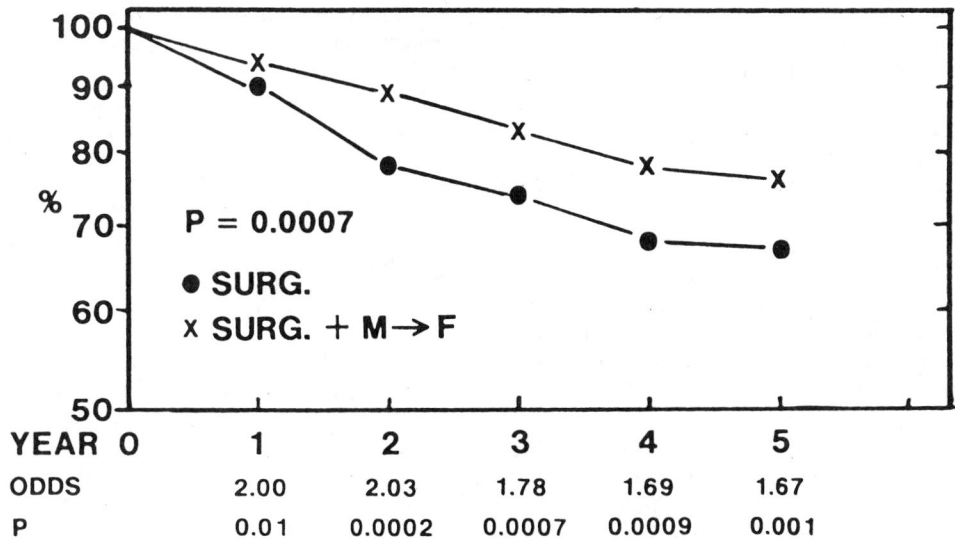

Figure 54.19.   The effect of M→F on disease-free survival of all patients with ER−, node-negative tumors. There were 372 patients treated with surgery alone having 111 events, and 365 patients receiving surgery + M→F having 71 events. *M*, methotrexate; *F*, 5-fluorouracil. (From Fisher B, Wickerham DL, Redmond C. Recent developments in the use of systemic adjuvant therapy for the treatment of breast cancer. Semin Oncol 1992;19:263–277.)

ment in 536 patients with high-risk (ER− tumor of any size or an ER+ tumor >3 cm), node-negative breast cancer. Disease-free survival was 84% in the CMFP-treated group and 69% in the control group ($p = .0001$) (418).

Local-Regional Failure after Adjuvant Therapy

The initial report of adjuvant CMF from Milan noted that CMF-treated patients had a significant decrease in local-regional and systemic recurrence (352). It is now apparent that a subset of women who have large primary lesions (>5 cm) or are multinode positive (four or more positive nodes) are at a high risk of local-regional recurrence despite adjuvant chemotherapy (419–421). Under these conditions, local-regional recurrence develops as the first sign of metastasis in 31 to 36% of cases. Postmastectomy radiation concurrent with or following adjuvant chemotherapy improves local control. However, there are no convincing data that postoperative radiation therapy improves overall survival.

Retrospective data on the proper sequencing of adjuvant chemotherapy and radiation have yielded conflicting results (422–424). The Joint Center for Radiation Therapy at Harvard states that those patients who received all chemotherapy prior to the radiation had a 41% local failure rate, while those who received the radiation first

had only a 4% local failure rate. The group at M. D. Anderson were unable to demonstrate that delaying radiation therapy until the completion of systemic chemotherapy had any effect on local control.

Since locoregional failure in breast cancer is often associated with a grave prognosis and generally heralds a systemic recurrence, better local control in high-risk cases might be expected to be associated with an overall improvement in survival (425, 426). Two prospective randomized trials have evaluated CMF, with or without radiation therapy, postmastectomy (427, 428). In each of these trials, there was an advantage in the radiation therapy group, especially in women with T3 or T4 lesions. It is now time to verify these results in a large, well-controlled and stratified clinical trial (429). Locoregional failure following lumpectomy plus radiation does not seem to be associated with an ominous prognosis, and many of these women can be rendered disease free with a mastectomy.

NEOADJUVANT CHEMOTHERAPY OF LOCAL-REGIONAL ADVANCED BREAST CANCER

The treatment of local-regional advanced (LRA), nonmetastatic breast cancer has undergone a major change in recent years, based upon the recognition that this condition is a systemic disease at the time of diagnosis. The emphasis of therapy has changed from local surgery and radiation therapy to primary systemic chemotherapy. With systemic chemotherapy as the initial therapeutic modality, inoperable tumors can frequently be converted to operable tumors, and many large, technically operable tumors can be reduced in size so that breast conservation may be possible (430–433).

LRA breast cancer is not a well-defined, solitary entity but, rather, a spectrum of disorders with divergent biologic behaviors. These range from indolent, slow-growing tumors that have been hidden by the patient for years prior to discovery to aggressive inflammatory cancers. This divergent biologic behavior requires individualization of therapy, but these tumors do have features in common. Basically, there are three subsets of LRA breast cancer: (a) *stage III_A*: large primary lesions (T3 ≥5 cm) or a tumor of any size with fixed ipsilateral axillary adenopathy (N₂); (b) *stage III_B*: tumors with direct extension to the chest wall, skin ulceration, satellite skin nodules, or breast edema (peau d'orange) (T₄), with or without fixed matted nodes (N₂), or any tumor associated with internal mammary adenopathy (N₃); and (c) *inflammatory carcinoma* (T₄d).

The multimodality approach to the management of LRA breast cancer is outlined in Table 54.16. This approach to the management of LRA breast cancer has been derived from the data of Perloff et al. (434), Lippman et al. (435), Swain et al. (436), Olson et al. (437), Loprinzi et al. (438), Hortobagyi et al. (439, 440), Bonadonna (353), Bonadonna et al. (441), and Smith et al. (442). With this approach to LRA breast cancer, an objective response with a 50% or greater reduction in the size of the primary tumor will occur in 70 to 90% of patients following the initial induction chemotherapy. From 16 to 40% of these responses will be clinically complete responses, but only 8 to 10% will be true pathologic complete responses. Mammography is a useful adjunct to physical examination in the evaluation of the response to induction chemotherapy (443). Fewer than 10% of patients will have no response to induction chemotherapy, and essentially none will progress during induction chemotherapy. More than 50% of previously inoperable patients will be converted to operable. Most patients with LRA breast cancer are disease-free after completion of induction chemotherapy and local treatment. Five-year survival rates exceed 80% for stage III_A but are only 30 to 40% for stage III_B. The prognosis in

Table 54.16. Multimodality Approach to Management of Local-Regional Advanced Breast Cancer

1. Confirm diagnosis of breast cancer by fine-needle aspiration cytology of the breast. Further fine-needle aspirations or core biopsies are performed for immunohistochemical assay for hormone receptors.
2. Rule out systemic metastases with a chest x-ray, bone scan, liver imaging procedure, basic blood chemistries, and blood count.
3. Initiate systemic Adriamycin-based chemotherapy with CAF, FAC, or AC (Table 54.10), unless there is a medical contraindication. If the patient has a prior history of cardiac disease, CMF, CMFVP, or a mitoxantrone-based regimen could be used.
4. Treat to maximal tumor response (three to five cycles).
5. Evaluate operability:
   (a) If the tumor has converted to operable, a modified radical mastectomy is performed. If there is minimal or no residual tumor in the surgical specimen, postoperative radiation is not recommended. If there is gross residual tumor, postoperative radiation is performed.
   (b) If the objective of therapy is to convert a T3 lesion to one <3 cm so breast-preserving surgery can be performed, the primary lesion should be outlined with punctate tattoos so the area can be located by the surgeon if a complete response occurs.
   (c) If the tumor has not converted to operable, local radiation is initiated.
6. Completion of systemic chemotherapy: three to five additional cycles of postoperative or postradiation chemotherapy (to a total of eight cycles) are administered.
7. If the patient is hormone receptor–positive, treatment with long-term tamoxifen is continued, after completion of the final cycle of chemotherapy, for a minimum of 5 years.

LRA breast cancer correlates well with the amount of residual disease following induction chemotherapy, with the patients achieving complete responses or near complete responses having the most durable remissions. The prognosis also correlates with axillary nodal involvement following induction chemotherapy, as would be expected (Table 54.17) (444). With multimodality therapy, local-regional recurrences have developed in only 15% of patients.

Inflammatory cancer is managed similarly to other LRA cancers of the breast. However, the addition of surgery following induction chemotherapy and radiation therapy has not had an impact on local or systemic control (445). Inflam-

Table 54.17. Prognostic Significance of Axillary Nodal Involvement after Preoperative Chemotherapy in Stage IIIA and IIIB Breast Cancer

Nodal Involvement	N	% Disease Free	% 10-Year Survival
0	100	63	65
1–3	96	40	44
4–10	93	23	32
>10	34	9	9

Modified from Frye D, Buzdar A, Hortobagyi G. Prognostic Significance of axillary nodal involvement after preoperative chemotherapy in stage III breast cancer (abstract). Proc Am Soc Clin Oncol, 1995;14:95.

matory carcinoma is a relatively rare, distinct clinicopathologic entity (1 to 6% of breast cancers). Clinically, it is associated with a seemingly inflamed, warm, tender, erythematous breast, usually without a distinct mass. Pathologically, tumor cells infiltrate dermal lymphatics. With local therapy alone, the 5-year survival rate is less than 5%. However, with the use of initial induction chemotherapy prior to local treatment, the 5-year survival rate has now increased to 30% (446, 447). Although most patients with inflammatory breast cancer are hormone-receptor negative, up to 30% are receptor positive. Long-term tamoxifen should be given in these cases after the completion of induction chemotherapy. There has been a definite improvement in the therapy of inflammatory breast cancer, but it remains a fertile area for clinical research (448).

MALE BREAST CANCER

Male breast cancer (MBC) is an uncommon disease accounting for less than 1% of all breast cancers (449–451). The median age of patients with MBC is approximately one decade older (64 to 71 years) than for female breast cancer patients. When MBC develops, its clinical course and metastatic pattern are similar to those of female breast cancers with a few notable exceptions: (a) overall, MBC is more hormonally responsive than female breast cancer, nearly 90% are ER+ and 75% are PR+ and (b) at presentation, MBC is locally advanced more frequently than female breast cancers with more than 30% of MBC patients having nipple ulceration, bloody nipple discharge, and/or nipple retraction at diagnosis (452–456).

Since MBC tends to present with locally advanced disease and since there is a paucity of tissue between the tumor and the chest wall, pa-

tients are at significant risk of chest wall recurrence following modified radical or radical mastectomy. It is therefore recommended that patients with MBC receive routine postoperative radiation therapy.

Hormone Therapy of Male Breast Cancer

MBC responds to both additive and ablative hormonal therapy, and as in female breast cancer, the response depends on hormone receptor status. ER− MBC is unresponsive to hormonal manipulation, while 80% or more of ER+ MBC is hormonally responsive. *Orchiectomy* has been the most frequent ablative procedure in MBC: 177 of 319 (55%) unselected patients with advanced MBC and 25 of 32 (78%) ER+ patients achieved a major response to orchiectomy (452, 457, 458).

In addition, MBC responds to a variety of additive hormonal agents (459). *Tamoxifen* is active in MBC, with a 49% (42 of 86) response in unselected patients and an 82% (18 of 22) response in ER+ patients (460). However, male patients may experience more side effects from tamoxifen than female patients, including hot flashes and decreased libido (461). Tamoxifen is equally active before or after an orchiectomy. The recommended dose of tamoxifen in MBC is the standard 20 mg daily. *Estrogens* (diethylstilbestrol, 1 mg three times daily) are active in advanced MBC, with a 32% (51 of 161) response rate. However, as in males treated with DES for advanced prostatic cancer, there is an increased risk of thromboembolic complications (462).

Other hormonal agents such as *progestins* (medroxyprogesterone acetate, 500–1500 mg i.m. daily), aminoglutethimide, and androgens (fluoxymesterone, 10 mg three times daily) have been reported to have activity in MBC in small groups of patients (463). LHRH agonists, with and without the antiandrogen flutamide, have been tested in MBC with promising results (464). Total androgen blockade with buserelin (an LHRH agonist) and cyproterone (an antiandrogen) seems effective in the treatment of advanced MBC, but its superiority as the standard means of androgen suppression remains to be demonstrated (465).

Chemotherapy in Male Breast Cancer

MBC responds to cytotoxic chemotherapy with the same frequency as female breast cancer. Also, MBC responds to the same basic regimens of CMF, CMFVP, CAF, and FAC (Tables 54.9 and

54.10) as female breast cancer (466). Chemotherapy in advanced MBC should be restricted to patients resistant to hormonal therapy.

Adjuvant Therapy in Male Breast Cancer

Degree of axillary nodal involvement, tumor size, and hormone receptor status have the same prognostic implications in MBC as in breast cancer in women. Since MBC is a rare disease, no large adjuvant trials have been possible. Bagley et al. (467) from the National Cancer Institute treated 24 stage II patients with adjuvant CMF. With a median follow-up of 46 months, four patients had developed recurrences and two of them had died. Patel et al. (468) from the M. D. Anderson Cancer Center treated 11 patients with stage II and III MBC with adjuvant FAC. With a median follow-up of 52 months, four had relapsed and seven remained disease free. Ribeiro (469, 470) treated 23 patients with stage II and III MBC with adjuvant tamoxifen for 1 year. At 5 years, 12 of 23 were disease free.

The data on the adjuvant therapy of MBC are sketchy, and it is difficult to make firm recommendations. However, it seems prudent to assume that since MBC is responsive to cytotoxic chemotherapy and even more responsive to hormonal therapy than female breast cancer, adjuvant therapy for stage II MBC may be beneficial.

For stage II MBC, the following seems reasonable:

1. For patients with positive axillary nodes: AC × 4 cycles
2. ER+ patients in addition to adjuvant chemotherapy, should also receive tamoxifen, 20 mg daily for 5 years
3. All patients should receive postoperative radiation therapy after completion of the 4 cycles of AC chemotherapy

Stage III MBC should be approached in the same manner as stage III breast cancer in women, using neoadjuvant chemotherapy. The treatment of stage III breast cancer is summarized in Table 54.14.

MBC remains a complex clinical problem and because of its rarity will remain an enigma.

FUTURE DIRECTIONS

Important advances have been and are being made in breast cancer therapy. Many of these advances are based upon the major conceptual change that breast cancer is frequently a systemic disease at diagnosis. This is the basis for the adjuvant therapy of stage I and II breast cancer and for neoadjuvant (up front) chemotherapy of stage III breast cancer. These techniques have resulted in improved survival of these groups of patients.

Since the last edition of this text, new nontoxic aromatase inhibitors have become available, which are destined to become first-line or second-line hormonal agents of choice. New pure antiestrogens are entering clinical trials and should be released for general use in the near future. The LHRH agonist goserelin will soon be approved for the therapy of metastatic breast cancer in both pre- and postmenopausal women.

Two new exciting chemotherapeutic drugs, paclitaxel and vinorelbine, are now available and are being evaluated in the adjuvant setting as well as for the treatment of advanced disease. Autologous bone marrow transplant (ABMT) in breast cancer was mentioned in the preceding edition, but it remains controversial with regard to its therapeutic efficacy in metastatic disease as well as in the adjuvant setting. Clinical trials of ABMT have been difficult to complete, since many patients have been unwilling to accept the risk of being randomized to a control group.

The inability to truly define the high-risk group stage I and the low-risk group with stage II breast cancer has been disappointing. In the last edition, a series of new markers were under investigation. None of these has yet proved to be truly predictive, and tumor size, nodal status, and hormone receptors remain the only reliable prognostic factors.

Lastly, the NSABP has launched a major Breast Cancer Prevention Trial (BCPT) based on the observation that women treated with long-term adjuvant tamoxifen have a significantly decreased risk of developing carcinoma of the opposite breast. Eleven thousand women (of the planned 16,000) at high risk of developing breast cancer have been enrolled. Subjects are randomized to tamoxifen (20 mg daily) or placebo for 5 years. The BCPT has been controversial to some activist groups. This has resulted in considerable negative publicity and hysteria. Many women have withdrawn their participation. Despite this, over 8000 women remain on study, and recruitment of new participants is continuing. One hopes that this important clinical trial will be completed and that breast cancer will prove to be a preventable disease.

REFERENCES

1. Kardinal CG, Yarbro JW. A conceptual history of cancer. Semin Oncol 1979;6:396–408.

2. Fisher B, Redmond C, Fisher ER. The contribution of recent NSABP clinical trials of primary breast cancer therapy to an understanding of tumor biology—an overview of findings. Cancer 1980;46:1009–1025.

3. Fisher B, Fisher ER. Transmigration of lymph nodes by tumor cells. Science 1966;152:1397–1399.

4. Fisher B, Fisher ER. Interrelationship of hematogenous and lymphatic tumor cell dissemination. Surg Gynecol Obstet 1966;122:791–799.

5. Fisher B. Cancer surgery: a commentary. Cancer Treat Rep 1984;68(1):31–41.

6. Fisher B. The surgical dilemma in the primary therapy of invasive breast cancer: a critical appraisal. Curr Probl Surg 1970;0ct:1–53.

7. Fisher B. A commentary on the role of the surgeon in primary breast cancer. Breast Cancer Res Treat 1981;1:17–26.

8. Fisher B. The evolution of paradigms for the management of breast cancer: a personal perspective [published erratum appears in Cancer Res 1992; 52(12):3512]. Cancer Res 1992;52:2371–2383.

9. Fisher B. Thoughts from a journey. J Clin Oncol 1993;11(12):2297–2305.

10. Fisher B, Ravdin RG, Ausman RK, et al. Surgical adjuvant chemotherapy in cancer of the breast: results of a decade of cooperative investigation. Ann Surg 1968;168:337–356.

11. Fisher B, Slack N, Katrych D, Wolmark N. Ten year follow-up results of patients with carcinoma of the breast in a co-operative clinical trial evaluating surgical adjuvant chemotherapy. Surg Gynecol Obstet 1975;140:528–534.

12. Fisher B, Bauer M, Wickerham L, et al. Relation of number of positive axillary nodes to the prognosis of patients with primary breast cancer: an NSABP update. Cancer 1983;52:1551–1557.

13. Fisher B, Redmond C, Fisher ER, et al. Ten-year results of a randomized clinical trial comparing radical mastectomy and total mastectomy with or without radiation. N Engl J Med 1985;312:674–681.

14. Fisher B, Redmond C, Poisson R, et al. Eight-year results of a randomized clinical trial comparing total mastectomy and lumpectomy with or without irradiation in the treatment of breast cancer. N Engl J Med 1989;320:822–828.

15. Fisher B, Redmond CK. Fraud in breast-cancer trials (letter). N Engl J Med 1994;330(20):1458–1460.

15a. Fisher B, Anderson S, Redmond CK, et al. Reanalysis and results after 12 years of follow-up in a randomized clinical trial comparing total mastectomy with lumpectomy with or without irradiation in the treatment of breast cancer. N Engl J Med 1995; 333:1456–1461.

15b. Christian MC, McCabe MS, Korn EL, et al. The National Cancer Institute audit of the National Surgical Adjuvant Breast and Bowel Project protocol B-06. N Engl J Med 1995;333:1469–1474.

16. Early Breast Cancer Trialists' Collaborative Group. Effects of adjuvant tamoxifen and of cytotoxic therapy on mortality in early breast cancer. An overview of 61 randomized trials among 28,896 women. N Engl J Med 1988;319:1681–1692.

17. Early Breast Cancer Trialists' Collaborative Group. Systemic treatment of early breast cancer by hormonal, cytotoxic, or immune therapy: 133 randomised trials involving 31 000 recurrences and 24 000 deaths among 75 000 women. Lancet 1992;339:1–15,71–85.

18. Jensen EY, Block GE, Smith S, et al. Estrogen receptors and breast cancer: response to adrenalectomy. Prediction of response in cancer therapy. Natl Cancer Inst Monogr 1971;34:55–70.

19. Wittliff JL. Specific receptors of the steroid hormones in breast cancer. Semin Oncol 1974;1:109–118.

20. Wittliff JL. Steroid-hormone receptors in breast cancer. Cancer 1984;53:630–643.

21. McGuire WL. Estrogen receptors in human breast cancer. J Clin Invest 1973;52:73–77.

22. McGuire WL, Carbone PO, Vollmer EP. Estrogen receptors in human breast cancer. New York: Raven Press, 1975.

23. Beatson GT. On the treatment of inoperable cases of carcinoma of the mamma: suggestions for a new method of treatment with illustrative cases. Lancet 1896;2:104–107,162–165.

24. Lett H. An analysis of 99 cases of inoperable breast cancer treated by oophorectomy. Lancet 1905; 1:227–230.

25. Yarbro JW. Cancer research and the development of cancer centers. In: Gross SC, Garb S, eds. Cancer treatment and research in humanistic perspective. New York: Springer, 1985:3–15.

26. Huggins C, Hodges CV. Studies on prostatic cancer. Cancer Res 1941;1:293–297.

27. Huggins C, Bergenstal DM. Inhibition of human mammary and prostatic cancer by adrenalectomy. Cancer Res 1952;12:134–140.

28. Taylor SG III, Slaughter DP, Smejkal W, et al. The effect of sex hormones on advanced carcinoma of the breast. Cancer 1948;1:604–617.

29. Taylor SG III, Morris RS. Hormones in breast metastasis therapy. Med Clin North Am 1951;35:51–61.

30. DeSombre ER, Kledzik G, Marshall S, Meites J. Estrogen and prolactin receptor concentrations in rat mammary tumors and response to endocrine ablation. Cancer Res 1976;36:354–358.

31. Allegra JC. Rational approaches to the hormonal treatment of breast cancer. Semin Oncol 1983; 10(Suppl 4):25–28.

32. Osborne CK, Yochmowitz MG, Knight WA, McGuire WL. The value of estrogen and progesterone receptors in the treatment of breast cancer. Cancer 1980;46:2884–2888.

33. Horwitz KB, McGuire WL, Pearson OH, Segaloff A. Predicting response to endocrine therapy in human breast cancer: a hypothesis. Science 1975;189:726–727.

34. Bezwoda WR, Esser JD, Dansey R, et al. The value of estrogen and progesterone receptor determinations in advanced breast cancer. Estrogen receptor level but not progesterone receptor level correlates with response to tamoxifen. Cancer 1991;68:867–872.

35. Clark GM, McGuire WL. Prognostic factors in primary breast cancer. Breast Cancer Res Treat 1983; 3(Suppl 1):S69–72.

36. McGuire WL, Clark GM. The prognostic role of progesterone receptors in human breast cancer. Semin Oncol 1983;10(Suppl 4):2–6.

37. Allegra JC. Role of hormone receptors in deter-

mining treatment of breast cancer. In: Allegra JC, ed. The management of breast cancer through endocrine therapies. Amsterdam: Excerpta Medica, 1984.

38. Godolphin W, Elwood JM, Spinelli JJ. Estrogen receptor quantitation and staging as complementary prognostic indicators in breast cancer: a study of 583 patients. Int J Cancer 1981;28:677–683.

39. Clark GM, McGuire WL, Hubay CA, et al. Progesterone receptors as a prognostic factor in stage II breast cancer. N Engl J Med 1983;309:1343–1347.

40. Clark GM, Sledge GW Jr, Osborne CK, McGuire WL. Survival from first recurrence: relative importance of prognostic factors in 1,015 breast cancer patients. J Clin Oncol 1987;5:55–61.

41. Clark GM, McGuire WL. Steroid receptors and other prognostic factors in primary breast cancer. Semin Oncol 1988;15(2):20–25.

42. Fisher ER, Sass R, Fisher B, et al. Pathologic findings from the National Surgical Adjuvant Breast Project. Correlations with concordant and discordant estrogen and progesterone receptors. Cancer 1987; 59:1554–1559.

43. Fisher B, Redmond C, Fisher ER, Caplan R. Relative worth of estrogen or progesterone receptor and pathologic characteristics of differentiation as indicators of prognosis in node negative breast cancer patients: findings from National Surgical Adjuvant Breast and Bowel Project protocol B-06. J Clin Oncol 1988; 6:1076–1087.

44. Pujol P, Hilsenbeck SG, Chamness GC, Elledge RM. Rising levels of estrogen receptor in breast cancer over 2 decades. Cancer 1994;74(5):1601–1606.

45. Lippman ME, Dickson RB, Bates S, et al. Autocrine and paracrine growth regulation of human breast cancer. Breast Cancer Res Treat 1986;7:59–70.

46. Fokete M, Wittlirt JL, Schally AV. Characteristics and distribution of receptors for [D-TRP⁶)]-luteinizing-hormone-releasing hormone, somatostatin, epidermal growth factor, and sex steroids in 500 biopsy samples of human breast cancer. J Clin Lab Anal 1989; 3(3):137–147.

47. Foekens JA, Portengen H, Janssen M, Klijn JGM. Insulin-like growth factor-1 receptors and insulin-like growth factor-1-like activity in human primary breast cancer. Cancer 1989;63:2139–2147.

48. Reubi J-C, Torhorst J. The relationship between somatostatin, epidermal growth factor, and steroid hormone receptors in breast cancer. Cancer 1989; 64:1254–1260.

49. Ben-David M, Kadar T, Schally AV. Micromethod for the determination of free and total prolactin receptors: measurement of receptor levels in normal and malignant mammary and prostate tissues. Med Sci 1986;83:8375–8379.

50. LeRoith D, Baserga R, Helman L, Roberts CT Jr. Insulin-like growth factors and cancer. Ann Intern Med 1995;122(1):54–59.

51. Castellani R, Visscher DW, Wykes S, et al. Interaction of transforming growth factor-alpha and epidermal growth factor receptor in breast carcinoma. An immunohistologic study. Cancer 1994;73(2):344–349.

52. Clark GM, Dressler LG, Owens MA, et al. Prediction of relapse or survival in patients with node-negative breast cancer by DNA flow cytometry. N Engl J Med 1989;320:627–633.

53. Muss HB, Kute TE, Case LD, et al. The relation of flow cytometry to clinical and biologic characteris-

tics in women with node negative primary breast cancer. Cancer 1989;64:1894–1900.

54. Witzig TE, Ingle JN, Cha SS, et al. DNA ploidy and the percentage of cells in S-phase as prognostic factors for women with lymph node negative breast cancer. Cancer 1994;74(6):1752–1761.

55. Meyer JS, Province MA. S-phase fraction and nuclear size in long term prognosis of patients with breast cancer. Cancer 1994;74(8):2287–2299.

56. Clark GM, Mathieu MC, Owens MA, et al. Prognostic significance of S-phase fraction in good-risk, node-negative breast cancer patients. J Clin Oncol 1992;10(3):428–432.

57. Tandon AK, Clark GM, Chamness GC, et al. HER-2/*neu* oncogene protein and prognosis in breast cancer. J Clin Oncol 1989;7:1120–1128.

58. Slamon DJ, Godolphin W, Jones LA, et al. Studies of the HER-2/neu proto-oncogene in human breast and ovarian cancer. Science 1989;244:707–712.

59. Paterson AHG, Lees AW, Jamil N, et al. Comparison of HER-2/neu oncogene amplification with other prognostic factors in node negative patients with breast cancer (abstract). Proc Am Soc Clin Oncol 1989; 8:24.

60. Hartmann LC, Ingle JN, Wold LE, et al. Prognostic value of c-*erb*B2 overexpression in axillary lymph node positive breast cancer. Results from a randomized adjuvant treatment protocol. Cancer 1994; 74(11):2956–2963.

61. Fung CY, Fisher DE. p53: from molecular mechanisms to prognosis in cancer (editorial). J Clin Oncol 1995;13(4):808–811.

62. Allred DC, Clark GM, Elledge R, et al. Association of p53 protein expression with tumor cell proliferation rate and clinical outcome in node-negative breast cancer. J Natl Cancer Inst 1993;85(3):200–2066.

63. Silvestrini R, Benini E, Daidone MG, et al. p53 as an independent prognostic marker in lymph node-negative breast cancer patients. J Natl Cancer Inst 1993; 85(12):965–970.

64. Friedrichs K, Gluba S, Eidtmann H, Jonat W. Overexpression of p53 and prognosis in breast cancer. Cancer 1993;72(12):3641–3647.

65. Rosen PP, Lesser ML, Arroyo CD, et al. p53 in node-negative breast carcinoma: an immunohistochemical study of epidemiologic risk factors, histologic features, and prognosis. J Clin Oncol 1995;13(4):821–830.

66. Watson PH, Safneck JR, Le K, et al. Relationship of c-myc amplification to progression of breast cancer from in situ to invasive tumor and lymph node metastasis. J Natl Cancer Inst 1993;85(11):902–907.

67. Pertschuk LP, Feldman JG, Kim DS, et al. Steroid hormone receptor immunohistochemistry and amplification of c-*myc* protooncogene. Relationship to disease-free survival in breast cancer. Cancer 1993; 71(1):162–171.

68. Kardinal CG. Endocrine therapy of breast cancer. In: Donegan WL, Spratt JS, eds. Cancer of the breast. 4th ed. Philadelphia: WB Saunders, 1995:534–580.

69. Miller WR, Hawkins RA, Forrest APM. Significance of aromatase activity in human breast cancer. Cancer Res 1982;42(Suppl):3365s–3368s.

70. Siiteri PK. Review on studies of estrogen biosynthesis in the human. Cancer Res 1982; 42(Suppl):3269s–3273s.

71. Frantz AG, Wilson JD. Endocrine disorders of the breast. In: Wilson JD, Foster DW, eds. Williams textbook of endocrinology. Philadelphia: WB Saunders, 1985:402–421.

72. Peyrat JP, Djiane J, Kelly PA, et al. Characterization of prolactin receptors in human breast cancer. Breast Cancer Res Treat 1984;4:275–281.

73. Freeman CS, Topper Y. Progesterone is not essential to the differentiative potential of mammary epithelium in the male mouse. Endocrinology 1978; 103:186–192.

74. Greenspan EM. Combination cytotoxic chemotherapy in advanced disseminated breast carcinoma. J Mt Sinai Hosp 1966;33:1–27.

75. Cooper R. Combination chemotherapy in hormone resistant breast cancer (abstract). Proc Am Assoc Cancer Res 1969;10:15.

76. Schally AV, Comaru-Schally AM, Redding TW. Antitumor effects of analogs of hypothalamic hormones in endocrine-dependent cancers (41797). Proc Soc Exp Biol Med 1984;175:259–281.

77. Kardinal CG. Cancer chemotherapy: historical aspects and future considerations. Postgrad Med 1985; 77(6):165–174.

78. Legha SS. Tamoxifen in the treatment of breast cancer. Ann Intern Med 1988;109:219–228.

79. Ingle JN, Ahmann DL, Green SJ, et al. Randomized clinical trial of diethylstilbestrol versus tamoxifen in postmenopausal women with advanced breast cancer. N Engl J Med 1981;304:16–21.

80. Vogel CL, East DR, Voigt W, Thomsen S. Response to tamoxifen in estrogen receptor-poor metastatic breast cancer. Cancer 1987;60(6):1184–1198.

81. Jordan VC, Phelps E, Lindgren JU. Effects of anti-estrogens on bone in castrated and intact female rats. Breast Cancer Res Treat 1987;10:31–35.

82. Turken S, Siris E, Soldin D, et al. Effects of tamoxifen on spinal bone density in women with breast cancer. J Natl Cancer Inst 1989;81:1086–1088.

83. Powles TJ, Hickish TF, Kanis JA, Ashley S. Tamoxifen preserves bone mineral density in postmenopausal women but causes loss of bone density in premenopausal women (abstract). Proc Am Soc Clin Oncol 1995;14:165.

83a. Powles TJ, Hickish T, Kanis JA, et al. Effect of tamoxifen on bone mineral density measured by dual-energy x-ray absorptiometry in healthy premenopausal and postmenopausal women. J Clin Oncol 1996; 14:78–84.

84. Love RR, Mazess RB, Barden HS, et al. Effects of tamoxifen on bone mineral density in postmenopausal women with breast cancer. N Engl J Med 1992; 326(13):852–856.

85. Love RR, Barden HS, Mazess RB, et al. Effect of tamoxifen on lumbar spine bone mineral density in postmenopausal women after 5 years. Arch Intern Med 1994;154(22):2585–2588.

86. Love RR, Wiebe DA, Feyzi JM, et al. Effects of tamoxifen on cardiovascular risk factors in postmenopausal women after 5 years of treatment. J Natl Cancer Inst 1994;86(20):1534–1539.

87. Thangaraju M, Kumar K, Gandhirajan R, Sachdanandam P. Effect of tamoxifen on plasma lipids and lipoproteins in postmenopausal women with breast cancer. Cancer 1994;73(3):659–663.

87a. Saarto T, Blomqvist C, Ehnholm C, et al. Antiatherogenic effects of adjuvant antiestrogens: a randomized trial comparing the effects of tamoxifen and toremifene on plasma lipid levels in postmenopausal women with node-positive breast cancer. J Clin Oncol 1996;14:429–433.

88. Pollak M, Costantino J, Polychronakos C, et al. Effect of tamoxifen on serum insulin-like growth factor I levels in stage I breast cancer patients. J Natl Cancer Inst 1990;82(21):1693–1697.

89. Lahti EI, Knip M, Laatikainen TJ. Plasma insulin-like growth factor I and its binding proteins 1 and 3 in postmenopausal patients with breast cancer receiving long term tamoxifen. Cancer 1994;74(2):618–624.

90. Noguchi S, Motomura K, Inaji H, et al. Down-regulation of transforming growth factor-α by tamoxifen in human breast cancer. Cancer 1993;72(1):131–136.

91. Jordan VC. Growth factor regulation by tamoxifen is demonstrated in patients with breast cancer (editorial). Cancer 1993;72(1):1–2.

92. Sutherland RL, Green MD, Hall RE, et al. Tamoxifen induces accumulation of MCF 7 human mammary carcinoma cells in the G_0/G_1 phase of the cell cycle. Eur J Cancer Oncol 1983;19:615–621.

93. Osborne CK, Boldt DH, Clark GM, Trent JM. Effects of tamoxifen on human breast cancer cell cycle kinetics: accumulation of cells in early G_1 phase. Cancer Res 1983;43:3583–3585.

94. Jordan VC, Allen KE, Dix CJ. Pharmacology of tamoxifen in laboratory animals. Cancer Treat Rep 1980;64:745–759.

95. Jordan VC. Laboratory studies to develop general principles for the adjuvant treatment of breast cancer with antiestrogen: problems and potential for future clinical applications. Breast Cancer Res Treat 1983; 3(Suppl 1):73–86.

96. Jordan VC, Mirecki DM, Gottardis MM. Continuous tamoxifen treatment prevents the appearance of mammary tumors in a model system. In: Jones SE, Salmon SE, eds. Adjuvant therapy of cancer IV. New York: Grune & Stratton, 1984:27–33.

97. Fisher B, Brown A, Wolmark N, et al. Prolonging tamoxifen therapy for primary breast cancer. Findings from the National Surgical Adjuvant Breast and Bowel Project clinical trial. Ann Intern Med 1987; 106:649–654.

98. Reid AD, Horobin JM, Newman EL, Preece PE. Tamoxifen metabolism is altered by simultaneous administration of medroxyprogesterone acetate in breast cancer patients. Breast Cancer Res Treat 1992; 22(2):153–156.

99. Loprinzi CL, Michalak JC, Quella SK, et al. Megestrol acetate for the prevention of hot flashes. N Engl J Med 1994;331(6):347–352.

100. Goldberg RM, Loprinzi CL, O'Fallon JR, et al. Transdermal clonidine for ameliorating tamoxifen-induced hot flashes. J Clin Oncol 1994;12(1):155–158.

101. Jordan VC, Fritz NF, Tormey DC. Long-term adjuvant therapy with tamoxifen: effects on sex hormone binding globulin and antithrombin III. Cancer Res 1987;47:4517–4519.

102. Auger MJ, Mackie MJ. Effects of tamoxifen on blood coagulation. Cancer 1988;61:1316–1319.

103. Rutqvist LE, Mattsson A for The Stockholm Breast Cancer Study Group. Cardiac and thromboembolic morbidity among postmenopausal women with early-stage breast cancer in a randomized trial

of adjuvant tamoxifen. J Natl Cancer Inst 1993; 85(17):1398–1406.

104. Mathew A, Chabon AB, Kabakow B, et al. Endometrial carcinoma in five breast cancer patients receiving tamoxifen (abstract). Proc Am Soc Clin Oncol 1989;8:26.

105. Fisher B, Costantino JP, Redmond CK, et al. Endometrial cancer in tamoxifen-treated breast cancer patients: findings from the National Surgical Adjuvant Breast and Bowel Project (NSABP) B-14. J Natl Cancer Inst 1994;86(7):527–537.

106. Fornander T, Hellstrom AC, Moberger B. Descriptive clinicopathologic study of 17 patients with endometrial cancer during or after adjuvant tamoxifen in early breast cancer. J Natl Cancer Inst 1993; 85(22):1850–1855.

107. Jordan VC. Tamoxifen and tumorigenicity: a predictable concern (editorial). J Natl Cancer Inst 1995; 87(9):623–626.

107a. Cuenca RE, Giachino J, Arredondo, et al. Endometrial carcinoma associated with breast carcinoma. Cancer 1996;77:2058–2063.

107b. Fisher B. Commentary on endometrial cancer deaths in tamoxifen-treated breast cancer patients. J Clin Oncol 1996;14:1027–1039.

108. Rutqvist LE, Johansson H, Signomklao T, et al. for the Stockholm Breast Cancer Study Group. Adjuvant tamoxifen therapy for early stage breast cancer and second primary malignancies. J Natl Cancer Inst 1995;87(9):645–651.

109. Conte CC, Nemoto T, Rosner D, Dao TL. Therapeutic oophorectomy in metastatic breast cancer. Cancer 1989;64:150–153.

110. Veronesi U, Cascinelli N, Greco M, et al. A reappraisal of oophorectomy in carcinoma of the breast. Ann Surg 1987;205:18–21.

111. Ingle JN, Krook JE, Green SJ, et al. Randomized trial of bilateral oophorectomy versus tamoxifen in premenopausal women with metastatic breast cancer. J Clin Oncol 1986;4:178–185.

112. Buchanan RB, Blamey RW, Durrant KR, et al. A randomized comparison of tamoxifen with surgical oophorectomy in premenopausal patients with advanced breast cancer. J Clin Oncol 1986;4:1326–1330.

113. Pritchard KI, Meakin JW, Boyd NF, et al. A randomized trial of adjuvant tamoxifen in postmenopausal women with axillary node positive breast cancer. In: Jones SE, Salmon SE, eds. Adjuvant therapy of cancer IV. New York: Grune & Stratton, 1984:339–347.

114. Sawka CA, Pritchard KI, Paterson AHG, et al. Role and mechanism of action of tamoxifen in premenopausal women with metastatic breast carcinoma. Cancer Res 1986;46:3152–3156.

115. Manni A, Pearson DH. Antiestrogen-induced remissions in premenopausal women with stage IV breast cancer: effects in ovarian function. Cancer Treat Rep 1980;64:779–785.

116. Buzdar AU, Hortobagyi GN, Frye D, et al. Bioequivalence of 20-mg once-daily tamoxifen relative to 10-mg twice-daily tamoxifen regimens for breast cancer [published erratum appears in J Clin Oncol 1994;12(6):1337]. J Clin Oncol 1994;12(1):50–54.

117. Plotkin D, Lechner JJ, Jung WE, Rosen PJ. Tamoxifen flare in advanced breast cancer. JAMA 1978; 240:2644–2646.

118. Brooks BJ, Lippman ME. Tamoxifen flare in advanced endometrial carcinoma. J Clin Oncol 1985; 3:222–223.

119. Legha SS, Powell K, Buzdar AU, Blumenschein GR. Tamoxifen-induced hypercalcemia in breast cancer. Cancer 1981;47:2803–2806.

120. Hall TC, Dederick MM, Nevinny HB. Prognostic value of hormonally induced hypercalcemia in breast cancer. Cancer Chemother Rep 1963;30:21–23.

121. Otteman LA, Long HJ. Hypercalcemic flare with megestrol acetate. Cancer Treat Rep 1984; 68:1420–1421.

122. Bradbeer JW, Kyngdon J. Primary treatment of breast cancer in elderly women with tamoxifen. Clin Oncol 1983;9:31–34.

123. Robertson JF, Todd JH, Ellis IO, et al. Comparison of mastectomy with tamoxifen for treating elderly patients with operable breast cancer. Br Med J Clin Res 1988;297:511–514.

124. Gazet JC, Markopoulos C, Ford HT, et al. Prospective randomized trial of tamoxifen versus surgery in elderly patients with breast cancer. Lancet 1988; 26:679–681.

125. Gaskell DJ, Hawkins RA, de Carteret S, et al. Indications for primary tamoxifen therapy in elderly women with breast cancer. Br J Surg 1992;79(12):1317–1320.

126. Martin LM, le Pechoux C, Calitchi E, et al. Management of breast cancer in the elderly. Eur J Cancer 1994;30(5):590–596.

127. Deschenes L. Droloxifene, a new antiestrogen, in advanced breast cancer. A double-blind dose-finding study. The Droloxifene 002 International Study Group. Am J Clin Oncol 1991;14(Suppl 2):S52–S55.

128. Hamm JT, Tormey DC, Kohler PC, et al. Phase I study of toremifene in patients with advanced cancer. J Clin Oncol 1991;9:2036–2041.

129. Pritchard KI, Paterson AH, Deschenes L, et al. A randomized double-blind trial of the antiestrogen droloxifene (3-OH tamoxifen) in previously untreated postmenopausal women with estrogen (ER)- or progesterone receptor (PGR)-positive or unknown metastatic or locally unresectable breast cancer (abstract). Proc Am Soc Clin Oncol 1991;10:A52.

130. Valavaara R, Tuominen J, Johansson R. Predictive value of tumor estrogen and progesterone receptor levels in postmenopausal women with advanced breast cancer treated with toremifene. Cancer 1990;66:2264–2269.

131. Wakeling AE, Dukes M, Bowler J. A potent specific pure antiestrogen with clinical potential. Cancer Res 1991;51:3867–3873.

132. DeFriend DJ, Howell A, Nicholson RI, et al. Investigation of a new pure antiestrogen (ICI 182780) in women with primary breast cancer. Cancer Res 1994;54(2):408–414.

133. Wärri AM, Huovinen RL, Laine AM, et al. Apoptosis in toremifene-induced growth inhibition of human breast cancer cells in vivo and in vitro. J Natl Cancer Inst 1993;85(17):1412–1418.

134. Vogel CL, Shemano I, Schoenfelder J, et al. Multicenter phase II efficacy trial of toremifene in tamoxifen-refractory patients with advanced breast cancer. J Clin Oncol 1993;11(2):345–350.

135. van Veelen H, Willemse PHB, Tjabbes T, et al. Oral high-dose medoxyprogesterone acetate versus tamoxifen. A randomized crossover trial in postmeno-

pausal patients with advanced breast cancer. Cancer 1986;58:7–13.

136. Ettinger DS, Allegra J, Bertino JR, et al. Megestrol acetate v tamoxifen in advanced breast cancer: correlation of hormone receptors and response. Semin Oncol 1986;l3(Suppl 4):9–14.

137. Muss HB, Wells HB, Paschold EH, et al. Megestrol acetate versus tamoxifen in advanced breast cancer: 5-year analysis—a phase III trial of the Piedmont Oncology Association. J Clin Oncol 1988;6:1098–1106.

138. Muss HB, Case LD, Atkins JN, et al. Tamoxifen versus high-dose oral medroxyprogesterone acetate as initial endocrine therapy for patients with metastatic breast cancer: a Piedmont Oncology Association study. J Clin Oncol 1994;12(8):1630–1638.

139. Allegra JC, Kiefer SM. Mechanisms of action of progestational agents. Semin Oncol 1985;12(Suppl 1):3–5.

140. Elizalde PV, Guerra FK, Gravano M, et al. Correlation of TGF-β_1 expression with medroxyprogesterone acetate responsiveness in mouse mammary adenocarcinomas. Cancer Invest 1995;13(2):173–180.

141. Johnson PA, Muss H, Bonomi P, et al. Megestrol acetate as primary hormonal therapy for advanced breast cancer. Semin Oncol 1988;15:34–37.

142. Loprinzi CL, Michalak JC, Schaid DJ, et al. Phase III evaluation of four doses of megestrol acetate as therapy for patients with cancer anorexia and/or cachexia. J Clin Oncol 1993;11(4):762–767.

143. Carpenter JT, Peterson L. Use of megestrol acetate in advanced breast cancer on a single daily dose schedule. Semin Oncol 1985;12(Suppl):40–42.

144. Cavalli F, Goldhirsch A, Jungi F, et al. Randomized trial of low- vs high-dose medroxyprogesterone acetate in the induction treatment of postmenopausal patients with advanced breast cancer. J Clin Oncol 1984;2:414–419.

145. Kornblith AB, Hollis DR, Zuckerman E, et al. for the Cancer and Leukemia Group B. Effect of megestrol acetate on quality of life in a dose-response trial in women with advanced breast cancer. J Clin Oncol 1993;(11):2081–2089.

146. Cash R, Brough AJ, Cohen MNP, Satoh PS. Aminoglutethimide (Elipten-Ciba) as an inhibitor of adrenal steroidogenesis: mechanism of action and therapeutic trial. J Clin Endocrinol Metab 1967;27:1239–1248.

147. Samojlik E, Santen RJ, Kirschner MA, Ertel NH. Steroid hormone profiles in women treated with aminoglutethimide for metastatic carcinoma of the breast. Cancer Res 1982;42:3349s–3352s.

148. Nemoto T, Rosner D, Patel JK, Dao TL. Aminoglutethimide in patients with metastatic breast cancer. Cancer 1989;63:1673–1675.

149. Santen RJ, Worgul TJ, Samojlik E, et al. A randomized trial comparing surgical adrenalectomy with aminoglutethimide plus hydrocortisone in women with advanced breast cancer. N Engl J Med 1981;305:545–551.

150. Ingle JN. Additive hormonal therapy in women with advanced breast cancer. Cancer 1984;53:766–777.

151. Höffken K, Jonat W, Possinger K, et al. Aromatase inhibition with 4-hydroxyandrostenedione in the treatment of postmenopausal patients with advanced breast cancer: a phase II study. J Clin Oncol 1990;8:875–880.

152. Lipton A, Harvey HA, Demers LM, et al. A phase I trial of CGS 16949A. A new aromatase inhibitor. Cancer 1990;65:1279–1285.

153. Lonning PE, Jacobs S, Jones A, et al. The influence of CGS 16949A on peripheral aromatisation in breast cancer patients. Br J Cancer 1991;63:789–793.

154. Raats JI, Falkson G, Falkson HC. A study of fadrozole, a new aromatase inhibitor, in postmenopausal women with advanced metastatic breast cancer. J Clin Oncol 1992;10:111–116.

155. Santen RJ, Demers LM, Lynch J, et al. Specificity of low dose fadrozole hydrochloride (CGS 16949A) as an aromatase inhibitor. J Clin Endocrinol Metab 1991;73:99–106.

156. Stein RC, Dowsett M, Hedley A, et al. The clinical and endocrine effects of 4-hydroxyandrostenedione alone and in combination with goserelin in premenopausal women with advanced breast cancer. Br J Cancer 1990;62:679–683.

157. Goss PE, Gwyn KMEH. Current perspectives on aromatase inhibitors in breast cancer. J Clin Oncol 1994;12(11):2460–2470.

158. Lipton A, Demers LM, Harvey HA, et al. Letrozole (CGS 20267). A phase I study of a new potent oral aromatase inhibitor of breast cancer. Cancer 1995;75(8):2132–2138.

159. Schulz J, Fox K, Conner G, et al. A phase II study of rogletimide (ROG) in females with advanced/metastatic breast cancer (A/M BrCa) (abstract). Proc Am Soc Clin Oncol 1995;14:93.

159a. Plourde PV, Dyroff M, Dowsett M, et al. Arimidex: a new oral, once-a-day aromatase inhibitor. J Steroid Biochem Molec Biol 1995;53:175–179.

159b. Buzdar AU, Smith R, Vogel C, et al. Fadrozole HCL (CGS-16949A) versus megestrol acetate treatment of postmenopausal patients with metastatic breast carcinoma: results of two randomized double blind controlled multiinstitutional trials. Cancer 1996;77:2503–2515.

160. Cocconi G, Bisagni G, Ceci G, et al. Low-dose aminoglutethimide with and without hydrocortisone replacement as a first-line endocrine treatment in advanced breast cancer: a prospective randomized trial of the Italian Oncology Group for Clinical Research. J Clin Oncol 1992;10:984–989.

161. Crivellari D, Galligioni E, Frustaci S, et al. Low-dose aminoglutethimide plus steroid replacement in advanced breast cancer patients resistant to conventional therapies. Cancer Invest 1989;7:113–116.

161a. Jonat W, Howell A, Blomqvist C, et al. on behalf of the Arimidex Study Group. A randomised trial comparing two doses of the new selective aromatase inhibitor anastrozole (Arimidex) with megestrol acetate in postmenopausal patients with advanced breast cancer. Eur J Cancer 1996;32A:404–412.

162. Kennedy BJ. Hormonal therapies in breast cancer. Semin Oncol 1974;1:119–130.

163. Garland L, Schpira DV. DES-JA vu: High-dose estrogen in advanced breast CA (abstract). Proc Am Soc Clin Oncol 1995;14:123.

164. Escher GC. Clinical improvement in inoperable breast carcinoma under steroid treatment. In: Council of Pharmacy and Chemistry, American Medical Association. Proceedings of the First Conference

on Steroid Hormone and Mammary Carcinoma. Chicago: American Medical Association 1949:92–99.

165. Baker LH, Vaitkevicius VK. Reevaluation of rebound regression in disseminated carcinoma of the breast. Cancer 1972;29:1268–1271.

166. Nestro RW, Cady B, Oberfield RA, et al. Rebound response after estrogen therapy for metastatic breast cancer. Cancer 1976;38:1834–1837.

167. Belani CP, Pearl P, Whitley NO, Aisner J. Tamoxifen withdrawal response. Report of a case. Arch Intern Med 1989;149:449–450.

168. Loeser A. Male hormone in the treatment of cancer of the breast. Acta Un Int Cancer 1939;4:375–385.

169. Ulrich P. Testosterone (hormone male) et son role possible dans le traitement de certains cancers du sein. Acta Un Gut Cancer 1939;4:377–385.

170. Rochefort H. Biochemical basis of breast cancer treatment by androgens and progestins. In: Gurpide E, Calandra R, Levy C, Soto RJ, eds. Hormones and cancer. New York: Alan R Liss, 1984:79–96.

171. Naeim F, Copper PH, Semion AA. Pelious hepatitis. Possible etiologic role of anabolic steroids. Arch Pathol 1973;95:284–285.

172. Bagheri SA, Boyer N. Peliosis hepatis associated with androgenic-anabolic steroid therapy. Ann Intern Med 1974;81:610–618.

173. Arafah BM. Decreased levothyroxine requirement in women with hypothyroidism during androgen therapy for breast cancer. Ann Intern Med 1994; 121(4):247–251.

174. Kelley RM. Hormones and chemotherapy in breast cancer. Cancer 1971;28:1686–1695.

175. Schell HW. Adrenal corticosteroid therapy in far-advanced cancer. Geriatrics 1972;27:131–134.

176. Bruera E, Roca E, Cedaro L, et al. Action of oral methylprednisolone in terminal cancer patients: a prospective randomized double-blind study. Cancer Treat Rep 1985;69:751–754.

177. Klijn JG, de Jong FH, Blankenstein MA, et al. Anti-tumor and endocrine effects of chronic LHRH agonist treatment (buserelin) with or without tamoxifen in premenopausal metastatic breast cancer. Breast Cancer Res Treat 1984;4:209–220.

178. Kaufmann M, Jonat W, Kleeberg U, et al. Goserelin, a depot gonadotrophin-releasing hormone agonist in the treatment of premenopausal patients with metastatic breast cancer. J Clin Oncol 1989;7:1113–1119.

179. Harvey HA, Lipton A, Max DT, et al. Medical castration produced by the GnRH analogue leuprolide to treat metastatic breast cancer. J Clin Oncol 1985; 3:1068–1072.

180. Buzzoni R, Bajetta E, Biganzoli L, et al. Combined goserelin plus tamoxifen treatment in premenopausal advanced breast cancer. A multicenter study by the Italian Trials in Medical Oncology (ITMO) group (abstract). Proc Am Soc Clin Oncol 1994;13:56.

181. Jonat W, Kaufmann M, Blamey RW, et al. A randomized trial comparing Zoladex (goserelin) with Zoladex plus Nolvadex (tamoxifen) as first-line treatment for premenopausal advanced breast cancer (abstract). Proc Am Soc Clin Oncol 1994;13:58.

182. Saphner T, Troxel AB, Tormey DC, et al. Phase II study of goserelin for patients with postmenopausal metastatic breast cancer. J Clin Oncol 1993;11(8):1529–1535.

183. Schally AV, Redding TW, Cai RZ, et al. Somatostatin analogs in the treatment of various experimental tumors. In: Klein J, ed. International symposium on hormonal manipulation in cancer: peptides, growth factors, and new (anti) steroidal agents. New York: Raven Press, 1987:431–440.

184. Schally AV. Oncological applications of somatostatin analogues. Cancer Res 1988;48:6977–6985.

185. Weckbecker G, Tolcsvai L, Stolz B, et al. The somatostatin analog octreotide enhances the antineoplastic actions of tamoxifen and ovariectomy on DMBA-induced mammary carcinoma (abstract). Proc Am Soc Clin Oncol 1995;36:492.

186. Davis HL Jr, Ramirez G, Ellerby RA, Ansfield FJ. Five-drug therapy in advanced breast cancer: factors influencing toxicity and response. Cancer 1974; 34:239–245.

187. Broder LE, Tormey DC. Combination chemotherapy of carcinoma of the breast. Cancer Treat Rev 1974;1:183–192.

188. Ramirez G, Klotz J, Strawitz JG, et al. Combination chemotherapy in breast cancer: a randomized study of 4 versus 5 drugs. Oncology 1975;32:101–108.

189. Brunner KW, Sonntag RW, Martz G, et al. A controlled study in the use of combined therapy for metastatic breast cancer. Cancer 1975;36:1208–1219.

190. Irwin LE, Pugh R, Sadoff L, et al. The influence on survival of continuous combination vs. sequential single agent chemotherapy in disseminated breast cancer (abstract). Presented at the American College of Physicians 56th annual meeting, San Francisco, 1975.

191. Ahmann DL, Bisel HF, Hahn PG, et al. An analysis of a multiple-drug program in the treatment of patients with advanced breast cancer utilizing 5-fluorouracil, cyclophosphamide, and prednisone with or without vincristine. Cancer 1975;36:1925–1935.

192. Canellos CP, De Vita VT, Gold GL, et al. Combination chemotherapy for advanced breast cancer: response and effect on survival. Ann Intern Med 1976; 84:389–392.

193. Canellos GP, Pocock SJ, Taylor SG III, et al. Combination chemotherapy for metastatic breast carcinoma: prospective comparison of multiple drug therapy with L-phenylalanine mustard. Cancer 1976; 38:1882–1886.

194. Otis PT, Armentrout SA. Combination chemotherapy in metastatic carcinoma of the breast: results with a three-drug combination. Cancer 1975; 36:311–317.

195. Creech RH, Catalano RB, Mastrangelo MJ, Engstrom PF. An effective low-dose intermittent cyclophosphamide, methotrexate, and 5-fluorouracil treatment regimen for metastatic breast cancer. Cancer 1975;35:1101–1107.

196. DeLena M, Brambilla C, Morabita A, Bonadonna G. Adriamycin plus vincristine compared to and combined with cyclophosphamide, methotrexate, and 5-fluorouracil for advanced breast cancer. Cancer 1975;35:1108–1115.

197. Kardinal CG. Chemotherapy. In: Donegan WL, Spratt JS, eds. Cancer of the breast. 2nd ed. Philadelphia: WB Saunders, 1979:405–447.

198. Livingston RB, Carter SE. Single agents in cancer chemotherapy. New York: IFI Plenum, 1970.

199. Anonymous: Compilation of phase II results with single antineoplastic agents (series). Cancer Treat Symp 1985;4:4.

200. Gasparini G, Caffo O, Barni S, et al. Vinorelbine is an active antiproliferative agent in pretreated advanced breast cancer patients: a phase II study. J Clin Oncol 1994;12(10):2094–2101.

201. Fumoleau P, Delgado FM, Delozier T, et al. Phase II trial of weekly intravenous vinorelbine in first-line advanced breast cancer chemotherapy. J Clin Oncol 1993;11(7):1245–1252.

202. Rowinsky EK, Donehower RC. Paclitaxel (Taxol) [published erratum appears in N Engl J Med 1995;333(1):75]. N Engl J Med 1995;332(15):1004–1014.

203. Torti FM, Bristow MR, Howes AE, et al. Reduced cardiotoxicity of doxorubicin delivered on a weekly schedule: assessment of endomyocardial biopsy. Ann Intern Med 1983;99:745–756.

204. Chlebowski RT, Paroly WS, Pugh RP, et al. Adriamycin given as a weekly schedule without a loading course: clinically effective with reduced incidence of cardiotoxicity. Cancer Treat Rep 1980;64:47–51.

205. Hortobagyi GN, Frye E, Buzdar AU, et al. Decreased cardiac toxicity of doxorubicin administered by continuous intravenous infusion in combination chemotherapy for metastatic breast carcinoma. Cancer 1989;63:37–45.

206. Legha SS. Infusional doxorubicin in the treatment of breast cancer. J Infus Chemother 1993;3:15–18.

207. Speyer JL, Green MD, Kramer E, et al. Protective effect of the bispiperazinedione ICRF-187 against doxorubicin-induced cardiac toxicity in women with advanced breast cancer. N Engl J Med 1988;319:745–752.

208. Speyer JL, Green MD, Zeleniuch-Jacquotte A, et al. ICRF-187 permits longer treatment with doxorubicin in women with breast cancer. J Clin Oncol 1992;10(1):117–217.

209. Carmo-Pereira J, Henriques E, Costa FO, et al. Epirubicin (E) as first line chemotherapy in disseminated breast carcinoma. A phase II study. Preliminary results (abstract). Proc Am Soc Clin Oncol 1989;8:31.

210. Twelves CJ, O'Reilly S, Coleman RE, et al. Weekly epirubicin for liver metastases in breast cancer (abstract). Proc Am Soc Clin Oncol 1989;8:32.

211. Shenkenberg TD, Von Hoff DD. Mitoxantrone: a new anticancer drug with significant clinical activity. Ann Intern Med 1986;105:67–81.

212. Weiss RB. Mitoxantrone: its development and role in clinical practice. Oncology 1989;3:135–148.

213. Henderson IC, Allegra JC, Woodcock T, et al. Randomized clinical trial comparing mitoxantrone with doxorubicin in previously treated patients with metastatic breast cancer. J Clin Oncol 1989;7:560–571.

214. Neidhart JA, Gochnour D, Roach R, et al. A comparison of mitoxantrone and doxorubicin in breast cancer. J Clin Oncol 1986;4:672–677.

215. Hainsworth JD. The use of mitoxantrone in the treatment of breast cancer. Semin Oncol 1995;22(Suppl 1):17–20.

216. Thompson P, Harvey V. Improved quality of life (QOL) in patients (PTS) with advanced breast cancer responding to treatment with mitoxantrone (MX) (abstract). Proc Am Soc Clin Oncol 1989;8:34.

217. Plowman PN, Harnett AN. Single agent mitoxantrone for metastatic breast cancer in the elderly (abstract). Proc Am Soc Clin Oncol 1989;8:29.

218. Benjamin RS. Rationale for the use of mitoxantrone in the older patient: cardiac toxicity. Semin Oncol 1995;22(1 Suppl 1):11–13.

218a. Capri G, Tarenzi E, Fulfaro F, Gianni L. The role of taxanes in the treatment of breast cancer. Semin Oncol 1996;23(Suppl 1):68–75.

219. Holmes FA, Walters RS, Theriault RL, et al. Phase II trial of Taxol, an active drug in the treatment of metastatic breast cancer. J Natl Cancer Inst 1991;83(24):1797–1805.

220. Reichman BS, Seidman AD, Crown JPA, et al. Paclitaxel and recombinant human granulocyte colony-stimulating factor as initial chemotherapy for metastatic breast cancer. J Clin Oncol 1993;11(10):1943–1951.

221. Gelmon K, Nabholtz JM, Bontenbal M, et al. Randomized trial of two doses of paclitaxel in metastatic breast cancer after failure of standard therapy (abstract). Ann Oncol 1994;5:198.

222. Seidman A, Crown J, Reichman B, et al. Lack of cross resistance of Taxol with anthracycline in the treatment of metastatic breast cancer (abstract). Proc Am Soc Clin Oncol 1993;12:63.

223. Gianni L, Capri G, Munzone E, et al. Paclitaxel (Taxol) efficacy in patients with advanced breast cancer resistant to anthracyclines. Semin Oncol 1994;21(Suppl 8):29–33.

223a. Hortobagyi GN, Holmes FA. Single-agent paclitaxel for the treatment of breast cancer: an overview. Semin Oncol 1996;23(Suppl 1):4–9.

224. Wilson WH, Berg SL, Bryant G, et al. Paclitaxel in doxorubicin-refractory or mitoxantrone-refractory breast cancer: a phase I/II trial of 96-hour infusion. J Clin Oncol 1994;12:1621–1629.

225. Sledge GW, Robert N, Sparano JA, et al. Paclitaxel (Taxol) doxorubicin combinations in advanced breast cancer: the Eastern Cooperative Oncology Group experience. Semin Oncol 1994;21(Suppl 8):15–18.

226. Gelmon K. Biweekly paclitaxel (Taxol) and cisplatin in breast and ovarian cancer. Semin Oncol 1994;21(Suppl 8):24–28.

227. O'Shaughnessy JA, Fisherman JS, Cowan KH. Combination paclitaxel (Taxol) and doxorubicin therapy for metastatic breast cancer. Semin Oncol 1994;21(Suppl 8):19–23.

227a. Dombernowsky P, Gehl J, Boesgaard M, et al. Paclitaxel and doxorubicin, a highly active combination in the treatment of metastatic breast cancer. Semin Oncol 1996;23(Suppl 1):13–18.

228. Fumoleau P, Chevallier B, Kerbrat P, et al. First line chemotherapy with Taxotere in advanced breast cancer: a phase II study of the EORTC clinical screening group (abstract). Proc Am Soc Clin Oncol 1993;12:56.

229. Chevallier B, Fumoleau P, Kerbrat P, et al. Docetaxel is a major cytotoxic drug for the treatment of advanced breast cancer: a phase II trial of the Clinical Screening Cooperative Group of the European Organization for Research and Treatment of Cancer. J Clin Oncol 1995;13:314–322.

230. Seidman AD, Hudis C, Crown JPA, et al. Phase II evaluation of Taxotere (rp56976, nsc628503) as initial chemotherapy for metastatic breast cancer (abstract). Proc Am Soc Clin Oncol 1993;12:63.

231. Trudeau ME, Eisenhauer E, Lofters W, et al. Phase II study of Taxotere as first line chemotherapy for metastatic breast cancer. A National Cancer Insti-

tute of Canada Clinical Trials Group study (abstract). Proc Am Soc Clin Oncol 1993;12:64.

231a. Trudeau ME, Eisenhauer EA, Higgins BP, et al. Docetaxel in patients with metastatic breast cancer: a phase II study of the National Cancer Institute of Canada—Clinical Trials Group. J Clin Oncol 1996; 14:422–428.

232. Dieras V, Fumoleau P, Chevallier B, et al. Second EORTC Clinical Screening Group phase II trial of Taxotere (docetaxel) as first line chemotherapy in advanced breast cancer (abstract). Proc Am Soc Clin Oncol 1994;13:78.

232a. Rittenberg CN, Gralla RJ, Cole JT, et al. Preventing docetaxel-induced fluid retention: the efficacy of corticosteroids (abstract). Proc Am Soc Clin Oncol 1996;15:531.

233. Valero V, Walters R, Theriault L, et al. Phase II study of docetaxel (Taxotere) in anthracycline-refractory metastatic breast cancer (abstract). Proc Am Soc Clin Oncol 1994;13:A1636.

234. Seidman AD, Reichman BS, Crown JPA, et al. Paclitaxel as second and subsequent therapy for metastatic breast cancer: activity independent of prior anthracycline response. J Clin Oncol 1995;13:1152–1159.

235. Langlois N, Gueritte F, Langlois Y, et al. Application of a modification of the Polonovski reaction to the synthesis of vinblastine type alkaloid. J Am Chem Soc 1976;22:7017–7024.

236. Weber B, Vogel C, Jones S, et al. A U.S. multicenter phase II trial of Navelbine in advanced breast cancer (abstract). Proc Am Soc Clin Oncol 1993;12:61.

237. Romero A, Rabinovich MG, Vallejo CT, et al. Vinorelbine as first line chemotherapy for metastatic breast carcinoma. J Clin Oncol 1994;12(2):336–341.

238. Spielmann M, Dorval T, Turpin F, et al. Phase II trial of vinorelbine/doxorubicin as first line therapy of advanced breast cancer. J Clin Oncol 1994; 12(9):1764–1770.

239. Hochster H, Vogel C, Blumenreich JG, et al. A multicenter phase II study of Navelbine and doxorubicin as first line chemotherapy of metastatic breast cancer (abstract). Proc Am Soc Clin Oncol 1994;13:100.

240. Chadjaa M, Izzo J, May-Levin F, et al. Preliminary data on 4 epiadriamycine-vinorelbine: a new active combination in advanced breast cancer (abstract). Proc Am Soc Clin Oncol 1993;12:88.

241. Ferrero JM, Wemdling JI, Hoch M, et al. Mitoxantrone-vinorelbine as first line chemotherapy in metastatic breast cancer: a pilot study (abstract). Proc Am Soc Clin Oncol 1993;12:108.

242. Scheithauer W, Kornek G, Halder K, et al. Effective second line chemotherapy of advanced breast cancer with Navelbine and mitomycin C. Breast Cancer Res Treat 1993;26:49–53.

243. Kardinal CG, Cole JT, Gralla RJ, et al. Navelbine (vinorelbine) and mitomycin C: combination therapy in advanced breast cancer (abstract). Proc Am Soc Clin Oncol 1995;14:131.

244. Heidelberger C, Chaudhuri NK, Danneberg P, et al. Fluorinated pyrimidines, a new class of tumor-inhibitory compounds. Nature 1957;179:663–666.

245. Carter SR. Single and combination nonhormonal chemotherapy in breast cancer. Cancer 1972; 30:1543–1555.

246. Bleyer WA. New vistas for leucovorin in cancer chemotherapy. Cancer 1989;63:995–1007.

247. O'Connell MJ. A phase III trial of 5-fluorouracil and leucovorin in the treatment of advanced colorectal cancer. A Mayo Clinic/North Central Cancer Treatment Group study. Cancer 1989;63:1026–1030.

248. Loprinzi CL. 5-Fluorouracil with leucovorin in breast cancer. Cancer 1989;63:1045–1047.

249. Arbuck SG. Overview of clinical trials using 5-fluorouracil and leucovorin for the treatment of colorectal cancer. Cancer 1989;63:1036–1044.

250. Swain SM, Lippman ME, Egan EF, et al. Fluorouracil and high-dose leucovorin in previously treated patients with metastatic breast cancer. J Clin Oncol 1989;7:890–899.

251. Jabboury K, Holmes F, Kau S, Hortobagyi G. Folinic acid modulation of low-dose fluorouracil (FU) infusion in refractory breast cancer: a dose optimization study (abstract). Proc Am Soc Clin Oncol 1989; 8:40.

252. Marini G, Simoncini E, Zaniboni A, et al. 5-Fluorouracil and high-dose folinic acid as salvage treatment of advanced breast cancer: an update. Oncology 1987;44:336–340.

253. Lokich J, Bothe A, Fine N, Perri J. Phase I study of protracted venous infusion of 5-fluorouracil. Cancer 1981;48:2565–2568.

254. Jabboury K, Holmes FA, Hortobagyi G. 5-Fluorouracil rechallenge by protracted infusion in refractory breast cancer. Cancer 1989;64:793–797.

255. Hatfield AK, Johnson PA, Egner JR, Long CA. Long-term continuous 5-fluorouracil (5-FU) infusion in the treatment of far advanced metastatic breast carcinoma (abstract). Proc Am Soc Clin Oncol 1989;8:35.

256. Huan S, Pazdur R, Singhakowinta A, et al. Low-dose continuous infusion 5-fluorouracil. Evaluation in advanced breast carcinoma. Cancer 1989; 63:419–422.

257. Cameron DA, Gabra H, Leonard RC. Continuous 5-fluorouracil in the treatment of breast cancer. Br J Cancer 1994;70(1):120–124.

258. Henderson IC. Chemotherapy for advanced disease. In: Bonadonna G, ed. Breast cancer: diagnosis and management. New York: John Wiley, 1984:274–280.

259. Christman K, Muss HB, Case LD, Stanley V. Chemotherapy of metastatic breast cancer in the elderly. The Piedmont Oncology Association experience. JAMA 1992;268(1):57–62.

260. Muss HB. Chemotherapy of breast cancer in the older patient. Semin Oncol 1995;22(1 Suppl 1):14–16.

261. Remvikos Y, Buezeboc P, Zajdela A, et al. Correlation of pretreatment proliferative activity of breast cancer with the response to cytotoxic chemotherapy. J Natl Cancer Inst 1989;81:1383–1386.

262. Osborne CK. DNA flow cytometry in early breast cancer: a step in the right direction. J Natl Cancer Inst 1989;81:1344–1345.

263. Ziegler LD, Connelly JH, Frye D, et al. Lack of correlation between histologic findings and response to chemotherapy in metastatic breast cancer. Cancer 1991;68(3):628–633.

264. Bonadonna G, Zambetti M, Valagussa P. Sequential or alternating doxorubicin and CMF regimens in breast cancer with more than three positive nodes. Ten-year results. JAMA 1995;273(7):542–547.

265. Fisher B, Brown AM, Dimitrov NV, et al. Two

months of doxorubicin-cyclophosphamide with and without interval reinduction therapy compared with 6 months of cyclophosphamide, methotrexate, and fluorouracil in positive-node breast cancer patients with tamoxifen-nonresponsive tumors: results from the National Surgical Adjuvant Breast and Bowel Project B-15. J Clin Oncol 1990;8(9):1483–1496.

266. Tormey DC, Weinberg VE, Leone LA, et al. A comparison of intermittent vs. continuous and of Adriamycin vs. methotrexate 5-drug chemotherapy for advanced breast cancer. A Cancer and Leukemia Group study. Am J Clin Oncol 1984;7:231–239.

267. Aisner J, Weinberg V, Perloff M, et al. Chemotherapy versus chemoimmunotherapy (CAF v CAFVP v CMF each ± MER) for metastatic carcinoma of the breast: a CALGB study. J Clin Oncol 1987; 5:1523–1533.

268. Smalley RV, Lefante J, Bartolucci A, et al. A comparison of cyclophosphamide, Adriamycin, and 5-fluorouracil (CAF) and cyclophosphamide, methotrexate, 5-fluorouracil, vincristine, and prednisone (CMFVP) in patients with advanced breast cancer. A Southeastern Study Group project. Breast Cancer Res Treat 1983;3:209–220.

269. Anonymous. CAF in metastatic breast cancer: standard therapy or another effective regimen? (editorial). J Clin Oncol 1987;5:1497–1499.

270. Bennett JM, Muss HB, Doroshow JH, et al. A randomized multicenter trial comparing mitoxantrone, cyclophosphamide, and fluorouracil with doxorubicin, cyclophosphamide, and fluorouracil in the therapy of metastatic breast carcinoma. J Clin Oncol 1988;6:1611–1620.

271. Follezou JY, Palangie T, Feuilhade F. Randomized trial comparing mitoxantrone with Adriamycin in advanced breast cancer. Presse Med 1987;16:765–768.

272. Gercovich FG, Negro A, Requejo H, et al. 5-Fluorouracil, cyclophosphamide and mitoxantrone (fucimix) vs fucimix-prednisone (PDN) for advanced breast cancer (ABC): a prospective and randomized trial. Preliminary report (abstract). Proc Am Assoc Cancer Res 1989;30:a1014.

273. Hainsworth JD, Andrews MB, Johnson DH, Greco FA. Mitoxantrone, fluorouracil, and high-dose leucovorin: an effective, well-tolerated regimen for metastatic breast cancer. J Clin Oncol 1991;9(10):1731–1735.

274. Jones SE, Mennel RG, Brooks B, et al. Phase II study of mitoxantrone, leucovorin, and infusional fluorouracil for treatment of metastatic breast cancer. J Clin Oncol 1991;9(10):1736–1739.

275. Hainsworth JD, Jolivet J, Hopkins LE, Greco FA. A randomized phase II trial of mitoxantrone, 5-FU, and high dose leucovorin (NFL) vs cyclophosphamide, methotrexate, 5-FU (CMF) in the first line treatment of metastatic breast cancer (abstract). Proc Am Soc Clin Oncol 1990;14:90.

276. Carmo-Pereira J, Costa FO, Henriques E. Mitoxantrone, folinic acid, 5-fluorouracil and prednisone as first-line chemotherapy for advanced breast carcinoma. A phase II study. Eur J Cancer 1993; 29A(13):1814–1816.

277. Sledge GW Jr, Roth BJ. Cisplatin in the management of breast cancer. Semin Oncol 1989;14(Suppl 6):110–115.

278. Cocconi C, Bisagni G, De List V, et al. Plati-

num (P) and etoposide (E) as a first-line chemotherapy (CT) for metastatic breast carcinoma (MBC). Preliminary results of a prospective randomized trial (abstract). Proc Am Soc Clin Oncol 1988;7:13.

279. Krook JE, Loprinzi CL, Schaid DJ, et al. Evaluation of the continuous infusion of etoposide plus cisplatin in metastatic breast cancer: a collaborative North Central Cancer Treatment Group–Mayo Clinic phase II study. Cancer 1990;65(3):418–421.

280. Cox EB, Burton GV, Olsen GA, Vugrin D. Cisplatin and etoposide: an effective treatment for refractory breast carcinoma. Am J Clin Oncol 1989;12(1):53–56.

281. Roth BJ, Sledge GW Jr, Williams SD, et al. Methotrexate, vinblastine, doxorubicin, and cisplatin (M-VAC) as first-line chemotherapy (CT) in metastatic breast cancer (MBC): a phase II trial of the Hoosier Oncology Group (abstract). Proc Am Soc Clin Oncol 1988; 7:31.

282. Langer CJ, Catalano R, Weiner LM, et al. Phase II evaluation of methotrexate, vinblastine, doxorubicin, and cisplatin (M-VAC) in advanced, measurable breast carcinoma. Cancer Invest 1995;13(2):150–159.

283. Goldie JH, Coldman AJ, Gudauskas GA. Rationale for the use of alternating non-cross-resistant chemotherapy. Cancer Treat Rep 1982;66:439–449.

284. Goldie JH. Arguments supporting the concept of non-cross-resistant combinations of chemotherapy. Cancer Invest 1994;12(3):324–328.

285. Goldie JH. Drug resistance and cancer chemotherapy strategy in breast cancer. Breast Cancer Res Treat 1983;3:129–136.

286. Henderson IC, Hayes DF, Come S, et al. New agents and new medical treatments for advanced breast cancer. Semin Oncol 1987;14:34–64.

287. Ahmann D, O'Fallon J, O'Connel MT, et al. Evaluation of a fixed alternating treatment in patients with advanced breast cancer. Cancer Clin Trials 1978; 1:219–226.

288. Kennealey GT, Boston B, Mitchell MS, et al. Combination chemotherapy for advanced breast cancer. Two regimens containing Adriamycin. Cancer 1978;42:27–33.

289. Tormey DC, Falkson G, Simon RM, et al. A randomized comparison of two sequentially administered combination regimens to a single regimen in metastatic breast cancer. Cancer Clin Trials 1979;2:247–256.

290. Nemoto T, Horton J, Simon R, et al. Comparison of four-combination chemotherapy programs in metastatic breast cancer. Comparison of multiple drug therapy with Cytoxan, 5-FU and prednisone versus Cytoxan and Adriamycin, versus Cytoxan, 5-FU and Adriamycin, versus Cytoxan, 5-FU and prednisone alternating with Cytoxan and Adriamycin. Cancer 1982; 49:1988–1993.

291. Tormey D, Gelman R, Falkson G. Prospective evaluation of rotating chemotherapy in advanced breast cancer. An Eastern Oncology Group trial. Am J Clin Oncol 1983;6:1–18.

292. Vogel CL, Smalley RV, Raney M, et al. Randomized trial of cyclophosphamide, doxorubicin, and 5-fluorouracil alone or alternating with a "cycle active" non-cross-resistant combination in women with visceral metastatic breast cancer: a Southeastern Cancer Study Group project. J Clin Oncol 1984;2:643–651.

293. Creagan ET, Green ST, Ahmann DL, et al. A phase III clinical trial comparing the combination cyclophosphamide, Adriamycin, cisplatin with cyclophosphamide, 5-fluorouracil, prednisone in patients with advanced breast cancer. J Clin Oncol 1984;2:1260–1265.

294. Cruciani G, Tienghi A, Molinari AL, et al. Cyclophosphamide, methotrexate, 5-fluorouracil, alternating with Adriamycin and mitomycin C in metastatic breast cancer: a pilot study. Tumori 1987;73:303–307.

295. Aisner J, Cirrincione C, Perloff M, et al. Combination chemotherapy for metastatic or recurrent carcinoma of the breast—a randomized phase III trial comparing CAF versus VATH versus VATH alternating with CMFVP: cancer and Leukemia Group B Study 8281. J Clin Oncol 1995;13:1443–1452.

296. Zambetti M, Giacobone A, Terenziani M, et al. Sequential treatment with Adriamycin-CMF in metastatic breast cancer (abstract). Proc Am Soc Clin Oncol 1995;14:116.

297. Kiang DT, Kennedy BJ, Younger J, et al. for Cancer and Leukemia Group B. Alternating chemotherapy regimens for patients with metastatic breast cancer. A pilot study based on tumor marker kinetics. Cancer 1995;75(3):826–380.

298. Norton L. Salvage chemotherapy of breast cancer. Semin Oncol 1994;21(4 Suppl 7):19–24.

299. Coates A, Gebski V, Stat M, et al. Improving the quality of life during chemotherapy for advanced breast cancer. A comparison of intermittent and continuous treatment strategies. N Engl J Med 1987;317:1490–1495.

300. Kardinal CG, Strnad BN. Confrontation with cancer: historical and existential aspects. In: Gross SC, Garb S, eds. Cancer treatment and research in humanistic perspective. New York: Springer, 1985:163–175.

301. Perloff M, Hart RD, Holland JF. Vinblastine, Adriamycin, thiotepa, and Halotestin (VATH). Therapy for advanced breast cancer refractory to prior chemotherapy. Cancer 1978;42(6):2534–2537.

302. Hart RD, Perloff M, Holland JF. One-day VATH (vinblastine, Adriamycin, thiotepa, and Halotestin) therapy for advanced breast cancer refractory to chemotherapy. Cancer 1981;48:1522–1527.

303. Tannir N, Yap H-Y, Hortobagyi GH, et al. Sequential continuous infusion with doxorubicin and vinblastine: an effective chemotherapy combination for patients with advanced breast cancer previously treated with cyclophosphamide, methotrexate, 5-FU, vincristine, and prednisone. Cancer Treat Rep 1984;68:1039–1041.

304. Ingle JN, Mailliard JA, Schaid DJ, et al. Randomized trial of doxorubicin alone or combined with vincristine and mitomycin C in women with metastatic breast cancer. Am J Clin Oncol 1989;12(6):474–480.

305. Oster MW, Park Y. Vincristine, Adriamycin, and mitomycin (VAM) therapy for previously treated breast cancer. A preliminary report. Cancer 1983; 51:203–205.

306. Luikart SD, Witman GB, Portlock CS. Adriamycin (doxorubicin), vinblastine, and mitomycin C combination chemotherapy in refractory breast carcinoma. Cancer 1984;54:1252–1255.

307. Yap H-Y, Blumenschein GR, Keating MJ, et al. Vinblastine given as a continuous 5-day infusion in the treatment of refractory advanced breast cancer. Cancer Treat Rep 1980;64:279–283.

308. Tannock I, Erlichman C, Perrault D, et al. Failure of 5-day vinblastine infusion in the treatment of patients with advanced refractory breast cancer. Cancer Treat Rep 1982;66(9):1783–1784.

309. Ingle JN, Ahmann DL, Gerstner JG, et al. Evaluation of vinblastine administered by 5-day continuous infusion in women with advanced breast cancer. Cancer Treat Rep 1984;68(5):803–804.

310. Hopkins JO, Jackson DV Jr, White DR, et al. Vincristine by continuous infusion in refractory breast cancer: a phase II study. Am J Clin Oncol (CCT) 1983; 6:529–532.

311. Konits PH, Aisner J, van Echo DA, et al. Mitomycin C and vinblastine chemotherapy for advanced breast cancer. Cancer 1981;48:1295–1298.

312. Garewal HS, Brooks RJ, Jones SE, Miller TP. Treatment of advanced breast cancer with mitomycin C combined with vinblastine or vindesine. J Clin Oncol 1983;1(12):772–775.

313. Rosner D, Nemoto T. Mitomycin C (MMC) and Velban (VLB) as fourth-line chemotherapy in metastatic breast cancer. A pilot trial (abstract). Proc Am Soc Clin Oncol 1987;6:a196.

314. Hryniuk W, Bush H. The importance of dose intensity in chemotherapy of metastatic breast cancer. J Clin Oncol 1984;2(11):1281–1288.

315. Henderson IC, Hayes DF, Gelman R. Dose-response in the treatment of breast cancer: a critical review. J Clin Oncol 1988;6(9):1501–1515.

316. Antman KH. Dose intensive therapy in breast cancer. In: Armitage JO, Antman KH, eds. High dose cancer therapy: pharmacology, hematopoietins, stem cells. Baltimore: Williams & Wilkins, 1992:701–718.

317. Peters WP, Shpall EJ, Jones RB, et al. High dose combination alkylating agents with bone marrow support as initial treatment for metastatic breast cancer. J Clin Oncol 1988;6:1368–1376.

318. Williams SF, Gilewski T, Mick R, et al. High dose consolidation therapy with autologous stem cell rescue in stage IV breast cancer: follow-up report. J Clin Oncol 1992;10:1743–1747.

319. Antman KH, Ayash L, Elias A, et al. A phase II study of high dose cyclophosphamide, thiotepa, and carboplatin with autologous marrow support in women with measurable advanced breast cancer responding to standard dose therapy. J Clin Oncol 1992; 10:102–110.

320. Elias A, Ayash L, Anderson KC, et al. Mobilization of peripheral blood progenitor cells by chemotherapy and granulocyte-macrophage colony stimulating factor for hematologic support after high dose chemotherapy for breast cancer. Blood 1992;79:3036–3044.

321. Ayash LJ, Elias A, Wheeler C, et al. Double dose intensive chemotherapy with autologous marrow and peripheral-blood progenitor-cell support for metastatic breast cancer: a feasibility study. J Clin Oncol 1994;12:37–44.

322. Patrone F, Ballestrero A, Ferrando F, et al. Four-step high dose sequential chemotherapy with double hematopoietic progenitor-cell rescue for metastatic breast cancer. J Clin Oncol 1995;13:840–846.

323. Shpall EJ, Jones RE, Bearman SI, et al. Transplantation of enriched CD34-positive autologous mar-

row into breast cancer patients following high dose chemotherapy: influence of CD34-positive peripheral-blood progenitors and growth factors on engraftment. J Clin Oncol 1994;12:28–36.

323a. Bearman SI, Shpall EJ, Jones RB, et al. High-dose chemotherapy with autologous hematopoietic progenitor cell support for metastatic and high-risk primary breast cancer. Semin Oncol 1996;23(Suppl 2):60–67.

324. Peters WP, Ross N, Vedenburgh J, et al. High dose chemotherapy and autologous bone marrow support as consolidation after standard-dose adjuvant therapy for high-risk primary breast cancer. J Clin Oncol 1993;11:1132–1143.

325. Lippman ME, Allegra JC, Thompson EB, et al. The relation between estrogen receptors and response rate to cytotoxic chemotherapy in metastatic breast cancer. N Engl J Med 1978;298:1223–1228.

326. Kiang DT, Frenning DH, Goldman AI, et al. Estrogen receptors and responses to chemotherapy and hormonal therapy in advanced breast cancer. N Engl J Med 1978;299:1330–1334.

327. Kardinal CG, Perry MC, Korzun AH, Wood W. Lack of differential response of estrogen receptor positive (ER+) vs. ER negative (ER−) breast cancer to Cytoxan + Adriamycin + 5-fluorouracil (CAF) chemotherapy (abstract). Proc Am Soc Clin Oncol 1986; 5:74.

328. Rosner D, Lane WW, Nemoto T. Differential response to chemotherapy in metastatic breast cancer in relation to estrogen receptor level. Results of a prospective randomized study. Cancer 1989;64:6–15.

329. Osborne CK, Kitten L, Arteaga CL. Antagonism of chemotherapy-induced cytotoxicity for human breast cancer cells by antiestrogens. J Clin Oncol 1989; 7(6):710–717.

330. Kardinal CG, Perry MC, Weinberg V, et al. Chemoendocrine therapy vs chemotherapy alone for advanced breast cancer in postmenopausal women: preliminary report of a randomized study. Breast Cancer Res Treat 1983;3:356–371.

331. Perry MC, Kardinal CG, Korzun AH, et al. Chemohormonal therapy in advanced carcinoma of the breast: Cancer and Leukemia Group B protocol 8081. J Clin Oncol 1987;5(10):1534–1545.

332. Krook JE, Ingle JN, Green SJ, et al. Randomized clinical trial of cyclophosphamide, 5-FU, and prednisone with or without tamoxifen in postmenopausal women with advanced breast cancer. Cancer Treat Rep 1985;69:355–361.

333. Allegra JC. Methotrexate and 5-fluorouracil following tamoxifen and Premarin in advanced breast cancer. Semin Oncol 1983;10(Suppl 2):23–28.

334. Eisenhauer EA, Bowman DM, Pritchard KI, et al. Tamoxifen and conjugated estrogens (Premarin) followed by sequenced methotrexate and 5-FU in refractory advanced breast cancer. Cancer Treat Rep 1984; 68:1421–1422.

335. Conte PF, Pronzato P, Rubagotti A, et al. Conventional versus cytokinetic polychemotherapy with estrogenic recruitment in metastatic breast cancer: results of a randomized cooperative trial. J Clin Oncol 1987;5(3):339–347.

336. Paridaens R, Heuson JC, Julien JP, et al. For the European Organization for Research and Treatment of Cancer Breast Cancer Cooperative Group. As-

sessment of estrogenic recruitment before chemotherapy in advanced breast cancer: a double-blind randomized study. J Clin Oncol 1993;11(9):1723–1728.

337. Ingle JN, Foley JF, Mailliard JA, et al. Randomized trial of cyclophosphamide, methotrexate, and 5-fluorouracil with or without estrogenic recruitment in women with metastatic breast cancer. Cancer 1994; 73(9):2337–2343.

338. Kuhajda FP, Piantadosi S, Pasternack GR. Haptoglobin-related protein (Hpr) epitopes in breast cancer as a predictor of recurrence of the disease. N Engl J Med 1989;321(10):636–640.

339. Bevilacqua G, Sobel ME, Liotta LA, Steeg PS. Association of low nm23 RNA levels in human primary infiltrating ductal breast carcinomas with lymph node involvement and other histopathological indicators of high metastatic potential. Cancer Res 1989; 49:5185–5190.

340. Gasparini G, Pozza F, Harris AL. Evaluating the potential usefulness of new prognostic and predictive indicators in node-negative breast cancer patients [published erratum appears in J Natl Cancer Inst 1993; 85(19):1605]. J Natl Cancer Inst 1993;85(15):1206–1219.

341. Fisher B, Redmond C, Fisher ER, Wolmark N. Systemic adjuvant therapy in treatment of primary operable breast cancer: National Surgical Adjuvant Breast and Bowel Project experience. NCI Monogr 1986;1:35–43.

342. Nissen-Meyer R, Høst H, Kjellgren K, et al. Treatment of node-negative breast cancer patients with short course of chemotherapy immediately after surgery. NCI Monogr 1986;1:125–128.

343. The Ludwig Breast Cancer Study Group. Combination adjuvant chemotherapy for node-positive breast cancer. Inadequacy of a single perioperative cycle. N Engl J Med 1988;319:677–683.

344. The Ludwig Breast Cancer Study Group. Prolonged disease-free survival after one course of perioperative adjuvant chemotherapy for node-negative breast cancer. N Engl J Med 1989;320:491–496.

345. Fisher B, Carbone P, Economou SG, et al. L-Phenylalanine mustard (L-PAM) in the management of primary breast cancer. A report of early findings. N Engl J Med 1975;292(3):117–122.

346. Fisher B, Redmond C, Wickerham DL, et al. Doxorubicin-containing regimens for the treatment of stage II breast cancer: the National Surgical Adjuvant Breast and Bowel Project experience. J Clin Oncol 1989; 7:572–582.

347. Fisher B, Rockette H, Robidoux A, et al. Effect of preoperative therapy for breast cancer (BC) on local-regional disease: first report of NSABP B-18 (abstract). Proc Am Soc Clin Oncol 1994;13:64.

348. Fisher B, Mamounas EP. Preoperative chemotherapy: a model for studying the biology and therapy of primary breast cancer (editorial). J Clin Oncol 1995;13(3):537–540.

349. Powles TJ, Hickish TF, Makris A, et al. Randomized trial of chemoendocrine therapy started before or after surgery for treatment of primary breast cancer. J Clin Oncol 1995;13(3):547–552.

350. Dimitrov N, Anderson S, Fisher B, et al. Dose intensification and increased total dose of adjuvant chemotherapy for breast cancer (BC): findings from NSABP B-22 (abstract). Proc Am Soc Clin Oncol 1994; 13:64.

351. DeCillis A, Anderson S, Wickerham DL, et al. and contributing investigators. Acute myeloid leukemia (AML) in NSABP B-25 (abstract). Proc Am Soc Clin Oncol 1995;14:98.

352. Bonadonna G, Brusamolino E, Valagussa P, et al. Combination chemotherapy as an adjuvant treatment in operable breast cancer. N Engl J Med 1976; 294:405–410.

353. Bonadonna G. Conceptual and practical advances in the management of breast cancer. J Clin Oncol 1989;7:1380–1397.

354. Bonadonna G, Valagussa P, Moliterni A, et al. Adjuvant cyclophosphamide, methotrexate, and fluorouracil in node-positive breast cancer: the results of 20 years of follow-up. N Engl J Med 1995;332(14):901–906.

355. Bianco AR, Del Mastro L, Gallo C, et al. Prognostic role of amenorrhea induced by adjuvant chemotherapy in premenopausal patients with early breast cancer. Br J Cancer 1991;63:799–803.

356. Brincker H, Rose C, Rank F, et al. Evidence of a castration-mediated effect of adjuvant cytotoxic chemotherapy in premenopausal breast cancer. J Clin Oncol 1987;5:1771–1778.

357. Dnistrian AM, Schwartz MK, Fracchia AA, et al. Endocrine consequences of CMF adjuvant therapy in premenopausal and postmenopausal breast cancer patients. Cancer 1983;51:803–807.

358. Fisher B, Sherman B, Rockette H, et al. L-Phenylalanine mustard (L-PAM) in the management of premenopausal patients with primary breast cancer. Lack of association of disease-free survival with depression of ovarian function. Cancer 1979;44:847–857.

359. Cooper RG, Holland JF, Glidewell O. Adjuvant chemotherapy of breast cancer. Cancer 1979; 44:793–798.

360. Cooper RG. Adjuvant chemotherapy for breast cancer: 20 years experience using CVFMP chemotherapy. Semin Oncol 1988;15(Suppl 3):29–34.

361. Wood WC. Cancer and Leukemia Group B adjuvant chemotherapy trials in postmastectomy breast cancer patients. Breast Cancer Res Treat 1983;3(Suppl 1):39–43.

362. Tormey DC, Weinberg VE, Holland JF, et al. A randomized trial of five and three drug chemotherapy and chemoimmunotherapy in women with operable node positive breast cancer. J Clin Oncol 1983; 1(2):138–145.

363. Korzun A, Norton L, Perloff M, et al. Clinical equivalence despite dosage differences of two schedules of cyclophosphamide, methotrexate, 5-fluorouracil, vincristine and prednisone (CMFVP) for adjuvant therapy of node-positive stage II breast cancer (abstract). Proc Am Soc Clin Oncol 1988;7:12.

364. Perloff M, Norton L, Korzun, et al. Advantage of an Adriamycin (A) combination plus Halotestin (H) after initial cyclophosphamide, methotrexate, 5-fluorouracil, vincristine and prednisone (CMFVP) for adjuvant therapy of node-positive stage II breast cancer (abstract). Proc Am Soc Clin Oncol 1986;5:70.

365. Wood WC, Budman DR, Korzun AH, et al. Dose and dose intensity of adjuvant chemotherapy for stage II, node-positive breast carcinoma. N Engl J Med 1994;330(18):1253–1259.

366. Henderson IC. Adjuvant systemic therapy for early breast cancer. Cancer 1994;74(1 suppl):401–409.

367. Love RR. Tamoxifen therapy in primary breast cancer. Biology, efficacy, and side effects. J Clin Oncol 1989;7:803–815.

368. Fisher B, Costantino J, Redmond C, et al. A randomized clinical trial evaluating tamoxifen in the treatment of patients with node-negative breast cancer who have estrogen-receptor-positive tumors. N Engl J Med 1989;320:479–484.

369. Baum M, Brinkley DM, Dossett JA, et al. Controlled trial of tamoxifen as adjuvant agent in management of early breast cancer: interim analysis at four years by Nolvadex Adjuvant Trial Organisation. Lancet 1983;1:257–261.

370. Baum M, Brinkley DM, Dossett JA, et al. Controlled trial of tamoxifen as single adjuvant agent in management of early breast cancer: analysis at six years by Nolvadex Adjuvant Trial Organisation. Lancet 1985;1:836–840.

371. Baum M, Brinkley DM, Dossett JA, et al. Controlled trial of tamoxifen as a single adjuvant agent in the management of early breast cancer: analysis at eight years by 'Nolvadex' Adjuvant Trial Organisation. Br J Cancer 1988;57:608–611.

372. Ribeiro G, Palmer MK. Adjuvant tamoxifen for operable carcinoma of the breast: report of clinical trial by the Christie Hospital and Holt Radium Institute. Br Med J 1983;286:827–830.

373. Ribeiro G, Swindell R. The Christie Hospital tamoxifen (Nolvadex) adjuvant trial for operable breast carcinoma—7-yr results. Eur J Cancer Clin Oncol 1985;21:897–900.

374. Ribeiro G, Swindell R. The Christie Hospital adjuvant tamoxifen trial–status at 10 years. Br J Cancer 1988;57:601–603.

375. Rutqvist LE, Cedermark B, Fornander T, et al. The relationship between hormone receptor content and the effect of adjuvant tamoxifen in operable breast cancer. J Clin Oncol 1989;7:1474–1484.

376. Fornander T, Rutqvist LE, Cedermark B, et al. Adjuvant tamoxifen in early-stage breast cancer: effects on intercurrent morbidity and mortality. J Clin Oncol 1991;9(10):1740–1748.

377. CRC Adjuvant Breast Trial Working Party (Abram WP, Baum M, Berstock DA, et al.). Cyclophosphamide and tamoxifen as adjuvant therapies in the management of breast cancer. Br J Cancer 1988; 57:604–607.

378. The Breast Cancer Trials Committee, Scottish Cancer Trials Office (MRC) (Bartlett K, Eremin O, Hutcheon A, et al.). Adjuvant tamoxifen in the management of operable breast cancer: the Scottish trial. Report from the Breast Cancer Trials Committee, Scottish Cancer Trials Office (MRC), Edinburgh. Lancet 1987;2:171–175.

379. Stewart HJ. The Scottish trial of adjuvant tamoxifen in node-negative breast cancer. Scottish Cancer Trials Breast Group. NCI Monogr 1992;11:117–120.

380. Fisher B, Redmond C, Wickerham DL, et al. Systemic therapy in patients with node-negative breast cancer: a commentary based on two National Surgical Adjuvant Breast and Bowel Project (NSABP) clinical trials. Ann Intern Med 1989;111:703–712.

381. Fisher B, Wickerham DL, Redmond C. Recent developments in the use of systemic adjuvant therapy for the treatment of breast cancer. Semin Oncol 1992; 19:263–277.

382. Fisher B, Costantino J, Redmond C, Wickerham DL, and other NSABP Investigators. Recent in-

formation from current NSABP trials of adjuvant therapy for breast cancer. In: Salmon SE, ed. Adjuvant therapy of cancer VII. Philadelphia: JP Lippincott, 1993:148–161.

383. Rose C, Thorpe SM, Andersen KW, et al. Beneficial effect of adjuvant tamoxifen therapy in primary breast cancer patients with high estrogen receptor values. Lancet 1985;1:16–19.

384. Pritchard KI. Current status of adjuvant endocrine therapy for resectable breast cancer. Semin Oncol 1987;14:23–33.

385. Rutqvist LE, Wallgren A, and Nilsson B. Is breast cancer a curable disease? A study of 14,731 women with breast cancer from the Cancer Registry of Norway. Cancer 1984;53:1793–1800.

385a. Fisher B, Dignam J, Wieand S, et al. Duration of tamoxifen (TAM) therapy for primary breast cancer: 5 versus 10 years (NSABP B-14) (abstract). Proc Am Soc Clin Oncol 1996;15:113.

386. Fisher B, Redmond C, Brown A, at al. Treatment of primary breast cancer with chemotherapy and tamoxifen. N Engl J Med 1981;305:1–6.

387. Fisher B, Redmond C, Brown A, et al. Influence of tumor estrogen and progesterone receptor levels on the response to tamoxifen and chemotherapy in primary breast cancer. J Clin Oncol 1983;1:227–241.

388. Fisher B, Redmond C, Brown A, et al. Adjuvant chemotherapy with and without tamoxifen in the treatment of primary breast cancer: 5-year results from the National Surgical Adjuvant Breast and Bowel Project trial. J Clin Oncol 1986;4:459–471.

389. Dombernowsky P, Zedeler K, Hansen M, et al. Randomized trial of adjuvant CMP + radiotherapy (RT) vs CMF alone vs CMF + tamoxifen (TAM) in pre- and menopausal stage II breast cancer (abstract). Proc Am Soc Clin Oncol 1992;11:54.

390. Ingle JN, Everson LK, Wieand HS, et al. Randomized trial of observation versus adjuvant therapy with cyclophosphamide, fluorouracil, prednisone with or without tamoxifen following mastectomy in postmenopausal women with node-positive breast cancer. J Clin Oncol 1988;6:1388–1396.

391. Ingle JN, Everson LK, Wieand HS, et al. Randomized trial to evaluate the addition of tamoxifen to cyclophosphamide, 5-fluorouracil, prednisone adjuvant therapy in premenopausal women with node-positive breast cancer. Cancer 1989;63:1257–1264.

392. Taylor SG IV, Knuiman MW, Sleeper LA, et al. Six-year results of the Eastern Cooperative Oncology Group trial of observation versus CMFP versus CMFPT in postmenopausal patients with node-positive breast cancer. J Clin Oncol 1989;7:879–889.

393. Tormey DC, Gray R, Gilchrist K, et al. Adjuvant chemohormonal therapy with cyclophosphamide, methotrexate, 5-fluorouracil, and prednisone (CMFP) or CMFP plus tamoxifen compared with CMF for premenopausal breast cancer patients: an Eastern Cooperative Oncology Group trial. Cancer 1990; 65:200–206.

394. Falkson HC, Gray R, Wolberg WH, et al. Adjuvant trial of 12 cycles of CMFPT followed by observation or continuous tamoxifen versus four cycles of CMFPT in postmenopausal women with breast cancer: an Eastern Cooperative Oncology Group phase II study. J Clin Oncol 1990;8:599–607.

395. Tormey DC, Gray R, Abeloff MD, et al. Adjuvant therapy with a doxorubicin regimen and long-term tamoxifen in premenopausal breast cancer patients: an Eastern Cooperative Oncology Group trial. J Clin Oncol 1992;10(12):1848–1856.

396. Fisher B, Redmond C, Legault-Poisson S, et al. Postoperative chemotherapy and tamoxifen compared with tamoxifen alone in the treatment of positive-node breast cancer patients aged 50 years and older with tumors responsive to tamoxifen: results from the National Surgical Adjuvant Breast and Bowel Project B-16. J Clin Oncol 1990;8:1005–1018.

397. Pearson OH, Hubay CA, Gordon NH, et al. Endocrine versus endocrine plus five-drug chemotherapy in postmenopausal women with stage II estrogen receptor-positive breast cancer. Cancer 1989;64:1819–1823.

398. Boccardo F, Amoroso D, Rubagotti A, et al. Chemotherapy versus tamoxifen versus chemotherapy plus tamoxifen in node positive, estrogen receptor positive breast cancer patients: an update at 8 years of the first GROCTA (Italian Cooperative Group for Adjuvant Chemohormonal Therapy of Breast Cancer) Trial. In: Salmon SE, ed. Adjuvant therapy of cancer VII. Philadelphia: JP Lippincott, 1993:181–192.

399. Pritchard KI, Zee B, Paul N, et al. CMF added to tamoxifen as adjuvant therapy in postmenopausal women with node-positve (+VE) estrogen (ER) and/or progesterone receptor (Pg R)+VE breast cancer negative results from a randomized clinical trial (abstract). Proc Am Soc Clin Oncol 1994;14:65.

400. Rivkin SE, Green S, Metch B, et al. Adjuvant CMFVP versus tamoxifen versus concurrent CMFVP and tamoxifen for postmenopausal, node-positive, and estrogen receptor-positive breast cancer patients: a Southwest Oncology Group study. J Clin Oncol 1994; 12(10):2078–2085.

401. Cummings FJ, Gray R, Tormey DC, et al. Adjuvant tamoxifen versus placebo in elderly women with node-positive breast cancer: long-term follow-up and causes of death. J Clin Oncol 1993;11(1):29–35.

402. Paik S, Hazan R, Fisher ER, et al. Pathologic findings from the National Surgical Adjuvant Breast and Bowel Project: prognostic significance of erbB-2 protein overexpression in primary breast cancer. J Clin Oncol 1990;8:103–112.

403. Tandon AK, Clark GM, Chamness GC, et al. Cathepsin D and prognosis in breast cancer. N Engl J Med 1990;322:297–302.

404. Sahin AA, Ro J, Ro JY, et al. Ki-67 immunostaining in node-negative stage I/II breast carcinoma: significant correlation with prognosis. Cancer 68:549–557.

405. Cote RJ, Rosen PP, Lesser ML, et al. Prediction of early relapse in patients with operable breast cancer by detection of occult bone marrow micrometastases. J Clin Oncol 1991;9:1749–1756.

406. Joensuu H, Toikleanen S, Klemi PJ. DNA index and S-phase fraction and their combination as prognostic factors in operable ductal breast carcinoma. Cancer 1990;66:331–340.

407. Keyhani-Rofagha S, O'Toole RV, Farrar WB, et al. Is DNA ploidy an independent prognostic indicator in infiltrative node-negative breast adenocarcinoma? Cancer 1990;65:1577–1582.

408. McGuire WL, Tandon AK, Allred DC, et al. How to use prognostic factors in axillary node-negative breast cancer patients. J Natl Cancer Inst 1990; 82:1006–1015.

409. McGuire WL, Clark GM. Prognostic factors and treatment decisions in axillary-node-negative breast cancer. N Engl J Med 1992;326:1756–1761.

410. Rosen PR, Groshen S, Saigo PE, et al. A long-term follow-up study of survival in stage I ($T_1N_0M_0$) and stage II ($T_1N_1M_0$) breast carcinoma. J Clin Oncol 1989;7:355–366.

411. Rosen PP, Groshen S, Saigo PE, et al. Pathological prognostic factors in stage I ($T_1N_0M_0$) and stage II ($T_1N_1M_0$) breast carcinoma: a study of 644 patients with median follow-up of 18 years. J Clin Oncol 1989; 7:1239–1251.

412. Rosen PP, Groshen S, Kinne DW. Prognosis in $T_2N_0M_0$ stage I breast carcinoma: a 20-year follow-up study. J Clin Oncol 9:1650–1661.

413. Rosen PP, Groshen S, Kinne DW, Norton L. Factors influencing prognosis in node-negative breast carcinoma: analysis of 767 $T_1N_0M_0/T_2N_0M_0$ patients with long-term follow-up. J Clin Oncol 1993; 11(11):2090–2100.

414. Tabar L, Fagerberg G, Day NE, et al. Breast cancer treatment and natural history: new insights from results of screening. Lancet 1992;339:412–414.

415. Quiet CA, Ferguson DJ, Weichselbaum RR, Hellman S. Natural history of node-negative breast cancer: a study of 826 patients with long-term follow-up. J Clin Oncol 1995;13(5):1144–1151.

416. Fisher B, Redmond C, Dimitrov NV, et al. A randomized clinical trial evaluating sequential methotrexate and fluorouracil in the treatment of patients with node-negative breast cancer who have estrogen-receptor-negative tumors. N Engl J Med 1989; 320(8):473–478.

417. Wolmark N. 1989: the year of adjuvant therapy in node-negative breast cancer. Princ Pract Oncol 1989;3(12):1–10.

418. Mansour EG, Gray R, Shatila AH, et al. Efficacy of adjuvant chemotherapy in high-risk node-negative breast cancer. An intergroup study. N Engl J Med 1989;320(8):485–490.

419. Stefanik D, Goldberg R, Byrne P, et al. Local-regional failure in patients treated with adjuvant chemotherapy for breast cancer. J Clin Oncol 1985; 3(5):660–665.

420. Fowble B, Gray R, Gilchrist K, et al. Identification of a subgroup of patients with breast cancer and histologically positive axillary nodes receiving adjuvant chemotherapy who may benefit from postoperative radiotherapy. J Clin Oncol 1988;6(7):1107–1117.

421. Buzdar AU, McNeese MD, Hortobagyi GN, et al. Is chemotherapy effective in reducing the local failure rate in patients with operable breast cancer? Cancer 1990;65(3):394–399.

422. Buchholz TA, Austin-Seymour MM, Moe RE, et al. Effect of delay in radiation in the combined modality treatment of breast cancer. Int J Radiat Oncol Biol Phys 1993;26(1):23–35.

423. Recht A, Come SE, Gelman RS, et al. Integration of conservative surgery, radiotherapy, and chemotherapy for the treatment of early-stage, node-positive breast cancer: sequencing, timing, and outcome. J Clin Oncol 1991;9(9):1662–1667.

424. Buzdar AU, Kau SW, Smith TL, et al. The order of administration of chemotherapy and radiation and its effect on the local control of operable breast cancer. Cancer 1993;71(11):3680–3684.

425. Pisansky TM, Ingle JN, Schaid DJ, et al. Patterns of tumor relapse following mastectomy and adjuvant systemic therapy in patients with axillary lymph node-positive breast cancer. Impact of clinical, histopathologic, and flow cytometric factors. Cancer 1993;72(4):1247–1260.

426. Kennedy MJ, Abeloff MD. Management of locally recurrent breast cancer. Cancer 1993;71(7):2395–2409.

427. Overgaard M, Christensen JJ, Johansen H, et al. Evaluation of radiotherapy in high-risk breast cancer patients: report from the Danish Breast Cancer Cooperative Group (DBCG 82) trial. Int J Radiat Oncol Biol Phys 1990;19(5):1121–1124.

428. Ragaz J, Jackson SM, Plenderleith IH, et al. Can adjuvant radiotherapy (XRT) improve the overall survival (OS) of breast cancer (BR CA) patients in the presence of adjuvant chemotherapy (CT)? 10-yr analysis of the British Columbia randomized trial (abstract). Proc Am Soc Clin Oncol 1993;12:60.

429. Pierce LJ, Lichter AS. Postmastectomy radiotherapy: more than locoregional control (editorial). J Clin Oncol 1994;12(3):444–446.

430. Jacquillat C, Weil M, Baillet F, et al. Results of neoadjuvant chemotherapy and radiation therapy in the breast-conserving treatment of 250 patients with all stages of infiltrative breast cancer. Cancer 1990; 66(1):119–129.

431. Singletary SE, McNeese MD, Hortobagyi GN. Feasibility of breast-conservation surgery after induction chemotherapy for locally advanced breast carcinoma. Cancer 1992;69:2849–2852.

432. Calais G, Berger C, Descamps P, et al. Conservative treatment feasibility with induction chemotherapy, surgery, and radiotherapy for patients with breast carcinoma larger than 3 cm. Cancer 1994;74(4):1283–1288.

433. Schwartz GF, Birchansky CA, Komarnicky LT, et al. Induction chemotherapy followed by breast conservation for locally advanced carcinoma of the breast. Cancer 1994;73(2):362–369.

434. Perloff M, Lesnick GJ, Korzun A, et al. Combination chemotherapy with mastectomy or radiotherapy for stage III breast carcinoma: a Cancer and Leukemia Group B study. J Clin Oncol 1988;6(2):261–269.

435. Lippman ME, Sorace RA, Bagley CS, et al. Treatment of locally advanced breast cancer using primary induction chemotherapy with hormonal synchronization followed by radiation therapy with or without debulking surgery. NCI Monogr 1986;1:153–159.

436. Swain SM, Sorace RA, Bagley CS, et al. Neoadjuvant chemotherapy in the combined modality approach of locally advanced nonmetastatic breast cancer. Cancer Res 1987;47(14):3889–3894.

437. Olson JE, Neuberg D, Pandya K, et al. The management of resectable stage III breast cancer: the Eastern Cooperative Oncology Group trial (abstract). Proc Am Soc Clin Oncol 1989;8:A85.

438. Loprinzi CL, Hass AC, Schray MF, et al. Response of local-regionally advanced breast cancer (LRABC) to initial combination chemotherapy. A pilot study of the North Central Cancer Treatment Group and Mayo Clinic (abstract). Proc Am Soc Clin Oncol 1989;8:42.

439. Hortobagyi GN, Ames FC, Buzdar AU, et al.

Management of stage III primary breast cancer with primary chemotherapy, surgery, and radiation therapy. Cancer 1988;62:2507–2516.

440. Hortobagyi GN. Comprehensive management of locally advanced breast cancer. Cancer 1990;66(6 Suppl):1387–1391.

441. Bonadonna G, Valagussa P, Brambilla C, et al. Adjuvant and neoadjuvant treatment of breast cancer with chemotherapy and/or endocrine therapy. Semin Oncol 1991;18(6):515–524.

442. Smith IE, Walsh G, Jones A, et al. High complete remission rates with primary neoadjuvant infusional chemotherapy for large early breast cancer. J Clin Oncol 1995;13(2):424–429.

443. Dershaw DD, Drossman S, Liberman L, Abramson A. Assessment of response to therapy of primary breast cancer by mammography and physical examination. Cancer 1995;75(8):2093–2098.

444. Frye D, Buzdar A, Hortobagyi G. Prognostic significance of axillary nodal involvement after preoperative chemotherapy in stage III breast cancer (abstract). Proc Am Soc Clin Oncol 1995;14:95.

445. Buzdar A, Hortobagyi G, Wasaff B, et al. Combined modality approach (CMA) for inflammatory carcinoma of breast (IBC): 20 year (yrs) experience of M. D. Anderson Cancer Center (abstract). Proc Am Soc Clin Oncol 1995;14:92.

446. Sherry MM, Johnson DH, Page DL, et al. Inflammatory carcinoma of the breast. Clinical review and summary of the Vanderbilt experience with multimodality therapy. Am J Med 1985;79:355–364.

447. Chevallier B, Asselain B, Kunlin A, et al. Inflammatory breast cancer. Determination of prognostic factors by univariate and multivariate analysis. Cancer 1987;60:897–902.

448. Jaiyesimi IA, Buzdar AU, Hortobagyi G. Inflammatory breast cancer: a review. J Clin Oncol 1992; 10(6):1014–1024.

449. Ajayi DOS, Osegbe DN, Ademiluyi SA. Carcinoma of the male breast in West Africans and a review of the literature. Cancer 1982;50:1664–1667.

450. Spence RAJ, Mackenzie G, Anderson JR, et al. Long-term survival following cancer of the male breast in North Ireland: a report of 81 cases. Cancer 1985; 55:648–652.

451. Siddiqui T, Weiner R, Morb J, Marsh RD. Cancer of the male breast with prolonged survival. Cancer 1988;62:1632–1636.

452. Griffith H, Muggia FM. Male breast cancer: update on systemic therapy. Rev Endocr Cancer 1989; 31:5–11.

453. Donegan WL. Cancer of the male breast. In: Donegan WL, Spratt JS, eds. Cancer of the breast. 4th ed. Philadelphia: WB Saunders, 1995:765–777.

454. Salvadori B, Saccozzi R, Manzari A, et al.

Prognosis of breast cancer in males: an analysis of 170 cases. Eur J Cancer 1994;30:930–935.

455. Guinee VF, Olsson H, Moller T, et al. The prognosis of breast cancer in males. A report of 335 cases. Cancer 1993;71:154–161.

456. Jaiyesimi IA, Buzdar AU, Sahin AA, Ross MA. Carcinoma of the male breast. Ann Intern Med 1992; 117:771–777.

457. Kantarjian H, Yap H-Y, Hortobagyi G, et al. Hormonal therapy for metastatic male breast cancer. Arch Intern Med 1983;143:237–240.

458. Bezwoda WR, Hesdorffer C, Dansey R, et al. Breast cancer in men: clinical features, hormone receptor status, and response to therapy. Cancer 1987; 60:1337–1370.

459. Patel JK, Nemoto T, Dao TL. Metastatic breast cancer in males: assessment of endocrine therapy. Cancer 1984;53:1344–1346.

460. Patterson JS, Battersby LA, Bach BK. Use of tamoxifen in advanced male breast cancer. Cancer Treat Rep 1980;64:801–804.

461. Moredo Anelli TF, Anelli A, Tran KN, et al. Tamoxifen administration is associated with a high rate of treatment-limiting symptoms in male breast cancer patients. Cancer 1994;74:74–77.

462. Tirelli U, Tumolo S, Talamini R, et al. Tamoxifen before and after orchiectomy in advanced male breast cancer (letter). Cancer Treat Rep 1982;66:1882–1883.

463. Pannuti F, Martoni A, Busutti L, et al. High-dose medroxyprogesterone acetate in advanced male breast cancer. Cancer Treat Rep 1982;66:1763–1765.

464. Doberauer C, Niederli N, Schmidt CG. Advanced male breast cancer treatment with the LH-RH analogue buserelin alone or in combination with the antiandrogen flutamide. Cancer 1988;62:474–478.

465. Lopez M, Natali M, Di Lauro L, et al. Combined treatment with buserelin and cyproterone acetate in metastatic male breast cancer. Cancer 1993; 72:502–505.

466. Lopez M, Di Laura L, Papaldo P, Lazzaro B. Chemotherapy in metastatic male breast cancer. Oncology 1985;42:205–209.

467. Bagley CS, Wesley MN, Young RC, Lippman ME. Adjuvant chemotherapy in males with cancer of the breast. Am J Clin Oncol 1987;10:55–60.

468. Patel HZ, Buzdar AU, Hortobagyi GN. Role of adjuvant chemotherapy in male breast cancer. Cancer 1989;64:1583–1585.

469. Ribeiro G. Male breast carcinoma—a review of 301 cases from the Christie Hospital and Holt Radium Institute, Manchester. Br J Cancer 1985;51:115–119.

470. Ribeiro G, Swindell R. Adjuvant tamoxifen for male breast cancer (MBC). Br J Cancer 1992;65:252–254.

55

Chemotherapy of Gastrointestinal Cancer

John Wilkes

Collectively, gastrointestinal cancers represent a large proportion of all malignancies diagnosed and treated in the United States each year. They are superseded by only genitourinary and respiratory tumors in incidence and mortality, respectively, with an estimated 223,000 new cases and 124,330 deaths in 1995 (1). While the incidence of gastric cancer in general and colorectal cancer in women appears to be on the decline, the age-adjusted death rates for other gastrointestinal sites remain constant or, as in the case of pancreatic cancer, are increasing. Surgical resection, when feasible, remains the only effective curative therapy, though combined modality approaches involving both induction and adjuvant strategies are under investigation. Radiotherapy and chemotherapy continue to play major roles in the palliation of advanced disease. This chapter reviews the current use of chemotherapy for advanced gastrointestinal malignancies as well as induction and adjuvant approaches for potentially curable disease.

ESOPHAGEAL CANCER

Systemic Therapy

There will be an estimated 12,100 new cases of esophageal cancer diagnosed in this country in 1995, with an anticipated 10,900 deaths (1). As the incidence:mortality ratio would suggest, the disease continues to have a dismal prognosis, with 5-year survival rates of 8% and a median survival of only 9 months (2). These statistics reflect the fact that most patients with esophageal cancer present with advanced disease, poor nutritional and performance status, and significant coexisting illnesses. Thus, the goals of therapy are often limited to palliation.

The evaluation of chemotherapeutic agents has been hampered by a number of factors, including variations in the extent of disease, prior and subsequent therapy, histologic subtypes, anatomic location, and varying response criteria. Nonetheless, at least 15 agents have been adequately evaluated against carcinoma of the esophagus, with demonstrated response rates of 15 to 38% (3). Active drugs include 5-fluorouracil (5-FU), cisplatin, mitomycin C, bleomycin, methotrexate, and vindesine (4–16). Used alone, these agents produce few complete responses and appear to have little impact on survival.

Combination regimens have been extensively studied over the past two decades, with cisplatin being a common component of many of these regimens (17–21). However, only the regimens of bleomycin + vindesine + cisplatin and 5-FU + cisplatin have been evaluated in a sufficient number of patients (18, 21). The former regimen has largely been abandoned because of the pulmonary toxicity associated with bleomycin, especially in this patient population. Despite the absence of published prospective trials comparing single agents with combinations or individual combination regimens, the combination of 5-FU + cisplatin has emerged as the "standard" chemotherapy for patients with squamous cell carcinoma of the esophagus. There currently exists no "standard" chemotherapy regimen for advanced adenocarcinoma of the esophagus, and efforts continue to identify effective and less toxic new agents and combined modality approaches.

Multimodality Therapy

Even in the minority of patients who present with localized carcinoma of the esophagus, the results of curative therapy remain disappointing, with median survivals of less than 12 months for patients treated either surgically or with radiotherapy alone (22, 23). As a result, the focus of many current clinical trials involves the use of chemotherapy in conjunction with radiotherapy and surgical resection.

Preoperative chemotherapy offers several advantages over adjuvant therapy, including the potential for improved efficacy and patient tolerability. Theoretically, this approach may also minimize the development of spontaneous drug resistance. Further, preoperative response in the primary tumor may facilitate resection and prolong survival. Finally, preoperative chemotherapy provides clinical investigators the best opportunity to assess the true biologic responses of the induction regimen.

At least three combined modality alternatives have been explored, including induction chemotherapy followed by surgery, preoperative chemoradiotherapy, and chemoradiotherapy without surgery.

Neoadjuvant chemotherapy has largely been studied in nonrandomized phase II trials (20, 21, 24–27). More recently, randomized comparison of cisplatin, vindesine, and bleomycin chemotherapy with preoperative radiotherapy (55 Gy) found similar response and resection rates, with 20% of patients alive and free of disease, and a median survival of 34 months (28). Other phase III trials have been unable to demonstrate an advantage to induction chemotherapy over surgery alone (29, 30).

Recent phase II and III trials have demonstrated a benefit to the addition of radiation therapy to induction chemotherapy. In a study by Forastiere et al., patients with locoregional esophageal cancer were treated with cisplatin, vinblastine, fluorouracil chemotherapy and concurrent radiation therapy over 21 days, followed by a planned transhiatal esophagectomy on day 42. Forty-one of 43 (95%) patients completed the preoperative regimen and went to surgery, and 36 (84%) were completely resected. Ten patients had no tumor in the resected specimen, for a 24% pathologic complete response rate. With a median 78.7-month follow-up, the median survival duration for all patients was 29 months, with 34% alive at 5 years. These results were a significant improvement

over their previous 14-month median survival duration (31).

An Intergroup phase III trial has evaluated chemotherapy with 5-FU and cisplatin and concurrent radiation therapy as primary treatment for patients with esophageal cancer. This prospective, randomized trial compared high-dose (6400 cGy) radiation alone with moderate-dose (5000 cGy) radiation plus four cycles of 5-FU and cisplatin chemotherapy initiated concurrently with radiation. One hundred twenty-one patients with either squamous cell carcinoma (n = 106) or adenocarcinoma (n = 15) of the thoracic esophagus entered this trial, which was closed prematurely because of a significant survival advantage seen in patients treated with the combined modalities. Updated results with a median follow-up of 40 months show that only 5% of patients treated with radiation therapy alone were alive, versus 33% of patients treated with combined-modality therapy, (32).

In conclusion, there remains no standard approach to patients with locally advanced and metastatic carcinoma of the esophagus. Efforts to identify new active chemotherapeutic and biologic agents are ongoing. Similarly, active phase II and III multimodality trials are attempting to answer the many schedule and dosing issues that remain in esophageal cancer.

GASTRIC CANCER

There will be approximately 24,000 cases of gastric cancer diagnosed in the United States in 1995. Although its incidence continues to decline, this malignancy remains the eighth leading cause of cancer death (1). The high mortality rates reflect the advanced stage of gastric cancer at presentation and the limitations of all current medical and surgical interventions.

Systemic Therapy

There are few adequately studied chemotherapeutic agents that have demonstrated any significant single-agent activity in advanced gastric cancer. 5-FU and mitomycin C have been most extensively studied and have reproducibly achieved responses of 15 to 35% (33, 34). Other agents that show some activity against locally advanced and metastatic gastric cancer include doxorubicin (Adriamycin), cisplatin, BCNU, etoposide, and epirubicin, which produce response rates of 12 to 19% (35–38). In general, the responses to any single agent are partial, are of brief duration, and have little or no clinical benefit. Combination chemotherapy, therefore, seemed a logical next step and produced improved response rates of 30 to 45% with survival of 6 to 9 months. 5-FU has been a constant in most of these regimens, combined with doxorubicin and mitomycin C (FAM), with doxorubicin and cisplatin (FAP), with doxorubicin and methyl-CCNU (FAMe), or with doxorubicin and BCNU (FAB) (39–44).

When compared in a randomized fashion in three sequential studies by the Gastrointestinal Tumor Study Group (GITSG), the FAMe combination was associated with a modest improvement in survival over that with FMe, FA, or FIMe (5-FU, razoxane, methyl-CCNU) (41, 45, 46). The Eastern Cooperative Oncology Group (ECOG) compared four combinations in a large randomized trial, with FAM achieving the highest overall response rate (47). In a randomized, prospective trial by the North Central Cancer Treatment Group (NCCTG), single-agent 5-FU was compared with 5-FU plus doxorubicin plus CCNU (FAMe), 5-FU plus doxorubicin plus cisplatin (FAP), and FAMe alternating with an investigational antifol, triazinate. None of the three combinations showed a significant advantage over single-agent 5-FU in terms of improvement in performance status, weight gain, or survival. The three combinations were also significantly more toxic than single-agent 5-FU (48).

Newer combinations of etoposide, doxorubicin, and cisplatin (EAP); 5-FU, doxorubicin, methotrexate, and leucovorin (FAMTX); and etoposide, leucovorin, and 5-FU have demonstrated complete response rates in metastatic disease of 10 to 15% (37, 49–53). A randomized trial comparing EAP with FAMTX demonstrated similar response rates (33% for FAMTX and 20% for EAP) and median survival rates (7 months for FAMTX and 6 months for EAP). However, the EAP regimen produced significantly more toxicity, including 17% treatment-related deaths (50). In a phase III EORTC trial, FAMTX was prospectively compared with FAM and proved superior in terms of response rates, survival, and toxicity, suggesting that FAMTX is currently the standard with which further regimens must be compared (54) .

As many patients with advanced gastric cancer are elderly and often have comorbid medical conditions, investigators are actively searching for less toxic combinations with activity in advanced disease. One such promising regimen, etoposide, leucovorin, and 5-FU (ELF), has demonstrated response rates of 32 to 52% in patients with advanced disease unsuitable for more aggressive therapy (55, 56). A randomized phase III trial comparing FAMTX, ELF, and 5-FU plus cisplatin is awaiting final analysis (57).

In summary, there are several combination programs capable of respectable response rates but with few complete responses. New combinations such as 5-FU, doxorubicin, and high-dose methotrexate with leucovorin rescue (FAMTX) or ELF appear to provide the best responses relative to their toxicities. The potential role of newer agents such as epirubicin, paclitaxel, gemcitabine, and the biologics is currently under active investigation.

Adjuvant Therapy

While the prognosis for patients with resectable gastric carcinoma limited to the mucosa is very good, with 5-year survival rates of 85 to 90%, these patients represent the vast minority of presentations. At this time, the prognosis for patients with resectable gastric carcinoma remains poor, and it is unclear that adjuvant therapy provides benefit. Of 14 major published trials using a variety of chemotherapeutic regimens in the adjuvant setting, only the Gastrointestinal Tumor Study Group (GTSG) trial demonstrated a survival advantage for adjuvant 5-FU and methyl-CCNU, while subsequent trials by the ECOG and the Veteran's Administration Surgical Adjuvant Group (VASAG) were nonconfirmatory (58–60). A recent metaanalysis of 14 randomized adjuvant trials in gastric cancer involving over 2000 patients failed to show a benefit to this approach (61). Currently, an Intergroup trial is under way evaluating adjuvant chemotherapy with 5-FU, leucovorin, and radiotherapy.

In an effort to improve resectability and overall survival, investigators have initiated clinical trials of neoadjuvant chemotherapy for patients with locally advanced or unresectable gastric cancer. In a small uncontrolled trial, neoadjuvant therapy with EAP produced a response rate of 70%, with a 21% complete response rate prior to surgery (62). Phase III trials will be necessary to establish the true value of such regimens.

HEPATIC CANCER
Systemic Therapy

The large number of available phase I and II protocols for unresectable hepatocellular cancer reflects our current lack of effective chemotherapy. Only a few single agents, including 5-FU, cisplatin, methotrexate, etoposide, and doxorubicin, have produced responses in unresectable hepatomas, and these have been infrequent (63–65). No single-agent or combination regimen given systemically has demonstrated any impact on patient survival, and there remains little if any justification for this approach outside of a clinical trial.

Intraarterial Therapy

As a result of increased hepatic extraction of certain chemotherapeutic agents, a number of studies have demonstrated better response rates with regional chemotherapy given via hepatic artery catheterization than with systemic therapy (66–69). Although these programs have reported improved response rates and survival in uncontrolled trials, the true impact of regional chemotherapy is difficult to determine, as many of these trials also involved embolization, ethanol injection, or ligature of the hepatic artery.

A variety of treatment approaches are under active investigation, including radioactive antibodies such as ^{131}I-antiferritin (70, 71), tamoxifen (72, 73), and biologics (74, 75). However, there remains no effective therapy for hepatoma, and any hopes of identifying new and active approaches will require enrollment of all eligible patients in ongoing clinical trials.

PANCREATIC CANCER

Most patients with carcinoma of the pancreas present with advanced unresectable disease in need of palliation. Despite intensive efforts, the utility of chemotherapy remains unproven in this unfortunate patient population. The identification of active agents is complicated by a variety of patient-related factors such as nutritional deficiencies, poor performance status, and the absence of bidimensional measurable disease. These factors combine to make the administration of aggressive chemotherapy difficult and hamper attempts to define and compare response rates.

Nevertheless, there are several chemotherapeutic agents available with response rates of 15% or greater. These include 5-FU, mitomycin, ifosfamide, and cisplatin (76–78). Lesser degrees of activity are seen with streptozotocin and doxorubicin. When used as single agents, these drugs produce few partial responses and virtually no complete responses.

Gemcitabine, an antimetabolite analogue of deoxycytidine, has recently been shown to have activity in pancreatic carcinoma. A prospective multicenter phase II trial that examined clinical benefit criteria identified a 27% clinical benefit response in 63 patients treated (79). A randomized multicenter comparison of gemcitabine and 5-FU has been reported in abstract. In this trial, gemcitabine demonstrated a small but significant improvement in overall survival and increased the proportion of 9-month survivors from 6% with 5-FU to 24% (80). Gemcitabine is available for compassionate use from the manufacturer and is currently awaiting FDA approval for this indication.

The somatostatin analogues such as octreotide are currently undergoing clinical investigation, as they have demonstrated in vitro activity against pancreatic adenocarcinoma cell lines (81). High-dose octreotide has shown some clinical benefit in small single-institution trials (82, 83).

Active single agents have been combined into several regimens, including FAM (5-FU, doxorubicin (Adriamycin), and mitomycin C (84), SMF (streptozotocin, mitomycin, and 5-FU) (85), FAM-S (FAM plus streptozotocin) (86), FAP (5-FU, doxorubicin, and cisplatin) (43), and FP (5-FU and cisplatin) (87). In small single-institution studies, encouraging response rates and median survivals have been reported with combination regimens, but these could not be reproduced by others (88–90).

The North Central Cancer Treatment Group (NCCTG) compared 5-FU, 5-FU plus doxorubicin, and the three-drug combination of 5-FU, doxorubicin, and mitomycin in 144 patients (88). With survival as the primary endpoint, the NCCTG found no likelihood that either FAM or FA would produce a 50% increase in survival compared with 5-FU alone. The Cancer and Leukemia Group B compared FAM with SMF in 196 patients with advanced pancreatic cancer, 133 of whom had measurable disease (89). There was no median difference in survival between regimens overall, although there was a slight survival benefit to FAM-treated patients with measurable disease. Response rates (in patients with measurable disease) were 14% for FAM and 4% for SMF.

Another initially promising regimen combining 5-FU, cyclophosphamide, methotrexate, vincristine, and mitomycin C (Mallinson regimen) was compared with 5-FU, doxorubicin, and cisplatin (FAP) and with 5-FU alone by the NCCTG (91). Objective response rates were 7% for 5-FU alone, 21% for the Mallinson regimen, and 15% for FAP. Both of the combination chemotherapy programs produced more toxicity, and no increase in median survival (4.5 months) was observed.

In a combined phase I-II study, 28 patients at Memorial Sloan-Kettering Cancer Center were treated with a combination of cisplatin, high-dose cytarabine, and caffeine (CAC) (92). A partial response rate of 39% was obtained. This regimen was then studied in a phase III randomized trial and proved to be inferior to SMF (93).

In contrast to metastatic colon cancer, attempts to modulate the activity of 5-FU with leucovorin have been largely unsuccessful to this point in patients with pancreatic carcinoma (94, 95). However, a recent report from UCLA suggests promising activity of a regimen combining continuous infusion 5-FU, leucovorin, mitomycin C, and dipyridamole (96). Of 41 evaluable patients, there were 4 complete responses (10%), 13 partial responses (31%), and a median survival of more than 15 months.

At this time, there is no standard effective single-agent or combination chemotherapy program for unresectable adenocarcinoma of the pancreas. Efforts must continue to enroll patients onto clinical trials investigating newer agents.

Locoregional Disease

For patients with disease confined to the pancreas and peripancreatic area, 5-FU and concomitant radiation therapy followed by weekly 5-FU was compared with radiation therapy alone (97). The median survival was 17.8 weeks for the radiation therapy alone group and 35 weeks for the combination arm. It appears that concurrent chemotherapy and radiation also increases the proportion of 1-year survivors from 10% with radiotherapy alone to 40% with the combined approach.

Adjuvant Therapy

In a small study, the GTSG randomized completely resected patients to receive either no further therapy or concurrent 5-FU and radiotherapy followed by weekly 5-FU (98, 99). Median survival was significantly longer in the treatment group (21 months) than in the control group (11 months). This study has been criti-

cized for its small size (43 patients) and long duration of accrual (8 years).

GALLBLADDER AND BILIARY DUCT CARCINOMAS

Biliary carcinomas represent a group of aggressive malignancies that are fortunately uncommon in Western countries, accounting for approximately 6000 deaths annually in the United States (1). As these patients often present with unresectable disease, the role for palliative chemotherapy has been investigated. However, the experience with chemotherapy for cancer of the biliary system remains limited by the small size of clinical trials. Highly variable response rates between clinical trials likely reflect patient selection as much as drug efficacy.

5-FU, mitomycin C, and doxorubicin are the most commonly used single agents, with response rates ranging from 10 to 20% (100, 101). Combination regimens have yielded similarly disappointing results. Responses to oral 5-FU plus streptozotocin or methyl-CCNU were uniformly poor, with only 3 of 34 patients responding in an ECOG trial (100). In the largest single series using combination chemotherapy, FAM produced a partial response rate of 29% (4 of 14 patients) (102). In the only randomized trial reported to date, the ECOG compared oral 5-FU, oral 5-FU plus streptozotocin, and oral 5-FU plus methyl-CCNU, with response rates of 11%, 12%, and 5%, respectively (100).

Regional chemotherapy with 5-FU, fluorodeoxyuridine (FUDR), or doxorubicin administered via hepatic artery infusion has, in general, produced higher response rates than systemic therapy. Pooled data from single-institution series suggest an overall response rate between 40 and 50% (103–105).

A recent trial from the ECOG suggests a role for the combination of radiotherapy and protracted venous infusion of 5-FU for patients with localized but unresectable pancreaticobiliary tumors. Median survival is reported to be 11.9 months, with 19% of patients alive at 2 years (106).

SMALL BOWEL CANCER

Malignant tumors of the small intestine are uncommon and account for only about 4600 cases yearly (1). The major histologic types are adenocarcinomas, sarcomas, lymphomas, and carcinoids (107). The chemotherapy for sarcomas, lymphomas, and carcinoids of the small bowel is the same as that for other primary sites and is discussed elsewhere.

Adenocarcinomas comprise approximately 45% of malignant tumors of the small intestine and are best treated with wide resection of the involved bowel segment and draining lymph nodes. There is no proven effective chemotherapy for either the metastatic or adjuvant settings, though regimens based on 5-FU have been reported (108).

COLORECTAL CANCER

Advanced Disease—Systemic Therapy

The chemotherapy of unresectable or metastatic colorectal cancer has lagged behind other areas in oncology. Thirty-seven years after its introduction into clinical medicine (109). the optimal dose and schedule of 5-FU (5-FU), the most effective and commonly used agent, has not been determined. Given intravenously 5-FU reliably produces a response rate of 10 to 20% (110–115). Although the minority of patients who respond to single agent 5-FU may have prolongation of survival, the overall impact on duration and quality of life has been negligible (116).

In addition to 5-FU and FUDR, the only other active drugs are the nitrosoureas and mitomycin (35). These drugs have response rates in the same range as 5-FU, with added toxicity.

The combination of 5-FU, vincristine, and methyl-CCNU was initially reported to produce response rates of 43% (117), but this could not be reproduced (118, 119). A similar combination of 5-FU, methyl-CCNU, vincristine, and a second nitrosourea, streptozotocin (MOF-Strep) also looked initially promising (120), but these results could not be replicated (121). Also, with longer follow-up, it has become apparent that the use of methyl-CCNU has been associated with an increased risk of leukemia and is no longer available (122). It appears that combination regimens produce moderately superior responses than 5-FU alone, with significantly increased toxicity and no tangible impact on survival.

In an attempt to improve the efficacy of 5-FU, investigators have studied alternative infusion schedules. As 5-FU has a very short half-life, it would seem ideally suited for protracted continuous infusion schedules, and significantly higher cumulative doses can be achieved with an acceptable toxicity profile (123, 124). The Mid-Atlantic Oncology Program randomized 187 patients to bolus 5-FU or a continuous infusion regimen and found the latter to produce significantly better response rates (30 vs. 7%). Unfortunately, the increased responses did not translate into a survival benefit (125).

Further efforts to improve upon the efficacy of 5-FU have involved attempts at biochemical modulation with a variety of agents such as leucovorin, methotrexate, PALA, allopurinol, and interferon. To date, the use of leucovorin (folinic acid) to modulate 5-FU has been most extensively studied. Pretreatment with leucovorin is thought to enhance the binding of 5-FU to its target enzyme, thymidylate synthetase, providing a greater inhibition of DNA synthesis (126).

Numerous trials evaluating different dosing and schedules of 5-FU and leucovorin have been carried out, with two different treatment strategies emerging as superior. The Roswell Park regimen involves weekly administration of high-dose 5-FU and leucovorin, and in three randomized trials comparing it with single-agent 5-FU, this regimen produced superior response rates (112, 127, 128). The dose-limiting toxicity of this regimen is diarrhea, which occurs in 30 to 40% of patients and may result in severe dehydration and even death if not properly recognized and aggressively treated.

The Mayo Clinic regimen involves low-dose leucovorin and 5-FU administered five consecutive days in a 4- to 5-week cycle. Three of six randomized prospective trials comparing this regimen with single-agent 5-FU have demonstrated significantly improved response rates with the addition of low-dose leucovorin (129–131). The most common toxicities associated with this regimen include stomatitis (28%), leukopenia (22%), and diarrhea (16%) (132) .

Currently, neither modulated 5-FU regimen shows clear superiority. In the only randomized comparison of the two regimens, conducted by the NCCTG and Mayo Clinic, it was concluded that the intensive-course 5-FU with low-dose leucovorin (Mayo regimen) had a superior therapeutic index, based on similar response rates, lower costs, and less need for hospitalization (133). Only 1 of the 10 randomized trials of 5-FU and leucovorin has demonstrated a continued survival advantage over 5-FU alone (131, 134). Physician choice often involves personal experience with a specific regimen, cost, and the patient tolerability of the distinctive toxicity profiles. Methotrexate, by increasing intracellular phosphoribosylpyrophosphate concentrations, can increase the conversion of 5-FU to the active FdUMP and may also increase the incorporation of fluorouracil into RNA. The clinical application of this potential modulation has been, for the most part, disappointing. A regimen combining high-dose methotrexate with 5-FU and leucovorin did demonstrate a 2.8-month improvement in survival over single-agent 5-FU but was inferior to the Mayo regimen in terms of survival, cost, response rates, and quality of life (131).

Preclinical data have suggested that the interferons also have the ability to modulate the activity of 5-FU. The combination of 5-FU plus recombinant α2a-interferon initially yielded a high partial response rate (76%) in previously untreated patients (135). The side effects were significant and included leukopenia, fever, and increased mucositis. A confirmatory trial conducted by the ECOG identified a response rate closer to 40%, with an acceptable toxicity profile (136).

A recent 5-armed Intergroup trial comparing high-dose 5-FU alone, 5-FU/PALA, 5-FU/oral leucovorin, 5-FU/high-dose leucovorin, and 5-FU/interferon has just completed accrual and will, one hopes, identify the most effective regimen.

Currently, there are intensive efforts to identify new agents with activity in colorectal carcinoma. Potential new agents under active investigation include the camptothecins (CPT-11 and 9-AC), alternative thymidylate synthase inhibitors (Tomudex, Tegafur, AG-331, LY231514), inhibitors of fluorouracil catabolism (UFT, 5-ethynyluracil), inhibitors of ribonucleotide reductase (gemcitabine), and monoclonal antibodies (Panorex).

Regional Therapy

Hepatic metastases from colorectal carcinomas derive most of their blood supply from the hepatic artery as opposed to the portal vein. Regional infusion of agents with high hepatic extraction such as FUDR also permits prolonged drug exposure at higher concentrations to the tumor cells (137). Thus, regional therapy via the hepatic artery (HAI) is a potentially attractive method of treating metastatic disease confined to the liver (138).

The most common toxicities associated with this approach include peptic ulcer disease and hepatic toxicity (139). The ulcer disease results from inadvertent perfusion of the stomach and duodenum via collateral vessels and can be prevented by dissection and ligation of these collaterals at the time of pump insertion (140). The

hepatic toxicity may be ameliorated by the co-administration of dexamethasone via HAI (141).

It is clear from at least 7 randomized trials comparing regional therapy with FUDR with systemic 5-FU alone that response rates are significantly better with hepatic arterial infusions (137, 138, 142–146). Crossover designs in earlier trials precluded a survival comparison, and the only two "pure" randomized trials comparing systemic 5-FU and HAI FUDR demonstrated no survival benefit. The Cancer and Leukemia Group B has recently initiated a prospective comparison of systemic 5-FU plus leucovorin and regional HAI therapy with FUDR, leucovorin, and dexamethasone for patients with hepatic metastases.

Adjuvant Therapy

Nearly 140,000 cases of colon and rectal cancer will be diagnosed in 1995, with approximately 40% of these patients dying of metastatic disease (1). The identification of an effective adjuvant strategy could obviously have a major impact. Initial attempts at adjuvant therapy focused on patients with stage II or III disease and compared 5-FU with surgery alone. In these trials, the adjuvant use of 5-FU added no benefit to surgery alone (147).

The first randomized trial to demonstrate a benefit for adjuvant therapy in patients with Dukes B and C colon carcinoma was reported by the National Surgical Adjuvant Breast and Bowel Project (NSABP) (148). In this trial, over 1100 patients were randomized to methyl-CCNU (semustine), vincristine, and 5-FU; BCG; or observation, with improved overall and disease-free survival in favor of the chemotherapy-treated patients. These results contrast with those of two earlier studies reported by the GITSG and VASOG (149, 150).

The mechanism of synergy between the antihelmintic drug, levamisole, and 5-FU continues to be a source of much speculation. Traditionally, levamisole's mechanism of action was thought to be related to its various immunomodulatory properties (151–155). More recent data from colon carcinoma cell lines suggest that the synergy between these two agents results from 5-FU incorporation into RNA with resultant accumulation of HLA class I mRNA, while levamisole augments the accumulation of these stable mRNAs (156).

Based on two preliminary trials from Europe that suggested a potential benefit for levamisole alone as a surgical adjuvant in patients with colon cancer, the NCCTG began a randomized trial of levamisole, 5-FU, the combination of 5-FU and levamisole, or observation alone in 401 patients with completely resected stage II and III colon cancer (157). There was no benefit to either the levamisole or 5-FU alone. However, the combination of 5-FU and levamisole demonstrated improved disease-free survival in all patients and overall survival for patients with stage III disease (Duke's C).

An Intergroup study was then designed attempting to confirm these results in a larger group of patients. In this trial, 1296 patients with resected stage II or III colon cancer were randomly assigned to observation or 1 year of chemotherapy with levamisole and 5-FU (158). In patients with stage III (Duke's C) colon cancer, the 5-FU plus levamisole regimen reduced the risk of cancer recurrence by 41% and the overall death rate by 33% over that of the control group. Survival at 3.5 years was 71% for the treatment arm and 55% for the surgery-alone controls. To date, there have been too few deaths or recurrences in the stage II (Duke's B) patients to demonstrate any benefit to adjuvant therapy. A National Institutes of Health Consensus Panel subsequently concluded that although optimal adjuvant therapy had not been devised, patients with stage III (Duke's C) colon cancer should be offered a clinical trial. Those unable to participate should be offered adjuvant 5-FU and levamisole (159).

The demonstration of improved responses to the combination of 5-FU and leucovorin in the metastatic setting led to clinical trials evaluating its potential as an adjuvant. The NSABP C-03 trial randomized over 1000 patients to either semustine, vincristine, and 5-FU (MOF) or 5-FU and leucovorin (160). Data from the NCCTG, NCI Canada, and two European trials comparing 5-FU and leucovorin with surgery alone demonstrated improved disease-free and overall survival for the treatment arms (161, 162).

Another approach to adjuvant therapy of colon cancer involves the use of short-term postoperative portal vein infusion of 5-FU plus heparin. In a randomized trial of 244 patients, Taylor et al. reported decreased hepatic metastases and improved overall survival (163). In an attempt to confirm these results, the NSABP C-02 trial randomized 1158 patients to surgery alone or to treatment with portal vein infusion with 5-FU plus heparin (164). Although a significant improvement in the disease-free survival was

noted, this did not translate into either an overall survival benefit or a reduction in liver recurrences.

The role for perioperative chemotherapy remains to be determined, and a current Intergroup study preoperatively randomizing patients to 7 days of perioperative 5-FU or observation followed by standard 5-FU and levamisole is actively accruing patients at this time. It is hoped that this trial will more clearly define the role of perioperative chemotherapy in colon cancer.

In contrast to colon cancer, the anatomic constraints of the pelvis may limit the surgeon's ability to obtain wide and clear margins, resulting in higher local recurrence rates in patients with rectal cancer. Radiation therapy alone has been able to significantly decrease the local recurrence rates but has not affected survival (147).

In 1988, the NSABP reported the preliminary initial results of the R-01 protocol comparing postoperative chemotherapy with semustine, vincristine, and 5-FU (MOF); postoperative radiation therapy; and observation alone for patients with resected stage II and III rectal cancer (165). In this trial, the chemotherapy group demonstrated both better disease-free and overall survival than those in the observation arm.

In the setting of combined chemotherapy and radiotherapy, the GTSG randomized 201 patients to radiotherapy and 5-FU with or without semustine (166). No difference was noted between the treatment groups, and it was concluded that semustine was not a necessary component of the adjuvant therapy of rectal cancer.

Similarly, an NCCTG study compared radiation alone with the combination of radiation therapy and chemotherapy with methyl-CCNU and 5-FU in patients with stage II and III rectal cancer (167). The combined-modality therapy treatment showed a clear advantage over radiation therapy alone, with reduced local recurrences, reduced distant metastases, and improved survival. There was a 46% reduction in pelvic recurrence, a 37% reduction in distant tumor spread, and a 29% reduction in patient deaths. An intergroup trial led by the NCCTG tested combined modality therapy with or without methyl-CCNU in a program identical to the study above (168). They found a recurrence rate 1.2 times higher for the methyl-CCNU arm, eliminating the possibility that methyl-CCNU is a vital component of this therapy.

In an effort to improve upon the efficacy of combined-modality therapy, the NCCTG conducted a randomized trial of 660 patients with stage II or III rectal carcinoma randomized to receive intermittent bolus or protracted venous infusion of 5-FU during radiotherapy. Systemic therapy with either 5-FU alone or 5-FU plus semustine was also administered. With a median follow-up of 46 months, there was no added benefit to semustine. More importantly, patients receiving the protracted 5-FU infusion during pelvic radiotherapy had better disease-free and overall survivals than patients receiving intermittent bolus 5-FU and radiotherapy (169).

An Intergroup trial is currently randomizing patients with stage II and III rectal cancer to either intermittent bolus 5-FU or protracted-infusion 5-FU before and after pelvic radiotherapy with protracted-infusion 5-FU. A third arm will determine the role, if any, of 5-FU modulation with levamisole and leucovorin.

APPENDICEAL CANCER

This extremely rare group of neoplasms includes several histologic types such as carcinoid tumors, mucinous cystadenocarcinomas, adenocarcinomas, and adenocarcinoids (170). There is insufficient information available to make specific recommendations regarding chemotherapy. The treatment of carcinoid tumors is covered elsewhere in this textbook.

ANAL CANCER

Epidermoid carcinomas of the anal region are uncommon, comprising 3 to 4% of all malignant lesions of the distal alimentary tract (171). The clinical course is characterized by local extension into contiguous soft tissues of the pelvis and by early lymphatic involvement. Hematogenous metastases are the exception. For these reasons, the early treatments of anal carcinoma involved surgery with either local resection or abdominoperineal resection.

In 1974, Nigro et al. reported results of using preoperative radiation and concurrent chemotherapy with 5-FU and mitomycin C in a small series of patients with anal cancer (172). Following completion of preoperative therapy, 84% of patients were rendered disease free. Impressive 5-year survival rates of 80% were obtained, with over 60% of patients alive with intact sphincter function (172, 178). These dramatic results quickly led to the adoption of chemoradiotherapy as the standard therapy despite the absence of a comparative trial.

Since the initial combined-modality study, a large number of clinical trials have been reported. Most of these trials use varying doses and schedules of 5-FU, mitomycin C, and radiotherapy, with the optimal regimen remaining to be defined (173–184). It appears that local control is improved with higher doses of radiation and concurrent schedules. Also, there is evidence to suggest that this approach may be significantly less effective for patients with tumors greater than 5 cm (183). For patients with incomplete responses or relapse, anecdotal reports suggest that cisplatin-based salvage regimens may have some utility (180, 186).

Advanced epidermoid anal carcinoma is much more likely to produce locoregional complications, which may be palliated with either surgery or radiotherapy. The optimal approach to the rare patient with systemic metastases is yet to be defined. Active agents include cisplatin, carboplatin, 5-FU, mitomycin, bleomycin, and methotrexate, either as single agents or in a variety of combinations. Response rates from small single-institution studies vary widely, with few complete responders and brief response durations (187–189).

ACKNOWLEDGMENT

The author gratefully acknowledges the expert assistance provided by Donna Hickman in the preparation of this manuscript.

REFERENCES

1. Wingo PA, Tong T, Bolden S. Cancer statistics, 1995. CA 1995;45:8–30.
2. Miller BA, Ries L, Hankey B, et al. Cancer statistics review 1973–1989. DHHS, NIH Publ. no. 92-2789, Bethesda, 1992.
3. Ajani J. Contributions of chemotherapy in the treatment of carcinoma of the esophagus: results and commentary. Semin Oncol 1994;21(4):474–482.
4. Tempero MA. Advances in the medical management of advanced gastrointestinal cancers. Curr Opin Oncol 1990;2:747–753.
5. Leichman L, Berry BT. Experience with cisplatin in treatment regimens for esophageal cancer. Semin Oncol 1991;18(Suppl 3):64–72.
6. Yagoda A, Mukherji B, Young C, et al. Bleomycin, an antitumor antibiotic: clinical experience in 274 patients. Ann Intern Med 1972;77:861–870.
7. Ravry M, Moertel CG, Schutt AJ, et al. Treatment of advanced squamous cell carcinoma of the gastrointestinal tract with bleomycin. Cancer Chemother Rep 1973;57:493–495.
8. Bedekian AY, Valdivieso M, Bodey GP, et al. Phase II evaluation of vindesine in the treatment of colorectal and esophageal tumors. Cancer Chemother Pharmacol 1979;2:263–266.
9. Edzinli EZ, Gelber R, Desai DV. Chemotherapy of advanced esophageal carcinoma: Eastern Coopera-

tive Oncology Group experience. Cancer 1980;46:2149–2153.

10. Bezwoda WR, Derman DP, Weaving A, et al. Treatment of esophageal cancer with vindesine. Cancer Treat Rep 1984;68:783–785.

11. Wittes RE, Adrianza ME, Parsons R, et al. Compilation of phase II results with single antineoplastic agents. Cancer Treat Symp 1985;4:91–130.

12. Leichman L, Berry BT. Experience with cisplatin in treatment regimens for esophageal cancer. Semin Oncol 1991;18(1 Suppl 3):64–72.

13. Coia LR. The use of mitomycin in esophageal cancer. Oncology 1993;50(Suppl 1):53–60.

14. Kelsen DP, Ilson DH. Chemotherapy and combined-modality therapy for esophageal cancer. Chest 1995;107(Suppl 6):224S–232S.

15. Kelsen D, Ajani J, Ilson D, et al. A phase II trial of paclitaxel (taxol) in advanced carcinoma of the esophagus. Semin Oncol 1994;21(5 Suppl 8):44–48.

16. Kelsen DP. The role of chemotherapy in the treatment of esophageal cancer. Chest Surg Clin North Am 1994;4(1):173–184.

17. Gisselbrecht C, Clavo F, Mignot L, et al. Fluorouracil (F), Adriamycin (A), and cisplatin (C) (FAP) combination chemotherapy of advanced esophageal carcinoma. Cancer 1983;52:974–977.

18. Kelsen DP, Coonley C, Hilaris B, et al. Cisplatin, vindesine, and bleomycin combination chemotherapy of local-regional and advanced esophageal carcinoma. Am J Med 1983;75:645–652.

19. Coonley CJ, Bains M, Hilaris B, Chapman R, Kelsen DP. Cisplatin and bleomycin in the treatment of esophageal carcinoma: a final report. Cancer 1984; 54:2351–2355.

20. Carey RW, Hilgenberg AD, Wilkins EW, Choi NC, Mathisen DJ, Grillo HL. Preoperative chemotherapy followed by surgery with possible postoperative radiotherapy in squamous cell carcinoma of the esophagus: evaluation of the chemotherapy component. J Clin Oncol 1986;4:697–701.

21. Kies MS, Rosen ST, Tsang T-K, et al. Cisplatin and 5-fluorouracil in the primary management of squamous esophageal carcinoma. Cancer 1987;60:2156–2160.

22. Earlham RJ, Johnson L. 101 Oesophageal cancers: a surgeon uses radiotherapy. Ann R Coll Surg Engl 1990;72:32–40.

23. Welvaart K, Caspers RJL, Verkes RJ, et al. The choice between surgical resection and radiation therapy for patients with cancer of the esophagus and cardia: a retrospective comparison between two treatments. J Surg Oncol 1991;47:225–229.

24. Kelsen DP, Cvitkovic E, Bains M, et al. Cisdichlorodiammine platinum II and bleomycin in the treatment of esophageal cancer. Cancer Treat Rep 1978; 62:1041–1046.

25. Schlag P, Hermann R, Fritze D, Buhr H, Herfarth C, Schettler G. Preoperative chemotherapy in localized cancer of the esophagus with cisplatinum, vindesine, and bleomycin. In: Wagner DJ, Blijhan GH, Smeets JBE, Wils JA, eds. Primary chemotherapy in cancer medicine. New York: Alan R Liss, 1985:253–258.

26. Kukla L, Lad T, McGuire W, Thomas P. Multimodality therapy of squamous carcinoma of the esophagus (abstract). Proc Am Soc Clin Oncol 1981; 22:449.

27. Kelsen DP. Chemotherapy-based multimodality therapy of esophageal cancer. In: Wagner DJ, Blijhan GH, Smeets JBE, Wils JA, eds. Primary chemotherapy in cancer medicine. New York: Alan R Liss, 1985:241–252.

28. Kelsen DP, Minsky B, Smith M, et al. Preoperative therapy for esophageal cancer: a randomized comparison of chemotherapy versus radiation therapy. J Clin Oncol 1990;8:1352–1361.

29. Roth JA, Pass HI, Flanagan MM, et al. Randomized clinical trial of preoperative and postoperative adjuvant chemotherapy with cisplatin, vindesine, and bleomycin for carcinoma of the esophagus. J Thorac Cardiovasc Surg 1988;96:242–248.

30. Maipang T, Vasinanukorn P, Petpichetchian C, et al. Induction chemotherapy in the treatment of patients with carcinoma of the esophagus. World J Surg 1994;56(3):191–197.

31. Forastiere AA, Orringer MB, Perez-Tamayo C, et al. Preoperative chemoradiation followed by transhiatal esophagectomy for carcinoma of the esophagus: final report. J Clin Oncol 1993;11(6):1118–1123.

32. Herskovic A, Martz K, al-Sarraf M, et al. Combined chemotherapy and radiotherapy compared with radiotherapy alone in patients with cancer of the esophagus. N Engl J Med 1992;326:1593–1598.

33. Comis RL, Carker SK. Integration of chemotherapy into combined modality treatment of solid tumors in gastric cancer. Cancer Treat Rev 1974;1:221–238.

34. Schein PS, MacDonald JS, Hoth D, et al. Mitomycin-c: experience in the United States with emphasis on gastric cancer. Cancer Chemother Pharmacol 1978; 1:73–75.

35. Haller DG. Chemotherapy in gastrointestinal malignancies. Semin Oncol 1988;15(Suppl 4):50–64.

36. Leichman L, Berry BT. Cisplatin therapy for adenocarcinoma of the stomach. Semin Oncol 1991; 18(Suppl 3):25–33.

37. Ajani JA, Ota DM, Jackson DE. Current strategies in the management of locoregional and metastatic gastric carcinoma. Cancer 1991;67:260–265.

38. Preusser P, Achterrath W, Wilke H, et al. Chemotherapy of gastric cancer. Cancer Treat Rev 1988; 15:257–277.

39. Kovach JS, Moertel CG, Schutt AJ, Hahn RG, Reitemeier RJ. A controlled study of 1–3-bis-(2-chlorethyl)-1-nitrosourea and 5-fluorouracil therapy for advanced gastric and pancreatic cancer. Cancer 1974; 33:563–567.

40. Moertel CG, Lavin PT. Phase II-III chemotherapy studies in advanced gastric cancer. Cancer Treat Rep 1979;63:1863–1869.

41. Gastrointestinal Tumor Study Group. Randomized study of combination chemotherapy studies in advanced gastric cancer. Cancer Treat Rep 1979;63:1871–1876.

42. Wadler S, Green M, Muggia F. The role of anthracyclines in the treatment of gastric cancer. Cancer Treat Rev 1985;12:105–132.

43. Moertel CG, Rubin J, O'Connell MJ, Schutt AJ, Wieand HS. A phase II study of combined 5-fluorouracil, doxorubicin, and cisplatin in the treatment of advanced upper gastrointestinal adenocarcinomas. J Clin Oncol 1986;4:1053–1057.

44. Levi JA, Fox RM, Tattersall MH, Woods RL, Thomson D, Gill G, for the Sydney Cooperative Oncology Group. Analysis of a prospectively randomized

comparison of doxorubicin versus 5-fluorouracil, doxorubicin, and BCNU in advanced gastric cancer: implications for future studies. J Clin Oncol 1986; 4:1348–1355.

45. Gastrointestinal Tumor Study Group. A comparative clinical assessment of advanced gastric carcinoma. Cancer 1982;49:1362–1366.

46. Gastrointestinal Tumor Study Group. Randomized study of combination chemotherapy in unresectable gastric cancer. Cancer 1984;53:13–17.

47. Douglass HO, Lavin PT, Goudsmit A, Klaasse DJ, Paul AR. An Eastern Cooperative Oncology Group evaluation of combination of MeCCNU, mitomycin C, Adriamycin, and 5-fluorouracil in advanced measurable gastric cancer (EST 2277). J Clin Oncol 1984; 2:1372–1381.

48. Cullinan SA, Moertel CG, Wieand HS, et al. Controlled evaluation of three drug combination regimens versus fluorouracil alone for therapy of advanced gastric cancer. J Clin Oncol 1994;12:412–416.

49. Preusser P, Wilke H, Achterrath W, et al. Phase II study with the combination etoposide, doxorubicin, and cisplatin in advanced measurable gastric cancer. J Clin Oncol 1989;7:1310–1317.

50. Kelsen D, Atiq OT, Saltz L, et al. FAMTX versus etoposide, doxorubicin, and cisplatin: a random assignment trial in gastric cancer. J Clin Oncol 1992; 10(4):541–548.

51. Klein HO, Dias Wickkramanayake P, Farrokh GR. 5-Fluorouracil (5-Fu), Adriamycin (ADM), and methotrexate (MTX)—a combination protocol (FAMTX) for treatment of metastasized stomach cancer (abstract). Proc Am Soc Clin Oncol 1986;5:84.

52. Wils J, Bleiberg H, Dalesio O, et al. An EORTC gastrointestinal group evaluation of the combination of sequential methotrexate and 5-fluorouracil, combined with Adriamycin in advanced measurable gastric cancer. J Clin Oncol 1986;4:1799–1803.

53. Preusser P, Wilke H, Achterrath W, et al. Phase II study with the combination of etoposide, doxorubicin, and cisplatin in advanced measurable gastric cancer. J Clin Oncol 1989;7:1310–1317.

54. Wils JA, Klein HO, Wagener DJ, et al. Sequential high-dose methotrexate and fluorouracil combined with doxorubicin—a step ahead in the treatment of advanced gastric cancer: a trial of the European Organization for the Treatment of Cancer Gastrointestinal Study Group. J Clin Oncol 1991;9(5):827–831.

55. di Bartolomeo M, Bajetta E, de Braud F, et al. Phase II study of the etoposide, leucovorin, and fluorouacil combination for patients with advanced gastric cancer unsuitable for aggressive therapy. Oncology 1995;52(1):41–44.

56. Wilke H, Preusser P, Fink U, et al. New developments in the treatment of gastric cancer. Cancer Treat Res 1991;55:363–373.

57. Wilke H, Wils J, Rougier A, et al. Preliminary analysis of a phase III trial of FAMTX versus ELF versus cisplatin/FU in advanced gastric cancer (GC). A trial of the EORTC Gastrointestinal Tract Cancer Cooperative Group and the AOI (Arbeitsgemeinschaft Internistische Onkologie) (abstract). Proc Am Soc Clin Oncol 1995;14:500.

58. Gastrointestinal Tumor Study Group. Controlled trial of adjuvant chemotherapy following curative resection for gastric cancer. Cancer 1982; 49:1116–1122.

59. Engstrom PF, Lavin PT, Douglass HO Jr, Brunner KW. Postoperative adjuvant 5-fluorouracil plus methyl CCNU therapy for gastric cancer patients. Eastern Cooperative Oncology Group study (EST 3275). Cancer 1985;55:1868–1873.

60. Higgins GA, Amadeo JH, Smith DE, et al. Efficacy of prolonged intermittent therapy with combined 5-FU and methyl CCNU following resection for gastric carcinoma. A Veterans Administration Surgical Oncology Group report. Cancer 1983;52:1105–1112.

61. Hermans J, Bonenkamp JJ, Boon ML, et al. Adjuvant therapy after curative resection for gastric cancer: meta-analysis of randomized trials. J Clin Oncol 1993;11:1441–1447.

62. Preusser HW, Fink U, Gunzer U, et al. Preoperative chemotherapy in locally advanced and non-resectable gastric cancer: a phase II study with etoposide, doxorubicin, and cisplatin. J Clin Oncol 1989;9:1318–1326.

63. Wanebo HJ, Falkson G, Order SE. Cancer of the hepatobiliary system. In: DeVita VT Jr, Hellman S, Rosenberg SE, eds. Cancer: principles and practice of oncology. 3rd ed. Philadelphia: JB Lippincott, 1989:836–874.

64. Falkson G, Ryan LM, Johnson LA. A randomized phase II study of mitoxantrone and cisplatin in patients with hepatocellular carcinoma: an ECOG study. Cancer 1987;60:2141–2145.

65. Melia WM, Westaby D, Williams R. Induction of remission in hepatocellular carcinoma. Cancer 1983; 51:206–210.

66. Epirubicin Study Group for Hepatocellular Carcinoma. Intra-arterial administration of epirubicin in the treatment of nonresectable hepatocellular carcinoma—a histopathologic study. Cancer 1984;54:387–392.

67. Onohara S, Kobayashi S, Itoh Y, et al. Intra-arterial cis-platinum infusion with sodium thiosulfate protection and angiotensin II induced hypertension for treatment of hepatocellular carcinoma. Acta Radiol 1988;29:197–202.

68. Toyoda H, Nakana S, Kumada T, et al. The efficacy of continuous local arterial infusion of 5-fluorouracil and cisplatin through an implanted reservoir for severe advanced hepatocellular carcinoma. Oncology 1995;52(4):295–299.

69. Patt YZ, Charnsangavej C, Yoffe B, et al. Hepatic arterial infusion of floxuridine, leucovorin, doxorubicin and cisplatin for hepatocellular carcinoma: effects of hepatitis B and C viral infection on drug toxicity and patient survival. J Clin Oncol 1994; 12(6):1204–1211.

70. Order SE, Stillwagon GB, Kelin JL, et al. Iodine 131 antiferritin, a new treatment modality in hepatoma: a Radiation Therapy Oncology Group study. J Clin Oncol 1985;3:1573–1582.

71. Order S, Pajak T, Leibel S, et al. A randomized prospective trial comparing full dose chemotherapy to ^{131}I antiferritin: an RTOG study. Int J Radiat Oncol Biol Phys 1991;20(5):953–963.

72. Martinez Cerezo FJ, Thomas A, Donoso L, et al. Controlled trial of tamoxifen in patients with advanced hepatocellular carcinoma. J Hepatol 1994;20(6):702–706.

73. Elba S, Giannuzzi V, Misciagna G, Manghisi OG. Randomized controlled trial of tamoxifen versus

placebo in inoperable hepatocellular carcinoma. Ital J Gastroenterol 1994;26(2):66–68.

74. Feun LG, Savaraj N, Hung S, et al. A phase II trial of recombinant leukocyte interferon plus doxorubicin in patients with hepatocellular carcinoma. Am J Clin Oncol 1994;17(5):393–395.

75. Yamamoto M, Iizuka H, Fujii H, et al. Hepatic arterial infusion of interleukin-2 in advanced hepatocellular cancer. Acta Oncol 1993;32(1);43–51.

76. O'Connell MJ. Current status of chemotherapy for advanced pancreatic and gastric cancer. J Clin Oncol 1985;3:1032–1039.

77. Loehrer P, Williams S, Einhorn L, Ansari R. Ifosfamide: an active drug in the treatment of adenocarcinoma of the pancreas. J Clin Oncol 1985;3:367–372.

78. Wils J, Kok T, Wagener D, et al. Activity of cisplatin in adenocarcinoma of the pancreas. Eur J Cancer 1993;29A(2):203–204.

79. Rothenberg ML, Burris HA, Andersen JS, et al. Gemcitabine: effective palliative therapy for pancreas cancer patients failing 5-FU (abstract). Proc Annu Meet Am Soc Clin Oncol 1995;14:470.

80. Moore M, Andersen J, Burris H, et al. A randomized trial of gemcitabine (GEM) versus 5FU as first-line therapy in advanced pancreatic cancer (abstract). Proc Annu Meet Am Soc Clin Oncol 1995; 14:473.

81. Perelli D, Mansi C, Savarino V, Celle G. Hormonal therapy of pancreatic cancer. Rationale and perspectives. Int J Pancreatol 1993;13(3):159–168.

82. Ebert M, Freiss H, Beger H, Buchler M. Role of octreotide in the treatment of pancreatic cancer. Digestion 1994;55(Suppl 1):48–51.

83. Cascinu S, Del Ferro E, Catalano G. A randomized trial of octreotide vs. best supportive care only in advanced gastrointestinal cancer patients refractory to chemotherapy. Br J Cancer 1995;71:97–101.

84. Smith FP, Hoth DF, Levin B, et al. 5-Fluorouracil, Adriamycin, and mitomycin C (FAM) chemotherapy for advanced adenocarcinoma of the pancreas. Cancer 1981;46:2014–2018.

85. Wiggans RG, Woolley PV, Mac Donald JS, et al. Phase II trial of streptozotocin, mitomycin c, and 5-fluorouracil (SMF) in the treatment of advanced pancreatic cancer. Cancer 1978;41:387–391.

86. Bukowski RM, Abderhalden RT, Hewlett JS, Weick JK, Groppe CW Jr. Phase II trial of streptozotocin, mitomycin c, and 5-fluorouracil in adenocarcinoma of the pancreas. Cancer Clin Trials 1980;3:321–324.

87. Rougier P, Zarba J, Ducreux M, et al. Phase II study of cisplatin and 120-hour continuous infusion of 5-fluorouracil in patients with advanced pancreatic adenocarcinoma. Ann Oncol 1993;4(4):333–336.

88. Cullinan SA, Moertel CG, Fleming TR, et al. A comparison of three chemotherapeutic regimens in the treatment of advanced pancreatic and gastric carcinoma. JAMA 1985;253:2061–2067.

89. Oster M, Gray R, Panasci L, Perry MC. Chemotherapy for advanced pancreatic cancer. A comparison of 5-fluorouracil, Adriamycin, and mitomycin (FAM) with 5-fluorouracil, streptozotocin, and mitomycin (FSM). Cancer 1986;57:29–33.

90. Takada T, Kato H, Matsushiro T, et al. Comparison of 5-fluorouracil, doxorubicin, and mitomycin-C with 5-fluorouracil alone in the treatment of pancreatic-biliary carcinomas. Oncology 1994;51(5):396–400.

91. Cullinan S, Moertel CG, Wieand Hs, et al. A phase II trial on the therapy of advanced pancreatic carcinoma: evaluations of the Mallinson regimen and combined 5-fluorouracil, doxorubicin, and cisplatin. Cancer 1990;65:2201–2212.

92. Dougherty JB, Kelsen D, Kemeny N, Magill G, Botet J, Niedzwiecki D. Advanced pancreatic cancer: a phase I-II trial of cisplatin, high-dose cytarabine, and caffeine. J Natl Cancer Inst 1989;81:1735–1738.

93. Kelson D, Hudis C, Niedzwiecki D, et al. A phase III comparison trial of streptozotocin, mitomycin, and 5-fluorouracil with cisplatin, cytosine arabinoside, and caffeine in patients with advanced pancreatic carcinoma. Cancer 1991;68(5):965–969.

94. DeCaprio J, Mayer R, Gonin R, Arbuck S. Flourouracil with high-dose leucovorin in previously untreated patients with advanced adenocarcinoma of the pancreas: results of a phase II trial. J Clin Oncol 1991; 9(12):2128–2133.

95. Crown J, Casper E, Botet J, et al. Lack of efficacy of high-dose leucovorin and fluorouracil in patients with advanced pancreatic adenocarcinoma. J Clin Oncol 1991;9(9):1682–1686.

96. Isacoff W, Reber H, Tompkins R, et al. Continuous 5-fluorouracil, calcium leucovorin, mitomycin-C, and dipyridamole; treatment for patients with locally advanced pancreatic cancer (abstract). Proc Annu Meet Am Soc Clin Oncol 1995;14:471.

97. Gastrointestinal Tumor Study Group. Comparative therapeutic trial of radiation with or without chemotherapy in pancreatic carcinoma. Int J Radiat Oncol Biol Phys 1979;5:1643–1647.

98. Kaiser MH, Ellenberg SS. Pancreatic cancer: adjuvant combined radiation and chemotherapy following curative resection. Arch Surg 1985;120: 899–903.

99. Gastrointestinal Tumor Study Group. Further evidence of effective adjuvant combined radiation and chemotherapy following curative resection of pancreatic cancer. Cancer 1987;59:2006–2010.

100. Falkson G, MacIntyre JM, Moretel CB. Eastern Cooperative Oncology Group experience with chemotherapy for inoperable gallbladder and bile duct cancer. Cancer 1984;54:965–969.

101. Crooke S, Bradner W. Mitomycin-c: a review. Cancer Treat Rev 1976;3:121–139.

102. Harvey JH, Smith FP, Schein PS. 5-Fluorouracil, mitomycin, and doxorubicin (FAM) in carcinoma of the biliary tract. J Clin Oncol 1984;2:1245–1250.

103. Oberfield RA, Rossi RL. The role of chemotherapy in the treatment of bile duct cancer. World J Surg 1988;12:105–108.

104. Warren K, Mountain J, Lloyd-Jones W. Malignant tumors of the bile ducts. Br J Surg 1972;59:501–503.

105. Watkins E, Oberfield R, Cady B, Clouse M. Arterial infusion chemotherapy of diffuse hepatic malignancies. Prog Clin Cancer 1978;7:235–237.

106. Whittington R, Neuberg D, Tester W, et al. Protracted intravenous fluorouracil infusion with radiation therapy in the management of localized pancreaticobiliary carcinoma: a phase I Eastern Cooperative Oncology Group trial. J Clin Oncol 1995;13(1):227–232.

107. Ashley SW, Wells SA Jr. Tumors of the small intestine. Semin Oncol 1988;15:116–128.

108. Jigyasu D, Bedikian A, Stroehlein J. Chemo-

therapy for primary adenocarcinoma of the small bowel. Cancer 1984;53:23–25.

109. Curreri A, Ansfield F, McIver F, et al. Clinical studies with 5-fluorouracil. Cancer Res 1958;18:748–784.

110. Hansen RM. Systemic therapy in metastatic colorectal cancer. Arch Int Med 1990;150:2265–2269.

111. Lokich J, Ahlgren J, Gullo J, et al. A prospective randomized comparison of continuous infusion fluorouracil with a conventional bolus schedule in metastatic colorectal carcinoma: a Mid-Atlantic Oncology Program study. J Clin Oncol 1989;7:425–432.

112. Petrelli N, Herrera L, Rustum Y, et al. A prospective randomized trial of 5-fluorouracil versus 5-fluorouracil and high dose leucovorin in previously untreated patients with advanced colorectal carcinoma. J Clin Oncol 1987;5:1559–1565.

113. Petrelli N, Douglass H, Herrera L, et al. The modulation of fluorouracil with leucovorin in metastatic colorectal carcinoma: a prospective randomized phase III trial. J Clin Oncol 1989;7:1419–1426.

114. Nobile M, Vidili M, Sobrero A, et al. 5-Fluorouracil alone or combined with high dose folinic acid in advanced colorectal cancer patients: a randomized trial (abstract). Proc Annu Meet Am Soc Clin Oncol 1988;7:371.

115. Advanced Colorectal Cancer Meta-Analysis Project. Modulation of fluorouracil by leucovorin in patients with advanced colorectal cancer: evidence in terms of response rate. J Clin Oncol 1992;10:896–903.

116. Carter SK. Large bowel cancer—the current status of treatment (editorial). J Natl Cancer Inst 1976; 56:3–10.

117. Moertel C, Schutt A, Hahn R, et al. Therapy of advanced colorectal cancer with a combination of 5-fluorouracil, methyl-1,3-cis(2-chloroethyl)-1-nitrosourea and vincristine. J Natl Cancer Inst 1975;36:675–682.

118. Posey L, Morgan L. Methyl-CCNU versus methyl-CCNU and 5-fluorouracil in carcinoma of the large bowel. Cancer Treat Rep 1977;61:1453–1458.

119. Kemeny N, Yagoda A, Braun D, et al. Randomized study of 2 different schedules of methyl-CCNU, 5-FU, and vincristine for metastatic colorectal carcinoma. Cancer 1979;43:78–82.

120. Kemeny N, Yagoda A, Braun D. Metastatic colorectal carcinoma: a prospective randomized trial of methyl CCNU, 5-fluorouracil (5-FU) and vincristine (MOF) versus MOF plus streptozotocin (MOF-Strep). Cancer 1983;51:20–24.

121. Gastrointestinal Tumor Study Group. Phase II study of methyl-CCNU, vincristine, 5-fluorouracil, and streptozotocin in advanced colorectal cancer. J Clin Oncol 1984;2:770–773.

122. Boice J, Greene M, Killen J, et al. Leukemia and pre-leukemia after adjuvant treatment of gastrointestinal cancer with semustine (methyl-CCNU). N Engl J Med 1983;309:1079–1083.

123. Carlson R, Sikic B. Continuous infusion or bolus injection in cancer chemotherapy. Ann Intern Med 1983;99:823–833.

124. Lokich J, Bothe A, Fine N, Perri J. Phase I study of protracted venous infusion of 5-fluorouracil. Cancer 1981;48:823–833.

125. Lokich J, Ahlgren J, Gullo J, et al. A prospective randomized comparison of continuous infusion fluorouracil with a conventional bolus schedule in metastatic colorectal carcinoma: a Mid-Atlantic Oncology Program study. J Clin Oncol 1989;7:425–432.

126. Grem JL, Hoth DF, Hamilton JM, King SA, Leyland-Jones B. Overview of current status and future direction of clinical trials with 5-fluorouracil in combination with folinic acid. Cancer Treat Rep 1987; 71:1249–1264.

127. Petrelli N, Douglass H, Herrera L, et al. The modulation of fluorouracil with leucovorin in metastatic colorectal carcinoma: a prospective randomized phase III trial. J Clin Oncol 1989;7:1419–1426.

128. Nobile M, Vidili M, Sobrero A, et al. 5-Fluorouracil alone or combined with high dose folinic acid in advanced colorectal cancer patients: a randomized trial (abstract). Proc Annu Meet Am Soc Clin Oncol 1988;7:371.

129. Doroshow J, Multhauf P, Leong L, et al. Prospective randomized comparison of fluorouracil and fluorouracil and high dose continuous infusion leucovorin calcium for the treatment of advanced measurable colorectal cancer in patients previously unexposed to chemotherapy. J Clin Oncol 1990;8:491–501.

130. Erlichman C, Fine S, Wong A, Elhakim T. A randomized trial of fluorouracil and folinic acid in patients with metastatic colorectal carcinoma. J Clin Oncol 1988;6:469–475.

131. Poon MA, O'Connell MJ, Moertel CG, et al. Biochemical modulation of fluorouracil: evidence of significant improvement of survival and quality of life in advanced colorectal carcinoma. J Clin Oncol 1989; 7:1407–1418.

132. Poon M, O'Connell M, Weiand H, et al. Biochemical modulation of fluorouracil with leucovorin: confirmatory evidence of improved therapeutic efficacy in advanced colorectal cancer. J Clin Oncol 1991; 9:1967–1972.

133. Buroker T, O'Connell M, Weiand S, et al. Randomized comparison of two schedules of fluorouracil and leucovorin in the treatment of advanced colorectal cancer. J Clin Oncol 1994;12:14–20.

134. Advanced Colorectal Cancer Meta-Analysis Project. Modulation of fluorouracil by leucovorin in patients with advanced colorectal cancer: evidence in terms of response rate. J Clin Oncol 1992;10:896–903.

135. Wadler S, Schwartz EL, Goldman M, et al. Fluorouracil and recombinant alpha-2a-interferon: an active regimen against advanced colorectal carcinoma. J Clin Oncol 1989;7:1769–1775.

136. Wadler S, Lembersky B, Atkins M, et al. Phase II trial of fluorouracil and recombinant interferon alfa-2a in patients with advanced colorectal carcinoma: an Eastern Cooperative Oncology Group study. J Clin Oncol 1991;9:1808–1810.

137. Chang AE, Schneider PD, Sugarbaker PH, Simpson C, Culnane M, Steinberg SM. A prospective randomized trial of regional versus systemic continuous 5-fluorodeoxyuridine chemotherapy in the treatment of colorectal metastases. Ann Surg 1987;206:685–693.

138. Neiderhuber J. Hepatic artery chemotherapy for colorectal cancer metastatic to the liver. Surg Annu 1987;19:263–277.

139. Kemeny N, Daly J, Oderman P, et al. Hepatic artery pump infusion toxicity and results in patients with metastatic colorectal carcinoma. J Clin Oncol 1984;2:595–600.

140. Hohn D, Stagg R, Price D, et al. Avoidance of

gastroduodenal toxicity in patients receiving hepatic arterial 5-fluoro-2'-deoxyuridine. J Clin Oncol 1985; 3:1257–1260.

141. Kemeny N, Canti J, Cohen A, et al. Phase II study of hepatic arterial floxuridine, leucovorin, and dexamethasone for unresectable liver metastases from colorectal carcinoma. J Clin Oncol;12:2288–2295.

142. Kemeny N, Daly J, Reichman B, Geller N, Botet J, Oderman P. Intrahepatic or systemic infusion of fluorodeoxyuridine in patients with liver metastases from colorectal carcinoma: a randomized trial. Ann Intern Med 1987;107:459–465.

143. Hohn DC, Stagg RJ, Friedman MA, et al. A randomized trial of continuous intravenous versus hepatic intra-arterial floxuridine in patients with colorectal cancer metastatic to the liver: the Northern California Oncology Group trial. J Clin Oncol 1989;7:1646–1654.

144. Martin JK Jr, O'Connell MJ, Wieand HS, et al. Intra-arterial floxuridine vs systemic fluorouracil for hepatic metastases from colorectal cancer: a randomized trial. Arch Surg 1990;125:1022–1027.

145. Wagman L, Kemeny M, Leong L, et al. A prospective randomized evaluation of the treatment of colorectal cancer metastatic to the liver. J Clin Oncol 1990; 8:1885–1893.

146. Rougier P, Laplanche A, Huguier M, et al. Hepatic arterial infusion of floxuridine in patients with liver metastases from colorectal carcinoma: long-term results of a prospective randomized trial. J Clin Oncol 1992;10:1112–1118.

147. Buyse M, Zeleniuch-Jacquotte A, Chalmers TC. Adjuvant therapy of colorectal cancer: why we still don't know. JAMA 1988;259:3571–3578.

148. Wolmark N, Fisher B, Rockette H, et al. Postoperative adjuvant chemotherapy or BCG for colon cancer: results from NSABP protocol C-01. J Natl Cancer Inst 1988;80(1):30–36.

149. Gastrointestinal Tumor Study Group. Adjuvant therapy of colon cancer—results of a prospectively randomized trial. N Engl J Med 1984;310:737–743.

150. Higgins G, Amadeo J, McElhinney J, et al. Efficacy of prolonged intermittent therapy with combined 5-fluorouracil and methyl-CCNU following resection for carcinoma of the large bowel: a Veterans Administration Surgical Oncology report. Cancer 1984; 53:1–8.

151. MacDonald JS, Schnall SF. The role of 5-FU plus levamisole in the therapy of colon cancer. Princ Pract Oncol Updates 1991;5(1):1–9.

152. Tripodi D, Parks L, Brugmans J. Drug-induced restoration of cutaneous delayed hypersensitivity in anergic patients with cancer. N Engl J Med 1973; 289:354–357.

153. Miwa H, Kawai T, Nakahara H, et al. Decrease in cell mediated immunity by surgical intervention and its prevention by levamisole. Int J Immunopharmacol 1980;2:31–36.

154. Davies N, Kynaston H, Yates J, et al. Reticuloendothelial stimulation: levamisole compared. Dis Colon Rectum 1993;36:1054–1059.

155. Holcombe R, Stewart R, Betzing K, Kannan K. Alteration of lymphocyte phenotype in patients receiving adjuvant 5-FU-levamisole (abstract). Proc Annu Meet Am Soc Clin Oncol 1993;12:295.

156. ElMuataz E, Abdalla G, Blair G, et al. Mecha-

nism of synergy of levamisole and fluorouracil: induction of human leukocyte antigen class I in a colorectal cancer cell line. J Natl Cancer Inst 1995;87(7):489–495.

157. Laurie JA, Moertel CG, Fleming TR, et al. Surgical adjuvant therapy for large bowel carcinoma: an evaluation of levamisole and the combination of levamisole and fluorouracil. J Clin Oncol 1989;7:1447–1456.

158. Moertel CB, Fleming TR, MacDonald JS, Haller DG, Laurie JA, Goodman PJ. Levamisole and fluorouracil for adjuvant therapy of resected colon carcinoma. N Engl J Med 1990;322:352–358.

159. NIH Consensus Conference: adjuvant therapy for patients with colon and rectal cancer. JAMA 1990; 264:1444.

160. Wolmark N, Rockette H, Fisher B, et al. The benefit of leucovorin-modulated fluorouracil as postoperative adjuvant therapy for primary colon cancer: results from National Surgical Adjuvant Breast and Bowel Project protocol C-03. J Clin Oncol 1993;11:1879–1887.

161. O'Connell M, Maillard J, Macdonald J, et al. An intergroup trial of intensive 5-FU and low dose leucovorin as surgical adjuvant for high risk colon cancer (abstract). Proc Annu Meet Am Soc Clin Oncol 1993; 12:190.

162. Erlichman C, Marsoni S, Seitz J, et al. Event free and overall survival is increased by FUFA in resected B and C colon cancer (abstract). Proc Annu Meet Am Soc Clin Oncol 1994;13:194.

163. Taylor I, Machin D, Mullee M, Trotter G, Cooke T, West C. A randomized controlled trial of adjuvant portal vein cytotoxic perfusion in colorectal cancer. Br J Surg 1985;72:359–363.

164. Wolmark N, Rockette H, Wickerham DL, et al. Adjuvant therapy of Duke's A, B, and C adenocarcinoma of the colon with portal vein fluorouracil hepatic infusion: preliminary results of National Surgical Adjuvant Breast and Bowel Project protocol C-02. J Clin Oncol 1990;8:1466–1475.

165. Fisher B, Wolmark N, Rockette H, et al. Postoperative adjuvant chemotherapy or radiation therapy for rectal cancer: results from NSABP protocol R-01. J Natl Cancer Inst 1988;80:21–29.

166. Gastrointestinal Tumor Study Group. Radiation therapy and fluorouracil with or without semustine for the treatment of patients with surgical adjuvant adenocarcinoma of the rectum. J Clin Oncol 1992; 10:549–557.

167. Krook JE, Moertel CG, Gunderson LL, et al. Effective surgical adjuvant therapy for high-risk rectal carcinoma. N Engl J Med 1991;324:709–715.

168. O'Connell MJ, Weiand H, Krook J, et al. Lack of value for methyl CCNU (MeCCNU) as a component of effective rectal cancer surgical adjuvant therapy: interim analysis of intergroup protocol 86-47-51 (abstract). Proc Am Soc Clin Oncol 1991;10:134.

169. O'Connell M, Martenson J, Wieand H, et al. Improving adjuvant therapy for rectal cancer by combining protracted-infusion fluorouracil with radiation therapy after curative surgery. N Engl J Med 1994; 331:502–507.

170. Lyss AP. Appendiceal malignancies. Semin Oncol 1988;15:129–137.

171. Borman B, Moertel C, O'Connell M. Carcinoma of the anal canal: a clinical and pathologic study of 188 cases. Cancer 1984;54:114–125.

172. Nigro ND, Vatikevicius VK, Considine B Jr. Combined therapy for cancer of the anal canal: a preliminary report. Dis Colon Rectum 1974;17:354–356.

173. Newman HK, Quan SHQ. Multimodality therapy for epidermoid carcinoma of the anus. Cancer 1976;37:12–18.

174. Bruckner HW, Spigelman MK, Mandel E, et al. Carcinoma of the anus treated with a combination of radiotherapy and chemotherapy. Cancer Treat Rep 1979;63:395–398.

175. Wanebo HJ, Futrell W, Constable W. Multimodality approach to surgical management of locally advanced epidermoid carcinoma of the anorectum. Cancer 1981;47:2817–2826.

176. Sischy B, Remington JH, Hinson EJ, Sobel SH, Woll JE. Definitive treatment of anal-canal carcinoma by means of radiation therapy and chemotherapy. Dis Colon Rectum 1982;25:685–688.

177. Cummings BJ, Rider WD, Harwood AR, et al. Combined radical radiation therapy and chemotherapy for primary squamous cell carcinoma of the anal canal. Cancer Treat Rep 1982;66:489–492.

178. Nigro ND, Seydel HG, Considine B Jr, Vaitkevicius VK, Leichman L, Kinzie JJ. Combined preoperative radiation and chemotherapy for squamous cell carcinoma of the anal canal. Cancer 1983;51:390–395.

179. Michaelson RA, Magill GB, Quan SHQ, Leaming RH, Nikrui M, Stearnes MW. Preoperative chemotherapy and radiation therapy in the management of anal epidermoid carcinoma. Cancer 1983;51:390–395.

180. Flam MS, John M, Lovalo LJ, et al. Definitive nonsurgical therapy for epithelial malignancies of the anal canal: a report of 12 cases. Cancer 1983;51:1378–1387.

181. Tiver KW, Langlands AO. Synchronous chemotherapy and radiotherapy for carcinoma of the anal canal—an alternative to abdominoperineal resection. Aust NZ J Surg 1984;54:101–108.

182. Sischy B. The use of radiation therapy combined with chemotherapy in the management of squamous cell carcinoma of the anus and marginally resectable adenocarcinoma of the rectum. Int J Radiat Oncol Biol Phys 1985;11:1587–1593.

183. Smith DE, Muff NS, Shetabi H. Combined preoperative neoadjuvant radiotherapy and chemotherapy for anal and rectal cancer. Am J Surg 1986;151:577–580.

184. Leichman L, Nigro N, Vaitkevicius VK, et al. Cancer of the anal canal: model for preoperative adjuvant combined modality therapy. Am J Med 1985;78:211–215.

185. Enker WE, Heilwell M, Janov AJ, et al. Improved survival in epidermoid carcinoma of the anus in association with preoperative multidisciplinary therapy. Arch Surg 1986;121:1386–1390.

186. Khater R, Frenoy M, Bourry J, et al. Cisplatin plus 5-fluorouracil in the treatment of metastatic anal squamous cell carcinoma. Cancer Treat Rep 1986;70:1345–1346.

187. Ajani J, Carrasco H, Jackson D, et al. Combination of cisplatin plus fluoropyrimidine chemotherapy effective against liver metastases from carcinoma of the anal canal. Am J Med 1989;87:221–224.

188. Salem P, Habboubi N, Naanasissie E, et al. Effectiveness of cisplatin in the treatment of anal squamous cell carcinoma. Cancer Treat Rep 1985;69:891–893.

189. Wilking N, Petrelli N, Herrera, et al. Phase II study of combination of bleomycin, vincristine, and high-dose methotrexate (BOM) with leucovorin rescue in advanced squamous cell carcinoma of the anal canal. Cancer Chemother Pharmacol 1985;15:300–302.

56

Chemotherapy of Endocrine Tumors

Richard J. McKittrick and Ronald L. Stephens

Few malignant neoplasms afford the significant managerial challenges of those associated with cancers arising in an endocrine organ. Not only do cancers of these organs require the usual spectrum of local and systemic therapies, they often produce hormones, which necessitates additional systemic treatment directed at counteracting excessive hormone secretion. It may even be necessary to counteract the hormone produced from the tumor before the primary cancer can be removed safely.

For many years there has been the recognition that the pathologic origins of many secretory cancers have a shared commonalty, being of neuroectodermal origin and referred to as *a*mine *p*recursor *u*ptake and *d*ecarboxylation tumors (APUD tumors or apudomas) (1). This notion of a common neuroectoderm origin has helped the medical community understand why tumors arising from such disparate anatomic origins as the adrenal gland and the bronchus (small cell tumors) may share an identical secretory potential and physiologic expression (i.e., excessive cortisone secretion). Additional treatment challenges are presented when some tumors fail to produce an otherwise expected secretory phenomenon even when liver metastases are present (i.e., rectal carcinoids). Endocrine cancers, even when metastatic, may have highly variable doubling times. Since many, although not all, of these patients with metastatic endocrine cancers may have many years of life left, the decision to treat must be balanced against several factors: the presence or absence of end-organ disability induced by hormone production, the local unresectable anatomic impingement on normal tissues, and the relative potential of cytotoxic therapy to be successful. This chapter explores the systemic management of endocrine neoplasms, leaving the more exotic descriptions of chemical diagnosis and detection to more comprehensive texts.

ADRENAL GLAND NEOPLASMS

As one might expect, the dual anatomic and physiologic nature of this gland gives rise to neoplasms with at least two distinct clinical patterns. Systemic treatment is largely dictated by whether or not the cancer arises from the cortical or medullary portion of the gland.

Adrenal Cortical Carcinomas

Although malignant neoplasms of either the cortex or medulla are rare, more work has been directed at the systemic therapy for those cancers arising in the cortex. Cortical adrenal neoplasms have an average survival of less than 3 months and may or may not produce hormones. The ability of a cortical cancer to produce hormones may have a modestly favorable impact on survival (2).

Once it was observed in 1947 that the insecticide DDD caused adrenal necrosis in canines, it was only a matter of time before some chemical relative would be tried in humans with adrenal cortical cancer (3, 4). The insecticide-related compound, o,p'DDD[1,1 dichloro-2(O-chlorophenyl)-2-(p-chlorophenyl) ethane] (mitotane), has been used for several decades in the treatment of this cancer and, in combination with 5-fluorouracil (5-FU), has even been credited with the isolated cure of a patient with cortical cancer metastatic to liver and lung (5). A dose of 8 to 10 g/day is frequently recommended, with the major limiting toxicities occurring in the gastrointestinal tract and the nervous system. Mitotane blocks adrenal steroid 11-β-hydroxylation, decreases cortisol production, and leads to cortical atrophy with chronic usage.

As a single agent, o,p'DDD has been used in humans with adrenal cortical cancer for three decades, and as a consequence, response criteria may vary from one study to another. Table 56.1 collates the reported series from a wide range of different clinical sources. In an era when response criteria were poorly defined, if at all, one of the first published series of patients with adrenal cortical carcinoma was a group of eight patients treated at the NCI (4). Bergenstal et al. reported a decrease in steroid production in all eight patients and "objective regression" in three of them.

Two important studies, with large numbers of patients, are those of Hutter and Kayhoe and Lubitz et al. (6, 7). These two reported series represent sequential reports on the NCI multiinstitutional trials, covering two periods in time, and sharing at least a common definition for steroid response (>30% decrease from baseline). The Hutter series (1960 to 1965) of patients demonstrated that 45 of 62 (73%) patients fulfilled this steroid response definition, and 20 of 59 (34%) showed an objective response in measurable tumor (6). The later series of Lubitz (1965 to 1969) revealed a steroid response in 52 of 61 (85%) patients and a measurable decrease in tumor size in 46 of 75 (61%) patients (7). These two trials seem to be among the most optimistic with regard to the effectiveness of o,p'DDD in patients with adrenal cortical carcinoma.

More recent studies include the two-part overlapping reports from M. D. Anderson, in which the last update of their patients reported o,p'DDD to be "moderately to very effective" in

Table 56.1. Adrenal Carcinoma: Pooled Response Rates Using Mitotane

Steroid Response (%)	Tumor Response (%)	Reference
8/8 (100)	3/8 (38)	(4)
45/62 (73)	20/59 (34)	(6)
52/61 (85)	46/75 (61)	(7)
?	8/34 (24)	(8)
?	9/47 (19)	(9)
?	21/72 (29)	(10)
?	8/36 (22)	(11)
Total 105/131 (80)	115/331 (35)	

9 of 47 (19%) patients (9, 12). A similar response rate of patients with measurable metastases was reported in Holland (8 of 34; 24%) (8). The Dutch report is somewhat difficult to interpret, since if one confines the analysis to only "measurable" disease patients, the denominator is reduced to 28, and with 8 responders the response rate increases to 29%. Regardless, the most important aspect of the Dutch study relates to the pharmacology data, in which serum levels of o,p'DDD exceeding 14 μg/mL seemed necessary to improve survival (8). During treatment with mitotane, the patient should receive glucocorticoid replacement and mineralocorticoid replacement if necessary.

To summarize by collating the o,p'DDD data from seven separate series, Table 56.1 shows an overall reported steroid response of 80% and a measurable tumor response rate of 35%. Many of these data were acquired in the era before standardized response criteria were used, and the largest number of the patients reported were studied by over 100 different investigators.

The published information about other agents in the treatment of adrenal cortical carcinoma usually reflect anecdotal reports or small series. Table 56.2 is a collation of some of the single agents and combination chemotherapy that have been used in adrenal cortical carcinoma. Cisplatin is a popular constituent (17, 19–25). Other agents tried without benefit (single case reports) include BCNU, methotrexate, and vinblastine.

The Eastern Cooperative Oncology Group (ECOG) reported their study comparing mitotane and Adriamycin in a crossover fashion (11). They concluded that mitotane or Adriamycin used initially can induce tumor regression in about 22% and 19% of selected patients, respectively. They also noted that Adriamycin is ineffective as second-line chemotherapy for patients with well-differentiated or functioning tumors for whom mitotane is ineffective. Schlumberger et al. reported a series of 16 patients treated with 5-fluorouracil, doxorubin, and cisplatin with an overall response rate of 23% (25). They observed one complete response and two partial responses; they also noted cardiotoxicity in three patients, myelotoxicity in four, and nephrotoxicity in one.

Because of earlier interest in cisplatin, the Southwest Oncology Group (SWOG) conducted a phase II study of mitotane and cisplatin in 42 patients (19). While the objective response rate was 30%, the toxicity of the regimen was consid-

Table 56.2. Adrenal Carcinoma: Response Rates Using Various Single Agents and Combination Chemotherapy

Drug(s)[a]	No. of Patients	Efficacy (PR or CR)	Reference
Single agents			
CDDP	1	1	(13)
CDDP	4	4	(14)
CDDP	4	1 CR, 1 PR	(15)
DOX	8	1	(16)
DOX	16	19% PR	(17)
Suramin	21	3 PR	(18)
Combination chemotherapy			
CDDP + mitotane	37	11 (30%) PR	(19)
CDDP + VP16	2	2 PR	(20)
CDDP + VP16 + DOX	2	2 PR	(18)
CDDP + VP16 + DOX + mitotane	7	3 PR	(21)
CDDP + VP16 + BLEO	4	1 CR, 2 PR	(22)
CDDP + VP16 + CTX + VCR	1	1	(23)
CDDP + DOX + CTX	11	18%	(24)
CDDP + DOX + 5FU	13	23%	(25)
CTX + VCR + mCCNU + BLEO	2	1 PR	(17)
CTX + MELPH or peptichemo	12	2 PR	(17)
STZ + mitotane	3	2 PR	(26)

[a]BLEO, bleomycin; CDDP, cisplatin; CTX, cyclophosphamide; DOX, doxorubicin; mCCNU, methylCCNU; MELPH, melphalan; STZ, streptozocin; VCR, vincristine; VP16, etoposide; 5FU, 5-fluorouracil.

ered moderate to severe. A total of 16 patients (47%) discontinued therapy because of the side effects. The current trial evaluates the combination of cisplatin and VP-16, and patients without prior exposure will receive o,p'DDD at the time of progression.

Forty percent of adrenocortical carcinomas produce excess steroid hormones, including glucocorticoid, androgen, mineralocorticoid, and estrogen (27). Palliative therapy has been attempted using such steroid inhibitors as aminoglutethimide and ketoconazole. Aminoglutethimide was originally marketed as an anticonvulsive but was found to produce adrenal insufficiency. The earliest case report of its successful use in a patient with adrenal cortical carcinoma was published by investigators from the University of Michigan in 1966 (28). This steroid inhibitor has found wider use in breast cancer patients than in patients with adrenal cortical carcinoma. Perhaps this is secondary to a gradual "escape" seen in the adrenal steroid suppression observed in this early case report (28).

A more recent agent noted for its broad suppression of steroidogenesis is ketoconazole, the oral antifungal agent recognized for its ability to block the conversion of lanosterol to ergosterol (29) as well as exhibiting cytotoxic in vitro activity against human cancer cell lines (30). With this dual action, ketoconazole would seem an ideal agent for future testing alone or in combination with cytotoxic chemotherapy. The most recent compound to be considered in the treatment of patients with adrenal cortical carcinoma is the polysulfonated naphthylurea antiparasitic drug, suramin. In a small series from the NCI, suramin achieved 2 partial responses out of 10 patients, but it has the potential for significant toxicity in the form of fever, hepatic injury, renal damage, rash, and a coagulopathy (18).

At this time, it would seem that patients with adrenal cortical carcinoma are candidates for investigative trials, studies that might include any of the compounds mentioned above or a new, untested phase II agent.

Adrenal Medulla Carcinomas (Pheochromocytomas)

Tumors arising in the medullary portion of the adrenal gland are very rare and may present a part of the syndrome of multiple endocrine neoplasias (MEN-2 a and b). The only series of any size in which patients with malignant pheochromocytomas have received consistent systemic treatment has been conducted at the NCI

(31). They used a combination of cyclophosphamide, vincristine, and dacarbazine; 11 of 14 (79%) patients demonstrated a decrease in catecholamine, and 8 patients (57%) showed actual tumor shrinkage (2 complete responses (CRs) and 6 partial responses (PRs)). Traditionally, clues for chemotherapeutic treatment of patients with pheochromocytoma have been found in the literature of neuroblastoma. Future clues for systemic therapy will likely continue to originate in leads from this more common tumor.

THYROID CANCER

Most patients with thyroid cancer are managed by surgery, thyroid replacement, thyroid-stimulating hormone (TSH) suppression, and, in many instances, ^{131}I. Cancers arising in this organ display a wide range of natural histories. There are slow-growing well-differentiated histologies such as papillary, follicular, and Hurthle cell types; a calcitonin-producing "C"-cell tumor that behaves more aggressively, medullary carcinoma; and finally, a frequently lethal tumor noted for locally aggressive behavior as well as vascular dissemination and early death, the anaplastic variation.

Two decades ago, two antibiotic antineoplastics, bleomycin and Adriamycin (doxorubicin), began to show early activity in patients with thyroid cancer (32, 33). Perhaps the latter agent, Adriamycin, has since received the greatest investigative attention, both as a single agent and in combination with other chemotherapy drugs. Three separate studies constitute the pooled data evaluation of Adriamycin found in Table 56.3 (34–36). This table reflects minimal activity in the anaplastic variety, with 5 of 35 (14%) responders but modest activity in well-differentiated histologies (12 of 38 (32%)) and in medullary cancers as well (4 of 13 (31%)). The pooled data in the anaplastic variety reflect a more disappointing activity for Adriamycin than previously thought, which may depend in part on the lower dose (60

Table 56.3. Adriamycin as a Single Agent in Thyroid Cancer: Pooled Data

	No.	PR(%)
Well differentiated	38	12 (32)
Medullary	13	4 (31)
Anaplastic	35	5 (14)

Data from references 34–36.

mg/m^2) used in 21 of the 35 (60%) pooled patients (36).

Regardless, the absence of meaningful phase II information about other agents in thyroid cancer leaves Adriamycin as not only the most studied of cancer drugs but also the most active compound around which to build other combinations. Frustrated by the poor outcome in high-risk anaplastic patients, the Arizona group resorted to an all-embracing approach that included surgery, ^{131}I therapy, Adriamycin, bleomycin, melphalan, vincristine, and bacillus Calmette-Guerin (BCG) immunotherapy (37). Although their patient population did not have evidence of distant metastases, all patients experienced massive local invasion, a typical finding in the anaplastic histology. Five of their 11 patients remained in complete remission for over 4 years, and it is surprising that a cooperative group has not picked up on this early favorable hint. Centralized histologic review of any trial attempting to study the aggressive anaplastic variety is necessary to separate it from histologies with which it can be confused, that is, lymphoma and the medullary subtype.

Combination chemotherapy in patients with advanced thyroid cancer has been systematically tested in only a few patients. There is only one meaningful randomized trial that compares a single agent (Adriamycin) with a combination (Adriamycin-cisplatin) (36). This ECOG trial is summarized, along with three other nonrandomized studies, in Table 56.4. The ECOG trial places the overall response rate to the combination of Adriamycin/cisplatin at only 28%. However, this trial, unlike the pooled data in Table 56.3, registered a few complete responders, something not recorded in the trial of Adriamycin as a single agent. Further analysis of the ECOG data reveals 2 CRs in the well-differentiated histologies, but most interesting are the 3 CRs in the anaplastic subset. A more exhaustive look at activity of the ECOG two-drug combination by cell type demonstrates 3 of 19 (16%) responses in the well-differentiated cell type, 2 of 6 (33%) in the medullary variety, and 6 of 18 (33%) in the anaplastic subset (36). The other reported CR was from Bukowski et al., where four drugs—Adriamycin, bleomycin, vincristine, and melphalan—also achieved an excellent response in a patient with anaplastic histology (42).

Three recent studies shed light on variations of commonly used chemotherapy. De Besi et al. used the three-drug regimen of Adriamycin, cisplatin, and bleomycin in 22 patients and re-

Table 56.4. Combination Chemotherapy for Thyroid Carcinoma

Agents[a]	No.	Efficacy (PR or CR)	Reference
DOX + CDDP	43	16% and 12%	(36)
DOX + CDDP	22	9% and 0%	(38)
DOX + CDDP + BLEO	22	32% and 9%	(39)
DOX + CDDP + VIND	18	6% and 0%	(40)
DOX + BLEO + VCR	14	50% and 0%	(41)
DOX + BLEO + VCR + MELPH	11	27% and 9%	(42)
MITOX + CDDP + VCR	15	40% and 27%	(43)
CTX + VCR + DTIC	7	29% and 0%	(44)
TOTAL	152	23% and 8% RR = 31%	

[a]BLEO, bleomycin; CDDP, cisplatin; CTX, cyclophosphamide; DOX, doxorubicin; DTIC, dacarbazine; MELPH, melphalan; MITOX, mitroxantrone; VCR, vincristine; VIND, vindesine.

ported 2 CRs (9%) and 7 PRs (32%) (39). Overall toxicity was described as "mild." Another group used Adriamycin, cisplatin, and vindesine in 18 patients with disappointing results, 1 PR (6%) (41). The third group treated patients with mitoxantrone, cisplatin, and vincristine and reported 4 CRs (27%) and 6 PRs (40%) (43). This was in a small group of 15 patients and bears repeating to confirm the level of activity.

In most thyroid studies, advanced thyroid cancer of other histologies and anaplastic thyroid cancer are studied together. One group of seven patients with advanced medullary thyroid carcinoma was treated with the cyclophosphamide, vincristine, and dacarbazine regimen (CVD) (44), a regimen reported to have activity in other advanced neuroendocrine tumors (31). CVD resulted in 2 PRs (tumor and biochemical responses), 1 biochemical-only PR, and 1 stable tumor and biochemical response for 14 months. This raises the question of whether medullary thyroid cancer should be treated differently than other advanced thyroid neoplasms.

Table 56.4 summarizes the overall reported response rate to combination chemotherapy in thyroid cancer at 31%. Although this percentage response is modest, leaving room to encourage new phase II trials, finding CRs from the combinations suggests that more than one drug may be indicated in patients with this cancer who are not eligible for research trials. Equally important in the care of these patients today is the small Arizona trial in anaplastic cancer patients ("high risk", locally invasive tumor), in which significant numbers of patients in their combination trial were free of disease after 4 years (37). Since there are small numbers of patients with this al-

most uniformly fatal subtype of thyroid cancer, it would seem that an intergroup study of combined aggressive therapy is overdue.

PANCREATIC ENDOCRINE CANCERS

There is a complex array of pancreatic endocrine cancers, each tumor type representing a unique challenge in primary management, anticipated hormonal production, clinical presentation, and potential responsiveness to systemic chemotherapy. In some instances, these tumors may not even arise in the pancreas itself, but rather in some adjacent intestinal site such as the stomach or small bowel. A knowledge of pancreatic endocrine cancers provides an excellent background for understanding the secretory endocrinology of the normal gland and vice versa.

Many endocrine pancreatic tumors secrete several hormones but are classified by the resultant clinical syndrome. The best-known neoplasms of the endocrine pancreas include gastrinomas (δ cells producing gastrin and the Zollinger-Ellison syndrome (ZES), of which 65% are malignant), functional islet cell tumors (α-cells, glucagonomas, 50% malignant; β-cell-insulinomas, 10% malignant), islet cell tumors producing excessive vasoactive intestinal polypeptide and pancreatic cholera (VIPomas, 50% malignant), islet cell tumors producing the 14–amino acid polypeptide inhibitor somatostatin (somatostatinomas), and the so-called nonfunctional islet cell carcinomas. The nonfunctional islet cell carcinomas include two tumors releasing hormones without clinical symptoms. This includes pancreatic polypeptide (PPomas) and neurotensin (neurotensinomas) secreting tumors. Histologically, they are indistinguishable from functional islet cell tumors.

Other uncommon hormone-producing tumors often arising in the pancreas include GHRFomas (release excess growth hormone releasing factor) (45). In one series of 30 cases, 30% began in the pancreas, 53% in the lung, 10% in the small intestine, and one case in the adrenal gland (46). Histologically, it is typical of other islet cell tumors, and it can metastasize. There are also reports of pancreatic endocrine tumors causing Cushing's syndrome (ACTHoma?) (47) and hyperparathyroidism (PTHoma?) (48).

All of these cancers are sufficiently rare that analysis of their individual sensitivities to chemotherapy is confounded by studies that lump the various types together. When they are separated, even a well-designed trial will possess such small numbers as to raise doubts about the usefulness of any recommended agent or agents. Table 56.5 represents a combination of studies investigating chemotherapy in pancreatic endocrine tumors. Objective response usually includes a 50% or more reduction in hormone levels and/or a 50% decrease in measurable tumor size.

One of the earliest successful chemotherapeutic agents to show promise in patients with functional β islet cell tumors, as well as in some nonfunctional islet cell cancers, was streptozocin. The first patient successfully treated with streptozocin suffered from what was perceived to be multiple hormone expression, including excessive secretion of insulin, gastrin, and glucagon (69). Liver metastases became smaller, and all excess secretory expression normalized. Later, another favorable objective and symptomatic response was recorded in a patient with a nonfunctional islet cell tumor, where a marked decrease in liver size and an increase in body weight occurred (70). In 1972, the NCI summarized the larger trial they had been supervising, reporting favorable biochemical responses in about 64% of 39 analyzed patients (49). In reality, 10 patients had complete biochemical responses, 11 a "good" partial biochemical response, and 4 a "poor" partial response. Patients with measurable disease showed 6 "good" partial responses and 5 complete responses, for an overall response rate in measurable patients of 11 of 30 (37%).

Since this first encouraging report with streptozocin, others have reported similar responses (51, 52, 71). Other single agents such as doxorubicin (53), carboplatin (58), and VP-16 have been

Table 56.5. Chemotherapy for Pancreatic Endocrine Tumors

Agent(s)[a]	No.	Objective Response	Reference
STZ	52	26 (50%)	(49)
STZ	42	14 (36%)	(50)
STZ	17	7 (41%)	(51)
STZ	16	10 (62%)	(52)
DOX	20	4 (20%)	(53)
CZT	13	7 (53%)	(54)
CZT	33	10 (30%)	(55)
DTIC	11	1 (9%)	(56)
DTIC	14	7 (50%)	(57)
CBCDA	9	0	(58)
VP16	2	0	(59)
STZ + DOX	38	26 (69%)	(55)
STZ + DOX	14	3 (21%)	(60)
STZ + DOX	25	9 (36%)	(61)
STZ + 5FU	40	25 (63%)	(50)
STZ + 5FU	31	17 (54%)	(62)
STZ + 5FU	34	15 (45%)	(55)
5FU + DOX + CDDP	5	1 (20%)	(63)
CDDP + VP16			
(anaplastic)	18	12 (67%)	(64)
(typical islet cell)	14	2 (14%)	
CZT + 5FU	44	14 (32%)	(65)
Octreotide	66	8 (11%)	(66)
Octreotide	46	8 (17%)	(67)
Octreotide	22	14 (64%)	(68)
Octreotide	19	6 (31%)	(62)
Interferon	57	29 (57%)	(62)
Interferon	22	17 (77%)	(63)

[a]CBCDA, carboplatin; CDDP, cisplatin; CZT, chlorozocin; DOX, doxorubicin; DTIC, dacarbazine; STZ, streptozocin; VP16, etoposide; 5FU, 5-fluorouracil.

used with limited success (61). Dacarbazine (56, 57) and chlorozotocin (54, 55) have shown promising results in some studies but not in others.

Of all the various combinations used, streptozocin plus 5-FU or streptozocin plus doxorubicin seem to be the most likely to produce objective responses in the larger studies (30, 55, 60–62, 71). The regimen of chlorozotocin plus 5-FU has shown modest activity (65). Moertel et al. generated interest with the combination of cisplatin and VP-16 in neuroendocrine tumors (64). Of note were the response rates of 67% in anaplastic neuroendocrine tumors but only 14% in typical islet cell tumors.

Use of the long-acting somatostatin-analogue octreotide has also shown modest activity (11–64% response rate) in pancreatic endocrine tumors (62, 66–68). Much of this "response" is actually a decrease in hormone excretion as compared with actual tumor shrinkage (67, 68). Somatostatin is a tetradecopeptide present throughout the gastrointestinal tract. It reduces plasma levels of insulin, glucagon, gastrin, secretin, motilin, and neurotensin (72).

α-Interferon has a good response rate (62, 73). In a review, Oberg averaged 11 studies for a biochemical response of 42% (range, 0–56%) and a tumor response of 11% (range, 0–21%) (74).

Should treatment of neuroendocrine pancreatic cancer be individualized by the clinical syndrome at diagnosis? (Should nonfunctioning tumors be treated differently than gastrimonas or insulinomas?) Because of the marked differences in biologic responses and tumor responses, octreotide and interferon are probably best reserved for functional neuroendocrine tumors or tumors not responding to chemotherapy (67, 75). Streptozocin and 5-FU or doxorubicin are standard regimens to use in treating unresectable symptomatic disease for all the pancreatic endocrine tumors (75). DTIC has shown promise in several patients with glucagonoma (57). Octreotide has been very helpful in managing symptoms of hormone excess in insulinomas, glucagonomas, and vipomas (68, 76).

MALIGNANT CARCINOID TUMORS

Malignant carcinoid tumors are rare neoplasms that may arise anywhere in the body but usually have their origin in the appendix (38%), ileum (23%), rectum (13%), or bronchus (11.5%) (77–84). Less common anatomic sites include the larynx, ovary, uterine, cervix, and mediastinum. Although rare, these neoplasms are also seen in children (85).

Morphologically and functionally, carcinoid tumors resemble the related, but more aggressive, small cell lung cancers and may even be confused with these tumors during microscopic analysis. Several authors have raised the possibility that in some series of small cell lung cancer, the long-term survivors may in fact be patients with carcinoids (86–88). Pathologists cannot differentiate carcinoids from pancreatic endocrine tumors, nor can they determine the malignant potential unless they see evidence of invasion or metastases. Although capable of producing many types of biologically active substances such as kinins (flushing), histamine, and prostaglandins, the most important substance from a chemical secretory standpoint is serotonin.

Metastatic liver involvement due to gastrointestinal midgut carcinoids can produce high levels of serotonin, which in turn produces diarrhea, retroperitoneal fibrosis, right-sided heart disease, and elevated urinary 5-hydroxyindolacetic acid (5-HIAA). Foregut and hindgut carcinoids are less likely to be associated with the carcinoid syndrome. Successful systemic treatment, or even anesthetic induction, can induce severe hypotension and death from the so-called carcinoid crisis (89). The relatively new secretory inhibitor and inhibitor of target organ hormonal expression, somatostatin, has been credited with protecting carcinoid patients during the life-threatening "carcinoid crisis" sometimes seen in surgery and anesthesia (90–93).

Surgery is regarded as the only curative therapy for carcinoid tumors. Chemotherapy for malignant carcinoid tumors has been less than satisfying. Because of this, most authors suggest palliation of symptoms by other means before chemotherapy (56, 94, 95). If the tumor causes the carcinoid syndrome, appropriate interventions directed at specific symptoms may be beneficial (i.e., diuretics for heart disease, avoiding alcohol and precipitating food to decrease flushing, antidiarrheal agents, and select bronchodilators for wheezing). Many would follow these interventions with octreotide, then interferon, then chemotherapy. See Table 56.6 for a tabulation of response rates.

In a report of 53 patients by Moertel, octreotide caused cessation of flushing in 53% and a 50% or more decrease in an additional 32% of patients (56). Diarrhea was completely resolved in 25% of patients and improved in 49% more patients. Other studies confirm this benefit and also mention a dramatic improvement in wheezing (105). Unfortunately, the objective tumor shrinkage with octreotide is in the range of 10 to 20% (101, 102).

Interferon also appears very useful in patients with carcinoid symptoms. It decreased symptoms for 5 of 9 patients (103), reduced rising 5-HIAA (76% of patients), but unfortunately, had minimal effect on tumor shrinkage, with a 0 to 20% objective response (97, 103, 106). Interferon regrettably causes flulike symptoms in 89% of patients, fatigue in 70%, weight loss in 59%, anemia in 31%, and increased liver enzymes and lipids in 31% (97). This same series by Oberg and Eriksson found an 80-month median survival in those treated with interferon versus an 8-month median survival for those receiving chemotherapy. This series would seem to suggest including interferon in a randomized trial.

Periodically over the past two decades of car-

Table 56.6. Chemotherapy for Carcinoid Tumors

Agent(s)[a]	No.	Objective Response	Reference
STZ	23	7 (30%)	(96)
STZ	6	1 (16%)	(56)
DOX	33	7 (21%)	(56)
5FU	19	5 (26%)	(56)
DTIC	18	3 (17%)	(56)
DACT	17	1 (6%)	(56)
CDDP	16	1 (6%)	(56)
STZ + 5FU	43	14 (33%)	(56)
STZ + 5FU	19	2 (11%)	(97)
STZ + CTX	47	12 (26%)	(98)
STZ + DOX	9	2 (22%)	(99)
STZ + CTX + 5FU	9	2 (22%)	(100)
STZ + CTX + 5FU + DOX	56	17 (31%)	(100)
Octreotide	25	4 (16%)	(101)
Octreotide	23	2 (9%)	(102)
Interferon	111	16 (15%)	(97)
Interferon	14	0 (0%)	(103)
Interferon	20	4 (20%)	(104)

[a]CBCDA, carboplatin; CDDP, cisplatin; CTX, cyclophosphamide; CZT, chlorozocin; DACT, dactinomycin; DOX, doxorubicin; DTIC, dacarbazine; STZ, streptozocin; VP16, etoposide; 5FU, 5-fluorouracil.

cinoid management, enthusiasm has been shown for resection of hepatic metastases (even when multiple), hepatic artery ligation, hepatic artery embolization, hepatic artery chemotherapy, or some combination of occlusion and chemotherapy (107–113). For those with symptomatic liver involvement, hepatic artery occlusion has shown high rates of improvement in symptoms. Eighty percent of patients had more than a 50% improvement (56). Hepatic artery occlusion with chemotherapy demonstrated an 86% objective response.

In any of these various approaches, most such treated patients achieve a considerable decrease in symptoms, and the vast majority of patients demonstrate an impressive decrease in the size of their liver metastases. Unquestionably, whatever the local approach, when applied enthusiastically, it almost always results in remarkable tumor control for some period of time. The availability of somatostatin will greatly diminish the risk of "carcinoid crisis" and the hypotensive deaths that would have been a threat to patients undergoing surgical manipulation of their liver metastases.

Tamoxifen is a miscellaneous agent used to treat carcinoid tumors and the carcinoid syndrome. Tamoxifen was reported to have eliminated the symptoms of carcinoid tumors in two

isolated case reports and even resulted in marked regression of liver metastases in one of the two patients (114, 115). Subsequently, a systematic trial using 30 mg/day of this antiestrogen in 16 carcinoid patients failed to achieve a single response (116).

The most studied antineoplastic agent in patients with carcinoids is streptozocin, which had its investigative debut in the early 1970s. Table 56.6 gives examples of the phase II single-agent data for this compound (55, 96). Smaller series report variable response rates of 0 to 100% but also have had few patients (two to eight) (117–120). In this table, responses refer to symptomatic and/or objective tumor shrinkage.

Although the early results with streptozocin alone were inconsistent, sufficient responses were seen to consider combining this drug with other antineoplastics. Table 56.6 summarizes a few select trials in carcinoid tumors with streptozocin used in combination (56, 97–100). Sample sizes varied considerably from one trial to another, although there seemed to be a response rate of 20 to 30% with streptozocin. This low response rate would certainly justify phase II trials of new agents in previously untreated patients with carcinoid tumors.

Several other agents have been studied in patients with carcinoid tumors, either alone or in combination. An initial report of actinomycin demonstrated three of three objective responders, but a much larger experience yielded a response in only 1 of 17 patients (56, 121, 122). Only a few patients have been treated with DTIC; in one series, 2 of 15 responded, and in another trial, 2 of 5 patients with carcinoid responded (122, 123). In a summary of the experience at the Mayo Clinic, Adriamycin yielded responses in 7 of 33 patients (21%), and with 5-FU, 5 of 19 patients (26%) responded (124). In a separate report from the Mayo Clinic, only one partial response was seen in 15 patients treated with cisplatin (125). Many years ago, the combination of cyclophosphamide and methotrexate was reported to show activity in a small group of carcinoid patients, but an enlarged trial of these two agents was negative (126, 127).

One can only conclude that chemotherapy achieves objective responses in about one-fifth to one-third of patients with carcinoid neoplasms and that combining apparently active single agents does not enhance response rates (Table 56.6). Obviously, new agents need to be tested. It is also important to recall that most patients treated with somatostatin achieve symptomatic control, and under certain conditions, this may save patients from life-threatening hypotension. Hence, part of the impetus to treat patients known to have slowly growing chemotherapeutically insensitive tumors with noncurative cytotoxics for relief of symptoms has been reduced by the availability of somatostatin.

PITUITARY ADENOMAS

Pituitary adenomas are very uncommon tumors, representing only 5% of primary intracranial brain tumors (128). Generally these tumors are classified as hormonally active or inactive. In a large series of 800 patients referred to the University of California San Francisco, 79% were hormonally active and 21% were inactive. Fifty-two percent of the active tumors secreted prolactin, 27% secreted growth hormone, 20% secreted corticotropin, and 0.3% secreted TSH (129). Surgery and radiation therapy are the primary treatment modalities used for these tumors. Bromocriptine has also been used to temporarily reduce prolactin levels in patients with incompletely treated macroadenomas.

The presence of somatostatin receptors on many pituitary adenomas has led to the use of scintigraphic scans to detect these tumors after injection of radionuclide-coupled somatostatin analogues (130, 131). The authors mention that prolactin- and ACTH-secreting tumors cannot be visualized in many instances but that a positive scan in patients with a GH- or TSH-secreting pituitary tumors is predictive of a good suppressive effect by octreotide. Octreotide almost always suppresses growth hormone levels because of suppression at the pituitary level (132). In general, GH-secreting tumors treated with octreotide have normalization of GH in 50% of patients and near normalization in another 30% of patients. Additionally, a decrease in tumor size occurs in approximately 50% of patients. In a series of 52 patients (133) octreotide reduced TSH secretion in almost all patients and normalized thyroid hormone levels in 73%. Partial tumor shrinkage was observed in 40% of those on long-term therapy. Octreotide appears to have had little effect on the few patients with prolactin- and ACTH-secreting adenomas who have been treated. This has been summarized nicely by Lamberts (133).

PARATHYROID CARCINOMA

Parathyroid carcinoma, a rare disease with a prevalence of 1 to 3% of all parathyroid tumors (134), is always associated with hypercalcemia and often with bone disease. Death is often at-

tributable to the metabolic disorder caused by the tumor and its metastases. In addition to treating the hypercalcemia medically with agents such as pamridonate, there are several reported responses to dacarbazine (135) and the combination of 5-FU, cyclophosphamide, and dacarbazine (136). The latter had a response duration of more than 5 months.

REFERENCES

1. Bolande PR. The neurocrestopathies: a unifying concept of disease arising from neural crest maldevelopment. Hum Pathol 1974;5:409–429.

2. Macfarlane DA. Cancer of the adrenal cortex: the natural history, prognosis and treatment in a study of fifty-five cases. Ann R Coll Surg Engl 1958;23:155–186.

3. Nelson AA, Woodard G. Severe adrenal cortical atrophy (cytotoxic) and hepatic damage produced in dogs by feeding 2,2-bis(parachlorophenyl)-1,1-dichloroethane (DDD or TDE). Arch Pathol 1949;48:387–394.

4. Bergenstal DM, Lipsett MB, Moy RH, Hertz R. Regression of adrenal cancer and suppression of adrenal function in man by o,p'DDD. Trans Assoc Am Physicians 1959;72:341–350.

5. Ostuni JA, Roginsky MS. Metastatic adrenal cortical carcinoma: documented cure with combined chemotherapy. Arch Intern Med 1975;135:1257–1258.

6. Hutter AM, Kayhoe DE. Adrenal cortical carcinoma: results of treatment with o,p'DDD in 138 patients. Am J Med 1966;41:581–592.

7. Lubitz JA, Freeman L, Okum R. Mitotane use in inoperable adrenal cortical carcinoma. JAMA 1973;223:1109–1112.

8. Van Slooten H, Moolenaar AJ, Van Seters AP, Smeenk D. The treatment of adrenocortical carcinoma with o,p'DDD: prognostic simplifications of serum level monitoring. Eur J Cancer Clin Oncol 1984;20:47–53.

9. Nader S, Hickey RC, Sellin RV, Samaan NA. Adrenal cortical carcinoma: a study of 77 cases. Cancer 1983;52:707–711.

10. Venkatesh S, Hickey RC, Sellin RV, Fernandez JF, Samaan NA. Adrenal cortical carcinoma. Cancer 1989;64:765–769.

11. Decker RA, Elson P, Hogan TF, et al. Eastern Cooperative Oncology Group study 1879: mitotane and Adriamycin in patients with advanced adrenocortical carcinoma. Surgery 1991;110:1006–1013.

12. Hajjar RA, Hickey RC, Samaan NA. Adrenal cortical carcinoma: a study of 32 patients. Cancer 1975;35:549–554.

13. Merrim CE. Treatment of genitourinary tumors with cisdichlorodiammineplatinum (II): experience in 250 patients. Cancer Treat Rep 1979;63:1579–1584.

14. Tattersall MHN, Lander H, Bain B, et al. Cisplatinum treatment of metastatic adrenal carcinoma. Med J Aust 1980;1:419–421.

15. Chun HG, Yagoda A, Kemeny N. Cisplatin for adrenal cortical carcinoma. Cancer Treat Rep 1983;67:513–514.

16. Hag MM, Legha SS, Samaan NA, et al. Cytotoxic chemotherapy in adrenal cortical carcinoma. Cancer Treat Rep 1980;64:909–913.

17. Berruti A, Terzolo M, Paccotti P, et al. Favorable response of metastatic adrenocortical carcinoma to

etoposide, Adriamycin, and cisplatin (EAP) chemotherapy. Report of two cases. Tumori 1992;78:345–348.

18. Stein CA, LaRocca RV, McAtee N, Myers CE. Suramin: an anticancer drug with a unique mechanism of action. J Clin Oncol 1989;7:499–508.

19. Bukowski RM, Wolfe M, Levine HS. Phase II trial of mitotane and cisplatin in patients with adrenal carcinoma: a Southwest Oncology Group study. J Clin Oncol 1993;11:161–165.

20. Johnson DH, Greco A. Treatment of metastatic adrenal cortical carcinoma with cisplatin and etoposide. Cancer 1986;58:2198–2202.

21. Pia A, Berruti A, Terzole M, Paccotti P, Letizia C, et al. Feasibility of the association of mitotane with etoposide, adriamycin and cisplatin combination chemotherapy in advanced adrenocortical cancer patients. Report on 7 cases. Ann Oncol 1995;6:509–510.

22. Heskith PJ, McCaffrey RP, Finkel HE, et al. Cisplatin-based treatment of adrenocortical carcinoma. Cancer Treat Rep 1987;71:222–224.

23. Crock PA, Clark ACL. Combination chemotherapy for adrenal carcinoma in a 5 1/2-year-old male. Med Pediatr Oncol 1989;17:62–65.

24. Van Slooten H, Van Oosterom AT. CAP (cyclophosphamide, doxorubicin, and cisplatin) regimen in adrenal cortical carcinoma. Cancer Treat Rep 1983;67:377–379.

25. Schlumberger M, Brugieres L, Gicquel C, Travagli JP, Droz JP, Parmentier C. 5-Fluorouracil, doxorubicin, and cisplatin as treatment for adrenal cortical carcinoma. Cancer 1991;67:2997–3000.

26. Eriksson B, Oberg K, Curstedt T, et al. Treatment of hormone-producing adrenocortical cancer with o,p'DDD and streptozocin. Cancer 1987;59:1398–1403.

27. Samaan NA, Hickey RC. Adrenal cortical carcinoma. Semin Oncol 1987;14(3):292–296.

28. Schteingart DE, Cash R, Conn JW. Amino-glutethimide and metastatic adrenal cancer: maintained reversal (six months) of Cushing's syndrome. JAMA 1966;198:143–146.

29. Pont A, Williams PL, Loose DS, et al. Ketoconazole inhibits adrenal steroid synthesis (abstract). Clin Res 1982;30:99A.

30. Rochlitz CF, Damon LE, Russi MB, Geddes A, Cadman EC. Cytotoxicity of ketoconazole in malignant cell lines. Cancer Chemother Pharmacol 1988;21:319–322.

31. Averbuch SD, Steakley CS, Young RC, et al. Malignant pheochromocytoma: effective treatment with a combination of cyclophosphamide, vincristine, and dacarbazine. Ann Intern Med 1988;109:267–273.

32. Harada T, Nishikawa Y, Suzuki T, Ito K, Baba S. Bleomycin treatment for cancer of the thyroid. Am J Surg 1971;122:53–57.

33. Gottlieb JA, Hill CS Jr, Ibanez MI, Clark RL. Chemotherapy of thyroid cancer: an evaluation of experience with 37 patients. Cancer 1972;30:848–853.

34. Gottlieb JA, Hill CS Jr. Adriamycin (NSC-123127) therapy in thyroid carcinoma. Cancer Chemother Rep 1975;6:283–296.

35. Husain M, Alsever RN, Lock JP, George WF, Katz FH. Failure of medullary carcinoma of the thyroid to respond to doxorubicin therapy. Hormone Res 1978;9:22–25.

36. Shimaoka K, Schoenfeld DA, DeWys WD, Creech RH, DeConti R. A randomized trial of doxo-

rubicin versus doxorubicin plus cisplatin in patients with advanced thyroid carcinoma. Cancer 1985;56:2155–2160.

37. Durie BGM, Hellman D, Woolfenden JM, O'Mara R, Kartechner M, Salmon SE. High-risk thyroid cancer: prolonged survival with early multimodality therapy. Cancer Clin Trials 1981;4:67–73.

38. Williams SD, Birch R, Einhorn LH. Phase II evaluation of doxorubicin plus cisplatin in advanced thyroid cancer: a Southeastern Cancer Study Group trial. Cancer Treat Rep 1986;70:405–407.

39. De Besi P, Busnardo B, Toso S, et al. Combined chemotherapy with bleomycin, Adriamycin, and platinum in advanced thyroid cancer. J Endocrinol Invest 1991;14:475–480.

40. Scherubl H, Raue F, Zeigler R. Combination chemotherapy of advanced medullary and differentiated thyroid cancer. J Cancer Res Clin Oncol 1990;116:21–23.

41. Sokal M, Harmer CL. Chemotherapy for anaplastic carcinoma of the thyroid. Clin Oncol 1978;4:3–10.

42. Bukowski RM, Brown L, Weick JK, Groppe CW, Purvis J. Combination chemotherapy of metastatic thyroid cancer: phase II study. Am J Clin Oncol 1983;6:579–581.

43. Kober F, Heiss A, Keminger K, Depsich D. Chemotherapy of highly malignant thyroid tumors. Wein Klin Wochenschr 1990;102:274–276.

44. Wu LT, Averbuch SD, Ball DW, De Bustros A, Baylin SB, McGuire WP. Treatment of advanced medullary thyroid carcinoma with a combination of cyclophosphamide, vincristine, and dacarbazine. Cancer 1994;73:432–436.

45. Rivier J, Spress J, Thorner M, Vale W. Characterization of a growth-hormone releasing factor from a human pancreatic islet cell tumor. Nature 1982;300:276–278.

46. Sano T, Asa SL, Kovacs K. Growth hormone releasing-producing tumors. Clinical, biochemical and morphological manifestations. Endocr Rev 1988;9(3):357–373.

47. Maton PN, Gardner JD, Jensen RT. Cushing's syndrome in patients with the Zollinger-Ellison syndrome. N Engl J Med 1986;315:1–5.

48. Bresler L, Boissel P, Conroy T, Grosdidier J. Pancreatic islet cell carcinoma with hypercalcemia: complete remission 5 years after surgical excision and chemotherapy. Am J Gastroenterol 1991;86(5):635–638.

49. Broder LE, Carter SK. Pancreatic islet cell carcinoma. II. Results of therapy with streptozotocin in 52 patients. Ann Intern Med 1973;79:108–118.

50. Moertel CG, Hanley JA, Johnson LA. Streptozotocin alone compared with streptozotocin plus fluorouracil in the treatment of advanced islet-cell carcinoma. N Engl J Med 1980;303:1189–1194.

51. Kvols LK, Buck M. Chemotherapy of the metastatic carcinoid and islet cell tumors: a review. Am J Med 1987;82:77–83.

52. Buchanan KD, O'Hare MMT, Russel CJF, Kennedy TL, Hadden DR. Factors involved in the responsiveness of gastrointestinal apudomas to streptozotocin (abstract). Dig Dis Sci 1986;31:511S.

53. Moertel CG, Lavin PT, Hahn RG. Phase II trial study of doxorubicin for advanced islet cell carcinoma. Cancer Treat Rep 1982;66:1567–1569.

54. Bukowski RM, McCracken JD, Balcerzak SP,

Fabian CJ. Phase II study of chlorozotocin in islet cell carcinoma. Cancer Chemother Pharmacol 1983;11:48–50.

55. Moertel CG, Lefkopoulo M, Lipsitz S, Hahn RG, Klassen D. Streptozocin-doxorubicin, streptozocin-fluorouracil, or chlorozotocin in the treatment of islet-cell carcinoma. N Engl J Med 1992;326:519–523.

56. Moertel CG. An odyssey in the land of small tumors. J Clin Oncol 1987;5(10):1503–1522.

57. Altimari AF, Badrinath K, Reisel HJ, Prinz RA. DTIC therapy in patients with malignant intra-abdominal neuroendocrine tumors. Surgery 1987; 102(6):1009–1017.

58. Saltz L, Lauwers G, Wiseberg J, Kelsen D. A phase II trial of carboplatin in patients with advanced APUD tumors. Cancer 1993;72:619–622.

59. Fiore JJ, Kelsen DP, Cheng E, Dukeman M. Phase II trial of VP-16 in apudomas (abstract). Proc AACR 1984;25:174.

60. Frame J, Kelsen D, Kemeny N, et al. A phase II trial of streptozotocin and Adriamycin in advanced APUD tumors. Am J Oncol 1988;11:490–495.

61. Eriksson B, Skogseid B, Lundqvist G, Wide L, Wilander E, Oberg K. Medical treatment and long-term survival in a prospective study of 84 patients with endocrine pancreatic tumors. Cancer 1990;65:1883–1890.

62. Eriksson B, Oberg K. An update of the medical treatment of malignant endocrine pancreatic tumors. Acta Oncol 1993;32(2):203–208.

63. Rougier P, Oliveira J, Ducreux M, Theodore C, Kac J, Droz JP. Metastatic carcinoid and islet cell tumours of the pancreas: a phase II trial of the efficacy of combination chemotherapy with 5-fluorouracil, doxorubicin and cisplatin. Eur J Cancer 1991;27(11):1380–1382.

64. Moertel CG, Kvols LK, O'Connell MJ, Rubin J. Treatment of neuroendocrine carcinomas with combined etoposide and cisplatin. Cancer 1991;68:227–232.

65. Bukowski RM, Tangen C, Lee R, et al. Phase II trial of chlorozotocin and fluorouracil in islet cell carcinoma: a Southwest Oncology Group study. J Clin Oncol 1992;10:1914–1918.

66. Maton PN. The use of long-acting somatostatin analogue, octreotide in patients with islet cell tumors. Gastroenterol Clin North Am 1989;18(4):897–922.

67. Maton PN, Gardner JD, Jensen RT. The use of long acting somatostatin analogue 201-995 in patients with pancreatic endocrine tumors. Dig Dis Sci 1989; 34(3S):28S–39S.

68. Kvols L, Buck M, Moertel CG, et al. Treatment of metastatic islet cell carcinoma with a somatostatin analogue (SMS 201-995). Ann Intern Med 1987; 107:162–168.

69. Murray-Lyon IM, Eddleston ALWF, Williams R, et al. Treatment of multiple-hormone-producing malignant islet-cell tumour with streptozotocin. Lancet 1968;2:895–898.

70. Moertel CG, Reitemeier RJ, Schutt AJ, Hahn RG. Phase II study of streptozotocin (NSC-85998) in the treatment of advanced gastrointestinal cancer. Cancer Chemother Rep 1971;55:303–307.

71. Moertel CG, Hanley JA, Johnson LA. Streptozotocin alone compared with streptozotocin plus fluorouracil in the treatment of advanced islet-cell carcinoma. N Engl J Med 1980;303:1189–1194.

72. Reichlin S. Somatostatin. N Engl J Med 1983; 309:1495–1501.

73. Oberg K, Eriksson B. Medical treatment of neuroendocrine gut and pancreatic tumors. Acta Oncol 1989;28(3):425–431.

74. Oberg K. Chemotherapy and biotherapy in neuroendocrine tumors. Curr Opin Oncol 1993; 5(1):110–120.

75. Modlin IM, Lewis JJ, Ahlman H, Bilchik AJ, Kumar RR. Management of unresectable malignant endocrine tumors of the pancreas. Surg Gynecol Obstet 1993;176(5):507–518.

76. Boden G, Ryan IG, Eisenschmid BL, et al. Treatment of inoperable glucagonoma with the long acting somatostatin analogue SMS 201–995. N Engl J Med 1986;314:1686–1689.

77. Snyderman C, Johnson JT, Barnes L. Carcinoid tumor of the larynx: case report and review of the world literature. Otolaryngol Head Neck Surg 1986; 95:158–164.

78. Harling H, Paulsen SM, Sorensen J. Primary malignant ovarian carcinoid. Gynecol Oncol 1986; 24:265–267.

79. Alenghat E, Okagaki T, Talerman A. Primary mucinous carcinoid tumor of the ovary. Cancer 1986; 58:777–783.

80. Louka MH, Danoff B, Brodovsky HS, Jahshan AE. Carcinoid tumors of the uterine cervix: response to combination chemotherapy and radiotherapy. Am J Clin Oncol 1982;5:487–493.

81. Seidel R, Steinfeld A. Carcinoid of the cervix: natural history and implications for therapy. Gynecol Oncol 1988;30:114–119.

82. Wick MR, Carney JA, Bernatz PE, Brown LR. Primary mediastinal carcinoid tumors. Am J Surg Pathol 1982;6:195–205.

83. Donovan PJ, Foley JF. Chemotherapy in invasive thymomas: five case reports. J Surg Oncol 1986; 33:14–17.

84. Godwin JD. Carcinoid tumors: an analysis of 2837 cases. Cancer 1975;36:560–569.

85. Chow CW, Sane S, Campbell PE, Carter RF. Malignant carcinoid tumors in children. Cancer 1982; 49:802–811.

86. Kennedy A. The diagnosis of pulmonary carcinoid tumours. Br J Dis Chest 1979;73:71–80.

87. Ibrahim N, Briggs J, Jeyasingham K, Forester-Wood CP, Andrianopoulos E. Chemotherapy for small cell lung cancer (letter). Br Med J (Clin Res) 1985; 290(6469):713.

88. Mooi WJ, van Zandwyk N, Dingemans KP, Koolen MGJ, Wagenvoort CA. The "grey area" between small cell and non-small cell lung carcinomas. Light and electron microscopy versus clinical data in 14 cases. J Pathol 1986;149:49–54.

89. Bonomi P, Hovey C, Dainauskas JR, Slayton R, Wolter J. Management of carcinoid syndrome. Med Pediatr Oncol 1979;6:77–83.

90. Thulin L, Samnegard H, Tyden G, Long DH, Efendic S. Efficacy of somatostatin in a patient with carcinoid syndrome (letter). Lancet 1978;2:43.

91. Roy RC, Carter RF, Wright PD. Somatostatin, anaesthesia, and the carcinoid syndrome. Anaesthesia 1987;42:627–632.

92. Marsh HM, Martin JK, Kvols LK, et al. Carcinoid crisis during anesthesia: successful treatment with a somatostatin analogue. Anesthesiology 1987; 66:89–91.

93. Kvols LK, Moertel CG, O'Connell MJ, Schutt

AJ, Rubin J, Hahn RG. Treatment of the malignant carcinoid syndrome: evaluation of a long-acting somatostatin analogue. N Engl J Med 1986;315:663–666.

94. Moertel CG, Johnson CM, McKusick MA, et al. The management of patients with advanced carcinoid tumors and islet cell carcinomas. Ann Intern Med 1994; 120(4):302–309.

95. Kvols LK, Buck M. Chemotherapy of endocrine malignancies: a review. Semin Oncol 1987;14(3):343–353.

96. Maton PN, Hodgson HJF. Carcinoid tumors and the carcinoid syndrome. In: Bouchier IAD, Allan RN, Hodgson HJF, Keighly MRB, eds. Textbook of gastroenterology. London: Bailliere-Tindall, 1984:620.

97. Oberg K, Eriksson B. The role of interferons in the management of carcinoid tumors. Acta Oncol 1991; 30(4):519–522.

98. Moertel CG, Hanley JA. Combination chemotherapy trials in metastatic carcinoid and malignant carcinoid syndrome. Cancer Clin Trials 1979;2:327–344.

99. Kelsen DP, Cheng E, Kemeny N, Magill CB, Yagoda A. Streptozotocin and Adriamycin in the treatment of APUD tumors (carcinoid, islet cell and medullary carcinomas of the thyroid) (abstract). Proc AACR 1982;23:111.

100. Bukowski R, Johnson K, Peterson RF, et al. A phase II trial of combination chemotherapy in patients with metastatic carcinoid tumors: a Southwest Oncology Group study. Cancer 1987;60:2891–2895.

101. Kvols LK, Moertel CG, O'Connell MJ, Schutt AJ, Rubin J, Hahn RG. Treatment of the malignant carcinoid syndrome: evaluation of a long-acting somatostatin analogue. N Engl J Med 1986;315:663–666.

102. Oberg K, Norheim I, Theodorsson E. Treatment of malignant midgut carcinoid tumours with a long-acting somatostatin analogue octreotide. Acta Oncol 1991;30(4):503–507.

103. Joensuu H, Kumpulainen E, Grohn P. Treatment of metastatic carcinoid tumour with recombinant interferon alfa. Eur J Cancer 1992;28A(10):1650–1653.

104. Moertel CG, Rubin J, Kvols LK. Therapy of metastatic carcinoid tumor and the malignant carcinoid syndrome with recombinant leukocyte A interferon. J Clin Oncol 1989;7:865–868.

105. Vinik AI, Moattari AR. Use of somatostatin analogue in management of carcinoid syndrome. Dig Dis Sci 1989;34:14S–27S.

106. Oberg K, Norheim I, Lind E, et al. Treatment of malignant carcinoid tumors with human leukocyte interferon: long-term results. Cancer Treat Rep 1986; 70:1297–1304.

107. Kune GA, Goldstein J. Malignant liver carcinoid: the place of surgery and chemotherapy: review and case presentation. Med J Aust 1974;2:777–780.

108. Jugdutt BI, Watanabe M, Turner FW. Hepatic artery ligation in treatment of carcinoid syndrome. Can Med Assoc J 1975;112:325–327.

109. Ensminger W, Niederhuber J, Dakhil S, Thrall J, Wheeler R. Totally implanted drug delivery system for hepatic arterial chemotherapy. Cancer Treat Rep 1981;65:393–400.

110. Martensson H, Nobin A, Bengmark S, Lunderquist A, Owman T, Sanden G. Embolization of the liver in the management of metastatic carcinoid tumors. J Surg Oncol 1984;27:152–158.

111. Mitty HA, Warner RRP, Newman LH, Train

JS, Parnes IH. Control of carcinoid syndrome with hepatic artery embolization. Radiology 1985;155:623–626.

112. Martin JK, Moertel CG, Adson MA, Schutt AJ. Surgical treatment of functioning metastatic carcinoid tumors. Arch Surg 1983;118:537–542.

113. Moertel CG, May GR, Martin JK, Rubin J, Schutt AJ. Sequential hepatic artery occlusion (HAO) and chemotherapy for metastatic carcinoid tumor and islet cell carcinoma (ICC) (abstract). Proc Am Soc Clin Oncol 1985;4:80.

114. Stathopoulos GP, Karvountzis GG, Yiotis J. Tamoxifen in carcinoid syndrome (letter). N Engl J Med 1981;305:52.

115. Myers CF, Ershler WB, Tannenbaum MA, Barth R. Tamoxifen and carcinoid tumor (letter). Ann Intern Med 1982;96:383.

116. Moertel CG, Engstrom PF, Schutt AJ. Tamoxifen therapy for metastatic carcinoid tumor: a negative study. Ann Intern Med 1984;100:531–532.

117. Moertel CG, Reitemeier RJ, Schutt AJ, Hahn RG. Phase II study of streptozotocin (NSC-85998) in the treatment of advanced gastrointestinal cancer. Cancer Chemother Rep 1971;55:303–307.

118. Stolinsky DC, Sadoff L, Braunwald J, Bateman JR. Streptozotocin in the treatment of cancer: phase II study. Cancer 1972;30:61–67.

119. Feldman JM, Quickel KE Jr, Marecek RL, Lebovitz HE. Streptozotocin treatment of metastatic carcinoid tumors. South Med J 1972;65:1325–1327.

120. Schein PS, O'Connell J, Blom J, et al. Clinical antitumor activity and toxicity of streptozotocin (NSC-85998). Cancer 1974;34:993–1000.

121. Dollinger M, Golbey R. Actinomycin D in the treatment of carcinoid tumors (abstract). Clin Res 1967; 15:335.

122. van Hazel GA, Rubin J, Moertel CG. Treatment of metastatic carcinoid tumor with dactinomycin or dacarbazine. Cancer Treat Rep 1983;67:583–585.

123. Dessinger A, Foley JF, Lemon HM. Therapy of malignant APUD cell tumors: effectiveness of DTIC. Cancer 1983;51:790–794.

124. Moertel CG. Treatment of the carcinoid tumor and the malignant carcinoid syndrome. J Clin Oncol 1983;1:727–740.

125. Moertel CG, Rubin J, O'Connell MJ. Phase II study of cisplatin therapy in patients with metastatic carcinoid tumor and the malignant carcinoid syndrome. Cancer Treat Rep 1986;70:1459–1460.

126. Mengel CE. The carcinoid syndrome. In: Holland JF, Frei E, eds. Cancer medicine. Philadelphia: Lea & Febiger, 1982:1818–1826.

127. Moertel CG, O'Connell MJ, Reitemeier RJ, Rubin J. Evaluation of combined cyclophosphamide and methotrexate therapy in the treatment of metastatic carcinoid tumor and the malignant carcinoid syndrome. Cancer Treat Rep 1984;68:665–667.

128. Norton JA, Levin B, Jensen RT. Cancer of the endocrine system. In: DeVita VT, Hellman S, Rosenberg SA, eds. Cancer principles & practice of oncology. 4th ed. Philadelphia: JB Lippincott, 1993: 1380–1382.

129. Wilson CB. Surgical management of endocrine-active pituitary adenomas. In: Walker MD, ed. Oncology of the nervous system. Boston: Martinus-Nijhoff, 1983:117–118.

130. Krenning EB, Bakker WH, Breeman WAP, et al. Localization of endocrine-related tumours with ra-

dioiodinated analogue of somatostatin. Lancet 1989; i:242–244.

131. Lamberts SWJ, Bakker WH, Reubi JC, Krenning EP. Somatostatin-receptor imaging in the localization of endocrine tumors. N Engl J Med 1990; 323:1246–1249.

132. Chanson P, Weintraub BD, Harris AG. Octreotide therapy for thyroid-stimulating hormone-secreting pituitary adenomas: a follow-up of 52 patients. Ann Intern Med 1993;119:236–240.

133. Lambert SWJ, Hofland LJ, De Herder WW, Kwekkeboom DJ, Reubi JC, Krenning EP. Octreotide and related somatostatin analogs in the diagnosis and treatment of pituitary disease and somatostatin receptor scintigraphy. Front Neuroendocrinol 1993;14(1):25–55.

134. Schantz A, Castleman B. Parathyroid carcinoma: a study of 70 cases. Cancer 1973;31:600–605.

135. Calandra DB, Chejfec G, Foy B, Lawrence AM, Paloyan E. Parathyroid carcinoma: biochemical and pathologic response to DTIC. Surgery 1984;96(6):1132–1137.

136. Bukowski RM, Sheeler L, Cunningham J, Esselstyn C. Successful combination chemotherapy for metastatic parathyroid carcinoma. Arch Intern Med 1984;144(2):399–400.

57

Chemotherapy of Genitourinary Cancers

Bruce E. Brockstein and Nicholas J. Vogelzang

PROSTATE CANCER

In 1996, it is projected that prostate cancer (PC) will be diagnosed in over 317,000 men, with 42,000 projected to die of the disease (1). PC is the most common cancer in males. In comparison, there are predicted to be 151,000 new cases of lung cancer (1). Lung cancer incidence is beginning to decline, while prostate cancer incidence continues to increase. One in 11 men will develop prostate cancer during his lifetime.

The etiology of PC is unknown, but racial and genetic factors have been identified (2). Vasectomy, which received much attention in the last several years as a risk factor, has not been proven to increase the risk of PC (3). At autopsy, latent microscopic foci of prostate cancer are equally common in all ethnic groups. However, clinical PC is far more common in African Americans than in Orientals. Evidence from Japanese migration analysis suggests that a western or high-fat diet may increase the risk of this disease in Japanese migrants to Hawaii or Brazil (4). Both these facts suggest that a high-fat diet acts as a promoter of prostate carcinogenesis.

Prostate-specific antigen (PSA) and transrectal needle core prostrate biopsies have become integral tools in the diagnosis, management, and treatment of PC. PSA was discovered and reported by the Roswell Park urologic research team in 1980 (5). It is a 35,000-kDa glycoprotein composed of 240 amino acids and is a serine protease of the kallikrein family (6). The protein is secreted into the seminal fluid and is localized to the prostatic acinar cells and ductal epithelium. It is found in no other organ. It has become widely used since 1987 and has revolutionized the diagnosis and management of local and ad-

vanced PC (7). Likewise, outpatient transrectal prostate biopsies with spring-loaded "guns" have equally revolutionized the field since 1987 to 1990. Their accuracy and safety have allowed ease of diagnosis of all prostate abnormalities.

Many reports have documented that PSA is proportional to the cancer volume in radical prostatectomy (RP) specimens (8–10). Furthermore, PSA is now accepted as the most sensitive and specific indicator of recurrent or residual PC. A PSA value that does not normalize postprostatectomy is highly suggestive of persistent or relapsed disease. Rare patients may have retained fragments of normal prostate tissue that produce PSA. Although the "normal" male range varies with age (11), a postprostatectomy PSA should enter the normal female range (<0.2 ng/mL). By this criterion, PC patients treated with RP can be divided into those potentially cured (patients with an undetectable PSA) and those destined to relapse (patients with a detectable PSA). The utility of PSA after radiotherapy (RT) is lower because the normal prostate gland continues to produce some PSA and because RT does not immediately eradicate all PC. The PSA level may decline gradually, reaching a nadir 18 to 24 months after RT (12). Similarly, failure to achieve a nadir PSA within the normal range or a rising PSA virtually assures local or distant relapse (13).

In locally advanced or metastatic disease, the PSA level is significantly higher than in localized PC. Stamey and Kabalin reported that the mean PSA value (Yang method) in 35 patients with overt metastatic disease (stage M-1) was 562 ± 103.7 ng/mL; 100% of patients had an elevated PSA (14). This value is based upon pre-1989 data. The mean PSA for patients with metastatic disease in 1995 is significantly lower, in the range of 100 to 120 ng/mL. The PSA values in patients with D_1 disease (mean PSA value, 100.6 ± 23.6) were not statistically different from those seen in patients with stage C disease (mean PSA value, 102.2 ± 28.4). PSA cannot reliably distinguish between locally advanced disease (T_3/T_4 or node+) and overt metastatic disease.

Schmid et al. (15) have shown that in untreated but nonmetastatic PC patients, PSA and tumor volume double approximately every 24 months. This can be used in decision making for the treatment of patients not committed to early intervention. Treatment of all kinds, however, interrupts this PSA natural history. Follow-up after treatment of localized PC should include a careful rectal examination every 3 to 6 months, a PSA every 3 to 12 months, and a general medical examination every year. Routine bone scans and acid phosphatase measurements are no longer indicated if the PSA is being followed routinely and if it was significantly elevated at the time of diagnosis. PSA should probably be measured every 3 to 6 months for stages B_2, C, and D_1, while every 12 months should suffice for patients with A_1, A_2, and B_1 disease.

An elevated or rising PSA after definitive local therapy requires a repeat value in 1 or 2 months. If the value is still elevated and/or rising, the patients should be restaged with a bone scan and pelvic computed tomography (CT) scan. If neither of these staging procedures discloses disease, the prostate should be rebiopsied if the patient had been treated with radiotherapy (16). If the patient had been treated with surgery, the prostatic fossa and urethra should be biopsied under color-flow Doppler and ultrasound guidance (17). A patient with a persistently elevated and/or rising PSA and negative staging procedures, including prostatic fossa and urethral biopsies, may benefit from adjuvant radiotherapy to the prostatic fossa if he had previously undergone surgery (18, 19). The role of salvage radical prostatectomy in patients who have previously undergone radiotherapy remains in doubt (20, 21). Most clinicians advocate androgen-deprivation therapy in these two situations. Various uses for the PSA in prostate cancer patients are shown in Table 57.1

Changes in the technology used to diagnose and stage prostate cancer patients have mandated changes in the staging system for prostate cancer. A comparison of historic and modern systems is shown in Table 57.2 (22). The American Joint Committee on Cancer and Union Internationale Contre le Cancer (UICC) TNM (tumor,

Table 57.1. Uses of the PSA in Prostate Cancer

1. Measuring the PSA doubling time in patients with T_1 or T_2 (A or B) disease who have elected observation prior to definitive local treatment or palliative hormonal therapy
2. Estimating the likelihood of locally advanced or metastatic disease in clinical stage T_1 or T_2 (A or B) disease
3. Monitoring the results of radical prostatectomy (PSA should be less than 0.2 mg/mL)
4. Monitoring the results of radiotherapy (PSA should return to "normal" male range over 19–24 months)
5. Predicting survival following endocrine ablation therapy (undetectable PSA levels are predictive of prolonged survival)
6. Detecting early relapse from primary androgen-deprivation therapy (this is of questionable value, since second-line therapies are of limited usefulness)
7. Estimating response to chemotherapy in hormone-refractory patients

node, metastasis) staging system probably more accurately reflects the pathologic stage of disease and prognosis (23, 24). Additionally it takes into account disease found by biopsy for an elevated PSA (T_{1c}) and found by transrectal ultrasound (TRUS) for an elevated PSA. Additionally, TRUS and other imaging techniques can modify the pretreatment staging, although the lower stage should be used (24).

Localized prostate cancer accounts for 80% of newly diagnosed cases. Many controversies in the diagnosis and treatment of localized prostate cancer stem from the prolonged natural history of the disease and from the asymptomatic nature of the cancer (the median time to death for localized prostate cancer is nearly 8 years).

Treatment of Localized Prostate Cancer

For localized prostate cancer, American Urologic Association staging system, A, B, C, and D_1, (or American Joint Committee T_{1-4} N_{0-3} M_0), there are differing opinions among surgical, medical and radiation oncologists as to the appropriate use and timing of the available modalities, i.e. radical radiotherapy, radical prostatectomy, hormone therapy, or observation. The pros and cons of each treatment modality are discussed for each stage of localized disease in the following sections.

Stage A_1 (T_{1a}) is classically defined as a benign gland on palpation plus the finding of three or fewer chips, or less than 5% of the tissue examined being composed of well-differentiated adenocarcinoma found incidentally at the time of

Table 57.2. A Comparison of Historic and Modern Staging Systems for Prostate Cancer.

Description			
Clinically localized disease	*Modified Whitmore*	*Modified Jewett*	*TNM*
Incidental TURP	A	A	T_1
Incidental TURP	A	A	T_1
• Focal, low-grade	A_1	A_1	T_{1a}
• Diffuse, high-grade	A_2	A_2	T_{1b}
Diagnosed on TRUS^a guided biopsy—prompted by elevated PSA only	—	—	T_{1c}
Clinically detected			
• Palpable tumor 1 lobe	B_1 (≤2 cm)	B_{1N} (≥1 cm)	T_{2a} (<½ lobe)
	B_1 (>2 cm)		T_{2b} (>½ lobe) but <1 lobe
• Palpable tumor both lobes	B_3	B_2	T_{2c} (both lobes)
• Palpable beyond capsule	C	C	T_{3-4}
• Extending to lateral sulcus	C_1	—	T_{3a} (unilat.)
			T_{3b} (bilat.)
• Extending to base of sem. vesicle(s)	C_2	—	T_{3c}
• Beyond base of sem. vesicle(s)	C_3	—	—
• Invades sphincter, bladder, neck, or rectum	—	—	T_{4a}
• Invades levator muscles or pelvic side wall	—	—	T_{4b}
Metastatic disease	D	D	$T_{1-4}N_{0-3}M_{0-1}$
• Pelvic lymph nodes only	D_1	D_1	$T_{1-4}N_{1-3}M_0$
• Bones	D_2	D_2	$T_{1-4}N_{1-3}M_1$
• Lung, liver, brain	—	—	$T_{1-4}N_{1-3}M_{1c}$
• Elevated acid phos. only	D_0	D_0	—
• Hormonally refractory	—	Commonly referred to as D_3	—

Adapted with permission from Mc Leod DG. Prostate cancer: past, present, and future. In: Dawson NA, Vogelzang NJ, eds. Prostate cancer. New York: Wiley-Liss, 1994.
^{a}TRUS, transrectal ultrasound.

transurethral resection of the prostate (TURP). A well-differentiated tumor is usually defined as a Gleason sum less than 4 (25). In addition, the acid phosphatase must be normal. The PSA level does not enter the staging system because benign prostatic hypertrophy (BPH) glands causing urinary obstruction frequently are associated with elevated PSA levels. When this strict definition is used, death from PC occurs in less than 2% of patients (26). Thus, stage A_1 PC is best treated with observation or repeat TURP. Bone scans and other radiographs need not be routinely performed. Epstein et al. reported that 16% of men (8 of 50) followed for 8 years or longer after diagnosis of A_1 disease experienced disease progression (27). They recommend radical prostatectomy in young men with stage A_1 disease. Caution is indicated in following such recommendations, as their definition of stage A_1 is not classical. Lowe and Listrom, in a study of 232 patients, support the classical management phi-

losophy but caution that median time to progression is 13 years, with some relapses occurring after 18 years (28)! Thus, long-term follow-up of these patients is mandatory.

Stage A_2 (T_{1b}) is defined classically as a benign gland on palpation, with more than three chips or more than 5% of the tissue examined consisting of moderately or poorly differentiated adenocarcinoma (Gleason sum, 4 or greater). Patients who have T_{1b} disease but a Gleason sum less than 4 probably have a prognosis similar to that of stage T_{1a} patients. The acid phosphatase must also be normal. When this definition is used, median time to disease progression is 4 to 5 years, and death from PC will occur in 50% of untreated patients within 10 years. Stage A_2 may be treated with either RT or RP, and survival improves to approximately 70 to 90% at 10 years (29). Surgery has an advantage over RT in that the subgroup of patients destined to die of PC will be identified. This subgroup contains those with occult lymph node involvement and possibly those with tumor outside the prostate capsule. TRUS and pre-TURP PSA levels may improve the clinical staging of patients who are recognized after TURP as having stage A_2 prostate cancer.

Stage T_{1c} is disease found on needle biopsy for an elevated PSA (usually 4 to 10 ng/mL) and is a new category in the 1992 TNM staging system. Though nonpalpable, many of these tumors have clinically aggressive features, including 52% with a Gleason's score ≥ 7 and location in the peripheral zone (10, 23). Twenty percent will be upgraded to pathologic stage T_3 ($_pT_3$), and 36% will be T_{2b} or greater on ultrasound ($_uT_{2b}$) (24). Recurrence rates following either RP or RT are low (10, 23, 24). The Johns Hopkins group has reported a 93% disease-free survival at 8 years in such patients treated with RP (10).

Stage B_1 (T_{2a}) is a palpable nodule in one lobe of the gland, with a normal serum acid phosphatase. The diagnosis is made by means of either fine-needle aspiration, biopsy, prostate ultrasound-directed biopsy, or the classical transperineal or transrectal core needle biopsy. RP or radical RT are approximately equivalent treatments, with a 50 to 60% relative survival at 10 years. Pathologically proven B_1 PC should have a 5-year survival rate approximately equivalent to that of stage A_2 PC. Interestingly, even in the presence of a dominant nodule, virtually all patients have bilateral multifocal disease.

Stage B_2(T_{2b}) is a palpable nodule involving both lobes of the gland but not obliterating the lateral sulcus, with a normal serum acid phosphatase. Considerable controversy exists about how to distinguish stage B_1 from B_2 pathologically. The percentage of gland involved using the whole mount approach appears to be the best current indicator of prognosis, but the PSA value may supplant tumor volume in the future. Tumor volume greater than 4.0 cm^3 conveys a worse prognosis (30). Pathologically proven B_2 PC treated with RP or RT has a 15-year relative survival of only 33%. RT and surgery appear to be equivalent modalities, with the choice between the two determined by subjective factors intrinsic to the patient and the physician (31). For example, the patient must be willing to undergo a 1-day major surgical procedure with a 10 to 20% risk of minor urinary incontinence or a 6- to 7-week course of RT with less than 5% risk of incontinence. In spite of the recent wave of enthusiasm for nerve-sparing, and thus potency-preserving, RPs (10, 31), impotence is less common with RT. Nerve-sparing procedures are generally feasible only for patients found to have organ-confined disease at surgery, and improvements in potency rates may in part be due to patient selection (32).

Stage C ($T_{3a}/T_{3b}/T_4$) is disease beyond the prostate capsule or involving the seminal vesicles, the pelvic side wall, the bladder, or rectum, with an elevated acid phosphatase. It has a fairly poor 15-year relative survival rate of about 15 to 30% (33, 34) because of occult metastases to nodes and distant organs. Most physicians who treat prostate cancer begin to suspect T_3/T_4 disease when the PSA is over 20 ng/mL. Since local disease can lead to significant clinical problems, most physicians treat these patients with RT, although the early use of hormone therapy has been advocated. Used prior to RT, hormonal therapy may decrease the volume of normal tissue irradiated (35). A randomized phase III study by the Radiation Therapy Oncology Group (RTOG) compared goserelin and flutamide, given for 2 months prior to and during RT, with RT alone for bulky primary lesions. Progression-free, but not overall, survival was significantly improved in the hormonally treated group (36). Similar results were found in a randomized study using RT with or without the same total androgen blockade for $_cT_3$, $_pT_3$, or D_1 patients (37). As neither study has fully matured, survival differences may surface with further follow-up.

Neutron particles are also available at a few radiation centers. When given alone or with standard x-rays as a mixed beam, neutrons may enhance local tumor control and improve survival (38). Unfortunately, late effects of neutrons (i.e. severe bladder and bowel toxicity) have also occurred, and thus funding for neutron-beam therapy centers is being severely curtailed.

An aggressive approach with surgery followed by adjuvant radiotherapy and hormone therapy has been advocated on the basis of improved outcome with combined-modality treatment in some studies (39–41). The role of neoadjuvant hormone therapy downstaging is under active clinical investigation (42–44). The current recommendation for clinical stage C (T_3/T_4) prostate cancer is RT, with a decision for or against hormone therapy to be made by the patient and his physician. In a related question, a large-scale Canadian/American study is randomizing men to hormone therapy with or without local radiation.

Clinical stage D_1 (T_{any}, N_{1-3}) cancer, defined

as clinically suspicious nodes found on the lymphangiogram or CT scan or pathologic stage D_1 found at the time of pelvic lymphadenectomy, carries a poor prognosis. Most patients will have a PSA of 40 ng/mL or more at diagnosis; 85 to 90% of clinically staged patients will develop metastases within 10 years (34, 45, 46). N_1 disease refers to a single lymph node less than 2 cm. N_2 describes a single lymph node between 2 and 5 cm or multiple lymph nodes less than 5 cm. N_3 disease refers to any metastasis more than 5 cm in its greatest dimension. The management of this stage of prostate cancer is very controversial. The main unresolved management questions are

1. Does RP improve local control in comparison to RT or expectant management? For example, Steinberg et al. (46) retrospectively showed improved local control and fewer complications in RP-treated patients than in those treated with RT or expectantly. A survival advantage has not been demonstrated for any method.
2. Does adjuvant hormonal therapy following RP improve outcome in pathologic stage D_1 patients? For example, both the Mayo Clinic (47, 48) and UCLA (49) experiences suggest a marginal benefit for immediate hormonal ablation.

Current approaches to patients with both clinical (decisions made preoperatively) and pathologic stage D_1 (decisions made intraoperatively or postoperatively) vary widely. The Southwest Oncology Group (SWOG) and Eastern Cooperative Oncology Group (ECOG) could not complete a randomized trial comparing immediate and delayed hormone therapy in such patients because of inadequate enrollment. Thus, most clinicians deal with each patient individually, using early combined androgen blockage in many.

New staging techniques, such as prostate ultrasound and PSA combined with precise surgical and pathologic staging result in stage migration (50). This phenomenon will result in more precise staging, more accurate prognosis, and an improved survival for patients with any given stage of the disease. Thus, patients with *pathologic* A_2 disease will have a better prognosis than those with *clinical* A_2 disease. Also, for example, pathologic stage D_1 with only a single node involved microscopically and a normal

Table 57.3. Prognosis and Treatment Recommendations by Stage for Prostate Cancer

Clinical Stage	Treatment Recommendations	Expected 10-Year Survival
A_1	Observation	90%
A_2	Surgery/radiotherapy	60–70%
B_1	Surgery/radiotherapy	50–60%
B_2	Radiotherapy/surgery	40–50%
C	Radiotherapy	30–40%
D_1	Hormones ± radiotherapy	10–15%

PSA, will have a substantially better prognosis than clinical D_1 with massive bilateral lymph node involvement and an elevated PSA. This warning is not meant to dissuade the use of the more accurate staging methods, it simply means that the prognostic meaning of a "clean" stage will be unclear for several decades. Only as sufficient numbers of patients are studied with these new staging techniques will the clinician have a clear prognostic picture.

In summary, the treatment approaches in Table 57.3 can be recommended for the management of localized PC. Each patient with localized prostate cancer should at least be seen by both a urologic and radiation oncologist. In this way, the patient can make an informed decision in what is often a very complicated, and emotionally charged, matter.

Treatment of Advanced Prostate Cancer

The therapy of metastatic or locally advanced prostate cancer has been hormone ablation since Huggins and Hodges reported the first clinical experience in 1941 (51). They performed orchiectomies in patients who had x-ray evidence of osteoblastic lesions. Most patients had relief of bone pain and an improved sense of well-being, with some patients experiencing prolonged survival. This initial report was greeted with widespread enthusiasm for hormone therapy, and therefore, no controlled randomized trials were performed comparing a group of patients who received hormone therapy with a group who did not. Thus, inferences regarding the survival advantage of hormone therapy can only be made on the basis of retrospective data. In 1950, Nesbit and Baum reported a series of 263 patients treated before, and 324 others treated after, the use of hormone therapy became widespread (52). Patients who received hormone therapy had a median survival approximately 18 months longer than those not treated with hormone therapy. Based on these data and the striking clinical benefit of hormone therapy, it is the widespread assumption of physicians that such therapy lengthens the life of patients with metastatic PC, and thus, a randomized trial can no longer be done.

Huggins and Hodges found that diethylstilbestrol (DES), an inexpensive synthetic compound with estrogenic activity, was apparently equivalent to orchiectomy in the treatment of metastatic PC (51). Since the Nesbit and Baum analysis suggested an advantage for the combination, the standard therapy in the United States for metastatic PC, from 1950 to 1970, was either orchiectomy, DES, or both. After a series of studies by the VA Cooperative Urologic Research Group (53) showed DES to be more toxic (excess cardiovascular toxicity, gynecomastia, and fluid retention) but no more effective than orchiectomy, DES use began to decline. However, the DES versus orchiectomy debate continued for many years. Orchiectomy had an advantage because it did not require ongoing compliance by the patient, produced no breast enlargement, induced maximum testosterone reduction, and had no excess cardiovascular morbidity. The only advantage of DES was that surgery was avoided.

In 1970, Schally and Guillemin in Louisiana and an independent group in Britain described the structure of the luteinizing-hormone-releasing hormone (LHRH) agonists (54). Schally's Nobel Prize–winning work led to the rapid development of LHRH agonists in clinical medicine. After binding of the LHRH agonist to the pituitary cells, there is an initial surge of luteinizing hormone (LH) and testosterone. The pituitary cells then become desensitized, and there is downregulation of the LHRH receptor, leading to a dramatic drop in LH and testosterone levels. This effect is the physiologic equivalent of castration, with anorchic levels of testosterone achieved by 1 month (55, 56). The first trial directly comparing an LHRH agonist, leuprolide (Lupron), with DES was reported in 1985 (55). This trial was underpowered by today's standards, but it enrolled 98 patients on leuprolide and 101 on DES (3 mg/day). There were no differences in survival or response. Hot flashes were more common in the LHRH agonist group, whereas gynecomastia and breast tenderness were more common in the DES group. Nausea and vomiting, edema, and thrombosis/phlebitis

were also more common in the DES group. The major disadvantages of the LHRH agonist were the cost and the cumbersome administration method, namely, daily subcutaneous injection. Lupron is now available as a monthly intramuscular injection of drug admixed with starch microspheres.

Goserelin (Zoladex), another LHRH agonist, became available as a monthly injection, releasing the drug from a subcutaneously placed copolymer pellet over a 30- to 40-day period. The first phase III trial of Zoladex was against orchiectomy, and the two were equivalent (56). In a subsequent trial patients, were offered either orchiectomy or Zoladex, a "patient choice" study. In that trial, over 80% of patients chose to undergo a monthly injection of Zoladex and avoid the psychologically damaging effects of castration (57). These randomized clinical trials with Zoladex and Lupron prove that they are comparable to (if not better than) other hormone therapies of PC.

With testosterone suppression by LHRH agonists proven to be an effective treatment of metastatic PC, factors prognostic for survival of metastatic PC could be identified. In a multivariate analysis, four factors were independently prognostic: baseline performance status, presence of absence of bone pain, and baseline testosterone and alkaline phosphatase levels (58). With all four factors unfavorable, median survival was less than 6 months, but if all four factors were favorable, median survival exceeded 3 years. To improve these results, two new approaches to hormonal therapy for PC were extensively studied in the mid-1980s. These included (a) "total androgen blockade" (TAB) with a nonsteroidal antiandrogen (flutamide) added to orchiectomy, DES, or LHRH agonist to block adrenal androgen induced stimulation of PC growth and (b) concomitant hormonal and chemotherapy. Chemohormonal therapy did not prove to be of benefit, but total androgen blockage has become the new paradigm.

Early enthusiasm for TAB was driven by a phase II trial by Labrie et al. in Quebec (59), in which 223 patients received flutamide in addition to an LHRH agonist or orchiectomy. Nonrandomized comparisons with orchiectomy, DES, or LHRH agonist studies showed an improved response rate (94 vs. 82%), an improved 2-year continued response rate (51 vs. near 0%), and an improved 4-year survival (43 vs. 10 to 28%). These provocative results led the United States National Cancer Institute to conduct a phase III trial comparing TAB with an LHRH agonist plus the antiandrogen flutamide with an LHRH agonist alone (leuprolide) (60). Crawford et al. reported the results of 603 randomized patients. The LHRH agonist plus flutamide was superior to the LHRH agonist alone ($p < .05$) in progression-free survival (16.5 vs. 13.9 months) and in overall survival (35.9 vs. 28.3 months). In a subset analysis of patients, it appeared that the benefit was primarily in those with a high performance status and minimal volume of disease. For the patient with advanced metastatic PC, the benefit was less. For example, patients with severe disease and a performance status of 3 (bedridden more than 50% of walking hours) had a median survival of 27.3 months with leuprolide and 23.9 months with leuprolide plus flutamide.

Many clinicians believed, as suggested by Kuhn et al., that the benefit of the antiandrogen was merely to prevent the transient worsening of disease that occurred with the testosterone release induced by the LHRH agonist (61). Thus a host of phase III trials were undertaken to further define the role of the antiandrogen in therapy. For example, the European Organization for the Research and Treatment of Cancer (EORTC) performed two randomized trials using the steroidal antiandrogen cyproterone acetate. There was no advantage for that antiandrogen in either study (62–63). Thrasher and Crawford recently reviewed this topic (64) and concluded that TAB may be of benefit but merits further study. A recent metaanalysis of 22 studies concluded that TAB was not superior to monotherapy with either orchiectomy or an LHRH agonist (65).

Another active area of investigation concerns the optimal antiandrogen for TAB. An early report of a large randomized study comparing once-daily bicalutamide (Casodex) and three-times-daily flutamide (Eulexin) showed an improved time to failure at 1 year and less diarrhea reported for the bicalutamide group (66). Bicalutamide may also be a more potent antiandrogen (67).

PSA plays a major role in the management of hormone-sensitive PC. The PSA level after TAB declines to normal in 71% of patients and to undetectable levels in approximately 22% of patients within 6 months of the start of antiandrogen therapy (66). Follow-up data are not yet available, but it is predicted that the subgroup of patients with undetectable levels will be those who have prolonged survival with hormone therapy (66, 68, 69).

In conclusion, the elderly male with metastatic PC detected by bone scan or physical examination requires reduction of the serum testosterone to the castrate range. Hormone ablation with an orchiectomy can be debilitating psychologically and will render all men impotent. Single monthly injections of a long-acting LHRH agonist results in similar side effects, but at an increased financial cost. This therapy, however, is well tolerated and is preferred by most patients with metastatic PC. TAB appears to offer a slight survival advantage over single-agent LHRH agonist therapy. The large-scale (>1300 patient) SWOG trial comparing monotherapy and TAB may answer the question.

The role of cytotoxic chemotherapy in the management of PC remains limited (70, 71) for many reasons: (a) methodologic difficulties, including the lack of reliable objective parameters for judging antitumor effects in bone metastases; (b) the generally older age of these patients and consequent susceptibility to severe toxicities with chemotherapy; (c) the variable natural history of hormone-refractory PC; and (d) the low growth rate of PC cells (72). Most clinical trials have failed to demonstrate an improvement in survival when multiple-agent chemotherapy is compared with single-agent chemotherapy in randomized trials in hormone-refractory patients (73) or when single- or multiple-agent chemotherapy is compared with controls. The only exception is the trial of cyclophosphamide (1 g intravenously every 3 weeks) versus placebo, which demonstrated a 3-month survival advantage for intravenous cyclophosphamide (74). Therefore, it has been suggested that the proper control for further studies continues to be a no-chemotherapy arm consisting of palliative treatment, such as RT, analgesics, or possibly a second-line hormonal manipulation. The endpoint for analysis should include survival, given the methodologic problems in assessing disease regression (70–72).

More recently, PSA has replaced the NPCP criteria as acceptable evidence of response to chemotherapy. Kelley et al. found a 50% decrease in PSA level after chemotherapy correlated with improved survival (75). Using PSA endpoints, several other regimens have recently been shown to have a potential role in the treatment of hormone-refractory PC. Tannock (71) and others have emphasized the importance of quality of life as a primary or secondary endpoint.

Many phase II chemotherapy studies have

been done in patients with hormonally resistant PC. Several drugs have shown activity with CR + PR rates of 5 to 30%. These numbers must be interpreted with caution, however, as the confidence intervals are wide and the response criteria vary widely. Higher response rates in earlier studies included patients with "stable disease." Active single agents include Adriamycin, cyclophosphamide, cisplatin, mitoxantrone, vinblastine, and trimetrexate (70, 73). Oral Cytoxan has shown activity in several recent studies (76). Estramustine phosphate (EMP) has shown poor activity as a single agent (77), but the combinations of EMP and vinblastine have shown non-PSA response rates of 25% (78, 79), and EMP and oral VP16, up to 50% (80). PSA responses (as defined by a PSA decrease of ≥50%) reach up to 60%, but median survival times in these groups do not exceed 10 months. Suramin, which probably acts as a growth factor inhibitor, has generated recent excitement. Objective response rates of 31% with PSA decreases of 50% or more in 63% of patients have correlated with clear improvements in survival in responders (81).

Presently, the goal of chemotherapy remains palliative. A recent randomized study examined pain and quality of life as endpoints in comparing mitoxantrone plus prednisone (M+P) with prednisone alone (P). The M+P group showed a statistically significant improvement in subjective pain control compared with the P group (27.5 vs. 13.6%, $p = .033$) (82).

Given these less than striking responses to any chemotherapeutic approaches, many clinicians continue to use second-line hormonal therapies (83, 84). These agents usually cause objective improvement in only 5 to 10% of patients, although 15 to 30% of patients will experience subjective improvement for 2 to 6 months. The agents most commonly used include ketoconazole, medroxyprogesterone acetate (Megace), and corticosteroids.

Recently, several investigators have reported a beneficial response to flutamide withdrawal in hormone-refractory patients (85, 86). Between 20 and 40% of patients treated with combined androgen blockade as initial treatment have shown a PSA decline of more than 50% after flutamide administration was discontinued, and these responses were durable for many months in some patients. Additionally, objective responses in bone scans and measurable disease have been seen. Symptomatic improvement correlated with PSA response, and the degree of PSA response correlated with duration of response to flutam-

ide withdrawal. This withdrawal response is felt to be due to mutations of the androgen receptor (AR) that allow the AR to be stimulated by the antiandrogen. Withdrawal of the antiandrogen from the AR induces cell death via apoptosis (87). This phenomenon of response to flutamide withdrawal is important not only as a modality for "treating" the hormone-refractory disease patient but also as a possible confounder in patients on clinical trials for hormone-refractory disease. For this reason, it is advisable that patients withdrawn from flutamide demonstrate a clear increase in PSA before initiating new treatments, either on or off study.

These disappointing responses to second-line hormone therapy and the lack of survival advantage demonstrated in the overall group of hormone-refractory patients have led many clinicians to recommend palliative radiation therapy, including intravenous radionuclides such as strontium (88, 89), as the most appropriate care for these patients. Other institutions offer these patients experimental or investigational chemotherapy.

TESTICULAR CANCER

Epidemiology

Testicular cancer is the most common cancer among young men between the ages of 15 and 34, and it is estimated that 7100 new cases will occur in 1995 (1). Testis cancer is also a sentinel disease because of its impact on a young and economically important group of patients.

Certain clinical clues may relate to the etiology of testicular cancer. Caucasians develop the disease at a rate that is four times that of African Americans. Certain Caucasian groups experience a substantial risk of testis cancer: in Denmark, there are almost 10 cases per 100,000 men (89), and Norway, Sweden, and the United Kingdom also have excessive rates. In contrast, Finland has a low incidence of the disease, and the disease is rare in Asian populations (90). There has also been a definite increase of the incidence of the disease since the 1960s; for example, the rate in Denmark in 1960 was about 4.2 per 100,000 males, whereas in 1982 the rate was over 10 per 100,000 (91).

Certain congenital anomalies seem to be associated with testicular cancer. One of the most frequent is cryptorchism (testicular maldescent). There is a 5- to 10-fold increased risk of testicular cancer in males with cryptorchism. The "normal" testicle is at a slightly increased risk as well, suggesting a "field defect" in the primitive germ cells (92). Ten to 14% of all patients with cancer of the testicle have a history of testicular maldescent (93), and carcinoma in situ was found in 5 of 300 men undergoing testicular biopsies for a history of cryptorchism (94). The cause of cryptorchism is unclear, but it is hypothesized to be an abnormality of the migration of the germ cells during the fifth to seventh week in utero. Abnormal embryogenesis in germ cell tumor patients may explain their increased risk of congenital anomalies of the urinary system (95). Renal agenesis, renal tract duplication, and medullary sponge kidney have been reported in excess in these patients. There is also an increased risk of testicular cancer in males with congenital inguinal hernias, supranummary nipples, spina bifida occulta, or a family history of testicular cancer (90, 96). The relationships between isochromosome 12p, the major chromosomal abnormality in germ cell cancer (97), cryptorchism, carcinoma in situ, and congenital anomalies is a subject for future research.

Differential Diagnosis

The differential diagnosis of testicular cancer must take into account all lesions within the scrotum such as hydroceles, epididymitis, orchitis, incarcerated hernias, epididymal cysts, and spermatoceles. In spite of the difficulties in diagnosis, physicians make the correct diagnosis on initial physical examination in about 60% of patients (93). Approximately 20% are diagnosed as having epididymitis or orchitis, 10% are diagnosed as having a hydrocele or traumatic problem, and 10% are misdiagnosed in a more significant way (i.e., no examination of the scrotum). Delay in the diagnosis of testis cancer can often be significant and may lead to poor outcome in some patients (93).

Radical orchiectomy is the principal procedure for the diagnosis and initial treatment of testicular cancer. This involves an incision over the spermatic cord and delivery of its distal contents through the incision. Since the primary lymphatic drainage of the testicle is to the periaortic nodes, any transscrotal procedure such as aspiration or biopsy will potentially allow malignant cells into the inguinal lymphatic drainage system and thus should be avoided. About 10% of patients with testicular cancer experience scrotal violation (98). In the past, it was felt that a hemiscrotectomy and inguinal lymph node

dissection was necessary to avoid a recurrence in the scrotum or inguinal nodes. With the recent advent of effective systemic chemotherapy, such approaches appear to be less necessary (98).

Histology and Examination

At the time of a radical orchiectomy, a histologic specimen is obtained. Seven to 13% of specimens will be non-germ-cell tumors, usually sex cord–stromal tumors or lymphomas. Recent advances in the treatment of testicular lymphoma have been reviewed (99). The reader is referred to a recent excellent textbook that discusses in detail the histologic subtypes of testicular tumors (100). This chapter is confined to a discussion of the treatment of testicular germ cell neoplasms. Histologically, approximately 50 to 60% of all germ cell tumors are seminomas, 20 to 30% are embryonal carcinomas, 10 to 20% are teratomas or teratocarcinomas, and less than 5% are choriocarcinomas. For treatment purposes, a major distinction must be made between seminoma and nonseminoma. A nonseminoma may contain areas of seminoma, but a seminoma may never contain nonseminoma components; that is, it must be histologically pure to be called seminoma.

On the physical examination of a testicular mass, a seminoma is commonly smooth, painless, and asymptomatic. A nonseminoma is commonly nodular, painful, and symptomatic. The mean age of all patients with testicular cancer is 31 years; the mean age of patients with seminoma is 37 years, the mean age of patients with mixed tumors (seminoma and nonseminoma) is 35 years, and the mean age of patients with pure nonseminomatous tumors is 28 years (93).

Tumor Markers

Both the human chorionic gonadotropin (HCG) and α-fetoprotein (AFP) tumor markers play a major role in the treatment and management of germ cell tumors. AFP, a protein with a molecular weight of 70,000, is synthesized by the fetal liver and yolk sac and is the major component of fetal serum. AFP shares considerable structural homology with human albumin, the major difference being that albumin is nonglycosylated and AFP is variably glycosylated (101). With complete surgical removal of a tumor producing AFP, the half-life of AFP is approximately 5 days. The 5-day half-life is a helpful and, at times, a definitive diagnostic test of the completeness of surgical excision of lesions. It is also a helpful and sometimes definitive marker of the degree of chemotherapy effectiveness (102).

HCG, in contrast to AFP, has a molecular weight of only 45,000 and a half-life of approximately 24 hours (102, 103). It also is used to test the completeness of surgical or chemotherapy treatment. It is normally synthesized by placental syncytiotrophoblasts. It shares α-chain homology with the pituitary hormones, luteinizing hormone (LH), follicle-stimulating hormone (FSH), and thyroid-stimulating hormone (TSH). Its β-chain shares 70% homology with the β-chain of LH. The major difference between LH and HCG is that the carboxy terminus portion of the HCG molecule from amino acid position 111 to amino acid position 145 is unique and not shared with LH. That portion of the amino acid chain is glycosylated at four distinct sites and accounts for four of the six glycosylation positions of the HCG molecule. Thus, antibodies raised against HCG most commonly recognize epitopes between positions 111 to 145, although certain antibodies recognize the glycosylation epitopes at the amino acid terminus of the molecule. This diversity of sites for antibody recognition is reflected clinically in that multiple different radioimmunoassays are commercially available to detect HCG (104). Comparability between assays may be poor because of the different epitopes recognized.

Ten to 15% of patients with seminoma will have a detectable level of HCG, but pure seminoma cannot produce AFP. There may be rare examples in which apparently pure seminoma histologically does produce AFP; however, one inevitably finds nonseminomatous components either through careful sectioning, by biopsies of metastatic lesions, or at autopsy. Such AFP-producing "seminomas" are treated as nonseminomas, since their prognosis is identical to that of nonseminomas. Nonseminomatous germ cell tumors are capable of producing both HCG and AFP. The choriocarcinoma component is an obligatory producer of HCG. The yolk sac tumor histologic component is an obligatory producer of AFP. Pure embryonal carcinoma may produce either or neither.

The management of germ cell tumors has been revolutionized since the markers AFP and HCG entered clinical practice between 1976 and 1978. The markers are highly concordant with the growth or regression of tumor and have been labeled as the prototype of tumor markers in human oncology. The clinical utility of these markers has been repeatedly demonstrated. Their utility may be declining, however, since the frequency of AFP elevation in metastatic nonseminoma has declined from approximately 70% in the late 1970s and early 1980s to 60% in the late 1980s. Likewise, HCG elevations have dropped from 70 or 80% to only 55% in a recent review (105).

A third serum marker for testicular cancer that is often ignored is lactate dehydrogenase (LDH). This tumor marker is produced by both seminoma and nonseminoma. Although not specific for histologic subtype, an elevated LDH is highly diagnostic for recurrent or residual disease. Its presence or absence does not reflect liver metastases but rather is a direct correlate of tumor volume and prognosis (106).

Staging

The most commonly used clinically relevant staging system is stage I (disease confined to the testicle), stage II (disease metastatic to the regional lymph nodes), and stage III (metastatic disease). This system does not integrate tumor volume or marker data and is likely to be revised shortly.

Treatment of Seminoma

The treatment of seminoma is straightforward. RT to the retroperitoneal lymph nodes in clinical stage I disease results in a 98% 5-year disease-free survival. The technique of radiotherapy for seminoma is well defined (107). In general, the port is known as a "hockey stick field"; the superior border is the diaphragm or top of T11, the inferior border is usually the inguinal incision, and the lateral borders are the renal hilar nodes. The contralateral testis is shielded, although 0.1% of the treatment dose still strikes that testis. The radiotherapy field usually encompasses the ipsilateral hemiscrotum in patients who have scrotal violations or large tumors.

Recently, some physicians have challenged the routine use of RT for stage I seminoma, since the great majority of patients may be cured with orchiectomy alone, while all patients are at risk for the delayed toxicities of RT. In a large Danish study, 261 patients were followed with tumor marker and radiologic observation only. With a median follow-up of 48 months, only 19% had relapsed. As a result of excellent salvage with RT in most and chemotherapy in some, only 3 patients (1%) died of seminoma. The 4-year re-lapse-free survival for patients with large (≥ 6 cm) tumors was 64%, compared with 82% for tumors 3 to 6 cm and 94% for tumors less than 3 cm. This prognostic factor may help physicians and patients choose between RT and observation for clinical stage I seminomas (108).

Patients with clinical stage II seminoma (en-larged retroperitoneal lymph nodes shown ei-ther on lymphangiogram or on CT scan) have a reduced 5-year disease-free survival rate of ap-proximately 79% with RT. As the volume of ret-roperitoneal disease increases, the disease-free survival decreases, yet data can be found sup-porting RT for all substages of stage II seminoma (109). Using the Royal Marsden Hospital (RMH) staging system (Table 57.4), stage IIA has a re-lapse rate of about 10% when treated with radio-therapy, while stages IIB, IIC, and IID have re-lapse rates of approximately 20%, 40%, and 60%, respectively (107). Thus, most physicians today recommend chemotherapy for stage IIC-D sem-inomas, with RT reserved for the stage IIA pa-tients. Opinion is divided on stage IIB. With this approach, virtually all patients will be cured of their disease. Management of RMH stage III and IV seminomas is identical to the management of stage III nonseminomas (see below).

The management of seminomas that produce HCG has been somewhat controversial. Recent data suggest that most HCG-producing semi-nomas do not have a worse prognosis, stage for stage, than non-HCG-producing seminomas. Since HCG-producing seminomas tend to be stage II or III at diagnosis, there has arisen the erroneous conclusion that it is a poor prognostic feature. In fact, HCG-positive or -negative stage I seminomas apparently have similar survival if treated by routine RT (110, 111).

Treatment of Stage I Nonseminoma

The management of clinical stage I nonsemi-nomas has recently been reviewed (112, 113, 114). To summarize, patients with a nonsemi-nomatous tumor whose clinical staging is nega-tive and whose markers have returned to normal are considered to be clinical stage I patients. The CT scan must be unequivocally negative, since the presence of a single enlarged lymph node defines the patient as a clinical stage II. A recent large study quantified the risk of pathologic stage II disease at 48% if an 8- to 9-mm lymph node is visible (115).

The traditional management of clinical stage

Table 57.4. Royal Marsden Hospital Staging System for Seminoma

Stage I	Tumor confined to the testis
Stage IIA	Retroperitoneal mass <2 cm or positive on lymphangiogram
Stage IIB	Retroperitoneal mass 2–4.9 cm
Stage IIC	Retroperitoneal mass 5–9.9 cm
Stage IID	Retroperitoneal mass >10 cm
Stage III	Tumor involving lymphatics above the diaphragm
Stage IV	Extranodal metastases

I patients has been a retroperitoneal lymph node dissection (RPLND). This allowed identification and treatment of the approximately 15 to 20% of patients who had microscopic or small-volume retroperitoneal disease not detectable with either CT scanning, lymphangiograms, or tumor marker tests. It also effectively "sterilized" the retroperitoneum, allowing follow-up to focus on the 6 to 14% risk of relapse, usually marker-pos-itive disease only or pulmonary metastasis (116). Surgical morbidity from the RPLND consisted primarily of postoperative complications (ileus, infections, etc.) and the long-term risk of retro-grade ejaculation. Retrograde ejaculation does not mean infertility, it simply means that the sperm, when ejaculated, are not emitted but rather are retained within the urinary bladder. This common and distressing event led physi-cians and patients to seek alternative approaches to the management of clinical stage I disease. One of the more successful ways to manage this problem has been the development of a nerve-sparing RPLND (117, 118). This technique has resulted in the virtual elimination of retrograde ejaculation. Nonetheless, many patients contin-ued to be concerned about the universal risk of surgical morbidity and mortality for a benefit of only 15%.

In Denmark and England, RT (40 to 50 cGy) to the retroperitoneum has been the standard treatment of clinical stage I nonseminoma since the 1940s. For example, in the Royal Marsden experience, only 2 of 84 patients relapsed in the retroperitoneum (107). Between 1980 and 1985, a Danish randomized trial compared RT with observation. Observation was defined as an ag-gressive follow-up of the patient, using CT scans, serum tumor markers, and physical examina-tions at 1- to 2-month intervals for 2 to 5 years. No survival differences were seen (119). Thus, close observation has become the standard management for clinical stage I nonseminoma in some European countries.

In surgically oriented countries and institutions, a number of "observation only" phase II trials have shown no decreased rate of survival as historically compared with standard RPLND (120, 113, 114). Both groups have a 98% 5-year overall survival (113). However, phase III trials have not been performed. There are concerns that small amounts of disease left in the retroperitoneal nodes will enlarge over a period of several years and lead to late retroperitoneal relapses (121). This has been documented in several patients. However, it is unlikely that a few late relapses will lead to abandonment of the observation approach.

Several models have been proposed to attempt to predict those stage I patients at highest risk of relapse. Vascular invasion is probably the most important predictor of relapse; 35% of patients in one surveillance study relapsed (113), and 49% of patients with vascular invasion in another study (122) had pathologic stage II disease noted from RPLND. Other poor prognostic factors include lymphatic invasion, percentage of embryonal carcinoma, and absence of yolk sac tumor. Decreases in the morbidity and mortality of RPLND, including the development of laparoscopic RPLND (123), could minimize the benefits of a surveillance program.

Adjuvant chemotherapy for clinical stage I disease could eliminate the risk of retroperitoneal lymph node relapse (15 to 20%) and distant relapse (6 to 14%) seen in patients treated with observation. This approach is attractive, although it would overtreat 75 to 80% of patients with stage I disease (112). Large-scale trials comparing observation with chemotherapy are being performed in Europe with encouraging preliminary data (124).

In conclusion, management of clinical stage I nonseminoma in the United States in 1995 includes offering the patient either an RPLND or observation with careful clinical follow-up. In some European countries, adjuvant chemotherapy is the standard of care, albeit with the potential for long-term toxicities and without long-term published outcome data. In these physicians' experience, approximately 75% of patients will continue to select the RPLND because of the precision and certainty that results. Among the 25% of patients who would select observation, certain patients should be excluded: patients with stage T_3 or T_4 tumors (i.e., tumors involving the spermatic cord or the scrotal wall

(125)), patients who have experienced a scrotal violation, and patients who are unreliable or who are geographically isolated and unable to return for regular visits.

Treatment of Stage II Nonseminoma

Clinical stage II testis cancer has been redefined by the advent of CT scanning and serum tumor markers. Before CT scans and markers were available, clinical stage II testis cancer was defined using lymphangiograms (LAGs) and intravenous pyelograms (IVPs). A definition of stage IA meant a normal LAG, while IB meant LAG-only evidence of involvement of the nodes. Stage IIA was defined by deviation of the ureters, and IIB was a clinically palpable mass. Patients who then received an RPLND for stage IA or IB disease and were found to have positive nodes had overall 10-year survival rates of approximately 70% (microscopic nodes) and 40% (macroscopic nodes), respectively (126). The 40 to 50% 10-year disease-free survival rate following an RPLND only for node-positive disease has been repeatedly confirmed.

The prognostic factors for relapse following the finding of a positive RPLND are relatively clear (116). With microscopic involvement of the lymph nodes (stage IIA) the relapse rate is 30 to 40%. In stage IIB disease, (macroscopic disease but <5 cm), the relapse rate is about 50%. Stage IIC (grossly evident disease >5 cm) seems to be associated with a relapse rate of 60% (127).

The role of adjuvant chemotherapy in the management of pathologically proven stage II disease emerged when several series (126–129) described a virtually 100% disease-free survival following adjuvant chemotherapy for pathologic stage II disease. As compelling as those data were, the role of adjuvant chemotherapy for pathologic stage II nonseminoma was firmly defined by the Testicular Cancer Intergroup Study (TCIS). In that trial, 195 patients were randomized to receive either no adjuvant chemotherapy (N = 98) or two cycles of cisplatin-based chemotherapy (N = 97). Of patients receiving two cycles of chemotherapy, only one died from testicular cancer, although there were six recurrences (only one of whom received adjuvant chemotherapy) and two deaths from other causes (127). Those patients randomized to no chemotherapy experienced a 49% recurrence rate, but only three died of testicular cancer. The authors concluded that two cycles of cisplatin-based adjuvant chemotherapy will "almost always prevent relapse in pathologic stage II testicular cancer." They also concluded that "when surgery, follow-up, and chemotherapy are optimal, observation with chemotherapy only for relapse will lead to equivalent cure rates." Most patients presented with these data prefer the certainty of virtual cure with two cycles of adjuvant chemotherapy and request immediate chemotherapy. Recently Motzer et al. treated 50 patients with pathologic stage II disease with two cycles of adjuvant cisplatin and etoposide, omitting bleomycin. At a median of 30 months of follow-up, all were alive and relapse free (130).

With the striking effectiveness of chemotherapy, the role of the RPLND in clinical stage II nonseminoma has declined. If patients have a strongly positive CT scan and/or positive markers, most physicians treat with three to four cycles of chemotherapy and reserve the RPLND for radiographically persistent retroperitoneal disease. Over 95% of patients undergoing an RPLND after chemotherapy are found to be free of tumor if there is no residual mass (131).

Therapy of Stage III Disease

Metastatic testicular cancer has been curable with chemotherapy since the report of "triple therapy" (actinomycin, L-phenylalanine mustard, and methotrexate) in 1960 by Li et al. (132). This model of combination chemotherapy provided a paradigm for the development of combination chemotherapy for Hodgkin's disease. Li et al. reported a cure rate of approximately 10 to 15%, and other reports were confirmative (133). With the development of vinblastine in 1970 and bleomycin in 1972, both active agents in germ cell tumors, a regimen known as VB-1 and subsequently VB-3 was developed at M. D. Anderson Hospital (134). With these two regimens, complete remission of disease was achieved in 33% and 48% of patients, respectively. The cost of complete remission was the pulmonary toxicity of bleomycin (which was eliminated or dramatically reduced by the use of the continuous infusion schedule) and the myelosuppression of vinblastine. From 1960 to 1972, other chemotherapeutic agents and regimens were tried with limited success. For example, single-agent methotrexate caused complete regressions in 4 of 10 patients (135).

All of these therapeutic endeavors were dwarfed by the discovery in 1974 of the activity of cis-diamminedichloroplatinum-II (cisplatin) as an active agent in germ cell tumors (136). Nine

of the first 11 germ cell testicular cancer patients treated with the drug experienced responses, 3 of which were complete. All of the patients treated at Roswell Park had far-advanced disease and were heavily pretreated with chemotherapy. This simple observation was the beginning of a revolution in the treatment of testicular cancer. Dr. Lawrence Einhorn at Indiana University, who trained at M. D. Anderson Hospital, combined cisplatin at the recommended phase II dose of 20 mg/m^2/day $\times$ 5 with a modification of the M. D. Anderson vinblastine and bleomycin regimen, using vinblastine at a dose of 0.15 mg/kg intravenously on days 1 and 2, and bleomycin 30 mg intravenously on days 2, 9, and 16. This PVB regimen repeated every 21 days became known as the "Einhorn" regimen and induced complete remissions in 70% of the first 47 patients treated (137). A long-term update of that group of patients demonstrated that 65% of the initial cohort of patients was alive and free of disease (138). The striking success of cisplatin in combination with vinblastine and bleomycin has been repeatedly confirmed throughout the world (139, 140).

At Memorial Sloan-Kettering Cancer Center in New York, where Dr. Li's work was carried out, the VAB regimens (vinblastine, actinomycin D, and bleomycin) were developed during the 1970s. VAB-1 (without cisplatin) cured between 10 and 15% of patients. VAB-2, VAB-3, and VAB-4, using cisplatin 120 mg/m^2 approximately every 3 to 4 months, were associated with 24%, 49%, and 50% complete remission rates (141). The VAB-6 regimen (using 120 mg/m^2 of cisplatin every month $\times$ 3 in addition to vinblastine, actinomycin, bleomycin and cyclophosphamide) had a complete remission rate equivalent to the PVB program. The Indiana regimen uses 20 mg/m^2/day $\times$ 5 days of cisplatin, whereas the Memorial regimen used 120 mg/m^2 of cisplatin as a single bolus. These two regimens differ somewhat in their clinical toxicity parameters; the VAB-6 regimen is slightly more nephrotoxic, and the PVB regimen is more myelotoxic (142). Nonetheless, since 1982, these two regimens have been viewed as clinically equal.

The importance of the dosage of cisplatin was defined by the SWOG in a randomized trial of over 100 testicular cancer patients (143). Patients received PVB with cisplatin 120 mg/m^2 as a single dose or cisplatin 15 mg/m^2/day for 5 days. Dose intensity of the cisplatin was the only variable in the randomized trial. Survival of patients receiving low-dose cisplatin was significantly inferior to that of patients receiving high-dose cisplatin. This pivotal study definitively established the value of high-dose cisplatin therapy. Thus, the management of stage III testicular cancer requires that high-dose cisplatin ($\geq$100 mg/m^2/cycle) be administered at 3- to 4-week intervals to these patients. Alternative regimens administering cisplatin at a dose-intensity of 50 to 60 mg/m^2/week are possibly equivalent to PVB or VAB-6, but no direct comparative trials have been reported.

As the striking success of the PVB and VAB-6 regimens was being reported, several new anti-germ-cell cancer drugs were also being developed. The most promising drug was etoposide, or VP-16, a semisynthetic derivative of the mitotic inhibitor podophyllotoxin, which inhibits the DNA-active enzyme topoisomerase II. The drug was highly synergistic with cisplatin in preclinical models. Small case series from the Charing Cross Hospital and the Royal Marsden Hospital (144) and, subsequently, larger trials from Minnesota (145) and Indiana (146) demonstrated its curative ability in approximately 20% of patients refractory to cisplatin-based chemotherapy. The activity of the drug was impressive enough to lead to phase III trials comparing PVB with bleomycin, etoposide, and platinum (BEP) in 244 patients. Patients with advanced disease treated with BEP had less neuromuscular toxicity and a better survival (p = .02) than those treated with PVB (147).

A similarly important trial (148) randomized 164 good-risk testicular cancer patients to three cycles of VAB-6 or four cycles of cisplatin and etoposide (EP). EP was less toxic than the VAB-6 regimen and induced a 93% complete remission rate, compared with 96% for VAB-6 (not significant). These two studies thus demonstrated the superiority of platinum/etoposide-based regimens to non-etoposide-based regimens.

As cure rates remained high for good-risk patients treated with only two or three drugs, focus changed to minimizing the toxicity of treatment. Cisplatin is associated with severe emesis, nephrotoxicity, ototoxicity, and peripheral nerve toxicity. Carboplatin, a cisplatin analogue, has substantially less toxicity, and several nonrandomized trials suggested equal efficacy. A large randomized trial of four cycles of EP versus etoposide and carboplatin (EC) showed EC to be inferior to EP (149). Those treated with EC had a 76% rate of durable CR versus 87% for the EP group at a median follow-up of almost 2 years. There was no difference in overall survival evident at 2 years. In this trial, EC was

given every 4 weeks and EP every 3 weeks, possibly accounting for the difference in outcome.

Again attempting to minimize treatment-related toxicity, a large randomized study was undertaken to address the question of the need for the fourth and most toxic cycle of BEP. Some 176 patients were randomized to either three or four cycles of BEP every 3 weeks. Disease-free survival was equivalent in each group. Based on this trial, it can be concluded that three cycles of BEP is adequate for favorable-risk disseminated germ cell tumor patients (150).

The role of bleomycin has been tested by the EORTC. This trial randomized patients to four cycles of PE or BEP. Ninety-one percent (140/153) of EP patients achieved CR versus 95% (154/160) of BEP patients. Seven EP patients had died as of the last update versus four BEP patients. Those differences were not statistically significant (151). Thus, the current standard chemotherapy for good-risk metastatic germ cell tumor must include cisplatin, (>100 mg/m^2/cycle) and etoposide (100 mg/m^2/day $\times$ 5) with either four cycles of EP or three cycles of BEP.

Another major advance has been the mathematically precise, quantifiable, and reproducible assignment of patients into "poor-risk" and "good-risk" categories (152–157). These studies, in general, identify the serum level of HCG, the serum level of LDH, and the volume of metastatic disease as the most important prognostic factors in achieving a complete remission. The AFP level and the size and number of lung metastases are important prognostic factors in some studies. Bajorin et al. found the Sloan-Kettering model (152) to be most precise and accurate (156).

A recent series by the Medical Research Council (MRC) examined the largest group of patients (N = 795) with metastatic nonseminomatous germ cell tumors. Based on seven clinical and pathologic features found to be independently prognostic, they developed a prognostic classification. Good-prognosis included those patients (67% of total) with none of the poor-risk factors (presence of liver, bone, or brain metastases, AFP above 1000 k units/L or HCG >10,000, mediastinal mass greater than 5 cm, or 20 or more lung metastases). These patients had a 93% 3-year survival compared with 68% for the group with one or more poor prognostic features (157).

Based on the inferior outcome of patients with high-risk disease, therapy must be more aggressive than that for good-risk patients. An intergroup trial randomized advanced-disease patients to BEP or to etoposide, cisplatin, and ifosfamide (VIP), asking whether ifosfamide is superior to bleomycin in the treatment of moderate-to-advanced-stage disease (by the Indiana University classification). There was no difference in survival, and VIP was more toxic (158). Thus, BEP × 4 remains the standard of care for initial treatment of high-risk disease. The current intergroup trial compares BEP × 4 with BEP × 2 plus two tandem cycles of high-dose chemotherapy (HDC) plus autologous bone marrow transplantation.

Despite all of the improvements in treatment in the past 20 years, approximately 25% of stage III patients will eventually relapse and require additional "salvage" chemotherapy. The most common approaches to initial treatment of these patients have been regimens containing both ifosfamide and cisplatin (159) or high-dose chemotherapy (HDC) with autologous stem cell rescue (ASCR). VIP or VeIP (VP-16 or vinblastine, ifosfamide, and cisplatin) followed by resection of residual mass will produce a complete response rate of 28 to 36% (160, 161). Approximately 15% will be free of disease after 1 to 2 years.

HDC regimens have generally incorporated carboplatin (1500 mg/m^2) and etoposide (1500 mg/m^2), with or without ifosfamide or cyclophosphamide. In heavily pretreated patients, a CR rate of 30% has been achieved, with 15 to 35% alive without disease at 2 years (162, 163). When used as an initial salvage regimen, both CR rates (55%) and continuous NED (no evidence of disease) rates (39%) may be higher, though some of these patients may have been cured by less intensive treatments (164). Motzer et al. (165) treated 22 poor-risk patients whose tumor markers were falling inappropriately slowly during initial therapy. In this group, 55% achieved a CR, with a 38% disease-free survival at 31 months. Droz et al. (166) examined prognostic factors for long-term response to HDC in 271 patients treated in 10 studies. The most important factor was disease status; cisplatin-responsive patients had a 35% NED rate, and refractory patients (progression during cisplatin treatment or within one month) had a 14% NED rate. Additionally, the dose of etoposide and ifosfamide (or cyclophosphamide) was found to be a significant predictor.

Patients who relapse following second- or third-line therapy should receive, when possible, treatment on a phase I or II study. This approach identified cisplatin and etoposide, the most im-

portant drugs used today. Recent studies have identified paclitaxel (CR rate, 10%; CR + PR, 26%) as an active agent (167). Daily oral etoposide has also shown efficacy in the setting of refractory disease, with a response rate of 14% (168).

The chronic toxicities of curative chemotherapy have recently been extensively reviewed (169). Mild irreversible loss of renal function has not progressed to renal failure, hypertension, or advanced renal disease (170–172). Chronic magnesium wasting has been identified in some of the patients treated with cisplatin (173) but does not appear to result in clinically significant toxicity (172). Approximately 40% of patients treated with bleomycin-containing regimens for testicular cancer experience Raynaud's phenomenon (174). These patients may notice reduction of the symptoms with time, while other patients are forced to alter their lifestyles to eliminate the cold-induced Raynaud's phenomenon. Finally, there is a transient infertility following platinum-based chemotherapy (175). The likelihood of infertility depends on prechemotherapy sperm counts (176). About 50% of patients recover sperm counts within 3 to 5 years following the completion of chemotherapy.

In conclusion, the management of stage I and II germ cell tumor of the testicle includes radical orchiectomy in all patients with RT to the retroperitoneum or observation in patients with clinical stage I seminoma. Either RPLND or observation are appropriate management of the patient with clinical stage I nonseminoma, with chemotherapy usually used for clinical stage II disease, and RPLND being reserved for resection of residual abnormalities. It is critical to stratify patients with metastatic stage III disease by the probability of complete remission. Patients who are identified as "good risk" (high probability of complete remission) should receive standard doses of cisplatin and etoposide-based chemotherapy (either three cycles of BEP or four cycles of EP). Patients identified as "poor risk" should receive intensification of standard chemotherapy, perhaps using ifosfamide or early bone marrow transplant. Such individualization of chemotherapy will lead to the cure of virtually all patients with this rapidly proliferating disease.

RENAL CARCINOMA

Cancer of the kidney is also called renal cell carcinoma (RCC), clear cell carcinoma, renal cortical carcinoma, kidney or renal adenocarcinoma, hypernephroma, or Grawitz tumor. All these names are synonyms for a cancer that arises from the proximal tubular cells of the human nephron (177). Kidney cancer has been known for centuries, and its histologic and clinical behavior is well documented (178).

Most cases of RCC are sporadic, but several well-defined inherited forms of kidney cancer have been described. Both the sporadic and hereditary forms frequently involve alterations of the short arm of chromosome three (3p). Familial kidney cancer is an autosomal dominant disease associated with a translocation or deletion at 3p14 (179, 180). Von Hippel-Lindau (VHL) is an autosomal disorder in which approximately one-third of patients develop RCC. In these patients, as well as in familial kidney cancer patients, tumors tend to be multifocal and occur at a younger age. In both VHL-associated RCC and sporadic RCC, mutations in the VHL gene at 3p25-6 are frequent and occur in about 56% of sporadic cases (179, 181). Conventional karyotypic analysis detects 3p abnormalities in 30% of patients (182). In addition, mutations of p53 can be commonly detected in RCC. Their reported incidence varies, and they are probably more frequent in advanced tumors (183). The existing evidence suggests that an accumulation of events including somatic mutations is necessary for the development and progression of RCC. Primary tumors are more commonly associated with 3p mutations and have a better prognosis than those with p53 or both p53 and 3p mutations, which portend more advanced disease with a worse prognosis (183, 184).

The most common histologic subtype of RCC is clear cell nuclear grade 1 to 2. Granular cell carcinoma is probably dedifferentiated nuclear grade 3 to 4 RCC. There is a third histologic subtype of RCC (accounting for less than 5% of cases) called the "sarcomatoid" variant. In most series, the survival of patients with the sarcomatoid variant is far below the median survival of either the clear cell or granular cell variants. The histologic subtypes may also constitute a spectrum, as evidenced by both molecular and clinical features. Clear cell carcinoma tends to be most commonly associated with 3p mutations (179, 185), whereas granular cell and sarcomatoid cancers tend to be more commonly associated with p53 mutations (186,187). The sarcomatoid variant probably represents a subtype with a greater degree of genetic change and a more advanced clinical picture.

There are two unusual histologic subtypes of RCC. One is an oncocytoma that has attracted considerable attention because of its virtually 100% survival and its unusual histologic appearance. The other unusual subtype of RCC is the papillary renal cell carcinoma, which has a slower clinical course than either the clear, granular, or sarcomatoid variants. Transitional cell carcinomas of the renal pelvis and collecting system must also be distinguished from renal parenchymal malignancies.

Clinical Features of Kidney Cancer

Approximately 29,000 new cases of kidney cancer are diagnosed every year in the United States, with 12,000 deaths per year from metastatic kidney cancer (1). There has been a slow, steady, increase in the incidence of the disease in both sexes over the past 30 years (188) (Fig 57.1). The male:female ratio is 2:1. The median age at diagnosis is 62 to 69 years. Metastases are present at diagnosis in about 18% of patients, as reported in a series of 2,473 patients from the American Cancer Society Illinois Division (189). The symptoms of kidney cancer are shown on Table 57.5.

Depending upon the selection criteria and the population base, an overall survival of 50% at 10 years is expected of patients with kidney cancer. The Robson kidney cancer staging system (190) is shown in Table 57.6. Other staging systems such as the TNM (191) are less able to discriminate between stages. Stage I patients have an excellent prognosis (80% or greater survival at 10 years). Stage II cancers (tumor invading the fat surrounding the kidney but confined within Gerota's fascia) have a 60 to 70% 10-year survival. Stage IIIA (tumor invading the vein or vena cava) has a 40 to 50% 5-year survival rate. Stage IIIB (tumor invading the lymph nodes) and stage IIIC (tumor invading both the nodes and the veins) have survival rates below 20% at 5 years. Stages IVA (tumor extending outside of Gerota's fascia and into the surrounding organs) and IVB (distant metastases) have median survivals of less than 1 year (189). For patients with metastatic disease, poor prognostic factors include poor performance status, multiple metastatic sites, and weight loss (192).

Therapy of Kidney Cancer

Treatment of kidney cancer must, if at all possible, be surgical, as metastatic disease is rarely curable. Through either an anterior transperitoneal, flank, or thoracoabdominal approach, the renal vessels are ligated, Gerota's fascia is in-

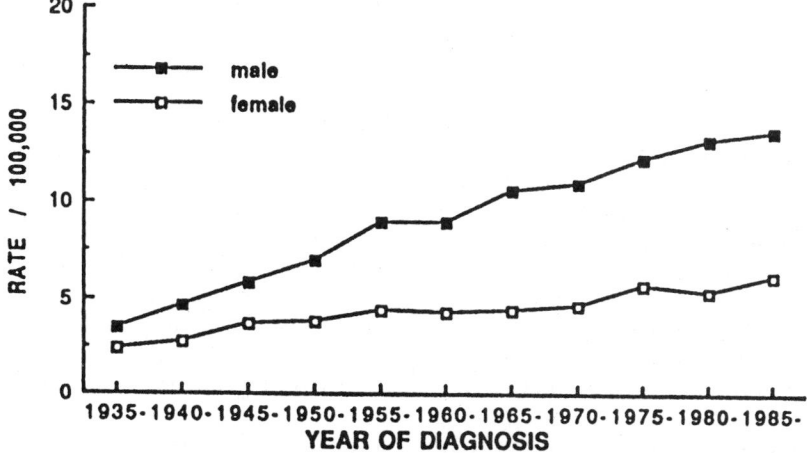

Figure 57.1. Standardized incidence rates of kidney cancer in Connecticut, 1935–1989. The incidence for both men and women has steadily increased. (Adapted with permission from Katz DL, Zheng T, Holford TR, Flannery J. Time trends in the incidence of renal cell carcinoma: Analysis of Connecticut Tumor Registry data: 1935–1989. Int J Cancer 1994;58:57–63.)

Table 57.5. Symptoms of Kidney Cancer

Symptom	% of Patients[a]
Pain	40
Hematuria	33
Weight loss	14
Other urinary	9
Fatigue	9
Metastatic	8
Fever	4

[a]Totals over 100% since patients could report more than one symptom.

Table 57.6. Robson Staging System for Kidney Cancer

Stage	Definition
I	Tumor limited to the kidney
II	Tumor invading perirenal fat but confined within Gerota's fascia
IIIA	Tumor invading renal vein or vena cava
IIIB	Tumor invading lymph nodes
IIIC	Combination of two preceding stages
IVA	Invasion of surrounding organs (other than adrenal glands)
IVB	Distant metastases

cised from its attachments, and the contents are removed en bloc. Regional lymphadenectomy is generally performed, though its benefits are disputed. Some authors have advocated an extended lymphadenectomy on the basis of a few reports of improved survival (mostly from single institutions) in these aggressively treated patients (193). These excellent results (a 5-year survival of 52% with lymph node involvement) may be partially a result of stage migration. Even with invasion into adjacent organs, a 5-year survival of approximately 5 to 10% can be achieved (189), arguing again for aggressive surgical management. Some patients who would otherwise require dialysis in the setting of a nephrectomy may be successfully treated with a partial nephrectomy (194).

RT for kidney cancer is commonly used for palliative control of painful bone metastases, brain metastases, or other painful lesions. Kidney cancer has a notorious reputation of being refractory to RT, yet in many series, RT has been shown to control painful lesions and lead to symptomatic improvement. Thus, judicious management and use of RT in the management of metastases is important (195).

Kidney cancer is one of the most common cancers undergoing spontaneous regression, but this event is still remarkably rare (196, 197). The operative risks of nephrectomy outweigh the potential benefit of a nephrectomy-associated spontaneous remission.

The observation that there is a male predominance of kidney cancer led early investigators to postulate a benefit of hormonal therapies. However, hormonal manipulations with progestational agents, antiestrogens, and antiandrogens have only rarely been successful (198–200) Thus, there is a minor role for nontoxic hormone therapy in metastatic kidney cancer.

The role of chemotherapy in metastatic kidney cancer has been widely explored. Single-agent chemotherapy of kidney cancer was recently reviewed, with the conclusion that no single agent was worthy to be considered "standard therapy" for metastatic kidney cancer (201). Although the list of drugs studied is extensive, continued persistence in studying new and old drugs in kidney cancer appears warranted. Recently, for example, FUDR has shown some evidence of activity (202–207). The best results with FUDR have been obtained using a continuous-infusion circadian treatment regimen, possibly with the addition of α-interferon to FUDR or 5-FU (208, 209) (Table 57.7). Response rates of 10 to 43% have been reported, but survival times may not be improved. Though FUDR may be an active drug for the treatment of RCC, chemotherapy for RCC should only be undertaken knowing the low response rate expected and so informing the patient.

A unique aspect of kidney cancer is that it contains among the highest concentrations of P-glycoprotein of any cancer. P-glycoprotein was discovered by Ling and Thompson on the surface of drug-resistant Chinese hamster ovary (CHO) cells (210). This 170,000-kDa protein has been characterized by Ronison et al. (211) and Safa et al. (212) as a "drug pump." The "pump" selectively binds chemotherapeutic agents with a ring-type structure and transports them out of the cells. The National Cancer Institute reported that 40 of 50 specimens of human renal cell carcinoma contained high or intermediate levels of P-glycoprotein (213). This suggests that P-glycoprotein is one of the major mechanisms by which renal cell cancer is resistent to chemotherapy. In vitro studies have shown several drugs to have the capacity to block the P-glycoprotein pump. Unfortunately, efforts to exploit this observation with drugs such as tamoxifen, cyclosporine, and verapamil have failed (214, 215).

Interferons, Interleukin-2, and Other Cytokines in the Therapy of Kidney Cancer

Renal carcinoma was singled out for interferon therapy because of its resistance to che-

Table 57.7. Results of Trials of Continuous Infusion FUDR or 5-FU for Metastatic Renal Cell Carcinoma

First Author	Year	No. of Patients	Regimen	Response rate CR%	PR%	Median (months) Survival
Hrushesky (204)	1990	63 (56)	Circadian FUDR 0.15 mg/kg/day × 14	7	13	15
		(7)	Intrahepatic FUDR 0.25 mg/kg/day × 14	14	42	
Dexeus (202)	1991	40	Circadian FUDR 0.15 mg/kg/day × 14	0	10	
Wilkinson (207)	1993	29	Constant/circadian FUDR 0.10 mg/kg/day × 14	3	17	15
Conroy (205)	1993	28	Circadian FUDR 0.15 mg/kg/day × 14	0	14	6
Falcone (206)	1993	16	Constant FUDR 0.125 mg/kg/day × 14 plus α2β 10MIU t.i.w.	6	25	
Small (203)	1994	15	Constant FUDR 0.10 mg/kg/day × 14 plus vinblastine 0.7 mg/m²/day	0	27	
Wadler (208)	1989	30	5-FU - 750 mg/m²/day × 5 →weekly bolus plus IFN-α_{2a} - 9 MU 3×/week	3	40	16+
Stadler (225)	1992	20	Constant FUDR 0.1 mg/kg/day × 5 plus oral leukovorin plus IFN-α_{2b} 30 MIU/m²/day × 6 days	0	0	

motherapy and the occurrence of spontaneous regression, suggesting an immune-mediated event. The first report of effectiveness of interferon in kidney cancer was by Quesada et al., who reported a 21% objective remission rate (216). The world's experience is well over 1000 patients treated and reported, with an objective regression rate of 16% (95% confidence interval of 13 to 19%) (217). No optimal dose, schedule, or species of interferon has been defined in the many trials conducted.

The most valuable information to emerge from the often conflicting interferon data came from the ECOG, who performed a prognostic factor analysis on 165 patients treated with the polyclonal α-interferon "Wellferon", with or without vinblastine (218). Overall survival, time to treatment failure, and response were significantly longer in patients with lung metastases only. Thus, it appears that the major determinant of response to, and survival after, interferon is probably patient selection criteria rather than the dose or schedule of interferon.

Other types of interferon have been tried in kidney cancer, with limited success. β-Interferon has a similar mechanism of action and is bound by a receptor similar to that of α-interferon. It has an approximately 20% response rate (219). Difficulties with formulation of the product and the volume that must be injected have limited interest in the drug. The role of γ-interferon in renal carcinoma has been somewhat controversial (220–222). Ellerhorst et al. recently reported a 15% response rate in a group of 35 patients treated with γ-interferon (223). Thus, while α-interferon remains a standard, γ-interferon may be modestly active as well.

Interferon in combination with chemotherapy has been tested in a number of different trials. All series have concluded that the combination is more toxic than either single agent alone and that the objective response rates are not superior to that expected with interferon. In one notable exception, Fossa et al. reported a randomized trial of interferon versus interferon plus vinblastine. The combination yielded a higher response rate (24 vs. 11%, $p = .07$), but no difference in survival (224). Trials of interferon with FUDR have yielded responses in 30% (0 to 43%) of 66 patients in three trials (206, 208, 225).

Although interleukin-2, discussed below, is presently the preferable first-line treatment for RCC, interferon continues to have a role in the treatment of this disease. While the optimal dose and schedule are not clear, if used as a single agent, 9 to 10×10^6 U should be given subcutaneously 2 to 3 days per week.

The therapy of metastatic kidney cancer was revolutionized with the introduction of interleukin-2 (IL-2), a true lymphokine produced by $CD4^+$ T lymphocytes. It was first identified in 1976 as a T cell growth factor by Morgan, Ruscetti, and Gallo (226). IL-2 exerts a variety of pleiotropic effects on the immune system. Its biology has recently been reviewed (227). Messenger RNA from a lymphoma cell line was cloned and subsequently expressed as a recombinant IL-2 product by Rosenberg et al. in 1983 (228). This led to the evaluation of IL-2 alone and in combination with other biologics in clinical trials that have continued to be spearheaded by Steven Rosenberg, M.D., Ph.D., at the National Cancer Institute. In initial phase I trials, neither Welte et al. at Memorial Sloan-Kettering (229) nor Atkins et al. from Tufts (230) reported responses. Meanwhile, Lotze et al. (231) reported that normal lymphocytes incubated with IL-2 could develop into lymphokine-activated killer (LAK) cells. These LAK cells, now known to be activated natural killer cells, became the subject of clinical trials in the mid-1980s.

Rosenberg et al. developed a clinical protocol for the immunotherapy of human cancer with IL-2 plus LAK cells. IL-2 was administered for 5 days, then therapy was interrupted while a rebound lymphocytosis occurred. These peripheral lymphocytes were then harvested by means of lymphocytopheresis for 3 to 5 days. The cells were cultured in the presence of high concentrations of interleukin-2 and then reinfused into the patient along with high doses of exogenous recombinant IL-2. Regression of disease was reported in over 35% of patients with metastatic kidney cancer. The results from the initial IL-2 plus LAK cell trials have been reviewed (232). In multiple subsequent studies, response rates for IL-2 plus LAK cells were consistently lower (232–233). Three subsequent, randomized trials studied IL-2 alone or with LAK cells (234–236). As a result of similar response rates for IL-2 with or without LAK at the NCI and other institutions, the use of costly and time-intensive LAK cells has been eliminated.

The Food and Drug Administration (FDA) approved IL-2 for the treatment of metastatic kidney cancer in early 1992. Standard high-dose IL-2 is given as a 600,000 to 720,000 IU/kg intravenous bolus every 8 hours for 15 doses over 5 days, repeated after a 7- to 10-day rest. The FDA review of eight similar clinical trials using high-dose IL-2 for RCC revealed an objective tumor response in 36 of 255 patients, including 12 complete responses, for an overall response rate of 14% and a CR rate of 5%. Responding patients were predicted to remain progression free for 18 months (237). More than 50% of the complete responses appeared to be durable. The serious toxicity of high-dose treatment (summarized below), however, beckoned a search for a less toxic, equally effective way to treat RCC patients with IL-2. This has included continuous infusion IL-2 (238), low-dose, bolus, inpatient IL-2 (239), intermittent outpatient intravenous bolus IL-2 (240), and outpatient subcutaneous IL-2 alone or with interferon (241–244).

Yang et al. reported the results of a randomized trial of high-dose bolus versus low-dose bolus IL-2. Some 125 patients were randomized to receive either 720,000 IU/kg intravenous bolus or 72,000 IU/kg every 8 hours for fifteen doses, repeated after a 7- to 10-day rest. The therapies were equally effective (high dose: CR rate 3%, PR 17%; low dose: CR 7%, PR 8%). Toxicity was markedly reduced in the low-dose group. Hypotension requiring vasopressors was reduced from 52 to 3%, and grade III thrombocytopenia from 9 to 1%. Treatable infections, however, were more common in the low-dose group (239).

Buter et al. (242) reported their experience with outpatient subcutaneous IL-2. Patients received 18 MIU subcutaneously daily × 5 for 4 to 6 weeks. Two complete responses and seven partial responses accounted for a response rate of 20%. Severe toxicities were infrequent, and responses were seen in patients more than 65 years old, making this regimen attractive despite its requirement for protracted administration. Inhalation IL-2 resulted in responses in 5 of 5 patients with lung metastases, but not in extrapulmonary sites. Toxicities were very mild (245).

Based on the demonstrated efficacy of IL-2 alone and interferon alone, multiple trials have examined the efficacy of combinations of the two biologics. A recent review of 596 patients reported in 21 studies demonstrated an overall response rate of 19% (243). Outpatient regimens reported response rates from 12 to 40% (243, 244). These outpatient regimens were well tolerated but not clearly superior to single-agent low-dose IL-2.

The toxicity of IL-2 therapy, particularly high-dose therapy, is myriad, and therefore, IL-2 requires an experienced physician for its administration. The toxicities resemble those of severe sepsis, with the attendant decrease in peripheral vascular resistance, capillary leak, and multiorgan system involvement (246–249). Fatigue, anorexia, fever, and chills are almost universal. Nausea, vomiting, and diarrhea are common. Up to half of patients treated on high-dose bolus regimens require vasopressors. Reversible azotemia, oliguria, and weight gain occur in most patients on treatment. Anemia and thrombocytopenia often require transfusions in high-dose patients. Infections, both line-related and others, are common. Death has consistently occurred in 1 to 2% of patients on treatment.

In conclusion, IL-2 alone, in spite of its toxicity, is the single most effective agent for treatment of metastatic RCC. The optimal dose is not yet defined, but the FDA-approved dose is 720,000 IU/kg every 8 hours for 5 days, repeated after a 7- to 10-day rest. Outpatient subcutaneous IL-2, with or without other cytokines or chemotherapy such as 5-FU or FUDR, especially in the context of a clinical trial, may be a preferable, cheaper, and better-tolerated means of administration. Further trials are needed to define more effective and safer regimens.

BLADDER CANCER

Bladder cancer will develop in 50,500 patients in 1995. Approximately 37,300 cases will occur in males and 13,200 in females. Bladder cancer, or transitional cell carcinoma of urothelium, was the 10th leading cause of cancer death in 1995, accounting for 11,200 deaths in the United States (1). Unlike other smoking-related cancers such as lung cancer, bladder cancer mortality is decreasing slightly each year (1).

Epidemiology and Molecular Biology

A full discussion of the epidemiology of bladder cancer is beyond the scope of this chapter, but it is important to recognize the carcinogens that cause bladder cancer. Aniline dyes were shown to be carcinogenic to bladder epithelium in 1885 by the German physician, Rehn. Subsequent epidemiologic studies have identified aromatic amines, particularly 2-naphthylamine (250) and benzidine, as a cause of bladder cancer in the dye, textile, printing, rubber, electrical cable, hair dressing, dry cleaning, and leather industries (251). Other risk factors for bladder cancer include heavy phenacetin exposure (252), cigarette smoking (253), prior cyclophosphamide exposure (254), and pelvic irradiation (255).

Bladder schistosomiasis is a risk factor for the development of squamous cell cancer of the bladder (256).

Emerging data are providing evidence that certain genetic alterations have a role in the development and/or progression of bladder cancer. Chromosome 9q deletions are found in carcinoma in situ (CIS), superficial bladder cancer, and invasive bladder cancer (257). This 9q deletion probably precedes the development of invasive disease (258). Other genetic alterations such as 3p, 5q, and 17q deletions are found in invasive but not papillary cancer, suggesting their role in progression of bladder cancer. Some invasive cancers lack 9q deletions, suggesting their emergence from a different early lesion (257). Overexpression of nuclear p53 has been associated with CIS (259). Further, its presence in both early and advanced cancers is clearly associated with recurrence of bladder cancer and decreased survival (260–262). Thus, measurement of p53 overexpression may have a role in selecting patients to receive adjuvant chemotherapy.

Histology

Bladder cancer histology is transitional cell carcinoma (TCC) in over 90% of biopsy specimens and can be graded as well, moderately, and poorly differentiated, or grades 1 to 3. The papillary, or well-differentiated, tumors are typically composed of a frondlike growth of transitional cells around a fibrovascular core. Poorly differentiated invasive bladder cancer may show evidence of squamous differentiation but is a highly aggressive and invasive cancer. Other histologic subtypes of bladder cancer include adenocarcinoma (typically occurring in patients with extrophy of the bladder), squamous cell cancer, and small cell cancer (263).

Staging

The staging of bladder cancer is either by the Jewett, Strong, Marshall categorization or by the American Joint Committee tumor, node, and metastases categorization, otherwise known as the TNM system (Table 57.8) (264).

Management of Superficial Bladder Cancer, (TIS, T_a or T_1)

The management of superficial bladder cancer has been and remains the subject of many reports. In 1983, Torti and Lum reviewed the ex-

Table 57.8. Staging Systems for Localized Bladder Cancer

Jewett, Strong, Marshall categorization	
Stage O	Epithelial tumor only
Stage A	Lamina propria invasion
Stage B_1	Superficial muscle invasion
Stage B_2	Deep-muscle invasion
Stage C	Perivesical fat invasion
Stage D_1	Lymph node involvement or pelvic sidewall involvement
TNM system	
TIS	Tumor in situ
T_x	Primary tumor cannot be assessed
T_a	Tumor confined to the mucosa
T_0	No evidence of primary tumor
T_1	Lamina propria invasion
T_2	Muscle-invasive tumor with no residual thickening in the bladder wall after resection
T_3	Muscle-invasive bladder cancer with residual thickening or a mass on bimanual examination after resection of the tumor transurethrally
T_{3a}	Invasion of deep muscle
T_{3b}	(Corresponding roughly to perivesical fat invasion) muscle-invasive tumor invasion through the bladder wall
T_4	Tumor fixed or extending to neighboring structures and/or microscopic evidence of such involvement
T_{4a}	Invasion of the prostate, uterus, or vagina
T_{4b}	Tumor fixed to the pelvic wall and/or the abdominal wall

tant literature and reported on 1676 patients (265). Median 5-year survival was 86%, and the median percentage of patients with superficial bladder tumor developing invasive bladder cancer was 10%, with a range from 6 to 25%. Thus, superficial bladder cancer has, in general, an excellent prognosis. Factors affecting prognosis of superficial bladder cancer have been recently reviewed (266). The most important prognostic factor appears to be grade, with high-grade lesions, regardless of stage, having a worse prognosis than similar stage low-grade lesions. Many other factors may affect the prognosis, including inability to completely excise the lesion, occult prostatic involvement, and/or continued exposure to carcinogens. Raghavan et al. have summarized 19 factors in bladder cancer that increased the risk of metastases or relapse (267).

Recently, nuclear p53 accumulation has emerged as one of the most important independent predictors of recurrence and survival in bladder cancer (260, 262).

The standard management of superficial disease has been transurethral resection of the bladder tumor (TURB) with electrocautery. Recurrent disease is treated either with TURB, intravesical chemotherapy, intravesical immunotherapy, or intravesical photodynamic therapy using the neodymium-YAG (yttrium-aluminum-garnet) laser (268). If surgical maneuvers are incomplete or unsuccessful, intravesical chemotherapy has been widely used. Its use may decrease tumor recurrence and delay the need for cystectomy (269–271). The utility of intravesicular chemotherapy to prevent progression to muscle invasive bladder cancer is less well proven (272–274). This is an important distinction, since many progressionless recurrences are asymptomatic and have little or no impact on survival. The agents most commonly used in the definitive treatment of superficial bladder tumor include thiotepa, epodyl, mitomycin C, Adriamycin, and bacillus Calmette-Guerin (BCG). In randomized controlled trials, the use of prophylactic chemotherapy with any of the above-mentioned agents will reduce the relapse rate by approximately 50%. Wide variations in effectiveness have been reported, and some series have reported no benefit of intravesical chemotherapy in a prophylactic setting (275).

Intravesical chemotherapy can be associated with both local and systemic toxicities. Thiotepa is reported to induce myelosuppression in 15 to 20% of patients, and acute leukemia has been reported as a late effect (269). Mitomycin C induces chemical cystitis in over 80% of patients, and 20% of patients develop contact dermatitis on the penis, scrotum, and hands. Doxorubicin also causes chemical cystitis in a substantial percentage of patients, as does Epodyl.

Intravesical BCG has recently emerged as probably the most effective intravesical agent (277). BCG, an attenuated strain of the tubercle bacillus, was first reported to be effective in eradicating CIS of the urinary bladder in small series by Morales et al. (278) and Lamm et al. (279). Both these small series reported complete disappearance of CIS in about 80% of patients. BCG has been directly compared with chemotherapy in randomized trials and appears to be superior (270, 280). In one of these trials, intravesicular and percutaneous BCG were compared with doxorubicin for recurrent T_a or T_1 cancer or TIS.

Significant advantages were seen for BCG in terms of decreased tumor recurrence, time to treatment failure, and complete response to CIS. Differences in survival were not significant (280).

CIS is a clinical-pathologic entity with a variable probability of progressing to invasive bladder cancer. In bladders removed for invasive cancer, multifocal CIS is commonly found. However, the frequency of progression and the interval over which such evolution may occur are relatively unpredictable. CIS has a prognostic continuum, with the management depending upon the prognosis. The most common presentation, a small focus at the base of or adjacent to a papilloma, is probably best treated by a TURB of the visibly involved area. Optimal management of CIS seen on random bladder biopsies for "irritable cystitis" now requires BCG therapy (see below). Diffuse macroscopic CIS is usually treated with immediate cystectomy, since the Mayo Clinic reported that over 70% of such patients eventually developed invasive bladder cancer (281).

The variable and poorly defined prognosis of CIS led Herr et al. to a randomized controlled trial of BCG plus TURB versus TURB alone for the treatment of superficial bladder cancer that was, in most cases, associated with CIS. This trial was conducted between 1978 and 1981, and 43 patients with CIS were randomized to TURB alone, while 43 underwent a TURB and 6 weeks of BCG therapy. Crossover to BCG therapy was allowed, and 18 patients who recurred with TURB alone crossed over to BCG at a median of 30 months. A final report of this study with at least 10 years of follow-up has been recently published (271). The 10-year progression free rate of BCG patients was 62%, compared with 38% with TURB alone (crossovers analyzed on TURB arm) ($p = .006$). Seventeen deaths from bladder cancer were reported on the TURB arm and 10 on the BCG arm ($p = .03$). These included 3 deaths from upper tract urothelial cancer (1 control, 2 on BCG) among 11 patients developing upper tract cancers. Of note, delayed BCG administration in the 18 crossover patients did not have an adverse effect on progression or survival.

In a second randomized trial, patients with superficial bladder cancer, with or without CIS, were randomized to receive either BCG (Connaught strain 120 mg/week × 6, then every 3 months) or intravesical Adriamycin (280). Outcome was analyzed separately for the 131 patients with CIS. The complete response rates of tumor were 70% in the BCG arm and 34% in the Adriamycin arm. The median times to treatment failure were 5 months and 39 months, respectively, for the Adriamycin and BCG groups. Five-year disease-free survival was 18 and 45%, respectively. There was not yet any survival advantage for the BCG group, though the total number of deaths was small.

These two trials have established BCG as the definitive therapy for CIS. The FDA recognized these data and approved BCG for the treatment of CIS in 1990. BCG has become the standard of care in the treatment of recurrent superficial disease and CIS of the urinary bladder.

BCG apparently requires an intact T-cell system, since substantial amounts of lymphokines and inflammatory mediators are released into the urine (282). It is unclear which cytokine in particular is responsible for the eradication of CIS. BCG may also directly bind to tumor cells, thereby allowing inflammatory cells to recognize them. BCG lacking the ability to bind to tumor cells is ineffective in eradicating CIS from the murine bladder (283).

In spite of this effectiveness, the toxicity of BCG remains considerable. The major dose-limiting toxicity of BCG is vesical irritability in over 90% of patients. Systemic "BCGosis" has been reported in up to 6% of patients treated (284), and a few deaths have occurred. This complication usually occurs in patients with a denuded urothelial surface secondary to a recent TURB. Therapy with isoniazid or many other antibiotics is highly effective.

Alternative therapies to eradicate CIS or superficial bladder tumors have been attempted. Torti et al., in a phase I-II study of 35 patients treated with recombinant α_{2b}-interferon, reported that 35% of patients had complete eradication of the disease with no systemic toxicity (285). Schering Inc. then conducted a randomized phase III trial of either 10 million (10^7) or 100 million (10^8) units of α_{2b}-interferon intravesically for CIS (286). Among 38 patients randomized to the low-dose arm, 2 (5%) had a complete response. Among 47 randomized to the high-dose arm, 20 (43%) had a complete response. The group concluded that 100 million units of α_{2b}-interferon had significant activity in the treatment of CIS.

Other inflammatory mediators, such as TNF and IL-2, have recently entered trials in this disease (287). Bropirimine, an oral inducer of interferon, produced complete responses in 5 of 12 patients with CIS treated on a phase I study.

Three of these patients had failed prior BCG (288).

Management of Muscle-Invasive Bladder Cancer

Radical cystectomy is the standard of care for muscle-invasive bladder cancer; however, pathologic upstaging postoperatively has fueled the debate about the relative value of radiotherapy and surgery in the treatment of bladder cancer. Remembering that the bladder wall is a thin muscular sack without a surrounding fascia, one can appreciate the mechanical ease with which tumor cells penetrate the muscular wall and invade the surrounding perivesical adipose tissue. In addition, common staging or noninvasive methods are often not accurate in determining the degree of penetration of the muscle wall. A number of large series have compared the clinical stage with the pathologic stage of bladder cancer (289–292). Most report that between 30 and 40% of patients clinically staged as T_2 or T_{3a} bladder cancer are pathologic T_{3b} or node positive. The clinical versus pathologic stage problem has persisted in spite of CT and MRI scans (289).

In the United States, surgical management with a radical cystectomy has become the standard therapy for muscle-invasive bladder cancer. This involves the removal of the bladder, the prostate or uterus, fallopian tubes, and ovaries (in females) along with the regional lymph nodes en bloc. This surgical technique allows precise surgical and pathologic staging. It has two long-lasting side effects: the need for permanent urinary diversion and total impotence (for both males and females). Both these problems have been approached with recent newer surgical techniques. First, the traditional ileostomy reservoir draining into an external collecting device has been replaced by a continent urinary diversion. Three commonly used types of diversions are the Kock pouch, which uses a segment of ileum; the Indiana pouch, which uses an ileal cecal segment; and the Studer pouch, a modification of the Kock pouch (293–295). In all procedures, the ostomy site is marsupialized to the skin, and the patient empties the pouch via a catheter every 4 to 8 hours. Recently, a technique has been developed in which the pouch, instead of being brought to the anterior abdominal interior wall, has been sutured to the urethra to form a neobladder (296–298).

These approaches have somewhat increased

the risk of complications of the radical cystectomy but have led to improved quality of life in most patients (299). The impotence problem has been ameliorated by "nerve sparing" cystectomies, since the neurovascular anatomy of the nerves required for penile and clitoral erection have been clearly defined (298). Sparing of even one of the bilateral neurovascular bundles allows preservation of potency, and thus in one series, 80% of men capable of having erections prior to cystectomy maintained potency (300). Long-term follow-up of patients treated with these newer techniques is lacking.

The historic 5-year survival expected with radical cystectomy is shown in Table 57.9 (301). The wide range of survivals (40 to 70%) reported for T_2 disease reflects the clinical staging error. Recent series of surgically treated T_2 lesions suggest a 5-year survival rate of 60 to 70%. Smith and Whitmore examined the impact of regional node metastases on survival from bladder cancer and found that essentially all 137 patients (except those with microscopic involvement of a single node) were dead of bladder cancer by 48 months (302). Even those with a single microscopic nodal focus had a survival of only 17% by 5 years. A recent series of 132 patients from the University of Southern California reported a 29% 5-year survival with node-positive bladder cancer when curative en bloc resection was performed. Retrospectively, radiation and chemotherapy had no impact on outcome (303). Modern combination chemotherapy, discussed below, may result in long-term complete remissions or cure in at least 20% of node-positive patients and 5 to 10% of D_2 patients with metastases (304).

There are numerous debates about the appropriate role of RT as a treatment for muscle-invasive bladder cancer. RT alone has a slightly inferior 5-year survival rate compared with surgery alone (305). Bloom et al. randomized 189 patients with T_3 bladder tumor to either 4000

Table 57.9. Historic 5-Year Survival for Bladder Cancer

TNM Stage	Jewett Stage	Survival
T_a	(O)	95–100%
T_1	(A)	85–90%
T_2	(B_1)	40–70%
T_{3a}	(B_2)	40–50%
T_{3b}	(C)	20–25%
T_4N+	(D_1)	5%

cGy in 4 weeks and immediate cystectomy or 6000 cGy in 6 weeks with salvage cystectomy as needed (305). A survival advantage was noted for the immediate cystectomy patients, but the difference was not statistically significant (survival at 5 years was 38% in the RT and cystectomy group and 29% in the RT-alone group). A confirmatory Danish series (306) randomized 183 patients in a manner identical to that of Bloom et al. Five-year survival in the cystectomy group was 35%, compared with 18% in the RT group ($p = .08$). This difference was most pronounced in the 5-year survival of the T_2 group (53 vs. 28%). Finally, a SWOG trial comparing preoperative RT plus cystectomy with cystectomy only showed no benefit to preoperative radiotherapy (307). These differences between surgery and RT may be due to inherent errors existing in clinical staging and to subtle selection biases (308). Nonetheless, a real advantage appears to exist for surgery.

Definitive RT with salvage cystectomy allows at least some patients to preserve bladder and sexual function, is associated with only a modest decrement in survival, and has become the standard of care in many centers. Several techniques have been used to increase the efficacy of RT. One technique is the interstitial insertion of radioisotope-containing needles (309). vander Weff-Messing has piloted and popularized this approach, which may be superior to external-beam RT only. Another technique adds systemic chemotherapy to RT, either concomitantly or sequentially (see below).

A number of studies have investigated new approaches for the treatment of locally advanced muscle-invasive bladder cancer. Most of these approaches have included the use of "preemptive" chemotherapy, or chemotherapy with concomitant RT or chemotherapy followed by either RT or cystectomy. There are several theoretical advantages to "up-front," "neoadjuvant" or "preemptive" chemotherapy: (a) downstaging of the bladder tumor allows preservation of the bladder or increases the ease of the cystectomy; (b) micrometastases present at diagnosis are most easily treated, thereby leading to improved survival; (c) treatment of an intact tumor allows an "in vivo assay" of chemosensitivity and may also provide prognostic significance; (d) chemotherapy prior to surgery or RT allows the drug access to the tumor before vascular sclerosis or fibrosis occurs secondary to RT or surgery; and (e) patients gain time to adapt to the medical necessity of an aggressive multimodality approach (including the possibility of a cystectomy).

Multiple uncontrolled studies have addressed the theoretical benefits discussed above, though no randomized trials have yet been reported. Although all studies differ in their design, all generally have included patients with T_2 through T_4 cancers. Cystoscopic biopsy or TURB has been followed by chemotherapy or chemotherapy plus RT. Cystectomy for nonresponding patients or partial cystectomy, RT, or observation generally followed as "definitive" local therapy. Conclusions from these trials can be summarized as follows:

1. Regarding downstaging of tumors and bladder preservation, cystectomy specimens have demonstrated complete responses in 10 to 43% of patients treated with neoadjuvant chemotherapy (310).
2. Bladder preservation is possible in a distinct subset of patients receiving neoadjuvant chemotherapy. In four studies with adequate follow-up, 4- to 5-year disease-free survival with an intact functioning bladder ranged from 13 to 45% (311–314). While this is encouraging, it must be interpreted in light of the fact that some patients treated without neoadjuvant chemotherapy may be able to preserve their bladders, and thus nonrandomized comparisons may be biased.
3. Regarding survival, the inherent biases in the selection of patients for these phase II studies makes any comparative statement dangerous. Reported survivals, however, do not seem dramatically worse and may be better than in traditionally treated patients.
4. Neoadjuvant therapy may provide important prognostic information. At least two studies have reported improved survival for patients who respond well to neoadjuvant chemotherapy, compared with those not responding (312).

In light of these conflicting and confusing data, the National Cancer Institute is currently sponsoring a trial of cystectomy alone versus neoadjuvant MVAC (methotrexate, vinblastine, Adriamycin, and cisplatin) chemotherapy for three cycles followed by cystectomy. This is entitled "Intergroup protocol 0080" (SWOG study 8710 or Cancer and Leukemia Group B (CALGB) study 8891). The projected number of patients required to determine the role of MVAC che-

motherapy is 232. The trial has been open for over 7 years, and patient accrual is still not complete. A similar randomized trial has been initiated in Europe, Canada, and Australia using MCV (methotrexate, cisplatin and vinblastine) or MVAC and allowing either surgery or RT as the means of local control. Finally, the Massachusetts General Hospital and the RTOG have initiated a study with or without two neoadjuvant cycles of MCV and combination cisplatin and RT (315). Thus, the exact role of neoadjuvant chemotherapy in the management of bladder cancer remains a subject of clinical investigation.

Another approach to this problem is with postoperative "adjuvant" chemotherapy. This approach, as opposed to the preoperative approach, allows treatment of patients based on pathologic grounds, thereby protecting a subset of patients with a high likelihood of surgical cure from the toxicities of chemotherapy. There is no time delay prior to definitive local treatment for those not responsive to chemotherapy. One large nonrandomized retrospective (316) and 3 smaller randomized trials (317–319) have formed the basis for the conclusions to be drawn regarding adjuvant chemotherapy.

The M. D. Anderson Hospital has reported a retrospective analysis of 338 patients treated between 1981 and 1986 using cyclophosphamide, doxorubicin and cisplatin as postoperative adjuvant chemotherapy (316). A total of 206 patients were considered to be low risk and received no adjuvant chemotherapy after cystectomy; 66% of those patients remain alive and free of disease. Some 61 patients were considered to have "high-risk" disease and were given adjuvant chemotherapy; 62% of that group remain free of disease. Another 71 patients also were considered to be high risk but for various reasons did not receive adjuvant chemotherapy. Only 37% of the "high-risk" patients remained alive and disease-free at the time of the report. The difference in survival between high-risk patients receiving chemotherapy and those not receiving chemotherapy was significant ($p = .001$).

Skinner (319) et al. reported positive results for a group of 91 patients randomized to undergo postoperative cisplatin, doxorubicin, and cyclophosphamide. Both median survival and time to progression were reported to be improved, but problems with the trial design, chemotherapy, and statistical methods may negate any reported benefits, and this trial must be interpreted cautiously. Studer et al. (318) reported no survival differences between 77 patients randomized to undergo adjuvant cisplatin or observation. Finally, Stockle et al. (317) from Mainz, Germany, reported impressively positive results in a small study of adjuvant chemotherapy; 49 patients were randomized to MVAC or MVEC (as MVAC, with etoposide replacing Adriamycin) versus observation. The study accrual was stopped prematurely when an interim analysis showed a significant advantage for the treatment group. Analyzed on an "intention to treat" basis, 7 of 26 chemotherapy patients and 18 of 23 surgery-only patients had recurred at about 2-year follow-up. Unfortunately, the patients who developed metastatic disease were not treated with MVAC. Although the study was small and reported only early follow-up, the results were encouraging.

A consistent theme in the randomized trials was the inability to treat ¼ to ⅓ of the patients randomized to chemotherapy. This remains an argument in favor of neoadjuvant chemotherapy. At this point, adjuvant chemotherapy is encouraging but should still be considered investigational.

Management of Metastatic Disease

The role of chemotherapy in the management of metastatic bladder cancer was definitively established by Yagoda (320). In an elegant series of phase II trials at Memorial Hospital in New York City between 1975 and 1980, groups of untreated patients received cisplatin (52% complete and partial response rate) or a combination of drugs with cisplatin, such as cyclophosphamide (Cytoxan) and Adriamycin (no apparent improvement in the response rate). Other drugs with activity in bladder cancer are shown on Table 57.10. These drugs include cisplatin, methotrexate, Adriamycin, vinblastine, cyclophosphamide, gallium nitrate, ifosfamide, and paclitaxel (Taxol). This list of active drugs has been used to develop numerous combination regimens for metastatic TCC (321). Highly active regimens include methotrexate and cisplatin, with a complete and partial response rate of 44% (322); methotrexate, cisplatin, and vinblastine (MCV), with an overall response rate of 56% (323); and MVAC, with a reported response rate of 69% (324).

In spite of these high response rates, the benefit of combination chemotherapy over single-agent chemotherapy remained unproven until 1992. A series of earlier trials comparing single-agent and multiple-agent chemotherapeutic reg-

Table 57.10. Single-Agent Chemotherapy Drugs with Activity in Bladder Cancer

Agent (Reference)	No. of Patients Reported	Response Rate
Cisplatin	320	30%
Methotrexate	236	29%
Adriamycin	274	17%
Vinblastine	38	16%
Vincristine	31	10%
Cyclophosphamide	98	31%[a]
5FU	141	17%[a]
Mitomycin	42	13%
Etoposide	47	8%
Bleomycin	102	6%
Carboplatin	46	22%
Gallium nitrate (336)	67	24%
10-Deaza-aminopterin	15	20%
Ifosfamide (339–341)	101	27%
Paclitaxel (334)	26	42%
Trimetrexate (344)	48	17%
Piritrexam (345)	29	38%
Gemcitabine (342, 343)	24	33%

[a]Older series with unclear criteria for response.

imens were unable to show a major survival advantage (325–327), although in each trial, the combination chemotherapy group had a slightly higher response rate and a slightly longer (2 to 3 month) median survival than to the patients receiving single-agent chemotherapy. Finally, Loehrer et al. reported that single-agent cisplatin, 70 mg/m^2 intravenously every 28 days, was inferior to MVAC in a randomized trial. Cisplatin-treated patients survived a median of 8.2 months, while MVAC-treated patients survived a median of 12.5 months (328). The overall response rates for the two groups were 39 and 12% for the MVAC and cisplatin groups, respectively. Toxicities, particularly myelosuppression, mucositis, and nausea and vomiting were more common with MVAC; five deaths occurred in MVAC-treated patients compared with none on cisplatin. This is the largest trial to date, and it has the statistical power to validate an advantage of combination chemotherapy. It provides a new standard for the treatment of metastatic bladder cancer. Not only is MVAC superior to cisplatin, but another trial from M. D. Anderson reported that MVAC chemotherapy was superior to CISCA (cisplatin, Cytoxan, and Adriamycin) chemotherapy (329). The response rate for MVAC was higher (65 vs. 46%; $p < .05$), and the survival duration was significantly longer (median 48 weeks vs. median 36 weeks; $p < .0003$).

The toxicity of the two regimens was comparable, except that nephrotoxicity was greater in the CISCA regimen, since cisplatin was administered at a dose of 100 mg/m^2 in the CISCA regimen and 70 mg/m^2 in the MVAC regimen.

The standard chemotherapy for advanced urothelial cancer is MVC or MVAC. Attempts to intensify the regimen with granulocyte or granulocyte-macrophage colony-stimulating factors have met with increased toxicity without improved outcome (330–332). Since only 5 to 10% of patients treated with MVAC are disease free at 3 to 5 years, new approaches are needed. In the past several years, several new single agents and combinations have shown activity in advanced bladder cancer, and these have recently been reviewed (333). Paclitaxel has shown a response rate of 42% (27% CR) in 26 previously untreated patients. Responses were seen mostly in lymph nodes and soft tissues, but some visceral responses were noted (334). Docetaxol has shown short-lived responses in 8 of 11 previously treated patients (335). Gallium nitrate has shown approximately 25% responses in MVAC-treated patients when administered by bolus (336) and slightly less when given as a continuous infusion (337, 338). Nephrotoxicity with bolus gallium and hypocalcemia and hypomagnesemia with continuous gallium were common. Ifosfamide resulted in a 21% response rate in second-line patients treated on an ECOG study (339) and 29 to 40% in two studies of first-line treatment (340, 341). Gemcitabine has shown excellent activity in two small studies (342, 343). Trimetrexate demonstrated a 17% (8 of 48) response rate in patients previously treated with methotrexate (344). Piritrexim in untreated patients resulted in 11 of 29 (38%) responses (345). Multidrug combinations using gallium, ifosfamide, or Taxol are in early use and are summarized in a recent review (333).

In conclusion, metastatic bladder cancer is a disease highly sensitive to chemotherapy. Much like small cell carcinoma of the lung, high initial response rates do not necessarily translate into long-term cure rates. Continued clinical trials are needed to explore new therapies for this disease.

ACKNOWLEDGMENTS

The authors would like to thank Helena Fleming, Deborah Stoit, and Joyce Trice for their assistance in the preparation of this manuscript. Supported in part by the Foster Schultz Memorial Fund for Cancer Research, by the Klein Tools Foundation, and by NIH Oncology Training Grant T32 CA09566.

REFERENCES

1. Wingo PA, Tong T, Bolden S. Cancer statistics, 1995. CA 1995;45:8–30.
2. Boyle P, Zaridze DG. Risk factors for prostate and testicular cancer. Eur J Cancer 1993;29A:1048–1055.
3. Guess HA. Is vasectomy a risk factor for prostate cancer? Eur J Cancer 1993;29A:1055–1060.
4. Severson RK, Nomura AMY, Grove JS, Stemmermann A. A prospective study of demographics, diet and prostate cancer among men of Japanese ancestry in Hawaii. Cancer Res 1989;49:1857–1860.
5. Kuriyama M, Wang MC, Papsidero LD, Killian CS, Shimaro T, et al. Quantitation of prostate-specific antigen in serum by a sensitive enzyme immunoassay. Cancer Res 1980;40:4658.
6. Watt KWK, Lee PJ, M'Timkulu T, Chan WP, Loor R. Human prostate-specific antigen: structural and functional similarity with serine protease. Proc Natl Acad Sci USA 1986;83:3166.
7. Andriole GL. Prostate cancer (editorial). J Urol 1955:154:1102.
8. Lange PH, Ercole CJ, Lightner DJ, Fraley EE, Vessella R. The value of serum prostate specific antigen determinations before and after radical prostatectomy. J Urol 1989;141:873–879.
9. Stamey TA, Kabalin JN, McNeal JE, Johnstone IM, Freiha F, Redwine EA, Yang N. Prostate specific antigen in the diagnosis and treatment of adenocarcinoma of the prostate. II. Radical prostatectomy treated patients. J Urol 1989;141:1076–1083.
10. Epstein JI, Walsh PC, Carmichael M, Brendler CB. Pathological and clinical findings to predict tumor extent of nonpalpable (stage T_{1c}) prostate cancer. JAMA 1994;271:368–374.
11. Oesterling JE, Jacobsen SJ, Chute CG, et al. Serum PSA in a community-based population of healthy men. JAMA 1993;270:860.
12. Ritter MA, Messing EM, Shanahan TG, Potts S, Chappell RJ, Kinsella TJ. Prostate specific antigen as a predictor of radiotherapy response and patterns of failure in localized prostate cancer. J Clin Onc 1992; 10:1208–1217.
13. Chauvet B, Felix-Favre C, Lupsascka N, et al. Prostate specific antigen decline: a major prognostic factor for prostate cancer treated with radiation therapy. J Clin Oncol 1994;12:1402–1407.
14. Stamey TA, Kabalin JN. Prostate specific antigen in the diagnosis and treatment of adenocarcinoma of the prostate. I. Untreated patients. J Urol 1989; 141:1070–1075.
15. Schmid HP, McNeal JE, Stamey TA. Observations on the doubling time of prostate cancer. The use of serial prostate-specific antigen in patients with untreated disease as a measure of increasing cancer volume. Cancer 1993;71:2031–2040.
16. Scardino PT, Wheeler TM. Local control of prostate cancer with radiotherapy: frequency and prognostic significance of positive results of postirradiation prostate biopsy. NCI Monogr 1988;7:95–103.
17. Salomon CG, Flisak ME, Olson MC, Podiak CM, Flanigan RC, Waters WB. Radical prostatectomy: transrectal sonographic evaluation to assess for local recurrence. Radiology 1993;189:713–719.
18. Eisburch A, Perez CA, Roessler EH, Lockett MA. Adjuvant irradiation after prostectomy for carci-

noma of the prostate with positive surgical margins. Cancer 1994;73:384–387.

19. Stein A, deKernion JB, Dorey F, Smith RB. Adjuvant radiotherapy in patients post radical prostatectomy with tumor extending through capsule or positive seminal vesicles. Urology 1992;39:59–62.

20. Rogers E, Ohori M, Kassabian VS, Wheeler TM, Scardino PT. Salvage radical prostatectomy: outcome measured by serum prostate specific antigen levels. J Urol 1995;153:104–110.

21. Stein A, Smith RB, deKernion JB. Salvage radical prostatectomy after failure of curative radiotherapy for adenocarcinoma of the prostate. Urology 1992; 40:197–200.

22. McLeod DG. Prostate cancer: past, present and future. In: Dawson NA, Vogelzang NJ, eds. Prostate cancer. New York: Wiley-Liss, 1994:1–18.

23. Ohori M, Wheeler TM, Scardino PT. The new American Joint Committee on Cancer and International Union against Cancer TNM classification of prostate cancer. Clinical pathologic correlations. Cancer 1994;73:104–114.

24. Zagers GK, Geara FB, Pollack A, von Eschenbach AC. The T classification of clinically localized prostate cancer. Cancer 1994;73:1904–1912.

25. Gleason DF. Histologic grade, clinical stage and patient age in prostate cancer. Consensus development conference on the management of clinically localized prostate cancer. NCI Monogr 1988;7:15–24.

26. Newman AJ Jr, Graham MD, Carlton CE Jr, Lieman S. Incidental carcinoma of the prostate at the time of transurethral resection: importance of evaluating every chip. J Urol 1982;128:948–951.

27. Epstein JI, Paull G, Eggleston JC, Walsh PC. Prognosis of untreated stage A_1 prostatic carcinoma: a study of 94 cases with extended follow-up. J Urol 1986; 136:837–841.

28. Lowe BA, Listrom MB. Incidental carcinoma of the prostate: an analysis of the predictors of progression. J Urol 1988;140:1340–1344.

29. Mohler JL, Partin AW, Epstein JI, et al. Prediction of prognosis in untreated stage A_2 prostatic carcinoma. Cancer 1992;69:511–519.

30. NcNeal JE, Price HM, Redwine EA, Freiha FS, Stamey TA. Stage A versus stage B adenocarcinoma of the prostate: morphological comparison and biological significance. J Urol 1988;139:61–65.

31. Walsh, PC. Radical retropubic prostatectomy with reduced morbidity: an anatomic approach. NCI Monogr 1988;7:133–137.

32. Talcott JA, Rieker P, Propert K, et al. Are the potency-sparing benefits of nerve-sparing radical prostatectomy due to patient selection (abstract 681). Proc Am Soc Clin Oncol 1995;14:252.

33. Bagshaw MA, Cox RS, Ray GR. Status of radiation treatment of prostate cancer at Stanford University. NCI Monogr 1988;7:47–60.

34. Perez CA, Pilepich MV, Garcia D, Simpson JR, Zivnuska F, Hederman MA. Definitive radiation therapy in carcinoma of the prostate localized to the pelvis: experience at the Mallinckrodt Institute of Radiology. NCI Monogr 1988;7:85–94.

35. Forman JD, Kumar R, Haas G, Montie J, Porter AT, Mesina CF. Neoadjuvant hormonal downsizing of localized carcinoma of the prostate effects on the volume of normal tissue irradiation. Cancer Invest 1995; 13:8–15.

36. Pilepich MV, Krall JM, Al-Sarraf M, et al. Androgen deprivation with radiation therapy compared with radiation therapy alone for locally advanced prostate carcinoma—a randomized comparative trial in the Radiation Therapy Oncology Group. Urology 1995; 45:616–623.

37. Pilepich MV, Caplan, Byhardt RW, et al. Phase III trial of androgen suppression using goserelin in unfavorable prognosis carcinoma of the prostate treated with definitive radiation therapy (report of the RTOG protocol 85-31) (abstract 631). Proc Am Soc Clin Oncol 1995;14:239.

38. Laramore GE, Griffin TW. Fast neutron radiotherapy: where have we been and where are we going? The jury is still out—regarding Maor MH, et al: IJROBP 1995;32:599–604. Int J Radiat Oncol Biol Phys 1995; 32:879–882.

39. Carter GE, Lieskovsky G, Skinner DG, Petrovich Z. Results of local and/or systemic adjuvant therapy in the management of pathological stage C or D1 prostate cancer following radical prostatectomy. J Urol 1989;142:1266–1271.

40. Lerner SE, Blute ML, Zincke H. Primary surgery for clinical T-3 adenocarcinoma of the prostate. In: Vogelzang NJ, Scardino PT, Shipley WU, Coffey D, eds. Comprehensive textbook of genitourinary oncology. Baltimore: Williams & Wilkins, 1996:803–811.

41. Cheng WS, Frydenberg M, Bergstrahl E, Larson-Keller JJ, Zincke H. Radical prostatectomy for pathologic stage C prostate cancer: influence of pathologic variables and adjuvant treatment on disease outcome. Urology 1993;42:283–291.

42. Labrie F, Dupont A, Cusan L, et al. Downstaging of localized prostate cancer by neoadjuvant therapy with flutamide and Lupron. The first controlled and randomized trial. Clin Invest Med 1993;16:499–509.

43. Cookson MS, Fair WR. Neoadjuvant hormonal therapy and radical prostatectomy for locally advanced prostate cancer. In: Vogelzang NJ, Scardino PT, Shipley WU, Coffey D, eds. Comprehensive textbook of genitourinary oncology. Baltimore: Williams & Wilkins, 1995:811–817.

44. Soloway MS, Sharifi R, Wajsman Z, et al. Randomized prospective study comparing radical prostectomy alone versus radical prostatectomy preceded by androgen blockage in clinical stage B2 ($T_{2b}N_xM_0$) prostate cancer. J Urol 1995;154:424–428.

45. Gerasi LA, Mata J, Easley JD, Wilbanks JH, Seale-Hawkins C, Carlton CE Jr, Scardino PT. Prognostic significance of lymph nodal metastases in prostate cancer. J Urol 1988;142:332–336.

46. Steinberg GD, Epstein JI, Pianatadosi S, Walsh PC. The management of stage D1 adenocarcinoma of the prostate: the Johns Hopkins experience 1974–1987. J Urol 1990;144:1425–1432.

47. Zincke H. Bilateral pelvic lymphadenectomy and radical retropubic prostatectomy for stage C or D1 adenocarcinoma of the prostate: possible beneficial effect of adjuvant treatment. NCI Monogr 1988;7:109–115.

48. Myers RP, Larson-Keller JJ, Bergstrahl EJ, Zincke H, Oesterling JE, Lieber MM. Hormonal treatment at the time of radical retropubic prostectomy for stage D1 prostate cancer: results of long-term follow up. J Urol 1992;147:910–915.

49. deKernion JB, Neuwirth H, Stein A, Dorey F,

Stenzi A, Hannah J, Blyth B. Prognosis of patients with stage D1 prostate carcinoma following radical prostectomy with and without early endocrine therapy. J Urol 1990;144:700–703.

50. Feinstein AR, Sosin DM, Wells CK. The Will Rogers phenomenon: stage migration and new diagnostic techniques as a source of misleading statistics for survival in cancer. N Engl J Med 1985;312:1604–1608.

51. Huggins C, Hodges CV. Studies on prostatic cancer. I: The effect of castration, estrogen and androgen injections on serum phosphatase in metastatic carcinoma of the prostate. Cancer Res 1941;1:293–297.

52. Nesbit RM, Baum WC. Endocrine control of prostatic carcinoma: clinical and statistical survey of 1818 cases. JAMA 1950;143:1317–1320.

53. Byar DP, Corle DK. Hormone therapy for prostatic cancer: results of the Veterans Administration Cooperative Urologic Research Group studies. NCI Monogr 1988;7:165–170.

54. Schally AV, Redding TW, Camura-Schally AM. Potential use of analogues of LHRH in the treatment of hormone sensitive neoplasms. Cancer Treat Rep 1984;68:281–289.

55. The Leuprolide Study Group. Leuprolide versus diethylstibesterol for metastatic prostatic cancer. N Engl J Med 1984;311:1281–1286.

56. Soloway MS, Chodak G, Vogelzang NJ, et al. Zoladex versus orchiectomy in treatment of advanced prostate cancer. Zoladex Prostate Study Group. Urology 1991;37:46–51.

57. Cassileth BR, Soloway MS, Vogelzang NJ, Schellhammer PS, Seidmon EJ, Hait HI, Kennealey GT. Patients' choice of treatment in stage D prostate cancer. Urology 1989;33(5 Suppl):57–62.

58. Chodak GW, Vogelzang NJ, Caplan RJ, Soloway M, Smith JA. Independent prognostic factors in patients with metastatic (stage D_2) prostate cancer. The Zoladex Study Group. JAMA 1991;265:618–621.

59. Labrie F, Dupont A, Belanger A, et al. New approach in the treatment of prostate cancer. Complete instead of only partial withdrawal of androgens. Prostate 1983;4:579–594.

60. Crawford ED, Eisenberg MA, McLeod DG, Spaulding JT, Benson R, et al. A controlled trial of leuprolide with and without flutamide in prostatic carcinoma. N Engl J Med 1989;321:419–424.

61. Kuhn J-M, Billebaud T, Navrath H, Moulonguet A, Fiet J, et al. Prevention of the transient adverse effects of a gonadotropin-releasing hormone analogue (buserelin) in metastatic prostatic carcinoma by administration of an antiandrogen (nilutamide). N Engl J Med 1989;321:413–418.

62. Pavone-Macaluso M, Pavone C, Serretta V, Caricello G. Antiandrogens alone or in combination for treatment of prostate cancer: the European experience. Urology Suppl 1989;34:27–36.

63. Schroeder FH, Lock TM, Chadha DR, et al. Metastatic cancer of the prostate managed with buserelin versus buserelin plus cyproterone acetate. J Urol 1987;137:192.

64. Thrasher B, Crawford ED. Combined androgen blockade. In: Vogelzang NJ, Scardino PT, Shipley WU, Coffey D, eds. Comprehensive textbook of genitourinary oncology. Baltimore: Williams & Wilkins, 1995:875–884.

65. Prostate Cancer Trialist's Collaborative Group.

Maximum androgen blockade in advanced prostate cancer: an overview of 22 randomized trials with 3283 deaths in 5710 patients. Lancet 1995;346:265–269.

66. Schellhammer P, Sharafi R, Block N, et al. A controlled trial of bicaluatamide (CASODEX) versus flutamide (Eulexin) each in combination with luteinizing hormone releasing hormone analog therapy in patients with advanced prostate cancer. Urology 1995;45:745–752.

67. Kennealey GT, Furr BJ. Use of the nonsteroidal anti-androgen casodex in advanced prostatic carcinoma. Urol Clin North Am 1991;18:99–110.

68. Miller JI, Ahmann FR, Droch GW, Emerson SS, Battagini MR. The clinical usefulness of serum prostate specific antigen after hormonal therapy of metastatic prostate cancer. J Urol 1992;147(3 part 2):956–961.

69. Eisenberger M, Crawford ED, McLeod D, Hussain M, Loehrer P, Blumenstein B. The prognostic significance of prostate specific antigen (PSA) in stage D_2 prostate cancer (PC). Interim evaluation of study 0105 (abstract 613). Proc Am Soc Clin Oncol 1995;14:235.

70. Eisenberger MA. Chemotherapy for prostate carcinoma. NCI Monogr 1988;7:151–163.

71. Tannock IF. Is there evidence that chemotherapy is of benefit to patients with carcinoma of the prostate? J Clin Oncol 1985;3:1013–1021.

72. Berges RR, Vukanovic J, Epstein JI, et al. Implications of cell kinetic changes during the progression of human prostatic cancer. Clin Cancer Res 1995;1:473–480.

73. Upadhyaya H, Vogelzang NJ. Chemotherapy of prostate cancer. In: Ernstoff MS, Heaney JA, Deschell RE, eds. Urologic cancer. New York: WW Norton, 1996, in press.

74. Scott WW, Gibbons RP, Johnson PE, et al. The continued evaluation of the effects of chemotherapy in patients with advanced carcinoma of the prostate. J Urol 1976;116:211–213.

75. Kelly WK, Scher HI, Muzamdar M, Vlamis V, Schwartz M, Fossa SD. Prostate-specific antigen as a measure of disease outcome in metastatic hormone-refractory prostate cancer. J Clin Oncol 1993;11:607–615.

76. Raghavan D, Cox K, Pearson BS, et al. Oral cyclophosphamide for the management of hormone-refractory prostate cancer. Br J Urol 1993;72:625–628.

77. Schmidt JD, Gibbons RP, Murphy GP, Bartolucci A. Adjuvant therapy for localized prostate cancer. Cancer 1993;71(3 Suppl):1005–1013.

78. Seidman AD, Scher HI, Petrylak D, et al. Estramustine and vinblastine: use of PSA as a clinical endpoint for hormone refractory prostatic cancer. J Urol 1992;147:931–934.

79. Hudes GR, Greenburg R, Krigel RL, et al. Phase II study of estramustine and vinblastine, two microtubule inhibitors, in hormone-refractory prostate cancer. J Clin Oncol 1992;11:1754–1761.

80. Pienta KJ, Redman B, Hussain M, et al. Phase II evaluation of oral estramustine and oral etoposide in hormone-refractory adenocarcinoma of the prostate. J Clin Oncol 1994;12:2005–2012.

81. Carducci M, Eisenberger MA, Kobayashi K, Reymo L, Egorin M. Suramin in advanced prostate cancer. In: Vogelzang NJ, Scardino PT, Shipley WU, Coffey D, eds. Comprehensive textbook of genitourinary oncology. Baltimore: Williams & Wilkins, 1996:897–907.

82. Tannock I, Osaha D, Ernst S, et al. Chemother-

apy with mitoxantrone (M) and prednisone (P) palliates patients with hormone-resistant prostate cancer (HRPC). Results of a randomized Canadian trial (abstract 653). Proc Am Soc Clin Oncol 1995;14:245.

83. Johnson DE, Babaian RJ, von Eschenbach AC, et al. Ketoconazole therapy for hormonally refractory metastatic prostate cancer. Urology 1988;31:1323–1134.

84. Dawson NA, Conaway M, Winer SP, et al. A randomized study comparing standard versus moderately high dose megesterol acetate in advanced prostate cancer. CALGB study (abstract 618). Proc Am Soc Clin Oncol, 1995;14:236

85. Scher HI, Kelly WK. Flutamide withdrawal syndrome: its impact on clinical trials and hormone-refractory prostate cancer. J Clin Oncol 1993;11:1566–1572.

86. Dupont A, Gomez JL, Cusan L, Koutsilieras M, Labrie F. Response to flutamide withdrawal in advanced prostate cancer in progression under combination therapy. J Urol 1993;150:908–913.

87. Taplin M, Rubley GJ, Shuster TD, et al. Mutation of the androgen receptor gene in metastatic androgen-independent prostate cancer. N Engl J Med 1995;132:1393–1398.

88. Crawford ED, Kozlowski JM, Debry A, et al. The use of strontium 89 for palliation of pain from bone metastases associated with hormone-refractory prostate cancer. Urology 1994;44:481–485.

89. Moller H. Decreased testicular cancer risk in men born in wartime. J Natl Cancer Inst 1989 81:1668–1669.

90. Oliver RTD. Epidemiology of testicular cancer. In: Vogelzang NJ, Scardino PT, Shipley WU, Coffey D, eds. Comprehensive textbook of genitourinary oncology. Baltimore: Williams & Wilkins, 1996:923–931.

91. Osterlind A. Diverging trends in incidence and mortality of testicular cancer in Denmark, 1943–1982. Br J Cancer 1986;53:501–555.

92. Depue RH, Pike ML, Henderson BE. Cryptorchidism and testicular cancer. J Natl Cancer Inst 1986; 77:830–833.

93. Bosl GJ, Vogelzang NJ, Goldman A, et al. Impact of delay in diagnosis on clinical stage of testicular cancer. Lancet 1981;1:970–973.

94. Giwercman A, Bruun E, Frimodt-Moller C, Skakkebaek NE. Prevalence of carcinoma in-situ and other histopathological abnormalities in testes of men with a history of cryptorchidism. J Urol 1989;142: 998.

95. Tollerud DJ, Blattner WA, Fraser MC, et al. Familial testicular cancer and urogenital developmental anomalies. Cancer 1985;55:1849–1854.

96. Aetiology of testicular cancer: association with congenital abnormalities, age at puberty, infertility, and exercise. United Kingdom Testicular Cancer Study Group. Br Med J 1994;308:1393–1399.

97. Bosl GJ, Dmitrovsky E, Reuter VF, et al. Isochromosome of chromosome 12: clinically useful marker for male germ cell tumors. J Natl Cancer Inst 1989;81:1874–1878.

98. Giguere J, Stablein DM, Spaulding JT, McLeod DG, Paulson DF, Weiss RB. The clinical significance of unconventional orchiectomy approaches in testicular cancer: a report from the testicular cancer intergroup study 1988;139:1225–1228.

99. Touroutoglou N, Dimopouos MA, Younes A, et al. Testicular lymphoma: late relapses and poor outcome despite doxorubicin-based therapy. J Clin Oncol 1995;13:1361–1367.

100. Vogelzang NJ, Scardino PT, Shipley WU, Coffey D, eds. Comprehensive textbook of genitourinary oncology. Baltimore: Williams & Wilkins, 1996.

101. Tomasi TB. Structure and function of alphafetoprotein. Annu Rev Med 1977;28:453–465.

102. Vogelzang NJ, Lange PH, Goldman A, Vessella RH, Fraley EE, Kennedy BJ. Acute changes of α-fetoprotein and human chorionic gonadotropin during induction chemotherapy of germ cell tumors. Cancer Res 1982;42:4855–4861.

103. Berger P, Schwartz S, Spotti O, Wick G, Mann K. Variants of human chorionic gonadotrophin from pregnant women and tumor patients recognized by monoclonal antibodies. J Clin Endocrinol Metab 1993; 77:347.

104. Schwarz S, Krude ZH, Nelboeck E, Berger P, Merz WE, Wick O. Relationship of orientation with affinity and activity of receptor-bound glycosylation variants of human chorionic gonadotropin (hCG) as visualized by monoclonal antibodies (MCA). J Recept Res 1991;11:437–458.

105. Bower M, Rustin GJS. Serum tumor markers and their role in monitoring germ cell cancer of the testis. In: Vogelzang NJ, Scardino PT, Shipley WU, Coffey D, eds. Comprehensive textbook of genitourinary oncology. Baltimore: Williams & Wilkins, 1996:968–980.

106. Vogelzang NJ, Lange PH, Goldberg E. Absence of sperm-specific lactate dehydrogenase in patients with testis cancer. Oncodev Biol Med 1982;3:269–272.

107. Einhorn LH, Crawford ED, Shipley WU, Loehrer PJ, Williams SD. Cancer of the testes. In: DeVita VT, Hellman S, Rosenberg SA, eds. Cancer: principles and practice of oncology. 3rd ed. Philadelphia: JB Lippincott, 1989:1071–1098.

108. von der Maase H, Specht L, Jacobsen GK, et al. Surveillance following orchidectomy for stage I seminoma of the testes. Eur J Cancer 1993;29A:1931–1934.

109. Smalley SR, Earle JD, Evans RG, Richardson RL. Modern radiotherapy results with bulky stage II and III seminoma. J Urol 1990;144:685–689.

110. Norgaard-Pedersen B, Schultz HP, Arends J, et al. Tumour markers in testicular germ cell tumors: five year experience from the DATECA study 1976–1980. Acta Radiol Oncol (Fasc) 1984;23:287–294.

111. Fung CY, Garnick MB. Clinical stage I carcinoma of the testis: a review. J Clin Oncol 1988;6:734–750.

112. Gressler VH, Levine LA, Vogelzang NJ. A third option in the management of patients with clinical stage I nonseminomatous germ cell tumor. J Clin Oncol 1990;8:4–8.

113. Read G, Stenning SP, Cullen MH, et al. Medical Research Council prospective study of surveillance for stage I testicular teratoma. J Clin Oncol 1992; 10:1762–1768.

114. Droz JP, van Oosterom AT. Treatment options in clinical stage I non-seminomatous germ cell tumours of the testes: a wager on the future? A review. Eur J Cancer 1993;29A:1038–1044.

115. Leibovitch I, Foster RS, Kopecky KK, Donohue JP. Is it possible to categorically define the "normal" and "abdominal" computed tomography in pa-

tients with low stage non-seminomatous germ cell cancer (abstract 783)? Proc Am Urol Assoc 1995; 153:424a.

116. McLeod DG, Weiss RB, Stablein DM, et al. Staging relationships and outcome in early stage testicular cancer: a report from the Testicular Cancer Intergroup study. J Urol 1991;145:1178–1183.

117. Donahue J. Testicular cancer, clinical stage 1. Ann Intern Med 1989;110:409–410.

118. Donohue JP, Thornhill JA, Foster RS, Rowland RG, Bihrle R. Retroperitoneal lymphadenectomy for clinical stage A testes cancer (1965–1989): modification of technique and impact on ejaculation. J Urol 1993; 149:237–243.

119. Rorth M, von der Maase H, Nielsen ES, et al. Orchiectomy alone versus orchiectomy plus radiotherapy in stage I non-seminomatous testicular cancer: a randomized study by the Danish Testicular Carcinoma Study Group. Int J Androl 1987;10:255–262.

120. Sturgeon JFG, Jewett MAS, Allison RE, et al. Surveillance after orchidectomy for patients with clinical stage I non-seminomatous testes tumors. J Clin Oncol 1992;10:564–568.

121. Baniel J, Foster RS, Gonin RG, Messener JE, Donohue JP, Einhorn LH. Late relapse of testicular cancer. J Clin Oncol 1995;13:1170–1176.

122. Klepp O, Olsson AM, Henrikson H, et al. Prognostic factors in clinical stage I non-seminomatous germ cell tumors of the testes: multivariant analysis of a prospective multicenter study. J Clin Oncol 1990;509–518.

123. Rukstalis DP, Chodak GW. Laparoscopic retroperitoneal lymph node dissection in a patient with stage I testicular carcinoma. J Urol 1992;148:1907–1910.

124. Cullen MH, Stenning SP, Parkinson MC, et al. Short course adjuvant chemotherapy in high risk stage I non-seminomatous germ cell tumors of the testis (NSGCTT): an MRC (UK) study report (abstract 650). Proc Am Soc Clin Oncol 1995;14:244.

125. Raghavan D, Vogelzang NJ, Bosl GJ, et al. Tumor classification and size in germ cell testicular cancer: influence on the occurrence of metastases. Cancer 1982;50:1591–1595.

126. Vogelzang NJ, Fraley EE, Lange PH, Torkelson J, Levitt S, Kennedy BJ. Stage II nonseminomatous testicular cancer: a 10-year experience. J Clin Oncol 1983;1:171–178.

127. Williams SD, Stablein DM, Einhorn LH, et al. Immediate adjuvant chemotherapy versus observation with treatment at relapse in pathological stage II testicular cancer. N Engl J Med 1987;317:1433–1438.

128. Socinski MA, Garnick MB, Stomper PC, Fung CY, Richie JP. Stage II non-seminomatous germ cell tumors of the testis: an analysis of treatment options in patients with low volume retroperitoneal disease. J Urol 1988;140:1437–1441.

129. Logothetis C, Swanson DA, Dexeus F, et al. Primary chemotherapy for clinical stage II non-seminomatous germ cell tumors of the testis: a follow-up of 50 patients. J Clin Oncol 1987;5:906–911.

130. Motzer RJ, Bajorin DF, Bosl GJ, et al. Etoposide (E) and cisplatin (P) is effective adjuvant chemotherapy (CT) in patients (pts) with stage II nonseminomatous germ cell tumors (NSGCT) following retroperitoneal lymph node dissection (RPLND) (abstract 605). Proc Am Soc Clin Oncol 1995;14:233.

131. Motzer R, Bosl GJ, Heelan R, et al. Residual mass: an indication for further treatment in patients with advanced seminoma following systemic chemotherapy. J Clin Oncol 1989;5:1064–1070.

132. Li MC, Whitmore WF, Golbey R, Grabstald H. Effects of combined drug therapy on metastatic cancer of the testis. JAMA 1960;174:1291–1299.

133. Mendelson D, Serpick AA. Combination chemotherapy of testicular tumors. J Urol 1971;103:619–623.

134. Samuels ML, Johnson DE, Holoye PV. Continuous intravenous bleomycin (NSC-125066) therapy with vinblastine (NSC-49842) in stage III testicular neoplasia. Cancer Chemother Rep 1975;59:563–570.

135. Wyatt J, McAninch LN. A chemotherapeutic approach to advanced testicular carcinoma. Can J Surg 1967;10:421–425.

136. Higby DJ, Wallace HJ, Albert DJ, Holland JF. Diamminodichloroplatinum II: a phase I study showing response in testicular and other tumors. Cancer 1974;33:1219–1225.

137. Einhorn LH, Donohue J. *Cis*-diamminedichloroplatinum, vinblastine and bleomycin combination chemotherapy in disseminated testicular cancer. Ann Intern Med 1977;87:293–298.

138. Roth BJ, Greist A, Kubilis PS, et al. Cisplatin based combination chemotherapy for disseminated germ cell tumors. Long-term follow-up. J Clin Oncol 1988;6:1239–1247.

139. Stoter G, Sleijfer DTH, Vendrik CPI, et al. Combination chemotherapy with *cis*-diamminedichloroplatinum, vinblastine, and bleomycin in advanced testicular non-seminoma. Lancet 1979;1:941–945.

140. Garnick MB, Canellos GP, Richie JP. Treatment and surgical staging of testicular and primary extragonadal germ cell cancer. JAMA 1983;250:1733–1741.

141. Bosl GJ. The treatment of germ cell tumors at Memorial Sloan-Kettering Cancer Center, 1960–1983. In: Garnick MB, ed. Contemporary issues in urologic cancer. New York: Churchill Livingstone, 1985:45–60.

142. Weiss RB, Stablein DEM, Muggia FM, et al. Toxicity comparisons between two chemotherapy regimens as adjuvant or salvage treatment in nonseminomatous testicular cancer. Cancer 1988;62:18–23.

143. Samson MK, Rivkin SE, Jones SE, et al. Dose-response and dose-survival advantage for high versus low-dose cisplatin combined with vinblastine and bleomycin in disseminated testicular cancer. A Southwest Oncology Group study. Cancer 1984;53:1029–1035.

144. Fitzharris BM, Kaye SB, Saverymuttu S, et al. VP16-213 as a single agent in advanced testicular tumors. Eur J Cancer 1980;17:245–249.

145. Vogelzang NJ, Kennedy BJ. "Salvage" chemotherapy for refractory germ cell tumors (abstract). Proc Am Soc Clin Oncol 1981;22:471.

146. Williams SD, Einhorn LH, Greco FA, et al. VP-16-213 salvage therapy for refractory germinal neoplasms. Cancer 1980;46:2154–2158.

147. Williams SD, Birch R, Einhorn LH, et al. Disseminated germ cell tumors: chemotherapy with cisplatin plus bleomycin plus either vinblastine or etoposide. A trial of the Southeastern Cancer Study Group. N Engl J Med 1987;316:1435–1440.

148. Bosl Gl, Geller NL, Bajorin D, et al. A randomized trial of etoposide and cisplatin versus vinblastine

+ bleomycin + cisplatin + cyclophosphamide + dactinomycin in patients with good-prognosis germ cell tumors. J Clin Oncol 1988;6:1231–1238.

149. Bajorin DF, Sarosdy MF, Pfister DG, et al. Randomized trial of etoposide and cisplatin versus etoposide and carboplatin in patients with good-risk germ cell tumors: a multi institutional study. J Clin Oncol 1993;11:598–606.

150. Einhorn LH, Williams SD, Loehrer PJ, et al. Evaluation of optimal duration of chemotherapy in favorable prognosis disseminated germ cell tumors; a Southeastern Cancer Study Group protocol. J Clin Oncol 1989;7:387–391.

151. Stoter G, Kaye S, Jones W, et al. Cisplatin (P) and VP16 (E) ± bleomycin (B), (BEP) vs (EP) in good risk patients with disseminated non-seminomatous testicular cancer; a randomized EORTC GU study group (abstract). Onkologie 1991;14(Suppl 4):17.

152. Bosl GJ, Geller NL, Cirrincione C, et al. Multivariate analysis of prognostic variables in patients with metastatic testicular cancer. Cancer Res 1983; 43:3402–3407.

153. Vogelzang NJ. Prognostic factors in metastatic testicular cancer. Int J Androl 1987;10:225–237.

154. Birch R, Williams S, Cone A, et al. Prognostic factors for favorable outcome in disseminated germ cell tumors. J Clin Oncol 1986;4:400–407.

155. Stoter G, Sylvester R, Sleijfer DT, et al. Multivariate analysis of prognostic factors in patients with disseminated nonseminomatous testicular cancer: results from a European Organization for Research on Treatment of Cancer multiinstitutional phase III study. Cancer Res 1987;47:2714–2718.

156. Bajorin D, Katz A, Chan E, et al. Comparison of criteria for assigning germ cell tumor patients to "good risk" and "poor risk" studies. J Clin Oncol 1988; 6:786–792.

157. Mead GM, Stenning SP, Parkinson MC, et al. The second Medical Research Council study of prognostic factors in non seminomatous germ cell tumors. J Clin Oncol 1992;10:85–94.

158. Nichols CP, Loehrer PJ, Einhorn LH, et al. Phase III study of cisplatin, etoposide and bleomycin (PVP$_{16}$B) or etoposide, ifosfamide and cisplatin (VIP) in advanced stage germ cell tumors; an intergroup trial (abstract 637). Proc Am Soc Clin Oncol 1995;14:241.

159. Loehrer PJ Sr, Lauer R, Roth BJ, Williams SD, Kalasinski LA, Einhorn LH. Salvage therapy in recurrent germ cell cancer: ifosfamide and cisplatin plus either vinblastine or etoposide. Ann Intern Med 1988; 109:540–546.

160. Harstrick A, Schmall HJ, Wilke H, et al. Cisplatin, etoposide, and ifosfamide salvage therapy for refractory or relapsing germ cell carcinoma. J Clin Oncol 1991;9:1549–1555.

161. Motzer RJ, Geller NL, Tan CCY, et al. Salvage chemotherapy for patients with germ cell tumors. The Memorial Sloan Kettering Cancer Center experience (1979–1989). Cancer 1991;67:1305–1310.

162. Siegart W, Beyer J, Strohscheer I, et al. High-dose treatment with carboplatin, etoposide and ifosfamide followed by autologous stem cell transplantation in relapsed or refractory germ cell cancer: a phase I/II study. J Clin Oncol 1994;12:1223–1231.

163. Broun ER, Nichols CR, Kneebone P, et al. Long-term outcome of patients with relapsed and refractory germ cell tumors treated with high-dose chemotherapy and autologous bone marrow rescue. Ann Intern Med 1992;117:124–128.

164. Broun ER, Nichols CR, Turns M, et al. Early salvage therapy for germ cell cancer using high dose chemotherapy with autologous bone marrow support. Cancer 1994;73:1716–1720.

165. Motzer RJ, Mazumdar M, Gulati SC, et al. Phase II trial of high-dose carboplatin and etoposide with autologous bone marrow transplantation in first-line therapy for patients with poor risk germ cell tumors. J Natl Cancer Inst 1993;85:1828–1835.

166. Droz JP, Kramar A, Pico JJ. Prediction of long-term response after high-dose chemotherapy with autologous bone marrow transplantation in the salvage treatment of non-seminomatous germ cell tumours. Eur J Cancer 1993;29A:818–821.

167. Motzer RJ, Bajorin DF, Schwartz LH, et al. Phase II trial of paclitaxel shows anti-tumor activity in patients with previously treated germ cell tumors. J Clin Oncol 1994;12:2277–2283.

168. Miller JC, Einhorn LH. Phase II study of daily oral etoposide in refractory germ cell tumors. Semin Oncol 1990;17(1 Suppl 2):36–39.

169. Aass N, Fossa SP, Raghavan D, Vogelzang NJ. Late toxicity after chemotherapy of testis cancer. In: Vogelzang NJ, Scardino PT, Shipley WU, Coffey D, eds. Comprehensive textbook of genitourinary oncology. Baltimore: Williams & Wilkins, 1996:1090–1096.

170. Stoter G, Koopman A, Vendrik CPJ, et al. Ten year survival and late sequelae in testicular cancer patients treated with cisplatin, vinblastine, and bleomycin. J Clin Oncol 1989;7:1099–1104.

171. Boyer M, Raghavan D, Harris PJ, et al. Lack of late toxicity in patients treated with cisplatin-containing combination chemotherapy for metastatic testicular cancer. J Clin Oncol 1990;8:21–26.

172. Bosl GJ, Leitner SP, Atlas SA. Increased plasma renin and aldosterone in patients treated with cisplatin-based chemotherapy for metastatic germ-cell tumors. J Clin Oncol 1986;4:1684–1689.

173. Vogelzang NJ, Torkelson JL, Kennedy BJ. Hypomagnesemia, renal dysfunction and Raynaud's phenomenon in patients treated with cisplatin, vinblastine and bleomycin. Cancer 1985;56:2765–2770.

174. Vogelzang NJ, Bosl GJ, Johnson K, Kennedy BJ. Raynaud's phenomenon: a common toxicity after combination chemotherapy of testicular cancer. Ann Intern Med 1981;95:288–292.

175. Lange PH, Narayan P, Vogelzang NJ, Schafer RB, Kennedy BJ, Fraley EE. Return of fertility after treatment for nonseminomatous testicular cancer: changing concepts. Urol 1983;129:1131–1135.

176. Horwich A, Lampe H, Norma A, Nicholas J, Jay O, Dearnaley D. Fertility after chemotherapy for metastatic germ cell tumors (abstract 620). Proc Am Soc Clin Oncol 1995;14:236.

177. Bander NH, Finstad CL, Cordon-Cardo C, et al. Analysis of a mouse monoclonal antibody that reacts with a specific region of the human proximal tubule and subsets of renal cell carcinomas. Cancer Res 1989;49:6774–6780.

178. Stenzl A, deKernion JB. Pathology, biology, and clinical staging of renal cell carcinoma. Semin Oncol 1989;16(Suppl):3–11.

179. Shuin T, Kondo K, Torigoe S, et al. Frequent somatic mutations and loss of heterozygosity of the

von Hippel-Lindau tumor suppressor gene in primary human renal cell carcinomas. Cancer Res 1994;54:2852–2855.

180. LaForgia S, Lasota J, Latif F, et al. Detailed genetic and physical map of the 3p chromosome region surrounding the familial renal cell carcinoma chromosome translocation, t(3;8)(p14.2;q4.1). Cancer Res 1993;52:3118–3124.

181. Gnarra JR, Lerman MI, Zbar B, Linehan WM. Genetics of renal-cell carcinoma and evidence for a critical role for von Hippel-Lindau in renal tumorigenesis. Semin Oncol 1995;22:3–8.

182. Presti JC Jr, Rao PH, Chen Q, et al. Histopathological, cytogenetic, and molecular characterization of renal cortical tumors. Cancer Res 1991;51:1544–1552.

183. Uhlman DL, Nguyen PL, Manivel C, et al. Association of immunohistochemical staining for p53 with metastatic progression and poor survival in patients with renal cell carcinoma. J Natl Cancer Inst 1994;86:1470–1475.

184. Reiter RE, Anglard P, Liu S, Gnarra JR, Linehan WM. Chromosome 17p deletions and p53 mutations in renal carcinoma. Cancer Res 1993;53:3092–3097.

185. Ogawa O, Kakehi Y, Ogawa K, Koshiba M, Sugiyama T, Yoshida O. Allelic loss at chromosome 3p characterizes clear cell phenotype of renal cell carcinoma. Cancer Res 1991;51:949–953.

186. Oda H, Nakatsura Y, Ishikawa T. Mutations of the p53 gene and p53 protein overexpression are associated with sarcomatoid transformation in renal cell carcinomas. Cancer Res 1995;55:658–662.

187. Ogawa O, Habuchi T, Kakehi Y, Koshiba M, Sugiyama T, Yoshida O. Allelic losses at chromosome 17p in human renal cell carcinoma are inversely related to allelic losses at chromosome 3p. Cancer Res 1992; 52:1881–1885.

188. Katz DL, Zheng T, Holford TR, Flannery J. Time trends in the incidence of renal cell carcinoma: analysis of Connecticut Tumor Registry data: 1935–1989. Int J Cancer 1994;58:57–63.

189. Guinan PO, Vogelzang NJ, Fregman AM, et al. Renal cell carcinoma: tumor size, stage and survival. J Urol 1995;153:901–903.

190. Robson CJ, Churchill BM, Anderson W. The results of radical nephrectomy for renal cell carcinoma. J Urol 1969;101:297–301.

191. Beahrs O, Henson D, Hutter R, Myers M, eds. Manual for staging of cancers. Philadelphia: JB Lippincott, 1988.

192. Elson PJ, Witte RS, Trump DL. Prognostic factors for survival in patients with recurrent or metastatic renal cell carcinoma. Cancer Res 1988;48:7310–7313.

193. Guiliani L, Giberti C, Martorina G, Rovida S. Radical extensive surgery for renal cell carcinoma: long-term results and prognostic factors. J Urol 1990; 143:468–474.

194. Moll V, Becht E, Ziegler M. Kidney preserving surgery in renal cell tumors; indications, techniques and results in 152 patients. J Urol 1993;150:319–323.

195. Halperin EC, Harisiadis L. The role of radiation therapy in the management of metastatic renal cell carcinoma. Cancer 1983;51:614–617.

196. Buzaid AC, Todd MB. Therapeutic options in renal cell carcinoma. Semin Oncol 1989;16(Suppl):12–19.

197. Vogelzang NJ, Priest ER, Borden L. Spontaneous regression of histologically proved pulmonary metastases from renal cell carcinoma: a case with 5-year follow-up. J Urol 1992;148:1247–1248.

198. Fuks JZ, Aisner J, Van Echo DA, Wiernik PH. Phase II study of medroxyprogesterone acetate with tamoxifen in advanced renal cell cancer. Cancer Treat Rep 1982;66:1773–1777.

199. Ahmed T, Benedetto P, Yagoda A, et al. Estrogen, progesterone, and androgen-binding sites in renal cell carcinoma: observations obtained in phase II trial of flutamide. Cancer 1984;54:477–481.

200. Al-Sarraf M, Eyre H, Bonnet J, et al. Study of tamoxifen in metastatic renal cell carcinoma and the influence of certain prognostic factors: a Southwest Oncology Group study. Cancer Treat Rep 1981;65:447–451.

201. Yagoda A, Abi Rached B, Petrylak D. Chemotherapy for advanced renal-cell carcinoma: 1983–1993. Semin Oncol 1995;22:42–60.

202. Dexeus FH, Logothetis CJ, Sella A, et al. Circadian infusion of floxuridine in patients with metastatic renal cell carcinoma. J Urol 1991;146:709–713.

203. Small EJ, Frye JW, Wilkinson MJ, Carroll PR, Ernst ML, Stagg RJ. A phase I/II study of alternating constant infusion floxuridine with constant infusion vinblastine for the treatment of metastatic renal cell carcinoma. Cancer 1994;73:2803–2807.

204. Hrushesky WJM, von Roemeling R, Lanning RM, Rabitan JT. Circadian-shaped infusion of floxuridine for progressive metastatic renal cell carcinoma. J Clin Oncol 1990;8:1504–1513.

205. Conroy T, Jeoffros L, Guillemin F, et al. Simplified chronomodulated continuous infusion of floxuridine in patients with metastatic renal cell carcinoma. Cancer 1993;72:2190–2197.

206. Falcone A, Cianci C, Ricci S, Brunetti I, Bertucceli M, Conte PF. Alpha-2b-interferon plus floxuridine in metastatic renal cell carcinoma. Cancer 1993; 72:564–568.

207. Wilkinson MJ, Frye JW, Small EJ, et al. A phase II study of constant-infusion floxuridine for the treatment of metastatic renal cell carcinoma. Cancer 1993;71:3601–3604.

208. Wadler S, Schwartz EL, Goldman M, et al. Fluorouracil and recombinant alpha-2a-interferon: an active regimen against advanced colorectal carcinoma. J Clin Oncol 1989;7:1769–1775.

209. Murphy BR, Rynard SM, Einhorn OH, Loehrer PJ. A phase II trial of interferon alpha-2A plus fluorouracil in advanced renal cell carcinoma. Invest New Drugs 1992;10:2125–2230.

210. Ling V, Thompson L. Reduced permeability in CHO cells as a mechanism of resistance to colchicine. J Cell Physiol 1974;83:103–116.

211. Roninson IB, Chin JE, Choi K, et al. Isolation of human mdr1 DNA sequences amplified in multidrug-resistance KB carcinoma cells. Proc Natl Acad Sci USA 1986;83:4538–4542.

212. Safa AR, Glover CJ, Meyers MB, Biedler JL, Felsted RL. Vinblastine photoaffinity labeling of a high molecular weight surface membrane glycoprotein specific for multidrug-resistant cells. J Biol Chem 1986; 261:6137–6140.

213. Fojo AT, Shen D-W, Mickley LS, Pastan I, Gottesman MM. Intrinsic drug resistance in human kidney cancer is associated with expression of a human multidrug-resistance gene. J Clin Oncol 1987;5:1922–1927.

214. Trump DL, Smith DC, Ellis PG, et al. High-dose oral tamoxifen, a potential multidrug-resistance-reversal agent: phase I trial in combination with vinblastine. J Natl Cancer Inst 1992;84:1811–1816.

215. Samuels BL, Mick R, Vogelzang NJ, et al. Modulation of vinblastine resistance with cyclosporin: a phase I study. Clin Pharmacol Ther 1993;54:421–429.

216. Quesada JR, Swanson DA, Trindade A, et al. Renal cell carcinoma: anti-tumor effects of leukocyte interferon. Cancer Res 1983;43:940–947.

217. Muss MB. Renal cell carcinoma, interferons in clinical applications. In: De Vita VT, Hellman S, Rosenberg SA eds, Biologic therapy of cancer. Philadelphia: JB Lippincott, 1991:298–310.

218. Neidhart JA, Anderson S, Harris JE, et al. Vinblastine fails to improve response of renal cancer to interferon alpha-N1: high response rate in patients with pulmonary metastasis. J Clin Oncol 1991;9:832–837.

219. Rinehart J, Malspeis L, Young D, et al. Phase I/II trial of human recombinant β-interferon serine in patients with renal cell carcinoma. Cancer Res 1986; 46:5364–5367.

220. Rinehart JJ, Malspeis L, Young D, Neidhart JA. Phase I/II trial of human recombinant interferon gamma in renal cell carcinoma. J Biol Response Mod 1986;5:300–308.

221. Garnick MB, Reich SD, Maxwell B, et al. Phase I/II study of recombinant interferon gamma in advanced renal cell carcinoma. J Urol 1988;139:251–255.

222. Aulitzky W, Gasti G, Aulitzky WE, et al. Successful treatment of metastatic renal cell carcinoma with a biologically active dose of recombinant interferon-gamma. J Clin Oncol 1989;7:1875–1884.

223. Ellerhorst JA, Kilbourn RG, Amato RJ, et al. Phase II trial of low dose gamma-interferon in metastatic renal cell carcinoma. J Urol 1994: 152:841–845.

224. Fossa SD, Martinelli G, Otto U, et al. Recombinant interferon alpha-2a with or without vinblastine in metastatic renal cell carcinoma: results of a European multi-center phase III study. Ann Oncol 1992; 3:301–305.

225. Stadler WM, Vogelzang NJ, Vokes EV, Charette J, Whitman G, et al. Continuous infusion fluorodeoxyuridine with leucovorin and high-dose interferon: a phase II study in metastatic renal-cell cancer. Cancer Chemother Pharmacol 1992:31:213–216.

226. Morgan DA, Rusceti FW, Gallo R. Selective in vitro growth of T-lymphocytes from normal human bone marrows. Science 1976;193:1007–1008.

227. Rubin JT. Interleukin-2: its biology and clinical application in patients with cancer. Cancer Invest 1993; 11:460–472.

228. Rosenberg SA, Grimm EA, McGrogan M, et al. Biological activity of recombinant human interleukin-2 produced in *Escherichia coli*. Science 1984; 223:1412–1415.

229. Welte K, Wang CY, Mertelsmann R, Venuta S, Feldman SP, Moore MAS. Purification of human interleukin 2 to apparent homogeneity and its molecular heterogeneity. J Exp Med 1982;156:454–464.

230. Atkins MB, Gould JA, Allegretta M, et al. Phase I evaluation of recombinant interleukin-2 in patients with advanced malignant disease. J Clin Oncol 1986;4:1380–1391.

231. Lotze MT, Grimm EA, Mazumder A, Straus-ser JL, Rosenberg SA. Lysis of fresh and cultured autologous tumor by human lymphocytes cultured in T-cell growth factor. Cancer Res 1981;41:4420–4425.

232. Rosenberg SA, Lotze MT, Yang JC, et al. Experience with the use of high-dose interleukin-2 in the treatment of 652 cancer patients. Ann Surg 1989; 210:474–485.

233. Linehan WM, Shipley WU, Parkinson DR. Cancer of the kidney and ureter. In: de Vita VT, Hellman S, Rosenberg SA eds. Cancer principles and practice of oncology. Philadelphia: JB Lippincott, 1993:1023–1051.

234. Figlin RA, Gitlitz BJ, Belldegrun A. Cellular and gene therapy. In: Vogelzang NJ, Scardino PT, Shipley WU, Coffey D, eds. Comprehensive textbook of genitourinary oncology. Baltimore: Williams & Wilkins, 1995:261–275.

235. McCabe M, Stablein D, Hawkins MJ. The modified group C experience—phase III randomized trials of IL-2 verus IL-2/LAK in advanced renal cell cancer and advanced melanoma (abstract 714). Proc Am Soc Clin Oncol 1991;10:213.

236. Bajorin D, Sell KW, Richards JM, et al. A randomized trial of interleukin 2 plus lymphokine-activated killer cells versus interleukin 2 alone in renal cell carcinoma (abstract 1106). Proc Am Assoc Cancer Res 1990;31:186

237. Fisher RI. Introduction; interleukin-2-advances in clinical research and treatment. Semin Oncol 1993;20(6 Suppl 9):1–2.

238. Dillman RO, Church C, Oldham RK, West WH, Schwartzberg L, Birch R. Inpatient continuous-infusion interleukin-2 in 788 patients with cancer. The National Biotherapy Study Group experience. Cancer 1993;71:2358–2370.

239. Yang JC, Topalian SL, Parkinson D, et al. Randomized comparison of high-dose and low-dose intravenous interleukin-2 for the therapy of metastatic renal cell carcinoma: an interim report. J Clin Oncol 1994; 12:1572–1576.

240. Bukowski RM, Goodman P, Crawford D, Sergi J, Redman BG, Whitehead RP. Phase II trial of high-dose intermittent interleukin-2 in metastatic renal cell carcinoma; a Southwest Oncology Group study. J Natl Cancer Inst 1990;82:143–146.

241. Atzpodien J, Kirchner H, Lopez Hänninen E, et al. European studies of interleukin-2 in metastatic renal cell carcinoma. Semin Oncol 1993;20(6 Suppl 9):22–26.

242. Buter J, Sleijfer DT, van der Graaf WTA, DeVries EGE, Willmese PHB, Mulder NH. A progress report on the outpatient treatment of patients with advanced renal cell carcinoma using subcutaneous recombinant interleukin-2. Semin Oncol 1993;20(6 Suppl 9):16–21.

243. Vogelzang NJ, Lipton A, Figlin RA. Subcutaneous interleukin-2 plus interferon alpha-2a in metastatic renal cell cancer: an outpatient multicenter trial. J Clin Oncol 1993;11:1809–1816.

244. Figlin RA, Pierce WC, Belldegrun A. Combination biologic therapy with interleukin-2 and interferon-alpha in the outpatient treatment of metastatic renal cell carcinoma. Semin Oncol 1993;20(6 Suppl 9):11–15.

245. Huland E, Huland H, Hinzer H. Interleukin-2 by inhalation: local therapy for metastatic renal cell carcinoma. J Urol 1992;147:344–348.

246. Pockaj BA, Topalain SL, Steinberg SM, White DE, Rosenberg SA. Infectious complications associated with interleukin-2 administration: a retrospective review of 935 treatment courses. J Clin Oncol 1993; 11:136–147.

247. Guleria AS, Yang JC, Topalain SL, et al. Renal dysfunction associated with the administration of high-dose interleukin-2 in 199 consecutive patients with metastatic melanoma or renal carcinoma. J Clin Oncol 1994;12:2714–2722.

248. Siegel JP, Puri RK. Interleukin-2 toxicity. J Clin Oncol 1991;9:694–704.

249. White Jr. RL, Schwartzentruber DJ, Guleria A. Cardiopulmonary toxicity of treatment with high dose interleukin-2 in 199 consecutive patients with metastatic melanoma or renal cell carcinoma. Cancer 1994; 74:3212–3222.

250. Hueper WC, Wiley FH, Wolfe HD. Experimental production of bladder tumors in dogs by administration of beta-naphthylamine. J Ind Hyg Toxicol 1938;20:46–55.

251. The BAUS Subcommittee on Industrial Bladder Cancer. Occupational bladder cancer: a guide for clinicians. Br J Urol 1988;61:183–191.

252. McCredie M, Stewart JH, Ford JM, Maclennan RA. Phenacetin-containing analgesics and cancer of the bladder or renal pelvis in women. Br J Urol 1983; 55:220–224.

253. Hartge P, Silverman D, Hoover R, et al. Changing cigarette habits and bladder cancer risk: a case control study. J Natl Cancer Inst 1987;78:1119–1125.

254. Levine LA, Richie JP. Urological complications of cyclophosphamide. J Urol 1989;141:1063–1069.

255. Silverman DT, Levine LI, Hoover RN. Occupational risks of bladder cancer in the United States: II. Non white men. J Natl Cancer Inst 1989;81:1480–1483.

256. Dimette RM, Sproat HF, Sayegh ES. The classification of carcinoma of the urinary bladder associated with schistosomiasis and metaplasia. J Urol 1956; 7:680–686.

257. Dalbagni G, Presti J, Reuter V, Fair WR, Cordon-Cardo C. Genetic alterations in bladder cancer. Lancet 1993;324:469–471.

258. Sidranski D, Frost P, Von Eschenbach A, Oyasu R, Preisinger AC, Vogelstein B. Clonal origin of bladder cancer. N Engl J Med 1992;326:737–740.

259. Sarkis AS, Dalbagani G, Cordon-Cardo C, et al. Alteration of p53 nuclear overexpression and tumor progression in carcinoma in situ of the bladder. J Urol 1994;152:388–392.

260. Esrig D, Elmajian D, Groshen S, et al. Accumulation of nuclear p53 and tumor progression in bladder cancer. N Engl J Med 1994;331:1259–1264.

261. Lipponen PK. Over-expression of p53 nuclear oncoprotein in transitional cell bladder cancer and its prognostic value. Int J Cancer 1993;53:365–370.

262. Sarkis AS, Bajorin DF, Reuter VE, et al. Prognositc value of p53 nuclear overexpression in patients with invasive bladder cancer treated with MVAC. J Clin Oncol 1995;13:1384–1390.

263. Young RH. Pathology of bladder cancer. In: Vogelzang NJ, Scardino PT, Shipley WU, Coffey D, eds. Comprehensive textbook of genitourinary oncology. Baltimore: Williams & Wilkins, 1996:326–337.

264. Denis CD. Clinical staging: its importance in therapeutic decisions and clinical trials. Hematol Oncol Clin North Am 1992;6:41–58.

265. Torti FM, Lum BL. The biology and treatment of superficial bladder cancer. J Clin Oncol 1983;2:505–531.

266. Kalish LA, Garnick MB, Richie JP. Appropriate endpoints for superficial bladder cancer clinical trials. J Clin Oncol 1987;5:2004–2008.

267. Raghavan D, Shipley WU, Garnick MB, Russell PJ, Richie JP. Biology and management of bladder cancer. N Engl J Med 1990;322:1129–1138.

268. Prout GR Jr, Lin C-W, Benson R Jr, et al. Photodynamic therapy with hematoporphyrin derivative in the treatment of superficial transitional-cell carcinoma of the bladder. N Engl J Med 1987;317:1251–1255.

269. Soloway MS. Rationale for intensive intravesical chemotherapy for superficial bladder cancer. J Urol 1980;123:461–466.

270. Melekos MD, Chionis HS, Paranychianakis GS, Dauaher HH. Intravesicle 4'-EPI-doxorubicin (epirubicin) versus bacillus Calmette-Guérin. A controlled perspective study on the prophylaxis of superficial bladder cancer. Cancer 1993;72:1749–1755.

271. Herr HW, Schwalb DM, Zhang ZF, et al. Intravesical bacillus Calmette-Guerin therapy prevents tumor progression and death from superficial bladder cancer: ten-year follow-up of a prospective randomized trial. J Clin Oncol 1995;13:1404–1408.

272. Kantoff P. Intravesical therapy for superficial bladder cancer: is it a wash? J Clin Oncol 1994;12:1–4.

273. Lum BL, Torti FM. Adjuvant intravesicular pharmacotherapy for superficial bladder cancer. J Natl Cancer Inst 1991;83:682–694.

274. Soloway MS. Editorial: intravesical therapy for bladder cancer. J Urol 1994;152:379–381.

275. MRC Working Party on Urological Cancer. The effect of intravesical thiotepa on the recurrence rate of newly diagnosed superficial bladder cancer: an MRC study. Br J Urol 1985;57:680–685.

276. Silverberg JM, Zarrabi MH. Acute nonlymphocytic leukemia after thiotepa instillation into the bladder: report of two cases and review of the literature. J Urol 1987;138:402–403.

277. Herr HW, Badalament RA, Amato DA, Laudone VP, Fair WR, Whitmore WF Jr. Superficial bladder cancer treated with bacillus Calmette-Guérin: a multivariate analysis of factors affecting tumor progression. J Urol 1989;141:22–29.

278. Morales A, Eidinger D, Bruce AW. Intracavitary bacillus Calmette-Guérin for the treatment of superficial bladder tumors. J Urol 1976;116:180–188.

279. Lamm DL, Tohr DE, Winters WD, Stogdill VD, Radwin HM. BCG immunotherapy of bladder cancer-inhibition of tumor recurrence and associated immune responses. Cancer 1981;48:82–94.

280. Lamm DL, Blumenstein BA, Crawford ED, et al. A randomized trial of intravesical doxorubicin and immunotherapy with bacille Calmette-Guérin for transitional cell carcinoma of the bladder. N Engl J Med 1991;325:1205–1209.

281. Utz DC, Hanash KA, Farrow GM. The plight of the patient with carcinoma in situ of the bladder. J Urol 1970;103:160–170.

282. Böhle A, Nowc CH, Ulmer AJ, et al. Elevations of cytokines interleukin-1, interleukin-2 and tumor necrosis factor in the urine of patients after intravesical bacillus Calmette-Guérin immunotherapy. J Urol 1990; 144:59–64.

283. Ratliff TL, Palmer JO, McGarr JA, Brown EF. Intravesical bacillus Calmette-Guërin therapy for murine bladder tumors: initiation of the response by fibronectin-mediated attachment of bacillus Calmette-Guërin. Cancer Res 1987;47:1762–1770.

284. Brosman SA, Lamm DL. The preparation, handling and use of intravesical bacillus Calmette-Guerin for the management of stage T_a, T_1, carcinoma-in-situ and transitional cell cancer. J Urol 1990;144:313–315.

285. Torti FM, Shortliffe LD, Williams RD, et al. Alpha-interferon in superficial bladder-cancer: a Northern California Oncology Group study. J Clin Oncol 1988;6:476–483.

286. Glashan RW. Randomized controlled study of intravesical α-2b interferon in carcinoma in situ of bladder. J Urol 1990;144:658–661.

287. Sternberg C, Arena M, Pansadora V, et al. Recombinant tumor necrosis factor for superficial bladder tumors. Ann Oncol 1992;3:741–745.

288. Sarosdy MF, Lamm DI, Williams RD. Phase I trial of oral bropirimine in superficial bladder cancer. J Urol 1992;147:31–33.

289. Voges GE, Tauschke E, Stöckle M, Alken P, Hohenfellner R. Computerized tomography: an unreliable method for accurate staging of bladder tumors in patients who are candidates for radical cystectomy. J Urol 1989;142:972–974.

290. Whitmore WF Jr, Marshall VF. Radical total cystectomy for cancer of the bladder: 230 consecutive cases five years later. J Urol 1962;87:853–861.

291. Johnson DE, Lamy SM. Complications of a single stage radical cystectomy and ileal conduit diversion: review of 214 cases. J Urol 1977;117:171–179.

292. Skinner DG, Lieskovsky G. Contemporary cystectomy with pelvic node dissection compared to preoperative radiation therapy plus cystectomy in management of invasive bladder cancer. J Urol 1984; 131:1069–1072.

293. Kock NG, Nilson AE, Nilsson LO, Norlen LJ, Philipson BM. Urinary diversion via a continent ileal reservoir: clinical results in 12 patients. J Urol 1982; 128:469–475.

294. Rowland RG, Mitchell ME, Bihrle P, Kahnoski RJ, Piser JE. Indiana continent urinary reservoir. J Urol 1987;137:1136–1139.

295. Studer UE. Continent urinary reservoirs. J Urol 1994;151:341–342.

296. Marshall F. Creation of an ileocolic bladder after cystectomy. J Urol 1988;139:1264–1268.

297. Wenderroth UK, Bachor R, Egghart G, Frohenberg D, Miller K, Hautmann RE. The ileal neobladder: experience and results of more than 100 consecutive cases. J Urol 1990;143(3):492–496.

298. Marshall FF, Mostwin JL, Radebaugh LC, Walsh PC, Brendler CB. Ileocolic neobladder post-cystectomy: continence and potency. J Urol 1991;145:502–504.

299. Boyd SD, Feinberg SM, Skinner DG, Lieskovsky G, Baron D, Richardson J. Quality of life survey of urinary diversion patients: comparison of ileal conduits versus continent Kock ileal reservoirs. J Urol 1987;138:1386–1389.

300. Schlegel PN, Walsh PC, Neuroanatomical approach to radical cystoprostatectomy with preservation of sexual function. J Urol 1987;138:1402–1406.

301. Ritchie JP, Radical cystectomy innovations and results. In: Raghavan D, ed. The management of bladder cancer. London: Edward Arnold, 1988:140–143.

302. Smith JA, Whitmore WF Jr. Regional lymph node metastasis from bladder cancer J Urol 1981; 126:591–595.

303. Lerner SP, Skinner DG, Lieskovsky G, et al. The rationale for en block pelvic lymph node dissection for bladder cancer patients with nodal metastases—long term results. J Urol 1993;149:758–764.

304. Roth BJ, Marks LB. Management of metastatic disease. In: Vogelzang NJ, Scardino PT, Shipley WU, Coffey D, eds. Comprehensive textbook of genitourinary oncology. Baltimore: Williams & Wilkins, 1996:540–556.

305. Bloom HJG, Hendry WF, Wallace DM, Skeet RG. Treatment of T_3 bladder cancer: controlled trial of pre-operative radiotherapy and radical cystectomy versus radical radiotherapy. (Second report and review) Br J Urol 1982;54:136–151.

306. Nerstrom B, and the Danish Bladder Cancer Group (DAVECA). Preoperative irradiation (40GY) and cystectomy versus radiotherapy (60GY) followed by salvage cystectomy in the treatment of advanced bladder cancer (T_2-T_{4a}). A randomized study (DAVECA 8201) (abstract). Eur Urol 1990;18(Suppl 1):6a.

307. Smith JA Jr, Crawford ED, Blumenstein B, et al. A randomized prospective trial of pre-operative irradiation plus radical cystectomy versus surgery alone for transitional cell carcinoma of the bladder. A Southwest Oncology Group study (abstract). J Urol 1988; 139:266A.

308. Gospodarowicz MK, Hawkins NV, Rawlings GA, et al. Radical radiotherapy for muscle invasive transitional cell carcinoma of the bladder: failure analysis. J Urol 1989;142:1448–1454.

309. vander Weff-Messing B, Menon RS, Hop WL. Cancer of the urinary bladder T_2, T_3, (N_xM_0) treated by interstitial radium: second report. Int J Radiat Oncol Biol Phys 1983;7:481–485.

310. Maffezini M, Torelli T, Villa E, et al. Systemic preoperative chemotherapy with cisplatin, methotrexate and vinblastine for locally advanced bladder cancer: local tumor response in early follow up response. J Urol 1991;145:741–743.

311. Herr HW, Scher HI. Neoadjuvant chemotherapy and partial cystectomy for invasive bladder cancer. J Clin Oncol 1994;12:975–980.

312. Srogi M, Simon SD. Primary methotrexate, vinblastine, doxorubicin and cisplatin chemotherapy and bladder preservation in locally invasive bladder cancer: a five year follow up. J Urol 1994;151:593–597.

313. Vogelzang NJ, Moormeier JA, Awan AM, et al. Methotrexate, vinblastine, doxorubicin and cisplatin followed by radiotherapy or surgery for muscle invasive bladder cancer: the University of Chicago experience. J Urol 1993;149:753–757.

314. Kaufman DS, Shipley WU, Griffin PP, Heney NM, Althausen AF, Efird JT. Selective bladder preservation by combination treatment of invasive bladder cancer. N Engl J Med 1993;329:1377–1382.

315. Shipley WU, Kaufman DS, Heney NM. Opportunities for bladder preservation in patients with localized invasive cancer using multimodality therapy. In: DeVita VT, Hellman S, Rosenberg SA, eds. Principles and practice of oncology updates. Philadelphia: JB Lippincott, 1990;4(4).

316. Logothetis CJ, Johnson DE, Chang C, et al. Adjuvant cyclophosphamide, doxorubicin and cisplatin chemotherapy for bladder cancer: an update. J Clin Oncol 1988;6:1590–1596.

317. Stöckle M, Meyenburg W, Wellek S. Advanced bladder cancer (stages pT3b, pT4a, pN1, pN2): improved survival after radical cystectomy and three adjuvant cycles of chemotherapy results of a controlled perspective study. J Urol 1992;148:302–307.

318. Studer UE, Bacchi M, Biedermann C. Adjuvant cisplatin chemotherapy following cystectomy for bladder cancer: results of a prospective randomized trial. J Urol 1994;152:81–84.

319. Skinner DG, Daniels JR, Russell CA. The role of adjuvant chemotherapy following cystectomy for invasive bladder cancer: a prospective comparative trial. J Urol 1991;145:459–467.

320. Yagoda A. Chemotherapy of metastatic bladder cancer. Cancer 1980;45(Suppl):1879–1888.

321. Logothetis CJ, Dexeus FH, Chang C, et al. Cisplatin, cyclophosphamide and doxorubicin chemotherapy for unresectable urothelial tumors: the MD Anderson experience. J Urol 1989;141:33–37.

322. Hillcoat BL, Raghavan D, Matthews, J, et al. A randomized trial of cisplatin versus cisplatin plus methotrexate in advanced cancer of the urothelial tract. J Clin Oncol 1989;7:706–709.

323. Harker WG, Meyers FJ, Freiha FS, et al. Cisplatin, methotrexate, and vinblastine (CMV): an effective chemotherapy regimen for metastatic transitional cell carcinoma of the urinary tract: a Northern California Oncology Group study. J Clin Oncol 1985;3:1463–1470.

324. Sternberg CN, Yagoda A, Scher HI, et al. M-VAC (methotrexate, vinblastine, doxorubicin and cisplatin) for advanced transitional cell carcinoma of the urothelium. J Urol 1988;139:461–469.

325. Khandekar JD, Elson PJ, DeWys WD, Slayton RE, Harris DT. Comparative activity and toxicity of cis-diamminedichloroplatinum (DDP) and a combination of doxorubicin, cyclophosphamide, and DDP in disseminated transitional cell carcinomas of the urinary tract. J Clin Oncol 1985;3:539–545.

326. Troner M, Birch R, Omura GA, Williams S. Phase III comparison of cisplatin alone vs. cisplatin, doxorubicin and cyclophosphamide in the treatment of bladder (urothelial) cancer: a Southeastern Cancer Study Group trial. J Urol 1987;137:660–665.

327. Soloway MS, Einstein A, Corder MP, Bonney W, Prout GR Jr, Coombs J. A comparison of cisplatin and the combination of cisplatin and cyclophosphamide in advanced urothelial cancer: a National Bladder Cancer Collaborative Group A study. Cancer 1983; 52:767–772.

328. Loehrer PJ, Einhorn LH, Elson PJ, et al. A randomized comparison of cisplatin alone or in combination with methotrexate, vinblastine and doxorubicin in patients with metastatic urothelial carcinoma: a cooperative group study. J Clin Oncol 1992;10:1066–1073.

329. Logothetis CJ, Dexeus FH, Finn L, et al. A prospective randomized trial comparing MVAC and CiSCA chemotherapy for patients with metastatic urothelial tumors. J Clin Oncol 1990;8:1050–1055.

330. Moore MJ, Iscoe N, Tannock IF. A phase II study of methotrexate, vinblastine, doxorubicin and cisplatin plus recombinant human granulocyte-macrophage colony stimulating factors in patients with advanced transitional cell carcinoma. J Urol 1993; 150:1131–1134.

331. Seidman AD, Scher HI, Gabrilove JL, et al. Dose-intensification of MVAC with recombinant granulocyte colony-stimulating factor as initial therapy in advanced urothelial cancer. J Clin Oncol 1993;11:408–414.

332. Loehrer PJ, Elson P, Dreicer R, et al. Escalated doses of methotrexate, vinblastine, doxorubicin and cisplatin plus recombinant human granulocyte colony-stimulating factor in advanced urothelial carcinoma: an Eastern Cooperative Oncology Group trial. J Clin Oncol 1994;12:483–488.

333. Roth BJ, Bajorin DF. Advanced bladder cancer: the need to identify new agents in the post M-VAC (methotrexate, vinblastine and cisplatin) world. J Urol 1995;153:894–900.

334. Roth BJ, Dreicer R, Einhorn LH, et al. Significant activity of paclitaxel in advanced transitional cell carcinoma of the urothelium: a phase II trial of the Eastern Cooperative Oncology Group. J Clin Oncol 1994;12:2264–2270.

335. Sadan S, Bajorin D, Amsterdam A, Scher H. Docetaxel in patients with advanced transitional cell cancer who failed cisplatin-based chemotherapy: a phase II trial (abstract 761). Proc Am Soc Clin Oncol 1994;13:244.

336. Crawford ED, Saiers JH, Baker LH, Costanzi JH, Bukowski RM. Gallium nitrate in advanced bladder carcinoma: Southwest Oncology Group study. Urology 1991;38:355–357.

337. Seligman PA, Crawford ED. Treatment of advanced transitional cell carcinoma of the bladder with continuous-infusion gallium nitrate. J Natl Cancer Inst 1991;83:1582–1584.

338. Seidman AD, Scher HI, Heinemann MII, et al. Continuous infusion gallium nitrate for patients with advanced refractory urothelial tract tumors. Cancer 1991;68:2561–2565.

339. Witte R, Loehrer P, Dreicer R, Williams S, Elson P. Ifosfamide in advanced urothelial carcinoma: an ECOG trial (abstract 707). Proc Am Soc Clin Oncol 1993;12:30.

340. Otaguro K, Ueda K, Niijima T, et al. Clinical evaluation of Z4942 (ifosfamide) for malignant urological tumors. Hinyokika Kiyo 1981;27:459–462.

341. Gad-el-Nawla N, Hamza MR, Zikri ZK, et al. Chemotherapy in invasive carcinoma of the bladder. A review of phase II trials in Egypt. Acta Oncol 1989; 28:73–76.

342. Pollera CF, Ceribelli A, Crecco M, Calabresi F. Weekly gemcitabine in advanced bladder cancer: a preliminary report from a phase I study. Ann Oncol 1994;5:182–184.

343. Stadler W, Kuzel T, Raghavan D, Levine E, Vogelzang NJ, Dorr F. A phase II study of gemcitabine in the treatment of patients with advanced transitional cell carcinoma (abstract 638). Proc Am Soc Clin Oncol 1995;14:241.

344. Witte RS, Elson P, Khandaker J, Trump DL. An Eastern Cooperative Oncology Group phase II trial of trimetrexate in the treatment of advanced urothelial carcinoma. Cancer 1994;73:688–691.

345. de Wit R, Kaye SB, Roberts JT, Stoter G, Scott J, Verweij J. Oral piritrexim, an effective treatment for metastatic urothelial cancer. Br J Cancer 1993;67:388–390.

58

Chemotherapy of Gynecologic Cancer

J. Tate Thigpen

Cancer of the female genital tract accounts for almost 80,000 cases of invasive cancer each year in the United States, with most of these being one of three neoplasms: endometrial carcinoma, carcinoma of the cervix, and celomic epithelial carcinoma of the ovary. Historically, with the exception of ovarian carcinoma, surgery, radiotherapy, or a combination of the two formed the primary management of most gynecologic malignancies. Success rates, particularly for carcinomas of the endometrium and cervix, were sufficiently high that little effort was expended in the development of systemic therapy until 1976 (1). Since 1976, significant information has been gained about the activity of cytotoxic and hormonal agents in a variety of neoplasms: endometrial carcinoma, uterine sarcomas, carcinoma of the cervix, and celomic epithelial carcinoma and germ cell tumors of the ovary. The following discussion focuses on the use of systemic therapy in these entities.

CARCINOMA OF THE ENDOMETRIUM

Carcinoma of the endometrium is the most common invasive neoplasm of the female genital tract. The most common presenting manifestation, dysfunctional uterine bleeding in the perimenopausal or postmenopausal woman, leads the patient to seek medical attention early in the course of the disease. As a result, the vast majority of patients are diagnosed when the disease is confined to the corpus of the uterus. The resultant relatively high cure rate of 66% gave the impression that this was a "benign" malignancy and actually slowed the development of effective systemic therapy. Data generated primarily

since 1976 form the basis for the use of systemic therapy in current management.

General Considerations

Carcinoma of the endometrium (2–5) consists mostly of adenocarcinoma (70% of all cases), with smaller numbers of adenosquamous carcinomas, adenoacanthomas, and clear cell and papillary serous carcinomas. The primary presenting manifestation is dysfunctional uterine bleeding, which occurs in patients who are perimenopausal or postmenopausal, who frequently are obese, hypertensive, and diabetic, and who characteristically demonstrate low parity. In the face of dysfunctional bleeding, endometrial sampling is mandatory. If sampling is negative, a dilation and curettage to establish the cause of the bleeding is the next step.

If endometrial carcinoma is found in the absence of evidence of distant spread, total abdominal hysterectomy should be done in conjunction with a careful assessment of extent of disease in the pelvis and abdomen. The resultant information should suffice to establish the surgical-pathologic stage of disease. The assignment of stage essentially divides the patient population into two groups: limited disease (stages I and II) and advanced disease (stages III and IV).

Management of Advanced or Recurrent Disease

Less than 15% of endometrial carcinomas present as advanced disease, and roughly 30 to 40% of patients with limited disease at presentation will recur. These two groups of patients are generally managed with systemic therapy, which includes both hormonal agents and cyto-toxic drugs.

HORMONAL THERAPY

Endometrial carcinoma is clearly a hormon-ally influenced disease process. Estrogens have been implicated in the etiology of the disease, but this discussion will focus on the therapeutic role of certain other hormonal agents, in partic-ular progestins (6). Older literature reports ob-jective regression of disease in 33% of patients with endometrial carcinoma treated with pro-gestational agents (Table 58.1) (7). Responses correlate with histologic grade and receptor sta-tus. Well-differentiated lesions are more likely to respond and are also more likely to be positive for estrogen and progesterone receptors than are poorly differentiated lesions. Lesions positive for estrogen and progesterone receptors appear more likely to respond to progestin therapy than lesions that are receptor negative (Table 58.2). Most of these trials were conducted with par-enteral progestins.

After an initial pilot study demonstrated that serum levels of progestin were comparable for oral and parenteral medroxyprogesterone ace-tate (MPA) (8), a large phase II study of oral MPA 150 mg/day in patients with advanced or recurrent endometrial carcinoma reported 32 complete (10%) and 26 partial (8%) responses among 331 patients with measurable disease not previously treated with systemic therapy (Table 58.3) (9). The median progression-free interval was 4 months, and median survival, 10.4 months. In the 102 patients with known receptor status, response to MPA occurred more fre-quently, and progression-free interval and sur-vival were longer, in patients with tumors posi-

Table 58.1. Progestins in the Management of Endometrial Carcinoma

Progestin	Patients	Response (%)
Earlier trials		
Medroxyprogesterone	151	34
Megestrol acetate	125	33
Medrogestone	56	30
Recent trials		
Delalutin and Depo-Provera	114	16

Data from Thigpen T, Vance R, Lambuth B, et al. Chemotherapy for advanced or recurrent gynecologic cancer. Cancer 1987; 60:2104–2116.

Table 58.2. Receptor Status and Response to Progestin Therapy

Series	ER+ PR+	ER− PR−
Creasman	3/5 (60%)	1/8 (12%)
Ehrlich	7/8 (80%)	1/16 (7%)
Benraad	5/6 (83%)	0/5 (0%)
Martin	13/13 (100%)	1/7 (14%)
McCarty	4/5 (80%)	0/8 (0%)
Total	32/37 (86%)	3/44 (7%)

Data from Thigpen T, Vance R, Lambuth B, et al. Chemotherapy for advanced or recurrrent gynecologic cancer. Cancer 1987; 60:2104–2116.

Table 58.3. Results of a Phase II Trial of Medroxyprogesterone Acetate 150 mg/day Orally in Advanced or Recurrent Endometrial Carcinoma with No Prior Systemic Therapy

Patients	Response	PFI[a] (Month)	Survival (Month)
Overall	58/331 (18%)	4.0	10.5
Receptor known			
ER[a] + PR + (29)	4/10 (40%)	8.5	13.5
ER + PR − (30)	2/16 (12%)	4.5	9.0
ER − PR − (43)	3/25 (12%)	2.5	9.5

Data from Thigpen T, Blessing J, DiSaia P, Ehrlich C. Oral me-droxyprogesterone acetate in advanced or recurrent endometrial carcinoma: results of therapy and correlation with estrogen and progesterone receptor levels. The Gynecologic Oncology Group experience. In: Baulier E, Iacobelli S, McGuire W, eds. Endocri-nology and malignancy. New York: Parthenon, 1986:446–454.
[a]ER, estrogen receptor; PFI, progression-free interval; PR, proges-terone receptor.

tive for both estrogen and progesterone recep-tors. The relatively small number of subjects with receptor data and the lack of quality control of laboratory techniques did not permit defini-tive conclusions. These results indicated clear-cut activity for progestins at a level somewhat less than that previously reported.

A follow-up study clarified several issues (Ta-ble 58.4) (10). The study randomized patients to receive either 200 or 1000 mg/day of MPA and required that blood levels of progestin be as-sessed. Blood levels confirmed patient compli-ance; surprisingly, the lower dose of MPA offered a marginal advantage in terms of progression-free interval with a higher response rate, although the difference was not statistically significant.

Table 58.4. Results of a Phase III Trial of Low-Dose versus High-Dose Medroxyprogesterone Acetate in Advanced or Recurrent Endometrial Carcinoma

Response	MPA 200 mg	MPA 1000 mg	Total
Complete response	24 (17%)	14 (10.0%)	38
Partial response	12 (9%)	10 (7%)	22
Stable disease	60 (44%)	53 (38%)	113
Increasing disease	42 (30%)	63 (45%)	105
Total	138	140	278

Data from Thigpen T, Brady M, Alvarez, et al. Oral medroxyprogesterone acetate in the treatment of advanced or recurrent endometrial carcinoma: a dose-response study by the Gynecologic Oncology Group. J Clin Oncol (in press).

Table 58.5. Results with Tamoxifen in Patients with Advanced or Recurrent Endometrial Carcinoma (7, 12)

Regimen	Patients	Response
60 mg/m^2/day	17	53%
20 mg/day	10	30%
20 mg/day	25	0%
20 mg/day	63	13%

Based on these two large trials, current use of hormonal therapy should be considered in advanced or recurrent disease, particularly for those patients with known receptor positivity or well-differentiated neoplasms. The hormones of choice are progestational agents.

The only other agent to be tested in a significant number of patients is tamoxifen, which demonstrated significant activity in two of four trials (7, 11–12) (Table 58.5). The most recent and largest of these four trials (12), conducted by the Gynecologic Oncology Group (GOG) in patients with no prior hormonal therapy, demonstrated only a 13% response rate among 63 patients. The weight of evidence thus suggests at best modest activity for tamoxifen.

CYTOTOXIC THERAPY

As of 1976, meaningful information on the use of cytotoxic drugs in the management of endometrial carcinoma was virtually nonexistent. Only three agents had been identified as potentially active on the basis of collected data from broad phase II trials: 5-fluorouracil, cyclophos-

phamide, and doxorubicin (1). Data concerning the use of combination chemotherapy were anecdotal.

A concerted effort to evaluate single agents in phase II trials has produced studies of 29 drugs over the last two decades (Table 58.6) (13–30). The anthracyclines doxorubicin and epirubicin, the platinum analogues cisplatin and carboplatin, paclitaxel, vincristine, and 5-fluorouracil have shown evidence of significant activity (defined as a response rate of 15% or greater). Phase II trials of new agents are a continuing part of the ongoing research effort of the cooperative groups.

Most attempts at evaluating potential combination regimens for endometrial carcinoma have consisted of small series with no control arm and hence no opportunity to assess the relative merits of combination and single-agent therapy (Table 58.7) (31). Three randomized attempts to identify effective combination chemotherapy have been conducted by the GOG in the last 17 years (Table 58.8). The first was based on two promising pilot studies and randomized patients to megestrol acetate plus either cyclophosphamide plus doxorubicin plus 5-fluorouracil (CAF) or melphalan plus 5-fluorouracil (MF) (32–34). Despite response rates of 94 and 75% respectively, in the pilot studies of 15 and 20 patients, no differences were observed in the phase III trial, with disappointing response rates of 38 and 36%, respectively, among the 155 measurable patients. Progression-free intervals and survivals were no different from those observed with doxorubicin alone (13).

The second GOG phase III trial randomized patients to doxorubicin with or without cyclophosphamide (35). Among 202 patients with measurable disease entered into study, doxorubicin yielded a response rate of 22% and median survival of 6.8 months, compared with 32% and 7.6 months for the combination. The response rate difference was marginally significant, but the survivals did not differ.

The third GOG phase II trial randomized patients to doxorubicin with or without cisplatin (36). The most recent analysis of this trial shows a superior response rate with the combination (46% vs. 27%) and a marginally better progression-free survival, with no difference in overall survival. The percentage of patients achieving a complete response on the combination was 21%, versus 9% with the single agent. These results do provide a basis for regarding this combination

Table 58.6. Single-Agent Activity in Endometrial Carcinoma

Drug	Schedule	Response
No prior chemotherapy		
Doxorubicin (13, 26)	60 mg/m^2/3 week	16/43 (38%)
	50 mg/m^2/3 week	4/21 (19%)
Epirubicin (28)	60 mg/m^2/3 week	7/27 (26%)
Cisplatin (14, 26)	50 mg/m^2/3 week	10/49 (20%)
	50 mg/m^2/3 week	4/11 (36%)
	50–100 mg/m^2/3 week	11/26 (42%)
Carboplatin (26)	400 mg/m^2/4 week	7/25 (28%)
	400 mg/m^2/4 week	9/27 (33%)
Hexamethylmelamine (16, 26)	280 mg/m^2 × 14 day/4 week	3/34 (9%)
	8 mg/kg/day	6/20 (30%)
Methotrexate (17)	40 mg/m^2/week	2/33 (6%)
Cyclophosphamide (26)	666 mg/m^2/3 week	0/19 (0%)
Ifosfamide (27)	1.2 g/m^2/day × 5 day/4 week	2/16 (13%)
Paclitaxel (30)	250 mg/m^2/3 week	10/28 (35%)
Vincristine (28)	60 mg/m^2/3 week	6/38 (16%)
Esorubicin (28)	60 mg/m^2/3 week	0/20 (0%)
Prior chemotherapy		
5-Fluorouracil (28)	–	7/34 (5%)
Piperazinedione (15)	9 mg/m^2/3 week	1/22 (5%)
Cisplatin (18)	50 mg/m^2/3 week	1/25 (4%)
	3 mg/kg/3 week	4/13 (31%)
Aminothiadiazole (19)	125 mg/m^2/week	0/21 (0%)
Teniposide (20)	100 mg/m^2/week	2/22 (9%)
AZQ (21)	22.5 mg/m^2/3 week	2/26 (8%)
Mitoxantrone (22, 28)	12 mg/m^2/3 week	1/19 (5%)
Razoxane (23)	1.5 g/m^2/week	0/24 (0%)
Etoposide (24)	100 mg/m^2 × 3 day/4 week	1/29 (3%)
Galactitol (25)	60 mg/m^2/week	1/17 (6%)
Vinblastine (26)	1.5 mg/m^2/day × 5 day/3 week CI[a]	4/34 (12%)
MGBG (26)	500 mg/m^2/day weekly	3/21 (14%)
AMSA (29)	- - - -	1/19 (5%)
Chlorambucil (28)	–	0/11 (0%)
Echinomycin (28)	–	1/21 (5%)
Cytembena (28)	–	10/30 (33%)
6-Mercaptopurine (28)	–	0/10 (0%)
Fludarabine (28)	–	0/19 (0%)
Semustine (MeCCNU) (28)	–	2/5 (40%)

[a]CI, continuous infusion.

(doxorubicin 60 mg/m^2 plus cisplatin 50 mg/m^2 every 3 weeks) as the treatment of choice for advanced or recurrent endometrial carcinoma.

CONCLUSIONS

Systemic therapy for advanced or recurrent disease offers some hope for disease remission. Initial treatment should consist of progestins in those patients with grade 1 or 2 disease and/or positive estrogen and progesterone receptors. Patients known to be receptor negative or to have failed on progestins should be managed with a combination of doxorubicin plus cis-

platin. In all cases, since systemic therapy offers only modest benefit, patients should be offered clinical trials if eligible.

Limited Disease

For patients with limited (stage I or II) disease, a number of pathologic factors determine the risk for recurrence: histologic grade, depth of myometrial invasion, extrauterine disease, nodal involvement, and peritoneal cytology (2–5). Most patients present with disease that is low risk for recurrence: grade 1 with no myo-

Table 58.7. Uncontrolled Trials of Combination Chemotherapy in Endometrial Carcinoma (31)

Regimen	Response	PFI/ Survival
Doxorubicin +		
Cisplatin	6CR[a],7PR/16	
	2CR,10PR/20	
Cisplatin + cytoxan + Megace	4CR,1PR/15	32 week/60 week
	5CR,4PR/15	8 month/12 month
Cisplatin + vinblastine	3CR,10PR/42	- - - -/8 month
Cytoxan + megace	4CR,11PR/56	
Cytoxan + 5-FU + Megace	3CR,6PR/58	
Cytoxan + 5-FU + tamoxifen	7CR,6PR/43	- - - -/20 month
Cytoxan + 5-FU + vincristine	5CR/20	- - - -/14.7 month
Melphalan + 5-FU + Megace	1CR,1PR/12	
	8CR/18PR/126	
	10CR,14PR/50	- - - -/5 month
Cisplatin + ifosfamide	3CR,1PR/4	

Data from Moore TD, Phillips PH, Nerenstone SR, Cheson BD. Systemic treatment of advanced and recurrent endometrial carcinoma: current status and future directions. J Clin Oncol 1991;9:1071–1088.
[a]- - - -, PFI not given; CR, complete response; PR, partial response; PRI, progression-free interval.

Table 58.8. Results of GOG Phase III Trials of Chemotherapy in Endometrial Carcinoma

Study and Regimen	Response	Survival
GOG protocol 28 (34)		
CAF + megestrol acetate	28/78 (36%)	10.1 months
MF + megestrol acetate	29/77 (38%)	10.6 months
GOG protocol 48 (35)		
Doxorubicin	22/97 (22%)	6.8 months
Doxorubicin + cytoxan	34/105 (32%)	7.6 months
GOG protocol 107 (36)		
Doxorubicin	37/137 (27%)	9.2 months
Doxorubicin + cisplatin	53/115 (46%)	8.8 months

metrial invasion, negative nodes, no extrauterine disease, and negative peritoneal cytology. These patients should have a 5-year disease-free survival that exceeds 90%; no systemic therapy should be considered.

For patients with one or more high-risk features, recurrence rates increase dramatically. It is reasonable to consider the use of some form of adjuvant therapy, but neither chemotherapy nor hormonal therapy has been shown to offer an improved survival. The GOG undertook a phase III trial in patients with one or more high-risk factors: grade 3 disease, deep myometrial invasion, positive nodes, or extrauterine spread (37). After initial total abdominal hysterectomy, bilateral salpingo-oophorectomy, and surgical staging followed by postoperative radiotherapy, patients were randomized to receive either no further therapy or doxorubicin 45 mg/m² every 3 weeks. With a median follow-up exceeding 4 years, 21% of the 139 evaluable patients had recurred; there were no significant differences between the two treatment arms.

No other controlled trials of adjuvant cytotoxic therapy have been reported in limited endometrial carcinoma. There is therefore no scientific basis for the use of adjuvant therapy in limited endometrial carcinoma at the present time.

Summary and Future Directions

The role of systemic therapy in endometrial carcinoma remains limited at the present time. For patients with advanced or recurrent disease, eight agents have been shown to have activity:

progestins, doxorubicin, epirubicin, the platinum analogues cisplatin and carboplatin, paclitaxel, vincristine, and 5-fluorouracil. Based on data from randomized trials, the combination of doxorubicin plus cisplatin yields a superior response rate (46 vs. 27%) along with a marginally superior progression-free survival. For patients with grade 1 or 2 disease or known receptor positivity, initial treatment should consist of progestins. For patients with grade 3 disease, known receptor negativity, or disease no longer responsive to hormones, a combination of doxorubicin plus cisplatin should be considered. There is no current documented role for systemic adjuvant therapy in limited disease.

UTERINE SARCOMAS

Uterine sarcomas, far less common than endometrial carcinoma, demonstrate a significant recurrence rate of at least 50%, even in stage I disease. This fact, plus their propensity to recur at distant sites, make these neoplasms prime candidates for the use of chemotherapy. The relative infrequency of these lesions, on the other hand, has limited the amount of meaningful information on the use of systemic therapy. Most clinical information comes from the studies of the GOG and includes trials conducted since 1973.

General Considerations

Uterine sarcomas are a heterogeneous group of neoplasms that includes mixed mesodermal sarcomas, leiomyosarcomas, endometrial stromal sarcomas, and certain rare histologic types. The mixed mesodermal sarcomas and the leio-

myosarcomas constitute 90% of the cases and are the only two types for which meaningful data are available. Because these two histologic types appear to respond differently to chemotherapy, they must be studied as separate patient populations. Within each population, there are two distinct situations in which chemotherapy has been studied: the management of advanced or recurrent disease and the adjuvant treatment of patients with stage I disease following complete surgical resection.

Advanced or Recurrent Disease

SINGLE AGENTS

Six drugs have been studied as single agents in uterine sarcomas. Among patients with mixed mesodermal sarcomas, two of these demonstrate clear-cut evidence of activity: ifosfamide and cisplatin (Table 58.9). Ifosfamide at a dose of 1.5 mg/m^2/day for 5 days every 4 weeks produced five complete and four partial responses among 28 patients with no prior chemotherapy (38). This agent appears to be the most active single agent studied to date.

Cisplatin was studied in patients with prior chemotherapy with evidence that the drug was active (18% response rate in 28 patients). A repeat trial in patients with no prior chemotherapy documented an essentially similar response rate of 19% among a larger group of 63 patients (39, 40). Both of these trials employed a relatively low dose of cisplatin of 50 mg/m^2 every 3 weeks. Investigators at M. D. Anderson Hospital used a higher dose, ranging from 75 to 100 mg/m^2 every 3 weeks (41). Only 12 patients with mea-

Table 58.9. Single-Agent Activity in Mixed Mesodermal Sarcoma of the Uterus

Drug	Prior Rx (Reference)	Schedule	Response
Ifosfamide	No (38)	1.5 g/m^2/day plus mesna 0.3 g/m^2/day for 5 days q 4 week	5CR,4PR/28 (32%)
Cisplatin	No (39)	50 mg/m^2 every 3 weeks	5CR,7PR/63 (19%)
	Yes (40)	50 mg/m^2 every 3 weeks	2CR,3PR/28 (18%)
	No (41)	75–100 mg/m^2 every 3 weeks	1CR,4PR/12 (42%)
Doxorubicin	No (42)	60 mg/m^2 every 3 weeks	4/41 (10%)
	No (43)	50–90 mg/m^2 every 3 weeks	0/9 (0%)
Etoposide	Yes (44)	100 mg/m^2/day for 3 days every 4 weeks	2PR/31 (6%)
Mitoxantrone	Yes (45)	12 mg/m^2 every 3 weeks	0/17 (0%)
Piperazinedione	Yes (46)	9 mg/m^2 every 3 weeks	0/6 (0%)

Table 58.10. Single-Agent Activity in Leiomyosarcomas of the Uterus

Drug	Prior Rx (Reference)	Schedule	Response
Doxorubicin	No (42)	60 mg/m² every 3 weeks	7/28 (25%)
Ifosfamide	No (47)	1.5 g/m²/day plus mesna 0.3 g/m²/day for 5 days q 4 week	4PR/28 (14%)
Cisplatin	No (39)	50 mg/m² every 3 weeks	1PR/33 (3%)
	Yes (48)	50 mg/m² every 3 weeks	1PR/19 (5%)
Etoposide	Yes (49)	100 mg/m²/day for 3 days every 4 weeks	1CR,2PR/28 (11%)
	No (50)	100 mg/m²/day for 3 days every 4 weeks	0/28 (0%)
Mitoxantrone	Yes (45)	12 mg/m² every 3 weeks	0/12 (0%)
Piperazinedione	Yes (46)	9 mg/m² every 3 weeks	1/11 (9%)

surable disease were entered into the study, but one complete and four partial responses were observed (42%). The small number of cases and the lack of a randomized trial make conclusions about the merits of the higher dose invalid.

Surprisingly, doxorubicin demonstrated relatively little activity in two trials of patients with mixed mesodermal sarcomas. The first, conducted as one arm of phase III trial with a dose of 60 mg/m² every 3 weeks, produced only four responses among 41 patients (42). The second used a range of doses from 50 to 90 mg/m² every 3 weeks, with most of the patients receiving either 75 or 90 mg/m² (43). No responses were seen among the nine patients with measurable disease.

Demonstrating negligible activity in phase II studies were etoposide (44), mitoxantrone (45), and piperazinedione (46).

Among patients with leiomyosarcomas, six single agents have been tested (Table 58.10). The most active single agent appears to be doxorubicin (42). Seven responses were observed among 28 patients treated with 60 mg/m² every 3 weeks. Ifosfamide demonstrated moderate activity, with four partial responses among 28 patients (47). Etoposide showed potential activity in a second-line trial (one complete and two partial responses among 28 patients) (49), but an attempted confirmatory trial in patients with no prior chemotherapy showed no responses among 28 patients (50). Essentially no activity was seen with cisplatin, mitoxantrone, and piperazinedione (45, 46, 48).

In summary, two drugs appear to possess significant activity in mixed mesodermal sarcomas of the uterus: ifosfamide and cisplatin. In leio-myosarcomas, only one significantly active agent has been identified to date, doxorubicin.

COMBINATION CHEMOTHERAPY

Adequate evaluation of combination chemotherapy requires randomized phase III trials, which have been completed in only two instances. These form the basis for any meaningful conclusions regarding the role of combination chemotherapy.

The first randomized trial compared doxorubicin with or without dimethyl triazinoimidazole carboxamide (DTIC) (Table 58.11) (42). No significant differences between the two regimens were noted, but the study was designed before the apparent differences in response to chemotherapy for leiomyosarcomas and mixed mesodermal sarcomas were observed. As a result, the total patient population supplied an insufficient number of each histologic type to permit subset analysis.

The second randomized trial studied doxorubicin with or without cyclophosphamide (Table 58.12) (51). The study was closed early because the likelihood of identifying differences was extremely small. The overall response rate for the combined data was similar to that seen in the first randomized trial.

With the subsequent recognition of the difference in response between leiomyosarcoma and mixed mesodermal sarcoma, future randomized trials will have to regard each of the two major histologic types as a separate patient population, which will increase the necessary time to completion for any study. An ongoing phase III trial takes this fact into account in that it involves only mixed mesodermal sarcomas; patients are ran-

Table 58.11. Randomized Trial of Doxorubicin with or without Dimethyl Triazinoimidazole Carboxamide in Advanced or Recurrent Uterine Sarcomas

Histologic Type	Doxorubicin	Doxorubicin + DTIC
Leiomyosarcoma	7/28 (25%)	6/20 (30%)
Mixed mesodermal sarcoma	4/41 (10%)	7/31 (23%)
Other sarcomas	2/11 (18%)	3/15 (20%)

Data from Omura GA, Major FJ, Blessing JA, et al. A randomized study of adriamycin with and without dimethyl triazinoimidazole carboxamide in advanced uterine sarcomas. Cancer 1983; 52:626–632.

Table 58.12. Randomized Trial of Doxorubicin with or without Cyclophosphamide in Advanced or Recurrent Uterine Sarcoma

	Response
Treatment	
Doxorubicin	1CR,4PR/26 (19%)
Doxorubicin + cyclophosphamide	2CR,3PR/26 (19%)
Cell type	
Leiomyosarcoma	3PR/23 (13%)
Mixed mesodermal sarcoma	3CR/2PR/20 (25%)
Other sarcoma	2PR/9 (22%)

Data from Muss HB, Bundy BN, DiSaia PJ, et al. Treatment of recurrent or advanced uterine sarcoma: a randomized trial of doxorubicin versus doxorubicin and cyclophosphamide (a phase III trial of the Gynecologic Oncology Group). Cancer 1985; 55:1648–1653.

domized to ifosfamide with or without cisplatin. The study is too early to permit any conclusions. In the population with leiomyosarcomas, single-agent trials are ongoing in an attempt to identify at least a second active agent.

In conclusion, there is no evidence to support the use of combination chemotherapy in advanced or recurrent uterine sarcomas at the present time.

Limited Disease

There is no defined role for adjuvant chemotherapy for stage I disease after complete surgical resection. Only one meaningful study has been conducted to date. This trial randomized patients to receive either doxorubicin 60 mg/m^2 every 3 weeks for eight cycles or no further ther-

apy (Table 58.13) (52). No significant differences in recurrence rate, progression-free interval, or survival were noted for either the overall patient population or either of the two major histologic subsets, although in each subset a 12% or greater difference in recurrence rate was noted, favoring the group receiving doxorubicin. In the overall population, the median survival was 73.7 months for the doxorubicin arm and 55.0 months for no further therapy.

Two factors limit further study of adjuvant therapy. The relatively low frequency of the disease makes it difficult to accrue sufficient patients to complete a study in a reasonable period of time. Additionally, the apparent difference in the way the two major histologic types respond to chemotherapy further complicates the problem of low disease incidence.

At the present time, there is no evidence that adjuvant chemotherapy is of any value in uterine sarcomas.

Conclusions and Future Directions

In conclusion, the role of chemotherapy in the management of uterine sarcomas is confined to the use of single-agent therapy in the treatment of patients with advanced or recurrent disease. In mixed mesodermal sarcomas, the drug of choice is either ifosfamide or cisplatin. An ongoing study is evaluating ifosfamide with or without cisplatin. Beyond this, efforts are directed to the identification of additional active agents. In leiomyosarcomas, only one conclusively active agent has been identified to date, doxorubicin. Efforts are directed to the identification of additional active drugs. No current role for chemotherapy has been defined in the adjuvant setting, and no studies are currently under way because of the lack of sufficiently active regimens in the advanced disease setting.

CARCINOMA OF THE CERVIX

Over the last 40 years, carcinoma of the uterine cervix has dramatically decreased as a cause of death, but still over 15,800 new cases are diagnosed annually, and over 4800 deaths are reported annually as a result of this disease (53). While radiotherapy and surgery form the basis of treatment of disease limited to the pelvis, patients who recur after initial locoregional therapy or who are unfortunate enough to present with advanced disease will depend upon systemic therapy for any hope of disease control.

Table 58.13. GOG Randomized Trial of Doxorubicin versus No Further Therapy in Completely Resected Stage I and II Uterine Sarcoma Showing Recurrence Rates

Cell Type	Doxorubicin	No Therapy	Total
Leiomyosarcoma	11/25 (44%)	14/23 (61%)	25/48 (52%)
Mixed mesodermal sarcoma	17/44 (39%)	25/49 (51%)	42/93 (45%)
Other sarcoma	3/6 (50%)	4/9 (44%)	7/15 (47%)
Total	31/75 (41%)	43/81 (53%)	74/156 (47%)

Data from Omura GA, Blessing JA, Major F, et al. A randomized clinical trial of adjuvant adriamycin in uterine sarcomas: a Gynecologic Oncology Group study. J Clin Oncol 1985;3:1240–1245.

General Considerations

The role of chemotherapy in carcinoma of the cervix has been limited for several reasons. First, excellent success with surgery and/or radiotherapy in limited-disease patients coupled with the high rate of early diagnosis as a result of the PAP smear yields good cure rates; thus, a minority of patients require systemic therapy. Second, a significant proportion of patients recur in the pelvis in the previous field of radiation; hence, delivery of drug to the cancer can be impaired by altered blood supply. In addition, the cells themselves may be resistant, particularly to alkylating agents, as a result of the prior radiation. Third, patients with prior pelvic radiotherapy have limited bone marrow reserve and are less tolerant of dose-intense chemotherapy; hence, doses of cytotoxic drugs are often less than optimal. Finally, recurrent or advanced cervix cancer is often associated with ureteral obstruction and resultant renal failure. This eliminates as therapeutic choices certain drugs that are nephrotoxic and complicates the use of other agents that are excreted at least in part by the kidneys.

Despite these limitations, a concerted effort to evaluate cytotoxic therapy has been ongoing since 1976. The results of this effort have provided evidence for a role of chemotherapy in two clinical situations: the management of advanced or recurrent disease no longer amenable to control with surgery and/or radiotherapy and concomitant use with radiation to sensitize carcinoma of the cervix to the effects of radiotherapy.

Advanced or Recurrent Disease

Studies of single cytotoxic agents in advanced or recurrent carcinoma of the cervix have, in most instances, distinguished between squamous cell carcinomas, which account for more than 80% of all cases, and nonsquamous carcinomas, which consist mostly of adenocarcinoma and adenosquamous tumors.

SQUAMOUS CELL CARCINOMA

A total of 52 cytotoxic agents have been tested in patients with advanced or recurrent squamous cell carcinoma of the cervix (Tables 58.14 and 58.15) (1, 54–113). While 19 of these agents have activity as defined by a response rate of 15% or greater, 4 are of particular interest because of relatively high response rates in carefully done trials.

The *platinum compounds* are the most extensively evaluated drugs in squamous cell carcinoma of the cervix: cisplatin, carboplatin, and iproplatin. First demonstrated to be active against carcinoma of the cervix by the GOG in 1978, the drug has been tested in a variety of doses and schedules (Table 58.16) (67–72). Several conclusions can be drawn from these extensive trials. First, the drug is clearly active against squamous cell carcinoma of the cervix at a dose of 50 mg/m^2 intravenously at a rate of 1 mg/min every 3 weeks. Secondly, there is a small but statistically significant increase in the response rate with a doubling of the dose to 100 mg/m^2, but no corresponding improvement in the progression-free or overall survival is seen. Thirdly, more prolonged infusions of the same dose over 24 hours have no effect on the response rate but do result in less nausea and vomiting, although the current availability of more potent antiemetic agents renders this observation less significant.

Other platinum compounds that have been tested in patients with squamous cell carcinoma of the cervix include carboplatin and iproplatin (65–66). In a GOG trial randomizing patients with advanced or recurrent squamous cell carcinoma of the cervix and no prior chemotherapy to one of these two agents, response rates of 15 and 11%, respectively, were observed. This ac-

Table 58.14. Single Agents Active in Squamous Cell Carcinoma of the Cervix (as defined by a response ≥ 15%)

Drug	Patients	Response (%)
Alkylating agents		
Cyclophosphamide (56, 57)	251	38 (15%)
Chlorambucil (56, 58)	44	11 (25%)
Dibromodulcitol (59, 60)	102	23 (23%)
Galactitol (61)	36	7 (19%)
Ifosfamide (62–64)	157	35 (22%)
Melphalan (55)	20	4 (20%)
Heavy metal complexes		
Carboplatin (65, 66)	175	27 (15%)
Cisplatin (67–72)	815	190 (23%)
Antibiotics		
Doxorubicin (73–79)	266	45 (17%)
Porfiromycin (55)	78	17 (22%)
Antimetabolites		
Baker's antifol (80)	32	5 (16%)
5-Fluorouracil (73, 81)	142	29 (20%)
Methotrexate (73, 74)	96	17 (18%)
Plant alkaloids		
Vincristine (55)	55	10 (18%)
Vindesine (55)	21	5 (24%)
Other agents		
CPT-11 (82)	55	13 (24%)
Hexamethylmelamine (55)	64	12 (19%)
Paclitaxel (30)	52	9 (17%)
Razoxane (83)	28	5 (18%)

Table 58.15. Single Agents Inactive in Squamous Cell Carcinoma of the Cervix (based on a response rate of <15%)

Drug	Patients	Response (%)
Aminothiadiazole (84)	21	1 (5%)
Amonafide (85)	20	1 (5%)
AMSA (86)	25	1 (4%)
Bleomycin (73)	172	17 (10%)
CCNU (56, 87)	63	3 (5%)
Diaziquone (88)	26	1 (4%)
Dichloromethotrexate (89)	No	3/37 (8%)
Didemnin (90, 91)	21	0 (0%)
Echinomycin (92)	28	2 (7%)
Edatrexate (93)	16	0 (0%)
Esorubicin (94)	28	0 (0%)
Etoposide (95)	31	0 (0%)
Fazarabine (96)	19	0 (0%)
5-Fluorouracil/leucovorin (97, 98)	66	6 (9%)
Gallium nitrate (99)	24	2 (8%)
Hydroxyurea (58)	14	0 (0%)
Iproplatin (66, 100)	177	19 (11%)
Maytansine (101)	29	1 (3%)
Menogaril (102)	22	0 (0%)
Merbarone (103)	21	2 (10%)
Mercaptopurine (73)	18	1 (5%)
Methyl-CCNU (56, 87)	94	7 (7%)
Mitomycin C (73, 104)	70	10 (14%)
Mitoxantrone (105)	26	2 (8%)
N-Methylformamide (106)	20	0 (0%)
PALA (107)	Yes	0/36 (0%)
Piperazinedione (108)	38	5 (13%)
Piroxantrone (109)	18	0 (0%)
Spirogermanium (55)	18	0 (0%)
Teniposide (110)	22	3 (14%)
TCN-P (111)	21	2 (10%)
Vinblastine (54, 112)	53	2 (4%)
Yoshi 864 (113)	18	0 (0%)

tivity appears to be of a lower order than that seen with cisplatin; hence, cisplatin remains the platinum compound of choice despite less toxicity noted with at least one of the other two drugs.

Ifosfamide is chemically similar to cyclophosphamide and acts as a classic alkylating agent. In carcinoma of the cervix, the drug has been given in a variety of doses and schedules (Table 58.17) (62–64). Five concerted phase II trials in patients with squamous cell carcinoma of the cervix, the overwhelming majority of whom had received prior radiotherapy, have been reported. In the three studies in patients with no prior chemotherapy, response rates of 33 to 50% were observed at three different dose levels and schedules. The two trials with patients with prior systemic treatment reflected much less activity, with only three partial responses among 36 patients (8%) with fractionated schedules over 5 days. Ifosfamide thus has clear activity in patients with no prior chemotherapy.

Dibromodulcitol is a halogenated sugar that acts primarily as an alkylating agent. The first

evidence of activity in carcinoma of the cervix came from collected phase II data that showed a response of 15% (7 responses among 47 patients) (60). A confirmatory trial by the GOG in patients with no prior chemotherapy showed significant activity, with 16 responses noted among 55 patients (29%) (59). Dibromodulcitol thus has significant activity in carcinoma of the cervix.

Doxorubicin has activity in squamous cell carcinoma of the cervix which was well documented in a phase III trial of the GOG in which the control arm of doxorubicin alone yielded a 20%) response rate in 61 patients (78). Other phase II trials confirm this activity and mark doxorubicin as a significant agent in these lesions (73–77, 79).

At least 15 other drugs are active (Table

Table 58.16. GOG Studies of Cisplatin in Squamous Cell Carcinoma of the Cervix

Dose and Schedule	Prior Rx	Response (%)
Protocol 26C (67)		
50 mg/m² q 3 week 2 hr infusion	No	11/22 (50%)
	Yes	2/12 (16%)
Protocol 43 (68)		
50 mg/m² q 3 week 2 hr infusion	No	31/150 (21%)
100 mg/m² q 3 week 2 hr infusion	No	52/166 (31%)
20 mg/m²/day × 5 day q 3 week 2 hr infusion	No	32/128 (25%)
Protocol 64 (69)		
50 mg/m² q 3 week 2 hr infusion	No	28/164 (17%)
50 mg/m² q 3 week 24 hr infusion	No	28/156 (18%)
Totals		184/798 (23%)

Table 58.17. Studies of Ifosfamide as a Single Agent in Carcinoma of the Cervix

Dose and Schedule[a]	Prior Rx	Response (%)
3.5 g/m²/day × 3 days q 4 weeks 8-hr infusion	No	9/18 (50%)
1.5 g/m²/day × 5 days q 4 weeks 1-hr infusion	No	12/30 (40%)
1.5 g/m²/day × 5 days q 4 weeks 1-hr infusion	No	5/24 (21%)
5 g/m²/day × 1 day q 4 weeks 1-hr infusion	No	10/30 (33%)
1.5 g/m²/day × 5 days q 4 weeks 1-hr infusion	No	8/51 (16%)
1.5 g/m²/day × 5 days q 4 weeks 1-hr infusion	Yes	0/9 (0%)
1.5 g/m²/day × 5 days q 4 weeks 1-hr infusion	Yes	3/27 (11%)

Data from Sutton GP, Blessing JA, Photopoulos G, et al. Phase II experience with ifosfamide/mesna in gynecologic malignancies: preliminary report of Gynecologic Oncology Group studies. Semin Oncol 1989;16(Suppl 3):68–72; Sutton GP, Blessing JA, Adcock L, et al. Phase II study of ifosfamide and mesna in patients with previously-treated carcinoma of the cervix: a Gynecologic Oncology Group study. Invest New Drugs 1989;7:341–343; and Thigpen T, Vance R, Khansur T, Malamud F. The role of ifosfamide and of systemic therapy in the management of carcinoma of the cervix. Semin Oncol (in press).
[a]Mesna was given with ifosfamide in each of the trials.

58.14). Among these, the greatest current interest is directed to paclitaxel, which to date has had limited testing (30). This wide range of active drugs opens the definite possibility for the development of effective combination chemotherapy.

Combination chemotherapy is essential if systemic treatment is to have a major impact on survival in patients with squamous cell carcinoma of the cervix. While multiple studies of combination chemotherapy have been reported (Tables 58.18, 58.19, 58.20, and 58.21) (114–141), most of these trials are relatively small, nonrandomized series that include patients with nonsquamous carcinoma of the cervix. It is impossible to draw definite conclusions about the relative merits of combination chemotherapy from these studies.

Despite the lack of definitive conclusions from these uncontrolled trials, several observations are worthy of note. First, platinum-based combinations have attracted the greatest amount of attention because the platinum compounds, particularly cisplatin, are the most extensively studied and consistently active drugs in squamous cell carcinoma of the cervix and because platinum-based combinations are consistently active and yield high response rates, particularly in patients who have not received radiation therapy. For combinations not including 5-flurouracil, doxorubicin, or ifosfamide, most trials of platinum-based combinations are small; hence, the value of these combinations is not clear (Table 58.18) (114–122).

Secondly, the combination of cisplatin plus 5-fluorouracil has been tested in five phase II trials (Table 58.19) (123–126). In patients not previously radiated, high response rates are reported (123–124). In previously radiated patients, however, response rates are lower and not significantly different from the response rate to single-agent cisplatin (123–126). Although the combination has never been evaluated in a phase III trial, there is little to suggest that it yields enhanced benefit.

Thirdly, combinations including a platinum compound and doxorubicin have been em-

Table 58.18. Studies of Platinum-Based Combination Chemotherapy without Ifosfamide, 5-Fluorouracil, or Doxorubicin in Squamous Cell Carcinoma of the Cervix

Regimen	Patients	Response (%)
Two-drug combinations		
Cisplatin + bleomycin (114, 115)	17	10 (59%)
	24	13 (54%)
	25	8 (32%)
Cisplatin + cyclophosphamide (116)	12	5 (42%)
Cisplatin + dichloromethotrexate (114)	13	10 (76%)
Cisplatin + galactitol (114)	18	7 (39%)
Cisplatin + methotrexate (117)	37	21 (57%)
Cisplatin + mitomycin C (114)	49	9 (18%)
	30	13 (43%)
Cisplatin + razoxane (118)	9	0 (0%)
Three- or four-drug combinations		
Cisplatin + bleomycin + methotrexate (119, 120)	9	8 (89%)
	19	10 (53%)
Cisplatin + bleomycin + vinblastine (114, 121)	23	15 (65%)
	10	6 (60%)
	33	22 (67%)
Cisplatin + bleomycin + etoposide + mitomycin C (122)	34	25 (74%)
	26	10 (39%)
Cisplatin + bleomycin + vinblastine + methotrexate (114)	5	0 (0%)
Cisplatin + bleomycin + vincristine + methotrexate (114)	15	10 (67%)
Cisplatin + bleomycin + vincristine + mitomycin C (114)	13	10 (78%)
	14	7 (50%)
	14	6 (43%)
	14	3 (21%)
	48	8 (17%)

Table 58.19. Studies of Combination Chemotherapy with Cisplatin plus 5-Fluorouracil in Squamous Cell Carcinoma of the Cervix

Regimen	Prior Radiotherapy	Response (%)
Cisplatin 100 mg/m^2/day × 1 day q 3 weeks + 5-Fluorouracil 1000 mg/m^2/day × 5 days 24-hr infusion q 3 weeks (123, 124)	No	20/29 (69%)
	No	13/19 (68%)
	No	3/16 (19%)
	Yes	2/13 (15%)
	Yes	12/55 (22%)
Cisplatin 100 mg/m^2/day × 1 day q 3 weeks + 5-Fluorouracil 1000 mg/m^2/day × 4 days 24-hr infusion q 3 weeks (125)	Yes	14/52 (27%)
Cisplatin 50 mg/m^2/day × 1 day q 3 weeks + 5-Fluorouracil 1000 mg/m^2/day × 5 days 24-hr infusion q 3 weeks (126)	Yes	12/55 (22%)
Cisplatin 20 mg/m^2/day × 5 days q 3 weeks + 5-Fluorouracil 200 mg/m^2/day × 5 days 24-hr infusion q 3 weeks (126)	Yes	11/18 (61%)

ployed widely outside clinical trials and have been regarded as highly active. Reported phase II trials with response rates ranging from 20 to 44% provide little support for this view (Table 58.20) (114, 127–130). No randomized studies of doxorubicin-based combinations have been conducted.

Fourthly, the most extensively studied platinum-based combinations include a platinum compound and ifosfamide (Table 58.21) (131–140). These combinations are of great interest because of the significant activity noted with each drug as a single agent. Three reports detail results with a two-drug combination of ifosfamide with either cisplatin or carboplatin (131–133). In two of these reports, ifosfamide is combined with cisplatin (131, 132). In one of the two trials, no patients had received prior radiotherapy

Table 58.20. Studies of Combination Chemotherapy Containing Both Cisplatin and Doxorubicin in Squamous Cell Carcinoma of the Cervix

Regimen	Patients	Response (%)
Cisplatin + doxorubicin (127)	19	6 (32%)
Cisplatin + doxorubicin + bleomycin (114)	21	8 (38%)
Cisplatin + doxorubicin + cyclophosphamide (114)	20	4 (20%)
Cisplatin + doxorubicin + methotrexate (128, 129)	48	18 (38%)
	28	8 (30%)
Cisplatin + doxorubicin + methyl CCNU (114)	23	7 (30%)
Cisplatin + doxorubicin + cyclophosphamide + bleomycin (130)	43	19 (44%)

Table 58.21. Studies of First-Line Combination Chemotherapy Including a Platinum Compound and Ifosfamide in Squamous Cell Carcinoma of the Cervix

Regimen*	Prior Rx	Response (%)
Two-drug combinations		
Ifosfamide 1.5 g/m²/day × 5 days q 4 weeks + cisplatin 20 mg/m²/day × 5 days q 4 weeks (131)	No	15/24 (62%)
Ifosfamide 2.5 g/m²/day × 5 days q 4 weeks + cisplatin 20 mg/m²/day × 5 days q 4 weeks (132)	No	15/30 (50%)
Ifosfamide 5 g/m²/day × 1 day q 4 weeks + carboplatin 300 mg/m²/day × 1 day q 4 weeks (133)	No	19/32 (59%)
Three-drug combinations		
Ifosfamide 5 g/m²/day × 1 day q 4 weeks + cisplatin 50 mg/m²/day × 1 day q 4 weeks + bleomycin 30 mg/day × 1 day q 4 weeks (136)	No	17/26 (65%)
Ifosfamide 1 g/m²/day × 5 days q 4 weeks + cisplatin 50 mg/m²/day × 1 day q 4 weeks + bleomycin 15 mg/day × 1 day (137)	No	9/9 (100%)
Ifosfamide 2 g/m²/day × 3 days q 4 weeks + carboplatin 200 mg/m²/day × 1 day q 4 weeks + bleomycin 30 mg/day × 1 day (138)	No	16/18 (89%)
Ifosfamide 5 g/m²/day × 1 day q 4 weeks + cisplatin 50 mg/m²/day × 1 day q 4 weeks + bleomycin 30 mg/day × 1 day (134)	Yes	3/24 (13%)
Ifosfamide 1.2 g/m²/day × 5 day q 4 weeks + cisplatin 50 mg/m²/day × 1 day q 4 weeks + bleomycin 30 mg/day × 1 day (135)	Yes	4/14 (29%)
Ifosfamide 5 g/m²/day × 1 day q 4 weeks + cisplatin 50 mg/m²/day × 1 day q 4 weeks + bleomycin 30 mg/day × 1 day (136)	Yes	26/36 (72%)
Ifosfamide 1 g/m²/day × 5 day q 4 weeks + cisplatin 50 mg/m²/day × 1 day q 4 weeks + bleomycin 15 mg/day × 1 day (137)	Yes	5/12 (42%)
Ifosfamide 2 g/m²/day × 3 day q 4 weeks + carboplatin 200 mg/m²/day × 1 day q 4 weeks + bleomycin 30 mg/day × 1 day (138)	Yes	5/17 (29%)
Ifosfamide 1 g/m²/day × 3 days q 4 weeks + cisplatin 25 mg/m²/day × 3 days q 4 weeks + etoposide 75 mg/day 3 days (139)	Yes	8/14 (57%)
Ifosfamide 1.5 g/m²/day × 3 days q 4 weeks + cisplatin 50 mg/m²/day × 1 day q 4 weeks + carboplatin 200 mg/m²/day × 1 day (140)	Yes	23/31 (74%)

*Mesna is given with ifosfamide in each regimen.

(131); in the other, only 17% of the patients had received prior radiation (132). Response rates of 62 and 50% were noted; hence, the combinations had high activity. The single trial employing ifosfamide with carboplatin concerned the use of neoadjuvant chemotherapy in newly diagnosed patients with no prior radiation (133). A similarly high response rate of 59% was observed.

Five reports provide results with a three-drug combination of bleomycin with ifosfamide plus a platinum compound (134–138). In patients with no prior radiotherapy, three series report response rates from 65 to 100% (136–138). In contrast, in the five reports that include patients with prior radiation, mixed results are noted, with response rates ranging from 13 to 72% (134–138). These data suggest that such three-drug combinations are highly active in patients with no prior radiation and less active if the patient has been previously radiated. The trials do not define a role for ifosfamide/platinum combina-

tions in the treatment of advanced or recurrent disease; but the facts that both ifosfamide and the platinum compounds are clearly active and that high response rates have been observed with two- and three-drug combinations, including ifosfamide and a platinum compound with or without bleomycin, provide reason for further study in randomized trials.

Two additional reports detail studies of platinum/ifosfamide-based combinations (139, 140). The first of these evaluated a combination of cisplatin 25 mg/m², ifosfamide 1.0 g/m², and etoposide 75 mg/m² daily for 3 days every 28 days (139). All patients had advanced or recurrent disease. Nine of the 14 had received prior radiation, and two had received prior chemotherapy including, in one instance, cisplatin. Eight patients (57%) achieved a complete response of 7 to 24 months duration. Three of the eight complete responses occurred in patients who had received no prior radiation. The second

Table 58.22. GOG Protocol 110, a Randomized Trial of Cisplatin Alone or with Either Ifosfamide or Dibromodulcitol (142): Ifosfamide plus Cisplatin Yields a Superior Response Rate, Compared with Cisplatin Alone

Regimen	Prior Radiotherapy	Response (%)
Cisplatin 50 mg/m^2/day × 1 day q 3 weeks	121/137 (88%)	10CR,16PR/137 (19%)
Cisplatin 50 mg/m^2/day on day 1 q 3 weeks + dibromodulcitol 180 mg/m^2/day orally on days 2–6 q 3 weeks	121/141 (86%)	14CR,17PR/141 (22%)
Cisplatin 50 mg/m^2 on day 1 q 3 weeks + ifosfamide 5 g/m^2 on day 1 q 3 weeks 24-hr infusion + mesna 6 g/m^2 on day 1 q 3 weeks 36-hr infusion	121/140 (86%)	19CR,28PR/140 (33%)

trial evaluated cisplatin 50 mg/m^2 plus ifosfamide 1.5 g/m^2 plus carboplatin 200 mg/m^2 every 28 days and reported 11 complete and 12 partial responses among 31 patients (74%), all of whom had received prior radiotherapy (140). These two trials suggest, not surprisingly, that the two combinations are active, but the merits relative to other combinations or single agents cannot be assessed.

Two randomized trials of ifosfamide-based combination chemotherapy have been conducted. The first, GOG protocol 110, randomized patients to one of three regimens (Table 58.22): cisplatin alone, cisplatin plus ifosfamide, or cisplatin plus dibromodulcitol (142). The ifosfamide/cisplatin regimen yielded a superior response rate (33% vs. 22% vs. 19%), but no differences were observed in progression-free and overall survival. The second, GOG protocol 149, randomizes patients with advanced or recurrent disease to ifosfamide plus cisplatin with or without bleomycin and is nearing completion of patient accrual, with no results available as yet.

In summary, based on current data, the regimen of choice for advanced squamous cell carcinoma of the cervix is a combination of ifosfamide and cisplatin. The two major thrusts of current investigation seek to identify other active agents and to assess the role of bleomycin in combination chemotherapy.

NONSQUAMOUS CARCINOMA

Available data on the use of chemotherapy in nonsquamous carcinomas of the cervix come from studies of the GOG (Table 58.23), which are single-agent trials involving mostly adenocarcinomas and adenosquamous carcinomas in patients who had received prior radiotherapy and, in some instances, prior chemotherapy. Of the 11 agents studied (142–151), only one is active as

Table 58.23. Studies of Single Agents in Nonsquamous Carcinoma of the Cervix

Drug	Prior Rx	Response (%)
Cisplatin (143)	No	4/20 (20%)
Piperazinedione (143)	Mixed	2/14 (14%)
VP-16 (144)	Mixed	1/19 (5%)
Galactitol (145)	Mixed	2/27 (7%)
ICRF-159 (146)	Mixed	1/25 (4%)
Mitoxantrone (147)	Mixed	2/25 (8%)
Diaziquone (148)	Mixed	2/26 (8%)
Aminothiadiazole (149)	Mixed	2/26 (8%)
VM-26 (150)	Mixed	1/23 (4%)
Ifosfamide (151)	Mixed	3/24 (12%)
Gallium nitrate (152)	Mixed	3/26 (12%)

defined by a response rate of 15% or greater, cisplatin (four responses among 20 patients) (142). There are no reported studies of combination chemotherapy in this patient population.

Locally Advanced Disease

The other significant role for chemotherapy is its use in combination with radiotherapy in patients with locally advanced disease (stages IIB through IVA). Because the intent of chemotherapy is to improve results achieved with radiotherapy, it is essential to evaluate the efficacy of such an approach through randomized phase III trials. Although the literature is replete with nonrandomized trials of approaches that evaluate concomitant single-agent or combination chemotherapy, neoadjuvant chemotherapy, intraarterial chemotherapy, and postradiation adjuvant chemotherapy, only randomized trials will be cited to form a basis for current practice.

Based on animal trials demonstrating that hydroxyurea enhances the effect of radiotherapy

(152), in 1970 the GOG initiated a trial of radiotherapy with either concomitant hydroxyurea or placebo in patients with stage IIIB or IVA disease (153). The study is tarnished by two criticisms. The patients were not surgically staged prior to study entry, and half of the 190 patients entered were inevaluable. These criticisms notwithstanding, the differences clearly favor the concomitant use of hydroxyurea (Table 58.24) and are confirmed by an independent study of the same regimens (154).

The second in a series of large randomized phase III trials of locally advanced carcinoma of the cervix included 283 stage IIB, IIIB, and IVA patients and required careful surgical staging of paraaortic node status (155). The trial randomized patients to radiation either alone or with *Corynebacterium parvum*. There were no differences between the two treatment arms, but a dramatic adverse impact of positive paraaortic nodes was noted on progression-free interval and survival.

As a result of the surgical staging data, the third large randomized trial of the GOG eliminated patients with positive paraaortic nodes (156). Two hundred ninety-six surgically staged patients with stage IIB through IVA disease and negative paraaortic nodes were randomized to radiation plus either hydroxyurea or misonidazole. The preliminary analysis of this completed trial shows a marginally superior progression-free interval for patients on the hydroxyurea arm ($p = .08$). Analysis of progression-free interval on each regimen by stage shows little difference among stage IIB patients treated with either arm. For patients with stage IIIB or IVA disease who received hydroxyurea, the progression-free interval curve is similar to that for the stage IIB

patients, but the curve for the misonidazole arm falls well below the others.

The results of these three large, randomized, phase III trials support the use of concomitant hydroxyurea and radiation in the management of locally advanced carcinoma of the cervix. Investigations of alternative approaches continue. A fourth completed GOG phase III trial randomized patients with stage IIB through IVA disease to radiation plus either hydroxyurea or cisplatin plus 5-fluorouracil. Preliminary results show no difference between the two arms of the study, but final conclusions await the definitive analysis of the trial.

In summary, there is solid evidence that chemotherapy given concomitantly with radiation in patients with locoregionally advanced disease yields superior results, compared with radiation alone. The regimen of choice is either hydroxyurea or a combination of cisplatin plus 5-fluorouracil. Benefit appears to be confined to those patients with the most advanced disease, those with stage IIIB or IVA disease.

Conclusions

Chemotherapy has two documented roles in the management of patients with carcinoma of the cervix. In the treatment of advanced or recurrent disease, the standard of care is the use of combination of ifosfamide plus cisplatin. In the management of patients with locally advanced disease, the standard of care for at least stage IIIB and IVA patients is concomitant hydroxyurea and radiotherapy. No evidence supports the use of chemotherapy in more limited disease; hence, such approaches to stages I-IIA should be confined to clinical trials.

Table 58.24. GOG Trial of Radiation with Either Hydroxyurea or Placebo in Patients with Stage IIIB or IVA Carcinoma of the Cervix (107) (Complete Response Rate, Progression-Free Interval and Survival Were Superior for Hydroxyurea) ($p < .05$)

Regimen	CR (%)	PFI[a]	Survival
Regimen I External radiation 5000 cGy/5–8 weeks Intracavitary radiation 3000 cGy point A Hydroxyurea 80 mg/kg every 3 days/12 weeks	32/47 (68%)	14 months	20 months
Regimen II External radiation 5000 cGy/5–8 weeks Intracavitary radiation 3000 cGy point A Placebo every 3 days/12 weeks	21/43 (49%)	8 months	11 months

[a]PFI, progression-free interval.

CELOMIC EPITHELIAL CARCINOMA OF THE OVARY

Cancer of the ovary includes three major categories of lesions: celomic epithelial carcinoma, germ cell neoplasms, and stromal tumors. Celomic epithelial carcinoma accounts for almost 90% of cases.

General Characteristics

A number of factors influence patient outcome: age, histologic type and grade, tumor DNA content, extent of disease at presentation, and, in the case of disease confined to the peritoneal cavity, volume of residual tumor. The most important is extent of disease at the time of diagnosis (FIGO stage) (157). Patients may be grouped into limited (stages I and II) disease, which accounts for 25% of all cases, and advanced (stages III and IV) disease, which accounts for 75% of all cases. A unique feature of ovarian carcinoma is its propensity to spread by the intraperitoneal route. For this reason, stage III is the most common stage at presentation and accounts for over half of all cases.

Precise identification of the stage is crucial to appropriate management and requires surgical exploration of the abdominal cavity through an incision sufficient to permit examination of the entire peritoneal surface. In the absence of gross extrapelvic disease, multiple biopsies should be taken. Finally, as the initial step in therapy, aggressive surgical cytoreduction should be attempted. Surgical cytoreduction is supported by retrospective studies that show an inverse correlation between volume of residual disease and both response to chemotherapy and survival (159–164). A recent randomized trial of interval surgical cytoreduction also supports the value of this procedure (165).

At the conclusion of the laparotomy, patients can be classified by stage, based on extent of disease at the time the abdomen is opened (Table 58.25). For those with advanced disease, stage III should be subdivided according to volume of disease at the time the abdomen was opened. From a more practical perspective, advanced disease patients are divided into those with small-volume residual disease after surgery (no nodule larger than 2 cm remaining) or those with large-volume residual disease. The small-volume patients constitute about 40 to 45% of advanced disease patients and have a better prognosis than the 55 to 60% who have large-volume disease.

Table 58.25. FIGO Staging System for Ovarian Carcinoma (158)

Stage		Description
I		Growth limited to the ovaries
	A	One ovary; no ascites; capsule intact; no tumor on external surface
	B	Two ovaries; no ascites; capsule intact; no tumor on external surface
	C	One or both ovaries with either: surface tumor; ruptured capsule; or ascites or peritoneal washings with malignant cells
II		Pelvic extension
	A	Involvement of uterus and/or tubes
	B	Involvement of other pelvic tissues
	C	IIA or IIB with factors as in IC
III		Peritoneal implants outside pelvis and/or positive retroperitoneal or inguinal nodes
	A	Grossly limited to true pelvis; negative nodes; microscopic seeding of abdominal peritoneum
	B	Implants of abdominal peritoneum 2 cm or less; nodes negative
	C	Abdominal implants greater than 2 cm and/or positive retroperitoneal or inguinal nodes
IV		Distant metastases

Advanced Disease

SINGLE-AGENT THERAPY

A number of cytotoxic agents as well as at least two biologicals and two hormonal agents have activity against celomic epithelial neoplasms (Table 58.26) (166–177). Of these, the platinum analogues appear to be the most important. *Cisplatin*, the most extensively studied platinum compound, demonstrates clear-cut activity in patients with no prior chemotherapy as well as in those refractory to prior alkylating agents (167, 168). *Carboplatin*, the second platinum compound to receive extensive testing in ovarian carcinoma, offers the advantage of less neurotoxicity and nephrotoxicity than cisplatin in exchange for thrombocytopenia as the dose-limiting adverse effect. The drug also has clear-cut activity (169–171) and, in comparative single-agent trials with cisplatin, appears to have similar activity in ovarian carcinoma (170, 171). A metaanalysis of three such trials comparing single-agent cisplatin 100 mg/m^2 with carboplatin 400 mg/m^2 reveals no significant difference in overall response rate, complete response rate,

Table 58.26. Cytotoxic Agents with Activity in Ovarian Carcinoma

Drug	Patients	Response Rate
Available agents		
Alkylating agents (166)	1371	33%
Cisplatin (166)	190	32%
Carboplatin (166)	82	24%
Paclitaxel (173–176)	189	29%
Docetaxel (180)	23	35%
Ifosfamide (181)	37	22%
Hexamethylmelamine (183–187)	215	24%
Doxorubicin (166)	102	33%
Liposomal doxorubicin (195)	35	20%
5-Fluorouracil (166)	126	29%
Methotrexate (166)	34	18%
Mitomycin (166)	49	16%
Oral etoposide (187–189)	31	26%
Gemcitabine (190)	42	19%
Progestins (166, 196)	176	12%
Tamoxifen (195)	105	18%
Investigational agents		
Topotecan (191–193)	255	18%
Prednimustine (166)	36	28%
Dihydroxybusulfan (166)	26	27%
Galactitol (166)	39	15%
Biologicals		
α-Interferon (166)	21	19%
γ-Interferon (166)	14	29%

or survival (171). Toxicity differed as expected: more neurotoxicity with cisplatin, more myelosuppression with carboplatin. There was very little nephrotoxicity in either arm.

Another important class of drugs is the taxanes. The first of these to undergo trials in ovarian carcinoma, paclitaxel (Taxol), is a natural product found in the bark of *Taxus brevifolia*, the western yew tree. The chemical structure is complex and is based on the taxane ring (172). Phase II studies of the drug in ovarian carcinoma employed Taxol in a range of doses from 135 mg/m^2 to 300 mg/m^2 over 24 hours every 3 weeks. Pretreatment with antihistamines, steroids, and H2 blockers was routinely given to prevent hypersensitivity reactions. Doses higher than 200 mg/m^2 required the use of granulocyte colony-stimulating factor (G-CSF).

Interest in Taxol as a part of the therapy of ovarian carcinoma is based on five phase II trials in which 189 patients with progressed, persistent, or relapsed ovarian carcinoma were treated with starting doses of Taxol ranging from 170 to 250 mg/m^2 over 24 hours every 3 weeks (173–176). Eleven complete and 43 partial responses were observed, for an overall response rate of

29%. Responses were observed in patients with progressed or persistent (clinically resistant) disease as well as those with relapsed (clinically sensitive) disease. This raises the possibility that Taxol is clinically non-cross-resistant with the platinum compounds and hence will enhance primary therapy.

Other studies of Taxol in previously treated patients have focused on dose and schedule. A coalition of the National Cancer Institute of Canada and the EORTC randomized patients with progressed or persistent disease to either 175 or 135 mg/m^2 every 3 weeks and to either a 24-hour infusion or a 3-hour infusion, in a bifactorial design (177). Two significant observations were made with regard to toxicity. The frequency of hypersensitivity reactions was low in both the 3- and 24-hour regimens. Neutropenia, on the other hand, was much less frequent in the 3-hour arm. No significant differences were observed in either the dose or infusion length comparisons with regard to response rate and survival. The higher dose and the shorter infusion each yielded superior progression-free survival, but the differences were 5 weeks and 1 week and hence clinically insignificant. This study demonstrates the feasibility of a shorter infusion time, which would facilitate outpatient administration of Taxol.

The issue of dose-response has been evaluated in two other settings. A metaanalysis of carefully audited data used as the basis for FDA approval of paclitaxel showed no relationship between dose or dose intensity and response over the range from 110 to 312 mg/m^2 (178). The GOG evaluated the possibility of a dose-response relationship for Taxol in a randomized phase III study comparing 175 and 250 mg/m^2 every 3 weeks, each given on a 24-hour schedule (179). The higher dose arm required the use of G-CSF. The results showed a superior response rate with the high dose (36 vs. 27%) (Table 58.27) but no difference in progression-free and overall survival. Toxicity was significantly greater with the higher dose schedule (thrombocytopenia, anemia, gastrointestinal toxicity, neurotoxicity, and myalgias).

The only other taxane in clinical trials currently is docetaxel (Taxotere). Results to date establish that the drug is active, but the relative merits of this agent as opposed to paclitaxel are not known (180). On this basis, the more established paclitaxel remains the taxane of choice.

Certain of the other active drugs are noteworthy because responses have been observed in patients clinically resistant to the platinum compounds, a rare phenomenon. These agents include: ifosfamide (181), hexamethylmelamine (182–186), oral etoposide (188–190), gemcitabine (190), topotecan (191–193), liposomal doxorubicin (194), and tamoxifen (195). These agents are important in the selection of salvage therapy for platinum-resistant patients.

EVOLUTION OF PLATINUM-BASED COMBINATION CHEMOTHERAPY

As of 1976, the chemotherapy of choice following initial surgery was a single alkylating agent, usually melphalan 0.2 mg/kg/day for 5 days every 4 to 6 weeks (197). Between 1976 and 1982, a series of two GOG studies (160, 197) in patients with large-volume advanced disease first compared melphalan versus doxorubicin plus cyclophosphamide and then doxorubicin plus cyclophosphamide versus the same two drugs plus cisplatin, a combination known as PAC. As treatment goes from the single agent to the two-drug combination to the platinum-based

three-drug regimen, significant improvements in clinical complete response rate, overall response rate, duration of response, and survival are observed (Table 58.28).

These two studies established platinum-based therapy as the treatment of choice for advanced ovarian carcinoma. Over the subsequent 6 years, trials were aimed at improving the therapeutic index of treatment. The GOG, in a study involving patients with small-volume stage III disease compared PAC with cisplatin plus cyclophosphamide, with the dose of cyclophosphamide escalated to maintain the dose intensity of the combination (198). Including all patients entered into the study, there was no difference between the two regimens in regard to pathologic complete response rate (as determined at second-look laparotomy, 24 vs. 26%), progression-free survival, and overall survival (Table 58.29). These results are supported by at least four other randomized trials (199–202) and established, as of 1986, the two-drug combination of cisplatin plus cyclophosphamide as the regimen of choice.

The introduction of a potentially less toxic platinum compound, carboplatin, prompted three comparisons of cisplatin versus carboplatin as single agents. These comparisons showed no significant difference in efficacy (171). Four subsequent randomized trials compared cisplatin-based combinations with carboplatin-based combinations (Table 58.30) (203–206). The only one of the four studies to find a difference compared two-drug regimens of cyclophosphamide plus either cisplatin or carboplatin (206). Survival was significantly better in the cisplatin arm, but the dose intensity of cisplatin in that arm was almost double that in the carboplatin arm. The weight of evidence from these

Table 58.27. Results of a Phase III Comparison of 175 mg/m² versus 250 mg/m² of Paclitaxel as Second-Line Therapy in Ovarian Carcinoma (179)

Regimen	Patients	Response Rate
Paclitaxel 175 mg/m²/day × 1 day q 3 weeks 24-hr infusion	163	28%
Paclitaxel 250 mg/m²/day × 1 day q 3 weeks 24-hr infusion[a]	171	36%

[a]G-CSF was given with the high-dose schedule. No differences in progression-free or overall survival were observed.

Table 58.28. Results of GOG Protocols 22 and 47 Evaluating Chemotherapy in Advanced Ovarian Carcinoma (160, 198)

Parameter	GOG 22		GOG 47	
	L-PAM[a]	AC[b]	AC[b]	PAC[c]
Patients	64	72	120	107
Complete response (CR)	20%	32%	26%	51%
Total response (CR + PR)	37%	49%	48%	76%
Pathologic CR			4/23	13/39
PRC/total			3%	12%
Duration	8 months	10 months	9 months	15 months
Median survival	12 months	14 months	16 months	20 months

[a]L-PAM, melphalan 0.2 mg/kg/day orally for 5 days every 4 to 6 weeks for ten courses.
[b]AC, doxorubicin 50 mg/m² plus cyclophosphamide 500 mg/m² both i.v. every 3 weeks for eight courses.
[c]PAC, cisplatin 50 mg/m² plus doxorubicin and cyclophosphamide as in AC all i.v. every 3 weeks for eight courses.

Table 58.29. Results of GOG Protocol 52, a Study of Minimal Residual Stage III Ovarian Carcinoma (198)

Parameter	PAC[a]	PC[b]
Patients	173	176
Early recurrence	19	30
Refused second look	36	37
Residual disease	73	67
Pathologic complete response (%)	45 (26%)	42 (24%)

[a]PAC, cisplatin 50 mg/m^2 plus doxorubicin 50 mg/m^2 plus cyclophosphamide 500 mg/m^2 all i.v. every 3 weeks for eight cycles.
[b]PC, cisplatin 50 mg/m^2 plus cyclophosphamide 1000 mg/m^2 both i.v. every 3 weeks for eight cycles.

seven studies favors the view that carboplatin and cisplatin are equivalent in efficacy against ovarian carcinoma. At this point, the regimen of choice was essentially cyclophosphamide plus a platinum compound, either cisplatin or carboplatin. The toxicity profile of the two drugs favored the use of carboplatin, which required no hydration or nephrotoxicity and caused less emesis and less neurotoxicity.

DOSE INTENSITY

Two themes have dominated clinical research in ovarian carcinoma in the 1990s: escalation of dose intensity and the role of paclitaxel. Dose intensity refers to the amount of chemotherapy to which a cancer is exposed per unit time; this is generally assumed to be reflected by the dose of drug in milligrams per square meter body surface area per unit time. This concept is well

Table 58.30. Randomized Trials of Cisplatin-Based vs. Carboplatin-Based Combination Chemotherapy in Advanced, Predominately Large-Volume Ovarian Carcinoma (203–206)

Study and Regimen	Response[a]	Survival
Alberts et al. (342 patients)		
Carboplatin 300 mg/m^2 q 4 weeks	cCR = 34%	20 months
Cyclophosphamide 600 mg/m^2 q 4 weeks	pCR = 12%	
Cisplatin 100 mg/m^2 q 4 weeks	cCR = 27%	17 months
Cyclophosphamide 600 mg/m^2 q 4 weeks	pCR = 7%	
ten Bokkel et al. (339 patients)		
Cyclophosphamide 100 mg/m^2 p.o. days 14–28	cCR = 24%	107 weeks
Hexamethylmelamine 150 mg/m^2 p.o. days 14–28		
Doxorubicin 35 mg/m^2 i.v. day 1		
Carboplatin 350 mg/m^2 i.v. day 1		
Cyclophosphamide 100 mg/m^2 p.o. days 14–28	cCR = 23%	108 weeks
Hexamethylmelamine 150 mg/m^2 p.o. days 14–28		
Doxorubicin 35 mg/m^2 i.v. day 1		
Cisplatin 20 mg/m^2 i.v. days 1–5		
Pater et al. (447 patients)		
Carboplatin 300 mg/m^2 q 4 weeks	pCR = 13%	24 months
Cyclophosphamide 600 mg/m^2 q 4 weeks		
Cisplatin 75 mg/m^2 q 4 weeks	pCR = 18%	23 months
Cyclophosphamide 600 mg/m^2 q 4 weeks		
Edmondson et al. (103 patients)		
Carboplatin 150 mg/m^2 q 4 weeks		20 months
Cyclophosphamide 1000 mg/m^2 q 4 weeks		
Cisplatin 60 mg/m^2 q 4 weeks		27 months
Cyclophosphamide 1000 mg/m^2 q 4 weeks		

[a]pCR, pathologic complete response; cCR, clinical complete response.

grounded in preclinical work, which shows that, as the concentration of drug in culture medium increases, the fraction of surviving cancer cells decreases logarithmically (207). A metaanalysis in 1987 (208) purported to show that dose intensity was important clinically. Data from over 60 published trials in ovarian carcinoma identified a correlation between the dose intensity of cisplatin and the observed response rate, but this correlation held only over a range of doses from 6 to 12 mg/m² week or up to 36 mg/m² every 3 weeks. This range falls below the usual range of clinical doses of 50 to 100 mg/m² every 3 weeks. A subsequent extension of these observations by the same investigators suggested that a correlation between dose intensity and therapeutic benefit was present up to a dose of 15 to 25 mg/m²/ week (45 to 75 mg/m² every 3 weeks) (209).

To determine whether dose intensity was important over a clinically relevant range of doses, the GOG randomized 458 patients with large-volume advanced disease to either low-dose cisplatin 50 mg/m² plus cyclophosphamide 500 mg/m² every 3 weeks for eight cycles or high-dose cisplatin 100 mg/m² plus cyclophosphamide 1000 mg/m² every 3 weeks for four cycles (Table 58.31) (210). Each regimen delivered the same total dose of chemotherapy, the high-dose schedule in half the time. Giving the prescribed low-dose regimen a dose intensity of 1, actual received dose intensity calculates to 1.90 for the high-dose arm and 0.95 for the low-dose schedule. On the low-dose arm, the overall response rate in the 130 measurable disease patients was 65%, versus 59% on the high-dose arm; clinical complete response rates were 26 and 27%, respectively. These differences were not significant. There was no difference in progression-free survival in either the measurable or nonmeasurable subset of patients; similarly no difference in overall survival in either patient subset was noted. The results of this study do not support the concept that enhanced dose intensity will produce greater therapeutic benefit.

The GOG results have been confirmed by a randomized trial in which patients with advanced disease were given either cisplatin 50 mg/m²/week for 9 weeks or cisplatin 75 mg/m² every 3 weeks for six cycles (211). The weekly arm delivered the same total of cisplatin in half the time, with each arm receiving 450 mg/m² of cisplatin. Within small-volume and large-volume patient subsets, no significant differences were observed with regard to either response rate or pathologic complete response rate. No overall differences were noted in either of these parameters, nor in regard to progression-free or overall survival.

While neither of these randomized trials of pure dose intensity showed an advantage for higher dose intensity across a clinically relevant range of doses, other lines of evidence have been cited to support the use of higher dose schedules. Trials of even higher dose intensities of cisplatin in conjunction with hypertonic saline to protect the kidneys, conducted by the National Cancer Institute of the United Stages, have been stated to yield higher response rates than more-standard doses (213). A closer examination of these data, however, shows a different story. In patients with large-volume disease, the NCI results can be compared with GOG results with PAC (160), regimens with a 3.3-fold difference in dose intensity of cisplatin. The pathologic complete response rates for the two regimens are 12 and 11% respectively, not different. In patients with small-volume disease, the NCI results can be compared with GOG results with a two-drug combination of cisplatin plus cyclophosphamide (198), regimens again with a 3.3-fold difference in dose intensity of cisplatin. The pathologic complete response rates for the two regimens are 38 and 30%, respectively, not significantly different. There thus appears to be no evidence from these data to support the importance of dose intensity or increased total dose of cisplatin over a 3.3-fold range of doses.

Table 58.31. Results of GOG Protocol 97, a Phase III Trial of Low-Dose versus High-Dose Cisplatin-Cyclophosphamide in Large-Volume Advanced Ovarian Carcinoma (210)

Regimen	Response Rate	PFI (months)	Survival (months)
Cisplatin 50 mg/m² Cytoxan 500 mg/m² Repeat every 3 weeks	CR 32%, RR 53%	12.2	23.9
Cisplatin 100 mg/ m² Cytoxan 1000 mg/ m² Repeat every 3 weeks	CR 26%, RR 45%	13.3	20.7

Higher doses of the same drug used in initial therapy have been cited as producing responses in the salvage setting. Many of these reports, however, fail to take into account whether the patient population under study responded to initial platinum-based therapy. One particular series that does report this factor provides a reason for these presumed responses to higher doses of the same drug (214). Thirty patients who had received platinum-based initial therapy and had either persistent, progressive, or relapsed disease were treated with high-dose carboplatin 800 mg/m^2 every 4 weeks. Eight responses were noted, for a response rate of 27%. All eight responses occurred, however, in patients who were still clinically platinum sensitive and who would be expected to demonstrate a response rate as high as 60% to retreatment with standard-dose platinum-based therapy. These data do not support the concept that responses result from higher dose intensity.

Intraperitoneal administration of drugs used in initial therapy to patients who have relapsed, persistent, or progressive disease is reported to yield responses as a result of exposure to higher doses of the drug because of the intraperitoneal route of administration. That enhanced exposure is possible is shown from data on mean peritoneal cavity to plasma concentration ratios for several drugs (215). The question is whether this enhanced exposure really yields responses in patients who were resistant to standard intravenous drug doses. A detailed examination of data does not support this concept. Virtually all responses to intraperitoneal platinum-based therapy in the salvage setting occur in those patients who responded to initial treatment and hence are considered platinum sensitive (216). Enhanced exposure, even by a factor of 12 to 20, thus does not appear to overcome platinum resistance. Recent results in a randomized phase III trial, however, lend at least some support to the value of this level of enhanced exposure to drug given by the intraperitoneal route (Table 58.32). Small-volume residual stage III patients receiving intraperitoneal cisplatin in combination with intravenous cyclophosphamide exhibited a superior survival to those receiving both drugs intravenously in the same dosage (median, 49 months vs. 41 months) (217).

Finally, claims have been made that regimens that combine enhanced dose intensity and greater total dose yield superior results. The primary basis for this is a randomized Scottish trial that compared cyclophosphamide 750 mg/m^2

Table 58.32. Results of a Phase III Comparison of IV Versus IP Cisplatin in Combination with IV Cyclophosphamide in Small-Volume Advanced Ovarian Carcinoma (217)

Regimen	Patients	Median Survival (months)
Cyclophosphamide 600 mg/m^2 i.v. Cisplatin 100 mg/m^2 i.v. Every 3 weeks for 6 cycles	279	41
Cyclophosphamide 600 mg/m^2 i.v. Cisplatin 100 mg/m^2 i.p. Every 3 weeks for 6 cycles	267	49

*p = .02; i.p./i.v. death hazard ratio = 0.76.

plus cisplatin either 50 mg/m^2 or 100 mg/m^2 every 3 weeks for six cycles (212). The higher dose regimen yielded a better response rate, progression-free survival, and overall survival. There are, however, several problems with this trial. One-third of the patients were stage IC or II and thus received adjuvant therapy. Less than half of all patients had measurable disease; hence, the response rate comparison was based on only 88 cases. Survival on the control arm is similar to that seen with single alkylating agent in GOG trials, despite the fact that one-third of the patients were stage IC or II. These facts raise serious doubts about the validity of the trial and the interpretation of the data.

A rational view of these data is that enhancing dose intensity is important until a threshold is reached. This is presumably the point at which all drug-sensitive cells have been eradicated. Further enhancement of dose intensity yields no greater benefit. In ovarian carcinoma, this point would appear to fall between 15 and 25 mg/m^2/ week for cisplatin. Whether dose can be escalated enough to overcome resistance and yield another gain is not known, but the results of the randomized phase III trial of intraperitoneal front-line therapy suggest that it might be possible. Further randomized trials of intraperitoneal therapy as well as randomized trials of standard-dose therapy versus high-dose chemotherapy plus stem cell support are needed to answer definitively the question of whether it is possible to reach a second threshold on the dose intensity curve. For now, doses of cisplatin higher than 75 mg/m^2 every 3 weeks should be avoided.

THE ROLE OF PACLITAXEL

While paclitaxel is an interesting drug as second-line single-agent therapy, its real promise is as a part of front-line therapy. To date, one major trial in previously untreated patients has been completed (218). This GOG study randomized patients with large-volume disease to six cycles of either cisplatin 75 mg/m^2 plus cyclophosphamide 750 mg/m^2 every 3 weeks or paclitaxel 135 mg/m^2 over 24 hours followed by cisplatin 75 mg/m^2 every 3 weeks. In the paclitaxel arm, administration of the paclitaxel prior to the cisplatin was important to optimize response and minimize toxicity (220).

A total of 388 patients were entered into the study (Table 58.33). The paclitaxel arm produced a significantly greater response rate (73 vs. 60%) and clinical complete response rate (51 vs. 31%). While the frequency of pathologic complete response was similar between the two arms (26% with the paclitaxel arm vs. 20%), the percentage of patients achieving a state of no gross residual disease on the paclitaxel arm was significantly higher (40%) than that seen with the control arm (24%). Progression-free interval (18 vs. 13 months) and overall survival (38 vs. 24 months) were significantly greater on the paclitaxel arm.

The dose-limiting toxicity, neutropenia, was more common in the paclitaxel arm, but the in-

Table 58.33. Results of GOG Protocol 111, a Comparison of Cisplatin plus Either Cyclophosphamide or Paclitaxel (218)

Response	Cis/Cyclo	Cis/Paclitaxel
Clinical response		
Complete response	37/111 (33%)	52/96 (54%)
Partial response	32/111 (29%)	22/96 (23%)
No response	42/111 (38%)	22/96 (23%)
Surgical response		
Pathologic complete response	35/178 (20%)	42/160 (26%)
Grossly disease free	42/178 (24%)	65/160 (40%)
Survival		
Progression-free survival (median)	13 months	18 months
Overall survival (median)	24 months	38 months

*Clinical response with cis/paclitaxel is superior ($p = .02$). Clinical complete response with cis/paclitaxel is superior ($p = .01$). Progression-free survival with cis/paclitaxel is superior ($p < .001$). Overall survival with cis/paclitaxel is superior ($p < .001$).

cidence of infection was the same in each arm. The frequency of hypersensitivity was very low, a reflection of the routine premedication used in the paclitaxel arm. Significant neurotoxicity was uncommon. Only seven patients on the paclitaxel arm experienced significant cardiac toxicity. One of the seven did have a fatal myocardial infarction, although the relationship of this event to the therapy was not clear. Other toxicities included first-degree heart block, asymptomatic ischemic events, hypotension with syncope, and arrhythmias including premature ventricular contractions.

To place these results into proper perspective, the relative risk of death on the cisplatin plus cyclophosphamide arm is set at 1.00. The resultant relative risk of progression or death on paclitaxel plus cisplatin is 0.6. This order of improvement is similar to the order of improvement seen when cisplatin was first added to therapy for advanced ovarian carcinoma.

These data establish paclitaxel plus cisplatin as the treatment of choice for advanced ovarian carcinoma. Current research efforts are further evaluating the role of paclitaxel in regard to dose and schedule (particularly 3- and 96-hour infusions), route of administration (intraperitoneal vs. intravenous), combination with other drugs (particularly carboplatin), and total duration of therapy (continuation beyond the six cycles). Although many questions remain to be answered, paclitaxel is firmly established as a part of front-line therapy in combination with a platinum compound.

In conclusion, the current recommendations for the management of newly diagnosed patients with advanced ovarian carcinoma are as follows. Treatment begins with an aggressive attempt to reduce the bulk of disease surgically. This should be followed by chemotherapy. At present, the regimen of choice is Taxol 135 mg/m^2 over 24 hours followed by cisplatin 75 mg/m^2 every 3 weeks for six cycles. A reasonable alternative would be either Taxol 135 mg/m^2 over 24 hours or 175 mg/m^2 over 3 hours followed by carboplatin dosed to an AUC of 7.5 every 3 weeks for six cycles, although it must be recognized that carboplatin combinations with Taxol have been studied only in phase I trial involving 20 patients. This approach should produce a response in 73%, clinical complete response in 51%, and gross disease-free state in 40% of patients with large-volume disease. Long-term survival may approach 20% in large-volume patients and a greater percentage with small-volume disease.

Limited Disease

Patients with limited (stages I or II) disease comprise a relatively small minority of patients with ovarian carcinoma. The great majority of such patients have stage I disease, which is discovered serendipitously at time of laparotomy for other reasons. The management of these patients begins with a careful staging laparotomy to ascertain that the patient has no microscopic disease within the peritoneal cavity. The definitive therapy is, of course, surgical resection, which should consist of a total abdominal hys-

terectomy and bilateral salpingo-oophorectomy plus omentectomy.

On the basis of the pathologic features of the primary neoplasm, patients can be divided into those at low risk and those at high risk for recurrence (Table 58.34) (220, 221). Factors of critical importance in assignment of risk include histologic grade, capsular rupture, surface excrescences, peritoneal cytology, ascites, and extraovarian spread. Patients at low risk for recurrence have a 5-year disease-free survival that exceeds 95% with surgical resection only (Table 58.35); hence, these patients require no adjuvant therapy (222).

Patients falling into the high-risk category have a sufficient risk of recurrence that further treatment should be considered. A randomized trial shows improved progression-free survival with cisplatin-based chemotherapy (Table 58.35) (222); final survival analysis awaits further follow-up. High-risk patients should therefore be treated with platinum-based adjuvant chemotherapy based on the improved progression-free survival.

Table 58.34. Criteria for Assignment of Patients to Groups at Low or High Risk for Recurrence (220, 221)

Group	Characteristics
Low risk	Grade 1 or 2 disease
	Intact capsule
	No tumor on external surface
	Negative peritoneal cytology
	No ascites
	Growth confined to ovaries
High risk[a]	Grade 3 disease
	Ruptured capsule
	Tumor on external surface
	Positive peritoneal cytology
	Ascites
	Growth outside ovaries

[a]Note: If any high-risk factors are present, the patient is considered high risk.

Salvage Therapy

While the literature reflects a pessimistic outlook for the patient who progresses or recurs after initial therapy, the proper approach to the patient can often result in prolonged remission of disease. The most critical factor to consider is the response of the patient to initial treatment (Table 58.36) (223). Patients who progress or recur are classified according to initial response to platinum-based chemotherapy. Those who are clinically platinum sensitive have an excellent chance to respond to further platinum-based treatment. Those who are clinically platinum re-

Table 58.35. Results of Randomized Trial of Adjuvant Platinum-Based Chemotherapy in High-Risk Limited Ovarian Carcinoma (222)

Regimen	Disease-Free at 5 Years
Low-risk patients (n = 92)	
Observation	90%
High-risk (grade 3) (n = 84)	
Observation	58%
Cisplatin 50 mg/m^2 q 4 weeks for 6 cycles	76%
High-risk (other reason) (174)	
Intraperitoneal ^{32}P	61%
Cisplatin 50 mg/m^2 q 4 weeks for 6 cycles	84%

*The differences between the two treatment arms in the two high-risk groups are statistically significant at $p < .05$ and $p < .01$, respectively. The reasons for classification as high risk are those given in Table 58.34.

Table 58.36. Definitions of Clinically Sensitive and Clinically Resistant Ovarian Carcinoma (224)

Classification	Definition
Platinum sensitive	Response to initial platinum-based chemotherapy and
	Minimum 6-month treatment-free interval before recurrence
Platinum resistant	Progression of disease while on platinum-based therapy or
	Best response to platinum-based therapy stable disease or
	Progression of disease within 6 months of initial therapy

sistant will respond less than 10% of the time to platinum-based treatment and should therefore be given drugs that exhibit at least some clinical non-cross-resistance: paclitaxel (173–179), docetaxel (180), ifosfamide (181), hexamethylmelamine (182–186), oral etoposide (187–189), gemcitabine (190), topotecan (191–193), liposomal doxorubicin (194), and tamoxifen (195).

Conclusions

The current approach to the management of ovarian carcinoma begins with an exploratory laparotomy to establish an accurate staging. This should be accompanied by an attempt at maximal surgical cytoreduction. Following completion of these steps, patients with advanced or recurrent disease should be treated with paclitaxel plus a platinum compound for six cycles. Patients with limited disease at low risk for recurrence require no further therapy. Those with high risk for recurrence need adjuvant therapy, which should consist of platinum-based chemotherapy.

GERM CELL CARCINOMAS OF THE OVARY

Approximately 10% of ovarian cancer consists of germ cell carcinomas. These neoplasms are classified into two broad groups: dysgerminomas and nondysgerminomas (Table 58.37) (224). Staging is that used for celomic epithelial carcinomas. The management of these patients begins with exploratory laparotomy, which serves to determine extent of disease and to permit surgical resection if possible. Subsequent therapy will depend on histology and the findings at laparotomy, on the basis of which patients can be placed into one of two groups: those

Table 58.37. Classification of Ovarian Germ Cell Carcinomas (228)

1. Dysgerminoma
2. Nondysgerminoma
    A. Teratoma
        1. Immature
        2. Mature
        3. Monodermal or specialized
    B. Endodermal sinus tumor
    C. Embryonal carcinoma
    D. Choriocarcinoma
    E. Polyembryoma
    F. Mixed cell tumors

with stages I–III disease that is completely resected and those with incompletely resected stage III and stage IV disease. Unlike the celomic epithelial carcinomas, however, therapeutic decisions have to be based on comparisons with historic controls, since these lesions are sufficiently uncommon that randomized trials are not feasible.

Stages I–III Completely Resected

Among patients with completely resected stage I, II, or III disease, those with endodermal sinus tumors, mixed cell tumors, embryonal carcinomas, choriocarcinomas, and immature teratomas appear to have a sufficiently high recurrence rate that adjuvant therapy should be considered. The largest experience with adjuvant chemotherapy is that of the GOG, whose studies have evaluated adjuvant VAC (vincristine, actinomycin D, and cyclophosphamide) or BEP (bleomycin, etoposide, and cisplatin) (225, 227).

Assessment of the relative value of these regimens is best accomplished by comparison with historic data on no adjuvant therapy (Table 58.38). Such a comparison shows a steady increase in the percentage of patients who remain disease-free at 16 months of follow-up as one goes from no adjuvant through VAC to BEP.

Table 58.38 Results of GOG Trials of Adjuvant Chemotherapy in Ovarian Germ Cell Carcinoma Expressed in Terms of the Percentage of Patients Remaining Disease Free at a Median Follow-Up of 16 Months following Completion of Therapy (225, 227)

Therapy	EST and MCT	Immature Teratoma
No adjuvant	34/165 (21%)	36/56 (64%)
VAC	53/82 (65%)	59/70 (84%)
BEP	30/31 (97%)	18/19 (95%)

VAC: Vincristine 1.5 mg/m^2 i.v. (max 2 mg) q 2 weeks × 12
Actinomycin D 350 μg/m^2 i.v. daily × 5 days q 4 weeks × 6
Cyclophosphamide 150 mg/m^2 i.v. daily × 5 days q 4 weeks × 6

BEP: Bleomycin 20 units/m^2 i.v. (max 30 units) weekly × 9
Etoposide 100 mg/m^2 i.v. daily × 5 q 3 weeks × 3
Cisplatin 20 mg/m^2 i.v. daily × 5 q 3 weeks × 3

These data suggest that for patients with completely resected stages I–III disease, adjuvant BEP is the treatment of choice for specific histologies: immature teratoma grades 2 and 3, endodermal sinus tumor, mixed cell tumor, and probably also embryonal carcinoma and choriocarcinoma. For other histologies, insufficient data exist to permit a definitive recommendation.

Stage III Incompletely Resected and Stage IV Disease

For patients with advanced ore recurrent disease, at least two chemotherapy regimens have been shown to be active by the GOG: VAC and PVB (cisplatin, vinblastine, and bleomycin) (Table 58.39) (226). While it is clear that both regimens are indeed active, the cisplatin-based combination yields higher response rates and a greater percentage of patients who remain disease-free for extended periods as a reflection of probable cure. The current study of the GOG evaluates a combination of bleomycin, etoposide, and cisplatin.

Tumor Markers

As is the case for testicular carcinomas, ovarian germ cell tumors do, in most cases, produce markers. α-Fetoprotein elevations have been noted in patients with endodermal sinus tumors, immature teratomas, mixed germ cell tumors, embryonal carcinomas, and polyembryomas. Elevations of human chorionic gonadotropin have been observed with choriocarcinomas, embryonal carcinomas, polyembryomas, mixed cell tumors, and less commonly dysgerminomas. These markers are useful in assessing response to chemotherapy and in following patients in complete remission for evidence of recurrence.

GESTATIONAL TROPHOBLASTIC DISEASE

Gestational trophoblastic disease includes a spectrum of neoplastic processes involving the placenta: molar pregnancy, invasive mole, and choriocarcinoma. While uncommon, the disease process is important because it is amenable to cure even in advanced stages of spread. The role of chemotherapy in management is major.

General Considerations

The diagnosis of gestational trophoblastic disease rests on the demonstration of a rising or plateauing human chorionic gonadotropin (HCG) level after evacuation of a hydatidiform mole, a histologic diagnosis of invasive mole or choriocarcinoma, or, following a pregnancy, a persistent elevation of HCG with or without objective

Table 58.39. Results of GOG Trials Employing Two Three-Drug Combinations in Incompletely Resected Stage III and Stage IV Germ Cell Carcinomas of the Ovary (226)

Histology and Therapy	CR	PR	Disease-Free
Immature teratoma			
VAC	—	—	4/8 (50%)
PVB	2/9 (22%)	2/9 (22%)	12/24 (50%)
Endodermal sinus tumor and mixed cell tumor			
VAC	—	—	3/14 (21%)
PVB	13/24 (54%)	8/24 (33%)	31/58 (53%)
Dysgerminoma			
PVB	3/4 (75%)	1/4 (25%)	7/8 (88%)
Choriocarcinoma			
PVB	2/3 (67%)	1/3 (33%)	2/3 (67%)

VAC: Vincristine 1.5 mg/m^2 i.v. (max 2 mg) q 2 weeks × 12
Actinomycin D 350 μg/m^2 i.v. daily × 5 days q 4 weeks × 6
Cyclophosphamide 150 mg/m^2 i.v. daily × 5 days q 4 weeks × 6
PVB: Vinblastine 12 mg/m^2 i.v. q 3 weeks × 4
Bleomycin 20 units/m^2 i.v. (max 30 units) weekly × 12
Cisplatin 20 mg/m^2 i.v. daily × 5 q 3 weeks × 3–4

evidence of metastases. Approximately 50% of all cases follow a hydatidiform mole, 25% an abortion, and 25% a normal pregnancy.

For purposes of decisions regarding the use of chemotherapy, it is important to separate the patient population into those at high risk and those at low risk. There are essentially three groups into which the patient population can be divided: nonmetastatic disease, metastatic disease at low risk, and metastatic disease at high risk. Assignment of a patient to one of these three groups requires that the patient be assessed for extent of disease. This evaluation should include the measurement of the β subunit of HCG and examination of the likely sites of spread: abdomen and pelvis, lungs, and brain.

These data permit the assignment of stage according to a system devised by the International Society for the Study of Trophoblastic Neoplasms (228) (Table 58.40). Stage I patients have disease confined to the uterus and comprise the group with nonmetastatic disease. Assignment of patients to the other two groups depends on additional variables: pretreatment HCG level, type of antecedent event, time from antecedent pregnancy or onset of symptoms to treatment, sites of metastases, and prior chemotherapy. Patients with one or more of the following are considered to be at high risk: pretreatment HCG greater than 100,000 IU/24 hours (urine) or 40,000 IU/mL (serum), time from antecedent event to treatment greater than 4 months, antecedent term pregnancy, metastases to sites other than lungs and vagina, and prior unsuccessful chemotherapy (229). These include all patients with stage IV disease and certain of those with stages II or III. Patients with stages II or III with none of these high-risk factors present are considered to be metastatic low-risk patients.

An alternative approach to categorizing patients is a scoring system that takes into account the same variables plus number and size of metastases and ABO blood group (Table 58.41). A score of seven or greater places the patient into a high-risk category (230). Regardless of which of these systems is used, the use of chemotherapy is determined by the group to which the patient is assigned.

Nonmetastatic Disease

The management of patients with nonmetastatic gestational trophoblastic disease depends on whether the patient wishes to preserve fertility. For those who have no such desire, hysterectomy is the initial therapeutic step. For those who do want to retain fertility and for those who have undergone hysterectomy, single-agent chemotherapy represents the standard of care (231). The two drugs most commonly employed are actinomycin D and methotrexate. In the case of actinomycin D, two different schedules have been employed at 2-week intervals: 10 to 13 mg/kg daily for 5 days and 1.25 mg/m² once every 2 weeks. Methotrexate has been given in two different schedules: 0.4 mg/kg daily for 5 days every 2 weeks and 1 mg/kg on days 1, 3, 5, and 7 followed by leucovorin 0.1 mg/kg on

Table 58.40. Staging System for Gestational Trophoblastic Disease (228)

Stage	Description
0	Molar pregnancy
I	Confined to uterine corpus
II	Metastasis to pelvis and vagina
III	Metastasis to lungs
IV	Other distant metastasis

Table 58.41. Prognostic Scoring System for Gestational Trophoblastic Disease (231) (Score <4 Low Risk, >7 High Risk)

Risk Factor	0	1	2	3
Age	<39	>39		
Antecedent event	Mole	Abortion	Term	
Event to therapy (month)	<4	4–6	7–12	>12
HCG at initial therapy	<10^3	10^3–10^4	10^4–10^5	>10^5
ABO blood group (female × male)		O × A; A × O	B or AB	
Largest tumor (cm)		3–5	>5	
Site of metastasis		Spleen; kidney	GI Tract; liver	Brain
Number of metastases		1–4	4–8	>8
Previous chemotherapy			One drug	Multiple drugs

days 2, 4, 6 and 8 every 15 to 18 days. More recently, a similar schedule of methotrexate 30 to 50 mg/m^2 weekly has been employed with similar success (232).

Cure is expected in essentially all patients. Between 85 and 90% should achieve this with the initial single-agent therapy. Should HCG levels plateau or rise after two courses or toxicity preclude adequate doses of therapy, treatment should be changed to the alternative single agent or hysterectomy in the case of those who did not undergo initial hysterectomy or both. Rarely, combination chemotherapy such as the regimens to be described for high-risk metastatic disease will be required.

Low-Risk Metastatic Disease

Patients with metastatic disease at low risk should be treated with the same single-agent chemotherapy as that used for nonmetastatic disease. In contrast to the nonmetastatic patients, however, almost half of the patients will develop resistance to the initial agent and will require a change to the alternative drug. Approximately 10 to 15% of all patients will fail on both single agents and require combination chemotherapy with or without surgery to eradicate persistent disease in the uterus. Determination of the need to change therapy is based on a plateau or rise in the HCG level on two consecutive samples or the appearance of new sites of metastases. This approach should yield essentially 100% cures (231).

High-Risk Metastatic Disease

For patients with high-risk metastatic disease, results with single-agent therapy are considerably poorer. Whereas virtually all patients with low-risk disease will respond to single agents, only 20% of high-risk patients respond. Combination chemotherapy, on the other hand, yields cure rates that approach 80% (234).

Two combination regimens have been studied extensively: (*a*) methotrexate, actinomycin D, and cyclophosphamide (MAC) (233–235) and (*b*) hydroxyurea, actinomycin D, methotrexate with leucovorin rescue, cyclophosphamide, vincristine, and doxorubicin (CHAMOCA) (237) (Table 58.42). A randomized clinical trial comparing MAC with a modified CHAMOCA (melphalan substituted for cyclophosphamide on day 8—CHAMOMA) included 42 patients, 22 randomized to MAC and 20 to CHAMOMA (237). Of the 22 patients receiving MAC, 16 (73%)

attained remission with primary therapy, and 5 more (23%) with secondary therapy. Only one patient died. In contrast, 6 (30%) of the 20 patients receiving CHAMOMA died of disease. A seventh who failed primary therapy did achieve remission with second-line therapy. Risk factors were reasonably balanced, with bias toward response, if any, appearing to favor the CHAMOMA regimen. This trial suggests that MAC is at least as effective as CHAMOMA, with similar toxicity, and is less complex to administer and would appear to be the treatment of choice of these two.

Recent results of uncontrolled studies of EMA-CO (etoposide, methotrexate-leucovorin, actinomycin D, cyclophosphamide, vincristine) have been interpreted to suggest that this regimen may offer a higher success rate (83% survival in 36 patients) than either MAC or CHAMOMA (238), but these observations need to be regarded in light of similarly uncontrolled trials suggesting that CHAMOCA was superior to MAC. The overall survival rate of 83%), moreover, does not appear superior to the 95% success rate observed with MAC in the randomized trial, although a randomized study would be required to assess the relative efficacy of each treatment. Three specific circumstances that require special considerations are treatment for resistant disease, management of hepatic metastases, and therapy for brain metastases. In the case of treatment for high-risk metastatic disease that has become resistant (231), complete remission rates are low (20% or less with combination chemotherapy such as MAC after failure on single-agent therapy). In patients who fail first-line combination therapy, the use of platinum-based regimens (together with etoposide if not a part of the initial therapy) yields at least some complete responses.

In regard to hepatic metastases, patients are at significant risk for hepatic bleeding with the first course of chemotherapy. Hepatic radiation and hepatic arterial infusion of chemotherapy have been recommended, but current data do not support the efficacy of such approaches as a routine part of therapy. If bleeding does occur, selective hepatic arterial occlusion with detachable silicon balloons has been reported to be effective (239).

Various measures have been recommended for the treatment of brain metastases. Some investigators have recommended the use of prophylactic intrathecal methotrexate for all patients with high-risk disease (240), but this has

Table 58.42. Three Regimens Employed in the Management of High-Risk Metastatic Gestational Trophoblastic Disease (233–237)

Regimen	Schedule and Doses	
MAC	Methotrexate 7 mg/m^2 i.v. or i.m. Actinomycin D 350 μg/m^2 i.v. Chlorambucil 5 mg/m^2 orally Repeat drugs daily for 5 days every 3 weeks	
CHAMOMA	Day 1: 12 MID 6:00 AM 12:00 NOON 6:00 PM Day 2: 7:00 AM Day 3: 7:00 PM Day 4: 1:00 AM 7:00 AM 1:00 PM 7:00 PM Day 5: 1:00 AM 7:00 PM Day 6: Day 7: Day 8: 7:00 PM Repeat every 3 weeks	Hydroxyurea 500 mg orally Hydroxyurea 500 mg orally Hydroxyurea 500 mg orally Actinomycin 0.2 mg i.v. Hydroxyurea 500 mg orally Vincristine 1 mg/m^2 i.v. Methotrexate 100 mg/m^2 i.v. Methotrexate 200 mg/m^2 i.v. over 12 hr Actinomycin 0.2 mg i.v. Actinomycin 0.2 mg i.v. Cyclophosphamide 500 mg/m^2 i.v. Leucovorin 14 mg i.m. Leucovorin 14 mg i.m. Leucovorin 14 mg i.m. Leucovorin 14 mg i.m. Leucovorin 14 mg i.m. Actinomycin 0.5 mg i.v. Leucovorin 14 mg i.m. Actinomycin 0.5 mg i.v. No treatment No treatment Melphalan 6 mg/m^2 orally Doxorubicin 30 mg/m^2 i.v.	
EMA-CO	Etoposide 100 mg/m^2 i.v. over 30 min days 1–2 Actinomycin D 0.5 mg i.v. days 1–2 Methotrexate 100 mg/m^2 i.v. push day 1 followed by 200 mg/m^2 i.v. infusion over 12 hr Leucovorin 15 mg i.m. every 12 hr for four doses 24 hr after starting metotrexate Vincristine 1 mg/m^2 i.v. day 8 Cyclophosphamide 600 mg/m^2 i.v. day 8 Repeat every 2 weeks	

not been shown to be necessary (241). In patients with documented brain lesions, escalated intravenous doses of methotrexate have been shown to achieve sustained complete remissions. The precise role of whole-brain radiation in conjunction with chemotherapy for these lesions is not clear (242).

Conclusions and Recommendations

Chemotherapy has a definite role in the management of patients with nonmetastatic as well as both low- and high-risk metastatic gestational trophoblastic disease. In those with nonmetas- tatic and low-risk metastatic disease, single-agent chemotherapy consisting of pulse-dose methotrexate or actinomycin D should yield high cure rates. Patients with high-risk metastatic disease require combination chemotherapy, with MAC or EMA-CO representing reasonable choices. The expected complete remission rate should exceed 80%.

OTHER GYNECOLOGIC MALIGNANCIES

Other nongestational gynecologic neoplasms including vulvar carcinoma, vaginal carcinoma, and fallopian tube carcinoma are sufficiently rare that no interpretable data are available to guide the use of systemic therapy in patient management.

REFERENCES

1. DeVita VT Jr, Wasserman T, Young RC, et al. Perspectives and research in gynecologic oncology. Cancer 1976;38:509–525.

2. Boronow RC, Morrow CP, Creasman WT, et al. Surgical staging in endometrial cancer. I. Clinical-pathologic findings of a prospective study. Obstet Gynecol 1984;63:825–832.

3. DiSaia PJ, Creasman WT, Boronow RC, Blessing JA. Risk factors and recurrence patterns in stage I endometrial cancer (for the Gynecologic Oncology Group). Am J Obstet Gynecol 1985;151:1009–1015.

4. Creasman WT, Morrow CP, Bundy BN, et al. Surgical pathological spread patterns of endometrial cancer (a Gynecologic Oncology Group study). Cancer 1987;60:2035–2041.

5. Morrow CP, Creasman WT, Homesley H, et al. Recurrence in endometrial carcinoma as a function of extended surgical staging data (a Gynecologic Oncology Group study). In: Morrow CP, Smart GE, eds. Gynaecologic oncology. New York: Springer-Verlag, 1985:147–153.

6. Food and Drug Administration. Estrogens and endometrial cancer. FDA Drug Bull 1976;6:18–20.

7. Thigpen T, Vance R, Lambuth B, et al. Chemotherapy for advanced or recurrent gynecologic cancer. Cancer 1987;60:2104–2116.

8. Sall S, DiSaia P, Morrow CP, et al. A comparison of medroxyprogesterone serum concentrations by the oral or intramuscular route in patients with persistent or recurrent endometrial carcinoma. Am J Obstet Gynecol 1979;135:647–650.

9. Thigpen T, Blessing J, DiSaia P, Ehrlich C. Oral medroxyprogesterone acetate in advanced or recurrent endometrial carcinoma: results of therapy and correlation with estrogen and progesterone receptor levels. The Gynecologic Oncology Group experience. In: Baulier E, Iacobelli S, McGuire W, eds. Endocrinology and malignancy. New York: Parthenon, 1986:446–454.

10. Thigpen T, Brady M, Alvarez R, et al. Oral medroxyprogesterone acetate in the treatment of advanced or recurrent endometrial carcinoma: a dose-response study by the Gynecologic Oncology Group. J Clin Oncol (in press).

11. Slavik M, Petty W, Blessing J, et al. Phase II clinical study of tamoxifen in advanced endometrial adenocarcinoma: a Gynecologic Oncology Group study. Cancer Treat Rep 1984;68:809–811.

12. Thigpen T. Personal communication.

13. Thigpen T, Buchsbaum H, Mangan C, Blessing J. Phase II trial of adriamycin in the treatment of advanced or recurrent endometrial carcinoma: a Gynecologic Oncology Group study. Cancer Treat Rep 1979; 63:21–27.

14. Thigpen T, Blessing J, Homesley H, Creasman W, Sutton G. Phase II trial of cisplatin as first-line chemotherapy in patients with advanced or recurrent endometrial carcinoma: a Gynecologic Oncology Group study. Gynecol Oncol 1989;33:68–70.

15. Thigpen T, Blessing J, Homesley H, Petty W. Phase II trial of piperazinedione in the treatment of advanced or recurrent endometrial carcinoma. Am J Clin Oncol 1986;9:21–23.

16. Thigpen T, Blessing J, Ball H, et al. Hexamethylmelamine as first-line chemotherapy in the treatment of advanced or recurrent carcinoma of the endometrium: a phase II trial of the Gynecologic Oncology Group. Gynecol Oncol 1988;31:435–438.

17. Muss H, Blessing J, Hatch K, et al. Methotrexate in advanced endometrial carcinoma: a phase II trial of the Gynecologic Oncology Group. Am J Clin Oncol 1990;13:61–63.

18. Thigpen T, Blessing J, Lagasse L, et al. Phase II trial of cisplatin as second-line chemotherapy in patients with advanced or recurrent endometrial carcinoma. Am J Clin Oncol 1984;7:253–256.

19. Asbury R, Blessing J, McGuire W, et al. Aminothiadiazole in patients with advanced carcinoma of the endometrium. Am J Clin Oncol 1990;13:39–41.

20. Muss H, Bundy B, Adcock L. Teniposide in patients with advanced endometrial carcinoma (a phase II trial of the Gynecologic Oncology Group). Am J Clin Oncol 1991;14:36–37.

21. Slayton R, Blessing J, DiSaia P, Phillips G. A phase II clinical trial of diaziquone in the treatment of patients with recurrent endometrial carcinoma. Am J Clin Oncol 1988;11:612–613.

22. Muss H, Bundy B, DiSaia P, Ehrlich C. Mitoxantrone for carcinoma of the endometrium: a phase II trial of the Gynecologic Oncology Group. Cancer Treat Rep 1987;71:217–218.

23. Homesley H, Blessing J, Conroy J, et al. ICRF-159 (Razoxane) in patients with advanced adenocarcinoma of the endometrium. Am J Clin Oncol 1986; 9:15–17.

24. Slayton R, Blessing J, Delgado G. Phase II trial of etoposide in the management of advanced or recurrent endometrial carcinoma: a Gynecologic Oncology Group study. Cancer Treat Rep 1982;66:1669–1671.

25. Stehman F, Blessing J, Delgado G, Louka M. Phase II evaluation of dianhydrogalactitol in the treatment of advanced endometrial adenocarcinoma: a Gynecologic Oncology Group study. Cancer Treat Rep 1983;67:737–738.

26. Thigpen T. Systemic therapy with single agents for advanced or recurrent endometrial carcinoma. In: Alberts D, Surwit E, eds. Endometrial carcinoma. Boston: Martinus Nijhoff, 1989.

27. Barton C, Buxton EJ, Blackledge G, et al. A phase II study of ifosfamide in endometrial cancer. Cancer Chemother Pharmacol 1990;26(Suppl):S4–S6.

28. Muss H. Chemotherapy of metastatic endometrial cancer. Semin Oncol 1994;21:107–113.

29. Hilgers R, Legha S, Johnston G, et al. m-AMSA and adenocarcinoma of the endometrium. Invest New Drugs 1984;2:335–338.

30. Thigpen T, Vance R, Khansur T. The platinum compounds and paclitaxel in the management of carcinomas of the endometrium and uterine cervix. Semin Oncol 1995;22:67–75.

31. Moore TD, Phillips PH, Nerenstone SR, Cheson BD. Systemic treatment of advanced and recurrent endometrial carcinoma: current status and future directions. J Clin Oncol 1991;9:1071–1088.

32. Bruckner H, Deppe G. Combination chemotherapy of advanced endometrial adenocarcinoma

with adriamycin, cyclophosphamide, 5-fluorouracil, and medroxyprogesterone acetate. Obstet Gynecol 1977;50(Suppl):10–12.

33. Cohen C, Deppe G, Bruckner H. Treatment of advanced adenocarcinoma of the endometrium with melphalan, 5-fluorouracil, and medroxyprogesterone acetate. Obstet Gynecol 1977;50:415–417.

34. Cohen C, Bruckner H, Deppe G, et al. Multidrug treatment of advanced and recurrent endometrial carcinoma: a Gynecologic Oncology Group study. Obstet Gynecol 1984;63:719–726.

35. Thigpen T, Blessing J, DiSaia P, et al. A randomized comparison of adriamycin with or without cyclophosphamide in the treatment of advanced or recurrent endometrial carcinoma (abstract). Proc Am Soc Clin Oncol 1985;4:115.

36. Thigpen T, Blessing J, Homesley H, Malfetano J, DiSaia P, Yordan E: Phase III trial of doxorubicin +/ − cisplatin in advanced or recurrent endometrial carcinoma. Proc Am Soc Clin Oncol 1993;12:261.

37. Thigpen JT, Morrow CP, Blessing J. Adjuvant chemotherapy in high-risk endometrial carcinoma. In: Bolla M, RAcinet C, Vrousos C, eds. Endometrial cancers. Basel: Karger, 1986;223–232.

38. Sutton GP, Blessing JA, Rosenheim N, Photopoulos G, DiSaia PJ. Phase II trial of ifosfamide and mesna in mixed mesodermal tumors of the uterus (a Gynecologic Oncology Group study). Am J Obstet Gynecol 1989;161:309–312.

39. Thigpen JT, Blessing JA, Beecham J, Homesley H, Yordan E. Phase II trial of cisplatin as first-line chemotherapy in patients with advanced or recurrent uterine sarcomas (a Gynecologic Oncology Group study). J Clin Oncol 1991;9:1962–1966.

40. Thigpen JT, Blessing JA, Orr JW Jr, DiSaia PJ. Phase II trial of cisplatin in the treatment of patients with advanced or recurrent mixed mesodermal sarcomas of the uterus: a Gynecologic Oncology Group study. Cancer Treat Rep 1986;70:271–274.

41. Gershenson DM, Kavanagh JJ, Copeland LJ, Edwards CL, Stringer CA, Wharton JT. Cisplatin therapy for disseminated mixed mesodermal sarcoma of the uterus. J Clin Oncol 1987;5:618–621.

42. Omura GA, Major FJ, Blessing JA, et al. A randomized study of adriamycin with and without dimethyl triazinoimidazole carboxamide in advanced uterine sarcomas. Cancer 1983;52:626–632.

43. Gershenson DM, Kavanagh JJ, Copeland LJ, Edwards CL, Freedman RS, Wharton JT. High-dose doxorubicin infusion therapy for disseminated mixed mesodermal sarcoma of the uterus. Cancer 1987; 59:1264–1267.

44. Slayton RE, Blessing JA, DiSaia PJ, Christopherson WA. Phase II trial of etoposide in the management of advanced or recurrent mixed mesodermal sarcomas of the uterus: a Gynecologic Oncology Group study. Cancer Treat Rep 1987;71:661–662.

45. Muss HB, Bundy BN, Adcock L, Beecham J. Mitoxantrone in the treatment of advanced uterine sarcoma. Am J Clin Oncol 1990;13:32–34.

46. Thigpen JT, Blessing JA, Homesley HD, Hacker N, Curry SL. Phase II trial of piperazinedione in patients with advanced or recurrent uterine sarcoma. Am J Clin Oncol 1985;8:350–352.

47. Sutton G, Blessing J, McGuire W, Photopoulos G, DiSaia P. Phase II trial of ifosfamide and mesna in leiomyosarcomas of the uterus. Gynecol Oncol 1990; 36:295.

48. Thigpen JT, Blessing JA, Wilbanks GD. Cisplatin as second-line chemotherapy in the treatment of advanced or recurrent leiomyosarcoma of the uterus. Am J Clin Oncol 1986;9:18–20.

49. Slayton R, Blessing J, Angel C, Berman M. Phase II trial of etoposide in the management of advanced or recurrent leiomyosarcoma of the uterus: a Gynecologic Oncology Group study. Cancer Treat Rep 1987;71:1303–1304.

50. Thigpen T. Personal communication.

51. Muss HB, Bundy BN, DiSaia PJ, et al. Treatment of recurrent or advanced uterine sarcoma: a randomized trial of doxorubicin versus doxorubicin and cyclophosphamide (a phase III trial of the Gynecologic Oncology Group). Cancer 1985;55:1648–1653.

52. Omura GA, Blessing JA, Major F, et al. A randomized clinical trial of adjuvant adriamycin in uterine sarcomas: a Gynecologic Oncology Group Study. J Clin Oncol 1985;3:1240–1245.

53. Wingo PA, Tong T, Bolden S. Cancer Statistics 1995. CA 1995;45:8–30.

54. Thigpen JT. Single agent chemotherapy in carcinoma of the cervix. In: Surwit E, Alberts D, eds. Cervix cancer. Boston: Martinus Nijhoff, 1987:119–136.

55. Thigpen T. Chemotherapy in the management of advanced or recurrent carcinoma of the cervix. In: Rubin S, Hoskins W, eds. Cervical cancer and preinvasive neoplasia. Philadelphia: Lippincott-Raven, 1996 (in press).

56. Muscato MS, Perry MC, Yarbro JW. Chemotherapy of cervical carcinoma. Semin Oncol 1982; 9:373–387.

57. Omura GA, Velez-Garcia E, Birch R, writing for the Southeastern Cancer Study Group. Phase II randomized study of doxorubicin, vincristine, and 5-FU versus cyclophosphamide in advanced squamous cell-carcinoma of the cervix. Cancer Treat Rep 1981;65:901–903.

58. Thigpen T, Vance RB, Balducci L, Blessing J. Chemotherapy in the management of advanced or recurrent cervical and endometrial carcinoma. Cancer 1981;48:658–665.

59. Stehman FB, Blessing JA, McGehee R, Barrett RJ. A phase II evaluation of mitolactol in patients with advanced squamous cell carcinoma of the cervix: a Gynecologic Oncology Group study. J Clin Oncol 1989; 7:1892–1895.

60. Lira-Puerto V, Piccart M, Wiernik P, et al. A comparison of US and Mexican experience with single drug therapy in advanced cervical cancer (NCI-PAHO and ECOG study). Proc Am Soc Clin Oncol 1985;4:117.

61. Stehman FB, Blom J, Blessing JA, et al. Phase II trial of galactitol 1,2:5,6-dianhydro in the treatment of advanced gynecologic malignancies: a Gynecologic Oncology Group study. Gynecol Oncol 1983;15:381–390.

62. Sutton GP, Blessing JA, Photopoulos G, et al. Phase II experience with ifosfamide/mesna in gynecologic malignancies: preliminary report of Gynecologic Oncology Group studies. Semin Oncol 1989; 16(Suppl 3):68–72.

63. Sutton GP, Blessing JA, Adcock L, et al. Phase II study of ifosfamide and mesna in patients with previously-treated carcinoma of the cervix: a Gynecologic

Oncology Group study. Invest New Drugs 1989;7:341–343.

64. Thigpen T, Vance R, Khansur T, Malamud F. The role of ifosfamide and of systemic therapy in the management of carcinoma of the cervix. Semin Oncol (in press).

65. Arseneau J, Blessing J, Stehman F, McGehee R. A phase II study of carboplatin in advanced squamous cell carcinoma of the cervix. Invest New Drugs 1986; 4:187–191.

66. McGuire WP, Arseneau J, Blessing JA, et al. A randomized comparative trial of carboplatin and iproplatin in advanced squamous carcinoma of the uterine cervix: Gynecologic Oncology Group study. J Clin Oncol 1989;7:1462–1468.

67. Thigpen T, Shingleton H, Homesley H, et al. Cis-platinum in treatment of advanced or recurrent squamous cell carcinoma of the cervix. Cancer 1981; 48:899–903.

68. Bonomi P, Blessing J, Stehman F, et al. Randomized trial of three cisplatin dose schedules in squamous-cell carcinoma of the cervix: a Gynecologic Oncology Group study. J Clin Oncol 1985;3:1079–1085.

69. Thigpen JT, Blessing JA, DiSaia PJ, et al. A randomized comparison of a rapid versus prolonged (24 hr) infusion of cisplatin in therapy of squamous cell carcinoma of the uterine cervix: a Gynecologic Oncology Group study. Gynecol Oncol 1989;32:198–202.

70. Cohen C, Castro-Marin A, Deppe G, Bruckner H, Holland J. Chemotherapy of advanced or recurrent cervical cancer with platinum II—a preliminary report. Proc Am Soc Clin Oncol 1978;19:401.

71. Baker L. Cisplatin in treatment of cervical and endometrial cancer patients. In: Prestayko J, Crooke S, Carter S, eds. Cisplatin: current status and new developments. New York: Academic Press, 1980:403–409.

72. Baker L, Boutselis J, Alberts D, et al. Combination chemotherapy for patients with disseminated carcinoma of the uterine cervix. Proc Am Soc Clin Oncol 1985;4:120.

73. Wasserman T, Carter S. The integration of chemotherapy into combined modality treatment of solid tumors. VIII. Cervical cancer. Cancer Treat Rev 1977; 4:25–46.

74. Cavins J, Geisler H. Treatment of advanced, unresectable, cervical carcinoma already subjected to complete irradiation therapy. Gynecol Oncol 1978; 6:256–260.

75. Piver M, Barlow J, Xynos F. Adriamycin alone or in combination in 100 patients with carcinoma of the cervix or vagina. Am J Obstet Gynecol 1978; 131:311–313.

76. Malkasian G, Decker D, Green S, Edmondson J, Jeffries J, Webb M. Treatment of recurrent and metastatic carcinoma of the cervix: comparison of doxorubicin with a combination of vincristine and 5-fluorouracil. Gynecol Oncol 1981;11:235–239.

77. Greenberg B, Kardinal C, Pajek T, Batemen J. Adriamycin versus adriamycin and bleomycin in advanced epidermoid carcinoma of the cervix. Cancer Treat Rep 1977;61:1383–1384.

78. Wallace H, Hreshchyshyn M, Wilbanks G, Boronow R, Fowler W, Blessing J. Comparison of the therapeutic effect of adriamycin alone versus adriamycin plus vincristine versus adriamycin plus cyclophosphamide in the treatment of advanced carcinoma of the cervix. Cancer Treat Rep 1978;62:1435–1441.

79. Freeman R, Herson J, Wharton T, Rutledge F. Single agent chemotherapy for recurrent carcinoma of the cervix. Cancer Clin Trials 1980;3:345–350.

80. Arseneau JC, Bundy B, Dolan T, et al. Phase II study of Baker's antifol in advanced squamous cell carcinoma of cervix. Am J Clin Oncol 1982;5:61–64.

81. Malkasian G, Decker D, Jorgensen E. Chemotherapy of carcinoma of the cervix. Gynecol Oncol 1977;5:109–120.

82. Takeuchi S, Noda K, Yakushiji M. Late phase II study of CPT-11, topoisomerse I inhibitor in advanced cervical carcinoma (abstract 708). Proc Am Soc Clin Oncol 1992;11:224.

83. Conroy JF, Lewis GC Jr, Blessing JA, et al. ICRF-159 in patients with advanced squamous cell carcinoma of the uterine cervix. Am J Clin Oncol 1984; 7:131–133.

84. Asbury RF, Blessing JA, Mortel R, et al. Aminothiadiazole in patients with advanced cervical carcinoma: a phase II study of the Gynecologic Oncology Group. Am J Clin Oncol 1987;10:299–301.

85. Asbury RF, Blessing J, Soper J. A Gynecologic Oncology Group phase II study of amonafide in squamous cell carcinoma of the cervix. Am J Clin Oncol 1994;17:125–128.

86. Bonomi P, Blessing JA, Sedlacek TV, et al. Phase II trial of AMSA in patients with advanced or recurrent squamous cell carcinoma of the cervix: a Gynecologic Oncology Group study. Cancer Treat Rep 1983;67:197–198.

87. Omura G, Shingleton H, Creasman W, Blessing J, Boronow R. Chemotherapy of advanced gynecologic cancer with nitrosoureas: a randomized trial of CCNU and methyl CCNU in carcinoma of the cervix, corpus, vagina, vulva and tube. Cancer Treat Rep 1978;62:833–835.

88. Slayton RE, Blessing JA, Stehman FB, Malfetano J. Phase II clinical trial of diaziquone in the treatment of patients with recurrent squamous cell carcinoma of the cervix: a Gynecologic Oncology Group study. Cancer Treat Rep 1986;70:1127–1128.

89. Roberts JA, Blessing JA, McGehee R, et al. Phase II trial of dichloromethotrexate in patients with advanced squamous cell carcinoma of the cervix: a Gynecologic Oncology Group study. Cancer Treat Rep 1987;71:1295–1296.

90. Jacobs A, Blessing J, Munoz A. A phase II trial of didemnin B in advanced or recurrent cervical carcinoma: a Gynecologic Oncology Group study. Gynecol Oncol 1991;44:268–270.

91. Weiss GR, Liu PY, O'Sullivan J, et al. A randomized phase II trial of trimetrexate or didemnin B for the treatment of metastatic or recurrent squamous carcinoma of the uterine cervix: a Southwest Oncology Group trial. Gynecol Oncol 1992;445:303–306.

92. Muss HB, Blessing JA, Malfetano J. Echinomycin in squamous-cell carcinoma of the cervix: a phase II trial of the Gynecologic Oncology Group. Am J Clin Oncol 1990;13:191–193.

93. Lincoln S. Personal communication of GOG data.

94. McGuire WP, Blessing JA, Yordan E, Beecham J. Phase II study of esorubicin in advanced or metastatic squamous carcinoma of the uterine cervix: a Gy-

necologic Oncology Group study. Invest New Drugs 1989;7:235–238.

95. Slayton RE, Creasman WT, Petty W, et al. Phase II trial of VP-16-213 in the treatment of advanced squamous cell carcinoma of the cervix and adenocarcinoma of the ovary: a Gynecologic Oncology Group study. Cancer Treat Rep 1979;63:2089–2092.

96. Manetta A, Blessing J, Mann W, Smith D. A phase II study of fazarabine in patients with advanced squamous cell carcinoma of the cervix: a Gynecologic Oncology Group study. Am J Clin Oncol 1995;18:156–157.

97. Look K, Blessing J, Muss H, et al. 5-Fluorouracil and leucovorin in the treatment of recurrent squamous cell carcinoma of the cervix: a phase II trial of the Gynecologic Oncology Group. Am J Clin Oncol 1992; 15:497–499.

98. Look K, Blessing J, Gallup D, et al. A phase II trial of 5-fluorouracil and high dose leucovorin in patients with recurrent squamous cell carcinoma of the cervix: a Gynecologic Oncology Group study. Am J Clin Oncol 1992;15:497–499.

99. Malfetano J, Blessing J, Homesley H, et al. A phase II trial of gallium nitrate in advanced or recurrent squamous cell carcinoma of the cervix. A Gynecologic Oncology Group study. Invest New Drugs 1991;9:109–111.

100. McGuire WP, Blessing JA, Hatch K, DiSaia PJ. A phase II study of CHIP in advanced squamous cell carcinoma of the cervix. Invest New Drugs 1986;4:181–186.

101. Thigpen JT, Ehrlich CE, Conroy J, Blessing JA. Phase II study of maytansine in the treatment of advanced or recurrent squamous cell carcinoma of the cervix. Am J Clin Oncol 1983;6:427–430.

102. Sutton G, Blessing J, Gallup D, Homesley H. Phase II trial of menogaril in patients with squamous carcinoma of the cervix: a Gynecologic Oncology Group study. Gynecol Oncol 1994;52:229–231.

103. Look K, Blessing J, Williams L, et al. A phase II trial of merebarone as salvage therapy for squamous cell carcinoma of the cervix: a Gynecologic Oncology Group study. Am J Clin Oncol 1995;18:441–443.

104. Thigpen T, Blessing J, Gallup D, et al. Phase II trial of mitomycin C in squamous cell carcinoma of the uterine cervix: a Gynecologic Oncology Group study. Gynecol Oncol (in press).

105. Muss HB, Sutton GP, Bundy B, Hatch KD. Mitoxantrone in patients with advanced cervical carcinoma: a phase II study of the Gynecologic Oncology Group. Am J Clin Oncol 1985;8:312–315.

106. McGuire WP, Blessing JA, Hatch KD, Berman ML. Phase II study of N-methylformamide in patients with advanced squamous cancer of the cervix. Invest New Drugs 1990;8:195–197.

107. Muss HB, Bundy B, DiSaia PJ, et al. PALA in advanced carcinoma of the cervix: a phase II study of the Gynecologic Oncology Group. Am J Clin Oncol 1984;7:741–744.

108. Thigpen JT, Blessing J, Homesley H, Adcock L. Phase II trial of piperazinedione in the treatment of advanced or recurrent squamous cell carcinoma of the cervix. Am J Clin Oncol 1983;6:423–426.

109. Lincoln S. Personal communication of GOG data.

110. Muss HB, Bundy BN, Yazigi R, Yordan E. Teniposide in squamous cell carcinoma of the cervix:

a phase II trial of the Gynecologic Oncology Group. Cancer Treat Rep 1987;71:873–874.

111. Feun L, Blessing J, Barrett R, Hanjani P. A phase II trial of tricyclic nucleoside phosphate (TCN-P) in patients with advanced squamous cell carcinoma of the cervix: a Gynecologic Oncology Group study. Am J Clin Oncol 1993;16:506–508.

112. Sutton GP, Blessing JA, Barnes W, Ball H. Phase II study of vinblastine in previously treated squamous carcinoma of the cervix: a Gynecologic Oncology Group study. Am J Clin Oncol 1990;13:470–471.

113. Slavik M, Muss H, Blessing JA. Phase II clinical study of Yoshi 864 in squamous cell carcinoma of the uterine cervix. Cancer Treat Rep 1983;67:195–196.

114. Brenner D. Combination chemotherapy of advanced cervix cancer. In: Surwit E, Alberts D, eds. Cervix cancer. Boston: Martinus Nijhoff, 1987:137–160.

115. Edmondson J, Johnson P, Wieand HS, et al. Phase II studies of bleomycin, cyclophosphamide, doxorubicin and cisplatin, and bleomycin and cisplatin in advanced cervical carcinoma. Am J Clin Oncol 1988; 11:149–151.

116. Jobson V, Homesley H, Muss H, Bundy B, Thigpen T. Chemotherapy of advanced squamous carcinoma of the cervix: a phase I-II study of high-dose cisplatin and cyclophosphamide. Am J Clin Oncol 1984;7:341–345.

117. Bezwoda WR, Nissenbaum M, Derman DP. Treatment of metastatic and recurrent cervix cancer with chemotherapy—a randomized trial comparing hydroxyurea with cis-diamminedichloroplatinum plus methotrexate. Med Pediatr Oncol 1986;14:17–19.

118. Bonomi P, Yordan E, Blessing J. Phase I trial of cisplatin and razoxane in advanced squamous cell carcinoma of the cervix. Am J Clin Oncol 1988;11:1–2.

119. Vogl S, Moukhtar M, Kaplan B. Chemotherapy for advanced cervical cancer with methotrexate, bleomycin, and cis-diamminedichloroplatinum. Cancer Treat Rep 1979;63:1005–1006.

120. Bonomi P, Yordan E. Chemotherapy of cervical carcinoma. In: Deppe G, ed. Chemotherapy of gynecologic cancer. 2nd ed. New York: Wiley-Liss, 1990:121–153.

121. Friedlander M, Kaye S, Sullivan A, et al. Cervical carcinoma: a drug-responsive tumor-experience with combined cisplatin, vinblastine, and bleomycin therapy. Gynecol Oncol 1983;16:275–281.

122. Chauvergne J, Heron J, Mayer F, et al. Chemotherapy of cancers of the uterine cervix with a combination of bleomycin, mitomycin, cisplatin and etoposide. Bull Cancer 1993;80:70–79.

123. Coleman R, Harper P, Gallagher C, et al. A phase II study of ifosfamide in advanced and relapsed carcinoma of the cervix. Cancer Chemother Pharmacol 1986;18:280–283.

124. Weiss G, Green S, Hannigan E, et al. A phase II trial of cisplatin and 5-fluorouracil with allopurinol for recurrent or metastatic carcinoma of the uterine cervix: a Southwest Oncology Group trial. Gynecol Oncol 1990;37:354–358.

125. Weiss GR, Green S, Hannigan E, et al. A phase II trial of cisplatin and 5-fluorouracil with allopurinol for recurrent or metastatic carcinoma of the uterine cervix. A Southwest Oncology Group trial. Gynecol Oncol 1990;37:354–358.

126. Bonomi P, Blessing J, Ball H, et al. A phase II evaluation of cisplatin and 5-fluorouracil in patients

with advanced squamous cell carcinoma of the cervix: a Gynecologic Oncology Group study. Gynecol Oncol 1989;34:357–359.

127. Omura G, Hubbard J, Hatch K. Limited tolerance for high dose cisplatin plus doxorubicin after radiotherapy for female pelvic cancer: a Gynecologic Oncology Group pilot study. Am J Clin Oncol 1985; 8:347–349.

128. Fine S, Sturgeon J, Gospodarowicz M, et al. Treatment of advanced carcinoma of the cervix with methotrexate, adriamycin, cisplatin. Proc Am Soc Clin Oncol 1983;2:154.

129. Wheelock J, Krebs H, Goplerud D, Myers N. Cisplatinum, doxorubicin, and methotrexate for recurrent cervical cancer. Obstet Gynecol 1985;66:410–412.

130. Edmondson J, Johnson P, Wieand HS, et al. Phase II studies of bleomycin, cyclophosphamide, doxorubicin and cisplatin, and bleomycin and cisplatin in advanced cervical carcinoma. Am J Clin Oncol 1988; 11:149–151.

131. Chiara S, Consoli R, Falcone A, et al. Cisplatin and 5-fluorouracil in advanced and recurrent cervical cancer. Tumori 1988;74:471–474.

132. Cervellino JC, Araujo CE, Sanchez O, Miles H, Nishihama A. Cisplatin and ifosfamide in patients with advanced squamous cell carcinoma of the uterine cervix. Acta Oncol 1995;34:257–259.

133. Kuhnle H, Meerpohl H, Eiermann W, et al. Phase II study of carboplatin/ifosfamide in untreated advanced cervical cancer. Cancer Chemother pharmacol 1990;26:S33–S35.

134. Ramm K, Vergote I, Kaern J, Trope C. Bleomycin-ifosfamide-cisplatinum (BIP) in pelvic recurrence of previously irradiated cervical carcinoma: a second look. Gynecol Oncol 1992;46:203–207.

135. Tay SK, Lai FM, Soh LT, Ang PT, Au E. Combined chemotherapy using cisplatin ifosfamide and bleomycin (PIB) in the treatment of advanced and recurrent cervical cancer. Aust NZ J Obstet Gynecol 1993;32:263–266.

136. Buxton E, Meanwell C, Hilton C, et al. Combination bleomycin, ifosfamide, and cisplatin chemotherapy in cervical cancer. J Natl Cancer Inst 1989; 81:359–361.

137. Kumar L, Bhargava V. Chemotherapy in recurrent and advanced cervical cancer. Gynecol Oncol 1991;40:107–111.

138. Murad AM, Triginelli SA, Ribalta JCL. Phase II trial of bleomycin, ifosfamide, and carboplatin in metastatic cervical cancer. J Clin Oncol 1994;12:55–59.

139. Kredentser DC. Etoposide, ifosfamide/mesna, and cisplatin chemotherapy for advanced and recurrent carcinoma of the cervix. Gynecol Oncol 1991; 43:145–148.

140. Filtenborg TA, Hansen HH, Aage ES, Rorth M. A phase II study of ifosfamide, carboplatin and cisplatin in advanced and recurrent squamous cell carcinoma of the uterine cervix. Ann Oncol 1993;4:485–488.

141. Omura G, Blessing J, Vaccarello L, Berman M, Mutch D, et al. A randomized trial of cisplatin versus cisplatin + mitolactol versus cisplatin + ifosfamide in advanced squamous carcinoma of the cervix by the Gynecologic Oncology Group (abstract). Gynecol Oncol (in press).

142. Thigpen JT, Blessing JA, Fowler WC Jr, Hatch K. Phase II trials of cisplatin and piperazinedione as single agents in the treatment of advanced or recurrent non-squamous cell carcinoma of the cervix: a Gynecologic Oncology Group study. Cancer Treat Rep 1986; 70:1097–1100.

143. Slayton RE, Blessing JA, Homesley HD. Phase II trial of etoposide in the management of advanced or recurrent non-squamous cell carcinoma of the cervix: a Gynecologic Oncology Group study. Cancer Treat Rep 1984;68:1513–1514.

144. Stehman FB, Blessing JA, Homesley HD, et al. Phase II evaluation of dianhydrogalactitol in the treatment of advanced non-squamous cervical carcinoma: a Gynecologic Oncology Group study. Invest New Drugs 1984;2:331–333.

145. Homesley HD, Blessing JA, Berman M. ICRF-159 in patients with advanced nonsquamous cell carcinoma of the cervix: a Gynecologic Oncology Group study. Am J Clin Oncol 1986;9:325–326.

146. Muss HB, Bundy BN, Homesley HD, Wilbanks G. Mitoxantrone in the treatment of advanced non-squamous carcinoma of the cervix. Invest New Drugs 1987;5:199–202.

147. Slayton RE, Blessing JA, Rettenmaier M, Ball H. A phase Ii clinical trial of diaziquone in the treatment of patients with recurrent adenocarcinoma and adenosquamous carcinoma of the cervix: a Gynecologic Oncology Group study. Invest New Drugs 1989; 7:337–340.

148. Asbury RF, Blessing JA, DiSaia PJ, Malfetano J. Aminothiadiazole in patients with advanced nonsquamous carcinoma of the cervix: a phase II study of the Gynecologic Oncology Group. Am J Clin Oncol 1989;12:375–377.

149. Muss HB, Bundy BN, Given FT, Stehman FB. Teniposide in patients with non-squamous-cell carcinoma of the cervix: a phase II trial of the Gynecologic Oncology Group. Am J Clin Oncol 1990;13:117–118.

150. Sutton G, Blessing J, Anderson B, et al. Phase II trial of ifosfamide and mesna in patients with recurrent or advanced nonsquamous carcinoma of the cervix. Proc Am Soc Clin Oncol 1990;9:167.

151. Malfetano J, Blessing J, Homesley H. A phase II trial of gallium nitrate in nonsquamous cell carcinoma of the cervix. Am J Clin Oncol 1995;18:495–497.

152. Sinclair W. The combined effect of hydroxyurea and x-rays in Chinese hamster cells in vitro. Cancer Res 1968;28:198–206.

153. Hreshchyshyn M, Aron B, Boronow R, et al. Hydroxyurea or placebo combined with radiation to treat stages IIIB and IV cervical cancer confined to the pelvis. Int J Radiat Oncol Biol Phys 1979;5:317–322.

154. Piver S. Hydroxyurea and radiation therapy in the treatment of carcinoma of the cervix. In: Surwit E, Alberts D, eds. Cervix cancer. Boston: Martinus Nijhoff, 1987;107–118.

155. DiSaia P, Bundy B, Curry S, et al. Phase III study on the treatment of women with cervical cancer, stage IIB, IIIBm, and IVA (confined to the pelvis and/or periaortic nodes), with radiotherapy alone versus radiotherapy plus immunotherapy with intraveous *Corynebacterium parvum*: a Gynecologic Oncology Group study. Gynecol Oncol 1987;26:386–397.

156. Stehman F, Bundy B, Keys H, et al. A randomized trial of hydroxyurea versus misonidazole adjunct to radiation therapy in carcinoma of the cervix. Am J Obstet Gynecol 1988;159:87–94.

157. Stehman F. Personal communication.

158. The new FIGO stage grouping for primary carcinoma of the ovary (1985). Gynecol Oncol 1986; 25:383–385.

159. Hoskins WJ. Surgical staging and cytoreductive surgery of epithelial ovarian cancer. Cancer 1993; 71:1534–1540.

160. Omura G, Blessing J, Ehrlich C, et al. A randomized trial of cyclophosphamide and doxorubicin with or without cisplatin in advanced ovarian carcinoma. Cancer 1986;57:1725–1730.

161. Ehrlich C, Einhorn L, Williams S, et al. Chemotherapy for stage III-IV epithelial ovarian cancer with *cis*-dichlorodiammine-platinum (II), adriamycin, and cyclophosphamide: a preliminary report. Cancer Treat Rep 1979;63:281–288.

162. Greco F, Julian C, Richardson R, et al. Advanced ovarian cancer: brief intensive combination chemotherapy and second-look operation. Obstet Gynecol 1981;58:199–205.

163. Young R, Howser D, Myers C, et al. Combination chemotherapy (CHex-UP) with intraperitoneal maintenance in advanced ovarian adenocarcinoma. Proc Am Soc Clin Oncol 1981;22:465.

164. Gall S, Bundy B, Beecham J, et al. Therapy of stage III (optimal) epithelial carcinoma of the ovary with melphalan or melphalan plus *Corynebacterium parvum* (a Gynecologic Oncology Group study). Gynecol Oncol 1986;25:26–36.

165. van der Burg MEL, van Lent M, Buyse M, et al. The effect of debulking surgery after induction chemotherapy on the prognosis in advanced epithelial ovarian cancer. Gynecologic Cancer Cooperative Group of the European Organization for Research and Treatment of Cancer. N Engl J Med 1995;332:675–677.

166. Thigpen JT. Single agent chemotherapy in the management of ovarian carcinoma. In: Alberts DS, Surwit EA, eds. Ovarian carcinoma. Boston: Martinus Nijhoff, 1985;115–146.

167. Wiltshaw E, Kroner T. Phase II trial of *cis*-dichlorodiammineplatinum (II) (NSC-119875) in advanced adenocarcinoma of the ovary. Cancer Treat Rep 1976;60:55–60.

168. Thigpen T, Lagasse L, Homesley H, et al. Cisplatinum in the treatment of advanced or recurrent adenocarcinoma of the ovary: a phase II study of the Gynecologic Oncology Group. Am J Clin Oncol 1983; 6:431–435.

169. Kjorstad K, Bertelsen K, Slevin M, et al. Phase II trial of carboplatin in ovarian cancer. Proc Am Soc Clin Oncol 1986;5:116.

170. Pecorelli S, Bolis G, Vassena L, et al. Randomized comparison of cisplatin and carboplatin in advanced ovarian cancer. Proc Am Soc Clin Oncol 1988; 7:136.

171. Rozencweig M, Martin A, Beltangady M, et al. Randomized trials of carboplatin versus cisplatin in advanced ovarian cancer. In: Bunn P, Ozols R, Canetta R, et al., eds. Carboplatin (JM-8): current perspectives and future directions. Philadelphia: WB Saunders, 1990:175–186.

172. Rowinsky EK, Donehower RC, Jones RJ, Tucker RW. Microtubule changes and cytotoxicity in leukemic cell lines treated with taxol. Cancer Res 1988; 48:4093–4100.

173. McGuire WP, Rowinsky EK, Rosenshein NB, Grumbine FC, Ettinger DS, et al. Taxol: a unique antineoplastic agent with significant activity in advanced

ovarian epithelial neoplasms. Ann Intern Med 1989; 111:273–279.

174. Thigpen T, Blessing J, Ball H, Hummel S, Barrett R. Phase II trial of paclitaxel in patients with progressive ovarian carcinoma after platinum-based chemotherapy: a Gynecologic Oncology Group study. J Clin Oncol 1994;12:1748–1753.

175. Einzig IA, Wiernik PH, Sasloff J, et al. Phase II study and long-term follow-up of patients treated with taxol for advanced ovarian adenocarcinoma. J Clin Oncol 1992;10:1748–1753.

176. Kohn E, Sarosy G, Bicher A, et al. Dose-intense taxol: high response rate in patients with platinum-resistant recurrent ovarian cancer. J Natl Cancer Inst 1994;86:18–24.

177. Swenerton K, Eisenhauer E, ten Bokkel Huinink W, et al. Taxol in relapsed ovarian cancer: high vs low dose and short vs long infusion: a European-Canadian study coordinated by the NCI Canada Clinical Trials Group (abstract). Proc Am Soc Clin Oncol 1993; 12:810.

178. Rowinsky E, Mackey M, Goodman S. Meta-analysis of paclitaxel dose-response and dose-intensity in recurrent or refractory ovarian cancer (abstract). Proc Am Soc Clin Oncol 1996;15:284.

179. Omura G, Brady M, Delmore J, et al. A randomized trial of paclitaxel at 2 dose levels and filgastrim at 2 doses in platinum pretreated epithelial ovarian cancer: a Gynecologic Oncology Group, SWOG, NCCTG and ECOG study. Proc Am Soc Clin Oncol (in press).

180. Francis P, Schneider J, Hann L, et al. Phase II trial of docetaxel in patients with platinum-refractory advanced ovarian cancer. J Clin Oncol 1994;12:2301–2308.

181. Sutton GP, Blessing JA, Photopoulos G, Berman ML, Homesley HD. Gynecologic Oncology Group experience with ifosfamide. Semin Oncol 1990; 17(Suppl 4): 6–10.

182. Blum RH, Livingston RB, Carter SK. Hexamethylmelamine—a new drug with activity in solid tumors. Eur J Cancer 1973;9:195–202.

183. Manetta A, MacNeill C, Lyter JA, et al. hexamethylmelamine as a single second-line agent in ovarian cancer. Gynecol Oncol 1990;36:93–96.

184. Moore D, Fowler W, Jones C, Crumpler L. Hexamethylmelamine chemotherapy for persistent or recurrent epithelial ovarian cancer. Am J Obstet Gynecol 1991;165:573–576.

185. Vergote I, Himmelmann A, Frankendal B, et al. Hexamethylmelamine as second-line therapy for platin-resistant ovarian cancer. Gynecol Oncol 1992; 47:282–286.

186. Rosen G, Lurain J, Newton M. Hexamethylmelamine in ovarian cancer after failure of cisplatin-based multiple-agent chemotherapy. Gynecol Oncol 1987;27:173–179.

187. Hoskins P, Swenerton K. Oral etoposide is active against platinum-resistant epithelial ovarian cancer. J Clin Oncol 1994;12:60–63.

188. DeWit R, van der Burg M, van den Gaast A, et al. Phase II study of prolonged oral etoposide in patients with ovarian cancer refractory to or relapsing within 12 months after platinum-containing chemotherapy. Ann Oncol 1994;5:656–657.

189. Rose P, Blessing J, Mayer A, Homesley H. Prolonged oral eroposide as second line therapy for plat-

inum resistant and platinum sensitive ovarian carcinoma: a Gynecologic Oncology Group study (abstract). Proc Am Soc Clin Oncol 1996;15:282.

190. Lund B, Hansen O, Theilade K, et al. Phase II study of gemcitabine in previously treated ovarian cancer patients. J Natl Cancer Inst 1994;86:1530–1533.

191. Carmichael J, Gordon A, Malfetano J, et al. Topotecan, a new active drug, vs paclitaxel in advanced epithelial ovarian carcinoma: International Topotecan Study Group trial (abstract). Proc Am Soc Clin Oncol 1996;15:283.

192. Gordon A, Bookman M, Malmstrom H, et al. Efficacy of topotecan in advanced epithelial ovarian cancer after failure of platinum and paclitaxel: International Topotecan Study Group trial (abstract). In press in Proc Am Soc Clin Oncol 1996;15:282.

193. ten Bokkel Huinink W, Gore M, Bolis G, Verweij J, et al. A phase II trial of topotecan for the treatment of relapsed advanced ovarian carcinoma (abstract). Proc Am Soc Clin Oncol 1996;15:284.

194. Muggia F, Hainsworth J, Jeffers S, et al. Liposomal doxorubicin is active against refractory ovarian cancer (abstract). Proc Am Soc Clin Oncol 1996;15:287.

195. Hatch K, Beecham J, Blessing J, et al. Responsiveness of patients with advanced ovarian carcinoma to tamoxifen: a Gynecologic Oncology Group study of second-line therapy in 105 patients. Cancer 1991; 68:269–271.

196. Malfetano J, Beecham J, Bundy B, Hatch K. A phase II trial of medroxyprogesterone acetate in epithelial ovarian cancers. A Gynecologic Oncology Group study. Am J Clin Oncol 1993;16:149–151.

197. Omura G, Morrow P, Blessing J, et al. A randomized comparison of melphalan versus melphalan plus hexamethylmelamine versus adriamycin plus cyclophosphamide in ovarian carcinoma. Cancer 1983; 51;783–789.

198. Omura GA, Bundy BA, Berek JS, et al. Randomized trial of cyclophosphamide plus cisplatin with or without doxorubicin in ovarian carcinoma: a Gynecologic Oncology Group study. J Clin Oncol 1989; 7:457–465.

199. Gruppo Interegionale Cooperativo Oncologico Ginecologia. Randomized comparison of cisplatin with cyclophosphamide/cisplatin and with cyclophosphamide/doxorubicin/cisplatin in advanced ovarian cancer. Lancet 1987;2:353–359.

200. Bertelsen K, Jakobsen A, Andersen JE, et al. A randomized study of cyclophosphamide and cisplatinum with or without doxorubicin in advanced ovarian carcinoma. Gynecol Oncol 1987;28:161–169.

201. Conte P, Bruzzone M, Chiara S, et al. A randomized trial comparing cisplatin plus cyclophosphamide versus cisplatin, doxorubicin and cyclophosphamide in advanced ovarian cancer. J Clin Oncol 1986; 4:965–971.

202. Hernadi Z, Juhasz B, Poka R, Lampe L. Randomized trial comparing combinations of cyclophosphamide and cisplatinum without or with doxorubicin or 4-epi-doxorubicin in the treatment of advanced ovarian cancer. Int J Gynecol Obstet 1988;27:199–204.

203. Alberts DS, Green SJ, Hannigan EV, et al. Improved therapeutic index of carboplatin plus cyclophosphamide versus cisplatin plus cyclophosphamide: final report by the Southwest Oncology Group of a phase III randomized trial in stages III and IV ovarian cancer. J Clin Oncol 1992;10:706–717.

204. ten Bokkel Huinink WW, van der Burg MEL, van Oosterom AT, Neijt JP, George M, et al. Carboplatin in combination therapy for ovarian cancer. Cancer Treat Rev 1988;15(Suppl B):9–15.

205. Pater J. Cyclophosphamide/cisplatin versus cyclophosphamide/carboplatin in macroscopic residual ovarian cancer. Initial results of a National Cancer Institute of Canada Clinical Trials Group trial (abstract). Proc Am Soc Clin Oncol 1990;9:155.

206. Edmondson JH, McCormack GM, Wieand HS, et al. Cyclophosphamide-cisplatin versus cyclophosphamide-carboplatin in stage III-IV ovarian carcinoma: a comparison of equally myelosuppressive regimens. J Natl Cancer Inst 1989;81:1500–1504.

207. Skipper H. Dose intensity versus total dose of chemotherapy: an experimental basis. In: De Vita VT Jr, Hellman S, Rosenberg S, eds. Important advances in oncology. Philadelphia: JB Lippincott, 1990:43–64.

208. Levin L, Hryniuk W. Dose intensity analysis of chemotherapy regimens in ovarian carcinoma. J Clin Oncol 1987;5:756–767.

209. Levin L, Simon R, Hryniuk W. Importance of multiagent chemotherapy regimens in ovarian carcinoma: dose intensity analysis. J Natl Cancer Inst 1993; 85:1732–1742.

210. McGuire WP, Hoskins WJ, Brady MF, Homesley H, Clarke-Pearson DI. A phase III trial of dose intense versus standard dose cisplatin and cytoxan in advanced ovarian cancer. Proc Am Soc Clin Oncol 1992;11:226.

211. Colombo N, Pittelli M, Parma G, et al. Cisplatin dose intensity in advanced ovarian cancer: a randomized study of conventional dose versus dose-intense cisplatin monochemotherapy. Proc Am Soc Clin Oncol 1993;12:255.

212. Kaye S, Lewis C, Paul J, et al. Randomized study of two doses of cisplatin with cyclophosphamide in epithelial ovarian cancer. Lancet 1992;340:329–333.

213. Rothenberg M, Ozols R, Glatstein E, et al. Dose-intensive induction therapy with cyclophosphamide, cisplatin, and consolidative abdominal radiation in advanced-stage epithelial ovarian cancer. J Clin Oncol 1992;10:727–734.

214. Ozols RF, Ostchega Y, Curt G, Young RC. High-dose carboplatin in refractory ovarian cancer patients. J Clin Oncol 1987;5:197–201.

215. Alberts DS, Young L, Mason NL, et al. In vitro evaluation of anticancer drugs against ovarian cancer at concentrations achievable by intraperitoneal administration. Semin Oncol 1985;12(Suppl):38–42.

216. Markman M, Reichman B, Hakes T, et al. Responses to second-line cisplatin-based intraperitoneal therapy in ovarian cancer: influence of a prior response to intravenous cisplatin. J Clin Oncol 1991;9:1801–1805.

217. Alberts D, Liu P, Hannigan E, et al. Phase III study of intraperitoneal cisplatin/intravenous cyclophosphamide vs IV cisplatin/IV cyclophosphamide in patients with optimal disease stage III ovarian cancer: a SWOG-GOG-ECOG intergroup study (abstract). Proc Am Soc Clin Oncol 1995;14:273.

218. McGuire WP, Hoskins WJ, Brady MF, et al. Cyclophosphamide and cisplatin compared with paclitaxel and cisplatin in patients with stage III and stage IV ovarian cancer. N Engl J Med 1996;334:1–6.

219. Rowinsky E, Gilbert M, McGuire W, et al. Sequences of taxol and cisplatin: a phase I and pharmacologic study. J Clin Oncol 1991;9:1691–1703.

220. Young R, Walton L, Decker D, et al. Early stage ovarian cancer: preliminary results of randomized trials after comprehensive initial staging. Proc Am Soc Clin Oncol 1983;2:148.

221. Thigpen JT, Blessing JA, Vance RB, Lambuth BW. Management of patients with stage I and II ovarian carcinoma. In: Proceedings of the Perugia International Cancer Conference II: recent advances in the treatment of testicular and ovarian cancer. New York: LP Communications, 1990:41–49.

222. Bolis G, Colombo N, Favalli G, et al. Randomized multicenter clinical trial in stage I epithelial ovarian cancer. Proc Am Soc Clin Oncol 1992;11:225.

223. Thigpen T, Vance R, Khansur T. Second-line chemotherapy for recurrent carcinoma of the ovary. Cancer 1993;71:1559–1564.

224. Gershenson DM, Malone JM Jr. Chemotherapy for malignant germ cell tumors of the ovary. In: Deppe G, ed. Chemotherapy of gynecologic cancer. 2nd ed. New York: Wiley-Liss, 1990:217–239.

225. Slayton RE, Park RC, Silverberg SG, Shingleton H, Blessing JA. Vincristine, dactinomycin and cyclophosphamide in the treatment of malignant germ cell tumors of the ovary: a Gynecologic Oncology Group study (a final report). Cancer 1985;56: 243–248.

226. Williams S, Blessing J, Slayton R, Homesley H, Photopoulos G. Ovarian germ cell tumors: adjuvant trials of the Gynecologic Oncology Group (GOG). Proc Am Soc Clin Oncol 1989;8:150.

227. Williams SD, Blessing JA, Moore DH, Homesley HD, Adcock L. Cisplatin, vinblastine, and bleomycin in recurrent ovarian germ cell tumors: a trial of the Gynecologic Oncology Group. Ann Intern Med 1989;3:22–27.

228. Goldstein DP, Berkowitz RS. Staging system for gestational trophoblastic tumors. J Reprod Med 1984;29:792–795.

229. Surwit EA, Alberts DS, Christian CD, Graham VE. Poor-prognosis gestational trophoblastic disease: an update. Obstet Gynecol 1984;64:21.

230. World Health Organization Scientific Group on Gestational Trophoblastic Disease. Gestational Trophoblastic Diseases, Technical Report Series #692. Geneva: World Health Organization, 1983.

231. Lurain JR. Chemotherapy of gestational trophoblastic disease. In: Deppe G, ed. Chemotherapy of gynecologic cancer. 2nd ed. New York: Wiley-Liss, 1990;273–301.

232. Homesley HD, Blessing JA, Rettenmaier M, Capizzi RL, Major FJ, Twiggs LB. Weekly intramuscular methotrexate for nonmetastatic gestational trophoblastic disease. Obstet Gynecol 1988;72:413–418.

233. Hammond CB, Borchert LG, Tyrey L, Creasman WT, Parker RT. Treatment of metastatic trophoblastic disease: good and poor prognosis. Am J Obstet Gynecol 1973;115:451–457.

234. Li MC, Whitmore WF Jr, Golbey R, Grabstald H. Effects of combined drug therapy on metastatic cancer of the testis. JAMA 1960;174:1291–1299.

235. Surwit EA, Hammond CB. Treatment of metastatic trophoblastic disease with poor prognosis. Obstet Gynecol 1980;55:565–570.

236. Bagshawe KD. Treatment of trophoblastic tumors. Recent Results Cancer Res 1977;62:192–199.

237. Curry SL, Blessing JA, DiSaia PJ, Soper JT, Twiggs LB. A prospective randomized comparison of methotrexate, dactinomycin, and chlorambucil versus methotrexate, dactinomycin, cyclophosphamide, doxorubicin, melphalan, hydroxyurea, and vincristine in poor prognosis metastatic gestational trophoblastic disease: a Gynecologic Oncology Group study. Obstet Gynecol 1989;73:357–362.

238. Bagshawe KD. Treatment of high-risk choriocarcinoma. J Reprod Med 1984;29:813–820.

239. Grumbine FC, Rosenshein NB, Brereton HD, Kaufman SL. Management of liver metastases from gestational trophoblastic neoplasia. Am J Obstet Gynecol 1980;137:959.

240. Athanassiou A, Begent RHJ, Newlands ES, Parker D, Rustin GJS, Bagshawe KD. Central nervous system metastases of choriocarcinoma: 23 years' experience at Charing Cross Hospital. Cancer 1983; 52:1728–1735.

241. Ausman JI, Levin VA, Brown WE, Rall DP, Femstermacel JD. Pharmacological principles derived from a monkey brain-tumor model. Brain tumor chemotherapy. J Neurosurg 1977;46:155–164.

242. Lurain JR, Brewer JI, Torok EE, Halpern B. Gestational trophoblastic disease. Treatment results at the Brewer Trophoblastic Disease Center. Obstet Gynecol 1982;60:354–360.

59

Chemotherapy of Sarcomas of Bone and Soft Tissue

Haralambos Raftopoulos and Karen H. Antman

Bone and soft tissue sarcomas currently represent 1% of adult malignancies and 15% of pediatric malignancies (1). Currently, there are 8070 newly diagnosed sarcomas and approximately 4880 deaths per year in the United States (2).

The predominant histologic type of sarcoma varies within different age groups (3). Embryonal rhabdomyosarcoma has a peak incidence in the orbit in 4 year olds and in the urinary tract in adolescence (4). Osteosarcoma has a biphasic pattern of incidence, with peaks in adolescents and again in the elderly, associated with Paget's disease or arising in prior radiotherapy ports (5). Ewing's sarcoma and synovial sarcoma typically develop between ages 15 and 30, while other sarcomas such as liposarcoma and leiomyosarcoma occur in middle age. Malignant fibrous histiocytoma (MFH) and chondrosarcoma generally arise in patients over age 55.

The principal sex affected differs within histologic variants. For example, 70% of patients with Kaposi's sarcoma are men, as are 58 to 62% of those with liposarcoma and embryonal rhabdomyosarcomas, while 65% of leiomyosarcomas occur in women. While the incidences of osteosarcoma by age in whites and nonwhites are virtually superimposable, for unknown reasons Ewing's sarcoma is predominantly a disease of Caucasians (5).

Etiology

About 5% of sarcomas are associated with prior radiotherapy, generally delivered 4 to 20 years prior to the diagnosis of sarcoma (5). Most radiation-associated sarcomas are osteosarcomas, but mixed mesodermal sarcomas of the uterus, mesotheliomas, and most other soft tissue sarcomas have been reported (6–9). The risk of a secondary sarcoma after radiation exposure has been quite low in most studies, except for patients with a prior diagnosis of retinoblastoma or Ewing's sarcoma or radium dial painters (5, 9). Sarcomas arising in radiation ports have been reported to respond less well to chemotherapy (10).

Chemical exposures have resulted in sarcomas. Sarcomas have also been causally associated with alkylating agents (particularly melphalan, procarbazine, nitrosoureas, and chlorambucil) given for prior childhood malignancies (9). Asbestos clearly causes mesothelioma (11). Polyvinyl chloride (plastic industries), androgens, and arsenic exposure, as well as iron overload (hemochromatosis), are associated with angiosarcoma of the liver (12). Dioxin (agent orange) exposure and agricultural herbicide use are associated with the development of soft tissue sarcomas and lymphomas in some, but not other, trials (13–15).

Immunosuppressed patients (because of prior renal transplantation, AIDS, chronic lymphocytic leukemia, or even autoimmune hemolytic anemia) have a higher than expected risk of developing soft tissue sarcomas, particularly Kaposi's sarcoma. Paget's disease of bone is associated with a 0.2% risk of developing osteosarcoma (16).

A viral etiology of sarcomas is well documented in other species (murine, simian, and avian sarcomas viruses). Circulating immune complexes in patients with sarcoma and their relatives suggest a viral etiology (17); however, there is no known causal association between viruses and human sarcomas. Kaposi's sarcoma commonly develops in patients with HIV (AIDS) and cytomegalovirus (CMV) infections, but in these settings, the sarcoma may result from the underlying immunosuppression (18). Recently, Lee et al. (19) and McClain et al. (20) have shown strong associations between the Epstein-Barr virus and the development of leiomyosarcomas in patients with AIDS and following organ transplantation, respectively.

Fibrosarcomas, particularly, have developed in scars of prior burns or major trauma, often after intervals of 30 years or more (3).

Genetics

Genetic conditions have been associated with the development of sarcoma. Children with familial retinoblastoma have about a 7% incidence of osteosarcoma 21, 22). Osteosarcomas carry a 13q⁻ chromosomal deletion originally observed in retinoblastoma (21, 22). These tumors develop both in radiation ports used for treatment of the initial retinoblastoma and in long bones clearly outside prior radiotherapy ports, thus suggesting a hereditary susceptibility to osteosarcoma (9). The deletion suggests the lack of a tumor suppressor gene (*RB*), and the role of the *RB* gene product in carcinogenesis.

Patients with neurofibromatosis have a 7 to 10% lifetime risk of developing a malignant sarcoma, generally histologically a neuro- or fibrosarcoma (23). (About half of all neurofibrosarcomas develop in patients with neurofibromatosis.) The neurofibromatosis gene (*NF-1*) is thought to be involved in the regulation of p21^{ras}. Those with familial or sporadic osteochondromas or fibrous dysplasia of bone develop osteosarcomas or chondrosarcoma within the preexisting lesion (5).

The identification of families with childhood sarcomas, breast cancer, and other tumors (Li-Fraumeni syndrome) was first described in 1969 (24). More than 50 kindreds have now been identified, and germ line *p53* mutations have been implicated (25).

A characteristic translocation between chromosome 11 and 22, seen in both Ewing's sarcoma and peripheral neuroectodermal tumors (PNETs) (26), is not merely of academic interest. PNETs, originally treated rather unsuccessfully on protocols for neuroblastoma, are currently treated more successfully with regimens for Ewing's sarcoma. The translocation results in the formation of a chimeric protein (EWS-FLI-1) with the characteristics of an aberrant transcription factor (27).

Synovial sarcomas (t(X;18)), alveolar rhabdomyosarcomas (t(2;13)), and myxoid liposarcomas (t(12;16)) are some further examples of sarcomas with characteristic cytogenetic abnormalities. The literature on additional abnormalities, as well as the elucidation of the molecular sequelae of such changes continues to expand (28, 29).

Classification

Sarcomas (fleshy tumors) were distinguished from carcinomas (crablike tumors) in antiquity. The term *sarcoma* is constructed from the Greek root *sarc* (flesh), as are sarcasm and sarcophagus. Most sarcomas develop in tissues of mesodermal embryologic origin and are thus related embryologically to leukemias and lymphomas. (Neurosarcomas, peripheral neuroectodermal tumors, and probably Ewing's sarcomas, however, arise from tissues of ectodermal embryologic origin.)

Sarcomas originating in bone are distinguished from those that derive from soft tissue. The most common sarcomas of bone are osteosarcoma, Ewing's sarcoma, and chondrosarcoma. Soft tissue sarcomas are further separated into the "classic" soft tissue sarcomas of trunk and extremities and the visceral sarcomas arising in the gastrointestinal (30) and gynecologic tracts (31). Miscellaneous sarcomas include Kaposi's sarcoma and mesotheliomas.

SARCOMAS OF BONE AND CARTILAGE

Bone lesions may be benign or malignant. Some benign lesions have the potential for malignant transformation. Primary malignant lesions (which arise de novo) and secondary malignancies (those arising from a prior benign tumor) must be distinguished from metastases. Radiographs of a lesion can help distinguish benign from malignant lesions and, in some cases, can suggest the histologic origin.

Osteosarcoma

The most common sarcoma of bone (and except for myeloma, the most common primary malignancy of bone), osteosarcoma is defined as a primary malignancy of bone that produces osteoid (3). About 900 new cases occur per year in the United States. The ratio of men to women affected is 1.5 to 2:1. The age distribution is bimodal, with the first peak in the second and third decades and the second in the sixth decade (5). Osteosarcoma classically arises in growth plates (i.e., around the epiphyses) of long bones during the adolescent growth spurt. Adolescent patients are taller than age-matched controls in some studies, and osteosarcoma is also found in large breeds of dogs (32).

In the second peak in incidence in older patients, osteosarcoma tends to develop in previously irradiated sites or in existing benign bone lesions such as pagetoid bone, solitary osteochondromas, or multiple enchondromatosis (Ollier's disease). The risk of sarcoma is 0.2% in patients with Paget's diseases. Axial lesions occur in less than 10% of pediatric patients but in 30 to 50% of adults. Extraosseous presentations are rare but occur in older adults.

Patients present with severe pain of relatively short duration, often with a firm-to-hard mass, stretched, shiny overlying skin, and prominent vascular markings. Patients with prior chronic radium ingestion such as watch dial painters (and occasionally those lacking any known risk factors, usually children under age 10) have developed multicentric osteosarcomas.

Patients with possible osteosarcoma should be referred to an institution with an experienced sarcoma service. In suspected cases, expert multimodal consultation is essential prior to biopsy. Radiographs, scans, and computerized tomography (CT) scans of primary lesions reveal osteolysis and periosteal new bone formation and late cortical destruction. Periosteal elevation may produce the classic "Codman's triangle" on x-ray. Slight, moderate, or densely sclerotic ossification transversing or radiating through an extracortical soft tissue extension may result in a characteristic "sunburst" appearance. A baseline angiogram may delineate the extent of invasion, define the vascular anatomy for limb-sparing surgery, and allow later evaluation of any response to preoperative chemotherapy (32).

STAGING AND DIAGNOSIS

Staging evaluation includes x-rays and CT of the primary and CT of the lungs to detect pulmonary metastases, the most likely site of metastases. Bone scans generally demonstrate intense uptake within the lesion and may detect skip lesions of bone, metastases, or a multicentric primary; uptake in the lungs suggests early pulmonary lesions. The generally elevated alkaline phosphatase level (except in very undifferentiated osteosarcoma) is of prognostic value. Ele-

vated values after amputation predict residual or relapsing disease (32).

The biopsy should be performed by the surgeon who will do the definitive resection. If the radiologic picture is virtually "diagnostic," a needle biopsy may be adequate to confirm the clinical diagnosis. An improperly placed biopsy, particularly of proximal tibial lesions, may render subsequent limb-sparing surgery impossible and may substantially compromise local control.

The formation of malignant osteoid is required for a histologic diagnosis of osteosarcoma. Osteosarcomas are further divided into osteoblastic (45% of cases), chondroblastic (27%), anaplastic (17%), fibroblastic (9%), and telangiectatic (1%) variants. Most authors have shown little prognostic value for the histologic subclassifications, although tumor grade appears to correlate with survival (32).

Superficial, low-grade variants (juxtacortical or parosteal osteosarcoma) are relatively uncommon (3 to 4% of osteosarcomas), arise equally in both sexes, and tend to affect adults (about a decade later than patients with high-grade osteosarcoma) with no prior risk factors. Grossly, these bulky tumors encircle the cortex of bone (generally, the distal femur; less commonly, the proximal humerus). Radiologically, the differential diagnosis includes osteochondroma and myositis ossificans (32).

PRIMARY THERAPY
Adjuvant Chemotherapy

Based on a consistent 20% 5-year disease-free survival of surgically treated patients, early adjuvant chemotherapy trials documented significantly improved disease-free survivals of 50 to 80%, compared with historic controls. However, the Mayo Clinic data from 1963 to 1974 demonstrated an improved disease-free survival for sequential cohorts of patients treated with surgery only: from 13%, for patients treated 1963 to 1968, to 42%, for 1972 to 1974, prompting the design of randomized trials (33).

Three small randomized trials have subsequently compared two- to six-drug chemotherapy regimens with observation (Table 59.1). In the Mayo Clinic study, adjuvant vincristine and high-dose methotrexate given after surgery did not significantly improve disease-free survival over observation alone (34). The Pediatric Oncology Group (POG) (35–37) and UCLA studies (38), however, showed a significantly improved 2-year disease-free survival after five- and six-

Table 59.1. Randomized Adjuvant Chemotherapy Trials in Osteosarcoma with an Observation Control Arm[a]

		Observation			Chemotherapy			
Institution	Regimen	No.	%DFS	%S	No.	%DFS	%S	p
Mayo Clinic	MV	18	44	62	20	40	80	NS
POG	MABCDP	18	11		18	61		<.001
UCLA	MABCD	28	39	65	27	59	86	.005

[a]M, high-dose methotrexate; P, cisplatin; V, vincristine; A, doxorubicin; C, cyclophosphamide; B, bleomycin; D, actinomycin D; DFS, disease-free survival; S, survival (2–5 years); NS, not significant; POG, Pediatric Oncology Group; UCLA, University of California at Los Angeles.

Table 59.2. Randomized Adjuvant Chemotherapy Trials in Osteosarcoma Assessing the Role of High-Dose Methotrexate[a]

		Drugs		% DFS		%S	
Institution	No.	1	2	1	2	1	2
EORTC	198	DPM	DP	41	57	64	50
Ontario	120	DM	D, M	49	53	NA	NA
CCSG	166	DM	Dm	40	40	NA	NA
Bologna	103	PM	P	78	62	NA	NA
CALGB	89	DM	D	40	52	57	82
Mayo Clinics	38	VM	Observation	40	43	52	55

[a]NA, not available; D, doxorubicin; P, cisplatin; m, moderate-dose methotrexate; M, high-dose methotrexate.

drug adjuvant regimens, respectively, and the UCLA study also demonstrated a significantly prolonged survival. Based on these randomized trials, doxorubicin- and cisplatin-based adjuvant chemotherapy is now accepted as standard treatment.

The optimal combination of agents and schedule is not yet established, however, one randomized trial has demonstrated an advantage for high-dose over standard-dose methotrexate (39,40), while five other trials show no advantage for high-dose methotrexate (Table 59.2). Two demonstrate a significant advantage for the group that received no methotrexate (41–43). Three other studies show no difference between the high-dose methotrexate arm and either low-dose (44) or no methotrexate (34) or delayed high-dose methotrexate (45). Because the dose rates of the other drugs were different, it is not possible to draw definitive conclusions from these data. The role of cyclophosphamide, bleomycin, and actinomycin D have not yet been defined.

Preoperative chemotherapy has many theoretical advantages over postoperative adjuvant chemotherapy. Early systemic treatment may more effectively eradicate microscopic metasta-

tic deposits. The response to preoperative chemotherapy can be evaluated histologically, and the regimen can be modified if the response is suboptimal. Patients with necrosis of more than 90% of the tumor in the resected specimen after preoperative chemotherapy have a significantly better survival. For patients with less than 90% tumor necrosis, switching to other effective agents postoperatively may increase the disease-free survival to 40%. Because resolution of tumor vascularity on angiography appears to correlate with histologic necrosis, following the angiogram to maximize the response prior to surgery may be reasonable (46).

Preoperative chemotherapy may facilitate limb-sparing surgery, allowing preservation of muscle groups and better limb function. The delay in surgery also allows procurement of the correct size internal prosthesis. Because of the potential for an increased local or distant failure rate for the few patients with a poor response to therapy, patients receiving preoperative chemotherapy require regular evaluation and prompt resection if response is suboptimal.

Preoperative chemotherapy delivered intra-arterially should provide a higher concentration of active drug to the tumor bed (38). However, the technique is technically time consuming, is associated with substantial toxicity, and has not been proven superior to the same agent given intravenously. UCLA investigators have demonstrated that preoperative intraarterial chemotherapy and postoperative intravenous chemotherapy results in a significantly improved survival, compared with preoperative therapy alone. The M. D. Anderson Hospital team has observed that intraarterial cisplatin is superior to intravenous high-dose methotrexate and that intraarterial cisplatin may also cause less vasculitis than intraarterial doxorubicin (47).

Osteosarcoma tends to be markedly radioresistant. Radiotherapy alone has not been shown to improve the rate of successful limb-sparing surgery or to decrease the risk of local recurrence for close or positive surgical margins. However, when given with doxorubicin, 3500 cGy preoperatively significantly increased the local complication rate compared with 1750 cGy (38).

Surgical Treatment

Either amputation or limb-sparing surgery may be appropriate. Lesions must be widely excised with several centimeters of pathologically documented uninvolved margins. Thus, patients with a significant soft tissue component or neurovascular involvement generally require amputation. Osteosarcomas arising in sites of prior Paget's disease or irradiation tend to be difficult to resect for cure due to their usual central location and vascularity. Combination chemotherapy and local resection are currently being studied in patients with borderline resectable lesions.

Limb-sparing surgery tends to be more successful for upper extremity lesions (because of the lack of weight bearing and dependent edema) and fully grown patients. Limb-length disparity resulting from surgery in childhood can be partially averted by the use of prostheses with a screw for lengthening the device every year. While functional results after limb-sparing procedures are excellent in 60 to 75% of patients, relapse or treatment complications may require later amputation. Fractures remain an important complication in active individuals (38). In appropriately selected patients, local control rates (90 to 97%) and survival are similar to those with amputation (38, 46).

Metastatic Osteosarcoma

Relapses tend to occur early, usually in the first 2 years after completion of primary therapy.

Major prognostic variables include grade and invasion through the bone cortex to involve soft tissue.

Metastases most frequently develop in lung and, less commonly, in bone. Combination chemotherapy and surgical resection should be considered for metastatic pulmonary nodules, particularly if there are five or fewer lesions and a disease-free interval of more than 12 months. Between 20 and 40% of these patients can be cured.

Most patients who develop metastases have already received a two- to six-drug adjuvant regimen. Readministration of the same drugs might achieve palliation if the metastases appeared 6 months or longer after the last adjuvant treatment. Active single agents include 60 to 90 mg/m^2 doxorubicin (responses in 39 of 183; response rate, 21%); 3 to 12 g/m^2 methotrexate with leucovorin rescue (58 of 97; 30 to 40%); 100 mg/m^2 cisplatin (12 of 48; 25%), and 5 to 10 g/m^2 ifosfamide (13 of 46; 28%). Cyclophosphamide, dacarbazine (DTIC), melphalan, and mitomycin C all have response rates of 15%. Patients who fail while receiving adjuvant therapy are candidates for phase II studies because significant palliation with standard agents is unlikely.

Ewing's Sarcoma

Ewing's sarcoma includes 10 to 14% of primary malignant bone tumors in whites but is rare in blacks (5). The incidence of Ewing's sarcoma peaks between ages 10 and 25 years (range, 2 to 65 years), with a 2:1 male:female ratio. Both Ewing's sarcoma and osteosarcoma occur in the same sex and age group, but they can usually be distinguished radiographically and histologically (5). Patients present with fever, weight loss, malaise, poorly localized bone pain, and a rapidly enlarging mass. Leukocytosis and an elevated erythrocyte sedimentation rate mimic osteomyelitis. Flat bones and the diaphyses of long bones are generally involved, with a prominent soft tissue component. The most common sites include femur (27%), pelvis (18%), and tibia and fibula (17%). Diagnosis of Ewing's sarcoma involving the pelvic bones is frequently delayed because of poorly localized pain and a clinically inapparent mass (32).

A primitive, small blue cell tumor of bone, cells in Ewing's sarcoma are arranged in clusters bordered by fibrous septa. In contrast to lymphoma, the reticulin stain outlines clusters of cells (32). The periodic acid–Schiff (PAS) diastase stain demonstrates large quantities of glycogen, also visible on electron microscopy. Cytogenetics reveal an 11:22 translocation in some cases, similar to that found in PNETs, suggesting a possible neurogenic origin of Ewing's sarcoma (26).

X-ray films and a CT scan of the primary and lungs are helpful in evaluating Ewing's sarcoma. Radiographically, Ewing's sarcoma forms a fusiform enlargement of the long bones, with "onion-skin" layering of the periosteum and central mottling ("cracked ice" appearance). A bone marrow aspirate and biopsy and a bone scan are also necessary for staging.

Clinically detectable metastases are present in about one-third of patients at diagnosis, most frequently in the lung, bone, bone marrow, and vertebrae (commonly leading to cord compression). However, Ewing's sarcoma is generalized at presentation, even in patients with no detectable metastases, as evidenced by a 90% mortality after surgical resection alone.

Current multimodality treatment results in cure of about 70% of children under 10 years of age with localized disease and about a third of children with metastases. Initial treatment consists of combination chemotherapy with doxorubicin, vincristine, and cyclophosphamide or ifosfamide prior to, and concurrent with, radiotherapy to the involved bone. Although dose schedules of other combinations vary, the Intergroup Ewing Sarcoma Study used 1.5 mg/m^2 vincristine per weeks 1 to 6 and 8 to 13; actinomycin D, 0.015 mg/kg daily, days 1 to 5 every 12 weeks; cyclophosphamide, 600 mg/m^2/ week; and doxorubicin, 30 mg/m^2 daily, days 1 to 3 every 3 weeks. Doxorubicin has significantly improved survival in randomized trials.

Radiotherapy of 6000 cGy to the primary (begun during the fourth or fifth cycle of chemotherapy) controls local disease in 70% of patients with good functional results. But because of the high local failure rate, expendable bones (rib, tibia, etc.) are sometimes resected rather than radiated. Resection seems particularly appropriate if Ewing's sarcoma arises in an expendable bone or if biopsy after radiotherapy and chemotherapy reveals residual viable tumor.

Survival rates correlate inversely with age (70% for patients <10 years old vs. 46% for those >16 years). Pelvic, humeral, and rib primaries carry a poor prognosis, as do a high lactate dehydrogenase (LDH), extensive soft tissue involvement, or metastases.

Surgical resection of pulmonary metastases has not been particularly useful in Ewing's sar-

coma. Areas of investigation for patients with a poor prognosis at diagnosis include the use of a standard induction regimen followed by high-dose chemotherapy with autologous bone marrow support.

Chondrosarcoma

Chondrosarcomas are the second most common sarcoma of bone, accounting for 17 to 22% of primary malignant tumors of bone (32). Rare extraskeletal chondrosarcomas arise totally within soft tissue. Primary chondrosarcomas occur in previously normal bone, while secondary chondrosarcomas arise in prior benign lesions, generally enchondromas. Malignant degeneration in patients with multiple enchondromatosis (Ollier's disease) generally results in low-grade tumors, while those in patients with associated soft tissue hemangiomas (Maffucci's disease) are frequently high grade. Chondrosarcomas comprise about a tenth of radiation-associated sarcomas and may arise in bone involved by Paget's disease.

The incidence of chondrosarcomas increases steadily with age (5). The most common sites of involvement are pelvis (31%), femur (21%), shoulder (13%), face (9%), and ribs (9%). Lesions can be painless or, if painful, rapidly increasing in size.

Radiographically, peripheral chondrosarcomas tend to have long, slightly calcified spicules radiating from the cortex to a flattened outer surface, with little evidence of cortical or medullary involvement and a faint "Codman's triangle" caused by lipping of the periosteum. Central chondrosarcomas have "popcorn"-shaped calcification. Bone scans generally demonstrate intense uptake within the lesion (32).

Chondrosarcomas are defined as malignant stromal tumors of bone that produce cartilage (but no osteoid). Grossly they have translucent, bluish white mucoid surfaces, with reactive new bone formation or cortical destruction. Histologically, the tumors have the appearance of cartilage with malignant chondrocytes. Low histologic grade is less reliable than patient age, site of origin, lesion size, and x-ray appearance in determining biologic behavior.

Histologic variants include mesenchymal chondrosarcoma, which tends to arise in the ribs, mandible, maxilla, skull, and in extraskeletal sites and is characterized by a small round cell histologic component and some sensitivity to chemotherapy (32).

Because chondrosarcomas are relatively resistant to both radiotherapy and chemotherapy and local recurrences tend to increase with histologic aggressiveness (48), they should be adequately resected at the time of diagnosis. Aggressive resection, particularly of eminently curable low-grade chondrosarcomas, is appropriate.

Giant Cell Tumor of Bone (Osteoclastoma)

The incidence of giant cell tumors, which constitute 5% of primary tumors of bone, peaks in the third decade, although patients range in age from 5 to 73 years. Half are located around the knee, arising in the distal femur, patella, or proximal tibia or fibula, occasionally associated with active Paget's disease. Fifty-five percent are women (32)

Radiographically, these tumors are generally eccentrically situated epiphyseal lesions with a central lucency and increasing density toward the periphery (with no new bone formation in actively growing lesions).

Grossly, the giant cell tumors may appear solid despite a cystic appearance on x-ray. Microscopically, prominent multinucleated giant cells are dispersed between well-vascularized stromal cells with nuclei identical to those in the giant cells. Large areas of dense collagen and prominent stroma with relatively few giant cells suggest malignant behavior.

Most patients require multiple therapeutic interventions before the disease is successfully eradicated. The prognosis of these tumors is often difficult to predict. A recurrence rate of 50% or more has been reported after curettage. While less than 10% are fully malignant on first presentation, after multiple recurrences up to 30% assume a malignant behavior. Sarcomatous transformation develops an average of 9 years after initial treatment and may be related to prior radiotherapy (32).

Other Bone Sarcomas

Fibrosarcoma, chordoma, angiosarcomas, and malignant fibrous histiocytomas (MFHs) of bone are less responsive to chemotherapy and are generally treated in the same way as soft tissue sarcomas.

SARCOMAS OF SOFT TISSUE

Soft tissue sarcomas are found in all age groups. Orbital rhabdomyosarcomas peak in in-

cidence in 4 year olds. MFH is the most common sarcoma in adults over 50 years old (3).

Patients usually present with a solitary, painless, palpable mass on the extremities or trunk. Forty percent of soft tissue sarcomas are found in the lower extremity, about 30% arise in the trunk and retroperitoneum, and 15% each in the upper extremity and head and neck. Intraabdominal and retroperitoneal primaries cause symptoms related to invasion or displacement of organs, weight loss, and pain. The duration of symptoms prior to diagnosis ranges from a few weeks to decades, with a median of 1 to 3 months.

Preoperative evaluation generally requires CT of the lungs and either a CT, or preferably nuclear magnetic resonance imaging, of the primary lesion for extent of involvement. If the lesion abuts bone, a bone scan may be helpful to determine if there is periosteal invasion or reaction. (Uptake does not document involvement and may only indicate reaction.) An incisional biopsy is generally optimal to allow multimodality consultation prior to the definitive resection.

The behavior and treatment of the histologic variants of soft tissue sarcoma as a group are generally similar grade for grade. The major exceptions of embryonal rhabdomyosarcoma, Kaposi's sarcoma, and mesothelioma are discussed elsewhere.

The goal of the treatment of soft tissue sarcomas is to achieve local control and to treat metastases (generally subpleural) if they are present. Wide excision (3 to 6 cm of normal tissue) is optimal, particularly for abdominal or low-grade lesions, to avoid the need for radiotherapy. Limb-sparing surgery is appropriate if uninvolved margins are documented pathologically and if adequate radiotherapy (6.6 Gy) can be delivered. Careful pathologic examination of the margins is essential to document adequate resection and the location of any involved margins for further resection.

Grading and Staging

A summary of the American Joint Committee staging system for soft tissue sarcomas (Table 59.3) is largely dependent on grade, based largely on the number of mitoses per 10 high power microscopic fields (1). Although the original series, based on 1215 patients from 13 university centers, observed a poor survival (26%) for high-grade primary lesions, more recent ad-

Table 59.3. Staging Schema for Soft Tissue Sarcomas

Stage	Grade	Comments	5-Year Survival % Patients treated 1954–1965
1	Low	<1 mitosis/10 HPF[a]	76
2	Intermediate	1–4 mitoses/10 HPF	56
3	High	>5 mitoses/10 HPF	26
4 A	Lymph node involvement		
4 B	Metastases		4
Grades 1–3	Lesion size:	A<5 cm B>5 cm	

Data from Russell WO, Cohen J, Enzinger FM, et al. A clinical and pathologic staging system for soft tissue sarcomas. Cancer 1977;40:1562–1570.
[a]HPF, high power microscopic field.

juvant studies have observed survivals of 50 to 70% for patients on the observation control arm. The 5-year survival rate for soft tissue sarcomas arising in various anatomic sites is similar when corrected for grade, except for intraabdominal and retroperitoneal tumors, which tend to be large and to have invaded vital organs.

Pathology

The gross appearance of soft tissue sarcomas is not particularly distinctive, although their microscopic appearance varies with their histologic origin. Soft tissue sarcomas are usually pseudoencapsulated fleshy tumors that grow along histologic planes, thus requiring wide excision (3 to 6 cm of normal tissue) for local control in the absence of radiotherapy. Low-grade tumors will push aside contiguous structures; high-grade tumors have prominent areas of necrosis with invasion of adjacent organs. Because of microscopic projections of tumor beyond the apparent "capsule," local recurrence follows a "shelling out" procedure in about 80% of cases.

Histologically, since osteosarcomas, rhabdomyosarcomas, and Ewing's sarcoma are treated routinely with combined-modality therapy including chemotherapy, it is most important to distinguish these from other sarcomas. The treatment of mesothelioma and Kaposi's sarcoma are also quite different from that of the classic sarcomas. Once these are excluded, the most important pathologic parameters are tumor grade, the extent of the surgical margins (and location

of any close margin), the size of the gross lesion in the unfixed pathology specimen, and the histologic type, in that order.

MALIGNANT FIBROUS HISTIOCYTOMA

MFH is the most common soft tissue sarcoma in patients aged 50 to 70 (3). The male:female ratio is 2:1. Deep lesions have a substantial likelihood of developing local recurrences and metastases, but histologically identical lesions that occur in the skin carry an excellent prognosis. Characterized in 1963 as a tumor with a storiform or cartwheel growth pattern mixed with pleomorphic areas, MFH is currently felt to be derived from cells of fibroblastic origin (based on immunohistochemical stains). An uncommon inflammatory variant is associated with fever, a high sedimentation rate, and a neutrophilia or eosinophilia resulting from a tumor-produced growth factor (49). Symptoms characteristically resolve if the tumor can be resected, and the prognosis for patients with a marked inflammatory infiltrate may be somewhat better. Myxoid lesions grow more slowly and behave somewhat less aggressively but are characterized by a substantial local failure rate, thus justifying wide local excision and radiotherapy or amputation. While initially described as having a higher propensity to involve lymph nodes than the approximately 10% reported for other sarcomas, lymph node involvement in larger, more recent series has ranged from 4 to 17% (3).

LIPOSARCOMA

The second most common soft tissue sarcoma in adults, liposarcomas vary considerably in behavior, ranging from low-grade well-differentiated and myxoid liposarcomas to high-grade round cell and pleomorphic liposarcomas. Most develop singly in the thigh or retroperitoneum, but some may be multicentric, particularly in the abdominal cavity and retroperitoneum. They rarely, if ever, arise from benign lipomas. Patients are generally in their sixth decade at diagnosis, with 55 to 60% of liposarcomas affecting men (3).

Histologically, almost half are myxoid liposarcomas, characterized by lipoblasts, branching thin-walled capillaries, and a myxoid matrix. Poorly differentiated myxoid liposarcomas comprised of small, round cells have an aggressive clinical course despite a paucity of mitotic activity. Well-differentiated liposarcomas are deceptively similar to lipomas histologically but vary more in cellular size and shape and may contain dedifferentiated areas or may be dedifferentiated in metastatic lesions. Inflammatory and sclerosing variants have been described. Pleomorphic liposarcomas are characterized by the presence of large giant cells, which may contain lipid droplets and frequent mitoses (3).

FIBROSARCOMA

Fibrous tumors range from benign encapsulated fibromas through locally invasive but borderline lesions such as fibromatosis and Dupytren's contracture to highly malignant sarcomas. Fibrosarcomas were formerly quite common; however, many lesions classified as fibrosarcomas in the past are now considered MFHs, spindle cell carcinomas, malignant schwannomas, or melanomas. Fibrosarcomas tend to originate from inter- and intramuscular fibrous tissue, fascia tendons, and aponeuroses. Males predominate (3).

SYNOVIAL SARCOMA

Synovial sarcomas develop predominantly in adolescents and young adults (median age 27) and are somewhat more common in men. A mass has often been present for more than a year. It arises most often in the extremities adjacent to a joint (particularly around the knee), involving the joint capsule, bursae, and tendon sheath but not the joint itself. Unlike other localized soft tissue sarcomas, only about half of synovial sarcomas cause pain or tenderness (3). One-third of these tumors contain calcification on x-ray, with fine stippling or even radiopaque tumor. Periosteal proliferation or invasion is less common. Histologically, synovial sarcomas are monophasic or biphasic, comprised of one or both epithelial and spindle cell components. Limb-sparing surgery is difficult because of the proximity and frequent fixation of this tumor to large joints.

NEUROSARCOMA

Comprising 5% of soft tissue sarcomas, malignant schwannomas differ from other sarcomas in that they arise from tissues of ectodermal embryologic origin. About half of neurosarcomas develop in patients with von Recklinghausen's neurofibromatosis (23). Pain or the sudden enlargement of a preexisting mass in a patient with neurofibromatosis should prompt immediate biopsy.

Because neurosarcomas tend to develop and extend for some distance within major nerve sheaths (resulting in a large fusiform mass along the nerve), they generally are found in the proximal extremity or trunk, and larger surgical and radiotherapy margins are required to ensure local control (3).

VASCULAR SARCOMAS

Malignancies of vascular endothelium, like their benign counterparts, may produce microangiopathic hemolytic anemia (Kasabach-Merritt syndrome), presumably as a result of traumatic injury of red blood cells traversing the tumor bed.

Hemangioendothelioma

These relatively rare vascular tumors of intermediate malignancy (between benign hemangiomas and conventional angiosarcomas) affect men and women about equally and rarely develop in childhood. The epithelioid variant differs from benign epithelioid hemangioma in that the vascular cells are more primitive with indistinct vascular channels (small intracellular lumina that occasionally contain erythrocytes). If the tumor contains areas with more than one mitosis per 10 high powered fields or significant necrosis, the course may be more aggressive. A spindle cell variant that occurs in younger patients, predominantly males, principally involves the skin of the hand and tends to be locally and regionally recurrent (3).

Angiosarcomas

These rare lesions (1% of sarcomas), described in the older literature under a variety of names, include tumors previously called hemangiosarcoma, lymphangiosarcoma, and hemangioblastoma, since immunoperoxidase stains suggest the same cell of origin.

One-third arise in the skin (e.g., as multicentric scalp lesions in elderly men or in edematous extremities, typically after mastectomy and lymph node dissection for breast cancer). A fourth each develop in soft tissue and in organs such as breast, liver, heart, and lungs. Angiosarcomas of the breast occur in young and middle-aged women (50), and those of the liver arise in adults previously exposed to thorium dioxide (for angiography), arsenic (insecticides), and vinyl chloride (plastics) (4). Angiosarcomas have also arisen in sites of prior radiotherapy (for breast cancer, Hodgkin's disease, cervical cancer, and others) and at the site of a foreign body or prior herpes zoster infection and are the most common primary malignant tumors of the myocardium (51).

Grossly, angiosarcomas of the skin appear to be single or, in half of the cases, clusters of bruises. Angiosarcomas in deeper locations have the consistency of a sponge rather than a distinct mass. Tumors infiltrate substantially beyond their apparent extent. Immunoperoxidase studies for factor VIII are rather variable; binding of the lectin Ulex europaeus is more common but less specific (3).

Even well-differentiated angiosarcomas metastasize widely and can be difficult to control locally (due to multifocality and extensive invasion). The prognosis is poor.

Kaposi's Sarcoma

The presentation of the classic variant is the development of multiple blue-red flat skin lesions that progress in an indolent manner to nodules and plaques up the lower legs in elderly men, particularly those of Mediterranean origin. These lesions generally respond to radiotherapy or low doses of vinblastine, doxorubicin, or α-interferon (52). Secondary tumors, especially lymphomas, are common.

A second form occurs in about 0.4% of renal transplant patients a mean of 16 months after the transplant, again more commonly in men of Mediterranean extraction. Kaposi's sarcoma may respond to a decreased immunosuppressive regimen.

A third aggressive variant of lymphadenopathic Kaposi's sarcoma of young children is endemic in some locations in Africa.

A highly aggressive Kaposi's sarcoma involving the mucous membranes of the mouth, stomach, lungs, skin, and lymph nodes is associated with acquired immune deficiency syndrome (AIDS) in homosexuals, but rarely in transfusion-associated AIDS. Coexistent opportunistic infections portend a short survival. α-Interferon or chemotherapy may palliate lesions in appropriate patients (18).

Hemangiopericytoma

Generally diagnosed in the fifth decade, hemangiopericytoma is a malignancy of vascular pericytes (normally found adjacent to the blood vessel endothelium, the cell of origin of angiosarcomas and hemangioendotheliomas). Thirty-five percent are found in the thigh and 25% in the retroperitoneum, often in a perirenal location, where these large tumors can be associated with substantial arterial venous shunting, bleeding, and even hypoglycemia. Intracranial hemangiopericytomas, formerly designated angio-

blastic meningiomas, grow along the sinuses, locally recur, and may metastasize. Dilated "antler" or "staghorn" configurations of anastomosing vascular channels are lined by a single layer of flattened endothelial cells. Surrounding tumor cells do not stain for factor VIII or Ulex europaeus lectin as do angiosarcomas (3).

COMMON SARCOMAS OF MUSCLE

Leiomyosarcoma

Derived from malignant smooth muscle, leiomyosarcomas are the most common soft tissue sarcoma in series that include sarcomas of the gastrointestinal (GI) tract and uterus. The median age of affected patients is 60 years. Of GI tract sarcomas, 62% occur in the stomach, but only 3% of gastric malignancies are sarcomas (30). Twenty-nine percent arise in the small bowel (20% of small intestinal malignancies) and 10% in the colon (0.1% of colorectal neoplasms). Patients with GI or uterine leiomyosarcomas present with life-threatening bleeding or pain. Distinctive upper GI series findings often suggest the diagnosis prior to histologic confirmation. Metastases develop in more than half of the patients with intraperitoneal seeding, liver metastases, and lung nodules (30). An epithelioid leiomyosarcoma, characterized by rounder, vacuolated (clear cell) features has also been called leiomyoblastoma. Gastric epithelioid leiomyosarcoma, functioning extraadrenal paragangliomas, and pulmonary hamartomas (chondromas) are recognized as a distinct triad (Carney's triad). Pulmonary lesions must be biopsied prior to the use of chemotherapy in these patients to establish the diagnosis (3).

Leiomyosarcomas of the retroperitoneum and the vena cava occur most commonly in women, and their growth may exacerbate during pregnancy. Tumors originating in other large veins affect men and women equally. Cutaneous and subcutaneous leiomyosarcomas generally affect men; perhaps because of their superficial location and small size at diagnosis, they carry a good prognosis. Multiple cutaneous leiomyosarcomas, however, should suggest metastases from an occult retroperitoneal or intraabdominal primary.

Rhabdomyosarcoma

Derived from striated muscle, rhabdomyosarcomas include embryonal, alveolar, and pleomorphic variants. The peak incidence for embryonal rhabdomyosarcomas of the orbit is age 4 years and for those of the GI tract, childhood and adolescence. Alveolar rhabdomyosarcomas arise most commonly in the extremities of adolescents and young adults and carry a more serious prognosis.

The disease is systemic at diagnosis, as evidenced by the 80% development of disseminated disease in the absence of chemotherapy despite local control. Patients are generally treated with combination chemotherapy including vincristine, actinomycin, and cyclophosphamide or ifosfamide. Doxorubicin is also frequently included. Lymph node metastases are common. Resection is followed by regional radiotherapy. While children with metastatic disease sometimes can be cured, the prognosis in adults, even with localized disease, is poor despite even excellent responses to primary aggressive chemotherapy (53).

While pleomorphic rhabdomyosarcomas are occasionally diagnosed, generally in older patients, they are frequently reinterpreted as MFHs when reviewed by a more experienced pathologist.

Primary Treatment

If preoperative evaluation reveals no evidence for metastasis on chest CT, the primary therapy for all localized soft tissue sarcomas (with the notable exceptions of rhabdomyosarcoma and Kaposi's sarcoma) is surgery. Wide excision (>3 cm of pathologically documented normal tissue) is optimal to avoid the need for radiotherapy. Should resection margins be pathologically uninvolved but less than 3 cm (generally a deep margin or one adjacent to a major nerve or bone), radiotherapy should be considered to increase the chance for local control without the need for amputation.

While many retroperitoneal and head and neck primaries are unresectable at presentation, superficial trunk lesions are frequently completely resectable. For extremity lesions, a combined-modality approach may be feasible, which would allow conservative (often limb-sparing) surgery preceded or followed by radiotherapy, without increasing the risk of locoregional recurrence (54, 55). The current standard of either limb-sparing surgery and radiotherapy or radical resection (often amputation) at experienced centers has dramatically improved the local control of soft tissue sarcomas from about 20% prior to 1950 to 90 to 95% for extremity lesions, 50 to 75% for trunk, but only 30–50% for retroperito-

neal primaries. Low-grade lesions with adequate local therapy are generally cured; thus, ensuring adequate local control is especially important.

RANDOMIZED ADJUVANT CHEMOTHERAPY TRIALS FOR SOFT TISSUE SARCOMA

Adjuvant chemotherapy is currently established in the treatment of rhabdomyosarcomas, osteosarcomas, and Ewing's sarcomas, but remains unproven in other adult soft tissue sarcomas.

The risks of adjuvant chemotherapy are not currently warranted in patients with low-grade lesions, given their low probability of metastatic spread. Initial pilot studies in adult soft tissue sarcomas comparing patients receiving adjuvant chemotherapy with historic controls were promising, with large statistically significant differences observed. However, as the survival of the control arms in subsequent randomized studies has been significantly better than that of historic controls, only randomized studies with nontreatment control arms are included in this analysis. (Table 59.4) Because surgical salvage of pulmonary metastases or recurrent local disease is possible in some patients, disease-free survival may be a less meaningful endpoint than overall survival.

Of the 12 reported adjuvant studies, only 2 (one from the Rizzoli Center in Bologna (56) and the other from the Foundation Bergonie in Bordeaux) show a significant overall survival advantage for chemotherapy. One study (European Organization for Research in the Treatment of Cancer (EORTC)) demonstrated a significant improvement in local control for adjuvant chemotherapy but no overall survival benefit (57). Subset analyses in two additional studies (from M. D. Anderson Hospital (58, 59) and the National Cancer Institute (NCI) (60)) currently indicate a significant disease-free survival advantage for adjuvant chemotherapy in extremity lesions but no significant improvement in survival. (While the NCI reported a significantly prolonged survival for the subset of chemotherapy-treated extremity primaries on initial reports (61–66), survival is no longer significantly different, due to late relapses (60). In the subset analysis of the same NCI study for retroperitoneal sarcomas, the survival of the control group is superior to the treatment group. Of the 12 randomized trials, the survival of the observation arm exceeds that of the chemotherapy arm in 3 studies (Mayo Clinic, Eastern Cooperative Oncology Group

Table 59.4. Randomized Adjuvant Trials in High Grade Soft Tissue Sarcomas[a]

Institute	Drugs	N	% DFS −	% DFS +	% DFS p	% S −	% S +	% S p
EORTC (57, 67, 68)								
	ACVD	468	43	56	.007	56	63	NS
Extremities		**233**	**64**	**64**	**NS**	**55**	**42**	**NS**
Bordeaux (69)								
	ACVD	59	16	57	<.01[b]	53	87	<.01
Extremities		**36**	**NA**	**NA**	**NA**	**NA**	**NA**	**NA**
Mayo Clinic (78, 79)								
	AVDAd	61	68	65	NS	70	70	NS
Extremities		**48**	**67**	**88**	**.08**	**83**	**63**	**NS**
MD Anderson (58, 59)								
	ACVAd	47	83	76	NS	NA	NA	NS
Extremities		**43**	**35**	**54**	**<.05**	**46**	**65**	**NS**
NCI (60–66, 70–72)								
	ACM							
non ext/non retroperitoneal		31	49	77	.075	58	68	NS
Trunk		22	47	92	<.01	61	82	NS
Retroperitoneal		15	NA	NA	NA	100	47	.06[c]
Extremities		**67**	**28**	**54**	**<.05**	**60**	**54**	**NS**
Scandinavia (81)								
	A	181	56	62	NS	70	75	NS
Extremities		**155**	**NS**	**NS**	**NS**	**NS**	**NS**	**NS**
Pooled DFCI/MGH, ISSG, ECOG (82)								
	A	168	53	66	NS	65	68	NS
Extremities		**72**	**64**	**79**	**NS**	**70**	**79**	**NS**
GOG (80)								
	A	156	47	59	NS	52	60	NS
UCLA (88)								
Extremities	A	**119**	**54**	**56**	**NS**	**74**	**78**	**NS**
Rizzoli (56, 87)								
Extremities	A	**77**	**45**	**73**	**<.05**	**70**	**91**	**<.05**

Modified with permission from Mazanet R, Antman KH. Sarcomas of soft tissue and bone. Cancer 1991;68:463–473.
[a]Abbreviations: DFS, disease-free survival; S, survival; −, without chemotherapy; +, with chemotherapy; EORTC, European Organization for the Research and Treatment of Cancer; DFCI/MGH, Dana Farber Cancer Institute/Massachusetts General Hospital; ISSG, Intergroup Sarcoma Study Group; ECOG, Eastern Cooperative Oncology Group; GOG, Gynecologic Oncology Group; UCLA, University of California at Los Angeles; NCI, National Cancer Institute; A, doxorubicin; V, vincristine; Ad, actinomycin D; C, cyclophosphamide; D, dacarbazine; NA, not available; NS, not significant.
[b]Authors reported metastatic-free survival.
[c]2-year survival inferior in chemotherapy arm.

(ECOG), Scandinavian study). Doxorubicin-associated cardiotoxicity has occurred in about 10% of treated patients, occasionally contributing to treatment-related deaths. Based on these data, adjuvant chemotherapy should be considered investigational for adult soft tissue sarcomas of any primary site.

European Organization for Research in the Treatment of Cancer (EORTC)

This largest study randomized 468 patients between observation versus CYVADIC (cyclophosphamide, vincristine, doxorubicin, and DTIC) given every 4 weeks (57, 67, 68). With a median follow-up of 80 months, there was no

significant difference between the observation and the chemotherapy arms in overall survival (56 vs. 63%). Disease-free survival (DFS) was superior for CYVADIC compared with controls (56 vs. 43%, $p = .007$), and local control of nonextremity lesions was significantly improved (22 vs. 12%) by chemotherapy.

Foundation Bergonie, Bordeaux

In a smaller study (59 patients) using identical doses of CYVADIC (initiated within 4 weeks of surgery and delivered every 3 weeks) followed for a median of 52 months, there was a significant advantage for chemotherapy in local recurrence rate (3 vs. 18%; $p = .03$), metastases-free suvival (16 vs. 57%; $p = .0003$), and overall survival (87 vs. 53%; $p = .002$). It is difficult to interpret this study because of its small size, an imbalance in histologies on the two arms, and an initial significant imbalance of patients with extremity primaries on the chemotherapy arm (69).

M. D. Anderson Hospital in Houston

Lindberg and colleagues randomized 47 patients with stage IIB and IIIB lesions (stratified for histology, but not for grade or size) to observation versus doxorubicin 60 mg/m², vincristine, and cyclophosphamide for seven cycles followed by the substitution of doxorubicin with actinomycin D for 18 months total therapy. An initial report at 18 months median follow-up reported unacceptable toxicity and poorer disease-free survival (76 vs. 83%) and survival for chemotherapy, presumably because of the imbalance of large high-grade lesions on this arm (grade III: 4/20 vs. 9/27; size >8 cm: 9/20 vs. 21/27; for observation vs. chemotherapy, respectively). However, with 10-year follow-up, the subset with extremity lesions on the chemotherapy arm had a significantly better disease-free survival, with a trend toward improved survival (DFS, 54 vs. 35%; survival, 65 vs. 36%, respectively) (58, 59).

National Cancer Institute (NCI)

Patients with sarcomas arising in both extremity and nonextremity sites were randomized to observation versus doxorubicin 50 to 70 mg/m² (550 mg/m² cumulative dose) and cyclophosphamide 500 to 700 mg/m² followed by 6 monthly cycles of 50 to 250 mg/kg of methotrexate with leucovorin rescue. In subset analysis, disease-free survival and initially survival of patients receiving chemotherapy for extremity primaries were significantly improved ($p < .01$) at a median follow-up of 5 years. However, with 2 additional years follow-up, there remains a difference in disease-free survival ($p = .04$), but survival is no longer significantly different ($p = .12$). An unexplained imbalance in patient numbers between the two arms suggests a problem with the randomization procedure or with exclusions; 41% of the chemotherapy group had distal lesions (forearm or below knee), compared with 25% of the control group. One-sided p values are used (60–66, 70).

In subset analysis of the 31 patients with truncal and head and neck primaries, there was a trend to a delay of recurrence, but no difference in survival. Of the 22 patients with trunk lesions,

12 received chemotherapy with a prolonged time to recurrence (3-year actuarial disease-free survival: 92 vs. 47%); however, survival was not significantly altered (82 vs. 61%). Of 15 patients with retroperitoneal primaries, however, the 2-year survival was inferior in the chemotherapy arm (100 vs. 46%; $p = .06$). Two patients developed cardiac toxicity, two developed cyclophosphamide cystitis, and three had severe bone marrow suppression (71, 72).

Fourteen percent of patients on the NCI trial developed clinical doxorubicin-associated congestive heart failure. An additional 56% had abnormal cardiac function on noninvasive testing after therapy (73). Up to 18% of patients withdrew from the study because of gastrointestinal and hematologic toxicity. The response rates for high-dose methotrexate and cyclophosphamide as single agents are low, and their contribution to doxorubicin-containing regimens in the metastatic setting have been minimal (60, 74–77).

Mayo Clinic

Sixty-one patients were randomized to observation versus eight cycles of doxorubicin, vincristine, and actinomycin D postoperatively. Radiotherapy was not given to the primary lesion, perhaps explaining the 28% local recurrence rate. Of 30 chemotherapy-treated patients, 3 required thoracotomy for pulmonary metastases, compared with 17 of 31 on the observation arm. Of the 48 patients with extremity lesions, 16 of 24 untreated patients remained disease-free (67%) compared with 21 of 24 (88%) of the treated patients at a median follow-up of 64 months ($p = .08$). However, survival was 82% for both study arms at 5 years because of aggressive salvage surgery and the deaths of several patients in the chemotherapy arm without relapse. Patients entered after first local failure had a higher subsequent local relapse rate but a similar rate of metastatic events and survival (78, 79).

Gynecologic Oncology Group (GOG)

International Federation of Gynecology and Obstetrics (FIGO) stage I and II uterine sarcomas were randomized after hysterectomy (stratified by stage and by prior radiotherapy) to doxorubicin 60 mg/m² versus observation for eight cycles. Of 225 patients entered, 156 patients were evaluable. No significant difference was observed between treatment groups. With a minimum follow-up of 24 months, disease-free and overall survivals were 47% and 42% for the observation arm, and 59% and 45% for the chemotherapy arm. Although pelvic radiotherapy reduced vaginal recurrences, overall survival and freedom from relapse remained unaffected. Single-agent doxorubicin had a 16% response rate in a prior GOG study in metastatic uterine sarcoma (80).

Scandinavia

Of 240 patients with high-grade excised soft tissue sarcomas randomized to either observation or 60 mg/m² doxorubicin every 4 weeks for nine cycles, 181 patients were evaluable. With a median of 40 months follow-up, the disease-free survival and survival were 56% and 70% for the observation arm, and 62% and 75% for the treatment arm, respectively. Local control was 92% in either arm following radical surgery alone or 88% for lesions marginally resected with postoperative radiotherapy. The conclusions were the same if all patients or only evaluable patients were analyzed. Tumor size greater than 5 cm and male sex were negative prognostic factors (81).

Pooled Studies

Three studies of adjuvant doxorubicin have been pooled for analysis: Intergroup Sarcoma Study Group (ISSG), Dana-Farber Cancer Institute/Massachusetts General Hospital (DFCI/MGH), and the Eastern Cooperative Oncology Group (ECOG) (82).

The ISSG began a trial in 1983 comparing six cycles of doxorubicin 35 mg/m²/day for 2 days versus observation. Of the 92 entered, 86 patients with stage IIB-IVA primaries stratified by size, grade, type of local therapy, and site of disease were available for analysis. No significant difference has been detected so far. Of the 41 patients receiving doxorubicin, 3 have developed congestive heart failure (83).

In the DFCI/MGH study, 46 stage IIB-IVA patients were stratified for stage, surgical margins, and primary size. Patients were randomized to five cycles of doxorubicin 90 mg/m² versus no further treatment. Doxorubicin was given entirely postoperatively at the DFCI. At the MGH, two cycles of doxorubicin were given preoperatively, and three cycles were given postoperatively. Of the 21 doxorubicin-treated patients, 2 developed congestive heart failure (84–86). At a median follow-up of 5 years, no significant difference in overall or disease-free survival was observed.

ECOG randomized 47 patients with stage IIB-IVA sarcoma between 7 cycles of 70 mg/m²

doxorubicin versus observation; 36 were eligible, the remainder were cancelled or ineligible, mostly due to staging errors (85, 86). There were no significant differences.

ADJUVANT TRIALS INITIALLY LIMITED TO EXTREMITY LESIONS

The survival of patients with even high-grade extremity lesions is currently 50 to 80% at various centers, and thus it is increasingly difficult to show a statistically significant difference in randomized adjuvant trials. More patients are required to show small differences, and a substantial fraction of patients who would not have relapsed without therapy are exposed to potential cardiotoxicity.

Instituto Ortopedico Rizzoli, Bologna

Of a total of 187 eligible patients with high-grade extremity lesions, 77 agreed to be randomized to six cycles of doxorubicin (total of 450 mg/m²) versus observation. Stratifications were age, site of primary, size, and stage. Local therapy consisted of radical surgery alone (28 patients); two cycles of doxorubicin 25 mg/m²/day for 3 days, 45 Gy preoperatively, followed by conservative surgery (29 patients); or reexcision for local recurrence (20 patients) with 45 Gy delivered postoperatively to the 10 with microscopic or gross residual disease. With a median follow-up of 28 months (range, 12–75), 20 of 44 (45%) in the observation arm and 24 of 33 (73%) in the chemotherapy arm remain disease free (p < .02) (3-year actuarial DFS, 42 vs. 68%; p < .05). Overall survival is 70% (31 of 44) and 91% (30 of 33) on the observation and control arms, respectively (3-year actuarial survival, 68 vs. 86%; p < .05). There was no difference in local control in the two arms (84 vs. 88%, respectively). The authors concluded that adjuvant doxorubicin seemed to increase both disease-free and overall survival in patients with resectable high-grade extremity soft tissue sarcomas (56, 87).

University of California at Los Angeles (UCLA)

Of 119 patients with grade III extremity sarcomas entered, 90% were greater than 5 cm in size. All received preoperative intraarterial doxorubicin and 17.5 Gy of local radiotherapy. Following limb-sparing surgery, patients were randomized to receive observation versus doxorubicin (45 mg/m²/day for 2 days every 4 weeks) for five cycles. Local recurrence occurred in 10%. With a median follow-up of 28 months,

Table 59.5. Commercially Available Agents in Soft Tissue Sarcoma by Class

	Author	References	Cases	% RR[a]			mg/m²
Anthracyclines							
Doxorubicin	**Total**		356	26			
	Blum	(98)	130	34			60–90 q 3 week
	O'Bryan et al.	(94)	49	31			60–75 q 3 week
	O'Bryan et al.	(93)	82	28			25–70 q 3 week
	Schoenfeld	(77)	66	27			70 q 3 week
	Borden et al.	(97)	93	19			70 q 3 week
	Borden et al.	(97)	92	16			15 q week
	Cruz et al.	(95)	15	13			20–25/day × 3 q week
Antimetabolites							
Methotrexate high-dose	**Total**		76	13			
	Rosen et al.	(117)	1	1/1			8,000/week
	Vaughan et al.	(118)	14	14			5–12,000/2 weeks
	Isacoff and Eilber	(119)	6	17			1.5–10,000
	Karakousis et al.	(120)	18	5			2–4,000/week
	Von Hoff et al.	(121)	26	20			Review
	Frei et al.	(122)	9	0/9			2–10,000/1–4 weeks
Methotrexate standard-dose	**Total**		81	21			
	Andrews	(123)	19	10			
	Subramanian	(124)	41	37			
	Buesa	(125)	21	0			
Bleomycin	Amato	(126)	32	6			
Actinomycin D	Golbey	(127)	30	17			
5-Fluorouracil	Gold	(128)	8	12			
Vincas							
Vincristine	**Total**		103	12			
	Selawry	(129)	15	40			
	Korbitz	(130)	7	0			
Etoposide	**Total**		40	8			
	Radice	(131)	34	6			
	Bleyer	(132)	6	16			
Alkylating Agents							
Ifosfamide (in adults by dose per course)							
High dose							
Elias (109, 133)	DFCI		20	35	2.5–4.5	1–4	10–18
Klein (134)			11	33	2.5–3.5	1–5	12–17
Chawla (135)			28	39	2.0	1–6	14.0
Czownicki (136)			13	38	1.25–2.5	1–5	12.5
Niederle (137)			57	46	1.6–2.5	1–5	12.5
Standard dose							
Antman (105)	DFCI		124	23	2.0–2.5	1–4	8–10
Wiltshaw (114)	Royal Marsden		67	24	5 or 8	1	8.0
Sutton (138)					1.5	1–5	7.5
Mixed mesodermal sarcoma	GOG		26	31			
Bramwell (75)	EORTC		68	18	5.0	d1	5.0
In children							
Pratt (139)	St. Jude's		24	33	1.6	1–5	8.0
Jurgens (140)	Dusseldorf				2	1–5	10
Ewing's			8	63			
Magrath (110, 141)	NCI		46	30	1.8	1–5	9.0
Ewing's			20	45			
Rhabdomyosarcoma			9	22			
Osteosarcoma			17	18			

Table 59.5—*continued.* Commercially Available Agents in Soft Tissue Sarcoma by Class

	Author	References	Cases	% RR[a]	mg/m²
Dacarbazine (DTIC)					
	Rosenberg	(65)	109	16	
	Buesa	(142)	44	18	
Cisplatin	**Total**		103	12	
	Bramwell	(143)	17	0	
	Karakousis	(144)	13	23	
	Samson	(145)	42	7	
	Thigpen	(146)	19	5	
	Budd	(147)	40	15	200 mg/m²
	Gershenson	(148)	12	42	GYN only
Carboplatin	Goldstein	(149)	50	12	3 CRs
Cyclophosphamide	**Total**		82	8	
	Bergsagel	(74)	12	16	
	Korst	(150)	3	0	
	Bramwell	(75)	67	8	

Updated with permission from Chang A, Rosenberg SA, Glatstein E, Antman K. Sarcomas of soft tissue. In: DeVita VT, Hellman S, Rosenberg SA, eds. Cancer principles & practice of oncology. 4th ed. Philadelphia: JB Lippincott, 1993:1436–1488.
[a]% RR, percent response when the denominator includes at least 10 cases.

there is no significant difference in disease-free or overall survival between the observation and chemotherapy arms (52 vs. 56% and 70 vs. 80%, respectively) (88).

There have been two randomized trials of two different preoperative or adjuvant chemotherapy schedules. One from UCLA compared intra-arterial and intravenous doxorubicin. End points were feasibility of limb salvage (98 vs. 100%, respectively), local recurrence (7 vs. 8%), incidence of complications (18 vs. 10%), and median tumor necrosis (70 vs. 60%) (89).

In the second study, 87 adults with extremity sarcomas treated at Memorial Sloan-Kettering Cancer Center in New York City received continuous infusion versus bolus doxorubicin. While fewer patients receiving continuous infusion had a decrease of more than 10% in ejection fraction (42 vs. 61% for bolus infusion), survival status was superior for those receiving bolus doxorubicin (90).

Therapy for Advanced Soft Tissue Sarcomas

RESECTION OF PULMONARY METASTASES

Resection of subpleural metastases in carefully selected patients results in disease-free survival in about 20% of patients. Patients with relatively slowly growing lesions (doubling time >20 days), a disease-free interval longer than 12

months, and fewer than five nodules have the best prognosis. Repeated thoracotomies in selected patients, if additional nodules appeared, rendered 72% of 43 such patients again disease free. Prolonged survival was associated with a disease-free interval of at least 18 months from prior thoracotomy (91).

A combined-modality approach (chemotherapy prior to resection) has yet to be evaluated in a randomized trial (92).

COMMERCIALLY AVAILABLE SINGLE AGENTS (TABLE 59.5)

Doxorubicin (Adriamycin) is the most active single agent in soft tissue sarcomas, with a response rate of 15 to 35% in various studies (77, 93–98). A dose-response relationship has been observed in nonrandomized trials (93, 94) and in combination with other agents in randomized trials (77, 99, 100), with dose rates of 60 to 70 mg/m² every 3 weeks generally superior to dose rates of 50 mg/m² or less.

Dacarbazine (DTIC) has a single-agent response rate of 16% and is particularly active in leiomyosarcomas. Nausea may be decreased by continuous infusion administration.

Ifosfamide is a cyclophosphamide analogue with one chloroethyl group shifted to the ring nitrogen atom. Preclinical and human phase I and II trials for sarcomas, lymphoma, and small cell lung cancer have shown an apparent lack of cross-resistance with cyclophosphamide (101–104). Ifosfamide has documented activity in patients with sarcoma who have failed doxorubicin-containing regimens (75, 105–115). Mesna is required for bladder protection and, in a randomized trial, was superior to N-acetylcysteine in preventing hematuria (116).

Investigational agent studies are shown in Table 59.6. Carminomycin is the only tested drug with a response rate above 20%.

RANDOMIZED CHEMOTHERAPY TRIALS IN ADVANCED SOFT TISSUE SARCOMAS

Most of the large randomized cooperative group studies report response rates of 17 to about 30%. The median survival in these trials is about 12 months, with no differences in survival generally observed (Table 59.7).

An improved response rate may be particularly important in the management of borderline resectable lesions, particularly in younger patients likely to tolerate the myelosuppression. Response might facilitate subsequent surgery and radiation to render the patient free of detectable disease. The role of chemotherapy before surgical resection of pulmonary nodules needs further exploration.

The addition of DTIC to doxorubicin has been evaluated in three randomized trials. The GOG and the ECOG evaluated doxorubicin as a single agent versus doxorubicin and DTIC (97, 218, 219). The response rate was higher for the combination in both studies, significantly in the ECOG study. In the third SWOG study, patients received doxorubicin, cyclophosphamide, and vincristine with either DTIC or actinomycin D. The DTIC-containing arm was significantly more active (220).

In contrast, SWOG, ECOG, and GOG studies evaluated the addition of cyclophosphamide to a doxorubicin-containing regimen, each showing no advantage for the addition of cyclophosphamide (76, 77, 221). In the ECOG trial, when the dose of doxorubicin was decreased from 70 mg/m^2 to 50 mg/m^2 to avoid myelosuppression from cyclophosphamide, the response rate for doxorubicin 70 mg/m^2 as a single agent was significantly higher than for the combination with the lower doxorubicin dose (77).

The EORTC randomized patients between 5 g/m^2 ifosfamide and 1.5 g/m^2 cyclophosphamide (75). The response rate was higher for the ifosfamide arm with less myelosuppression than with cyclophosphamide.

The EORTC evaluated doxorubicin alone, doxorubicin with ifosfamide, and doxorubicin, cyclophosphamide, DTIC, and vincristine (CYVADIC). There was significantly more myelosuppression and a trend but no significant advantage in response rate or survival for the two combinations.

An ECOG study of doxorubicin with or without ifosfamide observed a significant difference in response for the ifosfamide arm, with a trend for longer survival in the ifosfamide arm (222).

The SWOG/CALGB (Cancer and Leukemia Group B) study of doxorubicin and DTIC alone versus the addition of ifosfamide demonstrated response rates of 17 and 32%, respectively. Although the response rate and duration of response were significantly improved for the three-drug arm, myelosuppression (including fatal sepsis) was also significantly worse. Median survivals were 13 and 12 months, respectively (223).

Four studies randomized patients between different schedules of similar regimens. A SWOG study compared bolus versus continuous infusion doxorubicin and DTIC. The response rates were identical, but the toxicity (particularly doxorubicin-associated cardiotoxicity and nausea and vomiting from DTIC) was substantially less with the continuous infusion schedule (224). An adjuvant trial at Memorial Sloan-Kettering corroborated the decreased cardiotoxicity of continuous infusion doxorubicin, but patients receiving the continuous infusion had a higher incidence of relapse (90). M. D. Anderson compared CYVADIC at a high and intermediate dose (100), and the EORTC studied full-dose versus alternating half-dose therapy. Both studies documented a correlation of dose with response (99).

Thus, currently, the combination yielding the highest response rates in soft tissue sarcomas is doxorubicin (60 mg/m^2) and ifosfamide (7.5 g/m^2) with or without DTIC (1 g/m^2). The doses of doxorubicin and DTIC should be given by continuous infusion over 4 days to decrease the risk of cardiotoxicity and the severity of nausea and vomiting. Ifosfamide should be divided and given daily over 3 days and given with mesna for bladder protection. Physicians may choose single-agent doxorubicin or doxorubicin and DTIC for palliation for patients who may not tolerate the combination. Ifosfamide is currently the most active salvage agent for patients who have failed an Adriamycin-containing regimen.

In laboratory models of sarcomas and other

Table 59.6. Investigational Agents in Soft Tissue Sarcomas by Class

	Reference	Number Evaluable	Percentage Responding
Anthracyclines			
Carminomycin	(151)	48	27
Azotomycin	(152, 153)	28	18
AMSA	(154–157)	9	11
Iclarubicin	(158)	23	4
Diaziquone (AZQ)	(159–161)	108	2
Mitoxantrone	(162, 163)	115	1
Menogaril	(164)	21	5
Esorubicin	(165)	14	7
Epirubicin	(166)	32	19
Echinomycin	(167)	34	0
Antimetabolites			
Edatrexate	(168)	35	14
Trimetrexate	(169, 170)	36	8
Cycloleucine	(171–173)	118	11
Chlorozotocin	(126, 174–179)	160	4
Cytembena	(180, 181)	24	4
PALA/5 fluorouracil	(182, 183)	23	0
PALA/dipyridamole	(184, 185)	46	11
Baker's antifol	(186, 187)	30	0
Alkylating agents			
Nimustine	(188)	31	10
Methyl-CCNU	(189, 190)	85	6
Hexamethylmelamine	(191–193)	88	5
Dibromodulcitol	(194, 195)	34	3
Dianhydrogalacitol	(196)	28	0
Gallium nitrate	(197)	31	0
Vinca and related compounds			
VM-26	(131, 132, 198)	33	3
Vindesine	(199, 200)	3	0
Miscellaneous			
Docetaxel	(201)	29	17
DDMP	(202)	15	7
Piperazinedione	(203–205)	22	5
ICRF 159	(195)	29	5
MGBG	(126, 206)	54	2
Amonafide	(207)	18	0
MTP/PE	(208)	20	0
Miltefosine	(209)	18	0
Pyazofurin	(206, 210, 211)	47	0
Maytansine	(195, 212)	44	0
Bruceantin	(195, 212)	34	0
Homoharringtonin	(213)	16	0
Biologics			
Tumor necrosis factor	(214)	16	0
Tumor necrosis factor	(215)	1	0
α-Interferon	(216)	16	0
β-Interferon	(217)	20	1
IL2	(66)	6	0

Updated with permission from Chang A, Rosenberg SA, Glatstein E, Antman K. Sarcomas of soft tissue. In: DeVita VT, Hellman S, Rosenberg SA, eds. Cancer principles & practice of oncology. 4th ed. Philadelphia: JB Lippincott, 1993:1436–1488.

Table 59.7. Randomized Chemotherapy Trials in Measurable Soft Tissue Sarcoma

	Group[a]	Regimen[b]	No	% CR[c]	% RR[d]	Comments
Studies comparing the addition of DTIC						
Omura et al.	GOG	A	80	6	16	Uterine sarcoma only
(218)		AD	66	11	24	
Lerner	ECOG	A	34	3	18	
(219)		AD	32	3	44	Leiomyosarcomas only
Borden et al.	ECOG	A q 3 week	93	6	19	A 15 mg/m² week
(97)		A q week	92	4	16	A 70 mg/2 q 3 week
		AD	95	6	30	
Benjamin et al.	SWOG	ACVD	221	14	52	
(220)		ACVAd	224	12	40	
Studies evaluating the addition of cyclophosphamide						
Schoenfeld et al.	ECOG	A	66	6	27	A 70 mg/m²
(77)		ACV	70	4	19	A 50 mg/m²
		CVAd	64	2	11	A 0 mg/m²
Baker et al.	SWOG	AD	79	14	32	
(221)		ADC	95	13	35	
		ADAd	98	9	24	
Muss et al.	GOG	A	50	1	19	
(76)		AC	54	2	20	
Studies evaluating vindesine						
Borden et al.	ECOG	A Vindesine	149	4	17	
(225)		A	149	6	18	
Studies evaluating dose and schedule						
Zalupski et al.	SWOG	AD	135	7	19	Bolus
(224)		AD	143	10	18	Continuous infusion
Casper et al.	MSKCC	A	32			Bolus
(90)		A	39			Continuous infusion
Bodey et al.	SWOG	ADCV	27	15	67	A 50 mg/m² C 500 mg/m²
(100)		ADCV	24	33	71	A 80 mg/m² C 800 mg/m²
Pinedo et al.	EORTC	ADC	71	20	38	full dose rate
(99)		AD-CV	74	5	14	half dose rate
Studies evaluating ifosfamide						
Bramwell	EORTC	I	68	2	18	5 g/m²
(75)		C	67	1	8	1.5 g/m²
Antman	ISSG	AD	170	2	17	
(223)		ADI	166	4	32	Myelosuppression more severe
Santoro	EORTC	A	212	4	24	
(226)		AI	202	6	27	Myelosuppression more severe
		ACDV	135	8	28	Nausea vomiting more severe
Blum	ECOG	A	95	2	20	
(222)		AI	94	5	34	

Updated with permission from Chang A, Rosenberg SA, Glatstein E, Antman K. Sarcomas of soft tissue. In: DeVita VT, Hellman S, Rosenberg SA, eds. Cancer principles & practice of oncology. 4th ed. Philadelphia: JB Lippincott, 1993:1436–1488.

[a]GOG, Gynecologic Oncology Group; CALGB, Cancer and Leukemia Group B; ECOG, Eastern Cooperative Oncology Group; SWOG, Southwest Oncology Group; MSKCC, Memorial Sloan-Kettering Cancer Center; EORTC, European Organization for Research and Treatment of Cancer.

[b]A, doxorubicin; Ad, antinomycin D; C, cyclophosphamide; D, DTIC; I, ifosfamide; V, vincristine.

[c]CR, complete response.

[d]RR, response rate.

malignancies, delivery of the highest possible doses of chemotherapy is essential to achieving curative therapy. Theory and experimental and clinical data suggest that sarcomas recur despite an initial response to chemotherapy, because of resistance to the chemotherapy drugs. In the laboratory, resistance to alkylating agents can often be overcome by using a 5- to 10-fold higher dose (227). There is ample evidence of a correlation between doxorubicin dose and tumor response from 3 randomized trials (77, 99, 100).

Because the limiting toxicity of higher chemotherapy doses is myelosuppression, several authors have used hematopoietic growth factors to allow delivery of full dose on schedule (228–230).

Autotransplants have also been used to ensure prompt marrow recovery after high doses of chemotherapy. Ewing's sarcoma, rhabdomyosarcoma, and osteosarcoma are optimal tumors for studies of the role of high-dose therapy because of their sensitivity at conventional chemotherapy doses.

Forty-three children with malignant soft tissue sarcomas were treated at the Royal Marsden Hospital (Sutton, U.K.) with a rapid-dose-delivery chemotherapy schedule consisting six courses of vincristine, doxorubicin, and cyclophosphamide followed in 36 patients by high-dose melphalan with autologous bone marrow support. There was one toxic death due to infection and possible cardiomyopathy. International Society of Paediatric Oncology (SIOP) staging was 11 stage I, 13 stage II, 7 stage III, and 12 stage IV. Actuarial survival at 5 years was 57% and event-free survival was 44% for all stages; for patients with nonmetastatic diseases, 62 and 53%, respectively. This treatment strategy enables completion of all chemotherapy by 4 months. Radiation and surgery were conservative to minimize late sequelae (231).

Dumontet et al. treated a heterogeneous group of soft tissue sarcoma patients with high-dose chemotherapy followed by autologous bone marrow support and reported overall survival at 5 years of 32%, with 8 patients surviving free of disease (232).

Of 95 patients with sarcoma, collected in a review by Pinkerton for the European Bone Marrow Transplant registry, 64 received high-dose therapy as consolidation in first complete or partial response. About 20% remained in durable complete response at more than 40 months. However, 35% of the 40 patients transplanted in CR were disease free (233). At the Dana Farber

Cancer Institute, high-dose ifosfamide, carboplatin, and etoposide is being studied as consolidation in patients with sarcomas responding to conventional dose therapy (109, 133).

REFERENCES

1. Russell WO, Cohen J, Enzinger FM, et al. A clinical and pathologic staging system for soft tissue sarcomas. Cancer 1977;40:1562–1570.

2. Wingo P, Tong T, Bolden S. Cancer Statistics, 1995. CA 1995;45(1):8–30.

3. Enzinger FM, Weiss SW. Soft tissue tumors. St Louis: CV Mosby, 1988.

4. Tucker MA, Fraumeni JF. Soft tissue. In: Schottenfeld D, ed. Cancer epidemiology. Philadelphia: WB Saunders, 1982:827–836.

5. Fraumeni JF Jr, Boice JD Jr. Bone. In: Schottenfeld D, ed. Cancer epidemiology. Philadelphia: WB Saunders 1987:814–826.

6. Maurer R, Egloff B. Malignant peritoneal mesothelioma after cholangiography with thorotrast. Cancer 1975;36:1381–1385.

7. Falk H, Telles NC, Ishak KG, Thomas LB, Popper H. Epidemiology of thorotrast-induced hepatic angiosarcoma in the United States. Environ Res 1979;18:65–73.

8. Norris HJ, Roth E, Taylor HB. Mesenchymal tumors of the uterus. A clinical and pathologic study of 31 mixed mesodermal tumors. Obstet Gynecol 1966; 28:57–63.

9. Tucker M, D'Angio G, Boice J Jr, et al. Bone sarcomas linked to radiotherapy and chemotherapy in children. N Engl J Med 1987;317:588–593.

10. Kuten A, Sapir D, Cohen Y, Haim N, Borovik R, Robinson E. Postirradiation soft tissue sarcoma occurring in breast cancer patients: report of seven cases and results of combination chemotherapy. J Surg Oncol 1985;28(3):168–171.

11. Selikoff IF. Cancer risk of asbestos exposure. In: Hiatt HH, Watson JD, Winston JA, eds. Origins of human cancer. New York: Cold Spring Harbor, 1977:1964–1984.

12. Popper H, Thomas LB, Telles NC, Falk H, Selikoff IJ. Development of hepatic angiosarcoma in man induced by vinyl chloride, thorotrast, and arsenic. Am J Pathol 1978;92:349–376.

13. Sarma PR, Jacobs J. Thoracic soft-tissue sarcoma in Vietnam veterans exposed to agent orange. N Engl J Med 1986;306:1109.

14. Hoar SK, Blair A, Holmes FF, et al. Agricultural herbicide use and risk of lymphoma and soft-tissue sarcoma. JAMA 1986;256:1141–1147.

15. Constable JD, Timperi R, Clapp R, Antman K, Boynton B. Vietnam veterans and soft tissue sarcoma. Occup Med 1987;28:1215–1218.

16. Boyd JT, Doll R, Hill GB, et al. Mortality from primary tumours of bone in England and Wales. Br J Prev Soc Med 1969;23:12–22.

17. Huth JF, Gupta RK, Morton DL. Relationship between circulating immune complexes and urinary antigens in human malignancy. Cancer 1982;49:1150–1157.

18. Friedman-Kien AE, Laubenstein LJ, Rubinstein P, et al. Disseminated Kaposi's sarcoma in homosexual men. Ann Intern Med 1982;96:693–700.

19. Lee E, Locker J, Nalesnik M, et al. The association of Epstein-Barr virus with smooth-muscle tumors occurring after organ transplantation. N Engl J Med 1995;332(1):19–25.

20. McClain K, Leach C, Jensen HB, et al. Association of Epstein-Barr virus with leiomyosarcomas in young people with AIDS. N Engl J Med 1995;332(1):12–18.

21. Francois J. Retinoblastoma and osteogenic sarcoma. Ophthalmologica 1977;175:185–191.

22. Hansen M, Koufos A, Gallie B, et al. Osteosarcoma and retinoblastoma: a shared chromosomal mechanism revealing recessive predisposition. Proc Natl Acad Sci USA 1985;82:6216–6220.

23. Sorensen SA, Mulvihill JJ, Nielsen A. Long-term follow-up of von Recklinghausen neurofibromatosis, survival and malignant neoplasms. N Engl J Med 1986;314:1010–1015.

24. Li FP, Franmeni JF. Soft-tissue sarcomas, breast cancer, and other neoplasms: a familial syndrome? Ann Intern Med 1969;71:747–752.

25. Malkin D, Li F, Strong L, et al. Germ line p53 mutations in a familial syndrome of breast cancer, sarcomas, and other neoplasms. Science 1990;250:1233–1238.

26. Weng-Peng J, Triche TJ, Knutsen T, Miser J, Douglass EC, Israel MA. Chromosome translocation in peripheral neuroepithelioma. N Engl J Med 1984; 311:584–585.

27. May W, Lessnick S, Braun B, et al. The Ewing's sarcoma EWS/FLI-1 fusion gene encodes a more potent transcriptional activator and is a more powerful transforming gene than FLI-1. Mol Cell Biol 1993; 13(12):7393–7398.

28. Fletcher JA, Weidner N, Corson JM. Laboratory investigation and genetics in sarcomas. Curr Sci 1990; 2(3):467–473.

29. Shipley J, Crew J, Gusterson B. The molecular biology of soft tissue sarcomas. Eur J Cancer 1993; 29A(14):2054–2058.

30. Licht JD, Weissmann LB, Antman K. Gastrointestinal sarcomas. Semin Oncol 1988;15:181–188.

31. Antman KH. Uterine sarcomas. In: Knapp R, Bercowitz R, eds. Gynecologic oncology. New York: Macmillan, 1986:297–312.

32. Dahlin D. Bone tumors: general aspects and data on 6,221 cases. 3rd ed. Springfield, IL: Charles C Thomas, 1978.

33. Taylor W, Ivins J, Dahlin D, Edmonson J, Pritchard D. Trends and variability in survival from osteosarcoma. Mayo Clin Proc 1978;53:695–700.

34. Edmonson J, Green S, Ivins J, et al. A controlled pilot study of high-dose methotrexate as postsurgical adjuvant treatment for primary osteosarcoma. J Clin Oncol 1984;2:152–156.

35. Link M, Goorin A, Miser A, et al. The effect of adjuvant chemotherapy on relapse-free survival in patients with osteosarcoma of the extremity. N Engl J Med 1986;314:1600–1606.

36. Link M, Shuster J, Goorin A, et al. Adjuvant chemotherapy in the treatment of osteosarcoma: results of the multi-institutional osteosarcoma study. In: Ryan JR, Baker LO, eds. Recent concepts in sarcoma treatment. Dordrecht, Netherlands: Kluwer Academic Publishers, 1988:283–290.

37. Link M, Goorin A, Horowitz M, et al. Adjuvant chemotherapy of high-grade osteosarcoma of the extremity. Updated results of the multi-institutional osteosarcoma study. Clin Orthop 1991;270:8–14.

38. Eilber F, Guiliano A, Eckardt J, Patterson K, Moseley S, Goodnight J. Adjuvant chemotherapy for osteosarcoma: a randomized prospective trial. J Clin Oncol 1987;5:21–26.

39. Picci P, Bacci G, Campannacci R. Neoadjuvant chemotherapy for localized osteosarcoma of the extremities. Experience related to 103 cases treated between March 83–March 86. In: Salmon S, ed. Adjuvant therapy of cancer V. Orlando, FL: Grune & Stratton, 1987:711–718.

40. Picci P, Bacci G, Capanna R, et al. Neoadjuvant chemotherapy for osteosarcoma. Results of a prospective study. In: Ryan JR, Baker LO, eds. Recent concepts in sarcoma treatment. Dordrecht, Netherlands: Kluwer Academic Publishers, 1988:291–296.

41. Bramwell V, Burgers M, Sneath R, et al. Preliminary report of the first European osteosarcoma intergroup study (abstract). Proc Am Soc Clin Oncol 1988; 7:273.

42. Cortes E, Necheles T, Holland J, Carey R. Adjuvant chemotherapy for primary osteosarcoma: a Cancer and Leukemia Group B experience. In: Salmon S, Jones S, eds. Adjuvant chemotherapy of cancer IV. Orlando, FL: Grune & Stratton 1984:201–210.

43. Bramwell V, Burgers M, Sneath R, et al. A comparison of two short intensive adjuvant chemotherapy regimens in operable osteosarcoma of limbs in children and young adults: the first study of the European Osteosarcoma Intergroup. J Clin Oncol 1992;10(10):1579–1591.

44. Kraillo M, Ertel I, Makley J. A randomized study comparing high-dose methotrexate with moderate dose methotrexate as components of adjuvant chemotherapy in childhood nonmetastatic osteosarcoma: a report from the Childrens Cancer Study Group. Med Pediatr Oncol 1987;15:69–77.

45. Jenkin R, Biship A, Bourchard H. Osteosarcoma. A preliminary report of a trial of adjuvant chemotherapy (abstract). Am Soc Clin Oncol 1981; 22:525.

46. Murray J, Jessup K, Romsdahl M, et al. Limb-salvage study in osteosarcoma: early experience at M. D. Anderson Hospital and Tumor Institute. Cancer Treat Symp 1985;3:131–137.

47. Jaffe N, Robertson R, Ayala A, et al. Comparison of intra-arterial cis-diamminedicloroplatinum II with high-dose methotrexate and citrovorum factor rescue in the treatment of primary osteosarcoma. J Clin Oncol 1985;3:1101–1104.

48. Dahlin DC, Beabout JW. Dedifferentiation of low-grade chondrosarcomas. Cancer 1971;28:461–466.

49. Poon M-C, Durant JR, Norgard MJ, Chang-Poon V. Inflammatory fibrous histiocytoma: an important variant of malignant fibrous histiocytoma highly responsive to chemotherapy. Ann Intern Med 1982; 97:858–863.

50. Antman KH, Corson J, Greenberger JS, Wilson R. Multimodality therapy in the management of angiosarcoma of the breast. Cancer 1982;50:2000–2003.

51. Janigan DT, Husain A, Robinson NA. Cardiac angiosarcomas: a review and a case report. Cancer 1986;57:852–859.

52. Rybojad M, Borradori L, Verola O, Zeller J, Puissant A, Morel P. Non-AIDS-associated Kaposi's sarcoma (classical and endemic African types): treat-

ment with low doses of recombinant interferon-alpha. J Invest Dermatol 1990;95(6):176–179.

53. Russo P. Urologic sarcoma in adults. Urol Clin North Am 1991;18(3):581–588.

54. Suit HD, Russell WO, Martin RG. Sarcoma of soft tissue: clinical and histopathologic parameters and response to treatment. Cancer 1975;35:1478–1483.

55. Lindberg RD, Martin RG, Romsdahl MM, Barkley HT. Conservative surgery and postoperative radiotherapy in 300 adults with soft tissue sarcoma. Cancer 1981;46:2391–2397.

56. Picci P, Bacci G, Gherlinzoni F, et al. Results of a randomized trial for the treatment of localized soft tissue tumors of the extremities in adult patients. In: Ryan JR, Baker LO, eds. Recent concepts in sarcoma treatment. Dordrecht, Netherlands: Kluwer Academic Publishers, 1988:144–148.

57. Bramwell V, Rouesse J, Steward W, et al. Adjuvant CYVADIC chemotherapy for adult soft tissue sarcoma: reduced local recurrence but no improvement in survival. J Clin Oncol 1994;12(6):1137–1149.

58. Lindberg RD, Murphy WK, Benjamin RS, et al. Adjuvant chemotherapy in the treatment of primary soft tissue sarcomas: preliminary report. Management of bone and soft tissue tumors. Chicago: Year Book Medical Publishers, 1977:343–352.

59. Benjamin TO, Terjanian TO, Fenoglio CJ, et al. The importance of combination chemotherapy for adjuvant treatment of high-risk patients with soft-tissue sarcomas of the extremities. In: Salmon S, ed. Adjuvant therapy of cancer V. Orlando, FL: Grune & Stratton, 1987:735–744.

60. Baker AR, Chang AE, Glatstein E, Rosenberg SA. National Cancer Institute experience in the management of high-grade extremity soft tissue sarcomas. In: Ryan JR, Baker LO, eds. Recent concepts in sarcoma treatment. Dordrecht, Netherlands: Kluwer Academic Publishers, 1988:123–130.

61. Rosenberg SA, Tepper J, Glatstein E, et al. Prospective randomized evaluation of adjuvant chemotherapy in adults with soft tissue sarcomas of the extremities. Cancer 1983;52:424–434.

62. Rosenberg SA. Prospective randomized trials demonstrating the efficacy of adjuvant chemotherapy in adult patients with soft tissue sarcomas. Cancer Treat Rep 1984;68:1067–1078.

63. Rosenberg SA, Chang AE, Glatstein E. Adjuvant chemotherapy for treatment of extremity soft tissue sarcomas: review of National Cancer Institute experience. Cancer Treat Symp 1985;3:83–88.

64. Rosenberg SA. Adjuvant chemotherapy of adult patients with soft tissue sarcoma. In: DeVita V, Hellman S, Rosenberg S, eds. Important advances in oncology. Philadelphia: JB Lippincott, 1985:273–294.

65. Rosenberg SA, Suit HD, Baker LH. Sarcomas of soft tissue. In: DeVita V, Hellman S, Rosenberg S, eds. Cancer: principles & practice of oncology. 2nd. ed. Philadelphia: JB Lippincott, 1985:1243.

66. Rosenberg SA, Lotze MT, Muul LM, et al. A progress report on the treatment of 157 patients with advanced cancer using lymphokine-activated killer cells and interleukin-2 or high-dose interleukin-2 alone. N Engl J Med 1987;316:890–897.

67. Bramwell VHC, Rouesse J, Santoro A, et al. European experience of adjuvant chemotherapy for soft tissue sarcoma: preliminary report of randomized trial of cyclophosphamide, vincristine, doxorubicin, and dacarbazine. Cancer Treat Symp 1985;3:99–107.

68. Bramwell V, Rouesse J, Steward W, et al. European experience of adjuvant chemotherapy for soft tissue sarcoma: interim report of a randomized trial of CYVADIC versus control. In: Ryan JR, Baker LO, eds. Recent concepts in sarcoma treatment. Dordrecht, Netherlands: Kluwer Academic Publishers, 1988:157–164.

69. Ravaud A, Nguyen BB, Coindre JM, et al. Adjuvant chemotherapy with CyVADIC in high-risk soft tissue sarcoma: a randomized prospective trial. In: Salmon SE, ed. Adjuvant therapy of cancer VI. Philadelphia: WB Saunders, 1990:556–566.

70. Chang A, Kinsella T, Glatstein E, et al. Adjuvant chemotherapy for patients with high-grade soft-tissue sarcomas of the extremity. J Clin Oncol 1988;6:1491–1500.

71. Glenn J, Sindelar WF, Kinsella T. Results of multimodality therapy of resectable soft-tissue sarcomas of the retroperitoneum. Surgery 1985;97:316–325.

72. Glenn J, Kinsella T, Glatstein E, et al. A randomized, prospective trial of adjuvant chemotherapy in adults with soft tissue sarcomas of the head and neck, breast, and trunk. Cancer 1985;55:1206–1214.

73. Dresdale A, Bonow R, Wesley R, et al. Prospective evaluation of doxorubicin-induced cardiomyopathy resulting from postsurgical adjuvant treatment of patients with soft tissue sarcomas. Cancer 1983;52:51–60.

74. Bergsagel DE, Levin WC. A prelusive clinical trial of cyclophosphamide. Cancer Chemother Rep 1960;8:120–134.

75. Bramwell V, Mouridsen HT, Santoro A, et al. Cyclophosphamide vs ifosfamide: final report of a randomized phase II trial in adult soft tissue sarcoma. Eur J Cancer Clin Oncol 1987;23:311–321.

76. Muss HB, Bundy B, DiSaia PJ, et al. Treatment of recurrent advanced uterine sarcoma—a randomized trial of doxorubicin vs doxorubicin and cyclophosphamide. Cancer 1985;55:1648–1653.

77. Schoenfeld D, Rosenbaum C, Horton J, Wolter JM, Falkson G, DeConti RC. A comparison of Adriamycin versus vincristine and Adriamycin, and cyclophosphamide for advanced sarcoma. Cancer 1982;50:2757–2762.

78. Edmonson JH, Fleming TR, Ivins JC, et al. Randomized study of systemic chemotherapy following complete excision of nonosseus sarcomas. J Clin Oncol 1984;2:1390–1396.

79. Edmonson JH. Role of adjuvant chemotherapy in the management of patients with soft tissue sarcomas. Cancer Treat Rep 1984;68:1063–1066.

80. Omura GA, Major FJ, Blessing JA, et al. A randomized clinical trial of adjuvant Adriamycin in uterine sarcomas: a Gynecologic Oncology Group study. J Clin Oncol 1985;3:1240–1245.

81. Alvegard TA, Sigurdsson H, Mouridsen H, et al. Adjuvant chemotherapy with doxorubicin in high grade soft tissue sarcoma: a randomized trial of the Scandinavian Sarcoma Group. J Clin Oncol 1989;7:1504–1513.

82. Antman K, Ryan L, Borden E, et al. Pooled results from three randomized adjuvant studies of doxorubicin versus observation in soft tissue sarcoma: 10-year results and review of the literature. In: Salmon S,

ed. Adjuvant therapy of cancer VI. Philadelphia: WB Saunders, 1990:529–544.

83. Antman K, Amato D, Pilepich M, et al. A preliminary analysis of a randomized intergroup (SWOG, ECOG, CALGB, NCOG) trial of adjuvant doxorubicin for soft tissue sarcomas. In: Salmon S, ed. Adjuvant therapy of cancer IV. Orlando, FL: Grune & Stratton 1987:725–734.

84. Antman K, Suit H, Amato D, et al. Preliminary results of a randomized trial of adjuvant doxorubicin for sarcomas: lack of apparent difference between treatment groups. J Clin Oncol 1984;2:601–608.

85. Antman KH, Amato D, Lerner H, et al. Eastern Cooperative Oncology Group and Dana-Farber Cancer Institute/Massachusetts General Hospital Study. In: Jones S, Salmon S, eds. Adjuvant therapy of cancer IV. Orlando, FL: Grune & Stratton, 1984:611–620.

86. Antman K, Amato D, Lerner H, et al. Adjuvant doxorubicin for sarcoma: data from the ECOG and DFCI/MGH studies. Cancer Treat Symp 1985;3:109–115.

87. Gherlinzoni F, Bacci G, Picci P, et al. A randomized trial for the treatment of high-grade soft-tissue sarcomas of the extremities: preliminary observations. J Clin Oncol 1986;4:552–558.

88. Eilber FR, Giuliano AE, Huth JF, Morton DL. Adjuvant Adriamycin in high-grade extremity soft-tissue sarcomas—a randomized prospective trial (abstract C-488). Proc Am Soc Clin Oncol 1986;5:125.

89. Eilber FR, Giuliano AE, Huth JF, Weisenburger T, Eckardt J. Intravenous vs. intraarterial Adriamycin, 2800 r radiation and surgical excision for extremity soft tissue sarcomas: a randomized prospective trial (1194 abstract). Proc Am Soc Clin Oncol 1990;9:309.

90. Casper ES, Gaynor JJ, Hajdu SI, et al. A prospective randomized trial of adjuvant chemotherapy with bolus versus continuous infusion of doxorubicin in patients with high-grade extremity soft tissue sarcoma and an analysis of prognostic factors. Cancer 1991;68(6):1221–1229.

91. Pogrebniak HW, Roth JA, Steinberg SM, Rosenberg SA, Pass HT. Reoperative pulmonary resection in patients with metastatic soft tissue sarcoma. Ann Thorac Surg 1991;52(2):197–203.

92. Roth J, Putnam J Jr, Wesley M, Rosenberg S. Differing determinants of prognosis following resection of pulmonary metastases from osteogenic and soft tissue sarcoma patients. Cancer 1985;55:1361–1366.

93. O'Bryan RM, Baker LH, Gottlieb JB, et al. Dose response evaluation of Adriamycin in human neoplasia. Cancer 1977;39:1940–1948.

94. O'Bryan RM, Luce JK, Talley RW, Gottlieb JA, Baker LH, Bonadonna G. Phase II evaluation of Adriamycin in neoplasia. Cancer 1973;32:1–8.

95. Cruz AB, Thames EA, Aust JB, et al. Combination chemotherapy for soft tissue sarcomas: a phase III study. Surg Oncol 1979;11:313–323.

96. Creagan ET, Hahn RG, Ahmann DL, Bisel HF. A clinical trial of Adriamycin in advanced sarcomas. Oncology 1977;34:90–91.

97. Borden EC, Amato D, Enterline HT, Lerner H, Carrbone PP. Randomized comparison of Adriamycin regimens for treatment of metastatic soft tissue sarcomas. J Clin Oncol 1987;5:840–850.

98. Blum RH. An overview of studies in Adriamycin in the United States. Cancer Chemother Rep 1975;6:247–251.

99. Pinedo HM, Branwell VHC, Mouridsen HT, et al. CYVADIC in advanced soft tissue sarcoma: a randomized study comparing two schedules. A study of the EORTC Soft Tissue and Bone Sarcoma Group. Cancer 1984;53:1825–1832.

100. Bodey GP, Rodriquez V, Murphy WK, Burgess A, Benjamin RS. Protected environment–prophylactic antibiotic program for malignant sarcoma: randomized trial during remission induction chemotherapy. Cancer 1981;47:2422–2429.

101. Brock N. Pharmacological studies with ifosfamide—a new oxazaphosphorine compound. In: Semonsky M, Hejzler M, Masak S, eds. Advances in antimicrobial and antineoplastic chemotherapy. Proc 7th International Congress of Chemotherapy, vol 2, Prague 1971. Munchen: Urban and Schwarzenberg, 1972:749–756.

102. Cabanillas F, Hagemeister FB, Bodey GP, Freireich EJ. IMVP-16: an effective regimen for patients with lymphoma who have relapsed after initial combination chemotherapy. Blood 1982;60:693–697.

103. Antman KH, Montella D, Rosenbaum C, Schwen M. Phase II trial of ifosfamide with mesna in previously treated metastatic sarcoma. Cancer Treat Rep 1985;69:499–502.

104. Morgan LR, Posey LE, Rainey J, et al. Ifosfamide: a weekly dose fractionated schedule in bronchogenic carcinoma. Cancer Treat Rep 1981;65:693–695.

105. Antman KH, Ryan L, Elias A, Sherman D, Grier E. Response to ifosfamide and mesna: 124 previously treated patients with metastatic or unresectable sarcoma. J Clin Oncol 1989;7:126–131.

106. Bramwell V, Mouridsen H, Santoro A, et al. Cyclophosphamide versus ifosfamide: a randomized phase II trial in adult soft tissue sarcoma. Preliminary report of EORTC Soft Tissue and Bone Sarcomas Group (abstract). Proc Am Soc Clin Oncol 1985;4:143.

107. Czownicki Z, Utracka-Hutka B. Contributions to the treatment of malignant tumors with ifosfamide. In: Burkeret H, Voight HC, eds. Proc Int Holoxan Symposium. Dusseldorf: Asta-Werke AG, 1977:109–111.

108. de Kraker J, Voute PA. Ifosfamide and vincristine in pediatric tumors. A phase II study. Eur Paediatr Haematol Oncol 1984;1:47–50.

109. Elias AD, Eder JP, Shea T, Begg CB, Frei E III, Antman KH. High dose ifosfamide with mesna uroprotection: a phase I study. J Clin Oncol 1990;8:170–178.

110. Magrath IT, Sandlund JT, Rayner A, Rosenberg SA, Arasi V, Miser JS. Treatment of recurrent sarcomas with ifosfamide (abstract). Proc Am Soc Clin Oncol 1985;4:136.

111. Marti C, Kroner T, Remagen W, Berchtold W, Cserhati M, Vaarini M. High-dose ifosfamide in advanced osteosarcoma. Cancer Treat Rep 1985;69:115–117.

112. Otten J, Flamant F, Rodary C, et al. Effectiveness of combination of ifosfamide, vincristine and actinomycin D in inducing remission in rhabdomyosarcoma in children. For the RMS group of the International Society of Pediatric Oncology (abstract). Proc Am Soc Clin Oncol 1985;4:236.

113. Schutte J, Dombernowsky P, Santoro A, et al. Adriamycin and ifosfamide, a new effective combination in advanced soft tissue sarcoma: preliminary report of a phase II study of the EORTC Soft Tissue and

Bone Sarcoma Group (abstract). Proc Am Soc Clin Oncol 1986;5:145.

114. Stuart-Harris R, Harper PG, Kaye SB, Wiltshaw E. High-dose ifosfamide by infusion with mesna in advanced soft tissue sarcoma. Cancer Treat Rev 1983;10(Suppl A):163–164.

115. Wellens W, Donhuijsen-Ant R, Habets L, et al. Therapie progredienter Sarkome mit Etoposid und Ifosfamide. Aktuel Onkol 1981;4:159–164.

116. Legha S, Papadopoulos N, Plager C, et al. A comparative evaluation of the uroprotective effect of mercaptoethane sulfonate (mesna) and N-acetylcysteine in sarcoma patients treated with ifosfamide (abstract 1205). Proc Am Soc Clin Oncol 1990;9.

117. Rosen G, Caparros B, Nirenberg A, Cacavio A, Huvos AG. High dose methotrexate with citrovorum factor rescue in the treatment of radiation-induced sarcomas (abstract 771). Proc Am Assoc Cancer Res 1981; 22:194.

118. Vaugan C, McKelvey E, Balcerzak S, Loh K, Stephens R, Baker L. High dose methotrexate with leucovorin rescue plus vincristine in advanced sarcoma: a Southwest Oncology Group study. Cancer Treat Rep 1984;68:409–410.

119. Isacoff WH, Eilber F. Phase II clinical trial with high-dose methotrexate therapy and citrovorum factor rescue. Cancer Treat Rep 1978;62:1295–1304.

120. Karakousis CP, Rao U, Carlson M. High-dose methotrexate as secondary chemotherapy in metastatic soft-tissue sarcomas. Cancer 1980;46:1345–1348.

121. Von Hoff DD, Rozenceieg M, Louie AC, Bender RA, Muggia FM. "Single"-agent activity of high-dose methotrexate therapy with citrovorum factor rescue. Cancer Treat Rep 1978;62:233–235.

122. Frei E, Blum R, Pitman S, et al. High dose methotrexate with leuvovorin rescue, rationale and spectrum of antitumor activity. Am J Med 1979;68:370–375.

123. Andrews N, Wilson W. Phase II study of methotrexate in solid tumors. Cancer Chemother Rep 1967;51:471–474.

124. Subramanian S, Wiltshaw E. Chemotherapy of sarcoma—a comparison of three regimens. Lancet 1978;2:683–686.

125. Buesa JM, Mouridsen HT, Santoro A. Treatment of advanced soft tissue sarcomas with low-dose methotrexate: a phase II trial by the European Organization for Research on Treatment of Cancer (EORTC) Soft Tissue and Bone Sarcoma Group. Cancer Treat Rep 1984;68:683–694.

126. Amato DA, Borden EC, Shiraki M, et al. Evaluation of bleomycin, chlorozotocin, MGBG, and bruceantin in patients with advanced soft tissue sarcoma, bone sarcoma, or mesothelioma. Invest New Drugs 1985;3:397–401.

127. Golbey R, Li MC, Kaufman RF. Actinomycin in the treatment of soft part sarcomas. Proc James Ewing Society, 21st annual meeting, April 18th, 1968.

128. Gold G, Hall T, Shnider B, et al. A clinical study of 5-fluorouracil. Cancer Res 1959;19:935–939.

129. Selawry O, Holland J, Wolman I. Effect of vincristine (NSC-67574) on malignant solid tumors in children. Cancer Chemother Rep 1968;52:497–499.

130. Korbitzs BC, Davis HL, Ramirez G, Ansfield FJ. Low doses of vincristine (NSC-67574) for malignant disease. Cancer Chemother Rep 1969;53:249–254.

131. Radice PA, Bunn PAJ, Ihde DC. Therapeutic trials with VP-16 and VM-26. Cancer Treat Rep 1979; 63:1231–1239.

132. Bleyer WA, Chard RL, Krivit W, Hammond D. Epipodophyllotoxin therapy of childhood neoplasias. A comparative phase II analysis of VM26 and VP 16-213 (abstract). Proc Am Assoc Cancer Res 1978; 19:373.

133. Elias AD, Ayash LJ, Eder JP, et al. A phase I study of high-dose ifosfamide and escalating doses of carboplatin with autologous bone marrow support. J Clin Oncol 1991;9(2):320–327.

134. Klein HO, Wickramanayake PD, Coerper CL, Christian E, Pohl J, Brock N. High-dose ifosfamide and mesna as continuous infusion over five days—a phase I/II trial. Cancer Treat Rev. 1983;10(Suppl A):167–173.

135. Chawla SP, Rosen G, Lowenbraun S, Morton D, Eilber F. Role of high dose ifosfamide (HDI) in recurrent osteosarcoma (abstract). Proc Am Soc Clin Oncol 1990;9:310.

136. Czownicki Z, Utracka-Hutka B. Clinical studies with uromitexan—an antidote against urotoxicity of holoxan. Preliminary results. Nowotwory 1980; 30:377–383.

137. Niederle N, Scheulen ME, Cremer M, Schutte J, Schmidt CG, Seeber S. Ifosfamide in combination chemotherapy for sarcomas and testicular carcinomas. Cancer Treat Rev 1983;10(Supple A):129–135.

138. Sutton GP, Blessing JA, Photopulos G, Berman ML, Homesley HD. Early phase II Gynecologic Oncology Group experience with ifosfamide/mesna in gynecologic malignancies. Cancer Chemother Pharmacol. 1990;26(Suppl):S55–58.

139. Pratt CB, Green AA, Horowitz ME, et al. Central nervous system toxicity following the treatment of pediatric patients with ifosfamide/mesna. J Clin Oncol 1985;4:1253–1261.

140. Jurgens H, Exner U, Kuhl J, et al. High-dose ifosfamide with mesna uroprotection in Ewing's sarcoma. Cancer Chemother Pharmacol 1989:S40–44.

141. Magrath I, Sandlund J, Raynor A, Rosenberg S, Arasi V, Miser J. A phase II study of ifosfamide in the treatment of recurrent sarcomas in young people. Cancer Chemother Pharmacol 1986;18(Suppl 2):S25–28.

142. Buesa JM, Mouridsen HT, Oosterom ATV, et al. High-dose DTIC in advanced soft-tissue sarcomas in the adult. A phase II study of the EORTC soft tissue and bone sarcoma group. Ann Oncol 1991;2(4):307–309.

143. Bramwell VHC, Brugarols A, Mouridsen HT, et al. EORTC: phase II study of cisplatinum in CY-VADIC-resistant soft tissue sarcoma. Eur J Cancer 1979;15:1511–1513.

144. Karakousis CP, Holterman OA, Holyoke E. Cisdichlorodiamineplatinum (II) in metastatic soft tissue sarcomas. Cancer Treat Rep 1979;63:2071–2075.

145. Samson MK, Baker LH, Benjamin RS, Lane M, Plager C. Cisdichlorodiamineplatinum (II) in advanced soft tissue and bony sarcomas. A Southwest Oncology Group study. Cancer Treat Rep 1979; 63:2027–2028.

146. Thigpen JT, Blessing JA, Wilbanks GD. Cisplatin as second-line chemotherapy in the treatment of advanced or recurrent leiomyosarcoma of the uterus. Am J Clin Oncol 1986;9:18–20.

147. Budd GT, Metch B, Balcerzak SP, Fletcher WS, Baker LH, Mortimer JE. High-dose cisplatin for metastatic soft tissue sarcoma. Cancer 1990;65:866–869.

148. Gershenson DM, Kavanagh JJ, Copeland LJ, Edwards CL, Stringer CA, Wharton JT. Cisplatin therapy for disseminated mixed mesodermal sarcoma of the uterus. J Clin Oncol 1987;5:618–621.

149. Goldstein D, Cheuvart B, Trump DL, et al. Phase II trial of carboplatin in soft-tissue sarcoma. Am J Clin Oncol 1990;13(5):420–423.

150. Korst DR, Johnson D, Frenkel EP, Challener WL III. Preliminary evaluation of the effect of cyclophosphamide on the course of human neoplasms. Cancer Chemother Rep 1960;7:1–12.

151. Perevodchikova NI, Lichinister MR, Gorbunova VA. Phase II clinical study of carminomycin: its activity against soft tissue sarcomas. Cancer Treat Rep 1977;61:1705–1707.

152. Weiss AJ, Ramirez G, Grage T, Strawitz J, Goldman L, Downing V. Phase II study of azotomycin (NSC-56654). Cancer Chemother Rep 1968;52:611–614.

153. Chang P, Wiernik PHP. Phase II study of azotomycin in sarcomas. Cancer Treat Rep 1979;61:1719.

154. DeJager R, Body JJ, Dupong D, Klastersky J, Kenis Y. Phase I study of oral 4′ (9-acrindylamino-methanesulfon-anidide) M-AMSA (abstract). Proc Am Soc Clin Onc 1979;20:429(C-574).

155. Legha SS, Gutterman JU, Hall SW, et al. Phase I clinical investigation of 4′-(9-acridinylamino) methanesulfon-m-anisiside (NSC 249992), a new acridine derivative. Cancer Res 1978;38:3712–3716.

156. Von Hoff DD, Howser D, Gormley P, et al. Phase I study of methanesulfonamide, N-(4-9-acridinylamino)-3-methoxyphenyl-m-AMSA using a single-dose schedule. Cancer Treat Rep 1978;62:1421–1426.

157. Schneider R, Sklanoff R, Ochoa M. Phase I trial of AMSA (4′ acrindylamino)-methansulfon-manisidide (abstract). Proc Am Assoc Cancer Res 1979;20:114.

158. Bertrand M, Multhauf P, Bartolucci A, Ellison D, Gockerman J. Phase II study of aclarubicin in previously untreated patients with advanced soft tissue sarcoma. Cancer Treat Rep 1985;69:725–726.

159. Zidar B, Baker L, Rivkin S, Balcerzak SP, Stephens RL. A phase II study of diaziquone in advanced soft tissue and bony sarcoma. A Southwest Oncology Group study. Cancer Treat Rep 1985;69:1035–1036.

160. Chan C, Bartolucci A, Brenner D, et al. Phase II trial of diaziquone in anthracycline-resistant adult soft tissue bone sarcoma patients: a Southeastern Cancer Study Group trial. Cancer Treat Rep 1986;70:427–428.

161. Slayton RE, Blessing JA, Clarke-Pearson D. A phase II trial of diaziquone (AZQ) in mixed mesodermal sarcomas uterus. A Gynecologic Oncology Group study. Invest New Drugs 1991;9(1):93–94.

162. Presant C, Gams R, Bartolucci A. Treatment of metastatic sarcomas with mitroxantrone. Cancer Treat Rep 1984;68:813–814.

163. Bull FE, Von Hoff DD, Balcerzak SP, Stephens RL, Panettiere FJ. Phase II trial of mitoxantrone in advanced sarcomas. A Southwest Oncology Group study. Cancer Treat Rep 1985;69:231–233.

164. Buckner JC, Edmonson JH, Ingle JN, Schaid DJ. Evaluation of menogaril in patients with metastatic sarcomas and no prior chemotherapy exposure. Am J Clin Oncol 1989;12(5):384–386.

165. Giaccone G, Donadio M, Calciati A. Phase II study of esorubicin in the treatment of patients with advanced sarcoma. Oncology 1989;46(5):285–287.

166. Chevallier B, Montcuquet P, Fachini T, et al. Phase II study of epirubicin in advanced soft tissue sarcoma. Bull Cancer 1990;77(10):991–995.

167. Taylor SA, Metch B, Balcerzak SP, Hanson KH. Phase II trial of echinomycin in advanced soft tissue sarcomas. A Southwest Oncology Group study. Invest New Drugs 1990;8(4):381–383.

168. Casper E, Christman K, Schwartz G, Johnson B, Brennan M, Bertino J. Edatrexate in patients with soft tissue sarcoma. Activity in malignant fibrous histiocytoma. Cancer 1993;72(3):766–770.

169. Quirt I, Eisenhauer E, Knowling M, et al. A phase 2 study of trimetrexate in metastatic soft tissue sarcoma (abstract). Proc Am Soc Clin Oncol 1988;7:275.

170. Licht JD, Gonin R, Antman KH. Phase II trial of trimetrexate in patients with advanced soft tissue sarcoma. Cancer Chemother Pharmacol 1991;28(3):223–225.

171. Johnson R. Preliminary phase II trials with l-aminocyclopentane carboxylic acid (NSC-1026) (cycloleucine). Cancer Chemother Rep 1963;32:67–71.

172. Aust J, Andrews N, Schroeder J, Lawton RL. Clinical notes. Phase II study of l-aminocyclopentane-carboxylic acid (NSC 1026) in patients with cancer. Cancer Chemother Rep 1970;(pt 1)54:237–241.

173. Savlov ED, MacIntyre JM, Knight E, Woller J. Comparison of doxorubicin with cycloleucine in the treatment of sarcomas. Cancer Treat Rep 1981;65:21–27.

174. Mouridsen HT, Bramwell VH, Lacave J, et al. Treatment of advanced soft tissue sarcomas with chlorozotocin: a phase II trial of the EORTC Soft Tissue and Bone Sarcoma Group. Cancer Treat Rep 1981;65:509–511.

175. Kovach JS, Moertel CG, Schutt AF. A phase I study of chlorozotocin (NSC 178248). Cancer 1979;43:2189–2196.

176. Gralla RJ, Tan CTC, Young CW. Phase I trial of chlorozotocin. Cancer Treat Rep 1979;63:17–20.

177. Presant CA, Bartolucci AA. Phase II evaluation of chlorozotocin in metastatic sarcomas. Med Pediatr Oncol 1984;12:25–27.

178. Sordillo PP, Magill GB, Gralla RJ. Chlorozotocin: phase II evaluation in patients with advanced sarcomas. Cancer Treat Rep 1981;65:513–514.

179. Talley RW, Samson MK, Brownlee RW, Samhouri AM, Fraile RJ, Baker LH. Phase II evaluation of chlorozotocin in advanced human cancers. Eur J Cancer 1981;17:337–343.

180. Baker LH, Samson MK, Izbicki RM. Phase I and II evaluation of cytembena in disseminated epithelial ovarian cancer and sarcomas. Cancer Treat Rep 1976;60:1389–1391.

181. Matejovsky Z. Effects of cytembena in the treatment of malignant musculoskeletal tumors. Neoplasma 1971;18:473–480.

182. Kurzrock R, Yap BS, Plager C, et al. Phase II evaluation of PALA in patients with refractory metastatic sarcomas. Am J Clin Oncol (CCT). 1984;7:305–307.

183. Presant CA, Ardalan B, Multhauf P. Continuous five-day infusion of PALA and 5 FU: a pilot phase II trial. Med Pediatr Oncol 1983;11:162–163.

184. Baselga J, Magill GB, Curley T, Casper ES. Phase II trial of pala + dipyridamole in patients with metastatic soft tissue sarcoma (abstract 1187). Proc Am Assoc Cancer Res 1990;31.

185. Casper ES, Baselga J, Smart TB, Magill GB, Markman M, Ranhosky A. A phase II trial of PALA + dipyridamole in patients with advanced soft-tissue sarcoma. Cancer Chemother Pharmacol 1991;28(1):51–54.

186. Rodriquez V, Gottlieb J, Burgess MA, et al. Phase I studies with Baker's antifol (NSC 139105). Cancer 1976;38:690–694.

187. Thigpen JT, O'Bryan RM, Benjamin RS, Coltman CA Jr. Phase II trial of Baker's antifol in metastatic sarcoma. Cancer Treat Rep 1977;61:1485–1487.

188. Wagener D, Somers R, Santoro A, et al. Phase II study of nimustine in metastatic soft tissue sarcoma. European Organization for Research and Treatment of Cancer Soft Tissue and Bone Sarcoma Group. Eur J Cancer 1991;27(12):1604–1605.

189. Tranum BP, Haut A, Rivkin SE, et al. A phase II study of methyl CCNU in the treatment of solid tumors and lymphomas in the Southwest Oncology Group. Cancer 1974;35:1148–1153.

190. Creagan ET, Hahn JH, Ahmann DL, Edmonson JH, Bisel HF, Eagan RT. A comparative clinical trial evaluating the combination of actinomycin D, cyclophosphamide, and vincristine, and a single agent, methyl-CCNU, in advanced sarcomas. Cancer Treat Rep 1976;60:1385–1386.

191. Borden EC, Larson P, Ansfield FJ, et al. Hexamethylmelamine: treatment of sarcomas & lymphomas. Med Pediatr Oncol 1977;3:401–406.

192. Blum RH, Livingston RB, Carter SK. Hexamethylmelamine. A new drug with activity in solid tumors. Eur J Cancer 1973;9:195–202.

193. Sooriyaarachchi GS, Ramirez G, Roley EL. Hemangiopericytoma of the uterus. J Surg Oncol 1978;10:399–406.

194. Conroy JF, Roda PI, Prasavinichai S. Dibromodulcitol in the treatment of metastic hemangiopericytoma. Am J Clin Oncol (CCT) 1982;5:453–456.

195. Borden EC, Ash A, Enterline HT, et al. Phase II evaluation of dibromodulcitol, ICRF-159, and maytansine for sarcomas. Am J Clin Oncol (CCT) 1982;5:417–420.

196. Kimball JC, Cangir A. A phase II trial of dianhydrogalactitol in advanced soft tissue and bony sarcomas, a Southwest Oncology Group study. Cancer Treat Rep 1979;63:553–554.

197. Saiki J, Stephens R, Fabian C, Kraut E, Fletcher W. Phase II evaluation of gallium nitrate (NSC-15200) in soft tissue and bone sarcomas (abstract). Proc Am Assoc Cancer Res 1981;22:525.

198. Bleyer WA, Krivit W, Chard RL, Hammond D. Phase II study of VM-26 in acute leukemia, neuroblastoma, and other refractory childhood malignancies. A report from the Children's Cancer Study Group. Cancer Treat Rep 1979;63:977–981.

199. Currie VE, Wong PP, Krakoff IH, Young CW. Phase I trial of vindesine in patients with advanced cancer. Cancer Treat Rep 1978;62:1333–1336.

200. Rossof AH, Chandra G, Walter J, et al. Phase II trial of vindesine (desacetyl vinblastine amide sulfate) in advanced metastatic cancer. Proc Am Assoc Cancer Res 1979;20:146.

201. van Hoesel Q, Verweij J, Catimel G, et al. Phase II study with docetaxel (Taxotere) in advanced soft tissue sarcomas of the adult. EORTC Soft Tissue and Bone Sarcoma Group. Ann Oncol 1994;5(6):539–542.

202. Alberto P, DeJager RL, Brugarolas A, Hansen H, Cavalli F, Host H. Phase II study of diamino-dichlorophenyl-methylpyrimidine with folinic acid protection and rescue (abstract). Proc Am Assoc Cancer Res 1979;20:323.

203. Benjamin RS, Keating MJ, Valdivieso M, et al. Phase I-II study of piperazinedione in adults with solid tumors and acute leukemia. Cancer Treat Rep 1979;63:939–943.

204. LaGasse L, Thigpen T, Morrison F. Phase II trial of piperazinedione in treatment of advanced endometrial carcinoma, uterine sarcoma, and vulvar carcinoma (abstract). Proc Am Soc Clin Oncol 1979;20:388.

205. Thigpen T, Blessing JA, Homesley HD, Hacker N, Curry SL. Phase II trial of piperazinedione in treatment of advanced or recurrent uterine sarcoma, a GOG Study. Am J Clin Oncol 1985;8:350–352.

206. Sordillo PP, Magill GB. Phase II evaluation of pyrazofurin in patients with soft-tissue sarcomas. Am J Clin Oncol 1985;8:316–318.

207. Buys S, Metch B, Balcerzak S, Neefe J, Stuckey W. Phase II evaluation of amonafide in advanced sarcoma: a Southwest Oncology Group study. Cancer Invest 1994;12(4):399–402.

208. Verweij J, Judson I, Steward W, et al. Phase II study of liposomal muramyl tripeptide phosphatidylethanolamine (MTP/PE) in advanced soft tissue sarcomas of the adult. An EORTC Soft Tissue and Bone Sarcoma Group study. Eur J Cancer 1994;30A(6):842–843.

209. Verweij J, Krzemieniecki K, Kok T, et al. Phase II study of miltefosine (hexadecylphosphocholine) in advanced soft tissue sarcomas of the adult—an EORTC Soft Tissue and Bone Sarcoma Group study. Eur J Cancer 1993;29A(2):208–209.

210. Salem PA, Bodey GP, Burgess MA, Murphy WK, Freireich EJ. A phase I study of pyrazofurin. Cancer 1977;40:2806–2809.

211. Gralla RJ, Sordillo PP, Magill GB. Phase II evaluation of pyrazofurin in patients with metastatic sarcoma. Cancer Treat Rep 1978;62:1573–1574.

212. Blum R, Kahlert T. Maytansine: a phase I study of an ansamacrolide with antitumor activity. Cancer Treat Rep 1978;62:435–438.

213. Ajani JA, Dimery I, Chawla SP, et al. Phase II studies of homoharringtonine in patients with advanced malignant melanoma; sarcoma; and head and neck, breast, and colorectal carcinomas. Cancer Treat Rep 1986;70:375–379.

214. Rinehart J, Balcerzak SP, Hersh E. Phase II trial of tumor necrosis factor in human sarcoma: a Southwest Oncology Group study (abstract 1229). Proc Am Soc Clin Oncol 1990;9.

215. Robertson PA, Ross HJ, Figlin RA. Tumor necrosis factor induces hemorrhagic necrosis of a sarcoma. Ann Intern Med 1989;111:682–684.

216. Schuff-Werner P, Bartsch H, Schreml W, Nagel GA. Treatment of soft tissue sarcoma with recombinant alpha-interferon (abstract 1). Antiviral Res 1984;3:93.

217. Harris JE, Das Gupta T, Vogelzang M, et al.

Treatment of soft tissue sarcoma with fibroblast interferon—an American Cancer Society/Illinois Cancer Council Study. Cancer Treat Rep 1986;70:293–294.

218. Omura GA, Major FJ, Blessing JA, et al. A randomized study of Adriamycin with and without dimethyl trazenoimidazole carboxamide in advanced uterine sarcomas. Cancer 1983;52:626–632.

219. Lerner H, Amato D, Stevens C, Borden E, Enterline H. Leiomyosarcoma: the Eastern Cooperative Oncology Group experience with 222 patients (abstract C-561). Proc Am Assoc Cancer Res 1983;24:142.

220. Benjamin RS, Gottlieb JA, Baker LH. CYVADIC vs CYVADACT-A randomized trial of cyclophosphamide, vincristine and Adriamycin, plus either dacarbazine or actinomycin D in metastatic sarcomas (abstract). Proc Am Assoc Cancer Res 1976;17:256.

221. Baker LH, Frank J, Fine G, et al. Combination chemotherapy using Adriamycin, DTIC, cyclophosphamide, and actinomycin D for advanced soft tissue sarcomas: a randomized comparative trial. J Clin Oncol 1987;5(6):851–861.

222. Edmonson JH, Ryan L, Blum RH, et al. Randomized comparison of doxorubicin alone vs ifosphamide and doxorubicin or mitomycin, doxorubicin, cisplatin against advanced soft tissue sarcomas. J Clin Oncol 1993;11:1269–1275.

223. Antman K, Crowley J, Balcerzak SP, et al. An intergroup phase III randomized study of doxorubicin and dacarbazine with or without ifosfamide and mesna in advanced tissue and bone sarcomas. J Clin Oncol 1993;11:1276–1285.

224. Zalupski M, Metch B, Balcerzak S, et al. Phase III comparison of doxorubicin and dacarbazine given by bolus versus infusion in patients with soft-tissue sarcomas: a Southwest Oncology Group study. J Natl Cancer Inst 1991;83(13):926–932.

225. Borden EC, Amato DA, Edmonson JH, Ritch PS, Shiraki M. Randomized comparison of doxorubicin and vindesine to doxorubicin for patients with metastatic soft-tissue sarcomas. Cancer 1990;66(5):862–867.

226. Santoro A, Rouesse J, Steward W, et al. A randomized EORTC study in advanced soft tissue sarcomas: Adriamycin vs. Adriamycin and ifosfamid vs. cyvadic (abstract 1196). Proc Am Soc Clin Oncol 1990; 9:309.

227. Frei E III, Antman K, Teicher B, Eder P, Schnipper L. Bone marrow autotransplantation for solid tumors—prospects. J Clin Oncol 1989;7:515–526.

228. Antman KS, Griffin JD, Elias A, et al. Effect of recombinant human granulocyte-macrophage colony-stimulating factor on chemotherapy-induced myelosuppression. N Engl J Med 1988;319(10):593–598.

229. Steward WP, Verweij J, Somers R, et al. Doxorubicin plus ifosfamide with rhGM-CSF in the treatment of advanced adult soft tissue sarcomas—preliminary results of a phase II study from the EORTC Soft Tissue and Bone Sarcoma Group. J Cancer Res Clin Oncol 1991;117(Suppl 4 S1):43–47.

230. Steward WP, Verweij J, Somers R, et al. High dose chemotherapy with two schedules of recombinant human granulocyte-macrophage colony-stimulating factor in the treatment of advanced adult soft tissue sarcomas (abstract 1240). Proc Am Soc Clin Oncol 1991;10:349.

231. Pinkerton CR, Groot LJ, Barrett A, et al. Rapid VAC high dose melphalan regimen, a novel chemotherapy approach in childhood soft tissue sarcomas. Br J Cancer 1991;64(2):381–385.

232. Dumontet C, Biron P, Bouffet E, et al. High dose chemotherapy with ABMT in soft tissue sarcomas: a report of 22 cases. Bone Marrow Transplant 1992;10(5):405–408.

233. Pinkerton CR. Megatherapy for soft tissue sarcomas. EBMT experience. Bone Marrow Transplant 1991;3(120):120–122.

60

Chemotherapy of Carcinoma of Unknown Primary Site

John D. Hainsworth and F. Anthony Greco

Cancer of unknown primary site is a common clinical syndrome, accounting for 3 to 5% of all cancer diagnoses. The widespread nature of disease in most patients at the time of diagnosis precludes any consideration of curative surgical resection and has engendered widespread pessimism regarding treatment. Early attempts to devise effective empiric chemotherapy regimens were also largely unsuccessful, yielding low response rates and negligible effect on survival. The clinical heterogeneity of these patients also has made the design and clinical evaluation of uniform treatments for this entire group problematic.

As effective combination chemotherapy has developed for certain cancers, it is not surprising that some patients with carcinoma of unknown primary site are also benefited. The documentation of complete responses to chemotherapy in certain patient subsets has increased interest in the evaluation and treatment of patients with carcinoma of unknown primary site. Several clinical and pathologic features are now known to define potentially treatable subgroups of patients with carcinoma of unknown primary site. Therefore, optimal management requires appropriate clinical and pathologic evaluation, followed by application of specific treatment to patients in responsive subgroups.

Clinical Presentation

Due to the heterogeneity of this syndrome and the underlying diseases represented, clinical presentation is extremely variable. Typically, the patient develops symptoms at a site of metastatic cancer; routine history, physical examination, chest radiograph, laboratory studies, and selected radiologic evaluation based on symptoms fail to identify the primary site. At this point, a biopsy of the most accessible metastatic site is usually performed, and metastatic carcinoma is documented. The patient should initially be considered to have a "cancer of unknown primary site" if results of the relatively limited evaluation mentioned above does not suggest a primary site.

The initial light microscopic diagnosis provides a useful basis for further evaluation. The large majority of initial light microscopic diagnoses fall into one of four categories: adenocarcinoma, squamous carcinoma, poorly differentiated (anaplastic) neoplasm, and poorly differentiated carcinoma. A fifth category, recognized recently with increasing frequency and often requiring additional pathologic studies for complete definition, is the diagnosis of neuroendocrine carcinoma. These five patient groups are discussed separately, since they vary with respect to clinical characteristics, diagnostic evaluation, treatment, and prognosis.

ADENOCARCINOMA OF UNKNOWN PRIMARY SITE

Clinical Characteristics

Adenocarcinoma, the most frequent light microscopic diagnosis in patients with neoplasms of unknown primary site, accounts for approximately 60% of cases. As with most types of adenocarcinomas of known primary site, the incidence of adenocarcinoma of unknown primary site increases with advancing age. The typical patient with this diagnosis is therefore elderly and has metastatic tumor at several visceral sites. Common metastatic sites include the liver, lungs, and bones.

The sites of metastases determine the clinical presentation, and usually dominate the subsequent clinical course. It is unusual for the primary site to become clinically manifest during the patient's lifetime (only in 15–20%) (1). Even at autopsy, 20 to 30% of patients have no primary site detected. Occult primary sites in the lung and pancreas are the most commonly identified sites at autopsy, accounting for approximately 40% of all cases (2). Other gastrointestinal sites, including the stomach, colon, and liver are also frequent. Adenocarcinomas from a wide variety of other primary sites are also occasionally encountered. Adenocarcinomas of the breast and prostate, despite being relatively common cancers, are uncommon in this group of patients (2).

The prognosis for most patients with adenocarcinoma of unknown primary site is poor, with median survival times of 3 to 4 months in most large reported series. However, appropriate initial evaluation can identify certain subsets of patients with specific clinical syndromes; in these patient subgroups, treatment can have substantial impact on the clinical course.

Pathology

The diagnosis of adenocarcinoma is usually made without difficulty on the basis of light microscopic features and is based on the formation of glandular structures by neoplastic cells. However, adenocarcinomas from many sites share these histologic features, and therefore, the site of tumor origin is usually impossible to pinpoint. Certain histologic features can suggest specific primary sites, but even these are usually not specific enough to make a definitive diagnosis. Examples include "papillary features," typically seen in ovarian or thyroid cancers, and "signet ring cells," typically associated with gastric adenocarcinoma.

Additional pathologic studies, such as immunoperoxidase staining or electron microscopy, are unlikely to define a primary site in most adenocarcinomas of unknown primary site. One notable exception is the stain for prostate-specific antigen, which is quite specific for prostate cancer and should always be considered in males with adenocarcinoma of unknown primary site, particularly if bony involvement is dominant. In appropriate clinical settings, staining for estrogen receptor also may be considered, since positive staining supports the diagnosis of advanced breast cancer.

The diagnosis of "poorly differentiated adenocarcinoma" should be interpreted with cau-

tion, since patients with this diagnosis may be distinct from patients with well-differentiated adenocarcinoma in both tumor biology and responsiveness to systemic therapy. Criteria for the diagnosis of "poorly differentiated adenocarcinoma" may differ slightly among pathologists, since there is clearly a spectrum of differentiation, ranging from very well differentiated adenocarcinoma to completely anaplastic carcinoma that fails to show any differentiation. Minimal glandular formation or positive mucin staining in an otherwise poorly differentiated carcinoma often results in the diagnosis of poorly differentiated adenocarcinoma. Additional pathologic study in these patients is therefore appropriate, since immunoperoxidase staining can sometimes reveal unsuspected diagnoses. At present, patients with poorly differentiated adenocarcinoma of unknown primary site should be evaluated and treated according to the guidelines outlined for poorly differentiated carcinoma (see below).

Diagnostic Evaluation

If the primary site remains unidentified after routine history and physical examination, standard laboratory screening tests (complete blood count, chemistry profile, urinalysis), and chest radiograph, extensive additional testing is unlikely to be revealing. Specific symptoms should lead to directed radiologic evaluation, but a generalized evaluation of asymptomatic areas is nonproductive. A few additional diagnostic tests are probably appropriate. These include computerized tomographic (CT) scanning of the abdomen, which frequently reveals additional metastatic sites and identifies a primary site in a minority (<25%) of patients (3, 4). Serum prostate-specific antigen should be measured in all males, since this marker is quite specific for prostate cancer; all females with clinical presentation compatible with metastatic breast cancer should undergo mammography. Routine endoscopy of the upper and lower gastrointestinal tract is rarely productive in asymptomatic patients, and even the occasional finding of a small occult primary site does not aid in treatment decisions.

Treatment—Specific Subgroups

WOMEN WITH AXILLARY LYMPH NODE METASTASIS

Women who have axillary lymph node involvement with adenocarcinoma should be suspected of having metastatic breast cancer. Estrogen and progesterone receptors should always be measured in women presenting with isolated axillary lymph node metastases, since elevated levels provide strong evidence for the diagnosis of breast cancer (5). Mammograms often reveal an unsuspected occult primary in such patients.

In women with isolated axillary lymph node metastasis, treatment should proceed according to guidelines established for patients with stage II breast cancer. These patients are potentially curable with appropriate therapy. Modified radical mastectomy is the standard treatment for these patients, even when the physical examination and mammography are normal. The frequency of identifying an occult breast primary site in the mastectomy specimen has ranged from 44 to 82% in reported series but is usually in the 50 to 65% range (6–8). Occult primary tumors are usually less than 2 cm in diameter; in occasional patients, only "carcinoma in situ" is identified in the breast (9). Small numbers of patients have been treated with radiation therapy to the breast following axillary lymph node dissection, and results in these patients were similar to those achieved with mastectomy (7, 10). Axillary lymph node dissection alone is not recommended, since primary breast tumors will subsequently become manifest in approximately 50% of these patients (7, 10). The role of adjuvant therapy has not been studied; however, it seems reasonable to administer adjuvant therapy following guidelines established for stage II breast cancer. Prognosis following primary therapy is similar to that reported for stage II breast cancer (6, 8, 9).

Metastatic breast cancer should also be considered in women who have other sites of metastasis in addition to axillary lymph nodes. Determination of estrogen-receptor status is particularly important in these patients, since those with positive estrogen receptors may derive major palliative benefit from hormonal therapy.

Systemic chemotherapy, as used in the palliative treatment of metastatic breast cancer, may also benefit these patients.

WOMEN WITH PERITONEAL CARCINOMATOSIS

Women with adenocarcinoma involving the peritoneal surfaces usually have a primary tumor site in the ovary, although adenocarcinomas arising in the gastrointestinal tract or breast can occasionally produce this syndrome. The syndrome of peritoneal adenocarcinomatosis without a primary site in the ovaries is well described (11–17). Some of these patients have histologic features typical of ovarian carcinoma, such as psammoma bodies or papillary configuration. Others have poorly differentiated adenocarcinoma without distinctive features. When the histology suggests ovarian carcinoma, this syndrome has also been termed "peritoneal papillary serous carcinoma" or "multifocal extraovarian serous carcinoma." This syndrome has occurred in patients with previous bilateral oophorectomy, including some patients with familial ovarian carcinoma (18).

Several anecdotal reports in the early 1980s documented impressive responses to chemotherapy in women with peritoneal carcinomatosis. Most patients received cisplatin-based combination regimens similar to those used in the treatment of advanced ovarian cancer (11, 12, 14, 15). The results of treatment in several series of patients from single institutions have also been published (Table 60.1). The treatment approach in these patients varied slightly, but most patients underwent initial laparotomy with maximal surgical cytoreduction, followed by cisplatin-based combination chemotherapy. In all reported series, overall response rate was quite high, with a minority of complete responses and a few patients with long-term disease-free survival. Median survival ranged from 11 to 23

Table 60.1. Treatment of Women with Peritoneal Adenocarcinomatosis of Unknown Primary Site

| Investigator (Ref) | No. of Patients | Treatment | Response Rate (%) | | Median Survival (months) | % Disease-free Survivors >24 months |
			Overall	Complete		
Strnad et al. (16)	18	Surgical cytoreduction + cisplatin-based chemotherapy	39	39	23	17
Dalrymple et al. (13)	31	Surgical cytoreduction + chemotherapy[a]	32	10	11	6
Ransom et al. (17)	33	Surgical cytoreduction + cisplatin-based chemotherapy	—	13	17	9

[a]Patients received either chlorambucil alone or cisplatin-based therapy.

months, substantially different than the poor median survivals reported for other patients with adenocarcinoma of unknown primary.

The origin of these tumors is unknown, but some may arise from the peritoneal surface. Since the ovarian epithelium is an extension of the mesothelial surface, some carcinomas arising from the peritoneal (mesothelial) surface may share biologies similar to that of ovarian cancer. At present, these patients should be approached in the manner recommended for patients with stage III ovarian cancer. Although patients with this syndrome in previously reported series have received various cisplatin-based regimens, current treatment should probably include cisplatin and paclitaxel, since this combination has proven superior to others in the treatment of advanced ovarian cancer (19). Some of the patients in this group can be expected to have complete response to therapy, and a small percentage will have prolonged disease-free survival.

MEN WITH SKELETAL METASTASES

Male patients presenting with blastic bone metastases should be suspected of having metastatic prostate adenocarcinoma. Serum prostate-specific antigen (PSA) levels should be measured in all such patients, in addition to prostatic ultrasound examination with biopsy of any suspicious lesions. In addition, immunoperoxidase staining of the tumor for PSA should be considered. A positive staining for PSA confirms the diagnosis of prostate cancer in this clinical setting, and these patients should receive a trial of hormonal therapy as recommended for metastatic prostate cancer.

Occasional patients have been reported with PSA staining in adenocarcinoma at locations unusual for metastatic prostate cancer. In general, these patients have not had evidence of bone metastases, but have had lung, mediastinal lymph node, retroperitoneal lymph node, or brain metastases (20–22). Hormonal therapy was effective treatment for some of these patients.

ADENOCARCINOMA PRESENTING AS A SINGLE METASTATIC LESION

Occasionally, metastatic adenocarcinoma is identified at a single site (e.g., one lymph node group or a single mass). The possibility of an unusual primary site, rather than a metastatic lesion, should be considered (e.g., apocrine, sebaceous, eccrine carcinomas). However, these unusual carcinomas can usually be ruled out on the basis of the clinical and pathologic features. In most such patients, other sites of metastases

become evident in a relatively short time. However, local treatment with resection or radiation therapy sometimes results in meaningful palliation, and occasional long-term survivors have been reported.

Appropriate management depends on the site of involvement, but resection of a single lesion should be considered if technically feasible. In some instances, local radiation therapy alone or following surgical resection may improve local tumor control. The role of adjuvant chemotherapy following resection or radiation of a single metastatic site is undefined for patients with adenocarcinoma of unknown primary site. However, cisplatin-based therapy should be considered in patients with poorly differentiated adenocarcinoma (see following section).

Empiric Chemotherapy for Adenocarcinoma of Unknown Primary Site

Most patients with adenocarcinoma of unknown primary site do not fit into any of the specific subgroups described. Systemic chemotherapy is usually ineffective in these patients, producing relatively low response rates and few complete responses. The difficulty in treating this patient group is not surprising, since many of these patients have cancer types that respond poorly to therapy even when the primary site is known (i.e., lung, gastrointestinal primaries). The results of empiric chemotherapy trials containing 20 or more patients are summarized in Table 60.2. In many of these series, patients with poorly differentiated carcinoma, as well as those with adenocarcinoma, were included. 5-Fluorouracil (5-FU) is the only chemotherapeutic agent that has been well studied in this patient group as a single drug, and its activity is similar to that reported in various gastrointestinal primaries (response rates range from 0 to 16%) (1, 23, 24). A number of 5-FU-based regimens with demonstrated activity in the treatment of gastrointestinal malignancies have also been tested (25–30). Many of these are modifications of the FAM (5-FU, doxorubicin, mitomycin-C) regimen. As shown (Table 60.2), response rates have varied from 7 to 39%. However, median survival has remained in the 4- to 11-month range, and has not correlated well with reported response rate. Long-term disease-free survivors have not been reported with any of these regimens. Several recently reported regimens have included cisplatin in combination with other agents (26, 27, 33–36). Response rates with cisplatin-based regimens

Table 60.2. Results of Empiric Combination Chemotherapy in Patients with Adenocarcinoma of Unknown Primary Site

Regimen[a] (Ref)	Number of Patients	Response Rate (%)	Median Survival (months)
Combinations without cisplatin			
AM (25)	25	36	4
AM (26)	51	39	5
AM (27)	28	7	6
AMVi (28)	55	26	6
FAM (29)	43	30	11
FAM (30)	22	14	8
MFL (31)	21	5	2
CMeF (25)	22	5	3
CAV (32)	20	50	8
CAV (33)	34	24	5
Combinations with cisplatin			
CAFP (34)	47	28	7
AMP (27)	27	19	5
PVeB (26)	50	39	5
PEF (35)	36	22	11
PFL (36)	25	32	—
CAV/PE (33)	16	19	5

[a]Key: A, Adriamycin; M, mitomycin C; F, 5-fluorouracil; C, cyclophosphamide; Me, methotrexate; V, vincristine; P, cisplatin; Vi, vindesine; Ve, vinblastine; B, bleomycin; E, etoposide; L, leucovorin.

have been somewhat higher, but median survival has not been prolonged, and long-term disease-free survivors have not been reported. Since these regimens are usually more toxic, there is no current indication for their routine use in patients with adenocarcinoma of unknown primary site.

At present, patients with adenocarcinoma of unknown primary site should receive treatment designed to provide optimal palliation. For patients who are elderly or debilitated, such treatment may include symptomatic care only or palliative radiation therapy to a painful metastatic site. For patients with better performance status, a trial of systemic therapy is often reasonable, since a few patients will derive substantial palliative benefit. At present, no "best" chemotherapy combination regimen has been defined, and a clinician may choose from one of several regimens listed in Table 60.2, all having produced 20 to 30% response rates.

SQUAMOUS CARCINOMA OF UNKNOWN PRIMARY SITE

Squamous carcinoma at a metastatic site is unusual in the absence of an obvious primary

and accounts for only 5% of patients with carcinoma of unknown primary site. Most patients with squamous carcinoma of unknown primary site present with metastatic carcinoma limited to cervical lymph nodes. Less commonly, inguinal lymph nodes are the site of involvement. Effective treatment is available for both of these groups of patients.

Cervical Lymph Node Presentation

The cervical lymph nodes are the most common metastatic site for squamous carcinoma of unknown primary. Patients developing this syndrome share risk factors with patients who develop squamous cancers of the head and neck area and often have substantial histories of tobacco and alcohol use. In most instances, the upper or middle cervical lymph nodes are involved, and in these patients, a thorough search for a primary site in the head and neck area is an important part of the initial evaluation. Direct visualization of the oropharynx, hypopharynx, larynx, upper esophagus, and nasopharynx is recommended, with biopsy of any suspicious areas. When the lower cervical or supraclavicular lymph nodes are involved, primary lung cancer should be suspected, and fiberoptic bronchoscopy should be included in the diagnostic evaluation. In one large series of patients who developed cervical adenopathy as the initial sign of metastatic squamous carcinoma, this diagnostic workup revealed a primary site in 231 of 267 patients (87%) (37).

Recently, the Epstein-Barr viral genome has been identified in cervical lymph node metastases from nasopharyngeal carcinoma when DNA is analyzed by the polymerase chain reaction technique (38). This finding is not observed in metastatic squamous carcinomas from other head and neck primary sites or from the lung and, therefore, appears specific for nasopharyngeal carcinoma. Evaluation for the Epstein-Barr viral genome can be performed on tissue obtained by fine-needle aspiration and should be considered, particularly in young patients with poorly differentiated squamous histology. When the Epstein-Barr viral genome is found in cervical lymph node metastases, the patient should be treated according to recommendations for nasopharyngeal carcinoma.

When no primary site is identified after careful evaluation, appropriate treatment of the involved neck is potentially curative (Table 60.3). Five-year disease-free survivals of 30 to 50% have been consistently achieved. Not surpris-

Table 60.3. Squamous Carcinoma of Unknown Primary Site Involving Cervical Lymph Nodes: Summary of Treatment Results

Investigator (Ref)	Number of Patients	Treatment	5-Year Survival (%)
Barrie (39)	104	Surgery ± RT	31
Jesse (40)	184[a]	Surgery, RT, surgery + RT	43
Coker (41)	39	Surgery + RT	54
Jose (42)	54[a]	RT ± surgery	29
Nordstrom (43)	51[a]	Surgery, RT, surgery + RT	29
Fermont (44)	139[a]	RT	5
Leipzig (45)	32	Surgery, RT, surgery + RT	32 (3-year)
Pacini (46)	42	RT	23
Spiro (47)	79	Surgery, RT, surgery + RT	29
Mohit-Tabatabai (48)	46	Surgery, RT, surgery + RT	18
Yang (49)	80	RT	37
Carlson (50)	93	RT ± surgery	70+
McCunniff (51)	25	RT ± surgery	48
Bataini (52)	138	RT ± surgery	35
deBraud (53)	25	Surgery, RT, surgery + RT	44
	16	Chemotherapy + RT ± surgery	69 (3-year)

[a]Patients with adenocarcinoma, poorly differentiated carcinoma included.

ingly, outcome of treatment has depended on the extent of metastatic disease in the cervical lymph nodes, with N1 or N2 disease having a significantly higher cure rate than N3 or massive neck involvement.

The optimal treatment for patients with this syndrome is undefined, since no comparative studies have been performed. Similar results have been reported with radical neck dissection, radiation therapy, and a combination of these two modalities. When surgical therapy alone is used, a primary tumor in the head and neck subsequently becomes manifest in 20 to 40% of patients. This complication occurs much less frequently when radiation therapy is used, presumably because of the eradication of occult head and neck primary sites within the radiation field. Therefore, most authors recommend the use of radiation therapy, either alone or following radical neck dissection, using dosages and techniques similar to those used in patients with primary head and neck cancer. The nasopharynx, oropharynx, and hypopharynx should be included in the radiation portal (51).

Patients with low cervical or supraclavicular lymph nodes more frequently have an occult primary lung cancer, and treatment results are therefore inferior in this group of patients. However, if no other disease is detectable, the treatment approach should be similar in these patients, since occasional long-term survivors have been reported.

The role of chemotherapy in the treatment of patients with metastatic squamous carcinoma involving cervical lymph nodes is undefined. In one small nonrandomized comparison, patients treated with cisplatin and 5-FU in addition to local modalities showed a higher complete response rate (81 vs. 60%) and longer median survival time (>37 vs. 24 months) than did patients receiving local treatment alone (53). Until chemotherapy proves to play an integral role in the combined modality treatment of squamous carcinomas of the head and neck, it is unlikely to play a major role in patients with this syndrome.

Inguinal Lymph Node Presentation

Patients who develop squamous carcinoma in inguinal lymph nodes should be suspected of having a primary site in the perineal or anorectal areas, and appropriate evaluation is almost always successful in identifying the primary site. In females, careful examination of the vulva, vagina, and cervix is important, with biopsy of any suspicious areas. Uncircumcised males should have a careful penile examination. Anoscopy should be performed to exclude lesions in the anorectal area. Identification of a primary site in the perineal or anorectal areas is important, since curative treatment is available for carcinomas of the vulva, vagina, cervix, and anus, even after spread to the inguinal lymph nodes. For the occasional patient with no identifiable primary site, inguinal lymph node dissection with or without radiation therapy is the treatment of choice and is sometimes curative (54).

Squamous Carcinoma Metastatic to Other Sites

A primary lung carcinoma should be suspected when squamous cancer involves sites other than the cervical or inguinal lymph nodes. Computerized chest tomography and/or fiberoptic bronchoscopy should be considered. Chemotherapy with combination regimens effective in the treatment of non-small-cell lung cancer should be considered in patients with good performance status.

The pathologic diagnosis of metastatic squamous carcinoma is usually not difficult. Immunoperoxidase staining and electron microscopy are usually of no additional benefit in determining a primary site. However, patients with the diagnosis of "poorly differentiated squamous carcinoma" should be evaluated carefully, particularly if metastases occur at unusual sites and other clinical features are unusual for squamous lung cancer (e.g., young patient, nonsmoker). As with the diagnosis of "poorly differentiated adenocarcinoma," the diagnosis of poorly differentiated squamous carcinoma is sometimes based on minimal histologic criteria, and in these patients, additional pathologic evaluation is appropriate. Unless a more specific diagnosis is made, these patients should be considered for a trial of therapy as described for patients with poorly differentiated carcinoma (see below).

POORLY DIFFERENTIATED NEOPLASM

The diagnosis of poorly differentiated neoplasm by light microscopy implies the inability of the pathologist to distinguish between the major categories of malignant disease including carcinoma, lymphoma, and various mesenchymal tumors. Fortunately, additional pathologic techniques of tumor evaluation have become available so that a more specific diagnosis is almost always possible. In this group of patients, establishing a precise diagnosis is extremely important, since a variety of highly treatable cancers are poorly differentiated. The most frequent adult tumor for which specific, highly effective therapy is available is non-Hodgkin's lymphoma. When additional pathologic evaluation is performed, either with immunoperoxidase staining or electron microscopy, 34 to 66% of

poorly differentiated neoplasms are found to be intermediate- or high-grade non-Hodgkin's lymphoma (55–58). In children or young adults, a variety of highly treatable malignancies can be included, including various treatable sarcomas, neuroblastoma, Ewing's tumor, and germ cell tumors.

When the initial diagnosis is "poorly differentiated neoplasm," further pathologic evaluation is always required. Initial communication with the pathologist is important, since one common cause of a nonspecific light microscopic diagnosis is a small or poorly preserved biopsy specimen. Fine-needle aspiration biopsy usually provides an inadequate amount of tissue for optimal evaluation of poorly differentiated tumors, since histology is frequently difficult to evaluate, and the ability to perform special studies is limited. A larger biopsy specimen is recommended and is often adequate to make a more specific diagnosis. When the tumor type is still unclear, additional pathologic studies are required.

Immunoperoxidase Staining

The development of a large number of relatively sensitive and specific immunoperoxidase stains represents the major recent pathologic advance in the classification of poorly differentiated tumors. These stains, now widely available, can usually be reliably performed on formalin-fixed, paraffinized tissue. Immunoperoxidase reagents consist of either monoclonal or polyclonal antibodies directed at a variety of specific cell components or products, including enzymes, normal tissue components, hormones, oncofetal antigens, and other tumor markers. The results of immunoperoxidase staining must be interpreted in conjunction with the light microscopic appearance, since none of the stains is completely specific.

Table 60.4 summarizes the immunoperoxidase stains that are important in the diagnosis of specific tumor types. The diagnosis of lymphoma is usually possible, since the leukocyte common antigen stain is one of the most sensitive and specific immunoperoxidase stains available (59, 60). Most carcinomas can be identified by positive staining for cytokeratin (61–63). Neuroendocrine carcinoma is suggested by positive staining for neuron-specific enolase, chromogranin, or synaptophysin (64, 65). As discussed above, staining for PSA strongly suggests the diagnosis of prostate carcinoma in a male patient with metastatic adenocarcinoma (66). Melanoma

Table 60.4. Immunoperoxidase Staining Patterns Useful in the Differential Diagnosis of Neoplasms of Unknown Primary Site

Cancer Type	Immunoperoxidase Stain[a]
Carcinoma	Cytokeratin, EMA
Breast	ER, PR
Prostate	PSA
Germ cell	HCG, AFP[b]
Lymphoma	LCA
Melanoma	S-100 protein, HMB-45, NSE, vimentin
Sarcoma	Vimentin
Angiosarcoma	Factor VIII
Rhabdomyosarcoma	Desmin
Neuroendocrine tumor	Cytokeratin + NSE, chromogranin, synaptophysin

[a]Key: EMA, epithelial membrane antigen; ER, estrogen receptor; PR, progestrone receptor; PSA, prostate-specific antigen; HCG, human chorionic gonadotropin; AFP, α-fetoprotein; LCA, leukocyte common antigen; NSE, neuron-specific enolase.
[b]Typical histologic features also necessary to make this diagnosis.

is suggested by staining for S-100 protein, HMB-45 antigen, and vimentin; poorly differentiated sarcomas sometimes stain for either desmin, vimentin, or factor VIII antigen (67–69). Although germ cell tumors often stain for α-fetoprotein (AFP) or human chorionic gonadotropin (HCG), these stains are not specific enough to establish the diagnosis of germ cell tumor without the presence of typical histologic features (70, 71).

Care must be taken to avoid overinterpretation of immunoperoxidase stains, since no staining pattern is entirely specific. For example, some carcinomas stain positively with vimentin, some sarcomas stain with keratin, and a wide variety of nonneuroendocrine carcinomas stain with neuron-specific enolase.

Poorly differentiated neoplasms that are diagnosed as non-Hodgkin's lymphoma on the basis of immunoperoxidase staining can be treated effectively with combination chemotherapy. In a group of 35 such patients, treatment with standard lymphoma regimens resulted in an actuarial disease-free survival of 45% after a median follow-up of 30 months (58). Treatment outcome in this group was similar to a concurrently treated group of patients in whom the diagnosis was made definitively by light microscopy. Aggressive histology non-Hodgkin's lymphoma can therefore be reliably detected using immunoperoxidase staining techniques, and specific treatment can be administered with confidence in this patient group. Limited information exists concerning treatment of poorly differentiated neoplasms given diagnoses other than lymphoma on the basis of immunoperoxidase staining.

Electron Microscopy

Some poorly differentiated neoplasms have specific ultrastructural features, and identification of these features by electron microscopy allows specific diagnoses. This technique is less widely available and requires specific tissue preparation, so electron microscopy is usually reserved for neoplasms of uncertain lineage even after immunoperoxidase staining is completed. As with immunoperoxidase staining, the diagnoses of carcinoma and lymphoma can usually be reliably distinguished on the basis of electron microscopic features. Electron microscopy is probably superior to immunoperoxidase staining in the diagnosis of poorly differentiated neuroendocrine tumors (neurosecretory granules), melanoma (premelanosomes), and poorly differentiated sarcoma. However, undifferentiated tumors often lose their specific ultrastructural features in addition to their typical histology; therefore, the absence of a particular ultrastructural finding cannot be used to rule out a specific diagnosis.

Chromosomal Analysis

The chromosomal analysis of malignant tumors has not yet become a standard part of the pathologic evaluation. However, identification of specific chromosomal abnormalities in several solid tumors that frequently have poorly differentiated histology has stimulated recent interest in this technique. Two chromosomal rearrangements of sufficient specificity to enable diagnosis in poorly differentiated solid tumors have been identified. A specific chromosomal translocation (t11:22) has been found in all peripheral neuroepitheliomas and is also frequent in Ewing's tumor (72, 73). An isochromosome of the short arm of chromosome 12 (i12p) is found in a large percentage of testicular and extragonadal germ cell tumors in males (74).

The clinical relevance of molecular and cytogenic studies has been demonstrated in young patients with poorly differentiated carcinoma or adenocarcinoma involving primarily midline structures or with elevated serum levels of HCG or AFP (75, 76). In a group of 40 such patients, specific diagnoses were suggested by genetic studies in 17 (42%): germ cell tumor, 12; melanoma, 2; lymphoma, 1; peripheral neuroepithelioma, 1; desmoplastic small cell tumor, 1. Other pathologic techniques had not been diagnostic in any of the 12 patients with germ cell tumors. In these patients, cisplatin-based therapy produced a 75% overall response rate, with 45% complete responses. In other patients, similar therapy yielded only 17% overall response rates and no complete responders. Molecular genetic analysis was therefore useful in this patient group in identifying a chemotherapy-sensitive group of previously unsuspected extragonadal germ cell tumors.

Specific chromosomal abnormalities have also been well characterized in hematopoietic neoplasms, including leukemia, non-Hodgkin's lymphoma, and Hodgkin's disease (77). Because of the diagnostic accuracy of the immunoperoxidase stains in identifying lymphoma, molecular genetic analysis is rarely necessary in this patient group.

POORLY DIFFERENTIATED CARCINOMA OF UNKNOWN PRIMARY SITE

Approximately 20% of patients with carcinoma of unknown primary site have poorly differentiated carcinoma, and an additional 10% have poorly differentiated adenocarcinoma. Until relatively recently, these patient groups have not been separated from the larger group of patients with adenocarcinoma of unknown primary site and have been included in many of the empiric chemotherapy trials. It is now recognized that some of these patients have neoplasms that are highly sensitive to chemotherapy, and a small percentage are curable with appropriate therapy. Careful initial evaluation is therefore critical in this patient group, to ensure that patients with highly responsive neoplasms are identified and treated.

Pathologic Evaluation

Although the origin of these tumors is diverse, the histologic appearance is similar, showing cohesive sheets of malignant cells that fail to form any distinctive patterns. Even with careful retrospective review, some responsive tumors of well-defined types (e.g., germ cell tumor, lymphoma) could not be diagnosed with light microscopic examination alone (78). Therefore, additional pathologic examination with immu-noperoxidase staining and, in some cases, electron microscopy is required for optimal evaluation. Because the initial diagnosis of poorly differentiated carcinoma is somewhat more specific than "poorly differentiated neoplasm," the identification of unsuspected tumors of other types (particularly lymphoma) is much less frequent in this group. In a group of 87 patients with poorly differentiated carcinoma, a large battery of immunoperoxidase stains identified 16 patients (18%) with other diagnoses (79): melanoma, 8 patients; lymphoma, 4; neuroendocrine tumor, 3; and prostate carcinoma, 1. Patients with lymphoma were reliably identified and consistently had chemotherapy-sensitive neoplasms.

In most patients, the diagnosis of poorly differentiated carcinoma is confirmed by immunoperoxidase staining. Unfortunately, no histologic features or immunoperoxidase staining patterns have been identified in these patients that are useful in predicting chemotherapy responsiveness (78, 79). Immunoperoxidase staining with neuron-specific enolase was evaluated specifically in this respect, since "neuroendocrine differentiation" has been associated with increased tumor responsiveness in patients with non-small-cell lung cancer (80). In our patients with poorly differentiated carcinoma, 79 had immunoperoxidase staining with neuron-specific enolase performed, and 23 (29%) had positive staining (79). These patients had no other histologic or clinical features suggestive of neuroendocrine tumors. In this patient group, positive staining for neuron-specific enolase did not predict for higher response rate or improved survival.

Clinical Characteristics

Based on relatively limited clinical data, it appears that clinical characteristics differ somewhat in patients with poorly differentiated carcinomas and those with adenocarcinomas of unknown primary site (81). Although each group is heterogeneous with a great diversity of clinical features, patients with poorly differentiated carcinoma have a younger median age, frequently have a history of rapid progression of symptoms or rapid tumor growth, and more frequently have tumor location in the mediastinum, retroperitoneum, or peripheral lymph node areas. Some of these distinctive clinical features have proven useful in identifying chemotherapy-responsive subsets (see below).

Diagnostic Evaluation

The initial evaluation of these patients is similar to that described for patients with adenocarcinoma of unknown primary site. In addition to the workup previously described, all patients with poorly differentiated carcinoma should also have CT of the chest and abdomen and measurement of serum levels of HCG and AFP. The clinical utility of other tumor markers (e.g., CEA, CA-125, CA-19-9) has not been evaluated in this patient group.

Treatment

When a specific treatable neoplasm (e.g., lymphoma) is identified by specialized pathologic evaluation, therapy should be administered using established guidelines. Patients with elevated serum levels of AFP or HCG and clinical features suggestive of extragonadal germ cell tumor (i.e., mediastinal or retroperitoneal mass) should be treated according to recommendations for nonseminomatous extragonadal germ cell tumors, even when histologic examination does not render a specific diagnosis.

For patients in whom no specific diagnosis can be made other than "poorly differentiated carcinoma" or "poorly differentiated adenocarcinoma," a treatment trial with a cisplatin-based regimen is usually indicated. The first observations that some patients in this heterogeneous group have highly responsive tumors were made in the late 1970s, when several anecdotal reports appeared (82–84). Most of the patients in early reports were young males with tumor location in the mediastinum or retroperitoneum, many of whom also had elevated serum levels of HCG or AFP. Patients who had highly responsive tumors were thought initially to have histologically atypical extragonadal germ cell tumors. Most of the patients with long-term survival were treated with cisplatin-based regimens effective in the treatment of germ cell tumors.

Based on these encouraging results in a few patients, we prospectively studied the role of cisplatin-based therapy in patients with poorly differentiated carcinoma of unknown primary site. In a series of reports, we documented a high overall response rate and long-term disease-free survival in a minority of patients with this syndrome (81, 85, 86). Our experience in the treatment of 220 such patients, accumulated between 1978 and 1989, is summarized in Table 60.5. Most of the patients in this group did not have clinical characteristics strongly suggestive of extragonadal germ cell tumor. However, involvement of the mediastinum, retroperitoneum, and peripheral lymph node groups was relatively common. In the early years of this study, most patients received treatment with cisplatin, vinblastine, and bleomycin (PVB), then the most commonly used regimen for the treatment of advanced testicular cancer. More recently, as etoposide replaced vinblastine in the treatment of testicular cancer, our patients received cisplatin and etoposide, with or without bleomycin. All patients received an initial treatment trial of two courses of therapy, and responding patients received a total of four treatment courses. Major tumor responses were seen in 138 of 220 patients (62%), and 58 patients (26%) had complete response to treatment. Sixteen percent of the entire group remained free of tumor after a median follow-up of 61 months (range, 11 to 142 months) (86).

Table 60.5. Clinical Profile of 220 Patients with Poorly Differentiated Carcinoma or Poorly Differentiated Adenocarcinoma Treated with Cisplatin-Based Therapy

Clinical Characteristic	Number of Patients (%)
Median age (range)	39 (13–78)
Gender (male/female)	166/54
Light microscopic diagnosis	
Poorly differentiated carcinoma	142
Poorly differentiated adenocarcinoma	51
Poorly differentiated small cell carcinoma	12
Poorly differentiated neoplasm	11
Poorly differentiated squamous carcinoma	4
Dominant site of metastases	
Mediastinum	43 (20%)
Retroperitoneum	42 (19%)
Lung	29 (13%)
Peripheral lymph nodes	20 (9%)
Liver	11 (5%)
Other (9 sites represented)	26 (11%)
Multiple sites (no dominant site)	50 (23%)
Number of metastatic sites	
1	57 (36%)
2	67 (31%)
>2	96 (43%)
Elevated tumor markers (HCG or AFP)	40 (18%)
Treatment Results (216 evaluable)	
Complete response	58 (27%)
Partial response	80 (37%)
No response	78 (36%)
Long-term disease-free survival	36 (16%)

Similar results have recently been reported in patients selected by similar criteria and treated with cisplatin-based regimens (35, 87, 88). Van der Gaast et al. treated 40 patients with poorly differentiated carcinoma or poorly differentiated adenocarcinoma with cisplatin, etoposide, and bleomycin (87). Eighteen of 34 patients (53%) responded to therapy, with four complete responses (12%) and two long-term disease-free survivors. In a more heterogeneous patient group, Pavlidis et al. achieved a 16% complete response rate, including 3 of 11 complete responses (27%) in patients with undifferentiated carcinoma (88).

At present, patients with poorly differentiated carcinoma or poorly differentiated adenocarcinoma of unknown primary site should be treated initially with cisplatin-based combination chemotherapy. Although the optimal regimen is not defined, in our experience, cisplatin with etoposide and bleomycin produced results at least as good as those with cisplatin, vinblastine, and bleomycin, with less toxicity. The contribution of bleomycin to the regimen has not been evaluated. As in the treatment of germ cell tumors, four courses of such treatment is adequate, and all patients in our reports with long-term survival received only four courses. Unfortunately, patients who fail to achieve complete response or who are initially unresponsive to therapy usually have very resistant neoplasms. In these patients, response rates have been low regardless of which salvage therapy was used. In patients who have initial complete response and subsequently relapse, salvage therapy with regimens similar to those used in the treatment of refractory germ cell tumors (e.g., vinblastine, ifosfamide, cisplatin; VIP) produce excellent second responses in some.

Favorable Prognostic Factors

Since only a minority of patients have excellent treatment responses, we have analyzed our patients for clinical features predictive of treatment responsiveness and long-term survival (86). Prognostic features evaluated in a multivariate analysis included age, sex, smoking history, serum tumor marker status, number of metastatic sites, predominant site of tumor involvement, and light microscopic histology (poorly differentiated carcinoma vs. poorly differentiated adenocarcinoma). Several features were independently predictive of favorable treatment outcome, including tumor location in the retroperitoneum or peripheral lymph nodes, tumor limited to one or two metastatic sites, younger age, and negative smoking history.

Prognostic factors were also evaluated in a large series of patients reported from the M. D. Anderson Hospital (89). This group of 657 patients was heterogeneous, containing patients with all histologic subtypes. However, some of the same clinical features were found to be important, including a limited number of organ sites involved, tumor location in lymph nodes (including mediastinum and retroperitoneum) other than the supraclavicular lymph nodes, and female sex. In addition, the relatively poor outcome of patients with adenocarcinoma compared with other histologies was confirmed.

Although these prognostic features are useful, occasional excellent responses are seen even in patient groups with unfavorable clinical features. At present, even these patients should be considered for a brief trial of cisplatin-based chemotherapy.

NEUROENDOCRINE CARCINOMA OF UNKNOWN PRIMARY SITE

Improved pathologic methods for diagnosing neuroendocrine tumors have resulted in the recent recognition of a wider spectrum of these neoplasms. Most of the well-described adult neuroendocrine tumors have distinctive histology and indolent biologic behavior (Table 60.6). A second group of neuroendocrine tumors, typified by small cell lung cancer, has high-grade tumor biology and a typical "small cell" anaplastic appearance by light microscopy. A third group of neuroendocrine tumors, recently recognized, has high-grade biology and no distinctive neuroendocrine features by light microscopy. The initial diagnosis in this group is

Table 60.6. Adult Neuroendocrine Tumors

Indolent biology	Aggressive biology
Carcinoid tumor (many primary sites)	Small cell lung cancer
Islet cell tumor	Extrapulmonary small cell carcinoma (many primary sites)
Pheochromocytoma	Peripheral neuroepithelioma (usually in adolescents)
Medullary carcinoma, thyroid	Merkel cell tumor
Paraganglioma	? Adult neuroblastoma

usually poorly differentiated carcinoma, and neuroendocrine features are only recognized when immunoperoxidase staining or, more definitively, electron microscopy is performed. Neuroendocrine carcinomas of unknown primary site occur in each of these three categories and are briefly considered separately.

Low-Grade Neuroendocrine Carcinoma

Metastatic neuroendocrine tumors with histologic features typical of low-grade carcinoid or islet cell tumor are occasionally found without obvious primary site. In this situation, metastatic tumor almost always involves the liver and is sometimes associated with clinical syndromes produced by the secretion of bioactive substances (e.g., carcinoid syndrome, Zollinger-Ellison syndrome). In some of these patients, further evaluation reveals primary sites in the small intestine or pancreas.

As predicted by the histologic appearance, these neuroendocrine tumors usually exhibit an indolent biology, and management should follow guidelines established for metastatic carcinoid or islet cell tumors (see Chapter 56). These neoplasms are usually refractory to systemic chemotherapy, and cisplatin-based chemotherapy produces low response rates (90). Depending on the clinical situation, appropriate management may include local therapy (resection of isolated metastasis, hepatic artery ligation/embolization), treatment of associated syndromes with somatostatin analogues, 5-FU-based systemic therapy, or symptomatic management.

Small Cell Carcinoma

Patients with a history of cigarette smoking and small cell anaplastic carcinoma at a metastatic site usually have a bronchogenic primary. CT of the chest and fiberoptic bronchoscopy should be performed. If a pulmonary lesion is identified, the patient should be treated according to recommendations for extensive-stage small cell lung cancer. Small cell anaplastic carcinoma arising at a variety of extrapulmonary primary sites has also been described. Patients with localizing symptoms should have appropriate diagnostic studies performed.

When no primary site is identified, patients with small cell anaplastic carcinoma should be treated with combination chemotherapy as recommended for small cell lung cancer. These tumors are usually initially chemotherapy sensi-

tive, and major palliative benefit can be derived from treatment. In the rare instance when the tumor appears at a single metastatic site, the addition of radiation therapy to combination chemotherapy should be considered.

Poorly Differentiated Neuroendocrine Carcinoma

In approximately 10% of poorly differentiated carcinomas, electron microscopy reveals neurosecretory granules, a finding diagnostic of neuroendocrine carcinoma. These tumors have been called "poorly differentiated neuroendocrine tumors" or "primitive neuroectodermal tumors." In some of these tumors, neuroendocrine features are recognizable by light microscopy, while in others the light microscopic diagnosis is "poorly differentiated carcinoma." While electron microscopy is the most accurate means of pathologic diagnosis, most of the tumors also have typical immunoperoxidase staining patterns with positive staining for neuron-specific enolase, chromogranin, and synaptophysin.

We previously reported a group of 29 patients with poorly differentiated neuroendocrine tumors (91) and have recently updated our experience to include 43 patients treated with combination chemotherapy. Most of these patients had clinical evidence of high-grade tumor, and most had metastases in multiple sites. Thirty-three of 43 evaluable patients (77%) responded to chemotherapy with a platinum-based combination regimen. Thirteen patients (30%) had a complete response, and eight remain continuously disease-free more than 2 years after completion of therapy. An additional five patients with involvement at only one site received treatment with local modalities (surgical excision, 3; radiation therapy, 2), and four of these five patients had long-term survival.

The origin of these poorly differentiated neuroendocrine carcinomas remains unclear. In four of our patients, specific diagnoses were made either subsequently in their clinical course or at autopsy. Two patients had carcinoid tumors with "undifferentiated" growth pattern (both presented with abdominal carcinomatosis), one had small cell lung cancer, and one had extragonadal germ cell tumor with predominant neuroendocrine differentiation. It is likely that some additional patients had small cell lung cancer with occult primary tumor, but more than half of these patients had no smoking history, and the absence of overt pulmonary involvement makes this diagnosis unlikely in most patients. It is probable that some of these tumors are undifferentiated variants of well-recognized neuroendocrine tumors (e.g., carcinoid tumor), without a recognizable primary site. In the undifferentiated form, the clinical and pathologic characteristics no longer resemble the characteristics of the more differentiated counterpart. Anaplastic carcinoid tumors arising in the gastrointestinal tract are highly responsive to cisplatin-based chemotherapy, whereas carcinoid tumors with typical histology are usually resistant to cisplatin (90). A few case reports of patients with "extrapulmonary small cell carcinoma of unknown primary site" have also documented chemotherapy responsiveness and occasional long-term survival following systemic therapy (92, 93).

Although the nature of these tumors remains undefined, the presence of neurosecretory granules in patients with poorly differentiated carcinoma identifies a highly treatable subgroup. All patients in this group should be considered for a trial of combination chemotherapy with a platinum-based regimen. Some patients with a single site of tumor involvement may be curable with local treatment modalities alone; however, a course of adjuvant chemotherapy should also be considered in these patients if clinically feasible.

SUMMARY

Optimal treatment of patients with carcinoma of unknown primary site now requires awareness of the clinical and pathologic features defining specific treatable subsets of patients. Taken together, approximately 40% of patients fall into a defined subgroup with specific treatment implications (Fig. 60.1). These patients can be identified prospectively using the pathologic and clinical evaluation described in this chapter. All of these patients should receive a trial of specific therapy as described. Unfortunately, a large group of patients with relatively insensitive tumors remains. Current treatments have little impact on the course and survival of most of these patients, although a minority achieve palliative benefit with empiric chemotherapy. Improved therapy for these patients awaits advances in the treatment of non-small-cell lung cancer, pancreatic cancer, and other gastrointestinal malignancies, since most insensitive adenocarcinomas arise from these occult primary sites.

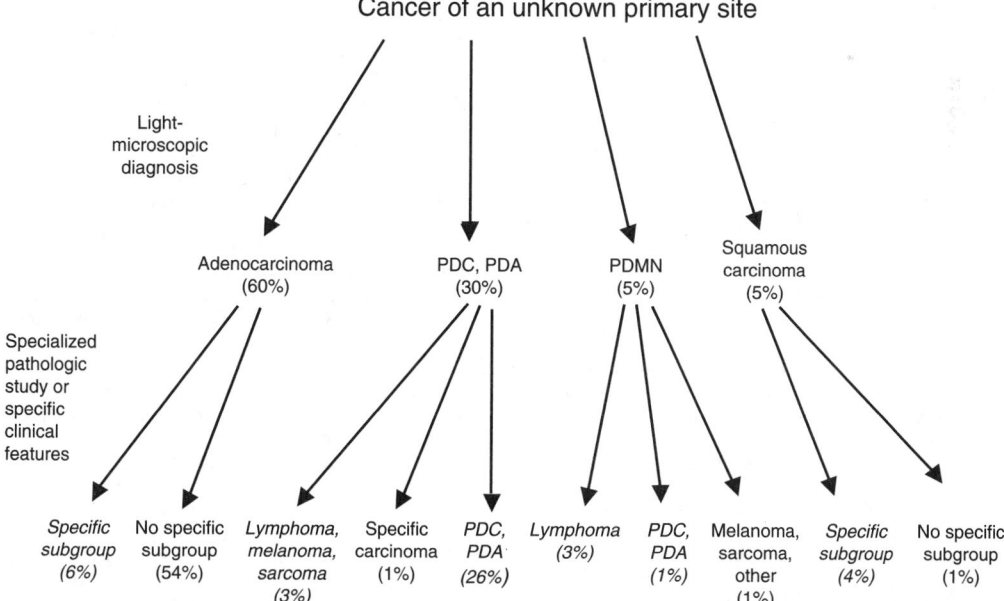

Figure 60.1.   Relative sizes of various clinical and histologic subgroups of patients with cancer of an unknown primary site as determined by optimal clinical and pathologic evaluation. Potentially treatable subgroups (described in the text) are indicated in italics and comprise approximately 40% of patients. *PDC*, poorly differentiated carcinoma; *PDA*, poorly differentiated carcinoma; *PDMN*; poorly differentiated malignant neoplasm. (Reprinted by permission of the New England Journal of Medicine from Hainsworth JD, Greco FA, 1993;329:258.)

REFERENCES

1. Shildt RA, Kennedy PS, Chen TT, Athens JW, O'Bryan RM, Balcerzak SP. Management of patients with metastatic adenocarcinoma of unknown origin: a Southwest Oncology Group study. Cancer Treat Rep 1983;67:77–79.

2. Nystrom JS, Weiner JM, Heffelfinger-Juttner J, Irwin LE, Bateman JR, Wolf RM. Metastatic and histologic presentations in unknown primary cancer. Semin Oncol 1977;4:53–58.

3. Karsell PR, Sheedy PF, O'Connell MJ. Computerized tomography in search of cancer of unknown origin. JAMA 1982;248:340–343.

4. McMillan JH, Levine E, Stephens RH. Computed tomography in the evaluation of metastatic adenocarcinoma from an unknown primary site. Radiology 1982;143:143–146.

5. Bhatia SK, Saclarides TJ, Witt TR, Bonomi PD, Anderson KM, Economou SG. Hormone receptor studies in axillary metastases from occult breast cancers. Cancer 1987;59:1170–1172.

6. Ashikari R, Rosen PP, Urban JA, Senoo T. Breast cancer presenting as an axillary mass. Ann Surg 1976; 183:415–417.

7. Merson M, Andreola S, Galimberti V, Bufalino R, Marchini S, Veronesi U. Breast carcinoma presenting as axillary metastases without evidence of a primary tumor. Cancer 1992;70:504–508.

8. Patel J, Nemoto T, Rosner D, Dao TL, Pickren JW. Axillary lymph node metastases from an occult breast cancer. Cancer 1981;47:2923–2927.

9. Rosen PP. Axillary lymph node metastases in patients with occult noninvasive breast carcinoma. Cancer 1980;46:1298–1306.

10. Ellerbroek N, Holmes F, Singletary E, Evans H, Oswald M, McNeese M. Treatment of patients with isolated axillary nodal metastases from an occult primary carcinoma consistent with breast origin. Cancer 1990;66:1461–1467.

11. August CZ, Murad TM, Newton M. Multiple focal extraovarian serous carcinoma. Int J Gynecol Pathol 1985;4:11–23.

12. Chen KT, Flam MS. Peritoneal papillary serous carcinoma with long-term survival. Cancer 1986; 58:1371–1373.

13. Dalrymple JC, Bannatyne P, Russell P, Solomon HJ, et al. Extraovarian peritoneal serous papillary carcinoma. A clinicopathologic study of 31 cases. Cancer 1989;64:110–115.

14. Gooneratne S, Sassone M, Blaustein A, Talerman A. Serous surface papillary carcinoma of the ovary: a clinicopathologic study of 26 cases. Int J Gynecol Pathol 1982;1:258–269.

15. Hochster H, Wernz JC, Muggia FM. Intra-abdominal carcinomatosis with histologically normal ovaries (letter). Cancer Treat Rep 1984;68:931–932.

16. Strnad CM, Grosh WW, Baxter J, Burnett LS, Jones HW III, Greco FA, Hainsworth JD. Peritoneal carcinomatosis of unknown primary site in women. Ann Intern Med 1989;111:213–217.

17. Ransom DT, Patel SR, Keeney GL, Malkosian GD, Edmonson JH. Papillary serous carcinoma of the peritoneum: a review of 33 cases treated with platin-based chemotherapy. Cancer 1990;66:1091–1094.

18. Tobacman JK, Greene MH, Tucker MA, Costa J, Kase R, Fraumeni JF. Intra-abdominal carcinomatosis after prophylactic oophorectomy in ovarian cancer-prone families. Lancet 1982;2:795–797.

19. McGuire WP, Hoskins WJ, Brady MF, Kucera PR, Look KY, Partridge EE, Davidson M. A phase III trial comparing cisplatin/cytoxan and cisplatin/Taxol in advanced ovarian cancer (abstract). Proc Am Soc Clin Oncol 1993;12:255.

20. Gentile PS, Carloss HW, Huang T-Y, Yam LT, Lam WK. Disseminated prostatic carcinoma simulating primary lung cancer. Cancer 1988;62:711–715.

21. Tell DT, Khoury JM, Taylor HG, Veasey SP. Atypical metastasis from prostate cancer: clinical utility of the immunoperoxidase technique for prostate specific antigen. JAMA 1985;253:3574–3575.

22. Kasabian NG, Previte SR, Kaloustian HD, Ganem EJ. Adenocarcinoma of the prostate presenting initially as an intracerebral tumor. Cancer 1992; 70:2149–2151.

23. Johnson RO, Castro R, Ansfield FJ. Response of primary unknown cancers to treatment with 5-fluorouracil. Cancer Chemother Rep 1964;38:63–64.

24. Moertel CG, Reitemeier RJ, Schutt AJ, Hahn RG. Treatment of the patient with adenocarcinoma of unknown origin. Cancer 1972;30:1469–1472.

25. Woods RL, Fox RM, Tattersall MHN, Levi JA, Brodie GN. Metastatic adenocarcinoma of unknown primary: a randomized study of two combination-chemotherapy regimens. N Engl J Med 1980;303:87–89.

26. Milliken ST, Tattersall MH, Woods RL, Coates AS, Levi JA, Fox RM, Raghaven D. Metastatic adenocarcinoma of unknown primary site. A randomized study of two combination chemotherapy regimens. Eur J Cancer Clin Oncol 1987;23:1645–1648.

27. Eagan RT, Therneau TM, Rubin J, Long HJ, Schutt AJ. Lack of value for cisplatin added to mitomycin-doxorubicin combination chemotherapy for carcinoma of unknown primary site. Am J Clin Oncol 1987;10:82–85.

28. Kambhus SA, Kelsen D, Niedzwiecki D, Ochoa M Jr. Phase II trial of mitomycin C, vindesine, and Adriamycin and predictive variables in the treatment of patients with adenocarcinoma of unknown primary site (abstract). Proc Am Assoc Cancer Res 1986;27:185.

29. Goldberg RM, Smith FP, Ueno W, Ahlgren JD, Schein PS. Fluorouracil, Adriamycin, and mitomycin in the treatment of adenocarcinoma of unknown primary. J Clin Oncol 1986;4:395–399.

30. van der Gaast AVD, Verweij J, Planting ASTH, Stoter G, van der Gaast A. 5-Fluorouracil, doxorubicin, and mitomycin C (FAM) combination chemotherapy for metastatic adenocarcinoma of unknown primary. Eur J Cancer Clin Oncol 1988;24:765–768.

31. Kelsen D, Martin DS, Colofiore J, Sawyer R, Coit D. A phase II trial of biochemical modulation using N-phosphonacetyl-L-aspartate, high-dose methotrexate, high-dose 5-fluorouracil, and leucovorin in patients with adenocarcinoma of unknown primary site. Cancer 1992;70:1988–1992.

32. Anderson H, Thatcher N, Rankin E, Wagstaff J, Scarfee JH, Crowther D. VAC (vincristine, Adriamycin and cyclophosphamide) chemotherapy for metastatic carcinoma from an unknown primary site. Eur J Cancer Clin Oncol 1983;19:49–52.

33. de Campos ES, Menasce LP, Radford J, Harris M, Thatcher N. Metastatic carcinoma of uncertain primary site: a retrospective review of 57 patients treated with vincristine, doxorubicin, cyclophosphamide,

(VAC) or VAC alternating with cisplatin and etoposide (VAC/PE). Cancer 1994;73:470–475.

34. Pasterz R, Savoraj N, Burgess M. Prognostic factors in metastatic carcinoma of unknown primary. J Clin Oncol 1986;4:1652–1657.

35. Raber MN, Faintuch J, Abbruzzese JL, Sumnull C, Frost P. Continuous infusion 5-fluorouracil, etoposide, and cis-diamminedichloroplatinum in patients with metastatic carcinoma of unknown primary origin. Ann Oncol 1991;2:519–520.

36. Lenzi R, Abbruzzese J, Amato R, Raber M, Frost P. Cisplatin, 5-fluorouracil and folinic acid for the treatment of carcinoma of unknown primary: a phase II study (abstract). Proc Am Soc Clin Oncol 1991; 10:301.

37. Jones AS, Cook JA, Phillips DE, Roland NR. Squamous carcinoma presenting as an enlarged cervical lymph node. Cancer 1993;72:1756–1761.

38. Feinmesser R, Miyazaki I, Cheung R, Freeman JL, Noyek AM, Dosch HM. Diagnosis of nasopharyngeal carcinoma by DNA amplification of tissue obtained by fine needle aspiration. N Engl J Med 1992; 326:17–21.

39. Barrie JR, Knapper WH, Strong EW. Cervical nodal metastases of unknown origin. Am J Surg 1970; 120:466–470.

40. Jesse RH, Perez CA, Fletcher GH. Cervical lymph node metastasis: unknown primary cancer. Cancer 1973;32:854–859.

41. Coker DD, Casterline PF, Chambers RG, Jacques DA. Metastases to lymph nodes of the head and neck from an unknown primary site. Am J Surg 1977;134:517–522.

42. Jose B, Bosch A, Caldwell WL, Frias Z. Metastasis to neck from unknown primary tumor. Acta Radiol Oncol 1979;18:161–170.

43. Nordstrom DG, Tewfik HH, Latourette HB. Cervical lymph node metastases from an unknown primary. Int J Radiat Oncol Biol Phys 1979;5:73–76.

44. Fermont AC. Malignant cervical lymphadenopathy due to an unknown primary. Clin Radiol 1980;31:355–358.

45. Leipzig B, Winter ML, Hokanson JA. Cervical nodal metastases of unknown origin. Laryngoscope 1981;91:593–598.

46. Pacini P, Olmi P, Cellai E, Chiavacci A. Cervical lymph node metastases from an unknown primary tumour. Acta Radiol Oncol 1981;20:311–314.

47. Spiro RH, DeRose G, Strong EW. Cervical node metastasis of occult origin. Am J Surg 1983;146:441–446.

48. Mobit-Tabatabai MA, Dasmahapatra KS, Rush BF Jr, Ohanian M. Management of squamous cell carcinoma of unknown origin in cervical lymph nodes. Am Surg 1986;52:152–154.

49. Yang ZY, Hu YH, Yan JH, Cai WM, Qin DX, Xu GZ, Wu XL. Lymph node metastases in the neck from an unknown primary. Report on 113 patients. Acta Radiol Oncol 1983;22:17–22.

50. Carlson LS, Fletcher GH, Oswald MJ. Guidelines for the radiotherapeutic techniques for cervical metastases from an unknown primary. Int J Radiat Oncol Biol Phys 1986;12:2101–2110.

51. McCunniff AJ, Raben M. Metastatic carcinoma of the neck from an unknown primary. Int J Radiat Oncol Biol Phys 1986;12:1849–1852.

52. Bataini JP, Rodriguez J, Jaulerry C, Brugere J,

Ghossein NA. Treatment of metastatic neck nodes secondary to an occult epidermoid carcinoma of the head and neck. Laryngoscope 1987;97:1080–1084.

53. de Braud F, Heilbrun LK, Ahmed K, Sakr W, Ensley JF, et al. Metastatic squamous cell carcinoma of an unknown primary localized to the neck. Advantages of an aggressive treatment. Cancer 1989;64:510–515.

54. Guarishci A, Keane TJ, Elhakim T. Metastatic inguinal nodes from an unknown primary neoplasm. A review of 56 cases. Cancer 1987;59:572–577.

55. Azar HA, Espinoza CG, Richman AV, Saba SR, Wang T. "Undifferentiated" large cell malignancies: an ultrastructural and immunocytochemical study. Hum Pathol 1982;13:323–333.

56. Gatter KC, Alcock C, Heryet A, Mason DY. Clinical importance of analysing malignant tumours of uncertain origin with immunohistochemical techniques. Lancet 1985;2:1302–1305.

57. Hales SA, Gatter KC, Heryet A, Mason DY. The value of immunocytochemistry in differentiating high-grade lymphoma from other anaplastic tumours. A study of anaplastic tumours from 1940 to 1960. Leuk Lymphoma 1989;1:59–63.

58. Horning SJ, Carrier EK, Rouse RV, Warnke RA, Michie SA. Lymphomas presenting as histologically unclassified neoplasms: characteristics and response to treatment. J Clin Oncol 1989;7:1281–1287.

59. Battifora H, Trowbridge IS. A monoclonal antibody useful for the differential diagnosis between malignant lymphoma and nonhematopoietic neoplasms. Cancer 1983;51:816–821.

60. Warnke RA, Gatter KC, Falini B, Hildreth P, Woolston RE, et al. Diagnosis of human lymphoma with monoclonal antileukocyte antibodies. N Engl J Med 1983;209:1275–1281.

61. Gabbiani G, Kapanci Y, Barazzone P, Franke WW. Immunochemical identification of intermediate-size filaments in human neoplastic cells. A diagnostic aid for the surgical pathologist. Am J Pathol 1981; 104:206–212.

62. Nagle RB, McDaniel KM, Clark VA, Payne CM. The use of antikeratin antibodies in the diagnosis of human neoplasms. Am J Clin Pathol 1983;79:458–465.

63. Schlegel R, Bank-Schlegel S, McLeod JA, Pinkus GS. Immunoperoxidase localization of keratin in human neoplasms. A preliminary survey. Am J Pathol 1980;101:41–48.

64. O'Connor DT, Burton D, Deftos LJ. Immunoreactive human chromogranin A in diverse polypeptide hormone producing human tumors and normal endocrine tissues. J Clin Endocrinol Metab 1983; 57:1084–1086.

65. Tapia FJ, Polak JM, Barbosa AJ, Bloom SR, Marangos PJ, Dermody C, Pearse AG. Neuron-specific enolase is produced by neuroendocrine tumors. Lancet 1981;1:808–811.

66. Allhof EP, Proppe KH, Chapman CM. Evaluation of prostate specific acid phosphatase and prostate specific antigen. J Urol 1983;129:316–319.

67. Denk H, Krepler R, Artlieb U, Gabbiani G, Rungger-Brandle E, Leoncini P, Franke WW. Proteins of intermediate filaments. An immunohistochemical and biochemical approach to the classification of soft tissue tumors. Am J Pathol 1983;110:193–208.

68. Kahn HJ, Marks A, Thom H, Baumal R. Role of

antibody to S-100 protein in diagnostic pathology. Am J Clin Pathol 1983;79:341–347.

69. Osborn M, Weber K. Biology of disease. Tumor diagnosis by intermediate filament type: a novel tool for surgical pathology. Lab Invest 1983;48:372–394.

70. Bosman FT, Giard RWM, Nieuwenhuijen-Kruseman AC, Knijnenburg G, Spaander PJ. Human chorionic gonadotrophin and alpha-fetoprotein in testicular germ cell tumors: a retrospective immunohistochemical study. Histopathology 1980;4:673–684.

71. Kurman KJ, Scardino PT, McIntire KR, Waldman TA, Javadpour N. Cellular localization of alpha fetoprotein and human chorionic gonadotropin in germ cell tumors of the testis using an indirect immunoperoxidase technique. A new approach to classification utilizing tumor markers. Cancer 1977; 40:2136–2151.

72. Whang-Peng J, Triche TJ, Knutsen T, Miser J, Douglass EC, Israel MA. Chromosome translocation in peripheral neuroepithelioma. N Engl J Med 1984; 311:584–585.

73. Turc-Carel C, Philip I, Berger MP, Philip T, Lenoir GM. Chromosomal translocation in Ewing's sarcoma. N Engl J Med 1983;309:497–498.

74. Bosl GJ, Ilson DH, Rodriguez E, Motzer RJ, Reuter VE, Chaganti RSK. Clinical relevance of the i(12p) marker chromosome in germ cell tumors. J Natl Cancer Inst 1994;86:349–358.

75. Motzer RJ, Rodriguez E, Reuter VE, Mazumdar M, Bosl GJ, Chaganti RSK. Molecular and cytogenic studies in the diagnosis of patients with midline carcinomas of unknown primary site. J Clin Oncol 1995; 13:274–282.

76. Motzer RJ, Rodriguez E, Reuter VE, Samaniego F, Dmitrovsky E, et al. Genetic analysis as an aid in diagnosis for patients with midline carcinoma of uncertain histologies. J Natl Cancer Inst 1983;83:341–346.

77. Arnold A, Cossman J, Bakhshi A, Jaffe ES, Waldmann TA, Korsmeyer SJ. Immunoglobulin-gene rearrangements as unique clonal markers in human lymphoid neoplasms. N Engl J Med 1983;309:1593–1599.

78. Hainsworth JD, Wright EP, Gray GF Jr, Greco FA. Poorly differentiated carcinoma of unknown primary site: correlation of light microscopic findings with response to cisplatin-based combination chemotherapy. J Clin Oncol 1987;5:1275–1280.

79. Hainsworth JD, Wright EP, Johnson DH, Davis BW, Greco FA. Poorly differentiated carcinoma of unknown primary: clinical usefulness of immunoperoxidase staining. J Clin Oncol 1991;9:1931–1938.

80. Graziano SL, Mazid R, Newman N, et al. The use of neuroendocrine immunoperoxidase markers to predict chemotherapy response in patients with nonsmall cell lung cancer. J Clin Oncol 1989;10:1398–1406.

81. Greco FA, Vaughn WK, Hainsworth JD. Advanced poorly differentiated carcinoma of unknown primary site: recognition of a treatable syndrome. Ann Intern Med 1986;104:547–556.

82. Richardson RL, Greco FA, Wolff S, Hande KR, Oldham RK. Extragonadal germ cell malignancy: value of tumor markers in metastatic carcinoma in young males (abstract). Proc Am Assoc Cancer Res 1979;20:204.

83. Richardson RL, Schoumacher RA, Fer MF, Hande KR, Forbes JT, Oldham RK, Greco FA. The unrecognized extragonadal germ cell cancer syndrome. Ann Intern Med 1981;94:181–186.

84. Fox RM, Woods RL, Tattersall MHN. Undifferentiated carcinoma in young men: the atypical teratoma syndrome. Lancet 1979;1:1316–1318.

85. Hainsworth JD, Greco FA. Poorly differentiated carcinoma of unknown primary site. In: Fer MF, Greco FA, Oldham R, eds. Poorly differentiated neoplasms and tumors of unknown origin. Orlando, FL: Grune & Stratton, 1986:189–202.

86. Hainsworth JD, Johnson DH, Greco FA. Cisplatin-based combination chemotherapy in the treatment of poorly differentiated adenocarcinoma of unknown primary site: results of a 12-year experience. J Clin Oncol 1992;10:912–922.

87. van der Gaast A, Verweij J, Henzen-Logmans SC, Rodenburg CJ, Stoter G. Carcinoma of unknown primary: identification of a treatable subset. Ann Oncol 1991;1:119–123.

88. Pavlidis N, Kosmidis P, Skaros D, Briassoulis E, Beer M, et al. Subsets of tumors responsive to cisplatin or carboplatin combinations in patients with carcinoma of unknown primary site. Ann Oncol 1992; 3:236–239.

89. Abbruzzese JL, Abbruzzese MC, Hess KR, Raber MN, Lenzi R, Frost P. Unknown primary carcinoma: natural history and prognostic factors in 657 consecutive patients. J Clin Oncol 1994;12:1272–1280.

90. Moertel CG, Kvols LF, O'Connell MJ, Rubin J. Treatment of neuroendocrine carcinomas with combined etoposide and cisplatin: evidence of major therapeutic activity in anaplastic variants of these neoplasms. Cancer 1991;68:227–233.

91. Hainsworth JD, Johnson DH, Greco FA. Poorly differentiated neuroendocrine carcinoma of unknown primary site: a newly recognized clinicopathologic entity. Ann Intern Med 1988;109:364–371.

92. Kasimis BS, Wuerker RB, Malefatto JP, Moran EM. Prolonged survival of patients with extrapulmonary small cell carcinoma arising in the neck. Med Pediatr Oncol 1983;11:27–32.

93. van der Gaast A, Verweij J, Prins E, Splinter TAW. Chemotherapy as treatment of choice in extrapulmonary undifferentiated small cell carcinomas. Cancer 1990;65:422–424.

61

Chemotherapy of Pediatric Solid Tumors

Donald K. Strickland and Nasrollah Hakami

In this chapter, four of the most common malignancies of the pediatric age group—neuroblastoma, Wilms' tumor, rhabdomyosarcoma, and retinoblastoma—are discussed. Together they account for nearly 20% of all the malignancies in children less than 15 years of age (1). For these malignancies, age, histology, and the extent of disease at diagnosis have a profound influence on treatment planning and outcome. Thus, the chemotherapy of each of these malignancies is discussed with these variables in mind.

NEUROBLASTOMA

Neuroblastoma, the most common extracranial solid tumor in children less than 5 years of age (1), arises from any site along the sympathetic nervous system chain. Most primary tumors occur in the abdomen, although infants more frequently have thoracic or cervical primaries. In addition, children are more likely than infants to present with regional lymph node spread or disseminated disease (2).

In addition to the history and physical examination, studies required for clinical staging include computed tomographic (CT) scan or magnetic resonance imaging (MRI) of the abdomen and pelvis, chest radiograph and CT scan, bone scan and radiographs, measurement of urinary catecholamine excretion, and bone marrow aspiration and biopsy. The most widely used staging system was reported by Evans et al. in 1971 (3). Subsequent studies from the St. Jude's Children's Research Hospital (SJCRH) and the Pediatric Oncology Group (POG) have also demonstrated the importance of resectability of the tumor as well as the extent of spread to regional lymph nodes (4, 5). These results have led to a staging system currently used by the POG (Table 61.1). Although comparable with respect to distinguishing patients with low-stage/good-prognosis and those with high-stage/poor-prognosis disease, substantial differences exist between these two staging systems. More recently, an International Neuroblastoma Staging System (INSS) was devised, incorporating important components from both the Evans and POG staging systems (2).

The age of the child and the extent of disease at diagnosis continue to be the most important predictors of prognosis. Additional prognostic factors have also been evaluated to assist in planning treatment and to enable separation of patients who need aggressive multimodal therapy from those who can be cured with minimal or no chemotherapy. Serum ferritin, neuro-specific enolase (NSE), G_{D2}, and lactate dehydrogenase (LDH) may have prognostic value (6). More recently, tumor DNA ploidy, N-myc oncogene amplification, and expression of P-glycoprotein have been recognized as potentially powerful tools for predicting outcome (7, 8).

Chemotherapy

STAGE A

Regardless of the age of the patient at diagnosis, more than 90% of the children with stage A are cured by complete resection of the tumor. Postoperative chemotherapy is not recommended (9).

STAGE B

By definition, complete resection of the malignancy cannot be accomplished in this group

Table 61.1. Pediatric Oncology Group Staging of Neuroblastoma

Stage	Description
A	Primary tumor: completely resected with or without microscopic residual
	Lymph nodes: intracavitary nodes not adherent to the tumor are histologically free of tumor
	Liver: histologically free of tumor in abdominal and pelvic primaries
B	Primary tumor: resected or biopsied with gross residual
	Lymph nodes and liver: as in stage A
C	Primary tumor: completely or incompletely resected
	Lymph nodes: intracavitary nodes not adherent to the tumor are histologically involved
	Liver: as in stage A
D	Malignancy has extended to extracavitary nodes, liver, skin, bone, bone marrow

of patients. Postoperatively, the goal of treatment is the eradication of residual disease with chemotherapy and/or radiation therapy. Recent POG studies suggest that complete control of residual disease can be achieved in most patients with 5 courses of cyclophosphamide (150 mg/m^2/day p.o. for 7 days) and doxorubicin (35 mg/m^2 i.v. on day 8) repeated every 3 to 4 weeks (10). A second-look operation is necessary at the conclusion of chemotherapy to confirm complete control of the disease or, if residual disease is present, to attempt to resect residual tumor. If residual disease is still present at the conclusion of the second-look surgery, another combination of agents that includes cisplatin and the epipodophyllotoxins, with or without radiation therapy, should be used.

STAGE C

In stage C, the primary tumor may or may not be completely resected; however, regional nodes have histologic evidence of involvement. The goal of postoperative treatment is complete control of the residual disease or, alternatively, reduction in size of the initially inoperable mass to make complete surgical resection of the primary tumor possible. This can be achieved using chemotherapy, with or without radiation therapy.

Age is an important prognostic indicator in this group of patients; infants less than 1 year of age fare significantly better than older children.

Five courses of sequential cyclophosphamide and doxorubicin as described for stage B produce remission, documented by second-look exploration, in most infants with stage C disease. Most of the remaining infants who fail to respond to this relatively less toxic regimen can be treated effectively with five courses of cisplatin (90 mg/m^2 i.v. on day 1) and tenoposide (100 mg/m^2 i.v. on day 3) repeated every 3 to 4 weeks (11).

In children older than 1 year of age with stage C disease, more aggressive chemotherapy is justified. Four-drug combinations of cyclophosphamide, doxorubicin, cisplatin, and epipodophyllotoxin used sequentially, or other combinations used for more advanced disease, are being used. Management of this group of patients is clearly challenging and requires careful coordinated use of surgery, chemotherapy, and radiation therapy to achieve disease control (12).

STAGE D

As in stage C disease, infants less than 12 months of age fare significantly better than older children, although those older than 6 months may require aggressive therapy (13). The regimens described in Table 61.2 are reported to produce excellent initial responses (14–20). However, the outlook remains grim for children with disseminated neuroblastoma. Autologous bone marrow transplantation is being used in a number of studies in an attempt to improve the outcome of this group of patients. The role of this modality has not yet been defined, however (21, 22).

Table 61.2. Combination Chemotherapy for Advanced Neuroblastoma

Regimen[a]	References
CDDP, CPM, VM (PCVm); DOX, CPM, VCR, DTIC (ACVD)	(14)
CPM, DOX, VCR (CAV); HID–CDDP, HID–VP (PVP)	(15, 16)
VCR, CDDP; HID–CDDP, HID–VP; HID–CPM, HID–VP	(17)
CBDCA, VP[b]	(18)
HID–CPM, VP[b]	(19)
IFOS, VP[b]	(20)

[a]VCR, vincristine; CPM, cyclophosphamide; CDDP, cisplatin; DOX, doxorubicin; VP, etoposide; VM, tenoposide; DTIC, dacarbazine; CBDCA, carboplatin; IFOS, ifosfamide; HID, high dose.
[b]Effective in refractory and recurrent neuroblastoma.

Special Cases

SPINAL CORD COMPRESSION

Intraspinal extension of intracavitary neuro-blastoma (dumbbell-shaped tumors), mostly in children with limited-stage disease, produces spinal cord compression and neurologic deficits. Laminectomy and radiation therapy have been the traditional treatment modalities; however, these approaches can be associated with serious long-term side effects. Excellent results with complete neurologic recovery have been reported with chemotherapy alone when instituted promptly after diagnosis (23). This approach should be considered as an effective alternative to radiation therapy and/or laminectomy.

EVANS STAGE IV-S DISEASE

Approximately 10% of patients, generally infants, with limited-stage neuroblastoma have remote metastases to liver, spleen, or bone marrow, without bone involvement. This intriguing group of patients, who may appear to have stage D disease, has an excellent survival. There is no general agreement as to the role of chemotherapy in these infants, in part because of frequent spontaneous regression and concerns about treatment-related morbidity and mortality (24, 25). Most investigators use chemotherapy in infants with stage IV-S disease with extensive liver and bone marrow involvement, as these infants have a higher tendency to develop progressive disease. In addition, patients diagnosed before age 2 months may have a worse prognosis than those with stage IV disease (13). Various biologic parameters, discussed above, have also been reported to be helpful in predicting the likelihood of disease progression, thus assisting in selection of those infants who might benefit from chemotherapy. When the decision is made to use chemotherapy, the potential for serious toxicity should influence both selection and dose of agents to be used. Five-day courses of cyclophosphamide (5 mg/kg/day i.v.), with or without vincristine (1.5 mg/m^2 i.v.) on the first day of each course, or sequential cyclophosphamide and doxorubicin described above, are appropriate.

WILMS' TUMOR

Wilms' tumor is the second most common abdominal malignancy in children under 15 years of age. Improvements in surgical techniques, advances in radiation therapy, and the introduction of multiagent chemotherapy have changed the outlook for children with Wilms' tumor from grim in the early part of this century to cure for more than two-thirds of the patients at present (26). These dramatic results are mainly due to the large-scale clinical trials of the National Wilms' Tumor Studies (NWTS). Since 1969, NWTS has completed four successive clinical trials; the most recent study was closed to accrual in 1994. A complete review of these studies is beyond the scope of this chapter. However, some of the major conclusions that form the basis of the current therapeutic approach to Wilms' tumor are summarized.

Clinicopathologic staging involves searching for distant metastases in lungs, liver, and bone, and eventually surgery and histologic evaluation. The NWTS demonstrated the importance of the extent of Wilms' tumor at diagnosis to outcome. The clinical groupings used in the first two studies were modified in the third study to a staging system underscoring the prognostic significance of regional lymph node involvement (27) (Table 61.3). Three histologic subtypes (tumors with anaplasia, clear cell sarcoma, and rhabdoid sarcoma) are associated with poor outcome and are designated as Wilms' with unfavorable histology (UH); the remainder are considered to be of favorable histology (FH). Anaplasia can be further categorized as focal or diffuse, the latter requiring intensification of chemotherapy (28). The clear cell sarcoma histology is associated with bone metastases (29), and rhabdoid tumors frequently metastasize to the brain (30).

Further refinement in the treatment of Wilms' tumor is certain to be made with longer follow-up of NWTS-III and -IV patients, so that no treatment regimen can be considered "standard." However, the control arms of the NWTS-III shown in Table 61.4 can be considered as an optimum treatment for patients with Wilms' tumor.

Wilms' Tumor with Favorable Histology

STAGE I

Patients in this group treated postoperatively with a combination of vincristine and dactinomycin for 6 months have an expected 2-year disease-free survival of over 90%.

STAGE II

The duration of postoperative chemotherapy with vincristine and dactinomycin is extended to 15 months, with an expected 2-year disease-free survival similar to that of patients with stage I FH.

STAGES III AND IV

These tumors are treated with radiation therapy and multiagent chemotherapy courses consisting of vincristine, dactinomycin, and doxorubicin for 15 months. In spite of this aggressive therapy, nearly a third of these patients will have disease recurrence.

Infants have a higher incidence of chemotherapy-induced toxicities. In NWTS-III, drug doses for infants with favorable-histology tumors and without metastatic disease were reduced, with a significant decrease in toxicity, while maintaining excellent relapse-free survival (31).

Wilms' Tumor with Unfavorable Histology

Patients with stage I anaplastic disease do just as well as those with stage I FH when treated with a combination of vincristine and dactinomycin for 6 months (32). Children with stage II-IV disease and focal anaplasia treated with vincristine, dactinomycin, and doxorubicin also have an excellent prognosis. The addition of cyclophosphamide to this regimen in patients with

diffuse anaplasia improves the 4-year relapse-free survival rate, although overall, the outlook is poorer than that for focal anaplasia (28). The prognosis for patients with clear cell sarcoma of the kidney has been improved with vincristine, dactinomycin, and doxorubicin, along with radiation therapy (33). Unfortunately, those with rhabdoid histology continue to fare poorly (26).

Table 61.4. Chemotherapy of Wilms' Tumor Based on the Results of NWTS-III

Stage	Histology[a]	Regimen[b]
I	FH/UH	VCR weekly (weeks 1–10), then on day 1 and 5 with DAC DAC (weeks 0, 5, 13, 24)
II	FH	VCR weekly (weeks 1–10, 15–20, 24–29, 33–38, 42–47, 51–56, 60–65) DAC (weeks 0, 5, 13, 22, 31, 40, 49, 58)
III–IV	FH	VCR weekly (week 1–10), then on day 1 and 5 with DAC DAC (weeks 0, 13, 26, 39, 52, 65) DOX (weeks 6, 19, 32, 45, 58)
II–IV	UH	Same as stage IV FH CYC for diffuse anaplasia

[a]FH, favorable histology; UH, unfavorable histology.
[b]VCR, vincristine (1.5 mg/m^2 i.v.); DAC, dactinomycin (15 µg/kg/day × 5 days i.v.); DOX, doxorubicin (20 mg/m^2/day × 3 days i.v.); CYC, cyclophosphamide (10 mg/kg/day × 3 days).

Table 61.3. National Wilms' Tumor Study Staging

Stage I   The tumor is limited to the kidney and completely excised. The surface of the renal capsule is intact. The tumor was not ruptured before or during removal. There is no residual tumor apparent beyond the margins of resection.

Stage II   The tumor extends beyond the kidney but is completely excised. There is regional extension of the tumor (that is, penetration of perirenal soft tissues). Blood vessels outside the kidney substance are infiltrated by or contain tumor thrombus. The tumor may have been biopsied or local spillage may have occurred, but the spillage was confined to the ipsilateral flank. No residual tumor is apparent at or beyond the margins of excision.

Stage III   Residual nonhematogenous tumor is present and confined to the abdomen. Any one or more of the following occur:
Lymph nodes (renal hilar, periaortic, or beyond) are found on biopsy to be involved by tumor.
There is diffuse peritoneal contamination by tumor, such as by spillage of tumor beyond the ipsilateral flank before or during surgery, or the tumor has penetrated through the peritoneal surface.
Tumor implants are found on the peritoneal surface.
Gross or microscopic tumor remains postoperatively.
The tumor is not completely resectable because of local infiltration into vital structures.

Stage IV   Hematogenous metastases are present (lung, liver, bone, brain, etc.).

Stage V   Bilateral renal involvement is present at diagnosis. An attempt should be made to stage each side according to the above criteria on the basis of the extent of the disease prior to biopsy.

Future goals include minimizing late effects and reducing iatrogenic complications. For the minority of patients who fail conventional therapy, additional active drugs are needed; carboplatin/cisplatin, ifosfamide, etoposide/tenoposide, bleomycin, melphalan, and thiotepa have been used successfully, alone or in combination (34–37).

RHABDOMYOSARCOMA

Rhabdomyosarcoma, the most common soft tissue sarcoma in children and young adults, appears in a wide anatomic area, including head and neck, thorax, retroperitoneal space, pelvis, and extremities. Accordingly, the clinical manifestations vary greatly, depending on the site of origin. Histologically, rhabdomyosarcomas are heterogeneous and may consist of embryonal, alveolar, differentiated/pleomorphic elements and sarcomas not otherwise characterized. The complex clinical manifestations and heterogeneous histology challenge the clinician with an array of diagnostic and therapeutic possibilities. Well-coordinated applications of surgery, radiation therapy, and multiagent chemotherapy in prospective randomized clinical trials have increased survival of children with rhabdomyosarcoma from 20% two decades ago to recent reports of 73% (38, 39). Although many cooperative groups and institutions have made significant contributions to diagnosis and treatment, the Intergroup Rhabdomyosarcoma Study Group (IRS), formed by all pediatric cooperative groups in the United States, Canada, and Europe, remains the largest source of data. Between 1972 and 1988, the IRS enrolled more than 2500 patients in three studies (38, 40, 41).

The most widely used staging system, the clinical grouping developed by IRS, is based on resectability of the mass, involvement of regional lymph nodes, and the presence or absence of distant metastases (Table 61.5). In addition to the information gathered by physical examination, size and extent of the primary tumor are determined by imaging studies, and metastases are sought in bone, bone marrow, lungs, and liver. In addition, for head and neck parameningeal primaries (nasal cavity, nasopharynx, paranasal sinuses, middle ear, mastoid, pterygopalatine, and infratemporal fossae), the base of skull and intracranial contents should be carefully examined by x-ray, CT scan, or MRI, and cerebral spinal fluid examined for the presence of malignant cells. For retroperitoneal and paraspinal tumors,

Table 61.5. IRS Clinical Grouping

Group	Findings
I	Localized disease, completely resected (regional nodes not involved); confined to muscle or organ of origin; contiguous involvement with infiltration outside the muscle or organ of origin, as through fascial planes.
II	Grossly resected tumor with microscopic residual disease; no evidence of gross residual tumor; no evidence of regional node involvement. Regional disease, completely resected (regional nodes involved and/or extension of tumor into an adjacent organ); all tumor completely resected with no microscopic residual tumor. Regional disease with involved nodes grossly resected but with evidence of microscopic residual.
III	Incomplete resection or biopsy with gross residual disease.
IV	Distant metastatic disease present at onset (lung, liver, bones, bone marrow, brain, and distant muscle and lymph nodes).

the spine and spinal cord should be examined by MRI or myelogram. Because of the high incidence of regional lymph node involvement, retroperitoneal nodes should be examined by CT scan in primaries involving lower extremity, inguinal, pelvic, and paratesticular regions (42).

The importance of the site of primary as a prognostic indicator is evident from IRS-I and -II studies. Orbital lesions have the best prognosis, while extremity, retroperitoneal, and pelvic lesions have the worst (43, 44). In current IRS studies, alveolar histology is considered to be unfavorable, whereas other histologic types, such as embryonal, pleomorphic/mixed, differentiated, and extraosseous Ewing's sarcoma, are favorable histologic variants. Identification of other prognostic features, such as tumor-cell DNA content (ploidy), may identify subgroups that require modification of therapy (45).

Chemotherapy

Chemotherapy is required in all stages and histologic variants of rhabdomyosarcoma, with more intensive regimens reserved for patients with poor prognostic indicators. Currently, multiagent chemotherapy regimens incorporate vincristine, dactinomycin, cyclophosphamide, doxorubicin, cisplatin, ifosfamide, etoposide, and dacarbazine in various combinations. Clearly, the chemotherapy of rhabdomyosar-

Table 61.6. Intergroup Rhabdomyosarcoma Study Group (IRS)-III Chemotherapy of Rhabdomyosarcoma

Group	Anatomic Location	Histology	Regimen
I	All	Favorable	31
I	All	Unfavorable	38
II	All except special group II[a]	Favorable	32 vs. 33
II	Special[a]	Favorable	32
II	All	Unfavorable	38
III	All except special[a], special pelvic[b]		34
III	Special[a]		32
III	Special pelvic[b]		37-A, 37-B
IV	All		34

[a]Orbit, scalp, parotid, oral cavity, larynx, oropharynx, and cheek primaries.
[b]Primary in bladder, vagina, uterus, prostate.

coma is evolving, and ongoing studies, including those being conducted by IRS-IV, promise to introduce further refinement. The treatment approach in IRS-III, based on stage, histology, and the site of primary as major prognostic factors (Table 61.6, 61.7), is used here as the basis for therapy.

CLINICAL GROUP I (FAVORABLE HISTOLOGY)

One year of vincristine and dactinomycin postoperatively results in a 5-year survival exceeding 90% (41). The addition of radiation therapy does not improve these results (38).

CLINICAL GROUP II (FAVORABLE HISTOLOGY)

Radiation therapy is combined with a more intensive postoperative regimen of vincristine and dactinomycin administered for 1 year. The benefit of adding doxorubicin to this regimen is unclear. The survival at 5 years for this group is over 80% (41).

CLINICAL GROUPS I AND II (UNFAVORABLE HISTOLOGY)

These patients benefit from vincristine, dactinomycin, and cyclophosphamide (VAC) in addition to doxorubicin and cisplatin. For this group, an 80% rate of survival has been achieved (41).

CLINICAL GROUP III

Intensive and repetitive courses of VAC produce a 5-year survival of approximately 80%. Special pelvic primary tumors (bladder, prostate, vagina, and uterus) benefit from VAC and the addition of doxorubicin and cisplatin, or dactinomycin plus etoposide (41).

CLINICAL GROUPS II AND III (ORBIT AND HEAD TUMORS)

One year of vincristine and dactinomycin, combined with radiation, achieves a 91% rate of survival (41).

PARAMENINGEAL

Cranial radiation, combined with intrathecal methotrexate, hydrocortisone, and cytarabine, has reduced the incidence of meningeal involvement in these patients. Patients who have evidence of overt meningeal involvement at the time of diagnosis are treated with more intensive intrathecal chemotherapy for 2 years. Patients with parameningeal disease had a 5-year survival rate of 69% in IRS-III, significantly higher than the 45% seen before the prophylactic regimen was instituted (38, 41).

CLINICAL GROUP IV

Pulsed VAC and radiation therapy produces a long-term survival of only 20 to 30%. The addition of doxorubicin and cisplatin or etoposide is of no benefit (38). Results from IRS-IV, which randomized this group of patients to receive vincristine/melphalan, ifosfamide/etoposide, or ifosfamide/doxorubicin, are not yet available.

Future prospects for the treatment of rhabdomyosarcoma should focus on further improving survival, while minimizing long-term effects of therapy. New treatment strategies are clearly needed, especially for patients with metastatic disease at diagnosis. Intensive chemotherapy followed by autologous marrow transplantation

Table 61.7. IRS-III Regimens[a]

Regimen 31
DAC weeks 0, 9, 18, 27, 36, 45
VCR weeks 3–8, 12–17, 21–26, 30–35, 39–45,
48–53
Regimen 38
VCR weeks 0–11
CDDP weeks 0, 3, 6, 9
DOX 24 hours after CDDP, weeks 0, 3
CYC 24 hours after CDDP, weeks 0, 6[b], 9[b]
RTX beginning week 6
VCR, CYC, and DOX alternating with DAC every 4
weeks, weeks 12–52
Regimen 32
Same as regimen 31, with RTX beginning on day 14
Regimen 33
Same as regimen 32, except DOX given weeks 3, 6,
12, 15, 21, 24
Regimen 34
VCR weeks 0–12, 16
DAC weeks 0, 12, 16
CYC weeks 0, 12, 16 (3-day infusion); weeks 3, 6[b],
9[b] (1-day infusion)
RTX week 6
VCR, DAC, CYC every 4 weeks after RTX if in
surgical or clinical CR, through week 104
Regimen 35
VCR weeks 0–12, 16
DOX weeks 0, 3, 12
CYC weeks 0, 12, 16 (3-day infusion); weeks 6[b], 9[b]
(1-day infusion)
CDDP week 0, 3, 6, 9
DAC week 16
RTX week 6
VCR, CYC, and DAC alternating with DOX every 4
weeks after RTX if in surgical or clinical CR,
through week 104

---

[a]Drug doses DAC 0.015 mg/kg/day i.v. × 5 days (maximum daily dose, 0.5 mg); VCR mg/m² /dose i.v. weekly (maximum dose, 2 mg); CDDP 90 mg/m² /dose i.v. over 8 hours; DOX 30 mg/m² /day × 2 days; CYC 10 mg/kg/day for 3 days or 20 mg/kg/day for 1 day.
[b]Delete CYC if bladder or extensive bone marrow irradiated.

is one possibility (46, 47), although one report of this approach did not show improved disease control (47).

RETINOBLASTOMA

Retinoblastoma is the most common intraocular malignancy, with an estimated incidence of one in 18,000 live births in the United States (48). The strong genetic influence and the increased risk for a second malignancy make retinoblastoma a unique childhood cancer (49, 50). Patients with nonhereditary retinoblastoma usually have unilateral disease with no family history of retinoblastoma. Those with bilateral disease or a family history of retinoblastoma typically have the less common heritable form, with an autosomal dominant pattern. The retinoblastoma gene has been located on the q14 band of chromosome 13 and is closely linked to the locus of the esterase gene (51).

Currently, more than 90% of children with retinoblastoma are surviving with such established treatment modalities as enucleation, photocoagulation, cryotherapy, and radiation therapy. Because of these excellent results, very few patients have been available for prospective randomized trials to determine the role of chemotherapy in patients with extraocular disease or systemic metastases. Very few clinical trials have been conducted within the pediatric cooperative groups, and the few studies reported have not provided conclusive evidence that chemotherapy is effective in children with extraocular retinoblastoma (52). A further obstacle to the design of clinical trials is the lack of a uniformly accepted staging system, which is necessary to draw a statistically valid conclusion on the effect of a therapeutic modality applied to a large number of patients. In the absence of a staging system, invasion of the optic nerve distal to the lamina cribrosa, involvement of choroid, retinal pigment epithelium, and the central nervous system, and distant metastases are indicators of poor outcome. Logically, these are the patients in whom chemotherapy might play an important role.

In the absence of any data, no definite recommendations for chemotherapy can be made. However, it is clear from various reports that retinoblastoma is sensitive to chemotherapy (53). Cyclophosphamide and its analogue ifosfamide are the most active single agents. Doxorubicin, the epipodophyllotoxins, vincristine, and cisplatin have been used in various combinations in retinoblastoma, primarily because of their effectiveness in other neuroectodermal tumors such as neuroblastomas (Table 61.8) (54–60). The effectiveness of these agents, either alone or in combination, is difficult to prove because they are frequently used with other treatment modalities, including radiation. Patients with evidence of meningeal involvement require intrathecal methotrexate, cytarabine, and hydrocortisone (56).

Clearly, well-organized clinical trials, similar

Table 61.8. Chemotherapy of Retinoblastoma

Drug[a]	Dose	Schedule
VCR	0.05 mg/kg	Every 3 weeks × 7 courses, then CYC/VCR every 3 weeks
DOX	0.67 mg/kg × 3 days	for 2 years
CYC	40 mg/kg	
CYC	300 mg/m² day 1	Every 3–4 weeks for 1 year
VM	100 mg/m² day 3	
CYC	150 mg/m² × 7 days	Every 3–4 weeks for 1 year
DOX	35 mg/m² day 8	
CYC	5 mg/m² × 5 days	Every 3–4 weeks for 1 year
VCR	1.5 mg/m² on day 1	
CTX IV	150 mg/m² days 1–7	Repeat 3 cycles
CTX PO	days 22–28, 43–49	
DOX	35 mg/m² days 10, 52	
CDDP	90 mg/m² days 8, 50, 71	
VP	150 mg/m²/24 hr, days 29–31, 73–75	

[a]VCR, vincristine; DOX, doxorubicin; CYC, cyclophosphamide; VM, tenoposide; CDDP, cisplatin; VP, etoposide.

to those described elsewhere in this chapter, are needed; because of the limited number of patients available, these studies need the involvement of the major pediatric cooperative groups in the United States and abroad. In this setting, promising new approaches, such as intensive chemotherapy followed by autologous bone marrow transplantation in patients with advanced disease, can be tested (61).

REFERENCES

1. Young JL, Miller RW. Incidence of malignant tumors in US children. J Pediatr 1975;86:254–258.

2. Brodeur GM, Castleberry RP. Neuroblastoma. In: Pizzo PA, Poplack DG, eds. Principles and practice of pediatric oncology. Philadelphia: JB Lippincott, 1993;739–767.

3. Evans AE, D'Angio GJ, Randolph J. A proposed staging for children with neuroblastoma. Cancer 1971; 27:374–378.

4. Ninane J, Pritchard J, Morris-Jones PH, et al. Stage II neuroblastoma: adverse prognostic significance of lymph node involvement. Arch Dis Child 1982;57:438–442.

5. Hayes FA, Green A, Hustu HO, Kumar M. Surgicopathologic staging of neuroblastoma: prognostic significance of regional lymph node metastases. J Pediatr 1983;102:59–62.

6. Evans AE, D'Angio GJ, Propert K, Anderson J, Hann H-WL. Prognostic factors in neuroblastoma. Cancer 1987;59:1853–1859.

7. Look AT, Hayes FA, Shuster JJ, et al. Clinical relevance of tumor cell ploidy and N-myc gene amplification in childhood neuroblastoma. A Pediatric Oncology Group study. J Clin Oncol 1991;9:581–591.

8. Chan HSL, Haddad G, Thorner PS, et al. P-glycoprotein expression as a predictor of the outcome of

therapy for neuroblastoma. N Engl J Med 1991; 325:1608–1614.

9. Nitschke R, Smith EI, Shochat S, et al. Localized neuroblastoma treated by surgery—a Pediatric Oncology Group study. J Clin Oncol 1988;6:1271–1279.

10. Nitschke R, Smith EI, Altshuler G, et al. Postoperative treatment of nonmetastatic visible residual neuroblastoma: a Pediatric Oncology Group study. J Clin Oncol 1991;9:1181–1188.

11. Castleberry RP, Shuster JJ, Altshuler G, et al. Infants with neuroblastoma and regional lymph node metastases have a favorable outlook after limited postoperative chemotherapy: a Pediatric Oncology Group study. J Clin Oncol 1992;10:1299–1304.

12. Castleberry RP, Kun L, Shuster JJ, et al. Radiotherapy improves the outlook for children older than one year with POG stage C neuroblastoma. J Clin Oncol 1991;9:789–795.

13. De Bernardi B, Pianca C, Boni L, et al. Disseminated neuroblastoma (stage IV and IV-S) in the first year of life. Cancer 1992;70:1625–1633.

14. Berthold F, Burdach S, Kremens B, et al. The role of chemotherapy in the treatment of children with neuroblastoma stage IV: the GPO (German Pediatric Oncology Society) experience. Klin Padiatr 1990; 202:262–269.

15. Kushner BH, O'Reilly RJ, LaQuaglia M, Cheung NKV. Dose-intensive use of cyclophosphamide in ablation of neuroblastoma. Cancer 1990; 66:1095–1100.

16. Kushner BH, LaQuaglia MP, Bonilla MA, et al. Highly effective induction therapy for stage 4 neuroblastoma in children over 1 year of age. J Clin Oncol 1994;12:2607–2613.

17. Pearson ADJ, Craft AW, Pinkerton CR, Meller ST, Reid MM. High-dose rapid schedule chemotherapy for disseminated neuroblastoma. Eur J Cancer 1992;28A:1654–1659.

18. Frappaz D, Michon J, Hartmann O, et al. Etoposide and carboplatin in neuroblastoma: a French So-

ciety of Pediatric Oncology phase II study. J Clin Oncol 1992;10:1592–1601.

19. Méresse V, Vassal G, Michon J, et al. Combined continuous infusion etoposide with high-dose cyclophosphamide for refractory neuroblastoma: a phase II study from the Société Francaise d'Oncologie Pédiatrique. J Clin Oncol 1993;11:630–637.

20. Kung FH, Pratt CB, Vega RA, et al. Ifosfamide/ etoposide combination in the treatment of recurrent malignant solid tumors of childhood. A Pediatric Oncology Group phase II study. Cancer 1993;71:1898–1903.

21. Lanino E, Boni L, Corciulo P, De Bernardi B. Did BMT change the clinical course of neuroblastoma? Bone Marrow Transplant 1991;3(Suppl 7):114–117.

22. Johnson FL, Goldman S. Role of autotransplantation in neuroblastoma. Hematol Oncol Clin North Am 1993;7:647–662.

23. Hayes FA, Green AA, O'Connor DM. Chemotherapeutic management of epidural neuroblastoma. Med Pediatr Oncol 1989;17:6–8.

24. Evans AE, Baum E, Chard R. Do infants with stage IV-S neuroblastoma need treatment? Arch Dis Child 1981;56:271–274.

25. McWilliams N. IV-S neuroblastoma—treatment controversy revisited. Med Pediatr Oncol 1986; 14:41–44.

26. National Wilms' Tumor Study Committee. Wilms' tumor: status report, 1990. J Clin Oncol 1991; 9:877–887.

27. Farewell VT, D'Angio GJ, Breslow N, Norkool P. Retrospective validation of a new staging system for Wilms' tumor. Cancer Clin Trials 1981;4:167–171.

28. Green DM, Beckwith JB, Breslow NE, et al. Treatment of children with stages II to IV anaplastic Wilms' tumor: a report from the National Wilms' Tumor Study Group. J Clin Oncol 1994;12:2126–2131.

29. Marsden HB, Lawler W, Kumar PM. Bone-metastasizing renal tumor of childhood. Morphological and clinical features, and differences from Wilms' tumor. Cancer 1978;42:1922–1928.

30. Bonnin JM, Rubinstein LJ, Palmer NF, Beckwith JB. The association of embryonal tumors originating in the kidney and in the brain. Cancer 1984;54:2137–2146.

31. Corn BW, Goldwein JW, Evans I, D'Angio GJ. Outcomes in low-risk babies treated with half-dose chemotherapy according to the third National Wilms' Tumor study. J Clin Oncol 1992;10:1305–1309.

32. Bonadio JF, Storer B, Norkool P, et al. Anaplastic Wilms' tumor: clinical and pathological studies. J Clin Oncol 1985;3:513–520.

33. Green DM, Breslow NE, Beckwith JB, Moksness J, Finklestein JZ, D'Angio GJ. Treatment of children with clear-cell sarcoma of the kidney: a report from the National Wilms' Tumor Study Group. J Clin Oncol 1994;12:2132–2137.

34. Pinkerton CR, Groot-Loonen JJ, Morris-Jones PH, Pritchard J. Response rates in relapsed Wilms' tumor. A need for new effective agents. Cancer 1991; 67:567–571.

35. Pein F, Pinkerton R, Tournade MF, et al. Etoposide in relapsed or refractory Wilms' tumor: a phase II study by the French Society of Pediatric Oncology and the United Kingdom Children's Cancer Study Group. J Clin Oncol 1993;11:1478–1481.

36. Pein F, Tournade MF, Zucker JM, et al. Etoposide and carboplatin: a highly effective combination in relapsed or refractory Wilms' tumor—a phase II study by the French Society of Pediatric Oncology. J Clin Oncol 1994;12:931–936.

37. de Camargo B, Melaragno R, Saba e Silva N, et al. Phase II study of carboplatin as a single drug for relapsed Wilms' tumor: experience of the Brazilian Wilms' Tumor Study Group. Med Pediatr Oncol 1994; 22:258–260.

38. Maurer HM, Beltangady M, Gehan E, et al. The intergroup rhabdomyosarcoma study I: a final report. Cancer 1988;61:209–220.

39. Crist WM, Garnsey L, Beltangady MS, et al. Prognosis in children with rhabdomyosarcoma: a report of the intergroup rhabdomyosarcoma studies I and II. J Clin Oncol 1990;8:443–452.

40. Maurer HM, Gehan EA, Beltangady M, et al. The intergroup rhabdomyosarcoma study—II. Cancer 1991;71:1904–1922.

41. Crist W, Gehan EA, Ragab AH, et al. The third intergroup rhabdomyosarcoma study. J Clin Oncol 1995;13:610–630.

42. Lawrence W, Hays DM, Moon TE (for the IRS Committee). Lymphatic metastasis with childhood rhabdomyosarcoma. Cancer 1977;39:556–559.

43. Neifeld JP, Maurer HM, Godwin D, et al. Prognostic variables in pediatric rhabdomyosarcoma before and after multimodal therapy. J Pediatr Surg 1979;1 4:699–703.

44. Gehan EZ, Glouer FN, Maurer HM, et al. Prognostic factors in children with rhabdomyosarcoma. NCI Monogr 1981;56:83–92.

45. Pappo AS, Crist WM, Kuttesch J, et al. Tumor-cell DNA content predicts outcome in children and adolescents with clinical group III embryonal rhabdomyosarcoma. J Clin Oncol 1993;11:1901–1905.

46. Kessinger A, Armitage JO. High dose therapy with autologous bone marrow transplantation for advanced soft tissue sarcoma (abstract). Proc Am Soc Clin Oncol 1987;6:126.

47. Horowitz ME, Kinsella TJ, Wexler LH, et al. Total-body irradiation and autologous bone marrow transplant in the treatment of high-risk Ewing's sarcoma and rhabdomyosarcoma. J Clin Oncol 1993; 11:1911–1918.

48. Pendergrass TW. Incidence of retinoblastoma in the United States. Arch Ophthalmol 1980;98:1204–1210.

49. Potluri VR, Helson L, Ellsworth RM, et al. Chromosomal abnormalities in human retinoblastoma. Cancer 1986;58:663–671.

50. Draper GJ, Saunders DM, Kingston JE. Second primary neoplasms in patients with retinoblastoma. Br J Cancer 1986;53:661–671.

51. Sparks RS, Murphree AL, Lingua RW, et al. Gene for hereditary retinoblastoma assigned to human chromosome 13 by linkage to esterase D. Science 1983; 219:971–973.

52. Wolff JA, Boesel GP, Dyment PG, et al. Treatment of retinoblastoma: a preliminary report. Int Congr Series 1981;570:364–368.

53. White L. Chemotherapy in retinoblastoma: current status and future directions. Am J Pediatr Hematol Oncol 1991;13:189–201.

54. Pratt CB, Crom DB, Howarth C. The use of chemotherapy for extraocular retinoblastoma. Med Pediatr Oncol 1985;13:330–333.

55. Zelter M, Gonzalez G, Schwartz L, et al. Treatment of retinoblastoma—results obtained from a prospective study of 51 patients. Cancer 1988;61:153–160.

56. Grabowski EF, Abramson DH. Intraocular and extraocular retinoblastoma. Hematol Oncol Clin North Am 1987;1:721–735.

57. Advani SH, Rao SR, Iyer RS, Pai SK, Kurkure PA, Nair CN. Pilot study of sequential combination chemotherapy in advanced and recurrent retinoblastoma. Med Pediatr Oncol 1994;22:125–128.

58. Nelson SC, Friedman HS, Oakes WJ, et al. Successful therapy for trilateral retinoblastoma. Am J Ophthalmol 1992;114:23–29.

59. Stannard C, Lipper S, Sealy R, et al. Retinoblastoma: correlation of invasion of the optic nerve and choroid with prognosis and metastasis. Br J Ophthalmol 1979;63:560–570.

60. Rootman J, Ellsworth RM, Hofhauer J, et al. Orbital extension of retinoblastoma: a clinicopathological study. Can J Ophthalmol 1978;13:72–80.

61. Saleh RA, Gross S, Casseno W, et al. Metastatic retinoblastoma successfully treated with immunomagnetic purged autologous bone marrow transplantation. Cancer 1988;62:2301–2303.

Section Seven

Chemotherapy of Hematologic Malignancies

62

Chemotherapy of Hodgkin's Disease

Dan L. Longo

Hodgkin's disease is a lymphoproliferative disorder that is diagnosed in about 8000 people per year in the United States. Age-adjusted incidence rates have not changed greatly overall but have declined in those over age 65 years. There is a bimodal distribution of risk as a function of age: the first peak incidence is in 20 to 24 year olds, and the second is in 80 to 84 year olds. The median age is 32 years. The incidence rate is 2.8 per 100,000; it is higher in whites than blacks and is higher in men than in women. With advances in treatment over the last 20 years, 5-year survival is 82% for those under age 65 years. The outlook is not so favorable in those over age 65 years: 5-year survival is only 40% (1).

CLINICAL PRESENTATION AND PATHOLOGY

Hodgkin's disease usually presents with a painless swelling of a lymph node, often in the cervical region. Some patients present with a mediastinal mass discovered incidentally on chest radiograph. Others present with unexplained fevers, weight loss, or night sweats, the classic B symptoms. An occasional patient will have periods of fever separated by 7- to 10-day afebrile periods (so-called Pel-Epstein fever). Pruritus is not uncommon; it is not a B symptom. Rare patients experience pain in sites of disease after ingestion of alcohol. Unusual presenting symptoms include superior vena cava syndrome, bone pain, splenomegaly, and paraneoplastic neurologic syndromes.

Histology

The diagnosis requires examination of a completely excised lymph node specimen. Hodg-

kin's disease effaces the normal lymph node architecture. The malignant cell is a Reed-Sternberg cell that may exist in several forms; classically, it is a large cell with a bilobed nucleus, with each lobe containing a prominent nucleolus. The nucleus has been said to resemble "owl's eyes." It is a rare cell in a pleiomorphic cellular infiltrate composed of T lymphocytes, plasma cells, macrophages, granulocytes, and eosinophils. There are several histologic subtypes of Hodgkin's disease. According to the recent revised European-American lymphoma (REAL) classification (2), the following subsets are defined (percentage of cases in parentheses): lymphocyte predominance (5%), nodular sclerosis (65%), mixed cellularity (25%), and lymphocyte depletion (5%). In addition, the REAL classification includes a provisional entity called lymphocyte-rich classical Hodgkin's disease, a subtype that was formerly considered a diffuse variant of lymphocyte predominance. Given the improvements in treatment in the last few decades, histologic subtype does not influence choice of treatment or treatment outcome.

The Reed-Sternberg Cell

The nature of the Reed-Sternberg cell remains largely undefined. The lymphocytic and histiocytic (L&H) variant seen in lymphocyte predominance is clearly a B cell; however, data regarding the cell of origin of most cases of Hodgkin's disease are not definitive (3). They often express CD30, CD15, CD71, and CD25; they may coexpress either B-cell or T-cell markers, and the pattern of marker expression may be different in distinct anatomic sites and at different times in the disease course. Efforts to define the clonality of the Reed-Sternberg cell have not yielded data that support a consensus (4–8). Data from interphase cytogenetics, immunoglobulin gene rearrangement, and Epstein-Barr virus episome structure support a contention of monoclonality, but other immunoglobulin gene rearrangement data argue against this notion.

Etiologic Factors

The causes of Hodgkin's disease are unknown. An infectious etiology has long been considered likely; the epidemiology of the disease has been said to be consistent with a rare consequence of a common infection (9). Epstein-Barr virus has been most commonly implicated. Serologic studies support a role for the virus in some cases, and evidence for the virus in Hodgkin's disease tissue can be obtained in 30 to 60% of cases, depending on the technique employed (10). In Central and South America, Epstein-Barr virus can be found in over 90% of cases of Hodgkin's disease (11). The disease occurs more frequently than expected in persons infected with HIV, but the role of this virus in the pathogenesis of Hodgkin's disease is unclear (12). The incidence is increased in woodworkers (13), in persons who have had infectious mononucleosis (14), and in those who have had tonsillectomy (15) and appendectomy (16).

Several observations favor a genetic contribution to the etiology. There are familial forms of Hodgkin's disease (17), and a weak linkage disequilibrium has been demonstrated for certain HLA haplotypes (18). Perhaps the strongest evidence for a genetic risk is the observation of Mack et al. (19) that monozygotic twins had a 99-fold increased risk compared with dizygotic twins. Among 187 pairs of dizygotic twins, one of whom had Hodgkin's disease, none of the unaffected twins developed the disease; among 179 pairs of monozygotic twins, one of whom had Hodgkin's disease, 10 of the twins developed Hodgkin's disease when 0.1 cases would have been expected.

It would appear that Hodgkin's disease is a final common morphologic pattern of response to diverse environmental influences superimposed on a genetic background of susceptibility.

STAGING AND PROGNOSTIC FACTORS

Hodgkin's disease usually originates in a lymph node and spreads to contiguous lymph node groups, not involving extranodal sites until late in the clinical course. Before the advent of effective combination chemotherapy programs, the prognosis of Hodgkin's disease was determined mainly by whether or not radiation therapy could be given with curative intent, which in turn depended on the extent of disease. Thus, an anatomic staging system emerged that separated patients into distinct prognostic groups based upon extent of disease. With advances in treatment, the outcomes of all stages of disease are remarkably similar, and staging is now used to determine the optimal treatment approach that is likely to lead to the 75 to 80% cure rate expected from state-of-the-art treatment.

The Cotswolds modification of the Ann Arbor staging system is provided in Table 62.1 (20). This modification acknowledges computed tomographic (CT) scanning in the staging evaluation and recognizes tumor bulk as an important prognostic factor; however, other changes have been less useful. In particular, the subdivision of patients with stage III disease into III_1 and III_2 subsets is of questionable importance because the outcome is similar in response to combination chemotherapy, the treatment of choice for patients with stage III and IV disease. In addition, using the designation [u], which stands for uncertain, for patients with residual radiographic abnormalities after treatment introduces needless complexity into the assessment of response. Most experts consider patients who have stable abnormalities for 1 month or longer after radiation therapy or for two successive cycles of combination chemotherapy to be in clinical complete remission. Because the relapse rate does not differ among subgroups of patients with or without residual radiographic abnormalities (21), there is no clear advantage in designating some patients as $CR_{[u]}$. We cannot predict accurately the 25 to 35% of complete responders who will relapse, and this special designation is unlikely to alter that fact.

The staging evaluation of patients with Hodgkin's disease is outlined in Table 62.2. Previously well patients with persistent lymphadenopathy should have an entire lymph node removed surgically. Fine-needle aspiration and incisional biopsies are not adequate procedures to make the diagnosis of Hodgkin's disease or to distinguish the many possible causes of adenopathy. The two areas of the staging evaluation most commonly misunderstood are (a) the requirement for lymphography and (b) the indications for staging laparotomy.

Table 62.1. Cotswolds Staging Classification

Stage	Definition
I	Involvement of a single lymph node region or lymphoid structure (e.g., spleen, thymus, Waldeyer's ring)
II	Involvement of two or more lymph node regions on the same side of the diaphragm (the mediastinum is a single site; hilar lymph nodes should be considered to be "lateralized" and when involved on both sides constitute stage II disease); the number of anatomic regions involved should be indicated by a subscript (e.g., II_3)
III	Involvement of lymph node regions or lymphoid structures on both sides of the diaphragm III_1: subdiaphragmatic involvement limited to spleen, splenic hilar nodes, celiac nodes, or portal nodes III_2: subdiaphragmatic involvement includes paraaortic, iliac, or mesenteric nodes plus structures in III_1
IV	Involvement of extranodal site(s) beyond that designated as "E." Involvement of liver or bone marrow
Subdesignations	
A:	No symptoms
B:	(a) unexplained weight loss of more than 10% of the body weight during the 6 months before staging investigation (b) unexplained, persistent, or recurrent fever with temperatures above 38°C during the previous month (c) recurrent drenching night sweats during the previous month
X:	Bulky disease: $\geq$10 cm maximum dimension of nodal mass Mediastinal mass maximum width $\geq$⅓ the internal transverse diameter of the thorax at the level of T5/6 on PA CXR
E:	Localized involvement of extralymphatic tissue, alone as the only site of disease (I_E), or by limited direct extension from (contiguous with) a known model site or proximal to a known nodal site (excluding liver and bone marrow)
CS:	Clinical stage
PS:	Pathologic stage, indicating staging biopsies

[a]CS or PS subscript designations for identified extranodal sites: M, bone marrow; H, liver; L, lung; O, bone; P, pleura; and D, skin.

Bipedal lymphography is essential to the management of patients with Hodgkin's disease if radiation therapy is considered to be a treatment option. Lymphography is the most reliable noninvasive method for detecting involvement of paraaortic lymph nodes (22). After the initial history, physical examination, and chest radiograph, about 90% of patients will have clinical stage I or stage II disease. After lymphography, ⅓ of those early-stage patients will be upstaged to stage III disease on the basis of paraaortic node involvement. Of the 60% of patients who remain stage I or II after lymphography, exploratory laparotomy will upstage ⅓. Thus, fewer than ½ of the patients who appear clinically to have early-stage disease will remain in early stage after sequential use of lymphography and laparotomy. The role played by lymphography cannot be fulfilled by abdominal CT scanning, a diagnostic test with a 35% false-negative rate. One cannot safely treat a patient with radiation

therapy when the risk of intraabdominal involvement is so great. Lymphography has the additional advantage of permitting a cheap and effective method of following the response to therapy.

Exploratory laparotomy includes splenectomy, wedge biopsy of the liver and the iliac crest, and sampling of lymph nodes from the periportal, perisplenic, mesenteric, paraaortic, and celiac regions. Because of the acute morbidity of the procedure and the lifelong increased infectious risk of spleen removal (reviewed in reference 22), it should only be undertaken when detection of intraabdominal disease would dictate a change from radiation therapy to combination chemotherapy as the treatment.

The gallium scan is not particularly useful in the staging evaluation; however, it can be very helpful during restaging evaluation at the completion of treatment. Any residual radiographic abnormality that is also detected on a gallium

Table 62.2. Staging Evaluation for Patients with Hodgkin's Disease

A. Mandatory procedures
 1. Biopsy, with interpretation by a qualified pathologist
 2. History, with recording of (a) age; (b) gender; (c) presence or absence of unexplained fever and its duration; (d) unexplained sweating, especially at night, and its severity; (e) unexplained loss of weight as a percentage of usual body weight and rapidity of loss; (f) unexplained pruritis
 3. Physical examination with special attention to evaluation of lymphadenopathy, size of liver and spleen and evaluation of bone tenderness
 4. Laboratory tests
    a. Complete blood count
    b. Erythrocyte sedimentation rate
    c. Liver and kidney function
    d. Alkaline phosphatase
 5. Radiographic examinations
    a. Chest x-ray, posteroanterior and lateral
    b. Abdominal and pelvis CT
    c. Bipedal lymphangiogram
 6. Bilateral bone marrow aspirates and biopsies
B. Contingent procedures
 1. Thoracic CT, *if* mediastinal, hilar, and/or mediastinal involvement is seen or suspected on CXR
 2. Laparatomy, *only if* decisions regarding management will be influenced
 3. Liver biopsy (percutaneous or CT-guided) *if* there is a clinical indication of hepatic involvement, or if there is evidence or splenic involvement
C. Optional ancillary procedures
 1. Gallium scanning
 2. Technetium bone scanning
 3. Magnetic resonance imaging (MRI)
 4. Ultrasonography
 5. Echocardiography
 6. Specialized serum tests: β_2-microglobulin, soluble CD30, soluble CD25, soluble CD4, soluble CD8

scan should be further evaluated for the presence of residual Hodgkin's disease.

As noted above, stage of disease dictates choice of treatment but is not necessarily important in determining prognosis when optimal therapy is used. Among patients of a particular stage, a number of prognostic factors may influence outcome, including B symptoms; age greater than 45 years (or 65 years); massive mediastinal involvement; bone marrow, liver, pleural, or multiple extranodal sites of involvement; low hematocrit; elevated lactate dehydrogenase levels; and a high erythrocyte sedimentation rate. In addition, recently, a number of other serum markers have been said to correlate with prognosis, including serum β_2-microglobulin levels, and levels of soluble CD30, CD25, CD8, and CD4. These tests have not yet been noted to be of value in selecting therapy or monitoring the course of treatment.

TREATMENT

The goal of Hodgkin's disease therapy is cure. Long-term disease-free survival is possible, even for patients in their fourth remission. Thus, it is particularly difficult to discern when the goal of treatment should switch from cure to palliation. Long-term control of disease is also possible with palliative therapy.

The optimal treatment approaches continue to be debated. In general, radiation therapy is used in the treatment of patients with early-stage disease, and combination chemotherapy is used in patients with advanced-stage disease. However, certain centers use combined-modality therapy for all stages of disease, and others use combination chemotherapy alone for all stages of disease. Several general principles should be applied to treatment planning. First, curative therapy, whether it is radiation therapy or chemotherapy, must be given in a technically rigorous fashion to maximize efficacy.

For radiation therapy, this means using linear accelerators that produce 6- to 10-MeV photons, large fields, evenly weighted opposed fields, careful treatment planning, precise simulation, and port film verification. Tumoricidal doses are 36 to 44 Gy and are generally given at a rate of 7.5 to 10 Gy/week in 1.5- to 2-Gy fractions, depending on field size and patient tolerance. Blocks are individually contoured to the patient's anatomy, and disease distribution and special additional blocking may be required to protect certain sites (e.g., spinal cord and heart).

For chemotherapy, optimal treatment involves delivering the drugs at the maximum tolerated dose. Modification of doses or schedule should not be made in anticipation of toxicity or to prevent short-term, non-life-threatening side effects (e.g., emesis). The granulocyte count is generally used as an in vivo biologic assay of the maximum tolerated dose of myelotoxic agents. If 100% of the dose does not lower the granulocyte count to 1000/mm³, the dose should be increased by 10% on the next cycle and should continue to be escalated in 10% increments until a nadir of less than 1000 cells/mm³ is reached. If the nadir granulocyte count is below 500/mm³ for 4 days or longer, the doses of myelotoxic agents should be decreased by 25% in the next cycle. If the granulocyte count has not recovered above 1500/mm^3 by day 1 of the next cycle, treatment may be delayed by up to 1 week. If the count has still failed to recover, the next cycle should begin 1 week late at a reduced dose.

Chemotherapy is given for at least six cycles. Patients should be restaged after cycle 4 and cycle 6. If sites of disease have continued to respond between cycles 4 and 6, two additional cycles of chemotherapy should be given. If radiographic abnormalities persist after cycle 4 and have not changed after cycle 6, a gallium scan should be performed. If the gallium scan is negative, two cycles of stable radiographic change can be interpreted as a complete response to therapy. If the gallium scan is positive, the positive site requires further diagnostic evaluation.

The second major principle of Hodgkin's disease treatment is that therapy must be selected on the basis of not only the efficacy against Hodgkin's disease but also the acute and chronic toxicities of the treatment. As discussed below in more detail, acute and chronic toxicities vary among treatment approaches. Alkylating agent–containing regimens produce infertility. Bleomycin and radiation therapy induce lung toxicity. Doxorubicin and radiation therapy can cause heart damage. Radiation therapy is associated with a serious risk of second solid tumors. Combined-modality therapy with large-field radiation therapy plus an alkylating agent–based chemotherapy program increases the risk of acute leukemia. These toxicities must be fully explained to patients and taken into account when treatment recommendations are made.

Chemotherapy Regimens Used in Primary Treatment

The most commonly used combination chemotherapy regimens and the expected treatment outcome for each are listed in Table 62.3. MOPP (mechlorethamine, vincristine, procarbazine, prednisone) (23, 24), ChlVPP (chlorambucil, vinblastine, procarbazine, prednisone) (25), and MVPP (vinblastine replaces vincristine in MOPP) (26) are similar in design and in efficacy. The complete response rate in patients with advanced-stage disease treated with these regimens is between 84 and 90%. About 25 to 35% of complete responders relapse. The long-term disease-free survival of patients with advanced-stage disease treated with these regimens is 60 to 65%. When patients with massive mediastinal involvement are separated from other patients with advanced-stage disease (such patients generally require combined modality therapy (see below)), the remaining advanced-disease patients have a 70% chance of being cured by these regimens (27). These regimens are often considered together as the alkylating agent–based programs.

ABVD (doxorubicin, bleomycin, vinblastine, dacarbazine) is a regimen designed by Bonadonna et al. to be effective in patients who no longer responded to MOPP (28). In a small randomized study comparing MOPP and ABVD (28), they showed that the two regimens were roughly comparable when used in previously untreated patients. The complete response rate to ABVD was 81%, and 64% of patients were alive and disease-free at 3 years of follow-up. Unfortunately, long-term follow-up is not available on this series of patients. However, there is no reason to think that ABVD-induced complete responses are not as durable as those obtained with alkylating agent–based regimens.

In the hope of improving the treatment outcome, Bonadonna et al. decided to alternate MOPP and ABVD in consecutive months (29), based largely on predictions made from the Goldie-Coldman hypothesis on drug resistance in cancer cells. In a randomized study in patients with stage IV disease, MOPP/ABVD induced complete remission in 89% of patients, and overall survival was 76% at 7 years (29). Using a similar strategy, Connors and Klimo (30) devised a regimen in which the MOPP drugs were given in the same monthly cycle with ABV, the dose of doxorubicin was increased, and dacarbazine was dropped (so-called MOPP-ABV hybrid program). Complete responses were obtained in 84% of patients treated with the MOPP-ABV hybrid program, and another 13% of patients who were partial responders became complete responders with the addition of involved-field radiation therapy. Survival at 7 years was 77%.

One important question in Hodgkin's disease treatment is whether the seven- or eight-drug regimens (i.e., MOPP/ABVD or MOPP-ABV hybrid) are superior to the four-drug regimens in antitumor effects. Prospective randomized trials have not led to consistent conclusions (reviewed in reference 31). In the Bonadonna et al. study of patients with stage IV disease (29), MOPP/ABVD was significantly more effective than MOPP. However, because the MOPP was projected to be given over 12 months instead of the usual six to eight cycles, dose modifications were made in the MOPP arm early in the course of

Table 62.3. Chemotherapy Regimens for Primary Treatment of Hodgkin's Disease

Drug Combination	Dose mg/m[2a]	Route[b]	Days Given[c]	Complete Remission (%)	Disease-Free Survival	Reference
MOPP				84	60% at 20 years	(23)
Mechlorethamine (nitrogen mustard)	6	IV	1, 8			
Vincristine	1.4	IV	1, 8			
Procarbazine	100	PO	1–14			
Prednisone	40	PO	1–14			
ChlVPP				85	65% at 10 years	(25)
Chlorambucil	6	PO	1–14			
Vinblastine	6	IV	1, 8			
Procarbazine	100	PO	1–14			
Prednisone	40[d]	PO	1–14			
MVPP				82	60% at 5 years	(26)
Mechlorethamine	6	IV	1, 8			
Vinblastine	6	IV	1, 8			
Procarbazine	100	PO	1–14			
Prednisone	40	PO	1–14			
ABVD				81	64% at 3 years	(28)
Doxorubicin	25	IV	1, 15			
Bleomycin	10	IV	1, 15			
Vinblastine	6	IV	1, 15			
Dacarbazine	375	IV	1, 15			
MOPP/ABVD				89	76% at 7 years	(29)
Alternating months of MOPP and ABVD						
MOPP/ABV hybrid				97	77% at 7 years	(30)
Mechlorethamine	6	IV	1	84% after drugs		
Vincristine	1.4 (max 2)	IV	1			
Procarbazine	100	PO	1–7	13% after RT		
Prednisone	40	PO	1–14			
Doxorubicin	35	IV	8			
Bleomycin	10	IV	8			
Vinblastine	6	IV	8			

[a]Milligrams per square meter of body surface area.
[b]IV, intravenous; PO, oral.
[c]Drug combinations were given over a 28-day cycle. Numbers shown refer to days of the cycle.
[d]Total dose, not mg/m^2

treatment in an effort to get patients through a full year of treatment. Thus, the more appropriate conclusion is that MOPP/ABVD is more effective than a dose-attenuated course of MOPP therapy.

The British National Lymphoma Investigation (BNLI) compared LOPP (chlorambucil (Leukeran) replaces mechlorethamine in MOPP) with LOPP alternating with EVAP (etoposide, vinblastine, doxorubicin, prednisone) (32). LOPP/EVAP was significantly more effective than LOPP, but both had response rates 20 to 25% lower than expected from state-of-the-art therapy. The regimens were given with maximum dose limits for vincristine, vinblastine, procarbazine, and etoposide independent of body sur-

face area. Thus, both regimens achieved substandard results; it may be that administration of more drugs compensates somewhat for delivering inadequate doses. Neither LOPP nor LOPP/EVAP are state-of-the-art regimens as reported.

In contrast to these two studies, which conclude that seven- or eight-drug regimens are superior to four-drug regimens, there are at least five other prospective randomized trials that fail to support this conclusion (see 31). In two of these studies, one from the Eastern Cooperative Study Group (33) and one from the European Organization for the Research and Treatment of Cancer (EORTC) (34), survival of MOPP/ABVD-treated patients was less than 10% better than that for patients treated with MOPP-like regimens, a difference that was not statistically significant given the numbers of patients on each study but could be significant in the population of Hodgkin's disease patients as a whole. However, in light of frequent ad hoc modifications in the delivery of MOPP-like regimens (also reviewed in 31), it is difficult to know whether the seven- or eight-drug regimens are truly better.

An interesting study conducted by Cancer and Leukemia Group B (CALGB) also cast some doubt on the superiority of seven- or eight-drug regimens (35). In a three-arm study comparing MOPP, ABVD, and MOPP/ABVD, MOPP/ABVD was significantly better than MOPP. However, the dose intensity of the MOPP arm was reduced. The important result of the study was that patients on the MOPP/ABVD and ABVD arms were nearly identical in their complete response rate and survival. Thus, it is not completely clear whether seven- or eight-drug regimens are superior in antitumor efficacy to four-drug regimens (correctly delivered). If they are more effective, the difference in antitumor effect is small.

Several studies are under way comparing administration of alternating MOPP and ABVD with hybrid programs in which all seven or eight drugs are administered in the same monthly cycle. So far, there are no significant differences between alternating and hybrid programs. In addition, two studies comparing 8-drug regimens to 10-drug regimens have failed to demonstrate any significant difference.

In conclusion, the regimens listed in Table 62.3 appear to be comparable in efficacy in the treatment of Hodgkin's disease, assuming they are delivered at their maximum tolerated dose. The alternating and hybrid seven- or eight-drug regimens may be somewhat more effective, but if they are, the difference is small.

Chemotherapy Regimens Used in Salvage Treatment

For patients who relapse from a radiation therapy-induced complete remission, any of the regimens in Table 62.3 is effective in inducing complete responses in 90% and long-term disease-free survival in about 67% of patients (23).

Patients in whom an initial course of combination chemotherapy is not curative fall into one of three groups: those who achieved an initial remission that lasted more than 1 year, those who achieved an initial remission that lasted less than 1 year, and those who failed to achieve a remission. The prognosis of each group is significantly different (36). Patients who do not achieve an initial complete remission are unresponsive to conventional-dose combination chemotherapy. Their only treatment option is high-dose therapy with bone marrow transplantation. Patients who relapse after an initial remission that lasted less than 1 year, a group that accounts for about ½ of all patients who relapse, have only a 10% long-term disease-free survival when treated with conventional dose salvage regimens. Patients who relapse after an initial remission that lasted a year or more are more responsive to conventional-dose salvage therapy. In our experience, about 85% of these patients respond to a second course of chemotherapy, and nearly half of the second remissions are durable. However, such patients often succumb to late treatment complications, and overall survival is only about 25%.

Almost everything we know about salvage therapy has been generated in patients in whom MOPP or a MOPP-like regimen failed to achieve cure. There are few data on patients treated initially with ABVD alone or with the seven- or eight-drug regimens. In the CALGB study (35), patients who relapsed after MOPP induction received ABVD, and those who relapsed after ABVD induction received MOPP. The results showed that MOPP was more effective in ABVD-relapsers than ABVD was in MOPP-relapsers. Although the p170 glycoprotein that mediates multidrug resistance (mdr) was not measured, it makes sense that patients relapsing after exposure to the natural products in ABVD might develop mdr and respond better to an alkylating agent–based regimen, the sensitivity to which should not be affected by mdr expression. By contrast, MOPP also contains a natural product, vincristine; thus, MOPP relapsers are also likely to express mdr and be resistant to the natural product–based ABVD regimen. Data on patients relapsing after MOPP/ABVD or MOPP/ABV hybrid are sparse; however, there is no convincing evidence that these patients relapse with disease that is more resistant to salvage therapy than patients initially treated with four-drug regimens (37, 38).

A large number of regimens have been explored for their ability to induce complete remissions in patients who have not been cured by their first course of combination chemotherapy (reviewed in reference 39). None of the second-line regimens have been established as the treatment of choice. Patients who were initially treated with an alkylating agent–based regimen generally receive ABVD as their second therapy; but this approach results in complete responses in only about 30% of patients and cures 10% or fewer of patients (40). In patients initially treated with ABVD, it appears that MOPP is the treatment of choice and may cure ⅓ of those who relapse (35). Patients initially treated with MOPP/ABVD or MOPP-ABV hybrid may also respond to MOPP alone. However, no relapsed patient should receive conventional-dose combination chemotherapy as the only salvage treatment unless high-dose therapy is medically contraindicated.

The advent of high-dose therapy with autologous stem cell transplantation has dramatically improved the outlook for patients who have not been cured by their initial course of combination chemotherapy (41, 42). About 40% of patients who failed to achieve an initial complete response will achieve long-term disease-free survival with high-dose therapy, and the cure rate for patients with short initial remissions is increased from 10% with conventional-dose chemotherapy to about 50% with high-dose therapy and stem cell support. Even the patients who had initial remissions longer than 12 months appear to benefit from high-dose salvage chemotherapy. Although this group is relatively responsive to conventional-dose regimens, Reece et al. (43) observed an 85% long-term progression-free survival after the use of high-dose therapy and autologous marrow transplantation, a survival rate at least twice as high as the best reported results with conventional-dose combination chemotherapy.

High-dose therapy works best (and lethal toxicity is lowest) when it is used early in the patient's course (i.e., as the treatment for patients in their first relapse) and in patients with good performance status. In patients who relapse or progress on therapy, it is reasonable to try one or two cycles of a conventional-dose salvage regimen to debulk the patient of tumor (outcome is also influenced by tumor burden). However, high-dose therapy should be given if the disease progresses or does not respond further to conventional-dose therapy. Selected conventional-dose regimens are listed in Table 62.4 (44–52). These regimens produce responses in most relapsed patients and complete responses in at least 30%. There are no data comparing various high-dose chemotherapy regimens. Those used most frequently are CBV (cyclophosphamide, BCNU, etoposide) and BEAM (BCNU, etoposide, cytarabine, melphalan). The doses and schedules of these and other selected regimens are listed in Table 62.4 (41, 42, 53–55). The original papers should be consulted for important details on administration. In addition to marrow toxicity, mucositis and pulmonary toxicity are common with these programs.

High-dose salvage therapy has become accepted as standard treatment because of its clear superiority over conventional-dose salvage therapy. Indeed, randomized studies are unlikely to be supported by either physicians or patients. The BNLI undertook a randomized comparison between BEAM plus autologous marrow and mini-BEAM, a regimen composed of the same agents given in doses not requiring stem cell support (56). In the first 40 randomized patients, high-dose BEAM was significantly more effective than mini-BEAM; however, the study could not be completed because patients and their physicians refused to participate in a randomization.

The source of the hematopoietic stem cells may be either autologous bone marrow or chemotherapy- or cytokine-mobilized peripheral blood stem cells. Allogeneic marrow transplantation has been undertaken in patients with relapsed Hodgkin's disease; however, allogeneic transplantation has not been shown to be superior to autologous stem cell support.

Late Complications of Treatment

SECOND MALIGNANCY

The major source of risk of second tumors in patients treated for Hodgkin's disease is from second solid tumors related to the use of radiation therapy (57). The risk is about 0.5 to 1%/year and appears to continue to increase well into the third decade of follow-up (58). Irradiated patients are at increased risk for melanoma; cancers of the salivary glands, head and neck, lung, breast, thyroid, stomach; and bone and soft tissue sarcomas (59, 60). Most solid tumors occur within the radiation field. Chemotherapy does not appear to add to the risk.

Acute leukemia occurs in about 2% of patients treated with an alkylating agent–based regimen. Unlike the risk of solid tumors, which increases with time, the risk of leukemia peaks at about 6 years after treatment and returns to normal after 10 years (61). This risk can be augmented by the concomitant use of large-field radiation therapy (about 15% risk), chronic-maintenance chemotherapy (about 15% risk), and nitrosoureas (about 10% risk). Splenectomy may increase the risk. Patients older than 40 years re-

Table 62.4. Chemotherapy Regimens for Salvage Treatment of Hodgkin's Disease

Regimen	No. of Patients	Complete Response No. (%)	Reference
Conventional dose regimens			
VABCD	18	8 (45)	(44)
vinblastine 6 mg/m² IV every 3 weeks			
doxorubicin 400 mg/m² IV every 3 weeks			
dacarbazine 800 mg/m² IV every 3 weeks			
CCNU 80 mg/m² PO every 6 weeks			
bleomycin 15 U IV every 1 week			
ABDIC	34	12 (35)	(45)
doxorubicin 45 mg/m² IV day 1			
bleomycin 5 U/m² IV days 1, 5			
dacarbazine 200 mg/m² IV days 1–5			
CCNU 50 mg/m² PO day 1			
prednisone 40 mg/m² PO days 1–5 every 28 days			
CBVD	20	9 (45)	(46)
CCNU 120 mg/m² PO day 1			
bleomycin 15 U IV days 1, 22			
vinblastine 6 mg/m² IV days 1, 22			
dexamethasone 3 mg/m² PO days 1–21 every 6 weeks			
PCVP	11	8 (72)	(47)
vinblastine 3 mg/m² IV every 2 weeks			
procarbazine 70 mg/m² PO every other day			
cyclophosphamide 70 mg/m² PO every other day			
prednisone 8 mg/m² PO every other day therapy lasts 1 year			
CEP	58	23 (40)	(48)
CCNU 80 mg/m² PO day 1			
etoposide 100 mg/m² PO day 1–5			
prednimustine 60 mg/m² PO day 1–5			
EVA	19	6 (32)	(49)
etoposide 200 mg/m² PO days 1–5			
vincristine 2 mg IV day 1			
doxorubicin 50 mg/m² IV day 1			
CEVD	32	14 (44)	(50)
CCNU 80 mg/m² PO day 1			
etoposide 120 mg/m² IV days 1–5, 22–26			
vindesine 3 mg/m² IV days 1, 22			
dexamethasone 3 mg/m² PO days 1–8, 1.5 mg/m² PO days 9–26 every 6 weeks			
EVAP	27	9 (33)	(39)
etoposide 120 mg/m² IV days 1, 8, 15			
vinblastine 4 mg/m² IV days 1, 8, 15			
cytarabine 30 mg/m² IV days 1, 8, 15			
cisplatin 40 mg/m² IV days 1, 8, 15 every 4 weeks			
mini-BEAM	44	14 (32)	(51)
BCNU 60 mg/m² day 1			
etoposide 75 mg/m² days 2–5			
cytarabine 100 mg/m² b.i.d. days 2–5			
melphalan 30 mg/m² day 6			

Table 62.4—*continued*. Chemotherapy Regimens for Salvage Treatment of Hodgkin's Disease

Regimen	No. of Patients	Complete Response No. (%)	Reference
dexa-BEAM	55	17 (31)	(52)
dexamethasone 8 mg/m^2 every 8 hours PO days 1–10			
BCNU 60 mg/m^2 day 2			
etoposide 75 mg/m^2 days 4–7			
cytarabine 100 mg/m^2 b.i.d. days 4–7			
melphalan 20 mg/m^2 day 3			
High-dose regimens[a]			
CBV			(41)
cyclophosphamide 1.5 g/m^2 days 1–4			
BCNU 300 mg/m^2 day 1			
etoposide 150 mg/m^2 days 1–3			
marrow day 7			
BEAM			(42)
BCNU 300 mg/m^2 day 1			
etoposide 100–200 mg/m^2 days 2–5			
cytarabine 200–400 mg/m^2 days 2–5			
melphalan 140 mg/m^2 day 6			
marrow day 7			
ICE			(53)
ifosfamide 4 g/m^2 days 1–4 (given with mesna uroprotection)			
carboplatin 600 mg/m^2/day 72-hour infusion days 1–3			
etoposide 250 mg/m^2 b.i.d. days 1–3			
marrow day 7			
EM			(54)
etoposide 60 mg/kg day 1			
melphalan 160 mg/m^2 day 2			
marrow day 5			
Augmented CBV			(55)
cyclophosphamide 1–8 g/m^2 days 1–4			
BCNU 600 mg/m^2 day 5			
etoposide 400 mg/m^2 b.i.d. days 1–3			
marrow day 7			

[a]Response rates are not provided due to heterogeneity in patient selection criteria; comparative trials have not yet been undertaken.

ceiving leukemogenic regimens have about three times the risk of younger patients.

ABVD does not appear to cause leukemia. MOPP/ABVD and the MOPP-ABV hybrid program both include alkylating agents; however, it appears that the total dose of alkylating agents in these regimens is below the threshold of leukemogenesis, because reports of leukemia after these regimens are rare.

CARDIAC AND PULMONARY DISEASE

Heart disease is second only to secondary cancer as a cause of death after treatment for Hodgkin's disease. The risk is nearly all related to the use of mantle-field radiation therapy. For children and adolescents treated with radiation therapy, the relative risk of fatal myocardial infarction was over 50-fold that of normal age-matched controls (62). In adults, there is more than a 3-fold increased risk of fatal myocardial infarction (63). Nonfatal cardiac disease has not been quantitated.

The doses of doxorubicin given in ABVD and the seven- or eight-drug regimens are too low to produce significant cardiac compromise unless preexisting heart failure is present. If incipient heart failure is a concern, alkylating agent–based regimens are safe; alternatively, epirubicin may be used instead of doxorubicin.

Bleomycin can produce serious pulmonary toxicity. In the CALGB study comparing MOPP, ABVD, and MOPP/ABVD (35), 3% of the patients treated with ABVD died from pulmonary toxicity, and with a median follow-up of only 3 years, other bleomycin-related deaths may occur. Thus, the risk of death from pulmonary failure after ABVD is at least as great as the risk of death from acute leukemia after MOPP. The total dose of bleomycin in MOPP/ABVD and MOPP-ABV hybrid regimens appears to be below the threshold of fatal lung toxicity, because toxic pulmonary deaths have not been reported with these regimens.

The use of bleomycin together with radiation therapy appears to result in an increased risk of pulmonary disease. Although the Stanford group has reported safely using vinblastine, bleomycin, and methotrexate together with radiation therapy in patients with early-stage disease (64), Bates et al. (65) found an unacceptably high level of pulmonary toxicity with this combination. Properly delivered mantle-field radiation therapy alone is rarely associated with clinically significant pulmonary compromise.

INFERTILITY

MOPP and similar regimens induce azoospermia in nearly 100% of men; women older than 26 years at the time of treatment generally lose menses permanently, and those younger than 26 years at the time of treatment experience recovery of menstrual cycles and fertility. Even in women whose cycles recover, menopause occurs prematurely (reviewed in reference 22). ABVD appears to have no permanent toxic effects on the gonads. MOPP/ABVD and MOPP-ABV hybrid data are just emerging; however, it appears that they induce roughly half the infertility associated with MOPP (66). Nevertheless, when patients in the CALGB three-arm study were surveyed for sexual problems, there were no significant differences among the three regimens in the frequency of complaints about sexual difficulties (67).

The gonads can usually be shielded from external-beam radiation therapy. However, direct or scatter radiation of more than 2 Gy to the testes can result in sterility in males, and depending on age at the time of treatment, 2 to 10 Gy to the ovaries can result in ovarian failure and sterility in women.

TREATMENT RECOMMENDATIONS IN SPECIFIC SETTINGS

Stage I, IIA Supradiaphragmatic Disease

Assuming that the patient has been staged with exploratory laparotomy, subtotal nodal radiation therapy is the treatment of choice, with 40 to 44 Gy to the mantle field followed by 36 to 40 Gy to the paraaortic nodes above the pelvis. If delivered accurately, 75% of patients will be cured. Certain patients are at very low risk for intraabdominal disease, including clinical stage IA patients with any of the following features: women, high cervical nodes, mediastinal mass only, lymphocyte-predominant histology. Such patients may be treated with radiation therapy without exploratory laparotomy. Another approach to the management of early-stage Hodgkin's disease is to do only clinical staging and treat the patients with combination chemotherapy (68) (Fig. 62.1). The long-term survival from this approach is at least as effective as that seen with subtotal nodal radiation therapy, and it avoids the late toxicity associated with laparotomy and radiation-related second tumors and cardiac disease.

Stage I, IIB Supradiaphragmatic Disease

Fifteen to 20% of patients with stage I or II disease present with B symptoms. If radiation therapy is contemplated, exploratory laparotomy must be performed. Some groups recommend adding chemotherapy to radiation therapy in these patients; however, this results in toxicities associated with both modalities. A preferable approach to management is to treat these patients with combination chemotherapy alone after clinical staging.

Stage I, IIA Subdiaphragmatic Disease

Ten percent of patients with stage I or II disease present with involvement limited to subdiaphragmatic sites. Patients with inguinal masses and a negative lymphogram may receive radiation therapy alone to an inverted Y-field without staging laparotomy. However, if the lymphogram is positive, laparotomy is required. About 40% of such patients will have splenic involvement. If an exploratory laparotomy confirms no involvement of the spleen, the patient should receive total nodal radiation therapy. Pa-

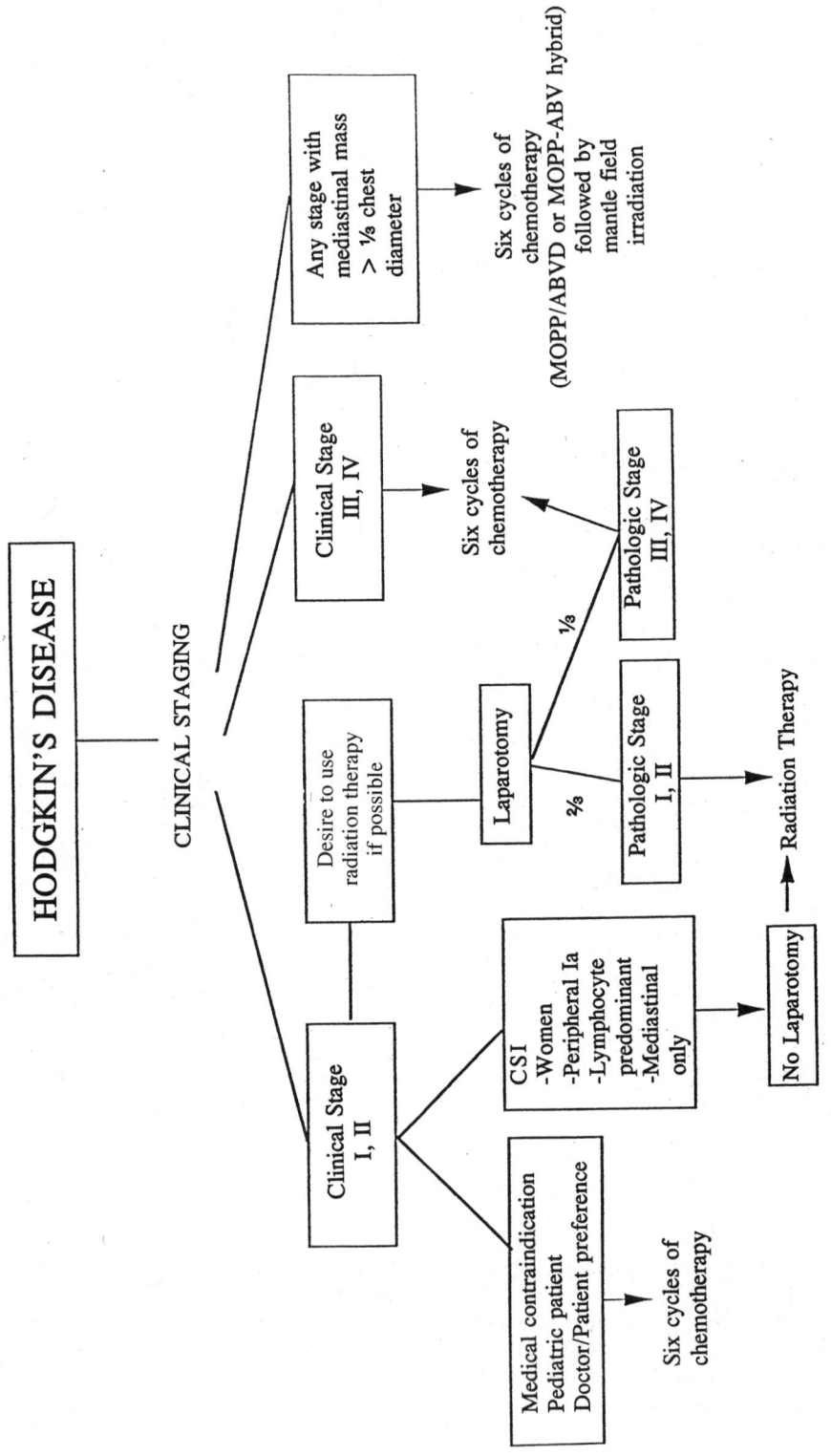

Figure 62.1.   Management algorithm for patients with Hodgkin's disease.

Treatment of MOPP-refractory Hodgkin's disease with vinblastine, doxorubicin, bleomycin, CCNU, and dacarbazine. Cancer 1982;51:1348–1352.

45. Tannir N, Hagemeister F, Velasqueez W, Cabanillas F. Long-term follow-up with ABDIC salvage chemotherapy of MOPP-resistant Hodgkin's disease. J Clin Oncol 1983;1:432–439.

46. Weiss J, Von Roemeling R, Peters HD, et al. Chemotherapy in pretreated Hodgkin's disease with lomustine, bleomycin, vinblastine, and dexamethasone. Dtsch Med Wochenschr 1983;108:1428–1432.

47. Mandelli F, Cimino G, Mauro FR, et al. Prognosis and management of patients affected by multi pre-treated Hodgkin's disease. Haematologia 1986; 71:205–208.

48. Santoro A, Viviani S, Valagussa P, et al. CCNU, etoposide and prednimustine in refractory Hodgkin's disease. Semin Oncol 1986;13(Suppl 1):23–26.

49. Richards MA, Waxman JH, Man T, et al. EVA treatment for recurrent or unresponsive Hodgkin's disease. Cancer Chemother Pharmacol 1986;18:51–53.

50. Pfreundschuh MG, Schoppe WD, Fuchs R, et al. Lomustine, etoposide, vindesine, and dexamethasone (CEVD) in Hodgkin's lymphoma refractory to cyclophosphamide, vincristine, procarbazine, and prednisone (COPP) and doxorubicin, bleomycin, vinblastine, and dacarbazine (ABVD): a multicenter trial of the German Hodgkin Study Group. Cancer Treat Rep 1987;71:1203–1207.

51. Colwill R, Crump M, Couture F, et al. Mini-BEAM as salvage therapy for relapsed or refractory Hodgkin's disease before intensive therapy and autologous bone marrow transplantation. J Clin Oncol 1995; 13:396–402.

52. Pfreundschuh MG, Rueffer U, Lathan B, et al. Dexa-BEAM in patients with Hodgkin's disease refractory to multidrug chemotherapy regimens: a trial of the German Hodgkin's Disease Study Group. J Clin Oncol 1994;12:580–586.

53. Wilson WH, Jain V, Bryant G, et al. Phase I and II study of high-dose ifosfamide, carboplatin, and etoposide with autologous bone marrow rescue in lymphomas and solid tumors. J Clin Oncol 1992;10:1712–1722.

54. Crump M, Smith AM, Brandwein J, et al. High-dose etoposide and melphalan, and autologous bone marrow transplantation for patients with advanced Hodgkin's disease: importance of disease status at transplant. J Clin Oncol 1993;11:704–711.

55. Reece DE, Barnett MJ, Connors JM, et al. Intensive chemotherapy with cyclophosphamide, carmustine, and etoposide followed by autologous bone marrow transplantation for relapsed Hodgkin's disease. J Clin Oncol 1991;9:1871–1879.

56. Linch DC, Winfield D, Goldstone AH, et al. Dose intensification with autologous bone marrow transplantation in relapsed and resistant Hodgkin's disease: results of a BNLI randomised trial. Lancet 1 1993;341:1051–1054.

57. Tucker MA, Coleman CN, Cox RS, Varghese A, Rosenberg SA. Risk of second cancers after treatment for Hodgkin's disease. N Engl J Med 1988;318:76–81.

58. Meadows AT, Obringer AC, Marrero O, et al. Second malignant neoplasms following childhood Hodgkin's disease: treatment and splenectomy as risk factors. Med Pediatr Oncol 1989;17:477–489.

59. Hancock SL, Tucker MA, Hoppe RT. Breast cancer after treatment of Hodgkin's disease. J Natl Cancer Inst 1993;85:25–31.

60. van Leeuwen FE, Klokman WJ, Hagenbeek A, et al. Second cancer risk following Hodgkin's disease: a 20-year follow-up study. J Clin Oncol 1994;12:312–325.

61. Blayney DW, Longo Dl, Young RC, Greene MH, Hubbard SM, et al. Decreasing risk of leukemia with prolonged follow-up after chemotherapy and radiotherapy for Hodgkin's disease. N Engl J Med 1987; 316:710–714.

62. Hancock SL, Donaldson SS, Hoppe RT. Cardiac disease following treatment of Hodgkin's disease in children and adolescents. J Clin Oncol 1993;11:1208–1215.

63. Hancock SL, Tucker MA, Hoppe RT. Factors affecting late mortality from heart disease after treatment of Hodgkin's disease. JAMA 1993;270:1949–1955.

64. Horning SJ, Hoppe RT, Hancock SL, Rosenberg SA. Vinblastine, bleomycin, and methotrexate: an effective adjuvant in favorable Hodgkin's disease. J Clin Oncol 1988;6:1822–1831.

65. Bates NP, Williams MV, Bessell EM, Vaughan Hudson G, Vaughan Hudson B. Efficacy and toxicity of vinblastine, bleomycin, and methotrexate with involved-field radiotherapy in clinical stage IA and IIA Hodgkin's disease: a British National Lymphoma Investigation pilot study. J Clin Oncol 1994;12:288–296.

66. Anselmo AP, Cartoni C, Bellantuono P, et al. Risk of infertility in patients with Hodgkin's disease treated with ABVD vs MOPP vs ABVD/MOPP. Haematologica 1990;75:155–158.

67. Kornblith AB, Anderson J, Cell DF, et al. Comparison of psychosocial adaptation and sexual function of survivors of advanced Hodgkin disease treated by MOPP, ABVD or MOPP alternating with ABVD. Cancer 1992;70:2508–2516.

68. Longo DL, Glatstein E, Duffey PL, et al. Radiation therapy vs combination chemotherapy in the treatment of early stage Hodgkin's disease: seven-year results of a prospective randomized trial. J Clin Oncol 1991;9:906–917.

69. Longo DL. To buzz or not to buzz, that is the question: the case against the routine use of radiation therapy in advanced stage Hodgkin's disease. Cancer Invest 1996, in press.

70. Fabian C, Dahlberg S, Miller T, et al. Efficacy of low dose involved field XRT in producing and maintaining CR following PR induction with MOP-BAP chemotherapy in Hodgkin's disease. Results of Southwest Oncology Group study 7808 (abstract 987). Proc Am Soc Clin Oncol 1989;8:253.

63

Non-Hodgkin's Lymphoma

James O. Armitage, Philip Bierman, and Julie Vose

The related group of malignancies of lympho-cytes known as non-Hodgkin's lymphomas has been steadily increasing in incidence in the United States for the last 40 years. It is estimated that there will be approximately 51,000 new cases diagnosed in the United States in 1995 (1). This is a common malignancy and one that will be seen regularly by primary care physicians as well as oncologists.

The non-Hodgkin's lymphomas present a wide spectrum of symptoms and signs at pres-entation, clinical aggressiveness, and response to therapy. Some non-Hodgkin's lymphomas are so indolent in their natural history that the "stan-dard" treatment is to observe the patient without therapy. On the other extreme, tumors such as Burkitt's lymphoma are among the most rapidly growing and highly aggressive malignancies known. Knowledge gained from the study of these disorders has had considerable impact on our approach to other malignancies. All non-Hodgkin's lymphomas are responsive to che-motherapy, and chemotherapy remains the treatment of choice for most patients with these disorders.

EPIDEMIOLOGY/ETIOLOGY

The incidence of non-Hodgkin's lymphoma varies considerably throughout the world (2–4). However, in the United States, the incidence has been steadily increasing by approximately 3 to 4% annually for the last 40 years (5). The rising incidence in the United States has been predom-inately in older patients and in men. The increas-ing frequency is primarily in the more aggres-sive, rather than the indolent, subtypes. In recent years, the incidence has increased because of the consequences of human immunodeficiency virus (HIV) infection. However, the impact of HIV in-fection on the frequency of non-Hodgkin's lym-phomas in the United States is still modest and does not account for the steady rise over the last several decades.

The etiology of non-Hodgkin's lymphoma in most patients with this disorder is unknown. Considerable evidence has accumulated that ex-posure to various chemicals increases the risk of developing non-Hodgkin's lymphoma (6–10). There is particularly strong evidence, developed in several states and other countries, that expo-sure to farm chemicals increases the risk of de-veloping non-Hodgkin's lymphoma (7–9). How-ever, the absolute incidence of non-Hodgkin's lymphomas related to farm chemicals must be fairly small because of the small proportion of people in the United States who make their liv-ing in farming.

A number of viruses have been associated with the development of non-Hodgkin's lym-phoma. Infection with HIV, as noted above, greatly increases the risk of developing non-Hodgkin's lymphoma (11–15). HIV depletes helper T-lymphocytes (i.e., CD4+ lymphocytes). However, the lymphomas that develop in these patients are almost invariably B-cell lymphomas that would be classified as diffuse large cell, im-munoblastic, or small non-cleaved cell lym-phoma in the working formulation (14, 15). Thus, the lymphomas in this situation are not directly caused by the HIV infection, but the in-fection seems to have a "permissive" effect.

Human T-cell leukemia virus-1 (HTLV-1) in-fection is common in the southern islands of Ja-pan and in certain regions in the Caribbean (16–20). A small proportion of patients infected by this virus develop T-cell non-Hodgkin's lympho-mas with a unique natural history and poor re-sponse to therapy (21). These lymphomas do seem to develop in direct response to infection by HTLV-1.

Finally, the Epstein-Barr virus has been associated with a number of lymphoproliferative disorders. These include Burkitt's lymphoma, lymphomas developing in organ and bone marrow transplant recipients, and lymphomas developing in patients infected with HIV (5). These lymphomas are almost always histologically aggressive and frequently contain genetic material from the Epstein-Barr virus incorporated into the nuclei of the lymphoma cells (23). However, the exact mechanism of lymphomagenesis remains obscure.

Lymphomas develop more frequently than would be expected in patients who have a variety of disorders of the immune system, not just immune defects associated with organ transplantation or infection by HIV. Patients with so-called autoimmune disorders such as rheumatoid arthritis have a higher incidence of lymphoma than would be expected (24, 25). Patients who have been successfully treated for Hodgkin's disease also are at increased risk of developing non-Hodgkin's lymphomas (26). The explanation for the development of lymphomas in these patients is unclear. This is also the case for lymphomas that develop in patients with certain inherited immune disorders such as ataxia telangiectasia, Wiskott-Aldrich syndrome, common variable immunodeficiency syndrome, agammaglobulinemia, and Chediak-Higashi syndrome (22, 27, 28). There is an unusual X-linked syndrome that leads to a characteristic lymphoproliferative disorder in certain families (29). Sometimes called the Purtillo syndrome, this condition leads to fatal lymphomas, infectious mononucleosis syndrome, or aplastic anemia in association with infection by Epstein-Barr virus in affected males.

CLINICALLY IMPORTANT SUBTYPES

Non-Hodgkin's lymphomas are malignancies of lymphocytes that generally grow as solid tumors. They can be classified in a great variety of ways, each of which can have some clinical utility. For example, lymphomas might be classified as nodal or extranodal, as localized or disseminated, or on the basis of immunologic or genetic characteristics. However, the diagnosis of non-Hodgkin's lymphoma is established by microscopic examination of a histologic specimen of the tumor by an experienced hematopathologist. Because different types of non-Hodgkin's lymphomas can be recognized by their histologic appearance and because they are associated with characteristic clinical responses to therapy, this is the starting point for evaluating patients with this disorder.

Establishing the histopathologic diagnosis of a specific type of non-Hodgkin's lymphoma is not trivial. Studies have shown that general surgical pathologists agree in their diagnosis with expert hematopathologists only slightly more than half the time (30, 31). Thus, before patients are treated for a non-Hodgkin's lymphoma, it is extremely important that their slides be evaluated by an expert in hematopathology. Even then, the diagnosis is not simple, and the pathologist should be provided with an adequate biopsy specimen. It is almost never appropriate for the diagnosis of non-Hodgkin's lymphoma to be established by a needle biopsy. Whenever possible, fresh material should be available to the pathologist to facilitate immunologic and genetic studies.

The labels applied to the various types of non-Hodgkin's lymphomas have varied dramatically over time and geographically. Whichever system is applied, the non-Hodgkin's lymphomas are divided into indolent disorders (usually with small cells), which are rarely cured with systemic therapy, and aggressive lymphomas (usually with large cells), in which systemic therapy can sometimes cure disseminated disease. The latter includes a group of very highly aggressive malignancies that sometimes present as leukemia.

The systems used to classify the various subtypes of non-Hodgkin's lymphomas have been purely morphologic (i.e., based on the size and shape of the cells), immunologic, or a combination of the two. A major advance in understanding these disorders came with the observation by Henry Rappaport that lymphomas could be subdivided on the basis of their pattern of growth (i.e., whether they grew in a follicular or diffuse pattern) and on the size and shape of the tumor cells (32). This led to the Rappaport classification. Unfortunately, about the time this system of classifying lymphomas came into widespread use, it became apparent that the large lymphocytes in the aggressive lymphomas were not histiocytes but transformed lymphocytes. At about the same time, it became widely recognized that lymphocytes could be divided into two categories (T cells or B cells), with widely differing biologic characteristics. Although the Rappaport classification had tremendous clinical relevance, these findings made it biologically less relevant.

Several other classifications were developed to take these findings into account. Two of these were particularly influential in the subsequent development of lymphoma classification. The Lukes-Collins classification was developed in the United States and was (33) based on the immunologic characteristics of the tumor cells in addition to their size and shape. In Europe, Karl Lennert developed the Kiel classification, which considered immunologic and morphologic characteristics but added the new observation of lymphoma "grade" (34), that is, the distinction between the slow-growing and rapidly growing lymphomas. The Kiel classification remains the most popular one in Europe.

To try to resolve the controversy over lymphoma nomenclature, the National Cancer Insti-

tute of the United States sponsored a study that led to the development of a compromise classification referred to as "the working formulation" (35). This classification, the most commonly used one in the United States today, incorporates the concept of grade level of malignancy along with cell size and shape (Table 63.1). All of these classification systems are highly clinically relevant and can be used to provide good care for patients with lymphoma.

Since the development of these classifications, a number of new lymphomas have been recognized by pathologists. In fact, it is unlikely that any classification will be permanent, since new

Table 63.1. Classification System for Lymphomas

Working Formulation	ILSG
Low grade	B-cell lymphomas
A. Malignant lymphoma, small lymphocytic	Low grade
Consistent with chronic lymphocytic leukemia	B-CLL/SLL
B. Malignant lymphomas, follicular	Lymphosplasmacytoid lymphoma
Predominantly small cleaved cell	Follicle center lymphomas
Diffuse areas	Marginal zone lymphomas (MALT)
Sclerosis	Mantle cell lymphoma
C. Malignant lymphoma, follicular mixed small	
cleaved and large cell	Aggressive
Diffuse areas	Diffuse large B-cell lymphoma
Sclerosis	Primary mediastinal large B-cell lymphomas
	Burkitt's lymphoma
Immediate grade	Precursor B-cell lymphoid lymphoma/leukemia
D. Malignant lymphoma, follicular	
Predominantly large cell	T-cell lymphomas
Diffuse areas	Low-grade
Sclerosis	T-CLL
E. Malignant lymphoma, diffuse small cleaved cell	Mycosis fungoides/Sezary syndrome
F. Malignant lymphoma, diffuse mixed, small and	Aggressive
large cell sclerosis	Peripheral T-cell lymphoma unspecified
Epithelioid cell component	Angioimmunoblastic T-cell unspecified
G. Malignant lymphoma, diffuse	Angiocentric lymphoma
Large cell	Intestinal T-cell lymphoma
Cleaved cell	Adult T-cell lymphoma/leukemia
Non-cleaved cell	Anaplastic large cell lymphoma
Sclerosis	Precursor T-lymphoid lymphoma/leukemia
High grade	
H. Malignant lymphoma large cell, immunoblastic	
Plasmacytoid	
Clear cell	
Polymorphous	
Polymorphous cell component	
Epithelioid cell component	
I. Malignant lymphoma lymphoblastic	
Convoluted cell	
Nonconvoluted cell	
J. Malignant lymphoma small non-cleaved cell	
Burkitt's	
Follicular areas	

understanding of the biology of lymphomas is likely to continue to lead to recognition of new subtypes. For example, a lymphoma of small and somewhat irregular cells has been recognized for some years and gone by the names diffuse intermediate lymphoma and centrocytic lymphoma (36–38). This lymphoma originates in B lymphocytes of the mantle zone (i.e., cells surrounding the follicle) and has a characteristic immunologic pattern (CD5+) and genetic makeup (t(11;14)). Currently termed mantle cell lymphomas, these tumors respond poorly to therapy and have a poor survival despite the small size of the tumor cells (39).

Another group of tumors that seems to originate from the marginal zone (i.e., outside the mantle zone) has recently been recognized. These tumors are also small lymphocytic B-cell lymphomas and have three recognized variants. Monocytoid B-cell lymphomas represent the lymph node variant (40, 41). Tumors that begin in the spleen are often called splenic lymphomas with villous lymphocytes (42). When these tumors originate in extranodal sites, they are referred to as mucosa-associated lymphoid tumors (MALTOMAs) (43, 44). These lymphomas also have a characteristic immunologic pattern (CD5−) but have an indolent natural history. MALTOMAs occurring in the stomach seem to be associated with infection by *Helicobacter pylori*, and eradication of *H. pylori* with antibiotics sometimes causes regression of localized gastric MALTOMAs (45).

The discovery of an antigen that frequently appears on the Reed-Sternberg cells of Hodgkin's disease (i.e., CD30 or Ki-1) led to the recognition of a particular subtype of large cell non-Hodgkin's lymphoma, called anaplastic large cell lymphoma, which characteristically stains for this antigen (46). Staining for CD30 is not diagnostic of this type of non-Hodgkin's lymphoma, since it is also seen in a variety of other types of non-Hodgkin's lymphoma. Anaplastic large cell lymphoma is associated with large, irregularly shaped tumor cells and frequently presents in extranodal sites (47). In the past, this particular type of lymphoma was frequently confused with undifferentiated carcinoma.

These and other new types of lymphomas have led to enthusiasm for an alternative system for diagnosing non-Hodgkin's lymphomas. The International Lymphoma Study Group has proposed a new system that recognizes many of these new types of lymphomas (48) (Table 63.1).

Table 63.2. Common Cytogenetic Abnormalities Seen in Non-Hodgkin's Lymphoma

Translocation	Histologic Type	Oncogene Involved
(1;14)(q24;q32)	Mantle cell	*bcl-1*
(4;18)(q32;q21)	All follicular lymphomas and some diffuse large cell lymphomas	*bcl-2*
(4;19)(q32;q13)	Small lymphocytic	*bcl-3*
(3;?)(q27;)	Diffuse large cell	*bcl-6*
(2;5)(p23;q35)	Anaplastic cell	*ALK*

"Biologic" Markers

It would be possible to develop other ways to classify lymphomas on the basis of biologic observations. For example, monoclonal antibodies that recognize a large number of surface antigens are widely available and could be used to develop a classification system. However, sufficient variation exists in staining patterns to make it unlikely that a system would be based entirely upon this approach. However, certain staining patterns (such as the presence or absence of CD5 on the surface of small lymphocytes, see above) can be very helpful to pathologists in reaching a diagnosis.

Cytogenetic or molecular genetic abnormalities that seem to be present in all lymphomas provide another potential method for classification. Certain cytogenetic abnormalities are highly associated with specific histopathologic subtypes of lymphomas (49, 50). It has been proposed that the genetic mistake might correlate better with the clinical course than does morphologic appearance in some circumstances. A list of genetic abnormalities associated with particular subtypes of non-Hodgkin's lymphomas is presented in Table 63.2.

FACTORS PREDICTING TREATMENT OUTCOME

Stage

The concept of staging a cancer is relatively new. Staging refers to observations about the patients and their disease that allows them to be divided into categories predictive of clinical course or the chances to benefit from one or another therapy. Staging systems only make sense when the natural histories or the chances to benefit from therapy vary by stage. Both are the case

Table 63.3. Outcome According to Risk Group Defined by the International Prognostic Index

Risk Group	No. of Risk Factors	Distribution of Patients (%)	CR Rate (%)	5-Year Survival Rate (%)
International index, all patients				
(n = 2031)				
Adverse factors (age >60 years, ↑ LDH, poor performance status, ≥2 extranodal sites, Ann Arbor stage III or IV)				
Low	0 or 1	35	87	73
Low intermediate	2	27	67	51
High intermediate	3	22	55	43
High	4 or 5	16	44	26
Age-adjusted index, patients ≤60 years old				
(n = 1274)				
Adverse factors (↑ LDH, poor performance status, Ann Arbor stage III or IV)				
Low	0	22	92	83
Low intermediate	1	32	78	69
High intermediate	2	32	57	46
High	3	14	46	32
Age-adjusted index, patients >60 years old				
(n = 761)				
Adverse factors (↑ LDH, poor performance status, Ann Arbor stage III or IV)				
Low	0	18	91	56
Low intermediate	1	31	71	44
High intermediate	2	35	56	37
High	3	16	36	21

with the staging systems used for patients with non-Hodgkin's lymphoma.

After a patient with non-Hodgkin's lymphoma has been definitively diagnosed, the next step in management is to complete a series of evaluations including a careful history and physical examination, laboratory studies, imaging studies, and sometimes further biopsies to allow assigning a stage. In a typical patient, the studies include a hemogram, a chemistry profile that includes a serum LDH, a serum β_2-microglobulin level, an erythrocyte sedimentation rate, chest x-ray, computed tomography (CT) scan of at least the abdomen and pelvis, and a bone marrow biopsy. More extensive studies might be used in individual patients. Results of these studies allow assignment of a stage.

For many years, the most popular staging system for patients with non-Hodgkin's lymphoma was the Ann Arbor classification (51), developed for the management of patients with Hodgkin's disease. More recently, it has become apparent that this is imperfect in staging patients with non-Hodgkin's lymphoma. A large international study recently developed a system, called the international index, which divides pa-

tients into prognostic categories (52). The international index includes the Ann Arbor stage and adds age, serum LDH level, number of extranodal sites of involvement by lymphoma, and performance status to better predict treatment outcome (Table 63.3). While originally developed for patients with large cell lymphoma, it has recently been demonstrated that this system also applies well to patients with small cell lymphoma (53).

Biologic Predictors of Treatment Outcome

The presence or absence of a number of molecules on the cell surface has been associated with a different therapeutic outcome in patients with non-Hodgkin's lymphoma. The most obvious and the most controversial immunologic subdivision is between T-cell and B-cell lymphomas. At least in patients with large cell lymphoma, there is some evidence that otherwise similar patients with T-cell lymphoma have a poorer outcome than those with B-cell lymphoma, but this remains very controversial (54–56). Patients whose tumors do not express molecules of the major histocompatibility complex also seem to be at a higher risk for treatment failure (57, 58). These findings might reflect the lack of recognition of the tumor by the normal immune system.

A number of cytogenetic abnormalities have been suggested to predict treatment outcome. The t(14;18) translocation is highly associated with follicular lymphomas but is also seen in approximately 25 to 30% of patients with large cell lymphoma (50). In large cell lymphoma, it has been associated with late relapse. One of the genes involved in this translocation is the BCL-2 gene (59). The protein produced by this gene inhibits apoptosis (i.e., programed cell death). This seems to lead to a new type of chemotherapy resistance, since most chemotherapeutic agents kill cells by activating apoptosis.

The rate of tumor proliferation also seems to be a prognostic factor in patients with non-Hodgkin's lymphoma. The rate of proliferation can be measured in a variety of ways, including the proportion of cells in the DNA synthesis phase of the cell cycle or by staining for the nuclear antigen Ki-67 (60, 61). Whichever method is used, lymphomas that have a higher proliferative fraction seem to be associated with a shorter survival and a higher treatment-failure rate (60–62). This presumably reflects the fact that rapidly proliferating tumors have more tumor regrowth between treatment cycles and might develop chemotherapy resistance more rapidly.

One mechanism of chemotherapy resistance that is now widely recognized is the expression of P-glycoprotein (the mediator of multidrug resistance) on the tumor cell surface. This molecule protects the cells from injury by natural products such as Adriamycin and vincristine. Non-Hodgkin's lymphomas seem to rarely express P-glycoprotein at the time of diagnosis but do so much more frequently at the time of treatment failure (63).

PRINCIPLES OF THERAPY

Patients with cancer are generally treated with surgery, radiotherapy, chemical treatments, or a combination of these approaches. As a general rule, surgery is a poor treatment for patients with non-Hodgkin's lymphomas. This presumably reflects the fact that these are tumors of the immune system, that is, cells that frequently circulate and are usually not confined to a single location. However, certain extranodal non-Hodgkin's lymphomas do seem to be cured sometimes with surgery alone (64).

Non-Hodgkin's lymphomas are highly sensitive to radiotherapy. However, the fact that radiotherapy must be used in a localized manner limits its effectiveness in the treatment of these patients. Even so, radiotherapy remains the most active single agent in the treatment of patients with non-Hodgkin's lymphoma and is probably underutilized in present treatment regimens.

Most patients with non-Hodgkin's lymphoma are treated with drugs that are usually referred to as "chemotherapy." A wide variety of agents are active in the management of patients with non-Hodgkin's lymphomas. When these drugs are used in combination, patients with some subtypes of non-Hodgkin's lymphoma can frequently be cured.

Non-Hodgkin's lymphomas vary greatly in the pace and aggressiveness of the illnesses they cause. Some patients with indolent lymphomas might be managed expectantly. That is, they might receive no initial therapy but be followed closely and treated when symptoms develop (65). This is especially appropriate for some patients with follicular small cleaved-cell lymphoma and marginal zone lymphomas. In elderly patients, this is frequently the treatment of choice. In contrast, patients with aggressive lymphomas require immediate therapy. Patients who present with apparently localized or widely disseminated disease have differing prognoses and varying treatment options. These are considered separately below.

LOCALIZED DISEASE

When considering tumors of the immune system, an "organ" system in which cells normally travel between different sites in the body, one might expect that anatomically localized cancers would be rare. In fact, most patients with non-Hodgkin's lymphomas do have widespread disease. Very few patients should be treated only with local therapy. However, patients with apparently localized lymphomas do have a better prognosis.

The definitions used in the literature for localized lymphomas have varied considerably. For the purposes of this chapter, localized lymphomas are those with the disease confined to one or two immediately adjacent sites (i.e., usually two lymph node sites or one extranodal site and the immediate draining lymph nodes), no tumor mass greater that 10 cm, and none of the systemic symptoms of lymphoma. Most of these patients do not have elevated serum LDH or serum β_2-microglobulin levels. Of course, the designation of a localized lymphoma must come after a careful staging evaluation. Most patients with Ann Arbor stage I or stage I_E lymphoma will meet this definition, as will a few patients with stage II lymphoma. Since definitions of localized lymphoma vary considerably in the literature, one needs to be certain of the definition used in a particular study if the results are to be applied to an individual patient.

Indolent (Low-Grade) Lymphoma

Most patients with indolent non-Hodgkin's lymphoma do not meet the above definition of localized disease. In fact, only a small minority of patients with follicular small cleaved-cell lymphoma, B-cell small lymphocytic lymphoma, or mantle cell lymphoma present with localized disease. The exception to this rule are the marginal zone lymphomas (66). In particular, the tumors sometimes referred to as MALTOMAs frequently present with apparently localized extranodal disease.

As is true for other clinical situations, the management of patients with localized low-grade lymphoma is controversial. In very elderly patients with asymptomatic disease, many would recommend observation without treatment. Patients who present with gastric MALTOMAs and infection with *H. pylori* can sometimes be treated by a combination of bismuth and antibiotics aimed at eradication of the bacteria (45). The most common treatment for patients with localized low-grade lymphoma has been involved or extended-field radiotherapy (67, 68). A significant proportion of patients thus treated achieve an extended disease-free survival, and some of these patients are almost certainly cured. However, the indolent nature of these disorders and the late relapses frequently seen preclude a definitive comment about the cure rate. Whether or not such patients benefit by chemotherapy before radiotherapy or as an adjunctive treatment after radiotherapy is uncertain. However, this might be a reasonable option, particularly in young patients.

Aggressive (Intermediate- and High-Grade) Lymphoma

Approximately 15 to 20% of patients with diffuse large cell lymphoma or similar histologic subtypes present with localized disease meeting the definition presented above. Treatment options in these patients do not include observation without therapy. These tumors disseminate rapidly, and survival is brief if they are untreated. However, a variety of treatments have been used.

An occasional elderly patient might be managed by surgical excision and close observation. However, most very elderly patients are treated with involved-field or extended-field radiotherapy. The chance of cure with radiotherapy depends upon the extent of the staging evaluation before treatment. In one study in which staging evaluation included a staging laparotomy, radiotherapy was associated with a cure rate of more than 50% (69). However, few physicians today would recommend this extensive staging evaluation. Previous series have demonstrated that the cure rate of patients with apparently localized diffuse large cell lymphoma is increased when adjuvant chemotherapy follows radiation (70, 71). However, the highly effective nature of combination chemotherapy in this disorder led other investigators to administer the chemotherapy initially and then add "adjuvant' radiotherapy to the original disease site. This led to a very high cure rate (in excess of 75%) in patients with stage I and nonbulky stage II diffuse large cell lymphoma (72–74)). A high cure rate can be achieved with chemotherapy alone (72, 75), and the amount of chemotherapy can be reduced to approximately one-half the usual number of courses by the addition of adjuvant radiotherapy (73, 74). More recently, a controlled trial compared a complete course of chemotherapy with a reduced course of chemotherapy followed by adjuvant radiotherapy in high-risk patients. The initial results of this study suggest a superior treatment outcome when chemotherapy and radiotherapy are combined (76).

The opimal regimen for individual patients must take into account the particular clinical setting. For most patients, the combination of an effective combination chemotherapy regimen followed by involved-field radiotherapy would seem to be optimal. However, occasional patients might choose to avoid the substantial complications associated with radiation of certain organs (e.g., a permanently dry mouth after radiation of the salivary glands). In these patients, a "full" course of chemotherapy is possibly the best choice. In some frail elderly patients, avoiding chemotherapy may be the best choice, and radiotherapy alone used.

DISSEMINATED DISEASE

Indolent (Low-Grade) Non-Hodgkin's Lymphomas

Most patients with disseminated low-grade lymphoma cannot be cured with presently available treatment. Because this remains an unpleasant reality, many physicians recommend observation without initial treatment to patients who are asymptomatic at the time of diagnosis (65). In some patients with low-grade non-Hodgkin's lymphoma, treatment may not be needed for months or years, and a substantial proportion of patients managed in this manner will have spontaneous regressions (77). However, the decision to observe without therapy does not mean that these patients can be seen infrequently. Patients must be followed closely to identify early signs of progression that could lead to serious and avoidable complications, such as ureteral obstruction. If the patient and the physician are not committed to very close follow-up, initial treatment should be used.

Many patients with low-grade non-Hodgkin's lymphoma present with symptoms that can be improved with therapy or are unwilling to be followed without therapy. For these patients, the treatment options include radiotherapy, single-agent chemotherapy, combination chemotherapy, new agents such as interferon, or a combination of these modalities (78–89). Because a complete or good partial remission can be achieved in most patients with disseminated low-grade lymphoma and because remissions can last for extended periods, achieving a complete remission is a reasonable goal when therapy is instituted. Patients treated with more aggressive chemotherapy regimens tend to achieve remission more rapidly, but the remissions do not last longer that those achieved more slowly with single-agent chemotherapy (86–89). In several studies, patients who received α-interferon in combination with their initial chemotherapy regimen or had the drug administered adjuvantly following a chemotherapy regimen had longer remissions than those treated with chemotherapy alone. However, the impact of this treatment approach on overall survival has been controversial.

A study is currently under way comparing an intensive combination chemotherapy regimen plus radiotherapy with no initial therapy but with the same chemotherapy regimen administered at the onset of progressive systemic disease (90). After a median follow-up of 4 years, a higher proportion of intensively treated patients were continuously free of disease (51 vs. 0%), but there was no difference in overall survival (84 vs. 83%). Because of the low cure rate in patients with indolent non-Hodgkin's lymphoma, trials of even more aggressive treatments such as autologous bone marrow transplantation have been undertaken. However, sufficient follow-up is not yet available to determine whether or not this increases the proportion of patients who might be cured.

Aggressive (Intermediate- and High-Grade) Non-Hodgkin's Lymphomas

It has been known for more then 20 years that patients with disseminated aggressive non-Hodgkin's lymphoma can be cured with combination chemotherapy regimens (91, 92). Unfortunately, while some regimens appear to be inferior, no one regimen has been demonstrated to be superior to others that are similarly intensive and contain active drugs. Numerous controlled clinical trials have been undertaken to identify an optimal chemotherapy regimen (93–106). The results from one of these, comparing four popular regimens, are presented in Table 63.4 (106). Some of the most popular regimens are detailed in Table 63.5. Most studies have focused on patients with diffuse large cell lymphoma. Effective chemotherapy regimens for diffuse large cell lymphoma seem to have in common the combination of an alkylating agent, an anthracycline, a vinca alkaloid, and a glucocorticoid. The addition of other agents known to be active, such as etoposide, bleomycin, cytarabine, procarbazine, etc. requires reducing the dose of the primary agents because of the limitations imposed by toxicity. Presumably, this "tradeoff" explains the lack of increased effec-

Table 63.4. Randomized Trial Comparing Four Major Chemotherapy Regimens For Diffuse Aggressive NHL

Regimen	Event-Free Survival	Overall Survival
CHOP	41%	54%
ProMACE/CytaBOM	46%	50%
m-BACOD	46%	52%
MACOP-B	41%	50%

Data from Fisher RI, Gaynor ER, Dahlberg S, et al. Comparison of CHOP vs m-BACOD vs ProMACE-CytaBOM vs MACOP-B in patients with intermediate or high-grade non-Hodgkin's lymphoma. N Engl J Med 1993;328:1002–1006.

Table 63.5. Selected Regimens Used to Treat Aggressive Non-Hodgkin's Lymphomas

Regimen	Dose	Administered on Day(s)
CHOP[a], 3-week cycles	Cyclophosphamide 750 mg/m² i.v.	1
	Adriamycin 50 mg/m² i.v.	1
	Vincristine 1.4 mg/m² i.v.	1
	Prednisone 100 mg p.o.	1–5
ProMACE/Cyta-BOM, 4-week cycles	Cyclophosphamide 650 mg/m² i.v. push	1
	Adriamycin 25 mg/m² i.v. push	1
	Etoposide (VP-116) 120 mg/m² i.v.	1
	Prednisone 60 mg/m² p.o.	1–14
	Cytarabine 300 mg/m² i.v. push	8
	Bleomycin 5 U/m² i.v. push	8
	Vincristine 1.4 mg/m² i.v. push	8
	Methotrexate 120 mg/m² i.v. push	8
	Folinic acid 25 mg/m² p.o. every 6 hr × 6 doses	9–10
ACVB, 2-week cycles	Cyclophosphamide 2,200 mg/m² i.v.	1
	Adriamycin 75 mg/m² i.v.	1
	Vindesine 2 mg/m² i.v.	1
	Bleomycin 5 U/m² i.v.	1
	Methyl-prednisone 60 mg/m² i.v.	1–5
	Methotrexate 15 mg intrathecal	1

[a]CNOP substitutes mitoxantrone at 12 mg/m² for Adriamycin.

tiveness of regimens with larger numbers of agents.

Certain principles do apply to the management of patients with diffuse large cell lymphoma with combination-chemotherapy regimens. One is that treatment with the full planned dose seems to be important. In two studies in which patients with certain adverse characteristics such as advanced age or previous extensive radiotherapy initially received reduced doses, the response rate was reduced, but treatment-related toxicity was not (107,108). In addition, increasing experience with a treatment regimen seems to be associated with reduced treatment-related mortality. For example, the treatment-related mortality in initial and subsequent groups of patients treated at the National Cancer Institute with a combination of Adriamycin, cyclophosphamide, etoposide, mechlorethamine, vincristine, procarbazine, and prednisone decreased from 13 to 8% (109), and in those treated with a combination of prednisone, Adriamycin, cyclophosphamide, etoposide, cytarabine, bleomycin, vincristine, and methotrexate, it decreased from 8 to 3% (110). In a similar experience at the University of Nebraska, we noted a reduction in the mortality rate from 9 to 4% in patients treated with cyclophosphamide, Adriamycin, bleomycin, procarbazine, vincristine, and prednisone

with increasing experience in the use of the regimen (111).

With currently available treatment programs, complete remissions can be achieved in 60 to 80% of adults with diffuse aggressive non-Hodgkin's lymphoma who have bulky stage II disease, stage III disease, and stage IV disease. Long-term disease-free survival is seen with no further treatment in 50 to 65% of the complete responders. Patients with aggressive non-Hodgkin's lymphoma seem to have higher response rates with increasing doses of chemotherapy regimens. However, toxicity limits the increase in doses. The intensity of treatment can be increased by the use of hematopoietic growth factors to allow an increased dose and/or shortened treatment interval and by the use of very high doses of chemotherapy, with or without total body radiotherapy, followed by autologous bone marrow or peripheral stem cell transplantation. Several pilot studies demonstrated a higher than expected cure rate in young patients with aggressive non-Hodgkin lymphomas and poor prognostic markers who were treated with the latter approach (112, 113). Recently, clinical trials have been undertaken using autologous bone marrow transplantation in the initial treatment of patients who did not respond rapidly to their initial chemotherapy regimen and as an adjuvant after achieving a complete remission. Initial results in patients in whom combination chemotherapy was combined with early bone marrow transplantation demonstrated a disease-free survival superior to that of patients treated with MACOP-B (114). However, overall survival was not increased. In another large study, patients who achieved a complete remission after an effective combination chemotherapy regimen (ACVBP, see Table 63.5 for drugs) were randomly allocated to a consolidative chemotherapy regimen or autologous bone marrow transplantation (115). Long follow-up has shown that patients with poor prognostic markers had a superior disease-free survival with adjuvant bone marrow transplantation. However, the use of bone marrow transplantation early in the treatment of these patients should be approached cautiously, because even in groups with a poor prognosis, some patients can be cured with standard chemotherapy regimens.

RELAPSED AND REFRACTORY DISEASE

The management of patients with relapsed or initially refractory non-Hodgkin's lymphoma also depends somewhat on the histologic subtype of the lymphoma. This is because of a different natural history after initial treatment failure. Patients with relapsed low-grade lymphoma often have prolonged survival after treatment failure—sometimes with minimal treatment. These disorders also are more likely to respond to second-line treatments.

It is very likely that young and elderly patients with relapsed low-grade lymphoma will be approached differently. In young patients, cure is likely to remain a goal of therapy even though it is not often achieved. Because of this, young patients with relapsed follicular low-grade lymphomas are often offered the opportunity to pursue bone marrow transplantation. These patients need to undergo HLA typing to see if they have a potential allogeneic bone marrow donor. In the absence of an allogeneic donor, autologous transplants can be performed if peripheral blood progenitor cells or bone marrow cells uncontaminated by tumor can be obtained or produced through in vitro marrow "purging" (116–118).

The experience with bone marrow transplantation in patients with marginal zone lymphomas or small lymphocytic lymphoma is minimal. However, there are reports of long-term survival

in patients undergoing allogeneic transplantation (119). Considerably more data are available for patients with low-grade follicular lymphomas undergoing bone marrow transplantation. Many patients have been treated, and disease-free survival for 5 years is an attainable treatment goal in a significant minority of patients who are transplanted after first relapse (116–118).

The only controlled data available for transplantation are from a study at St. Bartholomew's Hospital (116). The investigators compared the results of autologous bone marrow transplantation using purged marrow in patients in first relapse with the results of further chemotherapy at standard doses in historic controls. The authors found a significantly extended disease-free survival (but not overall survival) in the transplanted patients.

Patients selected for transplantation usually need to receive standard chemotherapy to achieve a complete or partial remission before the procedure. Patients with follicular lymphomas can often be treated with single-agent oral chemotherapy such as chlorambucil or cyclophosphamide or with a CHOP-like regimen. In patients who are refractory to these approaches, a cisplatin-based regime such as DHAP is often used (120). While similar regimens can also be used for patients with small lymphocytic and marginal zone lymphomas, fludarabine, alone or in combination, is more often used.

For older patients with low-grade lymphomas for whom transplantation is not considered to be an option, a very conservative approach is usually appropriate. If the patient is asymptomatic after a relapse, observation without treatment might be the best way to proceed. When patients are symptomatic because of local disease, involved-field radiotherapy might be the least morbid approach to resolving the problem. However, most of these patients will eventually require further treatment with chemotherapy. Once again, the simplest regimen given for the shortest period of time to achieve the goal of alleviating symptoms is generally the best approach. In these patients, in whom cure is not a realistic consideration, avoiding serious treatment complications seems paramount.

Patients with relapsed aggressive (i.e., intermediate- or high-grade) lymphomas have a much more serious outlook. These patients usually have a very short survival without successful intervention. Further treatment with standard chemotherapy does not usually succeed in producing long-term disease-free survival in these patients. Results for large numbers of patients have been reported in the literature, but the cure rate for second-line therapy is certainly less than 10% and probably less than 5% (120–122). However, patients often have an objective response to treatment (on the order of 50%).

Bone marrow transplantation produces long-term disease-free survival in a significant proportion of patients who are less than 60 to 70 years of age and sufficiently healthy (123–125). Transplant-related mortality has fallen from a previous 20–40% to less than 10% in experienced centers. Once again, patients usually undergo chemotherapy administered at standard doses in preparation for the transplant. In general, long-term disease-free survival can be achieved in 30 to 40% of patients who remain responsive to chemotherapy ("sensitive" relapse), while patients with chemotherapy-resistant disease (resistant relapse) are cured only 10% of the time (123).

The results of transplantation have been confirmed in a randomized trial. Patients were randomized in an international study to receive autologous bone marrow transplantation with a high-dose regimen incorporating carmustine, etoposide, cytarabine, and cyclophosphamide or continuing chemotherapy with DHAP (124). Only patients with sensitive relapse were included. Both disease-free survival and overall survival were superior in the patients undergoing transplantation (Table 63.6). It is also important to note that patients who underwent transplantation after failing DHAP did not fair well.

Patients with aggressive non-Hodgkin's lymphoma often do badly no matter what sort of salvage chemotherapy they receive for relapse. In these patients, there is a time when it is wise to accept the fact that the patient is not likely to be cured and attempt to minimize the morbidity of further treatments. For example, local radiotherapy might be less morbid than a new combination-chemotherapy regimen in a patient who has local symptoms. It is also worthwhile to remember that drugs such as naproxen or indomethacin can sometimes alleviate systemic symptoms such as fever with minimal morbidity.

SPECIAL SITUATIONS

Lymphoma in Childhood

Non-Hodgkin's lymphomas that occur in childhood are almost always histologically aggressive. Follicular lymphomas and other indolent non-Hodgkin lymphomas occur rarely. The histologic subtypes that are diagnosed most frequently are lymphoblastic lymphoma, small non-cleaved-cell lymphoma, and diffuse large cell lymphoma (127–129). Because these tumors tend to rapidly disseminate to the central nervous system (CNS) and bone marrow, evaluation and the initiation of treatment are generally undertaken expeditiously. While the international index can be applied to children with non-Hodgkin's lymphoma, different staging systems are often used (128).

In general, the cure rate for non-Hodgkin's lymphoma in children is higher than that in adults. This is not because children present more frequently with favorable clinical situations, but it is true, stage for stage and histologic subtype for histologic subtype. The explanation for this superior treatment outcome has been elusive and controversial. One explanation might be that children tolerate treatment better than adults and thus receive more intensive therapy. In fact, the typical regimens used in childhood do have a higher dose intensity. This might suggest the use of similar intensive regimens in young adults; this approach has been tested and is promising (130).

Another explanation for the superior outcome in children might be that non-Hodgkin's lymphomas in children are intrinsically different and more sensitive to chemotherapy. However, there is little evidence to support this. Non-Hodgkin's lymphomas that occur in children are different from similar subtypes in adults in their high propensity to disseminate to the CNS. For this reason, children generally receive CNS prophylaxis. This can be achieved with intrathecal chemotherapy alone, thereby avoiding the long-term complications of whole brain radiotherapy.

In adults, the treatment of localized lymphoma seems to be superior when radiotherapy is combined with chemotherapy (76). The same does not appear to be true in children. Randomized trials have demonstrated at least equal results with chemotherapy alone (131). This has

Table 63.6. The PARMA Study

Regimen	No. of Patients	Event-Free Survival	Overall Survival
ABMT	55	46%	53%
		$p = .001$	$p = .04$
DHAP	54	12%	32%

important implications for avoiding the long-term toxicity of radiotherapy in children.

Lymphoma in the Elderly

Elderly patients with non-Hodgkin's lymphoma are less likely to survive the disease than younger patients with similar histologic subtypes and stages (52). In almost all situations in which it has been examined, age is an important prognostic factor in non-Hodgkin's lymphoma. Whether this difference is related to more aggressive disease in elderly patients, a poorer tolerance of therapy, less intensive therapy being administered to elderly patients, an excess mortality from intercurrent illnesses, or a combination of these factors remains uncertain. However, when reasonably fit elderly patients are treated with a potentially curative combination-chemotherapy regimen, and intercurrent deaths are excluded, there does not seem to be a major difference in survival from that seen in young adults (80).

The treatment of elderly patients frequently presents a complicated problem to physicians. This is a situation in which effective communication between the patient, family, and physician is vital. Many elderly patients might not choose to undergo the rigors of intensive combination chemotherapy. This is particularly likely to be true in the very elderly and in patients with pre-existing serious illnesses. However, other elderly patients very much want to be cured and willingly accept the possibility of serious treatment-related complications. There is no one approach that can be adopted for all patients. One guiding principle should be that elderly patients must not be excluded from potentially curative therapy simply because of their age. In general, a CHOP-like chemotherapy regimen is preferable. However, a number of recent investigators have studied regimens adopted specifically for the management of the elderly (133, 134).

Most of the preceding comments apply best to the most common non-Hodgkin's lymphoma that occurs in elderly patients—diffuse large cell lymphoma. When elderly patients develop indolent non-Hodgkin's lymphoma such as follicular small cleaved-cell lymphoma, the treatment decision is often easier. Asymptomatic patients can frequently be followed expectantly. When therapy is required, it might be accomplished with involved-field radiotherapy to alleviate symptoms or "simple" chemotherapy such as oral chlorambucil.

Lymphoma in Patients with HIV Infection

As noted above, non-Hodgkin's lymphoma occurs with increased frequency in patients infected by HIV (11–15). The great majority of these lymphomas are of B-cell immunophenotype, and generally they are diffuse small noncleaved-cell lymphoma or diffuse large cell lymphoma. These patients can be divided into two groups. One group is represented by patients with known HIV infection and preceding opportunistic infections. These patients often develop non-Hodgkin's lymphomas in unusual extranodal sites. Intensive therapy in these patients is generally unrewarding, and treatment should be palliative in an attempt to avoid serious complications.

The other group of patients with HIV infection who develop non-Hodgkin's lymphoma contains those who are classified as having AIDS only because of the existence of the lymphoma. That is, they present with a lymphoma, are subsequently found to have HIV infection, but have had no opportunistic infections. The treatment in these patients should have an initial goal of curing the lymphoma. They should be treated with chemotherapy regimens that are capable of curing aggressive non-Hodgkin's lymphoma. However, there has been some debate about the optimal intensity (135–137). During the course of therapy, many of these patients will develop opportunistic infections. At this point, it is generally wise to become less aggressive, with a treatment approach aimed at avoiding treatment-related mortality.

Central Nervous System Lymphoma

Primary CNS lymphoma is increasing in incidence (138, 139). This is not just because of the frequent occurrence of lymphomas at this site in patients with HIV infection; it is also being seen increasingly in patients who are not immunocompromised. These tumors are usually B-cell non-Hodgkin's lymphoma and would be classified as diffuse large cell lymphoma.

The management of patients with primary CNS lymphoma is unsatisfactory (140). Cure remains unusual. At the present time, most patients are treated with a combination of radiation therapy to the brain and systemic chemotherapy. While regimens are sometimes chosen to include drugs that easily cross into the CNS, such as methotrexate and carmustine, it is unclear that any particular regimen produces better results. However, despite the long-term poor outlook, these patients almost always respond to therapy and frequently can achieve remission.

Lymphoblastic and Small Non-Cleaved-Cell Lymphoma in Adults

These lymphomas occur infrequently in adults (35). When they are diagnosed, prompt therapy with intensive regimens seems important. While the regimens for lymphoblastic lymphoma (141, 142) and small non-cleaved-cell lymphoma (143) vary, they share the use of CNS prophylaxis. Patients presenting with bone marrow involvement, CNS involvement, or a high serum LDH level have a poor outlook. Many oncologists would suggest bone marrow transplantation for the latter group in first remission, especially with lymphoblastic lymphoma (144, 145).

References

1. Wingo PA, Tong T, Bolden S. Cancer statistics, 1995. CA: Cancer J Clin 1995;45:8–30.
2. Devesa SS, Silverman DT, et al. Cancer incidence and mortality trends among sites in the United States, 1947–84. J Natl Cancer Inst 1987;79:701–745.
3. Leukemia Research Fund. Leukemia and Lymphoma: an atlas of distribution within areas of England and Wales 1984–1988. London: Leukemia Research Fund, 1990.
4. Devesa SS, Fears T. Non-Hodgkin's lymphoma time trends: United States and international data. Cancer Res 1992;52:5465s–5467s.
5. Boring CC, Squires TS, et al. Cancer statistics, 1991. CA: Cancer J Clin 1991;41:19–36.
6. Pearce N, Bethwaite P. Increasing incidence of non-Hodgkin's lymphoma: occupational and environmental factors. Cancer Res 1992;52:5496s–5500s.
7. Pearce NE, Smith AH, et al. Malignant lymphoma and multiple myeloma linked with agricultural occupations in New Zealand Cancer Registry based study. Am J Epidemiol 1985;121;225–237.
8. Pearce NE, Reif JS. Epidemiologic studies of cancer in agricultural workers. Am J Ind Med 1990;18:133–148.
9. Zahm SH, Blair A. Pesticides and non-Hodgkin's lymphoma. Cancer Res 1992;52:5485s–5989s.
10. Cantor KP, Blair A, et al. Hair dye use and risk of leukemia and lymphoma. Am J Public Health 1988;78:570–571.
11. Ross RK, Dwosky RL, et al. Non-Hodgkin's lymphomas in never married men in Los Angeles. Br J Cancer 1985;52:785–789.
12. Centers for Disease Control. Revision of the case definition of acquired immunodeficiency syndrome for national reporting—United States. Ann Intern Med 1985;103:402–403.
13. Levine AM, Shibata D, et al. Epidemiological and biological study of acquired immunodeficiency syndrome-related lymphoma in the county of Los An-

geles: preliminary results. Cancer Res 1992;52:5482s–5484s.
14. Levine AM. Lymphoma in acquired immunodeficiency syndrome. Semin Oncol 1990;17:104–112.
15. Karp JE, Broder S. Acquired immunodeficiency syndrome and non-Hodgkin's lymphomas. Cancer Res 1991;51:4743–4756.
16. Uchiyama T, Yodoi J, Sagawa, et al. Adult T-cell leukemia: clinical and hematologic features of 16 cases. Blood 1977;50:481–493.
17. Yoshida M, Miyoshi I, Hinuma Y. Isolation and characterization of retrovirus from cell lines of human adult T-cell leukemia and its implications in the disease. Proc Natl Acad Sci USA 1982;79:2031–2035.
18. Popovic M, Reitz MS, Sarngadharan MG, et al. The virus of Japanese adult T-cell leukemia is a member of the human T-cell leukemia virus group. Nature 1982;300:63–66.
19. Yoshida M, Seiki M, Yamagushi K, et al. Monoclonal integration of human T-cell leukemia provirus in all primary tumors of adult T-cell leukemia suggests causative role of human T-cell leukemia virus in the disease. Proc Natl Acad Sci USA 1984;81:2534–2537.
20. Blattner WA, Blayney DW, Robert-Guroff M, et al. Epidemiology of human T-cell leukemia/lymphoma virus. J Infect Dis 1983;147:406–416.
21. Broder S. Moderator T-cell lymphoproliferative syndrome associated with human T-cell leukemia/lymphoma virus. Ann Intern Med 1984;100:543–557.
22. Filipovich AH, Mathur A, et al. Primary immunodeficiencies: genetic risk factors for lymphoma. Cancer Res 1992;52:5465s–5468s.
23. Epstein MA, Achong BT, et al. Virus particles in cultured lymphoblasts from Burkitt's lymphoma. Lancet 1964;1:702–703.
24. Hoover RN. Lymphoma risks in populations with altered immunity. A search for mechanism. Cancer Res 1992;52:5477s–5479s.
25. Kinlen LJ. Incidence of cancer in rheumatoid arthritis and other disorders after immunosuppressive treatment. Am J Med Suppl 1A 1985;78:44–49.
26. Tucker MA, Coleman CN, Cox RS, et al. Risk of second cancers after treatment for Hodgkin's disease. N Engl J Med 1988;318:76–81.
27. Kinlen LJ. Immunosuppressive therapy and cancer. Cancer Surv 1982;1:565–583.
28. Filipovich AH, Mathur A, Kamat D, Shapiro RS. Primary immunodeficiencies: genetic risk factors for lymphoma. Cancer Res 1992;52(19 Suppl):5465s–5467s.
29. Purtillo DT, Grierson HL. Methods of detection of new families with X-linked lymphoproliferative disease. Cancer Genet Cytogenet 1991;51:143–153.
30. Jones SE, Butler JJ, Byrne GE, et al. Histopathologic review of lymphoma cases from Southwest Oncology Group. Cancer 1977;39:1071–1077.
31. Velez-Garcia E, Durant J, Gams R, et al. Results of a uniform histopathologic review system of lymphoma cases: a ten-year study from the Southeastern Cancer Study Group. Cancer 1983;52:675–680.
32. Rappaport H, Winter WJ, Hicks EB. Follicular lymphoma: a re-evaluating of its position in the scheme of a malignant lymphoma, based on a survey of 253 cases. Cancer 1956;9:792–821.
33. Lukes RJ, Collins RD. Immunologic characterization of human malignant lymphomas. Cancer 1974;34:1488–1503.

34. Lennert K, Mohri N, Stein H, Kaiserling E. The histopathology of malignant lymphoma. Br J Haematol 1975;31(Suppl):193–203.

35. The Non-Hodgkin's Lymphoma Pathologic Classification Project. National Cancer Institute sponsored study of classifications of non-Hodgkin's lymphomas: summary and description of a working formulation for clinical usage. Cancer 1981;49:2112–2135.

36. Weisenburger DD, Nathwani BN, Diamond LW, Winberg CD, Rappaport H. Malignant lymphoma, intermediate lymphocytic type: a clinicopathologic study of 42 cases. Cancer 1981;48:1415–1425.

37. Jaffe ES, Bookman MA, Longo DL. Lymphocytic lymphoma of intermediate differentiation—mantle zone lymphoma: a distinct subtype of B-cell lymphoma. Hum Pathol 1987;18:877–880.

38. Weisenburger DD, Sanger WG, Armitage JO, Purtillo DT. Intermediate lymphocytic lymphoma: immunophenotypic and cytogenetic findings. Blood 1987; 69:1617–1621.

39. Zucca E, Stein, Coiffer B. European Task Force (ELTF): report of the workshop on mantle cell lymphoma. Ann Oncol 1994;5:507–511.

40. Sheibani K, Sohn CC, Burke JS, Winberg CD, Wu AM, Rappaport H. Monocytoid B-cell lymphoma: a novel B-cell neoplasm. Am J Pathol 1986;124:310–318.

41. Ngan BY, Warnke RA, Wilson M, Takagi K, Cleary ML, Dorfman RF. Monocytoid B-cell lymphoma: a study of 36 cases. Hum Pathol 1991;22:409–421.

42. Matutes E, Catovsky D. Clinical and laboratory features of splenic lymphoma with villous lymphocytes. Haematol Oncol 1995;4:135–150.

43. Isaacson P, Wright DH. Malignant lymphoma of mucosa associated lymphoid tissue. Cancer 1983; 532:2515–2524.

44. Isaacson PF. Lymphomas of mucosa-associated lymphoid tissue (MALT). Histopathology 1990;16:617–619.

45. Roggero E, Zucca E, Pinotti G, Pascarella A, Capella C, et al. Eradication of *Helicobacter pylori* infection in primary low-grade gastric lymphoma of mucosa-associated lymphoid tissue. Ann Intern Med 1995; 122:767–769.

46. Stein H, Mason DY, Gerdes T, et al. The expression of the Hodgkin's disease associated antigen Ki-1 in reactive and neoplastic lymphoid tissue: evidence that Reed cells and histiocytic malignancies are derived from activated lymphoid cells. Blood 1985; 66:848–859.

47. Greer JP, Kinney MC, Collins RD, et al. Clinical features of 31 patients with Ki-1 anaplastic large-cell lymphoma. J Clin Oncol 1991;9:539–547.

48. Harris N, Jaffe E, Stein H, Banks P, Chan J, et al. A revised European-American classification of lymphoid neoplasms: a proposal from the International Lymphoma Study Group. Blood 1994;84:1361–1392.

49. Zech L, Harglund V, Nilsson K, et al. Characteristic chromosomal abnormalities in biopsies and lymphoid cell lines from patients with Burkitt's and non Burkitt's lymphoma. Int J Cancer 1976;17:47–56.

50. Rowley JD. Chromosome studies in non-Hodgkin's lymphomas. The role of the t(14;18) translocation. J Clin Oncol 1988;919–925.

51. Carbone PP, Kaplan HS, Musshoff K, Smitehres DW, Tubiana M. Report of the Committee on Hodgkin's Disease Staging Classification. Cancer Res 1971; 31:1860–1861.

52. Shipp M. Harrington D, Anderson J, et al. Development of a predictive model for aggressive lymphoma: the international NHL prognostic factors project. N Engl J Med 1993;329:997–1002.

53. Coiffier B, Bastion Y, Berger F, et al. Prognostic factors in follicular lymphomas. Semin Oncol 1993; 20:89–95.

54. Kwak LW, Wilson M, Weiss LM, et al. Similar outcome of treatment of B-cell and T-cell diffuse large-cell lymphomas: the Stanford experience. J Clin Oncol 1991;9:1426–1431.

55. Lippman SM, Miller TP, Spier CM, Slymen DJ, Grogan TM. The prognostic significance of the immunotype in diffuse large-cell lymphoma: a comparative study of the T-cell and B-cell phenotype. Blood 1988;72:436–441.

56. Coiffer B, Brouse N, Peuchmaur M, et al. Peripheral T-cell lymphomas have a worse prognosis than B-cell lymphomas: a prospective study of 361 immunophenotyped patients treated with the LNH-84 regimen. Ann Oncol 1990;1:45–50.

57. Miller TP, Lippman SM, Spier CM, Slymen DJ, Grogan TM. HLA-DR (Ia) immune phenotype predicts outcome for patients with diffuse large cell lymphoma. J Clin Invest 1988;82:370–372.

58. Swan F, Huh Y, Katz R, Cabanillas F, Rodriguez M, Epstein J. Beta-2-microglobulin (B2M) and HLA-DR cellular expression in relapsing large cell lymphomas (LCL): relationship to survival and serum B2M levels (abstract). Blood 1990;76(Suppl):375a.

59. Cleary ML, Sklar J. Nucleotide sequence of a t(14;18) breakpoint cluster in follicular lymphoma and demonstration of a breakpoint cluster near a transcriptionally active locus on chromosome 18. Proc Natl Acad Sci USA 1985;82:7439–7443.

60. Bauer KD, Merkel DE, Winter JN, et al. Prognostic implications of ploidy and proliferative activity in diffuse large cell lymphomas. Cancer Res 1986; 46:3173–3178.

61. Grogan TM, Lippman SM, Spier CM, et al. Independent prognostic significance of nuclear proliferation antigen in diffuse large cell lymphomas as determined by the monoclonal antibody Ki-67. Blood 1988; 71:1157–1160.

62. Woolridge TN, Grierson HL, Weisenburger DD, et al. Association of DNA content and proliferative activity with clinical outcome in patients with diffuse mixed cell and large cell non-Hodgkin's lymphoma. Cancer Res 1988;48:6608–6613.

63. Miller TP, Grogan TM, Dalton WS, Spier CM, Scheper FJ, Salmon SE. P-glycoprotein expression in malignant lymphoma and reversal of clinical drug resistance with chemotherapy plus high-dose verapamil. J Clin Oncol 1991;9:17–24.

64. Brooks JJ, Enterline HT. Primary gastric lymphomas: a clinicopathologic study of 58 cases with long-term follow-up and literature review. Cancer 1981;51:701–711.

65. Portlock CS, Rosenberg SA. No initial therapy for stage I and IV non-Hodgkin's lymphomas of favorable histological types. Ann Intern Med 1979;90:10–13.

66. Berger F, Felman P, Sonet A, Salles G, Bastion Y, et al. Nonfollicular small B-cell lymphomas: a het-

erogeneous group of patients with distinct clinical features and outcome. Blood 1994;83:2829–2835.

67. Richards MA, Gregory WM, Hall PA, et al. Management of localized non-Hodgkin's lymphoma: the experience at St. Bartholomew's Hospital 1972–1985. Haematol Oncol 1989;7:1–19.

68. Paryani SB, Hoppe RT, Cox RS, et al. Analysis of non-Hodgkin's lymphomas with nodular and favorable histologies, stages I and II. Cancer 1983;52:2300–2308.

69. Sweet DL, Kinzie J, Gaeke ME, Golomb HM, Ferguson DL, Ultmann JE. Survival of patients with localized diffuse histiocytic lymphoma. Blood 1981;58:1218–1223.

70. Carde P, Burgers JMV, van Glabbeke M, et al. Combination radiotherapy-chemotherapy for early stages non-Hodgkin's lymphoma: the 1975–1980 EORTC controlled lymphoma trial. Radiother Oncol 1984;2:301–312.

71. Nissen NI, Ersboll J, Hansen HS, et al. A randomized study of radiotherapy versus radiotherapy plus chemotherapy in stage I-II non-Hodgkin's lymphomas. Cancer 1983;52:1–7.

72. Connors JM, Klimo P, Fairey RN, Voss N. Brief chemotherapy and involved field radiation therapy for limited-stage, histologically aggressive lymphoma. Ann Intern Med 1987;107:25–30.

73. Jones SE, Miller TM, Connors JM. Long-term follow-up and analysis for prognostic factors for patients with limited-stage diffuse large-cell lymphoma treated with initial chemotherapy with or without adjuvant radiotherapy. J Clin Oncol 1989;7:1186–1191.

74. Longo DL, Glatstein E, Duffey PI, et al. Treatment of localized aggressive lymphomas with combination chemotherapy followed by involved-field radiation therapy. J Clin Oncol 1989;7:1295–1302.

75. Cabanillas F. Chemotherapy as definitive treatment of stage I-II large cell diffuse mixed lymphomas. Hematol Oncol 1985;3:25–31.

76. Glick J, Kim K, Earle J, O'Connell M. An ECOG randomized phase III trial of CHOP vs. CHOP + radiotherapy (XRT) for intermediate grade early stage non-Hodgkin's lymphoma (NHL) (abstract). Proc Am Soc Clin Oncol 1995;14:391

77. Krikorian JG, Portlock CS, Cooney P, Rosenberg SA. Spontaneous regression of non-Hodgkin's lymphoma: a report of nine cases. Cancer 1980;46:2093–2100.

78. Lister TA, Cullen MH, Beard MEJ, et al. Comparison of combined and single agent chemotherapy in non-Hodgkin's lymphoma of favorable histological sub-type. Br Med J 1978;1:533–538.

79. Kennedy BJ, Bloomfield CD, Kiang DT, et al. Combination versus successive single agent chemotherapy in lymphocytic lymphoma. Cancer 1978;41:23–29.

80. Hoppe RT, Kushlan P, Kaplan HS, et al. The treatment of advanced stage favorable histology non-Hodgkin's lymphoma: a preliminary report of a randomized trial comparing single agent chemotherapy, combination chemotherapy and whole body irradiation. Blood 1981;58:592–599.

81. Steward WP, Crowther D, McWilliam LJ, et al. Maintenance chlorambucil after CVP in the management of advanced stage, low grade histologic type non-Hodgkin's lymphoma. Cancer 1988;61:441–448.

82. Cabanillas F, Smith T, Bodey CP, et al. Nodular malignant lymphomas: factors affecting complete response and survival. Cancer 1979;44:1983–1990.

83. Dana BW, Dahlberg S, Bharat N, et al. Long term follow up of patients with low-grade lymphomas treated with doxorubicin-based chemotherapy or chemo-immunotherapy. J Clin Oncol 1993;11:644–651.

84. O'Connell MJ, Colgan JP, Oken MM, et al. Clinical trial of recombinant leukocyte A interferon as initial therapy for favorable histology non-Hodgkin's lymphomas and chronic lymphocytic leukaemia. J Clin Oncol 1986;4:128–136.

85. Foon KA, Roth MS, Bunn PA. Interferon therapy of non-Hodgkin's lymphoma. Cancer 1987;59:601–604.

86. Solal-Celigngy P, Lepage E, Brousse N, et al. Recombinant interferon alfa-2b combined with a regimen containing doxorubicin in patients with advanced follicular lymphoma. N Engl J Med 1993;329:1608–1614.

87. Price CGA, Pohatiner AZS, Steward W, et al. Interferon-alpha 2b in the treatment of follicular lymphoma: preliminary results of a trial in progress. Ann Oncol 1991;2:141–145.

88. Smalley RV, Andersen JW, Hawkins MJ, et al. Interferon alpha combined with cytotoxic chemotherapy for patients with non-Hodgkin's lymphoma. N Engl J Med 1992;327:1336–1341.

89. Andersen JW, Smalley RV. Interferon alfa plus chemotherapy for non-Hodgkin's lymphoma: five-year follow-up. N Engl J Med 1992;329:1821–1827.

90. Young RC, Longo DL, Glastein E, Ihde DC, Jaffe ES, DeVita VT Jr. The treatment of indolent lymphomas: watchful waiting vs aggressive combined modality treatment. Semin Hematol 1988;25(Suppl 2):11–16.

91. Levitt M, Marsh JC, DeConti R, et al. Combination sequential chemotherapy in advanced reticulum cell sarcoma. Cancer 1972;29:630–636.

92. DeVita VT Jr, Canellos GP, Chabner B, Schein P, Hubbard SP, Young RC. Advanced diffuse histiocytic lymphoma, a potentially curable disease. Lancet 1975;1:248–250.

93. Dupont J, Pavlovsky S, Woolley P, et al. A comparison of two chemotherapy regimens, C-MOPP and BACOP, for the treatment of diffuse mixed (DML) and histiocytic (DHL) lymphomas (abstract). Proc Am Soc Clin Oncol 1983;2:215.

94. O'Connell M, Anderson J, Earls J, Johnson G, Harrington D, Glick J. Combined modality therapy of advanced unfavorable non-Hodgkin's lymphoma (NHL): an ECOG randomized clinical trial (abstract). Proc Am Soc Clin Oncol 1984;3:241.

95. Hagberg H, Bjorkholm M, Glimelius B, Lindemalm CH, Mellstedt H, Killander A. CHOP vs MEV for the treatment of non-Hodgkin's lymphoma of favorable histopathology: a randomized clinical trial. Eur J Cancer Clin Oncol 1985;21:175–179.

96. Gordon LI, Harrington D, Andersen J, et al. Comparison of a second-generation combination chemotherapeutic regimen (m-BACOD) with a standard regimen (CHOP) for advanced diffuse non-Hodgkin's lymphoma. N Engl J Med 1992;327:1342–1349.

97. Cooper JA, Ding JC, Matthews JP, et al. A randomized comparison of MACOP-B and CHOP in in-

termediate grade non-Hodgkin's lymphoma (abstract). Proc Am Soc Clin Oncol 1991;10:271.

98. Garcia-Conde J, Vinolas N, Estape J. ProMACE-CytaBOM vs CHOP in the treatment of unfavorable lymphomas: a randomized trial (abstract). Blood 1991; 78(Suppl):127a.

99. Tura S, Zinzani PL, Mazza P, et al. F-MACHOP versus MACOP-B in the treatment of high grade malignant non-Hodgkin's lymphomas (abstract). Blood 1991;78(Suppl):109a.

100. Longo DL, DeVita VT Jr, Duffey PL, et al. Superiority of ProMACE-cytaBOM over ProMACE-MOPP in the treatment of advanced diffuse aggressive lymphoma: results of a prospective randomized trial. J Clin Oncol 1991;9:25. Erratum, J Clin Oncol 1991;9:25–38.

101. Gherlinzoni F, Guglielmi C, Mazza P, Amadori S, Mandelli F, Tura S. Phase III comparative trial (m-BACOD vs m-BNCOD) in the treatment of stage II to IV non-Hodgkin's lymphomas with intermediate- or high-grade histology. Semin Oncol 1990;17(Suppl 10):3–9.

102. Federico M, Moretti G, Gobbi PG, et al. Pro-MACE-cytaBOM versus MACOP-B in intermediate and high grade NHL: preliminary results of a prospective randomized trial. Leukemia 1991;5(Suppl 1):95–101.

103. Chisesi T, Santini G, Capnist G, et al. Pro-MACE-MOPP vs MACOP-B in high grade non-Hodgkin's lymphomas: a randomized study in a multicenter cooperative study group (NHLCSG). Leukemia 1991; 5(Suppl 1):107–111.

104. Koppler H, Pfluger KH, Eschenbach I, et al. Sequential versus alternating chemotherapy for high grade non-Hodgkin's lymphomas: a randomized multicenter trial. Hematol Oncol 1991;9:217–223.

105. Carde P, Meerwaldt JH, vanGlabbeke M, et al. Superiority of second over first generation chemotherapy in a randomized trial for stage III-IV intermediate and high-grade non-Hodgkin's lymphoma (NHL): the 1980–1985 EORTC trial. Ann Oncol 1991;2:431–435.

106. Fisher RI, Gaynor ER, Dahlberg S, et al. Comparison of CHOP vs m-BACOD vs ProMACE-CytaBOM vs MACOP-B in patients with intermediate or high-grade non-Hodgkin's lymphoma. N Engl J Med 1993;328:1002–1006.

107. Dixon DO, Neilan B, Jones SE, et al. Effect of age on therapeutic outcome in advanced diffuse histiocytic lymphoma: the Southwest Oncology Group experience. J Clin Oncol 1986;4:295–305.

108. Dana BW, Dahlberg S, Miller TP, et al. m-BACOD treatment for intermediate- and high-grade malignant lymphomas: a Southwest Oncology Group phase II trial. J Clin Oncol 1990;8:1155–1162.

109. Fisher RI, DeVita VT Jr, Hubbard SM, et al. Diffuse aggressive lymphomas: increased survival after alternating flexible sequences of ProMACE and MOPP chemotherapy. Ann Intern Med 1983;98:304–309.

110. Browne MJ, Hubbard SM, Longo DL, et al. Excess prevalence of *Pneumocystis carinii* pneumonia in patients treated for lymphoma with combination chemotherapy. Ann Intern Med 1986;104:338–349.

111. Vose JM, Armitage JO, Weisenburger DD, et al. The importance of age in survival of patients treated with chemotherapy for aggressive non-Hodgkin's lymphoma. J Clin Oncol 1988;6:1838–1844.

112. Gulati SC, Shank B, Black P, et al. Autologous bone marrow transplantation for patients with poor-prognosis lymphoma. J Clin Oncol 1988;6:1303–1313.

113. Gianni AM, Bregni M, Siena S, et al. Prospective randomized comparison of MACOP-B vs rhGM-CSF-supported high dose sequential myeloablative chemo-radiotherapy in diffuse large cell lymphomas (abstract). Proc Am Soc Clin Oncol 1991;10:274.

114. Gianni Am, Bregni M, Siena S, et al. Prospective randomized comparison of MACOP-B vs. rhGM-CSF supported high-dose sequential myeloablative chemo-radiotherapy in diffuse large cell lymphomas (abstract). Proc Am Soc Clin Oncol 1991;10:274.

115. Haioun C, Lepage E, Gisselbrecht C, Coiffier B, Bosly A, et al. Comparison of autologous bone marrow transplantation with sequential chemotherapy for intermediate-grade and high-grade non-Hodgkin's lymphoma in first complete remission: a study of 464 patients. J Clin Oncol 1994;12:2543–2551.

116. Rohatiner AZS, Johnson PWM, Price CGA, et al. Myeloablative therapy with autologous bone marrow transplantation as consolidation therapy for recurrent follicular lymphoma. J Clin Oncol 1994; 12:1177–1184.

117. Freedman AS, Rite J, Neuberg D, et al. Autologous bone marrow transplantation in 69 patients with a history of low grade B-cell non-Hodgkin's lymphoma. Blood 1991;77:2524–2530.

118. Bierman P, Vose J, Armitage J, et al. High-dose therapy followed by autologous hematopoietic rescue for follicular low grade non-Hodgkin's lymphoma (NHL) (abstract). Proc Am Soc Clin Oncol 1992; 11:1074.

119. Michallet M, Bandini G. High-dose therapy and bone marrow transplantation in chronic lymphocytic leukemia. High-Dose Cancer Ther 1992;2:715–727.

120. Velasquez WS, Cabanillas F, Salvador P, et al. Effective salvage therapy for lymphoma with cisplatin in combination with high-dose Ara-C and dexamethasone (DHAP). Blood 1988;71:117–123.

121. Cabanillas F, Hagemeister FB, McLaughlin P, et al. Results of MIME salvage regimen for recurrent or refractory lymphoma. J Clin Oncol 1987;5:407–415.

122. Cabanillas F. Experience with salvage regimens at M. D. Anderson Hospital. Ann Oncol 1991; 2(Suppl 1):31–33.

123. Phillip T, Armitage JO, Spitzer G, et al. High-dose therapy and autologous bone marrow transplantation after failure of conventional chemotherapy in adults with intermediate-grade or high-grade non-Hodgkin's lymphoma. N Engl J Med 1987;316:1493–1498.

124. Gribben JG, Goldstone AH, Linch DC, et al. Effectiveness of high-dose combination chemotherapy and autologous bone marrow transplantation for patients with non-Hodgkin's lymphomas who are still responsive to conventional-dose therapy. J Clin Oncol 1989;7:1621–1629.

125. Weisdorf DJ, Haake R, Miller WJ, et al. Autologous bone marrow transplantation for progressive non-Hodgkin's lymphoma: clinical impact of immunophenotype and in vitro purging. Bone Marrow Transplant 1991;8:135–142.

126. Phillip T, Guglielmi C, Chauvin F, Hagenbeek A, Van Der Lely J, et al. Autologous bone marrow

transplantation (ABMT) versus (VS) conventional chemotherapy (DHAP) in relapsed non-Hodgkin lymphoma (NHL): final analysis of the PARMA randomized study (216 patients). Proc Am Soc Clin Oncol 1995; 14:390.

127. Anderson JR, Wilson JF, Jenkin DT, et al. Childhood non-Hodgkin's lymphoma: the results of a randomized therapeutic trial comparing a 4-drug regimen (COMP) with a 10-drug regimen (LSA2-L2). N Engl J Med 1983;208:559–565.

128. Murphy SB, Rairclough DL, Hutchinson RE, Berad CW. Non-Hodgkin's lymphomas of childhood: an analysis of the histology, staging, and response to treatment of 338 cases at a single institution. J Clin Oncol 1989;7:186–193.

129. Patte C, Philip T, Rodary C, et al. Improved survival rate in children with stage III and IV B-cell non-Hodgkin's lymphoma and leukemia using multiagent chemotherapy: results of a study of 114 children from the French Pediatric Oncology Society. J Clin Oncol 1986;4:1219–1226.

130. Philip T. Lymphoblastic lymphoma and Burkitt's lymphoma in Caucasian adults: please don't forget the pediatric experience. Ann Oncol 1995;6:414–416.

131. Link MP, Donaldson SS, Berard CW, Shuster JJ, Murphy SB. Results of treatment of childhood localized non-Hodgkin's lymphoma with combination chemotherapy with or without radiotherapy. N Engl J Med 1990;322:1169–1174.

132. Vose JM, Armitage JO, Weisenburger DD, et al. The importance of age in survival of patients treated with chemotherapy for aggressive non-Hodgkin's lymphoma. J Clin Oncol 1988;6:1838–1844.

133. O'Reilly SE, Klimo P, Connors JM. Low-dose ACOP-B and VABE: weekly chemotherapy for elderly patients with advanced stage diffuse large-cell lymphoma. J Clin Oncol 1991;9:741–747.

134. Tirelli U, Zagonel V, Errante D, et al. A prospective study of a new combination chemotherapy regimen in patients older than 70 years with unfavorable non-Hodgkin's lymphoma. J Clin Oncol 1992; 10:228–236.

135. Bermucez MA, Grant KM, Rodvien R, Mendes F. Non-Hodgkin's lymphoma in a population with or at risk for acquired immunodeficiency syndrome: indications for intensive chemotherapy. Am J Med 1989; 86:71–76.

136. Levine AM, Sullivan-Halley J, Pike MC, et al. Human immunodeficiency virus-related lymphoma: prognostic factors predictive of survival. Cancer 1991; 68:2466–2472.

137. Kaplan LD, Abrams DI, Feigel E, et al. AIDS-associated non-Hodgkin's lymphoma in San Francisco. JAMA 1989;261:719–724.

138. Lettendre L, Banks PM, Reese DF, et al. Primary lymphoma of the central nervous system. Cancer 1992;49:939–944.

139. Hochberg FH, Miller DL. Primary central nervous system lymphoma. J Neurosurg 1988;68:835–853.

140. Fine HA, Mayer FJ. Primary central nervous system lymphoma. Ann Intern Med 1993;119:1093–1105.

141. Coleman CN, Picozzi VJ, Cox RS, et al. Treatment of lymphoblastic lymphoma in adults. J Clin Oncol 1986;4:1628–1637.

142. Levine AM, Forman SJ, Meyer PR, et al. Successful therapy of convoluted T-lymphoblastic lymphoma in adults. Blood 1983;61:92–99.

143. Bernstein JI, Coleman N, Strickler JG, et al. Combined modality therapy for adults with small noncleaved cell lymphoma (Burkitt's and non-Burkitt's type). J Clin Oncol 1986;4:847–858.

144. Verdonck LF, Dekker AW, deGast GC, et al. Autologous bone marrow transplantation for adult poor-risk lymphoblastic lymphoma in first remission. J Clin Oncol 1992;10:644–646.

145. Satini G, Congiu AM, Coser P, et al. Autologous bone marrow transplantation for adult advanced stage lymphoblastic lymphoma in 1st CR. A study of the NHL CSG. Leukemia 1991;5(Suppl 1):42–45.

64

Chemotherapy of Acute Leukemia in Adults

Clive S. Zent and Richard A. Larson

After two decades of incremental improvements in therapy, acute leukemia is now curable in approximately 50% of good-risk patients. An improved understanding of prognostic factors has allowed risk stratification, and more appropriate management strategies have led to better outcomes for patients with both acute myeloid leukemia (AML) and acute lymphoblastic leukemia (ALL). Recent trials have tested the concepts of dose intensification and the use of multiple non-cross-resistant agents. New drug development has had relatively little clinical impact, except for the introduction of all-*trans* retinoic acid (ATRA) for acute promyelocytic leukemia (APL). The appropriate role of bone marrow transplantation (BMT) remains to be defined, but progress has been made in elucidating the graft-versus-leukemia effect of donor lymphocytes. Improved antifungal and antiviral therapies have contributed to better supportive care. The ancillary role of hematopoietic growth factors in antileukemia treatment strategies and in supportive care remains investigational. New and improved technologies currently allow the identification in some cases of residual disease after treatment as well as earlier detection of leukemia relapse, and this capability will likely translate into improved survival in the near future.

Management of acute leukemia remains complex, requiring a multidisciplinary and dedicated team approach for optimal results. Therapy remains hazardous, unpleasant, and costly. Most adult patients with acute leukemia still die from the disease. Progress in understanding the molecular biology of leukemia has not yet translated into improved management and survival. Little progress has been made in improving the

survival of poor-prognosis groups, especially the elderly, those who develop leukemia after a myelodysplastic syndrome (MDS) or prior cytotoxic exposure (therapy-related leukemia; t-AML), and those with complex or unfavorable cytogenetic features. Nevertheless, considerable progress has been made. Initial response rates are high. Most patients achieve a remission and recover normal hematopoiesis, at least transiently. The current challenge has shifted to the ultimate eradication of the disease to prevent relapse.

DIAGNOSIS, CLASSIFICATION, AND PROGNOSTIC FACTORS

Acute leukemia is a malignant neoplasm of hematopoietic tissue characterized by the clonal accumulation of immature blood cells in the bone marrow. These abnormal cells are generally arrested in the blast stage of the normal maturation pathway. Aberrations in differentiation and function of blood cells are common, and normal hematopoiesis is suppressed.

The most precise diagnosis is made by examining the morphology, cytochemistry, immunophenotype and chromosomal abnormalities of bone marrow and peripheral blood cells. Bone marrow aspiration and biopsy are the standard diagnostic procedures. Aspiration may be difficult or impossible, (i.e., a "dry tap") in patients with very high marrow cellularity ("packed marrow"). The most widely used morphologic classification scheme, developed by the French-American-British Cooperative Group, is shown in Table 64.1 (1). Subgroups of AML and ALL are distinguished according to features of lineage differentiation. Flow cytometric analysis of cell surface markers is widely available and

Table 64.1. French-American-British (FAB) Classification of AML

FAB Subtype	Morphologic and Cytochemical Features	Frequency (%)
M0	Large, agranular myeloblasts, sometimes resembling lymphoblasts of FAB subtype L2; stain negative for myeloperoxidase and Sudan black; express CD13 or CD33 antigens on cell surface.	2–3
M1	Acute myeloblastic leukemia without maturation: large, poorly differentiated myeloblasts represent 90% or more of the nonerythroid cells; at least 3% of the myeloblasts stain positive for myeloperoxidase.	20
M2	Acute myeloblastic leukemia with maturation: between 30 and 89% of the nonerythroid cells are myeloblasts having abundant cytoplasm with moderate to many granules; Auer rods are often visible.	25–30
M3	Leukemia cells usually contain heavy azurophilic granulation; nuclear size varies greatly; nuclei are often bilobed or kidney-shaped; some cells contain bundles of Auer rods; leukemia cells stain strongly positive for myeloperoxidase; there is a microgranular variant; usually HLA-DR negative.	8–15
M4	Myeloblasts comprise over 30% of the nonerythroid cells but total granulocytic precursors do not exceed 80%; monocytic cells account for >20% of the nonerythroid cells; nonspecific esterase and chloroacetate stains are often positive; Auer rods may be present.	20–25
M4Eo	Myelomonoblasts plus morphologically and cytochemically abnormal eosinophils.	5
M5	Monoblasts, promonocytes, or monocytes comprise 80% or more of the nonerythroid cells; in one subtype (M5A), 80% or more of all the monocytic cells are monoblasts; in the well-differentiated subtype (M5B), less than 80% are monoblasts; α-naphthyl acetate positivity is extinguished by NaF.	10
M6	More than 50% of the nucleated marrow cells are erythroid; erythroblasts are usually strongly PAS positive; myeloblasts represent 30% or more of the nonerythroid cells.	5
M7	Large and small megakaryoblasts with high nucleus: cytoplasm ratio; cytoplasm is pale and agranular; standard cytochemical stains not definitive; platelet peroxidase and platelet-specific antibodies often positive.	1–2

can accurately distinguish myeloid from lymphoid leukemia (and B-cell lineage from T-cell) in most cases. A clear distinction between AML and ALL is not always possible. Rarely, null, biphenotypic, or bilineal acute leukemias occur.

Cytogenetic analysis of an individual patient's leukemia cells has become an increasingly important component of diagnosis prior to treatment in both AML and ALL (2). An adequate (>2 mL) sample of bone marrow aspirate from a fresh puncture site should be submitted for cytogenetic analysis in all patients suspected of having leukemia. Metaphase cells are stained, and the chromosome number and banding pattern are determined. Specific and well-characterized, recurring chromosomal abnormalities facilitate diagnosis, confirm subtype classification, and have major prognostic value for treatment planning (Table 64.2)

Cytogenetic data have been used to map chromosomal breakpoints at a molecular level, allowing the use of probes for fluorescence in situ hybridization (FISH) and of primers for reverse transcriptase polymerase chain reaction (RT-PCR) methods for the detection of tumor cells. FISH and RT-PCR can detect molecular genetic rearrangements not visible when examining chromosomal banding by conventional methods. However, both of the former methods test only for specific, defined genetic mutations and cannot be used initially for general screening or for a comprehensive evaluation. FISH analysis is more sensitive than conventional karyotypic analysis and can be performed on both metaphase and interphase cells. The morphology of the positive cells can be determined concurrently, and the proportional involvement by leukemia of all of the hematopoietic cells can be evaluated.

RT-PCR is the most sensitive method available for detecting occult leukemia cells (about 1 in 10^5 cells). As yet, however, the method is nonquantitative, and the results do not identify the cell type involved. The clinical significance of a

Table 64.2. Cytogenetic Subsets in AML

Karyotype	Complete Remission Rate	Remission Duration	Treatment Approach
t(8;21)	High	Long	Standard induction and intensive consolidation with chemotherapy alone
inv(16)(p13q22), t(16;16), or t(15;17)	High	Intermediate to long	Standard induction with an anthracycline; intensive consolidation chemotherapy with high-dose cytarabine; all-*trans* retinoic acid (ATRA) prior to chemotherapy for t(15;17)
t(9;11)	High	Short	Standard induction; consider BMT in first remission for most t(9;11) patients
del(5q), +13, +8, inv 3, del(12p), t(9;22), or complex abnormalities	Low	Short	New induction regimens, including use of growth factors during chemotherapy or modulators of drug resistance; BMT in first CR

positive result is currently being investigated. A positive assay confirms the presence of cells with the specific genetic abnormality but does not necessarily indicate the neoplastic growth potential of these cells. For example, a positive RT-PCR assay after treatment appears to predict leukemia relapse reliably in patients with APL and a t(15;17), but not in those with AML-M2 and a t(8;21) (2–4).

Several patient factors are known to be important in determining prognosis in acute leukemia (5). Most risk factors are not independent of advances in treatment, however, nor are they predictive across all of the specific biologic subsets of leukemia.

Age is the most important independent patient variable in determining outcome. Treatment results are best in young adults and are considerably poorer in patients older than 60 years. In addition, young or middle-aged adults may benefit from the availability of BMT to rescue patients after suffering a relapse. Elderly patients have a lower response rate to remission-induction chemotherapy and increased treatment toxicity, in part because of their high incidence of comorbid disorders. The poor survival of elderly patients, however, is not fully explained by their lower tolerance for intensive treatment. The disease itself appears to have a different natural history in this group. Elderly patients with AML are more likely to have had

a myelodysplastic syndrome (MDS) and are also more likely to have unfavorable cytogenetic features. Similarly, older patients with ALL have a higher incidence of the Philadelphia (Ph) chromosome, and this subgroup has a poor outcome.

Antecedent hematologic disorders such as MDS are a major adverse prognostic factor. Acute leukemia (t-AML) following treatment with alkylating agents, topoisomerase II inhibitors, or radiotherapy for a prior cancer has been well described and has a similarly poor outcome with conventional chemotherapy programs.

GENERAL PRINCIPLES OF THERAPY

The goal of remission induction chemotherapy is the rapid restoration of normal bone marrow function. The term complete remission (CR) is reserved for patients who have full recovery of normal peripheral blood counts and bone marrow cellularity with less than 5% residual blast cells. Induction therapy aims to reduce the total body leukemia cell population from approximately 10^{12} to below the cytologically detectable level of about 10^9 cells. This is followed by postinduction or consolidation therapy, usually comprising one or more courses of chemotherapy designed at eradication of residual leukemia, allowing the possibility of cure. Multiple chemotherapy drugs in high doses are typically used to prevent the emergence of resistant sub-clones and to limit cumulative and overlapping toxicities. Lower doses of prolonged mainte-nance therapy lasting 1 to 3 years have been used with some success in ALL, but this adjunctive therapy has uncertain value in AML.

BMT using an HLA-identical sibling donor is an established treatment modality in acute leu-kemia and is indicated for suitable high-risk pa-tients in first remission or for any young or mid-dle-aged patient in first relapse or second remission (6). Allogeneic BMT (alloBMT) has two therapeutic components. Intensive myeloab-lative therapy is used to eradicate all tumor cells, if possible. In addition, T cells in the donor mar-row can produce a graft-versus-leukemia (GvL) immune response that can destroy remaining leukemia cells; this effect has been correlated with improved disease-free survival. Unfortu-nately, this beneficial immune response is closely associated with acute and chronic graft-versus-host disease (GvHD), a major cause of morbidity and mortality following alloBMT. GvHD can be reduced by T-cell depletion from the donor mar-row, but only at the cost of increased rates of graft failure and leukemia relapse. Because the risk of treatment-related mortality increases with age, most centers restrict BMT to patients less than 60 years old. The use of alloBMT is also limited in part by donor availability. A patient has a 25 to 30% chance that each sibling will be HLA identical. Using siblings mismatched at only one HLA locus results in increased GvHD but may provide equivalent survival (6).

Allogeneic transplantation using a matched unrelated donor (MUD) is an option for younger adults who lack a sibling donor. The likelihood of finding a donor in the National Bone Marrow Donor Registry is related to the ethnic back-ground of the patient compared with the vol-unteer donor pool; the overall match rate is be-tween 40 and 50%. MUD BMT often involves prolonged delays until the transplant can be per-formed (median time, about 6 months), in-creased costs, and more severe complications. Nonengraftment and severe GvHD result in in-creased early mortality.

Autologous BMT allows the use of myeloab-lative therapy in patients who lack an allogeneic marrow donor as well as in older patients (7). The appropriate role for this treatment modality is controversial. Treatment-related morbidity and mortality (<5%) are relatively low, thus al-lowing its use in older patients, but relapse rates are high, and overall outcomes are not clearly better than those in patients who receive inten-sive but nonablative therapy. The relative con-tribution to relapse of (a) tumor cell contamina-tion in the reinfused cryopreserved marrow and (b) the failure of the high-dose therapy to eradi-cate all disease in vivo has not been determined. Purging leukemia cells from the harvested he-matopoietic cells in vitro using monoclonal an-tibodies or chemotherapy agents has been at-tempted. Purging techniques considerably delay engraftment without providing a proven benefit in decreasing the incidence of disease recur-rence. Hematopoietic cells capable of reconsti-tuting bone marrow function can be harvested for autologous transplantation by direct bone marrow aspiration or by apheresis of progenitor cells from peripheral blood. The yield from pe-ripheral blood can be augmented by mobiliza-tion following chemotherapy and/or growth factors. The use of peripheral blood stem cells has not been proven to decrease the risk of re-lapse, but it does accelerate the rate of hemato-poietic reconstitution.

Strategies to limit the toxicity and cost of BMT and yet capitalize on its ability to rescue patients who relapse are still under development. If mar-row transplantation were to be reserved for pa-tients who are not cured by standard therapy, then close surveillance during remission for early detection of relapse has increased impor-tance. High-dose chemoradiotherapy and BMT are most successful when minimal amounts of leukemia are present. Unfortunately, examina-tion of blood or bone marrow cytology detects relapse only when the patient again has a large tumor burden. Multiparameter flow cytometry may allow detection of recurrent disease at an earlier stage. In patients with well-character-ized molecular abnormalities, cytogenetics or Southern blot analysis may detect tumor cells at a level of 1 to 5% involvement of bone marrow cells. FISH analysis and RT-PCR are several or-ders of magnitude more sensitive.

ACUTE MYELOID LEUKEMIA (AML)

AML usually presents with the clinical fea-tures of bone marrow failure. Patients may have infection, anemia, and/or bleeding. Rare presen-tations include granulocytic sarcoma, or skin or central nervous system (CNS) manifestations. The blood usually shows a leukocytosis with normocytic anemia and thrombocytopenia. Cir-culating myeloblasts are often present. Some-times the leukocyte count may be low; this is a common feature in APL, for example. In rare cases, patients may present with thrombocytosis.

Remission Induction Therapy

The most common remission induction regimen used for patients with AML is cytarabine given by continuous intravenous (i.v.) infusion daily for 7 days plus daunorubicin given daily for 3 days (7+3 regimen). Depending on age and patient selection, 60 to 80% of patients achieve a CR (8). The outcome in general has not been improved by the substitution of other anthracyclines, increasing the dose of cytarabine, or adding a third or fourth drug (Table 64.3).

Daunorubicin was the first anthracycline of demonstrated value against AML. It has equivalent efficacy and less toxicity than doxorubicin. Idarubicin is a more lipophilic analogue of daunorubicin, and its active first metabolite, 13-hydroxyidarubicin, has a long half-life. Animal studies demonstrated greater activity against leukemia with less cardiotoxicity than daunorubicin (9). Evidence of the superiority of idarubicin compared with daunorubicin for AML is not compelling. Randomized trials showed nearly equivalent CR rates, survival, and cardiotoxicity (8–12). Two prospective studies showed better results with idarubicin plus cytarabine than with daunorubicin plus cytarabine, but there was no reduction in cardiotoxicity. A third trial showed equivalent CR rates overall, but the CR rate and survival were significantly better for patients less than 50 years old who received idarubicin (12). These studies have been criticized because the CR rates among the patients receiving daunorubicin were lower than expected, and the anthracycline doses used were not biologically equivalent. More recent data suggest that

Table 64.3. AML Remission Induction Chemotherapy Regimens

Drugs	Dose	Comment
1. Cytarabine	100 mg/m^2 daily as a continuous infusion for 7 days	"Standard" induction regimen resulting in approximately 60% to 80% remission rate and acceptable toxicity in patients under 60 years old
+ Daunorubicin	45 mg/m^2 intravenous push on each of the first 3 days of treatment	
2. Cytarabine	3 g/m^2 twice daily for a total of 12 doses	Yields a 90% remission rate; substantial toxicity precludes postremission therapy in a high proportion of patients
+ Daunorubicin	45 mg/m^2 intravenous push for 3 days following cytarabine	
3. Cytarabine	100 mg/m^2 daily as a continuous infusion for 7 days	Has produced a greater remission rate (88 vs. 70%) than cytarabine/daunorubicin in younger patients; appears superior to daunorubicin in patients with hyperleukocytosis; overall survival not clearly superior to "standard" regimen
+ Idarubicin	13 mg/m^2 intravenous push on each of first 3 days of treatment	
4. Cytarabine	100 mg/m^2 daily as a continuous infusion for 7 days	Remission rate similar to "standard" induction regimen; remission duration significantly improved, but overall survival comparable to "standard" regimen; may prolong survival in patients less than 55 years old but at expense of increased toxicity
+ Daunorubicin	50 mg/m^2 intravenous push on each of first 3 days of treatment.	
+ Etoposide	75 mg/m^2 daily for 7 days	

idarubicin may have greater cytotoxicity than daunorubicin against leukemia cells that express the multidrug resistance (MDR) phenotype (13).

Mitoxantrone, an anthracenedione, is a synthetic anthracycline analogue. It has been useful in combination with conventional and high doses of cytarabine, both for primary treatment and in relapsed disease (14, 15). Another agent, amsacrine is currently under investigation (16, 17).

Cytarabine in conventional doses of 100 to 200 mg/m^2/day is generally given by continuous intravenous infusion for 7 to 10 days (18). High-dose cytarabine (HDAC) regimens typically use 1000 to 3000 mg/m^2 given intravenously over 1 to 3 hours every 12 hours for 8 to 12 doses. HDAC increases the CR rate to 79 to 90% but at the cost of increased toxicity (19). Treatment mortality, the rate of early relapse, and overall survival are not clearly improved (20).

Attempts have been made to improve the CR rate of induction therapy by adding potentially non-cross-resistant drugs. Etoposide has activity as a single agent in approximately 25% of patients with previously treated AML. In a randomized trial among newly diagnosed patients, the addition of etoposide at 75 mg/m^2/day for 7 days to cytarabine and daunorubicin (7+3 regimen) produced increased toxicity but also prolonged remission duration in the etoposide arm (21). There was no survival benefit. A randomized comparison between cytarabine at standard doses and high doses, both in combination with daunorubicin and etoposide, showed no improvement in the CR rate or overall survival in the HDAC arm, although disease-free survival was significantly prolonged (22).

Acute Promyelocytic Leukemia

APL (FAB M3) is a biologically distinct disease with characteristic clinical, morphologic, and cytogenetic features (23, 24). The cytoplasmic granules in the leukemic blasts contain factors with procoagulant as well as fibrinolytic activity. Disseminated intravascular coagulation at presentation or soon after the initiation of cytotoxic chemotherapy can cause pulmonary or cerebrovascular hemorrhage in up to 40% of patients and produces a high mortality rate.

All-*trans* retinoic acid (ATRA; tretinoin) was first used in the treatment of APL in China in 1986 and has proved to be a highly effective remission induction agent (23, 24). ATRA acceler-

ates the terminal differentiation of malignant promyelocytes to mature neutrophils, leading to apoptosis and CR without bone marrow hypoplasia. This effect is a unique consequence of the rearranged *PML/RAR-α* gene resulting from the chromosomal abnormality t(15;17) that defines APL. ATRA induction therapy produces CR rates of 80 to 95% in both previously untreated and relapsed patients (24–26). Most treatment failure is due to early mortality. Primary resistance is rare. The median time to CR ranges from 38 to 44 days, but it may take as long as 90 days. As yet, the drug is only available as an oral preparation. The recommended daily dose is 45 mg/m^2. Doses from 15 to 100 mg/m^2 have been evaluated, and the optimal dose has not yet been determined.

ATRA does not have the usual toxicities associated with cytotoxic chemotherapy. Intrinsic drug toxicity is generally minor. Headache is common; pseudotumor cerebri has been described, but is rare. Nasal stuffiness, dry red skin, transient elevations in the transaminase levels and bilirubin, and hypertriglyceridemia are usually not treatment limiting (24, 25). ATRA is neither immunosuppressive nor myelosuppressive. The coagulopathy of APL typically improves rapidly with initiation of treatment.

Two specific and serious complications may occur with ATRA treatment of APL (27). In 25 to 40% of patients, the "retinoic acid syndrome" develops within 2 to 21 days after initiation of treatment and is characterized by fever, peripheral edema, pulmonary infiltrates and respiratory distress, hypertension, renal and hepatic dysfunction, and serositis resulting in pleural and pericardial effusions. The syndrome is possibly due to tissue infiltration by maturing malignant promyelocytes and the systemic effects of cytokine release. Many cases are associated with hyperleukocytosis, but the retinoic acid syndrome occurs with normal leukocyte counts in a third of cases. Early recognition and aggressive management with high-dose dexamethasone therapy (10 mg i.v. every 12 hr for 6 doses) has been effective. Cessation of ATRA therapy alone does not reverse the syndrome. However, once the complication resolves, ATRA can be restarted in most cases.

Hyperleukocytosis occurs in up to 50% of patients treated with ATRA and is probably secondary to the induction of cellular maturation (24). This may result in leukostasis, but complications are uncertain, and management is controversial. The European APL 91 Group instituted full doses of induction chemotherapy using cytarabine and daunorubicin in all patients showing a rapid rise in the leukocyte count after starting ATRA therapy (70% of patients) (25). In contrast, investigators at the Memorial Sloan-Kettering Cancer Center have reported that an increased leukocyte count is not intrinsically dangerous, and thus chemotherapy is not usually indicated (27). The leukocytosis has also been treated successfully with hydroxyurea.

Treatment of the coagulopathy associated with APL may be difficult, and patients should be managed expectantly. Coagulation parameters, including fibrinogen, D-dimer, and platelet levels, should be monitored closely. Platelet transfusions and cryoprecipitate or fresh frozen plasma are used to maintain the fibrinogen level above 100 mg/dL and the platelet count above 20,000/μL. The role of heparin is controversial. Continuous infusions of 5 to 10 U/kg/hr are widely used and appear effective at stopping the consumption of clotting factors. Inhibitors of fibrinolysis should be considered only for life-threatening hemorrhage.

The optimal role of ATRA in the treatment of APL is still evolving. The prospective randomized European APL 91 study failed to show a significant improvement in the CR rate with ATRA, compared with conventional 7+3 chemotherapy (25). However, patients treated with ATRA had longer remission durations and survivals. Investigators at Memorial Sloan-Kettering compared the success of ATRA induction therapy with their historic experience using the 7+3 regimen (26–27). There was no decrease in early mortality, but serious infections were decreased, and disease-free survival was prolonged. ATRA will undoubtedly have an important role as first-line therapy for remission induction in APL, either alone or in combination. The drug is also available for treatment of resistant and relapsed APL.

Complete hematologic remissions induced by ATRA alone are rarely associated with complete molecular remissions and have had a median duration of only 3.5 months (3, 24). Thus, remission consolidation using cytotoxic chemotherapy (generally daunorubicin and cytarabine) is required for long-term survival.

Postremission Therapy

Additional chemotherapy after a successful remission induction is mandatory to cure AML. The median disease-free survival for patients who receive no additional therapy is 4 to 8 months. When several courses of consolidation chemotherapy are given, survival at 2 to 3 years

Table 64.4. Options for Postremission Therapy for Adult AML Patients in First Remission

Option	Drug	Comment
High-dose consolidation therapy	Cytarabine 2–3 g/m² every 12 hours for a total of 12 doses; or twice/day on days 1, 3, and 5 for 6 doses	Very effective regimen administered monthly for two or more courses; causes significant toxicity in patients >60 years old
Standard consolidation therapy	Cytarabine 100 mg/m² daily as a continuous infusion for 5–7 days, plus daunorubicin 30–45 mg/m² intravenous push on each of the first 2–3 days of treatment	Myelosuppressive but has acceptable toxicity even in older patients; usually given monthly for 2–4 courses
Intensive maintenance therapy over 3 years	Cytarabine 100 mg/m² i.v. every 12 hours, plus 6-thioguanine 100 mg/m² orally every 12 hours, until severe marrow hypoplasia is achieved	Less toxic than high-dose consolidation chemotherapy, especially in older patients; bone marrow recovery is relatively rapid; requires continuous treatment for up to 3 years
Bone marrow transplantation	High-dose busulfan and cyclophosphamide; or total body irradiation and cyclophosphamide	Effective therapy for younger patients with a suitable donor; leukemia relapse is less frequent than in other forms of postremission therapy, but substantial toxicity results in comparable overall survival; autologous bone marrow transplantation may be employed in patients up to 60 years old

is 35 to 50% for young and middle-aged adults. For patients under 60 years old, consolidation therapy results in significantly longer survival than maintenance therapy alone (5, 28, 29).

The same induction therapy may be repeated for one or more cycles, with or without dose intensification, or non-cross-resistant drugs can be used for consolidation (Table 64.4). There is increasing evidence that HDAC provides the best survival for good- and intermediate-prognosis patients. Cytarabine has a favorable response relationship over a wide dose range. High intracellular drug concentrations saturate the deaminating metabolic enzyme pathway, leading to increased levels of the active agent ara-cytidine triphosphate. HDAC may be effective in eliminating resistant cell populations that survive induction therapy. The Cancer and Leukemia Group B (CALGB) conducted a randomized trial of consolidation therapy using four courses of cytarabine at low (100 mg/m^2/day) or intermediate doses (400 mg/m^2/day) as continuous intravenous infusions for 5 days or at high doses (3 g/m^2 every 12 hr on days 1, 3, and 5) (30). For patients less than 60 years old with a good or intermediate prognosis, disease-free survival in the HDAC arm was 46% at 3 years, compared with 35% for the intermediate-dose and 31% for the low-dose group ($p = .003$). There were relatively few relapses in the HDAC group more than 2 years after attaining CR. HDAC was considerably more toxic, however, and had a 5% treatment-related mortality. Among patients over 60 years old, the toxic death rate was even higher and contributed to the overall failure to improve outcome in this group. The age-related occurrence of cerebellar ataxia, which is irreversible in some patients, is of concern. The best results from consolidation therapy in patients over 60 years old are likely to be from two cycles of daunorubicin (30 to 45 mg/m^2 for 2 days) and cytarabine (100 mg/m^2/day for 5 days) (31). Alternating courses of other two-drug com-binations (e.g., etoposide/cyclophosphamide, mitoxantrone/etoposide, or mitoxantrone/diaziquone) are being tested.

Most studies reporting on allogeneic or autologous BMT for AML patients in first CR are nonrandomized, and many are retrospective. Considerable selection bias is generated by the delay between remission induction and transplantation and by the entry requirements for good performance status for most trials. Prospective randomized studies comparing intensive consolidation therapy and BMT have failed to show a clear survival advantage for BMT (Table 64.5). A European Organization for Research and Treatment of Cancer/Gruppo Italiano Malattie Ematologiche dell'Adulto (EORTC/ GIMEMA) trial demonstrated increased disease-free survival without improved overall survival (32, 33). Patients relapsing after consolidation chemotherapy had better survival than those relapsing after BMT. The British Medical Research Council (MRC) AML-10 study confirmed that autologous BMT in first CR does not presently confer a survival advantage (34). Consequently, for patients with AML, autologous BMT is often reserved as salvage therapy after relapse for suitable candidates without an allogeneic donor.

Maintenance therapy with relatively non-myelosuppressive doses of cytotoxic drugs has no proven benefit in the management of AML. Maintenance chemotherapy with low-dose cytarabine has been shown to be less effective than consolidation therapy. Continued therapy with ATRA does not prolong the remission duration of patients with APL. Relapses occurring in patients receiving ATRA maintenance are resistant to ATRA reinduction.

Salvage Therapy for Relapsed Patients

A limited number of agents are effective in the treatment of AML, and management of pa-

Table 64.5. A Randomized Trial Testing BMT in Adults with AML in First CR (32)

Subgroup	Ages (years)	No. of Patients[a]	4-Year Estimates (± SE)	
			DFS	Survival
Allogeneic BMT	<45	168	55 ± 4%	59 ± 4%
Autologous BMT	<60	128	48 ± 5%	56 ± 5%
Intensive chemotherapy	<60	126	30 ± 4%	46 ± 5%

Data from Zittoun RA, Mandelli F, Willemze R, et al. Autologous or allogeneic bone marrow transplant compared with intensive chemotherapy in acute myelogenous leukemia. N Engl J Med 1995;332:217–223.
[a]Intention-to-treat analysis (no. actually completing assigned treatment: allo = 144; auto = 95; intensive consolidation chemotherapy = 104); DFS denotes disease-free survival.

tients with resistant or relapsed disease is difficult (35). Patients with long initial remissions (>1 year) have a 50 to 60% reinduction rate with daunorubicin and cytarabine or with HDAC, but the duration of the second remission is usually shorter than the first. BMT should be considered for any patient who has relapsed after an intensive initial treatment program.

A HDAC regimen may be effective in 35 to 40% of patients resistant to conventional-dose cytarabine regimens (36). A regimen using etoposide and cyclophosphamide at high doses has produced CRs in 42% of similar patients (37). Mitoxantrone (10 to 12 mg/m^2/day) and etoposide (100 mg/m^2/day) given for 5 days is a commonly used relapse regimen (38, 39). Mitoxantrone has also been used in combination with diaziquone, a highly lipid-soluble aziridinylbenzoquinone (40). Patients failing all conventional drug protocols may elect to undergo experimental treatment with investigational drugs, such as amsacrine, diaziquone, 5-azacytidine, or carboplatin. Patients who relapse more than 1 year after alloBMT may benefit from a second alloBMT. Although transplant-related mortality is high (30 to 40%), a 4-year disease-free survival of 20 to 30% has been reported.

ELDERLY PATIENTS WITH ACUTE LEUKEMIA

Registry data indicate that the median age for patients with AML is 63 to 65 years old, nearly a decade older than the median ages of patients reported on in clinical trials. Older patients are clearly underrepresented in the literature, and the best treatment for elderly patients with AML (or ALL) remains controversial.

Two factors combine to explain in large part the poor outcome of elderly patients with leukemia. First and most obvious is the inability of many of these patients to withstand the rigors of intensive chemotherapy and its expected complications. Patients with age-related chronic cardiac, pulmonary, or renal disorders suffer greater acute toxicity from chemotherapy. Older patients may also have a lower bone marrow regenerative capacity, even after successful leukemia cytoreduction. Inability to tolerate long periods of pancytopenia and malnutrition, or the nephrotoxicity of aminoglycosides or amphotericin, remain major barriers to successful treatment.

At the same time, the genetic mutations most often associated with treatment failure in young patients (e.g., abnormalities of chromosomes 5 or 7 in AML or t(9;22) in ALL) are more common in older patients. Conversely, all of the "favorable" cytogenetic abnormalities, such as t(8;21), t(15;17), or inv(16) in AML, are more common in younger adults and are responsible in part for the better disease-free survival of young and middle-aged adults (2).

Myelodysplastic syndromes are also more common in older patients, and many cases of AML in elderly patients have presumably evolved through a myelodysplastic phase. The syndrome of myelodysplasia is characterized by the stepwise accumulation of genetic abnormalities, analogous to the evolution of new chromosomal abnormalities that occurs as chronic myelogenous leukemia accelerates into the blast phase. The multidrug-resistant phenotype may also emerge during this evolutionary process. At the same time, normal hematopoiesis is increasingly inhibited, and the normal stem cell compartment may be lost. The net result is ineffective hematopoiesis and dysfunctional blood cells. By the time that AML emerges, these patients are often colonized by pathogenic flora, threatened by recurrent bleeding episodes, and dependent on transfusions.

Primum Non Nocere

Not every patient benefits from intensive chemotherapy, and this is particularly true among elderly patients. Well-meaning attempts to induce remissions may actually shorten survival. Patients unlikely to survive treatment can be identified by their poor performance status or comorbid disorders. Case series from large referral institutions suggest that 25 to 50% of AML patients older than 60 years are not offered remission induction chemotherapy.

There are a few patients with "acute leukemia" by the usual quantitative criteria of more than 30% bone marrow blast cells whose disease has a much more smoldering course. These patients suffer from bone marrow failure and pancytopenia more than hyperleukocytosis. Their survival may be equally long, and their quality of life better, using transfusion support and antibiotics rather than intensive chemotherapy. This may be particularly true for "hypoplastic" AML.

The EORTC has reported on a randomized clinical trial for patients older than 65 years, comparing daunorubicin, cytarabine and vincristine treatment with a "watch and wait" strategy, using supportive care and resorting to cytoreductive chemotherapy only for relief of

AML-related symptoms (41). The 31 patients receiving remission induction chemotherapy survived significantly longer (median, 21 vs. 11 weeks; p = .015) than the "supportive care" group. The latter group first received hydroxyurea and cytarabine within a median of 9 days after diagnosis (range, 0 to 395 days) and spent a median of 50% of their remaining days in hospital, compared with 54% for the intensively treated cohort.

Many clinical trials have investigated the use of low doses of cytarabine, particularly in the elderly. Investigators in France randomized 46 AML patients older than 65 years to receive intensive chemotherapy with cytarabine and rubidazone (a daunorubicin analogue) and 41 patients to receive subcutaneous cytarabine at 10 mg/m^2/12 hours for 21 days (42). Although the number of complete remissions was greater with intensive chemotherapy, the early death rate was also higher, so that there were no differences in survival or remission duration between the two groups.

Several trials have evaluated the usefulness of oral idarubicin for elderly AML patients, partly in an attempt to diminish toxicity and avoid prolonged hospitalization if possible. The Finnish Leukemia Group randomized 26 patients over 65 years old to a conventional 5-day 6-thioguanine, ara-C, and daunorubicin (TAD) regimen and 26 patients to a completely oral regimen of etoposide, 6-thioguanine, and idarubicin (ETI) (43). After two courses, the CR rates were 23% for TAD and 60% for ETI, and the median survivals were 3.7 and 9.9 months, respectively.

Otherwise healthy older patients with acute leukemia, especially those with favorable cytogenetic features, should be offered curative chemotherapy. Although pilot studies have used more intensive initial chemotherapy, a reasonable standard regimen for many elderly patients is 7 days of continuous infusion cytarabine (100 mg/m^2/day) plus 3 days of daunorubicin (30 mg/m^2/day) (30). Using this regimen in 346 patients older than 60 years, the CALGB has reported a CR rate of 47%, with three-quarters of remissions occurring after one course. Unfortunately, even with postremission consolidation chemotherapy, the overall survival for this elderly group was only 9% after 4 years. More recent trials using higher anthracycline doses have reported CR rates of 55 to 65%, but the impact on overall survival is not yet known.

HEMATOPOIETIC GROWTH FACTORS

Improvements in supportive care, especially transfusions and antibiotics, have enhanced the outlook for both young and elderly leukemia patients. Uncontrolled trials using granulocyte-macrophage colony-stimulating factor (GM-CSF) or granulocyte colony-stimulating factor (G-CSF) suggested that the duration of neutropenia was decreased when growth factors were given after remission induction chemotherapy, and thus more intensive and effective chemotherapy could be given (44). At the same time, stimulation of leukemia regrowth by myeloid growth factors appears to be uncommon in vivo.

Preliminary data from several large controlled trials have recently been reported, but the issue remains unsettled. Differences in dose and schedule, and the specific growth factor and chemotherapy agents used, as well as the particular disease (i.e., AML or ALL) and the age group studied prevent firm conclusions. Even though a more rapid recovery of neutrophils has been observed in some trials, the nadir has not been affected, and thus, the incidence of severe infection remains high. As yet, growth factors have not had a marked impact on survival or remission duration for patients with AML.

ACUTE LYMPHOBLASTIC LEUKEMIA

Although ALL is the most common leukemia of childhood, it comprises only about 20% of acute leukemia in adults. During the past two decades, there has been marked progress in the treatment of both childhood and adult ALL, concomitant with considerable improvements in diagnostic and prognostic methods. Currently, 70 to 90% of adults achieve a CR, and 25 to 50% have long disease-free survivals (45).

ALL is diagnosed on the basis of characteristic cell morphology and cytochemistry and is subclassified by immunophenotypes. Approximately 20% are T cell in origin, 75% are precursor B cell, and 5% are more mature B cell. Acute undifferentiated leukemia (AUL) is often treated like ALL. ALL should be distinguished from minimally differentiated AML M0, which often has FAB-L2 morphology but does not express lymphoid-specific markers. In approximately 20% of cases of adult ALL, the lymphoblasts express both lymphoid and myeloid antigens. Myeloid-antigen positivity in adults was previously associated with a poorer prognosis, but the use of more intensive remission induction programs appears to have overcome the negative significance of this feature. Increasingly, classification based on immunophenotype and cytogenetic features is required for optimal treatment planning.

Prognostic Factors

Table 64.6 lists the important adverse prognostic factors that have a major influence on complete remission rates, and on remission durations and survivals in ALL (45, 46). In multivariate analyses, patients presenting with white blood cell (WBC) counts above 30,000/μL have had significantly shorter durations of remission than patients with lower leukocyte counts. However, among patients with T-cell ALL, extreme leukocytosis does not negatively affect outcome (46). Older age (>60 years) is another adverse characteristic. Remission duration and overall survival have decreased in almost every adult ALL trial as the ages of the patient groups have increased. Minor factors or those that have had some significance with certain treatment regimens are the percentage of circulating blast cells; the degree of bone marrow involvement; the presence of hepatomegaly, splenomegaly, or lymphadenopathy; lactate dehydrogenase (LDH) levels; CNS involvement at presentation; and the time required to achieve complete remission (e.g., >4 to 6 weeks).

Principles of Therapy

The aims of modern ALL treatment regimens are (a) the rapid restoration of normal bone marrow function, using multiple chemotherapy drugs at acceptable toxicities to prevent the emergence of resistant subclones; (b) the use of adequate prophylactic treatment of sanctuary sites such as the CNS; and (c) postremission con-

Table 64.6. Adverse Prognostic Features in Adult ALL

Remission Induction	Remission Duration/Survival
Age >60 years	Age >35 years
WBC >30,000/μL	WBC >30,000/μL
Non–T cell phenotype	Non–T cell phenotype
Lack of mediastinal	t(9;22) or BCR/ABL
adenopathy	rearrangement
Poor performance	t(4;11)
status	t(8;14) and variants
	Burkitt cell (L3)
	phenotype (Sig +)

solidation therapies to eliminate minimal (undetectable) residual disease. Postremission therapy has traditionally been categorized as intensification or consolidation treatment and prolonged maintenance.

A summary of large clinical trials using intensive induction and postremission therapies is provided in Table 64.7 (46 to 52). Four or five drugs are typically used for remission induction, followed by similar agents plus antimetabolites for remission consolidation treatment. There are data suggesting that high doses of cytarabine or cyclophosphamide may be particularly beneficial for patients with T-cell ALL and some high-risk subsets and that high-dose methotrexate may be particularly useful in B-lineage ALL. CNS prophylaxis is most often administered with intrathecal methotrexate plus either systemic methotrexate or cranial irradiation. Since some of the agents used systemically in the more intensive remission induction and consolidation programs do penetrate the leptomeninges, the need for additional CNS treatment may have diminished. The likelihood of an isolated CNS relapse for adults with ALL appears to be about 5%. For late intensification therapy, many approaches have been used, including BMT. Some period of maintenance chemotherapy has traditionally been given for 1 to 3 years, using 6-mercaptopurine and methotrexate, often with monthly pulses of vincristine and prednisone.

Critical appraisal of the impact of each component of postremission therapy on disease-free survival in any given trial is difficult for many reasons. There are few well-controlled randomized studies analyzing the importance of individual treatment components on outcome. Changes in treatment protocols have rarely been made in a stepwise fashion. Rather, changes in postremission therapy are often made simultaneously with new induction regimens. New drugs have been introduced along with other changes, making their impact on outcome difficult to discern. At present, the benefit of newer drugs such as etoposide or teniposide, high-dose cytarabine, or mitoxantrone cannot be critically evaluated.

Remission Induction

The use of vincristine and corticosteroids (prednisone or dexamethasone) plus an anthracycline (either doxorubicin or daunorubicin) forms the cornerstone of most modern induction regimens. The additional benefit of adding dau-

Table 64.7. Induction and Postremission Therapy Regimens for Adult Acute Lymphoblastic Leukemia[a]

Reference	Number of Patients	Median Age	Induction	Consolidation	Maintenance	CNS Prophylaxis	Complete Remission (%)	Median Survival (Months)
Hoelzer et al. (47)	368	25	V, P, D, A, C, Ara-C, 6-MP	Dex, V, Dox, C, Ara-C, TG	6-MP, MTX	IT MTX, XRT	74	28
Radford et al. (50)	59	37	V, P, Dox, A		V, P, Dox, 6-MP, MTX, ActD, C, BCNU	IT MTX, XRT	75	28
Hussein et al. (49)	168	28	V, P, Dox, C	Ara-C, MTX, TG, V, P, A, C	V, P, Dox, 6-MP, MTX, ActD, C, BCNU	IT MTX	68	18
Linker et al. (51)	109	25	V, P, A, D	V, P, A, D, Ara-C, VM26, MTX	6-MP, MTX	IT MTX, XRT	88	28[b]
Larson et al. (46)	197	32	V, P, A, D, C	C, Ara-C, 6-MP, V, A, Dox, Dex, TG	6-MP, MTX, V, P	IT MTX, XRT	85	36
Mandelli et al. (48)	541	30	V, P, D, A ± C	V, P, Mitox; V, Dex, MTX; VM26, Ara-C	6-MP, MTX, V, P	IT MTX	80	NR
Kantarjian et al. (52)	105	30	V, Dox, Dex ± C	MTX, A; Dox, Ara-C, V, P + AuBMT	MTX, D, 6-MP, P	None	84	19

[a]Abbreviations: A, L-asparaginase; Ara-C, cytarabine; BCNU, carmustine; Dox, doxorubicin; C, cyclophosphamide; D, daunorubicin; ActD, dactinomycin; Dex, dexamethasone; P, prednisone; TG, thioguanine; 6-MP, 6-mercaptopurine; MTX, methotrexate; IT, intrathecal; XRT, cranial irradiation; HDAC, high-dose cytarabine; Mitox, mitoxantrone; AuBMT, autologous bone marrow transplantation; NR, not reported.
[b]Median disease-free survival.

norubicin to vincristine, prednisone, and L-asparaginase was proven in a randomized trial conducted by the CALGB (study 7612) in which patients who also received daunorubicin had a CR rate of 83%, versus 47% for those who did not (53).

L-Asparaginase improves the CR rate when added as a third drug to vincristine and prednisone, but its value in improving either the CR rate or disease-free survival (DFS) when daunorubicin is included in the induction regimen is unclear. In childhood ALL, L-asparaginase appears to prolong DFS when given during consolidation.

Other agents that have been incorporated into induction regimens include cyclophosphamide, conventional and high-dose cytarabine, mercaptopurine, conventional and high-dose methotrexate, and mitoxantrone (45). The relative importance of individual drugs and drug schedules is difficult to discern, given the lack of randomized comparative trials. As yet, no modification involving the addition of a fourth or fifth drug to a three drug regimen has demonstrated reliably higher cure rates, although considerable benefit may accrue to certain subsets of patients.

Remission Consolidation

Postremission consolidation therapy is designed to eradicate the rapidly proliferating neoplastic cells that are thought to be responsible for early relapses. In general, drugs given during this period are cell-cycle-phase specific. The need for intensive consolidation therapy in achieving cure, unlike that of remission induction therapy, is, however, controversial. The relative benefit of any particular consolidation therapy is likely to be inversely proportional to the intensity of the initial induction therapy and its efficacy in rapidly reducing the leukemia cell mass.

Maintenance Therapy

A prolonged period of treatment with low doses of chemotherapy drugs, called remission maintenance therapy, is still standard in ALL. This approach stands in marked contrast to that with most other "curable cancers," such as Hodgkin's disease, large cell lymphoma, or testicular cancer, in which cure follows the initial intensive cytoreductive therapy, and low-dose maintenance chemotherapy provides no additional benefit. The necessity for prolonged maintenance therapy for adults with ALL may also be

a function of the intensity and the success of initial chemotherapy. As yet, the need for maintenance therapy has not been proven in adults.

The experience in childhood ALL has led to the use of methotrexate and 6-mercaptopurine in most maintenance regimens. Most adult trials have also used these two drugs, either alone or in combination with others. The duration of therapy has been derived empirically, and programs lasting 1 to 3 years are commonly used. The uncertainties regarding duration and even the necessity of maintenance therapy are due in part to our lack of knowledge about its mechanism of action. The continuous presence of low doses of antimetabolite drugs may kill drug-resistant leukemia cells or slowly dividing leukemia cells. Alternatively, maintenance therapy may modify the host immune response so that residual leukemia cells are destroyed, or it may suppress the proliferation of residual leukemia cells until senescence or apoptosis occurs, that is, until reinstitution of the normal regulation of lymphocyte survival. One or more of these mechanisms may be active in any individual patient. Clearly, much additional work remains to be done in this area.

Two trials in which maintenance therapy was omitted after consolidation therapy was completed demonstrated high relapse rates. In CALGB study 8513, all therapy ended after 29 weeks (54). Unfortunately, the median remission duration was found to be significantly shorter (11 vs. 21 months) than in the preceding trial that used 3 years of therapy. The median survival, however, was 19 months, compared with 16 months in the earlier trial. In a pilot study conducted by the Eastern Cooperative Oncology Group (ECOG 2483) in which no maintenance therapy was used after an intensive consolidation treatment lasting approximately 12 months, the median DFS was only 10 months, and the 4-year DFS was only 13% (55). Neither trial addressed the question of maintenance chemotherapy using a randomized design, and both trials are subject to the criticism that the initial induction and consolidation therapies were inadequate.

CNS Prophylaxis

The CNS is an important site of involvement by ALL. Although uncommonly found at diagnosis, CNS involvement is common at the time of relapse. The meninges may harbor leukemia cells, and the blood-brain barrier may shelter them from systemic chemotherapy. Recurrence within the CNS usually coincides with systemic relapse. Preventive treatment of the CNS during postremission therapy, termed CNS prophylaxis, has become an integral part of virtually all current adult ALL treatment protocols. Although the true value of CNS prophylaxis in adults is controversial, studies in which adult patients either refused or could not receive CNS prophylaxis have demonstrated a higher rate of CNS relapse compared with those receiving prophylaxis. CNS leukemia is more easily prevented than treated; once overt CNS leukemia has developed, there is a high likelihood of subsequent CNS relapse despite treatment.

CNS prophylaxis typically consists of cranial irradiation plus intrathecal methotrexate. Cytarabine and hydrocortisone are occasionally added to the methotrexate for "triple intrathecal therapy." In lieu of cranial irradiation, some investigators have substituted high-dose systemic chemotherapy with either methotrexate or cytarabine, since therapeutic levels of these drugs can be achieved in the cerebrospinal fluid when they are administered intravenously in high doses. Overall, the superiority of any one prophylactic therapy has not been established.

Modern Multiagent Clinical Trials

What is the expected outcome for patients with ALL treated with one of the modern multiagent chemotherapy regimens? The CALGB has recently reported on its 8811 trial, which evaluated 197 adults from 16 to 80 years old (median, 32 years) and used a dose-intense, multicourse 2-year treatment program (46). The CR rate was 85%, the median remission duration was 29 months, and the median survival overall was 36 months. The five-drug induction regimen used a single dose of cyclophosphamide, 3 days of daunorubicin, and 4 weeks of vincristine, prednisone, and L-asparaginase. The two myelosuppressive drugs (cyclophosphamide and daunorubicin) were given within the first 3 days, and the doses were reduced by one-third for patients over the age of 60. This was followed by early and late intensification courses.

The first intensification included 2 months of treatment using cyclophosphamide, intrathecal methotrexate, subcutaneous cytarabine, oral 6-mercaptopurine, intravenous vincristine, and more L-asparaginase. CNS prophylaxis was then completed with cranial irradiation and five weekly doses of intrathecal methotrexate together with daily 6-mercaptopurine. The late in-

tensification course lasted 6 weeks, followed by prolonged maintenance treatment with daily 6-mercaptopurine and weekly oral methotrexate plus monthly pulses of vincristine and prednisone until 2 years after diagnosis.

More recently, the CALGB has completed a trial (study 9111) using the same chemotherapy program but randomizing patients in a double-blind fashion to receive either filgrastim (G-CSF) or a placebo during the induction and early intensification courses (56). The CR rate among the patients who received G-CSF was 91%, compared with 83% for the placebo group, but this difference was not statistically significant. There was a significant shortening in the time to recover more than 1000 neutrophils/μL during the induction course from 22 days to 16 days. The shortening in the duration of neutropenia was more apparent in patients over 60 years old (16 days with G-CSF vs. 29 days on the placebo arm). Data from two other randomized trials suggest that concurrent use of G-CSF may improve the ability to deliver intensive chemotherapy more safely (57, 58). The follow-up periods for these trials are still short, however, and the full impact of the use of G-CSF during the treatment of adults with ALL remains to be determined.

Among the few large randomized trials in adults is the GIMEMA ALL 0288 trial (48). This multicenter Italian trial is one of the largest to date, enrolling 541 patients between 12 and 65 years old. Patients were randomly assigned to an induction regimen consisting of daunorubicin, vincristine, prednisone, and L-asparaginase, with or without a single dose of cyclophosphamide. Once in remission, patients were randomized to treatment with both consolidation and maintenance or to maintenance therapy alone. Preliminary results show no significant differences in the CR rates between patients who received cyclophosphamide and those who did not (80% on each arm). This calls into question the benefit of adding cyclophosphamide to the four-drug regimen of daunorubicin, vincristine, prednisone and L-asparaginase, although it is possible that its benefit will be on long-term relapse-free survival. As yet, the results of the second part of the study have not been reported, but one hopes they will shed light on the necessity for a consolidation phase once adequate intensive induction therapy is given.

The German ALL Group enrolled 368 patients into a multicenter study over a 5-year period, from 1978 to 1983 (47). The median age was

25 years. The CR rate was 74%, median remission duration was 24 months, and disease-free survival was 35% at 10 years. The remission induction treatment consisted of vincristine, prednisone, daunorubicin, and L-asparaginase during the first 4 weeks, and then cyclophosphamide, cytarabine, and 6-mercaptopurine during the next four. Favorable outcomes were observed for patients under 35 years old, those with T-ALL, and those with WBC under 30,000/ μL. In addition, delayed achievement of a CR (>4 weeks) was a poor prognostic factor for remission duration. Of interest, CNS involvement at presentation did not predict an adverse outcome, perhaps because effective therapy against CNS relapse was given with intrathecal methotrexate until the disappearance of all blast cells, together with 3000 cGy of irradiation to the skull and neuroaxis.

At the Memorial Sloan-Kettering Cancer Center, multiple courses of eight drugs were used in various combinations in the L-10 and L-10M protocols (59). A CR rate of 85% was reported among 72 patients. The median remission duration was 51 months, and disease-free survival at 5 years was estimated to be 45%. However, when the same chemotherapy program was evaluated in a multiinstitutional trial, investigators in the Southwest Oncology Group (SWOG) reported a CR rate of only 68% in 168 patients (49). The median remission duration was 23 months.

A similar chemotherapy program was evaluated at the University of Iowa (50). The HOP-L regimen produced a CR rate of 75% in 59 patients. The median remission duration was about 50 months, and 15 patients (34%) remained in continuous CR longer than 5 years. In contrast to other recent trials, patients with T-cell ALL had a poor outcome with this regimen.

An intensive consolidation chemotherapy program for adults with ALL has been evaluated by investigators at the University of California in San Francisco (51). After remission induction with daunorubicin, vincristine, prednisone, and L-asparaginase, cyclic courses of reinduction therapy, followed by cytarabine and teniposide, and then high-dose methotrexate, were given to 109 patients less than 50 years old. Maintenance therapy was given until 2.5 years in continuous CR. Forty-two percent of patients achieving a CR were projected to remain disease-free at 5 years, and the disease-free survival for all patients was 35%. Failure to achieve remission within 4 weeks and the presence of the Ph chromosome were

associated with 100% relapse. Fifty-nine percent of patients with T-ALL remained disease-free after achieving CR, compared with 31% of patients with blasts expressing the common ALL antigen (CD10).

A trial conducted at the M. D. Anderson Hospital using vincristine, Adriamycin, and dexamethasone (VAD) is notable for its low morbidity and mortality during the remission induction phase (52). Only 3% of the 105 patients died during induction, and only half of the patients required more than 1 week of hospitalization or prolonged use of intravenous antibiotics. The CR rate was 84%, and the median duration of remission was 22 months.

Burkitt Cell ALL

The first of the high-risk subsets that warrants special attention is Burkitt cell ALL, also known as FAB L3 or mature B-cell ALL. This subset makes up 3 to 5% of adult ALL cases. The ubiquitous biologic features are the presence of monoclonal surface immunoglobulin and the 8;14 translocation or one of its two variants. It is relatively easily recognized at diagnosis from the characteristic clinical findings of hepatosplenomegaly and lymphadenopathy. The LDH and uric acid levels are usually markedly elevated, and there is often leptomeningeal involvement. The lymphoblasts usually lack TdT reactivity. In the past, few if any of these patients survived following standard ALL treatment regimens of the type just reviewed.

More recently, there have been several reports of short intensive chemotherapy programs for B-cell ALL that yield a high CR rate and a survival plateau in the range of 30 to 40% (60, 61). These regimens, which may only require as few as 16 to 18 weeks of treatment, use high doses of methotrexate, cytarabine, and cyclophosphamide or ifosfamide together with other ALL drugs. Additional trials are under way to confirm these encouraging results.

Elderly Patients With ALL

A review of the annual age-specific leukemia incidence in the United States underscores the observation that ALL is relatively uncommon in the middle adult years but increases rapidly in incidence over the age of 60. These patients have only rarely been included in clinical trials, and as yet, there are no optimal treatment programs available (Table 64.8).

Table 64.8. ALL in Patients >60 Years Old

	No. of Patients	Median Age, years (Range)	Complete Remissions (%)	Median Survival, Months (Range)	3-Year Survival (%)
Newcastle, 1994 (62)					
No treatment	9	83 (67–91)	—	<1 (0–2)	0
Palliative	25	74 (63–88)	4 (16)	3 (0–27)	0
Curative	28	67 (60–80)	10 (36)	3 (0–84+)	20
MD Anderson, 1993 (63)					
VAD	52	(>60)	30 (58)	10 (0–48+)	<10
CALGB, 1994 (46, 56)					
8811/9111	55	65 (60–80)	36 (65)	10 (0–48+)	20

In a recent report from the northern counties of England, approximately one-third of ALL cases in adults occurred in patients over the age of 60 (62). Various treatment approaches have been taken in this elderly group of patients, but the outcomes are uniformly poor. Investigators at the M. D. Anderson Hospital have reported on 52 patients treated with infusional vincristine, Adriamycin, and dexamethasone (VAD). This regimen produced a high CR rate with relatively low toxicity in elderly patients (52, 63). In the most recent CALGB trials, a CR rate of 65% was observed in elderly patients (60 to 80 years old; median age, 65) (46, 56). Nevertheless, the 3-year survival in all three of these reports remains quite poor. The low tolerance of elderly patients for intensive chemotherapy remains one of the obstacles to increasing the overall cure rate in adults.

Philadelphia Chromosome–Positive ALL

Ph+ ALL is currently the major challenge in curing ALL, since it makes up approximately one-third of all adult cases and perhaps one-half of all B-lineage ALL (2, 64). Some progress has been made. Ph+ ALL has a high initial response rate but a short duration of remission (46). Shown in Table 64.9 are the outcomes of a group of 30 patients prospectively identified in a CALGB study (8811) to have a t(9;22) or the BCR/ABL rearrangement, compared with 83 patients known not to have this mutation. Although the complete remission rates were similar (70 vs. 84%), the remission durations were markedly shorter: 7 months (median) for the Ph+ cases versus more than 33 months for those known not to have a Ph chromosome ($p < .001$). This was also reflected in the median survival, which was

11 months versus 44 months ($p < .001$). As yet, no chemotherapy regimen alone appears to have the potential to cure this group of patients.

In contrast, the International Bone Marrow Transplant Registry has reported on the outcome after HLA-identical sibling marrow transplants for Ph+ ALL, either in first CR or with more advanced disease, and for a small number of Ph+ ALL patients with primary induction failure (65). The leukemia-free survival was approximately 35% for all three groups. The probability of relapse after transplantation was approximately 30 to 50% for the group overall, attesting in part to the therapy-resistant nature of this disease.

Thus, at this time, the treatment for Ph+ ALL should include an intensive remission induction

Table 64.9. Ph+ ALL Has a High Response Rate but Short Duration of Remission (CALGB 8811)

	Ph+ or BCR-ABL+	Not Ph+ ALL	
No. of patients	30	83	
Complete remission rate	70%	84%	$p = .11$
Median remission duration	7 months	>33 months	$p < .001$
3-Year remission rate	11%	56%	
Median survival duration	11 months	44 months	$p < .001$
3-Year survival rate	16%	56%	

Data from Larson RA, Dodge RK, Burns CP, et al. A five-drug remission induction regimen with intensive consolidation for adults with acute lymphoblastic leukemia: Cancer and Leukemia Group B study 8811. Blood 1995;85:2025–2037.

Table 64.10. A Randomized Trial Testing BMT in Adults with ALL in First CR

Subgroup	Age (median)	No. of Patients[a]	3-Year Estimates (± SE)	
			DFS	Survival
Allogeneic BMT	<40 (26)	116	43% ± 5%	55% ± 5%
Autologous BMT (purged, 81%)	<50 (25)	95	39% ± 5%	49% ± 5%
Chemotherapy	<50 (28)	96	32% ± 5%	42% ± 6%

Data from Fiere D, Lepage E, Sebban C, et al. Acute adult lymphoblastic leukemia: a multicentric randomized trial testing bone marrow transplantation as postremission therapy. J Clin Oncol 1993;11:1990–2001.
[a]Intention-to-treat analysis (actually transplanted: allo, 92; auto, 63).

chemotherapy program, followed by allogeneic BMT in the first CR if a donor is available. Alternatively, intensive postremission chemotherapy is being explored using high-dose cytarabine or methotrexate. There are preliminary data suggesting a possible benefit from the use of α-interferon during maintenance therapy. Considerable interest exists in investigating new agents including immunotoxins, modulators of multidrug resistance, and antisense molecules in this high-risk group of patients.

Relapsed or Refractory ALL

More than half of adult patients with ALL relapse despite modern chemotherapy (66). Most relapse within the first 2 years. Over 80% of relapses occur first in the bone marrow; the remainder occur in extramedullary sites, primarily the CNS. Relapses in other sites such as lymph nodes, skin, or testes occur much less frequently. Patients with an isolated extramedullary relapse have a very high risk for subsequent bone marrow relapse and should receive systemic chemotherapy following local treatment.

A variety of treatment protocols have been used in relapsed or refractory patients. High-dose cytarabine, with or without additional agents, produces complete remissions in about 50% of adult patients (67). However, in almost every instance, the median remission duration has been less than 6 months, and only a small fraction of these patients become long-term survivors. The best results for such patients have been obtained with allogeneic BMT in second remission.

FUTURE DIRECTIONS

Despite major advances in the treatment of adults with acute leukemia in the past decade, many patients continue to die either from their disease or the complications of its treatment. However, a number of novel experimental and clinical approaches hold promise for improving cure rates.

In recent years, the biologic heterogeneity of these diseases has been further defined. A variety of clinical and laboratory parameters convey useful prognostic information. The most consistently observed prognostic factors have been age and karyotype. Currently, detection of chromosomal abnormalities at the time of initial diagnosis provides the most useful means of identifying patients at risk of failing induction therapy as well as those likely to have short, intermediate, or prolonged remissions after achieving CR. In the future, such prognostic information will become valuable for assigning risk categories and in individualizing postremission therapy for a given patient.

Application of modern molecular technologies designed to detect minimal residual leukemia may aid clinicians in monitoring disease during and after chemotherapy. It could, therefore, lead to the early detection of patients likely to relapse, for whom further therapy may be necessary. Novel methods of circumventing multidrug resistance, exploiting immune mechanisms, or altering the control of malignant cell growth need to be investigated.

REFERENCES

1. Bennett JM, Catovsky D, Daniel MT, et al. Proposed revised criteria for the classification of acute myeloid leukemia. A report of the French-American-British cooperative group. Ann Intern Med 1985;103:620–625.

2. LeBeau MM, Larson RA. Cytogenetics and neoplasia. In: Hoffman R, Benz EJ Jr, Shattil SJ, Furie B, Cohen HJ, Silberstein LE, eds. Hematology basic principles and practice. 2nd ed. New York: Churchill Livingstone, 1995:878–898.

3. Miller WH, Levine K, DeBlasio A, et al. Detection of minimal residual disease in acute promyelocytic leukemia by a reverse transcription polymerase

chain reaction assay for the PML/RAR-α fusion mRNA. Blood 1993;82:1689–1694.

4. Nucifora G, Larson RA, Rowley JD. Persistence of the 8;21 translocation in patients with acute myeloid leukemia type M2 in long-term remission. Blood 1993; 82:712–715.

5. Devine SM, Larson RA. Acute leukemia in adults: recent developments in diagnosis and treatment. CA: Cancer J Clin 1994;44(6):326–352.

6. Christiansen NP. Allogeneic bone marrow transplantation for the treatment of adult acute leukemias. Hematol Oncol Clin North Am 1993;7:177–200.

7. Ball ED, Rybka WB. Autologous bone marrow transplantation for adult acute leukemia. Hematol Oncol Clin North Am 1993;7:201–231.

8. Stone RM, Mayer RJ. Treatment of the newly diagnosed adult with de novo acute myeloid leukemia. Hematol Oncol Clin North Am 1993;7:47–64.

9. Petti MC, Mandelli F. Idarubicin in acute leukemias: experience of the Italian cooperative group GIMEMA. Semin Oncol 1989;16(Suppl 2):10–15.

10. Vogler WR, Velez-Garcia E, Weiner RS, et al. A phase III trial comparing idarubicin and daunorubicin in acute myelogenous leukemia: a Southeastern Cancer Study Group study. J Clin Oncol 1992;10:1103.

11. Berman E, Heller G, Santorsa J, et al. Results of a randomized trial comparing idarubicin and cytosine arabinoside with daunorubicin and cytosine arabinoside in adult patients with newly diagnosed acute myelogenous leukemia. Blood 1991;77:1666–1674.

12. Wiernik PH, Banks PLC, Case DC Jr, et al. Cytarabine plus idarubicin or daunorubicin as induction and consolidation therapy for previously untreated adult patients with acute myeloid leukemia. Blood 1992;79:313–319.

13. Berman E, McBride M. Comparative cellular pharmacology of daunorubicin and idarubicin in human multidrug-resistant leukemia cells. Blood 1992; 79:3267.

14. Arlin ZA, Case DC Jr, Moore J, et al. Randomized multicenter trial of cytosine arabinoside with mitoxantrone or daunorubicin in previously untreated adults with acute nonlymphocytic leukemia. Leukemia 1990;4:177–183.

15. MacCallum PK, Davis CL, Rohatiner AZS, et al. Mitoxantrone and cytosine arabinoside as treatment for acute myelogenous leukemia at first recurrence. Leukemia 1993;7:1496–1499.

16. Larson RA, Day RS, Azarnia N, et al. The selective use of AMSA following high-dose cytarabine in patients with acute myeloid leukemia in relapse: a Leukemia Intergroup study. Br J Haematol 1992;82:337–346.

17. Berman E, Arlin ZA, Gaynor J, et al. Comparative trial of cytarabine and thioguanine in combination with amsacrine or daunorubicin in patients with untreated acute nonlymphocytic leukemia: results of the L-16M protocol. Leukemia 1989;3:115–121.

18. Dillman RO, Davis RB, Green MR, et al. A comparative study of two different doses of cytarabine for acute myeloid leukemia: a phase III trial of Cancer and Leukemia Group B. Blood 1991;78:2520–2526.

19. Phillips GL, Reece DE, Shepherd JD, et al. High-dose cytarabine and daunorubicin induction and postremission chemotherapy for the treatment of acute myelogenous leukemia in adults. Blood 1991;77:1429–1435.

20. Schiller G, Gajewski J, Nimer S, et al. A randomized study of intermediate versus conventional-dose cytarabine as intensive induction for acute myelogenous leukemia. Br J Haematol 1992;81:170–177.

21. Bishop JF, Lowenthal RM, Joshua D, et al. for the Australian Leukemia Study Group. Etoposide in acute nonlymphocytic leukemia. Blood 1990;75:27–32.

22. Bishop JF, Matthews JP, Young GA, et al. High dose cytarabine arabinoside in induction prolongs remission in acute myeloid leukemia: updated results of a randomized phase III trial (abstract). Blood 1994; 84(Suppl 1):232a.

23. Frankel SR. Acute promyelocytic leukemia. Hematol Oncol Clin North Am 1993;7:109–138.

24. Warrell RP, De The H, Wang Z, Degos L. Acute promyelocytic leukemia. N Engl J Med 1993;329:177–189.

25. Fenaux P, Le Deley MC, Castaigne S, et al. Effect of all *trans* retinoic acid in newly diagnosed acute promyelocytic leukemia. Results of a multicenter randomized trial. Blood 1993;82:3241–3249.

26. Warrell RP, Maslak P, Eardley A, et al. Treatment of acute promyelocytic leukemia with all-*trans* retinoic acid: an update of the New York experience. Leukemia 1994;8:929–933.

27. Vandat L, Maslak P, Miller WH, et al. Early mortality and the retinoic acid syndrome in acute promyelocytic leukemia: impact of leukocytosis, low-dose chemotherapy, PML/RAR-a isoform, and CD13 expression in patients treated with all-*trans* retinoic acid. Blood 1994;84:3843–3849.

28. Cassileth PA, Lynch E, Hines JD, et al. Varying intensity of postremission therapy in acute myeloid leukemia. Blood 1992;79:1924–1930.

29. Bishop JF. Intensified therapy for acute myeloid leukemia. N Engl J Med 1994;331:941–942.

30. Mayer RJ, Davis RB, Schiffer CA, et al. Intensive postremission chemotherapy in adults with acute myeloid leukemia. N Engl J Med 1994;331:896–903.

31. Stone RM, Mayer RJ. The approach to the elderly patient with acute myeloid leukemia. Hematol Oncol Clin North Am 1993;7:65–79.

32. Zittoun RA, Mandelli F, Willemze R, et al. Autologous or allogeneic bone marrow transplantation compared with intensive chemotherapy in acute myelogenous leukemia. N Engl J Med 1995;332:217–223.

33. Lowenberg B. Post-remission treatment of acute myelogenous leukemia. N Engl J Med 1995; 332:260–262.

34. Burnett AK, Goldstone AH, Stevens RF, et al. The role of BMT in addition to intense chemotherapy in AML in first CR—results of the MRC AML-10 trial (abstract). Blood 1994;84(Suppl 1):252a.

35. Schiffer CA, Lee EJ. Approaches to the therapy of relapsed acute myeloid leukemia. Oncology 1989; 3:23–27.

36. Herzig RH, Lazarus HM, Wolff SN, et al. High-dose cytosine arabinoside therapy with and without anthracycline antibiotics for remission reinduction of acute nonlymphoblastic leukemia. J Clin Oncol 1985; 3:992–997.

37. Brown RA, Herzig RH, Wolff SN, et al. High-dose etoposide and cyclophosphamide without bone marrow transplantation for resistant hematologic malignancy. Blood 1990;76:473–479.

38. Ho AD, Lipp T, Ehninger G, et al. Combination of mitoxantrone and etoposide in refractory acute my-

elogenous leukemia—an active and well tolerated regimen. J Clin Oncol 1988;6:213–217.

39. Daenen S, Lowenberg B, Sonneveld P, et al. Efficacy of etoposide and mitoxantrone in patients with acute myelogenous leukemia refractory to standard induction therapy and intermediate-dose cytarabine with amsidine. Leukemia 1994;8:6–10.

40. Amrein PC, Davis RB, Mayer RJ, Schiffer CA. Treatment of relapsed and refractory acute myeloid leukemia with diaziquone and mitoxantrone: a CALGB phase I study. Am J Hematol 1990;35:80–83.

41. Lowenberg B, Zittoun R, Kerkhofs H, et al. On the value of intensive remission-induction chemotherapy in elderly patients of 65+ years with acute myeloid leukemia: a randomized phase III study of the European Organization for Research and Treatment of Cancer Leukemia Group. J Clin Oncol 1989;7:1268–1274.

42. Tilly H, Castaigne S, Bordessoule D, et al. Low-dose cytarabine versus intensive chemotherapy in the treatment of acute nonlymphocytic leukemia in the elderly. J Clin Oncol 1990;8:272–279.

43. Ruutu T, Almqvist A, Hallman H, et al. Oral induction and consolidation of acute myeloid leukemia with etoposide, 6-thioguanine, and idarubicin in elderly patients: a randomized comparison with 5-day TAD. Leukemia 1994;8:11–15.

44. Stone RM. Hematopoietic growth factors and leukemia. Curr Opinion Oncol 1992;4:33–44.

45. Hoelzer D. Treatment of acute lymphoblastic leukemia. Semin Hematol 1994;31:1–15.

46. Larson RA, Dodge RK, Burns CP, et al. A five-drug remission induction regimen with intensive consolidation for adults with acute lymphoblastic leukemia: Cancer and Leukemia Group B study 8811. Blood 1995;85:2025–2037.

47. Hoelzer D, Thiel E, Loffler H, et al. Prognostic factors in a multicenter study for treatment of acute lymphoblastic leukemia in adults. Blood 1988;71:123–131.

48. Mandelli F, Annino L, Vegna ML, et al. GIMEMA ALL 0288. A multicentric study on adult acute lymphoblastic leukemia. Preliminary results. Leukemia 1992;6(Suppl 2):182–185.

49. Hussein KK, Dahlberg S, Head D, et al. Treatment of acute lymphoblastic leukemia in adults with intensive induction, consolidation, and maintenance chemotherapy. Blood 1989;73:57–63.

50. Radford JE Jr, Burns CP, Jones MP, et al. Adult acute lymphoblastic leukemia: results of the Iowa HOP-L protocol. J Clin Oncol 1989;7:58–66.

51. Linker CA, Levitt LJ, O'Donnell M, et al. Treatment of adult acute lymphoblastic leukemia with intensive cyclical chemotherapy: a follow-up report. Blood 1991;78:2814–2822.

52. Kantarjian HM, Walters RS, Keating MJ, et al. Results of the vincristine, doxorubicin, and dexamethasone regimen in adults with standard- and high-risk acute lymphocytic leukemia. J Clin Oncol 1990;8:994–1004.

53. Gottlieb AJ, Weinberg V, Ellison RR, et al. Efficacy of daunorubicin in the therapy of acute adult lymphocytic leukemia: a prospective randomized trial by the Cancer and Leukemia Group B. Blood 1984; 64:267–274.

54. Cuttner J, Mick R, Budman DR, et al. Phase III trial of brief intensive treatment of adult acute lymphocytic leukemia comparing daunorubicin and mitoxantrone: a CALGB study. Leukemia 1991;5:425–431.

55. Cassileth PA, Andersen JW, Bennett JM, et al. Adult acute lymphocytic leukemia: the Eastern Cooperative Oncology Group experience. Leukemia 1992; 6(Suppl 2):178–181.

56. Larson RA, Linker CA, Dodge RK, et al. Granulocyte-colony stimulating factor (filgrastim; G-CSF) reduces the time to neutrophil recovery in adults with acute lymphoblastic leukemia receiving intensive remission induction chemotherapy: Cancer and Leukemia Group B study 9111 (abstract 995). Proc Am Soc Clin Oncol 1994;13:305.

57. Ohno R, Tomonaga M, Kobayashi T, et al. Effect of granulocyte colony-stimulating factor after intensive induction therapy in relapsed or refractory acute leukemia. N Engl J Med 1990;323:871–877.

58. Ottmann OG, Hoelzer D, Gracien E, et al. Concomitant granulocyte colony-stimulating factor and induction chemoradiotherapy in adult acute lymphoblastic leukemia: A randomized phase III trial. Blood 1995;86:444–450.

59. Gaynor J, Chapman D, Little C, et al. A cause-specific hazard rate analysis of prognostic factors among 199 adults with acute lymphoblastic leukemia: the Memorial Hospital experience since 1969. J Clin Oncol 1988;6:1014–1030.

60. Fenaux P, Lai JL, Miaux O, et al. Burkitt cell acute leukemia (L3 ALL) in adults: a report of 18 cases. Br J Haematol 1989;71:371–376.

61. Hoelzer D, Ludwig W-D, Thiel E, et al. Improved outcome in adult B-cell acute lymphoblastic leukemia. Blood 1996;87:495–508.

62. Taylor PRA, Reid MM, Proctor SJ. Acute lymphoblastic leukemia in the elderly. Leuk Lymphoma 1994;13:373–380.

63. Preti A, O'Brien S, Robertson L, et al. Acute lymphocytic leukemia in the elderly: characteristics and outcome with the vincristine-Adriamycin-dexamethasone regimen (abstract 215). Blood 1993; 82(Suppl 1):57a.

64. Westbrook CA, Hooberman AL, Spino C, et al. Clinical significance of the BCR-ABL fusion gene in adult acute lymphoblastic leukemia: a Cancer and Leukemia Group B study (8762). Blood 1992;80: 2983–2990.

65. Barrett AJ, Horowitz MM, Ash RC, et al. Bone marrow transplantation for Philadelphia chromosome-positive acute lymphoblastic leukemia. Blood 1992; 79:3067–3070.

66. Preti A, Kantarjian HM. Management of adult acute lymphocytic leukemia: present issues and key challenges. J Clin Oncol 1994;12:1312–1322.

67. Giona F, Test AM, Annino L, et al. Treatment of primary refractory and relapsed acute lymphoblastic leukemia in children and adults: the GIMEMA/AIEOP experience. Br J Haematol 1994;86:55–61.

68. Fiere D, Lepage E, Sebban C, et al. Adult acute lymphoblastic leukemia: a multicentric randomized trial testing bone marrow transplantation as postremission therapy. J Clin Oncol 1993;11:1990–2001.

65

Chemotherapy of Chronic Lymphocytic Leukemia and Hairy Cell Leukemia

Kanti R. Rai and Dilip V. Patel

INCIDENCE

Chronic lymphocytic leukemia (CLL) is one of the diseases included in a diverse group termed chronic lymphoproliferative disorders (LPDs). Approximately 98% of all CLL cases manifest an accumulation of monoclonal B lymphocytes, and the remainder constitute T-cell CLL. Hairy cell leukemia (HCL), low-grade or indolent lymphoma, and prolymphocytic leukemia are the other chronic lymphoproliferative disorders. In the Western world, CLL is the commonest form of all leukemias. There is a higher incidence of CLL among males, with an overall M:F ratio of 1.7. Although CLL is a disease of the elderly, with a median age at diagnosis of 65 years, an increasing number of patients are being diagnosed at younger ages. About 10% of CLL patients are between 30 and 50 years of age. The incidence of disease is about 4 cases per 100,000 population of all ages, but in the 75- to 79-year-old group, the incidence is 22 per 100,000 (1). The disease occurs less frequently in Asian countries, and when it does occur in Japan or China, the phenotype usually is of T lymphocytes.

DIAGNOSIS

The diagnostic criteria for CLL are as follows:

1. A sustained, absolute lymphocytosis in the peripheral blood, composed of lymphocytes that morphologically appear mature. Although in most cases the number of lympho-

cytes exceeds $15 \times 10^9/L$, the minimum diagnostic threshold has been set at $5 \times 10^9/L$.
2. A majority of blood lymphocytes phenotypically reflects monoclonal B-cell lineage with certain characteristic features: low levels of surface membrane immunoglobulins, typically IgM or IgM and IgD; a single immunoglobulin light chain, either κ or λ; expression of one or more B-cell-associated antigens, CD19, CD20, CD21, and CD24; and coexpression of the T-cell-associated antigen CD5. CLL lymphocytes form rosettes when incubated with mouse erythrocytes.
3. When the absolute lymphocyte count is relatively low (i.e., between 5 and $10 \times 10^9/L$), an examination of bone marrow is advisable. This should demonstrate normal or hypercellularity with more than 30% lymphocytes among all nucleated cells. Morphologically, bone marrow lymphocytes (like those in the blood) also appear mature.

CLINICAL FEATURES

CLL patients may present with no symptoms at all (the diagnosis being made only accidentally, following a blood count performed for unrelated reasons) or they may have significant symptoms such as profuse night sweats, weight loss, fever without overt sepsis, and frequent infections. Many patients, however, have some symptoms that fall between these two extremes.

Similarly, upon physical examination, there may be no abnormality at all or, at the other end of the spectrum, there may be palpably large, bulky lymph nodes either in a single node-bearing area or generalized, with an enlarged spleen or liver or both. Such abnormal findings on physical examination are also often between the two extremes at the time of initial diagnosis.

LABORATORY FINDINGS

In addition to blood and bone marrow lymphocytosis and an abnormal phenotypic profile of lymphocytes which are characteristic of CLL, there are few abnormal laboratory findings. Neutropenia, anemia, and thrombocytopenia may occur at diagnosis or during the course of the disease, either as a result of the disease itself or from therapeutic intervention. A positive Coombs test is seen in about 25% of cases, but overt autoimmune hemolytic anemia is observed less frequently. Similarly, in a few cases, the thrombocytopenia may be explainable on an autoimmune basis. Hypercalcemia and increased serum levels of LDH and uric acid may be observed. Hypogammaglobulinemia frequently occurs because of loss of B-cell function in CLL.

PROGNOSIS AND CLINICAL STAGING

Using clinically measurable criteria, both the Rai (2, 3) and Binet (4) systems of staging separate CLL patients into three prognostic groups. According to the modified Rai staging, patients in the low-risk group (stage 0) have lymphocytosis without any other abnormality; patients in the intermediate-risk group (stages I and II) have, in addition to lymphocytosis, enlarged nodes and/or spleen or liver, and the high-risk group patients (stages III and IV) have anemia and/or thrombocytopenia. The median survival times for the low-, intermediate-, and high-risk groups are similar to Binet's stages A, B, and C: 12+, 8, and 2 years, respectively.

INDICATIONS FOR INITIATING TREATMENT

It is usually not necessary to initiate any therapy in a CLL patient immediately after the diagnosis has been established. It is advisable to allow a period of clinical observation (which may last from a few weeks to several years) and to start treatment upon the appearance of any of the following indications of "active" disease: (a) disease-related symptoms, such as profuse night sweats, weight loss, weakness, fever, and painfully enlarged lymph nodes; (b) hyperlymphocytosis, especially with total leukocyte counts exceeding $150 \times 10^9/L$; (c) bulky adenopathy or massive splenomegaly; (d) anemia or thrombocytopenia; or (e) frequent infections.

TREATMENT OF CLL: INTRODUCTION

As is the case with several other malignancies, radiation, surgery, and drug therapy are the standard therapeutic modalities in CLL. Radiation is effective for palliation, especially for an extremely large spleen or for a solitary lymph node–bearing area that has become very "bulky," disfiguring, or painful. Splenectomy has been found to be of considerable benefit when a massively enlarged spleen has become painful or nonresponsive to chemotherapy, steroids, or radiation or when there is clinical evidence of hypersplenism.

Drug therapy is the most frequently used modality in CLL. Although drug therapy has proven value in controlling various manifestations of activity of CLL, the best achievable responses have been partial remissions (PRs) with no major improvement in the natural history or in the overall survival during the past four decades. The goal of therapy, traditionally, has been palliation, but with the recent developments of improved and effective drugs and the supportive roles played by various hematopoietic growth factors, cytokines, and stem cells, the goal is gradually shifting toward achieving a complete remission (CR), with the hope that it will be long lasting.

Definition of CR and PR in CLL

The National Cancer Institute's Working Group (NCI-WG) (5) on CLL and the International Workshop on CLL (IWCLL) (6) have both developed the following criteria to assess response to therapy in a standardized manner. A CR requires the absence of symptoms attributable to CLL; normal findings upon physical examination; neutrophils, lymphocytes, platelets and hemoglobin of $\geq 1.5 \times 10^9/L$, $<4 \times 10^9/L$, $\geq 100 \times 10^9/L$, and ≥ 110 g/L, respectively, and a normocellular marrow with $<30\%$ lymphocytes. A PR requires a $\geq 50\%$ reduction in previously enlarged nodes, spleen, and liver; neutrophils, $\geq 1.5 \times 10^9/L$; platelets, $\geq 100 \times 10^9/L$; hemoglobin, ≥ 110 g/L, (or $\geq 50\%$ improvement over pretherapy decreased levels of platelets and hemoglobin). Although a presence of lymphoid nodule(s) in the bone marrow biopsy specimens is allowed in the NCI-WG definition of CR, in this discussion, only those patients whose marrow biopsy showed no residual lymphoid nodules are considered CRs; all others are included among "overall responses." NCI-WG is currently considering a proposal to include marrows with residual lymphoid nodules among PRs.

Drug Therapy

ALKYLATING AGENTS

Chlorambucil is the most commonly used drug as the initial therapy of CLL, with considerable variability in dose and schedule used by different clinicians. The two most frequent schedules are (*a*) pulsed-intermittent therapy 0.8 mg/kg orally in 1 day at intervals of 3 to 4 weeks (a 70-kg person receives 56 mg or 28 2-mg tablets) or (*b*) a daily dose schedule of 0.08 mg/kg orally (6 mg or 3 2-mg tablets). The drug dose is modified on an ongoing basis by monitoring blood counts and clinical response. If drug therapy is considered to be causing significant neutropenia, anemia, or thrombocytopenia, the frequency and dose of chlorambucil is reduced, provided there is evidence of clinical benefit, such as reduction in the size of enlarged lymph nodes and spleen and a trend of the absolute lymphocyte count returning to normal. In the absence of such evidence of clinical benefit, chlorambucil therapy is deemed ineffective after an adequate period of trial (usually about 2 months), and a second-line drug such as fludarabine is introduced. Most responses with chlorambucil are PRs (about 50 to 60%); CRs occur in only about 5% of cases. In a recently reported prospective intergroup randomized study (7) in which previously untreated patients with active CLL received 40 mg/m² chlorambucil at monthly intervals for up to 12 months (a more aggressive and intensive regimen than ever used before), a CR rate of 8% was obtained.

Cyclophosphamide is the second most commonly used drug as the initial therapy of CLL. There is also considerable variability in dose and schedule used by different clinicians prescribing cyclophosphamide in CLL. This drug is available for both oral and intravenous administration. The usual oral dose is 1 to 5 mg/kg daily (about 50 to 350 mg for a 70-kg person) or 10 to 15 mg/kg intravenously at intervals of 1 to 2 weeks. In the presence of continuing clinical benefit, the dose of cyclophosphamide is adjusted by monitoring blood counts as described for chlorambucil. The overall response profile of cyclophosphamide is similar to that of chlorambucil.

Chlorambucil and cyclophosphamide have mostly similar toxicity profiles, consisting mainly of myelosuppression, varying degrees of nausea and vomiting that are usually tolerable, and varying degrees of infertility, pulmonary fibrosis and interstitial pneumonia, drug fever, hypersensitivity reactions, seizures, and hepatotoxicity. Cyclophosphamide may infrequently cause hemorrhagic (chemical) cystitis or bladder carcinoma. Unlike chlorambucil, treatment with cyclophosphamide may produce alopecia.

GLUCOCORTICOSTEROIDS

Prednisone is the most commonly used corticosteroid. Prednisone is used as a single agent in the treatment of autoimmune hemolytic anemia or immune thrombocytopenia of CLL and in combination with an alkylating agent such as chlorambucil or cyclophosphamide as the initial therapy of active CLL. The starting dose of prednisone varies with the prescribing habits of clinicians, but usually it is 40 to 60 mg/m² orally daily. After 7 to 10 days, the dose is tapered gradually over a period of 2 weeks, and then a relatively smaller fixed dose (40 to 60 mg/day) is given for 5 to 7 days each month or in association with the intermittent schedule of chlorambucil or cyclophosphamide. Upon first usage of prednisone, it is not unusual to observe a steep increase in the blood lymphocyte count, but this count eventually decreases with continued therapy. As a single agent, prednisone results in 40 to 50% responses, usually all PRs.

The toxicity profile of prednisone therapy is well known. More noteworthy in CLL, which generally affects an elderly population, are an increased susceptibility to infections, hyperglycemia, fluid retention, euphoria, depression, osteoporosis, and cataracts.

NUCLEOSIDE ANALOGUES (8)

Three nucleoside analogues have been found effective in CLL: fludarabine, 2-chlorodeoxyadenosine (2-CdA), and pentostatin (deoxycoformycin). Of these, only fludarabine is FDA approved for therapy of CLL after alkylating agents are no longer effective; the other two have FDA approval for therapy of HCL, and clinicians use them for CLL patients when the standard therapies have failed.

Fludarabine

Fludarabine is given at a dose of 25 mg/m² daily intravenously for 5 days each month. The dose is modified on an ongoing basis by monitoring toxicity and benefit from therapy. Most of the systematic studies with fludarabine in CLL have been conducted at the M. D. Anderson Cancer Center (9). In 78 previously treated CLL patients, fludarabine resulted in 14% CRs and 57% overall responses. All 78 patients had previously received conventional therapy, and two-thirds of them had become refractory to such therapies. The overall median survival for those who had not become refractory to prior conventional therapy was about 3 years after response to fludarabine; it was only about 1 year for the refractory group. These results establish the value of fludarabine as a salvage therapy for CLL patients who have previously received conventional therapies with an alkylating agent. Usually, 4 to 6 cycles of fludarabine therapy are required to achieve maximal benefit.

The M. D. Anderson results in 35 previously untreated CLL patients given fludarabine show 37% CRs and 80% overall responses. With relatively few patients at risk on long-term follow-up, the overall survival appears superior to that of the previously treated but nonrefractory group (9).

In the recently reported prospective Intergroup study cited earlier (7), in which previously untreated patients with active CLL were randomly assigned to receive either chlorambucil or fludarabine, fludarabine induced 33% CRs, with an overall response rate of 71%. These results confirm the response data from the M. D. Anderson Cancer Center, but the results of relapse-free and overall survival from the Intergroup study will not be available until some time in 1998.

The toxicity associated with fludarabine is related to its myelosuppressive and immunosuppressive effects, resulting in episodes of fever and infection (8, 10). When prednisone was given in combination with fludarabine, there was an increased incidence of opportunistic infections with *Pneumocystis carinii* and *Listeria* organisms.

2-CdA

The dose and method of intravenous administration of 2-CdA was originally developed at the Scripps Clinic in La Jolla, California, where 0.1 mg/kg/day continuous infusion for 7 days was given every month. Subsequently, the same total dose was delivered in 5 days by giving 0.14 mg/kg by a 2-hour intravenous infusion each day (this regimen is easier to administer than continuous intravenous infusion). In previously treated CLL patients, Saven et al. (11) reported

4% CRs and 44% overall responses (PR + CR), while Tallman et al. (12) observed 31% PRs and no CR. Researchers from Sweden (13) observed a high incidence of CRs (39%) in previously treated patients, but these results could not be confirmed in other reported trials. Generally, about 4 to 6 cycles of therapy are necessary to obtain maximal beneficial responses with 2-CdA. The median duration of response in the Scripps Clinic trial was 4 months.

Although an early report (14) indicated that previously treated CLL patients who also had received fludarabine had excellent responses to 2-CdA, several investigators subsequently showed that fludarabine-resistant CLL patients are unlikely to respond to 2-CdA (12, 15–17). There is a higher response rate when 2-CdA is administered to previously untreated CLL patients, and an 85% overall response rate, including 10% CRs, was observed by investigators at Scripps Clinic (18).

The major toxicities of 2-CdA are from myelosuppression (thrombocytopenia can be dose limiting) and immunosuppression. Opportunistic infections, especially with *P. carinii*, *Listeria monocytogenes*, and *Cryptococcus neoformans*, have been reported (8, 10).

Pentostatin

Most of the clinical trials with pentostatin were performed over a decade ago and demonstrated some clinical activity in CLL, but this drug has not remained under active investigation in recent years. The usual dosage is 4 mg/m^2 intravenously weekly for 2 or 3 weeks, and then every 2 weeks for a few months. CRs have been relatively rare, but there were consistent reports of about 16 to 35% PRs in previously treated and untreated patients with CLL (19–21).

Toxicity with pentostatin is also related to its myelosuppressive and immunosuppressive effects (8, 10).

COMBINATION CHEMOTHERAPY REGIMENS

Before the emergence of nucleoside analogues, combination chemotherapy schedules used in non-Hodgkin's lymphoma were used as the second-line treatment after alkylating agents became ineffective in CLL patients. These combinations are the well-known COP or CVP (cyclophosphamide, vincristine, prednisone), CHOP (COP with doxorubicin in either standard or lower dosage, the M-2 protocol used for myeloma (vincristine, cyclophosphamide, prednisone, melphalan, and BCNU), CAP (cyclophosphamide, doxorubicin, prednisone), and POACH (prednisone, vincristine, cytosine arabinoside, cyclophosphamide, doxorubicin). Because of the proven effectiveness of fludarabine and 2-CdA in second-line therapy of CLL, the combination-drug regimens listed above are now being used as salvage attempts in individually selected refractory cases (22).

ALLOPURINOL

To prevent uric acid nephropathy and gouty complications, allopurinol is recommended in combination with other cytotoxic drugs when the initial tumor mass of CLL is high. The usual daily dose is 300 mg orally throughout the period while cytotoxic drugs are being administered.

CLL VARIANTS AND "TRANSFORMATIONS"

Prolymphocytic leukemia is a variant of CLL. There are no treatment methods for prolymphocytic leukemia that are distinct from those used for typical CLL. However, in CLL the first line of treatment is with chlorambucil or cyclophosphamide (with or without prednisone), but because the overall prognosis is worse with prolymphocytic leukemia, many clinicians use fludarabine or 2-CdA as the first-line therapy in the latter condition.

In some patients with CLL, after a variable period in the clinical course, the blood lymphocytes develop morphologic features of prolymphocytes; such patients are considered to have prolymphocytoid transformation. There is no known specifically effective therapy for this transformation, which is associated with poor prognosis. If not previously used in these patients, 2-CdA, pentostatin, or fludarabine should be tried when prolymphocytoid transformation occurs. Richter's transformation, another well-recognized terminal event in patients known to have CLL, is defined as the development of a large cell lymphoma over a background of CLL. This event represents a new malignancy in some patients and evolution of the preexisting CLL clone in others. There is no known effective therapy. Chemotherapy combination regimens generally used in advanced or refractory non-Hodgkins lymphoma are recommended for the treatment of Richter's transformation. The outlook for survival is poor.

ADJUNCTIVE THERAPY

Intravenous gamma globulin is recommended to provide protection from bacterial infections in CLL patients who are at high risk of developing such infections. Although the originally proposed dosage was 0.4 g/kg at 3-week intervals, a lower dosage of 0.1 to 0.2 g/kg at intervals of 4 to 6 weeks is adequate (22).

Recombinant α_{2B}- or α_{2A}-interferon can reduce the absolute lymphocyte count and shrink enlarged lymph nodes in early-stage CLL patients (23, 24). However, when used as maintenance therapy in patients who had achieved minimal residual disease status after chemotherapy, α-interferon did not eradicate residual disease or prolong the duration of remission (25). The usual dose of α-interferon is 3 million units subcutaneously 3 days each week.

Cyclosporin A has been found to be effective in controlling the autoimmune complications of CLL, especially pure red cell aplasia (26–30). The initial starting dose of cyclosporin A is 5 mg/kg/day orally to be tapered to a maintenance dose after 3 weeks.

HEMATOPOIETIC GROWTH FACTORS

Erythropoietin

In a placebo-controlled randomized trial (31), recombinant human erythropoietin (Epo) has been found to be effective in increasing the hematocrit by 6 points in about 50% of anemic CLL patients. The anemia in the patients studied was not due to hemolysis (either from autoimmune or nonimmune causes). A report from Greece reveals a similarly beneficial response with Epo in a smaller number of CLL patients with anemia (32). Another study has shown that endogenous Epo levels inappropriately low for the degree of anemia or an increase in hemoglobin by 5 g/L or more after 2 weeks of therapy strongly correlate with an eventual good response (33). The usual dose is 150 µg/kg subcutaneously three times a week.

Granulocyte Colony-Stimulating Factor (G-CSF)

Chemotherapy-induced severe neutropenia in CLL patients can be controlled with subcutaneous injections of G-CSF, 300 or 480 µg daily for 7 to 10 days. Such therapy can provide protection from infections in selected patients at risk.

Bone Marrow Transplantation

Allogeneic and autologous bone marrow or peripheral blood stem cell transplantation therapy is increasingly being considered in appropriately selected younger CLL patients whose disease is responsive to chemotherapy but who would not survive the necessarily high (myeloablative) doses of drugs without stem cell support. An adequate discussion of this subject is beyond the scope of this chapter.

HAIRY CELL LEUKEMIA

Hairy cell leukemia (HCL) is a rare form of leukemia, accounting for 2% of all adult leukemias, with a new-case occurrence of about 600 each year in the United States. The disease occurs predominantly in males, with a M:F ratio of 5:1. The median age of onset is about 50 years (37).

Diagnosis is suspected when characteristic morphologic features of prominent cytoplasmic projections of peripheral blood lymphocytes are observed. These are monoclonal B cells with certain phenotypic features that distinguish them from B lymphocytes of CLL; hairy cells are $CD19^+$, $CD20^+$, $CD22^+$ but, characteristically, CD5 negative, $CD11c^+$ and $CD25^+$. These cells are tartrate-resistant acid phosphatase positive (37). Palpable lymph nodes may be noted infrequently, but splenomegaly is observed in most patients. It is unusual to see hyperlymphocytosis; most often, a pancytopenia is noted upon peripheral blood count. The bone marrow biopsy specimen may be hyper- or hypocellular, showing a focal or diffuse lymphoid infiltrate with a characteristic halo of pale cytoplasm with hairy projections, round or slightly indented nuclei, and usually increased numbers of marrow reticulin fibers. Because of fibrosis, the marrow in HCL is frequently nonaspirable. The spleen pathology in HCL is distinct from that in other lymphoproliferative disorders and shows a diffuse infiltration of the red pulp by hairy cells (37).

Treatment

INDICATIONS FOR INSTITUTION OF TREATMENT

As is the case with CLL, in HCL it is also advisable to withhold definitive therapy after establishing the diagnosis, to observe the extent of disease activity in each individual patient. A minority of patients may have a stable course for several years, and it may be appropriate not to treat them until there is clear evidence of disease progression. Therapy is instituted if the patient develops a painfully enlarged spleen, the spleen has become massively enlarged, the cytopenias are worsening (hemoglobin <100 g/L, platelets $<100 \times 10^9$/L, or neutrophils $<1 \times 10^9$/L), or other complications of HCL, such as extralymphatic disease, autoimmune phenomena, or recurrent infections (37).

DIMINISHED ROLES FOR SPLENECTOMY AND CHLORAMBUCIL

A decade ago, splenectomy and chlorambucil were the choices available for HCL patients, and significant problems were associated with each. Today these patients can expect long-term control of their disease with any of three treatments developed within the past decade. The situation has changed to such an extent that chlorambucil and other alkylating agents do not merit inclusion in this discussion of therapy of HCL, and splenectomy is no longer considered a front-line treatment of choice in HCL but is reserved for situations when other agents have failed. Some clinicians favor splenectomy as first treatment for patients who present with a massively enlarged spleen and severe thrombocytopenia. Splenectomy is indicated when the spleen is very large and the diagnosis of HCL is in question; in such cases, besides its therapeutic value, spleen pathology is crucial for making a definitive diagnosis.

CURRENT THERAPEUTIC OPTIONS

2-CdA, pentostatin, and α-interferon are the three currently recognized and effective therapies for HCL.

2-CdA

A unique aspect of use of 2-CdA is that only a single (7-day) course induces a clinical complete remission in nearly 80% of HCL cases. There is no other example of similar results with a single drug in any other human malignancy. 2-CdA is given at 0.1 mg/kg/day by continuous intravenous infusion for 7 days. The incidence of CRs in published reports ranges between 75 and 85% (8, 39–44).

More than 50% of patients in the larger series had previously received other therapies such as α-interferon or pentostatin, and the incidence of CRs in these patients was as high as that in previously untreated (8). After the 7-day course, the cytopenia may worsen during the first few weeks, when along with neutropenia, some patients become febrile. In most cases, blood cultures are negative, and there is no clinical evidence of sepsis. However, when such instances of neutropenic-period fever do occur, it is considered advisable to place the patients on broad-spectrum antibiotics. 2-CdA has both myelosuppressive and immunosuppressive effects, as noted above (8, 10). It has been reported that although 2-CdA-induced CRs in HCL are durable, the Cd4$^+$ lymphocyte counts also may remain suppressed for prolonged periods after 2-CdA therapy (45). The enlarged spleen starts to shrink during the 7-day 2-CdA therapy and continues to do so after the treatment, so that by the end of 3 months, the spleen size returns to normal in more than 80% of cases. The blood counts are also normalized between 3 and 4 months after 2-CdA, and at this time, a repeat examination of the bone marrow shows a normal picture, confirming CR.

CdA-induced CRs in HCL are observed to be long lasting. In one reported series, at a median time of 30 months after 2-CdA, 77% of patients were still in CR (45). About 5% of patients show clinical relapse 1 to 3 years later and almost invariably have an excellent response again upon retreatment with 2-CdA. Although pharmacokinetics of subcutaneous administration of 2-CdA reveal a satisfactory bioavailability of the drug (46), we recommend continuous intravenous infusion in HCL because that is the method with which most of the reported series achieved CRs and because in HCL only one course of 2-CdA is required, and a patient may be willing to accept this inconvenience and remain with a proven effective method.

Although 2-CdA results in CRs, the patient is by no means considered to be cured of HCL. Occult disease or minimal residual disease can be detected by immunostaining techniques in some patients with CR (47). Evidence of such minimal or occult disease does not necessarily imply that more treatment should be administered. In most cases, these patients may remain in good health for a long time without further therapy. Only upon reappearance of any of the indications for treatment listed above should treatment with 2-CdA or other agents be considered.

Pentostatin

The usual pentostatin dosage is 4 mg/m^2 intravenously every 2 weeks. Maximally achievable responses are reached within 3 to 6 months

of therapy. The reported range of CR is between 64 and 89% (48–52), with lower CR rates of 33% (53) and 42% (54) in patients who were refractory to α-interferon. The toxicity profile of pentostatin is primarily due to its myelosuppressive and immunosuppressive effects (8, 10), but in general, the drug is well tolerated.

α-Interferon

A report of success with α-inteferon in a small number of patients in 1984 started a succession of further dramatic progress and identification of yet newer agents in the treatment of HCL (55). The product used initially was partially purified human α-interferon, but most subsequent and major studies were conducted with recombinant products α-2b and α-2a. The recommended dose is 3 million units by subcutaneous injection three times a week. A maximally achievable beneficial response is usually reached between 6 and 9 months. The incidence of CR in relatively recently published results of α-interferon therapy in a large number of patients in multiinstitutional studies ranges from 4 to 24%, and overall responses range from 49 to 81% (52, 56, 57). The median duration of α-interferon-induced responses in HCL has been reported to be about 18 months (57). Patients failing or relapsing after interferon therapy have a high likelihood of responding to 2-CdA or pentostatin. The toxicity profile of low-dose α-interferon therapy generally used in HCL is quite well known and consists of a mild-to-moderate flu like syndrome that abates spontaneously after a few weeks and is controllable with acetaminophen. Other toxicities are related to the myelosuppressive effects of α-interferon.

In summary, treatment of HCL is one of the major success stories in contemporary oncology. 2-CdA has become established as the first drug of choice for a patient a with active disease, and pentostatin is a close second choice. Both these drugs have very high rates of CR induction, and these are durable remissions. Many patients are now being followed several years after achieving CR, with no clinically evident disease, and it is tempting to consider them cured. Patients who fail to respond to one drug may respond to the other or to α-interferon. α-Interferon is clearly an effective agent in HCL, but it does not induce a high rate of CRs and is therefore used when 2-CdA and pentostatin are not available, not tolerated, or have failed. Splenectomy is no longer considered the treatment of choice in HCL, but it remains a very effective method of control of this disease in a few selected instances.

REFERENCES

1. Ries LAG, Miller BA, Hankey BF, Kosari CL, Harras A, Edwards BK, eds. SEER Cancer statistic review 1973–1991: titles and graphs, National Cancer Institute. NIH Publ. no. 94-2789. Bethesda, MD, 1994:232.

2. Rai KR, Sawitsky A, Cronkite EP, Chanana AD, Levy RN, Pasternack BS. Clinical staging of chronic lymphocytic leukemia. Blood 1975;46:219–234.

3. Rai KR. A critical analysis of staging in CLL. In: Gale RP, Rai KR, eds. Chronic lymphocytic leukemia: recent progress and future direction. 1987 UCLA symposia on molecular and cellular biology. New series, vol 59. New York: Alan R Liss, 1987:253–264.

4. Binet J-L, Auquier A, Dighiero G, Chastang C, Pignet H, et al. A new prognostic classification of chronic lymphocytic leukemia derived from a multivariate survival analysis. Cancer 1981;48:198–206.

5. Cheson BD, Bennett JM, Rai KR, Grever MR, Kay NE, et al. Guidelines for clinical protocols for chronic lymphocytic leukemia. Recommendations of the NCI-sponsored Working Group. Am J Hematol 1988; 29:152–163.

6. International Workshop on CLL. Chronic lymphocytic leukemia. Recommendations for diagnosis, staging and response criteria. Ann Intern Med 1989; 110:236–238.

7. Rai KR, Peterson B, Kolitz J, Elias L, Shepherd L, et al. for CALGB, SWOG, CTG/NCI-C, ECOG and NCI. Fludarabine induces a high complete remission rate in previously untreated patients with chronic lymphocytic leukemia. A randomized inter-group study (abstract 2414). Blood 1995;86 (Suppl 1):607a.

8. Tallman MS, Hakimian D. Purine nucleoside analogs: emerging roles in indolent lymphoproliferative disorders. Blood 1995;86:2463–2474.

9. Keating MJ, O'Brien S, Kantarjian H, Plunkett W, Estey E, et al. Long-term follow-up of patients with chronic lymphocytic leukemia treated with fludarabine as a single agent. Blood 1993;81:2878–2884.

10. Cheson BD. Infections and immunosuppressive complications of purine analog therapy. J Clin Oncol 1995;13:2431–2448.

11. Saven A, Carrera CJ, Carson DA, Buelter E, Piro LD. 2-Chlordeoxyadenosine treatment of refractory chronic lymphocytic leukemia. Leuk Lymph (Suppl) 1991;5:133–138.

12. Tallman MS, Hakimian D, Zanzig C, Hogan DK, Rademaker A, Rose E, Variakojis D. Cladribine in the treatment of relapsed or refractory chronic lymphocytic leukemia. J Clin Oncol 1995;13:983–988.

13. Juliusson G, Lilliemark J. High complete remission rate from 2-chloro-2-deoxyadenosine in previously treated patients with B-cell chronic lymphocytic leukemia response predicted by rapid decrease of blood lymphocyte count. J Clin Oncol 1993;11:679–689.

14. Juliusson G, Elmhorn-Rosenberg A, Lilliemark J. Response to 2-chlorodexoyadenosine in patients with B-cell chronic lymphocytic leukemia resistant to fludarabine. N Engl J Med 1992;327:1056–1061.

15. O'Brien S, Kantarjian H, Estey E, Koller C, Robertson B, et al. Lack of effect of 2-chlorodeoxyadenosine therapy in patients with chronic lymphocytic leukemia refractory to fludarabine therapy. N Engl J Med 1994;330:319–322.

16. Delannoy A, Hanique G, Ferrant A. 2-Chlorodeoxyadenosine for patients with B-cell chronic lymphocytic leukemia refractory to fludarabine (letter). N Engl J Med 1993;328:812.

17. Saven A, Lemon RH, Piro LD. 2-Chlorodeoxyadenosine for patients with B-cell lymphocytic leukemia resistant to fludarabine (letter). N Engl J Med 1993; 328:812–813.

18. Saven A, Lemon RH, Kosty M, Beutler E, Piro LD. 2-Chlorodeoxyadenosine activity in patients with untreated chronic lymphocytic leukemia. J Clin Oncol 1995;13:570–574.

19. Dillman RO, Mick R, McIntye OR. Pentostatin in chronic lymphocytic leukemia: A phase II trial of Cancer and Leukemia Group B. J Clin Oncol 1989; 7:433–438.

20. Ho AD, Thaler J, Stryckmans P, Coiffier B, Luciani M, Sonneveld P. Pentostatin in refractory chronic lymphocytic leukemia: a phase II trial of the European Organization for Research and Treatment of Cancer. J Natl Cancer Inst 1990;82:1416–1420.

21. Dearden C, Catovsky D. Deoxycoformycin in the treatment of mature B-cell malignancies. Br J Cancer 1990;62:4–5.

22. Rai KR, Patel DV. Chronic lymphocytic leukemia. In: Hoffman R, Benz EJ Jr, Shattil SJ, Furie B, Cohen HJ, Silberstein LE, eds. Hematology. Basic principles and practice. 2nd ed. New York: Churchill Livingstone, 1995:1308–1322.

23. Ziegler-Heitbrock HWL, Schlag R, Flieger D, Thiel E. Favorable response of early stage B-CLL patients to treatment with IFN-α_2. Blood 1989;73:1426–1430.

24. Molica S, Alberti A. Recombinant alpha-2a interferon in treatment of B-chronic lymphocytic leukemia. A preliminary report with emphasis on previously untreated patients in early stage of disease. Haematologica 1990;75:75–78.

25. O'Brien S, Kantarjian H, Beran M, Robertson LE, et al. Interferon maintenance therapy for patients with chronic lymphocytic leukemia in remission after fludarabine therapy. Blood 1995;86:1296–1300.

26. Chikkappa G, Pasquale D, Phillips PG, Mangan KF, Tsan MF. Cyclosporin-A for the treatment of pure red cell aplasia in patients with chronic lymphocytic leukemia. Am J Hematol 1987;26:179–183.

27. Tura S, Finelli C, Bandini G, Cavo M, Gobbi M. Cyclosporin A in the treatment of CLL associated with PRCA and bone marrow hypoplasia. Nouv Rev Fr Hematol 1988;30:479–481.

28. Bergui L, Gregoretti MG, Caligaris-Cappio F. Cyclosporin A in the treatment of B-chronic lymphocytic leukemia (letter). Leukemia 1994;8:1245–1246.

29. Emilia G, Messora C, Bensi L. The use of cyclosporin A in the treatment of B-chronic lymphocytic leukemia (letter). Leukemia 1995;9:357–358.

30. Reuss-Borst MA, Waller HD, Muller CA. Successful treatment of steroid-resistant hemolysis in chronic lymphocytic leukemia with cyclosporin-A. Am J Hematol 1994;46:375–376.

31. Rose E, Rai K, Revicki D, Brown R, Reblando J, and the Epo in Anemia of CLL Study Group. Clinical and health status assessments in anemic chronic lymphocytic leukemia patients treated with epoietin alfa. Blood 1994;84 (Suppl 1):526a.

32. Pangalis GA, Poziopoulos C, Angelopoulou MK, Siakantaris MP, Panayiotidis P. Effective treatment of disease related anaemia in B-chronic lymphocytic leukaemia patients with recombinant human erythropoietin. Br J Haematol 1995;89:627–629.

33. Cazzola M, Messinger D, Battistel V, Bron D, Cimino R, et al. Recombinant human erythropoietin in the anemia associated with multiple myeloma or non-Hodgkins lymphoma: dose finding and identification of predictors of response. Blood 1995;86:4446–4458.

34. Michallet M, Archimbaud E, Bandini G, Rowlings PA, Deeg HJ, et al. HLA-identical sibling bone marrow transplantation in younger patients with chronic lymphocytic leukemia. Ann Intern Med 1996; 124:311–315.

35. Khouri IF, Keating MJ, Vriesendorp HM, Reading CL, Przepiorka D, et al. Autologous and allogeneic bone marrow transplantation for chronic lymphocytic leukemia: preliminary results. J Clin Oncol 1994; 12:748–758.

36. Rabinow SN, Soiffer RJ, Gribben JG, Daley H, Freedman AS, et al. Autologous and allogeneic bone marrow transplantation for poor prognosis patients with B-cell chronic lymphocytic leukemia. Blood 1993; 82:1366–1376.

37. Hoffman M, Rai K. Hairy cell leukemia. In: Henderson ES, Lister TA, Greaves MF, eds. Leukemia. 6th ed. Philadelphia: WB Saunders, 1996:587–595.

38. Platanias L, Golomb HM. Hairy cell leukemia. Bailliere's Clin Haematol 1993;6:887.

39. Piro LD, Carrera CJ, Carson DA, et al. Lasting remissions in hairy cell leukemia induced by a single infusion of 2-chlorodeoxyadenosine. N Engl J Med 1990;332:1117–1120.

40. Estey EM, Kuzrock R, Kantargian HM, O'Brien SM, McCredie KB, Beran M. Treatment of hairy cell leukemia with 2-chlorodeoxyadenosine (2-CdA). Blood 1992;79:882–887.

41. Juliusson G, Liliemark J. Rapid recovery from cytopenia in hairy cell leukemia after treatment with 2-chloro-2-deoxyadenosine (CdA): relationship to opportunistic infections. Blood 1992;79:888–894.

42. Tallman MS, Hakimian D, Variakojis D, et al. A single cycle of 2-chlorodeoxyadenosine results in complete remission in the majority of patients with hairy cell leukemia. Blood 1992;80:2203–2209.

43. Lauria F, Benfenati D, Raspadori D, et al. Retreatment with 2-CdA of progressed HCL patients. Leuk Lymph (Suppl 1) 1994;14:143–145.

44. Hoffman M, Janson D, Aggarwal A, Rai KR. Long term results after treatment of hairy cell leukemia with 2-chlorodeoxyadenosine (abstract 1393). Blood 1995 (Suppl 1); 351a.

45. Seymour JF, Kurzrock R, Freireich EJ, Estey EH. 2-Chlorodeoxyadenosine induces durable remissions and prolonged suppression of CD4+ lymphocyte counts in patients with hairy cell leukemia. Blood 1994; 83:2906–2911.

46. Lilliemark J, Albertioni F, Hassan M, et al. On the bioavailability of oral and subcutaneous 2-chloro-2'-deoxyadenosine in humans: alternative routes of administration. J Clin Oncol 1992;10:1514–1518.

47. Hakimian D, Tallman MS, Kiley C, Peterson L. Detection of minimal residual disease by immunostaining of bone marrow biopsies after 2-chlorodeoxyadenosine for hairy cell leukemia. Blood 1993; 82:1798–1802.

48. Cassileth PA, Cheuvart B, Spiers ASD, et al. Pentostatin induces durable remissions in hairy cell leukemia. J Clin Oncol 1991;9:243–246.

49. Kraut EH, Bouroncle BA, Grever MR. Pentostatin in the treatment of advanced hairy cell leukemia. J Clin Oncol 1989;7:168–172.

50. Johnston JBV, Eisenhauer E, Corbett W, Scott JG, Zaentz SD. Efficacy of 2-deoxycoformycin in hairy cell leukemia: a study of the National Cancer Institute of Canada Clinical Trials Group. J Natl Cancer Inst 1988;80:765–769.

51. Catovsky D, Matutes E, Talavera JG, et al. Long-term results with 2-deoxycoformycin in hairy cell leukemia. Leuk Lymph 1994 (Suppl);14:109–113.

52. Grever M, Kopecky K, Foucar MK, et al. A randomized comparison of pentostatin vs. interferon alfa-2a in previously untreated patients with hairy cell leukemia: an intergroup study. J Clin Oncol 1994;13:974–982.

53. Ho AD, Thaler J, Mandelli F, et al. Response to pentostatin in hairy cell leukemia refractory to interferon-alpha. J Clin Oncol 1989;7:1533–1538.

54. Golomb HM, Dodge R, Mick R, et al. Pentostatin treatment of hairy cell leukemia patients who fail initial therapy with recombinant alpha-interferon: a report of CALGB study 8515. Leukemia 1994;8:2037–2040.

55. Quesada JR, Reuben J, Manning JT, et al. Alpha interferon for induction of remission in hairy cell leukemia. N Engl J Med 1984;310:15–18.

56. Golomb H, Fefer A, Golde D, Ozer H, et al. Update of a multi-institutional study of 195 patients with hairy cell leukemia treated with interferon alfa-2B (abstract). Proc Am Soc Clin Oncol 1990;9:215.

57. Rai KR, Davey F, Peterson B, Schiffer C, Silver RT, et al. Recombinant alpha-2b interferon in therapy of previously untreated hairy cell leukemia: long-term follow-up results of study for Cancer and Leukemia Group B. Leukemia 1995;9:1116–1120.

66

Chemotherapy of the Myelodysplastic Syndromes

Bruce D. Cheson

The myelodysplastic syndromes (MDS) are a heterogeneous group of hematopoietic disorders characterized, in most patients, by peripheral blood cytopenias with a hypercellular bone marrow (1). The incidence of MDS is difficult to estimate, since they are not included as a separate category within registries such as the NCI's Surveillance, Epidemiology and End Results (SEER) program. Older patients are most often affected; therefore, institutions with a higher proportion of elderly patients tend to encounter a greater number of cases. When patients are routinely screened (2), the frequency of MDS appears to be six times that of acute myeloid leukemia (AML), which is reported to be 2.2/100,000 population in the U.S (3).

MDS have historically been referred to as oligoblastic leukemia, refractory anemia, smoldering acute leukemia, or preleukemia. In 1982, the French-American-British (FAB) group presented a classification, modified in 1985, which currently is the most widely used (4, 5). MDS form a spectrum of diseases from those that are relatively indolent (i.e., refractory anemia with (RARS) or without (RA) ringed sideroblasts) to more aggressive disorders (i.e., refractory anemia with excess blasts (RAEB) and RAEB in transformation (RAEB-T). The distinction between RAEB-T and AML is based primarily on histopathology, rather than clinical features. As a result, patients with MDS may exhibit a clinical picture consistent with AML, with rapidly increasing numbers of blasts but without enough to fulfill the criteria for the diagnosis of AML. MDS are uniformly fatal disorders, the results of infection and bleeding, even for those who do not progress to AML (6, 7). The rate of transformation to AML varies by FAB subtype (8–11);

approximately 10 to 20% for RA or RARS, 20 to 30% for CMML, 40 to 50% for RAEB, and 60 to 75% for RAEB-T. CMML, the most variable of the MDS, may not have an associated pancytopenia and more closely resembles a myeloproliferative disorder (12, 13).

MDS may occur secondary to exposure to toxins or chemotherapy, but the cause remains unknown in 80 to 90% of patients. Secondary MDS have a higher frequency of transformation to AML and a worse outlook than de novo cases. Prognostic factors predicting poor survival include older age, anemia, neutropenia, thrombocytopenia, a high percentage of bone marrow blasts, extensive dyspoiesis, abnormal central clustering of immature precursors within the bone marrow (ALIP score), increased numbers of circulating $CD34^+$ cells (7, 8, 10, 12–19), abnormal cytogenetics (particularly involving chromosomes 5 and 7) (20), expression of the *mdr*-1 phenotype (21), and *RAS* oncogene mutations or activation (22–25). The relevance of *p53* mutations is under study (26).

THERAPY FOR MDS

Hormone Therapy

Corticosteroids have been used to treat most hematologic malignancies, and the MDS are no exception. Support for steroid treatment is based on limited in vitro data and anecdotal cases (27, 28). Bagby et al. (27) reported a correlation between in vitro and clinical resistance to steroid therapy in 29 cases; however, of the 3 responders, there were no complete remissions. Since these drugs further increase the susceptibility to infections in patients with MDS, they are contraindicated. Androgens do not appear to have a beneficial effect on the clinical course of MDS (29, 30). A preliminary report suggested activity for danazol, a semisynthetic attenuated androgen, in a small subset of patients with an associated immune-mediated cytopenia. This activity was not generalizable to other patients with MDS (31, 32).

Chemotherapy

Chemotherapeutic approaches evaluated in MDS have ranged widely in intensity, from single drugs to attenuated doses in multiagent regimens, standard-dose AML chemotherapy, and high-dose chemotherapy with bone marrow transplantation.

SINGLE AGENTS

Chemotherapy drugs have generally been selected for testing in MDS because they are active in AML. As a result, cytarabine has been the most extensively used. Ellison et al. (33) first reported complete remissions with doses of cytarabine as low as 10 mg/m^2/day, but response rates were clearly dose dependent, which encouraged the development of higher-dose regimens. Subsequently, however, an accumulation of anecdotal reports and small series suggested that cytarabine administered at 10 to 20% of the standard dose used in the treatment of AML (100 to 200 mg/m^2) given either every 12 hours subcutaneously or by a continuous intravenous infusion for 14 to 21 days might be effective therapy for MDS by inducing cellular differentiation (34–48), although other reports did not support the activity of this approach (30, 49–51). In a literature review of over 250 published cases of MDS treated with low-dose cytarabine, the complete remission rate was only 17%, with an additional 19% qualifying as partial remissions. No clinical or laboratory factors predicted response, and the data supported myelotoxicity rather than clinical differentiation. The median survival was 15 months, with no apparent prolongation of survival compared with the natural history of the disease. Myelosuppression was reported in 88% of cases, with 15% treatment-related deaths (50, 51).

In a randomized study conducted by the Eastern Cooperative Oncology Group and the Southwest Oncology Group (52), 125 eligible patients were randomized to receive either low-dose cytarabine or supportive care. The response rate to cytarabine of 23%, including 8 complete remissions, was comparable to the published data (50,

51). Responses were more common in RAEB-T, with 17% complete remissions and 25% partial remissions. However, the median duration of response was less than 8 months. Infections were more frequent in the treatment arm. There was a similar frequency of transformation to AML and no difference in survival. Therefore, low-dose cytarabine appears to have a limited role in the treatment of MDS. Combining low dose cytarabine with other putative differentiating agents (48, 53–55) or chemotherapy drugs (56) has not improved these results.

At the other end of the intensity spectrum are reports of high doses of cytarabine (e.g., 2 to 3 g/m^2 every 12 hours for 6 days) (57–60), which have resulted in a variable percentage of responses among series, generally of brief duration. Larson et al. (61) treated 17 patients with therapy-related MDS or AML with cytarabine at 1 to 3 g/m^2 every 12 hours for 12 doses, followed by intensive consolidation with similar doses. Death from treatment-induced marrow hypoplasia occurred in 5 patients (27%). Of eight patients who achieved a complete remission, cytogenetic analysis was repeated in seven, and the abnormality was no longer detectable in six of these. Nevertheless, the median remission duration of response was only 5 months, and seven of the eight patients relapsed within 8 months.

Anthracyclines and related compounds have had only limited evaluation as single agents in MDS. In one study using oral idarubicin, of 22 patients, there were 3 complete remissions and 3 partial remissions (response rate, 27%) (62), with a median response duration of 3.5 months. Low doses of aclarubicin (3 to 14 mg/m^2 daily for 7 to 10 days for two courses) induced 3 complete responses from 11 patients with MDS, but of brief duration (63).

Anecdotal activity has been noted with azathioprine (64), carboplatin, and other cisplatin analogues (65–67) and with etoposide, notably in patients with CMML (68, 69). Other agents including oral 6-thioguanine (6-TG) have not demonstrated sufficient promise to pursue in large-scale clinical trials (70).

Recent trials with topoisomerase I–inhibiting agents, such as topotecan, have shown activity in refractory acute leukemia (71, 72) and warrant evaluation in MDS. Further studies using these drugs alone and in combinations are planned.

COMBINATION CHEMOTHERAPY

Attenuated dose chemotherapy has been attempted in MDS, since patients tend to be elderly and more likely to die from marrow hypoplasia following intensive treatment. Letendre et al. (73) treated 18 patients (RAEB-9, RAEB-T-7, CMML-2) with 100 mg/m² of cytarabine and 60 mg/m² of VP-16 as a 1-hour infusion every 12 hours for 5 days, with two unspecified responses lasting 2 and 6 months, respectively; 3 patients progressed to AML within a month of therapy. All patients developed severe neutropenia and thrombocytopenia. Owens and Bennett (74) treated five elderly men (median age, 64 years) with RAEB or CMML with attenuated doses of daunomycin, cytarabine, and 6-TG, which, nevertheless, required hospitalization, with one early death. Improvements in blood counts occurred in four patients, although less than a partial remission, and lasted 1.5 to 9 months.

Intensive multidrug regimens generally induce lower rates in patients with MDS than in those with AML, and with greater toxicity (Table 66.1). Mertlesmann et al. (75) performed a retrospective analysis of 263 cases of AML treated with cytarabine, daunorubicin, and 6-thioguanine; 45 were reclassified as MDS, and 16 as

AML that had evolved from MDS. Of these 61 patients, 48% achieved a complete remission, similar to the 50% for the less differentiated cases of AML, but lower than the 59% for AML cases with differentiation. Duration of survival for patients with MDS or AML was similar. Armitage et al. (76) treated 20 patients with MDS with daunorubicin and cytarabine, with only three complete remissions and five treatment-related deaths. Compared with concurrent, but not randomized, patients treated with supportive care alone, chemotherapy appeared to be detrimental. Better results with chemotherapy in MDS are achieved in younger patients, in those with more aggressive subtypes of MDS (RAEB, RAEB-T), and those who have not received prior therapy for their MDS.

Treatment of patients with AML that has evolved from MDS has generally been unsuccessful, with lower response rates, higher mortality, and shorter survival than de novo AML (56, 61, 75, 79–82) (Table 66.2). Whether AML following an antecedent hematologic disorder has a different prognosis from AML secondary to cy-

Table 66.1. Intensive Chemotherapy Regimens for MDS

Investigator	Patients	Regimen[a]	CR (%)	Toxic Deaths (%)
Mertlesmann (75)	45	AT±D	51	NR
Armitage (76)	20	D/A	15	25
Kantarjian (7)	57	OAP;ROAP;AdOAP AMSA/OAP	15	NR
Preisler (57)	15	HiDAC	13	40+
Tricot (60)	15	HiDAC;D/A	53	33+
Fenaux (59)	20	R/A;HiDAC	50	30
Aul (49)	16	DAT	56	13
De Witte (77)	14	D or Ad/A	64	20
Estey (78)	74	FA;FLAG	58	23

[a]Abbreviations: A, cytarabine; T, 6-thioguanine; D, daunomycin; HiDAC, high-dose cytarabine; R, rubidazone; O, vincristine; P, prednisone; Ad, Adriamycin; AMSA, amsacrine; FA, fludarabine + cytarabine; FLAG, FA + G-CSF.

Table 66.2. Chemotherapy for AML following MDS

Investigator	Patients	Regimen[a]	CR (%)	Toxic Deaths (%)
Mertlesmann (75)	16	AT±D	31	NR
Keating (79)	32	ROAP	22	53
Preisler (80)	11	HiDAC	18	64
Martiat (83)	25	D/A	24	44
Fenaux (59)	9	R/A;HiDAC	44	44
Gajewski (82)	44	DAT	41	21
De Witte (77)	22	D or Ad/A	62	15
Hoyle (81)	36	DAT	42	25

[a]Abbreviations: A, cytarabine; T, 6-thioguanine; D, daunomycin; HiDAC, high-dose cytarabine; R, rubidazone; O, vincristine; P, prednisone; Ad, Adriamycin; AMSA, amsacrine; FA, fludarabine + cytarabine; FLAG, FA + G-CSF.

totoxic chemotherapy or other toxin exposure is controversial (80, 81). Keating et al. (79) used rubidazone, vincristine, cytarabine, and prednisone (ROAP) to treat 91 patients with AML, a third of whom had an antecedent hematologic disorder, mostly MDS. The complete remission rate for the primary AML group was 63%, compared with 22% for the secondary leukemias. Kantarjian et al. (7) described 112 patients who developed MDS or AML following chemotherapy or radiation therapy for a prior malignancy. In 51% of the patients, MDS was the first presentation, although 55% of these patients subsequently progressed to AML. The CR rate was 15% for patients with MDS and 37% for those with AML. The median survival was significantly shorter for patients with AML than for MDS at presentation (21 vs. 45 weeks) and did not appear to be different for those whose MDS progressed to AML. Martiat et al. (83) treated 25 patients with MDS that had transformed into AML, with no antecedent toxin exposure, using daunomycin and cytarabine. A complete remission was achieved in only 24% of patients, while 44% died of complications of treatment-induced myelosuppression. The median survival for this series was 5 months.

Gajewski et al. (82) treated 196 patients using daunomycin, cytarabine, and 6-thioguanine; complete response rates for the 44 patients with AML following a prior hematologic disorder and the 111 patients with primary AML were 41 and 73%, respectively. Moreover, bone marrow recovery took longer for the post-MDS patients. Aul and Schneider (49), treating 16 patients with MDS with daunomycin, cytarabine, and thioguanine, noted nine (56%) complete remissions and two (13%) partial remissions. All 5 RAEB-T patients achieved complete remissions, compared with 4 of 11 AML patients with prior MDS. The median duration of remissions was 5 (2 to 29) months. The Medical Research Council's 9th Acute Myeloid Leukemia trial (81) included 688 patients with primary AML and 66 with AML following either cytotoxic chemotherapy (n = 20), MDS (n = 36), or a myeloproliferative disorder (n = 10). Induction therapy involved daunorubicin, cytarabine, and 6-thioguanine, with a postremission randomization to either MAZE (amsacrine, 5-azacytidine, etoposide) or COAP (cyclophosphamide, vincristine, cytarabine, prednisolone). The complete remission rate for patients with primary AML was 66%, compared with 25% and 42% for the post-cytotoxic-

therapy and prior MDS patients, respectively. This difference was explained, in part, by a high rate of resistant disease in the latter two groups. Moreover, the median survival for the post-cytotoxic-therapy group was only 58.5 days, compared with 125.5 days in the post-MDS group. Nonetheless, neither the duration of remission nor the overall survival of the secondary AML patients were different from the those of the patients with primary AML when stratified for age. The negative influence of age has also been demonstrated by other investigators (77, 81, 82).

In contrast is the report by De Witte et al. (77), who treated 126 patients with primary AML, 22 patients with secondary AML, and 14 with MDS. Complete remission rates were 67%, 62%, and 64%, respectively. It is likely that the younger age of the patients (median age: AML, 44 years; secondary AML, 47 years; MDS, 42 years) was largely responsible for the favorable results in the latter two categories.

Newer regimens are in development to improve on these results. In vitro data suggest that fludarabine prior to cytarabine markedly augments incorporation of arabinosylcytosine $5'$-triphosphate (ara-CTP) into DNA (84–86). Pretreatment of cells with granulocyte- (G-) or granulocyte-macrophage colony stimulating factor (GM-CSF) may also increase their sensitivity to subsequent cytarabine (87). Estey et al. (78) developed combinations of fludarabine (30 mg/m^2 daily for 5 days) and cytarabine (2 g/m^2 over 4 hours beginning 3.5 hours after completion of fludarabine) (FA), or FA plus G-CSF (FLAG). The fludarabine dose was modified for serum creatinine levels of 2.0 mg/100 mL or greater (15 mg/m^2) and age of 60 years or older (20 mg/m^2). Of 43 patients with MDS (mostly RAEB and RAEB-T) with adverse cytogenetic abnormalities or an antecedent hematologic abnormality, the CR rates were 55 and 60% with FA and FLAG, respectively. Because of the short follow-up, an accurate prediction of response duration and survival was not possible.

Although patients with MDS most commonly fail to respond to therapy because of death from marrow hypoplasia, many exhibit clinical drug resistance. An interesting observation is that the gene that codes for the p-glycoprotein has been localized to the long arm of chromosome 7 (88), which is commonly involved in MDS and secondary leukemias. Evidence for multidrug resistance (mdr) is present in almost half the cases evaluated (21, 89); however, the clinical relevance of this observation remains to be determined.

Bone Marrow Transplantation

Allogeneic bone marrow transplantation (BMT) is the only curative therapy currently available for MDS in both adults and children, with a substantial proportion of patients remaining free of disease for longer than 10 years (60, 90–101) (Table 66.3). Unfortunately, most patients with MDS are elderly, and therefore, only a small fraction of patients are suitable candidates for this procedure. Anderson et al. (90) described 93 patients with a median age of 29 years (range, 4 to 54 years), most of whom were conditioned with cyclophosphamide and total body irradiation. Disease recurred in eight patients, between 14 days and 783 days following transplant, for an actuarial probability of relapse of 23%. Relapses occurred only in patients with RAEB and RAEB-T. At the time of the report, 28 of the 59 patients were alive and free of disease 12 to 215 months after transplant; 23 patients (39%) died from transplant-related complications, most often interstitial pneumonia and graft-versus-host disease (8 patients each).

O'Donnell et al. (99) treated 20 patients (age 4 to 48 years; median, 36); 45% died of transplant-related complications. Three patients relapsed at 67, 462, and 2922 days following transplant, one of whom underwent a second, successful transplant. Eight patients remained alive and well from 108+ to 3359+ days posttransplant. The European Bone Marrow Transplant Group (EBMTG) published their retrospective experience with 78 patients with MDS or secondary AML (94), using various preparative regimens. Disease status at the time of transplant was highly predictive for survival; patients transplanted while in complete remission had a 60% 2-year disease-free survival, compared with 18% for those who only partially responded to prior intensive chemotherapy. The disease-free survival at 2 years for previously untreated patients was 58% for RA or RARS, 74% for RAEB, 50% for RAEB-T, and 18% for secondary AML. Thirty-five of the 78 patients were disease-free at 2 to 91 months, 25 (32%) died of transplant-related complications, mainly interstitial pneumonitis (n = 9) and graft-versus-host disease (n = 7), and 18 patients relapsed.

Results following transplantation are particularly poor in the presence of extensive bone marrow fibrosis, age greater than 40 years, chemotherapy-resistant disease, longer disease duration, and the presence of excess blasts (90, 94).

As shown in Table 66.3, treatment-related deaths occur in almost 40% of patients with MDS. The use of hematopoietic growth factors and the donor peripheral blood stem cells, rather than bone marrow, may abbreviate the period of neutropenia and reduce the treatment-related morbidity from infections.

Sources of bone marrow other than HLA-identical sibling have also been used in MDS, including matched unrelated donors and partially matched family members (90, 93, 95, 103). In a recent report from the National Marrow Donor program of the first 462 cases of matched-unrelated donor transplants, 32 (7%) were for MDS. The median age of these patients was 24 years, with a median time to transplantation from diagnosis of less than a year. The probability of

Table 66.3. Bone Marrow Transplantation for MDS

Author	Regimen	Patients	DFS (months)	BMT-Related Deaths (%)
Tricot (102)	ARA-C/TBI+/-Cy	7	4(5+−32+)	29
O'Donnell (99)	Cy+/-Ara-C/TBI VP-16/TBI;BuCy	20	8(3+−120+)	45
Belanger (91)	Cy/TBI;BuCy	8	5(9+−35+)	25
Bunin (93)	Cy/Bu/Ara-C/MP/TBI	6	3(8+−18+)	33
Kolb (97)	Cy/TBI;BuCy	7	5(6−34)	29
Longmore (98)	Cy+/-Ara-C/TBI	23	12(6+−102+)	22
De Witte (94)	Variable	65	32(6+−91+)	31
Gajewski (95)	BuCy ± TBI	6	3(4−5)	50
Anderson (90)	Cy/TBI; BuCy	93	41%, 4 years	43

Abbreviations: DFS, disease-free survival; Ara-C, cytarabine; Cy, cyclophosphamide; Bu, busulfan; TBI, total body irradiation; MP, methylprednisolone.

survival at 2 years was 24%; however, the probability of disease-free survival was only 18%. A matched unrelated transplant is a therapeutic option to be considered for a younger patient (under 40 years) without a suitable family donor, who is experiencing progressive disease.

Autologous BMT has been used in only a few patients with MDS or AML and preexisting MDS. Gribben et al. (104) reported 5 cases of secondary AML, all of whom relapsed within 1 year of either a single or double graft. A recent study by the Children's Cancer Study Group identified 18 cases of MDS in a series of 137 patients with MDS or AML referred for allografting or autografting. Patients received induction with dexamethasone, cytarabine, 6-thioguanine, etoposide, and daunomycin, followed by busulfan and cyclophosphamide as a conditioning regimen. Thirteen of the 17 children with RAEB or RAEB-T or a secondary AML achieved a remission with induction chemotherapy; however, there were no data as to their outcome following ABMT (101). Autologous peripheral blood stem cell transplantation has been attempted in a few patients (105).

Biological Approaches

DIFFERENTIATING AGENTS

The availability of drugs capable of inducing cellular differentiation in vitro that can be safely administered in vivo has stimulated interest in applying this approach to clinical studies. The retinoids have been the most widely studied of the potential differentiating agents. Initial reports in MDS suggested response rates to 13-*cis*-retinoic acid or isoretinoin from 0% to approximately 20% (48, 106–113). Two randomized trials attempted to better characterize the role of 13-*cis*-retinoic acid in MDS. Clark et al. (55, 114) randomized 48 patients to treatment with 20 mg daily of oral 13-*cis*-retinoic acid, and 49 to supportive care; patients with more than 5% bone marrow blasts also received low-dose cytarabine. No difference in survival between the treated and control groups was detected. Koeffler et al. (115) randomized 68 patients to either 13-*cis*-retinoic acid (100 mg/m^2 by mouth daily) (n = 35) or placebo (n = 33). No responses were observed, and time to progression there was similar in the treatment arms. All-*trans* retinoic acid exhibits a high level of activity in patients with acute promyelocytic leukemia (116–118); however, studies in MDS have failed to demonstrate clinically meaningful activity (119–121).

Finally, both in vitro data and anecdotal reports suggest that the administration of retinoids may actually accelerate transformation to acute leukemia (122, 123).

5-Azacytidine, a pyrimidine analogue, is active in AML (124–128), but with considerable toxicity at doses required for response. Since the drug also induces in vitro cellular differentiation in association with hypomethylation of DNA, it was of interest for study in MDS. Chitambar et al. (129) used a relatively low dose (10 to 35 mg/m^2/day for 14 days) to treat 13 patients, 3 of whom achieved a partial response. Cancer and Leukemia Group B (CALGB) investigators (130) conducted a phase II trial of 5-azacytidine at 75 mg/m^2/day by continuous infusion for 7 days every 28 days in 48 patients with MDS and noted 11% complete remissions and 25% partial remissions. Major toxicities included nausea and vomiting; one patient died from neutropenic sepsis. Subcutaneous administration resulted in slightly lower response rates; 7% complete remissions, 17% partial remissions, and 14% with trilineage improvement but less than a partial response (131). These findings are similar to those achieved with low-dose cytarabine. A randomized trial is comparing 5-azacytidine with supportive care. 5-Aza-2'-deoxycytidine administered as an intermittent intravenous infusion achieved brief responses in a small series of patients with MDS; however, most experienced life-threatening neutropenia and/or thrombocytopenia (132).

Other potential differentiating agents have been tested; however, the results are either preliminary, controversial, or disappointing. Vitamin D$_3$ induces hypercalcemia but is without clinical activity (133, 134). Hexamethylene bisacetamide (HMBA) is a polar-planar solvent with potent in vitro differentiating activity. Clinical activity has been observed, with in situ hybridization studies suggesting differentiation of the malignant clone (135).

INTERFERONS

A number of clinical trials have evaluated the efficacy of α or γ interferons. Unfortunately, little activity has been observed with either agent, despite considerable treatment-related toxicity (136–143).

HEMATOPOIETIC COLONY-STIMULATING FACTORS

Myeloid growth factors have been extensively used in patients with MDS to decrease the

morbidity and mortality associated with prolonged neutropenia and, perhaps, to induce in
vivo cellular differentiation (144–157). To summarize the published data with G-CSF and GM-
CSF (Table 66.4), an improvement in the neutrophil count has been observed in 85%. Platelet
counts improve in 10%; however, a decrease in
platelet count, probably drug-induced, has also
been observed in a small number of patients, and
may be associated with clinical bleeding (158,
159). Increased reticulocyte counts in 38% have
rarely been accompanied by either an elevation
in hemoglobin or a decreased transfusion
requirement.

Interleukin-3 (IL-3) has also been evaluated in
MDS (145, 149, 152, 160) (Table 66.4). Ganser et
al. (149) treated nine patients in a phase I study;
leukocyte counts increased 1.3- to 3.6-fold in all
cases, and the neutrophil count increased in
seven. Minor increases in platelet counts were
observed in two of four severely thrombocytopenic patients. Gillio et al. (160) reported six
patients with RA, of whom two achieved an
increased neutrophil count, with a dramatic increase in the platelet count of one patient.

Neutrophil and platelet counts generally return to baseline within days to weeks of discontinuation of growth factor therapy. Therefore, it
is possible that continuous therapy may be advantageous. Negrin et al. (161) administered
G-CSF to 11 patients with MDS for periods of 3
to 16 months; maintaining the neutrophil count
above 1500/μL reduced the frequency of severe
infections and, perhaps, also transfusion requirements in a rare patient. However, this approach
remains a research question and should not be
considered standard care.

A critical issue is whether hematopoietic
growth factors may accelerate the progression
from MDS to AML. In more than a quarter of
cases of MDS treated with G- or GM-CSF, a significant increase in the percentage of bone marrow blasts has been observed, with AML developing in a similar number, often with rapid onset

and generally not reversible when growth factor
therapy was discontinued. Unfortunately, prognostic factors that consistently predict those
most likely to either respond or transform are
not available (148). Whether the transformation
to AML is drug-induced or part of the natural
history of the disease can only be determined by
a prospective randomized trial. Preliminary results have been published from a multicenter
trial in which 133 patients with MDS were randomized to a 90-day course of GM-CSF or observation, with a crossover to GM-CSF in the
event of an infection (162). Neutrophils were significantly higher in the treated group, with no
differences in hemoglobin level, platelet count,
or frequency of transfusions. Four patients in
each group transformed to AML during the
study. The crossover design of the study unfortunately confounds any comparison of survival.
The current recommendations for the use of myeloid growth factors is that they should be reserved for patients who are experiencing an infection in the setting of neutropenia (163).

Serum erythropoietin (EPO) levels are very
variable in patients with MDS and do not correlate with erythropoiesis (164, 165); therefore, it
is not clear that recombinant EPO will be effective in this disease. Schouten and coworkers
(166) treated 14 patients (RA 7, RAEB 2, RARS 2,
RAEB-T 3) with recombinant EPO; two responses were observed; however, both patients
transformed to AML while on therapy. Hellström et al. (167) reported 4 of 10 responses, but
without mention of disease acceleration. Other
series also support the low response rate to EPO
(168, 169). Whether combinations including EPO
and a myeloid growth factor can improve on
these results is an important research question
(170).

A number of strategies for integrating growth
factors with chemotherapy are being evaluated,
including the use of a growth factor to synchronize malignant cells followed by treatment with
S-phase-specific agents. The combination of GM-

Table 66.4. Hematopoietic Growth Factors in MDS

Factor	Pts	Percentage Increase				
		Neuts	Plts	Retics	BM Blasts	AML
GM-CSF	86	69	8	28	23	16
G-CSF	40	58	3	28	20	10
IL-3	26	65	19	32	9	5
EPO	61	—	—	23	—	—

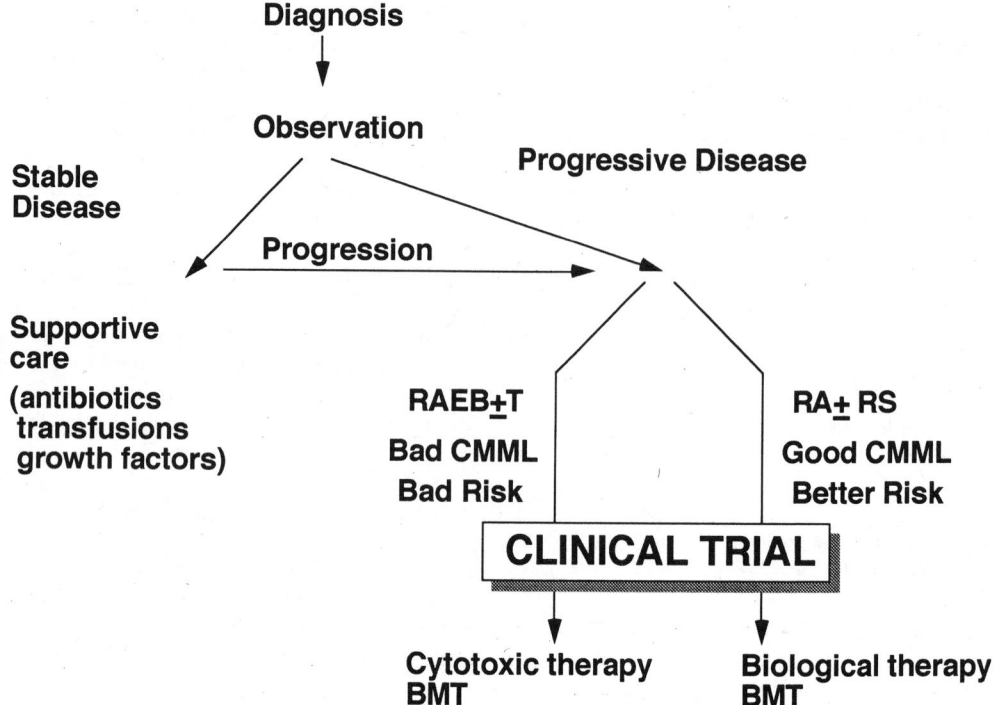

Figure 66.1.   The therapeutic approach to the patient with MDS depends on whether the disease is indolent or progressive. Patients can often be followed with only supportive measures, such as red blood cell or platelet transfusions, antibiotics, or hematopoietic growth factors, until there is evidence of clinical or hematologic deterioration. In the setting of progressive disease, therapy should be delivered, if possible, in the context of a clinical trial. For patients with more favorable MDS, studies evaluating new biologic therapies are appropriate. For those with more unfavorable characteristics, such as complex cytogenetic abnormalities or RAEB or RAEB-T histologies, more aggressive treatment programs may be more suitable. The option of allogeneic BMT should be offered to all patients under the age of 55 years with an HLA-identical sibling.

CSF and cytarabine leads to increased cell killing in vitro, with a differential effect on leukemic and nonleukemic cells (87, 171). Clinical trials are evaluating such combinations in patients with MDS (109).

Newer hematopoietic growth factors such as PIXY321 (GM-CSF/IL-3 fusion protein), stem cell factor, IL-6, IL-11, and IL-12 are still in early stages of clinical development (172–176). There has been considerable interest in the recent availability of thrombopoietin (177–180).

The optimal use of hematopoietic growth factors has not been defined. There are no data to suggest a survival advantage and minimal data to support long-term use. Intermittent administration may be considered in patients with severe neutropenia and recurrent infections.

CONCLUSIONS

New treatment approaches are urgently needed for patients with MDS. Current chemo-therapy agents achieve meaningful responses in a minority of cases and are associated with considerable morbidity and mortality. The results of published studies in MDS are often difficult to interpret because of difficulties in establishing an accurate diagnosis, heterogeneity within MDS subtypes, and the lack of standardized response definitions for MDS (181).

The standard therapy for MDS remains supportive care, with judicious use of red cell and platelet transfusions to minimize the risk of alloimmunization, and antibiotics when indicated (Fig. 66.1). Although growth factors such as erythropoietin, G-CSF, and GM-CSF are commercially available and clinical trials are ongoing using IL-3, PIXY321, IL-6, stem cell factor, thrombopoietin, and others, their initial promise has not yet been realized. Rational development of combinations of these agents may prove to be more effective. Most importantly, progress toward improved therapy for patients with MDS requires the rapid completion of carefully designed and conducted clinical trials addressing important biologic and therapeutic questions.

REFERENCES

1. Nand S, Godwin JE. Hypoplastic myelodysplastic syndrome. Cancer 1988;62:958–964.

2. Hamblin TJ, Oscier DG. The myelodysplastic syndrome—a practical guide. Hematol Oncol 1987; 5:19–34.

3. Miller BA, Linet MS, Cheson BD. Leukemias. In: Miller BA, Gloeckler Ries LA, Hankey BF, eds. SEER cancer statistics review: 1973–1990. Bethesda, MD: National Cancer Institute, 1993:XIII:1–23.

4. Bennett JM, Catovsky D, Daniel M-T, Flandrin G, Galton DAG, Gralnick H, Sultan C. Proposals for the classification of the myelodysplastic syndromes. Br J Haematol 1982;51:189–199.

5. Bennett JM, Catovsky D, Daniel MT, Flandrin G, Galton DAG, Gralnick HR, Sultan C. Proposed revised criteria for the classification of acute myeloid leukemia. A report of the French-American-British group. Ann Intern Med 1985;103:626–629.

6. Weisdorf DJ, Oken MM, Johnson GJ, Rydell RE. Chronic myelodysplastic syndrome: short survival with or without evolution to acute leukaemia. Br J Haematol 1983;55:691–700.

7. Kantarjian HM, Keating MJ, Walters RS, Smith TL, Cork A, McCredie KB, Freireich EJ. Therapy-related leukemia and myelodysplastic syndrome: clinical, cytogenetic, and prognostic features. J Clin Oncol 1986;4:1748–1757.

8. Tricot G, Vlietinck R, Boogaerts MA, Hendrickx B, De Wolf-Peeters C, Van den Berghe H, Verwilghen RL. Prognostic factors in the myelodysplastic syndromes: importance of initial data on peripheral blood counts, bone marrow cytology, trephine biopsy and chromosome analysis. Br J Haematol 1985;60:19–32.

9. Todd WM, Pierre RV. Preleukaemia: a long-term prospective study of 326 patients. Scand J Haematol 1986;45(Suppl):114–120.

10. Vallespi T, Torrabadella M, Julia A, Irriguible D, Jaen A, Acebedo G, Triginer J. Myelodysplastic syndromes: a study of 101 cases according to the FAB classification. Br J Haematol 1985;61:81–92.

11. Kerkhofs H, Hermans J, Maak HL, Leeksma CH. Utility of the FAB classification for myelodysplastic syndromes: investigation of prognostic factors in 237 cases. Br J Haematol 1987;65:83–92.

12. Fenaux P, Beuscart R, Lai JL, Jouet JP, Bauters F. Prognostic factors in adult chronic myelomonocytic leukemia: an analysis of 107 cases. J Clin Oncol 1988; 6:1417–1424.

13. Tefferi A, Hoagland HC, Therneau TM, Pierre RV. Chronic myelomonocytic leukemia: natural history and prognostic determinants. Mayo Clin Proc 1989;64:1246–1254.

14. Mufti GJ, Stevens JR, Oscier DG, Hamblin TJ. Myelodysplastic syndromes: a scoring system with prognostic significance. Br J Haematol 1985;59:425–433.

15. Foucar K, Langdon RM, Armitage JO, Olson DB, Carroll TJ Jr. Myelodysplastic syndromes. A clinical and pathologic analysis. Cancer 1985;56:553–561.

16. Sullivan SA, Marsden KA, Lowenthal RM, Jupe DM, Jones ME. Circulating CD34+ cells: an adverse prognostic factor in the myelodysplastic syndromes. Am J Hematol 1992;39:96–101.

17. Sanz GF, Sanz MA, Vallespi T, et al. Two regression models and a scoring system for predicting survival and planning treatment in myelodysplastic syndromes: a multivariate analysis of prognostic factors in 370 patients. Blood 1989;74:395–408.

18. Tricot G, De Wolf-Peeters C, Vlietinck R, Verwilghen RL. Bone marrow histology in myelodysplastic syndromes. II. Prognostic value of abnormal localization of immature precursors. Br J Haematol 1984; 58:217–225.

19. Varela BL, Chuang C, Woll JE, Bennett JM. Modifications in the classification of primary myelodysplastic syndromes: the addition of a scoring system. Hematol Oncol 1985;3:55–63.

20. Pierre RV, Catovsky D, Mufti GJ, Swansbury GJ, Mecucci C, et al. Clinical-cytogenetic correlations in myelodysplasia (preleukemia). Cancer Genet Cytogenet 1989;40:149–161.

21. List AF, Spier CM, Cline A, Doll DC, Garewal H, Morgan R, Sandberg AA. Expression of the multidrug resistance gene product (p-glycoprotein) in myelodysplasia is associated with a stem cell phenotype. Br J Haematol 1991;78:28–34.

22. Janssen JWG, Steenvoorden ACM, Lyons J, Anger B, Bohlke JU, et al. RAS gene mutations in acute and chronic myelocytic leukemias, chronic myeloproliferative disorders, and myelodysplastic syndromes. Proc Natl Acad Sci USA 1987;84:9228–9232.

23. Melani C, Haliasos A, Chomel JC, Miglino M, Ferraris AM, et al. Ras activation in myelodysplastic syndromes: clinical and molecular study of the chronic phase of the disease. Br J Haematol 1990;74:408–413.

24. Paquette RL, Landaw EM, Pierre RV, Kahan J, Lubbert M, et al. N-ras mutations are associated with poor prognosis and increased risk of leukemia in myelodysplastic syndrome. Blood 1993;82:590–599.

25. Yunis JJ, Boot AJM, Mayer MG, Bos JL. Mechanisms of ras mutation in myelodysplastic syndrome. Oncogene 1989;4:609–614.

26. Sugimoto K, Hirano N, Toyoshima H, Chiba S, Mano H, et al. Mutations of the p53 gene in myelodysplastic syndrome (MDS) and MDS-derived leukemia. Blood 1993;81:3022–3026.

27. Bagby GC Jr, Gabourel JD, Linan JW. Glucocorticoid therapy in the preleukemic syndrome (hemopoietic dysplasia). Ann Intern Med 1980; 92:55–58.

28. Motoji T, Teramura M, Takahashi M, Oshimi K, Okada M, et al. Successful treatment of refractory anemia with high-dose methylprednisolone. Am J Hematol 1990;33:8–12.

29. Najean Y, Pecking A. Refractory anaemia with excess of myeloblasts in the bone marrow: a clinical trial of androgens in 90 patients. Br J Haematol 1977; 37:25–33.

30. Najean Y, Pecking A. Refractory anemia with excess of blast cells: prognostic factors and effect of treatment with androgens or cytosine arabinoside. Cancer 1979;44:1976–1982.

31. Cines DB, Cassileth PA, Kiss JE. Danazol therapy in myelodysplasia. Ann Intern Med 1985;103:58–60.

32. Stadtmauer EA, Cassileth PA, Edelstein M, Abrahm J, Schreiber AD, Nowell PC, Cines DB. Danazol treatment of myelodysplastic syndrome. Br J Haematol 1991;77:502–508.

33. Ellison RR, Holland JF, Weil M, Jacquillat C, Boiron M, et al. Arabinosyl cytosine: a useful agent in

the treatment of acute leukemia in adults. Blood 1968; 32:507–523.

34. Baccarani M, Tura S. Differentiation of myeloid leukaemic cells: new possibilities for therapy. Br J Haematol 1979;42:485–490.

35. Baccarani M, Zaccaria A, Bandini G, Cavazzini G, Fanin R, Tura S. Low dose arabinosyl cytosine for treatment of myelodysplastic syndromes and subacute myeloid leukemia. Leuk Res 1983;7:539–545.

36. Griffin JD, Spriggs D, Wisch JS, Kufe DW. Treatment of preleukemic syndromes with continuous intravenous infusion of low-dose cytosine arabinoside. J Clin Oncol 1985;3:982–991.

37. Hoelzer D, Ganser A, Schneider W, Heimpel H. Low-dose cytosine arabinoside in the treatment of acute nonlymphoblastic leukemia and myelodysplastic syndromes. Semin Oncol 1985;12(Suppl 3):208–211.

38. Inbal A, Januszewicz E, Rabinowictz M, Shaklai M. A therapeutic trial with low-dose cytarabine in myelodysplastic syndromes and acute leukemia. Acta Haematol 1985;73:71–74.

39. Jehn U, De Bock R, Haanen C. Clinical trial of low-dose ara-C in the treatment of acute leukemia and myelodysplasia. Blut 1984;(48):255–261.

40. Maiolo AT, Foa P, Cortellaro M, Lambertenghi-Deliliers G, Colantoni A, et al. Low-dose cytosine arabinoside (ara-C) therapy in the myelodysplastic syndromes and acute myelogenous leukemia. Haematologica 1987;72:61–65.

41. Powell BL, Capizzi RL, Jackson DV, Richards F, Muss HB, et al. Low dose ara-C for patients with myelodysplastic syndromes. Leukemia 1988;2:153–156.

42. Roberts JD, Ershler WB, Tindle BH, Stewart JA. Low-dose cytosine arabinoside in the myelodysplastic syndromes and acute myelogenous leukemia. Cancer 1985;56:1001–1005.

43. Tricot G, De Bock R, Dekker AW, Boogaerts MA, Peetermans M, Punt K, Verwilghen RL. Low dose cytosine arabinoside (ara-C) in myelodysplastic syndromes. Br J Haematol 1984;58:231–340.

44. Vincent PC, Buck M, Young GAR, Benson WJ. Low dose cytarabine in acute non-lymphoblastic leukemia or myelodysplastic syndrome: report of six cases and review of the literature. Aust NZ J Med 1985; 15:10–15.

45. Winter JN, Variakojis D, Gaynor ER, Larson RA, Miller KB. Low-dose cytosine arabinoside (ara-C) therapy in the myelodysplastic syndromes and acute leukemia. Cancer 1985;56:443–449.

46. Wisch JS, Griffin JD, Kufe DW. Response of preleukemic syndromes to continuous infusion of low-dose cytarabine. N Engl J Med 1983;309:1599–1602.

47. Degos L, Castaigne S, Tilly H, Sigaux F, Daniel MT. Treatment of leukemia with low-dose ara-C: a study of 160 cases. Semin Oncol 1985;12(Suppl 3):196–199.

48. Letendre L, Levitt R, Pierre RV, Schroeder G, Krook JA, et al. Myelodysplastic syndrome treatment with danazol and cis-retinoic acid. Am J Hematol 1995; 48:233–236.

49. Aul C, Schneider W. The role of low-dose cytosine arabinoside and aggressive chemotherapy in advanced myelodysplastic syndromes. Cancer 1989; 64:1812–1818.

50. Cheson BD, Jasperse DM, Simon R, Friedman MA. A critical appraisal of low-dose cytosine arabi-

noside in patients with acute non-lymphocytic leukemia and myelodysplastic syndromes. J Clin Oncol 1986;4:1857–1864.

51. Cheson BD, Simon R. Low-dose ara-C in acute nonlymphocytic leukemia and myelodysplastic syndromes: a review of 20 years' experience. Semin Oncol 1987;14(Suppl 1):126–133.

52. Miller KB, Kyungmann K, Morrison FS, Winter JN, Bennett JM, Neiman RS, Head DR. The evaluation of low-dose cytarabine in the treatment of myelodysplastic syndromes a phase-III intergroup study. Ann Hematol 1992;65:162–168.

53. Hellström E, Robert K-H, Samuelsson J, Lindemalm C, Grimfors G, Treatment of myelodysplastic syndromes with retinoic acid and 1α-hydroxy-vitamin D3 in combination with low-dose ara-C is not superior to ara-C alone. Results from a randomized study. Eur J Haematol 1990;45:255–261.

54. Hellström E, Robert K-H, Gahrton G, Mellstedt H, Lindemalm C, et al. Therapeutic effects of low-dose cytosine arabinoside, alpha-interferon, 1α-hydroxyvitamin D3 and retinoic acid in acute leukemia and myelodysplastic syndromes. Eur J Haematol 1988;40:449–459.

55. Clark RE, Ismail SAD, Jacobs A, Payne H, Smith SA. A randomized trial of 13-cis retinoic acid with or without cytosine arabinoside in patients with the myelodysplastic syndrome. Br J Haematol 1987; 66:77–83.

56. Kusnierz-Glaz CR, Normann D, Weinberg R, Fuchs R, Flasshove M, et al. Subcutaneous low dose arabinosyl-cytosine and oral idarubicin in high risk adult acute myelogenous leukemia. Hematol Oncol 1993;11:73–80.

57. Preisler HD, Raza A, Barcos M, Azarnia N, Larson R, et al. High-dose cytosine arabinoside in the treatment of preleukemic disorders: a Leukemia Intergroup study. Am J Hematol 1986;23:131–134.

58. Richard C, Iriondo A, Garijo J, Baro J, Conde E, et al. Therapy of advanced myelodysplastic syndrome with aggressive chemotherapy. Oncology (Basel) 1989; 46:6–9.

59. Fenaux P, Lai JL, Jouet JP, Pollet JP, Bauters F. Aggressive chemotherapy in adult primary myelodysplastic syndromes. Blut 1988;57:297–302.

60. Tricot G, Boogaerts MA. The role of aggressive chemotherapy in the treatment of the myelodysplastic syndromes. Br J Haematol 1986;63:477–483.

61. Larson RA, Wernli M, Me Beau MM, Daly KM, Pape LH, Rowley JD, Vardiman JW. Short remission durations in therapy-related leukemia despite cytogenetic complete responses to high-dose cytarabine. Blood 1988;72:1333–1339.

62. De Bock R, Van Hoof A, Van Hove W, Zachee P, Mathijs R, et al. Oral idaraubicin (IDA) for RAEB, RAEBt, and acute leukemia (AL) post myelodysplastic syndrome (MDS). A phase II open study (abstract 794). Proc Am Soc Clin Oncol 1989;8:204.

63. Shibuya T, Teshima T, Harada M, Taniguchi S, Okamura T, Okamura S-I, Niho Y. Treatment of myelodysplastic syndrome and atypical leukemia with low-dose aclarubicin. Leuk Res 1990;14:161–167.

64. Zervas J, Geary CG, Oleesky S. Sideroblastic anemia treated with immunosuppressive therapy. Blood 1974;44:117–123.

65. Martinez JA, Martin G, Sanz GF, Sempere A, Jarque I, de la Rubia J, Sanz MA. A phase II clinical

trial of carboplatin infusion in high-risk acute non-lymphocytic leukemia. J Clin Oncol 1991;9:39–43.

66. Tamura K, Makino S, Araki Y. A phase I study of a new cisplatin derivative for hematologic malignancies. Cancer 1990;66:2059–2063.

67. Meyers FJ, Welborn J, Lewis JP, Flynn N. Infusion carboplatin treatment of relapsed and refractory acute leukemia: evidence of efficacy with minimal extramedullary toxicity at intermediate doses. J Clin Oncol 1989;7:173–178.

68. Doll D, Sun PCJ, List AF. Complete hematologic remission with oral etoposide in a patient with chronic myelomonocytic leukemia and profound dyserythropoiesis. Leuk Res 1994;18:381–384.

69. Oscier DG, Worsley A, Hamblin TJ, Mufti GJ. Treatment of chronic myelomonocytic leukaemia with low dose etoposide. Br J Haematol 1989;72:468–471.

70. Spitzer TR, Lazarus HM, Crum ED, Weissman R. Treatment of myelodysplastic syndromes with low-dose oral 6-thioguanine. Med Pediatr Oncol 1988; 16:17–20.

71. Rowinsky EK, Adjei A, Donehower RC, Gore SD, Jones RJ, et al. Phase I and pharmacodynamic study of the topoisomerase I-inhibitor topotecan in patients with refractory acute leukemia. J Clin Oncol 1994;12:2193–2203.

72. Kantarjian HM, Beran M, Ellis A, Zwelling L, O'Brien S, et al. Phase I study of topotecan, a new topoisomerase I inhibitor, in patients with refractory or relapsed acute leukemia. Blood 1993;81:1146–1151.

73. Letendre L, Levitt R, Pierre R, Therneau T. A pilot study of VP-16/ara-C in the treatment of unfavorable myelodysplastic syndrome (abstract 1119). Proc Am Soc Clin Oncol 1990;9:288.

74. Owens MR, Bennett JM. Effectiveness of attenuated chemotherapy in myelodysplastic syndromes: a preliminary report. Med Pediatr Oncol 1988;16:107–110.

75. Mertlesmann R, Thaler HT, To L, Gee TS, McKenzie S, et al. Morphological classification, response to therapy, and survival in 263 adult patients with acute nonlymphoblastic leukemia. Blood 1980; 56:773–781.

76. Armitage JO, Dick FR, Needleman SW, Burns CP. Effect of chemotherapy for the dysmyelopoietic syndrome. Cancer Treat Rep 1981;65:601–605.

77. De Witte T, Muus P, De Pauw B, Haanen C. Intensive chemotherapy for patients with myelodysplastic syndromes and acute myelogenous leukemia younger than 65 years. Bone Marrow Transplant 1989; 4(Suppl 3):33–35.

78. Estey E, Thall P, Andreef M, Beran M, Kantarjian H, et al. Use of granulocyte colony-stimulating factor before, during, and after fludarabine plus cytarabine induction therapy of newly diagnosed acute myelogenous leukemia or myelodysplastic syndrome: comparison with fludarabine plus cytarabine without granulocyte colony-stimulating factor. J Clin Oncol 1994;12:671–678.

79. Keating MJ, McCredie KB, Benjamin RS, Bodey GP, Zander A, Smith TL, Freireich EJ. Treatment of patients over 50 years of age with acute myelogenous leukemia with a combination of rubidazone and cytosine arabinoside, vincristine, and prednisone (ROAP). Blood 1981;58:584–591.

80. Preisler HD, Raza A, Barcos M, Azarnia N, Larson R, et al. High-dose cytosine arabinoside as the initial treatment of poor-risk patients with acute nonlymphocytic leukemia: a Leukemia Intergroup study. J Clin Oncol 1987;5:75–82.

81. Hoyle CF, De Bastos M, Wheatley K, Sherrington PD, Fischer PJ, et al. AML associated with previous cytotoxic therapy, MDS or myeloproliferative disorders: results from the MRC's 9th AML trial. Br J Haematol 1989;72:45–53.

82. Gajewski JL, Ho WG, Nimer SD, Hirji KF, Gekelman L, Jacobs AD, Champlin RE. Efficacy of intensive chemotherapy for acute myelogenous leukemia associated with a preleukemic syndrome. J Clin Oncol 1989;7:1637–1645.

83. Martiat P, Ferrant A, Michaux J-L, Sokal G. Intensive chemotherapy for acute non-lymphoblastic leukemia after primary myelodysplastic syndrome. Hematol Oncol 1988;6:299–305.

84. Gandhi V, Nowak B, Keating MJ, Plunkett W. Modulation of arabinosylcytosine metabolism by arabinosyl-2-fluoroadenine in lymphocytes from patients with chronic lymphocytic leukemia: implications for combination therapy. Blood 1989;74:2070–2075.

85. Gandhi V, Estey E, Keating MJ, Plunkett W. Synergistic combination of fludarabine and ara-C for AML therapy (abstract 198). Blood 1991;78(Suppl 1):52a.

86. Gandhi V, Kemena A, Keating MJ, Plunkett W. Fludarabine infusion potentiates arabinosylcytosine metabolism in lymphocytes of patients with chronic lymphocytic leukemia. Cancer Res 1992;52:897–903.

87. Bhalla K, Birkhofer M, Arlin Z, Grant S, Lutzky J, Graham G. Effect of recombinant GM-CSF on the metabolism of cytosine arabinoside in normal and leukemic human bone marrow cells. Leukemia 1988; 2:810–813.

88. Bell DR, Trent JM, Willard HF, et al. Chromosomal location of human p-glycoprotein gene sequence. Cancer Genet Cytogenet 1987;25:141–148.

89. Holmes J, Jacobs A, Cater G, Janowska-Wieczorek A, Padua RA. Multidrug resistance in haemopoietic cell lines, myelodysplastic syndromes and acute myeloblastic leukaemia. Br J Haematol 1989; 72:40–44.

90. Anderson JE, Appelbaum FR, Fisher LD, Schoch G, Shulman H, et al. Allogeneic bone marrow transplantation for 93 patients with myelodysplastic syndrome. Blood 1993;82:677–681.

91. Bellanger R, Gyger M, Perreault C, Bonny Y, St-louis J. Bone marrow transplantation for myelodysplastic syndromes. Br J Haematol 1988;69:29–33.

92. Bhaduri S, Kubanek B, Heit W, Pfleiger H, Kurrie E, Fliedner TM, Heimpel H. A case of preleukemia—reconstitution of normal marrow function after bone marrow transplantation (BMT) from identical twin. Blut 1979;38:145–149.

93. Bunin NJ, Casper JT, Chitambar C, Hunter J, Truitt R, Menitove J, Ash R. Partially matched bone marrow transplantation in patients with myelodysplastic syndromes. J Clin Oncol 1988;6:1851–1855.

94. De Witte T, Zwaan F, Hermans J, Vernant J, Kolb H, et al. Allogeneic bone marrow transplantation for secondary leukemia and myelodysplastic syndrome: a survey by the Leukaemia Working Party of the European Bone Marrow Transplantation Group (EBMTG). Br J Haematol 1990;74:151–155.

95. Gajewski JL, Ho WG, Feig SA, Hunt L, Kaufman N, Champlin RE. Bone marrow transplantation

using unrelated donors for patients with advanced leukemia or bone marrow failure. Transplant 1990;50:244–249.

96. Guinan E, Tarbell NJ, Tantravahi R, Weinstein HJ. Bone marrow transplantation for children with myelodysplastic syndrome. Blood 1989;73:619–622.

97. Kolb HJ, Holler E, Bender-Gotze C, Walther U, Mittermuller J, et al. Myeloablative conditioning for marrow transplantation in myelodysplastic syndromes and paroxysmal nocturnal haemoglobinuria. Bone Marrow Transplant 1989;4:29–34.

98. Longmore G, Guinan EC, Weinstein HJ, Gelber RD, Rappeport JM, Antin JH. Bone marrow transplantation for myelodysplasia and secondary acute non-lymphoblastic leukemia. J Clin Oncol 1990;8:1707–1714.

99. O'Donnell MR, Nademanee AP, Snyder DS, Schmidt GM, Parker PM, et al. Bone marrow transplantation for myelodysplastic and myeloproliferative syndromes. J Clin Oncol 1987;5:1822–1826.

100. Uderzo C, Locasciulli A, Rajnoldi AC, Mozzana R, Lambertenghi-Deliliers G, Masera G. Allogeneic bone marrow transplantation for myelodysplastic syndromes of childhood: report of three children with refractory anemia with excess blasts in transformation and review of the literature. Med Pediatr Oncol 1993; 21:43–48.

101. Woods WG, Kobrinsky N, Buckley J, Neudorf S, Sanders J, et al. Intensively timed induction therapy followed by autologous or allogeneic bone marrow transplantation for children with acute myeloid leukemia or myelodysplastic syndrome: a Childrens Cancer Group pilot study. J Clin Oncol 1993;11:1448–1457.

102. Tricot G, Boogaerts MA, Verwilghen RL. Treatment of patients with myelodysplastic syndromes: a review. Scand J Haematol 1986;36(Suppl 45):121–127.

103. Kernan NA, Bartsch G, Ash RC, Beatty PG, Champlin R, et al. Analysis of 462 transplantations from unrelated donors facilitated by the National Marrow Donor Program. N Engl J Med 1993;328:593–602.

104. Gribben JG, Goldstone AH, Linch DC, MacMillan AK, Richards JDM. Double autologous bone marrow transplantation in acute myeloid leukemia. Bone Marrow Transplant 1989;4(Suppl 1):209–211.

105. Demuynck H, Delforge M, Verhoef GEG, Vandenberghe P, Zachee P, Boogaerts MA. Autologous peripheral blood progenitor cell transplantation (PBSCT) as an alternative treatment option for patients with myelodysplastic syndromes (abstract 336). Blood 1994; 84(Suppl 1):87a.

106. Leoni F, Ciolli S, Longo G, Messori A, Ferrini PR. 13-Cis-retinoic acid treatment in patients with myelodysplastic syndrome. Acta Haematol 1988;80:8–12.

107. Kerndrup G, Bendix-Hansen K, Pedersen B, Ellegaard J, Hokland P. 13-Cis retinoic acid treatment of myelodysplastic syndromes. Leuk Res 1987;11:7–16.

108. Kerndrup G, Bendix-Hansen K, Pedersen B, Ellegaard J, Hokland P. Primary myelodysplastic syndrome: treatment of 6 patients with 13-cis retinoic acid. Scand J Haematol 1986;36(Suppl 45):128–132.

109. Hast R, Lauren SAL, Reizenstein P. Absent clinical effects of retinoic acid and isoretinoin treatment in the myelodysplastic syndrome. Hematol Oncol 1989;7:297–301.

110. Greenberg BR, Durie BGM, Barnett TC, Meyskens FL Jr. Phase I-II study of 13-cis retinoic acid in

myelodysplastic syndrome. Cancer Treat Rep 1985; 69:1369–1374.

111. Gold EJ, Mertlesmann RH, Itri LM, Gee T, Arlin Z, et al. Phase I clinical trial of 13-cis retinoic acid in myelodysplastic syndromes. Cancer Treat Rep 1983; 67:981–986.

112. Abrahm J, Besa EC, Hyzinski M, Finan J, Nowell P. Disappearance of cytogenetic abnormalities and clinical remission during therapy with 13-cis-retinoic acid in a patient with myelodysplastic syndrome: inhibition of the patient's malignant monocytoid clone. Blood 1986;67:1323–1327.

113. Besa EC, Abrahm JL, Bartholomew MJ, Hyzinski M, Nowell PC. Treatment with 13-cis-retinoic acid in transfusion-dependent patients with myelodysplastic syndrome and decreased toxicity with addition of alpha-tocopherol. Am J Med 1990;89:739–747.

114. Clark RE, Jacobs A, Lush CJ, Smith SA. Effect of 13-cis retinoic acid on survival of patients with myelodysplastic syndrome. Lancet 1987;1:763–765.

115. Koeffler HP, Heitjan D, Mertlesmann R, Kolitz JE, Schulman P, et al. Randomized study of 13-cis retinoic acid v placebo in the myelodysplastic disorders. Blood 1988;71:703–708.

116. Warrell RP Jr, Frankel SR, Miller WH, Scheinberg DA, Itri LM, et al. Differentiation therapy of acute promyelocytic leukemia with tretinoin (all-trans-retinoic acid). N Engl J Med 1991;324:1385–1393.

117. Meng-er H, Yu-chen Y, Shu-rong C, Jin-ren C, Jia-Xiang L, et al. Use of all-trans retinoic acid in the treatment of acute promyelocytic leukemia. Blood 1988;72:567–572.

118. Castaigne S, Chomienne C, Daniel MT, Ballerini P, Berger R, Fenaux P, Degos L. All-trans retinoic acid as a differentiation therapy for acute promyelocytic leukemia. I. Clinical results. Blood 1990;76:1704–1709.

119. Ohno R, Naoe T, Hirano M, Kobayashi M, Hirai H, Tubaki K, Oh H. Treatment of myelodysplastic syndromes with all-trans retinoic acid. Blood 1993; 81:1152–1154.

120. Kurzrock R, Estey E, Talpaz M. All-trans retinoic acid: tolerance and biologic effects in myelodysplastic syndrome. J Clin Oncol 1993;11:1489–1495.

121. Kahn MJ, Stadtmauer EA, Edelstein M, Salhaney K, Luger S, et al. Intermittent all-trans retinoic acid (ATRA) for the treatment of myelodysplasia (MDS) (abstract 2514). Blood 1994;84(Suppl 1):632a.

122. Lawrence HJ, Conner K, Kelly MA, Haussler MR, Wallace P, Bagby GC Jr. Cis-retinoic acid stimulates the clonal growth of some myeloid leukemia cells in vitro. Blood 1987;69:302–307.

123. Garewal H, Greenberg B, List A, Kummet T, Buzaid A, Meyskens F. N-(4-hydroxyphenyl) retinamide (4-HPR) therapy in myelodysplastic syndromes (MDS): possible disease acceleration by retinoids (abstract 767). Blood 1987;70(Suppl 1):228A.

124. Vogler WR, Miller DS, Keller JW. 5-Azacytidine (NSC 102816). A new drug for the treatment of myeloblastic leukemia. Blood 1976;48:331–337.

125. Saiki JH, Bodey GP, Hewlett JS, et al. Effect of schedule on activity and toxicity of 5-azacytidine in acute leukemia. A Southwest Oncology Group study. Cancer 1981;47:1739–1742.

126. Glover AB, Leyland-Jones BR, Chun HG, Davies B, Hoth DF. Azacytidine: 10 years later. Cancer Treat Rep 1987;71:737–746.

127. Larson RA, Sweet DL, Golomb HM, Testa JR, Rowley JD. Response to 5-azacytidine in patients with refractory acute nonlymphocytic leukemia and association with chromosome findings. Cancer 1982; 49:2222–2225.

128. Saiki JH, McCredie KB, Vietti TJ, Hewlett JS, Morrison FS, et al. 5-Azacytidine in acute leukemia. Cancer 1978;42:2111–2114.

129. Chitambar CR, Libnoch JA, Matthaeus WG, Ash RC, Ritch PS, Anderson T. Evaluation of continuous infusion low-dose 5-azacytidine in the treatment of myelodysplastic syndromes. Am J Hematol 1991; 37:100–104.

130. Silverman LR, Davis RB, Holland JF, Ellison RR, McIntyre OR, Carey RW, Frei E III. 5-Azacytidine (AZ) as a low dose continuous infusion is an effective therapy for patients with myelodysplastic syndromes (MDS) (abstract 768). Proc Am Soc Clin Oncol 1989; 8:198.

131. Silverman LR, Holland JF, Nelson D, Clamon G, Powell BL, et al. Trilineage (TLR) response of myelodysplastic syndromes (MDS) to subcutaneous (SQ) azacytidine (Aza C) (abstract 747). Proc Am Soc Clin Oncol 1991;10:222.

132. Zagonel V, Pinto A, Attadia V, Sorio R, Alosi M, et al. Phase I-II clinical-biological study of 5-aza-2′-deoxycytidine (5azaCdR) as a differentiation inducer in acute myeloid leukemia (AML) and myelodysplastic syndromes (MDS) of the elderly (abstract 767). Proc Am Soc Clin Oncol 1989;8:197.

133. Koeffler HP, Hirji K, Itri L. 1,25-Dihydroxy-vitamin D3: in vivo and in vitro effects on human preleukemic and leukemic cells. Cancer Treat Rep 1985; 69:1399–1407.

134. Mehta AB, Kumaran TO, Marsh GW. Treatment of advanced myelodysplastic syndrome with alfacalcidol (letter). Lancet 1984;2:761.

135. Andreef M, Stone R, Michaeli J, Young CW, Tong WP, et al. Hexamethylene bisacetamide in myelodysplastic syndrome and acute myelogenous leukemia: a phase II clinical trial with a differentiation-inducing agent. Blood 1992;80:2604–2609.

136. Elias L, Van Epps D, Smith KJ, Savage B. A trial of recombinant α_2 interferon in the myelodysplastic syndrome: II. characterization and response of granulocyte and platelet dysfunction. Leukemia 1987; 1:111–115.

137. Elias L, Hoffman R, Boswell S, Tensen L, Bonnem EM. A trial of recombinant α_2 interferon in the myelodysplastic syndromes: I. clinical results. Leukemia 1987;1:105–110.

138. Aul C, Gattermann N, Schneider W. Treatment of advanced myelodysplastic syndromes with recombinant interferon-alpha 2b. Eur J Haematol 1991; 46:11–16.

139. Rosti V, Carlo-Stella C, Pedrazzoli P, Cazzola M. In vitro and in vivo effects of recombinant interferon gamma on the growth of hematopoietic progenitor cells from patients with myelodysplastic syndrome. Haematologica 1989;74:435–440.

140. Gisslinger H, Chott A, Linkesch W, Fritz E, Ludwig H. Long-term α-interferon therapy in myelodysplastic syndromes. Leukemia 1990;4:91–94.

141. Beran M, Andersson B, Kantarjian H, Keating M, Rios A, et al. Hematologic response of four patients with smoldering acute myelogenous leukemia to partially pure gamma interferon. Leukemia 1987;1:52–57.

142. Maiolo AT, Cortelezzi A, Calori R, Polli EE. Recombinant γ-interferon as first line therapy for high risk myelodysplastic syndromes. Leukemia 1990; 4:480–485.

143. Stone R, Spriggs D, Arthur D, Griffin J, Mayer R, Kufe D. A phase I-II trial of recombinant human interferon gamma (rIFN-gamma) for acute myelocytic leukemia (AML) and myelodysplastic syndromes (MDS) (abstract 805). Proc Am Soc Clin Oncol 1989; 8:207.

144. Antin JH, Smith BR, Holmes W, Rosenthal DS. Phase I/II study of recombinant human granulocyte-macrophage colony-stimulating factor in aplastic anemia and myelodysplastic syndrome. Blood 1988; 72:705–713.

145. Brach M, Klein H, Platzer E, Mertlesmann R, Herrmann F. Effect of interleukin 3 on cytosine arabinoside-mediated cytotoxicity of leukemic myeloblasts. Exp Hematol 1990;18:748–753.

146. Estey EH, Kurzrock R, Talpaz M, McCredie KB, O'Brien S, et al. Effects of low dose recombinant human granulocyte-macrophage colony stimulating factor (GM-CSF) in patients with myelodysplastic syndromes. Br J Haematol 1991;77:291–295.

147. Ganser A, Volkers B, Greher J, Walther F, Hoelzer D. Recombinant human granulocyte-macrophage colony-stimulating factor in patients with myelodysplastic syndromes—a phase I/II trial. Onkologie 1988;11:53–55.

148. Ganser A, Volkers B, Greher J, Ottmann OG, Walther F, et al. Recombinant human granulocyte-macrophage colony-stimulating factor in patients with myelodysplastic syndromes—a phase I/II trial. Blood 1989;73:31–37.

149. Ganser A, Seipelt G, Lindemann A, Ottmann OG, Falk S, et al. Effects of recombinant human interleukin-3 in patients with myelodysplastic syndromes. Blood 1990;76:455–462.

150. Gradishar WJ, Le Beau MM, O'Laughlin R, Vardiman JW, Larson RA. Clinical and cytogenetic responses to granulocyte-macrophage colony-stimulating factor in therapy-related myelodysplasia. Blood 1992;80:2463–2470.

151. Hermann F, Lindemann A, Klein H, Lubbert M, Schultz G, Mertlesmann R. Effect of recombinant human granulocyte-macrophage colony-stimulating factor in patients with myelodysplastic syndrome with excess blasts. Leukemia 1989;3:335–338.

152. Nand S, Sosman J, Godwin JE, Fisher RI. A phase I/II study of sequential interleukin-3 and granulocyte-macrophage colony-stimulating factor in myelodysplastic syndromes. Blood 1994;83:357–360.

153. Negrin RS, Haeuber DH, Nagler A, Olds LC, Donlon T, Souza LM, Greenberg PL. Treatment of myelodysplastic syndromes with recombinant human granulocyte colony-stimulating factor. A phase I-II trial. Ann Intern Med 1989;110:976–984.

154. Thompson JA, Lee DJ, Kidd P, Rubin E, Kaufman J, Bonnem EM, Fefer A. Subcutaneous granulocyte-macrophage colony-stimulating factor in patients with myelodysplastic syndrome: toxicity, pharmacokinetics, and hematological effects. J Clin Oncol 1989; 7:629–637.

155. Vadhan-Raj S, Keating M, LeMaistre A, Hittelman WN, McCredie K, et al. Effects of recombinant human granulocyte-macrophage colony-stimulating

factor in patients with myelodysplastic syndromes. N Engl J Med 1987;317:1545–1552.

156. Vadhan-Raj S, Broxmeyer HE, Spitzer G, LeMaistre A, Hultman S, et al. Stimulation of non-clonal hematopoiesis and suppression of the neoplastic clone after treatment with recombinant human granulocyte-macrophage colony-stimulating factor in a patient with therapy-related myelodysplastic syndrome. Blood 1989;74:1491–1498.

157. Yoshida Y, Hirashima K, Asano S, Takaku F. A phase II trial of recombinant human granulocyte colony-stimulating factor in the myelodysplastic syndromes. Br J Haematol 1991;78:178–184.

158. Estey E, Kurzrock R, Talpaz M, Beran M, Kantarjian H, et al. Therapy of myelodysplastic syndromes (MDS) with GM-CSF (abstract 779). Proc Am Soc Clin Oncol 1989;8:200.

159. Rifkin RM, Hersh EM, Hultquist KN, Salmon SE. Therapy of the myelodysplastic syndrome (MDS) with subcutaneously (SC) administered recombinant human granulocyte-macrophage colony-stimulating factor (abstract 692). Proc Am Soc Clin Oncol 1989; 8:178.

160. Gillio AP, Castro-Malaspina H, Gasparetto C, Small TN, Childs B, et al. A phase I trial of recombinant human interleukin-3 in patients with myelodysplastic syndrome and aplastic anemia (abstract 571). Blood 1990;76(Suppl 1):145a.

161. Negrin RS, Haeuber DH, Nagler A, Kobayashi Y, Sklar J, et al. Maintenance treatment of patients with myelodysplastic syndromes using recombinant human granulocyte colony-stimulating factor. Blood 1990; 76:36–43.

162. Schuster MW, Larson R, Thompson JA, Coiffier B, Bennett JM, Israel RJ. Granulocyte-macrophage colony-stimulating factor (GM-CSF) for myelodysplastic syndrome (MDS): results of a multi-center randomized controlled clinical trial (abstract 1263). Blood 1990; 76(Suppl 1):318a.

163. American Society of Clinical Oncology. American Society of Clinical Oncology recommendations for the use of hematopoietic colony-stimulating factors: evidence-based clinical practice guidelines. J Clin Oncol 1994;12:2471–2508.

164. Jacobs A, Janowska-Wieczorek A, Caro J, Bowen DT, Lewis T. Circulating erythropoietin in patients with myelodysplastic syndromes. Br J Haematol 1989;73:36–39.

165. Bowen DT, Jacobs A, Cotes MP, Lewis TC. Serum erythropoietin and erythropoiesis in patients with myelodysplastic syndromes. Eur J Haematol 1990; 44:30–32.

166. Schouten HC, Vallenga E, van Rhenen D, de Wolf JTM, Coppens PJW, Blijham GH. Recombinant human erythropoietin (rhEPO) for patients with a myelodysplastic syndrome (MDS) (abstract 1280). Blood 1990;76(Suppl 1):317a.

167. Hellstrom E, Birgegard G, Lockner D, Helmers C, Wide L, Ost A. Treatment of myelodysplastic syndromes with recombinant human erythropoietin (abstract 1106). Blood 1990;76(Suppl 1):279a.

168. Stein RS, Abels RI, Krantz SB. Pharmacologic doses of recombinant human erythropoietin in the treatment of myelodysplastic syndromes. Blood 1991; 78:1658–1663.

169. Stebler C, Tichelli A, Dazzi H, Gratwohl A, Nissen C, Speck B. High-dose recombinant human erythropoietin for treatment of anemia in myelodysplastic syndromes and paroxysmal nocturnal hemoglobinuria: a pilot study. Exp Hematol 1990;18:1204–1208.

170. Negrin RS, Stein R, Vardiman J, Doherty K, Cornwell J, Krantz A, Greenberg PL. Treatment of the anemia of myelodysplastic syndromes using recombinant human granulocyte colony-stimulating factor in combination with erythropoietin. Blood 1993;82:737–743.

171. Cannistra SA, Groshek P, Griggin JD. Granulocyte-macrophage colony-stimulating factor enhances the cytotoxic effects of cytosine arabinoside in acute myeloblastic leukemia and in the myeloid blast crisis phase of chronic myeloid leukemia. Leukemia 1989; 3:328–334.

172. Witte ON. Steel locus defines a new multipotent growth factor. Cell 1990;63:5–6.

173. Asano S, Okano A, Ozawa K, Nakahata T, Ishibashi T, et al. In vivo effects of recombinant human interleukin-6 in primates: stimulated production of platelets. Blood 1990;75:1602–1605.

174. Demetri GD, Bukowski RM, Samuels B, Gordon M, Antman K, et al. Stimulation of thrombopoiesis by recombinant human interleukin-6 (IL-6) pre- and post-chemotherapy in previously untreated sarcoma patients with normal hematopoiesis (abstract 1452). Blood 1993;82(Suppl 1):367.

175. Teramura M, Kobayashi S, Hoshino S, Oshimi K, Mizoguchi H. Interleukin-11 enhances human megakaryocytopoiesis in vitro. Blood 1992;79:327–331.

176. Vadhan-Raj S, Papadopoulos NE, Burgess MA, Linke KA, Patel SR, et al. Effects of PIXY321, a granulocyte-macrophage colony-stimulating factor/interleukin-3 fusion protein, on chemotherapy-induced multilineage myelosuppression in patients with sarcoma. J Clin Oncol 1994;12:715–724.

177. Kaushansky K, Lok S, Holly RD, et al. Promotion of megakaryocyte progenitor expansion and differentiation by the c-Mpl ligand thrombopoietin. Nature 1994;369:568–571.

178. Lok S, Kaushansky K, Holly RD, et al. Cloning and expression of murine thrombopoietin and stimulation of platelet production in vivo. Nature 1994; 369:565–568.

179. Wendling F, Maraskovsky E, Debili N, et al. c-Mpl ligand is a humoral regulator of megakaryocytopoiesis. Nature 1994;369:571–574.

180. de Sauvage FJ, Hass PE, Spencer SD, et al. Stimulation of megakaryocytopoiesis and thrombopoiesis by the c-Mpl ligand. Nature 1994;369:533–538.

181. Cheson BD, Cassileth PA, Head DR, Schiffer CA, Bennett JM, et al. Report of the National Cancer Institute-sponsored workshop on definitions of diagnosis and response in acute myeloid leukemia. J Clin Oncol 1990;8:813–819.

67

Chemotherapy of Myeloproliferative Disorders

James K. Weick

In 1951, Damashek was the first to use the term "myeloproliferative syndrome" to characterize a group of bone marrow disorders with similar features of proliferation of blood cells of different lineages (1). The disorders described, then and now, include polycythemia vera, chronic myelogenous leukemia, myelofibrosis with myeloid metaplasia, and primary thrombocytosis. Numerous authors have concluded that these disorders are proliferative abnormalities of a pluripotent hematopoietic stem cell. Such information was derived both from chromosome analyses showing identical cytogenetic abnormalities in erythroid and myeloid precursors and from the descriptions of a single G6PD isoenzyme from all hematopoietic cell lines (2–4).

The therapies of myeloproliferative disorders (MPDs) have been advanced through the efforts of Dr. Louis Wasserman and the members of the Polycythemia Vera Study Group (PVSG), a cooperative group established in the mid-1960s to investigate the problems associated with the treatment of polycythemia vera. A natural outgrowth of this unique group was the inclusion of myelofibrosis and primary thrombocytosis among the diseases to be studied. Chronic myelogenous leukemia (CML) (or chronic granulocytic leukemia (CGL)) was not a disease felt to be in the purview of the PVSG, and contributions to the treatment of this disease have been made by cooperative groups and worldwide authors, alike.

POLYCYTHEMIA VERA

The Polycythemia Vera Study Group has established the standards for both the diagnosis and therapy of this relatively rare disease. The annual incidence is estimated to be approximately one case per 100,000 population, with a mean age of onset at 60 years and a slight male predominance (5). Realizing that there are complications that may be encountered and/or transitions to more aggressive myeloproliferative diseases, it may be expected that the overall survival of treated patients should be comparable to that of age-matched control groups drawn from the United States' population (6).

The goal of therapy for polycythemia vera (PV) is to establish normal hematologic blood counts; this can be accomplished either by phlebotomy or chemotherapy. All would agree that the initial objective of therapy is a hematocrit of 40 to 42%, obtained by phlebotomies of 250 to 500 mL approximately every other day. Obviously, such therapy does not control thrombocytosis, but subsequent therapy with myelosuppressive agents is much easier to achieve and maintain once the above mechanical action has been performed. The landmark study of the PVSG was the 01 study, which compared phlebotomy with chlorambucil with radioactive phosphorus (^{32}P) (7). Briefly, this study showed that patients treated with phlebotomy alone had excessive thrombotic complications in the first 3 to 4 years, whereas those treated with myelosuppression developed an increased incidence of acute leukemia and carcinomas of the skin and gastrointestinal tract at later times. The leukemia incidence was greatest in those persons treated with chlorambucil and became apparent by the 5th year. So high was this incidence that the chlorambucil arm of this study was discontinued and patients were randomized only to phlebotomy versus ^{32}P. A more recent update by Najean confirms the continued risk for developing cancers for myelosuppressive agents for at least 5 years after stopping therapy (8). The long-term risks for the phlebotomy group are those associated with myelofibrosis and subsequent agnogenic myeloid metaplasia, which may affect 50% of the patient population surviving 15 years or more.

No significant differences in survival were noted for the first 7 years of the 01 study. Attempts were made by the statistical center to determine factors defining the risk for thrombosis. While it was postulated that elevated platelet counts were a significant risk factor for thrombotic complications, a retrospective matched-pair study failed to show that either the level of the platelet count or hematocrits were associated with increased risks of thrombotic events. Elements that did appear to be contributing factors were high phlebotomy requirements, advanced age, and a history of prior thrombosis.

Phlebotomy has the advantage of rapidly decreasing the blood volume but also has the adverse effect of creating iron deficiency with its attendant ineffective erythropoiesis, cheilitis, glossitis, and other effects of tissue iron depletion (9). Along with the discomfort of repeated venesections, such measures also stimulate hematopoiesis, which increases platelet production and thus predisposes to further thrombotic problems. This latter complication prompted the PVSG to consider and complete a trial (PVSG-05) comparing radioactive phosphorus with phlebotomy plus the antiplatelet-aggregating agents aspirin and Persantine. The study was unable to demonstrate a decrease in thrombotic complications with the addition of aspirin (ASA) plus Persantine at the doses utilized. Additionally, an increase of hemorrhagic tendencies in patients treated with the antiplatelet agents was observed (10).

If chemotherapy agents are used in a maintenance phase, the most widely used and accepted is hydroxyurea; this is a ribonucleotide reductase inhibitor that has a wider therapeutic range in all MPDs than busulfan. In polycythemia, hydroxyurea therapy, supplemented by phlebotomy to maintain a normal hematocrit, diminishes the risk of thrombosis associated with phlebotomy alone (11, 12). Doses that are effective in the myeloproliferative disorders are generally in the range of 15 mg/kg per day, orally, both in PV as well as CML and primary thrombocytosis.

Radioactive phosphorus, administered either intravenously or orally, has proven efficacy in the management of polycythemia vera (13). As utilized in the initial 01 protocol, patients were phlebotomized to a normal hematocrit and then treated with 2.3 mCi/m^2 body surface intravenously to a maximum of 5 mCi per dose. Additional doses were possible after 12 weeks, with subsequent doses not to exceed a total yearly dose of 15 mCi. Using these parameters, control was accomplished in approximately 80% of all patients treated, and responses were long lasting. Overdosage can be seen with hypoplasia and possible leukemic evolution. In general, the toxicities of ^{32}P are intermediate between those of phlebotomy and chlorambucil.

The interferons have recently been introduced into the clinical armamentarium for myeloproliferative disorders. There is a long history of usage of this medicine in chronic myelocytic leukemia (see below), but only recently has this work been extended in the smaller numbers of patients for polycythemia vera. These advantages were seen in randomized trials as well as in pilot studies. In all instances, initial therapies were undertaken with phlebotomy to a normal hematocrit followed by maintenance therapy with α-interferon. Dosages employed varied from 3.0×10^6 U/m^2 subcutaneously three times a week to 3 million units daily for as long as 5 months (14, 15).

Thus, it may be seen that there is no single best therapeutic approach to the patient with PV. Repetitive phlebotomies are necessary initially to achieve normal values. The choice then becomes whether to use maintenance phlebotomy therapy or radioactive phosphorus in patients of non-child-bearing ages or myelosuppressive chemotherapy. Hydroxyurea and busulfan are probably more utilized in this country than the equally beneficial radioactive phosphorus, perhaps because of their ready availability.

The goal of therapy is to maintain the hematocrit levels below 45 because of the known inverse relationship between hematocrit and cerebral blood flow (16). With the dissolution of the PVSG, there have been few protocols dealing with the management of polycythemia vera, and the above represents the knowledge in 1987, which continues to date (17). Using follow-up data from the PVSG, long-term follow-up has determined that the median survival for phlebotomy-treated cases is 13.9 years, chlorambucil 9.1 years, and ^{32}P, 11.8 years.

AGNOGENIC MYELOID METAPLASIA (AMM)

This myeloproliferative disorder has been described with nearly as many different names as there are cases annually! The terms agnogenic myeloid metaplasia and idiopathic myelofibrosis are the two most commonly used in the literature. The syndrome has been recognized since the late 1800s and was initially characterized by reports of patients with splenomegaly, osteosclerosis, and a "leukemia-like" blood picture (18). It is likely that many of the early cases were in fact secondary myelofibrosis, incited by either infection or malignancy. Before the introduction by Damashek of the concept of myeloproliferative syndromes, Block in 1950 described myeloid metaplasia as an entity of its own, of unknown origin, closely related to polycythemia but with recognizable differences (19). A further contribution to the literature was established in 1975 with the description of studies of patients with myelofibrosis and G6PD heterozygosity who were shown to have only one type of G6PD in their red cells, white cells, and platelets (20). A book entirely devoted to the subject was published in that same year by Silverstein (21). Despite efforts to reverse the accompanying fibrosis of the marrow, the therapy of AMM remains supportive. Many efforts by well-intended clinicians have changed median survivals from an initial report of 7.5 years to later reports as low as 1.5 years, despite no seeming change in the clinical picture of this illness (22). Many patients are diagnosed in an asymptomatic condition and can remain so for many years; this should be a valuable lesson that no therapy may be required initially.

The principal problem involved in all patients with AMM is anemia: in at least 60% of patients, the hemoglobin value falls to less than 10 g/dL within 5 years of diagnosis, necessitating transfusion or therapy of any deficient hematinic (23). This anemia is often multifactorial and represents contributions from dyserythropoiesis, hemodilution from expanded blood volumes, hemolysis, both Coombs' positive and Coombs' negative, hypoproliferative anemia from the marrow fibrosis, and possibly iron deficiency from bleeding associated with portal hypertension (massive splenomegaly). Splenomegaly, which always accompanies this disorder, may be contributing in part to the anemia by shortening red cell life spans via overt hemolysis, and either prednisone and/or folic acid may be of some value (24).

Many clinicians would also begin a trial of androgen therapy, with an expected response rate of approximate 40% in these individuals. Such drugs and dosages could include oxymetholone 200 mg daily, danazol 200 mg three times daily, both given orally, or parenteral testosterone enanthate at a dose of 400 mg given intramuscularly weekly (25). The use of erythropoietin has largely been unsuccessful, and except for an occasional anecdotal report, it is not to be used on a regular basis (26).

Splenectomy should be considered in patients in whom it is felt that splenic hematopoiesis is contributing only a minor portion of total hematopoiesis (27). This can usually be estimated by some measurement of bone marrow imaging. Indications have been proffered for surgery in this disease: (a) painful or massive enlargement of the spleen, (b) refractory severe thrombocytopenia, (c) portal hypertension with varices, and (d) uncontrollable hemolytic or dilutional anemia severe enough to warrant this consideration (21). In published series, postoperative mortality ran as high as 10%, with the primary complication being hemorrhage in approximately one-third of cases and septicemia in an additional 10% of cases. When therapy is effective, the quality of life is markedly improved in survivors. Despite these possible benefits of surgery, life expectancy postoperatively averages 1 to 2 years.

Bone marrow transplantation is the only potential curative modality available today for AMM. Interest in this treatment was generated because of the successful transplantation and reversible marrow fibrosis following transplantation for CML with fibrosis as well as in cases of acute myelofibrosis (acute megakaryoblastic leukemia) (28). Because of the age of the patients involved and the lack of suitable donors, the possibility of transplantation is rare.

Because of the in vitro activity of α-interferon to suppress megakaryocytic and even collagen synthesis by murine fibroblasts as well as the reversibility of increased platelet levels of platelet-derived growth factor and transforming growth factor-β (TGF-β) in patients with myelofibrosis, authors have reported benefits, both in improving hematologic values as well as in shrinking spleens (29–31). To date, there is little information that other cytokines have any efficacy in the management of myelofibrosis. Several biologic agents, including suramin and tumor necrosis factor, can suppress TGF-β activity in vitro and offer a theoretical advantage to inhibit bone marrow fibrosis, but they have shown no clinical benefit in small reported series (32).

It remains clear that the essential supportive feature of therapy for AMM remains red cell transfusions as required. In most investigators' experience, the use of myelosuppressive agents such as busulfan, hydroxyurea, or even splenic artery cytosine arabinoside may reduce spleen size and control thrombocytosis, but with little effect on the anemia that is the major symptom (33–37). Similarly, focal radiation therapy may be of advantage in treating the pain of splenic infarction or splenic enlargement itself. This benefit is usually short-lived, and progressive disease is inevitable.

PRIMARY THROMBOCYTOSIS

Primary thrombocytosis, also called essential thrombocythemia or primary thrombocythemia, is the least common of the myeloproliferative disorders, and the PVSG is also responsible for establishing the criteria of this disease (38). These criteria include (a) platelet count in excess of 600,000/μL, (b) a hemoglobin below 13 g or a normal red cell mass, (c) stainable iron in the marrow or the failure of an iron trial to raise the hemoglobin after 1 month, (d) the absence of a Philadelphia chromosome, and (e) the relative paucity of any collagen fibrosis in the bone marrow with no other cause for reactive thrombocytosis. Such reactive disorders are legion and include iron deficiency, chronic inflammatory and infectious diseases, drugs, myelodysplasia, and prior splenectomy.

As in other myeloproliferative disorders, this disease typically presents in the 6th and 7th decades of life, without sex predilection, and has the propensity to both hemorrhage and thrombosis (39). Bleeding tends to involve mucous membrane surfaces, whereas thrombosis may involve both arterial and venous systems (40).

Although this disorder usually requires therapy upon diagnosis in elderly populations, Hoagland and Silverstein reported identical findings of a benign nature in patients under the age of 30, which may require no therapy (41). While morbidity is certainly a major concern in all patients diagnosed with primary thrombocytosis, normal life expectancy would be very common in this group of patients. Transformation and evolution into other myeloproliferative disorders is well established.

Therapies, when instituted, are geared toward reducing the platelet count toward normal. This may be required expeditiously because of hemorrhagic or thrombotic complications in which plateletpheresis is the quickest example of relief (42, 43). More often, time is not critical, and a more casual approach to therapy can be employed. Many of the agents proposed for either polycythemia vera or chronic myelogenous leu-

kemia are also beneficial in cases of thrombocytosis (44).

Despite the criteria for establishing the diagnosis, few criteria exist for timing the institution of therapy. Many will use the following criteria: for a platelet count of below 600,000/μL, no therapy; 600,000 to 1 million, therapy is "considered," and more than 1 million, most investigators will treat unless the patient is "very young." Results of the PVSG study for patients with between 600,000 and 1 million platelets/μL suggest that myelosuppressive therapy is much to be favored over platelet-antiaggregating agents (38). The use of these latter agents, including aspirin, dipyridamole, ticlopidine, and pyrimethamine, can normalize platelet aggregability but may lead to hemorrhagic complications (45, 46). Busulfan and hydroxyurea are probably equal in benefit, and the clinician must decide which of these agents would be helpful. Most would probably use hydroxyurea because of its rapid onset and offset of action. α-Interferon similarly has been of established efficacy in both decreasing platelet counts and resolving thrombocytosis-related symptoms (29, 47–52).

The most recent drug to be used in thrombocytosis disorders is anagrelide (55, 56). This drug has the unique ability to decrease platelet counts without markedly affecting either red blood cell activity or white cell count.

CHRONIC MYELOGENOUS LEUKEMIA

Chronic granulocytic leukemia (CGL), or chronic myeloid leukemia (CML), represents approximately 25% of all cases of adult leukemia and occurs with a slight male predominance at a median age of 50 years. Major advances noted in this disease involve the descriptions of the molecular biology of the Philadelphia chromosome and the therapies of this disease via bone marrow transplantation.

The description in 1960 of the Philadelphia chromosome has been greatly enhanced by the description of the abnormality at a narrow 5.8-kilobase fragment, also called the breakpoint cluster region (bcr) (55). There is translocation of genetic material between chromosomes 9 and 22, which places the Abelson protoncogene sequence from chromosome 9 to the bcr gene on chromosome 22 (56). This hybrid bcr-abl gene translates into a larger 8.5-kb mRNA and a 200-kDa protein with the potential to mediate oncogenesis (57).

The therapy of chronic-phase CML is very effective in obtaining a hematologic remission, but in only rare instances is there a conversion of the Philadelphia chromosome (58). The effective drug agents during this period include oral antimetabolites such as 6-mercaptopurine, 6-thioguanine, and hydroxyurea or oral alkylating agents such as busulfan, chlorambucil, cyclophosphamide, and alkeran; additional methods of treatment that have been successful have included splenectomy, splenic radiation, and radioactive phosphorus, all of which produce equivalent results (59–61). Attempts to use more severe myelosuppressive treatment with acute leukemia therapies have increased median survivals from the usual 36 to 42 months to an average of 50 to 60 months with these more intensive regimens (62–64). None, however, is equivalent to a cure.

Both α and γ interferons have been used extensively, and conversion to Philadelphia-negative disease has been reported (65–67). Current protocols in cooperative group settings are looking at the contribution of interferons to either hydroxyurea or alkylating agents.

The utility of busulfan has certainly been established in the 30 years of its existence (33). Historically, this has been the most popular agent for use in the chronic phase of CML, usually administered at doses of 4 to 6 mg daily from the time of diagnosis until the white blood cell count recedes below 20,000. Recognizing that the nadir of the white blood cell count generally occurs approximately 2 weeks after stopping busulfan, this can be a very safe drug as long as the above precautions are used. In general, the dose of busulfan should be reduced by 50% when the white count is reduced by 50%. Therapy is reinstituted whenever the white blood count exceeds 25,000 to 30,000 or there is any other attendant cytopenia. Such intermittent therapies can be managed with periodic office follow-ups until accelerated or blastic-phase CGL intervenes. The toxicities of busulfan are well detailed elsewhere in this volume and should be known to all treating physicians.

Many clinicians believe that the toxicities and difficulty of handling busulfan make hydroxyurea a much more desirable agent. This ribonucleotide reductase inhibitor, a cell cycle–specific antagonist of DNA synthesis, has a more rapid onset of action, and perhaps more importantly, the drug effect is gone much more rapidly upon discontinuing medication (38). As with alkylating agents, therapy is generally administered continuously. A standard starting oral dose in all myeloproliferative disorders is 15 to 30 mg/kg/day. Maintenance doses are generally on the order of 500 to 1500 mg daily, but this may be altered up or down depending on how sensitive or resistant the malignant clone is to the medication.

A rare complication of CGL is a hyperleukocytosis syndrome, which may require a leukapheresis similar to plateletpheresis for primary thrombocytosis (68). Such emergencies could conceivably occur in patients with neurologic symptoms, bleeding, or priapism.

Splenic irradiation can also dramatically reduce spleen size if it is painful or decrease blood counts rapidly. Similar efforts use hemibody radiation and total body radiation in an attempt to achieve one to two log cell kills.

Investigations are also in progress looking at new agents such as homoharringtonine, low-dose cytosine arabinoside, retinoic acids, and 2-CDA.

Any of the above measures are successful in establishing hematologic normalcy during chronic-phase CML. None has significantly changed the median survivals of this disease, which (as mentioned) vary from 36 to 42 months (69). Only the introduction of bone marrow transplantation has made cure a reasonable expectation in patients in whom such a procedure is possible (69–72). The transplant community would suggest that transplantation is desirable at the time of diagnosis, but often this is not realistic, and most agree that any time during the first year after diagnosis offers similar survival advantages. After the first year of diagnosis, the incidence of accelerated or blastic phase increases dramatically, and during these phases, transplant cures are less likely.

The best situation is with a syngeneic (identical twin) transplant, and second is a matched sibling donor allogeneic transplantation. Autologous transplantations are usually reserved for patients in blastic transformation, who are given samples of their own chronic phase bone marrow if hematologic control has been achieved with acute leukemia treatments (73). This approach is inferior to giving normal bone marrows of a donor population (74).

Investigative trials at transplant centers are looking at different preparatory regimens. Historically, these have used either a combination of busulfan plus Cytoxan or total body irradiation with Cytoxan. When bone marrow transplantation is performed in the chronic phase, survivals and remissions approach 70 to 75%;

this number is decreased to approximately 25 to 30% if transplantation is performed during blastic transformation of CGL. Clearly, marrow transplantation is the treatment of choice in chronic myelogenous leukemia.

REFERENCES

1. Damashek W. Some speculations on the myeloproliferative syndromes. Blood 1951;6:372–375.

2. Adamson JW, Fialkow PJ, Murphy S, et al. Polycythemia vera: stem-cell and probable clonal origin of the disease. N Engl J Med 1976;295:913–916.

3. Fialkow PJ, Faquet GB, Jacobson RJ, et al. Evidence that essential thrombocythemia is a clonal disorder with origin in a multipotent stem cell. Blood 1981;58:916–919.

4. Knuutila S, Ruutu T, Partanen S, Vuopio P. Chromosome lqt in erythroid and granulocyte-monocyte precursors in a patient with essential thrombocythemia. Cancer Genet Gytogenet 1983;9:245–249.

5. Berlin NI. Diagnosis and classification of the polycythemias. Semin Hematol 1975;12:339–351.

6. Wasserman LR. A cooperative study of polycythemia vera. Ann NY Acad Sci 1985;459:328–333.

7. Berk PD, Goldberg JD, Donovan PB, et al. Therapeutic recommendations in Polycythemia Vera Study Group Protocols. Semin Hematol 1986;23:132–143.

8. Najean Y, Dresch C, Rain J-D. The very-long-term course of polycythaemia: a complement to the previously published data of the Polycythemia Vera Study Group. Br J Haematol 1994;86:244–235.

9. Hutton RD. The effect of iron deficiency on whole blood viscosity in polycythaemic patients. Br J Haematol 1979;43:191–199.

10. Tartaglía AP, Goldberg JD, Berk PD, Wasserman LR. Adverse effects of antiaggregating platelet therapy in the treatment of polycythemia vera. Semin Hematol 1986;23:172–176.

11. Kaplan ME, Mack K, Goldberg JD, et al. Long-term management of polycythemia vera with hydroxyurea: a progress report. Semin Hematol 1986;23:167–171.

12. Boivin P. Indications, procedure and results for the treatment of polycythemia vera by bleeding, pipobroman and hydroxyurea. Nouv Rev FR Hematol 1993;35:491–498.

13. Hoffman R, Wasserman LR. Natural history and management of polycythemia vera. Adv Intern Med 1979;24:255–285.

14. Silver RT. Interferon-alpha-2b: a new treatment for polycythemia vera. Ann Intern Med 1993;119:1091–1092.

15. Sacchi S, Leoni P, Liberati M, et al. A prospective comparison between treatment with phlebotomy alone and with interferon alpha in patients with polycythemia vera. Ann Hematol 1994;68:247–250.

16. Thomas DJ, Marshall J, Russell RW, et al. Effect of haematocrit on cerebral blood-flow in man. Lancet 1977;2(8045):941–943.

17. Wasserman LR. Polycythemia Vera Study Group: a historical perspective. Semin Hematol 1986; 23:183–187.

18. Donhauser JL. The human spleen as an haematoplastic organ, as exemplified in a case of splenomegaly with sclerosis of the bone marrow. J Exp Med 1908;10:559–574.

19. Ward HP, Block MH. The natural history of agnogenic myeloid metaplasia (AMM) and a critical evaluation of its relationship with the myeloproliferative syndrome. Medicine (Baltimore) 1971;50(5):357–420.

20. Kahn A, Bernard JF, Cottreau D, Marie J, Boivin P. A deficient G-6PD variant with hemizygous expression in blood cells of a woman with primary myelofibrosis. Humangenetik 1975;30(1):41–46.

21. Silverstein MN. Agnogenic myeloid metaplasia. Acton, MA: Publishing Sciences Group, 1975.

22. Silverstein MN, Gomes MR, ReMine WH, Elveback LR. Agnogenic myeloid metaplasia. Natural history and treatment. Arch Intern Med 1967; 120(5):546–550.

23. Njoku OS, Lewis SM, Catovsky D, Gordon-Smith EC. Anaemia in myelofibrosis: its value in prognosis. Br J Haematol 1983;54(1):79–89.

24. Pettit JE, Lewis SM, Williams ED, Grafton CA, Bowring CS, Glass HI. Quantitative studies of splenic erythropoiesis in polycythaemia vera and myelofibrosis. Br J Haematol 1976;34(3):465–475.

25. Weinstein IM. Idiopathic myelofibrosis: historical review, diagnosis and management. Blood Rev 1991;5:98–104.

26. Iki S, Yagisawa M, Ohbayashi Y, Sato H, Urabe A. Adverse effect of erythropoietin in myeloproliferative disorders (letter). Lancet 1991;337(8734):187–188.

27. Benbassat J, Penchas S, Ligumski M. Splenectomy in patients with agnogenic myeloid metaplasia: an analysis of 321 published cases. Br J Haematol 1979; 42(2):207–214.

28. McGlave PR, Brunning RD, Hurd DD, Kim TH. Reversal of severe bone marrow fibrosis and osteosclerosis following allogeneic bone marrow transplantation for chronic granulocytic leukaemia. Br J Haematol 1982;52(2):189–194.

29. Appelbaum FR. Introduction and overview of interferon alfa in myeloproliferative and hemangiomatous diseases. Semin Hematol 1990;27(Suppl 4):1–5.

30. Furesi L, Pasini FL, Forconi S. Interferon alpha-2b in the treatment of myelofibrosis. Haematologica 1990;75(6):587–589.

31. Kanfer EJ, Price CM, Gordon AA, Barrett AJ. The in vitro effects of interferon-gamma, interferon-alpha and tumor necrosis factor-alpha on erythroid burst forming unit growth in patients with non-leukemic myeloproliferative disorders. Eur J Haematol 1993;50:250–254.

32. Tefferi A, Silverstein MN, Plumhoff EA, Reid JM, Ames MM. Suramin toxicity and efficacy in agnogenic myeloid metaplasia. J Natl Cancer Inst 1993; 8518;1520–1522.

33. Buggia I, Locatell F, Regazzi MB, Zecca M. Busulfan. Ann Pharmacother 1994;28:1055–1062.

34. Lofvenberg E, Nilsson T, Wahlin A, Jacobsson L. Hydroxyurea treatment of myeloproliferative disorders. Acta Med Scand 1987;222:169–174.

35. Lofvenberg E, Wahlin A, Roos G, Ost A. Reversal of myelofibrosis by hydroxyurea. Eur J Haematol 1990;44:33–38.

36. Manoharan A. Management of myelofibrosis with intermittent hydroxyurea. Br J Haematol 1991; 77(2):252–254.

37. Slocombe GW, Turner MJ, Newland AC. Massive splenomegaly in myeloproliferative disorders treated by splenic artery infusion of cytarabine. Clin Lab Haematol 1986;8(1):9–19.

38. Murphy S, Iland H, Rosenthal D, Laszlo J. Essential thrombocythemia: an interim report from the Polycythemia Vera Study Group. Semin Hematol 1986; 23:177–182.

39. Wehmeier A, Daum I, Jamin H, Schneider W. Incidence and clinical risk factors for bleeding and thrombotic complications in myeloproliferative disorders. Ann Hematol 1991;63:101–106.

40. Schafer AI. Essential thrombocythemia. Prog Hemost Thromb 1991;10:69–96.

41. Hoagland HC, Silverstein MN. Primary thrombocythemia in the young patient. Mayo Clin Proc 1978; 53:578–580.

42. Adami R. Therapeutic thrombocytopheresis: a review of 132 patients. Int J Artif Organs 1993;16:183–184.

43. Panlilio AL, Reiss RF. Therapeutic plateletpheresis in thrombocythemia. Transfusion 1979; 19(2):147–152.

44. Mitus AJ, Schafer AI. Thrombocytosis and thrombocythemia. Hematol Oncol Clin North Am 1990;4(1):157–178.

45. Bowcock SJ, Linch DC, Machin SJ, Stewart JW. Pyrimethamine in the myeloproliferative disorders: a forgotten treatment? Clin Lab Haematol 1987;9(2):129–136.

46. Ruggeri M, Castaman G, Rodeghiero F. Is Ticlopidine a safe alternative to aspirin for management of myeloproliferative disorders? Haematologica 1993; 78(Suppl):18–21.

47. Lazzarino M, Vitale A, Morra E, et al. Interferon alpha-2b as treatment for Philadelphia-negative chronic myeloproliferative disorders with excessive thrombocytosis. Br J Haematol 1989;72:173–177.

48. Ludwig H, Linkesch W, Gisslinger H, et al. Interferon-alpha corrects thrombocytosis in patients with myeloproliferative disorders. Cancer Immunol Immunother 1987;25:266–273.

49. Silver RT. Interferon in the treatment of myeloproliferative diseases. Semin Hematol 1990;27(Suppl 4):6–14.

50. Talpaz M, Kurzrock R, Kantarjian H, O'Brien S, Gutterman JU. Recombinant interferon alpha therapy of Philadelphia chromosome-negative myeloproliferative disorders with thrombocytosis. Am J Med 1989;86(5):554–558.

51. Tichelli A, Gratwohl A, Berger C, et al. Treatment of thrombocytosis in myeloproliferative disorders with interferon alpha-2a. Blut 1989;58:15–19.

52. Gisslinger H, Ludwig H, Linkesch W, Chott A, Fritz E, Radaszkiewicz T. Long-term interferon therapy for thrombocytosis in myeloproliferative diseases. Lancet 1989;8639:634–637.

53. Silverstein MN, Petitt RM, Solberg LA, Fleming JS, Knight RC, Schacter LP. Anagrelide: a new drug for treating thrombocytosis. N Engl J Med 1988;318:1292–1294.

54. Spencer CM, Brogden RN. Anagrelide: a review of its pharmacodynamic and pharmacokinetic properties, and therapeutic potential in the treatment of thrombocythaemia. Drugs 1994;47(6):809–822.

55. Heisterkamp N, Stam K, Groffen J. Structural organization of the bcr gene and its role in the Ph[1] translocation (letter). Nature 1985;315:758–761.

56. Shtivelman E, Lifshitz B, Gale RP, et al. Fused transcript of abl and bcr genes in chronic myelogenous leukemia. Nature 1985;315:550–554.

57. Clark SS, McLaughlin J, Crist WM, et al. Reports: unique forms of the abl tyrosine kinase distinguish Ph[1]-positive CML from Ph[1]-positive ALL. Science 1987;235:85–88.

58. Moloney WC. Natural history of chronic granulocytic leukemia. Clin Haematol 1977;6(1):41–53.

59. Kennedy BJ, Yarbro JW. Metabolic and therapeutic effects of hydroxyurea in chronic myelogenous leukemia. Cancer 1972;29:1052–1056.

60. Koeffler HP, Golde DW. Chronic myelogenous leukemia—new concepts (second of two parts). N Engl J Med 1981;304(21):1269–1274.

61. Reinhard EH, Neely L, Samples DM. Radioactive phosphorus in the treatment of chronic leukemias: long term results over a period of 15 years. Ann Intern Med 1959;50:942–958.

62. Cunningham I, Gee T, Dowling M, et al. Results of treatment of Ph1 + chronic myelogenous leukemia with an intensive treatment regimen (L5-protocol). Blood 1979;53:375–395.

63. Hester JP, Waddell CC, Coltman CA, et al. Response of chronic myelogenous leukemia patients to COAP-splenectomy: a Southwest Oncology Group Study. Cancer 1984;54:1977–1982.

64. Kantarjian HM, Vellekoop L, McCredie KB, et al. Intensive chemotherapy (ROAP 10) and splenectomy in patients with Philadelphia positive chronic myelogenous leukemia. J Clin Oncol 1985;3:192–200.

65. Kurzrock R, Talpaz M, Kantarjian H, et al. Phase II study of recombinant interferon gamma in chronic myelogenous leukemia (abstract). Blood 1986; 68:225a.

66. Talpaz M, Kantarjian HM, McCredie K, et al. Hematologic remission and cytogenetic improvement induced by recombinant human interferon alpha A in a chronic myelogenous leukemia. N Engl J Med 1986; 314:1065–1069.

67. Talpaz M, Kantarjian HM, McCredie KB, et al. Clinical investigation of human alpha interferon in chronic myelogenous leukemia. Blood 1987;69:1280–1288.

68. Lowenthal RM, Buskard NA, Goldman JM, et al. Intensive leukapheresis as initial therapy for chronic granulocytic leukemia. Blood 1975;46(6):835–844.

69. Fefer A, Cheever M, Thomas E, et al. Disappearance of Ph[1]-positive cells in four patients with chronic granulocytic leukemia after chemotherapy, irradiation and marrow transplantation from an identical twin. N Engl J Med 1979;300:333–337.

70. Goldman JM. Bone marrow transplantation for chronic myeloid leukaemia. Hematol Oncol 1987; 5:265–279.

71. McGlave PB, Arthur D, Haake R, et al. Therapy of chronic myelogenous leukemia with allogeneic bone marrow transplantation. J Clin Oncol 1987;5:1033–1040.

72. McCullough J, Scott EP, Halagan N, Strand R, McGlave P. Effectiveness of a regional bone marrow donor program in providing donors for unrelated bone marrow transplantation. JAMA 1988;259:3286–3289.

73. Marcus RE, Goldman JM. Autografting in chronic granulocytic leukemia. Clin Hematol 1986; 15:235–247.

74. Thomas ED, Clift RA, Fefer A, et al. Marrow transplantation for the treatment of chronic myelogenous leukemia. Ann Intern Med 1986;104:155–163.

68

Chemotherapy of Multiple Myeloma and Related Plasma Cell Dyscrasias

Mehdi Farhangi and Ali Khojasteh

TREATMENT OF MULTIPLE MYELOMA

The malignant cells in multiple myeloma have traditionally been thought of as terminally differentiated B cells that avidly synthesize and secrete immunoglobulin and characteristically exhibit low proliferative activity. The accumulation of large numbers of plasma cells in the bone marrow and other tissue sites supports this concept. Recent discoveries, however, seem to favor the existence of a heterogenous population of tumor cells (1). Aside from neoplastic plasma cells, there exist marrow cells bearing early B and T cell markers, the common acute lymphocytic leukemia antigen (CALLA), and myelocytic and monocytic markers (2–4). There is ample evidence that the malignant clone extends to the blood B lymphocytes (5–10) (Table 68.1). It has also become evident that the autonomous malignant clone is under the influence of various cytokines derived from autocrine or paracrine pathways. In this regard, the role of interleukin-6 (IL-6) is particularly important (11–12).

Further insight into the biology of myeloma can be derived from chemotherapy-induced tumor responses. Although most patients respond to currently available regimens, treatment failure may occur from the very outset (primary resistance). The hypodiploid tumors, comprising 10 to 20% of all newly diagnosed myelomas, are invariably resistant to chemotherapy (13). Drug resistance has also been observed in uncommon tumors exhibiting both kappa and lambda gene rearrangement (14).

Acquired drug resistance may be, but is not invariably, associated with the cell membrane expression of the multidrug-resistance (*MDR*-1) gene. In untreated myeloma, the *MDR*-1 gene is expressed in a small percentage of tumors (<5%); following chemotherapy, more than half will be positive (16–18).

The prognosis of myeloma depends on the biologic characteristics of the tumor (Table 68.2), with treatment affecting survival. Among prognostic factors, myeloma stages I–III (19), which correspond to the total body tumor burden and the presence or absence of renal failure, are important predictors of survival. The parameters of staging of myeloma are described in Table 68.3. The levels of serum β_2-microglobulin (20, 21) and the tumor labeling index (22) are also strong predictors of survival.

Other biologic factors that adversely influence the remission duration and overall survival are a rapid rate of response to chemotherapy (23), tumors with plasmablastic morphology (24), hypodiploidy, low RNA index (25), CALLA positivity (26), the expression of multiple my-

Table 68.1. Evidence for Clonal Extension in Multiple Myeloma

Biologic Observation	Reference
Blood B lymphocytes with surface idiotype shared by myeloma protein	(5, 6)
Blood B lymphocytes with clonal immunoglobulin gene rearrangement	(7)
Blood B lymphocytes with aneuploidy	(8)
Occurrence of CALLA-positive blood B cells	(9)
Correlation of blood B-lymphocyte labeling index with disease activity	(10)

eloid markers (3), elevated serum lactic dehy-drogenase (LDH) levels (27), and the expression of the *H-ras* oncogene (28).

Notable strides have been made in the treatment of myeloma since the introduction of alkylating agents in the 1960s. Prolongation of life with comfort is often produced by currently available treatment. Unfortunately thus far, with rare exception, no cures have been accomplished. Although the success in the treatment of myeloma, to a large extent depends on the judicial use of cytoreductive chemotherapy, famil-

iarity with certain pathophysiologic mechanisms can provide a rational basis for better management. For example, in recent years, the role of IL-6 as a promoter of malignant plasma cell proliferation has been recognized (12). The myeloma cell has abundant receptors for IL-6. In culture, it releases interleukin-1 (IL-1), lymphocytotoxin, tumor necrosis factor-β (TNF-β), IL-5, and IL-6 (13, 29, 30). IL-6 also augments the proliferation of osteoclasts, which is in part activated by IL-1, lymphocytotoxin, and TNF-β. The enhancement of osteoclastic activity appears to be responsible for osteopenia, osteolysis, pathologic fractures, and hypercalcemia (31). Thus, for hypercalcemic myeloma patients, aside from treatment of hypercalcemia per se, an effective therapy should include early cytoreductive chemotherapy. For the long term, moderate exercise should be encouraged, and drugs such as pamidronate (31a) that inhibit bone resorption should be used.

The immune deficiency (primarily humoral, but also cellular) makes the patients particularly susceptible to bacterial, fungal, and viral infections. Levels of normal immunoglobulins are profoundly depressed. Moreover, the response to immunization is suboptimal and short lasting (32). A decline in $CD4^+$ and an increase in $CD8^+$ T lymphocytes contribute to the immunodeficiency. Thus, early and appropriate use of antibiotics is imperative. The prophylactic use of intravenously administered immunoglobulin may be considered on a selective basis.

Table 68.2. Biologic and Clinical Factors Adversely Affecting Survival in Multiple Myeloma

Prognostic Factors	References
High myeloma stage	(19)
Renal failure	(19)
High serum β_2-microglobulin	(20, 21)
High tumor-labeling index	(22)
Rapidity of response to the primary chemotherapy	(23)
Old age	(22)
Low serum albumin	(20, 21)
Plasmablastic morphology	(24)
Hypodiploidy	(25)
Low RNA index	(25)
CALLA positivity	(26)
High serum LDH	(27)
H-ras oncogene expression	(28)
Myeloid phenotype expression	(3)

Table 68.3. Stages of Myeloma

Body Tumor Load	Corresponding Laboratory Requirements
Stage I: $<0.6 \times 10^{12}/m^2$	Should fulfill all the following criteria: Hb >10 g/dL Serum calcium <12.0 mg/dL No or solitary osteolytic lesion IgG M-component <5.0 g/dL or IgA <3.0 g/dL Bence Jones proteinuria <4.0 g/24 hr
Stage II: $0.6-1.2 \times 10^{12}/m^2$	Fulfilling criteria fitting neither those above nor below
Stage III: $>1.2 \times 10^{12}/m^2$	Having one or more of the following features: Hb <8.5 g/dL Serum calcium >12 mg/dL Advanced lytic bone lesions IgG M-component >7.0 g/dL IgA >5.0 g/dL Bence Jones proteinuria >12.0 g/24 hr

Substage A: BUN <30 mg/dL, creatinine <2.0 mg/dL.
Substage B: BUN ≥30 mg/dL, creatinine ≥2.0 mg/dL.

Table 68.4. Clinical and Laboratory Features of Smoldering Myeloma, Multiple Myeloma, and Monoclonal Gammopathy of Undetermined Significance (MGUS)

Clinical and Laboratory Features	Smoldering Myeloma	Multiple Myeloma	MGUS
Bone pain	−	±	−
Osteolytic bone lesion	+	+	−
Anemia (not attributable to other cause)	−	+	−
Hypercalcemia	−	±	−
M protein level	<3 g/dL	≥3 g/dL	<3 g/dL
Bone marrow plasmacytosis	≤15%	≥10%	<10%
Bence Jones proteinuria	±	±	−
Serum β_2-Microglobulin	Low	Low or high	Low
Plasma cell labeling index	Low	Elevated	Low

Certain Bence Jones proteins have been demonstrated to be nephrotoxic (33). The myeloma kidney and tubular cell dysfunctions are caused by Bence Jones proteins (34). Renal failure may be triggered by factors such as dehydration due to diarrhea or vomiting. The avoidance of body fluid loss and maintenance of good hydration cannot be underestimated. Some light chains by virtue of their structure can be amyloidogenic. In fact, symptoms referable to amyloidosis are observed in over 15% of myeloma patients and at times require appropriate therapeutic intervention.

Because of their physicochemical properties or biologic function, the myeloma proteins may account for a variety of clinical syndromes and laboratory abnormalities. These aspects of the disease are reviewed elsewhere and therapeutic recommendations made whenever applicable (35).

Treatment of Solitary Plasmacytoma

A small fraction (2 to 3%) of patients present with a solitary lesion of the skeleton or, rarely, of soft tissues. Such patients have little or no serum and urinary monoclonal immunoglobulin. In spite of an apparently solitary lesion revealed by x-ray, further study by computed tomography (CT) or magnetic resonance imaging (MRI) may identify additional lesions. Should there be no evidence for plasma cell tumor elsewhere after adequate studies, a curative radiation treatment using a tumor dose of at least 4500 cGy is recommended (15). Unfortunately, one-half to two-thirds of such patients will eventually develop generalized disease requiring systemic chemotherapy.

Treatment of Smoldering Multiple Myeloma

Asymptomatic or smoldering multiple myeloma (SMM) occurs in a minority of patients with plasma cell neoplasm. Table 68.4 compares the distinguishing clinical and laboratory features of SMM with those of multiple myeloma (MM) and monoclonal gammopathy of undetermined significance (MGUS). Presently, chemotherapy for SMM after diagnosis is not warranted. In a randomized trial, the deferral of treatment until the symptomatic, progressive phase of the disease had occurred did not adversely effect the overall survival (36).

Treatment of Multiple Myeloma

Response to treatment in myeloma is usually assessed by changes in serum and urinary monoclonal immunoglobulins. Decreases of 50% or more in serum M protein and 75% or more in urinary Bence Jones protein qualify the patient as a responder. Some investigators define response as a decline of 75% or more in the rate of M protein synthesis (37). A complete response (CR) is defined as the complete disappearance of M protein (by the immune fixation method) in serum and urine, together with a fall in bone marrow plasma cells below 5%. This definition does not indicate total eradication of the malignant clone. Recently, the reliance on M protein changes to indicate treatment efficacy has been questioned (38). Moreover, the decline in urinary Bence Jones protein in patients treated with glycocorticoids may not reflect reduced tumor load but a change in steroid-related Bence Jones protein catabolism (39). Presently, survival appears to be the most reliable criterion for comparison of various drug regimens.

A standard regimen of melphalan plus prednisone (MP) can produce 50 to 60% objective responses and a median survival of 30 to 40 months. Approximately 5 to 10% of patients survive 10 years or longer. Complete remissions occur in about 10% of treated patients. Prospectively randomized trials comparing MP with multidrug regimens such as M2, VCMP, VBAP, and ABCM (Table 68.5) have been completed by groups throughout the world (41–57). Except for two studies (42–43), no survival gain was obtained by using multidrug regimens. A meta-analysis of over 3800 patients (58) culled from randomized trials also found no survival advantage to multidrug regimens. Further analysis revealed that patients with good prognostic factors lived longer if MP was administered. The opposite was true for patients with poor prognostic determinants. In general, a higher response rate was observed in patients with stage III disease (Table 68.2) and those with poor prognosis when treated with polychemotherapy programs. It is ironic that based on available data, a more toxic regimen is the best choice for sicker patients.

At the present time, in our opinion, the MP regimen (40) outlined in Table 68.5, because of its simplicity, low toxicity, and cost, should be considered as primary treatment for most patients not enrolled in a clinical trial. Melphalan should be administered on an empty stomach to improve its intestinal absorption. A midcourse leukopenia should be documented, otherwise the drug dose should be raised as outlined (Table 68.5). A 6-week interval between treatment cycles is preferred over 3- to 4-week intervals, because more complete marrow recovery permits a higher dose of melphalan at each cycle. Several cycles of treatment are needed to attain a response. Patients exhibiting disease progression during the first two or three cycles should be regarded as refractory to alkylating agents (see below).

In patients with leukopenia and thrombocytopenia associated with a packed marrow, the melphalan dose may be reduced by 25 to 50% to avoid severe and prolonged cytopenia. The dose of melphalan should be raised in subsequent cycles. Alternatively, since most randomized trials have shown a trend toward higher response rates in stage III disease and patients with poor prognoses, a multidrug regimen such as M2 or VMCP/VBAP (Table 68.5) might be selected as the primary regimen.

Table 68.5. Drug Regimens for the Treatment of Multiple Myeloma

MP (40)
  Melphalan 0.15 mg/kg, p.o., for 7 days
  Prednisone 20 mg p.o., three times daily for 7 days
  Repeat this treatment every 6 weeks
  Increase daily dose of melphalan by 2 mg in the next
    cycle until midcycle cytopenia is produced
"M2" regimen: VBMCP (41)
  Vincristine 1.2 mg/m^2 i.v., day 1
  Carmustine 20 mg/m^2 i.v., day 1
  Cyclophosphamide 400 mg/m^2 i.v., day 1
  Melphalan 8 mg/m^2 p.o., days 1–4
  Prednisone 40 mg/m^2 p.o., days 1–7 and 20 mg/m^2
    p.o., days 8–14
  Repeat this treatment every 5 weeks
VMCP-VCAP (42)
  VMCP
    Vincristine 1 mg/m^2 i.v. bolus*, day 1
    Melphalan 6 mg/m^2 p.o., days 1–4
    Cyclophosphamide 125 mg/m^2 p.o., days 1–4
    Prednisone 60 mg/m^2 p.o., days 1–4 (prednisone
      dose is tapered)
    Alternate VMCP with VCAP (see below) every 3
      weeks for 6–12 months
  VCAP
    Vincristine 1 mg/m^2 i.v. bolus*, day 1
    Cyclophosphamide 125 mg/m^2 p.o., days 1–4
    Doxorubicin 30 mg/m^2 IVB, day 1
    Prednisone 60 mg/m^2 p.o., days 1–4 (prednisone
      dose is tapered)
    *Maximum 1.5 mg
VMCP-VBAP (42)
  VMCP
    As above
    Repeat every 3 weeks for three cycles to be
      followed by VBAP for three cycles
  VBAP
    Vincristine 1 mg/m^2 i.v. bolus*, day 1
    Carmustine 30 mg/m^2 i.v./1 hr, day 1
    Prednisone 60 mg/m^2 p.o., days 1–4 (prednisone
      dose is tapered)
    *Maximum 1.5 mg
    May repeat the entire cycle of VMCP-VBAP
ABCM (43)
  Doxorubicin 30 mg/m^2 i.v., on day 1
  Carmustine (BCNU) 30 mg/m^2 i.v., on day 1
  Cyclophosphamide 100 mg/m^2 p.o., on days 1–4
  Melphalan 6.0 mg/m^2 p.o., on days 1–4
  Alternating 3-week cycles of doxorubicin,
    carmustine, and Cytoxan melphalan
VAD (44)
  Vincristine 0.4 mg continuous i.v. infusion days 1–4
  Doxorubicin 9 mg/m^2 continuous i.v. infusion days
    1–4
  Dexamethasone 40 mg p.o., days 1–4, 9–12, 17–20
  Repeat cycles every 28 days
High-dose D (45)
  Dexamethasone 40 mg p.o., days 1–4, 9–12, 17–20
  Repeat cycles every 28 days

Maintenance Treatment

In most responders, a plateau phase occurs, characterized by stable levels of serum and urinary myeloma proteins, continued symptom relief, and hematologic improvement. About 10% of patients treated with MP and a higher percentage of patients treated by polychemotherapy enter into complete remission. The plateau phase is typically associated with low serum β_2-microglobulin levels and a low tumor labeling index. The necessity for continuing primary treatment after achieving a stable plateau is debatable. The major reason for drug discontinuation is fear of the development of myelodysplastic syndromes or acute nonlymphocyte leukemia, which occurs in patients who have received prolonged courses of alkylating agents (51). Moreover, in several randomized studies, discontinuation of the primary drug regimen after the attainment of remission did not adversely affect the overall survival, although a higher rate of relapse was observed. The resumption of treatment was associated with 40 to 60% response rates (59–63).

The Role of Interferon

α-Interferon (IFN-α) inhibits myeloma cell growth in vitro (64–67). The biologic mechanism for this inhibition is poorly understood. An anti-IL-6 function or downregulation of an IL-6 receptor are both suspected (68–69). In untreated patients, recombinant IFN-α produces remission in one-third of patients, with a median survival that is inferior to that of the MP regimen (70). Several attempts have been made to incorporate IFN-α into primary chemotherapy regimens in multiple myeloma. A study by Cancer and Leukemia Group B showed no improvement in response rate or survival when IFN-α was added to the MP regimen (71). In another trial, again no difference in response rate or survival was observed between the MP and MP + IFN-α regimens. Subgroup analysis, however, showed improved survival for patients with IgA myeloma and patients with Bence Jones myeloma (72).

IFN-α has been tried as a maintenance regimen with the hope of prolonging event-free survival and overall survival. The first randomized trial, by an Italian group (73), was quite promising. The median relapse-free and overall survivals (26 and 52 months, respectively) for patients treated with IFN-α were significantly better than those for untreated patients (14 and 39 months, respectively). A trial by the South West Oncology Group (74) and a German trial (75) did not confirm these results. Several other randomized studies are not yet mature.

Treatment of Advanced-Phase Myeloma

Reviews of this topic have been published (76, 77). Three separate groups of patients may be considered. The first includes patients who have relapsed after a period of unmaintained remission. Such patients stand a good chance of responding to the same primary treatment regimen, particularly if they have been off therapy for longer than 6 months. In one study, 57% of chemotherapy unmaintained relapses responded to the original MP regimen (62). Similarly, patients previously treated with the M2 regimen responded well to the same program given at the time of relapse (63).

The second group consists of patients who become refractory to treatment after an initial response. At this phase of the disease, at times, the biologic traits of aggressive tumors, such as a change in cell morphology, extraosseous plasmacytomas, plasma cell leukemia, lymphoma-like myeloma, and elevation of serum lactic dehydrogenase levels, may be encountered (13, 27). Several treatment regimens have been tried in late-phase myeloma (13, 78–85). IFN-α is effective in only 20% of such patients, producing short remissions (79). High-dose glucocorticoids, alone or in combination with other agents, are effective in a quarter to one-third of patients (13, 77, 86). Thus far, the VAD regimen (Table 68.5) appears to be the best second-line therapy (13, 44, 83). A response rate of 40 to 60% with a median survival of 1 to 1.5 years has been observed. The treatment is quite immunosuppressive; in one series, 37% of patients required hospitalization for treatment of infection (44).

The resistant relapse may be, but is not necessarily, associated with *MDR*-1 gene expression. Attempts have been made to overcome such resistance by addition of verapamil (89–91) or cyclosporine (92) to the VAD regimen. Only 10 to 20% of VAD-resistant patients responded when verapamil was added. In another study, cyclosporine (7.5 mg/kg/24 hours) added to the VAD regimen produced 58% responses in MDR-1-positive tumors and 31% responses in MDR-1-negative tumors (92).

Finally, a minority of patients are refractory to primary treatment. Such refractoriness is an ominous prognostic signal, since responses to alternate regimens are infrequent. Cytogenetic study has shown some patients in this group to have a hypodiploid karyotype (13). Data collected from the literature by Buzaid and Durie (77) confirmed that only 8% of primary refractory patients responded to alkylators. The VAD regimen was effective in 40%, and high-dose glucocorticoids in 30%.

High-dose therapy using melphalan 200 mg/m^2 with peripheral blood stem cells, with or without autologous bone marrow transplantation, was used in primary resistant or resistant relapse patients (93). The best results were obtained in primary resistant patients. Elevated β_2-microglobulin levels prior to transplantation and age above 50 had adverse effects on survival.

Irradiation, using the hemibody radiotherapy technique, can produce objective responses in about one-third of previously treated patients. The relief of pain is quite rewarding, and nearly 80% of patients may respond (77, 94, 95). The treatment is often associated with severe and, at times, irreversible myelotoxicity. Therefore, hemibody radiation should be reserved until all other therapeutic options are exhausted and the relief of pain is the sole therapeutic goal.

Allogeneic and Syngeneic Bone Marrow Transplantation for Treatment of Multiple Myeloma

Due to the older age of patients with multiple myeloma (median, 60 to 65 years), a small percentage of patients have been transplanted. Since the first report of syngeneic bone marrow transplantation (96), many centers have reported their results to the International Bone Marrow Transplantation Registry (IBMTR). In their most recent analysis (97), 257 patients were transplanted between 1981 and 1992; 87% of patients received marrow from HLA-identical siblings, 4% from identical twins, and 9% from alternative donors. The median age was 42 years (range, 22 to 59). The pretransplantation regimen consisted of total body irradiation (TBI) plus cyclophosphamide or melphalan. Some received busulfan and cyclophosphamide. The immunosuppression regime was cyclosporine with or without other agents. T-cell depletion was carried out in some cases. The early death toll was quite high; at 6 months posttransplant, 53 ± 7% of patients were alive. The long-term survival (24 ± 7%, 5-years posttransplant) appears to be slightly superior to that of conventional treatment. The report from the European Bone Marrow Transplantation Group (98) involving 122 patients, also indicated

a high early death rate of 53%. The long-term survival of 36% at 6 years was associated with a flattening of the survival curve beyond the third year posttransplantation. Patients achieving complete remission and those with grade I graft-versus-host disease did significantly better. Table 68.6 includes reports from other groups as well. In general, a select population of myeloma patients of young age (median, 42 to 43), with a history of 1 to 2 years of pretransplant therapy, have been transplanted. The improvement in long-term survival might, in part, be attributed to the selective nature of the population under study.

Allogeneic and syngeneic bone marrow transplantation, in spite of a heavy early loss of patients undergoing treatment, continue to be viable therapeutic options for patients younger than 55 years who have a donor available and no disqualifying factors for bone marrow transplantation.

High-Dose Therapy (HDT) with Autologous Bone Marrow (ABM) or Peripheral Blood Stem Cell (PBSC) Transplantation

HDT using melphalan at a dose of 140 mg/m^2, although quite toxic, was shown to induce a high rate of complete remission and better long-term survival. The long-term follow-up of a non-randomized selected group of patients showed a CR of 32% and a median survival of 47 months, with 35% surviving at 9 years (104). Since the mid-1980s, HDT in conjunction with autologous bone marrow transplantation has been tried by several centers to reduce early deaths and improve the chance for cure (Table 68.7). In earlier studies, ABM cells containing up to 30% myeloma cells were administered. In recent years, the methodology for harvesting of PBSCs (CD34+ cells) has matured. High-dose Cytoxan or other drug regimens and G-CSF or GM-CSF are administered prior to pheresis for collection of stem cells. In some studies, further enrichment of CD34+ cells has been carried out prior to transplantation (114, 147). PBSCs are not devoid of malignant B cells, although their number can be reduced by CD34 cell enrichment procedures. Theoretically, therefore, PBSCs are more suitable for transplantation than ABMs. Moreover, recovery from cytopenia occurs faster following PBSC transplantation (105). In previously untreated patients, prior to HDT and autologous cell transplantation, an induction regimen such as VAD is

Table 68.6. Allogeneic and Syngeneic Bone Marrow Transplantation in Multiple Myeloma

Group	Patients (No.)	Median Age	Early Death Rate (%)	Complete Response Rate (%)	Overall Survival
EBTG[a] (98)	122	43	53	42	36% at 6 years
IBMTR[b] (97)	257	42	No data	No data	24 ± 7% at 5 years
Bensinger et al. (99, 100)	62	44	No data	37	68% at 2 years
Vesole et al. (101)	35	43	26	34	43% at 2 years
Cario et al. (102)	33	43	64	33	36% at 19 months
Anderson et al. (103)	18	44	36	44	60% at 2.5 years

[a]EBTG, European Bone Marrow Transplantation Group.
[b]IBMTR, International Bone Marrow Transplantation Registry.

Table 68.7. High-Dose Therapy with Autologous Cell Transplantation in Multiple Myeloma[a]

Reference	Patients Treated (No.)	Age	Autologous Cell Source	Early Death Rate (%)	Complete Response (%)	Percentage Surviving (months)
Jagannath et al. (105)	112[b]	Median 50 (26–68)	PBSC ± ABM[c]	2	49	64% (42)
Harousseau et al. (106, 107)	168[d]	Median 52	ABM[e]	5	35	50% (41)
Attal et al. (108)	35[f]	<65	ABM[g]	3	43	81% (42)
Bjorkstrand et al. (109)	174[h]	Median 48 (27–64)	ABM (112) PBSC (45) Both (17)[i]	No data	No data	45% (36)
Anderson et al. (103)	32[j]	Median 45	Purged ABM[k]	3	34	70% (48)
Fermand et al. (110)	63[l]	Median 44	PBSC[m]	11	20	50% (59)
Fermand et al. (111)	199[n]	No data	PBSC[o]	No data	No data	71% (36)
Cunningham et al. (112)	53[p]	Median 52	ABM[q]	2	75	63% (54)
Cunningham et al. (113)	84[p]	Median 52	ABM[q]	0	77	87% (48)

[a]Abbreviations: ABM, autologous bone marrow; BCNU, carmustine; C, cyclophosphamide; E, etoposide; G-CSF, granulocyte colony-stimulating factor; GM-CSF, granulocyte-monocyte colony-stimulating factor; HDT, high-dose therapy; M, melphalan; PBSC, peripheral blood stem cell; TBI, total body irradiation.
[b]All previously untreated.
[c]M 200 mg/m^2 + G-CSF (86% received one autotransplant and 73% two autotransplants).
[d]130 patients treated ≤6 months and 38 patients >6 months prior to transplantation; 45% were refractory to previous treatment.
[e]M 140 mg/m^2 + TBI.
[f]Previously untreated patients.
[g]M 140 mg/m^2 + TBI 800 cGy.
[h]Details of pretransplant treatment not given.
[i]Details not given; some received TBI.
[j]Previously treated and untreated.
[k]M 70 mg/m^2 or C 60 mg/kg + TBI 1200–1400 cGy.
[l]Mixed refractory and sensitive.
[m]M 140 mg/m^2 + BCNU 120 mg/m^2 p.o., E 250 mg/m^2 i.v. ± C 60 mg/kg i.v. + TBI 1000–1200 cGy.
[n]Previously untreated, randomized to receive HDT or conventional therapy (VMCP regimen, Table 68.5). Primary resistant or relapse cases receiving conventional treatment were rescued by HDT.
[o]M 140 mg/m^2, BCNU 120 mg/m^2 p.o., E 250 mg/m^2 i.v., C 60 mg/kg i.v. + TBI 1200 cGy.
[p]Only responders to induction therapy were transplanted.
[q]M: 200 mg/m^2.

used. Table 68.7 shows data on several pilot studies. Although patients up to age 70 were entered in some studies, the median age of transplanted patients (42 to 52 years) was lower than that of patients in most randomized chemotherapy trials.

In contrast to allogeneic bone marrow transplantation, the early death rate has been low and the CR rate has been equally high. Most pilot studies have not been mature enough to provide long-term survival. The projected or actual median survival in these highly selected patients is reported to be between 3 to 5 years (105–113). It remains to be seen whether the survival curve will eventually flatten out and whether actual cure has been accomplished. In two small studies, both the disappearance and the persistence of a residual malignant clone was demonstrated using the polymerase chain reaction procedure in patients who were in complete remission (146, 148).

HDT with autologous cell transplantation, thus far available in only a few centers, is cumbersome and expensive. No definite conclusions can be drawn because of the highly selective nature of treated patients and the lack of long-term follow-up results. Prospectively randomized trials, in previously untreated patients, with meticulous attention to prognostic variables, are required to determine the role of such a regimen in the treatment of myeloma. Currently, two randomized studies are in progress (111, 115).

Treatment of Anemia

Immune-mediated hemolytic anemia is quite rare in myeloma. The causes of anemia in myeloma are often multifactorial: bone marrow replacement by malignant plasma cells, anemia of chronic disease, anemia associated with renal failure, and bone marrow failure due to chemotherapy can be cited. Fortunately, response to treatment is often associated with a rise in hemoglobulin concentration, and the need for blood transfusion is uncommon. In a subset of patients with low serum erythropoietin, treatment with erythropoietin may be rewarding (116).

Treatment of Bone Pain

Salicylates or acetaminophen with codeine are adequate for mild pain, but narcotic analgesics may be required for the treatment of severe pain. Diazapam is useful for interruption of painful muscle spasms associated with radiculopathy. Palliation of severe and well-localized bone pain can be accomplished by external-beam irradiation. A total radiation dose of 10 Gy is sufficient in most cases (117). Care must be taken to avoid the use of unnecessarily large radiation fields or the sequential treatment of painful areas to the detriment of an early start of chemotherapy. As noted above, hemibody radiation can be used in advanced-stage disease when cytoreductive chemotherapy is no longer an option and pain palliation is the sole purpose of treatment.

Treatment of Hypercalcemia

Mild hypercalcemia (serum calcium <12 mg/ dL) can be treated with saline infusion (3 to 4 L/ 24 hr) and furosemide (20 to 40 mg/day). Corticosteroids are quite effective for the treatment of hypercalcemia of myeloma. Prednisone at a dose of 1 to 1.5 mg/kg is adequate, with a rapid taper after the serum calcium level has normalized. Pamidronate disodium (60 to 90 mg in a single 24-hour intravenous infusion) or gallium nitrate (200 mg/m^2 dissolved in 1 L of saline for daily intravenous infusion for 5 days) are other alternatives. Calcitonin and corticosteroids used in combination are nearly always effective. Salmon calcitonin (4 IU/kg intramuscularly or subcutaneously every 12 hours) and prednisone (40 to 60 mg daily) are recommended.

Treatment of Osteolysis and Osteopenia

Orthopaedic intervention with irradiation may be required for management of threatened or actual fracture of long bones. Several attempts have been made to reduce bone resorption in myeloma. Fluoride and androgenic hormones were found ineffective. Gallium nitrate by continuous intravenous or subcutaneous infusion may inhibit bone resorption by blocking the biologic action of IL-1, TNF, and parathyroid hormone (118). Although the treatment can be given on an outpatient basis, it is unduly cumbersome. In a randomized trial by the Finnish Leukemia Group, Clodronate 2.4 g daily was found to delay the progression of osteolytic lesions (119). Pamidronate at a dose of 90 mg as a 4-hour intravenous infusion given every 4 weeks was found to reduce skeletal complications and improve the quality of life of patients with stage III multiple myeloma (31a).

Treatment of Renal Failure

Among the diverse causes of renal failure (hypercalcemia, hyperuricemia, infection, hyperviscosity, amyloidosis, etc.), the myeloma kidney (cast nephropathy) due to nephrotoxic Bence Jones proteins probably accounts for most cases of renal failure. Avoidance of precipitating factors such as dehydration, nephrotoxic antibiotics, and radiocontrast dye is quite important. Renal failure associated with hypercalcemia, unless long-standing, is mostly prerenal and thus can be reversed by fluid administration. The renal failure of myeloma kidney should be treated vigorously with hydration, alkalinization of the urine, and hemodialysis if necessary. Dialysis must be continued until an assessment of response to treatment for myeloma can be made. Dialysis is then maintained in responding patients. Substantial improvement in renal function may occur following chemotherapy, obviating the need for chronic dialysis (120). Plasmapheresis in conjunction with hemodialysis was reported to be more effective in patients with renal failure and Bence Jones proteinuria (121).

Treatment of Neurologic Complications

Myelopathy due to spinal cord impingement by an extradural plasmacytoma is an urgent problem. In patients without a previous diagnosis of myeloma, decompression laminectomy, with biopsy or excision, followed by radiation therapy, is recommended. In patients known to have myeloma, radiation alone may suffice. The clinical presentation of back pain associated with symptoms of radiculopathy can be very troubling and resistant to therapeutic measures. Adequate narcotic analgesics at appropriate intervals, diazepam as a spasmolytic, the use of a firm mattress, lumbar corsets or braces, and psychologic support are all necessary for successful management.

Meningeal myelomatosis occurs rarely and usually as a late event in the course of the illness. The diagnosis must be based on the demonstration of malignant cells in the spinal fluid and not myeloma proteins. Brain irradiation and intrathecal administration of methotrexate or cytosine arabinoside have been attempted with some success.

Rarely, retroorbital plasmacytoma associated with ocular proptosis can occur, requiring radiation treatment.

Treatment of Hyperviscosity Syndrome

The hyperviscosity syndrome occurs in myeloma less frequently than in Waldenström's macroglobulinemia. Several factors in addition to the monoclonal protein concentration contribute to the blood viscosity (35). The IgM monoclonal immunoglobulins, because of their large molecular size, and the IgAs, because of their occurrence in polymeric forms, cause more viscosity elevation than the IgGs. Plasmapheresis is the mainstay of treatment for symptomatic patients. The removal of 2 to 4 L of plasma can ameliorate symptoms; this may have to be repeated at weekly or biweekly intervals. The duration of pheresis is determined by the resolution of symptoms, which often correlates with a reduction of serum viscosity to less than 4.0 Ostwald units. Treatment of the underlying disease with chemotherapy usually obviates the need for continuing plasmapheresis. In patients with chemotherapy-unresponsive macroglobulinemia at a late stage of disease, plasmapheresis carried out at regular intervals is useful and quite necessary for palliation of symptoms.

TREATMENT OF WALDENSTRÖM'S MACROGLOBULINEMIA

Waldenström's macroglobulinemia is often an indolent lymphoproliferative disorder, characterized by the presence of plasmacytoid lymphocytes in blood and bone marrow and the production of monoclonal, pentameric IgM immunoglobulin. The clinical symptoms of the disease are often the consequence of the physicochemical properties of monoclonal immunoglobulin, resulting in the hyperviscosity syndrome and cryoglobulinemia. Symptoms are often temporarily relieved by reducing the serum concentration of M protein by plasmapheresis. The technical efficacy of this approach has recently been further refined (122). Durable disease control and sustained reduction of IgM production can be obtained by cytotoxic treatment including alkylating agents such as chlorambucil, melphalan, cyclophosphamide (123), and doxorubicin (124), often in combination with steroids. Recent clinical trails have demonstrated a relatively high and durable response to the nucleoside analogues fludarabine (125, 126) and 2-chlorodeoxyadenosine (127, 128), as a primary treatment and, to a lesser extent, as a second-line intervention. The benefits of other new antineoplastic agents such as paclitaxel (129) in macroglobulinemia are currently being investigated. The role of biologic modifiers with or without chemotherapeutic agents in the management of this disease is yet to be fully defined (130, 131).

The superiority of multiagent chemotherapy regimens (123) has not been shown.

TREATMENT OF HEAVY CHAIN DISEASES

The heavy chain disorders are a group of B-cell lymphoproliferative disorders with heterogenous clinical presentations, which commonly produce incomplete or deleted heavy chains of immunoglobulins. In light of the clinical and immunologic variabilities, the treatment approach to various heavy chain disorders must be individualized.

α Heavy Chain Disease

In the early prelymphomatous phase of the alimentary form of the disease, in which chronic diarrhea and malnutrition are the dominant features, antimicrobial therapy with tetracyclines, ampicillin, and metronidazole has led to a drastic improvement in symptoms and occasional histologic remission of the disease of the small intestine (132). The role of *Helicobacter pylori* and *Campylobacter jejuni* (133) in mediating the clinical expression has recently been debated. The response to antibiotics tends to decline with increasing alteration of intestinal lymphoplasmacytic infiltrates (134).

In the late prelymphomatous stage of the disease, variable responses have been reported with combined antimicrobial and antineoplastic chemotherapy (135). When frank lymphomatous evolution supervenes, antimicrobial therapy is universally ineffective. In this setting, the lymphoma is often of high-grade, large cell (immunoblastic) or undifferentiated subtype (132). In a prospective clinic trial, the CHOP (cyclophosphamide, doxorubicin, vincristine, prednisone) regimen has emerged as superior to the C-MOPP (cyclophosphamide, vincristine, procarbazine, prednisone) regimen (136). A high response rate and relatively prolonged survival have also been reported in patients in the advanced lymphomatous phase receiving CHOP or CHVP (cyclophosphamide, doxorubicin, etoposide, prednisone) followed by ABV (doxorubicin, bleomycin, vinblastine) (137).

The benefits of total abdominal irradiation in cases of α heavy chain disease–associated lymphoma confined to the abdomen have been shown (138). Resection of bulky lymphomatous deposits prior to chemotherapy or irradiation has enhanced the ultimate outcome of the treatment and has diminished the cata-strophic risk of intestinal perforation in these settings (135, 136). Nutritional interventions, management of the concurrent infections and opportunistic infestations, and correction of electrolyte disturbances are the cornerstones of supportive care in this disease.

γ Heavy Chain Disease

The clinical diversity of γ heavy chain disease has prompted a broad range of treatments from simple observation of the asymptomatic indolent subset of patients to aggressive multiagent chemotherapy regimens for patients with a high-grade lymphoma-like syndrome (139). In the latter group with lymphomatous foci threatening upper aerodigestive tract obstruction, irradiation of Waldeyer's ring has been recommended (140). Infection and autoimmune hemolysis may complicate the course of γ heavy chain disease, necessitating a prompt and aggressive intervention with antimicrobial and/or immunosuppressive agents, respectively (141).

μ Heavy Chain Disease

The variability of therapeutic options in μ heavy chain disease closely parallels the diversity of the clinical course of disease (141). Chemotherapeutic regimens, including alkylating agents with or without steroids, similar to those conventionally used in the treatment of chronic lymphocytic leukemia have led to some beneficial results (142).

TREATMENT OF MONOCLONAL IMMUNOGLOBULIN DEPOSITION DISEASE

Systemic light chain deposition disease was recognized first. In this disease, the monoclonal light chain, usually κ type, is found to involve the kidney and other organs such as liver and lung, by deposition at basement membranes. In contrast to primary amyloidosis, no amyloid fibrils are seen by electron-microscopic examination of the involved areas (143). It was subsequently noted that monoclonal heavy chain or heavy chain and light chain deposition can occur (144, 145). Renal disease in the form of renal failure, end-stage renal disease, with heavy or light proteinemia usually predominates the clinical presentation. Examination of a renal biopsy specimen with the immunofluorescent antibody technique may reveal the underlying pathologic processes. A clinical presentation of myeloma with skeletal manifestation occurs in a minority of patients. In such patients, cytotoxic chemotherapy may be beneficial, allowing additional therapy such as dialysis or kidney transplantation.

REFERENCES

1. King MA, Nelson DS. Tumor cell heterogeneity in multiple myeloma: antigenic morphologic, and functional studies of cells from blood and bone marrow. Blood 1989;73:1925–1935.

2. Grogran TM, Durie BGM, Lomen C, Spier C, Wirt DP, et al. Delineation of a novel pre-B cell component in plasma cell myeloma: immunochemical, immunophenotypic, genotypic, cytologic, cell culture and kinetic features. Blood 1987;70:932–942.

3. Grogran TM, Durie BGM, Spier CM, Richter L, Vela E. Myelomonocytic antigen positive multiple myeloma. Blood 1989;73:763–769.

4. Epstein J, Barlogie B, Katzmann J, Alexanian R. Phenotypic heterogeneity in aneuploid multiple myeloma indicates pre-B cell involvement. Blood 1988; 71:861–865.

5. Mellstedt H, Hammorstrom S, Holm G. Monoclonal lymphocyte population in human plasma cell myeloma. Clin Exp Immunol 1974;17:371–384.

6. Bast E, Van Camp B, Reynaert P, Wirniga G, Ballieux R. Idiotypic peripheral blood lymphocytes in monoclonal gammopathy. Clin Exp Immunol 1982; 47:677–682.

7. Berenson J, Wong R, Kim K, Brown N, Lichtenstein A. Evidence for peripheral blood B lymphocyte but not T lymphocyte involvements in multiple myeloma. Blood 1987;70:1550–1553.

8. Barlogie B, Alexanian R. Cellular aspects of myeloma. Biologic and clinical implications. In: Delamore IW, ed. Multiple myeloma and other paraproteinemias. Edinburgh: Churchill Livingstone, 1986:154–168.

9. Wearne AJ, Joshua DE, Brown RD, Kronenberg H. Multiple myeloma: the relationship between CALLA (CD10) positive lymphocytes in the peripheral blood and light chain isotype suppression. Br J Haematol 1987;67:39–44.

10. Witzig TE, Gonchoroff NJ, Katzmann JA, Therneau TM, Kyle RA, Greipp PR. Peripheral blood B cell labeling indexes are a measure of disease activity in patients with monoclonal gammopathies. J Clin Oncol 1988;6:1041–1046.

11. Klein B, Zhang X-G, Jourdan M, Content J, Houssiau F, et al. Paracrine rather than autocrine regulation of myeloma-cell growth and differentiation by interleukin-6. Blood 1989;73:517–526.

12. Zhang X-G, Klein B, Bataille R. Interleukin-6 is a potent myeloma-cell growth factor in patients with aggressive multiple myeloma. Blood 1989;74:11–13.

13. Barlogie B, Epstein J, Selvanayagam P, Alexanian R. Plasma cell myeloma—new biological insights and advances in therapy. Blood 1989;73:865–879.

14. Smith L, Barlogie B, Alexanian R. Biclonal and hypodiploid multiple myeloma. Am J Med 1986; 80:841–843.

15. Dimopoulos MA, Goldstein J, Fuller L, Delasalle K, Alexanian R. Curability of solitary bone plasmacytoma. J Clin Oncol 1992;10:587–590.

16. Dalton WS, Grogan TM, Meltzer PS, Scheper RJ, Durie BGM, et al. Drug-resistance in multiple myeloma: detection of p-glycoprotein and potential circumvention by addition of verapamil to chemotherapy. J Clin Oncol 1989;7:415–424.

17. Dalton WS, Salmon SE. Drug resistance in myeloma: mechanisms and approaches to circumstances. Hematol Oncol Clin North Am 1992;6:383–393.

18. Epstein J, Xlao H, Koba B. P-glycoprotein expression in plasma cell myeloma is associated with resistance to VAD. Blood 1989;74:913–917.

19. Durie BGM, Salmon SE. A clinical staging system for multiple myeloma. Correlation of measured myeloma cell mass with presenting clinical features, response to treatment and survival. Cancer 1975; 36:842–854.

20. Bataille R, Grenier J, Sany J. Beta-2-microglobulin in myeloma. Optimal use for staging, prognosis and treatment—a prospective study of 160 patients. Blood 1984;63:468–476.

21. Bataille R, Durie BGM, Grenier J, Sany J. Prognostic factors and staging in multiple myeloma: a reappraisal. J Clin Oncol 1986;4:80–87.

22. Greipp PR, Katzmann JA, O'Fallon WM, Kyle RA. Value of β_2-microglobulin level and plasma cell labeling indices as prognostic factors in patients with newly diagnosed myeloma. Blood 1988;72:219–223.

23. Farhangi M, Osserman EF. Biology, clinical patterns, and treatment of multiple myeloma and related plasma-cell dyscrasias. In: Twomey JJ, Good RA, eds. Comprehensive immunology 4, the immunopathology of lymphoreticular neoplasms. New York: Plenum 1978:684–686.

24. Greipp PR, Raymond NM, Kyle RA, O'Fallon WM. Multiple myeloma: significance of plasmablastic subtype in morphological classification. Blood 1985; 65:305–310.

25. Barlogie B, Alexanian R, Dixon D, Smith L, Smallwood L, Delasalle K. Prognostic implications of tumor cell DNA and RNA content in multiple myeloma. Blood 1985;66:338–341.

26. Durie BGM, Grogan TM. CALLA-positive myeloma: an aggressive subtype with poor survival. Blood 1985;66:229–232.

27. Barlogie B, Smallwood L, Smith T, Alexanian R. High serum levels of lactic dehydrogenase identify a high grade lymphoma-like myeloma. Ann Intern Med 1989;110:521–525.

28. Tsuchiya H, Epstein J, Selvanayagam P, Dedman JR, Gallick G, Alexanian R, Barlogie B. Correlated flow cytometric analysis of H-*ras* p21 and nuclear DNA in multiple myeloma. Blood 1988;72:796–800.

29. Lichtenstein A, Berenson J, Norman D, et al. Production of cytokines by bone marrow cells obtained from patients with multiple myeloma. Blood 1989; 74:1266–1273.

30. Bataille R, Jourdan M, Zhang X-G, et al. Serum level of interleukin-6, a potent myeloma cell growth factor as a reflection of disease severity in plasma cell dyscrasias. J Clin Invest 1989;84:2008–2011.

31. Mundy G, Bertolini DR. Bone destruction and hypercalcemia in plasma cell myeloma. Semin Oncol 1986;13:291–299.

31a. Berenson JR, Lichtenstein A, Porter L, et al. Efficacy of Pamidronate in reducing skeletal events in patients with advanced multiple myeloma. N Engl J Med 1996;334:488–493.

32. Jacobson DR, Zolla-Pazner S. Immuno-suppression and infection in multiple myeloma. Semin Oncol 1986;13:282–290.

33. Solomon A, Weiss DT, Kattine AA. Nephrotoxic potential of Bence Jones proteins. N Engl J Med 1991;324:1845–1850.

34. Solomon A. Clinical implications of monoclonal light chains. Semin Oncol 1986;13:341–349.

35. Farhangi M, Merlini G. The clinical implications of monoclonal immunoglobulins. Semin Oncol 1986;13:366–379.

36. Hjorth M, Hellquist L, Holmberg E, Magnusson B, Rodjer S, Westin J. Initial versus deferred melphalan-prednisone therapy for asymptomatic multiple myeloma stage I—a randomized study. Eur J Haematol 1993;50(2):95–102.

37. Alexanian R, Dimopoulos MA. The treatment of multiple myeloma. N Engl J Med 1994;330:484–489.

38. Palmer M, Belch A, Hanson J, et al. Reassessment of the relationship between M-protein decrement and survival in multiple myeloma. Br J Cancer 1989; 59:110–112.

39. Solomon A, McLaughlin CL, Capra JD. Bence Jones proteins and light chain of immunoglobulins. XI. A transient Bence Jones-related protein associated with corticosteroid therapy. J Clin Invest 1975;55:579–586.

40. Kyle RA, Greipp PA. Plasma cell dyscrasias. Current status. CRC Crit Rev Oncol Hematol 1988; 8:93–152.

41. Oken MM, Tsiatis A, Abramson N, Glick J. Evaluation of intensive (VBMCP) vs standard (MP) therapy for multiple myeloma (abstract). Proc Am Soc Clin Oncol 1987;6:A802.

42. Salmon SE, Haut A, Bonnet JD, et al. Alternating combination chemotherapy and levamisole improves survival in multiple myeloma: a SWOG study. J Clin Oncol 1983;1:453–461.

43. MacLennan ICM, Chapman C, Dunn J, et al. Combined chemotherapy with ABCM versus melphalan for treatment of myelomatosis. The Medical Resource Council Working Party for Leukemia in Adults. Lancet 1992;339:200–205.

44. Barlogie B, Smith L, Alexanian R. Effective treatment of advanced multiple myeloma refractory to alkylating agents. N Engl J Med 1984;310:1353–1356.

45. Alexanian R, Barlogie B, Dixon D. High-dose glucocorticoid treatment of resistant myeloma. Ann Intern Med 1986;105:8–11.

46. Kildahl-Andersen O, Bjark D, Bondevik A, Bull O, Burgess G, et al. Multiple myeloma in central and northern Norway 1981–1982: a follow-up study of a randomized trial of 5-drug combination therapy vs. standard therapy. Eur J Haematol 1988;41:47–51.

47. Pavlovsky S, Saslavsky J, Pinto MT, et al. A randomized trial of melphalan and prednisone versus melphalan, prednisone, cyclophosphamide, MeCCNU and vincristine in untreated multiple myeloma. J Clin Oncol 1984;2:836–840.

48. Finnish Leukemia Group, Palva IP, et al. Treatment of multiple myeloma with an intensive 5-drug combination or intermittent melphalan and prednisone; a randomized multi-centre trial. Eur J Haematol 1987;38:50–54.

49. Alexanian R, Dreicer R. Chemotherapy for multiple myeloma. Cancer 1984;53:583–588.

50. Bladé J, San Miguel JF, Alcalá A, et al. Alternating combination VCMP/VBAP chemotherapy versus melphalan/prednisone in the treatment of multiple myeloma: a randomized multicentric study of 487 patients. J Clin Oncol 1993;11:1165–1171.

51. Bergsagel DE, Bailey AJ, Langley GR, MacDonald RN, White DF, Miller AB. The chemotherapy of plasma-cell myeloma and the incidence of acute leukemia. N Engl J Med 1979;301:743–748.

52. Cooper MR, McIntyre OR, Propert KJ, et al. Single, sequential, and multiple alkylating agent therapy for multiple myeloma: a CALGB study. J Clin Oncol 1986;4:1131–1339.

53. Peest D, Deicher H, Coldewey R, Schmoll H-J, Schedel I. Induction and maintenance therapy in multiple myeloma: a multicenter trial of MP versus VCMP. Eur J Cancer Clin Oncol 1988;24:1061–1067.

54. Boccadoro M, Marmont F, Tribalto M, et al. Multiple myeloma: VMCP/VBAP alternating combination chemotherapy is not superior to melphalan and prednisone even in high-risk patients. J Clin Oncol 1991;9:444–448.

55. Durie BGM, Dixon DO, Carter S, et al. Improved survival duration with combination chemotherapy induction for multiple myeloma. A South West Oncology Group study. J Clin Oncol 1986;4:1227–1237.

56. Case DC, Lee BJ III, Clarkson BD. Improved survival times in multiple myeloma treated with melphalan, prednisone, cyclophosphamide, vincristine and BCNU: M2 protocol. Am J Med 1977;63:897–903.

57. Hjorth M, Hellquist L, Holmberg E, Magnussen B, Rödjer S, Westin J. Initial treatment in multiple myeloma: no advantage of multidrug chemotherapy over melphalan-prednisone. Br J Haematol 1990;74:185–191.

58. Gregory WM, Richards MA, Malpas JS. Combination chemotherapy versus melphalan and prednisone in the treatment of multiple myeloma: an overview of published trials. J Clin Oncol 1992;10:334–342.

59. Southwest Oncology Group. Remission maintenance therapy for multiple myeloma. Arch Intern Med 1976;294:17–23.

60. Alexanian R, Gehan E, Haut A, Saiki J, Weick J. Un-maintained remissions in multiple myeloma. Blood 1978;51:1005–1011.

61. Medical Research Council Working Party on Leukemia in Adults. Treatment comparisons in the third MRC myelomatosis trial. Br J Cancer 1980;42:823–830.

62. Belch A, Shelley W, Bergsagel D, Wilson K, Klimo P, White D, Willan A. A randomized trial of maintenance versus no maintenance melphalan and prednisone in responding multiple myeloma patients. Br J Cancer 1988;57:94–99.

63. Paccagnella A, Cartei G, Fosser V, et al. Treatment of multiple myeloma with M-2 protocol and without maintenance therapy. Eur J Cancer Clin Oncol 1983;19:1345–1351.

64. Salmon SE, Durie BGM, Young L, Liu RM, Trown PW, Stebbing N. Effects of cloned human leukocyte interferons in the human tumor stem cell assay. J Clin Oncol 1983;1:217–225.

65. Ludwig H, Fritz E. Individualized chemotherapy in multiple myeloma by cytostatic drug sensitivity testing of colony-forming stem cells. Anticancer Res 1981;1:329–335.

66. Browning G. The in vitro effect of leukocyte α-interferon on human myeloma cells in a semisolid agar culture system. Scand J Haematol 1985;35:178–181.

67. Brenning G, Ahre A, Nilsson K. Correlation between in vitro and in vivo sensitivity to human leukocyte interferon in patients with multiple myeloma. Scand J Haematol 1985;35:543–547.

68. Jernberg-Wiklund H, Pettersson M, Nilsson K. Recombinant interferon-gamma inhibits the growth of Il-6 dependent human multiple myeloma cell lines in vitro. Eur J Haematol 1991;46:231–234.

69. Jelinex DF, Aagaard-Tillery KM. Effect of interferon α on myeloma cell proliferation: mechanisms of interleukin-6 antagonism (abstract 691). Blood 1994; 84(Suppl 1):176a.

70. Bjorkholm M, Osterborg A, Brenning G, Gahrton G, Gyllenhammer H, et al. High doses of natural alpha-interferon (alpha-IFN) in the treatment of multiple myeloma—a pilot study from the Myeloma Group of Central Sweden (MGCS). Eur J Haematol 1988;41:123–130.

71. Cooper MR, Dear K, McIntyre OR, et al. A randomized clinical trial comparing melphalan/prednisone with or without interferon alfa-2b in newly diagnosed patients with multiple myeloma: a Cancer and Leukemia Group B study. J Clin Oncol 1993; 11:155–160.

72. Osterborg A, Bjorkholm M, Bjoreman M, et al. Natural interferon-α in combination with melphalan/prednisone versus melphalan/prednisone in the treatment of multiple myeloma stages II and III: a randomized study from the Myeloma Group of Central Sweden. Blood 1993;81:1428–1434.

73. Mandelli F, Avvisati G, Amador S, Boccadoro M. Genone A, et al. Maintenance treatment with recombinant interferon α-2b in patients with multiple myeloma responding to conventional induction chemotherapy. N Engl J Med 1990;322:1430–1434.

74. Salmon SE, Crowley JJ, Grogan TM, Finle P, Pugh RP, Barlogie B. Combination chemotherapy, glucocorticoids, and interferon alfa in the treatment of multiple myeloma: a South West Oncology Group study. J Clin Oncol 1994;12:2405–2414.

75. Peest D, Deicher N, Coldewey R, et al. Melphalan and prednisone (MP) versus vincristine, BCNU, Adriamycin, melphalan and dexamethasone (VBAM DeX) induction chemotherapy and interferon maintenance treatment in multiple myeloma. Current status of multicenter trial. The German Myeloma Treatment Group. Onkologie 1990;13:458–460.

76. Kyle RA, Greipp PR, Gertz MA. Treatment of refractory multiple myeloma and considerations for future therapy. Semin Oncol 1986;13:326–333.

77. Buzaid AC, Durie BGM. Management of refractory myeloma. A review. J Clin Oncol 1988;6:889–905.

78. Wilson K, Shelley W, Belch A, Brandes L, Bergsagel D, et al. Weekly cyclophosphamide and alternate-day prednisone. An effective secondary therapy in multiple myeloma. Cancer Treat Rep 1987;71:981–982.

79. Costanzi JJ, Cooper MR, Scarffe JH, Ozer H, Grubbs SS, et al. Phase II study of recombinant alpha-2b interferon in resistant multiple myeloma. J Clin Oncol 1985;3:654–659.

80. Ohno R, Kimura K. Treatment of multiple myeloma with recombinant interferon alfa 2A. Cancer 1986;57;1685–1688.

81. Bonnet J, Alexanian R, Salmon S, et al. Vincristine, BCNU, doxorubicin, and prednisone (VBAP)

combination in the treatment of relapsing or resistant multiple myeloma. A South West Oncology Group study. Cancer Treat Rep 1982;66:1267–1271.

82. Presant CA, Klahr C. Adriamycin, 1,3-bis (2-chloroethyl)-1 nitrosourea (BCNU, NSC#409962), cyclophosphamide plus prednisone (ABC-P) in melphalan-resistant multiple myeloma. Cancer 1978;42:1222–1227.

83. Scheithauer W, Cortelezzi A, Kutzmits R, Baldini L, Ludwig H. VAD protocol for treatment of advanced refractory multiple myeloma. Blut 1987;55:145–152.

84. Brandes LJ, Israel LG. Weekly low-dose cyclophosphamide and alternate-day prednisone. An effective low toxicity regimen for advanced myeloma. Eur J Hamematol 1987;39:362–368.

85. Barlogie B, Hall R, Zander A, Dicke K, Alexanian R. High dose melphalan with autologous bone marrow transplantation for multiple myeloma. Blood 1986;67:1298–1301.

86. Alexanian R, Dimopoulos AM, Delassale K, Barlogie B. Primary dexamethasone treatment for multiple myeloma. Blood 1992;80:887–890.

87. Collin R, Greaves M, Preston FE. Potential value of vincristine-Adriamycin-dexamethasone combination chemotherapy (VAD) in refractory and rapidly progressive myeloma. Eur J Haematol 1987; 39:203–208.

88. Lokhorst HM, Meuwissen OJA Th, Bast EJ, Dekker AW. VAD chemotherapy for refractory multiple myeloma. Br J Haematol 1989;71:25–30.

89. Salmon SE, Dalton WS, Grogan TM, Plezia P, Lehnert M, Roe DJ, Miller TP. Multidrug-resistant myeloma; laboratory and clinical effects of verapamil as a chemosensitizer. Blood 1990;78:44–50.

90. Gore ME, Selby PJ, Millar AB. The use of verapamil to overcome drug resistance in myeloma (abstract). Proc Am Soc Clin Oncol 1988;7:228.

91. Trumpe LH, Ho AD, Wulf G, Hunstein W. Addition of verapamil to overcome drug resistance in multiple myeloma: preliminary clinical observations in 10 patients (letter). J Clin Oncol 1989;7:1578–1579.

92. Sonneveld P, Durie BGM, Lokhorst HM, Marie JP, Solbu G, et al. Modulation of multidrug-resistant multiple myeloma by cyclosporin. Lancet 1992; 340:255–259.

93. Vesole DH, Barlogie B, Jagannath S, Cheson B, Tricot G, Alexanian R, Crowley J. High-dose therapy for refractory multiple myeloma: improved prognosis with better supportive care and double transplants. Blood 1994;84:950–956.

94. Tobias JS, Richards JDM, Blackman GM, et al. Hemibody irradiation in multiple myeloma. Radiother Oncol 1985;3:11–16.

95. McSweeney EN, Tobias JS, Blackman G, Goldstone AH, Richards JD. Double hemibody irradiation (DHBI) in the management of relapsed and primary chemoresistant multiple myeloma. Clin Oncol 1993; 5:378–383.

96. Osserman EF, DiRe LB, DiRe J, Sherman WH, Hersman JA, Storb R. Identical twin marrow transplantation in multiple myeloma. Acta Haematol 1982; 68:215–223.

97. Durie BGM, Gale RP, Horowitz MM. Allogeneic and twin transplantations for multiple myeloma: an IBMTR analysis (abstract 792). Blood 1994;84(Suppl 1):202a.

98. Gahrton G, Tura S, Ljungman P, et al. Allogeneic bone marrow transplantation in multiple myeloma. N Engl J Med 1991;325:1267–1273.

99. Bensinger WI, Buckner CD, Clift RA, et al. Phase one study of busulfan and cyclophosphamide in preparation for allogeneic marrow transplant for patient with multiple myeloma. J Clin Oncol 1992; 10:1492–1497.

100. Bensinger WI, Applebaum F, Clift R, et al. Allogeneic bone marrow transplantation for multiple myeloma, an analysis of risk factors for outcome (abstract). IV International Workshop on Multiple Myeloma, Rochester, MN, Oct 2–5, 1993:92.

101. Vesole DH, Jagannath S, Glenn LD, et al. Allogeneic bone marrow transplantation (Allo BMT) in multiple myeloma (abstract). Proc Am Soc Clin Oncol 1993;12:405.

102. Cavo M, Belardinelli A, Rosti G, et al. Busulfan and cyclophosphamide versus conditioning regimens including total body irradiation in preparation for allogeneic bone marrow transplantation in multiple myeloma. IV International Workshop on Multiple Myeloma, Rochester, MN, Oct 2–5, 1993:96–97.

103. Anderson KC, Andersen J, Soiffer R, et al. A monoclonal antibody purged bone marrow transplantation as consolidation in previously untreated multiple myeloma. J Clin Oncol 1994;12:759–763.

104. Cunningham D, Paz-Ares L, Gore ME, Malpas J, Hickish T, et al. High dose melphalan for multiple myeloma; long term follow-up data. J Clin Oncol 1994; 12(4):764–768.

105. Jagannath S, Vesole DH, Tricot G, Crowley J, Salmon SE, Barlogie B. Hematopoietic stem cell transplantations for multiple myeloma. Oncology 1994; 8(11):89–103.

106. Harousseau JL, Milpied N, Laporte JP, Collombat P, Facon T, et al. Double intensive therapy in high risk multiple myeloma. Blood 1992;79(11):2827–2833.

107. Harousseau JL, Attal M, Leblono V, et al. Autologous hematopoietic stem cell transplantation in multiple myeloma: a report of French Registry. IV International Workshop on Multiple Myeloma, Rochester, MN, Oct 2–5, 1993:105.

108. Attal M, Huguet F, Schlaifer D, Payen C, Laroche M, et al. Intensive combined therapy for previously untreated aggressive myeloma. Blood 1992; 79(5):1130–1136.

109. Björkstrand B, Ljungman P, Brand TL, Brunet S, Carlson K, et al. Autologous stem cell transplantation (ASCT) in multiple myeloma. A study of European BMT Registry (abstract 2124). Blood 1994; 84(Suppl 1):535a.

110. Fermand JP, Chevert S, Ravaud P, Divine M, Leblond V, et al. High-dose chemotherapy and autologous blood stem cell transplantation in multiple myeloma: result of a phase II trial involving 63 patients. Blood 1993;82(7):2005–2009.

111. Fermand JP, Ravaud P, Chevret S, et al. High dose therapy and autologous blood stem cell transplantation (ABSCT) versus conventional chemotherapy with HDT rescue in multiple myeloma (MM): results of a prospective randomized trial (abstract 808). Blood 1995;86(Suppl 1):205a.

112. Cunningham D, Paz-Ares L, Milan S, Powles R, Nicolson M, et al. High dose melphalan and autologous bone marrow transplantation as consolidation

in previously untreated myeloma. J Clin Oncol 1994; 12:759–763.

113. Cunningham D, Powles R, Malpas JS, et al. A randomized trial of maintenance therapy with interon-A following high dose melphalan and autologous bone marrow transplantation in myeloma (abstract). Proc Am Soc Clin Oncol 1994;12:759.

114. Lemoli RM, Fortuna A, Motta MR, Rizzi S, Amabile M, et al. Transplantation of enriched CD 34+ cells provides indirect purging of circulating tumor cell in multiple myeloma (MM) (abstract 1582). Blood 1994; 84(Suppl 1):399a.

115. Standard dose versus myeloablative therapy for previously untreated symptomatic myeloma (SW0G-9321, CALGB9312, ECOG-S9321).

116. Ludwig H, Fritz E. Kotzmann H, Höcker P, Gisslinger H, Barnas U. Erythropoietin treatment of anemia associated with multiple myeloma. N Engl J Med 1990;322:1693–1699.

117. Leigh BR, Kurtts TA, Mack CF, Matzner NB, Shimm DS. Radiation therapy for the palliation of multiple myeloma. Int J Radiat Oncol Biol Phys 1993; 25:801–804.

118. Warrell RP Jr, Lovett D, Dilmanian FA, et al. Low-dose gallium nitrate for prevention of osteolysis in myeloma: results of a pilot randomized study. J Clin Oncol 1993;11:2443–2450.

119. Lahtinen R, Laakso M, Palva I, Virkkunen P, Elomaa J. Randomized, placebo-controlled multicentre trial of clodronate in multiple myeloma. Finnish Leukemia Group. Lancet 1992;340(8827):1049–1052.

120. Coward RA, Mallick NP, Delmore IW. Should patient with renal failure associated with myeloma be dialysed? Br Med J 1983;287:1575–1578.

121. Zucchelli P, Pasquali S, Cagnoli L, Ferrari G. Controlled plasma exchange trial in acute renal failure due to multiple myeloma. Kidney Int 1988;33:1175–1180.

122. Busnach G, Mandelli E, Brando B, Brunati C. Clinical relevance of fractionation characteristics in cascade filtration. Department of Nephrology, Niguarda Ca; Granda Hospital, Milano, Italy. Int J Artif Organs 1993;16(Suppl 5):155–159.

123. Case DC Jr. Combination chemotherapy (M-2) protocol (BCNU, cyclophosphamide, vincristine, melphalan and prednisone) for Waldenstrom's macroglobulinemia. Blood 1982;59:934–937.

124. Clamon GH, Corder MP, Burns CP. Successful doxorubicin therapy of primary macroglobulinemia resistant to alkylating agents. Am J Hematol 1980; 9:221–223.

125. Keating MJ, O'Brien S, Plunkett W, Robertson LE, et al. Fludarabine phosphate: a new active agent in hematologic malignancies. Semin Hematol 1994; 31(1):28–39.

126. Binet JL. Fludarabine phosphate in chronic lymphoproliferative diseases. The French Group on CLL. Nouv Rev Fr Hematol 1993;35(1):5–7.

127. Dimopoulos MA, Kantarjian H, Weber D, et al. Primary therapy of Waldenstrom's macroglobulinemia with 2-clorodeoxyadenosine. J Clin Oncol 1994; 12:2694–2698.

128. Dimopoulos MA, O'Brien S, Kantarjian H, Estey EE, et al. Treatment of Waldenstrom's macroglobulinemia with nucleoside analogues. Leuk Lymphoma 1993;11(Suppl 2):105–108.

129. Dimopoulos MA, Luckett R, Alexanian R. Pri-

mary therapy of Waldenstrom's macroglobulinemia with paclitaxel (letter). J Clin Oncol 1994; 12(9):1998.

130. Mohammad RM, al-Katib A, Pettit GR, Sensenbrenner LL. Successful treatment of human Waldenstrom's macroglobulinemia with combination biological and chemotherapy agents. Cancer Res 1994; 154(1):165–168.

131. Rotoli B, DeRenzo A, Frigeri F, Buffardi S, et al. A phase II trial on alpha-interferon (alpha IFN) effect in patients with monoclonal IgM gammopathy. Leuk Lymphoma 1994;13(5–6):463–469.

132. Khojasteh A, Haghighi P. Immunoproliferative small intestinal disease. Portrait of a potentially preventable cancer from the third world. Am J Med 1990;89:483–490.

133. Puri AS, Aggarwal R, Khan EM, Naik S, et al. Explosive *Campylobacter jejuni* diarrhea in immunoproliferative small intestinal disease. Indian J Gastroenterol 1992;11(3):141–143.

134. Khojasteh A, Haghshenass M, Haghighi P. Current concepts: immunoproliferative small intestinal disease. A "third world lesion." N Engl J Med 1983; 308:1401–1405.

135. Khojasteh A. Immunoproliferative small intestinal disease (IPSID) in third world countries. In: Marsh MN, ed. Immunopathology of the small intestine. New York: John Wiley, 1987:121–150.

136. Shih LY, LIaw SJ, Dunn P, Kuo TT. Primary small-intestinal lymphomas in Taiwan: immunoproliferative small-intestinal disease and non-immunoproliferative small-intestinal disease. Department of Internal Medicine. J Clin Oncol 1994;12(7):1375–1382.

137. Ben-Ayed F, Halphen M, Najjar T, et al. Treatment of alpha chain disease. Results of prospective study in 21 Tunisian patients by the Tunisian-French Intestinal Lymphoma Study Group. Cancer 1989; 63:1251–1256.

138. Gray GM, Rosenberg SA, Cooper AD, Gregory PB, Stein DT, Herzenberg H. Lymphomas involving the gastrointestinal tract. Gastroenterology 1982; 82:143–152.

139. Kyle RA. The heavy-chain diseases. In: Wiernik PH, Canellas GP, Kyle RA, eds. Neoplastic diseases of the blood. New York: Churchill Livingstone, 1985:593–605.

140. Salmon SE, Cassady JR. Plasma cell neoplasms. In: DeVita T Jr, Hellman S, Rosenberg SA, eds. Cancer: principles and practice of oncology. Philadelphia: JB Lippincott, 1989:1853–1895.

141. Barlogie B, Alexanian R, Jagannath S. Plasma cell dyscrasias. JAMA 1992;268:2946–2951.

142. Brouet JC, Seligmann M, Danon F, Belpomme D, Fine J-M. μ-Chain disease: report of two new cases. Arch Intern Med 1979;139:672–674.

143. Buxbaum JN, Chuba JU, Hellman GC, et al. Monoclonal immunoglobulin deposition disease; light chain and light and heavy chain deposition disease and their relation to light chain amyloidosis: clinical features, immunology, and molecular analysis. Ann Intern Med 1990;112:455–464.

144. Aucouturier P, Khamlichi AA, Touchard G, et al. Brief report: heavy chain deposition disease. N Engl J Med 1993;329:1389–1393.

145. Solomon A, Weiss DT. Ominous consequences of immunoglobulin deposition (editorial). N Engl J Med 1993;329:1422–1423.

146. Corradini P, Voena C, Astolfi M, Ladetto M, Tarella C, Boccadoro M, Pileri A. High-dose chemoradiotherapy in multiple myeloma: residual tumor cells are detectable in bone marrow and peripheral blood cell harvests and after autografting (abstract 1583). Blood 1994;84(Suppl 1):399a.

147. Vesico R, Cao J, Hong C, Hua C, Lee C, Schiller G, et al. CD34-positive CEPRATE selection leads to a 4–5 log reduction in tumor burden in myeloma PBC autographs based on PCR and Poisson distribution analysis (abstract 1580). Blood 1994;84(Suppl 1):399a.

148. Björkstrand B, Lejungman P, Bird JM, Samson D, Gahrton G. Eradication of minimal residual disease, analyzed by PCR, after double high-dose chemoradiotherapy with autologous stem cell transplantation in multiple myeloma (abstract 817). Blood 1994; 84(Suppl 1):208a.

Appendix/WHO Toxicity Guidelines

Common Toxicity Criteria

Toxicity	Grade 0	Grade 1	Grade 2	Grade 3	Grade 4
Hematologic					
WBC	≥4.0	3.0–3.9	2.0–2.9	1.0–1.9	<1.0
PLT	WNL	75.0–normal	50.0–74.9	25.0–49.9	<25.0
Hgb g/100 mL	WNL	10.0–normal	8.0–10.0	6.5–7.9	<6.5
g/L	WNL	100–normal	80–100	65–79	<65
mmol/L	WNL	6.2–normal	4.95–6.2	4.0–4.9	<4.0
Granulocytes/bands	≥2.0	1.5–1.9	1.0–1.4	0.5–0.9	<0.5
Lymphocytes	≥2.0	1.5–1.9	1.0–1.4	0.5–0.9	<0.5
Hematologic—other	None	Mild	Moderate	Severe	Life threatening
Hemorrhage (Clinical)	None	Mild, no transfusion	Gross, 1–2 units transfusion per episode	Gross, 3–4 units transfusion per episode	Massive, >4 units transfusion per episode
Infection	None	Mild, no active treatment	Moderate, p.o. antibiotic	Severe, i.v. antibiotic, antifungal, or hospitalization	Life threatening
Gastrointestinal					
Nausea	None	Able to eat reasonable intake	Intake significantly decreased but can eat	No significant intake	—
Vomiting	None	1 episode in 24 hours	2–5 episodes in 24 hours	6–10 episodes in 24 hours	>10 episodes in 24 hours or requiring parenteral support
Diarrhea	None	Increase in 2–3 stools/day over pre-Rx	Increase of 4–6 stools/day, or nocturnal stools, or moderate cramping	Increase of 7–9 stools/day, or incontinence, or severe cramping	Increase of ≥10 stools/day, or grossly bloody diarrhea, or need for parenteral support
Gastrointestinal					
Stomatitis	None	Painless ulcers, erythema, or mild soreness	Painful erythema, edema, or ulcers, but can eat	Painful erythema, edema, or ulcers, and cannot eat	Requires parenteral or enteral support

	None/0	1	2	3	4
Esophagitis/dysphagia	None	Painless ulcers, erythema, mild soreness or dysphagia	Painful erythema, edema, or ulcers or moderate dysphagia but can eat without narcotics	Cannot eat solids, or requires narcotics to eat	Requires parenteral or enteral support or complete obstruction or perforation
Anorexia	None	Mild	Moderate	Severe	Life threatening
Gastritis/ulcer	No	Antacid	Requires vigorous medical management or nonsurgical treatment	Uncontrolled by medical management, requires surgery	Perforation or bleeding
Small bowel obstruction	No	—	Intermittent, no intervention	Requires intervention	Requires operation
Intestinal fistula	No	—	—	Yes	—
GI—other	None	Mild	Moderate	Severe	Life threatening
Other mucosal	None	Erythema, or mild pain not requiring treatment	Patchy and serosanguineous discharge or nonnarcotic for pain	Confluent fibrinous mucositis or ulceration or narcotic for pain	Necrosis
Liver					
Bilirubin	WNL	—	$<1.5 \times N$	$1.5–3.0 \times N$	$>3.0 \times N$
Transaminase (SGOT/AST, SGPT/ALT)	WNL	$\leq 2.5 \times N$	$2.6–5.0 \times N$	$5.1–20.0 \times N$	$>20.0 \times N$
Alk phos or 5' nucleotidase	WNL	$\leq 2.5 \times N$	$2.6–5.0 \times N$	$5.1–20.0 \times N$	$>20.0 \times N$
Liver, clinical	No change from baseline	—	—	Precoma	Hepatic coma
Liver, other	—	Mild	Moderate	Severe	Life threatening
Renal & bladder					
Creatinine	WNL	$<1.5 \times N$	$1.5–3.0 \times N$	$3.1–6.0 \times N$	$>6.0 \times N$
Proteinuria	No change	1+ or <0.3 g% or <3 g/L	2–3+ or 0.3–1.0 g% or 3–10 g/L	4+ or >1.0 g% or >10 g/L	Nephrotic syndrome

Common Toxicity Criteria—*continued*

Toxicity	Grade 0	Grade 1	Grade 2	Grade 3	Grade 4
Renal & bladder—continued					
Hematuria	Neg	Micro only	Gross, no clots	Gross + clots	Requires transfusion
BUN (mg%)	WNL, <20	21–30	31–50	>50	—
Urea (mmol/L)	WNL, <7.5	7.6–10.9	11–18	>18	—
Hemorrhagic cystitis	None	Blood on microscopic exam	Frank blood, no treatment required	Bladder irrigation required	Requires cystectomy or tranfusion
Renal failure	—	—	—	—	Dialysis required
Incontinence	Normal	With coughing, sneezing, etc.	Spontaneous, some control	No control	—
Dysuria	None	Mild pain	Painful or burning urination controlled by pyridium	Not controlled by pyridium	—
Urinary retention	None	Residue >100 mL or occ. catheter or difficulty initiating stream	Self-cath required for voiding	Surgery required (TUR or dilatation)	—
Increased frequency/ urgency	No change	Increase in frequency or nocturia up to 2 × normal	Increase > 2 × normal but < hourly	With urgency and hourly or more or requires catheter	—
Bladder cramps	None	—	Yes	—	—
Ureteral obstruction	None	Unilateral, no surgery required	Bilateral, no surgery required	Incomplete bilateral, but stents, nephrostomy tubes, or surgery needed	Complete bilateral obstruction
GU fistula	None	—	—	Yes	—
Kidney/bladder—other	—	Mild	Moderate	Severe	Life threatening
Alopecia	No loss	Mild hair loss	Pronounced or total hair loss	—	—

Pulmonary

	None or no change	Asymptomatic with abnormality in PFTs	Dyspnea on significant exertion	Dyspnea at normal level of activity	Dyspnea at rest
Dyspnea	None or no change	Asymptomatic with abnormality in PFTs	Dyspnea on significant exertion	Dyspnea at normal level of activity	Dyspnea at rest
pO_2/pCO_2	No change or $pO_2 > 85$ and $pCO_2 \leq 40$	pO_2 71–85, pCO_2 41–50	pO_2 61–70, pCO_2 51–60	pO_2 51–60, pCO_2 61–70	$pO_2 \leq 50$, $pCO_2 \geq 70$
DLCO	>90% of pretreatment	76–90% of pretreatment	51–75% of pretreatment	26–50% of pretreatment	≤25% of pretreatment
Pulmonary fibrosis	None	Radiographic changes, asymptomatic	—	Changes with symptoms	—
Pulmonary edema	None	—	—	Radiographic changes and diuretics needed	Requires intubation
Pneumonia (noninfectious)	None	Radiographic changes, no steroids needed	Steroids required	Oxygen required	Assisted ventilation required
Pleural effusion	None	Present	—	—	—
ARDS	None	Mild	Moderate	Severe	Life threatening
Cough	No change	Mild, relieved by OTC meds	Requires narcotic antitussive	Uncontrolled cough	—
Pulmonary—Other	—	Mild	Moderate	Severe	Life threatening

Cardiac

	None	Grade 1	Grade 2	Grade 3	Grade 4
Cardiac dysrhythmias	None	Asymptomatic, transient, no therapy required	Recurrent or persistent, no therapy required	Requires treatment	Requires monitoring; or hypotension, or ventricular tachycardia, or fibrillation
Cardiac function	None	Asymptomatic, decline of resting ejection fraction by less than 20% of baseline value	Asymptomatic, decline of resting ejection fraction by more than 20% of baseline value	Mild CHF, responsive to therapy	Severe or refractory CHF
Cardiac—ischemia	None	Nonspecific T-wave flattening	Asymptomatic, ST and T wave changes suggesting ischemia	Angina without evidence for infarction	Acute myocardial infarction

Common Toxicity Criteria—*continued*

Toxicity	Grade 0	Grade 1	Grade 2	Grade 3	Grade 4
Cardiac—continued					
Cardiac—pericardial	None	Asymptomatic effusion, no intervention required	Pericarditis (rub, chest pain, ECG changes)	Symptomatic effusion; drainage	Tamponade: drainage urgently required
Cardiac—other	—	Mild	Moderate	Severe	Life threatening
Blood pressure					
Hypertension	None or no change	Asymptomatic, transient increase by greater than 20 mm Hg (D) or to >150/100 if previously WNL; no treatment required	Recurrent or persistent increase by greater than 20 mm Hg (D) or to >150/100 if previously WNL; no treatment required	Requires therapy	Hypertensive crisis
Hypotension	None or no change	Changes requiring no therapy (including transient orthostatic hypotension)	Required fluid replacement or other therapy but not hospitalization	Requires therapy and hospitalization; resolves within 48 hours of stopping the agent	Requires therapy and hospitalization for >48 hours after stopping the agent
Phlebitis/thrombosis embolism	—	—	Superficial phlebitis (not local)	Deep vein thrombosis	Major event (cerebral/hepatic/pulmonary embolism)
Edema	None	1+ or dependent in evening only	2+ or dependent throughout day	3+	4+, generalized anasarca
Neurologic					
Neurosensory	None or no change	Mild paresthesias, loss of deep tendon reflexes	Mild or moderate objective sensory loss; moderate paresthesias	Severe objective sensory loss or paresthesias that interfere with function	—
Neuromotor	None or no change	Subjective weakness; no objective findings	Mild objective weakness without significant impairment of function	Objective weakness with impairment of function	Paralysis

	None	Mild	Moderate	Severe	
Neurocortical	None	Mild somnolence or agitation	Moderate somnolence or agitation	Severe somnolence, agitation, confusion, disorientation, or hallucinations	Coma, seizures, toxic psychosis
Neurocerebellar	None	Slight incoordination, dysdiadokinesis	Intention tremor, dysmetria, slurred speech, nystagmus	Locomotor ataxia	Cerebellar necrosis
Neuro—mood	No change	Mild anxiety or depression	Moderate anxiety or depression	Severe anxiety or depression	Suicidal ideation
Neuro—headache	None	Mild	Moderate or severe but transient	Unrelenting and severe	—
Neuro—constipation	None or no change	Mild	Moderate	Severe	ileus >96 hours
Neuro—hearing	None or no change	Asymptomatic hearing loss on audiometry only	Tinnitus	Hearing loss interfering with function but correctable with hearing aid	Deafness not correctable
Neuro—vision	None or no change	—	—	Symptomatic subtotal loss of vision	Blindness
Pain	None	Mild	Moderate	Severe	Intolerable
Behavioral change	None	Change, not disruptive to patient or family	Disruptive to patient or family	Harmful to others or self	Psychotic behavior
Dizziness/vertigo	None	Nondisabling	—	Disabling	—
Taste	Normal	Slightly altered taste, metallic taste	Markedly altered taste	—	—
Insomnia	Normal	Occasional difficulty sleeping, may need pills	—	Difficulty sleeping despite medication	—
Neurologic—other	—	Mild	Moderate	Severe	Life threatening

Common Toxicity Criteria—*continued*

Toxicity	Grade 0	Grade 1	Grade 2	Grade 3	Grade 4
Dermatologic					
Skin	None or no change	Scattered macular or papular eruption or erythema that is asymptomatic	Scattered macular or papular eruption or erythema with pruritus or other associated symptoms	Generalized symptomatic macular, papular, or vesicular eruption	Exfoliative dermatitis or ulcerating dermatitis
Local	None	Pain	Pain and swelling with inflammation or phlebitis	Ulceration	Plastic surgery indicated
Allergy	None	Transient rash, drug fever <38°C, 100.4°F	Urticaria, drug fever ≥38°C, 100.4°F, mild bronchospasm	Serum sickness, bronchospasm, req parenteral meds	Anaphylaxis
Flulike symptoms					
Fever in absence of infection	None	37.1–38.0°C 98.7–100.4°F	38.1–40.0°C 100.5–104.0°F	>40.0°C >104.0°F <24 hours	>40.0°C (104.0°F) >24 hours or fever with hypotension
Chills	None	Mild or brief	Pronounced or prolonged	—	—
Myalgia/arthralgia	Normal	Mild	Decrease in ability to move	Disabled	—
Sweats	Normal	Mild and occasional	Frequent or drenching	—	—
Malaise	None	Mild, able to continue normal activities	Impaired normal daily activity or bedrest <50% of waking hours	In bed or chair >50% of waking hours	Bedridden or unable to care for self
Flulike symptoms— other	—	Mild	Moderate	Severe	Life threatening
Weight gain/loss	<5.0%	5.0–9.9%	10.0–19.9%	≥20.0%	—

		Mild	Moderate	Severe	Life threatening
Metabolic					
Hyperglycemia	<116 mg/dL <6.2 mmol/L	116–160 6.2–8.9	161–250 9.0–13.9	251–500 14.0–27.8	>500 or ketoacidosis >27.8 or ketoacidosis
Hypoglycemia	>64 mg/dL >3.6 mmol/L	55–64 3.1–3.6	40–54 2.2–3.0	30–39 1.7–2.1	<30 <1.7
Amylase	WNL	<1.5 × N	1.5–2.0 × N	2.1–5.0 × N	> 5.1 × N
Hypercalcemia	<10.6 mg/dL <2.65 mmol/L	10.6–11.5 2.65–2.87	11.6–12.5 2.88–3.12	12.6–13.5 3.13–3.37	≥13.5 ≥3.37
Hypocalcemia	>8.4 mg/dL >2.1 mmol/L	8.4–7.8 2.1–1.95	7.7–7.0 1.94–1.75	6.9–6.1 1.74–1.51	≤6.0 ≤1.50
Hypomagnesemia	>1.4 mg/dL	1.4–1.2	1.1–0.9	0.8–0.6	≤0.5
Hyponatremia	WNL or >135 mmol/L	131–135	126–130	121–125	≤120
Hypokalemia	WNL or >3.5 mmol/L	3.1–3.5	2.6–3.0	2.1–2.5	≤2.0
Metabolic—other	—	Mild	Moderate	Severe	Life threatening
Coagulation					
Fibrinogen	WNL	0.99–0.75 × N	0.74–0.50 × N	0.49–0.25 × N	≤0.24 × N
Prothrombin time	WNL	1.01–1.25 × N	1.26–1.50 × N	1.51–2.00 × N	>2.00 × N
Partial thromboplastin time	WNL	1.01–1.66 × N	1.67–2.33 × N	2.34–3.00 × N	>3.00 × N
Coagulation—other	—	Mild	Moderate	Severe	Life threatening

Common Toxicity Criteria—*continued*

Toxicity	Grade 0	Grade 1	Grade 2	Grade 3	Grade 4
Endocrine					
Impotence/libido	Normal	Decrease in normal function	—	Absence of function	—
Sterility	—	—	Yes	—	—
Amenorrhea	No	Yes	—	—	—
Gynecomastia	Normal	Mild	Pronounced or painful	—	—
Hot flushes	None	Mild or <1/day	Moderate and ≥1/day	Frequent and interferes with normal function	—
Cushingoid	Normal	Mild	Pronounced	—	—
Endocrine—other	—	Mild	Moderate	Severe	Life threatening
Eye					
Conjunctivitis/keratitis	None	Erythema or chemosis, no steroids or antibiotics	Steroids or antibiotics required	Corneal ulceration or visible opacification	—
Dry eye	Normal	—	Requires artificial tears	—	Requires enucleation
Glaucoma	No change	—	—	Yes	—
Eye—other	—	Mild	Moderate	Severe	Life threatening

Index

Page numbers in *italics* denote figures; those followed by "t" denote tables.

Investigational Drugs

Generic Name	Common Name	Abbreviation
Acivicin	—	—
Aclarubicin (aclacinomycin-A)	—	—
Amonafide	Nafidimide	—
Amsacrine	Amsidyl (Parke-Davis)	*m*-AMSA
Anthracenedicarboxyaldehyde	Bisantrene	—
5-Azacytidine*	—	5-AZC
Aziridinylbenzoquinone	Diaziquone	AZQ
Buserelin	Suprefact	BSE
Buthionine sulfoximine	—	BSO
Bryostatin		
Caracemide	—	—
Chlorozotocin	—	—
4'-Deoxydoxorubicin	Esorubicin	DXDX
Diaziquone	—	AZQ
Dibromodulicitol	Elobromol	DBD
Didemin B	—	—
Droloxifene		
10-Edam	Edatrexate	10-EDAM
Ellipticinum	—	
Elsamicine	—	—
Epirubicin	Pharmarubicin	EPI
Etoposide phosphate	Etopophos	
Fazarabine	—	—
Flavone acetic acid	—	FAA
Fotemustine		
Ftorafur	Tegarfur	—
1-(2-Chloroethyl)-3-(4-methylcyclohexyl)-1-nitrosourea	Semustine	MeCCNU
Iproplatin	—	CHIP
Letrozole		
Lonidamine	—	LND